D0081191

Common Drug And Toxin Induced Vital Sign Changes

Hypothermia	Hyperthermia
Alpha adrenergic agonists (central)	Amphetamines
Barbiturates	Anticholinergics
Beta adrenergic antagonists	Cocaine and sympathomimetics
Carbon monoxide	Dinitrophenol
Ethanol	Hallucinogens
General anesthetics	Lithium
Hypoglycemics	Neuroleptics (NMS)
Opioids	Pentachlorophenol
Organophosphates	Phencyclidine
Sedative hypnotics	Salicylates

Hypotension	Hypertension
Antihypertensives	Amphetamine
Barbiturates	Anticholinergics
Beta adrenergic antagonists	Cocaine and sympathomimetics
Calcium channel blockers	Hallucinogens
Cyclic antidepressants	Lead
Diuretics	MAOI interaction
Ethanol	MAOI overdose
Iron	Phencyclidine
Opioids	
Phenothiazines	
Theophylline	

Hyperventilaton	
Amphetamines	Isoniazid
Anticholinergics	Methanol
Caffeine	Methemoglobin inducers
Camphor	Monomethyl hydrazine mushrooms *(Gyromitra esculenta)*
Carbon monoxide	Paraldehyde
Cocaine and symmpathomimetics	Pentachlorophenol
Cyanide	Phenformin
Dinitrophenol	Progesterone
Ethanol (ketoacidosis)	Salicylates
Ethylene glycol	Sodium monofluoroacetate
Hydrogen sulfide	Theophylline
Iron	

Bradycardia	Tachycardia
Beta adrenergic antagonists	Amphetamines
Calcium channel blockers	Anticholinergics
Central alpha agonists	Cocaine and sympathomimetics
Digitalis	Cyclic antidepressants
Opioids	Iron
Organophosphates	Phenothiazines
Phenylpropanol-amine	Theophylline

Hypoventilation	
Barbiturates	Nicotine
Botulism	Opioids
Clonidine	Organophosphates
Colchicine	Poison Hemlock *(Conium Maculatum)*
Elapid envenomation	Sedative-hypnotics
Ethanol	Strychnine
Isopropanol	Tetrodotoxin
Neuromuscular blockers	Tricyclic antidepressants

Goldfrank's

TOXICOLOGIC EMERGENCIES

Sixth Edition

Lewis R. Goldfrank, MD, FACP, FACEP, FAACT, FACMT
Director, Department of Emergency Medicine
Bellevue Hospital Center and New York University Medical Center
Associate Professor of Clinical Medicine
New York University School of Medicine
Medical Director, New York City Poison Center
New York, New York

Neal E. Flomenbaum, MD, FACP, FACEP
Emergency Physician-in-Chief
The New York Hospital
Professor of Clinical Medicine
Cornell University Medical College
Consultant, New York City Poison Center
New York, New York

Neal A. Lewin, MD, FACP, FACEP, FACMT
Director, Didactic Education, Department of Emergency Medicine
Bellevue Hospital Center and New York University Medical Center
Assistant Professor of Clinical Medicine
New York University School of Medicine
Consultant, New York City Poison Center
New York, New York

Richard S. Weisman, PharmD, ABAT
Director, Florida Poison Information Center/Miami
Research Associate Professor of Pediatrics
University of Miami School of Medicine
Miami, Florida

Mary Ann Howland, PharmD, ABAT
Clinical Professor of Pharmacy
St. John's University College of Pharmacy
Consultant, Department of Emergency Medicine
Bellevue Hospital Center and New York University Medical Center
Consultant, New York City Poison Center
New York, New York

Robert S. Hoffman, MD, FACEP, FAACT, FACMT
Bellevue Hospital Center and New York University Medical Center
Assistant Professor of Clinical Surgery/Emergency Medicine
New York University School of Medicine
Director, New York City Poison Center
New York, New York

With 87 contributors

APPLETON & LANGE
Stamford, Connecticut

The editors' and authors' royalties for this edition, as in the case of previous editions, are being donated to The New York City Poison Center to help care for poisoned patients.

98 99 00 01 02 / 10 9 8 7 6 5 4 3 2

Prentice Hall International (UK) Limited, *London*
Prentice Hall of Australia Pty. Limited, *Sydney*
Prentice Hall Canada, Inc., *Toronto*
Prentice Hall Hispanoamericana, S.A., *Mexico*
Prentice Hall of India Private Limited, *New Delhi*
Prentice Hall of Japan, Inc., *Tokyo*
Simon & Schuster Asia Pte. Ltd., *Singapore*
Editora Prentice Hall do Brasil Ltda., *Rio de Janeiro*
Prentice Hall, *Upper Saddle River, New Jersey*

Library of Congress Cataloging-in-Publication Data

Goldfrank's toxicologic emergencies / [edited by] Lewis R. Goldfrank . . . [et al.] ; with 86 contributors. — 6th ed.
p. cm.
Includes bibliographical references and index.
ISBN 0-8385-3148-2 (case : alk. paper)
1. Toxicological emergencies. 2. Toxicological emergencies—Case studies. I. Goldfrank, Lewis R., 1941- .
[DNLM: 1. Poisoning—case studies. 2. Poisoning—examination questions. 3. Emergencies—case studies. 4. Emergencies—examination questions. QV 600 G618 1998]
RA1224.5.G65 1998
615.9—dc21
DNLM/DLC
for Library of Congress 97-42664

ISBN 0-8385-3148-2
90000
9 780838 531488

Acquisitions Editor: Jane Licht
Developmental Editor: Beth P. Broadhurst
Production Editor: Jeanmarie M. Roche

PRINTED IN THE UNITED STATES OF AMERICA

DEDICATED TO . . .

The staffs of our hospital emergency departments,
who have worked with remarkable courage, concern, compassion, and understanding
in treating the patients discussed in this text and many thousands more like them

The staff of the New York City Poison Center,
who have quietly and conscientiously integrated their skill with ours
to serve these patients and many others who never needed a hospital visit
because of their efforts

The ambulance staff,
who taught us a great deal about toxicology
and who had faith in our ability

To my children, Rebecca and Andrew, to Jennifer and Charles,
to Michelle and James and my grandchildren, Benjamin, Adam, and Sarah
who have kept me acutely aware of the ready availability
of possible poisons, and
to my wife, partner, and best friend, Susan,
whose support was and is essential
and whose contributions will be found throughout the text (L.G.)

To my wife, Meredith, my children, Adam, David and Sari, and my parents and brother,
for all of the ways they made my participation in this edition possible (N.F.)

To my wife, Gail, and my children, Justin and Jesse, for their support and patience and
to my parents, who made it possible (N.L.)

To Diane and Robyn, for their support, patience, and understanding (R.W.)

To my husband, Bob, and children, Robert and Marcy, and
to my parents, family, friends, colleagues, and students for all their help and continuing inspiration (M.A.H.)

To my friends, family, and colleagues for their never-ending patience (R.H.)

Contributors

Cynthia K. Aaron, MD
Assistant Professor
Director, Toxicology Services
Division of Medical Toxicology
Department of Emergency Medicine
University of Massachusetts Medical Center
Worcester, Massachusetts
Chapter 87, "Insecticides: Organophosphates and Carbamates"
Antidotes in Depth, "Cyanide Antidotes"
Antidotes in Depth, "Pralidoxime"

Michael H. Allen, MD
Clinical Assistant Professor
Department of Psychiatry
New York University School of Medicine
Director, Comprehensive Psychiatric Emergency Program
Department of Psychiatry
Bellevue Hospital Center
New York, New York
Chapter 113, "Psychiatric Principles: Evaluating and Managing Suicidal and Violent Patients"

Judith C. Ahronheim, MD
Chief
Eileen E. Anderson Section of Geriatric Medicine
Department of Medicine
Saint Vincent's Hospital and Medical Center
New York, New York
Chapter 106, "Geriatrics"

Theodore I. Benzer, MD, PhD
Instructor
Division of Emergency Medicine
Department of Medicine
Harvard Medical School
Assistant in Emergency Medicine
Department of Emergency Medicine
Massachusetts General Hospital
Boston, Massachusetts
Chapter 102, "Prehospital and Interhospital Principles"

Jeffrey N. Bernstein, MD
Department of Pediatrics
University of Miami
Miami, Florida
Antidotes in Depth, "Antivenin (Scorpion and Spider)"

Kenneth O. Brambill, MSW, CSW
Associate Director of Social Work
Health and Hospitals Corporation
Department of Social Work
Bellevue Hospital Center
New York, New York
Chapter 112, "Psychosocial Principles in Assessment and Intervention"

Eddy A. Bresnitz, MD
Professor of Medicine and Community and Preventive Medicine
Division of Occupational and Environmental Health
Department of Community and Preventive Medicine
Allegheny University of the Health Sciences
MCP Hahnemann School of Medicine
Philadelphia, Pennsylvania
Chapter 91, "Industrial Poisoning: Information and Control"
Chapter 117, "Principles of Research Design"

Jeffrey R. Brubacher, MD
Clinical Instructor
Division of Medicine
Faculty of Surgery
University of British Columbia
Attending Physician
Department of Emergency Medicine
Vancouver Hospital and Health Sciences Centre
Vancouver, British Columbia, Canada
Chapter 49, "Beta-Adrenergic Antagonists"
Chapter 74, "Air and Water Pollution"

Paul Calabresi, MD
Professor of Medicine and Chairman Emeritus

Division of Clinical Pharmacology
Department of Medicine
Brown University
Director
Division of Clinical Pharmacology
Department of Medicine
Rhode Island Hospital
Providence, Rhode Island
Chapter 47, "Antineoplastic Agents"

Susan Callaghan-Montella, RN, MA
Director of Education and Development
Emergency Care Institute
Department of Emergency Medicine
Bellevue Hospital Center/New York University Medical Center
New York, New York
Chapter 114, "Nursing Principles"

William K. Chiang, MD
Assistant Professor of Clinical Surgery/Emergency Medicine
New York University School of Medicine
Department of Emergency Medicine
Research Director
Bellevue Hospital Center/New York University Medical Center
Consultant, New York City Poison Center
New York, New York
Chapter 27, "Otolaryngologic Principles"
Chapter 66, "Amphetamines"

James E. Cisek, MD
Associate Professor of Emergency Medicine
Medical Director, Poison Control Center
Department of Emergency Medicine
Medical College of Virginia
Richmond, Virginia
Chapter 108, "Substance Users"

Cathleen Clancy, MD
Medical Director
Maryland Poison Center
Clinical Assistant Professor
University of Maryland School of Pharmacy
Baltimore, Maryland
Attending Physician
Department of Emergency Medicine
Clinical Instructor
Georgetown University Medical Center
Medical Toxicologist
National Capital Poison Center
Adjunct Assistant Professor
Department of Emergency Medicine
George Washington University Medical Center
Washington, District of Columbia
Chapter 8, "Electrocardiographic Evaluation of the Poisoned or Overdosed Patient"

David E. Cohen, MD, MPH
Assistant Professor of Dermatology
Department of Dermatology
New York University School of Medicine
Director of Occupational and Environmental Dermatology
New York University Medical Center
New York, New York
Chapter 28, "Dermatologic Principles"

Steven C. Curry, MD
Director, Department of Medical Toxicology
Good Samaritan Regional Medical Center
Phoenix, Arizona
Chapter 10, "Neurotransmitters"

Kathleen A. Delaney, MD, FACP
Associate Professor of Surgery
Division of Emergency Medicine
University of Texas Southwestern Medical School
Dallas, Texas
Chapter 12, "Biochemical Principles"
Chapter 13, "Hepatic Principles"
Chapter 16, "Mutagens, Carcinogens, and Teratogens"
Chapter 18, "Thermoregulatory Principles"
Antidotes in Depth, "Dextrose"

Francis DeRoos, MD
Assistant Professor and Co-Director
Division of Toxicology
Department of Emergency Medicine
University of Pennsylvania
Attending Physician
Department of Emergency Medicine
Hospital of the University of Pennsylvania
Philadelphia, Pennsylvania
Chapter 50, "Calcium Channel Blockers"
Chapter 51, "Miscellaneous Antihypertensive Agents"

Suzanne Doyon, MD
Clinical Instructor
Division of Emergency Medicine
Department of Surgery
University of Maryland Medical Systems
Attending Physician
Department of Emergency Medicine
Mercy Hospital Center
Baltimore, Maryland
Chapter 41, "Anticonvulsants"

Donald A. Feinfeld, MD
Professor of Clinical Medicine
Division of Nephrology
Department of Medicine
State University of New York Health Science Center at Stony Brook
Stony Brook, New York
Associate Director
Division of Nephrology
Department of Medicine
Nassau County Medical Center
East Meadow, New York
Consultant, New York City Poison Center
New York, New York
Chapter 23, "Renal Principles"

Robert P. Ferm, MD, FAAP, FACEP, FACMT
Assistant Professor of Emergency Medicine
Division of Toxicology
Department of Emergency Medicine
University of Massachusetts Medical School
Director, Medical Toxicology Fellowship
Department of Emergency Medicine
University of Massachusetts Medical Center
Worcester, Massachusetts
Chapter 68, "Lysergic Acid Diethylamide and Other Hallucinogens"

Jeffrey S. Fine, MD
Assistant Professor of Pediatrics
New York University School of Medicine
Assistant Director
Pediatric Emergency Services
Department of Pediatrics and Emergency Medicine
Bellevue Hospital Center
Consultant, New York City Poison Center
New York, New York
Chapter 104, "Reproductive and Perinatal Principles"
Chapter 105, "Pediatric Principles"

Marsha D. Ford, MD
Clinical Associate Professor
Department of Emergency Medicine
University of North Carolina—Chapel Hill
Chapel Hill, North Carolina
Director, Division of Toxicology
Assistant Chairman
Department of Emergency Medicine
Medical Director, Carolinas Poison Center
Carolinas Medical Center
Charlotte, North Carolina
Chapter 78, "Arsenic"

E. John Gallagher, MD
Professor and Chair
Department of Emergency Medicine
Albert Einstein College of Medicine
Chief, Department of Emergency Medicine
Montefiore Medical Center
Bronx, New York
Chapter 19, "Neurologic Principles"

Frances A. Gautieri, MS, CSW, ACSW
Director, Department of Social Work
Health and Hospitals Corporation
Bellevue Hospital Center
New York, New York
Chapter 112, "Psychosocial Principles in Assessment and Intervention"

David S. Goldfarb, MD
Assistant Professor of Clinical Medicine and Urology
New York University School of Medicine
Director of Hemodialysis
Department of Nephrology
New York Department of Veteran Affairs Medical Center
Consultant, New York City Poison Center
New York, New York
Chapter 5, "Principles and Techniques Applied to Enhance Elimination of Toxins"

Kimberlie A. Graeme, MD
Toxicology Fellow
Department of Medical Toxicology
Good Samaritan Regional Medical Center
Phoenix, Arizona
Chapter 10, "Neurotransmitters"

Joseph H. Graziano, PhD
Professor of Public Health and Pharmacology
Head, Division of Environmental Health Sciences
Columbia University School of Public Health
New York, New York
Antidotes in Depth, "Succimer (2,3-Dimercaptosuccinic Acid, DMSA)"

Michael I. Greenberg, MD, MPH
Professor of Emergency Medicine and Public Health
Division of Occupational and Environmental Emergency Medicine
Department of Emergency Medicine
Allegheny University of the Health Sciences
MCP Hahnemann School of Medicine
Philadelphia, Pennsylvania
Chapter 109, "Healthcare Workers"

Richard J. Hamilton, MD
Attending Physician
Department of Emergency Medicine
Bellevue Hospital Center/New York University Medical Center
Instructor in Clinical Surgery/Emergency Medicine
Fellow in Medical Toxicology
New York City Poison Center
New York University School of Medicine
New York, New York
Chapter 36, "Vitamins"
Chapter 70, "Substance Withdrawal"

Fred M. Henretig, MD
Associate Professor of Pediatrics
Division of Emergency Medicine
Department of Pediatrics
University of Pennsylvania School of Medicine
Director, Section of Clinical Toxicology
Division of Emergency Medicine
Department of Pediatrics
Children's Hospital of Philadelphia
Philadelphia, Pennsylvania
Chapter 79, "Lead"

Glendon C. Henry, MD
Assistant Professor of Clinical Surgery/Emergency Medicine
New York University School of Medicine
Assistant Director

Department of Emergency Medicine
Bellevue Hospital Center/New York University Medical Center
Consultant, New York City Poison Center
New York, New York
Chapter 59, "Lithium"

Robert Hessler, MD
Assistant Professor of Clinical Surgery/Emergency Medicine
New York University School of Medicine
Assistant Director
Department of Emergency Medicine
Bellevue Hospital Center/New York University Medical Center
New York, New York
Chapter 21, "Cardiovascular Principles"

Judd E. Hollander, MD
Associate Professor and Clinical Research Director
Department of Emergency Medicine
University of Pennsylvania
Attending Physician
Department of Emergency Medicine
Hospital of the University of Pennsylvania
Philadelphia, Pennsylvania
Chapter 65, "Cocaine"

Christopher P. Holstege, MD
Medical Toxicology Fellow
Division of Medical Toxicology
Department of Emergency Medicine
Indiana Poison Center
Trauma Center at Methodist Hospital
Indianapolis, Indiana
Chapter 95, "Smoke Inhalation"

Oliver L. Hung, MD
Fellow in Medical Toxicology
Department of Emergency Medicine
Bellevue Hospital Center
New York City Poison Center
New York, New York
Chapter 76, "Herbal Preparations"

Paul A. James, MD
Assistant Professor
Associate Director for the Office of Research and Development
Department of Family Medicine
State University of New York at Buffalo
Buffalo, New York
Chapter 110, "Farmers"

Brian Kaufman, MD
Associate Clinical Professor of Anesthesiology and Medicine
New York University Medical Center
Director, Critical Care Section
Department of Anesthesiology
Medical Director Respiratory Therapy
Tisch University Hospital
New York, New York
Chapter 53, "Anesthetics and Neuromuscular Blocking Agents"

Debra Kennedy, MB, BS, FRACP
Fellow
Division of Pediatrics
Department of Clinical Pharmacology and Toxicology
The Hospital for Sick Children
Toronto, Ontario, Canada
Chapter 16, "Mutagens, Carcinogens, and Teratogens"

William P. Kerns II, MD, FACEP, FACMT
Clinical Assistant Professor
Division of Toxicology
Department of Emergency Medicine
Carolinas Medical Center
Charlotte, North Carolina
Chapter 97, "Cyanide and Hydrogen Sulfide"

Christopher Keyes, MD, MPH, FACMT
Chief, Section of Toxicology
Division of Emergency Medicine
University of Texas Southwestern Medical School
Dallas, Texas
Chapter 25, "Endocrine Principles"

Mark A. Kirk, MD
Medical Toxicology Fellowship Director
Department of Emergency Medicine
Indiana Poison Center
Trauma Center at Methodist Hospital
Indiana University School of Medicine
Indianapolis, Indiana
Chapter 95, "Smoke Inhalation"
Chapter 97, "Cyanide and Hydrogen Sulfide"
Chapter 103, "Use of the Intensive Care Unit"

Gideon Koren, MD
Professor
Division of Clinical Pharmacology and Toxicology
Departments of Pediatrics, Pharmacology, Pharmacy, and Medicine
University of Toronto
Director
Clinical Pharmacology, Toxicology, and Motherisk Program
Department of Pediatrics
The Hospital for Sick Children
Toronto, Ontario, Canada
Chapter 16, "Mutagens, Carcinogens, and Teratogens"

Ricky L. Langley, MD, MPH
Division of Occupational & Environmental Medicine
Duke University Medical Center
Durham, North Carolina
Chapter 110, "Farmers"

Walter LeStrange, RN, MPH, MS
Vice President

Faculty Practice Services, Inc
New York, New York
Chapter 116, "Risk Management and Legal Principles"

Michael McCann, PhD, CIH
New York, New York
Chapter 111, "Artists"

William J. Meggs, MD, PhD, FACEP
Associate Professor
Division of Toxicology
Department of Emergency Medicine
East Carolina University School of Medicine
Attending Physician
Department of Emergency Medicine
Pitt County Memorial Hospital
Greenville, North Carolina
Chapter 14, "Immunologic Principles"
Chapter 110, "Farmers"

Maria Mercurio, RPh, CSPI, MS
New York City Poison Center
Bureau of Laboratories
Department of Health
New York, New York
Chapter 82, "Thallium"

Sanford M. Miller, MD
Assistant Professor of Clinical Anesthesiology
New York University School of Medicine
Assistant Attending
Department of Anesthesiology
New York University Medical Center
Associate Attending
Department of Anesthesiology
Bellevue Hospital Center
New York, New York
Chapter 53, "Anesthetics and Neuromuscular Blocking Agents"

Kirk C. Mills, MD, FACEP
Associate Fellowship Director—Medical Toxicology
Department of Emergency Medicine
Wayne State University
Assistant Professor of Emergency Medicine
Department of Emergency Medicine
Detroit Receiving Hospital
Detroit, Michigan
Chapter 10, "Neurotransmitters"

Robert J. Nadig, MD
Assistant Professor
Department of Medicine
The Albert Einstein College of Medicine
Chief
Division of Occupational Medicine and Toxicology
Department of Medicine
The Beth Israel Health Care System
New York, New York
Chapter 81, "Cadmium and Other Metals and Metalloids"
Chapter 92, "Hazardous Materials Release and Decontamination"

Lewis S. Nelson, MD
Assistant Professor of Clinical Surgery/Emergency Medicine
New York University School of Medicine
Attending Physician
Department of Emergency Medicine
New York University Medical Center/Bellevue Hospital Center
Director, Medical Toxicology Fellowship Program
New York City Poison Center
New York, New York
Chapter 60, "Opioids"
Chapter 94, "Simple Asphyxiants and Pulmonary Irritants"

Sean Patrick Nordt, PharmD
Assistant Director
Division of Medical Toxicology
California Poison Control Center—San Diego Division
University of California, San Diego Medical Center
San Diego, California
Chapter 54, "Pharmaceutical Additives"

Harold H. Osborn, MD
Professor and Chairman
Department of Emergency Medicine
New York Medical College
Valhalla, New York
Director, Emergency Services
Department of Emergency Medicine
Lincoln Medical and Mental Health Center
Bronx, New York
Chapter 43, "Antituberculous Agents"
Chapter 44, "Antimalarial Agents"
Chapter 61, "Sedative-Hypnotic Agents"
Chapter 62, "Ethanol"

John D. Osterloh, MD, MS
Professor of Clinical Laboratory Medicine and Medicine
Department of Laboratory Medicine and Medicine
University of California, San Francisco
Associate Chief—Toxicology
Clinical Laboratories
San Francisco General Hospital
San Francisco, California
Chapter 6, "Laboratory Principles and Techniques to Evaluate the Poisoned or Overdosed Patient"

Edward J. Otten, MD
Professor of Emergency Medicine and Pediatrics
Director, Division of Toxicology
Department of Emergency Medicine
University of Cincinnati
Cincinnati, Ohio

Chapter 69, "Marijuana"
Chapter 99, "Snakes and Other Reptiles"
Antidotes in Depth, "Antivenin (Crotalid and Elapid)"

Mary E. Palmer, MD
Senior Fellow in Medical Toxicology
Department of Emergency Medicine
Bellevue Hospital Center
New York City Poison Center
New York, New York
Chapter 33, "Nonsteroidal Antiinflammatory Agents"

Jeanmarie Perrone, MD
Assistant Professor
Co-Director, Division of Toxicology
Department of Emergency Medicine
University of Pennsylvania
Attending Physician
Department of Emergency Medicine
Hospital of the University of Pennsylvania
Philadelphia, Pennsylvania
Chapter 35, "Iron"
Chapter 37, "Dieting Agents, Regimens, and Food Supplements"

Donald J. Pizzarello, PhD
Professor of Radiology, Retired
Department of Radiology
New York University Medical Center
New York, New York
Chapter 98, "Radiation"

Susan M. Pond, MD, FRACP
Adjunct Professor
University of Queensland
Brisbane, Australia
University of Sydney
Sydney, Australia
Chapter 5, "Principles and Techniques Applied to Enhance Elimination of Toxic Compounds"
Chapter 90, "Herbicides: Paraquat and Diquat"

Kevin Porter, Esq
Parker, Chapin, Slattau, Klompl
New York, New York
Chapter 116, "Risk Management and Legal Principles"

Dennis Price, MD
Assistant Professor of Clinical Surgery/Emergency Medicine
New York University School of Medicine
Attending Physician
Department of Emergency Medicine
Bellevue Hospital Center
New York, New York
Chapter 93, "Methemoglobinemia"

Rama B. Rao, MD
Fellow in Medical Toxicology
Department of Emergency Medicine
New York City Poison Center
Bellevue Hospital Center
New York, New York
Chapter 86, "Caustics and Batteries"

Kathleen M. Rest, PhD, MPA
Associate Professor
Division of Occupational and Environmental Health
Department of Family and Community Medicine
University of Massachusetts Medical Center
Worcester, Massachusetts
Chapter 91, "Industrial Poisoning: Information and Control"

Wendy Rives, MD
Clinical Instructor
Department of Psychiatry
New York University Medical Center
Comprehensive Psychiatric Emergency Program
Bellevue Hospital Center
New York, New York
Chapter 113, "Psychiatric Principles: Evaluating and Managing Suicidal and Violent Patients"

James R. Roberts, MD, FAAEM, FACMT
Professor and Vice Chair
Department of Emergency Medicine
Professor and Chief
Division of Toxicology
Director, Institute for the Treatment of Poisonous Bites and Stings
Allegheny University of the Health Sciences
MCP Hahnemann School of Medicine
Chairman
Director, Division of Toxicology
Department of Emergency Medicine
Mercy Health Systems
Philadelphia, Pennsylvania
Chapter 99, "Snakes and Other Reptiles"
Antidotes in Depth, "Antivenin (Crotalid and Elapid)"

Harriet Rubenstein, MPH, JD
Assistant Professor
Department of Community and Preventive Medicine
Allegheny University of the Health Sciences
MCP Hahnemann School of Medicine
Philadelphia, Pennsylvania
Chapter 91, "Industrial Poisoning: Information and Control"

Morton E. Salomon, MD, FACEP, FAAP
Vice Chairman and Associate Professor
Department of Emergency Medicine
Albert Einstein College of Medicine
Director
Department of Emergency Services
Montefiore Medical Center
Bronx, New York
Chapter 71, "Nicotine and Tobacco Preparations"

Miguel R. Sanchez, MD
Associate Professor of Clinical Dermatology
Department of Dermatology
New York University School of Medicine
Associate Director
Department of Dermatology
Bellevue Hospital Center
New York, New York
Chapter 28, "Dermatologic Principles"

Diane Sauter, MD, FACEP
Chairman
Department of Emergency Medicine
Greater Southeast Community Hospital
Washington, District of Columbia
Chapter 24, "Hematologic Principles"
Chapter 58, "Monoamine Oxidase Inhibitors"

David T. Schwartz, MD
Assistant Professor of Clinical Surgery and Emergency Medicine
New York University School of Medicine
Attending Physician
Department of Emergency Medicine
New York University Medical Center/Bellevue Hospital Center
New York, New York
Chapter 7, "Toxicologic Imaging"

Mark R. Serper, PhD
Assistant Professor of Psychology
Hofstra University
Hempsted, New York
Research Assistant Professor of Psychiatry
New York University School of Medicine
New York, New York
Chapter 113, "Psychiatric Principles: Evaluating and Managing Suicidal and Violent Patients"

Richard D. Shih, MD, FACEP, FAAEM
Residency Director
Department of Emergency Medicine
Morristown Memorial Hospital
Morristown, New Jersey
Attending Physician
New Jersey Poison Information and Education Systems
Newark Beth Israel Medical Center
Newark, New Jersey
Chapter 77, "Plants"
Chapter 85, "Hydrocarbons"

Martin J. Smilkstein, MD
Associate Professor of Emergency Medicine
Department of Emergency Medicine
Associate Director, Toxicology Fellowship Program
Oregon Poison Center
Oregon Health Sciences University
Portland, Oregon
Chapter 4, "Techniques Used to Prevent Gastrointestinal Absorption of Toxic Compounds"
Chapter 22, "Gastrointestinal Principles"
Chapter 26, "Ophthalmic Principles"
Chapter 31, "Acetaminophen"

Kevin Smothers, MD
Director
Emergency Department
Greenwich Hospital
Greenwich, Connecticut
Chapter 107, "AIDS—Pharmacology and Toxicology"

Jack W. Snyder, MD, JD, PhD
Associate Professor
Department of Emergency Medicine and Laboratory Medicine
Thomas Jefferson University
Philadelphia, Pennsylvania
Chapter 6, "Laboratory Principles and Techniques to Evaluate the Poisoned or Overdosed Patient"

Barbara E. Soppet, RN MA
Nurse Clinician
Division of Nursing
Emergency Department
Coney Island Hospital
Brooklyn, New York
Chapter 114, "Nursing Principles"

Christine M. Stork, PharmD, ABAT
Clinical Assistant Professor
Director, Central New York Poison Control Center
Department of Emergency Medicine
University Hospital, State University of New York Health Science Center
Syracuse, New York
Chapter 46, "Antibiotics"
Chapter 56, "Selective Serotonin Reuptake Inhibitors and Other Antidepressants"
Antidotes in Depth, "Dilution and Neutralization"

Young-Jin Sue, MD
Assistant Clinical Professor
Division of Pediatric Emergency Medicine
Department of Pediatrics
Albert Einstein College of Medicine
Attending Physician
Division of Pediatric Emergency Services
Department of Pediatrics
Montefiore Medical Center
Bronx, New York
Chapter 80, "Mercury"

Kenneth M. Sutin, MD
Assistant Professor of Clinical Anesthesiology and Clinical Surgery
Division of Critical Care Medicine
Department of Anesthesiology
New York University
Associate Director of Critical Care
Director of Recovery Room
Division of Critical Care Medicine
Department of Anesthesiology
Bellevue Hospital Center
New York, New York
Chapter 53, "Anesthetics and Neuromuscular Blocking Agents"

Stephen R. Thom, MD, PhD
Associate Professor of Emergency Medicine
Department of Emergency Medicine
Chief of Hyperbaric Medicine
Institute for Environmental Medicine
University of Pennsylvania
Philadelphia, Pennsylvania
Antidotes in Depth, "Hyperbaric Oxygen"

Christian Tomaszewski, MD
Clinical Assistant Professor
Department of Emergency Medicine
University of North Carolina—Chapel Hill
Chapel Hill, North Carolina
Toxicology Fellowship Director and Medical Director, Hyperbaric Medicine
Department of Emergency Medicine
Carolinas Medical Center
Charlotte, North Carolina
Chapter 96, "Carbon Monoxide"

Jeffrey R. Tucker, MD
Assistant Professor of Pediatrics
Division of Emergency Medicine
Department of Pediatrics
University of Connecticut School of Medicine
Farmington, Connecticut
Attending Physician
Division of Emergency Medicine
Department of Pediatrics
Connecticut Children's Medical Center
Hartford, Connecticut
Chapter 68, "Lysergic Acid Diethylamide and Other Hallucinogens"

Michael G. Tunik, MD
Assistant Professor of Clinical Pediatrics
Department of Pediatrics
New York University School of Medicine
Attending Physician
Department of Emergency Medicine
Bellevue Hospital Center
New York, New York
Chapter 72, "Food Poisoning"

Susi U. Vassallo, MD, FACEP, FACMT
Assistant Professor of Clinical Surgery/Emergency Medicine
New York University School of Medicine
Attending Physician
Department of Emergency Medicine
Bellevue Hospital Center/New York University Medical Center
Consultant, New York City Poison Center
New York, New York
Chapter 18, "Thermoregulatory Principles"

Staffan Wåhlander, MD
Assistant Professor of Clinical Anesthesiology and Surgery
Division of Critical Care
Department of Anesthesiology
New York University School of Medicine
Director, Critical Care Anesthesia
Associate Director, Surgical ICU
Bellevue Hospital Center
New York, New York
Chapter 53, "Anesthetics and Neuromuscular Blocking Agents"

Richard Y. Wang, DO, FACEP
Assistant Professor
Division of Emergency Medicine
Department of Medicine
Brown University School of Medicine
Director, Division of Medical Toxicology
Department of Emergency Medicine
Rhode Island Hospital
Providence, Rhode Island
Chapter 47, "Antineoplastic Agents"

Paul M. Wax, MD, FACMT
Associate Professor
Department of Emergency Medicine
University of Rochester School of Medicine
Department of Medicine
Strong Memorial Hospital
Rochester, New York
Chapter 1, "History"
Chapter 2, "Toxicologic Plagues and Disasters in History"
Chapter 83, "Antiseptics, Disinfectants, and Sterilants"
Antidotes in Depth, "Antiquated Antidotes"
Antidotes in Depth, "Sodium Bicarbonate"

Leslie R. Wolf, MD
Assistant Professor
Toxicology Coordinator
Department of Emergency Medicine
Wright State University School of Medicine
Dayton, Ohio
Chapter 29, "Genitourinary Principles"

Table of Antidotes in Depth

Readers of previous editions of Goldfrank's Toxicologic Emergencies *are undoubtedly aware that the editors have always felt that an emphasis on general management of poisoning or overdoses coupled with sound medical management is more important or as important as the selection and use of a specific antidote in the vast majority of cases. Nevertheless, there are some instances where nothing other than the timely use of a specific antidote or antagonist will save a patient. For this reason, and also because the use of such antidotes may be problematic, controversial, or unfamiliar to the practitioner (as new antidotes continue to emerge), we have included a section (or sections) at the end of each chapter where an in-depth discussion of such antidotes is relevant. The following "Antidotes in Depth" are included in this edition.*

Table of Contents

Preface

In this sixth edition of *Goldfrank's Toxicologic Emergencies*, we continue to proudly offer readers a case study approach to medical toxicology. Among the one dozen new chapters in this edition are discussions of toxicologic plagues, the use of electrocardiography in medical toxicology, and more detailed information on mutagens, carcinogens, teratogens, and radiation as well as immunologic principles. There are new chapters on genitourinary principles, thallium poisoning, water and airborne toxins, and the special populations of health care workers and substance abusers.

Expanded discussions of serotonin reuptake inhibitors, anesthetics, and neuromuscular blocking agents have also been included. The basic science chapters have been expanded and grouped together in a new section. In order to keep this expanded work in one volume, we moved the review material found at the end of previous editions to a newly created companion book, *Study Guide for Goldfrank's Toxicologic Emergencies*.

Goldfrank's Toxicologic Emergencies, originally a collection of clinical toxicology case discussions by two authors, is now a multi-authored text of close to 2,000 pages prepared under the direction of six author-editors who, until recently, all worked at the New York City Poison Center. As the text expanded in size and scope over the past two decades, we sought to address issues in medical toxicology in new ways that would make the book a valuable resource to the growing number of clinicians and researchers working in the field. In the second edition (1982), we expanded the case study material to make the work a more comprehensive clinical resource. In the third edition (1986), we added an organ-system approach to medical toxicology and also began a series of *antidotes-in-depth* to provide specific detailed information about newer and, in some cases, experimental antidotes. In the fourth edition (1990), we expanded both of these newer sections and began to address such subjects as nursing care, medical-legal issues, and the toxicology of AIDS treatments. For the fifth edition (1994), we added a section addressing the needs of special populations including reproductive, perinatal, pediatric, and geriatric principles and intensive care unit patients; we also began to seriously consider basic science issues such as neurotransmitters and biochemical and metabolic pathways.

Work on a new edition of this text literally begins the day the book is published. Although many of the chapters in this sixth edition may appear familiar to readers of previous editions, every chapter has been discussed, analyzed, criticized, and dissected at our weekly journal club and monthly editors' meetings. Although tearing down and reconstructing the text between each edition may seem like an extreme exercise to some, only in this manner can we hope to prevent ourselves from accepting and promulgating unfounded treatments and outdated concepts. We hope that you agree that this exercise is worthwhile and that each "new text" continues to serve you well. As always, we encourage your comments and thoughtful criticism, and we will do our best to incorporate your suggestions into future editions.

If this text helps to provide better patient care and stimulates interest in medical toxicology by students of medicine, nursing, and pharmacy; residents in emergency medicine, internal medicine, pediatrics, preventive health, and family practice; and, of course, fellows in medical toxicology, our efforts will have indeed been worthwhile.

Lewis R. Goldfrank
Neal E. Flomenbaum
Neal A. Lewin
Richard S. Weisman
Mary Ann Howland
Robert S. Hoffman

Preface to the First Edition

As attending emergency physicians in one of New York City's busiest emergency services, we have had to deal with some of the most amazing and complex problems that any physician could encounter, but in dealing with these problems we have had the pleasure of working with an enthusiastic and dedicated group of house officers who asked innumerable questions. It became obvious at Morrisania City Hospital the problems we saw most frequently involved those conditions that we were least adequately prepared to treat properly. We have noted, until very recently, almost complete neglect of toxicology in our medical schools. For example, as late as 1969 a classic textbook on pediatrics stated that the leading cause of childhood mortality was poisoning; yet only 12 pages in the text were devoted to toxicology. Only in the most recent editions have the standard texts on internal medicine begun to give comprehensive coverage of this field. Fortunately, the era in which toxicology was to seen but not heard has ended, but we would like to bring toxicology one step farther. We are attempting to make management of toxicologic problems exciting, so that these unfortunate patients will receive the same kind of care others without self-induced or iatrogenic disease receive. It is time we answered this question: Who is most responsible for the initiation of addiction or abuse? Is it not the health practitioner?

These case histories and their associated questions represent our attempts to respond to the house staff's needs. We have attempted to be practical yet pathophysiologic. These cases and questions have been used in teaching conferences for several years. When Peter Frishauf, the editor of *Hospital Physician,* proposed a monthly column, we saw that as a means of stimulation. Each of these cases appeared in our column "Toxicologic Emergencies" in the journal *Hospital Physician.*

The fact that 21 percent of the admissions to Morrisania City Hospital's adult medical service in 1974 were for toxicologic ingestion demonstrates the need for a competent clinical toxicologist. Alcoholism was found in more than 50 percent of those hospitalized at Morrisania City Hospital.

For the sake of structure, we have employed poetic license in some of the aspects of these cases. This has been done to emphasize certain issues and minimize others less relevant to the articles. (In an attempt to clarify a particular type of ingestion we have eliminated the "mixed overdose" component in several cases.)

In many instances drug ingestion mimics well-known diseases. In addition, the response to any ingestion is substrate-dependent. If the patient abuses other drugs, if he is ill, or if he has taken a massive ingestion, predictions are impossible. Drug ingestion must be considered when the patient's symptoms evolve without prodrome, when the varied manifestations do not fit any classic disease pattern and when the patient's history suggests drug ingestion.

We have deemphasized therapy other than that relating to the toxicologic ingestion; we have usually not followed the patient's hospital course; although it would be interesting to do so and we routinely do so in our practice. a number of our readers have criticized us for not being more detailed in our analyses. We have tried to limit our discussion to the necessary problem-solving and the initial therapeutic management in the emergency department. We think that the role of the emergency physician is to make the appropriate judgments rapidly and expedite and admission of seriously ill patients.

The first three chapters have been added to provide an overall plan for emergency management of any overdose. The introduction is meant to define the ground rules for the case assessments that follow. We have included an index so that the reader may study a differential diagnosis or a particular drug group. We have chosen not to create a table of syndromes but to present cases wherein we discuss the differential diagnosis. In recent years we have seen the development of several excellent handbooks in the field of toxicology and poisoning; yet our students and house officers have not mastered this body of knowledge. In an attempt to make toxicology attractive to the medical staff, we have chosen a problem-oriented approach. We have in no way tried to duplicate or compete with the outstanding works in the field of clinical pharmacology and toxicology. Each article has a number of important references relating to the problem being considered. . . .

Lewis R. Goldfrank
Robert H. Kirstein

Acknowledgments

We are grateful to Maryann Camisa, who not only helped manage this book's growth and development but also transformed scrawl into manuscript with precision and dedication for this sixth edition, as she did so faithfully for the fifth edition. We are also deeply appreciative of the secretarial efforts of Kristin Montella.

The many letters and verbal communications we have received with the reviews of the previous editions of this book continue to improve our efforts. We are deeply indebted to our friends, associates, and students who stimulated us to begin this book with their questions and then faithfully criticized our answers.

We thank the many volunteers, students, librarians, and particularly the St. John's University College of Pharmacy students and drug information staff who provide us with vital technical assistance in our daily attempt to deal with toxicologic emergencies.

We appreciate the artistic skills of John Ruggeri and Pamela Ryder, FNP, who have added line drawings of important plants and mushrooms to assist the reader in the understanding of these botanical species.

The conscientious and tireless work of James Semidy, who has found so many essential articles and prepared so many copies for the review by editors and authors, has been invaluable.

No words can adequately express our indebtedness to the many authors who worked on earlier editions of many of the chapters in this book. As different authors write and rewrite topics with each new edition, we recognize that without the foundation work of their predecessors this book would not be what it is today.

We greatly acknowledge the right to use extensive parts of "Rational Utilization of the Intensive Care Unit in Managing the Poisoned Patient," previously published in *Critical Care Toxicology* in the Contemporary Management in Critical Care series, Churchill Livingstone, New York, 1991.

CHAPTER 1

History

Paul M. Wax

The term *poison* first appeared in the English literature around the year 1230 to describe a potion or draught that had been prepared with deadly ingredients.[68,85] The history of poisons and poisoning, however, dates back thousands of years. Through the millennia, poisons have played an important role in human history—from political assassination in Roman times to contemporary environmental concerns.

This chapter offers a perspective on the impact of poisons (and poisoning) on history. It also provides a historic overview of human understanding of poisons and the development of toxicology. The chapter follows the important events in the evolution of toxicology from antiquity to the present. The development of the poison control center, as well as the genesis of the field of medical toxicology, are examined. An Antidote in Depth segment at the end of the chapter scrutinizes changes in poison management over the years, analyzing obsolete antidotes and other discarded therapeutic modalities. Chapter 2 will highlight some of the great poison plagues and disasters throughout history and examine societal consequences of these unfortunate events. An appreciation of past successes and mistakes should promote a keener insight and more critical evaluation of present-day toxicologic issues and help prepare us to tackle the problems of tomorrow.

The Poisons of Antiquity

The earliest poisons consisted of plant extracts, animal venoms, and minerals (Table 1–1). They were used for hunting, waging war, and official execution. The *Ebers Papyrus*, an ancient Egyptian text written about 1500 B.C., which is considered to be among the earliest medical records, describes many ancient poisons, including arsenic, antimony, lead, opium, mandrake, hemlock, aconite, wormwood, and cyanogenic glycosides.[52,85] These poisons were thought to have mystical properties and their use was surrounded by superstition and intrigue. Some agents, such as the calabar bean from the plant *Physostigma venenosum* (which contains physostigmine), were referred to as ordeal poisons. Ingestions of these substances were believed to be lethal to the guilty and harmless to the innocent.[52] The "penalty of the peach" involved the administration of crushed peach pits (containing amygdalin that is broken down to cyanide) as an ordeal poison. Magicians, sorcerers, and priests were the poison experts of antiquity. The Sumerians, in about 4500 B.C., were said to worship the deity Gula, who was known as the "mistress of charms and spells" and the "controller of noxious poisons" (Table 1–2).[85]

Arrow and Dart Poisons

The prehistoric Masai hunters of Kenya, who lived 18,000 years ago, may have utilized arrow and dart poisons to increase the lethality of their weapons used to kill animals and other humans.[11] One of these poisons may have consisted of extracts of *Strophanthus* species, an indigenous plant that contains strophanthin, a digitalis-like substance.[52] Cave paintings of arrowheads and spearheads reveal that these weapons may have been crafted with small depressions at the end to hold the poison.[86] In fact, the term *toxicology* appears to be derived from two Greek terms: *toxikos* ("bow") and *toxikon* ("poison into which arrowheads are dipped").[4,86]

References to arrow poisons are cited in a number of other important literary works. The ancient Indian text *Rg Veda*, written in the 12th century B.C., refers to the use of *Aconitum* species for arrow poisons.[11] In the *Odyssey*, Homer (ca. 850 B.C.) wrote about how Ulysses anointed his arrows with a variety of poisons, including extracts of *Helleborus orientalis* (thought to act as a heart poison) and snake venoms.[65] Aristotle (384–322 B.C.) described how the Scythians prepared and used arrow poisons.[87] In the Book of Job 6:04, arrow poisons are also cited: "For the arrows of the Almighty pierce men, and my spirit drinks in their poison."[10] Finally, reference to weapons poisoned with the blood of serpents can be found in the writings of Ovid (43 B.C.–A.D. 18).[93]

TABLE 1–1. POISONS KNOWN TO THE ANCIENT GREEKS AND ROMANS

Poisonous Animals and Fish
Cantharides (*Cantharis vesicatoria*)
Jellyfish (*Cnidaria*)
Puffer fish (*Tetraodontidae*)
Scorpions (*Scorpionida*)
Sea hare (*Aplysiidae*)
Snakes (*Serpentes*)
Stingrays (*Dasyatidae*)
Weeverfish (*Trachinidae*)

Poisonous Plants
Aconite (*Aconitum* species)
Cyanide (*Prunus* species)
Hellebore (*Veratrum album*)
Hemp (*Cannabis indica*)
Henbane (*Hyoscyamus niger*)
Mandrake (*Mandragora officinarum*)
Opium (*Papaver somniferum*)
Physostigmine (*Physostigma venenosa*)
Poison hemlock (*Conium maculatum*)
Strychnine (*Strychnos nux-vomica*)
Wormwood (*Artemisia absinthium*)

Poisonous Minerals
Antimony
Arsenic
Copper
Lead
Mercury

The first attempts at poison identification and classification, and the introduction of the first antidotes, took place during Greek and Roman times. An early categorization of poisons divided them into fast poisons such as strychnine, and slow poisons such as arsenic. In his treatise *Materia Medica*, the Greek physician Dioscorides (A.D. 40–80) categorized poisons by their origin: animal, vegetable, or mineral.[86] This remained the standard classification for the next 1500 years.[93]

Animal Poisons

Animal poisons usually referred to the venom from poisonous animals. While the venom from poisonous snakes has always been one of the most commonly found poisons, other poisonous animals of concern included toads, salamanders, jellyfish, stingrays, and sea hares. Nicander (204–135 B.C.), a Greek poet and physician, considered to be one of the earliest toxicologists, experimented with animal poisons using condemned criminals as subjects.[86] His poem "Theriaca" described the presentation and treatment of poisoning from animal toxins.[85] A notable fatality from the effects of an animal toxin was Cleopatra (69–30 B.C.), who reportedly committed suicide by deliberately falling on an African cobra.[41]

Vegetable Poisons

Theophrastus (ca. 370–286 B.C.) described vegetable poisons in his treatise *De Historia Plantarum*.[41] Notorious poisonous plants included aconite (*Aconitum* species), hellebore (*Veratrum album*), henbane (*Hyoscyamus niger*), mandrake (*Mandragora officinarum*), and hemlock (*Conium maculatum*). Aconite was among the most frequently encountered poisonous plants and was described as the "queen mother of poisons."[85] Hemlock was the official poison used by the Greeks and was employed in the execution of Socrates (ca. 470–399 B.C.) and many others.[64] Opium was also used by the ancients, both as a medicinal and as a poison. Poisonous plants used in India at this time included *Cannabis indica* (Tetrahydrocannabinol), *Croton tiglium* (Croton oil), and *Strychnos nux-vomica* (strychnine).[41]

Mineral Poisons

The mineral poisons of antiquity consisted of the heavy metals: lead, mercury, arsenic, and antimony. Undoubtedly the most famous of these was lead. Lead was discovered as early as 3500 B.C. Although controversy continues about whether an epidemic of lead poisoning among the Roman aristocracy contributed to the fall of the Roman empire, lead was extensively utilized during this period.[29,63] In addition to its considerable use in plumbing, lead was also utilized in the production of food and drink containers.[35] Not uncommonly, lead was added directly to wine, or the wine was intentionally prepared in a leaden kettle to improve its taste. Not surprisingly, chronic lead poisoning became widespread. Nicander is credited with describing the first case of lead poisoning in the second century B.C.[91] Dioscorides, writing in the first century A.D., noted that fortified wine was "most hurtful to the nerves."[91] Lead-induced gout ("saturnine gout") may have also been widespread among the Roman elite.[63]

Although not animal, vegetable, or mineral, the toxic effects of gases were also appreciated during antiquity. In the third century B.C. Aristotle commented that "coal fumes (carbon monoxide) lead to a heavy head and death."[39] Cicero (106–43 B.C.) referred to the use of coal fumes in suicide and execution, a practice that continues 2000 years later.

Poisoners

Intentional poisoning was common during the Roman times. In an attempt to curtail this practice, the Roman dictator Sulla issued the first law against poisoning, entitled the *Lex Cornelia*, in 81 B.C. According to its provisions, if convicted of poisoning, the perpetrator was sentenced to either loss of property and exile (if he or she was of high rank) or exposure to wild beasts (if he or she was of low rank). Members of the aristocracy employed a "taster" to shield themselves from potential poisoners.[93]

Locusta was one of the most infamous poisoners of all time. Hired by Nero's mother, Agrippina, as part of a scheme to make Nero emperor, Locusta reportedly used

TABLE 1–2. IMPORTANT FIGURES IN THE HISTORY OF TOXICOLOGY TO 1900

Person	Date	Importance
Gula	ca. 4500 B.C.	First deity associated with poisons
Shen Nung	ca. 2000 B.C.	Chinese emperor who experimented on poisons and antidotes and wrote treatise on herbal medicine
Ancient Greek and Roman Period		
Homer	ca. 850 B.C.	Wrote how Ulysses anointed arrows with the venom of serpents
Aristotle	384–322 B.C.	Described the preparation and use of arrow poisons
Theophrastus	ca. 370–286 B.C.	Referred to poisonous plants in *De Historia Plantarum*
Socrates	ca. 470–399 B.C.	Executed by poison hemlock
Nicander	204–135 B.C.	Wrote two poems that are among the earliest works on poisons: *Theriaca* and *Alexipharmaca*
King Mithridates VI	ca. 132–63 B.C.	Fanatical fear of poisons, developed mithridatum, one of first universal antidotes
Sulla	81 B.C.	Issued *Lex Cornelia,* first anti-poisoning law
Cleopatra	69–30 B.C.	Committed suicide from deliberate cobra snake envenomation
Locusta	First century A.D.	Poisoned Claudius (A.D. 54) and Britannicus (A.D. 55) with (most likely) arsenic
Andromachus	A.D. 37–68	Refined the mithridatum, known as the Theriaca of Andromachus
Dioscorides	A.D. 40–80	Wrote *Materia Medica,* which classified poison by animal, vegetable, and mineral
Galen	ca. A.D. 129–200	Prepared "Nut Theriac" for Roman Emperors, a remedy against bites, stings, and poisons; wrote *De Antidotis I and II,* which provided recipes for different antidotes including Mithridatum and Panacea
Medieval Period		
Maimonides	1135–1204	Wrote *Treatise on Poisons and their Antidotes*
Petrus Abbonus	1250–1315	Wrote *De Venenis,* major work on poisoning
Renaissance		
Paracelsus	1493–1541	Introduced dose concept to toxicology
Ambroise Pare	1510–1590	Spoke out against unicorn horns and bezoars as antidotes
Catherine de Medici	1519–1589	Introduced Italian poisoning techniques to France
William Piso	1611–1678	First to study emetic qualities of *ipecacuanha*
Hieronyma Spara	Died 1659	Taught women how to poison their husbands
Madame Giulia Toffana	Died 1719	Poisoned over 600 people with aqua Toffana
Marchioness de Brinvilliers	Died 1676	French poisoner who tested her poisons on hospitalized patients
Catherine Deshayes	Died 1680	Notorious French poisoner know as "La Voisin"
Age of Enlightenment		
Richard Mead	1673–1754	Wrote first book in English language dedicated to poisoning
Percivall Pott	1714–1788	First description of occupational cancer, relating the chimney sweep occupation to scrotal cancer
Felice Fontana	1730–1805	First scientific study of venomous snakes
Philip Physick	1767–1837	Early advocate of gastric lavage to remove poisons
Baron Guillaume Dupuytren	1777–1835	Early advocate of gastric lavage to remove poisons
Edward Jukes	1820	Self-experimented with gastric lavage apparatus known as Jukes's syringe
M. Bertrand	1813	Demonstrated charcoal efficacy in arsenic ingestion
P. Touery	1831	Demonstrated charcoal efficacy in strychnine ingestion
A. Garrod	1846	First systematic study of charcoal in an animal model
B. Howard Rand	1848	First charcoal efficacy study in humans
Bonaventure Orfila	1787–1853	Father of modern toxicology, wrote *Traite Des Poisons;* first to isolate arsenic from human organs
Robert Christison	1797–1882	Wrote *Treatise on Poisons,* one of the most influential texts in early 19th century
Francois Magendie	1783–1855	Discovered emetine and studied mechanism of cyanide and strychnine
Claude Bernard	1813–1878	Studied mechanism of toxicity of carbon monoxide and curare
O.H. Costill	1848	Wrote first book on symptoms and treatment of poisoning
Theodore Wormley	1826–1897	Wrote *Micro-chemistry of Poisons,* first American book devoted exclusively to toxicology
James Marsh	1794–1846	Developed reduction test for arsenic
Hugo Reinsch	1842	Developed qualitative test for arsenic and mercury
Max Gutzeit	1847–1915	Developed method to quantitate small amounts of arsenic
Albert Nieman	1860	Isolated cocaine alkaloid
Rudolf Kobert	1854–1918	Studied digitalis and ergot alkaloids
Louis Lewin	1850–1929	Studied many toxins including methanol, chloroform, snake venom, carbon monoxide, lead, opioids, and hallucinogenic plants

arsenic to poison Claudius, Nero's stepfather, in A.D. 54, and Britannicus, Nero's stepbrother, in A.D. 55.[41,86] In the latter case, Locusta managed to fool the taster by preparing an unusually hot soup that required additional cooling after the soup had been officially tasted. At the time of cooling, arsenic was unobtrusively slipped into the soup.

Ancient Antidotes

The recognition, classification, and use of poisons in Ancient Greece and Rome were accompanied by an intensive search for a universal antidote. In fact, many of the physicians from this period devoted significant parts of their careers to this endeavor.[85] Mystery and superstition surrounded the origin and source of these various agents. One of the earliest specific references to a protective agent can be found in Homer's *Odyssey*, where Ulysses is advised to protect himself by taking the antidote "moli." Recent speculation suggests that moli referred to *Galanthus nivalis*, a naturally occurring cholinesterase inhibitor. This agent could have been used as an antidote against poisonous plants such as *Datura stramonium*.[71]

Theriacs and the Mithridatum

The Greeks referred to the universal antidote as the *alexipharmica* or *theriac*.[85] The term *alexipharmica* was derived from the words *alexipharmakos* ("which keeps off poison") and *antipharmakon* ("antidote"). Over the years, *alexipharmica* was increasingly used to refer to a method of treatment, such as the induction of emesis by using a feather. *Theriac* (which had originally been used to refer to poisonous reptiles or wild beasts) was used to refer to the actual antidotes. Ingestion of the early theriacs (ca. 200 B.C.) was reputed to make people "poison-proof" against bites of all venomous animals except the asp. Their ingredients included wild thyme, apoponax, aniseed, fennel, parsley, meru, and anmi.[85]

The quest for the universal antidote was epitomized by the work of King Mithridates VI of Pontus (132–63 B.C.).[40] After repeatedly being subjected to poisoning attempts by his enemies during his youth, Mithridates channeled his fanatical fear of being poisoned into the development of universal antidotes. He performed acute toxicity experiments on criminals and slaves to find the best antidote. The preparation he concocted, known as the "mithridatum," contained a minimum of 36 ingredients and was considered the best antidote in the Roman pharmacy. This concoction was thought to be protective against spiders, scorpions, vipers, aconite, sea slugs, and all other poisonous substances.[40] Mithridates took his concoction every day. Ironically, as an old man, Mithridates attempted suicide by poison but supposedly was unsuccessful because he had become poison-proof. Having failed at self-poisoning, Mithridates was compelled to have a soldier kill him with a sword. Galen described Mithridates' experiences in a series of three books: *De Antidotis I*, *De Antidotis II*, and *De Theriaca ad Pisonem*.[40,89]

The theriac of Andromachus, also known as the "Venice treacle" or "galene," is probably the most famous theriac. According to Galen, this preparation, formulated during the first century A.D., was considered an improvement over the mithridatum.[89] It was prepared by Andromachus (A.D. 37–68), physician to emperor Nero. Andromachus added to the mithridatum ingredients such as the flesh of vipers, squills, and generous amounts of opium.[95] Other ingredients were removed. Altogether, 73 ingredients were required. It was advocated to "counteract all poisons and bites of venomous animals," as well as a host of other medical problems such as colic, jaundice, and dropsy.[85] It was used both therapeutically and prophylactically.[89] As evidence of its efficacy, Galen demonstrated that fowl receiving poison followed by theriac had a higher survival rate than fowl receiving poison alone.[85] It is likely, however, that the scientific rigor and methodology employed differed from current scientific practice.

By the Middle Ages, the theriac of Andromachus contained over 100 ingredients. Its synthesis was quite elaborate; the initial production period lasted months, followed by an aging process that lasted years (somewhat like vintage wine).[48] The final product was often more solid than liquid in consistency.

Other theriac preparations were named after famous physicians (Damocrates, Nicolaus, Amando, Arnauld, and Abano) who contributed additional ingredients to the original formulation. Over the centuries certain localities were celebrated for their own peculiar brand of theriac. Notable centers of theriac production included Cairo, Venice, Florence, Genoa, Bologna, and Istanbul. At times, theriac production was accompanied by great fanfare. For example, in Bologna, the mixing of the theriac could take place only under the direction of the medical professors at the university.[85]

Whether these preparations truly benefited anyone is debatable. It has been suggested that the theriac may have had an antiseptic effect on the gastrointestinal tract, while others have stated that theriac's sole benefit derived from its formulation with opium.[48] These agents remained very much in vogue throughout the Middle Ages and Renaissance. It was not until the 18th century that their efficacy was finally questioned by William Heberden in 1745, in *Antitheriaka: An Essay on Mithridatium and Theriaca*.[40] Nonetheless, pharmacopeias in France, Spain, and Germany continued to list these agents until the last quarter of the nineteenth century.[48] Theriac was still available in Italy and Turkey into the early twentieth century.

Sacred Earth

Beginning in the 5th century B.C., an adsorbent agent called *terra sigillata* was also promoted as a universal antidote. This agent, also known as the "sacred sealed earth," consisted of red clay that could be found on only one particular hill on the Greek island of Lemnos. Perhaps somewhat akin to the 20th-century "universal antidote," it was advocated as effective in counteracting all poisons.[85] With great ceremony, once per year, the terra sigillata was retrieved from this hill and prepared for subsequent use. According to Dioscorides, this clay was formulated with goat's blood to make it into a paste. At one time, it was included as part of the theriac of Andromachus. Demand for terra sigillata continued into the 15th century. Similar antidotal clays were found in Italy, Malta, Silesia, and England. Later analysis revealed these clays to be a combination of iron, aluminum, magnesium, and silicates.[85]

Charms

Charms, such as toadstones, unicorn horns, and bezoar stones, were also promoted as universal antidotes. Toadstones found in the heads of old toads were reputed to have the ability to extract poison from the site of a venomous bite or sting. In addition, the toadstone was supposedly able to detect the mere presence of poison by recognizing the heat characteristics of the poison.[85]

Much lore has surrounded the antidotal effects of the mythical unicorn horn. Ctesias, writing in 390 B.C., was the first to chronicle the wonders of the unicorn horn, claiming that drinking water or wine from the "horn of the unicorn" would protect against poison.[85] The horns were usually narwhal tusks or rhinoceros horns and were greatly valued. During the Middle Ages it was said that the unicorn horn was worth ten times the price of gold. Similar to the toadstone, the unicorn horn was used both to detect poisons and to neutralize them. It was said that a cup made of unicorn horn would sweat if a poisonous substance was placed in it.[47] To give further credence to its use, a 1593 study on arsenic-poisoned dogs reportedly showed that the horn was protective.[47]

Bezoar stones, also touted as universal antidotes, consisted of stomach or intestinal calculi formed by the deposition of calcium phosphate around a hair, fruit pit, or gallstone. They were removed from wild goats, cows, and apes and administered orally. The Persian name for the bezoar stone was *pad zahr* ("expeller of poisons"). The ancient Hebrews referred to them as *bel Zaard* ("every cure for poisons"). Over the years regional variations of bezoar stones were popularized, including an Asian variety from wild goat of Persia, an Occidental variety from llamas of Peru, and a European variety from chamois of the Swiss mountains.[28,85]

Early Attempts at Gastrointestinal Decontamination

Nicander wrote one of the earliest treatises on antidotes, entitled *Alexipharmaca* ("Antidotes for Poisons"). In this poem, he recommends induction of emesis by one of several different methods: (1) ingesting warm linseed oil, (2) tickling the hypopharynx with a feather, or (3) "emptying the gullet with a small twisted and curved paper."[51] Nicander also advocated the use of suction to limit envenomation.[86] The Romans referred to the feather as the "vomiting feather" or "pinna." Most commonly, it was utilized after a hearty feast. At times the pinna was dipped into a nauseating mixture to increase its efficacy.[51]

Toxicology During the Medieval and Renaissance Periods

The Scientists

From the fall of Rome until the lifetime of Moses Maimonides (1135–1204), the subject of poisons generated little documented attention. With the writing of Maimonides's *Treatise on Poisons and Their Antidotes* in 1198, the next stage in the development of toxicology began (see Table 1–2). Maimonides' treatise was one of the first works written on the treatment of poisons in over 1000 years. In part one of the treatise, Maimonides discussed the bites of snakes and mad dogs and stings of bees, wasps, spiders, and scorpions.[78] He also discussed the use of cupping glasses for bites (a progenitor of the modern suctioning device), and was one of the first to differentiate the hematotoxic (hot) from the neurotoxic (cold) effects of poison. In part two, he discussed mineral poisons and vegetable poisons and their antidotes. He described belladonna poisoning as causing a "redness and a sort of excitation."[78] He suggested that emesis should be induced by hot water, anethum, and oil, followed by fresh milk, butter, and honey. Although he rejected some of the popular treatments of the day, he advocated the use of the great theriac and the mithridatum as first and second-line agents in the treatment of snake bite.[78]

Paracelsus' (1493–1541) study on the dose–response relationship is usually considered the beginning of the scientific approach to toxicology. He was the first to emphasize the chemical nature of toxic agents.[69] Paracelsus stressed the need for proper observation and experimentation regarding the true response to chemicals. He underscored the need to differentiate between the therapeutic and toxic properties of chemicals when he stated in his "third defense," "What is there that is not poison? All things are poison and nothing [is] without poison. Solely the dose determines that a thing is not a poison."[23]

Whereas Paracelsus is the best known of the Renaissance toxicologists, Ambroise Pare (1510–1590) and William Piso (1611–1678) also contributed to the field. Pare argued against the use of the unicorn horn and bezoar stone.[50] He also wrote an early treatise on carbon monoxide poisoning. Piso is credited as one of the first to recognize the emetic properties of ipecacuanha.[76]

The Poisoners

Despite these advances in toxicologic treatment, the Renaissance is mainly remembered as the age of the poisoner, a time when the art of poisoning reached new stages. From the 15th to 17th centuries actual schools of poisoning existed in Venice and Rome. In Venice, poisoning services were provided by a group called the Council of Ten, whose members were hired to perform murder by poison.[87]

Members of the infamous Borgia family were credited with many poisonings during this period. They preferred using a poison called "la cantarella," a mixture of arsenic and phosphorus.[87] Rodrigo Borgia (1431–1503), who became Pope Alexander VI, and his son Cesare Borgia were reportedly responsible for the poisoning of cardinals and kings.

In the late 16th century, Catherine de Medici, wife of Henry II of France, introduced Italian poisoning techniques to France. She experimented on the poor, the sick, and the criminal. By analyzing the subsequent complaints of her victims, she is said to have learned the site of action and time of onset, the clinical signs and symptoms, and the efficacy of poisons.[30]

Murder by poison remained quite popular during the latter half of the 17th and early 18th centuries in Italy and France. One of the major centers for poison practitioners was Naples, the home of the notorious Madame Giulia Toffana. She reportedly poisoned more than 600 people, preferring a particular solution of white arsenic (arsenic trioxide), better known as "aqua toffana."[93] This concoction was dispensed under the guise of a cosmetic.[85] She was executed in 1719.

In France, the Marchioness de Brinvilliers (executed in 1676), and Catherine Deshayes (burned alive in 1680) were two of the most notorious poisoners.[93] The Marchioness tested her poison concoctions on hospitalized patients. Among her favorite poisons were corrosive sublimate (mercury bichloride), arsenic, lead, copper sulfate, and tartar emetic that contained antimony.[87] Deshayes, who was a fortuneteller and sorceress, was implicated in countless poisonings, including the killing of more than 2000 infants.[30] Better known as "La Voisin," she reportedly sold poisons to women wishing to rid themselves of their husbands. Her particular brand of poison was a concoction of arsenic, aconite, belladonna, and opium known as "la poudre de succession."[87]

Eighteenth- and Nineteenth-Century Developments in Toxicology

Groundwork for the development of toxicology as a distinct specialty took place during the 18th and 19th centuries (see Table 1–2). The poison mystique was gradually replaced with an increasingly rational and scientific approach to the study of these agents. Attention focused on the detection of poisons and the study of toxic effects of drugs and chemicals in animals.[62] Issues relating to adverse effects of industrialization and unintentional poisoning in the workplace and home environment were raised. Early experience and experimentation with methods of gastrointestinal decontamination took place.

Development of Analytical Toxicology and the Study of Poisons

The French physician Bonaventure Orfila (1787–1853) has been called the father of modern toxicology.[62] He emphasized toxicology as a distinct scientific discipline separate from clinical medicine and pharmacology.[8] He was an early medical-legal expert and championed the use of chemical analysis and autopsy material as evidence to prove that a poisoning had taken place. His treatise, *Traite des Poisons* (1814),[67] went through five editions and was regarded as the foundation of experimental and forensic toxicology.[92] It classified poisons into six groups: astringents, corrosives, acrids, septics or putrefiants, stupefacients and narcotics, and narcoticoacrids.

A number of other landmark works on poisoning also first appeared during this period. In 1829, Robert Christison (1797–1882), a professor of medical jurisprudence and Orfila's student, wrote *A Treatise on Poisons*.[16] This work simplified Orfila's poison classification schema by categorizing poisons into three groups: irritants, narcotics, and narcoticoacrids. Less concerned with jurisprudence than clinical toxicology, O. Costill's *A Practical Treatise on Poisons*, published in 1848, was the first modern clinically oriented text emphasizing the symptoms and treatment of poisoning.[19] In 1867 Theodore Wormley (1826–1897) published the first American book written exclusively on poisons. Entitled the *Micro-Chemistry of Poisons*,[94] this pioneering American contribution also expanded on methods of poison identification.[27]

Some of the early breakthroughs in the chemical analysis of poisons resulted from the search for a reliable assay for arsenic. Arsenic was widely available at this time and was suspected as the etiology in a large number of deaths. A reliable means of detecting arsenic was much needed by the courts. During the 19th century James Marsh (1794–1846), Hugo Reinsch, and Max Gutzeit (1847–1915) all worked on this problem; assays bearing their names were important contributions to the early history of analytic toxicology.[54,62] In an attempt to curtail criminal poisoning by arsenic, the Arsenic Act was passed by the British Parliament in 1851. This bill, which was one of the first modern day regulations on the sale of poisons, required that the retail sale of arsenic be confined to chemists, druggists, and apothecaries, and that a poison book record all arsenic sales.[9]

Systematic investigation into the underlying mechanisms of toxic substances also first took place during the 19th century. Much of this work was done in France and Germany. To cite just a few important accomplishments, Francois Magendie (1783–1855) studied the mechanisms of toxicity and sites of action of emetine, strychnine, and cyanide.[26] His student, Claude Bernard (1813–1878), the pioneering physiologist, made important contributions to the understanding of carbon monoxide and curare.[45] Rudolf Kobert (1854–1918) studied digitalis and ergot alkaloids and also authored a textbook on toxicology.[65] His fellow German, Louis Lewin (1850–1929), was the first person to intensively study the differences between the pharmacologic and toxicologic actions of drugs. He studied chronic opium intoxication as well as the toxicity of lead, carbon monoxide, snake venom, methanol, and chloroform. He also developed a classification system for psychoactive drugs, dividing them into euphorics, phantastics, inebriants, hypnotics, and excitants.[49]

Early Advances in Gastrointestinal Decontamination

Further experience with gastrointestinal decontamination also was gained during this period. A stomach pump was first designed by Munro Secundus in 1769 to administer neutralizing substances to sheep and cattle for the treatment of bloat.[12] The American surgeon Philip Physick (1768–1837) and the French surgeon Baron Guillaume Dupuytren (1777–1835) were two of the first physicians to advocate gastric lavage for the removal of poisons.[12] As early as 1805, Physick demonstrated the use of a "stomach tube" in this capacity. Using brandy and water as the irrigation fluid, he performed stomach washings in twins to wash out excessive doses of tincture of opium.[12] Dupuytren performed gastric emptying by first introducing warm water into the stomach via a large syringe attached to a long flexible sound and then withdrawing the "same water charged with poison."[12] Edward Jukes, a British surgeon, was another early advocate of poison removal by gastric lavage. Jukes first experimented on animals, performing gastric lavage after the oral administration of tincture of opium. Attempting to gain human experience, he experimented on himself, by first ingesting 10 drams (600 g) of tincture of opium and then performing gastric lavage using a 25-inch-long, 0.5-inch-diameter tube, which became known as Jukes's syringe.[57] Other than some nausea and a 3-hour sleep, he suffered no ill effects, and the experiment was deemed a success.

The principle of charcoal adsorption was first described by Scheele (1773) and Lowitz (1785), but the use of charcoal dates back to ancient times.[18] The earliest reference to the medicinal uses of charcoal is found in the Egyptian Papyrus of 1550 B.C.[18] The charcoal employed during Greek and Roman times, referred to as wood charcoal, was used to treat anthrax, chlorosis, vertigo, and epilepsy. By the late 18th century, topical application of charcoal was recommended for gangrenous skin ulcers and internal use of a charcoal-water suspension was recommended for use as a mouthwash and in the treatment of bilious conditions.[18]

The first hint that charcoal might have an antidotal role in the treatment of poisoning came about in a series of heroic self-experiments in France during the early 19th century. In 1813, the French chemist M. Bertrand publicly demonstrated the antidotal properties of charcoal by surviving a 5-g ingestion of arsenic trioxide that had been mixed with charcoal.[38] Eighteen years later, in 1831, before the French Academy of Medicine, the pharmacist P. F. Touery survived an ingestion consisting of 10 times the lethal dose of strychnine mixed with 15 g of charcoal.[38] One of the first reports of charcoal used in a poisoned patient was by the American Hort, who successfully treated a mercury bichloride-poisoned patient with large amounts of powdered charcoal in 1834.[5]

In the 1840s A. Garrod performed the first controlled study of charcoal when he examined its utility on a variety of poisons in animal models.[38] Using dogs, cats, guinea pigs, and rabbits, Garrod demonstrated the potential benefits of charcoal in the management of strychnine poisoning. He also emphasized the importance of early utilization of charcoal and the proper ratio of charcoal to poison. Other toxic substances, such as aconite, morphine, mercury bichloride, and hemlock, were also studied during this period. The first charcoal efficacy studies in humans were performed by the American physician B. Rand in 1848.[38]

It was not until the early 20th century that an activation process was added to the manufacture of charcoal. In 1900, the Russian Ostrejko demonstrated that treating charcoal with superheated steam significantly enhanced its adsorbing power.[18] Despite this improvement and the favorable reports mentioned, charcoal was only occasionally used in gastrointestinal decontamination until the early 1960s, when Holt and Holz repopularized its use.[36]

The Increasing Recognition of the Perils of Drug Abuse

Opioids

Although it was not until the mid-19th century that the peril of opiate addiction was first recognized, juice from the *Papaver somniferum* (opium) was known for its medicinal value in Egypt at least as early as the writing of the *Ebers Papyrus* in 1500 B.C. Egyptian pharmacologists of that time reportedly recommended opium as a pacifier for children who exhibited incessant crying in order to give the mother a rest.[80] As recently as the end of the 19th century, opium would still be extensively used to sedate infants due to the wide availability of opium-containing patent medications.[44] In Ancient Greece, Dioscorides and Galen were early advocates of opium as a therapeutic agent. During this time it was also used as a means of suicide. Mithridates' lack of success in his own suicidal poisoning may have been due to an opium tolerance that had developed from previous repetitive use.[80] One of the earliest descriptions of opium's abuse potential is attributed to Epistratos (304–257 B.C.), who criticized the use of opium for earache since it "dulled the sight and is a narcotic."[80]

Although the medical use of opium was promoted by Paracelsus in the 16th century, the popularity of this agent was given a significant boost when the distinguished British physician, Thomas Sydenham (1624–1689), invented laudanum (tincture of opium). In addition to opium, this preparation contained sherry, saffron, cinnamon, and cloves. Sydenham also formulated another opium concoction known as "syrup of poppies."[43] Another opium preparation that was used during this period, designed by Sydenham's protégé Thomas Dover, contained ipecac, as well as tartaric acid, saltpeter, licorice, and opium.

John Jones, the author of the 1700 text *The Mysteries of Opium Reveal'd,* was another enthusiastic advocate of the medicinal uses of opium.[43] A well-known opium user himself, Jones also provides one of the earliest descriptions of opiate addiction. He insisted that opium offered many benefits if the dose was moderate, but that discontinuation or a decrease in dose, particularly after "leaving off after long and lavish use," would result in symptoms such as sweating, itching, diarrhea, and melancholy. His recommendation for the treatment of these withdrawal symptoms included decreasing the dose of opium by 1% each day until the drug was totally withdrawn. During this period a number of English writers became well-known opium addicts including Samuel Taylor Coleridge, Elizabeth Barrett Browning, and

Thomas De Quincey, author of *Confessions of An English Opium Eater*. In many of these cases the initiation of opium use for medical reasons led to recreational use, tolerance, and dependence.[43]

Although opium was first introduced to Asian societies by Arabic physicians sometime after the fall of the Roman Empire, its use in Asian countries grew considerably during the 18th and 19th centuries. In one of the more deplorable chapters in world history, China's growing dependence on opium would be spurred on by the English desire to establish and profit from a flourishing drug trade.[80] Opium was grown in India and exported East. Despite Chinese protests and edicts against this practice, the importation of opium would persist throughout the 19th century, with the British going to war twice in order to maintain their right to sell opium. Not surprisingly, by the beginning of the 20th century, opium abuse in China was endemic.

In England, opium use continued to increase during the first half of the 19th century. During this period it was legal and freely available from the neighborhood grocer. To many, its use was considered no more problematic than alcohol.[32] With the discovery of Morphia in 1805 and the invention of the hypodermic syringe in the 1850s, parenteral administration of morphine would became the preferred route of opiate administration. Growing concerns about opiate abuse in England lead to the passing of the Pharmacy Act of 1868, restricting the sale of opium to registered chemists. But before the close of the century, in 1898, the Bayer Pharmaceutical Company of Germany would synthesize heroin from opium (Bayer also introduced aspirin that same year).[32] Although initially touted as a nonaddictive morphine substitute, problems with heroin use soon became evident. In the United States, the problems associated with uncontrolled use of opiates was also growing increasingly apparent. The 1914 Harrison Act was passed to forbid the use of opiates (and cocaine) without a prescription. A similar law, the Dangerous Drugs Act, was passed in the United Kingdom in 1920.[32]

Cocaine

Ironically, during the later part of the 19th century, the drug that would later compete with heroin for most notoriety, cocaine, was being enthusiastically recommended by Sigmund Freud and Robert Christison among others as a treatment for opiate addiction. Cocaine use dates back to at least 300 B.C., when South American Indians were reported to chew coca leaves during religious ceremonies.[58] Coca chewing has remained commonplace in some South American societies for thousands of years. It was used to increase work efficacy and elevate mood.

Recent study of an Egyptian mummy from about 950 B.C. revealed significant amounts of cocaine in the stomach and liver (as well as high amounts of tetrahydrocannabinol [THC] in the lung and muscle), suggesting oral use of cocaine during this time period.[61] In another investigation of 11 Egyptian (1079 B.C.–A.D. 395) and 72 Peruvian (A.D. 200–1500) mummies, cocaine (thought to be indigenous only to South America) and hashish (thought to be indigenous only to Asia) were found in both groups.[70] Such historical drug data challenges the assumptions about the lack of transatlantic contacts among ancient societies.

After Albert Niemann's isolation of cocaine alkaloid from coca leaf in 1860, growing enthusiasm for cocaine as a panacea ensued.[42] Some of the most important medical figures of the time, including William Halstead, the famed John Hopkins surgeon, enthusiastically promoted the use of cocaine. In 1884, Freud wrote *Uber Cocaine,*[13] advocating cocaine as an opium and morphine addiction cure and as a treatment for fatigue and hysteria. Halstead championed the anesthetic properties of this drug, although his own use of cocaine (and subsequent morphine use in an attempt to overcome his cocaine dependency) would later take a considerable toll.[66]

During the last third of the 19th century cocaine would be added to many popular over-the-counter tonics of the day. In 1863 a Frenchman, Angelo Mariani, introduced a new wine "Vin Mariani" that consisted of a mixture of cocaine and wine (6 mg of cocaine alkaloid per ounce) and was sold as a digestive and restorative.[58] In direct competition with the French tonic was the American-made Coca-Cola, developed by J.S. Pemberton. Coca-Cola was originally formulated with coca and caffeine and was marketed as a headache remedy and invigorator. With the public demand for cocaine increasing, patent medication manufacturers were adding cocaine to thousands of products. One such asthma remedy was "Dr. Tucker's Asthma Specific." Containing 420 mg of cocaine per ounce, this medication was applied directly to the nasal mucosa.[42] By the end of the 19th century, the first great American cocaine epidemic was underway.[59]

Similarly to what was occurring with opiates, the increasing use of cocaine led to a growing concern about its associated problems. In 1886 the first reports of cocaine-related cardiac arrest and stroke were published.[17] Reports of cocaine habituation occurring in patients using cocaine to treat their underlying opiate addiction also began to appear. In 1902 a popular book, *Eight Years in Cocaine Hell,* described some of these problems. *Century Magazine* called cocaine "the most harmful of all habit-forming drugs," and a report in the *New York Times* stated that cocaine was destroying "its victims more swiftly and surely than opium."[22] President William Taft in 1910 proclaimed cocaine Public Enemy Number 1, and in 1914 the Harrison Act was enacted calling for stringent control over the sale and distribution of cocaine.[22]

Hallucinogens

Other currently abused agents that were known to the ancients include peyote, hallucinogenic mushrooms, nutmeg, and cannabis. As early as 1300 B.C., Peruvian Indian tribal ceremonies included the use of mescaline-containing San Pedro cactus.[58] Peyote was well known to the American Indians and used in religious ceremonies from at least the 17th century. Hallucinogenic mushrooms, particularly *Psilocybe* mushrooms, were also used in the religious life of native Americans. These were called "teonanacatl," which means "God's sacred mushrooms" or "God's flesh."[72] Another hallucinogenic mushroom, *Amanita muscaria,* known as "fly agaric," was also used as a ritual drug and may have been known in India as "soma" around 2000 B.C. The use of cannabis dates back even further to around 2700 B.C., when it was used by the Chinese. Known as the "liberator of sin," cannabis use during that period may have been both therapeutic and recreational.[58] In India and Iran it was used as an intoxicant known as *bhang* as early as 1000 B.C.[60]

A more recent historical event that would have significant impact on modern-day hallucinogen use was the synthesis of lysergic acid diethylamide (LSD) by Albert Hofmann in 1938.[37] Working for Sandoz, Hofmann synthesized LSD while investigating the pharmacologic properties of ergot alkaloids. Subsequent self-experimentation by Hofmann led to the first description of its hallucinogenic effects and stimulated research into the use of LSD as a therapeutic agent. Hofmann is also credited with isolating psilocybin as the active ingredient in *Psilocybe Mexicana* mushrooms in 1958.[58]

Twentieth-Century Events

Early Regulatory Initiatives

The development of the specialty of medical toxicology and the role of poison control centers began shortly after World War II. Prior to this time, serious attention to the problem of household poisonings in the United States had been limited to a few federal legislative antipoisoning initiatives (Table 1–3). The 1906 Pure Food and Drugs Act was the first federal legislation that sought to protect the public from problematic and potentially unsafe drugs and food. The driving force behind this reform was Dr. Harvey W. Wiley, the chief chemist at the Department of Agriculture. Beginning in the 1880s Wiley investigated the problems of contaminated food. In 1902 he organized the "poison squad," which consisted of a group of volunteers who did self-experiments with food preservatives.[6] Revelations from the "poison squad" as well as the publication of Upton Sinclair's muckracking novel *The Jungle,*[82] exposing unhygienic practices of the meat-packing industry, led to growing support for legislative intervention. Samuel Hopkins Adams' reports about the patent (secret) medicine industry that some drug manufacturers added opiates to soothing syrups for infants also increased the call for reform.[75] Although the 1906 regulations were most concerned with protecting the public from adulterated food, regulations protecting against misbranded patent medications were also included.

The Federal Caustic Poison Act of 1927 was the first federal legislation specifically addressing household poisoning. Prior to this time, "poison" warning labels were not required on chemical containers regardless of their toxicity or availability. Spearheaded by the efforts of Dr. Chevalier Jackson, an otolaryngologist who showed that unintentional exposures to household caustic agents were an increasingly frequent cause of severe gastrointestinal burns, the act mandated that lye and acid-containing products clearly display a "poison" warning label.[84]

TABLE 1–3. PROTECTING OUR HEALTH: IMPORTANT UNITED STATES REGULATORY INITIATIVES PERTAINING TO POISONING AND TOXICOLOGY DURING THE 20TH CENTURY

Date	Federal Legislation
1906	Pure Food and Drugs Act
1914	Harrison Anti-Narcotic Act
1927	Federal Caustic Poison Act
1930	Food and Drug Administration (FDA) established
1938	Federal Food, Drug and Cosmetic Act
1948	Federal Insecticide, Fungicide and Rodenticide Act
1960	Federal Hazardous Substances Labeling Act
1962	Drug Amendments of 1962 to the Federal Food, Drug and Cosmetic Act
1963	Clean Air Act
1966	Child Protection Act
1970	Environmental Protection Agency established
1970	Occupational Safety and Health Act
1970	Poison Prevention Packaging Act
1972	Clean Water Act
1972	Consumer Product Safety Act
1972	Hazardous Material Transportation Act
1973	Lead-Based Paint Poison Prevention Act
1974	Safe Drinking Water Act
1976	Resource Conservation and Recovery Act
1976	Toxic Substance Control Act
1980	Comprehensive Environmental Response, Compensation and Liability Act (Superfund)
1986	Superfund Amendments and Reauthorization Act (SARA)
1988	Labeling of Hazardous Art Materials Act

The most pivotal regulatory initiative prior to World War II, and perhaps the most significant American regulation of the 20th century, was the Federal Food, Drug and Cosmetic Act of 1938. Although the Food and Drug Administration (FDA) had been established in 1930, and legislation to strengthen the 1906 regulations had been considered by Congress since President Franklin Roosevelt's first inauguration in 1933, by 1938 proposed revisions still had not been passed. The Elixir of Sulfanilamide tragedy in 1938 (see Chap. 2), in which 105 people died after taking a liquid preparation of sulfanilamide dissolved in diethylene glycol, provided the catalyst for legislative intervention.[56,90] Although the pending legislation at the time of the elixir disaster proposed banning false and misleading drug labeling and outlawing dangerous drugs, mandatory drug safety testing was not part of the proposal. The 1938 act would for the first time require assessment of drug safety prior to marketing.

The Development of Poison Control Centers

World War II led to the rapid proliferation of new drugs and chemicals into the marketplace and household.[21] At the same time, suicide became recognized as a leading cause of death from these agents.[83] These factors forced the medical community to develop a response to serious problems of unintentional and intentional poisonings. In Europe during the late 1940s, special toxicology wards were organized in Copenhagen and Budapest,[33] and a poison information service was begun in the Netherlands (Table 1–4).[88] An American Academy of Pediatrics study on pediatric accidents in 1952 revealed that over 50% of childhood accidents in the United States were due to potential poisonous ingestions.[34] This study led to the opening of the first U.S. poison control center in Chicago in 1953, under the leadership of Dr. Edward Press.[73] Press believed it had become extremely difficult for the individual physician to keep abreast of product information, toxicity, and treatment for the rapidly increasing number of potentially poisonous household products. This initial center was organized as a cooperative effort among the departments of pediatrics at several Chicago medical schools, with the goal of collecting and disseminating product information to inquiring physicians—mainly pediatricians.[73]

By 1957, 17 poison control centers were operating in the United States.[20] Using the Chicago center as a model, these first centers responded to physician callers by providing ingredient and toxicity information about drug and household products, and making treatment recommendations. Records were kept of the calls, and preventive strategies were introduced into the community. As more poison control centers opened, a second important function, providing information to callers from the general public, became increasingly commonplace. The physician pioneers in poison prevention and poison treatment were predominantly pediatricians who focused on childhood unintentional ingestions.[77]

During these early years in the development of poison control centers, each center had to collect its own product information, which was a laborious and often redundant task.[20] In an effort to coordinate poison control center operations and avoid unnecessary duplication, Surgeon General Dr. James Goddard responded to the recommendation of the American Public Health Service and established the National Clearinghouse for Poison Control Centers in 1957.[55] This organization, placed under the Bureau of Product Safety of the Food and Drug Administration, disseminated 5 by 8-inch index cards containing poison information to the various centers to help standardize poison center information resources. The Clearinghouse also collected and tabulated poison data from each of the centers.

Between 1953 and 1972 a rapid, uncoordinated proliferation of poison control centers occurred in the United States.[53] In 1962 there were 462 poison control centers.[1] By 1970 this number had risen to 590.[46] Six hundred sixty-one poison control centers existed in the United States in 1978, including 100 centers in the state of Illinois alone.[81] A change in the type of caller occurred, as lay public-generated calls began to outnumber physician-generated calls. Recognizing the publicity value and strong popular support associated with poison centers, some hospitals started poison control centers for public relations reasons without adequately recognizing or providing for the associated responsibilities. Unfortunately, many of these centers offered no more than a part-time telephone service located in the back of the emergency department or pharmacy, staffed by poorly prepared personnel.[81]

Despite the growing pains of the poison control services during this period, there were many significant achievements. A dedicated group of physicians and other health care professionals began devoting an increasing proportion of their time to matters pertaining to poisoning. In 1958, the American Association of Poison Control Centers (AAPCC) was founded to promote closer cooperation between poison centers, establish uniform standards, and develop educational programs for the general public and other health care professionals.[34] Annual research meetings were held and important legislative initiatives were stimulated by the organization's efforts.[55] Examples of such legislation include the Federal Hazardous Substances Labeling Act of 1960, which improved product labeling; the Child Protection Act of 1966, which extended labeling statutes to pesticides and other hazardous unlabeled substances; and the Poison Prevention Packaging Act of 1970, which mandated safety packaging. In 1961, in an attempt to heighten public awareness of dangers of unintentional poisoning, the third week of March was designated as Poison Prevention Week.

Another important organization, the American Academy of Clinical Toxicology (AACT), was founded in

TABLE 1–4. 20TH CENTURY MILESTONES IN THE DEVELOPMENT OF MEDICAL TOXICOLOGY

1949	First toxicology wards open in Budapest and Copenhagen
1949	First poison information service begins in the Netherlands
1952	American Academy of Pediatrics study showed 51% of children's accidents due to the ingestion of potential poisons
1953	First U.S. poison control center opens in Chicago
1957	17 poison control centers in operation in United States
1957	National Clearinghouse for Poison Control Centers established
1958	American Association of Poison Control Centers (AAPCC) founded
1961	First Poison Prevention Week
1962	462 poison control centers in United States
1963	Initial call for development of regional PCCs
1964	Creation of European Association for PCCs
1968	American Academy of Clinical Toxicology (AACT) established
1972	Introduction of microfiche technology to poison information
1974	American Board of Medical Toxicology (ABMT) established
1978	661 poison control centers in United States (100 in Illinois)
1978	AAPCC introduces standards of regional designation
1983	First examination given for Specialist in Poison Information (SPIS)
1985	American Board of Applied Toxicology (ABAT) established
1992	Medical Toxicology recognized by American Board of Medical Specialties (ABMS)
1994	First ABMS examination in Medical Toxicology
1997	75 poison control centers (including 48 regional centers) in United States

1968 by a diverse group of toxicologists. This group was "interested in applying principles of rational toxicology to patient treatment" and improving the standards of care on a national basis.[79] The journal *Clinical Toxicology*, initially sponsored by the AACT, also began publication in 1968. The first modern-day textbooks of clinical toxicology began to appear in the mid-1950s with the publication of Dreisbach's *Handbook of Poisoning* (1955),[25] Gleason, Gosselin, and Hodge's *Clinical Toxicology of Commercial Products* (1957),[31] and Arena's *Poisoning* (1963).[7]

Major advancements in the storage and retrieval of poison information took place during these years. As mentioned earlier, information regarding consumer products initially appeared on index cards distributed regularly to poison centers by the National Clearinghouse. By 1978, more than 16,000 individual product cards had been assembled.[81] The introduction of microfiche technology in 1972 enabled the storage of much larger amounts of data in a much smaller space of the individual poison center. Toxifile and POISINDEX, two large poison databases employing microfiche technology, were introduced at this time and gradually replaced the much more limited index card system.[81] During the 1980s, a fully computerized information retrieval system became standard at most poison centers when POISINDEX, which had become the standard database, was made more accessible using CD-ROM technology. Sophisticated information about the most esoteric of toxins was now instantaneously available everywhere.

In 1978 the poison control center movement entered an important new stage in its development when the AAPCC introduced standards for regional poison center designation.[53] By defining strict criteria, the AAPCC sought to upgrade poison center operations significantly and to offer a national standard of service. These criteria included employing poison specialists dedicated exclusively to operating the poison control center 24 hours per day and serving a catchment area of between 1 and 10 million people. Not surprisingly, this professionalization of the poison center movement led to a rapid consolidation of services, with the number of centers decreasing to 75 in 1997. Forty-eight (64%) have obtained regional certification. An AAPCC credentialing examination for poison information specialists was inaugurated in 1983 to help ensure the quality and standards of poison control centers.[15]

A poison control center movement has also evolved in Europe over the last 35 years, but unlike the movement in the United States, its growth from the beginning has focused on the development of strong centralized toxicology treatment centers. Beginning in the late 1950s, Dr. M. Gaultier in Paris developed an inpatient unit that was dedicated to the care of poisoned patients.[33] In Great Britain, the National Poison Information Service was developed at Guys Hospital in 1963 under Dr. Roy Goulding.[33] Dr. Henry Matthew initiated a regional poisoning treatment center in Edinburgh about the same time.[74] In 1964 the European Association for Poison Control Centers was formed at Tours, France.[33]

Further Regulatory Protection from Toxic Substances

The publication of Rachel Carson's *Silent Spring* in 1962, revealing the perils of an increasing toxic environment, heralded a drive for additional regulatory protection.[14] Starting with the Clean Air Act in 1963, laws were passed that would go a long way toward reducing the toxic burden on our environment (see Table 1–3). The establishment of the Environmental Protection Agency in 1970 spearheaded this attempt at protecting our environment, and during the next 10 years numerous regulations were introduced. Among the most important initiatives were the Occupational Safety and Health Act of 1970 that established the Occupational Safety and Health Administration (OSHA). This act mandated that employers provide safe work conditions for their employees. Specific exposure limits to toxic chemicals in the workplace were promulgated. The Consumer Product Safety Commission was created in 1972 to protect the public from consumer products that posed an unreasonable risk of illness or injury. Cancer-producing substances such as benzene, vinyl chloride, and asbestos have been banned from consumer products as a result of these new regulations. Toxic waste disasters at Love Canal, New York, and Time Beach, Missouri, led to the passing of the Comprehensive Environmental Response, Compensation and Liability Act (known as the Superfund) in 1980. This fund would help pay for cleanup of hazardous substance releases that posed a potential threat to public health.

Medical Toxicology Comes of Age

Over the last 25 years the specialty profile of medical toxicologists has changed. The recent development of emergency medicine and preventive medicine as medical specialties led to the training of more physicians with a dedicated interest in toxicology. By the early 1990s, emergency physicians accounted for more than half of medical toxicologists.[24] These developments have helped broaden the goals of poison control centers and medical toxicologists beyond the treatment of acute unintentional childhood ingestions to include a much wider array of toxic exposures—acute and chronic, adult and pediatric, unintentional and intentional, occupational and environmental.

The development of medical toxicology as a medical subspecialty began in 1974 when the AACT established the American Board of Medical Toxicology (ABMT) to recognize physician practitioners of medical toxicology.[3] From 1974 to 1992, 209 physicians obtained board certification from the ABMT. Formal subspecialty recognition of medical toxicology by the American Board of Medical Specialties (ABMS) was achieved in 1992 and a conjoint board with representatives from the specialties of emergency medicine, pediatrics, and preventive medicine was created. The first ABMS-sponsored examination in medical toxicology was offered in 1994. By 1997, 257 physicians were board certified in medical toxicology either by the ABMT and/or ABMS. The American College of Medical Toxicology was founded in 1994 as an organization designed to advance clinical, educational, and research goals in medical toxicology.

During the 1990s growing enthusiasm developed in the United States among some medical toxicologists to establish regional toxicology treatment centers. Adapting the model of more established European centers, toxicology treatment centers serve as referral centers for patients requiring advanced toxicology evaluation and treatment. Goals of such inpatient regional centers include enhancing care of the poisoned patient, strengthening toxicology training, and facilitating research. The evaluation of the clinical efficacy and fiscal viability of such programs is ongoing.

The professional maturation of nonphysicians with a primary interest in toxicology has also taken place over the past few years. In 1985 the AACT established the American Board of Applied Toxicology (ABAT), to administer a certifying examination for nonphysician practitioners of medical toxicology who have met certain rigorous standards.[2] By 1997 there were 58 toxicologists certified by this board, most of whom had either a PharmD in pharmacy or PhD in pharmacology.

Summary

Since the dawn of recorded history toxicology has had a great impact on human events. And although over the millennia the important poisons of the day have changed to some degree, toxic substances continue to challenge our everyday living. The era of poisoners for hire may have long ago reached its pinnacle, but environmental poisons confront all of us with no end of this poisoning menace in sight. Inevitably, knowledge acquired by one generation is often forgotten by the next, leading to a cyclical historical course. The ancients were undoubtedly much more knowledgeable than many of us about the benefits and drawbacks of medicinal and poisonous plants, lessons that would serve us well as additional herbal concoctions flood our marketplace leading to some of our more challenging present-day poisonings. Gastrointestinal decontamination strategies and drug abuse trends also appear to go in and out of favor in a cyclical course. This historic review is meant to not only remind us of our past, but to better prepare us for the future.

References

1. Adams WC: Poison control centers: Their purpose and operation. Clin Pharmacol Ther 1963;4:293–296.
2. American Board of Applied Toxicology: AACTion 1992;1:3.
3. American Board of Medical Toxicology: Vet Hum Toxicol 1987;29:510.
4. American Heritage Dictionary, 2nd college ed. Boston, Houghton Mifflin, 1991.
5. Anderson H: Experimental studies on the pharmacology of activated charcoal. Acta Pharmacol 1946;2:69–78.
6. Anderson OE: Pioneer statute: The pure food and drugs act of 1906. J Public Law 1964;13:189–196.
7. Arena JM: Poisoning: Chemistry, Symptoms, Treatments. Springfield, IL, Charles C. Thomas, 1963.
8. Arena JM: The pediatrician's role in the poison control movement and poison prevention. Am J Dis Child 1983;137:870–873.
9. Bartrip P: A "pennurth of arsenic for rat poison": The arsenic act, 1851 and the prevention of secret poisoning. Med Hist 1992;36:53–69.
10. Bible. Job 6:04.
11. Bissett NG: Arrow and dart poisons. J Ethnopharmacol 1989;25:1–41.
12. Burke M: Gastric lavage and emesis in the treatment of ingested poisons: A review and a clinical study of lavage in ten adults. Resuscitation 1972;1:91–105.
13. Byck R, ed: Cocaine papers by Sigmund Freud (English translation). New York, Stonehill Publishing, 1975, pp. 48–73.
14. Carson RL: Silent Spring. Boston, Houghton Mifflin, 1962.
15. Certification examination for poison information specialists. Vet Hum Toxicol 1983;25:54–55.
16. Christison R: A Treatise on Poisons. London, Adam Black, 1829.
17. Cocaine deaths reported for century or more. JAMA 1992;267:1045–1046.
18. Cooney DO: Activated Charcoal in Medical Applications. New York, Dekker, 1995.
19. Costill OH: A Practical Treatise on Poisons. Philadelphia, Grigg, Elliot, 1848.
20. Crotty J, Armstrong G: National clearinghouse for poison control centers. Clin Toxicol 1978;12:303–307.
21. Crotty JJ, Verhulst HL: Organization and delivery of poison information in the United States. Pediatr Clin North Am 1970;17:741–746.
22. Das G: Cocaine abuse in North America: A milestone in history. J Clin Pharmacol 1993;33:296–310.
23. Deichmann WB, Henschler D, Holmstedt B, Keil G: What is there that is not poison? A study of the Third Defense by Paracelsus. Arch Toxicol 1986;58:207–213.
24. Donovan JW, Goldfrank LR: Medical toxicologist practice characteristics, specialty certifications and manpower needs. Vet Hum Toxicol 1992;34:336. Abstract.
25. Dreisbach RH: Handbook of Poisoning: Diagnosis and Treatment. Los Altos, CA, Lange, 1955.
26. Earles MP: Early theories of mode of action of drugs and poisons. Ann Science 1961;17:97–110.
27. Eckert WG: Historical aspects of poisoning and toxicology. Am J Forensic Med Pathol 1981;2:261–264.
28. Elgood C: A treatise on the bezoar stone. Ann Med Hist 1935;7:73–80.
29. Gaebel RE: Saturnine gout among Roman aristocrats. N Engl J Med 1983;309:431.
30. Gallo MA: History and scope of toxicology. In: Klaassen CD, ed: Casarett and Doull's Toxicology: The Basic Science of Poisons, 5th ed. New York, McGraw-Hill, 1996, pp. 3–11.
31. Gleason MN, Gosselin RE, Hodge HC: Clinical Toxicology of Commercial Products: Acute Poisoning (Home and Farm). Baltimore, William & Wilkins, 1957.
32. Golding AMB: Two hundred years of drug abuse. J R Soc Med 1993;86:282–286.
33. Govaerts M: Poison control in Europe. Pediatr Clin North Am 1970;17:729–739.
34. Grayson R: The poison control movement in the United States. Industrial Medicine and Surgery 1962;31:296–297.

35. Green DW: The saturnine curse: A history of lead poisoning. South Med J 1985;78:48–51.
36. Greensher J, Mofenson HC, Caraccio TR: Ascendency of the black bottle (activated charcoal). Pediatrics 1987;80: 949–950.
37. Hofmann A: How LSD originated. J Psychedelic Drugs 1979;11:53–60.
38. Holt LE, Holz PH: The black bottle: A consideration of the role of charcoal in the treatment of poisoning in children. J Pediatr 1963;63:306–314.
39. Jain KK: Carbon Monoxide Poisoning. St. Louis, Warren H. Green, 1990, pp. 3–5.
40. Jarcho S: Medical numismatic notes. VII: Mithridates IV. Bull NY Acad Med 1972;48:1059–1064.
41. Jensen LB: Poisoning Misadventures. Springfield, IL, Charles C. Thomas, 1970.
42. Karch SB: The history of cocaine toxicity. Hum Pathol 1989;20:1037–1039.
43. Kramer JC: Opium rampant: Medical use, misuse, and abuse in Britain and the West in the 17th and 18th centuries. Br J Addiction 1979;74:377–389.
44. Kramer JC: The opiates: Two centuries of scientific study. J Psychedelic Drugs 1980;12:89–102.
45. Lee JA: Claude Bernard (1813–1878). Anaesthesia 1978; 33:741–747.
46. Lovejoy FH, Alpert JJ: A future direction for poison centers: A critique. Pediatr Clin North Am 1970;17:747–753.
47. Lucanie R: Unicorn horn and its use as a poison antidote. Vet Hum Toxicol 1992;34:563.
48. Lyons AS: Medicine: An Illustrated History. New York, Abradale Press, 1978.
49. Macht DI: Louis Lewin: Pharmacologist, toxicologist, medical historian. Ann Med Hist 1931;3:179–194.
50. Magner LN: A History of Medicine. New York, Marcel Dekker, 1992.
51. Major RH: History of the stomach tube. Ann Med Hist 1934;6:500–509.
52. Mann J: Murder, Magic, and Medicine. New York, Oxford University Press, 1992.
53. Manoguerra AS, Temple AR: Observations on the current status of poison control centers in the United States. Emerg Med Clin North Am 1984;2:185–197.
54. Marsh J: Account of a method of separating small quantities of arsenic from substances with which it may be mixed. Edinb New Phil J 1836;21:229–236.
55. McIntire M: On the occasion of the twenty-fifth anniversary of the American Association of Poison Control Centers. Vet Hum Toxicol 1983;25:35–37.
56. Modell W: Mass drug catastrophes and the roles of science and technology. Science 1967;156:346–351.
57. Moore SW: A case of poisoning by laudanum, successfully treated by means of Jukes's syringe. NY Med Phys J 1825;4:91–92.
58. Moriarty KM, Alagna SW, Lake CR: Psychopharmacology: An historical perspective. Psychiatr Clin North Am 1984;7:411–433.
59. Musto DF: America's first cocaine epidemic. Wilson Q 1989;13:59–64.
60. Nahas GG: Hashish in Islam 9th to 18th century. Bull NY Acad Med 1982;58:814–831.
61. Nerlich AG, Parsche F, Wiest I, et al: Extensive pulmonary haemorrhage in an Egyptian mummy. Virchows Arch 1995;427:423–429.
62. Niyogi SK: Historical development of forensic toxicology in America up to 1978. Am J Forensic Med Pathol 1980; 1:249–264.
63. Nriagu JO: Saturnine gout among Roman aristocrats: Did lead poisoning contribute to the fall of the empire? N Engl J Med 1983;308:660–663.
64. Ober WB: Did Socrates die of hemlock poisoning? NY State J Med 1977;77:254–258.
65. Oehme FW: The development of toxicology as a veterinary discipline in the United States. Clin Toxicol 1970;3:211–220.
66. Olch PD: William S. Halsted and local anesthesia. Anesthesiology 1975;42:479–486.
67. Orfila MP: Traite des Poisons. Paris, Ches Crochard, 1814.
68. Oxford English Dictionary, 2nd ed, vol 18. Oxford, Clarendon Press, 1989, p. 328.
69. Pachter HM: Paracelsus: Magic into Science. New York, Collier, 1961.
70. Parsche F, Balabanova S, Pirsig W: Drugs in ancient populations. Lancet 1993;341:503.
71. Plaitakis A, Duvoisin RC: Homer's moly identified as Galanthus nivalis: Physiologic antidote to stramonium poisoning. Clin Neuropharmacol 1983;6:1–5.
72. Pollock SH: The psilocybin mushroom pandemic. J Psychedelic Drugs 1975;7:73–84.
73. Press E, Mellins RB: A poisoning control program. Am J Public Health 1954;44:1515–1525.
74. Proudfoot AT: Clinical toxicology: Past, present and future. Hum Toxicol 1988;7:481–487.
75. Regier CC: The struggle for federal food and drugs legislation. Law and Contemporary Problems 1933;1:3–15.
76. Reid DHS: Treatment of the poisoned child. Arch Dis Child 1970;45:428–433.
77. Robertson WO: National organizations and agencies in poison control programs: A commentary. Clin Toxicol 1978; 12:297–302.
78. Rosner F: Moses Maimonides' treatise on poisons. JAMA 1968;205:98–100.
79. Rumack BH, Ford P, Sbarbaro J, et al: Regionalization of poison centers: A rational role mode. Clin Toxicol 1978; 12:367–375.
80. Sapira JD: Speculations concerning opium abuse and world history. Perspect Biol Med 1975;18:379–398.
81. Scherz RG, Robertson WO: The history of poison control centers in the United States. Clin Toxicol 1978;12:291–296.
82. Sinclair U: The Jungle. New York, Doubleday, 1906.
83. Suicide: A leading cause of death. JAMA 1952;150:696–697.
84. Taylor HM: A preliminary survey of the effect which lye legislation has had on the incidence of esophageal stricture. Ann Otol Rhinol Laryngol 1935;44:1157–1158.
85. Thompson CJ: Poisons and Poisoners. London, Harold Shaylor, 1931.
86. Timbrell JA: Introduction to Toxicology. London, Taylor & Francis, 1989.
87. Trestrail JH: The History of Poisoning and Poisoners Through the Ages. Grand Rapids, MI, Blodgett Regional Poison Center, 1989 (unpublished).
88. Vale JA, Meredith TJ: Poison information services. In: Vale

JA, Meredith TJ, eds: Poisoning: Diagnosis and Treatment. London, Update Books, 1981.
89. Watson G: Theriac and Mithridatium: A Study in Therapeutics. London, Wellcome Historical Medical Library, 1966.
90. Wax PM: Elixirs, diluents and the passage of the 1938 federal food, drug and cosmetic act. Ann Intern Med 1995; 122:456–461.
91. Wells C: Lead poisoning in the ancient world. Med Hist 1973;17:391–397.
92. Witthaus RA, Becker TC: Medical Jurisprudence: Forensic Medicine and Toxicology, vol. 1. New York, William Wood, 1894.
93. Witthaus RA: Manual of Toxicology, 2nd ed. New York, William Wood, 1911.
94. Wormley TG: Micro-Chemistry of Poisons. New York, William Wood, 1869.
95. Wright-St. Clair RE: Poison or medicine. NZ Med J 1970;71:224–229.

ANTIDOTES IN DEPTH

Antiquated Antidotes

Paul M. Wax

Although a perpetual search for better and improved antidotes features prominently in the history of toxicology, many of the so called "antidotal breakthroughs" over the years have not lived up to their promise (Table 1–5). A number of these antidotes have proven to be ineffective (eg, caffeine). Others were insufficiently tested (eg, propylene glycol) or replaced by "safer," more effective treatment (eg, paraldehyde).[11] Most troubling, the use of some of these agents actually worsened the clinical situation (eg, analeptics, copper sulfate). Unfortunately, just as the various classical theriac preparations remained popular into the 20th century, the use of many of these more "modern antidotes" has persisted long after scientific investigation demonstrated their ineffectiveness. An emphasis on physiologic antagonism with antidotes such as analeptics has often taken precedence over good supportive care. Finally, and not surprisingly, the use of modern-day theriacs such as the "universal antidote" persisted until quite recently, despite a lack of serious scientific support. This section highlights some of the critical changes in 20th-century poison management.

Analeptics

One of the most interesting changes in poison management took place during the 1940s and 1950s with regard to the use of analeptics in the treatment of barbiturate overdose.[44] Barbiturates, the first widely available sedative-hypnotics, were introduced in the early 20th century. Within a few years they became the most common cause of serious overdose.[5] In the 1920s barbiturate overdose management recommendations still included blood-letting techniques.[30] By the next decade, as interest in principles of antagonism between stimulants and depressants became widespread, much attention was focused on the use of analeptic agents to combat the sedative effects of barbiturates. Analeptic proponents argued that since the effects of cocaine intoxication appeared to be neutralized by barbiturates, a reciprocal approach—treating depressant overdose with stimulants—should also work.[30] The principle goal of analeptic therapy was to awaken the patient as soon as possible.

Numerous analeptic agents have been recommended over the years. Prior to the development of the first synthetic analeptics in the late 1920s, naturally occurring stimulants such as caffeine, lobeline, strychnine, cocaine, and camphor were utilized for this purpose. According to Leschke's *Clinical Toxicology*, a standard textbook published in 1934, the most effective remedy for the treatment of a sedative-hypnotic overdose was the intrathecal injection of 10% camphorated oil.[27] After a series of animal studies in the early 1930s, picrotoxin was enthusiastically endorsed as the analeptic of choice.[31] The subsequent introduction of synthetic analeptics such as nikethamide (Coramine) and pentylenetetrazol (Metrazol) increased the growing dependence on analeptics as the major treatment modality for barbiturate overdose.[22,25,32]

Analeptic treatment strategies were often referred to as "very energetic," because large doses of multiple analeptics were frequently utilized.[34] Even as recently as the 1950s, newer analeptics, such as bemegride, were being introduced and touted as the "real antidote" to barbiturate overdose.[41] During this time, methylphenidate was also used in the treatment of barbiturate overdose, decades prior to its popularization as a first-line agent in the treatment of attention deficit hyperactivity disorder. In 1967, one enthusiastic methylphenidate proponent emphasized: "Don't let comatose patients remain comatose [after barbiturate overdose]. Methylphenidate will waken them safely."[32] Toxicology textbooks published in the 1950s and 1960s continued to recommend caffeine, picrotoxin, and nikethamide as useful analeptic agents.[13,17,28] Subconvulsive electric shock therapy was also advocated as an alternative or adjunct to these chemical convulsants during this period.[38]

Unfortunately, many adverse effects were seen with the use of these analeptics, including hyperthermia, dysrhythmias, seizures, and psychosis.[24,32,37] It gradually became evident that analeptic therapy, despite the theoretical benefits, offered no real advantage, did not reduce mortality, and in fact placed the patient at risk for significant iatrogenic complications.[7] A different strategy was required.

Beginning in the mid-1940s a distinctive approach to barbiturate overdose was pioneered by Eric Nilsson and Carl Clemmesen at the Bispebjergs Hospital in Copenhagen, Denmark.[7,35] This treatment regimen, which became known as the Scandinavian method, abandoned the use of analeptics in the treatment of barbiturate overdose. Instead of primarily emphasizing the termination of coma, attention was directed at intensive supportive therapy with respiratory ventilation, oxygenation, and cardiovascular support. This strategy was analogous to the postanesthetic recovery room care provided to surgical patients. Using this "revolutionary"

TABLE 1–5. ANTIQUATED ANTIDOTES

Type of Antidote	Therapeutic Agent	Uses
Analeptic	Amphetamine	Sedative overdose
	Bemegride	Sedative overdose
	Caffeine	Sedative overdose
	Camphorated oil	Sedative overdose
	Lobeline	Sedative overdose
	Nikethamide (Coramine)	Sedative overdose
	Pentylenetetrazol (Metrazol)	Sedative overdose
	Picrotoxin	Sedative overdose
	Strychnine	Sedative overdose
Adsorbent	Universal antidote	GI decontamination
	Burnt toast	GI decontamination
Complexing agent	Sodium phosphate (Phospho-Soda)	Iron
Emetic	Apomorphine	Gastric emptying
	Copper sulfate	Gastric emptying
	Mechanical stimulation	Gastric emptying
	Mustard powder	Gastric emptying
	Salt water	Gastric emptying
	Tartar emetic	Gastric emptying
	Zinc sulfate	Gastric emptying
Heavy metal anitidote	Ascorbic acid	Lead, arsenic
	Calcium bromide	Lead
	Ferric hydroxide/magnesium hydroxide ("antidotum arsenici")	Arsenic
	Potassium ferrocyanide	Copper
	Potassium iodide	Lead
	Sodium formaldehyde sulfoxylate	Mercury bichloride
Miscellaneous	Acetazolamide	Salicylate
	Hypochlorites	Snake bites
	Potassium permanganate	Alkaloids (morphine, strychnine, aconitine)
	Propylene glycol	Phenolphthalein
	Raw rabbit brain	*Amanita phalloides*
Neutralizing agent	Calcium carbonate	Acid
	Hydrochloric acid	Alkali
	Lemon juice	Alkali
	Lime water	Acid
	Magnesium hydroxide	Acid
	Sodium bicarbonate	Acid
	Vinegar	Alkali
Sedative	Chloroform	Strychnine
	Digitalis	Delirium tremens
	Ethanol	Delirium tremens
	Ether	Agitation/seizures
	Paraldehyde	Delirium tremens
	Sodium bromide (used intrathecally)	Delirium tremens
	Tribromoethanol (Avertin)	Agitation/seizures

approach, barbiturate overdose mortality significantly dropped from about 20% using stimulation therapy to 1 to 2% using the Scandinavian method.[7]

Early Treatments of Opioid Overdose

Prior to the 1950s, opioid overdose was treated with many of the same analeptic agents, such as lobeline, nikethamide, pentylenetetrazol, and caffeine. In the early 1950s, an important development in the history of poison management took place when two specific opioid antidotes were introduced: nalorphine (Nalline) and levallorphan (Lorfan).[14] Both of these drugs were capable of reversing the respiratory effects of an opioid overdose by blocking a certain subset of opioid receptors. Nalorphine was also routinely administered to determine the presence or absence of opioids in suspected opioid abusers. This test, known as the Nalline test, was used as a monitoring tool in drug abuse programs.[19] The test was considered positive if it precipitated frank signs of opioid withdrawal or pupillary dilatation.

Unfortunately, neither nalorphine nor levallorphan was a pure opioid antagonist. Instead, the mixed agonist/antagonist properties of these drugs significantly limited their usefulness. Respiratory depression could be potentiated, especially in opioid-free patients. This was most likely to occur when these drugs were administered to unknown comatose patients with mild hypoventilation who had overdosed on sedative-hypnotics.

Naloxone, which was introduced in the 1970s, is a much safer drug because of its pure opioid antagonistic properties, and has replaced nalorphine and levallorphan in the treatment of opioid overdose.[15] Naloxone has no agonist properties, does not cause any additional respiratory depression, regardless of the ingestion, and is safe to use for an unknown overdose. In addition, it is useful in treating other mixed agonist-antagonist opioids, such as pentazocine, that do not respond to nalorphine.

Outdated and Dangerous Emetics

The role of emetics in poison management both in the home and at the hospital has undergone significant transformation over the years. The antimony salt, commonly known as tartar emetic, had a long history of use as an emetic as well as a sedative, expectorant, cathartic, and diaphoretic. During the 19th century tartar emetic was one of the three most widely prescribed drugs, along with opium and calomel (mercurous chloride).[20] Tartar emetic is no longer recommended for any purpose because of its toxicity and unreliability.[6]

Standard gastrointestinal decontamination recommendations during the 1960s included mechanical stimulation of the throat and the ingestion of saltwater emetics, or mustard water in the home, and copper sulfate, zinc sulfate, or apomorphine in the hospital.[1,23] Many authorities recommended mechanical stimulation of the pharynx (finger down the throat technique) as a quick and easy home remedy when induction of emesis was desirable.[1,9] This method, however, was found to be both ineffective and potentially traumatic, and is no longer encouraged.[9] Similarly, the use of saltwater emetics has been abandoned after numerous cases of severe salt intoxication resulted from its administration.[3,12] Mustard powder has not proved to be effective.[6]

The use of copper sulfate as an emetic[23] has also fallen out of favor due to its caustic properties, potential to cause acute copper poisoning, and unreliability.[21,42] Zinc sulfate is also no longer used as an emetic.[6]

Until the 1980s apomorphine was advocated as an emetic.[8,33] One reason for its use was because it was thought to be safer and more effective than copper sulfate.[21] It was supposed to be particularly useful for the combative or uncooperative patient because of its rapid onset of action and parenteral administration, and in this setting was frequently used instead of syrup of ipecac.[33] Apomorphine's propensity to cause central nervous system depression, however, increased the risk of subsequent aspiration and made its use potentially very dangerous. Moreover, a sterile injectable form of apomorphine has not been available in the United States for many years. For all of these reasons, enthusiasm for apomorphine gradually waned, leaving syrup of ipecac as the sole approved emetic.[29]

The Universal Antidote

Two other antidotes once commonly used for decontamination that have fallen into disfavor are the "universal antidote" and burnt toast. For many years the universal antidote, sold under the trade names Unidote and Res-Q, had become a medical tradition[36] and was advocated as part of the standard management of the poisoned patient in many textbooks.[13,17,28] Commercial preparations consisted of one part magnesium oxide, one part tannic acid, and two parts activated charcoal. An alternative home recipe consisted of milk of magnesia, strong tea, and burnt toast. Combination therapy of this sort was thought to offer a broader spectrum of action than activated charcoal alone. It was theorized that the magnesium oxide would neutralize acids and the tannic acid would precipitate alkaloids and metals.[28]

The use of the universal antidote declined by the mid-1980s and is no longer available. Studies demonstrated that activated charcoal was superior to the universal antidote in decreasing absorption[10,36] and that the decreased efficacy of the universal antidote was due to tannic acid interfering with activated charcoal's adsorbence of other toxins.[10] Furthermore, the potential hepatotoxicity of tannic acid was increasingly recognized.[36] Although burnt toast had been advocated as an activated charcoal substitute in the home,[2] its use was also abandoned due to its lack of significant adsorbent activity.[26]

Other Antiquated Antidotes

The use of drugs for the chemical restraint of agitated individuals has also undergone significant evolution during the past decades. Paraldehyde and ethanol, which were commonly used for the treatment of alcohol withdrawal,[18] have been replaced by the much safer and less toxic benzodiazepines. Likewise, depressant agents such as tribromoethanol (Avertin) and ether are no longer utilized because of the availability of safer alternative agents. The use of analeptics such as strychnine, picrotoxin, or pentylenetetrazol for the treatment of the depressive effects of ethanol has also become obsolete.[43]

Another change in treatment approach involves the use of neutralizing agents in the treatment of caustic ingestions. Until the 1970s, typical recommendations for the treatment of alkali ingestions included the use of vinegar (acetic acid), lemon juice, or, in some cases, dilute hydrochloric acid.[28] Suggestions for the neutralization of acid ingestions included the use of magnesium hydroxide, lime water, or calcium carbonate.[28] Because of the extremely rapid onset of action by a caustic agent, concerns arose over whether it was already too late to reverse the caustic process. Furthermore, the addition of neutralizing agents may increase the exothermic reaction and/or gas production.[39] Such reactions in an already weakened hollow viscus may be poorly tolerated and lead to extension of the tissue injury or perforation. For all of these reasons the use of neutralizing agents is no longer recommended.

Other abandoned antidotes include potassium iodide, used to enhance lead excretion, and ferric hydroxide (antidotum arsenici), used in the treatment of arsenic poisoning. Acetazolamide, which had been advocated for alkalinizing the urine in salicylate poisoning,[40] causes a systemic acidemia that can worsen the salicylate toxicity and is no longer employed. The use of sodium phosphate (Phospho-Soda) in the management of iron overdose in an attempt to create insoluble ferrous phosphate has also ceased due to problems with its marginal efficacy and hyperphosphatemia.[16]

Finally, enthusiasm has waned for raw rabbit brain, recommended as recently as the 1930s as offering a "chance of life" for patients with *Amanita phalloides* poisoning.[27] The raw brain approach was pioneered in the early 1800s after it was observed that rabbits could eat poisonous mushrooms without ill effects.[4] Postulating that rabbits had some sort of protective mechanism that neutralized the mushroom toxin, investigators formulated an antidotal concoction consisting of seven rabbit brains and three rabbit stomachs. The preparations was minced and grounded into pellets and administered with a sweetener. When patients who received the rabbit brain antidote survived the mushroom poisoning it was erroneously concluded that such an approach was effective.

Summary

While the judicious use of certain antidotes (eg, *N*-acetylcysteine, naloxone, pyridoxine) is critically important in the management of some poisoned patients, other antidotes do not necessarily offer a distinct clinical advantage and may create additional problems (eg, flumazenil, physostigmine). Many of our current antidotes have not undergone rigorous scientific evaluation regarding efficacy and safety. In time, some of these antidotes will undoubtedly join this ever-increasing list of antiquated antidotes. Lessons learned from the past (eg, the abandonment of analeptics) should help optimize present-day patient care and better prepare us to investigate and evaluate the next generation of antidotes.

References

1. Adams WC: Emetics in accidental poisoning. Pediatr Clin North Am 1961;8:351–352.
2. Arena J: Poisoning: Chemistry, Symptoms, Treatment. Springfield, IL, Charles C. Thomas, 1963.
3. Barer J, Hill L, Hill RM, Martinez WM: Fatal poisoning from salt used as an emetic. Am J Dis Child 1973;125:889–890.
4. Benjamin DR: Mushrooms: Poisons and Panaceas. New York, W.H. Freeman, 1995.
5. Berger FM: Drugs and suicide in the United States. Clin Pharmacol Therap 1967;8:219–223.
6. Cashman TM, Shirkey HC: Emergency management of poisoning. Pediatr Clin North Am 1970;17:525–534.
7. Clemmesen C, Nilsson E: Therapeutic trends in the treatment of barbiturate poisoning: The Scandinavian method. Clin Pharmacol Ther 1961;2:220–229.
8. Corby DG, Decker WJ, Moran MJ, Payne CE: Clinical comparison of pharmacologic emetics in children. Pediatrics 1968;42:361–364.
9. Dabbous IA, Bergman AB, Robertson WO: The ineffectiveness of mechanically induced vomiting. J Pediatr 1965; 66:952–954.
10. Daly JS, Cooney DO: Interference by tannic acid with the effectiveness of activated charcoal in "universal antidote." Clin Toxicol 1978;12:515–522.
11. Decker WJ: Antidotes: Some ineffective, insufficiently tested, outmoded, and potentially dangerous therapeutic agents. Vet Hum Toxicol 1983;25:10–15.
12. DeGenaro F, Nyhan WL: Salt: A dangerous "antidote." J Pediatr 1971;78:1048–1049.
13. Deichmann WB, Gerarde HW: Signs, Symptoms and Treatment of Certain Acute Intoxications, 2nd ed. Springfield, IL, Charles C. Thomas, 1958.
14. Eckenhoff JE, Funderburg LW: Observations on the use of the opiate antagonists nalorphine and levallorphan. Am J Med Sci 1954;228:546–553.
15. Evans LEJ, Roscoe P, Swainson CP, Prescott LF: Treatment of drug overdosage with naloxone, a specific narcotic antagonist. Lancet 1973;1:452–455.
16. Geffner ME, Opas LA: Phosphate poisoning complicating treatment for iron ingestion. Am J Dis Child 1980;134: 509–510.
17. Gleason MN, Gosselin RE, Hodge HC: Clinical Toxicology of Commercial Products: Acute Poisoning (Home & Farm), 2nd ed. Baltimore, Williams & Wilkins, 1963.
18. Gower WE, Kersten H: Prevention of alcohol withdrawal symptoms in surgical patients. Surg Gynecol Obstet 1980; 151:382–384.
19. Halbach H, Eddy NB: Tests for addiction of morphine type. Bull WHO 1963;28:139–173.
20. Haller JS: The use and abuse of tartar emetic in the 19th century materia medica. Bull Hist Med 1975;49:235–259.
21. Holtzman NA, Haslam RH: Elevation of serum copper following copper sulfate as an emetic. Pediatrics 1968;42: 189–193.
22. Jones AW, Dooley J, Murphy JR: Treatment of choice in barbiturate poisoning. JAMA 1950;143:884–888.
23. Karlsson B, Noren L: Ipecacuanha and copper sulfate as emetics in intoxications in children. Acta Pediatr Scand 1965;54:331–335.
24. Klaer-Larsen J: Delirious psychosis and convulsions due to Megimide. Lancet 1956;2:967–970.
25. Koppanyi T, Fazekas JF: Acute barbiturate poisoning: Analysis and evaluation of current therapy. Am J Med Sci 1950;220:559–576.
26. Lehman AJ: Substitution of burned toast for activated charcoal in the "universal antidote." Assoc Food Drug Official US Q Bull 1957;21:210–211.
27. Leschke E: Clinical Toxicology: Modern Methods in the Diagnosis and Treatment of Poisoning. Baltimore, William Wood, 1934.
28. Lucas GH: The Symptoms and Treatment of Acute Poisoning. Toronto, Clark Irwin, 1952.
29. MacLean WC: A comparison of ipecac syrup and apomorphine in the immediate treatment of ingestion of poisons. J Pediatr 1973;82:121–124.
30. Maloney AH, Fitch RH, Tatum AL: Picrotoxin as an antidote in acute poisoning by shorter acting barbiturates. J Pharmacol Exp Ther 1931;41:465–482.
31. Maloney AH: A comparative study of the antidotal action of picrotoxin, strychnine and cocaine in acute intoxication by the barbiturates. J Pharmacol Exp Ther 1933;49:133–140.
32. Mark LC: Analeptics: Changing concepts, declining status. Am J Med Sci 1967;254:296–302.
33. Meester WD: Emesis and lavage. Vet Hum Toxicol 1980; 22:225–234.
34. Nilsson E, Eyrich B: On treatment of barbiturate poisoning. Acta Med Scand 1950;137:381–389.
35. Nilsson E: On treatment of barbiturate poisoning: Modified clinical aspects. Acta Med Scand 1951;139(suppl 253):1–127.
36. Picchioni AL, Chin L, Verhulst HL, Dieterle B: Activated charcoal vs. "universal antidote" as an antidote for poisons. Toxicol Appl Pharmacol 1966; 8:447–454.
37. Reed CE, Driggs MF, Foote CC: Acute barbiturate intoxication: Study of 300 cases based on physiologic system of classification of severity of intoxication. Ann Intern Med 1952;37:290–303.
38. Robie TR: Treatment of acute barbiturate poisoning by nonconvulsive electrostimulation. Postgrad Med J 1951: 253–256.
39. Rumack BH, Burrington JD: Caustic ingestions: A rational look at diluents. Clin Toxicol 1977;11:27–34.
40. Schwartz R, Fellers F, Knapp J, Yaffe S: The renal response to administration of acetazolamide (Diamox) during salicylate intoxication. Pediatrics 1959;23:1103–1114.
41. Shulman A, Shaw FH, Cass NM, Whyte HM: A new treatment of barbiturate intoxication. Br Med J 1955;1:1238–1244.
42. Stein RS, Jenkins D, Korns ME: Death after use of cupric sulfate an emetic. JAMA 1976;235:801.
43. Taberner PV: Pharmacological treatment for alcohol dependence and withdrawal—An historical perspective. Alcohol Alcohol 1993;S2:259–262.
44. Wax PM: Analeptic use in clinical toxicology. A historical appraisal. J Toxicol Clin Toxicol 1997;35:203–209.

CHAPTER 2

Toxicologic Plagues and Disasters in History

Paul M. Wax

Mass poisonings have caused suffering and misfortune throughout history. From the ergot epidemics of the Middle Ages to contemporary industrial disasters, these plagues have had great political, economic, social, and environmental ramifications. Particularly within the last 100 years, as the number of toxins and potential toxins has risen dramatically, toxic disasters have become an increasingly common event. The sites of some of these events—Minamata Bay (Japan), Jonestown (Guyana), Love Canal (New York), Bhopal (India), Chernobyl (Ukraine)—have come to symbolize our increasingly toxic habitat. This chapter provides an overview of some of the most consequential and historically important toxin-mediated disasters.

Gas Disasters

Inhalation of toxic gases and oral ingestions resulting in food poisoning tend to subject the greatest number of people to adverse consequences of a toxic exposure. Toxic gas exposures may be the result of a natural disaster (eg, volcanic eruption), unintentional mishap (eg, industrial fire), or intentional homicidal or genocidal endeavor (eg, concentration camp gas chamber). Depending on the toxin, the clinical presentation may be acute, with a rapid onset of toxicity (cyanide gas), or subacute/chronic, with a gradual onset of toxicity (air pollution).

One of the earliest recorded toxic gas disasters resulted from the eruption of Mount Vesuvius near Pompeii, Italy, in A.D. 79 (Table 2–1). Poisonous gases generated from the volcanic activity reportedly killed thousands.[17] A much more recent natural disaster occurred in Cameroon in 1986, when excessive amounts of carbon dioxide were mysteriously vented from the volcanic crater lake, Lake Nyos.[5] Seventeen hundred fatalities reportedly resulted from exposure to this asphyxiant gas.

A toxic gas leak at the Union Carbide pesticide plant in Bhopal, India, in 1984 resulted in one of the greatest civilian toxic disasters in modern history.[84] An unintended exothermic reaction at this carbaryl-producing plant caused the release of over 24,000 kg of methyl isocyanate gas. This gas was quickly dispersed through the air over the densely populated area surrounding the factory, resulting in at least 2500 deaths and 200,000 injuries.[53] The initial response to this disaster was greatly limited by a lack of pertinent information about the toxicity of this agent. Calls for improvement in disaster preparedness and strengthened right-to-know laws regarding potential toxic exposures resulted from this tragedy.[17,84]

The release into the atmosphere of 26 tons of hydrofluoric acid at a petrochemical plant in Texas in October 1987 resulted in 939 people seeking medical attention at nearby hospitals. Ninety-four people were hospitalized but there were no deaths.[91]

More than any other toxin, carbon monoxide has been responsible for the largest number of toxic disasters. Fires, such as the Coconut Grove Night Club Fire in 1943, caused hundreds of deaths, many of them from carbon monoxide poisoning.[20] The 1990 fire at the Happy Land Social Club in the Bronx, New York claimed many victims including a large number of nonburn deaths.[47] Carbon monoxide was the most likely etiology in these deaths, although hydrogen cyanide gas and simple asphyxiation may also have contributed to the overall toxicity. Another notable toxic gas disaster involving a fire occurred at the Cleveland Clinic in 1929, where a fire in the radiology department resulted in 125 deaths.[16] The

TABLE 2–1. GAS DISASTERS

Toxin	Location	Date	Significance
Poisonous gas	Pompeii	A.D. 79	> 2000 died from eruption of Mt. Vesuvius
Chlorine, phosgene, mustard gas	Ypres, Belgium	1915–1918	100,000 dead, 1.2 million casualties from gas during WW I
NO_2, CO, CN	Cleveland Clinic	1929	Fire in radiology department, 125 deaths
Smog (SO_2)	Belgium, Meuse Valley	1930	64 deaths
CO, CN	Coconut Grove Night Club, Boston	1942	498 deaths from fire
CN, CO	Europe	1939–1945	Millions murdered by Zyklon-B (HCN) gas
CO	Salerno, Italy	1944	> 500 deaths on train stalled in tunnel
Smog (SO_2)	Donora, PA	1948	20 deaths, thousands ill
Smog (SO_2)	London	1952	4000 deaths attributed to the fog/smog
Mustard gas	Iraq-Iran	1982	New cycle of war gas casualties
Methyl isocyanate	Bhopal, India	1984	> 2000 deaths; 200,000 injuries
Carbon dioxide	Cameroon	1986	> 1700 deaths from release of gas from Lake Nyos
Hydrofluoric acid	Texas	1987	Atmospheric release, 94 hospitalized
CO, ? CN	Happy Land Social Club, Bronx, NY	1990	87 died in fire from toxic smoke
Toxic smoke?	Persian Gulf	1991	Gulf War syndrome—possible toxic etiology
Sarin	Matsumoto, Japan	1994	First of terrorist attacks in Japan using sarin
Sarin	Tokyo	1995	Subway exposure, 5510 people seek medical attention

burning of nitrocellulose radiographs produced nitrogen dioxide, cyanide, and carbon monoxide, gases thought to be responsible for many of the fatalities.

Air pollution is another source of toxic gases that has caused significant disease and death. Excessive smog in the Meuse Valley of Belgium in 1930 and in Donora, Pennsylvania, in 1948 was credited with excess morbidity and mortality. A dense smog in London in 1952 was responsible for 4000 deaths.[46] High levels of sulfur dioxide likely contributed to these outcomes.

Exposure to toxic gases with the deliberate intent to inflict harm has claimed an extraordinary number of victims during the 20th century. During World War I, chlorine, phosgene, and nitrogen mustard gases were used as weapons of war. Reportedly 100,000 deaths and 1.2 million casualties were attributed to these gas attacks in WWI.[17] Despite this deplorable use of known toxic agents, chemical weapons were used again in the 1980s during the Iraq-Iran war.

Mass murder and genocide by poisonous gas was utilized by the Nazis during World War II. Initially the Nazis used carbon monoxide to kill. To expedite the killing process, Nazi scientists developed Zyklon B gas (hydrogen cyanide gas). Up to 10,000 people per day were killed by the rapidly acting cyanide. Millions of innocent people were murdered using poisoning technology.

During recent wars, a variety of physical and neuropsychological ailments have been attributed to possible exposure to toxic agents.[35] Agent Orange was widely used as a defoliant during the Vietnam War. This herbicide consists of a mixture of 2,4,5-trichlorophenoxyacetic acid (2,4,5-T) and 2,4-dichlorophenoxyacetic acid (2,4-D) as well as small amounts of a contaminant 2,3,7,8-tetrachlorodibenzo-p-dioxin (TCDD), better known as dioxin. Although a higher incidence of skin cancers has been found in veterans who handled Agent Orange, other possible dioxin-related adverse health effects such as nonskin cancer, birth defects, and hepatic dysfunction have not been observed.[14] An increase in non-Hodgkin's lymphoma among Vietnam veterans has been seen, but this is not clearly attributable to herbicidal exposure.[71]

Gulf War syndrome is a constellation of chronic symptoms including fatigue, headache, muscle and joint pains, ataxia, paresthesias, diarrhea, skin rashes, sleep disturbances, impaired concentration, memory loss, and irritability that has been found in thousands of Persian Gulf War veterans without a clearly identifiable cause. A number of etiologies have been advanced to explain these varied symptoms, including exposure to the smoke from burning oil wells, chemical and biological warfare agents (eg, organophosphates), medical prophylaxis (pyridostigmine bromide, anthrax, and botulinum toxin vaccines), other pesticides (DEET), infectious agents (leishmaniasis), inhalation of sand contaminated with fungus, insect vectors, depleted uranium munitions, multiple chemical sensitivities, and posttraumatic stress disorder.[36] Although it has been recently speculated that organophosphate-induced delayed polyneuropathy may explain some of these clinical findings,[30] at present the true etiology of this mysterious illness remains unknown.[22,35,43]

Mass exposure to the very potent organophosphate nerve gas, sarin, did occur in March of 1995 when terrorists released this toxic agent in three separate subway lines in Tokyo.[60] Eleven people were killed and 5510 people sought emergency medical evaluation at more than 200 hospitals and clinics in the area.[74] Sarin gas exposure also resulted in several deaths and hundreds of casualties in Matsumoto, Japan in June 1994.

Food Disasters

Accidental contaminations of food and drink have led to numerous toxic disasters (Table 2–2). Over the centuries, ergot, produced by the fungus *Claviceps purpurea*, has caused a large number of deadly epidemics.[55] Epidemic ergotism occurred as the result of eating breads and cereals made from rye that had been contaminated by *C. purpurea*. In some epidemics convulsive manifestations predominated and in others gangrenous manifestations predominated. Ergot-induced severe vasospasm was thought responsible for both types of presentations.[54] Convulsive ergotism was initially described as a "fire which twisted the people," and the term St. Anthony's fire (Ignis sacer) was used to refer to the excruciating burning pain experienced in the extremities that is an early manifestation of gangrenous ergotism. In the year 994, 40,000 people died in Aquitania, France in such an epidemic.[45] The events surrounding the Salem witchcraft trials have also been attributed to the ingestion of contaminated rye. The bizarre and psychotic behaviors exhibited by some of the individuals associated with this event may have been caused by the hallucinogenic properties of ergotamine, an LSD congener.[10,51]

During the 20th century unintentional mass poisoning from food and drink contaminated with toxic chemicals has become all too common. One of the more unusual poisonings occurred in 1956 in Turkey, when wheat seed treated with the fungicide hexachlorobenzene and intended for planting was inadvertently used for human consumption. Four thousand cases of porphyria cutanea tarda were attributed to the ingestion of this wheat seed.[69]

Another example of chemical food poisoning took place in Epping, England, in 1965. In this incident, a sack of flour became contaminated with methylenedianiline when the chemical accidently spilled onto the flour during transport to a bakery. Subsequent ingestion of bread baked with the contaminated flour produced hepatitis in 84 people. This outbreak of toxic hepatitis became known as Epping jaundice.[42]

The manufacture of polybrominated biphenyls (PBBs) in a factory that also produced food supplements for livestock resulted in the unintentional contamination of a large amount of livestock feed in Michigan in 1973.[11] Significant morbidity and mortality among the livestock population resulted. Increased human tissue levels of PBBs were reported,[92] although human toxicity seemed limited to vague constitutional symptoms and abnormal liver function tests.[2]

The chemical contamination of a particular lot of rice oil in Japan in 1968 caused an illness called yusho ("rice oil disease"). This occurred when heat exchange fluid containing polychlorinated biphenyls (PCBs) and polychlorinated dibenzofurans (PCDFs) leaked from a heating pipe into the rice oil. More than 1600 people developed this new illness. Manifestations included chloracne, hyperpigmentation, increased incidence of liver cancer, and adverse reproductive effects. A similar illness after exposure to another batch of PCB-contaminated rice oil affected 2000 people in Taiwan in 1979. This latter epidemic was referred to as yu-cheng ("oil disease").[38]

In another oil contamination epidemic, consumption of an illegally marketed cooking oil in Spain in 1981 was responsible for a mysterious poisoning epidemic that affected more than 19,000 people and resulted in at

TABLE 2–2. FOOD DISASTERS

Toxin	Location	Date	Significance
Ergot	Aquitania, France	A.D. 994	40,000 died in the epidemic
Ergot	Salem, MA	1692	Bizarre behavior may be attributable to ergot
Lead	Devonshire, England	1700s	Colic from production of cider
Arsenious acid	France	1828	40,000 cases of polyneuropathy from contaminated wine and bread
Lead	Canada	1846	134 men died during Franklin expedition, possibly due to contamination of food stored in lead cans
Arsenic	Staffordshire, England	1900	Arsenic contaminated sugar used in beer production
Cadmium	Japan	1939–1954	Itai-itai disease
Hexachlorobenzene	Turkey	1956	4000 cases of porphyria cutanea tarda
Methyl mercury	Minamata Bay, Japan	1950s	Organic mercury poisoning from fish
Triorthocresylphosphate	Meknes, Morocco	1959	Cooking oil adulterated with turbojet lubricant
Cobalt	Quebec City and others	1960s	Cobalt beer cardiomyopathy
Methylenedianiline	Epping, England	1965	Epping jaundice
Polychlorinated biphenyls	Japan	1968	Yusho
Methyl mercury	Iraq	1971	> 400 deaths from contaminated grain
Polybrominated biphenyls	Michigan	1973	97% of state contaminated through food chain
Polychlorinated biphenyls	Taiwan	1979	Yu-Cheng
Rape seed oil (denatured)	Spain	1981	Toxic oil syndrome affected 19,000 people
Arsenic	Buenos Aires	1987	Malicious contamination of meat; 61 people underwent chelation

least 340 deaths. Exposed patients developed a multisystem disorder referred to as toxic oil syndrome (or toxic epidemic syndrome), characterized by pneumonitis, eosinophilia, pulmonary hypertension, scleroderma-like features, and neuromuscular changes. Although this syndrome was associated with the consumption of rapeseed oil denatured with 2% aniline, the exact etiologic agent was never definitively identified.[40,81]

Epidemics of heavy metal poisoning from contaminated food and drink have also occurred throughout history. Epidemic lead poisoning has been associated with many different vehicles of transmission, including leaden bowls, kettles, and pipes. A famous epidemic in the 18th century was known as the Devonshire colic. Although the exact etiology of this disorder was unknown for many years, later evidence suggested that the ingestion of lead-contaminated cider was responsible.[85]

Mass exposure to arsenic-contaminated food and drink has produced epidemics of polyneuropathy. Arsenical neuropathy developed in an estimated 40,000 people in France in 1828 when wine and bread were unintentionally contaminated by arsenious acid.[50] The use of arsenic-contaminated sugar in the production of beer in England in 1900 resulted in at least 6000 cases of peripheral neuropathy and 70 deaths (Staffordshire beer epidemic).[23]

A more recent arsenic mass poisoning occurred in Buenos Aires in 1987 when vandals broke into a butcher's shop and poured an unknown amount of acaricide (45% sodium arsenite solution) over 200 kg of partly minced meat.[66] The contaminated meat was purchased by 718 people. Of 307 meat purchasers who submitted to urine sampling, 49 had urine arsenic of 76 to 500 μg/dL and 12 had urine arsenic above 500 μg/dL.

A toxin-induced disorder associated with beer drinking involved the addition of cobalt as a foam stabilizer to several brands of beer in the 1960s. Certain local breweries in Quebec City, Minneapolis, Omaha, and Louvain, Belgium added 0.5 to 5.5 ppm cobalt to their beer. Epidemics of fulminant heart failure among heavy beer drinkers in these locales resulted (cobalt-beer cardiomyopathy).[1,57]

Methyl mercury, an organic mercurial, has been the etiologic agent for several recent poisoning epidemics. During the 1950s, a Japanese chemical factory that manufactured vinyl chloride and acetaldehyde routinely discharged mercury into Minamata Bay, resulting in contamination of the aquatic food chain. An epidemic of methyl mercury poisoning followed after the local people ate the poisoned fish.[64,82] Chronic brain damage, tunnel vision, deafness, and severe congenital defects were associated with this outbreak.[64] Another mass epidemic of methyl mercury poisoning occurred in Iraq in 1971 when the local population consumed homemade bread prepared from wheat seed treated with a methyl mercury fungicide.[3] Six thousand hospital admissions and over 400 hospital deaths were associated with this disaster. As with the hexachlorobenzene exposure in Turkey 25 years previously, the treated grain had been intended for use as seed but was instead used as food.

Contamination of the local water supply with the wastewater runoff from a zinc-lead-cadmium mine in Japan from 1939 to 1954 was believed responsible for causing itai-itai ("ouch-ouch") disease, an unusual chronic syndrome manifested by extreme bone pain and osteomalacia. The local water was used for drinking and irrigation of the rice fields. Approximately 200 people who lived along the banks of the Jintsu River developed these peculiar symptoms, which were thought most likely to be due to the cadmium.[9]

Therapeutic Drug Disasters

Toxic disasters have occurred in people using therapeutic amounts of pharmaceutical drugs (Table 2–3). These tragedies have generally occurred either unintentionally due to poor safety testing or a lack of understanding of diluents and excipients, or deliberately due to drug tampering. Complications from genetic engineering techniques may have contributed to a recent major disaster that involved tryptophan and eosinophilia–myalgia syndrome.

In September and October 1937, more than 100 deaths were associated with the use of one of the early sulfa preparations—elixir of sulfanilamide-Massengill—that contained 72% diethylene glycol as the vehicle for drug delivery. Little was known about diethylene glycol toxicity at the time, and many cases of renal failure and death occurred.[25] As a result of this catastrophe animal drug testing was mandated by the Food, Drug, and Cosmetic Act of 1938 to avoid similar tragedies in the future.[86] Unfortunately, diethylene glycol continued to be sporadically used in other countries as a medicinal diluent resulting in additional deaths in South Africa

TABLE 2–3. THERAPEUTIC DRUG DISASTERS

Toxin	Location	Date	Significance
Diethylene glycol	U.S.	1937	Elixir of sulfanilamide; renal failure
Thorotrast	U.S.	1930s–1950s	Hepatic angiosarcoma
Diethylstilbestrol	U.S., Europe	1940s–1950s	Vaginal adenocarcinoma in daughters
Stalinon	France	1954	Severe neurotoxicity from triethyltin
Thalidomide	Europe	1960	5000 cases of phocomelia
Benzyl alcohol	U.S.	1981	Gasping syndrome
Acetaminophen-cyanide	Chicago	1982	Tampering incident resulted in 7 homicides
Tryptophan	U.S.	1989	Eosinophilia–myalgia syndrome
Diethylene glycol	Haiti	1996	Acetaminophen elixir contaminated; renal failure; > 30 pediatric deaths

(1969), India (1986), Nigeria (1990), Bangladesh (1990 to 1992), and Haiti (1996).[87] In the most recent disaster in Haiti, at least 76 children died after ingesting an acetaminophen elixir formulated with glycerin contaminated with diethylene glycol.[19,68]

In the early 1960s, one of the greatest modern-day drug catastrophes occurred with the release of thalidomide. Its use as a sedative hypnotic by pregnant women resulted in about 5000 cases of severe congenital anomalies.[55] This tragedy was largely confined to Europe, Australia, and Canada where the drug was initially marketed. Only the length of time required for review and rigorous scrutiny of thalidomide's new drug application by the FDA prevented a concurrent disaster in the United States.[52]

Thorotrast (thorium dioxide 25%) is a radiologic contrast medium that was widely used between 1928 and 1955. Its use was associated with the development of hepatic angiosarcoma as well as skeletal sarcomas, leukemia, and "thorotrastomas"—malignancies at the site of extravasated thorotrast.[77,88]

Another major therapeutic drug misadventure involved the widespread use of diethylstilbestrol (DES) for the treatment of threatened and habitual abortions. Despite the lack of convincing efficacy data, as many as 10 million Americans received DES during pregnancy or in utero during a 30-year period until the drug's use in pregnancy was prohibited in 1971. Adverse health effects that have been associated with DES use include increased risk for breast cancer in "DES mothers" and increased risk of vaginal cancer, reproductive tract anomalies, and premature births in "DES daughters."[27,31]

The "Stalinon affair" in France in 1954 was another major toxicologic disaster that involved the unintentional contamination of a therapeutic agent. Stalinon was a proprietary oral medication that was marketed for the treatment of staphylococcal skin infections, osteomyelitis, and anthrax. Although it was supposed to contain diethyltin di-iodide and linoleic acid, triethyltin, a potent neurotoxin and most toxic of organotin compounds, and trimethyltin were present as impurities. Of the approximately 1000 people who received this medication, 217 patients developed symptoms and 102 patients died.[4,76]

In 1981 a number of premature neonates died with a "gasping syndrome" manifested by severe metabolic acidosis, respiratory depression with gasping, and encephalopathy.[26] Just prior to developing these findings, they had all received multiple injections of heparinized bacteriostatic sodium chloride solution (to flush their indwelling catheters) and bacteriostatic water (to mix medications), both of which contained 0.9% benzyl alcohol. Accumulation of large amounts of benzyl alcohol and its metabolite benzoic acid in the blood was thought responsible for this syndrome.[26]

In 1989 and 1990, eosinophilia–myalgia syndrome, a debilitating syndrome somewhat similar to toxic oil syndrome, developed in more than 1500 people who had taken L-tryptophan.[39,83] These patients presented with sclerodermalike features and eosinophilia. Intensive investigation revealed that all affected patients had ingested tryptophan produced by a single manufacturer. This manufacturer had recently introduced a new process involving genetically altered bacteria to improve tryptophan production. A contaminant produced by this process has been suggested as the etiologic agent of this syndrome.[6]

A different type of drug disaster resulted from the deliberate tampering with acetaminophen preparations in 1982. Seven Chicago residents died after ingesting acetaminophen capsules laced with potassium cyanide.[15] Because of this tragedy, packaging of over-the-counter medications was changed to decrease the possibility of future product tampering.[58] Despite these changes, however, deaths from product tampering continue to be reported.[13]

Alcohol and Illicit Drug Disasters

Unintended toxic calamities have resulted from the use of alcohol and other drugs of abuse (Table 2–4). During the early 20th century, and particularly during prohibition, the ethanolic extract of Jamaican ginger (also known as "the Jake") was a popular ethanol substitute in the southern and midwestern United States.[56] For years the Jake was sold adulterated with castor oil, but in 1930, as the price of castor oil rose, the Jake was reformulated with an alternative adulterant, triorthocresylphosphate (TOCP). Little was previously known about the toxicity of this compound, but TOCP proved to be a potent neurotoxin. At least 50,000 people who drank the Jake developed TOCP poisoning from 1930 to 1931, manifested by upper and lower extremity weakness ("ginger Jake paralysis") and gait impairment ("Jake walk" or "Jake leg").[56] Thirty years later in Morocco the dilution of cooking oil with a turbojet lubricant containing TOCP caused an additional 10,000 cases of TOCP-induced paralysis.[75]

Epidemic methanol poisoning among those seeking ethanol and other inebriants has also been well described. In one such incident in Atlanta in 1951, the ingestion of methanol-contaminated bootleg whiskey caused 323 cases of methanol poisoning, resulting in 41 deaths.[7] In another epidemic in 1979, 46 prisoners be-

TABLE 2–4. ALCOHOL AND ILLICIT DRUG DISASTERS

Toxin	Location	Date	Significance
Triorthocresyl-phosphate	U.S.	1930–1931	Ginger Jake paralysis
Methanol	Atlanta	1951	Epidemic from ingesting bootleg whiskey
Methanol	Jackson, MI	1979	Occurred in a prison
MPTP	San Jose, CA	1982	Drug-induced parkinsonism
3-Methyl fentanyl	Pittsburgh	1988	China white epidemic
Fentanyl	New York, NY	1990	"Tango and Cash" epidemic
Scopolamine/heroin	U.S. East Coast	1995–1996	325 cases of anticholinergic poisoning in heroin users

came ill after ingesting a methanol-containing diluent used in photocopy machines.[79]

So called "designer drugs" are a relatively new category responsible for several toxicologic disasters. In 1982 several intravenous drug abusers living in San Jose, California, who had been using MPTP (1-methyl-4-phenyl-1,2,3,6-tetrahydropyridine), a meperidine analog, developed a peculiar irreversible neurologic disease closely resembling parkinsonism.[44] Investigation revealed that these patients had unknowingly injected trace amounts of MPPP (1-methyl-4-phenyl-4-propionoxypiperidine), a contaminant of the amateur MPTP synthesis which had selectively destroyed cells in the substantia nigra, causing severe irreversible parkinsonism. As a result of the vigorous pursuit of the cause of this disaster, a better understanding of the pathophysiology of parkinsonism and possible future treatment modalities occurred.

Another example of a "designer drug" mass poisoning occurred in the New York metropolitan area in 1991, when a sudden epidemic of opioid overdoses occurred among heroin abusers who bought envelopes labeled "Tango and Cash."[21] Expecting to receive a new brand of heroin, the drug abusers instead purchased the much more potent fentanyl. Increased toxicity from fentanyl resulted from the inability of the dealer to adjust ("cut") the dose properly. Some purchasers presumably received little or no fentanyl while others received potentially lethal doses. A similar epidemic involving 3-methylfentanyl occurred in Pittsburgh in 1988.[48]

At least 325 cases of anticholinergic poisoning occurred among heroin users in New York City, Newark, Philadelphia, and Baltimore from 1995 to 1996.[70] The "street drug" used in these cases was contaminated with scopolamine. Whereas naloxone treatment was associated with increased agitation and hallucinations, physostigmine administration resulted in resolution of symptoms.

Occupational Toxin Epidemics

Occupation-related toxic epidemics have unfortunately become increasingly common (Table 2–5). These poisoning syndromes tend to have an insidious onset and may not be recognized clinically until years after exposure. The specific toxin may cause a myriad of problems; among the most worrisome concerns are their carcinogenic and mutagenic potential.

Although there was generally not a sound understanding of toxicologic mechanisms prior to the 20th century, several important occupational diseases were described during this time. The first description of an occupational cancer was by Sir Percivall Pott, in 1775, who noticed a high incidence of scrotal cancer in English chimney sweeps. Pott's belief that the scrotal cancer was caused by prolonged exposure to tar and soot was confirmed by work in the 1920s indicating that the polycyclic aromatic hydrocarbons contained in coal tar (including benzo[a]pyrene) are carcinogenic.[34]

The industrial revolution, which began during the 19th century, was accompanied by an increase in occupational diseases. During the 1860s a peculiar disorder attributed to the effects of inhaling mercury vapor was described among manufacturers of felt hats in New Jersey.[89] Mercury nitrate was used as an essential part of the felting process at this time. "Hatter's shakes" refers to the tremor that developed in an estimated 10 to 60% of hatters surveyed.[89] Extreme shyness, another manifestation of mercurialism, was also seen in many hatters in later studies. Five percent of hatters during this period died from renal failure. Other notable 19th- and early 20th-century occupational tragedies included an increased incidence of mandibular necrosis (phossy jaw) among workers in the match-making industry exposed to yellow phosphorus,[33] an increased incidence of bladder tumors among synthetic dye makers using beta-naphthylamine,[28] and an increased incidence of aplastic anemia among artificial leather manufacturers using benzene.[73]

Exposure to asbestos during the 20th century has become one of the largest and worst occupational and environmental disasters of all time.[12,59] Since the 1920s, millions of workers have been employed in industries that manufacture or utilize asbestos products. Individuals who worked in the shipyards during the 1940s, when asbestos was extensively used as an insulating and fireproofing material, have been at particular risk for asbestos-related diseases, which include mesothelioma, lung cancer, and asbestosis.

Other recent occupational poisonings involve expo-

TABLE 2–5. OCCUPATIONAL DISASTERS

Toxin	Location	Date	Significance
Polycyclic aromatic hydrocarbons	England	1700s	High incidence of scrotal cancer among chimney sweeps; first description of occupation-related cancer
Mercury	New Jersey	Mid- to late 1800s	Outbreak of mercurialism in hatters
Yellow phosphorus	Europe	Mid- to late 1800s	Phossy-jaw in match makers
Beta-naphthylamine	Worldwide	Early 1900s	Increased bladder cancer in dye makers
Benzene	Newark	1916–1928	Aplastic anemia among artificial leather manufacturers
Asbestos	Worldwide	1920s to present	Millions at risk for asbestos-related disease
Vinyl chloride	Louisville	1960s–1970s	Increased cases of hepatic angiosarcoma among polyvinyl chloride polymerization workers
Chlordecone	James River, Virgina	1973–1975	Increased incidence of neurologic abnormalities among insecticide workers
1,2-dibromo-chloropropane	California	1974	Infertility among pesticide makers

sure to a variety of newly synthesized chemicals. In Louisville, Kentucky, in 1974 an increased incidence of angiosarcoma of the liver was first noticed among polyvinyl chloride polymerization workers who were exposed to vinyl chloride monomer.[18] In 1975 chemical factory workers exposed to the organochlorine insecticide chlordecone (Kepone) experienced a high incidence of neurologic abnormalities, including tremor and chaotic eye movements.[80] An increased incidence of infertility among Californian pesticide workers exposed to dibromochloropropane (DBCP) was noted in 1977.[90]

Environmental Disasters

Although the incidence of significant human toxicity from dioxin (2,3,7,8-tetrachlorodibenzodioxin) and other similar polychlorinated compounds remains controversial, the lethality of this agent in an animal model has caused considerable concern for acute and latent injury from human exposure to this and other environmental toxins (Table 2–6). One of the most serious exposures to dioxin occurred in Seveso, Italy, in 1976, when an explosion at a factory producing the antiseptic hexachlorophene resulted in the release of a dioxin-containing chemical cloud into the atmosphere.[32] At 5-year follow-up, chloracne had been the only significant clinical finding related to the dioxin exposure.[72]

Large-scale toxic disasters have also increased due to mass exposure to toxic waste dumps. Previously inhabited but now deserted sites, such as Times Beach, Missouri, and Love Canal, New York, conjure up the very worst consequences of our toxic environment. Although little scientific evidence has been offered to confirm adverse health effects from the Love Canal toxic dump, this event has directed attention to the problems of how best to deal with environmental poisons and their disposal.[37,62]

TABLE 2–6. ENVIRONMENTAL AND RADIATION DISASTERS

Toxin	Location	Date	Significance
Radium	Orange, NJ	1910s–1920s	Increase in bone cancer in dial-painting workers
Radiation	Hiroshima and Nagasaki, Japan	1945	First atomic bombs dropped at end of WW II; clinical effects still evident today
Dioxin	Seveso, Italy	1976	Unintentional release of dioxin into environment; chloracne
Toxic waste	Times Beach, MO		Public alarm by dioxin containing toxic waste
Toxic waste	Love Canal, NY	1978	Further concern and intense debate about toxic waste
Radiation	Chernobyl, Ukraine	1986	Increase in childhood thyroid cancer; increase in other cancers anticipated
^{137}Cesium	Goiania, Brazil	1987	Acute radiation sickness and radiation burns

Radiation Disasters

A discussion of mass poisonings would be incomplete without mention of a growing number of radiation disasters that have occurred during the 20th century (Table 2–6). The first significant mass exposure to radiation occurred among several thousand teenage girls and young women employed in the dial-painting industry. These workers painted luminous numbers on watch and instrument dials with paint that contained radium. Exposure occurred by licking the paint brushes and inhaling radium-laden dust. Studies showed an increase in bone-related cancers as well as aplastic anemia and leukemia in exposed workers.[49,63]

Concerns about the health effects of radiation have continued to escalate since the dawn of the nuclear age in 1945. Long-term follow-up studies half a century after the atomic bombings at Hiroshima and Nagasaki have shown an increased incidence of leukemia, other cancers, radiation cataracts, hyperparathyroidism, delayed growth and development, and chromosomal anomalies in exposed individuals.[41]

The unintentional nuclear disaster at Chernobyl, Ukraine in April 1986 once again has forced us to confront the medical consequences of 20th-century scientific advances that brought us the atomic age.[24] The release of radioactive material resulted in the hospitalization of more than 200 people for acute radiation sickness and 31 deaths. In the long term many more people will undoubtedly be affected. The increase in childhood thyroid cancer has increased 100-fold in some areas with heavy contamination, and the total number of Chernobyl-associated cancers cases is likely to be high.[67]

Another serious radiation accident occurred in Goiania, Brazil in 1987. Two hundred and forty-four people were exposed to cesium^{137} when an abandoned radiotherapy unit was opened in a junkyard. One hundred and four people showed evidence of internal contamination, 28 had local radiation injuries, and 8 developed acute radiation syndrome. There were at least 4 deaths.[61,65]

Other Toxic Disasters

Toxic disasters have also manifested themselves as events of mass suicide and homicide. In 1978 in Jonestown, Guyana, 911 members of the Peoples Temple committed group suicide when they ingested a beverage containing cyanide.[29] More recently, in 1997, phenobarbital and ethanol (sometimes assisted by physical asphyxiation) was the suicidal method favored by 39 members of the Heavens Gate cult in Rancho Santa Fe, California. An epidemic of mysterious cardiopulmonary arrests at the Ann Arbor Veterans Administration Hospital in Michigan in July and August 1975 was attributed to the homicidal use of pancuronium by two nurses.[78] Intentional digoxin poisoning by hospital personnel may have explained some of the increase in deaths on a cardiology ward of a Toronto pediatric hospital in 1981, but the exact cause of the high mortality rate remained unclear.[8]

Summary

Toxicologic plagues and disasters have an all too prominent role in our history. Many critical concepts in toxicology and the management of poisoned patients can be learned from these events. Given the practical and ethical limitations in studying the effects of many specific toxins in humans, lessons from these unfortunate tragedies must be fully mastered and retained for future generations. Most importantly, as the stress on our health and environment from an ever-increasing array of toxins grows larger, an understanding of the pathogenesis of these toxic plagues (eg, issues pertaining to drug, food, and occupational safety) is critically important if future disasters are to be prevented.

References

1. Alexander CS: Cobalt-beer cardiomyopathy: A clinical and pathologic study of twenty-eight cases. Am J Med 1972; 53:395–417.
2. Anderson HA, Wolff MS, Lilis R, et al: Symptoms and clinical abnormalities following ingestion of polybrominated-biphenyl-contaminated food products. Ann NY Acad Sci 1979;320:684–702.
3. Baker F, Damluji S, Amin-Zaki L, et al: Methylmercury poisoning in Iraq. Science 1973;181:230–241.
4. Barnes JM, Stoner HB: The toxicology of tin compounds. Pharmacol Rev 1959;11:211–232.
5. Baxter PJ, Kapila M, Mfonfu D: Lake Nyos disaster, Cameroon, 1986: The medical effects of large scale emission of carbon dioxide? Br Med J 1989;298:1437–1441.
6. Belongia EA, Hedberg CW, Gleich GJ, et al: An investigation of the cause of the eosinophilia–myalgia syndrome associated with tryptophan use. N Engl J Med 1990;323: 357–365.
7. Bennett IL, Cary FH, Mitchell GL, Cooper MN: Acute methyl alcohol poisoning: A review based on experiences in an outbreak of 323 cases. Medicine 1953;32:431–463.
8. Buehler JW, Smith LF, Wallace EM, et al: Unexplained deaths in a children's hospital: An epidemiologic assessment. N Engl J Med 1985;313:211–216.
9. Cadmium pollution and itai-itai disease. Lancet 1971;2: 382–383.
10. Caporael LR: Ergotism: The Satan loosed in Salem. Science 1976;192:21–26.
11. Carter LJ: Michigan PBB incident: Chemical mix-up leads to disaster. Science 1976;192:240–243.
12. Corn JK, Starr J: Historical perspective on asbestos: Policies and protective measures in World War II shipbuilding. Am J Indust Med 1987;11:359–373.
13. Cyanide poisonings associated with over-the-counter medication, Washington State, 1991. MMWR 1991;40:161, 167–168.
14. DeStefano F: Effects of agent orange exposure. JAMA 1995; 273:1494.
15. Dunea G: Death over the counter. Br Med J 1983;286: 211–212.
16. Easton WH: Smoke and fire gases. Ind Med 1942;11: 466–468.
17. Eckert WG: Mass deaths by gas or chemical poisoning: A historical perspective. Am J Forensic Med Pathol 1991; 12:119–125.
18. Falk H, Creech JL, Health CW, et al: Hepatic disease among workers at a vinyl chloride polymerization plant. JAMA 1974;230:59–63.
19. Fatalities associated with ingestion of diethylene glycol-contaminated glycerin used to manufacture acetaminophen syrup—Haiti, November 1995–June 1996. MMWR 1996;45: 649–650.
20. Faxon NW, Churchill ED: The Coconut Grove disaster in Boston. JAMA 1942;120:1385–1388.
21. Fernando D: Fentanyl-laced heroin. JAMA 1991;265:2962.
22. Ficarra BJ: Medical mystery: Gulf war syndrome. J Med 1995;26:87–94.
23. Final report of the Royal Commission on Arsenical Poisoning. Lancet 1903;2:1674–1676.
24. Geiger HJ: The accident at Chernobyl and the medical response. JAMA 1986;256:609–612.
25. Geiling EHK, Cannon PR: Pathological effects of elixir of sulfanilamide (diethylene glycol) poisoning: A clinical and experimental correlation—Final report. JAMA 1938;111: 919–926.
26. Gershanik J, Boecler B, Ensley H, et al: The gasping syndrome and benzyl alcohol poisoning. N Engl J Med 1982; 307:1384–1388.
27. Giusti RM, Iwamoto K, Hatch EE: Diethylstilbestrol revisited: A review of the long-term health effects. Ann Intern Med 1995;122:778–788.
28. Goldblatt MW: Vesical tumours induced by chemical compounds. Br J Indust Med 1949; 6:65–81.
29. Guyana tragedy: An international forensic problem. INFORM Rep 1979;11:2–8.
30. Haley RW, Kurt TL: Self-reported exposure to neurotoxic chemical combinations in the Gulf War. JAMA 1997;277: 231–237.
31. Herbst AL, Ulfelder H, Poskanzer DC: Adenocarcinoma of the vagina. Association of maternal stilbestrol therapy with tumor appearance in young women. N Engl J Med 1971; 284:878–881.
32. Holmstedt B: Prolegomena to Seveso. Arch Toxicol 1979;44: 211–230.
33. Hughes JP, Baron R, Buckland DH, et al: Phosphorus necrosis of the jaw: A present day study. Br J Indust Med 1962;19: 83–99.
34. Hunter D: The Diseases of Occupations, 6th ed. London, Hodder & Stoughton, 1978.
35. Hyams KC, Wignall S, Roswell R: War syndromes and their evaluation: From the U.S. Civil War to the Persian Gulf War. Ann Intern Med 1996;125:398–405.

36. Iowa Persian Gulf Study Group: Self-reported illness and health status among gulf war veterans. JAMA 1997;277: 238–245.
37. Janerich DT, Burnett WS, Feck G, et al: Cancer incidence in the Love Canal area. Science 1981; 212:1404–1407.
38. Jones GRN: Polychlorinated biphenyls: Where do we stand now? Lancet 1989;2:791–794.
39. Kilbourne EM, de la Paz MP, Borda IA, et al: Toxic oil syndrome: A current clinical and epidemiologic summary, including comparisons with eosinophilia–myalgia syndrome. J Am Coll Cardiol 1991;18:711–717.
40. Kilbourne EM, Rigau-Perez JG, Heath C, et al: Clinical epidemiology of toxic-oil syndrome: Manifestations of a new illness. N Engl J Med 1983;309:1408–1414.
41. Kodama K, Mabuchi K, Shigematsu I: A long-term cohort study of the atomic-bomb survivors. J Epidemiol 1996;6: S95–105.
42. Koppelman H, Robertson MH, Saunders PG: The Epping jaundice. Br Med J 1966;1:514–516.
43. Landrigan PJ: Illness in gulf war veterans: Causes and consequences. JAMA 1997;277:259–261.
44. Langston JW, Ballard P, Tetrud JW, Irwin I: Chronic parkinsonism in humans due to a product of meperidine-analog synthesis. Science 1983;219:979–980.
45. Leschke E: Clinical Toxicology: Modern Methods in the Diagnosis and Treatment of Poisoning. Baltimore, William Wood, 1934.
46. Logan WPD: Mortality in the London fog incident, 1952. Lancet 1953;1:336–338.
47. Magnuson E: The devil made him do it. Time, April 9, 1990, p. 38.
48. Martin M, Hecker J, Clark R, et al: China white epidemic: An Eastern United States emergency department experience. Ann Emerg Med 1991;20:158–164.
49. Martland HS. Occupational poisoning in manufacture of luminous watch dials. JAMA 1929;92:466–473, 552–559.
50. Massey EW, Wold D, Heyman A: Arsenic: Homicidal intoxication. South Med J 1984;77:848–851.
51. Matossian MK: Ergot and the Salem witchcraft affair. Am Sci 1982;70:355–357.
52. McFadyen RE: Thalidomide in America: A brush with tragedy. Clin Med 1976;11:79–93.
53. Mehta PS, Mehta AS, Mehta SJ, Makjijani AB: Bhopal tragedy's health effects: A review of methyl isocyanate toxicity. JAMA 1990;264:2781–2787.
54. Merhoff GC, Porter JM: Ergot intoxication: Historical review and description of unusual clinical manifestations. Ann Surg 1974;180:773–779.
55. Modell W: Mass drug catastrophes and the roles of science and technology. Science 1967;156:346–351.
56. Morgan JP: The Jamaica ginger paralysis. JAMA 1982;248: 1864–1867.
57. Morin YL, Foley AR, Martineau G, Roussel J: Quebec beer-drinkers' cardiomyopathy: Forty-eight cases. Can Med Assoc J 1967;97:881–883.
58. Murphy DH: Cyanide-tainted Tylenol: What pharmacists can learn. Am Pharm 1986;26:19–23.
59. Murray R: Asbestos: A chronology of its origins and health effects. Br J Indust Med 1990;47:361–365.
60. Okumura T, Takasu N, Ishimatsu S, et al: Report on 640 victims of the Tokyo subway sarin attack. Ann Emerg Med 1996;28:129–135.
61. Oliveira AR, Hunt JG, Valverde NJL, et al: Medical and related aspects of the Goiania accident: an overview. Health Physics 1991;60:17–24.
62. Paigen B: Controversy at Love Canal. Hastings Center Rep 1982;12:29–37.
63. Polednak AP, Stehney AF, Rowland RE: Mortality among women first employed before 1930 in the U.S. radium dial-painting industry. Am J Epidemiol 1978;107:179–195.
64. Powell PP: Minimata disease: A story of mercury's malevolence. South Med J 1991;84:1352–1358.
65. Roberts L: Radiation accident grips Goiania. Science (news) 1987;238:1028–1031.
66. Roses OE, Fernandez JCG, Villaamil ED, et al: Mass poisoning by sodium arsenite. J Toxicol Clin Toxicol 1991;29: 209–213.
67. Rytomaa T: Ten years after Chernobyl. Ann Med 1996;28: 83–87.
68. Scalzo AJ: Diethylene glycol toxicity revisited: The 1996 Haitian Epidemic. J Toxicol Clin Toxicol 1996;34:513–516.
69. Schmid R: Cutaneous porphyria in Turkey. N Engl J Med 1960;263:397–398.
70. Scopolamine poisoning among heroin users—New York City, Newark, Philadelphia, and Baltimore, 1995 and 1996. MMWR 1996;45:457–460.
71. Selected Cancers Cooperative Study Group: The association of selected cancers with service in the U.S. military in Vietnam, I: non-Hodgkin's lymphoma. Arch Intern Med 1990; 150:2473–2483.
72. Seveso after five years. Lancet 1981;2:731–732.
73. Sharpe WD: Benzene, artifical leather and aplastic anemia: Newark, 1916–1928. Bull NY Acad Med 1993;69:47–60.
74. Sidell FR: Chemical agent terrorism. Ann Emerg Med 1996; 28:223–224.
75. Smith HV, Spalding JM: Outbreak of paralysis in Morocco due to ortho-cresyl phosphate poisoning. Lancet 1959;2: 1019–1021.
76. Stalinon: A therapeutic disaster. Br Med J 1958;1:515.
77. Stover BJ: Effects of thorotrast in humans. Health Physics 1983;44(S1):253–257.
78. Stross JK, Shasby M, Harlan WR: An epidemic of mysterious cardiopulmonary arrests. N Engl J Med 1976;295: 1107–1110.
79. Swartz RD, Millman RP, Billi JE, et al: Epidemic methanol poisoning: Clinical and biochemical analysis of a recent episode. Medicine 1981;60:373–382.
80. Taylor JR, Selhorst JB, Houff SA, Martinez AJ: Chlordecone intoxication in man. Neurology 1978; 28:626–630.
81. Toxic Epidemic Syndrome Study Group: Toxic epidemic syndrome, Spain, 1981. Lancet 1982;2:697–702.
82. Tsuchiya K: The discovery of the causal agent of Minimata disease. Am J Indust Med 1992;21:275–280.
83. Vargas J, Uitto J, Jimenez SA: The cause and pathogenesis of the eosinophilia–myalgia syndrome. Ann Intern Med 1992;116:140–147.
84. Varma DR, Guest I: The Bhopal accident and methyl isocyanate toxicity. J Toxicol Environ Health 1993;40:513–529.

85. Waldron HA: The Devonshire colic. J Hist Med 1970;25: 383–413.
86. Wax PM: Elixirs, diluents and the passage of the 1938 federal food, drug and cosmetic act. Ann Intern Med 1995; 122:456–461.
87. Wax PM: It's happening again—another diethylene glycol mass poisoning. J Toxicol Clin Toxicol 1996;34:513–516.
88. Weber E, Laarbai F, Michel L, Donckier J: Abdominal pain: Do not forget Thorotrast! Postgrad Med J 1995;7: 367–369.
89. Wedeen RP: Were the hatters of New Jersey "mad"? Am J Indust Med 1989;16:225–233.
90. Whorton MD, Krauss RM, Marshall S, Milby TH: Infertility in male pesticide workers. Lancet 1977;2:1259–1261.
91. Wing JS, Sanderson LM, Brender JD, et al: Acute health effects in a community after a release of hydrofluoric acid. Arch Environ Health 1991;46:155–160.
92. Wolff MS, Anderson HA, Selikoff IJ: Human tissue burdens of halogenated aromatic chemicals in Michigan. JAMA 1982;247:2112–2116.

PART A

General Approach to Medical Toxicology

CHAPTER 3

Principles of Managing the Poisoned or Overdosed Patient: An Overview

Lewis R. Goldfrank, Neal E. Flomenbaum, Neal A. Lewin, Richard S. Weisman, Mary Ann Howland, and Robert S. Hoffman

For almost three decades, medical toxicologists and poison centers have utilized a clinical approach to the poisoned or overdosed patient that emphasizes treating the patient rather than treating the poison. Too often in the past, patients were initially all but neglected while attention was focused on the list of ingredients on the container of the ingested product(s). Although the astute clinician must always be prepared to administer a specific antidote immediately in those uncommon instances when nothing else will save a patient, the overwhelming majority of poisoned or overdosed patients will benefit from an organized, rapid clinical management plan (Fig. 3–1).

The initial management of all seriously ill patients begins with attention to the ABCs: *a*irway compromise, *b*reathing difficulties, and *c*irculatory problems. When a patient's mental status is abnormal, the possibilities of head and cervical spine trauma must also be considered, and the cervical spine protected until injury can either be excluded or diagnosed and treated. The bedside assessment of the adequacy of respirations (frequency and depth) and a decision on the necessity of early intubation is followed by a determination of all of the vital signs and identification and treatment of life-threatening conditions such as hypotension, hypertension, bradycardia, tachycardia, dysrhythmias, hyperthermia, and hypothermia. Accurate identification and treatment of conduction disturbances and dysrhythmias necessitate obtaining a 12-lead ECG and cardiac monitoring early on. Similarly, an arterial blood gas analysis may be indicated early to more accurately assess ventilation, oxygenation, some toxic–metabolic etiologies of altered mental status (eg, a wide anion gap metabolic acidosis), and when appropriate, carbon monoxide poisoning (by co-oximetry).

With the initiation of an IV infusion, blood samples can be sent for CBC, BUN, glucose, electrolytes, and if indicated, Ca^{2+} and Mg^{2+}. If the patient has an altered mental status, samples can be obtained for CNS depressants and/or "drugs of abuse," although these tests rarely provide useful information. For the potentially suicidal patient, an acetaminophen level should be requested in addition to the tests already mentioned, and a test for any specific drug or toxin (such as salicylates or theophylline) suggested by the history, physical examination, or bedside diagnostic tests. Specimens may also be held or sent for levels of such other drugs or toxins as lithium, theophylline, iron, and digoxin as indicated.

Early treatment of a patient with a suspected drug overdose and an altered mental status should typically include consideration or administration of (1) hypertonic dextrose, 0.5 to 1.0 g/kg as D50W for an adult or D10–20W for a child; (2) thiamine, 100 mg IV for an adult; (3) naloxone, 2 mg IV bolus for adults and children with respiratory compromise; and (4) oxygen, 100% at 8 to 10 L/min. Dextrose administration may be omitted when hypoglycemia can be definitely excluded, but hypoglycemia may be the sole or contributing cause of coma even when the patient manifests focal findings.

The physical examination should be completed, searching carefully for any external signs of head, neck,

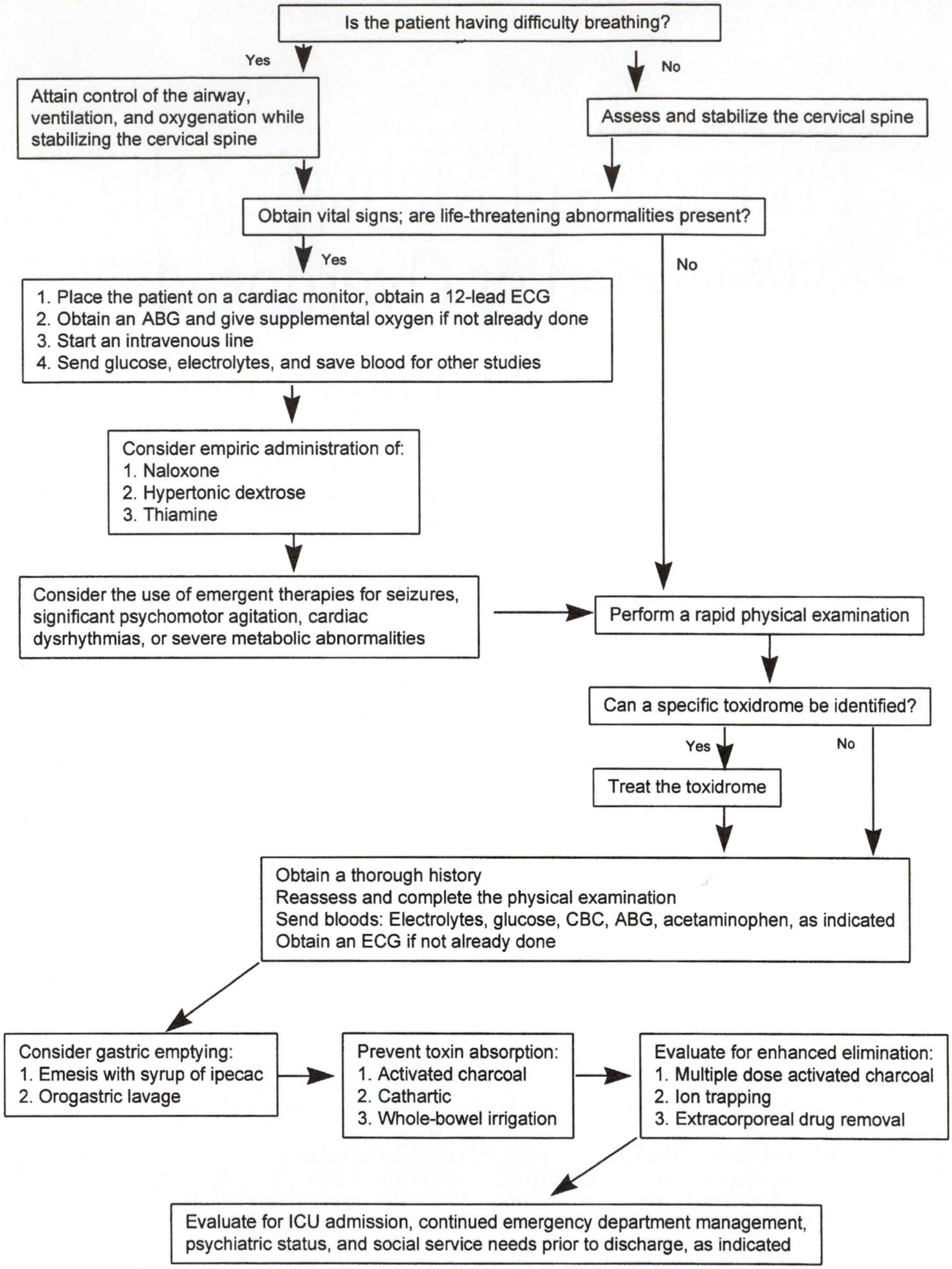

Figure 3–1. Basic guide to management of poisoned or overdosed patients. A fuller description of the steps in management may be found in the accompanying text and in Chapter 30. This algorithm is only a guide to actual management, and must of course take into consideration the clinical status of the patient.

TABLE 3–1. RECOMMENDED STOCK LIST OF THERAPEUTIC AGENTS FOR THE TREATMENT OF POISONINGS AND OVERDOSES[a]

Page in Text	Therapeutic Agent[b]	Uses
527	Activated charcoal	Toxin or drug adsorption
1620	Antivenin (*Crotalidae*), Polyvalent (Wyeth)	Crotalid snake envenomation
1620	Antivenin (*Elapidae*)	Elapid (Coral) snake envenomation
1635	Antivenin (*Latrodectus mactans*) (MSD)	Black widow spider envenomation
1434	Atropine	Bradydysrhythmias, beta-adrenergic antagonists, calcium channel blockers, cholinesterase inhibitors (organophosphates, physostigmine) exposure, digoxin and other cardiac glycosides, muscarinic muschrooms (*Clitocybe, Inocybe*)
1188	Botulinal antitoxin (ABE-trivalent)	Botulism (available from local health department or Centers for Disease Control and Prevention)
1424	Calcium chloride, calcium gluconate	Oxalates, fluoride, hydrofluoric acid, ethylene glycol, calcium channel blockers, beta-adrenergic antagonists, hypermagnesemia
1583	Cyanide kit (amyl nitrite, sodium nitrite, sodium thiosulfate)	Cyanide poisoning
628	Deferoxamine mesylate (Desferal)	Iron poisoning
683	Dextrose in water (50% adults), (20% pediatrics)	Hypoglycemia due to a variety of agents, to diagnose or treat patients with altered mental status
1078	Diazepam (Valium) or lorazepam (Ativan)	Seizures, severe agitation, stimulants
802	Digoxin specific antibody fragments (Digibind)	Digoxin, digitoxin, and cardiac glycosides of any origin (pharmaceuticals, plants, animals)
1274	Dimercaprol (BAL, British anti-lewisite)	Arsenic, mercury, gold, and lead poisoning
1310	Dimercaptosuccinic acid (DMSA, Succimer)	Lead, mercury, or arsenic poisoning
948	Diphenhydramine (Benadryl)	Extrapyramidal reactions (neuroleptics), allergic reactions
361	Dopamine HCl	Hypotension (rarely the preferred agent)
1064	Ethanol oral and parenteral dosage forms	Methanol and ethylene glycol poisoning
1315	Ethylenediaminetetraacetic acid (calcium disodium EDTA)	Lead, and other selected heavy metal poisoning
1017	Flumazenil	Reversal of pure benzodiazepine poisoning in a nonbenzodiazepine-dependent patient
1061	Folinic acid	Methanol poisoning, methotrexate toxicity
826	Glucagon	Beta-adrenergic antagonist and calcium channel blocker overdoses
523	Ipecac, syrup of	Emesis
535	Magnesium sulfate (Epsom salts) or magnesium citrate	Catharsis
798	Magnesium sulfate injection	Digitalis overdoses, hydrofluoric acid exposures, hypomagnesemia
1520	Methylene blue (1% solution)	Methemoglobinemia
1067	4-Methylpyrazole (Fomepizole)	Ethylene glycol and methanol poisoning
565	*N*-acetylcysteine (Mucomyst)	Acetaminophen overdoses
996	Naloxone hydrochloride (Narcan)	Opioid overdoses
1080	Nitroprusside	Hypertension and ergotamine overdoses
361	Norepinephrine (Levarterenol)	Hypotension (preferred for cyclic antidepressants), alpha adrenergic antagonist overdose
678	Octreotide	Hypoglycemia due to oral hypoglycemic agents
1564	Oxygen (oxygen, hyperbaric)	Carbon monoxide, cyanide, hydrogen sulfide poisoning
1269	d-Penicillamine	Copper poisoning
1133	Phenobarbital	Seizures, agitation
1080	Phentolamine	MAOI interactions, cocaine, epinephrine, ergot alkaloids
797	Phenytoin	Digitalis overdoses
614	Physostigmine salicylate (Antilirium)	Anticholinergic overdoses or poisoning
538	Polyethylene glycol electrolyte lavage solution	Gastrointestinal decontamination
1445	Pralidoxime chloride (2-PAM- chloride) (Protopam)	Cholinesterase inhibitor (organophosphates and carbamates) poisoning
722	Protamine sulfate	Heparin anticoagulation reversal
738	Pyridoxine hydrochloride	Isoniazid overdoses, ethylene glycol poisoning, monomethylhydrazine-containing mushroom ingestions
582	Sodium bicarbonate	1. Reversal of metabolic acidosis: cyanide, methanol, ethylene glycol 2. Enhanced elimination: salicylates, chlorpropamide, phenobarbital, methanol, chlorphenoxy herbicides 3. Reversal of type IA ECG effects: cyclic antidepressants, quinine, carbamazepine, type IA and IC antidysrhythmic agents, cocaine, select phenothiazines
535	Sorbitol	Catharsis
1361	Starch	Iodine poisoning
1038	Thiamine hydrochloride	Thiamine deficiency, ethylene glycol poisoning, alcoholism
719	Vitamin K_1 (Aquamephyton)	Warfarin anticoagulant or rodenticide toxicity

[a]Each emergency department should have all these agents readily available to its staff. Some of these antidotes may be stored in the pharmacy, and others may be available from the Centers for Disease Control and Prevention, but the precise mechanism for locating each agent must be known by the staff.
[b]A detailed analysis of each agent is found elsewhere in the text and in sections entitled Antidotes in Depth.

or blunt abdominal trauma; abnormal or focal neurologic findings; abnormal pupillary responses; unusual breath or skin odors (see Table 27–1); abnormal respiratory or cardiac sounds; and toxicologic syndromes or "toxidromes." Toxicologic etiologies of abnormal vital signs and physical findings are summarized in Tables 17–2 to 17–5. Toxidromes caused by particular drugs or toxins are summarized in Table 17–1 and other details of the physical assessment are provided in Chapter 30.

With stabilization of the patient's condition, attention can be addressed to the issues of gastrointestinal evacuation and prevention of drug or toxin absorption from the gastrointestinal tract. A detailed discussion of these issues may be found in Chapter 4. The indications, contraindications, precautions, and adverse effects associated with orogastric lavage, whole-bowel irrigation, administration of single or multiple dose activated charcoal, cathartics, and (in the conscious patient) emesis utilizing syrup of ipecac, are summarized in Tables 30–1 to 30–5. Fully referenced descriptions of whole-bowel irrigation, activated charcoal, cathartics, and syrup of ipecac may be found in the respective Antidotes in Depth sections immediately following Chapter 30.

At the next stage in the management of a poisoned or overdosed patient, it is appropriate to consider various methods of eliminating absorbed toxins. Currently, available methods range from raising urinary pH (also known as "ion trapping") to hemodialysis, hemoperfusion, hemofiltration, and exchange transfusion. All are described in Chapter 5.

Although the vast majority of toxicologic emergencies result from ingestion, injection or inhalation, the eyes and skin are occasionally the route of systemic absorption or are the organs at risk. The management of toxic cutaneous exposures and caustic eye injuries is described along with a more detailed management approach to the unknown or suspected overdose in Chapters 26, 28, and 30.

Typically in managing patients with toxicologic emergencies there is both a necessity as well as an opportunity to obtain various diagnostic studies and ancillary tests interspersed with stabilizing the patient's condition (when establishing intravenous access, for example), obtaining the history, and performing the physical examination. Chapters 5 to 8 discuss the timing and indications for qualitative and quantitative diagnostic laboratory studies, the use and interpretation of the electrocardiogram, and radiologic and imaging procedures in diagnosing and managing the poisoned or overdosed patient.

A recommended stock list of antidotes and therapeutic agents for the treatment of poisonings and overdoses appears in Table 3–1.

CHAPTER 4

Techniques Used to Prevent Gastrointestinal Absorption of Toxic Compounds

Martin J. Smilkstein

Limiting ongoing absorption of toxic compounds is one of the core principles of care for poisoned patients. Gastrointestinal decontamination is the most common issue considered and the topic of this chapter; however, an understanding of dermal, ocular, and respiratory decontamination is also important. Dermal decontamination is discussed in Chapter 28, decontamination of the eye in Chapter 26, and consideration for inhalation exposures in Chapter 94.

Although gastrointestinal decontamination has been a critical and familiar part of therapy of the poisoned patient for some time, no other area of medical toxicology has generated as much recent and continuing controversy. The controversy has arisen because the results of clinically relevant studies of gastric emptying, activated charcoal, and cathartics have challenged many of the assumptions on which previous therapy was based. Studies of gastric emptying have failed to show benefit, or found benefit only in limited circumstances.[4,91,112,132] Activated charcoal appears to be more effective than gastric emptying in many cases,[44,118,119] and often may enhance drug elimination in addition to decreasing absorption.[19,20,38] These findings are among many that have radically changed concepts about gastrointestinal decontamination.

Despite these ongoing controversies, a great deal of information is available that can form the basis for a rational approach to gastrointestinal decontamination. For specific information on dosages and technical aspects of delivering gastrointestinal decontamination modalities, see Chapters 3 and 30 and Antidotes in Depth: Syrup of Ipecac; Activated Charcoal; Cathartics; and Whole-Bowel Irrigation. It is the goal of this chapter to discuss a conceptual approach to the use of these modalities that can be modified as new data become available.

Because of variations in patient age, agent ingested, severity of symptoms, time since ingestion, presence of coingestants, and numerous other factors, it is not appropriate to create simplistic gastrointestinal decontamination guidelines. A single strategy may not always be logical, even in treating the same type of ingestion, in two different patients. It is more useful to understand each intervention and its limitations and then to consider each clinical situation individually using a logical approach. The first consideration is often whether or not to empty the stomach.

What Considerations Guide Appropriate Gastric Emptying Decisions?

The decision to utilize or forgo gastric emptying should be based on whether it is reasonable to expect that a beneficial amount of drug removal can be safely accomplished by gastric emptying. Several factors must be considered: (1) the risk or potential danger to the patient caused by the ingestion; (2) the likelihood that gastric emptying will remove a clinically significant amount of the ingestion; (3) the benefits of removing that amount of agent; (4) the risks of gastric emptying; and (5) the availability and utility of alternative methods to limit absorption.

What Factors Indicate That Ongoing Absorption May Be Dangerous?

An assessment of the risk to the patient includes a consideration of the amount and type of agent ingested and the clinical course since ingestion. If the clinician is confident that the ingestion was of a nontoxic agent or a nontoxic amount of a potentially toxic agent, then obviously gastric emptying is not indicated.

If the history obtained suggests a toxic ingestion but the clinical course excludes toxicity, then gastric emptying is again not appropriate. For example, consider an asymptomatic patient with a history of ingesting diazepam tablets 6 hours earlier, with no access to other agents, and observed by family members to have been asymptomatic throughout that 6 hour period. Regardless of the amount reported to have been ingested, such a patient does not require gastric emptying to treat the diazepam overdose. Absorption and clinical effects of diazepam occur rapidly, and the clinical course effectively excludes the ingestion. Such decisions require familiarity with the agent involved: 6 hours without symptoms is adequate to exclude significant iron toxicity, but it may be inadequate to exclude toxicity due to sustained-release verapamil or diltiazem, chlorpropamide, monoamine oxidase inhibitors, or Lomotil (diphenoxylate hydrochloride with atropine), which may cause delayed life-threatening symptoms.

Such an approach is appropriate only when other ingestants can be excluded. Because this is often not the case, many patients should be managed as though they have either a more recent, larger, or different (and potentially toxic) ingestion than that described to the health care practitioner. Another exception should be made for ingestions of extraordinarily high potential risk. Although the benefit of gastric emptying remains unproved for the majority of those, patients with high-risk ingestions have not specifically been studied, and as will be discussed, some data suggest evidence of benefit in this group. The safest course, therefore, at this time is to perform gastric emptying on patients with unknown, potentially lethal ingestions or known very high-risk ingestions (eg, cyanide, colchicine, chloroquine, aspirin, cyclic antidepressants, verapamil), sometimes even if the patient is asymptomatic beyond the time that onset of toxicity would be expected by history.

Can Gastric Emptying Remove a Clinically Significant Amount of the Agent Ingested?

The likelihood that gastric emptying will effectively remove a clinically significant amount of the agent depends on both whether any of the agent remains in the stomach and whether gastric emptying will successfully remove it. Absorption of many agents (eg, alcohols, most acetaminophen formulations) is so rapid that essentially no toxin remains in the stomach after a few hours[22] and gastric emptying is therefore not indicated. Even for the many toxins that are more slowly absorbed, the yield of delayed gastric emptying is often unimpressive.[42] Uncontrolled clinical studies[41,42] have suggested that drugs other than anticholinergics, sedative-hypnotics, and opioids (drugs that slow gastrointestinal motility) are unlikely to be recoverable by gastric emptying more than 2 to 4 hours after ingestion. These results, as in the case of other gastric emptying research, suggest little potential value of gastric emptying in most cases, but fail to resolve the question of benefit to the subset of individuals at very high risk.

Drugs with or without the ability to slow gut motility can also remain in the stomach if they tend to form adherent masses. Aspirin (especially enteric-coated),[21] iron,[58] meprobamate,[75] and phenobarbital[77] serve as examples of this phenomenon; that may also be true after massive ingestion of many agents. Drugs such as aspirin that may cause pylorospasm also cause prolonged gastric retention. Clinical anecdotes including postmortem information clearly show that, in some cases, large amounts of drug can remain in the stomach for hours to days. Even rapidly absorbed drugs may remain in the stomach for unusually long periods under certain clinical conditions.[149] These observations continue to stimulate the use of delayed gastric emptying despite the lack of proven clinical efficacy.

The occurrence of antecedent spontaneous vomiting is often considered another determinant of whether or not an agent remains in the stomach. Although it is true that some drug may remain in the stomach after repeated episodes of spontaneous vomiting, it is unlikely that a significant amount can subsequently be removed by either lavage or emesis. To induce further emesis or perform orogastric lavage is not only futile, it may increase the risk of further complications, and in the case of the use of syrup of ipecac, makes subsequent administration of activated charcoal more difficult.[44] Any attempt to determine how much antecedent vomiting is sufficient to obviate gastric emptying is clearly speculative and a matter of clinical judgment. As is the case for most issues related to gastrointestinal decontamination, the degree of risk to the patient from the ingestion must be considered along with the complications from the procedure. For example, it would be logical to forego gastric emptying after a codeine ingestion if the patient had vomited two or three times, but orogastric lavage might be appropriate after the same amount of vomiting following a massive colchicine overdose.

What Clinical Benefits of Gastric Emptying Have Been Demonstrated?

Gastric emptying can result in removal of drug from the stomach of poisoned patients,[13,24,41] and volunteer studies demonstrate that drug absorption can be decreased,[148] but neither of these observations proves clinical benefit. Although a difficult issue to study, clinical benefit from gastric emptying has been demonstrable only in patients with serious overdoses if gastric emptying is accomplished within 1 hour of the ingestion.[91] Other authors describe no benefit at all.[112,132] New guidelines have emphasized these studies, and concluded that gastric emptying should be entirely abandoned, or utilized only in extraordinary situations. While these studies do demonstrate that the majority of patients can be treated effectively with activated charcoal alone, they clearly do not prove that delayed gastric emptying is ineffective in all cases.

It is worthwhile to examine how the limitations of these studies should affect their interpretation. The decision to perform gastric emptying should be largely based on speculation that the ingestion may lead to a clinically unstable, life-threatening condition for which even a small decrease in toxic exposure may be critical. The impact of gastric emptying on the clinical outcome of patients with the most dangerous exposures is therefore of greatest interest. Studies thus far include patients with a wide variety of overdoses and possible overdoses, the vast majority of whom would be expected to do well with supportive care alone. Clearly, it is difficult to show any therapeutic benefit in such cases, and study of this heterogeneous group of cases does not resolve the question in the most important subset. Understandably, no controlled study to date has included enough patients with confirmed, life-threatening ingestions to adequately compare outcome with and without gastric emptying. It is also important to consider certain other drug subsets, such as sustained-release formulations, drugs likely to form aggregations or cause pylorospasm, amounts of drug large enough to exceed the adsorptive capacity of activated charcoal, and agents not well adsorbed to activated charcoal. Although gastric emptying would seem most logical after these ingestions, either they have not been studied separately or have been excluded from study altogether.[91,112]

In a recent study, in which the author concludes that gastric emptying is futile, the results actually appear to suggest benefit to gastric emptying in the highest-risk patients.[132] In 8 of 10 analyses of groups subdivided by severity or time to presentation and compared with regard to incidence of improvement and deterioration, results were better in the groups undergoing gastric emptying. Despite small subgroup size, these differences approached or achieved statistical significance in 4 of these analyses. The authors discount these observations as either due to other factors, or as not statistically significant. Power analysis indicated that the group size of the "severely" intoxicated group was only large enough to detect a twofold benefit from gastric emptying. Very few medical interventions provide a twofold benefit, and lesser degrees of benefit may be important, particularly in patients very close to life-threatening thresholds of toxicity.

An earlier study demonstrated benefit to gastric emptying among the most ill, despite the fact that 7 critically ill patients were excluded from the study.[91] Within any large sample of poisoned patients, the incidence of serious toxicity is low,[98–102] and the ability to demonstrate benefit despite exclusion of a significant portion of the sickest patients is noteworthy. In combination with the above-mentioned recent data, such observations suggest that gastric emptying will benefit a small, but critically important subset of patients.

An example of an analogous consideration is thrombolytic therapy for acute myocardial infarction. If thrombolytic therapy is assessed among all patients with chest pain, there is no evidence of benefit, and it is likely that harm will be evident due to treatment. If, instead, appropriate criteria are selected to define the patients at highest risk for consequential myocardial infarction and the conditions most likely to be associated with benefit, thrombolysis is an extraordinarily effective therapy. Similarly, no benefit is expected from gastric emptying if all overdose patients are considered, and this has been demonstrated in the above studies. What remains to be done is to define the characteristics of overdoses most likely to benefit from gastric emptying, and to study those cases.

It is unlikely that gastric emptying decisions will ever be amenable to strict predetermined criteria. Instead, a case-by-case analysis considering the factors that make gastric emptying more or less logical is appropriate (Table 4–1). In most cases, gastric emptying is only suggested for patients with ingestions matching several of the listed features. In some cases, however, the potential lethality of the ingestion is so great that a single feature might appropriately prompt orogastric lavage.

Until these issues are better evaluated, the value of gastric emptying will remain controversial. Studies clearly support the use of a selective approach and have resulted in decreased patient discomfort, complications, and cost from unnecessary gastric emptying. Nonetheless, it is inappropriate to generalize these findings to in-

TABLE 4–1. FACTORS THAT CUMULATIVELY INCREASE THE APPROPRIATENESS OF GASTRIC EMPTYING[a]

- Substantial risk of consequential toxicity: eg, ingestion of aspirin, chloroquine, colchicine, cyclic antidepressants, calcium channel blockers
- Evidence of consequential toxicity: eg, repeated seizures, hypotension, cardiac dysrhythmias, apnea, acid–base or other metabolic disturbances
- Antidotal or adjunctive therapy ineffective or non-existent: eg, calcium channel blockers, colchicine, iron, paraquat, selenious acid
- Recent ingestion (<1–2 hours)
- Ingestion exceeds adsorptive capacity of initial activated charcoal dosing: eg, >100 mg/kg of large pills such as aspirin, sustained-release verapamil, sustained-release theophylline
- Ingested agent not adsorbed by activated charcoal: eg, iron, lithium
- Ingested agent likely to form durable mass after overdose: eg, large amounts of aspirin, enteric coated agents, iron, meprobamate
- Ingestions of extended or sustained-release formulations: eg, calcium channel blockers, theophylline
- No antecedent vomiting
- Gastric tube placement required for activated charcoal administration
- No contraindications to gastric emptying

[a]The explanations and examples that follow each factor are meant only to illustrate the concepts, and are not intended to be comprehensive. See text for further discussion.

clude patients at highest risk. Based on current studies, it is neither scientifically nor logically sound to withhold gastric emptying from patients with overdoses of cyanide, colchicine, cyclic antidepressants, and many other potentially lethal ingestions; or after large ingestions of aspirin, beta-adrenergic antagonists, or calcium channel blockers and other agents with delayed and prolonged toxicity; or of lithium, iron, or other less-adsorbable agents (see individual chapters for expanded discussion). To establish the appropriate indications for gastric emptying in the context of these observations, it is critical to consider the possible risks.

What Are the Potential Complications of Gastric Emptying?

Gastric emptying is usually safe but can cause significant morbidity. Complications are very rare, and most are preventable by appropriate patient selection and the use of appropriate techniques (Chapters 3 and 30). Orogastric lavage can cause esophageal tears or perforation.[12,91,161] In addition, following lavage, nasal, oral, and pharyngeal injury, pyriform sinus and gastric perforation, and tracheal aspiration can occur.[107] Other complications described following nasogastric tube placement in settings other than poisoning management such as tracheal placement, pulmonary hemorrhage, pneumothorax, and empyema, are all potential complications of gastric lavage. Therapeutic use of syrup of ipecac has resulted in aspiration,[91,131] protracted vomiting,[35] Mallory–Weiss tears,[147] intracerebral hemorrhage,[87] pneumomediastinum and pneumoretroperitoneum,[163] and diaphragmatic rupture.[135] Attempts at gastric emptying may also propel ingested material beyond the pylorus, where many drugs are more readily absorbed.[138]

Perhaps the most common avoidable morbidity occurs in the somewhat combative patient who resists attempts at gastric emptying. If patient movement cannot be well controlled, alternatives to gastric lavage must be considered. In the majority of such cases there is little evidence for efficacy of gastric emptying, good evidence that activated charcoal will be effective (discussed later), and significant risk for injury to the patient or staff during the procedure. In the unusual case in which gastric emptying is deemed to be very important, persistent attempts at lavage may be indicated. Although the use of sedation or neuromuscular paralysis is common prior to gastric lavage,[48] except to obtain airway control, such measures are almost never indicated. Except in vanishingly rare circumstances, the risks of sedation and paralysis far outweigh the benefits of gastric emptying, and gastric lavage can be avoided or delayed until clinical findings permit the procedure without additional risk.

Contraindications to gastric emptying include any situation when it is unnecessary or ineffective (see the earlier discussion) or potentially dangerous. For example, gastric emptying is illogical after ingestion of alkaline caustics (Chap. 86), which cause consequential local injury but carry little risk from systemic absorption. Gastric emptying cannot be safely undertaken in these cases, and would not be expected to be of any value. The advisability of gastric emptying is more controversial after ingestion of agents such as phenols and acids, which although caustic can also cause systemic toxicity by absorption (Chap. 86). With some caustic agents, such as mercuric chloride, the potential systemic toxicity is so great that gastric emptying seems clearly warranted despite the presence of probable gastric injury.

What Are the Appropriate Alternatives to Gastric Emptying?

Assessment of the risk-to-benefit ratio of gastric emptying should take into account alternative treatments. Some have suggested the use of no gastrointestinal decontamination at all;[112] however, the most important alternative to gastric emptying is the use of activated charcoal alone. In volunteer studies following small ingestions of agents well adsorbed to activated charcoal, activated charcoal is more effective in preventing drug absorption than gastric emptying.[44,110,120,153] Studies of actual drug overdoses have found gastric emptying followed by activated charcoal to be no more effective than activated charcoal alone for the majority of poisoned patients.[91,112,132] Because the charcoal-to-drug ratio is one of the most important determinants of activated charcoal efficacy,[126] the amount of drug ingested may determine whether activated charcoal alone would be expected to be adequate. For patients with small ingestions of agents well adsorbed to activated charcoal, there is good support for the use of activated charcoal alone.

An activated charcoal-to-drug ratio of 10 to 1 can serve to illustrate this important concept. This commonly mentioned ratio is a midrange value from in vitro studies,[7] of uncertain clinical value, since ideal ratios vary by agent and GI conditions, but it serves as a useful conceptual guide. Using lorazepam (Ativan) as an example, to achieve a 10:1 charcoal-to-drug ratio in a patient who has ingested 100 tablets of 2 mg each requires only 2 g of activated charcoal. In an adult, a typical activated charcoal dose of 1 g/kg of body weight would then be expected to be quite effective in reducing further drug absorption. From another perspective, 2 g of activated charcoal would theoretically treat an ingestion of one thousand 0.2-mg clonidine tablets (200 mg total), whereas even 100 g of activated charcoal would be ineffective after an ingestion of only fifty 300-mg theophylline tablets (15 g total). Activated charcoal is still a critical part of management of patients with large ingestions, but gastric emptying may take on greater importance as an adjunct in these situations.

The availability of an antidote or adjunctive therapy may also affect the decision to forego gastric emptying. When there is no clear indication for gastric emptying, the risk of subsequent unexpected gastrointestinal absorption is more acceptable if there is a very effective treatment or antidote available. Antidotal therapy obviously should not replace gastric emptying if gastric emptying would clearly be effective, but this is not usually the case. Consider a patient who reportedly ingested 25 tablets of acetaminophen and codeine 4.5 hours earlier. Absorption would probably be complete even if possibly slowed by codeine. Since there would probably be little or no benefit of gastric emptying at this point, and since there are effective antidotes for both acetaminophen (*N*-acetylcysteine) and codeine (naloxone), it is appropriate to forego gastric emptying.

Summary: Gastric Emptying

The use of gastric emptying should be a selective (Table 4–1), not a routine procedure. Gastric emptying is largely an unproved therapy that is nevertheless useful in some situations when it can be accomplished safely. Rarely, if ever, should the patient be placed at additional serious risk to empty the stomach.

When Gastric Emptying Is Indicated, Which Technique Should Be Utilized?

Until 1985, syrup of ipecac was routinely administered after ingestions unless the patient was comatose or convulsing or had lost the gag reflex; under these circumstances orogastric lavage was recommended. Comparing the risks and benefits of these two methods, it became apparent that this approach was far too simplistic. While earlier debate focused primarily on which method removed more drug,[1,11,25] more recent work has attempted to view these modalities in the context of the whole patient. Determining relative benefit includes consideration of the amount of drug removed, whether that removal is consequential, comparison of the potential complications of each gastric emptying technique, and the impact of each upon the use of other important treatment methods such as activated charcoal and oral antidotes. In most circumstances, comparison of induced emesis and orogastric lavage is only of historical interest; however, the analysis is instructive.

Is Either Emesis or Orogastric Lavage Superior in Prevention of Toxin Absorption?

Attempts to determine conclusively whether emesis or lavage removes more drug have failed partly because of study design but more importantly because there may be no single correct answer. With respect to study design, studies of emesis or lavage recovery of liquid barium from puppies[1] or magnesium hydroxide solution from children[43] performed soon after ingestion may have little or no bearing on the potential to recover solid pill fragments 2 to 3 hours after most overdoses. Similarly, studies of lavage utilizing small-bore nasogastric tubes[25] do not provide useful information about the efficacy of lavage as practiced, using large-bore orogastric tubes. Other study design issues are evident in the literature and have led to a variety of conflicting and inaccurate conclusions.

Currently, no adequately controlled study has shown emesis or lavage to be clearly superior in drug removal.[137] Both are probably equivalent overall, but in the clinical setting of an actual specific ingestion, the overall results are not relevant. The results of several gastric emptying studies emphasize this fact. Although children given a standard dose of a magnesium hydroxide marker immediately before syrup of ipecac-induced emesis vomited an average of 28% of the marker, the range was 0 to 78%.[43] In another study, syrup of ipecac and lavage each resulted in average removal of about half of the ingested material, but the range of retained material in the gastrointestinal tract was 0 to 100%.[138] Similar variability has been noted in other controlled studies,[11] and the actual overdose setting certainly offers even more variables than these studies.

What Substances Will Pass Through an Orogastric Lavage Tube?

Another factor in considering whether emesis or lavage is preferable for a patient with a particular ingestion is the formulation of the substance (eg, liquid, tablet, capsule, enteric coating, size, shape) as it relates to the tube lumen size and the mechanics of gastric lavage. Large drug packets, pills, or pill fragments (particularly enteric-coated and sustained-release), adherent masses of pills, and plant or mushroom fragments will not pass through even a 40 French lavage tube.[2] If gastric emptying is appropriate, ipecac-induced emesis may be more logical for this group of ingestions. This issue is even more important when the patient is a small child. Passing a very large-bore tube in an infant is impossible, and a 24 French tube is probably the largest that can safely be used. As a result, substances that might be effectively removed by lavage in an adult cannot be lavaged from a child. However in many cases, although lavage may not return a substantial amount of solid material, syrup of ipecac-induced emesis may be contraindicated. In such cases, lavage should be considered to remove dissolved drug and small fragments as well as to administer activated charcoal.

When Is Emesis Contraindicated?

Deciding between syrup of ipecac-induced emesis and lavage is more often based on a consideration of potential risks than on efficacy. The most important of these risks is the aspiration of stomach contents into the tracheobronchial tree. Any patient who initially lacks the ability to protect his or her airway or is likely to lose airway protective reflexes during the duration of action of syrup of ipecac must not have emesis induced. Instead, if gastric emptying is indicated, such a patient should be lavaged, after endotracheal intubation. An ingestion of any substance causing or capable of rapidly causing a decreased level of consciousness, seizure, cardiovascular collapse, or neuromuscular paralysis should be managed this way. Examples of substances that may preclude the use of syrup of ipecac are cyclic antidepressants, isoniazid, propoxyphene, camphor, and propranolol, but many, if not most, serious overdoses may fit this description. The limited potential benefit offered by emesis does not justify placing the patient at risk for aspiration.

Induction of emesis is also contraindicated for ingestions of foreign bodies likely to cause mechanical injury or upper airway obstruction and in patients with certain structural lesions or bleeding diatheses. Contraindications to emesis are summarized in Table 30–4 and should be considered in addition to contraindications to gastric emptying in general.

How Does the Anticipated Use of Activated Charcoal or Other Oral Antidotes Impact Choice of Gastric Emptying Method?

The increasing appreciation of the efficacy of activated charcoal also has a profound effect on the approach to gastric emptying. In addition to replacing gastric emptying in many settings, activated charcoal is useful following gastric emptying in the vast majority of ingestions and is absolutely essential in some (see Antidotes in Depth: Activated Charcoal). Orogastric lavage can usually be accomplished rapidly and then followed quickly by administration of activated charcoal via the lavage tube. Syrup of ipecac results in significant delays in charcoal administration, due to the combination of delay to its onset of effect and a period of repeated emesis and subsequent nausea during recovery. Because delayed administration of activated charcoal clearly decreases its efficacy, emesis has been largely replaced by lavage in cases involving ingestions of toxic substances well-adsorbed to activated charcoal.

The effective use of oral *N*-acetylcysteine and other oral agents can also be delayed by the use of syrup of ipecac. Patients poisoned with acetaminophen are often nauseated from the ingestion itself, making the use of *N*-acetylcysteine difficult. Using syrup of ipecac in this situation will increase the tendency to vomit, further preventing or delaying effective use of *N*-acetylcysteine. In summary, if *N*-acetylcysteine or other oral agents are needed within 2 to 3 hours and gastric emptying is indicated, orogastric lavage would be the preferred method.

Are There Other Unique Considerations?

Use of syrup of ipecac at home for children not subsequently treated at a health care facility, as often recommended by poison centers, represents an important special issue. Thus far, activated charcoal is not a widely available, practical alternative,[32,47,50,69,88,94] and studies of gastric emptying efficacy are largely irrelevant in the assessment of this form of intervention. Due to the nature of such exposures, the potential benefit of emesis in this setting would likely be avoidance of an emergency department visit, rather than avoidance of consequential clinical deterioration. Without the use of ipecac, would symptoms occur from the exposure that are not dangerous, but are noticeable enough to prompt medical evaluation? Do such symptoms now occur, masked by, or misattributed to, ipecac-induced emesis? Does the induction of emesis provide reassurance to parents or poison center staff, facilitating home observation? Given the incidence of minor, unintentional pediatric exposures,[98–102] these questions are extraordinarily important to resolve.

A much rarer gastric emptying challenge is the problematic "body stuffer" (Chap. 65). Body stuffers are people who have quickly, and not carefully, ingested packets containing drugs of abuse, generally in an attempt to conceal evidence of drug possession. The amount ingested is often unclear, there is significant risk of drug container leakage, and there is no reliable early test to confirm and quantify the ingestion.[71] The drugs involved, typically cocaine or heroin, may cause abrupt clinical deterioration, but in the overwhelming majority of cases no identifiable toxicity occurs. Lavage is ineffective due to the size of the drug packages; syrup of ipecac induced emesis is potentially dangerous because of the possibility of clinical deterioration before or during emesis; and observation alone means a lengthy hospitalization that is most often unnecessary and for which there is no clear endpoint. There is certainly no consensus on the management of these patients, but in our opinion there is a role for syrup of ipecac-induced emesis in some cases, in combination with immediately delivered activated charcoal. This approach deserves consideration if the ingestion involves a small amount of drug, there is no evidence of drug leakage or drug effect by history or physical examination, the drug containers are crack vials or sealed water-resistant bags that are less likely to result in early massive leakage, and there is no contraindication to emesis. Others feel that the risk of subsequent deterioration can never be predicted and thus favor the use of activated charcoal and whole-bowel irrigation (described later in the chapter).

Some sustained-release pharmaceutical preparations present a special problem because the bulk of the pill matrix remains largely intact even as the active drug is released. This results in a pill that persists for many hours, too large to pass through a lavage tube.[2] In this case, lavage is ineffective and emesis will significantly complicate effective activated charcoal delivery, but such ingestions are often very serious and may be too massive to rely on activated charcoal alone. In many such cases, use of whole bowel irrigation is logical, but questions related to gastric emptying may be pertinent. For example, consider a patient who presents within an hour of a massive ingestion of persistent-matrix theophylline or verapamil, without antecedent vomiting. Would induction of emesis be a logical intervention?

A subset of the most problematic overdoses include those after which large amounts of drug, in a form too large to be effectively lavaged, may be present in the stomach. Sustained-release calcium channel blockers, aspirin and enteric-coated aspirin, theophylline, lithium, and many others are in this category. Theoretically, a "reversible" emetic might deserve investigation when lavage is ineffective, but emesis is problematic. The goal of this approach would be to induce rapid-onset emesis that could then be terminated by the physician to avoid the risks associated with persistent vomiting in case of clinical deterioration.

Apomorphine is a morphine derivative with diminished analgesic action and potent emetic effects mediated by stimulation of the chemoreceptor trigger zone and possibly the vestibular apparatus.[104] It generally induces emesis within 3 to 5 minutes of a single subcutaneous dose. Disadvantages include significant CNS and respiratory depression, and severe and protracted vomiting. It is currently unavailable in a premixed parenteral form. There are data to suggest that naloxone may reverse vomiting and at least some of the adverse effects associated with apomorphine,[23] but this has not been adequately studied. If, following emesis, the CNS, respiratory, and emetic effects of apomorphine could be safely reversed by naloxone, apomorphine could potentially be of value. A second approach would be to study the ability of newer potent antiemetics to reverse the effects of syrup of ipecac.[113] These approaches are mentioned only as areas of investigation that may relate to difficult treatment controversies. There are no data to support their use at this time.

Summary: Emesis Versus Gastric Lavage

In summary, when gastric emptying is indicated, orogastric lavage is preferable to syrup of ipecac-induced emesis in nearly all hospital cases. Settings where emesis continues to have a more important role include ingestions of objects too large to pass through a lavage tube, ingestions by infants and small children in whom large-bore tubes cannot be used safely, and home use. These guidelines are not absolute and always must be considered on an individual basis recognizing potential contraindications and alternatives for a particular patient and a particular ingestion.

What Is the Role of Activated Charcoal?

There is no question that activated charcoal has an important role in the management of toxicologic emergencies, but the description of that role is still being defined. Like other treatment modalities, the appropriate use of activated charcoal should be determined by analysis of the relative risks and benefits of its use. Rare potential adverse effects have become evident due to its widespread use, but without well-controlled studies in poisoned patients it has been difficult to accurately assess its clinical benefit.

How Beneficial Is Activated Charcoal?

It is necessary to consider separately the two potential benefits of activated charcoal: preventing the absorption of toxic agents from the gastrointestinal tract and enhancing the elimination of agents already absorbed. For activated charcoal to prevent systemic absorption of toxic substances from the gastrointestinal tract effectively, the substance must be adsorbed by activated charcoal and still be present in the gastrointestinal tract at the time of activated charcoal administration. When both of these conditions are met, there is no doubt that activated charcoal results in diminished absorption, lower peak serum concentration, and decreased area under the concentration versus time curve. Activated charcoal has been studied with hundreds of substances in vitro, in animals, in human volunteers, and in patients with actual overdoses.[26,38,130] Although controlled studies showing clinical benefit have not been done, these other data are convincing enough to warrant the use of activated charcoal soon after most ingestions.

Even substances not well adsorbed to activated charcoal may nevertheless be partially adsorbed, and thus activated charcoal may be beneficial even for these exposures. For example, based on in vitro studies, cyanide was categorized as not well adsorbed, since 1 g of activated charcoal bound only 35 mg of potassium cyanide, far less than other toxic agents studied.[7] If the same ratio were to hold in an actual patient, then delivery of 60 g of activated charcoal could adsorb 2.1 g of potassium cyanide, well above the expected lethal dose. In vivo efficacy of activated charcoal in the treatment of cyanide poisoning was demonstrated in an animal model,[93] suggesting that this logic is valid and that it may apply to other potentially lethal agents as well. As the amount ingested increases and the binding affinity decreases, the stoichiometric advantage is lost and this approach clearly becomes less effective. Typical ingestions of ethanol, lithium, or iron, for example, involve several grams of drug; thus, the very limited adsorption of each to activated charcoal makes this modality clinically insignificant. In fact, of commonly ingested substances, ethanol, lithium, and iron are the only ones for which activated charcoal has been documented to be completely ineffective.[123]

Other substances also often described as poorly adsorbed to activated charcoal are actually partially adsorbed or have not been studied. Hydrocarbons are said to be poorly adsorbed, yet activated charcoal decreased gastrointestinal absorption of kerosene, benzene, and dichloroethane in rats.[36,92] Metals have been similarly described, but significant activated charcoal adsorption of mercuric chloride was first noted in the 1940s,[7] and its therapeutic use in mercury poisoning dates to the 19th century. For many agents only in vitro data are available, which may or may not be applicable.

Regardless of the ingestion history, administration of activated charcoal may be appropriate due to the likelihood of inaccurate information or unrecognized co-ingestion of agents that are well adsorbed. For substances that are well adsorbed, activated charcoal not only decreases drug absorption from the gastrointestinal tract but also enhances elimination of drug already absorbed; thus, its use is often appropriate regardless of the interval since ingestion. Therefore, an initial dose of activated charcoal should be administered in nearly all cases of potentially toxic ingestions unless contraindicated.

Because of concerns that gastric lavage may delay activated charcoal administration, or increase drug absorption by dissolving drug or pushing it out of the stomach into the small intestine, it has been suggested that activated charcoal be administered prior to or during lavage.[30,138] Although theoretically appealing, this approach has obvious practical disadvantages. Its true role remains to be determined, but available studies suggest that there is no need to consider this method routinely. In a volunteer study, lavage resulted in no increase in drug passing the pylorus compared with untreated controls.[138] In addition, proper patient positioning[160] and proper lavage technique should limit drug passage beyond the pylorus. As a result, activated charcoal prior to or during lavage is rarely indicated, but it may be appropriate after particularly massive or dangerous ingestions.

Multiple-dose activated charcoal (MDAC) may also be indicated to prevent absorption in several circumstances when a significant amount of the agent is likely to remain in the gastrointestinal tract. Some ingestions are too massive to be effectively adsorbed by a single dose of activated charcoal. In other cases the continuous release of drug from a sustained-release formulation or concretion makes repeated doses of activated charcoal a logical choice. Only a few agents probably lead to formation of true concretions, but persistence of large quantities of undissolved drug in any form has similar clinical implications. Many substances slow gastrointestinal motility and are thus particularly likely to remain in the gastrointestinal tract, especially following large ingestions. Although cyclic antidepressants, calcium channel blockers, phenothiazines, anticholinergics, opioids, and sedative-hypnotics are usually associated with delayed gastrointestinal passage, many other substances are also capable of effectively delaying gastrointestinal passage directly or indirectly by altering electrolytes, changing blood pressure, causing mechanical obstruction, or pylorospasm, or by other mechanisms. As a result, MDAC is often appropriate regardless of whether or not the ingested substance is known to slow motility or cause concretions.

Multiple-dose activated charcoal is far more controversial as a method to enhance elimination of toxic substances (see Antidotes in Depth: Activated Charcoal).[33,38,123,130,155] For it to be effective in enhancing elimination of a given substance, the substance must either undergo enterohepatic recirculation or, more often, be present to a significant extent in circulating blood (enteroenteric recirculation, or "gut dialysis") and be well adsorbed to activated charcoal. For some substances, such as theophylline, there is good evidence that MDAC substantially limits absorption and enhances elimination. For many other substances, MDAC has been shown to alter drug kinetics favorably, but the change is small. In still other cases, despite in vitro adsorption, no effect has been noted in volunteers.

Applying the results of these studies to the overdose setting has been difficult. There are profound differences between drug pharmacokinetics at doses used in therapeutic or volunteer studies and "toxicokinetics" in poisoned or overdosed patients. Depending on whether drug is likely to persist in the gastrointestinal tract and whether the elimination of the drug is zero-order, first-order, or Michaelis-Menten, the effect of activated charcoal in overdose may be less than, equal to, or more than that seen at low drug dosage.[39] There is also uncertainty as to how much effect on drug kinetics is required to produce clinical benefit.[155] For example, many would argue that MDAC is not useful in treating saliclylate overdose because it either has no effect[76] or only slightly augments salicylate elimination.[85,109] On the other hand, proponents of MDAC in this setting would speculate that a small reduction in the area under the concentration versus time curve[80] might be enough to prevent some component of delayed clinical deterioration. On the basis of current information, utilization of MDAC is appropriate in many such potentially serious ingestions, when it can be accomplished safely.

Can Activated Charcoal Harm the Patient? Is It Ever Contraindicated?

Activated charcoal is generally safe and has few contraindications. Most patients with caustic ingestions who require endoscopy should not receive activated charcoal, since it does not effectively adsorb most caustics and in addition will then obscure the endoscopist's view. Although most patients tolerate activated charcoal well, at least some patients do vomit after receiving it. As a result, it is also contraindicated in patients with ingestions of pure petroleum distillates and other agents that are not well adsorbed to activated charcoal but that do carry a high risk of pulmonary aspiration. It should be noted that other toxic hydrocarbons (eg, benzene) and agents found in combination with hydrocarbons (eg, pesticides) have not been well studied and may be at least partially adsorbed by activated charcoal, making its administration appropriate.

Minor adverse effects of activated charcoal, including nausea, vomiting, and constipation, are common.[1,5,123] Pulmonary aspiration is the most serious complication that may occur in the overdose setting. Activated charcoal has been noted in the respiratory tract, and several cases of aspiration are described in the literature,[45,63,67,131,139] including fatalities.[18,51,68,102,111] It is not appropriate to consider these cases as the result of activated charcoal. Instead, they illustrate failure to secure adequate airway protection or direct instillation of activated charcoal into the trachea after improper nasogastric or orogastric tube placement. In addition to massive consequential aspiration, trivial charcoal aspiration is very common. An endotracheal tube cuff does not provide a perfect seal, and small amounts of black-tinged secretions are often suctioned from intubated patients with properly protected airways. There is no evidence that activated charcoal increases the risk of aspiration in patients with intact airway protective reflexes, or that it causes more severe sequellae than equivalent aspiration of gastric contents without activated charcoal. In summary, if appropriate standards of airway protection and activated charcoal administration techniques are observed, there is no increased risk of consequential pulmonary aspiration due to activated charcoal. This concern is therefore not an appropriate reason to forgo activated charcoal therapy.

Although there are few credible reports of other serious complications from a single dose of activated charcoal, cases of bowel obstruction or pseudo-obstruction have been described following MDAC.[27,57,65,66,103,133,162] Although extraordinarily rare, these cases deserve consideration. Features include decreased gut motility after 36 to 120 hours of repeated activated charcoal dosing at 3 to 6-hour intervals. As experience with MDAC continues, other cases may occur. This rare but serious risk should be weighed against the potential benefits. In a patient with decreased gastrointestinal motility, MDAC might be continued despite the risk if there were good evidence of enhanced toxin elimination (eg, massive phenobarbital overdose). On the other hand, if ileus were present, MDAC might not be warranted when there is little reason to expect much yield (eg, cyclic antidepressant overdose). Most reports of serious complications after MDAC have actually been the result of multiple cathartic doses. It is of critical importance to specify activated charcoal without cathartic when ordering MDAC for a patient (cathartics are discussed later).

Activated Charcoal: How Much, How Many Times, How Often?

There is no single correct dose of activated charcoal. As discussed, in some cases the expenditure of time, effort, and cost in administering large amounts or repeated doses of activated charcoal is not justified, but in other cases (eg, theophylline overdose) it should be considered a life-saving therapeutic maneuver of the highest priority.[124] The maximum amount of activated charcoal that can be safely and successfully given is unknown and certainly varies with the patient. To treat a severe theophylline overdose in an adult, as much as 100 g initially, followed by a continuous nasogastric tube infusion of 100 g/h may be appropriate. It is unusual for both patient and staff to tolerate such a regimen. It is certainly unnecessary and unreasonable to give most patients the maximum possible dosage, and although complications are rare, such dosing increases the risks. Although dosage has been largely dictated by convention or packaging, a more rational approach is possible. While it is certainly necessary to consider the age and size of the patient when determining activated charcoal dosage, it is also critical to consider the type of agent involved and the amount ingested.

The optimum activated charcoal dose would theoretically be the minimum dose that would completely adsorb the ingested toxic agent and, if relevant, maximize enhanced elimination. Because of variables such as the physical properties of the drug formulation ingested, the volume and pH of gastric and intestinal fluid, and the presence of other agents or foods adsorbed by activated charcoal,[8,9,105,121,125] the optimum dose cannot be known with certainty in any given patient. It is possible, however, to develop a logical approach to dosing based on available data. The results of in vitro studies show that ideal activated charcoal-to-drug ratios vary widely, but 10:1 is a representative value for many typical drugs and is therefore useful in theoretical consideration of optimal activated charcoal dosing.[7,126]

As noted, achieving a large activated charcoal-to-drug ratio is often quite feasible for ingestions of drugs dispensed in small formulations, such as digoxin (0.25 mg), clonidine (0.2 mg), or levothyroxine (0.025 to 0.3 mg), but impossible for agents such as adult aspirin (325 mg), sustained-release theophylline (200 to 400 mg), or sustained-release verapamil (up to 240 mg). This should not be interpreted to mean that activated charcoal dosage should be decreased significantly for small ingestions; it seems logical to use the largest dose that can be easily given (0.5 to 1 g/kg). Activated charcoal dosage should, however, be increased to treat certain ingestions. Maximal initial dosing (1.5 to 2 g/kg) is appropriate after massive ingestions of dangerous substances that are well adsorbed to activated charcoal (eg, theophylline, aspirin, sustained-release verapamil). Maximal activated charcoal dosing should also be used after ingestion of some lethal substances, even if they are poorly adsorbed, if a limited amount of adsorption to activated charcoal might be of significant clinical benefit (eg, cyanide).

The amount and frequency of MDAC dosing should vary based on considerations of risks and benefits as discussed. For cases less likely to benefit significantly from multiple doses, such as exposure to low-risk, rapidly absorbed, widely distributed substances, a low dose of MDAC, such as 0.5 to 1 g/kg every 4 to 6 hours, may be appropriate. More seriously poisoned patients should receive larger doses of activated charcoal, and patients for whom multiple-dose activated charcoal is critical, as in life-threatening overdoses of sustained-release theophylline, should be given as high a dose as they can tolerate, 1 g/kg or more per hour. Some patients tolerate "mini-boluses" or continuous nasogastric infusions better than large intermittent doses. In many cases, antiemetics are necessary to accomplish aggressive activated charcoal dosing in spite of theoretical undesirable effects of antiemetics such as decreased gastrointestinal motility or alteration in seizure potential. The appropriate endpoint for MDAC is also unstudied and may vary with the agent involved. The pharmacokinetics, toxicokinetics, and amount of the agent ingested all must be considered. In some cases, altered mental status or another toxic effect will persist long after activated charcoal's role has become minimal; in these cases multiple-dose therapy may be discontinued prior to clinical resolution. A number of studies have suggested that activated charcoal may unbind drug in the gastrointestinal tract (known as desorption), which then may become available for systemic absorption.[14,56,121] If desorption from activated charcoal is likely, such as after massive salicylate ingestion, it may be appropriate to continue MDAC even after clinical improvement is evident. In most cases, significant clinical improvement and the passage of activated charcoal stools are adequate criteria for termination of MDAC.

Summary: Activated Charcoal

A single dose of activated charcoal is appropriate after nearly all suspected toxic ingestions. Exceptions include confirmed, single-substance ingestions of lithium, iron, ethanol, simple hydrocarbons, or acid or alkali caustics. With adequate airway protection, there is no serious risk associated with single-dose therapy. Multiple-dose activated charcoal is warranted if there is evidence of a large amount of residual substance in the gastrointestinal tract or to enhance the elimination of a drug or toxin already absorbed. Strong clinical evidence supporting the use of MDAC exists for only a few types of drug overdoses, but its use is often appropriate even in unproved circumstances.

In most instances, 0.5 to 1 g/kg is an appropriate initial dose of activated charcoal; doses of 1.5 to 2 g/kg should be used following particularly massive or dangerous ingestions. Dosing varies when using MDAC. To treat exposures to substances for which there are less data or rationale to support multiple-dose activated charcoal, 0.5 g/kg every 4 to 6 hours is probably adequate. When multiple-dose therapy is felt to be critical, activated charcoal doses as high as 1.5g/kg per hour may be justified. Other exposures warrant dosing between these values, based on the factors discussed.

Should a Cathartic Be Used?

Are Cathartics Beneficial?

Although cathartics are routinely used in the treatment of the poisoned patient, their efficacy remains unproved. Cathartics are used to increase gastrointestinal transit speed and thus theoretically decrease the transit time during which drug absorption may occur. Cathartics may also counteract the constipating effect of activated charcoal. Another proposed reason to use cathartics is to promote rapid passage through the gastrointestinal tract to decrease time available for systemic absorption of drug that has "desorbed" from activated charcoal. Despite these theoretical advantages of cathartic use, it has been difficult to prove any consistent benefit.

No clinical benefit has been shown from the use of cathartics alone, and one study has even suggested that use of cathartics alone may be deleterious, perhaps by increasing drug dissolution.[3] Most studies have examined the possible effects of cathartics on the efficacy of activated charcoal. The addition of cathartic to activated charcoal has occasionally been of benefit,[37,62,64,82,128] but usually has no effect,[49,60,122,140] and has even been suggested to reduce the efficacy of activated charcoal according to two studies.[59,159]

Many cathartics are available, although only magnesium citrate, magnesium sulfate, and sorbitol are generally considered for use, and sorbitol is predominant in the United States (see Table 30–3). All are effective cathartics, as assessed by how quickly they produce a bowel movement.[89,145] Another clinically useful method of comparing cathartics would be to investigate how different cathartics affect activated charcoal adsorption. While the results of such studies thus far are often conflicting, no single cathartic has consistently been shown to increase or decrease drug absorption significantly, or to be superior with regard to either patient tolerance or time to first stool. Although several study design issues make interpretation difficult, some studies have suggested that sorbitol may be the most effective cathartic available,[74,89] and as a result it has gained tremendous popularity in recent years (see Antidotes in Depth: Cathartics).

Will Cathartics Harm the Patient? Are They Contraindicated?

In appropriate doses, and when contraindications to their use are excluded, there is no evidence that a single dose of cathartic is harmful. Following inadvertent overdosing (single or multiple dose), or following the use of repetitive (inappropriate) dosing in general, cathartics have been responsible for significant morbidity and mortality.

Use of sodium sulfate and sodium phosphate (Phospho-Soda) was associated with serious fluid and electrolyte disturbances.[46,95,108] The relative safety of magnesium cathartics may be a result of the limited absorption of magnesium compared to sodium.[1,15] Although limited, magnesium absorption does occur. There are no reports of magnesium toxicity following appropriate single-dose cathartic therapy in patients with normal renal function, but hypermagnesemia can be caused by magnesium cathartics. Cathartic-induced hypermagnesemia can occur even in patients with normal renal function after unintentional overdoses or after multiple "appropriate" doses of magnesium cathartics.[55,78,114,141,142]

In addition to electrolyte disturbances resulting from absorption of cathartic components, all cathartics can cause dehydration from water loss in the stool or intraluminal "third-spacing." An example of this phenomenon is sorbitol-induced fluid and electrolyte depletion. Sorbitol is not significantly absorbed but very effectively draws water into the gut lumen. As a result, severe fluid and electrolyte derangements, intravascular volume depletion, hypernatremia, shock, and acidosis have occurred after excessive sorbitol dosing. These abnormalities can occur in adults[5] or children,[54] but children presumably because of their size are at a particular risk. Sorbitol may also cause abdominal distention, usually without serious result but in one case massive enough to result in respiratory embarrassment and death.[10] Probably the result of gas production during sorbitol fermentation by gut flora,[53] distention appears to be most common and problematic when there is decreased gut motility.

The incidence of all cathartic-induced fluid and electrolyte disturbances is probably increased by slow gastrointestinal transit; thus, obstruction and ileus should be considered at least relative contraindications to cathartic use. The use of cathartics in patients with preexisting diarrhea is obviously also unnecessary and therefore contraindicated. Volume depletion should always be corrected before catharsis, and cathartic use should be minimized in infants because of the risk of causing significant fluid and electrolyte disorders. To avoid precipitating hypermagnesemia, magnesium-containing cathartics should not be used in patients with renal failure or decreased glomerular filtration rates from any cause, because of resultant impaired renal magnesium excretion.[115] These contraindications are summarized in Table 30–3.

What Is an Appropriate Cathartic Dosage?

Cathartic dosage is largely empirical. Appropriate goals of therapy are, first, to do no harm, and second, to use the minimum amount of cathartic needed to produce early and continued passage of stools. An initial dose of sorbitol, 1 g/kg, is reasonable in adults. Because of the risk of fluid and electrolyte disorders, cathartics should not be used for most low-risk ingestions in infants and very young children. For infants and children with potentially serious ingestions, a single dose of 0.5 g/kg of sorbitol may be given.

Guidelines for repeated cathartic dosing are even more speculative. The most important goal is to avoid the inadvertent use of multiple doses of cathartic during MDAC, which may result from the widespread use of combined activated charcoal and sorbitol products. An adult patient who is receiving MDAC occasionally requires a second sorbitol dose of 0.5 g/kg if stooling does not occur and no ileus is present. More than one additional dose of cathartic is rarely if ever necessary, and it is both inappropriate and dangerous to continue cathartic dosing repeatedly. In light of the lack of proven benefit and reports of rare but serious complications, additional cathartic doses should rarely, if ever, be given to small children, and then only with meticulous attention to vital signs, fluid intake and output (urinary, gastric, stool), and fluid and electrolyte status.

Summary: Cathartics

Single doses of cathartics are generally safe and appropriate, despite a lack of convincing evidence of efficacy. Although more than one dose of cathartic may sometimes seem logical, using multiple doses of any cathartic can cause significant toxicity, particularly in children. Repeat cathartic dosing should never be routinely ordered. If indicated in adults, repeat doses of cathartics should be used only with meticulous, frequent fluid and electrolyte monitoring.

When Should Whole-Bowel Irrigation Be Used?

Because cathartic dosage is limited by the risk of serious fluid and electrolyte disturbances, other methods of gastrointestinal decontamination have recently gained favor. One clinical advance has been the use of whole-bowel irrigation (WBI) using isotonic polyethylene glycol electrolyte lavage solutions such as CoLyte or Golytely.[1,6,150,154] These solutions were originally introduced for preoperative bowel preparations, and have only recently been used in the management of poisoned or overdosed patients. The components of these solutions are not absorbed, and since they are isotonic they cause no significant fluid shifts. As a result, large volumes can be used safely to "flush the gastrointestinal tract" unless the patient has an obstruction or ileus. Huge volumes over long durations have been used without any significant change in volume status, electrolytes, or other laboratory parameters.[72,79]

Rather than inducing diarrhea by drawing water into the stool or stimulating motility, whole-bowel irrigation washes bowel contents through the gastrointestinal tract mechanically by the use of large volumes of fluid. The first successful use of whole-bowel irrigation was in the management of iron overdose to treat patients with radiographic evidence of residual iron in the gastrointestinal tract.[151] Subsequently, studies of both human volunteers and animals show that whole-bowel irrigation reduces drug absorption after ingestion of ampicillin,[152] lithium,[143] and enteric-coated salicylates.[84] Other studies, however, have not shown whole-bowel irrigation to be effective.[29,127,136,146] Case reports have provided visually impressive radiographic or bedside evidence of gastrointestinal passage of arsenic,[96] iron,[52] lead,[116,134] and sustained-release calcium channel blockers.[28] Although visually impressive, these cases provide no useful data regarding the clinical benefits achieved with the procedure, nor do they demonstrate what would have occurred without whole-bowel irrigation.

The apparent safety and efficacy of whole-bowel irrigation make it an intriguing tool, but its role has yet to be defined. Delivering and retrieving the large volumes of solution required can present significant problems and is certainly not warranted routinely. The greatest utility of whole-bowel irrigation probably will be in the management of life-threatening ingestions of agents that are poorly adsorbed to activated charcoal (eg, iron, lithium); too massive for activated charcoal alone (eg, sustained-release calcium channel blockers, theophylline); or foreign bodies (eg, in body packers and stuffers) impossible to remove safely and effectively by other means.

Other than practical issues related to the administration of WBI, the most important concerns raised are about its effect on activated charcoal adsorption. Several studies have demonstrated that the most commonly used whole-bowel irrigation solutions interfere in vitro with activated charcoal's drug adsorption.[73,86,106,136] Whether the magnitude of benefit from whole-bowel irrigation outweighs the risk from slightly decreased activated charcoal adsorption remains to be shown. Perhaps simply increasing the amount, frequency, or duration of activated charcoal dosing would effectively compensate for any decreased adsorption. In cases involving iron or lithium, activated charcoal is unimportant. In other cases, such as massive ingestions of sustained-release drugs such as theophylline or verapamil where WBI may be of benefit and MDAC is essential, the potential for decreased efficiency of activated charcoal becomes an extremely important consideration. Other important considerations for study include effects of WBI-induced pH, intestinal fluid volume, and mechanical action on drug dissolution in massive overdose models.

Summary: Whole-Bowel Irrigation

WBI can reduce absorption and augment removal of toxic agents in the gastrointestinal tract, although like many other modalities, its actual clinical benefit remains undefined and unproved. Until the clinical benefit and potential adverse effects are better understood, its use should be limited to circumstances for which there are no adequate alternatives.

Are There Other Gastrointestinal Decontamination Modalities to Consider?

What Other Binding Agents May Be Utilized?

In rare cases, oral or enteral administration of binding resins may be useful. Cholestyramine adsorbs organochlorine pesticides such as chlordecone (Kepone) and lindane, and may limit their absorption or enhance their fecal elimination,[40,61,81] but it is not known whether this is clinically beneficial. Elimination of digoxin and digitoxin are also enhanced by use of cholestyramine[31,70,129] or colestipol,[16,83] but the availability of the far more effective digoxin-specific antibodies and activated charcoal probably makes these other forms of therapy unnecessary. Investigators have studied the possible efficacy of sodium polystyrene sulfonate (Kayexalate) to prevent gastrointestinal absorption and to increase elimination of lithium. Both effects have been demonstrated in human volunteer and animal studies,[17,97,157] but several study design issues limit the applicability of these results to poisoned patients. The resin-to-lithium ratios in these studies suggest that the value after actual poisoning will ultimately prove to be quite limited.

Gastrointestinal administration of Prussian blue (potassium ferricyanoferrate) has been advocated to exchange potassium for thallium, thus enhancing fecal thallium excretion. This unproved therapy is discussed in Chapter 82. Fuller's earth adsorbs paraquat and diquat, but there appears to be no reason to advocate its use over activated charcoal. Oral starch can be utilized diagnostically and therapeutically after ingestion of concentrated iodine solutions.

When Should Endoscopic Removal Be Utilized?

Endoscopic removal of gastric contents is often considered but is rarely of practical value. Endoscopic removal would be logical when a substance remains in the stomach, is a significant threat to the patient, cannot be removed by another less invasive means, and can be safely removed in this manner. Unfortunately, on a practical basis, many of the agents likely to be considered for endoscopic removal do not meet these criteria. Drug masses due to iron, enteric aspirin, meprobamate, and others, despite their solid appearance on radiographs, cannot be effectively grasped through an endoscope. When life-threatening deterioration is likely or evident, it remains unresolved whether these masses are best left alone, treated with whole-bowel irrigation, broken up, or surgically removed. There are no clinically relevant data regarding the use of these methods or others of theoretical value (eg, lithotripsy). In body packers and body stuffers (Chap. 65) only the most durable drug packets may be safely grasped in this manner;[72] others may rupture during removal, limiting the usefulness of endoscopy. In addition, removing multiple objects with an endoscope requires repeated passage of the endoscope and thus increases potential complications. Nonetheless, in rare circumstances meeting the criteria given, endoscopic removal may be of value.

When Is Surgery Indicated?

Although controversial, there are a few indications for surgical gastrointestinal decontamination. In rare instances, ingestion of drug-containing packets may require surgical removal. Mechanical bowel obstruction or bowel ischemia due to drug packets must be treated surgically.[34,117,158] Rupture of packets and resultant toxicity may be medically manageable if the amount of drug is small, the agent is not potentially lethal (marijuana), or an effective antidote is available (opioids). However, if packets containing a large amount of cocaine rupture, immediate surgical removal of remaining drug is warranted following appropriate stabilization.[144]

Other agents causing toxicity that form large masses or adhere to the gastrointestinal tract wall and are not removed by gastric emptying, activated charcoal, and cathartic or whole-bowel irrigation may also (rarely) require surgical removal. Although many agents are described as causing bezoar formation (eg, aspirin, bromide, meprobamate), in nearly all cases gastric emptying and aggressive activated charcoal are sufficient treatment. Patients with massive iron ingestions with iron still evident on radiograph after gastric emptying attempts and whole-bowel irrigation should be considered for gastrotomy if serious systemic toxicity or evidence of active gastrointestinal bleeding occurs.[58,156] Surgical intervention may also be indicated for patients who have ingested strong acids or bases, not for decontamination purposes, but to treat resultant gastrointestinal necrosis and perforation.

Summary

Gastrointestinal decontamination is far from an exact science, and controversy and change are expected. The issues discussed should provide a framework on which to build and refine a clinical approach. As in all areas of medicine, it is expected that thoughtful analysis of further research, clinical experience, and the unique features of each case will suggest appropriate modifications of current thinking and lead to improved patient care.

References

1. Abdallah AH, Tye A: A comparison of the efficacy of emetic drugs and stomach lavage. Am J Dis Child 1967; 113:571–575.
2. Agocha A, Wang R, Longmore W, et al: Drug disintegra-

tion time and its value in gastric lavage (abstract). Vet Hum Toxicol 1986;28:493–494.

3. Al-Shareef AM, Buss DC, Allen EM, Routledge PA: The effects of charcoal and sorbitol (alone and in combination) on plasma theophylline concentration after a sustained release formulation. Hum Exp Toxicol 1990;9: 179–182.
4. Albertson TE, Derlet RW, Foulke GE, et al: Superiority of activated charcoal alone compared with ipecac and activated charcoal in the treatment of acute toxic ingestions. Ann Emerg Med 1989;18:56–59.
5. Allerton JP, Strom JA: Hypernatremia due to repeated doses of charcoal-sorbitol. Am J Kidney Dis 1991;17: 581–584.
6. Ambrose N, Johnson M, Burdon D, et al: A physiologic approach of polyethylene glycol and a balanced electrolyte solution as bowel preparation. Br J Surg 1983;70: 428–430.
7. Anderson AH: Experimental studies on the pharmacology of activated charcoal: I. Adsorption power of charcoal in aqueous solutions. Acta Pharmacol 1946;2:69–78.
8. Anderson AH: Experimental studies on the pharmacology of activated charcoal: II. The effect of pH on the adsorption by charcoal from aqueous solutions. Acta Pharmacol 1947;3:199–218.
9. Anderson AH: Experimental studies on the pharmacology of activated charcoal: III. Adsorption from gastric contents. Acta Pharmacol 1948; 4:275–284.
10. Anker AL, Smilkstein MJ: Fatality from respiratory failure due to sorbitol-induced intestinal gas formation. Vet Hum Toxicol 1993;35:334. Abstract.
11. Arnold FJ, Hodges JB, Barta PA, et al: Evaluation of the efficacy of lavage and induced emesis in treatment of salicylate poisoning. Pediatrics 1959;23:286–301.
12. Askenasi R, Abramowicz M, Jeanmart J, et al: Esophageal perforation: An unusual complication of gastric lavage. Ann Emerg Med 1984;13:146.
13. Auerbach P, Osterloh J, Braun O, et al: Efficacy of gastric emptying: Gastric lavage versus emesis induced with ipecac. Ann Emerg Med 1986;15:692–698.
14. Augenstein WL, Kulig KW, Rumack BH: Delayed rise in serum drug levels in overdose patients despite multiple dose charcoal and after charcoal stools. Vet Hum Toxicol 1987;29:491. Abstract.
15. Bauer H: Constipating effect of charcoal. Arch Exp Pathol Pharmacol 1928;134:185.
16. Bazzano G, Bazzano GS: Digitalis intoxication: Treatment with a new steroid-binding resin. JAMA 1972;220:828–830.
17. Belanger DR, Tierney MG, Dickinson G: Effect of sodium polystyrene sulfonate on lithium bioavailability. Ann Emerg Med 1992;21:1312–1315.
18. Benson B, VanAntwerp M, Hergott T: A fatality resulting from multiple dose activated charcoal therapy. Vet Hum Toxicol 1989;31:335. Abstract.
19. Berg M, Berlinger W, Goldberg M, et al: Acceleration of the body clearance of phenobarbital by oral activated charcoal. Clin Pharmacol Ther 1983;33:351–354.
20. Berlinger WG, Spector R, Goldberg MJ, et al: Enhancement of theophylline clearance by oral activated charcoal. Clin Pharmacol Ther 1983;33:351–354.
21. Bogazc K, Caldron P: Enteric coated aspirin bezoar: elevation of serum salicylate level by barium study. Am J Med 1981;83:783–786.
22. Bond GR, Requa RK, Krenzelok EP, et al: Influence of time until emesis on the efficacy of decontamination using acetaminophen as a marker in a pediatric population. Ann Emerg Med 1993;22:1403–1407.
23. Bonuccelli U, Piccini P, Del Dotto P, et al: Naloxone partly counteracts apomorphine side effects. Clin Neuropharmacol 1991;14:442–449.
24. Bosse GM, Barefoot JA, Pfeifer MP, Rodgers GC: Comparison of three methods of gut decontamination in tricyclic antidepressant overdose. J Emerg Med 1995; 13:203–209.
25. Boxer L, Anderson F, Rowe D: Comparison of ipecac-induced emesis with gastric ravage in the treatment of acute salicylate ingestion. J Pediatr 1969; 74:800–803.
26. Bradberry SM, Vale JA: Multiple-dose activated charcoal: A review of relevant clinical studies. J Toxicol Clin Toxicol 1995;33:407–416.
27. Brubacher JR, Levine B, Hoffman RS: Intestinal pseudo-obstruction (Ogilvie's syndrome) in theophylline overdose. Vet Hum Toxicol 1996;38:368–370.
28. Buckley N, Dawson AH, Howarth D, Whyte IM: Slow-release verapamil poisoning. Use of polyethylene glycol whole-bowel lavage and high-dose calcium. Med J Australia 1993;158:202–204.
29. Burkhart KK, Wuerz RC, Donovan JW: Whole-bowel irrigation as adjunctive treatment for sustained-release theophylline overdose. Ann Emerg Med 1992; 21:1316–1320.
30. Burton BT, Bayer MJ, Barron L, Aitchison JP: Comparison of activated charcoal and gastric lavage in the prevention of aspirin absorption. J Emerg Med 1984;1:411–416.
31. Cady WJ, Rehder TL, Campbell J: Use of cholestyramine resin in the treatment of digitoxin toxicity. Am J Hosp Pharm 1979;36:92–94.
32. Calvert W, Corby D, Herbertson L, Decker W: Orally administered activated charcoal: Acceptance by children. JAMA 1971;215:641.
33. Campbell J, Chyka P: Physiochemical characteristics of drugs and response to repeat dose activated charcoal. Am J Emerg Med 1992; 10:208–210.
34. Caruana DS, Weinbach B, Goerg D, et al: Cocaine-packet ingestion: Diagnosis, management, and natural history. Ann Intern Med 1984; 100:73–74.
35. Chafee-Bahamon C, Lacouture PG, Lovejoy FH Jr: Risk assessment of ipecac in the home. Pediatrics 1985;75: 1105–1109.
36. Chin L, Picchioni AL, Duplisse BR: Comparative antidotal effectiveness of activated charcoal, Arizona montmorillonite, and evaporated milk. J Pharm Sci 1969;58: 1353–1358.
37. Chin L, Picchioni A, Gillespie T: Saline cathartics and saline cathartics plus activated charcoal as antidotal treatments. Clin Toxicol 1981; 18:865–871.
38. Chyka PA: Multiple-dose activated charcoal and enhancement of systemic drug clearance: summary of studies in animals and human volunteers. J Toxicol Clin Toxicol 1995;33:399–405.
39. Chyka PA, Holley JE, Mandrell TD, Sugathan P: Correlation of drug pharmacokinetics and effectiveness of multiple-dose activated charcoal therapy. Ann Emerg Med 1995;25:356–362.

40. Cohn WJ, Boylan JJ, Blanke RV, et al: Treatment of chlordecone (Kepone) toxicity with cholestyramine. N Engl J Med 1978;298:243–248.
41. Comstock EG, Faulkner TP, Boisaubin E, et al: Studies on the efficacy of gastric emptying as practiced in a large metropolitan hospital. Clin Toxicol 1981;18:581–597.
42. Comstock EG, Boisaubin EV, Comstock BS, et al: Assessment of the efficacy of activated charcoal following gastric lavage in acute drug emergencies. Clin Toxicol 1982;19: 149–165.
43. Corby D, Decker W, Moran M, et al: Clinical comparison of pharmacologic emetics in children. Pediatrics 1968;42: 361–364.
44. Curtis RA, Barone J, Giacona N: Efficacy of ipecac and activated charcoal and cathartic: Prevention of salicylate absorption in a simulated overdose. Arch Intern Med 1984; 144:48–52.
45. Dammann KZ, Wiley SH, Tominack RL: Aspiration pneumonia following activated charcoal: A case report. Vet Hum Toxicol 1988;30:353. Abstract.
46. Davis R, Eichner J, Bleyer W, et al: Hypocalcemia, hyperphosphatemia, and dehydration following a single hypertonic phosphate enema. J Pediatr 1977; 90:484–485.
47. Docksteder LL, Lawrence RA, Bresnick BL: Home administration of activated charcoal: Feasibility and acceptance. Vet Hum Toxicol 1986;28:471. Abstract.
48. Dronen SC, Merigian KS, Hedges JR, et al: A comparison of blind nasotracheal and succinylcholine-assisted intubation in the poisoned patient. Ann Emerg Med 1987;16: 650–652.
49. Easom JM, Caraccio TR, Lovejoy FH Jr: Evaluation of activated charcoal and magnesium citrate in the prevention of aspirin absorption in humans. Clin Pharm 1982;1:154–156.
50. Eisen TF, Lacouture PG, Woolf A: The palatability of a new milk chocolate charcoal mixture in children. Vet Hum Toxicol 1988;30:351–352. Abstract.
51. Elliot CG, Colby TV, Kelly TM, et al: Charcoal lung: Bronchiolitis obliterans after aspiration of activated charcoal. Chest 1989; 96:672–674.
52. Everson G, Bertaccini E, O'Leary J: Use of whole bowel irrigation in an infant following iron overdose. Am J Emerg Med 1991;9:366–369.
53. Falkaw S, Mekalanos J: The enteric bacilli and Vibrio. In: Davis BD, Dulbecco R, Eisen HN, Ginsberg HS, eds: Microbiology, 4th ed. Philadelphia, Lippincott, 1990, 561–587.
54. Farley TA: Severe hypernatremic dehydration after use of an activated charcoal-sorbitol suspension. J Pediatr 1986; 109:719–722.
55. Fassler CA, Rodriguez DB, Badesch WJ, et al: Magnesium toxicity as a cause of hypotension and hypoventilation: Occurrence in patients with normal renal function. Arch Intern Med 1985; 145:1604–1606.
56. Fillippone G, Fish S, Lacouture P, et al: Reversible adsorption (desorption) of aspirin from activated charcoal. Arch Intern Med 1987;147:1390–1392.
57. Flores F, Battle WS: Intestinal obstruction secondary to activated charcoal. Contemp Surg 1987;30:57–59.
58. Foxford R, Goldfrank LR: Gastrotomy: A surgical approach to iron overdose. Ann Emerg Med 1985;14:1223–1226.
59. Galey FD, Lambert RJ, Busse M, et al: Therapeutic efficacy of superactive charcoal in rats exposed to oral lethal doses of T-2 toxin. Toxicon 1987; 25:493–499.
60. Galinsky RE, Levy G: Evaluation of activated charcoal-sodium sulfate combination for inhibition of acetaminophen absorption and repletion of inorganic sulfate. J Toxicol Clin Toxicol 1984;22:21–30.
61. Garrettson LK, Guzelian PS, Blanke RV: Subacute chlordane poisoning. J Toxicol Clin Toxicol 1984–85;22:565–571.
62. Gaudreault P, Friedman PA, Lovejoy FH Jr: Efficacy of activated charcoal and magnesium citrate in the treatment of oral paraquat intoxication. Ann Emerg Med 1985;14: 123–125.
63. Givens T, Holloway M, Wason S: Pulmonary aspiration of activated charcoal: A complication of its misuse in overdose management. Pediatr Emerg Care 1992; 8:137–140.
64. Goldberg M, Spector R, Park G, et al: The effect of sorbitol and activated charcoal on serum theophylline concentrations after slow release theophylline. Clin Pharmacol Ther 1987; 41:108–111.
65. Gomez BIF, Brent JA, Munoz DC, et al: Charcoal stercolith with intestinal perforation in a patient treated for amitriptyline ingestion. J Emerg Med 1994; 12:57–60
66. Goulboume KB, Cisek JE: Small-bowel obstruction secondary to activated charcoal and adhesions. Ann Emerg Med 1994;24:108–110.
67. Harris CR, Filandrinos D: Accidental administration of activated charcoal into the lung: Aspiration by proxy. Ann Emerg Med 1993;22:143–146.
68. Harsh HH: Aspiration of activated charcoal. N Engl J Med 1986; 414:318.
69. Haulman J, Robertson WO: Syrup of ipecac in 1993. A personal perspective. Drug Safety 1993;9:79–84. Editorial.
70. Henderson KP, Solomon CP: Use of cholestyramine in the treatment of digoxin intoxication. Arch Intern Med 1988; 148:745–746.
71. Hoffman RS, Chiang WK, Weisman RS, et al: Prospective evaluation of "crack vial" ingestion. Vet Hum Toxicol 1990;32:164–167.
72. Hoffman RS, Smilkstein MJ, Goldfrank LR: Whole bowel irrigation and the cocaine body packer. Am J Emerg Med 1990;8:523–527.
73. Hoffman RS, Chiang WK, Howland MA, et al: Theophylline desorption from activated charcoal caused by whole bowel irrigation solution. J Toxicol Clin Toxicol 1991;29:191.
74. James LP, Nichols MH, King WD: A comparison of cathartics in pediatric ingestions. Pediatrics 1995;96:235–238.
75. Jenis EH, Payne RJ, Goldbaum LR: Acute meprobamate poisoning: A fatal case following a lucid interval. JAMA 1969;207:361–365.
76. Johnson D, Eppler J, Giesbrecht E, et al: Effect of multiple-dose activated charcoal on the clearance of high-dose intravenous aspirin in a porcine model. Ann Emerg Med 1996;26:569–574.
77. Johnson WE: Massive phenobarbital ingestion with survival. JAMA 1967;202:1106–1109.
78. Jones J, Heiselman D, Dougherty J, et al: Cathartic induced magnesium toxicity during overdose management. Ann Emerg Med 1986; 15:1214–1218.
79. Kaczorowski JM, Wax PM: Five days of whole-bowel irri-

gation in a case of pediatric iron ingestion. Ann Emerg Med 1996;27:258–263.
80. Karkkainen S, Neuvonen P: Pharmacokinetics of amitriptyline influenced by oral charcoal and urine pH. Int J Clin Pharmacol Ther Toxicol 1986;24:326–332.
81. Kassner JT, Maher TJ, Hull KM, Woolf AD: Cholestyramine as an adsorbent in acute lindane poisoning: A murine model. Ann Emerg Med 1993;22:1392–1397.
82. Keller RE, Schwab RA, Krenzelok EP: Contribution of sorbitol combined with activated charcoal in prevention of salicylate absorption. Ann Emerg Med 1990; 19:654–656.
83. Kilgore TL, Lehmann CR: Treatment of digoxin intoxication with colestipol. South Med J 1982;75:1259–1260.
84. Kirshenbaum LA, Mathews SC, Sitar DS, Tenenbein M: Whole bowel irrigation versus activated charcoal in sorbitol for the ingestion of modified release pharmaceuticals. Clin Pharmacol Ther 1989;46:264–271.
85. Kirshenbaum LA, Mathews SC, Sitar DS, et al: Does multiple dose charcoal therapy enhance salicylate excretion? Arch Intern Med 1990;150:1281–1283.
86. Kirshenbaum LA, Sitar DS, Tenenbein M: Interaction between whole bowel irrigation solution and activated charcoal: Implications for the treatment of toxic ingestions. Ann Emerg Med 1990;19:1129–1132.
87. Klein-Schwartz W, Gorman RL, Oderda GM, et al: Ipecac use in the elderly: The unanswered question. Ann Emerg Med 1984; 13:1152–1154.
88. Komberg AE, Dolgin J: Pediatric ingestions: Charcoal alone versus ipecac and charcoal. Ann Emerg Med 1991; 20:648–651.
89. Krenzelok EP, Keller R, Stewart RD: Gastrointestinal transit times of cathartics combined with charcoal. Ann Emerg Med 1985;14:1152–1155.
90. Krenzelok E, Heller M: Effectiveness of commercially available aqueous activated charcoal products. Ann Emerg Med 1987;16:1340–1343.
91. Kulig KW, Bar-Or D, Cantrill SV, et al. Management of acutely poisoned patients without gastric emptying. Ann Emerg Med 1985;14:562–567.
92. Laass W: Therapy of acute oral poisonings by organic solvents: Treatment by activated charcoal in combination with laxatives. Arch Toxicol 1980;4(suppl):406–409.
93. Lambert RJ, Kindler BL, Schaeff DJ: The efficacy of superactivated charcoal in treating rats exposed to a lethal oral dose of potassium cyanide. Ann Emerg Med 1988;17: 595–598.
94. Lamminpaa A, Vilska J, Hoppu K: Medical charcoal for a child's poisoning at home: Availability and success of administration in Finland. Hum Exp Toxicol 1993; 12:29–32.
95. Larson JE, Swigert SA, Angle CR: Laxative phosphate poisoning: Pharmacokinetics of serum phosphate. Hum Toxicol 1986;5:45–49.
96. Lee DC, Roberts JR, Kelly JJ, Fishman SM: Whole-bowel irrigation as an adjunct in the treatment of radiopaque arsenic. Am J Emerg Med 1995;13:244–245. Letter.
97. Linakis JG, Eisenberg MS, Lacouture PG, et al: Multiple-dose sodium polystyrene sulfonate in lithium intoxication: An animal model. Pharmacol Toxicol 1992; 70:38–40.
98. Litovitz TL, Holm KC, Clancy C, et al: 1992 Annual Report of the American Association of Poison Control Centers Toxic Exposure Surveillance System. Am J Emerg Med 1993;11:494–555.
99. Litovitz TL, Clark LR, Soloway RA: 1993 Annual Report of the American Association of Poison Control Centers Toxic Exposure Surveillance System. Am J Emerg Med 1994;12: 546–584.
100. Litovitz TL, Felberg L, Soloway RA, et al: 1994 Annual Report of the American Association of Poison Control Centers Toxic Exposure Surveillance System. Am J Emerg Med 1995;13:551–597.
101. Litovitz TL, Felberg L, White S, Klein-Schwartz W: 1995 Annual Report of the American Association of Poison Control Centers Toxic Exposure Surveillance System. Am J Emerg Med 1996;14:487–537.
102. Litovitz TL, Smilkstein MJ, Felberg L, et al: 1996 Annual Report of the American Association of Poison Control Centers Toxic Exposure Surveillance System. Am J Emerg Med 1997;15:447–500.
103. Longdon P, Henderson A: Intestinal pseudoobstruction following the use of enteral charcoal and sorbitol with mechanical ventilation with papaveretum sedation for theophylline poisoning. Drug Safety 1992;7:74–77.
104. MacLean W: A comparison of ipecac syrup and apomorphine in the immediate treatment of ingestion of poisons. J Pediatr 1973;82:121–124.
105. Makosiev F, Hoffman RS, Howland MA: Cocaine adsorption to activated charcoal: The effects of pH. Vet Hum Toxicol 1990;32:350. Abstract.
106. Makosiev FJ, Hoffman RS, Howland MA, Goldfrank LR: An in vitro evaluation of cocaine hydrochloride adsorption by activated charcoal and desorption upon addition of polyethylene glycol electrolyte lavage solution. J Toxicol Clin Toxicol 1993;31:381–395.
107. Mafiani PJ, Poole N: Gastrointestinal tract perforation with charcoal peritoneum complicating orogastric intubation and lavage. Ann Emerg Med 1993;22:606–609.
108. Martin R, Lisehora G, Braxton M, et al: Fatal poisoning from sodium phosphate enema: A case report and experimental study. JAMA 1987; 257:2190–2192.
109. Mayer AL, Sitar DS, Tenenbein M: Multiple dose charcoal and whole-bowel irrigation do not increase clearance of absorbed salicylate. Arch Intern Med 1992;152:393–396.
110. McNamara R, Aaron C, Gemborys M, Davidheiser S: Efficacy of charcoal versus ipecac in reducing serum acetaminophen in a simulated overdose. Ann Emerg Med 1988; 17:243–246.
111. Menzies DG, Busuttel A, Prescott LF: Fatal pulmonary aspiration of oral activated charcoal. Br Med J 1988;297: 459–466.
112. Merigian KS, Woodard Jr NM, Hedges JR, et al: Prospective evaluation of gastric emptying in the self poisoned patient. Am J Emerg Med 1990;8:479–483.
113. Minton NA: Volunteer models for predicting antiemetic activity of 5-HT3-receptor antagonists. Br J Clin Pharmacol 1994;37:525–530.
114. Mofenson H, Caraccio T: Magnesium intoxication in a neonate from oral magnesium hydroxide laxative. J Toxicol Clin Toxicol 1991;29:215–222.
115. Mordes JP, Wacker WEC: Excess magnesium. Pharm Rev 1978;239:273–300.

116. Murphy DG, Gerace RV, Peterson RG: The use of whole bowel irrigation in acute lead ingestion. Vet Hum Toxicol 1991;33:353. Abstract.
117. Nalbandian H, Sheth N, Dietrich R, et al: Intestinal ischemia caused by cocaine ingestion: Report of two cases. Surgery 1985;97:374–376.
118. Neuvonen PJ: Clinical pharmacokinetics of oral activated charcoal in acute intoxications. Clin Pharmacokinet 1982;7: 465–489.
119. Neuvonen PJ, Vartiainen M, Tokola O: Comparison of activated charcoal and ipecac syrup in prevention of drug absorption. Eur J Clin Pharmacol 1983;24:557–562.
120. Neuvonen PJ, Olkkola KT: Activated charcoal and syrup of ipecac in prevention of cimetidine and pindolol absorption in man after administration of metoclopramide as an antiemetic agent. J Toxicol Clin Toxicol 1984;22:103–114.
121. Neuvonen P, Oikkola K, Alanen T: Effect of ethanol and pH on the adsorption of drugs to activated charcoal: Studies in vitro and in man. Acta Pharmacol Toxicol 1984;54: 1–7.
122. Neuvonen PJ, Olkkola KT: Effect of purgatives on antidotal efficacy of oral activated charcoal. Hum Toxicol 1986;5: 255–263.
123. Neuvonen PJ, Olkkola KT: Oral activated charcoal in the treatment of intoxications: Role of single and repeated doses. Med Toxicol 1988;3:33–58.
124. Ohning B, Reed M, Blumer J: Continuous nasogastric administration of activated charcoal for the treatment of theophylline intoxication. Pediatr Pharmacol 1986;5: 241–245.
125. Olkkola KT, Neuvonen PJ: Do gastric contents modify antidotal efficacy of oral activated charcoal? Br J Clin Pharmacol 1984; 18:663–669.
126. Olkkola KT: Effect of charcoal-drug ratio on antidotal efficacy of oral activated charcoal in man. Br J Clin Pharmacol 1985;19:767–773.
127. Olsen KM, Ma FH, Ackerman BH, Stull RE: Low-volume whole bowel irrigation and salicylate absorption: A comparison with ipecac-charcoal. Pharmacotherapy 1993;13: 229–232.
128. Picchioni A, Chin L, Gillespie T: Evaluation of activated charcoal-sorbitol suspension as an antidote. Clin Toxicol 1982; 19:435–444.
129. Pieroni RE, Fisher JG: Use of cholestyramine resin in digitoxin toxicity. JAMA 1981;245:1939–1940.
130. Poisindex editorial staff: Activated charcoal/treatment. In: Rumack BH, ed: Poisindex Information System, Vol. 91. Denver, Micromedex, edition expires 2/28/97.
131. Pollack MM, Dunbar BS, Holbrook PR, et al: Aspiration of activated charcoal and gastric contents. Ann Emerg Med 1981;10:528–529.
132. Pond SM, Lewis-Driver DJ, Williams G, et al: Gastric emptying in acute overdose: a prospective randomised controlled trial. Med J Austral 1995;163:345–349.
133. Ray MJ, Padin DR, Condie JD, Halls JM: Charcoal bezoar: Small bowel obstruction secondary to amitriptyline overdose therapy. Dig Dis Sci 1988; 33:106–107.
134. Roberge RJ, Martin TG: Whole bowel irrigation in an acute oral lead intoxication. Am J Emerg Med 1992; 10:577–583.
135. Robertson WO: Syrup of ipecac associated fatality: A case report. Vet Hum Toxicol 1979;21:87–89.
136. Rosenberg PJ, Livingstone DJ, McLellan BA: Effect of whole-bowel irrigation on the antidotal efficacy of activated charcoal. Ann Emerg Med 1988;17:681–683
137. Saetta JP, Quinton DN: Residual gastric content after gastric lavage and ipecacuanha induced emesis in self poisoned patients: An endoscopic study. J R Soc Med 1991;84:35–38.
138. Saetta JP, March S, Gaunt ME, Quinton DN: Gastric emptying procedures in the self poisoned patient: Are we forcing gastric content beyond the pylorus? J R Soc Med 1991;84:274–277.
139. Silberman H, Davis SM, Lee A: Activated charcoal aspiration. NC Med J 1990;51:79–80.
140. Sketris IS, Mowry JB, Czajka PA, et al: Saline catharsis: Effect on aspirin bioavailability in combination with activated charcoal. J Clin Pharmacol 1982;22:59–64.
141. Smilkstein MJ, Smolinske SC, Kulig KW, et al: Severe hypermagnesemia due to multiple dose cathartic therapy. West J Med 1987;148:208–211.
142. Smilkstein MJ, Steedle D, Kulig KW, et al: Magnesium levels after magnesium-containing cathartics. J Toxicol Clin Toxicol 1988;26:51–65.
143. Smith SW, Ling LJ, Halstenson CE: Whole bowel irrigation as a treatment for acute lithium overdose. Ann Emerg Med 1991;20:536–539.
144. Suarez CA, Arango A, Lester JL: Cocaine-condom ingestion: Surgical treatment. JAMA 1977;238:1391–1392.
145. Sue YJ, Woolf A, Shannon M: Efficacy of magnesium citrate cathartic in pediatric toxic ingestions. Ann Emerg Med 1994;24:709–712.
146. Swanson-Brearman B, Dean BS, Krenzelok EP: Failure of whole bowel irrigation to decontaminate the GI tract following massive jequirity bean ingestion. Vet Hum Toxicol 1992;34:352. Abstract.
147. Tandberg D, Liechty EJ, Fishbein D: Mallory–Weiss syndrome: An unusual complication of ipecac-induced emesis. Ann Emerg Med 1981;10: 521–523.
148. Tandberg D, Diven BG, McLeod JW: Ipecac-induced emesis versus gastric lavage: A controlled study in normal adults. Am J Emerg Med 1986; 4:205–209.
149. Tarling MM, Toner CC, Withington PS, et al: A model of gastric emptying using paracetamol absorption in intensive care patients. Intens Care Med 1997;23:256–260.
150. Tenenbein M: Whole bowel irrigation for toxic ingestions. J Toxicol Clin Toxicol 1985;23:177–184.
151. Tenenbein M: Whole bowel irrigation in iron poisoning. J Pediatr 1987; 111:142–145.
152. Tenenbein M, Cohen S, Sitar DS: Whole bowel irrigation as a decontamination procedure after acute drug overdose. Arch Intern Med 1987; 147:905–907.
153. Tenenbein M, Cohen S, Sitar DS: Efficacy of ipecac induced emesis, orogastric lavage, and activated charcoal for acute drug overdose. Ann Emerg Med 1987;16: 838–841.
154. Tenenbein M: Whole bowel irrigation as gastrointestinal decontamination procedure after acute poisoning. Med Toxicol 1988;3:77–84.

155. Tenenbein M: Multiple doses of activated charcoal: Time for reappraisal? Ann Emerg Med 1991;20:529–531.
156. Tenenbein M, Wiseman N, Yatscoff RW: Gastrotomy and whole bowel irrigation in iron poisoning. Pediatr Emerg Care 1991;7:286–288.
157. Tomaszewski C, Musso C, Pearson JR, et al: Lithium absorption prevented by sodium polystyrene sulfonate in volunteers. Ann Emerg Med 1992;21:1308–1311.
158. Utecht MJ, Stone AF, McCarron MM: Heroin body packers. J Emerg Med 1993;11:33–40.
159. Van de Graaf W, Thompson WL, Sunshine I, et al: Adsorbent and cathartic inhibition of enteral drug absorption. J Pharmacol Exp Ther 1982;221:656–663.
160. Vance MV, Selden BS, Clark RF: Optimal patient position for transport and initial management of toxic ingestions. Ann Emerg Med 1992;21:243–246.
161. Wald P, Stern J, Weiner B, et al: Esophageal tear following forceful removal of an impacted oral-gastric lavage tube. Ann Emerg Med 1986;15:80–82.
162. Watson WA, Cremes KF, Chapman JA: Gastrointestinal obstruction associated with multiple dose activated charcoal. J Emerg Med 1986;4:401–407.
163. Wolowodiuk OJ, McMicken DB, O'Brien P: Pneumomediastinum and retropneumoperitoneum: An unusual complication of syrup of ipecac-induced emesis. Ann Emerg Med 1984;13:1148–1150.

CHAPTER 5

Principles and Techniques Applied to Enhance Elimination of Toxins

David S. Goldfarb and Susan M. Pond

Once techniques to inhibit absorption of a drug or toxin have been initiated, enhancing its elimination from the body is a logical next step in the treatment of poisoned patients. The methods that can be used are listed in Table 5–1. However, the use of any method to enhance elimination is tempered by the knowledge that, although many patients with overdoses are critically ill, current methods of intensive supportive care keep the overall mortality rate low in those who reach the hospital alive.[22,30] Moreover, since the elimination techniques are not without adverse effects and complications,[11,31,55] they are indicated in only a relatively small number of patients.[22,56] Although these figures are undoubtedly underestimates of the actual number of times the techniques were used, the percentages in which they were used in a cohort of 2 million patients in 1995 were low: alkalinization of the urine with or without diuresis, 0.35%; hemodialysis, 0.04%; hemoperfusion, 0.0003%.[30] Peritoneal dialysis has been utilized in less than half as many cases as hemoperfusion.

There have been very few prospective, randomized, controlled clinical trials to determine whether or not groups of patients benefit from enhanced elimination of various toxins. It is unlikely that these sorts of studies will be performed, given the relative scarcity of appropriate cases and the many variables that would have to be controlled. At present, we still must rely on our knowledge of the principles of the methods to identify the individual patients in whom enhanced elimination is indicated. Isolated case reports in which the kinetics are studied before, during, and after enhanced elimination are also very useful in establishing the efficacy of a method.

It should be noted that although methods to enhance elimination of toxins may be extremely effective, attention should never be diverted from the provision of comprehensive supportive care or maintenance of the normal routes of elimination while the procedure is performed. For example, if the patient becomes hypotensive during hemodialysis or hemoperfusion, reduced blood flow to the liver and kidneys would impair endogenous elimination pathways.

What Are the Clinical Indications to Enhance Elimination of a Toxin?

Enhanced elimination may be indicated in patients:

- Who fail to respond adequately to full supportive care. Such patients may have intractable hypotension, heart failure, seizures, metabolic acidosis or dysrhythmias.
- In whom the normal route of elimination of the toxin is impaired. Such patients may have renal or hepatic dysfunction, either preexisting or caused by the overdose. For example, a patient with chronic renal insufficiency associated with long-term lithium use, is more likely to develop toxic levels of the drug, and to require hemodialysis as therapy.
- In whom the amount of toxin absorbed or its concentration in blood or serum indicates that serious mor-

TABLE 5–1. METHODS OF ENHANCING ELIMINATION OF TOXIC COMPOUNDS

Diuresis
Manipulation of pH
Multiple doses of activated charcoal, cholestyramine, colestipol, kayexalate
Peritoneal dialysis
Hemodialysis
Sorbent hemoperfusion
Hemofiltration
Exchange transfusion
Plasmapheresis
Cerebrospinal fluid drainage and replacement
Toxin-specific antibody fragments
Prussian blue
Chelation
Nasogastric suction
Whole-bowel irrigation

bidity or mortality is likely. Such patients may not appear acutely ill on presentation. Toxins in this group include arsenic trioxide, ethylene glycol, lithium, mercuric chloride, methanol, paraquat, salicylate, and theophylline.

- Who have concurrent disease or are in an age group (very young or old) associated with increased risk of morbidity or mortality from the overdose. Such patients are intolerant of prolonged coma, immobility, and hemodynamic instability. An example is a patient with severe underlying respiratory disease and chronic theophylline intoxication.
- In whom the information available about the drug suggests that the various modalities of treatment will actually increase the toxin's removal.

Ideally, studies will have suggested an improvement in outcome in treated patients as compared to patients not treated with extracorporeal removal, but these data are rarely available.

Can the Toxin Be Removed?

Whether a toxin can be removed is determined both by the kinetics of the compound and by the mechanism of removal involved in each technique. Kinetic parameters after an overdose may differ from those after therapeutic or experimental doses.[49] For instance, carrier or enzyme-mediated elimination processes or plasma protein and tissue binding sites may be saturable, and thereby overwhelmed by higher levels of the drug or toxin in question. Thus, estimates of the expected endogenous rate of elimination of a substance in the setting of an overdose should be made, where possible, from knowledge of kinetics obtained in that setting, not after therapeutic doses.

Effective removal by any of the procedures listed in Table 5–1 is limited by a high endogenous clearance and large volume of distribution. The volume of distribution (Vd) relates the concentration of the toxin in the blood or serum to the total body burden. The larger the Vd, the less the compound is available to the blood compartment for elimination. For example, a substantial fraction of a dose of ethanol, which has a small volume of distribution (Vd = 0.6 L/kg body weight), is removed by hemodialysis, in contrast to an insignificant fraction of digoxin, with a large volume of distribution (Vd = 5 to 12 L/kg body weight). Lipid-soluble drugs and toxins and those that are highly protein bound have large volumes of distribution, which can exceed total body water, or total body weight. In addition to the alcohols, substances with low Vd include acetaminophen, phenobarbital, lithium, salicylates, and theophylline. Conversely those with a high Vd (up to 40 L/kg body weight), which would not be removed substantially by hemodialysis, include many beta-adrenergic antagonists (with the possible exception of atenolol[50]), diazepam, organophosphates, phenothiazines, quinidine, and the cyclic antidepressants.

When assessing the efficacy of any technique of enhanced elimination, a generally accepted principle is that the intervention is worthwhile only if the total body clearance of a toxin is increased by at least 30%.[11] This substantial increase is easier to achieve when the compound has a low endogenous clearance. Examples of substances with low endogenous clearance (< 4 mL/min per kg) include the alcohols, atenolol, sotalol, lithium, paraquat, phenytoin, salicylate, and theophylline. Drugs with high endogenous clearances include many beta-adrenergic antagonists, lidocaine, opioids, nicotine, and tricyclic antidepressants.

The efficacy of any technique of elimination can also be assessed by comparing the blood or plasma concentrations of the substance at the beginning and at the end of the procedure.[52] For example, a compound like theophylline, with one-compartment kinetics, is essentially limited to the extracellular space. The difference between the theophylline concentration before the procedure, minus the concentration at the end of the procedure, divided by the concentration at the beginning, is the fraction of the body burden of the compound that has been eliminated.

If the toxin, like lithium, distributes in part to the intracellular compartment as well as the extracellular compartment, an equilibrium is established for the compound between the intracellular and extracellular compartments. The latter includes the blood from which elimination occurs. An increase in the elimination rate from the extracellular compartment, such as by hemodialysis, disturbs this equilibrium. If the rate of redistribution of the compound from the intracellular compartment into the now-dialyzed extracellular compartment is slower than the rate of clearance across the dialysis membrane, the dialysis clearance, or total-body clearance rate can be limited. Thus, although plasma or blood concentrations may fall precipitously during the procedure, the total-body burden of the substance may not be affected significantly. This is demonstrated most clearly if the blood concentrations are monitored after discontinuation of the procedure and demonstrate re-

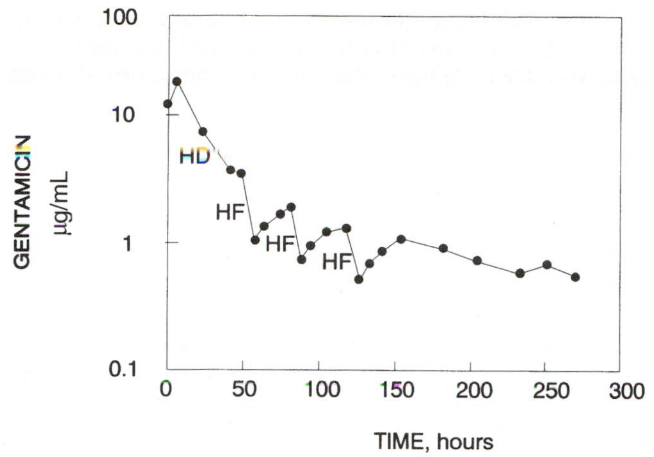

Figure 5–1. Serum concentrations of gentamicin before, during, and after hemodialysis (HD) and hemofiltration (HF). Note the rebound in concentrations after HF as the drug redistributes slowly from the peripheral tissues.

bounding serum levels, indicating postdialysis redistribution (Fig. 5–1).

Similarly, what appears to be efficient removal by hemodialysis or hemoperfusion may not indicate efficient removal of the total-body burden of a drug or toxin. Extraction ratios (discussed later) of 100% indicate that all of the substance passing through a hemoperfusion cartridge is removed. Yet if the compound fails to redistribute from intra- to extracellular compartment during the procedure, or is largely in the intracellular compartment to begin with, the total-body clearance may be quite low. An example is a 60-kg patient who ingests 100 tablets of 25 mg of a tricyclic antidepressant, such as amitriptyline.[18] Assuming the drug is fully absorbed, the 2500 mg distributes in an apparent volume of 40 L/kg body weight, to achieve a plasma level of 1000 ng/mL, a potentially toxic level. If charcoal hemoperfusion is performed with a blood flow rate of 350 mL/min (plasma flow rate of 200 mL/min), and the extraction ratio is 100%, the clearance of drug will be 200 mL/min or 200 μg/min. In 4 hours (240 minutes) of treatment, 48 mg (48,000 μg), or less than 2% of the drug ingested, will be removed. This will have no effect on prognosis.

When assessing efficacy, the clinical response must be considered in addition to the evidence of enhanced elimination. In some instances, improvement has been observed that would not be predicted from data on the kinetics of the parent compound. In the case of tricyclic antidepressants[53] unexpected improvement during hemoperfusion could have been fortuitous because the toxicity is manifested and ameliorates rapidly during the initial distribution phase. Alternatively, small amounts of the drug and active metabolites could have been removed from a shallow "toxic effect" compartment. This theory has been put forward to explain the response of individual patients overdosed with the neuroleptic chlorprothixene[26] and a combination of diltiazem and metoprolol.[1] Such effects can lead to transient improvements that are not sustained as drug redistributes from one pool to another, leading to recrudesence of symptoms. Much of the relevant literature fails to provide long-term follow-up to demonstrate prolongation of benefits after extracorporeal therapy ends. Finally, beginning the procedure during the initial distribution phase may increase the fraction of body burden that can be removed.

Conversely, in two studies, despite evidence of enhanced elimination of phenobarbital[43] or carbamazepine[54] produced by repeated oral administration of activated charcoal, there was no difference in the course of intoxication between patients so treated and overdosed, untreated controls. This is another limitation of the literature in the field: demonstration of removal of toxin is a poor surrogate for clinical benefit.

Techniques Available to Enhance Removal of Toxins

Though controversies remain about the efficacy of, or need for, removal for many toxins, a consensus regarding the indications for a number of procedures has been developed. This has led to consistent application of several techniques for some toxic exposures that occur relatively frequently. The techniques to enhance elimination most commonly applied over the last decade have been alkalinization of the urine for salicylate; hemodialysis for methanol, ethylene glycol, lithium, and salicylate; and hemoperfusion for theophylline.[22]

Manipulation of Urinary pH and Forced Diuresis

Many toxic compounds are weak acids or bases that are ionized in aqueous solution to an extent that depends on the pKa of the compound and the pH of the solution. Cell membranes are relatively impermeable to ionized (polar) molecules, whereas nonionized (nonpolar) forms can cross more easily. As compounds pass through the kidney, they may be filtered, secreted, and reabsorbed. If the urinary pH is manipulated to favor the ionized form, the drug is trapped in tubular fluid and not reabsorbed into the bloodstream; hence the rate and extent of its elimination are increased. To make manipulation of urinary pH worthwhile, the renal excretion of the compound must be sufficient to make increased clearance a major route of elimination.

Producing diuresis by volume expansion with sodium-containing solutions, such as normal saline or lactated Ringer's solution, may increase renal clearance. This would theoretically be most true for substances in which glomerular filtration is an important determinant of excretion, and particularly in instances where extracellular fluid volume is contracted. The significant risk of this therapy, however, is volume overload, manifested by pulmonary and cerebral edema. Administration of diuretics along with saline may diminish the risk, but complicates the therapy and increases the risk of metabolic alkalosis and hypokalemia. In addition, well-documented sources of morbidity are the urinary and intravascular catheters used to assess fluid balance. Most important, the unproven efficacy of forced diuresis in the management of any overdose has led most centers to abandon its use.

Acidification of the urine by systemic administration of HCl or NH_4Cl to enhance elimination of weak bases, such as phencyclidine or amphetamines, is no longer considered useful. The technique has been abandoned because it does not enhance removal of toxic compounds significantly and is complicated by systemic metabolic acidosis.

Alkalinization of the urine to enhance elimination of weak acids has a limited role for compounds such as salicylates,[38] phenobarbital,[29] chlorpropamide, formate, and the herbicide 2,4-dichlorophenoxyacetic acid [2,4-D].[45] These weak acids are ionized at alkaline urine pH and tubular reabsorption is thereby greatly reduced. Alkalinization is achieved by the intravenous administration of sodium bicarbonate, 1 to 2 mEq/kg every 3 to 4 hours. The goal is to increase urinary pH to 7 to 8.

This degree of alkalinization may be difficult, if not impossible, if metabolic acidosis and acidemia are present, as often is the case with salicylate poisoning. Administered sodium bicarbonate will be consumed by titration of plasma protons before appearing in the urine. On the other hand, salicylate poisoning often causes respiratory alkalosis as well. In that case, where PCO_2 is low, raising serum bicarbonate may lead to profound, life-threatening alkalemia. Finally, the risk of volume overload with sodium bicarbonate administration is the same as with the administration of NaCl. Hypernatremia after administration of hypertonic sodium bicarbonate may also ensue. Nonetheless, in one study, the renal clearance of salicylate increased fourfold as urine pH increased from 6.5 to 7.5 with alkalinization.[38] Increasing urine pH by administering carbonic anhydrase inhibitors such as acetazolamide is not recommended. Though elimination of the drug may be increased, metabolic acidosis will ensue unless ample sodium bicarbonate is administered as well. In the case of salicylates, acidemia may cause increased distribution of drug into the central nervous system. However it is achieved, bicarbonaturia is accompanied by urinary potassium losses; hypokalemia can be profound. The role of urinary alkalinization in the management of salicylate poisoning is further discussed in Chapter 32.

Alkalinization with or without diuresis is also used to maintain renal elimination of methotrexate in patients given high-dose folinic acid rescue therapy.[9] Extracellular fluid volume expansion with 0.9% NaCl and $NaHCO_3$ administration also protects the kidneys from the toxic effects of myoglobinuria in patients with extensive rhabdomyolysis.

Peritoneal Dialysis

Peritoneal dialysis can theoretically be performed to enhance the elimination of the few water-soluble, low-molecular-weight, poorly protein-bound compounds with a low volume of distribution.[20] Examples are the alcohols, lithium, salicylate, and theophylline.

Clearance of compounds in the aqueous dialysate is related to dialysate flow rate, the surface area of the peritoneum, and the molecular weight (MW) of the compound. Highest clearances are achieved for molecules with MW < 500 Daltons. The efficacy of peritoneal dialysis is markedly decreased when the patient is hypotensive.

Although peritoneal dialysis is a relatively simple method to enhance drug elimination, it is too slow to be useful. Peritoneal dialysis is therefore never the method of choice unless hemodialysis and hemoperfusion are unavailable.

Hemodialysis

During conventional hemodialysis, blood traverses a semipermeable membrane, bathed by a dialysis solution, or dialysate. Drugs and toxins diffuse across the membrane from blood into the dialysate along the concentration gradient (Fig. 5–2). In patients requiring acute dialysis, hemodialysis is usually performed by pumping blood from one lumen of a double-lumen catheter in the femoral or the subclavian vein. Blood is returned to the venous circulation through the second lumen. The appropriate catheter size is determined by the size of the patient. The blood lines and artificial kidney should be primed with an appropriate volume of fluid to reduce or avoid hypotension when the procedure is started. Full anticoagulation with heparin is usually required, although periodic flushes of the dialysis membrane with "heparinized saline" exposes the patient to low doses of heparin and little risk of systemic anticoagulation. Regional anticoagulation of the dialysis circuit with citrate or protamine is possible if heparin is completely contraindicated, although these agents complicate the procedure. In poisoned patients, hemodialysis is usually performed for 4 to 8 hours.

The characteristics of compounds that make them amenable to hemodialysis are listed in Table 5–2. These requirements greatly reduce the number of substances that can be expected to be cleared by dialysis. During hemodialysis, clearance of a drug or toxin (Cl_H) can be calculated according to

$$Cl_H = [Q_{in}(C_{in} - C_{out})]/C_{in}$$

where Q_{in} is the blood flow entering the dialyzer, C_{in} is the concentration of the drug or toxin in blood entering the system, and C_{out} is the concentration in blood leaving the system. The extraction ratio is a measure of the percentage of substance passing through the artificial kidney, or charcoal hemoperfusion cartridge. This can be calculated as:

$$ER = \frac{C_{in} - C_{out}}{C_{in}} \times 100$$

Hemodialysis is preferred to hemoperfusion to remove compounds such as bromide, chloral hydrate, trichloroethanol, ethanol, methanol and ethylene glycol, lithium, and salicylate. In addition to removing these compounds, hemodialysis can correct abnormalities such as metabolic acidosis or alkalosis, hyperkalemia, and fluid overload.

Several recent technological advances have allowed patients to tolerate dialysis with much less hemodynamic instability than in the past. These changes include

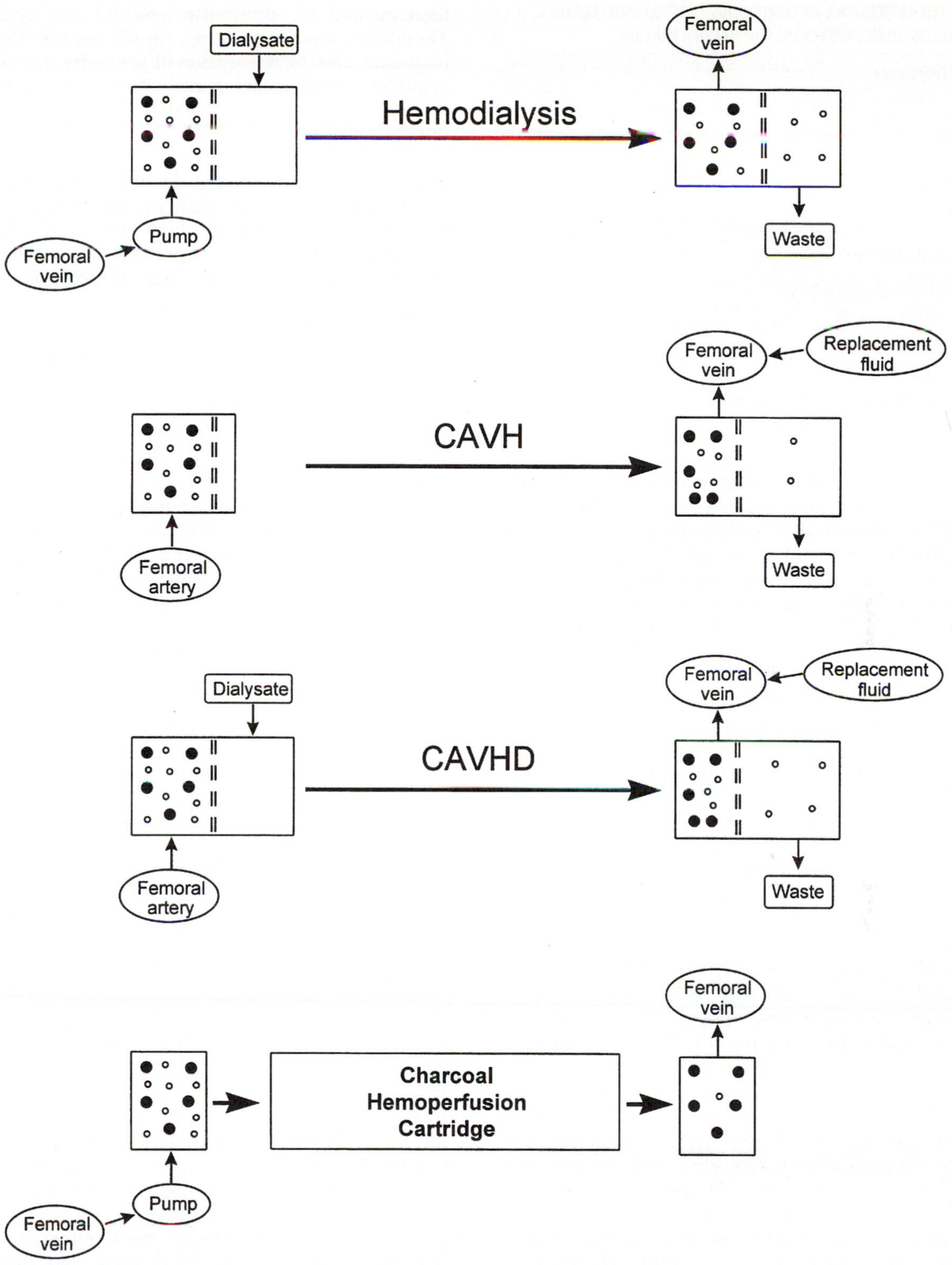

Figure 5–2. The comparative efficacy of hemodialysis, CAVH, CAVHD and charcoal hemoperfusion. Filled circles are high-molecular-weight substances such as plasma proteins; open circles are low-molecular-weight, diffusible solutes such as urea or methanol. In dialysis, solute moves across a semipermeable membrane (dashed lines) from a solution in which it is present in a high concentration (blood) to one in which it is at a low concentration (dialysate). In hemofiltration, plasma moves across a similar membrane in response to hydrostatic pressures. CAVH(D) is continuous arterio-venous hemofiltration without or with dialysis. CVVHD, continuous venovenous hemofiltration with dialysis, not pictured, is similar to CAVHD, but as it does not have arterial pressure to drive it, requires a blood pump. Charcoal hemoperfusion requires movement of blood through a sorbent-containing cartridge.

TABLE 5–2. CHARACTERISTICS OF COMPOUNDS THAT ALLOW CLEARANCE BY HEMODIALYSIS, HEMOPERFUSION, AND HEMOFILTRATION

For All Three Techniques
Low volume of distribution (<1 L/kg)
Single-compartment kinetics
Low endogenous clearance (<4 mL/min per kg)
For Hemodialysis
MW < 500 Daltons
Water soluble
Not bound to plasma proteins
For Activated Charcoal Hemoperfusion
Adsorption by activated charcoal
Plasma protein binding is not a contraindication
For Hemofiltration
MW <10,000 or 40,000 Daltons, depending on filter used

using dialysate in which the source of base is HCO_3 rather than acetate; computerized machines that allow fine control of ultrafiltration rates to limit volume losses; and the ability to manipulate, or "model" dialysate sodium concentrations. These innovations also allow treatment to be delivered in more instances than would have been previously possible. As a result, there are few patients in whom hemodialysis should not at least be instituted, if indicated. Hypotension may occur in the critically ill, particularly if the tubing dead space is not primed with blood or colloid. The procedure may be difficult or impossible to perform in patients with very low blood pressure or low cardiac output despite appropriate fluid and vasopressor therapy.

These innovations have permitted increases in dialysance. Better hemodynamic stability and better dual-lumen catheters allow use of higher blood flows up to 400 mL/min, while better ultrafiltration control allows the use of more permeable high-flux synthetic dialysis membranes with larger surface areas. Clearance rates reported in the literature of the 1970s and 1980s may significantly underestimate currently achievable clearance rates because of such developments. Nonetheless, a sound pharmacologic basis for the efficacy of dialysis must still be present; no amount of increased clearance will eliminate a drug or toxin with a large volume of distribution or significant tissue binding.

Complications of conventional hemodialysis are bleeding or thrombosis at the site used for vascular access; bleeding due to systemic anticoagulation with heparin; rare air embolus via central venous lines; and nosocomial infections. In addition, hemodialysis will increase the elimination of some drugs administered therapeutically, such as folic acid and other water soluble vitamins, ethanol, and antibiotics. Doses of these drugs therefore need to be increased during dialysis (see Antidote in Depth: Ethanol). Use of angiotensin-converting enzyme inhibitors is associated with angioedema when polyacrylonitrile (PAN) membranes are used for dialysis.[8]

The use of the REDY hemodialysis system in the management of poisonings should be discouraged. These units require no water supply because they regenerate dialysate by adsorption of solute by activated charcoal and exchange resins, and generate HCO_3 from urea by urease. This machine is still often used as a portable unit in some hospitals for the management of renal failure. However, dialysis clearance rates are too low for management of poisoning. Though the activated charcoal may be specifically useful in adsorbing theophylline, the absence of sufficiently high urea concentrations in most poisoned patients will prevent bicarbonate regeneration from urea and lead to metabolic acidosis.[5]

Charcoal Hemoperfusion

In general, if a compound is adsorbed by activated charcoal, charcoal hemoperfusion clearance will exceed that of hemodialysis. During hemoperfusion, blood is pumped much like in dialysis but through a cartridge containing a sorbent, either activated charcoal or carbon, both of which have a very large surface area (see Fig. 5–2). The sorbent is coated with a very thin layer of cellulose (Adsorba, made by Gambro), cellulose nitrate (Hemokart, made by Erika) or heparin-hydrogel (Biocompatible Hemoperfusion Systems, made by Clark), which prevents direct contact between blood and sorbent and helps prevent charcoal embolization. There may be a further theoretical advantage to the heparin-hydrogel coating, to diminish platelet aggregation. The adsorptive capacity of the cartridge is reduced with use because of deposition of cellular debris and blood proteins. The cartridge is therefore usually changed as often as every 2 to 4 hours.

As with hemodialysis, patients must be anticoagulated with heparin, and regional heparinization of the cartridge is possible if full anticoagulation is undesirable. The technique can be used in adults[13,41,57] or children.[10,35,40] Hemoperfusion is usually performed for 4 to 6 hours at flow rates of 250 to 400 mL/min.

The characteristics of compounds that make them amenable to hemoperfusion (see Table 5–2) differ from those for hemodialysis in the important respect that hemoperfusion is not limited by plasma protein binding. This is exemplified in a report in which hemoperfusion but not hemodialysis increased the elimination of the avidly protein-bound oral hypoglycemic agent chlorpropamide.[32] Some substances are poorly adsorbed by activated charcoal, including the alcohols, lithium, and many metals (see Antidote in Depth: Activated Charcoal), making hemoperfusion inappropriate in their management. Hemoperfusion clearance is calculated in a manner similar to that for hemodialysis. Hemoperfusion is the preferred method to enhance the elimination of carbamazepine, phenobarbital, phenytoin, and theophylline (Table 5–3). Hemodialysis and hemoperfusion have been performed in series for procainamide, thallium, and carbamazepine overdoses, with apparent clinical efficacy.[6,15,25] A hemoperfusion cartridge also has been inserted into an extracorporeal membrane oxygenation (ECMO) circuit through which the flow rate was > 3 L/min in a patient who ingested 2 g of propranolol.[51] The plasma concentrations of propranolol decreased more rapidly

TABLE 5–3. PROPERTIES OF TOXINS GROUPED BY EFFICACY OF EXTRACORPOREAL TECHNIQUES FOR ELIMINATION

Drug/Toxin	MW (Daltons)	Water Soluble	Vd (L/kg)	Protein Binding (%)	Endogenous Clearance (mL/min per kg)	Preferred method	Comments
Clinically Efficacious							
Bromide	35	Yes	0.7	0	0.1	HD	
Ethylene glycol	62	Yes	0.6	0	2.0	HD	Cl ↑ as dose ↓
Isopropanol	60	Yes	0.6	0	na	HD	
Lithium	7	Yes	0.6–1.0	0	0.4	HD	Cl ↓ in renal failure
Methanol	32	Yes	0.7	0	0.7	HD	
Salicylate	138	Yes	0.2	50	0.9	HD, HP	Cl and protein binding ↓ with ↑ dose; HD also corrects electrolytes, acid–base
Theophylline	180	Yes	0.5	56	0.7	HP>HD	HP & HD can also be combined
Possibly Clinically Efficacious							
Amanita toxin	373–990	Yes	0.3	0	2.7–6.2	HP	Possibly effective if performed in first 24 hours
Aminoglycosides	>500	Yes	0.3	1.5	<10	HD/HF	Cl ↓ with renal failure
Atenolol	255	Yes	1.0	2.5	<5	HD or HP	Useful if Cl↓ due to renal failure
Carbamazepine	236	No	1.4	74	1.3	HP	Cl ↑ in patients on long-term therapy
Disopyramide	340	No	0.6	1.2	90	HP	Protein binding ↓ as concentration ↑
Meprobamate	218	Yes	0.5–0.8	0–30	Low	HP	Most drug eliminated in 24–36 hours
Methotrexate	454	Yes	0.4–0.8	50	1.5	HF	
Paraquat	186	Yes	1.0	6	24.0	HP	Tight tissue binding precludes efficacy, unless early in course
Phenobarbital	232	No	0.5	24	0.1	HP	Only for prolonged coma
Phenytoin	252	No	0.6	90	0.3	HP	Cl ↓ as dose ↑
Procainamide	272	Yes	1.9	16	8.0	HF	Cl ↓ in renal failure
Sotalol	272	Yes	2.0	2.0	<5	HD or HP	
Trichlorethanol	149	Yes	0.6	0.4	0.7	HD	Metabolite of chloral hydrate

Cl = clearance; na = not available.

during extracorporeal membrane oxygenation than after it was discontinued. The high flow rate through the cartridge may have led to substantial clearance of the drug.

The complications of hemoperfusion are similar to those of hemodialysis. In addition, patients may develop thrombocytopenia, leukopenia, or hypocalcemia.[44] Better membrane encapsulation techniques have made embolization of charcoal particles extremely rare. As in the case of hemodialysis, doses of drugs used therapeutically may need to be increased if they are removed by hemoperfusion.

For theophylline toxicity, it may be advantageous to combine both hemoperfusion and hemodialysis by putting both the dialysis membrane and the activated charcoal cartridge "in series" in the blood circuit.[3,24] If blood traverses the dialysis membrane first, 50% of the drug will be dialyzed, and the activated charcoal cartridge will have less drug to adsorb. The activated charcoal cartridge will be exhausted more slowly, and higher extraction ratios will be maintained. The dialysis membrane will also allow correction of the acid–base and electrolyte disorders that frequently accompany theophylline toxicity.

Multiple-Dose Activated Charcoal: "Gastrointestinal Dialysis"

Oral administration of multiple doses of activated charcoal increases elimination of some drugs present in the blood. Avid adsorption of the drug by the charcoal maintains a concentration gradient across the intestinal epithelium. The drug then diffuses from blood where it is present in higher concentration, to the intestinal lumen, where no drug is left unbound.

This technique was first clearly demonstrated to enhance elimination after parenteral administration of phenobarbital.[4] As in the case of hemoperfusion, the technique would be expected to work with compounds that are avidly bound by activated charcoal, have low volumes of distribution with little binding by plasma proteins, and properties that allow transmembrane diffusion to proceed. Theophylline is another drug for which this technique appears to be especially useful. Valproic acid may be an example of a toxin cleared significantly by multiple-dose activated charcoal only when levels are high, as protein-binding sites become saturated and unbound drug in plasma becomes accessible to the enteric activated charcoal.[21] Multiple doses of activated charcoal, often administered with a single dose of cathartic, such as sorbitol, may lead to bowel obstruction if not carefully observed. This modality is discussed in more detail in Chapter 4.

Continuous Hemofiltration

Hemofiltration refers to the movement of plasma across a semipermeable membrane in response to hydrostatic pressure gradients. There is no dialysate solution on the other side of the membrane (see Fig. 5–2). Smaller solutes are transported across the membrane, following the water (bulk flow), while larger solutes, depending on permeability characteristics of the membrane, are excluded. The volume status of the patient determines whether replacement of all or some of the filtered plasma with physiologic electrolyte solution (lactated Ringer's solution or other commercially available preparations) is indicated. Although this technique can be done intermittently using a dialysis machine, it has been adapted for use in intensive care units as a continuous form of treatment. Continuous modalities of dialytic therapy are still relatively experimental for the treatment of poisoning. Clearances achieved with these techniques are significantly lower than those achieved with hemodialysis. Despite many anecdotal reports demonstrating significant drug clearance, there are no data demonstrating that these techniques affect prognosis or mortality.

There are several possible advantages. One is the ability to continue therapy for 24 hours each day. Therefore, hemofiltration can be instituted after hemodialysis or hemoperfusion to further remove a drug or toxin after it redistributes from tissue to blood.[42] This is an attractive modality for slow, continuous removal of drugs, like procainamide, or lithium, that distribute slowly from tissue binding sites or from the intracellular compartment.[16,28] Other drugs with volumes of distribution large enough to preclude use of dialysis or hemoperfusion might also be eliminated with longer courses. However, the rate of removal with this form of therapy may not be sufficient to benefit critically ill patients. Second, the technique may be best suited for patients with hypotension who cannot tolerate conventional hemodialysis or hemoperfusion.[12] Lastly, it may have the advantage over hemodialysis in being able to clear larger molecules such as methotrexate (MW 454.4).[16,19,37] There is growing evidence that a significant part of the clearance of many molecules occurs because of adsorption of the molecule to the synthetic membrane.[14]

Hemofiltration, like hemodialysis, requires that blood perfuse a hollow-fiber dialysis membrane, usually made of synthetic polysulfone or polyamide.[27,58] In most circumstances the patient must be fully anticoagulated for all of these procedures, but some hemofilters are available that may not require anticoagulation. In continuous arteriovenous hemofiltration (CAVH), blood is pumped through the filter by the patient's arterial pressure via a single-lumen femoral artery catheter returning to a femoral vein catheter. In continuous venovenous hemofiltration (CVVH), a blood pump is required to maintain adequate flow rates, but arterial puncture with large-bore catheters is avoided. However, the need for a blood pump also necessitates an experienced dialysis or ICU team to be continuously present for more than the 4 to 6 hours needed for acute hemodialysis or hemperfusion. Both the expense and the complexity of the drug-removal procedure are thereby increased.

In either technique, an ultrafiltrate is generated by the positive pressure on the blood side "pushing" plasma across the membrane. Ultrafiltrate flows of 100 to 6000 mL/h can be achieved. Clearance can be significantly enhanced by having a dialysis solution running countercurrent to the blood flow (hemodiafiltration, CAVHD, or CVVHD; see Fig. 5–2). Addition of dialysis will also usually suffice to treat supervening acute renal failure or preexisting chronic renal failure. In either of these modalities, fluid and electrolyte losses must be replaced carefully. Depending on the filter, compounds with molecular weight less than 10,000 or less than 40,000 Dalton, as well as water, urea, creatinine, and sodium, pass into the ultrafiltrate. Heparin, myoglobin, insulin, and vancomycin are examples of larger molecules cleared with relative efficiency.[17] The cellular components and molecules larger than the pore size of the membrane return to the circulation in the venous line. A hemofilter with a molecular weight cutoff of 40,000 Daltons cannot remove digoxin–antibody complexes (MW 45,000 to 50,000).[46] Essential electrolytes lost in the ultrafiltrate are replaced by IV fluids such as lactated Ringer's solution.

Attention must be paid to the possible, and undesired, removal of therapeutic drugs such as antibiotics via these continuous modalities. This is evident in managing patients with acute renal failure with these techniques. Data are slowly accumulating that allow estimation of clearances with different synthetic membranes, and doses necessary to maintain therapeutic drug levels.[7,14,48] Up to 50% of vancomycin doses may be removed by continuous hemofiltration.[34] Binding of the drug to ultrafiltration membranes may be of substantial importance to its clearance.

The properties of toxins that make them amenable to hemofiltration are listed in Table 5–2.

Plasmapheresis and Exchange Transfusion

Plasmapheresis and exchange transfusion are intended to eliminate molecules with large molecular weights that would not be dialyzable. This would include substances with molecular weight greater than 15,000 Daltons, typified by immunoglobulins. The substance should also have limited endogenous metabolism to make pheresis or exchange worthwhile. Both techniques, by removing plasma proteins, offer the consequent potential benefit of removal of protein-bound molecules, such as complexes of digoxin and antidigoxin antibodies, or thyroxine. However, there is little evidence that either technique affects the clinical course and prognosis. Thyroxine removal after intoxication, for example, is followed by significant rebound from tissue stores, so that reduction in serum levels is only transient.[23] While removal of digoxin–antibody complexes in patients with renal failure may lead to more rapid drug removal,[47] more simple effective therapy may be to repeat administration of *Fab* fragments.

Pheresis is particularly expensive, and both techniques expose the patient to the risks of infection with plasma- or blood-borne diseases. Replacement of removed plasma during plasmapheresis can be with fresh frozen plasma, albumin, or combinations of both. The former is associated with anaphylactic or allergic manifestations, such as fever, urticaria, wheezing, and hypotension in as many as 21% of cases.[36]

A different setting in which exchange transfusion may be appropriate is in the management of small infants or neonates in whom dialysis or hemoperfusion may be technically difficult. Anticoagulation and multiple-dose activated charcoal may be particularly contraindicated in the neonatal nursery where the risk of intracerebral bleeding and necrotizing enterocolitis are high. In premature neonates a single volume exchange has appeared to alleviate manifestations of theophylline toxicity.[2,39] The therapy has also been successfully used in this setting to treat salicylism.[33]

Summary

Further discussion of some of the techniques to enhance elimination is found in Chapters 105 (exchange transfusion), 47 (cerebrospinal fluid drainage and replacement), and 48 (toxin-specific antibodies). All of these techniques have limited, very specific indications, and the effect of these interventions on the overall body burden of the intoxicant is usually small. Interruption of the enterohepatic circulation and/or gastrointestinal dialysis (Chap. 4) can be used concurrently with the techniques discussed.

Multiple-dose activated charcoal, urinary alkalinization, and many of the other techniques listed in Table 5–1 can be instituted quickly in the emergency department. In contrast, the extracorporeal methods of toxin removal, including hemodialysis, sorbent hemoperfusion, and continuous hemofiltration, all require consultation with a nephrologist or intensivist. Timely utilization of these techniques requires mobilization of a competent team and preparation of the requisite equipment. Rapid identification of a toxic exposure for which these techniques are appropriate, and the presence of more ominous prognostic features, should lead to prompt notification of the appropriate consult services so that application of these techniques can proceed in an expeditious manner.

REFERENCES

1. Anthony T, Jastremski M, Elliott W, et al: Charcoal hemoperfusion for the treatment of a combined diltiazem and metoprolol overdose. Ann Emerg Med 1986; 15:1344–1348.
2. Assael BM, Caccamo ML, Gerna M et al: Effect of exchange transfusion in elimination of theophylline in premature neonates. J Pediatr 1977; 91:331–332.
3. Benowitz NL, Toffelmire EB: The use of hemodialysis and hemoperfusion in the treatment of theophylline intoxication. Semin Dial 1993; 6:243–252.
4. Berg M, Berlinger W, Goldberg M, et al: Acceleration of the body clearance of phenobarbital by oral activated charcoal. N Engl J Med 1982; 307:642–644.
5. Berns A, comment in Benowitz NL, Toffelmire EB: The use of hemodialysis and hemoperfusion in the treatment of theophylline intoxication. Semin Dial 1993; 6:243–252.
6. Bock E, Keller E, Heitz J, Heinemeyer G: Treatment of carbamazepine poisoning by combined hemodialysis/hemoperfusion. Int J Clin Pharmacol Ther Toxicol 1989;27: 490–492.
7. Bressolle F, Kinowski J, de la Coussaye JE, et al: Clinical pharmacokinetics during continuous haemofiltration. Clin Pharmacokinet 1994; 26:457–471.
8. Brunet P, Jaber K, Berland Y, Baz M: Analphylactoid reactions during hemodialysis and hemofiltration: Role of associating AN69 membrane and angiotensin 1-converting enzyme inhibitors. Am J Kidney Dis 1992; 19:444–447.
9. Chan H, Evans WE, Pratt CB: Recovery from toxicity associated with high-dose methotrexate: Prognostic factors. Cancer Treat Rep 1977; 61:797–804.
10. Chavers BM, Kjellstrand CM, Weigand C, et al: Techniques for use of charcoal hemoperfusion in infants: Experience in two patients. Kidney Int 1980; 18:386–389.
11. Cherskov M: Extracorporeal detoxification: Still debatable. JAMA 1992; 247:3047.
12. Christiansson LK, Kaspersson KE, Kulling PE, Ovrebo S: Treatment of severe ethylene glycol intoxication with continuous arteriovenous hemofiltration dialysis. J Toxicol Clin Toxicol 1995; 33:267–270.
13. Cutler RD, Forland SC, St. John PG, et al: Extracorporeal removal of drugs and poisons by hemodialysis and hemoperfusion. Ann Rev Pharmacol Toxicol 1987; 27:169–191.
14. Davies JG, Kingswood JC, Sharpstone P, Street MK: Drug removal in continuous haemofiltration and haemodialysis. Brit J Hosp Med 1995; 54:524–528.
15. DeBacker W, Zachee P, Verpooten GA, et al: Thallium intoxication treated with combined hemoperfusion-hemodialysis. J Toxicol Clin Toxicol 1982; 19:259–264
16. Domoto DT, Brown WW, Bruggensmith P: Removal of toxic levels of *N*-acetylprocainamide with continuous arteriovenous hemofiltration or continous arteriovenous hemodiafiltration. Ann Intern Med 1987; 106:550–552.
17. Forni LG, Hilton PJ: Continuous hemofiltration in the treatment of acute renal failure. N Engl J Med 1997;336: 1303–1309.
18. Garella S: Extracorporeal techniques in the treamtent of exogenous intoxications. Kidney Int 1988; 33:735–754.
19. Golper TA, Bennett WM: Drug removal by continuous arteriovenous haemofiltration: A review of the evidence in poisoned patients. Med Toxicol 1988; 3:341–349.
20. Golper TA: Drugs and peritoneal dialysis. Dial Transplant 1979; 8:41–43.
21. Graudins A, Aaron CK: Delayed peak serum valproic acid in massive divalproex overdose—Treatment with charcoal hemoperfusion. J Toxicol Clin Toxicol 1996; 34:335–341.
22. Henderson A, Wright DM, Pond SM: Experience with 732 acute overdose patients admitted to an intensive care unit over six years. Med J Aust 1993; 158:28–30.
23. Henderson A, Hickman P, Ward G, Pond SM: Lack of efficacy of plasmapheresis in a patient overdosed with thyroxine. Anaesth Intens Care 1994; 22:463:464.
24. Hootkins R, Lerman MJ, Thompson JR: Sequential and simultaneous "in series" hemodialysis and hemoperfusion in the management of theophylline intoxication. J Am Soc Nephrol 1990;1:923–926.
25. Kar PM, Kellner K, Ing RS, Leehey DJ: Combined high-efficiency hemodialysis and charcoal hemoperfusion in severe *N*-acetylprocainamide intoxication. Am J Kidney Dis 1992; 10:403–406.
26. Koppel C, Schirop Th, Ibe K, et al: Hemoperfusion in severe chlorprothixene overdose. Intensive Care Med 1987;13: 358–360.

27. Kramer P, ed: Arteriovenous Hemofiltration: A Kidney Replacement Therapy for the Intensive Care Unit. Berlin, Springer-Verlag, 1985, pp. 1–13.
28. Leblanc M, Raymond M, Bonnardeaux A, et al: Lithium poisoning treated by high-performance continuous arteriovenous and venovenous hemodiafiltration. Am J Kidney Dis 1996; 3:365–372.
29. Linton AL, Luke RG, Briggs JD: Methods of forced diuresis and its application in barbiturate poisoning. Lancet 1967; 2:377–379.
30. Litovitz TL, Felberg L, White S, Klein-Schwartz W: 1995 Annual Report of the American Association of Poison Control Centers Toxic Exposure Surveillance System. Am J Emerg Med 1996; 14:487–505.
31. Lorch JA, Garella S: Hemoperfusion to treat intoxications. Ann Intern Med 1979; 19:301–304.
32. Ludwig SM, McKenzie J, Faiman C: Chlorpropamide overdose in renal failure: Management with charcoal hemoperfusion. Am J Kidney Dis 1987; 10:457–460.
33. Manikian A, Stone S, Hamilton R, et al: Exchange transfusion as an alternative to hemodialysis in severe infant salicylism. J Toxicol Clin Toxicol 1996;34:585. Abstract.
34. Matzke GR, O'Connell MB, Collins AJ, et al: Disposition of vancomycin during hemofiltration. Clin Pharmacol Ther 1986; 40:425–430.
35. Mauer SM, Chabers BM, Kjellstrand CM: Treatment of an infant with severe chloramphenicol intoxication using charcoal-column hemoperfusion. J Pediatr 1980;96:136–139.
36. Mokrzycki MH, Kaplan AA: Therapeutic plasma exchange: Complications and management. Am J Kidney Dis 1994;23: 817–827.
37. Molina R, Fabian C Cowley B. Use of charcoal hemoperfusion with sequential hemodialysis to reduce serum methotrexate levels in a patient with acute renal insufficiency. Am J Med 1987; 82:350–352.
38. Morgan AG, Polak A: The excretion of salicylate in salicylate poisoning. Clin Sci 1971; 41:475–484.
39. Osborn HH, Henry G, Wax P, et al: Theophylline toxicity in a premature neonate—Elimination kinetics of exchange transfusion. J Toxicol Clin Toxicol 1993; 31:639–644.
40. Papadopoulou ZL, Novello AC: The use of hemoperfusion in children: Past, present, and future. Pediatr Clin North Am 1982; 29:1039–1052.
41. Park GD, Spector R, Roberts RJ, et al: Use of hemoperfusion for treatment of theophylline intoxication. Am J Med 1983; 74:961–966.
42. Pond SM, Johnston SC, Schoof DD, et al: Repeated hemoperfusion and continuous arteriovenous hemofiltration in a paraquat poisoned patient. J Toxicol Clin Toxicol 1987; 25:305–316.
43. Pond SM, Olson KR, Osterloh JD, Tong TC: Randomized study of the treatment of phenobarbital overdose with repeated doses of activated charcoal. JAMA 1984;251: 3104–3108.
44. Pond SM, Rosenberg J, Benowitz NL, et al: Pharmacokinetics of haemoperfusion for drug overdose. Clin Pharmacokinet 1979; 4:329–354.
45. Prescott L, Park J, Darrien T: Treatment of severe 2,4-D and mecoprop intoxication with alkaline diuresis. J Clin Pharmacol 1979; 7:11–116.
46. Quaife EJ, Banner W, Vernon DD, Christensen DW: Failure of CAVH to remove digoxin–Fab complex in piglets. J Toxicol Clin Toxicol 1990; 28:61–68.
47. Rabetoy GM, Price CA, Findlay JWA, Sailstad JM: Treatment of digoxin intoxication in a renal failure patient with digoxin-specific antibody fragments and plasmapheresis. Am J Nephrol 1990; 10:518–521.
48. Reetze-Bonorden P, Bohler J, Keller E: Drug dosage in patients during continuous renal replacement therapy. Clin Pharmacokinet 1993; 24:362–379.
49. Rosenberg J, Benowitz NL, Pond SM: Pharmacokinetics of drug overdose. Clin Pharmacokinet 1981; 6:161–192.
50. Saitz R, Williams BW, Farber HW: Atenolol-induced cardiovascular collapse treated with hemodialysis. Crit Care Med 1991; 19:116–118.
51. Smith B, Sullivan MJ: Lifesaving use of extracorporeal membrane oxygenation. Aust J Cardiovasc Perf 1990; 4:7–11.
52. Takki S, Gambertoglio JG, Honda DH, Tozer TN: Pharmacokinetic evaluation of hemodialysis in acute drug overdose. J Pharmacokinet Biopharm1978; 6:427–442.
53. Trafford JAP, Jones RK, Evans R, et al: Haemoperfusion with R–004 Amberlite resin for treating acute poisoning. Br Med J 1997; 2:1453–1455.
54. Wason S, Baker RC, Carolan P, et al: Carbamazepine overdose: The effects of multiple dose activated charcoal. J Toxicol Clin Toxicol 1992; 30:39–48.
55. Winchester JF: Evolution of artificial organs: Extracorporeal removal of drugs. Artif Organs 1986; 10:316–323.
56. Winchester JF: Poisoning: Is the role of the nephrologist diminishing? Am J Kidney Dis 1989;13:171–183.
57. Woo OF, Pond SM, Benowitz NL, et al: Benefit of hemoperfusion of theophylline intoxication. J Toxicol Clin Toxicol 1984; 22:411–424.
58. Zobel G, Trop M, Beitzke A, et al: Vascular access for continuous arteriovenous hemofiltration of infants and young children. Artif Organs 1988; 12:16–19.

CHAPTER 6

Laboratory Principles and Techniques to Evaluate the Poisoned or Overdosed Patient

John D. Osterloh and Jack W. Snyder

Although most toxicologic diagnoses and therapeutic decisions are based on clinical assessment, selective laboratory analyses of body fluids can be helpful in the management of patients exposed to toxic agents.[34] Practical considerations, however, may limit the utility of laboratory tests. Most importantly, the time required for analysis often exceeds the critical time course of a toxicologic episode. Furthermore, the cost of maintaining procedures, instruments, and appropriately trained personnel to detect or measure more than a few dozen agents cannot be justified in the current American healthcare environment.

Clinically useful interpretation of a toxicologic test typically requires a predictable relationship between the concentration (or presence) of an agent and its toxicologic effects and confidence that this knowledge will be useful in the management of the patient. For many drugs, knowledge of these relationships is derived from monitoring body fluid concentrations during the administration of therapeutic doses. However, predictions based on pharmacokinetics or pharmacodynamics at therapeutic doses may not always be appropriate in overdose cases (eg, theophylline elimination is first-order at therapeutic doses and zero-order in overdose). Among the well-studied and/or clinically important toxins, fewer than two dozen have demonstrated reliable correlations between body fluid concentrations and toxic effects. Hence, the clinical observation of signs and symptoms, together with other laboratory tests (eg, arterial blood gas) are still the best guide in the majority of cases.

What Are the Indications for Laboratory Testing?

Monitoring, diagnostic confirmation, and screening are the three basic reasons for requesting a laboratory test in the care of patients exposed to toxic agents. Each reason is associated with a different clinical setting, a different "prior probability" that the test condition exists, and a different analytic attribute necessary for analysis (Table 6–1). When *monitoring* a patient, the change in a highly prevalent test condition (ie, the body fluid concentration of a therapeutic drug) is being followed. Thus, analytic *precision*, or ability to detect a change, is required of the test. For example, to see whether a change in clinical status (eg, liver function) might alter a patient's theophylline concentration, a precise test is required.

By contrast, tests that *confirm a diagnosis* are performed when multiple diagnoses (including drug intoxication) are being considered. Analytic *specificity* is required to accurately categorize the patient's condition among a few diagnostic alternatives (moderate prior probabilities of these alternative conditions being pres-

TABLE 6–1. TYPES OF MEDICAL AND TOXICOLOGIC TESTS

Type of Test	Purpose	Preselection or Prior Suspicion	Prior Probability or Prevalence of Test Condition	Primary Attribute Required of Test	Toxicologic Example
Monitoring	Measure change	Yes	High	Precision	Therapeutic drug monitoring
Diagnostic	Sort, categorize	Yes	Medium	Specificity	Toxicology screen
Screening	Find	No	Low	Sensitivity	Employee drug testing

ent). Such diagnostic confirmatory testing may help answer the question: Is the patient's condition due, at least in part, to the presence of one or more drugs or toxic agents versus some other condition?

In the process of *screening*, there is no prior suspicion or preselection. All persons are tested for the presence of a low-prevalence condition (eg, phenylketonuria in all newborns; presence of illicit substances in employees), usually a disease or circumstance that is difficult to find by clinical means alone. Finding all cases of the test condition (ie, *sensitivity*) is important so that effective intervention is possible. Low rates of false positives (nonspecificity) are allowable, in that these can be excluded or confirmed by secondary testing.

The prevalence or prior probability of a drug's presence in body fluids strongly influences the reliability (ie, the predictive value of a positive or negative test) at a given sensitivity and specificity. For example, in employee populations with low prior probability of drug presence, screening methods are adapted to facilitate detection of low concentrations (increased sensitivity) with adequate specificity for only a small number of drugs.[18,39] Without such adaptations, the ratio of false positives to true positives would be unacceptably high in this low-prevalence setting. By contrast, in toxicologic emergencies with high prior probabilities of drug presence (based on clinical suspicion), testing is designed to identify a broader number of drugs at higher concentrations (increased specificity). Similarly, in medical examiner cases, the acquisition of drug paraphernalia or other nonlaboratory evidence often increases the prior probability of drug presence as a cause of death. Although postmortem tissue changes may influence analyte detection, body fluid concentrations of drugs or toxins are frequently very high in fatal cases, so sensitivity may not be given highest priority. Finally, in methadone maintenance programs, drug testing occurs in selected populations with high prior probabilities not only of a drug's presence, but also of high concentrations of a small number of drugs (eg, opioids).

Unfortunately, "tox-screen" terminology has been imprecisely applied to all of these testing situations (screening, diagnosis, monitoring). Therefore, to improve patient care and assure appropriate testing, physicians requesting a "tox-screen" should be aware of the intended use of the test (ie, not screening). In turn, laboratories should inform clinicians of the factors that contribute to analytic strategies in a particular locale (eg, which drugs are detectable, how many procedures and confirmatory methods are applied). The clinical reliability of any test is determined by its appropriate clinical use and prevalence of the test condition, together with its analytic validation, including precision, sensitivity, and specificity. In the absence of meaningful communication between clinicians and analysts, the toxicology screen will remain an imprecise, poorly understood, and potentially misleading term.

What Types of Methods Are Available in the Toxicology Laboratory?

Many toxicologic tests are already provided within the routine operation of the broader laboratory servicies (eg, co-oximetry, osmol gap, ethanol, ketones, lactate, organ enzymes, glucose, electrolytes). These will be discussed in the pertinent chapters where they apply. The future is likely to bring a more diffuse hospital toxicology laboratory. Because of increasing automation and cost reductions, more and more drug tests (especially therapeutic drug monitoring [TDM] and drugs of abuse testing) will continue to be consolidated onto larger core laboratory instruments. In addition, the current trend will continue for fewer hospital laboratories to provide full-service toxicologic analyses, using outside reference laboratories for justified tests. The reasons for this are the high labor and time costs of chromatographic methods compared with other laboratory tests and the costs associated with regulatory requirements in maintaining lesser used or rare test procedures.

Current methods of drug analysis include chromatography, immunoassay, chemical ("spot") tests, and spectrometry (Table 6–2).[15] Many of these types of methods can be developed or adapted either for detection of multiple substances or for individualized detection and quantitation of a single drug. Analysis is comparative, matching the properties or behavior of a substance with that of a valid reference compound (a laboratory must possess a valid reference agent for every substance that it identifies). Biologic samples frequently contain materials that interfere with drug detection, so isolation of drug from the biomatrix is typically required before characterization begins.

Immunoassays and gas chromatography currently have the widest applications for discrete and broad drug testing, respectively. Most broad testing methods are limited by sensitivity or by the range of drugs detectable in a single analysis or "run." For individual drugs, analytic methodology varies considerably. For example, in the absence of derivatization, morphine detection by immunoassay is easier and more sensitive than detection by

TABLE 6–2. A COMPARISON OF GENERIC TOXICOLOGIC METHODS FOR DRUGS

Method	Specificity[a]	Sensitivity[a]	Multidrug Detection Possible	Quantitative Adaptability	Turn around Time (h)	Labor Intensive	Technical Expertise
Chemical spot	+	+	No	No	<0.5	+	0
Spectrometric[b]	+	+	No	Yes	<2–4	++	++
IA[b]	++	++	Some	Some	<1	+	+
TLC	++	+	Yes	No	2–4	+++	++
GC	++	++	Yes	Yes	<4	++	++
HPLC	++	++	Yes	Yes	<4	++	++
GC-MS	+++	+++	Yes	Yes	<6	+++	++++

[a]Relative comparison for specific analyte: +, least; +++, most.
[b]Can be performed on analyzers widely used in clinical laboratory
IA = immunoassays, TLC = thin-layer chromatography, GC = gas chromatography, HPLC = high-performance liquid chromatography, GC-MS = gas chromatography–mass spectrometry

thin-layer chromatography, which in turn is easier than morphine detection by gas chromatography (without chemical derivatization). By contrast, the rank order of methods for ease of detection of desipramine is reversed (ie, GC > TLC > IA).

Chemical spot tests are often used for quick detection of specific substances. These tests rely on the chemical reactivity of the drug with specific reagents. Spot tests are seldom used where high sensitivity or specificity is required (eg, employee drug testing). By contrast, spot tests of urine can be quite useful in selected toxicologic emergencies because they are easily and rapidly performed and drug concentrations tend to be high.[20,21] Examples include Trinder's spot test for salicylate and the FPN test for phenothiazine type drugs (see Table 6–3).

Spectrophotometric assays may require a chemical reaction to convert the target drug into a light-absorbing species. In uncomplicated overdose cases, spectrophotometry provides acceptable accuracy for measurement of carboxyhemoglobin, methemoglobin, cyanide, salicylates, borate, and acetaminophen. Use of spectrophotometry has waned, however, as various interferences have been described (Tables 6–3 and 6–4). For example, sulfhemoglobin and methylene blue (the antidote for methemoglobin) falsely increase methemoglobin concentrations measured by co-oximetry. Renal failure, ketoacidosis, phenylketonuria, diflunisal, salicylamide, and phenothiazines may falsely increase salicylate concentrations measured by colorimetry.[12] Salicylates, salicylamide, hyperbilirubinemia, and renal failure interfere in the nitrosation reaction in acetaminophen colorimetry.[32] Today, many spectrometric methods have been replaced by automated immunologic or enzymatic assays.

Immunoassays currently measure serum concentrations of about 12 different drugs while 10 or more individual classes or specific drugs can be identified by individual urinary immunoassay. The dramatic surge in use of immunoassays can be attributed to ease of automation, rapid turnaround, and adaptability for use as presumptive tests in the emergency department. Immunoassays rely on drug-specific antibodies that bind either to drug in the patient's sample or to known concentrations of "labeled" drug added to that sample. (Labeled drug is bound to a solid matrix, to an enzyme, or to a fluorescent molecule.) Measurable endpoints in immunoassay include fluorescence polarization, products of enzymatic catalysis, aggregation-light transmission, and others. Table 6–3 lists urine immunoassays by drug class. Enzyme immunoassay (EIA) or EMIT (Syva. Co.) is most frequently used, but fluorescence polarization (TDX, Abbott) and immunoaggregation (KIMS, Roche) assays are also popular. Analytic sensitivity is usually more than sufficient for measurement of body fluid concentrations in overdose. In addition, disposable prepackaged manual devices have been marketed for bedside diagnosis, but the validity, reliability, and clinical utility of these tools are only now being established. For employee urine drug testing, immunoassays typically provide the initial screen, and a positive test must be confirmed by a nonimmunologic method (usually gas chromatography/mass spectrometry).

Chromatographic assays are widely used in emergency toxicology. Sensitivity is adequate for many common pharmaceuticals at concentrations seen in overdose. For most chromatographic procedures, drugs must first be extracted from the relevant body fluid. In addition, chemical derivatization may be necessary to produce molecules compatible with a chromatographic phase or detection system. For example, to detect morphine by gas chromatography, the extracted morphine must be *N*-acetylated to decrease its polarity, increase its volatility, and enhance its detectability. The derivatized extract is then separated from other solutes as the constituents of the mobile phase differentially interact with the chromatographic stationary phase.

Three types of chromatography are commonly used in toxicologic analyses: thin-layer chromatography (TLC), high-performance liquid chromatography (HPLC), and gas chromatography (GC). In TLC, extracted drugs are spotted and dried onto plates typically coated with silica gel. These plates are placed in a closed chamber containing a predetermined mixture of organic solvents. During migration of solvent up the plate, drugs in the extract are separated by differential interaction with silica gel and solvent. Drugs are then located (visualized) by spraying a series of chemical reactants on the plate

TABLE 6–3. TOXICOLOGIC METHODS USED IN URINE: DISCRETE QUALITATIVE TESTS

Drug/Group	Reagent/Method Name	Type of Method	Sensitivity[a] (Detection Interval)	Interferences, Nonspecificity[b]
Salicylate	Trinder's	Spot, SC	TD (< 1 d), OD	Salicylamide, diflunisal, ketonuria, phenylketonuria, proteinuria, sulfonamides, hippuric acids (toluene, xylene)[c]
Acetaminophen (*p*-aminophenol detected)	Ortho-cresol	Spot, SC	TD (< 1 d), OD	*N*-acetylcysteine, phenols from throat lozenges and mouthwashes,[c] proteinuria
Phenothiazines (metabolites)	Forrest or FPN (ferric-perchloratenitric)	Spot	TD for some (< 3 d), OD	Salicylates, desipramine, ketonuria,[c] proteinuria
Ethchlorvynol	Diphenylamine	Spot, SC	OD (< 3 d)	?
Phencyclidine, Methadone, TCAs	Tetrabromophenophthalein ethyl ester	Spot	OD	Other opioids, antihistamines, neuroleptics[c]
Chloral hydrate (trichloroethanol)	Fujiwara	Spot	TD (< 2 d), OD	Chlorinated hydrocarbons[c]
Opioids (morphine, codeine)	EMIT, FPIA, KIMS, CEDIA, RIA, CMI	IA	RD (< 3 d), OD	Other opiates (hydrocodone, hydromorphone, oxycodone, dihydrocodeine), morphine from poppy seeds, adulterants,[d,e] rifampin
Barbiturates	EMIT, FPIA, KIMS, CEDIA, RIA, CMI	IA	RD (< 4 d), OD	Other less used barbiturates,[c] NSAIDs,[b,e] adulterants[d,e]
Benzodiazepines (metabolites)	EMIT, FPIA, KIMS, CEDIA, CMI	IA	TD for some, OD (days to weeks)	Other less used benzodiazepines,[d] NSAIDs,[b,e] less sensitive to triazolam, lorazepam and alprazolam (diazepam, nordiazepam, chlordiazepoxide, temazepam, midazolam, oxazepam are typically detected)
Amphetamines (amphetamine/methamphetamine)	EMIT, FPIA, KIMS, CEDIA, RIA, CMI	IA	RD (< 2 d), OD	Newer generation assays react with MDA, MDMA, STP and *l*-methamphetamine (in Vick's inhaler). Older assays cross-reacted with many adrenergic amines,[f] chlorpromazine,[c] ranitidine, adulterants[d,e]
Marijuana metabolite (11-nor-9-carboxyl-tetrahydrocannabinol)	EMIT, FPIA, KIMS, CEDIA, CMI	IA	RD (< 2 wk), OD	NSAIDs in the past, adulterants[d]
Cocaine metabolite (benzoylecgonine)	EMIT, FPIA, KIMS, CEDIA, CMI	IA	RD (< 2 d), OD	Few, teas made from coca leaf, adulterants[d,e]
Phencyclidine	EMIT, FPIA, KIMS, CEDIA, CMI	IA	RD (< 1 wk), OD	PCP analogs, chlorpromazine, diphenhydramine, dextromethorphan, methadone
Ethanol	Ezymatic	SC	RD (< 1 d), OD	Microbiologic production of ethanol in poorly stored urine

[a]Method sensitive to overdose dosage (OD), therapeutic dosage (TD), "recreational dosage" (RD) for window of time detectable in parentheses.
[b]Not all reagent/methods cross-react to the same extent.
[c]Requires extremely large amounts.
[d]Adulterants such as soaps, acids, benzalkonium chloride, and glutaraldehyde are added to produce false negatives.
[e]Negative interference.
[f]Adrenergic amines such as phenylpropanolamine, ephedrine, pseudoephedrine, fenfluramine, phentermine, isometheptene, propylhexidrine. Also ranitidine, ritodrine, labetalol, tranylcypromine, trimethobenzamide, cyclamates and others in the past. Selegiline, famprozanone, and fenproporex are metabolized to amphetamines and can be detected.
EMIT = enzyme multiplied immunoassay technique, FPIA = fluorescent polarization immunoassay, KIMS = kinetic interaction of microparticle spheres, CEDIA = cloned enzyme donor immunoassay, RIA = radioimmunoassay, CMI = colloidal gold microparticle immunoassay, SC = spectrochemical, IA = immunoassay.

and comparing the location of sample spots with those of co-migrated reference drugs. Numerous modifications of the early Davidow procedure have been reported.[13] The combination of "staining" plus the migration distance of each drug (known as RF value) endows TLC with specificity that may not be achieved with more elaborate procedures. Analytical sensitivity, however, varies with the drug, detection method, and amount of starting material, and seldom falls below 1.0 mg/L. Hence, many potent drugs (eg, triazolam, fentanyl, and LSD) are not detected by TLC. Use of commercially prepared TLC systems (eg, Toxilab, Ansys, Inc.) has improved intralaboratory and interlaboratory validity and reproducibility. More than 30 standard drugs can be co-migrated on a single plate, permitting identification of these and many other drugs using information available in reference compendiums.

In HPLC, drugs are separated within tightly packed columns. High pressures (1000–6000 psi) must be applied to these columns to elute molecules for detection. Columns are typically packed with polar phases (silica gel) or nonpolar phases (alkyl groups) bonded to small particles. Polar phases are eluted with organic solvents whereas nonpolar phases are eluted with solvents miscible in aqueous buffers. As they leave the column, drugs are detected using refractometry, conductivity, electrochemical (redox) reactions, or the absorption of ultraviolet light. Drug identifications are based on *retention times*, which reflect the time required for a drug to elute from the column and pass the detector.

TABLE 6–4. POTENTIAL INTERFERENCES FOR QUANTITATIVE SERUM DRUG AND CHEMISTRY TESTS USED IN EMERGENCY TOXICOLOGY

Assay	Method	Causes of Falsely Increased Serum Level
Acetaminophen	SC	Salicylate, salicylamide, methyl salicylate (each will increase acetaminophen level by 10% of their level in mg/L); bilirubin; phenols; renal failure (each 1 mg/dL increase in creatinine = 30 mg/L acetaminophen).
	IA	Phenacetin.
	HPLC	Cephalosporins; sulfonamides.
Amitriptyline	HPLC, GC	Cyclobenzaprine.
Carboxyhemoglobin	SC	Fetal hemoglobin (neonates have false COHb of 4–5%).
Chloride	SC, EC	Bromide (0.8 mEq Cl = 1 mEq Br), much less in some EC methods.
Creatinine	SC	Ketoacidosis (may increase Cr up to 2–3 mg/dL); cephalosporins; creatine (eg, with rhabdomyolysis).
	EZ	Lidocaine metabolite, 5-fluorouracil.
Digoxin	IA	Endogenous digoxin-like substances in patients with renal failure, newborns, pregnancy, liver failure (up to 1 ng/mL). Cross-reaction of metabolites in renal failure (up to several ng/mL). Ingestion of oleander, red squill, Chan Su (other cardiac glycosides identified as digoxin). After digoxin antibody (Fab) administration.
Ethanol	EZ	Combination of lactate and increased serum LDH.
Ethylene glycol	EZ	Glycerol; elevated triglycerides.
	GC	Propylene glycol.
Glucose	EC	Acetaminophen and ascorbate on YSI and Medisense devices.
Iron	SC	Deferoxamine causes 15% lowering of total iron-binding capacity (TIBC). Lavender-top Vacutainer tube contains EDTA, which lowers total iron.
Isopropanol	GC	Skin disinfectant containing isopropyl alcohol used before venipuncture (highly variable, usually trivial, but up to 40 mg/dL).
Ketones	SC	*N*-acetylcysteine, valproate, captopril, levodopa.
Lithium	F, EC, SC	Green-top Vacutainer specimen tube (contains lithium heparin) may cause marked elevation (up to 6–8 mEq/L); benzamide.
	SC	Quinidine, procainamide.
Methemoglobin	SC	Sulfhemoglobin (cross-positive—10% by co-oximeter); methylene blue (2 mg/kg dose gives transient false positive up to 15% methemoglobin level); hyperlipidemia (triglyceride, 6000 mg/dL, may give false methemoglobin up to 28.6%). Falsely decreased level with in vitro spontaneous reduction to hemoglobin in Vacutainer tube (~ 10%/h). Analyze within 1 h.
Osmolality	Osm	Lavender-top (EDTA) Vacutainer specimen tube (15 mOsm/L); gray-top (fluoride-oxalate) tube (150 mOsm/L); bue-top (citrate) tube (10 mOsm/L); green-top (lithium heparin) tube (theoretically, up to 6–8 mOsm/L). Falsely normal if vapor pressure method used (most alcohols are volatilized, not ethylene glycol).
Salicylate	SC	Diflunisal, ketosis, salicylamide; accumulated salicylate metabolites in patients with renal failure (~ 10% increase).
	IA	Diflunisal.
	SC	Decreased or altered salicylate level from bilirubin; phenylketones.
Theophylline	HPLC	Acetazolamide; cephalosporins; endogenous xanthines and accumulated theophylline metabolites in renal failure (minor effect).
	IA	Caffeine; accumulated theophylline metabolites in renal failure.

GC = gas chromatography (interferences primarily with older methods), HPLC = high-pressure liquid chromatography, IA = immunoassay, SC = spectrochemical, TLC = thin-layer chromatography, F = flame emission, EC = electrochemical, EZ = enzymatic

The narrow range of drug polarity explored in a single "run" usually limits the use of HPLC in broad drug screening. The range of identifiable substances can be expanded, however, by using multiple columns and/or gradient systems that change the composition of eluting solvent during a single run. Although some automated HPLC systems can detect a wide variety of drugs at overdose concentrations, their utility in toxicologic emergencies has only recently been explored.[3] In its usual applications, the high selectivity (ie, resolving capacity) of HPLC makes it especially useful for screening classes of structurally similar compounds, for confirming the presence of selected agents, or for measuring the concentrations of specified drugs. Quantitation is achieved by comparing the amplitudes of sample peaks with those of "internal" standard compounds added in constant amounts to all samples. With extraction and preconcentration of analytes, HPLC can detect concentrations of 0.01–1.0 mg/L in serum and urine.

For GC, an extracted drug must be volatile at temperatures inside the column (80–300° C). Chemical derivatization can be performed to make a drug more volatile. As these drugs enter the column, they are heated to the gas phase, which then interacts with the "liquid" stationary phase to separate various molecules along the length of the column. Drugs eluting from the column can be detected using ionization, thermal conductivity, combustibility, electron donation, or capture of beta particles. Detection limits vary from 0.1 to 0.5 mg/L. Gas chromatography is frequently combined with detection by mass spectrometry (GC-MS), where effluent gases from the GC are ionized and fragmented during bombardment by electron beams or other methods. Gas chromatography–mass spectrometry provides great specificity because it produces a unique set of molecular fragments for each eluting drug. Moreover, when only these unique fragments are monitored, sensitivity may extend into the ng/L range.

Although classical GC or GC-MS can detect many agents associated with toxicologic emergencies, the clinical utility of these techniques is limited by labor intensiveness, by volatility and polarity requirements, and by the relatively small variety of drugs detected on a single chromatographic run. However, the introduction of capillary columns has improved resolution and specificity for many analytes. Examples of drug classes that are easily analyzed by GC are amphetamine-like drugs, opioids, antihistamines, and antidepressants.[17] A separate GC procedure can also be used for identification and quantitation of ethanol, methanol, isopropanol, and acetone. By contrast, analysis of ethylene glycol usually requires a dedicated procedure with a different preparative approach.

When Is the Measurement of Blood or Serum Concentrations Useful?

In overdose cases, drug concentrations in serum or blood are used: (1) to monitor the treatment or course of a patient, (2) to diagnose clinically inapparent or delayed toxicity, or (3) to define indications for unique interventions. Currently, measurements of acetaminophen, carboxyhemoglobin, digoxin, salicylates, ethylene glycol, iron, lithium, methanol, ethanol, methemoglobin, theophylline, and certain heavy metals (lead, arsenic, and mercury) can meet one or more of these goals (see Table 6–5).

For serum concentrations to be useful in toxicologic emergencies, the concentration–effect relationship should provide clinically useful information that would not otherwise be apparent from the patient's presentation. In most cases, clinical indicators of toxicity are sufficient to support diagnostic and therapeutic decisions. For example, the clinical manifestations of tricyclic antidepressant overdose are more informative than serum tricyclic antidepressant concentrations for predicting the course and severity of illness.[4,9]

TABLE 6–5. SUMMARY: WHEN BLOOD OR SERUM TOXICOLOGIC TESTS ARE USEFUL

Intoxications requiring concentrations to diagnose severity or monitor course

• Acetaminophen	• Iron
• Salicylate	• Methanol
• Theophylline	• Ethylene glycol
• Ethanol	• Methemoglobin
• Carbon monoxide (COHb)	

Intoxications requiring concentrations as criteria for therapy or to assess effectiveness of therapy

• All above (except ethanol)	• Phenobarbital
• Lithium	• Lead, mercury, arsenic
• Digoxin	• Organophosphates (cholinesterases)

Serum drug concentrations may help clinicians evaluate the role or effect of high-risk or expensive treatments designed to prevent life-threatening tissue concentrations or to shorten the period of coma induced by drugs with long residence times, as initially suggested many years ago.[35] For example, serum theophylline measurements can aid decisions to start or continue charcoal hemoperfusion. Similarly, serum digoxin and blood or urine metal concentrations can support decisions to start Digibind or metal chelation treatments, respectively. For selected toxicologic emergencies, Table 6–6 summarizes the clinical presentations, critical serum concentrations, and common rationales associated with hazardous or expensive treatments.

With the development of rapid, quantitative automated assays, serum concentrations of acetaminophen, digoxin, iron, salicylates, lithium, theophylline, ethanol, methanol, and whole blood concentrations of carboxyhemoglobin and methemoglobin should be readily available on an immediate basis in facilities that handle toxicologic emergencies. However, of all hospitals capable of routine chemistry tests, only 51% measured acetaminophen, 63% iron, 38% lithium, 51% salicylate, and 79% theophylline.[11] Accuracy (nearness to true values or target concentrations) and agreement between laboratories is greatest for drugs measured frequently and by uniform techniques (eg, anticonvulsants). Measurements of less common drugs are often performed by more varied methods, resulting in poorer accuracy and interlaboratory agreement. Interlaboratory coefficients of variation typically do not exceed 8% for commonly measured TDM-type drugs. [11]

Should Quantitative Serum Drug Screening Be Used for All Patients?

Some have advocated that routine serum screening for specific drugs (eg, acetaminophen, salicylate) should be performed on all patients suspected of *any* intoxication because the morbidity of a missed diagnosis is high, therapy is available, and such drugs are commonly compounded with other medications, such that they might be overlooked. The obvious limitation of this approach, currently, is that it could apply to only a few drugs where analysis is convenient and inexpensive. In three studies[1,33,40] where acetaminophen determinations were made in all presentations regardless of the suspected intoxicant, the incidence of finding a toxic concentration was quite low (<1%) in cases not already suspected of acetaminophen overdose. Although this represents a very low percentage of patients, routine acetaminophen testing is cost effective based on the potential severity of missed overdose and the failure to identify patients at risk by routine examination and other laboratory testing.

TABLE 6–6. QUANTITATION OF DRUGS: USE IN EVALUATION OF SPECIAL INTERVENTIONS

Drug/Toxin	Laboratory/Clinical Presentation	Concentration Criteria	Therapy	Rationale for Intervention
Acetaminophen	Hx, none	> 150 μg/mL @ 4 h, > 38 μg/mL @12 h	NAC	Prevent hepatotoxicity
Theophylline	Vomiting, tachycardia, hypotension, hypokalemia	> 90–100 μg/mL (in acute OD)	HP/HD	Avoid seizures
Phenobarbital	Coma	> 100 μg/mL	HP	Shorten coma time
Lithium	Altered mental status, tremor, choreoathetosis, or rigidity, consider renal insufficiency	> 4 mEq/L (in acute OD) > 2.5 mEq/L (in chronic OD)	HD	Reduce CNS effects, avoid seizures
Methanol Ethylene glycol	AG metabolic acidosis + osmol gap	> 25 mg/dL	HD	Avoid blindness, renal failure, fatality
Salicylate	AG metabolic acidosis	> 60 mg/dL	HD	Differential Dx of acidosis, avoid fatality
Digoxin	AV block, hyperkalemia, bradycardia (acute)	> 4 ng/mL (acute OD)	Digibind	Avoid cardiovascular failure
Iron	Hx, GI pain, vomiting	> 500 μg/dL	Deferoxamine	Avoid cardiovascular collapse, hepatic failure
Carboxyhemoglobin	Hx, headache, confusion, coma, acidosis, or no significant findings	>15%	Oxygen, possibly HBO	Avoid continued hypoxemia and CNS injury

Hx = history of exposure, HP = hemoperfusion, HD = hemodialysis, NAC = *N*-acetylcysteine, AG = anion gap, OD = overdose, AV = atrioventricular, CNS = central nervous system, HBO = hyperbaric oxygen

What Factors Alter the Interpretation of Serum or Blood Drug Concentrations?

The interpretation of serum drug concentrations can be influenced by the interaction of diseases and medication, interpersonal variations in pharmacodynamics, altered pharmacokinetics in overdose, and potential interferences in assays. For example, in overdose, salicylates are more toxic than would be predicted by linear extrapolation of the effects at therapeutic concentrations. With increased serum salicylate concentrations and acidemia, the rate of salicylate biotransformation and degree of protein binding reach a plateau (saturation kinetics) and increased amounts of free (unbound) drug cross the blood–brain barrier.

Multiple factors can simultaneously impact the interpretation of serum digoxin concentrations. The concentration of digoxin in a symptom-free patient with renal failure taking usual doses of the drug may rise to 4 ng/mL due to the false measurement of endogenous "digoxin-like" substances and the cross-reactivity of accumulated metabolites. By contrast, a patient with a serum concentration of 2 ng/mL may develop clinical signs of digoxin toxicity when hypokalemia is present. Thus, all drug concentrations need to be interpreted in light of clinical information.

For drugs not routinely quantitated in serum or blood (eg, risperidone), there is usually no substantiated concentration–effect relationship. One hazard of trying to interpret concentrations of such a drug is erroneously assuming that achieved levels during therapeutic dosing (often determined during clinical trials and mentioned in the *Physicians Desk Reference*) are equivalent to a "therapeutic range." Such data were not intended to and do not define concentrations associated with efficacy or toxicity.

What Is a "Tox Screen" and What Types Are Available?

A toxicology screen is any combination of analytic procedures designed to identify multiple common drugs encountered in overdose. Focused or "abbreviated screens" provide rapid detection of a few common, critical, or difficult-to-recognize drugs (eg, drugs of abuse). By contrast, "comprehensive screens" combine those procedures necessary to identify as many as 50 target substances. Complementary combinations of spot tests, immunoassays, thin-layer chromatography, and gas chromatography typically require 3–4 hours of intense labor.[20,25,34] The numbers and types of agents detected by these tests can be adapted to reflect regional differences in drug prevalence.[26] Comprehensive screens vary considerably among laboratories, and cost-containment frequently dictates the use of inexpensive commercial methods.

In most "screens," the presence of a drug should usually be confirmed by a second analytically distinct method. Indeed, laboratories should not report a drug identification unless the agent is detected by at least two methods or a single method known to be highly specific for a highly prevalent substance (eg, ethanol by gas chromatography). For example, preliminary or initial identification of codeine or morphine by immunoassay should be viewed only as presumptive evidence for the presence of those drugs. Subsequent confirmation by TLC or GC-MS would make the result reportable, whereas failure to confirm (as well as lack of initial identification) would lead to a report indicating "no detection." The necessity for confirmation in clinical (ie, nonforensic, nonsurveillance) settings depends on the prevalence of the drug in question, the specificity of the screening test, and the implications of a positive test. For illicit drugs, confirmation is preferred because the recording of a positive test may have consequences beyond the acute care episode. By contrast, the detection of benzodiazepines may not require confirmation because the immunoassays have adequate specificity for the class, because these agents are commonly found in hospitalized patients, and because their presence has little impact on immediate management.

Tables 6–7 and 6–8, respectively, list the drugs that are usually detectable and not usually detectable in comprehensive toxicology screens. By knowing which drugs are not detected, physicians can avoid the clinical false negatives that arise from ordering a test not capable of identifying particular drugs. With timely urine collections (see Table 6–3 for detection intervals of common illicit drugs), 98.4% of all drugs found in "positive" patients can be detected with a combination of immunoassay, TLC, spot tests, and GC/HPLC techniques.[20,34] Comprehensive drug testing capability is not widespread, however, since only 6% of clinical laboratories are enrolled in proficiency testing for comprehensive drug screening.[11]

A rapid limited screen for four to eight drugs of abuse is commonly offered (as an alternative or in addition to comprehensive drug screens) in facilities that manage toxicologic emergencies. Although this type of screen accounts for 80% of all clinical screening requests in our experience, and results are typically available within 45 minutes, most of the drugs identified do not significantly influence emergency care. For example, detection of marijuana metabolites is rarely helpful in acute care because these substances: (1) are rare causes of life-threatening illness, (2) are present in many overdose patients, and (3) may not indicate recent use because detectable marijuana metabolites are excreted in urine for days to weeks following the last exposure.

TABLE 6–7. DETECTABLE COMMON DRUGS INCLUDED ON MOST COMPREHENSIVE SCREENS

Alcohols—ethanol, methanol, isopropanol, acetone

Barbiturates/sedatives—amobarbital, secobarbital, pentobarbital, butalbital, butabarbital, phenobarbital, glutethimide, ethychlorvynol, methaqualone

Anticonvulsants—phenytoin, carbamazepine, primadone, phenobarbital

Benzodiazepines—chlordiazepoxide, diazepam, alprazolam, temazepam

Antihistamines—diphenhydramine, chlorpheniramine, brompheniramine, tripelennamine, trihexiphenidyl, doxylamine, pyrilamine, methapyrilene

Antidepressants—amitriptyline, nortriptyline, doxepin, imipramine, desipramine, trazodone, amoxapine, maprotiline, fluoxetine

Neuroleptics—trifluoperazine, perphenazine, prochlorperazine, chlorpromazine

Stimulants—amphetamine, methamphetamine, phenylpropanolamine, ephedrine, MDA, MDMA (other phenylethylamines), cocaine, phencyclidine

Opioids—heroin, morphine, codeine, oxycodone, hydrocodone, hydromorphone, meperidine, pentazocine, propoxyphene

Other analgesics—salicylates, acetaminophen

Cardiovascular drugs—lidocaine, propranolol, metoprolol, quinidine, procainamide, verapamil

Others—theophylline, caffeine, nicotine, sulfonylureas, strychnine

TABLE 6–8. TOXINS NOT DETECTABLE ON COMPREHENSIVE SCREENS CLASSIFIED BY AREA OF DIFFICULTY

Too Polar—antibiotics, diuretics, isoniazid, ethylene glycol, lithium, lead, iron

Too nonpolar—steroids, tetrahydrocannabinol, digoxin

Too nonvolatile—plant and fungal alkaloids, some phenothiazines

Too volatile—aromatic and halogenated hydrocarbon solvents, anesthetic gases, noxious gases (hydrogen sulfide, nitrogen dioxide, carbon monoxide)

Concentration too low—(potent drugs or drugs with large Vd)—clonidine, fentanyl, colchicine, ergot alkaloids, lysergic acid diethylamide, dioxin, digoxin, tetrahydrocannabinol

Toxic anions (too polar)—thiocyanate, cyanide, fluoride, bromide, borate, nitrite

New drugs—eg, buspirone

Currently, the screening of blood or serum cannot routinely be performed because sample sizes are often too small, drug concentrations are frequently too low or undetectable, and methods cannot be or have not been adapted for analysis of these body fluids. When emergency blood screens are requested and performed, they typically involve a series of single quantitative immunoassays usually reserved for therapeutic drug monitoring. For example, separate assays for digoxin, phenobarbital, theophylline, acetaminophen, and salicylate are offered as a group and called a "screen." The clinical utility of such an approach has not been established and its use is discouraged.

What Is the Relevance of Analytic Cutoff Concentrations Used in Qualitative Screening?

Analytic cutoff concentrations are concentrations above which a method can determine with certainty (> 95%) that the analyte drug is present and below which the probability decreases. Along with dose and pharmacokinetic variables, the cutoff concentrations will determine how long a drug is detectable in the urine or serum of a patient, that is, detection intervals (see Table 6–3 for some common detection intervals). A drug with a long half-life such as methadone can be detected for many days with a low detection limit. For patients with drug overdoses, the detection interval will be longer than the commonly stated detection intervals established in studies of "recreational doses."

What is the meaning of qualitatively detectable concentrations with overdose effects? Finding the presence of a drug on toxicologic testing is only that; it may or may not be related to the presenting clinical signs and symptoms. The criteria for the establishment of cutoff concentrations for many of the commonly used illicit drug immunoassays are analytical and not pharmacologic in nature. These are particularly established for use in surveillance drug testing programs, that is, low enough concentration cutoffs to expand the detection time interval and high enough to allow adequate confirmation by other methods. These are the same immunoassays used in hospital laboratory testing. Thus, qualitative urinary detection of some drugs may be too sensitive for the overdose situation. For example, the detection of methadone in an overdose patient may not explain the clinical presentation because the drug was ingested in therapeutic amounts or many days earlier. Furthermore, the relation between urinary concentrations or presence of any drug in the urine and clinical effects is often unclear due to variability in excretion patterns and renal dilution/concentration of the urinary fluid. Alternatively, not finding a potent drug included in a class of screened drugs may not indicate its absence (eg, a requested benzodiazepine screen that is insensitive for triazolam).

How Should Toxicology Tests Be Ordered?

To improve communication and decrease turnaround time, physicians requesting toxicologic tests should provide information on suspected drugs or diagnosis via a computerized order entry or a requisition form.[16] In addition, because of pending Health Care Financing Administration regulations pertaining to Medicare reimbursement and hospital/laboratory accreditation, the "medical necessity" of many laboratory tests will require documentation (usually only statement of diagnosis) on request forms. Further consultation with the laboratory, providing information about symptoms, working diagnoses, or suspected toxins, can be of help in narrowing the search for toxins only when the pathologist/analyst has a background in toxicology. For example, if the clinician states that he or she suspects clonidine as a cause of pinpoint pupils, the analyst can reply that screens identify many opiates, but will not typically detect the presence of clonidine. By contrast, when the clinician is confronted with a patient demonstrating "bizarre behavior" and requests only a urine amphetamine test, the analyst can suggest a more comprehensive screen that detects antihistamines, anticholinergics, and other drugs that commonly cause bizarre behavior or other psychiatric disturbances. In addition, the laboratory can provide information on expected detection intervals (see Table 6–3 also).

In emergency care, blood/serum for quantitation should be obtained as soon as the specified intoxicant becomes part of a differential diagnosis, only if results are likely to influence management or disposition. Although the results of comprehensive urine screening often do not influence emergency management, urine screening may be occasionally requested if the patient is admitted, since the findings may assist in-house physicians when diagnostic uncertainty persists. Specimens can also be refrigerated temporarily in the laboratory and can be analyzed if needed.

Urine is the preferred specimen for comprehensive, focused, or individual drug screens. The number of drugs detected and the rate of positives is consistently higher in urine than in serum or in gastric aspirates.[20,25,34] In one study, patients initially managed with gastric lavage showed the following percentage of positive specimens: gastric aspirate 38%, serum 54% (only sedative-hypnotics were measurable in serum) , and urine 93%.[2] In urine samples, the concentration of metabolites often exceeds that of the parent drug or very little parent drug remains (eg, phenothiazines), while in gastric aspirates, high concentrations of parent compounds occasionally facilitate drug identification. Serum is the preferred specimen for most quantitative tests of drugs demonstrating a concentration–effect relationship, though whole blood is used in instances of chemicals with low concentrations in serum and concentrated amounts in red blood cells.

What Drugs Are Most Commonly Found in Overdosed Patients?

Medical examiners report carbon monoxide, ethanol, sedatives, opioids, propoxyphene, and cyclic antidepressants (in decreasing order of frequency) as the most common substances involved in drug-related deaths.[10,31] Drug classes most frequently associated with mortality as reported by poison control centers include analgesics (opioid and nonopioid), antidepressants, stimulants (eg, amphetamines, cocaine, phencyclidine), sedative/hypnotics, cardiovascular agents, and alcohols.[27] In toxicologic emergencies, 50–80% of screens are positive. Cocaine metabolites and benzodiazepines are the most commonly detected substances. These agents together with opioids, other illicit stimulants, psychotropics, and antihistamines accounted for 70–90% of all agents found.[34,38] Pharmaceuticals are involved in less than 40% of pediatric exposures and Poison Control Center calls, but they are responsible for many serious intoxications, hospital admissions, and deaths, especially among teenagers. Children under six are typically exposed to a single agent, whereas 27–66% of adults ingest multiple substances.[14,22,27,43]

Are the Results of Toxicologic Screening Accurate?

Proficiency testing programs sponsored by the College of American Pathologists and the American Association for Clinical Chemistry are designed to assess the accuracy of toxicologic testing. In a random single round of testing of four specimens containing multiple drugs, the false-negative rate for carisoprodol (an unusual analyte) may reach 60% while the false-negative rate for cocaine metabolites (a common analyte) rarely exceeds 10%.[11] False positives, by contrast, rarely exceed 3–10% because concentrations in proficiency specimens are reasonably high and initial positives can be confirmed by a second method. The clinical impact of these few false positives is usually small because most false positives and some false negatives are the result of misidentification within a drug class (eg, pentobarbital for amobarbital).

When 26 specialty toxicology laboratories were challenged with a case history plus a urine containing four drugs that were difficult to detect, only two facilities identified all four drugs correctly.[8] Sixty-five percent identified dihydrocodeine, 54% identified methylenedioxyethylamphetamine (MDEA), 23% identified naloxone, and 23% identified aminoflunitrazepam (a metabolite of Rohypnol). Hence, false negatives are the major problem, averaging 10–30% across most laboratories and various drugs, and reinforce the concern that ordering physicians must be aware or consult with the performing laboratory regarding the content of the screen or detectability of a substance.

False negative results due to specimen manipulation or tampering are more likely to occur in forensic urine drug testing than in emergency drug screening. To increase the chances of a negative test, examinees may: (1) ingest weak acids or bases (eg, vinegar, bicarbonate of soda) to influence the excretion of acidic or basic drugs; (2) dilute the sample by ingesting fluids or directly adding water from the sink or commode; (3) substitute the urine of another person or animal; (4) add one or more interfering substances (eg, alcohol, ammonia, bleach, Drano, hydrogen peroxide, liquid handsoap, household cleaning solutions, salt, vinegar, NSAIDs, benzalkonium chloride [in Visine], glutaraldehyde, methylene blue, or Golden Seal tea). Most of these agents are used in an attempt to defeat the biologic basis of the immunoassay screening tests.[29]

How Often Do Cross-Reactive Drugs Cause False Positives?

Clearly, nonspecificity occurs (see Table 6–3). Most often, related drugs or derivatives are responsible, although in some assays quite different drugs may cross-react. In immunoassay type methods for phencyclidine, drugs such as methadone, diphenhydramine, and dextromethorphan have been reported to cross-react in different manufacturers' forms of the assay. Although Table 6–3 lists a number of cross-reactions that have been reported to occur, it is important to recognize that these do not occur in every commercial form of the assay and that manufacturers may have subsequently remedied the problem.

What Interpretative Considerations Should Apply to the Results of Qualitative Urine Tests?

To interpret the qualitative presence of a drug in the urine, all the above must be considered including: analytical sensitivity and specificity, pharmacologic variables, adulteration and clinical prior probability. The laboratory can assist with these considerations, but the physician must also be aware of clinical false positive and negatives. Clinical false positives arise from the detection of therapeutic medications not contributing to the clinical presentation. It is up to the physician to consider this, since qualitative results do not indicate the dosage, and the history may be lacking on medication use. Clinical false negatives are due to misapplication of the test or screen, that is, the ordered screen is not intended to detect the substance the physician has in mind. In some cases, this may result from not being aware of what was tested, for example, the metabolite is measured but the parent drug is not, or the drug is not included in the list of screened drugs. Also, selecting a drug test intended for use in the emergency situation, but applying it for screening or surveillance purposes, may result in insensitivity (ie, using a diagnostic test instead of a screening test).

The physician should also consider the prior likelihood that detectable drugs would explain the patient's condition. The prevalence of positive urine drug screens in suspected toxicologic emergencies ranges from 50–80% in busy settings.[34] Assuming a prior probability (of drug presence) of 50% and a sensitivity of 70–90% (averaged for all drugs), the predictive value of a negative comprehensive urine toxicologic screen is 63–83%. With a specificity of 90–100%, the predictive value of a positive screen is 83–100%. Thus, in high-prevalence settings, the "rule-in" value of the comprehensive toxicologic screen is greater than the "rule-out" value. This is a disconcerting observation since it is reported that physicians more often use comprehensive screens to "rule out" than to "rule in" drug toxicity.[24] However, in lower-prevalence settings (eg, in hospitals where physicians do not routinely see patients with overdoses), "rule-out" testing may occasionally be useful. For example, if the physician has a strong suspicion of metabolic coma (eg, hepatic encephalopathy), the prior probability of detectable drugs causing coma might be as low as 5–10%. With this lower prior probability and the same specificity and sensitivity of the toxicologic screen, the predictive value of a negative test is 76–90% while the predictive value of a positive test is only 33%.

Are the Results of Toxicologic Screening Clinically Useful?

In emergency care: (1) many diagnostic and management decisions are made before toxicologic tests results are reported; (2) patient responses to benign and diagnostic interventions (eg, naloxone) may preclude the need for testing; (3) few antidotal or other specific interventions are determined by toxicologic test results;[5] (4) overall morbidity and mortality are low in overdosed patients who are properly decontaminated and supported[23,27]; and (5) clinical features are often sufficient to diagnose a toxic episode and to predict its outcome.[5,30] For these reasons as well as analytical limitations described above, positive comprehensive drug screens have been found to influence diagnosis and treatment decisions in less than 15% of toxicologic emergencies.[5,7,19,24,28,44] While this impact rate is relatively high compared to many tests used in medicine, this fact and the other cited surveys suggest that the astute physician can establish the diagnosis in most cases on clinical grounds or successfully treat apparent toxic effects without knowing the specific toxin involved.

In 265 overdoses due to self-poisoning in Norway, the responsible drug or class of drug was correctly identified in 85% of patients using only the history, physical examination, and basic laboratory tests, including measurements of serum salicylate, acetaminophen, barbiturates, and lithium. Extra toxicologic screening was needed to identify other drugs in only 5% of the cases.[36] However, the physician diagnosis was incorrect or unknown in 14% when compared to follow-up testing and review. In another series, nurses, physicians, and pharmacists relied on classic descriptions of toxidromes to correctly identify the drug or class causing intoxication in more than 80% of the cases.[30] By contrast, information on drug intake has been reported to be unreliable or unavailable in 75% of toxicologic emergencies.[34,35] In reviewing a number of studies that compare the clinical diagnosis with results found on toxicologic screening, complete concordance of clinical predictions with comprehensive toxicologic screen results varies from 20–32%. Additional, unsuspected agents are detected in 20–48% of cases, while the clinically predicted substance is not found in 9–25% of cases.[34]

Why are toxicologic screens and individual tests still ordered if the impact is so low? One reason, asserted earlier, is that if the diagnosis remains unclear at a later point in time, the toxicologic testing requested earlier may help. A second reason is that even with an impact on decision making as low as a few percent, a life may be saved or morbidity avoided. A third reason is probably related to liability/documentation concerns. However, there may be an unassessed utility. Most past studies have focused on positive screen results and discrepancies in clinical and analytical findings.[6,41] The impact of negative test results have not been well examined. The disposition or transfer of a patient within the hospital (and associated costs) may be affected by negative "tox screen" results. For example, when physicians attempt to distinguish functional from drug-induced psychosis, a negative "tox screen" may help predict the need for more intense psychiatric care or transfer of the patient.[37] Future studies will be needed to examine the impact of toxicologic testing on patient disposition and costs. Also, with the advent of more rapid turnaround-time testing, such as "point-of-care" (bedside) devices,[42] investigations will be required to determine their impact at earlier time points on diagnosis, management, and patient disposition.

Is Toxicologic Testing Keeping Up With the Times?

As discussed above, toxicologic tests are unable or unavailable to detect the diverse world of chemical substances. With new drugs available to patients at ever increasing rates, the expectation might be that laboratories would keep up with detection of these new toxins. However, laboratories lag far behind in the analysis of new drugs introduced into the modern pharmacopoeia. For broad "tox screens," new drugs are not procedurally validated for testing as they become clinically available. Usually new drugs become incorporated into broad "tox screens" only after their notoriety and prevalence of abuse have increased, if such drugs are analytically detectable at meaningful concentrations. Felbamate, a recently introduced anticonvulsant, is not usually included along with other anticonvulsants on "tox screens." Even though felbamate is detectable, its frequency in use and incidence in overdose cases has been low. For specific drug testing, the labor in validating and maintaining chromatographic assays only for rare toxins is far too costly. Hospital laboratories will usually wait for less expensive immunoassays to be developed commercially. For example, LSD use is still fairly prevalent and psychiatric emergency departments often must discern LSD-induced psychosis from functional causes. Within the last few years convenient commercial immunoassays for LSD have been developed, supplanting testing performed by outside reference laboratories.

The contribution of metabolites to either pharmacologic activity or cross-reaction in immmunologic-based assays often is left unaddressed. Such studies are usually beyond the scope and budget of the hospital-based laboratory. Yet examples abound, where metabolites may cross-react and contribute to the total assay response, particularly in renal failure (digoxin, carbamazepine, phenytoin, theophylline, cyclosporine) or where metabolites are not measured, but contribute to the therapeutic and toxic effects (carbamazepine, tricyclic antidepressants).

In attemping to keep up with new toxins, many laboratories have purchased GC-MS equipment that is used to match mass spectral data of unknown compounds with extensive spectral libraries contained in CD-ROM archives. While this is an excellent first approach, it is insufficient documentation for the basis of a report to a physician. Such searches or matches can, in fact, identify the correct drug, but many cases of unusual or unlikely matches are also found. At a minimum, to report such a drug, the actual reference drug should be injected and compared, though a more complete validation of detection limits and precision is recommended. Physicians receiving reports specifying a rare or unusual toxin should check with the laboratory regarding the measures used to acquire confidence in that report.

Laboratories will usually send out requests for analysis of toxins that are not performed in-house. Because of slow turnaround times, tests are unlikely to affect emergency management and are likely to be challenged during reimbursement and restricted in the cost-contained managed care setting. For tests on unusual drugs, toxins of plant or animal origin, synthetic chemicals, environmental and occupational toxins (metals, solvents, and pesticides), consultation should be obtained from a toxicologist, the regional Poison Control Center, or the toxicology laboratory. Only a few such tests might be performed locally (eg, blood lead, blood cyanide, blood carboxyhemoglobin by co-oximeter, serum methanol, plasma and red blood cell cholinesterases, and urinary qualitative nicotine, atropine, and strychnine).

In summary, the patient's condition is usually the

best guide to diagnosis and mangement. In some cases, clinical observation alone is inadequate and testing for toxins will provide additional or better guidance.

References

1. Ashbourne JF, Olson KR, Khayam-Bashi H: Value of rapid screening for acetaminophen in all patients with intentional drug overdose. Ann Emerg Med 1989;18:1035–1038.
2. Auerbach PS, Osterloh JD, Braun O, et al: Efficacy of gastric emptying: gastric lavage vs. emesis induced with ipecac. Ann Emerg Med 1986;15:692–698.
3. Binder SR, Regalia M, Biaggi-McEachern, Mazhar M: Automated liquid chromatographic analysis of drugs in urine by on-line cleanup and isocratic multicolumn separation. J Chrom 1989;473:325–341.
4. Boehnert MT, Lovejoy FH Jr: Value of the QRS duration versus the serum drug level in predicting seizures and ventricular arrhythmias after an acute overdose of tricyclic antidepressants. N Engl J Med 1985;313:474–479.
5. Brett AS, Rothschild N, Gray R, et al: Predicting the clinical course in intentional drug overdose: Implications for use of the intensive care unit. Arch Intern Med 1987;147:133–137.
6. Brett AS: Implications of discordance between clinical impression and toxicology analysis in drug overdose. Arch Intern Med 1988;148:437–441.
7. Bury RW, Mashford ML: Use of a drug-screening service in an inner-city teaching hospital. Med J Aust 1981;1:132–133.
8. California Association of Toxicologists Newsletter–Summer. 1995; August:13–16.
9. Callaham M: Tricyclic antidepressant overdose. JACEP 1979;8:413–425.
10. Caplan YH, Ottinger WE, Park J, et al: Drug and chemical related deaths: incidence in the state of Maryland—1975 to 1980. J Forensic Sci 1985;30:1012–1021.
11. CAP Surveys: Urine Toxicology Survey 1995 Set UT-B; Therapeutic Drug Monitoring Survey 1995 Set Z-B; Chemistry Survey 1995 Set C4-B. College of American Pathologists, 1995.
12. Dalrymple RW, Sterns FM: Diflunisal interferes with determination of salicylate by Trinder, Abbott TDx and Dupont aca methods. Clin Chem 1986; 32:230.
13. Davidow B, Petri NL, Quame B: A thin-layer chromatographic screening procedure for detecting drug abuse. Am J Clin Pathol 1968;50:714–719.
14. Fazen LE, Lovejoy FH Jr, Crone RK, et al: Acute poisoning in a children's hospital: a 2-year experience. Pediatrics 1986;77:144–151.
15. Ferrara SD, Tedeschi L, Frison G, et al: Drugs-of-abuse testing in urine: statistical approach and experimental comparison of immunochemical and chromatographic techniques. J Anal Toxicol 1994;18:278–291.
16. Fligner CL, Robertson WO: Request and report forms in toxicology screening. Vet Hum Toxicol 1985;28:306. Abstract.
17. Forester EH, Hatchett D, Garriott JC: A rapid, comprehensive screening procedure for basic drugs in blood or tissues by gas chromatography. J Anal Toxicol 1978;2:50–55.
18. Griner PF, Glaser RJ: Misuse of laboratory tests and diagnostic procedures. N Engl J Med 1982;307:1336–1339.
19. Helliwell M, Hampel G, Sinclair E: Value of emergency toxicological investigations in differential diagnosis of coma. Br Med J 1979;2:819–821.
20. Hepler BR, Sutheimer CA, Sunshine I: The role of the toxicology laboratory in emergency medicine. II. Study of an integrated approach. J Toxicol Clin Toxicol 1984–85;22: 503–528.
21. Higgins G: Screening tests for common drugs. In: Clark EGC, ed: Isolation and Identification of Drugs in Pharmaceuticals, Body Fluids and Post-mortem Material, Vol. 1. London, The Pharmaceutical Press, 1974, pp. 3–15.
22. Jacobsen D, Halvorsen K, Marstrander J, et al: Acute poisonings of children in Oslo. Acta Paediatr Scand 1983;72: 553–557.
23. Jacobsen D, Fredericksen PS, Knutsen KM, et al: A prospective study of 1212 cases of acute poisoning: General epidemiology. Hum Toxicol 1984;3:93–106.
24. Kellermann AL, Fihn SD, Logerfro JP, et al: Impact of drug screening in suspected overdose. Ann Emerg Med 1987;16: 1206–1216.
25. Kellermann AL, Fihn SD, Logerfro JP, et al: Utilization and yield of drug screening in the emergency department. Am J Emerg Med 1988;6:14–20.
26. Lasky FD, Wesley JF, Marx AJ: Changes in the pattern of drugs detected in a toxicology screen in an upstate New York hospital. Pathol Annu 1985;20:161–187.
27. Litovitz TL, Felberg L, White S, Klein-Schwartz W: 1995 annual report of the American Association of Poison Control Centers. Toxic Exposure Surveillance System. Am J Emerg Med 1996;14:487–537.
28. Mahoney JD, Gross PL, Stern TA: The use of the toxic screen in the management of overdosed patients. Vet Hum Toxicol 1987;29:474. Abstract.
29. Mikkelsen SL, Ash KO: Adulterants causing false negatives in illicit drug testing. Clin Chem 1988;34:2333–2336.
30. Nice A, Leikin JB, Maturen A, et al: Toxidrome recognition to improve efficiency of emergency urine drug screens. Ann Emerg Med 1988;17:676–680.
31. Norton LE, Garriott JC, Di Maio VJM: Drug detection at autopsy: A prospective study of 247 cases. J Forensic Sci 1982; 27:61–71.
32. Osterloh JD: Limitations of acetaminophen assays. J Toxicol Clin Toxicol 1983;20:19–22.
33. Osterloh JD, Yu S: Simultaneous ion-pair and partition liquid chromatography of acetaminophen, theophylline and salicylate with application to 500 toxicologic specimens. Clin Chim Acta 1988;179:239–248.
34. Osterloh JD: Utility and reliability of emergency toxicologic testing. Emerg Med Clin North Am 1990;8:693–723.
35. Prescott LF: Limitations of hemodialysis and forced diuresis. In: Curry AS, ed: Symposium on the Poisoned Patient—Role of the Laboratory. CIBA Foundation Symposium, New York, Elsevier, 1974.
36. Rygnestad T, Berg KJ: Evaluation of benefits of drug analysis in the routine clinical management of acute self-poisoning. J Toxicol Clin Toxicol 1984;22:51–61.
37. Sanguineti VR, Samuel SE: Comorbid substance abuse and recovery from acute psychiatric relapse. Hosp Community Psychiatry 1993;44:1073–1076.

38. Schwartz JG, Stuckey JH, Prihoda TJ, et al: Hospital-based toxicology: Patterns of use and abuse. Texas Med 1990;86: 44–51.
39. Spiehler VR, O'Donnell CM, Gokhale DV: Confirmation and certainty in toxicologic screening. Clin Chem 1988;34: 1535–1539.
40. Sporer KA, Khayam-Bashi H: Acetaminophen and salicylate levels in patients with suicidal ingestion and altered mental status. Am J Emerg Med 1996;14:443-446.
41. Teitelbaum DT, Morgan J, Gray G: Nonconcordance between clinical impression and laboratory findings in clinical toxicology. Clin Toxicol 1977;10:417–422.
42. Tomaszewski C, Gibbs M, Runge J, et al: Impact of rapid bedside toxicology screen on workup of patients suspected of drug toxicity. J Toxicol Clin Toxicol 1996;34:580. Abstract.
43. Trinkoff AM, Baker SP: Poisoning hospitalizations and deaths from solids and liquids among children and teenagers. Am J Public Health 1986;76:657–660.
44. Wiltbank TB, Sine HE, Brody BB: Are emergency toxicology measurements really used? Clin Chem 1974;20:116–118.

CHAPTER 7

Toxicologic Imaging

David T. Schwartz

Radiographic imaging plays an important role in many aspects of clinical medicine and, in selected instances, can help in the management of toxicologic emergencies. Radiography can contribute in three ways to the care of the poisoned patient: (1) establishing a diagnosis; (2) assisting in therapeutic interventions; and (3) detecting complications of a poisoning or toxin exposure. The radiographic study must always be interpreted in light of the entire clinical situation. Most of the time, imaging will supplement the overall diagnostic impression. Occasionally, a radiographic study will suggest a toxicologic etiology when one was not originally suspected.

In some instances, radiographic studies are used to detect the toxin itself, whereas in others, the effect of the toxin on various organ systems is visualized. Conventional radiography is readily available in the Emergency Department (ED) and is the imaging modality most commonly used in acute patient management. However, the entire spectrum of imaging techniques has been employed in various toxicology problems, including enteric and intravascular contrast studies, computed tomography (CT), ultrasound, magnetic resonance imaging (MRI), and nuclear scintigraphy.

Visualizing the Toxin Itself

A number of toxins and medications are "radiopaque" and can potentially be detected radiographically. Radiopacity depends on several factors. First, the radiopacity of an object is relevant only in relation to the radiodensity of surrounding tissues. If the object is surrounded by material of similar radiodensity, it will not be detectable. Second, the intrinsic radiodensity of a substance is dependent on its physical density (g/cm^3) and the atomic numbers of its constituent atoms. Biologic tissues are composed mostly of carbon, in addition to hydrogen and oxygen, and have an average atomic number of approximately six. Substances that are significantly more radiodense than soft tissues include bone, which contains calcium (atomic number 20); radiocontrast agents containing iodine (atomic number 53) and barium (atomic number 56); iron (atomic number 26); and lead (atomic number 82). Some medications contain constituent atoms of high atomic number such as chlorine (atomic number 17), sulfur (atomic number 16), and potassium (atomic number 19). Although the atomic number contributes to making a medication radiodense, other determinants of radiodensity are usually more important and knowledge of atomic numbers is of little practical value in predicting radiodensity. Third, the thickness of an object also affects its radiodensity; small particles of a radiodense substance are often not visible. Last, the radiographic appearance of the surrounding area greatly affects the detectability of an object. A moderately radiodense tablet is easily seen against a uniform background in an in vitro study, but can be obscured by the shadows of overlying bone or bowel gas in a patient.

Most toxins gain entry into the body by ingestion, injection, or inhalation. If ingested, the toxin can potentially be visualized using an abdominal radiograph. Injected or inhaled toxins may also be amenable to radiographic detection. If the toxin itself is available for examination, it can be radiographed outside of the body to detect radiodense components.

Unknown Ingestion

A plain abdominal radiograph could theoretically be used to identify a certain ingested radiodense toxin; however, its role in screening patients who have ingested an unknown substance is controversial. It has been suggested that an abdominal film be obtained in the unresponsive overdose patient in an attempt to identify the involved toxin.[1] In reality, this approach has significant limitations. The number of potentially ingested substances that have consistently been shown to be radiodense is very limited. Furthermore, the radiographic appearance of ingested medications or toxins is not sufficiently distinctive to determine their composition in the absence of corroborating history (Fig. 7–1). Therefore,

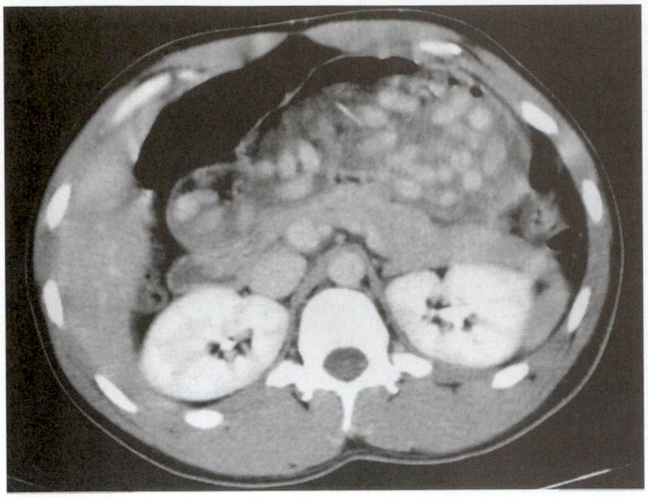

Figure 7–1. A 46-year-old male presented to the ED with abdominal pain. He had a depressed level of consciousness and a strong odor of alcohol on his breath. On physical examination, he had mild diffuse abdominal tenderness. Plain films of the chest and abdomen were negative. Because of his blunted mentation and abdominal pain, a CT scan of the abdomen was obtained. The CT revealed innumerable tablet-shaped densities within the stomach. The CT finding was interpreted as an overdose of some unknown medication, so orogastric lavage was attempted. The patient vomited a large amount of whole navy beans. Upon discharge from the Emergency Department several hours later, the patient was advised to chew his food fully before swallowing (and to reduce his consumption of alcohol). CT is able to detect small, nearly isodense structures such as these, which is not possible using conventional radiography. However, the radiographic detection of tablets, or tablet-like densities, does not permit their pharmacologic identification. *(Courtesy of Dr. Earl J. Reisdorff, Michigan State University, Lansing, Michigan.)*

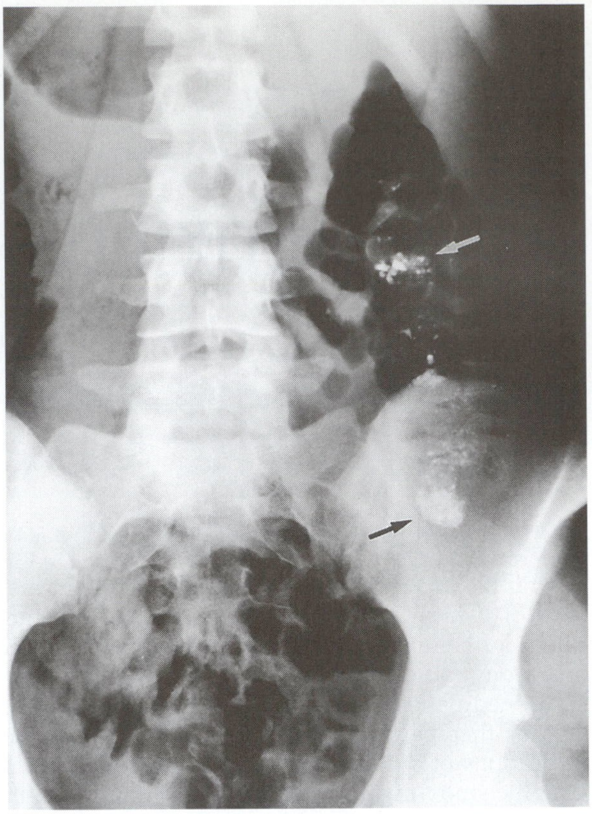

Figure 7–2. An abdominal radiograph obtained on a patient with upper abdominal pain revealed radiopaque material throughout the intestinal tract. Is his abdominal pain due to an overdose of iron tablets or to lead toxicity from eating paint chips? Further questioning of the patient revealed that he had been consuming bismuth subsalicylate (Pepto-Bismol) tablets in an attempt to treat his ulcer pain (bismuth, atomic number 83). The identification of radiopaque material does not allow determination of the nature of the substance.

the use of a plain film to screen patients in the hope of identifying an ingested toxin is not likely to be fruitful. However, when a specific ingestion is suspected and the substance is known to have consistent radiodensity, plain abdominal films can play a significant role in patient care. The plain film will both confirm the diagnosis, help estimate the amount ingested, and monitor the efficacy of gastrointestinal decontamination. Conversely, when an abdominal film is obtained for reasons other than a toxin ingestion (eg, to evaluate abdominal pain) and a radiodense substance is found, a knowledge of potentially radiodense substances is useful to generate a list of diagnostic possibilities (Fig. 7–2).[122,126]

A number of investigators have studied the radiopacity of various medications.[32,50,56,66,102,119,129,135] Most of these were in vitro experiments that used a water-bath model to simulate the overall radiodensity of the abdomen. These studies identified medications that possess greater or lesser radiodensity. A short list of the more consistently radiodense substances is summarized in the mnemonic: **CHIPS**—chloral hydrate, heavy metals, iron, psychotropics (phenothiazines), and sustained-release (enteric-coated) preparations.

Although the CHIPS mnemonic is widely known, it has several limitations that significantly reduce its usefulness in clinical practice.[119] First, it does not include all of the pills that have been shown to be radiodense in vitro, such as acetazolamide and busulfan. However, most of these medications are only mildly or moderately radiodense and are not reliably detected in vivo. Second, most of the medications that are radiodense in vitro, such as chloral hydrate, dissolve rapidly when ingested and become impossible to detect radiographically. Third, although heavy metals are very radiodense, they are no longer used in medications and would be unlikely to be associated with an unknown pill ingestion. Nevertheless, under certain circumstances, heavy metal exposure does remain a concern in the poisoned patient. For example, heavy metal contamination has been noted in some herbal medicine preparations.[148] Fourth, iron tablets are very radiodense and are usually very slow to dissolve but, in liquid or chewable form, may not be detected radiographically even when a large quantity has been ingested.[33,128] Fifth, psychotropics/phenothiazines include a wide variety of compounds of varying radiodensity. Trifluoperazine (containing fluorine, atomic number 9) is radiodense in vitro, whereas chlorpromazine (containing chlorine, atomic number 17) is not.[102,119] Lithium carbonate in the form of Lithobid had moderate radiodensity in one in vitro study, whereas a generic formulation did not.[102,119] Sixth, slow-release preparations and enteric coatings have variable composition and radiodensity. Pill formulations (fillers, binders, and coatings) vary between manufacturers and even a specific product can change depending on date of manufacture. The insoluble matrix of some sustained-release preparations is radiodense, and when seen on a radiograph, these pills may no longer contain active medication. Studies of newer sustained-release cardiac medications failed to show radiopacity.[127,135]

In summary, only a very limited number of medications and toxins can be reliably visualized radiographically, most notably iron preparations. Most radiodense medications have only moderate or minimal radiodensity and dissolve quickly in the stomach and intestinal tract. Therefore, plain abdominal radiography is not generally indicated for the detection or identification of ingested pills in a poisoned patient in whom the identity of the toxin is unknown.

In comparison to conventional radiography, ultrasound would theoretically be an ideal tool for detecting ingested pills because imaging depends on echogenicity rather than radiopacity. Solid pills should be sonographically detectable within the fluid-filled stomach. In one in vitro study using a water-bath model, virtually all intact pills could be seen.[2] These authors were also successful in a limited human experiment in detecting pills in the subject's stomach. Nevertheless, reliably finding pills scattered throughout the gastrointestinal tract, which often contains air that blocks the ultrasound beam, would be a formidable task and of limited if any clinical importance.

Known Toxin Exposure

When a particular substance that has been consistently shown to be radiodense in vivo is involved in the toxic exposure, radiography can play an important role in patient care. Radiography can confirm the exposure, quantify the amount of toxin involved, and monitor its removal from the body.

Iron Tablet Ingestion. Ferrous sulfate and ferrous gluconate tablets are radiodense and when ingested, fragment, and disintegrate slowly. In this specific situation, plain radiography has a well established role in patient care. If tablets are detected on an abdominal film, the iron ingestion is confirmed. Moreover, the quantity of tablets seen provides an indication of the amount ingested. Serial radiographs can be used to follow gastrointestinal decontamination (Fig. 7–3).[33,101] After gastrointestinal evacuation by whole bowel irrigation or gastric lavage, repeat radiographs help determine if further gastrointestinal decontamination or surgical or endoscopic removal is needed (see Fig. 22–3).[39,105,138] Nevertheless, caution must be exercised in using radiography to exclude the possibility of an iron ingestion because some iron preparations are not always radiographically detectable and the tablets may not be visible if they have already disintegrated. Liquid, chewable, or encapsulated ("Spansule") iron preparations rapidly fragment and disperse after ingestion and are less radiodense than ferrous sulfate tablets even when intact.[32]

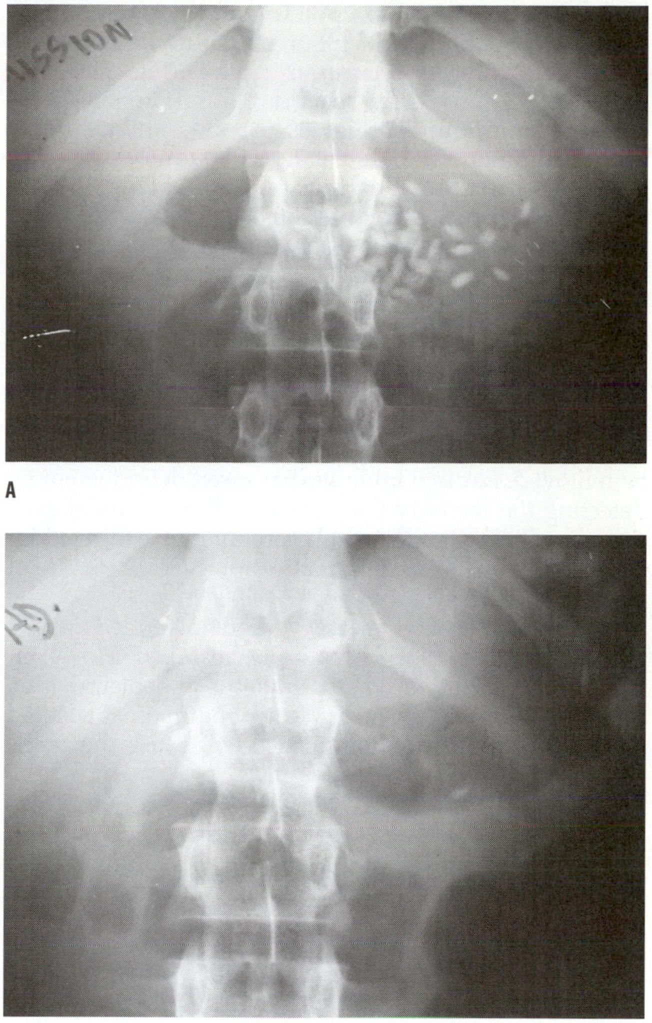

A

B

Figure 7–3. (**A**) The identification of a large number of radiopaque tablets confirms the diagnosis in a patient with a suspected iron overdose and permits rough quantification of the amount ingested. (**B**) Following emesis and whole bowel irrigation, a second radiograph revealed some remaining tablets and indicated the need for further intestinal decontamination. A third radiograph after additional bowel irrigation demonstrated clearing of the intestinal tract. *(Courtesy of the Toxicology Fellowship of the New York City Poison Center.)*

Heavy Metals. Heavy metals are very densely radiopaque and readily detected radiographically. "Heavy metal" is, in fact, a term that does not have a precise chemical definition. The medical toxicologist uses the term for metals of high atomic number that can be treated by chelation therapy, such as lead, mercury, arsenic, thallium, cadmium, and chromium. As with iron tablets, radiography can confirm the presence of heavy metal compounds and can be used to follow decontamination. Sources of heavy metal ingestions include leaded ceramic glaze (Fig. 111–1);[115] paint chips containing leaded paint (Fig. 79–8);[75,89] mercury compounds (Fig. 80–1); zinc sulfate (zinc, atomic number 30);[15] arsenic (atomic number 33) (Fig. 7–4);[78] and thallium (atomic number 81).[27,90] Enteral exposure to elemental mercury can occur when a glass thermometer or a long intestinal tube breaks. When the intestinal mucosa is intact, this poses little toxic risk (Fig. 7–5A). However, if the mucosa is disrupted, systemic absorption can occur.

Since elemental mercury is liquid at room temperature, it can be injected subcutaneously and intravenously for suicidal or other purposes. Subcutaneous deposits of elemental mercury are systemically absorbed and must be removed. Radiographic studies assist debridement by detecting the mercury that remains after the initial excision (Fig. 7–5B, C). Elemental mercury that is injected intravenously produces a dramatic radiographic picture of pulmonary embolization (Fig. 7–5D).[17,98]

Unlike elemental mercury, lead imbedded in soft tissues is usually not systemically absorbed. However, lead can be absorbed when a bullet is in contact with a synovial surface. Over many years, both mechanical and chemical action in the joint space will cause the bullet to fragment and gradually dissolve, allowing lead to enter the circulation and cause systemic toxicity. Bullets imbedded within joints should be removed to prevent joint deterioration and systemic absorption of lead (Fig. 7–6).[28,34,131,134]

Toxins in Containers. In some instances, toxins can be visualized even though they are of similar radiodensity to soft tissues. If a toxin is ingested in a container, the container itself may be visible. "Body packers" smuggle large quantities of drugs across international borders in securely sealed packets.[9,10,16,36,65,88,123] The many uniform oblong packets can be detected on plain abdominal radiographs either because the containers' walls contain a thin layer of air or metallic foil or because the packets are outlined by surrounding bowel gas (Fig. 7–7). In some cases, a "rosette" is seen representing the knot at the end of the packet.[123] Roughly 85–90% of body packers will have positive plain abdominal films.[10,16,88] Because rupture of a single container could be fatal, care must be taken to ensure that all packets are removed. Given the packets' great monetary value, the patient usually knows the exact number ingested. The number of packets retrieved from the fecal effluent after whole-bowel irrigation should be compared with the reported quantity in-

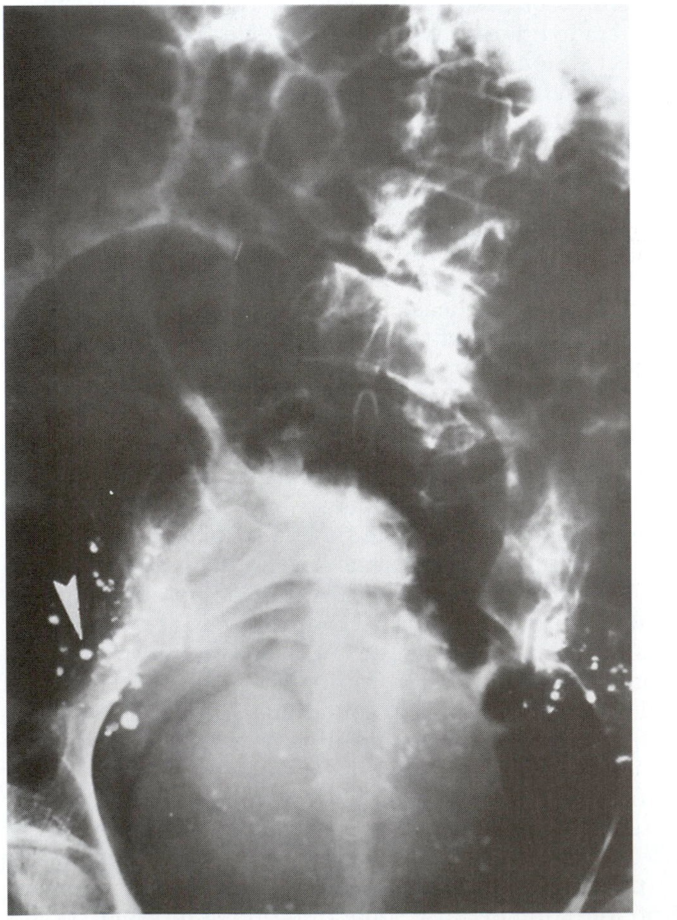

Figure 7–4. An abdominal radiograph in an elderly woman incidentally revealed radiopaque material in the pelvic region. This was residual from gluteal injection of antiluetic therapy she had received 35 to 40 years earlier. The injections may have contained bismuth or an arsenical. *(Courtesy of Dr. Emil J. Balthazar, Professor of Radiology, New York University, New York, New York.)*

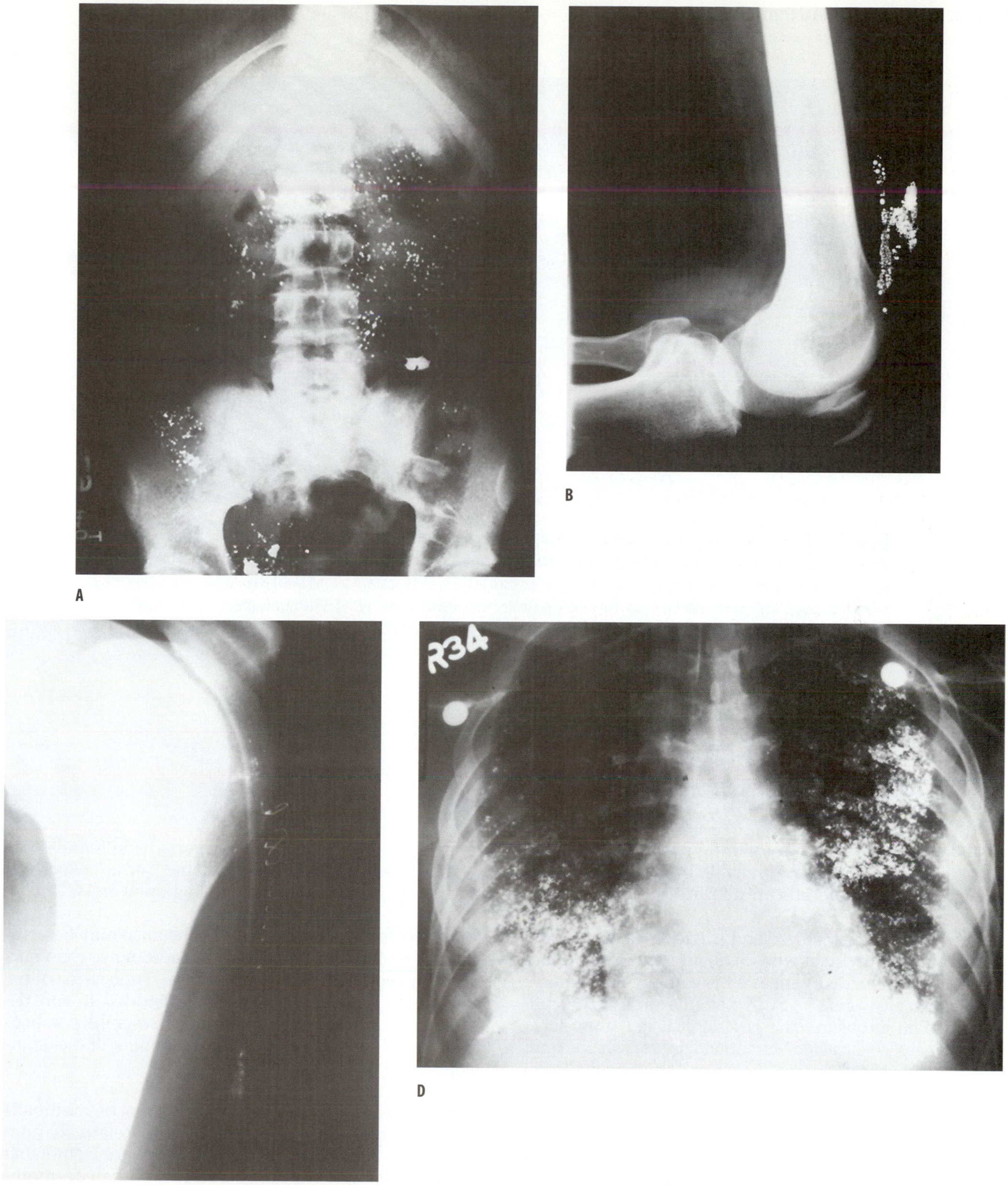

A

B

C

D

Figure 7–5. (**A**) Unintentional rupture of a Cantor intestinal tube distributed elemental mercury throughout the bowel. The mercury is not systemically absorbed if the intestinal mucosa is intact. *(Courtesy of Dr. Richard Lefleur, Associate Professor of Radiology, New York University, New York, New York.)* (**B**) Subcutaneous injection of liquid elemental mercury is readily detected radiographically. Since mercury is systemically absorbed from subcutaneous tissues, it must be removed by surgical excision. (**C**) A repeat radiograph after debridement reveals nearly complete removal of the mercury deposit. Surgical staples and a radiopaque drain are also visible. *(Courtesy of the Toxicology Fellowship of the New York City Poison Center.)* (**D**) The chest radiograph in a patient following intravenous injection of elemental mercury showing metallic pulmonary embolism. The patient developed respiratory failure, pleural effusions, and uremia and expired despite aggressive therapeutic interventions. *(Courtesy of Dr. N. John Stewart.)*

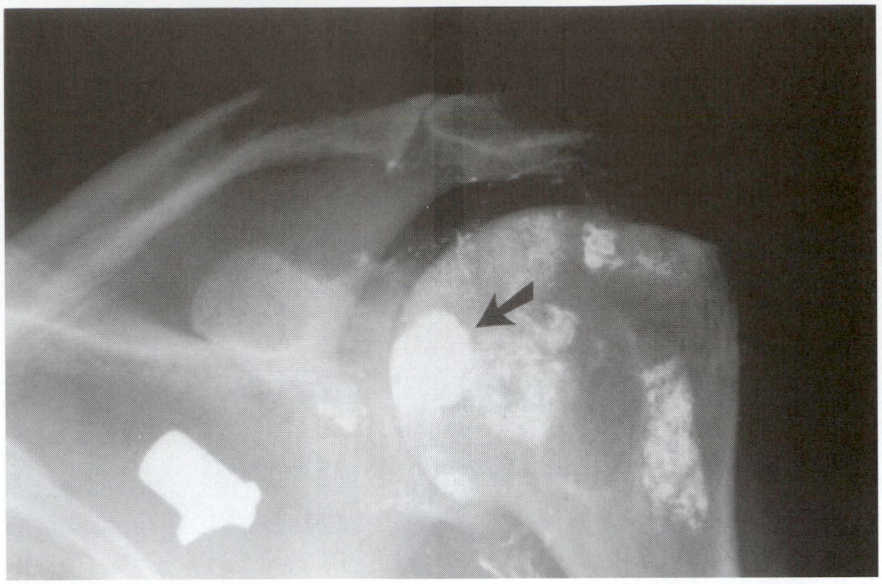

Figure 7–6. A "lead arthrogram" discovered many years after a bullet wound to the shoulder. At the time of the initial injury, the bullet was embedded in the articular surface of the humeral head (*arrow*). The portion of the bullet that protruded into the joint space was surgically removed, leaving a portion of the bullet exposed to the synovial space. A second bullet is embedded in the muscles of the scapula. Eight years after the injury, the patient presented with weakness and anemia. Extensive lead deposition throughout the synovium is seen. Lead level was 91 μg/dL. The patient was treated with dimercaptosuccinic acid (DMSA) chelation and surgical debridement of the synovium. *(Courtesy of the Toxicology Fellowship of the New York City Poison Center.)*

gested. Since one or two remaining packets can be difficult to visualize radiographically, the introduction of enteric contrast material can help detect any remaining containers (see Fig. 22–3).[60]

As opposed to the "body packer," the "body stuffer" is an individual who, in an attempt to avoid imminent arrest, hurriedly ingests his contraband in much less secure packaging.[116] Such patients pose a difficult management problem. The risk of leakage from such haphazardly constructed containers is very high, and information regarding the ingestion is generally completely unreliable. Radiographic studies cannot exclude the possibility of an ingestion, and in one series of 98 cases, no patient had a positive abdominal radiograph.[128] Occasionally a radiograph will confirm the ingestion (Fig. 7–8). If the material is in a glass or hard plastic crack vial, the container may be visualized on a plain film. However, only a minority of crack vials will be detected radiographically. In one series, crack vials were seen on abdominal radiographs in only 2 patients out of 23 suspected or 11 confirmed cases (9% or 18%, respectively).[59] If the person swallows soft plastic bags containing the drug, the containers will not be visible, although in three case reports, the "baggies" could be visualized by abdominal CT.[52,69,108] Occasional reports have found some degree of radiopacity of crack cocaine "rocks," which can therefore be detected on plain radiography and CT.[23,52]

Radiolucent Toxins. A radiolucent substance may be visualized by virtue of its being less radiodense than surrounding soft tissues. Hydrocarbons, such as gasoline, are relatively radiolucent when imbedded in soft tissues. The radiographic appearance resembles subcutaneous air that occurs in a gas-forming soft tissue infection (Fig. 7–9).

Mothballs. The content of different types of mothballs can be distinguished radiographically. Relatively nontoxic paradichlorobenzene mothballs are somewhat radiopaque, whereas more toxic naphthalene mothballs are radiolucent.[132] Radiographs of noningested mothballs outside of the patient can help distinguish these two types (see Chap. 84 and Fig. 84–2).

Halogenated Hydrocarbons. Some halogenated hydrocarbons have sufficient radiodensity to be visible on plain radiographs.[24] Radiopacity is proportionate to the number of chlorine atoms, and both carbon tetra-

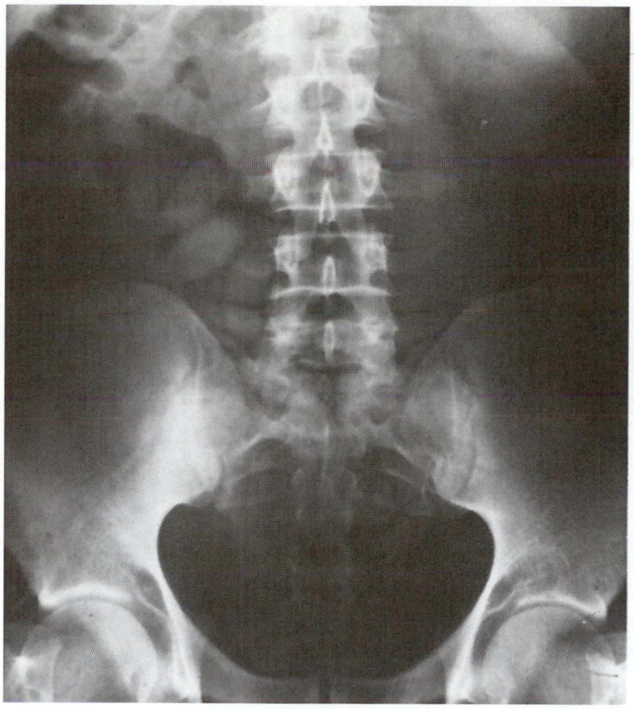

A

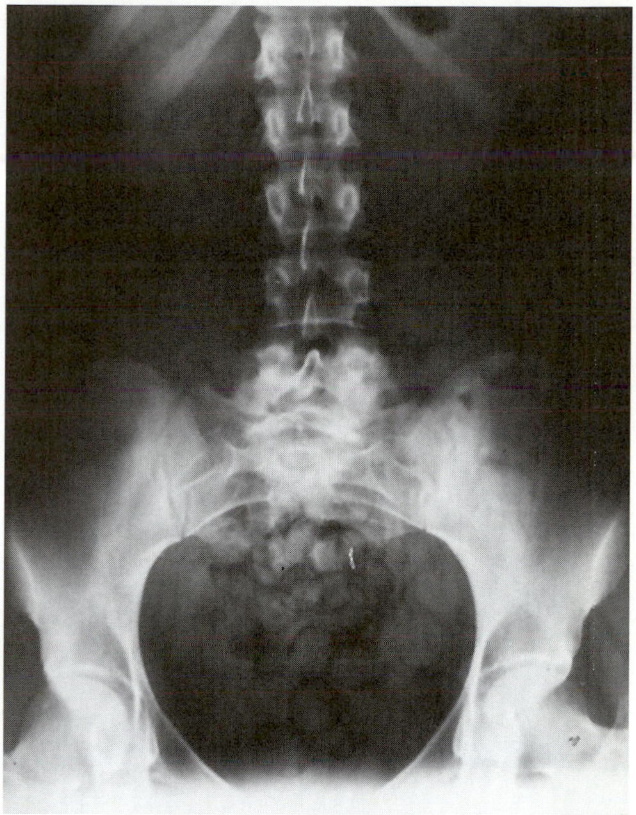

B

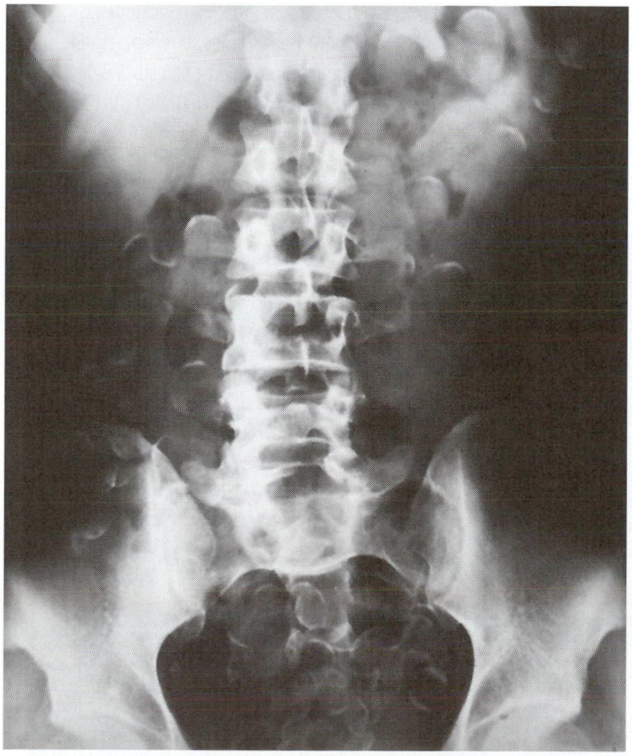

C

Figure 7–7. Three "body packers" showing the various radiographic appearances of the packets. Drug smuggling is accomplished by packing the gastrointestinal tract with large numbers of manufactured, well-sealed containers. (**A**) Multiple oblong packages are seen throughout the bowel. (**B**) The packets are visible in this patient because they are surrounded by a thin layer of air within the wall of the packet. (**C**) Metallic foil is part of the packet's container wall in this patient. *(Courtesy of Dr. Emil J. Balthazar, Professor of Radiology, New York University, New York, New York.)*

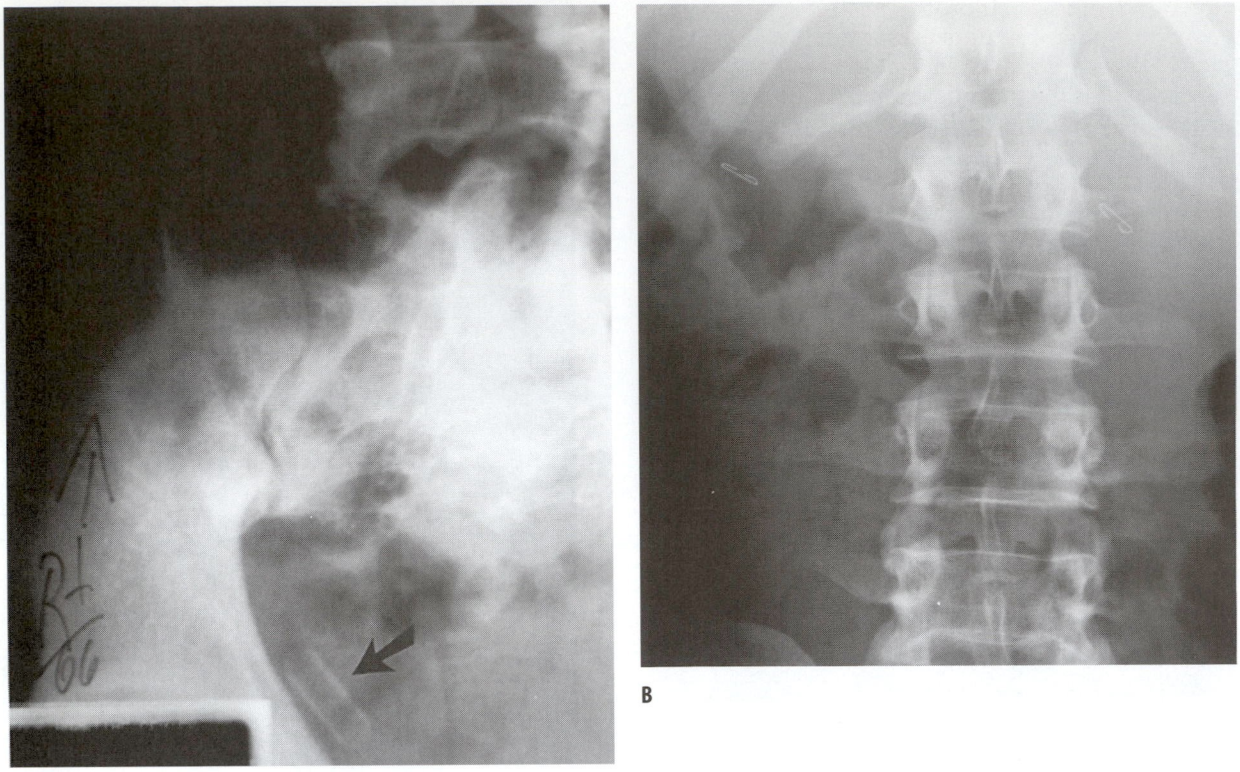

A B

Figure 7–8. Two "body stuffers." Radiography will help with the diagnosis only very infrequently. (**A**) An ingested glass crack vial is seen in the distal bowel (*arrow*). The patient had ingested his contraband several hours earlier at the time of a police raid. Only the tubular-shaped container, and not the drug, are visible radiographically. The patient did not develop signs of cocaine intoxication during 24 hours of observation. (**B**) Another patient in police custody was brought to the ED for allegedly ingesting his drugs. The patient repeatedly denied this. The radiographs revealed "nonsurgical" staples in his abdomen. When questioned again, the patient admitted that he has swallowed several plastic bags that were stapled closed. His chest radiograph revealed a bag stuck in his esophagus at the level of the aortic knob. This would have necessitated endoscopic removal, but a second film taken a short while later showed that the bag had passed into the abdomen. See also Figure 22–1—esophageal obstruction due to a hashish-filled toy balloon.

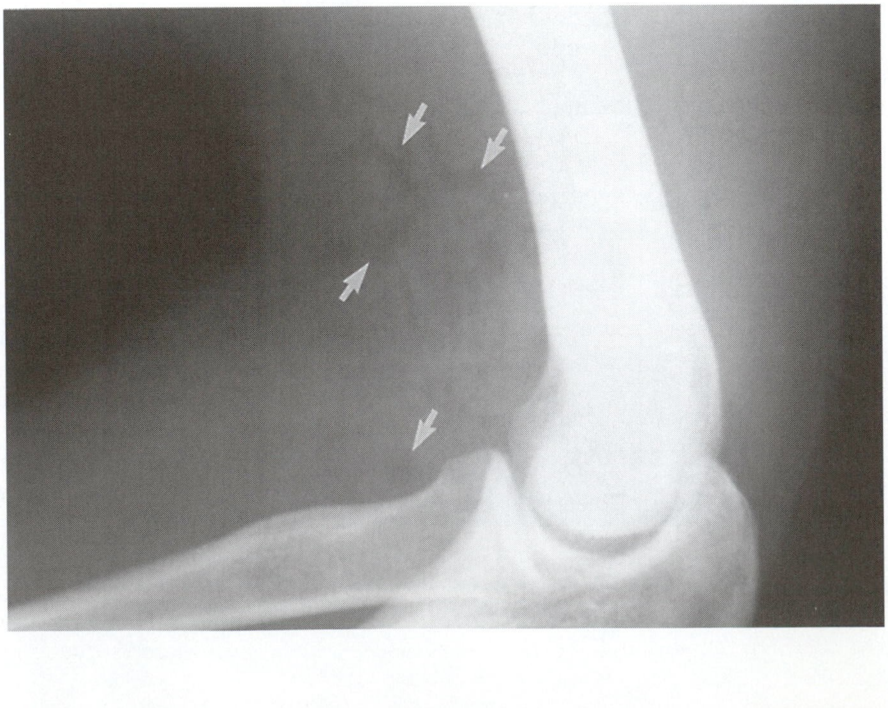

Figure 7–9. Subcutaneous injection of gasoline into the antecubital fossa. The radiolucent hydrocarbon mimics gas in the soft tissues as would be seen with a necrotizing soft-tissue infection such as necrotizing fasciitis or gas gangrene (*arrows*). The patient presented with localized redness, warmth, swelling, and fever. Sterile fluid collections without gas or purulence were found during surgical debridement. *(Courtesy of the Toxicology Fellowship of the New York City Poison Center.)*

chloride (CCl_4) and chloroform ($CHCl_3$) are radiopaque. Since these liquids are immiscible in water, they produce a triple layer in the stomach on an upright abdominal film: an uppermost air bubble, a middle radiodense chlorinated hydrocarbon layer, and a lower gastric fluid layer. However, these ingestions are rare, and even less frequently the quantity ingested is great enough to show this effect. A recent case report describes radiographic visualization of another halogenated hydrocarbon, methylene iodide[144] (see Chap. 85).

Summary

Obtaining an abdominal film in an attempt to identify pills or other toxins in a patient with an unknown ingestion is unlikely to be helpful and is, in general, not warranted. Radiography is most useful when the suspected substance is known to be consistently radiodense, such as is the case with iron compounds and heavy metals. The toxin can be radiographed either within the patient's abdomen, wherever else it might be located in the patient's body, or outside of the patient if uningested material is available. A "body packer" whose intestinal tract contains a large number of packets can also be reliably diagnosed by plain film radiography. Small numbers of radiolucent packets can be detected with the use of enteric radiographic contrast material.

Imaging the Effects of a Toxin on the Body

Imaging the effects of a toxin on the various organ systems of the body can assist in establishing a diagnosis, directing patient management, and detecting complications of the exposure. Although virtually any organ system can be affected, from an imaging standpoint, the most important are the lungs, the central nervous system, the gastrointestinal tract, and the skeleton. Many different imaging techniques can be used. The lungs and skeletal system are amenable to plain film visualization. Abdominal pathology can be detected to a limited extent on plain abdominal radiographs, although contrast studies and computed tomography are also useful. Imaging of the central nervous system involves the use of x-ray computed tomography, magnetic resonance imaging, and nuclear scintigraphy.

Skeletal Changes due to Toxins and Medications

Bone is readily visualized by conventional radiography because of its high content of calcium. Alterations in skeletal structure due to various pathologic processes are detectable radiographically, although such changes occur gradually and are usually not visible for at least 2 weeks. A number of medications and toxins affect bone mineralization and are therefore amenable to radiographic diagnosis. Toxicologic effects on bone can result in either increased or decreased bone mineralization (Table 7–1). Some toxins produce a characteristic radiographic picture, although the exact diagnosis usually depends on correlation with the clinical scenario.[5,100]

TABLE 7–1. TOXICOLOGIC CAUSES OF SKELETAL ABNORMALITIES

Toxins Causing Increased Bone Density	Toxins Causing Diminished Bone Density (diffuse osteoporosis or focal lesions)
Transverse Metaphyseal Bands (pediatric) Chondrosclerosis due to toxic effect on bone growth, not toxin deposition; may disappear. Distinguish from "growth arrest" or "stress," lines not toxin related and often persistent.	Corticosteroids: Osteoporosis: diffuse Osteonecrosis: focal eg, avascular necrosis of the femoral head. Loss of volume with both increased and decreased bone density. Osteonecrosis also occurs in alcoholism, bismuth arthropathy, Caisson's disease (dysbarism), etc.
Diffusely Increased Bone Density Fluorosis (adult and pediatric): Osteosclerosis, osteophytosis, ligament calcification. Usually involves the axial skeleton (vertebrae and pelvis) and can cause compression of the spinal cord and nerve roots. Hypervitaminosis A (pediatric): Cortical hyperostosis and subperiosteal new bone formation. Diaphysis of long bones may have an undulating appearance. Hypervitaminosis D (pediatric): Generalized osteosclerosis, cortical thickening, and metaphyseal bands.	Hypervitaminosis D (adult): Focal or generalized osteoporosis. Osteomyelitis (focal lytic lesions): Intravenous drug use causing septic emboli. Vertebral bodies and sterno-manubrial joint most commonly affected. Acro-osteolysis (distal phalanges): Vinyl chloride monomer.

In a young child who presents with anemia, neuropathy, or encephalopathy, lead poisoning should be suspected. Skeletal radiography can add support to the diagnosis of lead poisoning before a blood lead level or erythrocyte protoporphyrin measurement is determined. Lead lines are most often seen in children 2 to 9 years of age and are most prominent in rapidly growing tubular bones such as the distal femur and proximal tibia. The metaphyseal region of long bones develop layers of increased density along the growth plate (Fig. 7–10).[112] Flaring of the distal metaphysis also occurs with lead toxicity. Lead lines can be seen in the axial skeleton (vertebral bodies) and such flat bones as the iliac crest. Although an early report noted that lead lines did not appear below a blood lead level of 70 μg/dL,[118] a more recent study detected lead lines in approximately 80% of children with a mean lead level of 49 ± 17 μg/dL.[13] It generally takes several weeks for lead lines to appear, although in very young infants (2–4 months old) they can form within days of exposure.[147] After exposure ceases, the lead lines diminish and may eventually disappear.[118]

Lead lines are not due to the deposition of lead in bone, but are due to its toxic effect on bone growth. Lead impedes the remodeling of calcified cartilage in the zone

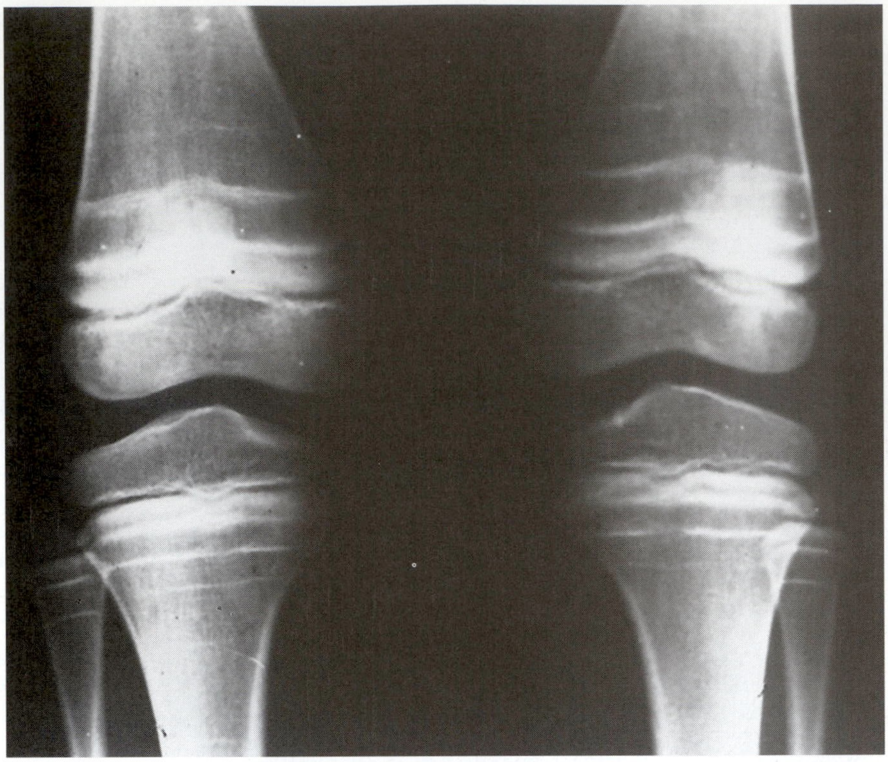

A

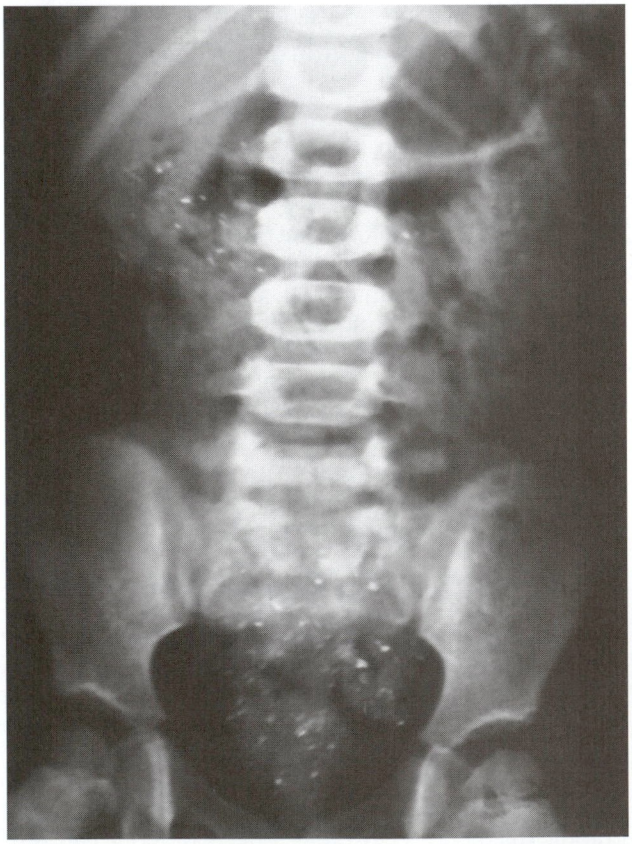

B

Figure 7–10. (**A**) A radiograph of a child's rapidly growing long bones, such as the bones about the knee, reveals several transverse bands of increased density representing bone growth abnormalities due to lead exposure. The multiplicity of lines implies repeated exposures to lead. (**B**) The abdominal radiograph of the child shows many intraluminal radiopaque flakes of leaded paint chips. *(Courtesy of Dr. Nancy Genieser, Professor of Radiology, New York University, New York, New York.)*

of provisional calcification just below the growth plate. This effect is termed chondrosclerosis.[13,30] Lead lines should be distinguished from the common "stress" lines or "growth arrest" lines. "Stress" lines are thin transverse lines seen in long bones and represent transient slowing of bone growth due to illness or trauma in childhood. "Stress" lines can persist into adulthood. Lead poisoning itself can leave residual "growth arrest" lines.

Other toxins that cause metaphyseal bands are yellow phosphorus and bismuth. Phosphorized cod liver oil was previously used to treat rickets and tuberculosis, while bismuth injections were used to treat syphilis. Today, exposures to yellow phosphorus and bismuth are usually the result of industrial exposures and suicide attempts. Other medical conditions that cause metaphyseal banding include transplacental infections, leukemia, hypothyroidism, and hypervitaminosis D (see Chap. 36).

Fluoride poisoning causes a diffuse increase in bone density. Endemic fluorosis occurs where drinking water contains very high levels of fluoride (at least two or more parts per million) or as an occupational exposure for aluminum workers handling cryolite (sodium-aluminum fluoride).[14] Fluorosis primarily affects the axial skeleton, especially the vertebral column and pelvis, and teeth. The skeletal changes associated with fluorosis are osteosclerosis, osteophytosis, and ligament calcification. Thickening of the vertebral column can cause compression of the spinal cord and nerve roots. Without a history of fluoride exposure, these clinical and radiographic findings can be mistaken for osteoblastic skeletal metastasis. The diagnosis of fluorosis is confirmed by histologic examination of the bone and measurement of fluoride levels in the bone and urine.[14]

Skeletal disorders that result in focal diminished bone density (or mixed sclerosis and rarefaction) include osteonecrosis, osteomyelitis, and osteolysis. There are many causes of osteonecrosis, also known as avascular necrosis, which most often affects the femoral head, the humeral head, and proximal tibia.[84] Toxicologic causes of osteonecrosis include long-term corticosteroid use and alcoholism. Osteonecrosis causes bone resorption due to necrosis resulting in skeletal lucencies and healing causing focal sclerosis. There is loss of bone volume and collapse (Fig. 7–11A). Acro-osteolysis refers to bone resorption of the distal phalanges and is associated with occupational exposure to vinyl chloride monomer. Protective measures have reduced its incidence since it was first described in the early 1960s.[113]

Osteomyelitis can complicate intravenous drug use and most often affects the axial skeleton, especially the vertebral bodies and intervertebral disks, and the sternum and sternoclavicular joints. Back pain or neck pain in these patients always merits serious consideration since vertebral osteomyelitis can be accompanied by a spinal epidural abscess and spinal cord compression (Fig. 7–11B).[62,71,94]

Pulmonary and Other Thoracic Complications

A large number of toxicologic disorders can cause abnormalities on chest radiographs.[4,8,40,96] These disorders most often involve the lungs, but the pleura, hilum, heart, and great vessels can also be affected (Table 7–2). Chest radiographs are most helpful in evaluating patients with respiratory distress and should be obtained in patients with dyspnea, tachypnea, rales or rhonchi, and hypoxemia.[1] Fever with or without respiratory symptoms can be caused by aspiration or by a medication reaction associated with lymphoid hyperplasia or a pleural effusion. Patients with chest pain may have a pneumothorax, pneumomediastinum, or aortic dissection, which can be diagnosed by chest radiography.

Many pulmonary disorders are radiographically detectable because they result in fluid accumulation within the air-filled lung. This fluid can be either edema, cellular material (inflammatory, fibrotic, or neoplastic), or blood. Most toxins are widely distributed throughout the lungs and produce a diffuse homogeneous or patchy radiographic abnormality rather than a focal opacity. The fluid accumulates within either the airspaces or interstitial tissues of the lung, and two major radiographic categories of pulmonary disease processes are airspace filling and interstitial lung disorders. Even though the disorders that cause these two radiographic patterns sometimes overlap, distinguishing airspace filling from interstitial abnormalities can help suggest certain diagnoses.

A chest radiograph is usually obtained when a specific toxic exposure is known or suspected. The radiograph can confirm the diagnosis, assess its severity, or detect complications. When the history of toxin exposure is obscure, a patient with an abnormal chest radiograph may initially be misdiagnosed as having pneumonia or another disorder that is more common than toxin-mediated lung disease.[113] Therefore, in all patients with chest radiographic abnormalities, a careful history must be obtained regarding possible exposures at work or at home and about the use of medications or other drugs.

In some cases, the chest radiograph will be negative despite significant pulmonary dysfunction. This can be because a delay often occurs between the time of exposure, the onset of symptoms, and the development of radiographic abnormalities. The initial radiograph may not reflect the full extent of the injury. If the pathologic insult does not cause intrapulmonary fluid accumulation, radiographic changes will not develop. Examples of this include reactive airways disease and emphysematous parenchymal destruction.

The lung is especially vulnerable to toxin exposure since lung tissue can have direct contact with a toxin by inhalation or aspiration. Toxins can also enter the lung via the pulmonary circulation. Last, toxins can exert systemic effects on the lung either by direct alveolar cell toxicity or by immunologically mediated lung damage. Other factors such as hypoxia, hypotension, hypoventilation, or aspiration of gastric contents due to CNS depression can contribute to pulmonary injury.

Diffuse Airspace Filling. Noncardiogenic pulmonary edema due to leaky, damaged capillary endothelium can be caused by overdose of salicylates, opioids, and cocaine (Fig. 7–12).[54,58,124,130,145] There are many other disorders that cause an acute respiratory distress syn-

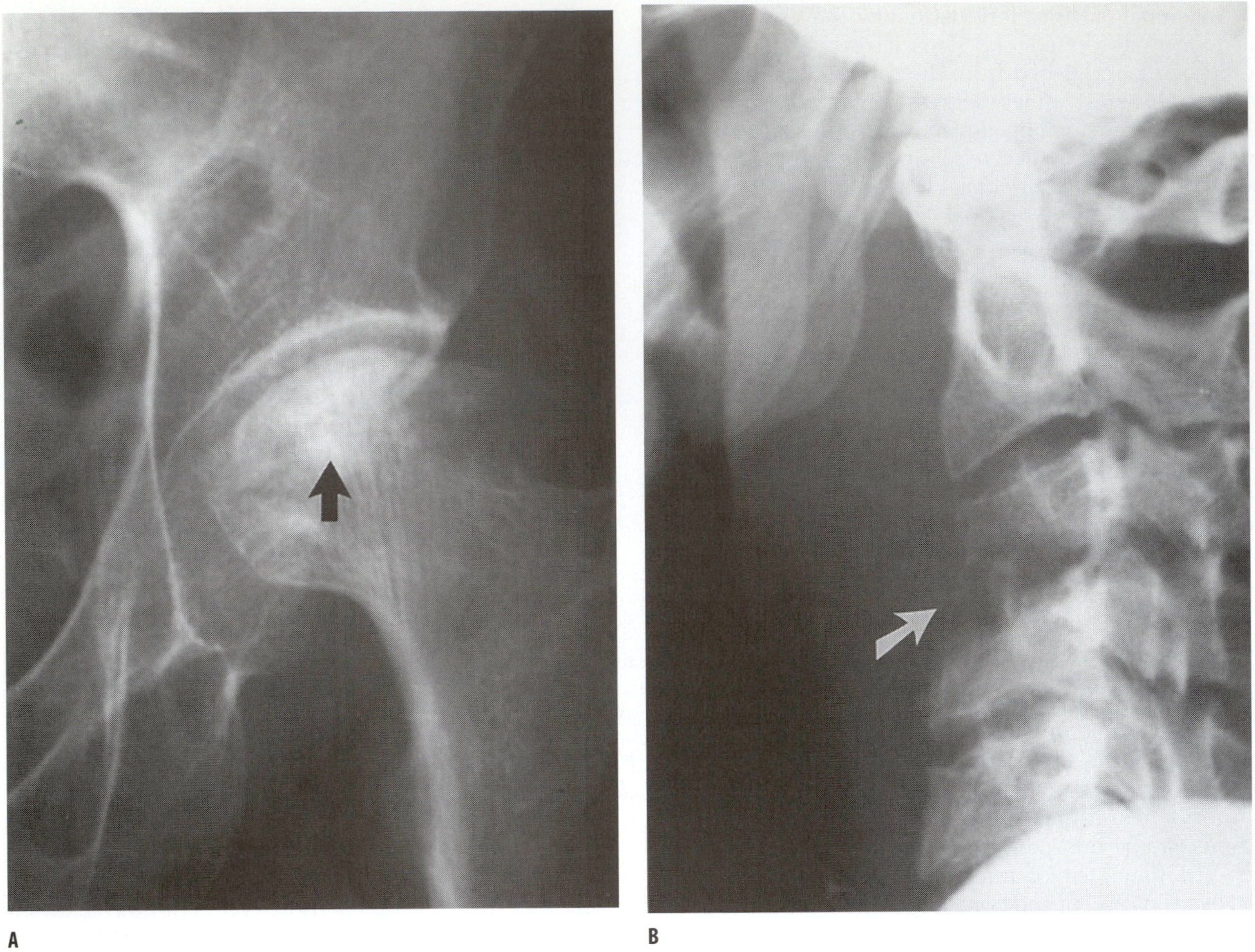

Figure 7–11. (**A**) Avascular necrosis causing collapse of the femoral head (*arrow*) in a patient with long-standing steroid-dependent asthma. (**B**) A patient with vertebral body osteomyelitis complicating intravenous drug use. He presented with neck pain, fever, and signs of spinal cord compression that developed over 1–2 weeks. Destruction of the endplates of C_3 and C_4 are seen (*arrow*). He underwent surgical decompression, iliac crest bone graft, and stabilization by plates and screws. Operative culture grew *Staphylococcus aureus.*

drome, including sepsis, anaphylaxis, near-drowning, major trauma, and pancreatitis. Noncardiogenic pulmonary edema must be distinguished from cardiogenic pulmonary edema, which can be due to alcoholic cardiomyopathy, and multilobar pneumonia. Smoking "crack" cocaine is also associated with diffuse intrapulmonary hemorrhage.[38] Other toxic exposures that result in diffuse airspace filling include inhalation of low- and intermediate-water solubility irritant gases, such as nitrogen dioxide (Silo Filler's Disease; Chap. 110), phosgene ($COCl_2$), chlorine, and sulfur dioxide (Chaps. 94–97). Organophosphate insecticide poisoning causes cholinergic hyperstimulation, resulting in bronchorrhea and diffuse airspace opacities (Chap. 87).

Focal Airspace Filling. Although focal lung infiltrates are most often due to bacterial pneumonia, aspiration can also cause localized airspace disease.[133] During aspiration, the most dependent portions of the lung are affected. When the patient is upright at the time of aspiration, the lower lung segments are involved. When the patient is recumbent, the posterior segments of the upper and lower lobes are affected. Aspiration of gastric contents can complicate a sedative drug or alcohol intoxication and also can occur during a seizure.

Ingestion of low-viscosity hydrocarbons is often accompanied by aspiration at the time the liquid is swallowed. This occurs in children with accidental ingestion of household products such as pine oil or kerosene, and in adults who have siphoned gasoline (Fig. 7–13). A chest radiograph obtained 6 hours after the ingestion will confirm the diagnosis of aspiration based on the patient's symptoms or physical examination findings. Patients with radiographic abnormalities and clinical signs of aspiration need to be hospitalized for close observation.[3]

Multifocal airspace filling occurs with septic pulmonary emboli, which can complicate intravenous drug

TABLE 7–2. CHEST RADIOGRAPHIC FINDINGS IN TOXIC EXPOSURES

Radiographic Pattern	Disease Processes	Responsible Agents	Other Diagnoses
Diffuse Airspace Filling	Acute respiratory distress syndrome Leaky capillaries	Salicylates Opioids Cocaine (also diffuse pulmonary hemorrhage)	Congestive heart failure Pneumonia: usually causes a focal infiltrate, but may be multifocal
	Cardiogenic pulmonary edema	Alcoholic cardiomyopathy, cocaine, cobalt	
	Cholinergic stimulation Bronchorrhea	Organophosphates, carbamates	
	Inhalant lung injury Low and intermediate water-solubility irritant gases	NO_2 (Silo Filler's Disease), Phosgene ($COCl_2$), Cl_2	
Focal Airspace Filling	Aspiration pneumonitis	Low-viscosity hydrocarbons Gastric contents: CNS depressants, alcohol, seizure	Pneumonia Septic emboli (IVDU)
Interstitial Patterns	Hypersensitivity pneumonitis:		
Fine reticular, nodular and reticulonodular	Medications	Nitrofurantoin, sulfa, etc	Asthma (clear chest film)
Coarse reticular fibrosis (honey comb)	Inhaled allergens (extrinsic allergic alveolitis)	Farmer's Lung, Pigeon Breeder's Lung, etc	Lymphangitic carcinomatosis Opportunistic infection, CHF
Patchy airspace filling may be seen in some cases	Cytotoxic lung damage	Chemotherapeutic agents (busulfan, bleomycin, methotrexate, etc)	CHF (interstitial)
	Phospholipidosis	Amiodarone	
	Injected particulates	Talcosis (illicit drug contaminant)	
	Pneumoconiosis	Asbestosis, silicosis, coal dust, beryllium	

use and right-sided bacterial endocarditis. The foci of pulmonary infection often undergo necrosis and cavitation (Fig. 7–14).

Interstitial Patterns. Interstitial lung diseases have an acute, subacute, or chronic course. Acute interstitial disorders include mild pulmonary edema or acute viral pneumonitis. Subacute interstitial lung disorders occur over days or weeks. They have a fine reticular, nodular, or reticulonodular pattern. Chronic interstitial disorders cause a coarse reticular pattern with loss of lung volume which, in its extreme form, results in "honeycomb" lung.

Hypersensitivity pneumonitis is a delayed-type hypersensitivity reaction to an ingested or inhaled substance.[25,114] When the allergen is inhaled, the disorder is also known as "extrinsic allergic alveolitis." Hypersensitivity pneumonitis occurs in sensitized persons who are exposed to various organic allergens such as those in moldy hay (Farmer's Lung) and bird droppings (Pigeon Breeder's Lung). There are two clinical syndromes: an acute, recurrent illness and a chronic, progressive form. The acute illness presents with fever and dyspnea that can mimic pneumonia or asthma. Symptoms abate when the patient is away from the allergen and recur with reexposure. In such cases, the chest radiograph is often normal or may show fine interstitial or alveolar infiltrates. The chronic form presents with insidious and progressive dyspnea, with the radiograph showing an interstitial fibrosis pattern. Diagnosis depends on a history of exposure that is usually related to certain occupations or hobbies.

The most common medication implicated in hypersensitivity pneumonitis is nitrofurantoin. The onset is 1 to 2 weeks into the course of the medication. Other medications that can cause hypersensitivity pneumonitis include sulfonamides and penicillins.

Many chemotherapeutic agents cause pulmonary injury by their direct toxic effect on alveolar and endothelial cells.[26,42] These agents include busulfan, bleomycin, cyclophosphamide, and methotrexate. The radiographic pattern is usually interstitial (reticular or nodular), but can include airspace filling or mixed patterns. The clinical course is progressive, beginning several weeks into therapy, and is related to the total cumulative dose. The patient presents with dyspnea, fever, and pulmonary infiltrates. The abnormality will often resolve with discontinuation of the offending medication. These clinical and radiographic findings must be distinguished from opportunistic infection, carcinomatosis, pulmonary edema, and intrapulmonary hemorrhage.

There are several other toxicologic causes of interstitial lung disease. Amiodarone toxicity causes phospholipid deposits to accumulate within alveolar cells. The radiographic appearance is interstitial, although airspace filling also occurs (Fig. 7–15). Injection of illicit drugs, which often have particulate contaminants such as talc, causes chronic interstitial lung disease.[35] Last, certain inhaled particulates such as asbestos, silica, and coal dust cause a pneumoconiosis, which is a chronic interstitial

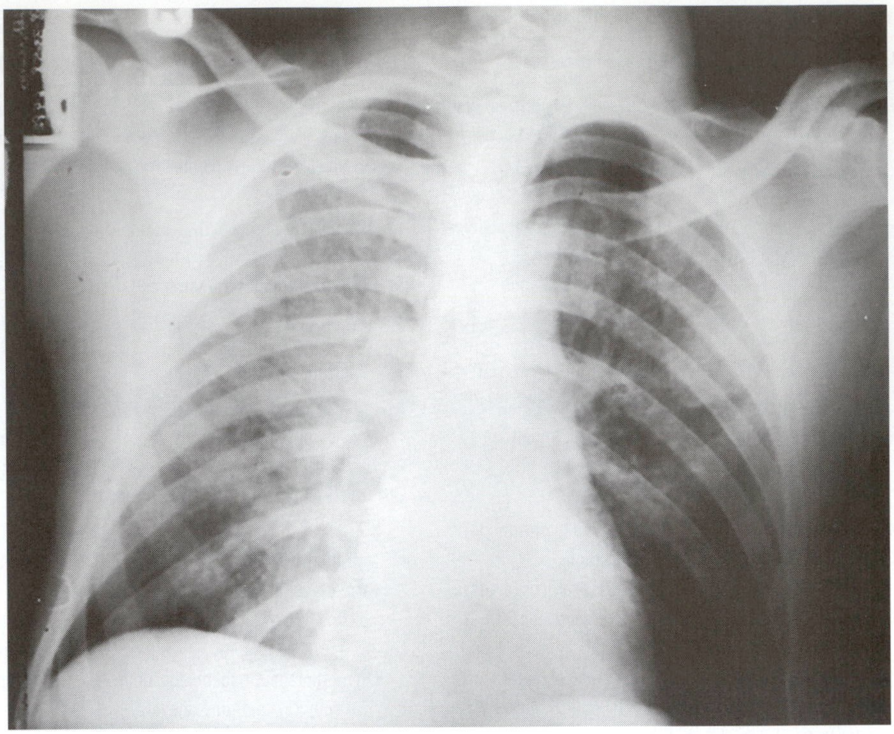

Figure 7–12. The chest radiograph of a patient who had recently injected heroin intravenously with resultant respiratory distress and pulmonary edema. The heart is of normal size, which makes cardiogenic pulmonary edema unlikely. Other diagnostic possibilities include pneumonia and aspiration of gastric contents. The rapid resolution with clearing of the radiograph in 2 days is typical of heroin-induced noncardiogenic pulmonary edema. Other overdoses that can produce this radiographic pattern include salicylates and cocaine.

lung disease[143] characterized by interstitial fibrosis and loss of lung volume. One of the clinical challenges in managing patients with a pneumoconiosis is to distinguish associated pulmonary conditions such as tuberculosis and carcinoma. Chest CT has greater sensitivity in detecting such lesions, although the final diagnosis depends on examination of sputum or lung tissue.[93]

Pleural Disease. Pleural effusions are seen in drug-induced lupus syndromes.[96] The most frequently implicated medications are procainamide, hydralazine, isoniazid, methyldopa, and chlorpropamide. The patient presents with fever and other symptoms of systemic lupus. Other disorders that can cause pleural effusions are neoplasia, congestive heart failure, and various infections.

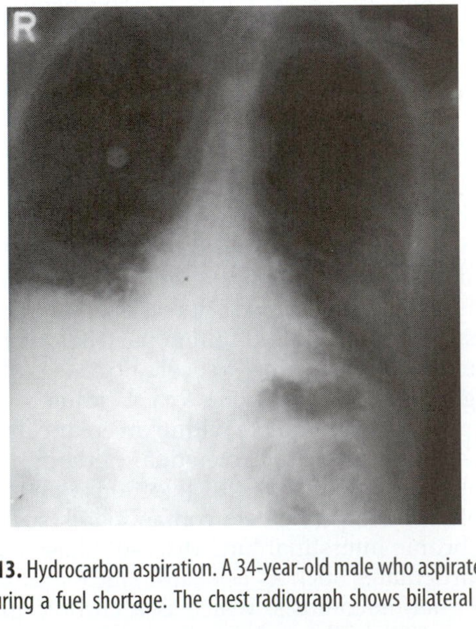

Figure 7–13. Hydrocarbon aspiration. A 34-year-old male who aspirated while siphoning during a fuel shortage. The chest radiograph shows bilateral lower lobe infiltrates.

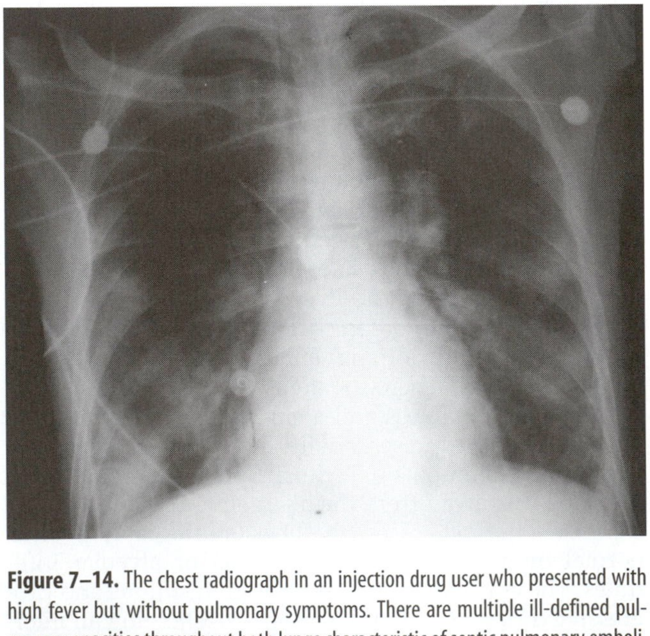

Figure 7–14. The chest radiograph in an injection drug user who presented with high fever but without pulmonary symptoms. There are multiple ill-defined pulmonary opacities throughout both lungs characteristic of septic pulmonary emboli. His blood cultures grew *Staphylococcus aureus*.

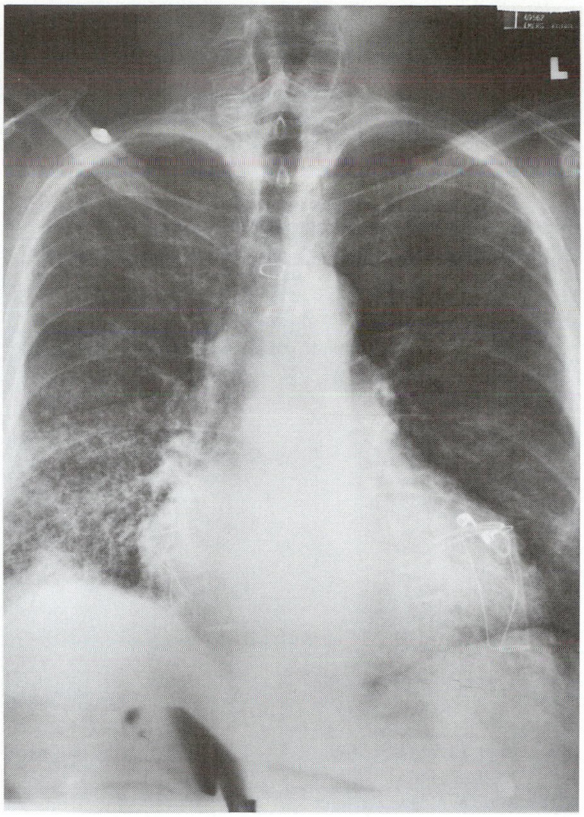

Figure 7–15. The chest radiograph of a patient with cardiac disease who presented to the ED with progressive dyspnea. The radiograph shows a reticular (interstitial) pattern. The initial diagnostic impression was pulmonary edema (interstitial). The patient was on amiodarone for malignant ventricular dysrythmias (note the implanted automatic defibrillator). The lack of response to diuretics and the high-resolution CT pattern suggested that this was actually toxicity to amiodarone. The drug was stopped and there was partial clearing over several weeks. *(Courtesy of Dr. Georgeann McGuinness, Department of Radiology, New York University, New York, New York.)*

Pneumothorax and pneumomediastinum are associated with illicit drug use. These findings are related to the route of administration rather than to the particular drug. Barotrauma caused by forceful inhalation of "crack" cocaine or marijuana results in pneumomediastinum (Fig. 7–16A).[31,104] A chest radiograph can therefore be helpful in a patient with cocaine-related chest pain. Forceful vomiting caused by syrup of ipecac or alcoholism can produce esophageal tears and pneumomediastinum.[146] Attempted intravenous injection into the subclavian and jugular veins is a common cause of pneumothorax in certain patient populations.[29]

Asbestos-related calcified pleural plaques develop many years after the exposure. These lesions are asymptomatic and have only a weak association with malignancy and interstitial lung disease. These pleural plaques should not be called "asbestosis" since that term refers to the interstitial lung disease caused by asbestos. Pleural plaques must be distinguished from mesothelioma, which is not calcified, enlarges at a more rapid rate and is associated with erosion into nearby structures such as the ribs (Fig. 7–17).

Lymphadenopathy. Phenytoin is a common cause of drug-induced lymphoid hyperplasia with hilar lymphadenopathy.[96] The patient presents with a febrile illness, often without respiratory symptoms.

Cardiovascular Abnormalities. The chest radiograph can provide a rough estimate of cardiac size and the anatomy of mediastinal great vessels. Cardiac enlargement due to dilated cardiomyopathy is seen in chronic alcoholism and with exposure to cardiotoxic medications such as adriamycin. Enlargement of the cardiac silhouette can also be due to a pericardial effusion, which can accompany a drug-induced lupus syndrome. Last, aortic dissection has been reported following use of cocaine and is another cause of cocaine-related chest pain.[43,111] The chest radiograph may show an enlarged or indistinct aortic knob as well as dilation of the ascending and descending aorta (Fig. 7–16B).

Abdominal Complications

Plain Abdominal Radiography. The plain abdominal radiograph has a limited ability to demonstrate abdominal complications in toxicologic emergencies. Depending on the diagnoses being considered, abdominal radiography can be helpful in evaluating patients with abdominal pain, vomiting, abdominal distention, or constipation. In particular, conventional radiography can detect upper alimentary tract perforation, intestinal obstruction, and adynamic ileus. An additional role of abdominal radiography is the identification of radiodense foreign bodies such as ingested pills and toxins, as described earlier in this chapter (Table 7–3).[49,81,85,92]

Gastrointestinal perforation is usually diagnosed by seeing free intraperitoneal air under the diaphragm on an upright chest radiograph. Esophageal perforation causes pneumomediastinum and mediastinitis. Esophageal and gastric perforation can occur following the ingestion of a highly caustic substance such as iron, alkali, or acid. Peptic ulcer perforation has been associated with crack cocaine use.[20,72] Esophageal or gastric perforation can complicate orogastric tube placement and lavage and syrup of ipecac–induced emesis (Fig. 7–18).[146]

Mechanical bowel obstruction can be caused by large intraluminal foreign bodies such as "body packer's" packets.[41] Adynamic ileus can complicate various drug ingestions such as opioids, anticholinergics, tricyclic antidepressants (especially amitriptyline and nortriptyline), and intestinal ischemia due to mesenteric vasospasm (Fig. 7–19).[9,45] Mechanical obstruction can usually be distinguished from adynamic ileus by plain abdominal films, even though both conditions cause distended air-filled loops of bowel. In adynamic ileus, the distention is relatively uniform throughout the entire bowel. With mechanical obstruction, there is a greater amount of intestinal gas and distention proximal to the point of obstruction and a relative paucity of gas and in-

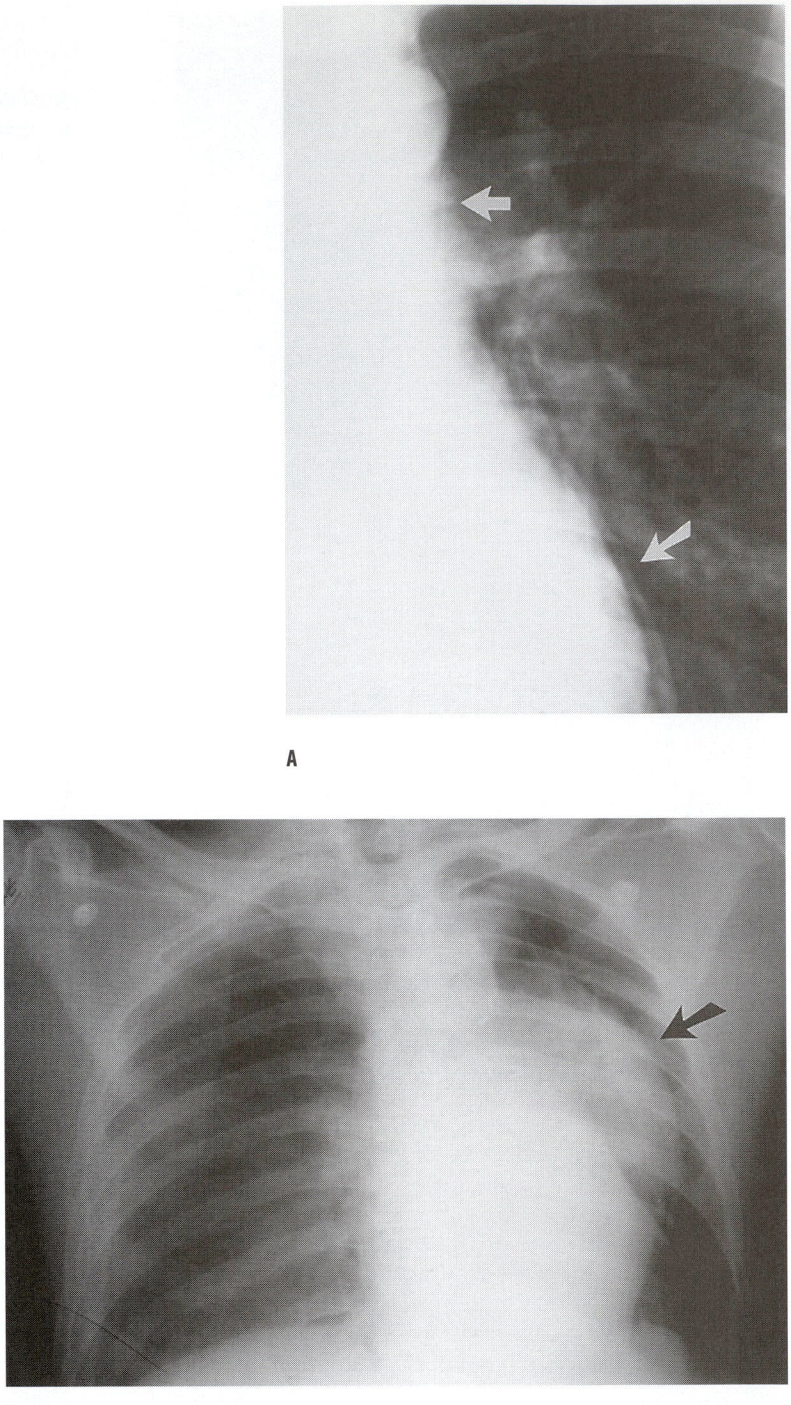

A

B

Figure 7–16. Two patients with chest pain following cocaine use. (**A**) Pneumomediastinum after forceful inhalation while smoking "crack" cocaine. A fine white line representing the pleura elevated from the mediastinal structures is seen (*arrows*). The patient's chest pain resolved over 24 hours of observation. There was no evidence of esophageal or tracheal injury. (**B**) Thoracic aortic dissection and rupture following cocaine use. The patient presented with chest pain radiating to the back. Chest radiography reveals a very wide and indistinct aortic contour (*arrow*). Hypotension and cardiac arrest occurred soon after arrival to the Emergency Department. *(Courtesy of the Toxicology Fellowship of the New York City Poison Center.)*

testinal collapse distal to the point of obstruction. On the upright abdominal radiograph, both intestinal obstruction and adynamic ileus show air–fluid levels. In mechanical obstruction, air–fluid levels are seen at different heights and produce a "step-ladder" appearance. When the diagnosis is uncertain (20–30% of cases), abdominal CT or GI contrast studies are of diagnostic value.[91]

Other abdominal complications of toxicologic exposures such as gastrointestinal bleeding and hepatotoxicity are not usually amenable to radiographic diagnosis. However, in certain circumstances, abdominal radiographs can be helpful. Although radiographs are usually not indicated in patients with gastrointestinal hemorrhage, they can reveal ingested iron pills as a cause of bleeding in a patient too young to give a reliable history.

The now obsolete radiocontrast agent thorium dioxide (Thorotrast) (thorium, atomic number 90) provides an interesting example of pharmaceutical-induced hepa-

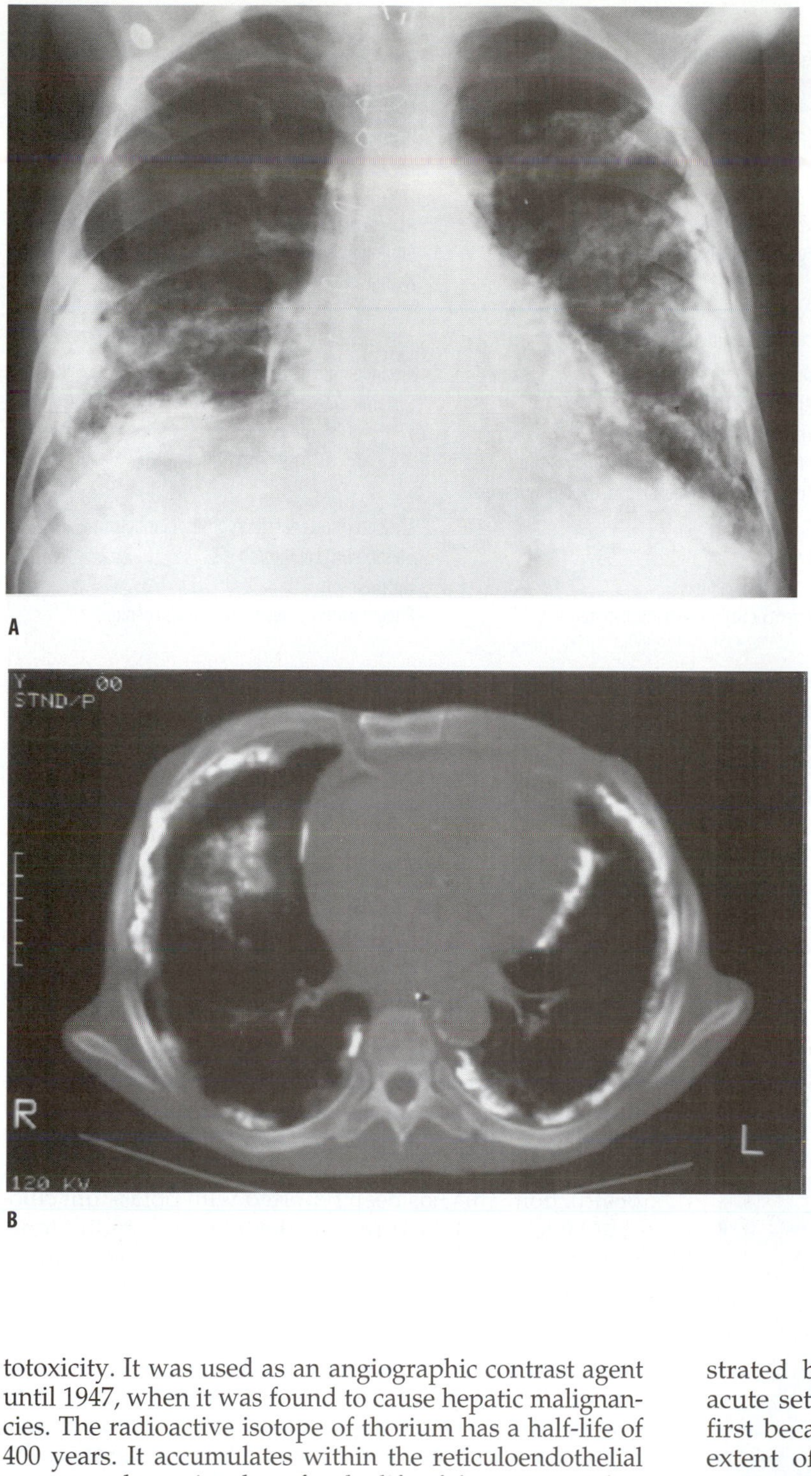

A

B

Figure 7–17. (**A**) Calcified pleural plaques typical of asbestos exposure are seen surrounding the lung and the surface of the diaphragm and heart. The patient was asymptomatic; this was an incidental radiographic finding. The fact that these radiographic opacities do not involve the lung is demonstrated by the patient's CT scan. (**B**) A lower thoracic CT image shows calcified pleural plaques (the diaphragmatic plaque is seen on the right), as well as the absence of any pleural-based tumor or interstitial lung disease ("asbestosis").

totoxicity. It was used as an angiographic contrast agent until 1947, when it was found to cause hepatic malignancies. The radioactive isotope of thorium has a half-life of 400 years. It accumulates within the reticuloendothelial system and remains there for the life of the patient. It has a characteristic radiographic appearance with multiple punctate densities in the liver, spleen, and lymph nodes (Fig. 7–20). These patients are at high risk for hepatic malignancies and pneumococcal sepsis due to their fibrotic spleens.[11,137]

Contrast Esophagram and Upper GI Series. The ingestion of caustic substances can cause severe damage to the mucosal lining of the esophagus. This can be demonstrated by a contrast esophagram, although in the acute setting, upper endoscopy should be performed first because it provides more information about the extent of injury and prognosis.[74] Administration of contrast prior to endoscopy will coat the mucosa, making the procedure difficult. For subsequent evaluation of these patients, a contrast esophagram will identify mucosal defects, scarring, and stricture formation (Fig. 7–21).[86] The choice between barium and a water-soluble contrast agent depends on the complication suspected. If the esophagus is severely strictured and there is risk of aspiration, barium should be used because aspirated water-soluble contrast material is damaging to the pulmonary parenchyma. If, on

TABLE 7–3. PLAIN ABDOMINAL RADIOGRAPHY

Radiographic Finding	Disease Process	Toxicologic Etiologies	Other Diagnoses
Pneumoperitoneum	Perforation of hollow viscus	Caustics: Iron, alkalis, acids Cocaine Syrup of ipecac Lavage tube	Peptic ulcer Cecal distention due to colonic obstruction or volvulus
Mechanical obstruction: Intestinal Gastric outlet	Intraluminal: Obturation Obstruction	Foreign body ingestion: Body packer, enteric-coated pills Bezoar: Gastric outlet obstruction	Adhesions Hernia, etc
Ileus	Diminished gut motility	Opioids Anticholinergics Tricyclic antidepressants Intestinal ischemia: Cocaine, oral contraceptives Toxin induced: Hypokalemia, hypomagnesemia	Intraabdominal disorders Systemic illness (sepsis, electrolyte disturbance, etc)
Intramural gas Also: Bowel wall thickening, thumb-printing, hepatic portal venous gas	Intestinal infarction: Vasospasm, thrombosis, embolization, or hypotension	Cocaine Ergots Oral contraceptives Agents causing systemic hypotension	Mesenteric arterial thrombosis or embolism Mesenteric vein thrombosis Hypotension Pneumatosis cystoides intestinalis (benign)
Radiodense foreign body	Ingestion Rectal or vaginal insertion	Iron pills Heavy metals Bismuth subsalicylate Calcium carbonate Pica (calcareous clay)	Intraabdominal calcifications (uterine fibroids, etc) Retained barium Telepaque

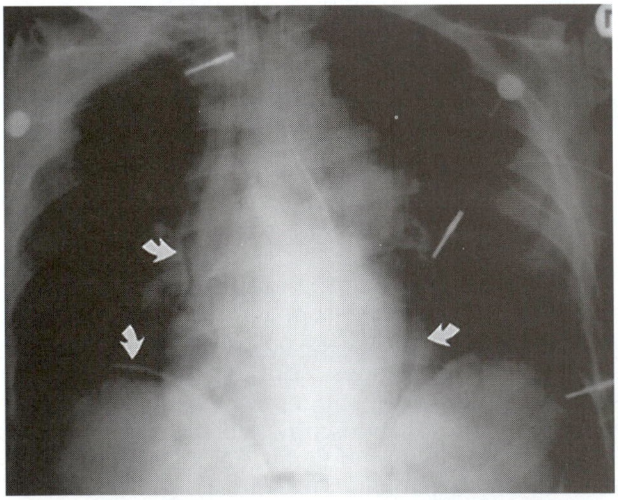

Figure 7–18. GI perforation following gastric lavage with a large bore orogastric tube. The upright chest radiograph shows air under the right hemidiaphragm and pneumomediastinum (*arrows*). An esophagram with water-soluble contrast did not locate the site of perforation. Laparotomy revealed a perforation of the anterior wall of the stomach. Gastric lavage can result in significant complications. This patient had had endotracheal intubation prior to lavage to prevent aspiration.

the other hand, esophageal or gastric perforation is suspected, water-soluble contrast is safer because extravasated barium is highly irritating to mediastinal and peritoneal tissues.

Esophageal and gastric outlet obstruction can be caused by ingested objects. Esophageal obstruction due to a drug packet can be demonstrated by a contrast esophagram (Fig. 22–1). Concretions of ingested material can form bezoars in the stomach, causing gastric outlet obstruction. This has been reported with potassium chloride tablets, sustained-release theophylline, and enteric-coated aspirin.[45,125] Mucosal ulcerations of the stomach and esophagus can be caused by numerous medications, most notably nonsteroidal antiinflammatory drugs.

Abdominal Computed Tomography. Abdominal CT serves an increasingly important role in the diagnosis of a wide variety of intraabdominal disorders. Certain toxicologic complications are amenable to CT diagnosis. Intestinal ischemia and infarction due to mesenteric arterial or venous thrombosis or vasospasm can be caused by cocaine, ergot alkaloids, and oral contraceptives. If there are clinical signs of bowel infarction, the patient should undergo emergency surgery without imaging studies. If the diagnosis is uncertain, an abdominal CT may help determine the etiology in a patient with abdominal pain out of proportion to the findings on physical examination. CT signs of intestinal ischemia are bowel wall thickening, intramural

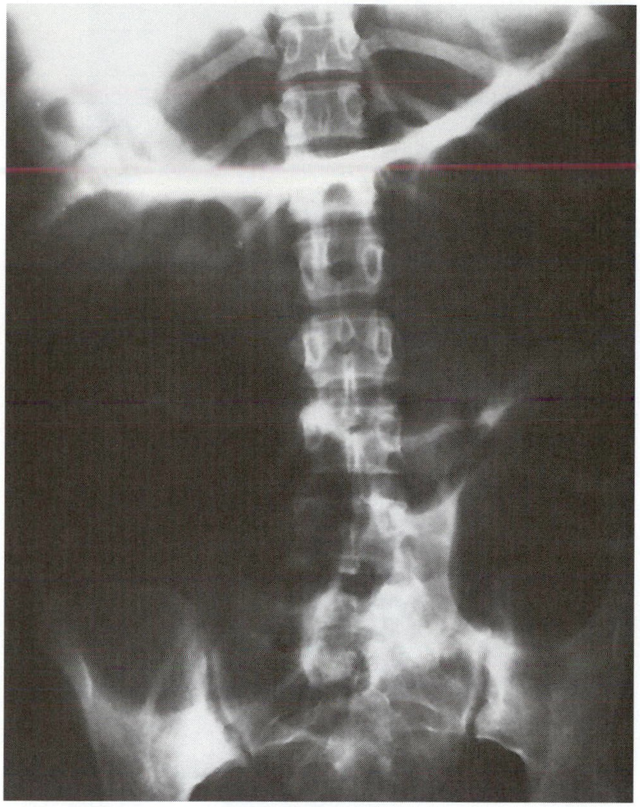

Figure 7–19. Methadone maintenance therapy causing abdominal distention. The radiograph reveals striking large bowel distention, termed colonic ileus or pseudo-obstruction, due to diminished gut motility caused by chronic opioid use. This must be distinguished from distal large bowel mechanical obstruction due to a stricture, volvulus, or an obstructing lesion such as a sigmoid carcinoma or fecal impaction. A contrast enema can help make the diagnosis. *(Courtesy of Dr. Emil J. Balthazar, Professor of Radiology, New York University, New York, New York.)*

hemorrhage, and, at a later stage, intramural gas and hepatic portal venous gas. In a small proportion of patients with ischemic bowel (5%), intramural gas will be visible on plain abdominal films.[9] In many patients with intestinal ischemia, the plain film and CT will show only a nonspecific ileus pattern, so the diagnosis must rest on the clinical presentation when imaging studies are not conclusive.

Some intraabdominal complications of intravenous drug use can be diagnosed on CT. These include splenic infarctions and localized infections such as splenic and psoas abscesses.[9]

Vascular Lesions. Angiography can demonstrate vascular complications of injection drug use such as venous thrombosis or arterial laceration with pseudoaneurysm formation (Figs. 108–3A, B and 108–4). Intravenous amphetamine use can cause necrotizing angiitis that is associated with microaneurysms, segmental stenosis, and thrombosis. Renal lesions are associated with severe hypertension and oliguric renal failure (Fig. 7–22). Fatal complications include aneurysm rupture, visceral infarction, and renal failure. Similar lesions can be demonstrated throughout the arterial tree, including the small bowel, liver, pancreas, and cerebral circulation.[22,110]

Neurologic Complications

Imaging studies have revolutionized the diagnosis of CNS disorders.[48] Both acute focal lesions and chronic degenerative changes can be detected. Central nervous system dysfunction can be caused by a wide variety of toxins.[80] In addition, neurologic injury can be an indirect sequela of toxin exposure related to hypoxia, hypotension, hypertension, cerebral vasospasm, head trauma, or infection (Table 7–4). Some toxins themselves can pro-

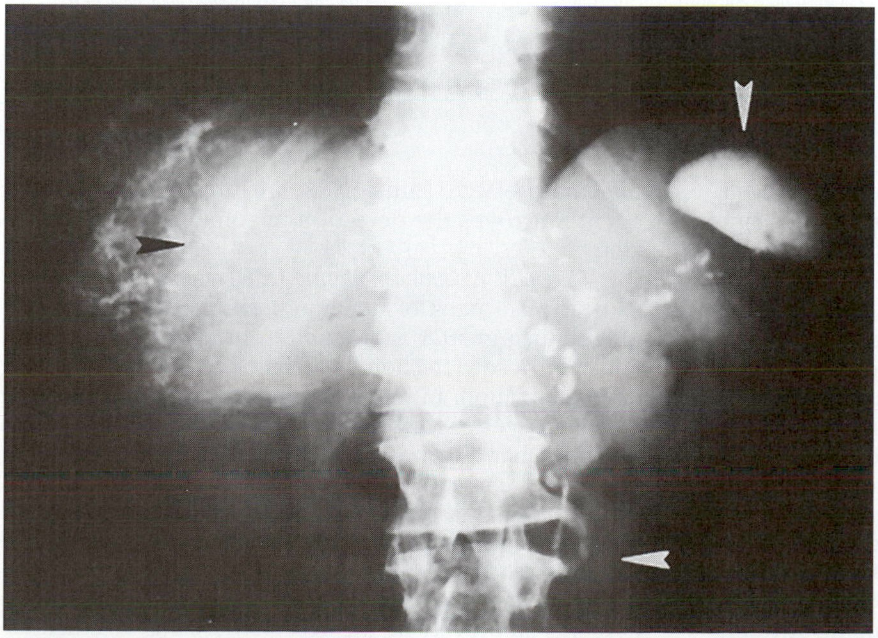

Figure 7–20. The abdominal radiograph of a patient who had received thorium dioxide (Thorotrast) for a radiocontrast study many years previously. The spleen (*vertical white arrow*), liver (*horizontal black arrow*), and lymph nodes (*horizontal white arrow*) are demarcated by thorium retained in the reticuloendothelial system. *(Courtesy of Dr. Emil J. Balthazar, Professor of Radiology, New York University, New York, New York.)*

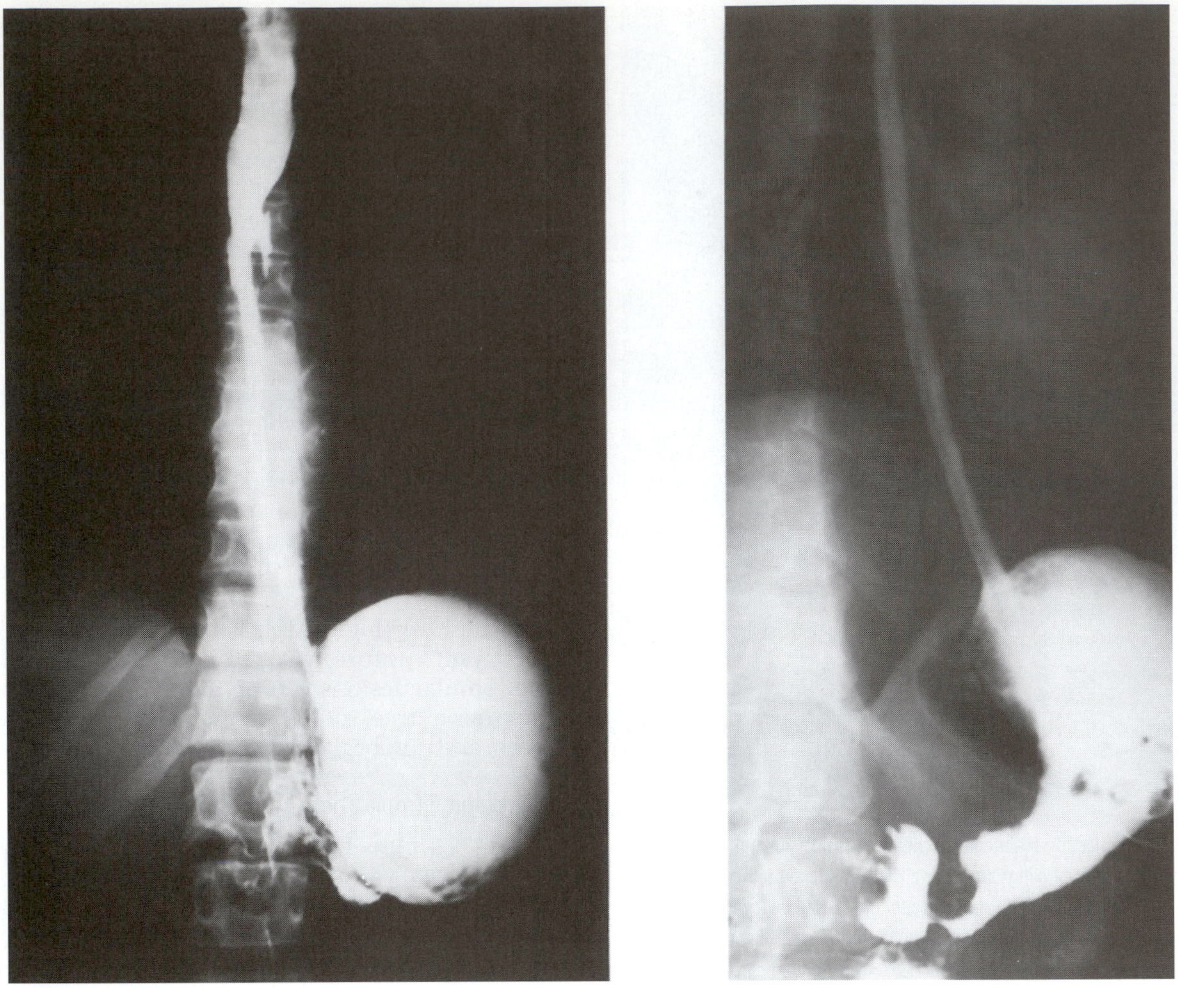

A B

Figure 7–21. (**A**) A barium swallow performed several days after ingestion of liquid lye showed intramural dissection and extravasation of barium with early stricture formation and hypomotility of the remainder of the esophagus. (**B**) At 3 weeks post-ingestion, there is an absence of peristalsis, diffuse narrowing of the esophagus, as well as scarring and reduction in size of the fundus and antrum of the stomach. *(Courtesy of Dr. Emil J. Balthazar, Professor of Radiology, New York University, New York, New York.)*

duce characteristic brain lesions. The medical toxicologist must be knowledgeable about these situations since they can provide a clue to the diagnosis or help assess the patient's prognosis.

Imaging Modalities. Introduced over 20 years ago, x-ray *computed tomography* (CT) was the first major advance in neuroimaging.[46] CT can directly visualize brain tissue and many intracranial lesions. CT is the study of choice in the emergency setting because it readily detects lesions that require emergency intervention, it is fast and widely available on an emergency basis, and it can accommodate invasive supportive and monitoring devices. CT is unsurpassed in its ability to diagnose acute intracranial hemorrhage. It can also detect parenchymal brain lesions that are causing intracranial mass effect. Infusion of an intravenous contrast agent improves the detection of some intracerebral lesions.

Magnetic resonance imaging (MRI) has supplanted CT in nearly all areas of nonemergency neurodiagnosis. It offers much greater anatomic resolution of brain tissues and improved detection of areas of cerebral edema and demyelinization. In the emergency setting, however, the disadvantages of MRI outweigh its strengths. MRI is less sensitive than CT in detecting acute blood collections. It is usually not readily available on an emergency basis. Image acquisition time is long and invasive support and monitoring devices are often incompatible with MR scanning machines.[82]

Nuclear scintigraphy that uses computed tomography is being employed in the research setting to elucidate

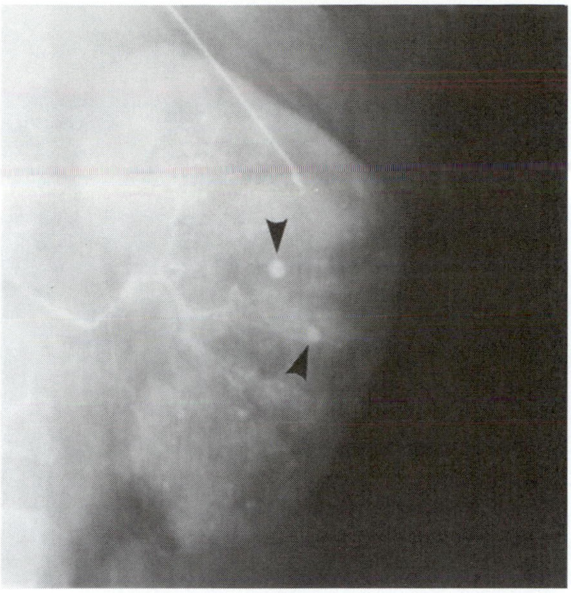

Figure 7–22. A selective renal angiogram in a methamphetamine user demonstrating multiple small and large aneurysms (*arrow*). *(Courtesy of Dr. Richard Lefleur, Associate Professor of Radiology, New York University, New York, New York.)*

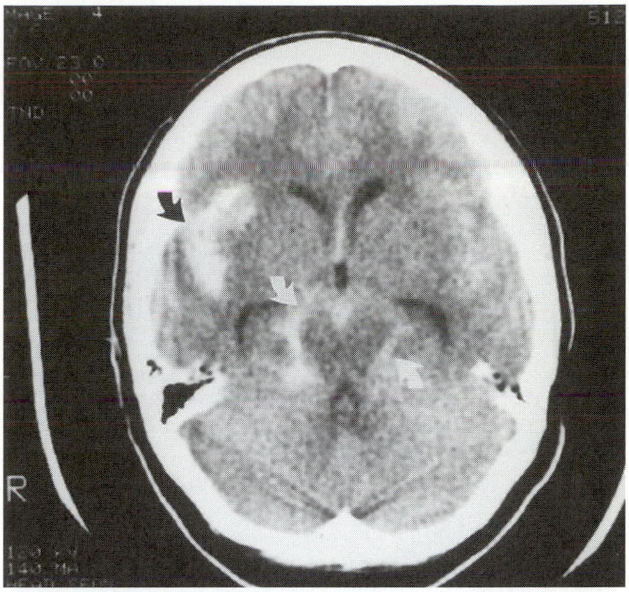

Figure 7–23. Subarachnoid hemorrhage following intravenous cocaine use. The patient had a sudden severe headache followed by a generalized seizure. Extensive hemorrhage is seen surrounding the midbrain at the level of the cerebral peduncles (*white arrows*) and in the right sylvian fissure (*black arrow*). Angiography revealed an aneurysm at the origin of the right middle cerebral artery. The aneurysm rupture was provoked by the acute elevation of blood pressure following a cocaine-induced catecholamine surge.

functional characteristics of the central nervous system. These include immediate and long-term effects of various drugs and toxins on regional brain metabolism, blood flow, and neurotransmitter distribution and function.[77,106]

Emergency Head CT Scanning. An emergency head CT scan is obtained primarily to detect acute intracranial hemorrhage and brain lesions causing mass effect. These lesions produce focal neurologic deficits, seizures, mental status changes, or headache. Toxicologic causes of intraparenchymal and subarachnoid hemorrhage include cocaine or other sympathomimetic drugs (Fig. 7–23). Drug-induced CNS depression predisposes the patient to head trauma, which can result in a subdural hematoma or cerebral contusion. Toxicologic causes of intracerebral mass lesions include septic emboli complicating intravenous drug use and HIV-associated CNS toxoplasmosis or lymphoma.[12,76,79,103] Acute hemorrhage is detected using a noncontrast scan. Tumors and focal infections are best demonstrated with a contrast CT and show a pattern of "ring-enhancement" (Fig. 7–24).

Altered mental status is the most common acute neurologic manifestation of a toxicologic emergency. In

TABLE 7–4. HEAD CT LESIONS

CT Finding	Brain Lesion	Toxicologic Etiology	Other Diagnoses
Hemorrhage	Intraparenchymal bleed Subarachnoid hemorrhage	Cocaine, amphetamine, phenylpropanolamine, phencyclidine, ephedrine, pseudoephedrine, mycotic aneurysm rupture (IVDU)	Hypertension A–V malformation Berry aneurysm
	Subdural hematoma	Trauma secondary to alcohol, sedative-hypotonics, seizure Anticoagulants	Head trauma
Brain lucencies	Basal ganglia focal necrosis (also subcortical white matter lucencies)	Carbon monoxide, cyanide, hydrogen sulfide, methanol	Hypoxia, hypoglycemia
	Stroke—vasospasm	Cocaine, sympathomimetics, ergotamine	Atherosclerotic cerebrovascular disease, embolism
	Mass lesion: tumor, abscess	Septic emboli	CNS tumor CNS abscess
Loss of brain tissue	Atrophy: cerebral, cerebellar	Alcoholism, toluene	Alzheimer's disease
Calcification	Basal ganglia	Carbon monoxide, lead	Physiologic (aging)

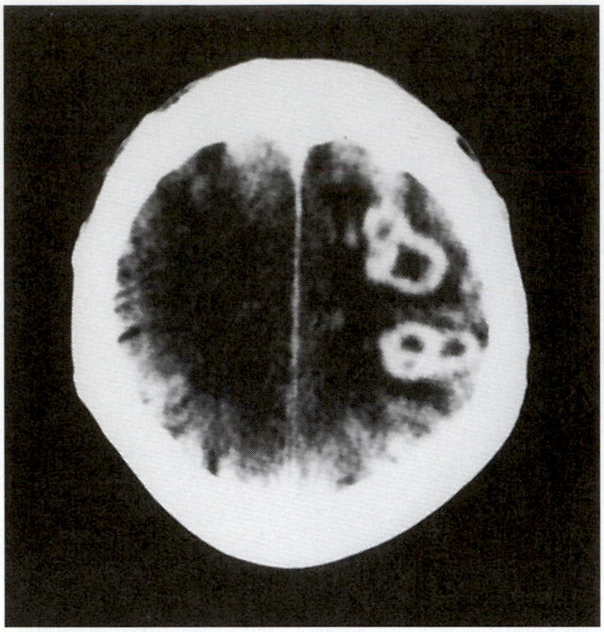

Figure 7–24. A patient with ring-enhancing intracerebral lesions complicating intravenous drug use. The patient presented with fever and altered mental status. In this patient, the lesions represent multiple septic emboli complicating acute *Staphylococcus aureus* bacterial endocarditis. A similar radiographic appearance is seen with lesions due to toxoplasmosis or primary CNS lymphoma in patients with AIDS. The patient was HIV negative and had negative serologic studies for toxoplasmosis.

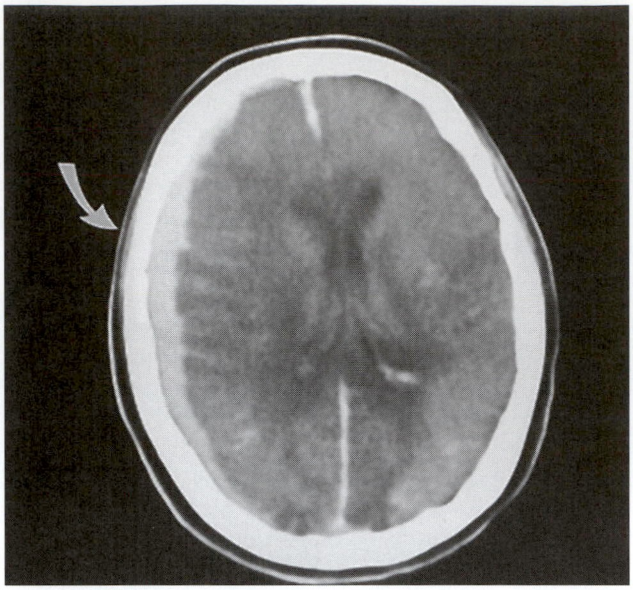

Figure 7–25. An acute subdural hematoma in an alcoholic patient following an alcohol binge. The patient's mental status did not improve during several hours of observation. There were no external signs of head trauma. A crescent-shaped blood collection is seen between the right cerebral convexity and the inner table of the skull (*arrow*).

most instances, imaging studies will be negative, and interrupting patient care to obtain an imaging study delays other, more important interventions. On the other hand, delayed diagnosis of an unsuspected intracranial mass lesion or hemorrhage could have disastrous consequences if imaging is deferred while the patient is being observed for clinical improvement because the altered level of consciousness was mistakenly attributed to an intoxication.

In some patients with altered mental status, an intracranial mass lesion can be present without causing a focal neurologic deficit. These situations include extra-axial lesions such as a subdural hematoma; mass lesions in "silent" areas of the brain; frontal lobe lesions that cause behavioral changes; and lesions that cause minor neurologic deficits that may not be detected in an obtunded patient. It is therefore important to obtain a head CT scan in patients who are at increased risk for an intracerebral mass lesion. Alcoholics, the elderly, and patients taking anticoagulant medications may have a subdural hematoma (Fig. 7–25); these persons have a high frequency of falls, cerebral atrophy, which stretches the bridging dural veins, and a coagulopathy or thrombocytopenia. Illicit drug users are also at great risk for intracranial mass lesions due to vascular or infectious disorders.

In summary, a cranial CT should be obtained in patients with altered mental status if there is a focal neurologic deficit, any evidence of head trauma, or failure to improve over time with frequent serial clinical examinations. Particular attention should be paid to certain patient groups that are at increased risk of intracerebral mass lesions such as alcoholics, injection drug users, and HIV-infected patients.

Toxin-mediated Structural Brain Injury. A number of toxins can directly damage the central nervous system and produce morphologic changes in the brain that are detectable with CT and MRI. These changes include generalized neuronal loss causing atrophy, focal areas of neuronal loss, demyelinization, and cerebral edema. The clinical importance of these imaging studies is not yet definitively established. Imaging abnormalities may help to estimate prognosis in a patient with neurologic dysfunction following a toxin exposure. In some cases, the imaging abnormality might suggest the correct diagnosis in a patient with neurologic disorder of uncertain etiology.[7,68,107]

The most widely used neurotoxin is *ethanol*. With long-term ethanol use, there is a general loss of neurons with resultant atrophy that can be seen with both CT and MRI. In some alcoholics, the loss of brain tissue is especially prominent in the cerebellum. However, the degree of cerebral or cerebellar atrophy does not always correlate with the extent of cognitive impairment or gait disturbance.[44,53,55,70,141,142]

Some toxins cause characteristic cerebral lesions that are detectable by CT and MRI. Carbon monoxide is one well-studied example. CT scans in about half of patients with severe neurologic dysfunction following carbon monoxide exposure show bilateral symmetrical lucencies in the basal ganglia, particularly the globus pallidus (Fig. 7–26).[19,64,68,97,109,120,121,139] Brain injury following carbon monoxide poisoning may be due to hypoxia, acidosis, hypoperfusion, and binding of carbon monoxide to neuronal cytochrome oxidase. The basal ganglia are especially sensitive to hypoxic damage because of their poorly anastomotic blood supply and high metabolic requirements. Subcortical white matter lesions also occur following carbon monoxide poisoning. Although these are less frequent than the basal ganglion lesions, white matter lesions have a greater association with poor neurologic outcome. Some patients with basal ganglion lesions and no white matter lesions experience significant clinical recovery. In general, patients with severe carbon monoxide poisoning who have normal CT scans have a better prognosis than those with imaging abnormalities. MRI is more sensitive than CT at detecting these CNS lesions, especially white matter abnormalities.

Occasionally, symmetrical globus pallidus lesions will be found on the CT scan of a patient with altered mental status in whom carbon monoxide poisoning was not suspected as a potential cause. Although this is an indirect approach to the diagnosis, occult carbon monoxide poisoning continues to be a difficult diagnostic challenge since it can mimic many other, more common diseases. In one reported case, an infant who presented with an unknown encephalopathy was found to have bilateral globus pallidus lesions on CT. This prompted measurement of the child's carboxyhemoglobin level, which was elevated. Investigation revealed a faulty exhaust system in the family car.[107] In another report, an elderly patient suspected of having had a stroke had actually been poisoned by his newly installed wood-burning stove. The CT scan showed bilateral basal ganglion lesions that led to the diagnosis of carbon monoxide poisoning.[68]

CT and MRI have identified cerebral lesions in other cases of toxin-mediated neurologic degeneration, including methanol (putamenal lesions),[6,51] ethylene glycol, cyanide,[37,95] hydrogen sulfide, inorganic and organic mercury,[87] manganese,[7] heroin,[73] barbiturates, solvents such as toluene (in both occupational and illicit use),[63,117] and podophyllin.[18,99] The lesions are usually nonspecific and include basal ganglion lucencies, white matter lesions, and atrophy. They represent demyelinization, ischemia, or necrosis. Nontoxicologic disorders can also cause similar imaging abnormalities including hypoxia, hypoglycemia, and infectious encephalitis.[51,57]

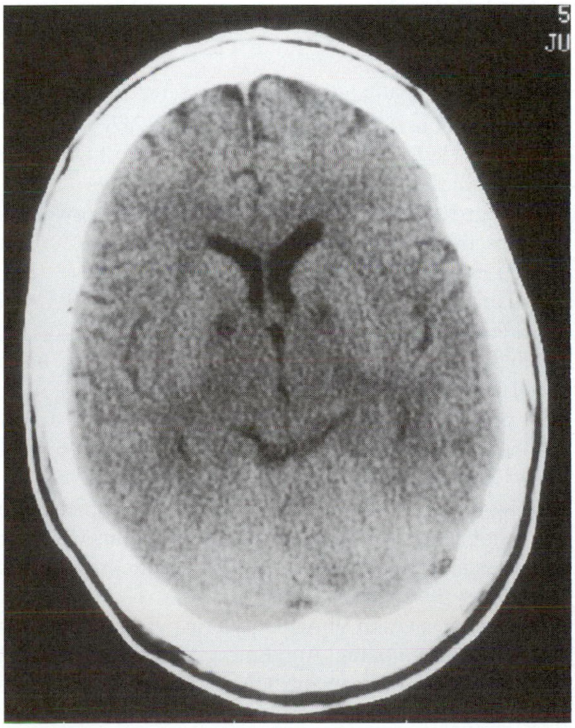

Figure 7–26. A head CT of a patient with mental status changes following carbon monoxide poisoning. The scan shows characteristic symmetrical lucencies of the globus pallidus bilaterally. *(Courtesy of Dr. Paul Blackburn, Maricopa Medical Center, Phoenix, Arizona.)*

Functional Brain Imaging. Both CT and MRI provide anatomic information, whereas nuclear medicine studies demonstrate aspects of cerebral function. These studies use radioactive isotopes that are bound to carrier molecules (ligands). The particular ligand chosen depends on the biologic function being studied. The labeled carrier molecule is taken up by certain cells in proportion to their physiologic activity or is distributed in the brain in proportion to regional blood flow. The radioactive emission of the isotope is detected by a scintigraphic camera and an image is formed showing the quantity and distribution of the tracer. Better anatomic detail is provided by computed tomographic techniques to generate cross-sectional images. This is termed *emission computed tomography* (ECT) because the image is formed by radiation emitted from an isotope located within the patient. There are two technologies: *single photon emission computed tomography* (SPECT) and *positron emission tomography* (PET). These imaging techniques are used in the research setting to visualize the neurologic effects of a particular toxin and to elucidate the mechanisms of toxin-induced neurologic derangement.

SPECT employs conventional isotopes such as technetium-99m and iodine-123.[77] These isotopes are bound to ligands that are taken up in the brain in proportion to regional blood flow (reflecting local metabolic rate) or neurotransmitter receptor location. PET scanning uses radioactive isotopes of biologic elements such as carbon-11, oxygen-15, nitrogen-13, and fluoride-18 (a substitute for hydrogen).[106] These radioisotopes have very short half-lives so that PET scanning requires an on-site cyclotron to produce the isotope. The isotopes are incorporated into molecules such as glucose, oxygen, water, and various neurotransmitters and drugs. Labeled glucose is taken up in proportion to the local metabolic rate for glucose. Uptake of labeled oxygen demonstrates the local metabolic rate for oxygen. A number of neurotransmitters can be labeled to generate images reflecting their concentration and distribution within the brain.

Both PET and SPECT have been used to study functional aspects of the brain that are affected by toxin exposure. In chronic alcoholics, both CT and MRI can visualize cerebellar atrophy; however, there is a poor correlation between the magnitude of cerebellar atrophy and the clinical signs of cerebellar dysfunction. PET scans can demonstrate diminished cerebellar metabolic rate for glucose, which seems to correlate more accurately with the patient's clinical status.[47,141]

SPECT and PET imaging have been used to study the neurologic effects of cocaine and carbon monoxide.[21,67,83] SPECT blood flow scintigraphy has demonstrated focal cortical perfusion defects in patients who chronically use cocaine. The extent of perfusion defect correlates with the frequency of drug use. The focal perfusion defects probably represent local vasculitis or small areas of cerebral infarction.[61,136]

PET scanning has been used to demonstrate the effects of cocaine on cerebral blood flow and regional glucose metabolism. PET neurotransmitter studies show promise in elucidating potential mechanisms of action of cocaine. Using labeled dopamine analogs, a down-regulation of dopamine (D_2) receptors is noted following a binge of cocaine use. This finding may correlate with the cocaine craving that occurs during early cocaine withdrawal. Using ^{11}C-labeled cocaine, uptake of cocaine can be demonstrated in the basal ganglia, a region rich in dopamine receptors.[140]

Much remains to be learned about these imaging modalities before they can be applied to patient care. They are able to demonstrate abnormalities in many patients with toxin exposures, although other patients with significant cerebral dysfunction have normal studies. It is hoped that in the future, these techniques will assist in diagnosis, management, and prognosis of the neurologic complications of a toxin exposure.

Summary

This chapter has highlighted some of the situations in which imaging studies are useful in toxicologic emergencies. Imaging can be an important tool in establishing a diagnosis, assisting in patient management, or detecting various complications of a toxicologic emergency. However, the intelligent use of any clinical test requires a thorough knowledge of its capabilities and limitations, an appreciation of whether it is indicated in a particular situation, and an understanding of how its results should be applied to the care of an individual patient.

References

1. American College of Emergency Physicians: Clinical policy for the initial approach to patients presenting with acute toxic ingestion or dermal or inhalation exposure. Ann Emerg Med 1995;25:570–585.
2. Amitai Y, Silver B, Leikin JB, Frischer H: Visualization of ingested medications in the stomach by ultrasound. Am J Emerg Med 1992;10:18–23.
3. Anas N, Namasonthi V, Ginsberg CM: Criteria for hospitalizing children who have ingested products containing hydrocarbons. JAMA 1981;246:840–843.
4. Ansell G: The Chest. In: Radiology of Adverse Reactions to Drugs and Toxic Hazards. Rockville, MD, Aspen Publications, 1985, pp. 1–99.
5. Ansell G: The Chest. In: Radiology of Adverse Reactions to Drugs and Toxic Hazards. Rockville, MD, Aspen Publications, 1985, pp. 254–326.
6. Aquilonius SM, Bergstrom K, Enolesson P, et al: Cerebral computed tomography in methanol intoxication. J Comput Assist Tomogr 1980;4:425–428.
7. Arjona A, Mata M, Bonet M: Diagnosis of chronic manganese intoxication by magnetic resonance imaging. N Engl J Med 1997;336:964–965.
8. Aronchick JM, Gefter WB: Drug-induced pulmonary disorders. Semin Roentgenol 1995:30;18.
9. Balthazar EJ, Lefleur R: Abdominal complications of drug addiction: radiologic features. Semin Roentgenol 1983;18: 213–214.
10. Beerman R, Nunez D, Wetli C: Radiographic evaluation of the cocaine smuggler. Gastrointest Radiol 1986;11:351–354.
11. Bensinger TA, Keller AR, Merrell LF, O'Leary DS: Thorotrast-induced reticuloendothelial blockade in man. Am J Med 1971;51:663–668.
12. Berger JR, Donovan-Post MJ, Levy RM: The acquired immunodeficiency syndrome. In: Greenberg JO, ed: Neuroimaging: A Companion to Adams and Victor's Principles of Neurology. New York, McGraw-Hill, 1995, chap. 18, pp. 413–434.
13. Blickman JG, Wilkinson RG, Graef JW: The radiologic "lead band" revisited. AJR 1986;146:245–247.
14. Bruns BR, Tytle T: Skeletal fluorosis: A report of two cases. Orthopedics 1988;11:1083–1087.
15. Burkhart KK, Kulig KW, Rumack B: Whole-bowel irrigation as treatment for zinc sulfate overdose. Ann Emerg Med 1990;19:1167–1170.
16. Caruana DS, Weinbach B, Goerg D, Gardner LB: Cocaine-packet ingestion. Ann Intern Med 1984;100:73–74.
17. Celli B, Khan MA: Mercury embolism of the lung. N Engl J Med 1976;295:883–885.
18. Chan YW: Magnetic resonance imaging in toxic encephalopathy due to podophyllin poisoning. Neuroradiology 1991;33:372–373.
19. Chang KH, Han MH, Kim HS, et al: Delayed encephalopathy after acute carbon monoxide intoxication: MR imaging features and distribution of cerebral white matter lesions. Radiology 1992;184:117–122.
20. Cheng CLY, Svesko V: Acute pyloric perforation after prolonged crack smoking. Ann Emerg Med 1994;23:126–128.
21. Choi IS, Kim SK, Lee SS, Choi YC: Evaluation of outcome of delayed neurologic sequelae after carbon monoxide poisoning by technetium-99m hexamethylpropylene amine oxime brain single photon emission computed tomography. Eur Neurol 1995;35:137–142.
22. Citron BP, Halpern MM, McCarron M, et al: Necrotizing angiitis associated with drug abuse. N Engl J Med 1970; 283:1003–1011.

23. Cranston PE, Pollack CV, Harrison RB: CT of crack cocaine ingestion. J Comput Assist Tomogr 1992:16;560–563.
24. Dally SL, Garnier R, Bismuth C: Diagnosis of chlorinated hydrocarbon poisoning by x-ray examination. Br J Indus Med 1987; 44:424–425.
25. Dee P, Armstrong P: Inhalational lung diseases. In: Armstrong P, Wilson AG, Dee P, Hansell DM, eds: Imaging of Diseases of the Chest, 2nd ed. St. Louis, Mosby–Year Book, 1995, pp. 426–460.
26. Dee P: Drug and radiation induced lung disease. In: Armstrong P, Wilson AG, Dee P, Hansell DM, eds: Imaging of Diseases of the Chest, 2nd ed. St. Louis, Mosby–Year Book, 1995, pp. 461–483.
27. Desenclos JA, Wilder MH, Coppenger GW, et al: Thallium poisoning: An outbreak in Florida, 1988. South Med J 1992;85:1203–1206.
28. Dillman RO, Crumb CK, Lidsky MJ: Lead poisoning from a gunshot wound. Am J Med 1979;66:509–514.
29. Douglass RE, Levison MA: Pneumothorax in drug abusers: An urban epidemic? Am Surg 1986;52:377–380.
30. Edeiken J, Dalinka M, Karasick D: Edeiken's Roentgen Diagnosis of Diseases of Bone, 4th ed. Baltimore, Williams & Wilkins, 1990, pp. 1401–1406.
31. Eurman DW, Potash HI, Eyler WR, et al: Chest pain and dyspnea related to "crack" cocaine smoking: Value of chest radiography. Radiology 1989;172:459–462.
32. Everson GW, Oudjhane K, Young LW, Krenzelok EP: Effectiveness of abdominal radiographs in visualizing chewable iron supplements following overdose. Am J Emerg Med 1989;7:459–463.
33. Everson GW, Bertaccini EJ, O'Leary J: Use of whole bowel irrigation in an infant following iron overdose. Am J Emerg Med 1991;9:366–369.
34. Farber JM, Rafii M, Schwartz D: Lead arthropathy and elevated serum lead levels after a gunshot wound of the shoulder. AJR 1994;162:385–386.
35. Feigen DS: Talc: understanding its manifestations in the chest. AJR 1986;146:295–301.
36. Felson B, Spitz HB: Unusual foreign bodies in bowel. JAMA 1977;237:2225–2226.
37. Finelli PF: Changes in the basal ganglia following cyanide poisoning. J Comput Assist Tomogr 1981;5:755–756.
38. Forrester JM, Steele AW, Waldron JA, Parsens PE: Crack lung: an acute pulmonary syndrome with a spectrum of clinical and histopathological findings. Am Rev Respir Dis 1990;142:462–467.
39. Foxford R, Goldfrank L: Gastrotomy—A surgical approach to iron overdose. Ann Emerg Med 1985;14:1223–1226.
40. Fraser RO, Pare JAP, Pare PD, Fraser RS, Genereux GP: Drug and poison induced pulmonary disease. In: Diagnosis of Diseases of the Chest, 3rd ed. Philadelphia, Saunders, 1991, pp. 2417–2479.
41. Freed TA, Sweet LN, Gauder PJ: Balloon obturation bowel obstruction: A hazard of drug smuggling. AJR 1976;127: 1033–1034.
42. Fulkerson WJ, Gockerman JP: Pulmonary disease induced by drugs. In: Fishman AP, ed: Pulmonary Diseases and Disorders, 2nd ed. New York, McGraw-Hill, 1988, pp. 793–811.
43. Gadaleta D, Hall MH, Nelson RL: Cocaine induced acute aortic dissection. Chest 1989;96:1203–1205.
44. Gallucci M, Amicarelli I, Rossi A, et al: MR imaging of white matter lesions in uncomplicated chronic alcoholism. J Comput Assist Tomogr 1989;13:395–398.
45. Gatenby RA: The radiology of drug-induced disorders in the gastrointestinal tract. Semin Roentgenol 1995:30;62–76.
46. Gibby WA, Zimmerman RA: X-ray computed tomography. In: Mazziotta JG, Gilman S, eds: Clinical Brain Imaging: Principles and Applications. Philadelphia, Davis, 1992, pp. 3–34.
47. Gilman S, Adams K, Koeppe RA, et al: Cerebellar and frontal hypometabolism in alcoholic cerebellar degeneration studied with positron emission tomography. Ann Neurol 1990;28:775–785.
48. Gilman S: Advances in neurology. N Engl J Med 1992; 326:1608–1616.
49. Ginaldi S: Geophagia: An uncommon cause of acute abdomen. Ann Emerg Med 1988;17:979–981.
50. Handy CA: Radiopacity of oral non liquid medications. Radiology 1971;98:525–533.
51. Hantson P, Duprez T, Mahieu P: Neurotoxicity to the basal ganglia shown by magnetic resonance imaging (MRI) following poisoning by methanol and other substances. J Toxicol Clin Toxicol 1997;35:151–161.
52. Harchelroad F: Identification of orally ingested cocaine by CT scan. Vet Hum Toxicol 1992;34:350. Abstract.
53. Haubek A, Lee K: Computed tomography in alcoholic cerebellar atrophy. Neuroradiology 1979;18:77–79.
54. Heffner JE, Harley RA, Schabel SI: Pulmonary reactions from illicit substance abuse. Clin Chest Med 1990;11: 151–162.
55. Hillbom M, Mulronen A, Holm L, Hindmarsh T: The clinical versus radiological diagnosis of alcoholic cerebellar degeneration. J Neurol Sci 1986;73:45–53.
56. Hinkel CL: The significance of opaque medications in the gastrointestinal tract, with special reference to enteric coated pills. Am J Roentgenol 1951;65:575–581.
57. Ho VB, Fitz CR, Chuang SH, Geyer CA: Bilateral basal ganglia lesions: Pediatric differential considerations. Radiographics 1993;13:269–292.
58. Hoffman CK, Goodman PC: Pulmonary edema in cocaine smokers. Radiology 1989;172:463–465.
59. Hoffman RS, Chiang WK, Weisman RS, Goldfrank LR: Prospective evaluation of "crack-vial" ingestion. Vet Hum Toxicol 1990;32:164–167.
60. Hoffman RS, Smilkstein MJ, Goldfrank LR: Whole bowel irrigation and the cocaine body-packer. Am J Emerg Med 1990;8:523–527.
61. Holman BL, Mendelson J, Garada B, et al: Regional cerebral blood flow improves with treatment in chronic cocaine polydrug users. J Nucl Med 1993;34:723–727.
62. Holzman RS, Bishko F: Osteomyelitis in heroin addicts. Ann Intern Med 1971;75:693–696.
63. Hormes JT, Filley CM, Rosenberg NL: Neurologic sequelae of chronic solvent vapor abuse. Neurology 1986;36: 698–702.
64. Horowitz AL, Kaplan R, Sarpel O: Carbon monoxide toxicity: MR imaging in the brain. Radiology 1987;162: 787–788.
65. Horrocks AW: Abdominal radiography in suspected "body packers." Clin Radiol 1992;45:322–325. 1993;47:219. Comment.

66. Jaeger RW, Decastro FJ, Barry RC, et al: Radiopacity of drugs and plants: In vivo limited usefulness. Vet Hum Toxicol 1981:23:2–4 (suppl).
67. Jibiki I, Kurokawa K, Yamaguchi N: ^{123}I-MP brain SPECT imaging in a patient with the interval form of CO poisoning. Eur Neurol 1991;31:149–151.
68. Jones JS, Lagasse J, Zimmerman G: Computed tomographic findings after acute carbon monoxide poisoning. Am J Emerg Med 1994;12:448–451.
69. Keys N, Wahl M, Aks S, et al: Cocaine body stuffers: A case series. J Toxicol Clin Toxicol 1995;33:517. Abstract.
70. Koller WC, Glatt SL, Perlik S, et al: Cerebellar atrophy demonstrated by computed tomography. Neurology 1981;31:405–412.
71. Koppel BS, Tuchman AJ, Mangiardi JR, et al: Epidural spinal infection in intravenous drug abusers. Arch Neurol 1988;45:1331–1337.
72. Kram HB, Hardin E, Clark SR, Shoemaker WC: Perforated ulcers related to smoking "crack" cocaine. Am Surg 1992;58:293–294.
73. Kreigstein AR, Armitage BA, Kim PK: Heroin inhalation and progressive spongiform leukoencephalopathy. N Engl J Med 1997;336:589–590.
74. Kuhn JR, Tunell WP: The role of cine-esophagography in caustic esophageal injury. Am J Surg 1983;146:804–806.
75. Kulshrestha MK: Lead poisoning diagnosed by abdominal x-rays. J Toxicol Clin Toxicol 1996;34:107–108.
76. Landi JL, Spickler EM: Imaging of intracranial hemorrhage associated with drug abuse. Neuroimaging Clin North Am 1992;2:187–194.
77. Lassen NA, Holm, S: Single photon emission computerized tomography. In: Mazzotta JG, Gilman S, eds: Clinical Brain Imaging: Principles and Applications. Philadelphia, Davis, 1992, pp. 108–134.
78. Lee DC, Roberts JR, Kelly JJ, Fishman SM: Whole-bowel irrigation as an adjunct in the treatment of radiopaque arsenic. Am J Emerg Med 1995;13:244–245.
79. Levine SR, Brust JCM, Futrell N, et al: Cerebrovascular complications of the use of the "crack" form of alkaloidal cocaine. N Engl J Med 1990;323:699–704.
80. Lexa FJ: Drug-induced disorders of the central nervous system. Semin Roentgenol 1995:30;7–17.
81. Litovitz TL: Button battery ingestions: A review of 56 cases. JAMA 1983;249:2495–2500.
82. Lufkin RB: Magnetic resonance imaging. In: Mazziotti JG, Gilman S, eds: Clinical Brain Imaging: Principles and Applications. Philadelphia, Davis, 1992, pp. 36–69.
83. Maeda Y, Kawasaki Y, Jibiki I, et al: Effect of therapy with oxygen under high pressure of regional cerebral blood flow in the interval form of carbon monoxide poisoning: Observation from subtraction of technetium-99m HMPAO SPECT brain imaging. Eur Neurol 1991;31:380–383.
84. Mankin HJ: Nontraumatic necrosis of bone (osteonecrosis). N Engl J Med 1992;326:1473–1479.
85. Maravilla AM, Berk RN: The radiographic diagnosis of pica. Am J Gastroenterol 1978;70:94–99.
86. Martel W: Radiographic features of esophagogastritis secondary to extremely caustic agents. Radiology 1972; 103:31–36.
87. Matsumoto SC, Okajima T, Inayoshi S, Ueno H: Minamata disease demonstrated by computed tomography. Neuroradiology 1988;30:42–46.
88. McCarron MM, Wood JD: The cocaine "body packer" syndrome. JAMA 1983;250:1417–1420.
89. McElvaine MD, DeUngria EG, Mattte TD, et al: Prevalence of radiographic evidence of paint chip ingestion among children with moderate to severe lead poisoning, St. Louis, Missouri, 1989 through 1990. Pediatrics 1992;89: 740–742.
90. Meggs WJ, Hoffman RS, Shih RD, et al: Thallium poisoning from maliciously contaminated food. J Toxicol Clin Toxicol 1994;32:723–730.
91. Megibow AJ, Balthazar EJ, Cho KC, et al: Bowel obstruction: evaluation with CT. Radiology 1991;180:313–318.
92. Mengel CE, Carter WA: Geophagia diagnosed by roentgenograms. JAMA 1964;187:955–956.
93. Merchant JA, Schwartz DA: Chest radiography for assessment of the pneumoconioses. In: Rom WN, ed: Environmental and Occupational Medicine, 2nd ed. Boston, Little Brown, 1992.
94. Messer HD, Litvinoff J: Pyogenic cervial osteomyelitis. Arch Neurol 1976;33:571–576.
95. Messing B, Storch B: Computer tomography and magnetic resonance imaging in cyanide poisoning. Eur Arch Psychiatr Neurol Sci 1988;237:139–143.
96. Miller WT: Pleural and mediastinal disorders related to drug use. Semin Roentgenol 1995:30;35–48.
97. Miura T, Mitomo M, Kawi R, Harada K: CT of the brain in acute carbon monoxide intoxication: Characteristic features and prognosis. AJNR 1985;6:739–742.
98. Naidich TP, Bartlett D, Wheeler PS, Stern WZ: Metallic mercury emboli. AJR 1973;117:886–891.
99. Nelson DL, Batnitzky S, McMillan JH, et al: The CT and MRI features of acute toxic encephalopathies. AJNR 1987; 8:951.
100. Neustadter LM, Weiss M: Medication-induced changes of bone. Semin Roentgenol 1995:30;88–95.
101. Ng RCW, Perry K, Martin DJ: Iron poisoning: Assessment of radiography in diagnosis and management. Clin Pediatr 1979;18:614–616.
102. O'Brien RP, McGeehan PA, Helmeczi AW, Dula DJ: Detectability of drug tablets and capsules by plain radiography. Am J Emerg Med 1986;4:302–312.
103. Olsen WL, Cohen W: Neuroradiology of AIDS. In: Federle M, Megibow A, Nadich DP, eds: Radiology of Acquired Immune Deficiency Syndrome. New York, Raven Press, 1988, pp. 21–45.
104. Palat D, Denson M, Sherman M, Matz R: Pneumomediastinum induced by inhalation of alkaloidal cocaine. NY State J Med 1988;438–439.
105. Peterson CD, Fifield GC: Emergency gastrotomy for acute iron poisoning. Ann Emerg Med 1980;9:262–264.
106. Phelps ME: Positron emission tomography. In: Mazziotti JS, Gilman S, eds: Clinical Brain Imaging: Principles and Applications. Philadelphia, Davis, 1992, pp. 71–106.
107. Piatt JP, Kaplan AM, Bond RO, Berg RA: Occult carbon monoxide poisoning in an infant. Pediatr Emerg Care 1990;6:21–23.
108. Pollack CV, Biggers DW, Carlton FB, et al: Two crack cocaine body stuffers. Ann Emerg Med 1992;21:1370–1380.

109. Pracyk JB, Stolp BW, Fife CE, et al: Brain computerized tomography after hyperbaric oxygen therapy for carbon monoxide poisoning. Undersea Hyperb Med 1995;22:1–7.
110. Ramchandani P, Pollack HM: Radiology of drug-related genitourinary disease. Semin Roentgenol 1995:30;77–87.
111. Rashid J, Eisenberg MJ, Topol EJ: Cocaine-induced aortic dissection. Am Heart J 1996;132:1301–1304.
112. Resnick D: Heavy metal poisoning and deficinecy. In: Resnick D, ed: Diagnosis of Bone and Joint Disorders, 3rd ed. Philadelphia, Saunders, 1995, chap. 76, pp. 3353–3364.
113. Resnick D, Niwayama G: Osteolysis and Chondrolysis. In: Resnick D, ed: Diagnosis of Bone and Joint Disorders, 3rd ed. Philadelphia, Saunders, 1995, pp. 4467–4469.
114. Richerson HB: Hypersensitivity pneumonitis (extrinsic allergic alveolitis). In: Fishman AP, ed: Pulmonary Diseases and Disorders, 2nd ed. New York, McGraw-Hill, 1988, pp. 667–674.
115. Roberge RJ, Martin TG: Whole bowel irrigation in an acute oral lead intoxication. Am J Emerg Med 1992;10:577–583.
116. Roberts JR, Price D, Goldfrank LR, Hartnett L: The bodystuffer syndrome: A clandestine form of drug overdose. Am J Emerg Med 1986;4:24–27.
117. Rosenberg NL, Kleinschmidt-DeMasters BK, Davis KA, et al: Toluene abuse causes diffuse central nervous system white matter changes. Ann Neurol 1988;23:611–614.
118. Sachs HK: The evolution of the radiologic lead line. Radiology 1981;139:81–85.
119. Savitt DL, Hawkins HH, Roberts JR: The radiopacity of ingested medications. Ann Emerg Med 1987;16:331–339.
120. Sawada Y, Ohashi N, Maemura K, et al: Computerized tomography as an indication of long term outcome after acute carbon monoxide poisoning. Lancet 1980;2:783–784.
121. Sawada Y, Sakamoto T, Nishide, et al: Correlation of pathological findings with computed tomographic findings after acute carbon monoxide poisoning. N Engl J Med 1983;308:1296.
122. Schabel SI, Rogers CI: Opaque artifacts in a health food faddist simulating ovarian neoplasm. Am J Roentgenol 1978;130:789–790.
123. Sinner WN: The gastrointestinal tract as a vehicle for drug smuggling. Gastrointest Radiol 1981;6:319–323.
124. Smith DA, Leake L, Loflin JR, Yealy DM: Is admission after intravenous heroin overdose necessary? Ann Emerg Med 1992;21:1326–1330. Ann Emerg Med 1993;22: 1638–1639. Comment.
125. Sogge MR, Griffith JL, Sinar DR, Mayes GR: Lavage to remove enteric-coated aspirin and gastric outlet obstruction. Ann Intern Med 1977;87:721–722.
126. Spitzer A, Caruthers S, Stables DP: Radiopaque suppositories. Diagnostic Radiol 1976;121:71–73.
127. Sporer KA, Manning JJ: Massive ingestion of sustained-release verapamil with a concretion and bowel infarction. Ann Emerg Med 1993;22:603–605.
128. Sporer KA, Firestone J: Clinical course of crack cocaine body stuffers. Ann Emerg Med 1997;29:596–601.
129. Staple TW, McAlister WH: Roentgenographic visualization of iron preparations in the gastrointestinal tract. Radiology 1964;83:1051–1056.
130. Stern WZ, Spear PW, Jacobson HG: The roentgen findings in acute heroin intoxication. AJR 1968;103:522–532.
131. Stromberg BV: Symptomatic lead toxicity secondary to retained shotgun pellets: Case report. J Trauma 1990;30: 356–357.
132. Sue YJ, Saperstein A, Zawin J, et al: Radiopacity of paradichlorobenzene containing household products. Vet Hum Toxicol 1992;34:350. Abstract.
133. Swartz MN: Approach to the patient with pulmonary infections. In: Fishman AP, ed: Pulmonary Diseases and Disorders, 2nd ed. New York, McGraw-Hill, 1988, pp. 1375–1759.
134. Switz DM, Elmorshidy ME, Deyerle WM: Bullets, joints and lead intoxication. Arch Intern Med 1976;136: 939–941.
135. Tillman DJ, Ruggles DL, Leiken JB: Radiopacity study of extended-release formulations using digitized radiography. Am J Emerg Med 1994;12:310–314.
136. Tumeh SS, Nagel JS, English RJ, et al: Cerebral abnormalities in cocaine abusers: Demonstration by SPECT perfusion brain scintigraphy. Radiology 1990;176:821–824.
137. Velasquez G, Ward CF, Bohrer SP: Thorium dioxide: Still around. South Med J 1985;78:743–745.
138. Venturelli J, Kwee Y, Morris N, Cameron O: Gastrotomy in the management of acute iron poisoning. J Pediatr 1982;100:768–769.
139. Vieregge P, Klostermann W, Blumm RG, Borgis KJ: Carbon monoxide poisoning: Clinical, neurophysiological, and brain imaging observations in acute disease and follow-up. J Neurol 1989;236:478–481.
140. Volkow ND, Fowler JS, Wolf AP: Use of positron emission tomography to investigate cocaine. In: Nahas GG, Latour C, eds: Physiopathology of Illicit Drugs: Cannabis, Cocaine, Opiates. Oxford, Pergamon Press, 1991, pp. 129–141.
141. Wang GJ, Volkow ND, Roque CT, et al: Functional importance of ventricular enlargement and cortical atrophy in healthy subjects and alcoholics as assessed with PET, MR imaging, and neuropsychologic testing. Radiology 1993; 186:59–65. Radiology 1993;186:13–15. Comment.
142. Warach SJ, Charness ME: Imaging the brain lesions of alcoholics. In: Greenberg JO, ed: Neuroimaging: A Companion to Adams and Victor's Principles of Neurology. New York, McGraw-Hill, 1995, chap. 18, pp. 503–515.
143. Weill H, Jones RN: Occupational pulmonary diseases. In: Fishman AP, ed: Pulmonary Diseases and Disorders, 2nd ed. New York, McGraw-Hill, 1988, pp. 1465–1474.
144. Weimerskirch PJ, Burkhart KK, Bono MJ, et al: Methylene iodide poisoning. Ann Emerg Med 1990;19:1171–1176.
145. Williams MH: Pulmonary complications of drug abuse. In: Fishman AP, ed: Pulmonary Diseases and Disorders, 2nd ed. New York, McGraw-Hill, 1988, pp. 819–860.
146. Wolowodiuk OJ, McMicken DB, O'Brien P: Pneumomediastinum and pneumoperitoneum: An unusual complication of syrup of ipecac induced emesis. Ann Emerg Med 1984;13:1148–1151.
147. Woolf DA, Riach CF, Derweesh A, Vyas H: Lead lines in young infants with acute lead encephalopathy: A reliable diagnosic test. J Tropic Pediatr 1990;36:90–93.
148. Zimmers T: Heavy metal herbs. Ann Emerg Med 1985; 14:486–487.

CHAPTER 8

Electrocardiographic Evaluation of the Poisoned or Overdosed Patient

Cathleen Clancy

The electrocardiogram (ECG) is one of the few diagnostic procedures that reveals immediate, useful clinical information. This has far-reaching implications in toxicology, where other diagnostic test results often return too late to effectively impact the care of an acutely poisoned patient.

History

The knowledge of a relationship between electricity and muscular movement can be traced back to 1790, when Luigi Galvani electrically stimulated an in vitro preparation of the legs of a frog, and made them "dance." In 1887, Waller developed a "capillary electrometer" that transmitted electrical impulses from a man's skin to a capillary tube. Pulsations similar to the patient's heartbeat were visible in the tube.[141] In 1903, Willem Einthoven graphically displayed the electrical activity of the heart and even named the different waves, "P," "QRS," and "T." He called this tracing an "elektrokardiogramme."[38] The term "EKG," still employed by some authors, was derived from Einthoven's spelling. The term "ECG," which is consistent with our current spelling of electrocardiogram, is used in this text.

Normal Electrocardiogram

Basic Electrophysiology of the Myocardial Cell

The normal, resting, myocardial cell (myocyte) is polarized, or electrically charged. The outside of the cell is positive and the inside of the cell carries a –90-mV charge. When the myocardial cells in the sinus node become depolarized, ion channels in the nearby myocardium open and there is a net influx of positive sodium and calcium ions that propagate depolarization. Depolarization precipitates the contraction of the myocyte and initiates the slow outward potassium currents that will allow the now refractory sodium, calcium, and potassium channels to respond to the subsequent stimulus. The depolarization spreads throughout the myocardium, causing the coordinated contraction known as systole. After a well-defined time period the myocardial membrane becomes repolarized by an outward current of potassium and an inward current of chloride (Table 8–1) and returns to the relaxed, polarized state (diastole).

Figure 8–1 shows schematically the relationship of the major ion fluxes across the myocardial cell membrane, the phases of the action potential, and the surface ECG recording. The action potential describes electric

TABLE 8–1. IONS AS CHARGE CARRIERS ACROSS CELL MEMBRANES

Ion	Charge	Direction of Passive Flux	Current Generated	Effect of Membrane Potential
Calcium	Positive	Inward	Inward	Depolarization
Sodium	Positive	Inward	Inward	Depolarization
Potassium	Positive	Outward	Outward	Repolarization
Chloride	Negative	Inward	Outward	Repolarization

Reproduced, with permission, from Katz AM: Cardiac ion channels. N Engl J Med 1993;328:1245.

potentials monitored from outside the cell. It is divided into five phases: phase 0, depolarization; phase 1, overshoot; phase 2, plateau; phase 3, repolarization; and phase 4, resting. When the cell is excited by a stimulus from another cell or by spontaneous depolarization (pacemaker cells), selective channels in the membrane open allowing sodium and calcium to enter the cell. Sodium enters the cell via fast sodium channels and calcium enters through L-type (slow) and T-type (fast) calcium channels. During phase 1, these sodium channels begin to close, but the initial repolarization immediately after the overshoot is mediated by activation of the transient outward current carried by potassium ions.[55,131] The plateau (phase 2) results from a balance between inward currents (primarily the slowly decaying L-type calcium channels, possibly a sodium–potassium exchange current, and a small inward chloride flux) and the outward potassium currents. The slow inward calcium current maintains the early plateau phase and is partially responsible for the increase in intracellular calcium that initiates contraction of the muscle cell during phase 2. During repolarization (phase 3), the outward potassium currents overwhelm the decaying inward currents. This outward potassium current is often called the "delayed rectifier current," since it returns the interior of the cell to electronegativity. Four separate types of potassium channels contribute to the repolarization phase.[55] Phase 4 is a resting state, with a persistent inward potassium current

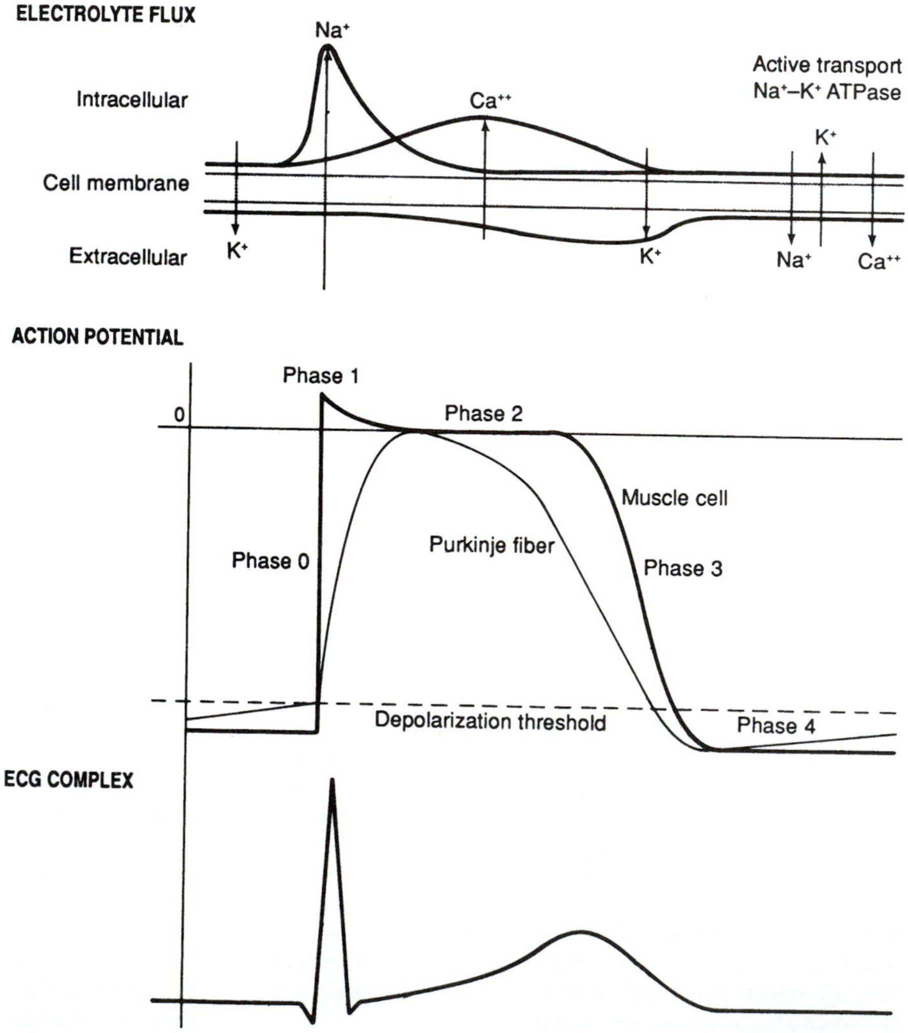

Figure 8–1. Relationship of electrolyte movement across the cell membrane to the action potential and the surface ECG recording.

that maintains membrane polarization. Finally, in pacemaker cells, a decay in the outward potassium and an inward leaking background sodium current leads to a spontaneous, gradual increase in the resting potential, and eventually, spontaneous depolarization. The ion currents are regulated by a complex system of channels (receptor-operated and voltage-operated), pumps and carriers (sodium–potassium pump, calcium pump, sodium–calcium countertransport system, sodium–hydrogen exchanger), receptors (adrenergic, muscarinic, and purinergic), and cytoplasmic regulators of second messengers (cyclic AMP-phosphodiesterase).

During phases 0–2, a normal cell cannot normally be depolarized again by another stimulus. The cell is refractory. During phase 3 (repolarization), an electrical stimulus of greater magnitude may cause another depolarization. The cell is *relatively* refractory. During phase 4, a stimulus that reaches the threshold level causes depolarization, and the cycle begins again.

An impulse that reaches the myocardial cell before repolarization is complete, and causes a depolarization, is called an "early afterdepolarization" (Fig. 8–2). Early afterdepolarizations occur when the membrane potential is decreased during phase 2 (type 1) and phase 3 (type 2) of the cardiac action potential. An impulse that occurs after completion of repolarization (phase 4) is called a "delayed afterdepolarization" (Fig. 8–2). The delayed afterdepolarizations generally arise when the membrane potential is more negative than when early afterdepolarizations are recorded. Early afterdepolarizations may be responsible for the lengthened repolarization time and ventricular tachydysrhythmias in acquired and congenital forms of the long QT syndrome, and in patients with drug-induced torsades de pointes (Table 8–2 and page 116: QT prolongation section). The ionic basis of early afterdepolarizations is unclear but may be via the L-type calcium channel. Early afterdepolarizations are suppressed by magnesium.[9,138] Delayed afterdepolarizations are postulated to be the cause of some dysrhythmias induced by digoxin poisoning (Fig. 8–3).[76] The mechanism seems to be related to increases in intracellular calcium that activate a nonselective cation channel or an electrogenic sodium–calcium exchanger that causes a transient inward current carried primarily by sodium ions. This inward sodium current generates the delayed afterdepolarizations. The increased calcium concentrations may come from extensive sympathetic stimulation,[84] or large doses of digoxin, or other abnormal physiologic conditions.

The toxicity and mechanism of action of many drugs and toxins is based on their ability to block either individual or multiple ion channels.[55]

TABLE 8–2. CLASSIFICATION AND CAUSES OF THE LONG QT INTERVAL SYNDROMES

The acquired long QT interval syndromes (pause-dependent)
Antidysrhythmic drugs
Class IA drugs with class III properties
Class III drugs
Severe bradycardia
Complete atrioventricular block
Sinus node dysfunction
Electrolyte disturbances
Hypokalemia
Hypomagnesemia
Nonantidysrhythmic drugs
Psychotropic agents: phenothiazines, haloperidol
Tricyclic and tetracyclic antidepressants
Antihypertensive agents: bepridil, lidoflazine, prenylamine, ketanserin
Antimicrobial agents: erythromycin, trimethoprim-sulfamethoxazole, pentamidine, amantidine, chloroquine
Antifungal agents: ketoconazole, itraconazole
Antihistaminic agents: terfenadine, astemizole
Other drugs: cocaine, organophosphate insecticides, arsenic, vasopressin
Other conditions
Cardiac disorders: myocarditis, ventricular tumor
Endocrine disorders: hypothyroidism, hypoparathyroidism, pheochromocytoma, hyperaldosteronism
Intracranial disorders: subarachnoid hemorrhage, cerebrovascular accident, encephalitis, head injury
Nutritional disorders: liquid protein diet, starvation
The hereditary long QT interval syndromes (adrenergic-dependent)
Jervell and Lange-Nielsen syndrome
Romano-Ward syndrome

Modified, with permission, from Tan HL, Hou CJ, Lauer MR, Sung RJ: Electrophysiologic mechanisms of the long QT interval syndromes and torsades de pointes. Ann Intern Med 1995;122:702.

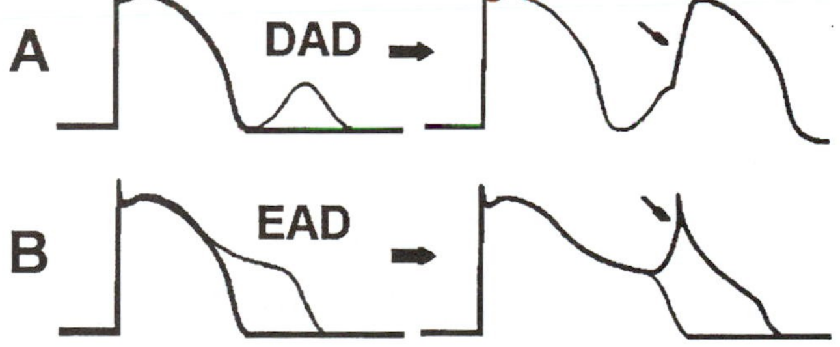

Figure 8–2. (**A**) Delayed afterdepolarization (DAD) arising after full repolarization. A delayed afterdepolarization that reaches threshold results in a triggered upstroke (*arrow, right*). (**B**) Early afterdepolarization (EAD) interrupting phase 3 repolarization. Under some conditions, a triggered beat can arise from an early afterdepolarization (*arrow, right*). *(Reproduced, with permission, from Roden DM: Antiarrhythmic drugs. In: Hardman JG, Limbird LE, Molinoff PB, Ruddon RW, Gilman AG, eds: Goodman and Gilman's The Pharmacological Basis of Therapeutics, 9th ed. New York, McGraw-Hill, 1996, pp. 845.)*

Basic Physiology of an ECG

The pattern that appears on the ECG paper is a recording of the sum of electrical activities that are taking place in the heart during depolarization and repolarization. The

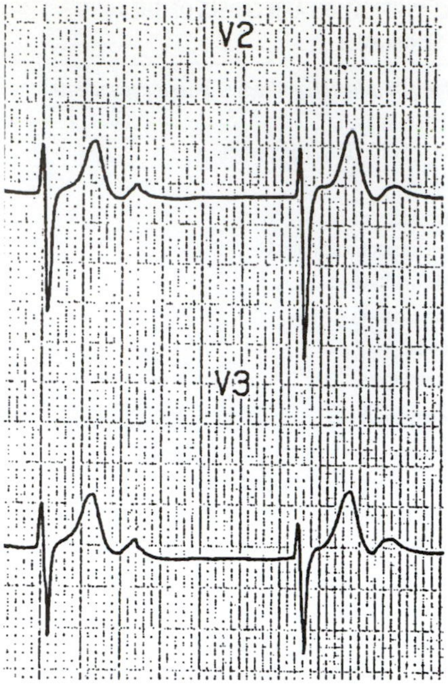

Figure 8–3. This ECG was recorded from a 20-year-old man who ingested an unknown quantity of digoxin. Delayed afterdepolarizations can be seen following the T waves.

cardiac monitor and the ECG screen are both types of oscilloscopes that convert the electrical activity in the heart into a light pattern displayed on a screen. The modern ECG machinery is computerized to provide a written interpretation of time intervals and rhythms. A tracing is recorded on heat-sensitive graph paper to produce "the ECG," the hard copy of the original tracing. The X-axis records time and the Y-axis records voltage. Each small square on the graph paper is 1 mm^2. Horizontally, on the X-axis, each small box denotes 0.04 seconds of elapsed time. Five small boxes (bold lines) represents 0.2 seconds. On the Y-axis, most ECG machines are calibrated so that a 1 mV signal produces a 10-mm deflection.

Leads. The lead placement that was described in 1913 has become the basis for the bipolar leads I, II, and III (Fig. 8–4).[38] For lead I the left arm electrode is the positive pole and the right arm electrode is the negative pole. Lead II has a positive pole on the left leg and a negative pole on the right arm. Lead III has a positive pole on the left leg and the negative pole on the left arm. Einthoven's triangle is an equilateral triangle formed by the sum of these leads. Unipolar extremity leads and precordial leads have since been added to our standard ECG. Wilson and colleagues connected limb leads, called VR, VL, and VF, to a common point where the sum of the potentials from leads I, II, III was zero. A unipolar potential was measured.[146] The voltage of the currently used, augmented (a) leads (aVR, aVL, and aVF) is based on these unipolar leads (VR, VL, and VF) but amplified $1\frac{1}{2}$ times from Wilson's original concept (Fig. 8–5).[53]

The precordial leads (V_1, V_2, V_3, V_4, V_5, V_6) are also unipolar measurements of the change in electric potential measured from a central point to the six anterior and left lateral chest positions (Fig. 8–6). For example, if V_2 is placed over the right ventricle, part of the initial positive ventricular deflection (QRS complex) reflects right ventricular activation, with electrical forces moving toward the electrode. Then the majority of the terminal negative deflection reflects activation of other muscle tissue (sep-

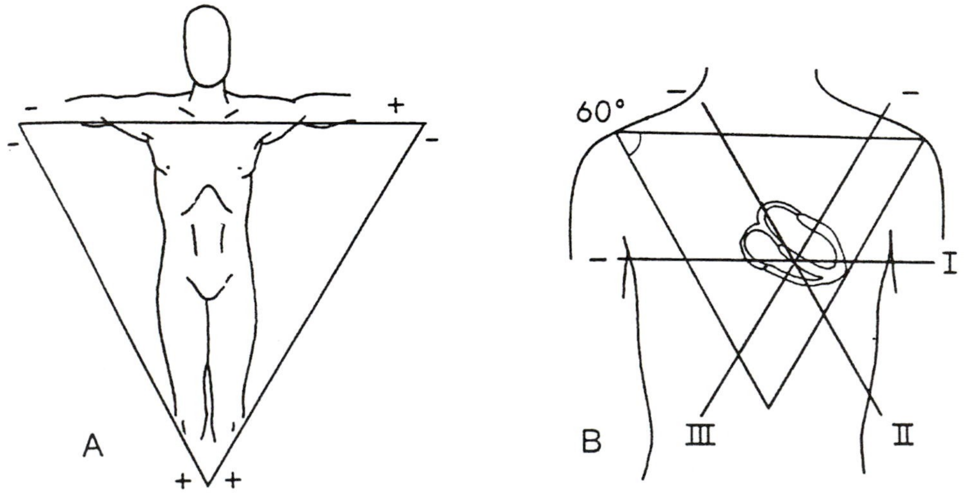

Figure 8–4. The relationships of the original three limb leads are illustrated. (**A**) The equiangular (60 degrees) Einthoven triangle formed by leads I, II, and III is shown with positive and negative poles of each of the leads indicated. (**B**) The Einthoven triangle is shown in relation to a schematic view of the heart. Leads I, II, and III are also presented as a triaxial reference system that intersects in the center of the ventricles. *(Reproduced, with permission, from Wagner GS: Cardiac electrical activity, recording the normal electrocardiogram. In: Wagner GS: Marriott's Practical Electrocardiography, 9th ed. Baltimore, Williams & Wilkins, 1994, p. 21.)*

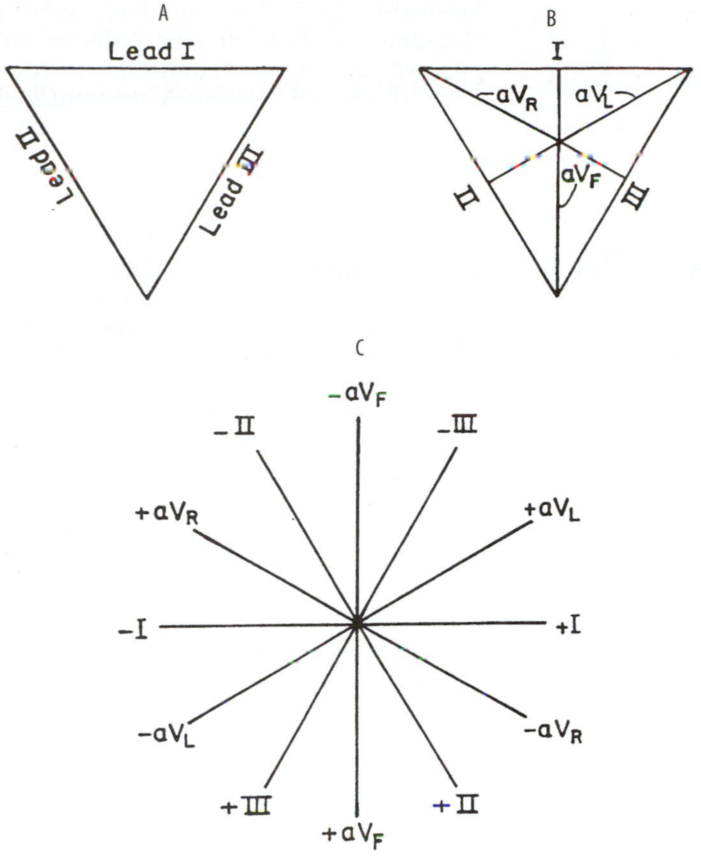

Figure 8–5. (**A**) Einthoven's equilateral triangle formed by leads I, II, and III. (**B**) The unipolar limb leads are added to the equilateral triangle. (**C**) The hexaxial reference system derived from B. *(Reproduced, with permission, from Electrocardiography. In: Chou T, Knilans TK, eds: Clinical Practice Adult and Pediatric, 4th ed. Philadelphia, Saunders, 1996, p. 7.)*

tum, left ventricular wall) when the electrical forces are moving away from the electrode (Fig. 8–7).

The electrical potential vectors defined by the limb leads project in the frontal plane and record forces moving either superiorly or inferiorly and to the left or the right. The vectors defined by the chest leads project in the horizontal plane and exclusively record forces directed anteriorly or posteriorly, and to the left or the right. Recordings from each of these 12 leads (I, II, III, aVR, aVL, aVF, V_1, V_2, V_3, V_4, V_5, V_6) evaluate the heart from two different planes in 12 different positions, yielding a three-dimensional "picture" of the electrical potentials that govern the function of the heart, with respect to time and voltage.

A continuous cardiac monitor usually relies on recordings from one of two bipolar leads. The leads are either a *m*odified *l*eft chest lead with the positive electrode in the V_1 position (lead MCL_1) or a lead II (Fig. 8–8). The recording from an MCL_1 lead is similar in appearance to a V_1 recording on a 12-lead ECG and is commonly used in routine monitoring. The positive electrode is placed over the fourth intercostal space just to the right of the sternum. The negative electrode is placed at the second intercostal space, midline on the upper left chest

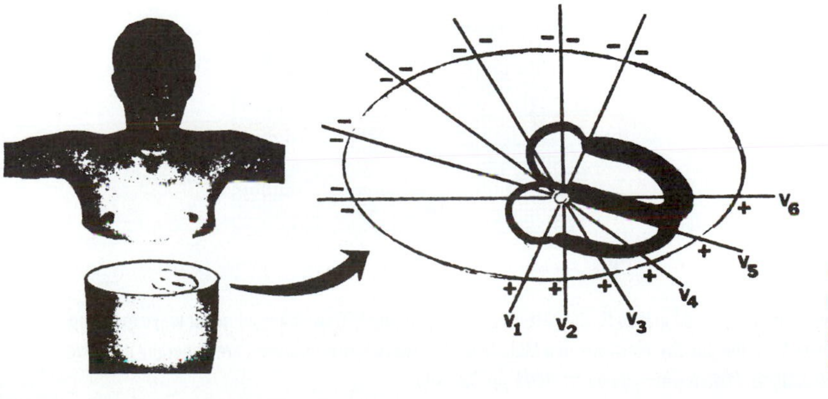

Figure 8–6. Each of the chest leads is oriented through the AV node and exits through the patient's back, which is negative. *(Reproduced, with permission, from Dubin D: Rapid Interpretation of EKG's, ed. V, Tampa, FL, Cover Publishing Co, 1996, p. 47.)*

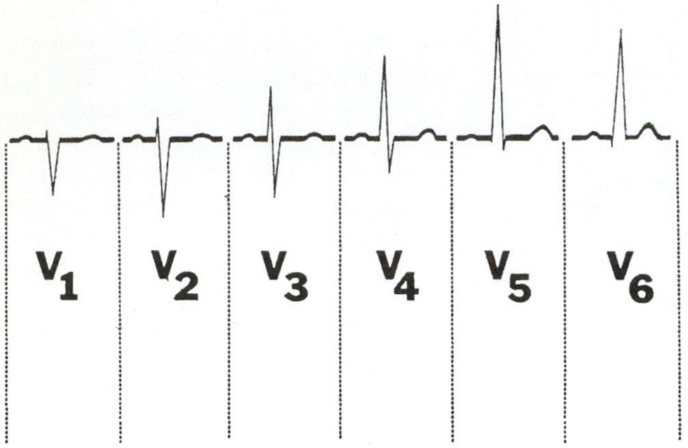

Figure 8–7. By examining an ECG you will notice that the waves of the six chest leads show progressive changes from V_1 to V_6. *(Reproduced, with permission, from Dubin D: Rapid Interpretation of EKG's, ed. V, Tampa, FL, Cover Publishing Co, 1996, p. 49.)*

or on the outer third of the left clavicle. This lead visualizes ventricular activity well; however, lead II shows atrial activity (ie, the P wave) much more clearly. Electrode placement for lead II has the positive electrode on the lower extreme left side of the left chest and the negative electrode on the second intercostal space in the midline of the upper right chest.

The Tracing. The ECG tracing has specific nomenclature to define the characteristic patterns. Waves refer to positive or negative deflections from baseline (P wave, T wave, U wave). A segment is defined as the distance between two waves (ST), and an interval measures the duration of a wave plus a segment (QT, PR). Complexes are a group of waves without intervals or segments between them (QRS). Electrophysiologically, the P wave and PR interval on the ECG tracing represent the depolarization of the atria. The QRS complex represents the depolarization of the ventricles. Repolarization is depicted by the ST segment, the T wave, the QT interval, and the U wave (Fig. 8–9).[29]

The P wave. The early, middle, and late portions of the P wave are represented sequentially by the electrical potential generated by the right atrium, both atria combined, the interatrial septum, and the left atrium. The sinus node or an ectopic focus located in the right atrium are the most common pacemakers. A normal P wave usually has a duration 0.08 to 0.11 seconds; axis, +45 degrees to +60 degrees (upright in leads I and II and inverted in aVR); amplitude, less than 0.25 mV; and a rounded or notched appearance. A notched P wave suggests delayed conduction across the atrial septum. In normal individuals this delay should not exceed 0.04 seconds.

Clinically, abnormalities of the P wave are seen with

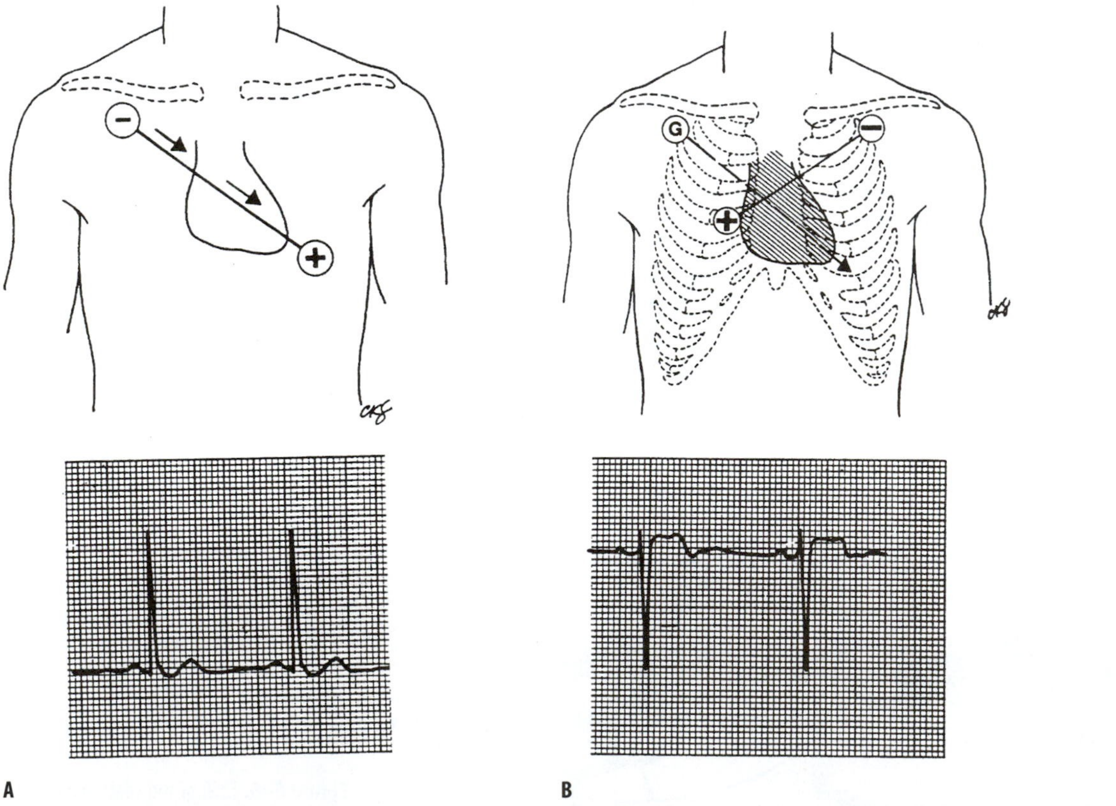

Figure 8–8. (**A**) The current flow in the heart is toward the positive electrode in lead II. The pattern produced on the ECG will have all major wave forms upright, positive. (**B**) The main current flow in the heart is away from the positive electrode in a MCL_1 lead. The wave forms produced are generally negative. *(Reproduced, with permission, from Catalano JT: Guide to ECG analysis. Philadelphia, Lippincott, 1993, pp. 38–39.)*

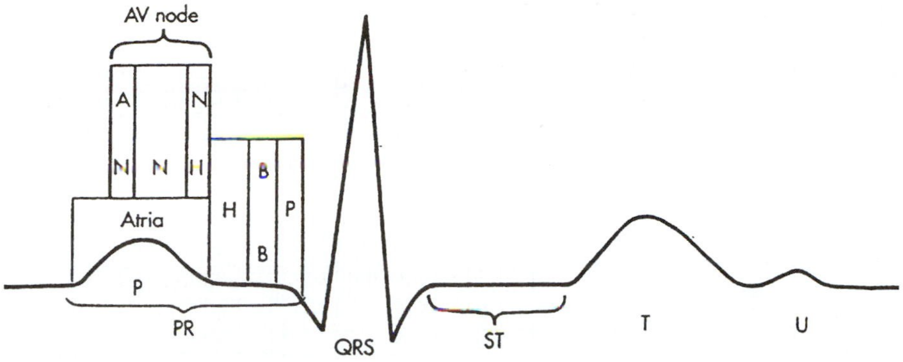

Figure 8–9. The normal ECG: P wave, atrial depolarization; QRS, ventricular depolarization; ST segment and T wave, ventricular repolarization. The U wave is a small positive deflection. The PR interval reflects not only atrial depolarization, but also the conduction time through the AV node, His bundle (H), bundle branches (BB), and Purkinje fibers (P). AN, atrionodal; N, compact AV node; NH, nodal His. *(Reproduced, with permission, from Conover MB: Understanding Electrocardiography, 7th ed. St. Louis, Mosby-Year Book, 1996, p. 17.)*

agents that depress automaticity, causing sinus arrest and nodal or ventricular escape rhythms (adrenergic antagonists, calcium channel blockers, hypokalemia). The P wave would be absent in rhythms with sinus arrest. P waves decrease in amplitude as hyperkalemia becomes more severe until they become indistinguishable from the baseline.

The PR Interval. The PR interval is measured from the beginning of the P wave to the beginning of the QRS complex, and thus is actually a PQ interval. Electrically the PR interval represents the interval between the onset of atrial depolarization and the onset of ventricular depolarization. During this interval the electrical impulse must travel from the atria through the AV node, bundle of His, bundle branches, and the Purkinje fibers until the ventricular myocardium begins to depolarize. The normal PR interval in adults is 0.12 to 0.20 seconds. Children usually have more rapid conduction and a shorter PR interval and older adults generally have a longer PR interval. The segment between the end of the P wave and the beginning of the QRS complex reflects atrial repolarization and is usually isoelectric. However, in some normal patients this segment may be displaced (usually less than 0.8 mm) in the opposite direction of the P wave due to atrial repolarization. The larger the P wave the greater the magnitude of the depression. In these patients the PR interval would be depressed in all leads except AVR. This depression can interfere with using the PR interval as a baseline to determine ST segment elevation. In this setting the TP segment (between the end of the T wave and the beginning of the P wave) can be used to define a baseline.

Agents that decrease conduction would initially cause marked lengthening of the PR segment until conduction from the pacemaker cells completely ceases and the P wave is no longer related to the QRS complex (complete heart block). Some agents affect conduction by blocking calcium channels (calcium channel blockers) or adrenergic receptors (beta-adrenergic antagonists) or the sodium–potassium pump (digoxin).

The QRS Complex. The QRS complex reflects the electrical forces generated by ventricular depolarization. The depolarization of the left ventricle contributes most of the forces reflected by the QRS complex because of its larger muscle mass. However, when a right bundle branch block is present, the two ventricles will depolarize sequentially, first left then right, and will be distinguishable on the ECG. The normal QRS duration in adults varies between 0.06 and 0.10 seconds. The normal range for the QRS axis in the frontal plane is between –30 degrees and +105 degrees, although most people will have values between +30 and +75. The axis will vary with the weight and age of the patient. Overweight individuals will have a more leftward axis (closer to 0 degrees, or negative) and thin people will have a more vertical axis (closer to 90 degrees). People over the age of 40 will have a more rightward axis (between –30 degrees and +90 degrees) and people under the age of 40 will have an axis closer to 0 degrees (usually between 0 degrees and +105 degrees).

The axis of the terminal 40-msec (0.04 seconds) of the QRS complex, which is the last box of the QRS complex on the electrocardiogram paper, can be considered separately. A rightward deflection (> 120 degrees) of this small segment (R wave in lead aVR and S wave in aVL) is correlated with toxicity from cyclic antidepressant agents[98,147] and some other toxins, including cocaine, Type IA and IC antidysrhythmic agents, phenothiazines, amantadine, and carbamazepine (Fig. 8–10).

Widening of the QRS complex is seen with agents that cause sodium channel blockade, like cyclic antidepressants and quinidine. Abnormalities in the serum concentrations of potassium may also cause widening and distortion of the QRS complex. Hypothermia may cause an abnormality at the junction of the QRS complex with the ST segment, the J-point, causing an apparent widening of the QRS complex.

The ST Segment. The ST segment is the distance between the end of the QRS complex and the beginning of the T wave. This segment reflects the period of time between depolarization and the start of repolarization. Both the length of this segment and the degree of displacement from the baseline are important. The segment between the end of the T wave and the start of the P wave or the PR interval is often used for reference as the isoelectric baseline. The J-point refers to the junction of the QRS complex with the ST segment, and is typically a 90 degree angle.

Prolongation or shortening of the ST segment is

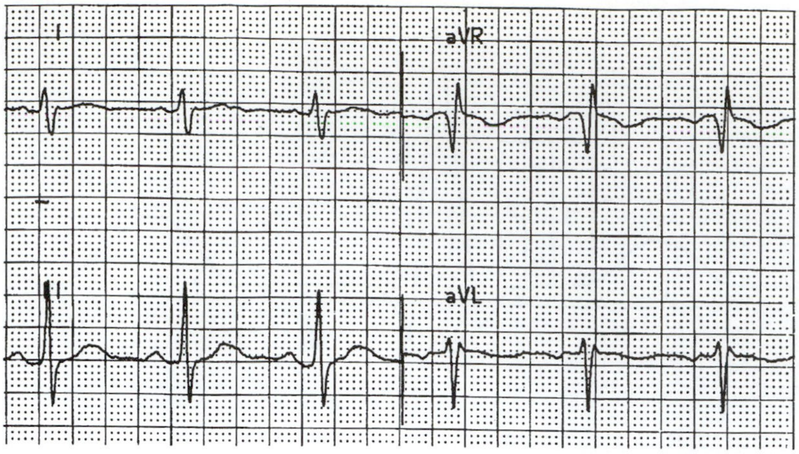

Figure 8–10. ECG showing leads I, II, aVR, and aVL of a patient with a tricyclic antidepressant overdose. The prominent S wave in leads I and aVL and R wave in aVR demonstrate the terminal 40-msec rightward axis shift.

most often caused by abnormalities in the serum calcium concentration. Hypercalcemia, which shortens the ST segment, is often caused by malignancy and such drugs and toxins as antacids (milk alkali syndrome), hydrochlorothiazide, cholecalciferol (vitamin D), vitamin A, and other retinoids. Hypocalcemia, which prolongs the ST segment, is caused by a number of agents, including fluoride, calcitonin, ethylene glycol, mithramycin, and phosphates.

The T Wave. The T wave represents ventricular repolarization. The polarity of repolarization generally proceeds in the same direction as depolarization and thus the deflection is usually in the same direction as the QRS complex. The normal T wave is asymmetric. The first half is concave and has a more gradual slope than the second half. The amplitude is greatest in lead II and is normally less than 6 mm, although it may reach as high as 12 mm in some normal adults.

A peaked T wave is usually evidence of hyperkalemia. Hyperkalemia may be seen following exposure to numerous agents (see Chap. 15, Table 15–8).

The QT Interval. The QT interval represents the entire duration of ventricular systole and is measured from the end of the QRS complex to the end of the T wave. The lead with the largest T wave should be used for this measurement. With slow heart rates a prominent U wave can obscure the terminal portion of the T wave, and with fast heart rates the P wave can obscure the terminal portion of the T wave. In these cases the QT interval should be estimated by following the downslope of the T wave. The normal QT interval varies with the heart rate, and numerous formulas and tables to obtain the corrected QT interval (QTc) are available. At a heart rate of 70 beats/min the upper limit of normal for the QT interval is approximately 0.40 seconds.

There is a brief moment in the middle of repolarization, during the T wave on the ECG, when some myocardial fibers are refractory but others are not. This time interval has been called the vulnerable period (Fig. 8–11).[29] An electrical stimulus from a pacemaker cell, from a premature ventricular contraction, or from an external or internal pacemaker that reaches the myocardium at this time can cause depolarization leading to electrical chaos. This chaos may manifest as ventricular tachycardia, ventricular fibrillation, or torsades de pointes. Early and delayed afterdepolarizations (see page 107: basic electrophysiology of the myocardial cell) are terms used to describe these extra depolarizations. Agents that cause sodium channel blockade, Vaughan-Williams Class I antidysrhythmic agents (see Chap. 52), prolong the duration of this vulnerable period. Agents that cause potassium channel blockade, Class III antidysrhythmic agents, enhance the possibility of reentrant dysrhythmias. Although at a cellular level these agents are antidysrhythmic, the multicellular effects may be prodysrhythmic. The probability of ventricular dysrhythmias and torsades de pointes is increased by both sodium and potassium channel blockade.[127] Prolongation of the QT interval may be caused by numerous agents that affect ventricular repolarization (Table 8–2).

The U Wave. The U wave is a small deflection that occurs after the T wave and usually with a similar orientation. The exact electrophysiologic etiology is unclear and, be-

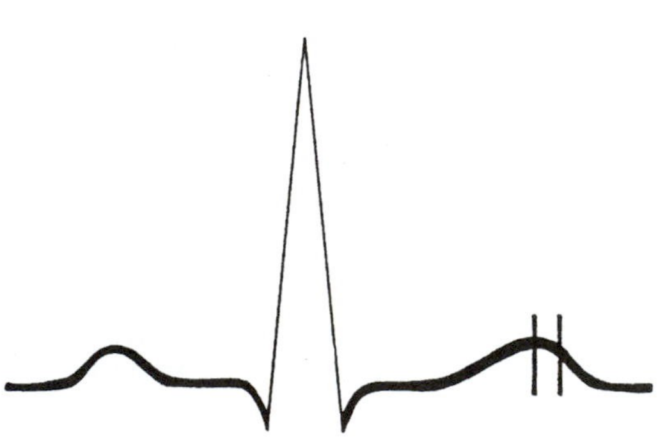

Figure 8–11. Approximate location of the vulnerable period. *(Reproduced, with permission, from Conover MB: Understanding Electrocardiography, 7th ed. St. Louis, Mosby-Year Book, 1996, p. 28.)*

cause of its low voltage, usually goes unnoticed. The amplitude is usually about 5–25% smaller than the amplitude of the T wave. One theory is that the U wave represents afterpotentials, or incomplete repolarization, of the ventricular myocardium. Another proposed mechanism is that the U wave is caused by repolarization of the Purkinje fibers.[75] The U wave is largest in leads V_2 and V_3, with an average height of 0.33 mm, although normal U waves may reach 2.0 mm in height. Distinguishing a U wave from a notched T wave is difficult. The apices of a notched T wave are usually less than 0.15 seconds apart, and the peaks of a T-U complex are greater than 0.15 seconds apart. Transient U wave inversion can be caused by myocardial ischemia or systemic hypertension.[93]

Hypokalemia is the most common cause of prominent U waves (see Chap. 15 and Table 15–8).

The Normal Pediatric ECG

The cardiac electrophysiology of infants and children is different from that of adults. Not surprisingly, the normal pediatric ECG is also different in many ways from the normal adult ECG (Table 8–3). The resting heart rate of infants and children is substantially higher than that of adults, and conduction, in general, is faster. The amplitude of the QRS complex depends on the relative masses of the right and left ventricles and the impedance of the body tissues, and thus is very variable in the early years. In a term infant the right ventricle is substantially larger than the left, and the ECG demonstrates prominent R waves in the right precordium and deep S waves in the left lateral precordium. An R wave up to 26 mm and an S wave up to 22 mm may be normal in a newborn.[34] An adult ratio of left–right ventricular size is usually reached by the age of 6 months. The more vertical orientation of the heart in the chest produces a higher voltage in the mid-precordial leads. In infants, Q waves are commonly seen in the inferior and lateral precordial leads, but are abnormal in leads I and aVL. The T waves are the most notable difference between pediatric and adult electrocardiograms. The T waves in the right precordial leads in children are deeply inverted until age 7 and sometimes beyond (persistent juvenile T wave pattern).

While congenital heart disease is the most common cause of electrocardiographic abnormalities in children, electrolyte disorders and drugs may also cause changes in electrophysiology that are reflected on the ECG. Abnormalities that are useful markers on the adult ECG may not always be as useful in the pediatric population. A rightward deviation of the terminal 40-msec QRS axis is helpful in assessing adults for tricyclic antidepressant toxicity (see Chap. 55); however, in children, this marker is not predictive of toxicity.[13]

Abnormal Electrocardiogram

Abnormalities in the rate or pattern of the electrocardiogram tracing can provide the clinician with immediate information about a patient's cardiovascular status. A rate that is too fast (eg, supraventricular tachycardia, ventricular tachycardia, ventricular fibrillation) or too slow (eg, conduction abnormalities, sinus bradycardia) may not provide adequate cardiac output to maintain a reasonable blood pressure. Any rhythm other than normal sinus rhythm is referred to as a dysrhythmia in this text. Initially, abnormalities of the pattern seen on the ECG may be localized to one wave or interval but often will rapidly progress to involve all elements of the ECG tracing including the rate and interfere with maintenance of cardiac output. Agents that effect the pattern, agents that primarily cause a slowing of the heart rate, and those that cause a rapid heart rate will be discussed. Of course most affected ECGs will fall into all three categories (abnormal pattern, fast rate, slow rate) at some point. Ischemia is seen on the ECG as a current of injury that is localized to one or two areas of the heart (inferior,

TABLE 8–3. NORMAL VALUES FOR PEDIATRIC ECG

Age	Heart Rate (beats/min)	QRS Axis (degrees)	PR Interval (msec)	QRS Duration (msec)	Q (III) (mV)	R (V_1) (mV)	S (V_1) (mV)	R (V_4) (mV)	S (V_4) (mV)	R (V_6) (mV)	S (V_6) (mV)
0–1 d	93–155	59–163	79–161	21–76	0.01–0.34	0.5–2.6	0.1–2.3	0.3–3.0	0.3–2.8	0.–1.2	0–1.0
1–3 d	91–158	64–161	81–139	22–67	0.01–0.33	0.5–2.7	0.1–2.1	0.6–3.0	0.2–2.7	0.–1.2	0.–1.0
3–7 d	90–166	77–163	73–136	21–68	0.01–0.35	0.3–2.4	0.1–1.7	0.6–2.9	0.3–2.6	0–1.2	0–1.0
7–30 d	106–182	65–161	72–138	22–79	0.01–0.35	0.3–2.1	0.1–1.1	0.8–2.9	0.3–2.3	0.2–1.7	0–1.0
1–3 mo	120–179	31–113	72–130	23–75	0.01–0.34	0.3–1.8	0.1–1.3	1.3–3.8	0.5–2.2	0.5–2.2	0–0.7
3–6 mo	106–186	7–104	73–146	22–79	0–0.32	0.3–2.0	0.1–1.7	1.1–4.3	0.3–2.3	0.6–2.2	0–1.0
6–12 mo	108–169	6–99	72–157	23–76	0–0.33	0.2–2.0	0.1–1.8	1.2–3.6	0.2–2.3	0.6–2.3	0–0.7
1–3 y	90–151	7–101	81–148	27–75	0–0.32	0.3–1.8	0.1–2.1	1.1–3.5	0.3–2.0	0.6–2.3	0–0.7
3–5 y	72–138	6–104	83–161	30–72	0–0.29	0.2–1.8	0.2–2.2	1.3–4.5	0.2–1.8	0.8–2.4	0–0.5
5–8 y	64–132	11–143	90–163	32–79	0–0.25	0.1–1.4	0.3–2.3	1.2–4.4	0.2–1.9	0.8–2.7	0–0.4
8–12 y	62–130	9–114	88–171	32–85	0–0.27	0.1–1.2	0.3–2.5	1.1–4.2	0.2–1.9	0.9–2.6	0–0.4
12–16 y	61–120	11–130	92–176	34–88	0–0.19	0.1–1.0	0.3–2.2	0.7–3.9	0.1–1.8	0.7–2.3	0–0.4

Reproduced, with permission, from Chou T, Knilans TK, eds: Electrocardiography. In: Clinical Practice Adult and Pediatric, 4th ed. Philadelphia, Saunders, 1996, pp. 650, as adapted from Davignon A, Rautabarjo P, Boiselle E, et al: Normal ECG standards for infants and children. Pediatr Cardiol 1979;1:123.

anterior, or lateral). When ECG abnormalities are detected, therapy must be appropriately defined.

Abnormal Pattern

A medication or toxin that causes a gradual change in the pattern on the ECG may provide the clinician with the opportunity to intervene before the patient suffers significant morbidity. These agents also cause a tachycardia or bradycardia at some point in their toxicity.

Electrolytes. The transmembrane shifts of ions are affected by the concentration gradients of serum electrolytes and the function of specific channels; sodium, potassium, and the sodium–potassium ATPase pump. The ion concentration, particularly of potassium and calcium, determines the configuration, duration, and amplitude of the action potential and causes characteristic changes in the surface ECG recording.

Potassium. The total body potassium content of an average adult is about 53–55 mEq/kg, of which only 2% is located in the intravascular space. The range of normal for extracellular serum potassium is 3.5–5.0 mEq/L, but intracellular potassium concentrations are about 140 mEq/L.[18] The large intracellular store of potassium is maintained by a variety of systems, the most important of which is sodium–potassium ATPase. The relationship between total body stores and serum potassium is not linear. A small change in the total body potassium may result in dramatic alterations in serum concentrations. As the serum potassium concentrations vary, a progression of characteristic changes is seen on the ECG. The exact numeric serum concentration at which these changes occurs varies widely from patient to patient.

HYPERKALEMIA. Hyperkalemia at levels less than 6.5 mEq/L causes tall, tented T waves with normal QRS, QTc, and P wave durations (Fig. 8–12). As the measured potassium rises to 6.5–8 mEq/L, the QRS complex begins to widen and a deep S wave may be seen in the precordial leads. The P wave diminishes in amplitude and duration. The ST segment seems to disappear as the terminal S wave becomes contiguous with the tented T wave and forms a sine wave.

Hyperkalemia may be seen following exposure to numerous agents (see Chap. 15 and Table 15–8).

HYPOKALEMIA. As the serum potassium declines from the normal range, ECG findings include ST depression and a progressive decrease in the amplitude of the T wave (Fig. 8–13). When the serum potassium decreases further, the amplitude of the U wave increases and eventually the U and T waves fuse. The amplitude and duration of both the QRS complex and the P wave increase as the PR interval lengthens. Ventricular tachycardia, torsades de pointes, ventricular fibrillation, and asystole may develop if proper therapy is not instituted.

Hypokalemia is a common adverse effect of many medications and toxins (see Chap. 15 and Table 15–8).

Calcium. Calcium is the most abundant mineral in the human body; however, 98–99% is located in bone. About half of the extraosseous calcium is protein bound, leaving very small concentrations of free calcium. The levels of free calcium, or ionized calcium, are carefully regulated by a complex interaction between dietary intake, renal elimination, vitamin D activity, parathyroid hor-

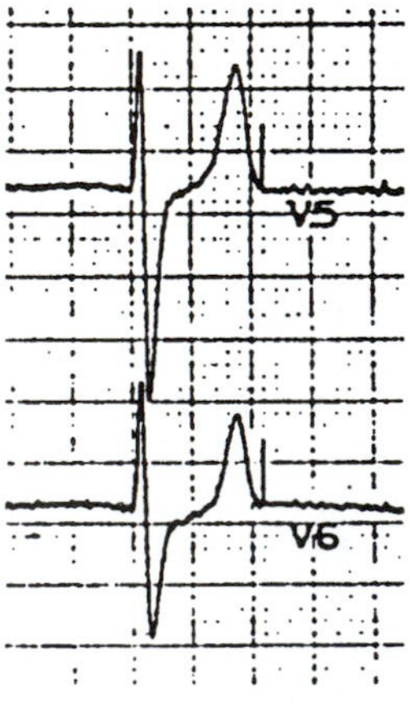

Figure 8–12. A 51-year-old sanitation worker suffered inhalation and dermal exposure to hydrofluoric acid. This ECG was recorded approximately $1\frac{1}{2}$ hours after exposure and demonstrates marked hyperkalemic changes with peaked T waves, absent P waves, and prolongation of the QRS complex.

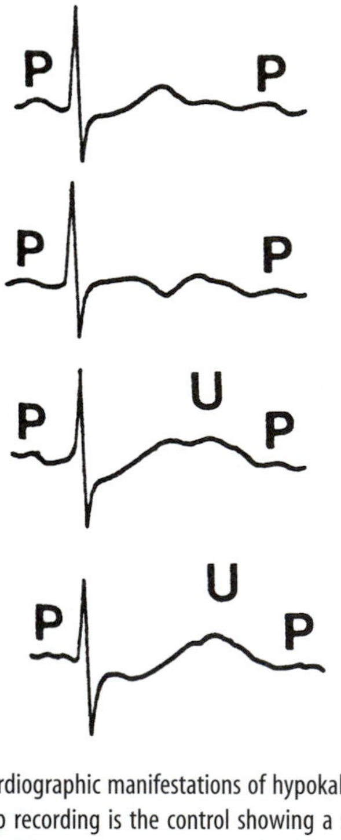

Figure 8–13. Electrocardiographic manifestations of hypokalemia (intermediate precordial lead). The top recording is the control showing a small but normal U wave. The remaining recordings are arranged to show increasing degrees of hypokalemia. *(Adapted, with permission, from Castellanos A, Myerburg RJ: The resting electrocardiogram. In: Hurst JW, Logue RB, Rackley CE, et al, eds: The Heart: Arteries and Veins, 6th ed. New York, McGraw-Hill, 1986, p. 225.)*

mone, and calcitonin. Normal values of ionized calcium in an adult are usually 4.52–5.28 mg/dL, whereas total calcium usually ranges from 8.5 to 10.5 mg/dL.

HYPERCALCEMIA. The ECG findings of hypercalcemia are a decrease in the QTc interval, which is actually a shortening of the ST segment (Fig. 8–14). The duration of the QTc interval is inversely proportional to the serum calcium level. The morphology and duration of the QRS and T and P waves remain essentially unchanged. Malignancy is a common cause of hypercalcemia. Agents that might cause hypercalcemia include antacids (milk alkali syndrome), hydrochlorothiazide, cholecalciferol (vitamin D), vitamin A, and other retinoids (see Chap. 15 and Table 15–9).

HYPOCALCEMIA. The major effect of hypocalcemia is prolongation of the QTc interval (Fig. 8–14). This effect is caused by prolongation of the ST segment and is unique to hypocalcemia. The T wave remains unchanged. The prolongation of the ST segment is approximately proportional to the decrease in ionized calcium. Hypocalcemia is caused by a number of agents, including fluoride, calcitonin, ethylene glycol, mithramycin, and phosphates (see Chap. 15 and Table 15–9).

Magnesium. About 50% of total body magnesium is stored in the bone and the remainder is located in the soft tissues. Normal serum magnesium levels range from 0.75 to 1.0 mmol/L. Only about 1–2% of the total body magnesium (average 2000 mEq or 24 g) is located in the extracellular fluid. Magnesium is required for DNA and protein synthesis and is essential for all biologic activities involving adenosine triphosphate. Serum magnesium levels correlate poorly with total body stores.[54]

Isolated changes in serum magnesium do not seem to cause specific ECG manifestations, although multiple ECG abnormalities have been reported.[54] When hypomagnesemia coexists with hypokalemia, as is usually the case, QU prolongation and torsades de pointes may be seen.[55,138] The QU interval is the distance between the end of the Q wave and the end of the U wave. Differentiation between the QU and the QT intervals is difficult if the T and U waves are superimposed. Hypokalemia and hypomagnesemia alone do not usually prolong the QT interval. Longstanding and marked magnesium deficiency lowers the amplitude of the T wave and causes depression of the ST segment. A slight narrowing of the QRS and tall, peaked T waves with a normal QT interval may also be seen.[106] Hypomagnesemia may also potentiate digoxin toxicity.[119] Hypermagnesemia has been associated with a prolongation of the QT or QU interval[26] and an increase in the PR interval and QRS duration. Occasionally sinus and AV node block occurs when intravenous magnesium is administered.[50,92,125]

Some toxins that are known to alter serum magnesium are listed on Table 15–10 and discussed in that chapter. However, alterations in the other cations (sodium, potassium, and calcium) can also alter the serum magnesium.

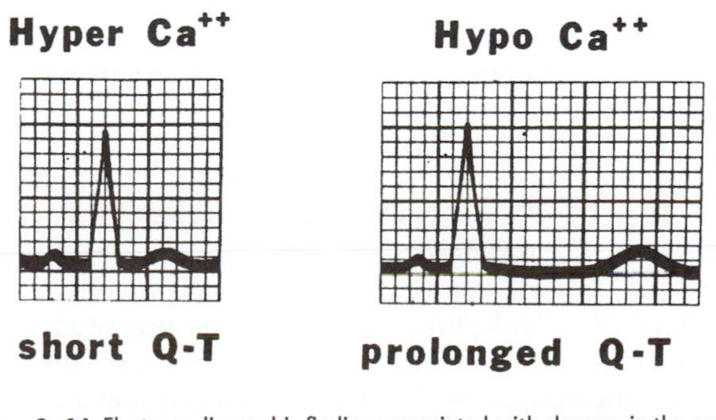

Figure 8–14. Electrocardiographic findings associated with changes in the serum calcium. *(Reproduced, with permission, from Dubin D: Rapid Interpretation of EKG's, ed. V. Tampa, FL, Cover Publishing Co, 1996, p. 297.)*

Digoxin

ECG Findings. Cardiac glycosides profoundly alter the electrophysiology of the heart. After therapeutic doses of digoxin, the ECG can reveal a "digoxin effect" demonstrating a slow heart rate from increased vagal tone and repolarization abnormalities, including sagging ST segments, inverted T waves, and normal or shortened QT intervals. As the dose of digoxin increases, clear manifestations of toxicity will appear (see Chap. 48).

These manifestations of digoxin toxicity vary with the dose and differ depending on the specific type of cardiac tissue involved. The atria and ventricles exhibit increased automaticity and excitability, resulting in extrasystoles and tachydysrhythmias. Conduction velocity is reduced in both myocardial and nodal tissue, resulting in an increased PR interval and AV block.[152] The AV node becomes more refractory while the myocardium becomes less refractory, resulting in a prolonged PR interval and AV block, accompanied by a decrease in the QT interval. (See Antidotes in Depth: Digoxin–Specific Antibody Fragments [Fab].)

Ectopic rhythms appear as the first sign of digitalis poisoning in 10–15% of cases. Ectopic rhythms, such as nonparoxysmal junctional tachycardia, ventricular premature extrasystoles, ventricular flutter and fibrillation, atrial flutter and fibrillation, and bidirectional ventricular tachycardia, are due to enhanced automaticity, reentry, or both.[115] (See Tables 48–2 and 48–3.)

Bidirectional ventricular tachycardia (Fig. 8–15) is particularly characteristic of severe digitalis toxicity and results from alterations of intraventricular conduction, junctional tachycardia with aberrant intraventricular conduction, or, on rare occasions, alternating ventricular pacemakers. Depression of the atrial pacemakers causing sinus node arrest may also be seen. Other features include sinoatrial block, AV block, and sinus exit block resulting from depression of normal conduction. When conduction and the normal pacemaker are both depressed, ectopic pacemakers may take over, producing atrial tachycardia with AV block (Fig. 8–16). Atrioventricular dissociation may occur due to suppression of the dominant pacemaker with escape of a subsidiary pace-

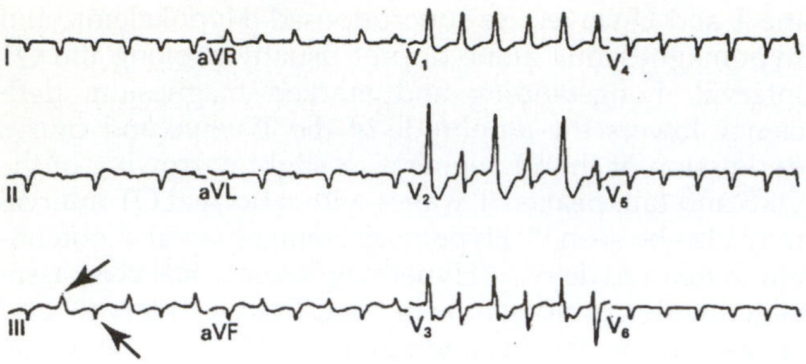

Figure 8–15. Digoxin-induced bidirectional ventricular tachycardia. A 71-year-old woman had recently undergone mitral-valve replacement after being treated with digoxin for 12 years for atrial fibrillation. After the operation, the same dose of digoxin was administered intravenously, despite rising creatinine levels. The 12-lead electrocardiogram shows an alternating QRS axis that is characteristic of bidirectional ventricular tachycardia (*arrows*), a dysrhythmia virtually diagnostic of digitalis toxicity. The serum digoxin level at the time of the electocardiogram was 4.5 ng/mL (normal, 0.8–2.0 ng/mL). *(Reproduced, with permission, from Valent S, Kelly P: Images in clinical medicine: digoxin-induced bidirectional ventricular tachycardia. N Engl J Med 1997;336:550.)*

maker or to an inappropriate acceleration of a ventricular pacemaker. Hypotension, shock, and cardiovascular collapse can ensue.

While there are marked differences in symptomatology between acute and chronic cardiac glycoside poisoning, the electrocardiographic manifestations are similar (see Chap. 48).

QT Prolongation

ECG Findings. Long QT syndromes are classified as acquired or hereditary based on the conditions that appear to trigger the polymorphic ventricular tachycardia and torsades de pointes associated with these syndromes. Both the hereditary and acquired forms of prolonged QT syndrome may have similar morphology on the surface electrocardiogram: the typical short–long–short initiating sequence (more common in the acquired form), abnormal U waves, prolongation of the QT or QU interval, and facilitation by hypokalemia. Clinically, however, hereditary but not acquired, long QT syndromes are clearly related to adrenergic stimulation or enhancement of sympathetic nervous system tone. Typically, bizarre and dynamic long QT or long QTU segments are observed during periods of beta$_1$-adrenergic stimulation or excitement associated with intense sympathetic activation.

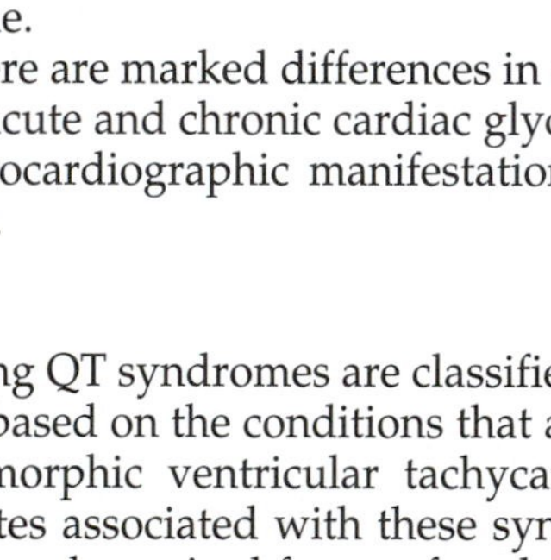

Figure 8–16. This ECG demonstrates atrial tachycardia with AV block in a patient with digoxin toxicity.

Patients have variable susceptibility to prolongation of the QT interval by drugs and a variable response to a prolonged QT interval. Factors that contribute to the development of torsades de pointes include hypokalemia, hypomagnesemia, hypocalcemia, bradycardia, ischemia, and tissue hypoxia.

Mechanisms. Many of the mechanisms for the long QT syndromes, acquired or hereditary, have not been fully elucidated. The acquired syndromes are referred to as pause-dependent because the torsades de pointes associated with them generally occurs at slow heart rates or in response to short–long–short RR interval sequences. The hereditary long QT syndromes are typically considered adrenergic-dependent because the torsades de pointes associated with them is generally triggered by adrenergic-activation or enhancement of sympathetic nervous system tone. There is some overlap between these two syndromes. Patients with adrenergic-dependent forms are more likely to develop dysrhythmias during episodes of bradycardia or when electrolyte abnormalities are also present.

The hereditary long QT syndrome, Jervell-Lange-Nielsen (autosomal recessive), is associated with deafness, while patients with Romano-Ward syndrome (autosomal dominant) have normal hearing. These syndromes seem to be related to a defect in the Harvey *ras*-1 gene on chromosome 11. Evidence suggests that this gene may help to modulate potassium channel function, especially in response to beta$_1$-adrenergic activation. This defect may also lead to an inappropriate adaptive response in the duration of the action potential in response to changes in heart rate.[7,79,150]

The initiation of torsades de pointes in patients with acquired, pause-dependent, long QT syndrome often involves a premature ventricular contraction, closely coupled with the last normal QRS complex and then followed by a pause. The next sinus beat initiates another closely coupled premature ventricular contraction, which is the first beat of the torsades de pointes. In the hereditary forms, enhanced sympathetic tone alone may initiate dysrhythmias.

Early afterdepolarizations develop because of the failure of normal repolarization and may have a role in the genesis of QT prolongation in acquired and congenital forms of the long QT syndrome and the dysrhythmias. Scenarios that enhance the net outward potassium current during repolarization or that enhance the net inward sodium or L-type calcium currents prevent normal repolarization and allow the membrane potential to oscillate at the plateau phase level. Patients with the idiopathic congenital long QT syndrome may have a myocardial defect in repolarization involving an outward potassium current or an inward slow calcium current, rather than a "sympathetic imbalance." Sympathetic

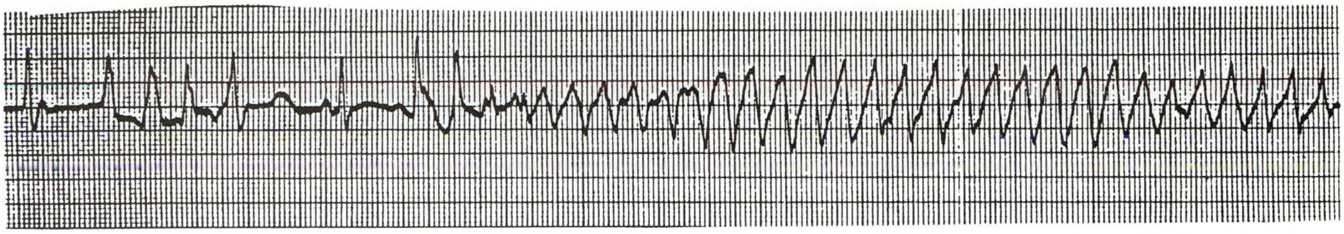

Figure 8–17. Torsades de pointes in a patient who ingested an unknown amount of thioridazine.

stimulation could periodically increase the early afterdepolarization amplitude to provoke ventricular tachydysrhythmias. Alpha-adrenergic receptor stimulation also increases the amplitude of early afterdepolarizations, and this effect may be blocked by alpha-adrenergic receptor blockade and by magnesium.[9]

Antidysrhythmic drugs are responsible for most of the patients presenting with the acquired long QT syndrome. Classes IA and III in the Vaughan-Williams classification of antidysrhythmic drugs are most commonly involved, although class IC agents have also caused torsades de pointes (see Chap. 52). Class IA antidysrhythmic agents (disopyramide, procainamide, quinidine) depress the rapid action potential upstroke, decrease conduction velocity by sodium channel blockade, and significantly prolong repolarization by potassium channel blockade. Class III agents (amiodarone, bretylium, *N*-acetylprocainamide, sotalol) primarily block potassium channels and slow repolarization but have little or no effects on sodium channels. Torsades from sotalol exposure seems to be dose dependent and dysrhythmias from amiodarone are rare.[74,96] Class IC agents (encainide, flecainide, moricizine, propafenone) markedly depress the rapid action potential upstroke and decrease conduction velocity by sodium channel blockade but exert little effect on repolarization. They have little or no potassium channel blocking properties and yet also cause QT prolongation. Class IB agents (lidocaine, mexiletine, moricizine, tocainide) effect predominantly abnormal tissue and enhance repolarization. They have minimal effect on the QT duration.

The electrophysiologic effects of phenothiazines are similar to those of quinidine (see Chap. 57). The most common ECG changes caused by the phenothiazines include widening, flattening, notching, or inversion of the T wave; prolongation of the QTc interval; and prominence of the U wave. Early afterdepolarizations may trigger ventricular dysrhythmias and are difficult to distinguish from the other T-wave abnormalities. These repolarization abnormalities are seen more frequently in patients receiving thioridazine (Mellaril) (see Fig. 8–17) and mesoridazine (Serentil)[86] than in those receiving chlorpromazine (Thorazine) or, even less, trifluoperazine (Stelazine).[10] Haloperidol, a butyrophenone, can also cause ventricular dysrhythmias. The ECG abnormalities are dose related. With thioridazine, repolarization abnormalities are usually not seen when the dose is less than 100 mg/day. Such abnormalities are present in about half of the patients when the dose is between 100 and 300 mg/day and in about three-fourths when the dosage is above 300 mg/day. The effects usually appear within 1 or 2 days after the beginning of therapy and reach their maximum in 4 or 5 days.[65] The combination of thioridazine and desipramine at therapeutic doses caused sustained ventricular tachycardia in an otherwise healthy 38-year-old woman.[145] Although intraventricular conduction defects may be seen, they are not common. Supraventricular and ventricular tachycardia may be observed in patients who take high doses of the drug.[48] Ventricular tachycardia and ventricular fibrillation were responsible for sudden death in some of these patients.[4,62,68]

Pentamidine isethionate, an antiparasite agent used in the treatment of *Pneumocystis carinii* in AIDS patients, is associated with ventricular tachydysrhythmias and torsades de pointes[41,83,110,132] that may persist for weeks after discontinuation.[14,31,143] The similarity between the structures of pentamidine and procainamide probably accounts for these pentamidine-induced dysrhythmias.[31]

QT prolongation and torsades de pointes also occur with the "nonsedating" antihistamines, astemizole (Hismanal)[16,126] and terfenadine (Seldane).[88,94] Terfenadine was voluntarily withdrawn from the market because of this cardiotoxicity (see Chap. 34).

Cyclic Antidepressants

ECG Findings. A 12-lead ECG is an invaluable adjunct in the evaluation of all overdose patients but particularly in the cyclic antidepressant overdose patient. Potential findings include sinus tachycardia, prolongation of the PR and QTc intervals, QRS complex widening, nonspecific ST-T wave changes, bundle branch blocks, second- or third-degree AV block, supraventricular dysrhythmias, ventricular dysrhythmias, rightward deviation of the terminal 40-msec QRS axis in the frontal plane, and asystole (see Table 8–4).[56,61,95]

A prospective analysis of ECGs from cases reported to a poison center demonstrated that the maximal limb lead QRS duration was prognostic of seizures and cardiac dysrhythmias following acute tricyclic antidepressant ingestions.[17] Seizures occurred in 30% of patients with QRS complexes greater than 100 msec, and cardiac

TABLE 8–4. ELECTROCARDIOGRAPHIC ABNORMALITIES ASSOCIATED WITH CYCLIC ANTIDEPRESSANT OVERDOSES

Sinus tachycardia
Prolonged PR, QRS, QTc intervals
ST-T wave changes
Bundle branch blocks
Second- or third-degree AV block
Supraventricular dysrhythmias
Atrial and AV junctional tachycardias
Atrial fibrillation
Atrial flutter
Sinus bradycardia
Ventricular dysrhythmias
PVCs
Idioventricular rhythm
Ventricular tachycardia
Ventricular fibrillation
Torsades de pointes
Terminal 40-ms frontal QRS vector between 130 and 270 degrees
Asystole

Reproduced, with permission, and modified from Groleau G, Jotte R, Barish R: The electrocardiographic manifestations of cyclic antidepressant therapy and overdose: a review. J Emerg Med 1990;8:599.

dysrhythmias occurred in 50% of patients with QRS complexes wider than 160 msec. None of the 49 patients studied had either a seizure with a QRS complex less than 100 msec or a cardiac dysrhythmia with a QRS complex less than 160 msec. Other studies have confirmed the prognostic value of the QRS duration.[47,64,73,121]

The combination of a rightward axis shift in the terminal 40-msec of the QRS complex (Fig. 8–10) along with a prolonged QTc and a sinus tachycardia is highly specific and sensitive for cyclic antidepressant poisoning, but the absence of these findings is not exclusionary.[23,98,147] The axis of the terminal 40-msec of the QRS complex is determined by observing the last box (0.04 seconds) of the QRS complex on the electrocardiogram paper. An R wave (positive deflection) in lead AVR and S wave (negative deflection) in leads I and aVL suggest there is a rightward deflection, greater than 120 degrees, of this small segment.

Another study retrospectively reviewed the ECGs of first-generation cyclic antidepressant overdose patients and noncyclic antidepressant overdose patients with respect to the character of the terminal 40-msec frontal plane QRS axis.[147] The authors concluded that a patient with a cyclic antidepressant overdose was 8.6 times more likely to have a terminal 40-msec axis of more than 120 degrees than a patient cohort without a cyclic antidepressant overdose, and that the terminal 40-msec axis was a better indicator of first-generation cyclic antidepressant overdosage than the QRS complex. No correlation was found between QRS complexes and cyclic antidepressant plasma concentrations. This study confirmed an earlier study that demonstrated that the terminal 40-msec frontal plane QRS vector was a sensitive and specific marker for cyclic antidepressant toxicity.[98] This marker may not be reliable in pediatric patients. A rightward deflection of the terminal QRS forces following tricyclic antidepressant overdose has been reported in a 17-year-old pediatric patient.[109] However, in one retrospective chart review of 37 children diagnosed with tricylic antidepressant overdose and 35 controls (all less than 11 years old) there was such interpatient variability, unrelated to age, that a rightward deviation of the terminal 40-msec QRS axis could not distinguish between poisoned and healthy children.[13]

A recent prospective study suggests that an absolute height of the terminal portion of aVR that is greater than 3 mm predicted seizures or dysrhythmias in tricyclic antidepressant poisoned patients.[77]

Mechanisms. The cyclic antidepressants exert a membrane depressant, local anesthetic effect on the myocardium by blocking the fast sodium channels and slowing sodium influx into cells during phase 0 of the action potential.[51,85,140] This "quinidine-like" effect causes intraven-

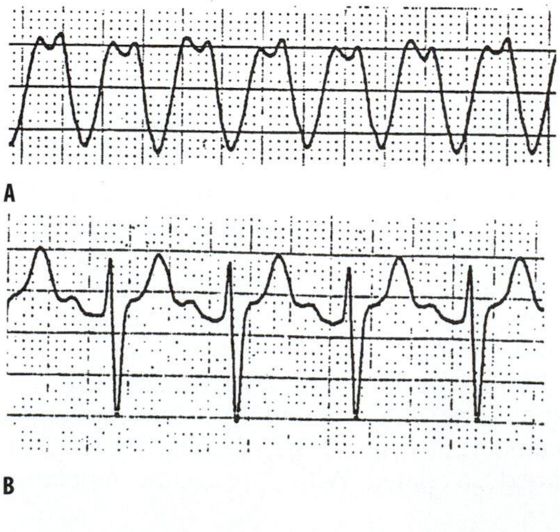

Figure 8–18. (**A**) Rhythm strip of a 15-year old girl with an amitriptyline overdose, demonstrating the patient's initial wide complex dysrhythmia noted on presentation. (**B**) Rhythm strip demonstrating the immediate response to intravenous sodium bicarbonate administration.

tricular conduction delays (Fig. 8–18A), ventricular dysrhythmias and negative inotropy with decreased cardiac output, decreased coronary perfusion, and hypotension. Sodium bicarbonate therapy can ameliorate the cardiovascular toxicity (Fig. 8–18B).

Hypothermia

ECG findings. Hypothermia is commonly associated with overdoses. The most common ECG abnormality in hypothermia is generalized, progressive depression of myocardial conduction. This general decrease in conduction is seen as progressive slowing of the sinus rate, prolongation of the PR and QTc intervals, and an apparent increase in QRS duration. The increase in QRS duration is actually an elevation or distortion of the J-point and has been called a J wave, or an Osborn wave (Fig. 8–19).[100] Osborn waves are commonly seen when the core temperature is less than 30°C (85°F), but do not seem to have specific prognostic significance.[136] A constant or intermittent oscillation of the baseline as a result of muscle tremors may also be present, even though shivering may not be clinically evident. Profound hypothermia is associated with atrial fibrillation, ventricular dysrhythmias, ventricular fibrillation, and asystole. Electrocardiographic abnormalities that persist after rewarming suggest underlying heart disease[101] or are the result of myocardial damage during hypothermia.

Mechanisms. The electrophysiologic basis for the development of Osborn waves is unclear. Possible mechanisms include a current of injury or delayed ventricular depolarization. Early repolarization may be occurring in a portion of the ventricle before delayed depolarization is completed in another portion. Small J waves may also be seen in normal patients with the early repolarization pattern, in cerebral injuries, and even in patients with Prinzmetal's angina.

Rapid Rate

The distinction between toxins that cause a rapid rate and those that cause a slow rate on the ECG is somewhat artificial, since many agents can do both. Table 21–10 lists a wide variety of agents that often cause tachydysrhythmias. Agents that cause supraventricular tachycardia early in their clinical course (sympathomimetics, phosphodiesterase inhibitors, cyclic antidepressants, antihistamines, anticholinergics), also cause ventricular tachycardia in more serious cases of poisoning. Some agents (digoxin, propoxyphene, chloroquine) cause ventricular tachycardia by other mechanisms (QT prolongation, blockade of the sodium–potassium pump) and only rarely cause supraventricular tachycardia.

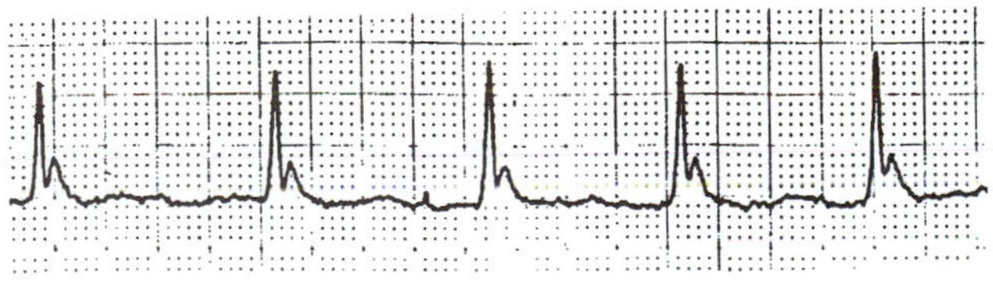

Figure 8–19. Typical ECG seen in hypothermia. This patient was a 69-year-old man with a core temperature of 24°C (75.2°F). Note the typical J wave abnormalities (Osborn waves) in the terminal phase of the QRS complex. This patient's ECG returned to its premorbid state on rewarming.

The rate of impulse formation at the sinus node is regulated by a balance between parasympathetic and sympathetic parts of the autonomic nervous system. Sympathomimetic agents increase sympathetic tone, producing sinus tachycardia and enhanced AV nodal conduction. Sinus tachycardia may be the first manifestation of exposure to a sympathomimetic agent, but other supraventricular or ventricular dysrhythmias may also develop. Common agents that result in a tachycardia include anticholinergics, antihistamines, alpha- and beta-adrenergic agonists, cocaine, and amphetamines.

Anticholinergics and Antihistamines. Poisoning by diphenhydramine and other over-the-counter antihistamines is usually associated with marked anticholinergic effects (see Chap. 34). Tachycardia is the predominant cardiac effect. However, wide complex tachycardias can also occur.[27] The mechanism is similar to that of other local anesthetics with inhibition of the fast sodium channels. At very high concentrations the potassium channels are also inhibited. The newer nonsedating antihistamines, terfenadine and astemizole, cause tachycardia and lengthening of the QT interval resulting in torsades de pointes (see page 107: QT prolongation section).

Adrenergic Agonists. The $beta_2$-adrenergic agonists (metaproterenol, terbutaline, albuterol, salmeterol, salbutamol) in high doses can also cause ventricular dysrhythmias.[25,63,67] The mechanism involves cAMP and also stimulation of sodium–potassium ATPase causing hypokalemia.[18]

Phosphodiesterase Inhibitors. The methylxanthines include theophylline (1,3-dimethylxanthine), caffeine (1,3,7-trimethylxanthine), and theobromine (3,7-dimethylxanthine) and are all structurally similar (see Fig. 38–1). Common cardiac manifestations of theophylline overdose include supraventricular tachycardia (Fig. 8–20), atrial fibrillation or flutter, and ventricular dysrhythmias.[122] Theophylline is a potent phosphodiesterase inhibitor and also acts as an adenosine receptor antagonist (see Chap. 39). Another complication of theophylline overdose is hypokalemia, which may contribute to the cardiac toxicity.[18,123] Catecholamine activity rises more than 10-fold following theophylline intoxication, and some evidence indicates that this catecholamine surge may be responsible for the hypokalemia and the myocardial irritability.[123]

Amrinone is used therapeutically as an ionotrope and acts by inhibiting phosphodiesterase III and thus inhibits cAMP degradation in the myocardium. Increased cAMP favors calcium influx and delivery to the contractile system. It may enhance sinoatrial node automaticity

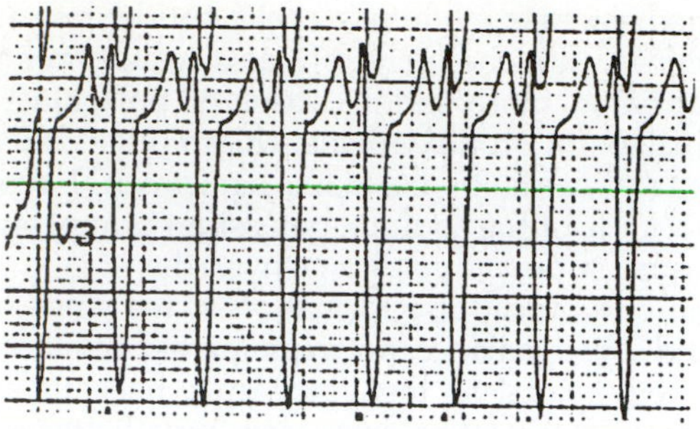

Figure 8–20. Supraventricular tachycardia in an 18-year-old female with a serum theophylline level of 97 μg/mL. This rhythm was effectively treated with intravenous diltiazem.

and atrioventricular conduction as a result of the calcium influx.[60,118]

Caffeine is probably the most widely available sympathomimetic agent. It is found in many prescription and nonprescription pharmaceuticals (weight-loss preparations), in beverages, and as an adulterant in central nervous system stimulants. In addition to sympathomimetic effects that can cause cardiovascular toxicity ranging from sinus tachycardia to ventricular fibrillation and asystole, caffeine has numerous multisystem effects[108] (see Chap. 38). The mechanism of toxicity involves inhibition of phosphodiesterase causing an accumulation of cAMP, adenosine receptor blockade,[49] increased norepinephrine, and effects on intracellular calcium.[120]

Diet Agents. Anorectic agents often contain sympathomimetic agents other than caffeine. A transiently recommended regimen containing phenteramine, with amphetamine-like effects, and fenfluramine (*N*-ethyl-alpha methyl-*m*-trifluromethyl-phenethylamine), with amphetamine and serotonin effects, has caused a number of fatal dysrhythmias, and both agents have been withdrawn from the market.[22,46,52,139] Pulmonary hypertension has also been linked to chronic use of fenfluramine,[1] although a specific mechanism for the pulmonary hypertension has not been elucidated. Phencyclidine, although not a dieting agent, is an agent that has both stimulant and depressant effects (see Chap. 67); however, the prominent cardiovascular effects include sinus tachycardia and hypertension.[36,89]

Botanical Agents. Some botanical agents (see Chap. 77) are known for their sympathomimetic properties including khat (*Catha edulis*) and ginseng (*Panax ginseng* or *P. quinquefolium*). Cathinone is the active ingredient in khat. Methcathinone with a similar chemical structure to cathinone is synthesized in clandestine laboratories from ephedrine and causes cardiac toxicity that is similar to amphetamines.[40,114,144] The betel nut (*Areca catechu*) also has stimulant and depressant properties.

Thyroid Hormone. Death or serious toxicity is rarely reported following acute overdose of thyroid hormone.[80,137] Cardiac manifestations are more common following chronic overdosage and may include sinus tachycardia, congestive heart failure, and dysrhythmias.[15]

Metals. Arsenic poisoning causes multisystem organ failure. The cardiac manifestations include sinus tachycardia, nonspecific ST-T wave abnormalities that may mimic hyperkalemia or ischemia, prolongation of the QT interval, and torsades de pointes.[105] Dysrhythmias may occur 1 to 4 weeks after presentation.[12] The mechanism is unknown, although either a direct dysrhythmogenic effect or an immunologic myocarditis has been postulated.

Lithium affects ion flux in myocardial cells, perhaps by affecting the sodium–potassium pump, and causes reversible changes on the electrocardiogram.[148] Some of these changes may mimic mild hypokalemia, although documentation of low cellular potassium levels is lacking.[30,133] T-wave flattening is the most commonly reported electrocardiographic abnormality.[19] Chronically poisoned patients seem to have more T-wave abnormalities than acutely poisoned patients.[78] Other findings include T-wave inversion, ST segment depression or elevation, and conduction abnormalities. The clinical significance of these reversible ECG findings is unclear. More serious cardiovascular manifestations including ventricular dysrhythmias[35,148,149] and myocardial infarction[104] are rare but have been reported following serious overdose.

Other. Sinus tachycardia and unusual ST-T wave changes have been reported in a patient following overdose with minoxidil. A 20-year-old woman developed ST depressions (leads II, III, and aVF) and inverted T waves (leads I, II, III, and aVF, and V_3 through V_6) in the absence of hypotension or documented electrolyte abnormalities. The ECG abnormalities were resolving 10 hours after admission.[107]

Envenomation by scorpions can cause a wide variety of electrocardiographic abnormalities including sinus tachycardia and ST-T wave abnormalities that can simulate an acute myocardial infarction.[57,58]

Hydralazine has been associated with sinus tachycardia and diffuse, marked ST depression.[124] The mechanism is unclear.

Baclofen is a lipid-soluble derivative of the inhibitory neurotransmitter gamma-aminobutyric acid (GABA) and binds to the $GABA_B$ receptor. Tachydysrhythmias (atrial fibrillation, atrial flutter), bradycardia, and conduction defects (widening of the QRS complex and lengthening of the PR interval) have been reported following overdose.[113]

Dipyridamole is an antithrombotic agent used to modify platelet function and is also used intravenously as a non-nitrate coronary vasodilator for noninvasive stress thallium cardiac imaging. Overdosage of oral dipyridamole caused ST depression and inversion of the T waves in an otherwise healthy 23-year-old woman who presented with a blood pressure of 70/30 mm Hg. The ECG changes were reversed following therapy with aminophylline and dopamine.[24]

Ventricular Tachycardia

Ventricular tachycardia is the final common pathway for many agents that cause cardiovascular toxicity. Some agents (antidysrhythmic agents, astemizole, terfenadine, phenothiazines, and pentamidine) that cause ventricular tachycardia and torsades de pointes by prolonging the QT interval are discussed in detail above (see page 116).

Chloral Hydrate. Halogenated hydrocarbons increase the release of endogenous catecholamines and also "sensitize" the myocardium to the effects of catecholamines. The sedative-hypnotic chloral hydrate (2,2,2-trichloroethane–1,1-diol) also causes reduced myocardial contractility and a shortened refractory period (see Chap. 61). Ventricular tachycardia or ventricular fibrillation may occur with much lower levels of endogenous epinephrine in the presence of halogenated hydrocarbons (Fig. 8–21).[71] Persistent cardiac dysrhythmias are common terminal events in severe overdoses.

Propoxyphene. Propoxyphene causes a blockade of the fast sodium channels as do the Type IA and IC antidysrhythmics agents. In overdose, propoxyphene has been reported to cause seizures and dysrhythmias.[82] Sodium bicarbonate has been used successfully to reverse conduction disturbances (junctional rhythm with a widened QRS complex) that were evident on the ECG of a poisoned patient.[128] The mechanism is postulated to be related to both serum alkalinization and increases in sodium ion concentration.[72,129]

Phenothiazines. The electrophysiologic effects of phenothiazines are similar to those of quinidine, with widening, flattening, notching, or inversion of the T wave; prolongation of the QTc interval; and prominence of the U wave (see page 117). These repolarization abnormalities are seen more frequently in patients receiving thioridazine (Mellaril) and mesoridazine (Serentil).[10] Early afterdepolarizations may trigger ventricular dysrhythmias and are difficult to distinguish from the other T-wave abnormalities (see page 116).

Risperidone is a newer antipsychotic agent that causes both dopamine and serotonin antagonism. At therapeutic doses there are no significant cardiovascular effects; however, in overdose, widening of the QRS complex and marked prolongation of the QTc interval have been seen.[21]

Amantadine. Amantadine is a tricyclic amine that inhibits the reuptake of dopamine and norepinephrine. Although central nervous system depression is the predominant toxicity seen following amantadine overdose, cardiac dysrhythmias also occur. QT prolongation and ventricular dysrhythmias may be exacerbated by isoproterenol and dopamine infusion.[117] In one reported patient, QT prolongation and sinus bradycardia was associated with marked hyperthermia (42°C).[20]

Chloroquine. Chloroquine is a potent cardiac toxin that causes profound negative ionotropy, vasodilation, and decreased intraventricular conduction. Electrocardiographic changes associated with overdosage resemble changes seen with the Type IA agents (quinidine), including a widened QRS complex, flattened or inverted T waves, bradycardia, and ventricular dysrhythmias (Fig. 8–22A,B).[33,112] Chloroquine reversibly blocks potassium channels, causing hypokalemia.[18,70] The degree of hypokalemia closely correlates with the clinical features observed and the dose of chloroquine ingested.[28] Treatment includes appropriate airway management, decontamination, diazepam, epinephrine, potassium repletion, and good supportive care.[11,60,90,112]

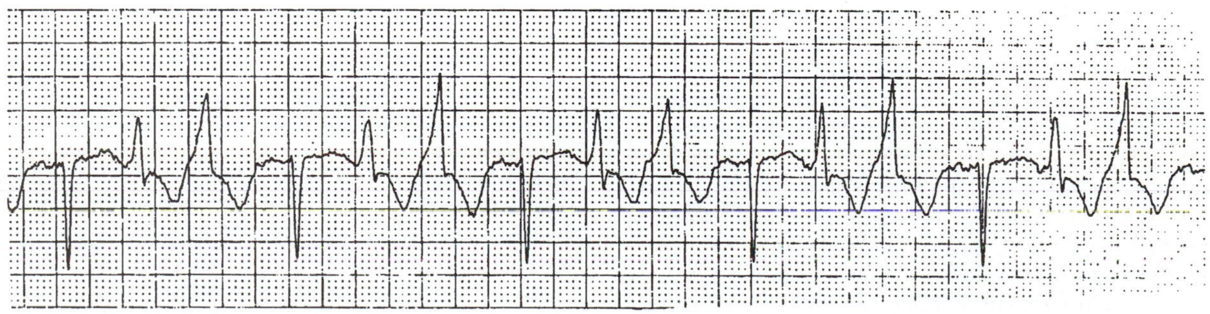

Figure 8–21. This rhythm strip shows ventricular ectopy in a patient following a chloral hydrate overdose. Following the administration of propranolol the ectopy resolved.

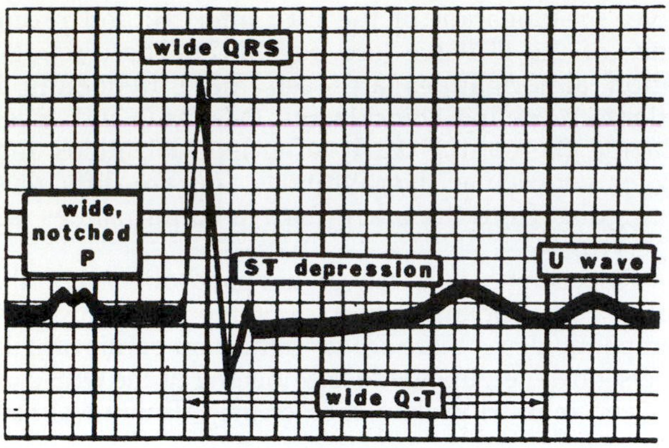

A

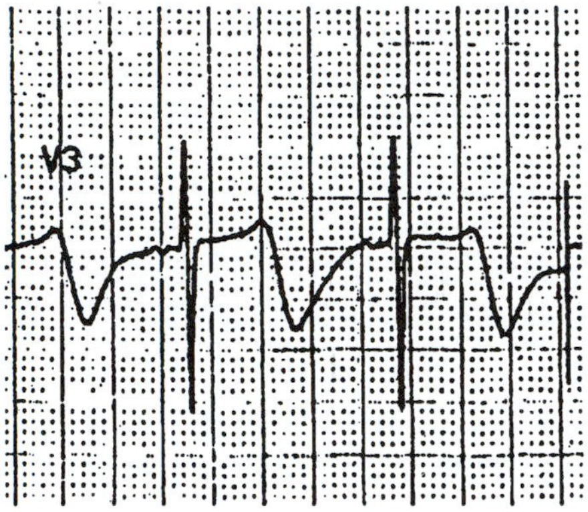

B

Figure 8–22. (**A**) Quinidine effects. Quinidine causes widening of the P wave and widening of the QRS complex. There is often ST depression with a prolonged QT interval. The presence of U waves is typical as well. *(Reproduced, with permission, from Dubin D: Rapid Interpretation of EKG's, ed. V. Tampa, FL, Cover Publishing Co, 1996, p. 229.)* (**B**) This patient presented following a quinidine overdose. Notable features on his electrocardiogram include a notched P wave and QT prolongation. The U wave may be obscured by the deep T-wave inversion.

Botanicals. Plants can also cause ventricular tachydysrhythmias. Commonly known as monkshood or wolfbane, *Aconitum napellus* has cardiac effects that have been described as similar to digoxin[81] and similar to quinidine.[2,69,87] Although the mechanism is unclear, bradycardia and conduction defects have been described on the initial ECG. The final fatal dysrhythmia is often ventricular tachycardia or ventricular fibrillation.[42,130] The yew (*Taxus baccata, Taxus canadensis*) can cause cardiac toxicity similar to that caused by the cardiac glycosides by blocking the activity of the sodium–potassium pump. Third-degree AV block, sinus bradycardia, ventricular tachycardia, ventricular fibrillation, and torsades de pointes have all been reported following the ingestion of yew.[66,142,151] Some patients seem to respond to administration of atropine.[43] Some authors have even empirically utilized digoxin-specific antibody fragments (Fab) to treat the refractory bradycardia and conduction defects.[32]

Slow Rate

Bradycardia and asystole are the terminal events following fatal ingestions of many drugs, but some agents tend to cause sinus bradycardia (Table 21–8) and conduction abnormalities (Table 21–7) early in the course of toxicity. Bradycardia may be caused by effects on the central or peripheral nervous system, directly or indirectly influencing the sinus node. Conduction abnormalities are caused by agents that affect ion flux across the myocardial cell membrane. Calcium channel blockers, beta-adrenergic antagonists (see Chaps. 49–51 on antihypertensive agents), and digoxin are the leading causes of sinus bradycardia and conduction disturbances.

Calcium Channel Blockers. The electrocardiographic manifestations of calcium channel blocker and beta-adrenergic antagonist overdoses are difficult to distinguish (see Table 8–5). In general both types of agents cause decreased ionotropy and decreased conduction. The pharmacologic actions of the drugs in each group differ significantly depending on their individual chemical structure (see Chaps. 49, 50).

There are three structural classes of calcium channel blocking agents: papaverine derivatives (verapamil), benzothiazepines (diltiazem), and the dihydropyridine group, including nifedipine and the newer agents (nicardipine, isradipine, felodipine, amlodipine, bepridil, mibefradil, and nimodipine). All of these agents block the slow, L-type, calcium channels, which are found primarily at the sinus and AV nodes. The cardiovascular toxicity and ECG manifestations vary tremendously from one class to another. The dihydropyridine group has more profound peripheral smooth muscle vasodilatory effects and the verapamil group tends to have more potent central cardiac effects that decrease atrioventricular node conduction and myocardial contractility. Diltiazem has both central and peripheral circulatory effects. In the overdose patient, the central effects often predominate and the toxicity is more similar to that of verapamil. Diltiazem and verapamil also have negative inotropic ef-

TABLE 8–5. ELECTROPHYSIOLOGIC AND CARDIOVASCULAR EFFECTS OF CALCIUM CHANNEL BLOCKERS AND BETA-ADRENERGIC ANTAGONISTS

	Nifedipine	Verapamil	Diltiazem	Beta-Adrenergic Antagonists
Coronary vasodilation	↑	↑	↑	0
Peripheral vasodilation	↑↑	↑	↑	↓↓
Myocardial contractility	↓/0	↓	↓/0	↓↓
RR interval	↓	↑↓	↑	↑
QRS complex	0	0	0	0
QTc interval	0	0	0	0
PR interval	0	↑	↑	↑

↑ = increase, ↓ = decrease, ↑↓ = variable, 0 = no change

Modified from Frishman WH: β-Adrenergic blockers. Med Clin North Am 1988;72:41; and Weiner BA: Calcium channel blockers. Med Clin North Am 1988; 72:88–89.

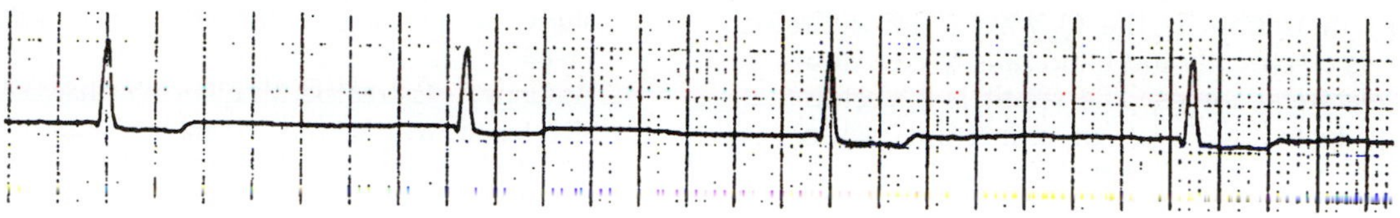

Figure 8–23. This rhythm strip was taken 8 hours after an 18-year-old female intentionally ingested 2400 mg of verapamil in a suicide attempt. At the time the ECG was recorded, her blood pressure was 80/30 mm Hg and her pulse was 38 beats/minute.

fects, although diltiazem has more prominent peripheral vasodilatory effects.[91,102] The onset and duration of their effects vary considerably with the formulation: extended release versus rapid release. Sustained-release verapamil can cause severe conduction delays, including first-degree heart block and AV block, more than 12 hours after exposure.[134] Figure 8–23 shows a rhythm strip from a patient with a verapamil overdose.

Beta-adrenergic Antagonists. The ECG manifestations of beta-adrenergic antagonists include sinus bradycardia, complete heart block, and ventricular dysrhythmias and resemble those seen with calcium channel blocker toxicity (see Chap. 49). The toxicity of the beta-adrenergic antagonists differs significantly from each other in their selectivity for the $beta_1$ receptor, their intrinsic sympathomimetic activity, and their membrane stabilizing activity. The properties of a drug at therapeutic doses are helpful in predicting toxicity in an overdose setting. Agents with membrane-stabilizing effects include acebutolol,[97] alprenolol, metoprolol, oxprenolol,[6] pindolol,[99] and propranolol.[5] These agents have Type IA antidysrhythmic effects like quinidine. Agents known to have a partial agonist effect at the beta-adrenergic receptor, called intrinsic sympathomimetic activity, include pindolol, oxprenolol, and alprenolol. Sotalol acts more like a Vaughan-Williams Class III antidysrhythmic agent, causing prolongation of the action potential and of the refractory period. Torsades de pointes with QT prolongation is not uncommon following sotalol overdose.[3,37,39,59,116,135]

Ischemia

The ECG changes demonstrating ischemia, injury, and cellular death are reflected by T-wave changes, ST segment displacement, and the appearance of Q waves. Repolarization normally proceeds from the epicardium to the endocardium, the reverse direction of depolarization, and an upright T wave is recorded. In subendocardial ischemia the polarity of the T wave would be unchanged. In the presence of subepicardial ischemia, depolarization in the epicardium is prolonged and the normal order of repolarization is reversed, proceeding from endocardium to epicardium, causing T-wave inversion.

The proposed mechanisms for the displacement of the ST segment during myocardial injury are a diastolic current of injury and a systolic current of injury, or a combination of both. The diastolic current of injury is associated with a flow of current from the uninjured to the injured area that causes a downward displacement of the ST segment. This downward displacement is automatically shifted toward the baseline by the capacitor-coupled amplifier of the ECG. When the entire heart (including the injured area) is depolarized, the ST segment appears elevated compared to baseline. The concept of the systolic current of injury proposes that during the time period defined by the ST segment, the normal heart is depolarized but the injured area undergoes early repolarization. The result is a current flow from the more positive, injured, area to a more negative, uninjured, area. The result is true elevation of the ST segment. Similarly, if rather than repolarizing early, the injured area fails to depolarize with the normal myocardium, a current of injury would exist and an elevated ST segment would be recorded (Fig. 8–24). The diagnostic feature of myocar-

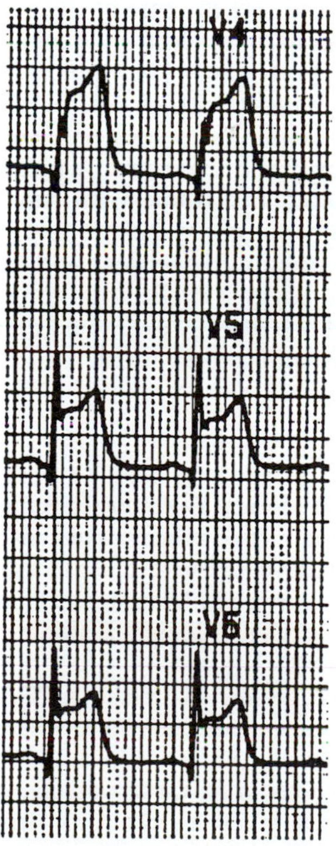

Figure 8–24. Leads V_4–V_6 are shown from the ECG of a 27-year-old with substernal chest pain after using crack cocaine.

dial necrosis, infarction, is the Q wave. The infarcted myocardium is electrically inert and fails to contribute to the normal electrical forces. The result is a vector that points away from the area of infarction, which is recorded on the ECG as a Q wave.[44]

Any poisoning that results in hypotension and hypoxia may result in ECG changes of ischemia, injury, and cellular death. Patients who are poisoned by agents that commonly cause vasospasm, including cocaine (see Chap. 65) and the ergot alkaloids, are particularly prone to myocardial ischemia and infarction.

The cardiovascular effects of the ergot alkaloids are complex. The cardiovascular toxicity varies widely depending on the particular alkaloid structure, the chronicity, and the dose. The mechanisms of coronary vasospasm include peripheral vasoconstriction, arteriolar constriction, and damage to the capillary endothelium.[103] There are also some alpha-adrenergic antagonist effects of some ergot alkaloids that may ameliorate the toxicity. Valvular fibrosis, with thickening and immobility, has also been reported in patients following chronic use of ergotamines, although the mechanism is unclear.[8,45,111] The combination of ergotamine and caffeine is commonly used to treat migraine headaches.

Summary

The ECG is an invaluable source of information and has the potential to redirect the care of the poisoned patient. ECGs can demonstrate electrolyte abnormalities and suggest specific poisonings, before blood is even drawn. For example, a patient with caustic burns who has evidence of hyperkalemia or hypocalcemia on the ECG suggests hydrofluoric acid exposure. A patient manifesting signs of the opioid toxidrome with runs of ventricular tachycardia might suggest exposure to propoxyphene. A patient with an unknown overdose and evidence of QRS widening might suggest cyclic antidepressant exposure. An ECG should be critically examined early in the initial evaluation of any poisoned patient.

References

1. Abenhaim L, Moride Y, Brenot F: Appetite-suppressant drugs and the risk of primary pulmonary hypertension. N Engl J Med 1996;325:609–615.
2. Agarwa B, Agarwal R, Misra D: Malignant arrhythmias induced by accidental aconite poisoning. Indian Heart J 1977;29:246–248.
3. Alderfliegel F, Leeman M, Demaeyer PH, et al: Sotalol poisoning associated with asystole. Intensive Care Med 1993;19:57–58.
4. Alexander CS, Nini A: Cardiovascular complications in young patients taking psychotropic drugs. Am Heart J 1969;78:757–769.
5. Andersson T, Heath A, Mattsson H: Prenalterol as an antidote to massive doses of metoprolol—A cardiovascular study in the dog. Acta Med Scand 1982;659(suppl): 71–88.
6. Anthony T, Jastremski M, Elliot W: Charcoal hemoperfusion for the treatment of a combined diltiazem and metoprolol overdose. Ann Emerg Med 1986;15:1344–1348.
7. Attwell D, Lee JA: A cellular basis for the primary long Q-T syndromes. Lancet 1988;1:1136–1138.
8. Austin SM, El-Hayek A, Comianos M, Tamulonis DU: Mitral valve disease associated with long-term ergotamine use. South Med J 1993;86:1179–1181.
9. Baillie DS, Inoue H, Kaseda S, et al: Magnesium suppresses early depolarizations and ventricular tachyarrhythmias induced in dogs by cesium. Circulation 1989; 77:1395–1402.
10. Banta TA, St Jean A: The effect of phenothiazines on the electrocardiogram. Can Med Assoc J 1964;91:537.
11. Bauer P, Maire B, Wever M, et al: Full recovery after a chloroquine suicide attempt. J Toxicol Clin Toxicol 1991; 29:23–30.
12. Beckman KJ, Bauman JS, Pimental PA, et al: Arsenic-induced torsades de pointes. Crit Care Med 1991;19:290–292.
13. Berkovitch M, Matsui D, Fogelman R, et al: Assessment of the terminal 40-millisecond QRS vector in children with a history of tricyclic antidepressant ingestion. Pediatr Emerg Care 1995;11:75–77.
14. Bibler MR, Chou TC, Toltzis RJ, et al: Recurrent ventricular tachycardia due to pentamidine-induced cardiotoxicity. Chest 1988;94:1303–1306.
15. Binimelis J, Bassas L, Marruecos L, et al: Massive thyroxine intoxication: Evaluation of plasma extraction. Intensive Care Med 1987;13:33–38.
16. Bishop RO, Gaudry PL: Prolonged QT interval following astemizole overdose. Arch Emerg Med 1989;6:63–65.
17. Boehnert M, Lovejoy FH Jr: Value of the QRS duration versus the serum drug level in predicting seizures and ventricular arrhythmias after an acute overdose of tricyclic antidepressants. N Engl J Med 1985;313:474–479.
18. Bradberry SM, Vale AJ: Disturbances of potassium homeostasis in poisoning. J Toxicol Clin Toxicol 1995;33: 295–310.
19. Brady HR, Horgan JH: Lithium and the heart: Unanswered questions. Chest 1988;93:166–169.
20. Brown CR, Hernandez S, Kelly MT: Hyperthermia and death from amantadine overdose. Vet Hum Toxicol 1987;29:463. Abstract.
21. Brown K, Levy H, Brenner C: Overdose of risperidone. Ann Emerg Med 1993;22:1908–1910.
22. Campbell DB, Moore BR: Fenfluramine overdosage. Lancet 1969;2:1306–1307.
23. Caravati EM, Bossart PJ: Demographic and electrocardiographic factors associated with severe tricyclic antidepressant toxicity. J Toxicol Clin Toxicol 1991;29:31–43.
24. Chen ZC, Kwan CM, Chen JH: Profound shock resulting from a large dose of dipyridamole. Int J Cardiology 1994;46:75–78.
25. Chew WC, Lew LC: Ventricular ectopics after salbutamol infusion for preterm labour. Lancet 1979;2:1383–1384.
26. Chou T, Knilans TK, eds: Electrocardiography. In: Clinical Practice Adult and Pediatric, 4th ed. Philadelphia, Saunders, 1996, pp. 3–17, 506, 533, 541–545, 650.

27. Clark RF, Vance M: Massive diphenhydramine poisoning resulting in a wide-complex tachycardia: Successful treatment with sodium bicarbonate. Ann Emerg Med 1992;21: 318–321.
28. Clemessy J-L, Favier C, Borron SW, et al: Hypokalemia related to acute chloroquine ingestion. Lancet 1995;346: 877–880.
29. Conover MB: Understanding Electrocardiography, 7th ed. St. Louis, Mosby–Year Book, 1996, pp. 3–28.
30. Cooper R, LeGrady D, Nanas S, et al: Increased sodium-lithium countertransport in college students with elevated blood pressure. JAMA 1983;249:1030–1034.
31. Cortese LM, Gasser RA Jr, Bjornson DC, et al: Prolonged recurrence of pentamidine-induced torsades de pointes. Ann Pharmacother 1992;26:1365–1369.
32. Cummins RO, Haulman J, Quan L: Near-fatal yew berry intoxication treated with external cardiac pacing and digoxin-specific FAB antibody fragments. Ann Emerg Med 1990;19:77–82.
33. Czajka PA, Flynn OF: Nonfatal chloroquine poisoning. Clin Toxicol 1978;13:361–369.
34. Davignon A, Rautabarjo P, Boiselle E, et al: Normal ECG standards for infants and children. Pediatr Cardiol 1979; 1:123.
35. Demers RG, Heninger G: Electrocardiographic changes during lithium therapy. Dis Nerv Syst 1970;31:674–677.
36. Eastman JW, Cohen SN: Hypertensive crisis and death associated with phencyclidine poisoning. JAMA 1975;231: 1270–1271.
37. Edvardsson N, Varnauskas E: Clinical course, serum concentrations and elimination rate in a case of massive sotalol intoxication. Eur Heart J 1987;8:544.
38. Einthoven W: Die galvanometrische Registrirung des menschlichen Elecktrokardiogramms, zugleich eine Beurteilung der Anwendung des Capillar-Elektrometers in der Physiologie. Arch f d g Physiol 1903;99:472.
39. Elonen E, Neuvonen PJ, Tarssanen L, et al: Sotalol intoxication with prolonged QT interval and severe tachyarrhythmias. Br Med J 1979;1:1184.
40. Emerson TS, Cisek JE: Methcathinone: A Russian designer amphetamine infiltrates the rural Midwest. Ann Emerg Med 1993;22:1897–1903.
41. Engrav MB, Coodley G, Magnusson AR: Torsades de pointes after inhaled pentamidine. Ann Emerg Med 1992;21:1403–1405.
42. Fatovich DM: Aconite: A lethal Chinese herb. Ann Emerg Med 1992;21:309–311.
43. Feldman R, Szajewski JM, Chrobak J: Four cases of self-poisoning with extract of yew (Taxus baccata) needles. Pol Arch Med Wewn 1988;79:26–29.
44. Fisch C: Electrocardiography. In: Braunwald E: Heart Disease: A Textbook of Cardiovascular Medicine, 5th ed. Philadelphia, Saunders, 1997, pp. 128–129.
45. Flaherty KR, Bates JR: Mitral regurgitation caused by chronic ergotamine use. Am Heart J 1996;131:603–606.
46. Fleisher MR, Campbell DB: Fenfluramine overdosage. Lancet 1969;2:1306–1307.
47. Foulke GE: Identifying toxicity risk early after antidepressant overdose. Am J Emerg Med 1995;13:123–126.
48. Fowler NO, McCall D, Chou TC, et al: Electrocardiographic changes and cardiac arrhythmias in patients receiving psychotropic drugs. Am J Cardiol 1976;37:223.
49. Fredholm BB, Abbracchio MP, Burnstock G, et al: Nomenclature and classification of purinoceptors. Pharmacol Rev 1994;46:143–156.
50. Frohna WJ: Iatrogenic magnesium overdose in a patient with suspected acute myocardial infarction. Am J Emerg Med 1995;13:436–437.
51. Glassman AH: Cardiovascular effects of tricyclic antidepressants. Annu Rev Med 1984;35:503–511.
52. Gold RG, Gordon HE, Da Costa RD, et al: Fenfluramine overdosage. Lancet 1969;2:1306.
53. Goldberger E: A simple, indifferent, electrocardiographic electrode of aero potential and a technique of obtaining augmented, unipolar, extremity leads. Am Heart J 1942;23: 483–492.
54. Graber TW, Yee AS, Baker FJ: Magnesium: Physiology, clinical disorders, and therapy. Ann Emerg Med 1981;10: 49–57.
55. Grant HI, Yeston NS: Cardiac arrest secondary to emotional stress and torsade de pointes in a patient with associated magnesium and potassium deficiency. Crit Care Med 1991;19:292–293.
56. Groleau G, Jotte R, Barish R: The electrocardiographic manifestations of cyclic antidepressant therapy and overdose: A review. J Emerg Med 1990;8:597–605.
57. Gueron M, Yarom R: Cardiovascular manifestations of severe scorpion sting. Chest 1970;57:156–162.
58. Gueron M, Ilia R, Sofer S: The cardiovascular system after scorpion envenomation. A review. J Toxicol Clin Toxicol 1992;30:245–258.
59. Gupta K: Hazards of β-blockers in the elderly: Severe bradycardia due to sotalol overdose. Br J Clin Pract 1985;39:116.
60. Hantson P, Ronveau JS, Coninck BD, et al: Amrinone for refractory cardiogenic shock following chloroquine poisoning. Intensive Care Med 1991;17:430–431.
61. Hermsdoef MK, Oerlinghausen BM: Tricyclic neuroleptic and antidepressant overdose: Epidemiological, electrocardiographic, and clinical features—a survey of 92 cases. Pharmacopsychiatr 1990;23:17–22.
62. Hollister LE, Kosek JC: Sudden death during treatment with phenothiazine derivatives. JAMA 1965;192:93.
63. Hudgens DR, Conradi SE: Sudden death associated with terbutaline sulfate administration. Am J Obstet Gynecol 1993;169:120–121.
64. Hulten B-A, Adams R, Askenasi R, et al: Predicting severity of tricyclic antidepressant overdose. J Toxicol Clin Toxicol 1992;30:161–170.
65. Huston JR, Bell GE: The effect of thioridazine hydrochloride and chlorpromazine on the electrocardiogram. JAMA 1966;198:134–138.
66. Ingen GV, Visser R, Peltenburg H, et al: Sudden unexpected death due to Taxus poisoning. A report of five cases with review of the literature. Forensic Sci Int 1992; 56:81–87.
67. Ingrams GJ, Morgan FB: Transcutaneous overdose of terbutaline. Br Med J 1993;307:484.
68. Irons GV, Orgain ES: Digitalis-induced arrhythmias and their management. Prog Cardiovasc Dis 1966;8:539–569.

69. Kapoor S, Sen A: Cardiovascular aspects of aconite poisoning in human beings. Indian Heart J 1969;21: 329–338.
70. Kelly JC, Wasserman GS, Bernard WD, et al: Chloroquine poisoning in a child. Ann Emerg Med 1990;19:91–94.
71. King K, England JF: Chloral hydrate overdose. Med J Aust 1983;2:260.
72. Kulling PJ: Treatment of cardiac membrane stabilizing dysrhythmias. J Toxicol Clin Toxicol 1996;34:131–132.
73. Lavoie FW, Gansert GG, Weiss RE: Value of initial ECG findings and plasma drug levels in cyclic antidepressant overdose. Ann Emerg Med 1990;19:696–699.
74. Lazzara R: Amiodarone and torsade de pointes. Ann Intern Med 1989;111:549–551.
75. Lepeschkin E: Physiological basis of the U wave. In: Schlant RC, Hurst JW, eds: Advances in Electrocardiography, Vol. 2, Chap. VII. New York, Grune & Stratton, 1976, p. 353.
76. Lerman BB: Response of nonreentrant catecholamine-mediated ventricular tachycardia to endogenous adenosine and acetylcholine: Evidence for myocardial receptor-mediated effects. Circulation 1993;87:382–390.
77. Liebelt EL, Francis PD, Woolfe AD: ECG lead aVR versus QRS interval in predicting seizures and arrhythmias in acute tricyclic antidepressant toxicity. Ann Emerg Med 1995;26:195–201.
78. Linakis J, Woolf A: Clinical features of acute versus chronic lithium intoxication. Vet Hum Toxicol 1989;31:370. Abstract.
79. Lindemann JP, Watanabe AM: Sympathetic control of cardiac electrical activity. In: Sipes DP, Jalife J, eds: Cardiac Electrophysiology: From Cell to Bedside. Philadelphia, Saunders, 1990, pp. 277–283.
80. Litovitz TL, White D: Levothyroxine ingestion in children: An analysis of 78 cases. Am J Emerg Med 1985;4: 297–300.
81. Mack R: Play it again Voltaire—Aconite (monkshood) poisoning. NC Med J 1985;46:518–519.
82. Madfsen PS, Strom J, Reiz S: Acute propoxyphene poisoning in 222 consecutive cases. Acta Anaesth Scand 1984; 28:661–665.
83. Mani S, Kocheril AG, Andriole VT: Case report: Pentamidine and polymorphic ventricular tachycardia revisited. Am J Med Sci 1993;305:236–240.
84. Marchi S, Szabo B, Lazzara R: Adrenergic induction of delayed afterdepolarizations in ventricular myocardial cells: Beta induction and alpha modulation. J Cardiovasc Electrophysiol 1991;2:476.
85. Marshall JB, Forker AD: Cardiovascular effects of tricyclic antidepressant drugs: Therapeutic usage, overdose, and management of complications. Am Heart J 1982;103: 401–414.
86. Marrs-Simon P, Zell-Kanter M, Kendzierski DL, et al: Cardiotoxic manifestations of mesoridazine overdose. Ann Emerg Med 1988;17:1074–1078.
87. Martens PR, Vandevelde K: A near lethal case of combined strychnine and aconitine poisoning. J Toxiol Clin Toxicol 1993;31:133–138.
88. Mathews DR, McNutt B, Odkerholm R, et al: Torsade de pointes occurring in association with terfenadine use. JAMA 1991;266:2375–2376. Letter.
89. McMahon B, Ambre J, Ellis J: Hypertension during recovery from phencyclidine intoxication. Clin Toxicol 1978; 12:37–40.
90. Meeran K, Jacobs MG: Chloroquine poisoning: Rapidly fatal without treatment. Br Med J 1993;307:49–50.
91. Mitchell LB, Schroeder JS, Mason JW: Comparative clinical electrophysiologic effects of diltiazem, verapamil and nifedipine. A review. Am J Cardiol 1982;49:629–635.
92. Miller JR, Van Dellen TR: Electrocardiographic changes following the intravenous administration of magnesium sulfate. J Lab Clin Med 1941;26:1116–1120.
93. Miwa K, Miyagi Y, Fujita M, et al: Transient terminal U wave inversion as a more specific marker for myocardial ischemia. Am Heart J 1993;125:981–986.
94. Monahan BP, Ferguson CL, Killeavy ES, et al: Torsade de pointes occurring in association with terfenadine use. JAMA 1990;264:2788–2790.
95. Newton EH, Shih RD, Hoffman RS: Cyclic antidepressant overdose: A review of current management strategies. Am J Emerg Med 1994;12:376–379.
96. Nguyen PT, Scheinman MM, Seger J: Polymorphous ventricular tachycardia: Clinical characterization, therapy, and the QT interval. Circulation 1986;74:340–349.
97. Nicolas F, Villers D, Rozo L, et al: Severe self-poisoning with acebutolol in association with alcohol. Crit Care Med 1987;15:173–174.
98. Niemann JT, Bessen HA, Rothstein RJ, et al: Electrocardiographic criteria for tricyclic antidepressant overdose. Ann Emerg Med 1986;57:1154–1159.
99. Offenstadt G, Hericord PH, Amstutz PH: Intoxication volontaire par le pindolol. Nouv Presse Med 1976;5:1539.
100. Osborn JJ: Experimental hypothermia: Respiratory and blood pH changes in relation to cardiac function. Am J Physiol 1953;175:389.
101. Paton BC: Accidental hypothermia. Pharmacol Ther 1983; 22:331–377.
102. Pearigen PD, Benowitz NL: Poisoning due to calcium antagonists. Experience with verapamil, diltiazem and nifedipine. Drug Safety 1991;6:408–430.
103. Peroutka SJ: Drugs effective in the treatment of migraine. In: Hardman JG, Limbird LE, Molinoff PB, Ruddon RW, Gilman AG, eds: Goodman and Gilman's The Pharmacological Basis of Therapeutics, 9th ed. New York, McGraw-Hill, 1996, pp. 491–496.
104. Perrier A, Martin P-Y, Fuvre H, et al: Very severe self-poisoning: Lithium carbonate intoxication causing a myocardial infarction. Chest 1991;100:863–865.
105. Peterson RG, Rumack BH: D-Penicillamine therapy of acute arsenic poisoning. J Pediatr 1977;91:661–666.
106. Pollick C, Cujec B, Parker S, et al: Left ventricular wall motion abnormalities in subarachnoid hemorrhage: An echocardiographic study. J Am Coll Cardiol 1988;12: 600–605.
107. Pott SW, Rose SR: Minoxidil overdose with ECG changes: Case report and review. J Emerg Med 1992;10:53–57.
108. Price KR, Fligner DJ: Treatment of caffeine toxicity with esmolol. Ann Emerg Med 1990;19:85–87.

109. Probst BD: The utility of a 12-lead electrocardiogram in diagnosing a suspected antidepressant overdose. Clin Pediatr 1992;10:622–625.
110. Quadrel MA, Atkin SH, Jaker MA: Delayed cardiotoxicity during treatment with intravenous pentamidine: Two case reports and a review of the literature. Am Heart J 1992;123:1377–1379.
111. Redfield MM, Nicholson WJ, Edwards WD, Tajik AJ: Valve disease associated with ergot alkaloid use: Echocardiographic and pathologic correlations. Ann Intern Med 1992;117:50–52.
112. Riou B, Barriot P, Rimailho A, Baud FJ: Treatment of severe chloroquine poisoning. N Engl J Med 1988;318:1–6.
113. Roberge RJ, Martin TG, Hodgman M, et al: Supraventricular tachyarrhythmia associated with baclofen overdose. J Toxicol Clin Toxicol 1994;32:291–297.
114. Rockhold RW, Carlton FB, Corkern R, et al: Methcathinone intoxication in the rat: Abrogation by dextrorphan. Ann Emerg Med 1997;29:383–391.
115. Rosen MR, Wit A, Hoffman BF: Cardiac antiarrhythmic and toxic effects of digitalis. Am Heart J 1975;89: 391–399.
116. Salzberg MR, Gallagher EJ: Propranolol overdose. Ann Emerg Med 1980;9:26–27.
117. Sartori M, Pratt CM, Young JB: Torsade de pointes: malignant cardiac arrhythmia induced by amantadine poisoning. Am J Med 1984;77:388–391.
118. Sati Y, Wada Y, Taira N: Comparative studies of cardiovascular profiles of milrinone and amrinone by use of isolated, blood-perfused dog heart preparations. Heart Vessels 1986;2:213–220.
119. Seller RH, Cangiano J, Kim KE, et al: Digitalis toxicity and hypomagnesemia. Am Heart J 1970:79;57–68.
120. Serafin WE: Drugs used in the treatment of asthma. In: Hardman JG, Limbird LE, Molinoff PB, Ruddon RW, Gilman AG, eds: Goodman and Gilman's The Pharmacological Basis of Therapeutics, 9th ed. New York, McGraw-Hill, 1996, pp. 672–678.
121. Shannon M: Duration of QRS disturbances after severe tricyclic antidepressant intoxication. J Toxicol Clin Toxicol 1992;30:377–386.
122. Shannon M: Predictors of major toxicity after theophylline overdose. Ann Intern Med 1993;119:1161–1167.
123. Shannon M: Hypokalemia, hyperglycemia and plasma catecholamine activity after severe theophylline intoxication. J Toxicol Clin Toxicol 1994;32:41–47.
124. Smith BA, Ferguson DB: Acute hydralazine overdose: Marked ECG abnormalities in a young adult. Ann Emerg Med 1992;21:326–330.
125. Smith PK: Pharmacologic actions of parenterally administered magnesium salts. Anesthesiology 1942:3;323.
126. Snook J, Boothman-Burrell D, Watkins J, Colin-Jones D: Torsade de pointes ventricular tachycardia associated with astemizole overdose. Br J Clin Pract 1988;42: 257–259.
127. Starmer FC: The cardiac vulnerable period and reentrant arrhythmias: Targets of anti- and proarrhythmic processes. PACE 1997;20(pt II):445–454.
128. Stork CM, Redd JT, Fine K, Hoffman RS: Propoxyphene-induced wide QRS complex dysrhythmia responsive to sodium bicarbonate—A case report. J Toxicol Clin Toxicol 1995;33:179–183.
129. Stork CM: Treatment of cardiac membrane stabilizing dysrhythmias—Author's reply. J Toxicol Clin Toxicol 1996; 34:133–134.
130. Tai YT, But PP-H, Young K, Cau C-P: Cardiotoxicity after accidental herb-induced aconite poisoning. Lancet 1992; 340:1254–1256.
131. Tan HL, Hou CJ, Lauer MR, Sung RJ: Electrophysiologic mechanisms of the long QT interval syndromes and torsades de pointes. Ann Intern Med 1995;122: 701–714.
132. Thalhammer C, Bogner JR, Lohmoller G: Chronic pentamidine aerosol prophylaxis does not induce QT prolongation. Clin Invest 1993;71:319–322.
133. Tilkian AS, Schroeder JS, Kao JJ: Cardiovascular effects of lithium in man: A review of the literature. Am J Med 1976;61:665–670.
134. Tom PA, Morrow CT, Kelen GD: Delayed hypotension after overdose of sustained release verapamil. J Emerg Med 1994;12:621–625.
135. Totterman KJ, Turto H, Pellinen T: Overdrive pacing as treatment of sotalol induced ventricular tachyarrhythmias (torsade de pointes). Acta Med Scand 1982;(suppl)668: 28–32.
136. Trevino A, Razi B, Beller BM: The characteristic electrocardiogram of accidental hypothermia. Arch Intern Med 1971;127:470.
137. Tunget CL, Clark RF, Turchen SG: Raising the decontamination level for thyroid hormone ingestion. Am J Emerg Med 1995;13:9–13.
138. Tzivoni D, Keren A, Cohen AM, et al: Magnesium therapy for torsade de pointes. Am J Cardiol 1984;53:528–530.
139. Veltri JC, Temple AR: Fenfluramine poisoning. J Pediatr 1975;87:119–121.
140. Vohra J, Burrows G, Hunt D, et al: The effect of toxic and therapeutic doses of tricyclic antidepressant drugs on intracardiac conduction. Eur J Cardiol 1975; 3:219–227.
141. Waller AD: Demonstration on man of the electromotive changes accompanying the heart's beat. J Physiol 1887; 8:229.
142. Werth J, Murphy JJ: Cardiovascular toxicity associated with yew leaf ingestion. Br Heart J 1994;72:92–93.
143. Wharton JM, Demopulos PA, Goldschlager N: Torsade de pointes during administration of pentamidine isethionate. Am J Med 1987;83:571–576.
144. Widler P, Mathys K, Brenneisen R, et al: Pharmacodynamics and pharmacokinetics of khat: A controlled study. Clin Pharmacol Ther 1994;55:556–562.
145. Wilens TE, Stern TA: Ventricular tachycardia associated with desipramine and thioridazine. Psychosomatics 1990;31:100–103.
146. Wilson FN: Foreward. In: Barker JM: The Unipolar Electrogram: A Clinical Interpretation. New York, Appleton-Century-Crofts, 1952, p. xii.
147. Wolfe TR, Caravati EM, Rollins DE, et al: Terminal 40-ms frontal plane QRS axis as a marker for tricyclic antidepressant overdose. Ann Emerg Med 1989;18:348–351.

148. Woods JW, Parker JC, Watson BS: Perturbation of sodium-lithium countertransport in red cells. N Engl J Med 1983;308:1258–1261.
149. Worthley L: Lithium toxicity and refractory cardiac arrhythmias treated with intravenous magnesium. Anesth Intensive Care 1974;2:357–360.
150. Yatani A, Okabe K, Polakis P, et al: ras p21 and GAP inhibit coupling of muscarinic receptors to atrial potassium channels. Cell 1990;61:769–776.
151. Yersin B, Frey JG, Schaller MD, et al: Fatal cardiac arrhythmias and shock following yew leaves ingestion. Ann Emerg Med 1987;16:1396–1397.
152. Zimmers T, Golomb RI: Cases in electrocardiography. Am J Emerg Med 1991;9:588–591.

CHAPTER 9

Identifying the Nontoxic Exposure

Richard S. Weisman

A large number of calls received by poison centers throughout the United States are for nontoxic exposures. During the past 5 years, greater than 40% of the exposures reported to the American Association of Poison Centers were judged by poison information specialists to be nontoxic exposures.[5–9] One of the most important skills that an emergency physician, poison information specialist, or medical toxicologist can develop is the ability to identify and appropriately triage exposures that are not likely to result in toxicity. This may prevent an unnecessary visit to the ED (or physician's office), or if the patient is in the ED, it may prevent unnecessary testing. Allowing patients with nontoxic exposures to be evaluated, observed, and followed up outside of the emergency department or physician's private office, is cost effective and a major justification for governmental funding for poison centers. Poison Centers also render a substantial public health service in that they relieve the overcrowding common to many large inner-city emergency departments by keeping patients at home who do not require medical evaluation or interventions.

The patient with a potentially nontoxic exposure who telephones an emergency department, paramedic base station, or a poison center requires extensive evaluation by a health care provider with specialized training in toxicology. The analysis of nontoxic exposures can be divided into two major categories. The first and least problematic category is exposure to products unlikely to result in toxicity at any dose. In such a situation, the physician or information specialist must only establish by history an absolute identity of the product and the route of administration. The latter information is important because a product that may be harmless at any dose by a particular route of exposure (dermal, oral, ocular, inhalation) may be toxic by another route. An example of this concept would be pure talcum powder. This product never causes a problem if applied dermally or if unintentional inhalation occurs. If, however, during intentional ingestion or substantial inhalation the patient aspirates the powder, severe pulmonary complications or death may occur.[14]

The second type of nontoxic exposure is an exposure to a product in a quantity that is not toxic. An example of this is a 50 mg/kg exposure to acetaminophen.[16] The discussion that follows is devoted to developing strategies for reliably determining whether exposure to a potentially toxic drug or product is at a safe amount.

When Can an Exposure Be Considered Nontoxic?

The decision to consider an exposure nontoxic is largely dependent on how much history can be gathered with regard to the exposure, how reliable the information is, and what the probability is that the exposure might result in toxicity if the quantity of the exposure was significantly underestimated. Before an exposure is considered nontoxic, all of the following criteria (Table 9–1) should be met.[11–13]

Absolute Product Identification

The product must be absolutely and completely identified. The product name, manufacturer, ingredients, quantities, concentrations, and production date are all essential in assessing the toxicity of the product. The health care provider must be cognizant of the fact that manufacturers often change product ingredients (both active and inactive) without changing the product name. If there are

TABLE 9–1. GENERAL GUIDELINES FOR CATEGORIZING AN EXPOSURE AS NONTOXIC

1. The product must be absolutely identified.
2. Only a single product can be involved in the exposure.
3. The exposure must be unintentional.
4. The Consumer Product Safety Commission's "signal words" (CAUTION, WARNING, DANGER) must not be found on the label.
5. A reliable approximation of the quantity of substance involved in the exposure must be possible.
6. The route(s) of exposure can be accurately assessed from the available history.
7. The exposed individual is symptom free.
8. Follow-up consultation must be possible; in the case of a child, the parent must appear to be reliable.

Adapted from Mofenson HC, Greensher J, Caraccio TR: Ingestions considered nontoxic. Emerg Med Clin North Am 1984;2:159–174; and Mofenson HC, Greensher J. The nontoxic ingestion. Pediatr Clin North Am 1970; 17:583–590.

any inconsistencies or missing information in the patient's exposure history, the ingestion cannot be classified as being nontoxic. The clinician should always consider that patients often transfer medications into different containers. When unexplained symptoms are noted, the remote possibility that a manufacturing or labeling error or product tampering has occurred must be considered. Recently over 70 children in Haiti developed acute renal failure and neurologic toxicity when diethylene glycol was used instead of propylene glycol as the vehicle in acetaminophen syrup.[18]

Single Product Exposure

Only a single product can be involved in the exposure. Synergistic or additional toxicity and/or toxic interactions may occur if multiple substances are involved and additional care must therefore be used in trying to assess this type of exposure. An evaluation of such a patient at either the physician's office or an emergency department is almost always the safer course to follow. Most unintentional exposures, particularly in children, involve exposure to small amounts of one product. Concurrent exposure to multiple products should alert the physician to the possibility that the ingestion was intentional or the result of abuse or neglect.[11,17] A history indicating that the current problem is not the patient's first "unintentional" poisoning may also be a clue to a psychiatric disorder in the adult patient or neglect or abuse in the pediatric patient.

Unintentional Exposure

An adult who has intentionally ingested a drug or toxin almost always requires evaluation in a health care facility. With the exception of therapeutic errors and mistakes from confusion, or mental, linguistical, or visual impairment, most ingestions in adults result from misuse, abuse, or suicidal intent. Identifying over the telephone adults who may require psychiatric or social stabilization is not possible. Unintentional toxic exposures in adults may include therapeutic errors and drug-interactions, occupational or environmental exposures and food poisonings.

Suicide gestures and ingestions by drug and alcohol users comprise the largest proportion (> 90%) of intentional exposures.[5–9] Both of these types of patients may be difficult to adequately assess over the telephone; they give the least accurate histories and they have a high probability of having a life-threatening exposure. Every effort should be made to expedite their transfer to a health care facility capable of providing medical, psychiatric, and social assistance. The emergency physician should be extremely reluctant to categorize an exposure in an adult as being an unintentional, nontoxic exposure unless a meticulous history and appropriate physical examination can be performed.

Consumer Product Safety Commission Signal Words

The product label must not contain a Consumer Product Safety Commission signal word indicating a potential hazard of toxicity. The Consumer Product Safety Commission (CPSC) is one of four federal agencies that protects the public from the hazards of unrecognized toxins. The other agencies are the Environmental Protection Agency (EPA), the Food and Drug Administration (FDA), and the Occupational Safety and Health Administration (OSHA). The CPSC has developed a series of signal words that must be clearly and prominently displayed on the label of any consumer product when potentially hazardous chemicals are present. These signal words include Caution, Warning, and Danger.[1] An ingestion should never be judged to be nontoxic if a CPSC signal word is found on the product in question. Patients who have been exposed to a product containing a signal word require assessment by a health care provider knowledgeable in toxicology and capable of providing both basic and advanced poison management.

Amount of Exposure

A reliable approximation of the amount of product or toxin ingested must be possible. The history of the amount ingested is often the key determinant as to whether an ingestion can be considered nontoxic. The detail required in the history of the amount ingested is directly related to the potential toxicity of the product. A much more precise history will be required for the patient who unintentionally ingests digoxin tablets than for the patient who unintentionally ingests oral contraceptives. The margin of error acceptable in quantifying the amount ingested is inversely related to the product's toxicity.

Several logical conclusions can be reached from the magnitude of the ingestion: The patient who ingests 4 ounces of automotive motor oil may require psychiatric evaluation and counseling, whereas the patient who unintentionally takes a sip of the same motor oil may not require any care.

Although the 4-ounce ingestion will probably not result in significantly greater toxicity than the sip, one is unintentional and the other is probably not and may represent either grave psychiatric impairment or suicidal intent. The likelihood is greater that other substances have been concurrently ingested with the automotive motor oil if it appears that the ingestion was intentional. The larger ingestion requires referral to an ED or health care facility, evaluation, and ultimately psychiatric evaluation. Little if any poison management would be required for either ingestion unless aspiration occurred. If it can be established that an ingestion is unintentional, the amount ingested can often be used to calculate the nontoxic nature of the exposure. For example, if a 3-year-old (15 kg) drank liquid acetaminophen (160 mg/5 mL) from a bottle containing 60 mL, an accurate analysis can be made of the maximum possible exposure based upon the adult's statement about how much acetaminophen remains.[15]

In this example, knowing that 30 mL remains of a 60-mL bottle containing 32 mg/mL of acetaminophen enables the health care provider to determine that a total of 960 mg of acetaminophen was ingested. A dose-per-body-weight-exposure calculation analysis (mg/kg) enables the determination of an ingestion of 64 mg/kg of acetaminophen.

$$\text{Amount ingested} = 30\ \text{mL} \times 32\ \text{mg/mL} = 960\ \text{mg}$$

$$\text{mg/kg dose} = 960\ \text{mg}/15\ \text{kg} = 64\ \text{mg/kg}$$

Approximate toxic dose for acetaminophen = 150 mg/kg

The toxicity datFa for pediatric acetaminophen poisonings clearly indicate that an acute ingestion of less than 150 mg/kg has not been associated with hepatotoxicity in a 3 year-old child;[16] therefore, the clinician can confidently categorize this ingestion as nontoxic. To ensure that no toxicity ensues, it is also necessary to consider any other acetaminophen the child may have ingested during the previous 12 to 24 hours. If these questions can be answered with confidence, gastric decontamination would not be necessary, nor would a visit to a health care facility for an acetaminophen blood level be necessary. The child would have had to ingest approximately 2.5 times the amount reported by history to reach the threshold for anticipated hepatotoxicity. The clinician's or poison information specialist's only intervention should be to counsel the child's parents about the basic skills necessary to poison-proof the child's environment.

The quantitative assessment of an exposure or ingestion is difficult or impossible when two children share a toxic ingestion. It is also difficult to assess the actual amount ingested when a large amount of a liquid product has been partially ingested and partially spilled on or around the child. For both of these situations the only safe approach is to develop a "worst case scenario." If it is possible to determine exactly how much of the product is unaccounted for, it is necessary to assume that each child ingested the entire amount that is missing. In the situation where a product has been partially spilled and partially ingested, it is again necessary to assume that the entire missing amount was ingested. It is extremely difficult to estimate how much liquid has been absorbed by the child's clothing or how much liquid is present in a puddle on the bathroom or kitchen floor. If the product is well absorbed through the skin, the contribution it may play in a combined ingestion and dermal exposure is impossible to predict. The problem can be further complicated if the product contains highly volatile substances such as acetone, ethyl acetate, or ethyl or isopropyl alcohol, which may lead to toxicity not only by gastric absorption but also by dermal absorption and inhalation.[4]

In summary, if an accurate estimate of the amount of the ingestion cannot be established, the prudent approach is to assume the worst case scenario and to provide a higher level of care and surveillance than may intuitively seem necessary.

Route of Exposure

The route(s) of exposure can often be accurately assessed from the available history. Determination of the amount of toxicity that is likely to occur from an exposure is largely dependent on how the patient was exposed.[10] Household products such as bleach, laundry detergents, ammonia, or rubber cement are generally nontoxic following a dermal exposure, minimally toxic following an oral exposure, but can cause considerable morbidity following prolonged inhalation or upon ocular exposure. As in the case of most other products, if such household products are aspirated, the consequences may be significant. A routine part of the assessment of a patient with a nontoxic exposure should include careful questioning to exclude the possibility of multiple routes of exposure.

An Absence of Clinical Effects

The presence of symptoms (related to the exposure) is a clue that some toxic effect is occurring and that further assessment may be warranted. If symptoms are present, the exposure cannot be considered nontoxic, but this does not necessarily mean that a patient must be evaluated in a health care facility. If the symptoms are minor in severity and not likely to result in further illness or complications, further medical evaluation may not be needed. The ingestion of products such as household bleach (2–5% sodium hypochlorite) are usually not associated with significant toxicity such as burns of the skin, oropharynx, or esophagus.[3] Following an ingestion of household bleach, the patient should not have pain, dysphagia, drooling, or dyspnea (see caustics and batteries, Chap. 86). It would not be considered unusual if the patient vomited once following the ingestion of household bleach. Visual inspection of the oropharynx should reveal no erythema or bullae. If the child continues to vomit or shows any involvement of the respiratory tract such as coughing, shortness of breath, or any other difficulty in breathing, immediate medical care is needed. If this assessment cannot be reliably performed by the caller, the patient should be evaluated in an ED or by a physician.

TABLE 9–2. HOUSEHOLD ITEMS GENERALLY REGARDED AS NONTOXIC

Personal-use items	***Medications***
Bath oils	Antacids
Body conditioners	Antibiotics (with some exceptions)
Bubble bath	Calamine lotion
Cologne (low alcohol content)	Birth control pills
Cosmetics	Corticosteroids
Deodorant	Hydrogen peroxide 3%
Eye makeup	Mineral oil
Hair spray & tonic	Zinc oxide
Hand lotions	Zirconium oxide
Lipstick	***Miscellaneous***
Petroleum jelly	Book matches (one book)
Rouge	Candles
Shampoo (small amounts)	Cigarettes
Shaving cream	Grease, motor oil
Suntan lotion	Incense
Thermometer (elemental mercury not toxic if ingested)	Latex paint
Toothpaste	Lubricating oil
	Newspaper
Art supplies	Putty
Ballpoint pen ink	Silica gel
Chalk	Spackle
Charcoal	
Clay	***Cleaning products***
Crayons (marked A.P., C.P.)	Fabric softener
Felt-tip pens (water base)	Household bleach 2–5%
Pencils (graphite)	Laundry detergent
Watercolors	
White glue, paste	
Toys	
Bathtub toys	
Caps (for toy guns)	
Etch-a-sketch	
Play-doh	
Silly-putty	
Teething rings	
Toy cosmetics	

Follow-up Consultation

All of these triage decisions are based on the premise that follow-up consultation is possible and that the parent or guardian is reliable. Care must be taken in establishing that an exposure is nontoxic or minimally toxic. There is always the possibility that an error in judgment can occur. The option of care in the home is only possible if the poison center, physician's office, or emergency service is able to make a follow-up call to ascertain that the victim has remained asymptomatic or that minor symptoms are resolving. A parent, guardian, or other responsible adult (not the victim) must be capable of recontacting the health care provider when there is either a change in the history or a change in the patient's clinical condition. At the time of the initial contact it is extremely important to assess the caller's reliability and capacity to understand and comply with the directions needed to monitor the exposed individual. Whenever a failure in communications occurs or when there is a high probability of a communications breakdown, the patient should be brought to the health care environment.

What Are the Most Common Poison Center Consultations for Nontoxic or Minimally Toxic Exposures?

The list of household items that generally do not result in toxicity appears in Table 9–2.[2] The products can be conveniently divided into six major categories: personal-use items, art supplies, toys, medications, miscellaneous household items, and cleaning products.

References

1. Craft AW, Lawson CR, Williams H, Sibert JR: Accidental childhood poisoning with household products. Br Med J 1984;288:682.
2. Done AK: Poisoning from common household products. Pediatr Clin North Am 1970;17:569–581.
3. Edwards JN, Jenkins HL, Volans GN: Hazards of household cleaning products. Hum Toxicol 1982;1:403–409.
4. Litovitz TL: The alcohols: ethanol, methanol, isopropanol, ethylene glycol. Pediatr Clin North Am 1986;33:311–323.
5. Litovitz TL, Holm KC, Bailey KM, Schmidtz BF: 1991 Annual Report of the American Association of Poison Control Centers, National Data Collection System. Am J Emerg Med 1992;10:452–505.
6. Litovitz TL, Holm KC, Clancy C, et al: 1992 Annual Report of the American Association of Poison Control Centers Toxic Exposure Surveillance System. Am J Emerg Med 1993;11:494–555.
7. Litovitz TL, Clark LR, Soloway RA: 1993 Annual Report of the American Association of Poison Control Centers Toxic Exposure Surveillance System. Am J Emerg Med 1994; 12:546–584.
8. Litovitz TL, Felberg L, Soloway RA, et al: 1994 Annual Report of the American Association of Poison Control Centers Toxic Exposure Surveillance System. Am J Emerg Med 1995;13:551–597.
9. Litovitz TL, Felberg L, White S, Klein-Schwartz W: 1995 Annual Report of the American Association of Poison Control Centers Toxic Exposure Surveillance System. Am J Emerg Med 1996;14:487–537.
10. Lovejoy FH Jr, Flowers J, McGuigan MA: The epidemiology of poisoning from household products. Vet Hum Toxicol 1979;21(suppl):33–34.
11. McGuigan MA: Poisoning in childhood. Emerg Med Clin North Am 1983;1:187–200.
12. Mofenson HC, Greensher J, Caraccio TR: Ingestions considered nontoxic. Emerg Med Clin North Am 1984;2: 159–174.
13. Mofenson HC, Greensher J: The nontoxic ingestion. Pediatr Clin North Am 1970;17:583–590.

14. Motomatsu K, Adachi H, Uno T: Two infant deaths after inhaling baby powder. Chest 1979;75:448–450.
15. Osborne SC, Garrettson LK: Perception of toxicity and dose by 3- and 4-year-old children. Am J Dis Child 1985;139:790–792.
16. Peterson RG, Rumack BH: Toxicity of acetaminophen overdose. JACEP 1978;7:202–205.
17. Rogers J: Recurrent childhood poisoning as a family problem. J Fam Pract 1981;13:337–340.
18. Scalzo AJ: Diethylene glycol toxicity revisited: The 1996 Haitian epidemic. J Toxicol Clin Toxicol 1996;34:513–516.

PART B

The Biochemical and Molecular Basis of Medical Toxicology

CHAPTER 10

Neurotransmitters

Steven C. Curry, Kirk C. Mills, and Kimberlie A. Graeme

Many poisonous substances produce their primary toxic effects by affecting neurotransmission. This chapter briefly reviews normal physiology of neurotransmission, the molecular action and biochemistry of several major neurotransmitters and their receptors, and toxicologic mechanisms by which numerous substances act at the molecular level. Neurotransmitters and neuromodulators of particular toxicologic interest are acetylcholine, norepinephrine, epinephrine, dopamine, serotonin, γ-aminobutyric acid, γ-hydroxybutyrate, glycine, glutamate, and adenosine.

When studying the molecular actions of drugs and toxins on neurotransmitter systems, it is apparent that substances rarely have single pharmacologic actions. For example, doxepin, in part, blocks voltage-gated sodium channels, blocks histaminic H_1 and H_2 receptors, blocks α-adrenergic receptors, blocks muscarinic acetylcholine receptors, blocks dopamine D_2 receptors, blocks $GABA_A$ receptors, prevents potassium efflux, and inhibits norepinephrine and serotonin uptake. For obvious reasons, then, this chapter cannot include every action of every drug or toxin on the nervous system. Nor is it meant to be a complete discussion of toxic syndromes produced by various agents, as these are covered in specific chapters. Rather, the intent is to provide a general and basic understanding of the mechanisms of action of various toxic agents affecting neurotransmitter function and receptors, especially in the central nervous system. With this focus, the clinical effects produced by various toxins are more easily understood and predicted, and specific treatments aimed at reversing pharmacologic effects of the offending agents can be rationally undertaken.

Given the complexity of the nervous system and the numerous actions of a given drug, it is not always clear which neurotransmitter system is producing an observed effect during a particular intoxication. Therefore, pharmacologic agents discussed in this chapter may be found in several sections. In each section, an attempt is made to note what appears to be a drug or toxin's main mechanism of action, although other actions are noted when possible.

Neuron Physiology and Neurotransmission

Membrane Potentials, Ion Channels, and Nerve Conduction

Sodium–potassium ATPase moves three sodium ions (Na^+) from inside the cell to the interstitial space while pumping two potassium ions (K^+) into the cell. Because the cell membrane is not freely permeable to large negatively charged molecules on the inside of the cell, such as proteins, an equilibrium results in which the inside of the neuron is negative with respect to the outside. Typical neuronal resting membrane potential is –65 mV.

Sodium, calcium (Ca^{2+}), K^+, and chloride (Cl^-) ions move into and out of neurons through ion channels.[62] Ions always move passively down electrochemical gradients through ion channels, which are long polypeptides comprising several subunits that span the plasma membrane several times. Many different ion channels are structurally comparable, sharing similar amino acid sequences.[23,62] Channels for a specific ion can also vary in structure, depending on the specific subunits that have combined to form the channel. Because of structural similarity of different channels, it is not surprising that many drugs or toxins are able to bind to more than one type of ion channel.

Most ion channels fall into two general classes: voltage-gated (voltage-dependent) ion channels, and ligand-gated ion channels. Voltage-gated channels open or close in response to changes in membrane potential. Ligand-gated channels open or close when a ligand (eg, neurotransmitter) binds to the channel to change its configuration.

A commonly accepted model describes voltage-gated Na^+ channels (and other voltage-dependent channels) in three possible states. At rest, the Na^+ channel is closed and impermeable to sodium, preventing Na^+ from moving into the cell. When the channel undergoes activation, the channel opens, allowing Na^+ to move intracellularly, down its electrochemical gradient. The channel then undergoes a third conformational change by becoming inactivated, preventing further influx of Na^+. The term "recovery" describes the conversion of inactive channels back to the resting state, a process that requires repolarization of the cell membrane.

Depolarization of a neuron usually results from an initial inward flux of cations (Na^+ or Ca^{2+}), or prevention of K^+ efflux. The fall in membrane potential (movement toward 0) results in further activation of these voltage-dependent Na^+ channels, allowing yet a greater influx of cations. When the membrane potential falls to threshold, Na^+ channels are activated en masse and there is a large influx of Na^+.

Depolarization of a segment of the neurolemma causes the adjacent neuronal membrane to reach threshold, resulting in the propagation of an action potential down the neuron. Sodium channel activation is quickly followed by inactivation. Over the short term, repolarization of the neuron occurring after inactivation of Na^+ channels mainly results from efflux of K^+ and some influx of Cl^-. Most drugs that block voltage-gated Na^+ channels (eg, tricyclic antidepressants, quinidine, local anesthetics) do so by binding to inactive channels, slowing recovery.

Neurotransmitter Release

Neurotransmitters are chemicals that are released from nerve endings into the synapse, where they produce effects by binding to receptors on postsynaptic and/or presynaptic cell membranes. The receptors may be on other neurons or effector organs such as smooth muscle. Concentrations of neurotransmitters in cytoplasm are usually low because of rapid degradation by various enzymes and because they diffuse out of the nerve ending. To provide a source of neurotransmitter that is protected from degradation and that can be rapidly released, neurotransmitters are pumped into and stored in vesicles in the axonal nerve terminal for release. As a wave of depolarization from Na^+ influx reaches the nerve ending, the membrane depolarization causes voltage-dependent Ca^{2+} channels to open, allowing Ca^{2+} to move rapidly into the cell. This influx of Ca^{2+} triggers exocytosis of vesicle contents into the synapse. The voltage-dependent Ca^{2+} channels responsible for inward Ca^{2+} currents that trigger neurotransmitter release are mainly of the N subtype.[100] Calcium channel blockers used in clinical practice (eg, verapamil, nifedipine) do not block this subtype of voltage-dependent Ca^{2+} channel, but rather block the L type. However, L subtype Ca^{2+} channels reside elsewhere on neurons, explaining the ability of these drugs to affect some neurologic functions.

Vesicle Transport of Neurotransmitters

The pH inside neurotransmitter vesicles is about 5.5, much lower than that in the cytoplasm. Transporter proteins in the vesicle membrane that are responsible for moving neurotransmitters into the vesicle are powered by ATP hydrolysis and by the voltage gradient from differing H^+ ion concentrations on each side of the membrane.[23,62]

Neurotransmitters are confined in the vesicle, to a great extent, by ion trapping, as they are more ionized and less able to diffuse back out of the vesicle at the lower pH. Anything that causes a decrease in the pH gradient across the vesicle membrane will result in the movement of neurotransmitter into the cytoplasm.[121] For example, amphetamines move into vesicles, where they buffer H^+ ions, causing the movement of biogenic amine neurotransmitters out of vesicles, raising cytoplasmic concentrations of neurotransmitters.[121,122]

Neurotransmitter Uptake

While acetylcholine is inactivated in the synapse by enzymatic degradation, most neurotransmitters have their synaptic effects terminated by active uptake into neurons and, frequently, into glial cells. These transporters are distinct from those responsible for movement of neurotransmitters into vesicles within the cytoplasm. Cell membrane transporters (uptake pumps) for different neurotransmitters are structurally similar (up to 70% amino acid homology) and part of a superfamily of Na^+-dependent transport proteins.[49,128] They generally comprise 600–700 amino acids and form loops spanning the plasma membrane 12 times. The uptake of neurotransmitters is powered by the simultaneous movement of Na^+ into the neuron by the transporter protein.

Several properties make transporter proteins of particular toxicologic significance. First, they are capable of moving neurotransmitters in either direction; when cytoplasmic neurotransmitter concentrations are significantly elevated, neurotransmitters can be transported back into the synapse. Second, these transporters are not always completely specific for a particular substance. For instance, the uptake transporter for norepinephrine can pump dopamine and other biogenic amines into the neuron. Third, a drug or toxin that acts at the level of the membrane transporter may affect functions of several different neurotransmitters, depending on its specificity for a particular transporter. As an example, fluoxetine is fairly specific at inhibiting uptake of serotonin, while cocaine inhibits the uptake of serotonin, norepinephrine, and dopamine.

Neurotransmitter Receptors

Channel Receptors. The first general class of neurotransmitter receptors is ligand-gated ion channels (channel receptors or ionotropic receptors) in which the receptor for the neurotransmitter is part of an ion channel. By binding to its receptor, the neurotransmitter allosterically changes the configuration of the ion channel so that ions can more easily traverse the channel and enter or leave the cell. As an example, the acetylcholine nicotinic receptor is a ligand-gated Na^+ channel. When acetylcholine binds to the nicotinic receptor, the channel's configuration changes, allowing Na^+ to move into the cell and trigger an action potential. (The action potential then propagates down muscle via voltage-gated Na^+ channels.) Other examples of channel receptors are found in Table 10–1.

G Protein Receptors. The second general class of neurotransmitter receptors is linked to G proteins, which are part of a superfamily of proteins with GTPase activity responsible for signal transduction across plasma membranes.[14] G proteins comprise three polypeptide subunits: α, β, and γ chains. These chains span the plasma membrane several times, and they associate with a separately transcribed neurotransmitter receptor that spans the cell membrane seven times, with an external binding site for neurotransmitters.

The α subunit of a G protein accounts for much of its activity resulting from neurotransmitter binding to its receptor. The α chain normally binds GDP in the cytoplasm and is inactive. When a neurotransmitter binds to its receptor on the outside of the cell membrane, GDP dissociates from the α chain and GTP binds in its place, activating the α subunit. The activated α chain dissociates from the β and γ chains and moves to an effector in the membrane to produce a physiologic effect. The effector may be an enzyme that the activated α chain stimulates or inhibits (eg, adenyl cyclase) or an ion channel that it opens or closes directly or through other chemical reactions (eg, channel phosphorylation).[24] Intrinsic GTPase activity in the α chain converts the GTP to GDP, inactivating the α subunit and allowing it to reassociate with the β and γ chains at the neurotransmitter receptor.

G proteins are categorized by the type of α chain they contain. For examples, G_s (containing the α subunit, α_s) is a positive allosteric effector of membrane-bound adenyl cyclase; activation of a neurotransmitter receptor coupled to G_s causes a rise in intracellular 3′,5′-cyclic adenosine monophosphate (cAMP) concentration. Neurotransmitter receptors activating G_i (containing α_i) inhibit adenyl cyclase and can open K^+ channels to cause K^+ efflux. These and other types of G proteins produce other effects as well.

TABLE 10–1. TYPES OF NEUROTRANSMITTER AND NEUROMODULATOR RECEPTORS

Ion channel	Linked to G protein
ACh nicotinic	ACh muscarinic
$GABA_A$, $GABA_C$	$GABA_B$
Glycine (inhibitory)	Dopamine
Glutamate AMPA	Norepinephrine
Glutamate NMDA	$5\text{-}HT_{1,2,4}$
Glutamate kainate	Adenosine
$5\text{-}HT_3$	Glutamate metabotropic

ACh = acetylcholine; GABA = γ-aminobutyric acid; 5-HT = serotonin; AMPA = α-amino-3-hydroxy-5-methyl-4-isoxazole proprionate; NMDA = *N*-methyl-*d*-aspartate.

Neurotransmitter receptors coupled to G proteins are noted in Table 10–1. A given neurotransmitter can activate different classes of receptors (eg, channel and G protein) or different types of receptors in the same class. For example, $GABA_A$ receptors are Cl^- channels while $GABA_B$ receptors are coupled to G proteins. Dopamine$_1$ (D_1) receptors are linked to G_s while D_2 receptors can be linked to G_i or G_0.

Neuronal Excitation and Inhibition

Excitatory neurotransmitters usually act postsynaptically by causing Na^+ or Ca^{2+} influx, or by preventing K^+ efflux, triggering depolarization and an action potential (Fig.

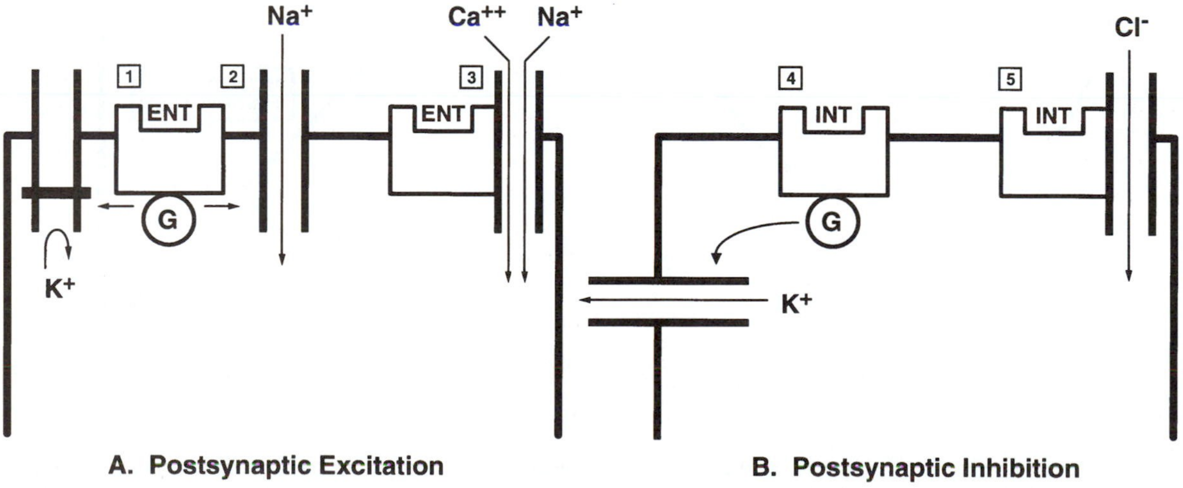

Figure 10–1. Common mechanisms of postsynaptic excitation and inhibition. In panel A, an excitatory neurotransmitter (ENT) binds to receptors linked to G proteins to prevent K^+ efflux [1] or to allow Na^+ influx [2], producing membrane depolarization. An ENT may also agonize and open a cation channel [3] to allow Na^+ and/or Ca^{2+} influx with resultant membrane depolarization. In panel B, an inhibitory neurotransmitter (INT) hyperpolarizes the membrane (causes the inside of the neuron to become more negative) by binding to receptors linked to G proteins to enhance K^+ efflux [4], or by binding to Cl^- channel receptors to allow Cl^- influx [5]. G = G protein.

10–1). These effects may be mediated by channel or G protein–coupled receptors.

Postsynaptic inhibition can be mediated by channel receptors or by receptors coupled to G proteins (Fig. 10–1). Inhibition is usually accomplished by movement of Cl^- into the neuron or by movement of K^+ out of the neuron. Both processes hyperpolarize the neuron and move membrane potential farther away from threshold, making it more difficult for a given stimulus to depolarize the membrane to threshold voltage.

Presynaptic inhibition, the prevention of neurotransmitter release, is usually mediated by receptors coupled to G proteins. When a neurotransmitter released from a neuron binds to a receptor on that same neuron to limit further neurotransmitter release, the receptor is termed an "autoreceptor."[108] Autoreceptors reside on dendrites, cell bodies, axons, and presynaptic terminals. Autoreceptors on dendrites and cell bodies (somatodendritic autoreceptors) usually inhibit further neurotransmitter release by increasing K^+ efflux, hyperpolarizing the neuron away from threshold (Fig. 10–2). Conversely, activation of autoreceptors found on presynaptic terminals (terminal autoreceptors) usually limits rises in intracellular Ca^{2+} concentration by limiting Ca^{2+} influx or preventing release from intracellular Ca^{2+} stores, impairing exocytosis of neurotransmitter vesicles (Fig. 10–2). Types of neurotransmitter receptors that serve as autoreceptors also usually reside postsynaptically, where they may mediate different physiologic effects.

Presynaptic nerve terminal inhibition of neurotransmitter release is not limited to actions by autoreceptors. Presynaptic terminal inhibitory receptors for various neurotransmitters may be found on a single neuron. For example, not only does stimulation of an α_2 autoreceptor on a noradrenergic nerve limit norepinephrine release, but stimulation of presynaptic α_2 receptor found on postsynaptic parasympathetic nerve terminals prevents acetylcholine release (Fig. 10–3).

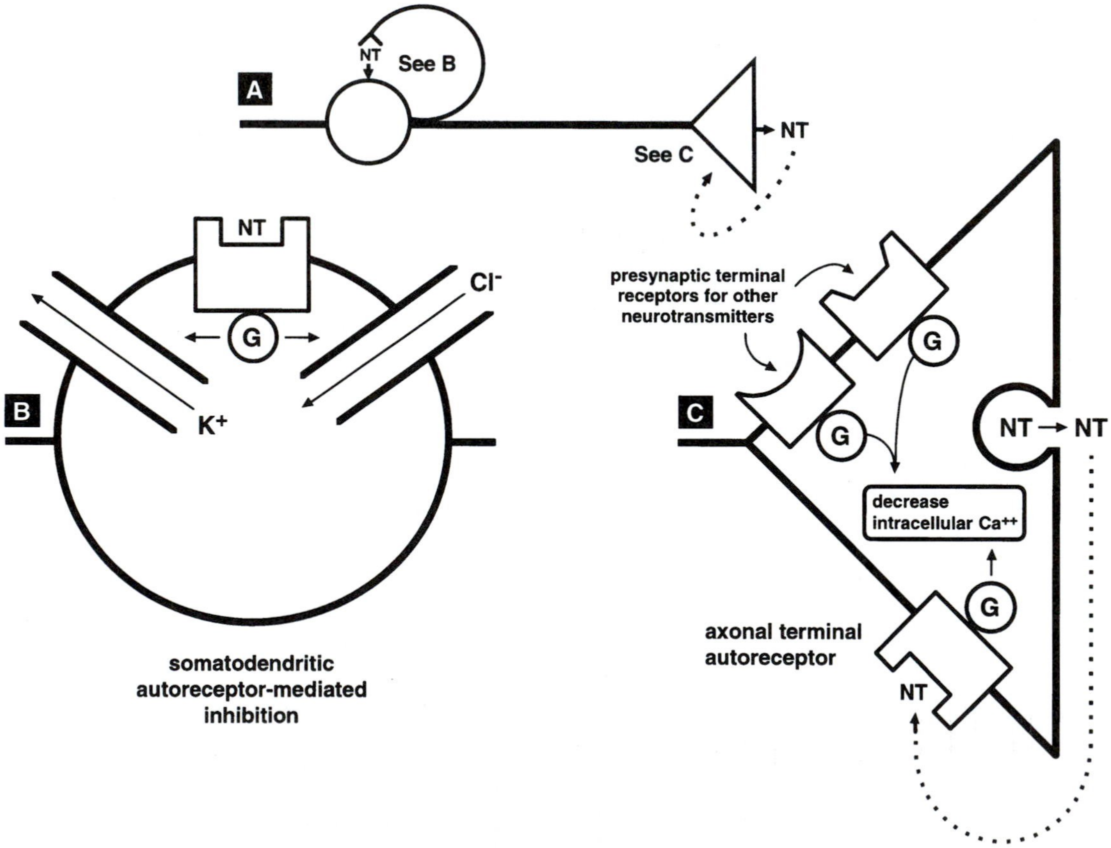

Figure 10–2. Common mechanisms of presynaptic inhibition (the inhibition of neurotransmitter release). Neuron A releases neurotransmitter, which returns to activate receptors on the cell body or dendrites (somatodendritic autoreceptors) or on the axonal terminal (terminal autoreceptors). Such activation limits further release of neurotransmitter by completing a negative feedback loop. At somatodendritic autoreceptors (panel B), neurotransmitter binding results in activation of G proteins, which promote either K^+ efflux or Cl^- influx; both processes hyperpolarize the neuron away from threshold. At terminal autoreceptors (panel C), NT binding activates G proteins, which, through various mechanisms, lower intracellular Ca^{2+} concentration to prevent exocytosis of neurotransmitter vesicles, despite depolarization. Presynaptic inhibitory receptors (panel C) for other types of neurotransmitters that are also commonly found on nerve endings. NT = neurotransmitter; G = G protein.

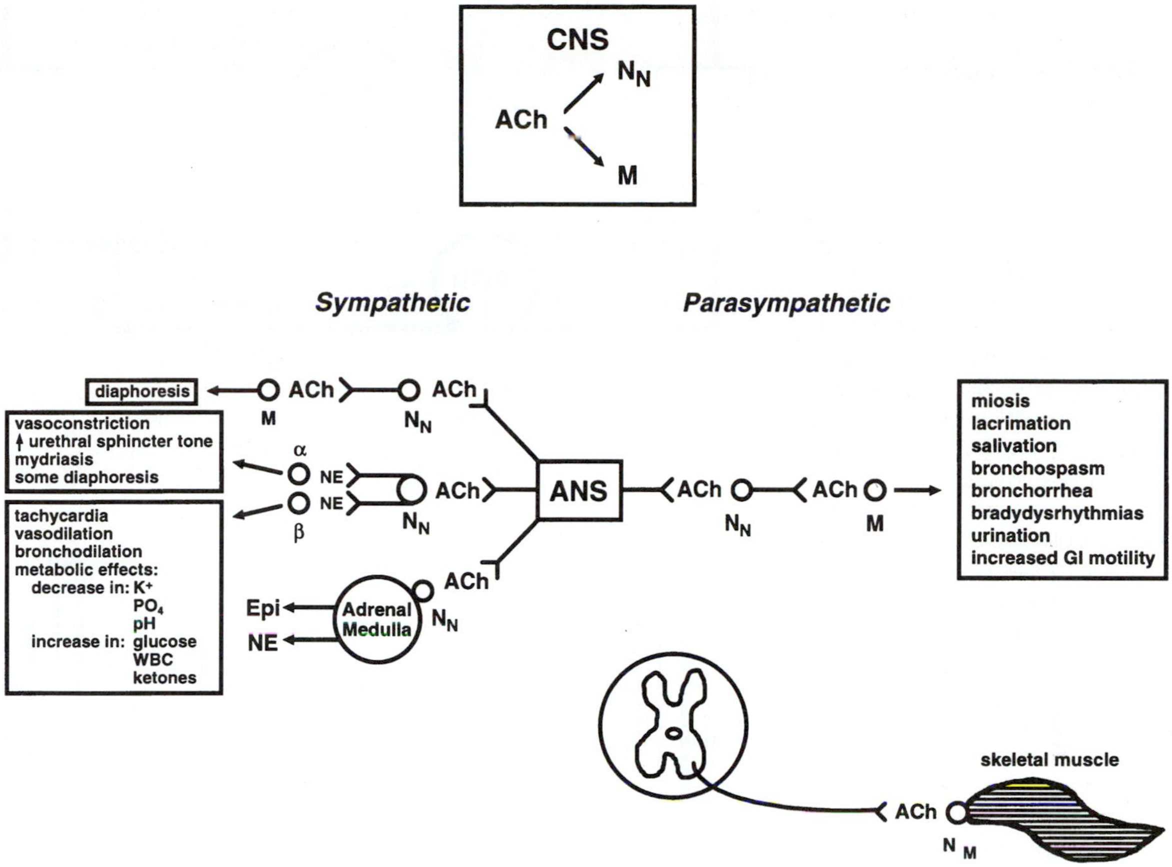

Figure 10–3. Schematic diagram of the cholinergic nervous system, including adrenergic involvement in the autonomic nervous system. ACh binds to CNS, ganglionic, and adrenal nicotinic receptors (N_N) and to nicotinic receptors on skeletal muscle (N_M). ACh also binds to various subtypes of muscarinic (M) receptors in the CNS and on effector organs innervated by postganglionic parasympathetic neurons and most sweat glands. NE and/or EPI released in response to ganglionic ACh stimulation of N_N receptors stimulates α- and β-adrenergic receptors. CNS = central nervous system; ACh = acetylcholine; NE = norepinephrine; EPI = epinephrine; ANS = autonomic nervous system.

Finally, stimulation of receptors on presynaptic nerve endings may enhance, rather than inhibit, neurotransmitter release. Such receptors also are usually coupled to G proteins. For example, stimulation of a β_2 receptor on an adrenergic nerve terminal enhances norepinephrine release. Activation of some presynaptic metabotropic glutamate receptors increases neuronal calcium concentrations to enhance release of glutamate or other neurotransmitters.

Acetylcholine

Acetylcholine (ACh) is a neurotransmitter of the central and peripheral nervous system. Centrally, it is found in both brain and spinal cord; cholinergic fibers project diffusely to the cerebral cortex. Peripherally, ACh serves as a neurotransmitter in autonomic and somatic motor fibers (Fig. 10–3).

Synthesis, Release, and Inactivation

Acetylcholine is synthesized from acetyl coenzyme A and choline. Acetylcholine moves into synaptic vesicles, where it is stored before release into the synapse by Ca^{2+}-dependent exocytosis. Acetylcholine undergoes degradation in the synapse to choline and acetic acid by acetylcholinesterase. A Na^+-dependent transporter in the neuronal membrane then pumps choline back into the cytoplasm to be used again as a substrate for ACh synthesis (Fig. 10–4). Pseudocholinesterase (plasma cholinesterase) is made in the liver and plays no role in the degradation of synaptic ACh metabolism. However, it does metabolize some drugs, including cocaine and succinylcholine.

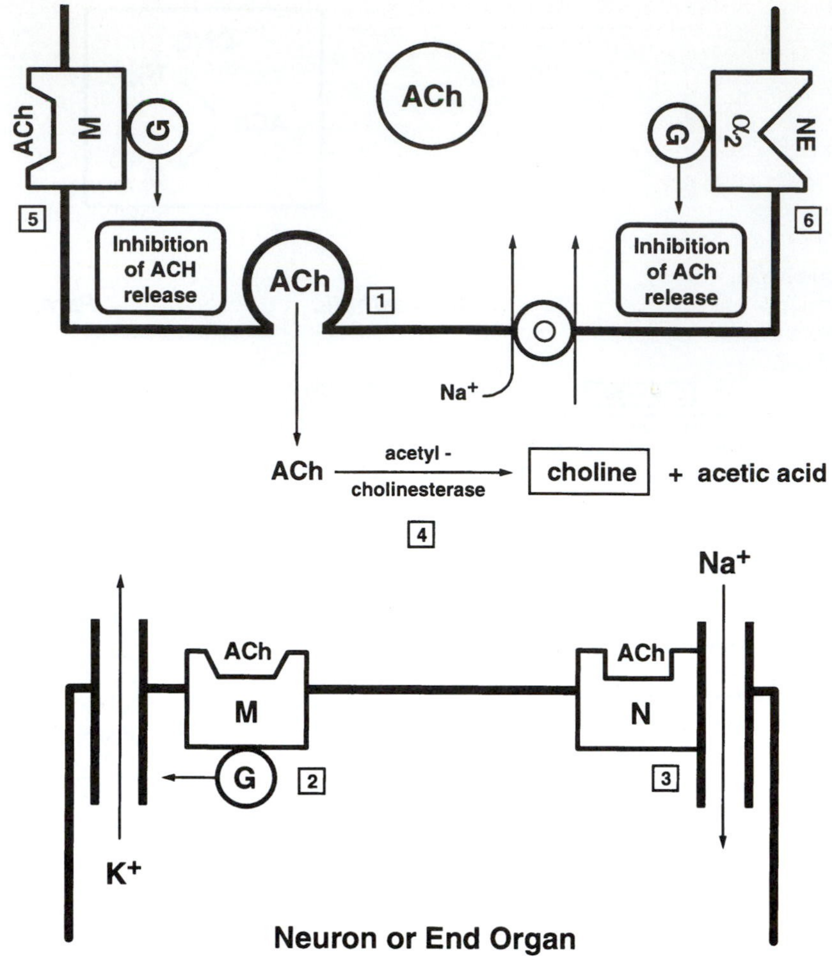

Figure 10–4. Cholinergic nerve ending. Activation of postsynaptic muscarinic receptors hyperpolarizes the postsynaptic membrane through G protein–mediated enhancement of K^+ efflux. (Several subtypes of muscarinic receptors exist and may be coupled to various G proteins. A muscarinic receptor coupled to a G protein that opens K^+ channels is shown only as an example.) Postsynaptic nicotinic receptor activation causes Na^+ influx and membrane depolarization. Presynaptic muscarinic and α_2 adrenergic receptor activation prevents ACh release through lowering of intracellular Ca^{2+} concentration. Agents in Table 10–2 may act to enhance or prevent release of ACh [1]; stimulate or block postsynaptic muscarinic (M) receptors [2]; stimulate or block nicotinic (N) receptors [3]; inhibit acetylcholinesterase [4]; prevent ACh release by stimulating presynaptic muscarinic autoreceptors [5] or adrenergic α_2 receptors (on parasympathetic postganglionic terminals) [6]; or enhance ACh release by antagonizing presynaptic muscarinic receptors [5] or α_2 receptors (on parasympathetic postganglionic terminals) [6]. ACh = acetylcholine; NE = norepinephrine; G = G protein.

Acetylcholine Receptors

Nicotinic Receptors. After release from cholinergic nerve endings, ACh binds to two main types of receptors, nicotinic and muscarinic.[62,74] Nicotinic receptors are found in the central nervous system (CNS; mainly in spinal cord), on postganglionic autonomic neurons (both sympathetic and parasympathetic), and at skeletal neuromuscular junctions, where they mediate muscle contraction (Fig. 10–3). Nicotinic receptors are part of a Na^+ channel and are thus channel receptors. Stimulation of these receptors by ACh results in Na^+ influx, depolarization of the neuron or effector (eg, skeletal muscle), and triggering of an action potential. Nicotinic receptors vary in structure and comprise various subunits, resulting in at least two main subtypes of nicotinic receptors: N_M receptors found mainly on skeletal muscle; N_N receptors found at the autonomic ganglia, in the adrenal medulla, and in the CNS.

Muscarinic Receptors. Muscarinic receptors are found in the CNS (mainly in brain), as receptors for postganglionic parasympathetic nerve endings, and as postganglionic sympathetic receptors for most sweat glands (Fig. 10–4). There are at least five subtypes of muscarinic receptors, which are linked to several G proteins. For example, in the heart, ACh released from the vagus nerve binds to a muscarinic receptor linked to G_i. G_i opens K^+ channels, allowing efflux of K^+ down its concentration gradient, which makes the inside of the cell more negative and more difficult to depolarize, slowing heart rate. Different subtypes of muscarinic receptors also act as autoreceptors in various locations; M_1 is the most common.

Chemical Agents (Table 10–2)

Modulators of Acetylcholine Release. Figure 10–4 illustrates sites of actions of numerous agents that act on the cholinergic nervous system. Botulism toxin, some neurotoxins from pit vipers, and elapid β-neurotoxins prevent release of ACh from peripheral nerve endings.[53] This results in ptosis, other cranial nerve signs, weakness, and respiratory failure. Hypermagnesemia also inhibits acetylcholine release, probably by inhibiting Ca^{2+} influx into the nerve ending.[74]

Guanidine, aminopyridines, and black widow spider venom enhance the release of ACh from nerve endings. Guanidine has been tried as a treatment for botu-

TABLE 10–2. AGENTS AFFECTING CHOLINERGIC NEUROTRANSMISSION*

Cholinomimetic Agents

Cause ACh release

- α_2 Adrenergic antagonists[a]
- Aminopyridines
- Black widow spider venom
- Carbachol
- Guanidine

Anticholinesterases

- Echothiophate iodide
- Edrophonium
- Galanthamine
- *N*-Methylcarbamate insecticides
- Neostigmine
- Organophosphates
- Physostigmine
- Pyridostigmine
- Tacrine

Direct nicotinic agonists

- Arecoline
- Carbachol (weak)
- Coniine
- Cytisine
- Decamethonium (initial)[b]
- Lobeline
- Methacholine (weak)
- Nicotine
- Succinylcholine (initial)[b]

Direct muscarinic agonists

- Bethanechol
- Carbachol
- Methacholine
- Muscarine
- Pilocarpine

Cholinolytic Agents

Direct nicotinic antagonists

- α-Bungarotoxin[c]
- Arecoline
- Atracurium[d]
- Coniine
- Cytisine
- Decamethonium[b]
- Doxacurium[d]
- Gallamine[d]
- Hexamethonium[e]
- Lobeline
- Mecamylamine[e]
- Mivacurium[d]
- Nicotine
- Pancuronium[d]
- Pentolinium[e]
- Pipecuronium[d]
- Succinylcholine[b]
- Trimethaphan[e]
- Tubocurarine[d]
- Vecuronium[d]

Direct muscarinic antagonists

- Amantadine
- Antihistamines
- Atropine
- Benztropine
- Carbamazepine
- Clozapine
- Cyclobenzaprine
- Cyclopentolate
- Glutethimide
- Orphenadrine
- Phenothiazines
- Pirenzepine
- Procainamide
- Quinidine
- Scopolamine
- Tricyclic antidepressants
- Trihexyphenidyl
- Tropicamide

Inhibit ACh release

- α_2 Adrenergic agonists[f]
- Botulinum toxins
- *Crotalidae* venoms
- *Elapidae* β-neurotoxins
- Hypermagnesemia

*Direct agonists and antagonists bind to ACh receptors to mimic or block the effects of ACh, respectively.

ACh = acetylcholine.

[a]Antagonism of α_2 receptors enhances ACh release from the parasympathetic nerve endings.

[b]Depolarizing neuromuscular (N_M) blocking agent.

[c]α-Bungarotoxin is representative of many elapid (snake) α-neurotoxins that block N_M receptors to produce paralysis and death from respiratory failure in a manner similar to curare.

[d]Nondepolarizing neuromuscular blocking agent.

[e]Relatively specific for N_N receptors.

[f]Stimulation of presynaptic α_2-adrenergic receptors on parasympathetic nerve endings prevents ACh release.

lism. Aminopyridines block voltage-gated K^+ channels to prevent K^+ efflux; the resultant action potential widening (delayed repolarization) causes prolongation of Ca^{2+} channel activation, enhancing influx of Ca^{2+} and promoting neurotransmitter release. Aminopyridines have been used therapeutically in Lambert-Eaton syndrome, myasthenia gravis, multiple sclerosis, and experimentally in calcium channel blocker overdose. Black widow spider venom causes acetylcholine release with resultant muscle cramping and diaphoresis.[6] Carbachol, a nicotinic and muscarinic agonist, also probably causes ACh release.

Nicotinic Receptor Agonists and Antagonists. Agents that bind to and stimulate nicotinic receptors may stimulate postganglionic sympathetic and parasympathetic neurons, skeletal muscle endplates, and the neurons within the CNS (Fig. 10–3). Prolonged depolarization at the receptor eventually causes blockade of nicotinic receptors.[89] For example, poisoning by nicotine (a nicotine receptor agonist) produces hypertension, tachycardia, vomiting, diarrhea, muscle fasciculations, and convulsions (excitation), followed by hypotension, bradydysrhythmias, paralysis, and coma (blockade). Nicotinic agonists include nicotine alkaloids (eg, nicotine, coniine, arecoline, lobeline), carbachol (although mainly muscarinic), and methacholine (slight). Succinylcholine is a neuromuscular blocking agent that first stimulates and then blocks N_M receptors.

Agents that block nicotinic receptors without stimulation at skeletal neuromuscular junctions (N_M receptors) produce weakness and paralysis. Examples include curare and atracurium. Alpha-neurotoxins from elapids (eg, α-bungarotoxin) are direct nicotinic antagonists, producing ptosis, weakness, and respiratory failure from paralysis.[134]

Chemicals blocking N_N receptors (eg, nicotine) produce autonomic ganglionic blockade and may produce CNS effects as well. Trimethaphan is used as a pharmacologic ganglionic blocker. However, trimethaphan is not entirely specific for N_N receptors; occasional patients develop weakness and paralysis from its N_M blockade.

Muscarinic Receptor Agonists and Antagonists. Peripheral muscarinic agonists produce bradycardia, miosis, salivation, lacrimation, vomiting, diarrhea, bronchospasm, bronchorrhea, and micturition. Central muscarinic agonists produce sedation, extrapyramidal dystonias and rigidity, coma, and convulsions. Examples of direct muscarinic agonists are muscarine (from mushrooms), bethanechol, pilocarpine, carbachol, and methacholine.

Anticholinergic poisoning syndrome results from blockade of muscarinic receptors and is more appropriately referred to as antimuscarinic poisoning syndrome.[111] Central nervous system muscarinic blockade produces confusion, agitation, myoclonus, tremor, picking movements, abnormal speech, hallucinations, and coma. Peripheral antimuscarinic effects include mydriasis, anhidrosis, tachycardia, urinary retention, and ileus. Muscarinic antagonists number in the hundreds. Examples are listed in Table 10–2.

Acetylcholinesterase Inhibition. Agents inhibiting acetylcholinesterase raise ACh concentrations at both nicotinic and muscarinic receptors, producing a variety of CNS, sympathetic, parasympathetic, and skeletal muscle signs and symptoms.[26] Anticholinesterases include organophosphates and *N*-methylcarbamates. Organophosphates are usually encountered as insecticides, although a topical medicinal organophosphate (echothiophate iodide) is used for the treatment of glaucoma. *N*-methylcarbamates are found as insecticides and pharmaceuticals. Medicinal *N*-methylcarbamates include physostigmine, pyridostigmine, and neostigmine. Edrophonium, galanthamine, and tacrine are noncarbamate, reversible anticholinesterases.

Alpha$_2$ Agonists and Antagonists. Agonists and antagonists of α_2-adrenergic receptors are discussed in detail below. Briefly, stimulation of presynaptic α_2 receptors on postganglionic parasympathetic nerve endings decreases ACh release. Conversely, presynaptic α_2 antagonism increases ACh release (Fig. 10–4).

Norepinephrine and Epinephrine

Norepinephrine (NE), epinephrine (EPI), dopamine (DA), and serotonin (5-hydroxytryptamine; 5-HT) have historically been referred to as biogenic amines and their neurotransmitter systems are similar in many respects. Neurotransmitter synthesis, vesicle transport and storage, uptake, and degradation share many enzymes and structurally similar transport proteins. All four types of neurons are affected by cocaine, reserpine, amphetamines, and monoamine oxidase inhibitors (MAOIs). In addition, these agents produce several different effects in the same system. For example, in the noradrenergic neuron, amphetamines work mainly by causing the release of cytoplasmic NE, but they also inhibit NE uptake and their metabolites inhibit monoamine oxidase. Actions of drugs that affect all biogenic amine neurotransmission are described in the most detail for noradrenergic neurons. For the sake of brevity, similar mechanisms of action are simply noted in discussions of dopaminergic and serotonergic neurotransmission.

Norepinephrine is released from postganglionic sympathetic fibers (Fig. 10–3) and is also found in the CNS. The adrenal gland, acting as a modified sympathetic ganglion, releases EPI and lesser amounts of NE in response to stimulation of ACh nicotinic (N_N) receptors. Epinephrine-containing neurons also reside in the brainstem.

The locus ceruleus is the main noradrenergic nucleus in the brain.[62] Axons radiate from this nucleus out to all layers of the cerebral cortex, to the cerebellum, and to other structures. Norepinephrine demonstrates both excitatory and inhibitory actions in the CNS. Norepinephrine released from locus ceruleus projections in the hippocampus increases cortical neuron activity through β receptor activation and G protein–mediated inhibition of K^+ efflux. Norepinephrine released in outer cortical areas has an inhibitory effect mediated by α receptor agonism. At this level, NE produces slow cortical neuron hyperpolarization and decreased rates of spontaneous firing. Consistent with this, NE demonstrates anticonvulsant actions in animals; carbamazepine's anticonvulsant action may be due in part to inhibition of NE uptake.[41] Despite antagonistic actions on different cortical neurons, electrical stimulation of the locus ceruleus produces widespread cortical activation and excitation. This overall effect probably explains a great deal of the hyperattentiveness and lack of fatigue that accompanies intoxications with agents that mimic or increase noradrenergic activity in the brain.

Synthesis, Release, and Uptake

A schematic representation of a noradrenergic neuron is shown in Fig. 10–5. Tyrosine hydroxylase is the rate-limiting enzyme in NE synthesis and is sensitive to negative feedback by NE. Dopa undergoes decarboxylation by L-amino acid decarboxylase to DA. L-Amino acid decarboxylase (dopa decarboxylase) is not specific for dopa. For example, it also catalyzes the formation of serotonin from 5-hydroxytryptophan.

About one-half of cytoplasmic dopa is actively pumped into vesicles containing the enzyme dopamine-β-hydroxylase. The remaining DA is quickly deaminated. In the vesicle, dopamine-β-hydroxylase converts DA to NE. Vesicles isolated from nerve endings contain DA, NE, dopamine-β-hydroxylase, and ATP. All of these substances are released into the synapse during Ca^{2+}-dependent exocytosis triggered by neuronal firing.[62]

In neurons containing EPI as a neurotransmitter, NE is released from vesicles into the cytoplasm, where it is converted to EPI. Epinephrine is then transported back into vesicles before synaptic release.[74]

Norepinephrine is removed from the synapse mainly by uptake into the presynaptic neuron by a norepinephrine transporter. While this transporter has great affinity for NE, it also transports other amines, including DA, tyramine, MAOIs, and amphetamines. Once pumped back into the cytoplasm, NE can either be transported back into vesicles for further storage and release or can be quickly enzymatically degraded by monoamine oxidase (MAO), an enzyme found on the outer mitochondrial membrane.

Monoamine oxidase can be found in sympathetic postganglionic neurons, intestinal mucosa, liver, kidney, lung, and brain. It comprises two isoenzymes, MAO-A and MAO-B,[78] each with relatively separate affinities for various substrates (Table 10–3). Monoamine oxidase has two main actions. First, neuronal MAO degrades cytoplasmic amines, including neurotransmitters, to prevent elevated cytoplasmic concentrations of biogenic amines. Second, hepatic and intestinal MAO prevents large quan-

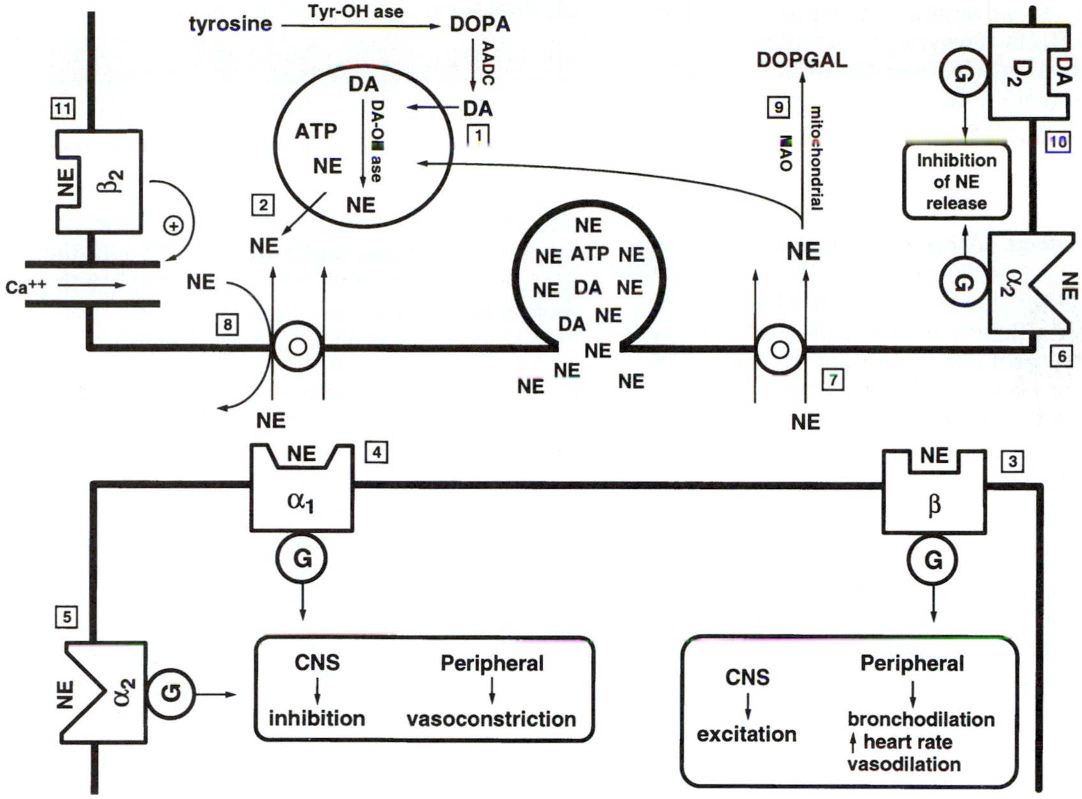

Figure 10–5. Noradrenergic nerve ending. The postsynaptic membrane may represent an end organ or another neuron in the CNS. Brief examples of effects resulting from postsynaptic receptor activation are shown. Agents in Tables 10–4 and 10–5 produce effects by inhibiting transport of DA or NE into vesicles [1]; causing movement of NE from vesicles into the cytoplasm [2]; stimulating or blocking postsynaptic α and β receptors [3–5]; modulating NE release by stimulating or blocking presynaptic α_2 autoreceptors [6] or presynaptic dopamine (D_2) receptors [10]; blocking uptake of NE [7]; causing reverse transport of NE out of cytoplasm into the synapse by raising cytoplasmic NE concentrations (indirect action) [8]; inhibiting MAO to prevent NE degradation [9]; or modulating NE release through stimulation or blockade of presynaptic β_2 receptors [11]. Tyr-OHase = tyrosine hydroxylase; AADC = L-aromatic amino acid decarboxylase; DA = dopamine; DA-OHase = dopamine-β-hydroxylase; NE = norepinephrine; G = G protein; MAO = monoamine oxidase; DOPGAL = 3,4-dihydroxyphenylglycoaldehyde; ATP = adenosine triphosphate; CNS = central nervous system.

tities of dietary bioactive amines from entering the circulation and producing systemic effects.

Catechol-*O*-methyltransferase (COMT) also metabolizes NE and EPI. However, little COMT resides in neurons. In other tissue, COMT metabolizes catecholamines, including those that have entered the systemic circulation.

Adrenergic Receptors

The two main types of adrenergic receptors are α–adrenergic receptors and β–adrenergic receptors. All adrenergic receptors are linked to G proteins.

Beta–adrenergic Receptors. Beta–adrenergic receptors are linked to G_s, and their stimulation raises cAMP concentration, which in turn may produce several effects, including regulation of ion channels. Beta–adrenergic receptors are divided into three major subtypes (β_1, β_2, and β_3) depending on their affinity for various agonists and antagonists.[38,47,57,62] In general, peripheral β_1–adrenergic receptors are found mainly in the heart,

TABLE 10–3. CHARACTERISTICS OF MONOAMINE OXIDASE (MAO) ISOENZYMES

	MAO Isoenzymes	
	MAO-A	*MAO-B*
Location		
Brain	+	+++
Intestine	+++	+
Liver	++	++
Platelets	0	++++
Placenta	++++	0
Substrates		
Norepinephrine	++++	+
Epinephrine	++	++
Dopamine	++	++
Serotonin	++++	+
Tyramine	++	++

while peripheral β_2–adrenergic receptors mediate other adrenergic effects. Presynaptic β_2–adrenergic receptor activation causes release of NE from nerve endings (positive feedback). Beta$_3$–adrenergic receptors reside mainly in fat, where they regulate metabolic processes, but are also found in the gallbladder and colon.

Alpha–adrenergic Receptors. Alpha–adrenergic receptors are linked to other G proteins that inhibit adenyl cyclase and lower cAMP levels, affect ion channels, increase intracellular calcium through inositol triphosphate and diacylglycerol production, or produce other actions. These receptors are divided into two main types (α_1 and α_2) and at least six subtypes.[19,57]

Alpha$_1$–adrenergic receptors reside on the postsynaptic membrane in continuity with the synaptic cleft. Stimulation of these receptors on vasculature results in vasoconstriction.

Alpha$_2$–adrenergic receptors reside on both sides of the synapse. Stimulation of presynaptic α_2–adrenergic receptors mediates negative feedback, limiting further release of NE (Fig. 10–5). Postganglionic parasympathetic neurons (cholinergic) also contain presynaptic α_2–adrenergic receptors that, when stimulated, prevent release of ACh (Fig. 10–4).

Postsynaptic α_2–adrenergic receptors on vasculature also mediate vasoconstriction.[21] Norepinephrine released from nerve endings mainly produces vasoconstriction by stimulating postsynaptic α_1–adrenergic receptors, while circulating epinephrine and norepinephrine (eg, adrenal in origin or exogenously administered) mainly produce vasoconstriction through stimulation of postsynaptic α_2–adrenergic receptors.[63] This distinction is important when choosing α adrenergic antagonists for therapeutic use. A patient with hypertension from high circulating catecholamine concentrations (eg, pheochromocytoma or clonidine withdrawal) or from extravasation of norepinephrine from an IV line needs both α_1 and α_2 blockade to vasodilate (eg, phentolamine), while the patient with essential hypertension may do well with a selective α_1 adrenergic antagonist (eg, prazosin). Stimulation of postsynaptic α_2–adrenergic receptors in the brainstem inhibit sympathetic output and produce sedation (Fig. 10–6).

Chemical Agents (Tables 10–4 and 10–5)

Chemicals producing pharmacologic effects that result in or mimic increased activity of the adrenergic nervous system are called sympathomimetics (Table 10–4). Those with the opposite effect are sympatholytics (Table 10–5).

Sympathomimetics

Direct-acting Agents. Drugs or chemicals whose sympathomimetic actions result from direct binding to α- or β-adrenergic receptors are called direct-acting sympathomimetics. Most of these drugs do not cross the blood–brain barrier in significant quantities.

Indirect-acting Agents. Agents that produce sympathomimetic effects by causing the release of cytoplasmic NE from the nerve ending in the absence of vesicle exocytosis are called indirect-acting sympathomimetics. Amphetamine is the prototype of indirect-acting agents and is used for the discussion of what is known about their mechanism of action. In general, mechanisms of indirect release of NE by amphetamines, cocaine, phencyclidine, MAOIs, and mixed-acting agents noted in Table 10–4 are similar in that their actions depend on their ability to produce elevated cytoplasmic NE concentrations.

Amphetamine and structurally similar indirectly acting agents move into the neuron by the membrane transporter that pumps NE into the neuron. (Lipophilic indirectly acting agents move into the neuron by diffusion.) From the cytoplasm, amphetamines are transported into neurotransmitter vesicles, where they buffer hydrogen ions to raise intravesicle pH. As noted earlier, much of the vesicle's ability to concentrate NE (and other neurotransmitters) is due to ion trapping of NE at the lower pH. The rise in intravesicle pH produced by amphetamines causes NE to leave the vesicle and move into the cytoplasm.[121,122] Such movement may be due to diffusion and/or reverse transport of NE by the vesicle membrane transporter. In the cytoplasm, amphetamines also compete with NE and DA for transport into vesicles, which further contributes to elevated cytoplasmic NE concentrations. In the case of amphetamines, the rise in cytoplasmic concentrations of NE is enhanced by the ability of amphetamine metabolites to inhibit MAO, which impairs NE degradation.

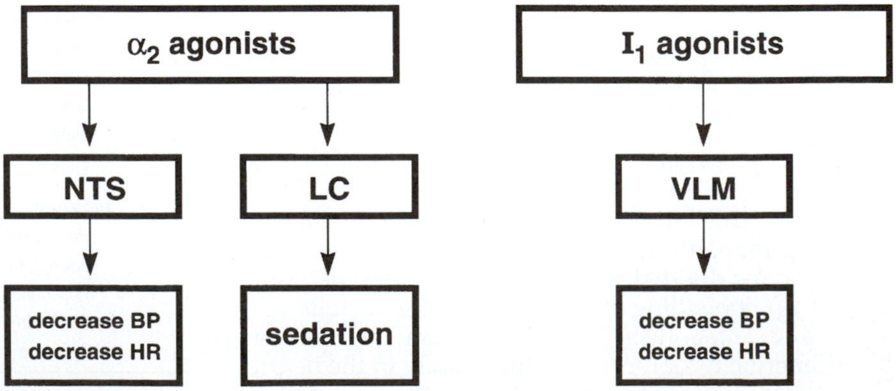

Figure 10–6. Central actions of agents that activate adrenergic α_2 and/or activate imidazoline (I_1) receptors. NTS = nucleus tractus solitarius; LC = locus ceruleus; VLM = rostral ventrolateral medulla.

TABLE 10–4. SYMPATHOMIMETICS*

Direct-acting

β–Adrenergic Agonists

- Albuterol
- Dobutamine
- Epinephrine
- Isoetharine
- Isoproterenol
- Metaproterenol
- Norepinephrine
- Ritodrine
- Terbutaline

α–Adrenergic Agonists

- Dobutamine
- Epinephrine
- Ergot alkaloids
- Methoxamine
- Norepinephrine
- Phenylephrine

Indirect-acting

- Amphetamines
- Cocaine
- Fenfluramine
- MAOIs
- Methylphenidate
- Pemoline
- Phencyclidine
- Phendimetrazine
- Phenmetrazine
- Propylhexedrine
- Tyramine

Mixed-acting

- Dopamine
- Ephedrine
- Mephentermine
- Phenylpropanolamine
- Pseudoephedrine

Selective α_2–Adrenergic Antagonists

- Idazoxan
- Yohimbine

Imidazoline Receptor Antagonists

- Idazoxan

MAOIs

- Amphetamine metabolites
- Clorgyline[a]
- Isocarboxazid
- Moclobemide[a]
- Pargyline
- Phenelzine
- Selegiline[b]
- Tranylcypromine

Inhibit NE Uptake

- Amitriptyline
- Amoxapine
- Amphetamines
- Benztropine
- Carbamazepine
- Cocaine
- Desipramine
- Diphenhydramine
- Doxepin
- Imipramine
- Maprotiline
- Nortriptyline
- Orphenadrine
- Pemoline
- Tramadol
- Trihexyphenidyl
- Venlafaxine

*Direct-acting sympathomimetics bind to and activate adrenergic receptors in a manner similar to norepinephrine. Indirect-acting agents increase cytoplasmic NE concentrations, resulting in reverse transport of NE from cytoplasm into the synapse. Mixed-acting agents act both directly and indirectly, although one action usually prevails. α_2–Adrenergic antagonists bind to presynaptic adrenergic nerve terminals to enhance release of norepinephrine as well as to increase sympathetic nervous system activity through central postsynaptic α_2–adrenergic receptors.

MAOIs = monoamine oxidase inhibitors; NE = norepinephrine.

[a]Mainly inhibit MAO-A at low doses.

[b]Mainly inhibit MAO-B at low doses.

TABLE 10–5. SYMPATHOLYTICS*

α–Adrenergic Antagonists

- Clozapine
- Doxazosin
- Droperidol
- Ergot alkaloids
- Labetalol
- Mirtazapine
- Phenothiazines
- Phenoxybenzamine
- Phentolamine
- Prazosin
- Quinidine
- Risperidone
- Terazosin
- Trazodone
- Tricyclic antidepressants
- Urapidil

Inhibit Dopamine-β-Hydroxylase

- Diethyldithiocarbamate
- Disulfiram
- MAOIs

β–Adrenergic Antagonists

- Acebutolol[a]
- Alprenolol[a]
- Atenolol
- Betaxolol
- Bisoprolol
- Carteolol[a]
- Carvedilol
- Esmolol
- Labetalol
- Metipranolol[a]
- Metoprolol
- Nadolol
- Oxprenolol[a]
- Penbutolol[a]
- Pindolol[a]
- Practolol[a]
- Propranolol
- Sotalol
- Timolol

Prevent NE Release with Depolarization

- Bretylium[b]
- Guanethidine
- Reserpine[b]

α_2–Adrenergic Agonists

- α-Methyldopa[c]
- Clonidine
- Guanabenz[d]
- Guanfacine[d]
- Moxonidine[e]
- Naphazoline
- Oxymetazoline
- Rilmenidine[e]
- Tetrahydralazine
- Xylometazoline

Imidazoline Receptor Agonists

- Clonidine
- Guanabenz[d]
- Guanfacine[d]
- Moxonidine[e]
- Naphazoline
- Oxymetazoline
- Rilmenidine[e]

Inhibitors of Vesicle Uptake

- Guanethidine
- Reserpine[b]
- Tetrabenazine

*Antagonists prevent NE binding to α and β–adrenergic receptors. Activation of peripheral presynaptic α_2–adrenergic receptors limits release of NE. Activation of central postsynaptic α_2–adrenergic receptors decreases sympathetic output.

NE = norepinephrine; MAOIs = monoamine oxidase inhibitors.

[a]Partial β agonist.

[b]Causes transient NE release after initial dose.

[c]Metabolized to α-methylnorepinephrine, which activates α_2 receptors.

[d]Mainly activates α_2 receptors.

[e]Mainly activates imidazoline receptors.

Every time the Na^+-dependent transporter moves a bioactive amine (eg, tyramine) into the neuron where it is then released, a binding site for NE on the transporter transiently faces inward and becomes available for reverse transport of NE out of the neuron. The normally low concentration of cytoplasmic NE prevents significant reverse transport. In the face of elevated cytoplasmic NE concentrations produced by indirect-acting agents as described above, the Na^+-dependent neuronal membrane transporter moves NE out of the neuron and back into the synapse, where the neurotransmitter stimulates adrenergic receptors (indirect action). This process is sometimes referred to as facilitated exchange diffusion, or "displacement" of NE from the nerve ending. Evidence for reverse transport by amphetamines is that inhibitors of the transporter (eg, tricyclic antidepressants) prevent amphetamine-induced NE release.

While all indirect-acting agents cause reverse NE transport by increasing cytoplasmic NE concentrations, those that move into the neuron by the membrane transporter (eg, amphetamines, MAOIs, dopamine, tyramine) further enhance reverse transport because their uptake causes more NE binding sites on the transporter to face inward per unit time.

While cocaine's main adrenergic effect results from inhibition of the membrane uptake transporter, cocaine also causes some NE release. In fact, cocaine similarly lessens pH gradients across vesicle membranes[122] to raise cytoplasmic concentrations of NE. The fact that cocaine produces less NE release than amphetamines is explained by cocaine-induced inhibition of the membrane transporter and by the fact that cocaine does not move into the neuron by active uptake (ie, does not increase the number of NE binding sites facing inward), but diffuses into the neuron.

Phencyclidine (PCP) is a hallucinogen that has multiple pharmacologic actions. Like intoxications from many hallucinogens, PCP intoxication is accompanied by increased adrenergic activity, which results from PCP-induced decreases in pH gradients across the vesicle membrane[122] and indirect release of NE. Like cocaine, PCP moves into the neuron by diffusion rather than uptake through the membrane transporter, at least partly explaining less PCP-induced NE release than is typically seen in amphetamine poisoning.

Reserpine, guanethidine, and bretylium cause neurotransmitter release with initial doses or early in overdose before their primary sympatholytic effects are observed. Presumably this is due to transient rises in cytoplasmic NE concentrations.

In addition to causing acetylcholine release, black widow spider venom causes vesicle exocytosis of NE, producing hypertension and diaphoresis over the palms, soles, upper lip, and nose.[96] All of the aforementioned indirectly acting agents, except black widow spider venom, enter the CNS.

Mixed-acting Agents. Mixed-acting sympathomimetics act directly and indirectly.[74] For example, phenylpropanolamine indirectly causes NE release and acts directly as an α agonist. Intravenously administered dopamine indirectly causes NE release, explaining most of its vasoconstricting activity, but also directly stimulates dopaminergic and β-adrenergic receptors. Direct α agonism is seen at high doses. Except for dopamine, these agents also cross the blood–brain barrier to produce central effects.

Uptake Inhibitors. Inhibitors of NE uptake raise concentrations of NE in the synapse to produce excessive stimulation of adrenergic receptors. Cocaine's main adrenergic effect is by this mechanism.

There are two main mechanisms of action for inhibitors of biogenic amine uptake: competitive and noncompetitive. Noncompetitive inhibitors such as cyclic antidepressants, carbamazepine, methylphenidate, and cocaine bind at or near the carrier site on the transporter to prevent the transporter from moving NE and other agents into or out of the neuron. These inhibitors are not transported into the neuron by this mechanism; lipophilic agents diffuse into the neuron. Various drugs used for their antimuscarinic effects also block NE uptake noncompetitively. These include benztropine, diphenhydramine, trihexyphenidyl, and orphenadrine.[82]

The second mechanism, competitive inhibition of uptake, characterizes most indirect-acting agents, including amphetamines and structurally similar compounds (eg, mixed-acting agents, MAOIs). These agents prevent NE uptake by competing with synaptic NE for binding to the carrier site on the membrane transporter, the mechanism by which these agents move into the neuron. In fact, an additional adrenergic action of amphetamines, mixed-acting agents, MAOIs, and tyramine is to raise synaptic NE concentrations by competing with NE for uptake, thereby compounding their indirect and/or direct actions.

MAO Inhibitors. MAO inhibitors are transported by the NE transporter into the neuron, where they have several actions.[78] Inhibition of MAO, their main pharmacologic effect, results in increased cytoplasmic concentrations of NE and some indirect release of neurotransmitter into the synapse. As a more minor effect they also may displace NE from vesicles by raising pH in a manner similar to amphetamines. These actions explain the initial hyperadrenergic findings following MAOI overdose and probably also account for occasional and unpredictable adrenergic crises in patients taking these agents, despite the patients' compliance with diet.

Nonspecific MAOIs inhibit both isozymes of MAO, preventing intestinal and hepatic degradation of bioactive amines as well. A person taking such an MAOI who then ingests food or receives drugs containing indirect-acting sympathomimetics (eg, tyramine, phenylpropanolamine, DA, amphetamines) has a much larger cytoplasmic concentration of NE to transport into the synapse and may therefore develop central and peripheral hyperadrenergic findings. While MAO inhibitors specific for the MAO-B isozyme may be less likely to predispose to food or drug interactions by maintaining significant hepatic MAO activity, any isoenzyme specificity is lost as the dose of the MAOI is increased. In fact, selegiline, currently marketed as a selective MAO-B inhibitor, partially inhibits MAO-A activity at therapeutic doses. Specificity may lack importance when indirect-acting agents are administered systemically (eg, intravenous dopamine or amphetamines). Several amphetamine metabolites are capable of inhibiting MAO, contributing to their sympathomimetic activity.

Occasionally patients suffering from refractory depression respond to a combination of MAOIs and tricyclic antidepressants. This combination therapy is usually unaccompanied by excessive adrenergic activity because the inhibition of the membrane uptake transporter by the tricyclic antidepressant prevents excessive reverse transport of elevated cytoplasmic NE concentrations produced by MAOIs. In animals, tricyclic antidepressants that prevent NE uptake or cocaine, also an NE uptake inhibitor, protect against drug and food interactions with MAOIs by inhibiting the uptake transporter, thus inhibiting reverse transport. Nevertheless, some patients suffer severe toxicity and death when MAOIs and tricyclic antidepressants are combined.

Alpha$_2$–adrenergic Antagonists. Yohimbine blocks α_2–adrenergic receptors to produce a mixed clinical picture. Peripheral postsynaptic α_2 blockade produces vasodilation. Blockade of presynaptic α_2–adrenergic receptors on cholinergic nerve endings (Fig. 10–4) enhances ACh release, occasionally producing bronchospasm[67] and contributing to diaphoresis. Similar presynaptic actions on peripheral noradrenergic nerves enhance catecholamine release (Fig. 10–5). Blockade of central α_2–adrenergic receptors in the locus ceruleus results in CNS stimulation, while blockade of postsynaptic α_2–adrenergic receptors in the nucleus tractus solitarius may enhance sympathetic output (Fig. 10–6). The final result includes hypertension, tachycardia, agitation, mania, mydriasis, diaphoresis, and bronchospasm.[70] Yohimbine does not block imidazoline receptors (see discussion of imidazoline receptors below).

Sympatholytics

Direct Antagonists. Direct α and β–adrenergic receptor antagonists are noted in Table 10–5. In overdose, and sometimes at therapeutic doses, any β–adrenergic receptor selectivity becomes insignificant. Some β–adrenergic antagonists also are partial agonists.

Drugs that Prevent NE Release. Drugs that prevent the release of NE, despite membrane depolarization, include guanethidine and bretylium. Both drugs initially cause release of NE and can produce transient sympathomimetic effects. Drugs that block the vesicle uptake transporter prevent the movement of NE into vesicles and deplete the nerve ending of this neurotransmitter, also preventing NE release after depolarization. Examples include rauwolfia alkaloids (reserpine), tetrabenazine, and guanethidine (in part). Like guanethidine, reserpine causes transient NE release with initial dosing or early in overdose. Beta-adrenergic antagonists block presynaptic β_2–adrenergic receptors to limit catecholamine release from nerve endings, although this does not appear to be their main mechanism of action.

Imidazoline and Alpha$_2$–adrenergic Agonists. Numerous imidazoline derivatives (eg, clonidine) and structurally similar compounds have been used as centrally acting antihypertensive agents or long-acting topical vasoconstrictors. Historically, their hypotensive actions were attributed entirely to α_2–adrenergic agonism since stimulation of postsynaptic α_2–adrenergic receptors in the nucleus tractus solitarius (NTS) of the brainstem decreases sympathetic output (Fig. 10–6). Recent studies demonstrate, however, that despite high affinity of clonidine and similar drugs for α_2-adrenergic receptors, their antihypertensive actions are also dependent on activation of specific imidazoline receptors (also known as imidazole receptors) in the rostral ventrolateral medulla (VLM) that are distinct from α-adrenergic receptors.[35,106]

Imidazoline receptors have been subdivided into I_1 and I_2 (with subtypes) and are found in peripheral tissues (eg, kidney) as well as in the brain. Catecholamines such as norepinephrine do not bind to imidazoline receptors, and the naturally occurring ligand(s) for these receptors has yet to be elucidated. The molecular consequences of receptor activation also remain unclarified. However, recent data indicate that mitochondrial MAO may serve as one of the I_2 receptors.[88]

Most agents that bind to imidazoline receptors also have significant affinity for α_2–adrenergic receptors (Table 10–5).[35,40,51] Researchers have generally concluded that sedation, coma, and respiratory depression seen after ingestion of many clonidine-like drugs result from activation of α_2–adrenergic receptors in the locus ceruleus. Hypotension and bradycardia result from activation of I_1 receptors in the VLM and agonism of postsynaptic α_2–adrenergic receptors in the NTS.[130] Depending on relative affinities for I_1 and α_2–adrenergic receptors, pharmacologic explanations for sympatholytic activity of various drugs vary. For example, α-methylnorepinephrine (the metabolite of α-methyldopa) activates α_2–adrenergic receptors, but does not bind to imidazoline receptors; central sympatholytic effects result from postsynaptic α_2 adrenergic agonism in the NTS. Rilmenidine has much greater affinity for I_1 than α_2–adrenergic receptors. Most of its sympatholytic effect results from imidazoline receptor agonism in the VLM and it is not as sedating as clonidine. Undoubtedly, many agents such as clonidine produce sympatholytic activity through activation of both central I_1 and α_2–adrenergic receptors.

Ingestion of agents that activate α_2 and imidazoline receptors (eg, clonidine) produces a mixed picture. Peripheral postsynaptic α_2 stimulation produces vasoconstriction, pallor, and hypertension, often with reflex bradycardia (Fig. 10–5). Impaired ACh release from cholinergic nerve endings (Fig. 10–4) produces dry mouth, even with therapeutic doses. Peripheral presynaptic α_2 stimulation prevents NE release (Fig. 10–5), while central α_2 stimulation in the locus ceruleus accounts for CNS and respiratory depression (Fig. 10–6). Stimulation of postsynaptic α_2–adrenergic receptors in the NTS and/or stimulation of central I_1 receptors in the VLM is thought to inhibit sympathetic output and enhance parasympathetic tone, explaining hypotension with bradycardia (Fig. 10–6).

Dopamine-β-Hydroxylase Inhibition. Inhibition of dopamine-β-hydroxylase (Fig. 10–5) prevents the conversion of DA to NE, resulting in less NE release and less α and β stimulation with neuronal firing. Disulfiram produces such inhibition.[39] Because most of dopamine's ability to cause vasoconstriction is mediated by NE release, NE may be the vasopressor of choice in a hypotensive patient taking disulfiram. Diethyldithiocarbamate, used in metal chelation and in some AIDS patients, is a disulfiram metabolite that has a similar action. MAOIs and α-methyldopa also inhibit dopamine-β-hydroxylase, although this is not their main mechanism of action.[78]

Dopamine is relatively contraindicated in hypotensive patients who have overdosed on MAOIs. First, DA acts indirectly and its administration may produce an adrenergic storm. Second, even if an adrenergic storm does not occur, most of dopamine's α-mediated vasoconstriction is secondary to NE release. In the presence of MAOIs, NE synthesis may be impaired from concomitant dopamine-β-hydroxylase inhibition, and DA may not reliably raise blood pressure if cytoplasmic and vesicular stores have been depleted. In the presence of impaired NE release or α blockade by any cause, unopposed DA-induced vasodilation from action on peripheral DA and β receptors may paradoxically lower blood pressure further. Norepinephrine and EPI can be used to support blood pressure relatively safely in patients taking MAOIs, since these vasopressors have little or no direct action and are metabolized by COMT when given intravenously.

Dopamine

Because dopamine is the direct precursor for NE, noradrenergic vesicles contain DA. The release of NE from peripheral sympathetic nerves therefore always results in release of some DA (Fig. 10–5), as does the release of NE and EPI from the adrenal gland, explaining the normal presence of DA in systemic blood. In peripheral tissues, DA receptors cause vasodilation of mesenteric, renal, and coronary vascular beds. Dopamine can also stimulate β-adrenergic receptors and, at high doses, directly stimulate α-adrenergic receptors. When DA is administered intravenously, most vasoconstriction is due to DA-induced NE release.

Dopamine accounts for about one-half of all catecholamines in the brain and is present in greater quantities than NE or 5-HT. In contrast to the diffuse projection of noradrenergic neurons, dopaminergic neurons and re-

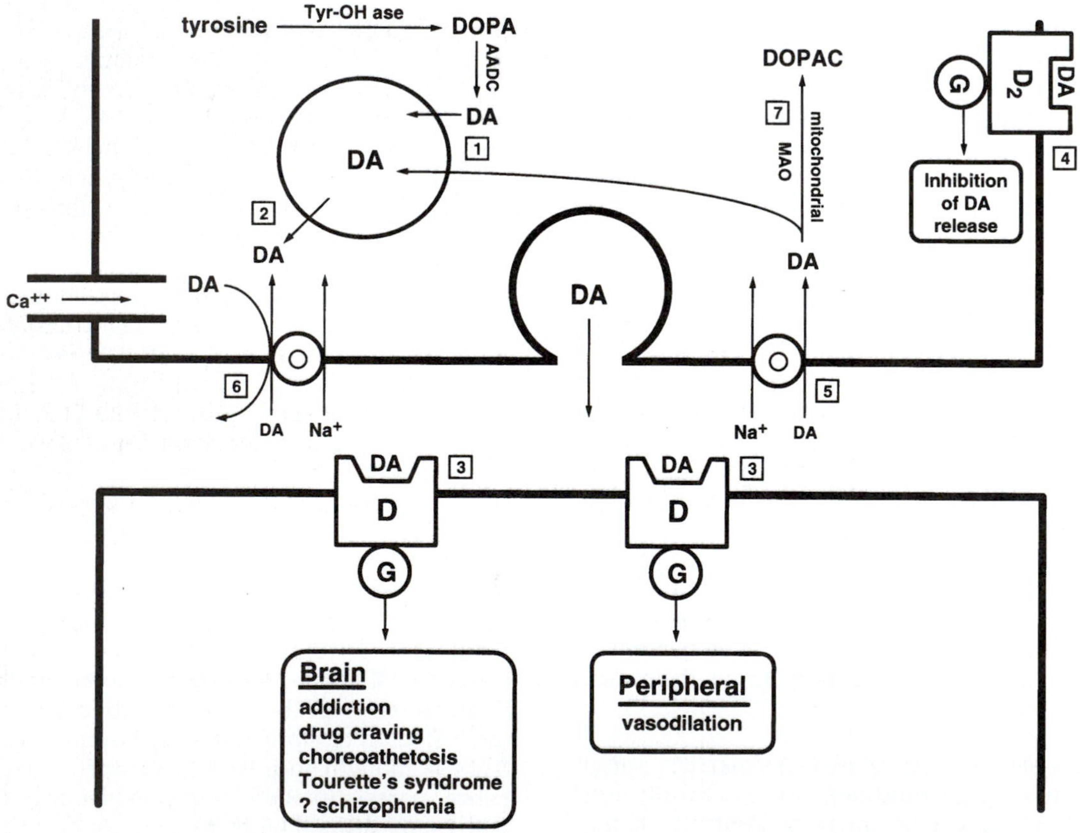

Figure 10–7. A dopaminergic nerve ending and postsynaptic membrane. DA released from nerve endings binds to various postsynaptic DA receptors (D) on neurons or peripheral end organs. Stimulation of presynaptic D_2 receptors [4] prevents further DA release. Agents in Table 10–6 may act to inhibit vesicle uptake [1]; cause DA to leave the vesicle and move into the cytoplasm [2]; stimulate or block dopamine receptors [3,4]; inhibit DA uptake [5]; cause reverse transport of cytoplasmic DA into the synapse by raising cytoplasmic DA concentrations (indirect action) [6]; or prevent DA degradation by inhibiting MAO [7]. Tyr-OHase = tyrosine hydroxylase; AADC = l-aromatic amino acid decarboxylase; MAO = monoamine oxidase; DOPAC = 3,4-dihydroxyphenylacetic acid; DA = dopamine; G = G protein.

ceptors are highly organized and concentrated in several areas, especially in the basal ganglia and limbic system.[62]

Excessive dopaminergic activity in the striatum and/or other areas from any cause (eg, increased release, impaired uptake, increased receptor sensitivity) may produce acute choreoathetosis[64] and acute Gilles de la Tourette syndrome, with tics, spitting, and cursing. Excessive dopaminergic activity in the limbic system and, perhaps, other areas produces paranoid psychosis indistinguishable from paranoid schizophrenia and is thought responsible for much of the drug craving and addictive behavior in patients abusing sympathomimetic drugs. Diminished dopaminergic tone (eg, impaired release, receptor blockade) in the basal ganglia produces various extrapyramidal disorders such as acute dystonias and parkinsonism.

TABLE 10–6. AGENTS AFFECTING DOPAMINERGIC NEUROTRANSMISSION*

Dopamine Agonism

Direct stimulation of dopamine receptors
- Apomorphine
- Bromocriptine
- L-Dopa[a]
- Lisuride
- Pergolide

Inhibit dopamine metabolism (MAOIs)
- Clorgyline
- Isocarboxazid
- Moclobemide
- Pargyline
- Phenelzine
- Selegiline
- Tranylcypromine

Indirectly acting
- Amantadine
- Amphetamines
- Benztropine
- Decongestants
- Diphenhydramine
- MAOIs
- Methylphenidate
- Orphenadrine
- Pemoline
- Phencyclidine
- Trihexyphenidyl

Inhibit dopamine uptake
- Amantadine
- Amphetamines
- Benztropine
- Bupropion
- Cocaine
- Diphenhydramine
- Methylphenidate
- Orphenadrine
- Pemoline
- Trihexyphenidyl

Increase dopamine receptor sensitivity
- Amphetamines
- Metoclopramide
- Neuroleptics
- Phenytoin

Dopamine Antagonism

Block dopamine receptors
- Amoxapine
- Clozapine
- Droperidol
- Haloperidol
- Loxapine
- Maprotiline[b]
- Metoclopramide
- Molindone
- Phenothiazines
- Pimozide
- Risperidone
- Thioxanthenes
- Trazodone[b]
- Tricyclic antidepressants[b]

Destroy dopaminergic neurons
- MPTP

Prevent vesicle dopamine uptake
- Reserpine
- Tetrabenazine

*Direct agonists and antagonists bind to dopamine receptors to mimic or block the effects of dopamine, respectively.

MAOIs = monoamine oxidase inhibitors; MPTP = 1-methyl-4-phenyl-1,2,3,6-tetrahydropyridine.

[a]Metabolized to dopamine, which acts as agonist.

[b]Relatively weak D_2 receptor antagonists.

Synthesis, Release, and Uptake

The steps of DA synthesis and vesicle storage are the same as those for NE, except that DA is not converted to NE after transport into vesicles (Fig. 10–7). Dopamine is removed from the synapse via uptake by a neuronal membrane DA transporter. Like the NE transporter, this pump is not completely specific for DA, but transports drugs such as amphetamines and other structurally similar sympathomimetics.

Cytoplasmic DA has a fate similar to NE. It is pumped back into vesicles or degraded by MAO. Catechol-*O*-methyltransferase degrades DA that has entered the systemic circulation.

Dopamine Receptors

All DA receptors are linked to G proteins and are divided into two main groups, depending on whether they raise or lower cAMP concentrations.[109,116] Dopamine$_1$-like receptors (D_1 and D_5) are linked to G_s and raise cAMP concentrations. Numerous variants of each receptor type (eg, $D_{5pseudo-1}$, $D_{5pseudo-2}$) exist. Dopamine is 10 times more potent at D_5 as compared to D_1 receptors.

D_2-like receptors (D_2, D_3, D_4) are linked to G_i, G_0, and perhaps other G proteins that have several actions, including inhibition of adenyl cyclase and lowering of cAMP levels.[62] Again, numerous subtypes of receptors exist (eg, D_{2s}, D_{2L}, D_{2Ala96}, $D_{4.1}$ through $D_{4.9}$).[109] D_2 receptors are especially prevalent in the basal ganglia and limbic system, while D_3 and D_4 receptors are concentrated in the limbic system and cerebral cortex. Schizophrenia is associated with elevated densities of D_2-like receptors, particularly D_4. Some D_2 receptors also are found on presynaptic membranes, where they mediate inhibition of further neurotransmitter release, including the peripheral release of NE (Figs. 10–5 and 10–7).

Chemical Agents (Table 10–6)

Dopamine Agonism

Indirect and Mixed-acting Agents. Most indirect- and mixed-acting sympathomimetics cause DA release. The mechanism of action is similar to NE, except that DA transporters are involved. Benztropine, diphenhydramine, trihexyphenidyl, and orphenadrine cause DA release, perhaps contributing to their abuse potential noted below.[82] Excessive dopaminergic activity following therapeutic doses or overdoses of decongestants (eg, pseudoephedrine), amphetamines, methylphenidate, and pemoline can produce acute choreoathetosis and Tourette syndrome.[16,71] Parkinsonian patients ingesting excessive doses of L-dopa (which is converted to DA) may present with similar symptoms.

Direct Agonists. Bromocriptine is an ergot derivative that is a direct DA receptor agonist. Toxic effects include those described above for indirect-acting agents. Apomorphine directly activates D_2 receptors. Such action at the chemoreceptive triggering zone produces vomiting, while agonism in the basal ganglia explains the former's use in the treatment of Parkinson's disease.

Uptake Inhibition. Agents that inhibit DA uptake include cocaine, amphetamines, methylphenidate, and probably amantadine. Increased dopaminergic activity from cocaine intoxication may produce choreoathetosis ("crack dancing") and Tourette syndrome. In general, antidepressants are not strong dopamine uptake blockers. However, bupropion appears to be more active in this regard.[105]

As noted above, much of the drug craving and addiction produced by sympathomimetics probably results from excessive dopaminergic activity. Interestingly, the anticholinergic drugs, benztropine, diphenhydramine, trihexyphenidyl, and orphenadrine are also DA uptake inhibitors, possibly explaining their abuse.[82,115] In fact, benztropine is one of the most potent DA uptake inhibitors known. Amantadine, an antiparkinsonian agent that causes DA release and some inhibition of DA uptake (as well as being anticholinergic) is also abused.

Increase of Receptor Sensitivity. Several drugs are thought to increase sensitivity of DA receptors, resulting in choreoathetosis, even with therapeutic doses (eg, phenytoin). Evidence exists that increased DA receptor sensitivity may be responsible for movement disorders resulting from amphetamines.[27] Tardive dyskinesia (discussed below) may also result from increased dopamine receptor sensitivity.

MAO Inhibition. Monoamine oxidase inhibitors inhibit the breakdown of cytoplasmic DA. Part of food and drug interactions with MAOIs results from excessive release of DA from nerve endings.

Dopamine Antagonism

Direct Receptor Blockade. Blockade of DA receptors is the specific aim when using many therapeutic agents. The neuroleptic action of butyrophenones, phenothiazines, and other antipsychotics mainly correlate with their ability to block D_2 receptors, probably in the limbic system. Many phenothiazines block both D_1 and D_2 receptors, while haloperidol mainly blocks D_2 receptors. Unfortunately, neuroleptics and metoclopramide also block DA receptors in the striatum, producing various extrapyramidal symptoms, including acute parkinsonism and dystonias. Clozapine, a neuroleptic agent that usually does not produce extrapyramidal effects, demonstrates low affinity for D_2 receptors (such as those in the basal ganglia) but blocks limbic D_3 and D_4 receptors. Risperidone antagonizes D_2, D_3, and D_4 receptors with equal affinity.[56] Buspirone, an antianxiety agent, antagonizes D_2 receptors, explaining occasional extrapyramidal reactions. Various tricyclic antidepressants, especially amoxapine, block D_2 receptors to some extent.

The chronic use of DA blocking agents causes upregulation of DA receptors. The continued use or, especially, withdrawal of DA antagonists (neuroleptics, metoclopramide, occasionally antidepressants) may result in excessive dopaminergic activity and tardive dyskinesia that are characterized by choreiform movements typical of excessive dopaminergic influence in the striatum.

The blockade of DA receptors by numerous agents, including butyrophenones, phenothiazines, and metoclopramide can produce a poorly understood disorder called neuroleptic malignant syndrome. Neuroleptic malignant syndrome also follows acute withdrawal of DA agonists (eg, stopping L-dopa or bromocriptine in a patient prior to surgery). Neuroleptic malignant syndrome is characterized, in part, by mental status changes, autonomic instability, rigidity, and hyperthermia.

Indirect Antagonism. Reserpine and tetrabenazine prevent transport of DA into storage vesicles and deplete nerve endings of DA. 1-Methyl-4-phenyl-1,2,3,6-tetrahydropyridine (MPTP), a meperidine analog, undergoes activation by MAO to a metabolite that causes neuronal death. That MPTP causes isolated destruction of dopaminergic neurons is explained by its selective transport by the membrane DA transporter. Both MAOIs and inhibitors of DA transporters prevent MPTP-induced destruction of dopaminergic neurons.

Serotonin

Serotonin (5-HT, 5-OH-tryptamine) is a ubiquitous indole alkylamine found in nature (animals, plants, venoms) that acts as a neurotransmitter centrally, but is also found peripherally. In fact, less than 2% of the body's 5-HT is found within the CNS. Serotonergic neurons lie in or in juxtaposition to numerous midline nuclei in the brainstem (nine raphe nuclei), from which they project to various parts of the brain, including the basal ganglia.[81] Serotonin is involved with mood, personality, affect, appetite, motor function, temperature regulation, sexual activity, pain perception, sleep induction, and other basic functions. Serotonin is not essential for any of these processes but modulates their quality and extent. The serotonergic system is extremely diverse, with over 14 types of receptors that act to stimulate or inhibit neurons, including those of other neurotransmitter systems.[107] Serotonin is also the precursor for the pineal hormone melatonin.

Peripherally, 5-HT is produced mainly in the enterochromaffin cells of the intestine. Local release may contribute to peristalsis, but the co-release of numerous other mediators makes its exact action difficult to discern. Platelets take up 5-HT while passing through the enteric circulation. Serotonin is released from activated platelets to interact with other platelet membranes (promotes aggregation) and with vascular smooth muscle (vasoconstriction in most vascular beds). Experimentally, 5-HT has diverse effects on the cardiovascular and peripheral nervous system, although the importance of these actions is uncertain in the normal physiologic state. Serotonin produces vasoconstriction (stimulation of

5-HT_2 receptors) in all vascular beds except for coronary arteries and skeletal muscle, where it produces vasodilation in the presence of intact endothelium.

Centrally, it is particularly difficult to ascribe a specific symptom or physical finding to serotonergic neurons because of the diversity of their physiologic actions. However, serotonin definitely is important in the action of many hallucinogenic drugs.

Synthesis, Release, and Uptake

Figure 10–8 illustrates 5-HT synthesis. Tryptophan-5-hydroxylase is the rate-limiting enzyme of 5-HT synthesis. L-Amino acid decarboxylase (dopa decarboxylase) converts 5-hydroxytryptophan to 5-HT. Cytoplasmic 5-HT is transported into vesicles, where it is concentrated by ion trapping before release by Ca^{2+}-dependent exocytosis. After release into the synapse, a transporter in the neuronal membrane transfers 5-HT back into the neuron, where it reenters vesicles or is degraded by MAO.[104]

Serotonergic Receptors

Serotonin receptor classification is controversial and changing.[52] Most authors identify four major types of functioning receptors (5-HT_1 through 5-HT_4) and numerous subtypes. Additional 5-HT receptors (5-HT_{51E}, 5-HT_{1F}, 5-HT_{2B}, $5HT_5$, $5HT_6$, and $5HT_7$) have been cloned, but their role in normal human neurotransmission remains unclear.[107]

5-HT_1 Receptors. Receptors in the 5-HT_1 class are coupled to G proteins and commonly increase K^+ efflux and decrease cAMP concentrations. 5-HT_1 receptors comprise several subtypes. 5-HT_{1A} receptors reside predominantly on raphe nuclei, where they act as somatodendritic au-

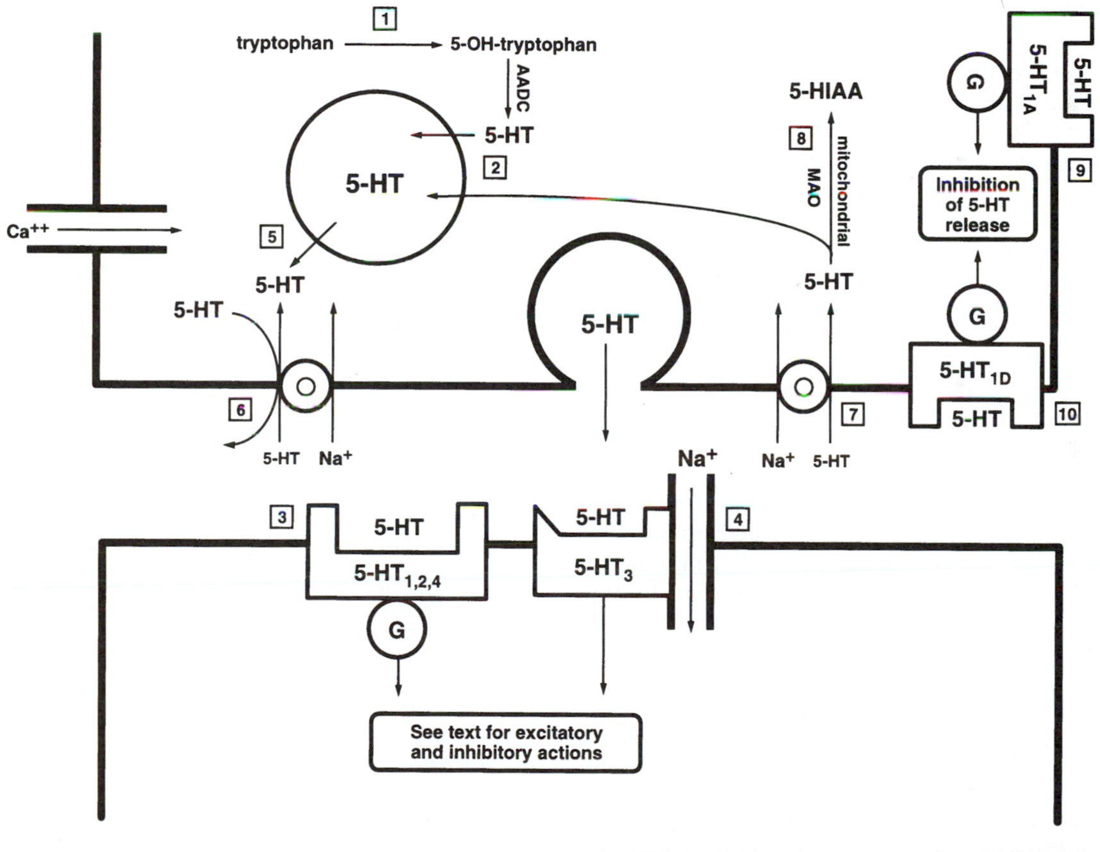

Figure 10–8. A serotonergic nerve ending and postsynaptic membrane. Tryptophan hydroxylase converts tryptophan to 5-OH-trytophan [1]. In mitochondria, 5-HT is degraded by MAO to an intermediate compound, which is converted to 5-OH-indoleacetic acid (5-HIAA) [8]. Most if not all 5-HT receptors are found in both the CNS and periphery. 5-HT_1, 5-HT_2, and 5-HT_4 receptors are coupled to G proteins. 5-HT_3 receptors are ligand-gated Na^+ channels. In addition to being found on the postsynaptic membrane, 5-HT_{1A} and 5-HT_{1D} receptors serve as presynaptic autoreceptors that, when stimulated, decrease further release of 5-HT [9, 10]. Presynaptic 5-HT_{1A} receptors serve as somatodendritic autoreceptors, whereas presynaptic 5-HT_{1D} receptors act as terminal autoreceptors. Agents in Table 10–7 act to prevent vesicle uptake of 5-HT [2]; stimulate or block 5-HT receptors [3,4,9,10]; cause 5-HT to move from the vesicle into the cytoplasm [5]; cause reverse transport of 5-HT from the cytoplasm into the synapse by raising cytoplasmic 5-HT concentrations [6]; inhibit 5-HT uptake [7]; or prevent 5-HT degradation by inhibiting MAO [8]. 5-HT = 5-OH-tryptamine (serotonin); MAO = monoamine oxidase; 5-HIAA = 5-OH-indoleacetic acid; AADC = l-amino acid decarboxylase; G = G protein.

toreceptors.[104] Some 5-HT$_{1A}$ receptors are located postsynaptically, where they also inhibit through similar mechanisms.

Central 5-HT$_{1D}$ receptors act as inhibitory terminal autoreceptors. Cranial blood vessels possess 5-HT$_{1D}$ receptors that produce vasoconstriction and decrease inflammation when activated. The 5-HT$_{1B}$ subclass is found predominantly in rodents and is functionally equivalent to the human 5-HT$_{1D}$ receptor, differing by only one amino acid.[36]

5-HT$_2$ Receptors. The three subtypes of 5-HT$_2$ receptors are coupled to G proteins thus serving to decrease K^+ efflux and/or increase intracellular Ca^{2+} concentration by raising concentrations of inositol triphosphate and diacylglycerol.[104] 5-HT$_{2A}$ receptors are most concentrated in the cerebral cortex, where they serve as excitatory postsynaptic receptors. They also reside on platelets, where their activation leads to platelet aggregation. 5-HT$_{2C}$ receptors (previously 5-HT$_{1C}$) reside on the choroid plexus, where they regulate cerebral spinal fluid production. While 5-HT$_{2B}$ receptors have been identified, their role remains ill-defined.

5-HT$_3$ Receptors. Like the ACh nicotinic receptor, 5-HT$_3$ receptors are ligand-gated Na^+ channels.[4] Upon activation, they stimulate the neuron by opening the channel to cause depolarization through Na^+ influx. Centrally, they are found diffusely, but are especially concentrated in the chemoreceptive triggering zone, where their activation induces emesis. In the cerebral cortex, their activation leads to increased release of dopamine and decreased release of ACh. In contrast to cerebral actions, activation of peripheral 5-HT$_3$ receptors on cholinergic nerves in the gut enhance ACh release to increase gastrointestinal motility.

5-HT$_4$ Receptors. These receptors are coupled to G proteins (G_s). Their activation leads to increased cAMP concentrations. 5-HT$_4$ receptors are scattered diffusely throughout the brain, and their exact role remains undefined. Peripheral 5-HT$_4$ receptors reside in the heart and intestines, where they serve to produce tachycardia and contraction of gut smooth muscle, respectively.

Chemical Agents (Table 10–7)

Serotonin Agonists. The ingestion of tryptophan is thought to increase 5-HT production and was commonly used as an unproved sleep aid until removal from the market because of associated eosinophilia myalgia syndrome. The antianxiety agents buspirone, gepirone, and ipsapirone act as partial agonists at somatodendritic and postsynaptic 5-HT$_{1A}$ receptors.[107] Sumatriptan, an antimigraine agent, mainly agonizes 5-HT$_{1D}$ receptors, but crosses the blood–brain barrier poorly, if at all.[107]

Metoclopramide and cisapride, prokinetic drugs, activate 5-HT$_4$ receptors to increase gut motility.[131] Activation of 5-HT$_4$ receptors on the heart explains tachycardia sometimes seen at therapeutic doses. Perhaps cisapride's ability to lessen K^+ efflux (through G proteins) also accounts for occasional reports of torsades de pointes.

TABLE 10–7. AGENTS AFFECTING SEROTONERGIC NEUROTRANSMISSION*

Serotonin Agonism
Enhance 5-HT synthesis
L-Tryptophan
Direct 5-HT agonists
Buspirone
Cisapride
Ergots and indoles (LSD, etc)[a]
Gepirone
Ipsapirone
mCPP
Metoclopramide
Phenylalkylamines (eg, mescaline)[a]
Sulpride
Sumatriptan
Urapidil
Increase 5-HT release
Amphetamines
Cocaine
Codeine derivatives
Dexfenfluramine
Dextromethorphan
Fenfluramine
MDMA
Reserpine (initial)
Nonspecific 5-HT agonists
Lithium
Inhibit 5-HT breakdown (MAOIs)
Clorgyline
Isocarboxazid
Moclobemide
Pargyline
Phenelzine
Tranylcypromine
Selegiline
Inhibit 5-HT uptake
Amitriptyline
Amphetamines
Cocaine
Desipramine
Dextromethorphan
Doxepin
Fluoxetine
Fluvoxamine
Imipramine
Meperidine
Nefazodone
Nortriptyline
Sertraline
Tramadol
Trazodone
Venlafaxine
Serotonin Antagonism
Direct 5-HT antagonists
Chlorpromazine
Clozapine
Cyproheptadine
Ergots and indoles (eg, LSD)[a]
Granesitron
Haloperidol
Ketanserin
Mainserin
Methysergide
Metoclopramide
Mirtazapine
Nefazodone
Ondansetron
Phenothiazines
Phentolamine
Phenylalkylamines (eg, mescaline)[a]
Pindolol
Propranolol
Risperidone
Ritanserin
Trazodone
Tricyclic antidepressants
Tropisetron
Inhibit vesicle uptake
Reserpine
Tetrabenazine

*Direct agonists and antagonists bind at 5-HT receptors to mimic or inhibit the action of 5-HT, respectively. The mechanism by which lithium enhances serotonergic tone remains unclear.

5-HT = serotonin; mCPP = *m*-chlorphenylpiperazine (metabolite of trazodone and nefazodone); LSD = lysergic acid diethylamide; MAOIs = monoamine oxidase inhibitors; MDMA = methylenedioxymethamphetamine.

[a]Hallucinogenic indoles and phenylalkylamines antagonize and stimulate various 5-HT receptors. Their hallucinatory action mainly results from partial agonism at 5-HT$_2$ receptors.

Numerous indoles and phenylalkylamines, including ergot alkaloids, LSD, psilocybin, and mescaline, exhibit both agonistic and antagonistic effects at multiple 5-HT receptors. Their hallucinogenic action is best explained by partial agonism at 5-HT$_{2A}$ receptors. Some substituted amphetamines (eg, methylenedioxymethamphetamine) may directly stimulate serotonin receptors.

Cocaine and indirect-acting sympathomimetics, especially amphetamines, cause serotonin release as previously described. Other releasing agents are dextromethorphan and codeine derivatives. Centrally, dopamine undergoes uptake into serotonergic neurons to displace 5-HT from the neuron. Ingestion of L-dopa or other agents that increase CNS dopamine concentrations can cause 5-HT release.[81]

Inhibitors of 5-HT uptake include amphetamines, cocaine, various antidepressants, meperidine, and dextromethorphan. Several antidepressants are specific for inhibiting 5-HT uptake. Examples of selective serotonin reuptake inhibitors (SSRIs) include fluoxetine, sertraline, paroxetine, and fluvoxamine. The use of SSRIs sometimes produces extrapyramidal side effects[5] for reasons that remain unclear because of 5-HT numerous actions in the basal ganglia: prevention of the release of DA, glutamate, and ACh. Again, reserpine and tetrabenazine prevent 5-HT uptake into vesicles.

Monoamine oxidase-A accounts for most 5-HT degradation, and nonspecific MAOIs and MAO-A inhibitors (clorgyline, moclobemide) both raise 5-HT levels and, through indirect action, probably cause 5-HT release.[11]

Serotonin Antagonists. Trazodone and nefazodone act mainly as antagonists at 5-HT_2 receptors, but are also weak uptake inhibitors. Both undergo metabolism to *m*-chlorophenylpiperazine (mCPP), which activates most 5-HT receptors but is especially active at 5-HT_{2C} receptors.[131] Methysergide and cyproheptadine are antagonists at 5-HT_1 and 5-HT_2 receptors.

Most neuroleptics and tricyclic antidepressants antagonize 5-HT_{2A} and, to a lesser extent, 5-HT_{2C} receptors.[104] In fact, investigators are interested in developing antipsychotic agents similar to risperidone that possess potent antagonistic properties at 5-HT_2 receptors without potent dopamine receptor blockade, to limit extrapyramidal side effects.

Ondansetron and granisetron antagonize 5-HT_3 receptors.[42] Their antiemetic action is thought to be explained by several mechanisms. Central antagonism at the chemoreceptor triggering zone lessens vomiting. Peripheral antagonism in the gut prevents ACh release, decreasing gut motility. Finally, antagonism of 5-HT_3 receptors on the vagus nerve decrease vagal stimulation of the vomiting center in the brainstem. Ondansetron and other experimental 5-HT_3 antagonists are being studied in the treatment of schizophrenia because of their ability to prevent dopamine release.

Serotonin Syndrome. Excessive stimulation of 5-HT_{1A} receptors and, to a lesser extent, 5-HT_2 receptors causes serotonin syndrome.[48,119] Briefly, this disorder is characterized by shivering, myoclonus, tremor, and rigidity (especially of legs), along with hyperthermia, tachycardia, diaphoresis, confusion, agitation, convulsions, and coma.[81] This iatrogenic, idiosyncratic syndrome results most commonly from the combined use of two serotonergic drugs (eg, SSRI and lithium, SSRI and MAOI, MAOI and clomipramine). Recent reports indicate that serotonin syndrome may occur following the isolated use or overdose of a single serotonergic agent (eg, venlafaxine or fluvoxamine). Drugs that act to increase CNS DA concentrations, such as levodopa and bromocriptine, have potential to precipitate serotonin syndrome by indirect serotonin release.[81] Sumatriptan is unlikely to produce serotonin syndrome because it is several times less effective at agonizing 5-HT_{1A} than 5-HT_{1D} receptors and penetrates the blood–brain barrier poorly.[94]

Adverse effects (eg, rigidity, hyperthermia) resulting from interactions between MAOIs and meperidine, dextromethorphan, or codeine derivatives may result from excessive serotonergic activity, since all of these agents have agonistic actions on serotonergic neurotransmission (Table 10–7).[7,17,61]

Gamma-Aminobutyric Acid

Gamma-aminobutyric acid (GABA) is one of two main inhibitory neurotransmitters of the central nervous system (glycine is discussed separately, below). Drugs that enhance GABA activity are generally used as anticonvulsants, sedative-hypnotics, and general anesthetics. Agents that antagonize GABA activity typically have the opposite effect, producing CNS excitation and convulsions. GABA is synthesized from glutamate, the brain's main inhibitory neurotransmitter.

In general, GABA inhibition predominates in the brain. In the spinal cord, through mono- and polysynaptic reflex pathways, GABA mediates a number of physiologically minor peripheral effects outside the CNS (eg, vasodilation, bladder relaxation).[15] Spinal cord GABA is important in attenuating skeletal muscle reflex arcs.

Synthesis, Release, and Uptake

GABA synthesis is illustrated in Figure 10–9. Glutamic acid decarboxylase (GAD) requires pyridoxal phosphate (PLP) as a cofactor. Pyridoxal phosphate is synthesized from pyridoxine (vitamin B_6) by the enzyme pyridoxine kinase (PK).[80]

GABA is transported into vesicles and later released through Ca^{2+}-dependent exocytosis into the synapse. Uptake of GABA from the synapse is mediated by a Na^+-dependent transporter. Evidence also suggests that GABA is released into the synapse from cytoplasm by reverse transport under some conditions. Cytoplasmic GABA can be transported back into vesicles or degraded by GABA-transaminase (GABA-T) to succinate semialdehyde (SSA), part of which then undergoes oxidation to succinate. GABA-T also requires PLP as a cofactor.[86]

GABA Receptors

There are three main types of GABA receptors[112] (Table 10–8). GABA_A receptors are Cl^- channels that mediate postsynaptic inhibition by allowing Cl^- to move into and hyperpolarize the postsynaptic neuron. Situated at various sites in relation to the GABA recognition site on the Cl^- channel are sites for exogenous and endogenous

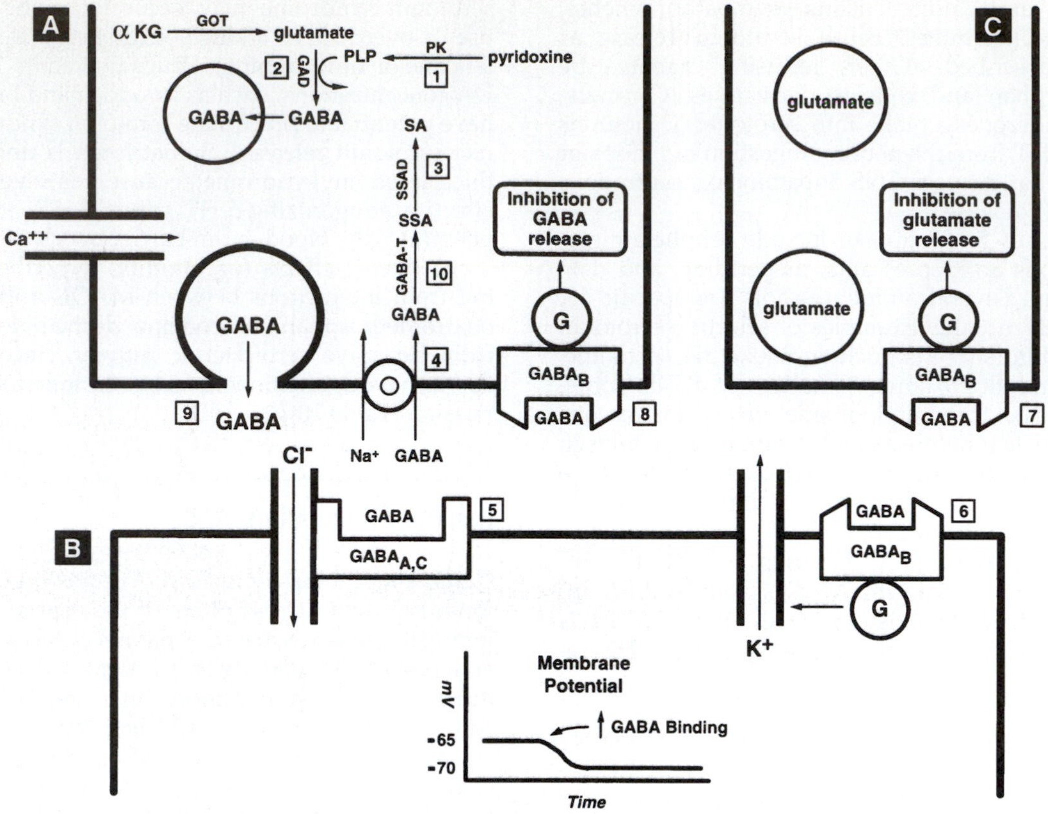

Figure 10–9. GABAergic neurotransmission. GABA released from neuron A binds to postsynaptic $GABA_A$, $GABA_B$, or $GABA_C$ receptors to hyperpolarize and inhibit neuron B [5,6] or to presynaptic $GABA_B$ receptors on neuron C [7] to inhibit neurotransmitter release by blocking Ca^{2+} influx (an excitatory glutaminergic neuron is shown as an example). Stimulation of $GABA_B$ autoreceptors on neuron A [8] also reduces further release of GABA. Acute falls in PLP lead to impaired GAD activity and low GABA concentrations. Though GABA-T also requires PLP, acute falls in PLP do not affect this enzyme significantly because of tight PLP binding to the GABA-T complex. Agents in Table 10–9 act to impair PLP formation by inhibiting PK [1]; to increase GABA concentrations by either stimulating GAD [2] or inhibiting SSAD [3]; to inhibit GABA uptake [4]; to stimulate or block GABA receptors [5–8]; to cause GABA release [9], or to inhibit GABA-T [10]. GOT, GABA-T, and SSAD are mitochondrial enzymes. GABA = γ-aminobutyric acid; α KG = α-ketoglutarate; GAD = glutamic acid decarboxylase; PLP = pyridoxal phosphate; PK = pyridoxine kinase; GABA-T = GABA-transaminase; SSA = succinate semialdehyde; SSAD = succinate semialdehyde dehydrogenase; SA = succinic acid; GOT = glutamic-oxaloacetic transaminase; G = G protein.

modulatory agents (Fig. 10–10) where numerous excitatory and depressant drugs bind and through which $GABA_A$ receptor responsiveness is regulated under normal physiologic conditions.[114,135] The common denominator for modulation at the $GABA_A$ complex is an increase or decrease in inward Cl^- current.

Throughout the CNS there is regional variation in the expression of multiple subunit genes for the $GABA_A$ complex. $GABA_A$ receptors exist as pentamers, composed of at least an α, β, and γ subunit. At least 13 distinct subunits have been identified (six α, three β, three γ, and one δ), and these combine to form various pentameric $GABA_A$ Cl^- channels with different pharmacologic affinities for certain ligands, including anesthetics, benzodiazepines, and GABA itself.[79]

The second type of GABA receptor, $GABA_B$, was fortuitously discovered when baclofen, a GABA analog now known to be a $GABA_B$-specific agonist, was surprisingly found to bind to presynaptic membranes. $GABA_B$ receptors exist as at least two subtypes[12] and are coupled to G proteins that mediate both presynaptic and postsynaptic inhibition.[83] Presynaptic inhibition is mediated by preventing Ca^{2+} influx so as to impair exocytosis of neurotransmitter vesicles, including those containing excitatory amino acids (eg, glutamate). Postsynaptic inhibition is mediated by increasing K^+ efflux through K^+ channels, resulting in hyperpolarization of the membrane away from threshold. Through presynaptic actions, $GABA_B$ re-

TABLE 10–8. GABA RECEPTORS AND THEIR CHARACTERISTICS

	$GABA_A$	$GABA_B$	$GABA_C$
Receptor	Cl^- channel	G-protein coupled	Cl^- channel
Bicuculline antagonism	Yes	No	No
Baclofen agonism	No	Yes	No
Benzodiazepine agonism	Yes	No	No
Barbiturate agonism	Yes	No	No
Picrotoxin atagonism	Yes	No	Slight

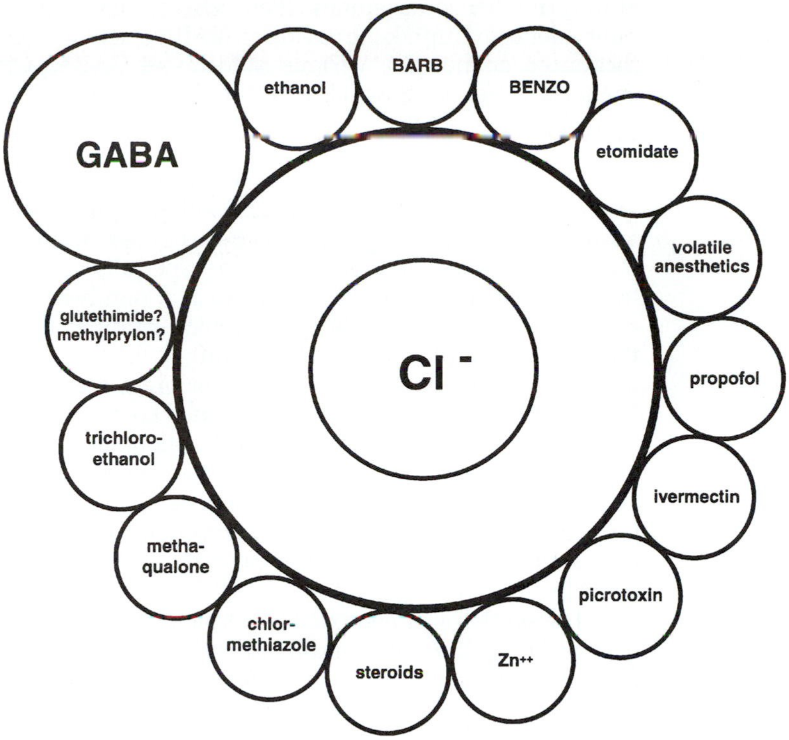

Figure 10–10. Schematic representation of the $GABA_A$ Cl^- channel receptor complex. Benzodiazepines (BENZO), barbiturates (BARB), picrotoxin, and steroids clearly bind to different sites around the channel. Although separate circles represent different binding sites for other agents, this distinction is not always apparent. For example, general anesthetics and ethanol may produce their effects by interacting with the steroid binding site. Given their structural similarity to barbiturates, it is reasonable to suspect that glutethimide and methyprylon may bind to the $GABA_A$ complex, but this has not been clarified. Chloral hydrate undergoes metabolism to trichloroethanol, which interacts with the $GABA_A$ receptor complex.

ceptors also serve as autoreceptors, where their activation in response to synaptic GABA provides feedback inhibition of further neurotransmitter release (Fig. 10–9).

Most recently a third GABA receptor, $GABA_C$, has been found in the mammalian retina and hippocampus; its function outside of the retina remains vague.[59,133,138] Like $GABA_A$, the $GABA_C$ receptor is a Cl^- channel that, when activated, allows increased Cl^- influx. Unlike $GABA_A$ receptors, $GABA_C$ receptors are insensitive to bicuculline, benzodiazepines, barbiturates, and neuroactive steroids and are less sensitive to picrotoxin (Table 10–8). $GABA_C$ receptors are activated at 40-fold lower GABA concentrations than $GABA_A$ receptors, are less liable to desensitization, and remain open longer than $GABA_A$ Cl^- channels.

Chemical Agents (Table 10–9)

Modulation of GABA Production. Isoniazid (INH) and other hydrazines (eg, monomethylhydrazine from mushrooms) lower CNS GABA concentrations by several mechanisms. Most important, they compete with pyridoxine for binding to PK, impairing PLP production.[80] Pyridoxal phosphate binding to the glutamic acid decarboxylase (GAD) complex is easily reversible.[86] The acute decrease in PLP concentration, then, is rapidly accompanied by impaired GABA synthesis and a decrease in GABA concentration. Lack of normal GABA inhibition produces seizures typical of hydrazine intoxications. While PLP is also required for GABA degradation by GABA-T, acute decreases in PLP do not affect this enzyme nearly as much, since PLP is more tightly bound to the GABA-T complex and remains associated with the enzyme.[86] To a lesser extent, INH binds to the GAD-PLP complex to prevent GABA formation.

Cyanide inhibits numerous enzymes besides cytochrome oxidase. Inhibition of GAD with a resultant fall in GABA concentration may partly explain seizures seen in cyanide poisoning. Domoic acid (see section on glutamate) may inhibit GAD.[31]

The exact mechanism of valproate's anticonvulsant action is unknown. In vitro studies demonstrate its ability to increase brain GABA concentrations either by inhibition of succinate semialdehyde dehydrogenase or by activation of GAD.[60] Vigabatrin, an anticonvulsant, acts by inhibiting GABA-T.

$GABA_A$ Agonism. The $GABA_A$ receptor complex is illustrated in Figure 10–10. In general, substances that increase $GABA_A$ complex activity cause CNS depression, ranging from mild sedation and nystagmus to ataxia, stupor, coma, and even general anesthesia. Most indirect agonists that bind to the $GABA_A$ complex have no activity in the absence of GABA. With some exceptions, their pharmacologic actions require the binding of GABA to its receptor and do not result from a direct effect on Cl^- conductance exclusive of GABA binding. Many of these drugs have additional actions that are not mediated through the $GABA_A$ complex.

Direct GABA Agonists. The main direct GABA agonist of toxicologic interest is muscimol, found in some poisonous mushrooms. Muscimol binds to the GABA receptor on the $GABA_A$ complex to mimic the action of GABA.[87] Ibotenic acid, a direct glutamate agonist found in the

TABLE 10–9. AGENTS AFFECTING GABAERGIC NEUROTRANSMISSION*

GABA Agonism	GABA Antagonism
Enhance GABA synthesis	*Direct $GABA_A$ antagonists*
Valproate	Bicuculline
Direct $GABA_A$ agonists	Cephalosporins
Muscimol	Ciprofloxacin
Progabide[a]	Enoxacin
Indirect $GABA_A$ agonists	Imipenem
Avermectin	Nalidixic acid
Barbiturates	Norfloxacin
Benzodiazepines	Ofloxacin
Chloral hydrate	Penicillin
Chlormethiazole	*Indirect $GABA_A$ antagonists*
Ethanol	Aztreonam
Etomidate	Clozapine
Felbamate	Flumazenil
General anesthetics	Lindane
Glutethimide(?)	MAOIs
Ivermectin	Maprotiline
Meprobamate	Organochlorine insecticides
Methaqualone	Penicillin
Methyprylon(?)	Pentylenetetrazol
Propofol	Picrotoxin
Steroids	Steroids
Trichloroethanol	Tricyclic antidepressants
Zolpidem	*Inhibit GAD*
Direct $GABA_B$ agonists	Cyanide
Baclofen	Domoic acid
Progabide[a]	Hydrazines
Inhibit GABA-T	Isoniazid
Vigabatrin	*Direct $GABA_B$ antagonists*
Inhibit GABA uptake	Phaclofen[b]
Guvacine	Saclofen[b]
Tiagabine	*Inhibit PK*
Valproate	Hydrazines[c]
	Isoniazid[c]

*Direct agonists and antagonists bind to the GABA binding site on GABA receptors to mimic or inhibit the action of GABA, respectively. Because of structural similarity to barbiturates, it is possible that glutethimide and methyprylon act on $GABA_A$ receptors, although this has not been confirmed. GABA = γ-aminobutyric acid; GABA-T = GABA transaminase; GAD = glutamic acid decarboxylase; PK = pyridoxine kinase; MAOIs = monoamine oxidase inhibitors.

[a]Directly agonizes $GABA_A$ and $GABA_B$ receptors as well as being metabolized to GABA.

[b]Though not thought to cross blood–brain barrier in meaningful amounts.

[c]Major site of action is PK inhibition, although some GAD inhibition occurs.

same mushrooms, is decarboxylated to muscimol just as glutamate is decarboxylated to GABA.

Indirect GABA Agonists. Benzodiazepines bind to the benzodiazepine receptor on the $GABA_A$ complex to increase the affinity of GABA for its receptor and to increase the frequency of Cl^- channel opening in response to GABA binding.[114] GABA also increases benzodiazepine receptor affinity for benzodiazepines. (Benzodiazepines also inhibit adenosine uptake apart from $GABA_A$ activity; see section on adenosine). Various isoforms of $GABA_A$ Cl^- channels differ in their affinity for different benzodiazepines. Investigators have divided these benzodiazepine binding sites on the $GABA_A$ complex into at least two different types, depending on their affinity for various compounds. BZ_1 receptors exhibit high affinity for quazepam, cinolazepam, some β-carbolines, and imidazopyridines (eg, zolpidem) and are especially concentrated in the cerebellum.[113] Zolpidem is a non-benzodiazepine that binds to the benzodiazepine-binding site of the $GABA_A$ complex to enhance Cl^- influx. BZ_2 receptors are rich in the hippocampus and other brain areas, but have a low affinity for the aforementioned compounds.

Numerous steroids, such as alphaxalone and naturally occurring analogs, bind to more than one site on the $GABA_A$ complex to inhibit or enhance the action of GABA.[46,114] Even large doses of intravenous cholesterol (containing a steroid nucleus) produce general anesthesia.

The synthesis of neuroactive steroids is regulated, in part, by benzodiazepine binding to mitochondrial benzodiazepine receptors (MBR) apart from the $GABA_A$ complex.[66,113,114] These mitochondrial benzodiazepine binding sites are found both inside and outside the CNS and were originally called peripheral benzodiazepine receptors. Mitochondrial benzodiazepine binding sites comprise three subunits: a voltage-dependent anion channel; an adenine nucleotide carrier; and a binding site for PK 11195, an isoquinoline carboxamide derivative.[45] Benzodiazepines vary with their affinity for mitochondrial binding. Upon binding, benzodiazepines appear to enhance the movement of cholesterol into mitochondria to begin steroid synthesis. Some of carbamazepine's action may be due to binding at mitochondrial benzodiazepine receptors.[41]

Barbiturates bind to the $GABA_A$ complex to produce several effects.[114] All barbiturates enhance the action of GABA. That is, they produce more Cl^- influx for a given amount of GABA binding by increasing the duration of Cl^- channel opening. Whereas phenobarbital does not change the affinity of GABA or benzodiazepines for their binding sites, depressant barbiturates, such as pentobarbital, do increase GABA and benzodiazepine receptor affinities for their ligands, further enhancing inward Cl^- currents. At high concentrations, at least some barbiturates directly open Cl^- channels to cause Cl^- influx. In addition, barbiturates have other actions that depress all excitable membranes, including cardiac and smooth muscle.

The intravenous anesthetics propofol and etomidate enhance inward $GABA_A$ Cl^- currents to produce their anesthetic actions.[2,91] Volatile general anesthetics also act as indirect agonists at the $GABA_A$ complex.[69,114]

Some of ethanol's action is mediated through binding to the $GABA_A$ complex.[114,135] At low concentrations, ethanol enhances the effect of GABA on Cl^- influx. In mouse neurons, ethanol concentrations as low as 230 mg/dL directly open the Cl^- channel. Methaqualone produces at least part of its pharmacologic effect through indirect $GABA_A$ activity. Little is known of glutethimide's and methyprylon's mechanisms of action. Their structural similarity to barbiturates suggests that much or most of it resides at the $GABA_A$ receptor. Trichloroethanol, a metabolite of chloral hydrate, and chlormethiazole interact at the $GABA_A$ complex in a manner similar to barbiturates, although it is not clear if they are binding to an identical site on the Cl^- channel.[135] Ivermectin, an anthelminthic, activates $GABA_A$ Cl^- channels by increasing GABA binding in rat brains.

Meprobamate displays barbiturate-like action at the $GABA_A$ receptor and, at high concentrations, is able to cause Cl^- influx in the absence of GABA.[101a] High concentrations of felbamate also cause inward Cl^- currents in the presence of GABA, although this seems unimportant at therapeutic doses.[101a]

Inhibition of GABA Uptake. Valproate and the anticonvulsants guvacine and tiagabine work, in part, by inhibiting GABA uptake.[85] Although valproate is structurally similar to GABA, its inhibition of the GABA transporter does not appear to be competitive, suggesting that valproate moves into the neuron by a different mechanism (eg, diffusion).

$GABA_A$ Antagonism

Direct $GABA_A$ Antagonists. Substances that act by any mechanism to decrease $GABA_A$ activity can cause CNS excitation and convulsions by preventing inhibitory inward Cl^- currents. Direct antagonists bind to the same site as GABA to prevent GABA binding, the prototype being the convulsant bicuculline. Various antibiotics interact with the $GABA_A$ receptor to antagonize the action of GABA. In a dose-dependent manner, both imipenem and cephalosporins appear to directly antagonize GABA binding and can produce seizures at high doses or at therapeutic doses in susceptible individuals.[44] Evidence suggests that penicillin may also directly antagonize GABA binding. Electrophysiologic and radioligand binding studies indicate that norfloxacin, ciprofloxacin, ofloxacin, and enoxacin all combine with the GABA binding site to prevent GABA binding, with ofloxacin being the weakest antagonist.[50] Theophylline and at least some nonsteroidal antiinflammatory agents markedly enhance GABA antagonism by some fluoroquinolones in vitro.[1,110] Excluding patients with neurologic disease, most patients reported to suffer seizures while taking therapeutic doses of ciprofloxacin are also taking theophylline and/or nonsteroidal antiinflammatory agents (ciprofloxacin can also raise theophylline levels to produce seizures).[1,110]

Indirect $GABA_A$ Antagonists. Penicillin is well-known for producing convulsions at high doses (eg, > 20 million units penicillin/day with renal insufficiency), and both penicillin and aztreonam, a monobactam, appear to block the Cl^- channel to prevent GABA-mediated inward Cl^- currents.[44,127]

Picrotoxin, from *Anamirta cocculus* (fish berries), and the experimental convulsant pentylenetetrazol bind to the picrotoxin site of the $GABA_A$ receptor complex to inhibit the action of GABA. Excessive doses produce CNS excitation and convulsions. Organochlorine insecticides (eg, lindane, chlordane, heptachlor) inhibit the action of GABA also by binding to what appears to be the picrotoxin site.[72] Convulsions characterize acute intoxications by these agents.

Flumazenil antagonizes benzodiazepines and zolpidem at their receptor to reverse their pharmacologic effects. Paradoxically, large doses of flumazenil exhibit anticonvulsant activity in animals. This is explained by flumazenil's ability to inhibit adenosine uptake, not by its partial agonism at the benzodiazepine receptor (see below).[95]

It has been suggested that the efficacy of most antidepressants may be due to antagonism at the $GABA_A$ complex.[118] Cyclic antidepressants, including amoxapine and maprotiline, and at least two MAOIs (isocarboxazid and tranylcypromine) inhibit GABA-mediated Cl^- influx at $GABA_A$ receptors.[75,118] Their potency at inhibiting Cl^- influx correlates with the frequency of seizures seen in patients taking therapeutic doses of these medications. Impaired $GABA_A$ activity may contribute to or be primarily responsible for seizures seen in patients who overdose on these agents. The exact binding site of these drugs on the $GABA_A$ receptor complex is not yet known, although some evidence suggests at least indirect activity at the picrotoxin binding site.

Some subtypes of $GABA_A$ receptors are susceptible to inhibition by zinc ions.[114] What role this plays in normal physiology or toxicology is not established.

$GABA_A$ Withdrawal. Chronic use of $GABA_A$ complex agonists leads to down-regulation of $GABA_A$ complex activity. Acute withdrawal from all $GABA_A$ direct and indirect agonists appears almost identical except for time course; in all cases, the common mediator is impaired Cl^- influx. Withdrawal of all $GABA_A$ agonists can cause tremor, hypertension, tachycardia, diaphoresis, agitation, hallucinations, and convulsions. Conversely, any $GABA_A$ complex agonist can stop withdrawal from another, since all increase Cl^- influx. One exception might be that withdrawal from a triazolobenzodiazepine appears controllable only with a similar drug because of actions on certain subtypes of benzodiazepine receptors (ie, particular subtypes of $GABA_A$ chloride channels). Because of their $GABA_A$ action, benzodiazepines and barbiturates are effective in controlling $GABA_A$ withdrawal seizures. Phenytoin and carbamazepine do not stop $GABA_A$ withdrawal seizures since their anticonvulsant actions are due to other pharmacologic effects independent from GABA.

$GABA_B$ Agonists. The main $GABA_B$ receptor agonist of toxicologic significance is baclofen.[83] Intoxication is characterized by coma, hypothermia, hypotension, bradydysrhythmias, and seizures. The convulsions seen in patients with baclofen overdose are thought to result from dysinhibition inhibition of inhibitory neurons. That is, baclofen may be inhibiting the release of GABA by presynaptic agonism at autoreceptors.

Carbamazepine has some action on $GABA_B$ receptors, although this is not thought to explain most of its anticonvulsant action. As noted below, some of γ-hydroxybutyrate's actions may be mediated through activation of $GABA_B$ receptors.

$GABA_B$ Withdrawal. Baclofen withdrawal is similar clinically to $GABA_A$ withdrawal. It is mainly characterized by hallucinations, agitation, tremor, increased sympathetic activity, and convulsions. Withdrawal is treated by reinstituting baclofen therapy.

Gamma-hydroxybutyrate

Gamma-hydroxybutyrate (GHB; γ-hydroxybutyric acid) was first synthesized in the 1960s as a water-soluble sedative agent able to cross the blood–brain barrier and only later found to be naturally present in the mammalian brain.[22] Toxicologic interest in this compound stems mainly from its abuse. Controversy exists as to whether GHB should be considered a neurotransmitter or simply a neuromodulator since it is unclear whether this substance is concentrated within vesicles for synaptic release, although there has been described a GHB sodium-dependent uptake transporter.[54] While evidence exists for GHB-induced generalized neuronal inhibition, large doses of GHB injected into animals produce convulsions.

Several proposed pathways for endogenous GHB formation exist.[22,76] Most interest is directed at the reduction of succinate semialdehyde to GHB (Fig. 10–11). Several lines of evidence suggest that GHB undergoes conversion back to succinate semialdehyde before being oxidized to succinate.

Little is known of GHB receptors. Receptors appear to be heterogeneously distributed in the brain, with highest concentrations in the hippocampus and lowest in the cerebellum. At least two general receptors have been described thus far, based on binding affinity for GHB or other ligands.

High-affinity receptors for GHB do not respond to GABA, GABAergic agonists, γ-butyrolactone, or dopamine. Similarly, GHB does not activate $GABA_A$ Cl^- channels. GHB's actions are not antagonized by flumazenil.

Some low-affinity receptors may actually be $GABA_B$ receptors.[22,76] While normal endogenous GHB concentrations are probably not high enough to activate $GABA_B$ receptors, high GHB concentrations seen after overdose may be.

Evidence exists for GHB's metabolism back to GABA (Fig. 10–11). Thus, pharmacologic effects resulting from GHB administration may result, in part, from secondary GABA formation.[22]

Intoxication resulting from ingestion of GHB is explained by GHB receptor and possibly $GABA_B$ receptor activation, and comprises rapid onset of coma, vomiting, bradycardia, hypotension, convulsions, and apnea that usually resolves within several hours. Patients with congenital deficiency of succinate semialdehyde dehydrogenase (SSAD) shunt more succinate semialdehyde to GHB, resulting in accumulation of GHB in the CNS (Fig. 10–11). Clinically these patients exhibit severe psychomotor retardation, ataxia, and seizures.[58,101] Valproic acid similarly elevates endogenous GHB concentrations by inhibiting SSAD.

Glycine as an Inhibitory Neurotransmitter

Glycine acts as a postsynaptic inhibitory neurotransmitter in the spinal cord and lower brainstem. Glycine's most important action is to inhibit reflex arcs, thus suppressing excessive firing by lower motor neurons, preventing inordinate and uncontrollable muscle action.

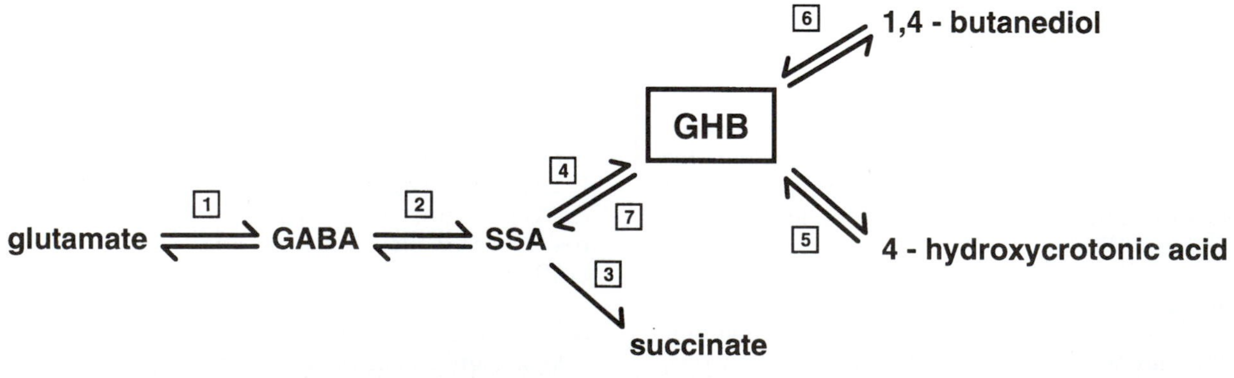

Figure 10–11. Potential pathways of GHB (γ-hydroxybutyrate) synthesis and degradation. GABA = γ-aminobutyric acid; SSA = succinate semialdehyde; [1] = glutamic acid decarboxylase; [2] = GABA-transaminase; [3] = succinate semialdehyde dehydrogenase; [4] = specific succinate semialdehyde reductase and/or NADPH-dependent aldehyde reductase 2; [5] = mitochondrial beta oxidation; [6] = alcohol dehydrogenase and aldehyde dehydrogenase; [7] NADPH-dependent aldehyde reductase 1 or mitochondrial pyridine nucleotide independent oxido-reductase.

Release and Uptake

Glycine is transported into storage vesicles and undergoes Ca^{2+}-dependent exocytosis upon neuronal depolarization (Fig. 10–12). Glycine is removed from the synapse through uptake by a Na^+-dependent transporter.

Glycine Receptors

Like $GABA_A$, the glycine receptor is a Cl^- channel on the postsynaptic membrane.[9,13] $GABA_A$ Cl^- channels and glycine Cl^- channels share significant amino acid homology. Also analogous to GABA, glycine receptor activation causes an inward Cl^- current that hyperpolarizes the membrane. More than one glycine molecule must bind to sites on the Cl^- channel to produce inhibitory Cl^- influx.

Chemical Agents (Table 10–10)

Strychnine is the main toxicologic agent affecting glycinergic transmission. Strychnine binds near the glycine receptor to prevent glycine's action on Cl^- influx,[3] at least in part by decreasing glycine's binding to its receptors. Glycine and strychnine receptors may overlap. Since glycine must bind to more than one site on the Cl^- channel for successful agonism, a plausible explanation is that strychnine may bind to one of glycine's binding sites. This physiologic antagonism of glycine's action produces increased muscle tone, rigidity, opisthotonus, trismus, and death from respiratory failure and rhabdomyolysis. Given the similarity in Cl^- channels, it is not surprising that strychnine binds to the $GABA_A$ complex in vitro. However, strychnine's affinity for this complex is less than that for glycine receptors, and most of its toxicologic action is due to physiologic antagonism of glycine's inhibitory action.

TABLE 10–10. AGENTS AFFECTING INHIBITORY GLYCINE CHLORIDE CHANNELS*

Glycine agonists	*Glycine antagonists*
Ethanol	Strychnine
Propofol	Picrotoxin

*Ethanol and propofol enhance Cl^- influx through glycine Cl^- channels, although they do not appear to be direct agonists. Evidence exists for picrotoxin's direct antagonism at the glycine binding site in contrast to $GABA_A$ Cl^- channels, where it acts at a site separate from where GABA binds.

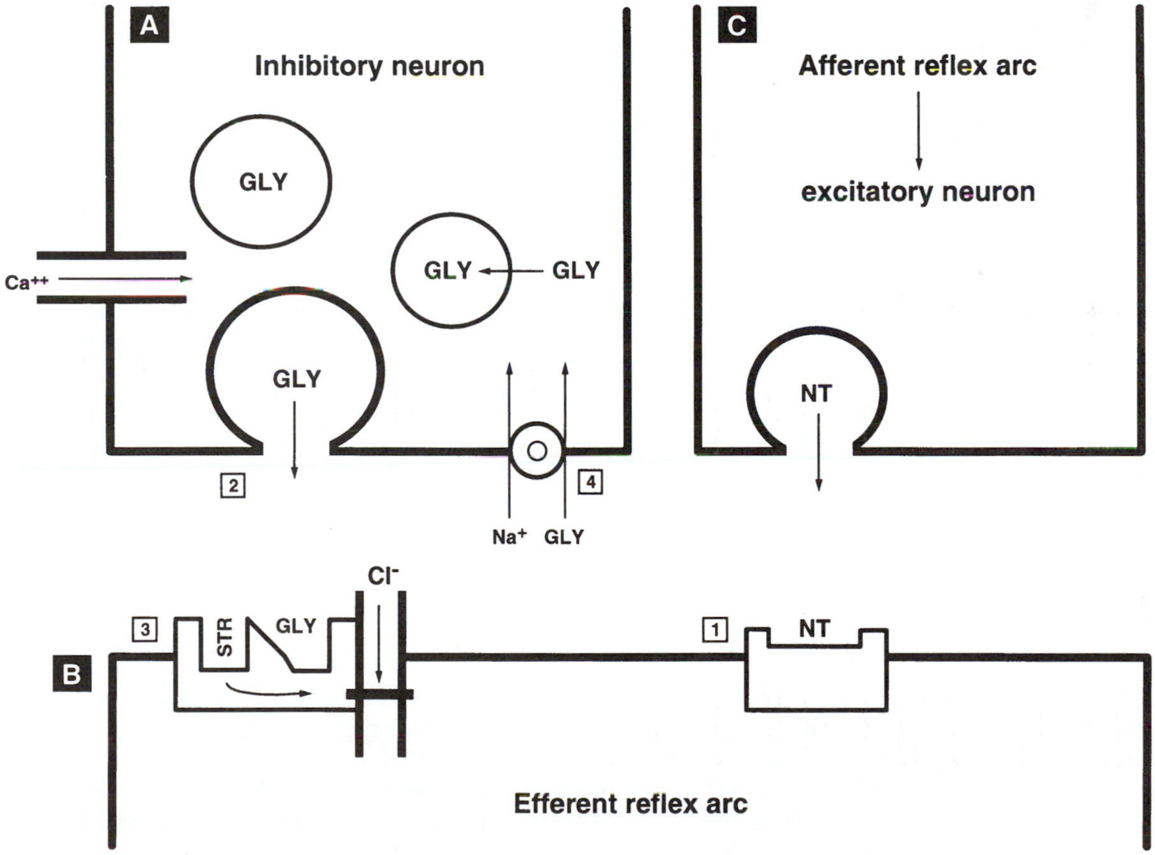

Figure 10–12. Inhibitory glycinergic neurotransmission. Signals from the afferent limb of a reflex arc (neuron C) cause the release of an excitatory neurotransmitter (NT) that crosses the synapse to bind to neuron B in the efferent limb of the reflex arc [1]. To prevent excessive neuronal firing and motor activity, glycine (GLY) released from inhibitory neuron A [2] binds to glycine Cl^- channel receptors on neuron B [3] and causes inhibition by hyperpolarization. Synaptic glycine is transported back into the neuron [4]. Strychnine (STR) binds to the glycinergic Cl^- channel [3] to decrease glycine's binding, which prevents Cl^- influx. While strychnine is shown binding to a separate site from glycine, there is evidence that these sites may overlap.

Numerous other agents act on glycinergic Cl^- channels. Picrotoxin binds to the glycine receptor to impair Cl^- influx.[73] Tetanus toxin produces rigidity and trismus by preventing glycine release from nerve endings in the spinal cord and brainstem. Both ethanol and propofol potentiate glycine-mediated inward Cl^- currents through action at the α subunit of the glycine receptor, just as they do at $GABA_A$ Cl^- channels.[77] The seizure-like rigidity seen in some patients during induction of anesthesia with propofol, which occurs despite an electroencephalogram devoid of seizure activity, is not yet satisfactorily explained by propofol's action at $GABA_A$ or glycine receptors.

Glutamate

Glutamate is the main excitatory neurotransmitter in the CNS. Aspartate has similar actions, although its exact role as a neurotransmitter is not as well-defined. Glutamate and aspartate are commonly referred to as excitatory amino acid neurotransmitters. Glutaminergic neurotransmission has been a subject of intense research because of its role in mediating neuronal damage in degenerative neurologic diseases and during times of trauma, ischemia, hypoglycemia, and status epilepticus.[30] While glutamate receptor stimulation is necessary

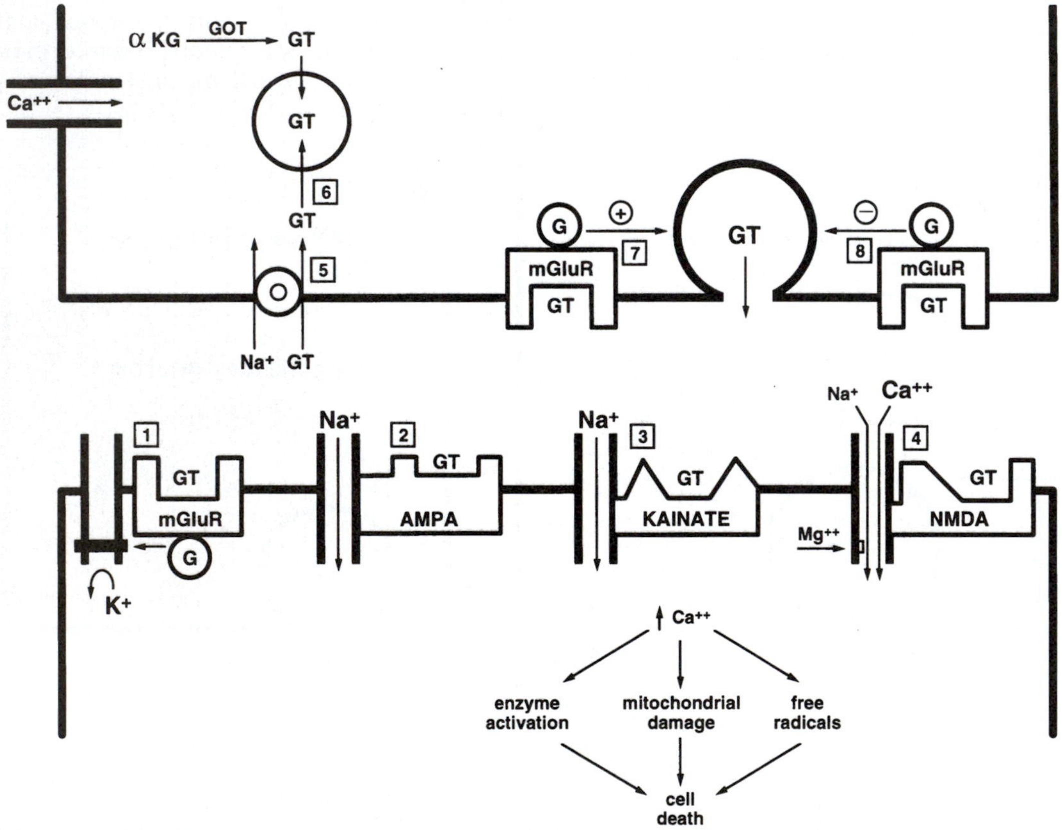

Figure 10–13. Glutaminergic neurotransmission. GOT converts α-ketoglutarate (α KG) to glutamate in the mitochondria. Synaptic glutamate binds to four main types of receptors. AMPA [2], kainate [3], and NMDA [4] receptors are cation channels. Membrane depolarization in response to agonism at any of the channel receptors causes neuronal excitation through cation influx. Metabotropic receptors (mGluR) [1,7,8] are coupled to G proteins and exist on pre- and postsynaptic membranes. Postsynaptic metabotropic receptors [1] excite by preventing K^+ efflux or inhibit by enhancing K^+ efflux (only excitation is illustrated). Presynaptic metabotropic receptors act to inhibit [8] or enhance [7] glutamate (and other neurotransmitters) release through modulating intracellular Ca^{2+} concentrations. A more detailed illustration of the NMDA receptor is found in Figure 10–14. Excessive influx of Ca^{2+} through NMDA receptors causes neuronal damage and death. A Mg^{2+} ion normally blocks the NMDA receptor channel to prevent Ca^{2+} influx despite GT binding. However, depolarization of the neuronal membrane by Na^+ influx resulting from activation of any of the other receptors will cause Mg^{2+} to dissociate from the NMDA receptor and allow potentially damaging inward Ca^{2+} currents. Various agents in Table 10–11 affect glutaminergic neurotransmission, in part, by stimulating or blocking the various GT receptors [1–4,7,8]; by preventing glutamate uptake [5]; or by preventing vesicle uptake of GT [6]. α KG = α-ketoglutarate; GOT = glutamic-oxaloacetic transaminase; GT = glutamate; mGluR = metabotropic glutamate receptor; G = G protein.

for normal brain activity (eg, memory), excessive glutamate receptor activation endogenously or by glutamate agonists can produce convulsions, neuronal damage, and death. Glutamate antagonists demonstrate anticonvulsant activity and neuroprotective action in animal models of brain and spinal cord injury.

Synthesis, Release, and Uptake

Glutamate is synthesized, in part, from α-ketoglutarate before transportation into storage vesicles, prior to release into the synapse by Ca^{2+}-dependent exocytosis (Fig. 10–13). After stimulating glutamate receptors, glutamate undergoes uptake by a Na^{+}-dependent transporter. As in GABAergic neurons, reverse transport of glutamate from the cytoplasm into the synapse by the membrane transporter may occur under some circumstances.[30] Glutamate serves as the substrate for GABA synthesis.

Glutamate Receptors

Glutamate receptors exist as ion channels and as receptors linked to G proteins.[124] A single neuron may possess numerous types of glutamate receptors. Postsynaptic glutamate receptors are usually excitatory, though some inhibitory actions have been demonstrated. Presynaptic terminal glutamate receptors may inhibit or enhance release of various neurotransmitters, including glutamate (Fig. 10–13).[97]

Ion Channel Glutamate Receptors. Three ion channel glutamate receptors have been identified. All allow for excitation through cation influx. These receptors are further categorized and named by their abilities to be agonized or antagonized by various substances: kainate, AMPA (α-amino-3-hydroxy-5-methyl-4-isoxazole propionate), and NMDA (*N*-methyl-*d*-aspartate).[124]

The kainate receptor for glutamate is named after its affinity for kainic acid found in seaweed. It is an ion channel receptor whose activation allows Na^{+} influx and small amount of K^{+} efflux. When stimulated, this postsynaptic receptor produces excitation by triggering neuronal depolarization.

The AMPA receptor is an ion channel structurally similar to the kainate receptor and also mediates Na^{+} influx on postsynaptic membranes, triggering neuronal depolarization.[8] The AMPA receptor is the most common ion channel glutamate receptor found in the brain and appears to account for most glutaminergic excitation under normal conditions.

The most studied glutamate receptor is the NMDA receptor (Fig. 10–14). This is a Ca^{2+} channel whose activation allows for inward Ca^{2+} and Na^{+} currents (and some K^{+} efflux), resulting in neuronal depolarization and triggering of an action potential. Excessive stimulation of NMDA receptors by glutamate released during times of ischemia, trauma, hypoglycemia, or convulsions triggers damaging rises in intracellular Ca^{2+} concentrations, acti-

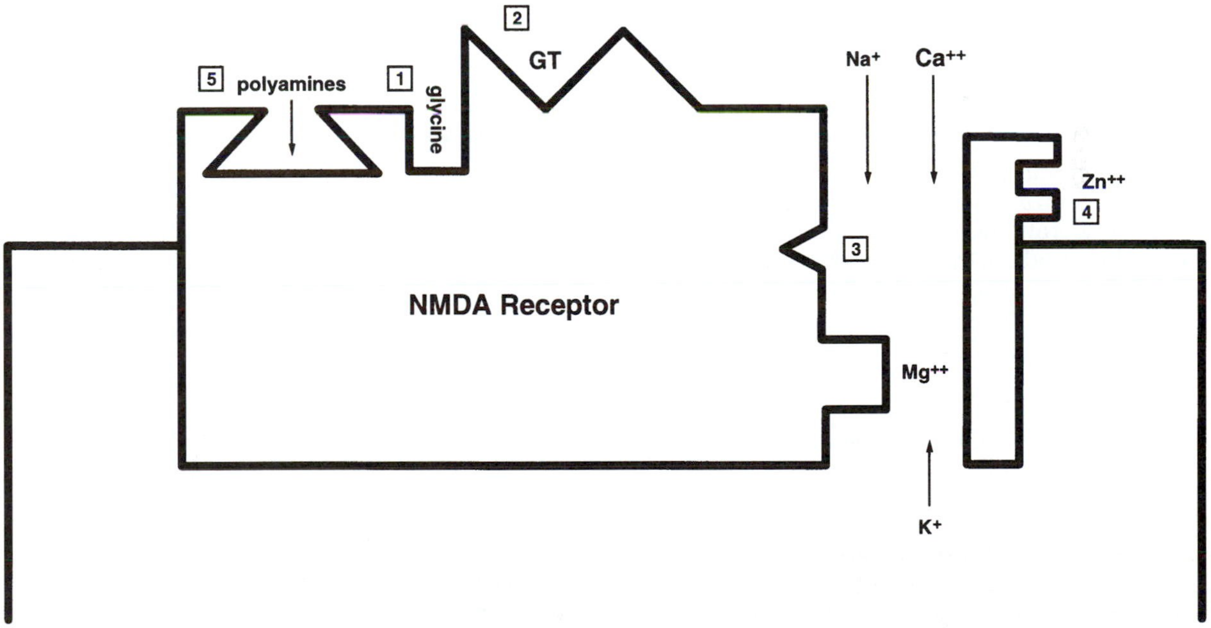

Figure 10–14. Schematic drawing of the NMDA receptor for glutamate (GT). The NMDA receptor is a voltage-gated and ligand-dependent Ca^{2+} channel. GT binds to its receptor on the channel [2] to open the Ca^{2+} channel and allow Ca^{2+} and Na^{+} influx and lesser amounts of K^{+} efflux. Mg^{2+} normally blocks the Ca^{2+} channel, preventing cation influx in response to GT binding. Mg^{2+} leaves the channel when the membrane is depolarized by 20–30 mV. Glycine must also bind to its site on the receptor complex [1] for successful GT agonism. Polyamines bind on the extracellular surface of the receptor [5]. Zn^{2+} binds [4] to inhibit Ca^{2+} influx. The phencyclidine (PCP) binding site [3] lies within the channel. Agents in Table 10–11 can block glycine's binding [1], block the Ca^{2+} channel by binding to the PCP binding site [3], or directly stimulate the glutamate binding site [2].

vation of numerous enzymes, and free radical formation, all of which incite cell death.[124] Antagonists of NMDA Ca^{2+} channels are anticonvulsants and provide neuroprotection during times of neuronal insult.

The Ca^{2+} channel of the NMDA receptor is normally blocked by Mg^{2+} in a voltage-dependent manner, preventing Ca^{2+} influx despite glutamate binding (Fig. 10–14).[62,103] Only when the neuronal membrane is depolarized by at least 20–30 mV through some other mechanism (eg, activation of another receptor) will Mg^{2+} leave the channel and allow Ca^{2+} influx in response to glutamate binding. Thus, the NMDA glutamate receptor is both a ligand-gated and voltage-gated ion channel. Many neurons have both NMDA and non-NMDA receptors for glutamate. Stimulation of kainate or AMPA receptors by glutamate indirectly causes cell damage through Na^+ influx, since the membrane depolarization they produce causes Mg^{2+} to leave the NMDA receptor and allows for potentially damaging inward Ca^{2+} currents.[34] Calcium ion influx through voltage-gated ion channels (including L subtype) on cell bodies that open in response to depolarization also contributes to accumulation of intracellular calcium and cell damage. Therefore, excessive activation of any glutamate receptor has the potential to produce neuronal cytotoxicity.

Glutamate alone is incapable of opening Ca^{2+} channels after binding to its receptor, even after Mg^{2+} has dissociated from the ion channel. Glycine also must bind to its specific receptor on the NMDA receptor complex for successful glutamate agonism (Fig. 10–14), making glycine an indirect agonist of excitatory neurotransmission.[68] In fact, two molecules of glutamate and two molecules of glycine are required for successful agonism. Strychnine does not antagonize glycine's excitatory action at NMDA receptors, explaining why glycine NMDA receptors are also known as strychnine-insensitive glycine receptors.

Zinc ions normally bind to the NMDA receptor complex to antagonize the action of glutamate. Binding of spermine or spermidine to a polyamine binding site on the extracellular side of the NMDA receptor results in increased affinity of glycine and glutamate for their binding sites. However, polyamine agonism is not essential for glutamate activation of NMDA receptors.[102]

Metabotropic Glutamate Receptors. Metabotropic glutamate receptors are linked to various G proteins on post- and presynaptic membranes (Fig. 10–13) and are the least understood glutamate receptors. Eight different receptors have been isolated to date.[97] In contrast to ion channel glutamate receptors, metabotropic receptors may excite or inhibit pre- and postsynaptic membranes. Data thus far indicate that excitatory postsynaptic receptors are linked to G proteins that block K^+ efflux. On presynaptic membranes, these receptors may prevent neurotransmitter release by lowering intracellular calcium concentrations, or may enhance neurotransmitter release through the generation of inositol triphosphate (IP_3) and mobilization of intracellular Ca^{2+} stores. Postsynaptic inhibition appears to result through opening of K^+ channels with resultant K^+ efflux.[98]

Chemical Agents (Table 10–11)

Glutamate Agonism. Domoic acid produces amnestic shellfish poisoning, partly characterized by confusion, agitation, convulsions, memory disturbance, neuronal damage, and death.[93,123] The structural similarity between domoic acid and glutamate is thought to explain excessive activation of kainate receptors with secondary NMDA receptor activation and neuronal damage.[120]

Investigators hypothesize that other naturally occurring glutamate receptor agonists produce additional neurologic diseases. The neurogenic form of lathyrism results from using chickling peas (*Lathyrus sativus*) as a food staple. Chickling peas contain β-*N*-oxalylamino-l-alanine (BOAA), an agonist of AMPA receptors.[28,65] Neurogenic lathyrism was common in German concentration and prisoner of war camps in World War II and still occurs regularly in some parts of the world. A similar illness, Guam amyotrophic lateral sclerosis–parkinsonism–dementia (Guam ALS-PD), results from ingestion of the false sago palm (*Cycas circinalis L.*), which contains α-amino-β-methylaminopropionic acid (β-*N*-methylamino-l-alanine; BMAA), also a potent AMPA receptor agonist.[28,65,117] This illness prevailed on Guam and Rota during food shortages brought on by World War II.

Ibotenic acid, from poisonous mushrooms, activates NMDA and some metabotropic glutamate receptors.[65] It undergoes decarboxylation to muscimol, a direct agonist at $GABA_A$ receptors.

Because NMDA receptor antagonism reproduces many signs and symptoms of schizophrenia, investigators are directing efforts at increasing glutamate's activity at NMDA channels in an effort to treat the disease. After crossing the blood–brain barrier, milacemide un-

TABLE 10–11. AGENTS AFFECTING GLUTAMINERGIC NEUROTRANSMISSION*

Glutamate Agonism	*NMDA receptor antagonists*
Direct glutamate receptor agonists	Amantadine
BMAA	Dextrorphan[b]
BOAA	Dizocilpine (MK801)
Domoic acid	Ketamine
Ibotenic acid[a]	Memantine
Willardine	Pentamidine
	Phencyclidine
Glycine NMDA receptor agonists	*NMDA glycine antagonism*
d-Cycloserine	Ethanol
Milacemide	Felbamate
Glutamate Antagonism	Kynurenic acid
Prevent glutamate release	Meprobamate
Lamotrigine	*Polyamine antagonists*
Nimodipine	Ifenprodil
Riluzole	Eliprodil

*Direct glutamate agonists bind in place of glutamate to various receptors to mimic glutamate's action. Glycine agonists mimic the action of glycine at NMDA glutamate receptors.

NMDA = *N*-methyl-*d*-aspartate; BOAA = β-*N*-oxalylamino-l-alanine; BMAA = α-amino-β-methylaminopropionic acid.

[a]The only direct agonist to activate metabotropic glutamate receptors. Also decarboxylated in vivo to muscimol, a direct $GABA_A$ agonist.

[b]Metabolite of dextromethorphan.

dergoes conversion to glycine, which stimulates NMDA receptors. D-Cycloserine also crosses the blood–brain barrier to stimulate glycine NMDA receptors.[137]

Glutamate Antagonism

Prevention of Glutamate Release. Riluzole, used for the treatment of amyotrophic lateral sclerosis, indirectly prevents release of glutamate. Lamotrigine diminishes glutamate release through blockade of voltage-gated Na^+ channels. Blockade of voltage-gated calcium channels by nimodipine appears to impair glutamate release as well.[124]

NMDA Receptor Antagonists. While some experimental agents and pharmaceuticals antagonize the action of glutamate, most of our knowledge concerns antagonism at NMDA receptors. Phencyclidine and ketamine appear to bind within the ion channel (PCP binding site) to block Ca^{2+} influx following glutamate binding (Fig. 10–14).[125] Both agents have other pharmacologic actions and can produce convulsions in overdose. However, in animal models of seizures and neuronal insult, both drugs are neuroprotective and anticonvulsant.

Dextromethorphan and its first-pass metabolite, dextrorphan, exhibit anticonvulsant activity in animals. Dextrorphan's anticonvulsant activity results, in part, from blockade of NMDA receptor Ca^{2+} channels by binding to the PCP site.[126] Dextromethorphan does not bind to the NMDA complex but, like dextrorphan, can directly block N- and L-type voltage-dependent Ca^{2+} channels.[21]

Dizocilpine (MK-801) is a NMDA receptor antagonist that binds to the PCP binding site in the NMDA Ca^{2+} channel. Human trials of dizocilpine resulted in adverse effects similar to those produced by phencyclidine, preventing further use in humans as a neuroprotective agent. Amantadine binds to the PCP binding site in NMDA Ca^{2+} channels to block cation influx; this is thought to explain some of its efficacy in the treatment of Parkinson's disease. Pentamidine also antagonizes glutamate binding at NMDA channels.[124]

Glycine Antagonists. Ethanol competitively prevents glycine's binding to the NMDA receptor, resulting in up-regulation of this glutaminergic system.[124] Although glycine antagonism is not the main mechanism by which ethanol produces intoxication, the acute withdrawal of ethanol is accompanied by excessive NMDA activity and may explain some of the characteristic agitation, hallucinations, and convulsions. In some animal models of ethanol withdrawal seizures, NMDA receptor antagonists are better anticonvulsants than $GABA_A$ agonists.[55]

Felbamate's anticonvulsant activity may result, in part, from antagonism of glycine at NMDA channels.[124] Kynurenic acid, a metabolite of L-tryptophan, prevents NMDA activation through glycine antagonism.

Meprobamate also antagonizes NMDA glutamate receptors by a yet-to-be determined mechanism. However, given the structural similarity to felbamate, meprobamate may act by antagonizing the action of glycine.[101a]

Polyamine Antagonism. Ifenprodil and eliprodil antagonize glutamate's action at NMDA channels by preventing polyamine binding.[102]

Adenosine

There exist two main types of purine receptors: P_1 receptors possess highest affinity for adenosine; P_2 receptors exhibit highest affinity for ATP and adenosine diphosphate (ADP).[18] The overall action of adenosine throughout the body is to lessen oxygen requirements and to increase oxygen and substrate delivery.[132] In keeping with this paradigm, adenosine functions in the CNS as an extremely important inhibitory neuromodulator and vasodilator.

Adenosine Receptors

P_1 receptors are currently divided into A_1, A_2, and A_3 receptors (and subtypes), with evidence that A_4 may also exist.[18,129,136] In the central and autonomic nervous systems, A_1 receptors reside on presynaptic and postsynaptic membranes, where they serve as inhibitory modulators for numerous neurotransmitter systems; they are particularly prevalent in association with glutaminergic neurons in the CNS.

In the CNS, A_2 receptors are concentrated on cerebral vasculature and produce vasodilation when stimulated. Additionally, A_2 receptors are especially prevalent on neurons in the striatum and other areas of the brain rich in dopamine where they have only been identified postsynaptically. A_3 receptors are found diffusely in the CNS, with an unclear role.

A_1, A_2, and A_3 receptors are coupled to G proteins.[84] Postsynaptic A_1 stimulation results in K^+ channels opening and K^+ efflux with subsequent hyperpolarization of the neuron (Fig. 10–15). Evidence suggests that G protein–mediated Cl^- influx may explain postsynaptic hyperpolarization by A_1 activation in some cases. Presynaptic A_1 stimulation modifies voltage-dependent Ca^{2+} channels, lessening Ca^{2+} influx during depolarization, which limits exocytosis of neurotransmitter. Therefore, activation of A_1 receptors prevents release of neurotransmitters presynaptically and inhibits their response postsynaptically. Presynaptic A_1 activation also increases glutamate uptake from the synapse.

A_2 receptors are known to be coupled only to G_s. The rise in cAMP concentration resulting from their activation on cerebral vasculature and elsewhere produces vasodilation. Activation of striatal A_2 receptors decreases postsynaptic D_2 receptor sensitivity, limiting postsynaptic responses to dopamine.[132]

Synthesis, Release, and Uptake

An equilibrium between adenosine, adenosine monophosphate (AMP), ADP, and ATP exists in the living cell. Normal intracellular concentrations of adenosine range from 50 to 300 nM. During times of adequate oxygen de-

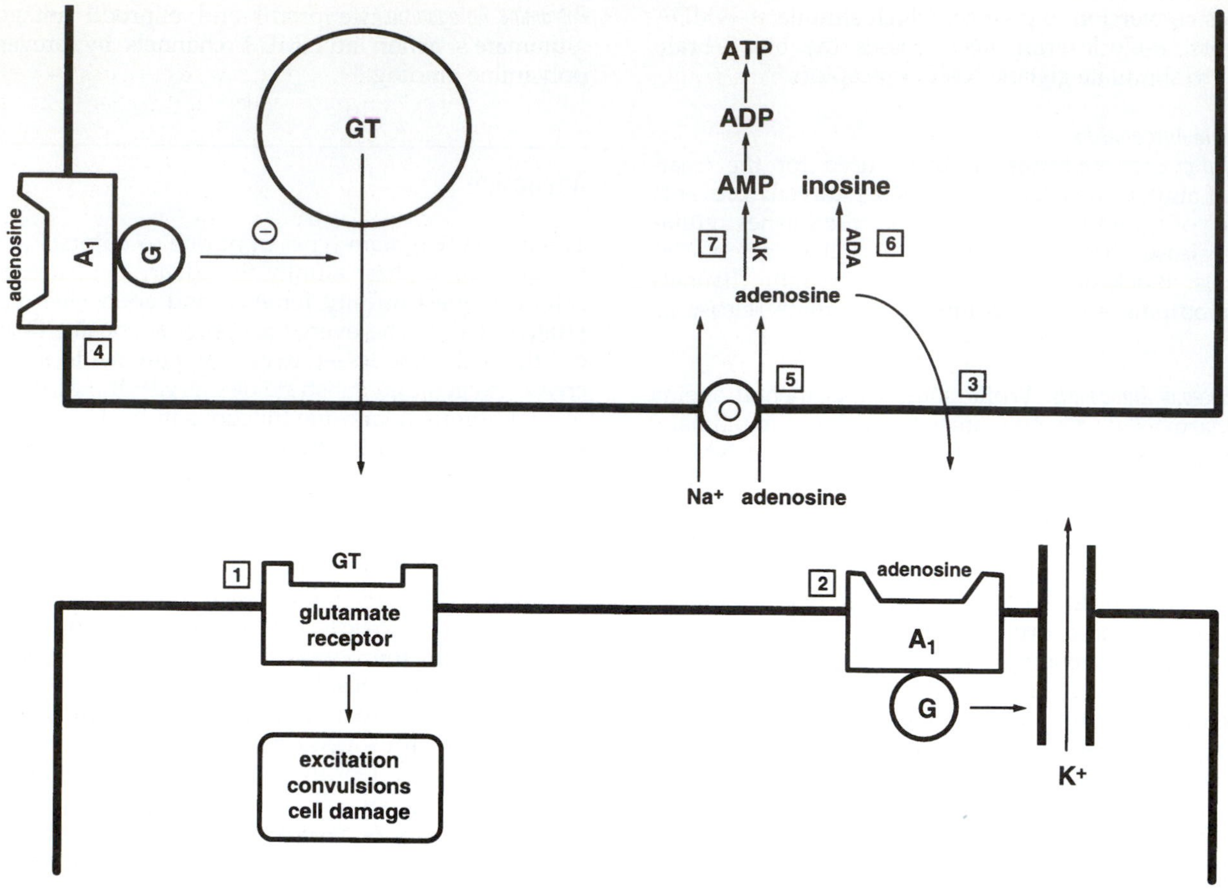

Figure 10–15. Adenosine's role in regulating excitatory neurotransmission, using glutamate as an example. In this example, GT stimulates receptors on the postsynaptic neuron to cause excitation and damaging inward Ca^{2+} currents [1]. Adenosine enters the synapse when GT is released, although the exact mechanism of adenosine's release is not clear [3]. Adenosine binds to postsynaptic A_1 receptors [2] to open K^+ channels and inhibit the neuron by hyperpolarization. Adenosine also stimulates presynaptic A_1 receptors [4] to lower intracellular Ca^{2+} concentrations, thereby impairing further release of GT. After uptake, adenosine is acted on either by AK [7] to form AMP, or by ADA [6] to form inosine. When metabolic activity exceeds oxygen delivery, adenosine concentrations rise from excessive metabolism of ATP. Not shown is adenosine's binding to vascular A_2 receptors to cause G protein–mediated vasodilation. Agents in Table 10–12 act to block adenosine receptors [2,4], including vascular A_2 receptors (not shown); to prevent adenosine uptake [5]; to inhibit ADA [6]; to inhibit AK [7]. GT = glutamate; ADA = adenosine deaminase; AK = adenosine kinase; AMP = adenosine monophosphate; ADP = adenosine diphosphate; ATP = adenosine triphosphate; G = G protein.

livery and oxidative phosphorylation, adenosine is used to produce ATP. During increased cellular catabolism, especially during inadequate oxygen delivery, adenosine concentrations rise as phosphorylated adenosine species are degraded to adenosine without rapid conversion of adenosine to ATP. When oxygen delivery is adequate to meet metabolic demands, neuronal adenosine mainly arises from *S*-adenosyl homocysteine hydrolase's action on *S*-adenosyl homocysteine.

Adenosine undergoes release from the neuron into the synapse during depolarization (Fig. 10–15). It is not agreed upon whether adenosine is actually stored in vesicles or released in another manner. Adenosine may be better described as a neuromodulator than a neurotransmitter for this reason. A minority of synaptic adenosine arises from degradation of ATP released with neurotransmitters from vesicles.

Adenosine undergoes uptake back into neurons and glial cells by a Na^+-dependent purine transporter. Intracellular adenosine is metabolized to inosine by adenosine deaminase. Conversely, adenosine kinase (AK) phosphorylates adenosine to begin ATP formation.[32]

Adenosine and Seizure Termination

In humans and in animal models of status epilepticus, including those from drugs and toxins, there are two alternating phases of electrical activity noted on electroencephalography.[37] Periods of high-frequency spike activity accompanied by marked increases in cerebral oxygen consumption and metabolic requirements alternate with interictal periods of isolated spike waves during which metabolic demands are less. The high-frequency phase lasts only a few minutes before suddenly terminating, sometimes with a few seconds of electrocerebral silence. A gradual increase in electrical activity during the interictal phase eventually leads to a recurrence of high-frequency spike activity.

These periodic spontaneous self-terminations of high-frequency electrical activity initially occur before neurons exhaust oxygen and energy supplies. These punctuations result from adenosine release from depolarizing neurons (and probably glial cells). Adenosine acts on presynaptic receptors to prevent further release of excitatory neurotransmitters and acts on postsynaptic receptors to inhibit their actions.

Any agent that directly or indirectly enhances adenosine's action at A_1 receptors in the brain will usually exhibit anticonvulsant activity. An agent that antagonizes A_1 receptors in the brain will have two main effects. First, A_1 antagonists will trigger seizure onset by causing excessive release of and responsiveness to excitatory neurotransmitters (eg, glutamate). Second, A_1 antagonism will impair seizure self-termination, making seizures from any etiology more likely to persist and less likely to respond to anticonvulsants.

Agents that antagonize A_2 receptors produce cerebral vasoconstriction and may limit oxygen delivery during times of increased demand. Antagonism of A_2 receptors in the striatum may theoretically increase dopamine-mediated motor activity.

Chemical Agents (Table 10–12)

Indirect Adenosine Agonists. Papaverine and dipyridamole inhibit adenosine uptake.[92] Like all agonists of adenosine's action, papaverine and dipyridamole demonstrate anticonvulsant activity when injected into the CNS. Such actions are not achievable with safe systemic doses.

Benzodiazepines inhibit adenosine uptake,[29,95] in addition to their actions at $GABA_A$ receptors. This explains observations that methylxanthines, potent adenosine receptor antagonists, reverse benzodiazepine-induced sedation in humans. The potencies of benzodiazepines as inhibitors of adenosine uptake show good correlation with clinical anxiolytic and anticonflict potencies, suggesting that such inhibition plays an important role in their action. The anticonvulsant effect of large doses of flumazenil also results from inhibition of adenosine uptake. Carbamazepine inhibits adenosine uptake ex vivo.

An increasing number of studies indicate that adenosine mediates many of the acute and chronic motor effects of ethanol on the brain. Ethanol, probably through its metabolite, acetate, prevents adenosine uptake, raising synaptic adenosine concentrations.[20] Excessive stimulation of several adenosine receptors in the cerebellum may explain much of the motor impairment from low ethanol concentrations. In fact, animals made tolerant to ethanol develop cross-tolerance to adenosine agonists. In mice, adenosine receptor agonists increase ethanol-induced incoordination while adenosine antagonists decrease this intoxicating response.[33]

Numerous other agents are now recognized as inhibitors of adenosine uptake, including propentofylline, nimodipine, and other calcium channel blockers.[90,92]

Dipyridamole inhibits adenosine deaminase, raising adenosine concentrations. During times of elevated adenosine levels that occur with cardiac or cerebral ischemia, acadesine further enhances adenosine's beneficial actions by three mechanism: inhibition of AK; inhibition of ADA; and inhibition of adenosine uptake.[84]

Adenosine Antagonists. The main adenosine antagonists of toxicologic concern are methylxanthines. Theophylline and caffeine are selective P_1 antagonists, blocking both A_1 and A_2 receptors.[132] A_3 receptors appear resistant to blockade by methylxanthines. Peripherally, methylxanthines produce excessive release of catecholamines from peripheral nerve endings (and probably the adrenal gland) by blocking presynaptic A_1 receptors. In turn, catecholamine-mediated responses are exaggerated by blockade of inhibitory postsynaptic A_1 receptors on end organs.[43]

Centrally, enhanced release and actions of excitatory neurotransmitters (eg, glutamate) and resultant lack of periodicity probably explain convulsions that are frequently refractory to anticonvulsants. Reasons that theophylline convulsions carry such a high mortality stem from a lack of self-termination (continual high-frequency spike activity and large metabolic demands) that has resulted from A_1 antagonism, compounded by A_2-blockade-mediated cerebral vasoconstriction.[37,99] $GABA_A$ receptor agonism, especially by barbiturates, most effectively prevents and terminates methylxanthine-induced seizures. Phenytoin not only is ineffective in treating theophylline-induced seizures but actually increases likelihood of seizures and mortality.[10]

Like phenytoin, carbamazepine's major anticonvulsant effect results from Na^+ channel blockade. Unlike phenytoin, carbamazepine appears to antagonize A_1 receptors.[25,29] This may explain the higher frequency of

TABLE 10–12. AGENTS AFFECTING ADENOSINE AND RECEPTORS

Adenosine Agonism	*Inhibit ADA*
Inhibit uptake	Acadesine
Acadesine	Dipyridamole
Benzodiazepines	Pentostatin
Carbamazepine	*Inhibit AK*
Dipyridamole	Acadesine
Flumazenil	***Adenosine Antagonism***
Indomethacin	*A_1 blockade*
Nifedipine	Caffeine
Nimodipine	Carbamazepine
Nitrendipine	Theophylline
Papaverine	*A_2 blockade*
Propentofylline	Caffeine
Verapamil	Theophylline

ADA = adenosine deaminase; AK = adenosine kinase.

seizures after carbamazepine overdose than after phenytoin overdose. The absence of A_2 blockade by carbamazepine theoretically allows for increases in cerebral blood flow to meet metabolic demands of the seizing brain.

References

1. Akahane K, Sekiguchi M, Une T, Osada Y: Structure-epileptogenicity relationship of quinolones with special reference to their interaction with gamma-aminobutyric acid receptor sites. Antimicrob Agents Chemother 1989;33:1704–1708.
2. Albertson TE, Walby WF, Joy RM: Modification of GABA-mediated inhibition by various injectable anesthetics. Anesthesiology 1992;77:488–499.
3. Aprison MH, Lipkowitz KB, Simon JR: Identification of a glycine-like fragment on the strychnine molecule. J Neurosci Res 1987;17:209–213.
4. Apud JA: The 5-HT3 receptor in mammalian brain: A new target for the development of psychotropic drugs? Neuropsychopharmacology 1993;8:117–130.
5. Arya DK: Extrapyramidal symptoms with selective serotonin reuptake inhibitors. Br J Psychiatry 1994;165: 728–733.
6. Baba A, Cooper JR: The action of black widow spider venom on cholinergic mechanisms in synaptosomes. J Neurochem 1980;34:1369–1379.
7. Bem JL, Peck R: Dextromethorphan: An overview of safety issues. Drug Saf 1992;7:190–199.
8. Bettler B, Mulle C: AMPA and kainate receptors. Neuropharmacology 1995;34:123–139.
9. Betz H, Schmitt B, Becker CM, et al: The vertebrate glycine receptor protein. Biochem Soc Symp 1986;52: 57–63.
10. Blake KV, Massey KL, Hendeles L, et al: Relative efficacy of phenytoin and phenobarbital for the prevention of theophylline-induced seizures in mice. Ann Emerg Med 1988;17:1024–1028.
11. Blier P, de Montigny C, Chaput Y: A role for the serotonin system in the mechanism of action of antidepressant treatments: Preclinical evidence. J Clin Psychiatry 1990;51(suppl 4):14–20.
12. Bonanno G, Raiteri M: Multiple $GABA_B$ receptors. Trends Pharmacol Sci 1993;14:259–261.
13. Bormann J, Hamill OP, Sakmann B: Mechanism of anion permeation through channels gated by glycine and gamma-aminobutyric acid in mouse cultured spinal neurones. J Physiol (Lond) 1987;385:243–286.
14. Bourne HR, Sanders DA, McCormick F: The GTPase superfamily: Conserved structure and molecular mechanism. Nature 1991;349:117–127.
15. Bowery NG, Pratt GD: $GABA_B$ receptors as targets for drug action. Arzneimittelforschung 1992;42:215–223.
16. Briscoe JG, Curry SC, Gerkin RD, Ruiz RR: Pemoline-induced choreoathetosis and rhabdomyolysis. Med Toxicol Adverse Drug Exp 1988;3:72–76.
17. Browne B, Linter S: Monoamine oxidase inhibitors and narcotic analgesics: A critical review of the implications for treatment. Br J Psychiatry 1987;151:210–212.
18. Burnstock G: Current state of purinoceptor research. Pharm Acta Helv 1995;69:231–242.
19. Bylund DB: Subtypes of $alpha_1$- and $alpha_2$-adrenergic receptors. FASEB J 1992;6:832–839.
20. Carmichael FJ, Orrego H, Israel Y: Acetate-induced adenosine mediated effects of ethanol. Alcohol Alcohol Suppl 1993;2:411–418.
21. Carpenter CL, Marks SS, Watson DL, Greenberg DA: Dextromethorphan and dextrorphan as calcium channel antagonists. Brain Res 1988;439:372–375.
22. Cash CD: Gammahydroxybutyrate: An overview of the pros and cons for it being a neurotransmitter and/or a useful therapeutic agent. Neurosci Behav Rev 1994;18: 291–304.
23. Bloom FE: Neurotransmission and the central nervous system. In: Hardman JG, Limbird LE, Molinoff PB, Ruddon RW, Gilman AG, eds: The Pharmacological Basis of Therapeutics, 9th ed. McGraw-Hill, New York, 1995, pp. 267–293.
24. Clapham DE: Direct G protein activation of ion channels? Annu Rev Neurosci 1994;17:441–464.
25. Clark M, Post RM: Carbamazepine, but not caffeine, is highly selective for adenosine A_1 binding sites. Eur J Pharmacol 1989;164:399–401.
26. Clark RF, Curry SC: Organophosphates and carbamates. In: Reisdorff EJ, Roberts MR, Wiegenstein JG, eds: Pediatric Emergency Medicine. Philadelphia, Saunders, 1993, pp. 684–693.
27. Clements MR, Hamilton DV, Siklos P: Thyrotoxicosis presenting with choreoathetosis and severe myopathy. J R Soc Med 1981;74:459–460.
28. Couratier P, Hugon J, Sindou P, et al: Cell culture evidence for neuronal degeneration in amyotrophic lateral sclerosis being linked to glutamate AMPA/kainate receptors. Lancet 1993;341:265–268.
29. Czuczwar SJ, Szczepanik B, Wamil A, et al: Differential effects of agents enhancing purinergic transmission upon the antielectroshock efficacy of carbamazepine, diphenylhydantoin, diazepam, phenobarbital, and valproate in mice. J Neural Trans Gen Sect 1990;81:153–166.
30. Dagani F, D'Angelo E: Glutamate metabolism, release, and quantal transmission at central excitatory synapses: Implications for neural plasticity. Funct Neurol 1992;7: 315–336.
31. Dakshinamurti K, Sharma SK, Sundaram M: Domoic acid induced seizure activity in rats. Neurosci Lett 1991;127: 193–197.
32. Deckert J, Gleiter CH: Adenosine—An endogenous neuroprotective metabolite and neuromodulator. J Neural Transm Suppl 1994;43:23–31.
33. Diamond I, Gordon AS: The role of adenosine in mediating cellular and molecular responses to ethanol. EXS 1994;71:175–183.
34. Doble A: Excitatory amino acid receptors and neurodegeneration. Therapie 1995;50:319–337.
35. Dominiak P: Historic aspects in the identification of the I_1 receptor and the pharmacology of imidazolines. Cardiovasc Drugs Ther 1994;8(suppl):21–26.
36. Dubovsky SL, Thomas M: Beyond specificity: Effects of

serotonin and serotonergic treatments on psychobiological dysfunction. J Psychosom Res 1995;39:429–444.
37. Eldridge FL, Paydarfar D, Scott SC, Dowell RT: Role of endogenous adenosine in recurrent generalized seizures. Exp Neurol 1989;103:179–185.
38. Emorine LJ, Feve B, Pairault J, et al: Structural basis for functional diversity of beta$_1$-, beta$_2$- and beta$_3$-adrenergic receptors. Biochem Pharmacol 1991;41:853–859.
39. Eneanya DI, Bianchine JR, Duran DO, Andresen BD: The actions and metabolic fate of disulfiram. Annu Rev Pharmacol Toxicol 1981;21:575–596.
40. Ernsberger P, Haxhiu MA, Graff LM, et al: A novel mechanism of action for hypertension control: Moxonidine as a selective I$_1$-imidazoline agonist. Cardiovas Drugs Ther 1994;8 (suppl):27–41.
41. Faingold CL, Browning RA: Mechanisms of anticonvulsant drug action. I. Drugs primarily used for generalized tonic-clonic and partial epilepsies. Eur J Pediatr 1987; 146:8–14.
42. Figg WD, Graham CL, Hak LJ, Dukes GE: Ondansetron: A novel antiemetic agent. South Med J 1993;86:497–502.
43. Fredholm BB, Duner-Engstrom M, Fastbom J, et al: Role of G proteins, cyclic AMP, and ion channels in the inhibition of transmitter release by adenosine. Ann NY Acad Sci 1990;604:276–288.
44. Fujimoto M, Munakata M, Akaike N: Dual mechanisms of GABA$_A$ response inhibition by β-lactam antibiotics in the pyramidal neurones of the rat cerebral cortex. Br J Pharmacol 1995;116:3014–3020.
45. Gavish M: Hormonal regulation of peripheral-type benzodiazepine receptors. J Steroid Biochem Mol Biol 1995; 53:57–59.
46. Gee KW, McCauley LD, Lan NC: A putative receptor for neurosteroids on the GABA$_A$ receptor complex: The pharmacological properties and therapeutic potential of epalons. Crit Rev Neurobiol 1995;9:207–227.
47. Giacobino JP: β$_3$-Adrenoceptor: An update. Eur J Endocrinol 1995;132:377–385.
48. Glennon RA, Darmani NA, Martin BR: Multiple populations of serotonin receptors may modulate the behavioral effects of serotonergic agents. Life Sci 1991;48:2493–2498.
49. Graham D, Langer SZ: Advances in sodium-ion coupled biogenic amine transporters. Life Sci 1992;51:631–645.
50. Halliwell RF, Davey PG, Lambert JJ: Antagonism of GABA$_A$ receptors by 4-quinolones. J Antimicrob Chemother 1993;31:457–462.
51. Hamilton CA: The role of imidazoline receptors in blood pressure regulation. Pharmacol Ther 1992;54:231–248.
52. Harrington MA, Zhong P, Garlow SJ, Ciaranello RD: Molecular biology of serotonin receptors. J Clin Psychiatry 1992;53 (suppl 10):8–27.
53. Hawgood B, Bon C: Snake venom presynaptic toxins. In: Tu AT, ed: Reptile Venoms and Toxins: Handbook of Natural Toxins, Vol. 5. New York, Marcel Dekker, 1991, pp. 3–52.
54. Hechler V, Peter P, Gobaille S, et al: γ-Hydroxybutyrate ligands possess antidopaminergic and neuroleptic-like activities. J Pharmacol Exp Ther 1993;264:1406–1414.
55. Hoffman PL, Grant KA, Snell LD, et al: NMDA receptors: Role in ethanol withdrawal seizures. Ann NY Acad Sci 1992;654:52–60.
56. Huttunen M: The evolution of the serotonin-dopamine antagonist concept. J Clin Psychopharmacol 1995;15 (suppl 1):4S–10S.
57. Insel PA: Adrenergic receptors—Evolving concepts and clinical implications. N Engl J Med 1996;334:580–585.
58. Jakobs C, Bojasch M, Monch M, et al: Urinary excretion of gamma-hydroxybutyric acid in a patient with neurological abnormalities. The probability of a new inborn error of metabolism. Clin Chim Acta 1981;111:169–178.
59. Johnston GA: GABA$_C$ receptors: Relatively simple transmitter-gated ion channels. Trends Pharmacol Sci 1996;17: 319–323.
60. Joy RM, Albertson TE: In vivo assessment of the importance of GABA in convulsant and anticonvulsant drug action. Epilepsy Res 1992;8(suppl):63–75.
61. Kamei J, Mori T, Igarashi H, Kasuya Y: Serotonin release in nucleus of the solitary tract and its modulation by antitussive drugs. Res Commun Chem Pathol Pharmacol 1992;76:371–374.
62. Kandel ER, Schwartz JH, Jessell TM, eds: Principles of Neural Science, 3rd ed. New York, Elsevier, 1991.
63. Kiowski W, Hulthen UL, Ritz R, Buhler FR: α_2 Adrenoceptor-mediated vasoconstriction of arteries. Clin Pharmacol Ther 1983;34:565–569.
64. Klawans HL, Weiner WJ: The pharmacology of choreatic movement disorders. Prog Neurobiol 1976;6:49–80.
65. Krogsgaard-Larsen P, Hansen J: Naturally-occurring excitatory amino acids as neurotoxins and leads in drug design. Toxicol Lett 1992;64/65:409–416.
66. Krueger KE, Papadapoulos V: Mitochondrial benzodiazepine receptors and the regulation of steroid biosynthesis. Annu Rev Pharmacol Toxicol 1992;32:211–237.
67. Landis E, Shore E: Yohimbine-induced bronchospasm. Chest 1989;96:1424.
68. Leeson PD, Iversen LL: The glycine site on the NMDA receptor: Structure-activity relationships and therapeutic potential. J Med Chem 1994;37:4053–4067.
69. Lin LH, Whiting P, Harris RA: Molecular determinants of general anesthetic action: Role of GABA$_A$ receptor structure. J Neurochem 1993;60:1548–1553.
70. Linden CH, Vellman WP, Rumack B: Yohimbine: A new street drug. Ann Emerg Med 1985;14:1002–1004.
71. Lowe TL, Cohen DJ, Detlor J, et al: Stimulant medications precipitate Tourette's syndrome. JAMA 1982;247: 1168–1169.
72. Lummis SC, Buckingham SD, Rauh JJ, Sattelle DB: Blocking actions of heptachlor at an insect central nervous system GABA receptor. Proc R Soc Lond [Biol] 1990; 240:97–106.
73. Lynch JW, Rajendra S, Barry PH, Schofield PR: Mutations affecting the glycine receptor agonist transduction mechanism convert the competitive antagonist, picrotoxin, into an allosteric potentiator. J Biol Chem 1995;270: 13799–13806.
74. Lefkowitz RJ, Hoffman BB, Taylor P: The autonomic and somatic motor nervous systems. In: Hardman JG, Limbird LE, Molinoff PB, Ruddon RW, Gilman AG, eds: The

Pharmacological Basis of Therapeutics, 9th ed. McGraw-Hill, New York, 1995, pp. 105–139.

75. Malatynska E, Knapp RJ, Ikeda M, Yamamura HI: Antidepressants and seizure-interactions at the GABA-receptor chloride-ionophore complex. Life Sci 1988;43:303–307.
76. Mamelak M: Gammahydroxybutyrate: An endogenous regulator of energy metabolism. Neurosci Biobehav Rev 1989;13:187–198.
77. Mascia MP, Mihic SJ, Valenzuela CF: A single amino acid determines differences in ethanol actions on strychnine-sensitive glycine receptors. Mol Pharmacol 1996;50: 402–406.
78. McDaniel KD: Clinical pharmacology of monoamine oxidase inhibitors. Clin Neuropharmacol 1986;9:207–234.
79. McKernan RM, Whiting PJ: Which $GABA_A$-receptor subtypes really occur in the brain? Trends Neurosci 1996; 19:139–143.
80. Miller J, Robinson A, Percy AK: Acute isoniazid poisoning in childhood. Am J Dis Child 1980;134:290–292.
81. Mills KC: Serotonin syndrome. Am Fam Physician 1995;52:1475–1482.
82. Modell JG, Tandon R, Beresford TP: Dopaminergic activity of the antimuscarinic antiparkinsonian agents. J Clin Psychopharmacol 1989;9:347–351.
83. Mott DD, Lewis DV: The pharmacology and function of central $GABA_B$ receptors. Int Rev Neurobiol 1994;36: 97–223.
84. Muller CE, Scior T: Adenosine receptors and their modulators. Pharm Acta Helv 1993;68:77–111.
85. Nilsson M, Hansson E, Rohnback L: Transport of valproate and its effects on GABA uptake in astroglial primary culture. Neurochem Res 1990;15:763–767.
86. Oja SS, Kontro P: Neurochemical aspects of amino acid transmitters and modulators. Med Biol 1987;65:143–152.
87. Olsen RW: The GABA postsynaptic membrane receptor-ionophore complex. Mol Cell Biochem 1981;39:261–279.
88. Parini A, Moundanos CG, Pizzinat N, Lanier SM: The elusive family of imidazoline binding sites. Trends Pharmacol Sci 1996;17:13–16.
89. Palmer T: Agents acting at the neuromuscular junction and autonomic ganglia. In: Hardman JG, Limbird LE, Molinoff PB, Ruddon RW, Gilman AG, eds: The Pharmacological Basis of Therapeutics, 9th ed. McGraw-Hill, New York, 1995, pp. 177–197.
90. Parkinson FE, Rudophi KA, Fredholm BB: Propentofylline: A nucleoside transport inhibitor with neuroprotective effects in cerebral ischemia. Gen Pharmacol 1994; 25:1053–1058.
91. Peduto VA, Concas A, Santoro G, et al: Biochemical and electrophysiologic evidence that propofol enhances GABAergic transmission in the rat brain. Anesthesiology 1991;75:1000–1009.
92. Pelleg A, Porter RS: The pharmacology of adenosine. Pharmacotherapy 1990;10:157–174.
93. Perl TM, Bedard L, Kosatsky T, et al: An outbreak of toxic encephalopathy caused by eating mussels contaminated with domoic acid. N Engl J Med 1990;322:1775–1780.
94. Peroutka SJ: VI. Serotonin receptor subtypes and neuropsychiatric diseases: Focus on $5\text{-}HT_{1D}$ and $5\text{-}HT_3$ receptors agents. Pharmacol Rev 1991;43:579–586.
95. Phillis JW, O'Regan MH: The role of adenosine in the central actions of the benzodiazepines. Prog Neuropsychopharmacol Biol Psychiatry 1988;12:389–404.
96. Picotti GB, Bondiolotti GP, Meldolesi J: Peripheral catecholamine release by alpha-latrotoxin in the rat. Naunyn Schmiedebergs Arch Pharmacol 1982;320:224–229.
97. Pin JP, Bockaert J: Get receptive to metabotropic glutamate receptors. Curr Opin Neurobiol 1995;5:342–349.
98. Pin JP, Duvoisin R: The metabotropic glutamate receptors: Structure and functions. Neuropharmacology 1995; 34:1–26.
99. Pinard E, Riche D, Puiroud S, Seylaz J: Theophylline reduces cerebral hyperaemia and enhances brain damage induced by seizures. Brain Res 1990;511:303–309.
100. Pucilowski O: Psychopharmacological properties of calcium channel inhibitors. Psychopharmacology (Berl) 1992; 109:12–29.
101. Rating D, Hanefeld F, Siemes H, et al: 4-Hydroxybutyric aciduria: A new inborn error of metabolism I. Clinical review. J Inherit Metab Dis 1984;7(suppl 1):90–92.
101a. Rho JM, Donevan SD, Rogawski MA: Barbiturate-like actions of the propanediol dicarbamates felbamate and meprobamate. J Pharmacol Exp Ther 1997;280:1383–1391.
102. Rock DM, Macdonald RL: Polyamine regulation of *N*-methyl-*d*-aspartate receptor channels. Annu Rev Pharmacol Toxicol 1995;35:463–482.
103. Rogawski MA: The NMDA receptor, NMDA antagonists and epilepsy therapy. Drugs 1992;44:279–292.
104. Roth BL: Multiple serotonin receptors: clinical and experimental aspects. Ann Clin Psychiatry 1994;6:67–78.
105. Rudorfer MV, Potter WZ: Antidepressants: A comparative review of the clinical pharmacology and therapeutic use of the "newer" versus the "older" drugs. Drugs 1989;37: 713–738.
106. Sannajust F, Head GA: Involvement of imidazoline-preferring receptors in regulation of sympathetic tone. Am J Cardiol 1994;74:7A–19A.
107. Saxena PR: Serotonin receptors: Subtypes, functional responses and therapeutic relevance. Pharmacol Ther 1995; 66:339–368.
108. Scholz KP: Introductory perspective. In: Dunwiddie TV, Lovinger DM, eds: Presynaptic Receptors in the Mammalian Brain. Birkhauser, Boston, 1993, pp. 1–11.
109. Seeman P, Van Tol HM: Dopamine receptor pharmacology. Trends Pharmacol Sci 1994;15:264–270.
110. Segev S, Rehavi M, Rubinstein E: Quinolones, theophylline, and diclofenac interactions with the gamma-aminobutyric acid receptor. Antimicrob Agents Chemother 1988;32:1624–1626.
111. Selden BS, Curry SC: Anticholinergics. In: Reisdorff EJ, Roberts MR, Wiegenstein JG, eds: Pediatric Emergency Medicine. Philadelphia, Saunders, 1993, pp. 693–700.
112. Shefner SA, Osmanovic SS: $GABA_A$ and $GABA_B$ receptors and the ionic mechanism mediating their effects of locus coeruleus neurons. Prog Brain Res 1991; 88:187–195.
113. Sieghart W: Pharmacology of benzodiazepine receptors: An update. J Psychiatr Neurosci 1994;19:24–29.
114. Sieghart W: Structure and pharmacology of γ-aminobutyric $acid_A$ receptor subtypes. Pharmacol Rev 1995;47: 181–234.
115. Smith MJ: Abuse of the antiparkinson drugs: A review of the literature. J Clin Psychiatry 1980;41:351–354.

116. Sokoloff P, Schwartz JC: Novel dopamine receptors half a decade later. Trends Pharmacol Sci 1995;16:270–275.
117. Spencer PS, Nunn PB, Hugon J, et al: Guam amyotrophic lateral sclerosis-parkinsonism-dementia linked to a plant excitant neurotoxin. Science 1987;237:517–522.
118. Squires RF, Saederup E: Antidepressants and metabolites that block $GABA_A$ receptors coupled to 35S-*t*-butylbicyclophosphorothionate binding sites in rat brain. Brain Res 1988;441:15–22.
119. Sternbach H: The serotonin syndrome. Am J Psychiatry 1991;148:705–713.
120. Stewart GR, Zoromski CF, Price MT, et al: Domoic acid: A dementia-inducing excitotoxic food poison with kainic acid receptor specificity. Exp Neurol 1990;110:127–138.
121. Sulzer D, Maidment NT, Rayport S: Amphetamine and other weak bases act to promote reverse transport of dopamine in ventral midbrain neurons. J Neurochem 1993;60:527–535.
122. Sulzer D, Rayport S: Amphetamine and other psychostimulants reduce pH gradients in midbrain dopaminergic neurons and chromaffin granules: A mechanism of action. Neuron 1990;5:797–808.
123. Teitelbaum JS, Zatorre RJ, Carpenter S, et al: Neurologic sequelae of domoic acid intoxication due to the ingestion of contaminated mussels. N Engl J Med 1990;332: 1781–1787.
124. Thomas RJ: Excitatory amino acids in health and disease. J Am Geriatr Soc 1995;43:1279–1289.
125. Thornberg SA, Saklad SR: A review of NMDA receptors and the phencyclidine model of schizophrenia. Pharmacotherapy 1996;16:82–93.
126. Tortella FC, Ferkany JW, Pontecorvo MJ: Anticonvulsant effects of dextrorphan in rats, possible involvement in dextromethorphan-induced seizure protection. Life Sci 1988;42:2509–2514.
127. Tsuda A, Ito M, Kishi K, et al: Effect of penicillin on GABA-gated chloride ion influx. Neurochem Res 1994;19: 1–4.
128. Uhl GR: Neurotransmitter transporters (plus): A promising new gene family. Trends Neurosci 1992;15:265–268.
129. van Galen PJ, Stiles GL, Michaels G, Jacobson KA: Adenosine A_1 and A_2 receptors: Structure-function relationships. Med Res Rev 1992;12:423–471.
130. van Zwieten PA, Chalmers JP: Different types of centrally acting antihypertensives and their targets in the central nervous system. Cardiovasc Drugs Ther 1994;8:787–799.
131. Villalon CM, Terron JA, Ramirez-San Juan E, Saxena PR: 5-Hydroxytryptamine: Considerations about discovery, receptor classification and relevance to medical research. Arch Med Res 1995;26:331–344.
132. von Lubitz DK, Carter MF, Beenhakker M, Lin RC, Jacobson KA: Adenosine: A prototherapeutic concept in neurodegeneration. Ann NY Acad Sci 1995;765:163–178.
133. Wang TL, Hackam AS, Guggino WB, et al: A single amino acid in gamma-aminobutyric acid p1 receptors affects competitive and noncompetitive components of picrotoxin inhibition. Proc Natl Acad Sci USA 1995;92: 11751–11755.
134. Watt G, Theakston RDG, Hayes CG, et al: Positive response to edrophonium in patients with neurotoxic envenoming by cobras (*Naja naja philippinensis*). N Engl J Med 1986;315:1444–1448.
135. Whiting PJ, McKernan RM, Wafford KA: Structure and pharmacology of vertebrate $GABA_A$ receptor subtypes. Int Rev Neurobiol 1995;38:95–138.
136. Williams M: Purine nucleosides and nucleotides as central nervous system modulators. Adenosine as the prototypic paracrine neuroactive substance. Ann NY Acad Sci 1990;603:93–107.
137. Wood PL: The co-agonist concept: Is the NMDA-associated glycine receptor saturated in vivo? Life Sci 1995; 7:301–310.
138. Woodward RM, Polenzani L, Miledi R: Characterization of bicuculline/baclofen-insensitive gamma-aminobutyric acid receptors expressed in *Xenopus* oocytes. I. Effects of Cl^- channel inhibitors. Mol Pharmacol 1992;42:165–173.

CHAPTER 11

Pharmacokinetics and Toxicokinetics

Mary Ann Howland

Pharmacokinetics is the study of the behavior of drugs including absorption, distribution, metabolism, and excretion. Mathematical models and equations are used to describe and then to predict this behavior. Pharmacodynamics is the investigation of the relationship of drug concentration to clinical effect. Toxicokinetics is the study of the absorption, distribution, metabolism, and excretion of a xenobiotic under circumstances that produce toxicity or excessive exposure. Xenobiotics are foreign, natural, or man-made chemicals, including drugs, pesticides, environmental agents, and industrial agents.[28] Toxicodynamics is the study of the relationship of toxic concentrations of xenobiotics to clinical effect.

Humans with overdoses provide many challenges to the mathematical precision of toxicokinetics and toxicodynamics because many variables (dose, time of ingestion, presence of vomiting, etc) are often unknown. In contrast to the therapeutic setting, atypical solubility characteristics are noted and saturation of enzymatic processes occur. Alterations in enzymatic saturation and protein binding may lead to enhanced absorption (decreased first-pass effect), more free drug available in the serum due to saturation of plasma protein binding, or prolonged elimination due to saturation of hepatic enzymes or active tubular secretion. In addition, age, gender, genetics, chronopharmacokinetics, and the effects of being critically ill with poor organ perfusion all add to the lack of precision.[3,8,24,45,48] Poison management interventions may alter one or more kinetic parameters. There are numerous approaches to these obstacles that include obtaining historical information from the patient's family and friends, doing drug counts, procuring sequential serum concentrations during the toxic phases, and occasionally repeating a pharmacokinetic evaluation during therapeutic dosing of that same agent to obtain comparative data.

Toxicokinetic principles can, however, be applied to facilitate our understanding and to make certain gross predictions. These principles can help evaluate whether a certain antidote or extracorporeal method is appropriate for use, when the serum concentration might be expected to drop into the therapeutic range, what ingested dose might be considered potentially toxic, what the onset and duration of toxicity might be, and what the importance is of a specific serum concentration. With all of this in mind, the clinical status of the patient is paramount, and mathematical formulas and equations can never substitute for evaluating the patient! The goal of this chapter is to explain the principles, present the mathematics in a "user friendly" fashion,[53] and demonstrate the application of these principles and mathematics by way of examples and case illustrations.

Absorption

Absorption is defined as the process by which a xenobiotic enters the body. In order for an agent to cause an effect, it must reach the bloodstream and then be distributed to the site or sites of action. Both the rate (k_a) and extent of absorption (F) are measurable and important determinants of toxicity. The rate of absorption often predicts the onset of action, while the extent of absorption (bioavailability) often predicts the intensity of the effect.[22,23] Figure 11–1 depicts how changes in the rate of absorption may affect toxicity when the bioavailability is held constant versus how toxicity may be affected by changes in bioavailability when the rate of absorption is held constant.

The route by which the xenobiotic enters the body significantly affects both the rate and extent of absorp-

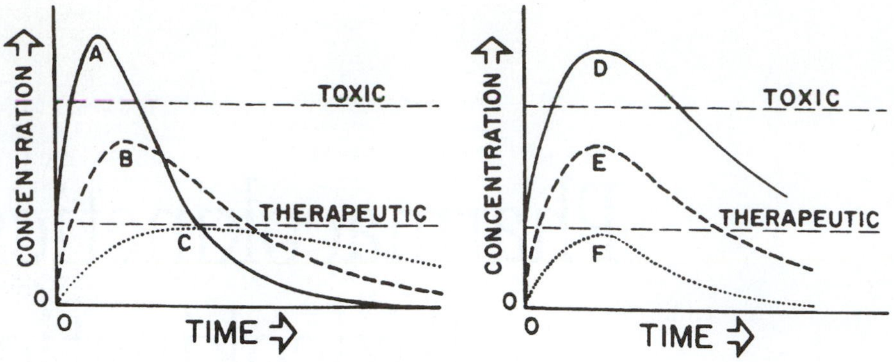

Figure 11–1. Effects of changes in k_a (rate of absorption) and *F* (bioavailability) on the blood concentration time graph and achieving a toxic threshold. In curves A, B, and C, *F* is constant as k_a is decreased. In curves D, E, and F, k_a is constant as *F* is decreased. *(Reprinted, with permission, from Riviere JE: Absorption and distribution. In: Hodgson E, Levi P, eds: Introduction to Biochemical Toxicology. Norwalk, CT, Appleton & Lange, 1994, p. 22.)*

tion. As an approximation, the rate of absorption proceeds in the following order from fastest to slowest: intravenous ≈ inhalation > intramuscular, subcutaneous, intranasal, oral > cutaneous, rectal. Following the oral administration of 200 mg of cocaine hydrochloride, the onset of action is 20 minutes, with an average peak concentration of 200 ng/mL.[47] This compares with smoking 200 mg of cocaine freebase, which has an onset of action of 8 seconds and a peak level of 640 ng/mL, or IV administration of 200 mg cocaine hydrochloride, which has an onset of action of 30 seconds and a peak level of 100 ng/mL.[47]

A xenobiotic must diffuse through a number of membranes before it can reach its site of action. Figure 11–2 shows the number of membranes through which a xenobiotic typically diffuses. Membranes are predominantly composed of phospholipids and cholesterol in addition to other lipid compounds.[33] A phospholipid is composed of a polar head and a fatty acid tail. Membranes are composed of the phospholipids arranged so that the fatty acid tails are inside and the polar heads face outward in a mirror image.[37] Proteins (in a 1:5 ratio with lipids) are found within and on the outside and may traverse the membrane.[33] Pores are found throughout the membrane. The principles relating to diffusion apply to absorption, distribution, certain aspects of elimination and to each instance when a xenobiotic is transported through a membrane.

Transport through membranes occurs via passive diffusion, filtration (the bulk flow with water through pores of small molecules with MW < 100), active transport or facilitated transport, and rarely endocytosis (see Fig. 11–3). Most xenobiotics transverse membranes via simple passive diffusion. The rate of diffusion is determined by Fick's Law of Diffusion. See Equation 11–1.

$$\text{Rate of diffusion} = \frac{dQ}{dt} = \frac{DAK(C_1 - C_2)}{h}$$

Where:
D = diffusion constant
A = surface area of the membrane
K = partition coefficient
h = membrane thickness
C_1-C_2 = difference in concentrations of the xenobiotic at each side of the membrane

(Eq. 11–1)

The driving force for passive diffusion is the difference in concentration of the xenobiotic on both sides of the membrane. *D* is a constant for each xenobiotic and derived when the differences in concentration between the two sides of the membrane is 1. The larger the surface area *A*, the higher the rate of diffusion. Most xenobiotics are absorbed faster in the small intestine compared to the stomach because of the tremendous surface area created by the presence of microvilli. The partition coefficient *K* represents the lipid to water partitioning of the xenobiotic. To a substantial degree, the more lipid soluble an agent, the more easily it crosses membranes.

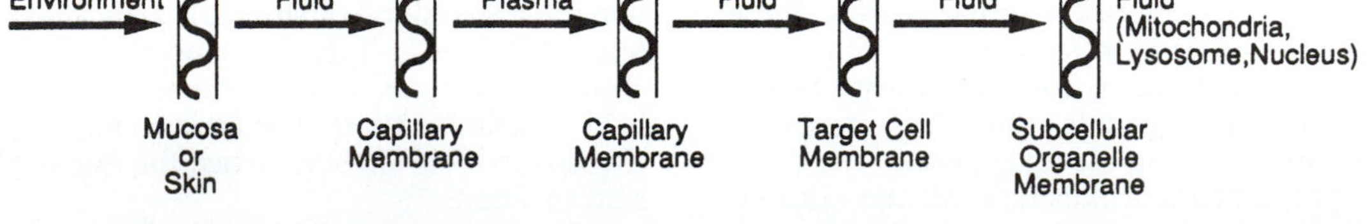

Figure 11–2. Illustration of the number of membranes encountered by a xenobiotic in the processes of absorption and distribution. *(Reprinted, with permission, from Riviere JE: Absorption and distribution. In: Hodgson E, Levi P, eds: Introduction to Biochemical Toxicology. Norwalk, CT, Appleton & Lange, 1994, p. 12.)*

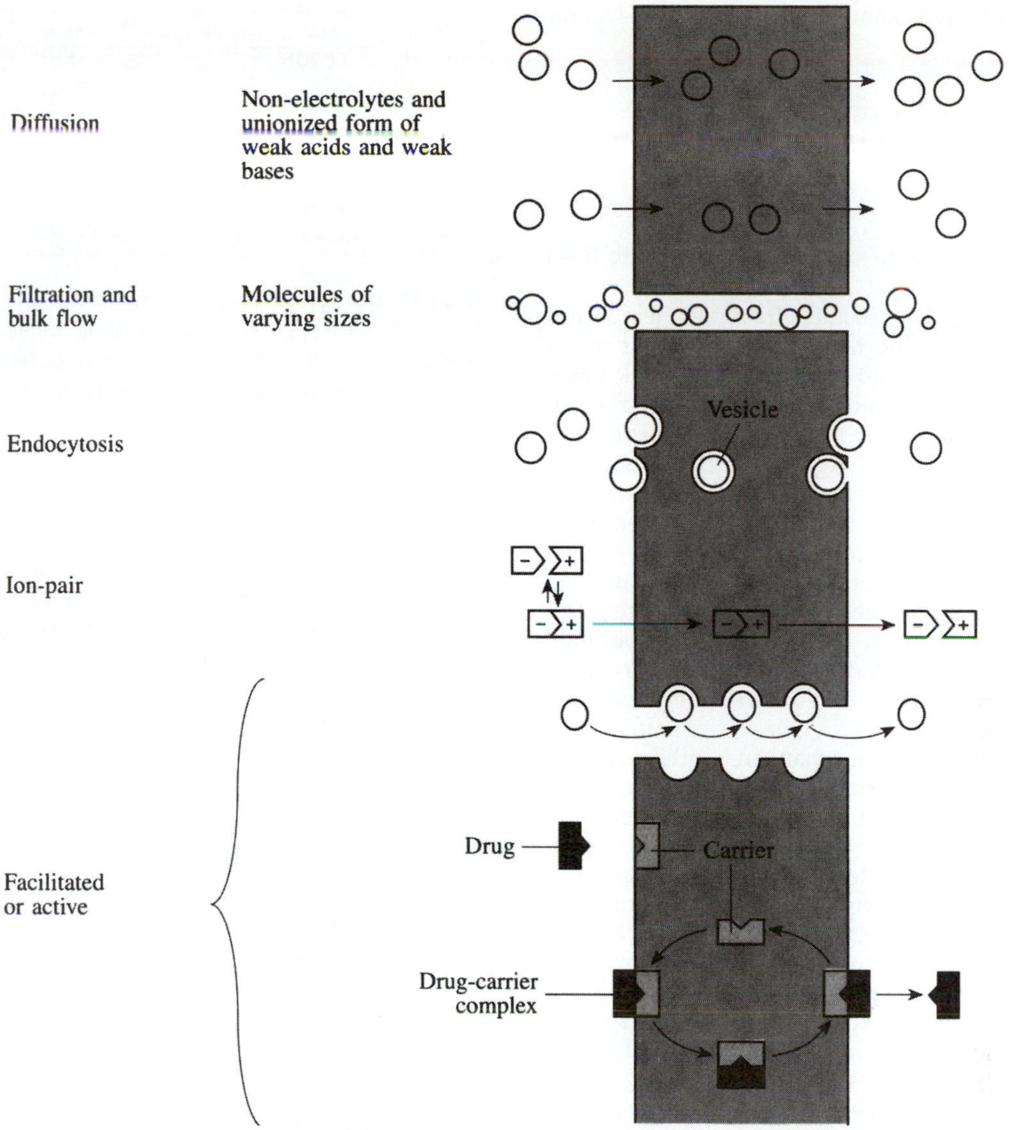

Figure 11–3. Illustration of transport mechanisms involved in the passage of xenobiotics across membranes. *(Reprinted, with permission, from Gram TE: Drug absorption and distribution. In: Craig CR, Stitzel RE, eds: Modern Pharmacology With Clinical Applications. Boston, Little, Brown, 1997, p. 17.)*

Membrane thickness (h) is inversely proportional to the rate at which a xenobiotic diffuses through the membrane. Xenobiotics that are uncharged, nonpolar, are of low molecular weight, and have sufficient lipid solubility have the highest rates of diffusion.

The extent of ionization of weak electrolytes (weak acids and weak bases) affects their rate of diffusion. Nonpolar and uncharged molecules penetrate faster. The Henderson-Hasselbalch relationship is used to determine the degree of ionization. An acid, by definition, gives up a hydrogen ion and a base accepts a hydrogen ion. $RCOOH(HA)$ and $RNH_3^+(BH^+)$ are acids and $RCOO^-(A^-)$ and $RNH_2(B)$ are bases. The equilibrium dissociation constant K_a can then be described by Equations 11–2A and 11–2B.

$$\text{For weak acids: } HA = H^+ + A^- \qquad Ka = \frac{[H^+]\,[A^-]}{[HA]}$$

(Eq. 11–2A)

$$\text{For weak bases: } BH^+ = B + H^+ \qquad Ka = \frac{[H^+]\,[B]}{[BH^+]}$$

(Eq. 11–2B)

In order to work with the numbers in a more comfortable fashion the negative log of both sides is determined and results in Equations 11–3A and 11–3B.

$$\text{For weak acids: } -\log Ka = -\log [H^+] - \frac{\log [A^-]}{[HA]}$$

(Eq. 11–3A)

$$\text{For weak bases: } -\log Ka = -\log [H^+] - \frac{\log [B]}{[BH^+]}$$

(Eq. 11–3B)

By definition the negative log of $[H^+]$ is expressed as pH and the negative log of K_a is pK_a. Rearranging the equations gives the familiar forms of the Henderson-

Hasselbalch equations as shown in Equations 11–4A and 11–4B.

$$\text{For weak acids: } pH = pKa + \frac{\log [A^-]}{[HA]} \quad \text{(Eq. 11–4A)}$$

$$\text{For weak bases: } pH = pKa + \frac{\log [B]}{[BH^+]} \quad \text{(Eq. 11–4B)}$$

Since noncharged molecules traverse membranes faster, it can be understood that weak acids cross membranes faster in an acidic environment and weak bases achieve the same result in a basic environment. In addition, when the pH equals the pK_a, half of the xenobiotic is charged and half is noncharged. The pH of selected body fluids is given in Table 11–1 and the extent of charged versus noncharged xenobiotic is represented in Figure 11–4 at different pH and pK_a values.

Lipid solubility and ionization both have a distinct influence on absorption. These characteristics are demonstrated in Figure 11–5 for three different xenobiotics. Although the three agents have similar pK_as their different partition coefficients result in different degrees of absorption from the stomach.

Specialized transport mechanisms either require energy to transport xenobiotics against a concentration gradient (active transport) or they can be non-energy requiring and lack the ability to transport against a concentration gradient (facilitated transport). These transport mechanisms are of importance in the renal and biliary systems. These same principles apply to a small number of lipid-insoluble molecules that resemble endogenous agents.[15,42] For example, 5-fluorouracil resembles pyrimidine and is transported by the same system, whereas thallium and lead are actively absorbed by endogenous transport mechanisms that normally absorb iron and calcium, respectively.[15] Filtration is generally considered to be unimportant for the absorption of most xenobiotics, but it is more important with regard to elimination. Endocytosis, where a cellular membrane encircles a xenobiotic, is responsible for the absorption of large macromolecules such as the oral Sabin polio vaccine.[42]

TABLE 11–1. pH OF SELECTED BODY FLUIDS

Fluids	pH
Gastric secretions	1.0–3.0
Small intestinal secretions: duodenum	5.0 to 6.0
Small intestinal secretions: ileum	8
Large intestinal secretions	8
Plasma	7.4
Cerebrospinal fluid	7.3
Urine	4.0–8.0

Reprinted, with permission, from Brody TM: Absorption, distribution, metabolism and elimination. In: Brody TM, Larner J, Minneman KP, Neu HC, eds: Human Pharmacology: Molecular to Clinical, 2nd ed. St. Louis, Mosby, 1994, p. 51.

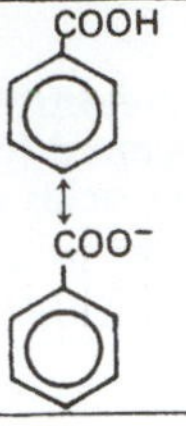

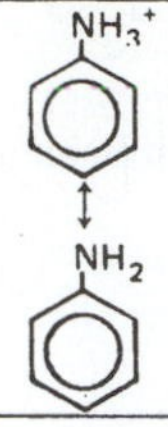

pH	Benzoic Acid % Nonionized	Aniline % Nonionized
1	99.9	
2	99	0.1
3	90	1
4	50	10
5	10	50
6	1	90
7	0.1	99

Figure 11–4. Effect of pH on the ionization of benzoic acid ($pK_a = 4$) and aniline ($pK_a = 5$). *(Reprinted, with permission, from Rozman KK, Klaassen CD: Absorption, distribution and excretion of toxicants. In: Klaassen CD, ed: Casarett & Doull's Toxicology: The Basic Science of Poisons. New York, McGraw-Hill, 1996, p. 93.)*

Numerous factors affect the gastrointestinal absorption of xenobiotics. These include xenobiotic-related characteristics such as dosage form, degree of ionization, and partition coefficient and patient factors such as gastrointestinal blood flow, gastrointestinal motility, and the presence or absence of food, ethanol, or other interfering substances. See Figure 11–6.

The formulation of a xenobiotic is extremely important in predicting GI absorption. Disintegration and dissolution must precede passive absorption. Sustained release (eg, calcium channel blockers) and enteric-coated (eg, ASA) formulations resist disintegration and delay the time to onset of effect. Dissolution is affected by ionization and the partition coefficient, as noted above. In the overdose setting the formation of concretions (eg, meprobamate) and bezoars (eg, bromide) significantly delay the time to onset of toxicity.[16,17] See Table 11–2.

Most xenobiotics are primarily absorbed in the small intestine due to the large surface area and extensive blood flow of the small intestines.[36] Critically ill patients who are hypotensive, have a reduced cardiac output, or are receiving vasoconstrictors such as norepinephrine will have a decreased perfusion of vital organs including the GI tract, kidney, and liver.[3] Not only will absorption be delayed, but elimination will also be diminished.[36] Extremely short gastrointestinal transit times will reduce absorption. This has been the unproven rationale for the use of cathartics and is currently the highly conceivable theoretical basis for the use of whole bowel irrigation. Anything that delays emptying of the stomach delays absorption due to delay in delivery to the small intestine. Delays in gastric emptying occur due to the presence of food, especially fatty meals, agents with anticholinergic (atropine, diphenhydramine, phenothiazines), opioid (methadone, morphine), or antiserotonergic (ondansetron) properties, ethanol, and any agent that results in pylorospasm (salicylates, iron).

Bioavailability is defined as the extent of absorption. See Equation 11–5. The fractional absorption (F) of a xenobiotic is defined by the area under the curve (AUC) of the designated route of absorption as compared to the AUC of the intravenous route. The plasma concentration versus time curve (AUC) for each route represents the amount absorbed.

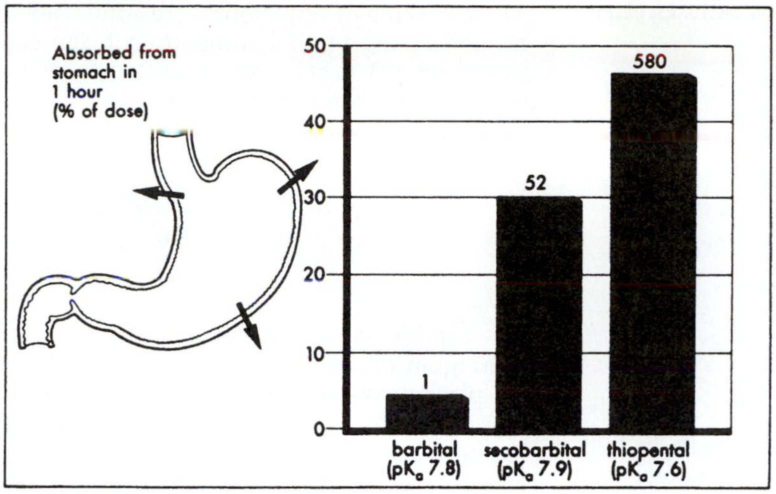

Figure 11–5. Influence of increasing lipid solubility on the amount of xenobiotic absorbed from the stomach for three xenobiotics with similar pK_a values. The number above each column is the oil/water equilibrium partition coefficient. *(Reprinted, with permission, from Brody T: Absorption, distribution, metabolism and elimination. In: Brody TM, Larner J, Minneman KP, Neu HP, eds: Human Pharmacology: Molecular to Clinical, 2nd ed. St. Louis, Mosby, 1994, p. 50.)*

$$F = \frac{(AUC)_{\text{route under study}}}{(AUC)_{IV}}$$

(Eq. 11–5)

Gastric emptying (orogastric lavage, syrup of ipecac) and activated charcoal are used to decrease the bioavailability of ingested xenobiotics. The oral administration of certain chelators (deferoxamine, *d*-penicillamine) actually enhances the bioavailability of the complexed xenobiotic, while some such as succimer have had no effect on the toxin's absorption.[18] The concept of creating a less soluble form of iron to inhibit absorption by administration of sodium bicarbonate has been studied, but shown to be ineffective.[7]

Presystemic elimination may decrease or increase the bioavailability of a xenobiotic. The GI tract contains microbial organisms that can metabolize or degrade xenobiotics such as penicillin by acid hydrolysis, digoxin and oral contraceptives by microbial metabolism, and insulin by peptidases.[33] However, in rare cases, gastrointestinal hydrolysis can convert a xenobiotic into a toxic metabolite such as amygdalin into cyanide, a metabolic step that does not occur with intravenous delivery.[14] Venous drainage from the stomach and intestine delivers orally administered xenobiotics directly to the liver via the portal vein and avoids direct delivery to the systemic circulation. This venous drainage is referred to as the first-pass effect.[2,50] The hepatic extraction ratio is the percentage of xenobiotic metabolized in one pass of blood through the liver.[32] Drugs that undergo significant first-pass metabolism (eg, propranolol, verapamil) are used at much lower IV doses than oral doses. Some drugs are not administered by the oral route because of significant first-pass effect (eg, lidocaine, nitroglyerin).[4] Sublingual administration of agents such as nitroglyerin bypasses the portal circulation and avoids first-pass metabolism. In the overdose setting, presystemic elimination may be saturated, leading to an increased bioavailability of xenobiotics such as cyclic antidepressants, phenothiazines, opioids, and many beta-adrenergic antagonists.[35] Hepatic metabolism usually transforms the xenobiotic into

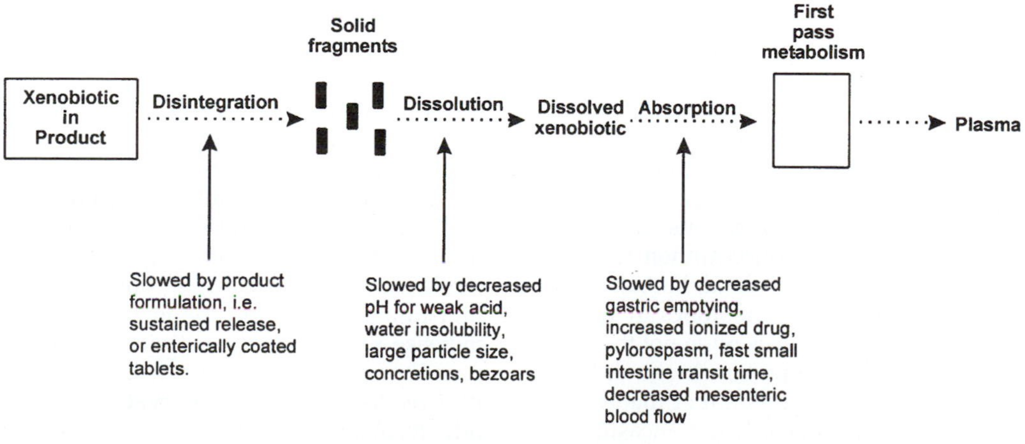

Figure 11–6. Determinants of absorption.

TABLE 11–2. DRUGS THAT COMMONLY FORM CONCRETIONS, BEZOARS, DELAY GASTRIC EMPTYING, AND/OR RESULT IN PYLOROSPASM

Anticholinergic agents
Barbiturates
Bromides
Enteric-coated tablets
Glutethimide
Iron
Meprobamate
Methaqualone
Opioids
Salicylates

a less active metabolite, but occasionally results in the formation of a more toxic agent such as parathion to paraoxon. Biliary excretion into the small intestine usually occurs for these transformed xenobiotics of molecular weights > 350 D (daltons) and may result in a xenobiotic appearing in the feces, although it has not been given orally.[20,33,44] Hepatic conjugated metabolites such as glucuronides may be hydrolyzed in the intestines to the parent or an active form to be reabsorbed through what is called the enterohepatic circulation (eg, nitrobenzene).[25,28,31,33] The enterohepatic circulation may result in a double-peak phenomenon with regard to a xenobiotic's availability.[42]

Distribution

Once the xenobiotic reaches the systemic circulation or central compartment, it is available for transport to peripheral tissue compartments. Both the rate and extent of distribution depend on many of the same principles discussed with regard to diffusion. Additional factors include affinity of the xenobiotic for plasma and tissue proteins, acid–base status of the patient (which affects ionization), and physiologic barriers to distribution (blood–brain barrier, placental transfer, blood–testis barrier).[11,21,37] Blood flow accounts for the initial phase of distribution, whereas xenobiotic affinities determine the final distribution pattern.

Volume of distribution (V_d) is the proportionality term used to relate the dose of the xenobiotic the individual receives and the resultant plasma concentration. Plasma and serum concentrations are used essentially interchangeably. When a reference or calculation is made with regard to a concentration in the body, it is actually a plasma concentration. When concentrations are measured in the laboratory, a serum concentration (clotted and centrifuged blood) is often determined. In reality the laboratory measurements of most xenobiotics in serum or plasma are nearly equivalent. This is often not the case for whole blood determination if the xenobiotic distributes into the erythrocyte. V_d is an apparent or theoretical volume into which drug distributes. It is a measure of how much drug is located inside and outside of the plasma compartment, since only the plasma compartment is assayed. In a 70-kg adult the plasma volume is 3 L. If 1000 mg of xenobiotic were administered and it remained in the plasma compartment, the concentration would be 333 mg/L and calculated by Equation 11–6, where S equals the percent pure drug if a salt form is used.

$$Vd = \frac{S \times F \times \text{Dose (mg)}}{C_0} \qquad \text{(Eq. 11–6)}$$

Experimental determination of a V_d involves administering an IV dose of the xenobiotic and extrapolating the plasma concentration time curve back to time zero (C_0). If the determination takes place after steady state has been achieved, the volume of distribution is then referred to as the V_{dss}. For many xenobiotics the V_d is already known and is available in the literature. See Table 11–3. When V_d is known and the dose ingested is known, a maximum plasma concentration can be predicted, assuming all of the xenobiotic is absorbed and no elimination has taken place. This assumption usually overestimates the plasma concentration. The V_d does not describe where the xenobiotic is distributed in the body. Distribution is complex, and differential affinities for various storage sites (plasma proteins, liver, kidney, fat, and bone) in the body determine where a xenobiotic resides. In a 70-kg person the total body water (TBW) is about 0.6 L/kg or 42 L. One thousand milligrams of a xenobiotic existing solely in TBW would have a plasma concentration of about 24 mg/L. A low V_d is often considered to be < 1 L/kg. For some xenobiotics such as digoxin (V_d = 5 L/kg) or the cyclic antidepressants (V_d = 10–15 L/kg), the V_d is much larger than the actual volume of the body. A large V_d indicates that the xenobiotic resides outside of the plasma compartment, but it does not describe the site of distribution.

The site of accumulation of a xenobiotic may or may not be its site of action or toxicity. If the site of accumulation is not its site of toxicity, then the storage depot may be inactive and the accumulation may be protective.[37] Selective accumulation of xenobiotics occurs in certain areas of the body because of affinity for certain tissue-binding proteins. The kidney contains metallothionein, which has a high affinity for metals such as cadmium, lead, and mercury.[11] The retina contains the pigment melanin, which binds and accumulates chlorpromazine, thioridazine, and chloroquine.[11] Other examples of xenobiotics accumulating in at least one primary site of toxicity are carbon monoxide combining with hemoglobin and paraquat distributing to the lungs.[34] DDT, chlordane, and polychlorinated biphenyls are stored in fat,[51] while lead is sequestered in bone. Lead in bone[19] is not immediately toxic, but mobilization of bone through an increase in osteoclastic activity[37] (hyperparathyroidism, possibly pregnancy) may distribute lead to sites of toxicity (soft tissues, blood). Starvation can mobilize xenobiotics from fat.

Several plasma proteins bind xenobiotics and act as carriers and storage depots. The percentage of protein binding varies as do the affinities and reversibility. Once

TABLE 11–3. PHARMACOKINETIC CHARACTERISTICS OF AGENTS ASSOCIATED WITH THE LARGEST NUMBER OF TOXICOLOGIC DEATHS

	Vd L/kg	Protein Binding %	Renal Elimination % Unchanged	Hepatic Metabolism % (CYP)	Active Metabolite	Enterohepatic
Analgesics						
Acetaminophen	0.8–1	5–20	2	95 (CYP2E1-3–8)	results in NAPQI	27–42% excreted in bile
Aspirin	0.15–0.2	50–80 (salicylic acid) saturable	10 (pH dependent)	Majority	Salicylic acid	None
Methadone	3.59	71–87	5–50	Yes	None?	Yes
Morphine	3–4	35	8.5–12	*n*-Demethylation	75% Morphine-6-glucuronide	Yes
Propoxyphene	12–26	80	<10	>90 (3A4)	Norpropoxyphene	Yes?
Antidepressants						
Amitriptyline	8.3±2	96	5	Yes (2C9)	Nortriptyline (2D6)	Yes
Desipramine	33–42	92	0.3–2.6	Yes (2D6)	None	Yes
Doxepin	20±8	—	0	Yes	Desmethyldoxepin	Yes
Imipramine	15±6	85	0–1.7	Yes (2D6)	Desipramine	Yes
Lithium	0.79	None	89–98	None	None	None
Cardiovascular Drugs						
Digoxin	5.1–7.4	20–25	57–80 in 6–12 hrs.		Minor amount	Yes
Diltiazem	5.3	70–80	1–3	60 deacetylated 35 other	Desacetyldiltiazem	No
Nifedipine	0.8–1.4	92–98	?	98 oxidation (3A4)	No	No
Propranolol	3.6	93	<0.5	>95 (2C19, 2D6)		No
Verapamil	4.7	83–92	?	97 dealkylated	Norverapamil	No
Stimulants and Drugs of Abuse						
Amphetamine	6.11 in drug dependent 3.5–4.6	16	45 (pH dependent)	50	Conjugated *p*-hydroxynorephedrine 0.3% Conjugated *p*-hydroxyamphetamine 2–4%	No
Cocaine	1.96–2.7	8.7	9.5–20 (pH dependent)	29–49	Norcocaine; (?) Others	No
Heroin	25	40	Minor		β-acetylmorphine 1.3% Morphine 4.2%	No
Methamphetamine	3.2–3.7	pH dependent			Amphetamine 4–7% *p*-hydroxymethamphetamine 15%	No
Sedative/Hypnotics						
Chloral hydrate	0.75	70–80	Minor	Alcohol dehydrogenase	Trichloroethanol	No
Phenobarbital	0.88	40–50	78–87 pH dependent	Yes	None	No
Alcohols						
Ethanol	0.5–0.6	None	Very little	95 alcohol dehydrogenase	Acetaldehyde	No
Ethylene glycol	0.6–0.8	None	20		Many (oxalic acid)	No
Methanol	0.6–0.7	None	3–5	95–80 alcohol dehydrogenase	Formic acid	No
Miscellaneous						
Cyanide	~0.4	~60	0		None	None
Theophylline	~0.5	50–60	7	90 (3A4) (2E1)	1,3 dimethyluric acid Caffeine (in neonates)	No
Organophosphates						
Malathion	?	None		Metabolized by microsomal enzymes		No
Chlorpyrifos	?	None		Yes	3,5,6-Trichloro-2-pyridonol	No
Rodenticides						
Brodifacoum	0.985 (rats)	None		Yes		No
Strychnine	13	None	10–20 24 h	Yes		No

bound to plasma protein, the xenobiotic is transported through the circulation. If binding affinity is very strong it will remain largely confined to the plasma until elimination occurs. However, dissociation and reassociation occur if another carrier is available with a higher binding affinity. Most plasma measurements of xenobiotic concentration reflect total drug (bound plus unbound). Only the unbound drug is free to diffuse through membranes for distribution or for elimination. Albumin binds primarily to weakly acidic, usually poorly water soluble, xenobiotics, which include salicylates, phenytoin, and warfarin. Alpha$_1$ acid glycoprotein (a globulin, MW 44,000 D) usually binds basic xenobiotics including lidocaine, imipramine, and propranolol.[40] Transferrin, a beta$_1$ globulin, transports iron, and ceruloplasmin carries copper.

Phenytoin is an example of a drug whose effects are significantly influenced by changes in concentration of plasma albumin. When albumin concentrations are in the normal range, approximately 90% of phenytoin is bound to albumin. As the albumin concentration decreases, however, more drug is free for distribution and a greater response to the same phenytoin dose is often observed. The actual plasma phenytoin concentration can be adjusted based on albumin concentrations to achieve an appropriate interpretation of free or unbound phenytoin within the conventional therapeutic range of 10–20 mg/L of free plus bound phenytoin. It is this free form of phenytoin that is active. See Equation 11–7.

$$\text{Adjusted phenytoin concentration} = \frac{\text{actual phenytoin concentration}}{\left(\frac{0.9 \times [\text{albumin}]}{4.4}\right) + 0.1} \qquad \text{(Eq. 11–7)}$$

The clinical implications are that a malnourished patient with an albumin of 2 g/dL receiving phenytoin can manifest toxicity with a plasma phenytoin concentration of 12 mg/L. This measurement is total phenytoin (bound + unbound). Since the patient has a reduced albumin concentration, this actually represents a substantially higher proportion and absolute amount of active unbound phenytoin. Substitution into the above equation of 12 mg/L for actual plasma phenytoin concentration and 2 g/dL for albumin gives an adjusted plasma phenytoin concentration of 23.86 mg/L (therapeutic range 10–20 mg/L).

Although drug interactions are often attributed to the displacement of xenobiotics, the significance is overestimated. Displacement transiently increases the amount of unbound drug , but this same drug is then available for elimination as well as distribution. Many of the instances where protein displacement was previously thought to be responsible for toxicity are now attributed to the simultaneously occurring inhibition of metabolism.[38]

Saturation of plasma proteins may occur in the therapeutic range for agents such as valproic acid. Acute saturation of plasma protein binding following an overdose often leads to consequential effects because of the large amounts encountered. Salicylates and iron are examples of xenobiotics where saturation of plasma protein binding in the overdose setting becomes an important factor increasing toxicity due to increased distribution to the CNS (salicylates) or to the liver, heart, and other tissues (iron).

Specific therapeutic maneuvers in the overdose setting are designed to alter the distribution by often simultaneously inactivating and or enhancing elimination of the xenobiotic to limit toxicity. These therapeutic maneuvers include (1) manipulation of pH to alkalinize plasma to keep the salicylate molecule charged and out of CNS while limiting renal reabsorption, (2) use of chelators (succimer, dimercaprol, and EDTA for lead), and (3) the use of antibody fragments (Digibind).

The V_d not only permits predictions about plasma concentrations but also assists in defining whether an extracorporeal method of removal is beneficial for a particular toxin. If the V_d is large (> 1 L/kg), it is unlikely that hemodialysis, hemoperfusion, or exchange transfusion would be effective since most of the xenobiotic resides outside of the plasma compartment. Plasma protein binding also influences this decision. If the xenobiotic is more tightly bound to plasma proteins than to activated charcoal, then hemoperfusion is unlikely to be beneficial even if the V_d is small. In addition, high plasma protein binding limits the effectiveness of hemodialysis, since only unbound xenobiotic will freely cross the dialysis membrane. Exchange transfusion can be effective for a xenobiotic with a small V_d and substantial plasma protein binding, because both bound and free xenobiotic are removed simultaneously.

Elimination

Removal of a parent compound from the body (elimination) begins as soon as the xenobiotic is delivered to clearance organs such as the liver, kidney, and lungs. Elimination begins immediately but may not be the predominant process until absorption and distribution are diminishing. As expected, the functional integrity of the major organ systems (cardiovascular, renal, hepatic) are major determinants of the efficiency of xenobiotic removal and of therapeutically administered antidotes. The xenobiotics themselves may cause renal or hepatic failure (ie, acetaminophen), subsequently limiting their own elimination. Other factors influencing elimination include age (enzyme maturation), competition or inhibition of elimination processes by interacting xenobiotics, saturation of enzymatic processes, gender, genetics, and the physiochemical properties of the xenobiotic.[26]

Elimination can be accomplished by metabolism (biotransformation) to one or more metabolites, or by excretion from the body of unchanged xenobiotic. Excretion can occur via the kidneys, lungs, feces, and body secretions (sweat, tears, milk). Hydrophilic (polar) xenobiotics and their metabolites are generally excreted via the kidney. The majority of metabolism occurs in the liver but can also take place in the blood or in other tissues (skin, GI tract, nasal mucosa, eye, placenta, or kidneys). Lipophilic (noncharged or nonpolar) xenobiotics are usually metabolized in the liver to hydrophilic metabolites. These metabolites are often inactive, but may be active and contribute to toxicity such as amitriptyline to nortriptyline, procainamide to *N*-acetylprocainamide, and meperidine to normeperidine, all of which are then excreted by the kidney[12,30] (see Table 11–4).

Metabolic reactions catalyzed by enzymes are generally divided into two categories called phase I and phase II. Phase I or preparative metabolism may or may not precede phase II and is responsible for introducing polar groups onto nonpolar xenobiotics by oxidation, reduction, and hydrolysis or by dealkylation to expose polar groups.[10,28] Phase II or synthetic reactions conjugate the polar group with glucuronide, sulfate, acetate (often a less polar metabolite, which is reabsorbed), methyl groups, glutathione (mercapturic acid synthesis), and amino acids (glycine, taurine, and glutamic acid).[6,10,28] Comparatively, phase II reactions produce a much larger increase in hydrophilicity than phase I reactions. The enzymes involved in these reactions have low substrate specificity, and those in the liver are usually localized to either the endoplasmic reticulum (microsomes) or the soluble fraction of the cytoplasm (cytosol).[28] The location of the enzymes becomes important if they form reactive metabolites that are then concentrated there and cause toxicity (see Table 11–5). Acetaminophen causes centrilobular necrosis because the cytochrome P450 2E1 isoenzymes, which form NAPQI, the toxic metabolite, are located there.

The enzymes that metabolize the largest variety (over 300 different substrates) of xenobiotics are heme-containing proteins referred to as cytochrome P450 monoxygenase enzymes.[15,28] These enzymes were formerly called the mixed function oxidase system and are found in abundance in the liver's microsomal endoplasmic reticulum. These enzymes catalyze the oxygenation of xenobiotics. They require oxygen and a cofactor, the NAD(P)H-containing flavoprotein, which acts as a source of electrons. In the reduced state (Fe^{2+}), cytochrome P450 binds oxygen or carbon monoxide. The discovery and initial name resulted from spectral identification of the CO-bound cytochrome P450, which binds light maximally at 450 nm. The cytochrome P450 system is composed of many enzymes grouped into families, subfamilies, and individual genes (over 20 isoenzymes) based on the similarity of their amino acid sequencing. Toxicity may result from induction or inhibition of cytochrome P450 isoenzymes by another xenobiotic, resulting in a consequential drug interaction (see Table 11–6). Many of these interactions are predictable based on the known xenobiotic affinities and their ability to induce or inhibit the system.[5,28,29,43] However, polymorphism (individual genetic expression of isoenzymes),[1] stereoisomer variability[49] (enantiomers with different potencies and isoenzyme affinities), and the ability of a xenobiotic's metabolism to be performed by alternate pathways contributes to unexpected outcomes.

TABLE 11–4. EXAMPLES OF XENOBIOTICS ACTIVATED BY HUMAN P450

CYP1A1	
	Benzo[*a*]pyrene and other polycyclic aromatic hydrocarbons
CYP1A2	
	Acetaminophen
	2-Acetylaminofluorene
	4-Aminobiphenyl
	2-Aminofluorene
	2-Naphthylamine
	NNK[a]
	Amino acid pyrolysis products
CYP2A6	
	N-Nitrosodiethylamine
	NNK[a]
CYP2B6	
	6-Aminochrysene
	Cyclophosphamide
	Ifosphamide
CYP2C 8, 9, 18, 19	
	None known
CYP2D6	
	NNK[a]
CYP2EI	
	Acetaminophen
	Acrylonitrile
	Benzene
	Carbon tetrachloride
	Chloroform
	Dichloromethane
	1,2-Dichloropropane
	Ethylene dibromide
	Ethylene dichloride
	Ethyl carbamate
	N-Nitrosodimethylamine
	Styrene
	Trichloroethylene
	Vinyl chloride
CYP3A4	
	Acetaminophen
	Aflatoxin B, and G,
	6-Aminochrysene
	Benzo[*a*]pyrene 7,8-dihydrodiol
	Cyclophosphamide
	Ifosphamide
	l-Nitropyrene
	Sterigmatocystin
	Senecionine
	Tris(2,3-dibromopropyl) phosphate
CYP4A9/11	
	None known

[a]NNK. 4-(methylnitrosamino)-1-(3-pyridyl)-*l*-butanone; a tobacco-specific nitrosamine.

Adapted from Guengerich, FP: Reactions and significance of cytochrome P450 enzymes. J Biol Chem 1991;266:10019–10022.

Reprinted, with permission, from Parkinson A: Biotransformation of xenobiotics. In: Klaassen C, ed: Casarett & Doull's Toxicology: The Basic Science of Poisons, 5th ed. New York, McGraw-Hill, 1996, p. 154.

TABLE 11–5. GENERAL PATHWAYS OF XENOBIOTIC BIOTRANSFORMATION AND THEIR MAJOR SUBCELLULAR LOCATION

Reaction	Enzyme	Localization
	Phase I	
Hydrolysis	Carboxylesterase	Microsomes cytosol
	Peptidase	Blood, lysosomes
	Epoxide hydrolase	Microsomes, cytosol
Reduction	Azo-and nitro-reduction	Microflora, microsomes, cytosol
	Carbonyl reduction	Cytosol
	Disulfide reduction	Cytosol
	Sulfoxide reduction	Cytosol
	Quinone reduction	Cytosol, microsomes
	Reductive dehalogenation	Microsomes
Oxidation	Alcohol dehydrogenase	Cytosol
	Aldehyde dehydrogenase	Mitochondria, cytosol
	Aldehyde oxidase	Cytosol
	Xanthine oxidase	Cytosol
	Monoamine oxidase	Mitochondria
	Diamine oxidase	Cytosol
	Prostaglandin H synthase	Microsomes
	Flavin-mono-oxygenases	Microsomes
	Cytochrome P450	Microsomes
	Phase II	
	Glucuronide conjugation	Microsomes
	Sulfate conjugation	Cytosol
	Glutathione conjugation	Cytosol, microsomes
	Amino acid conjugation	Mitochondria, microsomes
	Acylation	Mitochondria, cytosol
	Methylation	Cytosol

Reprinted, with permission, from Parkinson A: Biotransformation of xenobiotics. In: Klaassen CD, ed: Casarett & Doull's Toxicology: The Basic Science of Poisons, 5th ed. New York, McGraw-Hill, 1996, p. 114.

Excretion is primarily accomplished by the kidneys, although as mentioned earlier, biliary, pulmonary, and body fluid secretions contribute to lesser degrees. Urinary excretion occurs through glomerular filtration, tubular secretion, and passive tubular reabsorption. The glomerulus filters unbound xenobiotics of a particular size and shape in a nonsaturable way. Passive tubular reabsorption accounts for the reabsorption of noncharged, lipid-soluble xenobiotics and is therefore influenced by the pH of the urine and the pK_a of the xenobiotic. The principles of diffusion discussed above, for example, permit the ion trapping of salicylate (pK_a = 3.5) in the urine through urinary alkalinization. Tubular secretion is an active process subject to saturation and drug interactions (see Table 11–7). Tubular secretion is often less developed in the neonate.

Classical Versus Physiologic Compartment Toxicokinetics

Models have been developed to study the movement of xenobiotics in the body and to allow description of this movement with mathematical equations. Classical compartmental models (traditionally one or two compartments) are data based and assume that changes in plasma concentrations mirror tissues concentrations.[27] More recently, advances in computer technology have facilitated the utilization of concepts developed in the late 1930s.[46] Physiologically based models consider the movement of xenobiotics based on known or theorized biologic processes and have the advantages of being unique for each xenobiotic, allowing the prediction of tissue concentrations, incorporating the effects of changing physiologic parameters, and affording better extrapolation from laboratory animals.[53] Unfortunately, physiologic modeling is still in its infancy and the mathematical modeling is often exceedingly complex[9] (see Figs. 11–7, 11–8, and 11–9). The most commonly used mathematical equations are based on classical compartmental modeling and are explained and used in the following discussions.

The one-compartment model is the simplest for analytic purposes and is applied to xenobiotics that rapidly enter and distribute throughout the body. This model assumes that changes in plasma concentrations will result in and reflect proportional changes in tissue concentrations. Many xenobiotics do not instantaneously equilibrate with the tissues and are better described by a two-compartment model (ie, digoxin, lithium, lidocaine). In the two-compartment model, a xenobiotic is distributed instantaneously to highly perfused tissues (central compartment) and then is secondarily and more slowly distributed to a peripheral compartment. Elimination is assumed to take place from the central compartment.

The rate of a reaction is characterized by whether it is directly proportional to the concentration of xenobiotic. Many reactions are directly proportional and are termed first order or linear. Processes that are capacity limited or saturable are termed nonlinear (not proportional to the concentration of xenobiotic) and are described by the Michaelis-Menten equation, which is derived from enzyme kinetics.

Calculus is used to derive the first-order equation, but this need not be intimidating and is easily understood if explained in a stepwise fashion, as done by Yang and Andersen.[53]

Rate is directly proportional to concentration of xenobiotic as in Equation 11–8.

$$\text{Rate } \alpha \text{ Concentration (C)} \qquad \text{(Eq. 11–8)}$$

An infinitesimal change in concentration of a xenobiotic (dC) with respect to an infinitesimal change in time (d*t*) is directly proportional to the concentration (*C*) of the xenobiotic as in Equation 11–9.

$$\frac{dC}{dt} \ \alpha \ C \qquad \text{(Eq. 11–9)}$$

The proportionality constant *k* is added to the right side of the expression to mathematically allow the intro-

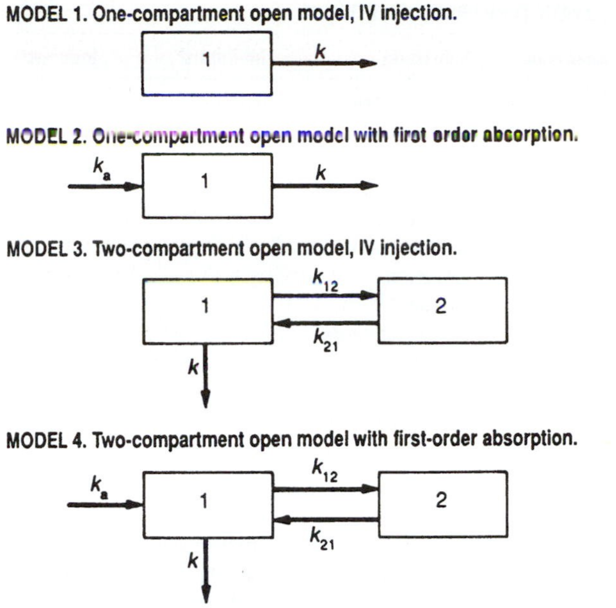

Figure 11–7. Various classical compartmental models. K = pharmacokinetic rate constants; 1 = plasma or central compartment; 2 = tissue compartment; K_{12} = rate constant into tissue from plasma; K_{21} = rate constant into plasma from tissue; K_a = absorption rate constant. *(Reprinted, with permission, from Shargel L, Yu A: Introduction to Pharmacokinetics: Applied Biopharmaceutics and Pharmacokinetics, 3rd ed. Norwalk, CT, Appleton & Lange, 1993, p. 40.)*

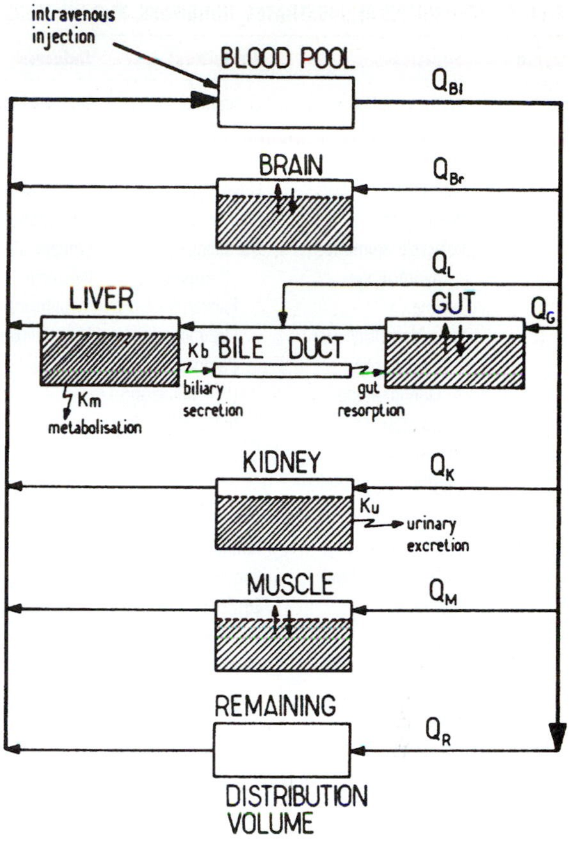

Figure 11–9. Illustration of a physiologic model specific for phenobarbital. Q = blood flow. *(Reprinted, with permission, from Engasser JM, Sarhan F, Falcoz C, et al: Distribution, metabolism and elimination of phenobarbital in rats: physiologically based pharmacokinetic model. J Pharmaceutical Sci 1981;70:1235.)*

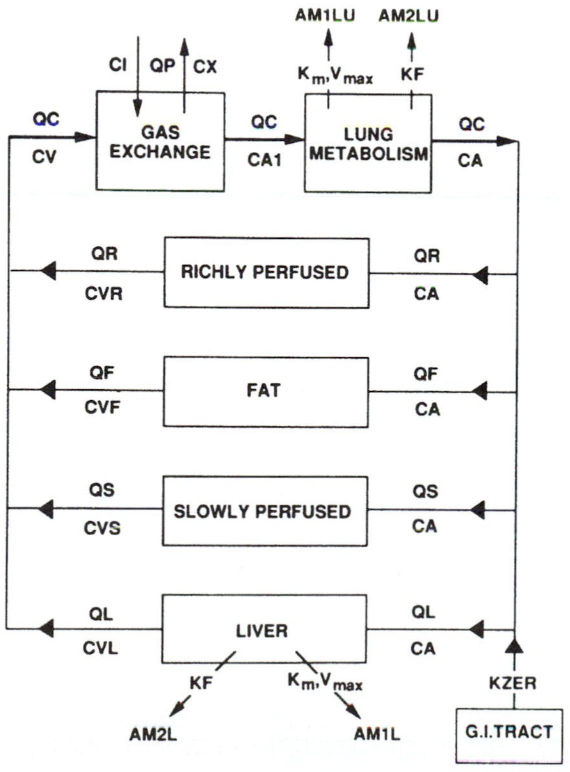

Figure 11–8. A graphical representation of a physiologically based pharmacokinetic model, where *C* equals the concentration of the xenobiotic, *Q* the flow rate, and the arrows indicate the movement of the xenobiotic. Additional details are found in the original article. CA = concentration in arterial blood; CV = concentration in mixed venous blood; AM 1(2)LU = amount metabolized in the lung; AM 1(2)L = amount metabolized in the liver. *(Reprinted, with permission, from Yang R, Andersen M: Pharmacokinetics. In: Hodgson E, Levi P, eds: Introduction to Biochemical Toxicology. Norwalk, CT, Appleton & Lange, 1994, p. 59.)*

TABLE 11–6. XENOBIOTICS AS SUBSTRATES, INHIBITORS, AND INDUCERS OF VARIOUS HEPATIC CYTOCHROME ISOENZYMES*

Isoenzyme	Substrates	Inhibitors[b]	Inducers[c]
CYP1A2	Acetaminophen Aromatic amines Caffeine Clozapine Phenacetin Polycyclic aromatic hydrocarbons Tacrine TCAs (demelthylation) Amitriptyline Clomipramine Imipramine Theophylline Triorthocresylphosphate R-warfarin	Cimetidine Diltiazem Erythromycin Fluvoxamine Mexiletine Quinolone antibiotics Enoxacin Ciprofloxacin Perfloxacin (NOT Ofloxacin or lomefloxacin)	Charcoal broiled foods Cigarette smoke (not pure nicotine) Omeprazole Piperonyl butoxide TCDD (dioxin)
CYP2C9[a]	Amitriptyline (demethylation) Diclofenac Ibuprofen Imipramine Phenytoin (4-OH) Piroxicam S-warfarin	Amiodarone Cimetidine Cotrimoxazole Fluconazole Metronidazole	Rifampin
CYP2C19[a]	Diazepam Impiramine Omeprazole Pentamidine Phenytoin Propranolol	Felbamale Fluoxetine Fluvoxamine Omeprazole Tranylcypromine	Rifampin
CYP2D6[a]	Amitriptyline Captopril Clomipramine Clozapine Codeine (to morphine) Debrisoquine Deprenyl Desipramine Dextromethorphan Encainide Flecainide Fluoxetine Haloperidol (reduced) Imipramine (OH) Metoprolol Mexiletine Nevirapine Nortriptyline (OH) Ondansetron Paroxetine Perphenazine Propafenone Propranolol (4-OH) Risperidone Thioridazine Venlafaxine	Amiodarone Fluoxetine Haloperidol Paroxetine Propafenone Quinidine (not quinine) Thioridazine Yohimbine	
CYP2E1	Acetaminophen Acrylonitrile Alcohols Aniline Benzene Caffeine Chloroform Dapsone Ethylene dibromide Halothane Isoniazid Theophylline Vinyl chloride	Disulfiram DMSO Fomepizole	Ethanol Isoniazid
CYP3A4 (previously known as nifedipine oxidase)	Acetaminophen Aflatoxin B_1 & G_1 Aldrin Amiodarone Astemizole Budesonide Carbamazepine Cisapride Cyclosporine Dapsone Delavirdine Diazepam Diltiazem Erythromycin Felodipine Indinavir Imipramine Lidocaine Losartin Lovastatin Midazolam Nevirapine Nifedipine Omeprazole Quinidine Saquinavir Tacrolimus Tamoxifen Taxol Terfenadine Theophylline Verapamil Warfarin	Cimetidine Clotrimazole Clarithromycin Diltiazem Erythromycin Fluconazole (large dose) Fluoxetine (norfluoxetine) Grapefruit juice (flavonoids) Itraconazole Ketoconazole Miconazole Nefazodone Omeprazole Propoxyphene (?) Quinidine	Carbamazepine Dexamethasone Glucocorticoids Nevirapine (auto) Phenobarbital Phenytoin Rifampin

*Refer to following page for table footnotes.

TABLE 11–7. XENOBIOTICS SECRETED BY RENAL TUBULES

Organic Anion Transport	Organic Cation Transport
Acetazolamide	Acetylcholine
Bile salts	Amiodarone
Cephalosporins	Atropine
Indomethacin	Cimetidine
Hydrochlorothiazide	Digoxin
Furosemide	Diltiazem
Methotrexate	Dopamine
Penicillin G	Epinephrine
Probenecid	Morphine
Prostaglandins	Neostigmine
Salicylate	Procainamide
	Quinidine
	Quinine
	Triamterene
	Trimethoprim
	Verapamil

duction of an equal sign. The constant k represents all of the bodily factors such as metabolism and excretion that contribute to the determination of concentration. See Equation 11–10.

$$\frac{dC}{dt} = kC$$

(Eq. 11–10)

Introducing a negative sign to the left-hand side of the equation describes the "decay" or decreasing xenobiotic concentration. See Equation 11–11.

$$-\frac{dC}{dt} = kC$$

(Eq. 11–11)

This equation is impractical because of the difficulty in measuring infinitesimal changes in C or t. Therefore, the use of calculus allows the integration or summing of all of the changes from one concentration to another beginning at time zero and going to time t. This is mathematically represented by the integration sign "∫". ∫ means to integrate the term from concentration at time zero (C_0) to concentration at a given time t (C_t). ∫ means the same with respect to time, where t_0 = zero. Before this application, the previous equation is first rearranged. See Equation 11–12.

$$-\frac{dC}{C} = kdt$$

$$\int_{C_0}^{C_t} -\frac{dC}{C} = k\int_{t_0}^{t} dt$$

(Eq. 11–12)

The integration of dC divided by C is the natural logarithm of C (ln C) and the integration of dt is t. See Equation 11–13.

$$-\ln C\Big|_{C_0}^{C_t} = kt\Big|_{t_0}^{t}$$

(Eq. 11–13)

[a]2C subfamily subject to polymorphism. Genetic factors are responsible for producing poor metabolizers (5–10% of North American population), normal metabolizers (vast majority), and fast metabolizers (very minor). Antipyrine is used experimentally to define the genotype of poor metabolizers.

[b]Inhibitors reduce the metabolism of substrates and lead to elevated blood levels of substrates. The onset for inhibition occurs quickly in contrast to induction. Inhibitors may or may not be substrates for the enzyme they inhibit (competitive), or they may be noncompetitive (mechanism based or suicidal).

[c]Administration of inducers causes the creation of quantitatively more enzymes that can metabolize substrates leading to reduced blood levels of substrates. Induction is dose dependent and time dependent. Time is required for increased synthesis of the enzyme (delaying onset) and time is required for the inducers to be eliminated. Cigarette smoking is known to have an effect on theophylline metabolism for as long as 4 mo after cessation. Inducers do not necessarily cause autoinduction.

This is not meant to be an exhaustive listing and is adapted from references 5, 28, 29, 43.

CYP	→	Cytochrome
Arabic numeral	→	Family
Capital letter	→	Subfamily
Arabic numeral	→	Individual gene
eg, CYP1A2		

The vertical straight lines dictate evaluating the terms between those two limits. The following series of manipulations are then performed. See Equation 11–14.

$$-(\ln C_t - \ln C_0) = k(t-0)$$

(Eq. 11–14A)

$$-\ln C_t + \ln C_0 = kt$$

(Eq. 11–14B)

$$-\ln C_t = -\ln C_0 + kt$$

(Eq. 11–14C)

$$\underset{\text{Can be measured}}{\ln C_t} = \underset{\text{Constant}}{\ln C_0} - \underset{\text{Can be selected}}{kt}$$

(Eq. 11–14D)

Equation 11–14D can be recognized as taking the form of an equation of a straight line (Equation 11–15), where the slope is equal to the rate constant k and the intercept is C_0.

$$y = b + mx$$

(Eq. 11–15)

Instead of working with natural logarithms, an exponential form (the antilog) of Equation 11–14D may be used. See Equation 11–16.

$$C_t = C_0 e^{-kt}$$

(Eq. 11–16)

Graphing the ln (natural logarithm) of the concentration of the xenobiotic at various times for a first-order reaction is a straight line. The above equation describes the events when there is only one first-order process occurring. This is appropriate for a one-compartment model (see Fig. 11–10).

In this model regardless of the concentration of the xenobiotic, the rate (percentage) of decline is constant. The absolute amount of xenobiotic eliminated changes continuously while the percent eliminated remains constant. k is reported in h^{-1}. A k of 0.10 h^{-1} means the xenobiotic is being processed (eliminated) at a rate of 10% per hour. k is often designated as k_e to refer to it as the elimination rate constant. The time it takes the xenobiotic concentration to be reduced by 50% is called the half-life. The half-life is determined by rearrangement of Equation 11–14D and let C_2 be the C at time t_2 and C_1 be the C at t_1 and rearrange to give Equation 11–17.

$$(t_1 - t_2) = \frac{(\ln C_1 - \ln C_2)}{k_e}$$

(Eq. 11–17)

Substitution of 2 for C_1 and 1 for C_2 or 100 for C_1 and 50 for C_2 gives Equations 11–18A and 11–18B.

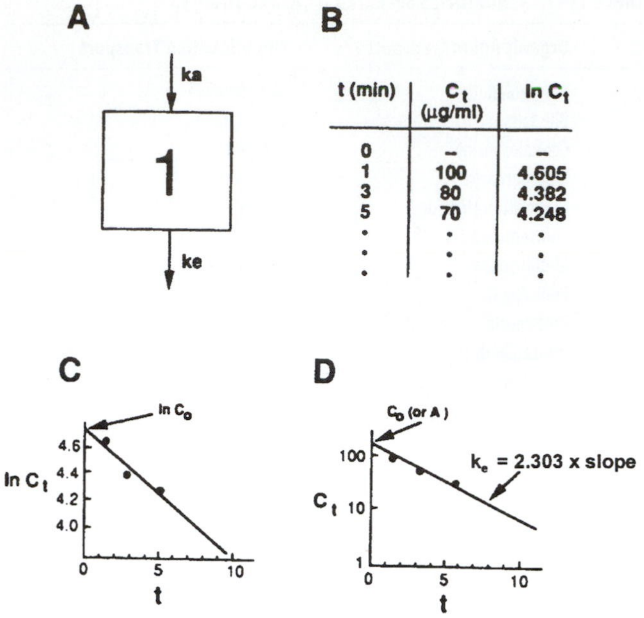

Figure 11–10. A one-compartment pharmacokinetic model demonstrating (**A**) Graphical illustration. (**B**) Hypothetical data set. (**C**) Linear plot. (**D**) Semilogarithmic plot. *(Modified and reprinted, with permission, from Yang R, Andersen M: Pharmacokinetics. In: Hodgson E, Levi P, eds: Introduction to Biochemical Toxicology. Norwalk, CT, Appleton & Lange, 1994, p. 54.)*

$$t_{1/2} = \frac{(\ln 2 - \ln 1)}{k_e}$$

(Eq. 11–18A)

$$t_{1/2} = \frac{0.693}{k_e}$$

(Eq. 11–18B)

The use of semilog paper facilitates graphing the first-order equation. However, semilog paper plots log (not ln) versus time. Therefore when using semilog paper, to keep the mathematics correct, the rate constant or slope (k) must be divided by 2.303 (see Fig. 11–10).

The mathematical modeling becomes more complex when more than one first-order process is contributing to the overall elimination process. The equation that incorporates two first-order rates is used for a two-compartment model and is Equation 11–19.

$$C_t = Ae^{-\alpha t} + Be^{-\beta t}$$

(Eq. 11–19)

Figure 11–11 demonstrates a two-compartment model. Alpha (α) often represents the distribution phase, while beta (β) is the elimination phase.

The rate of reaction of a saturable process is not linear (not proportional to the concentration of xenobiotic) when saturation occurs (see Fig. 11–12). It is best described by the Michaelis-Menten equation used in enzyme kinetics. See Equation 11–20.

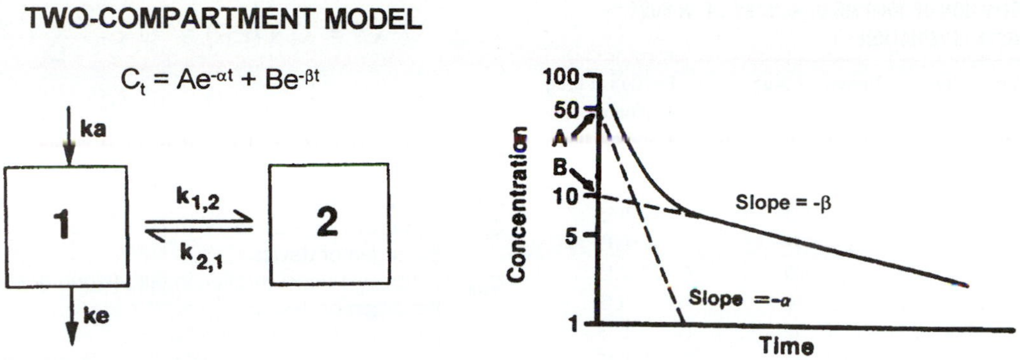

Figure 11–11. Mathematical and graphical forms of a two-compartment classical pharmacokinetic model. k_a represents the absorption rate constant, k_e represents the elimination rate constant, α represents the distribution phase, and β the elimination phase. *(Reprinted, with permission, from Yang R, Andersen M: Pharmacokinetics. In: Hodgson E, Levi P, eds: Introduction to Biochemical Toxicology. Norwalk, CT, Appleton & Lange, 1994, p. 55.)*

$$v = \frac{Vmax \times C}{Km + C}$$

(Eq. 11–20)

where v is the velocity or rate of the enzymatic reaction, C is the concentration of the xenobiotic, V_{max} is the maximum velocity of the reaction between the enzyme and the xenobiotic, and K_m is the affinity constant between the enzyme and the xenobiotic.[53]

Application of this equation to toxicokinetics requires v to become the infinitesimal change in concentration of a xenobiotic (dC) with respect to an infinitesimal change in time (dt) as previously discussed (see Equation 11–10), and V_{max} and K_m to represent the culmination of many biologic processes. The Michaelis-Menten equation then becomes Equation 11–21 where the negative sign again represents decay.

$$-\frac{dC}{dt} = \frac{Vmax \times C}{Km + C}$$

(Eq. 11–21)

When the concentration of the xenobiotic is very low ($C <<<<< K_m$), it can be dropped from the bottom right of the equation because its contribution becomes negligible. The resulting equation is then recognized as a first-order process. See Equations 11–22A and 11–22B. Conceptually this is understandable, since at a very low xenobiotic concentration the process is not saturated.

$$-\frac{dC}{dt} = \frac{Vmax \times C}{Km}$$

(Eq. 11–22A)

Since Vmax divided by Km is a constant, k

$$-\frac{dC}{dt} = kC$$

(Eq. 11–22B)

However, when the concentrations of the xenobiotic are extremely high and exceed the capacity of the system ($C >>>>> K_m$), the rate becomes fixed at a constant maximal rate regardless of the exact concentration of the xenobiotic. This is termed a zero-order reaction. Tables 11–8A and 11–8B compare a first-order reaction to a zero-order reaction. A half-life calculation on a xenobiotic displaying zero-order behavior is inappropriate since metabolic rates are continuously changing. Enzyme saturation is a common occurrence following overdose as the capacity of an enzyme system is overwhelmed.

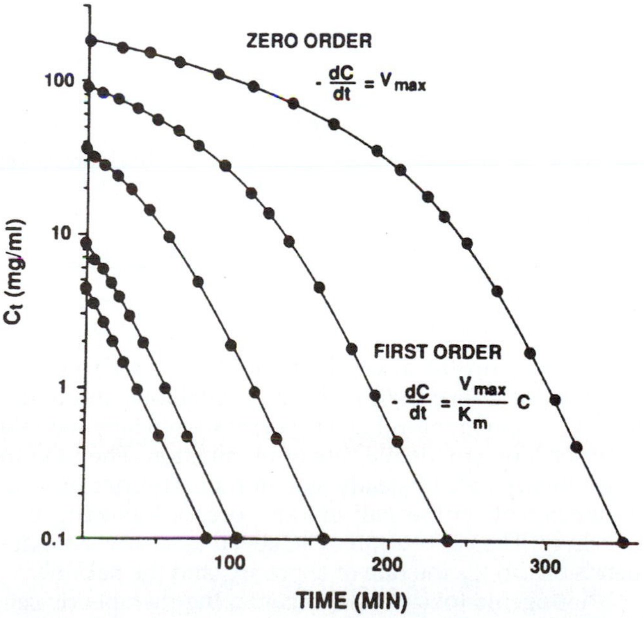

Figure 11–12. Concentration versus time curve for a xenobiotic showing nonlinear pharmacokinetics. *(Reprinted, with permission, from Yang R, Andersen M: Pharmacokinetics. In: Hodgson E, Levi P, eds: Introduction to Biochemical Toxicology. Norwalk, CT, Appleton & Lange, 1994, p. 57.)*

Clearance

Clearance (Cl) relates the rate of transfer or elimination of a xenobiotic from a reference fluid (usually plasma) to the plasma concentration of the xenobiotic and is ex-

TABLE 11–8A. ILLUSTRATION OF 1000 MG OF XENOBIOTIC IN BODY FOLLOWING FIRST-ORDER ELIMINATION

Time after Drug Administration (h)	Amount of Drug in Body (mg)	Amount of Drug Eliminated over Preceding Hour (mg)	Fraction of Drug Eliminated over Preceding Hour
0	1000	—	—
1	850	150	0.15
2	723	127	0.15
3	614	109	0.15
4	522	92	0.15
5	444	78	0.15
6	377	67	0.15

pressed in units of volume per unit time (ie, mL/min). See Equation 11–23.[13,27,39]

$$Cl = \frac{\text{Rate of elimination}}{C}$$

(Eq. 11–23)

The determination of creatinine clearance is familiar and is a well-known example of the concept of clearance. Creatinine clearance ($Cl_{creatinine}$) is determined by Equation 11–24.

$$Cl_{creatinine} = \frac{U \times V}{C}$$

(Eq. 11–24)

where *U* is the concentration of creatinine in urine (ie, mg/mL), *V* is the volume flow of urine (ie, mL/min), *C* is the plasma concentration of creatinine (ie, mg/mL), and the units for clearance would be mL/min. A creatinine clearance of 100 mL/min means that 100 mL of plasma is completely cleared of creatinine in each minute.

Clearance for a particular eliminating organ or for extracorporeal elimination is calculated with Equation 11–25.

TABLE 11–8B. ILLUSTRATION OF 1000 MG OF XENOBIOTIC IN BODY FOLLOWING ZERO-ORDER ELIMINATION

Time after Drug Administration (h)	Amount of Drug in Body (mg)	Amount of Drug Eliminated over Preceding Hour (mg)	Fraction of Drug Eliminated over Preceding Hour
0	1000	—	—
1	850	150	0.15
2	700	150	0.18
3	550	150	0.21
4	400	150	0.27
5	250	150	0.38
6	100	150	0.60

$$Cl = Q \times (ER) = Q \times \frac{(C_{in} - C_{out})}{C_{in}}$$

(Eq. 11–25)

Where:
Cl = clearance for the eliminating organ or extracorporeal device
Q = blood flow to the organ or device
ER = extraction ratio
C_{in} = xenobiotic concentration in fluid (blood or serum) entering the organ or device
C_{out} = xenobiotic concentration in fluid (blood or serum) leaving the organ or device

Clearance can be applied to any elimination process independent of the precise mechanisms (ie, first order, Michaelis-Menten), and will represent the sum total of all of the rate constants for xenobiotic elimination. Total body clearance ($Cl_{total\ body}$) is the sum of clearances of all of the individual eliminating processes, as seen in Equation 11–26.

$$Cl_{total\ body} = Cl_{renal} + Cl_{hepatic} + Cl_{intestinal} + Cl_{chelation} + \ldots$$

(Eq. 11–26)

For a first-order process (one-compartment model), clearance is given by Equation 11–27.

$$Cl = k_eVd$$

(Eq. 11–27)

Experimentally the clearance can be derived by examining the intravenous dose of xenobiotic in relation to the area under the plasma concentration (AUC) versus time curve from time zero to time *t*. See Equation 11–28. The AUC is calculated using the trapezoidal rule or through integral calculus (units: eg, mg h/mL). (See Figs. 11–13 and 11–14.)

$$Cl = \frac{Dose_{IV}}{AUC_{0\text{-}t}}$$

(Eq. 11–28)

Steady State

When exposure to a xenobiotic occurs at a fixed rate, the plasma concentration of the xenobiotic gradually achieves a plateau level at a concentration where the rate of absorption equals the rate of elimination. The time to reach nearly 95% of steady state for a first-order process is dependent on the half-life and occurs following five half-lives. The concentration achieved at steady state depends on the V_d, the rate of exposure, and the half-life.

Iatrogenic toxicity can occur in the therapeutic setting when dosing decisions are based on plasma concentrations determined prior to achieving a steady state. This is especially true for drugs that have long half-lives such as digoxin[52] and phenytoin.

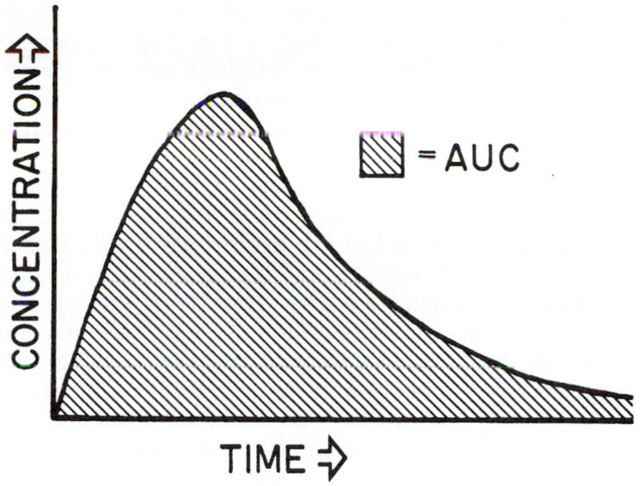

Figure 11–13. The area under the curve (AUC) of a concentration versus time profile obtained after extravascular administration of a xenobiotic. *(Reprinted, with permission, from reference Riviere JE: Absorption and distribution. In: Hodgson E, Levi P, eds: Introduction to Biochemical Toxicology. Norwalk, CT, Appleton & Lange, 1994, p. 21.)*

Peak Plasma Concentrations

Peak plasma concentrations (C_{max}) of a xenobiotic occur at the time of peak absorption. At this point in time, absorption rate is equal to the elimination rate. Thereafter, the elimination rate predominates and plasma concentrations begin to decline. Whereas the C_{max} depends on the dose, the rate of absorption (k_a), and the rate of elimination (k_e), the time to peak (t_{max}) is independent of dose and only depends on the k_a and k_e. For the same dose of xenobiotic, if the k_e remains constant and the rate of absorption increases, then the t_{max} will occur sooner and the C_{max} will be higher. The AUC will remain the same. However if the k_a remains constant and the k_e is increased, then the t_{max} occurs sooner, the C_{max} decreases, and the AUC decreases[41] (see Table 11–9).

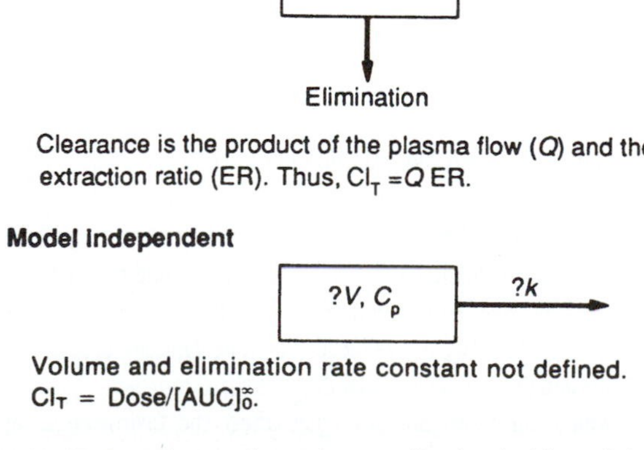

Plasma flow is not considered. $Cl_T = k\ V_D$.

Clearance is the product of the plasma flow (Q) and the extraction ratio (ER). Thus, $Cl_T = Q$ ER.

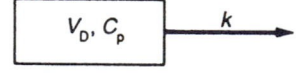

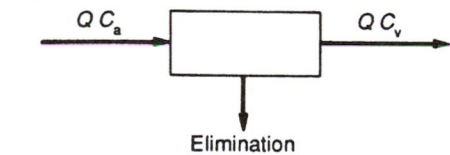

Cl_T = Dose/$[AUC]_0^\infty$.

Figure 11–14. General approaches to clearance. *(Reprinted, with permission, from Shargel L, Yu A: Introduction to pharmacokinetics. In: Applied Biopharmaceutics and Pharmacokinetics, 3rd ed. Norwalk, CT, Appleton & Lange, 1993, p. 280.)*

In the overdose setting, gastric emptying, single-dose activated charcoal, and whole bowel irrigation decrease k_a. Multiple-dose activated charcoal, manipulation of pH to promote ion trapping to facilitate elimination, and certain chelators (ie, DMSA, deferoxamine) increase k_e and are likely to decrease C_{max}, t_{max}, and AUC.

Interpretation of Plasma Concentrations

In order for plasma concentrations to be of more value than just demonstrating presence, there must be an established relationship between effect and plasma concentration. For many drugs used therapeutically, there is an established therapeutic range (eg, phenytoin, digoxin, carbamazepine, theophylline). However, there are also many drugs for which there is no established therapeutic range (eg, diazepam, propranolol, verapamil). Some agents exhibit hysteresis (the effect increases as the plasma concentration is decreasing; eg, physostigmine). For many xenobiotics, there is very little information on toxicodynamics. Often sequential plasma concentrations are collected for retrospective analysis to attempt a correlation between plasma concentrations and toxicity. Tolerance to drugs such as ethanol also influences the interpretation of plasma concentrations. Tolerance is an example of a pharmacodynamic or toxicodynamic effect due to cellular adaptation.

Other factors that influence the interpretation of plasma concentrations include chronicity of dosing (single acute dose vs chronic dosing), whether absorption is still ongoing and therefore concentrations are still rising, whether distribution is still ongoing and therefore concentrations are uninterpretable, or whether the value is a peak or trough or steady-state concentration (see Figure 11–15). Clinical examples where interpretation varies dependent on the dosing pattern of a single acute dose versus chronic dosing include theophylline, digoxin, lithium, and acetaminophen. Sustained-release preparations and those xenobiotics that delay gastric emptying or form concretions would have prolonged absorptive phases and require serial plasma concentrations, if plasma concentrations are to be meaningful (see Chap. 7). Peak and trough values are often consequential for monitoring of certain antibiotics (eg, gentamicin).

Pitfalls in interpretation also arise when the units for a particular plasma concentration are not obtained or are unfamiliar (ie, mmol/L) to the clinician. In those cases, the normal range should be sought. Often in the overdose setting the type of analysis utilized is not generally applied to such large concentrations, and the laboratory may make errors in dilution or errors become inherent in

TABLE 11–9. PHARMACOKINETIC EFFECTS OF THE ABSORPTION RATE CONSTANT AND ELIMINATION RATE CONSTANT[a]

Absorption Rate Constant K_a (h^{-1})	Elimination Rate Constant K_e (h^{-1})	t_{max} (h)	C_{max} (μg/mL)	AUC (μg h/mL)
0.1	0.2	6.93	2.50	50
0.2	0.1	6.93	5.00	100
0.3	0.1	5.49	5.77	100
0.4	0.1	4.62	6.26	100
0.5	0.1	4.02	6.69	100
0.6	0.1	3.58	6.99	100
0.3	0.1	5.49	5.77	100
0.3	0.2	4.05	4.44	50
0.3	0.3	3.33	3.68	33.3
0.3	0.4	2.88	3.16	25
0.3	0.5	2.55	2.79	20

[a] t_{max} = time to peak plasma concentration, C_{max} = peak xenobiotic concentration, AUC = area under the curve. Values are based on a single oral dose (100 mg) that is 100% bioavailable ($F = 1$) and has an apparent V_d of 10 L. The drug follows a one-compartment open model. The AUC is calculated by the trapezoidal rule from 0 to 24 h.

Reprinted, with permission, from Shargel L, Yu A: Pharmacokinetics of drug absorption. In: Applied Biopharmaceutics and Pharmacokinetics, 3rd ed. Norwalk, CT: Appleton & Lange, 1993, p. 183.

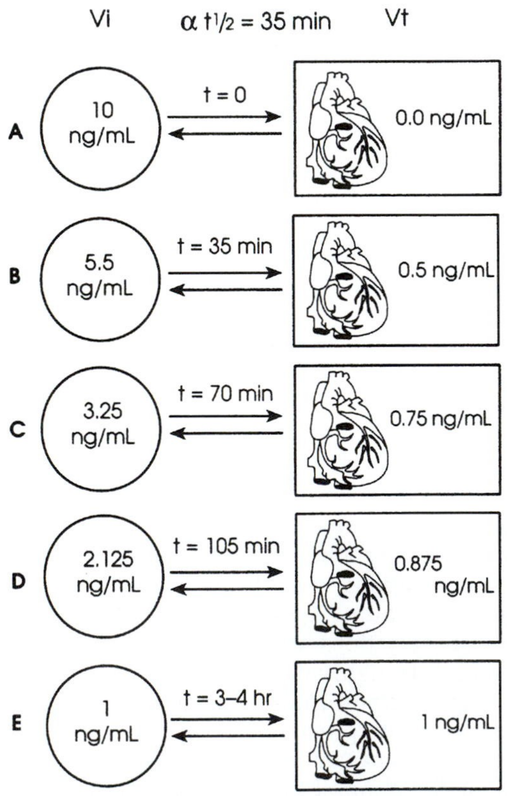

Figure 11–15. A theoretical two-compartment model for digoxin. *(Reprinted, with permission, from Winter ME: Digoxin in Basic Clinical Pharmacokinetics. 3rd ed. Koda-Kimble MA, Young LY, eds: Vancouver, Washington, Applied Therapeutics Inc. 1994, p. 202.)*

the assay (see Chap. 7). In those cases the director of the laboratory should be consulted and perhaps a reference laboratory used. The type of collection tube (ie, plasma or serum instead of whole blood for certain metals) or receptacle or the conditions during delivery of the sample may give rise to inaccurate or inadequate information. When in doubt, call the laboratory prior to sample collection. The laboratory usually measures total xenobiotic (free plus bound), and for agents that are highly plasma protein bound, reductions in albumin increase free concentrations and alter the interpretation of the reported value (ie, phenytoin; see Equation 11–7). Active metabolites may contribute to toxicity and may not be measured. Collection of accurate data for analysis requires at least 4 data points during one elimination half-life, and during extracorporeal methods of elimination, ideal criteria for determining amount removed requires assay of the dialysate or charcoal cartridge and not just plasma concentrations. Patient weight and height and, when indicated, hemoglobin, creatinine, albumin, and other parameters to assess elimination pathways may be helpful.

Case Illustrations

The following cases are designed to illustrate a number of pharmacokinetic and toxicokinetic principles. They readily demonstrate the application of many of the mathematics previously explained.

CASE 1. A 23-year-old, 90-kg female is seen in the emergency department 2 hours after ingestion of 50 of her brother's Theodur (300 mg) tablets. She is alert and oriented with a BP 130/75 mm Hg, HR 110 beats/min, RR 20 breaths/min, T 99.7°F rectally. Her initial theophylline serum concentration is 40 mg/L.

1. Estimate a peak serum concentration knowing that theophylline has a V_d of 0.5 L/kg, an $S = 1$ (not a salt form), and an $F = 1$ (100% bioavailable). Rearrange Equation 11–6.

$$V_d = \frac{S \times F \times \text{Dose (mg)}}{C_0}$$

$$0.5\ \text{L/kg} \times 90\ \text{kg} = \frac{1 \times 1 \times 50 \times 300\ \text{mg}}{C_0} = 333\ \text{mg/L}$$

2. Why would this serum concentration not be achieved if the history were correct?

   Increasing the number of tablets of sustained-release dosage forms may alter their release characteristics, delay absorption, and reduce k_a (absorption rate constant). Elimination (k_e) is occurring during the absorptive phase so C_{max} and AUC are reduced. Vomiting typically occurs with theophylline and decreases bioavailability.

3. How would our treatment strategies affect the toxicokinetics of theophylline?

   Activated charcoal and whole bowel irrigation decrease bioavailability. Multiple-dose activated charcoal, charcoal hemoperfusion, and hemodialysis enhance elimination.

4. Can the patient be considered medically clear at this time?

   No. Serum concentrations may continue to rise and may not peak for 12–24 hours. Therefore, sequential serum concentrations should be analyzed frequently until concentrations have started to fall, and then less frequent determinations are necessary as the concentration approaches the therapeutic range (see Chap. 39).

CASE 2. A 63-year-old, 60-kg female is brought to the emergency department by her family after ingesting 25 (0.25 mg) digoxin tablets 1/2 hour ago. The patient complains of nausea, but is otherwise asymptomatic. Her physical examination is normal. BP 130/85 mm Hg, HR 76 beats/min and irregular, RR 17 breaths/min, and T 98°F rectally. The ECG shows controlled atrial fibrillation at a rate of 76.

1. Estimate this patient's plasma digoxin concentration. Assume a V_d = 5 L/kg, an $S = 1$, and an $F = 0.8$ (80%).

$$C_0 = \frac{S \times F \times \text{Dose}}{V_d}$$

$$C_0 = \frac{1 \times 0.8 \times 25 \times 0.25\text{ mg} \times 1000000\text{ ng/1 mg}}{5\text{ L/kg} \times 1000\text{ mL/L} \times 60\text{ kg}} = 16.7\text{ ng/mL}$$

2. Her serum digoxin concentration returns at 15 ng/mL (therapeutic = 0.8–2 ng/mL). Why does this patient not show more severe signs of digoxin toxicity?

   This patient does not show serious signs and symptoms of toxicity from digoxin because digoxin fits a two-compartment model with a long distribution half-life. Toxicity is related to the concentration in the peripheral (heart) compartment. However, in several hours she may show severe signs of toxicity. See Figure 11–15.

3. How does Digibind alter the toxicokinetics of digoxin?

   Digibind reduces the V_d of digoxin by binding digoxin in the plasma, thereby establishing a concentration gradient to pull digoxin from reversible tissue (eg, heart) binding sites. All digoxin bound to Digibind is inactive. The Digibind–digoxin complex is eliminated slightly faster than digoxin alone due to a reduced V_d.

4. How would you calculate the dose of Digibind?

   If the ingested dose is known:

$$\text{Total body load (TBL)} = S \times F \times \text{Dose}$$

$$= 1 \times 0.8 \times 25 \times 0.25\text{ mg} = 5\text{ mg}$$

1 vial of Digibind binds 0.5 mg of digoxin

$$\#\text{ vials Digibind} = \frac{\text{TBL (5 mg)}}{0.5\text{ mg digoxin/vial Digibind}} = 10\text{ vials}$$

If serum concentration is known:

$$\text{TBL (mg)} = C\text{(ng/mL)} \times (1\text{ mg/1000000 ng})$$

$$\times V_d(\text{L/kg})(1000\text{ mL/L}) \times \text{Weight of patient (kg)}$$

$$= \frac{15\text{ ng/mL} \times 5\text{ L/kg} \times 60\text{ kg}}{1000} = 45\text{ mg}$$

$$\#\text{vials Digibind} = \frac{\text{TBL (45 mg) of digoxin}}{0.5\text{ mg digoxin/vial Digibind}} = 9\text{ vials Digibind}$$

OR a simplified version:

$$\#\text{ vials Digibind} = \frac{C\text{(ng/mL)} \times \text{Weight of patient (kg)}}{100}$$

$$= 9\text{ vials Digibind}$$

The numbers of vials of Digibind calculated either by using the history of the amount ingested or based on the serum concentration are usually different because each formula has independent inherent errors.

CASE 3. A patient receives a continuous infusion of pentobarbital for 3 days. He is taken off the infusion and has not awakened after 6 hours. The reported duration of hypnotic action after a single IV dose is 1–4 hours. Is there a toxicokinetic explanation for this?

Yes. The short duration of action after a single dose of IV pentobarbital is attributed to redistribution following the dose. With chronic dosing, accumulation occurs and the elimination half-life becomes 15–48 hours.This patient may require several days to awaken.

CASE 4. A 70-kg man with no history of alcoholism ingests enough methanol to achieve a serum concentration of 100 mg/dL (1 g/L). The following information is available:

Methanol: molecular weight 32 daltons; water soluble;
Specific gravity (sp gr) of absolute ethanol and methanol: 0.8 g/mL
V_d of ethanol and methanol = 0.6 L/kg
Protein binding of ethanol and methanol = negligible
Bioavailability for ethanol and methanol = 100%
Hemodialysis clearance of ethanol and methanol = 150 mL/min; assume hemodialysis is a first-order process
Hemodialysis extraction ratio of ethanol and methanol = 100%
V_{max} = 0.15 g/kg/h for ethanol for naive person

1. How much methanol did the patient drink if gasline antifreeze is 95% methanol?

$$C_0 = \frac{S \times F \times \text{Dose}}{V_d} \qquad \text{Rearranging: } S \times F \times \text{Dose} = C_0 \times V_d$$

$$1 \times 1 \times \text{Dose} = 1\text{ g/L} \times 0.6\text{ L/kg} \times 70\text{ kg}$$

$$= 42\text{ g of 100\% concentration}$$

(S = 1; there is no salt form of an alcohol)

$$42\text{ g} \times 1\text{ mL/0.95 g (95\% conc)} \times 1\text{ mL/0.8 g (sp gr)}$$

$$= 55\text{ mL of 95\% of methanol}$$

2. How much ethanol as vodka (80 proof = 40%) should be given to the patient as a loading dose to achieve a serum concentration of 100 mg% (100 mg/dL or 1 g/L)?

$$C_0 = \frac{S \times F \times \text{Dose}}{V_d} \qquad \text{Rearranging: } S \times F \times \text{Dose} = C_0 \times V_d$$

$$1 \times 1 \times \text{Dose} = 1\text{ g/L} \times 0.6\text{ L/kg} \times 70\text{ kg} = 42\text{ g}$$

$$42\text{ g} \times 1\text{ mL/0.4 g (40\% conc)} \times 1\text{ mL/0.8 g (sp gr)}$$

$$= 131\text{ mL of 40\% ethanol}$$

3. What maintenance dose of ethanol should be given to the patient to maintain an ethanol serum concentration of 100 mg/dL (1 g/L)?

The V_{max} of 0.15 g/kg/h is the maximum rate of elimination for a patient not tolerant to ethanol. The maintenance dose is designed to replace the amount of ethanol eliminated. Therefore:

$$0.15\,\text{g/kg/h} \times 70\,\text{kg} = 10.5\,\text{g/h} \times 1\,\text{mL}/0.1\,(10\%) \times 1\,\text{mL}/0.8\,(\text{sp gr}) = 131.25\,\text{mL/h of }10\%\text{ ethanol (can be given po or IV)}$$

4. How many hours of hemodialysis would be necessary to achieve a methanol serum concentration of 10 mg/dL (1 g/L)?

$K_e = Cl/V_d$; $Cl_{total\ body} = Cl_{HD} + Cl_{endogenous} = Cl_{HD} + 0$ (minimal endogenous clearance when methanol metabolism is blocked with ethanol)

$$\frac{150\,\text{mL/min} \times 60\,\text{min/h} \times 1\,\text{L}/1000\,\text{mL}}{0.6\,\text{L/kg} \times 70\,\text{kg}}$$

$$= 0.214\,\text{h}^{-1} = 21.4\%\text{ per hour eliminated}$$

$$t_{1/2} = 0.693/k_e = 0.693/0.214\,\text{h}^{-1} = 3.22\,\text{h}$$

$$t_1 - t_2 = \frac{\ln C_1 - \ln C_2}{k_e} = \frac{\ln 100 - \ln 10}{0.214\,\text{h}^{-1}}$$

$$= 10.74\text{ hours to go from }100\,\text{mg/dL to }10\,\text{mg/dL}$$

CASE 5. A 70 kg-male is brought to the hospital with a serum concentration of phenytoin of 80 μg/mL (mg/L). Assume the ingestion occurred 2 days earlier and there is no ongoing absorption. Estimate how long it might take this patient to reach 20 μg/mL. The following information is available:

$$V_d = 0.7\,\text{L/kg}$$

$$V_m\ (\text{maximum metabolic capacity}) = 7\,\text{mg/kg/d}$$

$$K_m\ (\text{serum concentration at which the metabolic rate is at one-half the maximum metabolic rate} = 4\,\text{mg/L}$$

$$v = \frac{V_{max} \times C}{K_m + C} = \frac{7\,\text{mg/kg/d} \times 70\,\text{kg} \times 80\,\text{mg/L}}{4\,\text{mg/L} + 80\,\text{mg/L}}$$

$$= 466.6\,\text{mg/day eliminated at zero order}$$

Estimate the initial amount of phenytoin in body:

$$\text{Dose} = C \times V_d = 80\,\text{mg/L} \times 0.7\,\text{L/kg} \times 70\,\text{kg} = 3920\,\text{mg}$$

Estimate amount of phenytoin in body at 20 mg/L:

$$\text{Dose} = C \times V_d = 20\,\text{mg/L} \times 0.7\,\text{L/kg} \times 70\,\text{kg} = 980\,\text{mg}$$

$$3920\,\text{mg} - 980\,\text{mg} = 2940\,\text{mg as the amount that needs to be eliminated}$$

At an elimination rate of 466.6 mg/day, it will take about 6.3 days to go from a serum phenytoin concentration of 80 mg/dL to 20 mg/dL assuming neither ongoing absorption nor enhanced elimination from repeat dose activated charcoal.

Using the formula

$$t = \frac{[(K_m)(\ln Cp_1/\ln Cp_2)] + (C_1 - C_2)}{V_m/V_d}$$

$$= \frac{(4\,\text{mg/L}) \times (4.38 - 3) + (80 - 20)}{7\,\text{mg/kg/d} \times 70\,\text{kg} \times 0.7\,\text{L/kg} \times 70\,\text{kg}}$$

$$= 6.55\text{ days}$$

CASE 6. Compare the utility of exchange transfusion, peritoneal dialysis, hemodialysis, and hemoperfusion for ingestion of 2 g of either amitriptyline or theophylline in a 15-kg child.

The following information is available:

$$V_d\text{ of amitriptyline} = 30\,\text{L/kg; protein binding} = \text{high}$$

$$V_d\text{ of theophylline} = 0.5\,\text{L/kg; protein binding} = \text{moderate}$$

$$\text{Blood volume} = 85\,\text{mL/kg; a double volume exchange} = 85\,\text{mL/kg} \times 2$$

Estimate that 300 mL of peritoneal fluid is administered over 10 min, that the equilibration time is 20 min, and that 300 mL is removed over 30 min for a total time of 60 min.

Assume HP clearance of 200mL/min for theophylline.

1. Would exchange transfusion be reasonable for amitriptyline or theophylline removal?

$$\text{Double volume exchange} = 85\,\text{mL/kg} \times 2$$

$$\text{In this child} = 85\,\text{mL/kg} \times 15\,\text{kg} \times 2 = 2550\,\text{mL} = 2.55\,\text{L}$$

$$V_d\text{ for amitriptyline in this child} = 30\,\text{L/kg} \times 15\,\text{kg} = 450\,\text{L}$$

$$450\,\text{L}/2.55\,\text{L} = 176\text{ double-exchange transfusions, an unrealistic number!}$$

$$V_d\text{ for theophylline in this child} = 0.5\,\text{L/kg} \times 15\,\text{kg} = 7.5\,\text{L}$$

$$7.5\,\text{L}/2.55\,\text{L} = \text{about 3 double exchanges, a reasonable number!}$$

2. Would peritoneal dialysis be reasonable for amitriptyline or theophylline removal?

No for both amitriptyline and theophylline.

For amitriptyline:

$$300\,\text{mL/h} = 0.3\,\text{L/h} = 7.2\,\text{L/d}$$

$$450\,\text{L}/7.2\,\text{L/d} = 62.5\text{ days}$$

For theophylline:

$$7.5\,\text{L}/7.2\,\text{L/h} = 25\,\text{h; too long in a life-threatening situation}$$

3. Would hemodialysis be reasonable for amitriptyline or theophylline removal?

No, for amitriptyline. Yes, for theophylline.

For hemodialysis:

There is unlikely to be any benefit for amitriptyline removal because of high protein binding and large V_d.

Moderate protein binding of theophylline would be limiting but a small V_d would be advantageous. Result would be acceptable for theophylline.

4. Would activated charcoal hemoperfusion be reasonable for amitriptyline or theophylline removal?

No, for amitriptyline. Yes, for theophylline.

For hemoperfusion:

Protein binding may be of less importance if binding to activated charcoal is stronger than binding to protein.

For amitriptyline:

$$200\ \text{mL/min} \times 60\ \text{min/h} = 1.2\ \text{L/h; assume complete clearance}$$

$$k_e = \text{Cl}/V_d = 1.2\ \text{L/h}/30\ \text{L/kg} \times 15\ \text{kg} = 0.00266\text{h}^{-1} = 0.266\%/\text{h}$$

$$t_{1/2} = 0.693/k_e = 0.693/0.002666 = 260\ \text{hours; totally unreasonable}$$

For theophylline:

$$k_e = \text{Cl}/V_d = 1.2\ \text{L/h}/7.5\ \text{L} = 0.16/\text{h}$$

$$t_{1/2} = 0.693/k_e = 0.693/0.16 = 4.33\ \text{hours; perfectly reasonable!}$$

Some of theses cases were used at workshops given at the NYCPCC and Christine Stork, Pharm D, assisted with some of these.

Acknowledgment

Richard S. Weisman, PharmD, Candace Smith, PharmD, and John R. Reynolds, PharmD, contributed to this chapter in a previous edition.

References

1. Bertilsson L: Geographical/interracial differences in polymorphic drug oxidation. Clin Pharmacokinet 1995;29: 192–209.
2. Blaschke TF, Rubin PC: Hepatic first-pass metabolism in liver disease. Clin Pharmacokinet 1979;4:423–432.
3. Bodenham A, Shelly MP, Park GR: The altered pharmacokinetics and pharmacodynamics of drugs commonly used in critically ill patients. Clin Pharmacokinet 1988;14:347–373.
4. Boyes RN, Scott DB, Jebson PJ, et al: Pharmacokinetics of lidocaine in man. Clin Pharmacol Ther 1971;12:105–116.
5. Ciummo PE, Katz NL: Interactions and drug metabolizing enzymes. Am Pharm 1995;9:41–51.
6. Dauterman WC: Metabolism of toxicants: Phase II reactions. In: Hodgson E, Levi P, eds: Introduction to Biochemical Toxicology. Norwalk, CT, Appleton & Lange, 1994, pp. 113–132.
7. Dean B, Oehme FW, Krenzelok E: A study of iron complexation in a swine model. Vet Hum Toxicol 1988;30:313–315.
8. DeGeorge JJ: Food and drug administration viewpoints on toxicokinetics: The View from Review. Toxicol Pathol 1995; 220–225.
9. Engasser JM, Sarhan F, Falcoz C, et al: Distribution, metabolism and elimination of phenobarbital in rats: Physiologically based pharmacokinetic model. J Pharmaceutical Sci 1981;70:1233–1238.
10. Gillette JR: Factors affecting drug metabolism. Ann NY Acad Sci 1971;179:43–66.
11. Gram TE: Drug absorption and distribution. In: Craig CR, Stitzel RE, eds: Modern Pharmacology With Clinical Applications. Boston, Little, Brown, 1997, pp. 13–24.
12. Guengerich FP, Liebler DC: Enzymatic activation of chemicals to toxic metabolites. CRC Crit Rev Toxicol 1985;14: 259–307.
13. Gwilt PR: Pharmacokinetics. In: Craig CR, Stitzel RE, eds: Modern Pharmacology with Clinical Applications. Boston, Little, Brown, 1997, pp. 49–58.
14. Hill HZ, Backer R, Hill GJ: Blood cyanide levels in mice after administration of amygdalin. Biopharm Drug Dispos 1980;1:211–220.
15. Hodgson E, Levi PE: Metabolism of toxicants phase I reactions. In: Hodgson E, Levi P, eds: Introduction to Biochemical Toxicology. Norwalk, CT, Appleton & Lange, 1994, pp. 75–111.
16. Iberti T, Patterson B, Fisher C: Prolonged bromide intoxication resulting from a gastric bezoar. Arch Intern Med 1984; 144:402–403.
17. Jenis EH, Payne RJ, Goldbaum LR: Acute meprobamate poisoning: A fatal case following a lucid interval. JAMA 1969;207:361–365.
18. Kapoor SC, Wielopolski L, Graziano JH, LoIacono NJ: Influence of 2,3-dimercaptosuccinic acid on gastrointestinal lead absorption and whole body lead retention. Toxicol Appl Pharmacol 1989;97:525–529.
19. Klaassen CD, Shoeman DW: Biliary excretion of lead in rats, rabbits and dogs. Toxicol Appl Pharmacol 1974;29:436–446.
20. Klaassen CD, Watkins JB: Mechanisms of bile formation, hepatic uptake, and biliary excretion. Pharmacol Rev 1984; 36:1–67.
21. Klotz U: Pathophysiological and disease-induced changes in drug distribution volume: pharmacokinetic implications. Clin Pharmacokinet 1976;1:204–218.
22. Koch-Weser J: Bioavailability of drugs. Part I. N Engl J Med 1974;291:233–237.
23. Koch-Weser J: Bioavailability of drugs. Part II. N Engl J Med 1974;291:503–506.
24. Lemmer B, Bruguerolle B: Chronopharmacokinetics, are they clinically relevant? Clin Pharmacokinet 1994;26: 419–427.
25. Levine WG: Biliary excretion of drugs and other xenobiotics. Ann Rev Pharmacol Toxicol 1978;18:81–96.
26. McCarthy J, Gram TE: Drug metabolism and disposition in pediatric and gerontological stages of life. In: Craig CR, Stitzel RE, eds: Modern Pharmacology with Clinical Applications. Boston, Little, Brown, 1997, pp. 43–48.
27. Medinsky MA, Klaassen CD: Toxicokinetics. In: Klaassen CD, ed: Casarett & Doull's Toxicology: The Basic Science of Poisons, 5th ed. New York, McGraw-Hill, 1996, pp. 187–198.
28. Parkinson A: Biotransformation of xenobiotics. In: Klaassen C, ed: Casarett & Doull's Toxicology: The Basic Science of Poisons, 5th ed. New York, McGraw-Hill, 1996, pp. 113–186.
29. Pharmacist's Letter, ed: Stockton, CA, document #120507.
30. Pirmohamed M, Kitteringham NR, Park BK: The role of active metabolites in drug toxicity. Drug Safety 1994;11: 114–144.
31. Plaa OL: The enterohepatic circulation. In: Gillette JR, Mitchell JR, eds: Handook Experimental Pharmacology. New York, Springer, 1975, pp. 28, 130–140, 480.

32. Pond SM, Tozer TN: First-pass elimination: basic concepts and clinical consequences. Pharmacokinetics 1984;9:1–25.
33. Riviere JE: Absorption and distribution. In: Hodgson E, Levi P, eds: Introduction to Biochemical Toxicology. Norwalk, CT, Appleton & Lange, 1994, pp. 11–48.
34. Rose MS, Lock EA, Smith LL, Wyatt I: Paraquat accumulation: Tissue and species specificity. Biochem Pharmacol 1976;25:419–423.
35. Rosenberg J, Benowitz NL, Pond S: Pharmacokinetics of drug overdose. Clin Pharmacokinet 1981;6:161–192.
36. Rowland M, Tozer TN: Clinical Pharmacokinetics Concepts & Applications, 2nd ed. Philadelphia, Lea & Febiger, 1989.
37. Rozman KK, Klaassen CD: Absorption, distribution and excretion of toxicants. In: Klaassen CD, ed: Casarett & Doull's Toxicology: The Basic Science of Poisons. New York, McGraw-Hill, 1996, pp. 91–112.
38. Sansom LN, Evans AM: What is the true clinical significance of plasma protein binding displacement interactions? Drug Safety 1995;12:227–233.
39. Shargel L, Yu A: Drug clearance. In: Applied Biopharmaceutics and Pharmacokinetics, 3rd ed. Norwalk, CT, Appleton & Lange, 1993, pp. 265–292.
40. Shargel L, Yu A: Drug distribution and protein binding. In: Applied Biopharmaceutics and Pharmacokinetics, 3rd ed. Norwalk, CT, Appleton & Lange, 1993, pp. 77–110.
41. Shargel L, Yu A: Pharmacokinetics of drug absorption. In: Applied Biopharmaceutics and Pharmacokinetics, 3rd ed. Norwalk, CT, Appleton & Lange, 1993, pp. 169–192.
42. Shargel L, Yu A: Physiologic factors related to drug absorption. In: Applied Biopharmaceutics and Pharmacokinetics, 3rd ed. Norwalk, CT, Appleton & Lange, 1993, pp. 111–134.
43. Slaughter RL, Edwards DJ: Recent advances: The cytochrome P450 enzymes. Ann Pharmacother 1995;29: 619–623.
44. Stowe CM, Plaa GL: Extrarenal excretion of drugs and chemicals. Annu Rev Pharmacol 1968;8:337–356.
45. Sue Y, Shannon M: Pharmacokinetics of drugs in overdose. Clin Pharmacokinet 1992;23:93–105.
46. Teorell T: Kinetics of distribution of substances administered to the body. Depart Med Chem Univ of Uppsala, Sweden 1937;205–225.
47. Verebey K, Gold MS: From coca leaves to crack: The effect of dose and routes of administration in abuse liability. Psychiatr Ann 1988;18:513–520.
48. Vesell ES: The model drug approach in clinical pharmacology. Clin Pharmacol Ther 1991;50:239–248.
49. Welling PG: Differences between pharmacokinetics and toxicokinetics. Toxicol Pathol 1995;23:143–147.
50. Wilkinson GR: Influence of hepatic disease on pharmacokinetics. In: Evans WE, Schentag J, Justo W, eds: Applied Pharmacokinetics: Principles of Therapeutic Drug Monitoring. Spokane, Applied Therapeutics, 1986, pp. 116–138.
51. Wilkinson GR: Plasma and tissue binding considerations in drug disposition. Drug Metab Rev 1983;14:427–465.
52. Winter ME: Digoxin in Basic Clinical Pharmacokinetics, 3rd ed. Koda-Kimble MA, Young LY, eds: Vancouver, Washington, Applied Therapeutics Inc 1994;pp198–235.
53. Yang R, Andersen M: Pharmacokinetics. In: Hodgson E, Levi P, eds: Introduction to Biochemical Toxicology. Norwalk, CT, Appleton & Lange, 1994, pp. 49–73.

CHAPTER 12

Biochemical Principles

Kathleen A. Delaney

Toxins injure living organisms by interfering with critical metabolic processes, causing structural injury to cells, or altering the cellular genetic material. The specific biochemical sites of actions that disrupt metabolic processes are well characterized for many toxins, although mechanisms of cellular injury are not. This chapter focuses on those general biochemical principles that are relevant to an understanding of the injurious effects of toxins, with references to a few well-characterized toxins whose mechanisms of action illustrate basic principles. Mutagens and carcinogens are discussed in Chapter 16.

Knowing what a toxin does at the site of injury, for example, enzyme inhibition, DNA alteration, or lipid peroxidation, contributes only partly to understanding the injurious interaction between a toxin and a living organism. How the toxic substance is absorbed, distributed, and eliminated and where it is activated or detoxified all affect the form and concentration of the toxin in different tissues, and its capacity to produce injury. Damage may be confined to one organ by the mechanism of exposure, such as gastrointestinal or dermal injury by a caustic agent, hepatocellular injury following ingestion of a toxin selectively delivered to the liver by the portal venous system, or pulmonary injury by an inhaled toxin. In addition, the ability of a toxin to enter a particular organ is an important factor in toxicity. As an example, many potential central nervous system (CNS) toxins fail to produce injury because they cannot cross the blood–brain barrier. The negligible CNS effects of the mercuric salts when compared with organic mercury compounds are related to their inability to penetrate the CNS. Two potent biologic toxins, ricin (from *Ricinus communis*) and alpha amanitin (from *Amanita phalloides*), block protein synthesis through the inhibition of RNA polymerase. Their very different clinical effects are related to tissue accessibility. Ricin has a special binding protein that allows it to gain access to the endoplasmic reticulum in gastrointestinal (GI) mucosal cells, causing severe diarrhea.[45] Alpha amanitin is transported into hepatocytes by the bile salt transport systems, where inhibition of protein synthesis leads to cell death.[40,48] Unlike ionized toxins, uncharged, lipophilic substances pass easily through lipid cell membranes to enter the systemic circulation (See Chap. 11 for a more extensive discussion of basic principles of pharmacokinetics.)

Toxins That Inhibit Specific Enzymes

Like ricin and the cyclopeptide amanita toxins that block the synthetic function of RNA polymerase, many toxins disrupt metabolic processes by inhibiting specific cellular enzymes. Warfarin inhibits vitamin K 2,3-epoxide reductase, blocking synthesis of the reduced quinol form of vitamin K that is required to activate clotting factors II, VII, IX, and X (see Chap. 42).[34,83] The presence of lead blocks several enzymes that are critical for hemoglobin synthesis[35] (see Chap. 79). Organophosphate insecticides bind to esterases that contain a serine hydroxyl group at their active site. Binding to the serine moiety of acetylcholinesterase leads to enzyme inhibition and accumulation of acetylcholine, resulting in characteristic signs of excessive cholinergic stimulation[52] (see Chap. 87). Organophosphate insecticides also bind avidly to and irreversibly inhibit the active site of the serum enzyme beta-carboxylesterase, while alpha-carboxylesterases cleave organophosphates but are not inhibited by them.[4] These same carboxylesterases are responsible for the formation of cocaethylene in the presence of ethanol, an ethyl ester of cocaine that may increase its toxicity.[41]

Toxins That Inhibit Critical Biochemical Pathways: Glycolysis, the Krebs Cycle, and Oxidative Phosphorylation

When inhibition of a specific enzyme disrupts critically important biochemical processes, rapid cellular death occurs. Such important metabolic pathways include glycolysis, the tricarboxylic acid or Krebs cycle, and oxidative phosphorylation.

Glycolysis results in the oxygen-independent, or anaerobic, metabolism of glucose. The tricarboxylic acid cycle and oxidative phosphorylation are the major pathways of oxidative metabolism. These pathways are primarily responsible for the synthesis of adenosine triphosphate or ATP: the metabolic fuel required for synthetic functions, active transport, and maintenance of electrolyte balance and membrane integrity. Oxidative phosphorylation also disposes of electrons or "reducing equivalents" generated by the oxidative metabolism of cellular fuels such as sugars and lipids. Oxidative metabolism is highly energy efficient, producing 36 moles of ATP for each mole of glucose metabolized, compared to the 2 moles of ATP produced by glycolysis.[44] The following sections review the basics of cellular metabolism and those toxins that affect critical metabolic functions.

Roles of NADH and NADPH in Metabolism

The pyridine nucleotides NADPH/$NADP^+$ (nicotinamide adenine dinucleotide phosphate) and NADH/NAD^+ (nicotinamide adenine dinucleotide) function in their reduced and oxidized forms to transport electrons in oxidation–reduction reactions. Oxidation involves the extraction of electrons from a substrate and their transfer to molecular oxygen or to another electron-seeking (electrophilic) substance. Reduction involves the transfer of electrons to a substrate. The reduction of NAD^+ to NADH (or $NADP^+$ to NADPH) requires two electrons plus a hydrogen ion (H^+):

$$2e^- + H^+ + NAD^+ = NADH$$

$$2e^- + H^+ + NADP^+ = NADPH$$

An example of how pyridine nucleotides are used in oxidation–reduction reactions is illustrated by the oxidation of ethanol[46] (Fig. 12–1).

NADPH, which serves primarily to carry electrons from the oxidative reactions of catabolism to the synthetic (anabolic) reactions of biosynthesis, is present in significant amounts only in cells that are actively synthesizing new molecules, such as proteins, steroids, and fatty acids. The primary source of NADPH in the cell is the pentose phosphate pathway (also called the hexose–monophosphate shunt), an alternative pathway for the oxidation of glucose that produces NADPH and 5-ribose phosphate as a by-product[44] (see Fig. 12–2). Ultimately, electrons extracted from catabolic processes by the two-electron reduction of NAD^+ to NADH are transferred to molecular oxygen through the mitochondrial cytochrome–mediated electron transport system. The ability to recycle NADH by "dumping" electrons picked up during the oxidation of various cellular fuels allows oxidative metabolism to proceed. This is the metabolic point where hypoxia exerts its deleterious effect.

Glycolysis

Glycolysis is the biochemical pathway responsible for the initial metabolism of glucose. Other sugars enter the glycolytic pathway after conversion to glycolytic intermediates (Fig. 12–3). Glycolysis results in the anaerobic production of two molecules of ATP for each molecule of glucose metabolized to pyruvate. Under anaerobic conditions, pyruvate is enzymatically reduced to lactate by lactate dehydrogenase in an NADH-requiring step. When NAD^+ and oxygen are available, pyruvate is converted by pyruvate decarboxylase to acetyl-CoA, which condenses with oxaloacetate to form citrate and enter the Krebs cycle[44] (Fig. 12–4).

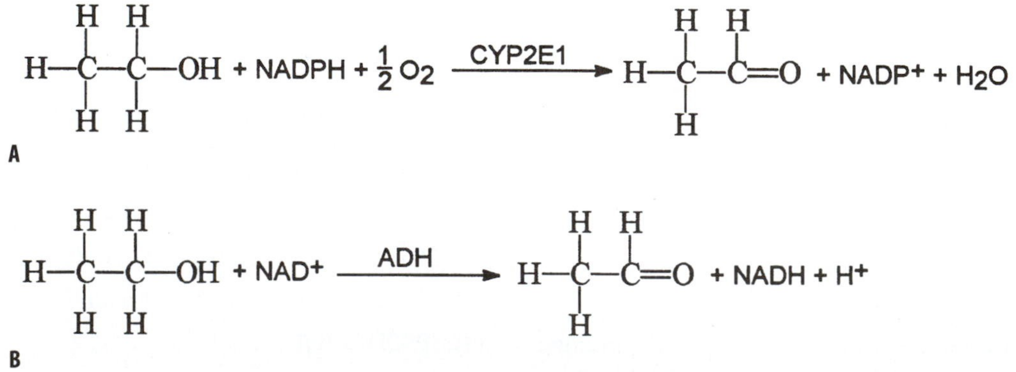

Figure 12–1. Enyzmatic conversion of ethanol to acetaldehyde. **A.** Conversion of ethanol to acetaldehyde by the P450 mixed function oxidase system using reduced NADPH and oxygen. **B.** Conversion of ethanol to acetaldehyde by alcohol dehydrogenase using oxidized NAD^+. This figure illustrates how NAD and NADP can function in oxidation reactions in both their oxidized and reduced forms.

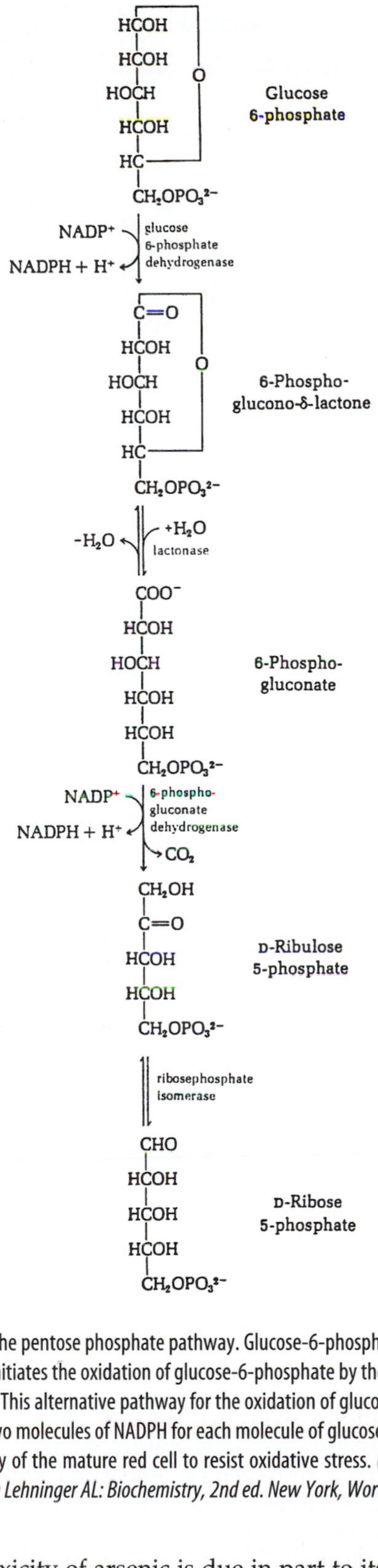

Figure 12–2. The pentose phosphate pathway. Glucose-6-phosphate dehydrogenase (G-6-PD) initiates the oxidation of glucose-6-phosphate by the pentose phosphate pathway. This alternative pathway for the oxidation of glucose results in the production of two molecules of NADPH for each molecule of glucose. NADPH is critical to the ability of the mature red cell to resist oxidative stress. *(Reprinted, with permission, from Lehninger AL: Biochemistry, 2nd ed. New York, Worth, 1975.)*

The toxicity of arsenic is due in part to its effects on glycolysis. It is a powerful inhibitor of 3-phosphoglyceraldehyde dehydrogenase (3-PGA), which catalyzes the oxidation of glyceraldehyde-3-phosphate to 3-phosphoglycerol-phosphate, resulting in the preservation of a high-energy phosphate bond that is used to synthesize ATP in the next step of glycolysis.[14] Arsenic substitutes for phosphate in the synthesis of 3-phosphoglycerol-phosphate, forming 3-phosphoglycerol-arsenate. This unstable compound is rapidly hydrolyzed, resulting in interruption of glycolysis[56] (see Fig. 78–2).

The Krebs Cycle

Mitochondria contain all the enzymes essential to the function of the tricarboxylic acid or Krebs cycle (Fig. 12–4). These reactions are a major source of NADH and are critical to the aerobic production of ATP. The Krebs cycle oxidizes pyruvate, the end product of glycolysis, to ultimately form one molecule of CO_2, one molecule of GTP (guanosine triphosphate), and five molecules of NADH, which feed into the electron–cytochrome transport chain and produce 15 molecules of ATP. In addition, the tricarboxylic acid cycle provides intermediates for amino acid synthesis and for gluconeogenesis.

Inhibitors of the Krebs cycle are potent toxins. Two powerful rodenticides, sodium fluoroacetate and fluoroacetamide, become incorporated into fluoroacetyl coenzyme A and enter the Krebs cycle by condensation with oxaloacetate, forming fluorocitrate. This substance blocks the conversion of citrate to isocitrate by aconitase, resulting in the accumulation of large amounts of citrate in the mitochondria and inhibition of the cycle[81] (Fig. 12–5).

Thiamine is an important cofactor for Krebs cycle enzymes that carry out decarboxylation reactions. It is required for the conversion of pyruvate to acetyl-CoA by pyruvate decarboxylase and for the conversion of alpha-ketoglutarate to succinyl-CoA by alpha-ketoglutarate dehydrogenase. It is also essential to the function of transketolase, an enzyme involved in the synthesis of complex sugars, and has a role in neuronal conduction.[44,84] The life-threatening effects of thiamine deficiency are likely related to impairment of these three enzyme functions (see Antidotes in Depth: Thiamine).

Electron Transport and Oxidative Phosphorylation

The oxidative phosphorylation of adenosine diphosphate (ADP) to ATP occurs during the transport of electrons down a series of membrane-bound iron-containing cytochromes, ultimately resulting in the reduction of molecular oxygen to water (Fig. 12–6). These reactions take place in the mitochondria.

Toxins that inhibit electron transport lead to rapid depletion of cellular energy stores, followed by failure of ATP-dependent active transport pumps, loss of essential electrolyte gradients, and increases in cell volume. Well characterized toxins include cyanide and hydrogen sulfide, which block the cytochrome aa_3 mediated reduction of O_2 to H_2O. Carbon monoxide also combines with cytochrome aa_3, although its major toxic effect is related to displacement of oxygen from hemoglobin and myoglobin. Other agents less commonly involved in poisoning also inhibit cytochromes: azide at cytochrome aa_3, antimycin A at the cytochrome bc_1 step, and rotenone

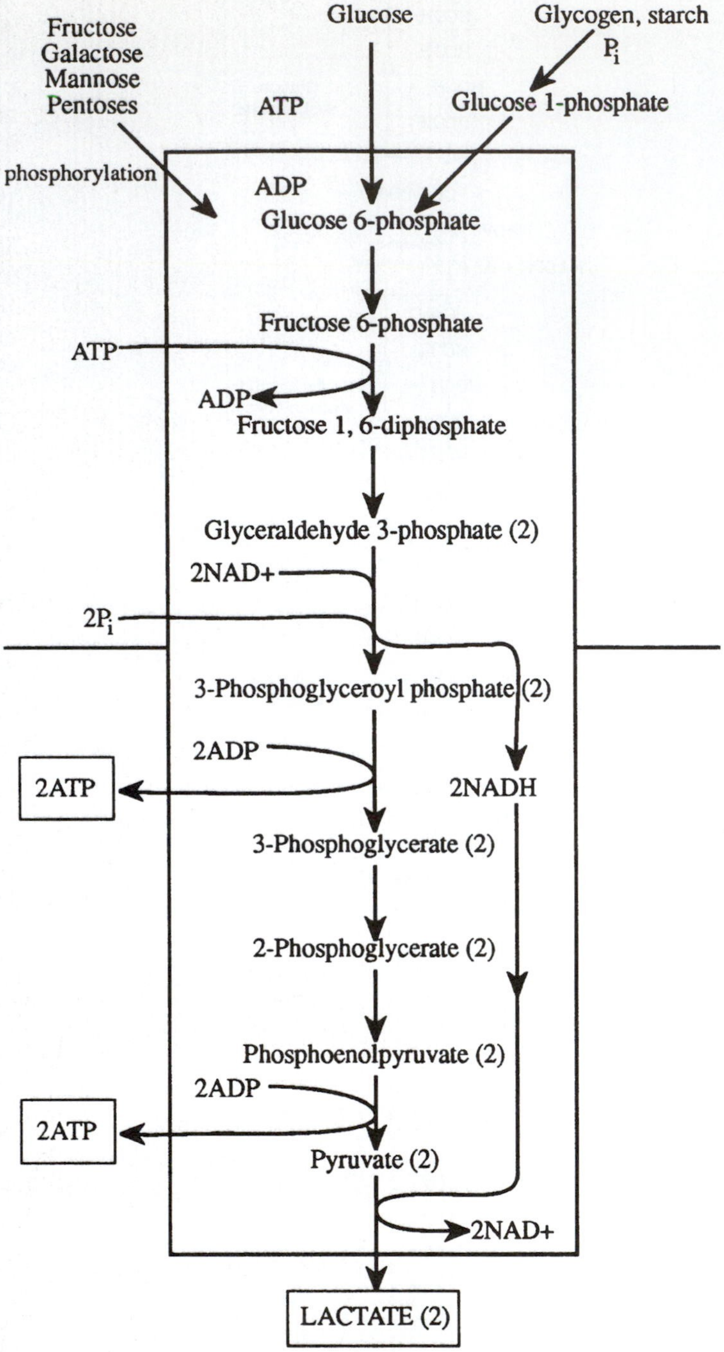

Figure 12–3. Glycolysis. The anaerobic metabolism of carbohydrates. *(Reprinted, with permission, from Lehninger AL: Biochemistry, 2nd ed. New York, Worth, 1975.)*

(a toxic plant substance used by South American Indians to poison fish) at the NADH dehydrogenase–ubiquinone step.[3,5,71]

A substantial amount of energy is generated by electron transport that is normally captured in the stable high-energy phosphate bonds of ATP. If ATP synthesis is blocked but electron transport continues, the electron transport is said to be "uncoupled" from oxidative phosphorylation. When this occurs, the energy obtained from the oxidation of NADH and reduction of O_2 is released as heat. Various toxins act as "uncouplers." In in vitro mitochondrial preparations, dinitrophenol stimulates increased glutamate oxidation associated with decreased ATP synthesis and no change in oxygen utilization, suggesting an uncoupling of oxidative phosphorylation from ATP synthesis.[60] Fatal exposures of workers to dinitrophenol compounds used as weed killers and to pentachlorophenol (a wood preservative) are associated with severe hyperthermia.[49,51] Fatalities in rats following acute oral ingestion of dinitrophenol are also associated

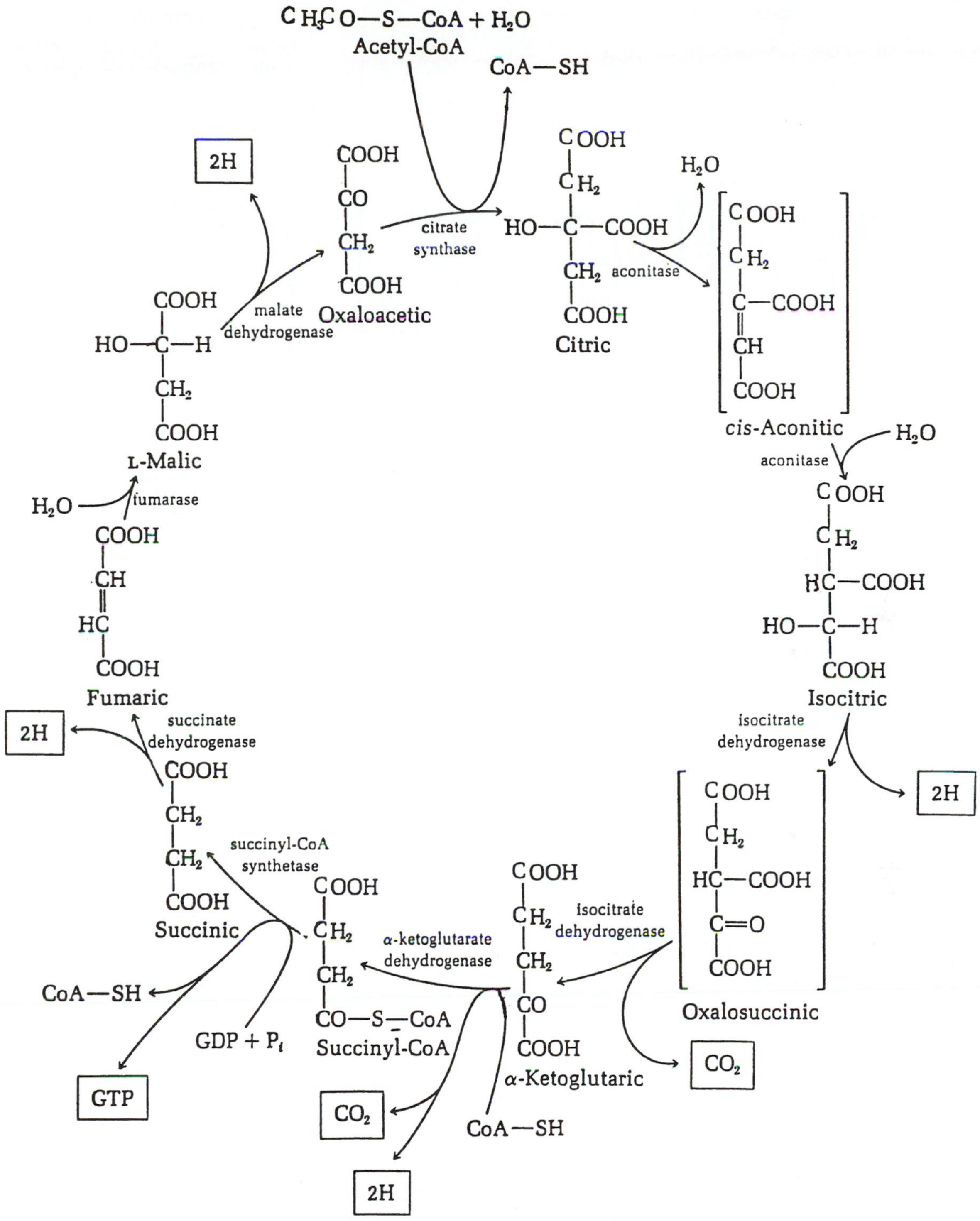

Figure 12–4. The Krebs (tricarboxylic acid) cycle. *(Reprinted, with permission, from Lehninger AL: Biochemistry, 2nd ed. New York, Worth, 1975.)*

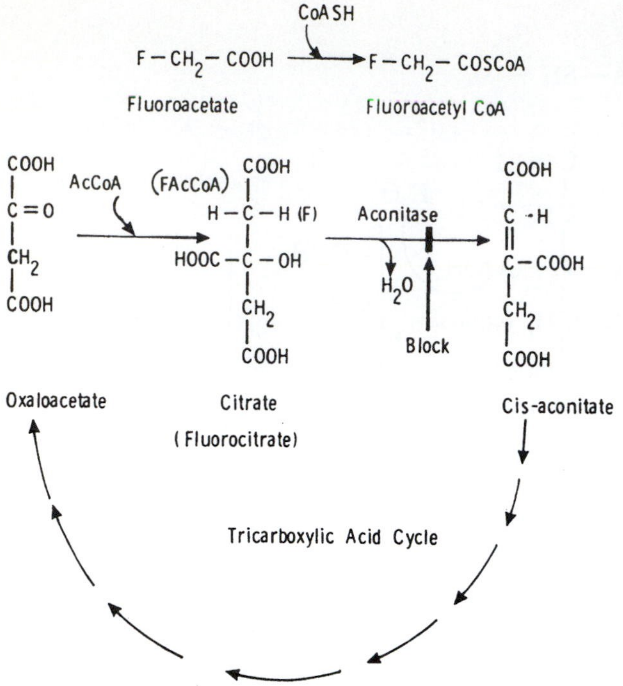

Figure 12–5. Metabolism of fluoroacetic acid to fluoroacetyl-CoA and mechanism underlying the blockade of the Krebs cycle. Fluorocitrate cannot be dehydrated to *cis*-aconitate by aconitase and therefore blocks the cycle at this point. *(Reprinted, with permission, from Timbrell JA: Principles of Biochemical Toxicology. London, Taylor & Francis, 1987.)*

with significant hyperthermia.[77] The hyperthermia and lactic acidosis resulting from severe salicylate poisoning are also attributed to an uncoupling of oxidative phosphorylation by salicylates.[74]

Other Metabolic Pathways: The Pentose Phosphate Pathway and Gluconeogenesis

The Pentose Phosphate Pathway

The main purpose of the pentose phosphate pathway in most tissues is the production of NADPH for biosynthetic reactions (Fig. 12–2). This pathway also provides important protection against oxidative stress in the mature red cell. Two enzymes in the pathway, glucose-6-phosphate dehydrogenase (G–6–PD) and 6-phosphogluconate dehydrogenase use NADP+ as a cofactor and reduce it to NADPH.[73] Persons with G–6–PD deficiency have a reduced capability to synthesize NADPH and may develop hemolysis following exposure to oxidant chemicals. Hemolysis in persons with G–6–PD deficiency is now thought to be related to the requirement of NADPH for the maximal functioning of both glutathione peroxidase and catalase, enzymes that scavenge toxic peroxides produced by encounters of erythrocytes with oxidant chemicals.[26] Another manifestation of oxidative

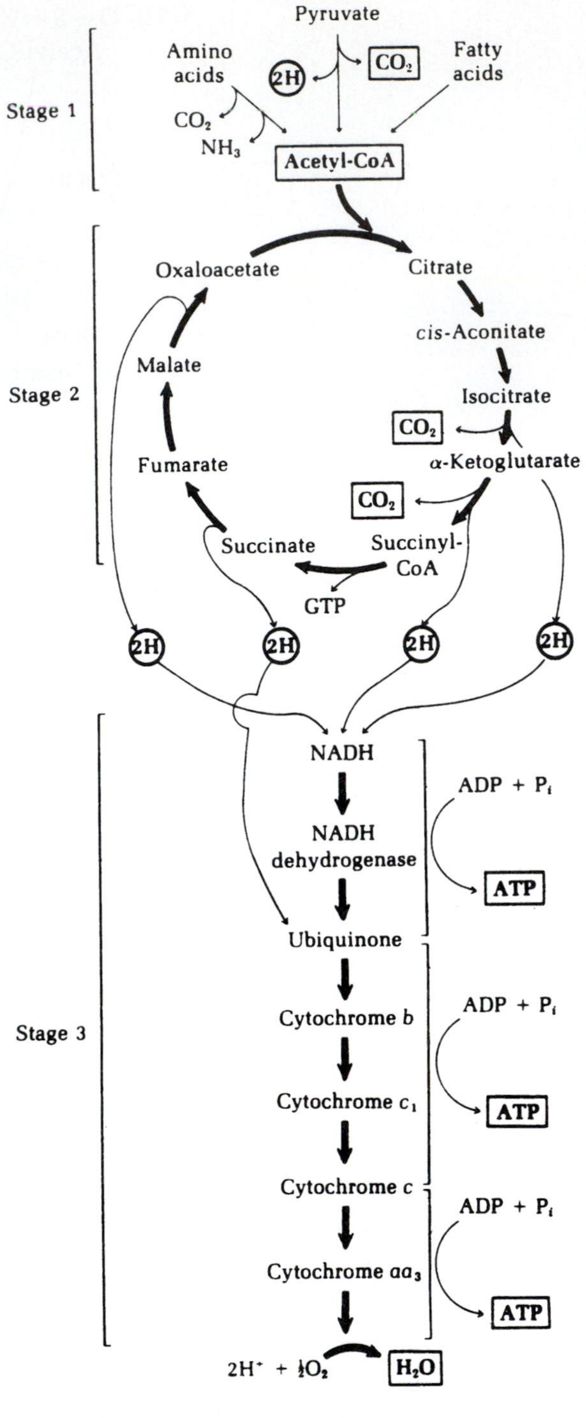

Figure 12–6. Stages in cell respiration. Stage 1: Mobilization of acetyl-CoA from glucose, fatty acids, and some amino acids. Stage 2: The citric acid cycle. Stage 3: Electron transport and oxidative phosphorylation. *(Modified, with permission, from Lehninger AL: Principles of Biochemistry, New York, Worth, 1982.)*

stress is the oxidation of the iron in hemoglobin from Fe^{2+} to Fe^{3+} producing methemoglobin, which occurs both spontaneously and as a response to toxins such as nitrites and aminophenols. Persons who have G-6-PD deficiency have limited ability to utilize the alternative NADPH-dependent methemoglobin reductase that reduces methemoglobin following the administration of methylene blue (see Chap. 93). These patients have adequate levels of NADH-dependent methemoglobin reductase and do not develop methemoglobinemia under normal conditions.

Gluconeogenesis

Gluconeogenesis is the biochemical pathway that facilitates the conversion of amino acids and intermediates of the Krebs cycle to glucose. It is an important source of glucose during fasting, and allows maintenance of glycogen stores. The pathway is illustrated in Figure 12-7. Most of the steps in the synthesis of glucose-6-phosphate from pyruvate are simply the reverse of glycolysis, with three exceptions: (1) the conversion of glucose-6-phospate to glucose, (2) the conversion of fructose-1,6-biphosphate (FDP) to fructose-6-phosphate, and (3) the synthesis of phosphoenolpyruvate from pyruvate. These three reactions are catalyzed by irreversible enzyme steps in the direction of glycolysis. While the first two gluconeogenic bypasses simply use different enzymes, the synthesis of phosphoenolpyruvate from pyruvate is more complex, requiring several steps to bypass the irreversible pyruvate kinase step of glycolysis. Pyruvate is first converted to oxaloacetate within the mitochondria, then to malate, which is transported out of the mitochondria. In the cytosol malate is reconverted back to oxaloacetate, then to phosphoenolpyruvate. Certain amino acids, notably alanine, glutamate, and aspartate, are readily converted to Krebs cycle intermediates and can be transformed to glucose through this cycle.[44] The cycle depends on the presence of NAD^+ in the cytosol, which is necessary to oxidize lactate to pyruvate. It also requires the presence of NADH within the mitochondria. Under conditions when the reducing potential (the NADH/NAD^+ ratio) in the cytosol outside the mitochondria is high, gluconeogenesis is impaired.

A number of toxins impair gluconeogenesis, resulting in hypoglycemia when glycogen stores are depleted. Ethanol is associated with hypoglycemia by this mechanism. The proposed mechanism is based on the observation that the metabolism of ethanol results in an increase in the cytosolic NADH/NAD^+ ratio. This affects two important steps that require the availability of NAD^+: the conversion of lactate to pyruvate and the conversion of extra-mitochondrial malate to oxaloacetate.[2,47] Significant hypoglycemia occurs in fasting glycogen-deficient patients who are intoxicated with ethanol.[2,23]

Hypoglycin A, an unusual amino acid from the unripe Akee fruit that is the cause of Jamaican vomiting sickness, also inhibits gluconeogenesis. Ingestion of this agent causes profound hypoglycemia associated with the accumulation of amino acid metabolites.[21,79] Hypoglycin A is metabolized to an intermediate MCPA (methylenecyclopropylacetic acid), which has metabolic effects that indirectly inhibit gluconeogenesis. It blocks the oxidation of long-chain fatty acids, an important source of NADH in the mitochondria. It also inhibits the metabolism of several glycogenic amino acids, including leucine, isoleucine, and tryptophan, and blocks their en-

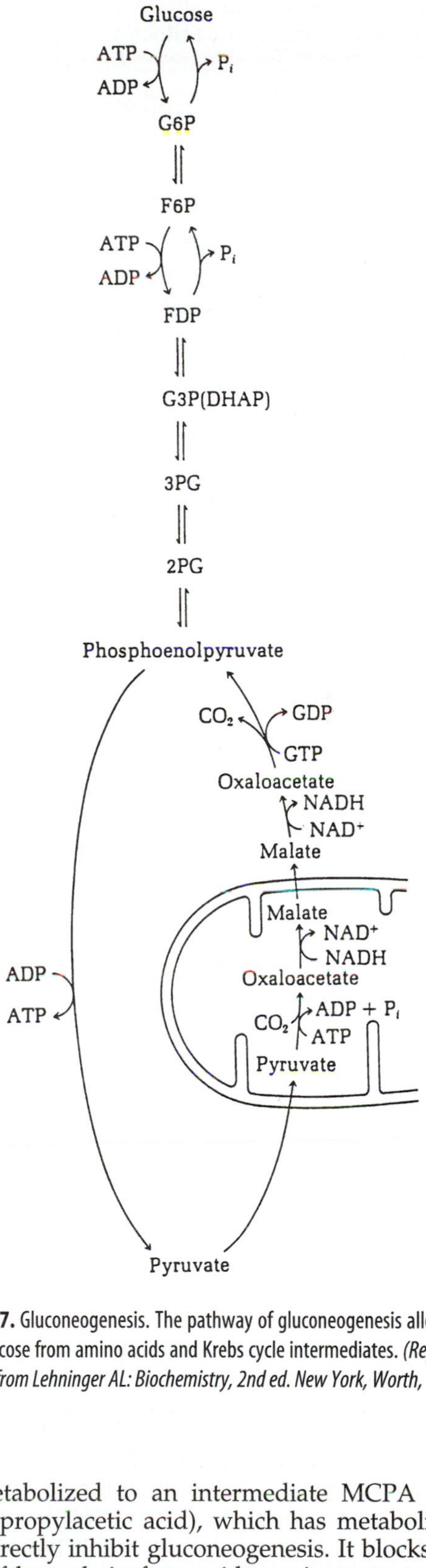

Figure 12-7. Gluconeogenesis. The pathway of gluconeogenesis allows the synthesis of glucose from amino acids and Krebs cycle intermediates. *(Reprinted, with permission, from Lehninger AL: Biochemistry, 2nd ed. New York, Worth, 1975.)*

trance into the Krebs cycle. MCPA may also block the transport of malate out of the mitochondria.[69,78,79,80]

Toxins That Are Substrates for Synthetic Enzymes

Sometimes a toxin is mistaken for a natural substrate by synthetic enzymes, which act on it and facilitate its injurious effect. The suicidal incorporation of fluoroacetate into the Krebs cycle described above is an example of this mechanism of toxic injury (Fig. 12–5). This mechanism is also illustrated by analogs of purine and pyrimidine bases, which are phosphorylated by cellular enzymes and incorporated into growing RNA or DNA chains, producing point mutations or breakage of the cellular genetic material (see Chap. 16 on mechanisms of mutagenesis). For example, the pyrimidine analog 5-fluorouracil (5-FU) used in the treatment of adenocarcinomas of the intestine is phosphorylated to 5-fluoro-dUTP and incorporated into growing DNA chains. This results in structural instability of the growing tumor cell. It is also a potent inhibitor of thymidylate synthetase, the enzyme which converts the RNA precursor uridine monophosphate (UMP) to the DNA precursor thymidine monophosphate (TMP). This limits TMP availability and inhibits the synthesis of normal DNA.[16,70]

Toxins With Specific Receptor Binding Affinities

A toxin may undergo high-affinity binding to specific protein receptors, disrupting neurosynaptic transmission or membrane transport processes. Drugs such as atropine, antihistamines, and tricyclic antidepressants gain access to and block postsynaptic muscarinic acetylcholine receptors in the eyes, bladder, skin, and bowel, resulting in a characteristic anticholinergic syndrome.[25] Pancuronium selectively blocks postsynaptic nicotinic acetylcholine receptors in muscle, resulting in paralysis. The toxicity of opioids is mediated by binding to specific receptors in the CNS. The high affinity of carbon monoxide for hemoglobin or cyanide for cytochrome aa_3 accounts for some of their injurious effects.

Biotransformation: Detoxification and Activation of Xenobiotics

The ability to detoxify and eliminate both endogenous and environmental toxins (xenobiotics) is crucial to the maintenance of physiologic homeostasis and normal metabolic functions for all organisms. A simple example is the necessity of detoxifying cyanide, a potent cellular poison that is ubiquitous in the environment and is also a product of normal metabolism. Mammals have evolved the enzyme rhodanese that combines cyanide with thiosulfate to create the less toxic, renally excreted compound, thiocyanate.[82] Enzymes like rhodanese whose function is to biotransform and detoxify xenobiotics are ubiquitous in the body. Many of them facilitate the biotransformation of broad classes of substrates such as alcohols, aldehydes, esters, or amines, acting on many different substrates within these groups. The locations of these enzymes are often related to their function. Enzymes that act on more fat-soluble, lipophilic toxins are commonly found embedded in lipid membranes such as the endoplasmic reticulum. When cells are mechanically disrupted and centrifuged, these membrane-bound enzymes are found in the pellet or microsomal fraction; hence they are called microsomal enzymes. Enzymes located in the liquid matrix of cells are called cytosolic enzymes and are found in the supernatant when disrupted cells are centrifuged. Microsomal enzymes are found primarily in the liver, but also exist in the kidney, lung, gut, and urinary bladder. Cytosolic biotransformation enzymes are found in all tissues.[39]

Many xenobiotics that gain access to the body have lipophilic properties that facilitate absorption through the skin, lungs, or mucosal surfaces. The essence of detoxification reactions is to convert lipophilic substances to less active, more soluble, readily excretable substances. Sometimes in the course of these metabolic transformations the process goes awry, and a more toxic metabolite may be formed. This is the mechanism whereby many toxins, some of which may initially be chemically innocuous, cause injury. Many examples of agents that are transformed to more toxic agents by biotransformation are described in the following sections.

Injury by Metabolites at Distant Sites

Toxic metabolites may be synthesized at one site and transported to other target sites, where they cause injury. This appears to be the case for benzene, which is metabolized by hepatic microsomal enzymes to benzoquinone and dihydroxybenzene intermediates, which subsequently injure the bone marrow.[85] Two commonly used industrial solvents, *n*-hexane and methyl-*n*-butyl ketone, produce peripheral neuropathy. Their common hepatic metabolite, 2,5-hexanedione, is the postulated neurotoxic agent[18] (Fig. 12–8). Acetonitrile (CH_3CN), a solvent product used to remove artificial fingernails, is converted by hepatic enzymes to cyanide, resulting in fatal systemic poisoning hours after ingestion.[15] The toxic alcohols methanol and ethylene glycol must be converted by ADH and aldehyde dehydrogenase (ALDH) to toxic metabolites in order to exert their toxic effects (see Chap. 64).

The toxicity of ingested compounds may be altered by enzymatic activity or bacterial flora in the GI tract. Amygdalin, the cyanogenic glycoside that is the active toxic component of laetrile, must be hydrolyzed in the gut to cyanide to exert its toxicity (see Fig. 97–1). Intravenous forms of laetrile do not cause toxicity in animal studies.[33] Nitrates present in well water in farming communities can be converted to nitrites by gut bacteria, leading to methemoglobinemia. A high gastric pH in very young infants allows the growth of enteric organisms in the stomach and makes them particularly susceptible to the toxic effects of ingested nitrates.[68]

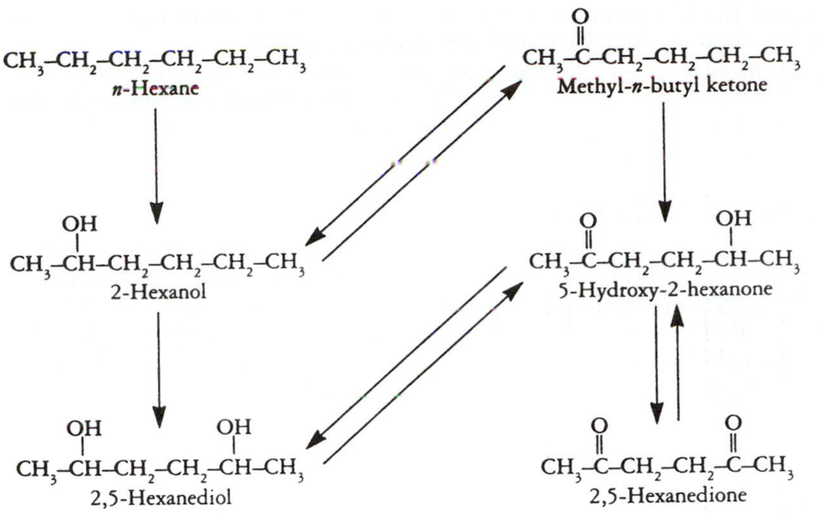

Figure 12–8. The metabolism of methyl-*n*-butyl ketone and *n*-hexane. 2,5-Hexanedione is thought to be the common neurotoxic metabolite. *(Reprinted, with permission, from Rom WN: Environmental and Occupational Medicine. Boston, Little, Brown, 1992, p. 567. Modified from DiVincenzo GD, Kaplan CJ, DeDinas J: Toxicol Appl Pharmacol 1976;36:511–522.)*

In Situ Injury by Metabolites of Biotransformation Reactions

The capacity of a tissue to metabolize certain toxins may be essential to the production of injury in that tissue. Highly reactive metabolites, such as epoxide intermediates and free radicals, exert damage at the site where they are synthesized. Structural examples of the formation of reactive epoxides during the metabolism of vinyl chloride and trichloroethylene are given in Figure 12–9. Tissue injury by reactive metabolites occurs commonly in the liver, the major site of metabolism of foreign compounds, but occurs in other organs as well.[29,75,87] The lungs, skin, kidneys, and gastrointestinal tract have the capacity to metabolize xenobiotics.[39] Even the nasal mucosa converts xenobiotics to metabolites that result in local injury.[13] Cycasin, a naturally occurring carcinogen, is harmless when administered parenterally to animals. However, when administered orally, it is hydrolyzed by gut bacteria to methylazoxymethanol, a powerful carcinogen that causes colon cancers at the site of biotransformation.[22,72,87] Ipomeanol, a fungal toxin associated with pulmonary injury in rats, specifically causes necrosis of alveolar epithelial cells following its activation by enzymes in those cells.[11] Acute tubular necrosis is occasionally seen in patients with overdose of acetaminophen.[38] This has recently been attributed to metabolism by prostaglandin H synthase (PHS), levels of which are much higher in the kidney compared to levels of P450 enzymes. PHS normally mediates the conversion of arachadonic acid to prostaglandin by way of a highly reactive intermediate. It has been proposed that renal PHS converts acetaminophen to a highly reactive semiquinoneimine that binds and damages renal tubular cells.[20] Following selective concentration in lung tissue, paraquat is transformed to a free radical in an oxgen-dependent reaction by enzymes in the nonciliated alveolar epithelial cells. The free radical then selectively injures those cells.[66]

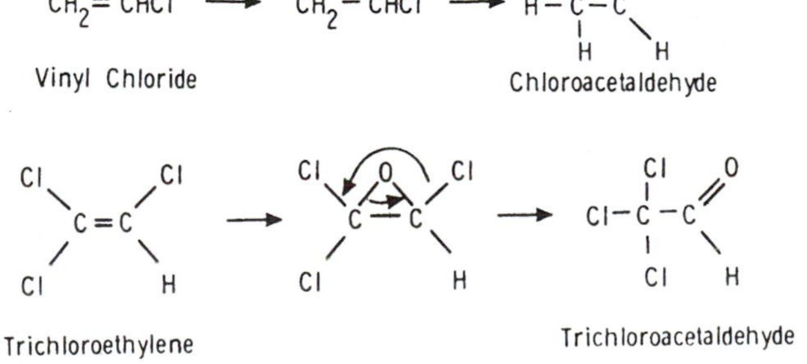

Figure 12–9. The metabolism of vinyl chloride and trichloroethylene via epoxide intermediates. *(Modified, with permission, from Timbrell JA: Principles of Biochemical Toxicology. London, Taylor & Francis, 1987.)*

Monoamine oxidases (MAO) are mitochondrial enzymes present in many tissues. They oxidize a large number of different amines, including dopamine, epinephrine, and serotonin, and xenobiotics such as primaquine and haloperidol. The metabolic activity of MAO was responsible for the outbreak of parkinsonism associated with the use of MPTP (methylphenyltetrahydropyridine), an unintended product of an attempt to synthesize a "designer" analog of meperidine, methylphenylpropionoxypiperidine (MPPP) (see Chap. 60). After crossing the blood–brain barrier, MPTP is transformed by MAO to $MPDP^+$ (methylphenyldihydropyridine), which is thought to be nonenzymatically converted to MPP^+. The MPP^+ is taken up by specific dopamine transport systems into dopaminergic neurons in the substantia nigra, resulting in neuronal death by a still unclear mechanism.[27]

Mechanisms of Biotransformation of Toxins

Phase I Reactions

The metabolism of xenobiotics is mediated by phase I and phase II biotransformation reactions. Phase I reactions result in the synthesis of a more chemically reactive metabolite of a lipophilic xenobiotic. In most cases, these are followed by phase II reactions that conjugate the product produced in the phase I reaction with another molecule that detoxifies it, renders it significantly more soluble, and facilitates its elimination.

Phase I reactions are primarily oxidation–reduction reactions. Oxidation involves the extraction of electrons from a substrate and their transfer to molecular oxygen or to another electron-seeking (electrophilic) substance such as NAD^+. Reduction involves the transfer of electrons to a substrate. Phase I reactions result in the addition of more polar, reactive groups such as hydroxyl (-OH), sulfhydryl (-SH), amino ($-NH_2$), aldehyde (-COH), or carboxyl (-COOH).[39] The most common biochemical oxidation–reduction reactions are mediated by three types of enzyme systems: (1) membrane-bound iron-containing P450 cytochromes that are oxidized (Fe^{3+}) or reduced (Fe^{2+}) during their transfer of electrons from one substrate to another; (2) membrane-bound flavin-associated NADPH dependent monoxygenases; and (3) cytosolic NADH or NADPH-linked dehydrogenases, which oxidize or reduce substrates by transfer of electrons between the oxidized (NAD^+, $NADP^+$) and reduced (NADH, NADPH) forms of these nucleotides.[29,42,46]

The most important example of a phase I enzyme system is the microsomal cytochrome P450 mono-oxygenase system, or mixed-function oxygenase system. Cytochrome P450 enzymes are heme proteins located mainly in the endoplasmic reticulum. The cytochrome gets its name from its spectrophotometric characteristics. When reduced cytochrome P450 (Fe^{2+}) binds to carbon monoxide, its maximal absorption spectrum occurs at 450 nm.[30] The cytochrome P450 mixed-function oxygenase system is actually a coupled system containing an NADPH-dependent reductase that facilitates the transfer of electrons from NADPH to the enzyme-substrate complex and a heme-containing cytochrome that then allows oxidation of the complex by molecular oxygen and transfer of electrons to oxygen to form a water molecule. These enzymes mediate many different types of oxidation reactions. A general example is the oxidation of a foreign compound R-H to R-OH. The stoichiometric illustration of this reaction is the following:

$$RH + NADH + O_2 \rightarrow NAD^+ + H_2O + ROH$$

This reaction occasionally proceeds through a reactive radical intermediate:

$$(FeO)^{3+} + RH \rightarrow (FeOH)^{3+}R \rightarrow Fe^{3+} + ROH$$

In other cases, electron transfer may result in the production of an activated metabolite.[30]

$$Fe^{3+} + ROOH \rightarrow RO^- + (FeOH)^{3+}$$

$$Fe^{3+} + ROOH \rightarrow RO + (FeOH)^{2+}$$

Reductive biotransformation is facilitated by the P450 system when the electrons donated by NADPH are transferred to the substrate, rather than to molecular oxygen. The reduction of a nitro group $R-NO_2$ to an amine $R-NH_2$ is an example of reductive biotransformation by the mixed-function oxidases.

Another important phase I system is the alcohol, aldehyde, and ketone oxidation system. These are predominantly cytosolic enzymes that depend on NAD^+ for oxidation reactions. A clinically familiar example is the metabolism of ethanol to acetaldehyde by alcohol dehydrogenase, followed by the rapid metabolism of acetaldehyde to acetic acid by aldehyde dehydrogenase (Fig. 12–1). Alcohol dehydrogenase is a cytosolic enzyme found in the liver, lungs, kidney, and gastric mucosa that oxidizes many different alcohols.[1,46] Gender based differences in the activity of ADH in gastric mucosa account for the greater observed toxicity of ethanol in women.[24] Atypical forms of ADH are responsible for the rapid oxidation of ethanol in Japanese and Chinese peoples, resulting in a characteristic flush as acetaldehyde, the product of ADH, accumulates.[1] These persons may also be deficient in ALDH, an enzyme that converts aldehydes to carboxylic acids, or in this case converts acetaldehyde to acetic acid.[28]

Liver ADH has a very low K_m for ethanol. The K_m is the substrate concentration at which 50% of the maximal rate of activity of the enzyme occurs. A low K_m indicates that ADH is capable of catalyzing the oxidation of ethanol at very low concentrations of ethanol and is therefore the primary metabolic enzyme for ethanol. The acute metabolism of ethanol to acetaldehyde alters the "redox" potential of the cell by raising the ratio of NADH to NAD^+. This makes it harder for the cell to carry out important oxidation reactions such as the conversion of lactate to pyruvate, the oxidation of fatty acids, and gluconeogenesis.[46]

Ethanol may also be metabolized by a microsomal oxygen and NADPH-dependent cytochrome P450. The enzyme that specifically metabolizes ethanol is inducible, that is, its concentration and activity increase in persons who chronically consume large amounts of ethanol.[46] The gene for this enzyme is named CYP2E1. The enzyme has been purified and named P4502E1. P4502E1 has a high K_m for ethanol, which means that it is functional only when ethanol levels are high. It also metabolizes other substrates such as acetaminophen and carbon tetrachloride.[46] The microsomal enzyme accounts for only a small fraction of ethanol metabolism in those who drink modestly but accounts for a significant fraction of ethanol metabolism in alcoholics.[46]

The oxidation of ethanol to acetaldehyde by alcohol dehydrogenase and the microsomal mixed-function oxidase system illustrates how NAD^+ and $NADP^+$ can function in oxidation reactions in both their oxidized and reduced forms (see Fig. 12–1).

The P450 Enzymes

The P450 enzymes are the most numerous and important of the enzymes involved in phase I oxidation reactions. More than 200 genes coding for P450 enzymes have been identified and classified into more than 30 families based on their amino acid sequences.[31] Information from research in this field is accumulating rapidly. Enzymes that share less than 40% of their amino acid sequences are classified into different gene families (CYP1, CYP2, CYP3, etc). Enzymes that share 40–55% of their sequences are in different subfamilies (CYP1A, CYP1B, CYP1C, etc). Those that have greater than 55% homology of their amino acid sequences are in the same subfamilies (CYP1A1, CYP1A2, CYP1A3, etc). All of the P450 enzymes that have been shown to have a role in metabolism of xenobiotics in humans belong to three gene families, CYP1, CYP2, CYP3.[58] A great deal of information about the substrate selectivity and catalytic activity of the different P450 enzymes has also been obtained.[29] Most of these enzymes have low substrate specificity and can enzymatically alter a variety of substances.[29] The amount of the enzyme and the sensitivity of the enzyme for the substrate (its K_m) often confers more specificity and makes one P450 enzyme dominant over another in terms of substrate selectivity.[29,31] Since many different P450 enzymes may catalyze the same reaction, it is sometimes difficult to determine which enzyme has the major role in vivo, that is, which has the lowest K_m and the fastest rate. The effect of the K_m for ethanol on its metabolism by ADH and the P450 system has been discussed above. As another example, diazepam is metabolized by both P4502C19 and P4503A4. However, the affinity of P4503A4 for diazepam is so low (that is, the K_m is high) that the majority of diazepam is metabolized by P4502C19.[37] Omeprazole, which is metabolized by P4502C19, blocks the metabolism of diazepam and significantly prolongs its half-life.[62] Other P450 enzymes are highly selective. This is the case for P45021A2, a mitochondrial enzyme that specifically catalyzes the 21-hydroxylation of progesterone, an important step in steroid synthesis.[30]

The functional heterogeneity exhibited by these different enzymes has considerable impact on the potential toxicity of drugs and other xenobiotics on an individual. Different persons metabolize drugs differently. Functional differences are due in some cases to the considerable genetic polymorphism that exists among human P450 systems. In addition, activity levels of enzymes may be altered by concomitant exposure to other agents. Some examples of recently defined forms of P450 enzymes follow.

P4503A4. An excellent example of functional heterogeneity of the P450 enzymes is the recent discovery that some patients taking terfenidine develop very high levels, resulting in spontaneous ventricular tachycardia. This has been related to blockade of P4503A4 by concomitant use of ketoconazole or erythromycin.[63] In addition to its role in the catabolism of terfenidine, P4503A4 also metabolizes dihydropine calcium channel blockers, cyclosporine, some benzodiazepines, and some macrolide antibiotics. Table 12–1 lists a few of the defined human P450 enzymes and their substrates. Most pharmaceuticals are metabolized by P4502D6 or P4503A4. A substance in grapefruit juice has also been associated with a decreased ability to metabolize dihydropine calcium channel blockers.[19,63] CYP3A4 does not exhibit genetic polymorphism.[63]

P4502D6. An important example of the impact of genetic polymorphism of the P450 system is the effect of decreased levels of P4502D6 on drug toxicity. This enzyme was first detected as the enzyme responsible for the metabolism of the antihypertensive debrisoquine, hence it is sometimes referred to as debrisoquine hydrolase. About

TABLE 12–1. OXIDATION OF DRUGS AND TOXINS BY HUMAN P450s

1A1	1A2	2B6	2C8	2C9, 10	2C19	2D6	2E1	3A4
Polycyclic aromatic hydrocarbons	Phenacetin	Cyclophosphamide	Tolbutamide	Hexobarbital	Diazepam	Debrisoquine	Chlorzoxazone	Nifedipine
	Theophylline			Tienilic acid		Sparteine	Acetaminophen	Warfarin
	Acetaminophen			Warfarin		Bufuralol	Methadone	Quinidine
				Phenytoin		Encainide	Isoniazid	Ethinyl estradiol
				Tolbutamide		Propranolol	CCl_4	Terfenadine
						Phenformin	Aniline	Cyclosporine
						Captopril	*p*-Dinitrophenol	FK506
						Metropolol	Ethanol	Rapamycin
						Nortriptyline		Midazolam
						Guanoxan		Triazolam
						Perhexiline		Lovastatin
						4-Methoxyamphetamine		Erythromycin
						Propafenone		Benzphetamine
						Dextromethorphan		Troleandomycin
						Codeine		Lidocaine
						Imipramine		Dapsone
								Taxol
								Alfentanil
								Acetaminophen

Adapted, with permission, from Guengerich FP: Catalytic selectivity of human cytochrome P450 enzymes: relevance to drug metabolism and toxicity. Toxicol Lett 1994;70:133–138.

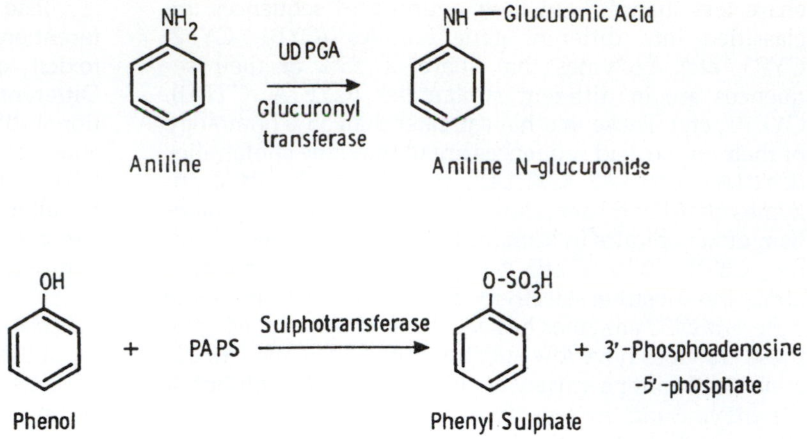

Figure 12–10. Examples of phase II conjugation reactions; aniline conjugation with glucuronic acid, and phenol with sulfate. UDPGA = uridine diphosphate glucuronic acid; PAPS = 3′-phosphoadenosine-5′-phosphosulfate. *(Reprinted, with permission, from Timbrell JA: Principles of Biochemical Toxicology. London, Taylor & Francis, 1987, pp. 73–74.)*

8% of Caucasians are deficient in this enzyme, which is also important in the metabolism of phenformin, several tricyclic antidepressants, the newer selective serotonin reuptake inhibitors (SSRIs), antidysrhythmics, and many others[29,63] (See Table 12–1). Decreased activity of P4502D6 was implicated in the development of severe lactic acidosis in some patients taking phenformin.[59] This enzyme is inhibited by any substance that it metabolizes, an effect that resulted in a 10-fold decrease in the clearance of desipramine when co-administered with fluoxetine in one study. The toxic implications of this are clear.[8] Quinidine also inhibits P4502D6, although it is not a substrate for the enzyme.[8,63]

P4502E1. P4502E1 is a form of P450 that has significant toxicologic implications. It is inducible by a number of substances including ethanol, phenobarbital, isoniazid, phenytoin, and cigarette smoke.[43,86] It also actively produces free radicals such as hydroxyl ($OH^\bullet$), superoxide ($O_2^{\bullet-}$), hydroperoxyl radical ($HO_2^\bullet$), and other reactive metabolites associated with adduct formation and lipid peroxidation. Free radical production has been extensively demonstrated in rat and rabbit livers and in cultured human hepatocytes. It occurs during the metabolism of a number of substrates including carbon tetrachloride, ethanol, acetaminophen, paranitrophenol, aniline, and *N*-nitrosomethylamine.[17] Induction of this enzyme is associated with increased liver injury by reactive metabolites of carbon tetrachloride (see Chap. 13). It also increases liver injury by bromobenzene in rats.[32] Acute elevations of ethanol inhibit this enzyme. This effect is illustrated by the capacity of acute administration of ethanol to inhibit the metabolism of methadone by P4502E1, resulting in higher brain levels, while chronic ingestion hastens its metabolism.[10] Cimetidine also inhibits P4502E1 and is protective against liver injury by acetaminophen in rats.[43,64,76] Acute ethanol ingestion inhibits the metabolism of acetaminophen by cytochrome P450 and may also be protective.[9]

For the reader who wishes more depth in this subject, Parkinson has written a highly comprehensive review of the P450 enzymes and their roles.[61]

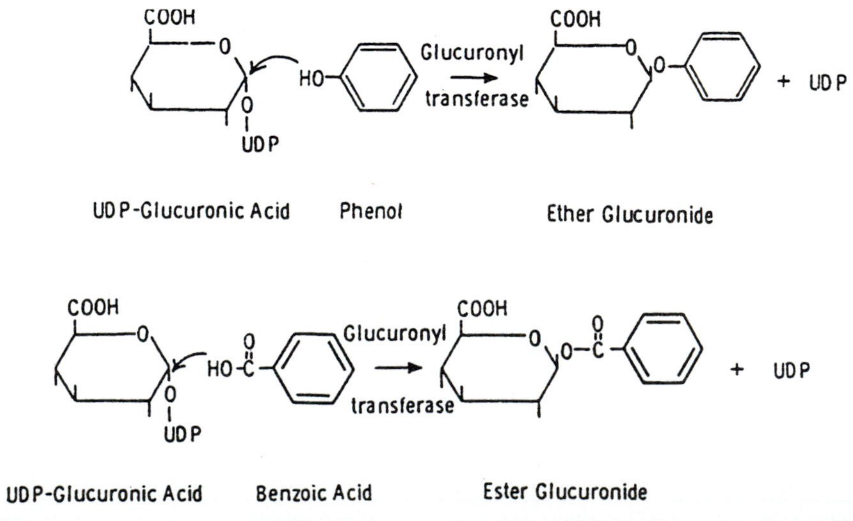

Figure 12–11. Formation of ether and ester glucuronides of phenol and benzoic acid, respectively. *(Reprinted, with permission, from Timbrell JA: Principles of Biochemical Toxicology. London, Taylor & Francis, 1987.)*

Conjugation (Phase II) Reactions

Conjugation with endogenous molecules such as glucuronic acid, glutathione, or sulfate terminates pharmacologic activity and greatly increases the water solubility of the activated molecules resulting from phase I biotransformation reactions. The resulting molecules are more readily excretable.[36,81] Phase II reactions are synthetic in nature and require energy provided by the hydrolysis of high-energy phosphate compounds such as ATP.

Glucuronide formation is an important conjugation reaction. It occurs via glucuronyl transferase through conjugation of glucuronic acid donated by uridine diphosphate glucuronic acid (UDPG) with the nitrogen, sulfhydryl, hydroxyl, or carboxyl groups of foreign or endogenous compounds. The conjugated compounds are readily eliminated in the urine or bile, not only because they are more polar but because glucuronidation confers an ionized carboxyl group that is recognized by biliary and renal active transport systems for organic acids. The glucuronidation of aniline is illustrated in Figure 12–10 and of phenol and benzoic acid in Figure 12–11. Glucuronidation is an important mechanism for the detoxification of acetaminophen (see Chap. 31).

Transfer of an inorganic sulfate group to the hydroxyl group of phenols or alcohols is another common mechanism for detoxification of compounds. The major donor for this reaction is oxidized cysteine. The sulfation of phenol illustrates an important concept in biotransformation (Fig. 12–10). The affinity of sulfate for phenol is very high, so that when low doses of phenol are administered the predominant excretion product is the sulfate ester. However, the capacity of this reaction is readily saturated, so that when high doses of phenol are administered, glucuronidation becomes the main method of detoxification. Alternative biochemical pathways of metabolism are utilized when primary pathways are inaccessible because of overwhelming concentrations of the toxin, depletion of important cofactors, or inhibition of the favored pathway by another agent. This can result in the production of toxic metabolites that are not normally generated. A familiar example of this is the generation of the injurious electrophilic metabolite NAPQI during the metabolism of large amounts of acetaminophen (see Chap. 31).

The glutathione-S transferases catalyze the conjugation of the tripeptide glutathione (glycine-glutamate-cysteine) with a diverse group of toxic compounds. The reactive compounds are electrophilic metabolites of the P450 microsomal enzymes that initiate an electrophilic attack on the sulfur group of cysteine. The glycine and glutamate residues are then cleaved and the molecule acetylated, resulting in an *N*-acetylcysteine (mercapturic acid) conjugate that is readily excreted in the urine. This mechanism effectively detoxifies many reactive electrophiles produced by the P450 system, such as the epoxide metabolite of naphthalene (Fig. 12–12) or bromobenzene (Fig. 12–13). NAPQI, the highly reactive product of acetaminophen metabolism, is also avidly bound by glutathione.[6,12] The importance of glutathione conjugation in the prevention of acetaminophen-induced liver injury is well appreciated[53,54,55] (see Fig. 31–1).

Mechanisms of Cellular Injury

Free Radical Formation

The mechanisms that lead to cellular injury by reactive metabolites are less well defined than those that result in metabolic impairment. Several mechanisms have been postulated. Free radicals are highly reactive molecules

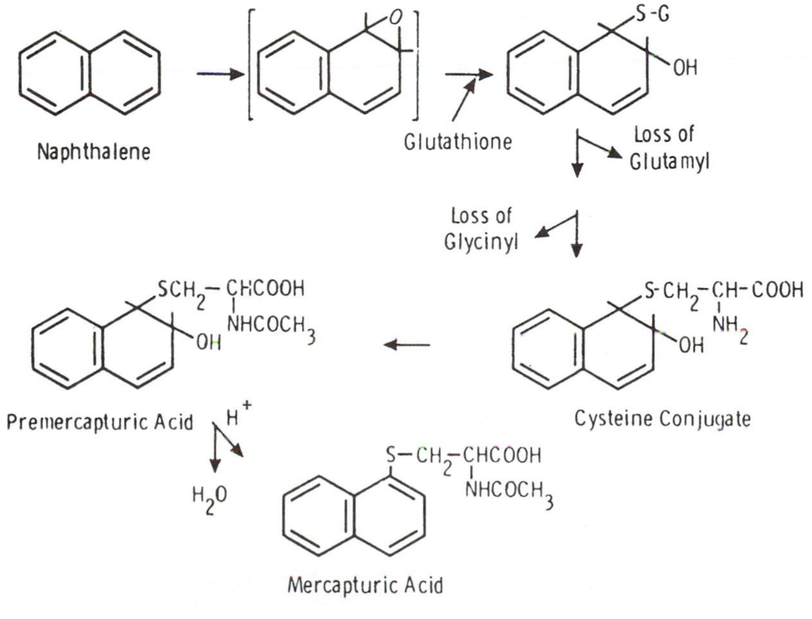

Figure 12–12. Conjugation of naphthalene-1,2 oxide with glutathione and formation of naphthalene mercapturic acid. *(Reprinted, with permission, from Timbrell JA: Principles of Biochemical Toxicology. London, Taylor & Francis, 1987.)*

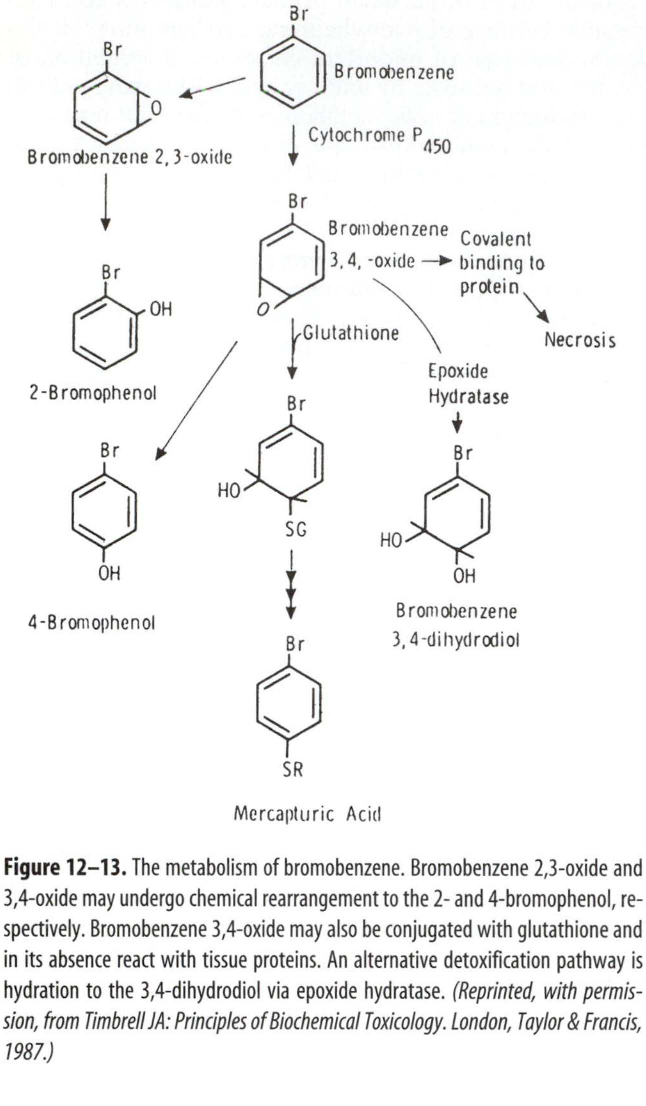

Figure 12–13. The metabolism of bromobenzene. Bromobenzene 2,3-oxide and 3,4-oxide may undergo chemical rearrangement to the 2- and 4-bromophenol, respectively. Bromobenzene 3,4-oxide may also be conjugated with glutathione and in its absence react with tissue proteins. An alternative detoxification pathway is hydration to the 3,4-dihydrodiol via epoxide hydratase. *(Reprinted, with permission, from Timbrell JA: Principles of Biochemical Toxicology. London, Taylor & Francis, 1987.)*

that have an unpaired electron in their outer orbits. They can be formed by homolytic cleavage of a covalent bond, illustrated by the reaction

$$AB \rightarrow A^{\bullet} + B^{\bullet} \qquad \text{or} \qquad O_2 \rightarrow O^{\bullet} + O^{\bullet}$$

Oxygen is frequently involved in the production of free radicals. The free radical species of oxygen are illustrated in Table 12–2. Free radicals are too reactive to be directly measured, but their presence is implied by the products of their reactions. Oxygen free radicals are common products of metabolism, and "scavenging" enzymes such as superoxide dismutase and peroxidase are abundant in cells. In the presence of oxygen certain toxins generate highly reactive free radicals that cause injury at the site of their formation. The ethanol-inducible CYP2E1 likely has a significant role in the production of toxic injury by its substrates, including carbon tetrachloride, ethanol, and acetaminophen.[17] It produces significant amounts of superoxide and peroxide and, in the presence of iron, produces a hydroxyl free radical that readily initiates lipid peroxidation.[17] The most destructive oxygen free radical is the hydroxyl free radical, $OH^{\bullet}$, which will react with any biologic molecule in the vicinity, causing damage to proteins, DNA, lipids, or carbohydrates. Free radicals are most destructive when they initiate chain reactions, such as occurs when a free radical attacks polyunsaturated fatty acids in cellular membranes, resulting in lipid peroxidation. Free radical attack on an unsaturated fatty acid in a lipid membrane removes a hydrogen atom from a methylene carbon and leaves an unpaired electron, causing the formation of a lipid radical that attacks other unsaturated fatty-acid chains and results in a chain reaction, destroying the cellular membrane (Fig. 12–14). In addition, destruction of the membrane produces degradation products that initiate inflammatory reactions in the cell.[75] The formation of free radicals is implicated in the pulmonary injury caused by paraquat, the myocardial injury caused by doxorubicin, and the liver injury caused by carbon tetrachloride.[57,66,75] Paraquat reacts with NADPH to form a pyridinyl free radical, which in turn reacts with oxygen to generate the superoxide anion radical (Fig. 12–15). In the presence of iron these superoxide radicals are converted to hydroxyl radicals that initiate lipid peroxidation in the lungs. Adriamycin is metabolized to a semiquinone free radical in the cardiac mitochondria, which in the presence of oxygen forms a superoxide anion radical that initiates myocardial lipid peroxidation.[57] Carbon tetrachloride (CCl_4) is metabolized by the cytochrome P450 system to the trichloromethyl radical $^{\bullet}CCl_3$, which binds covalently to cellular macromolecules. In the presence of oxygen, this is converted to $^{\bullet}CCl_3O_2$, which can initiate lipid peroxidation (see Fig. 12–16).[67]

TABLE 12–2. FREE RADICAL SPECIES OF OXYGEN

$O_2^{\bullet}$	Superoxide anion
$O^{\bullet}$	Singlet oxygen
$OH^{\bullet}$	Hydroxyl radical
$HO_2^{\bullet}$	Hydroperoxyl radical
$R\text{-}OOH^{\bullet}$	Lipid-peroxide radical

Adduct Formation

Activated toxins formed by phase I biotransformation reactions may also injure cells by binding, or forming adducts with cellular molecules. This occurs with hepatocellular injury by acrolein and by acetaminophen. How the binding of an activated toxin to a cellular macromolecule causes injury to the cell is not known. Interference with enzyme activity due to alteration of the conformational structure of adduct-bound proteins has been postulated.[6] Suicidal alkylation of P450 enzymes by activated substrates may stimulate lysosomal proteolysis.[31] In the case of acetaminophen-induced hepatotoxicity, cellular injury does not occur in the absence of demonstrable binding of APAP to cellular protein constituents,

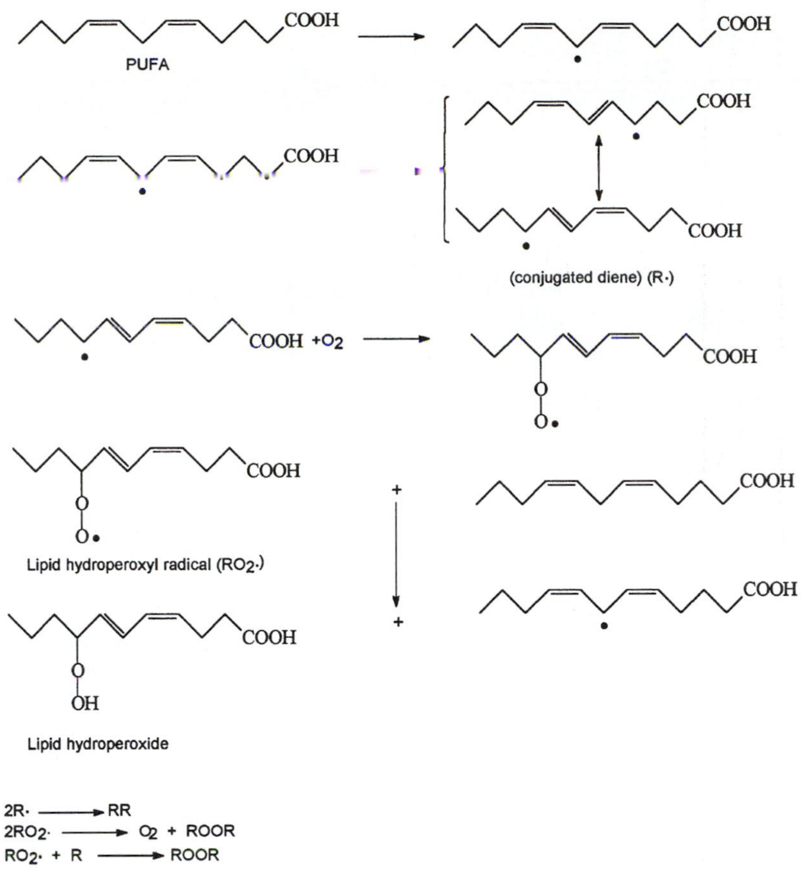

Figure 12–14. Lipid peroxidation initiated by hydroxyl radical. PUFA = polyunsaturated fatty acids. *(Reprinted, with permission, from Southorn PA, Powis G: Free radicals in medicine: I. Chemical nature of biologic reactions. Mayo Clin Proc 1988;63:381–389.)*

but again the exact mechanism of injury by adducts is not known.[7] Autoimmune mechanisms have been demonstrated in some cases. The most likely mechanism by which a drug precipitates autoimmune injury is through the formation of an adduct with a cell, which then induces an immune response against the drug macromolecule or against an immunologically altered cellular macromolecule. Cell destruction might then be mediated by complement- or antibody-directed lysis; by specific cell-mediated cytotoxicity; or by an inflammatory response induced by immune complexes and complement.[50,65] Activated polymorphonucleocytes have been shown to release cytotoxic lysosomal enzymes and oxygen free radicals in response to immune activation.[50]

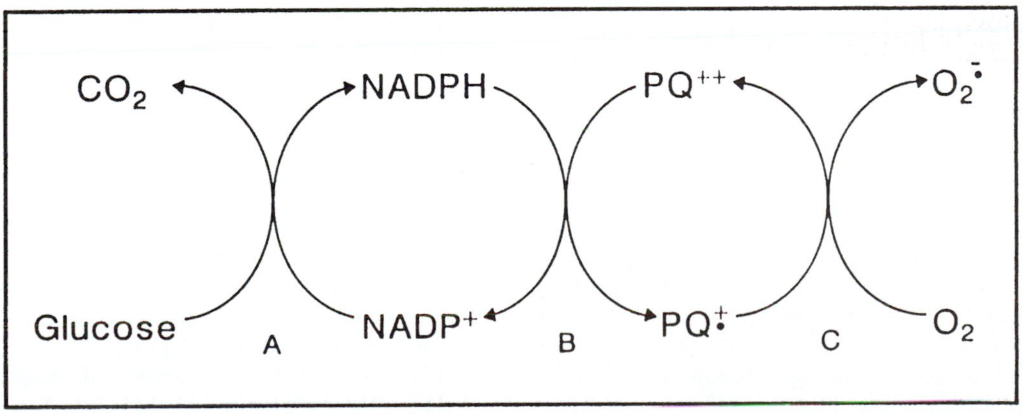

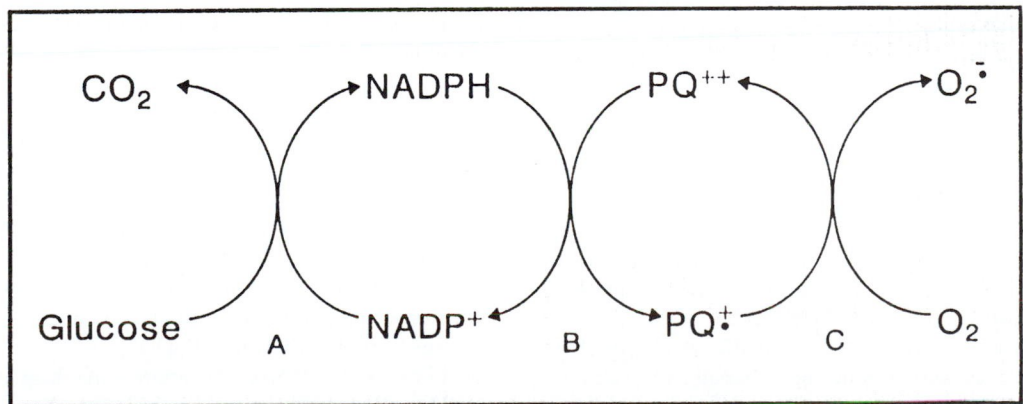

Figure 12–15. Formation of superoxide anion radical by oxidation–reduction cycling of paraquat pyridynyl cation. The following reactions are involved in paraquat toxicity. (**A**) Hexose-monophosphate shunt provides reducing equivalents in the form of NADPH. (**B**) Paraquat pyridinyl cation (PQ^{++}) is reduced to cation radical ($^{\bullet}PQ^{+}$). This reaction proceeds continuously being catalyzed by NADPH cytochrome P450 reductase. (**C**) Oxidation–reduction cycling of pyridinyl cation radical reacting with molecular oxygen forms superoxide anion radical and pyridinyl cation. *(Reprinted, with permission, from Southorn PA, Powis G: Free radicals in medicine: I. Chemical nature of biologic reactions. Mayo Clin Proc 1988;63:381–389.)*

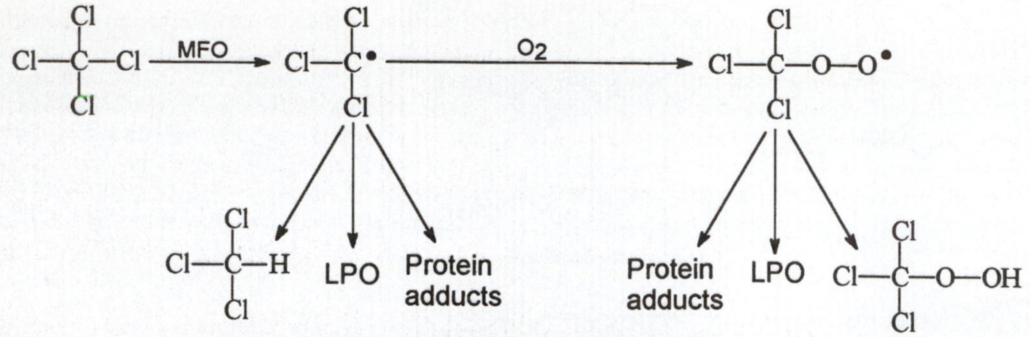

Figure 12–16. Carbon tetrachloride metabolism by the hepatocyte. Under hypoxic conditions, the CCl_3 radical is the predominant species formed. At higher oxygen tensions, CCl_3 is oxidized to CCl_3OO. LPO = lipid peroxidation; MFO = mixed-function oxidation. *(Reprinted, with permission, from Brent JA, Rumack BH: Role of free radicals in toxic hepatic injury. II. Are free radicals the cause of toxin induced liver disease? J Toxicol Clin Toxicol 1993;31:175.)*

Summary

Humans and animals living in a modern environment are exposed to a wide variety of potential toxins. Some substances, including therapeutic drugs, are harmless at low doses and toxic only at high doses. The toxicity of those agents that interrupt important biologic functions or that result in cellular injury is dose-related and is manifested acutely. The diverse mechanisms of toxic injury have been discussed in general terms. The capacity of foreign chemicals to cause injury is clearly a function of many factors specific to the toxin, the tissue injured, and the individual animal or species.

References

1. Agarwal DP, Goedde HW: Pharmacogenetics of alcohol dehydrogenase. In Kalow W, ed: Pharmacogenetics of Drug Metabolism. New York, Pergamon, 1992, pp. 263–280.
2. Arky RA, Freinkel N: Alcohol hypoglycemia. Arch Intern Med 1964;114:501–507.
3. Albert A: Fundamental aspects of selective toxicity. Ann NY Acad Sci 1965;123:5–18.
4. Aldridge WN: Serum esterases: I. Two types of esterase (A and B) hydrolysing *p*-nitrophenyl acetate, propionate and butyrate, and a method for their determination. Biochem J 1953;53:110–117.
5. Ariens EJ, Wius EW, Veringa EJ: Stereoselectivity of bioactive xenobiotics. Biochem Pharmacol 1988;37:9–18.
6. Badr MZ, Belinsky SA, Kauffman FC, Thurman RG: Mechanism of hepatoxicity to periportal regions of the liver lobule due to allyl alcohol: role of oxygen and lipid peroxidation. J Pharmacol Exp Ther 1986;238:1138–1142.
7. Bartolone JB, Beierschmitt WP, Birge RB, et al: Selective acetaminophen metabolite binding of hepatic and extrahepatic proteins: An *in vivo* and *in vitro* analysis. Toxicol Appl Pharmacol 1989;99:240–249.
8. Bergstrom RF, Peyton AL, Lemberger L: Quantification and mechanism of the fluoxetine and tricyclic antidepressant interaction. Clin Pharmacol Ther 1992;51:239–248.
9. Black M, Raucy J: Acetaminophen, alcohol and cytochrome P450. Ann Intern Med 1986;104:427–429.
10. Borowsky SA, Lieber CS: Interaction of methadone and ethanol metabolism. J Pharmacol Exp Ther 1978;207: 123–129.
11. Boyd MR, Burka LT: In vivo studies on the relationship between target organ alkylation and the pulmonary toxicity of a chemically reactive metabolite of 4-ipomeanol. J Pharmacol Exp Ther 1978;20:687–689.
12. Boyland E, Chasseaud LF: The role of glutathione *S*-transferase in mercapturic acid biosynthesis. Adv Enzymol 1969; 2:173–219.
13. Brittebo EB: Metabolism of xenobiotics in the nasal olfactory mucosa: Implications for local toxicity. Pharmacol Toxicol 1993;72:50–52.
14. Brown MM, Rhyne BC, Goyer RA, Fowler BA: Intracellular effects of chronic arsenic administration on renal proximal tubule cells. J Toxicol Environ Health 1976;1:505–514.
15. Caravati EM, Litovitz TL: Pediatric cyanide intoxication and death from an acetonitrile-containing cosmetic. JAMA 1988;260:3470–3473.
16. Cheng YUC, Nakayama K: Effects of 5-fluoro–2-doxyuridine on DNA metabolism in HeLa cells. Mol Pharmacol 1983;23:171–174.
17. Dai Y, Rashba-Step J, Cederbaum AI: Stable expression of human cytochrome P4502E1 in HepG2 cells: Characterization of catalytic activities and production of reactive oxygen intermediates. Biochemistry 1993;32:6928–6937.
18. DiVincenzo G, Kaplan CJ, DeDinas J: Characterization of the metabolites of methyl *n*-butyl ketone, methyl *iso*-butyl ketone, and methyl ethyl ketone in guinea-pig serum and their clearance. Toxicol Appl Pharmacol 1976;36:511–518.
19. Edgar B, Bailey D, Bergstrand R, et al: Acute effects of drinking grapefruit juice on the pharmacokinetics and dynamics of felodipine, and its potential clinical relevance. Eur J Clin Pharmacol 1992;42:313–317.
20. Eling TE, Thompson DC, Foureman GL, et al: Prostaglandin H synthase and xenobiotic oxidation. Annu Rev Pharmacol Toxicol 1990;30:1–45.
21. Feng PC, Patrick SJ: Studies of the action of hypoglycin-A, an hypoglycaemic substance. Br J Pharmacol 1958;13: 125–130.
22. Fiala ES, Caswell N, Sohn OS, et al: Non alcohol dehydrogenase-mediated metabolism of methylazoxymethanol in

the deer mouse, *Peromyscus maniculatus.* Cancer Res 1984; 44:2885–2891.

23. Freinkel N, Singer DL, Arky RA, et al: Alcohol hypoglycemia. I. Carbohydrate metabolism of patients with clinical alcohol hypoglycemia and the experimental reproduction of the syndrome with pure ethanol. J Clin Invest 1963;42:1112–1133.
24. Frezza M, di Padova C, Pozzato G, et al: High blood alcohol levels in women: The role of decreased gastric alcohol dehydrogenase activity and first-pass metabolism. N Engl J Med 1990;322:95–99.
25. Frommer DA, Kulig KW, Marx JA, Rumack BH: Tricyclic antidepressant overdose. JAMA 1987;257:521–526.
26. Gaetani GF, Galiano S, Canepa L, et al: Catalase and glutathione peroxidase are equally active in detoxification of hydrogen peroxide in human erythrocytes. Blood 1989; 73:334–339.
27. Gerlach M, Riederer P, Przuntek H, et al: MPTP mechanisms of neurotoxicity and their implications for Parkinson's disease. Eur J Pharmacol 1991;208:273–286.
28. Goedde HW, Agarwal DP: Pharmacogenetics of aldehyde dehydrogenase. In: Kalow W, ed: Pharmacogenetics of Drug Metabolism. New York, Pergamon, 1992, pp. 281–311.
29. Guengerich FP: Catalytic selectivity of human cytochrome P450 enzymes: relevance to drug metabolism and toxicity. Toxicol Lett 1994;70:133–138.
30. Guengerich FP: Reactions and significance of cytochrome P450 enzymes. J Biol Chem 1991;266:10019–10022.
31. Halpert JR, Guengerich FP, Bend JR, et al: Selective inhibitors of cytochromes P450. Toxicol Appl Pharmacol 1994;125:163–175.
32. Hétu C, Dumont A, Joly JG: Effect of chronic ethanol administration on bromobenzene liver toxicity in the rat. Toxicol Appl Pharmacol 1983;67:166–177.
33. Hill HZ, Backer R, Hill GJ: Blood cyanide levels in mice after administration of amygdalin. Biopharm Drug Dispos 1980;1:211–220.
34. Hirsh J: Oral anticoagulant drugs. N Engl J Med 1992; 324:1865–1868.
35. Ibels LS, Pollock CA: Lead intoxication. Med Toxicol 1986;1:387–390.
36. Jakoby WB, Bend JR, Caldwell J: Metabolic Basis of Detoxification: Metabolism of Functional Groups. New York, Academic, 1982.
37. Kato R, Yamazoe Y: The importance of substrate concentration in determining cytochromes P450 therapeutically relevant in vivo. Pharmacogenetics 1994;4:359–362.
38. Kleinman JG, Breittenfield RV, Roth DA: Acute renal failure associated with acetaminophen ingestion: Report of a case and review of the literature. Clin Nephrol 1980;14: 201–205.
39. Krishna DR, Klotz U: Extrahepatic metabolism of drugs in humans. Clin Pharmacokinet 1994;26:144–160.
40. Kroncke KD, Fricker G, Meier PJ, et al: Alpha-amanitin uptake into hepatocytes. J Biol Chem 1986;261:12562–12567.
41. La Du BN: Human serum paraoxonase/arylesterase. In: Kalow W, ed: Pharmacogenetics of Drug Metabolism. New York, Pergamon, 1992, pp. 51–91.
42. Lawton MP, Cashman JR, Cresteil T, et al: A nomenclature for the mammalian flavin-containing monooxygenase gene family based on amino acid sequence identities. Arch Biochem Biophys 1994;308:254–257.
43. Lee WM: Drug-induced hepatotoxicity. N Engl J Med 1995;333:1118–1127.
44. Lehninger AL: Glycolysis in Biochemistry: The molecular basis of cell structure and function, 2nd ed. New York, Worth Publishers, Inc, 1979, pp. 417–439.
45. Lewis MS, Youle RJ: Ricin subunit association: Thermodynamics and the role of the disulfide bond in toxicity. J Biol Chem 1986;261:11571–11577.
46. Lieber CS: Alcohol and the liver: 1994 update. Gastroenterology 1994;106:1085–1105.
47. Lieber CS: Metabolic derangement induced by alcohol. Annu Rev Med 1967;18:35–54.
48. Lindell TJ, Weinberg F, Morris PW: Specific inhibition of nuclear RNA polymerase II by alpha-amanitin. Science 1970;170:447–449.
49. Mason MF, Wallace SM, Forster E, et al: Pentachlorophenol poisoning: Report of two cases. J Forensic Sci 1965; 10:136–147.
50. Mehendale HM, Roth RA, Gandolfi AJ: Novel mechanisms in chemically induced hepatotoxicity. FASEB J 1994;8: 1285–1295.
51. Menon JA: Tropical hazards associated with the use pentachlorophenol. Br Med J 1958;1:1156.
52. Minton NA, Murray VSG: A review of organophosphate poisoning. Med Toxicol 1988;3:350–375.
53. Mitchell JR, Jollow DJ: Progress in hepatology. Metabolic activation of drugs to toxic substances. Gastroenterology 1975;68:392–410.
54. Mitchell JR, Thorleinsson SS, Potter WZ, et al: Acetaminophen-induced hepatic injury: Protective role of glutathione in man and rationale for therapy. Clin Pharmacol Ther 1974;16:676–683.
55. Mitchell JR, Jollow DJ, Potter WZ, et al: Acetaminophen induced hepatic necrosis. IV: Protection role of glutathione. J Pharmacol Exp Ther 1973;187:211–217.
56. Mitchell RA, Chang BF, Huang CH, DeMaster EG: Inhibition of mitochondrial energy-linked functions by arsenate: Evidence for a nonhydrolytic mode of inhibitor action. Biochemistry 1971;10:2049–2053.
57. Myers CD, McGuire WP, Liss RH: Adriamycin: The role of lipid peroxidation in cardiac toxicity and tumor response. Science 1977;197:165–167.
58. Nelson DR, Kamataki T, Waxman DJ, et al: The P450 superfamily: Update on new sequences, gene mapping, accession numbers, early trivial names, and nomenclature. DNA Cell Biol 1993;12:1–51.
59. Oates NS, Shah RR, Idle JR, Smith RL: Influence of oxidation polymorphism on phenformin kinetics and dynamics. Clin Pharmacol Ther 1983;34:827–834.
60. Parker VH: Effect of nitrophenols and halogenophenols on the enzymatic activity of rat liver mitochondria. Biochem J 1957;69:306–310.
61. Parkinson A: Biotransformation of xenobiotics. In: Klaassen CD, ed: Casarett & Doull's Toxicology: The Basic Science of Poisons, 5th ed. New York, McGraw-Hill, 1996, pp. 151–156.
62. Parkinson A, Hurwitz A: Omeprazole and the induction of

human cytochrome P450: A response to concerns about potential adverse effects. Gastroenterology 1991;100:1157–1164.
63. Peck CC, Temple R, Collins JM: Understanding consequences of concurrent therapies. JAMA 1993; 269:1550–1552.
64. Pirotte JH: Apparent potentiation of hepatotoxicity from small doses of acetaminophen by phenobarbital. Ann Intern Med 1984;101:403. Letter.
65. Pohl LR: Drug-induced allergic hepatitis. Semin Liver Dis 1990;10:305–315.
66. Rose MS. Lock EA, Smith LL, Wyatt I: Paraquat accumulation: Tissue and species specificity. Biochem Pharmacol 1976;25:419–423.
67. Rosen GM, Rauckman EJ: Carbon tetrachloride induced lipid peroxidation: A spin trapping study. Toxicol Lett 1982;10:337–344.
68. Rosenfield AB, Huston R: Infant methemoglobinemia in Minnesota due to nitrates in well water. Minn Med 1950;33:787–796.
69. Ruderman N, Shafrir E, Bressler R: Relation of fatty acid oxidation to gluconeogenesis: Effect of pentenoic acid. Life Sci 1968;7:1083–1089.
70. Santi DV, McHenry CS, Sommer A: Mechanism of interactions of thymidylate synthetase with 5-fluorodeoxyuridylate. Biochemistry 1974;13:471–480.
71. Shimkin MB, Anderson NN: Acute toxicities of rotenone and mixed pyrethrins in mammals. Proc Soc Exp Biol Med 1936;34:135–138.
72. Sohn OS, Fiala ES, Puz C, et al: Enhancement of rat liver microsomal metabolism of azoxymethane to methylazoxymethanol by chronic ethanol administration: Similarity to the microsomal metabolism of *N*-nitrosodimethylamine. Cancer Res 1987;47:3123–3129.
73. Smith JE, Beutler E: Methemoglobin formation and reduction in man and various animal species. Am J Physiol 1966;210:347–350.
74. Smith MHG, Jeffrey SW: The effects of salicylate on oxygen and carbohydrate metabolism in the isolated rat diaphragm. Biochem J 1956;63:524–529.
75. Southorn PA, Powis G: Free radicals in medicine: I. Chemical nature of biologic reactions. Mayo Clin Proc 1988;63: 381–389.
76. Speeg KV, Mitchel MC, Maldonado AL: Additive protection of cimetidine and *N*-acetylcysteine treatment against acetaminophen induced hepatic necrosis in the rat. J Pharmacol Exp Ther 1985;234:550–554.
77. Spencer HC, Rowe VK, Adams EM, Irish DD: Toxicological studies on laboratory animals of certain alkyldinitrophenols used in agriculture. J Indian Hyg Toxicol 1948;30:10–25.
78. Tanaka K: On the mode of action of hypoglycin A. J Biol Chem 1972;247:7465–7478.
79. Tanaka K, Kean EA, Johnson B: Jamaican vomiting sickness. N Engl J Med 1976;295:461–467.
80. Tanaka K, Miller EM, Isselbacher KJ: Hypoglycin A: A specific inhibitor of isovaleryl CoA dehydrogenase. Proc Natl Acad Sci 1971;68:20–24.
81. Timbrell JA: Principles of Biochemical Toxicology. London, Taylor & Francis, 1987.
82. Way JL: Cyanide intoxication and its mechanism of antagonism. Annu Rev Toxicol 1984;24:451–481.
83. Whitlon DS, Sadowski JA, Suttie JW: Mechanisms of coumarin action: Significance of vitamin K epoxide reductase inhibition. Biochemistry 1978;17:1371–1377.
84. Wilson JD: Vitamin deficiency and excess: In: Isselbacher KJ, Braunwald E, Wilson JD, et al, eds: Harrison's Principles of Internal Medicine, 13th ed. New York, McGraw-Hill, 1994, pp. 472–479.
85. Yager JW, Eastmond DA, Robertson ML, et al: Characterization of micronuclei induced in human lymphocytes by benzene metabolites. Adv Cancer Res 1990;50:393–399.
86. Zand R, Nelson SD, Slattery JT, et al: Inhibition and induction of cytochrome P4502E1-catalyzed oxidation by isoniazid in humans. Clin Pharmacol Ther 1993;54:142–149.
87. Zedeck MS, Grab DJ, Sternberg S: Differences in the acute responses of the various segments of rat intestine to treatment with the intestinal carcinogen, methoxyazomethanol acetate. Cancer Res 1977;37:32–36.

CHAPTER 13

Hepatic Principles

Kathleen A. Delaney

The liver has an essential role in the maintenance of physiologic homeostasis. Its functions include the synthesis, storage, and breakdown of glycogen; the metabolism of lipids; the synthesis of albumin, clotting factors, and other important proteins; the synthesis of bile acids necessary for the absorption of lipids and fat-soluble vitamins; the metabolism of cholesterol; the excretion of metals, most importantly iron, copper, zinc, manganese, mercury, and aluminum; and the detoxification of products of metabolism such as bilirubin and ammonia.[44,92] Generalized disruption of these important functions results in familiar manifestations of liver failure: hyperbilirubinemia, coagulopathy, hypoalbuminemia, hyperammonemia, and hypoglycemia. Disturbances of more specific functions result in accumulation of toxic metals, fat-soluble vitamin deficiencies, hypercholesterolemia, and steatosis.[91]

The liver, which contains the highest concentration of enzymes involved in phase I oxidation–reduction reactions, is also the primary site of biotransformation and detoxification of exogenous toxins or xenobiotics.[28,50] Its interposition between the gut and systemic circulation makes it the first-pass recipient of toxins absorbed from the gastrointestinal tract into the portal vein, including endotoxins produced by gut bacteria. The liver also receives blood from the systemic circulation and participates in the detoxification and elimination of substances that reach the bloodstream through other routes, such as inhalation or cutaneous absorption. The biliary tract provides an important route for the excretion of detoxified xenobiotics and products of metabolism.[45]

Owing to its location at the end of the portal system and its substantial complement of biotransformation enzymes, the liver is especially vulnerable to toxic injury. Many toxins that are readily absorbed by the gut are lipophilic, chemically inert substances that require chemical activation to make them sufficiently soluble to be eliminated. Although phase I activation followed by phase II conjugation usually results in detoxification of these compounds, it occasionally leads to the production of compounds with increased toxicity, which is often manifest at the site of their synthesis. (See Chaps. 11 and 12, for a more in-depth discussion of the biotransformation reactions.)

Morphology and Function of the Liver

Approximately 75% of the blood supply to the liver is derived from the portal vein, which drains the alimentary tract, spleen, and pancreas. This blood is enriched with nutrients and other absorbed agents and is poor in oxygen. The remainder of the hepatic blood flow comes from the hepatic artery, which delivers well-oxygenated blood from the systemic circulation.[40]

Blood from the hepatic artery and portal vein mixes in the sinusoids, where it comes in close contact with the cords of hepatocytes.[40] Oxygen content diminishes several-fold as blood flows from the portal area to the central vein.[3] The sinusoidal lining formed by endothelial cells is thin and fenestrated, allowing transfer of fluid, chylomicrons, and proteins across the space of Disse between the sinusoids and hepatocytes. Macrophages (Kupffer cells) within the sinusoids scavenge particulate materials and cell debris. When immunologically activated by toxins, Kupffer cells contribute to the generation of oxygen free radicals and may also participate in the production of autoimmune injury to hepatocytes.[22] Ito cells or "fat storage cells" found between the endothelial cells and hepatocytes are a primary site for the storage of vitamin A and fat.[27]

Bile acids, organic anions, bilirubin, phospholipids, xenobiotics, and other constituents of bile are transported through the hepatocytes into the bile canaliculi by active transport systems that have specificity for acids, bases, and neutral compounds.[41,44,45,75] The hepatocyte plasma membranes have three active transport systems for bile acids: a sodium-dependent bile salt transporter in the sinusoidal membrane; an ATP-dependent bile salt carrier across the canalicular membrane; and a potential-driven canalicular membrane transport site.[7] Glucuronidated xenobiotics are substrates for the bile acid transport systems and are actively secreted into bile. Compounds with molecular weights greater than 350 daltons are also preferentially secreted into bile. Bile formation involves the production of a flow of fluid, in addition to the transport and concentration of constituents from the sinusoids and hepatocytes.[61] Bile flow is an active process facilitated by ATP-dependent contractions of actin filaments that encircle the canaliculi.[127] Tight junctions separate the contents of the bile canaliculi from the sinusoids and hepatocytes, maintaining a rigid and functionally necessary compartmentalization. Bile flows from tiny canaliculi through increasingly larger conduits, finally into the common duct, gall bladder, and duodenum.[49] While most detoxified xenobiotics that are secreted into bile are eliminated in the feces, some are reabsorbed back into the systemic circulation, resulting in an enterohepatic circulation. Compounds most likely to be reabsorbed have a low molecular weight and are non-ionized at intestinal pH. Examples of toxins that undergo enterohepatic recirculation include nortriptyline and chlorpromazine.[41,67] Methyl mercury also recirculates between the gall bladder and the systemic circulation, resulting in decreased clearance and prolonged toxicity.[20] A physiologically necessary enterohepatic circulation facilitates the conservation of bile acids and some vitamins.

The basic histologic structural unit of the liver is the hepatic lobule, a hexagon with the central vein at the center and the portal triads at the angles (Fig. 13–1). The lobule has classically been used to describe the location of hepatic injury. Hepatocellular injury that occurs near the central vein is called centrilobular necrosis whereas necrosis near the portal area is called periportal necrosis.

The acinus is a functional unit of the liver. It is located between two central veins and is bisected by branches of the hepatic artery and portal vein. Cords of hepatocytes radiate from these vessels toward the central vein. The acinus is divided into three zones, which reflect the metabolic and functional activity of the acinus. Zone 1 has a twofold higher oxygen content than zone 3.[2,3] Zone 1 has a higher concentration of glutathione, whereas zone 3 has a greater capacity for glucuronida-

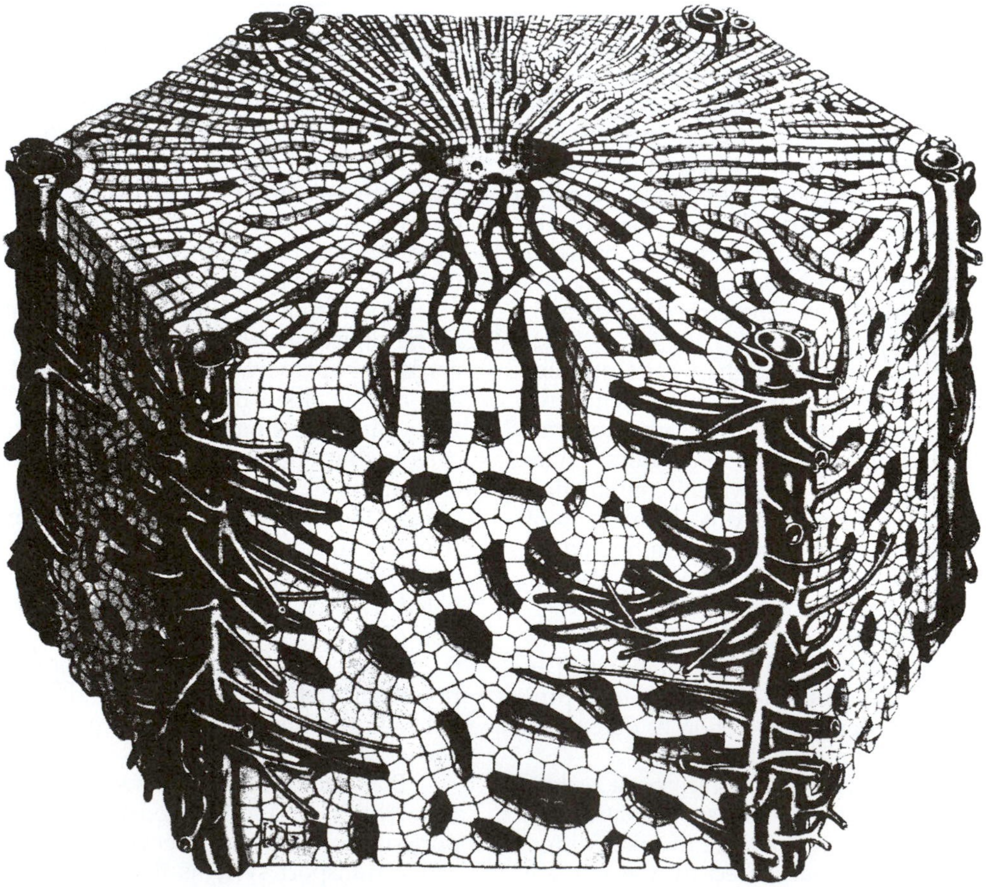

Figure 13–1. Liver lobule, schematic view. The central vein lies in the center of the figure, surrounded by anastomosing cords of blocklike hepatocytes. Around the periphery of the schema are six evenly spaced "triads" lying at an angle in the polyhedron lobule. Each triad consists of branches of the portal vein, hepatic artery, and bile duct. *(Reprinted, with permission, from Weiss L: Cell and Tissue Biology. A Textbook of Histology, 6th ed, Baltimore: Urban & Schwarzenberg Fig. 22–1, 1988, p. 687.)*

tion and sulfation.[29,123] Zone 3 also has higher levels of alcohol dehydrogenase and of the ethanol-inducible P4502E1 cytochrome oxidase.[59,60,123] Zone 2 is intermediate in activity. There is fortunately some correlation between these two schematic efforts to conceptualize the liver (Fig. 13–2). Centrilobular or perivenular necrosis describes injury in zone 3 of the liver acinus, whereas periportal necrosis describes injury in zone 1.

Which Factors Affect the Localization of Hepatic Injury?

These functional and anatomic characteristics have important relevance to the production of liver injury by toxins. The oxygen gradient between zones 1 and 3 affects the distribution of injury caused by some toxins. Allyl alcohol, for example, is metabolized in the liver to acrolein, its hepatotoxic metabolite. Despite the observation that the rate of metabolism of allyl alcohol to acrolein is greater in the central vein areas, hepatocellular damage occurs preferentially in the zone 1 or periportal areas. The extent of damage done in isolated rat livers exposed to allyl alcohol is dependent on the oxygen content of the perfusates, suggesting that the mechanism of injury may be related to oxygen-mediated free radical injury.[3] The tendency for centrilobular or zone 3 accumulation of fat in patients with alcoholic steatosis is attributed to the effect of relative hypoxia in the central vein area on the oxidation potential of the hepatocyte.[59]

The localization of enzymes involved in biotransformation also affects the site of injury in the hepatic lobule. In addition to acetaminophen, nitrosamines, and benzene, the P4502E1 has a significant capacity to convert carbon tetrachloride (CCl_4) to a reactive intermediate. Selective injury to the centrilobular (zone 3) area caused by CCl_4 is postulated to be due to the greater concentration of P4502E1 in cells in those areas. Cultures of cells from the centrilobular area (zone 3) are much more susceptible to injury by CCl_4 than are cultures from zone 1. The observed effects of isoniazid (an inhibitor of the enzyme P4502E1) and chronic ethanol intake (an inducer of the gene CYP2E1) on cellular injury in cultures of cells from the periportal and central vein areas exposed to CCl_4 also supports the association of CCl_4 injury with the localization of P4502E1 activity. Although this may be the most appropriate terminology, CYP and P450 are used interchangeably throughout this text. Isoniazid significantly decreases the injury associated with exposure of cultured zone 3 cells to CCl_4, whereas chronic treatment with ethanol significantly enhances it.[60]

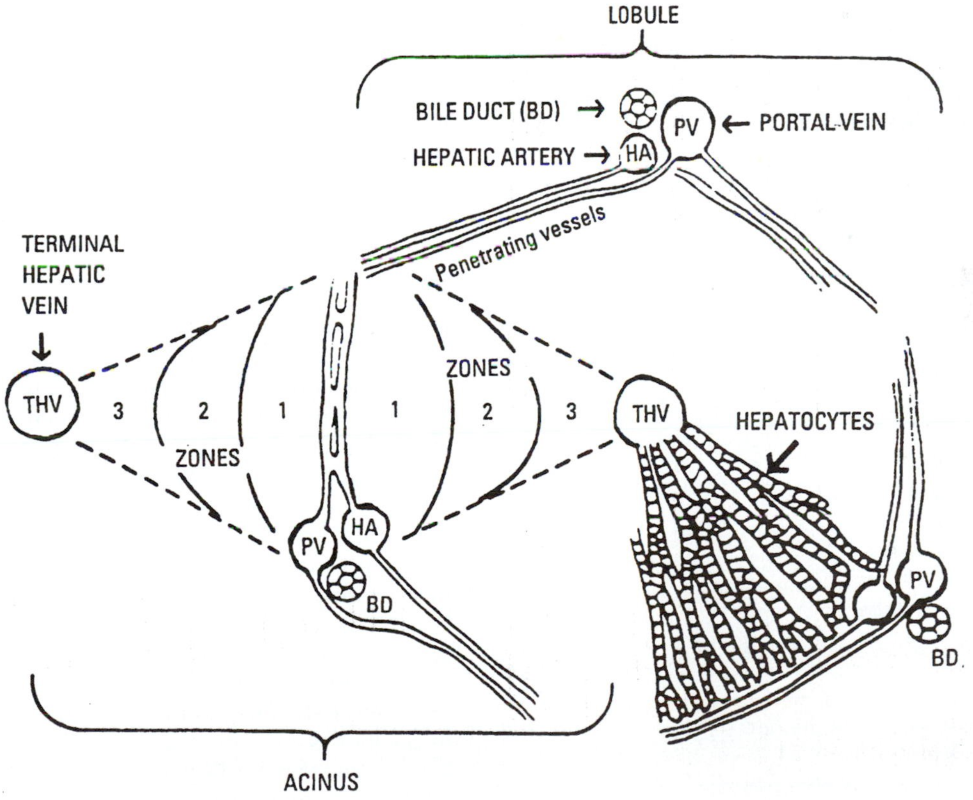

Figure 13–2. The liver lobule and the acinus. The hepatic lobule is a hexagonal structure with the hepatic vein at the center. The acinus has at its base the hepatic artery and portal vein. Blood flows from the base of the acinus through the sinusoids across zones 1, 2, and 3 of the acinus to exit in the hepatic vein. Zone 1 of the acinus corresponds with the periportal area of the lobule, while zone 3 of the acinus corresponds with the centrilobular area. *(Reprinted, with permission, from Moslen MT: Toxic responses of the liver. In: Klaassen C, ed: Casarett & Doull's Toxicology: The Basic Science of Poisons, 5th ed. New York, McGraw-Hill, 1996, pp. 403–416.)*

Which Factors Affect the Development of Hepatotoxicity?

Agents such as acetaminophen (APAP), phosphorous, or *Amanita* toxin that produce liver damage in all humans in a predictable and dose-dependent manner are known as intrinsic hepatotoxins. Those that cause liver damage in a small number of individuals and whose effect is not dose dependent or predictably reproducible are known as idiosyncratic hepatotoxins (Table 13–1). The majority of hepatotoxins are idiosyncratic.[93] Some cause hepatotoxicity very rarely, whereas others produce it commonly. A mild degree of hepatitis occurs in as many as 20% of patients exposed to the inhaled anesthetic agent halothane. This form of halothane hepatitis is likely due to direct toxicity as it can be induced in animals who are pretreated with P450 inducers and then subjected to hypotension or hypoxia during treatment.[21,83,107] An individual's susceptibility to a hepatotoxin depends on numerous factors, including the activity of biotransformation enzymes, the availability of substrates, and the immunocompetence of the individual. These in turn are affected by age, gender, diet, underlying diseases, concurrent exposure to other drugs or toxins, and genetic factors. Sporadic unpredicted hepatotoxicity is less likely to be truly "idiosyncratic" than the result of the combined effects of genetic and other factors that result in the overproduction or decreased clearance of toxic metabolites.[55]

TABLE 13–1. HEPATOTOXINS

Examples of intrinsic hepatotoxins
Acetaminophen
Carbon tetrachloride
Cyclopeptide-containing mushrooms
Yellow phosphorus
Examples of idiosyncratic hepatotoxins
Allopurinol
Alpha-methyldopa
Amiodarone
Bromobenzene
Cereulin
Chlorpromazine
Chlorpropamide
Diclofenac
Dimethylformamide
Disulfiram
Erythromycin estolate
Ethanol
Halothane
Isoniazid
Methotrexate
Nitrofurantoin
Nucleoside analogs (fialuridine, zidovudine, etc)
Oral contraceptives
Phenylbutazone
Phenytoin
Propylthiouracil
Tetracycline
Valproic acid

Enzyme Polymorphism

Many enzymes involved in biotransformation show genetic polymorphism. Patients with low levels of *N*-acetyl transferase are more likely to develop "lupus-like" reactions to procainamide, hydralazine, or isoniazid.[88] Approximately 8% of Caucasians are deficient in the enzyme P4502D6 (formally called debrisoquine hydroxylase), which is responsible for the metabolism of a number of drugs including debrisoquine (an antihypertensive identified as the first substrate of this enzyme), several antidepressants and antidysrhythmics, some opioids, and phenformin.[55,88] Perihexilene, an antianginal agent that was marketed in Europe in the 1980s, caused severe liver disease and peripheral neuropathy in persons with a demonstrated inability to metabolize debrisoquine.[115] Patients with Gilbert's syndrome, a congenital disorder that results in impairment of glucuronyltransferase, are at increased risk of hepatic injury following ingestions of APAP. Studies of therapeutic dosing of APAP in these patients demonstrate decreased glucuronidation and increased bioactivation.[17] Until recently, genetic factors were thought to contribute to the hepatotoxicity of isoniazid (INH).[77,79] Rapid acetylators of INH form monoacetylhydrazine, a substrate for P450 conversion to an active metabolite, at a faster rate than slow acetylators. Epidemiologic studies have shown that both rapid and slow acetylators are at similar risk of INH hepatotoxicity, probably because rapid acetylators detoxify monoacetylhydrazine at a faster rate.[30]

Effects of Other Drugs or Toxins on Enzyme Function

Increased susceptibility to hepatic injury in humans may theoretically result from increased formation of hepatotoxic metabolites following alteration of the activities of biotransformation enzymes. The chronic ingestion of ethanol induces the CYP2E1 gene, which results in a 5–10-fold increase in P4502E1 activity in the endoplasmic reticulum of chronic alcoholics.[16,59] Chronic administration of INH to slow acetylators also induces P4502E1 activity and, conversely, ethanol use may increase the hepatotoxicity of INH.[55,135] Anecdotal reports contend that hepatic injury may occur following therapeutic doses of APAP in alcoholics.[71,85,113] If this does occur it is extremely rare. The inability to demonstrate a significantly increased risk of hepatotoxicity due to ingestion of APAP in alcoholics may be related to the observation that at least three forms of P450 contribute to the metabolism of APAP by humans and the contribution of P4502E1 varies considerably among individuals.[135] Animal studies of bromobenzene toxicity, an agent whose metabolism is similar to that of APAP, show that chronic ethanol administration causes an earlier onset of bromobenzene hepatotoxicity in rats, with only a small increase in the extent of hepatic necrosis. The dose of bromobenzene required for hepatic injury to occur is not altered by pretreatment with ethanol.[34] Chronic administration of phenobarbital to rats results in a very significant increase in the hepatotoxic effects of bromobenzene.[100] The cultured hepatocytes of ethanol-treated rats show increased in vitro susceptibility to the hepatotoxic effects of carbon tetrachloride (CCl_4), which is also metabolized by P4502E1.[60] (see Chap. 12). In addition to CCl_4, other solvents such as dimethylformamide, bromobenzene, and benzene potentially have increased toxicity in the worker who is a chronic alcoholic.[34,82,98]

Some drug combinations increase the possibility of hepatotoxic reactions, probably because one agent alters the metabolism of the other, leading to the production of toxic metabolites. This is the case with combinations of rifampin and isoniazid; amoxacillin and clavulanic acid; and trimethoprim and sulfamethoxazole.[1,26,33,38,52,55,57,76,109,129]

Immune Responses

Several types of hypersensitivity reactions result in different forms of liver injury. An immune mechanism is implied by the demonstration of autoantibodies, antibodies against the drugs, or activated T lymphocytes (see Chap. 14). The presence of eosinophilia, atypical lymphocytosis, fever, and rash are interpreted as indicating a hypersensitivity mechanism. A history of repeated exposure followed by illness that resolves with withdrawal of the agent and recurs with reexposure also suggests hypersensitivity. An autoimmune etiology of hepatic toxicity is only implied and not proven for many suspected agents. Phenytoin induces both hepatic necrosis and cholestasis in association with a systemic response that includes rash, eosinophilia, atypical lymphocytosis, and demonstrated serum IgG antibodies against phenytoin.[46] The clinical presentation associated with liver injury by chlorpromazine also suggests a hypersensitivity reaction. Jaundice associated with fever, chills, rash, and eosinophilia occurs in 1% of treated patients 1–5 weeks after exposure. Readministration of the drug results in recurrence.[35,116] Erythromycin estolate also causes fever, rash, and eosinophilia beginning 2–21 days after initiation of the drug and recurring with readministration.[9,19,134] Similar reactions occur following administration of sulfonamides and diclofenac[55,108] (see Chap. 46).

The most likely mechanism by which a drug precipitates autoimmune injury to the liver is through the formation of an adduct with the hepatic cell. An adduct is an activated metabolite that becomes covalently bonded following a chemical attack on a cellular macromolecule. This then acts like a hapten, inducing an immune response against the drug macromolecule or against an immunologically altered cellular macromolecule. The formation of adducts requires activation of the drug since most are chemically inert in their ingested forms. Destruction of the hepatocyte might then be mediated by complement- or antibody-directed lysis; by specific cell-mediated cytotoxicity; or by an inflammatory response induced by immune complexes and complement.[74,93]

An immune mechanism predominates in the liver injury caused by alpha-napthylisothiocyanate (ANIT), a toxin that causes acute cholangitis associated with polymorphonuclear cell (PMN) infiltration in a rat model.[15] In in vitro studies PMNs release cytotoxic lysosomal enzymes and oxygen free radicals in response to activation by ANIT.[15,74] Additionally, antibodies directed against circulating neutrophils decrease the extent of liver damage caused by ANIT, supporting the proposal that PMN activation is an important factor in liver injury caused by this toxin.[15] Lymphocyte sensitization occurs in hepatitis caused by a number of drugs including isoniazid, erythromycin, and floxacillin.[93,125] In rare cases multiple exposures to the anesthetic agent halothane result in fulminant hepatic failure, which is associated with autoantibodies against a neoantigen formed by an adduct of halothane with an hepatoprotein, which may be a microsomal carboxylesterase[21,74,83,93,124] (See Chap. 53). Neoantigens directed against a drug or metabolite-protein adducts have also been demonstrated in hepatitis caused by ethanol and alpha-methyldopa.[59,93]

A long list of drugs has been associated with the development of granulomatous hepatitis, an entity associated with chronic fatigue and histologic characteristics including caseating granulomata that resemble sarcoidosis[55] (Table 13–2).

Availability of Substrates

The availability of substrates for detoxification may significantly affect the likelihood of hepatic injury. The metabolism of APAP illustrates the delicate balance that exists between detoxification and the production of injurious metabolites. In healthy adults taking therapeutic amounts of APAP, elimination occurs primarily through glucuronidation and secondarily through sulfa-

TABLE 13–2. SOME DRUGS ASSOCIATED WITH GRANULOMATOUS LIVER DISEASE

Allopurinol
Aspirin
Carbamazepine
Cephalexin
Diazepam
Diltiazem
Halothane
Hydralazine
Isoniazid
Methyldopa
Nitrofurantoin
Penicillin
Phenytoin
Procainamide
Procarbazine
Quinidine
Sulfonamides
Sulfonylureas

Adapted, with permission, from Lee WM: Drug-induced hepatotoxicity. N Engl J Med 1995;333:1118–1127.

tion.[17] Under normal circumstances less than 10% undergoes oxidative metabolism, resulting in the production of the electrophilic metabolite *N*-acetyl-*p*-benzoquinoneimine (NAPQI). In most cases NAPQI is rapidly detoxified by conjugation with glutathione.[78] Excessive amounts of APAP saturate the pathways of sulfation and glucuronidation, resulting in increased synthesis of NAPQI, which reacts avidly with hepatocellular macromolecules if glutathione is not available.[14,78,94,96] An inverse correlation exists between the cellular concentration of glutathione and the demonstration of injurious covalent binding of APAP metabolites to liver cells.[14] Glutathione may be depleted during the course of metabolism of APAP by otherwise normal livers, or it may be depleted prior to the administration of APAP in starved patients or certain patients with liver disease.[53,117] Prior administration of other drugs that induce cytochrome P450 activity such as phenobarbital or isoniazid may also predispose to toxicity at lower doses, while prior administration of cytochrome P450 inhibitors, such as cimetidine, may be protective.[55,90,119] Acute ethanol ingestion competes for the metabolism of APAP by cytochrome P450 and may also be protective.[6]

Pathologic and Biochemical Manifestations of Hepatic Injury

Toxic hepatic injury is manifested in a variety of pathologic ways, including acute necrosis, steatosis, and cholestasis, all of which are discussed below. In addition, vascular injuries may cause obstruction to venous or arterial flow. Table 13–3 lists various morphologies of toxic hepatic injury and associated toxins.

Acute Hepatocellular Necrosis

Acute necrosis of the hepatocyte disrupts all aspects of its function. It may be focal, involving scattered hepatocytes; zonal, localized to the periportal or central vein area; or panacinar, extending across the acinus. Significant inflammation reflected by an invasion of neutrophils is apparent[55,99,109] (Fig. 13–3). Extensive necrosis results in functional liver failure. Cell death is preceded by the formation of blebs in the lipid membrane and leakage of cytosolic enzymes, primarily aminotransferases and lactate dehydrogenase. Coalescence of blebs leads to rupture of the cellular membrane and acute irreversible cell death with disintegration of the nucleus and termination of all cellular function. Prior to membrane rupture, this injury is reversible by membrane repair processes.[74] The formation of activated metabolites that bind to cell macromolecules as well as the potential for immune-mediated cell injury is described (see above, and Chap. 12). How these interactions, particularly the binding of electrophilic metabolites (adducts), lead to cell necrosis is not well known. The most clearly defined mechanism of rapid injury to the cell is that of initiation of a cascading lipid peroxidation reaction following attack by a free radical. The P4502E1 enzyme has a significant potential to produce oxygen free radicals that are important in the production of hepatic injury by CCl_4 and APAP.[16] In addition, activated polymorphonuclear cells and Kupffer cells produce oxygen free radicals that may contribute to cellular injury.[22,74,93]

TABLE 13–3. EXAMPLES OF AGENTS ASSOCIATED WITH DIFFERENT MORPHOLOGIES OF LIVER INJURY

Acute hepatocellular injury
Acetaminophen
Alpha-methyldopa
Arsenic
Carbon tetrachloride
Disulfiram
Ethanol
Halothane
Iron
Isoniazid
Methotrexate
Phenytoin
Procainamide
Propylthiouracil
Tetracycline
Troglitazone
Yellow phosphorus
Cholestasis
Alpha-napthylthiocyanate (ANIT)
Chlorpromazine
Chlorpropamide
Ethanol
Erythromycin estolate
Floxacillin
Nitrofurantoin
Rifampin
Steatosis
Amiodarone
Cereulin
Ethanol
Nucleoside analogs (fialuridine, zidovudine, etc)
Sodium valproate
Tetracycline
Chronic active hepatitis
Isoniazid
Methyldopa
Nitrofurantoin
Trazodone

Several common drugs and toxins produce hepatic necrosis. Carbon tetrachloride, halothane, and APAP have been previously described. Isoniazid (INH) is an important antituberculous drug that can cause extensive necrosis. Asymptomatic transient elevation in aminotransferases occurs in 10–20% of patients using INH during the first 2 months of therapy. Approximately 1% develop overt hepatitis and 0.1% die.[5,25,63,64,76,80,111,129] Risk factors for the development of hepatotoxicity are female

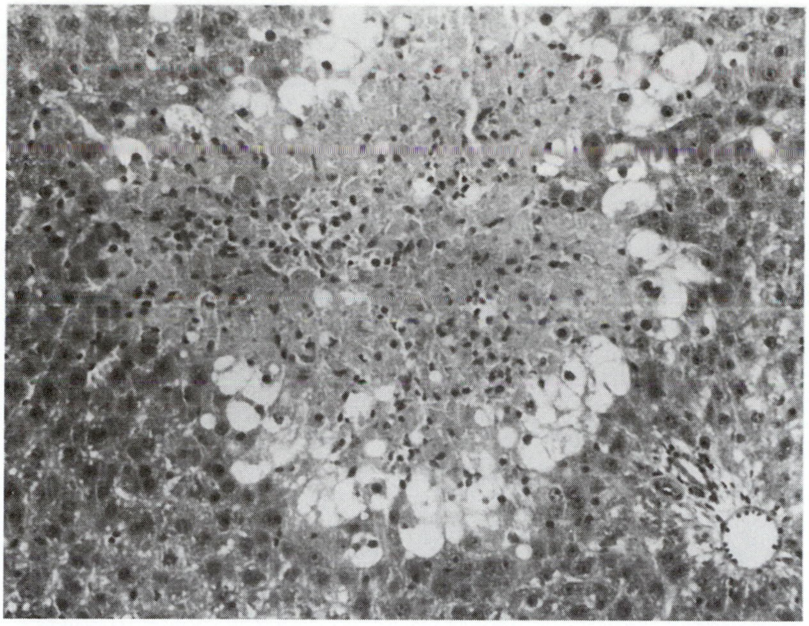

Figure 13–3. Centrilobular necrosis in a rat liver caused by bromobenzene administration. Note the polymorphonuclear infiltrate in the necrotic area surrounded by vacuolated hepatocytes. *(Reprinted, with permission, from Hetu C, Dumont A, Joly J-G: Effect of chronic ethanol administration on bromobenzene liver toxicity in the rat. Toxicol Appl Pharmacol 1983;67: 166–167.)*

gender, increasing age, coadministration with rifampin, and alcoholism[18,26,48,57,118] (see Chaps. 43, 62)

Steatosis

Steatosis is a condition associated with the abnormal accumulation of fat in hepatocytes (Figs. 13–4, 13–5) Two forms of steatosis are described; macrovesicular steatosis, in which the nucleus is displaced by accumulation of intracellular fat, and microvesicular steatosis, characterized by fat droplets that do not displace the nucleus. The intracellular fat accumulation reflects abnormal hepatocellular metabolism and may occur due to any one or more of the following mechanisms: impaired synthesis of lipoproteins; increased mobilization of peripheral adipose stores; increased uptake of circulating lipids; increased triglyceride production; decreased binding of triglycerides to lipoprotein; decreased release of very-low-density lipoproteins from the hepatocytes, and decreased beta-oxidation of fatty acids. Steatosis in nonfatal cases is reversible following withdrawal of the causative agent. Cell injury and death are a reflection of underly-

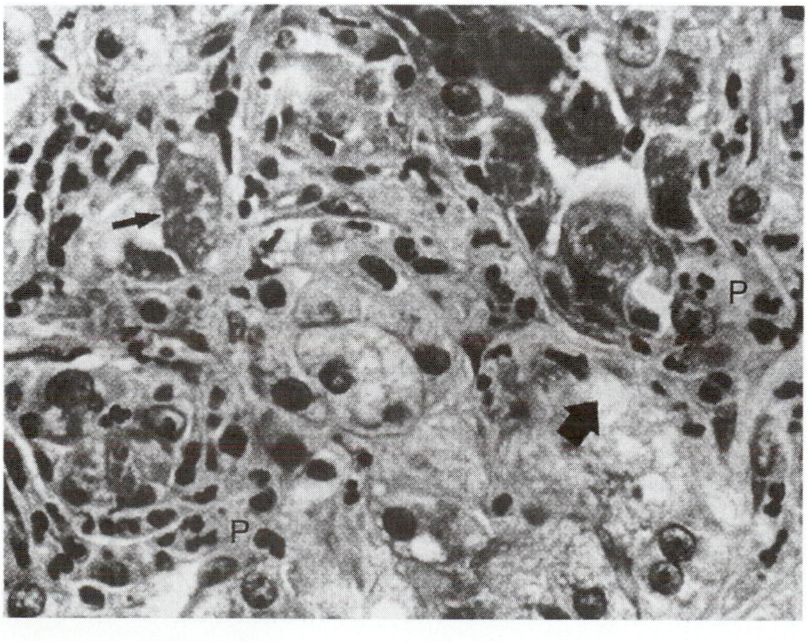

Figure 13–4. This specimen is taken from a patient with nonalcoholic macrovesicular steatosis associated with the administration of amiodarone. The small arrow indicates the presence of Mallory bodies. The large arrow points to accumulated intracellular fat. Polymorphonuclear leukocytes are indicated by the letter P. Note that the nuclei are eccentric, displaced by the accumulated intracellular fat *(Reprinted, with permission, from Lee WM: Drug-induced hepatotoxicity. N Engl J Med 1995;333:1118–1127.)*

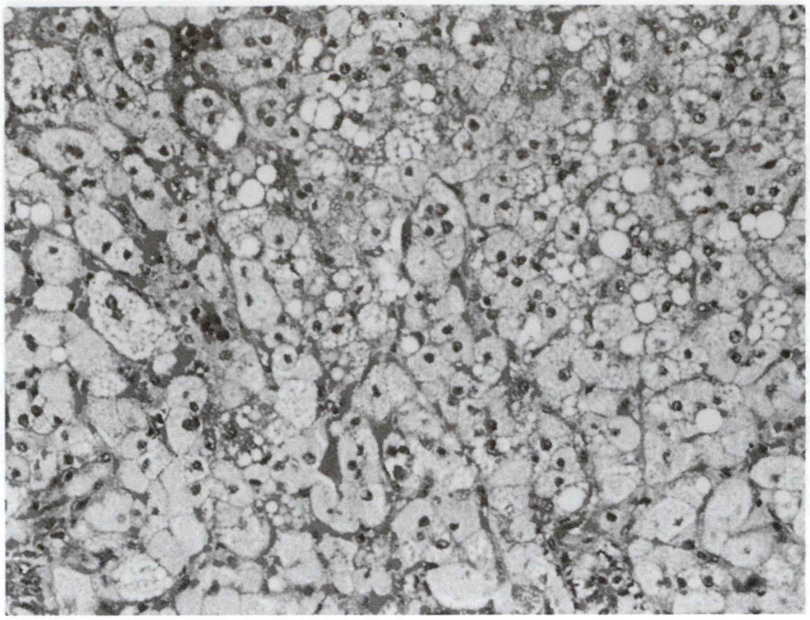

Figure 13–5. This specimen shows severe microvesicular steatosis in a patient treated with fialuridine. Note the central location of the nuclei. *(Reprinted, with permission, from McKenzie R, Fried MW, Sallie R, et al: Hepatic failure and lactic acidosis due to fialuridine (FIAU), an investigational nucleoside analogue for chronic hepatitis B. N Engl J Med 1995;333: 1099–1105.)*

ing metabolic dysfunction. Causes of macrovesicular steatosis include ethanol and amiodarone. Amiodarone hepatic toxicity pathologically resembles that of alcoholic hepatitis, with steatosis, Mallory bodies, and potential of progression to cirrhosis. Lamellated intralysosomal inclusion bodies were found in all cases in one study and thought to be specific for amiodarone toxicity.[104]

Microvesicular steatosis is often associated with a more severe form of hepatocellular dysfunction. High doses of tetracycline produce a microvesicular form of hepatic steatosis. This is associated with moderately elevated aminotransferase and alkaline phosphatase concentrations and markedly prolonged prothrombin times with progression to fulminant hepatic failure. Steatosis associated with tetracycline toxicity appears to be the result of inhibition of lipoprotein synthesis.[112]

Recently, microvesicular steatosis has been reported in patients taking antiviral nucleoside analogs (zidovudine, zalcitabine, and didanosine) for the treatment of HIV infection.[55,73] The nucleoside analog fialuridine caused severe hepatotoxicity and several deaths during a study of its use in the treatment of chronic hepatitis B infection. Microscopic examinations of liver specimens showed marked accumulation of fat with minimal necrosis or structural injury. In these cases severe acidosis with minimal elevation of hepatocellular enzymes and bilirubin and failure of hepatic synthetic function suggested injury localized to the mitochondria, which was supported by the abnormal electron-microscopic appearance of hepatocellular mitochondria.[73] Microvesicular steatosis associated with defective beta-oxidation of fatty acids and also attributed to mitochondrial failure was reported very recently in a fatal case of *Bacillus cereus* food poisoning, where high levels of the bacterial emetic toxin cereulide were found in the bile and liver. Microvesicular steatosis was associated with extensive hepatocellular necrosis.[66] In these cases, lactic acidosis is the biochemical manifestation of impaired energy production while microvestibular steatosis reflects failure of fatty acid metabolism, which is likely also related to impairment of energy production.[24,110] In addition to cereulin, other toxins associated with mitochondrial failure are hypoglycin, the cause of Jamaican vomiting sickness; aflatoxin; and margosa oil.[110] Microvesicular steatosis is also seen with Reye's syndrome and acute fatty liver of pregnancy.[55]

The initial pathologic lesion seen in alcoholic liver disease is the development of reversible macrovesicular steatosis. Ethanol increases the uptake of fatty acids into hepatocytes and decreases lipoprotein secretion. Most important, the increased $NADH/NAD^+$ ratio associated with hepatic metabolism of ethanol results in decreased oxidation of fatty acids and promotion of fatty acid synthesis.[59]

Sodium valproate causes mild elevations of aminotransferases in about 11% of patients, usually during the first few months of therapy.[95] The earliest pathologic lesion is the production of microvesicular steatosis, which occurs in the absence of necrosis.[58] A small percentage of patients progress to fulminant hepatic failure characterized by microvesicular steatosis and necrosis in the centrilobular area (zone 3).[136] The mechanism of toxicity is suspected to be related to inhibition of oxidation of long-chain fatty acids by the metabolite 2-propyl pentenoic acid.[43,136]

Steatosis also occurs following exposure to the industrial solvent dimethylformamide. The mechanism of hepatotoxicity in humans is unknown, but in animal models dimethylformamide is metabolized to monomethyl formamide; both compounds are hepatotoxic.[62] Liver biopsies in patients with acute illness show focal hepatocellular necrosis and microvesicular steatosis. More prolonged, less symptomatic exposures result in significant macrovesicular steatosis with mild aminotransferase elevations.[99]

Cholestasis

Cholestasis results from a number of toxic pathogenic mechanisms. Acute jaundice following hepatic necrosis is a manifestation of general failure of liver function. More specific mechanisms that have been postulated to result in cholestasis include (1) impairment of the integrity of tight membrane junctions that functionally isolate the canaliculus from the hepatocyte and sinusoids; (2) failure of transport of bile components across the hepatocytes; (3) blockade of specific membrane active transport sites; (4) decreased membrane fluidity resulting in altered transport; and (5) decreased canalicular contractility resulting in decreased bile flow (Fig. 13–6).

A well-studied example of drug-induced cholestasis is seen in rats exposed to alpha-napthylisothiocyanate (ANIT). A specific injury localized to the tight junctions that separate the hepatocyte from the canaliculi results in reflux of bile constituents into the sinusoidal space and increased access of sinusoidal molecules to the biliary tree.[49] Rifampin impedes the uptake of bilirubin into hepatocytes.[129] Methyltestosterone and C–17 alkylated anabolic steroids impair the secretion of bilirubin into canaliculi.[41] Estrogens cause intrahepatic cholestasis by altering the composition of the lipid membrane and inhibiting the rate of secretion of bile into the canaliculi.[41,49] Cholestasis with periductal inflammation is seen with exposure to chlorpromazine and may be caused by inhibition of Na-K ATPase, which results in decreased canalicular contractility.[37,97,106] Cyclosporine inhibits sodium-dependent uptake of bile salts across the sinusoidal membrane and blocks ATP-dependent bile salt transport across the canalicular membrane.[7] Floxacillin, rifampin, and erythromycin cause cholestasis with minimal inflammation or evidence of hepatocellular injury.[125,129]

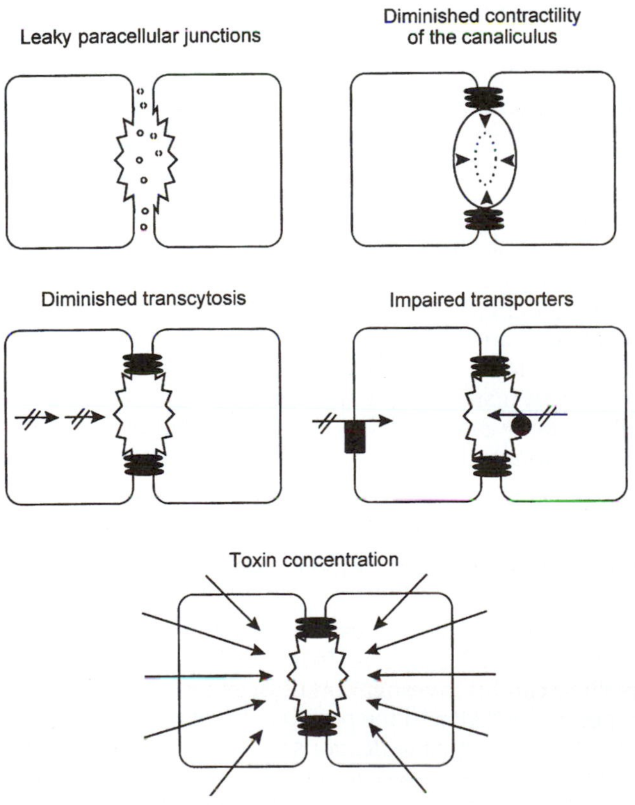

Figure 13–6. Potential mechanisms of toxin-induced cholestasis. *(Reprinted, with permission, from Moslen MT: Toxic responses of the liver. In: Klaassen CD, ed: Casarett & Doull's Toxicology: The Basic Science of Poisons. New York, McGraw-Hill, 1996, pp. 403–416.)*

Veno-occlusive Disease

Hepatic veno-occlusive disease, which clinically resembles the Budd-Chiari syndrome, results in massive hepatic congestion and ascites. It is associated with the use of oral contraceptives and cytotoxic drugs.[51,103] It occurs sometimes in epidemic proportions after exposure to pyrrolizidine alkaloids found in herbal teas and a variety of other plant preparations, primarily from the Boraginaceae, Compositae, and Leguminosae families.[132] Outbreaks of hepatotoxicity have been reported in South Africa after the ingestion of flour contaminated with Senecio (ragwort); in Jamaica after the ingestion of "bush teas"; and in India and Afghanistan when food was contaminated with *Heliotropium lasiocarpium* and *Crotolaria*.[8,81,114,121] Cases are also reported following the ingestion of Russian comfrey tea.[103,128,133] The injury is caused by an activated pyrrole derivative produced by the cytochrome P450 system.[68,69,130,132] There is intense sinusoidal dilation in the centrilobular areas associated with liver cell atrophy and necrosis. Central and sublobular hepatic veins may also be narrowed by intimal edema and fibrosis. The gross appearance is that of a "nutmeg" liver.[51] A rapidly progressive form of veno-occlusive disease attributed to endothelial injury is also seen following high-dose treatment with cyclophosphamide.[72]

Peliosis hepatis is characterized by large blood-filled cavities associated with sinusoidal dilation. It is most frequently associated with the use of androgenic steroids[4] (see Chap. 25). Most patients are asymptomatic, but occasionally these dilated sinusoids rupture and result in hemoperitoneum.

Chronic Active Hepatitis

A form of chronic hepatitis clinically resembling that produced by viral infections occurs with the chronic administration of some drugs such as alpha-methyldopa, nitrofurantoin, trazodone, diclofenac, and phenytoin.[36,41,55,56,65,70,101,102,105,108] In some cases gamma globulins are elevated and there is a positive test for antinuclear antigens, suggesting an immune mechanism for chronic active hepatitis. Jaundice is prominent in these patients, with liver biopsy commonly revealing intrahepatic cholestasis as well as centrilobular inflammation. Hepatocellular enzymes are elevated 5–60-fold.[108]

Cirrhosis

Cirrhosis is a condition caused by progressive fibrosis and scarring of the liver. It results in progressive irreversible hepatic dysfunction and portal hypertension. Fibrosis is related to the increased production of collagen. In alcoholic cirrhosis, "activated" lipocytes in the centrilobular area appear to play a major role in the production of septal and perivenular collagen, which correlates with collagen deposition in the space of Disse. Acetaldehyde also stimulates collagen production by lipocytes, as do other aldehydes that are products of lipid peroxidation.[59] Chronic ingestion of excessive amounts of vitamin A (25,000 U/day × 6 years or 100,000 U/day × $2\frac{1}{2}$ years) results in cirrhosis. The earliest lesions in vitamin A toxicity are a characteristic increase in the fat content of the sinusoidal fat-storing cells, or Ito cells with increasing degrees of fibrosis caused by collagen formation by the Ito cells. The presence of portal hypertension is early and striking.[27,55] Like vitamin A, alpha-methyldopa and methotrexate cause a slow progressive development of cirrhosis with minimal clinical symptoms.[41,55,56]

Hepatic Tumors

The anabolic steroids are associated with the development of malignant tumors such as angiosarcoma and hepatocellular carcinoma in addition to hepatic adenomas.[13,23,39] The contraceptive steroids are more frequently associated with the development of hepatic adenoma.[47] Vinyl chloride is also associated with the development of angiosarcoma.

What Are the Clinical Presentations of Patients With Toxin-induced Liver Disease?

The patient with liver injury related to a toxin may present in a variety of ways, ranging from an asymptomatic clinical state with mild elevation of aminotransferases, or jaundice and pruritus with minimal symptoms, to acute hepatomegaly with ascites or fulminant hepatic failure. Symptoms of liver disease include anorexia, nausea, vomiting, right upper quadrant discomfort, and fatigue. Signs include hepatomegaly, spider angiomata, percussion tenderness in the right upper quadrant, ascites and abdominal venous distension (so called *caput medusa*), jaundice, gynecomastia, and testicular atrophy.

Some agents used therapeutically over longer periods of time, such as isoniazid, may manifest delayed onset of toxicity over several weeks to months prior to the development of symptoms.[54] Chronic drug-induced hepatitis may smolder for long periods, sometimes eluding diagnosis.[55] An indolent progression to cirrhosis with minimal symptoms is seen in some chronic exposures to vitamin A, methotrexate, and alpha-methyldopa.[55] Cholestatic injury is manifested primarily by jaundice and pruritus. Aminotransferases may be mildly elevated. Alkaline phosphatase may be normal or increased.[125,129]

Patients with significant acute occupational exposure to dimethylformamide present with abdominal pain, anorexia, and disulfiram-type reactions.[126] Aminotransferase concentrations are elevated 2 to 30 times normal, and ALT is usually greater than AST. Bilirubin and alkaline phosphatase concentrations are often normal.[99] Acute intentional exposures have resulted in fulminant hepatic failure.[84]

The presentations of certain drugs and toxins that induce acute liver failure follow an orderly progression. Rapid development of portal hypertension, ascites, and death follows the onset of some cases of veno-occlusive disease.[51] Patients with acute, large exposures to carbon tetrachloride, yellow phosphorus, acetaminophen, and cyclopeptide-containing mushrooms present first with GI symptoms. This is followed by a period of well-being (1–3 days) and then signs of acute hepatic and renal failure with fatigue, anorexia, and nausea followed by profound jaundice, hemorrhage, ascites, hepatic encephalopathy, and death. Fulminant hepatic failure is defined as impaired liver function progressing to encephalopathy within 8 weeks of onset of illness.[54,89] Most cases of fulminant hepatic failure are associated with toxins or viral hepatitis. In these cases a patient may progress from health to death in as little as 2–10 days.[54] Fulminant hepatic failure is usually associated with extensive necrosis, although it may occur in the absence of demonstrable necrosis, such as seen in Reye's syndrome or fialuridine toxicity.[54,73] It is caused by a number of toxic agents, which include *Amanita phalloides* mushrooms, APAP, tetracycline, phosphorus, halogenated hydrocarbons, isoniazid, alpha-methyldopa, and valproate.[54]

Complications from fulminant hepatic failure include encephalopathy, cerebral edema, coagulopathy, renal dysfunction, hypoglycemia, hypotension, pulmonary edema, sepsis, and death. Fulminant hepatic failure is best managed in a specialized liver unit. The overall mortality rate for fulminant hepatic failure is 80–94% but is variable depending on the etiologic agent.[54]

What is the Evaluation of the Patient With Liver Disease?

The history is critical in establishing the diagnosis of the patient with liver disease. A medication history should include careful investigation of over-the-counter agents, especially APAP and the possible use of herbal therapies. Nearly all chronic medications should be suspect. An occupational history may indicate exposure to vinyl chloride (plastics industry), dimethylformamide (leather industry), or other industrial solvents. Alcohol abuse is a common cause of acute hepatitis and the most common cause of cirrhosis.[59] A history of male homosexual contacts, recent transfusion, or intravenous drug use indicates the possibility of hepatitis B. Recent travel to an underdeveloped country suggests the possibility of hepatitis A. A history of recurrent episodes of pain and vomiting should suggest the possibility of cholelithiasis.

Laboratory tests are helpful and certain patterns may point toward the etiology (Table 13–4). Macrocytic anemia, thrombocytopenia, and hypoalbuminemia suggest a more chronic process. Elevation of the aminotransferases indicates hepatocellular injury, although elevations of the AST or ALT as high as 1000 IU occur in acute obstruction of the biliary tract. In alcoholic liver disease the AST level is two to three times greater than the ALT. Elevation of either of these enzymes above 300 IU suggests another cause.[92] In other forms of hepatitis the ALT level is generally greater than the AST. Elevations of alkaline phosphatase and glutamyl transferase transpeptidase (GGTP) result from obstruction to bile flow, either in the liver or as a result of mechanical obstruction in the biliary tract. Serologic studies for the presence of markers of hepatitis A, B, and C should be done routinely in patients with hepatitis.

Although elevated aminotransferase levels suggest hepatocellular injury, their degree of elevation does not always reflect the severity of injury. Hepatic failure occurs in the absence of elevation of the aminotransferases, although very dramatic elevations are seen in most cases where necrosis is prominent. The AST and ALT values may be increased up to 500 times normal in these cases, while alkaline phosphatase will increase only one- to threefold.[54,73] In previously healthy patients, the serum albumin, with a half-life of 21 days, is a good measurement of the acuity of liver dysfunction. The albumin concentration is usually normal in acute hepatitis unless there is preexisting liver disease or malnutrition. The short half-lives (hours to a few days) of the vitamin K–dependent clotting factors II, VII, IX, and X make the prothrombin time a good indicator of the severity of acute hepatic dysfunction. Abnormally low levels of factors II, VII, IX, and X, reflected as an elevation in the prothrombin time (or INR), may result from ingestion of anticoagulants, vitamin K deficiency, or severe hepatic dysfunction (see Chap. 42). Elevation of the prothrombin time in acute hepatitis suggests severe necrosis and a higher risk of fulminant hepatic failure.[31,54,73]

In the patient with severe liver injury, hypoglycemia is a major concern. The arterial blood gas most commonly shows a respiratory alkalosis. Severe metabolic acidosis is seen in patients with hepatic failure due to mitochondrial injury, such as Reye's syndrome, acute fatty liver of pregnancy, or poisoning with a nucleoside analog.[54,73]

The CT and MRI scans are reasonable tests for evaluating metastatic disease in the liver and will demonstrate obstruction of the biliary tract. An ultrasound examination is useful in excluding extrahepatic etiologies of hyperbilirubinemia. The radionucleotide liver scan has been used to diagnose cirrhosis and veno-occlusive disease, although MRI and CT scans are now used more commonly. Liver biopsy may be helpful but is not specifically diagnostic in drug-induced hepatic injury.

Management of Patients With Liver Disease Due to Toxins

In many cases the liver injury resolves with simple withdrawal of the offending toxin.[54,98,99] In cases of severe injury, good supportive care in an intensive care environment is essential. Liver transplantation is now a practical therapeutic modality.[131] Overall 1-year survival for liver transplantation in the 1980s was 80% and 5-year survival was 60–70%.[116] Since complications that make transplantation difficult or contraindicated may develop quickly in toxin-induced hepatic failure, the decision to transplant needs to be made early and clinical criteria are needed to predict which patients will benefit. This prediction is extremely difficult. Patients who survive acute hepatic necrosis often recover completely so that hepatic transplantation should only be offered to those patients who have little chance for survival without the procedure. A figure of less than 20% chance of survival is an accepted cutoff point for this risk–benefit decision.[86,87] Currently, well-developed transplant criteria have been formulated only for acetaminophen toxicity. Patients with serum pH < 7.30 or a combination of stage III or IV encephalopathy (Table 13–5), creatinine > 3.3 mg/dL,

TABLE 13–4. LABORATORY ABNORMALITIES

Disorder	Alkaline Phosphatase, Glutamyl Transferase, 5′ Nucleotidase (AlkPhos/GGTP/5′NT)	Alanine Aminotransferase, Aspartate Aminotransferase (ALT, AST)	Albumin	Prothrombin Time	Bilirubin	Lactate
Acute hepatocellular injury	↑	↑↑↑	N	N→↑↑↑	↑↑	N
Cirrhosis	↑	N or ↑	↓	↑	N or ↑	N
Mitochondrial injury	N or ↑	↑	N	↑↑	N or ↑	↑↑↑
Cholestatic injury	↑	N or ↑	N	N	↑↑	N
Chronic infiltrative disease (granuloma, tumor)	↑↑	↑	N	N	N	N
Biliary Obstruction	↑	N or ↑	N	N	↑↑	N

Key: ↑ = Increased, ↓ = Decreased, N = Normal, ↑↑↑ = Greatly increased

TABLE 13–5. CLINICAL STAGES OF ACUTE HEPATIC ENCEPHALOPATHY

Stage	Level of Consciousness Intellectual Function	Neuromuscular Abnormalities	Electroencephalography
I	Personality changes: Euphoria; occasionally depression; forgetful; slowness of mentation and affect; untidiness; slurred speech; disorder in sleep rhythm; restlessness	Slight tremor; incoordination; asterixis; handwriting changes	Usually normal; rarely symmetric slowing 5–6 cycles/second, triphasic waves
II	Accentuation of stage I; drowsiness; inappropriate behavior; lethargy; disorientation, memory loss	Tremor; dysarthria; asterixis; abnormal reflexes; loss of sphincter control	Abnormal: generalized symmetric slowing; triphasic waves
III	Somnolence, stupor, delirium, incoherent speech; confusion (marked)	Tremor present (if patient can cooperate), asterixis; muscle rigidity; abnormal reflexes; incontinent	Abnormal: symmetric slowing, triphasic waves
IV	Coma; patient may (stage IVA) or may not (stage IVB) respond to painful stimuli	Tremor usually lacking; plantar extension; decerebate; pupillary responses preserved	Abnormal: very slow 2–3 cycles/second; delta activity

Modified, with permission from Trey C, Burns DG, Saunders SJ: Treatment of hepatic coma by exchange blood transfusion. N Engl J Med 1966;274:474 and Schafer DF, Jones EA: Hepatic encephalopathy in Zakim D, Boyer TD: Hepatology. A Textbook of Liver Disease. Philadelphia, Saunders, 1990. (Second Edition), vol 1, p. 450.

and prothrombin time > 1.8 times control are at increased risk of a poor outcome in acetaminophen ingestions.[87] Patients with rapidly progressive hepatic failure related to exposure to a toxin should be referred at an early stage to a transplant center for evaluation.[54]

Other Therapies

Intravenous *N*-acetylcysteine benefits patients with fulminant hepatic failure caused by different etiologies and is also beneficial in both the early and late phase of APAP toxicity[32,42] (see Antidotes in Depth: Acetylcysteine).

Hyperbaric oxygen protects rats from CCl_4 poisoning.[12] Under these conditions, the $^{\bullet}CCl_3$ that is produced by P450 metabolism is rapidly oxidized to the trichloromethyl radical, which is highly reactive but is less toxic because it is detoxified by reduced glutathione.[10,120] The administration of glutathione has also been shown to protect the rat liver against injury by CCl_4.[11] Hyperbaric oxygen was used in one human poisoning with a good outcome.[122]

Summary

The primary role of the liver in the biotransformation of xenobiotics results in an increased risk of hepatotoxicity. The spectrum of liver injury includes combinations of cholestasis, steatosis, and hepatocellular necrosis. Injury may be due to immunologic mechanisms, free radical initiation of lipid peroxidation, mitochondrial injury, and other less well defined mechanisms related to the formation of adducts. Drug-induced liver injury can be dose dependent and predictable or idiosyncratic and unpredictable. Idiosyncratic injury is affected by host characteristics that include genetic makeup, concomitant or previous exposure to drugs and toxins, and the underlying condition of the liver.

Acknowledgment

Charles Maltz, MD and Todd Bania, MD contributed to this chapter in a previous edition.

References

1. Alberti-Flor JJ, Hernandez ME, Ferrer JP, et al: Fulminant liver failure and pancreatitis associated with the use of sulfamethoxazole-trimethoprim. Am J Gastroenterol 1989; 84:1577–1579.
2. Arber N, Zajick G, Areil I: The streaming liver: II. Hepatocyte life history. Liver 1988;8:80–87.
3. Badr MZ, Belinsky SA, Kauffman FC, Thurman RG: Mechanism of hepatoxicity to periportal regions of the liver lobule due to allyl alcohol: Role of oxygen and lipid peroxidation. J Pharmacol Exp Ther 1986;238:1138–1142.
4. Bagheri SA, Boyer JL: Peliosis hepatis associated with androgenic-anabolic steroid therapy. Ann Intern Med 1974;81:610–618.
5. Black M, Mitchel JR, Zimmerman HJ: Isoniazid-associated hepatitis in 114 patients. Gastroenterology 1975;69: 289–302.
6. Black M, Raucy J: Acetaminophen, alcohol and cytochrome P450. Ann Intern Med 1986;104:427–429.
7. Bohme M, Muller M, Leier I, et al: Cholestasis caused by inhibition of the adenosine triphosphate-dependent bile salt transporter in rat liver. Gastroenterology 1994;107: 255–265.
8. Bras G, Jellife DB, Stuart KL: Veno-occlusive disease of liver with non-portal type of cirrhosis, occurring in Jamaica. Arch Pathol 1954;57:285–300.

9. Braun P: Hepatotoxicity of erythromycin. J Invest Dis 1969;119:300–306.
10. Burk RF, Lane JM, Patel K: Relationship of oxygen and glutathione in protection against carbon tetrachloride-induced hepatic microsomal lipid peroxidation and covalent binding in the rat: Rationale for the use of hyperbaric oxygen to treat carbon tetrachloride ingestion. J Clin Invest 1984;74:1996–2001.
11. Burk RF, Patel K, Lane JM: Reduced glutathione protection against rat liver microsomal injury by carbon tetrachloride: Dependence on O_2. Biochem J 1983;215:441–445.
12. Burk RF, Reiter R, Lane JM: Hyperbaric oxygen protection against carbon tetrachloride hepatotoxicity in the rat. Gastroenterology 1986;90:812–818.
13. Carrasco D, Prieto M, Pallardo L: Multiple hepatic adenomas after long-term therapy with testerone enenthate. J Hepatol 1985;1:573–578.
14. Corcoran GB, Racz WJ, Smith CV, Mitchell JR: Effects of *N*-acetylcysteine on acetaminophen covalent binding and hepatic necrosis in mice. J Pharmacol Exp Ther 1985;232: 864–872.
15. Dahm LJ, Schultze AE, Roth RA: An antibody to neutrophils attenuates α-napthylisothiocyanate-induced liver injury. J Pharmacol Exp Ther 1991;256:412–420.
16. Dai Y, Rashba-Step J, Cederbaum AL: Stable expression of human cytochrome P4502E1 in HepG2 cells: Characterization of catalytic activities and production of reactive oxygen intermediates. Biochemistry 1993;32:6928–6937.
17. deMorais SMF, Uetrecht JP, Wells PG. Decreased glucuronidation and increased bioactivation of acetaminophen in Gilbert's syndrome. Gastroenterology 1992;102: 577–586.
18. Dickinson DS, Bailey WC, Hirschowitz BI: Risk factors for isoniazid (INH)-induced liver dysfunction. J Clin Gastroenterol 1981;3:271–279.
19. Diehl AM, Latham P, Boitnott JK: Cholestatic hepatitis from erythromycin ethylsuccinate. Am J Med 1984;76: 931–934.
20. Dutczak WJ, Clarkson TW, Ballatori N: Biliary-hepatic recycling of a xenobiotic: Gallbladder absorption of methyl mercury. Am J Physiol 1991;261:G873-G880.
21. Elliott RH, Strunin L: Hepatotoxicity of volatile anaesthetics. Br J Anaesth 1993;70:339–348.
22. ElSisi AED, Earnest DL, Sipes IG: Vitamin A potentiation of carbon tetrachloride hepatotoxicity: Role of liver macrophages and active oxygen species. Toxicol Appl Pharmacol 1993;119:295–301.
23. Falk H, Thomas LB, Popper H, et al: Hepatic angiosarcoma associated with androgenic-anabolic steroids. Lancet 1979;2:1120–1122.
24. Fromenty B, Pessayre D: Inhibition of mitochondrial beta-oxidation as a mechanism of hepatotoxicity. Pharmacol Ther 1995;67:101–154.
25. Garibalde RA, Drusin RE, Ferebee SH, Gregg MB: Isoniazid-associated hepatitis: Reports of an outbreak. Am Rev Respir Dis 1972;106:357–365.
26. Gronhagen-Riska C, Hellstrom PE, Froseth B: Predisposing factors in hepatitis induced by isoniazid-rifampin treatment of tuberculosis. Am Rev Respir Dis 1978;118: 461–466.
27. Guebel AP, DeGalocsy C, Alves N, et al: Liver damage caused by therapeutic vitamin A administration: Estimate of dose-related toxicity in 41 cases. Gastroenterology 1991;100:1701–1709.
28. Guengerich FP: Catalytic selectivity of human cytochrome P450 enzymes: Relevance to drug metabolism and toxicity. Toxicol Lett 1994;70:133–138.
29. Gumucio J: Hepatocyte heterogeneity: The coming of age from the description of a biological curiosity to a partial understanding of its physiological meaning and regulation. Hepatology 1989;9:154–160.
30. Gurumurthy P, Krishnamurthy MS, Nazareth O, et al: Lack of relationship between hepatic toxicity and acetylator phenotype in three thousand South Indian patients during treatment with isoniazid for tuberculosis. Am Rev Respir Dis 1984;129:58–61.
31. Harrison PM, O'Grady JG, Keays RT, et al: Serial prothrombin time as prognostic indicator in paracetamol induced fulminant hepatic failure. Br Med J 1990;301: 964–966.
32. Harrison PM, Wendon AE, Grimson AE: Improvement by *N*-acetylcysteine of hemodynamics and oxygen transport in fulminant hepatic failure. N Engl J Med 1991;324: 1852–1857.
33. Hebbard GC, Smith KG, Gibson PR, Bhathal PS: Augmentin-induced jaundice with a fatal outcome. Med J Aust 1992;156:285–286.
34. Hetu C, Dumont A, Joly J-G: Effect of chronic ethanol administration on bromobenzene liver toxicity in the rat. Toxicol Appl Pharm 1983;67:166–167.
35. Hollister LE: Allergy to chlorpromazine manifested by jaundice. Am J Med 1957;23:870–879.
36. Hoyumpa AM, Connell AM: Methyldopa hepatitis: Report of three cases. Am J Dig Dis 1973;18:213–222.
37. Ishak KG, Irey NS: Hepatic injury associated with phenothiazines: Clinicopathologic and follow-up study of 36 patients. Arch Pathol 1972;93:283–304.
38. Jenner PJ, Ellard GA: Isoniazid-related hepatotoxicity: A study of the effect of rifampicin administration on the metabolism of acetylisoniazid in man. Tubercle 1989;70: 93–101.
39. Johnson FL, Lerner KG, Siegel M: Association of androgenic-anabolic steroids therapy with development of hepatocellular carcinoma. Lancet 1972;2:1273–1276.
40. Jones AL, Spring-Mills E: The liver and gallbladder. In Weiss L, ed: Cell and Tissue Biology. A Textbook of Histology, 6th ed. Baltimore, Urban & Schwarzenberg, 1988, pp. 687–714.
41. Kaplowitz N, Aw TY, Simon FR, et al: Drug-induced hepatotoxicity. Ann Intern Med 1986;104:826–839.
42. Keays R, Harrison PM, Wendon JA: Intravenous acetylcysteine in paracetamol induced fulminant hepatic failure: A prospective controlled trial. Br Med J 1991;303: 1026–1029.
43. Kesterson JW, Grannehan GR, Machinist JM: The hepatotoxicity of valproic acid and its metabolites in rats: I. Toxicologic, biochemical and histopathologic studies. Hepatology 1984;4:1143–1152.
44. Klaassen CD: Biliary excretion of metals. Drug Metab Rev 1976;5:165–193.

45. Klaassen CD, Watkins JB: Mechanisms of bile formation, hepatic uptake, and biliary excretion. Pharmacol Rev 1984;36:1–67.
46. Kleckner HB, Yakulis V, Heller P: Severe hypersensitivity of diphenylhydantoin with circulating antibodies to the drug. Ann Intern Med 1975;83:522–523.
47. Knowles DM, Casarella WJ, Johnson PM, et al: The clinical, radiologic, and pathologic characterization of benign hepatic neoplasms. Medicine 1978;57:223–239.
48. Kopanoff DE, Snider D, Caras GJ: Isoniazid-related hepatitis. Am Rev Respir Dis 1978;117:991–1001.
49. Krell H, Metz J, Jaeschke H, et al: Drug-induced intrahepatic cholestasis: Characterization of different pathomechanisms. Arch Toxicol 1987;60:124–130.
50. Krishna DR, Klotz U: Extrahepatic metabolism of drugs in humans. Clin Pharmacokinet 1994;26:144–160.
51. Kumana CR, Ng M, Lin HJ, et al: Herbal tea induced veno-occlusive disease: Quantification of toxic alkaloid exposure in adults. Gut 1985;26:101–104.
52. Larrey D, Vial T, Micaleff A, et al: Hepatitis associated with amoxicillin-clavulanic acid combinations: Report of 15 cases. Gut 1992;33:368–371.
53. Lauterburg BH, Velez ME: Glutathione deficiency in alcoholics. Risk factor for paracetamol hepatotoxicity. Gut 1988;29:1153–1157.
54. Lee WM: Acute liver failure. N Eng J Med 1993;329: 1862–1872.
55. Lee WM: Drug-induced hepatotoxicity. N Engl J Med 1995;333:1118–1127.
56. Lee WM, Denton WT: Chronic hepatitis and indolent cirrhosis due to methyldopa. The bottom of the iceberg? JCS Med Assoc 1989;85:75–79.
57. Lees AW, Allan GW, Smith J: Toxicity from rifampicin plus isoniazid and difampin plus ethambutol therapy. Tubercle 1971;52:182–190.
58. Lewis JH, Zimmerman HJ, Garrett CT, et al: Valproate-induced hepatic steatogenesis in rats. Hepatology 1982;2: 870–873.
59. Lieber CS: Alcohol and the liver: 1994 update. Gastroenterology 1994;106:1085–1105.
60. Lindros KO, Cai Y, Penttila KD. Role of ethanol-inducible cytochrome P–450 IIE1 in carbon tetrachloride-induced damage to centrilobular hepatocytes from ethanol-treated rabbits. Hepatology 1990;5:1092–1097.
61. Lira M, Schteingart CD, Steinbach JH, et al: Sugar absorption by the biliary ductular epithelium of the rat: Evidence for two transport systems. Gastroenterology 1992;102: 563–571.
62. Lundberg I, Lundberg S, Kroneri T: Some observations on dimethylformamide hepatotoxicity. Toxicology 1981;22: 1–7.
63. Maddrey WC: Isoniazid-induced liver disease. Semin Liver Dis 1981;1:129–133.
64. Maddrey WC, Boitnott JK: Isoniazid hepatitis. Ann Intern Med 1973;79:1–12.
65. Maddrey WC, Boitnott JK: Severe hepatitis from methyldopa. Gastroenterology 1975;68:351–360.
66. Mahler H, Pasi A, Kramer JM, et al: Fulminant liver failure in association with the emetic toxin of *Bacillus cereus*. N Engl J Med 1997;336:1142–1148.
67. Manoguerra AS, Weaver LC: Poisoning with tricyclic antidepressant drugs. Clin Toxicol 1977;10:149–157.
68. Mattocks AR: Pyrrolic and *N*-oxide metabolites formed from pyrrolizidine alkaloids by hepatic microsomes in vitro: Relevance to in vivo hepatoxicity. Chemobiol Interaction 1983;43:209–222.
69. Mattocks AR: Toxicity of pyrrolizidine alkaloids. Nature 1968;217:723–728.
70. Mazuryk H, Kastenberg D, Rubin R, Munoz SJ: Cholestatic hepatitis associated with the use of nafcillin. Am J Gastroenterol 1993;88:1960–1962.
71. McClain CJ, Kromhout JP, Peterson FJ, Holtzman JL: Potentiation of acetaminophen hepatotoxicity by alcohol. JAMA 1980;244:251–253.
72. McDonald GB, Hinds MS, Fisher LD, et al: Veno-occlusive disease of the liver and multiorgan failure after bone marrow transplantation: A cohort study of 355 patients. Ann Intern Med 1993;118:255–267.
73. McKenzie R, Fried MW, Sallie R, et al: Hepatic failure and lactic acidosis due to fialuridine (FIAU), an investigational nucleoside analogue for chronic hepatitis B. N Engl J Med 1995;333:1099–1105.
74. Mehendale HM, Roth RA, Gandolfi AJ: Novel mechanisms in chemically induced hepatotoxicity. FASEB J 1994;8:1285–1295.
75. Meier PJ: Canalicular membrane transport process. In: Tavoloni N, Berk PD, eds: Hepatic Transport and Bile Secretion. Physiology and Pathophysiology. New York. Raven, 1993, pp. 587–596.
76. Mitchell I, Wendon J, Fett S, et al: Anti-tuberculous therapy and acute liver failure. Lancet 1995;345:555–556.
77. Mitchell JR, Jollows DJ: Metabolic activation of drugs to toxic substances. Gastroenterology 1975;68:392–410. Review.
78. Mitchell JR, Thorgeirsson SS, Potter WZ: Acetaminophen induced hepatic injury: Protective role of glutathione in man and rationale for therapy. Clin Pharmacol Ther 1974;16:676–684.
79. Mitchell JR, Thorgeirsson VP, Black M: Increased incidence of isoniazid hepatitis in rapid acetylators: Possible relation to hydrazine metabolites. Clin Pharmacol Ther 1975;18:70–78.
80. Mitchell JR, Zimmerman HJ, Ishak KG: Isoniazid liver injury: clinical spectrum, pathology and probable pathogenesis. Ann Intern Med 1976;84:181–189.
81. Mohabbat O, Younos MS, Merzad AAA, et al: An outbreak of hepatic veno-occlusive disease in North Western Afghanistan. Lancet 1976;2:269–271.
82. Nakajima T, Okino T, Sato A: Kinetic studies on benzene metabolism in the rat liver—possible presence of three forms of benzene metabolizing enzymes in the liver. Biochem Pharm 1987;36:2799–2804.
83. Neuberger J, Williams R: Halothane anesthesia and liver damage. Br Med J 1984;289:1136–1139.
84. Nicolas F, Rodineau P, Rouzioux JM: Fulminant hepatic failure in poisoning due to ingestion of T 61, a veterinary euthanasia drug. Crit Care Med 1990;18:573–575.
85. O'Dell JR, Zetterman RK, Burnett DA: Centrilobular hepatic fibrosis following acetaminophen-induced hepatic necrosis in an alcoholic. JAMA 1986;255:2636–2637.

86. O'Grady JG, Tan KC, Williams R: Selection criteria and results of orthotopic liver transplantation in the UK. In: Williams R, Hughes RD, eds: Acute Liver Failure. Improved Understanding and Better Therapy. London, Miter Press, 1991, pp. 77–80.
87. O'Grady JG, Wendon J, Tan KC: Liver transplantation after paracetamol overdose. Br Med J 1991;303:221–223.
88. Peck CC, Temple R, Collins JM: Understanding consequences of concurrent therapies. JAMA 1993;269: 1550–1552.
89. Pimstone NR, Goldstein LI, Ward R, et al: Liver transplantation. In: Zakim D, Boyer TD, eds: Hepatology. A Textbook of Liver Disease, 2nd ed. Philadelphia, Saunders, 1990, pp. 1459–1475.
90. Pirotte JH: Apparent potentiation of hepatotoxicity from small doses of acetaminophen by phenobarbital. Ann Intern Med 1984;101:403. Letter.
91. Podolsky DK, Isselbacher KJ: Alcoholic liver disease and cirrhosis. In: Isselbacher KJ, Braunwald E, Wilson JD, eds: Harrison's Principles of Internal Medicine, 13th ed. New York, McGraw-Hill, 1994, pp. 1483–1495.
92. Podolsky DK, Isselbacher KJ: Derangements of hepatic metabolism. In: Isselbacher KJ, Braunwald E, Wilson JD, eds: Harrison's Principles of Internal Medicine, 13th ed. New York, McGraw-Hill, 1994, pp. 1448–1453.
93. Pohl LR: Drug-induced allergic hepatitis. Semin Liver Dis 1990;10:305–315.
94. Potter WZ, Davis DC, Mitchell JR, et al: Acetaminophen-induced hepatic necrosis: III. Cytochrome P–450 mediated covalent binding *in vitro*. J Pharmacol Exp Ther 1973;187: 203–210.
95. Powel-Jackson PR, Tredger JM, Williams R: Progress report: Hepatotoxicity to valproate—a review. Gut 1984;25: 673–681.
96. Prescott LF: Paracetamol toxicity: Pharmacological consideration and clinical management. Drugs 1983;25:290–314.
97. Read AE, Harrison CV, Sherlock S: Chronic chlorpromazine jaundice: With particular reference to its relationship to primary biliary cirrhosis. Am J Med 1961;31: 249–258.
98. Redlich CA, Beckett WS, Sparer J, et al: Liver disease associated with occupational exposure to the solvent dimethylformamide. Ann Intern Med 1988;108:680–686.
99. Redlich CA, West AB, Fleming L: Clinical and pathological characteristics of hepatotoxicity associated with occupational exposure to demethylformamide. Gastroenterology 1990;99:748–757.
100. Reid WD, Christie B, Krishna G, et al: Bromobenzene metabolism and hepatic necrosis. Pharmacology 1971;6: 41–55.
101. Reynolds TB, Peters RL, Yamada S: Chronic active and lupoid hepatitis caused by a laxative, oxyphenisatin. N Engl J Med 1971;285:813–820.
102. Rheinhart HH, Reinhart E, Korlipara P, Peleman R: Combined nitrofurantoin toxicity to liver and lung. Gastroenterology 1992;102:1396–1399.
103. Ridker PM, Phkuma S, McDermott W, et al: Hepatic venocclusive disease associated with the consumption of pyrrolizidine-containing dietary supplements. Gastroenterology 1985;88:1050–1054.
104. Rigas B, Rosenfeld LE, Barwick KW, et al: Amiodarone hepatotoxicity: A clinicopathologic study of five patients. Ann Intern Med 1986;104:348–351.
105. Rodman JS, Deutsch DJ, Grutman SI: Methyldopa hepatitis: A report of six cases and review of the literature. Am J Med 1976;60:941–948.
106. Ros E, Small DM, Carey MC: Effects of chlorpromazine hydrochloride on bile salt synthesis, bile formation and biliary lipid secretion in the rhesus monkey: A model for chlorpromazine-induced cholestasis. Eur J Clin Invest 1979;9:29–33.
107. Ross WT Jr, Daggy BP: Hepatic necrosis caused by halothane and hypoxia in phenobarbital-treated rats. Anethesiology 1979;51:321–326.
108. Sallie RW, McKenzie T, Reed WD, et al: Diclofenac hepatitis. Aust NZ J Med 1991;21:251–255.
109. Sarma GR, Immanuel C, Kailasam S, et al: Rifampin-induced release of hydrazine from isoniazid: A possible cause of hepatitis during treatment of tuberculosis with regimens containing isoniazid and rifampin. Am Rev Respir Dis 1985;133:1072–1075.
110. Schafer F, Sorrell MF: Power failure, liver failure. N Engl J Med 1997;336:1173–1174.
111. Scharer L, Smith JP: Serum transaminase elevations and other hepatic abnormalities in patients receiving isoniazid. Ann Intern Med 1969;71:1113–1120.
112. Schultz JC, Adamson JS, Workman WW, et al: Fatal liver disease after intravenous administration of tetracycline in high dosage. N Engl J Med 1963;269:999–1004.
113. Seef LB, Cuccherini BA, Zimmerman HJ, et al: Acetaminophen hepatotoxicity in alcoholics. Ann Intern Med 1986;104:399–404.
114. Selzer G, Parker RGF: Senecio poisoning exhibiting as Chiari's syndrome: A report on twelve cases. Am J Pathol 1951;27:885–907.
115. Shah RR, Oates NS, Idle JR, et al: Impaired oxidation of debrisoquine in patients with perhexilene neuropathy. Br Med J 1982;284:295–299.
116. Sherlock S. Drugs and the liver. In: Diagnosis of the Liver and Biliary System, 8th ed. Oxford, Blackwell Scientific, 1989, pp. 372–409.
117. Slattery JG, Wilson JM, Kalhorn TF, Nelson SD: Dose-dependent pharmacokinetics of acetaminophen: Evidence of glutathione depletion in humans. Clin Pharmacol Ther 1987;41:413–418.
118. Snider DE, Caras GJ: Isoniazid-associated hepatitis deaths. A review of available information. Am Rev Resp Dis 1992;145:494–497.
119. Speeg KV, Mitchel MC, Maldonado AL: Additive protection of cimetidine and *N*-acetylcysteine treatment against acetaminophen induced hepatic necrosis in the rat. J Pharmacol Exp Ther 1985;234:550–554.
120. Stacey NH, Ottenwilder H, Kappus G: CCl_4-induced lipid peroxidation in isolated rat hepatocytes with different oxygen concentration. Toxicol Appl Pharmacol 1982;62: 421–427.
121. Tandon BN, Tandon HD, Tandon RK, et al: An epidemic of veno-occlusive disease of liver in Central India. Lancet 1976;2:271–272.
122. Truss CD, Killenberg PG: Treatment of carbon tetrachlo-

ride poisoning with hyperbaric oxygen. Gastroenterology 1982;82:767–769.

123. Tsutsumi M, Lasker JM, Shimizu M, et al: The intralobular distribution of ethanol-inducible P450IIE1 in rat and human liver. Hepatology 1989;10:437–446.
124. Vergani D, Mieli-Vergani G, Alberti A: Antibodies to the surface of halothane-altered rabbit hepatocytes in patients with severe halothane associated hepatitis. N Engl J Med 1980;303:66–71.
125. Victorino RMM, Maria VA, Correia AP, et al: Floxacillin-induced cholestatic hepatitis with evidence of lymphocyte sensitization. Arch Intern Med 1987;147:987–989.
126. Wang JD, Lai MY, Chen JS: Dimethylformamide-induced liver damage among synthetic leather workers. Arch Environ Health 1991;46:161–166.
127. Watanabe M, Tsukada N, Smith CR, et al: Permeabilized hepatocyte couplets: Adensosine triphosphate-dependent bile canalicular contractions and a circumferential pericanalicular microfilament belt demonstrated. Lab Invest 1992;65:203–213.
128. Weston CF, Cooper BT, Davies JD, et al: Veno-occlusive disease of the liver secondary to ingestion of comfrey. Br Med J 1987;295:183.
129. Westphal JF, Wvtter D, Brogard JM: Hepatic side-effects of antibiotics. J Antimicrob Chemother 1994;33:387–401.
130. Williams DE, Reed RL, Kezierski B, et al: Bioactivation and detoxication of the pyrrolizidine alkaloid senecionine by cytochrome P–450 enzymes in rat liver. Drug Metab Dispos 1989;17:387–392.
131. Woodle ES, Woody RR, Cox KL: Orthotopic liver transplantation in a patient with amanita poisoning. JAMA 1985;253:69–70.
132. Yeong ML, Clark SP, Waring JM, et al: The effects of comfrey derived pyrrolizidine alkaloids on rat liver. Pathology 1991;23:35–38.
133. Yeong ML, Swinburn B, Kennedy M, et al: Hepatic veno-occlusive disease associated with comfrey ingestion. J Gastroenterol Hepatol 1990;5:211–214.
134. Zafrani ES, Ishak KG, Rudzki C: Cholestatic and heptatocellular injury associated with erythromycin ester. Dig Dis Sci 1979;24:385–396.
135. Zand R, Nelson SD, Slattery JT, et al: Inhibition and induction of cytochrome P4502E1-catalyzed oxidation by isoniazid in humans. Clin Pharmacol Ther 1993;54:142–149.
136. Zimmerman HJ, Ishak KG: Valproate-induced hepatic injury: Analysis of 23 fatal cases. Hepatology 1982;2: 591–597.

CHAPTER 14

Immunologic Principles

William J. Meggs

The explosive growth of knowledge of the immune system and concomitant development of immunotechnology in recent decades has had impact on virtually every area of medicine, and medical toxicology has not been exempt from this impact. Immune deficiency syndromes and diseases manifest as an inability of an organism to hold the world of microorganisms at bay, and a number of toxins can selectively damage parts or all of the immune system and lead to life-threatening infections. Autoimmune diseases, in which the immune system attacks "self" to damage one or more organ systems, can be triggered by toxic exposures through several mechanisms. Allergic diseases may also be induced by toxins through a variety of mechanisms, and it can be argued that the increasing incidence of allergic diseases such as asthma may be due to environmental toxins. Research has elucidated the interactions between the immune system and the nervous system, and neurogenic inflammation results from the interaction of chemical irritants with sensory nerves. Immunotoxicology has emerged as an interdisciplinary field that studies the effects of toxins on the immune system.[17,18]

Technological developments in laboratory immunology have had an impact on the diagnosis and treatment of toxic diseases. Toxin-specific monoclonal antibodies can be used to neutralize poisons ranging from colchicine and digoxin to snake venoms. Immune assays can provide rapid identification of the etiology of poisoning and are used to determine the species of a snake bite by analyzing toxins in the blood or urine. In this chapter a brief overview of the immune system will be given, including a discussion of the interaction of the immune system and the nervous system. The role of toxins in immune deficiency, autoimmunity, and allergy will be discussed. Finally, the role of the immunology laboratory in diagnosing and treating poisonings will be presented.

The Immune System, an Overview

The immune system is an intricate and dispersed organ system that consists of an interacting web of cells, antibodies, and mediators. It is now known that the immune system is organized in separate but overlapping branches, and activation of one branch can actually suppress activity of another. Each branch has a unique function and can have pathologic manifestations from both inappropriate activation and malfunction.

Anti-Parasite System

The eosinophil is a white blood cell that migrates into tissues and destroys parasites by releasing major basic protein, eosinophil cation protein, and eosinophil protein-X.[28] These proteins can also damage host tissues, as observed in the hypereosinophil syndrome.[100] IgE antibody specific for parasite antigens is produced by plasma cells and binds to receptors on the surface of mast cells and basophils. Mast cells reside in tissues in close proximity to blood vessels and nerves.[34,91] Antigen cross-linking of surface IgE molecules on mast cells leads to the extrusion of mast cell granules and pre-formed mediators into the extracellular space and the production of nonstored mediators. These mediators include the vasoactive amine histamine and chemotactic factors for neutrophils and eosinophils. Activation of this system by environmental antigens can produce asthma attacks, rhinosinusitis, urticaria, angioedema, gastrointestinal symptoms, and systemic anaphylaxis.

Anti-Encapsulated Bacteria System

This system destroys encapsulated bacteria. Opsonization refers to the coating of the bacteria with immunoglobulin molecules of the IgG and IgM classes, which are produced by plasma cells. The bacteria are then identified as foreign by neutrophils and macrophages, which engulf them by phagocytosis and destroy them with oxidants. In tissues, chemotactic factors lead to the migration of neutrophils and macrophages to sites of tissue invasion by bacteria. Opsonized bacteria are removed from the bloodstream by the reticuloendothelial system, which consists of Kupffer cells (macrophages lining splenic and hepatic sinusoids). Opsonized bacteria activate the complement system. This system is responsible for the adverse effects noted in immune complex diseases such as serum sickness.[110] Immune complexes are found in systemic lupus erythematosus and other collagen vascular diseases and are implicated in lupus nephritis.[47]

Anti-Cell System

This system seeks and destroys abnormal cells, including cancer cells, mycobacteria, cells infected by viruses, and fungi. T lymphocytes are produced that have receptors specific for given antigens. Cytotoxic T lymphocytes and natural killer cells differentiate from lymphocytes. These T cells are specialized to seek out and destroy tumor and other unwanted cells.

Control System

The immune system is controlled by T lymphocytes. T-helper cells potentiate the response to a specific antigen, and T-suppressor cells suppress the response. T cells secrete protein messengers called cytokines that regulate the immune system and modulate the inflammatory response. Activation of one branch of the immune system shuts down the other branches through the production of inhibitory cytokines. One adverse effect of this inhibition is the disease chronic candida vulvovaginitis. Women with this disease make IgE against candida, so that low-grade infections produce severe inflammation with swelling and pruritis. Cellular immunity, the only defense humans have against candida, is inhibited, so the candida infection cannot be cleared.[113] Immunotherapy with injections of candida antigen has been demonstrated to cure chronic candida vaginitis, presumably by the inhibition of IgE production and a concomitant activation of cellular immunity against candida.[87]

Neurogenic Inflammation and the Immune System–Nervous System Interaction

Neurogenic inflammation occurs when mediators are released from sensory nerve C-fibers. The most important of these mediators is substance P. Sensory nerve C-fibers are found in subepithelial tissues of the respiratory tract, gastrointestinal tract, and skin. These fibers contain chemoreceptors that are triggered by chemical irritants. Examples of chemical irritants are cigarette smoke, gases such as sulfur dioxide and chlorine, solvents such as toluene diisocyanate and formaldehyde, and some fragrances, perfumes, and pesticides. When the irritants bind to the nerve fiber chemoreceptors, chemical mediators including substance P, calcitonin gene–related peptide, and neurokinin A are released. These substances produce vasodilatation and edema. In addition, the binding of irritants to the chemoreceptors triggers a nerve impulse that travels to the central nervous system.[73,75]

Crossover Network

Immunogenic and the neurogenic inflammation are related. Human skin mast cells contain receptors for substance P,[11] and the binding of substance P to mast cells triggers mast cell degranulation and the release of mast cell mediators. Sensory nerve C-fibers have surface receptors for histamine, and when histamine binds to the nerve fibers, substance P is released and an impulse is transmitted up the nerve fiber.[9] Figure 14–1A depicts the relationship between nerve fibers and mast cells.

Neurogenic Switching

Most commonly, clinical symptoms appear at the site of inoculation with antigen or chemical irritant. It is known that in certain instances the site of response can be switched to another site.[66] Examples include systemic anaphylaxis to ingestions of food and drugs, in which there is a rapid development of signs and symptoms in many organ systems. Food allergy most commonly causes gastrointestinal symptoms of diarrhea, nausea, vomiting, abdominal bloating, and cramping, but it can result in urticaria, asthma, laryngeal edema, and systemic anaphylaxis. The site switching is thought to occur at the level of the central nervous system, with the response to the sensory nerve signal from the site of inoculation being rerouted to another peripheral location, leading to substance P release at the other location, as depicted in Figure 14–1B. Evidence for neurogenic switching comes from animal studies, in which systemic anaphylaxis can be blocked by ablating nerve pathways, even though histamine release still occurs at the inoculation site.[49,50]

The Toxic Induction of Immune Deficiencies

The hallmark of immune deficiency is a susceptibility to infections. A number of immune deficiency syndromes are defined, and the types of infections associated with each syndrome correlates with the branch of the immune system that is deficient. Many immune deficiency syndromes are genetic in origin and are manifested in early childhood. Examples include severe combined immune deficiency syndrome (SCIDS), an autosominal recessive deficiency of adenosine deaminase in which there is an absence of both B and T lymphocytes. Both cellular and antibody deficiencies occur, and death occurs in early childhood in the absence of a bone marrow transplant or extreme environmental isolation. Bruton's disease is X-linked with B-lymphocyte lineage failure, no antibodies are produced, and infections with encapsulated bacteria are common. Common variable immunodeficiency syn-

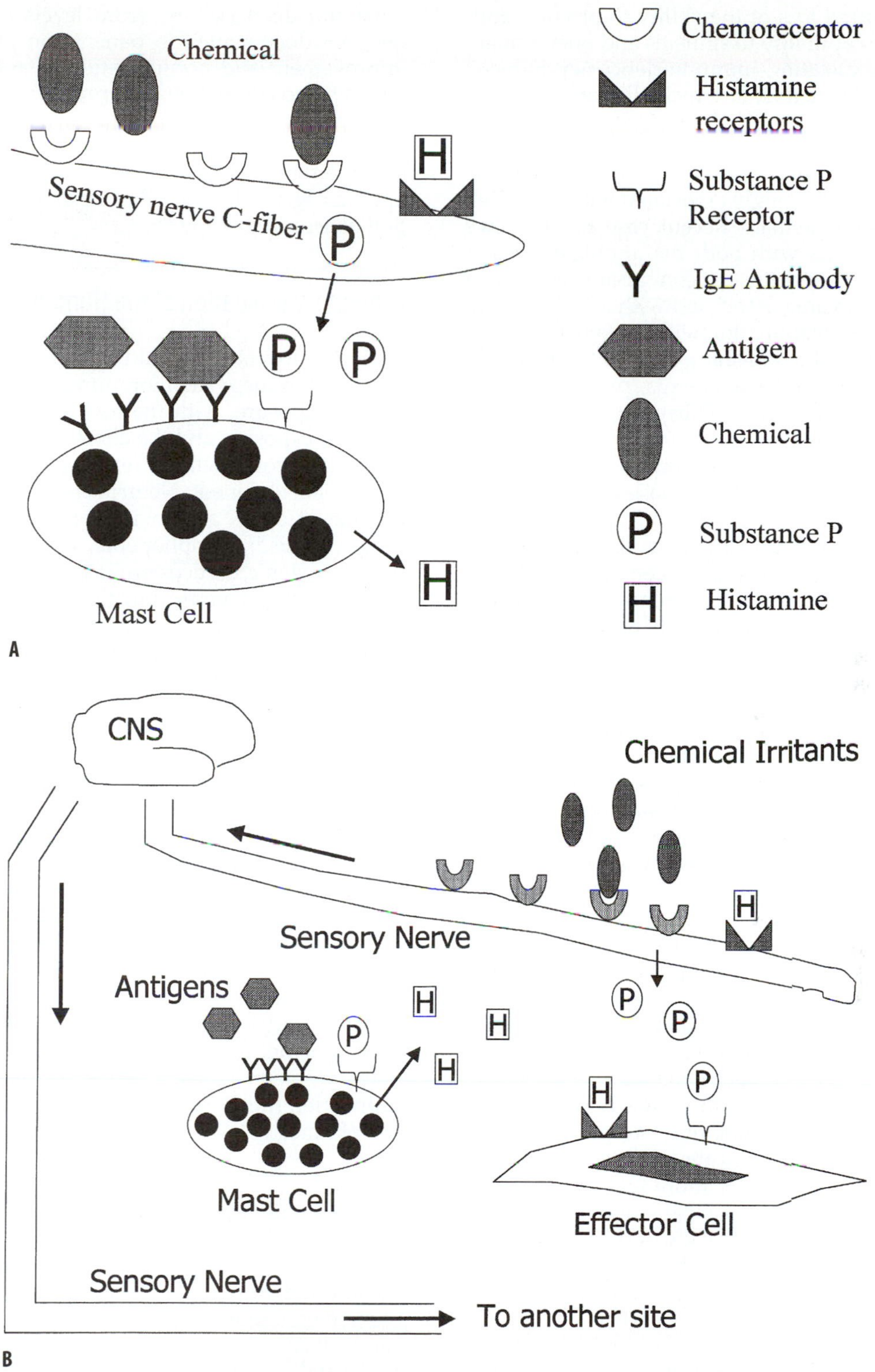

Figure 14–1. The mechanisms of neurogenic inflammation triggered by chemical irritants, immunogenic inflammation triggered by allergens, and their relationship are depicted. (**A**) Chemical irritants bind sensory nerve C-fibers to release substance P and other inflammatory mediators, whereas antigen binds IgE molecules on mast cell surfaces to produce mast cell degranulation and the release of histamine and other mediators. Mast cells have receptors for substance P, whereas sensory nerve fibers have histamine receptors. (**B**) Sensory nerve fibers communicate an inflammatory response to the central nervous system.

drome is an acquired loss of the ability to produce antibodies, with a susceptibility to sinusitis and pneumonia.

The most devastating immune deficiency induced by toxins is aplastic anemia, in which all branches of the immune system are destroyed. A recent study of aplastic anemia in the United States, Europe, Israel, and Thailand found penicillamine, gold, and carbamazepine to be the pharmaceuticals most strongly associated with the development of aplastic anemia.[37] Recent case reports have linked aplastic anemia with both the antiplatelet agent ticlopidine[21,56,92,101,111] and the anticonvulsant felbamate.[2] A case of aplastic anemia associated with a herbal medicine was linked to contamination with phenylbutazone.[74] A French study found a vanishing role for toxins previously known to cause aplastic anemia, presumably due to preventive measures.[58] In 1897 benzene was reported to cause aplastic anemia with chronic occupational inhalational exposure.[97] Following benzene exposure the estimated incidence is 1 per 100 exposed individuals at 100 ppm and 1 per 10,000 exposed individuals at 10–20 ppm.[58] Inhalation exposure to burning oil in Kuwait during the Persian Gulf war has also been associated with aplastic anemia,[93,99] and the organochlorine pesticide lindane has also been associated with aplastic anemia.[6] Agranulocytosis is most strongly associated with procainamide, antithyroid drugs, and sulfasalazine.[37]

Dioxins and furans may suppress cellular immunity in humans. The compound 2,3,7,8-tetrachlorodibenzo-*p*-dioxin (TCDD) suppresses T-helper cell function in exposed workers up to 20 years after exposure.[106] Workers exposed to a mixture of phenoxy herbicides contaminated with dioxins and furans have an increased total and respiratory cancer mortality relative to controls[3]. An increased total cancer mortality, and in particular cancer mortality from digestive and respiratory cancers, was found in workers exposed to TCDD.[77] This increase in cancer mortality may be due to impaired cellular immunity against tumors.

The toxic suppression of antibody production leads to bacterial infections. IgG deficiency is associated with sinusitis, bronchitis, and pneumonia. IgA deficiency is associated with upper respiratory infections and gastroenteritis. A number of xenobiotics suppress antibody production, and in many cases the association has been verified by rechallenge. One or more IgG subclass deficiencies are observed in 66.7% of asthmatics treated with chronic corticosteroids but only 6.7% of those not treated with chronic corticosteroids.[45] Carbamazepine produces hypogammaglobulinemia with absent B lymphocytes accompanied by agranulocytosis.[98] In workers occupationally exposed to lead, there is a decrease in immunoglobulin levels with increasing lead levels.[8] Sulfasalazine depresses IgG, IgM, and IgA in patients with inflammatory arthritis, with an incidence of 2%, 5%, and 3%, respectively.[22] Suppression of serum immunoglobulins by cigarette smoking and exposure to industrial solvents is synergistic.[71]

A number of studies have linked phenytoin to selective IgA deficiency, and the link was verified in some reports by rechallenge.[33,95,104] Recurrent respiratory infections and decreases in serum levels of IgA, IgG_2, and IgG_4 are documented in patients on phenytoin; clinical improvement and normalization of antibody levels followed discontinuation of phenytoin.[5] Selective IgA deficiency has been reported in association with captopril[29,109] and penicillamine.[31,82] Three patients with juvenile rheumatoid arthritis treated with aspirin developed an IgA deficiency that resolved with discontinuation of aspirin therapy.[46]

Laboratory Evaluation of the Human Immune System

A tiered approach should be used in evaluating the human immune system for immune deficiency following a toxic exposure, with the tests ordered determined by the toxic exposure and the clinical consequences. A complete blood count with differential screens for cytopenias should be obtained. Neutropenia from exposure to a number of drugs and toxins can result in bacterial and fungal sepsis.[44] Lymphopenia, most notably associated with iatrogenic corticosteroid administration, results in susceptibility to viral, fungal, and mycobacterial infections.[13] Recurrent respiratory infections including sinusitis is associated with hypogammaglobulinemia, which is assessed by ordering immunoglobulin levels. A total IgG level is not sufficient to exclude IgG subclass deficiencies, which are associated with infections.

Integrity of cellular immunity can be assessed with delayed hypersensitivity skin tests to mumps, measles, and candida. Intradermal injections of antigen should lead to erythema and induration at 24–48 hours. In vitro evaluation of cellular immunity may be determined by lymphocyte proliferation assays to specific antigens and mitogens. Deficiencies of cellular immunity are associated with viral, fungal, and mycobacterial infections and are thought to impart an increased risk of cancer. Some toxins selectively decrease T-helper cell counts, and total T-helper and T-suppressor cell counts, as well as the ratio of helper to suppressor cells, can be determined by flow cytometry. Dioxin exposure lowers the helper to suppressor ratio[106] and is associated with an increased risk of cancer.[77]

The Toxic Induction of Autoimmunity

Autoimmune diseases are due to an immune response to noninfected host tissues, leading to inflammation and tissue destruction. The toxic induction of autoimmunity has been associated with some pharmaceutical and environmental chemicals. Examples of toxins associated with the induction of autoimmune diseases are given in Tables 14–1 and 14–2.

There are several mechanisms by which a xenobiotic can induce autoimmune disease.

1. A chemical can bind to host tissue so that modified host tissue antigens are recognized as foreign and the tissue is destroyed. Autoimmune hemolytic anemia

TABLE 14–1. XENOBIOTICS IMPLICATED IN THE INDUCTION OF IMMUNOSUPPRESSION

Agranulocytosis
Angiotensin converting enzyme inhibitors, antithyroid agents, phenothiazines
Aplastic Anemia
Antineoplastic agents, arsenic, benzene, bismuth, carbamazepine, chlordane, chloramphenicol, DDT, felbamate, gold compounds, mercury, penicillamine, phenylbutazone, phenytoin, silver, sulfonamides, ticlopidine, trimethadione, zidovudine
Cellular Immune Impairment
Chlordane, DDT, lindane, malathion, 1,2,3,6,7,8-hexachlorodibenzo-*p*-dioxin (HCDD), polybrominated biphenyls (PBBs), 2,3,7,8-tetrachlorodibenzo-*p*-dioxin (TCDD), 2,3,7,8-tetrachlorodibenzofuran (TCDF), phencyclidine
Hypogammaglobulinemia
Carbamazepine, cigarette smoking, corticosteroids, phenytoin, sulfasalazine, solvents

associated with penicillin results if an immune response is mounted against penicillin bound to red blood cell membranes.[25]

2. In a process termed molecular mimicry, an immune response can be mounted against an agent that is chemically similar to host tissue, and the host tissue can be secondarily destroyed. Examples in which infectious agents can induce autoimmunity by molecular mimicry include type I diabetes mellitus[27,36,105] and rheumatic heart disease.[15]
3. A chemical can alter the regulatory system that prevents the immune system from attacking self-antigens. Examples of this mechanism include autoimmune hemolytic anemia induced by the antihypertensive methyldopa,[43] which inhibits T-suppressor cell function. Procainamide stimulates T-helper cell function[69] and induces autoimmunity.

TABLE 14–2. XENOBIOTIC INDUCTION OF AUTOIMMUNITY

Autoimmune hemolytic anemia
Alpha-methyldopa, penicillin, penicillamine
Autoimmune thyroid disease
Polybrominated biphenyls, polychlorinated biphenyls, lithium, penicillamine, amiodarone
Autoimmune hepatitis
Alpha-methyldopa, oxyphenacetin, halothane
Immune complex glomerulonephritis
Cadmium, gold, mercury
Myasthenia gravis
Penicillamine, tiopronine, trimethadione
Pemphigus
Alpha-mercaptopropionylglycine, captopril, penicillamine, pyrithioxine
Polymyositis
Penicillamine
Scleroderma
Rape seed oil contaminated with anilines, silica dust, vinyl chloride
Systemic lupus erythematosis
Hydralazine, procainamide, phenytoin, hydrazine, tartrazine, alfalfa sprouts

Epidemics of autoimmune disease have occurred when populations were exposed to an environmental chemical that induced autoimmunity. The Spanish Toxic Oil Syndrome of 1981 began when street vendors in the region of Madrid, Spain, sold bottles of cooking oil that were later found to be rapeseed oil contaminated with anilines. Of approximately 100,000 exposed individuals, some 20,000 developed a disease with arthralgias and myalgias, gastrointestinal symptoms, fever, rash, pruritis, and pneumonitis with dyspnea, often with laboratory abnormalities of eosinophilia and thrombocytopenia.[76] The disease was self-limited in most individuals, but approximately 15% of those with illness developed a progressive collagen vascular disease with features of progressive systemic sclerosis, Sjögren's syndrome, Raynaud's phenomena, and pulmonary hypertension.[1,23] A revealing feature of this epidemic was that those who developed progressive autoimmune disease from the exposure were more likely to have HLA haplotypes associated with collagen vascular disease.[35,108] These data suggest that a combination of environmental exposure and genetic susceptibility can lead to the onset of some cases of autoimmune disease.

In 1960 an epidemic of erythema multiforme was associated with a margarine preparation, with approximately 20,000 of some 600,000 exposed individuals developing the disease.[54]

Systemic lupus erythematosus is commonly associated with xenobiotic exposure. Pharmaceuticals that can induce lupus include hydralazine and procainamide, and less commonly phenytoin and isoniazid.[112] Inhalation of the laboratory reagent hydrazine has led to lupus as well.[85] Ingestion of alfalfa sprouts[55] and tartrazine[80] can also induce lupus. It has been suggested that many cases thought to represent idiopathic lupus may indeed be related to environmental chemicals that induce the disease.[85]

Allergic Diseases and Toxins

Disorders that may be triggered by exposure to allergens include asthma, rhinitis, sinusitis, gastroenteritis, migraine,[70,107] urticaria, and angioedema. Disease results from the combination of allergy and end-organ sensitivity (see Table 14–3). For example, an attack of allergic asthma occurs with a combination of exposure to an allergen in a host with hyperreactive airways.[51] Toxic exposures may induce both antibody production against previously benign substances and induce end-organ sensitivity to allergic stimuli.

The reactive airways dysfunction syndrome (RADS) is described as an asthmalike illness occurring after a single high-dose irritant exposure that persists long after the initial exposure.[7,38,52,62] Some substances inducing asthma include acetic acid,[83] ammonia,[24] chlorine,[26,30,40] ethylene oxide,[16] sulfur dioxide,[10] glacial acetic acid,[41] smoke,[7] dust,[7] and toluene diisocyanate.[53] Patients with RADS have asthma attacks as well as constitutional symptoms associated with previously tolerated levels of chemical irritants.[67] Chronic inflammation with lymphocytic infiltrates is seen on pulmonary biopsy.[30]

Reactive upper-airways dysfunction syndrome (RUDS) refers to the induction of chronic rhinitis following an irritant exposure, and these individuals have a persistent intolerance to chemical irritants.[64] Nasal biopsy findings in patients with RADS and RUDS include proliferation of peripheral nerves, basement membrane thickening, chronic inflammation with lymphocytic infiltrates, and gaps in tight junctions.[67] These findings suggest a mechanism for the persistent reactivity to chemicals and inflammation seen in this patient population.[68]

Another mechanism by which toxins induce allergic diseases is as environmental adjuvants. In immunology, an adjuvant is a substance that enhances the development of immunity to a second substance. The branch of the immune system activated is specific for each adjuvant. Examples include alum, which induces IgE antibody to a co-injected protein. Killed mycobacteria in oil (Freund's complete adjuvant) induces cellular immunity to a co-injected protein. Environmental adjuvants are chemicals that induce immune responses to other substances in the environment, and environmental adjuvants are thought to be responsible for the increasing prevalence of respiratory allergy in industrialized countries.[72] Diesel exhaust particles,[72] sulfur dioxide,[59,60,61,86] nitrogen dioxide,[59,60,61] and ozone[4,59,60,61] are verified inducers of IgE antibody to simultaneously inhaled proteins in experimental models.

Polyaromatic hydrocarbons in diesel exhaust particles enhance the production of IgE antibodies by B cells in vitro[102] and enhance the in vivo IgE production in the human upper airway.[19] After in vivo nasal challenge with diesel exhaust particles, cytokine production is increased in the human upper airway.[20] It is suggested that diesel exhaust particles may play a role in the world wide increase in allergic respiratory disease.[81]

TABLE 14–3. HYPERSENSITIVITY ASSOCIATED WITH DRUGS AND CHEMICALS

Cardiovascular
Myocarditis: cyclic antidepressants, hydrochlorothiazide, vaccines
Vasculitis: barbiturates, cephalosporins, dapsone, griseofulvin, hydantoins, insulin, penicillin, phenylbutazone, sulfonamides, vaccines, antivenins
Hematologic
Hemolytic anemia: cephalosporins, alpha-methyldopa, procainamide, sulfonamides
Hepatic
halothane, *p*-aminosalicylic acid, alpha-methyldopa, sulfonamides
Renal
Interstitial nephritis: methicillin, penicillins, phenytoin
Respiratory
Asthma: aspirin, cephalosporins, penicillin, sulfonamides, diisocyanates, phthalic anhydrides, trimellitic anhydrides, formaldehyde, cobalt salts, nickel salts, platinum salts
Skin
Contact dermatitis: benzocaine, beryllium salts, chlorpromazine, chromium salts, isoniazid, neomycin, nickel salts, phenols, pyrethrins, quinidine
Exanthems: numerous pharmaceuticals
Erythema multiforme: penicillin, salicylates, phenytoin, phenylbutazone, sulfonamides
Fixed drug eruptions: barbiturates, phenolphthalein, phenylbutazone, quinine, sulfonamides, tetracycline
Cutaneous vasculitis: penicillins, phenytoin, pyrazalones, sulfonamides
Purpura: phenytoin, quinine, quinidine, sulfonamides
Erythema nodosum: birth control pills
Toxic epidermal necrolysis: allopurinol, mithramycin, phenytoin, sulfonamides

Chemical Sensitivity

Individuals with a heightened response to chemical irritants such as the products of combustion (cigarette smoke, wood fires, gasoline and diesel vehicle exhaust), perfumes, fragrances, cleaning products such as ammonia and disinfectants, and pesticides are said to have chemical sensitivity. Chemical sensitivity differs from allergy in that it ocurrs due to the fact that small molecular weight chemical irritants interact with chemoreceptors on sensory nerves to release substance P and other mediators of neurogenic inflammation.[75] Allergy ocurrs as larger molecular weight proteins react with IgE antibodies on mast cell surfaces to release histamine and other allergic mediators. Respiratory symptoms are very prominent in these individuals,[64] and the majority of individuals with asthma or rhinitis have some degree of chemical sensitivity.[63,94] Although chemical sensitivity is not as well understood as allergy, neurogenic inflammation is thought to play an important role in this type of sensitivity.[65,73,75] A possible mechanism of chemical sensitivity currently under investigation is the dysregulation of neurogenic inflammation.[73]

Immunologic Therapy of Poisonings

In principle, antibodies against specific toxins can be administered to bind and neutralize these toxins, and some antibody therapies are currently available in the United States (Table 14–4). *Immunotoxicotherapy* has been defined[88] as the procedure to sequester, extract or redistribute, and eliminate a toxin from the body by the use of antibody molecule entities with *specific active binding sites* (SABS). A schematic of an antibody molecule is given in Figure 14–2. The variable region V is the site on the antibody molecule that binds specific antigens. A fragment of an antibody molecule that contains a variable region should be as effective in neutralizing a toxin as the entire molecule. The nomenclature for possible fragments of antibiotic molecules is given in Figure 14–2.

Polyvalent serums are produced by immunizing an animal so immunoglobulin is produced against either a single toxin or a complex mixture of toxins such as found in venoms. The serum is collected, and the globulin fraction is extracted for injection. This serum contains antibody against a host of substances, as well as other serum proteins. Monovalent serum, which contains antibody to a specific substance, may be purified from polyvalent serum by affinity chromatography. Monoclonal antibody may be produced by a hybridoma, which is the fusion product of a plasma cell producing specific antibody and a tumor cell. These hybrid cells produce large quantities of specific antibody in culture and have provided a source of previously unimaginable quantities of specific antibody. Recombinant DNA technology can be used to insert the gene for a specific antibody into a bacterial cell, which then manufactures the antibody.

Electrophoresis of four different antibody products is depicted in Figure 14–3. An affinity-purified or monoclonal antibody against a single epitope would appear as a monoclonal spike in the gamma region of the electrophoretic spectrum. It can be seen from the figure that increasing levels of purification lead to a predominance of gamma globulins.

TABLE 14–4. IMMUNOTOXICOTHERAPY FOR POISONINGS CURRENTLY AVAILABLE IN THE UNITED STATES

Toxin	Type of Sera	Manufacturer/Supplier
Elapid venin	horse serum	Wyeth
Bark scorpion venin	goat serum	University of Arizona
Black widow venin	horse serum	Merck
Botulinum toxin	horse serum	Centers for Disease Control
Brown recluse venin (experimental)[a]	rabbit immunoglobulin isolated with affinity	Vanderbilt University
Crotalid venin[b]	horse serum	Wyeth
Digoxin	Fab fragment of sheep antibody	Glaxo Wellcome
Tetanus toxin	human serum	Bayer Biological

[a]Rees R, Campbell D, Reiger E, et al: The diagnosis and treatment of brown recluse spider bites. Ann Emerg Med 1987;16:945–949.

[b]Antivenin for nonnative snakes, scorpions, and spiders can be obtained from zoological parks. Consult Poison Centers for sources. (See Chapters 99 and 100 and associated Antidotes in Depth.)

Antibody fragments may be produced by cleaving the antibody molecules with an enzyme and harvesting the fragment that contains the variable region specific for a toxin. Advantages of antibody fragments are the reduced molecular weight and lack of adverse effects associated with the Fc portion of the antibody molecule. In a rat model, doses of Fab fragments up to several grams per kilograms were well tolerated.[42] Humanized antibodies, prepared by combining an antibody fragment from a nonhuman species containing the variable region with a human antibody molecule fragment, may have greatest utility in the treatment of infectious diseases where the human Fc portion is needed.

Adverse reactions to autologous sera include allergic reactions and serum sickness. Anaphylactic shock, urticaria, and bronchospasm can occur during the administration of the serum. A positive skin test to the sera increases the probability of an allergic reaction. Treatment is with epinephrine, antihistamines, oxygen, fluid support, and corticosteroids. If a patient with known allergy to a sera has to be treated, the patient can be desensitized by beginning therapy with a dose too small to produce a reaction, and then progressively increasing the dose.

Serum sickness occurs 7–14 days after initial exposure to foreign protein such as those contained in sera, with urticaria, vasculitis, arthralgias, myalgias, fever, and in some cases glomerulonephritis. With prior exposure, onset may be as early as 2 days. Serum sickness can be effectively treated with corticosteroids and plasmapheresis, which is seldom needed. Both anaphylaxis and serum sickness can be prevented by the use of antibody fragments rather than whole antibody molecules.

Factors that determine the clinical utility of an antibody or fragment specific for a toxin are the size of the product, the volumes of distribution of the toxin and antibody product, the kinetics of the binding of the toxin to the variable region, the kinetics of the binding of the toxin to active sites such as receptors, the stability of the product in vivo, and the elimination kinetics of the toxin–antibody complex.[90] The volume of distribution of IgM and IgG in humans is 5 L, while the volume of distribution of Fab fragments is 30 L. Volume of distribution of toxins varies greatly, and ideally the volume of distribution of the antibody product should equal that of the toxin. The rate at which the antibody product is distributed in tissue can also influence efficacy. IgG and $(Fab)_2$ equilibrates with interstial fluid in 12–24 hours, while Fab equilibrates in 2–4 hours.[103]

To reverse toxicity, the specific antibody must have a high affinity for the toxin. Treatment of digoxin toxicity with monoclonal antibodies results in a marked redistribution of toxin, with total digoxin in plasma increasing by approximately sixfold while free plasma digoxin falls dramatically.[90]

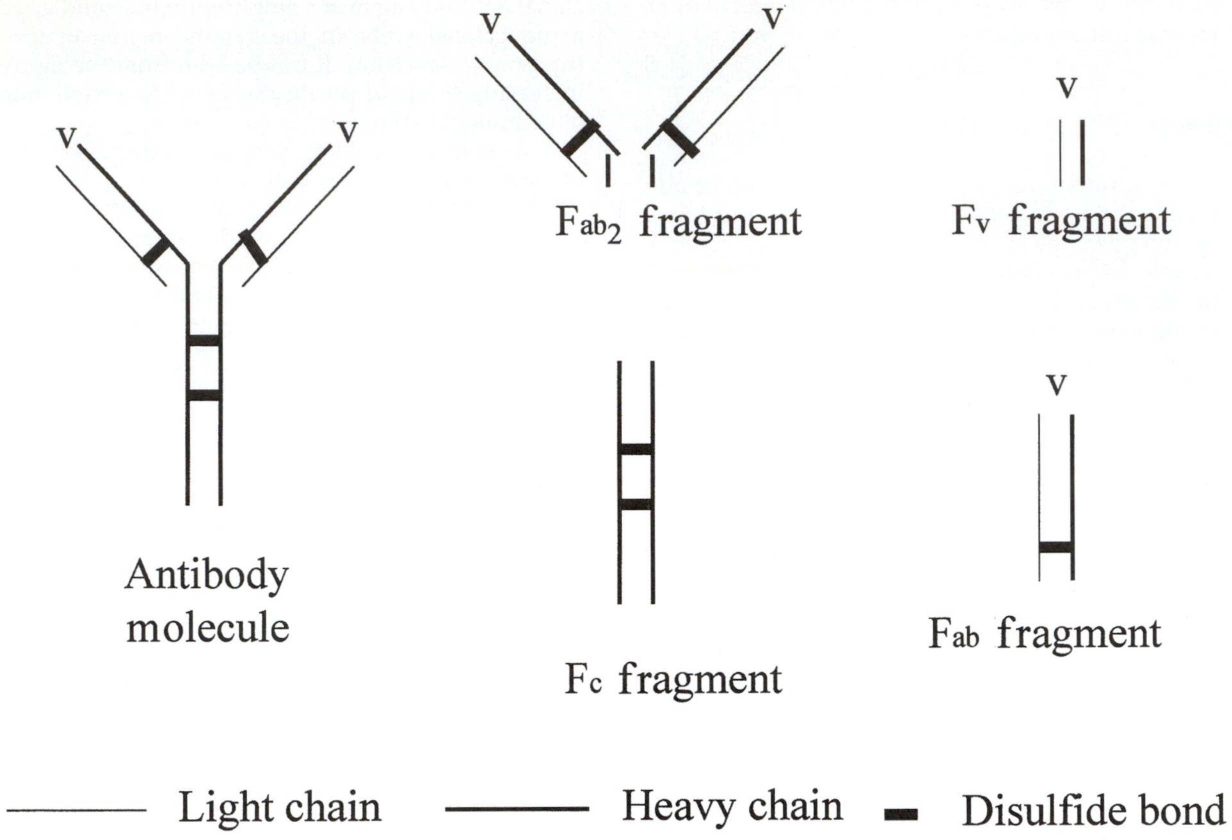

Figure 14–2. An antibody molecule can be broken into fragments by enzymatic digestion. The antigen binding site (variable region) is denoted by V.

The high molecular weight and small volume of distribution of antibody molecules limit their use to those substances that do not require large amounts of neutralizing antibody. Though factors in addition to stoichiometry play a role in determining the effective dose of an antibody or fragment, toxins with small lethal doses will generally require less neutralizing antibody. One antibody molecule has two binding sites for antigen, so from the standpoint of stoichiometry one antibody molecule must be administered to neutralize two molecules of drug.

Immunotoxicotherapy of Drug Overdoses

The first available commercial product for treating drug or toxin overdoses is Digibind (Glaxo Wellcome), which is an Fab fragment of specific antibody to digoxin from the sera of immunized sheep. The digoxin-specific antibody is purified by affinity chromatography, and the Fab fragment is obtained by digestion of the antibody with papain. The molecular weight is 46,200 daltons. Digibind is a safe and effective treatment for digoxin poisoning (see Chap. 48 and Antidotes in Depth: Digoxin–Specific Antibody Fragments (Fab)). Colchicine poisoning has also been effectively treated with Fab antibody fragments.[89] Antibodies have been developed against and demonstrated to be effective in animal models for poisonings with desipramine.[14,79] Ricin toxicity has been reversed by neutralizing monoclonal antibodies in a mouse model,[48] while phencyclidine has been studied in dogs.[78]

For substances like theophylline in which ingestions of a large mass of drug occur, antibody therapy would be possible only if a small variable-region fragment could be developed. Consider a 100-kg patient who ingests enough theophylline to develop a toxic blood level of 100 μg/mL. The amount of drug ingested would be

$$\text{Total drug (mg)} =$$

$$\text{serum drug concentration} \times V_d \times \text{weight in kg}$$

$$= 100\ \mu\text{g/mL} \times 0.5\ \text{L/kg} \times 100\ \text{kg}$$

$$= 5\ \text{g}$$

The molecular weight of Fab needed to stoichiometrically bind 5 g of theophylline would be

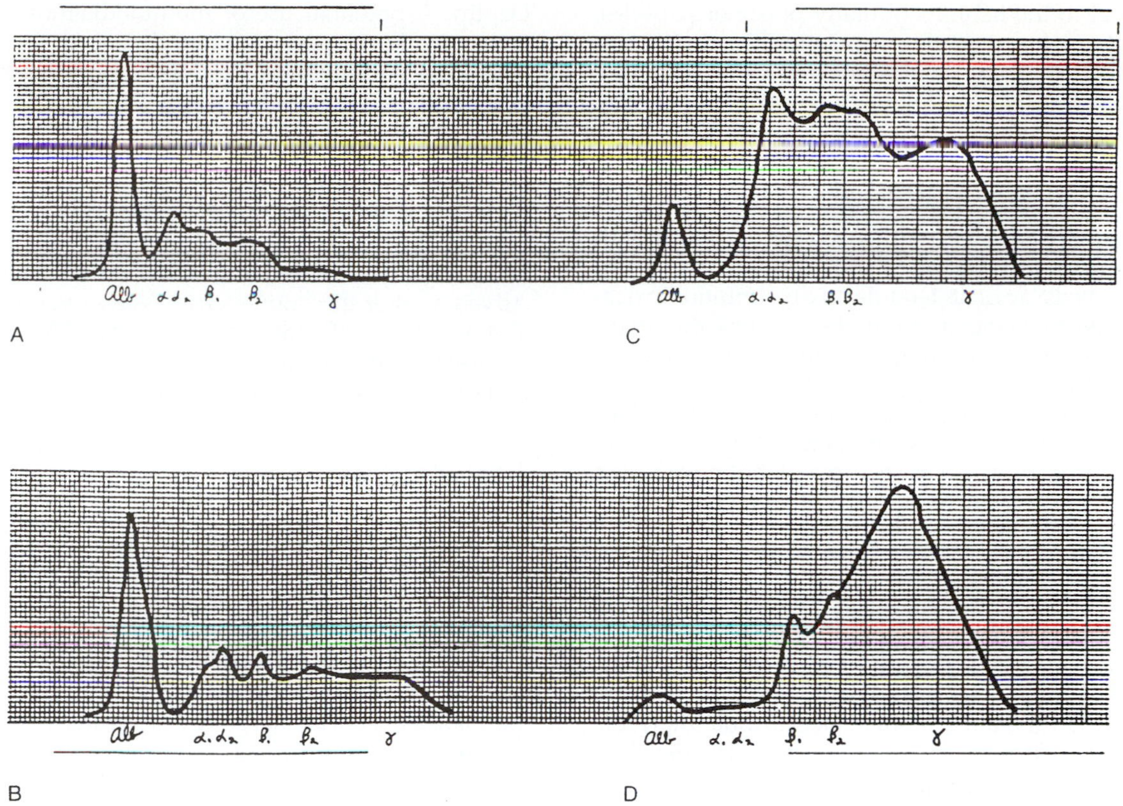

Figure 14–3. Protein electrophoresis of equine-derived (**A**) skin test material (normal serum, Merck Sharpe & Dohme); (**B**) *Latrodectus* antivenin (crude hyperimmune serum; Merck Sharpe & Dohme); (**C**) *Crotalid* antivenin (ammonium sulfate precipitation, filtration; Wyeth); (**D**) *Latrodectus* antivenin (pepsin digestion, ammonium sulfate precipitation, filtration; Commonwealth Serum Laboratories). With increasing purification, a relative increase in immunoglobulins and decrease in other fractions can be seen.

$$\text{Ratio of Fab to drug needed} = (\text{molecular weight of Fab})/(\text{mol wt of drug}) = 261{:}1$$

$$\text{The mass of Fab needed} = 261 \times 5\ \text{g} = 2.81\ \text{kg}$$

Clearly it would be impossible to infuse this amount of Fab fragment into a person and the cost would be prohibitive. This example illustrates that immunotoxicotherapy will probably be limited to those situations where milligram amounts of the substance is toxic, unless small fragments containing variable regions can be developed.

Technical problems can impede the development of an antibody to specific drugs. The molecular weight of most drugs is too small for them to be immunogenic, so the drug must be conjugated to a protein. Antibodies have to be raised against the drug–protein conjugate. The affinity for antibody molecules raised against a drug–protein adduct to the drug alone varies with the specific epitope on the adduct that the antibody recognizes.

Immunotoxicotherapy of Envenomations

The venom of pit viper species in the United States is sufficiently similar that one product, Antivenin (Crotalidae) Polyvalent (equine origin), (ACP, Wyeth Laboratories, Philadelphia, PA) is used for all pit viper envenomations. This antivenin is derived from horse sera, contains whole antibody molecules, and has greater than 75% rate of hypersensitivity reactions.[12] Antivenin Polyvalent Crotalid (Ovine) Fab (Crotab, Therapeutic Antibodies, Inc., Nashville, TN) is an affinity-purified sheep Fab fragment that has been developed but is not commercially available at this writing. In a murine model using lethality as an outcome, the Fab product was found to be 3.1 to 9.6 times more potent than the whole-antibody product when tested against the venom of nine pit vipers endogenous to the United States.[12] Experience with other Fab products suggests that incidence of hypersensitivity reactions will be greatly reduced with the Fab product.

Internationally, a host of antivenins are available in

regions local to the habitats of many poisonous species. Envenomations by nonnative species occurs due to importation for research, display in zoos, and pets. Antivenin is stocked by zoos and other institutions and may be located by consulting a regional poison center.

Immunotoxicotherapy for Bacterial Toxins

Antibody products are currently used for poisoning with botulinum toxin (see Chap. 73 and Antidotes in Depth) and prophylaxis against tetanus toxin. Immunotoxicotherapy using monoclonal antibodies against the toxins and mediators of septic shock have not to date been successful.[57] Immunotoxicotherapy directed against *Clostridium difficile* toxoids is successful against *C. difficile* enteritis for both in vitro and in vivo models.[39] A case of severe pertussis treated with specific gamma globulin with high titers of anti-pertussis toxin antibody had a good clinical outcome.[32]

Immune Techniques for Detecting Toxins

A number of techniques have been developed that use specific antibody against a substance to quantitate the amount of substance present in a specimen. The development of radioimmunoassay (RIA) by Berson and Yalow, for which Yalow won the 1977 Nobel Prize in physiology or medicine, heralded a new era in laboratory medicine. Techniques that followed include the enzyme-linked immunosorbent assay (ELISA), the enzyme-multiplied immunoassay (EMIT), and the fluorescence polarization immunoassay (FPIA). In the RIA method, a known amount of antibody against the substance to be measured (analyte) is incubated with the specimen, and then radiolabeled analyte of known quantity is added to the specimen. Determination of the amount of radioactivity bound to antibody allows a calculation of the amount of analyte in the original specimen. Disadvantages of RIA are expense, hazards of radioisotope use and disposal, and the long time required to complete assays. Its uses are limited to hormone assays, for which it was originally developed, and measurement of therapeutic drug levels.

In the ELISA assay, specific antibody against the analyte is congugated to an enzyme that changes the optical characteristics of a reagent. The specimen with unknown amount of analyte is mixed with the antibody–enzyme complex , the solution is cleansed by removal of excess complex, the reagent that undergoes an optical change in the presence of the enzyme is added, and quantitation of the color change allows a calculation of the amount of analyte in the original specimen. ELISA assays are used in Sweden to measure plasma levels of viper venom before and after administration of Fab fragment antivenin.[96]

Such technology is not as essential in the United States as in other countries, because the two groups of poisonous snakes found in the United States are easily distinquished clinically (see Chap. 99 and Antidote in Depth). A potential use of immunodiagnosis following envenomation is determining the need for treatment after bites with delayed toxicity such as the coral snake and Mohave rattlesnake. Since brown recluse spider bites have delayed toxicity and the spider is not always identified, the simultaneous availability of an antivenin and diagnostic test would also have great impact on treatment (see Chap. 100 and Antidote in Depth).

EMIT and FPIA are similar to RIA, but fluorescene labeled analyte is used instead of radiolabeled analyte. Advantages of the fluorescence assays over RIA are cost and avoidance of radioactive reagents. EMIT and FPIA are used in toxicologic screens to detect drugs of abuse and drugs associated with overdoses.

Acknowledgment

Martin J. Smilkstein, MD and Mary Ann Howland, Pharm D contributed to this chapter in a previous edition.

References

1. Alonso-Ruiz A, Zea-Mendoza AC, Salazar-Vallinas JM, et al: Toxic oil syndrome: a syndrome with features overlapping those of various forms of scleroderma. Semin Arthritis Rheum 1986;15:200–212.
2. Felbamate use linked to aplastic anemia. Warning issued on drug's use. Am J Hosp Pharm 1994;51:23–24.
3. Becher H, Flesch-Janys D, Kauppinen T, et al: Cancer mortality in German male workers exposed to phenoxy herbicides and dioxins. Cancer Causes Control 1996;7:302–304.
4. Biagini RE, Moorman WJ, Lewis TR, et al: Ozone enhancement of platinum asthma in a primate model. Am Rev Respir Dis 1986;134:719–725.
5. Blanco A, Palencia R, Solis P, et al: Transient phenytoin induced IgA deficiency and permanent IgE increase. Allergol Immunopathol 1986;14:535–538.
6. Brahams D: Lindane exposure and aplastic anaemia. Lancet 1994;343:1092.
7. Brooks SM, Weiss MA, Bernstein IL: Reactive airways dysfunction syndrome (RADS): Persistent asthma syndrome after high level irritant exposure. Chest 1985;88:376–384.
8. Castillo Mendez A, Rodriguez Diaz T, Leon Lobeck A, et al: Effect of occupational lead exposure on the immunoglobulin concentration and cellular immune function in man. Rev Alerg 1993;40:95–97.
9. Cavagnaro J, Lewis RM: Bidirectional regulatory circuit between the immune and neuroendocrine systems. Year Immunol 1989;4:241–252.
10. Charan NB, Myers CG, Lakshminarayan S, et al: Pulmonary injuries associated with acute sulfur dioxide inhalation. Am Rev Respir Dis 1979;119:555–560.
11. Church MK, el-Lati S, Caulfield JP: Neuropeptide-induced secretion from human skin mast cells. Int Arch Allergy Appl Immunol 1991;94:310–318.
12. Consroe P, Egen NB, Russell FE, et al: Comparison of a new ovine antigen binding fragment (Fab) antivenin for United States Crotalidae with the commercial antivenin for protection against venom-induced lethality in mice. Am J Trop Med Hyg 1995;53:507–510.

13. Craddock CG: Corticosteroid induced lymphopenia, immunosuppression, and body defense. Ann Intern Med 1978; 88:564–566.
14. Dart, RC, Sidki A, Sullivan JB, et al: Ovine desipramine antibody fragments reverse desipramine cardiovascular toxicity in the rat. Ann Emerg Med 1996;27:309–315.
15. Dell A, Antoine SM, Gaunt CJ, et al: Autoimmune determinants of rheumatic carditis: localization of epitopes in human cardiac myosin. Eur Heart J 1991;12 (suppl D): 155–162.
16. Deschamps D, Rosenberg N, Soler P, et al: Persistent asthma after accidental exposure to ethylene oxide. Br J Ind Med 1992;49:523–525.
17. Descotes J: Immunotoxicology of Drugs and Chemicals, 2nd ed. Amsterdam, Elsevier, 1988.
18. Descotes J: Drug-Induced Immune Disease. Amsterdam, Elsevier, 1990.
19. Diaz-Sanchez D, Dotson AR, Takenaka H, Saxon A: Diesel exhaust particles induce local IgE production in vivo and alter the pattern of IgE messenger RNA isoforms. J Clin Invest 1994;94:1417–1425.
20. Diaz-Sanchez D, Tsien A, Casillas A, et al: Enhanced nasal cytokine production in human beings after in vivo challenge with diesel exhaust particles. J Allergy Clin Immunol 1996;98:114–123.
21. Dunn P: Aplastic anemia with ticlopidine therapy in two Chinese patients. Ann Pharmacother 1996;30:547. Letter.
22. Farr M, Kitas GD, Tunn EJ, et al: Immunodeficiencies associated with sulphasalazine therapy in inflammatory arthritis. Br J Rheum 1991;30:413–417.
23. Fernandez-Segoviano P, Esteban A, Martinez-Cabruja R: Pulmonary vascular lesions in the toxic oil syndrome in Spain. Thorax 1983;38:724–729.
24. Flury KE, Ames DE, Rodarte JR, et al: Airway obstruction due to inhalation of ammonia. Mayo Clin Proc 1983;58: 389–393.
25. Garratty G: Immune cytopenia associated with antibiotics. Transfusion Med Rev 1993;7:255–267.
26. Gautrin D, Boulet L-P, Boutet M, et al: Is reactive airways dysfunction syndrome a variant of occupational asthma? J Allergy Clin Immunol 1994;93:12–22.
27. Gianani R, Sarvetnick N: Viruses, cytokines, antigens, and autoimmunity. Proc Natl Acad Sci USA 1996;93: 2257–2259.
28. Gleich GG, Adolphson CR: The eosinophilic leukocyte structure and function. Adv Immunol 1986;39;137–253.
29. Hammarstrom L, Smith CI, Berg CI: Captopril-induced IgA deficiency. Lancet 1991;337:435. Letter.
30. Hasan FM, Geshman A, Fuleihan FJD: Resolution of pulmonary dysfunction following acute chlorine exposure. Arch Environ Health 1983;38:76–80.
31. Hjalmarson O, Hanson LA, Nilsson LA: IgA deficiency during D-penicillamine treatment. Br Med J 1977;1:549.
32. Ichimaru T, Ohara Y, Hojo M, et al: Treatment of severe pertussis by administration of specific gamma globulin with high titers antitoxin antibody. Acta Paediatr 1993; 82:1076–1078.
33. Ishizaka A, Nakinishi M, Kasahara E, et al: Phenytoin-induced IgG_2 and IgG_4 deficiencies in a patient with epilepsy. Acta Paediatr 1992;81:646–648.
34. Kaliner MA: Late phase reactions. N Engl Reg Allergy Proc 1986;7:236–240.
35. Kammuler ME, Bloksma N, Seinen W: Chemical-induced autoimmune reactions and Spanish toxic oil syndrome. Focus on hydantoins and related compounds. J Toxicol Clin Toxicol 1988;26:157–174.
36. Karges WJ, Ilonen J, Robinson BH, et al: Self and non-self antigens in diabetic autoimmunity: Molecules and mechanisms. Mol Aspect Med 1995;16:79–213.
37. Kaufman DW, Kelly JP, Jurgelon JM, et al: Drugs in the aetiology of agranulocytosis and aplastic anemia. Eur J Haem 1996;60 (suppl):23–30.
38. Kava T: Acute respiratory infection, influenza vaccination and airway reactivity in asthma. Eur J Respir Dis 1987; 150:1–38.
39. Kelly CP, Pothoulakis C, Vavva F, et al: Anti-*Clostridium difficile* bovine immunoglobulin concentrate inhibits cytotoxicity and enterotoxicity of *C. difficile* toxins. Antimicrob Agents Chemother 1996;40:373–379.
40. Kennedy SM, Enarson DA, Janssen RG, et al: Lung health consequences of reported accidental chlorine gas exposures among pulpmill workers. Am Rev Respir Dis 1991; 143:74–79.
41. Kern DG: Outbreak of the reactive airways dysfunction syndrome after a spill of glacial acetic acid. Am Rev Respir Dis 1991;144:1058–1064.
42. Keyler DE, Shelver WL, Landon J, et al: Toxicity of high doses of polyclonal drug-specific antibody Fab fragments. Int J Immunopharm 1994;16:1027–1034.
43. Kirtland HH, Mohler DN, Horowitz DA: Methyldopa inhibition of suppressor-lymphocyte function: A proposed cause of autoimmune hemolytic anemia. N Engl J Med 1980;302:825–832.
44. Klastersky J: Febrile neutropenia. Supportive Care Cancer 1993;1:233–239.
45. Klaustmeyer WB, Gianos ME, Kurchara ML, et al: IgG subclass deficiencies associated with corticosteroids in obstructive lung disease. Chest 1992;102:1137–1142
46. Kondo N, Takao A, Ori T: Case report: Immunoglobulin A deficiency in patients with juvenile rheumatoid arthritis treated with aspirin. Biotherapy 1993; 7:59–62.
47. Lefkowith JB, Gildeson GS: Nephrogenic autoantibodies in lupus: Current concepts and continuing controversies. Arthritis Rheum 1996;39:894–903.
48. Lemley PV, Amanatides P, Wright DC: Identification and characterization of a monoclonal antibody that neutralizes ricin toxicity in vitro and in vivo. Hybridoma 1994;13: 417–421.
49. Leslie CA, Mathe AA: Modification of guinea pig lung anaphylaxis by central nervous system (CNS) pertubations. J Allergy Clin Immunol 1989;83:94–101.
50. Levy RM, Rose JE, Johnson JS: Effect of vagotomy on anaphylaxis in rat. Clin Exp Immunol 1976;24:96–101.
51. Li JT, O'Connell EJ: Clinical evaluation of asthma. Ann Allergy Asthm Immunol 1996;76:1–13.
52. Lieberman P: Anaphylactoid reactions to radiocontrast material. Clin Rev Allergy 1991;9:319–338.
53. Luo JC, Nelsen KG, Fischbein A: Persistent reactive airways dysfunction syndrome after exposure to toluene diisocyanate. Br J Ind Med 1990;47:239–241.

54. Mali JW, Malten KE: The epidemic of polymorph toxic erythema in the Netherlands in 1960. The so-called margarine disease. Acta Derm Venereol 1966;46:123–135.
55. Malinow MR, Bardana EJ, Pirofsky B, et al: Systemic erythematosis in monkeys fed alfalfa sprouts: Role of a nonprotein amino acid. Science 1982;216:415–417.
56. Mallet L, Mallet J: Ticlopidine and fatal aplastic anemia in an elderly woman. Ann Pharmacother 1994;28:1169–1171.
57. Manzullo EF: Sepsis: The role of steroids and monoclonal antibodies in treatment. Oncology 1994;8:115–120.
58. Mary JY, Guiguet M, Baumelou E: Drug use and aplastic anaemia: The French experience. French Cooperative Groups for the epidemiological study of aplastic anemia. Eur J Haem 1996;60 (suppl):35–41.
59. Matsumura Y: The effects of ozone, nitrogen dioxide, and sulfur dioxide on the experimentally induced allergic respiratory disorder in guinea pigs. I. The effects of sensitization with albumin through the airway. Am Rev Respir Dis 1970;102:430–437.
60. Matsumura Y: The effects of ozone, nitrogen dioxide, and sulfur dioxide on the experimentally induced allergic respiratory disorder in guinea pigs. II. The effects of ozone on the absorption and the retention of antigen in the lung. Am Rev Respir Dis 1970;102:438–443.
61. Matsumura Y: The effects of ozone, nitrogen dioxide, and sulfur dioxide on the experimentally induced allergic respiratory disorder in guinea pigs. III. The effect on the recurrence of dyspnea attacks. Am Rev Respir Dis 1970; 102:444–447.
62. McFadden ER Jr: Exercise-induced airway obstruction. Clin Chest Med 1995;16:671–682.
63. Meggs WJ: Health effects of indoor air pollution. NC Med J 1992;53:354–358.
64. Meggs WJ, Cleveland CH Jr: Rhinolaryngoscopic examination of patients with the multiple chemical sensitivity syndrome. Arch Environ Health 1993;48:14–18.
65. Meggs WJ: Neurogenic inflammation and sensitivity to environmental chemicals. Environ Health Perspect 1993; 101:234–238.
66. Meggs WJ: Neurogenic switching: A hypothesis for a mechanism for shifting the site of inflammation in allergy and chemical sensitivity. Environ Health Perspect 1995; 103:54–56.
67. Meggs WJ, Elsheik T, Metzger WJ, et al: Nasal pathology and ultrastructure in patients with chronic airway inflammation (RADS and RUDS) following an irritant exposure. J Toxicol Clin Toxicol 1996;34:383–396.
68. Meggs WJ: Hypothesis for the induction and propagation of chemical sensitivity based on biopsy studies. Environ Health Perspect 1997;105(suppl 2):473–481.
69. Miller KB, Salem K: Immune regulatory disorders produced by procainamide. Transplant Proc 1982;73:487–492.
70. Monro J: Food-induced migraine. In: Brostoff J, Challacombe SJ, eds: Food Allergy and Intolerance. London, Bailliere Tindall, 1987, Chapter 37, p. 633.
71. Moszczynski P, Slowinski S, Moszczynski P: Synergistic effect of organic solvents and tobacco smoke on the indicators of humoral immunity in humans. Gig Tr Prof Zabol 1991;3:34–36
72. Muranaka M, Suzuki S, Koizumi S, et al: Adjuvant activity of diesel-exhaust particulates for the production of IgE antibody in mice. J Allergy Clin Immunol 1986;77:616–623.
73. Nadel JA: Neutral endopeptidase modulates neurogenic inflammation. Eur Respir J 1991;4:745–754.
74. Nelson L, Shih R, Hoffman R: Aplastic anemia induced by an adulterated herbal medication. J Toxicol Clin Toxicol 1995;33:467–470.
75. Nielsen GD: Mechanisms of activation of the sensory irritant receptor by airborne chemicals. Crit Rev Toxicol 1991;21:183–208.
76. Noriega AR, Gomez-Reino J, Lopez-Encouentra A, et al: Toxic epidemic syndrome, Spain, 1981. Lancet 1982;2: 697–702.
77. Ott MG, Zober A: Cause specific mortality and cancer incidence among employees exposed to 2,3,7,8-TCDD after a 1953 reactor accident. Occup Environ Med 1996;53:606–612.
78. Owens SM, Mayersohn M: Phencyclidine-specific Fab fragments alter phencyclidine disposition in dogs. Drug Metab Dispos 1986;14:52–58.
79. Pentel PR, Ross CA, Landon J, et al: Reversal of desipramine toxicity in rats with polyclonal drug-specific antibody Fab fragments. J Lab Clin Med 1994;123:387–393.
80. Pereyo N: Hydrazine derivatives and induction of systemic lupus erythematosis. J Am Acad Dermatol 1986; 14:514–515.
81. Peterson B, Saxon A: Global increases in allergic respiratory disease: The possible role of diesel exhaust particles. Ann Allergy Asthma Immunol 1996;77:26308.
82. Proesmans W, Jaeken J, Eeckels R: D-Penicillamine-induced IgA deficiency in Wilson's disease. Lancet 1976; 2:804–805.
83. Rajan KG, Davies BH: Reversible airways obstruction and interstitial pneumonitis due to acetic acid. Br J Ind Med 1989;46:67–68.
84. Rees R, Campbell D, Reiger E, et al: The diagnosis and treatment of brown recluse spider bites. Ann Emerg Med 1987;16:945–949.
85. Reidenberg MM, Durant PJ, Harris RA, et al: Lupus erythematosis-like disease due to hydrazine. Am J Med 1983;75:365–370.
86. Riedel F, Kramer M, Scheibenbogen C, et al: Effects of SO_2 exposure on allergic sensitization in the guinea pig. J Allergy Clin Immunol 1988;82:527–534.
87. Riggs D, Miller MM, Metzger WJ: Recurrent allergic vulvoganitis. Treatment with *Candida albicans* allergen immunotherapy. Am J Obstet Gynecol 1990;162:332–336.
88. Scherrmann JM, Terrien N, Urtizberea M, et al: Immunotoxicotherapy: Present status and future trends. J Toxicol Clin Toxicol 1989;27:1–35.
89. Scherrmann JM, Sabouraud AE, Urtizberea M, et al: Clinical use of colchicine-specfic Fab fragments in colchicine poisoning. Vet Hum Tox 1992;34:334. Abstract.
90. Scherrmann JM: Antibody treatment of toxin poisoning—recent advances. J Toxicol Clin Toxicol 1994;34:363–375.
91. Schwartz L, Huff T: Biology of mast cells and basophils. In: Middleton E Jr, Reed CE, Ellis EF, et al, eds: Allergy Principles and Practice. St Louis, Mosby, 1993, Chapter 8, p. 135.
92. Shapiro CD, Walk D: Aplastic anemia associated with ticlopidine. Neurology 1996;47:300.

93. Shem SC, Kumar R, Roberts IA: Aplastic anaemia after exposure to burning oil. Lancet 1995;346:183.
94. Shim C, Williams MH Jr: Effect of odors in asthma. Am J Med 1986;80:18–22.
95. Shindo K, Kono T, Kitajima J, et al: Crusted scabies in acquired selective IgA deficiency. Acta Derm Venereol 1991;71:250–251.
96. Sjostrom L, Karlson-Stiber C, Persson H, et al: Development and clinical application of immunoassays for European adder (*Vipera berus berus*). Toxicon 1996;34:91–98.
97. Smith MT: Overview of benzene-induced aplastic anaemia. Eur J Haem 1996;60(suppl):107–110.
98. Spickett GP, Gompeis MM, Saunders PW: Hypogammaglobulinaemia with absent B-lymphocytes and agranulocytosis after carbamazepine treatment. J Neurol Neurosurg Psychiatry 1996;60:459.
99. Stern MA, Eckman J, Otterman MK: Aplastic anemia after exposure to burning oil. N Engl J Med 1994;331:58. Letter.
100. Straetmans N, Ferrant A, Martiat P, et al: Hypereosinophilia syndrome. A propos of 2 cases and literature review. Acta Clin Belg 1992;47:90–99.
101. Su CC, Tseng CD, Hwang JJ, et al: Severe aplastic anemia induced by ticlopidine: report of a case. J Formosan Med Assoc 1995;94:689–691.
102. Takenaka H, Zhang K, Diaz-Sanchez D, et al: Enhanced IgE production results from exposure to the aromatic hydrocarbons from diesel exhaust: Direct effects on B-cell IgE production. J Allergy Clin Immunol 1995;95:103–115.
103. Talesnik E, Rivero SJ, Gonzalez B: Serum IgA deficiency induced by prolonged phenytoin treatment. Rev Invest Clin 1989;41:331–335.
104. Thanh-Barthet CV, Urtizberea M, Sabouraud AE, Cano NJ, et al: Development of a sensitive radioimmunoassay for Fab fragments: Application to Fab pharmacokinetics in humans. Pharmacol Res 1993;10:692–696.
105. Tisch R, McDevitt H: Insulin dependent diabetes mellitus. Cell 1996;85:291–297.
106. Tonn T, Esser C, Schneider EM, et al: Persistence of decreased T-helper cell function in industrial workers 20 years after exposure to 2,3,7,8-tetrachlorodibenzo-*p*-dioxin. Environ Health Perspect 1996;104:422–426
107. Vaughn R, Lyndon E: Neurologic reactions to foods and food additives. In: Metcalfe DD, Sampson HA, Simon RA, eds: Food Allergy. Oxford, Blackwell Scientific, 1991, pp. 355–369.
108. Vicario JL, Serrano-Rios M, San Andres F, et al: HLA-DR3, DR4 increase in chronic stage of Spanish oil disease. Lancet 1982;1:276. Letter.
109. Vil'chinskaia M, Nasonov EL, Zharova EA, et al: Immunological effects of captopril and ramipril in patients with hypertension. Klin Med 1990;68:61–64.
110. Virella G: Immune complex diseases. Immunol Ser 1990; 50:395–414.
111. Weiner P, Zidan F, Paz R: Severe aplastic anemia due to ticlopidine. Isr J Med Sci 1995;31:444–445.
112. Weinstein A: Drug-induced lupus erythematosis. In: Schwartz RS, ed: Progress in Clinical Immunology, Vol. 4. New York, Grune & Stratton, 1980, pp. 1–21.
113. Witkens SS, Jeremias J, Ledger WJ: A localized allergic response to Candida in woman with recurrent vaginitis. J Allergy Clin Immunol 1988;81:412–416.

CHAPTER 15

Fluid, Electrolyte, and Acid–Base Principles

Robert S. Hoffman

Selected Normal Laboratory Values

Electrolyte	Conventional Units	S.I. Units
Sodium	135–145 mEq/L	135–145 mmol/L
Potassium	3.5–5.0 mEq/L	3.5–5.0 mmol/L
Calcium	8.4–10.2 mg/dL (4.2–5.1 mEq/L)	2.10–2.55 mmol/L
Magnesium	1.3–2.1 mEq/L	0.65–1.05 mmol/L

Although many discussions of fluid, electrolyte, and acid–base abnormalities present guidelines for evaluating blood chemistries strictly on a numerical basis, a meaningful analysis must be based on the clinical characteristics of each patient. Specifically, while a rigorous appraisal of these laboratory parameters will often yield the correct differential diagnosis, useful information can be gained from the history and physical examination, and this information will often provide the data necessary to refine the differential diagnosis appropriately. Thus the evaluation always begins with an overall assessment of the patient's status. (Many of the issues discussed here overlap with Chaps. 20–23).

Initial Patient Assessment

History

The history should include clinical complaints associated with fluid and electrolyte abnormalities. Common manifestations of toxin exposure result in fluid losses through the respiratory system (hyperpnea and tachypnea), the gastrointestinal system (vomiting and diarrhea), the skin (diaphoresis and fever), and the kidneys (polyuria). Patients with volume depletion may complain of thirst or even polydipsia.

A history of exposure to over-the-counter and prescription medications, toxins, and premorbid conditions is important to assess volume status. Also, the time of year, ambient temperature, and humidity should always be considered.

Physical Examination

The vital signs offer the first markers of gross alterations in volume status. While hypotension and tachycardia may herald life-threatening volume depletion, an initial increase of the heart rate and a narrowing of the pulse pressure may be earlier findings. Patient abnormalities may be recognized through a dynamic evaluation, realizing that the measurement of a single set of supine vital signs offers useful information only when grossly abnormal. The addition of orthostatic pulse and blood pressure measurements provides a more meaningful determination of functional volume status (Chap. 21).

The respiratory rate and pattern can give clues to the patient's metabolic status. When metabolic acidosis is present, hyperventilation (manifested as tachypnea, hyperpnea, or both) usually is noted. Though hypoventilation (bradypnea or hypopnea) will be present during metabolic alkalosis, it is rarely clinically significant and must be detected by arterial blood gas analysis.

The skin should be evaluated for turgor, moisture content, and presence of edema. The moisture content of the mucous membranes can also provide valuable information. These are general parameters and may not necessarily directly correlate with the status of hydration. This dissociation is especially true with toxin exposure, as many drugs and toxins alter skin and mucous membrane findings without necessarily altering volume status. Antihistamines and anticholinergics commonly dry mucous membranes and skin without producing volume depletion. Conversely, patients exposed to sympathomimetic agents (cocaine) or cholinergic agents (organophosphate insecticides) may have quite moist skin and mucous membranes even in the setting of significant fluid losses. These dissociative characteristics further reinforce the need to assess the patient in entirety to identify a single responsible agent or unifying perspective for the clinical presentation.

The physical findings associated with electrolyte abnormalities are often nonspecific. Hypo- and hypernatremia, hypercalcemia, and hypermagnesemia all can produce a depressed mental status. Neuromuscular excitability (tremor, hyperreflexia, etc) is noted with hypocalcemia, hypomagnesemia, hyponatremia, and hypo- and hyperkalemia. Multiple electrolyte disorders can produce confusing clinical presentations, or patients may appear normal. Rarer diagnostic findings, such as Chvostek and Trousseau signs (found in hypocalcemia), may be useful in assessing known toxin exposures.

Rapid Diagnostic Tools

The electrocardiogram (ECG) is a useful tool for emergency department (ED) screening of some common electrolyte abnormalities (Chap. 8). It is easy to perform, rapid, inexpensive, and routinely available. In this context, the ECG is used most often for evaluation of changes in potassium and calcium (see below). Unfortunately, the sensitivity and specificity of ECG findings associated with hyperkalemia appear to be of limited value. Both poor sensitivity (0.43) and specificity (0.86) were demonstrated when ECGs were used to diagnose hyperkalemia.[144]

In most medical conditions bedside assessment of urine specific gravity can provide valuable information about volume status.[81] A high urine specific gravity, greater than 1.020 (signifying concentrated urine), usually correlates with volume depletion. However, when the kidney is the source of the volume loss, the specific gravity is usually normal, 1.010. Many toxins, however, interfere with this test's utility. Examples of this phenomenon include the patient with lithium-induced diabetes insipidus whose urine remains dilute (low specific gravity) despite consequential volume depletion and the patient with chlorpropamide-induced syndrome of inappropriate antidiuretic hormone secretion whose urine remains concentrated (high specific gravity) in the presence of a normal to high volume status.

Other rapid tests include the urine dipstick and the urine ferric chloride test. The urine dipstick may be useful for rapidly determining the presence of ketones, which are often associated with specific toxicologic problems (eg, salicylates, alcoholic ketoacidosis) and common causes of metabolic acidosis (eg, diabetic ketoacidosis, salicylates, alcoholic ketoacidosis). The ferric chloride test rapidly detects exposure to salicylates with a high sensitivity and specificity (Chap. 32).

Laboratory Studies

A simultaneous determination of the serum electrolytes, blood urea nitrogen (BUN), glucose, and arterial blood gas is adequate to determine most common acid–base, fluid, and electrolyte abnormalities. More complex clinical problems may require determinations of urine and serum osmolalities, urine electrolytes, serum ketones, lactic acid concentrations, or other tests to assist in diagnosis. A systematic approach to common problems is discussed below.

Acid–Base Abnormalities

Definitions

The terminology of acid–base disorders often leads to confusion and error. The following definitions provide the appropriate frame of reference for the remainder of the chapter.

The terms *acidosis* and *alkalosis* refer to processes that tend to change pH in a given direction. By definition a patient is said to have:

- A *metabolic acidosis* if his or her serum bicarbonate (HCO_3) is less than 24 mEq/L. Because compensation is inherent, metabolic acidosis is accompanied by a PCO_2 less than 40 mm Hg and a pH less than 7.40 unless another process is present.
- A *metabolic alkalosis* if his or her serum HCO_3 is more than 24 mEq/L. Because of inherent compensation, metabolic alkalosis is accompanied by a PCO_2 greater than 40 mm Hg and a pH greater than 7.40 unless another process is present.
- A *respiratory acidosis* if his or her partial pressure of carbon dioxide (PCO_2) is greater than 40 mm Hg. Because of inherent compensation, respiratory acidosis is accompanied by a serum HCO_3 greater than 24 mEq/L and a pH less than 7.40 unless another process is present.
- A *respiratory alkalosis* if his or her PCO_2 is less than 40 mm Hg. Once again, because of inherent compensation, respiratory alkalosis is accompanied by a serum HCO_3 less than 24 mEq/L and a pH greater than 7.40 unless another process is present.

Any combination of acidoses and alkaloses can be present in any one patient at any given time.

The terms *acidemia* and *alkalemia* refer only to the resultant pH of blood (acidemia being less than 7.40 and alkalemia being greater than 7.40). These terms do not describe the process or processes that led to the alteration in pH. Although in reality a range exists for normal pH values, serum bicarbonate concentration, and partial pressure of carbon dioxide, accepting a single value as normal greatly simplifies the analysis without distorting the results.

The following case discussion illustrates the approach to acid–base disorders.

PATIENT 1. A 27-year-old man was found unconscious at home with a suicide note and some empty pill containers. A history of IV drug use was assumed by the paramedics because of the presence of track marks on his skin. The initial assessment was notable for a blood pressure of 140/90 mm Hg, a pulse of 120 beats/min, and a respiratory rate of 18 breaths/min. The patient was placed on high-flow oxygen and transported to the emergency department (ED). On route to the ED, an IV line was inserted and blood samples were obtained for later analysis. The patient then was given 2 mg of naloxone, 25 g of dextrose, and 100 mg of thiamine IV without clinical response.

On arrival in the ED the patient was intermittently agitated and deeply lethargic with a blood pressure of 120/90 mm Hg, a pulse rate of 110 beats/min, labored respirations of 18 breaths/min, and a rectal temperature of 38.1°C (100.6°F). His skin was slightly diaphoretic and was notable for multiple track marks of various ages. His head was without signs of trauma. Pupils were 4 mm in size, equal, and round, but sluggishly reactive to light. His neck was supple, without signs of meningeal irritation. His chest was clear to auscultation and percussion, and heart sounds were normal. His abdomen was soft, without organomegaly, and with good bowel sounds. Rectal tone was normal, and stool was negative for occult blood. Neurologic assessment revealed good motor strength, intact corneal and oculocephalic reflexes, and brisk but symmetric deep tendon reflexes. Plantar flexion was present.

The blood specimens obtained by the paramedics were sent to the laboratory for electrolytes, glucose, BUN, CBC, and acetaminophen level. Two serum tubes were placed aside for future studies as indicated. An arterial blood gas analysis was obtained on room air, and an ECG showed sinus tachycardia with no evidence of PR, QRS, or QT abnormalities. After a gag reflex was confirmed, the patient was placed in the left lateral decubitus position and was lavaged with a 40 French orogastric tube. When the lavage fluid was clear, a slurry of 60 g of activated charcoal in water and 70 g of sorbitol was instilled and the tube was removed.

The arterial blood gas analysis showed a pH of 7.30, PCO_2 of 15 mm Hg, and PO_2 of 120 mm Hg.

What Is the Patient's Acid–Base Abnormality?

By definition, the low PCO_2 is indicative of a respiratory alkalosis, which can be either primary or in response to a metabolic acidosis. In an acute respiratory alkalosis the relationship between the fall in PCO_2 and the rise in pH is described as follows:[100]

For every fall of 10 mm Hg in the PCO_2 there should be a rise of 0.08 units in the pH.

Thus for this patient, the fall in the PCO_2 of 25 mm Hg (from 40 mm Hg to 15 mm Hg) would be expected to produce a rise of 0.20 in the pH (2.5×0.08). Since the pH is lower than the predicted value of 7.60, a metabolic acidosis is present. If only one primary process affecting acid–base balance is present (meaning the other is compensatory), the primary process can be identified by the pH. Specifically, it is generally assumed that overcompensation from either a renal or a pulmonary perspective cannot occur.[96,100] That is, if the primary process is a metabolic acidosis, a respiratory alkalosis will tend to raise the pH toward normal, but never to greater than 7.40. If the primary process is a respiratory alkalosis, a compensatory metabolic acidosis will tend to lower the pH toward normal, but never to less than 7.40. The same is true for primary metabolic alkalosis and primary respiratory acidosis. Further assessment requires an evaluation of the serum electrolytes.

The laboratory studies of patient 1 returned as follows: sodium (Na), 133 mEq/L; potassium (K), 3.6 mEq/L; chloride (Cl), 99 mEq/L; bicarbonate (HCO_3), 12 mEq/L; BUN, 12 mg/dL; creatinine (Cr), 0.9 mg/dL; and glucose (Glu), 120 mg/dL.

The next step in the analysis involves a calculation of the anion gap.

What Is the Anion Gap, and How Is It Calculated?

The law of electroneutrality states that the net positive and negative charges of the serum must be equal. Although the concept of the anion gap is said to have arisen from the "Gamblegram" originally described in 1939,[45] its use was not popularized until the determination of serum electrolytes became routinely available. Simply put, since all of the negative charges present in the serum must equal all of the positive charges present in the serum, then the sum of the positive charges minus the sum of the negative charges would have to equal zero.

The problem that immediately arises is that all charged species are not routinely measured. Normally present but unmeasured cations consist of calcium and magnesium, while normally present but unmeasured anions consist of phosphate, sulfate, albumin, and organic acids.[36,43,102] Sodium and potassium normally account for 95% of extracellular cations, while chloride and bicarbonate account for 85% of extracellular anions.[36] Thus since more cations than anions are measured, subtracting the anions from the cations normally yields a positive number, known as the anion gap. The anion gap is therefore derived as follows:

$$\text{Na} + \text{K} + \text{unmeasured cations } (U_c) = \text{Cl} + \text{HCO}_3 + \text{unmeasured anions } (U_a)$$

$$\text{Anion gap} = U_a - U_c$$

or

$$\text{Anion gap} = (\text{Na} + \text{K}) - (\text{Cl} + \text{HCO}_3)$$

Since potassium is largely an intracellular cation and rarely alters the anion gap, it is often deleted from the equation for simplicity. Most authors[36,43,102] prefer this approach, yielding the equation:

$$\text{Anion gap} = Na - (Cl + HCO_3)$$

Using the equation shown above, the normal anion gap had previously been determined to be 12 ± 4 mEq/L.[36,142] More recent work in the 1990s, however, has demonstrated that as a result of a change in laboratory instrumentation and higher chloride values than previously reported, the range for a normal anion gap has fallen to 7 ± 4 mEq/L.[141]

A variety of pathologic conditions may result in a rise or fall of the anion gap. High anion gaps result from increased presence of unmeasured anions or decreased presence of unmeasured cations (Table 15–1).[36,43,121] Similarly, a low anion gap results from an increase in unmeasured cations or a decrease in unmeasured anions (Table 15–2).[36,43,57,129]

The popularity of the anion gap revolves around its ability to help diagnose disorders responsible for the generation of a metabolic acidosis. When a metabolic acidosis is present, as in the case described above, it should be further categorized as being a high- or normal-anion-gap type. A high-anion-gap metabolic acidosis results from the absorption or generation of an acid pair with an unmeasured anion (eg, lactic acid). Normal-anion-gap acidoses result from processes that produce bicarbonate loss and chloride retention (eg, diarrhea). Causes of high- and normal-anion-gap metabolic acidoses are shown in Tables 15–3 and 15–4. The patient described above has an anion gap of 22 mEq/L [133 – (99 + 12)], and thus is said to have a high-anion-gap metabolic acidosis.

How Reliable Is the Anion Gap?

Several authors have considered the utility of the anion gap determination.[17,44,68] When 57 hospitalized patients were studied to determine the cause of elevated anion gaps, in those patients whose anion gap was greater than 30 mEq/L the cause was always lactic acidosis or ketoacidosis.[44] In patients with smaller elevations of the anion gap, the ability to define the cause of the elevation diminished; in only 14% of patients with anion gaps of 17–19 mEq/L could the etiology be defined. Another study determined that although the anion gap is often used as a screening test for hyperlactatemia (as a sign of poor perfusion), only those patients with the highest serum lactate concentrations were found to have elevated anion gaps.[68] Finally, in a sample of 571 patients, those with higher anion gaps tended to have an increased severity of illness, resulting in a higher admission rate, a greater percentage of whom required admission to intensive care units, and a higher mortality.[17] Thus although the absence of an anion gap does not exclude significant illness, when the anion gap is very elevated it usually is attributed to a given etiology and associated with consequential illness.

TABLE 15–1. CAUSES OF A HIGH ANION GAP

Increased unmeasured anions
Metabolic acidosis (see Table 15–3)
Dehydration
Therapy with sodium salts of unmeasured anions
sodium citrate
sodium lactate
sodium acetate
Therapy with certain antibiotics
carbenicillin
sodium penicillin
Alkalosis
Decrease in unmeasured cations
Simultaneous hypomagnesemia, hypocalcemia, and hypokalemia

TABLE 15–2. CAUSES OF A LOW ANION GAP

Increase in unmeasured cations
Hypercalcemia
Hypermagnesemia
Hyperkalemia
Lithium intoxication
Multiple myeloma
Decrease in unmeasured anions
Hypoalbuminemia
Dilution
Overestimation of the chloride
Bromism
Iodism
Nitrate excess

TABLE 15–3. CAUSES OF A HIGH ANION GAP METABOLIC ACIDOSIS

Carbon monoxide
Cyanide
Ethylene glycol
Hydrogen sulfide
Isoniazid
Iron
Ketoacidoses (diabetic, alcoholic, and starvation)
Lactate
Metformin
Methanol
Paraldehyde
Phenformin
Salicylates
Sulfur (inorganic)
Theophylline
Toluene
Uremia

Note: Many clinicians rely on the mnemonic **MUDPILES** to help remember this differential diagnosis where M represents Methanol, U (Uremia), D (Diabetic Ketoacidosis), P (Paraldehyde), I (Iron), L (Lactic Acidosis), E (Ethylene Glycol), and S (Salicylates).

TABLE 15–4. CAUSES OF A NORMAL-ANION-GAP METABOLIC ACIDOSIS

Drugs
Acetazolamide
Acidifying agents
Ammonium chloride
Arginine hydrochloride
Hydrochloric acid
Lysine hydrochloride
Cholestyramine
Sulfamylon
Gastrointestinal bicarbonate loss
Diarrhea
Pancreatic fistula
Miscellaneous
Hyperalimentation
Post-hypocapnia
Rapid IV hydration with 0.9% NaCl
Renal tubular acidosis
Ureteroenterostomy

How Can the Differential Diagnosis of a High-Anion-Gap Metabolic Acidosis Be Narrowed?

The ability to diagnose the etiology of a high-anion-gap metabolic acidosis is an essential skill in clinical medicine. The following discussion provides a rapid and cost-effective approach to the problem. As always, the clinical history and physical examination may provide essential clues to the diagnosis. Iron intoxication is associated with significant GI symptoms. The absence of these symptoms virtually excludes the diagnosis of iron intoxication (Chap. 35). Furthermore, when iron overdose is suspected, an abdominal radiograph may show the presence of tablets. The acidosis associated with isoniazid (INH) intoxication results from seizures, the absence of which excludes INH as the cause of a metabolic acidosis (Chap. 43). Methanol intoxication, and to a lesser extent ethylene glycol intoxication, may be associated with visual complaints or an abnormal funduscopic examination (Chap. 64). Paraldehyde has a characteristic odor (Chap. 27). When these findings are absent, the laboratory analysis must be relied on.

1. Begin with the electrolytes: an elevated BUN and creatinine are essential to diagnose uremia. Similarly, hyperglycemia should raise the possibility of diabetic ketoacidosis. The absence of an elevated glucose does not, however, exclude the possibility of euglycemic diabetic ketoacidosis,[70] or alcoholic or starvation ketoacidosis, which are often associated with normal or even low serum glucose concentrations. If the electrolytes are not available, a glucose reagent test should be performed to help confirm or exclude the possibility of hyperglycemia.
2. Proceed to the urinalysis: do not wait for the laboratory results, as all of these studies are easily accomplished. In addition, if there is a suspicion of high-anion-gap metabolic acidosis, and only the arterial blood gas analysis is completed, the evaluation may begin here, while the electrolyte determination is pending. A urine dipstick for glucose and ketones will help with the diagnosis of diabetic ketoacidosis and other ketoacidoses. Note that the absence of urinary ketones does not exclude a diagnosis of alcoholic ketoacidosis (Chap. 62) and ketones are often present in severe salicylism (Chap. 32). The urine of a patient who has ingested fluorescein-containing antifreeze (ethylene glycol) may fluoresce when exposed to a Wood's lamp. Also, since ethylene glycol is metabolized to oxalate, calcium oxalate crystals may be present in the urine of a poisoned patient. Both of these findings are useful if present, but their absence does not exclude poisoning (Chap. 64). Finally, a urine ferric chloride test should be performed. This test is unfortunately neither 100% sensitive nor specific for the diagnosis of salicylism (Chap. 32). When the ferric chloride test is positive, a serum salicylate level must be obtained, but a negative ferric chloride test may not definitively exclude salicylism in the correct clinical setting.
3. An arterial or central venous blood lactate level can be helpful. In theory, if the lactate (measured in mmol/L or mEq/L) can entirely account for the fall in serum bicarbonate, then the cause of the anion gap can be attributed to lactic acidosis.

When the above analysis is not productive, the diagnosis is usually toxic alcohol ingestion, starvation, or alcoholic ketoacidosis (with minimal urine ketones) or a multifactorial process involving small amounts of lactate and other anions. One approach is to provide the patient with 1–2 hours of hydration, dextrose, and thiamine. If the acidosis resolves, the etiology is either keto- or lactic acidosis. Alternatively, a more detailed search for the toxic alcohols, involving either the osmol gap or specific levels, should be initiated (see below).

In patient 1, urinalysis revealed trace amounts of protein, small ketones, and large glucose (after dextrose administration). There were no crystals or fluorescence, but a ferric chloride test was positive. A lactate level was not obtained.

Would Further Acid–Base Analysis Help Limit the Differential Diagnosis?

The most striking laboratory abnormality in this patient is the HCO_3 of 12 mEq/L. This value not only confirms the presence of a significant metabolic acidosis, but also allows for a better definition of the nature of the disturbance.

Winters' equation allows for a prediction of the degree of the respiratory compensation (fall of the PCO_2) in acute metabolic acidosis if the serum bicarbonate is known, as follows:[3]

$$PCO_2 = [1.5 \times (HCO_3)] + 8 \pm 2$$

Thus, since this patient has a HCO_3 of 12 mEq/L, it can be predicted that the PCO_2 should be:

$$(1.5 \times 12) + 8 \pm 2 \quad \text{or} \quad 26 \pm 2 \text{ mm Hg}$$

Since the PCO_2 of patient 1 was substantially lower than would have been predicted by Winters' equation, it can be concluded that both a primary metabolic acidosis and a primary respiratory alkalosis were present. As shown by Narins and Emmett, it is empirically true that in a pure compensated metabolic acidosis, the PCO_2 is usually the same as the last two digits of the pH.[100] For example, a pH of 7.26 would correlate with a PCO_2 of 26 mm Hg. In this case the PCO_2 of 15 mm Hg is much lower than would be predicted from the last two digits of the pH (7.30 or 30), suggesting a second primary process.

The single disorder in the differential diagnosis of a high-anion-gap metabolic acidosis that is commonly associated with the presence of primary metabolic acidosis and primary respiratory alkalosis is salicylism (Chap. 32). Thus with the positive ferric chloride test, the presence of urinary ketones, and the acid–base abnormalities noted, salicylate intoxication is essentially confirmed.

The patient's serum salicylate level was later reported as 97 mg/dL, and he underwent hemodialysis with complete recovery.

What Is the Osmol Gap, and How Should it Be Used?

The osmol gap is defined as the difference between the measured osmolality and the calculated osmolarity.[129] Osmolarity is a measure of the total number of particles in one liter of solution. Osmolality differs from osmolarity only in that the number of particles is expressed per kilogram of solution. Thus osmolarity and osmolality represent molar and molal concentrations of solutes, respectively.[50] Also, in clinical medicine, osmolarity is usually calculated, whereas osmolality is usually measured.

Calculating osmolarity requires a summing of the known particles in solution. Since, as opposed to weight or concentration, molarity and miliequivalents are particle-based measurements, the known constituents of serum have to be converted to molar values. Assumptions are required based on the extent of dissociation of polar compounds (such as sodium chloride), the water content of serum, and present but rarely included species (calcium, magnesium, etc). The nature and limitations of these assumptions is beyond the scope of this chapter. The reader is referred to several reviews for more details.[53,62,104] Many equations have been used and evaluated for calculating osmolarity. One investigation that used 13 different methods to evaluate sera from 715 hospital patients[31] concluded that the most accurate equation was:

$$1.86\,(\text{Na in mEq/L}) + (\text{glucose in mg/dL})/18 + (\text{BUN in mg/dL})/2.8$$

Obvious sources of potential error in this calculation include laboratory error in determining any of the measured parameters and the failure to account for a number of osmotically active particles.

The measurement of serum osmolality is not without potential error as well, and stems from the use of different laboratory techniques. One survey of clinical laboratory methodology demonstrated that while over 80% of facilities studied offered osmometry, 11% used the vapor pressure method exclusively (as opposed to the freezing point method).[35] Furthermore, half of the laboratory supervisors questioned failed to recognize that the vapor pressure technique was likely to produce an erroneously low serum osmolality for serum containing methanol, ethanol, or isopropanol.[35] This error results from the fact that these alcohols will boil out of solution before the boiling point of water is reached.

The mathematical and theoretical errors in determining osmolarity and osmolality are potentially additive when the two values are mathematically combined to determine the osmol gap. In addition, a conceptual error is also present. The uncharged particle (eg, methanol) has osmotic activity that is not calculated, but does not produce an anion gap until it is metabolized (eg, to formate). Although the metabolite also has osmotic activity, its activity is accounted for by sodium in the osmolarity calculation, because it is largely dissociated, existing as sodium formate. Thus, at least in theory, an early ingestion is marked by an elevated osmol gap and a normal anion gap, whereas later, the anion gap increases and the osmol gap decreases. This effect is highlighted by several case reports.[5,132] Despite these limitations, a determination of the osmol gap is commonly proposed as a diagnostic adjunct when considering ingestions of toxic alcohols. To qualify as a good screening test, the osmol gap should predict toxic alcohol ingestion with a low frequency of false-negative results (have a high sensitivity). To exclude a diagnosis of toxic alcohol ingestion, the determination of an osmol gap should have a low frequency of false-positive results (high specificity). As a first step, the range of normal values (and its variability) must be known. Using the formula for osmolarity shown above, the previously mentioned study determined that the "normal" osmol gap was 10 ± 6 mOsm.[31] However, when studied in over 300 samples, the more commonly used equation:

$$2(\text{Na in mEq/L}) + (\text{glucose in mg/dL})/18 + (\text{BUN in mg/dL})/2.8$$

yielded normal values of −2 ± 6 mOsm and ranged from −5 to +15 mOsm with other commonly used equations.[62] While the concept of a negative osmol gap might be disconcerting, the numerous approximations used to calculate osmolarity may not be valid. Also, although ethanol is the most common cause of elevated osmolality in varied groups of patients,[18,21,105,114] a serum ethanol measurement was not included for any of the patients used in the reference that serves as the standard to define osmol gaps.[31] The relatively recent inclusion of ethanol in the osmolarity formula in a systematic evaluation of normal values predictably increased the calculated osmolarity in patients in whom ethanol was present, making the osmol gap smaller than previously suggested, or even negative.[62] Furthermore, recent work has shown a slight rise in measured sodium.[141] If this is related to changes in laboratory determination, it will also lead to a lowering of the osmol gap. In fact, other investigations have concluded that the mean osmol gap in control (presumably ethanol-free) populations was a negative value.[53,69,120] Thus the commonly used "normal" value of less than 10 mOsm, often attributed to two earlier works,[50,129] is clearly "arbitrary" in the authors' own words, erroneous, and should be abandoned.

The largest limitation of the osmol gap calculation comes from the documented large standard deviation around a small "normal" number.[31,62,69,120] This variability may result from true population variability, in which case the standard deviation will never be reduced. Alternatively, an error of 1 mEq/L in the determination of the serum sodium may result in an error of 2 mOsm in the calculation of the osmol gap. As a result of this variability, the molecular weight of the toxins in question (ethylene glycol level of 50 mg/dL would contribute only 7.8 mOsm/L), and the predicted fall in osmol gap as metabolism occurs, small or even negative osmol gaps will never exclude toxic alcohol ingestion.[52,62] This overall concept is illustrated by the case of a patient with an osmol gap of 7.2 mOsm who ultimately required hemodialysis for a severe ethylene glycol intoxication.[132] Furthermore, though large osmol gaps may be suggestive of toxic alcohol ingestions, common conditions such as alcoholic ketoacidosis, lactic acidosis, renal failure, and shock are all associated with elevated osmol gaps.[69,120,126] Since lactate and ketones should not account for any increase in the osmol gap because they are charged, these conditions are probably associated with the accumulation of small uncharged molecules in the serum. Thus, because both the negative and positive predictive values of this test are inadequate, its utility as a screening tool must be questioned.

Can Any Tests Be Used to Differentiate the Causes of a Normal-Anion-Gap Metabolic Acidosis?

Although the differential diagnosis for a normal-anion-gap metabolic acidosis is extensive (Table 15–4), most cases result from either urinary or GI bicarbonate losses: renal tubular acidosis (RTA) or diarrhea, respectively. When the history and physical examination are unable to narrow the differential diagnosis, the use of a urinary anion gap has been suggested.[11]

The urinary anion gap [(Na + K) – (Cl)], correlates with ammonium (NH_4) excretion.[56] As ammonium elimination increases, the urinary anion gap narrows, since ammonium serves as an unmeasured cation and is accompanied by chloride. The normal-anion-gap metabolic acidosis that is associated with diarrhea results from GI bicarbonate loss. During this process the kidney's ability to eliminate ammonium is undisturbed and in fact increases as a normal response to the acidosis. Thus with GI bicarbonate losses the urinary anion gap should be low. Alternatively, the patient with RTA has lost the ability either to resorb bicarbonate or to increase ammonium excretion in response to an acidosis, and the urinary anion gap should be elevated. When the urinary anion gap was calculated in patients with diarrhea or RTA, it was found that those patients with diarrhea had a mean negative gap (–20 ± 5.7 mEq/L), as compared to a positive gap (23 ± 4.1 mEq/L) in those with RTA.[56] Therefore, when evaluating the patient with a normal-gap metabolic acidosis, the determination of a urinary anion gap should help determine the source of the disorder.

Metabolic Alkalosis

PATIENT 2. A 2-week-old boy was brought to the ED by his parents because of a 36-hour history of fever, diarrhea, and lethargy. The child was born at 39 weeks gestation via normal spontaneous vaginal delivery and had Apgar scores of 9 and 10. The baby and the mother were discharged from the hospital at the usual time, and the baby remained well until 36 hours prior to presentation in the ED. Physical examination was remarkable for an irritable child who was unconsolable, even by his parents. Vital signs were a blood pressure of 60/40 mm Hg, an irregular pulse at 160 beats/min, a respiratory rate of 28 breaths/min, and a rectal temperature of 38.3°C (100.9°F). His skin was dry and without a rash. His anterior fontanel was depressed, and his capillary refill was delayed. The remainder of the physical assessment was unremarkable.

The patient was placed on a cardiac monitor that showed frequent premature ventricular contractions (confirmed by 12-lead ECG). An intravenous catheter was inserted, and blood was drawn for culture, electrolytes, glucose, and CBC. An arterial blood gas sample was obtained on room air and supplemental oxygen was administered. The child was given dextrose (1 g/kg) and a 20 mL/kg bolus of normal saline IV. A lumbar puncture was performed and immediately afterward the child was started on broad-spectrum antibiotics.

The laboratory studies returned. Arterial blood gas values were: pH, 7.76; PCO_2, 40 mm Hg; PO_2, 96 mm Hg. Electrolytes were: Na, 154 mEq/L; K, 3.1 mEq/L; Cl, 86 mEq/L; HCO_3, 43 mEq/L; BUN, Cr, and Glu, were normal. The lumbar puncture revealed a normal cell count and chemistry, with a negative Gram stain.

What Are the Adverse Effects of Metabolic Alkalosis?

Life-threatening metabolic alkalosis is rare but can result in tetany (from decreased ionized calcium),[86] weakness (from decreased potassium),[92] altered mental status leading to coma,[82] seizures,[54] and cardiac dysrhythmias.[76] In addition, metabolic alkalosis shifts the oxyhemoglobin dissociation curve to the left, impairing tissue oxygenation (Chap. 20). The expected compensation for a metabolic alkalosis is a respiratory acidosis, which is produced by hypoventilation and increased PCO_2. Standard discussions of metabolic alkalosis suggest that the respiratory compensation is irregular and inadequate at best, invoking a teleological argument to suggest that hypoventilation and hypoxia would be more undesirable than metabolic alkalosis.[100] However, several authors have demonstrated that cases of severe hypoventilation and respiratory failure can occur in response to metabolic alkalosis, suggesting a real, although uncommon risk.[92,107]

What Is the Approach to a Patient with Metabolic Alkalosis?

Metabolic alkalosis results from GI or urinary loss of acids, administration of exogenous bases, or renal bicarbonate retention (impaired bicarbonate loss). Causes of metabolic alkalosis are listed in Table 15–5. By comparison, metabolic alkalosis is less common and less toxicologically consequential than high-anion-gap metabolic acidosis.

The etiologies of metabolic alkalosis can be characterized therapeutically as chloride-responsive or chloride-resistant. Chloride-responsive etiologies (diuretics, vomiting and nasogastric suction, chloride diarrhea, etc) are usually associated with a low urinary chloride excretion (<10 mEq/L).[60,76] These disorders respond rapidly to infusion of sodium chloride when concomitant therapy addresses the underlying problem. Chloride-resistant disorders (hyperaldosteronism, severe potassium depletion, etc) are characterized by urinary chlorides greater than 10 mEq/L and tend to be resistant to sodium chloride therapy.[47,60] These disorders often require potassium repletion or agents that reduce mineralocorticoid effects (spironolactone) before correction can occur.[47] When volume loading (sodium chloride repletion) is ineffective, or emergent correction of the alkalosis is required, some authors have suggested infusions of lysine or arginine hydrochloride, or dilute hydrochloric acid.[92]

TABLE 15–5. CAUSES OF A METABOLIC ALKALOSIS

Gastrointestinal acid loss
- Chloride diarrhea (congenital)
- Nasogastric suction (protracted)
- Vomiting (protracted)

Urinary acid loss
- Common
  - Diuretics
- Rare
  - Adrenogenital syndrome
  - Bartter's syndrome
  - Cushing's syndrome
  - Hyperaldosteronism (primary)
  - Hypercalcemia
  - Licorice (glycyrrhizic acid)
  - Little's syndrome
  - Magnesium deficiency

Base administration
- Acetate (dialysis or hyperalimentation)
- Bicarbonate
- Carbonate (antacids)
- Citrate (posttranfusion)
- Milk alkali syndrome

Renal bicarbonate retention
- Hypercapnia (chronic)
- Hypochloremia
- Hypokalemia
- Volume contraction

Further history revealed that patient 2 was being fed oral baking soda several times per day as part of a folk remedy. Urinary chloride was 6 mEq/L. He was treated with intravenous normal saline with a subsequent resolution of clinical and laboratory abnormalities. The parents were educated about the risks of all prescription and nonprescription medications and folk remedies.

What Is the Delta Gap (Δ Gap) and How Is It Used?

Many patients have mixed acid–base disorders such as a simultaneous metabolic acidosis and metabolic alkalosis. Depending on their relative effects, the patient may have significant acidemia or alkalemia, minor alterations in pH, or even a "normal" pH.

A typical example might be the patient with diabetic ketoacidosis (DKA) and vomiting. While DKA would be expected to produce a classic high-anion-gap metabolic acidosis, the vomiting could raise the serum bicarbonate producing a normal value. The toxicologic clinical correlate of the patient with a mixed acid–base disorder might be the iron-poisoned patient with refractory vomiting and a multifactorial high-anion-gap metabolic acidosis (Chap. 35). Another example might be the patient with alcoholic ketoacidosis and vomiting. In both cases it is conceivable that the patient with two clinically obvious disorders could have a pH of 7.40, a PCO_2 of 40 mm Hg, and a serum bicarbonate level of 24 mEq/L. In most circumstances, one process predominates, and its significance is minimized if the second process goes undiagnosed.

In the patient with a simple anion-gap metabolic acidosis, each decrease of 1 mEq/L in the serum bicarbonate should be associated with a rise of 1 mEq/L in the anion gap.[100] This occurs because the unmeasured anion is paired with the acid that is titrating the bicarbonate. Any deviation from this direct relationship may be an indication of a mixed acid–base disorder.[58,100,106] Thus the ratio of the change in the anion gap (ΔAG) to the change in the serum bicarbonate (shown below) evolved:

$$\text{Anion gap ratio} = \Delta AG/\Delta HCO_3$$

A ratio of close to 1 would suggest a pure high-anion-gap metabolic acidosis. When the ratio is greater than 1 there is a relative increase in bicarbonate (suggesting a mixed disorder) that can result only from a concomitant metabolic alkalosis or a respiratory acidosis. Alternatively, when the ratio is less than 1, the added presence of either hyperchloremic (normal anion gap) metabolic acidosis or compensated (chronic) respiratory alkalosis is suggested. One author[143] suggested the use of the gap in the anion gap, or the following equation:

$$\text{Gap of the gap} = \Delta AG - \Delta HCO_3$$

where a gap greater than 6 mEq/L would suggest metabolic alkalosis and a gap less than 6 mEq/L would suggest hyperchloremic acidosis.

The utility of the relationship between the change in the anion gap and the change in the serum bicarbonate has been evaluated by several authors.[29,103,106,117] Although supported strongly by some authors,[103,106] others suggest that it is often flawed and frequently misleading.[29,117] The section below summarizes the discussion.

For the fall in bicarbonate to be either proportionally or linearly related to the rise in the anion gap the following criteria should be met:

1. All of the acid formed should be titrated by bicarbonate. In fact, there are many nonbicarbonate buffer systems, and the duration of acidosis relates to the relative contributions of these systems.[122]
2. The volumes of distribution of the proton, its associated anion, and bicarbonate should be the same. This is not always true. For example, in the case of lactic acidosis, lactate remains extracellularly while some of the acid is buffered intracellularly, such that the increase in the anion gap (from lactate) is less than the decrease in bicarbonate.[116]
3. Elimination of the anion and regeneration of bicarbonate should be equal. For example, in the patient with a ketoacidosis, the ketone moieties are often cleared quickly when renal function is normal and poorly when renal function is impaired.[2]
4. Acidosis and alkalosis should not alter the anion gap themselves. As pH changes, the charges on serum proteins change, such that acidemia tends to decrease the anion gap and alkalemia tends to increase the gap.[1] This change is related to the generation of lactate and a change in the charges on albumin (an unmeasured anion).
5. There must be no concurrent process other than the anion gap metabolic acidosis that affects the anion gap.

For these reasons we support the statements of one author,[29] who appears to be correct in concluding that "the exact relationship between the ΔAG and ΔHCO_3 in a high anion gap acidosis is not readily predictable and deviation of the $\Delta AG/\Delta HCO_3$ ratio from unity does not necessarily imply the diagnosis of a second acid–base disorder." However, very large deviations from a value of 1 probably suggest the presence of a second disorder.

How Do Drugs and Toxins Alter Fluid Balance?

Significant fluid abnormalities occur commonly in the setting of toxin exposure. Gastrointestinal losses in the form of vomiting, diarrhea, GI bleeding, and third spacing (from GI burns) result from a variety of toxic exposures and their management (emetics and cathartics). Renal losses result from the ability of many toxins to increase glomerular filtration rate (inotropes), impair resorption (diuretics), or enhance urine volume in response to an obligate solute load (salicylates). Finally, insensible losses occur through increased sweating (sympathomimetics, cholinergics, and uncouplers of oxidative phosphorylation) and pulmonary losses as a result of increased minute ventilation (salicylates and sympathomimetics) or bronchorrhea (cholinergics). This section focuses on two specific entities: the syndrome of inappropriate secretion of antidiuretic hormone (SIADH) and diabetes insipidus (DI). Other specific fluid issues are found in Chapters 22 and 23 and chapters relating to individual toxins.

What Is Diabetes Insipidus, and What Toxins Produce This Disorder?

Plasma osmolality is maintained through a complex interaction between the hypothalamus, pituitary gland, and kidney. Extensive discussions of these mechanisms[10,97,98,137] are summarized below. Osmolality is sensed by a group of neurons (known as osmoreceptors) located in the anterior hypothalamus. Changes in osmolality are mediated through changes in thirst and urinary concentration of solutes; the latter is controlled by the hormone arginine vasopressin (antidiuretic hormone; ADH). Antidiuretic hormone is synthesized in the hypothalamus and released by the posterior pituitary gland in response to stimulation from the osmoreceptors. As plasma osmolality rises, ADH is released, reaching its maximum at a serum osmolality of about 295 mOsm/kg. Antidiuretic hormone is transported to the kidney via the bloodstream, where it increases the synthesis of cyclic adenosine monophosphate (cAMP). This increase in cAMP increases the permeability of the distal convoluted tubule and collecting duct such that water is reabsorbed and urine becomes more concentrated (urine osmolality may be as high as 800 mOsm/kg). Alternatively, as plasma osmolality falls, ADH release is diminished. This results in a decrease in renal cAMP generation, with the distal convoluted tubule and collecting duct becoming less permeable to water, and a net production of dilute urine.

Diabetes insipidus (hypotonic polyuria) may be termed neurogenic (resulting from failure to sense a rising osmolality or failure to release ADH) or nephrogenic (resulting from failure of the kidney to respond appropriately to ADH). Although there are many nontoxicologic causes for DI (eg, trauma, tumor, sarcoid, idiopathic, vascular, and congenital), toxins have the ability to interfere with ADH effects through both central and peripheral mechanisms. Ethanol, opioid antagonists, and alpha-adrenergic agonists all suppress ADH release.[7,97] Lithium,[24,88,125] demeclocycline,[124] methoxyflurane,[90] propoxyphene,[15] foscarnet,[101] mesalazine,[89] streptozotocin,[28] amphotericin,[64] lobenzarit,[116] rifampin,[110] and colchicine[137] are all associated with nephrogenic DI (see Table 15–6).

Of these agents, lithium has been the most extensively evaluated. Although polyuria is a common finding with lithium therapy (occurring in 20–70% of patients on maintenance therapy),[12] the exact incidence of DI is unclear. Estimates range from 10–20%[88] to as high as 80%.[21]

What Are the Signs and Symptoms of Diabetes Insipidus, and How Is it Diagnosed?

Patients with DI complain of polyuria and polydipsia. Urine volumes typically exceed 30 mL/kg/day[137] and may be as high as 9 L/day with nephrogenic DI[88] and

12–14 L/day with neurogenic (central) DI.[99] Nocturia, fatigue, and decreased work performance are noted.[137] With neurogenic DI resulting from hypothalamic or pituitary damage, other signs of neuroendocrine dysfunction may also be present.[99]

Urine specific gravity is low (less than 1.010) and serum sodium is usually elevated. Nephrogenic DI may be associated with hypokalemia and hypercalcemia.[137] Further diagnostic evaluation should begin with simultaneous determination of the urine and serum osmolality. The diagnosis of diabetes insipidus is established by the occurrence of dilute urine (urine osmolality < 300 mOsm/kg) in the presence of concentrated electrolytes (plasma osmolality > 295 mOsm/kg).[137] Following this determination, a trial of desmopressin (DDAVP), an arginine vasopressin analog, will help to differentiate between neurogenic and nephrogenic DI. If the etiology of the DI is neurogenic, the patient will promptly respond to DDAVP and urine osmolality will increase.[137]

What Is the Treatment for Diabetes Insipidus?

The initial approach to the patient with DI involves the repletion of intravascular volume and the restoration of electrolyte balance. If a reversible cause for the DI can be established, it should be corrected. Patients with neurogenic DI should be maintained on either vasopressin or DDAVP. The latter is usually preferred because of the lack of vasopressor effects. In the past, patients were occasionally treated with oral agents known to produce SIADH (see below). Patients with nephrogenic DI can be treated with thiazide diuretics,[32] prostaglandin inhibitors,[28,64,83] or amiloride.[12]

What Is SIADH, and What Toxins Produce It?

In a sense, the syndrome of inappropriate secretion of antidiuretic hormone may be thought of as the opposite of diabetes insipidus. In SIADH hyponatremia and plasma hypotonicity result from continued production or release of ADH in the setting of low plasma osmolality.[10] Early reviews claimed that SIADH was a disorder of volume overload, based largely on evidence of weight gain.[97] The consistent absence of edema, however, and the fact that the decrease in sodium cannot be accounted for by the fluid gain (weight gain) suggest that fluid retention is only a minor part of the mechanism.[79]

The clinical presentation of SIADH is that of hyponatremia.[10,99] Symptoms are related to both the absolute fall in serum sodium concentration and its rate of decline. Irritability, lethargy, weakness, and muscle cramps may be noted.[99] In more severe cases, coma and seizures will develop.[10,99]

There are many nontoxicologic etiologies of SIADH, most of which involve pulmonary or intracranial processes. Common causes include infections, malignancies, and surgery.[10,79,97,99] Table 15–6 summarizes drugs and toxins known to produce SIADH. The oral hypoglycemics, including agents from both the sulfonylurea (eg, chlorpropramide) and biguannide (eg, phenformin) classes produce hyponatremia more commonly than the other agents.[98] Their actions are multifactorial and can include both the potentiation of endogenous ADH and the stimulation of ADH release.[98] Many psychiatric medications including the selective serotonin reuptake inhibitors, cyclic antidepressants, neuroleptics, and others are implicated in causing SIADH.[20,22,77,85,131,136] Evidence suggests that complex interactions between the dopaminergic and noradrenergic systems control ADH release.[131] Additional evidence supports a role of serotonin in drug induced SIADH. Serotonin (specifically 5-HT_2 and/or 5-HT_{1c}) stimulates ADH release[6,72] and stimulates water intake.[67] An important role of serotonin is supported by the occurrence of SIADH with hallucinogenic amphetamine (MDMA) use.[66,140]

TABLE 15–6. CAUSES OF SIADH AND DIABETES INSIPIDUS (DI)

SIADH	DI
Amiloride	Amphotericin
Amitriptyline	Colchicine
Biguanides	Demeclocycline
Carbamazepine (oxcarbamazepine)	Ethanol
Cisplatin	Foscarnet
Clofibrate	Lithium
Cyclophosphamide	Lobenzarit disodium
Desmopressin	Methoxyflurane
Diazoxide	Mesalazine
Imipramine	Propoxyphene
Indapamide	Rifampin
Indomethacin	Streptozotocin
MDMA	
Oxytocin	
Nicotine	
Selective serotonin reuptake inhibitors	
Sulfonylureas	
Thioridazine	
Tranylcypromine	
Vasopressin	
Vincristine (vinblastine)	

How Is SIADH Diagnosed and Treated?

The diagnosis of SIADH is based on establishing the presence of hyponatremia, low plasma osmolality, and impaired urinary dilution. More simply stated, SIADH is present when urine osmolality is high in the setting of low plasma osmolality. In addition, evidence of edema, hypotension, hypovolemia, and adrenal or thyroid deficiency must be lacking.[79] Other atypical causes of hyponatremia such as psychogenic polydipsia need to be excluded.[113] Uric acid also falls and is a good marker of SIADH in cases where the diagnosis is unclear.[26,130]

Treatment begins with fluid restriction.[10] Since the goal of this therapy is to establish a negative fluid balance, careful attention to intake and output is required. If an offending agent can be identified, it should be eliminated. Although many cases will resolve in 1–2 weeks,[10,79,99] the syndrome may persist. If this occurs, therapy with demeclocycline or lithium may be helpful, since severe fluid restriction is often intolerable. One author[42] suggested that demeclocycline was more efficacious than lithium when the two agents were compared in a small series of patients with SIADH. When hyponatremia is associated with life-threatening clinical presentations, most authorities recommend the careful infusion of hypertonic (3%) saline.[10,79]

What Are Common Causes of Drug- and Toxin-induced Electrolyte Abnormalities?

Sodium

Sodium concentration in the extracellular space is intrinsically related to extracellular fluid balance. Since serum sodium concentration is greater than that of any other electrolyte, it serves as the major osmotic agent. Thus the osmoreceptors mentioned above used to maintain fluid balance are, in a practical sense, sodium receptors. As a free water deficit increases, the serum sodium rises. This results in an increase in serum osmolality, which releases antidiuretic hormone in an attempt to restore fluid balance by minimizing urinary water losses. Sodium balance is maintained by complex interactions between dietary intake, obligate losses in urine and stool, natriuretic factors, overall fluid balance, and effects of hormones such as antidiuretic hormone and adrenal mineralocorticoids.[16] Any perturbation in these normal regulatory pathways can potentially result in the development of hypo- or hypernatremia (depressed or elevated serum sodium concentration).

Hyponatremia results from sodium loss, fluid retention in excess of sodium retention, or both mechanisms. Since ADH controls the relative relationship between the amount of fluid and sodium in the urine, all drugs and toxins associated with SIADH produce hyponatremia. In addition to these agents, drugs such as the thiazide diuretics reduce the serum sodium through ADH effects. Although patients with diuretic-induced hyponatremia have elevated levels of ADH, the presence of a metabolic alkalosis and hypokalemia distinguishes them from patients with classic SIADH.[41] A complex mechanism for this effect is proposed, including interference with maximal urinary dilution and free water retention in response to decreased extracellular fluid volume.[41] Lithium also produces a renal sodium-wasting syndrome that seems to be unrelated to ADH effects.[93]

Other, non-ADH systems can contribute to hyponatremia. Ingestion of licorice, containing glycyrrhizic acid, produces a syndrome of hyponatremia, hypokalemia, and hypertension resembling mineralocorticoid excess. Although the exact mechanism is debated, one report suggested that a glycyrrhizic acid–induced reduction in 11-beta-hydroxysteroid dehydrogenase activity could account for the findings.[34,37]

Although psychogenic polydipsia has been well described,[55,113] drug- and toxin-induced free water excess is quite uncommon. One example of this occurs during urologic procedures, such as transurethral prostatic resection (TURP), where large volumes of irrigation solution are required. Because of the need to cauterize wounds electrically, these fluids cannot contain conductive electrolytes, such as sodium. Although sorbitol, dextrose, and mannitol have been used to maintain the osmolality of irrigating solutions, their optical characteristics are undesirable. Thus, it is currently common to irrigate with a glycine-containing solution. When this solution is absorbed through the prostatic venous plexus, a rapid reduction in sodium results in an attempt to maintain a normal osmolality (the glycine solution has significant osmotic activity, but no sodium).[61,94]

Finally, sodium loss via nonrenal or GI mechanisms is also uncommon. Hyponatremia in burn patients treated with the topical applications of silver nitrate creams results from the diffusion of sodium through permeable skin into the hypotonic dressing.[23] These and other causes of hyponatremia are summarized in Table 15–7.

The clinical manifestations of hyponatremia are dependent on both the absolute sodium concentration and its rate of decline.[8] Chronic, slow depression of sodium is usually well tolerated, while rapid decline may be associated with catastrophic events. Symptoms include lethargy, depression, apathy, and mental status changes that result from swelling of cells in the CNS. Although treatment is usually as described above, concern exists over rapid correction of hyponatremia and the risk of irreversible CNS damage (central pontine myelinolysis).[9,133]

Drug- and toxin-induced hypernatremia results from relative free water losses (DI and agents that produce significant GI and dermal fluid loss), the parenteral administration of sodium-containing drugs, and excessive oral sodium intake. Toxins that cause hypernatremia are summarized in Table 15–7.

Oral sodium chloride and oral sodium citrate have been used as emetics and antiemetics, respectively. As might be expected, both have produced severe hypernatremia.[16] One case of fatal hypernatremia resulted from gargling with a supersaturated salt solution.[95]

Agents that produce significant diarrhea, such as lactulose or cholestyramine, can cause hypernatremia through free water loss. This is of grave concern with the use of cathartics in the management of poisonings. Multiple doses of sorbitol have been reported to produce se-

TABLE 15–7. CAUSES OF ALTERED SERUM SODIUM

Hyponatremia	Hypernatremia
Agents that cause SIADH: see Table 15–6	Agents that cause DI: see Table 15–6
Captopril and other ACE inhibitors	Antacids (baking soda)
Desmopressin	Cholestyramine
Diuretics	Glycerol
Glycine (transurethral prostatectomy syndrome)	Lactulose
Licorice (glycyrrhizic acid)	Mannitol
Lithium	Povodine–iodine
Nonsteroidal antiinflammatory drugs	Sodium salts (bicarbonate, chloride, citrate)
Silver nitrate	Sorbitol
	Urea

vere hypernatremic dehydration and death in both children and adults.[19,38,49] Given the limited evidence in support of routine administration of cathartics, the risk of diarrhea should contraindicate the use of multiple doses of cathartics in all but the rarest of situations. One survey demonstrated that a large percentage of EDs stocked only premixed activated charcoal preparations containing sorbitol.[138] The presence of sorbitol in this preparation creates the potential for iatrogenic cathartic poisoning from multiple-dose activated charcoal.

Water loss can also occur through the skin. Although diffuse diaphoresis resulting from cocaine or organophosphate intoxication has the potential to produce hypernatremia, this rarely, if ever, occurs. However, application of a burn remedy containing hyperosmolar povodine–iodine to the skin of burn patients has been reported to produce significant water losses and hypernatremia.[123]

The symptoms of significant hypernatremia consist largely of altered mental status ranging from confusion to coma and neuromuscular weakness resulting in respiratory paralysis and eventually death. If hypernatremia is associated with volume depletion, cardiovascular findings consisting of tachycardia and orthostatic and eventually supine hypotension can occur. Treatment consists of replacing the relative water deficit. As with hyponatremia, rapid correction of hypernatremia is potentially dangerous, resulting in cerebral edema. Most sources suggest that 0.9% saline infusion is adequate regardless of the magnitude of the free water deficit.

Potassium

Drug- and toxin-induced alterations in serum potassium probably occur more commonly than do alterations in the other electrolytes, due to potassium's critical role in a variety of homeostatic processes and its large intracellular store. Potassium balance is complicated.[108,118] The total body potassium content of an average adult is about 53–55 mEq/kg, of which only 2% is located in the intravascular space. The large intracellular store of potassium is maintained by a variety of systems, the most important of which is the Na^+-K^+-ATPase pump. The relationship between total body stores and serum potassium is not linear, such that small changes in the total body potassium may result in dramatic alterations in serum concentrations.

Americans ingest 50–150 mEq/day of potassium, about 90% of which is subsequently eliminated in the urine. Although potassium undergoes free glomerular filtration, the majority is reabsorbed by the time the urine reaches the proximal tubule. The body has two major defenses against a potassium load: the ability to increase urinary elimination by decreased resorption and increased distal tubular secretion (to a maximum of 600–700 mEq/day), and the ability to transfer potassium intracellularly. In addition, GI absorption of potassium is decreased as serum potassium increases.

Hypokalemia (a decrease in serum potassium) results from decreased oral intake, GI losses secondary to repeated vomiting or diarrhea, urinary losses through increased secretion or decreased resorption, and processes that shift potassium into the intracellular compartment.[16] Table 15–8 summarizes drugs and toxins commonly associated with hypokalemia.

TABLE 15–8. CAUSES OF ALTERED SERUM POTASSIUM

Hypokalemia	Hyperkalemia
Amphotericin	Amiloride
Barium (soluble salts)	Angiotensin-converting enzyme inhibitors
Beta-adrenergic agonists	Beta-adrenergic antagonists
Bicarbonate	Cardiac glycosides
Caffeine	Fluoride
Carbonic anhydrase inhibitors	Heparin
Cathartics	Nonsteroidal antiinflammatory drugs
Dextrose	Penicillin (potassium)
Insulin	Spironolactone
Licorice (glycyrrhizic acid)	Succinylcholine
Loop diuretics	Triamterene
Oral hypoglycemics	
Osmotic diuretics	
Salicylates	
Sodium polystyrene sulfate	
Sympathomimetics	
Theophylline	
Thiazide diuretics	
Toluene	

The neuromuscular manifestations of hypokalemia are extensively reviewed elsewhere.[78] Patients with hypokalemia are often asymptomatic when the decrease in serum potassium is mild (serum levels of 3.0–3.5 mEq/L). Occasionally, polyuria is noted, as hypokalemia interferes with renal concentrating mechanisms. With more significant potassium deficits (serum levels of 2.0–3.0 mEq/L), generalized malaise and weakness become evident. As potassium levels fall (to less than 2 mEq/L), weakness becomes prominent and areflexic paralysis and respiratory failure may occur, necessitating intubation and mechanical ventilation.[78,139] Rhabdomyolysis is also likely. These neuromuscular manifestations are so prominent that prior to obtaining the serum electrolytes, these manifestations of hypokalemia may be erroneously attributed to a primary neuromuscular syndrome such as Guillain-Barré. Other findings may include GI symptoms (hypoperistaltism) or symptoms related to associated electrolyte abnormalities (depending on the etiology).

Electrocardiographic changes are common, even with mild potassium depletion, although the absence of ECG changes should never be used to exclude significant hypokalemia. Common ECG findings of hypokalemia include sagging of the ST segment, decreased T-wave amplitude, and increased U-wave amplitude (Chap. 8). These findings may herald life-threatening rhythm disturbances.[65,84]

Treatment of hypokalemia involves removing the offending agent and correcting the potassium deficit. Potassium supplementation may be given orally or intravenously or both. The debate over the maximum safe infusion rate for intravenous potassium is summarized elsewhere.[80] Based on experience with more than 1300 infusions, one group concluded that under intensive care monitoring, intravenous administrations of 20 mEq/h (by central or peripheral vein) were well tolerated. They also found that each 20 mEq of potassium administered correlated with an average increase in serum potassium of 0.25 mEq/L. Other authors have used significantly larger doses (up to 100 mEq/h) in life-threatening circumstances.[27,91]

Hyperkalemia (an increase in serum potassium) results from decreased elimination (renal insufficiency, potassium sparing diuretics, hypoaldosteronism), increased intake (either oral or IV), or redistribution from tissue stores.[16] The last mechanism is of major toxicologic importance: in overdose both the cardiac glycosides (Chap. 48) and the beta-adrenergic antagonists (Chap. 49) cause hyperkalemia by allowing potassium to be released from its intracellular reservoir. Blockade of the Na^+-K^+-ATPase pump with digitalis intoxication produces hyperkalemia that may be not only diagnostic but also of prognostic importance[13] (Chap. 48). Intracellular potassium concentration is maintained in part through catecholamine-mediated uptake of potassium in liver and muscle cells.[87,115] Thus, with overdose of a beta-adrenergic antagonist some of the stores are released, producing a moderate rise of serum potassium (usually to the level of 5.0–5.5 mEq/L) (Chap. 49). Other drugs and toxins that cause hyperkalemia are listed in Table 15–8.

After oral ingestions of potassium salts, patients routinely present complaining of nausea and vomiting. Ileus, local irritation with bleeding, and GI perforation may complicate the clinical course.[118] In the absence of ingestion, GI symptoms of hyperkalemia are usually very mild. Neuromuscular manifestations include weakness with an ascending flaccid paralysis and respiratory compromise, with intact sensation and cognition.[78,108]

The cardiac manifestations of hyperkalemia are the most prominent and life-threatening. Electrocardiographic patterns progress through characteristic changes.[118,119] Although the progression of ECG changes is very reproducible, there is tremendous individual variation with respect to the absolute potassium concentration at which these ECG findings occur. Initially, the only ECG finding may be the presence of tall, peaked T waves. As the potassium increases, the QRS complex tends to blend into the T waves, the P-wave amplitude decreases, and the PR-interval prolongs. Next, the P wave is lost and ST-segment depression occurs. Finally, the distinction between the S and T waves becomes blurred and the ECG takes on a sine wave configuration (Chap 8). Hemodynamic instability and cardiac arrest result. As the patient's potassium falls, these ECG changes resolve in a reverse fashion.

The treatment of severe hyperkalemia includes standard airway management, methods to reverse the ECG effects, methods to move potassium intracellularly, and methods to enhance potassium elimination. Pharmacologic interventions, extensively discussed elsewhere,[118] are summarized here. Calcium works almost immediately to protect the myocardium against the effects of hyperkalemia but does not change the serum potassium concentration. A potentially life-threatening interaction occurs, however, when the patient with cardiac glycoside toxicity is given calcium (Chap. 48), and therefore this modality should be used with some caution. The administration of insulin and hypertonic dextrose or of sodium bicarbonate moves potassium intracellularly. Cationic exchange resins, such as sodium polystyrene sulfonate, work slowly to enhance GI potassium loss. Hemodialysis or peritoneal dialysis may be useful, especially when significant renal impairment is present. Beta-adrenergic agonist inhalation therapy is also suggested to increase the intracellular potassium concentration.[4]

Calcium

Although calcium is the most abundant mineral in the human body, 98–99% of it is located in bone. Approximately half of the remaining calcium is bound to plasma proteins (mostly albumin) and most of the rest is complexed to various anions, with free calcium representing a very small fraction of extraosseous stores. Calcium concentration is maintained through interactions between dietary intake and renal elimination, modulated by vitamin D activity, parathyroid hormone, and calcitonin. More extensive discussions of calcium physiology are found elsewhere.[109]

Drug- and toxin-induced hypercalcemia is uncommon and usually relates to agents that increase calcium in the diet (antacids) or decrease its elimination (thiazides).[16] Cholecalciferol, available as a rodenticide, can increase serum calcium by increasing its release from bone, increasing GI absorption, and decreasing renal elimination (Chap. 89). Vitamin D intoxication from excessive supplementation of milk can also cause hypercalcemia.[73] Other causes of hypercalcemia are listed in Table 15–9.

Symptoms of hypercalcemia consist of lethargy, muscle weakness, nausea, vomiting, and constipation. Life-threatening manifestations include complications

TABLE 15–9. CAUSES OF ALTERED SERUM CALCIUM

Hypocalcemia	Hypercalcemia
Aminoglycosides	Aluminum
Bicarbonate	Androgens
Calcitonin	Antacids (magnesium containing)
Ethanol	Antacids (calcium containing)
Ethylene glycol	Cholecalciferol
Fluoride	Glucocorticoids
Furosemide	Tamoxifen
Mithramycin	Thiazide diuretics
Neomycin	Lithium
Phenobarbital	Vitamin A
Phenytoin	
Phosphate	
Theophylline	

from altered mental status (aspiration), ECG changes (Chap. 8), and cardiac dysrhythmias. Treatment of clinically significant hypercalcemia focuses on removing the offending agent when possible, decreasing GI absorption, increasing distribution into bone, and enhancing elimination through forced diuresis.[109,134]

Drug- and toxin-induced hypocalcemia is more common than hypercalcemia. Minor, often clinically insignificant, decreases in serum calcium occur in association with anticonvulsant and aminoglycoside therapy.[16] Severe, life-threatening hypocalcemia can occur, however, as a manifestation of fluoride toxicity from hydrofluoric acid (Chap. 86).[33,135] Direct complexation with fluoride ion is responsible for the rapid production of hypocalcemia in this setting. This mechanism is distinct when compared to other drugs and toxins (Table 15–9) that produce hypocalcemia by decreased absorption, enhanced renal loss, or redistribution.

Symptoms of hypocalcemia consist largely of neuromuscular findings, including paresthesias, cramps, carpopedal spasm, tetany, and seizures. Although ECG abnormalities are common (Chap. 8), life-threatening dysrhythmias are rare. Treatment strategies focus on calcium replacement. When hypomagnesemia or hyperphosphatemia is present, these abnormalities must be corrected or calcium replacement will fail.[109]

Magnesium

Magnesium is the fourth most abundant cation in the body (after calcium, sodium, and potassium), with a normal total body store of about 2020 mEq in a 70-kg human.[111] Like calcium, a substantial percentage of magnesium (about 50%) is stored in bone, with most of the remainder distributed in the soft tissues. Only about 1–2% of magnesium is located in the extracellular fluid; therefore, serum levels correlate poorly with total body stores.[112] Magnesium homeostasis is maintained through dietary intake and renal and GI losses, modulated by hormonal effects.

Clinically significant hypermagnesemia is uncommon in the absence of renal failure, except when massive parenteral infusions of magnesium salts overwhelm renal compensatory mechanisms. This has been reported with inadvertent intravenous infusion,[14,63] urologic procedures involving irrigation with magnesium salts,[39,74] and ingestion of large quantities of magnesium-containing cathartics.[40,46,51] The greatest concern is iatrogenic overdose from the use of magnesium-containing cathartics as part of routine poison management.[48,75,127] In a series of poisoned patients, single-dose magnesium cathartic failed to produce any demonstrable rise in serum magnesium concentrations.[128] However, patients who received three doses of magnesium sulfate over 8 hours had a statistically significant increase in their magnesium concentration.[128] Thus, as with sorbitol use, the potential for iatrogenic toxicity exists, mandating cautious use of magnesium-containing cathartics, especially in patients with renal insufficiency. Other causes of hypermagnesemia are listed in Table 15–10.

TABLE 15–10. CAUSES OF ALTERED SERUM MAGNESIUM

Hypomagnesemia	Hypermagnesemia
Aminoglycosides	Antacids (magnesium containing)
Amphotericin	Cathartics (magnesium containing)
Cisplatin	Lithium
DDT	
Ethanol	
Fluoride	
Laxatives	
Loop diuretics	
Methylxanthines	
Osmotic diuretics	
Phosphates	
Strychnine	
Theophylline	
Thiazide diuretics	

The symptoms of hypermagnesemia correlate roughly with serum concentrations but depend somewhat on the rate of increase and host factors. At magnesium concentrations of about 3–10 mEq/L, patients feel weak, nauseated, flushed, and thirsty. Bradycardia, hypotension, and decreased deep tendon reflexes are noted. As levels increase, hypoventilation, muscle paralysis, and ventricular dysrhythmias occur. Magnesium levels greater than 10 mEq/L, especially those greater than 15 mEq/L, are often associated with fatal events.

Hypermagnesemia should be considered a life-threatening disorder. When significant neuromuscular or ECG manifestations are noted, parenteral administration of calcium will reverse some of the toxicity.[59] Further therapy should focus on enhancing elimination with fluid resuscitation and loop diuretics.[59] Hemodialysis will rapidly correct hypermagnesemia when renal function is inadequate.

Drug- and toxin-induced hypomagnesemia is common, but rarely life-threatening. Renal losses (from diuretics and renal tubular acidosis), GI losses (from ethanol), and complexation (from fluoride or hyperphosphatemia) are common. Other causes of hypomagnesemia are listed in Table 15–10. These are the same mechanisms that produce other electrolyte abnormalities, so when hypomagnesemia is suspected or discovered, other electrolyte abnormalities are usually present.

The symptoms of hypomagnesemia are lethargy, weakness, fatigue, neuromuscular excitation (tremor and hyperreflexia), nausea, and vomiting.[25,30] Dysrhythmias can occur, especially during therapy with cardiac glycosides. Signs and symptoms consistent with hypocalcemia and hypokalemia may also be present.

Treatment involves removing the offending agent (if it can be identified) and restoring magnesium balance. Although either oral or parenteral supplementation is usually acceptable for mild hypomagnesemia, parenteral therapy is required when significant clinical effects are present. Most authors suggest that in the absence of renal insufficiency a safe dose of magnesium sulfate in the adult is 16 mEq (2 g) infused over several minutes,[25,71] to a maximum of 1 mEq/kg of magnesium in a 24-hour period (1 g of magnesium sulfate contains about 8 mEq of magnesium). During this time, frequent serum magnesium determinations should be obtained and the presence of reflexes documented. If hyporeflexia occurs, the magnesium infusion should be discontinued.

Summary

The evaluation of fluid, electrolyte, and acid–base status is a fundamental component of the management of the poisoned or overdose patient. A clear appreciation of the pathophysiologic causes of these abnormalities and a rational approach to their correction is essential for reducing the mortality and morbidity from poisoning. In addition, many fluid and electrolyte abnormalities result from adverse drug reactions and therefore become part of the routine patient evaluation.

References

1. Adrogue HJ, Brensilver J, Madias NE: Changes in the plasma anion gap during chronic metabolic acid–base disturbances. Am J Physiol 1978;235:291–297.
2. Adrogue HJ, Wilson H, Boyd AE, et al: Plasma acid–base patterns in diabetic ketoacidosis. N Engl J Med 1982;307: 1603–1610.
3. Albert MD, Dell RB, Winters RW: Quantitative displacement of acid–base equilibrium in metabolic acidosis. Ann Intern Med 1967;66:312–322.
4. Allon M, Dunlay R, Copkney C: Nebulized albuterol for acute hyperkalemia in patients on hemodialysis. Ann Intern Med 1989;110:426–429.
5. Ammar KA, Heckerling PS: Ethylene glycol poisoning with a normal anion gap caused by concurrent ethanol ingestion: importance of the osmolal gap. Am J Kidney Dis 1996;27:130–133.
6. Anderson IK, Martin GR, Ramage AG: Central administration of 5-HT activates 5-HT_{1A} receptors cause sympathoexcitation and 5-HT_2/5-HT_{1C} receptors to release vasopressin in anaesthetized rats. Br J Pharmacol 1992;107: 1020–1028.
7. Andreoli TE: The posterior pituitary. In: Wyngaarden JB, Smith LH, eds: Cecil Textbook of Medicine, 18th ed. Philadelphia, Saunders, 1988, pp. 1305–1313.
8. Ayus JC, Arieff AI: Symptomatic hyponatremia: Making the diagnosis rapidly. J Crit Ill 1990;5:846–856.
9. Ayus JC, Krothapalli RK, Arieff AI: Treatment of symptomatic hyponatremia and its relation to brain damage: A prospective study. N Engl J Med 1987;317:1190–1195.
10. Barter FC: The syndrome of inappropriate secretion of antidiuretic hormone (SIADH). Disease of the Month 1973; Nov:1–47.
11. Battle DC, Hizon M, Cohen E, et al: The use of the urinary anion gap in the diagnosis of hyperchloremic metabolic acidosis. N Engl J Med 1988;318:594–599.
12. Battle DC, von Riotte AB, Aviria M, Grup M: Amelioration of polyuria by amiloride in patients receiving long-term lithium therapy. N Engl J Med 1985;312:408–414.
13. Bismuth C, Gaultier M, Conso F, et al: Hyperkalemia in acute digitalis poisoning: Prognostic significance and therapeutic implications. Clin Toxicol 1973;6:153–162.
14. Bourgeois FJ, Thiagarajah S, Harbert GM, et al: Profound hypotension complicating magnesium therapy. Am J Obstet Gynecol 1986;154:919–920.
15. Bower BR, Wegienka LC, Forsham PH: In vitro studies of mechanism of polyuria induced by dextropropoxyphene (Darvon). Proc Soc Exp Biol Med 1965;120:155–157.
16. Brass EP, Thompson WL: Drug-induced electrolyte abnormalities. Med Toxicol 1982;24:207–228.
17. Brenner BE: Clinical significance of the elevated anion gap. Am J Med 1985;79:289–296.
18. Britten JS, Myers RA, Benner C, et al: Blood ethanol and serum osmolality in the trauma patient. Am Surg 1982; 48:451–455.
19. Caldwell JW, Nava AJ, DeHaas DD: Hypernatremia associated with cathartics in overdose management. West J Med 1987;147:593–596.
20. Catalano G, Kanfer SN, Catalano MC, Alberts VA: The role of sertraline in a patient with recurrent hyponatremia. Gen Hosp Psychiatry 1996;18: 278–283.
21. Champion HR, Baker SP, Benner C, et al: Alcohol intoxication and serum osmolality. Lancet 1975;1:1402–1404.
22. Chan TY: Indapamide-induced severe hyponatremia and hypokalemia. Ann Pharmacother 1995;29:1124–1128.
23. Connelly DM: Silver nitrate, ideal burn wound therapy? NY State J Med 1970;70:1642–1644.
24. Cox M, Singer I: Lithium and water metabolism. Am J Med 1975;59:153–157.
25. Cronin RE, Knochel JP: Magnesium deficiency. Adv Intern Med 1983;28:509–533.
26. Decaux G, Schlesser M, Coffernils M, et al: Uric acid, anion gap and urea concentration in the diagnostic approach to hyponatremia. Clin Nephrol 1994;42:102–108.
27. DeFronzo RA, Bia M: Intravenous potassium chloride therapy. JAMA 1981;245:2446. Letter.
28. Delaney V, de Pertuz Y, Nixon D: Indomethacin in streptozocin-induced nephrogenic diabetes insipidus. Am J Kidney Dis 1987;9:79–83.
29. DiNubile MJ: The increment in the anion gap: Overextension of a concept. Lancet 1988;2:951–952.
30. Dirks JH: The kidney and magnesium regulation. Kidney Int 1983;23:771–777.
31. Dorwart WV, Chalmers L: Comparison of methods for calculating serum osmolality from chemical concentrations, and the prognostic value of such calculations. Clin Chem 1975;21:190–194.
32. Earley LE, Orloff J: The mechanism of antidiuresis associated with administration of hydrochlorothiazide to patients with vasopressin resistant diabetes insipidus. J Clin Invest 1962;41:1988–1997.
33. Edelman P: Hydrofluoric acid burns: State of the art review. Occup Med 1986;1:89–103.
34. Edwards CRW: Lessons from licorice. N Engl J Med 1991; 325:1242–1243.
35. Eisen TF, Lacouture PG, Woolf A: Serum osmolality in alcohol ingestions: Differences in availability among laboratories of teaching hospital, nonteaching hospital, and commercial facilities. Am J Emerg Med 1989;7:256–259.
36. Emmet M, Narins RG: Clinical use of the anion gap. Medicine 1977;56:38–54.

37. Farese RV, Biglieri EG, Shackleton CHL: Licorice induced hypermineralocorticoidism. N Engl J Med 1991;325: 1223–1227.
38. Farley TA: Severe hypernatremic dehydration after use of an activated charcoal–sorbitol suspension. J Pediatr 1986;109:719–722.
39. Fassler CA, Rodriguez M, Badesch DB, et al: Magnesium toxicity as a cause of hypotension and hypoventilation: Occurrence in patients with normal renal function. Arch Intern Med 1985;145:1604–1606.
40. Ferdinandus J, Pederson JA, Whang R: Hypermagnesemia as a cause of refractory hypotension, respiratory depression, and coma. Arch Intern Med 1981;141:669–670.
41. Fichman MP, Vorherr H, Kleeman CR, et al: Diuretic-induced hyponatremia. Ann Intern Med 1971;75:853–863.
42. Forrest JN, Cox M, Hong C, et al: Superiority of demeclocycline over lithium in the treatment of chronic syndrome of inappropriate secretion of antidiuretic hormone. N Engl J Med 1978;298:173–177.
43. Gabow PA: Disorders associated with an altered anion gap. Kidney Int 1985;27:472–483.
44. Gabow PA, Kaehny WD, Fennessey PV, et al: Diagnostic importance of an increased serum anion gap. N Engl J Med 1980;303:854–858.
45. Gamble JL: Chemical Anatomy, Physiology, and Pathology of Extracellular Fluids: A Lecture Syllabus, 6th ed. Cambridge, MA, Harvard University Press, 1960, p. 131.
46. Garcia-Webb P, Bhagat C: Hypermagnesaemia and hypophosphataemia after ingestion of magnesium sulfate. Br Med J 1984;288:759.
47. Garella S, Chazan JA, Cohen JJ: Saline-resistant metabolic alkalosis or "chloride wasting nephropathy." Ann Intern Med 1970;73:31–38.
48. Garrelts JC, Watson WA, Holloway KD, et al: Magnesium toxicity secondary to catharsis during management of theophylline poisoning. Am J Emerg Med 1989;7:34–37.
49. Gazda-Smith E, Synhawsky A: Hypernatremia following treatment of theophylline toxicity with activated charcoal and sorbitol. Arch Intern Med 1990;150:689–690.
50. Gennari FJ: Serum osmolality: Uses and limitations. N Engl J Med 1984;310:102–105.
51. Gerard SK, Hernandez C, Khayam-Bashi H: Extreme hypermagnesemia caused by an overdose of magnesium-containing cathartics. Ann Emerg Med 1988;17:728–731.
52. Glasser DS: The utility of the serum osmol gap in the diagnosis of methanol or ethylene glycol ingestion. Ann Emerg Med 1996;27:343–346.
53. Glasser L, Sternglanz PD, Combie J, Robinson A: Serum osmolality and its applicability to drug overdose. Am J Clin Pathol 1973;60:695–699.
54. Goldman MA, Lisak R, Matz R, et al: Hypochloremic alkalosis with symptoms of seizure disorder. NY State J Med 1970;70:306–308.
55. Goldman MB, Luching DJ, Robertson GL: Mechanisms of altered water metabolism in psychotic patients with polydipsia and hyponatremia. N Engl J Med 1988;318:397–403.
56. Goldstein MD, Bear R, Richardson RMA, et al: The urine anion gap: A clinically useful index of ammonium excretion. Am J Med Sci 1986;292:198–202.
57. Goldstein RJ, Lichtenstein NS, Souder D: The myth of the low anion gap. JAMA 1980;243:1737–1738.
58. Goodkin OH, Krishna GG, Narins RG: The role of the anion gap in detecting and managing mixed acid–base disorders. Clin Endocrinol Metab 1984;13:333–349.
59. Graber TW, Yee AS, Baker FJ: Magnesium: Physiology, clinical disorders and therapy. Ann Emerg Med 1981;10: 49–57.
60. Harrington JT: Metabolic alkalosis. Kidney Int 1984;26: 88–97.
61. Hoekstra PT, Kahnoski R, McCamish MA, et al: Transurethral prostatic resection syndrome—A new perspective: encephalopathy with associated hyperammonemia. J Urol 1983:130:704–707.
62. Hoffman RS, Smilkstein MJ, Howland MA, Goldfrank LR: Osmol gaps revisited: normal values and limitations. J Toxicol Clin Toxicol 1993;31:81–93.
63. Hoffman RS, Smilkstein MJ, Rubenstein F: An "amp" by any other name: The hazards of intravenous magnesium dosing. JAMA 1989;261:557. Letter.
64. Hohler T, Teuber G, Wanitschke R: Indomethacin treatment in amphotericin B induced nephrogenic diabetes insipidus. Clin Invest 1994;72:769–771.
65. Hohnloser SH, Verrier RL, Lown B, et al: Effect of hypokalemia on susceptibility to ventricular fibrillation in the normal and ischemic canine heart. Am Heart J 1986; 112:32–35.
66. Holden R, Jackson MA: Near-fatal hyponatraemic coma due to vasopressin over-secretion after "ecstasy" (3,4-MDMA). Lancet 1996;347:1052. Letter.
67. Hubbard JI, Lin N, Sibbald JR: Subfornical organ lesions in rats abolish hyperdipsic effects of isoproterenol and serotonin. Brain Res Bull 1989;23:41–45.
68. Iberti TJ, Leibowitz AB, Papadakos PJ, Fischer EP: Low sensitivity of the anion gap as a screen to detect hyperlactatemia in critically ill patients. Crit Care Med 1990;18: 275–277.
69. Inaba H, Hirasawa H, Mizuguchi T: Serum osmolality gap in postoperative patients in intensive care. Lancet 1987; 1:1331–1335.
70. Ireland JT, Thomson WS: Euglycemic diabetic ketoacidosis. Br Med J 1973;3:107.
71. Iseri LT, Freed J, Bures AR: Magnesium deficiency and cardiac disorders. Am J Med 1975;58:837–845.
72. Ivoino M, Steardo L: Effect of substances influencing brain serotonergic transmission on plasma vasopressin levels in the rat. Eur J Pharmacol 1985;113:99–103.
73. Jacobus CH, Holick MF, Shao Q, et al: Hypervitaminosis D associated with drinking milk. N Engl J Med 1992;326: 1173–1177.
74. Jenny DB, Goris GB, Urwiller RD, et al: Hypermagnesemia following irrigation of renal pelvis: cause of respiratory depression. JAMA 1978;240:1378–1379.
75. Jones J, Heiselman D, Dougherty J, et al: Cathartic-induced magnesium toxicity during overdose management. Ann Emerg Med 1986;15:1214–1218.
76. Kassirer JP, Berkman PM, Lawrenz DR, Schwartz WB: The critical role of chloride in the correction of hypokalemic alkalosis in man. Am J Med 1965;38:172–189.
77. Kessler J, Samuels SC: Sertraline and hyponatremia. N Engl J Med 1996;335:524. Letter.
78. Knochel JP: Neuromuscular manifestations of electrolyte disorders. Am J Med 1982;72:521–535.

79. Kovacs L, Robertson GL: Syndrome of inappropriate antidiuresis. Endocrinol Metab Clin North Am 1992;21: 859–875.
80. Kruse JA, Carlson RW: Rapid correction of hypokalemia using concentrated intravenous potassium chloride infusions. Arch Intern Med 1990;150:613–617.
81. Kulberg A: Urinalysis and urine culture. In: Flomenbaum N, Goldfrank LR, eds: Diagnostic Testing in the Emergency Department. Rockville, MD, Aspen, 1984, pp. 19–29.
82. Lavie CH, Crocker EF, Key KJ, et al: Marked hypochloremic metabolic alkalosis with severe compensatory hypoventilation. South Med J 1986;79:1296–1299.
83. Libber S, Harison H, Spector D: Treatment of nephrogenic diabetes insipidus with prostaglandin synthesis inhibitors. J Pediatr 1986;108:305–311.
84. Lichstein E, Chadda K, Fenig S: Atrial pacing in the treatment of refractory ventricular tachycardia associated with hypokalemia. Am J Cardiol 1972;30:550–553.
85. Liu BA, Mittmann N, Knowles SR, Shear NH: Hyponatremia and the syndrome of inappropriate secretion of antidiuretic hormone associated with the use of selective serotonin reuptake inhibitors: a review of spontaneous reports. Can Med Assoc J 1996;155:519–527.
86. Lubash GD, Cohen BD, Young CW, et al: Severe metabolic alkalosis with neurologic abnormalities. N Engl J Med 1958;258:1050–1052.
87. Lundberg P: The effect of adrenergic blockade on potassium concentrations in different conditions. Acta Med Scand 1983;672(suppl):121–152.
88. Lydiard RB, Gelenberg AJ: Hazards and adverse effects of lithium. Annu Rev Med 1982;33:327–344.
89. Masson EA: Mesalazine associated nephrogenic diabetes insipidus presenting as weight loss. Gut 1992;33:563–564.
90. Mazze RI, Trudell JR, Cousins MJ: Methoxyflurane metabolism and renal dysfunction: Clinical correlation in man. Anesthesiology 1971;35:247–252.
91. McCarron D: Correcting potassium depletion. Drug Ther 1979;4:65–72.
92. Mennen M, Slovis CM: Severe metabolic alkalosis in the emergency department. Ann Emerg Med 1988;17:354–357.
93. Mercado R, Michelis MF: Severe sodium depletion syndrome during lithium carbonate therapy. Arch Intern Med 1977;137:1731–1733.
94. Mizutani AR, Parker J, Katz J, et al: Visual disturbances, serum glycine levels and transurethral resection of the prostate. J Urol 1990;144:697–699.
95. Moder KG, Hurley DL: Fatal hypernatremia from exogenous salt intake: Report of a case and review of the literature. Mayo Clin Proc 1990;65:1587–1594.
96. Morganroth ML: Six steps to acid–base analysis: Clinical applications. J Crit Ill 1990;5:460–469.
97. Moses AM, Miller M, Streeten DHP: Pathophysiologic and pharmacologic alterations in the release and action of ADH. Metabolism 1976;25:697–721.
98. Moses AM, Miller M: Drug-induced dilutional hyponatremia. N Engl J Med 1974;291:1234–1239.
99. Moses AM, Notman DD: Diabetes insipidus and syndrome of inappropriate antidiuretic hormone secretion (SIADH). Adv Intern Med 1982;27:73–100.
100. Narins RG, Emmett M: Simple and mixed acid–base disorders: A practical approach. Medicine 1980;59:161–187.
101. Navarro JF, Quereda C, Quereda C, et al: Nephrogenic diabetes insipidus and renal tubular acidosis secondary to foscarnet therapy. Am J Kidney Dis 1996;27:431–434.
102. Oh MS, Carroll HJ: Current concepts: The anion gap. N Engl J Med 1977;297:814–817.
103. Oster JR, Perez GO, Masterson BJ: Use of the anion gap in clinical medicine. South Med J 1988;81:229–237.
104. Osterloh JD, Kelly TJ, Khayam-Bashi H, Romeo R: Discrepancies in osmolal gaps and calculated alcohol concentrations. Arch Pathol Lab Med 1996;120:634–641.
105. Pappas AA, Gadsden RH, Taylor EH: Serum osmolality in acute intoxication: A prospective study. Am J Clin Pathol 1985;84:74–79.
106. Perez GO, Oster JR: Acid–base disorders: II. Use of $\Delta AG/\Delta HCO_3$ in evaluating mixed acid–base disorders—A patient management problem. South Med J 1986;79: 882–886.
107. Perrone J, Hoffman RS: Compensatory hypoventilation in metabolic alkalosis. Acad Emerg Med 1996;3:981–982.
108. Ponce SP, Jennings AE, Madias NE, et al: Drug-induced hyperkalemia. Medicine 1985;64:357–370.
109. Potts JT: Diseases of the parathyroid gland and other hyper- and hypocalcemic disorders. In Wilson JD, Braunwald E, Isselbacher KJ, et al, eds: Harrison's Principles of Internal Medicine, 12th ed. New York, McGraw-Hill, 1991, pp. 1902–1921.
110. Quinn BP: Nephrogenic diabetes insipidus and tubulointerstitial nephritis during continuous therapy with rifampin. Am J Kidney Dis 1989;14:217–220.
111. Randall RE, Cohen MD, Spray CC, et al: Hypermagnesemia in renal failure: Etiology and toxic manifestations. Ann Intern Med 1964;61:73–88.
112. Reinhart RA: Magnesium metabolism: a review with special reference to the relationship between intracellular content and serum levels. Arch Intern Med 1988;148: 2415–2420.
113. Riggs AT, Dysken MW, Kim SW, Opsahl JA: A review of disorders of water homeostasis in psychiatric patients. Psychosomatics 1991;32:133–148.
114. Robinson AG, Loeb JN: Ethanol ingestion: Commonest cause of elevated plasma osmolality? N Engl J Med 1971;284:1253–1255.
115. Rosa RM, Silva P, Young JB, et al: Adrenergic modulation of extrarenal potassium disposal. N Engl J Med 1980; 302:431–434.
116. Sakane N, Yoshida T, Umekawa T, Miyazaki R: Nephrogenic diabetes insipidus induced by lobenzarit disodium treatment in patients with rheumatoid arthritis. Intern Med 1996;35:119–122.
117. Salem MM, Mujais SK: Gaps in the anion gap. Arch Intern Med 1992;152:1625–1629.
118. Saxena K: Clinical features and management of poisoning due to potassium chloride. Med Toxicol Adverse Drug Exp 1989;4:429–433.
119. Saxena K: Death from potassium chloride overdose. Postgrad Med 1988;84:97–102.
120. Schelling JR, Howard RL, Winter SD, Linas SL: Increased osmolal gap in alcoholic ketoacidosis and lactic acidosis. Ann Intern Med 1990;113:580–582.
121. Schwartz SM, Carroll HM, Scharschmidt LA: Sublimed (inorganic) sulfur ingestion. A cause of life-threatening

metabolic acidosis with a high anion gap. Arch Intern Med 1986;146:1437–1438.
122. Schwartz WB, Orning KJ, Porter R: The internal distribution of hydrogen ions with varying degrees of metabolic acidosis. J Clin Invest 1957;36:373–382.
123. Scoggin C, McClellan JR, Cary JM: Hypernatraemia and acidosis in association with topical treatment of burns. Lancet 1977;1:959. Letter.
124. Singer I, Rotenberg D: Demeclocycline-induced nephrogenic diabetes insipidus. Ann Intern Med 1973;79:679–683.
125. Singer I, Rotenberg D: Mechanisms of lithium action. N Engl J Med 1973;289:254–260.
126. Sklar AH, Linas SL: The osmolal gap in renal failure. Ann Intern Med 1983;98:481–482.
127. Smilkstein MJ, Smolinske SC, Kulig KW, et al: Severe hypermagnesemia due to multiple-dose cathartic therapy. West J Med 1988;148:208–211.
128. Smilkstein MJ, Steedle D, Kulig KW, et al: Magnesium levels after magnesium-containing cathartics. J Toxicol Clin Toxicol 1988;26:51–65.
129. Smithline N, Gardner KD: Gaps: Anionic and osmolal. JAMA 1976;236:1594–1597.
130. Sonnenblick M, Rosin A: Increased uric acid clearance in the syndrome of inappropriate secretion of antidiuretic hormone. Isr J Med Sci 1988;24:20–23.
131. Spigset O, Hedenmalm K: Hyponatremia and the syndrome of inappropriate antidiuretic hormone secretion (SIADH) induced by psychotropic drugs. Drug Safety 1995;12:209–225.
132. Steinhart B: Case report: Severe ethylene glycol intoxication with normal osmolal gap—"A chilling thought." J Emerg Med 1990;8:583–585.
133. Sterns RH, Riggs JE, Schochet SS: Osmotic demyelination syndrome following correction of hyponatremia. N Engl J Med 1986;314:1535–1542.
134. Suki WN, Yium JJ, Von Minden M, et al: Acute treatment of hypercalcemia with furosemide. N Engl J Med 1970; 283:836–840.
135. Tepperman PB: Fatality due to acute systemic fluoride poisoning following a hydrofluoric acid skin burn. J Occup Med 1980;22:691–692.
136. Van Amelsvoort T, Bakshi R, Devaux CB, Schwabe S: Hyponatremia associated with carbamazepine and oxcarbamazepine therapy: A review. Epilepsia 1994;35:181–188.
137. Vokes TJ, Robertson GL: Disorders of antidiuretic hormone. Endocrinol Metab Clin North Am 1988;17:281–299.
138. Wax PM, Wang R, Mercurio M, et al: The prevalence of sorbitol in repetitive dose activated charcoal regimens in emergency departments. Ann Emerg Med 1993;22: 1807–1812.
139. Wetherill SF, Guarino MJ, Cox RW: Acute renal failure associated with barium chloride poisoning. Ann Intern Med 1981;95:187–188.
140. Wilkins B: Cerebral oedema after MDMA ("ecstasy") and unrestricted water intake. Hyponatraemia must be treated with low water input. Br Med J 1996;313:689–690. Letter.
141. Winter SD, Pearson R, Gabow PA, et al: The fall of the serum anion gap. Arch Intern Med 1990;150:311–313.
142. Witte DL, Rodgers JL, Barrett DA: The anion gap: Its use in quality control. Clin Chem 1976;22:643–646.
143. Wrenn K: The delta gap: An approach to mixed acid–base disorders. Ann Emerg Med 1990;19:1310–1313.
144. Wrenn KD, Slovis CM, Slovis BS: The ability of physicians to predict hyperkalemia from the ECG. Ann Emerg Med 1991;20:1229–1232.

CHAPTER 16

Mutagens, Carcinogens, and Teratogens

Debra Kennedy, Kathleen A. Delaney, and Gideon Koren

Toxins injure living organisms by interfering with critical metabolic processes, causing structural injury to cells, or altering the cellular genetic material. Many specific types of injury to the genome that may result in genetic mutations are well described. Mechanisms of tumor formation or carcinogenesis are less clearly understood and documented. The general principles relevant to an understanding of the mechanisms of mutagenesis and carcinogenesis are outlined.

The teratogenesis section of the chapter focuses on the different ways that the extent of fetal xenobiotic exposure can be more accurately determined. The various biologic markers of fetal exposure that are currently available and the ways in which they may be used to counsel couples at risk as well as to gain a more quantitative estimate of the true extent of fetal xenobiotic exposure are discussed.

The Chemistry of the Genome: A Brief Review

DNA (deoxyribonucleic acid) is the primary genetic material of eukaryotic cells. It is composed of chains of nucleotide bases that pair with a second, complementary chain to form a double-stranded structure known as a double helix. The human genome is incorporated into 23 pairs of chromosomes (22 autosomes and 1 pair of sex chromosomes). All somatic cells contain a diploid number of chromosomes (46), while germ cells contain a haploid number (23).

DNA is transcribed into RNA (ribonucleic acid), which is then translated into amino acids. In DNA, the purine bases adenine and guanine always pair with the pyrimidine bases thymine and cytosine, respectively. In RNA the pyrimidine base uracil substitutes for thymine. The structures of the nucleotide base precursors are illustrated in Figure 16–1.

A typical hypothetical DNA sequence might be:

5′-AAATTGGGCCTACGGCTA-3′

3′-TTTAACCCGGATGCCGAT-5′

The 3′–5′ section of this sequence would be transcribed into single-stranded messenger RNA (mRNA) with the following sequence:

5′-AAAUUGGGCCUACGGCUA-3′

When the messenger RNA strand is translated into protein, each set of three bases will code for a specific amino acid. The code is redundant, so that several different triplets may code for the same amino acid. This hypothetical segment of mRNA would code for a protein with the following amino acid sequence:

5′-AAA UUG GGC CUA CGG CUA-3′

lysine–leucine–glycine–leucine–threonine–leucine

Mutagens

Mutagens are agents that produce alterations in DNA. They may interact with the DNA molecule in a number of ways to produce chemical injury. Not every alteration or mutation in DNA will have an effect on gene expression.

For example, a DNA alteration such that the third base of mRNA in the above sequence is changed from A to G would have no effect on the protein synthesized, as both AAA and AAG code for the amino acid lysine. However, a change of the second base to guanine (A to

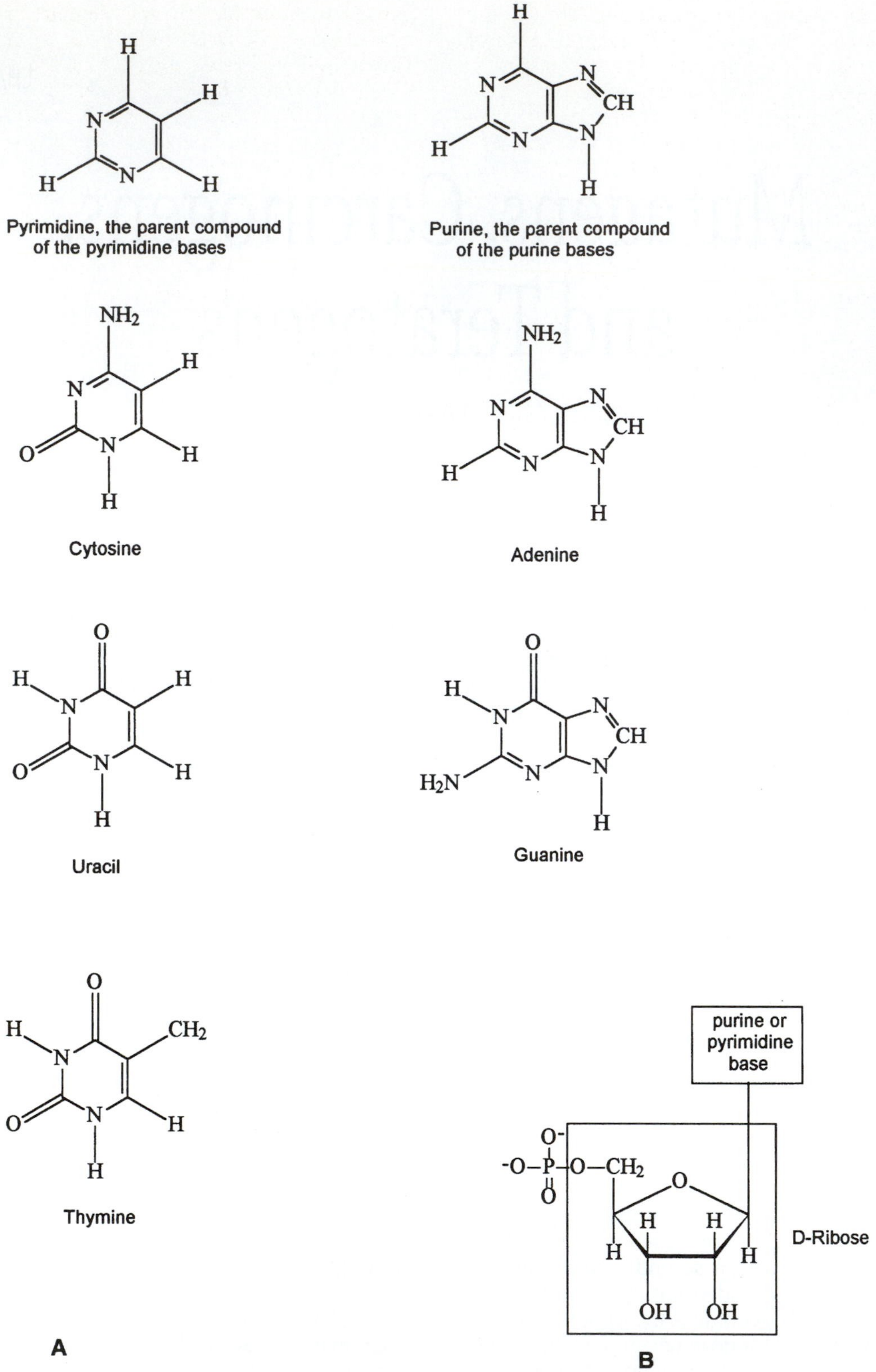

Figure 16–1. (**A**) The structures of the purine and pyrimidine bases. (**B**) The general structure of a nucleotide. *(Reprinted, with permission, from Lehninger AL: Principles of Biochemistry. New York, Worth, 1982.)*

G) would result in arginine being incorporated into the protein, as AGA codes for arginine. The significance of this change depends on the importance of that particular amino acid alteration on protein structure and function. Some amino acid changes have no clinical effect at all and are known as polymorphisms. Other changes will have profound clinical effects and result in absent or abnormal protein (gene product). For example, one of the commonest genetic disorders in the world is sickle cell disease, which results from a single amino acid change in the hemoglobin molecule, producing an abnormal hemoglobin called hemoglobin S.

In the above mRNA, a mutation that would cause the fifth base (uracil) to change to adenine (U to A) would result in the codon UAG, which is a "stop codon" and signals the termination of protein synthesis. Clearly, this could have a deleterious effect on the final protein product depending upon the part of the sequence where it occurred.[40] Deletion or addition of a DNA base pair causes a "frame-shift mutation," which puts the triplet code out of sequence. Again, depending on where in the sequence it occurs, a frame shift may have a significant impact on the final protein product.

The following simple linguistic example illustrates the effect of a frame-shift mutation:

CAN THE CAT EAT THE RAT

becomes:

CAN HEC ATE ATT HER AT

This makes no sense at all. A comparable effect would be seen in the protein product of messenger RNA transcribed from a frame-shift mutation.

Other mutagens act on the chromosomes during cell division, causing large breaks and consequently deletions and rearrangements at the time of crossover during mitosis.[40] Mutations can occur both in somatic (body) cells and in germ (gonadal) cells. The implications of germ cell mutations are that these errors may be passed on to the individual's offspring and hence to subsequent generations.

A number of biochemical mechanisms may lead to the above-mentioned alterations in cellular DNA. Base pair changes can result from a direct chemical action on a base. For example, nitrous acid (HNO_2) deaminates adenine to form hypoxanthine, which pairs with cytosine. This leads to an A:T to G:C mutation (Fig. 16–2). Alkylation of the N7 or O6 positions of guanine may cause a G:C to A:T change[40] (Fig. 16–2).

Incorporation of abnormal analogs into DNA occurs only when the cell is dividing and DNA is being replicated. These abnormal analogs may result in single base pair mutations. For example, the keto form of 5-bromouracil closely resembles thymine and may be inserted as a nucleotide in place of thymidine triphosphate during DNA replication. It may then spontaneously convert to its enol form, which pairs more readily with guanine. Further replication would therefore result in an A:T to G:C base pair mutation.[40] Frame-shift mutations may be caused by intercalation of a foreign molecule such as acridine into the DNA chain prior to replication. When the chain is replicated, an additional base is inserted opposite acridine. Alkylating agents may cause alteration of bases so that they cannot pair, leading to deletion of a base pair and a frame-shift mutation. Alkylation and cross-linking of DNA strands during replication may also result in disruption of the chromosome during mitosis. These effects are more prominent in growing tissues, and this ability of alkylating agents is responsible for their therapeutic action of killing cancer cells as well as their carcinogenic property.

A simple in vitro measure of mutagenicity is the Ames test, which uses *Salmonella* bacteria that are unable to synthesize histidine. Mutagenic chemicals increase the likelihood of back mutations, which allow these bacteria to grow on histidine-free media. The number of colonies of altered bacteria growing on histidine-free media gives a quantitative measure of the capacity of the tested chemical to alter DNA.[2]

Mutagens that require metabolic activation are identified by the addition of liver homogenate to the Ames test. The Ames test is a good screening technique to determine whether a chemical has the potential to interact with DNA. However, it is clear that a simple in vitro test such as the Ames test cannot take into account all the complexities of the intact organism.

Not all mutagens are carcinogens: when used as a predictor of carcinogenicity, approximately 90% of known carcinogens react positively.

Carcinogens

Carcinogens are agents that cause neoplastic change. Most (but not all) classical carcinogens are also mutagens in that they alter DNA. While the biochemical mechanisms of alteration of DNA by foreign chemicals are fairly well characterized, the ultimate events leading to the unregulated growth of cells is not well understood.

Carcinogens such as estrogen and asbestos, which do not appear to affect DNA, are called epigenetic carcinogens. Their mechanisms of carcinogenicity are poorly understood and are not further addressed here. This section focuses on the toxicology of a number of well-studied mutagenic compounds known to be carcinogens.

It is clear from the list of agents in Table 16–1 that carcinogens are found in a wide variety of chemical classes and that they may be naturally occurring or synthetic agents.[3] For example, aflatoxin B1 is a potent liver carcinogen that is formed by molds that contaminate improperly stored foodstuffs; polycyclic aromatic amines such as benzo(*a*)pyrene are generated by partial combustion processes such as the charcoal cooking of food and burning wood.[52]

There are no simple structure–activity rules that can be applied to determine whether a given compound can be designated as a carcinogen (or noncarcinogen) solely on the basis of its chemical structure.

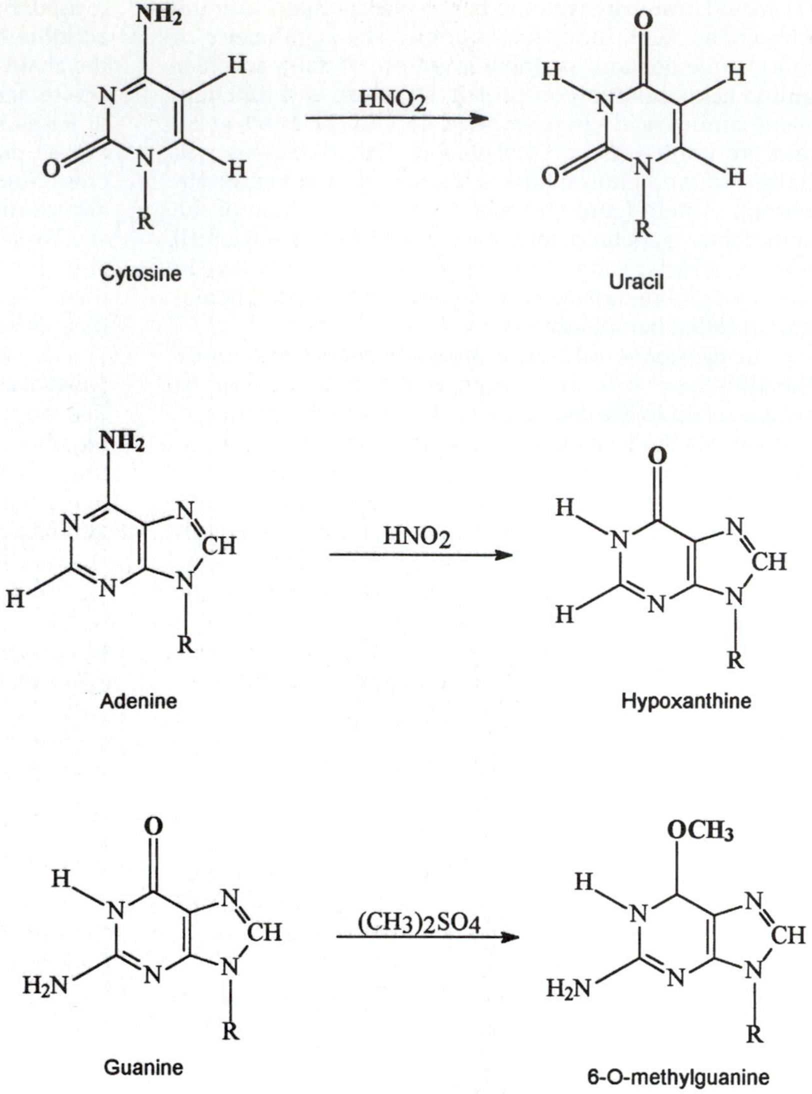

Figure 16–2. Deamination of cytosine and adenine by nitrous acid, a metabolite of nitrosamines. Methylation of guanine leads to faulty base pairing. *(Reprinted, with permission, from Lehninger AL: Principles of Biochemistry. New York, Worth, 1982.)*

Most mutagenic carcinogens interact with DNA in a way that may lead to persistent alteration of the cell's genome and its ability to normally regulate cell division. Whether or not the cellular DNA is permanently altered depends on a number of factors, including distribution, access to tissues, and biotransformation. Many mutations in DNA strands are recognized by the cell and are repaired before the damaged DNA is replicated and incorporated into new DNA or transcribed into RNA. The availability and efficiency of DNA repair systems in a particular tissue is an important factor influencing carcinogenicity. Replication of the cell with the unrepaired DNA still present is a requirement for permanent alteration of the genome.[70] Many DNA mutations are probably lethal to the cell carrying them. Individuals with conditions such as xeroderma pigmentosum where there is a genetic deficiency of DNA-repair enzymes exhibit an increased risk for the development of some, but not all, forms of cancer.

Carcinogenesis is a multistage biochemical and biologic process. In its simplest form the process can be divided into two major events: initiation and promotion. Initiation or neoplastic transformation involves the covalent binding of the ultimate carcinogen to DNA, resulting in alteration of the genetic code. Initiation can occur after a single exposure to the putative agent. Many chemicals known to cause cancer are not carcinogenic in the form in which they enter the body and require biotransformation to convert them from an inactive state into their ultimate carcinogenic form.[47] For example, polycyclic aromatic hydrocarbons such as benzo(*a*)-pyrene are chemically inert in their parent form and are unable to form covalent bonds with DNA. Enzyme systems biotransform these unreactive pro- or pre-carcinogens into chemically reactive (electron-deficient) products that can covalently bind with nucleophilic sites on cellular macromolecules. Metabolic activation generally requires more than one enzymatic step. Initial activation

TABLE 16–1. AGENTS IMPLICATED IN HUMAN CARCINOGENESIS

Acetophenitidin (phenacetin)	Cyclophosphamide
Aromatic amines	Diethylstilbestrol (DES)
Arsenic	Ionizing radiation
Aflatoxins	Melphalan
Benzene	Phenytoin
Benzidine	Tars, soots, mineral oils
Cadmium	Tobacco smoke
Carbon tetrachloride	Ultraviolet radiation
Chloramphenicol	Vinyl chloride
Chromium	

Modified, with permission, from Okey AB: Carcinogenesis and mutagenesis by xenobiotic chemicals. In: Kalent H, Roschlau WHE, eds: Principles of Medical Pharmacology, 5th ed. Toronto, Decker, 1989, pp. 632–643.

is often carried out by different enzymes of cytochrome P450, but activation by enzymes in the prostaglandin synthesis pathway as well as by reductases and peroxidases is also well established.[52]

Promotion refers to a poorly defined series of events that allow initiated cells to proliferate into tumors. Several chemicals that are not in themselves carcinogens are able to promote the development of tumors that have been initiated by other agents. Examples in experimental animals include phenol, DDT, cigarette smoke extracts, and polychlorinated biphenyls (PCBs). In contrast to initiating agents, promoting agents do not appear themselves to be mutagens.

In experimental settings, promoting agents must be given after treatment with the initiator and need to be given repeatedly over a prolonged period of time. The actions of promoters, unlike those of initiators, appear to be reversible, at least in the early stages of the process.

In recent years there has been great interest in "cancer genes." As a general model, it has been proposed that the conversion of proto-oncogenes into oncogenes is a key event in the initiation of tumors. Proto-oncogenes are normal cellular genes, most of which appear to code for cellular growth factors or growth factor receptors. When a proto-oncogene is damaged by a carcinogen (for example undergoes mutation or chromosomal breakage and translocation) the resulting oncogene drives the abnormal cell division and differentiation that is typical of neoplasia.

The site of tumor development is determined by the tissue and species-specific DNA repair systems, tissue activation and deactivation, the structure of the carcinogen, as well as the dosage. For example, the symmetric dialkylnitrosamines (Fig. 16–3) cause tumors in rats according to the chemical structure of the R group. The dimethyl and diethyl compounds cause liver cancer, while the dibutyl compound causes bladder cancer, and lung cancer is associated with the diamyl compound.

Large single doses of dimethylnitrosamine in rats lead to renal rather than hepatic carcinomas. Hamsters are deficient in a specific liver enzyme that repairs alkylated guanine bases in DNA and are thus highly susceptible to the hepatic carcinogenic effects of dimethylnitrosamine. In contrast, diethylnitrosamine primarily causes lung tumors in hamsters. Asymmetric nitrosamines cause cancer of the esophagus in rats.[77] These effects are specific to the structure of the carcinogen, the tissue affected, and the species, and in a very general way illustrate the enormous complexity of the interaction between living tissues and potential carcinogens.

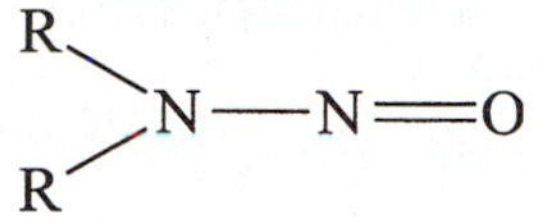

Figure 16–3. These symmetric dialkylnitrosamines cause tumors in rats, the type of which depends on the chemical structure of the R group.

Teratogens

Environmental insults that result in structural defects after fertilization are known as *teratogens*. The term is derived from the Greek words *teratos* (monster) and *gen* (producing). Those environmental influences that produce abnormalities of function rather than visible structural anomalies have been termed *hadegens* (derived from Hades, the Greek god of the underworld, who wore a helmet to render himself invisible). A third term, *trophogen*, is used to describe environmental agents that alter growth, because growth may be considered either morphologic or functional. A given environmental agent may cause all three types of effects, or may cause different effects according to the gestational timing of the exposure.[26] For example, rubella infection is teratogenic, hadegenic, and trophogenic in the first trimester, whereas after 20 weeks' gestation it is only hadegenic.

For both medical-legal and scientific reasons, there has been increasing interest in the field of teratology, particularly with regard to the relatively new field of neurobehavioral teratology (hadegenic agents). There has also been increased emphasis on providing "proof" of human teratogenicity. Unfortunately it may be difficult to prove that a particular insult or agent (xenobiotic) is teratogenic, hadegenic, or trophogenic. A number of approaches may be used to try and delineate potentially harmful fetal exposures.[8]

Qualitative Criteria for Proof of Teratogenicity

The first approach is to establish certain qualitative criteria for the proof of human teratogenicity.[69] Many recognized human teratogens do not fulfill all of the criteria shown in Table 16–2. For example, thalidomide, one of the major human teratogens, was not shown to be teratogenic in animal models. Therefore these criteria can be used only as guidelines, and need to be considered in conjunction with other relevant data.

TABLE 16–2. COMPILATION OF CRITERIA FOR PROOF OF HUMAN TERATOGENICITY

1. There should be proof of exposure to the agent having occurred at a critical stage(s) in prenatal development (evidence from prescriptions, physicians' records, dates of ingestion).
2. There should be findings from appropriately controlled epidemiologic studies that show that exposure to the agent produces an increase in the occurrence of specific phenotypic effects, and a recognizable pattern of both major and minor malformations. A particular defect (eg, Ebstein's anomaly in association with lithium exposure) or constellation of defects (eg, fetal hydantoin syndrome) is particularly helpful.
3. There should be animal models of the exposure that mimic the effects in humans, ideally at clinically comparable doses.
4. There should be a dose–response relationship that has been demonstrated in either animal models or human exposures, such that the greater the exposure, the more severe the fetal phenotypic effects. It should be noted that dose–response has not been shown for any of the well-known human teratogens, including retinoic acid, thalidomide, and diethylstilbestrol.
5. There should be biologic plausibility for the mechanism of action of the putative teratogenic agent (eg, retinoic acid appears to interfere with normal neural crest cell function and migration).
6. There may be a subset of exposed individuals who are intrinsically predisposed to the teratogenic effects of a particular agent due either to an inborn error of metabolism or to some other genetic polymorphism. This would provide a biologic explanation for the clinically well-recognized variability of teratogenic effects.

From references 6, 26, 69.

Another approach to attempt to qualify and/or quantify fetal exposure is to measure biologic markers of the putative teratogen in the fetus or neonate (or even in the mother), thereby gaining a semiquantitative estimate of the extent of teratogen exposure in utero. This approach may also yield a "fetal dose response" by estimating the dose and timing of a particular exposure.[6]

However, this approach is obviously not universally applicable for a number of reasons:

1. Exposure may be too early in gestation to be measured at a later stage of pregnancy.
2. Appropriate biologic markers may not exist for the particular xenobiotic.
3. Suitable body fluid samples may not be readily obtainable.

There are also a number of ethical issues that go beyond the scope of this text involved in the measurement, particularly in neonates, of biologic markers of in utero exposure, especially to illicit drugs such as cocaine and opioids.

It is clear that neither documentation of the extent of fetal exposure nor measurement of biologic markers alone can prove teratogenicity in a particular situation. A rational approach is to combine both the qualitative criteria and the biologic markers where available in an attempt to provide the mother with the best possible information and risk estimate.

Problems in Assessing Possible Fetal Exposure

Recall Bias

Often one of the major limitations in risk assessment is the mother's recall of her xenobiotic exposure. There may be a number of reasons for this, including genuine inability to recall details, guilt, denial, and the fact that in some instances the substances involved are illicit and admission of their use may result (in the mother's perception at least) in prosecution or the involvement of children's welfare agencies.

Case-control studies of teratogenic effects based on maternal recall have highlighted the inaccuracy of maternal recall, particularly in cases of adverse outcome. It has been shown that there is a recall bias in reporting gestational alcohol consumption in that women who have given birth to children with congenital defects tend to retrospectively minimize their history of alcohol ingestion compared with their reported consumption when questioned antenatally.[16]

It has also been shown that there is a less than optimal recall not only of drug dosages and gestational timing of the exposure, but also of the actual agents, especially when there are multiple exposures. In addition the manner in which the mother is questioned may alter her responses.[49] With regard to substance abuse, it has been shown that maternal history does not reliably predict fetal exposure, although actual drug abusers are more likely to admit use than infrequent drug users.[19,54]

Health care professionals have also been shown to be poor at accurately predicting maternal substance abuse,[64] so that reliance on their "gut feelings" will fail to identify a significant proportion of infants at risk.

Biologic Variability

It is well known that most human teratogens (including alcohol and thalidomide) affect only some of the fetuses exposed and that there is considerable variability in phenotypic effects. Causes of this variability may include differences in placental transfer and metabolism as well as genetic polymorphisms in enzymatic function and expression. It has been observed that once a mother has had a child affected by in utero exposure to phenytoin, for example, she is more likely to have a second affected child than another mother whose first infant was not similarly affected. It has been proposed that the reason for this is that the child has inherited from at least one parent a gene that results in a diminished ability to metabolize the drug, and therefore increases the likelihood of the drug's teratogenic effects.[70] In the future it may be possible to predict which fetuses are at highest risk of teratogenicity, based on their drug-metabolizing genotype.[8] By performing analysis on neonatal samples such as hair, urine, blood, meconium, and amniotic fluid, a better understanding of the sources of mother–infant variability may be gained.[59] This can be useful, not only in the study of environmental agents and drugs of abuse, but also in the study of prescribed drugs and medicinal teratogens, such as warfarin and valproic acid as well as fetotoxins such as captopril.[30]

Biologic Markers of Fetal Exposure

Blood

Cord blood is a readily available biologic fluid, collection of which does not entail ethical implications. Frequently, however, cord blood levels of a xenobiotic may have a very limited clinical applicability and the potential for analytic value may be restricted. For example, measurement of carboxyhemoglobin from cord blood samples in the neonate reflects exposure to carbon monoxide only over the few hours immediately prior to delivery, a time when most women are in a hospital and therefore do not smoke. Similarly, measurement of blood and urine levels of nicotine and cotinine reflect only very recent exposure.

It has been documented that tissue hypoxia causes increased production of erythropoietin, and that elevated cord blood erythropoietin levels have been seen in chronic fetal hypoxia in association with conditions such as maternal preeclampsia, diabetes, and Rh isoimmunization. Because maternal smoking affects fetal hemodynamics and increases the level of fetal carboxyhemoglobin, it is likely that a proportion of fetuses of smoking mothers are chronically hypoxic in utero. Erythropoietin and hemoglobin levels have been used as indirect biologic markers of fetal exposure to maternal cigarette smoking.[74] In this study about 20% of neonates whose mothers smoked during pregnancy had mean cord blood erythropoietin concentrations higher than in infants whose mothers were nonsmokers, suggesting chronic hypoxia. There was also a positive correlation between cord blood hemoglobin and erythropoietin concentrations.[74]

Lead has long been recognized as a neurodevelopmental toxin[50] but it is only relatively recently that concerns have been raised about its teratogenic effects. An association between cord blood lead levels greater than 0.48 mmol/L and low Bayley Mental Development Index (MDI) scores at 6, 12, 18, and 24 months of age has been demonstrated.[5] Of note, postnatal blood lead levels were not associated with low MDI scores or with low Bayley Psychomotor Index (PDI) scores.[5]

Obstetric complications associated with elevated lead exposure include spontaneous abortion, premature rupture of the membranes, and preterm delivery.[51] Lead is known to cross the placenta freely, probably by both passive and active transport mechanisms. Transplacental transfer of lead has been shown from as early as 12–14 weeks' gestation with increasing amounts of lead being detected in fetal tissues with advancing gestation.[60] Lead has also been shown to accumulate in fetal liver and bones. It is important to detect babies potentially exposed in utero to excess lead as early as possible. There have been several studies that have shown good correlation between maternal and cord blood lead levels.[4,23,48] However, lead exposure throughout pregnancy cannot be assumed from a single blood measurement, because of changes in maternal blood levels and placental permeability to lead. Thus neonatal hair analysis (as discussed below) may be a more accurate way of assessing cumulative in utero lead exposure.[38]

Urine

Urine reflects only a very small window of time in terms of fetal exposure. For example, the cocaine metabolite, benzoylecognine, is measurable in urine only 96–120 hours after the last exposure to cocaine, and thus urine analysis alone may underestimate the true extent of prenatal cocaine exposure. One group of researchers found that when sufficiently sensitive analytic methods were used, maternal urine, neonatal urine, and meconium analyses yielded similar results for detection of prenatal cocaine exposure.[10] Rapid mass screening techniques with high sensitivity and specificity (96% and 100%, respectively) have been developed to test urine and to identify neonates exposed in utero to cocaine.[76]

Meconium

Opioids and cannabinoids as well as cocaine and nicotine and their metabolites can all be measured in meconium, and several different analytic methods have recently been validated.[11,46,53,55] Meconium is formed from a composite of desquamated intestinal and cutaneous epithelial cells, bile, pancreatic and intestinal secretions, and swallowed amniotic fluid. Fetal swallowing first occurs at around 12 weeks' gestation so that the accumulation of drugs in meconium via fetal urine production and swallowing of amniotic fluid should theoretically be demonstrable after this time.

Postmortem analysis of meconium from a fetus that was spontaneously aborted at 17 weeks' gestation revealed the presence of cocaine, at a concentration that could be related to the amount and timing of maternal cocaine use during the pregnancy.[57] Meconium is an ideal specimen for analysis of drugs and metabolites in the newborn period for the following reasons:

1. The collection of meconium is simple and noninvasive.
2. Drugs in meconium are present for up to 3 days after delivery.
3. Initial testing can be performed with common laboratory techniques for mass screening, with confirmatory testing using gas chromatography–mass spectrometry (GC-MS).
4. Testing is sensitive and specific.
5. Analysis of serial meconium samples may reflect the type, timing, and amount of in utero drug exposure.

A study of 59 infants showed that the analysis of newborn infants' hair by radioimmunoassay or of meconium by GC-MS was more sensitive than analysis by immunoassay of urine and can detect fetal exposure to cocaine during the last 2 trimesters of pregnancy.[9]

Another study of 1201 mother–infant pairs showed that meconium testing detected an additional 33% of exposed infants compared with urine testing.[67] Furthermore, cocaethylene, a metabolite of both cocaine and ethanol, has been shown to accumulate in greater concentrations in meconium than in urine and thus is a useful analyte for identifying both cocaine and ethanol exposure.[41]

A large-scale prospective drug screening study of over 3000 neonates using analysis of meconium for morphine (opioids), cocaine, and cannabinoid showed a fourfold increase in the incidence of drug exposure in newborns compared to maternal self-report. This was found to be particularly significant in the less heavily exposed group of neonates with no obvious manifestations at birth and whose mothers denied drug use during pregnancy, compared with the more heavily exposed group who either had obvious clinical signs and/or mothers who were drug abusers (consistent and substantial users) and who were more likely to admit to drug use.[54]

Adaptation of the meconium test for large-scale use in mass screening programs has important implications in attempting to identify additional neonates at risk of intrauterine cocaine exposure as well as for its research and epidemiologic purposes.[54]

The nicotine metabolites cotinine and *trans*-3'-hydroxycotinine can be measured in the meconium of infants of active smokers, and their concentrations are directly related to the degree of smoking by the mother. Similarly, metabolite levels are detected in the meconium of infants of passive smokers, with concentrations found to be comparable to those of infants whose mothers were light smokers.[56]

There are, however, a number of limitations to using meconium as opposed to hair samples to determine intrauterine drug exposure in a clinical setting. As yet no dose–response curves have been established with meconium (as opposed to hair). Meconium is present in only the first few days of life, so that if the exposure is not initially suspected or if the first specimen(s) of meconium are discarded, then analysis cannot be performed. It is also not clear how much of the drugs and their metabolites that are present in meconium result from the swallowing of amniotic fluid and how much from the enterohepatic circulation.

Results of meconium analysis may not be accurate if there is in utero passage of meconium and the infant is meconium-stained at birth (often a sign of fetal distress, which may or may not be related to the particular in utero exposure). In these situations the first postnatal meconium specimen may contain less drug than the initial meconium, which was unaffected by exogenous feeding, but was passed in utero and therefore unable to be analyzed.[57] After birth, the amount of drug measurable in meconium may be diluted as the baby feeds and new stool is formed. It has been shown that although measurable in the first three meconium stools, the amount of cocaine metabolite diminishes significantly after the second stool.[64]

Another confounding issue is contamination of meconium specimens by neonatal urine. It has been shown that high concentrations of drug metabolites in meconium may result from extracorporeal urinary contamination.[42]

Hair

The hair that neonates are born with grows during the last 3–4 months of pregnancy. Thus the presence of drugs or environmental toxins in neonatal hair reflects the xenobiotic milieu over the last trimester of gestation.

Adult hair grows at a rate of approximately 1.5 cm per month and therefore analysis of hair may detect not only the presence and level of exposure but also time-dependent changes in drug use over a period of several months. Measurements in hair are several times more sensitive for cocaine exposure than either maternal history or urine measurements and can give an estimate of the time frame of the exposure.[24]

Animal and human studies demonstrate that both maternal and fetal accumulation of cocaine and its major metabolite, benzoylecognine, follow a linear pattern within clinically used doses, and thus hair measurements may be used to estimate maternal use.[18] Benzoylecognine can also be measured in neonatal hair.[32] Pyrolysis of crack cocaine results in hair accumulation of cocaine, but not its benzoylecognine metabolite. However, after admitted systemic use, both cocaine and benzoylecognine are detectable in hair. Also, external contamination with crack smoke is washable, whereas systemic exposure is not. In the context of the neonate, "external contamination" is not relevant, as fetal hair is in contact with amniotic fluid, which is swallowed and excreted via the urinary tract of the unborn baby.[34] Thus, measurement of hair benzoylecognine can distinguish between passive and active maternal crack cocaine exposure.

Another study of the prevalence of fetal exposure to cocaine in the years 1990–1991 in Toronto ascertained 37 neonates out of a total of 600 (6.2%) who tested positive to cocaine. Of these babies, 33 were detected by the hair test, while 4 infants, who had low urine concentrations, were not identified. The urine test failed to identify 76% of the cases.[17]

Both morbidity and mortality may be increased when alcohol and cocaine are used together.[61] The simultaneous use of alcohol and cocaine is believed to result in enhanced feelings of euphoria, significant improvement in alcohol-related changes in psychomotor performance, as well as cardiovascular changes such as a marked increase in heart rate.[15] A 1990 survey indicated that approximately 12 million Americans use cocaine and alcohol concurrently.[22]

One of the substances associated with the increased effects is cocaethylene, a product formed in the liver by the combination of alcohol and cocaine and which has a half-life approximately four times longer than that of cocaine. In one study, 18 women who presented for delivery without antenatal care were randomly selected. Of these, 10 women admitted to using alcohol and 13 reported using cocaine during the pregnancy. Out of the 9 women who admitted using both alcohol and cocaine during pregnancy, 8 were positive for cocaethylene in hair, while the ninth one was positive for cocaine and benzoylecognine. One patient who denied using alcohol was positive for cocaethylene, while 7 patients who denied alcohol use on history were negative for cocaethylene. Of the patients whose hair tested positive for cocaethylene, 88% gave a positive alcohol history. Thus hair analysis for cocaine as well as cocaethylene can be used to evaluate the use of alcohol as well as cocaine during pregnancy.[12]

Maternal cigarette smoking is associated with negative obstetric outcome, including decreased birth weight, prematurity, spontaneous abortions, perinatal mortality, and the sudden infant death syndrome.[1] Infants of passive smokers are also at risk of measurable exposure to cigarette smoke.

Cigarette smoke emits numerous toxins, including nicotine, carbon monoxide, hydrogen cyanide, and benzo(a)pyrene. Because of its oxygen dissociation properties, fetal hemoglobin has a higher affinity for carbon monoxide than does normal adult hemoglobin and thus levels of carboxyhemoglobin are higher in fetal than in maternal blood. This results in lower amounts of oxygen reaching developing fetal tissues as well as reduced function of cytochrome enzymes and impaired cellular respiration.[43] There is also increasing evidence that intrauterine exposure to cigarette smoke and its toxic metabolites may result in neurobehavioral teratogenicity.[20,21,66] Accumulation of nicotine and cotinine in neonatal hair reflects chronic systemic exposure to these toxins and therefore may correlate with neonatal risks.

Because it is lipid soluble, nicotine has a large volume of distribution (2–3 L/kg) and readily permeates cell membranes. It is absorbed through the lungs and skin, as well as the mucous membranes of the gastrointestinal tract and nasal passages. Once absorbed, nicotine disappears rapidly from the bloodstream because of both widespread tissue uptake and hepatic metabolism.[37,58] Nicotine is filtered and actively secreted by the renal tubules. Nicotine's elimination half-life in adult humans is between 1 and 3 hours, and thus monitoring in the blood is unlikely to reflect the true extent of chronic smoking. Cotinine is the major metabolite of nicotine, formed by a double oxidation reaction catalyzed by cytochrome P450 and then by cytosolic aldehyde oxidase. Cotinine has a considerably longer elimination half-life than nicotine (10–14 hours) and is predominantly excreted in the urine. Accumulation of nicotine and its major metabolite, cotinine, may be measured in neonatal hair to estimate fetal exposure to maternal cigarette smoking.[14,28] A study measuring hair concentrations of both cotinine and nicotine in 94 mother–infant pairs, including mothers who were smokers, nonsmokers, and passive smokers, found significantly higher concentrations of nicotine and cotinine in the hair of smokers and their infants when compared with nonsmoking mothers and their infants. Concentrations in passive smokers and their infants were also significantly higher than in nonsmokers and their infants. There was also a significant correlation between maternal and neonatal hair concentrations of both nicotine and cotinine.[14]

Unfortunately, maternal reporting of cigarette use in pregnancy is often inaccurate, because of guilt, perception of fetal risk, and fear. It is probably for these reasons that reported use has been shown to correlate poorly with hair accumulation of both nicotine and cotinine in both mother and infant. This highlights the importance of an independent biologic marker such as hair nicotine and cotinine measurement to more accurately evaluate fetal exposure to cigarette smoke.

Because one of the major problems encountered in the analysis of neonatal hair is the frequently small amount of hair available for analysis, a method to detect both cocaine and nicotine in the same hair sample was developed.[29] This has clear benefits in quantifying specific exposures and correlating potential neonatal effects, particularly as the majority of mothers who use cocaine also smoke cigarettes.

The tragic experience from Minamata Bay, Japan, revealed the devastating neurotoxicity of methylmercury, with fetuses and infants showing particular susceptibility. Research supports that the developing nervous system is particularly vulnerable during the last 2 trimesters of pregnancy and during early postnatal life. Other studies have shown that methylmercury crosses the placental barrier and achieves higher concentrations in the fetus than in the mother.[62]

Methylmercury is distributed evenly through the body and is also incorporated into growing hair. Based on toxicokinetic and practical considerations, hair is the optimal biomarker of methylmercury exposure, in both mothers and infants. Mercury levels in cord blood and in maternal scalp hair correlate well. However, dose–response relationships, particularly with regard to developmental neurotoxicity, are not completely known.[25,45] Methylmercury may also be transferred to neonates via breast milk, thus representing a further potential neurotoxic risk. Urinary mercury excretion is a good marker of inorganic mercury exposure but does not reflect methylmercury exposure.

Amniotic Fluid

It is well documented in both animals and humans that drugs may be detected in amniotic fluid after maternal drug administration.[7,72] The appearance of drug in the amniotic fluid is usually delayed after a single dose of drug to the mother. However, with chronic drug use, the concentration in amniotic fluid gradually increases. Peak concentrations may greatly exceed simultaneously obtained concentrations in maternal and fetal plasma.[71,72] Many drug metabolites as well as the parent compound also appear in amniotic fluid, for example cocaine and its metabolites benzoylecognine, ecognine methyl ester, and cocaethylene.[63] The fetus may therefore be repeatedly exposed to the effects of these drugs via contact with amniotic fluid that contains these substances.[44]

In one study, amniotic fluid and urine samples were obtained from 23 subjects with documented cocaine abuse. Cocaine and benzoylecognine were detected in 74% of amniotic fluid samples taken from the known cocaine abusers, while in the same subjects, conventional maternal and neonatal urine toxicology screens were positive in only 61% and 35%, respectively.[27] Other data suggest that measurement of cocaine and its metabolites in amniotic fluid offers no benefits over urinary drug evaluation.[10] Cotinine may be measured in amniotic fluid collected during routine second trimester amniocentesis. Although the mechanism is not understood, it appears that nicotine and its metabolites accumulate both in the fetus and in the amniotic fluid, as levels in neonatal cord blood and in amniotic fluid are found to be higher than in maternal blood.[65]

Ultrasonography

One further prenatal biologic marker of fetal exposure is ultrasound examination with particular emphasis on fetal biometry and specific structural defects, such as neural tube defects (for example in association with valproic acid or carbamazepine exposure). With improved ultrasound technology over the past decade, there has been an increased awareness and reporting of fetal anomalies associated with known or potential teratogen exposures detected on midtrimester ultrasound examination.[35]

There are recent reports of specific fetal anomalies being detected on midtrimester ultrasound, for example, radial ray defects, following valproic acid exposure,[39,68,78] as well as a major cardiac defect and hydrocephalus associated with first trimester retinoic acid exposure.[73]

Cocaine is implicated in a number of obstetric complications and birth defects. One recent report describes the antenatal sonographic detection of two fetuses with limb–body wall complex in mothers who smoked large amounts of cocaine during the first trimester of pregnancy.[75]

New techniques such as three-dimensional ultrasound may further revolutionize prenatal diagnosis, particularly of craniofacial and cerebral malformations.

Counseling Issues

The main aim of counseling women following potential teratogenic exposure is to present an accurate, up-to-date estimate of their specific risk in an easily understood, nondirective manner. Different women will perceive and interpret the same data very differently, partly because of their educational, ethnic, and social backgrounds, and partly because of their levels of fear, anxiety, and possibly guilt. Hence the counseling they receive should be specifically tailored to their needs, so that they are able to understand the particular issues concerning the teratogenic exposure during their pregnancy and in particular what should be done regarding the future of the pregnancy.

Perception of Risk and Decision Making

The major decision to be made by women exposed to a xenobiotic is whether or not to continue with their pregnancy. Clearly there may be several possible reasons why a woman (and her partner) would want to terminate a pregnancy, but incorrect perception of teratogenic risk is an important factor.[31]

Since the tragedy of thalidomide in the 1960s there has been increased public and media awareness of the possibility of teratogenic effects of drugs and environ-

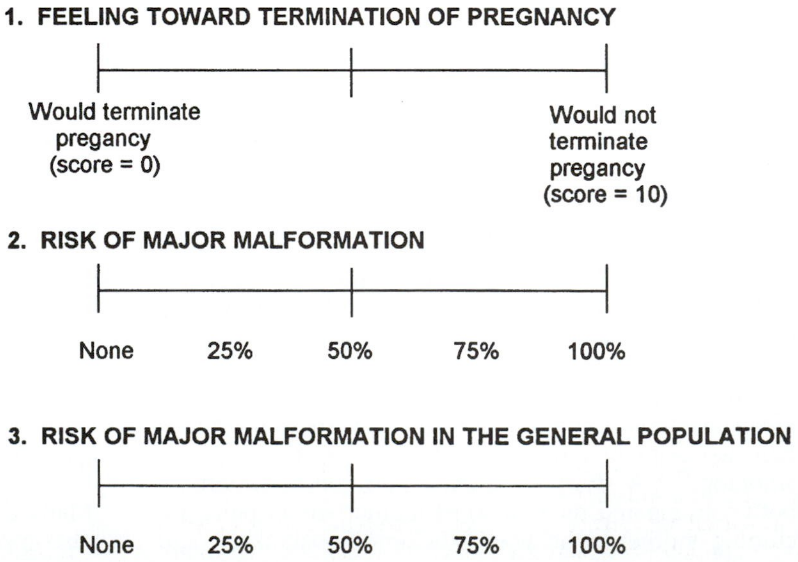

Figure 16–4. A visual analog scale depicting an individual's feeling about the need for termination of pregnancy and the individual's perception of the teratogenic risk for drug or chemical exposure.

mental agents, even though there are relatively few proven human teratogens. Not only the mass media but even reputable scientific publications tend to publish and emphasize the positive findings (ie, fetal abnormalities) and potentially harmful effects of xenobiotics rather than their safety and lack of documented teratogenicity.[13,33]

One study, using the visual analog scale depicted in Figure 16–4, assessed the perception of teratogenic risk of 80 women attending an antenatal consultation clinic for drug and chemical exposure and found that women exposed to agents not known to be teratogenic assigned themselves a risk of 24% ± 2.8% (comparable to the risk of one of the major known teratogens—thalidomide). Once they received appropriate counseling their perception of risk was reduced to 14.5% ± 3%, and their tendency to terminate the pregnancy also decreased significantly after the consultation. In contrast, women exposed to known teratogens perceived their risk as being 36.2% ± 11.7% before the interview and did not change their perception afterwards.They also did not change their tendency toward terminating the pregnancy.[36]

Thus appropriate intervention (counseling) in early pregnancy can prevent unnecessary termination of pregnancy by correcting misinformation and misconceptions and thereby decreasing the unrealistically high perception of risk by women exposed to nonteratogens.

Summary and Future Directions

Increasingly and predominantly because of medical-legal influences, it will become necessary to determine as precisely as possible the nature of fetal xenobiotic exposure. The use of biologic markers is a way to semiquantitatively determine exposure to a number of these agents. In the future it is likely that there will be more substances, both environmental and medicinal, that will be amenable to this form of analysis and new techniques that will result in increased accuracy and thus improved quantification of the exposure.

Most human teratogens and fetotoxins affect some fetuses while sparing others. It is possible that interpatient variability in the rate and extent of placental transfer of drugs is one source of variability in toxicologic response. Thus, neonatal hair and meconium analysis may allow a better understanding of the sources of variability that clearly exist between some mother–infant pairs. This approach may well have relevance not just for environmental agents and drugs of abuse, but also for medicinal teratogens (eg, phenytoin) and fetotoxins (eg, captopril).

References

1. Abel EL: Smoking and pregnancy. J Psychoactive Drugs 1984;16:327–328.
2. Ames BN: Identifying environmental chemicals causing mutations and cancer. Science 1979;204:587–593.
3. Ames BN, Magaw R, Gold LS: Ranking possible carcinogenic hazards. Science 1987;236:271–280.
4. Angell NF, Lavery JP: The relationship of blood lead levels to obstetric outcome. Am J Obstet Gynecol 1982;142:40–46.
5. Bellinger D, Leviton A, Waternauz C, et al: Longitudinal analyses of prenatal and postnatal lead exposure and early cognitive development. N Engl J Med 1987;316: 1037–1043.
6. Brent R: Evaluating the alleged teratogenicity of environmental agents. Clin Perinatol 1986;13:609–613.
7. Brien JF, Clarke DW, Smith GN, et al: Disposition of acute, multiple-dose ethanol in the near-term pregnant ewe. Am J Obstet Gynecol 1987;157:204.
8. Buehler BA, Delimont D, van Maes M, Finnell RH: Prenatal prediction of risk for the fetal hydantoin syndrome. N Engl J Med 1990;322:1567–1572.
9. Callahan CM, Grant TM, Phipps P, et al: Measurement of gestational cocaine exposure: Sensitivity of infants' hair, meconium, and urine. J Pediatr 1992;120:763–768.
10. Casanova OQ, Lombardero N, Behnke M, et al: Detection of cocaine exposure in the neonate. Analyses of urine, meconium, and amniotic fluid from mothers and infants exposed to cocaine. Arch Pathol Lab Med 1994;118:988–993.
11. Clark GD, Rosenweig IB, Raisys VA, et al: The analysis of cocaine and benzoylecognine in meconium. J Anal Toxicol 1992;16:261–263.
12. DiGregorio GJ, Barbieri EJ, Ferko AP, Ruch EK: Prevalence of cocaethylene in the hair of pregnant women. J Anal Toxicol 1993; 7:445–446. Letter.
13. Easterbrook PJ, Berlin JA, Copalan R, Matthews DR: Publication bias in clinical research. Lancet 1991;337:867–872.
14. Eliopoulos C, Klein J, Phan MK, et al: Hair concentrations of nicotine and cotinine in women and their newborn infants. JAMA 1994;271:621–623.
15. Farre M, de la Torre R, Llorente M, et al: Alcohol and cocaine interactions in humans. J Pharmacol Exp Ther 1993; 266:1364–1373.
16. Feldman Y, Koren G, Mattice D, et al: Determinants of recall and recall bias in studying drug and chemical exposure in pregnancy. Teratology 1989;40:37–45.
17. Forman R, Klein J, Meta D, et al: Prevalence of fetal exposure to cocaine in Toronto, 1990–1991. Clin Invest Med 1994;17:206–211.
18. Forman R, Schneiderman J, Klein J, et al: Accumulation of cocaine in maternal and fetal hair: The dose-response curve. Life Sci 1992;50:1333–1341.
19. Frank DA, Zuckerman BS, Amaro H, et al: Cocaine use during pregnancy: Prevalence and correlates. Pediatrics 1988; 82:888–895.
20. Fried PA, O'Connel CM, Watkinson B: Sixty and 72-month follow-up of children prenatally exposed to marijuana, cigarettes and alcohol: Cognitive and language assessment. Dev Behav Pediatr 1992;13:383–391.
21. Fried PA, Watkinson B, Gray BA: A follow-up study of attentional behavior in 6-year-old children exposed prenatally to marijuana, cigarettes and alcohol. Neurotoxicol Teratol 1992;14:299–311.
22. Gerschanick J, Brooks G, Little J: Blood lead values in pregnant women and their offspring. Am J Obstet Gynecol 1974; 119:508–511.
23. Graham K, Koren G, Klein J, et al: Determination of gestational cocaine exposure by hair analysis. JAMA 1989;262: 3328–3330.
24. Grandjean P, Weihe P, Nielsen JB: Methylmercury: Signifi-

cance of intrauterine and postnatal exposures. Clin Chem 1994;40:1395–1400.
25. Grant BF, Harford TC: Concurrent and simultaneous use of alcohol with cocaine: Results of a national survey. Drug Alcohol Depend 1990;25:97–104.
26. Holmes L: Fetal environmental toxins. Pediatr Rev 1992; 13:364–370.
27. Jain L, Meyer W, Moore C, et al: Detection of fetal cocaine exposure by analysis of amniotic fluid. Obstet Gynecol 1993;81:787–790.
28. Klein J, Chitayat D, Koren G: Hair analysis as a marker for fetal exposure to maternal smoking. N Engl J Med 1993; 2328:66–67.
29. Klein J, Forman R, Eliopoulos C, Koren G: A method for simultaneous measurement of cocaine and nicotine in neonatal hair. Ther Drug Monitoring 1994;16:67–70.
30. Koren G: Measurement of drugs in neonatal hair: A window to fetal exposure. Forensic Sci Intl 1995;70:77–82
31. Koren G, Bologa M, Long D, et al: Perception of teratogenic risk by pregnant women exposed to drugs and chemicals during the first trimester. Am J Obstet Gynecol 1989; 160:1190–1194.
32. Koren G, Ben David S: Measurement of drugs in neonatal hair—A window of fetal exposure. Harefuah 1995;129: 336–338.
33. Koren G, Klein N: Bias against negative studies in newspaper reports of medical research. JAMA 1991;266:1824–1826.
34. Koren G, Klein J, Forman R, Graham K: Hair analysis of cocaine: Differentiation between systemic exposure and external contamination. J Clin Pharmacol 1992;32:671–675.
35. Koren G, Nulman I: Antenatal visualization of malformations associated with drugs and chemicals. Dev Brain Dysfunct 1993;6:305–316.
36. Koren G, Pastuszak A: Prevention of unnecessary pregnancy terminations by counselling women on drug, chemical, and radiation exposure during the first trimester. Teratology 1990;41:657–661.
37. Kyerematen GA, Vesel E: Metabolism of nicotine. Drug Metab Rev 1991;23:3–41.
38. Laker M: On determining trace element levels in man: The uses of blood and hair. Lancet 1982;2:260–262.
39. Langer B, Haddad J, Gasser B, et al: Isolated fetal bilateral radial ray reduction associated with valproic acid usage. Fetal Diag Ther 1994;9:155–158.
40. Lehninger AL: Principles of Biochemistry. New York, Worth, 1982, pp. 879–886.
41. Lewis DE, Moore CM, Leikin JB: Cocaethylene in meconium specimens. J Toxicol Clin Toxicol 1994;32:697–703.
42. Lombardero N, Casanova O, Behnke M, et al: Comparison of specimens for GC/MS detection of prenatal cocaine exposure. Ann Clin Lab Sci 1993;23:385–394.
43. Longo L: The biological effects of carbon monoxide on the pregnant woman, fetus and newborn infant. Am J Obstet Gynecol 1977;129:69–103.
44. Mahone PR, Scott K, Sleggs G, et al: Cocaine and metabolites in amniotic fluid may prolong fetal drug exposure. Am J Obstet Gynecol 1994;171:465–469.
45. Marsh DO, Clarkson TW, Cox C, et al: Fetal methylmercury poisoning, relationship between concentrations in single strand of maternal hair and child effects. Arch Neurol 1987;44:1017–1022.
46. Maynard EC, Amuroso LP, Oh W: Meconium for drug testing. Am J Dis Child 1991;145:650–652.
47. Miller EC: Some current perspectives on chemical carcinogenesis: Presidential address. Cancer Res 1978;8:1479–1496.
48. Milman N, Christensen JM, Ibsen KK: Blood lead and erythrocyte zinc protoporphyrin in mothers and newborn infants. Eur J Pediatr 1988;147:71–73.
49. Mitchell AE, Cottler LB, Shapira SP: Effect of questionnaire design on recall of drug exposure in pregnancy. Am J Epidemiol 1986;123:670–676.
50. Moore MR, McIntosh MJ, Bushnell JWR: The neurotoxicity of lead. Neurotoxicology 1986;7:541–546.
51. Nogaki K: On action of lead on body of lead refinery workers: particularly conception, pregnancy and parturition in case of females and on vitality of their newborn. Excerpta Med 1958;4:2176.
52. Okey AB: Carcinogenesis and mutagenesis by xenobiotic chemicals. In: Kalant H, Roschlau WHE, eds: Principles of Medical Pharmacology, 5th ed. Toronto, Decker, 1989, pp. 632–643.
53. Ostrea EM, Brady MJ, Parks PM, Asencio DC, Naluz A: Drug screening of meconium in infants of drug dependent mothers: An alternative to urine testing. J Pediatr 1989; 115:474–477.
54. Ostrea EM, Brady M, Gause S, et al: Drug screening of newborns by meconium analysis: A large-scale, prospective, epidemiologic study. Pediatrics 1992;89:107–113.
55. Ostrea EM, Martier S, Welch R, Brady M: Sensitivity of meconium drug screen in detecting intrauterine drug exposure of infants. Pediatr Res 1990;27:219. Abstract.
56. Ostrea EM, Knapp DK, Romero A, et al: Meconium analysis to assess fetal exposure to nicotine by active and passive maternal smoking. J Pediatr 1994;124:471–476.
57. Ostrea EM, Romero A, Knapp DK, et al: Postmortem drug analysis of meconium in early-gestation human fetuses exposed to cocaine: Clinical implications. J Pediatr 1994;125: 477–479.
58. Pilotti A: Biosynthesis and mammalian metabolism of nicotine. Acta Physiol Scand 1980;479(suppl):13–17.
59. Potter S, Klein J, Valiante G, et al: Maternal cocaine use without evidence of fetal exposure. J Pediatr 1994;125: 652–654.
60. Rajegowda BK, Glass L, Evans HE: Lead concentration in newborn infants. J Pediatr 1972;80:116–117.
61. Randall T: Cocaine, alcohol mix in body to form even longer lasting, more lethal drug. JAMA 1992;267:1043–1044.
62. Reynolds WA, Pitkin RM: Transplacental passage of methylmercury and its uptake by primate fetal tissues. Proc Soc Exp Biol Med 1975;148:523–526.
63. Ripple MG, Goldberger BA, Caplan YH, et al: Detection of cocaine and its metabolites in human amniotic fluid. J Anal Toxicol 1992;16:328–331.
64. Rosengren S, Longobucco D, Bernstein B, et al: Meconium testing for cocaine metabolite: Prevalence, perceptions, and pitfalls. Am J Obstet Gynecol 1993;168:1449–1456.
65. Ruhle W, Graf von Ballestrem CL, Pult HM, Gnirs J: Correlation of cotinine levels in amniotic fluid, umbilical artery

blood and maternal blood (in German). Geburtshilfe und Frauenheilkunde 1995;15:156–159.
66. Rush D, Callahan KR: Exposure to passive cigarette smoking and child development. Ann NY Acad Sci 1989;562: 74–100.
67. Ryan RM, Wagner CL, Schultz JM, et al: Meconium analysis for improved identification of infants exposed to cocaine in utero. J Pediatr 1994;125:435–440.
68. Sharony R, Garber A, Viskochil D, et al: Preaxial ray reduction defects as part of valproic acid embryofetopathy. Prenat Diag 1993;13:909–918.
69. Shephard TH: "Proof" of human teratogenicity. Teratology 1994;50:97–98.
70. Strickler SM, Dansky LV, Miller MA, et al: Genetic predisposition to phenytoin-induced birth defects. Lancet 1985;2: 746–749.
71. Szeto HH: Kinetics of drug transfer to the fetus. Clin Obstet Gynecol 1993;36:246–254.
72. Szeto HH, Umans JG, McFarland JW: A comparison of morphine and methadone disposition in the maternal–fetal unit. Am J Obstet Gynecol 1982;143:700–706.
73. Van Maldergem L, Jauniaux E, Gillerot Y: Morphological features of a case of retinoic acid embryopathy. Prenat Diag 1992;12:699–701.
74. Varvarigou A, Beratis NG, Makri M, Vagenakis AG: Increased levels and positive correlation between erythropoietin and hemoglobin concentrations in newborn children of mothers who are smokers. J Pediatr 1994;124:480–482.
75. Viscarello RR, Ferguson DD, Nores J, Hobbins JC: Limb-body wall complex associated with cocaine abuse: Further evidence of cocaine's teratogenicity. Obstet Gynecol 1992; 80:523–526.
76. Welch E, Fleming LE, Peyser I, et al: Rapid cocaine screening of urine in a newborn nursery. J Pediatr 1993;123: 468–470.
77. Williams GM, Weisburger JH: Chemical carcinogens. In: Amdur MO, Doull J, Klaassen CD, eds: Casarett and Doull's Toxicology: The Basic Science of Poisons. New York, Macmillan, 1991, pp. 127–200.
78. Ylagan LR, Budorick NE: Radial ray aplasia in utero: A prenatal finding associated with valproic acid exposure. J Ultrasound Med 1994;13:408–411.

PART C

The Pathophysiologic Basis of Medical Toxicology: The Organ System Approach

CHAPTER 17

Vital Signs and Toxic Syndromes

Lewis R. Goldfrank, Neal E. Flomenbaum, Neal A. Lewin, Richard S. Weisman, Mary Ann Howland, and Robert S. Hoffman

Normal Vital Signs by Age

Age	Systolic BP mm Hg	Diastolic BP mm Hg	Pulse bpm	Respiratory Rate/min
Adult	90–140	< 90	60–100	8–14
16 years	120	70	80	12–16
12 years	110	70	85	15–20
10 years	110	70	90	15–20
6 years	100	60	100	20–25
4 years	100	60	100	20–25
2 years	100	60	110	25–30
1 year	95	60	120	25–30
6 months	90	60	120	30
4 months	85	50	120	30–35
2 months	80	45	120	30–35
Newborn	60	40	125	35–40

The normal temperature is defined at 95–100.4°F or 35–38°C

For over 200 years the American medical community has attempted to standardize its approach to the assessment of patients.[2] At New York Hospital in 1865, temperature, pulse, and respiratory rate were incorporated into the bedside chart and called "vital signs." However, only in the early part of the 20th century did the determination of the blood pressure also become routine.[7] In addition to its more widely appreciated role, the vital signs can provide valuable physiologic clues pointing to the toxicologic etiology of an illness. Many toxic substances affect the autonomic nervous system, which is responsible for changes in vital signs mediated by the sympathetic and parasympathetic pathways. Meticulous attention to initial as well as repeat determinations of these clinical signs is of extreme importance in identifying a pattern of changes suggesting a particular drug or group of drugs. A description of the vital signs as "normal" or "stable" is too nonspecific to be meaningful and therefore should never be accepted. Moreover, no patient should be considered too agitated for determination of a complete set of vital signs; indeed, the agitated patient is urgently in need of a thorough evaluation.

The value of continually monitoring the vital signs is best demonstrated by a patient who presents with an anticholinergic overdose and is then given physostigmine or, conversely, a patient poisoned by organophosphates who is given atropine. It is important to recognize when a sinus tachycardia becomes a sinus bradycardia (anticholinergic followed by physostigmine use or excess) or when a sinus bradycardia becomes a normal sinus rhythm or progresses to a sinus tachycardia (organophosphate overdose followed by atropine use). More common, perhaps, is the patient who overdoses on an opioid and is given the opioid antagonist naloxone (bradypnea to tachypnea and then to a more normal pattern). These analyses become exceedingly complicated when a patient has taken two or more substances, such as an opioid and cocaine. The effects of cocaine may be "unmasked" by the use of naloxone, and the clinician is then forced to differentiate opioid withdrawal from cocaine toxicity by using a combination of history, vital signs, and physical examination. Careful observation will help determine the success of a therapeutic intervention and guide the clinician in making the necessary adjustments to the initial therapy.

The most typical toxic syndromes are described in Table 17–1. These autonomic syndromes are best described by a combination of the vital signs (blood pressure, pulse, respiratory rate, temperature) and clinically obvious end organ manifestations. The end-organ and organ system signs that prove most clinically useful are those of the central nervous system (mental status), ophthalmologic (pupil size), gastrointestinal (peristalsis), skin (dryness vs diaphoresis), mucous membranes (salivation vs dryness), and genitourinary systems (urinary retention). Among the vital signs the most clinically sensitive indicators are typically the pulse and blood pressure. A detailed analysis of each toxic syndrome will be found in the appropriate chapter of the text. In this chapter, the syndromes will be considered in their broadest sense to enable the reader to initiate the assessment and differential diagnosis.

Mofenson and Greensher[6] coined the term "toxidrome" from toxic syndromes to describe the groups of signs and symptoms that tend to consistently result from particular toxins. The original toxidromes on their list along with those of other medical toxicologists appear as Table 17–2. This table reviews many of the most commonly encountered toxins and their typical clinical manifestations. However, the reader should note that the actual clinical manifestations of an ingestion or exposure are far more variable than the syndromes described in the table. Toxidromes are most useful when thinking about a clinical presentation and formulating the framework for assessment. Although some patients may present as "classic" cases, others will manifest combinations or formes frustes and have fewer signs, but nevertheless provide at least a partial clue as to the correct diagnosis. Partial presentations do not necessarily imply less severe disease and, therefore, are no less important to appreciate.

A table of normal values for the vital signs is particularly valuable in assessing children. Knowing the variations in values that are termed normal during this period of aging is essential in the evaluation of children. The adult normal values are defined as a blood pressure of 90–140 mm Hg systolic and < 90 mm Hg diastolic; a pulse of 60–100 beats per minute; a respiratory rate between 8 and 14 respirations per minute; and a temperature of 95–100.4° F or 35–38° C. The broad range of values termed normal in adults serves only as a guide. The assessment of the individual human being will be essential to determine if a value is truly numerically or clinically normal, rapid, or slow; high or low. The very young as well as the geriatric individual may have thermoregulatory abnormalities that either inhibit responses or promote excessive responses. Blood pressure and pulse may have significant variations associated with change in receptor responsiveness as well as fitness, the presence of atherosclerosis, and general cardiovascular function.

In some instances, an unexpected combination of findings may be particularly helpful in identifying a toxin or a combination of toxins. For example, a dissociation between such typically paired changes as an increase in pulse with a decrease in blood pressure (cyclic antidepressants or phenothiazines), a decrease in pulse with an increase in blood pressure (phenylpropanolamine), may be extremely helpful diagnostically, as the etiologies for this unexpected dissociation may include only a few possibilities. The use of these unexpected or atypical clinical findings is demonstrated in Chapter 21.

TABLE 17–1. TOXIC SYNDROMES

	Vital Signs								
Group	***BP,***	***P,***	***RR,***	***T,***	**Mental Status**	**Pupil size**	**Peristalsis**	**Diaphoresis**	**Other**
Adrenergic (α, β) agonists	↑	↑	↑	↑	Altered	↑	↑	↑	Flush
Anticholinergic agents	±	↑	±	↑	Altered	↑	↓	↓	Dry mucous membranes, flush, urinary retention
Cholinergic (muscarinic, nicotinic) agents	±	±	—	—	Altered	±	↑	↑	Salivation, lacrimation, urination, bronchorrhea, fasciculations
Opioids	↓	↓	↓	↓	Altered	↓	↓	↓	Hyporeflexia
Withdrawal of opioids	↑	↑	—	—	Normal	↑	↑	Present	Nausea, vomiting, hyperactivity, rhinorrhea, piloerection
Sedative-hypnotics or ethanol	↓	↓	↓	↓	Altered	±	↓	↓	Hyporeflexia
Withdrawal of sedative-hypnotics or ethanol	↑	↑	↑	↑	Altered	↑	Normal to ↑	Present	Nausea, tremor, seizures

↑ = increases; ↓ = decreases; ± = variable; — = change unlikely.

TABLE 17–2. SPECIFIC DRUGS OR TOXINS AND THEIR TOXIC SYNDROMES

Toxin	Vital Signs	Mental Status	Signs and Symptoms	Clinical Findings
Acetaminophen	Normal (early)	Normal	Anorexia, nausea, vomiting	RUQ tenderness, jaundice (late)
Amphetamines	Hypertension, tachycardia, tachypnea, hyperthermia	Hyperactive, agitated, toxic psychosis	Hyperalertness, panic, anxiety, diaphoresis	Mydriasis, hyperactive peristaltism diaphoresis
Antihistamines	Hypotension, hypertension, tachycardia, hyperthermia	Altered (agitation, lethargy to coma), hallucinations	Blurred vision, dry mouth, inabilitiy to urinate	Dry mucous membranes, mydriasis, flush, diminished peristaltism, urinary retention
Arsenic (acute)	Hypotension, tachycardia	Alert to coma	Abdominal pain, vomiting, diarrhea, dysphagia	Dehydration
Barbiturates	Hypotension, bradypnea, hypothermia	Altered (lethary to coma)	Slurred speech, ataxia	Dysconjugate gaze, bullae, hyporeflexia
Beta-adrenergic antagonists	Hypotension, bradycardia	Altered (lethargy to coma)	Dizziness	Cyanosis, seizures
Botulism	Bradypnea	Normal unless hypoxia	Blurred vision, diplopia, dysphagia, sore or dry throat, diarrhea	Ophthalmoplegia, mydriasis, ptosis, cranial nerve abnormalities, descending paralysis
Carbamazepine	Hypotension, tachycardia, bradypnea, hypothermia	Altered (lethargy to coma)	Hallucinations, extrapyramidal movements, seizures	Mydriasis, nystagmus
Carbon monoxide	Often normal	Altered (lethargy to coma)	Headache, dizziness, nausea, vomiting	Seizures
Clonidine	Hypotension, hypertension, bradycardia, bradypnea	Altered (lethargy to coma)	Dizziness, confusion	Miosis
Cocaine	Hypertension, tachycardia, tachypnea, hyperthermia	Altered (anxiety, agitation, delirium)	Hallucinations, paranoia, panic, anxiety, restlessness	Mydriasis, nystagmus
Cyclic antidepressants	Hypotension, tachycardia	Altered (lethargy to coma)	Confusion, dizziness, dry mouth, inability to urinate	Mydriasis, dry mucous membranes, distended bladder, flush, seizures
Digitalis	Hypotension, bradycardia	Normal to altered, visual distortion	Nausea, vomiting, anorexia, visual disturbances	None
Disulfiram/ethanol	Hypotension, tachycardia	Normal	Nausea, vomiting, headache, vertigo	Flush, diaphoresis, tender abdomen
Ethylene glycol	Tachypnea	Altered (lethargy to coma)	Abdominal pain	Slurred speech, ataxia
Iron	Hypotension, tachycardia	Normal or lethargy	Nausea, vomiting, diarrhea, abdominal pain, hematemesis	Tender abdomen
Isoniazid	Often normal	Normal or altered (lethargy to coma)	Nausea, vomiting	Seizures
Isopropanol	Hypotension, tachycardia, bradypnea	Altered (lethargy to coma)	Nausea, vomiting	Hyporeflexia, ataxia, acetone odor on breath
Lead	Hypertension	Altered (lethargy to coma)	Irritability, abdominal pain (colic), nausea, vomiting, constipation	Peripheral neuropathy, seizures, gingival pigmentation
Lithium	Hypotension (late)	Altered (lethargy to coma)	Diarrhea, tremor, nausea	Weakness, tremor, ataxia, myoclonus, seizures
Mercury	Hypotension (late)	Altered (psychiatric disturbances)	Salivation, diarrhea, abdominal pain	Stomatitis, ataxia, tremor
Methanol	Hypotension, tachypnea	Altered (lethargy to coma)	Blurred vision, blindness, abdominal pain	Hyperemic disks, mydriasis
Opioids	Hypotension, bradycardia bradypnea, hypothermia	Altered (lethargy to coma)	Slurred speech, ataxia	Miosis, decreased peristaltism
Organophosphates/ carbamates	Hypotension/hypertension bradycardia/tachycardia, bradypnea/tachypnea	Altered (lethargy to coma)	Diarrhea, abdominal pain, blurred vision, vomiting	Salivation, diaphoresis, lacrimation, urination, bronchorrhea, defecation, miosis, fasciculations, seizures
Phencyclidine	Hypertension, tachycardia, hyperthermia	Altered (agitation, lethargy to coma)	Hallucinations	Miosis, diaphoresis, myoclonus, blank stare, nystagmus, seizures
Phenothiazines	Hypotension, tachycardia, hypothermia or hyperthermia	Altered (lethargy to coma)	Dizziness, dry mouth, inability to urinate	Miosis or mydriasis, decreased bowel sounds, dystonia
Salicylates	Hypotension, tachycardia, tachypnea, hyperthermia	Altered (agitation, lethargy to coma)	Tinnitus, nausea, vomiting	Diaphoresis, tender abdomen, pulmonary edema
Sedative-hypnotics	Hypotension, bradypnea, hypothermia	Altered (lethargy to coma)	Slurred speech, ataxia	Hyporeflexia, bullae
Theophylline	Hypotension, tachycardia, tachypnea, hyperthermia	Altered (agitation)	Nausea, vomiting, diaphoresis, anxiety	Diaphoresis, tremor, seizures, dysrhythmias

Blood Pressure

Blood pressure and pulse should initially be assessed with the patient in the supine position. Following this determination, a more dynamic evaluation of cardiovascular integrity can be made by obtaining orthostatic vital signs—both blood pressure and pulse. This is one of the most helpful bedside examinations that can be performed to assess a patient for either actual volume depletion or relative volume depletion secondary to peripheral vasodilation (see Chap. 21, Table 21–3). A rough estimation of volume deficits can be correlated with these changes. However, the response is also dependent on other factors such as advanced age,[4] autonomic nervous system dysfunction (diabetes mellitus, tabes dorsalis, thiamine depletion, postsympathectomy states), and medication use. The groups of medications most commonly associated with orthostatic hypotension are the antidepressants, antihypertensives, antiparkinsonians, neuroleptics, diuretics, and CNS depressant agents (see Table 17–3; Chap. 21).

Drugs and toxins can produce hypotension by four major mechanisms: decreased peripheral resistance, decreased myocardial contractility, dysrhythmias, and intravascular volume depletion. Many drugs and toxins can initially cause severe orthostatic hypotension, without marked supine hypotension, and any drug or toxin that affects autonomic control of the myocardium or peripheral capacitance vessels may lead to orthostatic hypotension. Hypotension may result from many drugs, such as alpha-adrenergic antagonists, beta-adrenergic antagonists, calcium channel blockers, diuretics, nitrates, ethanol, opioids, cyclic antidepressants, phenothiazines, and sedative hypnotics (see Table 17–4; Chap. 21).

Drugs and toxins associated with hypertension include CNS stimulants, such as amphetamines, cocaine, and phencyclidine, and monoamine oxidase inhibitors (MAOI) in overdose or in combination with a contraindicated food or drug. Excessive amounts of nicotine and thyroid hormone typically result in hypertension. Hypertension and a concomitant decrease in heart rate is a common presentation noted with phenylpropanolamine ingestion. As a rule, hypertension resulting from drug overdoses is followed by hypotension.

Changing patterns of blood pressure often assist in the diagnostic evaluation: an MAOI overdose or an MAOI interaction with a contraindicated drug or food characteristically causes an initially normal blood pressure, then severe hypertension followed abruptly in the former by severe hypotension. Accurate, consistently performed repetitive blood pressure determinations are essential to identify and, if necessary, treat these rapidly changing conditions. Proper cuff sizes for the obese and

TABLE 17–3. COMMON DRUG GROUPS AND TOXINS THAT CAUSE ORTHOSTATIC HYPOTENSION

Antihypertensives	***Ciguatera***
Alpha-adrenergic antagonists	***Diuretics***
Central $alpha_2$-adrenergic agonists	Thiazides
Angiotensin converting enzyme inhibitors and antagonists	Loop diuretics
Ganglionic blockers	***CNS depressants***
Trimethaphan	Ethanol
Miscellaneous	Opioids
Reserpine	Sedative-hypnotics
Vasodilators	***Neuroleptics***
Hydralazine	Phenothiazines
Nitrates	Butyrophenones
Antianginals	***Drugs or toxins causing volume depletion***
Beta-adrenergic antagonists	See Table 21–2 for a detailed listing of drugs and toxins.
Calcium channel blockers	
Antidepressants	
Cyclic antidepressants	
MAO inhibitors	
Antiparkinson agents	
Bromocriptine	
L-Dopa	
Pergolide mesylate	

TABLE 17–4. COMMON DRUGS AND TOXINS THAT AFFECT BLOOD PRESSURE

Hypotension	Hypertension
Alpha-adrenergic antagonists	Amphetamines
Angiotensin converting enzyme inhibitors and antagonists	Anticholinergics
Antidysrhythmic agents	Cocaine
Anticholinergics	Ephedrine/pseudoephedrine
Arsenic (acute)	Ergotamine and derivatives
Beta-adrenergic antagonists	Epinephrine
Calcium channel blockers	Lead
Ciguatera	Monoamine oxidase inhibitors (overdose and drug interaction)
Clonidine	Nicotine (early)
Cyanide	Phencyclidine
Cyclic antidepressants	Phenylpropanolamine
Disulfiram/ethanol	Thallium
Ethanol	
Iron	
Isopropanol	
Mercury	
Methanol	
Nitrates and nitrites	
Nitroprusside	
Opioids	
Organophosphates and carbamates	
Phenothiazines	
Sedative-hypnotic agents	
Theophylline	

See Chapter 21, Cardiovascular Principles, for additional agents that affect hemodynamic function.

for children must be used and examination of blood pressures in both arms and legs, if indicated, will prevent serious diagnostic errors.

Pulse

Extremely useful clinical information can be obtained by evaluating the pulse for rate, regularity, and amplitude (see Table 17–5; Chap. 21). The carotid artery is usually easily palpated in children and young adults; however, for reasons of safety and reliability the brachial artery is preferred in infants and elderly adults. A direct correlation exists in that heart rate increases approximately 8 beats/min for each 1° C elevation in temperature.[3]

The pulse rate is the net result of a balance between adrenergic and cholinergic (muscarinic and nicotinic) tone. It follows that any substance that exerts a therapeutic or toxic effect on these components can result in pulse abnormalities. Beta-adrenergic antagonists, calcium channel blockers, clonidine, digitalis, and related compounds cause bradycardia. Mushrooms with varying quantities of muscarine (*Clitocybe* and *Inocybe* spp.) may have the same effect. Organophosphate and carbamate insecticides, by inhibiting acetylcholinesterase, usually produce a bradycardia through muscarinic effects, although due to their nicotinic effects and the potential for causing hypoxia and hypovolemia, may also produce tachycardia.

TABLE 17–5. COMMON DRUGS AND TOXINS THAT AFFECT PULSE

Bradycardia	Tachycardia
Antidysrhythmics	Amphetamines
Alpha-adrenergic agonists	Antihistamines
Beta-adrenergic antagonists	Atropine and other anticholinergics
Calcium channel blockers	Arsenic (acute)
Ciguatera	Caffeine
Clonidine	Carbon monoxide
Digitalis glycosides	Cocaine
Opioids	Cyanide
Organophosphates and carbamates	Cyclic antidepressants
	Disulfiram/ethanol
	Ephedrine/pseudoephedrine
	Epinephrine
	Ethylene glycol
	Iron
	Organophosphates and carbamates
	Phencyclidine
	Phenothiazines
	Sedative hypnotic withdrawal
	Thallium
	Theophylline
	Thyroxine

See Chapter 21, Cardiovascular Principles, for additional agents affecting heart rate.

Bradycardia also quite commonly results from many drugs that cause CNS depression, including sedative-hypnotics, opioids, and clonidine. Substances that directly affect the myocardial pacemaker and conduction pathways can result in the most profound bradycardias.

Tachycardia commonly results from stimulants such as amphetamines, caffeine, cocaine, nicotine, theophylline, sympathomimetic agents, and withdrawal from ethanol or sedative-hypnotic agents. Antihistamines and anticholinergic agents such as atropine, scopolamine, and the cyclic antidepressants may cause a marked tachycardia. The inability to differentiate easily between the adrenergics and anticholinergics by vital signs alone illustrates the principle that no single vital sign abnormality can definitively establish a toxicologic diagnosis. As previously noted, an abnormal vital sign can be much more helpful in establishing a diagnosis when it is part of a group of signs or symptoms. In trying to differentiate between adrenergic and anticholinergic exposure, remember that although a rapid pulse rate (and several other vital sign abnormalities) commonly results from both adrenergics and anticholinergics, diaphoresis and/or increased bowel sounds suggest adrenergic toxicity, whereas decreased sweating, absent bowel sounds, and urinary retention help diagnose or point to anticholinergic toxicity (Table 34–3).

Assessment of the amplitude of the pulse can be helpful in evaluating cardiac output. For example, the alternating force known as pulsus alternans results from extrasystoles and myocardial dysfunction due to digitalis poisoning.

Respiratory Rate

As always, establishment of an airway and evaluation of respiratory status are the initial priorities in patient stabilization. Although respiration is usually assessed initially for rate, careful observation of the depth and pattern is essential (see Table 17–6) in establishing the etiology of a systemic illness or toxic exposure.

Tachypnea, an increase in rate, may result from the direct effect of a CNS stimulant, salicylates acting on the brainstem, or aspiration of gastric contents, a common complication of toxic exposures to hydrocarbon products or CNS depressants. Pulmonary injury from any source may lead to hypoxemia with initial increase of the tachypnea but later depression of the respiratory rate and depth. In the case of CNS depressants, bradypnea, or a decrease in rate, may occur sooner as an effect of the drug on the brainstem. Progression from fast to slow breathing may also be seen with increasing levels of cyanide or carbon monoxide.

As a result of CNS depression, the alcohols methanol or ethylene glycol, may transiently cause hypoventilation due to bradypnea (a decreased rate of breathing) or hypopnea (a decrease in tidal volume). In time, however, hyperventilation (tachypnea or hyperpnea) will become predominant as late-onset metabolic

TABLE 17–6. COMMON DRUGS AND TOXINS THAT AFFECT RESPIRATORY RATE

Bradypnea	Tachypnea
Barbiturates	Carbon monoxide
Clostridium botulinum	Cyanide
Clonidine	Ethylene glycol
Ethanol	Hydrogen sulfide
Isopropanol	Isopropanol
Neuromuscular blockers	Methanol
Opioids	Methemoglobin producing agents
Organophosphates and carbamates	Nicotine
Sedative-hypnotics	Organophosphates and carbamates
	Salicylates
	Sympathomimetics
	Theophylline

See Chapter 20, Respiratory Principles, for additional agents affecting respiratory rate.

acidosis develops. In general, metabolic acidosis is ordinarily accompanied by hyperventilation as a compensatory mechanism to maintain (or attempt to maintain) a normal pH. Drugs and toxins that routinely produce a metabolic acidosis include salicylates, methanol, ethylene glycol, and sometimes ethanol when it results in alcoholic ketoacidosis: "Hyperventilation" may be characterized by tachypnea (an increased rate of breathing) or hyperpnea (an increase in tidal volume), or both. Salicylate poisoning may result in only an increased tidal volume or hyperpnea and may not necessarily result in tachypnea. When hyperventilation results solely or predominantly from hyperpnea, the less-astute clinician may miss this important finding entirely and even incorrectly describe such a hyperventilating patient as "hypoventilating" if the rate is slow.

Cluster breathing, which may appear similar to the normal periodic breathing seen in many young infants, is characterized by normally grouped respirations followed by apnea. It may occur with significant respiratory center dysfunction associated with CNS depressant or clonidine overdose.

Other respiratory patterns, such as central neurogenic hyperventilation or apneustic and ataxic breathing, may result from neurologic catastrophes and do not specifically implicate a toxicologic etiology. Central hyperventilation or rapid deep respirations often evolve into apneustic respirations, manifested by prolonged inspiration associated with slow, short expiratory movements. Ataxic or chaotic, irregular rhythms imply failure of respiratory control at the level of the medulla and often precede respiratory arrest. The progression from Cheyne-Stokes breathing, characterized by an increase in depth and sometimes rate of respiration followed by apnea, to ataxic breathing is evidence of a rostrocaudal deterioration of neurologic function from any etiology. Specific causes of this progressive deterioration include posttraumatic herniation, hypoxia, cerebrovascular accidents, and meningitis. It is important to note, however, that toxin- or drug-induced CNS dysfunction classically presents with a rostrocaudal *dissociation of neurologic signs* not corresponding to a well-defined lesion affecting a single locus or contiguous loci. The combination of ataxic breathing with intact pontine reflexes such as reactive pupils is a good example of the dissociative neurologic character of toxin-induced coma in contradistinction to a pontine hemorrhage (Chap. 19).

Temperature

Temperature evaluation and control are critical. However, temperature assessment can be done only if safe and reliable equipment is used. The risks of inaccuracy are substantial when an oral temperature is taken in the tachypneic patient, an axillary temperature is taken in the patient found outdoors, or a tympanic temperature is taken in a patient with cerumen. A rectal temperature with a rubber protective probe is essential when dealing with an agitated individual. In this text temperature determinations are performed per rectum unless stated otherwise.

Both hypothermia (T < 35°C; < 95°F) and hyperthermia (T > 38°C; > 100.4°F) are common manifestations of overdose, and unless immediately recognized and managed appropriately they can result in grave complications and inappropriate or inadequate resuscitation efforts. Hyperthermia from any cause can lead to extensive muscle breakdown and myoglobinuric renal failure as well as direct brain injury.

Fever can result from a distinct neurologic response to a signal demanding thermal up-regulation or from an externally imposed hyperthermia as seen in heat stroke, in cancer chemotherapy, or in an infant excessively swaddled in clothing.[10] Fevers higher than 41.1°C (106°F) are extremely rare unless normal feedback mechanisms are overwhelmed.[1] Hyperthermia of this extreme nature is usually attributed to heat stroke, malignant hyperthermia, or drug-related temperature disturbances.

Fever patterns accompanying diverse medical problems have been documented extensively over the years but appear to have only a limited value in medical toxicology. Fever patterns have been studied with regard to infectious diseases, and even in this field of specialization the patterns are not specific enough to be of substantial assistance.[8]

Drug-induced fevers coincide with the administration of a drug and disappear within 48–96 hours of its discontinuation.[5,9] One of the most common drug-related fever patterns in the emergency department is defervescence after an acute episode of hyperthermia associated with agitation or a seizure. In the case of a seizure, fever persists for several hours, even in the absence of an infectious etiology for the elevation in body temperature. One-third of the patients may still be febrile at 48 hours,[11] substantially longer than the duration of the associated lactic acidosis, which usually dissipates within 1 hour.[9]

Table 17–7 is a representative list of toxins that affect body temperature (see Chap. 18 for greater detail). The

TABLE 17–7. COMMON DRUGS AND TOXINS THAT AFFECT BODY TEMPERATURE

Hyperthermia	Hypothermia
Amphetamines	Carbon monoxide
Anticholinergics	Ethanol and other alcohols
Antihistamines	Hypoglycemic agents
Arsenic (acute)	Opioids
Cocaine	Phenothiazines
Cyclic antidepressants	Sedative-hypnotic agents
Dinitrophenol	
Lithium	
Monoamine oxidase inhibitors	
Phencyclidine	
Phenothiazines	
Salicylates	
Sedative-hypnotic withdrawal	
Theophylline	
Thyroxine	

See Chapter 18, Thermoregulatory Principles, for a more complete listing.

CNS stimulants, such as the amphetamines, cocaine, and phencyclidine, cause hyperthermia, predominantly on the basis of hyperactivity and extreme muscle hypertonicity as well as by peripheral and central thermogenic mechanisms. Antihistamines, anticholinergic agents, and cyclic antidepressants produce hyperthermia by central and peripheral mechanisms. Salicylates and dinitrophenol can produce hyperthermia by uncoupling oxidative phosphorylation (see Chap. 32).

Excessive exogenous thyroid hormone can increase the basal metabolic rate, thereby raising a patient's temperature. Any phase of ethanol or sedative-hypnotic withdrawal may produce increased motor activity and hyperthermia (Chap. 70).

Hypothermia will impair the metabolism of many drugs at both toxic and therapeutic levels, leading to unpredictable delayed effects when the patient is warmed. Most importantly, a hypothermic patient should never be declared dead without both an extensive assessment, as well as a full resuscitative effort, particularly if the body temperature remains less than 95°F (35°C). Hypothermia is most commonly caused by environmental exposure, but drugs and toxins that cause metabolic failure or impairment, such as carbon monoxide, cyanide, hydrogen sulfide, sulfonylureas, and insulin, can also produce hypothermia. Drugs and toxins such as phenothiazines, butyrophenones, barbiturates, ethanol, opioids, and sedative-hypnotics may cause hypothermia by direct central hypothalamic and/or peripheral effects (vasodilation). In addition, all of these drugs and toxins impair judgment and CNS function, thereby placing patients at great risk for hypothermia resulting from exposure to the cold of northern winter climates.

Continuous monitoring of the vital signs is as essential in medical toxicology as in any other type of emergency or critical care medicine. For this reason not only are the vital signs an essential part of the initial evaluation of every case, but repeated values are almost always necessary throughout the subsequent case management.

Acknowledgment

Alan G. Kulberg, MD contributed to this chapter in a previous edition.

References

1. Dubois EF: Why are fever temperatures over 106° F rare? Am J Med Sci 1949;217:361–368.
2. Fiore MC: The new vital signs: Assessing and documenting smoking status. JAMA 1991;266:3183–3189.
3. Karajalainen J, Vitassalo M: Fever and cardiac rhythm. Arch Intern Med 1986;146:1169–1171.
4. Lipsitz LA: Orthostatic hypotension in the elderly. N Engl J Med 1989;321:952–957.
5. Lipsky BA, Hirschman JV: Drug fever. JAMA 1981;245:851–854.
6. Mofenson HC, Greensher J: The nontoxic ingestion. Pediatr Clin North Am 1970;17:583–590.
7. Musher DM, Dominguez EA, Bar-Sela A: Edouard Seguin and the social power of thermometry. N Engl J Med 1987;316:115–117.
8. Musher DM, Fainstein V, Young EJ, Pruett TL: Fever patterns: their lack of clinical significance. Arch Intern Med 1979;139:1225–1228.
9. Orringer CE, Eustace JC, Wunsch CD, Gardner LB: Natural history of lactic acidosis after grand mal seizures: A model for the study of an anion gap acidosis not associated with hyperkalemia. N Engl J Med 1977;297:796–799.
10. Styrt B, Sugarman B: Antipyresis and fever. Arch Intern Med 1990;150:1589–1597.
11. Wachtel TJ, Steele GH, Day JA: Natural history of fever following a seizure. Arch Intern Med 1987;147:1153–1155.

CHAPTER 18

Thermoregulatory Principles

Susi U. Vassallo and Kathleen A. Delaney

Despite exposure to wide fluctuations of environmental temperature, human body temperature is maintained within a narrow range.[15,104] Elevation or depression of body temperature occurs when (1) thermoregulatory mechanisms are overwhelmed by exposure to extremes of environmental heat or cold; (2) endogenous heat production is either inadequate, resulting in hypothermia, or exceeds the physiologic capacity for dissipation, resulting in hyperthermia; or (3) disease processes or drug effects interfere with normal thermoregulatory responses to heat or cold exposure.

Methods of Heat Transfer

Heat is transfered to or away from the body through radiation, conduction, convection, and evaporation. *Radiation* involves the transfer of heat from a body to the environment and from warm objects in the environment, for example the sun, to a body. *Conduction* involves the transfer of heat to solid or liquid media in direct contact with the body. Water immersion or wet clothing in contact with the body conducts significant amounts of heat away from the body. This effect facilitates cooling in a swimming pool on a hot summer day, or may lead to hypothermia despite moderate ambient temperatures on a rainy day. The amount of heat lost through conduction and radiation depends on the temperature gradient between skin and surroundings, cutaneous blood flow, and insulation such as subcutaneous fat, hair, clothing, or fur in lower animals.[118] In the respiratory tract, heat is lost by conduction to water vapor or gas. In animals unable to sweat, this represents the primary method of heat loss. The amount of heat lost through the respiratory tract depends on the temperature gradient between inspired air and the environment, as well as the rate and depth of breathing.[118] *Convection* is the transfer of heat to the air surrounding the body. Wind velocity and ambient air temperature are the major determinants of convective heat loss. *Evaporation* is the process of vaporization of water, or sweat. Large amounts of heat are dissipated from the skin during this process, resulting in cooling. Ambient temperature, rate of sweating, air velocity, and relative humidity are important factors in determining how much heat is lost through evaporation. On a very humid day, sweat may pour off, rather than evaporate from a person exercising in a hot environment, thereby accomplishing little heat loss. In very warm environments, thermal gradients may be reversed, leading to transfer of heat to the body by radiation, conduction, or convection.[130,154]

Physiology of Thermoregulation

In the normal human, stimulation of peripheral and hypothalamic temperature-sensitive neurons results in autonomic, somatic, and behavioral responses that lead to the dissipation or conservation of heat. Thermoregulation is the complex physiologic process that serves to maintain hypothalamic temperature within a narrow range of 37 ± 0.4°C known as the set point.[256] This hypothalamic set point is influenced by diurnal variation and the menstrual cycle. Maintaining, raising, or lowering the set point results in many outwardly visible physiologic manifestations of thermoregulation such as sweating, shivering, flushing, or panting. In the central nervous system, thermosensitive neurons are located predominantly in the preoptic area of the anterior hypothalamus, although some are found in the posterior hypothalamus. Warming of the hypothalamus in conscious animals results in vasodilation, hyperventilation, salivation, and increases in evaporative water loss as well as a reduction of cold-induced shivering and vasoconstriction.[102] Cooling of the hypothalamus in conscious animals causes shivering, vasoconstriction, and increased metabolic rate, even if the environment is hot.[94] How these temperature-sensitive neurons of the hypothalamus detect change and effect neuronal transmission is unclear. Altered action potential initiation and propagation due to temperature-dependent changes in membrane potential, changes in the ratios of Na^+ to Ca^{2+} ions, which alter neuronal excitability and neurotransmitter release, or effects on the Na^+ K^+-ATPase pump, may be involved.[118] In the brainstem, warm- and cold-sensitive neurons are located in the medullary reticular formation, where information from cutaneous receptors, spinal cord, and preoptic area of the anterior hypothalamus is processed and relayed from the periphery to the hypothalamus.[104,107,110,177]

The spinal cord also manifests thermosensitivity. Heat- and cold-sensitive ascending spinal impulses are conducted in the spinothalamic tract. As in the hypothalamus, heating or cooling of the spinal cord locally causes thermoregulatory responses to occur.[102] In addition to the hypothalamus, brainstem, and spinal cord, there is evidence of thermosensitivity in the deep abdominal viscera.[90,102,201] Intraabdominal heating or cooling results in thermoregulatory responses. Cold- and warm-sensitive afferent impulses can be recorded from the splanchnic nerves in animals.[90,203] Finally, the skin also contains heat and cold thermosensitive neurons. Cold receptors are free nerve endings that protrude into the basal epidermis, while warm-sensitive receptors protrude into the dermis.[101,103] Cutaneous thermoreceptor output is effected by the absolute temperature of the skin, rate of temperature change, and area of stimulation.[102] Cutaneous cold receptors are Aδ and C nocioreceptor afferent fibers. Aδ-fibers are small-diameter thinly myelinated fibers that conduct at 5–30 m/s, and C-fibers are small-diameter unmyelinated fibers that conduct at 0.5–2 m/s.[122] Afferents from heat receptors are primarily C-fibers. Cutaneous thermoreceptive neurons respond to external temperature change as well as rate of temperature change, sending early warning to the CNS via afferent impulses, allowing rapid and transient thermoregulatory responses before brain temperature changes (Fig. 18–1).

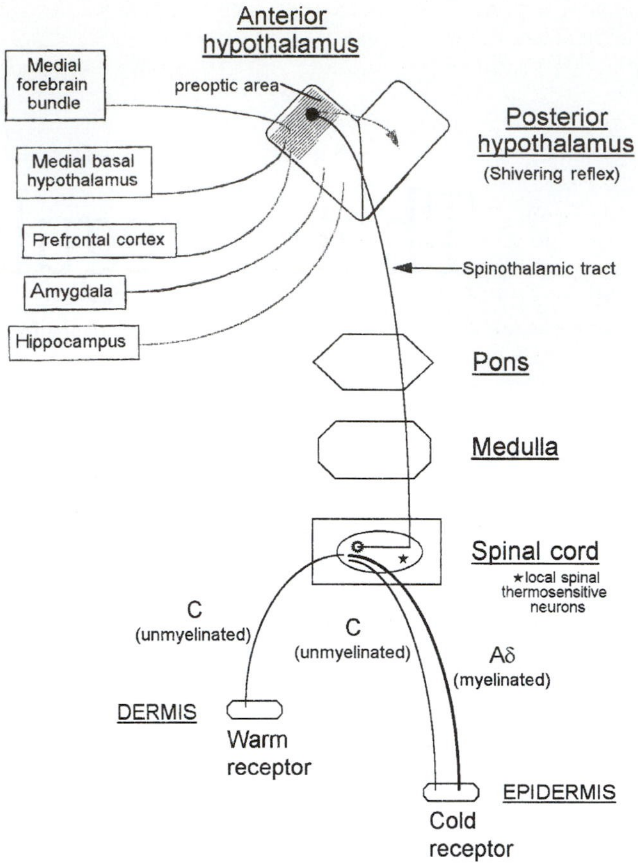

Figure 18–1. A schematic representation of the response of cutaneous thermoreceptive neurons to external temperature change as an early warning to the central nervous system.

Vasomotor and Sweat Gland Function

Vasomotor responses to thermoregulatory input differ according to location. The normal thermoregulatory response to heat stress is mediated primarily by heat-sensitive neurons in the hypothalamus. Increased body core temperature results in active dilation in the extremities and is under noradrenergic control; increasing sympathetic stimulation results in vasoconstriction, and decreasing sympathetic control results in vasodilation. Vasodilation in the head, trunk, and proximal limbs is due not to decreased sympathetic tone but rather to an active process that is under the influence of cholinergic sudomotor nerves and local effects of temperature on venomotor tone. Sweat glands release local transmitters such as vasoactive intestinal polypeptide (VIP) or bradykinins and vasodilation results. Areas of the body such as the forehead, where sweating is most prominent during heat stress, correspond to areas where active vasodilation is greatest. The neurotransmitters involved in the relationship between vasodilation and sweating as a reponse to heat stress are not fully elucidated, but animal evidence suggests the presence of specific vasodilator nerves.[102]

Sweat glands are controlled by sympathetic postganglionic nerve fibers, which are cholinergic, and large amounts of acetylcholinesterase as well as other peptides involved in neural transmission such as VIP are found in sudomotor nerve terminals.[101,102]

Neurotransmitters and Thermoregulation

The neurotransmitters involved in thermoregulation include serotonin, norepinephrine, acetylcholine, dopamine, prostaglandins, β-endorphins, and intrinsic hypothalamic peptides such as arginine vasopressin, adrenocorticotrophic hormone, thyrotropin releasing hormone, and α-melanocyte stimulating hormone.[38,188] Studies on the effects of individual neurotransmitters in thermoregulation yield contradictory results, depending on the animal species and the route of administration of the exogenous neurotransmitter. Refinements in techniques of microinjection of neurotransmitters into the hypothalamus of animals, rather than intraventricular instillation, have elucidated microanatomic sites where neurotransmitters are active. However, more research is necessary with regard to stimulation of thermoregulatory responses by individual neurotransmitters. Interspecies variation and theoretical differences in response to exogenous versus endogenous peptides makes this study difficult.

Apomorphine is a mixed dopamine agonist that has been shown to cause hypothermia in animals; studies using selective D_1 and D_2 receptor agonists and antagonists suggest the hypothermic effect of apomorphine is due to its effects on D_2 receptors, with some modulation by D_1 receptors in the hypothalamus.[164] Stimulation of D_2 receptors appears to mediate the hypothermia induced by the peptide sauvagine.[25] Dopamine D_3 receptors undoubtedly play a role as well; stimulation of D_3 by specific agonists caused hypothermia in an animal model.[165,166] There appears to be a link between dopamine D_2 receptors and norepinephrine receptors in the hypothalamus, perhaps leading to vasodilation and hypothermia. The effect of clozapine in producing hypothermia in the rat was demonstrated to be due to D_1 and D_3 stimulation.[165,212] Lesser-known peptides appear to be involved in thermoregulation. For example, neuropeptide Y is an amino acid neurotransmitter that occurs in high concentrations in the preoptic area of the anterior hypothalamus. Administration of neuropeptide Y caused a reduction in core temperature when administered with adrenoceptor antagonists such as prazosin, an α_1 antagonist, propranolol, a β-adrenergic antagonist, and clonidine, a central α_2-adrenergic agonist.[66,211] The administration of synthetic cannabinoids induces hypothermia in animals, an effect which is antagonized by adrenergic agonists and enhanced by adrenergic antagonists.[196] Finally, studies on muscarinic receptors suggests the involvement of muscarinic M_2 and M_3 receptors in the production of hypothermia when agonists to these receptors are administered centrally.[213] Blockers of ATP-sensitive K^+ channels can reverse the effect of cholinomimetic drugs in producing hypothermia.[198]

Furthur research into the relationship of neurotransmitters and thermoregulatory responses will clarify the complex interaction of neurotransmitters, receptors, and hypothermia. When elucidated, the effects of pharmacologic agents on thermoregulation will be better understood.

Drug Effects on Thermoregulation

Many drugs and toxins have pharmacologic effects that interfere with thermoregulatory responses[152,155,245] (Tables 18–1, 18–2). Alpha-adrenergic agonist agents (eg, phenylephrine, phenylpropanolamine, cocaine) prevent vasodilation in response to heat stress. Increased endogenous heat production in the setting of increased motor activity also occurs in patients poisoned with cocaine or amphetamines. Life-threatening hyperthermia has been associated with the use of these agents. Beta-adrenergic antagonists and calcium channel blockers diminish the

TABLE 18–1. EFFECTS OF DRUGS AND TOXINS THAT PREDISPOSE TO HYPERTHERMIA

I. Impaired cutaneous heat loss
- A. Vasoconstriction through α-adrenergic stimulation
  - Amphetamine
  - Cocaine
  - Ephedrine
  - Phenylpropanolamine
  - Pseudoephedrine
- B. Sweat gland dysfunction by anticholinergic effects
  - Antihistamines
  - Belladonna alkaloids
  - Cyclic antidepressants
  - Phenothiazines

II. Myocardial depression
- A. Decreased cardiac output
  - Antidysrhythmic agents
  - β-adrenergic antagonists
  - Calcium channel blockers
- B. Reduced cardiac filling by dehydration
  - Diuretics
  - Ethanol

III. Hypothalamic depression
- Neuroleptic agents

IV. Impaired behavioral response
- Ethanol
- Opioids
- Phencyclidine
- Sedative-hypnotics
- Cocaine

V. Uncoupling of oxidative phosphorylation
- Pentachlorophenol
- Dinitrophenol
- Salicylates

VI. Increased muscle activity through agitation, seizures, or rigidity
- Amphetamine
- Caffeine
- Cocaine
- Isoniazid
- Lithium
- Monoamine oxidase inhibitors
- Phencyclidine
- Strychnine
- Sympathomimetic agents

VII. Dystonia
- Butyrophenones
- Phenothiazines

VIII. Withdrawal
- Dopamine agonist
- Ethanol
- Sedative-hypnotic

TABLE 18–2. EFFECTS OF DRUGS AND TOXINS THAT PREDISPOSE TO HYPOTHERMIA

Impaired nonshivering thermogenesis
β-Adrenergic antagonists
Cholinergic agents
Hypoglycemic agents
Impaired perception of cold
Carbon monoxide
Ethanol
Hypoglycemic agents
Opioids
Sedative-hypnotics
Impaired shivering by hypothalamic depression
Carbon monoxide
Ethanol
General anesthetic agents
Opioids
Phenothiazines
Sedative-hypnotics
Impaired vasoconstriction
α-Adrenergic antagonists
Ethanol
Phenothiazines

cardiac reserve available to compensate for heat-induced vasodilation, whereas diuretics decrease cardiac reserve through their effects on intravascular volume.[50] Beta-adrenergic antagonists also interfere with the capacity to maintain euthermia under conditions of cold stress, possibly related to their interference with the mobilization of substrates required for thermogenesis.[102,155] Opioids, and diverse sedative-hypnotics, depress hypothalamic function and predispose to hypothermia in the overdose setting.[68] Carbon monoxide poisoning must also be considered in the hypothermic patient. Organophosphate insecticides and other agents that cause cholinergic stimulation cause hypothermia by stimulation of inappropriate sweating and possibly through depression of the endogenous utilization of calorigenic substrates.[155] Drugs with anticholinergic effects decrease sweating and predispose to hyperthermia during environmental heat exposure or exercise. Phenothiazines appear to interfere with normal response to both heat and cold. Severe hyperthermia associated with the absence of sweating has been frequently described in patients on phenothiazines and may be a consequence of their anticholinergic effects.[214,258] Effects on cold tolerance have been attributed to their α-adrenergic antagonist effects, which prevent vasoconstriction in response to cold stress.[153] In addition, hyperthermia associated with severe extrapyramidal rigidity may occur in patients on neuroleptic agents.[145] This rigidity is attributed to the dopamine-blocking effects of this class of drugs.

Ethanol

The most common variable related to the occurrence of hypothermia in an urban setting is the use of ethanol.[47,251] The mechanism by which ethanol predisposes to hypothermia is said to be by virtue of its effects on CNS depression, by vasodilation, and by blunting of behavorial responses to cold. However, thermoregulatory dysfunction in ethanol intoxication is undoubtedly more complex.

In animal models, ethanol leads to hypothermia, the extent of which depends in part on ambient temperature.[182,204,205] In mice, as the dose of ethanol increased, body temperature decreased and the rate of this decline in body temperature was faster at higher ethanol doses.[176] The decline in body temperature could be reversed by increasing ambient temperature; increasing ambient temperature to 36°C caused an immediate rise in the body temperature.[176] The poikilothermic effect of ethanol was not due to hypoglycemia, and hypoglycemia was not the reason for the thermolytic action of ethanol. Rats treated with equipotent amounts of sodium pentobarbital showed the same effects on body temperature as rats treated with ethanol, suggesting a similar central mechanism of depression of brain function resulting in altered thermoregulation.[176]

What mechanisms are involved in the "ethanol-induced depression of brain function"? A number of issues are currently under investigation. Genetic factors influence the effects of ethanol in producing hypothermia.[208] Mouse strains bred for sleep times differed in sensitivity to ethanol's effect on temperature.[78,169,176] Mice can be selectively bred for genetic sensitivity or insensitivity to acute ethanol-induced hypothermia, and the differences appear to be mediated by the serotonergic systems.[69] Another neurotransmitter found in many animal species, known as Histidyl-proline dike-topiperazine (cyclo His-Pro or CHP) acts at the preoptic-anterior hypothalamus to modulate body temperature in many animal species.[31,111] Exogenous administration of this neuropeptide produced a dose-dependent decrease in ethanol-induced hypothermia. Attenuation of hypothermia resulted from passive immunization with CHP antibody.[31,111] Ethanol effects may be mediated through modulation of endogenous opioid peptides, as high dose (10 mg/kg) naloxone reverses ethanol-induced hypothermia in animals.[193]

Pharmacokinetic parameters of ethanol metabolism change in hypothermia. Hypothermic piglets infused with ethanol showed slower ethanol metabolism and a smaller volume of distribution and, as a result, higher ethanol levels than normothermic controls. Ethanol elimination and metabolism decreased as temperature fell.[135]

Tolerance develops to the effect of ethanol in producing hypothermia in all species.[70,182] The degree of tolerance is proportional to the dose and duration of treatment with ethanol and is not accounted for by the increased rate of metabolism with chronic exposure.[118] Age is a factor in the development of tolerance; older animals do not display this same degree of tolerance to the hypothermic effects of chronic ethanol administration as do younger animals.[173,192,255] The development of tolerance to ethanol-induced hypothermia is affected by genetic factors. Experimentally, tolerance to ethanol-induced hypothermia increases the incorporation of certain amino acids into proteins in the rat brain. The formation of new proteins in ethanol-tolerant rats suggests stimulation of gene expression related to the tolerant state.[118,247] In addition to genetic factors, perhaps deficits in NMDA receptor systems occur, one mechanism implicated in the development of ethanol tolerance. In addition, altered NADH oxidation to NAD^+, diminished blood flow to the liver, or slowing of metabolism through the P450 microsomal enzyme system may be involved.[208]

Hypothermia alters the breath–ethanol partition in the alveolus, and the temperature of expired breath alters breath alcohol analysis results. Breath alcohol analysis of ethanol yields lower values by 7.3% per degree centigrade decrease in the patient with mild hypothermia.[73] Whether breath alcohol analysis is also affected by hyperthermia in the test subject remains to be studied.[73]

Disease Processes and Thermoregulation

Many disease processes interfere with normal thermoregulation, limiting an individual's capacity to prevent hypothermia or hyperthermia. Extensive dermatologic disease or burns impair sweating and vasomotor responses to heat stress.[27] Patients with autonomic disturbances (primarily diabetes) or peripheral vascular disease also have altered vasomotor responses that impair vasodilation and sweating.[202] Extensive surgical dressings may preclude the evaporation of sweat in an otherwise normal patient. Heat-stressed persons with poor cardiac reserve may not be able to sustain a skin blood flow high enough to maintain normothermia.[61,233] Intense motor activity may lead to excessive endogenous heat production in patients with Parkinson's disease or hyperthyroidism. Patients with agitated delirium or seizures also have significantly elevated rates of endogenous heat production. Hypothalamic injury caused by cerebrovascular accidents, trauma, or infection may disturb thermoregulation.[59,148] Hypothalamic dysfunction can lead to high, unremitting fevers and insufficient stimulation of heat loss mechanisms such as sweating. Hypothalamic damage may predispose to hypothermia by interference with centrally mediated heat conservation.[59,148,215,216] Fever, the normal response to stimulation of the hypothalamus by pyrogens, results in an elevated physiologic temperature set point and is a disadvantage in the heat-stressed individual.[102]

Hypothermia

Epidemiology

Hypothermia is defined as a lowering of the core body temperature to less than or equal to 95°F (35°C). From 1979 to 1992, at least 10,550 people died of hypothermia in the United States.[33] Approximately half of these deaths occurred in persons greater than age 64 years. Medical factors increased the risk in this group, including limited mobility, impaired shivering, chronic illness, confusion, decreased protective fat, and slower metabolic rates. Social isolation and deprivation, poor nutrition, and inadequate access to or utilization of indoor heating, often due to financial concerns, were additional factors associated with hypothermia.[34,105,126] Other risks associated with hypothermia in all groups were ethanol use, mental illness, use of neuroleptic medication, hypothyroidism, starvation, immobilization, dehydration, poverty, and homelessness[33] (Table 18–3).

Most hypothermic deaths occur in the winter months; however, mildly cool environments and windy wet conditions are also frequently associated with hypothermia. Of the 10 states with the greatest rate of hypothermia-related deaths, in only two, Illinois and Alaska, are the deaths associated with severe winter weather. The other states that led the nation in hypothermia-related deaths from 1979 to 1982 are not commonly associated with severe winter conditions and include Alabama, Arizona, New Mexico, North Carolina, Oklahoma, South Carolina, Tennessee, and Virginia.[33]

Response to Cold

The normal physiologic response to cold is precipitated by stimulation of cold-sensitive neurons in the skin, so that the onset of the body's response to cold occurs prior to cooling of central blood. Cold-sensitive neurons in the skin send afferent impulses to the hypothalamus, resulting in shivering and piloerection. Shivering is the main thermoregulatory response to cold in humans, except in neonates, where nonshivering thermogenesis prevails. Shivering arises in the posterior hypothalamus when impulses from cold-sensitive thermoreceptors are integrated in the anterior hypothalamus and communicated to the posterior hypothalamus, or when cold-sensitive neurons in the posterior hypothalamus are activated directly. Efferent stimuli from the posterior hypothalamus travel through the midbrain tegmentum, pons, and lateral medullary reticular formation to the motor pathways of the tectospinal and rubrospinal tracts, resulting in shivering.[18] In addition, local cooling of the spinal cord leads to shivering by increasing excitability of motor neurons, and this mechanism of stimulation of shivering may occur later, when core temperature drops.

Heat produced without muscle contraction is known as nonshivering thermogenesis.[26,102] Nonshivering thermogenesis is mediated by the sympathetic nervous system.[42] Catecholamines activate adenylate cyclase, increasing cAMP, resulting in mobilization of fat and glucose stores (β-adrenergic receptors).[155,210] It is blocked by β-adrenergic receptor blockade and increased by administration of norepinephrine. Brown adipose tissue is the most important site of nonshivering thermogenesis. In humans, brown fat is found primarily in neonates, although in cold-acclimatized people there may be small amounts found on autopsy.[26]

TABLE 18–3. FACTORS PREDISPOSING TO HYPOTHERMIA

Advanced age
Decreased metabolic rate
Decreased temperature discrimination
Decreased ability to shiver
Reduced peripheral blood flow
Central nervous system depression
Ethanol
Hypothalamic dysfunction
Infection
Intracranial bleeding
Stroke
Toxins
Endocrine
Diabetic ketoacidosis
Hyperosmolar coma
Hypopituitarism
Hypothyroidism
Environmental
Homelessness
Unintentional
Hepatic failure
Immobilization
Central nervous system dysfunction
Illness
Spinal cord injury
Trauma
Nutritional
Hypoglycemia
Glycogen depletion
Starvation
Thiamine deficiency
Sepsis
Social
Failure to use indoor heating
Homelessness
Inadequate indoor heating
Poverty
Social isolation
Uremia

In addition to shivering and nonshivering thermogenesis, efferent sympathetic fibers from the hypothalamus stimulate peripheral vasoconstriction (α-adrenergic receptors). Piloerection and vasoconstriction result in decreased heat loss from the body. Intense vasoconstriction shunts blood away from the periphery to the core and antidiuretic hormone antagonism results in increased urine output and hemoconcentration.

Disease Processes and Hypothermia

Several disease processes commonly result in an inability to maintain a normal body temperature in a cool environment. Hypothermia may develop in association with sepsis,[146] hypothyroidism, hypoglycemia, uremia, hepatic failure, or poor nutrition.[199,202] Hypothalamic injury may result in chronic poikilothermia, defined as variation in body temperature > ± 2°C upon exposure to environmental temperature changes.[153] Thiamine deficiency adversely affects the hypothalamus, perhaps because of inefficient glucose metabolism, and leads to hypothermia.[134] Spinal cord transections above the first thoracic segment interrupt hypothalamic–sympathetic outflow pathways, resulting in hypothermia.[202] The elderly are at greater risk of hypothermia because of decreased vasomotor responses and decreased capacity to shiver.[43,45] Mentally and physically impaired patients may be unable to make appropriate behavioral responses to heat or cold.

Evaluation for underlying disease is often difficult in the hypothermic patient.[71,146] The mental status may be markedly altered by hypothermia but is not usually abnormal until the temperature falls below 32°C (90°F). If normal mental status is not regained when the temperature reaches 90°F during rewarming, underlying CNS structural, toxic, or metabolic problems must be considered.[71,199] Failure of the patient to rewarm quickly suggests the presence of underlying disease. Hypothermic patients without underlying disease are reported to rewarm at a rate of 1.0–3.7°F/h (average, 2.1°F/h) while patients with significant underlying disease (sepsis, GI hemorrhage, diabetic ketoacidosis, pulmonary embolus, myocardial infarction) in one study warmed at a rate of 0.25–1.8°F/h (average, 1°F/h).[250]

Alteration of Drug Metabolism in Hypothermia

Metabolism of drugs is altered in the setting of hypothermia. In hypothermic piglets, volume of distribution and total body clearance of fentanyl is decreased.[137] Similarly, in piglets given gentamycin, the volume of distribution and clearance rate decreased linearly to the decrease in cardiac output and glomerular filtration rate.[136] Hypothermic puppies given intravenous lidocaine showed slower rate of disappearance of the drug than in normothermia.[170] Humans and animals given propranolol showed a reduced volume of distribution and decreased total body clearance, resulting in higher than expected propranolol levels.[159,179] Decreased hepatic metabolism of propranolol during hypothermia has been shown in vitro.[160]

Hypothermia prolongs neuromuscular blockade with *d*-tubocurarine[92] and increases neuromuscular blockade with suxamethonium.[253] Phenobarbital metabolism and volume of distribution decreased with hypothermia in children.[117] The lethal dose of digoxin was doubled in hypothermic dogs.[16]

The reasons for altered drug metabolism in hypothermia have yet to be elucidated. Volume of distribution changes, in part due to peripheral vasoconstriction. Cardiac output decreases,[189] leading to decreased liver perfusion and decreased delivery of drug to hepatic microsomal enzymes.[92,119,120,121] Plasma volume decreases as free water moves intracellularly, causing hemoconcentration and further decreasing organ perfusion.[254] Biliary excretion of atropine, procaine, and sulfanilamide has been demonstrated to decrease in vitro.[119,120,121] Glomerular filtration rate decreases in hypothermia.[23] In vitro, metabolic pathways including acetylation and hydrolysis decrease with cooling.[119,121] Reasons for altered metabolism include delayed distribution of the drug and altered enzyme function with temperature and pH changes.

Clinical Findings

The minimum temperature (>31.7°C; >90°F) on a standard clinical thermometer requires that the temperature be checked using a thermal probe. One such instrument, with a range of 20–42°C, is manufactured. This thermocouple has a pliable rubber-covered probe and allows for continuous temperature monitoring throughout the hospital course.

The clinical effects of hypothermia are related to the membrane-depressant effects of cold, which result in ionic and electrical conduction disturbances in the brain, heart, peripheral nerves, and other major organs[106] (Table 18–4). Cold tissues are protected by decreases in tissue oxygen requirements. As body temperature decreases, metabolic activity will decline at about 7% per 1°C.[254] This effect provides significant protection to vital organs despite the potentially deleterious effects of membrane suppression.

Effects on the central nervous system are temperature-dependent and predictable. Mild hypothermia (32–35°C ; 90–95°F) is usually relatively benign. Ataxia, slight clumsiness, slowed response to stimuli, and dysarthria are common.[71] As cooling continues, mental status slowly declines. In moderate hypothermia (27–32°C; 80–90°F), the patient is usually lethargic but still likely to respond verbally. In severe hypothermia (20–27°C; 68–80°F) the patient is unlikely to respond verbally but will react purposefully to noxious stimuli.[71] In profound hypothermia (<20°C; 68°F) the patient is unresponsive to stimuli. Pupils may be fixed and dilated and the patient may appear dead.[98] However, standard criteria of brain death do not apply to hypothermic patients. The hypothermia itself protects against cerebral hypoxic damage.[106] Temperature drop inhibits the release of the excitatory neurotransmitter glutamate and attenuates the release of dopamine in brain ischemia models, suggesting a protective effect of hypothermia in brain injury.[30] Ventricular cerebrospinal fluid glutamate concentrations were lower in patients showing benefit from mild induced hypothermia after brain injury when compared to brain injured patients kept normothermic. Under controlled circumstances patients have survived with temperatures as low as 9°C (48.2°F).[74] Vigorous resuscitation is required for these patients. In particular, cardiac resuscitation should not be terminated in the field, where temperatures are seldom taken. The adage that a patient cannot be considered dead until he or she is warm and dead is critical to providing appropriate management. This approach may lead to hours of cardiopulmonary resuscitation in hypothermic patients with ventricular fibrillation, ventricular tachycardia, or asystole but will be ultimately successful in certain patients initially presumed to be dead.[231]

The cardiac and hemodynamic effects of cold correlate closely with the temperature. As cooling begins there is a transient increase in cardiac output. Tachycardia develops secondary to shivering and sympathetic stimulation. At about 81°F (27°C) shivering ceases. Bradycardia develops with maintenance of a normal cardiac stroke volume.[28] This bradycardia is responsible for the decreased myocardial oxygen demand that is protective in the setting of hypothermia.[28] In profound hypothermia,

TABLE 18–4. PHYSIOLOGIC AND CLINICAL MANIFESTATIONS OF HYPOTHERMIA

Cardiovascular
Normal, decreased, or increased cardiac output
Normal heart rate or tachycardia, then bradycardia
Vasoconstriction and central shunting of blood
ECG
Prolongation of intervals
Atrial fibrillation
Increased ventricular irritability
J-point elevation
Central nervous system
Mild: 32–35°C (90–95°F)
Normal mentation or slightly slowed
Moderate: 27–32°C (80–90°F)
Lethargic but verbally responsive
Severe: 20–27°C (68–80°F)
Unlikely to respond verbally, purposeful to noxious stimuli
Profound: < 20°C (< 68°F)
Unresponsive, may appear dead
Gastrointestinal tract
Decreased motility
Depressed hepatic metabolism
Hematologic
Hemoconcentration
Left shift of oxyhemoglobin dissociation curve
Kidneys
Cold-induced diuresis
Antidiuretic hormone antagonism
Lungs
Respiratory rate variable
Bronchorrhea
Metabolic
Metabolic acidosis
Increased glycogenolysis
Increased serum free fatty acids
Normal thyroid and adrenal function

bradycardia may progress to asystole and death. Unlike cerebral circulation, where autoregulation is preserved during cooling, coronary autoregulation is disturbed during hypothermia, and myocardial injury may ensue.[28] Attempts to maximize myocardial oxygenation through administration of oxygen and volume replacement to increase diastolic filling pressure are worthwhile. Pharmacologic or electrical attempts to increase heart rate may dangerously increase myocardial oxygen demand.

The initial respiratory response to hypothermia is hyperventilation. As temperature continues to decrease, hypoventilation develops, which may progress to apnea and death. In animal models, this has been attributed to cold-induced failure of phrenic nerve conduction.[128]

Management

After blood specimens have been drawn, the hypothermic patient should be given 0.5–1.0 g glucose/kg body weight as $D_{50}W$ and 100 mg of thiamine IV. If hypoglycemia is the cause of the hypothermia, the response to glucose may be dramatic, heralded by the onset of shivering and rapid return to normal body temperature. Wernicke's encephalopathy is uncommon but may be associated with mild hypothermia; thermoregulation and normal ocular motion may return after the initiation of thiamine therapy.[134]

Hypothermia shifts the oxygen dissociation curve to the left (see Chap. 20), resulting in decreased oxygen unloading to tissues; therefore, oxygen administration may be of benefit.[52] If clinically indicated for airway protection or inadequate ventilation or oxygenation, endotracheal intubation should be performed and can be done without complication.[47,142,167] However, there are examples in the literature of ventricular fibrillation occurring during endotracheal intubation.[12,77,98,195,252] Every effort should be made to limit patient activity and stimulation during the acute rewarming period, which may increase myocardial oxygen demand or alter myocardial temperature gradients, increasing the risk of iatrogenic ventricular fibrillation. Although Swan-Ganz catheters and central venous lines have been placed without complications,[96,142] they should be avoided unless absolutely essential, so as not to precipitate ventricular dysrhythmias.[240] If a central venous catheter is considered necessary, it should not be allowed to touch the myocardium.[242] Patients who develop ventricular fibrillation are difficult to manage. In these instances, CPR should be initiated, and the patient intubated and ventilated to maintain a pH of 7.40 uncorrected for temperature. Aggressive rewarming should be instituted because standard therapy for ventricular fibrillation is often unsuccessful until rewarming is achieved. Patients should be supported, then defibrillated; if unsuccessful, defibrillation should not be attempted again until the patient has been warmed several degrees centigrade. Defibrillation may not be successful until the temperature exceeds 30°C (86°F); however, defibrillation occurring successfully in animals and patients with temperatures of less than 30°C is reported.[4,12, 49,172] The oxygen-powered "thumper" and cardiopulmonary bypass devices have been successfully used during prolonged hypothermic cardiopulmonary arrests.[12,41,144,232,240]

Hypotension

When hypotension occurs in hypothermia, it is usually due to the slowed heart rate and commonly associated volume depletion. Fluid depletion in hypothermia occurs due to a variety of mechanisms, including central shunting of blood by vasoconstriction and cold-induced diuresis. Cold diuresis occurs when increases in central blood volume result in inhibition of antidiuretic hormone. Impairment of renal enzyme activity and decreased renal tubular reabsorption contributes to the large quantities of dilute urine known as cold diuresis.[93,97,142,254] Normal saline should be given to expand intravascular volume. Urine output is an important indicator of organ perfusion and the adequacy of intravascular volume in the hypothermic patient, although the initial cold diuresis may lead to underestimation of fluid needs.[254]

Pharmacologic Interventions

Bretylium. Bretylium tosylate is a benzyl quarternary ammonium compound with a biphasic action, initially causing release of norepinephrine and then blocking its release. This may cause transient hypertension, but hypotension most commonly results.[172,193] Hypothermic dogs given bretylium had significantly lower mean arterial pressures and systemic and pulmonary vascular resistance as compared to control.[193] The mechanism of the antidysrhythmic effect of bretylium in normothermia may be related to its ability to increase the myocardial refractory period.[193]

Bretylium may be of benefit in the treatment of ventricular fibrillation during hypothermia. The antidysrhythmic effect of bretylium is poorly understood. It prolongs the cardiac action potential and reduces heterogeneity of repolarization times.[207] The net effect seems to be stabilization of the cardiac rhythm. Bretylium is found to increase the fibrillation threshold in hypothermic cats given 50 mg/kg bretylium[181] and in dogs given 15 mg/kg bretylium[29] and 7.5 mg/kg prior to cooling.[193] In a canine study[172] cooling occurred and either a saline placebo or bretylium 40 mg/kg were administered prior to attempted induction of ventricular fibrillation by manuevers. Six dogs out of 11 given placebo developed ventricular fibrillation with manipulation, whereas only 1 of the 11 dogs pretreated with bretylium developed ventricular fibrillation with manipulation. However, 3 dogs receiving pretreatment with bretylium fibrillated during the infusion, before manuevers were begun. Of the 6 dogs given placebo who fibrillated, all were successfully resuscitated, although 4 required bretylium to do so. This study did not attain statistical significance, and bretylium infusion both resulted in ventricular fibrillation and was effective in chemical defibrillation of ventricular fibrillation.[172] A single case of chemical defibrillation with bretylium has been reported in an unintentional hypothermia victim at 29.5°C.[48]

Dopamine. Dopamine increases cardiac output, mean arterial pressure, heart rate, and stroke volume in dogs cooled to 25°C, and stabilizes pulmonary arterial wedge pressure.[178] In a canine hypothermia model, dopamine infusions provided some protection from ventricular fibrillation. Dopamine lowered the temperature at which ventricular fibrillation occurred and reduced the incidence of ventricular fibrillation, as did infusion of norepinephrine.[7] The added benefit of dopamine in hypothermia may be due to its renal and splanchnic vasodilating properties, increasing renal perfusion and supporting urine output.[80] Dopamine increases myocardial oxygen demand and decreases peripheral perfusion, potentially detrimental effects in the hypothermic patient.[7]

Rewarming

Three types of rewarming modalities are used in the management of hypothermic patients.[44,147] Passive external rewarming involves covering the patient with blankets and protecting from further heat loss. Passive external rewarming uses the patient's own endogenous heat production for rewarming and is most successful in healthy patients with mild to moderate hypothermia whose capacity for endogenous heat production is intact.[97] Passive external rewarming has been reported to be successful in hypothermic patients with temperatures as low as 20.6°C (69°F).[238] Advocates of passive external rewarming argue that it allows vasoconstriction to persist and it decreases the incidence of core temperature "afterdrop" and shock from vasodilation associated with active skin rewarming.[97,167,238]

Active external rewarming involves the external application of heat to the patient. The use of this modality is controversial. Complications associated with active external rewarming are attributed to acute vasodilation of peripheral vessels, resulting in hypotension and an increased peripheral demand on the persistently cold myocardium. Skin warming may also lead to a physiologically detrimental suppression of shivering.[97] The return of cold blood from the extremities to the heart is suggested to exacerbate intramyocardial temperature gradients, which cause ventricular irritability in hypothermia.[151] Some authors advocate application of heat to the trunk only, rather than to the trunk and extremities, in an attempt to avoid these complications.[139] Despite this approach, in pigs, blood returning to the heart was found to be warm before warming of central organs occurred.[82] Active external rewarming is often used successfully.

Complete submersion is available in some institutions. Eighteen patients with temperatures of 26–33°C were successfully warmed in a Hubbard tank, although one fatality not associated with rewarming occurred.[257] Submersion must be used with caution, however, due to the inherent difficulties of controlling agitated patients and monitoring and resuscitating patients in water.

Mortality rates for active external rewarming are frequently reported to be higher than for passive external rewarming,[202] but case selection has not been controlled in these series. It is possible that sicker patients who fail to rewarm passively are then actively rewarmed and have a higher mortality rate due to their underlying disease rather than the method of therapy selected. The published series and case reports do not allow for an analysis of this hypothesis. Selection of either passive or active external rewarming in treatment of mild to moderate hypothermia does not appear to influence the prognosis as much as the presence or absence of underlying disease.[109,167,250] In our experience, passive rewarming has not resulted in mortality except in patients with severe underlying disease. We have had several patients with initial temperatures less than 21°C (69.8°F) who survived passive rewarming without lethal ventricular dysrhythmias. Studies with well controlled patient populations will be essential to resolve the debate over the merits of passive versus active rewarming.

Active core rewarming involves attempts to increase central core temperature directly, by warming the heart prior to the extremities or periphery. Minimally invasive modalities include the administration of heated, humidified oxygen delivered by face mask or endotracheal tube,[99] and gastric lavage with warmed fluids. Transcutaneous pacing was successful in improving hemodynamic parameters and speeding rewarming in an animal model.[57] Peritoneal lavage with warmed dialysate is another easily instituted, effective modality.[115,184] More invasive techniques involve the rerouting of blood through external blood rewarming equipment via cardiopulmonary or femoral–femoral bypass. Hemodialysis is also of benefit in rewarming and is effective in correcting acid–base disturbances.[32,104,174] Heparin-coated bypass systems are available, thereby avoiding systemic anticoagulation and thus decreasing the risk of bleeding complications. Extracorporeal venovenous rewarming and continuous arteriovenous rewarming show improved rewarming rates when compared to standard techniques such as saline lavage of the bladder, stomach, or peritoneal cavity.[76] Active core rewarming is generally reserved for severely hypothermic patients or those with unstable cardiac rhythms (ventricular fibrillation or tachycardia, or asystole) attributed to hypothermia.[4,51,98]

Afterdrop

Afterdrop is the continuing decrease in core temperature once rewarming begins. Afterdrop has been demonstrated in cooling experiments of inanimate objects and reflects continued cooling of central structures before heat from external sources reaches the core. There is no evidence to suggest that this drop in temperature is more dangerous than that same temperature arrived at during the original cooling.[150] Afterdrop is greater when rectal temperatures are measured than when myocardial temperatures are obtained.[99] Concern for afterdrop is frequently given as the reason that peripheral warming should be delayed in order that core temperature is not lowered by cooler blood returning from the extremities. However, there is no evidence of pooling of blood in the periphery nor of increased flow during surface rewarming.[150,217] Flow studies in the hand, arm, calf, and foot demonstrate that afterdrop has already occurred and is completed before any increase in blood flow occurs in the limbs.[150,249]

The Electrocardiogram

The most common ECG abnormality in hypothermia is generalized, progressive depression of myocardial conduction. Because myocardial oxygen demands remain unchanged in spite of cooling, and stroke volume is preserved, the number of beats per minute decreases as a means of decreasing myocardial oxygen requirements. PR, QRS, and QTc intervals are all prolonged, and increasingly profound hypothermia may lead to gradual progression to asystole.[243] Ventricular fibrillation occurs most commonly at temperatures less than 30°C (86°F) and is a high O_2 consumption dysrhythmia occurring in an irritable myocardium. Atrial fibrillation is the most common dysrhythmia occurring in hypothermia.[72,191,244] Shivering may not be clinically evident, but a fine muscular tremor frequently produces a mechanical artifact in the baseline of the electrocardiogram.[62] A deflection occurring at the junction of the QRS and ST segment is invariably present in patients with temperatures <30°C (86°F)[63] (Fig. 18–2). First described in a single patient in 1938,[239] the J-point deflection is commonly known as the Osborn wave.[194] The J-point deflection, thought to be a "current of injury" associated with CO_2 retention under hypothermic conditions, was believed to be a poor prognostic sign.[194] Subsequent study has refuted its prognostic significance, as the J-point deflection is invariably found in the hypothermic patient when multiple electrocardiographic leads are obtained.[62,63,241,244] The size of the J-point deflection increases as body temperature decreases.[190,244] Dysrhythmias that occur in the absence of underlying heart disease invariably disappear with rewarming alone.

Interpretation of Arterial Blood Gas Physiochemistry

Assessment of the adequacy of ventilation and oxygenation in the hypothermic patient often poses a dilemma to clinicians, as chemical effects of cold on arterial pH and blood gases lead to confusion in the interpretation of arterial blood gas values. Cold inhibits the dissociation of water molecules, causing pH to increase as cooling occurs. In vitro, the pH change of blood as it is cooled increases parallel to the pH change of neutral water. The partial pressures of CO_2 and O_2 decrease as cooling occurs, even as the blood content of those gases remains unchanged. Blood in a syringe taken from a patient whose body temperature is 98.6°F (37°C) yields a pH 7.40 and a PCO_2 40 mm Hg in the blood gas machine at 37°C but would yield a pH 7.72 and a PCO_2 14 mm Hg if the blood were cooled to 61°F (16°C) and the values were measured at that temperature. Specially calibrated laboratory equipment, not routinely available, is required to measure blood gas values directly at other than normal body temperature. A patient whose body temperature is 61°F (16°C) and whose actual in vivo blood gas values are pH 7.72 and PCO_2 14 mm Hg would have values of pH 7.40 and PCO_2 40 mm Hg when the blood was warmed to 37°C and measured in the standard laboratory blood gas machine. Because the machine measures pH and blood gas pressures only in blood warmed to 37°C (the uncorrected values), the actual in vivo values in hypothermic patients can be approximated using mathematically derived corrected values. Since the pH of neutrality has increased also, it is unclear what clinical meaning these corrected values have. The uncorrected values indicate what the pH and PCO_2 would be if the patient were euthermic. At first glance the clinician might be content to learn that a hypothermic patient at 16°C has a corrected pH of 7.47 and PCO_2 of 40 mm Hg. However, the uncorrected values of pH 7.18 and PCO_2 111 mm Hg indicate that the patient has a significant respiratory acidosis. Attempts to maintain a corrected pH of 7.40 may lead to hypoventilation and risk alveolar collapse and impairment of oxygenation. The preponderance of evidence in the anesthesia and cardiovascular surgery literature suggests that maintenance of ventilation is associated with a decreased incidence of myocardial injury and a decreased incidence of ventricular fibrillation.[52] Blood gas values of pH and PCO_2 should be left uncorrected after the blood sample is warmed in the blood gas machine and interpreted in the same way as in the euthermic patient.[52]

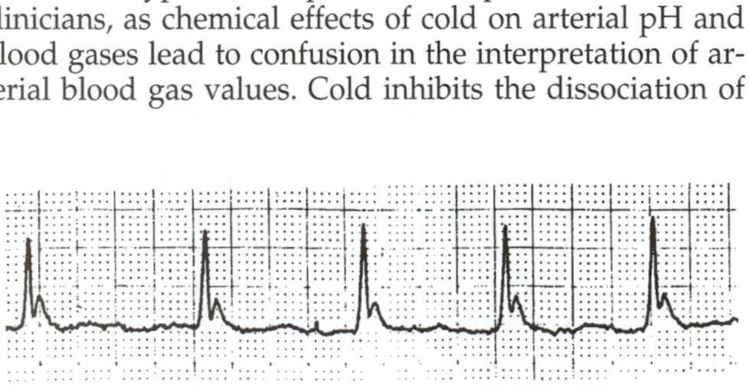

Figure 18–2. A characteristic electrocardiographic finding in the patient with profound hypothermia. The terminal phase of the QRS complex shows a typical elevation of the J-point or Osborn wave.

Prognosis in Hypothermia

Except in cases of profound hypothermia,[98] the prognosis is most closely correlated with the presence or absence of underlying disease.[109,167,187,250,251] In patients with hypothermia alone and no underlying disease mortality is 0–10%. In the presence of an underlying disease, mortality rises to 75–90%. Morbidity results from associated frostbite and trauma.

Prolonged cardiorespiratory arrest and absolute temperature do not predict poor outcome.[4,49,141,240,243] In severely hypothermic patients, profound hyperkalemia (K^+ >10 mmol/L) has been associated with unsuccessful resuscitation.[98,156,219]

Frostbite. Hypothermia may be accompanied by frostbite when patients are exposed to environmental temperatures that are less than –6.7°C (20°F).[168] Frostbite should be managed by rapid rewarming. The extremity involved may be placed in a large, soft basin of warm water (38–43°C; 100–108°F) for 30 minutes. The water temperature must be frequently adjusted, as the frozen extremity will have the effect of ice cubes, and with time cool the water in the basin. Analgesia may be necessary, as the rewarming process is often painful. Frostbitten areas should never be rubbed, as the tissue is particularly sensitive to trauma. Dextran, alcohol, vasodilators, and anticoagulants have not proven useful. Sympathectomy in this situation is also of unproven benefit and remains highly controversial.[129,140,162]

Prevention. Because many patients may not wear (and may not possess) adequate clothing, it is essential that they be assessed for social services support once the acute episode has been resolved. In addition, many of these patients live in substandard, inadequately heated (often unheated) housing. Patients should be advised to wear comfortable, warm clothing to prevent future episodes of hypothermia. Adequate clothing is particularly important for patients traveling by automobile in inclement weather. Multiple layers of loose-fitting, lightweight garments are warmer than bulky, dense, clothing. The importance of adequate nutrition should also be stressed.

Hyperthermia

Definition of Heatstroke

Heatstroke is defined by a rectal temperature greater than 106°F (41.1°C) in the setting of a neurologic disturbance manifested by psychosis, delirium, stupor, coma, and/or convulsions.[130] Temperature criteria cannot be absolute, as information regarding the patient's temperature is rarely available at the time of onset of heatstroke. In some instances the temperature may not be measured for several hours, during which time cooling may have been instituted or occurred spontaneously.[124,125] When appropriate environmental conditions prevail, the diagnosis of heatstroke should be made liberally. Although the absence of sweating was once thought to comprise part of the definition of heatstroke,[39,185] many patients with heatstroke have been noted to maintain the ability to sweat on presentation.[46,157,225,226]

Epidemiology of Heatstroke

Hundreds of Americans die annually of heatstroke, and 80% of the victims are older than 50 years. Heatstroke is the second most common cause of death among high school athletes, exceeded only by spinal injuries. Several studies have shown mortality rates from heatstroke to be 30%–80%. Thousands of others survive with significant heat-related morbidity.[6,58,116,127] The high morbidity and mortality of heatstroke markedly contrast with those of profound hypothermia, where the prognosis is related not to the temperature itself, but to the underlying etiology. The overall prognosis in heatstroke depends primarily on how long the temperature has been elevated prior to cooling, the maximum temperature reached, and the affected individual's health.

Heat-related deaths are preventable, and preparedness of cities and health care workers essential. Mortality during heat waves is increased in urban areas where there has not been a heat wave for several years.[37,60,116,221] Socially isolated individuals or those with preexisting illness, as well as the frail and elderly, are at greatest risk of death during heat waves. Confinement to bed was the strongest predictor of death in the Chicago heat wave of 1995, and living alone doubled the risk of death. There were fewer deaths among people with working air conditioners or access to an air-conditioned place.[222] In times of heat waves, preventive public health programs should encourage visiting nurses, housekeepers, and community service programs such as Meals-on-Wheels to increase the awareness of the danger of heat and identify those individuals most at risk.[222] A decreased risk of death was found among people contacted in this way during the Chicago heat wave.[222] The media must alert the public and provide information on avoiding heat illness, as well as encourage individuals to help one another to stay cool by assuring access to cooling measures.

Thermoregulation and Heat Stress

The normal thermoregulatory response to heat stress is mediated primarily by heat-sensitive neurons in the hypothalamus. Increased body core temperature results in active dilation of cutaneous vessels, and skin blood flow increases.[102,210] Increased skin blood flow is attained primarily by an increase in heart rate and stroke volume; therefore, the capacity to increase cardiac output is critical to cooling. Compensatory shifting of blood flow from the splanchnic and renal vessels to the skin furthur increases skin blood flow.[108,210] Sweat gland function is activated by parasympathetic stimulation, and the combination of vasodilation, increased skin blood flow, and increased sweating results in heat loss through convection and evaporation. Dehydration after profuse sweating increases plasma osmolarity. Heat-sensitive neurons in the preoptic anterior hypothalamus are inhibited by locally increased osmolarity and by input from distal hepatoportal osmoreceptors. The inhibition of heat-sensitive neurons results in decreased heat dissipation response.[38,188]

Types of Heatstroke

Heatstroke is commonly divided into two types: exertional and nonexertional. Nonexertional, or classical, heatstroke describes heatstroke occurring in the absence of extreme exertion. Nonexertional heatstroke is most commonly described during heat waves, and the victims are predominantly those persons least able to tolerate heat: infants,[10] the aged,[43] the psychiatrically impaired, and the chronically ill.

Exertional heatstroke occurs as a result of increased motor activity. It may occur in young, healthy individuals who are exercising or in individuals whose increased motor activity results from other causes, such as seizures or agitation. Often a period of significant heat stress in exercising individuals precedes the development of heatstroke. Military recruits who develop heatstroke may sometimes present to the camp infirmary with vague complaints prior to collapse.[225] Published studies of heatstroke in miners, athletes, and military recruits describe several precipitating factors in heatstroke: fatigue associated with a recent deficit in sleep, poor physical conditioning, a recent febrile illness, recent heat-related symptoms such as thirst or weakness, relative volume depletion, failure to allow for acclimatization, and obesity. Symptoms of nausea, weakness, headache, diarrhea, or irritability often precede the development of heatstroke. Although rapid onset of symptoms and acute loss of consciousness are frequently reported in exertional heatstroke, the preceding period of heat stress and insidious symptoms may go unrecognized. While exertional heatstroke is more likely to occur during intense exertion in a hot, humid environment, it may also occur with moderately intense exercise early in the morning, when environmental conditions do not usually represent a thermoregulatory stress.[8]

Infants may suffer heatstroke under circumstances that do not appear unusual. Well-meaning parents sometimes overinsulate children with clothing and blankets, inhibiting their cutaneous heat loss.[10,112,113,180]

Differential Diagnosis of Hyperthermia

In addition to exposure and exertion, conditions that predispose to severe hyperthermia include primary hypothalamic lesions, intracranial hemorrhage, agitation, alcohol and sedative-hypnotic withdrawal, seizures, and the use of therapeutic and illicit drugs[79,85,86,87,138,158,236] (Table 18–5). Included in the differential diagnosis of severe hyperthermia are the serotonin syndrome, malignant hyperthermia, and neuroleptic malignant syndrome, all of which may result in high temperature, altered mental status, and increased muscle tone.

TABLE 18–5. DIFFERENTIAL DIAGNOSIS OF HYPERTHERMIA

I. Increased heat production
- A. Increased muscle activity
  - Agitation
  - Catatonia
  - Ethanol withdrawal
  - Exercise
  - Infectious diseases
  - Malignant hyperthermia
  - Monoamine oxidase inhibitor drug interactions
  - Neuroleptic malignant syndrome
  - Parkinson's disease
  - Sedative-hypnotic withdrawal
  - Seizures
  - Serotonin syndrome
  - Toxins
- B. Increased metabolic rate
  - Hyperthyroidism
  - Pheochromocytoma
  - Sympathomimetic agents

II. Impaired heat loss
- A. Environmental
  - Heat
  - Humidity
  - Lack of acclimatization
- B. Social disadvantage
  - Isolation
  - Poverty
  - Lack of air conditioning
  - Confinement to bed
- C. Medical illness
  - Cardiac insufficiency
  - Diabetes
  - Hypertension
  - Pulmonary
  - CNS dysfunction
- D. Dehydration
- E. Fatigue
- F. Limited behavioral response
  - Extremes of age
  - Psychiatric impairment
  - Mental retardation
  - Toxin-induced

Serotonin Syndrome. The serotonin syndrome results from excess stimulation of the serotonin receptor, primarily the 5-HT_{1A} subtype.[235] Drug interactions are most commonly the cause of the syndrome. Monoamine oxidase inhibitors used in conjunction with tricyclic antidepressants,[14] selective serotonin reuptake inhibitors,[67] L-tryptophan,[11,237] meperidine,[95] dextromethorphan,[206] amphetamines,[138,229] and sumatriptan have all been reported to lead to serotonergic hyperstimulation and severe symptoms.[81,235] The clinical condition resulting from excess serotonin includes alterations in conciousness, restlessness, increased muscle tone, tremor, gastrointestinal disturbance, and hyperthermia. Treatment of the syndrome focuses on control of hyperthermia using aggressive cooling, muscle relaxation using primarily benzodiazepines, or, in severe cases, endotracheal intubation and paralysis (see Chap. 53).

Malignant Hyperthermia. Malignant hyperthermia is a very rare disorder associated with a congenital disturbance of calcium regulation in striated muscle. Malignant hyperthermia was first reported in 1960. Ten deaths occurred in a single family following general anesthesia.[55] Exposure to anesthetics, depolarizing muscle relaxants or, rarely, severe exertion precipitates uncontrolled calcium influx into the sarcoplasmic reticulum leading to severe muscle rigidity and hyperthermia.[88,114] The clinical setting of severe muscle rigidity and hyperthermia following general anesthesia usually is adequate to define the syndrome (see Chap. 53).

Neuroleptic Malignant Syndrome. A severe extrapyramidal syndrome associated with muscle rigidity, autonomic dysfunction, and altered mental status was first described in 1968.[53] This disorder develops during the administration of neuroleptic drugs or the withdrawal of dopaminergic agents. Increased muscle tone due to dopaminergic blockade of the striatum, as well as central altered hypothalamic thermoregulation, leads to hyperthermia.[100] Temperature elevation and alteration of mental status occur after the onset of muscle rigidity.[17,53,91] Laboratory findings are not specific and include marked elevation of CPK in some patients and leukocytosis with a left shift. Neuroleptic malignant syndrome must be distinguished from the much more common cases of heatstroke in psychiatric patients that are due to heat intolerance caused by the anticholinergic effects of neuroleptic drugs or antihistamines prescribed to control extrapyramidal symptoms[214,258] (see Chap. 57).

Pathophysiologic Characteristics of Heatstroke

Hypotension and tachycardia in heatstroke are caused by a number of factors. The heatstroke patient may have a reduced plasma volume secondary to dehydration. There is peripheral pooling of blood associated with an increase in cutaneous blood flow from 0.5 L/min to 7–8 L/min.[108,210] In addition, patients may manifest primary myocardial insufficiency.[131] Clinically, patients exhibit either a hypo- or hyperdynamic circulatory response. The observed circulatory response to heat stress is a function of the patient's cardiac reserve, volume status, and degree of myocardial heat injury. The hyperdynamic condition is characterized by increased cardiac index and decreased systemic vascular resistance.[186] These hemodynamic characteristics are seen in patients who are able to maintain a significantly increased cardiac output in response to the circulatory demand of heat stress.

Dehydrated patients or those with primary myocardial insufficiency may exhibit a hypodynamic response. These patients have a decreased cardiac index and increased systemic vascular resistance.[186,234] Whether or not pulmonary vascular resistance is affected is unclear. High central venous pressures have been found in some patients, with evidence of right heart failure and right heart dilation on autopsy.[157] This has led to the suggestion that pulmonary vascular resistance may be elevated.[186] In 64% of 34 patients with heatstroke, central venous pressures were greater than 3 cm H_2O. Twelve patients had a CVP ≤ 0 and 10 were > 10 cm H_2O. These authors cautioned against injudicious infusion of large quantities of intravenous fluids and resulting complications of congestive heart failure and fluid overload. In the study, only three patients required more than 2 L of normal saline during cooling. Crystalloid infusion ranged from 500 to 2500 mL, and none of the patients developed associated fluid overload problems.[223]

A study of 13 cases of heatstroke in Mecca pilgrims monitored with pulmonary artery (Swan-Ganz) catheters demonstrated a good correlation of CVP with pulmonary capillary wedge pressures.[3] A pulmonary artery catheter study in elderly patients with heatstroke showed that pulmonary vascular resistance was low or normal. Pulmonary capillary wedge pressures were not elevated.[233] Serial electrocardiograms in 51 religious pilgrims suffering from heatstroke showed normal sinus rhythm in 25%, sinus tachycardia in 52%, atrial fibrillation in 16%, and sinus bradycardia in 6%. ST segment depression and other ST-T wave changes were reported. The QT interval showed no abnormality. In some patients, echocardiography showed pericardial effusions and regional wall motion abnormalities, asymmetric septal hypertrophy, right ventricular dilation, and left ventricular dilation with impaired function.[2]

In addition to right heart dilation, autopsy studies of the heart have shown pericardial effusions, interstitial edema, degeneration and necrosis of myocardial fibers, and subendocardial hemorrhage.[125,157] Postmortem examination of the lungs has revealed vascular congestion, pleural effusions, and parenchymal hemorrhages.[157,186]

Gastrointestinal hemorrhage, vomiting, and diarrhea occur frequently.[225] At autopsy, edema and hemorrhage of the bowel wall are seen.[35] Liver injury occurs commonly and is not clinically manifest until the second or third day following the temperature increase.[124,225] Centrilobular changes, such as widening of central veins and adjacent sinusoids and pooling of blood, can be seen on liver biopsy. Repeat biopsies demonstrated that these changes, in addition to varying degrees of hepatocellular degeneration, resolve as the patient recovers.[124] In other cases, only congestion and fatty infiltration are seen.[35]

Neuropsychiatric impairment is, by definition, present in all cases of heatstroke. Length of coma correlates significantly with mortality.[9,225] Autopsy studies demonstrate a variety of structural and microscopic CNS injuries. Edema and venous congestion are evident. The number of cortical neurons is reduced, with concomitant glial proliferation. Striking cerebellar Purkinje cell deterioration occurs. The hypothalamus appears to be relatively spared, with limited edema of the neuronal nuclei. Hemorrhages occur throughout the brain.[35,157,225] Persistent cerebellar dysfunction occurs, as does lower motor neuron damage, manifested by areflexia and muscle wasting.[54,143] Higher cortical functions are spared in survivors.[163] Permanent neurologic sequelae are correlated with degree and duration of hyperthermia.

Acute renal failure was the major cause of death in heatstroke victims before the advent of hemodialysis.[220,246] In addition to the direct effects of heat, volume depletion, and hypotension, myoglobinuria secondary to rhabdomyolysis results in further renal tubular injury. This is especially common in the agitated or exercising patient.[40,79,197] The mechanism by which myoglobin contributes to renal failure remains controversial. At autopsy the kidneys are enlarged, with numerous petechial hemorrhages.[157] Acute tubular necrosis is seen on biopsy.

Frank bleeding is associated with significant morbidity and mortality in many cases of heatstroke. Coagulation disturbances seen in patients with heatstroke appear to be multifactorial. Elevation of the prothrombin time may occur within 30 minutes of temperature elevation and has been attributed to direct heat injury of clotting factors.[13] Liver damage may significantly contribute to the coagulation disturbances, although this would not be manifest as acutely.[13,175,200] Evidence of diffuse capillary basement-membrane injury has been demonstrated by electron microscopy and is thought to precipitate consumptive coagulopathy in severe cases of heatstroke.[35,230]

Thrombocytopenia is very common and occurs within 30 minutes of onset of heatstroke, frequently in the absence of other evidence of disseminated intravascular coagulation. Direct thermal injury leading to decreased platelet survival and megakaryocyte damage may play a role[157,175] (Table 18–6).

Clinical Findings in Heatstroke

Clinical evaluation of the hyperthermic patient begins with careful assessment of the vital signs. Heart rates greater than 130 beats/min are common. Hypotension is frequently noted. Other vital sign abnormalities include an elevation of the respiratory rate, often above 30 breaths/min. Most importantly, temperature is elevated. After cooling, there is often a secondary rise in temperature that suggests persistent disturbances of thermoregulation.[157]

Physical examination demonstrates findings consistent with the diagnosis of heatstroke. Neurologic examination reveals a confused, delirious, comatose, or seizing patient. Pupils may be normal, fixed and dilated, or pinpoint. Decerebrate or decorticate posturing may be evident. Muscle tone is increased, normal, or flaccid. The skin may be hot and dry or diaphoretic. Nasal and oropharyngeal bleeding may be present as a consequence of the acute coagulopathy seen in heatstroke. Examination of the lungs is often nonspecific, although heatstroke victims are at risk of pulmonary edema as a primary event associated with capillary endothelial damage or following overly aggressive fluid resuscitation. Cardiac auscultation may reveal a flow murmur secondary to high cardiac output or a right ventricular gallop. Neck vein distension indicates increased central venous pressure. Jaundice suggests hepatic injury and occurs on the second or third day following the onset of heatstroke.[36] Nasogastric aspiration or rectal examination may demonstrate gross bleeding. A petechial rash can be seen on examination of the skin, probably secondary to capillary endothelial damage.

Laboratory Findings of Heatstroke

Lactic acid dehydrogenase (LDH) rises as a consequence of diffuse tissue injury. Early rises in aminotransferases (ALT, AST) which peak at 48 hours, are indicators of the liver damage that occurs during heatstroke.[124] Elevation of muscle enzymes was noted in all patients in one study of exertional heatstroke[225] and in 86% of patients in one study of nonexertional heatstroke.[84] Nonspecific ST and T wave changes on ECG are common. Myocardial enzyme elevation occurs and correlates with ECG changes.[125] Results of lumbar puncture are nonspecific, are often normal, or may demonstrate elevated CSF protein and lymphocytosis.[225]

Other laboratory parameters are affected by heatstroke. Dehydration leads to hemoconcentration in patients exposed to elevated temperatures for a period of time. Hypokalemia is common, with potassium deficits as great as 500 mEq occurring during the early period of heat exposure.[133] Arterial blood gas analysis may show a respiratory alkalosis secondary to direct stimulation of the respiratory center by heat[234] or a metabolic acidosis secondary to lactic acid production.[46,234] Hypophosphatemia is common and has been attributed to respiratory alkalosis, which causes intracellular shifts of phos-

TABLE 18–6. PHYSIOLOGIC AND CLINICAL MANIFESTATIONS OF HEATSTROKE

Cardiovascular
Hypodynamic states in elderly
Hyperdynamic states in young healthy individuals
Electrocardiogram
Nonspecific
Widening of QRS due to underlying abnormality (eg, cocaine toxicity, hyperkalemia associated with rhabdomyolysis)
Central nervous system
Altered mental status
Irritability, confusion ataxia, seizures, coma
Weakness, dizziness, headache
Plantar extension, pupillary abnormalities, decorticate posturing
EEG
Normal or diffuse slowing
CSF
Normal or increased protein
Lymphocytosis
Gastrointestinal
Vomiting, diarrhea, hematemesis
Hematologic
Bleeding diathesis
Prolonged PT and PTT
Disseminated intravascular coagulation
Thrombocytopenia
Petechiae
Purpura
Leukocytosis
Hepatic
Hepatic insufficiency at 12–36 h
Elevated AST, ALT, LDH
Metabolic
Metabolic acidosis and respiratory alkalosis
Electrolyte disturbance
Hypernatremia
Hypokalemia
Hypocalcemia
Hypophosphatemia
Muscle
Rhabdomyolysis
Elevated CPK
Renal
Decreased renal perfusion
Myoglobinuria
Proteinuria
Oliguria
Acute tubular necrosis
Interstitial necrosis

phate.[132] Renal tubular damage may also lead to phosphate depletion;[89] however, in 8 of 10 heatstroke patients with hypophosphatemia none were alkalemic.[22] The hypophosphatemia in these cases was associated with increased phosphaturia and decreased tubular reabsorption of phosphorus, a finding reversed after cooling. Parathyroid hormone levels were normal in 7 of 9 patients and serum calcium was normal in 9 of 10, suggesting that parathyroid hormone depression was not the cause of phosphaturia of heatstroke. All patients had normal fractional excretion of sodium.[22] Phosphate and potassium are elevated when significant muscle injury has occurred. Calcium is normal or low, the latter secondary to binding to damaged muscle tissue. Later, hypercalcemia occurs, possibly due to release of this bound calcium.[75,149]

Significant alterations occur in leukocyte subsets in heatstroke victims. One study reported an increased ratio of T-suppressor to T-cytotoxic cells, as well as increased natural killer cells. There was a significant decrease in the percentages of T, B, and T-helper cells. These changes correlated with the degree of hyperthermia.[20] Catecholamines are increased in heatstroke[1] and may affect the distribution of the lymphocyte subsets.[20] It is possible that the increased susceptibility to infection described in heatstroke and the alterations in lymphocyte populations are related.[20]

Effects of Drugs in Heatstroke

Drugs predispose the individual to heatstroke by two primary mechanisms: increased production of heat as a result of drug action and interference with the body's ability to dissipate heat due to pharmacologic effects on thermoregulatory centers. Increased production of heat due to agitation, seizures, or increased muscle tone may result from phencyclidine, cyclic antidepressants, monoamine oxidase inhibitors, strychnine, lithium, neuroleptics, and cocaine, amphetamines, and other sympathomimetics. Drug–drug interactions may cause life-threatening increases in temperature, such as the combination of monoamine oxidase inhibitors with meperidine or dextromethorphan resulting in the hyperserotonin syndrome. The uncoupling of oxidative phosphorylation by salicylate, pentachlorophenol, or dinitrophenol leads to the release of metabolic energy as heat, rather than trapping that energy in the form of high-energy phosphate bonds in ATP. Increased heat production occurs as a result of the stimulation of hepatic metabolism by sympathomimetic drugs and, of course, by the increased physical activity often associated with sympathomimetic drug use.

During heat stress, vasodilation leads to increased cutaneous blood flow, demanding a higher cardiac output. Parasympathetic stimulation results in increased sweating. Drugs that impair these physiologic mechanisms for heat dissipation predispose the individual to heatstroke. Drugs with anticholinergic actions, such as antihistamines, cyclic antidepressants, and neuroleptics interfere with sweating. Sympathomimetic drugs stimulate α-adrenergic receptors, impairing vasodilation. Antihypertensives and antianginal drugs (most notably calcium channel blockers and β-adrenergic antagonists) with negative inotropic and chronotropic effects impair the heart's ability to meet the output requirements of increased skin blood flow. Volume depletion by diuretics also limits cardiac output. Neuroleptics cause hypothalamic depression, altering the normal CNS response to heat stress. Finally, drugs such as ethanol, opioids, and sedative-hypnotics impair normal behavioral responses, and heat-related discomfort is unnoticed.

Heatstroke and Subsequent Heat Intolerance

Whether heatstroke victims are subsequently unable to adapt to exercise in a hot environment remains unclear. Is the heatstroke victim genetically predisposed to heat intolerance, or does heatstroke occur as a result of environmental and host factors? Several studies have suggested that heatstroke leads to persistent heat intolerance. These studies have often used a single heat intolerance test.[65,224,227,228] A study of 10 previous heatstroke victims showed no difference in acclimatization responses, thermoregulation, whole-body sodium and potassium balance, sweat gland function, and blood values when compared with controls.[8] The rate of recovery from exertional heatstroke probably differs among individuals. In this study, 1 of 10 patients was found to have recurrent heat intolerance 12 months after the study.[8] Resolution of heat intolerance was delayed for 5 months in an individual who had experienced heatstroke twice.[123]

Treatment of Heatstroke

Body temperatures > 106°F place the patient at great risk for end-organ injury. Rapid cooling is the first priority. Successful treatment requires adequate preparation. Equipment needed for rapid cooling (eg, fans, ice and tubs for submersion) should be readily available in the ED. En route to the hospital, the patient's clothes should be removed and he or she should be covered with ice- and water-soaked sheets. Respiration and cardiovascular status should be stabilized and monitored. Oxygen should be administered.

Management must also focus on the early recognition of hyperthermia. The cause should be determined and appropriate measures initiated immediately. Pharmacologic agents (eg, antihistamines, butyrophenones, phenothiazines) and physical restraints (eg, camisoles, strait jackets) that interfere with heat dissipation should not be used.[87] Light hand and foot restraints should be used to protect the patient from harming himself or herself if necessary. If light restraints are used, the patient should be monitored continuously. The patient who is hyperthermic in the setting of ethanol or sedative-hypnotic withdrawal should be treated with a benzodiazepine.[86] The patient should never be confined to a small, unventilated seclusion room. Adequate cooling, hydration, sedation, and electrolytes and substrate repletion should be ensured.[84]

In the ED, appropriate laboratory studies should be drawn and an IV line placed. Administration of 0.5–1.0 g/kg glucose as $D_{50}W$ and 100 mg of thiamine should be considered. A rectal probe should be placed for continuous temperature monitoring. The patient should be immersed in an ice bath with a fan blowing over the patient if possible. In addition to the ice bath, iced gastric lavage may be effective.

Agitation, seizures, and cardiac dysrhythmias must be managed while cooling is accomplished. Benzodiazepines are the treatment of choice for agitation and seizures. Heatstroke patients may have significant volume needs, depending on the amount of fluid lost prior to the onset of heatstroke. Hypotension should be treated with fluids and cooling. Volume repletion should be monitored carefully by parameters such as blood pressure, pulse, central venous pressure, pulmonary wedge pressure, and urine output. As the temperature returns to normal, the hypotension may resolve if significant volume deficits are not present.[39,131,133] In patients with myoglobinuria, an attempt should be made to increase renal blood flow and urine output. The use of sodium bicarbonate and mannitol in the prevention of acute tubular necrosis in these cases is controversial.[64,75,209]

Despite the possible causative role of phenothiazines, some clinicians have recommended their use in heatstroke.[39,83] However, although phenothiazines may theoretically reduce shivering and the possibility of rebound hyperthermia, their onset of action is slow.[185] In addition, phenothiazines depress an already altered mental status, may produce hepatotoxicity in a compromised liver, may lower the seizure threshold,[19] may cause acute dystonic reactions, may exacerbate hypotension, and interfere with thermoregulation and cooling by affecting the hypothalamus. Most authorities believe there is no indication for neuroleptics in the treatment of hyperthermia. When shivering occurs during cooling, we recommend the judicious use of a benzodiazepine. In addition, benzodiazepines treat ethanol and sedative-hypnotic withdrawal and cocaine intoxication, common causes of hyperthermia.

There is no role for antipyretic agents in the management of heatstroke. Aspirin and acetaminophen lower temperature by reducing the hypothalamic set point, which is only altered in a patient febrile from inflammation or endogenous pyrogens.[56] Heatstroke, however, occurs when cooling mechanisms are overwhelmed, and the hypothalamic thermoregulatory set point is not disturbed.[15,102]

Dantrolene sodium is the preferred drug in the treatment of malignant hyperthermia.[88,114,248] It acts directly on skeletal muscle and either inhibits the release of calcium or increases calcium uptake through the sarcoplasmic reticulum.[24] Its utility has not been demonstrated in other conditions associated with hyperthermia, and there is no evidence to support its administration for other conditions.[5] In a prospective, randomized double-blind, placebo-controlled study of 52 patients with heatstroke, IV dantrolene sodium at 2 mg/kg body weight did not alter cooling time.[21] There was no significant difference in the mean number of hospital days necessitated by heatstroke victims who received dantrolene and cooling versus those who received cooling alone. It has been proposed that dantrolene may influence central dopaminergic metabolism in patients with neuroleptic malignant syndrome by affecting calcium-triggered neurotransmitter release in the central nervous system; however, further study is required.[183] Anecdotal reports of the efficacy of dopamine agonist agents such as bromocriptine and amantadine have appeared in descriptions of neuroleptic malignant syndrome.[161] No drug therapy should delay the institution of aggressive external cooling (Table 18–7).

Prevention of Heatstroke

In the young, active population, prophylaxis should be accomplished by gradual acclimatization. Active persons should select the coolest and least humid time of day to be outdoors. Exposure should be increased slowly, and work paced. Breaks should be frequent initially and later may be decreased in number and length. Overweight and underconditioned persons require even longer periods of acclimatization. Airy and cool clothing should be chosen. The practice of exercising in unventilated plastic clothing to increase weight loss leads to the loss of fluid, not fat, and defeats the body's cooling mechanisms, resulting in hyperthermia.

Athletes performing during hot, humid weather should increase drinking beyond their thirst.[171,218] For example, those preparing for a marathon should drink ap-

TABLE 18–7. MANAGEMENT OF HEATSTROKE

Preparation
- Ice and cooling fans available in ED
- Monitor weather reports
- Alert media

Arrival

Rapid cooling
- Clear airway and administer oxygen
- Cover with ice- and water-soaked sheets
- Stabilize respiratory and cardiovascular status
- Cool as rapidly as possible

Intravenous access
- NaCl or Ringer's lactate, based on CVP
- Administration of 0.5–1.0 g/kg dextrose, and 100 mg thiamine
- Benzodiazepines for agitation, shivering, seizures

Continuous monitoring
- Remove from ice bath at 38.3°C (101°F)
- Watch for rebound hyperthermia

Cautions
- Neuroleptics may have serious adverse effects
- Antipyretic agents do not work
- Cooling blankets alone are inadequate

proximately 250 mL of water 10–15 minutes prior to the race and continue to drink that amount every 3–4 km. Water is a safe and effective mechanism for maintaining fluid balance. All individuals who fatigue easily or manifest nausea, vomiting, cramps, weakness, dizziness, or collapse should limit their activity and must be watched carefully.

Anyone who takes illicit drugs, medications, or has a medical condition that may interfere with thermoregulation should be monitored closely for signs of heat intolerance or hyperthermia. Stopping or at least decreasing the dose of high-risk medications during heatstroke season should be strongly considered.

References

1. Al-Haramy MS: Catecholamines in heat stroke. Milit Med 1989;154:263–264.
2. Al-Harthi SS, Nouh MS, Qaranquish A, et al: Non-invasive evaluation of cardiac abnormalities in heat stroke pilgrims. Int J Cardiol 1992;37:151–154.
3. Al-Harthi SS, Sharaf El-Deen MS, Aktar J, Nouh MS: Hemodynamic changes and intravascular hydration state in heat stroke. Ann Saudi Med 1989;9:378–383.
4. Althaus U, Aeberhard P, Schupbach P, et al: Management of profound accidental hypothermia with cardiorespiratory arrest. Ann Surg 1982;195:492–495.
5. Amsterdam JT, Syverud SA, Barker WJ, et al: Dantrolene sodium for treatment of heatstroke victims: Lack of efficacy in a canine model. Am J Emerg Med 1986;4:399–405.
6. Anderson RJ, Reed G, Knochel J: Heatstroke. Ann Intern Med 1983;28:115–140.
7. Angelakos ET, Daniels JB: Effect of catecholamine infusions on lethal hypothermic temperatures in dogs. J Appl Physiol 1969;26:194–196.
8. Armstrong LE, De Luca J, Hubbard RW: Time course of recovery and heat acclimation ability of prior exertional heatstroke patients. Med Sci Sports Exerc 1990;22:36–48.
9. Austin MG, Berry JW: Observations on one hundred cases of heat stroke. JAMA 1956;161:1525–1529.
10. Bacon C, Scott D, Jones P: Heatstroke in well-wrapped infants. Lancet 1979;1:422–425.
11. Baloh RW, Dietz J, Spooner JW: Myoclonus and ocular oscillations induced by L-tryptophan. Ann Neurol 1982;11:95–97.
12. Baumgartner F, Janusz, MT, Jamieson WRE, et al: Cardiopulmonary bypass for resuscitation of patients with accidental hypothermia and cardiac arrest. Can J Surg 1992;35:184–187.
13. Beard ME, Hickton CM: Haemostasis in heatstroke. Br J Haematol 1982;52:269–274.
14. Beaumont G: Drug interactions with clomipramine (Anafranil). J Int Med Res 1973;1:480–484.
15. Bernheim HA, Block LH, Atkins E: Fever: Pathogenesis, pathophysiology and purpose. Ann Intern Med 1979;91:261–270.
16. Beyda EJ, Jung M, Bellet S: Effect of hypothermia on the tolerance of dogs to digitalis. Circ Res 1961;9:129–135.
17. Birkhimer LJ, DeVane CI: The neuroleptic malignant syndrome: Presentation and treatment. Drug Intell Clin Pharm 1984;18:462–465.
18. Birzis L, Hemingway A: Descending brain stem connections controlling shivering in cat. J Neurophysiol 1956;19:37–43.
19. Blum K, Eubanks, JD, Wallace JE, Hamilton H: Enhancement of alcohol withdrawal convulsions in mice by haloperidol. Clin Toxicol 1976;9:427–434.
20. Bouchama A, Al Hussein K, Adra C, et al: Distribution of peripheral blood leukocytes in acute heatstroke. J Appl Physiol 1992;73:405–409.
21. Bouchama A, Cafege A, Devol EB, et al: Ineffectiveness of dantrolene sodium in the treatment of heatstroke. Crit Care Med 1991;19:176–180.
22. Bouchama A, Cafege A, Rovertson W, et al: Mechanisms of hypophosphatemia in humans with heatstroke. J Appl Physiol 1991;71:328–332.
23. Boylan JW, Hong SK: Regulation of renal function in hypothermia. Am J Physiol 1966;211:1371–1378.
24. Britt BA: Dantrolene. Can Anaesth Soc J 1984;31:61–75.
25. Broccardo M, Improta G: Sauvagine-induced hypthermia: Evidence for an interaction with the dopaminergic system. Eur J Pharmacol 1994;258:179–184.
26. Bruck K: Non-shivering thermogenesis and brown adipose tissue in relation to age, and their integration in the thermoregulatory system. In: Lindberg O, ed: Brown Adipose Tissue. New York, Elsevier, 1970, pp. 117–154.
27. Buchwald I, Davis PJ: Scleroderma with fatal heatstroke. JAMA 1967;201:124–125.
28. Buckberg GD, Brazier JR, Nelson RL, et al: Studies of the effects of hypothermia on regional myocardial blood flow and metabolism during cardiopulmonary bypass. I. The adequately perfused beating, fibrillating and arrested heart. J Thorac Cardiovasc Surg 1977;73:87–95.
29. Buckley JJ, Bosch OK, Bacaner MB: Prevention of ventricular fibrillation during hypothermia. Anesth Analg 1971;50:587–593.
30. Busto R, Globus M, Dietrich W, et al: Effect of mild hypothermia on ischemia-induced release of neurotransmitters and free fatty acids in rat brain. Stroke 1989;20:904–910.
31. Carlton J, Khan S, Hao W, et al: Attenuation of alcohol-induced hypothermia by Cyclo(His-Pro) and its analogs. Neuropeptides 1995;28:351–355.
32. Carr ME Jr, Wolfert AI. Rewarming by hemodialysis for hypothermia: Failure of heparin to prevent DIC. J Emerg Med 1988;6:277–280.
33. CDC. Hypothermia-related deaths—New Mexico, October 1993–March 1994. MMWR 1995;44:933–935.
34. CDC. Hypothermia-related deaths—Vermont, October 1994–February 1996. MMWR 1996;45:1093–1095
35. Chao TC, Sinniah R, Pakiam JE: Acute heatstroke deaths. Pathology 1981;13:145–156.
36. Chobanian SJ: Jaundice occurring after resolution of heatstroke. Ann Emerg Med 1983;12:102–103.
37. Clark JF: Some effects of the urban structure on heat mortality. Environ Res 1972;5:93–104.
38. Clark WG, Lipton JM: Brain and pituitary peptides in thermoregulation. Pharmacol Ther 1983;22:249–297.
39. Clowes GHA, O'Donnell TF: Current concepts: Heatstroke. N Engl J Med 1974;291:564–566.
40. Cogen FC, Rigg G, Simmons JL, Domino EF: Phencycli-

dine-associated acute rhabdomyolysis. Ann Intern Med 1978;88:210–212.

41. Cohen DJ, Cline JR, Lepinski SM, et al: Resuscitation of the hypothermic patient. 1988;6:475–478.
42. Collins KJ: The autonomic nervous system and the regulation of body temperature. In: Bannister R, ed: Autonomic Failure: A Textbook of Clinical Disorders of the Autonomic Nervous System, 3rd ed. Oxford University Press, 1992, pp. 212–230.
43. Collins, KJ, Exton-Smith AN: Thermal homeostasis in old age. J Am Geriatr Soc 1983;31:519–524.
44. Collis ML, Steinman AM, Chaney RD: Accidental hypothermia: An experimental study of practical rewarming methods. Aviat Space Environ Med 1977;48:625–632.
45. Cooper KE, Ferguson AV: Thermoregulation and hypothermia in the elderly. In: Pozos RS, Wittmers LE, eds: The Nature and Treatment of Hypothermia. Minneapolis, University of Minnesota, 1983, pp. 35–45.
46. Costrini AM, Pitt MA, Gustafson AB: Cardiovascular and metabolic manifestations of heat stroke and severe heat exhaustion. Am J Med 1979;66:296–302.
47. Danzl DF, Pozos RS: Multicenter hypothermia survey. Ann Emerg Med 1987;16:1042–1055.
48. Danzl DF, Sowers MB, Vicario SJ, et al: Chemical ventricular defibrillation during hypothermia with bretylium tosylate. Ann Emerg Med 1982;11:698–699.
49. DaVee TS, Reineberg EJ: Extreme hypothermia and ventricular fibrillation. Ann Emerg Med 1980;9:100–102.
50. DeGaravilla L, Durkot MJ, Ihley TM, et al: Adverse effects of dietary and furosemide-induced sodium depletion on thermoregulation. Aviat Space Environ Med 1990;61: 1012–1017.
51. Delaney KA: Hypothermic sudden death. In: Paradis NA, Halaperin HR, Nowak RM, ed: Cardiac Arrest. The Science and Practice of Resuscitation. Williams and Wilkins, 1996, pp. 745–760.
52. Delaney KA, Howland MA, Vassallo S, Goldfrank LR: The assessment of acid–base disturbances in hypothermia and their physiological consequences. Ann Emerg Med 1989; 18:72–82.
53. Delay J, Deniker P: Drug-induced extrapyramidal syndromes. In: Vinkin PJ, Bruyn GW, eds: Handbook of Clinical Neurology: Diseases of the Basal Ganglia, Vol. 6. Amsterdam, North Holland, 1969, pp. 248–266.
54. Delgado G, Tunon T, Gallego J, et al: Spinal cord lesions in heatstroke. J Neurol Neurosurg Psychiatry 1985;48: 1065–1067.
55. Denborough MA, Lovell RRH: Anesthetic deaths in a family. Lancet 1969;2:45. Letter.
56. Dinarello CA, Wolff SM: Pathogenesis of fever in man. N Engl J Med 1978;298:607–612.
57. Dixon RG, Dougherty JM, White LJ, et al: Transcutaneous pacing in a hypothermic-dog model. Ann Emerg Med 1997;29:602–606.
58. Eichler AC, McFee AS, Root HD: Heatstroke. Am J Surg 1969;118:855–861.
59. El-Gamal N, Frank S: Perioperative thermoregulatory dysfunction in a patient with a previous traumatic hypothalamic injury. Anesth Analg 1995;80:1245–1247.
60. Ellis FP. Mortality from heat illness and heat-aggravated illness in the United States. Environ Res 1972;5:1–58.
61. El Sherif N, Shahwan L, Sorour AH: The effect of acute thermal stress on general and pulmonary hemodynamics in the cardiac patient. Am Heart J 1979;79:305.
62. Emslie-Smith D: Accidental hypothermia: A common condition with a pathognomonic electrocardiogram. Lancet 1958;2:492–495.
63. Emslie-Smith D, Sladden GE, Stirling GR: The significance of changes in the electrocardiogram in hypothermia. Br Heart J 1959;21:343–351.
64. Eneas JF, Schoenfeld PY, Humphreys MH: The effect of infusion of mannitol-sodium bicarbonate on the clinical course of myoglobinuria. Arch Intern Med 1979;139: 801–805.
65. Epstein Y, Shapiro Y, Brill S: Role of surface area to mass ratio and work efficiency in heat tolerance. J Appl Physiol 1983;54:831–836.
66. Esteban J, Chover AJ, Sanchez P, et al: Central administration of neuropeptide Y induces hypothermia in mice. Possible interaction with central noradrenergic systems. Life Sci 1989;45:2395–2400.
67. Feighner JP, Boyer WF, Tyler DL, Neborsky RJ: Adverse consequences of fluoxetine–MAOI combination therapy. J Clin Psychiatry 1990;51:222–225.
68. Fell RH, Gunning AJ, Bardhan KD, Triger DR: Severe hypothermia as a result of barbiturate overdose complicated by cardiac arrest. Lancet 1968;1:392–394.
69. Feller DJ, Young ER, Riggan JP, et al: Serotonin and genetic differences in sensitivity and tolerance to ethanol hypothermia. Psychopharmacology (Berlin) 1993;112: 331–338.
70. Finn DA, Boone DC, Alkana RL: Temperature dependence of ethanol depression in rats. Psychopharmacology (Berlin) 1986;90:185–189.
71. Fischbeck KH, Simon RP: Neurological manifestations of accidental hypothermia. Ann Neurol 1981;10:384–387.
72. Fleming PR, Muir FH: Electrocardiographic changes in induced hypothermia in man. Br Heart J 1957;19:59–66.
73. Fox GR, Hayward JS: Effect of hypothermia on breath-alcohol analysis. J Forensic Sci 1987;32:320–325.
74. Fruehan AE: Accidental hypothermia. Arch Intern Med 1960;106:218–229.
75. Gabow PA, Kaehny WD, Kelleher SP: The spectrum of rhabdomyolysis. Medicine 1982;61:141–152.
76. Gentilello LM, Cobean RA, Offner PJ, et al: Continuous arteriovenous rewarming: Rapid reversal of hypothermia in critically ill patients. J Trauma 1992;32:316–327.
77. Gillen, JP, Vogel MF, Holterman RK, Skiendzielewski JJ: Ventricular fibrillation during orotracheal intubation of hypothermic dogs. Ann Emerg Med 1986;15:412–416.
78. Gilliam DM, Collins AC: Concentration-dependent effects of ethanol in long-sleep and short-sleep mice. Alcohol Clin Exp Res 1983;7:337–342.
79. Ginsberg MD, Hertzman M, Schmidt-Nowara WV: Amphetamine intoxication with coagulopathy, hyperthermia and reversible renal failure. Ann Intern Med 1970;73: 81–85.
80. Goldberg LI: Cardiovascular and renal actions of dopamine: potential clinical applications. Pharmacol Rev 1972; 24:1–30.
81. Goldberg LI: Monoamine oxidase inhibitors: Adverse reactions and possible mechanisms. JAMA 1964;190:132–138.

82. Golden F St C, Hervey GR: The "after-drop" and death after rescue from immersion in cold water. In: Adam JM, ed: Hypothermia Ashore and Afloat. Aberdeen, Scotland, Aberdeen University Press, 1981, pp. 37–56.
83. Gottschalk PG, Thomas JE: Heat stroke. Mayo Clin Proc 1966;41:470–482.
84. Graham GS, Lichtenstein MJ, Hinson JM, Theil GB: Nonexertional heatstroke: Physiologic management and cooling in 14 patients. Arch Intern Med 1986;146:87–90.
85. Granoff AL, Davis JM: Heat illness syndrome and lithium intoxication. J Clin Psychiatry 1978;39:103–107.
86. Greenblatt DJ, Gross PL, Harris J, et al: Fatal hyperthermia following haloperidol therapy of sedative hypnotic withdrawal. J Clin Psychiatry 1978;39:673–675.
87. Greenland P, Southwick WH: Hyperthermia associated with chlorpromazine and full sheet restraint. Am J Psychiatry 1978;135:1234–1235.
88. Gronert GA: Controversies in malignant hyperthermia. Anesthesiology 1983;59:273–274.
89. Guntupalli KI, Sladen A, Selker RG, et al: Effects of induced total-body hyperthermia on phosphorous metabolism in humans. Am J Med 1984;77:250–254.
90. Gupta BN, Nier K, Hensel H: Cold-sensitive afferents from the abdomen. Pflueggers Arch 1979;380:203–204.
91. Guze BH, Baxter LR: Current concepts: Neuroleptic malignant syndrome. N Engl J Med 1985;313:163–166.
92. Ham J, Miller RD, Benet LZ, et al: Pharmacokinetics and pharmacodynamics of d-tubocurarine during hypothermia in the cat. Anesthesiology 1978;49:324–329.
93. Hamlet MP: Fluid shifts in hypothermia. In: Pozos RS, Wittmers LE, eds: The Nature and Treatment of Hypothermia. Minneapolis, University of Minnesota Press, 1983, pp. 94–99.
94. Hammel HT: Regulation of internal body temperature. Annu Rev Physiol 1968;30:641–710.
95. Hanson TE, Dieter K, Keepers GA: Interaction of fluoxetine and pentazocine. Am J Psychiatry 1990;147:949–950.
96. Harari A, Regnier B, Rapin M: Haemodynamic study of prolonged deep accidental hypothermia. Eur J Intensive Care Med 1975;1:65–70.
97. Harnett RM, Pruitt JR, Sias FR: A review of the literature concerning resuscitation from hypothermia: I. The problem and general approaches. Aviat Space Environ Med 1983;5:425–434.
98. Hauty MG, Esrig BC, Hill JG, Long WB: Prognostic factors in severe accidental hypothermia: Experiences from the Mt. Hood tragedy. J Trauma 1987;27:1107–1112.
99. Hayward JS, Steinman AM: Accidental hypothermia: An experimental study of inhalation rewarming. Aviat Space Environ Med 1975;46:1236–1240.
100. Heiman-Patterson TD: Neuroleptic malignant syndrome and malignant hyperthermia. Med Clin North Am 1993; 77:477–492.
101. Hensel H: Cutaneous thermoreceptors. In: Hensel H (ed): Handbook of Sensory Physiology, Vol. 2. Berlin, Springer–Verlag 1972, pp. 79–110.
102. Hensel H: Neural processes in thermoregulation. Physiol Rev 1973;53:948–1007.
103. Hensel H, Andres KH, During MV: Structure and function of cold receptors. Pflueggers Arch 1974;352:1–10.
104. Hernandez E, Praga M, Alcazar JM, et al: Hemodialysis for treatment of accidental hypothermia. Nephron 1993;63: 214–216.
105. Hislop LJ, Wyatt JP, McNaughton GW, et al: Urban hypothermia in the west of Scotland. Br Med J 1995;311:725.
106. Hochachka PW: Defense strategies against hypoxia and hypothermia. Science 1986;231:234–241.
107. Hori T, Harada Y: Responses of midbrain raphe neurons to local temperature. Pflueggers Arch 1976;364:205–207.
108. Hubbard RW: An introduction: The role of exercise in the etiology of exertional heatstroke. Med Sci Sports Exerc 1990;21:2–5.
109. Hudson LD, Conn RD: Accidental hypothermia: Associated diagnoses and prognosis in a common problem. JAMA 1974;227:37–40.
110. Inoue S, Murakami N: Unit responses in the medulla oblongata of rabbit to changes in local and cutaneous temperature. J Physiol 1976;259:339–356.
111. Jacobs JJ, Prasad C, Wilber J: Cyclo-(His-Pro): Mapping hypothalamic sites for its hypothermic action. Brain Res 1982;250:205–209.
112. Jardine DS: A mathematical model of life-threatening hyperthermia during infancy. J Appl Physiol 1992;73: 329–339.
113. Jardine DS, Haschke RH: An animal model of life-threatening hyperthermia during infancy. J Appl Physiol 1992; 73:340–345.
114. Jardon OM: Physiologic stress, heat stroke, malignant hyperthermia: A perspective. Milit Med 1982;147:8–14.
115. Jessen K, Hagelsten JO: Peritoneal dialysis in the treatment of profound accidental hypothermia. Aviat Space Environ Med 1978;49:426–429.
116. Jones TS, Liang AP, Kilbourne EM, et al: Morbidity and mortality associated with the July 1980 heat wave in St. Louis and Kansas City, Mo. JAMA 1982:247:3327–3331.
117. Kadar D, Tang BK, Conn AW: The fate of phenobarbitone in children in hypothermia and at normal body temperature. Can Anaesth Soc J 1982;29:16–33.
118. Kalant H, Le AD: Effects of ethanol on thermoregulation. Pharmacol Ther 1984;23:313–364.
119. Kalser SC, Kelvington EJ, Kunig R, Randolph MM: Drug metabolism in hypothermia. Uptake, metabolism and excretion of C^{14}-procaine by the isolated, perfused rat liver. J Pharmacol Exp Ther 1968;164:396–404.
120. Kalser SC, Kelvington EJ, Randolph MM: Drug metabolism in hypothermia. Uptake, metabolism and excretion of S^{35}-sulfanilamide by the isolated, perfused rat liver. J Pharmacol Exp Ther 1968;159:389–398.
121. Kalser SC, Kelvington EJ, Randolph MM, Santomenna DM: Drug metabolism in hypothermia. II. C^{14}-atropine uptake, metabolism and excretion by the isolated, perfused rat liver. J Pharmacol Exp Ther 1965;147:260–269.
122. Kandel, ER, Schwartz JH, Jessell TM: Principles of Neural Science, 3rd. ed. New York, Elsevier, 1991.
123. Keren G, Epstein Y, Magazanik A: Temporary heat intolerance in a heatstroke patient. Aviat Space Environ Med 1981;52:116–117.
124. Kew M, Bersohn I, Seftel H, Dent G: Liver damage in heatstroke. Am J Med 1970;49:192–202.
125. Kew MC, Tucker RBK, Bersohn I, Seftel HC: The heart in heatstroke. Am Heart J 1972;77:324–335.
126. Kilbourne EM: Illness due to thermal extremes. In: Last

JM, ed: Maxcy-Rosenau Public Health and Preventive Medicine, 12th ed. Norwalk, CT, Appleton-Century-Crofts, 1986, pp. 711–714.

127. Kilbourne EM, Choi K, Jones TS, Thacker SB: Risk factors for heatstroke: A case-control study. JAMA 1982;247: 3332–3336.
128. Kiley JP, Eldridge FL, Millhorn DE: Synaptic transmission of phrenic nerve stimuli fail in hypothermic cats. Respir Physiol 1984;58:295–312.
129. Killian H: Cold and frost injuries. In: Frey R, Safar P, eds: Disaster Medicine, Vol. 3. New York, Springer-Verlag, 1981, p. ix.
130. Knochel JP: Environmental heat illness: An eclectic review. Arch Intern Med 1974;133:841–863.
131. Knochel JP, Beisel WR, Herndon EG, et al: The renal, cardiovascular, hematologic and serum electrolyte abnormalities of heatstroke. Am J Med 1961;30:299–309.
132. Knochel JP, Caskey JH: The mechanism of hypophosphatemia in acute heatstroke. JAMA 1977;238:425–426.
133. Knochel JP, Dotin LN, Hamburger RJ: Pathophysiology of intense physical conditioning in a hot climate. J Clin Invest 1972;51:242–255.
134. Koeppen AH, Daniels JC, Barron KD: Subnormal body temperatures in Wernicke's encephalopathy. Neurology 1969;21:493–498.
135. Koren G, Barker C, Bohn D, et al: Effect of hypothermia on the pharmacokinetics of ethanol in piglets. Ann Emerg Med 1989;18:118–121.
136. Koren G, Barker C, Bohn D, et al: Influence of hypothermia on the pharmacokinetics of gentamycin and theophylline in piglets. Crit Care Med 1985;13:844–847.
137. Koren G, Barker C, Goresky G, et al.: The influence of hypothermia on the disposition of fentanyl—Human and animal studies. Eur J Clin Pharmacol 1987;32:373–376.
138. Krisko I, Lewis E, Johnson JE: Severe hyperpyrexia due to tranylcypromine–amphetamine toxicity. Ann Intern Med 1969;70:559–564.
139. Kuehn LA: Introduction. In: Pozos RS, Wittmers LE, eds: The Nature and Treatment of Hypothermia. Minneapolis, University of Minnesota Press, 1983.
140. Lapp NL, Juergens JL: Frostbite. Mayo Clin Proc 1965; 40:932–938.
141. Laufman H: Profound accidental hypothermia. JAMA 1951;147:1201–1212
142. Ledingam IM, Mone JG: Treatment of accidental hypothermia: A prospective clinical study. Br Med J 1980; 280:1102–1105.
143. Lefkowitz D, Ford CS, Rich C, et al: Cerebellar syndrome following neuroleptic induced heatstroke. J Neurol Neurosurg Psychiatry 1983;46:183–185.
144. Letsou, GV, Kopf, GS, Elefteriades JA, et al: Is cardiopulmonary bypass effective for treatment of hypothermic arrest due to drowning or exposure? Arch Surg 1992; 127:525–528.
145. Levinson DF, Simpson GM: Neuroleptic-induced extrapyramidal symptoms with fever. Arch Gen Psychiatry 1986;43:839–848.
146. Lewin S, Brettman LR, Holzman RS: Infections in hypothermic patients. Arch Intern Med 1981;141:920–924.
147. Lilja GP: Emergency treatment of hypothermia. In: Pozos RS, Wittmers LE, eds: The Nature and Treatment of Hypothermia. Minneapolis, University of Minnesota Press, 1983, pp. 143–151.
148. Lipton JM, Rosenstein J, Sklar FH. Thermoregulatory disorders after removal of a craniopharyngioma from the third cerebral ventricle. Brain Res Bull 1981;7:369–373.
149. Llach F, Felsenfeld AJ, Haussler MR: The pathophysiology of altered calcium metabolism in rhabdomyolysis-induced acute renal failure. N Engl J Med 1976;305:117–123.
150. Lloyd EL: The cause of death after rescue. Int J Sports Med 1992;13 (suppl 1):196–199.
151. Lloyd EL: Factors affecting the onset of ventricular fibrillation in hypothermia. Lancet 1974;2:1294–1296.
152. Lomax P: Neuropharmacological aspects of thermoregulation. In: Pozos RS, Wittmers LE, eds: The Nature and Treatment of Hypothermia. Minneapolis, University of Minnesota Press, 1983, pp. 81–94.
153. MacKenzie MA, Hermus ARMM, Wollersheim HCH, et al: Poikilothermia in man: Pathophysiology and clinical implications. Medicine 1991;70:257–268.
154. Maclean D, Emslie-Smith D: Accidental Hypothermia. London, Blackwell, 1977.
155. Maickel RP: Interaction of drugs with autonomic nervous function and thermoregulation. Fed Proc 1970;29: 1973–1979.
156. Mair P, Kornberger E, Furtwaengler W, et al: Prognostic markers in patients with severe accidental hypothermia and cardiocirculatory arrest. Resuscitation 1994;27: 47–54.
157. Malamud N, Haymaker W, Custer RP: Heatstroke: A clinico-pathologic study of 125 fatal cases. Milit Surg 1946;99:397–444.
158. McAllister RG: Fever, tachycardia and hypertension with acute catatonic schizophrenia. Arch Intern Med 1978;138: 1154–1156.
159. McAllister RG, Bourne DW, Tan TG, et al: Effects of hypothermia on propranolol kinetics. Clin Pharmacol Ther 1979;25:1–7.
160. McAllister RG, Tan TG: Effect of hypothermia on drug metabolism. In vitro studies with propranolol and verapamil. Pharmacology 1980;20:95–100.
161. McCarron MM, Boettger ML, Peck JJ: A case of neuroleptic malignant syndrome successfully treated with amantadine. J Clin Psychiatry 1982;43:381–382.
162. McCauley RL, Hing DN, Robson MC, Heggers JP: Frostbite injuries: A rational approach based on the pathophysiology. J Trauma 1983;23:143–147.
163. Mehta AC, Baker RN: Persistent neurological deficits in heatstroke. Neurology 1979;20:336–340.
164. Menon MK, Fordon LI, Kodama CK, Fitten J: Influence of D-1 receptor system on the D-2 receptor mediated hypothermic response in mice. Life Sci 1988;43:871–881.
165. Millan M, Audinot V, Melon C, Newman-Tancredi A, et al: Evidence that dopamine D3 receptors participate in clozapine-induced hypothermia. Eur J Pharmacol 1995; 280:225–229.
166. Millan MJ, Audinot V, Rivet J, et al: S14297, a novel selective ligand at cloned human dopamine D_3 receptors, blocks 7-OH-DPAT-induced hypothermia in rats. Eur J Pharmacol 1994;260:37–38.

167. Miller JW, Danzl DF, Thomas DM: Urban accidental hypothermia: 135 cases. Ann Emerg Med 1980;9:456–461.
168. Mills WJ: Accidental hypothermia. In: Pozos RS, Wittmers LE, eds: The Nature and Treatment of Hypothermia. Minneapolis, University of Minnesota Press, 1983, pp. 182–193.
169. Moore JA, Kakihana R: Ethanol-induced hypothermia in mice: influence of genotype on development of tolerance. Life Sci 1978;23:2331–2338.
170. Morishima HO, Mueller-Heubach E, Shnider SM: Body temperature and disappearance of lidocaine in newborn puppies. Anesth Analg 1971;50:938–942.
171. Moroff SV, Bass DE: Effects of overhydration on man's physiological responses to work in the heat. J Appl Physiol 1965;20:267–270.
172. Murphy K, Nowak RM, Tomlanovich MC: Use of bretylium tosylate as prophylaxis and treatment in hypothermic ventricular fibrillation in the canine model. Ann Emerg Med 1986;15:1160–1166.
173. Murphy MT, Lipton JM: Effects of alcohol on thermoregulation in aged monkeys. Exp Gerontol 1983;18:19–27.
174. Murray PT, Fellner SK. Efficacy of hemodialysis in rewarming accidental hypothermia victims. J Am Soc Nephrol 1994;5:422A. Abstract.
175. Mustafa KY, Omer O, Khogali M, et al: Blood coagulation and fibrinolysis in heatstroke. Br J Haematol 1985;61: 517–523.
176. Myers RD: Alcohol's effect on body temperature: Hypothermia, hyperthermia or poikilothermia? 1981;7: 209–220.
177. Nakayama T, Hardy JD: Unit responses in the rabbit's brain stem to changes in brain and cutaneous temperature. J Appl Physiol 1969:27:848–857.
178. Nicodemus HF, Chaney RD, Herold R: Hemodynamic effects of inotropes during hypothermia and rapid rewarming. Crit Care Med 1981;9:325–328.
179. Nicodemus HF, Chaney RD, Herold R: Lidocaine/propranolol: hemodynamic effects during hypothermia and rewarming. J Surg Res 1981;30:6–13.
180. Nicoll KA, Davies L: How warm are babies kept at home? Health Visit 1986;59:113–114.
181. Nielsen KC, Owman C: Control of ventricular fibrillation during induced hypothermia in cats after blocking the adrenergic neurons with bretylium. Life Sci 1968;7: 159–168.
182. Nikki P, Vapaatolo H, Karppanen H: Effect of ethanol on body temperature, postanesthetic shivering and tissue monoamines in halothane-anaesthetized rats. Ann Med Exp Biol Fenn 1971;49:157–161.
183. Nisijima K, Ishiguro T: Does dantrolene influence central dopamine and serotonin metabolism in the neuroleptic malignant syndrome: a retrospective study. Biol Psychiatry 1993;33:45–48.
184. O'Connor JP: Use of peritoneal dialysis in severely hypothermic patients. Ann Emerg Med 1986;15:162–163. Letter.
185. O'Donnell TF: Acute heatstroke. JAMA 1975;234:824–828.
186. O'Donnell TF, Clowes GHA: The circulatory abnormalities of heatstroke. N Engl J Med 1972;287:734–737.
187. O'Keefe KM: Accidental hypothermia: A review of 62 cases. JACEP 1977;6:491–496.
188. Ogawa T, Low PA: Autonomic regulation of temperature and sweating. In: Low PA, ed: Autonomic Disorders. Evaluation and Management. Little, Brown, 1993, pp. 79–91.
189. Ohmura A, Wong KC, Westenkow DR, Shaw L: Effects of hypocarbia and normocarbia on cardiovascular dynamics and regional circulation in the hypothermic dog. Anesthesiology 1979;50:293–298.
190. Okada M: The cardiac rhythm in accidental hypothermia. J Electrocardiol 1984;17:123–128.
191. Okada M, Nishimura F, Yoshino H, et al: The J wave in accidental hypothermia. J Electrocardiol 1983;16:23–28.
192. Okulicz-Kozaryn I, Mikolajczak P, Kaminska E: Tolerance to hypothermia and hypnotic action of ethanol in 3 and 14 month old rats. Pharmacol Res 1992;25:63–64.
193. Orts A, Alcaraz C, Goldfrank L, Turndorf H, Puig M: Morphine–ethanol interaction on body temperature. Gen Pharmacol 1991;22:111–116.
194. Osborn JJ: Experimental hypothermia: respiratory and blood pH changes in relation to cardiac function. Am J Physiol 1953;175:389–398.
195. Osborne L, Kamal El-Din AS, Smith JE: Survival after prolonged cardiac arrest and accidental hypothermia. Br Med J 1984;289:881–882.
196. Ovadia H, Wohlman A, Mechoulam R, Weidenfeld J: Characterization of the hypothermic effect of the synthetic cannabinoid HU-210 in the rat. Relation to the adrenergic system and endogenous pyrogens. Neuropharmacology 1995;34:175–180.
197. Patel R, Das M, Palazzolo M, et al: Myoglobinuric acute renal failure in phencyclidine overdose: report of observations in eight cases. Ann Emerg Med 1980;9:549–553.
198. Patel S, Hutson PH: Hypothermia induced by cholinomimetic drugs is blocked by galanin: possible involvement of ATP-sensitive K channels. Eur J Pharmacol 1994;255:25–32.
199. Paton BC: Accidental hypothermia. Pharmacol Ther 1983;22:331–377.
200. Perchick JS, Winkelstein A, Shadduch RK: Disseminated intravascular coagulation in heatstroke. JAMA 1975;231: 480–483.
201. Rawson RO, Quick KP: Evidence of deep-body thermoreceptor response to intraabdominal heating of the ewe. J Appl Physiol 1970;28:813–820.
202. Reuler JB: Hypothermia: Pathophysiology, clinical settings and management. Ann Intern Med 1978;89:519–527.
203. Riedel W: Warm receptors in the dorsal abdominal wall of the rabbit. Pflueggers Arch 1976;361:205–206.
204. Ritzmann RF, Tabakoff B: Body temperature in mice: A quantitative measure of alcohol tolerance and physical dependence. J Pharmacol Exp Ther 1976;199:158–170.
205. Ritzmann RF, Tabakoff B: Dissociation of alcohol tolerance and dependence. Nature 1976;263:418–420.
206. Rivers N, Horner B: Possible lethal reaction between Nardil and dextromethorphan. Can Med Assoc J 1970; 103:85. Letter.
207. Roden DM: Antiarrhythmic drugs. In: Hardman JG, Limbird LE, Molinoff PB, Ruddon RW, Gilman AG, eds: Goodman and Gilman's The Pharmacological Basis of Therapeutics, 9th ed. New York, McGraw-Hill, 1996, p. 862.

208. Romm E, Collins AC: Body temperature influences on ethanol elimination rate. Alcohol 1987;4:189–198.
209. Ron D, Taitelman U, Michaelson M, et al: Prevention of acute renal failure in traumatic rhabdomyolysis. Arch Intern Med 1984;144:277–280.
210. Rowell LB: Cardiovascular aspects of human thermoregulation. Circ Res 1983;52:367–379.
211. Ruiz de Elvira MC, Coen CW: Centrally administered neuropeptide Y enhances the hypothermia induced by peripheral administration of adrenoceptor antagonists. Peptides 1990;11:963–967.
212. Salmi P, Karlsson T, Ahlenius S: Antagonism by SCH23390 of clozapine-induced hypothermia in the rat. Eur J Pharmacol 1994;253:67–73.
213. Sanchez C, Lembol H: The involvement of muscarinic receptor subtypes in the mediation of hypothermia, tremor and salivation in male mice. Pharmacol Toxicol 1994; 74:35–39.
214. Sarnquist F, Larson CP: Drug-induced heatstroke. Anesthesiology 1973;39:348–350.
215. Satinoff E. Disruption of hibernation caused by hypothalamic lesions. Science 1966;155:1031–1033.
216. Satinoff E: Impaired recovery from hypothermia after anterior hypothalamic lesions in hibernators. Science 1964; 148:399–400.
217. Savard GK, Cooper KE, Veale WL, Malkinson TJ: Peripheral blood flow during rewarming from mild hypothermia in humans. J Appl Physiol 1985;58:4–13.
218. Sawka MN, Young AJ, Latzka WA, et al: Human tolerance to heat strain during exercise: Influence of hydration. J Appl Physiol 1992;73:368–375.
219. Schaller MD, Fischer AP, Perret CH: Hyperkalemia: A prognostic factor during acute severe hypothermia. JAMA 1990;264:1842–1845.
220. Schrier RW, Henderson HS, Tisher CC, Tannen RL: Nephropathy associated with heat stress and exercise. Ann Intern Med 1967;67:356–366.
221. Schuman SH. Patterns of urban heat-wave deaths and implications for prevention: Data from New York and St. Louis during July, 1966. Environ Res 1972;5:59–75.
222. Semenza JC, Rubin CH, Falter KH, et al: Heat-related deaths during the July 1995 heat wave in Chicago. N Engl J Med 1996;335:84–90.
223. Seraj MA, Channa AB, Harthi SS, et al: Are heat stroke patients fluid depleted? Importance of monitoring central venous pressure as a simple guideline for fluid therapy. Resuscitation 1991;21:33–39.
224. Shapiro Y, Magazanik A, Udassin R, et al: Heat intolerance in former heatstroke patients. Ann Intern Med 1979;90:913–916.
225. Shibolet S, Coll R, Gilat T, Sohar E: Heatstroke: Its clinical picture and mechanism in 36 cases. Q J Med 1967; 36:525–548.
226. Shibolet S, Lancaster MC, Danon Y: Heatstroke: A review. Aviat Space Environ Med 1976;47:280–301.
227. Shvartz E, Shapiro Y, Magazanik A, et al: Heat acclimation, physical fitness, and responses to exercise in temperate and hot environments. J Appl Physiol 1977;43:678–683.
228. Shvartz E, Shibolet S, Merez A, et al: Prediction of heat tolerance from heart rate and rectal temperature in a temperate environment. J Appl Physiol 1977;43:684–688.
229. Smilkstein MJ, Smolinske SC, Rumack BH: A case of MAO inhibitor/MDMA interaction: agony after ecstasy. 1987; 25:149–159.
230. Sohal RS, Sun SC, Colcolough HL, Burch GE: Heatstroke: an electron microscopic study of endothelial cell damage and disseminated intravascular coagulation. Arch Intern Med 1968;122:43–47.
231. Southwick FS, Preston DH: Recovery after prolonged asystolic cardiac arrest in profound hypothermia. JAMA 1980;243:1250–1253.
232. Splittgerber FH, Talbert JG, Sweezer WP, Wilson RF: Partial cardiopulmonary bypass for core rewarming in profound accidental hypothermia. Am Surg 1986;52:407–411.
233. Sprung CL: Hemodynamic alterations of heatstroke in the elderly. Chest 1979;75:362–366.
234. Sprung CL, Portocarrero CJ, Fernaine AV, Weinberg PF: The metabolic and respiratory alterations of heat stroke. Arch Intern Med 1980;140:665–669.
235. Sternbach H: The serotonin syndrome. Am J Psychiatry 1991;148:705–713.
236. Tavel ME, Davidson W, Batterton TD: A critical analysis of mortality associated with deliruim tremens: Review of 39 fatalities in a 9-year period. Am J Med Sci 1961; 242:58–69.
237. Thomas JM, Rubin EH: Case report of a toxic reaction from a combination of tryptophan and phenelzine. Am J Psychiatry 1984;141:281–283.
238. Tolman KG, Cohen A: Accidental hypothermia. Can Med Assoc J 1970;103:1357–1361.
239. Tomaszewski W: Changements electrocardiographiques. Observes chez un homme mort de froid. Arch Mal Coeur 1938;31:525–528.
240. Towne WD, Geiss P, Yanes HO, Rahimtoola SH: Intractable ventricular fibrillation associated with profound accidental hypothermia—Successful treatment with partial cardiopulmonary bypass. N Engl J Med 1972;287: 1135–1136.
241. Trevino A, Razi B, Beller BM: The characteristic electrocardiogram of accidental hypothermia. Arch Intern Med 1971;127:470–473.
242. Truscott DG, Firor WB, Clein LJ: Accidental profound hypothermia Arch Surg 1973;106:216–218.
243. Tysinger DS, Grace JT, Gollan F: The electrocardiogram of dogs surviving 1.5° centigrade. Am Heart J 1955;50: 816–822.
244. Vassallo S, Delaney KA, Hoffman R, et al: A prospective evaluation of the electrocardiographic manifestations of hypothermia. Acad Emerg Med 1995;2:344. Abstract.
245. Vassallo SU, Delaney KA: Pharmacologic effects on thermoregulation: Mechanisms of drug-related heatstroke. J Toxicol Clin Toxicol 1989;27:199–224.
246. Vertel RM, Knochel JP: Acute renal failure due to heat injury. Am J Med 1967;43:435–451.
247. Walczak DD: Biochemical correlates of alcohol tolerance: Role of cerebral protein synthesis. Ph.D. Thesis, University of Toronto.
248. Ward A, Chaffman MO, Sorkin EM: Dantrolene: A review of its pharmacodynamic and pharmacokinetic properties and therapeutic use in malignant hyperthermia, the neuroleptic malignant syndrome and an update of its use in muscle spasticity. Drugs 1986;32:130–167.

249. Webb P: Afterdrop of body temperature during rewarming: an alternative explanation. J Appl Physiol 1986; 60:385–390.
250. Weyman AE, Greenbaum DM, Grace WJ: Accidental hypothermia in an alcoholic population. Am J Med 1974; 56:13–20.
251. White JD: Hypothermia: The Bellevue experience. Ann Emerg Med 1982;11:417–424.
252. Wickstrom P, Ruiz E, Lilja GP, et al: Accidental hypothermia core rewarming with partial bypass. Am J Surg 1976;131:622–625.
253. Wislicki L: Effects of hypothermia and hyperthermia on the actions of neuromuscular blocking agents. I. Suxamethonium. Arch Int Pharmacodyn Ther 1960;126:68–78.
254. Wong KC: Physiology and pharmacology of hypothermia. West J Med 1983;138:227–232.
255. York JL, Chan AW: Age effects on chronic tolerance to ethanol hypnosis and hypothermia. Pharmacol Biochem Behav 1994;49:371–376.
256. Young AA, Dawson NJ: Evidence for on-off control of heat dissipation from the tail of rat. Can J Physiol Pharmacol 1982;60:392–398.
257. Zachary L, Kucan JO, Robson MC, Frank DH: Accidental hypothermia treated with rapid rewarming by immersion. Ann Plast Surg 1982;9:238–241.
258. Zelman S, Guillan R: Heatstroke in phenothiazine-treated patients: A report of three fatalities. Am J Psychiatry 1970;126:1787–1790.

CHAPTER 19

Neurologic Principles

E. John Gallagher and Neal A. Lewin

General Concepts

Neurotoxicology

One of the cardinal principles of neurotoxicology is localization. A careful history, including detailed information about unintentional and intentional exposure to medications and occupational exposures, combined with the neurologic examination, can help identify the level of the neuraxis involved. This anatomic approach divides the nervous system into two highly interactive components: the central nervous system (CNS) and peripheral nervous system (PNS).

The CNS and PNS are differentially affected by toxins for several reasons. Although both are protected compartments, the characteristics of the blood–brain barrier and blood–nerve barrier differ. Thus, certain toxins that are able to gain access to one compartment may fail to gain access to the other, resulting in differential vulnerabilities. In addition, recovery from neurotoxic insult differs in the CNS and PNS. Although the entire nervous system is postmitotic, axon regrowth following nerve injury is much more extensive in the PNS than in the CNS. Finally, CNS toxicity and PNS toxicity have different clinical presentations. Whereas CNS toxins commonly cause altered mental status, movement disorders, headache, or seizures, PNS toxicity characteristically presents as altered sensory and/or motor function together with normal cognition. Unfortunately, many toxins do not adhere to simple efforts at anatomic or histologic classification. A thorough understanding of neurotoxicology requires knowledge of the biochemical affinities of particular toxins for specific classes of neurons and glia and a comprehension of the interactions of these toxins with neural tissue at the molecular level. These basic considerations are discussed in subsequent chapters targeted at specific toxins. The intent of this chapter is to focus on general clinical neurologic principles that are particularly relevant to toxicology.

Central Nervous System

Central nervous system toxicity presenting as an acute change in mentation may be characterized as abnormalities in either the level or content of consciousness. Alterations in level of consciousness, which represent quantitative abnormalities, may reflect a toxin-induced depression of consciousness, from lethargy through stupor to coma. In contrast, alterations in the content of consciousness represent qualitative abnormalities, typically presenting as confusion or delirium, often with superimposed agitation. Because altered mental status is such a common component of a toxicologic emergency, the first part of this chapter will focus on a comprehensive approach to this clinical problem. This section is followed by a discussion of drug- and toxin-induced movement disorders, which are divided into the akinesias and the dyskinesias. Finally, other manifestations of CNS toxicity, such as seizures and headache, are discussed.

Central Nervous System

Altered Mental Status

The practical problem confronting the physician in the evaluation of a patient with an acute change in mental status is determining whether the cause is toxicologic, metabolic (including infectious), neurologic (structural), psychiatric, or a combination of one or more of these groups.[193] For example, an agitated and apparently confused patient might be suffering from a sympathomimetic ingestion, hypoglycemia, subarachnoid hemorrhage, or acute schizophrenia. A patient presenting in coma might be suffering from a sedative-hypnotic ingestion, hepatic encephalopathy, or intracerebral hemorrhage. Only through the systematic application of basic neurologic principles can the differential diagnosis be narrowed to the point where reasonable management decisions can be made.

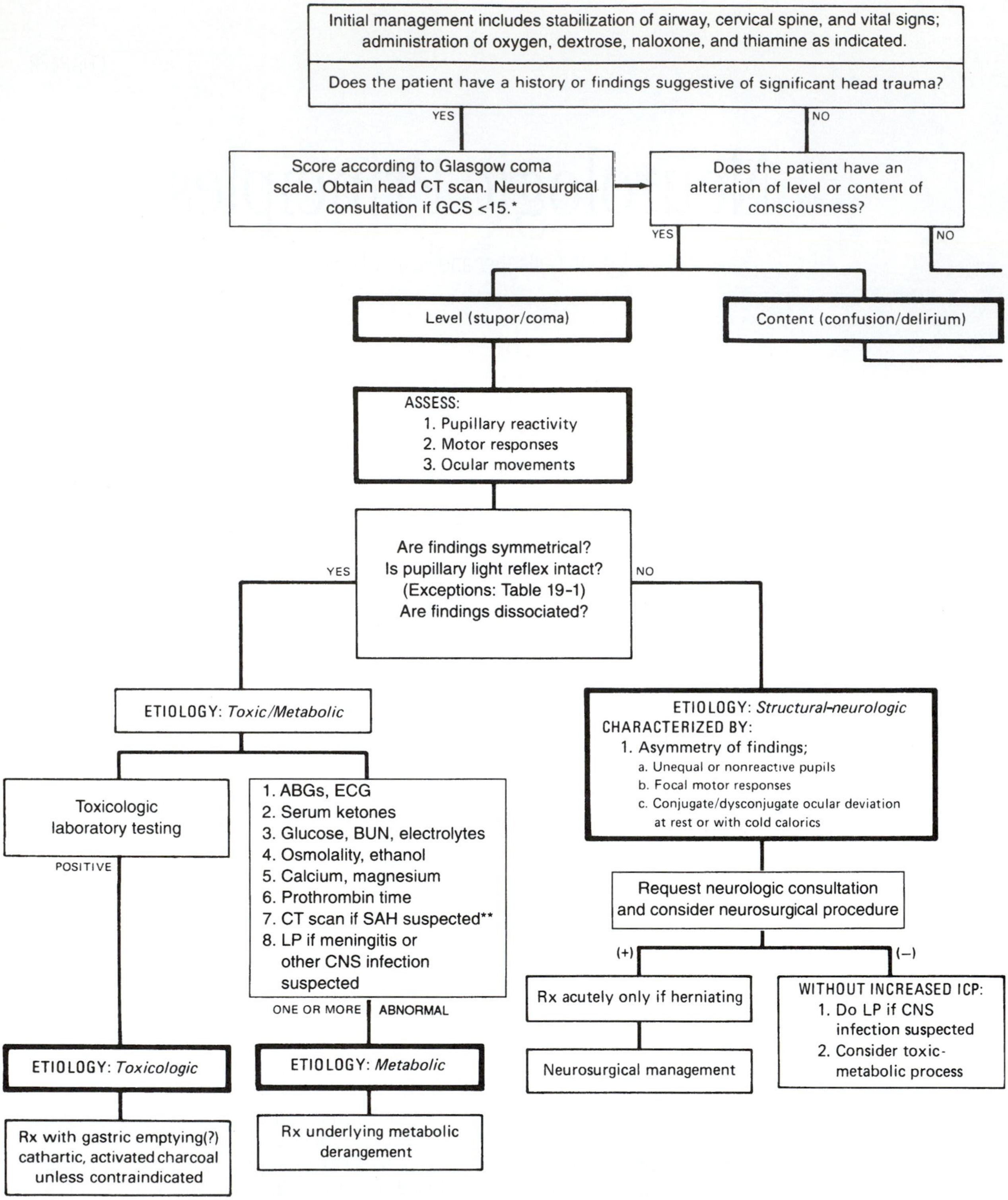

Figure 19–1. Assessment of the patient with an altered level or content of consciousness. *Always consider that a patient may have multiple etiologies for his/her altered consciousness. **SAH behaves much like toxic-metabolic etiologies, although it is a structural–neurologic entity.

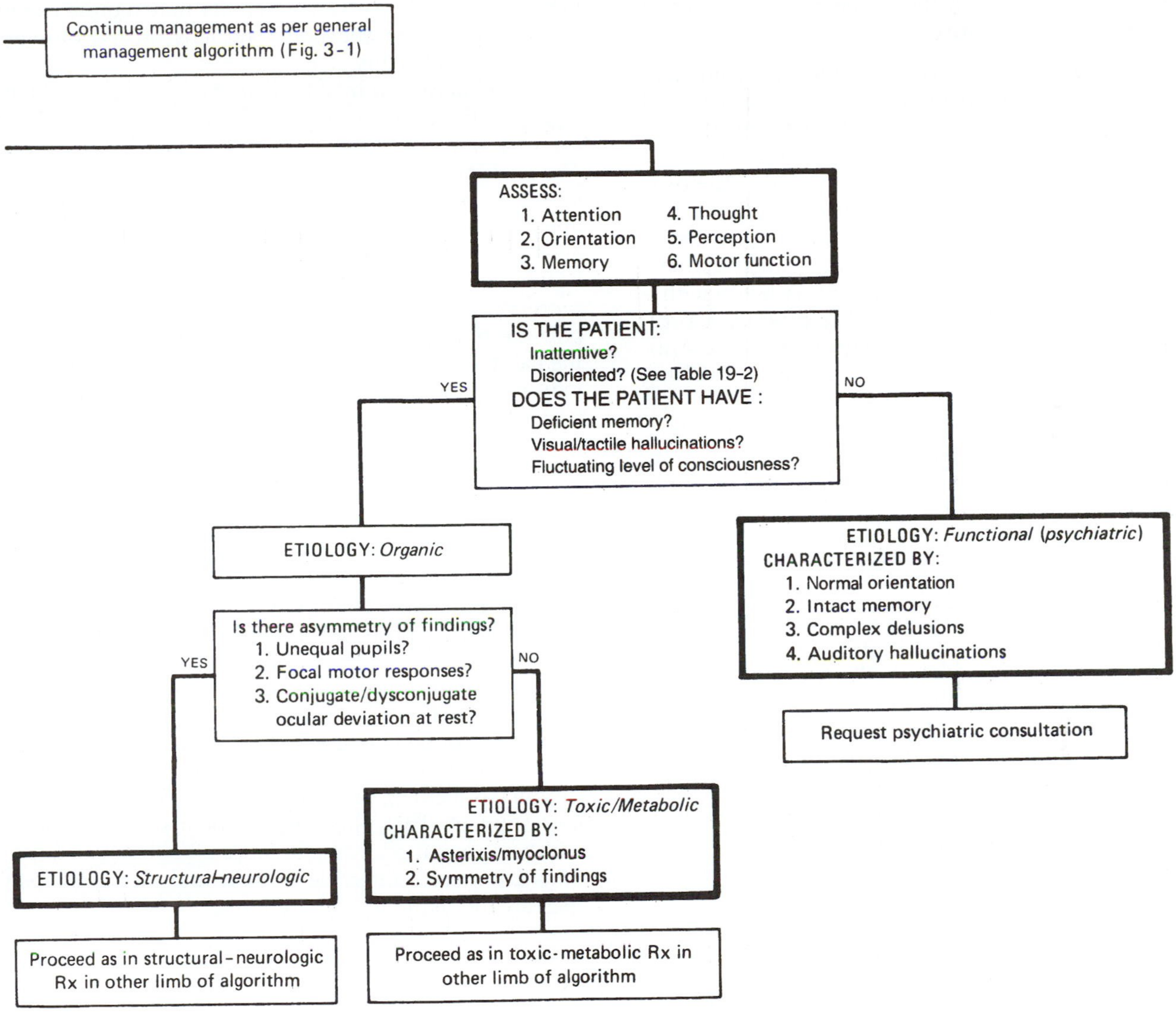
Continue management as per general management algorithm (Fig. 3-1)
ASSESS:
1. Attention
2. Orientation
3. Memory
4. Thought
5. Perception
6. Motor function
IS THE PATIENT:
Inattentive?
Disoriented? (See Table 19-2)
DOES THE PATIENT HAVE :
Deficient memory?
Visual/tactile hallucinations?
Fluctuating level of consciousness?
YES
NO
ETIOLOGY: Organic
ETIOLOGY: Functional (psychiatric)
CHARACTERIZED BY:
1. Normal orientation
2. Intact memory
3. Complex delusions
4. Auditory hallucinations
Request psychiatric consultation
Is there asymmetry of findings?
1. Unequal pupils?
2. Focal motor responses?
3. Conjugate/dysconjugate ocular deviation at rest?
YES
NO
ETIOLOGY: Toxic/Metabolic
CHARACTERIZED BY:
1. Asterixis/myoclonus
2. Symmetry of findings
ETIOLOGY: Structural-neurologic
Proceed as in structural-neurologic Rx in other limb of algorithm
Proceed as in toxic-metabolic Rx in other limb of algorithm

The first portion of this section discusses these basic principles, with the intent of assigning patients with altered mental status to one of the four major categories listed above and displayed in Figure 19–1. It is appropriate that this discussion should be undertaken in a toxicology text, since approximately 30% of all patients presenting with coma of unknown etiology will, on further investigation, turn out to have been exposed to a toxin.[172] Overdoses also commonly induce organic confusion or delirium. For both of these reasons, the physician must always consider a toxin in the differential diagnosis of acutely altered mental status.

Initial Management. The first priority in the management of any patient with altered mental status is assessment and stabilization of the airway and vital signs (Chap. 3). Oxygen saturation should be measured by pulse oximetry and oxygen administered to any patient who is hypoxic. If there is any suspicion of carbon monoxide poisoning or methemoglobinemia, the pulse oximeter may be unreliable and a blood gas specimen should be analyzed on a co-oximeter (see Chaps. 20, 93 and 96). Patients with a depressed level of consciousness and respiratory depression should receive 0.1–2.0 mg of naloxone IV (see Antidotes in Depth: Opioid Antagonists). Thiamine, 100 mg IV, can be given safely to any patient with an altered mental status but is especially indicated for those who appear undernourished, particularly those who are chronic alcoholics, and 0.5–1.0 g/kg of dextrose should be administered to patients with or without focal findings.[32] (see Antidotes in Depth: Opioid Antagonists, Thiamine Hydrochloride, and Dextrose). All patients should be placed on a cardiac monitor.

Additional tests that may be helpful in a patient with altered mental status include an ECG, blood glucose, electrolytes, BUN, blood ethanol, calcium, prothrombin time, and serum ketones. Specific toxicologic tests are determined by the clinical findings (Chap. 6).

After these initial interventions and stabilization are accomplished, a "circumstantial" history is obtained (see detailed discussion in Chaps. 3 and 30). The patient is then examined as described below and categorized as probable toxicologic, metabolic, structural neurologic, or psychiatric. From this initial categorization, further management logically follows.

Alterations in the Level of Consciousness

The Comatose Patient. A significant alteration in the level of consciousness precludes a meaningful evaluation of the content of consciousness. Coma, defined as unarousable unresponsiveness, is the prototypical alteration in level of consciousness. Stupor is defined as arousability only in response to a noxious stimulus. Although stupor and coma are often discussed as a single entity, the general principles mentioned below strictly pertain only to patients who are unarousable and therefore truly comatose. Much of the discussion that follows is a distillation of Plum and Posner's work on the classification of disorders of consciousness.[172]

In a patient presenting to the ED in coma, it is of primary importance to distinguish between structural neurologic causes, such as cerebrovascular accidents and epidural/subdural hematomas and toxic-metabolic causes such as sedative-hypnotic ingestions or hyperosmolarity. This can be accomplished with reasonable accuracy by the assessment of three clinical parameters: pupillary equality and reactivity to light, ocular position at rest and in response to provocative maneuvers, and motor response to noxious stimuli.[170]

PUPILLARY REFLEXES. Assessing the pupils requires a strong light source, and assessing reactivity may require examination under magnification. The lens on the otoscope may be useful for this.

In coma caused by a toxic-metabolic process, the integrity of the pupillary light reflex remains intact. There are very few exceptions to this principle[148] (Table 19–1). The vast majority of toxic and metabolic processes preserve the pupillary light reflex until the terminal (near apneic) stages of coma. The commonly used depolarizing agents, such as succinylcholine,[167] and nondepolarizing agents, such as pancuronium[52] and vecuronium,[27] do not represent exceptions to this general rule and do not impair the pupillary light reflex. Asymmetric findings are the hallmark of structural neurologic disease. The pupils may react unequally to light. In striking contrast to the vast majority of overdoses, coma caused by structural neurologic disease may be accompanied by pupillary abnormalities at some point in its evolution.

The hallmark of toxicologic coma, and indeed of all toxic-metabolic coma, is a dissociation of findings. This means the pupils are "dissociated from" other neuraxis dysfunction in a fashion that is not characteristic of structural brain disease. Thus, in addition to symmetric findings, patients whose coma results from a toxicologic or metabolic etiology will typically have an intact and equal pupillary light reflex (see exceptions in Table 19–1) that may be paired with an absent oculovestibular response, no ocular motion in response to cold water irrigation (see below), an absent (flaccid) motor response to noxious stimuli (see below), or hypoventilation requiring ventilatory support. This phenomenon of dissociation occurs with toxic-metabolic coma because other brainstem functions are more vulnerable to toxic and metabolic insult than are the pupillary light reflexes.

TABLE 19–1. TOXIC-METABOLIC ENCEPHALOPATHIES THAT MAY CAUSE COMA AND NONREACTIVE PUPILS

	Large/Fixed[a]	Small/Fixed[b]	Midvariable/Fixed
Anoxia	X		
Anticholinergics	X		
Barbiturates[c]			X
Glutethimide			X
Hypothermia (< 28°C)			X
Opioids		X	

[a]Although it does not cause coma, dopamine may cause fixed and dilated pupils.
[b]Pilocarpine eyedrops are common causes of fixed, small pupils.
[c]Seen only with very large doses of barbiturates.

PROVOCATIVE MOVEMENTS IN ASSESSING EYE MOVEMENTS. Two provocative maneuvers are involved in assessing eye movements, the oculocephalic maneuver ("doll's eyes") and cold caloric testing. The reader is referred to standard neurology texts for detailed description of these maneuvers. If extraocular eye movements are full and equal bilaterally to these maneuvers, the brainstem is intact. If asymmetry exists, structural disease should be strongly considered. With structural disease, the position of the eyes at rest may be asymmetric, demonstrating either conjugate or dysconjugate gaze deviation. In contrast, in toxic-metabolic processes the eyes are positioned within a few degrees of the midline, unless the patient is seizing or postictal or has an underlying strabismus. If these entities can be excluded with reasonable certainty, significant ocular divergence in a comatose patient is indicative of a structural brainstem lesion.[172]

In contrast, in coma caused by a toxic-metabolic process the eyes either respond or do not respond to provocative maneuvers, but in either case there is bilateral symmetry.

MOTOR RESPONSE TO NOXIOUS STIMULI. Stimuli that are noxious but not harmful, in ascending order of noxiousness, include nasal tickle with cotton wisp or swab, pressure on the lunula of the nailbed with the side of a pen or tongue depressor, and pinching the loose skin on the inner aspect of the upper arm. The use of more noxious stimuli is unnecessary.

The motor responses to a noxious stimulus in structural neurologic disease are often asymmetric or focal. When a comatose patient is given a noxious stimulus, one of three motor responses occurs: "appropriate," flaccid, or stereotypic. Stereotypic responses take one of two forms, abnormal flexor (decorticate posturing) or abnormal extensor (decerebrate posturing). Use of the abnormal flexor/extensor terminology is preferred, since this is less misleading anatomically and affords better interobserver concordance.[199] A comatose patient with a structural lesion might show abnormal flexion in one upper extremity and flaccidity or abnormal extension in the other. Alternatively, a patient with a toxicologic cause for coma may demonstrate any of the various motor responses, but in general should do so symmetrically and without evidence of focality.

Thus, by observing the pupillary reactivity, eye movements, and motor responses for evidence of asymmetry or dissociation, it is usually possible to decide whether a patient's coma is based on a structural neurologic or toxic-metabolic etiology, respectively. From this decision, subsequent management logically follows.

There are exceptions to the above generalizations. Structural disease does not always produce focality. Mass lesions of the brain may cause compression of the brainstem bilaterally. In this dynamic process, neurologic signs that were originally asymmetric may become bilateral and symmetric by the time the physician sees the patient. Conversely, toxic-metabolic conditions such as hyperosmolar nonketotic hyperglycemia[172] or hypoglycemia[155] may produce focal deficits.

Alteration in the Content of Consciousness: The Patient With Delirium or Psychiatric Illness. Clinical assessment of the content of consciousness presupposes a certain arousability or level of consciousness. Acute alterations in the content of consciousness may be caused by either organic or "functional" etiologies. The term *organic* is used here to denote toxic-metabolic or structural neurologic disease, and *functional* refers to the major psychiatric disorders. The term *psychotic* is used here in a restricted sense to describe patients with a nonorganic psychosis who are suffering from serious psychiatric illness.

This division between organic and functional disease is an artificial dichotomy that reflects our limited knowledge regarding the neurochemistry of psychiatric disorders. The psychoses are a diverse set of diseases of unknown etiology that are almost certainly organic in origin (perhaps reflecting defects in neurotransmission) but have not yet been metabolically characterized.

Unlike the partitioning of coma into structural and toxic-metabolic categories, the organic versus functional construct has no firm anatomic or physiologic substrate. The basis for this division is that currently the management of these two groups of illnesses is very different.[126]

In approaching a patient with an alteration in the content of consciousness, the physician must decide first whether the etiology is organic or functional, and if organic, whether toxic-metabolic or structural neurologic (see Fig. 19–1). This problem is analogous to that presented by the comatose patient. The major difference in the evaluation of the patient with an alteration in content (psychosis, delirium) rather than level of consciousness (coma) is that in the case of altered content, the clinical examination places great emphasis on meticulous assessment of the mental status. In the case of a severely altered level of consciousness, a mental status examination is not possible and attention is therefore directed toward the assessment of pupils, ocular movements, and motor response. The major difference is that psychiatric disease, which only rarely causes coma (1–2%),[172] typically presents as an alteration in content of consciousness (Table 19–2).

In general, any middle-aged or elderly person presenting with acutely altered mentation, without an antecedent psychiatric history, should be presumed to have an organic etiology until proved otherwise. The components of the mental status examination used for evaluating the patient with an alteration in content of consciousness are listed in Table 19–2.

Level of Alertness. Initially, level of alertness is assessed by simple observation. Typically, a delirious patient demonstrates a clouded sensorium and fluctuating level of consciousness over time, whereas a patient with primary psychiatric illness generally has a more stable level of consciousness.

Attention. Before evaluating higher cognitive function, the patient's attention span must be assessed. Just as a depressed level of consciousness precludes further testing of mental status, inattention makes it difficult to test orientation, memory, and other cognitive processes. Num-

TABLE 19–2. TYPICAL DISTINGUISHING FEATURES OF ALTERATIONS IN THE CONTENT OF CONSCIOUSNESS

	Organic		Psychiatric	
Clinical Feature	**Delirium**	**Dementia**	**Mood Disorder (Unipolar or Bipolar)**	**Schizophrenia**
Onset	Acute	Insidious	Gradual/subacute	Gradual/subacute
Short-term temporal profile	Fluctuating	Stable	Stable	Stable
Age at onset	Any age	≥ 50 y	< 40 y unless situational or involutional	< 30 y
Level of alertness	Clouded (may be depressed or hyperalert)	Normal unless far advanced	Normal, slightly depressed or hyperalert	Normal or hyperalert
Attention	Impaired	Unimpaired unless far advanced	Unimpaired unless severe	Unimpaired unless distracted by hallucinations
Orientation	Disoriented	Disoriented unless early and mild	Oriented	Oriented
Memory	Globally impaired	Short-term more impaired than long-term	Intact	Intact
Thought processes	Disorganized, incoherent, rambling	Disorganized but less evident than in delirium	Delusions may be self-deprecatory or grandiose	Delusions typical, fixed, elaborate, paranoid, or grandiose
Perceptual distortions	Hallucinations commonly visual, tactile, or auditory	None	Hallucinations uncommon	Auditory hallucinations common
Asterixis	Suggestive of toxic-metabolic encephalopathy	None	None	None
Outcome	Mortality or resolution	Deterioration if no treatable cause found	Resolution and recurrence; mortality associated with suicide	Resolution and recurrence, often with deterioration; mortality associated with command hallucinations

ber repetition is the simplest means of testing attention, using a nonsequential, nonrepeating string of seven digits (eg, 9185072). The numbers should be given to the patient at a rate of one per second. Inability to repeat at least five of the digits in the correct sequence is indicative of inattention,[197] an essential feature of delirium.[96] Attention may be impaired in patients with psychiatric disease who are actively hallucinating or severely depressed but is more characteristically diminished in patients with organic confusion. A selective inattention toward one side of the body—usually the left—due to a nondominant parietal lobe lesion is virtually diagnostic of structural neurologic disease.

Orientation. Disoriented patients must be assumed to have organic pathology until proved otherwise. Organically disturbed patients are typically disoriented to time and place but only rarely to person. It is important to ask the patient to state as precisely as possible the day, month, and year, rather than infer his or her degree of orientation from conversation. Many patients, especially those with slowly progressive organic confusion such as dementia, can obscure their deficit quite skillfully in casual conversation. Unlike inattentiveness, disorientation is not an essential feature of delirium.[96]

Memory. Memory is a complex process, involving reception, retention, and retrieval of information. Short-term memory can be most readily assessed by asking the patient to recall three unrelated words after the passage of 3–5 minutes. Ability to recall two of three objects is the best cutpoint but is only about 80% sensitive and 75% specific for the diagnosis of organic confusion.[61] Impairment of memory is characteristically seen only in organic conditions, although a severely psychotic patient may occasionally do poorly on memory testing because of preoccupation with intrusive hallucinations. Similarly, a severely depressed "pseudodemented" patient may appear to have poor recall simply because of a failure to make the required effort.

Thought. Assessment of the patient's thought process and content should be directed toward a search for delusions, often paranoid or grandiose in nature. Specific questions asked in a matter-of-fact manner—"Are you afraid someone is out to hurt you? Is anyone trying to control your mind? Do you have thoughts you cannot get out of your head? Do you possess any special powers?"—are often met with a surprisingly direct response. Patients with organic disease may be paranoid, but generally their delusions are not as intricate as those of schizophrenic patients.

It is also important to distinguish between a thought disorder and a language disorder. A true language disturbance (aphasia) represents a focal neurologic finding, usually localizing the pathology to the dominant hemisphere. When the aphasia is characterized by a paucity of speech (nonfluent aphasia), there is often an accompanying right-sided hemiparesis, and the diagnosis of a structural lesion is not difficult. Fluent aphasia, however, can easily be confused with delirium or psychosis. Typically, fluent aphasia can be distinguished from organic confusion by the presence of frequent agrammatical paraphasic errors that are not a prominent feature of most cases of delirium or dementia. Fluent aphasia can also be distinguished from psychosis by the frequency of neologisms, which tend to appear in agrammatically constructed sentences and, unlike the occasional neologisms of acute psychosis, are nonrepetitive (since they essentially represent random output of language). A psychotic neologism may have some symbolic meaning to the patient and is repeated over and over. Although an extensive discussion of the various forms of aphasia is beyond the scope of this chapter, it is important to remember that disjointed speech does not necessarily reflect disjointed thought.

Perception. To determine whether the patient is actively hallucinating, the examiner must observe him or her carefully for repeated head turning, directed eye movements, staring, or incoherent mumbling. As in the assessment of thought content, the direct approach is often most rewarding. For example, one might ask: "Do you sometimes see things that you think may not be real? Do you ever feel things, like bugs, crawling on your skin? Do you sometimes hear voices calling you names or telling you to do something you do not want to do? Have you ever heard your name called and turned to find no one there?"

Well-formed auditory hallucinations are indicative of schizophrenia, although they are also sometimes seen in major affective disorders. Poorly formed auditory hallucinations are not diagnostically distinctive. Visual hallucinations are suggestive, but not diagnostic, of delirium. Tactile, gustatory, and olfactory hallucinations, while relatively rare, usually indicate organic disease. A differential diagnosis of common causes of drug-induced delirium is presented in Table 19–3.

Motor. Just as in coma, focal motor findings here suggest structural neurologic disease until proved otherwise. Asterixis is an extremely helpful finding since it is highly suggestive of a toxic-metabolic cause of altered mentation. Movement disorders associated with drugs or toxins are discussed later in this chapter.

In practice, it is sometimes difficult to distinguish toxic-metabolic from structural neurologic disease. This occurs when a toxic-metabolic process produces focal findings (which is relatively uncommon)[126,155,197] or when an "extraaxial" structural lesion, such as a subdural hematoma or subarachnoid hemorrhage, produces minimal focality because the pathologic process is located outside brain parenchyma. In the former case, usually the patient undergoes an unnecessary CT or MRI scan but little harm is done. In the latter case, however, failure to perform a CT or MRI scan may have dire consequences.[53,76,102,130] It is for this reason that even the slightest suggestion of focality in an apparent overdose should prompt a neuroimaging procedure, as should any degree of diagnostic uncertainty generated either by the circumstances under which the patient was found (eg, at the foot of a flight of stairs) or by evidence of head trauma on examination. If structural disease is suspected in a comatose or confused patient, a CT scan should be obtained immediately.

With the application of basic neurologic principles,

TABLE 19–3. DIFFERENTIAL DIAGNOSIS OF DRUG-INDUCED DELIRIUM

Substance	Psychiatric Examination
Amphetamines	Clear sensorium
Amphetamine, methamphetamine, phenmetrazine, mephentermine	Auditory and visual hallucinations
	Paranoia
	Suicidal
	Homicidal
	Similar to cocaine
Anticholinergics	Disorientation
Belladonna alkaloids, antihistamines, cyclic antidepressants	Hyperexcitability
	Mania
	Paranoia
	Auditory and visual hallucinations
Cocaine	Normal sensorium or paranoia
	Tactile sensations (cocaine bugs)
	Hallucinations
Ethanol withdrawal	Aggression, depression, or anxiety
	Disorientation
Hallucinogens	Oriented to time, place, and person
LSD (lysergic acid diethylamide), peyote, indolealkylamines (psilocybin, morning glory seeds)	Perceptual and cognitive distortion
	Mild apprehension to panic, hyperalert
	Feelings of worthlessness or omnipotence
Phencyclidine	Unresponsive
Ketamine	Extreme agitation
	Violence
	Schizophreniform behavior
	Homicidal
	Suicidal
	Elevated pain threshold
Sedative-hypnotic withdrawal	Anxiety
Barbiturates, benzodiazepines, diverse others	Disorientation
	Hallucinations

it should be possible to determine, on the basis of history, clinical examination, and readily obtainable laboratory[111] and radiographic data, whether a patient with an altered mental status is suffering from structural neurologic disease, a psychiatric disorder, or a toxic-metabolic derangement. On the basis of a categorical rather than specific diagnosis, a rational plan of management and further evaluation can then be formulated.[77,78]

Movement Disorders

Virtually all of the movement disorders caused by primary neurologic disease can be induced by a drug or toxin.[75,150] The drugs that are most frequently implicated in movement disorders are the neuroleptics, calcium channel blockers,[22,37,44,49–51,57,68,69,79,82,114,119,132,137,144,146,153,155,162,166,186,200] orthopramides and substituted benzamides,[12,19,20,62,67,84,85,95,98,145,147,149,151,161,187,188,220] CNS stimulants,[4,26,36,47,72,73,97,101,133,152,198,201] antidepressants, anticonvulsants,[8,63,80,182,206] antiparkinsonian drugs, and lithium.[65,91,103,131,203] It is possible for one drug or toxin to induce two or more types of movement disorders in the same patient.[99] These disorders can be classified[213] as a decrease in movement (akinesia) and or an increase in movement (dyskinesia).[213] The akinesias that occur secondary to drugs and toxins primarily include the family of drug-induced parkinsonian syndromes. The dyskinesias that are most relevant to toxicology include tremor, chorea, ballismus, dystonia, akathisia, tardive dyskinesia, myoclonus, and asterixis.

Akinesia. Parkinson's disease is characterized by tremor, rigidity, akinesia, and postural instability. Other common features include lack of spontaneous smiling and decreased frequency of blinking, giving the patient an expressionless appearance. Stooped posture, a shuffling gait, drooling, and micrographia are also common features.[154]

Drug-induced parkinsonism may be caused by agents that either destroy cells in the substantia nigra (eg, manganese, 1-methyl-4-phenyl-1,2,3,6-tetrahydropyridine [MPTP]) or, much more commonly, agents that antagonize the effects of dopamine, either pre- or postsynaptically (see Table 19–4).

MPTP-induced parkinsonism has been reported almost exclusively in individuals using a synthetic opioid.[48,118] The syndrome differs from that of idiopathic Parkinson's disease in its rapidity of onset. In most patients, the effects appear to be permanent.[117] Because of the insights that MPTP toxicity has provided into the pathophysiology, treatment, and prevention of idiopathic Parkinson's disease, it has received a great deal of attention (Chap. 60).

TABLE 19–4. DRUG AND TOXIN-INDUCED PARKINSONISM

Neuroleptics	Other Drugs	Toxins
Chlorpromazine	Alpha-methyldopa	Alcohol withdrawal
Chlorprothixene	Calcium channel blockers	Carbon disulfide
Clozapine	Captopril[a]	Carbon monoxide[b]
Droperidol	Lithium[a]	Cyanide
Fluphenazine	Metoclopramide	Manganese
Haloperidol	Phenytoin[a]	Methanol
Loxapine	Prochlorperazine	MPTP[c]
Mesoridazine	Reserpine	
Molindone	Tetrabenazine	
Perphenazine		
Pimozide		
Thioridazine		
Thiothixene		
Trifluoperazine		

[a]Equivocal evidence
[b]Both acute and postanoxic carbon monoxide toxicity
[c]Methyl-4-phenyl-1,2,3,6-tetrahydropyridine
Modified, with permission, from Weiner WJ, Lang AE: Movement Disorders: A Comprehensive Survey. Mt. Kisco, NY, Futura, 1989, p. 600.

Neuroleptic drugs are the most common reversible cause of parkinsonism. The development of parkinsonism is dose dependent and seems to be related to the blockade of D_2 receptors and is correlated with the degree of D_2 receptor occupancy in the striatum. The halogenated and piperazine phenothiazines and butyrophenones are most likely to produce parkinsonism.[99] Some of the commonly used neuroleptics and other agents causing parkinsonism are listed in Table 19–4.

Parkinsonism due to the neuroleptics and other drugs may be treated either by the addition of an anticholinergic medication, such as benztropine, or by discontinuation of the neuroleptic.[13,23,63,71,74,80,93,100,128,138,139,140,150,159,169,182,202,206,216] However, onset or aggravation of parkinsonian signs has occurred with withdrawal of neuroleptics perhaps by causing degeneration of vulnerable nigrostriatal neurons by generating cytotoxic free radicals or accelerating neuronal firing rates.[99] There is some evidence that the use of amantadine may be more effective than anticholinergics in the treatment of drug-induced parkinsonism.[18,175,208] Because it has fewer adverse effects, and because of its efficacy in preventing recurrent dystonia, amantadine may be the treatment of choice for all extrapyramidal syndromes due to the neuroleptics.[25]

The use of adjunctive anticholinergic drugs to prevent the development of parkinsonism is controversial. A consensus statement by the World Health Organization did not recommend the use of these drugs because they potentially increase the risk of tardive dyskinesia.[18,175]

Toxins that damage the basal ganglia such as carbon monoxide (see Chap. 96) often result in cell death, with variable symptomatic response to dopaminergic medications such as levodopa and bromocriptine. Other treatment modalities, such as long-term chelation for patients whose parkinsonism is due to manganese poisoning, have been used with some success but remain controversial.[46]

Dyskinesias

Tremor. Tremor, an involuntary rhythmic oscillating movement resulting from contractions of reciprocally innervated antagonistic muscles,[110] is traditionally categorized into three groups: resting, postural, and kinetic. These three categories of tremor due to primary neurologic disease are distinguished, in part, because the management of each is different. For example, the treatment of Parkinson's disease is not at all similar to management strategies for essential tremor (the most common form of tremor encountered in practice). However, when the cause of tremor is a drug or toxin, there is often a great deal of overlap among the three varieties of tremor. In particular, a drug-induced resting tremor often has a component of postural tremor as well. Thus, virtually all of the neuroleptic medications listed in Table 19–5 are capable of producing postural tremor. Likewise, many of the agents (eg, phenytoin, mercury) that cause postural tremor also cause kinetic tremor. Conversely, drugs that

TABLE 19–5. CAUSES OF DRUG- AND TOXIN-INDUCED POSTURAL TREMOR

Drugs
Amiodarone
Amphetamines
Beta-adrenergic agonists
Caffeine
Cocaine
Corticosteroids
Cyclic antidepressants
Ergotamine
Levodopa
Lithium
MAOIs (toxic interaction with food or drug)
Monosodium glutamate
Neuroleptic agents[a]
Phenytoin
Theophylline
Valproic acid
Toxins
Arsenic
Bismuth
Carbon disulfide
Carbon monoxide
Lead
Mercury
Methylbromide
Phencyclidine
Withdrawal
Ethanol
Sedative-hypnotics

[a]Virtually all those listed in Table 19–4 can produce postural tremor.

cause postural tremor as a manifestation of withdrawal typically cause a kinetic tremor and ataxia at toxicity (eg, alcohol, benzodiazepines, barbiturates).

RESTING TREMOR. The most characteristic feature of a resting tremor (static or parkinsonian tremor) is that it is most marked with the limb at rest and decreases with voluntary movement. It is typically seen in association with the akinetic movement disorders and is often produced by the drugs and toxins listed in Table 19–4.

POSTURAL TREMOR. Postural tremor (action or sustention tremor) is present when the limbs are maintained in an outstretched position and during movement, and may increase slightly at the endpoint of a goal-directed motion. This type of tremor is much less apparent at rest and disappears entirely if the patient completely relaxes the limb. Table 19–5 lists the drugs and toxins most commonly responsible for the induction of a postural tremor.

KINETIC TREMOR. Kinetic tremor (intention, ataxic, or cerebellar tremor) is absent when the extremity is at rest and during the first part of voluntary movement, but it increases markedly in amplitude as the goal is approached.

Alcoholic cerebellar degeneration is among the most common toxic causes of kinetic tremor and ataxia.[210] This tremor is often made worse by an accompanying sensory peripheral neuropathy that impairs proprioception. When seen initially, recent-onset ataxia should be treated with thiamine, since the tremor may be a manifestation of Wernicke's encephalopathy.

Lithium is another common cause of tremor in which multiple mechanisms are probably involved. Although tremor is a frequent sign of toxicity, patients with therapeutic lithium levels may exhibit both postural and kinetic tremors,[207] which respond to dosage reduction. However, grossly irregular kinetic and resting tremors should be regarded as a sign of severe toxicity until proved otherwise.[173]

Although most patients with tremor secondary to valproic acid have a mild postural tremor, the drug may also cause a resting or kinetic tremor, including a marked tremor of the head.[107] Similar to tardive dyskinesias seen with psychotropic agents, the tremor may not begin until months after the drug has been started, and it may worsen over time.[94] Tremor severity is not closely related to valproate blood levels, but it does respond to reduction or cessation of the drug.[106]

Exposure to methyl mercury causes destruction of the small internal granular cell neurons of the cerebellar cortex, producing atrophy, marked ataxia, and kinetic tremor[191] (see Chap. 80). Amiodarone, a potent ventricular antidysrhythmic, commonly causes resting, postural, and kinetic tremors.[213] The associated ataxia is worsened by a concomitant distal polyneuropathy that affects proprioception.[168]

Finally, toxicity associated with ethanol, phenytoin, carbamazepine, barbiturates, chloral hydrate, ethchlorvynol, glutethimide, methaqualone, or any benzodiazepine can produce a syndrome of dysarthria, horizontal and vertical nystagmus, ataxia, kinetic tremor, and asterixis. Peripheral neuropathies may also cause tremor, known as neuropathic tremor, attributable to either weakness[180] or loss of proprioception[3] (see the section on peripheral neurotoxicity). Causes of kinetic tremor are summarized in Table 19–6.

Chorea. Chorea is a series of abrupt, random, excessive, spontaneous movements and is associated with the drugs and toxins listed in Table 19–7. It is also associated with a variety of electrolyte and endocrine disorders, such as hyperglycemia, hypoglycemia, hypernatremia, hyponatremia, hypocalcemia, hypomagnesemia, hyperthyroidism, hypoparathyroidism, and Wernicke's encephalopathy. The prototypic neurologic diseases associated with chorea are Huntington's chorea and Wilson's disease.

Dystonia

Acute Dystonia. Acute dystonias are slower than choreiform movements and include a wide array of sustained spasms of muscle groups. Some of the more common of these are oculogyric crisis (eyes are forced into upward or upward/lateral gaze), blepharospasm, involuntary

TABLE 19–6. CAUSES OF DRUG- AND TOXIN-INDUCED KINETIC TREMOR

Alcoholic cerebellar degeneration
Amiodarone
Barbiturates
Benzodiazepines
Carbamazepine
Chloral hydrate
Colistin
Ethanol
Ethchlorvynol
Glutethimide
Lithium
Methaqualone
Methyl mercury
Phenytoin
Piperazine
Valproic acid

TABLE 19–7. CAUSES OF DRUG- AND TOXIN-INDUCED CHOREA

Drugs
Anticholinergics
Antihistamines
Benztropine
Cyclic antidepressants
Anticonvulsants
Carbamazepine
Phenobarbital
Phenytoin
Antiparkinsonians
Amantadine
Bromocriptine
Levodopa
Pergolide
Corticosteroids
Lithium
Metoclopramide
Neuroleptics
Butyrophenones
Phenothiazines
Oral contraceptives
Sympathomimetics
Amphetamines
Caffeine
Cocaine
Methylphenidate
Theophylline
Toxins
Carbon monoxide
Ethanol
Manganese
Thallium
Toluene

Modified, with permission, after Weiner WJ, Lang AE: Movement Disorders: A Comprehensive Survey. Mt. Kisco, NY, Futura, 1989, p. 600.

tongue movements, torticollis (head twisted to the side), retrocollis (neck hyperextended), dysphagia, dysarthria, opisthotonos (a particularly severe form, characterized by hyperextension of the spine and retrocollis), and, occasionally, stridor.[134] Acute dystonias appear early. Half of them present within 2 days of starting the drug and the vast majority within the first week[15] (see Chap. 57 and Table 57–4). Any of the neuroleptic or antiemetic drugs listed in Table 19–8 can produce acute dystonias. They are also seen rarely as an adverse effect of the 4-aminoquinolone antimalarials, such as chloroquine and hydroxychloroquine.[204] The pathophysiology of acute dystonias appears to be linked, in part, to an increase in cholinergic tone, but the role of dopaminergic transmission remains obscure.[163]

These movement disorders are often extremely uncomfortable and frightening to patients. Unfortunately, because they occur in psychiatric patients, many of whom are psychotic, and because the movements appear at times to be under voluntary control, acute dystonias are frequently misdiagnosed as "hysterical." A reasonable approach to treatment is to give patients who have a dystonic reaction (and who do not appear to have anticholinergic toxicity) 1 mg/kg of diphenhydramine IV. If the dystonia resolves with the diphenhydramine, an additional dose of 1 mg/kg IM may be given, followed by 1 mg/kg orally every 6 hours for 48 hours. As noted above, there is some evidence that amantadine may be superior to the anticholinergics in preventing recurrence of dystonias.[25]

In addition to the neuroleptics, several other drugs and toxins produce opisthotonos. These include tricyclic antidepressants, phenytoin, metaldehyde, brucine, water hemlock, tremetol (a plant chemical), phencyclidine, cocaine, lithium, delphene (an insect repellent), and strychnine. Some of these dystonias may be short-lived, episodic seizures with a predominantly tonic phase.

Tardive Dystonia. As its name implies, tardive dystonia typically occurs following continuous use of neuroleptic drugs for months to years. It is also seen with use of metoclopramide, levodopa, and other antiparkinsonian medications, such as bromocriptine, and occasionally is a presenting feature of phenytoin or carbamazepine toxicity. Like acute dystonia, tardive dystonia primarily involves the craniocervical musculature and may respond to anticholinergic drugs.[34] Like tardive dyskinesia, with which it is often grouped, it is a delayed complication of neuroleptic medication and is a chronic illness, with only about 10% of patients returning to baseline after discontinuation of the drug[104] (see Chap. 57 and Table 19–8).

Tardive Dyskinesia. One simple working definition of tardive dyskinesia is all involuntary movement disorders, other than tremor, that occur as a complication of chronic neuroleptic treatment. The movements of tardive dyskinesia are choreiform in frequency and amplitude, although they tend to be more stereotypic than other choreiform movements. The muscles of the mouth, face, and

TABLE 19–8. DRUGS ASSOCIATED WITH INDUCTION OF ACUTE AND/OR TARDIVE DYSTONIA/DYSKINESIA

Drug	Dystonia	Dyskinesia
Anticonvulsants:		
carbamazepine, phenytoin	X	
Antidepressants:		
fluvoxamine	X	X
Calcium channel blockers:		
flunarizine, cinnarizine		X
Dopamine agonists:		
levodopa	X	
Neuroleptic agents		X
Orthopramides and substituted benzamides:		
metoclopramide	X	X
clebopride		X
sulpride		X
veralipride		X

TABLE 19–9. DRUGS ASSOCIATED WITH INDUCTION OF AKATHISIA

Drug
Neuroleptic drugs
Metoclopramide, prochlorperazine
Dopamine storage and transport inhibitors:
α-methytyrosine, reserpine, tetrabenazine
Levodopa and dopamine agonists
Antidepressants:
selective serotonin-reuptake inhibitors
tricyclic antidepressants
phenelzine
Calcium channel blockers:
flunarizine, cinnarizine

especially the tongue are involved early, producing the characteristic lingual-facial-buccal dyskinesia. Other components of tardive dyskinesia include chewing, sucking, or lip smacking movements, which are frequently audible. Because tardive dyskinesia is so polymorphous, the following three criteria have been suggested as prerequisites to the establishment of the diagnosis: (1) minimum of 3 months cumulative exposure to a neuroleptic; (2) moderate abnormal involuntary movements in at least one body part or mild abnormal involuntary movements in at least two body parts; and (3) absence of any other explanation for the movement disorder[185] (see Table 19–8).

Because treatment of established tardive dyskinesia is extremely difficult, early identification is particularly important.[66] If a tardive dyskinesia develops, the patient should be immediately referred to his or her psychiatrist for withdrawal of any anticholinergic medication and for dose reduction of the patient's neuroleptic medication, if possible. Other medications used to control debilitating tardive dyskinesias include benzodiazepines and dopamine antagonists.

Akathisia. Akathisia is a form of involuntary motor restlessness that results in an inability to remain still for any sustained period.[31] The common causes of akathisia are the neuroleptics and antiemetics listed in Table 19–9 as well as antiparkinsonian agents and the sympathomimetics. Akathisia is one of the most common types of extrapyramidal adverse effects caused by neuroleptics and typically occurs within 2–3 months of starting oral medication.[34] In contrast, depot injections may produce akathisia within a few days.[14]

Patients with akathisia do not manifest any particular movement and may often appear merely restless, making it easy to confuse this entity with psychotic agitation. Indeed, it may be possible to distinguish newly developed akathisia from worsening psychosis only by increasing the dose of neuroleptic medication.[157] If the agitation worsens, this suggests that the problem is akathetic. Because this is a common and troubling symptom to many patients, it is important to consider akathisia in the differential diagnosis of agitation in any patient on neuroleptics.

Myoclonus and Asterixis. Myoclonic movements are shock-like, jerking, involuntary movements of muscle groups. They are usually caused by sudden contractions of muscles ("positive" myoclonus), but in the case of asterixis, a related movement disorder, the cause is a transient relaxation of a muscle group resulting in a momentary loss of posture or position ("negative" myoclonus) (see Table 19–10).

Myoclonus. Myoclonus can be classified in several different ways, based on clinical findings, presumed anatomic locus of the pathology in the nervous system, the neurotransmitters thought to mediate the movement disorder, or etiology. The most useful classification scheme in toxicology is an etiologic one that focuses on the toxic-metabolic cause.

Asterixis. Asterixis is most easily elicited by asking the patient to extend the elbow and dorsiflex the wrist with the fingers extended and abducted, as if stopping traffic. After a brief latent period, the fingers begin to flex and extend involuntarily at the metacarpal–phalangeal joints, as posture is alternately lost and regained. This is followed by sudden palmar flexion at the wrist, with a slower return to dorsiflexion.[120,189] Although asterixis was first described in patients with hepatic failure,[2] it has since been found in association with a large number of toxic-metabolic encephalopathies. It has also been associated with structural disease, but far less commonly.[135]

Multifocal Myoclonus. Multifocal myoclonus is a dysrhythmic contraction of various muscle groups throughout the body, especially affecting the facial and proximal muscles. Although myoclonus represents muscle contraction

TABLE 19–10. TOXIC-METABOLIC CAUSES OF ASTERIXIS AND MULTIFOCAL MYOCLONUS

Metabolic
Hepatic failure
Hyperosmolarity
Hypoosmolarity
Postanoxic encephalopathy
Renal failure
Ventilatory failure
Toxic
Anticholinergics
Anticonvulsants
Benzodiazepines
Bismuth
Crotalid venom
Cyclic antidepressants
DDT
Ethanol
Lead
Levodopa
Mercury
Methylbromide
Sedative-hypnotics

Modified, with permission, from Fahn S, Marsden CD, Van Woert MH: Definition and classification of myoclonus. Adv Neurol 1986;43:1–5.

TABLE 19–11. TOXICOLOGIC CAUSES OF FASCICULATIONS

Amphetamines
Arsenic
Barium salts
Black widow spider envenomation
Brucine
Caffeine
Camphor
Cholinergic agents (including organophosphates and carbamates)
Cocaine
Ergotamines
Fluorides
Hypoglycemic agents
Lead
Lithium
Manganese
Mercury
Nicotine
Phencyclidine
Quaternary ammonium compounds (including muscarinic mushrooms)
Scorpion envenomation
Shellfish poisoning (saxitoxin)
Strychnine
Tetrodotoxin poisoning (puffer fish)

and asterixis represents muscle relaxation, when asterixis begins to spread and the patient appears to be twitching all over, it may be difficult to distinguish severe asterixis from multifocal myoclonus. Fortunately, it may not be necessary to do so, since either usually implies a toxic-metabolic encephalopathy, such as those listed in Table 19–10. These encephalopathies are typically accompanied by an alteration of mental status, although in mild cases the movement disorder, in particular asterixis, may be more prominent than the altered mental status.

Fasciculations. Fasciculations are contractions of muscle fibers within an individual motor unit; a single motor nerve cell and the several hundred muscle fibers it innervates. Fasciculations, which appear as a visible twitch, frequently occur when a muscle is fatigued or the patient is cold. In this setting, fasciculations are not pathologic. When associated with a primary neurologic disorder, fasciculations may be attributable to disease of the motor neuron (amyotrophic lateral sclerosis), nerve root, peripheral nerve, neuromuscular junction, or the skeletal muscle itself.[178]

Fasciculations are not well understood. Although there is disagreement regarding their origin,[178,215] it appears that a low excitability threshold of the axonal membrane plays a role in their production.[178] Consequently, augmentation of cholinergic "tone" at the neuromuscular junction (as is seen with organophosphate or nicotine toxicity) or increase in the irritability of skeletal muscle (eg, caffeine, theophylline) both produce fasciculations. See Table 19–11 for a complete listing of toxicologic causes of fasciculations.

Neuroleptic Malignant Syndrome. The signs of neuroleptic malignant syndrome can be divided into four major categories: autonomic instability (thermoregulation), altered mental status, movement disorder, and other neurologic dysfunction.[38,113] The movement disorders include tremor in about half of patients, severe akinetic rigidity in about one-third, and dystonia or chorea in about half.[156] Some patients have a combination of movement disorders. For further discussion see Chapters 18 and 57.

Headache

The 1990 International Headache Society Classification divides headache into 13 categories, with 129 subtypes.[165] Two sections of this classification are relevant to toxicology: "Headache associated with substances or their withdrawal" represents a primary toxic effect and is divided into headaches induced by acute exposure, chronic exposure, acute withdrawal, chronic withdrawal, and unknown mechanism. "Headache associated with metabolic disorder" includes metabolic derangements such as hypoxia, hypercarbia, and hypoglycemia, which may represent secondary effects of drugs or toxins.

Most headaches associated with toxic-metabolic disorders are poorly understood, but may be secondary to vasodilation of cranial vessels, abrupt or substantial elevations in blood pressure (>130 mm Hg diastolic), or an increase in intracranial pressure.[16,86] Because the pathogenesis of vascular headache is currently being challenged on both clinical and epidemiologic grounds, it can no longer be presumed that agents that produce the common toxic vascular headache necessarily act directly on the vasculature to produce pain. It is at least equally plausible that the headache is secondary to a toxin-induced alteration in the relationship between neurotransmitters—in particular, serotonin—and their receptors.[181] Table 19–12 lists the most common chemicals, drugs, and toxins that, by either a primary or secondary effect on the pain-sensitive structures of the cranium and its contents, appear to produce headache as a prominent symptom.

Seizures

Seizures represent episodic pathologic electrical activity in the brain that causes an array of short-lived neurologic signs and symptoms.[45] Seizures are classified into generalized and partial, according to an international taxonomy. Generalized seizures are further subdivided into tonic-clonic (grand mal, major motor, or convulsive), tonic, clonic, absence (minor motor, nonconvulsive, or petit mal), atonic, and myoclonic. Partial seizures are classified as simple or complex (psychomotor or temporal lobe), either of which may evolve into the other or secondarily generalize to a grand mal seizure.[45]

Unless there is underlying focal neurologic disease or epilepsy, most seizures caused by drugs and toxins are of the generalized tonic-clonic variety. Depending on the degree of toxicity, the seizures may be isolated, recurrent, or continuous (ie, without an interictal period of regaining consciousness, which is a definition of status epilepticus).[55,179]

Status epilepticus represents a true emergency, because brain metabolism is markedly increased at the

TABLE 19–12. CHEMICALS, DRUGS, AND TOXINS ASSOCIATED WITH HEADACHE

Analgesics and nonprescription (OTC) preparations
Alpha-adrenergic agonists (eg, pseudoephedrine)
Butyl nitrite
Caffeine withdrawal (in many OTC medications)
Indomethacin
Isobutyl nitrite
Vitamin A

Prescription medications
Amyl nitrite
Anesthetics (halothane, ketamine, enflurane, *d*-tubocurare)
Antibiotics (nalidixic acid, tetracycline, minocycline, nitrofurantoin, metronidazole, sulfamethoxazole, griseofulvin)
Antihypertensives (hydralazine, nifedipine, prazosin, reserpine)
Corticosteroids and steroid withdrawal
Danocrine (Danazol)
Ergotamines
Hypoglycemic agents
Isoamyl nitrite
Isosorbide dinitrate
Nitroglycerin (oral, transdermal)
Oral contraceptives
Quinine (cinchonism)
Theophylline

Psychopharmacologic agents
Monoamine oxidase inhibitors when ingested with:
  Tyramine-containing foods (red wine, aged cheese, bananas)
  Medication (phenylephrine, ephedrine)
Phenothiazines

Alcohol and drugs of abuse
Amphetamines
Cocaine
Disulfiram (when mixed with ethanol)
Ethanol withdrawal ("hangover")
Ethylene glycol
Methanol
Phencyclidine

Food and drink
Aged cheese (cheddar, mozzarella, Gruyere, Stilton, brie, Camembert)
Caffeine
Chocolate
Ethanol
Fermented or pickled foods (herring, sour cream, yogurt, vinegar, marinated meats, smoked fish)
Fruits (bananas, plantain, avocado, figs, passion fruit, raisins, pineapple, oranges, citrus fruits)
Monosodium glutamate
Nitrite-containing meat (hot dogs, bologna, pepperoni, salami, pastrami, bacon, sausages, corned beef)
Sugar substitutes (diet drinks)
Sulfites (salad bars, shrimp, soft drinks, some wines)
Vegetables (onions, pods of broad beans [lima, navy], nuts)
Yeast products (yeast extract, fresh bread, doughnuts)

Botanicals
Coprinus spp (disulfiramlike reaction if ingested with ethanol) (see Chap. 75)
Herbal preparation (Lobelia, Galega) (see Chap. 76)
Nicotine
Various plants (see Chap. 77)

Heavy metals
Lead, especially tetraethyl lead
Metal fume fever (caused by welding or smelting of brass, cadmium, chromium, cobalt, copper, iron, magnesium, manganese, nickel, tin, zinc)

Pesticides
Carbamates
Organophosphates

Occupational and environmental
Carbon monoxide
Cyanide
Hydrocarbons
Hydrogen sulfide
Methemoglobin inducers
Toxic inhalants (and simple asphyxiants)

Toxic envenomation and marine animal ingestion
Arthropods (bite: *Rickettsia rickettsii*)
Lyme disease
Marine animals (Ciguatoxin [vertebrate fish], Scombroid [mahimahi flush], Gymnothorax poisoning [eels], Tetrodon [puffer fish]) (see Chap. 72)

same time oxygen supply is reduced by recurrent apneic periods.[55] In addition, status epilepticus produces dysfunctional autoregulation, shunting blood away from ischemic-sensitive areas.[55] Excessive muscle activity can cause hyperthermia and myoglobinuric acute renal failure.

The most common form of drug-induced seizures are alcohol related. These usually present as withdrawal seizures ("rum fits") and can occur in the withdrawal phase after as little as 6 hours of abstinence from drinking.[192] Sympathomimetics such as cocaine (especially crack) commonly cause drug-induced seizures by producing an abrupt decrement in the seizure threshold [72] and by its effect on sodium channels. Some anticonvulsant drugs prolong the inactivation of the sodium channels, thereby reducing the ability of neurons to fire at high frequencies. The activated channel remains open but it is blocked by an inactivation gate. Carbamazepine, phenytoin, and valproate act by this mechanism. Some anticonvulsant drugs reduce the metabolism of GABA, others act at the $GABA_A$ receptor, enhancing chloride influx in a response to GABA, thus increasing membrane polarization and decreasing seizures. Gabapentin acts presynaptically to promote GABA release; benzodiazepines and barbiturates act at $GABA_A$ receptors, enhancing chloride influx by opening the chloride channels. Some anticonvulsant drugs such as valproate and ethosuximide reduce the flow of calcium through T-type calcium channels, reducing current that may trigger generalized absence seizures (see Chaps. 40 and 65).

Table 19–13 lists the drugs and toxins that commonly cause seizures as a primary (direct reduction of seizure threshold) or secondary (eg, cellular hypoxia due to carbon monoxide) event. Virtually any drug can cause seizures as a terminal event.

Peripheral Nervous System

It is imperative that a rigorous history of exposure to infectious agents as well as toxins be obtained in any patient presenting with a peripheral neuropathy. Diseases of peripheral nerves can be categorized in at least two ways. The first classification is based on distribution of the neuropathy: focal or diffuse. Focal neuropathies include both unifocal (mononeuropathy) and multifocal neuropathy, usually attributable to injury, ischemia, infiltration, or autoimmune disease. In diffuse neuropathies (polyneuropathy), signs and symptoms tend to be symmetric and generalized rather than focal. Toxins almost invariably cause polyneuropathy and are only rarely implicated in focal neuropathy.

The second classification scheme is based on anatomic locations of the pathologic process within the peripheral nerve and is therefore divided into four subtypes: (1) axonopathies, characterized by early involvement of the axon; (2) myelinopathies, characterized by initial involvement of the myelin sheath or Schwann cell, causing demyelination of the peripheral nerve; and (3) neuronopathies, characterized by the presence of early pathologic changes in the nerve cell body. The neuronopathies can be further subdivided into (a) motor (anterior horn cell), (b) sensory (dorsal root ganglion), and (c) autonomic neuropathies. (4) Transmission neuropathies are characterized by toxins interfering with the release of neurotransmitters from the nerve or propagation of electrical impulses.[183] This classification serves as the basis for Table 19–14.

Axonopathies

Axonopathies are the most common form of drug- or toxin-induced peripheral neuropathy. They typically begin distally, where the axons are most vulnerable, and proceed proximally.[83] For unclear reasons, long and large-diameter fibers are preferentially affected. Clinically there is symmetric, diffuse, stocking–glove sensorimotor loss. Withdrawal of the toxic exposure is followed by a period of coasting, during which the clinical findings continue to worsen before improvement begins. Because axons regenerate at a rate of about 2 mm/day, recovery is prolonged and is often complicated by denervation atrophy.

Toxin-Induced Axonopathies. Acrylamide monomer is generally regarded as an experimental model for toxin-induced axonopathies.[194] The chemical is used in grouting and, through occupational exposure, produces weakness of the extremities distally, hyperhidrosis, and numbness of the hands and feet.[70] Features that are not typical of distal axonopathy include diffuse loss of reflexes (rather than initial loss of ankle jerks alone) and ataxia that is out of proportion to proprioceptive loss, perhaps attributable to cerebellar toxicity. Because the exposure is often transdermal, there may be an associated contact dermatitis of the hands. Removal from exposure in the early stages results in complete recovery. If exposure is prolonged, residual weakness, sensory abnormalities, and ataxia may persist.

Chronic alcoholism causes a distal, symmetric, sensorimotor polyneuropathy with a predilection for the lower extremities, producing dysesthesias, weakness, and decreased reflexes. The ataxia often seen in chronic alcoholics should always be treated as thiamine deficiency, although it is usually due to a combination of diminished proprioception and midline cerebellar degeneration. The pathologic process of alcoholic peripheral neuropathy shows features of axonopathy accompanied by demyelination. It is probably related to nutritional deficiency rather than to a direct effect of alcohol, although this has not been established with certainty.[209]

Allyl chloride, used in the manufacture of epoxy resin, produces a characteristic distal axonopathy with stocking–glove sensory deficit and loss of ankle jerks.[88]

Inorganic arsenic produces two different clinical findings, depending on the nature of the exposure. Massive but sublethal exposure, as in attempted suicide or homicide, causes vomiting, diarrhea, and shock. In individuals who survive, a distal, sensorimotor, symmetric axonopathy characterized by severe paresthesias develops within 1–3 weeks of ingestion.[123] Chronic exposure,

TABLE 19–13. DRUG- OR TOXIN-INDUCED SEIZURES

Analgesics and nonprescription (OTC) preparations

Antihistamines
Caffeine
Mefenamic acid
Phenylbutazone
Salicylates

Prescription medications

Antihistamines
Carbamazepine
Chlorambucil
Chloroquine
Clonidine
Digoxin
Ergotamines
Fenfluramine
Isoniazid
Lidocaine
Methotrexate
Phenytoin
Procarbazine
Quinine (cinchonism)
Sulfonylureas
Theophylline

Psychopharmacologic medications

Antiemetics
Cyclic antidepressants
Lithium
Methylphenidate
Monoamine oxidase inhibitors (esp w/food or drug reaction)
Neuroleptics
Opioids (propoxyphene, meperidine)
Pemoline
Sedative-hypnotics (W)
  Barbiturates
  Benzodiazepines
  Other nonbarbiturate sedative-hypnotics

Alcohols and drugs of abuse

Amphetamines
Cocaine
Disulfiram reaction
Ethanol (W)
Ethylene glycol
MDMA (methylenedioxymethamphetamine)
Methanol
Phencyclidine

Botanicals

Ackee fruit
Coprinus spp (disulfiramlike reaction w/alcohol)
Daphne
Herbal preparations (lobelia, jimson weed, gaiega, pokeweed, mandrake, passion flower, periwinkle, wormwood) (see Chaps. 76, 77)
Mistletoe
Nicotine
Rhododendron

Heavy metals

Arsenic
Copper
Lead
Manganese
Nickel

Household toxins

Benzalkonium chloride
Boric acid (chronic)
Camphor
Fluoride
Hexachlorophene
Phenol

Pesticides

Diquat
Organochlorines (lindane)
Organophosphates
Paraquat
Pyrethrins
Rodenticides (thallium, sodium monofluoroacetate, strychnine, zinc phosphide, arsenic)

Occupational and environmental toxins

Carbon disulfide
Carbon monoxide
Chlorphenoxy herbicides
Cyanide
Hydrocarbons
  Simple asphyxiants (methane, ethane, propane, butane, natural gas)
  High volatility (benzene, toluene, gasoline, naphtha, mineral spirits, light gas oil)
  Halogenated (carbon tetrachloride, trichloroethane)
Hydrogen sulfide
Methyl bromide
Toxic inhalants (simple asphyxiants producing hypoxia—helium, nitrogen, nitrous oxide)
Triazine

Toxic envenomation and marine animal ingestion

Marine animals (Gymnothorax, saxitoxin [shellfish])
Pit viper
Scorpion
Tick bite (*Rickettsia rickettsii*)

W = withdrawal seizure.
Phenytoin may also cause seizures with chronic toxicity.

TABLE 19–14. CLASSIFICATION OF SELECTED TOXIN- OR DRUG-INDUCED PERIPHERAL NEUROPATHIES

Neuronopathy	Axonopathy	Myelinopathy	Transmission Neuropathy
Acute toxic neuropathies			
Pyridoxine (S)	Hexacarbons (SMA)	Arsenic (SM)	Blackwidow spider
	Thallium (SM)	Diphtheria (SM)	Botulism
	Triorthocresyl phosphate (SM)		Ciguatoxin
	Vacor (MA)		Elapid and crotalid venoms
			Gymnothoratoxin
			Saxitoxin
			Scorpion venom
			Tetradotoxin
			Tick paralysis
Subacute/chronic toxic neuropathies			
None convincingly demonstrated	Acrylamide (SM)	Amiodarone (SM)	
	Allyl chloride (SM)	Buckthorn	
	Arsenic (SM)	Diphtheria (SM)	
	Buckthorn (M)	Gold (SM)	
	Carbon disulfide (SM)	Trichlorethylene (SM)	
	Colchicine (S)		
	Disulfiram (SM)		
	Dapsone (M)		
	2′-3′-dideoxycytidine (ddC), ddI		
	Ethanol (M)		
	Ethambutol (S)		
	Ethionamide (S)		
	Ethylene oxide (SM)		
	Glutethimide (S)		
	Gold (SM)		
	Hexacarbons (SM)		
	Hydralazine (SM)		
	Isoniazid (SM)		
	Methyl bromide (SM)		
	Mercury (M)		
	Metronidazole (SM)		
	Misonidazole (SM)		
	Nitrofurantoin (SM)		
	Nitrous oxide (S)		
	Nucleosides (S)		
	Organophosphorous esters (SM)		
	Polychlorinated biphenyls (SM)		
	Phenytoin (SM)		
	Platinum (S)		
	Podophylin (SM)		
	Taxol (S)		
	Thallium (SM)		
	Vincristine (SM)		

S = sensory; M = motor; A = autonomic

as occurs in copper and lead smelters and in miners, is characterized by the development of gastrointestinal upset and constitutional symptoms, followed by mucocutaneous changes, and finally by a predominantly sensory distal neuropathy with dysesthesias of the hands and feet (see Chap. 78).

Carbon disulfide (CS_2), used in the manufacture of rayon and cellophane, produces a distal axonopathy with numbness and loss of reflexes in the lower extremities, extending to the upper limbs with continued exposure.[211] Recovery is gradual and may be incomplete.

Ethylene oxide produces a distal sensorimotor axonopathy marked by numbness, weakness, and absent or diminished reflexes throughout.[59] Because ethylene oxide is used in gas sterilization and may be retained in dialysis tubing following the sterilization process, it is

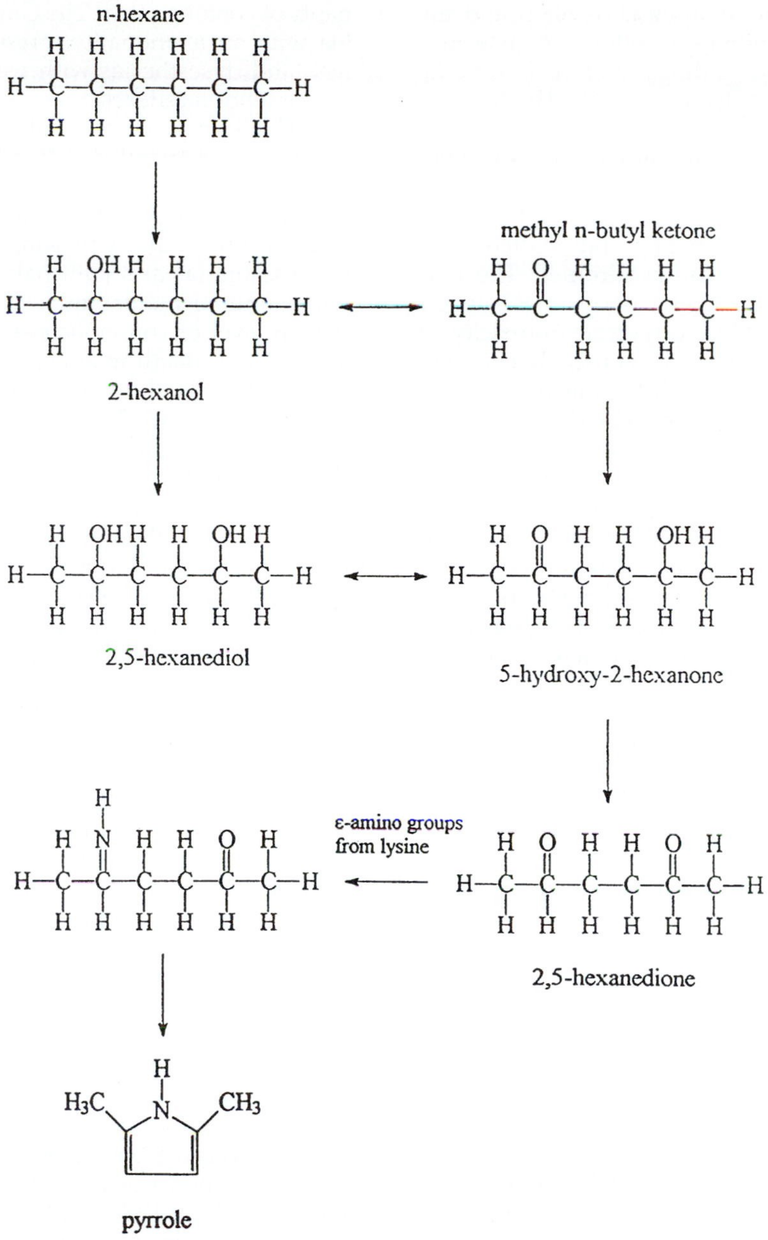

Figure 19–2. Metabolism of *N*-hexane. *(Reprinted, with permission, from Hoffman RS: Approach to the poisoned patient with peripheral neuropathy. In: Ford M, Delaney K, Ling L, Erickson T, eds: Clinical Toxicology. Philadelphia, Saunders, 1998.)*

considered a potential contributor to neuropathy in long-term dialysis patients.[218]

Hexacarbons that produce axonopathy include *n*-hexane and methyl *n*-butyl ketone, both of which are metabolized to 2,5-hexanedione (Fig. 19–2), which is thought to be the neuropathic agent, decreasing phosphorylation of neurofilaments and destroying the normal cytoskeletal matrix. The neurofilament proteins cause axonal swelling and thereby cause the axonopathy.[1,92] Hexane is a common solvent used in lacquers and glues. Analogous to arsenic neurotoxicity, there is a relatively acute form seen with large, short-term exposures (glue sniffing) and a more chronic form associated with industrial exposure. In both varieties, distal sensory symptoms predominate initially, with less reflex loss than is seen in other polyneuropathies.[195] As the neuropathy progresses, motor symptoms develop and migrate proximally. Glue sniffers, in whom toluene may also play a role, may have findings of cranial nerve involvement and autonomic disturbances, such as excessive sweating of the hands and feet. In some patients who have massive exposures due to chronic glue sniffing, a quadraparesis may develop over a period of months, presenting a clinical picture similar to that of acute inflammatory demyelinating polyradiculoneuropathy (AIDP or Guillain-Barré syndrome).[7] The phenomenon of coasting seen in other axonopathies is an extremely common feature of hexacarbon neurotoxicity. In mild industrial exposures, recovery is usually complete within a year. In glue sniffers with high-level exposure, residual neurologic deficits may persist indefinitely.

Most of the neurotoxicity of mercury involves the CNS rather than PNS. Mercury vapor and metallic mercury only rarely cause peripheral neuropathy.[5] Mercury vapor can cause an AIDP-like picture dominated by motor abnormalities.[219] Whether organic mercury causes peripheral neuropathy is unknown, although alkyl mercury can produce severe arm and leg dysesthesias (as in the Minamata Bay outbreak) through a CNS mechanism[122] (see Chap. 80).

Methyl bromide is used as a refrigerant, insecticide, fumigant, and fire extinguisher. Exposure may produce both CNS and PNS disease. In the PNS, the findings are typical of an axonopathy with stocking–glove numbness, distal weakness, and loss of ankle jerks.[105] Ataxia of the upper and lower limbs may be due to cerebellar toxicity, rather than a sensory ataxia secondary to peripheral neuropathy.

Organophosphorus esters are used in plastics manufacturing, petroleum additives, flame retardants, and insecticides. Most of these agents interfere with the action of acetylcholinesterase. Those with potent anticholinesterase properties may produce fatal cholinergic poisoning. Others, of which triorthocresyl phosphate (TOCP) is the prototype, interfere only slightly with the action of acetylcholinesterase and produce a delayed polyneuropathy of the distal axonopathy type. Earlier in the 20th century there were outbreaks of polyneuropathies in the United States due to misuse of TOCP as an adulterant in Jamaican ginger extract (Jake leg paralysis).[11] With a single large exposure, a transient mild cholinergic syndrome occurs, followed in approximately 1 week by distal paresthesias and later by weakness and reflex loss, which may migrate proximally. In contrast to the relatively gradual development of most other axonopathies, the neuropathy produced by TOCP becomes full-blown within 2 weeks of symptom onset. Although there is sensory involvement, the predominant symptom is marked weakness. As the peripheral neuropathy resolves, signs of previously masked CNS toxicity become apparent with the development of lower-extremity spasticity. Prognosis is related to severity of exposure, with some patients recovering fully and others remaining relatively disabled with a characteristic combination of upper and lower motor neuron findings.

Polychlorinated biphenyls (PCBs) have been reported to cause a neuropathy when ingested as contaminants of cooking oils.[43] The clinical findings are compatible with an axonopathy, presenting with distal numbness and dysesthesias with weakness and decreased or absent tendon reflexes.

Thallium produces acute, subacute, and chronic axonopathies, depending primarily on the quantity of the initial toxic exposure and the time elapsed since the exposure (see Chap. 82). The acute variety begins within hours to a few days of poisoning. This is followed by distal dysesthesias and joint pain in the lower extremities, with minimal motor and reflex abnormalities. Depression in level of consciousness reflects concomitant CNS toxicity, and death may occur within weeks due to cardiorespiratory failure[17] (see Chap. 82). The subacute form develops a few weeks after exposure and, in contrast to acute toxicity, is characteristically accompanied by alopecia.[42] Severe, sometimes disabling dysesthesias dominate the clinical presentation, accompanied by mild weakness and preserved, though diminished, reflexes. Complete recovery can be expected. Chronic thallium toxicity is not well described, but it appears that tremor, chorea, and ataxia overshadow the signs and symptoms of the peripheral axonopathy. Most thallium toxicity that was seen in the United States was related to unintentional, suicidal, or homicidal ingestion, rather than occupational exposure to a thallium-containing rodenticide or insecticide.

Ingestion of rodenticides containing Vacor (*N*-3-pyridylmethyl-*N*-*p*-nitrophenyl urea; PNU) produces an acute axonopathy, marked by weakness and autonomic dysfunction, complicated by development of diabetes, often within hours of exposure[125] (see Chap. 89).

Colchicine, when used as chronic prophylaxis against recurrent gouty arthritis, may cause a mild sensory distal axonopathy. However, an accompanying necrotizing myopathy with proximal muscle weakness and creatine kinase elevations usually dominates the clinical presentation, especially when the medication is given in patients with chronic renal failure.[176]

Dapsone has been used in the treatment of pneumocystis pneumonia (see Chap. 107), brown recluse spider bites (see Chap. 100), and leprosy and for certain dermatologic conditions (see Chap. 28). Prolonged treatment or massive ingestion produces a symmetric, distal, pure motor axonopathy followed by atrophy.[87] Use of the drug in pneumocystis and leprosy has not resulted in neuropathy.

Disulfiram, used in the treatment of alcoholism, may produce a sensorimotor distal axonopathy characterized by plantar dysesthesias, gait unsteadiness, weakness, and loss of ankle jerks. Return to baseline usually follows discontinuation of the drug.[29]

Isoniazid (see Chap. 43), one of the most widely used antituberculous medications, commonly produces a distal sensorimotor axonopathy through interference with pyridoxine and other vitamins of the B group.[21] For this reason, any patient taking isoniazid should also receive 50 mg of pyridoxine daily, as prophylaxis against isoniazid neuropathy. (See Chap. 36 and Antidotes in Depth: Pyridoxine.)

Ethambutol, another antituberculous medication,

appears to cause a mild sensory distal axonopathy characterized by numbness of the fingers and toes.[160] The optic neuropathy produced by ethambutol at doses exceeding 20 mg/kg/day is generally of greater concern, due to the variable recovery of visual acuity following drug withdrawal.[171]

Ethionamide, which is much less widely used in treatment of tuberculosis than isoniazid or ethambutol, appears to produce a peripheral neuropathy similar to that caused by ethambutol, but has not been reported to produce optic neuropathy.[121]

Glutethimide is a sedative-hypnotic that causes a distal axonopathy in chronic, high-dose users, characterized by impairment of all sensory modalities, calf tenderness, mild ataxia, and loss of ankle jerks.[164]

Hydralazine, used to reduce afterload in the management of severe congestive heart failure, rarely produces a distal, predominantly sensory axonopathy. There is some evidence that this neuropathy is related to pyridoxine deficiency.[174]

Metronidazole, commonly used in the treatment of anaerobic and protozoal infections, causes a predominantly sensory axonopathy marked by distal dysesthesias and sensory ataxia due to large-fiber proprioceptive involvement. Most cases have followed prolonged exposure.[30]

Misonidazole, which is used to sensitize cancer cells in radiotherapy, causes a distal, predominantly sensory axonopathy, characterized by painful dysesthesias of the lower extremities.[142]

Nitrofurantoin is primarily used in the treatment of urinary tract infections. Peripheral neuropathy of the axonal type occurs within weeks to months of instituting the drug, beginning with distal numbness, followed by an unusually rapid development of severe motor and sensory symptoms.[54] Patients with diabetes or renal disease may be especially prone to develop nitrofurantoin neuropathy, although it has also been reported in patients without these underlying diseases.[221]

Nitrous oxide, widely used in emergency departments and dental offices as an analgesic, may produce a myeloneuropathy if abused. Moderate abuse produces a symmetric sensory axonopathy, sometimes accompanied by ataxia of the upper and lower extremities, presumably due to proprioceptive loss. Prolonged, high-level exposure causes, in addition to a severe peripheral neuropathy, lower-extremity spasticity, reflecting CNS involvement in the form of a myelopathy.[90] There is some evidence that this toxicity may be mediated through interference with vitamin B_{12} metabolism, thus accounting for the similarity between full-blown nitrous oxide toxicity and combined system disease.[9]

Nucleoside neuropathy is caused by a number of agents used to treat AIDS, particularly dideoxyinosine (ddI). The distal axonopathy is characterized by severe plantar dysesthesias that extend to the upper extremities if the drug is continued. There appears to be minimal motor involvement[143] (see Chap. 107).

Phenytoin may rarely cause a mild peripheral neuropathy, characterized by stocking–glove dysesthesias and mild weakness that responds to drug withdrawal.[129]

Cisplatin (*cis*-diamine-dichlorplatinum II), a commonly used chemotherapeutic agent, produces a predominantly large-fiber sensory axonopathy, with marked diminution of proprioception and vibration sense, accompanied by minimal weakness with relative preservation of pain and temperature sense.[177]

Pyridoxine produces both acute and chronic forms of peripheral neuropathy by two different mechanisms. The acute form is a neuronopathy (discussed below). The chronic form is associated with high doses of pyridoxine and begins with acral numbness. This is followed by predominantly large-fiber proprioceptive involvement, producing an impairment of manual dexterity and a gait disturbance. Motor fibers appear to be spared. Distal tendon reflexes are diminished or absent because the afferent loop of the reflex arc is affected. In contrast to the acute pyridoxine-induced neuropathy, recovery is usually satisfactory following discontinuation of the drug[184] (see Chap. 36 and Antidotes in Depth: Pyridoxine).

Organic gold, used in the treatment of rheumatoid arthritis, rarely causes a peripheral neuropathy with features of both axonopathy and myelinopathy. The clinical picture is one of distal numbness and, later, weakness in the lower extremities accompanied by loss of ankle jerks.[108]

Taxol is used in the treatment of solid tumors. Intravenous injection is followed by acral dysesthesias, loss of all sensory modalities, absent tendon reflexes, proximal spread, and preserved motor function. The neuropathy, which has pathologic features of both axonopathy and myelinopathy, worsens and then resolves in a few weeks.[127]

Vincristine is also used as chemotherapy for a variety of malignancies. The axonopathy that this agent produces is unusual in that it begins with paresthesias in the hands prior to the feet, followed by weakness, which is initially more marked in the upper extremities. In general, motor abnormalities dominate the clinical picture and tend to resolve slowly following discontinuation of the drug.[40]

Podophyllin resin, used in the treatment of condylomata acuminata, appears to produce a severe distal axonopathy as well as CNS dysfunction. Neurotoxicity from a lipid-soluble mitotic spindle binder seems plausible, but it is rare and supported primarily by anecdotal case reports.[58]

A number of other drugs or toxins have been associated with peripheral neurotoxicity but have not convincingly been demonstrated to cause peripheral neuropathy. These include lithium, amitriptyline, phenobarbital, penicillamine, cytosine arabinoside, and styrene.[183]

Myelinopathies

Myelinopathies are characterized by diffuse demyelination that usually spares the axon. There is generalized weakness with mild sensory loss, presumably because the heavily myelinated, large motor axons are more severely affected than the small-diameter myelinated and unmyelinated sensory fibers. For this reason, the large sensory fibers that mediate proprioception, vibration, and touch are impaired, while pain, temperature, and autonomic function are relatively preserved. Because both the afferent and efferent limbs of the reflex arc are involved, the reflexes are symmetrically absent. Usually, areflexia in the lower extremities precedes reflex loss in the upper extremities. Because remyelination is a relatively rapid process compared to axonal regeneration, recovery may be dramatic once the toxin is removed.

Diphtheria neuropathy results from an exotoxin produced by *Corynebacterium diphtheriae*, usually following infection of the throat or skin. Diphtheria toxin inhibits the ability of Schwann cells to synthesize myelin, producing demyelination of the dorsal and ventral roots, with involvement of the dorsal root ganglion itself.[60] The disease produces two distinct forms of peripheral neurotoxicity. There is an early phase, characterized by weakness adjacent to the site of infection, due to local effects of the toxin. The pharyngeal variant of this syndrome follows throat infections. It is a cranial neuropathy characterized by palatal weakness, nasal speech, and palatal sensory loss, with a predominance of motor over sensory abnormalities. Blurred vision may develop as a consequence of paralysis of ocular accommodation, although the pupillary light reflexes are spared. In cutaneous diphtheria, weakness and numbness also occur contiguous to the site of infection. Both pharyngeal and cutaneous variants of the early phase have an excellent prognosis. The late manifestations include a generalized demyelinating neuropathy of rapid onset occurring about 5–8 weeks after infection, with distal sensorimotor findings and hyporeflexia. Recovery is usually complete in cases without myocardial involvement.[141]

Fruit from the buckthorn shrub, which is indigenous to the southwest United States, produces a subacute motor polyneuropathy that may cause death. One to 3 weeks following ingestion, survivors develop a diffuse segmental demyelination causing a rapidly ascending motor neuropathy, with minimal sensory findings.[35]

Lead polyneuropathy is now rare in the United States. Although it is difficult to classify, experimental models argue most strongly for a direct toxic effect on Schwann cells, leading to a myelinopathy.[196] Plumbism is a predominantly motor neuropathy with minimal sensory complaints. The previously reported focal motor variants of lead poisoning (wrist-drop, shoulder girdle weakness, hand intrinsic-muscle atrophy, peroneal muscle weakness, and laryngeal paralysis) have become rare.[24] Current presentations are more often characterized by gastrointestinal complaints and constitutional symptoms associated with generalized distal weakness and atrophy, reflex loss, mild sensory abnormalities, and fasciculations[33] (see Chap. 79).

Trichlorethylene is used in the rubber and dry cleaning industries and was once used as a general anesthetic. Industrial exposure produces a characteristic syndrome confined to the cranial nerves, especially the trigeminal nerve, producing loss of sensation on the face and difficulty chewing due to motor involvement. Cranial nerves III and VII are also sometimes involved. Trichlorethylene exposure is often associated with herpes simplex infection, suggesting that exposure reactivates the latent virus.[41] Although the neuropathology for this isolated neuropathy is unclear, the weight of evidence favors a myelinopathy.[56]

Amiodarone is a ventricular antidysrhythmic that produces a distal polyneuropathy, with weakness of the lower extremities followed by dysesthesias.[168] Both postural and kinetic tremor have been reported, accompanied by ataxia. Although there are findings of both axonopathy and demyelination, nerve biopsies support histopathologic findings of a predominantly symmetric myelinopathy.

Neuronopathies

Toxic neuronopathies directly affect the neuron itself, especially the dorsal root ganglion.[112] The cell bodies for the trigeminal nerve, the sensory nerve for the face, have much in common with the dorsal root ganglion cells and often have similar vulnerabilities to neurotoxins. Because of this, the clinical findings are segmental; that is, they follow the course of a nerve root, either a dermatome or myotome. Abnormalities may be entirely sensory (if only the dorsal root ganglion is affected, as in herpes zoster), entirely motor (as in poliomyelitis, where only the anterior horn cell is affected), or mixed, with autonomic features. The neuronopathies are the least common and most poorly understood of the three types of peripheral neuropathy.

Acute pyridoxine neuronopathy is caused by massive doses of pyridoxine, which disrupts the cellular metabolism of the dorsal root ganglion. Presumably the fenestrated blood vessels at this site account for the selective vulnerability. The clinical findings demonstrate rapid to subacute development of widespread sensory loss with appendicular ataxia and autonomic instability. Because the pathologic process involves only the dorsal root ganglion, motor function is unimpaired. In contrast to the chronic form, the prognosis in the few patients studied is poor, with persistent, incapacitating sensory ataxia[6] (see Chap. 36 and Antidotes in Depth: Pyridoxine).

Neuromuscular Junction Toxicity (Transmission Neuropathy)

Toxins Affecting the Neuromuscular Junction. Botulism is the most toxic substance known. The exotoxin of *Clostridium botulinum* binds to the presynaptic portion of the neuromuscular junction, preventing release of acetylcholine. The neurotoxic signs and symptoms are anticholinergic, with a predilection for involvement of the cranial neuromuscular junctions. Specific findings include abnormalities of extraocular movement, pupillary dilation, ptosis, dysphagia, dysphonia, diplopia, descending motor paralysis, and respiratory failure, with preservation of mental status and sensation. Reflexes are also usually preserved until the end stage of the illness. Because the binding is irreversible, clinical recovery occurs slowly and only with the formation of new neuromuscular junctions. The presentation and management are discussed in greater detail in Chapter 73.

Tetanus is a neurotoxin that involves the neuromuscular junction, sympathetic pathways, spinal cord, and brain. Tetanospasmin, the clinically important exotoxin of *Clostridium tetani*, travels from the point of entry, largely via the axon, to the central nervous system. There it blocks release of inhibitory neurotransmitters, producing disinhibited, widespread muscular spasm and autonomic instability. Tetanospasmin's effect on the neuromuscular junction, which is similar to that of botulism, is usually overshadowed by its central effects. Trismus is the most common presenting symptom, followed by generalized muscle spasm, which can be triggered by uninhibited afferent stimuli such as a noise, bright light, or touch. These spasms are produced by simultaneous and sustained contraction of agonist/antagonist muscles and may lead to laryngospasm, respiratory paralysis, and death. There are often accompanying fluctuations in vital signs and dysrhythmias, but the mental status is generally clear and unaltered.[214]

Among indigenous North American snakes, envenomation from the coral snake and Mojave rattlesnake can cause postsynaptic neuromuscular blockade. This produces ptosis (often the first sign of systemic toxicity), dysarthria, dysphagia, dysesthesias, and generalized weakness, which may culminate in death from respiratory failure.[109] Other Elapidae toxins may act presynaptically to prevent acetylcholine release or postsynaptically to produce competitive or noncompetitive acetylcholine receptor blockade. The majority of snakebites in the United States, however, are due to pit vipers and in these bites the neurotoxic symptoms are overshadowed by hematologic effects and local soft tissue reaction (see Chap. 99).

Black widow spider venom (see Chap. 100) acts at the neuromuscular junction, causing release of acetylcholine from presynaptic vesicles.[81] This produces severe skeletal muscle cramping, frequently involving the chest or abdomen, depending on the site of envenomation. Fatalities are uncommon and tend to occur primarily in small children.

Tick paralysis is thought to be due to presynaptic block of acetylcholine release at the neuromuscular junction.[158] The characteristic picture is one of an ascending paralysis, with reflex loss and intact sensation, closely resembling Guillain-Barré syndrome (AIDP). If the tick is not discovered and removed, death may occur secondary to paralysis of respiratory muscles. An unexplained ataxic variant of this syndrome has been reported that appears to implicate a separate central cerebellar effect of the toxin elaborated by the tick[115] (see Chap. 100).

A number of marine neurotoxins interfere with neuromuscular transmission. These include ciguatoxin, gymnothoratoxin, tetrodotoxin, and saxitoxin. Initial symptoms of dysesthesias of the mouth, tongue, and perioral area are common to all four toxins, indicating that poisoning of the neuromuscular junction is neither the sole, nor, in many instances, the dominant effect of these toxins. Interference with neuromuscular transmission does, however, account for the mortality, which is attributable to respiratory paralysis. Ciguatoxin, the most commonly reported vertebrate fish-borne toxin, and gymnothoratoxin, found in certain eels, produce a similar clinical picture, dominated by sensory complaints. Ciguatoxin causes a unique, unexplained symptom of cutaneous temperature inversion (ie, warm feels cold and cold feels warm). Mortality is rare in both ciguatoxin and gymnothorax poisoning. In contrast, tetrodon poisoning, which is secondary to ingestion of puffer-type fish, carries a high mortality. It is characterized by oral dysesthesias, followed by a rapidly ascending paralysis, which may culminate in respiratory failure. Saxitoxin is transmitted by shellfish, usually during the summer months when a red tide is present. Following onset of the characteristic dysesthesias described above, the patient may manifest several movement disorders, including both kinetic and postural tremor, ataxia, lower cranial neuromuscular dysfunction, and cardiorespiratory symptoms, which may be fatal. Marine toxins are discussed in greater detail in Chapters 72 and 101.

Organophosphates and carbamates, which are frequently used as insecticides, produce cholinergic toxicity by binding to acetylcholinesterase, resulting in muscarinic (parasympathetic), nicotinic (striated muscle and autonomic ganglia), and CNS effects, producing a diffuse and often fatal neurotoxicity (see Chap. 87).

TABLE 19–15. DRUGS AND TOXINS THAT ACT AT THE NEUROMUSCULAR JUNCTION (TRANSMISSION NEUROPATHY)

Presynaptically acting drugs and toxins
ACTH, Corticosteroids
Azathioprine
Botulinum toxins
Crotalidae venin
Elapidae beta neurotoxins
Lactrodectus mactans venin
Magnesium
Tick paralysis
Verapamil
Postsynaptically acting drugs and toxins
d-Penicillamine
Neuromuscular blockers
Nicotine alkaloids
Organophosphates, carbamates
Phenothiazines
Trimethaphan
Pre- and postsynaptically acting drugs
Antibiotics
Aminoglycosides
Clindamycin
Polymyxins
Beta-adrenergic antagonists
Chloroquine
Lithium
Phenytoin
Procainamide
Quinidine

Drugs Affecting the Neuromuscular Junction. Drugs that act at the neuromuscular junction are listed in Table 19–15, according to whether they are thought to act presynaptically, postsynaptically, or simultaneously at both sites.

Myopathies

Diffuse Toxic Myopathies. Myopathies can be diffuse or focal. Diffuse myopathies present clinically with weakness, which must be distinguished from neuropathic weakness since further evaluation, management, and prognosis are quite different. Myopathic weakness typically is proximal, lacks sensory findings, and preserves deep tendon reflexes unless the myopathy is very far advanced.

Drugs and toxins may cause injury to skeletal muscle through a variety of mechanisms. The drugs and mechanisms are listed in Table 19–16 and are discussed in detail elsewhere.[136]

Necrotizing myopathy is due to direct toxic action of a drug on muscle. The characteristic presentation is proximal weakness and myalgia, accompanied by creatine kinase elevations and, in severe cases, myoglobinuria. Toxins associated with a necrotizing myopathy include aminocaproic acid, clofibrate, lovastatin, heroin, phencyclidine, syrup of ipecac, vincristine, colchicine, and zidovidine.[10]

Chloroquine and amiodarone cause a relatively mild, painless, proximal "autophagic" myopathy with normal or slightly elevated creatine kinase. Both are associated with neuropathy, which usually dominates clinically, especially in the case of amiodarone-associated demyelination.[10]

Prolonged use of corticosteroids will produce a painless proximal myopathy. In asthmatics, systemic steroids produce both skeletal muscle and diaphragmatic weakness,[28] whereas inhaled steroids may produce a localized myopathy of laryngeal muscles.[217]

Alcohol is among the most common causes of toxic myopathy. The acute form, which presents as widespread myalgia and proximal weakness with creatine kinase elevations, is less common than chronic alcoholic myopathy and is associated with binge drinking. In both animal models and humans there is a correlation between blood ethanol levels and creatine kinase elevations.[116] The chronic form of alcoholic myopathy is painless and proximal, with a predilection for the pelvic and shoulder girdles. It is accompanied by atrophy, normal creatine kinase levels, and, frequently, an alcoholic neuropathy. The pathology is not completely understood.

Hypokalemia may produce a myopathy ranging from mild to severe. When weakness is marked, there may be associated creatine kinase elevations and loss of reflexes. Causes include gastrointestinal losses due to chronic vomiting or diarrhea, often related to emetic or cathartic abuse. Patients with anorexia nervosa or bulimia may develop hypokalemic myopathy secondary to self-induced vomiting. Urinary losses occur with the use of diuretics and in individuals consuming large amounts of licorice, which contains glycyrrhizic acid, an aldosterone-like substance.[205] Glycyrrhizic acid may also be found in traditional Chinese herbal medicines, snuff, and chewing tobacco.

TABLE 19–16. MYOPATHIES CAUSED BY DRUGS AND TOXINS

Diffuse toxic myopathies
Necrotizing myopathy
Aminocaproic acid
Clofibrate
Heroin
Ipecac
Lovastatin and other HMG-CoA reductase inhibitors
Phencyclidine
Vincristine
Zidovidine
Autophagic myopathy
Amiodarone
Chloroquine
Corticosteroids
Ethanol
Hypokalemia caused by
Barium salts
Cathartic abuse
Emetic abuse
Glycyrrhizic acid
Inflammatory myopathy (myositis)
D-penicillamine
Eosinophilia-myalgia syndrome (L-tryptophan)
Other drugs
Beta-adrenergic antagonists
Cimetidine
Cyclosporine
Doxylamine
Ethchlorvynol
Penicillin
Propylthiouracil
Rifampin
Sulfonamides
Envenomation (species indigenous to North America)
Snakes
Copperhead
Rattlesnake
Water moccasin
Spiders
Brown recluse spider
Insects
Hornets
Wasps
Microbial myotoxins
Clostridium perfringens
Focal toxic myopathies
Needle myopathy
Opioids

A variety of agents may produce an inflammatory myopathy or myositis. These include D-penicillamine, which may produce a polymyositis-like picture in some patients.[39]

Other drugs that have rarely been associated with

myopathy include beta-adrenergic antagonists, rifampin, sulfonamides, penicillin, propylthiouracil, cimetidine, ethchlorvynol, and cyclosporin.

Eosinophilia-myalgia syndrome described in 1990 has been associated with ingestion of a particular preparation of the amino acid L-tryptophan. The clinical picture is that of sudden onset of severe myalgia, cutaneous involvement, and peripheral eosinophilia. An ascending polyneuropathy has also been reported in some patients. Pathologically, this is an eosinophilic myositis and fasciitis.[89]

Envenomation with snakes, spiders, and wasps may produce serious myotoxicity. Among snakes indigenous to North America, pit viper venom (*Crotalidae sp,* including the rattlesnake, copperhead, and water moccasin) produces more severe myonecrosis and rhabdomyolysis than the more neurotoxic coral snake venom (*Elapidae sp*). This is discussed in further detail in Chapter 99. Among arthropods, brown recluse spider envenomation has been associated with myonecrosis and rhabdomyolysis,[64] as have stings by wasps and hornets.[190]

Of the microbial myotoxins, those elaborated by *Clostridium perfringens* are among the best characterized. At least one of these toxins causes focal myonecrosis and gas gangrene, which is rapidly progressive and frequently fatal.

Focal Myopathies. Focal myopathies are due to the combined effects of needle insertion and the local effects of the injected drug. Although many drugs have been associated with focal myopathy, opioids are among the most important, especially in patients with sickle cell disease. Because many of these patients lack venous access, they are given repeated intramuscular injections of opioids for painful crises, causing abscess formation, fibrosis, and muscle atrophy.

Acknowledgment

Richard B. Lipton, MD contributed to this chapter in a previous edition.

References

1. Abou-Donia MB: Solvents. In: Abou-Donia MB, ed: Neurotoxicology. Boca Raton, CRC Press, 1992, pp. 395–421.
2. Adams RD, Foley JM: The neurological disorder associated with liver disease. Res Publ Assoc Res Nerv Ment Dis 1953;32:198.
3. Adams RD, Shahani BT, Young RR: A severe pansensory familial neuropathy. Trans Am Neurol Assoc 1972;98: 67–69.
4. Albanese A, Rossi P, Altavista MC: Can trazodone induce parkinsonism? Clin Neuropharmacol 1988;11:180–182.
5. Albers JW, Cavender GD, Levine SP, et al: Asymptomatic sensorimotor polyneuropathy in workers exposed to elemental mercury. Neurology 1982;32:1168–1174.
6. Albin RL, Albers JW, Greenberg HS, et al: Acute sensory neuropathy-neuronopathy from pyridoxine overdose. Neurology 1987;37:1729–1732.
7. Altenkirch HJ, Mager J, Stoltenburg G, et al: Toxic polyneuropathies after sniffing a glue thinner. J Neurol 1977;214:137–152.
8. Alvarez-Gómez MJ, Vaamonde J, Narbona J, et al: Parkinsonian syndrome in childhood after sodium valproate administration. Clin Neuropharmacol 1993;16:451–455.
9. Amess JA, Burman JF, Rees GM, et al: Megaloblastic haematopoiesis in patients receiving nitrous oxide. Lancet 1978;1:339–342.
10. Argov Z, Mastaglia FL: Drug-induced neuromuscular disorders in man. In: Walton JN, ed: Disorders of Voluntary Muscle, 5th ed. Edinburgh, Churchill Livingstone, 1988, p. 981.
11. Aring CD: The systemic nervous affinity of triorthocresyl phosphate (Jamaican ginger palsy). Brain 1942;65:34.
12. Avorn J, Bohn RL, Mogun H, et al: Neuroleptic drug exposure and treatment of parkinsonism in the elderly: A case-control study. Am J Med 1995;99:48–54.
13. Avorn J, Gurwitz JH, Bohn RL, et al: Increased incidence of levodopa therapy following metoclopramide use. JAMA 1995;274:1780–1782.
14. Ayd FJ: Side effects of depot fluphenazines. Compr Psychiatry 1974;15:277–284.
15. Ayd FJ: A survey of drug-induced extrapyramidal reactions. JAMA 1961;175:1054–1060.
16. Badran RH, Weir RJ, McGuiness JB: Hypertension and headache. Scot Med J 1970;15:48–51.
17. Bank WJ, Pleasure DE, Suzuki K, et al: Thallium poisoning. Arch Neurol 1972;26:456–464.
18. Barnes TRE, McPhillips MA: Antipsychotic-induced extrapyramidal symptoms. Role of anticholinergic drugs in treatment. CNS Drugs 1996;6:315–330.
19. Bateman DN, Darling WM, Boys R, et al: Extrapyramidal reactions to metoclopramide and prochlorperazine. Q J Med 1989;71:307–311.
20. Bateman DN, Rawlins MD, Simpson JM: Extrapyramidal reactions with metoclopramide. Br Med J 1985;291: 930–932.
21. Blakemore WF: Isoniazid. In: Spencer PS, Schaumburg HH, eds: Experimental and Clinical Neurotoxicology. Baltimore, Williams & Wilkins, 1980, p. 476.
22. Benvenuti F, Baroni A, Bandinelli S, at al: Flunarizine-induced parkinsonism in the elderly. J Clin Pharmacol 1988;28:600–608.
23. Binder RL, Kazamatsuri H, Nishimura T, et al: Tardive dyskinesia and neuroleptic-induced parkinsonism in Japan. Am J Psychiatry 1987;144:1494–1496.
24. Boothby JA, DeJesus PV, Rowland LP: Reversible forms of motor neuron disease. Arch Neurol 1974;31:18–23.
25. Borison RL: Amantadine in the management of extrapyramidal side effects. Clin Neuropharmacol 1983;6(suppl 1):57–63.
26. Bouchard RH, Pourcher E, Vincent P: Fluoxetine and extrapyramidal side effects. Am J Psychiatry 1989;146: 1352–1353. Letter.
27. Bowman WC: Non-relaxant properties of neuromuscular blocking drugs. Br J Anaesth 1982;54:147–160.
28. Bowyer SL, La Monthe MP, Hollister JR: Steroid myopathy: Incidence and detection in a population with asthma. J Allergy Clin Immunol 1985;76:234–242.

29. Bradley WG, Hewer RL: Peripheral neuropathy due to disulfiram. Br Med J 1966;2:449–450.
30. Bradley WG, Karlsson IJ, Rasso ICG: Metronidazole neuropathy. Br Med J 1977;2:610–611.
31. Braude WM, Barnes TR, Gore SM: Clinical characteristics of akathisia: A systematic investigation of acute psychiatric inpatient admissions. Br J Psychiatry 1983;143: 139–150.
32. Browning RG, Olson DW, Steuven HA, Mateer JR: 50% dextrose: Antidote or toxin? Ann Emerg Med 1990;19: 683–687.
33. Buchthal F, Behse F: Electrophysiological studies and nerve biopsy in men exposed to lead. Br J Ind Med 1979;36:135–147.
34. Burke RE, Fahn S, Jankovic J, et al: Tardive dystonia: Late-onset and persistent dystonia caused by antipsychotic drugs. Neurology 1982;32:1335–1346.
35. Calderon-Gonzalez R, Rizzi-Hernandez H: Buckthorn polyneuropathy. N Engl J Med 1967;277:69–71.
36. Caley CF, Friedman JH: Does fluoxetine exacerbate Parkinson's disease? J Clin Psychiatry 1992;53:278–282.
37. Capella D, Laporte JR, Castel JM, et al: Parkinsonism, tremor, and depression-induced by cinnarizine and flunarizine. Br Med J 1988;297;722–723. Letter.
38. Caroff SN: The neuroleptic malignant syndrome. J Clin Psychiatry 1980;41:79–83.
39. Carroll GJ, Will RK, Peter JB, et al: Penicillamine induced polymyositis and dermatomyositis. J Rheumatol 1987;14: 995–1001.
40. Casey EB, Jellife AM, LeQuesne PM, et al: Vincristine neuropathy: Clinical and electrophysiological observations. Brain 1973;96:69–86.
41. Cavanagh JB, Buxton PH: Trichlorethylene cranial neuropathy: Is it really a toxic neuropathy or does it activate latent herpes virus? J Neurol Neurosurg Psychiatry 1989;52:297–303.
42. Cavanagh JB, Fuller NH, Johnson HR, et al: The effects of thallium salts, with particular reference to the nervous system changes. Q J Med 1974;43:293–319.
43. Chia L, Chu F: Neurological studies on polychlorinated biphenyl (PCB)-poisoned patients. Am J Ind Med 1984;5: 117–126.
44. Chouza C, Scarameli A, Caamaño JL, et al: Parkinsonism, tardive dyskinesia, akathisia, and depression-induced by flunarizine. Lancet 1986;1:1300–1304.
45. Commission on Classification and Terminology of the International League Against Epilepsy: Proposal for the revised clinical and electroencephalographic classification of epileptic seizures. Epilepsia 1981;22:489.
46. Cook DG, Fahn S, Brait KA: Chronic manganese intoxication. Arch Neurol 1974;30:59–64.
47. Daric C, Dollfus S, Mihout B, et al: Fluoxetine et symptomes extrapyramidaux. A propos de deux observations. Encephale 1993;19:61–62.
48. Davis GC, Williams AC, Markey SP, et al: Chronic parkinsonism secondary to intravenous injection of meperidine analogues. Psychiatry Res 1979;1:249–254.
49. De Michele G, Filla A, Coppola N, et al: Extrapyramidal side-effects of flunarizine. Acta Neurol (Napoli) 1987;9:230–233.
50. Dick RS, Barold SS: Diltiazem-induced parkinsonism. Am J Med 1989;87:95–96. Letter.
51. Di Rosa AE, Morgante L, Meduri M, et al: Parkinson-like side effects during prolonged treatment with flunarizine. Funct Neurol 1987;2:47–50.
52. Durant NN, Marshall IG, Savage DS, et al: The neuromuscular and autonomic blocking activities of pancuronium, Org NC 45 and other pancuronium analogues. J Pharm Pharmacol 1979;31:831–836.
53. Edelman RR, Warach S: Magnetic resonance imaging (first of two parts). N Engl J Med 1993;328:708–716.
54. Ellis FG: Acute polyneuritis after nitrofurantoin therapy. Lancet 1962;2:1136–1138.
55. Engel J Jr, Troupin AS, Crandall PH, et al: Recent developments in the diagnosis and therapy of epilepsy. Ann Intern Med 1982;97:584–598.
56. Feldman RG, White RF, Currie JN, et al: Long-term follow-up after single toxic exposure to trichlorethylene. Am J Ind Med 1985;8:119–126.
57. Fernández-Pardal M, Fernández-Pardal J, Micheli F: Aggravation of Parkinson's disease by cinnarizine. J Neurol Neurosurg Psychiatry 1988;51:158–159. Letter.
58. Filley CM, Graff-Richard NR, Lacy JR, et al: Neurologic manifestations of podophyllin toxicity. Neurology 1982; 32:308–311.
59. Finelli PF, Morgan TF, Yaar I, et al: Ethylene oxide induced polyneuropathy. A clinical and electrophysiologic study. Arch Neurol 1983;40:419–421.
60. Fisher CM, Adams RD: Diphtheritic polyneuritis: A pathological study. J Neuropathol Exp Neurol 1956;15: 243–268.
61. Folstein MF, Folstein SE, McHugh PR: The "Mini-Mental State": A practical method for grading the cognitive state of patients for the clinician. J Psychiatry Res 1975;12: 189–198.
62. Franchignoni FP, Tesio L: Sindrome parkinsoniana indotta da veralipride. Minerva Ginecol 1995;47:277–279.
63. Froomes PR, Stewart MR: A reversible parkinsonian syndrome and hepatotoxicity following addition of carbamazepine to sodium valproate. Aust NZ J Med 1994;24: 413–414.
64. Gabow PA, Kaehny WD, Kelleher SP: The spectrum of rhabdomyolysis. Medicine 1982;61:141–152.
65. Gajkowski K, Werkowicz-Pelczyk D, Masiak I, et al. Neurologic symptoms in lithium poisoning. Neurol Neurochir Pol 1987;21:412–414.
66. Ganzini L, Casey DE, Hoffman WF, et al: The prevalence of metoclopramide-induced tardive dyskinesia and acute extrapyramidal movement disorders. Arch Intern Med 1993;153:1469–1475.
67. Ganzini L, Heintz R, Hoffman WF, et al: Acute extrapyramidal syndromes in neuroleptic-treated elders: A pilot study. J Geriatr Psychiatry Neurol 1991;4:222–225.
68. García-Ruiz P, García de Yébenes, J, Jiménez-Jiménez FJ, et al: Parkinsonism associated to calcium channel blockers (CCB). A prospective follow-up study. Clin Neuropharmacol 1992;15:19–26.
69. García-Albea E, Jiménez-Jiménez FJ, Ayuso-Peralta L, et al: Parkinsonism unmasked by verapamil. Clin Neuropharmacol 1993;16:263–265.

70. Garland TO, Patterson MW: Six cases of acrylamide poisoning. Br Med J 1967;4:134–138.
71. Gatto EM, Fernández-Pardal M, Micheli F: Agravación del parkinsonismo por fluoxetine. Medicina (B Aires) 1994;54: 182. Letter.
72. Gawin FH, Ellinwood EH: Cocaine and other stimulants. Actions, abuse and treatment. N Engl J Med 1988;318: 1173–1182.
73. Gernaat HBPE, Van de Woude J, Touw DJ: Fluoxetine and parkinsonism in patients taking carbamazepine. Am J Psychiatry 1991;141:118–119. Letter.
74. Gershanik OS. Drug-induced parkinsonism in the aged: recognition and prevention. Drugs Aging 1994;5:127–132.
75. Gershanik OS. Drug-induced movement disorders. Curr Opin Neurol Neurosurg 1993;6:369–376.
76. Gibby WA, Zimmerman RA: X-ray computed tomography. In: Mazziotta JC, Gilman S, eds: Clinical Brain Imaging: Principles and Applications. Philadelphia, Davis, 1992, p. 3.
77. Gilman S: Advances in neurology, Part I. N Engl J Med 1992;326:1608–1616.
78. Gilman S: Advances in neurology, Part II. N Engl J Med 1992;326:1671–1676.
79. Giménez-Roldán S, Mateo D: Cinnarizine-induced parkinsonism. Susceptibility related to aging and essential tremor. Clin Neuropharmacol 1991;14:156–164.
80. Goñi M, Jiménez M, Seijoo M: Parkinsonism-induced by phenytoin. Clin Neuropharmacol 1985;8:383–384.
81. Gorio A, Mauro A: Reversibility and mode of action of black widow spider venom on the vertebrate neuromuscular junction. J Gen Physiol 1979;73:245–263.
82. Graham DF, Stewart-Wynne EG: Diltiazem-induced acute parkinsonism. Aust NZ J Med 1994;24:70. Letter.
83. Griffin JW, Watson DF: Axonal transport in neurological disease. Ann Neurol 1988;23:3–13.
84. Grimes JD: Parkinsonism and tardive dyskinesia associated with long-term metoclopramide therapy. N Engl J Med 1981;305:1417. Letter.
85. Grimes JD, Hassan MN, Preston DN: Adverse neurologic effects of metoclopramide. Can Med Assoc J 1982;126: 23–25.
86. Gucer G, Vierstein: Long-term intracranial pressure recording in the management of pseudotumor cerebri. J Neurosurg 1978;49:256–263.
87. Gutmann L, Martin JD, Welton W: Dapsone motor neuropathy: an axonal disease. Neurology (Minneap) 1976;26: 514–516.
88. He F, Lu B, Zhang S, et al: Chronic allyl chloride poisoning: An epidemiological, clinical, toxicological, and neuropathological study. G Ital Med Lav 1985;7:5–15.
89. Hertzman PA, Blevins WL, Mayer J, et al: Association of the eosinophilia-myalgia syndrome with the ingestion of tryptophan. N Engl J Med 1990;322:869–873.
90. Heyer EJ, Simpson DM, Bodis-Wollner I, et al: Nitrous oxide: Clinical and electrophysiologic investigation of neurologic complications. Neurology 1986;36:1618–1622.
91. Hoffman RS: Approach to the poisoned patient with peripheral neuropathy. In: Ford M, Delaney K, Ling L, Erickson T, eds: Clinical Toxicology. Philadelphia, Saunders, 1998 (in press).
92. Holroyd S, Smith D: Disabiling parkinsonism due to lithium: a case report. J Geriatr Psychiatry Neurol 1995;8:118–119. Letter.
93. Hubble JP: Drug-induced parkinsonism. In: Stern MB, Koller WC, eds: Parkinsonian Syndromes. New York: Marcel Dekker, 1993, pp. 111–122.
94. Hyman NM, Dennis PD, Sinclair KG: Tremor due to sodium valproate. Neurology 1979;29:1177–1180.
95. Indo T, Ando K: Metoclopramide-induced parkinsonism. Clinical characteristics of ten cases. Arch Neurol 1982;39:494–496.
96. Inouye SK, van Dyck CH, Alessi CA, et al: Clarifying confusion: The confusion assessment method. Ann Intern Med 1990;113:941–948.
97. Jansen Steur ENH: Increase of parkinson disability after fluoxetine medication. Neurology 1993;43:211–213.
98. Jiménez-Jiménez FJ, Cabrera-Valdivia F, Ayuiso-Peralta L, et al: Persistent parkinsonism and tardive dyskinesia-induced by clebopride. Mov Disord 1993;8:246–247.
99. Jiménez-Jiménez FJ, Garcia-Ruis PJ, Molina JA: Drug-induced movement disorders. Drug Safety 1997;16:180–204.
100. Jiménez-Jiménez FJ, Ortí-Pareja M, Ayuso-Eralta L, et al: Drug-induced parkinsonism in a movement disorders unit. A four-year survey. Parkinsonism Rel Disord 1996;2:145–149.
101. Jiménez-Jiménez FJ, Tejeiro J, Martínez-Junquera G, et al: Parkinsonism exacerbated by paroxetine. Neurology 1995;45:2406.
102. Jones KM, Mulkern RV, Schwartz RB, et al: Fast spin-echo MR imaging of the brain and spine: Current concepts. Am J Roentgenol 1992;158:1313–1320.
103. Kane J, Rifkin A, Quitkin F, et al: Extrapyramidal side effects with lithium therapy. Am J Psychiatry 1978;135: 851–853.
104. Kang UJ, Burke RE, Fahn S: Natural history and treatment of tardive dystonia. Mov Disord 1986;1:193–208.
105. Kantarjian AD, Shaheen AS: Methyl bromide poisoning with nervous system manifestations resembling polyneuropathy. Neurology (Minneap) 1963;13:1054–1058.
106. Karas BJ, Wilder BJ, Hammind EJ, et al: Treatment of valproate tremors. Neurology 1983;33:1380–1382.
107. Karas BJ, Wilder BJ, Hammond EJ, et al: Valproate tremors. Neurology 1982;32:428–432.
108. Katrak SM, Pollock M, O'Brien CP, et al: Clinical and morphological features of gold neuropathy. Brain 1980;103: 671–693.
109. Kitchens CS, Van Mierop LH: Envenomation by the eastern coral snake (*Micrurus fulvius fulvius*). JAMA 1987; 258:1615–1618.
110. Koller WC: Diagnosis and treatment of tremors. Neurol Clin 1984;2:499–514.
111. Korein J, Cravioto H, Leicach ML: Reevaluation of lumbar puncture: A study of 129 patients with papilledema or intracranial hypertension. Neurology 1959;9:290–299.
112. Krinke G, Schaumburg HH, Spencer P, et al: Pyridoxine megavitaminosis produces degeneration of peripheral sensory neurons (sensory neuronopathy) in the dog. Neurotoxicology 1980;2:13–21.
113. Kurlan R, Hamill R, Shoulson I: Neuroleptic malignant syndrome. Clin Neuropharmacol 1984;7:109–120.

114. Kuzuhard S, Kohara N, Ohkawa Y, et al: Parkinsonism, depression and akathisia induced by flunarizine, a calcium entry blockade. Report of 31 cases. Rinsho Shinkeigaku 1989;29:681–686.
115. Lagos JC, Thies RE: Tick paralysis without muscle weakness. Arch Neurol 1969;21:471–474.
116. Lane RJM, Radoff FM: Alcohol and serum creatine kinase levels. Ann Neurol 1981;10:581–583.
117. Langston JW, Ballard P: Parkinsonism induced by MPTP: Implication for treatment and the pathogenesis of PD. Can J Neurol Sci 1984;11:160–165.
118. Langston JW, Ballard P, Tetrud JW, et al: Chronic parkinsonism in humans due to a product of meperidine-analog synthesis. Science 1983;219:979–980.
119. Laporte JR, Capellà D: Useless drugs are not placebos: Lessons from flunarizine and cinnarizine. Lancet 1986;I:853–854. Letter.
120. Leavitt S, Tyler HR: Studies in asterixis. Arch Neurol 1964;10:360–368.
121. Leggat PO: Ethionamide neuropathy. Tubercule 1962; 43:95.
122. LeQuesne PM, Damluji SF, Rustam H: Electrophysiological studies of peripheral nerves in patients with organic mercury poisoning. J Neurol Neurosurg Psychiatry 1974;37:333–339.
123. LeQuesne PM, McLeod JG: Peripheral neuropathy following a single exposure to arsenic. J Neurol Sci 1977;32: 437–451.
124. Levin BE: The clinical significance of spontaneous pulsations of the retinal vein. Arch Neurol 1978;35:37–40.
125. Lewitt P: The neurotoxicity of the rat poison Vacor. N Engl J Med 1980;302:73–77.
126. Lipowski J: Update on delirium. Psychiatr Clin North Am 1992;15:335–346.
127. Lipton RB, Appel SC, Dutcher JP, et al: Taxol produces a predominantly sensory neuropathy. Neurology 1989;39: 368–373.
128. Llau ME, Nguyen L, Senard JM, et al. Syndromes parkinsoniens de pharmacovigilance sur dix ans. Rev Neurol (Paris) 1994;150:757–756.
129. Lovelace RE, Horwitz SJ: Peripheral neuropathy in long term diphenylhydantoin therapy. Arch Neurol 1968;18: 69–77.
130. Lufkin RB: Magnetic resonance imaging. In: Mazziotta JC, Gilman S, eds: Clinical Brain Imaging: Principles and Applications. Philadelphia, Davis, 1992, p. 39.
131. Lutz EG: Acute lithium-induced parkinsonism precipitated by liquid protein diet. J Med Soc N J 1978;75:165–166. Letter.
132. Malaterre HR, Lauribe P, Paganelli F, et al: Syndrome parkinsonien, effet indesirable possible des inhibiteurs calciques. Arch Mal Coeur 1992;85:1335–1337.
133. Malek-Ahmadi P, Allen SA: Paroxetine-molindone interaction. J Clin Psychiatry 1995;56:82–83. Letter.
134. Marsden CD, Tarsy D, Baldessarini RJ: Spontaneous and drug-induced movement disorders in psychotic patients. In: Benson DF, Blemer D, eds: Psychiatric Aspects of Neurologic Disease. New York, Grune & Straton, 1975, p. 219.
135. Masey EW, Goodman JC, Stewart C, et al: Unilateral asterixis: Motor integrative dysfunction in focal vascular disease. Neurology 1979;29:1180–1182.
136. Mastaglia RL, Walton LWD, eds: Skeletal Muscle Pathology, 2nd ed. Edinburgh, Churchill Livingstone, 1992, pp. 511, 599.
137. Martí-Massó JF, Carrera N, de la Puente E: Posible parkinsonismo por cinaricina. Med Clin (Barc) 1985;85:614–616.
138. Martí-Massó JF, Carrera N, Urtasun M: Drug-induced parkinsonism: A growing list. Mov Disord 1993;8:125. Letter.
139. Martí-Massó JF, Carrera N, Urtasun M: Newer drugs inducing parkinsonism. Ninth International Symposium on Parkinson's Disease: 1988 June 5–9; Jerusalem, Israel, p. 137. Abstract.
140. Martí-Massó JF, Poza JJ: Parkinsonismo inducido o agravado por fármacos: Características clínicas y evolución histórica de los fármacos implicados. Neurología (Spain) 1996;11:10–5.
141. McDonald WI, Kocen RS: Diphtheritic neuropathy. In: Dyck PJ, Thomas PK, Lambert EH, eds: Peripheral Neuropathy, Vol 2. Philadelphia, Saunders, 1984, p. 2010.
142. Melgaard B, Hansen HS, Kamieniecka Z, et al: Misonidazol neuropathy: A clinical electrophysiological and histological study. Ann Neurol 1982;12:10–17.
143. Merigan T, Skowron G, Bozette SA, et al: Circulating p24 antigen levels and responses to dideoxycytidine in human immunodeficiency virus (HIV) infections. Ann Intern Med 1989;110:189–194.
144. Micheli FE, Fernández-Pardal M, Giannaula R, et al: Movement disorders and depression due to flunarizine and cinnarizine. Mov Disord 1989;4:139–146.
145. Micheli F, Gatto E, Fernández-Pardal M, et al: Domperidona y enfermedad de parkinson. Medicina (B Aires) 1988;48:218. Letter.
146. Micheli F, Pardal MF, Gatto M, et al: Flunarizine- and cinnarizine-induced extrapyramidal reactions. Neurology 1987;7:881–884.
147. Milandre L, Ali-Cherif A, Khalil R: Syndrome parkinsonien au cours d'un traitement par le veralipride. Rev Med Intern 1991;12:157–158.
148. Miller NR: Walsh and Hoyt's Clinical Neuro-Ophthalmology, 4th ed. Baltimore, Williams & Wilkins, 1982, p. 175.
149. Miller LG, Jankovic J: Neurologic approach to drug-induced movement disorders: A study of 125 patients. South Med J 1990;8:525–532.
150. Miller LG, Jankovic J: Metoclopramide-induced movement disorders. Clinical findings with a review of the literature. Arch Intern Med 1989;149:2486–2492.
151. Montagna P, Gabellini AS, Monari L, et al: Parkinsonian syndrome after long-term treatment with clebopride. Mov Disord 1992;7:89–90.
152. Montastruc JL, Fabre N, Blin O, et al: Does fluoxetine aggravate Parkinson's disease? A pilot prospective study. Mov Disord 1995;10:355–357.
153. Moretti A, Lucantoni C: Flunarizine-induced parkinsonism: Clinical report. Ital J Neurol Sci 1988;9:295–297.
154. Morgante L, Rocca WA, Di Rosa AE, et al: Prevalence of Parkinson's disease and other types of parkinsonism: A

door-to-door survey in three Sicilian municipalities. The Sicilian neuro-epidemiologic study (SNES) group. Neurology 1992:42:1901–1907.
155. Montgomery BM, Pinner CA: Transient hypoglycemic hemiplegia. Arch Intern Med 1964;114:680–684.
156. Morris HH, McCormick WF, Reinarz JA: Neuroleptic malignant syndrome. Arch Neurol 1980;37:462–463.
157. Munetz MR, Cornes CL: Distinguishing akathisia and tardive dyskinesia: A review of the literature. J Clin Psychopharmacol 1983;3:343–350.
158. Murnaghan MF: Site and mechanism of tick paralysis. Science 1960;131:418–419.
159. Murphy JE, Stewart RB: Efficacy of antiparkinsonian agents in preventing antipsychotic-induced extrapyramidal symptoms. Am J Hosp Pharm 1979;36:641–646.
160. Nair VS, LeBrun M, Kass I: Peripheral neuropathy associated with ethambutol. Chest 1980;77:98–100.
161. Naito Y, Kuzuhara S: Parkinsonism-induced or worsened by cisapride. Nippon Ronen Igakkai Zasshi 1994;31: 899–902.
162. Nakashima K, Shimoda M, Kuno N, et al: Temporary symptom worsening caused by manidipine hydrochloride in two patients with Parkinson's disease. Mov Disord 1994;9:106–107.
163. Neale R, Gerhardt S, Leibman JM: Effects of dopamine agonists, catecholamine depletors and cholinergic and GABAergic drugs on acute dyskinesias in squirrel monkeys. Psychopharmacology 1984;82:20–26.
164. Nover R: Persistent neuropathy following chronic use of glutethimide. Clin Pharmacol Ther 1967;8:283–285.
165. Oleson J: The classification and diagnosis of headache disorders. Neurol Clin 1990;8:793–799.
166. Padrell MD, Navarro M, Faura CC, et al: Verapamil-induced parkinsonism. Am J Med 1995;99:436. Letter.
167. Paton WDM: The effects of muscle relaxants other than muscular relaxation. Anesthesiology 1959;20:453–463.
168. Pellissier JF, Pouget J, Cros D, et al: Peripheral neuropathy induced by amiodarone chlorohydrate. J Neurol Sci 1984;63:251–266.
169. Pérez-Gilabert Y, Mateo D, Giménez-Roldán S: Actividad asistencial en una consulta hospitalaria especializada en enfermedad de Parkinson y transtornos del movimiento: Un estudio prospectivo durante a os. Neurología (Spain) 1994;9:317–323.
170. Peterson J: Coma. In: Rosen P, Barkin RM, Braen GR, et al, eds: Emergency Medicine Concepts and Clinical Practice, 3rd ed. St. Louis, Mosby–Year Book, 1992, p. 1728.
171. Petrera JE, Fledelius HC, Trojaborg W: Serial pattern evoked potential recording in a case of toxic optic neuropathy due to ethambutol. Electroencephalogr Clin Neurophysiol 1988;71:146–149.
172. Plum F, Posner J: The Diagnosis of Stupor and Coma, 3rd ed. Philadelphia, Davis, 1982, pp 2, 64, 255.
173. Prien RF: Lithium in the treatment of affective disorders. Clin Neuropharmacol 1978;3:113.
174. Raskin NH, Fishman RA: Pyridoxine-deficiency neuropathy due to hydralazine. N Engl J Med 1965;273: 1182–1185.
175. Remington G, Bezchlibnyk-Butler K: Management of acute antipsychotic-induced extrapyramidal syndromes. CNS Drugs 1996; 5 (suppl 1): 21–35.
176. Riggs JE, Schochet SS Jr, Gutman L, et al: Chronic human colchicine neuropathy and myopathy. Arch Neurol 1986;43:521–523.
177. Roelofs RI, Hruskesky W, Rogin J, et al: Peripheral sensory neuropathy and cisplatin chemotherapy. Neurology 1984;34:934–938.
178. Roth G: The origin of fasciculations. Ann Neurol 1982;12:542–547.
179. Rothner AD, Morris HH III: Generalized status epilepticus. In: Lueders H, Lesser R, eds: Epilepsy: Electroclinical Syndrome. New York, Springer-Verlag, 1987, p. 207.
180. Said G, Bathien N, Cesaro P: Peripheral neuropathies and tremor. Neurology 1982;32:480–485.
181. Saper JR, Silberstein SS, Gordon CD, Hamel RL: Handbook of Headache Management. Baltimore, Williams & Wilkins, 1993, pp. 6, 16.
182. Sasso E, Delsoldato S, Negrotti A, et al: Reversible valproate-induced extrapyramidal disorders. Epilepsia 1994;35:391–393.
183. Schaumburg HH, Berger AR, Thomas PK: Disorders of Peripheral Nerves, 2nd ed. Philadelphia, Davis, 1992, pp. 3, 257, 274, 314.
184. Schaumburg H, Kaplan J, Windelbank A, et al: Sensory neuropathy from pyridoxine abuse. N Engl J Med 1983;309:445–448.
185. Schooler NR, Kane JM: Research diagnoses for tardive dyskinesia. Arch Gen Psychiatry 1982;39:486–487.
186. Semperé AP, Duarte J, Cabezas C, et al: Parkinsonism induced by amlodipine. Mov Disord 1995;10:115–116.
187. Semperé AP, Duarte J, Palomares JM, et al: Parkinsonism and tardive dyskinesia after chronic use of clebopride. Mov Disord 1994;9:114–115.
188. Sethi KD, Patel B, Meador KJ: Metoclopramide-induced parkinsonism. South Med J 1989;82:1581–1582. Letter.
189. Shahani BT, Young RR: Asterixis: a disorder of the neural mechanisms underlying sustained muscular contraction. In: Shahani M, ed: The Motor System: Neurophysiology and Muscle Mechanisms. New York, Elsevier, 1976, p. 301.
190. Shilkin KB, Chen BT, Khoo OT: Rhabdomyolysis caused by hornet venom. Br Med J 1972;1:156–157.
191. Shiraki H: Neuropathological aspects of organic mercury intoxication, including Minimata disease. In: Vinken PJ, Bruyn GW, eds: Handbook of Clinical Neurology, Vol. 36. Amsterdam, North-Holland, 1979, p. 83.
192. Simon RP: Alcohol and seizures. N Engl J Med 1988;319:715–716. Editorial.
193. Smith J: Organic brain syndrome. In: Rosen P, Barkin RM, Braen GR, et al, eds: Emergency Medicine Concepts and Clinical Practice, 3rd ed. St. Louis, Mosby–Year Book, 1992, p. 1766.
194. Spencer PS, Schaumburg HH: Central-peripheral distal axonopathy: The pathology of dying-back polyneuropathies. In: Zimmerman HM, ed: Progress in Neuropathology, Vol. 3. New York, Grune & Stratton, 1976, p. 253.
195. Spencer PS, Schaumburg HH, Sabri MI, et al: The enlarg-

ing view of hexacarbon neurotoxicity. CRC Crit Rev Toxicol 1980;7:279–356.
196. Sobue G, Pleasure D: Experimental lead neuropathy: Inorganic lead inhibits proliferation but not differentiation of Schwann cells. Ann Neurol 1985;17:462–468.
197. Strub RL, Black FW: The Mental Status Examination in Neurology, 2nd ed. Philadelphia, Davis, 1985, p. 43.
198. Tate JL: Extrapyramidal symptoms in a patient taking haloperidol and fluoxetine. Am J Psychiatry 1989;146: 399–400.
199. Teasdale G, Jennett B: Assessment of coma and impaired consciousness. Lancet 1974;2:81–84.
200. Teasdale G, Knill-Jones R, Van Der Sande J: Observer variability in assessing impaired consciousness and coma. J Neurol Neurosurg Psychiatry 1978;41:603–610.
201. Teusink JP, Alexopoulos GS, Shamoian CA: Parkinsonian side effects induced by a monoamine oxidase inhibitor. Am J Psychiatry 1984;141:118–119. Letter.
202. Trenkwalder C, Schwartz J, Gebhard J, et al: Starnberg trial on epidemiology of parkinsonism and hypertension in the elderly. Prevalence of Parkinson's disease and related disorders assessed by a door-to-door survey of inhabitants older than 65 years. Arch Neurol 1995;52: 1017–1022.
203. Tyrer P, Alexander MS, Regan A, et al: An extrapyramidal syndrome after lithium therapy. Br J Psychiatry 1980;136: 191–194.
204. Umez-Eronini EM, Eronini EA: Chloroquine-induced involuntary movements. Br Med J 1977;1:945–946.
205. Valeriano J, Tucker P, Kattah J: An unusual cause of hypokalemic muscle weakness. Neurology (Cleveland) 1983;33:1242–1243.
206. van der Zwan Jr A: Transient Parkinson syndrome and tremor caused by the use of sodium valproate. Ned Tijdschr Geneeskd 1989;133:1230–1232.
207. Van Putten T: Lithium-induced disabling tremor. Psychosomatics 1978;19:27–31.
208. Van Putten T, Gelenberg AJ, Lavoie PW: Anticholinergic effects on memory: benztropine vs. amantidine. Psychopharmacol Bull 1987;23:26–29.
209. Victor M: Polyneuropathy due to nutritional deficiency and alcoholism. In: Dyck PJ, et al, eds: Peripheral Neuropathy. Philadelphia, Saunders, 1984, p. 1899.
210. Victor M, Adams RD, Mancall E: A restricted form of cerebellar degeneration occurring in alcoholic patients. Arch Neurol 1959;1:579–688.
211. Vigliani EB: Carbon disulfide poisoning in viscose rayon factories. Br Med J 1954;2:235.
212. Walsh TJ, Garden JW, Gallagher B: Obliteration of retinal venous pulsations. Am J Ophthalmol 1969;67:954–956.
213. Weiner WJ, Lang AE: Movement Disorders: A Comprehensive Survey. Mt. Kisco, NY, Futura, 1989, p. 600.
214. Weinstein L: Tetanus. N Engl J Med 1973;289:1293–1296.
215. Wettstein A: The origin of fasciculations in motor neuron disease. Ann Neurol 1979;5:295–300.
216. Werner EG, Olanow CW: Parkinsonism and amiodarone therapy. Ann Neurol 1989;25:630–632.
217. Williams AJ, Baghat MS, Stableforth DE, et al: Dysphonia caused by inhaled steroids: Recognition of a characteristic laryngeal abnormality. Thorax 1983;38:813–821.
218. Windebank AJ, Blexrud MD: Residual ethylene oxide in hollow fiber hemodialysis units is neurotoxic in vitro. Ann Neurol 1989;26:63–68.
219. Windebank AJ, McCall JT, Dyck PJ: Metal neuropathy. In: Dyck PJ, Thomas PK, Lambert EH, Bunge RP, eds: Peripheral Neuropathy, Vol. 2, 2nd ed. Philadelphia, Saunders, 1984, p. 2148.
220. Yamamoto M, Ujike H, Ogawa N: Metoclopramide-induced parkinsonism. Clin Neuropharmacol 1987;10: 287–289.
221. Yiannikas C, Pollard JD, McLeod JG: Nitrofurantoin neuropathy. Aust NZ J Med 1981;11:400–405.

CHAPTER 20

Respiratory Principles

Robert S. Hoffman

Essential Abbreviations	
PO_2	Partial pressure of oxygen (in mm Hg; 1 mm Hg = 1 torr)
PAO_2	Alveolar PO_2
PaO_2	Arterial PO_2
PCO_2	Partial pressure of carbon dioxide (in mm Hg)
O_2 Sat	Hemoglobin oxygen saturation (in percent)
FIO_2	Percent oxygen in inspired air
CO	Carbon monoxide
COHb	Carboxyhemoglobin
MetHb	Methemoglobin

The primary function of the lung is to exchange gases. Specifically, this role can be divided into the transport of oxygen (O_2) into the blood, and the elimination of carbon dioxide (CO_2) from the blood. In addition, the lungs serve as minor organs of metabolism and elimination for a number of compounds, a source of insensible water loss, and a means of temperature regulation. Cellular oxygen utilization is dependent on many factors, including respiratory drive, percent oxygen in inspired air, airway patency, chest wall and pulmonary compliance, diffusing capacity, ventilation/perfusion mismatch, hemoglobin content, hemoglobin oxygen loading and unloading, cellular oxygen uptake, and cardiac output. Toxins have the unique ability to inhibit or impair each of these factors necessary for oxygen utilization and result in respiratory dysfunction. This chapter will illustrate how toxins interact with the mechanisms of gas exchange and oxygen utilization, and conclude with a practical approach to assessing the poisoned patient.

Pulmonary Manifestations of Toxin Exposures

Respiratory Drive

Respiratory rate and depth are regulated by the need to maintain a normal PCO_2 and pH.[39] Most of the control for ventilation occurs at the level of the medulla, although this is modulated both by involuntary input from the pons and voluntary input from the higher cortex. Changes in PCO_2 are measured primarily by a central chemoreceptor, located near the exit for cranial nerves IX and X, which measures CSF pH, and secondarily by peripheral chemoreceptors in the carotid and aortic bodies, which actually measure PCO_2. Input with regard to PO_2 is obtained from carotid and aortic chemoreceptors. Stretch receptors relay information about pulmonary dynamics, such as the volume and pressure.

Toxins can affect respiratory drive in one of several ways: direct suppression of the respiratory center, alteration in the response of chemoreceptors to changes in PCO_2, direct stimulation of the respiratory center, increase in metabolic demands due to agitation or fever, which in turn increases total body oxygen consumption, or indirectly due to the creation of acid–base disorders. For example, opioids (see Chap. 60) depress respiration both by decreasing the responsiveness of chemoreceptors to CO_2 and by direct suppression of the pontine and medullary respiratory centers.[25,69,94] Any toxin that causes a decreased respiratory drive or a decreased level of consciousness can produce bradypnea (a decreased respiratory rate), hypopnea (a decreased tidal volume), or both, resulting in hypoventilation (see Chap. 17).

Methylxanthines, cocaine, and other sympathomimetics may cause an increase in respiratory drive as well as an increase in oxygen consumption. Salicylates produce hyperventilation by both central and peripheral effects (ie, respiratory alkalosis and acidemia) (see Chaps. 15, 32, 38, 39, 65). The net consequence of increased respiratory drive, increased oxygen consumption, or metabolic acidosis is the generation of either tachypnea (an elevated respiratory rate), hyperpnea (an increased tidal volume), or both. Whether alone or in combination, tachypnea and hyperpnea produce hyperventilation. Toxins that commonly produce hypo- or hyperventilation are listed in Tables 20–1 and 20–2.

Decreased Inspired FIO_2

Barometric pressure at sea level ranges near 760 mm Hg. At this pressure, 21% of ambient air is comprised of oxygen (FIO_2 = 21%), and after subtracting for the water vapor normally present in the lungs, the PAO_2 is about 150 mm Hg. Any reduction in FIO_2 decreases the PAO_2, thereby producing signs and symptoms of hypoxemia (a low PaO_2). At an FIO_2 of 12–16%, patients will experience tachypnea, tachycardia, and impaired coordination. A further decrease to an FIO_2 of 10–14% will produce severe fatigue, and decreases to between 6% and 10% will be associated with nausea, vomiting, and lethargy. An FIO_2 less than 6% is incompatible with life.[63]

This effect on FIO_2 is typically observed as elevation increases above sea level, because barometric pressure falls. By 18,000 feet, barometric pressure is only 380 mm Hg, and the PAO_2 falls to below 70 mm Hg. At 63,000 feet, the barometric pressure falls to 47 mm Hg, a level where the PAO_2 equals 0 mm Hg. While it is important to remember this relationship, altitude-induced decreases in FIO_2 are rarely important in clinical medicine, even in commercial airline flights, where the cabins are pressurized to a maximum of several thousand feet above sea level. However, in closed (mines, sewers, silos) or low-lying (swamps) spaces, oxygen may be replaced or displaced by other gases that intrinsically have no direct toxicity. Common examples of these gases, referred to as simple asphyxiants (Table 20–3), are found in swamps, mines, sewers, and silos, alone or in combination with more toxic gases. Since they have little or no toxicity other than their ability to replace oxygen, removal of the victim from exposure and administration of supplemental oxygen are curative if permanent injury due to hypoxia has not already developed (see Chap. 94).

The potential magnitude of toxicity from simple asphyxiants was best exemplified by the disasters in Cameroon near the Lakes of Monoun and Nyos, in 1984 and 1986, respectively. For unclear reasons, Lake Nyos, a volcanic lake, released a cloud of carbon dioxide (CO_2) gas of approximately a quarter of a million tons. Because CO_2 is 1.5 times heavier than air, the gas cloud flowed into the surrounding low-lying valleys, killing by asphyxia over 1700 people, and affecting countless more due to hypoxia. Most survivors recovered without complications.[4,29,50]

TABLE 20–1. DRUGS AND TOXINS THAT PRODUCE HYPOVENTILATION

Barbiturates	Electrolyte abnormalities	Sedative-hypnotics
Botulinum toxin	Ethanol	Strychnine
Carbamates	Neuromuscular blocking agents	Tetanus toxin
Clonidine	Nicotine	Tetrodotoxin
Colchicine	Opioids	Toxic alcohols
Cyclic antidepressants	Organophosphates	
Elapid envenomation	Poison hemlock (coniine)	

TABLE 20–2. DRUGS AND TOXINS THAT PRODUCE HYPERVENTILATION

Amphetamines	Gyrometra mushrooms (monomethyl hydrazine)	Phenformin
Anticholinergics		Progesterone
Caffeine	Hydrogen sulfide	Salicylates
Camphor	Iron	Sodium monofluoroacetate
Carbon monoxide	Isoniazid	Theobromine
Cocaine	Methanol	Theophylline
Cyanide	Metformin	
Dinitrophenol	Methemoglobin inducers	
Ethanol (ketoacidosis)	Paraldehyde	
Ethylene glycol	Pentachlorophenol	

Chest Wall

Hypoventilation can occur as a result of a decrease in either respiratory rate or tidal volume. Thus, even when the stimulus to breath is normal, adequate ventilation is dependent on the coordination and function of the muscles of the diaphragm and chest wall. Changes in this function can result in hypoventilation by two separate mechanisms; both muscle weakness and muscle rigidity may impair the patient's ability to expand the chest wall. Toxicologic causes of muscle weakness include botulinum toxin,[79] electrolyte abnormalities such as hypokalemia[51,95] or hypermagnesemia,[22] organophosphates,[61,80] and neuromuscular blocking agents.[8,44] Patients with hypoventilation due to muscle weakness respond well to assisted ventilation and correction of the underlying problem (see Chaps. 15, 53, 73, 87). Chest wall rigidity impairing ventilation can be seen in strychnine poisoning,[9,55] tetanus toxin,[14,48,85] and fentanyl use[13,16] (see Chaps. 60, 89). Often these patients are difficult to ventilate despite intubation and may require muscle relaxants, neuromuscular blocking agents, or naloxone (for fentanyl).

Airway Patency

The airway itself may be compromised in several ways. As a patient's mental status becomes impaired, the airway is often obstructed by the tongue.[33] Alternatively,

TABLE 20–3. SIMPLE ASPHYXIANTS

Argon	Hydrogen
Carbon dioxide	Methane
Ethane	Nitrogen
Helium	Propane

drug- or toxin-induced vomitus, or aspiration of activated charcoal or a foreign body, can directly obstruct the trachea or major bronchi with resultant hypoxia.[33,57,72,78] Obstruction may also result from increased secretions produced during organophosphate poisoning. Laryngospasm may occur either as a manifestation of systemic reactions, such as anaphylaxis, or as a result of edema from thermal or caustic injury[58] (see Chaps. 86 and 95). Similarly, the tongue can become swollen in response to thermal[58] or caustic injury or toxic exposure to plants such as *Dieffenbachia* spp,[19] or as a result of reactions to drugs such as angiotensin converting enzyme inhibitors[24] (see Chaps. 51, 77, 86, 95). Regardless of the mechanism, upper airway obstruction results in hypoventilation, hypoxemia, and hypercapnia (hypercarbia) with the persistence of a normal A–a gradient (see A–a gradients below). Upper airway obstruction is often acute and severe and requires immediate therapy to prevent further clinical compromise. Bronchospasm may be a manifestation of anaphylaxis, as well as exposure to pyrolyzed cocaine,[35,77] smoke,[58] irritant gases[36,42,67] (Table 20–4), or dust (eg, cotton in byssinosis), or a result of occupational asthma[54] and hypersensitivity pneumonitis[98] (see Chaps. 94, 95).

Airway collapse may result from pneumothorax caused by barotrauma, which more commonly results from the manner of administration of illicit drugs than from actual drug overdose. One remarkable form of pneumothorax or hydropneumothorax results from an attempt to inject heroin or cocaine into the internal jugular vein, commonly referred to as a "pocket shot." A patient who attempts to direct a needle into the depression in the neck lateral to the sternocleidomastoid above the clavicle may instead lacerate the apical pleura. A predominance of left-sided pneumothoraces from pocket shots probably is related to the fact that most people are right-handed.[33] Barotrauma may also result from nasal insufflation or inhalation of drugs. This form of barotrauma is seen most often in cocaine (particularly in the form of "crack") and marijuana users, who either smoke or insufflate these drugs and then perform prolonged Valsalva maneuvers in an attempt to enhance the drug's effects[6,11,65,81,96] (see Chaps. 65, 69). The increased airway pressure leads to rupture of an alveolar bleb, and free air dissects along the peribronchial paths into the mediastinum and pleural cavities. The use of nitrous oxide, which originally gained popularity in the 1970s as a drug of abuse, is also noted to cause barotrauma.[46] The medical profession has not been immune to this widespread abuse. Indeed, a study of medical and dental students from the 1970s found that between 8.5% and 20% of each enrolled class used nitrous oxide in social situations.[46] Although people who have access to nitrous oxide in the hospital or laboratory may siphon the agent from tanks meant for inhalation, at parties they inhale nitrous oxide that is used as a propellant in whipped cream cans. Tremendous pressure generated by the escaping gas is then transmitted to the airways, sometimes resulting in severe barotrauma.

TABLE 20–4. IRRITANT GASES

Ammonia	Isocyanates
Chloramine	Nitrogen dioxide
Chlorine	Ozone
Chloracetophenone (CN)	Phosgene
Chlorobenzylidene-malonitrile (CS)	Phosphine
Fluorine	Sulfur dioxide
Hydrogen chloride	

Under these circumstances a chest tube is inserted for a pneumothorax greater than 10–20% and/or when gas exchange is compromised.[30,37] Alternatively, insertion of a 14-gauge catheter into the pleural space with aspiration of the air may successfully treat the pneumothorax and avoid the occasional morbidity associated with chest tube insertion.[30] When hypoxia, hypotension, absent breath sounds, and tracheal deviation suggest tension pneumothorax, immediate intervention is required, prior to radiographic confirmation.

Ventilation–Perfusion Mismatch

Ventilation–perfusion (V/Q) mismatch is manifested at the extremes by aeration of the lung without arterial blood supply (as in pulmonary embolism from injected contaminants) and by a normal blood supply to the lung without any ventilation. Impaired blood supply to a normal lung and normal blood supply to an inadequately ventilated lung constitute an infinite number of gradations that exist between the extremes. The normal response to regional variations in ventilation is to shunt blood away from an area of lung that is poorly ventilated, thereby preferentially delivering blood to an area of the lung where gas exchange is more efficient. An hypoxia-induced reduction in local nitric oxide production appears to be responsible for the regional vasoconstriction that occurs.[1] This effect, commonly known as hypoxic pulmonary vasoconstriction, is best described in patients with chronic obstructive lung disease and helps compensate for the V/Q mismatch associated with that disorder. Although it is unclear whether toxin-induced alterations in pulmonary nitric oxide production play a major role in the V/Q mismatch seen in poisoning, research in this area is just beginning.

Toxin-induced V/Q mismatch more commonly results from perfusion of an abnormally ventilated lung, as may occur following aspiration of gastric contents, a frequent complication of many types of drug overdoses.[33] Although alterations in consciousness and loss of protective airway reflexes are predisposing factors, certain toxins, such as hydrocarbons, directly predispose to aspiration pneumonitis due to their specific characteristics of volatility, viscosity, and surface tension[32] (see Chap. 85).

The diagnosis of aspiration pneumonitis often relies on the chest radiograph for confirmation. The location of the infiltrate depends on the patient's position when the aspiration occurred. Most commonly, aspiration occurs in the right mainstem bronchus, because the angle with the carina is not as acute as it is on the left side. When aspiration occurs in the supine position, the subsequent infiltrate is usually manifest in the posterior segments of the upper lobe and superior segments of the lower lobe. Aspiration not only involves vomitus, as secretions, activated charcoal, teeth, dentures, food, and other foreign bodies are also frequently aspirated.

Diffusing Capacity Abnormalities

Severe impairment in diffusing capacity commonly results from local injury to the lungs in disorders such as interstitial pneumonia, aspiration, toxic inhalations, and near drowning, and from systemic effects of sepsis, trauma, and various other medical disorders.[5] When this process is acute and associated with clinical criteria including rales, hypoxemia (unspecified degree), and bilateral involvement on a chest radiograph demonstrating a normal heart size, it is commonly referred to as noncardiogenic pulmonary edema. It may also be defined as the presence of increased intraalveolar fluid in the lungs with a normal cardiac output.[73,99] More rigid criteria, such as a PaO_2/FIO_2 ratio < 300 mm Hg (regardless of PEEP), bilateral infiltrates on the chest radiograph, and either the pulmonary artery wedge pressure ≤ 18 mm Hg or no clinical evidence of left atrial hypertension, are used to define the term acute lung injury (ALI).[5] When these same criteria are met, but the patient's PaO_2/FIO_2 ratio is < 200 mm Hg (regardless of PEEP), the term acute respiratory distress syndrome (ARDS) is used.[5,52] Approximately 150,000 Americans develop ARDS annually, many as a result of toxins, and with a fatality rate of almost 50%.[12]

Commonly, patients are chronically exposed to toxins associated with reduced diffusing capacity by smoking tobacco and other substances, or working with asbestos, silica, and coal, which cause slow pulmonary fibrosis or promote emphysema. Recent work has emphasized the ability of chronically smoked cocaine to alter pulmonary function.[87] More acutely, noncardiogenic pulmonary edema from opioids, salicylates, or phosgene and severe fibrosis from paraquat can cause profound alterations in diffusion[62,73,99] (see Chaps. 32, 60, 90, 94). Associated parenchymal damage is almost always present and causes both reduction in lung volumes and ventilation–perfusion mismatch. Intravenous injection of street drug contaminants such as talc[66] and septic emboli from right-sided endocarditis[45] may result in isolated vascular defects with reduction in diffusion capacity. Similarly, cocaine-induced pulmonary spasm can obstruct vascular channels and alter pulmonary function, creating ventilation–perfusion mismatch.[18]

Noncardiogenic pulmonary edema, a common cause of ARDS from drug overdose, is by no means a new phenomenon. The edema fluid (and the resulting hypoxia, pulmonary rales, and radiographic abnormalities) may develop in part because of increased permeability of the alveolar and capillary basement membrane.[12,17,56,73,99] Proteinaceous fluid leaks from the capillaries into the alveoli and interstitium of the lung. Several mechanisms have been proposed as the cause for noncardiogenic pulmonary edema, although there is no single unifying mechanism for all of the drugs that have been implicated. Noncardiogenic pulmonary edema may result from exposure to toxins that produce hypoventilation by three different mechanisms: hypoxia may injure the vascular endothelial cells; autoregulatory vascular redistribution may cause localized capillary hypertension; or alveolar microtrauma may occur as alveolar units collapse, only to be reopened suddenly during reventilation.[73,99] Other agents may be directly toxic to the capillary epithelial cells or may be partly responsible for the release of vasoactive substances.[73,99] The effects of salicylates and other nonsteroidal antiinflammatory agents may be mediated via effects on prostaglandin synthesis. Finally, sympathomimetic stimulants may cause "neurogenic" pulmonary edema, which is thought to be mediated by massive catecholamine discharge. Elevated catecholamine levels are also noted in experimental opioid overdose, possibly supplying a link between hypoxia, hypercarbia, and the catecholamine hypothesis of noncardiogenic pulmonary edema.[60]

In the 1880s, Sir William Osler described pulmonary edema in an opium user.[64] We have since learned that there are many types of drugs that can cause noncardiogenic pulmonary edema. The opioids, such as morphine, heroin, codeine, propoxyphene, and methadone, are still the most common causes (see Chap. 60), but such diverse agents as the sedative-hypnotic agents, salicylates, cocaine, carbon monoxide, diuretics, and calcium channel blockers have all been associated with this entity.[20,21,23,27,28,34,40,43,49,68,70,76,82,84,100] Table 20–5 summarizes the causes of noncardiogenic pulmonary edema. The route of administration is not usually the determining factor. Pulmonary edema has resulted from oral, intravenous, and inhalational use of drugs. Because the source of the problem is increased pulmonary capillary permeability, patients with noncardiogenic pulmonary edema have a normal pulmonary-capillary wedge pressure, unlike patients with cardiogenic pulmonary edema.

Cardiogenic pulmonary edema may also occur as the result of a drug overdose. Etiologies for this phenome-

TABLE 20–5. TOXICOLOGIC CAUSES OF NONCARDIOGENIC PULMONARY EDEMA

Amiodarone	Irritant gases
Amphetamines	Lidocaine
Amphotericin	Opioids
Bleomycin	Protamine
Calcium channel blockers	Salicylates
Carbon monoxide	Smoke inhalation
Chlordiazepoxide	Streptokinase
Cocaine	Terbutaline
Colchicine	Thiazide diuretics
Cytosine arabinoside	Tricyclic antidepressants
Ethchlorvynol	Vinca alkaloids
Haloperidol	

non include the ingestion of large amounts of a negative inotrope (beta-adrenergic antagonists, type IA antidysrhythmics, etc), myocardial infarction (from cocaine), and, theoretically, the use of digoxin-specific antibodies to treat digoxin overdose in a patient with congestive heart failure. Since many overdoses are mixed overdoses, the distinction between cardiogenic and noncardiogenic pulmonary edema is often difficult to establish by physical examination and requires invasive monitoring techniques.

Although the treatments for cardiogenic and noncardiogenic pulmonary edema have similarities, critical aspects of the therapy differ, and therefore an accurate diagnosis must be established. Most diagnostic tests may not be helpful in differentiating between these two diseases. Physical examination will reveal the presence of rales with both entities. An S_3 gallop if present suggests a cardiac cause of pulmonary edema, but its absence does not establish the diagnosis of noncardiogenic pulmonary edema. In both entities the arterial blood gas analysis demonstrates hypoxia and the chest radiograph shows perihilar, basilar, or diffuse alveolar infiltrates. The presence of "vascular redistribution" on the chest radiograph, however, is suggestive of a cardiogenic etiology; a normal-sized heart is more commonly associated with noncardiogenic pulmonary edema, whereas an enlarged heart is more typical of cardiogenic pulmonary edema (see Fig. 7–12). Three diagnostic tests that may be useful in establishing the correct diagnosis are radionucleotide ventriculography ("gated pool" scan), echocardiography, and pulmonary artery (Swan-Ganz) catheter pressure measurements. The radionucleotide scan, while accurately measuring cardiac output, is not routinely available in the ED or ICU and usually requires transporting a critically ill patient to the nuclear medicine suite. Although echocardiography can be performed as a portable "bedside" technique, it is less sensitive and less specific for determinations of cardiac output. Therefore, the most definitive diagnostic procedure in the emergency setting is the insertion of a pulmonary artery catheter for hemodynamic monitoring. Cardiogenic pulmonary edema results from an elevated left atrial filling pressure (elevated pulmonary-capillary wedge pressure) and a decreased cardiac output (measured by a thermodilution catheter). In patients with noncardiogenic pulmonary edema, the pulmonary artery, pulmonary artery wedge pressure, and cardiac output will all be normal (Table 20–6).

The basic treatment for noncardiogenic pulmonary edema, ALI, and ARDS is supportive care while the toxin is eliminated and healing occurs in the pulmonary capillaries.[52] The most critically ill patients require a pulmonary artery catheter for management. The pulmonary arterial wedge pressure should be kept below 10 mm Hg, and probably in the range of 2–4 mm Hg. However, an adequate cardiac output, blood pressure, and urine output must be maintained. Infusions of albumin or dextran to increase the plasma oncotic pressure and prevent fluid from exuding into the alveoli are not effective, unless the patient is hypoalbuminemic. Although low tidal volume ventilation with lower airway pressures may "rest" the lung and allow healing, the efficacy of jet ventilators or membrane oxygenators has not yet been well studied. Some studies suggested a potential role for extracorporeal membrane oxygenation in the treatment of noncardiogenic pulmonary edema.[47] Positive end-expiratory pressure (PEEP) may be particularly beneficial. The PEEP should be maintained as low as possible, in the range of 5–20 cm H_2O, to maintain a PO_2 of approximately 65 mm Hg with an inspired oxygen concentration of 40% or less. In patients who do not have a pulmonary artery catheter, the dynamic lung capacitance [tidal volume/(end inspiratory pressure–end expiratory pressure)] seems to correlate with the best PEEP for oxygenation. Higher PEEP settings are not always beneficial and may cause an increased incidence of pneumothorax or hypotension. An increase in PEEP may result in a modest increase in PO_2 but a larger decrease in venous return and decreased cardiac output. Therefore, with each change in PEEP, the resulting actual increase (or perhaps decrease) in oxygen delivery to the body should be determined. A discussion of the treatment of cardiogenic pulmonary edema is found in Chapter 21.

Hemoglobin and the Chemical Asphyxiants

Disorders of hemoglobin oxygen content as well as hemoglobin loading and unloading all result in cellular hypoxia, which in turn results in hyperventilation. Anemia is a common complication of the infections associated with parenteral drug abuse. In addition, many toxins result in hemolysis or direct bone marrow suppression.

TABLE 20–6. PULMONARY ARTERY CATHETER VALUES

	RA Mean (mm Hg)	RV S/D (mm Hg)	PA S/D (mm Hg)	PA Mean (mm Hg)	PAW (mm Hg)	CI (L/min/m²)
Normal	5	20/5	20/10	16	4–12	2.5–4.0
Cardiogenic pulmonary edema	N–H	N–H/H	H/H	H	H	L
Noncardiogenic pulmonary edema, ALI and ARDS	N	N/N	N/N	N	N	N

RA = right atrium; RV = right ventricle; PA = pulmonary artery; PAW = pulmonary capillary wedge; CI = cardiac index; S = systolic; D = diastolic; N = normal; H = high; L = low.

Among the latter group are the heavy metals, lead, benzene, and ethanol. Hemolysis may be seen in individuals exposed to lead or arsine gas and in patients with G6PD deficiency exposed to oxidants (see Chap. 24).

The oxygen-carrying capacity of blood declines in almost direct proportion to hemoglobin content, as seen in Figure 20–1. As shown in Figure 20–1A, under most normal conditions the dissolved oxygen content of the blood contributes little, and thus the last portion of the equation can be eliminated. Anemia resulting in a decrease of the hemoglobin content to 7.5 g/dL (a hematocrit of approximately 22%) would decrease the oxygen content of the blood to about 10.2 mL O_2/dL, as shown in Figure 20–1B. Since, unless an abnormal hemoglobin is present, central cyanosis will only be visible with a concentration of reduced (deoxy-) hemoglobin of at least 5 g/dL, anemia can significantly impair oxygen-carrying capacity without the development of this common physical manifestation (see Chap. 93).

Similarly, as the PO_2 reaches higher values (as in hyperbaric oxygen chambers), the dissolved oxygen content becomes significant and may be of therapeutic value, particularly when the oxygen-carrying content of hemoglobin is compromised. The PO_2 corresponding to an FIO_2 of 100% is approximately 600 mm Hg. At 3 atmospheres and 100% oxygen, PO_2 values in excess of 1500 mm Hg can be achieved. Under these conditions the dissolved oxygen content of the blood rises dramatically (to as much as 4.5 mL O_2/dL) and may be adequate to sustain life even in the absence of any contribution from hemoglobin, as shown in Figure 20–1C.

The chemical asphyxiants that produce methemoglobin, carboxyhemoglobin, and sulfhemoglobin all interfere with oxygen loading and/or unloading to various

Oxygen content (O_2 content) = hemoglobin bound oxygen + dissolved oxygen

A. Normal conditions: hemoglobin (Hb)=15g/dL; PO_2=100 mm Hg, oxygen saturation (O_2 Sat)=95%

O_2 content = [(Hb)(O_2 sat)(constant) + (another constant)(PO_2)

= [(Hb)(O_2 sat)(1.39 mL O_2/g%) + (0.003 mL O_2/dL/mm Hg)(PO_2)

= [(15gm/dL)(95%)(1.39 mL O_2/g%) + (0.003 mL O_2/dL/mm Hg)(100 mm Hg)]

= [(19.8 mL O_2/dL) + (0.3 mL O_2/dL)]

= 20.1 mL O_2/dL = 20.1 volumes percent

B. Anemia: Hb=7.5g/dL; PO_2=100 mm Hg, O_2 Sat=95%

O_2 content = [(Hb)(O_2 sat)(1.39 mL O_2/g%) + (0.003 mL O_2/dL/mm Hg)(PO_2)

= [(7.5gm/dL)(95%)(1.39 mL O_2/g%) + (0.003 mL O_2/dL/mm Hg)(100 mm Hg)]

= [(9.9 mL O_2/dL) + (0.3 mL O_2/dL)]

= 10.2 mL/dL = 10.2 volumes percent

C. Hyperbaric oxygen: Hb=15g/dL; PO_2=1500 mm Hg, O_2 Sat=100%

O_2 content = [(Hb)(O_2 sat)(1.39 mL O_2/g%) + (0.003 mL O_2/dL/mm Hg)(PO_2)

= [(15gm/dL)(100%)(1.39 mL O_2/g%)+(0.003 mL O_2/dL/mm Hg)(1500 mm Hg)]

= [(20.9 mL O_2/dL) + (4.5 mL O_2/dL)]

= 25.4 mL/dL = 25.4 volumes percent

Figure 20–1. Oxygen content of the blood.

degrees. Methemoglobin inhibits oxygen loading, producing cyanosis that is unresponsive to supplemental oxygen (see Chap. 93). In addition, the oxyhemoglobin saturation curve is shifted to the left, interfering with unloading (see Fig. 20–2). Carboxyhemoglobin has similar effects on oxygen loading and unloading, but carboxyhemoglobin is not associated with cyanosis (see Chap. 96). Sulfhemoglobin has similar effects on oxygen loading, but actually shifts the oxyhemoglobin saturation curve to the right, favoring unloading. Cyanide, hydrogen sulfide, and sodium azide primarily affect oxygen utilization by interfering with the cytochrome oxidase system (see Chap. 97).

Cardiac Output

Any toxin that causes a decreased cardiac output or hypotension may result in tissue hypoxia and tachypnea. This is seen most frequently with overdoses of beta-adrenergic antagonists and calcium channel blockers, antidysrhythmics, cyclic antidepressants, and phenothiazines (see Chap. 21).

Approach to the Poisoned Patient

The initial assessment of every patient must involve the evaluation of upper airway patency. Adequacy of ventilation should then be determined. Care must be taken to protect the cervical spine, if concomitant injury is suspected. When airway patency is in question, maneuvers to establish and protect the airway are of prime importance. Often this may simply involve repositioning the chin, jaw, or head, or suctioning secretions or vomitus from the airway. However, insertion of an oral or nasopharyngeal airway, or nasopharyngeal or endotracheal intubation, or surgical cricothyroidotomy may all be required as clinically indicated. Once the airway is secured, high-flow supplemental oxygen should be provided and the depth, rate, and rhythm of respirations evaluated. An acceptable tidal breath is one that transports 12–15 mL of air/kg body weight.[89] Hypoventilation resulting from an inadequate respiratory rate or tidal volume is arbitrarily defined as PCO_2 greater than 44 mm Hg and leads to hypoxia and ventilatory failure.[31] The symptoms of hypoxia and or hypercarbia are nonspecific and resemble toxicity from many agents. Initially, patients appear restless and confused. Signs of sympathetic discharge, such as tachycardia and diaphoresis, may be noted. Later, patients may complain of headache, only to become sedated and subsequently comatose, as further deterioration occurs. Because these signs and symptoms are nonspecific, arterial blood gas analysis must be used early in the assessment of patients who present with drug overdose and possible ventilatory failure (see section below).

A trial of naloxone, hypertonic dextrose, and thiamine may be indicated for the patient with an altered mental status and or respiratory compromise (see Chap. 3). Since opioid overdose and hypoglycemia are rapidly reversible, potential causes of respiratory failure, these diagnoses should be addressed before most other interventions are considered. Failure to identify and reverse these conditions may result in unnecessary diagnostic and therapeutic interventions in addition to irreversible neurologic sequelae.

Having assured an acceptable airway, the remainder of the evaluation can proceed. A rapid assessment of the remainder of the vital signs (see Chap. 17) should then occur. Obtaining a history and physical examination, pulse oximetry, arterial blood gas analysis, measured oxygen saturation, and a chest radiograph are sufficient to determine the diagnosis of pulmonary pathology in most cases. However, adjuncts, such as in-

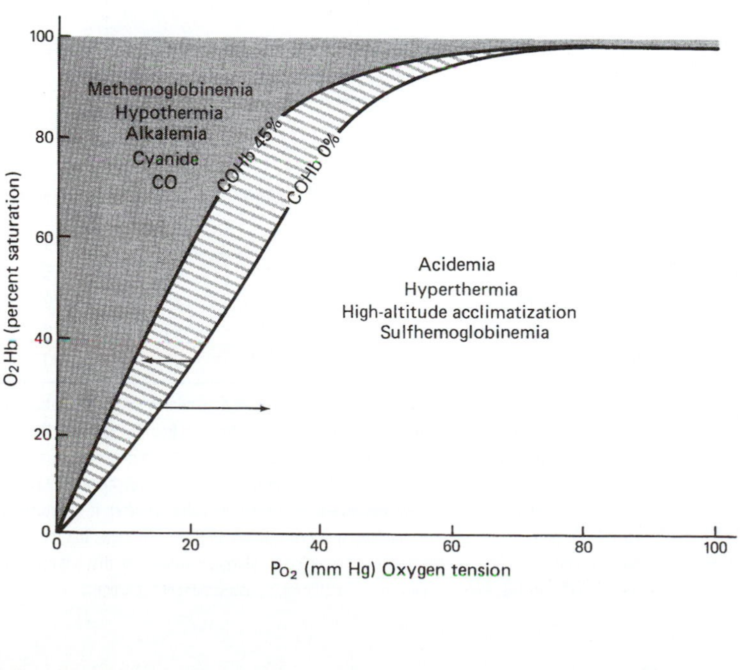

Figure 20–2. Oxyhemoglobin dissociation curve at 37°C and pH 7.40. (Hematocrit does not alter this relationship.)

vasive hemodynamic monitoring, evaluation of the arterial-venous oxygen difference, and xenon ventilation and technetium scanning, may be required.

History

A directed history must include questions on the nature, onset, and duration of symptoms, drug use and abuse, home and occupational exposures, and underlying pulmonary pathology. If the patient is suffering from a significant degree of respiratory compromise, most or all of the history may have to be obtained from friends, relatives, paramedics, co-workers, or others.

Physical Examination

The physical evaluation must include a detailed assessment of depth, rate, and rhythm of respirations, use of accessory muscles, direct evaluation of the oropharynx, position of the trachea, and presence and quality of breath sounds. Skin and nail-bed color must be observed for pallor or cyanosis. Funduscopic examination is a useful adjunct to the examination. Papilledema may be noted in the presence of acute hypercapnia. Additionally, since cyanide poisoning interferes with oxygen delivery to tissue, the venous oxygen saturation remains high. During the funduscopic examination this may appear as arteriolization of the retinal veins, where the veins take on a color more characteristic of arteries (see Chap. 97).

Pulse Oximetry

Pulse oximeters have gained widespread acceptance as rapid, noninvasive indicators of hemoglobin oxygen saturation. As defined, hemoglobin oxygen saturation is the ratio of oxyhemoglobin to total hemoglobin. By using two light-emitting diodes, the pulse oximeter is able to measure absorbance at the peak wavelengths for oxy- and deoxyhemoglobin (940 and 660 nm, respectively). Thus the ratio of oxyhemoglobin to oxy- plus deoxyhemoglobin (total hemoglobin) can be calculated.[74] The clinician may then estimate the PO_2 from the oxygen saturation.

Some limitations of this approach require elaboration. Since the oxyhemoglobin saturation curve becomes quite flat above 90% saturation (Fig. 20–2), small changes in saturation over 90% may represent very large changes in PO_2. Thus a decrease from 97% saturation to 95% saturation might represent a substantial change in PO_2. Although a low saturation is an early indicator of hypoxic hypoxia, this is only one of many causes of tissue hypoxia. If total hemoglobin is low, oxygen-carrying capacity is inadequate even with good saturation, as shown in Figure 20–1. Dyshemoglobinemias, such as carboxyhemoglobin, methemoglobin, and possibly sulfhemoglobin, interfere with the accuracy of pulse oximeter determinations and are of particular concern in the poisoned patient.[88,90] Specifically, using a standard pulse oximeter, the presence of elevated concentrations of methemoglobin will tend to make the saturation approach 84–86%.[3,75] Carboxyhemoglobin is falsely interpreted by the pulse oximeter as mostly oxyhemoglobin, and thus readings tend to appear normal even with significant carbon monoxide poisoning. This concept is shown in Table 20–7.

Accurate response by the pulse oximeter also requires adequate blood pressure, lack of strong venous pulsations (as might occur in a patient with tricuspid regurgitation), translucent nails (no nail polish), absence of circulating dyes (methylene blue), and a near normal temperature.[74] Finally, we are often more interested in PCO_2 than PO_2 as it is a better measure of ventilation. The pulse oximeter gives no information with regard to PCO_2. While the pulse oximeter may give early clues to the presence of hypoxic hypoxia, extrapolation of oxygen saturation to standard arterial blood gas values may be difficult because of the many possible sources of error. Pulse oximetry is therefore best used as an initial screening tool for hypoxic hypoxia and later in combination with the initial arterial blood gas measurement, as a determination of the patient's response to therapy.

Arterial Blood Gas

Arterial blood gas analysis is an easy and rapid means of evaluating both acid–base status and the quality of gas exchange. Attention must be paid to the method for determining oxygen saturation, specifically whether it is measured or calculated from PO_2. If the measured O_2 saturation is lower than would be predicted from the PO_2 (the calculated O_2 saturation), the presence of carboxyhemoglobin or methemoglobin must be suspected. A normal calculated O_2 saturation does not exclude these disorders (see section on co-oximetry).

Because it is easier to obtain, venous blood gas analysis is occasionally used as a substitute for arterial blood gas analysis. When compared to arterial values,

TABLE 20–7. INTERPRETATION OF OXYGEN SATURATIONS REPORTED FROM VARIOUS SOURCES

		% Oxygen Saturation		
Condition	PO_2 (mm Hg)	ABG	Pulse oximeter	Co-oximeter
Normal	95	95	95	95
Anemia	95	95	95	95*
Methemoglobinemia (30%)	95	95	85	70
Carboxyhemoglobinemia (30%)	95	95	93	70
Hypoxemia	60	90	90	90

The table demonstrates limitations of the various methods for determining oxygen saturation (O_2 saturation). The arterial blood gas (ABG) calculates the O_2 saturation from the dissolved oxygen content (PO_2) and becomes abnormal only when the PO_2 falls. The pulse oximeter uses only two wavelengths of light and produces substantial errors in the presence of a dyshemoglobinemia. Since the co-oximeter uses more wavelengths of light than the pulse oximeter, it can correctly identify the presence of carboxyhemoglobin and methemoglobin. The co-oximeter has the additional advantage (*) of calculating the total hemoglobin and oxygen content, so that it is useful in the setting of anemia. All techniques are acceptable for the assessment of hypoxemia.

venous pH and PO_2 are lower, while PCO_2 is higher. Errors can be introduced by increased muscle activity of the extremity being tested (eg, seizures) or placement of a tourniquet. Mixed venous blood, however, is required for accurate determination of the arterial-venous oxygen extraction (see below) and is an excellent indicator of acid–base status, cardiovascular function, and oxygen utilization. Unfortunately, a central venous catheter is required for sampling. When performing a peripheral venous blood gas analysis, it is usually assumed that this is only an approximation of mixed venous blood.

The PO_2 is generally considered adequate only if it lies within the flat portion at the upper right of the sigmoidal-shaped oxyhemoglobin dissociation curve (Fig. 20–2). That portion of the curve includes the PO_2 range from 60 to 100 mm Hg, which corresponds to oxygen saturations greater than 90%. As mentioned previously, within this flat portion there can be discernible changes in PO_2 with little change in oxygen saturation. For instance, an arterial PO_2 of 80 mm Hg corresponds roughly to an oxygen saturation of 95%. If the PO_2 falls to 60 mm Hg, the oxygen saturation falls to 90%, and this insignificant decrease in the oxygen-carrying capacity of the blood is of minimal clinical concern. If the PO_2 falls another 20 mm Hg, however, there is a more significant reduction in oxygen saturation, to about 70%. Thus, changes in PO_2 above 60 mm Hg are usually not of therapeutic significance, because the O_2 saturation is above 90%. These changes are, however, frequently of diagnostic significance.[31]

An exception to this concept applies to the patient who is under metabolic stress, as might result from low cardiac output, impaired vascular flow, anemia, or dyshemoglobinemia. Under these circumstances even the modest gain achieved by increasing both dissolved oxygen content and hemoglobin saturation above 90% may be desirable, as discussed in the section on hemoglobin and chemical asphyxiants. Also, even if a PO_2 greater than 60 mm Hg or an O_2 saturation greater than 90% is considered acceptable in most acute settings, it is still desirable to achieve greater values, when feasible, to create a safety zone in case of clinical deterioration.

What Is the Significance of a Decreased PO_2?

In a patient with a diminished PO_2, five clinically relevant mechanisms for the hypoxemia should be considered: (1) alveolar hypoventilation, (2) ventilation–perfusion mismatch or imbalance, (3) shunting, (4) diffusion abnormality, and, rarely, (5) a decrease in inspired FIO_2. In most clinical circumstances, diffusion defects cannot be distinguished from ventilation–perfusion mismatch. Usually the responsible mechanism can be identified by calculating the alveolar–arterial oxygen (A–a) gradient (shown later in the chapter). In patients with alveolar hypoventilation, the A–a gradient is completely normal (15 mm Hg or less when breathing room air). Patients with ventilation–perfusion imbalance have an A–a gradient that is increased but normalizes when 100% oxygen is administered for at least 20 minutes. A normal A–a gradient is less than 100 mm Hg on 100% oxygen. The arterial PO_2 on 100% oxygen reaches approximately 575 mm Hg. In contrast, a patient with a shunt will also have an increased A–a gradient while breathing room air, but when 100% oxygen is administered the arterial PO_2 falls substantially below 575 mm Hg and the A–a gradient does not normalize. Finally, in the case of a patient with hypoxia resulting from breathing in an environment where the FIO_2 is less than 21%, the PO_2 should correct rapidly when the patient is removed from the environment or supplemental oxygen is delivered.

In general, as discussed previously, a low PO_2 can be improved by supplying supplemental oxygen. Although in this instance the patient's laboratory values correct, the underlying process still remains. It is important to remember that the laboratory correlate of hypoventilation is hypercapnia on the arterial blood gas analysis. If hypercapnia is associated with a low arterial pH (less than 7.35), manual assistance or mechanical ventilation should be considered, regardless of whether the PO_2 corrects with supplemental oxygen.[31]

Use of the Co-oximeter

Routine analysis of an arterial blood gas yields a measured pH, measured PO_2, and measured PCO_2. Ordinarily, the serum HCO_3, base excess, and percent oxygen saturation of hemoglobin are all calculated values. The oxygen saturation is of clinical significance because it usually correlates with the oxygen content of the blood, and thus the oxygen available to the tissues. However, implied in this relationship is a normal amount of functional hemoglobin. Since the oxygen saturation is calculated from the measured PO_2 using the oxyhemoglobin dissociation curve, it represents only the saturation of normal hemoglobin. Thus, in the presence of even a small percentage of abnormal hemoglobin, the calculated oxygen saturation will overestimate the total oxygen content of the blood. For example, a patient with PO_2 of 95 mm Hg has a calculated oxygen saturation of 95%. If this patient also has a 30% methemoglobinemia, only 70% of the total hemoglobin is saturated to 95% and the actual saturation is only 67%. This is clinically important because, as stated above, hemoglobin saturations of less than 90% do not provide adequate oxygen delivery to the tissues. The co-oximeter measures total hemoglobin, oxyhemoglobin, deoxyhemoglobin, carboxyhemoglobin, and methemoglobin spectrophotometrically, as shown in Figure 20–3. The resultant saturation is a measured oxygen saturation of the total hemoglobin by including four common hemoglobin variants, and thus correlates with the total oxygen content of the blood.

The difference between measured and calculated oxygen saturation represents the percentage of abnormal hemoglobin present. This gap is helpful in the diagnosis of methemoglobin and carboxyhemoglobin and useful in assessing the adequacy of therapy for these disorders. Common indications for co-oximetry include cyanosis that is unresponsive to oxygen (methemoglobin), smoke inhalation (carboxyhemoglobin and possibly methemo-

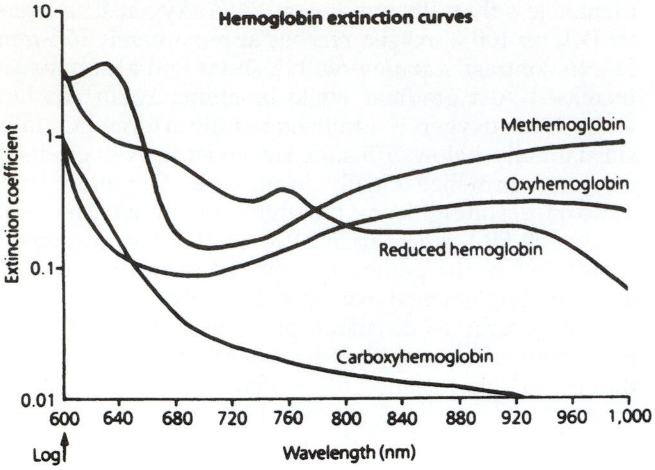

Figure 20–3. Normal and abnormal co-oximetry curves. Transmitted light absorbance spectra are shown for four hemoglobin species: oxyhemoglobin, reduced (deoxy) hemoglobin, carboxyhemoglobin, and methemoglobin. *(Adapted, with permission, from International Anesthesiology Clinics. Boston, Little Brown & Co., 1987; 25(3):138. Tremper KK, Barker SJ: Using pulse oximetry when dyshemoglobin levels are high. J Crit Illness 1988; 3:103–107.)*

globin), and evaluation of therapy for cyanide toxicity (methemoglobin).

Like so many other tools, the co-oximeter is not perfect. Its biggest limitation occurs when dealing with uncommon hemoglobins. Since only four wavelengths of light are used by most co-oximeters, they have the ability to define only four hemoglobin variants. Rare dyshemoglobinemias, such as sulfhemoglobin, are therefore interpreted as one or a combination of the four common hemoglobin variants, giving erroneous results. This phenomenon is commonly noted in neonates, where fetal hemoglobin may be interpreted as carboxyhemoglobin.[92,97] Although this error rarely adds more than 10% to the true carboxyhemoglobin value, this amount may become significant because of the difficulties in assessing the neuropsychiatric status of infants possibly exposed to carbon monoxide. Some newer co-oximeters are not affected by fetal hemoglobin, and should be used in neonatal cases of suspected carbon monoxide poisoning.[93] Additionally, co-oximeters tend to interpret low levels (< 2.5%) of carboxyhemoglobin inconsistently.[59] Fortunately this rarely has clinical implications.

Chest Radiograph

Radiographic detection of a pneumothorax or pneumomediastinum, cardiogenic pulmonary edema, noncardiogenic pulmonary edema, ALI and ARDS, aspiration pneumonitis, or the presence of a foreign body is crucial, but can usually be delayed until the initial evaluation is completed. Confirmation of endotracheal tube placement is necessary but initially can be ascertained by auscultating bilateral breath sounds following compression of a bag valve mask. For patients with occupational disorders, the chest radiograph is essential to confirm and stage exposures to asbestos, silica, coal, and other causes of pneumoconiosis.

Therapeutic Options

Supplemental Oxygen

Supplemental oxygen is indicated for all patients with suspected or confirmed respiratory insufficiency. While it is generally advisable to begin with high flow (12 L/min) via a nonrebreather mask, lower concentrations of oxygen may be used in more stable patients. It is important to remember that a normal saturation on pulse oximetry does not imply that there is no need for supplemental oxygen. This can be determined only after a more complete assessment. Initially there should be little concern over worsening hypercapnia in patients with COPD and respiratory failure, as many of these patients will require intubation for their hypoventilation. If time and the patient's clinical condition permit, an arterial blood gas analysis should be obtained prior to administering supplemental oxygen or mechanical ventilation so that the patient's respiratory status can be adequately defined. In many situations the patient's condition will not permit delay, and subsequent arterial blood gas analyses will be needed to determine the ability to decrease the FIO_2 or the need for intubation. Hyperbaric oxygen is indicated for carbon monoxide poisoning and other exposures (see Antidotes in Depth: Hyperbaric Oxygen).

Additional respiratory support can be offered from a newer techniques. Bilevel positive airway pressure (BiPAP) is well known for its beneficial effects in patients with COPD. Recent work has demonstrated some utility for patients with acute respiratory dysfunction in the emergency department.[71] Although this technique may be useful in overdose patients, it should be considered only a temporizing measure for patients who are expected to recover rapidly, or while preparing for intubation.

Intubation

Once the decision for mechanical ventilation has been made, the route needs to be selected. We prefer oral intubation because it permits the use of a larger endotracheal tube—usually 8 mm or larger—than does nasal intubation. If the patient later needs bronchoscopy, it can be done through the endotracheal tube. Some data suggest that bronchoscopy with bronchoalveolar lavage may have both diagnostic[91] and therapeutic[53,58] implications for poisoned patients. However, in an awake patient, nasotracheal intubation done blindly or with the aid of a flexible fiberoptic laryngoscope may be more easily performed. One advantage of nasotracheal intubation over oral intubation is that orogastric lavage can be performed more easily when the oral cavity is unimpeded. Once the trachea is intubated, the tube should be checked to ensure that it is correctly positioned. If a patient breathing 100% oxygen has a PO_2 of 50 mm Hg, a 50% shunt exists. This may be due to ARDS, but could also result from an endotracheal tube that is in the right mainstem bronchus and a left lung that is not being ventilated.[7] If the left lung is not being ventilated, the arterial blood gas values can be restored to normal simply by pulling the endotracheal tube back above the level of the carina.

All patients who sustain drug overdoses and show signs or symptoms or respiratory insufficiency should have chest radiographs performed. Unfortunately, intubated patients usually have portable radiographs and the carina may be difficult to visualize because of the poor quality of portable radiographs. When seen, the carina is visualized between T-5 and T-7 in most patients. Thus, the tip of the endotracheal tube should be above T-5 for proper (safe) placement. When a portable chest radiograph is obtained, the patient's neck may be extended or flexed, altering the location of the endotracheal tube tip. The tip of the endotracheal tube may move up (with flexion) or down (with extension) by almost 2 cm. It is therefore essential to note the position of the neck during the examination.[7,83,87]

Mechanical Ventilation

Once a patient is intubated for ventilatory support, the respirator mode—assist, control, or intermittent mandatory ventilation (IMV)—is selected. Patients with pure hypoventilation usually require a controlled fixed rate; an arterial blood gas analysis is drawn and the rate adjusted accordingly. Patients with pulmonary parenchymal processes, such as ALI, ARDS, or severe pneumonia, usually do well when placed on either assist or IMV mode. With the IMV mode, a given number of mandatory breaths is administered at the set tidal volume. The patient may take additional breaths without assistance, permitting lower mean airway pressure, which theoretically may reduce the risk of barotrauma and hemodynamic compromise.[39] Although the lower airway pressures associated with IMV are desirable, many authorities recommend the use of the assist mode because it eliminates the patient's work of breathing.[52]

The next decision concerns the FIO_2 that should be provided. A number of formulas have been devised. One approach is to intubate a patient, control breathing, administer 100% oxygen, and decrease to an FIO_2 of less than 50% as quickly as possible in an attempt to prevent oxygen toxicity.[52] Although the toxic effects of oxygen are well known for paraquat (see Chap. 90), evidence suggests that oxygen may be an important mediator of other toxin-induced pulmonary injuries, such as with iron.[41] A PO_2 of 60 mm Hg or a measured oxygen saturation greater than 90% is acceptable, and therefore there is little reason to expose patients to much higher concentrations of oxygen once these conditions have been met. Many clinicians feel more comfortable establishing a "buffer" against deterioration by increasing the PO_2 somewhat above 60 mm Hg, but prolonged exposure to higher values is rarely indicated. The tidal volume should be set at 12–15 mL/kg/breath. If oxygenation cannot be maintained with FIO_2 of 50% or less, PEEP may be used, with careful reassessment of serial arterial blood gas analyses, changes in effective compliance, and hemodynamic data with each increment in PEEP.

Pharmacologic Adjuncts

Only a few pharmacologic agents have a significant place in reversing toxin-induced respiratory dysfunction. Naloxone as discussed above may have the greatest role. Atropine and pralidoxime may be useful for respiratory dysfunction from cholinesterase inhibitors (see Antidotes in Depth: Pralidoxime and Chap. 87). Elapid antivenin and botulism antitoxin are rarely used but may be lifesaving. Neostigmine can reverse muscle weakness from nondepolarizing neuromuscular blocking agents (see Chap. 53). More commonly, clinicians are required to treat bronchospasm from exposure to pulmonary irritants. The use of $beta_2$-selective adrenergic agonist bronchodilators is demonstrated to be effective in these cases.[26] The role of corticosteroids remains controversial. An inhaled solution of 2% sodium bicarbonate may provide symptomatic relief for patients with exposure to hydrogen chloride or chlorine.[15]

Recent investigations suggest a potential role for the use of exogenous nitric oxide in a variety of pulmonary conditions. Specifically, nitric oxide may be useful as a bronchodilator,[10] a means to reverse hypoxic pulmonary vasoconstriction,[2] and as a treatment for ARDS.[1] Because of the difficulties of administering this agent and its potential toxicities (including methemoglobinemia), further research is required before routine administration of nitric oxide can be suggested in even a select subset of disorders.

How Can These Principles Be Applied to Poisoned Patients?

Two 30-year-old patients who overdosed were brought to the ED. Both have ingested substantial amounts of barbiturates and diazepam. An arterial blood gas drawn from patient 1 while he was breathing room air revealed a pH of 7.18, PCO_2 of 70 mm Hg, PO_2 of 50 mm Hg, and a calculated bicarbonate of 24 mEq/L. An arterial blood gas drawn from patient 2, also breathing room air, revealed a pH of 7.31, PCO_2 of 50 mm Hg, PO_2 of 50 mm Hg, and a calculated bicarbonate of 25 mEq/L. Quick analysis showed that patient 1 was hypercapnic with a significant respiratory acidosis. Patient 2 did not appear as ill; his PCO_2 was not very elevated and his pH was not significantly reduced. The A–a gradients are calculated to be 12.5 mm Hg for patient 1 and 37.5 mm Hg for patient 2 (see Fig. 20–4A,B).

The A–a gradient should be no more than one-third of a patient's age.[38] Patient 1 has a normal A–a gradient

A. Arterial PCO_2 approximates alveolar PCO_2 and is substituted as:

$$PAO_2 = PIO_2 - \frac{PCO_2}{R}$$

$$PIO_2 = (FIO_2)(PB - PH_2O)$$

where PAO_2 is alveolar PO_2, PIO_2 is partial pressure of inspired O_2, $PaCO_2$ is arterial PCO_2, and R is the respiratory exchange ratio. Therefore:

$$PAO_2 = [(FIO_2)(PB - PH_2O)] - \frac{PCO_2}{R}$$

where FIO_2 is the inspired O_2 fraction, PH_2O is water vapor pressure, and PB is barometric pressure. On room air at sea level, FIO_2 = 21%. At steady state, R = 0.8. At sea level, PB = 760 mm Hg and PH_2O = 47 mm Hg. Therefore:

$$PAO_2 = [(FIO_2)(PB - PH_2O)] - \frac{PCO_2}{R}$$

$$= [(0.21)(760 - 47)] - \frac{PCO_2}{R}$$

$$= 150 - [(1.25)(PCO_2)]$$

Since the A-a gradient is equal to $PAO_2 - PaO_2$ it can be expressed as:

$$150 - [(1.25)(PCO_2)] - PaO_2 \quad \text{or} \quad 150 - [(1.25)(PCO_2) + PaO_2]$$

A normal A–a gradient is 10–15 mm Hg, but this increases with age. A rough estimate of the normal A–a gradient is one-third the patient's age.

B. Referring to the two overdosed patients above, the A-a gradient for patient 1 is:

$$150 - [(1.25)(70) + 50] = 12.5 \text{ mm Hg}$$

This calculation reveals a normal gradient, indicating that the etiology for hypoxemia and hypoventilation is extrinsic to the lung itself.

In patient 2 the A-a gradient is:

$$150 - [(1.25)(50) + 50] = 37.5 \text{ mm Hg}$$

This abnormally high A-a gradient is consistent with the pneumonia seen on the patient's chest radiograph.

Figure 20–4. (A) Derivation of the definition of alveloar–arterial (A–a) oxygen gradients. **(B)** Using the (A–a) gradients.

(12.5 mm Hg). Therefore, the mechanism for his hypoxemia must be purely alveolar hypoventilation, because that is the only mechanism that does not disrupt gas exchange. The treatment is to reverse the hypoventilation by assisting the patient's ventilation. Mechanical ventilation will reduce the PCO_2, increase the PO_2, and stabilize the patient until he is no longer under the influence of the drugs he has ingested.

Alternatively, the A–a gradient of patient 2 (37.5 mm Hg) is significantly elevated. There are two possible mechanisms for this hypoxemia: ventilation–perfusion mismatch or shunting. To discern which of these two mechanisms is responsible, the patient should be given 100% oxygen. In either case, however, the increased A–a gradient suggests that there is intrinsic pulmonary pathology causing the hypoxemia. On finding an increased A–a gradient, a chest radiograph should be examined for an intrinsic pulmonary cause of the gas exchange abnormality. Patient 2 had a significant right lower lobe infiltrate. He had aspirated and a pneumonia developed, which contributed to his hypoxemia. His treatment, therefore, included antibiotic therapy and respiratory support.

Acknowledgment

Stuart Garay, MD, contributed to this chapter in a previous edition.

References

1. Adnot S, Raffestin B, Eddahibi S: NO in the lung. Respir Physiol 1995;101:109–120.
2. Albertson TE, Walby WF, Allen RP, et al: The pharmacology and toxicology of three new biologic agents used in pulmonary medicine. J Toxicol Clin Toxicol 1995;33: 427–438.
3. Barker SJ, Tremper KK, Hyat J: Effects of methemoglobin on pulse oximetry and mixed venous oximetry. Anesthesiology 1989;70:112–117.
4. Baxter PJ, Kapila, Mfonfu D: Lake Nyos disaster, Cameroon, 1986: The medical effects of large scale emission of carbon dioxide? Br Med J 1989;298:1437–1441.
5. Bernard GB, Artigas A, Brigham KL: The American-European consensus conference on ARDS: Definitions, mechanisms, relevant outcomes, and clinical trial coordination. Am J Respir Care Med 1994;149:818–824.
6. Birrer RB, Calderon J: Pneumothorax, pneumomediastinum, and pneumopericardium following Valsalva's maneuver during marijuana smoking. NY State J Med 1984;84:619–620.
7. Blanc VF, Tremblay NA: The complications of tracheal intubation. Anesth Analg 1974;53:202–212.
8. Book WJ, Abel M, Eisenkraft JB: Adverse effects of depolarising neuromuscular blocking agents: Incidence, prevention and management. Drug Safety 1994;10:331–349.
9. Boyd RE, Brennan PT, Deng JF, et al: Strychnine poisoning: Recovery from profound lactic acidosis, hyperthermia, and rhabdomyolysis. Am J Med 1983;74:507–512.
10. Brett SJ, Evans TW: Nitric oxide: Physiologic roles and therapeutic implications in the lung. Br J Hosp Med 1996; 55:487–490.
11. Bush MN, Rubenstein R, Hoffman I, Bruno MS: Spontaneous pneumomediastinum as a consequence of cocaine use. NY State J Med 1984;84:618–619.
12. Byrne K, Sugarman HJ: Experimental and clinical assessment of lung injury by measurement of extravascular lung water and transcapillary protein flux in ARDS: A review of current techniques. J Surg Res 1988;44:185–203.
13. Caspi J, Klausner JM, Safadi T, et al: Delayed respiratory depression following fentanyl anesthesia for cardiac surgery. Crit Care Med 1988;16:238–240.
14. Cherubin CE: Epidemiology of tetanus in narcotic addicts. NY State J Med 1970;70:267–271.
15. Chisholm CD, Singletary EM, Okerberg CV, et al: Inhaled sodium bicarbonate therapy for chlorine inhalational injuries. Ann Emerg Med 1989;18;466.
16. Christian CM, Waller JL, Moldenhauer CC: Postoperative rigidity following fentanyl anesthesia. Anesthesiology 1983;58:275–277.
17. Cope DK, Grimbert F, Downey JM, Taylor AE: Pulmonary capillary pressure: A review. Crit Care Med 1992;20: 1043–1056.
18. Delaney K, Hoffman RS: Pulmonary infarction associated with crack cocaine use in a previously healthy 23 year old woman. Am J Med 1991;91:92–94.
19. Drach G, Maloney WH: Toxicity of the common houseplant *Dieffenbachia*. JAMA 1963;184:1047.
20. Duberstein JL, Kaufman DM: A clinical study of an epidemic of heroin intoxication and heroin-induced pulmonary edema. Am J Med 1971;51:704–714.
21. Ettinger NA, Albin RJ: A review of the respiratory effects of smoking cocaine. Am J Med 1989;87:664–668.
22. Fassler CA, Rodriguez N, Badesch DB, et al: Magnesium toxicity as a cause of hypotension and hypoventilation: Occurrence in patients with normal renal function. Arch Intern Med 1985;145:1604–1606.
23. Fein A, Grossman RF, Jones JG, et al: Carbon monoxide effect on alveolar epithelium permeability. Chest 1980;78: 726–731.
24. Finley CJ, Silverman MA, Nunez AE: Angiotensin-converting enzyme inhibitor-induced angioedema is unrecognized. Am J Emerg Med 1992;10:550–552.
25. Florez J, McCarthy LE, Borison HL: A comparative study in the cat of the respiratory effects of morphine injected intravenously and into the cerebrospinal fluid. J Pharmacol Exp Ther 1968;163:448–455.
26. Flury KE, Dines DE, Rodarte JR, et al: Airway obstruction due to inhalation of ammonia. Mayo Clin Proc 1983; 53:389–393.
27. Frand UI, Shim CS, Williams MH: Heroin-induced pulmonary edema. Ann Intern Med 1972;77:29–35.
28. Frand UI, Shim CS, Williams MH: Methadone-induced pulmonary edema. Ann Intern Med 1972;76:975–979.
29. Freeth KJ, Kay RLF: The Lake Nyos gas disaster. Nature 1987;325:104–105.
30. Frumkin K, Wright SW: Tube thoracostomy. In: Roberts JR, Hedges JR, eds: Clinical Procedures in Emergency Medicine, 2nd ed. Philadelphia, Saunders, 1991, pp. 128–149.

31. Garay SM: Arterial blood gas analysis and pulmonary testing. In: Flomenbaum N, Goldfrank L, eds: Diagnostic Testing in the Emergency Department. Rockville, MD, Aspen, 1984, pp. 85–103.
32. Gerarde HW: Toxicological studies on hydrocarbons. IX: Aspiration hazard and toxicity of hydrocarbons and hydrocarbon mixtures. Arch Environ Health 1963;6:35–47.
33. Glassroth J, Adams GD, Schnoll S: The impact of substance abuse on the respiratory system. Chest 1987;91: 596–602.
34. Glauser FL, Smith WR, Caldwell A, et al: Ethchlorvynol (Placidyl) induced pulmonary edema. Ann Intern Med 1976;84:46–48.
35. Gordon K: Case report: Freebased cocaine smoking and reactive airway diseases. J Emerg Med 1989;7:145–147.
36. Griffith DE, Levin JL: Respiratory effects of outdoor air polution. Postgrad Med J 1989;86:111–117.
37. Guenter CA: Chest trauma. In: Guenter CA, Welch MH, eds: Pulmonary Medicine, 2nd ed. Philadelphia, Lippincott, 1982, pp. 512–554.
38. Guenter CA: Respiratory function of the lungs and blood. In: Guenter CA, Welch MH, eds: Pulmonary Medicine, 2nd ed. Philadelphia, Lippincott, 1982, pp. 153–191.
39. Hedley-Whyte J, Burgess GE, Feeley TW, Miller MG: Applied Physiology of Respiratory Care. Boston, Little Brown, 1976.
40. Heffner JE, Sahn SA: Salicylate-induced pulmonary edema. Ann Intern Med 1981;95:405–409.
41. Howland MA: Risks of parenteral deferoxamine for acute iron poisoning. J Toxicol Clin Toxicol 1996;34:491–497.
42. Hu H, Fine J, Epstein P, et al: Tear gas: Harassing agent or toxic chemical weapon. JAMA 1989;262:660–663.
43. Humbert VH, Munn NJ, Hawkins RF: Noncardiogenic pulmonary edema complicating massive diltiazem overdose. Chest 1991;99:258–260.
44. Hunter JM: New neuromuscular blocking agents. N Engl J Med 1995;332:691–699.
45. Hussey HH, Katz S: Septic pulmonary infarction. Ann Intern Med 1945;22:526–542.
46. Joseph WL, Fletcher HS, Giordano JM: Pulmonary and cardiovascular implications of drug addiction. Ann Thorac Surg 1973;15:263–274.
47. Katz NM, Buchholz BJ, Howard E, et al: Venovenous extracorporeal membrane oxygenation for noncardiogenic pulmonary edema after coronary bypass surgery. Ann Thorac Surg 1988;46:462–464.
48. King WW, Cave DR: Use of esmolol to control autonomic instability of tetanus. Am J Med 1991;91:425–428.
49. Klein MD: Noncardiogenic pulmonary edema following hydrochlorothiazide ingestion. Ann Emerg Med 1987;116: 901–903.
50. Kling GW, Clark MA, Compton HR, et al: The 1986 Lake Nyos gas disaster in Cameroon, West Africa. Science 1987;236:169–175.
51. Knochel JP: Neuromuscular manifestations of electrolyte disorders. Am J Med 1982;72:521–535.
52. Kollef MH, Schuster DP: The acute respiratory distress syndrome. N Engl J Med 1995;332:27–37.
53. Kulling P: Hospital treatment of victims exposed to combustion products. Toxicol Lett 1992;64–65:283–289.
54. Lam S, Chan-Yeung M: Occupational asthma: Natural history, evaluation and management. In: Rosenstock L, ed: Occupational Medicine: State of the Art Reviews. Philadelphia, Hanley & Belfus, 1987, pp. 373–381.
55. Lambert JR, Byrick RJ, Hammeke MD: Management of acute strychnine poisoning. Can Med Assoc J 1981;124: 1268–1270.
56. Leeman D: The pulmonary circulation in acute lung injury: A review of some recent advances. Int Care Med 1991;17:354–360.
57. Little JW, Smith LH: Pulmonary aspiration. West J Med 1979;131:122–129.
58. Liu D, Olson KR: Smoke inhalation. In: Hoffman RS, Goldfrank LR, eds: Contemporary Management in Critical Care: Critical Care Toxicology. New York, Churchill Livingstone, 1991, pp. 203–224.
59. Mahoney JJ, Vreman HJ, Stevenson DK, Van Kessel AL: Measurement of carboxyhemoglobin and total hemoglobin by five specialized spectrophotometers (co-oximeters) in comparison with reference methods. Clin Chem 1993; 39:1693–1700.
60. Mill CA, Flacke JW, Miller JD, et al: Cardiovascular effects of fentanyl reversed by naloxone at varying arterial carbon dioxide tensions in dogs. Anesth Analg 1988;67: 730–736.
61. Minton NA, Murray SG: A review of organophosphate poisoning. Med Toxicol 1988;3:350–375.
62. Onyeama HP, Oehme FW: A literature review of paraquat toxicity. Vet Hum Toxicol 1984;26:494–502.
63. Osern LN: Simple asphyxiants. In: Rom WN, ed: Environmental and Occupational Medicine. Boston, Little, Brown, 1983, pp. 285–288.
64. Osler W: Edema of the left lung: Morphia poisoning. Mont Gen Hosp Rep 1880;1:291–292.
65. Palat D, Denson M, Sherman M, Matz R: Pneumomediastinum induced by inhalation of alkaloidal cocaine. NY State J Med 1988;88:438–439.
66. Pare JAP, Fraser R, Hogg JC, et al: Pulmonary "mainline" granulomatosis: Talcosis of intravenous methadone abuse. Medicine 1979;58:229–239.
67. Park S, Giammona ST: Toxic effects of tear gas on an infant following prolonged exposure. Am J Dis Child 1972; 123:245–246.
68. Parsons PE: Respiratory failure as a result of drugs, overdoses, and poisonings. Clin Chest Med 1994;15:93–102.
69. Pentiah P, Reilly F, Borison HL: Interactions of morphine sulfate and sodium salicylate on respiration in cats. J Pharmacol Exp Ther 1966;154:110–118.
70. Persky VW, Goldfrank LR: Methadone overdoses in a New York City hospital. J Am Coll Emerg Phys 1976; 5:111–113.
71. Pollack C, Torres MT, Alexander L: Feasability study of the use of bilevel positive airway for respiratory support in the emergency department. Ann Emerg Med 1996;27: 189–192.
72. Pollack M, Dunbar B, Holbrook P, Fields A: Aspiration of activated charcoal and gastric contents. Ann Emerg Med 1981;10:528–529.
73. Reed CR, Glauser FL: Drug-induced noncardiogenic pulmonary edema. Chest 1991;100:1120–1124.

74. Reinhard M, Cuxem G: Pulse oximeters. Med Focus Int 1992;5:36–37.
75. Reynolds KJ, Palayiwa, E, Moyle JTB, et al: The effect of dyshemoglobins on pulse oximetry: Part I, theoretical approach and Part II, experimental results using an in vitro test system. J Clin Monitoring 1993;9:81–90.
76. Richman SR, Harris RD: Acute pulmonary edema associated with librium abuse. Radiology 1972;103:57–58.
77. Rubin RB, Neugarten J: Cocaine-associated asthma. Am J Med 1990;88:438–439.
78. Saba GP, James AE, Johnson BA, et al: Pulmonary complications of narcotic abuse. Am J Roentgenol 1974;122: 733–739.
79. Schmidt-Nowara WW, Samet JM, Rasario PA: Early and late pulmonary complications of botulism. Arch Intern Med 1983;143:451–456.
80. Senanayake N, Karalliede L: Neurotoxic effects of organophosphorous insecticides: An intermediate syndrome. N Engl J Med 1987;316:761–763.
81. Shesser R, Davis D, Edelstein S: Pneumomediastinum and pneumothorax after inhaling alkaloidal cocaine. Ann Emerg Med 1981;10:213–215.
82. Sklar J, Timms RM: Codeine-induced pulmonary edema. Chest 1977;72:230–231.
83. Sladen A: Emergency endotracheal intubation. Chest 1979;75:535–536. Editorial.
84. Stern WZ: Roentgenographic aspects of narcotic addiction. JAMA 1976;236:963–965.
85. Sun KO, Chan YW, Cheung RTF, et al: Management of tetanus: a review of 18 cases. J R Soc Med 1994;87:11–13.
86. Taryle DA, Chandler JE, Good JT Jr, et al: Emergency room intubation: Complications and survival. Chest 1979; 75:541–543.
87. Thadani PV: NIDA conference report on the cardiopulmonary complications of "crack" cocaine use: Clinical manifestations and pathophysiology. Chest 1996;110: 1072–1076.
88. Tremper KK, Barker SJ: Using pulse oximetry when dyshemoglobin levels are high. J Crit Illness 1988;3: 103–107.
89. Trunkey DD: Initial assessment and management. In: The American College of Surgeons Committee on Trauma, eds: Advanced Trauma Life Support Course. Chicago, American College of Surgeons, 1985, pp. 9–30.
90. Vegfors M, Lennmarken C: Carboxyhaemoglobinaemia and pulse oximetry. Br J Anaesth 1991;66:625–626.
91. Vijayan VK, Pandey VP, Sankaran K, et al: Bronchoalveolar lavage study in victims of toxic gas leak at Bhopal. Indian J Med Res 1989;90:407–414.
92. Vreman HJ, Ronquillo RB, Ariagno RL, et al: Interference of fetal hemoglobin with the spectrophotometric measurement of carboxyhemoglobin. Clin Chem 1988;34:975–977.
93. Vreman HJ, Stevenson DK: Carboxyhemoglobin determined in neonatal blood with a co-oximeter unaffected by fetal oxyhemoglobin. Clin Chem 1994;40:1522–1527.
94. Weil JV, McCullough RE, Kline JS, Sodal IE: Diminished ventilatory response to hypoxia and hypercapnia after morphine in normal man. N Engl J Med 1975;292: 1103–1106.
95. Wetherill SF, Guarino MJ, Cox RW: Acute renal failure associated with barium chloride poisoning. Ann Intern Med 1981;95:187–188.
96. Wiener MD, Putman CE: Pain in the chest in a user of cocaine. JAMA 1987;258:2087–2088.
97. Wimberley PD, Siggaard-Anderson O, Fogh-Anderson N: Accurate measurements of hemoglobin oxygen saturation, and fractions of carboxyhemoglobin and methemoglobin in fetal blood using radiometer OSM3: Corrections for fetal hemoglobin fraction and pH. Scan J Clin Lab Invest 1990;50(suppl 203):235–239.
98. Woodard ED, Friedlander B, Lesher RJ, et al: Outbreak of hypersensitivity pneumonitis in an industrial setting. JAMA 1988;259:1965–1969.
99. Zachariades N, Agouridakis P, Parker J: Adult respiratory distress syndrome: A review. J Oral Maxillofac Surg 1993;51:402–407.
100. Zimmerman GA, Clemmer TP: Acute respiratory failure during therapy for salicylate intoxication. Ann Emerg Med 1981;10:104–106.

CHAPTER 21

Cardiovascular Principles

Robert Hessler

Toxins frequently produce deleterious effects on the cardiovascular system. The maintenance of adequate tissue perfusion depends on the volume status and vascular resistance, cardiac contractility, and cardiac rhythm. These components of the hemodynamic system are all vulnerable to the effects of drugs and toxins. Cardiovascular toxicity may therefore be manifested by the development of (1) hypotension or hypertension, (2) congestive heart failure and pulmonary edema, or (3) cardiac conduction abnormalities or dysrhythmias. The presence of these specific cardiovascular abnormalities may be helpful in determining the type of toxic exposure. Even when multiple cardiovascular abnormalities occur, the specific pattern of the anomalies may suggest a particular class or type of drug or toxin.

Mechanisms of Cardiovascular Toxicity

An alteration in hemodynamic functioning may be due to either indirect metabolic effects or to direct effects on the nervous system, heart, or blood vessels. A poisoning may lead to hemodynamic changes secondary to development of acidemia, alkalemia, hypoxia, or electrolyte abnormalities. In these cases, supportive care with ventilation, oxygenation, and fluid and electrolyte repletion will usually improve the cardiovascular status. The cardiovascular abnormalities are frequently due to metabolic changes and are generally not useful in identification of a specific toxic substance.

A drug or toxin may also cause specific hemodynamic abnormalities due to direct effects on the nervous system, heart, or blood vessels. Frequently, these effects are mediated by the autonomic nervous system. Drugs and toxins may (1) interfere with synthesis of neurotransmitters, (2) affect the release of neurotransmitters into the synapse, (3) interfere with the normal degradation of transmitters, (4) mimic neurotransmitters at the postsynaptic receptors, or (5) block the postsynaptic receptors. (A detailed discussion of the normal physiology of neurotransmission, neurotransmitters and receptors, and their interaction with toxins, is found in Chap. 10.)

The parasympathetic nervous system utilizes acetylcholine as the neurotransmitter. Stimulation of the parasympathetic nervous system causes minimal dilation of arterioles and minimal effects on blood pressure. However, the effects on lacrimation, salivation, and diaphoresis, and on the internal organs (including the heart), are more profound. Parasympathetic effects on the heart include decrease in heart rate, contractility, conduction velocity, and development of various degrees of heart block. These effects of cholinomimetic drugs (and of acetylcholine) at the autonomic effector organs are termed muscarinic effects. Other toxins may stimulate or block the nicotinic receptors of the autonomic ganglia and cause hemodynamic changes.

The sympathetic nervous system is primarily responsible for the maintenance of arteriolar resistance and blood pressure. Norepinephrine is the primary neurotransmitter of the sympathetic nervous system. Substances that affect the synthesis or degradation of norepinephrine or interact with adrenergic receptors may have profound effects on blood pressure. The sympathetic receptors are divided into alpha- and beta-adrenergic receptors. The alpha$_1$-adrenergic receptors are located on the postsynaptic membrane and primarily cause constriction of arterioles when stimulated. The alpha$_2$-adrenergic receptors are primarily located on the presynaptic membrane and are "autoregulatory" receptors. Binding of norepinephrine (or an analog drug) to these alpha$_2$-adrenergic receptors decreases the amount of norepinephrine released into the synapse. All beta-adrenergic receptors stimulate adenyl cyclase via interaction with the G_s membrane protein. Activation of adenyl cyclase leads to elevation of cyclic AMP and activation of specific protein kinases (discussed in detail in Chap. 49). The beta$_1$-adrenergic receptors are primarily located in the heart. Stimulation of beta$_1$-adrenergic receptors increases heart rate, contractility, conduction velocity, and automaticity. Beta$_2$-adrenergic receptors are located primarily on smooth muscle (including in the arterioles). Stimulation of beta$_2$-adrenergic receptors relaxes smooth muscle and dilates arterioles. The more recently identified beta$_3$ receptor is located primarily on adipocytes. This receptor plays a role in lipolysis.[46,92] Beta$_3$-adrenergic receptors in the heart may also increase contractility.[169]

A drug's cardiovascular toxicity may also be mediated by effects on the central nervous system (CNS). The peripheral effects of the drug (including hypotension, dysrhythmias, or even pulmonary edema) are caused by effects on the sympathetic and parasympathetic pathways. For example, "centrally acting" antihypertensive medications (eg, clonidine) interact with presynaptic alpha$_2$-adrenergic receptors in cardiovascular centers in the medulla and elsewhere in the CNS. This results in decreased sympathetic outflow from the CNS, decreased peripheral vascular resistance, decreased heart rate, and decreased blood pressure.

Other drugs may exert cardiovascular toxicities through effects on the peripheral nervous system. In particular, the synaptic junctions (with their chemically mediated transmission of the nerve impulse) are particularly vulnerable to drug-induced toxicities. For example, phenylephrine (Neo-Synephrine) interacts with the postsynaptic alpha$_1$-adrenergic receptors of the sympathetic nervous system to produce hypertension. As another example, organophosphate insecticides inhibit the degradative enzyme cholinesterase and cause accumulation of acetylcholine in parasympathetic synapses. This effect on the nerve endings in the sinoatrial (SA) and atrioventricular (AV) nodes of the heart causes bradycardia and heart block.

Hemodynamic compromise can also occur when an ingested substance directly affects the heart or blood vessels. This includes toxins with negative ionotropic properties. An overdose of a calcium channel blocking agent would lead to a decrease in the intracellular calcium concentration and to changes in the transmembrane potential. The resulting hemodynamic effects are decreased myocardial cell contractility (congestive heart failure), decreased conductivity in the electrical system of the heart (heart block), and relaxation of vascular smooth muscle (hypotension).

A toxin that acts directly on the cardiovascular or nervous system may cause a characteristic alteration of blood pressure, heart rate, and cardiac rhythm. Initial therapy is often directed at normalizing life-threatening abnormalities in vital signs. However, the identification of a particular class of drugs or toxins as the causative agent may lead to more specific and appropriate therapy.

Blood Pressure Abnormalities

The majority of agents that affect blood pressure modulate the normal chemical interactions at the postganglionic sympathetic neurons. The interaction between these nerve endings and receptors on blood vessels largely determines the vascular tone and blood pressure. Toxins may initiate complex interactions resulting in hypotension or hypertension. In fact, a single drug can cause either hypotension or hypertension, depending on the dose and time.

Figure 21–1 is a diagram of a postganglionic sympathetic neuron's synapse with a blood vessel. Norepinephrine is synthesized and stored in vesicles in the nerve ending. In response to depolarization of the sympathetic nerve, the vesicles fuse with the cell membrane and norepinephrine is released into the synapse. The norepinephrine may be metabolized by catechol-*O*-methyltransferase (COMT) or monoamine oxidase (MAO), may be actively pumped back into the neuron, or may bind to the postsynaptic alpha$_1$-adrenergic receptors on the blood vessel. Norepinephrine binding to the alpha$_1$-adrenergic receptors causes constriction of the blood vessel. Beta-adrenergic receptors that can bind circulating catecholamines or drugs are also present on the blood vessel. The beta-adrenergic receptors cause dilation of the blood vessel and thus a decrease in blood pressure.

Hypertension

The majority of agents that cause an elevation in blood pressure exert their effects through interaction with the postsynaptic alpha-adrenergic receptors. Indirect-acting agents achieve these effects by increasing the release of norepinephrine storage granules or decreasing the active reuptake of norepinephrine into the presynaptic neuron. These indirect-acting agents cause initial hypertension as the norepinephrine is released into the synapse. However, since the norepinephrine is rapidly depleted from the nerve ending, the blood vessel no longer constricts, and the blood pressure decreases. Thus, indirect-acting agents often cause transient hypertension followed by persistent hypotension. Direct-acting agents either decrease the degradation of norepinephrine or directly interact with the alpha-adrenergic receptors. Direct-acting agents cause more persistent hypertension.

Can the Causative Toxic Agent Be Determined? Table 21–1 lists the drugs and toxins that cause hypertension along with their pharmacologic activities. Physical examination alone will seldom identify the single causative agent in any toxic exposure. However, often a clinical constellation of signs and symptoms can be identified that is associated with a particular class of agents. Nearly all of the agents that cause hypertension are beta-adrenergic receptor agonists, cyclic antidepressants, or sympathomimetic drugs. Physical examination frequently can distinguish between the effects of these three classes of medications (see Table 17–1). Differences among these agents are also seen in the mental status examination. Sympathomimetic agents, including cocaine and amphetamines, rarely cause a depressed mental status but rather cause agitation. The presence of lethargy or coma in a patient suspected of a cocaine or amphetamine overdose should suggest other possible diagnoses, including multiple drug overdose, alternative drug ingestions,

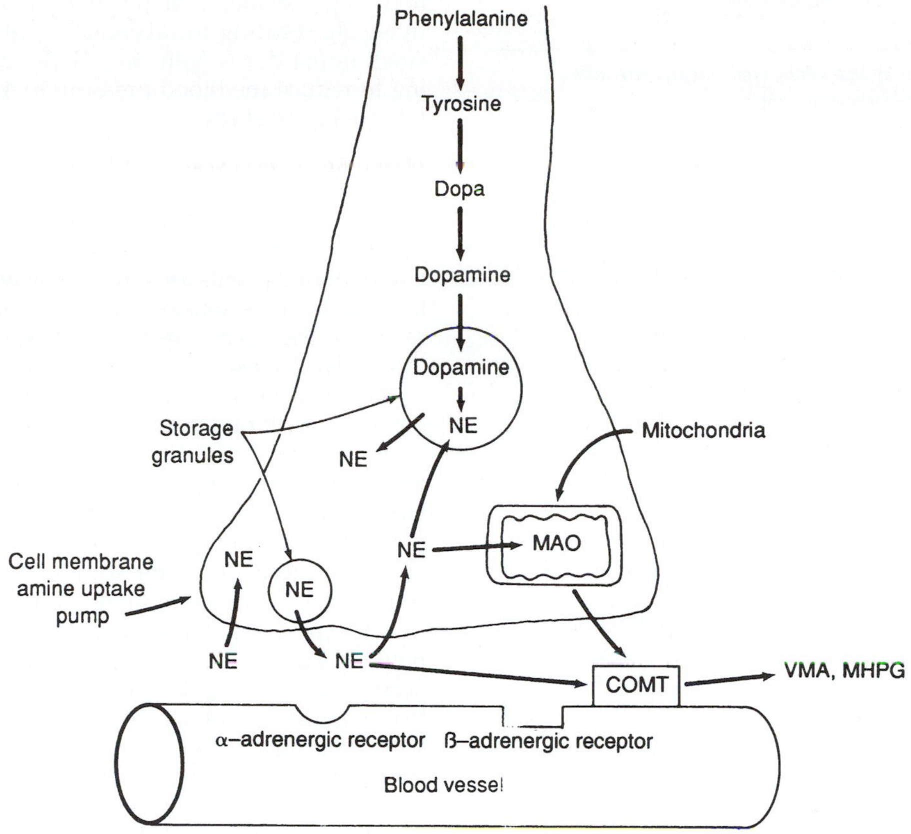

Figure 21–1. Postganglionic sympathetic neuron. Shown is the synthesis storage in granules, release, reuptake, and degradation of norepinephrine (NE). Norepinephrine is synthesized in storage vesicles in the nerve ending. These vesicles fuse with the nerve ending in response to stimulation and release the NE into the synaptic space. The NE then binds to postsynaptic receptors, undergoes active reuptake into the nerve ending, or is metabolized. (MAO = monoamine oxidase; COMT = catechol-*O*-methyltransferase; VMA = 3-methoxy-4-hydroxymandelic acid; MHPG = methoxyhydroxyphenylglycol.)

metabolic disorders, a postictal state, or central nervous system infection or hemorrhage.

In contrast, patients with cyclic antidepressant overdoses often present confused and agitated initially. However, as increasing amounts of the drug are absorbed into the bloodstream and the tissue levels increase, the patient may quickly become lethargic or stuporous. In addition, anticholinergic findings such as mydriasis, urinary retention, flushed skin color, decreased bowel sounds, and dry skin and mucous membranes may suggest cyclic antidepressant overdose.

The pattern of blood pressure elevation may sometimes be helpful in determining the class of agent ingested. Cyclic antidepressants and drugs such as cocaine and amphetamines produce hypertension due to increased release of norepinephrine from the presynaptic vesicles and inhibition of reuptake into the nerve ending. However, the hypertensive effect of a cyclic antidepressant is usually very transient. As the alpha-adrenergic antagonist and the myocardial depressant properties of the drug become more significant, the blood pressure decreases and the patient becomes normotensive or even hypotensive.

Beta-adrenergic receptor agonists may cause hypertension or hypotension, or even relatively normal blood pressure. The result of an overdose depends on the specific agent ingested and the relative action on the various types of beta-adrenergic receptors. Beta$_1$-adrenergic receptors cause lipolysis and cardiac stimulation (increased inotropy and chronotropy), whereas beta$_2$-adrenergic receptors mediate bronchodilation and vasodilation.[84] This would suggest that only agents with a predominant beta$_1$-adrenergic effect could cause hypertension. However, recent work has demonstrated that 10 to 50% of the heart's beta-adrenergic receptors are actually beta$_2$-adrenergic.[20–22,179] Thus, even beta$_2$-adrenergic selective agents may cause increased inotropy and chronotropy. The resulting blood pressure would depend on the relative affinities of the drug for receptors in the heart (increased cardiac output) and the vasculature (decreased peripheral resistance).

Should Toxin-Induced Hypertension Be Treated? Knowledge of the mechanism and duration of a toxin's activity is important for choosing the appropriate antihypertensive agent. First, those indirect acting agents that act only by

TABLE 21–1. DRUGS AND TOXINS THAT COMMONLY CAUSE HYPERTENSION

Hypertensive Effect Mediated by Alpha-Adrenergic Receptor Interaction

- Direct alpha-adrenergic receptor binding agents
  - Epinephrine
  - Norepinephrine (Levophed)
  - Phenylephrine (Neo-Synephrine)
  - Ergotamines
  - Methoxamine (Vasoxyl)
- Indirect-acting alpha-adrenergic agents[a]
  - Amphetamines
  - Bretylium
  - Cocaine
  - Monoamine oxidase inhibitors
  - Phencyclidine
  - Cyclic antidepressants
  - Noncyclic antidepressants
  - Cyclobenzaprine (Flexeril)
  - Yohimbine (Locon)
  - Dexfenfluramine
- Direct- and indirect-acting alpha-adrenergic agents
  - Dopamine
  - Ephedrine
  - Metaraminol (Aramine)
  - Naphazoline (Privine)
  - Oxymetazoline (Afrin)
  - Tetrahydrozoline (Visine)
  - Phenylpropanolamine[a]
  - Pseudoephedrine

Hypertensive Effects Not Mediated by Alpha-Adrenergic Receptor Interaction

- Angiotensin
- Beta-adrenergic receptor agonist agents[b]
  - Nonselective
    - Isoproterenol (Isuprel)
    - Isoxsuprine (Vasodilan)
    - Nylidrin (Arlidin)
  - Relatively $beta_2$-adrenergic receptor selective
    - Albuterol (Proventil, Ventolin)
    - Metaproterenol (Alupent)
    - Terbutaline (Brethine)
- Cholinomimetics[a]
- Nicotine[a]
- Renal toxic agents
- Steroids
- Thromboxane A_2
- Vasopressin

[a]These agents may cause transient hypertension followed by hypotension.
[b]These agents may also cause hypotension.

causing an increase in norepinephrine release and a decrease in reuptake often cause only transient hypertension. The initial hypertension may be followed by norepinephrine depletion and hypotension. Hypertension accompanying overdoses such as cyclic antidepressant or even cocaine frequently requires no specific therapy because the blood pressure often soon normalizes. Treatment may be required if the blood pressure is severely elevated or if the patient experiences cardiac, renal, or neurologic sequelae of the hypertension. Then, a relatively short-acting intravenous agent should be used in small initial doses with careful blood pressure monitoring to reduce the blood pressure to a safe level until the toxic drug effect resolves.

What Is the "Drug of Choice" for Treatment of Toxin-Induced Hypertension? A sedative agent, such as a benzodiazepine, should be used early in the treatment of hypertension due to a sympathomimetic agent such as cocaine. Sedative hypnotic agents are almost always successful in controlling the hypertension (and possible dysrhythmias) by reducing the central sympathetic stimulus[28,41,56] and the catecholamine excess.[75]

Beta-adrenergic antagonists should be avoided in the treatment of hypertension due to any sympathomimetic drug. Sympathomimetic agents interact with the alpha-adrenergic receptors on the peripheral vasculature. Additionally blocking the $beta_2$-adrenergic receptors on these arterioles may lead to "unopposed" alpha-adrenergic receptor stimulation, increased arterial constriction, and increased blood pressure.

The potential for adverse interaction between sympathetic stimulants and beta-adrenergic antagonists has been most thoroughly studied in cocaine intoxication. Beta-adrenergic antagonists have reportedly been used with some clinical success.[53,125,126] However, recent pharmacologic studies have elucidated the potential for adverse reactions. In experimental models of cocaine-induced hemodynamic dysfunction and mortality, propranolol (and other beta-adrenergic antagonists) has been shown to be protective,[40] to have no effect,[152] or to increase mortality.[17,105,139] In the squirrel monkey, propranolol or atenolol potentiated cocaine's hypertensive effects but antagonized the cocaine-mediated increase in heart rate.[135] The reasons for the differences in these experimental results are unclear but may be related to the dose of cocaine or beta-adrenergic antagonist utilized. In a study of the hemodynamic effects of cocaine in dogs, propranolol resulted in an increase in systemic vascular resistance, but the blood pressure did not increase. The dose of cocaine in this study resulted in decreased myocardial contractility and the propranolol further decreased the contractility. The cardiac output and blood pressure decreased.[76]

The exacerbation of hypertension and coronary vasospasm when beta-adrenergic antagonists are administered to cocaine-intoxicated patients probably results from "unopposed" peripheral alpha-adrenergic stimulation.[86] In actual clinical use, propranolol has been shown to potentiate cocaine-induced coronary vasoconstriction.[4] Beta-adrenergic antagonists have resulted in increased hypertension when used in the treatment of clinical cocaine intoxication.[43,120,131] Therefore, labetalol (Normodyne, Trandate), with both alpha- and beta-adrenergic antagonist activity, has been suggested as a theoretically safer medication.[43,51] However, labetalol's alpha-blocking activity is relatively weak. The beta-adrenergic antagonist potency of labetalol is approximately seven times greater than its alpha-antagonist potency. The experimental data in animal models of cocaine toxicity are contradictory and demonstrate either hemodynamic improvement,[19] no hemodynamic effects,[135] decreased mortality,[40] no change in mortality,[153] or increased mortality.[105,139] Labetalol has been used with clinical success in individual cases.[43,51,74] However, treatment of a patient with a pheochromocytoma,[19] unintentional epinephrine overdosage,[88] or cocaine-induced coronary vasoconstriction[16] has resulted in increased hypertension and clinical signs of alpha-adrenergic stimulation. Since clinical experience is limited and clinical deterioration may occur, labetalol should probably be avoided in treatment of sympathomimetic agent toxicity (see Chap. 65).

If the hypertension is not controlled with the use of a sedative agent alone, the safest agents would be either a direct arteriolar-dilating agent (eg, nitroprusside or nitroglycerin) or a pure alpha-adrenergic blocking agent (eg, phentolamine). Clinical experience with calcium channel blocking agents is limited; and contradictory results of their use in experimental animal models have shown the agents to be either protective[153] or harmful.[42]

In the treatment of hypertensive overdoses not involving the peripheral $alpha_1$-adrenergic receptors, beta-adrenergic antagonists may be utilized. In these cases, either esmolol as a continuous infusion or propranolol in 1 mg IV boluses (to a maximum of 8 to 10 mg) could be used. However, either nitroprusside or labetalol would probably be more effective.

Hypotension

An extremely large number of toxins are reported to cause hypotension. Frequently the cause of hypotension is coexisting hypoxia, acidosis, anaphylaxis, volume depletion, or dysrhythmias. In addition, the terminal event in any massive poisoning may be cardiovascular collapse and hypotension.

How Is Hypotension Defined? Typically, hypotension is arbitrarily defined as a systolic blood pressure of less than 90 mm Hg. However, this is not an adequate clinical parameter. Young children (and adults with a small body habitus) may have a normal systolic pressure less than 90 mm Hg (see Chap. 17). Patients with hypothermia have decreased metabolic demands, and a lower blood pressure may be considered "normal" for these patients as well (see Chap. 18). Most importantly, patients with long-standing hypertension may have inadequate tissue perfusion even with systolic pressures greater than 90 mm Hg. These usually hypertensive patients require a higher perfusion pressure due to narrowing of their arteries and arterioles secondary to atherosclerotic disease, arteriolar hypertrophy, or arteriolar smooth muscle constriction (with loss of the normal autoregulatory circulatory mechanisms).

Hypotension is best defined as inadequate tissue perfusion. The clinical assessment of tissue perfusion must be based on the vital signs (pulse pressure), skin color, capillary refill, mental status, urine output and concentration, and acid–base balance. However, frequently a toxin may directly affect one or more of these clinical parameters. In these patients, the clinical assessment of volume and hemodynamic status may be difficult. Measurement of central venous pressure, cardiac filling pressure, cardiac output, systemic vascular resistance, and more precise arterial pressures may be necessary in critically ill patients.

What Is the Pathophysiology of Hypotension? Poor tissue perfusion may result from hypovolemia, decreased peripheral vascular resistance, myocardial depression, or dysrhythmias. A single toxin may exert several effects on the hemodynamic system. Appropriate treatment of the hypotension requires an understanding of the pathophysiologic consequences of the toxic ingestion and the resultant hemodynamic derangement.

The most common mechanism responsible for hypotension in a poisoned patient is intravascular volume depletion. Intravascular volume may decrease due to gastrointestinal, urinary, or insensible losses. Additionally, fluid may redistribute from the intravascular space into the intracellular, interstitial, pleural, or peritoneal spaces ("third spacing" of fluid). Finally, the central venous pressure may be relatively decreased due to venodilation and increased venous capacitance.

Intravascular volume depletion in the poisoned patient most frequently occurs due to gastrointestinal fluid losses. Vomiting and/or diarrhea are extremely common sequela of toxic exposures. Additionally, the management of these exposures also may result in significant fluid losses. For example, syrup of ipecac is frequently used to produce vomiting to remove toxin from the patient's gastrointestinal tract. Unfortunately, this may result in excessive fluid losses without clearly being beneficial for removal of many toxins. Volume depletion can also result from excessive use of cathartic agents (magnesium salts or sorbitol) used with activated charcoal in standard poison management protocols. While a single appropriate dose of a cathartic agent is generally safe, multiple doses are rarely, if ever, indicated and should be given only with careful fluid and electrolyte monitoring.

Table 21–2 lists common toxins that may cause significant intravascular volume depletion.

Insensible fluid losses from the lungs and skin may become significant in poisoning. Massive diaphoresis requiring volume resuscitation frequently occurs after intoxications with cocaine, sympathomimetic agents, and cholinergic agents. Uncoupling of oxidative phosphorylation by salicylate or dinitrophenol poisoning can produce hyperthermia and significant diaphoresis. Pulmonary fluid losses are increased by the increased respiratory rate seen in salicylate and sympathomimetic ingestions and by bronchorrhea associated with cholinergic toxicity.

Intravascular fluid may move into the interstitial and intercellular spaces, leading to hemodynamic compromise. This fluid shift results from cellular membrane damage and capillary disruption or from direct injury to the tissue beds. Toxicologically, this most commonly results from gastrointestinal tract burns from ingestion of agents such as strong acid or alkali, phenol, or iron.

TABLE 21–2. TOXINS THAT CAUSE INTRAVASCULAR VOLUME DEPLETION

Gastrointestinal Losses	Insensible Losses	Urinary Losses	Interstitial Redistribution	Vascular Dilation
Antibiotics	Amphetamines	Diabetes insipidus[a]	Caustics	Alcohols
Arsenic salts	Carbamate insecticides	Diuretics	Crotalid envenomation	Antihypertensives
Carbamate insecticides	Chlorphenoxy herbicides (2-4 D)	Ethanol	Iodine	Anticholinergic agents
Castor bean (ricin)	Cocaine	Lithium	Iron	Calcium channel blockers
Colchicine	Dinitrophenol	Mercury salts	Phenol	Cyclic antidepressants
Cyclopeptide mushroom toxin	Methylxanthines	Methylxanthines	Salicylates	Disulfiram reaction
Disulfiram reaction	Organophosphate insecticides	Salicylates		Diuretics
Iodine	Salicylates	Tetracycline (outdated)		Hydralazine
Iron		Vacor		Iron
Laxatives and cathartics				Methylxanthines
Lithium				Nitrates and nitrites
Mercury salts				Opioids
Methylxanthines				Phenothiazines
Nonsteroidal antiinflammatory drugs				Sedative-hypnotic agents
Opioid withdrawal				
Organophosphate insecticides				
Podophyllin				
Pokeweed (saponins)				
Rosary pea (abrin)				
Zinc phosphate				

[a]See Chapter 15 for toxins causing diabetes insipidus.

Adapted and modified from Bania T, Hoffman R: Management of hemodynamic compromise in the poisoned patient. In: Hoffman RS, Goldfrank LR, eds: Contemporary Management in Critical Care. *New York, Churchill Livingstone, 1991, pp. 181–183.*

Increased urinary losses may occur by several toxic mechanisms. These include osmotic diuresis from an obligate solute load (salicylates, Vacor-induced diabetes), direct effects on the renal tubules (diuretics, mercury salts), increased glomerular filtration (inotropic agents), and development of diabetes insipidus (lithium). (Table 15–6 includes information on toxin-induced diabetes insipidus.)

Hypotension may also be caused by toxins that affect the venous tone. These agents result in an increase in venous capacitance, decrease in the venous pressure, and relative hypovolemia. The effects may be mediated via central effects on the sympathetic nervous system or direct effects on the peripheral vasculature. Sedative-hypnotic agents and central alpha$_2$-adrenergic agonists (eg, clonidine) decrease the central sympathetic outflow. The decrease in venous tone and peripheral vascular resistance may result in hypotension. Other toxins block peripheral alpha$_1$-adrenergic receptors or stimulate beta$_2$-adrenergic receptors to produce vascular smooth muscle relaxation and venodilation. Cyclic antidepressants, phenothiazines, theophylline, and cocaine may also deplete catecholamines in the presynaptic nerve endings. Other agents, such as nitrites, nitrates, and ethanol, may act as direct vasodilators and cause hypotension.

Assessment of Volume Status in the Poisoned Patient. Assessment of volume status may be particularly difficult in the patient with a toxic exposure. The usual signs of dehydration include dry mucous membranes, dry skin, low blood pressure, tachycardia, narrowed pulse pressure, clouded sensorium, and decreased urine output. Unfortunately, various toxins can mimic any of these clinical findings in a euvolemic poisoned patient (see Table 17–1). Moreover, hypovolemic patients may present with diaphoresis, flushed skin, hypertension, bradycardia, or increased urine output due to the effects of a toxic ingestion. This is particularly of concern in sympathomimetic agent or cocaine ingestions, where inadequate initial fluid resuscitation may contribute to an eventual adverse outcome.

A central venous or pulmonary artery pressure catheter may be required in some critically ill patients. But in most cases, clinical assessment of central venous pressures is adequate. The patient's upper body should be placed at the best degree of trunk elevation for visualization of the neck veins. The position of the top of the venous column of blood is noted. The vertical distance from the top of this column to a point on the midaxillary line directly posterior to the fourth anterior interspace (the approximate location of the center of the right atrium) is estimated.[175] This distance corresponds to the central venous pressure. Alternatively, the vertical distance from the top of the blood column in the neck vein to the sternal angle is determined. The sternal angle in the average patient is approximately 5 cm above the center of the right atrium. Therefore, the central venous pressure can be estimated simply by adding 5 cm to the vertical height of the venous blood column above the sternal angle.[18]

Orthostatic Hypotension from Toxins. Even with a 30% or greater volume loss, the supine blood pressure may remain normal in young, previously healthy patients. Additional information about the adequacy of the patient's volume status may be obtained by orthostatic vital sign testing. Normally, the cardiovascular system responds to sitting or standing with vasoconstriction and a slight increase in heart rate. Patients with hypovolemia will be unable to maintain adequate intravascular pressure when upright and will have either an exaggerated increase in heart rate or a drop in blood pressure. Toxins may also prevent adequate vasoconstriction or heart rate increase, resulting in "positive" orthostatic vital sign testing.

The approach to orthostatic vital sign testing and interpretation of the results has not been standardized. Table 21–3 describes a generally accepted approach for testing orthostatic vital sign changes.[94,174]

A variety of toxins can produce orthostatic blood pressure changes (Table 21–4).[94,174] Volume depletion is the most common cause of toxin-induced orthostatic vital sign changes. However, other toxins may prevent an adequate vasoconstrictor response, or may block the normal slight heart rate increase. In these cases, cardiac output and blood pressure decrease when the patient is upright.

Can the Toxic Agent Causing Hypotension Be Determined? Identification of a specific toxin causing hypotension in an overdosed or poisoned patient requires the integration of a detailed history, complete physical examination, and laboratory studies. The presence of volume depletion or orthostatic vital sign changes may be helpful. Other substances may produce a classic toxicologic syndrome (toxidrome).

Some medications exert their toxic hypotensive effects simply as their therapeutic effects are carried to an excessive degree. For example, the beta-adrenergic antagonists cause decreased contractility and decreased heart rate with a resultant drop in cardiac output and blood pressure. The calcium channel blocking agents cause decreased contractility, decreased heart rate, and arterial dilation.

Opioids and Sedative-Hypnotic Agents. The cardiovascular changes that occur with an overdose of an opioid or a sedative-hypnotic agent (not including antihistamines or other anticholinergic medications) are remarkably similar. The sedative-hypnotic agents include such structurally diverse compounds as benzodiazepines, barbiturates, ethanol, ethchlorvynol (Placidyl), chloral hydrate, meprobamate (Miltown), and glutethimide (Doriden). CNS depression is probably the common action of these drugs, and also accounts for most of their hypotensive effects. Sedation results in a paralysis of neurocardiovascular regulation with a marked decrease in sympathetic impulses to the heart and peripheral vasculature. The heart rate decreases, cardiac contractility decreases, peripheral vasculature dilates, and hypotension results. In addition, some of these medications have mild direct effects on cardiac contractility, further contributing to the decreased blood pressure.

In addition to their sedative effects, opioids have two activities that may increase their potential to produce hypotension. First, opioids act directly on local vasculature to increase venous capacitance. This property is useful in the treatment of congestive heart failure, but potentiates the hypotensive effects of opioids. Second, opioids induce vagal stimulation. This blocks the reflex sympathetic stimulation of the heart rate that would normally occur as a result of hypotension. Thus, a hemodynamically inappropriate bradycardia will frequently accompany the low blood pressure. The bradycardia

TABLE 21–4. TOXINS THAT CAUSE ORTHOSTATIC HYPOTENSION

Antihypertensives	***Antidepressants***
Adrenergic antagonists	Cyclic antidepressants
Guanethidine	MAO inhibitors
Bretylium	
Angiotensin-converting enzyme inhibitors	***Antiparkinson Agents***
	Bromocriptine
Central alpha$_2$-adrenergic antagonists	L-dopa
	Pergolide mesylate
Alpha-methyldopa	
Clonidine	***Diuretics***
Guanabenz	Thiazides
Guanfacine	Loop diuretics
Ganglionic blockers	
Trimethaphan	***CNS Depressants***
Miscellaneous	Ethanol
Reserpine	Opioids
Peripheral alpha$_1$-adrenergic antagonists	Sedative-hypnotics
Prazosin	***Neuroleptics (Antipsychotics)***
Phenoxybenzamine	Phenothiazines
Vasodilators	Butyrophenones
Hydralazine	
Nitrates	***Toxins Causing Volume Depletion***
	See Table 21–2
Antianginals	
Beta-adrenergic antagonists	
Calcium channel blockers	

TABLE 21–3. ORTHOSTATIC VITAL SIGNS ("TILT" TESTING)

1. After the patient is supine for 2 minutes, determine the blood pressure and pulse rate.
2. Stand the patient *for at least 1 minute* and determine the blood pressure and pulse rate again and observe for any orthostatic symptoms, such as dizziness or lightheadedness. If it is impossible for the patient to stand, have the patient sit up with feet dangling *for at least 2 minutes* before determining vital signs.

The test is positive if any *one* of the following is true:

- Systolic blood pressure decreases ≥ 20 mm Hg
- Diastolic blood pressure decreases ≥ 10 mm Hg
- Pulse increases ≥ 10 beats/min
- Development of clinical symptoms of hypovolemia (dizziness, syncope, lightheadedness)

Significance of a positive test: 10–15 mL/kg volume loss.

Adapted and modified from Williams T, Knopp R: The clinical use of orthostatic vital signs. In: Roberts JR, Hedges JR, eds: Clinical Procedures in Emergency Medicine. Philadelphia, Saunders, 1991, p. 445.

results from specific interaction of opioids with μ_2 opioid receptors in the brain,[63,111,122] resulting in vagal afferent-mediated cardiovascular effects.

The physical findings associated with either an opioid or a sedative-hypnotic overdose are remarkably similar. Patients present with a depressed mental status, ranging from lethargic to obtunded to comatose. Moreover, either drug overdose can cause hypotension, decreased respirations, and small reactive pupils. Fortunately, the initial management of patients with both classes of overdoses is identical and consists largely of supportive measures. The administration of naloxone (Narcan) would seem to be a diagnostic and possibly therapeutic measure. The sedative, respiratory, and cardiovascular effects of opioids can be completely reversed by the antagonist effect of naloxone (see Antidotes in Depth: Opioid Antagonists).

Often the identification of the toxin responsible for hypotension is based on other physical findings associated with the drug. Some toxins that produce hypotension also exert specific cardiac effects that may help identify them as the causative agent (Table 21–5). The various medications may be separated into groups depending on their effects on the heart rate and the ECG. The presence of cardiac conduction abnormalities or dysrhythmias could implicate a particular class or group of medications. Likewise, the absence of specific pulse or ECG changes may help exclude a particular agent as the cause for the hypotension (although not completely eliminating the possibility). However, although Table 21–5 lists the most common ECG manifestations associated with particular toxins, individual toxins in specific cases may demonstrate different heart rate or ECG findings.

Chloroquine and quinine ingestions demonstrate the QRS prolongation and cardiac conduction defects seen with membrane-stabilizing agents. However, these agents also may cause depressed mental status, hypokalemia, an ill-defined cardiovascular collapse, cardiac arrest, and apnea.[99] Mortality seems to be associated with ingestion of greater than 5 g, hypotension, or prolongation of the QRS. Toxicity usually occurs within 6 to 8 hours of ingestion, but may rarely be delayed.[14] The recommended therapy is mechanical ventilation, aggressive supportive care, diazepam,[34,119] and epinephrine or amrinone for inotropic support.[31,32,58,99] Administration of thiopental was temporally associated with cardiac arrest in 7 patients, probably due to additive vasodilatory and negative ionotropic effects.[32]

TABLE 21–5. HEART RATE AND ECG ABNORMALITIES OF DRUGS THAT CAUSE HYPOTENSION

	Characteristic ECG Abnormalities[a]		
Heart Rate	***No Change***	***Heart Block or Prolonged Intervals***	***Dysrhythmias***
Bradycardia	Alpha$_1$-adrenergic antagonists	Beta-adrenergic antagonists	Digoxin
	Alpha$_2$-adrenergic agonists	Calcium channel blockers	Propafenone
	Ciguatera	Cholinomimetic agents	Propoxyphene
	Misoprostol	Magnesium	Sotalol
	Opioids	Propafenone	
	Plant toxins (Table 77–4)	Sotalol	Aconitine
	Andromedotoxin		
	Veratrine		
	Sedative hypnotics		
	Vancomycin		
Tachycardia	ACE inhibitors	Anticholinergic agents	Anticholinergic agents
	Arsenic	Antidysrhythmic agents	Antidysrhythmic agents
	Arterial dilators	Antihistamines	Antihistamines
	Belladonna alkaloids	Cocaine	Arsenic
	Buproprion	Cyclic antidepressants	Chloral hydrate
	Cocaine	Digoxin	Cocaine
	Cyclic antidepressants	Phenothiazines	Cyclic antidepressants
	Disulfiram		Methylxanthines
	Diuretics		Noncyclic antidepressants
	Ganglionic blockers		Phenothiazines
	Iron		Stonefish venom
	Noncyclic antidepressants		Sympathomimetics
	Sedative-hypnotics (rare)		
	Stonefish venom		
	Yohimbine		

[a]The toxic ingestion of an agent does not always produce the characteristic ECG changes.

Treatment of Drug-Induced Hypotension. As with any significant abnormality in vital signs, hypotension must often be treated before the exact cause is known. The history, physical examination, laboratory evaluation, and treatment must proceed concomitantly. Treatment may include removal of the toxic agent from the gastrointestinal tract with orogastric lavage and activated charcoal (if effective for the particular toxin) and supportive care. Diagnostic studies should include an arterial blood gas analysis, determinations of serum electrolytes and hematocrit, cardiac monitoring and a 12-lead ECG, chest radiography, and appropriate blood and urine toxicologic studies. If possible, orthostatic vital signs should be determined. A central venous pressure measurement may be useful in patients whose neck veins cannot be visualized. Patients who do not respond to clinical management may require insertion of a pulmonary artery catheter for accurate determination of cardiac filling pressures and cardiac output.

As shown in Figure 21–2, an algorithm for the management of toxin-induced hypotension usually proceeds with the administration of intravenous fluids. However, in patients who have evidence of fluid overload or congestive heart failure, a vasopressor agent should be administered while further diagnostic studies are performed. A chest radiograph or measurement of pulmonary artery pressures may determine that the hypotension is not directly related to a toxin. For patients with distended neck veins, other diagnoses must be carefully considered, such as congestive heart failure (possibly related to the drug), myocardial infarction, cardiac tamponade, pulmonary embolism, tension pneumothorax, and valvular heart disease.

Which Vasopressor Agent Should Be Used for a Poisoned Patient? In general, if the precise toxin is unknown and if the hypotension is not responsive to fluid infusion and other measures, a vasopressor must be used. The first choice of vasopressor agent in this situation is either norepinephrine (Levophed) or phenylephrine (Neo-Synephrine). Choosing the most appropriate vasopressor requires an

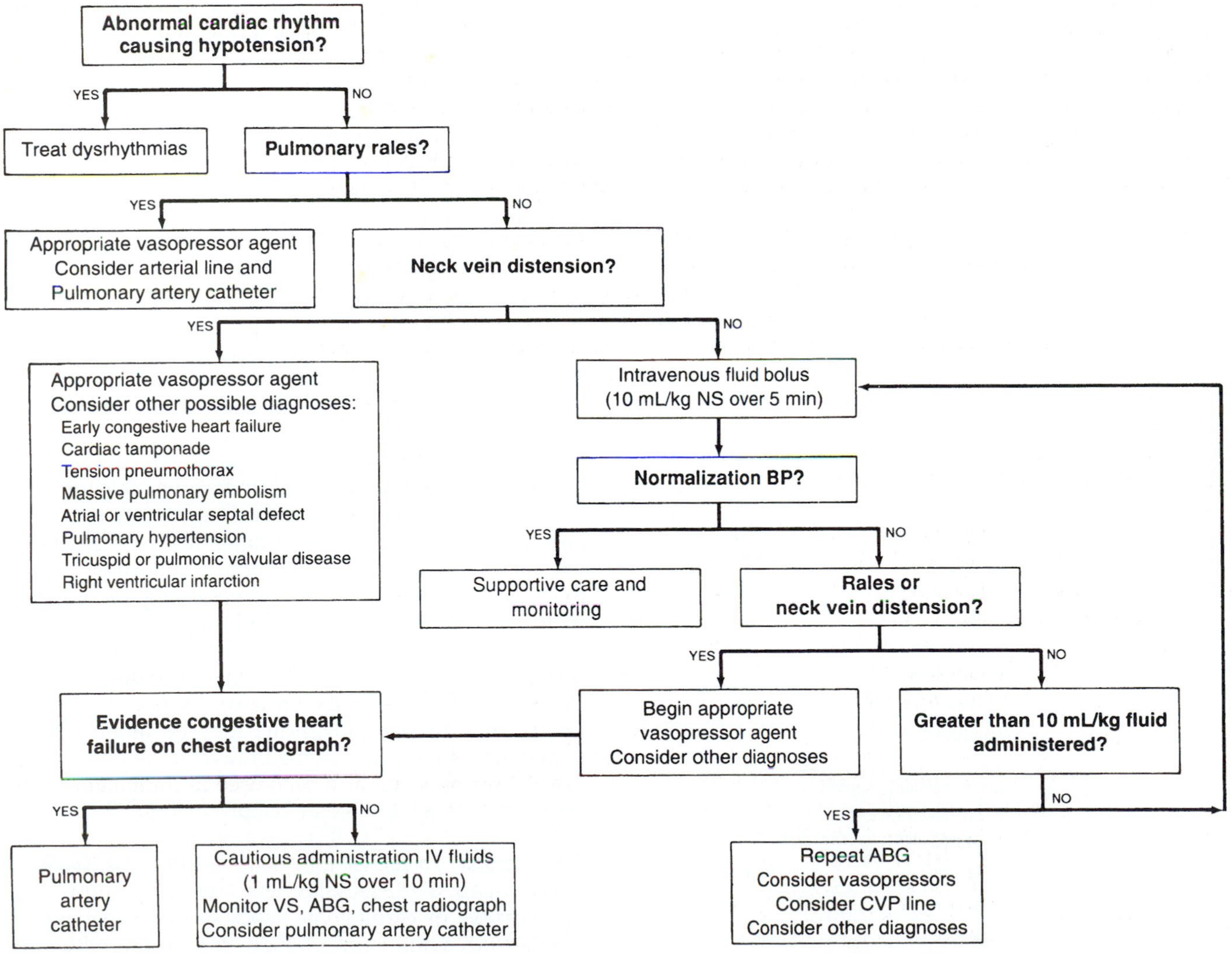

Figure 21–2. Management of drug-induced hypotension.

understanding of the physiologic mechanisms causing the decrease in blood pressure. In cyclic antidepressant or phenothiazine toxicity, dopamine may be ineffective or may cause clinical deterioration. However, in other overdoses (Table 21–6), dopamine is the vasopressor of choice, because at low doses it preserves renal and gastrointestinal circulation via specific dopamine vasodilatory receptors in these organs.

Cyclic Antidepressants, Phenothiazines, and Cocaine. Norepinephrine or phenylephrine should be used to treat persistent hypotension in overdose of drugs with alpha-adrenergic antagonist effects (eg, cyclic antidepressants, phenothiazines, or $alpha_1$-adrenergic receptor antagonists such as prazosin or phenoxybenzamine). Dopamine may be less efficacious and may have adverse effects. Dopamine, an indirect-acting agent, is dependent on stimulating the endogenous release of norepinephrine from the presynaptic nerve ending vesicles. When norepinephrine stores are depleted, dopamine may be relatively ineffective in the treatment of hypotension. In addition, the beta-adrenergic stimulatory effects of dopamine may predominate and lead to dysrhythmias and worsening of the hypotension (due to peripheral beta-adrenergic receptor-mediated vasodilatation).[1,7,24]

Beta-Adrenergic Antagonists. Logic would suggest that a beta-adrenergic receptor-stimulating drug (such as isoproterenol) might be the antidote for a beta-adrenergic antagonist overdose. However, isoproterenol stimulates the arterial $beta_2$-adrenergic receptors and may decrease the blood pressure. For this reason, a vasopressor with both alpha- and beta-adrenergic stimulating properties is a safer choice. Epinephrine has greater beta-adrenergic stimulant properties than dopamine and would be the preferred vasopressor. Dopamine or norepinephrine could also be used in combination with a beta-adrenergic stimulating drug such as isoproterenol or dobutamine. Glucagon is the most effective antidote and should be given first.[52,71,72,81,115,127,149,164] Glucagon presumably works by circumventing the beta-adrenergic antagonist agent-induced decrease in intracellular cAMP.[52,167] An initial bolus of 3 to 10 mg IV should be given immediately and, if effective, a continuous infusion of 2 to 5 mg/h is required (see Antidotes in Depth: Glucagon).

Amrinone may also be an effective treatment for the cardiovascular toxicity of beta-adrenergic antagonists and other toxins. Amrinone is a phosphodiesterase inhibitor and probably exerts at least some of its inotropic activity by increasing intracellular cAMP and by enhancing calcium movement into the cell. In a canine model, amrinone significantly increased inotropy, stroke volume, and cardiac output.[93] However, amrinone does not reverse the heart rate depression caused by beta-adrenergic antagonists, such as propranolol. Therefore, it probably should be used together with either glucagon or a chronotropic agent. In a case of chloroquine poisoning, the addition of amrinone successfully treated cardiogenic shock that was refractory to epinephrine, dopamine, and bicarbonate.[58] Patients with severe verapamil poisoning who do not respond to calcium and catecholamines may responded to the addition of amrinone or isoproterenol.[53,82] However, amrinone has significant vasodilatory properties and may result in worsening of hypotension. Therefore, until there is further clinical experience in toxin exposures, amrinone should only be used with caution in poisoned patients, and only in combination with appropriate additional chronotropic and vasopressor medications.

TABLE 21–6. AGENTS USEFUL IN THE TREATMENT OF HYPOTENSION

Toxic Ingestion	Suggested Vasopressor Agent (in order of choice)[a]	Specific Indicated Therapy
Beta-adrenergic antagonist	Epinephrine Dopamine Dobutamine Isoproterenol	Glucagon Amrinone
Calcium channel blocker	Dopamine Dobutamine Isoproterenol	Calcium Glucagon Amrinone
Clonidine	Dopamine	Naloxone
$Alpha_1$-adrenergic antagonist or phenothiazine	Avoid dopamine Norepinephrine (Levophed) Phenylephrine (Neo-Synephrine)	
Cyclic antidepressants	Avoid dopamine Norepinephrine (Levophed) Phenylephrine (Neo-Synephrine)	Sodium bicarbonate
Cholinomimetic agents	Dopamine	Atropine
Opioids	Dopamine	Naloxone
Magnesium	Dopamine	Calcium

[a]Norepinephrine (Levophed) or phenylephrine (Neo-Synephrine) should be used as a pressor agent if the patient does not rapidly respond to one of the other vasopressor agents.

Calcium Channel Blocking Agents. Intravenous calcium gluconate or calcium chloride has been shown to reverse the negative inotropic effect of verapamil.[4,26,39,50,100,103] However, the atrioventricular conduction abnormalities and bradycardic effects of verapamil poisoning are only partially reversed by calcium.[59,121] Glucagon has also been used for calcium channel blocker overdose, in combination with calcium.[4,112,121,144] Atropine is seldom effective for treatment of the bradycardia or AV nodal block.[69,121] Epinephrine or norepinephrine may be more effective than dopamine for improving bradycardia and hypotension.[65] Amrinone has also been used in combination with calcium, catecholamines, and isoproterenol.[53,82]

CPR, Temporary Pacemaker, Intra-aortic Balloon Pump, Cardiopulmonary Bypass. Patients with hemodynamic compromise, bradycardia, or cardiogenic shock must receive aggressive hemodynamic support. Patients whose condition results from drug toxicity have a potentially completely reversible process. Every effort should be made to support the patient's hemodynamic status until the toxin can either be removed or metabolized. If the patient is bradycardic, a pacemaker may be indicated.[2,97,142,166] Patients have recovered completely even after prolonged CPR.[2,85] Extracorporeal membrane oxygenation[54,173] or an intraaortic balloon pump can support life while specific therapy directed at the toxin is instituted.[24,35,48,64,85] In cases of severe cardiogenic shock or electromechanical dissociation, cardiopulmonary bypass[64,166] may sustain life until the toxin can be degraded by the normal metabolic pathways or removed by hemodialysis, hemofiltration, or the use of activated charcoal in the gastrointestinal tract.

Congestive Heart Failure

Toxins may produce cardiogenic or noncardiogenic pulmonary edema. In noncardiogenic pulmonary edema there is increased intraalveolar fluid in the lungs despite a normal cardiac output. The fluid, hypoxia, rales, and chest radiograph abnormalities result from increased permeability of the alveolar and capillary basement membrane. Proteinaceous fluid leaks from the capillaries into the alveoli and interstitium of the lung. Noncardiogenic pulmonary edema results from exposure to solvents, salicylates, sedative-hypnotics, stimulants, nonsteroidal antiinflammatory agents, and opioids. (The mechanisms, etiologic agents, and treatment of noncardiogenic pulmonary edema are discussed in Chap. 20.)

Cardiogenic pulmonary edema occurs as a result of the toxin's direct effects on the contractility (inotropy) of the heart. Acute cardiogenic pulmonary edema, resulting from a decreased cardiac output, occurs primarily in patients with calcium channel blocking agent or beta-adrenergic receptor antagonist overdoses. Other agents that can exert depressant effects on cardiac contractility include antihistamines, phenothiazines, antidysrhythmics, anticholinergics, and anesthetics. Pulmonary edema may also result from the ingestion of large quantities of sodium-containing drugs (eg, sodium penicillin) or as a late consequence of drugs that cause renal failure. In addition, chronic exposure to some chemotherapeutic agents (eg, doxorubicin [Adriamycin]) and other drugs (eg, ethanol) may result in long-term cardiac toxicities.

What Diagnostic Tests Are Useful?

The treatments for cardiogenic and noncardiogenic pulmonary edema ultimately differ, and therefore an accurate diagnosis is essential. Most diagnostic tests will not be helpful in differentiating between these two conditions. Arterial blood gas analysis demonstrates hypoxia and the chest radiograph shows perihilar, basilar, or diffuse alveolar infiltrates. The presence of "vascular redistribution" on the chest radiograph is highly suggestive of a cardiogenic etiology, but this is a somewhat nonspecific sign and may not always be seen. Normal heart size on chest radiograph is also not helpful in differentiating between etiologies, but an enlarged heart develops only with chronic causes of congestive heart failure. In acute toxicity the heart is normal in size but does not contract normally (see Chap. 20).

How Should Acute Cardiogenic Pulmonary Edema Be Treated in the Poisoned Patient?

In general, initial management of toxin-induced cardiogenic pulmonary edema is identical to that in pulmonary edema of purely cardiac origin (eg, valvular or ischemic heart disease). The treatment modalities include agents to decrease preload and afterload and to increase cardiac output.

Three unique factors must be considered in the treatment of toxin-induced pulmonary edema. First, interactions between the toxin and therapeutic agents (especially inotropic agents) may occur. Second, drugs that precipitate cardiogenic edema (eg, calcium channel blocking agents and antihistamines) may also cause noncardiogenic pulmonary edema.[17,69,70] And third, early aggressive or invasive diagnostic and therapeutic interventions may be necessary.

Patients with toxin-induced congestive heart failure or cardiogenic shock must receive aggressive hemodynamic support. Patients with cardiac disease and resultant pulmonary edema may have underlying structural or intrinsic myocardial abnormalities that are frequently irreversible. However, acutely toxic patients have a potentially completely reversible process. Every effort must be made to support the patient's vital signs until the toxin can be removed or metabolized.

Cardiac Dysrhythmias and Conduction Abnormalities

Toxins may produce adverse effects on the electrical activity of the heart. These effects may be mediated by the sympathetic and parasympathetic nervous system, or the toxin may act directly on the myocardial conduction system or other myocardial cells. Metabolic abnormalities (especially acidemia, hypotension, hypoxia, and electrolyte abnormalities) may further exacerbate the toxicity or may be the sole cause of the cardiovascular abnormalities. Therefore, correction of metabolic abnormalities must be a high priority in the treatment of patients with drug toxicity.

The terminal phase of serious drug ingestions may include nonspecific hemodynamic abnormalities and cardiac dysrhythmias. However, many substances directly or primarily affect cardiac rhythm or conduction.

Mechanisms for Conduction Abnormalities and Dysrhythmias

Drugs that cause dysrhythmias or cardiac conduction abnormalities usually affect the myocardial cell membrane. They may act indirectly via the nervous system or directly on the myocardial cells, but the final result is an alteration in the functioning of the cellular membrane. The spontaneous generation of a normal or abnormal rhythm, and the conduction of the rhythm within the heart, depends on the maintenance of appropriate transmembrane potentials.

In most cases, the underlying mechanism responsible for a drug's toxicity is unknown. For some medications, such as calcium channel blocking agents and some antidysrhythmic agents, the toxicity appears to result from the same mechanism as their therapeutic effects. For other toxins, the mechanism seems to be an entirely unrelated effect on the cellular electrophysiology.

To understand the toxicity of drugs and to plan appropriate therapy, an understanding of the basic electrophysiology of the myocardial cell is essential. Figure 21–3 shows a typical action potential of myocardial cell depolarization, the electrolyte fluxes responsible for the action potential, and the resulting ECG complex. The action potential is divided into five phases: phase 0, depolarization; phase 1, overshoot; phase 2, plateau; phase 3, repolarization; and phase 4, resting. When the cell is excited (by stimulus from another cell or by spontaneous depolarization), selective channels in the membrane open, allowing sodium to enter the cell. During phase 1, these sodium channels begin to close, and the change in membrane potential opens specific calcium channels. During phase 2, the inward depolarizing calcium current is balanced by an outward repolarizing potassium current. The outward potassium currents are termed "delayed rectifier" currents. The current through the delayed rectifier channels increases and the inward calcium current decreases at the end of phase 2. Phase 3 occurs as the permeability of the membrane to sodium (Na^+) and potassium (K^+) returns to resting levels. Phase 4 is a resting state, with active transport of sodium, potassium, and calcium to reestablish the "predepolarization" concentrations and membrane potential. In pacemaker cells during phase 4, changes in potassium and sodium channels lead to a spontaneous, gradual increase in the resting potential and eventual spontaneous depolarization. Recent electrophysiologic studies of individual ion chan-

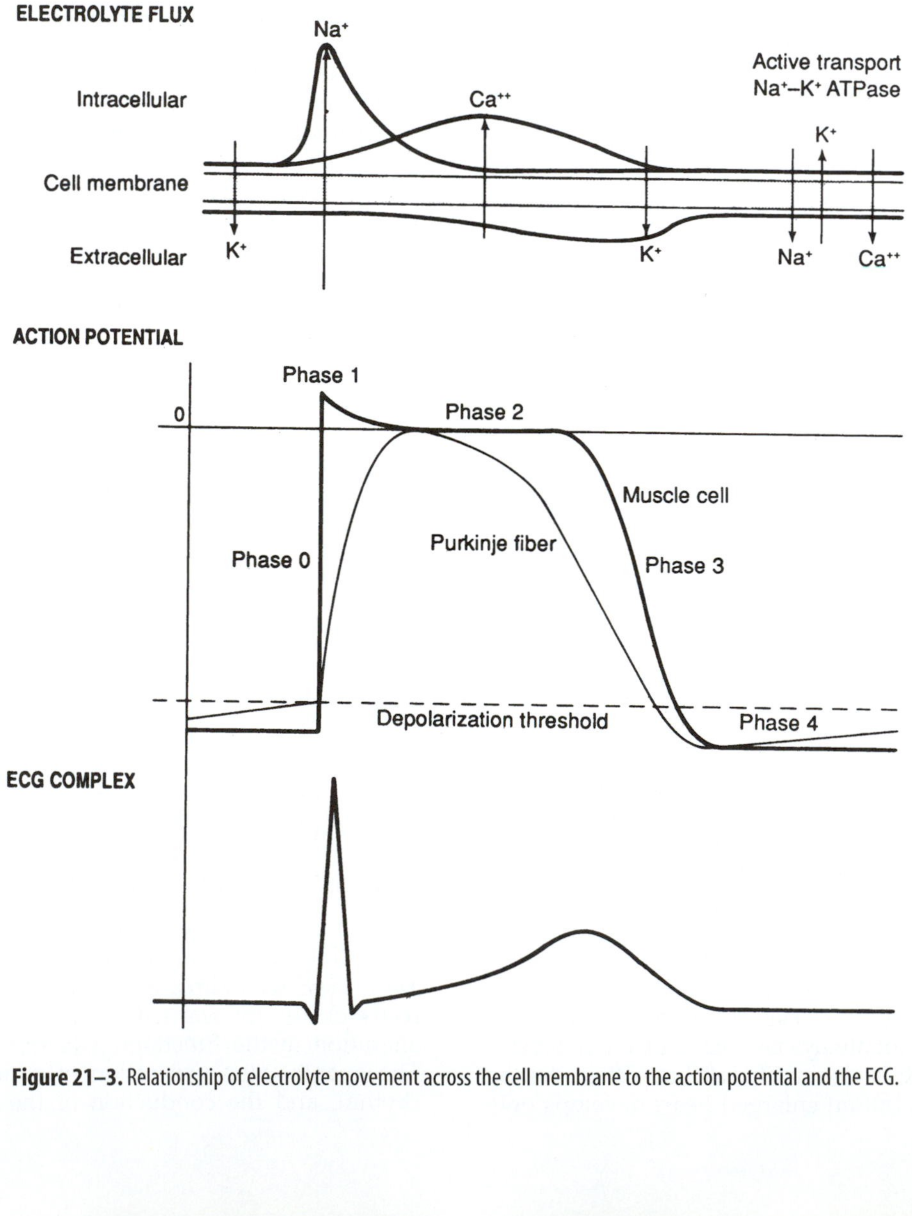

Figure 21–3. Relationship of electrolyte movement across the cell membrane to the action potential and the ECG.

nels have identified multiple subtypes of the sodium, potassium, and calcium channels.[128]

During phases 0 to 2, the cell cannot be depolarized again with another stimulus (the cell is refractory). During phase 3 (repolarization), an electrical stimulus of greater magnitude may cause another depolarization (the cell is relatively refractory). During phase 4, a stimulus that reaches the threshold level causes depolarization (see Chap. 8).

Mechanisms of Rhythm (and Dysrhythmia) Initiation

Cardiac rhythms can be produced by three mechanisms: spontaneous depolarization (automaticity), reentry pathways, and afterdepolarization ("triggered automaticity"). In normal cardiac conduction system cells (eg, Purkinje fiber cells), the sodium channels play a much less significant role in generating the action potential (Fig. 21–3). During phase 4, the potassium current out of the cell and the inward sodium current gradually and spontaneously increase until the threshold potential is reached (and the membrane undergoes depolarization). In normal myocardium, this spontaneous depolarization occurs most rapidly in the sinus node, the pacemaker for the heart. However, toxins can affect the membrane and cause other myocardial pacemaker cells or even muscle cells spontaneously to depolarize more rapidly. This mechanism, increased automaticity, accounts for many of the dysrhythmias seen with cardiac glycoside and catecholamine toxicity.

Other dysrhythmias result from reentry phenomena. The dysrhythmias are usually generated when an early impulse (atrial premature contraction or ventricular premature contraction) reaches a branch point with a partial block to conduction in one of the branches (Fig. 21–4). The impulse is carried through only one of the branches and then spreads through the myocardial cells. After a short delay, the impulse reaches the distal end of the previously blocked pathway. By this time, the region is no longer refractory and conducts the impulse in a retrograde fashion. The impulse continues in a continuous circuit, depolarizing the heart with each passage. Reentry mechanisms appear to be responsible for most of the dysrhythmias attributable to overdose of antidysrhythmic agents.

Triggered dysrhythmias (or "afterdepolarizations") result from oscillations and instability in the membrane potential during phase 4. The normal action potential is followed by an abnormal depolarization of lower amplitude. However, if the oscillation reaches the threshold potential, the membrane depolarizes and another action potential is generated. The initial normal action potential acts as a "trigger" for the abnormal oscillations. The mechanism is often termed "triggered automaticity."

Two major types of triggered automaticity occur. In delayed afterdepolarization (DAD), the normal action potential is followed by an oscillation during phase 4. Delayed afterdepolarizations occur primarily under conditions of increased intracellular calcium. These triggered rhythms are responsible for many of the dysrhythmias of cardiac glycoside toxicity. DAD amplitude increases with increased heart rate or cardiac pacing. This may explain why pacing may initiate dysrhythmias in digoxin-toxic patients.[147] The second type of afterdepolarization is termed early afterdepolarization (EAD). The abnormal afterdepolarization occurs during the downslope of phase 3 of the action potential. EADs occur when the cardiac action potential is markedly prolonged. Specifically, antidysrhythmic and other drugs that prolong the action potential duration may result in EADs (see Chap. 52). Torsades de pointes, discussed later in the chapter, is probably also caused by early afterdepolarizations.

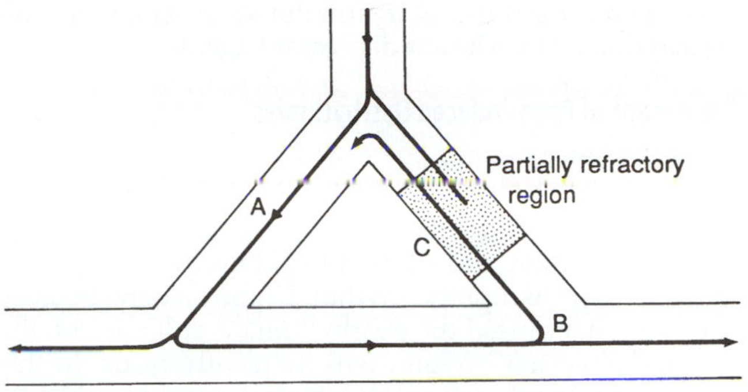

Figure 21–4. Mechanism of reentry dysrhythmias. An impulse traveling down a conduction pathway reaches a branch point with one branch refractory (C). The impulse is conducted down the other branch (A), and spreads through the myocardium eventually to reach B, the distal end of the originally refractory branch. However, branch C is no longer refractory, and the impulse is conducted retrograde up through branch C again to be conducted down branch A. The myocardium is depolarized during each loop around the circuit as the impulse spreads from the distal end of branch A.

The cardiac toxicity of some drugs results from their effects on the propagation of the electrical impulse through the conduction system of the heart. These drugs may cause conduction blocks, including first, second, and even third-degree (complete) heart block. The ECG abnormalities of these toxins are due to effects on the AV node or His bundle. Other drugs affect conduction by their action on the left bundle or right bundle branches by delaying repolarization of the myocardial cells. These effects are seen on the ECG as a widening of the QRS complex or prolongation of the QT interval. Toxins that cause conduction blocks usually affect phases 0 or 2 of the action potential, prolonging the action potential, and increasing the refractory period. These effects frequently result from overdoses of antidysrhythmic drugs such as encainide or flecainide. Drugs and toxins that may cause conduction abnormalities are listed in Table 21–7. Frequently, drugs that cause conduction blocks may also cause an increase in reentry dysrhythmias. Indeed, the presence of QRS or QT prolongation may portend the development of significant dysrhythmias from either antidysrhythmic or cyclic antidepressant agents.

Treatment of Drug-Induced Dysrhythmias

Patients with hypotension, ischemic chest pain, or congestive heart failure should be treated with electrical conversion where applicable. In less critically ill patients, fluid boluses may correct mild hypotension or vagal maneuvers may disrupt the rhythm. Unfortunately, because the drug that caused the dysrhythmia is still present, the original abnormal rhythm will frequently recur. In this case, carefully selected antidysrhythmic agents (based on the rhythm and toxin) may be helpful. In the absence of hemodynamic compromise, the dysrhythmia (especially if supraventricular) can often be monitored until specific therapy directed at the precise toxin and rhythm can be instituted. Indeed, for drug-induced supraventricular dysrhythmias that are not hemodynamically significant, the safest therapy is often observation and monitoring until the drug is eliminated from the body.

Bradycardic Dysrhythmias

Bradycardia, heart block, and eventually asystole are frequently the terminal events in a massive overdose of any drug. In many cases, these effects are due to the accompanying metabolic changes. For instance, severe hyperkalemia (that may accompany any acidosis) results in a wide complex, sinusoidal bradycardic rhythm. Other drugs that usually produce tachycardia may, in massive overdoses or as a terminal event, produce bradycardia. These drugs include cyclic antidepressant, anticholinergic, and sympathomimetic agents. The bradycardia in these cases usually results from profound depletion of norepinephrine from peripheral sympathetic nerves.

What Toxins Cause Bradycardia? Several classes of drugs typically produce bradycardia (Table 21–8). Several different mechanisms may account for drug-induced bradycardia. The toxin may effect the central or peripheral nervous system, or effect rhythm generation or conduction in the heart. Central nervous system-mediated bradycardia is probably the most common drug-induced cause for mild sinus bradycardia. Most agents that cause CNS sedation will usually decrease sympathetic outflow to the heart and produce a heart rate in the range of 40 to 60 beats/min. This includes the sedative-hypnotic agents, opioids, and alpha$_2$-adrenergic receptor agonist ("cen-

TABLE 21–7. DRUGS AND TOXINS THAT CAUSE CONDUCTION ABNORMALITIES AND/OR HEART BLOCK

Alpha$_1$-adrenergic antagonists
Alpha$_2$-adrenergic agonists
Amantidine
Antidysrhythmics
Astemizole
Beta-adrenergic antagonists
Bupivacaine
Calcium channel blockers
Carbamazepine
Cardiac glycosides
Chloroquine and quinine
Cholinomimetics
Cocaine
Cyclic antidepressant agents
Cyclobenzaprine
Electrolytes
Potassium
Magnesium
Heavy metal salts
Arsenic
Pentamidine
Phenothiazines
Propoxyphene
Sympathomimetics
Terfenadine

TABLE 21–8. DRUGS AND TOXINS THAT CAUSE BRADYCARDIA

Alpha$_1$-adrenergic agonists
(reflex bradycardia)
Alpha$_2$-adrenergic agonists
Alpha-methyldopa
Clonidine
Guanfacine
Guanabenz
Yohimbine
Antidysrhythmics
Beta-adrenergic antagonists
Cardiac glycosides (digoxin)
Cholinomimetics
Carbamates or organophosphates
Edrophonium (Tensilon)
Neostigmine (Prostigmin)
Physostigmine (Antilirium)
Ciguatera
Misoprostol
Opioids
Phenylpropanolamine
Plant toxins (Chap. 77)
Aconitine
Andromedotoxin
Cardiac glycosides
Jin bu huan[29]
Veratrine
Sedative-hypnotic agents
Late presentations or massive exposures to:
Anticholinergics
Cocaine
Cyclic antidepressants
Sympathomimetics

trally acting") antihypertensive drugs. Blockade of the peripheral $alpha_1$-adrenergic receptors may also cause a relative bradycardia by decreasing sympathetic input to the heart. Drugs with these properties such as alpha-methyldopa would be expected to cause only a mild bradycardia (in the range of 40 to 60 beats/min).

The most profound bradycardias result from overdoses of drugs that have direct effects on the myocardial pacemaker and conduction system cells. These drugs depress phase 4 spontaneous depolarization and result in reduced pacemaker activity. Examples of drugs with these effects include calcium channel blockers, beta-adrenergic antagonists, and class Ia, Ib, and Ic antidysrhythmics (Table 21–9). The antidysrhythmics are divided into four classes based on their general properties: class I, membrane stabilizers; class II, beta-adrenergic antagonists; class III, potassium channel blocker agents; and class IV, calcium channel blockers.[157,159] The class I antidysrhythmic agents have been further divided into three classes based on their effects on the membrane ion channels and the action potential (Table 21–9).[61,158]

Asystole typically is the end result of progressive bradycardia and conduction system block. In massive overdoses, any toxin causing bradycardia could potentially cause asystole. Beta-adrenergic antagonists, calcium channel blockers, cardiac glycosides, and the other antidysrhythmics have all been reported to cause asystole and death. Cyclic antidepressants and cholinesterase inhibitors (eg, physostigmine) in large doses also may cause asystole.

What Is the Treatment for Toxin-Induced Bradycardia? The general treatment of toxin-induced nonsinus bradycardia of unknown etiology includes following the standard advanced cardiac life support (ACLS) guidelines. Symptomatic patients should initially be treated with atropine. Patients who do not respond to atropine should be treated with an intravenous infusion of epinephrine or dopamine. Isoproterenol should be avoided, due to the potential for stimulation of vascular $beta_2$-adrenergic receptors with resulting arteriolar dilatation and hypotension. Obviously, if the causative agent is known, specific

TABLE 21–9. CLASSES OF ANTIDYSRHYTHMIC AGENTS: PHARMACOLOGIC EFFECTS

	Site of Action				Effects on the ECG		
Class	***Sodium Channels***	***Potassium Channels***	***Calcium Channels***	**Examples**	***PR***	***QRS***	***QT***
Sodium Channel Blockers							
Ia	++/+++	++	0	Diisopyramide Procainamide Quinidine	±	↑	↑
Ib	+/++	±	0	Lidocaine Phenytoin Mexiletine Tocainide	±	±	±
Ic	+++	++/+++	0	Encainide Flecainide Propafenone Moricizine	↑	↑	↑↑
Beta-Adrenergic Antagonists							
II	0	0	+ (indirect)	Propranolol Atenolol Esmolol Metoprolol Timolol	↑	±	±
Potassium Channel Blockers							
III	+	++	0	Amiodarone Bretylium Sotalol	↑	±	↑
Calcium Channel Blockers							
IV	0	0	+++	Verapamil Diltiazem Nifedipine Nicardipine	↑	±	±

+ = mild blockade; ++ = moderate blockade; +++ = marked blockade; ↑ = increases; ± = no significant effect.

therapy directed at removal or neutralization of the drug may be indicated. For example, glucagon and amrinone (Inocor) may be beneficial in beta-adrenergic antagonist or calcium channel blocker overdoses, and calcium may be beneficial for calcium channel blocker overdose. Digoxin-specific Fab antibodies (Digibind) should be administered to patients with digoxin toxicity.

All patients with bradycardia due to a toxic ingestion should have an external transcutaneous demand pacemaker placed. For severe symptomatic bradycardia, insertion of a transvenous pacemaker should be considered early. However, use of a temporary pacemaker must not delay or be substituted for more specific and effective therapy. For instance, in digitalis intoxication, cardiac pacing has a higher mortality than the use of Digibind (digoxin-specific antibodies), due to iatrogenic accidents associated with pacemaker placement, pacing-induced dysrhythmias, and limited effectiveness of the pacemaker in treating the underlying intoxication.[147] Patients who present with bradycardia or conduction delays must be considered to be at risk of progressing to asystole or third-degree heart block if more drug is absorbed from the gastrointestinal tract or tissue concentrations increase.

Conduction Abnormalities and Heart Block. The drugs and medications that cause cardiac conduction abnormalities are listed in Table 21–7. Most of these toxins are the same agents that cause bradycardia. The drugs and medications that decrease sympathetic tone usually only produce first-degree or second-degree Mobitz type I heart block via effects on innervation of the atrioventricular node. Rarely, these agents can produce second-degree Mobitz type II or even third-degree heart block. Anticholinergic and antihistaminic agents may also cause conduction delays.

The more profound ECG interval abnormalities and the more serious degrees of heart block usually accompany overdoses with cardiac glycosides, cyclic antidepressants, or antidysrhythmic drugs. The cyclic antidepressants possess quinidine-like "membrane-stabilizing" activity similar to the class I antidysrhythmic agents. Figure 21–3 shows the action potential and the contribution of each phase to the ECG complex. Agents that depress phase 0 (sodium influx) produce widening of the QRS complex and slowing of conduction. Agents that prolong phase 2 or 3 produce prolongation of the QT interval and refractory period. Table 21–9 lists the classes of antidysrhythmic agents, their effects on action potential, and the ECG abnormalities they cause.

Surprisingly, antidysrhythmic agents increase the occurrence of dysrhythmias in 5 to 25% of patients, even at what are considered therapeutic serum levels. By prolonging the refractory period, the drug may increase the likelihood of the unidirectional block required to initiate reentry dysrhythmias. Class Ia and Ic antidysrhythmics, the agents with the greatest effects on the refractory period, are those most commonly reported to induce dysrhythmias.[30,78,80,104] Overdose of class Ib antidysrhythmics can produce bradycardia[108] or other dysrhythmias.[9] Propafenone (Rythmol) and sotalol (Betapace) are class III antidysrhythmic agents that also have beta-adrenergic antagonist properties. Overdose may produce coma and seizures in addition to bradycardia, hypotension, conduction delays, and dysrhythmias.[2,77] Amiodarone (Cordarone), another class III antidysrhythmic, has minimal beta-adrenergic antagonist properties but does not cause coma or seizures. Acute overdose of amiodarone is rare due to the poor bioavailability, and the large volume of distribution limits peak serum levels. However, dysrhythmias may result, especially if hypokalemia or other antidysrhythmic agents are present.[89]

Tachycardic Dysrhythmias

Both supraventricular and ventricular tachydysrhythmias may occur in poisoning. Common medications and toxins that may cause tachydysrhythmias are listed in Table 21–10.

Sinus tachycardia is the most common tachycardic rhythm seen in the poisoned patient. Sinus tachycardia may result from such toxic effects as fever, stress, hypovolemia, catecholamine excess, or from direct effects of the toxin on the sinoatrial node. In general, the patient with sinus tachycardia is treated with supportive care and correction of any underlying metabolic or hemodynamic abnormalities. The tachycardia will resolve as the toxin is metabolized or removed from the body. In stimulant drug and sympathomimetic agent exposures, the sinus tachycardia may be extremely fast (greater than 150 beats/min) and may require treatment. In this case, sedation with benzodiazepines will usually control the tachycardia effectively.

Supraventricular tachycardias occur frequently in poisoned patients. The most common agents are medications or toxins with anticholinergic activity, the antidysrhythmics, and the sympathomimetic drugs. The tachydysrhythmias often are mediated by the drug's sympathomimetic effects. Cocaine and amphetamines stimulate the beta$_1$-adrenergic receptors on the myocardial cells. Much of the dysrhythmic potential of cyclic antidepressants, antihistamines, and theophylline appears to be mediated through indirect effects on the sympathetic system. Halogenated hydrocarbons including chloral hydrate increase the release of endogenous catecholamines and also "sensitize" the myocardium to the effects of catecholamines. In the presence of halogenated hydrocarbons, ventricular tachycardia or ventricular fibrillation may occur with much lower levels of endogenous epinephrine or exogenous beta-adrenergic stimulants.

The toxic effects of antidysrhythmics (and other agents with "quinidine-like" activity, such as the cyclic antidepressants) are primarily due to their effects on the myocardial cell membrane. The supraventricular dysrhythmias that result from overdose of antidysrhythmics or cyclic antidepressants are associated with prolonged QRS complexes and QT intervals. In patients with cyclic antidepressant ingestions, the duration of the QRS complex is of prognostic value. None of 49 patients who in-

TABLE 21–10. DRUGS AND TOXINS THAT CAUSE VENTRICULAR AND SUPRAVENTRICULAR DYSRHYTHMIAS

Amantidine
Antidysrhythmics class I, II, III, and IV
Anticholinergics
Antihistamines
Baclofen
Botanicals and plants (Chap. 77)
Carbamazepine
Cardiac glycosides
Catecholamines
Chloroquine and quinine
Cholinomimetics
Physostigmine
Cyclic antidepressant agents
Cyclobenzaprine
Flumazenil
Halogenated hydrocarbons
Inhalational anesthetics
Hydrocarbons and solvents
Jellyfish venom
Metal salts
Arsenic
Lithium
Magnesium
Mercury
Potasssium
Pentamidine
Phenothiazines
Phosphodiesterase inhibitors
Amrinone
Methylxanthines
Propoxyphene
Sedative hypnotic agents
Chloral hydrate
Ethanol
Sympathomimetics
Alpha agonists
Amphetamines
Beta-adrenergic agonists
Cocaine
Phencyclidine
Thyroid hormone preparations

gested TCAs and had a QRS less than 160 msec had dysrhythmias, but 50% of patients with a QRS greater than or equal to 160 msec had dysrhythmias.[15] Identification of a cyclic antidepressant ingestion is critical.

The presence of a rightward axis in the terminal 40 msec of the QRS complex (R wave in AVR and S wave in AVL) frequently occurs with cyclic antidepressant toxicity. In fact, the combination of a rightward terminal QRS axis (between 130 and 270 degrees) together with a prolonged QTc and sinus tachycardia is highly suggestive of cyclic antidepressant toxicity.[110,176] In one study, a patient with a cyclic antidepressant had an increased risk of major toxicity if any of the following were present: terminal 40 msec QRS axis > 135 degrees, QTc > 480 msec, heart rate > 120, ingestion of amitriptyline, cyclic antidepressant level > 800 ng/mL, age > 30 years, QRS > 100 msec, or QRS axis > 90 degrees.[27]

However, estimating the axis of the terminal 40 msec is difficult. More simply, ECGs with an abnormal rightward terminal QRS axis have a small S wave in I and aVL and a small R wave in aVR (Chap. 8).[55] However, these ECG findings may not always occur. And, especially in children, a rightward terminal QRS axis may occur in ECG of nonpoisoned patients.[8] Ingestion of other medications (eg, phenothiazines and antidysrhythmics) also frequently prolong the QRS complex and QT interval.[78,83,96,165] In fact, the coingestion of a neuroleptic agent with a cyclic antidepressant significantly increases the likelihood of ECG abnormalities and possibly increases the risk of adverse cardiac events.[171] Sodium bicarbonate has also been used successfully for treating patients with these ECG abnormalities due to noncyclic antidepressant ingestions.

Patients with suspected cyclic antidepressant overdoses must be carefully observed in spite of negative ECG criteria. The presence of an R wave in aVR greater than 3 mm, the R/S ratio in aVR greater than 0.7, and a QRS duration greater than 100 msec may correlate with development of seizures and ventricular dysrhythmias.[90] However, the negative predictive value of these criteria is still only about 92%. Combining other clinical criteria with the ECG criteria will probably be more sensitive for identifying those patients most at risk of life-threatening toxicity. One recent study divided patients into high- and low-risk groups based upon ECG and clinical symptoms present 6 hours after ingestion (or ED presentation if ingestion time was not known). The patients were classified as high risk if any of the following were present: QRS > 0.10 msec, dysrhythmias, altered mental status, seizures, respiratory depression, or hypotension. Of the 67 patients in the study, 13 of the 39 patients in the high-risk group, but none of the 28 patients in the low-risk group, developed subsequent complications after the 6-hour period.[47] An ECG from a patient who ingested a cyclic antidepressant is shown in Chap. 8, Figure 8–10.

Administration of sodium bicarbonate to cyclic antidepressant toxic patients narrows the QRS complexes, shortens the QT interval, and suppresses ventricular dysrhythmias.[23,107,109,113,116,132,133] The arterial pH should be maintained at 7.45 to 7.55. If the patient has cerebral or pulmonary edema and administration of the large sodium load in sodium bicarbonate is contraindicated, hyperventilation may also be effective.[44,50,79,113] In the future, non-sodium-containing buffers may be available and effective.[143] Seizures lead to hypoxia and increasing acidosis; patients may develop widening of the QRS, hypotension, dysrhythmias, and cardiac arrest in the immediate post-ictal period.[91,148] Administration of calcium should be avoided, because animal studies have shown an increased risk of ventricular dysrhythmias and seizures with no improvement in blood pressure.[162] In one case report, glucagon improved the blood pressure and narrowed the QRS complexes.[137] The most potentially beneficial future treatment for cyclic antidepressant toxicity is the use of drug-specific antibody fragments currently being tested in animal models (Chap. 55).[114]

How Should Toxin-Induced Supraventricular Tachycardia Be Treated? If the patient is unstable (hypotension, chest pain, or congestive heart failure), an attempt should usually be made to treat toxin-induced supraventricular tachycardia (SVT) immediately with electrical cardioversion. Unfortunately, because the toxic agent is still present, the supraventricular dysrhythmia may recur. In these cases, repeated cardioversion will not be effective, and pharmacologic therapy for the dysrhythmia should be considered.

Adenosine (Adenocard) would seem to be a potentially effective agent for toxin-induced supraventricular dysrhythmias. The drug has no hemodynamic effects when given as a 6 to 12-mg bolus, and the short half-life (less than 10 seconds) limits the duration of any adverse reactions. However, the short half-life could lead to rapid recurrence of the rhythm as the adenosine is quickly metabolized while the toxin is still present. If the dysrhythmia recurs, repeated boluses of adenosine would serve no useful purpose and should not be used. In this case, an agent with a longer half-life should then be considered. Additionally, a few potential drug interactions exist that must be considered when using adenosine for toxin-induced supraventricular tachycardia. Most importantly, dipyridamole (Persantine) inhibits the uptake of adenosine into cells and prolongs and potentiates the effects of adenosine. Prolonged complete heart block or asystole may result. Adenosine also potentiates the dysrhythmic effects of carbamazepine (Tegretol). Finally, adenosine may not be effective for dysrhythmias caused by methylxanthines, such as caffeine or theophylline. Methylxanthines competitively inhibit the effects of adenosine. Doses of adenosine higher than the usually recommended 6 or 12 mg may be effective in these cases. However, no clinical studies have been performed to assess the effectiveness or safety of higher doses of adenosine in methylxanthine toxicity.

Other antidysrhythmics may be employed, if necessary. Calcium channel blockers and beta-adrenergic antagonists must not be administered to patients with wide-complex dysrhythmias unless the rhythm is clearly demonstrated not to be ventricular tachycardia. Patients with ventricular tachycardia who are erroneously treated with verapamil for presumed supraventricular tachycardia with aberrancy develop profound hypotension in 44 to 100% of cases.[25,123,141] In suspected poisonings with a prolonged QRS or QT interval, the patient should be assumed to have ingested a cyclic antidepressant,[11,15,23,79,107,110,113,132,133] antidysrhythmic,[78,80,165] or phenothiazine.[83,96] Sodium bicarbonate (1 to 2 mEq/kg) should be administered and the ECG should be monitored. If the QRS intervals improve, additional sodium bicarbonate should be infused to maintain the serum pH at approximately 7.50 to 7.55. (See Antidotes in Depth: Sodium Bicarbonate.)

If the patient is hemodynamically stable, frequently the best action is simply careful monitoring until the toxin is removed or metabolized. Obviously, if the toxin is known, specific therapy may be indicated. For instance, if cardiac glycoside toxicity is suspected, digoxin-specific antibodies should be administered. (See Antidotes in Depth: Digoxin–Specific Antibody Fragments.)

Possible interactions between the ingested toxin and pharmacologic treatment must be considered before antidysrhythmic therapy is instituted. The antidysrhythmic should be given cautiously, with careful hemodynamic monitoring. In particular, class Ia and Ic antidysrhythmics should never be used in the treatment of any toxin ingestion (eg, cyclic antidepressants or phenothiazines) that may potentially cause conduction abnormalities. And, calcium channel blocking or beta-adrenergic antagonist agents should be used with extreme caution in poisoned patients who have conduction abnormalities or hypotension.

In the vast majority of poisonings, supraventricular dysrhythmias require no specific therapy other than close monitoring and general supportive care. The dysrhythmia will resolve as the toxin is eliminated from the body. The presence of dysrhythmias may suggest a more severe toxic ingestion and may indicate the need for more aggressive removal of the toxic agent.

Which Drugs Cause Ventricular Tachycardia? Ventricular dysrhythmias frequently accompany hypotension, hypoxia, acidemia, electrolyte abnormalities, and other metabolic derangements that occur in critically ill patients. It is often impossible to determine whether the dysrhythmia is due to the toxin or to other underlying metabolic abnormalities. Some common drugs clearly can cause ventricular dysrhythmias; they are listed in Table 21–10. The rarity of published reports detailing a particular drug's toxicity may reflect either the rarity of toxicity or infrequency of the drug's exposure. For example, although rare cases of sudden death with pentamidine isethionate have been reported, the first documentation of pentamidine-related torsades de pointes (a type of polymorphic ventricular tachycardia) occurred in 1987 during treatment of *Pneumocystis carinii* pneumonia in two patients with acquired immunodeficiency syndrome (AIDS).[168] With the increased use of pentamidine isethionate to treat AIDS-related *P. carinii* pneumonia, multiple reports appeared implicating the drug in torsades de pointes syndrome (discussed later in the chapter). However, some common drugs clearly can cause ventricular dysrhythmias; they are listed in Table 21–10.

Ventricular dysrhythmias rarely occur in patients after ingesting only opioid or sedative-hypnotic agents. However, alcohol, chloral hydrate, and propoxyphene may more commonly cause dysrhythmias. Ethanol usually causes atrial dysrhythmias (holiday heart syndrome) but also may cause ventricular extrasystoles. The cardiovascular effects of propoxyphene (Darvon) are unique among the opioids. Propoxyphene is metabolized in the liver to norpropoxyphene, which has less analgesic effect, a much longer half-life, and local anesthetic properties similar to those of the class I antidysrhythmic agents.[38] The marked QRS widening and dysrhythmias of propoxyphene toxicity may respond to naloxone,[57] sodium bicarbonate,[145] or lidocaine.[170] Similarly, chloral hydrate is metabolized to produce the toxic compound, trichloroethanol. This halogenated hydrocarbon causes catecholamine release and also sensitizes the myocardium to the effects of catecholamines. For this reason, chloral hydrate should not be used for the sedation of pediatric patients with stimulant agent ingestions.[136] Lidocaine may be effective for the ventricular dysrhythmias of chloral hydrate (and halogenated hydrocarbons). However, an intravenously administered beta-adrenergic antagonist, such as propranolol, is the preferred antidysrhythmic.[55,138] The cardiovascular toxicity of inhalational anesthetics and halogenated solvents (eg, carbon tetrachloride) is also thought to result from this same effect on catecholamine sensitivity.

Management of Drug-Induced Ventricular Dysrhythmias. Ventricular dysrhythmias should be managed much like those occurring in association with a myocardial infarction. In addition to the usual supportive measures (including oxygen, ECG monitoring, and blood tests such as hematocrit, electrolytes, and BUN), antidysrhythmic drugs are frequently indicated. The choice of agent depends somewhat on the toxin. Class Ia and Ic and possibly class III antidysrhythmics should be avoided if the patient is poisoned with any drug with quinidine-like activities or if the ECG shows any conduction delays (other than first- or second-degree Mobitz type I). Using these drugs would only potentiate the conduction system toxicity of the drug originally ingested. If the QRS or QT interval is prolonged, the dysrhythmia should be presumed to be secondary to the quinidine-like activity of a cyclic antidepressant,[11,15,23,79,107,110,113,132,133] phenothiazine,[83,96] chloroquine,[32] or antidysrhythmic.[78,80,165] If bicarbonate is ineffective for these dysrhythmias, a class Ib agent, such as lidocaine, would be an appropriate therapeutic agent and may be effective for treating cyclic antidepressant-induced ventricular dysrhythmias.[5,87]

What Is Torsades de Pointes? Torsades de pointes is a unique type of ventricular tachycardia in which the ECG resembles a sinusoidal wave of increasing and decreasing magnitude, undulating above and below the baseline. The dysrhythmia propagates from numerous simultaneous ventricular tachycardia reentry foci scattered throughout the ventricles. The QRS complexes change as these various foci compete to depolarize the ventricle. The pathophysiology of torsades de pointes is usually related to development of early afterdepolarizations (EAD). (Early afterdepolarization is discussed in more detail above.) Myocardial cells with long refractory periods (phases 2 and 3 of the action potential curve, Fig. 21–3) are most predisposed to EADs.

Patients with either hereditary prolonged QT syndrome or acquired prolongation due to drugs or metabolic effects are at increased risk of developing torsades de pointes. The QT interval corresponds to phases 2 and 3 of the action potential curve. Agents that affect the potassium or calcium channels and currents would be expected to cause torsades de pointes. Indeed, one of the hereditary prolonged QT syndromes is due to a defect in a gene HERG that encodes a potassium channel.[37] However, drugs and antidysrhythmic agents that effect primarily sodium channels also may prolong the QT intervals and cause torsades de pointes. Some sodium channels may remain open during phase 2 and contribute to the plateau phase duration of the action potential. A defect in a protein that controls sodium channel inactivation is responsible for another form of the congenital long QT syndrome.[163] A typical torsades de pointes dysrhythmia is shown in Figure 8–17.

Metabolic and electrolyte abnormalities, particularly hypocalcemia, hypomagnesemia, and hypokalemia, may interfere with the ion channel currents and may cause of torsades de pointes. However, the most common cause is drug toxicity. Any drug that causes ventricular tachycardia may cause torsades de pointes. But the most frequent causes are drugs that prolong the QT interval, such as class Ia and Ic antidysrhythmics, cyclic antidepressants, and phenothiazines. Although the newer class Ic antidysrhythmics (such as encainide and flecanide) usually cause greater QT interval prolongation, class Ia agents (such as quinidine and procainamide) are responsible for more reported cases. This is probably simply due to the relatively infrequent use of class Ic antidysrhythmics (due in part to concerns about the higher risk of prodysrhythmic effects). Of the other antidysrhythmics, sotalol and amiodarone (class III) have also been reported to cause torsades de pointes. Class Ib agents such as lidocaine have no significant effect on QT interval and would not be expected to cause torsades de pointes.

Pentamidine isethionate is associated with ventricular tachydysrhythmias and torsades de pointes[45,95,150,118] that may persist for weeks after discontinuation.[12,33,168] The similarity of pentamidine's structure to that of procainamide (Fig. 21–5) probably accounts for the pentamidine-induced torsades de pointes and ventricular dysrhythmias.[33]

Torsades de pointes has also been reported to occur with the "nonsedating" antihistamines astemizole (Hismanal)[13,62,68,124,134,140,151,172] and terfenadine (Seldane).[98,102] The large number of reports may be due to the very frequent use of these antihistamines. Nearly all reported cases of terfenadine-induced torsades de pointes result from changes in the parent drug's metabolism. Normally, more than 99% of terfenadine undergoes first-pass metabolism in the liver to a clinically active carboxy metabolite and an inactive dealkylated metabolite.[73] Unchanged terfenadine is usually not even detectable in serum. However, studies have shown that the unchanged parent drug (but not the active or inactive metabolites) has a quinidine-like action that is responsible for inducing dysrhythmias.[177] Agents that prevent metabolism of terfenadine would lead to the accumulation of the unchanged parent compound in the serum and increased risk of dysrhythmia. Terfenadine is metabolized by CYP3A4, a specific cytochrome P-450. Eryth-

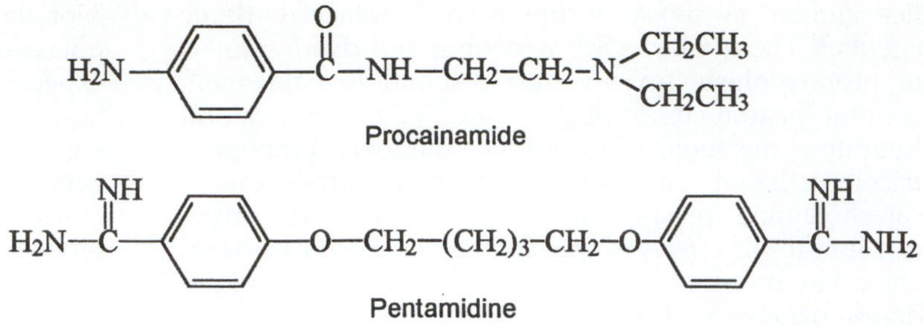

Figure 21–5. Structure of pentamidine isethionate and procainamide. Similarity in the chemical structure probably accounts for occurance of pentamidine-induced torsades de pointes.

romycin,[66] clarithromycin,[3,106] itraconazole,[73,156] and ketoconazole[98,117,180] decrease the liver metabolism of the terfenadine, lead to increased levels of the parent compound, and cause increased toxicity. Azithromycin (Zithromax) and fluconazole (Diflucan) are not metabolized via CYP3A4 and do not increase the risk of developing torsades de pointes.[60,161] Cimetidine and ranitidine also do not cause accumulation of the unmetabolized terfenadine parent compound.[67]

Terfenadine and astemizole interact with the potassium channels to prolong the QT interval and induce torsades de pointes.[10,130] Terfenadine enters the mouth of the delayed rectifier potassium channel after it opens.[178] Terfenadine may block multiple subclasses of the delayed rectifier potassium channel[36] or may actually block calcium and sodium channels in addition to the delayed rectifier channels.[101] There is some evidence that the blockade actually occurs at the HERG channel, the same site involved in one form of the congenitally prolonged QT syndrome.[129,146] In any case, inhibition of the currents during phase 2 of the action potential prolongs the plateau phase, results in EADs, and predisposes to torsades de pointes.

Treatment of Torsades de Pointes. Whether torsades de pointes is hereditary, metabolic, or drug induced, the treatment must not include medications that could further prolong the QT interval. In particular, class Ia and Ic antidysrhythmics must never be used. Torsades de pointes complicated by hypotension, ischemia, or heart failure should be treated initially with electrical cardioversion. However, cardioversion is often ineffective, or the rhythm quickly recurs. In such cases, lidocaine should be given immediately and cardioversion repeated. Unfortunately, lidocaine is also often ineffective, as are other class Ib agents. Other therapies that may be effective for treatment of torsades de pointes are listed in Table 21–11.

TABLE 21–11. THERAPY FOR TORSADES DE POINTES SYNDROME

Correct electrolyte and metabolic abnormalities
Lidocaine
Magnesium
Isoproterenol infusion
Overdrive pacing
Bretylium
Cardioversion
Beta-adrenergic antagonists (for nontoxin etiology)

Magnesium sulfate seems to be the most effective treatment.[155] Magnesium may be given as an infusion of 2 to 6 g IV over 10 to 40 minutes or administered as a constant infusion of 5 to 20 mg/min.[6,154] Magnesium infusions have been associated with respiratory arrest and asystole when inappropriate dosage or infusion rates have been used or when administered to patients with severe renal insufficiency.[49,160] Therefore, the patient receiving magnesium must be observed carefully for changes in rhythm, respirations, reflexes, or blood pressure. Magnesium treatment seems to be effective even in patients who have normal serum magnesium levels. If a total infusion of 4 to 8 g of magnesium is ineffective (or magnesium is contraindicated, or the patient cannot tolerate the infusion), overdrive pacing or an isoproterenol infusion can be tried. As the heart rate increases, the refractory period decreases. This change could interrupt the dysrhythmia. Bretylium, although a class III antidysrhythmic agent, does not usually prolong the QRS complex. It is frequently ineffective for torsades de pointes, however, and should be used only with caution.

Summary

Drugs and toxins may interact with the heart or blood vessels to produce hypotension or hypertension, congestive heart failure, dysrhythmias, or cardiac conduction delays. The occurrence of these abnormalities, individually or in combination, may suggest a particular toxin or class of drugs as the etiologic agent and may dictate initial treatment. Often, significant abnormalities in vital signs must be corrected even before the toxin is identified. Only by understanding both the pharmacology of the toxic drug and the physiology of the heart and vasculature can appropriate treatment be delivered.

Definitive care of the poisoned patient with hemodynamic compromise or a dysrhythmia begins with recognition that a toxic agent may be present. Although structural and metabolic etiologies must always be considered, the toxic effects of drugs must also be included in the differential diagnosis. A variety of clinical clues, when present, should heighten the physician's suspicion

TABLE 21–12. CLUES THAT AN UNANTICIPATED TOXIN MAY BE THE CAUSE OF HEMODYNAMIC COMPROMISE OR DYSRHYTHMIAS

History

New-onset, concomitant seizure
Gastrointestinal disturbances (colicky pain, nausea, vomiting, diarrhea)
Prior ingestion of medications (consider possibility that container may have been mislabeled or misidentified)
Depression (even if patient denies toxin ingestion)
Suspected myocardial ischemia in patient < 35 years old

Past Medical History

Treatment with *any* cardiac medications (especially antidysrhythmics or digoxin)
History of psychiatric illness, asthma, or hypertension
History of drug use or abuse

Physical Examination Vital Signs

Heart rate
- Sinus tachycardia with rate < 140 beat/min
- Sinus tachycardia without apparent identified cause
- Sinus bradycardia

Respiratory rate
- Any unexplained depression or elevation in rate

Temperature
- Elevation but especially if > 106° F (> 41.1 °C)
- Hypothermia

Dissociation between typically paired changes, for example:
- Hypotension and bradycardia (tachycardia expected)
- Fever and dry skin (diaphoresis expected)
- Hypertension and tachycardia (reflex bradycardia anticipated)
- Depressed mental status and tachypnea (decreased respirations common)

Relatively rapid changes in vital signs
- Initial hypertension becomes hypotension
- Increasing sinus tachycardia or hypertension

General

Alteration in consciousness, such as depressed mental status, confusion, or agitation
Findings usually not associated with cardiovascular diseases
- Ataxia, bullae, dry mucous membranes, lacrimation, miosis or mydriasis, nystagmus, unusual odor, flushed skin, salivation, tinnitus, tremor, visual disturbances

Findings consistent with a toxidrome (Table 17–2)
- Especially findings consistent with anticholinergic, sympathomimetic, or sedative-hypnotic agents

Laboratory Tests

Any unexpected or unexplained laboratory result, especially:
- Metabolic acidosis
- Respiratory alkalosis
- Hypokalemia or hyperkalemia
- Hyperglycemia

ECG
- Prolonged QRS complex or QT interval
- Any heart block
- Supraventricular tachycardia rate > 240 beat/min
- Occurrence of any uncommon dysrhythmia
- Occurrence of more than one type or class of dysrhythmia

that a toxic drug effect may be responsible for the hemodynamic or dysrhythmic problem. Some of these clues are listed in Table 21–12.

References

1. Addy JA: Dopamine not effective for treatment of hypotension in chlorpromazine overdose: First case report. J Emerg Nurs 1995;21:99–101.
2. Alderfliegel P, Leeman M, Demaeyer P, Kahn RJ: Sotalol poisoning associated with asystole. Intensive Care Med 1993;19:57–58.
3. Amsden GW: Erythromycin, clarithromycin, and azithromycin: Are the differences real? Clin Ther 1996;18: 56–72.
4. Ashraf M, Chaudhary K, Nelson J, Thompson W: Massive overdose of sustained-release verapamil: A case report and review of literature. Am J Med Sci 1995;310:258–263.
5. Bain DJG, Turner T: Imipramine poisoning. Arch Dis Child 1971;46:887.
6. Banai S, Tzivoni D, Schuger C: Effectiveness of magnesium sulfate in torsades de pointes: A study of nine patients. J Am Coll Cardiol 1987;9:245A. Abstract.
7. Benowitz NL, Rosenberg J, Becker CE: Cardiopulmonary catastrophes in drug-overdosed patients. Med Clin North Am 1979;63:127–140.
8. Berkovitch M, Matsui D, Fogelman R, et al: Assessment of the terminal 40-millisecond QRS vector in children with a history of tricyclic antidepressant ingestion. Pediatr Emerg Care 1995;11:75–77.
9. Berman MF, Lipka LJ: Relative sodium block by bupivacaine and lidocaine in neonatal rat myocytes. Anesth Analg 1994;79:350–356.
10. Berul CI, Morad M: Regulation of potassium channels by nonsedating antihistamines. Circulation 1995;91: 2220–2225.
11. Bessen HA, Niemann JT, Haskell RJ, et al: Effect of respiratory alkalosis in tricyclic antidepressant overdose. West J Med 1983;139:373–376.
12. Bibler MR, Chou TC, Toltzis RJ, Wade PA: Recurrent ventricular tachycardia due to pentamidine-induced cardiotoxicity. Chest 1988;94:1303–1306.
13. Bishop RO, Gaudry PL: Prolonged QT interval following astemizole overdose. Arch Emerg Med 1989;6:63–65.
14. Bodenhamer JE, Smilkstein MJ: Delayed cardiotoxicity following quinine overdose: A case report. J Emerg Med 1993;11:279–285.
15. Boehnert M, Lovejoy FH: Value of the QRS duration versus the serum drug level in predicting seizures and ventricular arrhythmias after an acute overdose of tricyclic antidepressants. N Engl J Med 1985;313:474–479.
16. Boehrer DB, Moliterno DJ, Willard JE, et al: Influence of labetalol on cocaine-induced coronary vasoconstriction in humans. Am J Med 1993;94:608–610.
17. Brass BJ, Winchester-Penny S, Lipper BL: Massive verapamil overdose complicated by noncardiogenic pulmonary edema. Am J Emerg Med 1996;14:459–461.
18. Braunwald E: Approach to the patient with heart disease. In: Isselbacher KJ, Adams RD, Braunwald E, Petersdorf

RG, Wilson JD, eds: Harrison's Principles of Internal Medicine. New York, McGraw-Hill, 1980, p. 995.

19. Briggs RSJ, Birtwell AJ, Pohl JEF: Hypertensive response to labetalol in pheochromocytoma. Lancet 1978;1: 1045–1046.
20. Bristow MR: The beta adrenergic receptor: Configuration, regulation, mechanism of action. Postgrad Med 1988;29: 19–26.
21. Bristow MR, Ginsberg R: Beta 2 receptors on myocardial cells in human ventricular myocardium. Am J Cardiol 1986;57:3F–6F.
22. Brown JE, McLeod AA, Shand DG: In support of cardiac chronotropic beta 2 adrenoceptors. Am J Cardiol 1986; 57:11F–16F.
23. Brown TCK, Barker GA, Dunlop ME, et al: The use of sodium bicarbonate in the treatment of tricyclic antidepressant induced arrhythmias. Anesth Int Care 1973;1: 203–210.
24. Buchman AL, Dauer J, Geiderman J: The use of vasoactive agents in the treatment of refractory hypotension seen in tricyclic antidepressant overdose. J Clin Psychopharmacol 1990;10:409–413.
25. Buxton AE, Marchlinski FE, Doherty JU, Flores B: Hazards of intravenous verapamil for sustained ventricular tachycardia. Am J Cardiol 1987;59:1107–1110.
26. Candell J, Valle V, Soler M, Rius J: Acute intoxication with verapamil. Chest 1979;75:200–201.
27. Caravati EM, Bossart PJ: Demographic and electrocardiographic factors associated with severe tricyclic antidepressant toxicity. J Toxicol Clin Toxicol 1991;29:31–43.
28. Catravas JD, Waters IW: Acute cocaine intoxication in the conscious dog: Studies on the mechanism of lethality. J Pharmacol Exp Ther 1981;217:350–356.
29. Centers for Disease Control and Prevention (CDC). Jin bu huan toxicity in adults—Los Angeles, 1993. MMWR 1993;42:920–922.
30. Chung PK, Tuso P: The electrocardiographic changes in a case of flecainide overdose. Conn Med 1990;54:183–185.
31. Clemessy JL, Angel G, Borron SW, et al: Therapeutic trial of diazepam versus placebo in acute chloroquine intoxiations of moderate gravity. Intensive Care Med 1996;22: 1400–1405.
32. Clemessy JL, Taboulet P, Hoffman JR, et al: Treatment of acute chloroquine poisoning: A 5-year experience. Crit Care Med 1996;24:1189–1195.
33. Cortese LM, Gasser RA Jr, Bjornson DC, et al: Prolonged recurrence of pentamidine-induced torsades de pointes. Ann Pharmacother 1992;26:1365–1369.
34. Croes K, Augustijns P, Sabbe M, et al: Diminished sedation during diazepam treatment for chloroquine intoxication. Pharm World Sci 1993;15:83–85.
35. Crome P: Poisoning due to tricyclic antidepressant overdosage: Clinical presentation and treatment. Med Toxicol 1986;1:261–285.
36. Crumb WJ, Wible B, Arnold DJ, et al: Blockade of multiple human cardiac potassium currents by the antihistamine terfenadine: Possible mechanism for terfenadine associated cardiotoxicity. Mol Pharmacol 1995; 47:181–190.
37. Curran ME, Splawski I, Timothy KW, et al: A molecular basis for cardiac arrhythmia: HERG mutations cause long QT syndrome. Cell 1995;80:795–803.
38. Darvon product insert. In: Physicians Desk Reference, 49th ed. Oradell, NJ, Medical Economics, 1995, pp. 1322–1324.
39. DaSilva O, DeMelo E, Filho D: Verapamil acute self-poisoning. Clin Toxicol 1979;14:361–367.
40. Derlet RW, Albertson TE: Acute cocaine toxicity: Antagonism by agents interacting with adrenoceptors. Pharmacol Biochem Behav 1990;36:225–231.
41. Derlet RW, Albertson TE: Diazepam in the prevention of seizures and death in cocaine-intoxicated rats. Ann Emerg Med 1989;18:542–546.
42. Derlet RW, Albertson TE: Potentiation of cocaine toxicity with calcium channel blockers. Am J Emerg Med 1989; 7:464–468.
43. Dusenberry SJ, Hicks MJ, Mariani PJ: Labetalol treatment of cocaine toxicity. Ann Emerg Med 1987;16:235. Letter.
44. Dziukas LJ, Vohra J: Tricyclic antidepressant poisoning. Med J Aust. 1991;154:244–250.
45. Engrav MB, Coodley G, Magnusson AR: Torsades de pointes after inhaled pentamidine. Ann Emerg Med 1992;21:1403–1405.
46. Enocksson S, Shimizu M, Lonnqvist F, et al: Demonstration of an in vivo functional beta 3-adrenocepter in man. J Clin Invest 1995;95:2239–2245.
47. Foulke GE: Identifying toxicity risk early after antidepressant overdose. Am J Emerg Med 1995;13:123–126.
48. Frierson J, Bailly D, Shultz T, et al: Refractory cardiogenic shock and complete heart block after unsuspected verapamil SR and atenolol overdose. Clin Cardiol 1991;14: 933–935.
49. Frohna WJ: Iatrogenic magnesium overdose in a patient with suspected acute myocardial infarction. Am J Emerg Med 1995;13:436–437.
50. Gay GR: Clinical management of acute and chronic cocaine poisoning. Ann Emerg Med 1982;11:562–572.
51. Gay GR, Loper KA: The use of labetalol in the management of cocaine crisis. Ann Emerg Med 1988;17: 282–283.
52. Glick G, Parmley W, Wechsler A, Sonnenblick E: Glucagon: Its enhancement of cardiac performance in the cat and dog and persistence of its inotropic action despite beta receptor blockade with propranolol. Circ Res 1968;22:789–799.
53. Goenen M, Col J, Compere A, et al: Treatment of severe verapamil poisoning with combined amrinone-isoproterenol therapy. Am J Cardiol 1986;58:1142–1143.
54. Goodwin DA, Lally KP, Null DM Jr: Extracorporeal membrane oxygenation support for cardiac dysfunction from antidepressant overdose. Crit Care Med 1993;21:625–627.
55. Graham SR, Day RO, Lee R, Fulde GW: Overdose with chloral hydrate: A pharmacological and therapeutic review. Med J Aust 1988;149:686–688.
56. Guinn MM, Bedford JA, Wilson MC: Antagonism of intravenous cocaine lethality in nonhuman primates. Clin Toxicol 1980;16:499–508.
57. Hantson P, Evenepoel M, Ziade D, et al: Adverse cardiac manifestations following dextropropoxyphene overdose:

Can naloxone be helpful? Ann Emerg Med 1995;25: 263–266.
58. Hantson P, Ronveau JL, DeConinck B, et al: Amrinone for refractory cardiogenic shock following chloroquine poisoning. Intensive Care Med 1991;17:430–431.
59. Hariman RJ, Mangiardi LM, McAllister RG Jr, et al: Reversal of the cardiovascular effects of verapamil by calcium and sodium: Differences between electrophysiologic and hemodynamic responses. Circulation 1979;59: 797–804.
60. Harris S, Hilligoss DM, Colangelo PM, et al: Azithromycin and terfenadine: Lack of drug interaction. Clin Pharmacol Ther 1995; 58:310–315.
61. Harrison DC: Current classification of antiarrhythmic drugs as a guide to their rational clinical use. Drugs 1986;31:93–95.
62. Hasan RA, Zureikat GY, Nolan BM: Torsades de pointes associated with astemizole overdose treated with magnesium sulfate. Pediatr Emerg Care 1993;9:23–25.
63. Hassen AH, Broudy EP: Selective autonomic modulation by mu- and kappa-opioid receptors in the hindbrain. Peptides 1988;9:63–67.
64. Hendren WG, Schieber RS, Garrettson LK: Extracorporeal bypass for the treatment of verapamil poisoning. Ann Emerg Med 1989;18:984–987.
65. Hofer CA, Smith JK, Tenholder MF: Verapamil intoxication: A literature review of overdoses and discussion of therapeutic options. Am J Med 1993;95:431–438.
66. Honig PK, Woosley RL, Zamani K, et al: Changes in the pharmacokinetics and electrocardiographic pharmacodynamics of terfenadine with concomitant administration of erythromycin. Clin Pharmacol Ther 1992;52: 231–238.
67. Honig PK, Wortham DC, Zamani K, et al: Effect of concomitant administration of cimetidine and ranitidine on the pharmacokinetics and electrocardiographic effects of terfenadine. Eur J Clin Pharmacol 1993;45:41–46.
68. Hoppu K, Tikanoja T, Tapanainen P, et al: Accidental astemizole overdose in young children. Lancet 1991;338: 538–540.
69. Howarth DM, Dawson AH, Smith AJ, et al: Calcium channel blocking drug overdose: An Australian series. Hum Exp Toxicol 1994;13:161–166.
70. Humbert VH, Munn NJ, Hawkins RF: Noncardiogenic pulmonary edema complicating massive diltiazem overdose. Chest 1991;99:258–260.
71. Ilingworth R: Glucagon for beta blocker poisoning. Lancet 1980;1:86.
72. Jacobsen D, Helgeland A, Koss A: Treatment of beta blocker poisoning. Lancet 1980;2:1031–1032.
73. Jurima-Romet M, Crawford K, Cyr T, Inaba T: Terfenadine metabolism in human liver. In vitro inhibition by macrolide antibiotics and azole antifungals. Drug Metab Dispos 1994; 22:849–857.
74. Karch SB: Managing cocaine crisis. Ann Emerg Med 1988;18:228–229. Letter.
75. Karch SB: Serum catecholamines in cocaine intoxicated patients with cardiac symptoms. Ann Emerg Med 1987;16: 481–483.
76. Kenny D, Pagel PS, Warltier DC: Attenuation of the systemic and coronary hemodynamic effects of cocaine in conscious dogs. Basic Res Cardiol 1992;87:465–477.
77. Kerns W, English B, Ford M: Propafenone overdose. Ann Emerg Med 1994;24:98–103.
78. Kim SY, Benowitz NL: Poisoning due to class Ia antiarrhythmic drugs quinidine, procainamide, and diisopyramide. Drug Saf 1990;5:393–420.
79. Kingston ME: Hyperventilation in tricyclic antidepressant poisoning. Crit Care Med 1979;7:550–551.
80. Koppel C, Oberdisse U, Heinemeyer G: Clinical course and outcome in class Ic antiarrhythmic overdose. J Toxicol Clin Toxicol 1990;28:433–444.
81. Kosinski E, Malindzak G: Glucagon and isoproterenol in reversing propranolol toxicity. Arch Intern Med 1973;132: 840–843.
82. Koury SI, Stone CK, Thomas SH: Amrinone as an antidote in experimental verapamil overdose. Acad Emerg Med 1996;3:762–727.
83. Krikler DM, Curry PVL: Torsades de pointes, an atypical ventricular tachycardia. Br Heart J 1968;38:117–120.
84. Lands AM, Arnold A, McAuliff SP: Differentiation of receptor systems activated by sympathomimetic amines. Nature 1967;214:597–598.
85. Lane AS, Woodward AC, Goldman MR: Massive propranolol overdose poorly responsive to pharmacologic therapy: Use of the intra-aortic balloon pump. Ann Emerg Med 1987;16:1381–1383.
86. Lange RA, Cigarroa RG, Flores DC, et al: Potentiation of cocaine-induced coronary vasoconstriction by beta adrenergic blockade. Ann Intern Med 1990;112:897–903.
87. Langou RA, Van Dyke C, Tahan SR, et al: Cardiovascular manifestations of tricyclic antidepressant overdose. Am Heart J 1980;100:458–464.
88. Larsen LS, Larsen A: Labetalol in the treatment of epinephrine overdose. Ann Emerg Med 1990;19:680–682.
89. Leatham EW, Holt DW, McKenna WJ: Class III antiarrhythmics in overdose. Presenting features and management principles. Drug Saf 1993;9:450–462.
90. Liebert EL, Francis PD, Woolf AD: ECG lead aVR versus QRS interval in predicting seizures and arrhythmias in acute tricyclic antidepressant toxicity. Ann Emerg Med 1995; 26:195–201.
91. Lipper B, Bell A, Gaynor B: Recurrent hypotension immediately after seizures in nortriptyline overdose. Am J Emerg Med 1994;12:452–453.
92. Lonnqvist F, Krief S, Strosberg AD, et al: Evidence for a functional $beta_3$ adrenoceptor in man. Br J Pharmacol 1993;110:929–936.
93. Love JN, Leasure JA, Mundt DJ, Janz TG: A comparison of amrinone and glucagon therapy for cardiovascular depression associated with propranolol. J Toxicol Clin Toxicol 1992;30:399–412.
94. Mader SL: Orthostatic hypotension. Med Clin North Am 1989;73:1337–1349.
95. Mani S, Kocheril AG, Andriole VT: Case report: Pentamidine and polymorphic ventricular tachycardia revisited. Am J Med Sci 1993;305:236–240.
96. Marrs-Simon P, Zell-Kanter M, Kendzierski DL, et al: Car-

diotoxic manifestations of mesoridazine overdose. Ann Emerg Med 1988;17:1074–1078.

97. Marshall JB, Forker AD: Cardiovascular effects of tricyclic antidepressant drugs: Therapeutic usage, overdose, and management of complications. Am Heart J 1982;103: 401–414.
98. Mathews DR, McNutt B, Okerholm R, et al: Torsades de pointes occurring in association with terfenadine use. JAMA 1991;266:2375–2376. Letter.
99. McKenzie AG: Intensive therapy for chloroquine poisoning. A review of 29 cases. S Afr Med J 1996;86:597–599.
100. McMillan R: Management of acute severe verapamil intoxication. J Emerg Med 1988;6:193–196.
101. Ming Z, Nordin C: Terfenadine blocks time-dependent Ca^{2+}, Na^{+}, and K^{+} channels in guinea pig ventricular myocytes. J Cardiovasc Pharmacol 1995; 26:761–769.
102. Monahan BP, Ferguson CL, Killeavy ES, et al: Torsades de pointes occurring in association with terfenadine use. JAMA 1990;264:2788–2790.
103. Morris DL, Goldschlager N: Calcium infusion for reversal of adverse effects of intravenous verapamil. JAMA 1983;249:3212–3213.
104. Mortensen ME, Bolon CE, Kelley MT, et al: Encainide overdose in an infant. Ann Emerg Med 1992;21:998–1001.
105. Murphy DJ, Walker ME, Culp DA, Francomacaro DV: Effects of adrenergic antagonists on cocaine-induced changes in respiratory function. Pulm Pharmacol 1991;4: 127–134.
106. Nahata M: Drug interactions with azithromycin and the macrolides: An overview. J Antimicrob Chemother 1996; 18:133–142.
107. Nattel S, Mittleman M: Treatment of ventricular tachyarrhythmias resulting from amitriptyline toxicity in dogs. J Pharmacol Exp Ther 1984;231:430–435.
108. Nelson LS, Hoffman RS: Mexiletine overdose producing status epilepticus without cardiovascular abnormalities. J Toxicol Clin Toxicol 1994;32:731–736.
109. Newton EH, Shih RD, Hoffman RS: Cyclic antidepressant overdose: A review of current management strategies. Am J Emerg Med 1994;12:376–379.
110. Niemann JT, Bessen HA, Rothstein RH, et al: Electrocardiographic criteria for tricyclic antidepressant cardiotoxicity. Am J Cardiol 1986;57:1154–1159.
111. Paakkari P, Paakkari I, Peuerstein G, Siren AL: Evidence for differential opioid mu 1- and mu 2-receptor mediated regulation of heart rate in the conscious rat. Neuropharmacology 1992;31:777–782.
112. Pearigen PD, Benowitz NL: Poisoning due to calcium antagonists. Drug Saf 1991;6:408–430.
113. Pentel PR, Benowitz NL: Tricyclic antidepressant poisoning: Management of arrhythmias. Med Toxicol 1986; 1:101–121.
114. Pentel PR, Ross CA, Landon J, et al: Reversal of desipramine toxicity in rats with polyclonal drug-specific antibody Fab fragments. J Lab Clin Med 1994;123:387–393.
115. Peterson C, Leeder S, Sterner S: Glucagon therapy for beta blocker overdose. Drug Intell Clin Pharm 1984;18:394–398.
116. Pimentel L, Trommer L: Cyclic antidepressant overdoses. A review. Emerg Med Clin North Am 1994;12:533–547.
117. Pohjola-Sintonen S, Viitasalo M, Toivonene L, Neuvonen P: Torsades de pointes after terfenadine-itraconazole interaction. Br Med J 1993;306:186.
118. Quadrel MA, Atkin SH, Jaker MA: Delayed cardiotoxicity during treatment with intravenous pentamidine: Two case reports and a review of the literature. Am Heart J 1992; 123:1377–1379.
119. Rajah A: The use of diazepam in chloroquine poisoning. Anaesthesia 1990;45:955–957.
120. Ramoska E, Sacchetti AD: Propranolol-induced hypertension in treatment of cocaine intoxication. Ann Emerg Med 1985;14:112–113.
121. Ramoska EA, Spiller HA, Winter M, Borys D: A one-year evaluation of calcium channel blocker overdoses: Toxicity and treatment. Ann Emerg Med 1993;22:196–200.
122. Randich A, Robertson JD, Willinghan T: The use of specific opioid agonists and antagonists to delineate the vagally mediated antinociceptive and cardiovascular effects of intravenous morphine. Brain Res 1993;603:186–200.
123. Rankin AC, Rae AP, Cobbe SM: Misuse of intravenous verapamil in patients with ventricular tachycardia. Lancet 1987;2:472–474.
124. Rao KA, Adlakha A, Verma-Ansil B, et al: Torsades de pointes ventricular tachycardia associated with overdose of astemizole. Mayo Clin Proc 1994;69:589–593.
125. Rappolt RT, Gay G, Inaba DS: Use of inderal (propranolol—Ayerst) in 1a (early stimulative) and 1b (advanced stimulative) classification of cocaine and other sympathomimetic reactions. Clin Toxicol 1978;13:325–332.
126. Rappolt RT, Gay G, Inaba DS, Rappolt NR: Propranolol in cocaine toxicity. Lancet 1976;2:640–641. Letter.
127. Robson R: Glucagon for beta blocker poisoning. Lancet 1980;2:1356–1357.
128. Roden DM: Antiarrhythmic drugs. In: Hardman JG, Limbird LE, Molinoff PB, et al, eds: Goodman & Gilman's Pharmacological Basis of Therapeutics, 9th ed. New York, McGraw-Hill, 1996, pp. 839–843.
129. Roy M, Dumaine R, Brown AM: HERG, a primary human ventricular target of the nonsedating antihistamine terfenadine. Circulation 1996; 94:817–823.
130. Salata JJ, Jurkiewicz NK, Sallace AA, et al: Cardiac electrophysiological actions of the histamine H1-receptor antagonists astemizole and terfenadine compared with chlorpheniramine and pyrilamine. Circ Res 1995; 76:110–119.
131. Sand IC, Brody SL, Wrenn KD, Slovis CM: Experience with esmolol for the treatment of cocaine associated cardiovascular complications. Am J Emerg Med 1991;9: 161–163.
132. Sasyniuk BI, Jhamandas V: Mechanism of reversal of toxic effects of amitriptyline on cardiac purkinje fibers by sodium bicarbonate. J Pharmacol Exp Ther 1984;231: 387–394.
133. Sasyniuk BI, Jhamandas V, Valois M: Experimental amitriptyline intoxication: Treatment of cardiac toxicity with sodium bicarbonate. Ann Emerg Med 1986;15: 1052–1059.
134. Saviuc P, Danel V, Dixmerias F: Prolonged QT interval and torsades de pointes following astemizole overdose. J Toxicol Clin Toxicol 1993;31:121–125.

135. Schindler CW, Tella SR, Goldberg SR: Adrenoceptor mechanisms in the cardiovascular effects of cocaine in conscious squirrel monkeys. Life Sci 1992;51:653–660.
136. Seger D, Schwartz G: Chloral hydrate: A dangerous sedative for overdose patients? Pediatr Emerg Care 1994;10: 349–350.
137. Sener EK, Gabe S, Henry JA: Response to glucagon in imipramine overdose. J Toxicol Clin Toxicol 1995;33: 51–53.
138. Sing K, Erickson T, Amitai Y, Hryhorczuk D: Chloral hydrate toxicity from oral and intravenous administration. J Toxicol Clin Toxicol 1996;34:101–106.
139. Smith M, Garner D, Niemann JT: Pharmacologic interventions after an LD50 cocaine insult in a chronically instrumented rat model. Are beta blockers contraindicated? Ann Emerg Med 1991;20:768–771.
140. Snook J, Boothman-Burrell D, Watkins J, Colin-Jones D: Torsades de pointes ventricular tachycardia associated with astemizole overdose. Br J Clin Pract 1988;42:257–259.
141. Stewart RB, Bardy GH, Greene HL: Wide complex tachycardia: Misdiagnosis and outcome after emergent therapy. Ann Intern Med 1986;104:766–771.
142. Stinson J, Walsh M, Feely J: Ventricular asystole and overdose with atenolol. Br Med J 1992;305:693.
143. Stone CK, Kraemer CM, Carroll R, Low R: Does a sodium-free buffer affect QRS width in experimental amitriptyline overdose? Ann Emerg Med 1995;26:58–64.
144. Stone CK, May WA, Carroll R: Treatment of verapamil overdose with glucagon in dogs. Ann Emerg Med 1995; 25:369–374.
145. Stork CM, Redd JT, Fine K, Hoffman RS: Propoxyphene-induced wide QRS complex dysrhythmia responsive to sodium bicarbonate—A case report. J Toxicol Clin Toxicol 1995;33:179–183.
146. Suessbrich J, Waldegger S, Lang F, Busch AE: Blockade of HERG channels expressed in *Xenopus* oocytes by the histamine receptor antagonists terfenadine and astemizole. FEBS Lett 1996;385:77–80.
147. Taboulet P, Baud FJ, Bismuth C, Vicaut E: Acute digitalis intoxication: Is pacing still appropriate? J Toxicol Clin Toxicol 1993;31:261–273.
148. Taboulet P, Michard F, Muszynski J, et al: Cardiovascular repercussions of seizures during cyclic antidepressant poisoning. J Toxicol Clin Toxicol 1995;33:205–211.
149. Tai YT, Lo CW, Chow WH, Cheng CH: Successful resuscitation and survival following massive overdose of metoprolol. Br J Clin Pract 1990;44:746–747.
150. Thalhammer C, Bogner JR, Lohmoller G: Chronic pentamidine aerosol prophylaxis does not induce QT prolongation. Clin Invest 1993;71:319–322.
151. Tobin JR, Doyle TP, Ackerman Ad, Brenner JI: Astemizole-induced cardiac conduction disturbances in a child. JAMA 1991;266:2737–2740.
152. Trouve R, Nahas GG: Antidotes to lethal cocaine toxicity in the rat. Arch Int Pharmacodyn Ther 1990;305:197–207.
153. Trouve R, Nahas GG, Maillet M: Nitrendipine as an antagonist to the cardiac toxicity of cocaine. J Cardiovasc Pharmacol 1987;9:S49–S53.
154. Tzivoni D, Banai S, Schuger C, et al: Treatment of torsades de pointes with magnesium sulfate. Circulation 1988;77: 392–397.
155. Tzivoni D, Keren A, Cohen AM, et al: Magnesium therapy for torsades de pointes. Am J Cardiol 1984;53:528–530.
156. Varhe A, Olkkola KT, Neuvonen PJ: Oral trizolam is potentially hazardous to patients receiving systemic antimycotics ketoconazole or itraconazole. Clin Pharmacol Ther 1994; 56:601–607.
157. Vaughan-Williams EM: A classification of antiarrhythmic actions reassessed after a decade of new drugs. J Clin Pharmacol 1984;24:129–147.
158. Vaughan-Williams EM: Subgroups of class I antiarrhythmic drugs. Eur Heart J 1984;5:96–98.
159. Vaughan-Williams EM: Classification of antiarrhythmic drugs. In: Sandoe E, Ellen FJ, Olesen KH, eds: Symposium on Cardiac Arrhythmias. Helsingor, Denmark, Sodertalje Press, 1970.
160. Vissers RJ, Purssell R: Iatrogenic magnesium overdose: Two case reports. J Emerg Med 1996;14:187–191.
161. Von Rosensteil NA, Adam D: Macrolide antibacterials. Drug interactions of clinical significance. Drug Saf 1995; 18:105–122.
162. Wananukul W, Keyler DE, Pentel PR: Effect of calcium chloride and 4-aminopyridine therapy on desipramine toxicity in rats. J Toxicol Clin Toxicol 1996;34:499–506.
163. Wang Q, Shen J, Splawski I, et al: SCN5A mutations associated with an inherited cardiac arrhythmia, long QT syndrome. Cell 1995;80:805–811.
164. Ward DE, Jones B: Glucagon and beta blocker toxicity. Br Med J 1976;1:151.
165. Wasserman F, Brodsky L, Dick MM, et al: Successful treatment of quinidine and procainamide intoxication. N Engl J Med 1958;259:797–802.
166. Watling SM, Crain JL, Edwards TD, Stiller RA: Verapamil overdose: Case report and review of the literature. Ann Pharmacother 1992;26:1373–1378.
167. Wei J, Spotnitz H, Spotnitz W, et al: Pharmacologic antagonism of propranolol in dogs. J Thorac Cardiovasc Surg 1984;87:732–742.
168. Wharton JM, Demopulos PA, Goldschlager N: Torsades de pointes during administration of pentamidine isethionate. Am J Med 1987;83:571–576.
169. Wheeldon NM, McDevitt DG, Lipworth BJ: Investigation of putative beta$_3$ adrenoceptors in man. Q J Med 1993;86: 255–261.
170. Whitcomb DC, Gilliam FR, Starmer CF, Grant AO: Marked QRS complex abnormalities and sodium channel blockade by propoxyphene reversed with lidocaine. J Clin Invest 1989;84:1629–1636.
171. Wilens TE, Stern TA, O'Gara PT: Adverse cardiac effects of combined neuroleptic ingestion and tricyclic antidepressant overdose. J Clin Psychopharmacol 1990;10:51–54.
172. Wiley JF, Gelber JL, Henretig FM, et al: Cardiotoxic effects of astemizole overdose in children. J Pediatr 1992;120: 799–802.
173. Williams JM, Hollingshed MJ, Vasilakis A, et al: Extracorporeal circulation in the management of severe tricyclic antidepressant overdose. Am J Emerg Med 1994;12: 456–458.

174. Williams T, Knopp R: The clinical use of orthostatic vital signs. In: Roberts JR, Hedges JR, eds: Clinical Procedures in Emergency Medicine. Philadelphia, Saunders, 1991, pp. 445–449.
175. Winson T, Burch GE: Clinical assessment of central venous pressure. Am Heart J 1946;31:387.
176. Wolfe TR, Caravati EM, Rollins DE: Terminal 40-ms frontal plane QRS axis as a marker for tricyclic antidepressant overdose. Ann Emerg Med 1989; 18:348–351.
177. Woosley RL, Chen Y, Freiman JP, Gillis RA: Mechanism of the cardiotoxic actions of terfenadine. JAMA 1993;269: 1532–1536.
178. Yang T, Prakash C, Roden DM, Snyders DJ: Mechanism of block of a human cardiac channel by terfenadine racemate and enantiomers. Br J Pharmacol 1995; 115:267–274.
179. Zerkowski HR, Ikezono K, Rohm N, et al: Human myocardial beta adrenoceptors: Demonstration of both beta 1 and beta 2 adrenoceptors mediating contractile responses to beta agonists on the isolated right atrium. Arch Pharmacol 1986;332:142–147.
180. Zimmermann M, Duruz H, Guiand O, et al: Torsades de pointes after treatment with terfenadine and ketoconazole. Eur Heart J 1992;13:1002–1003.

CHAPTER 22

Gastrointestinal Principles

Neal E. Flomenbaum and Martin J. Smilkstein

The role of the gastrointestinal (GI) tract in toxicologic emergencies is usually defined by its relationship to the absorption of toxic agents; as a result, GI decontamination is a major focus of clinical practice, research, and controversy (see Chap. 4). However, the GI tract should also be recognized as an important *site* of toxic effects, both as a result of decontamination procedures (Table 22–1) and, more importantly, the action of certain drugs and poisons. GI manifestations of toxic exposures range from incidental to life-threatening and result from both direct and indirect mechanisms.[5] Direct effects alter GI tract function and/or structure. Direct effects that disrupt function without causing immediate structural changes may do so by extrinsic (eg, cholinergic excess) or by intracellular (eg, colchicine) mechanisms; direct effects that do cause immediate structural changes inevitably result in functional impairment (eg, caustics). An example of an *indirect* effect is vomiting caused by an agent that only stimulates the chemoreceptor trigger zone, and has no direct effect on the gastric mucosa (as with digoxin or apomorphine).[36]

In some cases of altered GI function, such as increased gut motility from opioid withdrawal, function is not seriously impaired and the change is often useful in establishing a diagnosis. Conversely, decreased gut motility caused by cyclic antidepressants or other anticholinergics; the severe constipation or obstipation sometimes caused by opioids;[36] and the pseudo-obstruction caused by the neuroleptics butyrophenones and phenothiazines can harm the patient or complicate management. Because there are no structural changes associated with either of these types of altered GI function, there is no significant local injury. Such agents as salicylates, iron, and other metals, however, are capable of causing both serious systemic effects and life-threatening GI hemorrhage, perforation, or delayed stricture. Finally, alkalis typify substances that result in little or no systemic absorption or toxicity while causing morbidity or mortality from direct GI injury.

Toxins With Widespread Effects on the Gastrointestinal Tract

Caustics, ionizing radiation, and ethanol and other alcohols constitute a group of toxins that adversely affect the GI tract in many locations and sometimes by a variety of mechanisms. Before considering specific sections of the GI tract, the gastrointestinal toxicity of these three classes of agents will be reviewed.

Caustics

Without question, caustics are the major source of toxicity to the upper GI tract from lips to small intestines. Although caustics are discussed extensively in Chapter 86, it is worth reviewing briefly the patterns of destruction associated with the two main types of caustics, alkalis and acids. Alkaline caustics such as sodium hydroxide (NaOH), also known as lye, drain cleaner, and oven cleaner, produce a liquifactive destruction of the mucosa that may destroy and perforate all layers, depending on the strength, form (liquid, crystal), amount, and duration of contact. The primary sites of destruction after ingestion of an alkaline caustic are the lips, mouth, oropharynx, and esophagus. When perforation does not occur, healing is characterized by scarring and strictures that sometimes cannot be treated except by replacement of the affected esophagus by colon interposition.[28,92]

In contrast to the alkalis, strong acids are said to be most damaging to the stomach and duodenum and to skip or spare the esophagus. However, in one study of a large number of acid ingestions from India, where strong acids are commonly available as toilet cleansers, the esophagus was as frequently involved as the stomach and duodenum. The author noted that in western studies of caustic ingestions, acids only account for about 5% of reported cases and that this may explain, in part, the misconception.[99]

TABLE 22–1. GASTROINTESTINAL COMPLICATIONS OF GASTRIC DECONTAMINATION MEASURES

Procedure	Adverse Effect
Orogastric lavage	Emesis
	Esophageal tears or perforation (Mallory-Weiss or Boerhaave syndromes)
	Gastric perforation
	Hemorrhage
Activated charcoal	Constipation
	Diarrhea
	Intestinal obstruction or pseudo-obstruction (especially after repetitive doses in the setting of dehydration or prior bowel adhesions)
	Vomiting and aspiration
Cathartics	Abdominal cramping (sorbitol)
	Diarrhea and frequent watery stools (sorbitol)
	Electrolyte imbalance: increased Mg^{2+}, decreased K^+ and Na^+, (also increased PO_4^{3+} and decreased Ca^{2+} and K^+ from phosphate enemas)
	Nausea and vomiting
	Rectal prolapse
	Volume depletion and consequent metabolic alkalosis
Emesis with syrup of ipecac	Delayed emesis after loss of gag reflex
	Diarrhea
	Electrolyte imbalance with chronic use
	Esophageal (Mallory-Weiss) tears
	Gastric rupture or herniation
	Intractable vomiting and aspiration
Whole-bowel irrigation	Bloating
	Colonic perforation (in the presence of severe diverticulitis)
	Rectal itching (from excessive wiping)
	Vomiting, especially with rapid administration

When the esophagus is injured by acids, the damage may not be as great as when strong alkalis are involved, perhaps as a result of the coagulation necrosis produced by acids there. However, the damage to the stomach and the systemic effects of acid ingestion may be devastating. Strong acids produce acidemia—normal anion gap type initially in the case of hydrochloric acid, and wide anion gap type in all other cases. Because of its tendency to perforate the stomach, acid ingestions result in widespread damage to other abdominal organs such as the spleen, pancreas, and biliary tract (see Chap. 86 and Fig. 8–21). In addition to causing the same type of late effects seen after alkaline ingestions, acid ingestions may cause esophageal pseudodiverticuli, gastric atony, decreased acid secretion, and gastric outlet obstruction.[12,41,67] Both acid and alkali ingestions have been linked to squamous cell carcinoma of the esophagus and stomach, particularly at the gastroesophageal junction, years after the ingestion.[2,18,33,40]

Hydrofluoric acid (HF) differs from other acids. Although its pKa would suggest that it is a weak acid, its ability to penetrate tissues and other unique properties of HF make it the deadliest of all acids. HF primarily affects the stomach initially, but systemic absorption is rapid and ingestions of large amounts of highly concentrated solutions are almost always fatal (see Chap. 86).[9,49,90]

Other commonly available substances that are corrosive to the GI tract include ammonium hydroxide ("ammonia"), automatic dishwasher detergents, sodium hypochlorite (bleach),[3] alcohols, and phenol.

Ionizing Radiation

The acute radiation syndrome is a symptom complex that develops after whole-body radiation exposure and is divided into four phases, two of which involve the gastrointestinal tract.[14,72] An initial phase of nausea, vomiting, intestinal cramps, diarrhea, salivation, and dehydration follows exposures to over 1 Gy. Onset of vomiting within 2 hours indicates exposure to doses over 6 Gy. Vomiting that begins within minutes usually indicates a lethal exposure; within 1 hour, a near-lethal dose; and within 1 to 5 hours, a significant dose. Following the initial period of toxic effects, there is a latent period of days to weeks, unless the exposure is massive. The third phase is characterized by the additional gastrointestinal effects of electrolyte disturbances and dehydration and by such hematopoietic effects as pancytopenia (see Chaps. 24 and 98). Death can occur within 2 weeks of an exposure to more than 10 Gy and within 2 days of an exposure to doses exceeding 20 Gy. The fourth phase is characterized by long-term effects such as neoplasms, sterility, and cataract formation.[72]

The acute pathologic changes of the GI tract associated with acute radiation syndrome have been most extensively studied in the large bowel and consist of crypts with bizarre-appearing nuclei, mucin depletion, eosinophils in the lamina propria, and eosinophilic crypt abscesses.[7,65,75,97] In the small bowel, exposure to more than 30 Gy results in loss of villi and inflammatory cells in the lamina propria.[75,91]

Late pathologic changes include mucin depletion, telangiectatic vessels in the mucosa and submucosa, mucosal atrophy, decreased number and distorted architecture of crypts, edema, fibrinous exudates, and fibrosis.[75]

Ethanol and Other Alcohols

Ethanol is often painful to the oropharynx and esophagus upon ingestion, but its major gastrointestinal toxicity occurs in the stomach (Table 22–2). Alcohol-induced lesions tend to occur after acute ingestions of 8% or higher concentrations,[75] and alcohol-induced erosive gastritis (sometimes with the concomitant use of aspirin) may be responsible for more than half the cases of upper GI hemorrhages in some series.[15,39,75] As commonly used, the term "alcoholic gastritis" describes the gastric erosions and subepithelial hemorrhages with or without inflammatory cell infiltrates seen (endoscopically) in alcoholics.[44,96] When *H. pylori* is identified in alcoholics

TABLE 22–2. GASTROINTESTINAL EFFECTS OF ALCOHOL

Mouth
Nutritional stomatitis
Cheilosis

Esophagus
Esophagitis
Diffuse esophageal spasm
Mallory-Weiss tear
Rupture with mediastinitis

Stomach
Acute gastritis
Chronic hypertrophic gastritis
Peptic ulcer
Hematemesis

Small and Large Intestines
Malabsorption
Diarrhea

Liver
Steatosis
Alcoholic hepatitis
Cirrhosis

Pancreas
Acute pancreatitis
Chronic pancreatitis
Pancreatic pseudocyst

Adapted from West LF, Maxwell DS, Noble EP, Solomon DH: Alcoholism. Ann Intern Med 1984; 100:412–420.

with chronic antral gastritis, eradication of the organism, and not abstinence or antacid treatment alone, is necessary to eliminate the lesions.[95]

Alcohol increases the secretion of gastric juice[61,75]; reduces the transmucosal potential difference, allowing back diffusion of hydrogen ions[24,75]; and increases gastric mucosal permeability.[87] Microscopically, alcohol-induced lesions initially alter cell cytoplasm and nuclei[17] followed by widening of the intracellular space, focal separation of the tight junctions, and disruption of the apical membrane.[16,75]

Although most studies of small intestinal mucosa show only minimal light microscopic changes induced by alcohol,[57,75,80] patients who drink large amounts of alcohol acutely or chronically, typically experience diarrhea for several reasons: rapid transit from enhanced propulsive movements,[22,50] decreased intestinal disaccharidase activity,[22,68] decreased bile secretion from alcoholic liver disease,[22,47,78] and decreased pancreatic exocrine function or steatorrhea.[22,57] Markedly decreased absorption of fluid and electrolytes[22,42] together with ileal and colonic fluid malabsorption are also partly responsible for the diarrhea.[22]

Other gastrointestinal effects of ethanol include reflex esophagitis resulting from reduced lower esophageal sphincter pressure,[37] esophageal and gastric tears from vomiting (Mallory-Weiss and Boerhaave syndromes) after acute alcohol ingestion, and pancreatitis, hepatitis, and cirrhosis.

Lips, Mouth, and Oropharynx

Edema and Obstruction

The loose connective tissue and rich vascularity of the lips, mouth, and oropharynx predispose this region to edema formation from both local and systemic exposures (Table 22–3). Angioedema caused by many agents may present in this manner.[25] Because swelling about the

TABLE 22–3. TOXIC EFFECTS ON THE LIPS, MOUTH, AND OROPHARYNX

Type of Effect	Mechanism	Example
Gingivitis, stomatitis (loose teeth)	Inflammation and irritation	Caustics Chemotherapeutic agents Ciguatera (tooth pain) Ionizing radiation Metals (arsenic trioxide, mercuric chloride, lead, thallium, zinc chloride) Oxalates Phenol Phenytoin Phosphorous
Edema	Allergic Angioedema Mechanical irritation and injury	Penicillin ACE inhibitors Caustics Oxalate-containing plants
Pain and ulceration	Early	Caustics Paraquat
	Delayed	Daunorubicin Fluorouracil Methotrexate
Drooling	Increased saliva	Aminopyridine Cholinesterase inhibitors Nicotine Phencyclidine
	Dysphagia	Foreign bodies (drug packets, batteries)
Dry mouth	Decreased saliva	
	Direct	Anticholinergics Botulism
	From hypovolemia	
	Diuresis	Diuretics Lithium
	Insensible loss	Salicylates CNS stimulants
	Decreased fluid intake	CNS depressants
	Increased GI fluid losses	Cathartics Colchicine
Tongue discoloration	Direct toxic effects	Blue—methylene blue Brown—bromide, bismuth Green—vanadium

mouth may be the first recognized symptom of a systemic immediate hypersensitivity reaction, it is important to consider and prepare for the possibility of impending systemic anaphylaxis in addition to assessing the local findings.[4] Angioedema of the face, tongue, soft palate, and uvula is a fairly common adverse reaction to angiotensin-converting enzyme (ACE) inhibitors. Most cases of ACE inhibitor-induced angioedema may be successfully managed without airway intervention, but airway compromise has been described.[86]

In addition to reactions following systemic exposures, substances that directly injure the mucosa or submucosa may also cause localized edema. Edema of the lips, mouth, and tongue is common after ingestion of caustic chemicals[92] or irritants such as oxalate-containing plants.[54] The latter category should not be regarded lightly, as deaths have occurred as a result of such ingestions, particularly by infants.[54] It is obviously imperative to establish and maintain an airway when there is evidence of obstruction, but endotracheal intubation is also often indicated for patients without current airway compromise who may be expected to experience rapid swelling and consequent airway compromise.

Ulceration and Pain

Probably the most common sign of toxic exposure to the mouth and oropharynx is ulceration from the ingestion of caustic substances, which the patient experiences as pain. In addition to the caustics already mentioned, paraquat ingestions result in lip, tongue, and pharyngeal pain and ulceration. A unique feature of paraquat ingestions is the formation of a pseudomembrane in the pharynx said to resemble that of diphtheria.[89] Lip, mouth, and pharyngeal ulcerations may also occur several days after exposure to agents that prevent regeneration of normal mucosa by interfering with the epithelial cell cycle. Examples of this second group include methotrexate[34] and ionizing radiation.

Drooling and Dry Mouth

Toxicologic causes of drooling include agents such as organophosphates and carbamates that lead to increased production of saliva,[62] as well as those that prevent normal swallowing because of pain (caustics),[20,26] obstruction (body stuffers),[63,77] or neurologic dysfunction (tetrodotoxin poisoning).[93]

Dry mouth may result from decreased production of saliva due to anticholinergic drugs (Chap. 34), exposure to other agents such as botulism[81] and, of course, intravascular volume depletion resulting from other sequellae of toxic exposures such as decreased liquid intake during periods of altered consciousness, increased insensible water loss during fever or hyperpnea, increased GI or urinary losses, or a combination.

Tongue Discoloration

Discoloration of the mouth and tongue is associated with many conditions and exposures,[70] but few of these associations are specific or consistent enough to be of diagnostic value. Disturbances of normal taste are very common either from local oral exposure (eg, cocaine) or systemic effects (eg, crotalid envenomation). Extensive lists of taste alterations attributed to toxic exposures are available.[71,79] Again, a lack of specificity limits the applicability of these observations in the setting of toxicologic emergency care (see Chap. 27).

Esophagus

The normal esophagus acts primarily as a conduit between the mouth and stomach. To accomplish this function, the esophagus consists of a layer of inner stratified squamous cell epithelium with mucous glands to provide lubrication, surrounded by layers of smooth muscle that contract in a coordinated manner to propel food distally into the stomach by peristalsis.[27] Afferent nerve pain fibers sense injury to the protective mucosa and submucosa, while fibers within and around the muscular layer sense excessive stretch or tension. As a result of this relatively simple structure and function, pain and difficulty swallowing are essentially the only esophageal signs and symptoms resulting from toxic exposures (Table 22–4).

Pain

Retrosternal pain from endothelial or submucosal injury is most often burning in quality and fairly well localized. Regardless of cause, direct stimulation of afferent

TABLE 22–4. DRUGS AND TOXINS THAT EFFECT THE ESOPHAGUS

Type of Effect	Mechanism	Examples
Pain—retrosternal	Pain fiber stimulation	Alcohol Caustics
	Increased muscle tension due to:	
	Obstruction	Foreign body/drug packets
	Spasm	Caustics
	Mediastinitis/esophageal perforation	Caustics Emetics Foreign body
Dysphagia/odynophagia	Neuromuscular	Botulism Diphtheria Strychnine Thallium Tetrodotoxin Paralytic shellfish
	Mechanical—obstruction	Diphtheria Foreign body (drug packets) Large pill size or large number of pills
	Mechanical—irritation and injury	Caustics Iodine Mercuric chloride Paraquat, diquat

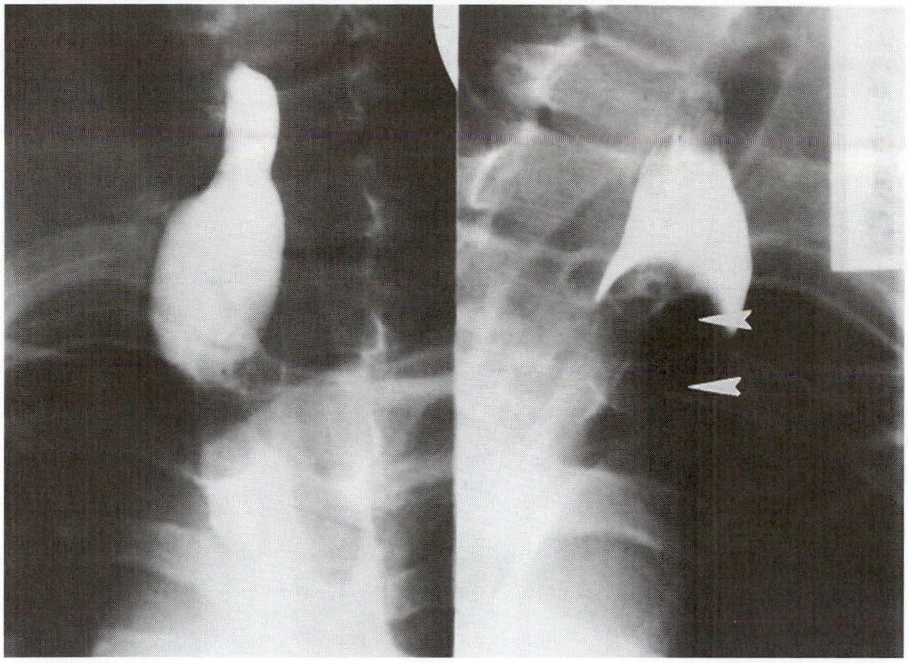

Figure 22–1. This barium swallow demonstrates an esophageal obstruction. It is part of a study done on a prisoner who had a contact visit with his wife. Shortly thereafter he became short of breath with severe neck pain and was unable to swallow water. After the barium study, a large toy balloon (*arrows*) filled with hashish was removed by endoscopy.

esophageal pain fibers results in this "heartburn" perception.[27] Intermittent periods of sharp, severe chest pain often indicate alterations in esophageal muscle tension from spasm, contraction against resistance, or mechanical stretch from foreign bodies. Esophageal injury causes local spasm. Serious injury to the mucosa and submucosa can stimulate sustained, diffuse spasm,[27] without any obvious intermittent or waxing and waning character. Acids, alkalis, and other caustics, corrosives, and solvents are the most common causes of significant esophageal injury (Chap. 86), and may cause any combination of these pain patterns.

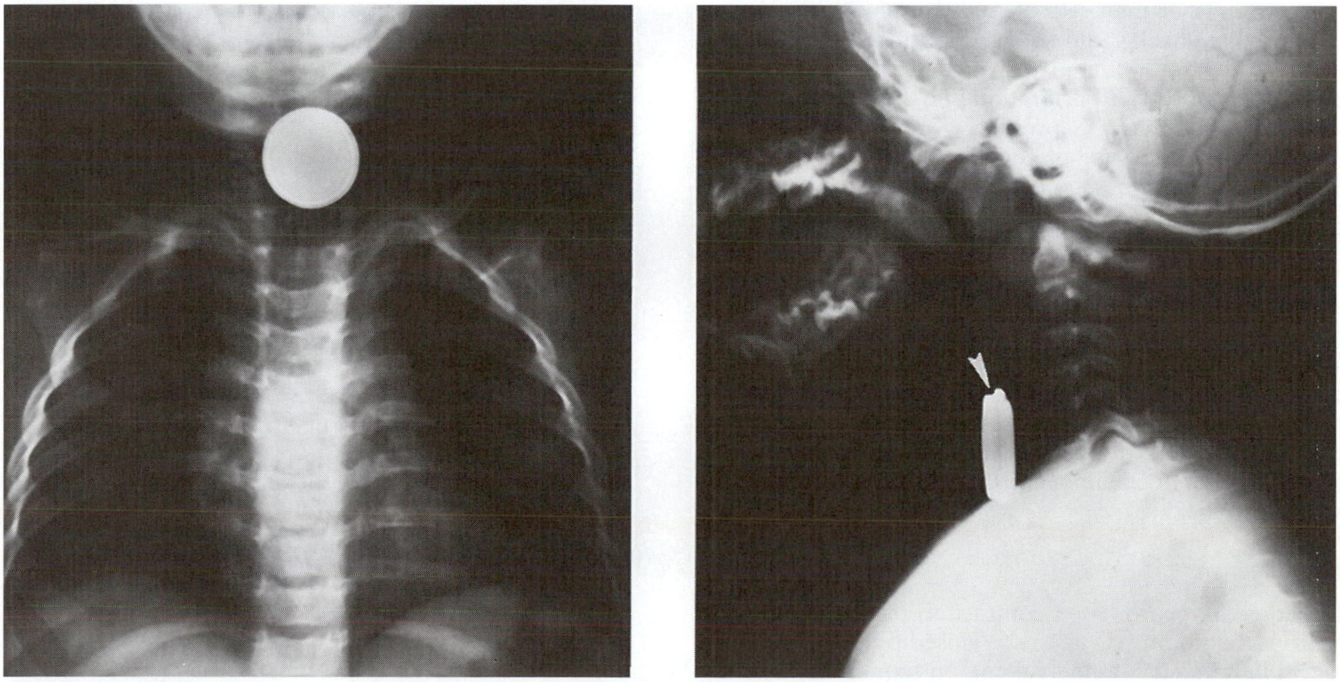

A B

Figure 22–2. A. Posterior-anterior view. **B.** Lateral neck view. The large button battery demonstrated here (notice crimp [*arrow*]) provoked significant pain and was lodged in the esophagus at the level of the cricopharyngeus. Endoscopic removal of the battery was possible. *(Courtesy of Nancy Genieser, MD, Professor of Radiology, New York University.)*

Dysphagia and Obstruction

Toxicologic causes of difficulty swallowing related to the esophagus include foreign body obstruction,[63,77] such as from hastily swallowed drug packets (Fig. 22–1) or batteries (Fig. 22–2), both of which may leak with disasterous consequences.[48,51] Dysphagia may also be due to esophageal spasm from local injury,[20,26,92] primarily from caustics. The normal swallowing function of the striated muscle of the hypopharynx can be similarly affected and cause dysphagia by interference with normal transfer of swallowed material into the esophagus.[27] In addition, striated muscle function can be altered by agents that disrupt normal neuromuscular transmission, such as botulism.[81] Esophageal stricture is a late complication of caustic exposure, which may also result in pain and difficulty swallowing.[27] Because of its delayed occurrence, it is not an important immediate treatment consideration but it is important to anticipate this possibility and evaluate the patient for stricture development during follow-up (Chap. 86). Esophageal stricture may occur after unrecognized esophageal injury from a variety of medications.[8]

Stomach

Pain and Ulceration

In general, the results of direct chemical injury to the stomach are similar to those of esophageal injury,[56] although several features make the clinical presentation somewhat different (Table 22–5). The location of pain is epigastric rather than retrosternal. Unremitting pain radiating to the back should suggest posterior penetration; severe diffuse abdominal pain and tenderness suggest possible gastric wall perforation and peritonitis,[46,66] but serious injury may be present without early tenderness.[64,73] Because of its horizontal position and restricted outlet at the pylorus, substances that pass quickly through the esophagus without significant injury may pool in the stomach and cause damage after prolonged contact. In addition, the unique chemical and structural environment may make the gastric mucosa more susceptible to injury by acids and other agents (Chap. 86). Probably all gastric mucosal injury is compounded by the back-diffusion of gastric acid after disruption of the normal mucosal barrier.[27,85] Ingested foreign bodies may become obstructed throughout the GI tract as demonstrated both by plain radiography and/or contrast studies[53] (Fig. 22–3).

Vomiting

The forceful, coordinated contraction of circumferential gastric smooth muscle against a closed pylorus results in regurgitation, an extremely common sequela of toxic exposure. Vomiting results from stimulation of the vomiting center in the floor of the fourth ventricle.[27] The vomiting center may be stimulated by either of two separate mechanisms. The first is direct afferent nerve input to the

TABLE 22–5. DRUGS AND TOXINS THAT EFFECT THE STOMACH

Type of Effect	Mechanism	Examples
Pain	Epigastric pain fiber stimulation	Alcohols Antimetabolites Arsenic Caustics Colchicine Iron Mercuric chloride NSAIDs Podophyllin Salicylates
	Perforation (Peritonitis)	Caustics Salicylates Pill concretions
	Obstruction	Bezoars Foreign body NSAIDs Salicylates
Vomiting	Local stimulation	Caustics Colchicine Detergents/soap (strong) Fluoride Metals (iron, mercury, thallium, arsenic) Mushrooms Salicylates Solvents Staphylococcal exotoxin Zinc chloride
	Central chemoreceptor trigger zone	Cardiac glycosides CO (?) Opioids Nicotine
	Local and central	Methylxanthines (theophylline, caffeine) Syrup of ipecac
	Increased intracranial pressure	
	Toxin-induced hemorrhage	Amphetamine Cocaine Phenylpropanolamine
	Edema	Vitamin A Postanoxic brain injury
	Hemorrhage or infarct Hypertension Hypotension Coagulopathy	Anticoagulants
Hematemesis	Direct mucosal injury	Alcohols (ethanol, isopropyl) Caustics Metals Plants Radiation Salicylates and NSAIDs Zinc chloride
	Coagulopathy	Anticoagulants Hepatic failure

vomiting center from any of several areas. The GI tract, particularly the first part of the duodenum, gives rise to many such fibers. Many drugs and chemicals cause vomiting by direct action on these GI tract fibers.[27] The second mechanism is stimulation of the chemoreceptor trigger zone also in the area postrema of the fourth ventricle. This area lacks afferent fibers, and its electrical stimulation does not cause vomiting. Rather, the chemoreceptors respond to certain agents in blood or cerebrospinal fluid, resulting in efferent stimulation of the vomiting center. Some substances are capable of stimulating vomiting by stimulating both GI tract fibers and the chemoreceptor trigger zone. Also, secondary effects of toxic exposure may include increased intracranial pressure or brainstem ischemia or hemorrhage, all of which are very potent causes of vomiting.

The color of the emesis often has diagnostic value. In most cases, the color of the ingested agent determines the color of the emesis; occasionally, however, the emesis may have a characteristic color not reflective of the ingestant itself. Examples include blue-green emesis after ingestion of copper sulfate, blue-brown emesis if starch is present in the stomach after ingestion of iodine, and the smoking, luminescent stools with a "garlic-like" odor after a yellow-phosphorus ingestion.

Hematemesis

Hematemesis, sometimes massive, may occur after ingestion of any agent that disrupts the gastric mucosa such as caustics, mercuric chloride, or iron,[55,66] or as a result of toxic coagulopathy.[13,29,32]

Small and Large Intestines

Normal intestinal function includes secretion of digestive enzymes, gentle mechanical mixing and propulsion of intestinal contents, and absorption of nutrients and water.[27] Each of these functions can be impaired by toxic exposures and result in signs and symptoms (Table 22–6).

Pain

Abdominal pain most commonly results from abnormally forceful or frequent intestinal smooth muscle contractions, which in turn results from local irritation, cholinergic stimulation, or contraction against a foreign body.[94] This type of pain is colicky and variable in intensity, frequency, and location. The frequency of intestinal contraction and the site of pain referral varies depending on the region of intestine affected.[84] Persistent pain associated with reproducible abdominal tenderness should suggest serosal or peritoneal involvement from intestinal perforation. Another form of pain, ischemic pain, results from cocaine use.[11,31,58,60] Gastrointestinal perforation may follow, particularly with the use of crack cocaine,[19,45] although bowel obstruction may be easier to demonstrate than perforation on plain radiography (Fig. 22–4).

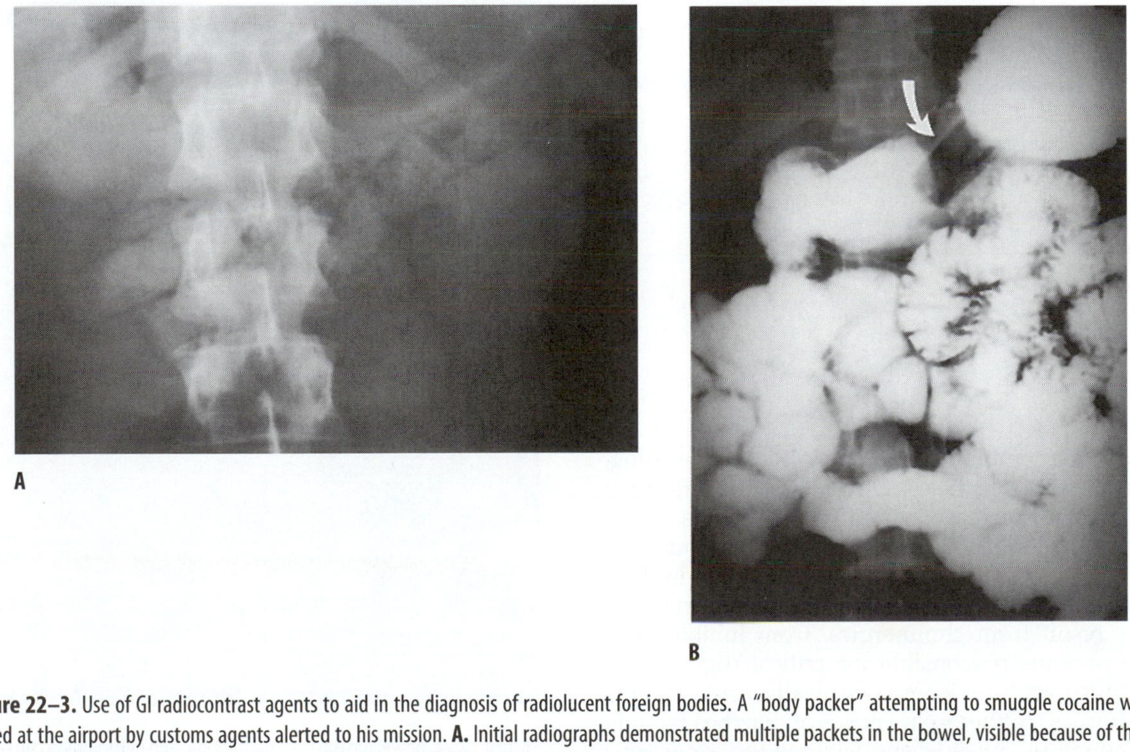

A

B

Figure 22–3. Use of GI radiocontrast agents to aid in the diagnosis of radiolucent foreign bodies. A "body packer" attempting to smuggle cocaine was arrested at the airport by customs agents alerted to his mission. **A.** Initial radiographs demonstrated multiple packets in the bowel, visible because of the thin layer of air trapped between layers of latex in the packet wall. Whole-bowel irrigation eliminated multiple packets in the fecal effluent and repeat plain radiographs were "negative." **B.** However, a subsequent upper GI contrast study with small bowel follow-through revealed one remaining packet in the stomach (*arrow*), which was then removed using flexible endoscopy.

TABLE 22–6. DRUGS AND TOXINS THAT EFFECT THE SMALL AND LARGE INTESTINES

Type of Effect	Mechanism	Examples
Pain	Increased contraction	
	Local irritation	Caustics
		Colchicine
		Metals
		Mushrooms
		Solanine-containing plants
		Stimulant cathartics
	Cholinergic stimulation	Cholinesterase inhibitors
		Opioid withdrawal
	Obstruction	Foreign body/drug-containing packets
Diarrhea	Mechanical irritation and injury	Bacterial endo- and exotoxins (food poisoning)
		Cathartic stimulants
		Caustics
		Colchicine
		Metals
		Mushrooms
		Solanine-containing plants
	Failure of mucosal regeneration	Colchicine
		Daunorubicin
		Etoposide
		Fluorouracil
		Ionizing radiation
		Podophyllin
	Cholinergic stimulation	Cholinesterase inhibitors
		Nicotine
		Opioid withdrawal
	Other mechanisms	Theophylline
Constipation	Local effects	Fluid and electrolyte depletion
	Central effects	Anticholinergics
		Infant botulism
		Opioids and other CNS depressants

Diarrhea

Diarrhea is also a common GI manifestation of poisoning, resulting from several causes. Direct injury to intestinal mucosa stimulates increased motility and results in impaired secretion of digestive enzymes as well as impaired absorption across the mucosa, all of which result in diarrhea.[1,21] Toxin-related diarrhea in the absence of structural injury may result from cholinergics, from inhibition of membrane proteins responsible for critical digestive or transport functions,[21] or from osmotically active agents such as cathartics.[43] Other toxic causes of diarrhea include colchicine, mercuric chloride, endogenous and exogenous bacterial toxins (food poisoning), and plants such as pokeweed. Malabsorption can result from changes in intraluminal pH or binding of nutrients in a nonabsorbable form.

Melena

Melena and hematochezia result from the same substances that cause hematemesis but may also follow cocaine-related bowel ischemia[19,45,58,60,98] or antimetabolite poisoning. Many forms of stool discoloration have been described.[6,69] As in emesis, the color of the feces results from the color of the ingested material or from upper or lower GI bleeding. Black stools do not always indicate bleeding, however, but may instead result from iron ingestion, senna, or bismuth subsalicylate (Pepto-Bismol) use. Rarely, a unique color change in the stools occurs, such as pink stools from phenolphthalein in alkaline medium or smoking, phosphorescent stools with a garlic odor after phosphorus ingestion.

Constipation

Constipation results from several types of poisoning such as opioids, cyclic antidepressants and infant botu-

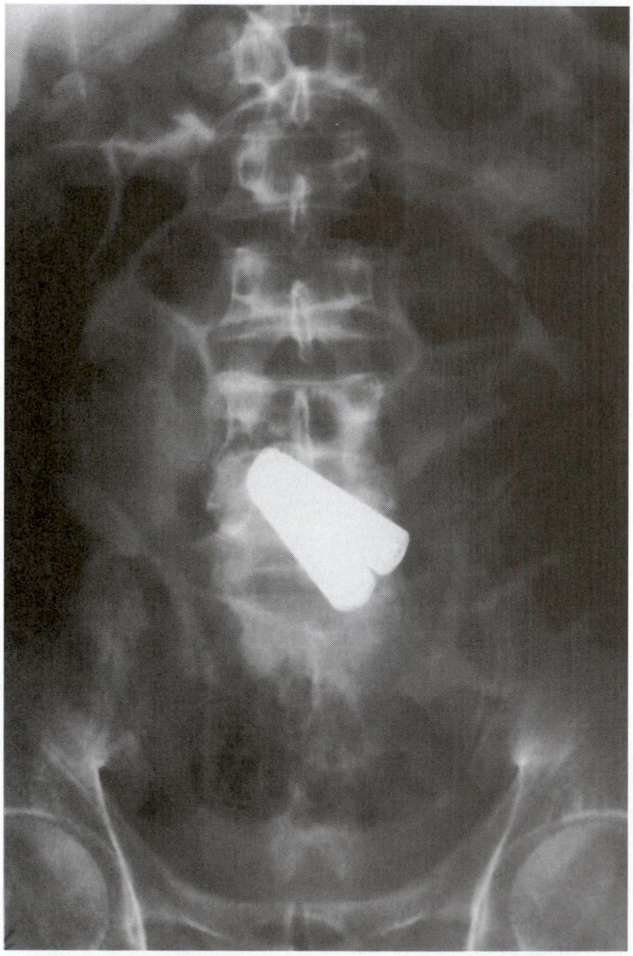

Figure 22–4. Bowel obstruction, perforation, and peritonitis occurred after ingestion of two "AA" batteries by a patient who had prior abdominal surgery. Plain films demonstrate the batteries and distended loops of bowel, but there is no evidence of free intraperitoneal air.

lism, which cause decreased GI motility[23,82]; phenothiazines, causing pseudoobstruction; and such indirect causes as drug-induced electrolyte disorders.[52]

Pancreas

The remaining components of the digestive system include the liver, gallbladder, and pancreas. Hepatobiliary principles are considered in Chapter 13, and pancreatic toxicity will be considered briefly here (Table 22–7). Although the definitive diagnosis of acute pancreatitis is pathologic and therefore only possible after surgical intervention or postmortem examination, the combination of abdominal pain, elevated pancreatic enzymes (serum amylase, serum lipase), and perhaps diagnostic and ultrasound or CT findings is usually sufficient to establish a clinical diagnosis.[35,88] Acute pancreatitis may occur either as isolated or recurrent attacks; it is distinguished from chronic pancreatitis by the absence of continuing inflammation, irreversible structural changes, or permanent impairment of exocrine and endocrine function.[88] Pancreatic duct stenosis that results from necrosis and disruption of the pancreatic duct during acute pancreatitis is known as chronic obstructive pancreatitis.

The substance most commonly responsible for acute toxicity to the exocrine pancreas is ethanol. When acute pancreatitis is induced by alcohol, small amounts of activated trypsin associated with disproportionately high concentrations of protein, zymogens, and trypsin inhibitor may be found within the ducts[74,76] along with hypertriglyceridemia.[76] Alcoholic pancreatitis is considered a form of chronic pancreatitis, but clinically an acute exacerbation more typically resembles and is treated as an acute pancreatitis.[88]

Unless further defined, the term "pancreatitis" tends to be used to describe dysfunction of the *exocrine* pancreas. The drugs and substances that are toxic to the exocrine pancreas differ from those that damage the *endocrine* pancreas. Agents that reduce or destroy B cells include the poisons alloxan, streptozocin, and vacor[38] and the antimicrobial pentamidine.[10,30,59,83] All of these substances may cause permanent diabetes mellitus. Other medications toxic to the endocrine pancreas include sulfonamides and diazoxide. A list of drugs and substances toxic to both the exocrine and endocrine pancreas may be found in Table 22–7.

TABLE 22–7. DRUG AND TOXINS ASSOCIATED WITH PANCREATITIS

Exocrine Pancreas	Endocrine (Islets of Langerhans) Pancreas
Alcohols	***Alpha Cells***
Ethanol	Cobalt salts
Methanol	Decamethylene diquaindine
	Phenylethyldiquanide
Analgesics and NSAIDs	
Acetaminophen	***Beta Cells***
Opioids	Alloxan
Salicylates[a]	Androgens
Sulindac	Cyclizine
Antibiotics	Cyproheptadine
Pentamidine	Diazoxide
Rifampin	Dihydromorphanthridine
Sulfonamides	Epinephrine
Tetracycline	Glucagon
Anticonvulsants	Glucocorticoids
Valproic acid	Growth hormone
	Pentamidine
Antihypertensives	Streptozocin
ACE inhibitors	Sulfonamides
Alpha-methyldopa[a]	Vacor
Diazoxide[a]	Zinc chelators
Antimitotics	***Delta Cells***
Azathioprine	None known
L-asparaginase	
Mercaptopurine	
Diuretics	
Chlorthalidone[a]	
Ethacrynic acid[a]	
Furosemide	
Thiazides	
Hormones	
Corticosteroids	
Estrogens	
Others	
Organophosphates	
Phenformin	

[a]Based on single or rare case reports.

From: Riddell RH, Strauss FH: The Pancreas. In: Riddell RH, ed: Pathology of Drug-Induced and Toxic Diseases. New York, Churchill Livingstone, 1982, pp. 611–629.

Summary

Except when injured or perforated by agents such as caustics, ionizing radiation, and alcohol, or obstructed by drug-containing packets or batteries, the gastrointestinal tract is typically not regarded as a significant site of drug toxicity. Nevertheless, because of both its potential as a site of severe local or systemic effects and the role that gastrointestinal signs and symptoms play in various diagnostic toxidromes, the gastrointestinal tract is an important consideration in almost any toxicologic emergency.

Acknowledgments

Howard Mofenson, MD and Thomas Carraccio, Pharm D contributed material to Table 22–3.

References

1. Anderson WM, Mason RE, Brinson RR, Schwartz GR: Diarrhea. In: Schwartz GR, Cayten CG, Mangelsen MA, et al, eds: Principles and Practice of Emergency Medicine, 3rd ed. Philadelphia, Lea & Febiger, 1992, pp. 463–471.
2. Appleqvist P, Salmo S: Lye corrosion carcinoma of the esophagus: A review of 63 cases. Cancer 1980;45: 2655–2685.
3. Ashcraft KW, Padula RT: The effect of dilute corrosives on the esophagus. Pediatrics 1974; 53:226–232.
4. Austen KF: The anaphylactic syndrome. In: Samte M, Talmage DW, Frank MM, et al, eds: Immunological Disease, 4th ed. Boston, Little, Brown, 1988, pp. 1119–1133.
5. Balthazar EJ, Lefleur R: Abdominal complications of drug addiction: Radiologic features. Semin Roentgenol 1983; 18:213–220.
6. Baran RB, Rowles B: Factors affecting coloration of urine and feces. J Am Pharm Assoc 1973; 13:139–142.
7. Berthrang M, Fajardo LF: Radiation injury in surgical pathology. Part II: Alimentary tract. Am J Surg Pathol 1981; 5:153–178.
8. Bonavina L, DeMeester TR, McChesney L, et al: Drug-induced esophageal stricture. Ann Surg 1987; 206:173–183.
9. Bost RO, Springfield A: Fatal Hydrofluoric acid ingestion: A suicide case report. J Analyt Toxicol 1995; 19:535–536.
10. Bouchard P, Sai P, Reach G, et al: Diabetes mellitus following pentamidine-induced hypoglycemia in humans. Diabetes 1982; 31:40–45.
11. Caruana DS, Weinbach B, Goerg D, Gardner LB: Cocaine packet ingestions: Diagnosis, management and natural history. Ann Intern Med 1984; 100:73–74.
12. Chaudhary A, Puri AS, Dhar P, et al: Elective surgery for corrosive-induced gastric injury. World J Surg 1996; 20:703–706.
13. Clark R, Rake MO, Flute PT, Williams R: Coagulation abnormalities in acute liver failure; pathogenetic and therapeutic implications. Scand J Gastroenterol 1973; 8(suppl 19):63–70.
14. Conklin JJ, Walker RL, Hirsch EF: Current concepts in the management of radiation injuries and associated trauma. Surg Gynecol Obstet 1985; 156:809–826.
15. Dagradi AE, Lee ER, Brosco DL, Stampien SJ: The clinical spectrum of hemorrhagic erosive gastritis. Am J Gastroenterol 1973; 60:30–46.
16. Dinoso VP, Chuarg J, Marthy SNS: Changes in mucosal and venous histamine concentrations during installation of ethanol in the canine stomach. Am J Digest Dis 1976; 21: 93–97.
17. Eastwood ME, Erdmann KR: Effects of ethanol on canine gastric epithelial ultra structure and transmucosal potential difference. Am J Digest Dis 1978; 23:429–435.
18. Eaton H, Tennekoon GE: Squamous carcinoma of the stomach following corrosive acid burns. Br J Surg 1972; 59:382–387.
19. Endress C, Kling GA: Cocaine-induced small bowel perforation. Am J Radiol 1990; 154: 1346–1347.
20. Estrera A, Taylor W, Mills LJ, Platt MR: Corrosive burns of the esophagus and stomach: A recommendation for an aggressive surgical approach. Ann Thorac Surg 1986; 41:276–283.
21. Field M, Rao MC, Chang EB: Intestinal electrolyte transport and diarrheal disease. N Engl J Med 1989; 321:800–806, 879–883.
22. Fine KD, Guenter JK, Fordtran JS: Diarrhea. In: Sleisinger MH, Fordtran JS, eds: Gastrointestinal Disease, 5th ed. Philadelphia, WB Saunders, 1993, p. 1062.
23. Frommer DA, Kulig KW, Marx JA, Rumack BH: Tricyclic antidepressant overdose. JAMA 1987; 257:521–526.
24. Geall MG, Phillips SF, Summerskill WHJ: Profile of gastric potential difference in man. Effects of aspirin, alcohol, bile, and endogenous acid. Gastroenterology 1970; 58:437–443.
25. Gigli I, Sheffer AL, Austen KF: Angioedema. In: Samte M, Talmage DW, Frank MM, et al, eds: Immunological Disease, 4th ed. Boston, Little, Brown, 1988, pp. 1205–1220.
26. Gorman RL, Khin-Maung-Gyi MT, Klein-Schwartz W, et al: Initial symptoms as predictors of esophageal injury in alkaline corrosive ingestions. Am J Emerg Med 1992; 10:189–194.
27. Greenberger NJ: Gastrointestinal Disorders: A Pathophysiologic Approach, 4th ed. Chicago, Year Book, 1990.
28. Haller JA, Andrews HG, White JJ, et al: Pathophysiology and management of acute corrosive burns of the esophagus: Results of treatment in 285 children. J Pediatr Surg 1971; 578–584.
29. Hardy DL: Fatal rattlesnake envenomation in Arizona: 1969–1984. J Toxicol Clin Toxicol 1986; 24:1–10.
30. Hauser L, Sheehan P, Simpkins H: Pancreatic pathology in pentamidine-induced diabetes in acquired immunodeficiency syndrome patients. Hum Pathol 1991;22: 926–929.
31. Hoffman RS, Smilkstein MJ, Goldfrank LR: Whole bowel irrigation and the cocaine "body packer": A new approach to a common problem. Am J Emerg Med 1990; 8:523–527.
32. Hoffman RS, Smilkstein MJ, Goldfrank LR: Evaluation of coagulation factor abnormalities after long-acting anticoagulant overdose. J Toxicol Clin Toxicol 1988; 26:233–248.
33. Hopkins RA, Postlethwait RW: Caustic burns and carcinoma of the esophagus. Ann Surg 1981; 194:146–148.
34. Hung DZ, Deng JF, Tsai WJ, et al: Methotrexate intoxication in a uremic patient. European Association of Poison Centers and Clinical Toxicologists XV congress, Istanbul, May 24–27, 1992, p. 95. Abstract.
35. Jacobson S: Gastrointestinal testing. In: Flomenbaum N, Goldfrank L, Jacobson S, eds: Emergency Diagnostic Testing, 2nd ed. St. Louis, Mosby-Yearbook, 1995, pp. 258–264.
36. Jaffe JH, Martin WR: Opioid analgesics and antagonists. In: Gilman AG, Rall TW, Nies AS, Taylor P, eds: The Pharmacological Basis of Therapeutics, 8th ed. New York, Pergamon, 1990, pp. 485–521.
37. Kaufman SE, Kaye MD: Induction of gastro-oesophageal reflux by alcohol. Gut 1979; 19:336–338.
38. Kenney RM, Michaels IAL, Flomenbaum NE, Yu GSM: Poisoning with N-3-Pyridylmethyl-N^1-P-nitrophenyl urea (vacor). Arch Pathol Lab Med 1981; 105:367–370.
39. Khodadoost J, Glass GBJ: Erosive gastritis and acute gastroduodenal ulceration as source of upper gastrointestinal bleeding in liver cirrhosis. Digestion 1972; 7:129–138.
40. Kivrianta VK: Corrosion carcinoma of the esophagus. Acta Otolaryngol 1952; 42:89–95.
41. Kocchar R, Mehta SK, Nagi B, Goenka MK: Corrosive

acid-induced esophageal intramural pseudodiverticulosis—A study of 14 patients. J Clin Gastroenterol 1991; 13:371–375.
42. Krasner N, Cochran KM, Russell RI, et al: Alcohol and absorption from the small intestine. I: Impairment of absorption from the small intestine in alcoholics. Gut 1976; 17:245–248.
43. Krenzelok EP, Keller R, Stewart RD: Gastrointestinal transit times of cathartics combined with charcoal. Ann Emerg Med 1985; 14:1152–1155.
44. Laine L, Weinstein WM: Histology of alcoholic hemorrhagic "gastritis." A prospective evaluation. Gastroenterology 1988; 94:1254–1262.
45. Lee HS, LaMaute HR, Prizzi WF, et al: Acute gastrointestinal perforations associated with use of crack. Ann Surg 1990; 211:15–17.
46. Lewin KJ, Riddell RH, Weinstein WM: Stomach and proximal duodenum: Inflammatory and miscellaneous disorders. In: Lewin KJ, Riddell RH, Weinstein WM, eds: Gastrointestinal Pathology and Its Clinical Implications. New York, Igaku-Shoin, 1992, p. 506.
47. Linscheer WG: Malabsorption in cirrhosis. Am J Clin Nutr 1970;23:488–492.
48. Litovitz T, Schmitz BF: Ingestion of cylindrical and button batteries: An analysis of 2382 cases. Pediatrics 1992;89: 747–757.
49. Manoguerra AS, Neuman TS: Fatal poisoning from acute hydrofluoric acid ingestion. Am J Emerg Med 1986; 4:362–363.
50. Martin JL, Justus PG, Mathias JA: Altered mutility of the small intestine in response to ethanol (ETOH): An explanation for the diarrhea associated with the consumption of alcohol. Gastroenterology 1980; 78:1218. Abstract.
51. Maves MD, Carithers JS, Birck HG: Esophageal burns secondary to disc battery ingestion. Ann Otol Rhinol Laryngol 1984; 93:364–369.
52. McAlister NH, Abrams HB, Schlosser R, Sturtridge W: Unintentional self-intoxication with inorganic calcium. J Intern Med 1990; 228:193–195.
53. McCarron MM, Wood JD: The cocaine body packer syndrome. JAMA 1983; 250:1417–1420.
54. McIntire MS, Guest JR, Porterfield JF: Philodendron: An infant death. J Toxicol Clin Toxicol 1990; 28:177–183.
55. McLauchlan GA: Acute mercury poisoning. Anaesthesia 1991; 46:110–112.
56. Meredith JW, Kon ND, Thompson JN: Management of injuries from liquid lye ingestion. J Trauma 1988; 28:1173–1180.
57. Mezey E, Jow E, Slavin RE, Tobon F: Pancreatic function and intestinal absorption in chronic alcoholism. Gastroenterology 1970; 59:657–664.
58. Mizrahi S, Laor D, Stamler B: Intestinal ischemia induced by cocaine abuse. Arch Surg 1988; 123:394. Letter.
59. Murphey SA, Josephs AS: Acute pancreatitis associated with pentamidine therapy. Arch Intern Med 1981; 141:56–58.
60. Nalbandian H, Sheth N, Dietrich R, et al: Intestinal ischemia caused by cocaine ingestion: Report of two cases. Surgery 1985; 97:374–376.
61. Nalin DR, Levine MM, Rhead J, et al: Cannabis, hydrochlrohydria and cholera. Lancet 1978; 2:859–861.
62. Namba T, Nolte C, Jackrel J, Grob D: Poisoning due to organophosphate insecticides. Am J Med 1971; 50:475–492.
63. Nandi P, Ong GB: Foreign body in the esophagus: Review of 2,394 cases. Br J Surg 1978; 65:5–9.
64. Nicosia JF, Thronton JP, Folk FA, Saletta JD: Surgical management of corrosive gastric injuries. Ann Surg 1974; 180:139–143.
65. Novak JM, Collins JT, Donowitz M, et al: Effects of radiation on the human gastrointestinal tract. J Clin Gastroenterol 1979; 1:9–39.
66. Oakes DD, Sherck JP, Mark JBD: Lye ingestion: Clinical patterns and therapeutic implications. J Thorac Cardiovasc Surg 1982; 83:194–204.
67. Ochi K, Ohashi T, Sato S, et al: Surgical treatment for caustic ingestion injury of the pharynx, larynx and esophagus. Acta Otolaryngol 1996; 522(suppl):116–119.
68. Perlow W, Baraona E, Lieber CS: Symptomatic intestinal disaccharidase deficiency in alcoholics. Gastroenterology 1977; 72:680–684.
69. Poisindex editorial staff: Feces colors. In: Rumack BH, Spoerke DG, eds: Poisindex Information System, Vol. 77, edition expired 8/31/93. Denver, Micromedex, 1993.
70. Poisindex editorial staff: Oral changes. In: Rumack BH, Spoerke DG, eds: Poisindex Information System, Vol. 77, edition expired 8/31/93. Denver, Micromedex, 1993.
71. Poisindex editorial staff: Taste disturbance. In: Rumack BH, Spoerke DG, eds: Poisindex Information System, Vol 77, edition expired 8/31/93. Denver, Micromedex, 1993.
72. Pons P, Sullivan JB: Radiation and radioactive emergencies. In: Sullivan JB, Krieger GR, eds: Hazardous Materials Toxicology. Baltimore, Williams & Wilkins, 1992 pp. 441–450.
73. Ray JF III, Myers WO, Lawton BR, et al: The natural history of liquid lye ingestion. Arch Surg 1974; 109:436–439.
74. Renner IG, Rinderknecht H, Douglas AP: Profiles of pure pancreatic secretions in patients with acute pancreatitis: The possible role of proteolytic enzymes in pathogenesis. Gastroenterology 1978; 75:1090–1098.
75. Riddell RH: The gastrointestinal tract. In: Riddell RH, ed: Pathology of Drug-Induced and Toxic Diseases. New York, Churchill-Livingstone, 1982, p. 515–606.
76. Riddell RH, Strauss FH: The pancreas. In: Riddell RH, ed: Pathology of Drug-Induced and Toxic Diseases. New York, Churchill-Livingstone, 1982, pp. 607–629.
77. Roberts J, Price D, Goldfrank L, Hartnett L: The body stuffer syndrome: A clandestine form of drug overdose. Am J Emerg Med 1986; 4:21–27.
78. Roggin GM, Iber FL, Linscheer WG: Intraluminal fat digestion in the chronic alcoholic. Gut 1972; 13:107–111.
79. Rollin H: Drug-related gustatory disorders. Ann Otol Rhinol Laryngol 1978; 87:37–42.
80. Rubin G, Rybak BJ, Linden J, et al: Ultrastructural changes in the small intestine induced by ethanol. Gastroenterology 1972; 63:801–814.
81. Schmidt-Nowara WW, Samet JM, Rosario PA: Early and late pulmonary complications of botulism. Arch Intern Med 1983; 143:451–456.
82. Schmidt RD, Schmidt TW: Infant botulism: A case series and review of the literature. J Emerg Med 1992; 10:713–718.
83. Schwartz MS, Cappell MS: Pentamidine-associated pancreatitis. Dig Dis Sci 1989; 34:1617–1620.
84. Silen W: Cope's Early Diagnosis of the Acute Abdomen,

18th ed. New York, Oxford University Press, 1991, pp. 146–153.

85. Silen W, Skillman JJ: Stress ulcer, acute erosive gastritis and the gastric mucosal barrier. Adv Intern Med 1974; 19:195–212.
86. Slater EE, Merrill DD, Guess HA, et al: Clinical profile of angioedema associated with angiotensin converting-enzyme inhibition. JAMA 1988; 260:967–970.
87. Smith BM, Skillman JJ, Edwards BG, Silen W: Permeability of the human gastric mucuosa. Alteration by acetylsalicylic acid and ethanol. N Engl J Med 1971; 285:716–721.
88. Soergel KH: Acute pancreatitics. In: Sleisinger MH, Fordtran JS, eds: Gastrointestinal Disease, 5th ed. Philadelphia, Saunders, 1993, pp. 1628–1655.
89. Stephens DS, Walker DH, Schaffer W, et al: Pseudodiphtheria. Ann Intern Med 1981; 94:202–204.
90. Stremski ES, Grande GA, Ling LJ: Survival following hydrofluoric acid ingestion. Ann Emerg Med 1992;21: 1396–1399.
91. Tarpila S: Morphological and functional response of human small intestine to ionizing radiation. Scand J Gastroenterol, 1971; 6(suppl):9–48.
92. Thompson JN: Corrosive esophageal injuries. I. A study of nine cases of concurrent accidental caustic ingestion. Laryngoscope 1987; 97:1060–1068.
93. Torda TA, Sinclair E, Ulyatt DB: Puffer fish (tetrodotoxin) poisoning: Clinical record and suggested management. Med J Aust 1973; 1:599–602.
94. Trent MS, Kim U: Cocaine packet ingestions: Surgical or medical management. Arch Surg 1987; 122:1179–1181.
95. Uppal R, Lateef SK, Korsten MA, et al: Chronic alcoholic gastritis. Roles of alcohol and *Helicobacter pylori*. Arch Intern Med 1991; 151:760–764.
96. Weinstein WM: Gastritis and gastropathies. In: Sleisinger MH, Fordtran JS, eds: Gastrointestinal Disease, 5th ed. Philadelphia, Saunders, 1993, p. 547.
97. Weisbrot IM, Liber AF, Gordon BS: The effects of therapeutic radiation on colonic mucosa. Cancer 1975; 36:931–940.
98. Yang RD, Han MW, McCarthy JH: Ischemic colitis in a crack abuser. Dig Dis Sci 1991; 36:238–240.
99. Zargar SA, Kochar R, Nagi B, et al: Ingestion of corrosive acids: Spectrum of injury to upper gastrointestinal tract and natural history. Gastroenterology 1989;97:702–707.

CHAPTER 23

Renal Principles

Donald A. Feinfeld

Many substances cause or aggravate renal dysfunction. The kidneys are particularly susceptible to toxic injury for four reasons.[126] They receive 20 to 25% of cardiac output yet make up less than 1% of total body mass. They are metabolically active, and thus vulnerable to agents that disrupt metabolism. They remove water from the filtrate and may build up a high concentration of toxic substances. Finally, the glomeruli and interstitium are susceptible to activation of the immune system. Many factors, such as renal perfusion, may affect an individual's reaction to a particular nephrotoxin.[11] The clinician should be aware of these factors and, when possible, alter them to minimize the adverse effect after a toxic exposure.

Major Toxic Syndromes of the Kidney

Although toxins may injure any part of the nephron (Fig. 23–1), there are three major syndromes of toxic renal injury: chronic renal failure, nephrotic syndrome, and especially, acute renal failure (which for purposes of continuity will be discussed last) (Table 23–1). Nephrotoxins usually affect the most metabolically active segment of the nephron—the tubules; therefore, most nephrotoxicity involves either acute or chronic tubular injury, although glomerular injury may sometimes result from drugs or chemicals.

Chronic renal failure is identified as any disease process that causes progressive decline of renal function over a period of years. The most common lesion of nephrotoxic chronic renal failure is chronic interstitial nephritis (Table 23–2), which involves destruction of tubules over a prolonged period,[65] with tubular atrophy, fibrosis, and a variable cellular infiltrate (Fig. 23–2), sometimes accompanied by papillary necrosis. The onset is usually insidious and relatively asymptomatic, often presenting as secondary hypertension or unexplained chronic renal failure. The major symptom is nonspecific nocturia. Papillary necrosis may lead to ureteral colic. There is mild to moderate proteinuria that remains well under the nephrotic range. Unlike other chronic renal disorders, interstitial nephritis is characterized by failure of the diseased tubules to adapt to the renal impairment, resulting in metabolic imbalances such as hyperchloremic metabolic acidosis, sodium wasting, and hyperkalemia early in the course.[61] Injury to erythropoietin-secreting cells may lead to a disproportionate anemia.

Nephrotic syndrome is characterized by massive proteinuria (> 3 g/day in the adult), hypoalbuminemia, edema, and hyperlipidemia. Although the relationships among these findings are not completely understood, the underlying event is injury to the glomerular barrier that normally prevents macromolecules from passing from the capillary lumen into the urinary space. Albumin loss usually exceeds urinary excretion, due to renal tubular catabolism of filtered protein. The tubules also retain sodium, causing expansion of the extracellular space and edema. The glomerular lesion may progress to renal failure if the pathologic process continues. Toxins induce nephrotic syndrome (Table 23–3) either (1) by releasing hidden antigens into the blood, leading to immune deposits in the glomerular basement membrane and to changes in the basement membrane (eg, gold, Fig. 23–3); or (2) by upsetting immunoregulatory balance (eg, nonsteroidal antiinflammatory drugs). A less common glomerular lesion is hypersensitivity vasculitis.

Acute renal failure is defined as any abrupt decline in renal function that impairs the kidney's capacity to maintain metabolic balance. It may involve prerenal factors that impair renal perfusion, such as volume depletion, shock, or congestive heart failure. Hence, toxic events that cause bleeding (overdose of anticoagulants), volume depletion (diuretics, cathartics, or emetics), cardiac dysfunction (beta-adrenergic antagonists), or hypotension may lead to acute prerenal failure.[59] Urinary tract obstruction from crystalluria (eg, oxalosis in ethylene glycol poisoning) also causes acute renal failure. However, the most common nephrotoxic lesions are intrinsic renal in-

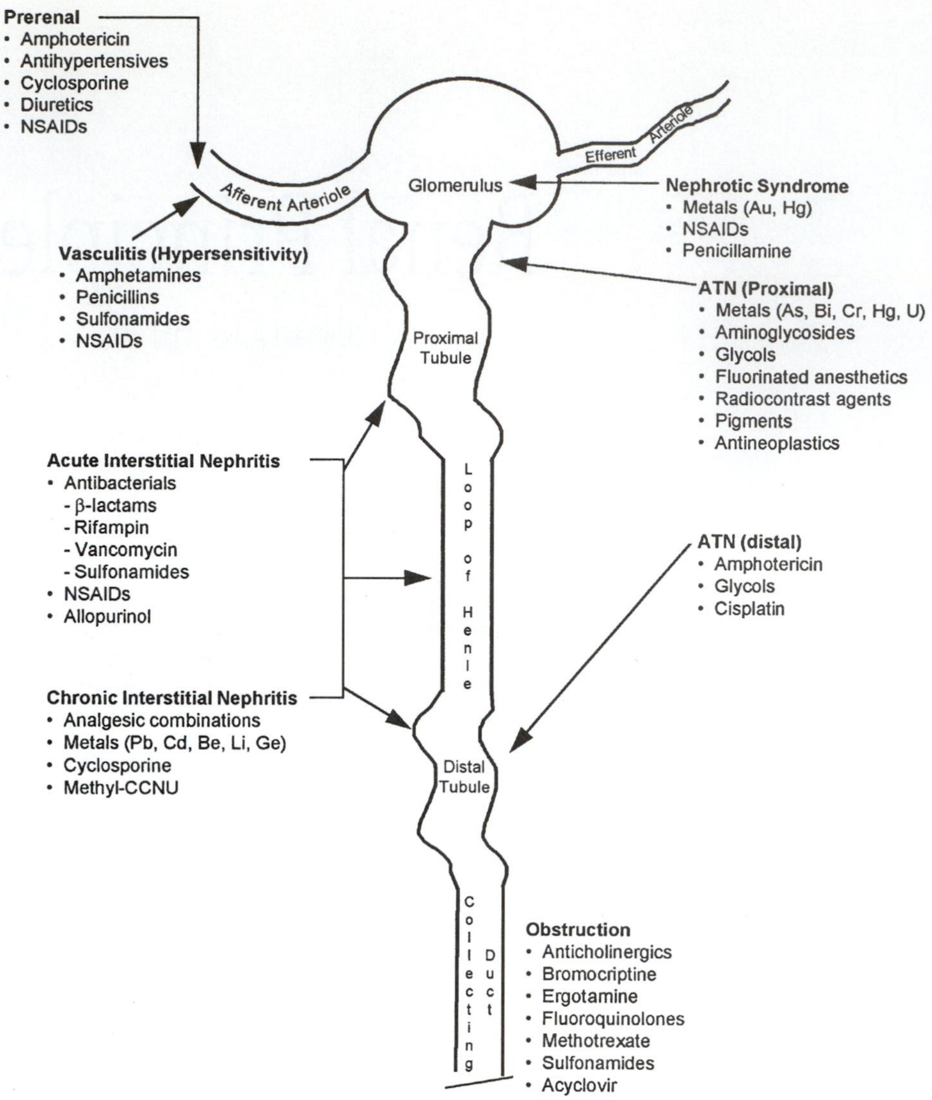

Figure 23–1. Schematic diagram showing the major nephrotoxic processes and the sites on the nephron that they chiefly affect.

TABLE 23–1. MAJOR NEPHROTOXIC SYNDROMES

Chronic Renal Failure
Chronic interstitial nephritis
Papillary necrosis
Chronic glomerulosclerosis
Nephrotic Syndrome
Minimal glomerular change
Membranous nephropathy
Focal segmental glomerulosclerosis
Acute Renal Failure
Acute prerenal failure
Acute urinary tract obstruction
Acute tubular necrosis
Acute interstitial nephritis
Acute vasculitis

TABLE 23–2. SUBSTANCES THAT COMMONLY CAUSE CHRONIC INTERSTITIAL NEPHRITIS

Analgesic combinations (aspirin + phenacetin or acetaminophen)
Cyclosporine
Metals (beryllium, cadmium, lead, lithium, platinum [as cisplatin])
Nitrosoureas (BCNU, methyl-CCNU)

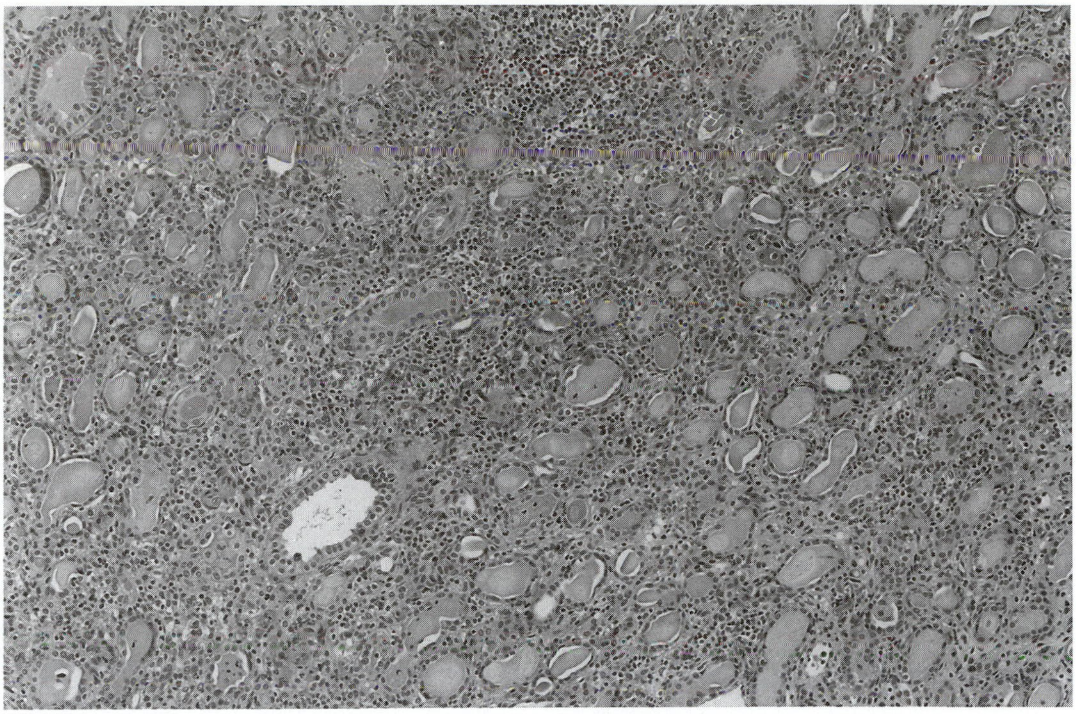

Figure 23–2. Chronic interstitial nephritis (secondary to NSAID). Interstitial fibrosis, lymphocytic infiltration, and tubular atrophy. (H&E × 225.) *(Courtesy of Dr. Rabia Mir.)*

juries, particularly acute tubular necrosis and acute interstitial nephritis (see Table 23–1).[4]

Acute tubular necrosis (Table 23–4), the most common nephrotoxic event, is characterized pathologically by patchy necrosis of tubules, usually the proximal segments (Fig. 23–4).This lesion is associated with three different processes: direct toxic injury, ischemic injury from renal hypoperfusion, and pigmenturia.[149] Direct toxins affect different segments; for example, uranium attacks the proximal tubule and amphotericin the distal tubule (see Fig. 23–1). However, the clinical pattern of rapidly declining renal function, often accompanied by oliguria, is identical in all forms of tubular necrosis. Direct toxicity accounts for about 35% of all cases of acute tubular necrosis.[110,198] Poisoning may also lead to tubular necrosis from hypotension or cardiac failure with ischemia of nephron segments that are particularly vulnerable to hypoxia. Pigmenturia means either myoglobinuria from rhabdomyolysis (skeletal muscle necrosis) or hemoglobinuria from massive hemolysis.[54] Either pigment may cause tubular injury and necrosis by precipitating in the tubular lumen.[63,149] Although there is controversy as to how a tubular lesion leads to glomerular shutdown, it is generally felt that tubular obstruction, back-leak of filtrate across injured epithelium, renal hypoperfusion, and decreased glomerular filtering surface combine to impair glomerular filtration.[193]

TABLE 23–3. SUBSTANCES THAT COMMONLY CAUSE NEPHROTIC SYNDROME

Captopril
Drugs of abuse
Metals (gold, mercury)
NSAIDs
Penicillamine
Probenecid
Trimethadione/paramethadione

Clinically, acute tubular necrosis presents as a rapid deterioration of renal function, usually first noted as azotemia. Muddy brown casts or renal tubular cells may be seen in the urinary sediment, but hematuria and leukocyturia are unusual. Disorders of metabolic balance, such as hyperkalemia and metabolic acidosis, are also common. Although tubular sodium reabsorption is decreased, the fall in glomerular filtration usually leads to positive sodium and water balance.[130]

Acute interstitial nephritis (Table 23–5) is clinically similar to acute tubular necrosis and often must be diagnosed by renal biopsy, which shows a cellular infiltrate separating tubular structures (Fig. 23–5). Nearly all acute interstitial nephritis is due to hypersensitivity.[197] In many cases the renal failure is accompanied by manifestations of systemic allergy such as fever, rash, or eosinophilia, and finding eosinophils in the urine is consistent with this disorder.[147] However, about 25% of patients with drug-induced interstitial nephritis have no signs of hypersensitivity. Unlike those with tubular necrosis, most patients with acute interstitial nephritis have hematuria and leukocyturia.[10]

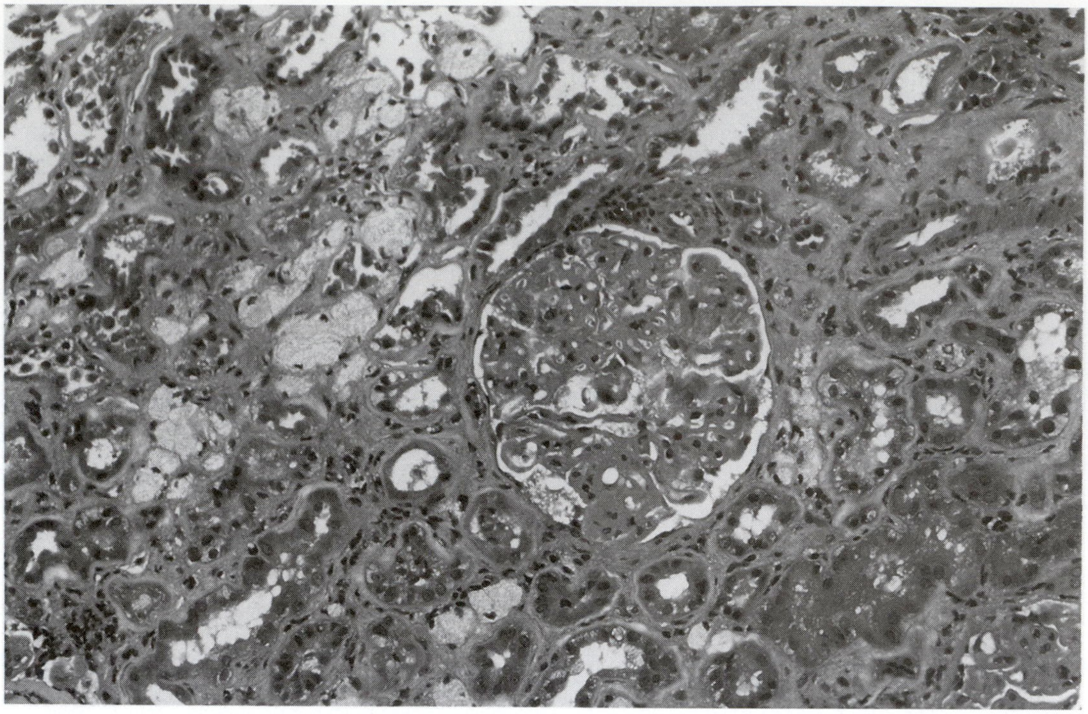

Figure 23–3. Membranous glomerulonephropathy (secondary to gold), a cause of nephrotic syndrome. Globally thickened glomerular capillaries, and interstitial foam cells are seen. (H&E × 450.) *(Courtesy of Dr. Rabia Mir.)*

TABLE 23–4. SUBSTANCES THAT COMMONLY CAUSE ACUTE TUBULAR NECROSIS

Acetaminophen
Antibacterials
Aminoglycosides
Amphotericin
Pentamidine
Polymyxins
Antineoplastic drugs
Cisplatin
Iphosphamide
Methotrexate
Mithramycin
Streptozocin
Fluorinated anesthetics
Glycols
Halogenated hydrocarbons
Iodinated radiocontrast media
Metals
Arsenic
Bismuth
Chromium
Mercury
Mushrooms
Cortinarius spp
Amanita spp
Pigments
Myoglobin
Hemoglobin
Toxins that cause hypotension or volume depletion

Differentiating Among the Causes of Acute Renal Failure

Patients who present with acutely deteriorating renal function often represent a difficult diagnostic challenge. Not only are there three major etiologic categories, but each category has several subdivisions; and more than one factor may be present. For example, a patient with an opioid overdose may have neurogenic hypotension (prerenal) together with muscle necrosis causing myoglobinuric renal failure (intrinsic renal) and opioid-induced urinary retention (postrenal). Because renal, prerenal, and postrenal processes are not mutually exclusive and require different interventions, all three should always be considered, even when one appears to be the most obvious cause of the renal failure.

Prerenal failure (renal hypoperfusion) initiates a sequence of events leading to renal salt and water retention.[13] Renin is released, causing production of angiotensin, which both enhances proximal tubular sodium reabsorption and stimulates adrenal aldosterone release to effect distal sodium reabsorption. Prerenal failure is therefore accompanied by low urinary sodium excretion (Table 23–6). Release of antidiuretic hormone increases water and urea retention.

Drugs may cause prerenal failure without necessarily causing intrinsic renal injury (Table 23–7). Blood volume can be decreased by diuretics or cathartics, and blood pressure reduced excessively by antihypertensive agents. Some drugs (eg, cyclosporine, amphotericin,

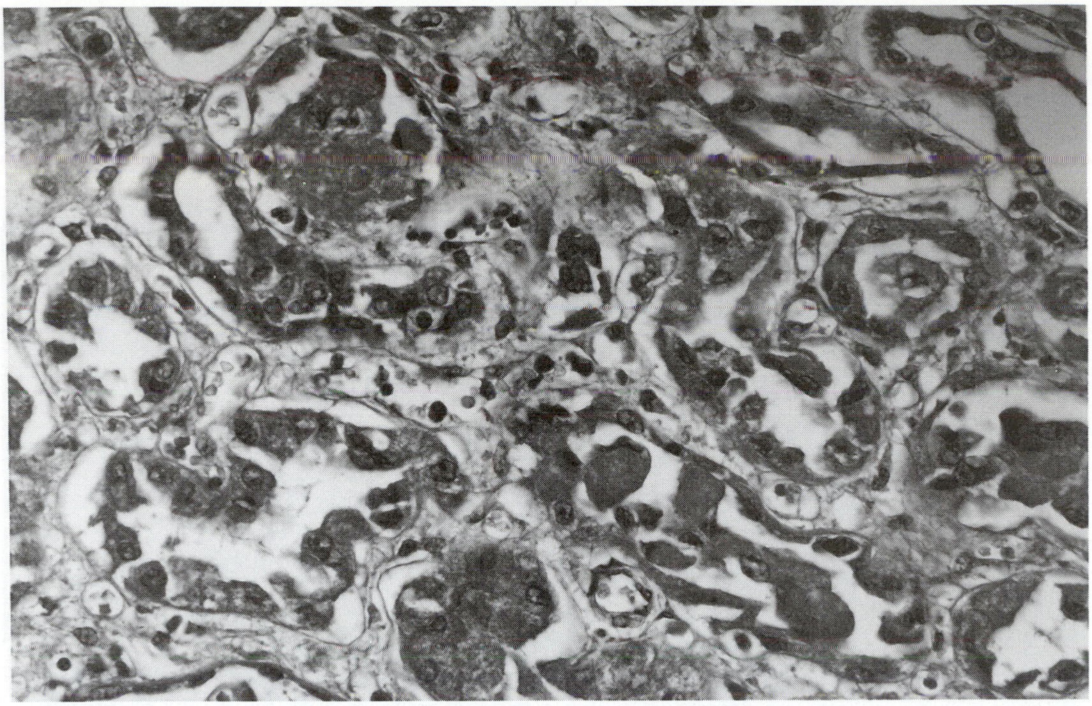

Figure 23–4. Acute tubular necrosis (secondary to mercury). Proximal tubular epithelial necrosis and sloughing are associated with interstitial edema. (H&E × 450.) *(Courtesy of Dr. Rabia Mir.)*

methotrexate) cause prerenal vasoconstriction. NSAIDs lower filtration rate by inhibiting production of vasodilatory prostaglandins in the afferent arteriole. Finally, cardiotoxic substances such as doxorubicin may cause severe heart failure. Some drugs cause a hypersensitivity vasculitis (Table 23–8). Urinary tract obstruction should always be considered when the kidneys fail rapidly. Although complete obstruction leads to anuria, partial obstruction, which is more common, is usually associated with alternating oliguria and polyuria. Continued production of urine in the presence of obstruction leads to distension of the urinary tract above the blockage. Calyceal dilation is common. Obstruction of the bladder outlet or urethra may distend the bladder.

Obstruction may be caused by medications (Table 23–9).[65] Most do so by impairing contraction of the bladder through anticholinergic action (atropine, tricyclic antidepressants). Rarely, certain drugs, particularly methysergide,[191] have been associated with retroperitoneal fibrosis and ureteral constriction. Finally, a few drugs lead to crystalluria and intratubular obstruction. Sometimes the drug itself forms precipitates (sulfonamides or methotrexate) or causes excretion of a precipitating chemical such as oxalate (fluorinated anesthetics).

TABLE 23–5. SUBSTANCES THAT COMMONLY CAUSE ACUTE INTERSTITIAL NEPHRITIS

More Common	Less Common
Allopurinol	Anticonvulsant drugs
Antibacterials	Carbamazepine
Beta-lactams, especially ampicillin, methicillin, penicillin	Phenobarbital
	Phenytoin
	Captopril
Azathioprine	Diuretics
NSAIDs	Furosemide
Rifampin	Thiazides
Sulfonamides	
Vancomycin	

Patient Evaluation

Evaluation of a patient with suspected toxic renal injury should include extrarenal as well as renal factors. The kidney's response to toxins is affected by previous renal function, renal blood flow, and the presence of urinary tract obstruction that can exert back pressure on the nephrons, all of which must be taken into consideration.

History

A past history of renal disease or other conditions that can affect the kidney (eg, diabetes, hypertension, cardiovascular disease) should be noted. Flank pain, hematuria, or any abnormal pattern of urine output are important symptoms. The patient's intravascular volume status affects renal perfusion. Thus, a history of heart disease or a disorder that lowers plasma volume such as vomiting or diarrhea is important. Prior cancer chemotherapy with drugs such as cisplatin or methyl-CCNU should be noted. All current medications should

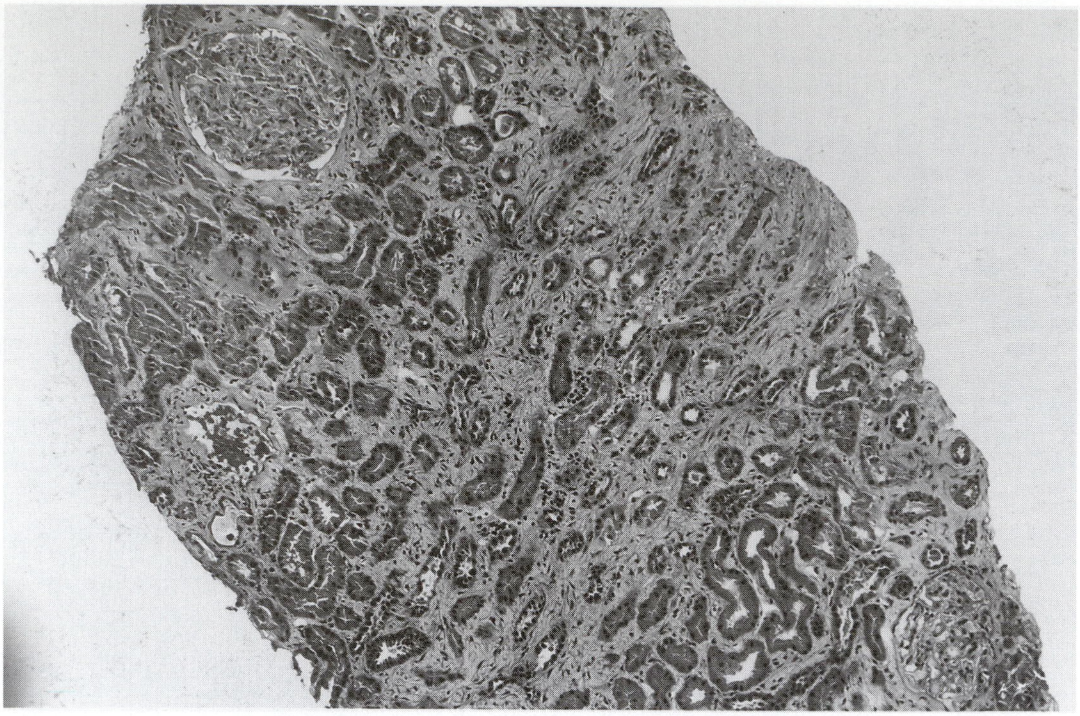

A

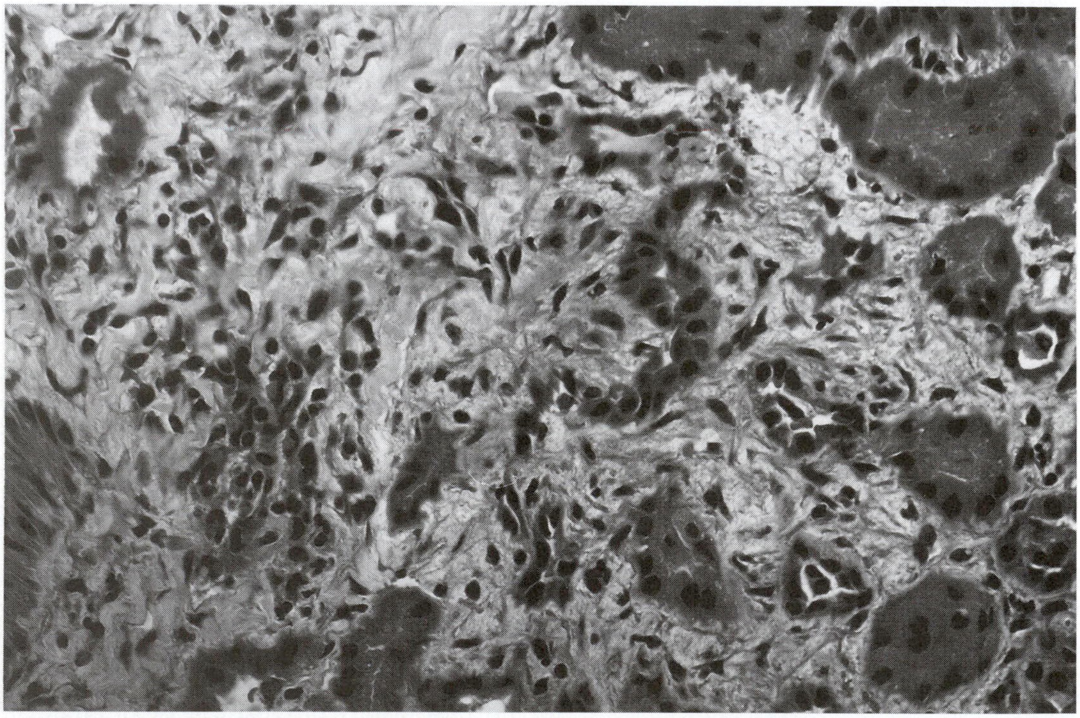

B

Figure 23–5. Acute interstitial nephritis (secondary to rifampin). Interstitial edema and patchy lymphocyte, plasma cell, and eosinophil infiltration occurs without fibrosis. Tubular epithelium shows degenerative and regenerative changes, and mononuclear cell infiltration (tubulitis). (**A,** H&E × 112; **B,** H&E × 450.) *(Courtesy of Dr. Rabia Mir.)*

TABLE 23–6. TESTS OF RENAL FUNCTION

Acute

To differentiate prerenal failure from acute tubular necrosis:

1. BUN:Creatinine ratio: usually > 20:1 in prerenal failure.
2. Urine sodium: usually < 20 mEq/L in prerenal failure; usually > 40 mEq/L in acute tubular necrosis.
3. Fractional sodium excretion (FE_{Na}) is the most reliable test[12,13]:

$$\left(\frac{\text{Urine[Na]}/\text{Plasma[Na]}}{\text{Urine[creatinine]}/\text{Plasma[creatinine]}}\right) \times 100$$

$FE_{Na} < 1\%$ (ie, normal) in prerenal failure if the patient has not received diuretics or large infusions of sodium, which increase fractional sodium excretion despite normal tubular function. In tubular necrosis or interstitial nephritis, renal sodium reabsorption is decreased, and $FE_{Na} > 1\%$. This is correct except in the case of pigmenturia or iodinated radiocontrast media-associated renal failure, when the test is of no benefit.

Chronic

Creatinine clearance: $U \times V/P$

(normal range: 90–130 mL/min), where U is urine creatinine concentration, V is urine flow per unit time (usually mL/min), and P is plasma creatinine. Urine collection must be complete; U and P must be in the same units.

be evaluated for potential renal effects, not only directly toxic drugs but also drugs such as diuretics that may enhance the toxicity of other substances.[82] The patient's intake of alcohol (especially "moonshine," which often contains lead) and drugs of abuse should be explored. Careful occupational history and assessment of hobbies and lifestyle are crucial, with emphasis on exposure to nephrotoxic chemicals, metals, and solvents.

Physical Examination

The patient's hemodynamics should be carefully assessed. Postural changes in pulse and blood pressure and either engorgement or decreased filling of the neck veins give important information about the intravascular volume. Funduscopy may reveal evidence of chronic hypertension or diabetes. All aspects of cardiac function should be noted. Injuries or scars in the suprapubic area or evidence of past urologic or retroperitoneal surgery may suggest obstruction, as may a palpable or percussible bladder.

TABLE 23–7. SUBSTANCES THAT COMMONLY CAUSE ACUTE PRERENAL FAILURE

Amphotericin
Antihypertensive agents
Cathartics
Cyclosporine
Diuretics
Doxorubicin
Iron
Methotrexate
NSAIDs
Toxins that cause hypotension or volume depletion

TABLE 23–8. DRUGS THAT MAY CAUSE HYPERSENSITIVITY VASCULITIS

Amphetamines
Fenoprofen
Naproxen
Penicillins
Sulfonamides

Laboratory Evaluation

Nephrotoxic injury is not always apparent clinically, so the laboratory becomes exceedingly important. Acute depression of renal function may be suspected if urine output decreases, but oliguria is not universal. The most important parameter of renal function is glomerular filtration. Since urea and creatinine are largely excreted by this route, serum levels of these substances are used as markers of renal function. However, the blood level of any substance depends on both production and excretion. Azotemia—elevation of blood urea nitrogen (BUN) or creatinine—is a standard indication of renal insufficiency. However, BUN or creatinine in the normal range does not exclude a substantial degree of renal impairment. The relationship between these parameters and glomerular filtration rate is hyperbolic, so blood levels usually do not exceed the upper limits of normal until more than 50% of kidney function is lost. In addition, decreased production of urea (starvation or liver failure) or creatinine (amputation, muscle wasting) may result in a normal-appearing BUN or creatinine in the presence of significant renal impairment. Since many nephrotoxic drugs are associated with nonoliguric acute renal failure (urine volume > 400 mL/day), progressive azotemia without oliguria should always raise suspicion of a drug-related cause.

TABLE 23–9. SUBSTANCES THAT MAY CAUSE URINARY OBSTRUCTION

Bladder Dysfunction

- Anticholinergics
  - Antihistamines
  - Antidepressants (tricyclic)
  - Atropine
  - Scopolamine
- Bromocriptine
- CNS depressants
- Neuroleptics

Crystal Deposition

- Ethylene glycol
- Fluorinated anesthetics
- Fluoroquinolone antibacterials
- Methotrexate
- Heme pigments
- Phenylbutazone
- Sulfonamides

Retroperitoneal Fibrosis

- Ergotamines

Certain drugs alter measured levels of urea and creatinine in the absence of any change in renal function.[142] Cefoxitin and ketones absorb light at the same frequency as the creatinine reaction product, thus artifactually increasing the measured level. Serum creatinine may also be increased by drugs that block renal creatinine secretion, such as cimetidine and trimethoprim. Blood urea nitrogen may be raised independent of renal function by tetracycline or corticosteroids, which increase protein catabolism.

In chronic renal insufficiency or failure it is necessary to assess the remaining renal function in order to manage the patient properly. Clearance measurements are generally used to determine glomerular filtration rate. The most common is endogenous creatinine clearance (see Table 23–6).

In acute renal failure it is not helpful to determine clearance, as the accuracy is dependent on the presence of a steady state. Changing glomerular function during a clearance time period makes the resulting estimation inaccurate. There is also a lag period between changes in kidney function and changes in BUN or creatinine levels. In general, a patient with acute renal failure should be treated as if glomerular filtration were below 10 mL/min. In acute renal failure a random sample of urine should be sent promptly for sodium and creatinine measurements to determine fractional sodium excretion (see Table 23–6).

Examination of the urine is of paramount importance in cases of poisoning. Even if urine is sent to the laboratory, it should also be examined carefully by the physician. Standard dipsticks will detect albumin and glucose. The dipstick test for blood is useful for confirming the presence of small amounts of blood or myoglobin but is not a substitute for careful microscopic examination of the sediment. The physician should look not only for red or white cells but also for crystals, tubular elements, casts, and bacteria. If acute interstitial nephritis is a consideration, a fresh urine sample should be stained for eosinophils.[147]

Further evaluation of the patient with acute renal failure should include tests for obstruction, which can be caused by a number of substances (see Table 23–9). Postvoiding residual urine volume should be measured by catheterization; a volume in excess of 75 to 100 mL should prompt urologic consultation. Renal ultrasonography should be performed to look for hydronephrosis.

Nephrotoxicity of Specific Substances

Metals

Table 23–10 summarizes the nephrotoxic effects of metals. *Antimony* caused transient acute renal failure in a child treated with high doses of the metal.[33]

Arsenic commonly causes acute renal failure by binding to sulfhydryl-containing proteins, forming arsenate, a multisystem toxin. Renal failure may be due in part to circulatory collapse or volume depletion from diarrhea, but arsenate is a direct distal tubule toxin.[202] Arsine gas attacks both proximal and distal tubules, causing interstitial inflammation[138] and inducing hemolysis; the resultant hemoglobinuria contributes to the renal failure.[113] Very severe arsenic-induced acute renal failure leads to chronic interstitial fibrosis.[201]

TABLE 23–10. NEPHROTOXIC EFFECTS OF METALS

	Toxic ATN	Shock ATN	Hemolysis	AIN	CIN	Tub Dys	NS	GN
Antimony	+							
Arsenic	+++	+++	++	+	+			
Barium	+							
Beryllium					++			
Bismuth	++			+		+	+	
Cadmium					+++	+++		
Chromium	+++							
Copper		+	+					
Germanium					+			
Gold	+						+++	
Iron		++			+			
Lead	+		+		+++	+++		
Lithium	+				++	++		
Mercury	+++	+				+	+	
Platinum (cisplatin)	++				++	++		
Silicon								+
Silver	+							
Thallium	+			+				
Uranium	+							

ATN = acute tubular necrosis; AIN = acute interstitial nephritis; CIN = chronic interstitial nephritis, Tub Dys = tubular dysfunction (renal glycosuria, electrolyte wasting, etc); NS = nephrotic syndrome; GN = glomerulonephritis. +++ = common; + = uncommon.

Barium may cause acute renal failure.[211] As this metal inhibits potassium exit from cells,[172] barium nephropathy is accompanied by hypokalemia (sometimes severe), which is unusual in acute renal failure (see Chap. 89).

Beryllium, a known pulmonary toxin, may also cause chronic interstitial nephritis, with granulomas and glomerulosclerosis.[17]

Bismuth causes dose-related injury to the proximal tubule. Low doses lead to tubular dysfunction; higher doses cause oliguric acute renal failure from tubular necrosis with interstitial inflammation.[21,195] Nephrotic syndrome is reported after medicinal administration of bismuth.[20]

Cadmium toxicity is mediated by a hepatic binding protein, metallothionein. Although binding of cadmium by this protein may protect other organs, the cadmium–metallothionein complex is readily taken up by the kidneys and cumulatively damages proximal tubular segments.[209] Initial changes are functional; pathologic changes occur after chronic exposure. Up to 80% of individuals exposed chronically to cadmium develop low-molecular-weight proteinuria[71] or Fanconi syndrome (amino aciduria, phosphaturia, renal glycosuria, proximal renal tubular acidosis, and hyperuricosuria).[1,102] The latter may be associated with urolithiasis.[102] Eventually, chronic interstitial nephritis with progressive renal failure supervenes.

Chromium is nephrotoxic as chromate or dichromate ion; it injures the proximal segments of the proximal tubule.[149] Very low doses may lead to hyposthenuria or glycosuria.[206]

Copper (as copper sulfate) was linked to two fatal cases of acute tubular necrosis secondary to volume depletion from vomiting, diarrhea, and sulfhemoglobinemic hemolysis.[176]

Germanium may cause chronic interstitial nephritis.[148]

Gold may cause nephrotic syndrome, often with hematuria, which usually reverses over several months after gold is discontinued and chelation instituted. Pathologic examination shows membranous glomerulopathy (see Fig. 23–3) with subepithelial immune deposits.[200] Gold deposits in proximal tubular cells and occasionally in glomerular epithelium.[7] This lesion may be a human counterpart to experimental Heymann nephritis, where reaction to a tubular antigen leads to epimembranous immune complex nephropathy[200]; this has been reproduced by injecting gold salts into rats.[144] Gold-induced tubular necrosis is also reported.[51]

Iron poisoning, particularly in children, may cause acute renal failure from renal ischemia due to GI bleeding, vomiting, diarrhea, and shock.[39,199] Large doses of iron are not nephrotoxic in animals, but chronic interstitial nephritis occurs in patients with hemochromatosis,[126] so long-term tubular iron deposition may have a toxic effect.

Lead inhibits sulfhydryl-dependent enzymes and replaces calcium in biochemical systems; its effect is cumulative. Lead slowly injures mitochondria in proximal tubular cells,[6,98] causing chronic interstitial nephritis with fibrosis, exacerbated by hypertension. Since progression of the disease is insidious, it is important to evaluate for prior or current lead exposure in patients with unexplained renal failure.

Like cadmium, lead causes functional impairment of proximal tubules, with Fanconi syndrome and tubular proteinuria.[36] Subclinical tubular impairment is reported in lead workers, some of whom had tubular fibrosis on biopsy.[210] Impaired uric acid secretion is characteristic of lead nephropathy, with hyperuricemia and clinical gout.[15] The combination of gout, hypertension, and chronic renal failure should raise the suspicion of lead exposure.[19,58] Confirmatory studies include whole blood lead levels, evaluation of heme synthesis (eg, δ-aminolevulinic acid levels), and lead mobilization studies (24-hour urine lead excretion before and after 0.5 to 1 g of IV calcium disodium EDTA).[32,42,58] Acute lead poisoning, characterized by jaundice, colic, and hemolytic anemia, is also reported to cause acute renal failure.[45]

Lithium commonly causes polyuria without pathologic changes,[184] from increased thirst or nephrogenic diabetes insipidus (Chap. 15). Some patients develop distal renal tubular acidosis (inability to lower urine pH < 5.4 after an acid load). These derangements usually disappear when lithium is discontinued. A few patients treated chronically with lithium may develop decreased renal function,[92] with chronic interstitial nephritis on biopsy.[91] The role of lithium in this disease was challenged by a study that showed a high incidence of interstitial nephritis in psychiatric patients not receiving the drug, for unclear reasons.[49] However, rats given lithium develop distal tubular lesions,[69] suggesting that there may be a risk of this complication in humans. There are occasional reports of both acute renal failure[114] and nephrotic syndrome[3] associated with lithium therapy.

Mercury has a strong affinity for renal tissue, especially as mercuric ion, although organic mercury and mercury vapor are also nephrotoxic. Mercury necroses proximal tubular cells[149] (see Fig. 23–4) by attacking sulfhydryl groups of mitochondrial proteins.[167] Swelling of poisoned tubular cells may be a factor in renal failure.[74] Oliguric acute renal failure with tubular cell casts is typical. Tubular functional abnormalities (glycosuria, aminoaciduria) may occur rarely.

Animals given very low doses of mercury develop nephrotic syndrome[2] due to low-grade tubular injury, which releases sequestered tubular antigens into the circulation and triggers an immune nephritis. A human equivalent is the membranous nephropathy reported in a few patients using topical mercury-containing preparations,[23] probably analagous to that seen with gold toxicity.

Platinum metal is relatively innocuous, but some of its compounds, such as the antitumor drug cisplatin, are nephrotoxic, predominantly to distal tubules.[80,173] Functional renal defects related to cisplatin include loss of urinary concentrating ability and renal magnesium wasting, which precede acute renal failure from tubular necrosis. Pretreatment hydration with saline or mannitol ameliorates this,[85] but there is still a risk of renal failure; the dose must be carefully adjusted and the patient closely followed after treatment. The newer congener carboplatin is less nephrotoxic, but may injure the kidneys,[186] as can the industrial chemical carboplatinite.[213]

Chronic renal failure from tubulointerstitial disease has been reported in patients previously treated with cisplatin.[80] Even with hydration, enough cisplatin may be taken up by tubular cells to produce subsequent tubular atrophy.[173]

Exposure to *silicon* is felt to be a risk factor for development of rapidly progressive glomerulonephritis.[101]

Silver salts cause tubular lesions in animals[126] and (rarely) acute tubular necrosis in humans.[123]

Thallium poisoning is associated with loss of urinary concentrating ability and albuminuria and sometimes acute renal failure with tubular necrosis and interstitial inflammation.[180]

Uranium selectively injures the middle segment of the proximal tubule in experimental models of acute tubular necrosis,[149] but human cases of uranium-induced acute renal failure are rare.[155]

Solvents

Carbon tetrachloride (CCl_4), known for hepatotoxicity, is also a nephrotoxin. Acute liver failure associated with CCl_4 poisoning may cause renal shutdown via the hepatorenal syndrome, but direct renal tubular injury is also common, with necrosis of the proximal tubule and loop of Henle.[149] Swelling of the glomerular basement membrane and parietal epithelial cells is also frequently seen.[188] CCl_4 is converted to trichloromethoxyl free radicals by cytochrome P450 enzymes in proximal tubules. These free radicals are quickly metabolized to chloroform and phosgene, the probable causes of cell necrosis.[185] The findings demonstrate oliguric acute renal failure, hematuria with red cell casts, moderate proteinuria, and crystalluria.[126] The lesion is usually reversible if the patient recovers from the hepatic injury.

Tetrachloroethylene poisoning resembles that of CCl_4, with hepatotoxicity predominating but occasionally acute renal failure from tubular necrosis.[180]

Trichloroethylene can cause acute tubular necrosis when sniffed.[14]

Toluene is associated with myoglobinuric acute renal failure.[166]

Glycols

Ethylene glycol is itself non-nephrotoxic and is cleared fairly well by the kidneys.[34] However, it is metabolized to glycolic acid and then oxalic acid. Subsequent deposition of oxalate crystals in the tubules causes obstruction and acute renal failure.[154] The crystals also provoke severe interstitial inflammation, which adds to the renal impairment and causes hematuria and proteinuria, followed by oliguria or anuria. The renal shutdown worsens the metabolic acidosis produced by the metabolites. Flank pain is a common complaint.

Diethylene glycol directly causes necrosis of proximal and distal tubular cells.[149] Hyperoxaluria may also complicate poisoning with this chemical.[86] Renal failure is often severe, especially if bilateral cortical necrosis supervenes.

Ethylene glycol dinitrite may cause renal tubular damage by producing methemoglobinemia.[126]

Propylene glycol is relatively nontoxic but may cause acute hemolysis when injected and has caused hemoglobinuric acute renal failure in animals.[105]

Antimicrobial Agents

Aminoglycosides are still a leading cause of drug-induced renal failure. With the exception of streptomycin, all antibiotics in this group cause tubular necrosis and renal failure. Aminoglycosides are taken up by proximal tubular cells, and incorporated into lysosomes, forming myeloid bodies.[26] Dose-related tubular necrosis is attributed to lysosomal failure[77] or damage to mitochondria.[183]

The incidence of nephrotoxicity in patients treated with aminoglycosides such as gentamicin varies from 1 to 30%. Risk factors for this complication include preexisting renal impairment, renal hypoperfusion, rising trough levels of the drug, and frequent dosage.[152] Infants are particularly at risk: a misplaced decimal point in a child's gentamicin order may lead to administration of a toxic dose. Tubular uptake of gentamicin appears to be saturable; hence, administration of infrequent large doses gives less net renal accumulation than more frequent, smaller doses.[50]

Gentamicin is probably more nephrotoxic than tobramycin[189] or amikacin[115]; however, all of these drugs can cause renal failure. Aminoglycoside nephropathy presents clinically as nonoliguric acute renal failure,[96] which usually resolves 1 to 3 weeks after the drug is discontinued. Renal magnesium and potassium wasting may occur. In addition to tubular necrosis, aminoglycosides may rarely cause allergic acute interstitial nephritis.[135,174]

The *penicillins* are not nephrotoxic but can cause acute interstitial nephritis. This is most frequent with methicillin, followed by ampicillin and penicillin, but may occur with any drug in this group.[10] The hypersensitivity reaction is not dose related, although the majority of patients have received the drug for 10 days or more.[10] Many patients with penicillin-associated interstitial nephritis have no prior history of penicillin allergy.

The clinical picture of acute interstitial nephritis often includes such allergic manifestations as rash or eosinophilia. Secondary fever at the onset of azotemia is common, and flank pain or arthralgia may be present. Nearly all patients have hematuria; most have leukocyturia, often with eosinophils.[11] The lesion usually improves once the drug is discontinued. A course of corticosteroids may hasten recovery;[8,79,119] many physicians use this treatment only if the renal failure does not improve promptly when the drug is stopped.

The penicillins may rarely cause hypersensitivity vasculitis, leading to acute glomerular inflammation and renal failure.[140]

Cephalosporins, like penicillins, can cause allergic interstitial nephritis, either directly[11] or from cross-sensitivity to penicillins.[107]

Some cephalosporins have intrinsic nephrotoxicity. Cephaloridine, the most toxic, is transported into tubular cells, becomes trapped, and causes necrosis[68]; it is no longer used in the United States. Cephalothin, the first available cephalosporin, rarely caused acute tubular necrosis, usually with additional risk factors (excessive dosage or concomitant use of other nephrotoxic agents).[68] The newer cephalosporins are much less nephrotoxic; acute renal failure with their use is nearly always hypersensitivity.

Sulfonamides were the first drugs associated with acute interstitial nephritis.[133] There is a cellular infiltrate, sometimes with granulomas. Trimethoprim/sulfamethoxazole also causes acute interstitial nephritis.[119]

Early reports of sulfonamide-associated renal failure were due to tubular obstruction from precipitation of the drug in the urine.[53] Newer sulfonamides such as sulfisoxazole and sulfamethoxazole are much more soluble than their predecessors, and crystalluria is now exceedingly rare. The sulfonamides, like the penicillins, are occasionally associated with hypersensitivity vasculitis.[140]

Tetracyclines may elevate BUN due to their catabolic activity, which leads to breakdown of endogenous proteins and excess production of urea.[160] There are scattered reports of acute tubular necrosis associated with tetracycline in patients with prior renal dysfunction, which decreases excretion of the drug, causing excessively high blood and tissue levels.[181] The most notorious functional renal defect associated with tetracyclines is Fanconi syndrome, reported during the 1960s[72] after exposure to outdated medication containing citric acid stabilizer, which is no longer used; hence, this complication is historical. Tetracyclines may also, rarely, cause allergic acute interstitial nephritis.[207]

Vancomycin was once a common cause of acute tubular necrosis. It is now felt that much of the early toxicity from vancomycin was due to incomplete purification of the drug.[9] Vancomycin-associated renal failure is relatively uncommon and is due to allergic interstitial nephritis.[56]

Rifampin is also associated with acute interstitial nephritis (see Fig. 23–5) but nearly always occurs either with intermittent dosage (eg, twice weekly)[162] or after the drug is stopped and resumed,[145] such as when a patient with tuberculosis is lost to follow-up after discharge and restarted on rifampin when recrudescence occurs. The nephritis is often accompanied by systemic symptoms such as fever, flank pain, and nausea, and patients frequently develop hematuria and oliguria.[145] The pathologic lesion usually resolves after the drug is stopped and may not respond to steroid treatment.[165]

Polymyxins (polymyxin B and colistin), now rarely used, are potent renal tubular toxins that often caused nonoliguric acute tubular necrosis.[109] Acute interstitial nephritis is also reported with polymyxin.[24]

Amphotericin has many adverse effects on the kidney.[35] It creates channels in the luminal membrane of the distal nephron,[5] which allows back-leakage of secreted H^+ and leakage of cellular K^+ into the lumen. Nearly all patients given the drug develop distal renal tubular acidosis and hypokalemia.[127] Renal magnesium wasting, seen in patients receiving more than 200 mg of amphotericin, exacerbates potassium loss.[18] Equally common is loss of urinary concentrating ability, which can cause dehydration.

Decreased renal function is also frequent with amphotericin. Following intravenous infusion of the drug there is an acute reduction in glomerular filtration rate, due to prerenal vasoconstriction, with transient oliguria followed by a short polyuric phase.[35] Renal dysfunction may persist for days. Acute tubular necrosis, due to both toxic and hemodynamic effects on the kidney, is common after administration of amphotericin and is both dose-related and cumulative. Permanent renal damage occurs in many patients receiving more than 4 g of amphotericin. Amphotericin nephrotoxicity may be prevented by limiting the dosage and correcting volume deficits promptly. Prophylactic volume expansion with saline may ameliorate amphotericin toxicity,[87] but vasodilators and mannitol are felt to be ineffective.

Fluoroquinolones (norfloxacin, ciprofloxacin, ofloxacin, and cinoxacin) may potentially cause acute tubular necrosis or interstitial nephritis.[78] In addition, there is a risk of crystalluria from these drugs.

Nitrofurantoin may rarely cause acute interstitial nephritis.[139]

Pentamidine, used to treat *Pneumocystis carinii* infections, can cause acute renal failure, often associated with hypoglycemia.[190]

Phenazopyridine is not antibacterial but is used to relieve dysuria in urinary tract infections. Overdose of the drug can cause acute tubular necrosis, accompanied by a yellow tinge to the skin.[67]

Acyclovir may cause acute renal failure due to precipitation of the drug in the renal tubules[29] or, rarely, acute tubular necrosis.[22]

Foscarnet can cause nephrotoxic acute renal failure.[30]

Nonsteroidal Antiinflammatory Agents

Widely used, nonsteroidal antiinflammatory drugs (NSAIDs) range from over-the-counter agents such as aspirin, acetaminophen, naproxen, and ibuprofen to prescription drugs. Much of the toxicity of these medications is renal.[41] Because this toxicity is related to their common mechanism of action, they are discussed as a group.

The NSAIDs inhibit cyclooxygenase, the enzyme that produces precursors to the prostaglandins, a family of 20-carbon fatty acids that act as local regulators of tissue function. As prostaglandin production decreases, production of leukotrienes, derived from the same fatty acid source but with different actions, is enhanced.[178]

A number of functional renal abnormalities accompany the use of NSAIDs. Prostaglandins dilate afferent renal arterioles in the presence of renal vasoconstrictor substances like angiotensin. Patients with high angiotensin levels (eg, in chronic renal failure, volume depletion, or congestive heart failure) may have hemodynamically mediated decreases in renal perfusion when given NSAIDs,[75] causing not only prerenal azotemia but also retention of sodium, with edema or aggravated heart failure. Prostaglandins mitigate the effect of antidiuretic hormone on the collecting duct, so water retention and hyponatremia may result from NSAID use.[41] Prostacyclin, a renal prostaglandin, stimulates renin, and the NSAIDs compete with aldosterone for binding sites. These events make hyperkalemia a common complication of NSAID use[178]; this is usually well tolerated but may become life threatening, particularly in the elderly or in those with chronic renal disease or hypoaldosteronism.[75]

NSAIDs also cause parenchymal renal disease, possibly due to loss of the antiinflammatory effects of prostaglandins, which attenuate lymphokine activity.[41] The most common renal disease from NSAIDs is acute interstitial nephritis. The pathology closely resembles that of allergic interstitial nephritis (discussed earlier), but without eosinophilia.[28] The resulting renal failure is usually exacerbated by the hemodynamic effects of prostaglandin deficiency. Nephritis usually occurs after the drug has been used for several months or more but may happen after shorter exposure. It generally resolves after the drug is discontinued, although prolonged exposure may lead to chronic interstitial nephritis (see Fig. 23–2).

Nephrotic syndrome often accompanies the interstitial nephritis caused by NSAIDs if the proteinuria is massive,[28] and may also occur as an isolated complication of NSAID use.[66,208] The glomerular lesion resembles "minimal-change" nephropathy: No abnormalities are seen on light or immunofluorescence microscopy. In addition to the renal toxicity described, *naproxen* and *fenoprofen* may also cause hypersensitivity vasculitis, which usually improves within a few weeks after the drug is stopped.

Acetaminophen (APAP) can be directly nephrotoxic. APAP overdose is usually associated with hepatocellular necrosis. However, because the cytochrome P450 enzymes that convert the drug to a toxic metabolite are also present in kidney (CYP, 1A2, 2E1), tubular cell injury leading to renal failure may result from APAP overdose.[31] It has been suggested that APAP's nephrotoxicity, unlike its hepatotoxicity, may not respond to *N*-acetylcysteine.[48]

Sulindac may be less nephrotoxic than other NSAIDs because of a weaker effect on renal prostaglandins.[38] It has not been associated with interstitial nephritis but can cause nephrotic syndrome.[208]

Chronic interstitial nephritis with papillary necrosis is a major complication of chronic NSAID use (analgesic nephropathy), particularly aspirin–phenacetin combinations.[175] The toxicity of these drugs is cumulative: A minimum of 2 kg is needed to cause renal injury. The lesion begins as inflammation around the renal papillae and culminates in nephron loss and interstitial fibrosis.[126] The papillae may slough and cause ureteral colic; more often there is insidious progressive renal failure with mild low-molecular-weight proteinuria and leukocyturia. As patients are often reluctant to admit taking large quantities of nonprescription drugs, not only is a careful history important, but other clues, such as gastric irritation from aspirin or methemoglobinemia from phenacetin, must be sought. In addition to aspirin, other NSAIDs may rarely cause papillary necrosis.[178] Combinations of these drugs are far more nephrotoxic than individual agents, although caution should be observed whenever any NSAID is prescribed. It was reported that daily consumption of APAP, the first metabolite of phenacetin, may be a risk factor for chronic renal failure.[175] However, a recent position paper on analgesic use concludes that the main risk for analgesic nephropathy is the use of combinations, and that usual doses of APAP are probably safe.[88]

Other Antiarthritis Agents

Allopurinol, which lowers uric acid, is a potent allergen and may cause interstitial nephritis.[76]

Sulfinpyrazone, a uricosuric agent, also causes allergic interstitial nephritis with nonoliguric acute renal failure and eosinophilia.[94,119]

Probenecid, another uricosuric drug, may cause nephrotic syndrome; pathology shows membranous nephropathy.[90]

Penicillamine, used to treat rheumatoid arthritis as well as to chelate toxic metals, is a well-documented cause of membranous nephropathy and nephrotic syndrome.[170]

Colchicine may cause acute renal failure, possibly due to muscle necrosis and myoglobinuria.[192]

Diuretics

The commonly used diuretics are usually categorized as *loop diuretics*, which act at the loop of Henle (ethacrynic acid, furosemide, bumetanide, and torasemide); *distal tubule diuretics* (thiazides and quinazolones); and *potassium-sparing diuretics* (spironolactone, triamterene, and amiloride). Although these drugs are not generally nephrotoxic, they may cause functional or parenchymal renal injury.

Loop diuretics and distal tubule diuretics cause prerenal failure by contracting extracellular fluid volume. Both groups of diuretics may also be associated with allergic acute interstitial nephritis, often accompanied by drug fever and eosinophilia.[119,124] A renal granuloma was found in one such case.[125]

Potassium-sparing diuretics are minimally nephrotoxic but may cause life-threatening hyperkalemia and acidosis by inhibiting renal K^+ and H^+ secretion.[62] *Mannitol*, the most commonly used osmotic diuretic, may cause acute renal failure when given in prolonged high doses, probably due to prerenal vasoconstriction.[83]

Antihypertensive Agents

Antihypertensive drugs rarely cause nephrotoxicity and are generally given to protect the kidneys from hypertensive nephropathy. Excessive dosage, of course, will cause prerenal failure due to decreased renal perfusion from the low blood pressure.

Captopril may rarely cause nephrotic syndrome,[164] with membranous nephropathy. This complication has not been reported to date with the newer angiotensin-converting enzyme inhibitors, which lack captopril's sulfhydryl group. Captopril may also cause allergic interstitial nephritis.[194]

Methyldopa rarely causes acute interstitial nephritis and acute renal failure.[212] There is a single reported case of urinary obstruction from retroperitoneal fibrosis associated with methyldopa.[99]

Anticonvulsant Agents

Phenytoin is a well-documented cause of acute interstitial nephritis.[10] One such case was associated with antibodies to tubular basement membrane.[97]

Carbamazepine can cause interstitial nephritis; it was shown to activate the patient's cultured lymphocytes.[93]

Phenobarbital has rarely been associated with interstitial nephritis and acute renal failure.[150]

Trimethadione and *paramethadione*, used to treat petit mal epilepsy, may cause membranous nephropathy with nephrotic syndrome,[16] which usually regresses when the drug is discontinued.

Anesthetic Agents

General anesthesia may cause acute renal failure by producing hypotension. However, the fluorinated hydrocarbons are directly nephrotoxic because of the release of fluoride from the parent molecule.

Methoxyflurane is the most nephrotoxic anesthetic. Two functional renal disturbances are seen following prolonged methoxyflurane anesthesia. Nephrogenic diabetes insipidus is characterized by postanesthesia polyuria and hyperoxaluria, which may worsen the renal injury. Acute tubular necrosis with renal failure and oliguria may follow the polyuria after 2 to 3 days.[153] Although this process is usually reversible, repeated exposure to methoxyflurane can lead to chronic renal failure with interstitial fibrosis and calcification, accompanied by distal renal tubular acidosis.[84]

Halothane is much less nephrotoxic than methoxyflurane, as it releases less fluoride, but is associated with acute renal failure.[77]

Enflurane is less lipid soluble than methoxyflurane but may also rarely cause acute renal failure.[55]

Antineoplastic Agents

Of all the antineoplastic medications, cisplatin (see the "Metals" section earlier in the chapter) is the most nephrotoxic. However, a number of other drugs in this category can also cause renal damage.

Methotrexate, a folic acid analog, can cause dose-related acute renal failure. During administration of methotrexate, there is a transient fall in glomerular filtration rate, particularly in pediatric patients.[118] Although vasospasm is usually the cause, methotrexate may also precipitate in renal tubules, causing obstruction.[161] At low doses of methotrexate, this problem can usually be prevented by adequate hydration and alkalinization of the urine. However, direct tubular toxicity from methotrexate is also reported, with proximal tubular necrosis and interstitial infiltration.[43]

Streptozocin can damage kidney cells as well as pancreatic islets. The first indication of the drug's nephrotoxicity is proteinuria.[179] If the drug is continued, tubular injury ensues, starting as Fanconi syndrome and loss of urinary concentrating ability, followed by azotemia and oliguric acute renal failure,[177] which usually resolves if the drug is stopped.

The *nitrosoureas (BCNU, CCNU,* and *methyl-CCNU)* are associated with long-term cumulative nephrotoxicity, most frequently in patients receiving more than 1.5 to 2 g/m^2 of the drug.[57,177] Methyl-CCNU is the most toxic of the three. The pathologic lesion is chronic interstitial nephritis, with irreversible fibrosis and glomerulosclerosis.

Mithramycin toxicity often includes acute tubular necrosis and renal failure.[104]

Mitomycin C primarily injures the glomerulus, and high doses are associated with glomerulosclerosis.[120] The drug may also cause hemolytic–uremic syndrome with microangiopathic hemolytic anemia.[156]

Azacytidine is a tubular toxin and can give rise to Fanconi syndrome as well as acute proximal and distal tubular necrosis.[159]

Iphosphamide may cause acute renal failure, particularly in young children.[182]

Immunosuppressive Agents

Azathioprine is not directly nephrotoxic but is associated with acute allergic interstitial nephritis.[187]

Cyclosporine is nephrotoxic. The earliest renal effect is prerenal vasoconstriction, with decreased glomerular filtration from renal hypoperfusion,[95,157] which usually responds to reduction of the dose. Some patients treated with cyclosporine develop acute renal failure, unrelated to rejection, that does not resolve with decreased dosage. Renal biopsy shows tubular injury with inclusion bodies,[129] confirmed by urinary appearance of a tubular cytosolic enzyme.[64] The renal ischemia may exacerbate this lesion. In kidney transplant patients, an interstitial infiltrate is reported.[129]

Chronic renal failure in patients receiving long-term cyclosporine treatment is from selective damage to medullary segments, fibrosis, and atrophy of the outer stripe that may then progress to end-stage disease.[143] This lesion is reported both in patients with renal homografts and with nonrenal transplants where the kidneys were initially normal.

Tacrolimus (FK–506) causes acute and chronic nephrotoxicity similar to that of cyclosporine, also related to prerenal vasoconstriction.[146] A recent animal study suggests that both drugs, although chemically different, have a common toxic pathway due to their binding of the intracellular enzyme calcineurin phosphatase.[196]

Radiocontrast Agents

Acute renal failure due to iodinated radiocontrast media usually begins within 24 hours of administration, often followed by an oliguric phase. Renal function usually begins to improve within a week, but dialysis is sometimes necessary.

Contrast agents deliver an osmotic load, and their injection leads to a period of volume expansion and diuresis,[137] accompanied by profound vasodilation. This is followed by intense vasoconstriction, which suggests that ischemia plays a role in the pathogenesis of contrast nephropathy.[136] During the oliguric phase fractional excretion of sodium is often low,[60] despite the fact that the pathologic lesion is acute tubular necrosis, with vaculization and cell swelling.[205] This lesion has been called "osmotic nephropathy," as it may be seen after injection of other hyperosmotic substances. A review article suggests that lower-osmolality contrast agents may be less nephrotoxic than the older high-osmolality dyes.[163] However, lower-osmolality contrast media can cause similar pathologic lesions[134] and severe renal failure.[12] The osmolality may be less important than a direct toxic or ischemic effect on tubular cells.

Conditions that increase the risk of acute renal failure after radiocontrast agents include preexisting renal insufficiency, particularly from diabetes, Bence Jones proteinuria, renal hypoperfusion, and injection of a large amount of dye. As with cisplatin, prevention of hypovolemia and saline or mannitol loading appear to reduce the risk of radiocontrast nephropathy.[163]

Miscellaneous Drugs and Substances

A number of other drugs may cause allergic interstitial nephritis, including *cimetidine*,[119,128] *ranitidine*,[70] *phenylpropanolamine*,[25] *clofibrate*,[46] and *ticlopidine*.[169]

Paraquat and *diquat*, two toxic herbicides, may cause acute renal failure in addition to damaging other organs (see Chap. 90).[204]

Bromate poisoning may cause acute renal failure and deafness in children.[81]

Bromocriptine causes urinary tract obstruction due to retroperitoneal fibrosis.[27]

Aluminum phosphide, used as a pesticide in granaries, is associated with acute renal failure.[106]

Deferoxamine overdose is reported to cause acute renal failure.

Inhaled *mycotoxins*, such as *ochratoxin*, may cause acute renal failure.[52]

Overdose of *epinephrine* may lead to acute renal failure in the neonate.[116]

The bisphosphonate *etidronate* is associated with acute renal failure when given intravenously.[151]

Extremely high consumption of *Worcestershire sauce* was reported to cause renal stones and aminoaciduria.[141]

Drug Abuse Nephropathy

Chronic self-injection of *heroin* or *cocaine* is recognized as a cause of chronic renal failure (CRF) and nephrotic syndrome, which has been confirmed epidemiologically.[47] There is generally a history of years of daily drug injections, most often with heroin. Renal biopsy shows focal segmental glomerulosclerosis,[47,121] but unlike patients with idiopathic focal sclerosis, drug abusers usually present with renal insufficiency or failure and progress rapidly to end-stage renal disease. Rare patients with drug abuse nephropathy may improve or stabilize after discontinuing the drug.[121]

There is much speculation as to the etiology of drug abuse nephropathy. It has been suggested that the contaminants, rather than the drug, cause the damage. In one study, animals injected with pure heroin had no renal lesions while those injected with street heroin developed glomerulosclerosis.[132] Drug abuse nephropathy is associated with marked interstitial fibrosis in addition to the glomerular lesion, which may explain the rapid progression to renal failure.[111]

Addicts who inject drugs subcutaneously may develop renal amyloidosis secondary to chronic skin abscesses and granulomas with lymphedema and suppuration, similar to amyloid in patients with other chronic inflammatory conditions.[100] Like those addicts with focal segmental glomerulosclerosis, they often present with advanced renal dysfunction. One patient with renal amyloidosis due to drug abuse improved when the addiction was terminated.[44]

Lysergic acid diethylamide (LSD) is not nephrotoxic but has been linked to retroperitoneal fibrosis, like the related ergotamines methysergide and bromocriptine.[191]

Amphetamines may cause a polyvasculitis that leads to proteinuria, hematuria, and chronic renal failure.[40] Intravenous injection of amphetamines[89,103] or cocaine[171] may also cause myoglobinuric acute renal failure.

Pigment Nephropathy

Both myoglobinuria and hemoglobinuria can cause acute renal failure, and either of these conditions may complicate poisoning or overdose. Tubular injury results from precipitation of the pigment in the renal tubules.[149] However, the conditions that produce them may be different.

Myoglobinuria sufficient to cause renal damage usually occurs following necrosis of striated muscle. Alcohol can be directly myotoxic in some individuals.[158] Drugs that produce profound hypokalemia (eg, diuretics and laxatives) or predispose to hyperthermia (neuroleptics) can cause muscle necrosis on this basis. Most commonly, poisoning leads to muscle breakdown from pressure necrosis following prolonged unconsciousness (opioids and sedative-hypnotics), excessive muscle contraction (cocaine), or grand mal seizures (alcohol withdrawal, theophylline).[73] Myoglobinuric acute renal failure has also accompanied poisoning with carbon monoxide, copper sulfate, and zinc phosphate.[32,108,122]

Myoglobin passes the glomerular filter and is normally excreted without causing toxicity. A study of patients with rhabdomyolysis suggested that the actual concentration of myoglobin in the urine may be a factor in the development of acute renal failure.[63] If myoglobin becomes inspissated in the lumen due to renal hypoperfusion and high tubular water absorption, the myoglobin molecule dissociates in an acidic environment, releasing hematin, which is tubulotoxic.[54] Because many intoxications are associated with intravascular volume depletion and acidosis, the poisoned patient is at risk to develop this complication.

Myoglobinuric renal failure is diagnosed by the development of acute renal failure in the presence of a condition causing muscle breakdown and a simultaneous elevation of muscle enzymes in the serum, especially creatinine kinase and aldolase. A positive orthotolidine test of the urine is seen in the absence of erythrocytes in the sediment, and urine myoglobin may be detected by radioimmunoassay. However, because primary renal failure may itself result in detectable myoglobinuria that does not worsen renal function,[61] finding myoglobin in the urine does not necessarily establish the diagnosis.

The renal failure associated with myoglobinuria can be prevented by early intervention. Volume expansion is quite effective provided renal injury has not yet occurred.[168] Alkalinizing the urine may prevent dissociation of the myoglobin molecule and minimize tubular necrosis. However, massive rhabdomyolysis may be associated with severe hypocalcemia due to the release of large amounts of phosphorus from necrosing muscle into the blood. Alkalemia in this setting may cause tetany or seizures, which would worsen the muscle injury.[108] Hence, the risk of alkalinization must be weighed against the benefit. Early alkalinization, before the renal failure becomes irreversible and before electrolyte abnormalities occur, is more likely to be of benefit.

Hemoglobinuria follows hemolysis, which can follow exposure to a number of poisons, including snake and spider venoms and many chemicals, such as cresol, phenol, analine, arsine, and methylene chloride. Sensitivity reactions to drugs (hydralazine, quinine) may also cause hemolysis.[254]

The pathophysiology of hemoglobinuric renal failure is similar to that seen with myoglobinuria. The pigment deposits in the tubules and dissociates, and necrosis occurs.[149] Volume depletion and acidosis are also precipitating factors in this disorder. Conversely, volume expansion may help prevent renal failure in hemolysis, as in myoglobinuria. Because phosphate release does not occur significantly with hemoglobinuria, the urine should be alkalinized as well.

Mushroom Poisoning

Two kinds of mushrooms have been reported to cause acute tubular necrosis. *Cortinarius spp* mushrooms may cause oliguric acute renal failure.[112] *Amanita spp* poisoning has also been associated with renal failure, in addition to its hepatic and GI toxicity (see Chap. 75).[131]

Alternative Medical Treatments

In recent years there has been an interest in so-called "alternative" or "complementary" medical treatments; the National Institutes of Health have established a Branch of Alternative Medicine. However, some of these remedies may have toxic effects on the kidneys.

Chinese herbal medicine sometimes employs the herbs *Stephania tetrandra* and *Magnolia officinalis* in weight-loss programs. Both have caused irreversible interstitial nephritis and fibrosis.[203]

Gallbladder of the grass carp, eaten by Chinese hoping to promote well being, causes acute tubular necrosis and toxic hepatitis.[117]

Disodium edetate (EDTA) is injected intravenously to chelate calcium in the hope of leaching the calcium out of atheromatous plaques. Although the major adverse effect of disodium edetate is profound hypocalcemia, there is one report of an acute fall in renal function associated with "chelation therapy,"[32] a complication more commonly seen with calcium disodium edetate.[42]

References

1. Adams RG, Harrison JF, Scott P: The development of cadmium-induced proteinuria, impaired renal function and osteomalacia in alkaline battery workers. Q J Med 1969; 38:425–443.
2. Albini B, Glurich I, Andres GA: Mercuric chloride-induced immunologically mediated diseases in experimental animals. In: Porter GA, ed: Nephrotoxic Mechanisms of Drugs and Environmental Toxins. New York, Plenum, 1982.
3. Alexander F, Martin J: Nephrotic syndrome associated with lithium therapy. Clin Nephrol 1981;15:267–271.
4. Anderson HL Jr, Feinfeld DA: Mechanisms of drug-induced renal failure. Hosp Physician 1987;23:27–40.
5. Andreoli T: On the anatomy of amphotericin B-cholesterol pores in lipid bilayer membranes. Kidney Int 1973;4: 337–345.
6. Angevine JM, Kappas A, DeGowin RL, et al: Renal tubular nuclear inclusions of lead poisoning: A clinical and experimental study. Arch Pathol 1962;73:486–494.
7. Antonovych TT: Gold nephropathy. Ann Clin Lab Sci 1981;11:386–391.
8. Appel GB: A decade of penicillin-related interstitial nephritis: More questions than answers. Clin Nephrol 1980;13:151–154.
9. Appel GB, Given DB, Levine LR, et al: Vancomycin and the kidney. Am J Kidney Dis 1986;8:75–80.
10. Appel GB, Kunis CL: Acute tubulo-interstitial nephritis. Contemp Issues Nephrol 1983;10:151–185.
11. Appel GB, Neu HC: Acute interstitial nephritis induced by beta-lactam antibiotics. In: Fillastre JH, Whelton A, Tulkens P, eds: Antibiotic Nephrotoxicity. Paris, INSERM, 1982.
12. Aron NB, Feinfeld DA, Peters AT, et al: Acute renal failure associated with ioxaglate, a low-osmolality radiocontrast agent. Am J Kidney Dis 1989;13:189–193.
13. Badr KF, Ichikawa I: Prerenal failure: A deleterious shift from renal compensation to decompensation. N Engl J Med 1988;319:623–629.
14. Baerg RD, Kimberg DV: Centrilobular hepatic necrosis and acute renal failure in "solvent sniffers." Ann Intern Med 1970;73:713–720.
15. Ball BU, Sorensen LB: Pathogenesis of hyperuricemia in saturnine gout. N Engl J Med 1969;280:1199–1202.
16. Bar-Khayim Y, Teplitz C, Garella S, et al: Trimethadione

(Tridione) induced nephrotic syndrome. Am J Med 1973; 54:272–280.
17. Barnett RN, Brown DS, Cadorna CB, et al: Beryllium disease with death from renal failure. Conn Med 1961;25: 142–147.
18. Barton CH, Pahl M, Vaziri N, et al: Renal magnesium wasting associated with amphotericin B therapy. Am J Med 1984;77:471–474.
19. Batuman V, Maesaka JK, Haddad B, et al: The role of lead in gouty nephropathy. N Engl J Med 1981;304:520–523.
20. Beattie JW: Nephrotic syndrome following sodium bismuth tartrate therapy in rheumatoid arthritis. Ann Rheum Dis 1953;12:144–146.
21. Beaver DL, Burr RE: Bismuth inclusions in the human kidney: A long-term autopsy study. Arch Pathol 1963;76: 89–94.
22. Becker BN, Fall P, Hall C, et al: Rapidly progressive acute renal failure due to acyclovir: Case report and review of the literature. Am J Kidney Dis 1993;22:611–615.
23. Becker CG, Becker EF, Maher JF, et al: Nephrotic syndrome after contact with mercury: A report of five cases, three after the use of ammoniated mercury ointment. Arch Intern Med 1962;110:178–186.
24. Beirne GJ, Hansing CE, Octaviano GW, et al: Acute renal failure caused by hypersensitivity to polymyxin B sulfate. JAMA 1967;202:156–158.
25. Bennett WM: Hazards of the appetite suppressant phenylpropanolamine. Lancet 1979;2:42–43. Letter.
26. Bennett WM, Gilbert DN, Houghton D, et al: Gentamicin nephrotoxicity: Morphologic and pharmacologic features. West J Med 1977;126:65–68.
27. Bowler JV, Ormerod IE, Legg NJ: Retroperitoneal fibrosis and bromocriptine. Lancet 1986;2:466. Letter.
28. Brezin JH, Katz SM, Schwartz AB, et al: Reversible renal failure and nephrotic syndrome associated with nonsteroidal anti-inflammatory drugs. N Engl J Med 1979; 301:1271–1273.
29. Brigden D, Rosling AE, Woods NC: Renal function after acyclovir intravenous injection. Am J Med 1982;73: 182–185.
30. Cacoub P, Deray G, Baumelou A, et al: Acute renal failure induced by foscarnet. Clin Nephrol 1988;29:315–318.
31. Campbell NR, Baylis B: Renal impairment associated with an acute paracetamol overdose in the absence of hepatotoxicity. Postgrad Med J 1992;68:116–118.
32. Catsch A, Harmuth-Hoene AE: The chelation of heavy metals. In: International Encyclopedia of Pharmacology and Therapeutics. New York, Pergamon, 1979, pp. 111–224.
33. Charlas R, Benabadji A: Néphrite azotémique au cours du traitement par l'antimoine d'un cas de leishmaniase viscérale infantile. Maroc Méd 1962;41:1180–1182.
34. Cheng JT, Beysolow TD, Kaul B, et al: Clearance of ethylene glycol by kidneys and hemodialysis. J Toxicol Clin Toxicol 1987;25:95–108.
35. Cheng JT, Feinfeld DA: Amphotericin B and the kidney. Hosp Physician 1988;24:68–72.
36. Chisolm JJ Jr, Harrison HC, Eberlein WR, et al: Aminoaciduria, hypophosphatemia, and rickets in lead poisoning. Am J Dis Child 1955;89:159–168.
37. Chugh KS, Nath IV, Ubroi HS, et al: Acute renal failure due to non-traumatic rhabdomyolysis. Postgrad Med J 1979;55:386–392.
38. Ciabbatoni G, Cinotti GA, Pierucci A, et al: Effects of sulindac and ibuprofen in patients with chronic glomerular disease. N Engl J Med 1984;310:279–283.
39. Cianciulli P, Sorrentino F, Forte L, et al: Acute renal failure occurring during intravenous desferrioxamine therapy: Recovery after hemodialysis. Haematologica 1992;77: 514–515.
40. Citron BP, Halpern M, McCarron M, et al: Necrotizing angiitis associated with drug abuse. N Engl J Med 1970;283:1003–1011.
41. Clive DM, Stoff J: Renal syndromes associated with nonsteroidal anti-inflammatory drugs. N Engl J Med 1984;310: 563–572.
42. Collet JT: EDTA-chelation therapy. Ned Tijdschr Geneeskd 1992;136:191–192.
43. Condit PT, Chanes PE, Joel W: Renal toxicity of methotrexate. Cancer 1969;23:126–131.
44. Crowley S, Feinfeld DA, Janis R: Resolution of nephrotic syndrome and lack of progression of heroin-associated renal amyloidosis. Am J Kidney Dis 1989;13:333–335.
45. Crutcher JC: Clinical manifestations and therapy of acute lead intoxication due to the ingestion of illicitly distilled alcohol. Ann Intern Med 1963;59:707–715.
46. Cumming A: Acute renal failure and interstitial nephritis after clofibrate treatment. Br Med J 1980;281:1529–1530.
47. Cunningham EE, Brentjens JR, Zielezny MA, et al: Heroin nephropathy: A clinicopathologic and epidemiologic study. Am J Med 1980;68:47–53.
48. Davenport A, Finn R: Paracetamol (acetaminophen) poisoning resulting in acute renal failure. Nephron 1988;50: 55–56.
49. Davies B, Kincaid-Smith P: Renal biopsy studies of lithium and pre-lithium patients and comparison with cadaver transplant kidneys. Neuropharmacology 1979;18: 1001–1002.
50. DeBroe ME, Giuliano R, Verpooten G: Choice of drug and dosage regimen: Two important risk factors for aminoglycoside nephrotoxicity. Am J Med 1986;80:115–118.
51. Derot M, Kahn J, Mazalton A, et al: Néphrite anurique aigue mortelle après traitement aurique, chrysocyanose associée. Bull Mém Soc Méd Hôp Paris 1954;70:234–239.
52. Di Paolo N, Guarnieri A, Loi F, et al: Acute renal failure from inhalation of mycotoxins. Nephron 1993;64:621–625.
53. Dorfman LE, Smith JP: Sulfonamide crystalluria: A forgotten disease. J Urol 1970;104:482–483.
54. Dubrow A, Flamenbaum W: Acute renal failure associated with myoglobinuria and hemoglobinuria. In: Brenner BM, Lazarus JM, eds: Acute Renal Failure, 2nd ed. New York, Churchill Livingstone, 1988, pp. 279–293.
55. Eichhorn JH, Hedley-White J, Steinman TI, et al: Renal failure following enflurane anesthesia. Anesthesiology 1976;45:557–560.
56. Eisenberg ES, Robbins N, Lenci M: Vancomycin and interstitial nephritis. Ann Intern Med 1981;95:658. Letter.
57. Ellis ME, Weiss RB, Kuperminc M: Nephrotoxicity of lomustine. Cancer Chemother Pharmacol 1985;15:174–175.

58. Emmerson BT: Chronic lead nephropathy: The diagnostic use of calcium EDTA and the association with gout. Australas Ann Med 1963;12:310–324.
59. Espinel CH, Gregory AW: Differential diagnosis of acute renal failure. Clin Nephrol 1980;13:73–77.
60. Fang LS, Sirota RA, Ebert TH, et al: Low fractional excretion of sodium with contrast media-induced acute renal failure. Arch Intern Med 1980;140:531–533.
61. Feinfeld DA, Briscoe AM, Nurse HM, et al: Myoglobinuria in chronic renal failure. Am J Kidney Dis 1986;8:111–114.
62. Feinfeld DA, Carvounis CP: Fatal hyperkalemia and hyperchloremic acidosis: Association with spironolactone in the absence of renal impairment. JAMA 1978;240:1516.
63. Feinfeld DA, Cheng JT, Beysolow TD, et al: A prospective study of urine and serum myoglobin levels in patients with acute rhabdomyolysis. Clin Nephrol 1992;38: 193–195.
64. Feinfeld DA, D'Agati V, Benvenisty A, et al: Cyclosporin A and urine glutathione-*S*-transferase. Proc EDTA-ERA 1985;22:561–565.
65. Feinfeld DA, Nurse HM, Hotchkiss JL, et al: The clinical spectrum of chronic interstitial nephritis. Hosp Physician 1985;21:102–104.
66. Feinfeld DA, Olesnicky L, Pirani CL, et al: Nephrotic syndrome associated with the use of non-steroidal anti-inflammatory drugs. Nephron 1984;37:174–179.
67. Feinfeld DA, Ranieri R, Lipner HI, et al: Renal failure in phenazopyridine overdose. JAMA 1978;240:2661.
68. Foord RD: Cephaloridine, cephalothin and the kidney. J Antimicrob Chemother 1975;1(suppl 3):119–133.
69. Forrest JN Jr, Marcy TW, Biemesderfer D, et al: Cytoskeletal defect in cortical collecting duct cells in lithium-induced polyuria. Kidney Int 1981;19:200. Abstract.
70. Freeman HJ: Ranitidine-associated interstitial nephritis in a patient with celiac sprue. Can J Gastroenterol 1988;2:35.
71. Friberg L: Chronic cadmium poisoning. Arch Ind Health 1959;20:401–407.
72. Frimpter GW, Timpanelli AE, Eisenmenger WJ, et al: Reversible "Fanconi syndrome" caused by degraded tetracycline. JAMA 1963;184:111–113.
73. Gabow PA, Kaehny WD, Kelleher SP: The spectrum of rhabdomyolysis. Medicine (Balt) 1982;61:141–152.
74. Gade R, Feinfeld DA, Gade MF: A microradiographic study of nephrons in mercuric chloride-induced acute renal failure in the rabbit. Invest Radiol 1983;18:183–188.
75. Galler M, Folkert VW, Schlondorff D: Reversible acute renal insufficiency and hyperkalemia following indomethacin therapy. JAMA 1981;246:154–155.
76. Gelbart DR, Weinstein AB, Fajardo LF: Allopurinol-induced interstitial nephritis. Ann Intern Med 1977;86: 196–198. Letter.
77. Gelman ML, Lichtenstein N: Halothane-induced nephrotoxicity. Urology 1981;17:323–327.
78. Gerritsen WR, Peters A, Henny FC, et al: Ciprofloxacin-induced nephrotoxicity. Nephrol Dial Transplant 1987;2: 382–383. Letter.
79. Gilbert DN, Gourley R, d'Agostino A, et al: Interstitial nephritis due to methicillin, penicillin, and ampicillin. Ann Allergy 1970;28:378–385.
80. Goldstein RS, Mayor GH: The nephrotoxicity of cisplatin. Life Sci 1983;32:685–690.
81. Gradus D, Rhoads M, Bergstrom LB, et al: Acute bromate poisoning associated with renal failure and deafness presenting as hemolytic-uremic syndrome. Am J Nephrol 1984;4:188–191.
82. Greven J, Klein H: Renal effects of furosemide in glycerol-induced acute renal failure of the rat. Pflügers Arch 1976; 365:81–87.
83. Gudallah MF, Lynn M, Work J: Case report: Mannitol nephrotoxicity syndrome. Am J Med Sci 1995;309:219–222.
84. Halpren BA, Kempson RC, Coplon NS: Interstitial fibrosis and chronic renal failure following methoxyflurane anesthesia. JAMA 1973;233:1239–1242.
85. Hayes DM, Cvitkovic E, Golbey RB, et al: High dose cisplatinum diammine dichloride: Amelioration of renal toxicity by mannitol diuresis. Cancer 1977;39:1372–1381.
86. Hébert JL, Auzépy P, Durand A: Acute human and experimental poisoning with diethylene glycol. Sém Hôp Paris 1983;59:344–349.
87. Heidemann HT, Gerkens JF, Spickard WA, et al: Amphotericin B nephrotoxicity in humans decreased by salt repletion. Am J Med 1983;75:476–481.
88. Henrich WL, Agodoa LE, Barrett B, et al: Analgesics and the kidney: summary and recommendations to the scientific advisory board of the National Kidney Foundation from an ad hoc committee of the National Kidney Foundation. Am J Kidney Dis 1996;27:162–165.
89. Henry JA, Jeffreys KJ, Dawling S: Toxicity and deaths from 3,4-methylenedioxyamphetamine ("ecstasy"). Lancet 1992;340:384–387.
90. Hertz P, Yager H, Richardson JB: Probenecid-induced nephrotic syndrome. Arch Pathol 1972;94:241–243.
91. Hestbech J, Aurell M: Lithium induced uremia. Lancet 1979;1:212–213. Letter.
92. Hestbech J, Hansen HE, Amdisen A, et al: Chronic renal lesions following long-term treatment with lithium. Kidney Int 1977;12:205–213.
93. Hogg RJ, Sawyer M, Hecox K, et al: Carbamazepine induced acute tubulointerstitial nephritis. J Pediatr 1981;98: 830–832.
94. Howard T, Hoy RH, Warren S, et al: Acute renal dysfunction due to sulfinpyrazone therapy in post-myocardial infarction: Cardiomegaly, reversible hypersensitivity, interstitial nephritis. Am Heart J 1981;102:294–295.
95. Humes HD, Jackson NM, O'Connor RP, et al: Pathogenetic mechanisms of nephrotoxicity: Insights into cyclosporine nephrotoxicity. Transplant Proc 1985;17(suppl 1):51–62.
96. Humes HD, Weinberg JM, Knauss TC: Clinical and pathophysiologic aspects of aminoglycoside toxicity. Am J Kidney Dis 1982;2:5–29.
97. Hyman LR, Ballow M, Knieser MR: Diphenylhydantoin interstitial nephritis: Roles of cellular and humoral immunologic injury. J Pediatr 1978;92:915–920.
98. Inglis JA, Henderson DA, Emmerson BT: The pathology and pathogenesis of chronic lead nephropathy occurring in Queensland. J Pathol 1978;124:65–76.
99. Iversen BM, Nordahl E, Thunold S, et al: Retroperitoneal

fibrosis during treatment with methyldopa. Lancet 1975;2: 302–304.

100. Jacob H, Charytan C, Rascoff JH, et al: Amyloidosis secondary to drug abuse and chronic skin suppuration. Arch Intern Med 1978;138:1150–1151.
101. Kallenberg CGM: Renal disease—another effect of silica exposure. Nephrol Dial Transplant 1995;10:1117–1119.
102. Kazantzis G: Renal tubular dysfunction and abnormalities of calcium metabolism in cadmium workers. Environ Health Perspect 1979;28:155–159.
103. Kendrick WC, Hull, AR, Knochel JP: Rhabdomyolysis and shock after intravenous amphetamine administration. Ann Intern Med 1977;86:381–387.
104. Kennedy BJ: Metabolic and toxic effects of mithramycin during tumor therapy. Am J Med 1970;49:494–503.
105. Kesten HD, Mulinos MG, Pomerantz L: Pathologic effects of certain glycols and related compounds. Arch Pathol 1939;27:447.
106. Khosla SN, Nand N, Khosla P: Aluminium phosphide poisoning. J Tropic Med Hyg 1988;91:196–198.
107. Kleinknecht D, Vanhille P, Morel-Maroger L: Acute interstitial nephritis due to drug hypersensitivity: An up-to-date review with a report of 19 cases. Adv Nephrol 1983;12:277–308.
108. Knochel JP: Rhabdomyolysis and myoglobinuria. In: Suki WN, Eknoyan G, eds: The Kidney in Systemic Disease, 2nd ed. New York, Wiley, 1981, pp. 263–284.
109. Koch-Weser J, Sidel V, Federman ER, et al: Adverse effects of sodium colistimethate: Manifestations and specific reaction rates during courses of therapy. Ann Intern Med 1970;72:857–868.
110. Koren G: The nephrotoxic potential of drugs and chemicals: Pharmacologic basis and clinical relevance. Med Toxicol 1989;4:59–72.
111. Kunis C, Olesnicky L, Nurse H, et al: Heroin nephropathy: Clinical–pathological correlations. Ninth International Congress on Nephrology, Los Angeles CA, June 11–16, 1984. Abstract 102A.
112. Lampe KF: Toxic effects of plant toxins. In: Klaassen CD, Amdur MO, Doull J, eds: Casarett and Doull's Toxicology, 3rd ed. New York, Macmillan, 1986, pp. 757–770.
113. Landrigan PJ: Arsenic. In: Rom WN, ed: Environmental and Occupational Medicine. Boston, Little, Brown, 1983, pp. 473–480.
114. Lavender S, Brown JN, Berrill WT: Acute renal failure and lithium intoxication. Postgrad Med J 1973;49:277–279.
115. Lerner SA, Schmitt B, Seligsohn R, et al: Comparative study of ototoxicity and nephrotoxicity in patients randomly assigned to treatment with amikacin or gentamicin. Am J Med 1986;80:90–104.
116. Levine DH, Levkoff AH, Pappu LD, et al: Renal failure and other serious sequelae of epinephrine toxicity in neonates. South Med J 1985;78:874–877.
117. Lim PS, Lin JL, Hu SA, et al: Acute renal failure due to ingestion of the gallbladder of grass carp: Report of 3 cases with review of literature. Renal Failure 1993;15: 639–644.
118. Link DA, Fosburg MT, Ingelfinger JR, et al: Renal toxicity of high dose methotrexate. Pediatr Res 1976;10:455. Abstract.
119. Linton AL, Clark WF, Drieger AA, et al: Acute interstitial nephritis due to drugs: Review of the literature with a report of nine cases. Ann Intern Med 1980;93:735–741.
120. Liu K, Mittelman A, Sproul EE, et al: Renal toxicity in men treated with mitomycin C. Cancer 1971;28:1314–1320.
121. Llach F, Descoeudres C, Massry SG: Heroin associated nephropathy: Clinical and histological studies in 19 patients. Clin Nephrol 1979;11:7–12.
122. Loughridge LW, Leader LP, Brown DAL: Acute renal failure due to muscle necrosis in carbon monoxide poisoning. Lancet 1958;2:349–351.
123. Lucké B: Lower nephron nephrosis: The renal lesions of crush syndrome of burns, transfusions and other conditions affecting the lower segment of the nephrons. Mil Surg 1946;99:371–396.
124. Lyons H, Pinn VW, Cortell S, et al: Allergic interstitial nephritis causing reversible renal failure in four patients with idiopathic nephrotic syndrome. N Engl J Med 1973;288:124–128.
125. Magil AB, Ballon HS, Cameron ECC, et al: Acute interstitial nephritis associated with thiazide diuretics: Clinical and pathological observations in three cases. Am J Med 1980;69:939–943.
126. Maher JF: Toxic nephropathy. In: Brenner BM, Rector FC Jr, eds: The Kidney. Philadelphia, Saunders, 1976.
127. McCurdy DK, Frederic M, Elkinton JR: Renal tubular acidosis due to amphotericin B. N Engl J Med 1968;278: 124–130.
128. McGowan WR, Vermillion SE: Acute interstitial nephritis related to cimetidine therapy. Gastroenterology 1980;79: 746–749.
129. Mihatsch MJ, Thiel G, Spichtin HD, et al: Morphological findings in kidney transplants after treatment with cyclosporine. Transplant Proc 1983;15:2821–2835.
130. Miller TJ, Anderson RJ, Linas SL, et al: Urinary diagnostic indices in acute renal failure: A prospective study. Ann Intern Med 1978;89:47–50.
131. Mitchel DH: Amanita mushroom poisoning. Annu Rev Med 1980;31:51–57.
132. Moody C, Kaufman R, McGuire D, et al: The role of adulterants in heroin nephropathy. Abstr Natl Kidney Found 1985;15:A12.
133. More RH, McMillan GC, Duff GL: The pathology of sulfonamide allergy in man. Am J Pathol 1946;22:703–705.
134. Moreau JF, Droz D, Noel LH: Tubular nephrotoxicity of water soluble iodinated contrast media. Invest Radiol 1980;15 (suppl 6): S54–S60.
135. Morin JP, Viotte G, Vandewalle A, et al: Gentamicin-induced nephrotoxicity: A cell biology approach. Kidney Int 1980;18:583–590.
136. Mudge GH, Meier FA, Ward KK: Pathogenesis of renal impairment induced by radiocontrast drugs. In Solez K, Whelton A, eds: Acute Renal Failure. New York, Marcel Dekker, 1984.
137. Mudge GH: Nephrotoxicity of urographic radiocontrast drugs. Kidney Int 1980;18:540–552.
138. Muehrcke RC, Pirani CL: Arsine induced anuria: A correlative clinicopathologic study with electron microscopic observations. Ann Intern Med 1968;68:853–866.
139. Muehrcke RC, Pirani CL, Kark RM: Interstitial nephritis: A

clinicopathological renal biopsy study. Ann Intern Med 1967;66:1052.

140. Mullick FG, McAllister HA Jr, Wagner BM, et al: Drug-related vasculitis: Clinicopathologic correlations in 30 patients. Hum Pathol 1979;10:313–325.

141. Murphy KJ: Bilateral renal calculi and aminoaciduria after excessive intake of Worcestershire sauce. Lancet 1967;2: 401–403.

142. Muther RS: Drug interference with renal function tests. Am J Kidney Dis 1983;3:118–120.

143. Myers BD, Ross J, Newton L, et al: Cyclosporine-associated chronic nephropathy. N Engl J Med 1984;311:699–705.

144. Nagi AH, Alexander F, Barbas AZ: Gold nephropathy in rats: Light and electron microscopic studies. Exp Mol Pathol 1971;15:354–362.

145. Nessi R, Bonoldi GL, Redaelli B, et al: Acute renal failure after rifampicin: A case report and survey of the literature. Nephron 1976;16:148–159.

146. Neylan J, Whelchel J, Laskow D, et al.: Adverse events in the comparative dose finding trial of FK-506 in primary renal transplantation. Am Soc Transplant Phys 1993;12: 154.

147. Nolan CR, Anger MS, Kelleher SP: Eosinophiluria: A new method of detection and definition of the clinical spectrum. N Engl J Med 1986;315:1516–1519.

148. Obara K, Saito T, Sato H, et al: Germanium poisoning: Clinical symptoms and renal damage caused by long-term intake of germanium. Jpn J Med 1991;30:67–72.

149. Oliver J, MacDowell M, Tracy A: The pathogenesis of acute renal failure associated with traumatic and toxic injury: Renal ischemia, nephrotoxic damage and the ischemuric episode. J Clin Invest 1951;30:1307–1351.

150. Ooi BS, First MR, Pesce AJ, et al: IgE levels in interstitial nephritis. Lancet 1974;1:1254–1256.

151. O'Sullivan TL, Akbari A, Cadnapaphornchai P: Acute renal failure associated with the administration of parenteral etidronate. Renal Failure 1994;16:767–773.

152. Paller MS: Drug-induced nephropathies. Med Clin North Am 1990;74:909–916.

153. Panner BJ, Freeman, RB, Roth-Mayo VA, et al: Toxicity following methoxyflurane anesthesia. JAMA 1970;214:86–90.

154. Parry MF, Wallach R: Ethylene glycol poisoning. Am J Med 1974;57:143–150.

155. Pavlakis N, Pollack CA, McLean G, et al: Deliberate overdose of uranium: Toxicity and treatment. Nephron 1996; 72:313–317.

156. Pavy MD, Wiley EL, Abeloff MD: Hemolytic-uremic syndrome associated with mitomycin therapy. Cancer Treat Rep 1982;66:457–461.

157. Perico N, Ruggenenti P, Gaspari P, et al: Daily renal hypoperfusion induced by cyclosporine in patients with renal transplantation. Transplantation 1992;54:56–60.

158. Perkoff GT, Dioso MM, Bleisch V, et al: A spectrum of myopathy associated with alcoholism. I. Clinical and laboratory features. Ann Intern Med 1967;67:493–510.

159. Peterson BA, Collins AJ, Vogelzang NJ, et al: 5-Azacytidine and renal tubular dysfunction. Blood 1981;57: 182–185.

160. Phillips ME, Eastwood JB, Curtis JR, et al: Tetracycline poisoning in renal failure. Br Med J 1974;2:149–151.

161. Pitman SW, Parker LM, Tattersall MHN, et al: Clinical trials of high dose methotrexate with citrovorum factor: Toxicologic and therapeutic observations. Cancer Chemother Rep 1975;6:43–49.

162. Poole G, Stradling P, Worlledge S: Potentially serious side effects of high-dose twice-weekly rifampicin. Br Med J 1971;3:343–347.

163. Porter GA: Radiocontrast-induced nephropathy. Nephrol Dial Transplant 1994;9(suppl 4):146–156.

164. Prins EJL, Hoorntje SJ, Weening JJ, et al: Nephrotic syndrome in patients on captopril. Lancet 1979;2:306–307. Letter.

165. Qunibi WY, Godwin J, Eknoyan G: Toxic nephropathy during continuous rifampin therapy. South Med J 1980; 73:791–792.

166. Reisin E, Teicher A, Jaffe R, et al: Myoglobinuria and renal failure in toluene poisoning. Br J Ind Med 1975;32:163–164.

167. Rodin AE, Crowson CN: Mercury nephrotoxicity in the rat. II. Investigation of the intracellular site of mercury nephrotoxicity by correlated serial time histologic and histoenzymatic studies. Am J Pathol 1962;41: 485–499.

168. Ron D, Taitelman MD, Michaelson MD, et al: Prevention of acute renal failure in traumatic rhabdomyolysis. Arch Intern Med 1984;144:277–280.

169. Rosen H, El-Hennawy AS, Greenberg S, et al: Acute interstitial nephritis associated with ticlopidine. Am J Kidney Dis 1995;25:934–936.

170. Ross JH, McGinty F, Brewer DG: Penicillamine nephropathy. Nephron 1980;26:184–186.

171. Roth D, Alarcon FJ, Fernandez JA, et al: Acute rhabdomyolysis associated with cocaine intoxication. N Engl J Med 1988;319:673–677.

172. Roza O, Berman LB: The pathophysiology of barium: Hypokalemic and cardiovascular effects. J Pharmacol Exp Ther 1971;177:433–439.

173. Safirstein R, Winston J, Goldstein M, et al: Cisplatin nephrotoxicity. Am J Kidney Dis 1986;8:356–367.

174. Saltissi D, Pulsey CD, Rainford DJ: Recurrent acute renal failure due to antibiotic-induced interstitial nephritis. Br Med J 1979;1:1182–1183.

175. Sandler DP, Smith JC, Weinberg CR, et al: Analgesic use and chronic renal disease. N Engl J Med 1989;320: 1238–1243.

176. Sanghvi LM, Sharma R, Mirsa SN, et al: Sulfhemoglobinemia and acute renal failure after copper sulfate poisoning: Report of two fatal cases. Arch Pathol 1957;63:172–175.

177. Schacht RG, Feiner HD, Gallo GR, et al: Nephrotoxicity of nitrosoureas. Cancer 1981;38:1328–1334.

178. Scharschmidt LA, Feinfeld DA: Renal effects of nonsteroidal antiinflammatory drugs. Hosp Physician 1989; 25:29–33.

179. Schein PS, O'Connell MJ, Blom J, et al: Clinical antitumor activity and toxicity of streptozotocin. Cancer 1974;34: 993–1000.

180. Schreiner GE, Maher JF: Toxic nephropathy. Am J Med 1965;38:409–449.

181. Shils ME: Renal disease and the metabolic effects of tetracycline. Ann Intern Med 1963;58:389–408.

182. Shore R, Greenberg M, Geary D, et al: Iphosphamide-

induced nephrotoxicity in children. Pediatr Nephrol 1992; 6:162–165.

183. Simmons CF, Bogusky RT, Humes HD: Inhibitory effects of gentamicin on renal mitochondrial oxidative phosphorylation. J Pharmacol Exp Ther 1980;214:709–715.
184. Singer I: Lithium and the kidney. Kidney Int 1981;19: 374–387.
185. Sipes IG, Krishna G, Gillette JR: Bioactivation of carbon tetrachloride, chloroform, and bromotrichloromethane: Role of cytochrome. Life Sci 1977;20:1541–1548.
186. Sleijfer DTH, Smit EF, Meijer S, et al: Acute and cumulative effects of carboplatin on renal function. Br J Cancer 1989;60:116–120.
187. Sloth K, Thomsen AC: Acute renal insufficiency during treatment with azathioprine. Acta Med Scand 1971;189: 145–148.
188. Smetana H: Nephrosis due to carbon tetrachloride. Arch Intern Med 1939;63:760–777.
189. Smith CR, Lipsky JJ, Laskin OL, et al: Double-blind comparison of the nephrotoxicity and auditory toxicity of gentamicin and tobramycin. N Engl J Med 1980;302: 1106–1109.
190. Stahl-Bayliss CM, Kalman CM, Laskin OL: Pentamidine-induced hypoglycemia in patients with the acquired immune deficiency syndrome. Clin Pharmacol Ther 1986;39: 271–275.
191. Stecker JF Jr, Rawls HP, Devine CJ, et al: Retroperitoneal fibrosis and ergot derivatives. J Urol 1974;112:30–32.
192. Stefanidis I, Bohm R, Hagel J, et al: Toxic myopathy with kidney failure as a colchicine side effect in familial Mediterranean fever. Dtsch Med Wochenschr 1992;117: 1237–1240.
193. Stein JH, Lifschitz MD, Barnes LD: Current concepts of the pathophysiology of acute renal failure. Am J Physiol 1978;234:F171–181.
194. Steinman TI, Silva P: Acute renal failure, skin rash, and eosinophilia associated with captopril therapy. Am J Med 1983;75:154–156.
195. Sterne TL, Whitaker C, Webb CH: Fatal cases of bismuth intoxication. J Louisiana State Med Soc 1955;107:332–335.
196. Su Q, Weber L, Lettir M, et al: Nephrotoxicity of cyclosporin A and FK–506: Inhibition of calcineurin phosphatase. Renal Physiol Biochem 1995;18:128–139.
197. Ten RM, Torres VE, Milliner DS, et al: Acute interstitial nephritis: Immunologic and clinical aspects. Mayo Clin Proc 1988;63:921–930.
198. Thadhani R, Pascual M, Bonventre J: Medical progress: Acute renal failure. N Engl J Med 1996;334:1448–1460.
199. Thompson J: Ferrous sulfate poisoning: Its incidence, symptomatology, treatment, and prevention. Br Med J 1950;1:645–646.
200. Tornroth T, Skrifvars B: Gold nephropathy prototype of membranous glomerulonephritis. Am J Pathol 1974;75: 573–590.
201. Uldall PR, Khan HA, Ennis JE, et al: Renal damage from industrial arsine poisoning. Br J Ind Med 1970;27:372–377.
202. Vallee BL, Ulmer DD, Wacker WEC: Arsenic toxicology and biochemistry. Arch Ind Health 1960;21:132–151.
203. Vanherweghem JL, Depierreux M, Tielemans C, et al: Rapidly progressive interstitial renal fibrosis in young women: Association with slimming regimen including Chinese herbs. Lancet 1993;341:387–391.
204. Vanholder R, Colardyn F, De Reuck J, et al: Diquat intoxication: Report of two cases and review of the literature. Am J Med 1981;70:1267–1271.
205. VanZee BE, Hoy WE, Talley TE, et al: Renal injury associated with intravenous pyelography in nondiabetic and diabetic patients. Ann Intern Med 1978;89:51–54.
206. Varma A, Jha V, Ghosh AK, et al: Acute renal failure in a case of fatal chromic acid poisoning. Renal Failure 1994;16:653–657.
207. Walker RG, Thomson NM, Dowling JP, et al: Minocycline-induced acute interstitial nephritis. Br Med J 1979;1:524.
208. Warren GV, Korbet SM, Schwartz MM, et al: Minimal change glomerulopathy associated with nonsteroidal anti-inflammatory drugs. Am J Kidney Dis 1989;13:127–130.
209. Wedeen RP, Batuman V: Tubulo-interstitial nephritis induced by heavy metals and metabolic disturbances. Contemp Issues Nephrol 1983;10:211–241.
210. Wedeen RP, Maesaka JK, Weiner B, et al: Occupational lead nephropathy. Am J Med 1975;59:630–641.
211. Wetherill SF, Guarine MJ, Cox RW: Acute renal failure associated with barium chloride poisoning. Ann Intern Med 1981;95:187–188.
212. Wilson M, Brown DJ, Brown RW, et al: Renal failure from alpha-methyldopa therapy. Aust NZ J Med 1974;4: 415–416.
213. Woolf AD, Ebert TH: Toxicity after self-poisoning by ingestion of potassium chloroplatinite. J Toxicol Clin Toxicol 1991;29:467–472.

CHAPTER 24

Hematologic Principles

Diane Sauter

The physiologic role of every organ system is dependent upon the normal function of blood. Blood transports the substances required for energy production, removes the waste products of respiration, and defends against the invasion of a nearly infinite variety of potential microbial and chemical pathogens. Additional functions include transport of hormones to end organs, metabolism of certain drugs, provision of the mediators of inflammation, and maintenance of vascular integrity through coagulation.

Exposure of the blood and blood-forming organs to toxins may interfere with any morphologic or functional aspect of blood. Depressed cell formation, increased destruction, desaturation of hemoglobin, and impairment of coagulation can all result from exposure to a large variety of toxic agents. The response to an exogenous toxin depends upon the nature and quantity of the agent, and the capacity of the system to respond to the insult. Due to individual variation, often no clear and predictable dose–response relationship can be determined. For example, exposure to naphthalene, a known toxin, may be tolerated in low doses by healthy individuals, whereas individuals with glucose-6-phosphate dehydrogenase (G-6-PD) deficiency may develop massive hemolysis when exposed to the same dose. When a substantial exposure occurs, even the ability of healthy individuals to detoxify naphthalene may be overwhelmed, resulting in hemolysis.

Marrow

The mature cellular elements of blood lack the capacity for self-replication. They have finite life expectancies and the turnover rate is quite high. The replenishment of senescent cells is accomplished by the bone marrow.

All cellular components of the hematopoietic system appear to arise from a single pluripotent lymphoid stem cell[143] that gives rise to B and T cells directly (Fig. 24–1).[229] In addition, it engenders another pluripotent stem cell from which other committed cell lines develop, including those that result in mature erythrocytes, neutrophils, monocytes eosinophils, basophils, and platelets.[2,34,38,229]

The least differentiated of these cells is slow growing, and therefore relatively resistant to chromosomal damage from radiation, for example, but capable of self-replication.[90,211] Derivative cells are more committed and cannot produce more than one cell type. The most highly diferentiated cells lack the capacity for self-renewal.[2] At least 13 cytokines that are essential for the normal growth, differentiation, and function of the cellular elements of the blood are identified and characterized.[172–174] These glycoproteins are essential for a diversity of functions such as phagocytosis, the induction of T-lymphocyte cytotoxicity, chemotaxis, the maturation of B cells into antibody-producing cells, and the enhancement of cellular responsiveness to various microbial and parasitic agents.[89,172–174] They also regulate the cellular release of various mediators of inflammation such as prostaglandins, tumor necrosis factor, and plasminogen activator.[174] Deficiencies of the hematopoietic growth factors may result in a failure of development or function. The use of erythropoietin for the treatment of anemia associated with renal failure represents the first therapeutic use of these hematopoietic growth factors.[174] Additional uses may include therapy for postchemotherapeutic myelosuppression, or the enhancement of engraftment following bone marrow transplantation.[174] Concerns have been voiced with regard to the surreptitious use of these agents by athletes wishing to enhance their performance.[174]

The integrity of the hematopoietic microenvironment (including fibroblasts, endothelial cells, macrophages, and adventitial reticulum cells of the marrow) is essential to normal hematopoiesis.[38,76,172] Injury to either the matrix of the marrow or to the stem cells may result in significant loss of certain cell lines or pancytopenia.[76]

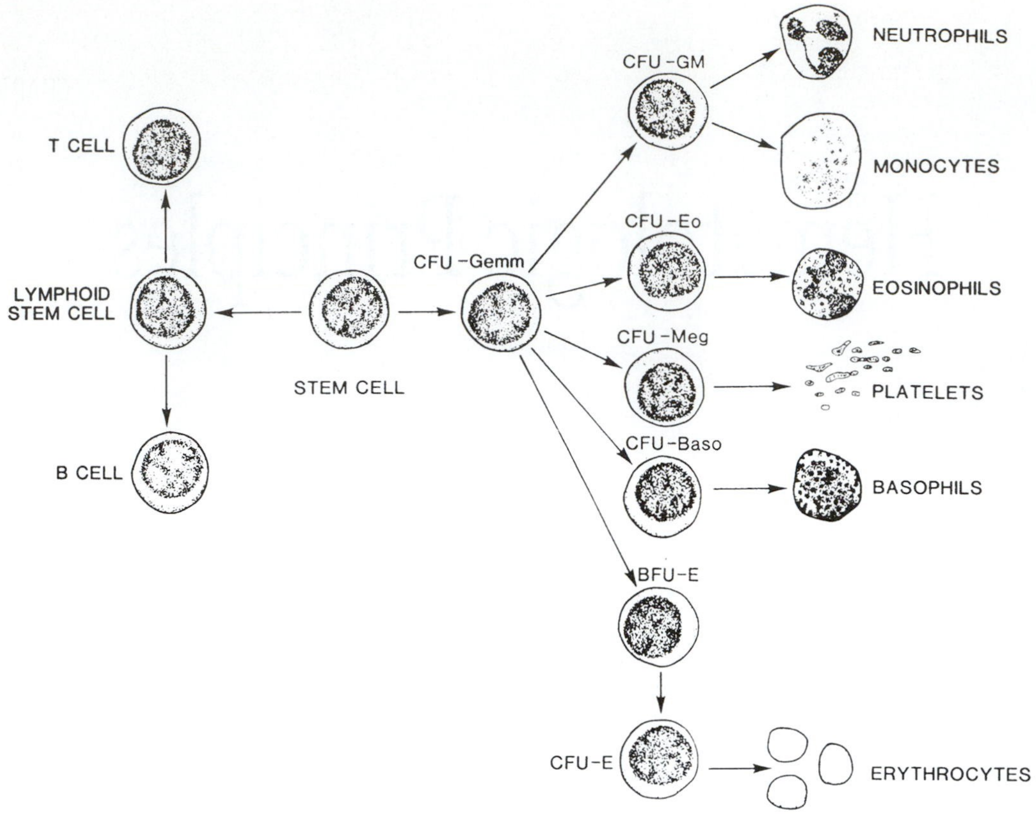

Figure 24–1. Hierarchy of hematopoiesis. The various progenitors are schematically represented. CFU-GEMM = multipotential progenitor for granulocytes, macrophages, erythroid cells, megakaryocytes; CFU-GM = progenitor for neutrophils and monocytes; CFU-Eo = progenitor for eosinophils; CFU-Baso = progenitor for basophils; CFU-Meg = progenitor for megakaryocytes; BFU-E = most primitive committed progenitor for erythroid line; CFU-E = more mature progenitor for erythroid line. *(Reprinted with permission from Lee GR, Bithell TC, Foerster J, et al, eds: Wintrobe's Clinical Hematology, 9th ed. Philadelphia, Lea & Febiger, 1993, Vol. 1, p. 51.)*

Pediatric Considerations

Erythropoiesis begins in the liver of the fetus at about the 6th week of gestation. By the 12th week the spleen participates in hematopoiesis. At about the 16th week the bone marrow becomes active, although erythropoiesis continues in the liver and spleen until the last trimester. By the time birth takes place, hematopoiesis occurs exclusively in the bone marrow. In the neonate as well as the adult, blood formation occurs largely in the hollow cavities of the long bones, the sternum, calvarium, vertebrae, and ribs.[132]

The hemoglobin of the fetus and neonate (HbF) differs from that of adults in important ways. It has an increased affinity for oxygen that results from the poor binding of 2,3-diphosphoglycerate (2,3-DPG). HbF confers an advantage in utero by allowing fetal hemoglobin to compete effectively with maternal hemoglobin for oxygen.[15]

Beginning at about 12 weeks of gestation, the percentage of HbF in fetal red cells declines.[160] There is a corresponding increase in HbA. The percentage of HbA reaches adult levels by about 6 months of age.[158] The persistence of HbF after birth is, however, a potential hazard, as it may impair the unloading of oxygen to the tissues. This places the neonate at particular risk of hypoxic insult that may occur with the development of any of the toxic dyshemoglobinemias.[132]

Toxins Affecting Hematopoiesis: Aplastic Anemia

Interference with the production of cellular elements by toxins may occur through multiple mechanisms.[187,227] Certain toxins are known to damage the hematopoietic microenvironment directly,[76] or cause injury directly to stem cells (benzene).[197] Various nutritional deficiencies (folate and vitamin B_{12}), or agents that antagonize the activity of essential enzymes may result in the impairment of DNA synthesis (antimetabolites).[87] DNA duplication may be blocked by the alkylating agents, which bind the component bases (nitrogen mustard).[29] Other agents interfere with cellular division by disrupting the microtubules of the mitotic spindle (colchicine, vinblastine, vincristine).[29,202] Another mechanism of toxicity is the interference with protein synthesis (chloramphenicol).[222]

A variety of toxins, including many with therapeutic uses, are harmful to bone marrow.[187,227] The toxicity may be reversible or irreversible, and may affect cells in various stages of differentiation.[187,227] Damage to the most primitive cellular elements or to the hematopoietic microenvironment will affect the development of all cell lines.[76] Injury to more mature committed cells may result in the deficiency of a single cellular element such as occurs with pure red cell aplasia[108,222] or pure white cell aplasia.[164]

Benzene

The causal relationship between benzene exposure and a variety of hematologic abnormalities has been recognized since the early 1900s.[159,187,197,227] Exposure results from the industrial use of benzene as a solvent in glues, inks, resins, and varnishes[4–6,43,179,215] and its use in the home as an insecticide.[129] Benzene is a significant toxic component of cigarette smoke.[219] While the availability of benzene for industrial use has been greatly restricted, many commercially available solvents, paint removers, and degreasers still contain benzene as a contaminant.[197] Benzene is a colorless liquid that is highly volatile and explosive. It is obtained as a product of coal tar distillation.[179]

Although the primary route of exposure is through inhalation,[179] transcutaneous absorption is significant.[159] Approximately half of an absorbed dose is excreted unchanged through the pulmonary route.[159] The remainder is hepatically metabolized, conjugated with sulfate and glucuronide, and excreted in the urine.[159,198]

Benzene is metabolized primarily in the liver via the cytochrome P4502E1 mixed-function oxidase system.[104,189] Metabolites include benzene epoxide, which exists in equilibrium with benzene oxepin and spontaneously rearranges to form phenol (Fig. 24–2).[96] It is believed that oxidative metabolites formed in the liver such as catechol and hydroquinone are transported through the blood to target organs, of greatest significance, the bone marrow. An aryl hydrocarbon hydroxylase, a form of mixed-function oxidase (MFO) involved in benzene hydroxylation in liver, is active in bone mar-

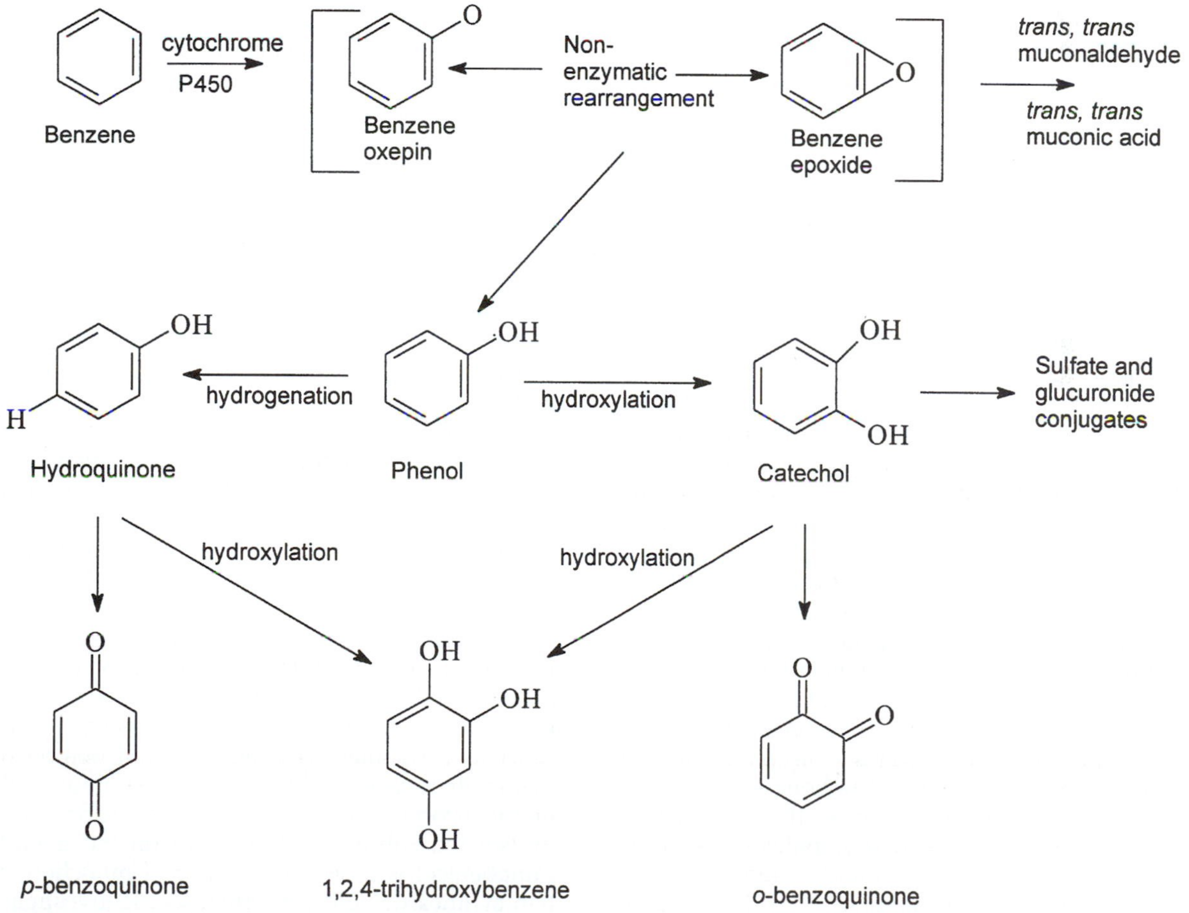

Figure 24–2. Benzene is metabolized by hepatic cytochrome P450 mixed function oxidase to oxepins and oxides. Benzene oxide may be further oxidized to the opened ring products *trans, trans* muconaldehyde and *trans, trans* muconic acid. Benzene metabolites are hydroxylated to phenol, catechol, hydroquinone, and 1,2,4 trihydroxybenzene, which may be excreted in the urine as ethereal sulfates and glucuronides.

row as well. This MFO may be responsible for the production of the metabolites toxic to the marrow.[10] In the marrow, benzene derivatives are further metabolized by myeloperoxidase to toxic quinones and semiquinones.[64,184,189] Phase I metabolites (phenol and hydroquinone) also serve as substrates for phase II reactions (conjugation with sulfate and glucuronide). The products of phase II metabolism, as well as the open-ring products (*trans, trans* muconic acid), are excreted in the urine.[70] The rate of metabolism and the relative proportion of by products depends upon the dose, the duration, and chronicity of exposure, and the presence of other aromatic hydrocarbons.[159] Simultaneous exposure to other aromatics slows the metabolism of benzene.[159]

The toxicity of benzene is complex. The mechanism of toxicity was elucidated in part from the study of the bone marrow of rabbits following the daily subcutaneous injection of benzene.[147] Tritiated thymidine was used to examine the effects of benzene on DNA and RNA synthesis. Severe pancytopenia occurred in all animals, and a profoundly hypocellular marrow resulted. Animals that survived developed hypercellular marrows. The myeloid cell line demonstrated a greater degree of depression than did the erythroid cell line. In addition, effects on single cell lines as well as pancytopenias are described. Aplastic anemias occurred following the serious depletion of cellular precursors. The administration of benzene resulted in the formation of DNA derivatives that may predispose to mutation. Extensive chromosomal aberrations have been observed in patients who develop leukemia following benzene exposure. The individual cell lines affected as well as the severity of the injury to the blood depends on the extent of exposure as well as individual susceptibility.[219] Studies in 1977 demonstrated that the causative agent was a metabolite of benzene rather than the parent compound.[197] In fact, the toxic agent is the first hepatic metabolite, benzene oxide.[96] This metabolic product is a potent electrophile capable of binding to nucleophilic sites on cellular macromolecules such as proteins and nucleic acids.[197] Semiquinones, quinones, and perhaps *trans, trans* muconaldehyde are now believed to be the ultimate toxic species.[104] Disease may result, in part from the covalent binding of reactive benzene metabolites to cellular macromolecules such as DNA. Genetic damage, including damage to both the number and structure of chromosomes, occurs as the result of the generation in bone marrow of active oxygen species such as superoxide anion radicals, hydrogen peroxide, hydroxyl radicals, and singlet oxygen.[104] These species are highly clastogenic, producing chromosome aberrations, sister chromatid exchanges and micronuclei.[196,197] The bone marrow production of these toxic species damages the stromal cells of the hematopoietic microenvironment.[76] These cells support and regulate the growth and differentiation of lymphoid and myeloid precursors.[64,196–198] Interference with the production of the hematopoietic growth factors that support the colony-forming units[153] is responsible for the development of the characteristic hematologic toxicity associated with benzene exposure. In addition, the structural chromosomal injuries are very likely related to the development of myelodysplastic syndrome and ultimately the leukemias.[196]

Clinically, benzene toxicity is associated with a variety of hematologic abnormalities. The development of disease depends upon the production of numerous metabolites, and does not result from the administration of any individual toxic metabolite.[198] The most frequently reported dyscrasia is aplastic anemia. Acute myeloblastic leukemia and other forms of acute nonlymphocytic leukemia are noted frequently in survivors of aplastic anemia.[5,6,43,179,196,216] Other reported abnormalities include pancytopenia accompanied by a hypoplastic marrow, hemolytic anemia, marrow hyperplasia, myeloid metaplasia, and lymphopenia.[179,203] Additional related information may be found in Chapter 85.

Chloramphenicol

Another agent unquestionably linked to the development of aplastic anemia is chloramphenicol.[7,107,188,217,230,231] Chloramphenicol (CAP) is an antimicrobial agent originally isolated from the species of actinomycetes called *Streptomyces Venezuela.*[231] It was chemically synthesized, introduced as a pharmaceutical agent in 1948,[107] and rapidly became widespread for multiple, often minor, indications. An analysis of deaths following the use of CAP demonstrated that the incidence of death from aplastic anemia was 13 times that of the general population.[217]

Chloramphenicol is an antimicrobial agent with a nitrobenzene moiety. It is bacteriostatic in some cases, and possibly bactericidal against a wide range of gram-negative and rickettsial organisms. Its major site of degradation is the liver. The half-life is significantly prolonged in severe liver and renal disease.[230]

Two distinct clinical syndromes of toxicity are associated with the use of CAP. The first is dose-related bone marrow toxicity producing anemia.[188] It is associated with a normocellular marrow and is reversible when CAP is withheld.[230]

The second syndrome is aplastic anemia. It is not dose related, generally occurs within 5 months of treatment, and is characterized by the development of an aplastic marrow and death. These two types of toxicity are apparently unrelated. Toxicity is direct, rather than immune mediated.[230,231]

Chloramphenicol inhibits the binding of messenger RNA to ribosomes, thus preventing protein synthesis in bacterial cell-free systems.[169,170,222,224] This results from an inhibition of the transfer of amino acids from soluble RNA to ribosomes. This effect is not demonstrable in mammalian cells.[221] The effect of CAP in animal cells is on the incorporation of labeled amino acids into proteins by isolated subcellular fractions from rat liver.[169] Chloramphenicol is a potent inhibitor of mitochondrial protein synthesis.[195] Electron microscopic investigations revealed altered mitochondrial ultrastructure in bone marrow cells including an increased density of the mitochondrial matrix without the derangement of cristae. This disruption of mitochondrial functioning is now felt to be the etiology of CAP-related aplastic anemia.[195] Additional related information may be found in Chapter 46.

Colchicine

Colchicine, a drug used primarily as a potent antiinflammatory, is a natural plant product of the autumn crocus, *Colchicum autumnale*. It is an antimitotic agent, blocking mitosis in metaphase and in the G_1 phase, preventing DNA synthesis. Following acute or chronic poisoning from colchicine, leukopenia and thrombocytopenia are observed, along with other symptoms such as gastrointestinal hemorrhage and disseminated intravascular coagulation.[53,202] Other hematologic effects include anisocytosis, poikilocytosis, and anemia, even in the absence of hemolysis. Recently, a few case reports have described the successful treatment of the leukopenia resulting from colchicine toxicity with granulocyte colony-stimulating factor. Intravenous doses of 300 μg/day have been associated with a normalization in leukocyte numbers beginning within a day of the initiation of therapy.[58,100,167] Additional related information may be found in Chapter 47.

Ionizing Radiation

The risk of unintentional exposure to ionizing radiation is a significant public health concern. Sources of irradiation that are of concern include x-rays, gamma rays, and fast and slow neutrons. Beta and alpha particles do not penetrate tissue enough to result in acute hematologic injury.[93] Following an acute exposure to a given dose of ionizing radiation, the absorbed dose (D) may be described as the mean energy (e) transferred to matter of mass (m). This relationship can be summarized as $D = e/m$. The unit for the absorbed dose is the Gray (Gy), which equals 1 J/kg^{-1}. The older unit, the rad, is equivalent to 1/100 Gy.[79] Considering that the transfer of energy from different types of radiation varies with the mass and velocity of the particle or ray in question, an attempt has been made to normalize the biologic cellular effects of a given dose. This has been done with reference to the gamma dose required to produce certain predictable effects. The energy transferred along the path of ionizing particles or rays to tissue is referred to as the linear energy transfer (LET). The ratio of the LET for a particular type of radiation to the LET for gamma radiation in water is the radiation weighting factor (Wr). The equivalent dose is defined as H = DWr (Fig. 24–3).

Following radiation exposures of 10 to 15 Gy all proliferating cells will be affected. At doses of 80 to 100 Gy, no stem cells will remain.[56] Ionizing radiation directly damages cellular DNA preventing cellular replication.[214] Rapidly proliferating cells, such as cells lining the gastrointestinal tract and bone marrow, are at greatest risk from the effects of ionizing radiation. Mature erythrocytes, neutrophils, and platelets do not divide, so their qualitative assessment will initially be normal following radiation exposure.[56] Progenitor cells are injured and fail to proliferate to replace those lost from natural senescence. Mature cells will then disappear from the circulation at a rate that is determined by their natural life span.

$$H = DWr$$

where

H = equivalent dose in Seivert (older unit is rem)

D = dose in Gray

Wr = radiation weighting factor

Figure 24–3. The radiation equivalent dose.

Neutrophils will remain at or above normal values for 4 days, and then disappear with a half-life of about 7 hours. Platelets will disappear within 7 days, and red blood cells within 120 days.[56]

Morphologic changes that have been described in lymphocytes following an acute exposure to ionizing radiation include the clumping of nuclear chromatin, free chromatin masses within the nuclear membrane, and split and fragmented nuclei.[93] In addition, giant neutrophils and neutrophils with multilobed nuclei, degenerative changes in platelets and eosinophils, and giant platelets have been described.[93]

An investigation of the effects of very low dose radiation (equivalent to a single chest radiograph) on whole blood demonstrated the generation of inflammatory mediators (products of the arachidonic acid cascade).[216] The researchers thus postulated inflammation as a mechanism of hematologic injury, in addition to direct chromosome breakage from exposure to ionizing radiation.

A prolongation of the clotting time unrelated to platelet loss or dysfunction is described following acute, but not chronic radiation exposure.[93] This effect appears to be due to an increase in the amount of a circulating heparin-like substance, and is a major cause of death from acute radiation injury in experimental animals.[93] This abnormality can be reversed with the administration of protamine sulfate.

In cases of inhomogeneous or partial irradiation, stem cells will migrate from the less severely affected marrow sites to repopulate the more severely affected sites.[56] In this situation, the liklihood of spontaneous recovery and survival is much greater than in cases of homogeneous total body irradiation. One of the most sensitive indicators of exposure is the decrease in the total lymphocyte pool.[55,93] With an exposure of 1/4 Gy, lymphocyte counts will decrease initially and then normalize within 24 to 48 hours. Following doses of greater than 1 Gy, lymphocyte counts will decrease within 3 hours and return to normal over 30 days. Animal studies have demonstrated a predictable course of cellular depletion, allowing for laboratory indicators to be of prognostic value.[56] If granulocytes can be measured at 4 to 6 days following exposure, and platelets do not decline steadily within 10 days, then survival of the stem cell pool and spontaneous recovery is likely. Replacement of individual cellular elements may be necessary. If, however, granulocytes disappear between 4 and 6 days following exposure (<300 × 10^6 cells/L), platelet counts decrease with a slope that predicts zero cells by day 10, and lymphocytes are low within one day, then it is likely that the hematopoietic stem cells were affected. Spontaneous recovery is unlikely to occur and a bone marrow transplant may be indicated.[56] The link between the exposure to ionizing radiation and the development of hematologic malignancies has been well established. Studies of the survivors of large nuclear explosions have shown an increase in the frequency of all types of leukemia with the exception of chronic lymphocytic leukemia.[12]

Therapy for the acute effects of this potentially lethal exposure may represent a future application for the use of cloned hematopoietic growth factors. Additional information on the toxic effects of ionizing radiation may be found in Chapter 98.

Other Agents

Another agent of historical interest implicated in the development of aplastic anemia is neoarsphenamine, an antisyphyllitic arsenical associated with the development of multiple blood dyscrasias including agranulocytosis.[60,97,131]

Quinacrine, an antimalarial agent, has been associated with the development of aplastic anemia in one in 30,000 patients.[187] The mechanism of toxicity is unknown but thought to relate to the suppression of leukocyte respiration.[57,187,227]

The anticonvulsant agents mesantoin and trimethadione have been implicated in the development of aplastic anemia through an unknown mechanism.[1]

Phenylbutazone,[141,200] a nonsteroidal antiinflammatory; gold therapy for rheumatoid arthritis[78]; the inhalation of kerosene,[83] possibly contaminated with benzene; and other agents (Table 24–1) have been associated with aplastic anemia.

Clinical Features

The clinical development of aplastic anemia is typically insidious. Although initial symptoms generally result from anemia or hemorrhage (purpura or bleeding gums),[187,227,231] occasionally, fever or infection heralds the onset of aplastic anemia.[187] Due to the relatively long life span of the red cells, bone marrow depression is manifested by neutropenia and thrombocytopenia prior to the onset of anemia.[147] One of the first manifestations of bone marrow depression of the erythroid line is reticulocytopenia.[147,227] The course of aplastic anemia is typically relentless, with death occurring from sepsis or hemorrhage within 18 months of diagnosis.[231]

TABLE 24–1. AGENTS ASSOCIATED WITH THE DEVELOPMENT OF APLASTIC ANEMIA

Acetazolamide	Methotrexate, low dose
Acetophenetidin	Methylphenylhydantoin
Acetylsalicylic acid	Methylprylon
Alpha-methyldopa	Methylthiouracil
Amodiaquine hydrochloride	Metolazone
Amphotericin B	Naproxen
Azothymidine	Oxyphenbutazone
Bismuth	Oxytetracycline
Carbamazepine	Parathion
Carbimazole	Penicillamine
Carbon tetrachloride	Penicillin
Carbutamide	Pentachlorophenol
Chloramphenicol	Phenacemide
Chlordane	Phenantoin
Chlordiazepoxide hydrochloride	Phenylbutazone
Chlorophenothane (DDT)	Piperacetazine
Chloroquine	Potassium perchlorate
Chlorothiazide	Primidone
Chlorpheniramine	Prochlorperazine
Chlorpromazine	Promazine
Chlorpropamide	Propylthiouracil
Chlortetracycline	Pyrimethamine
Cimetidine	Pyrilamine maleate
Colbutamide	Quinacrine hydrochloride
Colchicine	Quinidine
Colloidal silver	Salicylamide
Dinitrophenol	Solvents
Diphenylhydantoin sodium	Streptomycin
Epinephrine	Sulfadimethoxine
Ethosuximide	Sulfamethoxazole-trimethoprim
Flucytosine	Sulfamethoxypyridazine
Gamma benzene hexachloride	Sulfaphenazole
Gold salts	Sulfathiazole
Ibuprofen	Sulfisoxazole
Indomethacin	Sulfonamides
Lithium	Sulindac
Mepazine	Thiacetazone
Meprobamate	Thiocyanate
Mercurochrome	Tolbutamide
Methazolamide	Trimethadione
Methicillin sodium	Tripelennamine
Methimazole	

Adapted from Williams WJ, Beutler E, Erslav AJ, Lichtman MA, eds: Hematology, *4th ed. New York, McGraw-Hill, 1990; and Lee RG, Bithell TC, Foerster J, et al, eds:* Wintrobe's Clinical Hematology, *9th ed. Philadelphia, Lea & Febiger, 1993.*

Disorders Resulting in Toxicity to the Erythrocyte

The development of the erythrocyte from the erythroid precursor cells involves the production of heme and globin with the loss of the nucleus and cytoplasmic organelles once these functions are completed.

The mature erythrocyte is a highly specialized cell lacking cytoplasmic organelles. Its predominant function is that of oxygen transport. Since the mature cell lacks a nucleus it is incapable of protein (or lipid) synthesis and division. The erythrocyte is a solution of protein and electrolytes enclosed in a phospholipid bilayer membrane. Ninety five percent of its protein is hemoglobin. The remainder includes enzymes required to maintain hemoglobin in its functional or reduced state. The red cell membrane contains multiple ATP-dependent enzyme pumps that maintain the stratification of electrolytes and include Na-K-ATPase, Ca-Mg-ATPase, Mg-ATPase, and a glucose transport protein.[207]

Ninety percent of the dry weight of the red cell is hemoglobin. Hemoglobin is a conjugated protein with a molecular weight of 64,500 daltons. Hemoglobin is composed of four separate peptide (globin) chains: two alpha and two beta chains. Each globin chain encloses a heme group in a hydrophobic pocket. The heme group is the product of the condensation and cyclization of four porphobilinogen molecules. The final step is the insertion of iron into the center of the porphyrin ring.[45]

Hemoglobin variants may occur as a result of nucleotide replacement in the gene that is encoded for hemoglobin (as in sickle cell disease) or through a post-transcriptional modification resulting from pathologic processes including toxin exposure (hemoglobin A1C, methemoglobin, or sulfhemoglobin).[134]

The red cell produces energy through two pathways: anaerobic (Embden-Meyerhoff pathway) and aerobic (pentose phosphate or hexose monophosphate shunt). Anaerobic metabolism results in the formation of NADH, which is a cofactor necessary for methemoglobin reduction. In addition, this pathway produces ATP necessary to power Na-K-ATPase, which maintains the integrity of the limiting lipid membrane, and 2,3-diphosphoglycerate, which regulates the binding of O_2 to hemoglobin.

The product of the aerobic pathway is NADPH, which serves as an electron donor and cofactor in the reduction of oxidized glutathione. Reduced glutathione is the major reducing agent of the RBC and is the main source of protection against oxidative attack.

Multiple abnormalities in the development, structure, and function of the red cell or its component parts may result from exposure to pharmaceutical agents or toxins. In addition, subclinical biochemical or structural abnormalities may be exacerbated and become manifest following the exposure to various agents (as with patients with G-6-PD deficiency or porphyria).

Dyshemoglobinemias

Exposure to a number of toxins may result in abnormalities of hemoglobin that interfere with its ability to bind, transport, and release oxygen.

Methemoglobin

Methemoglobin is hemoglobin in which the heme has been oxidized to the ferric (+3) state rendering it incapable of oxygen transport. Ninety-seven percent of the iron in normal hemoglobin is present in the (+2) or ferrous state, and is slowly but continuously oxidized to the +3 or ferric state. Methemoglobin exerts its toxicity in two ways. It is incapable of oxygen transport and thus reduces the oxygen-carrying capacity of the blood. In addition, it shifts the oxyhemoglobin dissociation curve to the left, interfering with the unloading of oxygen and exacerbating any preexistent hypoxia.[39,41]

Two intracellular mechanisms function to maintain the level of methemoglobin at less than 3%.[38] One mechanism reduces potential oxidants to inactive substances. This mechanism includes catalase[206] (which reduces hydrogen peroxide), glutathione with or without glutathione peroxidase,[52,176] and to a small degree ascorbic acid. These enzymes, which would prevent the formation of methemoglobin, are evident in vitro but play only a minor role in vivo. Individuals who are deficient in these enzymes do not manifest methemoglobinemia.[38] Secondly, specific enzyme systems exist whose function is to reduce methemoglobin to oxyhemoglobin. The major pathway of red blood cell methemoglobin reduction depends on the presence of reduced nicotine adenine dinucleotide (NADH)-dependent methemoglobin reductase. To a lesser degree, reduced NADPH-dependent methemoglobin reductase contributes to the maintenance of normal oxyhemoglobin levels.[181,182]

Certain congenital defects in both activity of NADH-dependent methemoglobin reductase and the structure of the hemoglobin molecule combine to produce the clinical picture of congenital methemoglobinemia. Levels of methemoglobin that may be well tolerated in the congenital form of the disease may be devastating when acquired acutely. This is because the patient who experiences acute elevations of methemoglobin lacks the compensatory mechanisms that develop with protracted exposure. In addition, the same substances that cause acute elevations of methemoglobin exert other effects that exacerbate the toxicity. Children are more sensitive than adults to oxidative stress, because they have lower levels of NADH-dependent methemoglobin reductase.[26,133] For more detail see Chapter 93 and Antidotes in Depth: Methylene Blue.

Carboxyhemoglobin

Carbon monoxide (CO) exposure is a serious problem encountered throughout the year in all parts of the country. From 1991 to 1995, approximately 67,000 exposures to CO were reported in the United States, resulting in 179 deaths.[124–128] The majority of these exposures were unintentional. Carbon monoxide is an odorless, colorless, nonirritating gas produced by the incomplete combustion of carbonaceous materials.[68] Common sources include smoke from fires, hydrocarbon, and coal burning stoves; automobile exhaust systems; smoke from cigars, cigarettes, and pipes; and the exposure to methylene chloride through its in vivo hepatic metabolism to carbon monoxide.[68] Molecular oxygen is reversibly bound to iron in the ferrous (+2) state. Interactions occur among the four globin–heme units that facilitate the binding and unbinding of oxygen.[207] This effect is referred to as cooperativity.

The toxicity of carbon monoxide results from its binding to hemoglobin, myoglobin, and the cytochrome oxidase chain. The formation of carboxyhemoglobin (COHb) decreases hemoglobin oxygen saturation, depriving tissues of oxygen. Another result of exposure to carbon monoxide is that hemoglobin will be partially bound to carbon monoxide and partially bound to oxygen. This leads to a decrease in the cooperativity that normally facilitates the unbinding of oxygen at tissue sites.[194] The oxyhemoglobin dissociation curve will be shifted to the left, reflecting the fact that oxygen is more tightly bound by hemoglobin, depriving tissues of oxygen. The binding of carbon monoxide to the cytochrome chain interferes with cellular respiration, further exacerbating tissue hypoxia. For details regarding the clinical presentation and treatment of patients with carbon monoxide poisoning see Chapter 96.

Sulfhemoglobin

Sulfhemoglobin is a green-pigmented molecule containing a sulfur atom rather than an iron atom in one or more of the porphyrin rings.[18,149] It is formed upon exposure of hemoglobin to hydrogen sulfide gas (sewer gas),[144,224] and has been seen with other exposures as well. Sulfhemoglobin is ineffective in oxygen transport.[114] The clinical findings that result from exposure include mucous membrane irritation, headache, nausea, cough, dizziness, dyspnea, pulmonary edema, seizures, coma, and death.[224] Treatment is controversial. It is usually not a fatal disorder. Some have recommended the use of the Lilly cyanide antidote kit or hyperbaric oxygen.[224] No therapy has proven to be of benefit.

Disorders of Porphyrin Production

Porphyria

The porphyrias are characterized by the excessive production and excretion of porphyrins, porphyrin precursors, or both. The congenital porphyrias result from inherited enzymatic defects in heme biosynthesis. Multiple congenital syndromes exist and vary with respect to the particular enzymatic defect. Typically the syndromes include various combinations of cutaneous photosensitivity and neurologic abnormalities, resulting in apparent psychosis or autonomic neuropathies producing abdominal pain. Ineffective erythropoiesis and hemolysis are also part of this syndrome. Laboratory evaluation demonstrates the excretion of large amounts of porphyrin and porphyrin precursors in the urine and stool.[46,112] Multiple drugs and toxins are known to exacerbate the symptoms of porphyria through the induction of enzymes active in porphyrin production (Table 24–2).

TABLE 24–2. AGENTS ASSOCIATED WITH THE EXACERBATION OF THE PORPHYRIAS

Unsafe	Potentially Unsafe
Aminoglutethimide	Alfadolone
Barbiturates	Alfaxolone
Carbamazepine	Alkylating agents
Carbromal	2-Allyloxy-3-methylbenzamide
Chlorpropamide	Alpha-methyldopa
Cyclosporine	Bemegride
Danazol	Chloroquine
Diclofenac	Clonazepam
Diphenylhydantoin	Clonidine
Ergotamines	Etomidate
Estrogens	Hydralazine
Ethanol	Ketamine
Ethchlorvynol	Metapyrone
Glutethimide	Nikethamide
Griseofulvin	Pargyline
Hydrochlorthiazide + triamterene	Pentazocine
Iron salts	Pentylenetetrazole
Isopropylmeprobamate	Rifampin
Mephenytoin	Spironolactone
Meprobamate	Theophylline
Methprylon	Tolazamide
Novobiocin	Tranylcypromine
Primidone	
Progestins	
Pyrazolone preparations	
Sulfonamides	
Tolbutamide	
Trimethadione	
Valproic acid	

Adapted from Lee RG, Bithell TC, Foerster J, et al, eds: Wintrobe's Clinical Hematology, *9th ed. Philadelphia, Lea & Febiger, 1993; and Dukes MNG, ed:* Meyler's Side Effects of Drugs, *12th ed. Amsterdam, Elsevier, 1992.*

Lead

Lead toxicity is associated with an inhibition of several of the enzymes involved in porphyrin synthesis. Metal smelters, foundry workers, welders, solderers, printers, and those engaged in storage battery manufacturing are exposed to lead through dermal, pulmonary, and gastrointestinal routes.[102] Nonindustrial exposures occur frequently. Childhood lead poisoning due to the ingestion of leaded paint or, uncommonly, by living in proximity of lead-producing industries is a serious public health problem. These lead exposures are additive to the background lead levels generated in the greatest part by leaded gasoline.

The clinical effects of lead poisoning are multiple and include central and peripheral nervous system, gastrointestinal, rheumatologic, hepatic, renal, endocrine, and hematologic manifestations.[91] These clinical effects are described in more detail in Chapter 79. Chronic lead intoxication results in a hypochromic, microcytic anemia, more commonly seen in children than adults.[102,225] Basophilic stippling of the red cells is a prominent, although not specific finding. This anemia is morphologically similar to that of iron deficiency anemia and is thought to result from both a decrease in red cell life span and an inhibition of hemoglobin synthesis.[102] Extraerythrocytic iron metabolism is not affected. For further details the reader is referred to Chapter 79.

Sideroblastic Anemias

The sideroblastic anemias are characterized by the presence of amorphous iron deposits in the form of ferric phosphate and ferric hydroxide in the erythroblast mitochondria.[23,74] The iron-laden mitochondria assume a perinuclear distribution resulting in the appearance of the ring sideroblast on stained bone marrow aspirates. In general, extra-erythrocytic iron transport is normal: it is the incorporation of iron into heme that is impaired.[23] It is believed to result from the inadequate synthesis of heme in turn due to the inhibition of various enzymes in porphyrin synthesis including alpha levulinic acid dehydratase (ALAD), uroporphyrinogen decarboxylase, coproporphyrinogen oxidase, and ferrochelatase.[74,105] Ineffective heme synthesis impairs globin synthesis through a feedback mechanism. Sideroblastic anemia may be seen in nutritionally deprived and anemic alcoholic patients. It is often associated with pyridoxine deficiency.[85] In addition it has been associated with the use of chloramphenicol,[16] isoniazid, pyrazinamide, and cycloserine[23] and is noted in hypothermic patients[154] and copper-deficient patients.[232] It is reversible on withdrawal of the offending agent.

Sideroblastic anemia is a frequent accompaniment of ethanol abuse and occurs in approximately 25% of cases.[9,48,85,162,183] It appears to be related to the abnormal mitochondrial metabolism of iron.[143] Of note is the coexistence of a decrease in the activity of ALA synthetase, ALA dehydratase, and ferrochelatase, three enzymes essential to the normal synthesis of heme. Ineffective erythropoiesis is associated with the development of the sideroblastic morphology.[109,143,148]

Megaloblastic Anemia

Two forms of vitamin B_{12} are cofactors in two essential reactions in mammalian cells: 5′-deoxyadenosylcobalamin is a cofactor in hydrogen ion transfer reactions and methylcobalamin catalyzes the transfer of single carbon fragments. These processes are required for the synthesis of methionine from homocysteine.[42] 5′-methyltetrahydrofolate is also required in this process and for the conversion of deoxyuridilate to thymidylate. Both processes produce essential precursors for nucleic acid synthesis. In addition, acetylcholine and other important amines such as epinephrine and creatine are synthesized from methionine.[42]

Megaloblastic anemia results when DNA synthesis is impaired by the depletion of B_{12} or folate. The rapid turnover of the cellular elements of blood requires the synthesis of massive amounts of protein. Thus, impaired protein synthesis due to impaired DNA synthesis is manifested first by anemia and atrophic gastritis.[87] Megaloblastic anemia is a known complication of the administration of various chemotherapeutic agents. In particular, the drugs that inhibit tumor growth because they interfere with DNA synthesis, such as 6-mercaptopurine, 5-fluorouracil, cyclophosphamide, cytosine arabinoside, azathioprine, and the folate antagonists, predictably produce this toxic effect.[87]

Ethanol is toxic to each cellular component of blood. Multiple morphologic and functional abnormalities have been documented in alcoholic patients or in those acutely intoxicated.[47,48,81,85,122,116,162,168,187] Some abnormalities are the result of the direct effects of ethanol or the first metabolite, acetaldehyde, on blood.[122] Some abnormalities result from the nutritional deprivation characteristic of alcohol abuse,[121,122] and some result from alcoholic hepatotoxicity.[28,183]

Chronic ethanol abuse is well known to be associated with megaloblastic changes and the hypersegmentation of granulocytes.[121,183] This is known to occur secondary to folate deficiency.[84] Many alcoholic patients consume their entire daily calorie requirements through the ingestion of ethanol.[48] They therefore lack essential vitamins necessary as cofactors for many synthetic and metabolic processes.[8,59,121,162] Not only is the diet of many alcoholic patients deficient in folate, but alcohol damages the intestinal mucosa, resulting in an inability to absorb folate.[122] Furthermore, enterohepatic recirculation of folate is impaired, exacerbating the inhibition of folate-dependent processes and manifesting first as megaloblastic anemia.[122,123]

Glucose-6-Phosphate Dehydrogenase Deficiencies

Glucose-6-phosphate dehydrogenase (G-6-PD) catalyzes the first step of the pentose phosphate shunt: the conversion of G-6-PD to phosphogluconolactone. In the process, NADP is reduced to NADPH, which is necessary to maintain the supply of reduced glutathione. This provides the red cells' main defense against oxidation. In the presence of powerful oxidant drugs or chemicals, the supply of glutathione becomes exhausted and an attack on free sulfhydryl groups occurs. Intermediates implicated in this process include H_2O_2 and superoxide anion radicals.[35,94] Hemoglobin and other cellular elements may become denatured. Heme is released from globin, and the protein chain unfolds and precipitates as insoluble aggregates or Heinz bodies. The Heinz bodies attach to red cell membranes, compromising deformability and resulting in removal by liver or spleen reticuloendothelial cells.[19]

A large number of variants of G-6-PD exist, resulting in differences in enzyme activities among individuals. Deficient activity of G-6-PD may result from decreased enzyme synthesis, altered catalytic activity, or reduced stability of the enzyme. The gene that encodes for G-6-PD is X-linked, and therefore males are affected more severely than females. In females, due to the random nature of X-chromosome inactivation, the blood of heterozygotes may have a range of G-6-PD activity between zero and 100%, and the severity of hemolysis varies.[99]

Clinically, hemolysis may ensue in susceptible indi-

TABLE 24–3. DRUGS AND CHEMICALS CAUSING HEMOLYTIC ANEMIA IN PATIENTS WITH G-6-PD DEFICIENCY

Acetanilid	Phenylhydrazine
Diphenylsulfone (Dapsone)	Primaquine
Methylene blue	Sulfacetamide
Nalidixic acid	Sulfamethoxazole
Naphthalene	Sulfanilamide
Niridazole	Sulfapyridine
Nitrofurantoin	Thiazolesulfone
Pamaquine	Toluidine blue
Pentaquine	Trinitrotoluene

Adapted from Williams WJ, Beutler E, Erslav AJ, Lichtman MA, eds: Hematology, *4th ed. New York, McGraw-Hill, 1990; and Lee RG, Bithell TC, Foerster J, et al, eds:* Wintrobe's Clinical Hematology, *9th ed. Philadelphia, Lea & Febiger, 1993.*

viduals beginning from 2 to 4 days following the ingestion of an offending agent. Jaundice, pallor, and dark urine may occur with abdominal and back pain. A decrease in the concentration of hemoglobin will occur. The peripheral smear will demonstrate cell fragments, and cells that have had Heinz bodies "bitten" from them. Bone marrow stimulation will result in a reticulocytosis and an increased red cell mass. Newly formed cells will have the highest activity of G-6-PD, and therefore be more resistant to hemolysis. In general, a normal bone marrow will be able to compensate for ongoing hemolysis, and return the hemoglobin concentration back to normal. During an episode of hemolysis, the cells with the least G-6-PD activity (those with a genetically determined deficiency and those that are senescent) will be hemolyzed first. The cells with adequate G-6-PD activity will survive. Therefore, the measurement of the activity of G-6-PD following a hemolytic episode may be misleading.[82]

Drugs and toxins that represent oxidative stressors for red cells are listed in Table 24–3.

Immune-Mediated Hemolytic Anemia

The immune-mediated hemolytic anemias occur when ingested drugs or environmental toxins trigger an antigen antibody reaction. In general, drug molecules are too small to be sensitizing agents. Antigenicity is acquired following the binding of drug molecules to carrier proteins in blood. The particulars of the drug carrier immune activation sequence form the basis for the classification of this group of hemolytic anemias.[191]

The first class of reaction occurs when the drug acts as a hapten and binds to membrane proteins on the surface of the red cell. This results in the fixation of complement by IgG, and subsequent splenic sequestration and hemolysis.[191] The hemolytic anemia triggered in certain patients by penicillin represents the prototype of this reaction.[62]

The second type of this reaction is mediated by immune complexes and occurs with drugs that have a low affinity for cellular membranes. Small doses of drugs result in hemolysis, and red cell injury is primarily mediated by complement. Complexes of drug and IgM are implicated as the complement trigger in this second process.[191]

The third process occurs when the presence of drug induces the formation of antibody to cellular components (as with alpha-methyldopa). This is a true autoantibody reaction directed against red cell surface antigen.[13]

The severity of hemolysis is variable. In certain cases transfusion will be required to replace red cells. In general, resolution of the hemolytic process is complete with withdrawal of the responsible agent.

Non-Immune-Mediated Nonoxidant Causes of Hemolysis

Arsine

Arsine is a colorless, odorless, nonirritating gas that is 2.5 times denser than air. It is produced by the action of water on a metallic arsenide. Poisonings are associated with the admixture of acids and crude metals that contain arsenic as an impurity. Workers involved in galvanizing, soldering, etching, lead plating, and computer microchip processing are at risk for poisoning. Acute toxicity is associated with a 25% mortality rate.[13] Clinical signs and symptoms appear 2 to 24 hours after exposure and may include headache, malaise, dyspnea, abdominal pain with nausea and vomiting, hepatomegaly, hemolysis with hemoglobinuric renal failure, and death.[13,27,95,163] The peripheral smear of arsine-poisoned patients shows all of the typical abnormalities associated with hemolytic anemia.

The mechanism of hemolysis is believed to involve the fixation of arsine by hemoglobin.[72] The oxidation of arsine apparently yields arsenic dihydride as an intermediate, and finally elementary arsenic. Either of these products could be the hemolytic agent.

All heavy metals, including arsenic, have an affinity for sulfhydryl groups. One author[116] proposed that the complexing of arsenic derivatives with red cell sulfhydryl groups results in an impairment of the Na-K-ATPase that is necessary for cell membrane stability.

The treatment of choice is cessation of exposure and possibly exchange transfusion in severe cases. Adequate hydration and possibly alkalinization of the urine may be useful to protect against hemoglobin cast formation.

Chronic low-grade hemolysis is reported in workers exposed to arsine during the cyanide extraction of gold.[27] It appears that chronic exposure to low levels of arsine can produce clinically significant disease. Arsine poisoning should, therefore, be included in the differential diagnosis of hemolytic anemia.

Copper Sulfate

Copper sulfate is widely used in India in the whitewashing and leather industries. Although no data are available on the incidence of this poisoning in the United States, in India its availability results in its frequent ingestion both accidentally and in suicide attempts.

Symptoms following ingestion include a metallic taste, nausea, vomiting, epigastric burning, and gastrointestinal hemorrhage.[33,151,209] Methemoglobinemia, hemolysis, renal failure, and death are frequently reported.[33,151,209]

An in vitro study[51] in which human erythrocytes were incubated with copper sulfate showed a tenfold enhancement in oxidation of NADPH, inhibition of glycolysis in the pentose phosphate shunt, and inhibition of G-6-PD. Similar results were found after incubating red cells with cupric acetate.[44] Each of these phenomena probably contributes to the hemolytic effect of copper sulfate. No proven therapy exists for this poisoning. Treatment is supportive with transfusions, volume replacement, and hemodialysis performed as indicated. Table 24–4 summarizes the causes of immune and nonimmune-mediated hemolysis.

Venoms

The toxicity to the blood of snake and spider venoms is discussed in Chapters 99 and 100.

White Blood Cell Series

The neutrophilic, eosinophilic, and basophilic granulocytes develop from a common progenitor cell, the myeloblast. They follow similar patterns of proliferation, differentiation, maturation, storage, and delivery. These cells are critical in the defense against a wide variety of invading pathogens.

Polymorphonuclear Leukocytes

The production and function of PMNs is supported and controlled by various hematopoietic growth factors, opsonins, humoral factors such as antigen–antibody complexes, bacterial toxins, and components of complement. Polymorphonuclear leukocytes use both aerobic and anaerobic mechanisms for energy production.[11] Basophils and eosinophils contain high-affinity receptors for IgE as well as receptors for complement. The granules of these cells contain large amounts of histamine and leukotrienes.[11] Eosinophils defend the organism against the larval stages of parasitic infections and serve as the modulators of hypersensitivity reactions.[11]

Leukopenia, or a depression of the white cell count, is the most commonly reported blood dyscrasia resulting from the exposure to physical or chemical agents. Typically various combinations of leukopenia, neutropenia, and pancytopenias are reported.[11,60,90,115,117,136,216,218]

Granulocytopenia develops as a result of a hypersensitivity reaction in patients previously exposed to the inciting antigen.[50,80,171,186,205,223] Multiple mechanisms have been postulated including direct cell lysis, agglutination, and splenic sequestration and destruction.[80]

The onset of the disorder may be abrupt or may develop insidiously. It is twice as common in females as in males.[80] Typically the patient develops a severe pharyngitis followed in rapid succession by prostration, agranulocytosis, sepsis, and death.[80,159,186] The largest number of cases of agranulocytosis reported have been associated with the use of aminopyrine and dipyrone.[40,106,135,165,201,220] Other agents that may be associated with this syndrome are listed in Table 24–5.

The use of lithium salts is known to be associated with the production of neutrophilic granulocytes.[14,30,36,77,103,150,178,185,190,212] Dose–response investigations have demonstrated the clonal proliferation of granulo-

TABLE 24–4. ETIOLOGIES OF HEMOLYSIS

Immune Mediated
Type I: Drug–red cell complex, IgG triggers complement
Type II: Immune complex mediated, IgM triggers complement
Type III: True autoimmune to red cell membrane
Non-Immune Mediated
Arsine gas
Copper sulfate
G-6-PD deficiency
Hypoosmolality
Hypophosphatemia
Lead
Snake venins
Spider venins

TABLE 24–5. DRUGS ASSOCIATED WITH THE DEVELOPMENT OF AGRANULOCYTOSIS

Acetylsalicylic acid	Neuroleptics
Aminopyrine	Nifedipine
Amodiaquine	Niflumic acid
Antihistamines	NSAIDs
Beta-lactams	Oral hypoglycemics
Captopril	Paracetamol
Carbamazepine	Penicillamine
Cephalosporins	Penicillins
Chloroquine	Pentazocine
Clofibrate	Piroxicam
Clozapine	Pyrimethamine
Co-trimoxazole	Pyrimethamine + dapsone
Diclofenac	Rifampicin
Dipyrone	Salazosulfapyridine
Enalapril	Spironolactone
Furosemide	Sulfonamides
Ibuprofen	Sulindac
Indomethacin	Suramin
Levamisole	Thiouracils
MAO-inhibitors	Tricyclic antidepressants
Mebendazole	Trimethoprim
Mianserin	Vancomycin

Adapted from Williams WJ, Beutler E, Erslav AJ, Lichtman MA, eds: Hematology, *4th ed. New York, McGraw-Hill, 1990; and Dukes MNG, ed:* Meyler's Side Effects of Drugs, *12th ed. Amsterdam, Elsevier, 1992.*

cyte precursors with nanomolar levels of lithium.[14] This effect is not specific to any one cell line. In vitro murine studies have demonstrated megakaryocytosis in response to lithium.[31] Lithium appears to serve a specific role in the metabolism of phosphoinositides, which are essential to cell membrane receptor activation.[140] This effect may be mediated by suppressor T-lymphocytes, and has led to the suggestion that lithium may play a role in the stimulation of leukocyte production in patients with various immunodeficiencies.[65]

One of the hematologic abnormalities noted consistently in studies of alcoholic patients is the vacuolization of granulocyte and erythrocyte precursors.[122,173] Although not associated with aplastic anemia, these findings are apparent on bone marrow aspiration within hours of the ingestion of ethanol. This change is exceedingly characteristic and occurs in the absence of folate deficiency, sideroblastic changes, megaloblastic changes, or thrombocytopenia.[122] Granulocytopenia occurs frequently in alcoholic patients.[48,183] It is associated with impaired leukocyte mobilization in response to inflammation and impaired adherence of leukocytes to vessel walls.[24,67,161] This effect is noted immediately following a single dose of ethanol and does not persist through periods of abstinence.[121] Chemotaxis and phagocytosis are unaffected.

Platelets

Platelets are morphologically heterogeneous, highly complex cells that play an essential role in hemostasis. Microscopically, they contain multiple storage granules with nucleotides, calcium ions, catecholamines, inorganic pyrophosphate and orthophosphate, and other proteins vital to platelet functioning. In addition, platelets possess abundant metabolic equipment and more than 90 enzymes. Platelets posses the capacity to synthesize, and to contract and secrete biologically active substances when stimulated. They conduct glycolysis as well as glycogen synthesis. Like muscle cells, they are equipped to expend a large amount of energy over a short period of time. Primarily this occurs during aggregation, the release reaction, and clot retraction.[21,86] When exposed to damaged vascular surfaces, platelets adhere and become activated. The formation of the platelet plug involves a complex series of steps resulting in blood coagulation, fibrin deposition, and clot retraction.[21,86]

Thrombocytopenia is the most common manifestation of an acquired bleeding disorder.[21] The mechanism generally is immune mediated. Drug-induced platelet antibodies are reported to occur in 1 out of 100,000 drug exposures.[20]

The development of antiplatelet antibodies occurs in association with the use of multiple medications including quinine (cocktail purpura), quinidine,[111] stibophen,[98] ampicillin,[25] cephalothin,[73] and allyl isopropylcarbamide.[98] Most commonly, IgG is the antibody implicated, although some reports have identified IgA[49] (associated with acetaminophen use) and IgM (associated with the use of clonazepam,[213] rifampin,[22] and sodium valproate.[180]

As in the case of immune-mediated red cell destruction, multiple immune mechanisms may operate.[17,98,110,204] Drugs may act as haptens.[17] Subsequent interactions between drug, antibody, and platelets result in platelet damage and removal by the reticuloendothelial system.[204] Alternatively, drugs may complex with plasma proteins or another carrier. Antibody forms to the complex, complement becomes fixed, and "innocent bystander" destruction of platelets ensues.[32,110]

Thrombocytopenia develops within 12 hours of a repeated exposure to a sensitizing agent.[192] In patients ingesting the drug for the first time, 7 days are required for the development of the immune response.[63] Clinically, fever, chills, pruritis, and lethargy may occur.[98] The onset of bleeding may be abrupt.[192] Hemorrhagic vesicles may be seen in the oral mucosa.[49,98] Life-threatening hemorrhage may develop.[98,157] Laboratory investigations will demonstrate an absence of platelets on peripheral smear,[98,110,157] high MPV prolongation of the bleeding time,[111] deficient clot retraction, and an abnormal prothrombin consumption test.[98] Bone marrow aspiration will demonstrate normal or increased numbers of megakaryocytes and immature forms will be seen.[98] Various laboratory methodologies are available for confirmation of the presence of antiplatelet antibodies. Other than general supportive measures, treatment includes the transfusion of blood products as indicated, the use of steroids, as well as withdrawal of the involved agent.[98]

Platelet destruction that is not immunologically mediated was seen in association with the use of ristocetin, an antituberculous drug no longer in clinical use.[199] It promotes the attachment of von Willebrand factor to a platelet receptor and initiates direct platelet to platelet interactions and agglutination. Table 24–6 lists the drugs that are associated with the development of antiplatelet antibodies.

Impaired platelet function occurs as a result of the use of acetylsalicylic acid. Thromboxane A2 is one of the mediators active in normal platelet aggregation. Normally, thromboxane A2 is produced in activated platelets by the oxygenation of arachidonate liberated from phospholipids. The formation of thromboxane A2 is catalyzed by cyclooxygenase and thromboxane synthetase. In the presence of nonsteroidal antiinflammatory drugs (cyclooxygenase inhibitors) such as acetylsalicylic acid, indomethacin, and imidazole derivatives, platelet cy-

TABLE 24–6. DRUGS ASSOCIATED WITH THE DEVELOPMENT OF ANTIPLATELET ANTIBODIES

Acetaminophen
Ampicillin
Cephalosporin
Clonazepam
Quinidine
Quinine
Rifampin
Sodium valproate
Stibophen

clooxygenase becomes acetylated, producing a blockade of thromboxane A2 and thus interfering with platelet aggregation.[63,177]

Thrombocytopenia is a frequent accompaniment of chronic alcohol abuse.[48,121,183] The etiology is poorly understood. It occurs unassociated with folate deficiency, sepsis, hypersplenism, or disseminated intravascular coagulation. It may be associated with granulocytopenia.[81,121,183] It is apparently unrelated to poor nutrition.[122] Bone marrow aspiration may be normal or demonstrate increased numbers of megakaryocytes.[122] In mice, ethanol has been found to inhibit both primary ADP induced aggregation and the platelet release reaction.[37] Impaired platelet aggregation can be demonstrated in human subjects during the intravenous administration of ethanol.[81]

Anticoagulants

Tissue-type plasminogen activator is a physiologic plasminogen activator present in human blood. It is synthesized principally in the vascular endothelium. Its action on plasminogen is enhanced in the presence of fibrin. The administration of genetically engineered tissue plasminogen activator (or other potent thrombolytics) induces a hemostatic deficit through its activity on the clotting factors in blood, the vascular endothelium, and the platelet plug.[138,139] Not unexpectedly, the major risk of thrombolytic therapy is hemorrhage.[69,208,211] The risk is greatest in patients who have undergone recent vascular procedures such as phlebotomy, arteriotomy, and intramuscular injection.[3,92,101,193,226] The risk of intracranial hemorrhage is significant and is increased in patients with untreated hypertension, a longer duration of thrombolysis,[152] advanced age,[71] and with high dose t-PA.[71] Life threatening hemorrhage is controlled by reversing the hemostatic defect by discontinuing the administration of the thrombolytic agent and infusing either whole plasma or cryoprecipitate, and by providing platelets that have not been exposed to a plasminogen activator or aspirin.[137] Persistent anticoagulation may be reversed by the administration of epsilon aminocaproic acid (5 g IV over 30 to 45 minutes, then 1 g every 2 hours, as needed).[138] Other reported adverse effects of thrombolytic therapy have included hypotension and allergic reactions. The allergic reactions were minor and had no influence on mortality. About half of patients experiencing hypotension required pharmacologic therapy.[208]

Bleeding disorders associated with the use of warfarin and agents with warfarin like effects are discussed in Chapter 42.

Natural coumarins occur in plants such as sweet clover (*Melilotus* species), tonka beans (*Dipteryx odorata* and *D. oppositfolia*), sweet woodruff (*Asperula odorata*), and vanilla leaf (*Trilisa odoratissima*).[120] One report exists of a patient who developed a hemorrhagic diathesis manifested by menometrorrhagia from drinking tea made from these plants.[88]

Acquired inhibitors of individual coagulation factors have resulted from the use of various pharmacologic agents.[54,66,75,113,118,119,130,145,155,156,166,175] The development of acquired inhibitors of factor VIII are reported in conjunction with the use of penicillin,[155] nitrofurantoin, sulfanilamide, arsenicals, and horse serum.[113] A patient died of hemorrhage from a factor VIII inhibitor that developed shortly after the initiation of chlorpromazine therapy.[66] A patient developed a circulating inhibitor of factor VIII in association with the use of phenytoin.[166] The inhibitor was felt to be polyclonal IgG antibodies.

Acquired inhibitors of factor XIII resulting in defective clot stabilization and hemorrhage have been reported in multiple patients using isoniazid (INH).[119,130,145] Serious hemorrhage including one death has resulted.[118] Values for prothrombin time, partial thromboplastin time, and thrombin time were normal. Measurements of factor XIII were abnormal. The inhibitor was found to disappear following the withdrawal of INH.

Summary

The toxins that adversely effect the blood form a diverse group. In addition to the metals, animal venoms, oxidizing agents, and asphyxiants discussed, hydrocarbons such as phenol suppress hematopoiesis, and excessive amounts of oral anticoagulants may result in bleeding abnormalities due to the inhibition of vitamin K-dependent clotting factors. The list of possibilities is virtually endless. Although hemolysis has been commonly attributed to certain plant ingestions such as castor beans (*Ricinus communis*), rosary pea beans (*Abrus precatorius*), and the false morel (*Gyromitra esculenta*), no evidence of this is found in the literature. The variety and ubiquitous nature of many of the toxins effecting the blood necessitate consideration of toxic exposures in the differential diagnosis of hematologic disease.

References

1. Abbott JA, Schwab RS: The serious side effects of the newer antiepileptic drugs: Their control and prevention. N Engl J Med 1950;242:943–949.
2. Abramson S, Miller RG, Phillips RA: The identification in adult bone marrow of and restricted stem cells of the myeloid and lymphoid systems. J Exp Med 1977;145: 1567–1579.
3. AIMS Trial Study Group: Long-term effects of intravenous antistreplase in acute MI: Final report of the AIMS study. Lancet 1990;335:427–431.
4. Aksoy M, Dincol K, Akgun T, et al: Haematological effects of chronic benzene poisoning in 217 workers. Br J Ind Med 1981;28:296–302.
5. Aksoy M, Dincol K, Erdem S, et al: Acute leukemia due to chronic exposure to benzene. Am J Med 1972;52:160–166.
6. Aksoy M, Erdem S, Dincol G: Leukemia in shoe workers exposed chronically to benzene. Blood 1974;44:837–841.
7. Alavi JB: Aplastic anemia associated with intravenous chloramphenicol. Am J Hematol 1983;15:375–379.
8. Ali MAM, Brain MC: Ethanol inhibition of haemoglobin synthesis: In vitro evidence for a haem correctable defect in normal subjects and alcoholics. Br J Haematol 1974; 28:311–316.

9. Ali MAM, Sweeney G: Erythrocyte coproporphyrin and protoporphyrin in ethanol-induced sideroblastic erythropoiesis. Blood 1974;43:291–295.
10. Andrews LS, Sonawane BR, Yaffe SJ: Characterization and induction of aryl hydrocarbon [Benzo(a)pyrene] hydroxylase in rabbit bone marrow. Res Commun Chem Pathol Pharmacol 1976;15:319–330.
11. Athens JW: Granulocytes and neutrophils. In: Lee RG, Bithell TC, Forester J, et al, eds: Wintrobe's Clinical Hematology, 9th ed. Philadelphia, Lee & Febiger, 1993, pp. 223–266.
12. Badman DG, Jaffe ER: Blood and air pollution: State of knowledge and research needs. Otolaryngol Head Neck Surg 1996;114:205–208.
13. Bakemeier RF, Leddy JD: Erythrocyte autoantibody associated with alpha-methyldopa: Heterogeneity of structure and specificity. Blood 1968;32:1–14.
14. Barr RD, Koekebakker M, Brown EA, Falso MC: Putative role for lithium in human hematopoiesis. J Lab Clin Med 1987;109:159–163.
15. Bauer C, et al: Different effects of 2-3 diphosphoglycerate and adenosine triphosphate on oxygen affinity of adult and fetal human hemoglobin. Life Sci 1969;7:271–277.
16. Beck EA, Ziegler G, Schmid R, Ludin H: Reversible sideroblastic anemia caused by chloramphenicol. Acta Haematol 1967;38:1–10.
17. Belkin GA: Cocktail purpura: An unusual case of quinine sensitivity. Ann Intern Med 1967;66:583–586.
18. Berzofsky JA, Peisach J, Horecher BL: Sulfheme proteins. IV. The stoichiometry of sulfur incorporation on the isolation of sulfhemin, the prosthetic group of sulfmyoglobin. J Biol Chem 1972;247:3783–3791.
19. Beutler E: The mechanism of glutathione destruction and protection in drug-sensitive and non-sensitive erythrocytes. J Clin Invest 1957;36:617–628.
20. Bithell TC: Thrombocytopenia caused by immunologic platelet destruction: Idiopathic thrombocytopenic purpura (ITP), drug-induced thrombocytopenia, and miscellaneous forms. In: Lee RG, Bithell TC, Foerster J, et al, eds: Wintrobe's Clinical Hematology, 9th ed. Philadelphia, Lee & Febiger, 1993, pp. 1329–1355.
21. Bithell TC: Thrombocytopenia: Pathophysiology and classification. In: Lee RG, Bithell TC, Foerster J, et al, eds: Wintrobe's Clinical Hematology, 9th ed. Philadelphia, Lee & Febiger, 1993, pp. 1325–1328.
22. Blajchman J, Lowry RC, Pettit JE, et al: Rifampin-induced immune thrombocytopenia. Br Med J 1970;3:24–26.
23. Bottomley SS: Sideroblastic anemia. In: Jacobs A, ed: Iron in Biochemistry and Medicine. London, Academic Press, 1980, pp. 363–392.
24. Brayton RG, Stokes PE, Schwartz MS, et al: Effect of alcohol and various diseases on leukocyte mobilization, phagocytosis, and intracellular bacterial killing. N Engl J Med 1970;282:123–128.
25. Brooks AP: Thrombocytopenia during treatment with ampicillin. Lancet 1974;2:723.
26. Bucklin R, Myint MK: Fatal methemoglobinemia due to well water nitrates. Ann Intern Med 1960;52:703–705.
27. Bulmer FMR, Rothwell HE: Chronic arsine poisoning among workers employed in the cyanide extraction of gold: A report of fourteen cases. J Ind Hygiene Tox 1940;22:111.
28. Burke JP, Rubin E: The effects of ethanol and acetaldehyde on the products of protein synthesis by liver mitochondria. Lab Invest 1979;41:393–400.
29. Calabresi P, Chabner BA: Chemotherapy of neoplastic diseases. In: Hardman JG, Limbird LE, Molinoff PB, et al, eds: Goodman and Gilman's The Pharmacological Basis of Therapeutics, 9th ed. New York, McGraw-Hill, 1996, pp. 1225–1232.
30. Catane R, Kaufman J, Mittelman A, Murphy GP: Attenuation of myelosuppression with lithium. N Engl J Med 1977;297:452–453.
31. Chatelain C, Burstein SA, Harker LA: Lithium enhancement of megakaryocytopoiesis in culture: Mediation via accessory marrow cells. Blood 1983;62:172–176.
32. Christie DJ, Aster RH: Drug–antibody–platelet interaction in quinine and quinidine-induced thrombocytopenia. J Clin Invest 1982;70:989–998.
33. Chuttani HK, Gupta PS, Gulati S, Gupta DN: Acute copper sulfate poisoning. Am J Med 1965;39:849–854.
34. Clark SC, Kamen R: The human hematopoietic colony-stimulating factors. Science 1987;236:1229–1237.
35. Cohen G, Hochstein P: Generation of hydrogen peroxide in erythrocytes by hemolytic agents. Biochemistry 1964;3: 895–900.
36. Cohen MS, Zakhirch B, Metcalf JA, Roof RK: Granulocyte function during lithium therapy. Blood 1979;53:913–915.
37. Cooper GW, Dinowitz H, Cooper B: The effects of administration of ethyl alcohol to mice on megakaryocyte and platelet development. Thrombosis Haemostasis 1984;52: 11–14.
38. Curry JL, Trentin JT, Wolf N: Hemopoietic spleen colony studies II. Erythropoiesis. J Exp Med 1967;125:703–720.
39. Curry S: Methemoglobinemia. Ann Emerg Med 1982; 11:214–221.
40. Dameshek W, Claus A: The effect of drugs in the production of agranulocytosis with particular reference to amidopyrine hypersensitivity. J Clin Invest 1936;15:85–97.
41. Darling RC, Roughton FJR: The effect of methemoglobin on the equilibrium between oxygen and hemoglobin. Am J Physiol 1942;137:56–66.
42. Das KC, Herbert V: Vitamin B_{12}-folate interrelations. Clin Haematol 1976;5:697–745.
43. DeGowin RL: Benzene exposure and aplastic anemia followed by leukemia fifteen years later. JAMA 1963; 185:748–751.
44. Deiss A, Lee GR, Cartwright GE: Hemolytic anemia in Wilson's disease. Ann Intern Med 1970;73:413–418.
45. Dessypris EN: Erythropoiesis. In: Lee RG, Bithell TC, Foerster J, et al, eds: Wintrobe's Clinical Hematology, 9th ed. Philadelphia, Lee & Febiger, 1993, pp. 134–157.
46. Dowdle E, Mustard P, Spong N, Eales L: The metabolism of [5-^{14}C] delta-aminolaevulinic acid in normal and porphyric human subjects. Clin Sci 1968;34:233–251.
47. Doyle K: Alterations in complete blood counts due to low to moderately high levels of dietary ethanol. Vet Hum Toxicol 1988;30:423–425.
48. Eichner ER, Hillman RS: The evolution of anemia in alcoholic patients. Am J Med 1971;50:218–232.

49. Eisner EV, Shahidi NT: Immune thrombocytopenia due to a drug metabolite. N Engl J Med 1972; 287:376–381.
50. Evans RS, Ford WP: Studies of the bone marrow in immunological granulocytopenia. Arch Intern Med 1958;101: 244–251.
51. Fairbanks VF: Copper sulfate-induced hemolytic anemia. Arch Intern Med 1967;120:428–432.
52. Finch CA: Methemoglobinemia and sulfhemoglobinemia. N Engl J Med 1948;239:470.
53. Finkelstein M, Goldman L, Grace ND, Foley M, Randall N: Granulocytopenia complicating colchicine therapy for primary biliary cirrhosis. Gastroenterology 1987;93: 1231–1235.
54. Fiore PA, Ellis LD, Dameshek HL, et al: XIII inhibition and antituberculous therapy. Clin Res 1971;19:418.
55. Fliedner TM, Andrews GA, Cronkite EP, Bond VP: Early and late cytologic effects of whole body irradiation on human marrow. Blood 1964;23:471–487.
56. Fliedner TM, Nothdurft W, Steinbach KH: Blood cell changes after radiation exposure as an indicator for hemopoietic stem cell function. Bone Marrow Transplant 1988;3:77–84.
57. Follette JH et al: The effect of chloramphenicol and other antibiotics on leukocyte respiration. Blood 1956;11: 234–242.
58. Folpini A, Furfori P: Colchicine toxicity-clinical features and treatment. Massive overdose case report. J Toxicol Clin Toxicol 1995;33:71–77.
59. Freedman ML, Cohen HS, Rossman J, et al: Ethanol inhibition of reticulocyte protein synthesis: The role of haem. Brit J Haematol 1975;30:351–363.
60. Freeman HE: Aplastic anemia with thrombopenic purpura and agranulocytosis complicating mapharsen therapy. Arch Dermatol Syphil 1944;50:320–322.
61. Freston JW: Cimetidine and granulocytopenia. Ann Intern Med 1979;90:264–265.
62. Funicella T, et al: Penicillin-induced immunohemolytic anemia associated with circulatory immune complexes. Am J Hematol 1977;3:219–223.
63. Gangarosa EJ, Johnson TR, Ramos HS: Ristocetin-induced thrombocytopenia: Site and mechanism of action. Arch Intern Med 1960;105:83–89.
64. Ganousis LG, Goon D, Zyglewska T, et al: Cell-specific metabolism in mouse bone marrow stroma: Studies of activation and detoxification of benzene metabolites. Molec Pharmacol 1992;42:1118–1125.
65. Gelfand EW, Dosch HM, Hastings D, Shore A: Lithium: A modulation of cyclic AMP-dependent events in lymphocytes? Science 1979;203:365–367.
66. Glazier RL, Crowell EB: Factor VIII inhibitor associated with chlorpromazine-induced hepatic injury. Thromb Haemost 1977;37:523–526.
67. Gluckman SJ, MacGregor RR: Effect of acute alcohol intoxication on granulocyte mobilization and kinetics. Blood 1978;52:551–559.
68. Goldfrank L, Weisman RS, Bresnitz EA, Lewin NA: The inhaled agents and other disorders of oxygen transport. In: Hanson WJ, ed: Clinics in Emergency Medicine, Vol. 5. Toxic Emergencies. New York, Churchill Livingstone, 1984, pp. 196–225.
69. Goldhaber SZ, Heit J, Sharma GVRK, et al: Randomised controlled trial of recombinant tissue plasminogen activator versus urokinase in the treatment of acute pulmonary embolism. Lancet 1988;2:293–298.
70. Goldstein BD, Benzene toxicity. Occup Med 1988;3: 541–554.
71. Gore JM, Sloan M, Price TR, et al: Intracerebral hemorrhage, cerebral infarction, and subdural hematoma after acute myocardial infarction and thrombolytic therapy in the thrombolysis in myocardial infarction study. Circulation 1991;83:448–459.
72. Graham AF, Crawford TBB, Marrian GF: The action of arsine on blood. Biochem J 1946;40:256.
73. Gralnick HR, et al: Thrombocytopenia with sodium cephalothin therapy. Ann Intern Med 1972;77:401–404.
74. Grasso JA, Hines JD: A comparative electron microscopic study of refractory and alcoholic sideroblastic anemia. Br J Haematol 1969;17:35–44.
75. Green D: Spontaneous inhibitors of factor VIII. Br J Haematol 1968;15:57–75.
76. Greenberger JS: Toxic effects on the hematopoietic microenvironment. Exp Hematol 1991;19:1101–1109.
77. Hammond WP, Dale DC: Cyclic hematopoiesis: Effects of lithium on colony-forming cells and colony-stimulating activity in gray collie dogs. Blood 1982;59:179–184.
78. Hansen RM, Csuka ME, McCarty DJ, Saryan LA: Gold induced aplastic anemia. Complete response to corticosteroids, plasmapheresis, and *N*-acetylcysteine infusion. J Rheum 1985;12:794–797.
79. Harley NH. Toxic effects of radiation and radioactive materials. In: Klaassen CD, ed: Casarett and Doull's Toxicology: The Basic Science of Poisons, 5th ed. New York, McGraw-Hill, 1996, pp. 773–800.
80. Hartl W: Drug allergic agranulocytosis (Schultz's disease). Semin Hematol 1965;2:313–337.
81. Haut MJ, Cowan DH: The effect of ethanol on hemostatic properties of human platelets. Am J Med 1974; 56:22–33.
82. Herz F, Kaplan E, Scheye ES: Diagnosis of erythrocyte glucose-6-phosphate dehydrogenase deficiency in the Negro male despite hemolytic crisis. Blood 1970;35:90–93.
83. Hiebel J, Grant HL, Friedman IV: Bone marrow depression following exposure to kerosene. A report of 3 cases. Am J Med Sci 1963;246:185–191.
84. Hillman RS, McGuffin R, Campbell C: Alcohol interference with the folate enterohepatic cycle. Trans Assoc Am Physicians 1977;90:145–156.
85. Hines JD: Reversible megaloblastic and sideroblastic marrow abnormalities in alcoholic patients. Br J Haematol 1969;16:87–101.
86. Hirsch J, Doery JCG: Platelet function in health and disease. Prog Hematol 1971;7:185–234.
87. Hoffbrand AV, Ganeshaguru K, Hooton JWL, Tripp F: Megaloblastic anemia: Initiation of DNA synthesis in excess of DNA chain elongation as the underlying mechanism. Clin Haematol 1976;5:727–745.
88. Hogan RP III: Hemorrhagic diathesis caused by drinking an herbal tea. JAMA 1983;249:2679–2680.
89. Holbrook ST, Christensen RD: Hematopoietic growth factors. Adv in Pediatr 1991;38:23–49.

90. Homayouni H, Gross P, Setia U, Lynch TJ: Leukopenia due to penicillin and cephalosporin bandages. Arch Intern Med 1979;139:827–828.
91. Ibels LS, Pollock CA: Lead intoxication. Med Toxicol 1986;1:387–410.
92. ISAM Study Group: A prospective trial of intravenous streptokinase in acute myocardial infarction. Mortality, morbidity and infarct size at 21 days. N Engl J Med 1986;314:1465–1471.
93. Jacobson LO, Marks EK, Lorenz E: The hematological effects of ionizing radiation. Radiology 1949;52:371–395.
94. Jain SK, Hochstein P: Generation of superoxide radicals by hydrazine its role in phenylhydrazine-induced hemolytic anemia. Biochim et Biophys Acta 1979;586:128–136.
95. Jenkins GC, Kazontis G, Owen R: Arsine poisoning: Massive hemolysis with minimal impairment of renal function. Br Med J 1965;2:78–80.
96. Jerina DM, Daley JW: Arene oxides: A new aspect of drug metabolism. Science 1974;185:573–582.
97. Kadin M: Aplastic anemia following use of neoarsphenamine. Arch Dermatol Syphil 1938;37:787–796.
98. Karpatkin S: Drug-induced thrombocytopenia. Am J Med Sci 1971;262:68–78.
99. Kattamis CA: Glucose-6-phosphate dehydrogenase deficiency in female heterozygotes and the X-inactivation hypothesis. Acta Pediatr Scand 1967;172(suppl):103–109.
100. Katz R, Chuang LC, Sutton JD: Use of granulocyte colony-stimulating factor in the treatment of pancytopenia secondary to colchicine overdose. Ann Pharmacother 1992; 26:1087–1088.
101. Kay P, Ahmad A, Floten S, et al: Emergency coronary bypass surgery after intracoronary thrombolysis for evolving myocardial infarction. Br Heart J 1985;53:260–264.
102. Klaassen CD: Heavy Metals and heavy metal antagonists. In: Hardman JG, Limbird LE, Molinoff PB, et al, eds: Goodman and Gilman's The Pharmacological Basis of Therapeutics, 9th ed. New York, McGraw-Hill, 1996, pp. 1649–1672.
103. Klutman NE: Lithium carbonate therapy for zidovudine-associated neutropenia in patients with acquired immunodeficiency syndrome. Am J Med 1985;85:428–431.
104. Kolachana P, Subrahmanyam VV, Meyer KB, et al: Benzene and its phenolic metabolites produce oxidative DNA damage in HL60 cells in vitro and in the bone marrow in vivo. Cancer Res 1993;53:1023–1026.
105. Konopka L, Hoffbrand AV: Haem synthesis in sideroblastic anaemia. Br J Haematol 1979;42:73–83.
106. Kracke RR: Relation of drug therapy to neutropenic states. JAMA 1938;111:1255–1259.
107. Krakoff IH, Karnofsky DA, Burchenol JH: Effects of large doses of chloramphenicol on human subjects. N Engl J Med 1955;253:7–10.
108. Krantz SB: Diagnosis and treatment of pure red cell aplasia. Med Clin North Am 1976;60:945–958.
109. Krasner N, Moore MR, Thompson GG, et al: Depression of erythrocyte delta-aminolaevulinic acid dehydratase activity in alcoholics. Clin Sci Molec Med 1974;46:415–418.
110. Kulis, J: Chemically induced, selective thrombocytopenic purpura. Arch Intern Med 1965;116:559–561.
111. Kunicki TJ, Christie DJ, Aster RH: The human platelet receptor(s) for quinine/quinidine-dependent antibodies. Blood Cells 1983;9:293–301.
112. Larson AW, Wasserstrom WR, Felsher BF, Shih JC: Post-traumatic epilepsy and acute intermittent porphyria: Effects of phenytoin, carbamazepine, and clonazepam. Neurology 1978;28:824–828.
113. Lechner K: Acquired inhibitors in nonhemophiliac patients. Haemostasis 1974;3:65–93.
114. Lemberg R, Legge JW: Hematin Compounds and Bile Pigments. New York, Interscience, 1949, p 490.
115. Lesses MF, Gargill SL: Thiouracil as a cause of neutropenia and agranulocytosis. N Engl J Med 1945;233 :803–811.
116. Levinsky WJ, Smalley RV, Hillger PN: Arsine hemolysis. Arch Environ Health 1970;20:436–440.
117. Levitt, LJ: Chlorpropamide-induced pure white cell aplasia. Blood 1987;69:394–400.
118. Lewis JH: Homorrhagic disease associated with inhibitors of fibrin cross-linkage. Ann NY Acad Sci 1972;202:213–219.
119. Lewis JH, Szeto ILF, Ellis LD, et al: An acquired inhibitor to coagulation factor XIII. Johns Hopkins Med J 1967; 120:401–407.
120. Lewis WH: Medical Botany: Plants Affecting Man's Health. New York, Wiley-Interscience, 1977, p. 192.
121. Lindenbaum J: Folate deficiency and alcohol. In: Lindenbaum J, ed: Nutrition in Hematology. New York, Churchill Livingstone, 1983 pp. 33–59.
122. Lindenbaum J, Leiber CS: Alcohol-induced malabsorption of vitamin B_{12} in man. Nature 1969;224:80.
123. Lindenbaum J, Leiber CS: Hematologic effects of alcohol in man in the absence of nutritional deficiency. N Engl J Med 1969;281:334–338.
124. Litovitz TL, Clark LR, Soloway RA: 1993 annual report of the American Association of Poison Control Centers Toxic Exposure Surveillance System. Am J Emerg Med 1994; 12:546–555.
125. Litovitz TL, Felberg L, Soloway RA, et al: 1994 annual report of the American Association of Poison Control Centers Toxic Exposure Surveillance System. Am J Emerg Med 1995;13:551–597.
126. Litovitz TL, Felberg L, White S, et al: 1995 annual report of the American Association of Poison Control Centers Toxic Exposure Surveillance System. Am J Emerg Med 1996; 14:487–537.
127. Litovitz TL, Holm KC, Bailey KM, Schmitz BF: 1991 annual report of the American Association of Poison Control Centers National Data Collection System. Am J Emerg Med 1992;10:452–505.
128. Litovitz TL, Holm KC, Clancy C, et al: 1992 annual report of the American Association of Poison Control Centers Toxic Exposure Surveillance System. Am J Emerg Med 1993;2:494–555.
129. Loge PJ: Aplastic anemia following exposure to benzene hexachloride (Lindane). JAMA 1965;193:104–114.
130. Lorand L, Maldonado N, Fradera J, et al: Hemorrhagic syndrome of autoimmune origin with a specific inhibitor against fibrin stabilizing factor (factor XIII). Br J Haematol 1972;23:17–27.
131. Loveman AB: Toxic granulocytopenia, purpura hemorrhagica and aplastic anemia following arsphenamines. Ann Intern Med 1938;5:1238–1256.
132. Lukens JN: Blood formation in the embryo, fetus, and newborn. In: Lee RG, Bithell TC, Foerster J, eds: Win-

trobe's Clinical Hematology, 9th ed. Philadelphia, Lee & Febiger, 1993, pp. 79–100.
133. Lukens JN: Methemoglobinemia and other disorders accompanied by cyanosis. In: Lee RG, Bithell TC, Foerster J, et al, eds: Wintrobe's Clinical Hematology, 9th ed. Philadelphia, Lee & Febiger, 1993, pp. 1262–1271.
134. Lukens JN, Lee GR: Unstable hemoglobin disease. In: Lee RG, Bithell TC, Foerster J, eds: Wintrobe's Clinical Hematology, 9th ed. Philadelphia, Lee & Febiger, 1993, pp. 1054–1060.
135. Magis C, Barge A, Dausset J: Serologic study of an allergic agranulocytosis due to noramidopyrine. Clin Exp Immunol 1968;3:989–1003.
136. Mamus SW, Burton JD, Groat JD, et al: Ibuprofen-associated pure white-cell aplasia. N Engl J Med 1986;314: 624–625.
137. Marder VJ: The use of thrombolytic agents: Choice of patient, drug administration, laboratory monitoring. Ann Intern Med 1979;90:802–808.
138. Marder VJ, Hirsh J, Bell WR: Rationale and practical basis of thrombolytic therapy. In: Colman RW, Hirsh J, Marder VJ, Salzman EW, eds: Hemostasis and Thrombosis: Basic Principles and Clinical Practice, 3rd ed. Philadelphia, Lippincott,1994, p. 1526.
139. Marder VJ, Sherry S: Thrombolytic therapy: Current status. N Engl J Med 1988;318:1512–1518, 1585–1595.
140. Marx JL: A new view of receptor action. Science 1984;224:271–274.
141. Mauer EF: The toxic effects of phenylbutazone (butazolidin). N Engl J Med 1955;253:404–410.
142. Maximow AA: Relation of blood cells to connective tissues and endothelium. Physiol Rev 1924;4:533–563.
143. McColl KEL, Thompson GG, Moore MP, et al: Acute ethanol ingestion and haem biosynthesis in healthy subjects. Eur J Clin Invest 1980;10:107–112.
144. McCutcheon AD, Melb MD: Sulphhaemoglobinemia and glutathione. Lancet 1960;1:240–242.
145. McGehee W, Feinstein DI, Carpenter G, et al: Factor XIII inhibitor in a patient receiving INH. Clin Res 1971;19:180.
146. Meagher RC, Sieber F, Spivak JL: Suppression of hematopoietic-progenitor-cell proliferation by ethanol and acetaldehyde. N Engl J Med 1982;307:845–849.
147. Moeschlin S, Speck B: Experimental studies on the mechanism of action of benzene on the bone marrow (radioautographic studies using ^{3}H-thymidine). Acta Haematol 1967;38:104–111.
148. Moore MR, Beattie AD, Thompson GG, et al: Depression of delta-aminolaevulinic acid dehydrase activity by ethanol in man and rat. Clin Sci 1971;40:81–88.
149. Morell DB, Chang Y: The structure of the chromophore of sulphmyoglobin. Biochim Biophys Acta 1967;136:121–130.
150. Morley DC, Galbraith PR: Effect of lithium on granulopoiesis in culture. Can Med Assoc J 1978;118:288–290.
151. Nagaraj MV, Rao PV, Susarala S: Copper sulphate poisoning, hemolysis and methemoglobinemia. J Assoc Physicians India 1985;33:308–309.
152. National Institutes of Health Consensus Panel: Thrombolytic therapy in thrombosis. Ann Intern Med 1980;93: 141–144.
153. Niculescu R, Bradford HN, Colman RW, et al: Inhibition of the conversion of pre-interleukins-1 alpha and 1 beta to mature cytokines by p-benzoquinone, a metabolite of benzene. Chem Biol Interact 1995;98:211–222.
154. O'Brien H, Amess JAL, Mollin DL: Recurrent thrombocytopenia erythroid hypoplasia and sideroblastic anemia associated with hypothermia. Br J Haematol 1982;51: 451–456.
155. Orris DJ, Lewis JH, Spero JA: Blocking coagulation inhibitors in children taking penicillin. J Pediatr 1980, 97:426–429.
156. Otis PT, Feinstein DI, Rappaport SI, et al: An acquired inhibitor of fibrin stabilization associated with isoniazid therapy: Clinical and biochemical observations. Blood 1974;44:771–781.
157. Packham MA, Mustard JF: Pharmacology of platelet-affecting drugs. Circulation 1980;62(suppl V):26–41.
158. Paes B, Andrew M, Milner R, Ali MAM: Developmental changes in red cell creatine and free erythrocyte protoporphyrin in healthy full-term infants during the first 6 months of life. J Pediatr 1986;108:745–747.
159. Paustenbach DJ, Bass RD, Price P: Benzene toxicity and risk assessment, 1972–1992: Implications for future regulation. Environ Health Perspect 1993;101(suppl 6): 177–200.
160. Phillips HM, Holland BM, Jones JA, et al: Definitive estimate of rate of hemoglobin switching: Measurement of percent hemoglobin F in neonatal reticulocytes. Pediatr Res 1988;23:595–597.
161. Pickrell KL: The effect of alcoholic intoxication and ether anesthesia on resistance to pneumococcal infection. Bull Johns Hopkins Hosp 1938;63:238.
162. Pierce HI, McGuffin RG, Hillman RS: Clinical studies in alcoholic sideroblastosis. Arch Intern Med 1976;136: 283–289.
163. Pinto SS: Arsine poisoning: Evaluation of the acute phase. J Occup Med 1976;18:633–635.
164. Piscotta AV, Ebbe S, Lennon EJ, et al: Agranulocytosis following administration of phenothiazine derivatives. Am J Med 1958;25:210–223.
165. Plum P: Etiology of Agranulocytosis in Clinical and Experimental Investigations in Agranulocytosis. London, 1937, p. 95.
166. Poon MC, Saito H, Ratnoff OD, et al: Techniques for demonstration of the specificity of circulating anticoagulants against antihemophilic factor (factor VIII), with studies of two cases possibly related to diphenylhydantoin therapy. Blood 1977;49:477–482.
167. Putterman C, Chetrit EB. Colchicine intoxication: Clinical pharmacology, risk factors, features and management. Semin Arthritis Rheum 1991;21:143–155.
168. Rand ML, Packham MA, Kinlough-Rathbone RL, et al: Effects of ethanol on pathways of platelet aggregation in vitro. Thromb Haemost 1988;59:383–387.
169. Rendi R: The effect of chloramphenicol on the incorporation of labeled amino acids into proteins by isolated subcellular fractions from rat liver. Exp Cell Res 1959; 18:187–189.
170. Rendi R, Ochou S: Effect of chloramphenicol on protein synthesis in cell-free preparations of *Escheria coli*. J Biol Chem 1962;237:3711–3713.
171. Ritz ND: Agranulocytosis due to administration of salicylazosulfa-pyridine (azulfidine). JAMA 1960;172:237–239.
172. Robinson BE, Quesenberg PJ: Hematopoietic growth factors: Overview and clinical applications, part II. Am J Med Sci 1990;300:237–244.

173. Robinson BE, Quesenberg PJ: Hematopoietic growth factors: Overview and clinical applications, part III. Am J Med Sci 1990;300:311–321.
174. Robinson BE, Quesenberg PJ: Review: Hematopoietic growth factors: Overview and clinical applications, part I. Am J Med Sci 1990;300:163–170.
175. Rosenberg RD, Coleman RW, Lorand L: A new haemorrhagic disorder with defective fibrin stabilization and cryofibrinogenaemia. Br J Haematol 1974; 26:269–284.
176. Rossi-Fanelli A, Antonini E, Mondovi B: Ferrihemoglobin reduction in normal and methemoglobinemic subjects. Clin Chem Acta 1957;2:476–480.
177. Roth GJ, et al: Acetylation of prostaglandin synthetase by aspirin. Proc Natl Acad Sci USA 1975;72:3073–3076.
178. Rothstein G, Clarkson DR, Larsen W, et al: Effect of lithium in neutrophil mass and production. N Engl J Med 1978;298:178–180.
179. Saita G: Benzene induced hypoplastic anemias and leukaemias. In: Gridwood RH, ed: Blood Disorders Due to Drugs and Other Agents. Amsterdam, Excerpta Medica, 1973, pp. 127–146.
180. Sandler RM, et al: IgM platelet autoantibody due to sodium valproate. Br Med J 1958;2:1502–1505.
181. Sass MD, Caruso CJ, Axelrod R: Mechanism of the TPNH-linked reduction of methemoglobin by methylene blue. Clin Chem Acta 1969;24:77–85.
182. Sass MD, Caruso CJ, Farhanji M: TPNH-methemoglobin reductase deficiency: A new red cell enzyme deficiency. J Lab Clin Med 1967;70:760–767.
183. Savage D, Lindenbbaum J: Anemia in alcoholics. Medicine 1986;65:322–338.
184. Schattenberg DG, Stillman WS, Gruntmeir JJ, et al: Peroxidase activity in murine and human hematopoietic progenitor cells: Potential relevance to benzene-induced toxicity. Molec Pharmacol 1994;46:346–351.
185. Schubert T, Muller WE: Lithium but not cholinergic ligands influence guanylate cyclase activity in intact human lymphocytes. Biochem Pharmacol 1990;3:439–444.
186. Schultz W: Verh Deutsch Ges Ann Med 1935;47:179–192.
187. Scott JL, Cartwright GE, Wintrobe MM: Acquired aplastic anemia: An analysis of thirty-nine cases and review of the pertinent literature. Medicine 1959;38:119–172.
188. Scott JL, Finegold SM, Belkin GA, Lawrence JS: A controlled double-blind study of the hematologic toxicity of chloramphenicol. N Engl J Med 1965;272:1137–1142.
189. Seaton MJ, Schlosser PM, Medinsky MA: In vitro conjugation of benzene metabolites by human liver: Potential influence of interindividual variability on benzene toxicity. Carcinogenesis 1995;16:1519–1527.
190. Shopsin B, Friedman K, Gershon S: Lithium and leukocytosis. Clin Pharmacol Ther 1971;12:923–928.
191. Shulman NR: A mechanism of cell destruction in individuals sensitized to foreign antigens and its implications in auto-immunity. Ann Intern Med 1964;60:506–521.
192. Shulman NR, Jordon JV: Platelet immunology. In: Colman RW, Hirsh J, Marder VJ, Salzman EW, eds: Hemostasis and Thrombosis, 3rd ed. Philadelphia, Lippincott, 1994, pp. 414–468.
193. Skinner JR, Phillips SJ, Zeff RJ, et al: Immediate coronary bypass following failed streptokinase infusion in evolving myocardial infarction. J Thorac Cardiovasc Surg 1984; 87:567–70.
194. Smith RP: Toxic responses of the blood. In: Klaassen CD, Amduk MO, Doull J, eds: Casarett & Doull's Toxicology, 5th ed. McGraw-Hill, New York, 1996, pp. 335–354.
195. Smith U, Smith DS, Yunis AA: Chloramphenicol-related changes in mitochondrial ultrastructure. J Cell Sci 1970; 7:501–521.
196. Snyder R, Kalf GF: A perspective on benzene leukemogenesis. Crit Rev Toxicol 1994;24:177–209.
197. Snyder R, Lee EW, Kocsis JJ, Witmer CM: Bone marrow depressant and leukemogenic actions of benzene. Life Sci 1977;21:1709–1721.
198. Snyder R, Witz G, Goldstein BD: The toxicology of benzene. Environ Health Perspect 1993;100:293–306.
199. Sorensen B: Case of fatal thrombopenia about 10 months after treatment with a gold preparation. Acta Med Scand 1951;141:27–35.
200. Sperling IL: Adverse reactions with long-term use of phenyl-butazone and oxyphenbutazone. Lancet 1969;2: 535–537.
201. Squier T, Madison FW: Primary granulocytopenia due to hypersensitivity to amidopyrine. J Allergy 1934;6:9–16.
202. Stanley MW, Taurog JD, Snover DC: Fatal colchicine toxicity: Report of a case. Clin Exper Rheumatol 1984;2: 167–171.
203. Steinberg B: Bone marrow regeneration in experimental benzene intoxication. Blood 1949;4:550–556.
204. Stricker RB, Shuman MA: Quinidine purpura: Evidence that glycoprotein V is a target platelet antigen. Blood 1986;67:1377–1381.
205. Taetle R, Lane TA, Mendelsohn: Drug-induced agranulocytosis: In vitro evidence for immune suppression of granulopoiesis and a cross-reacting lymphocyte antibody. Blood 1979;54:501–512.
206. Takahara S, Hamilton HB, Neel JV: Hypocatalasemia: A new genetic carrier state. J Clin Invest 1960;39:610–619.
207. Telen MJ: The mature erythrocyte. In: Lee RG, Bithell TC, Foerster J, et al, eds: Wintrobe's Clinical Hematology, 9th ed. Philadelphia, Lea & Febiger, 1993, pp. 101–133.
208. Third International Study of Infarct Survival Collaborative Group. ISIS–3: A randomised comparison of streptokinase vs aspirin alone among 41,299 cases of suspected acute myocardial infarction. Lancet 1992;339:753–770.
209. Thirumalaikorlundusubramanian P, Chandramomohan M, Johnson ES: Copper sulphate poisoning. J Indian Med Assoc 1984;82:6–8.
210. Till JE, McCulloch EA: A direct measurement of the radiation sensitivity of normal mouse bone marrow cells. Rad Res 1961;14:213–222.
211. TIMI Research Group: Immediate vs delayed catheterization and angioplasty following thrombolytic therapy for acute MI: TIMI IIA results. JAMA 1988;260:2849–2858.
212. Tisman G, Herbert V, Rosenblatt S: Evidence that lithium induces human granulocyte proliferation: Elevated serum vitamin B_{12} binding capacity in vivo and granulocyte colony proliferation in vitro. Br J Haematol 1973;24: 767–771.
213. Veall RM, Hogarth HC: Thrombocytopenia during treatment with clonazepam. Br Med J 1975;4:462.
214. Vicker MG, Bultmann H, Glade U, Hafker T: Ionizing ra-

diation at low doses induces inflammatory reactions in human blood. Radiat Res 1991;128:251–257.
215. Vigliani EX, Saita G: Benzene and leukemia. N Engl J Med 1964;271:872–876.
216. Walker JG: Fatal Agranulocytosis complicating treatment with ethacrynic acid. Ann Intern Med 1966;64:1303–1305.
217. Wallerstein RO, Condit PK, Kasper CK, et al: Statewide study of chloramphenicol therapy and fatal aplastic anemia. JAMA 1969;208:2045–2050.
218. Wang RIH, Schuller G: Agranulocytosis following procainamide administration. Am Heart J 1969;78:282–284.
219. Wantanabe KH, Bois FY, Daisey JM, et al: Benzene toxicokinetics in humans: Exposure of bone marrow to metabolites. Occup Environ Med 1994;51:414–420.
220. Watkins CH: The possible role of barbiturates and amidopyrine in causation of leukopenic states. Proc Mayo Clin 1933;8:713–714.
221. Weisberger AS: Mechanism of action of chloramphenicol. JAMA 1969;209:97–103.
222. Weisberger AS, Wolfe S, Armentront S: Inhibition of protein synthesis in mammalian cell-free systems by chloramphenicol. J Exp Med 1964;120:161–181.
223. Weitzman SA, Stossel TP: Drug-induced immunological neutropenia. Lancet 1978;2:1068–1072.
224. Whitcraft III DD, Bailey TD, Hart GB: Hydrogen sulfide poisoning treated with hyperbaric oxygen. J Emerg Med 1985;3:23–25.
225. White JM, Selhi HS: Lead and the red cell. Br J Haematol 1975;30:133–138.
226. Wilcox RG, vonDer Lippe G, Olsson CG, et al: Trial of tissue plasminogen activator for mortality reduction in acute myocardial infarction: Anglo-Scandinavian Study of Early Thrombolysis (ASSET). Lancet 1988;2:525–528.
227. Williams DM, Lynch RE, Cartwright GE: Drug-induced aplastic anemia. Semin Hematol 1973;10:195–223.
228. Wright CS, Doan CA, Haynie HC: Agranulocytosis occuring after exposure to a DDT pyrethrum aerosol bomb. Am J Med 1946;1:562–567.
229. Wu AM, Till JE, Siminovich L, McCulloch EA: A cytological study of the capacity for differentiation of normal hemopoietic colony-forming cells. Cell Physiol 1967;69: 177–184.
230. Yunis AA: Chlorampherical-induced bone marrow suppression. Semin Hematol 1973;10:225–234.
231. Yunis AA, Bloomberg GR: Chloramphenicol toxicity: Clinical features and pathogenesis. Prog Hematol 1964;4: 138–159.
232. Zidar BL, Shadduck RK, Zeigler Z, Winkelstein A: Observations on the anemia and neutropenia of human copper deficiency. Am J Hematol 1977;3:177–185.

CHAPTER 25

Endocrine Principles

Christopher Keyes

The endocrine glands produce substances secreted into the systemic circulation to regulate activities in various parts of the body. These substances are hormones, which include steroids, prostaglandins, catecholamines, and proteins or polypeptides. Hormones act primarily by modulating protein synthesis or activating cyclic AMP at receptor sites located on the cell walls of the target organs. An exhaustive discussion of the field of endocrinology is not the scope of this chapter. Instead, the focus will be on the topics of hypoglycemic agents, thyroid toxicology, and steroid and androgenic agents that are important toxicologic concerns.

Endocrine physiology is best described as a delicate homeostasis of hormone antagonists and corresponding feedback mechanisms. Toxins usually impact the endocrine system by changing the effect that a hormone has on a target organ, changing the response of that organ or substituting for it, or altering the feedback mechanism necessary for homeostasis. Understanding basic organ function is necessary to predict the response evoked by a toxin.

Approach to the Patient With Endocrine Toxicity

Managing a patient's potential endocrine toxicity begins with obtaining a thorough medical history including the pharmaceutical agents to which the person has been exposed. Particular attention should be given to previous or ongoing endocrine therapy. This history may reveal important information about hormonal supplementation or other medications that the patient is receiving. Drug interactions may result as one health practitioner is unaware of the agents prescribed by another. A patient may not know the importance of these interactions. Diagnostic measures may include laboratory testing, an electrocardiogram, and other methods with regard to the specific agents that will be discussed. Pregnancy testing is always prudent in patients who are of childbearing potential, both for consideration of the health of the fetus and the hormonal effects specific to pregnancy.

Hypoglycemia and Hypoglycemic Agents

The most common endocrinopathy in the United States is diabetes mellitus. Agents used in the treatment of this disease are therefore commonly prescribed, usually with the objective of long-term lowering of blood glucose.

Treatment of chronically increased blood glucose is an important objective to prevent the complications of diabetes mellitus. The Diabetes Control and Complications Trial (DCCT)[18] was a multicenter trial that provided evidence of the benefits of maintaining closer control of blood sugar for patients with insulin-dependent diabetes mellitus. Patients who maintained an intensive treatment regimen had a reduced incidence of microvascular and neuropathic complications. As a result of this study, many clinicians are also attempting to achieve stricter control of blood sugar in non-insulin-dependent diabetics. In this study diabetics who monitored blood sugar by home glucose monitoring had dramatically lower rates of vascular complications. This cohort unfortunately had approximately a threefold increase in hypoglycemic episodes. Many diabetic patients now emphasize closer control of blood glucose, and hypoglycemic reactions are becoming commonplace in emergency departments. Some elderly patients, or those who are not intellectually competent or responsible, are particularly at risk to suffer hypoglycemia due to errors in the control of their own treatment.

Medications designed to lower blood glucose are a frequent cause of emergency treatment. A hypoglycemic episode commonly is referred to as an "insulin reaction" by patients taking this hormonal replacement. Oral agents designed to control hyperglycemia are in common use today, and often require a different management from an overdose of insulin. The sulfonylureas usually have a much longer duration of action as compared to regular insulin, and hence require prolonged observation and admission to the hospital. The specific characteristics of these agents will be discussed in Chapter 40. Here the discussion will focus on principles that guide the treatment of toxicity from this pharmaceutical class.

Hypoglycemia effects all tissues, but clinically the most evident site of toxicity is the brain. This organ utilizes almost two-thirds of the circulating glucose. The CNS is particularly vulnerable to hypoglycemia because unlike muscle, the brain is not able to make use of free fatty acids as an energy substrate. Synthesis of glucose is essential during the early phases of hypoglycemia in order to preserve the integrity of the central nervous system. Amino acids are the primary precursors of gluconeogenesis, which takes place in the liver. In the event of prolonged hypoglycemia, acetoacetic acid and beta hydroxybutyric acid can be used as energy substrates by the brain, but these substances require time to synthesize and are not available in the early phases of hypoglycemia.[75] Symptoms of neuroglycopenia may be mistaken for neuropsychiatric disease.[15]

Glucose Metabolism and Endocrine Regulation

Carbohydrates constitute more than half of the usual dietary caloric intake. Starches are hexose polymers, and these are broken down to oligosaccharides and disaccharides by pancreatic amylase. Disaccharides are broken down to single hexose units by the *disaccharidases*. The *alpha-glucosidases* are disaccharidases that break down maltose and sucrose to their component monomers fructose and glucose. These glucosidases are located in the brush border of the small intestine. Glucose is readily absorbed across the intestinal lining. Facilitated by insulin, glucose is taken up into the bloodstream, and utilized by tissues throughout the body. It is then either oxidized by the glycolytic pathway (see Fig. 12–2) and the Krebs cycle (see Fig. 12–4) to provide energy for cellular metabolism, or saved by conversion to adipose tissue or by incorporation into glycogen.

Gluconeogenesis

When blood sugar is decreased below normal levels, glucose production is stimulated. This occurs through the conversion of glycogen into glucose, or by the process of gluconeogenesis. Stimulated by glucagon, gluconeogenesis is the process of creating glucose by conversion from various substrates. In the gluconeogenic pathway, the reactions of glycolysis are reversed, with the exception of three steps that are irreversible. These irreversible metabolic reactions of glycolysis include those catalyzed by specific enzymes: the *hexokinases*, *phosphofructokinase* and *pyruvate kinase* (see Fig. 12–3). The first bypass step is from pyruvate to phosphoenolpyruvate (PEP). To accomplish this, pyruvate enters the Krebs cycle through conversion to oxaloacetate (OAA), a reaction catalyzed by *pyruvate carboxylase*. OAA is then converted to PEP by the enzyme *phosphoenolpyruvate carboxykinase*. The second bypass step occurs when fructose 1,6 diphosphate is converted to fructose 6 phosphate. This hydrolysis is catalyzed by *fructose 1,6-diphosphatase*. Finally, glucose-6-phosphate is converted to glucose, catalyzed by *glucose-6-phosphatase*. (see Fig. 12–2)

A variety of substrates are used for glucose synthesis via gluconeogenesis. A prominent source is lactate, generated by anaerobic metabolism in the muscle tissues. Here pyruvate is reduced to lactate by *lactate dehydrogenase*. The lactate diffuses into the bloodstream traveling to the liver, where it is extracted and converted via gluconeogenesis to glucose. The glucose then enters the bloodstream and is available for use by brain, muscle, and other tissues. This process of lactate being formed by tissues and converted to glucose by the liver is called the Cori cycle. The gluconeogenic portion of the cycle requires net utilization of ATP. Any amino acid that can be converted to pyruvate, oxaloacetate, or alpha-ketoglutarate may serve as a glucose substrate in this pathway.

Triglycerides are made up of fatty acids and glycerol. Fatty acids enter the citric acid cycle via acetyl coenzyme A, but cannot be used to synthesize glucose. Glycerol, however, can be utilized by metabolism to dihydroxyacetone phosphate (DHAP).

Glycogen Utilization

The liver is able to store approximately 70 g of glucose in the form of glycogen. A much greater amount is stored in skeletal muscle. Glycogenolysis occurs between meals, and particularly during relatively long fasting periods such as sleep. Glucose residues are removed from alpha-1-4 linkages by *phosphorylase*. Activation of *glycogen phosphorylase* is subject to important hormonal regulation and will be discussed later. Branches in glycogen require a *debranching enzyme* to remove further glucose residues. The resulting glucose-1-phosphate is catalyzed to glucose-6-phosphate by the enzyme *phosphoglucomutase*, then by the action of *glucose-6-phosphatase* to glucose. Although muscle contains the bulk of glycogen in the body, it lacks this last enzyme, hence glucose is not released into the bloodstream by this tissue.[61] Liver and intestine, however, have *glucose-6-phosphatase*, permitting them to release glucose to the circulation.

When there is a decrease in blood glucose, the liver is able to initiate glycogenolysis and gluconeogenesis to provide this essential substrate to the circulation. This process of glucose generation is inhibited by the presence of large amounts of insulin, but stimulated by the action of epinephrine, norepinephrine, and glucagon.

Insulin: A Key Modulator of Anabolic Metabolism

Glucose permeability normally occurs in the brain even in the absence of insulin. Insulin, secreted by the beta cells of the pancreatic islets, promotes glucose utilization by muscle, adipose tissue, and liver. Insulin causes these tissues to utilize more glucose by increasing their cellular permeability to this substrate while promoting glycogen formation and fatty acid synthesis (Fig. 25–1a). The enzyme *insulinase*, present in liver, kidney, and muscle, rapidly degrades insulin,[74] causing it to have a normal half-life of only 5 to 6 minutes. This time may be prolonged in diabetic individuals who have developed anti-insulin antibodies.[41]

Insulin acts somewhat differently in each of the major tissues. Glycogen formation and fatty acid synthesis are enhanced by insulin in adipose tissue. The conversion of glucose to glycerol, a precursor to triglyceride formation, is also promoted. Breakdown of triglycerides is blocked by insulin's inhibition of *hormone-sensitive lipase*, the enzyme responsible for hydrolysis of these molecules.[51]

Glucose transport into muscle tissue is enhanced by insulin (Fig. 25–1b). Insulin also increases *hexokinase* activity, which phosphorylates glucose to glucose-6-phos-

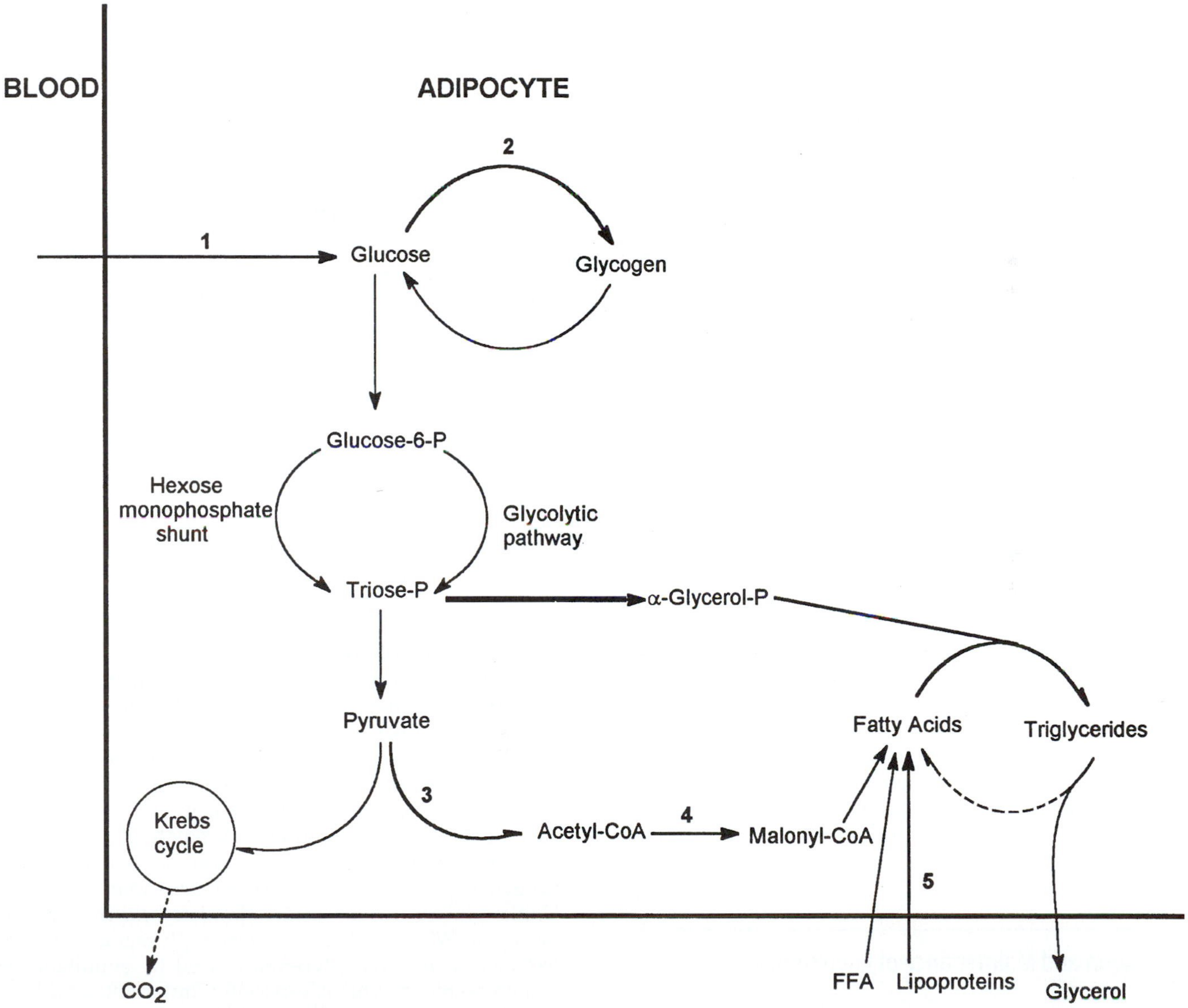

Figure 25–1. A. Carbohydrate and lipid metabolism in adipose tissue. Heavy arrows indicate reactions enhanced by insulin as follows. 1. Transport of glucose into adipose cell. 2. Conversion of excess glucose to glycogen. 3. Decarboxylation of pyruvate. 4. Initiation of fatty acid synthesis. 5. Uptake of fatty acids from circulating lipoproteins. The breakdown of triglycerides is inhibited by insulin (broken arrow).

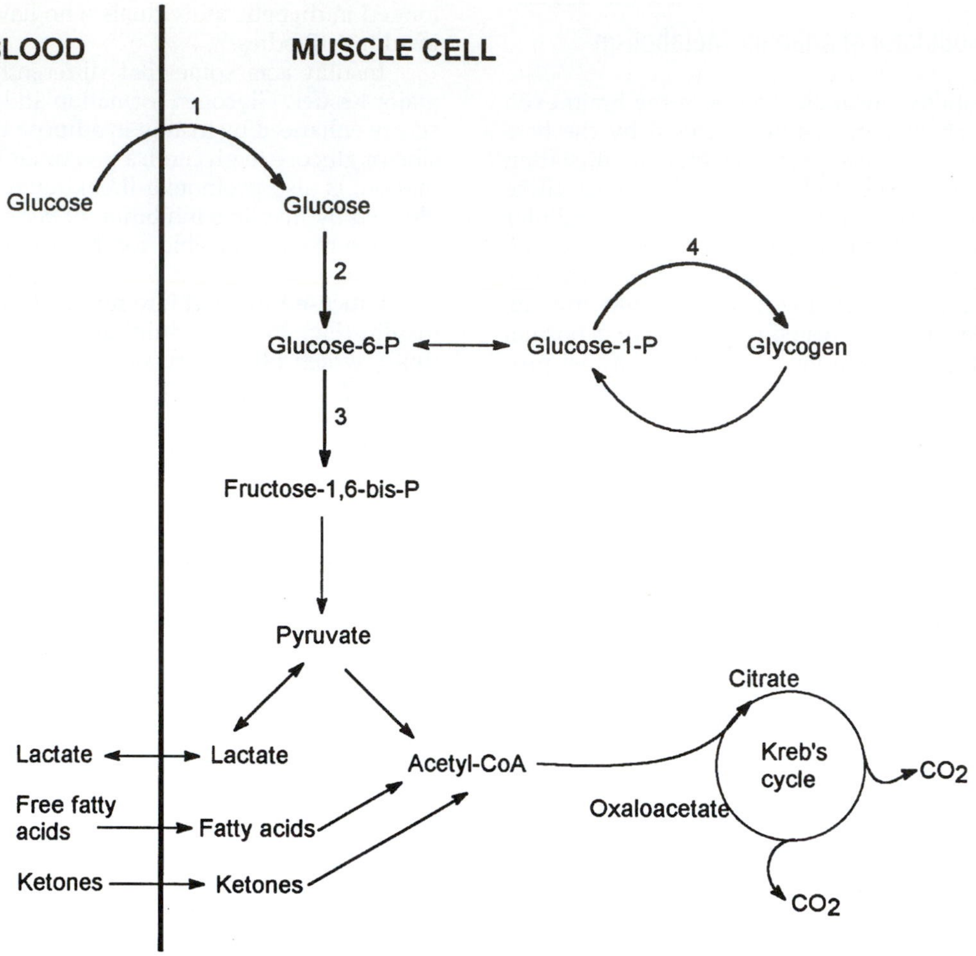

Figure 25–1. B. Carbohydrate and lipid metabolism in a muscle. Rate-limiting reactions accelerated by insulin are indicated by heavy arrows as follows. 1. Transport of glucose into muscle cells. 2. Phosphorylation of glucose by hexokinase. 3. Addition of the second phosphate by phosphofructokinase. 4. Storage of glucose as glycogen. *(Reprinted with permission from Johnson LR, ed: Essential Medical Physiology. New York, Raven, 1992, pp. 612–613.)*

phate, transiently trapping the glucose inside the cell. Glycogen formation is then enhanced. The remainder of glucose is oxidized with the formation of energy for cellular metabolism. Protein synthesis is stimulated.

In the setting of insulin hypersecretion and hypoglycemia, glucose utilization by muscle, adipose, and other tissues is enhanced even at the expense of the brain. Glycogenolysis is suppressed, as is intrahepatic gluconeogenesis.

Glucagon and Maintenance of Euglycemia

Glucagon is a polypeptide containing 29 amino acids. It is secreted by the alpha cells of the pancreatic islets and serves to *maintain* adequate blood glucose in the setting of hypoglycemia, an effect opposite to that of insulin. Its metabolic action is almost entirely limited to the liver. Glucagon initiates a chain of events, through cyclic AMP, to activate *phosphorylase*, the rate-limiting enzyme in the degradation of glycogen to glucose-1-phosphate. After dephosphorylation, glucose is released from the liver into the bloodstream. In addition, glucagon promotes glucose synthesis via gluconeogenesis.

Glucagon secretion is greatly stimulated by hypoglycemia, epinephrine, and norepinephrine. Conversely, insulin, glucose, and free fatty acids inhibit alpha cell release of glucagon. In addition to stimulating glucagon release, epinephrine also directly stimulates liver gluconeogenesis, although to a lesser extent than glucagon. Unlike glucose, amino acids stimulate *both* insulin and glucagon. When protein is ingested, glucagon may protect against the hypoglycemia caused by simultaneous insulin secretion. This is especially important for a low-carbohydrate meal. The balance of insulin and glucagon in the serum determines which processes will prevail intrahepatically: glucose utilization and storage (insulin effect predominates) or glucose production (glucagon effect predominates).[70,97]

Another hormone, somatostatin, inhibits the release of both alpha-cells (glucagon) and beta-cells (insulin) of the pancreas, growth hormone, TSH, and gastrointestinal peptide hormones.[76] Somatostatin's suppression of glucagon is much more potent than with insulin, but it is also much more transient. Somatostatin is secreted by the delta cells of the pancreas, which appear to be downstream with respect to blood circulation from the alpha and beta cells in this tissue. It is thought, therefore, that somatostatin must exert its effects through the systemic circulation.[81] The precise role of somatostatin remains to be elucidated. Its effects in different tissues are mediated by a variety of receptors. Researchers are seeking somatostatin analogues with more specific end-organ effects. This polypeptide is also found in other tissues of the body.[22]

In the diabetic patient, duration of illness is an important factor when considering the response to hypoglycemia. Early in the course of the disease, both glucagon and epinephrine action remain intact, and the response to hypoglycemia is effective.[78,79] Later in the illness, even secretion of epinephrine is diminished in response to hypoglycemia. There is evidence that with very strict control of type I diabetes, as evidenced by maintenance of glycosylated hemoglobin close to normal levels, brain uptake of glucose may be normal even in the setting of hypoglycemia, thus preserving cerebral metabolism.[9] Also the type of diabetes is important. Patients with non-insulin-dependent diabetes mellitus retain the glucagon response as compared with insulin-dependent diabetics.[6,7] Hence, glucagon may be relatively less effective in treatment of sulfonamide-induced hypoglycemia, because these patients may have near-maximal stimulation of glucagon prior to the initiation of therapy.

Autonomic Nervous System and Carbohydrate Metabolism

The autonomic nervous system (ANS) has important interactions with carbohydrate metabolism. Substances activate the ANS by interacting with proteins on the cell membrane. These occur in a specific sequence: the receptor is stimulated, a G protein is activated, and cell messenger enzymes or ion channels are "switched on."[80] G-proteins are membrane bound structures that allow very versatile and varied responses through complex interactions on the cell membrane.[33–35,91] Activated by the receptors, these proteins then regulate various cellular effectors such as adenyl cyclase and ion channels on the cell membrane.

Beta-adrenergic agonist action stimulates insulin secretion, as does parasympathetic stimulation. Alpha-adrenergic receptor stimulation inhibits secretion. Epinephrine stimulates glucagon secretion and can also directly increase gluconeogenesis, although not as strongly as glucagon. The catecholamines also increase substrate availability for gluconeogenesis, and inhibit insulin secretion.[73] The catecholamines are dependent on a basal level of cortisol in order to exert their gluconeogenic action.[83] This is also true of glucagon. Cortisol therefore has a permissive effect on the action of these hormones.

Therapy with beta-adrenergic antagonists can worsen hypoglycemia in diabetic patients. Epinephrine's effect on increasing hepatic glucose release is mediated by beta$_2$-adrenergic stimulation.[19,72] When diabetics are given beta-adrenergic antagonists, catecholamine induced gluconeogenesis and glycogenolysis are impaired. These agents are to be avoided whenever possible in diabetic patients on insulin or sulfonylurea therapy. A newly recognized beta$_3$-adrenergic receptor exists, which may enhance breakdown of adipose tissue; the exact function of this receptor remains to be elucidated.[55,60]

Causes of Hypoglycemia

Insulin and the sulfonylureas commonly are associated with episodes of hypoglycemia (see Chap. 40 for an extensive discussion of this topic). Many diabetics are accustomed to recognizing these reactions, and are able to initiate replacement of glucose rapidly. Some individuals are not able to do so, and are therefore at greater risk of prolonged hypoglycemia if, for example, insulin control is too aggressive. The sulfonylureas have afforded an alternative to injection therapy, and are used primarily by patients who have decreased responsiveness to insulin. The latter condition is commonly associated with obesity. The biguanides work by decreasing production of glucose by the liver[89] and increasing peripheral utilization.[3] Currently the only available biguanide is metformin. Ciglitazone and thiolidazone are two examples of a new thiazolidinedione class of agents that work primarily by increasing end-organ response to insulin.[30,52,54] Neither the biguanides nor the thiolidazones cause hypoglycemia when used independently of the sulfonylureas or insulin. Metformin can cause lactic acidosis particularly when used in patients with renal or liver failure, but traglitazone has not been reported to have this effect.

Other Pharmaceutical Agents and Toxins Causing Hypoglycemia

Many drugs may cause hypoglycemia (see Table 40–1). The mechanisms vary considerably, but attention to the basic principles discussed earlier in this chapter will help in understanding how a decrease in circulating glucose occurs.

Ethanol may cause a decrease in serum glucose, particularly in the setting of previously depleted glycogen stores. Clinically significant hypoglycemia is uncommon, however.[24,86,90] Ethanol inhibits hepatic gluconeogenesis by decreasing the $NAD^+/NADH$ ratio, thus promoting oxaloacetate transformation to malate. This blocks the gluconeogenic step leading to phosphoenolpyruvate, stopping glucose synthesis. It is therefore understandable that hypoglycemia only occurs when glycogen stores are depleted. This may be the principal mechanism involved in the development of alcohol-induced hypoglycemia of children under the age of 5 years.[5,17,102]

Pentamidine causes hypoglycemia, and later hyperglycemia by destroying pancreatic islet beta cells.[82] Patients with renal failure are at particular risk of pentamidine-induced hypoglycemia.[2] Acetaminophen is not a direct inducer of hypoglycemia; however, in the event of extensive liver necrosis of any cause, glucose storage and metabolism are impaired, making glucose monitoring essential. Salicylates cause increased glucose utilization and may cause hypoglycemia, especially in children (see Chap. 32). This may occur within the CNS even without peripheral hypoglycemia. For this reason it is recommended that serum glucose be determined with initial laboratory assessment and also whenever alteration in mental status is noted. Propranolol has an effect opposite to that of epinephrine, causing hypoglycemia and hyperkalemia in overdose.

Treatment of Hypoglycemia

Treatment of hypoglycemia is discussed in Chapter 40. Administration of dextrose is the mainstay of such treatment. Glucagon is sometimes used as a temporizing measure to treat hypoglycemia in patients who have no intravenous access because it can be administered intramuscularly.[94] It acts rapidly, and can maintain serum glucose at life-sustaining levels while glycogen stores continue to be available. When administered intravenously, glucagon action is transient, with a plasma half-life of only 3 to 6 minutes.[50,71] When used for the treatment of hypoglycemia usually 1 to 2 mg are administered parenterally. Glucagon's action to raise serum glucose is largely dependent on adequate glycogen stores in the liver. These stores may be depleted in chronic alcoholism, prolonged fasting, or with certain hormonal deficiencies (eg, cortisol, growth hormone) and hence glucagon may be ineffective in these circumstances.[10,12] Glucose supplementation should always follow its use. In the presence of high insulin levels, the ability of glucagon to raise blood glucose is decreased. Glucagon should not be used when intravenous glucose is available in these situations.

Diazoxide is not recommended for treatment of hypoglycemia, since it is minimally effective and is associated with hypotension. Somatostatin, which inhibits glucose-stimulated beta-cell insulin release, has been used to control hypoglycemia, but it is not practical due to its short half-life (4 to 5 minutes). More recently, octreotide, a long-acting somatostatin analogue (half-life of 72 minutes), has been shown to be effective in preventing recurrence of hypoglycemia in patients with sulfonylurea overdoses.[8] Octreotide also prevented hypoglycemia in patients with quinine overdoses[71] and in those with insulinomas.[45] Patients should be admitted and monitored with serial blood sugar measurements for a minimum of 1 to 2 days as clinically warranted.[8,68]

Thyroid Toxicology

Physiology

To properly understand the impact of thyroid supplements and inhibitory agents on the function of the human body, the interaction of these hormones with the following sites must be examined: (1) the hypothalamus, (2) the pituitary gland, (3) the thyroid gland, and (4) the target organs for the thyroid hormones (Fig. 25–2a). As in the case of many other endocrine relationships, feedback loops are very important in determining the function of these organs.

The hypothalamus is an intermediate between cerebral centers and the pituitary gland. When the hypothalamus receives specific neurotransmitter stimulation, thyroid-releasing hormone (TRH) is produced. Thyroid-releasing hormone is transported through the venous sinusoids to the pituitary, where thyroid-stimulating hormone (TSH) is released. When this hormone enters the circulation, it stimulates thyroid hormone production and its release.

Thyroid physiology is an excellent example of the concept of feedback control of hormonal function. Most endocrine organs tend to produce an excess of hormone. When the desired effect is achieved, inhibition of the secretory gland occurs. When thyroid hormones are released, they exert an inhibitory influence on the pituitary gland, which diminishes the production of TSH. This suppression of TSH is a frequently used laboratory marker in the evaluation of hyperthyroidism.

Thyroid hormones consist of tyrosine molecules with iodine substitutions. Two forms of the hormone are physiologically active, triiodothyronine and tetraiodothyronine (Fig. 25–2b). The synthesis of thyroid hormones is a multiple-step process. Tyrosine is concentrated in the follicles of the thyroid gland, which consist of an epithelial layer surrounding a proteinaceous colloidal substance called thyroglobulin. Thyroglobulin contains a large amount of tyrosine. After iodide is absorbed from the circulation, it is concentrated in the thyroid cells that surround the follicles, by a process of active transport. It is thought that the enzyme *iodide peroxidase* catalyzes the formation of tyrosine and iodide free radicals, which then combine to form monoiodotyrosine (MIT) and diiodotyrosine (DIT). The substituted tyrosine molecules thus formed combine to form triiodothyronine (T_3) and tetraiodothyronine (T_4). T_3 and T_4 are taken up by the endothelial cells by endocytosis and broken down in the lysosomes. T_3 and T_4 (thyroxine), the thyroid hormones, are subsequently released into the circulation. Of the two thyroid hormones, T_3 is the more active, having approximately three times as great a thyroid hormonal effect as thyroxine (T_4). Only 15% of T_3 is secreted directly by the thyroid. The remaining T_3 is formed by the peripheral deiodonation of T_4, which occurs mainly in the liver and kidney by the enzyme, 5′-deiodonase. The action of T_4 may be explained com-

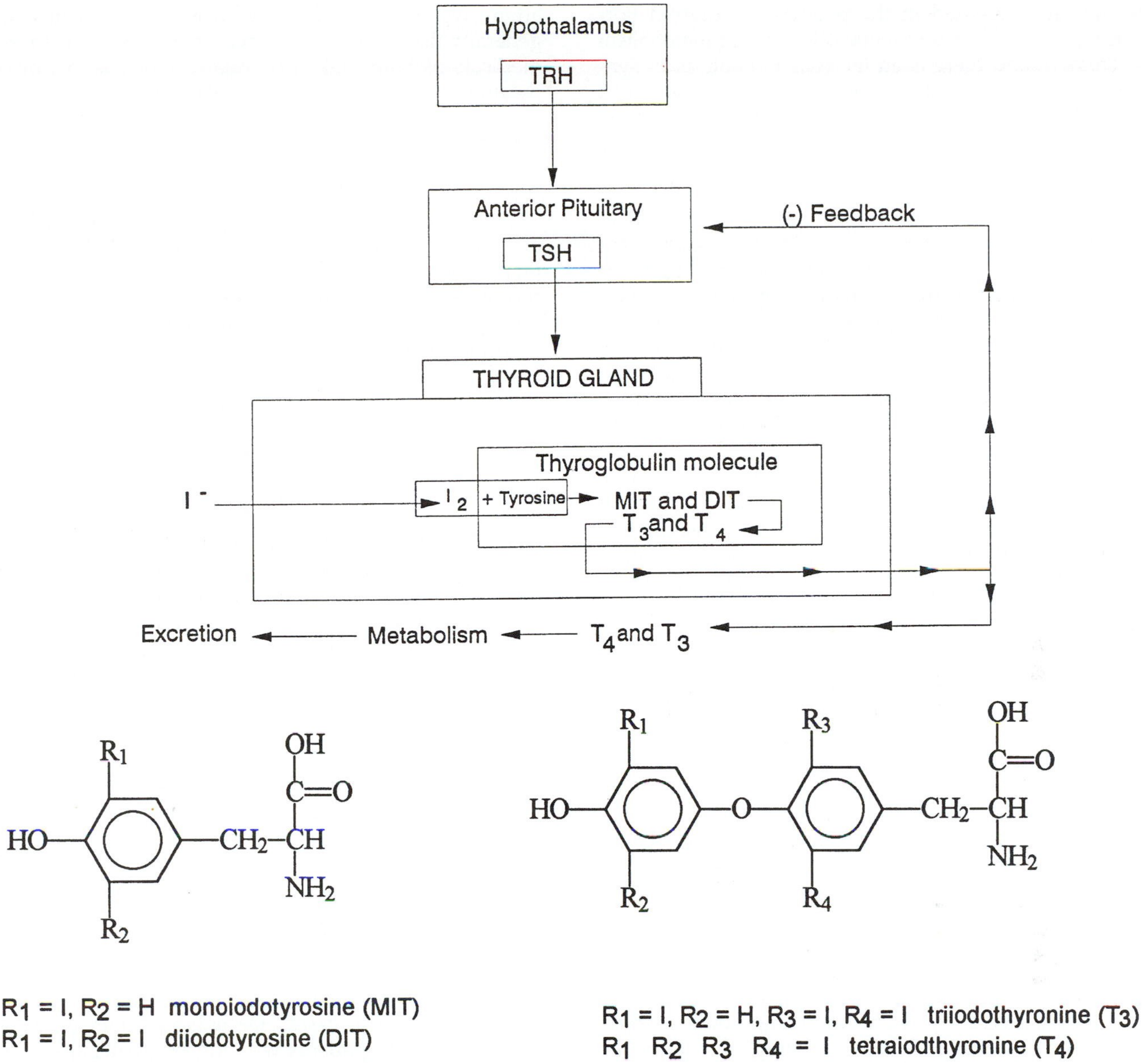

A

B

Figure 25–2. A. Hypothalamic–pituitary–thyroid axis and the control of thyroid hormone synthesis and metabolism. **B.** Structures of thyroid hormones. Left, monoiodotyrosine and diiodotyrosine. Right, triiodothyronine and tetraiodothyronine. *(Reprinted with permission from Van Leeuwen FXR, Krajnc-Franken MAM, Loeber JG: Endocrinotoxicology: Methodological aspects. In: Neisink, RJM, De Vries J, Hollinger MA, eds: Toxicology: Principles and Applications. New York, CRC Press, p. 891.)*

pletely by its conversion to T_3 outside of the thyroid gland.

Thyroid Hormone Function and Hyperfunction

Thyroxine and T_3 exert their action intracellularly, where they are ultimately metabolized. Sequential deiodonation accounts for approximately two thirds of hormonal inactivation. Most of the remaining hormone is eliminated intrahepatically by glucuronidation or sulfation. Cytochrome P-450 inducers such as phenobarbital and phenytoin increase the rate of clearance of thyroid hormones, but there is no perceptible decrease in circulating hormone, presumably due to feedback stimulation of thyroid secretion.

Thyroid hormones act through nuclear receptors, regulating gene transcription and synthesis of specific proteins. These proteins act by stimulating Na^+/K^+-ATPase, thereby increasing oxygen consumption. Thyroid function is the most important determinant of basal metabolic rate (BMR). Most aspects of carbohydrate metabolism are increased in the presence of thyroid hormone excess, as is protein metabolism. Lipid metabolism is increased, and there is an increase in cholesterol synthesis. Cholesterol levels are actually lowered, however, due to thyroxine stimulation of bile acid secretion. Thyroid action exercises a permissive effect on many hormones to exert their action, including the catecholamines and insulin.

Thyroxine and T_3 are highly bound to proteins in the serum, approximately 99.97% in the nonpregnant adult. Thyroxine-binding globulin (TBG) binds approximately two thirds of the circulating thyroid hormones, while albumin and other proteins bind the remainder. The amount of hormone bound to proteins can vary greatly, increasing in pregnancy and decreasing in chronic disease, for example. Such changes in protein binding must be considered when measuring total thyroxine in the blood.

When an excess of active thyroid hormone exists, the condition is known as hyperthyroidism. The clinical picture consists of the manifestations of increased metabolism, along with tachycardia, tremor, anxiety and other behavioral changes, and sometimes cardiovascular effects such as atrial fibrillation.[32] This constellation of symptoms is called *thyrotoxicosis*, and may result from overproduction of the hormone, activation of circulating hormone from T_4 to T_3, or from exogenous administration of thyroid supplements. The most common condition causing the thyroid to secrete excess hormone is Graves' disease, a diffuse increase in thyroid gland volume which accounts for approximately two-thirds of cases. Graves' disease is often accompanied by exophthalmos and is autoimmune in nature. Hyperfunction of the thyroid can be manifested by thyrotoxicosis, described previously. If it is especially severe and accompanied by decompensation of the patient, it is called *thyroid storm* or *thyrotoxic crisis*. The most common causes of this condition involve primary pathology of the thyroid gland itself.

Chronic excess thyroid hormone ingestion is a relatively common occurrence. Thyroid supplementation for treatment of hypothyroidism is widespread. It is estimated that Synthroid, the commercial name of the most common form of levothyroxine (T_4), is the fifth most commonly prescribed drug in the United States. Generic substitutes have been shown to be bioequivalent in one study.[20,21] Acute overdoses with this agent are also common, particularly among children, but they are almost universally benign[59] and no deaths have been reported. Significant ingestions of levothyroxine will not usually be manifest clinically until a week after the exposure. This is a result of the delay in peripheral conversion of thyroxine to the metabolically active T_3. Overdoses of preparations containing T_3 will often manifest in the first several days.

Chronic exposures to thyroid supplementation can lead to more severe disease, and may present with thyrotoxicosis or thyroid storm. *Thyrotoxicosis facticia* is a chronic ingestion of thyroid hormone, often by healthcare workers.[42] The objective of such ingestion may be to attain weight loss. This syndrome of thyrotoxicosis generally occurs in patients who have access to thyroid medications being taken by relatives or friends, or can obtain the medications at their place of employment.[62,92] Ground meat from the neck of animals has resulted in symptoms of thyroid excess, dubbed *hamburger thyrotoxicosis*.[46] Administration of excessive thyroid supplement chronically may also result in accelerated osteoporosis.[67]

Persons who ingest these hormones chronically may develop severe manifestations such as cardiac dysrhythmias, including atrial flutter or atrial fibrillation, tachycardia, and even cardiac failure. Thyroid storm may occur as a result of intercurrent illness in the setting of thyrotoxicosis. Tachycardia is often out of proportion to fever. The patient may become unresponsive and death can occur in up to 20% of patients with thyroid storm.

Thyroid Laboratory Testing

Until recently, thyroid testing has been undertaken using combinations of measurements of total T_3 and/or T_4 and some measurement of hormone binding. Recently, direct measurement of free hormone concentrations using radioimmunoassay has been developed for commercial use. A newer, rapid TSH test with very increased sensitivity is now widely available, using monoclonal antibodies. This supersensitive TSH test may be used in the emergent diagnosis and management of thyroid disorders. The most common application is in thyroid excess, where TSH is usually nondetectable (<0.1 mU/L) in most assays.

Management of Thyroid Excess

In patients who overdose acutely with thyroid supplement medications, the management consists of home observation in most cases. Decontamination is recommended in those patients who ingest greater than 5 mg of levothyroxine.[96] In cases where children have ingested larger doses, syrup of ipecac is usually recommended within the first hour after the ingestion. In cases where the levothyroxine dose is greater than 4 mg, it has been suggested that the patient be followed by regular telephone contact for 10 days.[54] Thyroxine levels may be elevated but provide no clinically useful information. Treatment should be based on the development of symptoms. Beta-adrenergic antagonist therapy and acetaminophen are usually sufficient treatment for these cases.[37]

Treatment for thyroid storm includes hydration, antipyretics, antithyroid drugs, and addressing the underlying causes. Beta-adrenergic antagonists are the usual treatment for suppression of the symptoms of thyrotoxicosis, and are successful in reducing heart rate, palpitations, anxiety, and tremor. Propranolol is the most commonly employed agent, but this is based on tradition. Other beta-adrenergic antagonists may be used, except in those instances where they are contraindicated, such as in asthma and congestive heart failure. Verapamil may be considered in such situations.[44]

Antithyroid Drugs

Antithyroid drugs are used to decrease the amount of thyroid hormone in hyperthyroidism, most commonly for Graves' disease. Methimazole (MMI) is a thionamide derivative that decreases production of thyroid hormone, most likely by inhibiting the activity of *thyroid peroxidase*.[93] Propylthiouracil (PTU), also a thionamide, is a more commonly used agent which in addition to this diminution of thyroid hormone synthesis also inhibits conversion of T_4 to the metabolically more active T_3. This results from PTU inactivation of 5′-deiodonase, an effect that methimazole does not have.[26,58] Methimazole can cause agranulocytosis, an effect not reported with PTU.[65] Agranulocytosis is apparently dose related. This potentially life-threatening adverse effect can now be treated by administration of granulocyte colony-stimulating factor.[4] No other serious sequelae have been associated with thionamides in acute overdose.

Other Drugs That Alter Thyroid Function

A variety of drugs have secondary effects on thyroid physiology. It is uncommon for these agents to cause clinically significant disease related to thyroid function. Lithium therapy is an exception to this, causing goiter in as many as 37% of patients, and hypothyroidism in 5 to 15% of patients.[36] Thyroid function tests should be performed upon initiation of lithium treatment, and at regular intervals thereafter. Iodine can have a substantial impact on thyroid function, but this is usually transient. Small doses may stimulate thyroid hormone secretion. With larger iodine exposure (over 10 mg/day), thyroid hormone release is decreased, usually within the first day. This effect is maximal after about 2 weeks, but with time this effect does not continue.[44] Iodinated contrast media has also been reported to have this effect. Amiodarone may induce thyrotoxicosis by providing iodine in doses that stimulate thyroid production.[11,40]

Steroids and Anabolic Supplements

When corticotropin-releasing factor (CRF) is produced by the hypothalamus, it results in the release of adrenocorticotropin (ACTH), a polypeptide from the anterior pituitary gland. ACTH is produced from a larger precursor molecule, pro-opiomelanocortin (POMC), from which other important peptides are produced. Other peptides derived from POMC include the endorphins and melanocyte stimulating hormones.[56] ACTH stimulates adrenal steroid synthesis, a process initiated by uptake of cholesterol to form an undifferentiated steroid nucleus. Three divergent metabolic pathways may then follow to produce C-19 steroids with androgenic function and 17-ketosteroids, or C-21 steroids with mineralocorticoid or glucocorticoid properties (Fig. 25–3). The more central zone is the *fasciculata-reticularis,* where cortisol and androgen synthesis occurs, whereas peripherally aldosterone and adrenal androgens are formed in the *glomerulosa.* As in the case of the thyroid hormones, steroid hormones circulate largely bound to serum proteins. Metabolism of the steroids occurs in the liver, largely by glucuronidation.

The major adrenally secreted androgen is dehydroepiandrosterone (DHEA). Other androgenic steroids secreted include 11-beta-hydroxyandrostenedione, and testosterone. In the male, the testes produce a smaller, yet significant proportion of androgenic steroids, whereas in the female almost all are derived from the adrenals.

Steroids exert their action through a cyclic AMP-mediated cascade, after diffusing passively across cell membranes. The action that results depends on the initiating molecule. Glucocorticoids are so named because they tend to increase blood glucose levels by promoting gluconeogenesis. The glucocorticoid receptor has been delineated, and amino acid sequences in the binding domain are now identified. DNA enhancement of transcription is normally inhibited by the receptor. When the glucocorticoid binds, the receptor is disinhibited.[31,48] Levels of hydrocortisone respond rapidly to stressors such as trauma or hypoglycemia. When hydrocortisone levels are diminished, stresses such as these may cause hypotension and death, hence the importance of substitution of this steroid agent in the setting of adrenal insufficiency. Levels of both the carrier proteins and free cortisol also increase in pregnancy.

Glucocorticoid effects are well known to most practitioners due to their widespread use. These effects are dependent upon the relative potency of a given agent being administered, and to the duration of therapy. Potency of some representative corticosteroids are listed in Table 25–1. They modulate carbohydrate, lipid, and nucleic acid metabolism. The most important role of glucocorticoids is in carbohydrate metabolism, where they act to preserve glucose availability to the brain. Gluconeogenesis is enhanced, while peripheral utilization is inhibited. This is particularly noticeable in the setting of starvation, where the absence of glucocorticoids results in hypoglycemia. With long-term exposure to supraphysiologic doses of glucocorticoids, a condition resembling diabetes ensues. This is manifested by fasting hyperglycemia and insulin resistance.[63] Cushing's syndrome is the manifestation of glucocorticoid excess, which also effects lipid metabolism. Fat deposits in a specific pattern in the back of the neck, referred to as "buffalo hump," and in the face, known as "moon facies." With acute administration of glucocorticoids, an increase in circulating polymorphonuclear leukocytes is seen, resulting from demargination from vessel walls. Over time, there is a decrease in the number of circulating eosinophils, lymphocytes, monocytes, and basophils. Leukocyte function is also impaired, which is the major reason that glucocor-

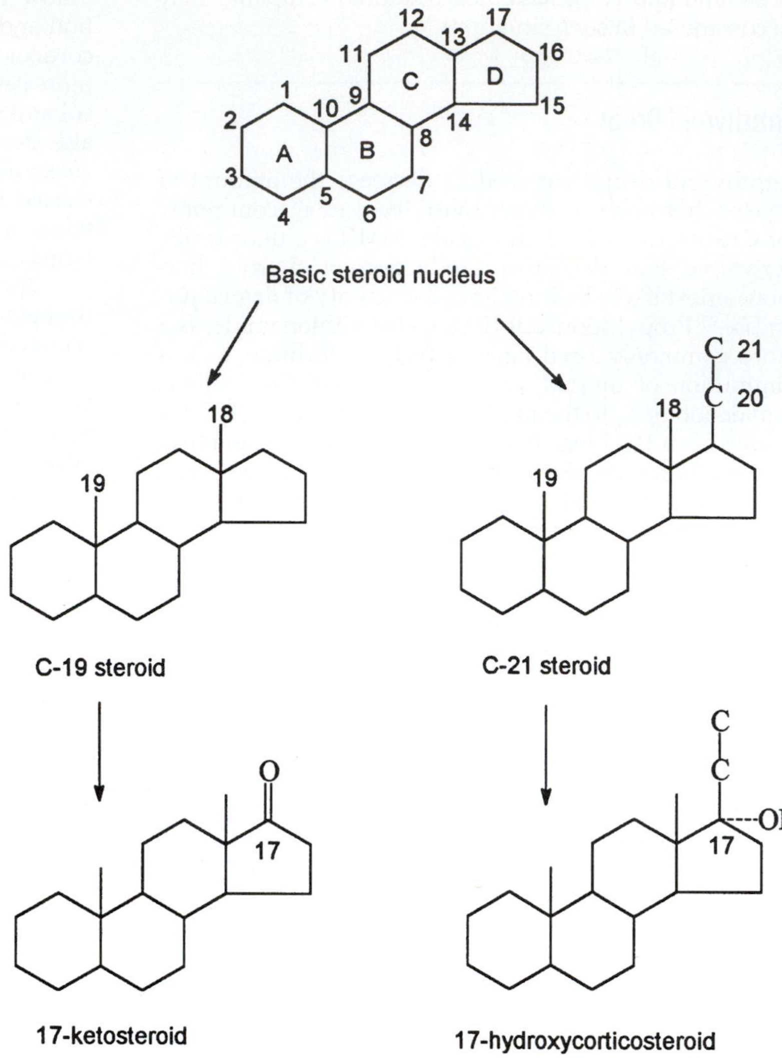

Figure 25–3. Basic steroid structure and nomenclature. *(Reprinted with permission from Wartofsky L, in: Isselbacher KJ, Braunwald E, Wilson JD, et al, eds: Harrison's Principles of Internal Medicine, 13th ed. New York, McGraw-Hill, 1994, p. 1931.)*

TABLE 25–1. RELATIVE POTENCIES OF COMMONLY USED CORTICOSTEROIDS

	Relative Potency[a] (mg)	
Corticosteroid	***Glucocorticoid (Antiinflammatory)***	***Mineralocorticoid (Sodium-Retaining)***
Hydrocortisone	1	1
Cortisone	0.8	0.8
Desoxycorticosterone	0	30–50
Fludrocortisone	10	125
Prednisone	4	0.8
Prednisolone	4	0.8
Methylprednisolone	5	0.5
Triamcinolone	5	0
Dexamethasone	25	0
Betamethasone	25	0

[a]Hydrocortisone expressed as unity

ticoids possess immunosuppressive and antiinflammatory effects.[13] In contrast, the red blood cell mass increases in Cushing's syndrome, while a normochromic, normocytic anemia is characteristic of Addison's disease (hypoadrenal state).

Patients with glucocorticoid excess may develop mood elevation and CNS excitability. Some may become overtly psychotic. The mechanism of this "steroid psychosis" is unknown, but these agents may play a role in the control of local neuronal excitability.[64]

Mineralocorticoids increase extracellular fluid volume by causing renal distal tubular reabsorption of sodium. Aldosterone is the most important mineralocorticoid, which also acts to increase the secretion of potassium. Its major stimulus is the renin–angiotensin system. If angiotensin-converting enzyme (ACE) inhibitors are taken, activation of angiotensin is blocked, and synthesis of aldosterone is decreased. This has the effect of lowering blood pressure and retaining potassium. Treatment of ACE inhibitor overdose is undertaken primarily by intravenous volume repletion. Steroid genesis can also be inhibited by other agents. One such agent used frequently in the emergency department is etomidate. Etomidate has occasionally been associated with suppression of the adrenal axis and decreased serum cortisol, especially when sedation with this agent has been prolonged. Hydrocortisone should be administered in these cases.[98]

Androgenic and Anabolic Steroid Use

Androgens stimulate male secondary sexual characteristics by binding to receptors in target tissue cytoplasm. As early as 1938 it was observed that removing the testes in guinea pigs abolished the larger skeletal muscle size in males.[69] Plasma concentrations of testosterone are increased in males during the neonatal period and remain elevated after puberty.[39] Feedback inhibition of the pituitary becomes minimal at puberty.[100]

Anabolic steroids are used for medical purposes for such indications as osteoporosis, anemia, breast cancer treatment, or hypogonadism.[16] There is a continual pursuit of newer agents that minimize the androgenic (masculinizing) effects while maintaining the anabolic (growth) effects. Use of anabolic steroids by athletes has become an epidemic in the United States. Estimates based on the National Household Survey on Drug Abuse suggest that there are more than one million current or former users of anabolic steroids in the United States.[103] The users typically wish to increase athletic performance or muscle mass by using these agents. Muscle mass may be increased by use of these agents in some cases, but aerobic capacity is probably not increased.[1,43]

The method of use of these agents varies considerably among individuals. Testosterone has had a resurgence in recent years due to the difficulty in distinguishing this molecule from endogenous hormone. It has a very short duration of action, however, and is not practical for those seeking the presumed benefits of anabolic steroids. Other agents fall into two general classes, based on the substitutions at the 17-alpha-position with alkyl or carboxylic acid side groups. The alkyl substitution results in agents that are well absorbed orally, due to their resistance to hepatic first-pass metabolism. These agents are associated with hepatotoxicity.[25,29,66] The 17-alpha-carboxylic acid substitution results in agents that are poorly absorbed orally, and are used parenterally. The carboxylic side group must be hydrolyzed prior to becoming active biologically. Agents are often taken in large doses for short periods of time, and several different agents may be taken simultaneously. The latter phenomenon is referred to as *stacking*.[92] Other patterns of use include *plateauing*, where different steroids are taken in overlapping patterns to prevent tolerance. *Pyramiding* is the practice whereby anabolic steroids are taken for finite periods of time alternating with periods of abstinence.[38] These drugs have been taken in cycles of 12 to 18 weeks to minimize adverse effects such as testicular atrophy.

Numerous side effects have been attributed to the anabolic steroids, and these have been reviewed elsewhere.[47] In males, these hormones result in a negative feedback, causing a decrease in testosterone, luteinizing hormone (LH), and follicle-stimulating hormone (FSH).[14,77,84] This occurs even with long-term low-dose use of an agent such as the very commonly used methandrostenolone (Dianabol).[77] Testicular atrophy,[88] decreased spermatogenesis,[49] and gynecomastia often ensues, and may be the result of inadequate breakdown of estrogen by a less-efficient liver.[101]

Premature epiphyseal closure is an important musculoskeletal system effect in children. An increased susceptibility to cartilaginous and ligamentous injury has also been described with the use of these agents.[85] Levels of LDL cholesterol are increased, with simultaneous decreases in HDL. These findings may explain a relationship between anabolic steroid use and an increased risk of stroke and myocardial infarction in athletes using these agents.[27,28]

In women, a variety of androgenic effects—including amenorrhea, acne, hirsutism, and reduction in breast size—become evident even at therapeutic doses.[47] Baldness, clitoral hypertrophy, deepening of the voice, and facial hairs are usually irreversible.

The most serious toxicity of the anabolic steroids is associated with the 17-alpha-alkylated (oral) agents, which may cause severe hepatotoxicity. Elevated aminotransferase levels are often transient, but may persist and culminate in severe liver disease.[27] Hepatic cholestasis is occasionally fatal.[95] *Peliosis hepatis* is a common finding following anabolic steroid use, consisting of blood-filled sacks in the peripheral zone of the hepatic lobule.[57]

Hepatic neoplasms have been reported extensively in association with anabolic steroid use. In one review, the majority of these were hepatocellular carcinomas or angiosarcomas, with the remaining being hepatomas or other benign tumors.[47] Although most patients with hepatocellular carcinoma rapidly succumb, some of these neoplasms may remit with cessation of the drug.[99]

Testing for anabolic steroid use has been an ongoing concern by those responsible for competitive athletic events. The International Olympic Committee has issued standards for such testing, indicating that gas chromatography/mass spectrometry (GC/MS) analysis is the only method that consistently does not report false-positive results.[47,50,85]

Other hormonal agents have also been used by athletes in an effort to enhance performance. Growth hormone is one such agent that has been used, due to the inability of urine tests to detect this protein. No problems with short-term use have been noted, but no benefits are derived from such misuse of this hormone.

Estrogenic Agents and Oral Contraceptives

The estrogens are the hormones responsible for female secondary sexual characteristics. They exert their actions mostly on specific tissues that respond to their presence. These include the mammary glands, vagina, uterus, and fallopian tube. Of greatest importance, estrogens cause endometrial hyperplasia. Along with progesterone, estrogen regulates the reproductive cycle in females. Estrogen supplementation is very common. It is frequently prescribed in postmenopausal women to manage symptoms of menopause and later to prevent osteoporosis. Approximately one of five women in their childbearing years uses combinations of estrogens with progesterone to prevent conception.

Estrogens contain the cyclopentanophenanthrene ring characteristic of steroids, with an essential phenol present in the A ring. Nonsteroidal estrogens exist that also possess the phenol structure. The most widely known of these nonsteroidal agents is diethylstilbestrol (DES). Estradiol is produced in the liver and adipose tissue by oxidation of estradiol-17-beta, secreted by the ovary. Estradiol is subsequently hydrated to form estriol. Androstenedione is converted to estradiol-17-beta-alpha through conversion to testosterone, and aromatization of the A ring. This accounts for up to one third of estrogen production after menopause. In addition to conversion to estriol, estrogens can undergo glucuronidation and sulfation. These mechanisms increase their water solubility and renal excretion.

Estrogens taken in large quantities frequently cause nausea. Gynecomastia and feminization may be seen in males, especially after prolonged administration. If estrogens are administered for a long period and then withdrawn, uterine bleeding may be severe as a result of endometrial hyperplasia. Endometrial hyperplasia is also considered a risk factor for adenocarcinoma.

The nonsteroidal stilbene derivates such as DES are metabolized via quinone and semiquinone intermediates, which may be related to the teratogenic and carcinogenic effects of these drugs. These agents are orally active and have a relatively long duration of action. DES has been associated with vaginal clear-cell adenocarcinoma in the offspring of women who received DES during their first trimester of pregnancy. Other vaginal and cervical structural abnormalities have also been identified in these daughters of DES users.

In addition to the physiologic role of the estrogens, they are often used in combination with progestins to inhibit ovulation. Progestins are substances related to progesterone, the endogenous hormone produced by the corpus luteum during pregnancy (by the placenta) and during the normal menstrual cycle (by the corpus luteum). Numerous synthetic derivatives of progesterone have been developed.

The tissue targets of progesterone action include the mammary gland and uterus. Receptors for progesterone in these tissues are dependent on a permissive effect of estrogen. This hormone is responsible for maintaining pregnancy and decreasing the contractility of the endometrium. Progesterone is necessary for breast development and postpartum lactation, mediated by prolactin. The progestins are used principally in conjunction with estrogen as oral contraceptive agents. These agents can cause androgenic sequelae when used in large doses, including hirsutism and acne. Progestins are thought to decrease the risk of endometrial cancer and perhaps breast cancer when used with estrogen in postmenopausal women.

Oral contraceptive pill (OCP) use results in an increased risk of thromboembolic phenomena.[53] Carbohydrate and lipid metabolism are also influenced in many patients. Glucose intolerance may occur, especially in those patients who develop diabetes during their gestation. Serum triglyceride levels increase markedly, and depend on the progestin content of the preparation. Perhaps through this increase in triglycerides, HDL cholesterol levels are reduced. Estrogens tend to increase HDL levels.

Overdose with oral contraceptive pills (OCP) is rarely reported, perhaps due to the benign nature of the increased dosage. Vaginal spotting may be seen, and edema of the thighs has been reported with estradiol implant overdose.[23,87]

Acknowledgements

Donna Seger, MD contributed to this chapter in a previous edition.

References

1. American College of Sports Medicine: Position stand on the use of anabolic-androgenic steroids in sports. Am J Sports Med 1984;12:13–18.
2. Assan R, Perronne C, Assan D, et al: Pentamidine-induced derangements of glucose homeostasis. Determinant roles of renal failure and drug accumulation. A study of 128 patients. Diabetes Care 1995;18:47–55.
3. Bailey CJ: Biguanides and NIDDM. Diabetes Care 1992;15:755–772.
4. Bartalena L , Bogazzi F , Martino E: Adverse effects of thyroid hormone preparations and antithyroid drugs. Drug Saf 1996;15:53–63.
5. Beattie JO, Hull D, Cockburn F: Children intoxicated by alcohol in Nottingham and Glasgow, 1973–84. Br Med J 1986;292:519–521.
6. Boden G, Soriano M, Hoeldke R, et al: Counterregulatory hormone release and glucose recovery after hypoglycemia in noninsulin-dependent diabetic patients. Diabetes 1983; 32:1055–1059.
7. Bolli G, Tsahkian E, Haymond M, et al: Defective glucose counterregulation after subcutaneous insulin in noninsulin-dependent diabetes mellitus. J Clin Invest 1984; 73:1532–1541.
8. Boyle PJ, Justice K, Krenz AJ, et al: Octreotide reverses hyperinsulinemia and prevents hypoglycemia induced by sulfonylurea overdoses. J Clin Endocrinol Metab 1993; 76:752–756.
9. Boyle PJ, Kempers SF, O'Connor AM, et al: Brain glucose uptake and unawareness of hypoglycemia in patients with insulin-dependent diabetes mellitus. N Engl J Med 1995; 333:26, 1726–1731.
10. Cahill GF: Action of adrenal cortical steroids on carbohydrate metabolism. In: Christy NP, ed: The Human Adrenal Cortex. New York, Harper & Row, 1971, pp. 205–240.

11. Cappiello E, Boldorini R, Tosoni A, et al: Ultrastructural evidence of thyroid damage in amiodarone-induced thyrotoxicosis. J Endocrinol Invest 1995;18:862–868.
12. Cherrington AD: Gluconeogenesis: Its regulation by insulin and glucagon. In: Brownlee M, ed: Handbook of Diabetes Mellitus. Vol. 3. Intermediary Metabolism and Its Regulation. New York, Garland STPM Press, 1981, pp. 49–117.
13. Chrousos GP: The hypothalamic–pituitary–adrenal axis and immune-mediated inflammation. N Engl J Med 1995;332:1351–1362.
14. Clerico A, Ferdeghini M, Palombo C, et al: Effect of anabolic treatment on the serum levels of gonadotropins, testosterone, prolactin, thryoid hormones and myoglobin of male athletes under physical training. J Nuclear Med Allied Sci 1981;23:79–88.
15. Cortesao L, Saraiva AM, Guerreiro L: The endocrine pancreas. Acta Med Port 1995;8(suppl 1):S47–S53.
16. Council on Scientific Affairs, American Medical Association: Drug abuse in athletes. Anabolic steroids and human growth hormone. JAMA 1988;259:1703–1705.
17. Cummins LH: Hypoglycemia and convulsions in children following alcohol ingestion. J Pediatr 1961;58:23–26.
18. DCCT Research Group: The effect of intensive treatment of diabetes on the development and progression of long-term complications in insulin-dependent diabetes mellitus. N Engl J Med 1993;333:541–549.
19. DeFeo P, Bolli G, Periello G, et al: The adrenergic contribution to glucose counterregulation: Dependency on alpha-cell function and mediation through beta-adrenergic receptors. Diabetes 1983;32:887–893.
20. Dong BJ, Hauck WW, Gambertoglio JG, et al: Bioequivalence of generic and brand-name levothyroxine products in the treatment of hypothyroidism. JAMA 1997;277: 1205–1213.
21. Drummond R: Thyroid storm. JAMA 1997;277:1238–1243. Editorial.
22. Dubois MP: Immunoreactive somatostatin is present in discrete cells of the endocrine pancreas. Proc Natl Acad Sci USA 1975;72:1340–1344.
23. Eden J: Too much of a good thing? Two cases of oestrogen overdosage associated with oestradiol implants. Med J Aust 1990;152:558. Letter.
24. Ernst AA, Jones K, Nick TG, et al: Ethanol ingestion and related hypoglycemia in a pediatric and adolescent emergency department population. Acad Emerg Med 1996;1: 46–49.
25. Farrell GC, Joshua DE, Uren RF, et al: Androgen-induced hepatoma. Lancet 1975;1:430–432.
26. Farwell AP, Braverman LE: Thyroid and antithyroid drugs. In: Hardman JG, Limbird LE, Molinoff PB, Ruddon RW, eds: Goodman & Gilman's The Pharmacological Basis of Therapeutics, 9th ed. New York, McGraw-Hill, 1996, pp. 1383–1409.
27. Ferenchick GS: Drug abuse and stroke. Ann Internal Med 1991;114:431–432.
28. Ferenchick GS: Are androgenic steroids thrombogenic? N Engl J Med 1990;322:476–477.
29. Foss GL, Simpson SL: Oral methyltestosterone and jaundice. Br Med J 1959;1:259.
30. Fujita T, Sugiyama Y, Taketomi S, et al: Reduction of insulin resistance in obese and/or diabetic animals by 5-[4-(1-methylcyclonhexylmethoxy) benzyl]-thiazolidine-2,4-dione IADD–3878, U-63,287, ciglitazone), a new antidiabetic agent. Diabetes 1983:32;804–810.
31. Funder JW: Adrenal steroids: New answers, new questions. Science 1987;237:236–237.
32. Gavin LA: Thyroid crisis. Med Clin North Am 1991; 75:179–193.
33. Gilman AG: Nobel lecture. G proteins and regulation of adenyl cyclase. Biosci Rep 1995;15:65–97.
34. Gilman AG: G proteins: Transducers of receptor-generated signals. Annu Rev Biochem 1987;56:615–649.
35. Gilman AG: G proteins and dual control of adenylate cyclase. Cell 1984;36:577–579.
36. Gittoes NJ , Franklyn JA: Drug-induced thyroid disorders. Drug Saf 1995;13:46–55.
37. Golightly LK, Smolinske SC, Kulig KW, et al: Clinical effects of accidental levothyroxine ingestion in children. Am J Dis Child 1985;141:1025–2110.
38. Graham W, Kennedy M: Recent developments in the toxicology of anabolic steroids. Drug Saf 1990;5:548–476.
39. Griffin JE, Wilson JP: The testes. In: Bondy PK, Rosenberg LE, eds: Metabolic Control and Disease, 7th ed. Philadelphia, Saunders, 1980, pp. 1535–1578.
40. Guyetant S, Wion-Barbot N, Rousselet MC: C-cell hyperplasia associated with chronic lymphocytic thyroiditis: A retrospective quantitative study of 112 cases. Hum Pathol 1994;25:514–521.
41. Hachiya HL, Treves ST, Kahn CR, et al: Altered insulin distribution and metabolism in type I diabetics assessed by I-insulin scanning. J Clin Endocrinol Metab 1987;64: 801–808.
42. Hamolsky MW: Truth is stranger than factitious. N Engl J Med 1982;307:436–437.
43. Haupt HA: Anabolic steroids: A review of the literature. Am J Sports Med 1984;12:469–484.
44. Haynes RC: Thyroid and antithyroid drugs. In: Gilman, AG, Rall TW, Nies AS, Taylor P, eds: Goodman and Gilman's The Pharmacological Basis of Therapeutics, 8th ed. New York, McGraw-Hill, 1990, pp. 1376.
45. Hearn PR, Ahmed M, Woodhouse NJY: The use of SMS 201–995, (somatostatin analogue) in insulinomas. Horm Res 1988;29:211–213.
46. Hedbert CW: An outbreak of thyrotoxicosis caused by the consumption of bovine thyroid gland in ground beef. N Engl J Med 1987;316:993–998.
47. Hickson RC, Ball KL, Falduto MT: Adverse effects of anabolic steroids. Med Toxicol Adverse Drug Exp 1989;4: 254–271.
48. Hollenberg SM, Giguere V, Segui P, et al: Co-localization of DNA binding and transcriptional activation functions in the human glucocorticoid receptor. Cell 1987;49:39–46.
49. Holma P: Effect of an anabolic steroid (metandienone) on central and peripheral blood flow in well-trained male athletes. Ann Clin Res 1977;9:215–221.
50. Johnson FL: The association of oral androgenic-anabolic steroids and life-threatening disease. Med Sci Sports 1975;7:284–286.
51. Kahn RC, Shecter Y: Insulin, oral hypoglycemic agents and the pharmacology of the endocrine pancreas. In:

Gilman AG, Rall TW, Nies AS, Taylor P, eds: Goodman and Gilman's The Pharmacological Basis of Therapeutics, 8th ed. New York, McGray-Hill, 1990, p. 1488.
52. Kellerer M, Kroder G, Tippmer S, et al: Troglitazone prevents glucose-induced insulin resistance insulin receptor in Rat–1 fibroblasts. Diabetes 1994;43:447–453.
53. Kleiner SM: Performance-enhancing aids in sports: Health consequences and nutritional alternatives. J Am Coll Nutr 1991;10:163–176.
54. Kosaka K, Kuzuya K, Akanuma Y, et al. Clinical evaluation of a new oral hypoglycemic drug CS–045 in patients with non insulin-dependent diabetes mellitus poorly controlled by sulfonylureas: A double-blind, placebo-controlled study. J Clin Ther Med 1993;3:61–93.
55. Krief S, Lonnqvist F, Raimbault S, et al: Tissue distribution of b3-adrenergic receptor mRNA in man. J Clin Invest 1993;91:344–349.
56. Krieger DT, Martin JB: Brain Peptides. N Engl J Med 1981;304:944–951.
57. Lamb DR: Anabolic steroids in athletics: How well do they work and how dangerous are they? Am J Sports Med 1984;12:31–38.
58. Leonard JL, Visser TJ: Biochemistry of iodination. In: Hennemann G, ed: Thyroid Hormone Metabolism. New York, Marcel Dekker, 1986, pp. 189–230.
59. Litovitz TL, White J: Levothyroxine ingestions in children: An analysis of 78 cases. Am J Emerg Med 1985;3:297–300.
60. Lonqvist F, Krief S, Strosberg AD, et al: Evidence for a functional β_3-adrenergic receptor in man. Br J Pharmacol 1993;110:929–936.
61. Luckner R, Challis A, West D, et al: A problem in the radiochemical assay of glucose-6-phosphate in muscle. Biochem J 1984;218:649–651.
62. Mariotti S, Marino E, Cupin C, et al: Low serum thyroglobulin as a clue to the diagnosis of thyrotoxicosis factictia. N Engl J Med 1982;307:410–412.
63. McMahon M, Gerich J, Rizza R: Effects of glucocorticoids on carbohydrate metabolism. Diabetes Metab Rev 1988;4: 17–30.
64. Mellon SH: Neurosteroids: Biochemistry, modes of action, and clinical relevance. J Clin Endocrinol Metab 1994;78: 1003–1008.
65. Meyer-Gessner M, Bender G, Lederbogen S, et al: Antithyroid drug-induced agranulocytosis: Clinical experience with ten patients treated at one institution and review of the literature. J Endocrinol Invest 1994;17:29–36.
66. Mosbach EH, Shefer S, Abell LL: Identification of the fecal metabolites of 17α-methyltestosterone in the dog. J Lipid Res 1968;9:93–97.
67. Nuovo J, Ellsworth A, Christensen DB, et al: Excessive thyroid hormone replacement therapy. J Am Board Fam Pract 1995;8:435–439.
68. Moore DF, Wood DF, Volans GN: Features, prevention and managment of acute overdose due to antidiabetic drugs. Drug Saf 1993;9:218–229.
69. Papanicolau GN, Falk EA: General muscular hypertrophy induced by androgenic hormones. Science 1938;87: 238–239.
70. Peterson DR, Carone FA, Oparil S, et al: Differences between renal tubular processing of glucagon and insulin. Am J Physiol 1989;38:1217–1229.
71. Philips RE, Looareesuwan S, Bloom SR, et al: Effectiveness of SMS 210–995, a synthetic long-acting somatostatin analogue, in treatment of quinine-induced hyperinsulinemia. Lancet 1986;1:713–714.
72. Popp D, Shah S, Cryer P: Role of epinephrine mediated adrenergic mechanisms in hypoglycemic glucose counterregulation and posthypoglycemic hyperglycemia in insulin-dependent diabetes mellitus. J Clin Invest 1982;69: 315–326.
73. Porte D: A receptor mechanism for the inhibition of insulin release by epinephrine in man. J Clin Invest 1967;45:86–94.
74. Rabkin R, Hamik A, Yagil C, et al: Processing of ^{125}I-insulin by polarized cultured kidney cells. Exp Cell Res 1996;224:136–142.
75. Randle P, Hales C, Garland P, et al: The glucose fatty acid cycle. Its role in insulin sensitivity and the metabolic disturbances of diabetes mellitus. Lancet 1963;1:785–789.
76. Reichlin S: Somatostatin (parts I and II.) N Engl J Med 1983;309:1495–1503, 1556–1563.
77. Remes K, Vuopio P, Jarinenen M, et al: Effect of short-term treatment with an anabolic steroid (methandienone) and dehyroepiandrosterone sulphate on plasma hormones, red cell volume and 2,3-diphosphoglycerate in athletes. Scand J Clin Lab Invest 1977;37:577–586.
78. Rizza RA, Cryer PE, Gerich JE: Role of glucagon, catecholamines and growth hormone in human glucose counterregulation. Effect of somatostatin and combined alpha- and beta adrenergic blockade on plasma glucose recovery and glucose flux rates after insulin-induced hypoglycemia. J Clin Invest 1979;64:62–71.
79. Rizza R, Cryer P, Haymond M, et al: Adrenergic mechanism for the effect of epinephrine on glucose production and clearance in man. J Clin Invest 1980;65:682–689.
80. Ross EM: G proteins and receptors in neuronal signaling. In: Hall ZW, ed: An Introduction to Molecular Neurobiology. Sunderland, Mass, Sinaver, 1992, pp. 181–206.
81. Samols E, Bonner-Weir S, Weir GC: Intra-islet insulin-glucagon somatostin relationships. J Clin Endocrinol Metab 1986;15:53–58.
82. Sands M, Kron MA, Brown RB: Pentamidine: A review. Rev Infect Dis 1985;7:625–634.
83. Scully R: Case records of the Massachusetts General Hospital. N Engl J Med 1984;310:580–587.
84. Shephard RJ, Killinger D, Fried T: Responses to sustained use of anabolic steroids. Br J Sports Med 1977;11:170–173.
85. Smith DA, Perry PJ: The efficacy of ergogenic agents in athletic competition. I: Androgenic-anabolic steroids. Ann Pharmacother 1992;26:520–528.
86. Sporer KA, Ernst AA, Conte R, et al: The incidence of ethanol-induced hypoglycemia. Am J Emerg Med 1992;10:403–405.
87. Stadel BV: Oral contraceptives and cardiovascular disease. N Engl J Med 1981;305: 672–677.
88. Strauss RH: Anabolic steroids. Clin Sports Med 1984; 3:743–748.
89. Stumvoll M, Nurjan N, Perillo G, et al: Metabolic effects of

metformin in non-insulin-dependent diabetes mellitus. N Engl J Med 1995;33:550–554.
90. Sucov A, Woolard RH: Ethanol-associated hypoglycemia is uncommon. Acad Emerg Med 1995;2:185–189.
91. Tang WJ, Gilman AG: Type-specific regulation of adenyl cyclase by G protein beta gamma subunits. Science, 1991;254:1500–1503.
92. Tatro DS: Use of steroids by athletes. Drug Newsletter 1985;4:33–34.
93. Taurog A, Dorris ML: Peroxidase-catalyzed bromination of tyrosine, thyroglobulin, and bovine serum albumin: Comparison of thyroid peroxidase and lactoperoxidase. Arch Biochem Biophys 1991;287:288–296.
94. Taylor JR, Sherratt HJA, Davies DM: Intramuscular or intravenous glucagon for sulphonylurea hypoglycemia. Eur J Clin Pharmacol 1978;14:125–127.
95. Taylor WN: Anabolic Steroids and the Athlete. Jefferson, NC, Mcfarland, 1982.
96. Tunget CL, Clark RF, Turchen SG, et al: Raising the decontamination level for thyroid hormone ingestions. Am J Emerg Med 1995;13:9–13.
97. Unger RH: Glucagon physiology and pathophysiology in the light of new advances. Diabetologia 1985;28: 574–578.
98. Wagner RL, White PF, Kan PB, et al: Inhibition of adrenal steroidogenesis by the anesthetic etomidate. N Engl J Med 1984;310:1415–1421.
99. Wakabayashi T, Onda H, Tada T, et al: High incidence of peliosis hepatis in autospy cases of aplastic anemia with special reference to anabolic steroid therapy. Acta Pathologica Japonica 1984;34:1079–1086.
100. Wilson JD: Androgens. In: Hardman JG, Limbird LE, Molinoff PB, Ruddon RW, eds: Goodman & Gilman's The Pharmacological Basis of Therapeutics, 9th ed. New York, McGraw-Hill, 1996, p 1442.
101. Wilson JD, Griffin JE: The use and misuse of androgens. Metabolism 1980;29:1278–1295.
102. Wright J: Alcohol induced hypoglycemia. Br J Alcohol Alcoholism 1979;14:174–176.
103. Yesalis CE, Kennedy NJ, Kopstein AN, et al: Anabolic-androgenic steroid use in the United States. JAMA 1993;270: 1217–1221.

CHAPTER 26

Ophthalmic Principles

Martin J. Smilkstein

Effective management of potentially poisoned patients must involve consideration of the ophthalmic system. Examination of the eye not only provides clues to the diagnosis of certain toxic exposures but may also lead to timely detection of life-threatening nontoxicologic problems, such as intracranial hemorrhage. In addition, the importance of the components of the visual system as targets of toxicity is well known. The eye may be injured by direct contact with a number of agents, may provide a portal of entry for agents with systemic toxicity, and may itself be adversely affected by many systemic exposures. Understanding these principles can be lifesaving or sightsaving, and allows for a more efficient, systematic approach to toxicologic emergency care.

Ophthalmic Examination Findings

Before considering specific toxic exposures in detail, it is important to consider briefly normal function and how dysfunction leads to clinical signs and symptoms pertaining to the eye and visual function.

Visual Acuity and Color Perception

Decreased acuity can result from abnormalities anywhere in the optic system that affect either light transmission or neural elements.[18,31] Corneal injury or edema from any cause may cause blurring of vision, characteristically described as "halos" around lights. Toxicologic causes of corneal abnormalities include direct exposure to chemicals, failure of corneal protective reflexes due to local anesthetic effects or a profoundly decreased level of consciousness, and incomplete eyelid closure during coma. Mydriasis, also a common feature of acute drug and chemical exposure (Table 26–1), may interfere with the pupillary constriction component of the near reflex, resulting in decreased acuity for near objects. Lens clouding or cataract formation causes blurred vision and decreased light perception, as does blood or other deposits in the aqueous or vitreous humors. Drug-induced lens abnormalities due to chronic exposures are well described[25,31] (Table 26–2), but are not important in the evaluation of toxicologic emergencies. Even if light reaches the retina without distortion, abnormal reception or transmission can result from ischemia or injury to any neural element from the retina to the optic cortex. Direct, acute visual neurotoxic injury is rare and is caused almost exclusively by methanol or quinine. Indirect injury following drug-induced central nervous system (CNS) ischemia or hypoxia is far more common. Alterations in color perception generally result from abnormalities in retinal or optic nerve function. Color vision abnormalities are attributed to hundreds of agents, but unlike those due to chronic drug exposure such abnormalities are rare and inconsistent features of acute toxicity.[25]

Pupil Size and Reactivity

Normally, the pupils are equal to each other in size, 3 to 4 mm under typical light conditions, round, and react directly and consensually to increased light intensity by constricting. Pupillary constriction also occurs as part of the near reflex when a person attempts to focus on near objects. All of these characteristics result from the balance between cholinergic innervation of the iris sphincter (constrictor) by cranial nerve III and sympathetic innervation of the radial muscle of the iris (dilator).[18] Pupillary dilation (mydriasis) can result from increased sympathetic stimulation by endogenous catecholamines or from systemic (eg, cocaine, amphetamines) or ocular (eg, phenylephrine) exposures to sympathomimetic drugs. Mydriasis can also result from inhibition of cholinergic-mediated pupillary constriction and is the mechanism for mydriasis caused by systemic or ocular exposures to anticholinergic agents (Chap. 34). Neurologic injury resulting in either midbrain or cranial nerve III dysfunction (eg, increased intracranial pressure) is a more ominous etiology of the mydriasis, caused by loss of constrictor function. Because pupillary constriction in response to

TABLE 26–1. OPHTHALMIC FINDINGS DUE TO ACUTE TOXIC EXPOSURES

Miosis
- Increased cholinergic tone
  - Anticholinesterases (carbamates, organophosphates, physostigmine)
  - Carbachol
  - Muscarine
  - Nicotine
  - Opioids
  - Pilocarpine
- Decreased sympathetic tone
  - Clonidine
  - Guanabenz
  - Methyldopa
- Coma from sedative-hynotic agents (barbiturates, benzodiazepines, ethanol)
- Pontine hemorrhage

Mydriasis
- Decreased cholinergic tone
  - Antihistamines
  - Belladonna alkaloids
  - Cyclic antidepressants (inconsistent finding)
  - Postanoxic encephalopathy (many causes)
- Increased sympathetic tone
  - Amphetamines
  - Cocaine
  - Phenylephrine and other sympathomimetics
  - Ethanol and sedative-hypnotic withdrawal

Nystagmus
- Carbamazepine
- Ethanol
- Phencyclidine
- Phenytoin
- Sedative-hypnotic agents

Disconjugate Gaze
- Botulism
- Elapid envenomation
- Neuromuscular blocking agents
- Paralytic shellfish poisoning
- Tetrodotoxin
- Secondary to decreased level of consciousness (many causes)

Funduscopic Abnormalities
- Carbon monoxide (red)
- Cocaine (vasoconstriction)
- Cyanide (retinal vein arteriolization)
- Ergot alkaloids (vasoconstriction)
- IV drug use (embolic)
- Methanol (disc and retinal pallor or hyperemia)
- Methemoglobin (cyanotic)

TABLE 26–2. EXAMPLES OF OCULAR ABNORMALITIES CAUSED BY CHRONIC SYSTEMIC EXPOSURES[a]

Corneal/Conjunctival Inflammation
- Cytosine arabinoside (Ara-C)
- Isotretinoin[b]
- Mercury (acrodynia)
- Practolol[c]

Corneal Deposits
- Amiodarone[b]
- Chloroquine
- Chlorpromazine
- Copper[d]
- Gold
- Mercury[d]
- Silver (argyria)[d]
- Vitamin D

Cataracts
- Busulfan[c]
- Corticosteroids[b]
- Dinitrophenol (internal use)[d]
- Trinitrotoluene[c,d]

Lens Deposits
- Amiodarone[b]
- Chlorpromazine
- Copper[d]
- Iron
- Mercury[d]
- Silver[d]

Myopia[c]
- Acetazolamide
- Diuretics (chlorthalidone, thiazides, spironolactone)
- Sulfonamides

Retinal Injury
- Carbon disulfide[d]
- Carmustine[c]
- Chloramphenicol[c]
- Chloroquine
- Cinchona alkaloids (quinine)[b]
- Deferoxamine[c]
- Digitalis[c]
- Ethambutol
- Thallium
- Vincristine[c]

Retrobulbar and Optic Neuropathy
- Carbon disulfide[d]
- Chloramphenicol[d]
- Dinitrobenzene[d]
- Dinitrochlorobenzene[d]
- Dinitrotoluene[c,d]
- Disulfiram
- Ethambutol[b]
- Isoniazid[c]
- Lead[c]
- Thallium
- Vincristine[c]

Cortical Blindness
- Cisplatin
- Cyclosporin A
- Interleukin[c]
- Tacrolimus (FK506)
- Methylmercury compounds[d]

[a]This list includes only selected examples and is not intended to be comprehensive.
[b]Particularly important example.
[c]Reported, but extremely rare from this exposure.
[d]Mostly historical interest—associated with patterns of use no longer common.

light is a major determinant of normal pupil size, blindness from ocular, retinal, or optic nerve disorders also leads to mydriasis (eg, methanol, quinine). Reactivity of mydriatic pupils to light varies with the etiology of the mydriasis.[31] Although often difficult to appreciate, constriction to light can usually be elicited after sympathomimetic exposures because constrictor function is preserved, whereas this is often not the case when mydriasis results from anticholinergic excess. Light reactivity is absent in cases of complete blindness due to retinal or optic neurologic injury, but may be preserved if there is some remaining light perception.

Pupillary constriction (miosis) can result from increased cholinergic stimulation (eg, opioids, pilocarpine, anticholinesterases such as organophosphates) or inhibition of sympathetic dilation (eg, clonidine, pontine hemorrhage). There are conflicting reports regarding the pupillary effects of many drugs. Depending on the stage and severity of toxicity, the presence of coingestants or coexistent hypoxemia, and numerous other factors, many individual substances (eg, phencylidine, barbiturates) are reported to cause both mydriasis and miosis.[31,40] For some substances, the pupillary examination provides consistent information (Table 26–1), but many factors are involved and the significance of the pupil size and reactivity must always be considered in the context of the remainder of the patient evaluation.

Extraocular Movement, Diplopia, and Nystagmus

Maintenance of normal eye position and movement requires coordinated function of a complex circuit involving bilateral frontal and occipital cortices, multiple brainstem nuclei, cranial nerves, extraocular muscles, and connecting fibers between each.[2,18] Because of the many elements necessary for normal function, abnormalities of eye movement can result from several causes and are extremely common.[31] Probably the most common abnormality is reversible nystagmus (Table 26–1). Drug-induced nystagmus may take many forms, but is most commonly jerk nystagmus, as opposed to pendular, or horizontal and symmetric. The nystagmus may be evident at rest but is accentuated by visual pursuit and extreme lateral gaze. These features are unique to drug-induced causes. Drug-induced vertical nystagmus is rarely seen, except as a result of phencyclidine toxicity, and when present should always suggest a structural lesion of the CNS. Loss of conjugate gaze commonly results from CNS depression of any cause, including many overdoses. Except after extremely rare neurotoxin exposures (Table 26–1), diplopia without decreased level of consciousness should not be attributed to acute toxicologic causes. In addition to the transient effects of some overdoses, other agents (eg, thallium, carbon disulfide, carbon monoxide) may cause sustained gaze disorders due to residual cranial nerve and CNS injury.[31] Nystagmus and ophthalmoplegia due to thiamine deficiency usually improve after therapy, but nystagmus may not resolve completely.[70]

Ocular Caustic Exposures: First Aid and Initial Approach

The initial approach to all patients with ocular chemical exposures should be immediate decontamination by irrigation, using copious amounts of the most immediately available safe aqueous solution.[14,46,51] Irrigation is intended to accomplish at least four objectives: immediate dilution of the offending agent, removal of the agent, removal of any foreign body, and in some cases, normalization of anterior chamber pH. Water, normal saline, lactated Ringer's solution, and balanced salt solution (BSS) are all appropriate choices. In theory, BSS is ideal, because it is both isotonic and buffered to physiologic pH. Lactated Ringer's solution (pH 6 to 7.5) and normal saline (pH 4.5 to 7) are also isotonic and therefore theoretically preferable to water. There is no convincing evidence that the choice significantly affects outcome, and although lactated Ringer's solution, normal saline, and water cause more discomfort than BSS,[34] an ocular topical anesthetic is usually required for effective irrigation, thus negating this concern. As delays of even seconds can dramatically affect outcome,[31] there is no justification for waiting for another solution if water is the first available agent. Irrigation must include the conjunctival recesses, internal and external palpebral surfaces, and cornea and bulbar conjunctiva. Effective irrigation includes lid retraction and eversion or use of a scleral shell irrigating device. After irrigation, visual acuity testing, inspection of the eye, and slit-lamp examination should be completed. Fluorescein examination demonstrates corneal epithelial defects but not depth of the burn, corneal edema, or anterior chamber involvement, and by itself is therefore not an acceptable alternative to slit-lamp examination.

Should Exposure-Specific Irrigating Solutions Be Used?

Much literature has been written about ideal irrigating agents and specific antidotes, but it is clear that simple dilution and mechanical removal by immediate, copious irrigation with water or other safe aqueous solutions is always appropriate.[14,46,51,61] Despite theoretical concern, there is probably no toxic exposure for which standard aqueous solutions are contraindicated. Of greatest theoretical concern are agents such as white or yellow phosphorus, metallic sodium, and metallic potassium that may react violently in the presence of water, leading to heat, mechanical injury, and in the latter two cases, generation of sodium hydroxide and potassium hydroxide, respectively.[31] In one such case, after noting smoke coming from ocular phosphorus particles, copper sulfate solution (3%) was used after standard irrigation to decrease the reactivity of residual embedded phosphorus.[31] Conjunctival lesions healed quickly and recovery was rapid and complete, although there is no way to evaluate whether the use of copper sulfate improved the result. Although not well studied, irrigation with large amounts of water probably dissipates the heat of the initial hydration reaction with conjunctival moisture more than it initiates a thermochemical reaction. In addition to removing the offending material, irrigation serves to dilute and remove the alkaline byproducts formed by reaction with conjunctival water.

The use of irrigating solutions for more common exposures, including hydrofluoric acid and phenols, is also debated. For treatment of experimental hydrofluoric acid exposures (Chap. 86), calcium salt solutions are too irritating to the eye, but isotonic magnesium chloride solutions are effective in reducing injury and are not irritating.[41,42] Fortunately, from a practical standpoint, normal saline is equally effective, and thus there is no reason to use less readily available solutions. For phenol exposure, topical low-molecular-weight polyethylene glycol (PEG) solutions are effective for treatment of experimental skin exposure; for eyes, copious water irrigation appears to be as effective as PEG.[12] There is, however, a report of superior efficacy of PEG-400 over water in treatment of human phenol eye burns.[37] Although PEG-400 may be readily available at work sites where phenols are used, it is not a realistic option in the emergency department, and there should be no hesitation to use water, normal saline, lactated Ringer's solution, or BSS as lavage solutions. Ocular exposures to cyanoacrylate adhesives (eg, Super Glue, Krazy Glue) commonly result in rapid adherence between upper and lower eyelids that may persist for days. Such occurrences may be associated with corneal abrasions[19] but are otherwise relatively harmless. Management is problematic, as acetone or ethanol, which are often effective in dermal-to-dermal adhesions caused by cyanoacrylates, cannot be used safely on the eye.[60] Application of gauze pads soaked with mineral oil is successful but requires 36 hours of treatment.[10] Specific treatments of varying value, to be used after copious irrigation, are recommended for other unusual exposures. Consultation with a regional poison center or use of a comprehensive information source[31,60] should be considered in any case of suspected ocular toxic exposure involving unusual agents.

How Long Should Irrigation Be Continued?

In order to accomplish the goals of irrigation, as described, the appropriate duration will vary with the exposure. Most solvents, for example, do not penetrate deeper than the superficial cornea, and brief (10 to 20 minutes) irrigation is generally sufficient.[31] After exposure to acids or bases, normalization of the conjunctival pH is often suggested as a useful endpoint. Although theoretically sound, this practice has not been assessed in the clinical setting. When measured by sensitive experimental methods, normal pH of the conjunctival surface is 6.5 to 7.6.[1] This is highly method-dependent, however, and normal values in the literature range from 5.2 to 8.6.[15] When measured by touching pH-sensitive paper to the moist surface of the conjunctival cul-de-sac, normal pH is most often near 8.[3] Therefore, after irrigation following alkali burns, pH should not be expected to reach 7 and is more likely to stabilize near 8.[31] In this setting, lower pH values may indicate the pH of the irrigant, rather than the ocular surface. Waiting for an interval of several minutes between irrigation and pH testing will allow washout of any residual irrigant.[16] Choice of testing paper is important, as some are intended for use at extremes of pH and lack sensitivity in the clinically useful range.

Despite these limitations, a logical role for pH assessment can be described: probably a minimum of 2 L of irrigant per affected eye should be used before any assessment of pH; and then, after 7 to 10 minutes, the pH of the lower fornix conjunctiva should be checked. Thereafter, cycles of 10 to 15 minutes of irrigation followed by rechecks should be continued until the pH is 7.5 to 8. This is certainly adequate for exposures to weak acids, which do not penetrate well, and for apparently minor alkaline exposures.

For alkaline exposures with obvious severe symptomatology, and after burns from concentrated acids, normal surface pH is not an adequate endpoint (see the section on Alkali later in the chapter). After serious alkali burns, irrigation should be continued for at least 2 hours, regardless of surface pH, in an attempt to correct anterior chamber pH.[31,51,61] Following this lengthy irrigation, it is then logical to verify that conjunctival pH has normalized, and to continue irrigation if needed. This plan is also advisable for severe acid burns. In such cases, immediate ophthalmologic consultation is mandatory and irrigation should be continued until the consultant advises discontinuation. There is no evidence that prolonged irrigation helps prevent the effect of intraocular fluoride after hydrofluoric acid exposure; in fact, prolonged irrigation may actually lead to increased corneal disruption. Although not well studied, the same guidelines discussed for other acids are probably appropriate for irrigation after hydrofluoric acid exposures.

Other General Measures

There is a great deal of controversy regarding appropriate adjunctive therapy for chemical burns of the eye. In all cases in which serious injury is evident, the treatment plan should include discussion with an ophthalmologist. Generally, patients with corneal injury should be treated with an ocular topical antibiotic providing antistaphylococcal and antipseudomonal coverage. Cycloplegics not only reduce pain from ciliary spasm, but also decrease the likelihood of posterior synechiae formation. Eye patches and systemic analgesics also improve patient comfort. It is never appropriate to dispense topical ophthalmic anesthetic agents, because repeated use of these agents leads to further corneal disruption both by direct chemical effects and by eliminating corneal protective reflex sensation.

Ocular Caustic Exposures: Specific Agents

The effect of any chemical on the eye depends on the inherent properties of the agent (eg, solvents, detergents); the amount, concentration and pH of the agent; and the duration of exposure. The end result of ocular exposure to these agents depends on the extent of damage to the cornea, particularly the integrity and function of the stroma; chemical penetration into the anterior chamber and the resulting injury to its structures; and resultant inflammatory reaction.[31,46,51,52,54] Because similar chemicals tend to produce similar reactions, they can be conveniently grouped for discussion into acids, alkalis, and others.

Acids

Fortunately, weak acids do not penetrate the cornea well.[31,51] The hydrogen ion precipitates ocular proteins on contact, causing coagulation and thereby somewhat limiting the extent of penetration. The dehydrating effect of some acids, the heat of hydration, and the affinity of each anion for corneal tissues all affect the extent of injury. Intense pain usually results from stimulation of exposed nerve endings in the corneal epithelium. Corneal defects are common, but in many cases the damaged epithelium is swept away, revealing healthy underlying stroma to support normal repair of the epithelium. Strong acids can penetrate and damage deeper corneal tissue and structures of the anterior chamber and lead to the more serious sequelae, such as those often seen after alkali burns.[31,51] Prolonged exposure to weaker acids may result in significant extension of the injury and thus immediate irrigation is mandatory.

Hydrofluoric acid may cause unexpectedly severe injury due to its ability to penetrate deep into the eye.[8,41,42,59] Although 1% calcium gluconate eye drops have been advocated[8] to bind free fluoride, there is no evidence that this is beneficial. This treatment requires further study before it can be recommended, particularly because excess calcium has been suggested to be detrimental after alkali burns.[33]

Alkali

Alkali burns of the eye represent an ophthalmic emergency. A rational approach to care is based on an understanding of the complex pathophysiology of these injuries. In a minor burn, injury may be limited to destruction and lysis of corneal epithelium, causing a lesion similar to a corneal abrasion. If the amount is large or the concentration high, if the agent is a strong base (eg, sodium hydroxide) or has a tendency to penetrate (eg, ammonium hydroxide), or if the exposure is prolonged, deeper injury occurs.[31,54,58] Penetration into corneal stroma may destroy keratocytes, alter collagen structure, and damage the endothelium.[54] Paradoxically, more extensive burns may be less painful, due to destruction of corneal nerve endings and resultant anesthesia. In addition to indicating an increased depth of the burn, these stromal and endothelial injuries often impair the ability of the cornea to regenerate later and to maintain an adequate epithelium. Further penetration can cause the pH of the anterior chamber to rise significantly within 2 to 3 minutes.[49,54] Ammonium hydroxide is especially destructive by this mechanism, as it penetrates far more rapidly than other alkalis. Experimentally, 8.5% ammonium hydroxide increases anterior chamber pH within 15 seconds.[31] As a result, the sequelae of these exposures are severe and may be out of proportion to both pH and the degree of surface injury.

The increase in intraocular pH is injurious to the trabecular meshwork, iris, lens, and ciliary body and also triggers a sudden contraction of corneal and scleral collagen, leading to increased intraocular pressure and exacerbation of pain. A less dramatic but more sustained increase in intraocular pressure then ensues, resulting from intraocular prostaglandin release.[54]

In addition to these direct effects, further injury results from the inflammatory response to the initial injury. Dysfunction of the normal blood–aqueous humor barrier results in exudation of protein and inflammatory cells into the anterior chamber, leading to a severe fibrinous reaction. Fibrosis in turn can lead to permanent angle closure and glaucoma. On the opposite extreme, permanent dysfunction of the ciliary body can result in visual loss due to collapse of the eye (phthisis bulbi).[54]

The initial ocular examination may not reveal the full extent of injury, which may not be evident for 48 to 72 hours.[54] In the ensuing days to weeks, the balance between degradation of injured tissue and reconstruction and reepithelialization determines the outcome. After severe burns, normal repair is distinctly rare and extensive scarring is common. The goal of therapy is to prevent corneal ulceration, ocular perforation, and glaucoma while preserving the eye for possible secondary surgical revision or repair.

The mainstay of treatment is immediate and copious irrigation following the guidelines discussed. After exposures to calcium hydroxide (lime) from mortar or cement splashes, any adherent material must be found and removed. A sterile cotton-tipped applicator soaked in 0.05 molar disodium edetate (EDTA) may aid this process.[31,51,58] Follow-up is essential in all cases of alkali eye burns. Emergent consultation with an ophthalmologist should be obtained for all suspected severe burns. For isolated, very superficial corneal defects this is not necessary; however, if there is pain unrelieved by topical anesthetics, grossly evident corneal opacification, increased intraocular pressure, or any slit-lamp examination evidence of deep corneal burn, corneal edema, or anterior chamber cell or flare, immediate consultation is essential. These signs or symptoms suggest the possibility of serious corneal injury or penetration of alkali to deeper ocular structures.

Not only is comprehensive early evaluation important, but the advisability of several experimental or controversial treatments should be determined in conjunction with the ophthalmologist. Emergent needle paracentesis and lavage of the anterior chamber, when done early, removes alkali and returns pH to normal and also decreases intraocular pressure.[31,49,54] Animal studies suggest that this technique is useful, but its benefit has not been proved in human exposures, possibly due to delay in patient presentation and limited availability of expertise in the technique. In addition to antibiotics, and cycloplegics, topical steroids, citrate, and ascorbate may be advised. Early steroid treatment may decrease the inflammatory response, but continued use inhibits fibroblast function and healing.[21,54] Some ophthalmologists therefore suggest steroids only for the first 7 days. Well-controlled research supports the use of topical and systemic ascorbate and citrate.[50,53,55–57] The aqueous humor has ascorbate concentrations 15 to 20 times higher than blood. After alkali exposure, intraocular ascorbate concentrations decrease precipitously, suggesting that the local deficiency might result in impaired collagen synthesis and poor healing. In animals, both topical and systemic administration of ascorbate decreases the incidence of corneal ulceration after alkali burns. By a different mechanism of action, citrate is also effective in animal models. Apparently by chelation of calcium and magnesium,[33] citrate appears to inhibit chemotaxis, phagocytosis, and enzyme release by polymorphonuclear neutrophils. In rabbits, the combination of topical citrate and ascorbate was more effective against corneal ulceration than citrate alone.[53] Clinical trials of combinations of oral and topical ascorbate, citrate, and placebo have been initiated, but no results have yet been reported.

Other proposed early treatments have included chelators (cysteine, acetylcysteine, penicillamine) to inhibit collagenase and the use of dimethylsulfoxide, epidermal growth factor, fibronectin, hyaluronate, hypertonic ointments, immunosuppressants, platelet activating factor antagonists, progestins, superoxide dismutase, synthetic matrices, vasoconstrictors, and vasodilators.[5,6,17,31,65,66] Other than acetylcysteine, most are either experimental or have been abandoned. Newer efforts have focused on regeneration of adequate corneal support through delayed autologous conjunctival transplantation as a method to supply limbal stem cells.[63]

Other Chemical Exposures

Most solvents cause immediate pain and superficial injury due to dissolution of corneal epithelial fat, but do not penetrate or react significantly with deeper tissue.[31] The epithelial defect may be large or complete, but the limited depth of injury usually allows rapid regeneration. Detergents and surfactants cause variable injury, ranging from minor irritation from soaps to extensive injury from cationic agents such as concentrated benzalkonium chloride.[31] Fortunately, most agents do not effectively penetrate the cornea. Ocular exposure to A-200 pyrinate pediculocide shampoo causes typical detergent-surfactant injury, leading to extensive loss of corneal epithelium but with normal underlying stroma, and therefore complete healing within days.[31] Lacrimators (tear gas), such as chloracetophenone, stimulate corneal nerve endings and cause pain, burning, and tearing but produce no structural injury at low concentrations. At high concentrations, these agents can produce significant corneal injury.[31] Specific information on thousands of agents is readily available if necessary.[31,60]

Systemic Absorption and Toxicity from Ocular Exposures

Systemic absorption from ocular exposures has caused serious toxicity, morbidity, and death.[4,35] Although the patterns of toxicity are characteristic of the agents involved, recognition may be delayed due to a failure to appreciate the eye as a significant route of absorption. There is limited transcorneal diffusion and some mucosal absorption after nasolacrimal drainage, but most absorption is via conjunctival capillaries and lymphatics, and is markedly increased during conjunctival inflammation. Unlike the gastrointestinal route of absorption, there is no significant first-pass hepatic removal after ocular absorption and, therefore, bioavailability is much greater.[35,64] By the time toxicity is apparent, there is no role for ocular decontamination to prevent further absorption. After instillation of eye drops, absorption is generally complete within 7 minutes.

Children appear to be at greatest risk, possibly because of the higher relative drug dose they experience when systemic absorption does occur.[9,35,48] Diligent attempts to comply with prescribed dosing in a struggling, crying infant may result in excessive dosing. Also, as doses of ocular medications are typically not adjusted based on patient weight, the consequences of equivalent degrees of systemic absorption are much greater for an infant than for an adult. Toxicity from eye drops is also a problem among the elderly, probably due to the combination of greater use of potentially toxic ophthalmic medications and the presence of comorbid conditions.

Prevention of systemic toxicity from topical ophthalmic medications requires recognition of the risk, careful history taking before prescribing, use of the lowest effective concentration and dose, patient education, and proper administration. To minimize inadvertant absorption, the following is recommended: instillation of no more than two drops of any eye drop solution at one time in the superolateral corner of the eye, and gentle finger compression of the medial canthus.[35]

Mydriatics

Mydriatics are used almost exclusively to dilate the pupils prior to diagnostic evaluation of the eyes. This extraordinarily common practice is not generally considered to be potentially dangerous; however, the risk may be substantial if the precautions outlined are not considered. Anticholinergic poisoning (Chap. 34), including florid manifestations and fatalities, is well described after ocular use of atropine (Isopto Atropine), cyclopentolate (Cyclogyl), and scopolamine (eg, Isopto Hyoscine) eyedrops, especially in infants.

The use of the alpha-adrenergic agonist phenylephrine (Neo-Synephrine) eyedrops, in a 10% solution, has caused severe hypertension, subarachnoid hemorrhage, ventricular dysrhythmias, and myocardial infarction. Fortunately, these effects are rare if the 2.5% ocular phenylephrine is used. All phenylephrine preparations should be avoided in patients taking MAO inhibitors (Chap. 58). Mydriatics can also precipitate acute angle-closure glaucoma in susceptible individuals.

Miotics and Other Antiglaucoma Drugs

Maintaining miosis to prevent angle closure is an important part of glaucoma therapy. Anticholinesterase agents used for this purpose, such as echothiopate (Phospholine), exacerbate asthma, Parkinsonism, peptic ulcer, and cardiac disease. If neuromuscular blockade is required for patients using ocular anticholinesterases, an agent not metabolized by plasma cholinesterase (eg, atracurium, pancuronium, vecuronium, or tubocurarine) must be used. Succinylcholine and mevacurium are cleared by plasma cholinesterase and have profoundly prolonged effects when an anticholinesterase is present.[35] Because of their long duration of action and resultant risk of accumulation after repeated dosing, anticholinesterase agents are associated with the highest incidence of adverse reactions among susceptible patients.

Miosis can also be produced by use of direct cholinergic agonists, such as pilocarpine (Isopto Carpine), which have a much shorter duration of action. Although absorption is limited, nausea and abdominal cramps can occur at recommended doses. After excessive dosing, salivation, diaphoresis, bradycardia, and hypotension have occurred.

Beta-adrenergic antagonists, such as timolol (Timoptic), are used to lower intraocular pressure but have caused a variety of adverse effects, including bradycardia, hypotension, myocardial infarction, syncope, transient ischemic attacks, congestive heart failure, exacerbation of asthma, status asthmaticus, and respiratory arrest. Timolol has exacerbated symptoms in patients with myasthenia gravis and is implicated in both causing and masking symptoms of hypoglycemia in diabetics. Nonspecific complaints of anorexia, anxiety, depression, fatigue, hallucinations, headache, and nausea are also described after use of timolol eyedrops.

An ophthalmic formulation of a highly selective alpha-$_2$-adrenergic agonist, brimonidine (Alphagan), has now been introduced to treat glaucoma.[71] Systemic absorption of these eye drops in a child has led to bradycardia, hypotension, and decreased level of consciousness, similar to the central effects of other alpha-$_2$-adrenoceptor agonists (eg, clonidine).[9] Brimonidine, clonidine, and several imidazolines share similar signs of toxicity, apparently mediated through both alpha-$_2$-adrenoceptors and imidazoline receptors.[13]

Antimicrobials

Life-threatening reactions to ophthalmic antimicrobials are unusual but do occur. Episodes of aplastic anemia have occurred after prolonged use of chloramphenicol (Chloromycetin) eye preparations,[24] and Stevens-Johnson syndrome was reported after short-term use of ophthalmic sulfacetamide (Sulamyd) in a patient with a history of allergy to sulfa drugs.[30]

Toxicity to Ocular Structures from Nonocular Exposures

Ocular toxicity from systemic agents is almost always the result of chronic exposure, and the manifestations develop over a prolonged period of time. Thousands of substances are implicated, affecting every element of the visual system from the cornea to the optic cortex. Thorough discussion of this topic is beyond the scope of this text, but examples of causative agents are listed in Table 26–2.[20,22,25,31,36,69] Because many of these are commonly prescribed medications, adverse drug reactions should always be considered when patients present with visual abnormalities or unusual ocular findings on examination.

In the setting of emergency care, toxin-induced disturbances of normal vision from systemic exposures take many forms. Impaired near-vision from mydriasis, and diplopia or nystagmus from interference with normal control of extraocular movements, are examples of common, usually harmless, visual effects. Serious effects generally result from injury or dysfunction of the neural elements from the retina to the cortex. Such toxicity can be direct (neurotoxic) or indirect (hypoxia, ischemia). Many agents historically reported to cause acute visual loss directly are no longer available (Table 26–3).[31] Methanol and quinine are currently the most important agents that cause direct visual toxicity after acute oral poisoning. Many agents capable of causing vasospasm, hypotension, or embolization also cause acute visual loss (Table 26–3).[67] Hypoxia or ischemia can cause visual impairment, and many instances are reported after serious toxic exposures. Blindness and other visual defects are described following recovery from severe intoxication with barbiturates and other sedative-hypnotics, opioids, carbon monoxide, and many other drugs and toxins.[31]

TABLE 26–3. AGENTS REPORTED TO CAUSE VISUAL LOSS AFTER ACUTE EXPOSURES

Direct Causes
Methanol
Quinine
Lead[a]
Mercuric chloride[a]
Indirect Causes[b]
Amphetamines
Cocaine
Embolization of foreign material (parenteral steroids)
Cisplatinum
Combined endocrine agents (TRH with GNRH and glucagon)
Combined antihypertensive agents (alpha-methyldopa with propranolol, diazoxide with furosemide and atenolol)
Deferoxamine
Ergot alkaloids
Agents No Longer in Use[c]
Arsanilates
Arsenicals (organic)
Aspidium (*Dryopteris filix-mas*)
Cinchona derivatives (cinchonine, cinchonidine, ethyl hydrocupriene, isoamyl hydrocupriene)
Cortex granati (pomegranate bark)
Hexamethonium
Iodates
Phenazone (antipyrine)
Phodomyrtus (finger cherries)

[a]Distinctly rare with these poisonings.
[b]Distinctly rare with use of these agents; visual loss often instantaneous, secondary to sudden hypotension, vascular spasm, or embolization.
[c]Well-documented causes of visual loss, but no cases in recent decades.
Adapted, with permission, from Smilkstein MJ, Kulig KW, Rumack BH: Acute toxic blindness: Unrecognized quinine poisoning. Ann Emerg Med 1987;16:98–101.

Methanol

Formate, the byproduct of methanol metabolism (Chap. 64), appears to be the cause of visual toxicity from methanol poisoning. Evidence is accumulating that the primary event in ocular toxicity is the metabolism of methanol by retinal glial cells, which results in local elevation of formate concentration.[23,28,29,39,47] The exact effects of formate remain to be defined, but formate has been postulated to interfere with cytochrome oxidase and with the Na^+-K^+-ATPase system in the fibers of the optic nerve head.[38] Although the retina is the likely primary site of toxicity,[23,28,29,39,45,47] injury to the retinal ganglion cells and the retrobulbar optic nerve are also described, possibly as secondary effects. The visual signs and symptoms of methanol-induced visual disturbance include blurred or misty vision, "snowfield" vision, spots, central and peripheral scotomata, decreased light perception, and complete blindness.[7] The physical examination is consistent with the mechanism described: although in many patients with only mild visual impairment the examination may be normal, the most consistent finding in severe cases is initial hyperemia of the optic head, which later becomes edematous. The extension of the edema to the surrounding retina correlates with central scotomata, which are common. In severe cases, the edema may extend to large areas of the retina. In the most severe cases, when light perception is lost, the pupils may be widely dilated and unreactive.

In severe cases histopathologic examination reveals injury to the retinal ganglion cell layer and extension of the optic nerve injury to the retrobulbar nerve fibers.[29]

Optic atrophy often follows, and although central scotomata and peripheral visual field constriction are common, more complete visual loss may then occur. It is not currently possible to predict which patients will develop residual visual impairment, but the constellation of severe initial impairment, dilated and unreactive pupils, and widespread retinal edema implies a particularly poor visual prognosis.

The concentration and duration of formate exposure appears to be critical to the development of retinal toxicity, but there are not yet reliable estimates or practical methods of determining these variables after human poisoning. Therefore, any patient with acidemia after methanol poisoning is assumed to be at risk for retinal damage. As discussed in Chapter 64, the risk can be reduced by the administration of folate or folinic acid to enhance the elimination of formate and to prevent retinal folate depletion[28,29] (see Antidote in Depth: Folic Acid and Leucovorin [Folinic Acid]).

Quinine

The mechanism of quinine-induced visual impairment is less well understood, but it is known to involve neurotoxic injury to the optic nerve and perhaps retinal ganglion cells.[32] Visual symptoms may include blurred vision, central and peripheral scotomata, and complete blindness.[11] The onset of visual impairment varies, but sudden visual loss can occur as late as 14 hours or more after overdose.[67] Physical examination reveals pupils that are dilated and unreactive in proportion to the degree of visual impairment. Funduscopic examination is often completely normal but may show edema of the optic nerve, retina, or both, and retinal arteriolar constriction.[31] Retinal vasoconstriction was previously thought to be the cause of visual injury, and therapies such as vasodilators and stellate ganglion block were used in an attempt to reverse the vasospasm.[68] Further study has clearly shown complete blindness with normal vessels and recovery in patients with vasospasm.[27,67] Retinal vasoconstriction is therefore no longer thought to be of primary importance, although there is still speculation that vasospasm may have a modifying effect on outcome. Currently, there is no role for vasodilator therapy in these cases. Recovery is often very rapid, but residual impairment is common in severe cases. In a study of 225 cases of quinine poisoning, 70 patients developed visual impairment. Of 31 patients whose worst ocular manifestation was blurred vision, all had complete visual recovery. However, of 39 patients who developed complete blindness, only 17 had full recovery.[11] The most common residual effects are peripheral field defects and central scotomata. Impaired color vision and complete blindness may also persist, but this is less common. Varying degrees of visual impairment (quinine amblyopia) have resulted from quinine exposure in many forms, but complete blindness is reported only after oral ingestion of large amounts of quinine. As in methanol poisoning, it is difficult to predict which patients will develop quinine amblyopia, but it does appear to be dose related. Although it certainly occurs at lower levels, complete blindness should be expected if quinine serum levels exceed 20 mg/mL in the first 10 hours after ingestion (Chap. 44).[11]

Ocular Complications of Drug Abuse

In addition to the well-known ocular signs of opioid, cocaine, amphetamine, and phencyclidine intoxication, a number of complications may result from short- or long-term abuse of these and other agents.[43] Quinine amblyopia (see the preceding section) due to intravenous use of quinine-containing heroin is one of many ocular complications caused by injection of contaminants. Talc retinopathy was first described after prolonged intravenous abuse of methylphenidate (Ritalin),[26] but has subsequently been noted after intravenous use of heroin, methadone,[44] codeine, meperidine (Demerol), and pentazocine (Talwin). Talc retinopathy develops only after extensive drug abuse. In one study of intravenous methadone abusers, only patients who had injected more than 9000 tablets developed this complication. Infectious complications, such as fungal (*Candida, Aspergillus*) or bacterial (*Staphylococcus spp, Bacillus cereus*) endophthalmitis are well known as both direct effects of intravenous drug abuse and secondary complications of acquired immunodeficiency syndrome (AIDS). In addition to AIDS-related ophthalmic infections such as cytomegalovirus, cryptococcus, toxoplasmosis retinitis, and choroidal *Mycobacterium avium intracellulare*, other disorders include retinal cotton-wool spots, conjunctival Kaposi's sarcoma, and ocular motility disorders due to infectious or neoplastic meningitis. Corneal defects have been noted after smoking cocaine alkaloid ("crack eye").[62] Cocaine that is either volatilized or inadvertently introduced by direct contact, probably results in corneal anesthesia and loss of corneal protective reflex sensation. Minor trauma, such as eye rubbing, then leads to corneal epithelial defects. In addition, there appears to be an increased incidence of infectious keratitis and corneal ulceration in these patients. The ability of local anesthetics to interfere with corneal epithelial adhesion may also play a role.

References

1. Abelson MB, Udell IJ, Weston JH: Normal human tear pH by direct measurement. Arch Ophthalmol 1981;99:301.
2. Adams RD, Victor M: Disorders of ocular movement and pupillary function. In: Adams RD, Victor M, eds: Principles of Neurology, 3rd ed. New York, McGraw-Hill, 1985, pp. 194–210.
3. Adler IN, Wlodyga RJ, Rope SJ: The effects of pH on contact lens wearing. J Am Optom Assoc 1968;39:1000–1001.
4. Anonymous: Adverse systemic effects from ophthalmic drugs. Med Lett Drugs Ther 1982;24:53–54.
5. Bazan HE, Braquet P, Reddy ST, Bazan NG: Inhibition of the alkali burn-induced lipoxygenation of arachidonic acid in the rabbit cornea in vivo by a platelet activating factor antagonist. J Ocular Pharmacol 1987;3:357–365.

6. Ben-Hanan I, Landshman N, Assia E, Belkin M: Further evidence for the involvement of immunoregulatory processes in corneal alkali burns: Effects of immunosuppression and convalescent serum. Ophthalmic Res 1986;18:288–291.
7. Benton CD, Calhoun FP: The ocular effects of methyl alcohol poisoning: Report of a catastrophe involving 320 persons. Am J Ophthalmol 1953;36:1677–1685.
8. Bentur Y, Tannenbaum S, Yaffe Y, Halpert M: The role of calcium gluconate in the treatment of hydrofluoric acid eye burn. Ann Emerg Med 1993;22:1488–1490.
9. Berlin R, Sing K, Lee U, Steiner R: Toxicity from the use of brimonidine ophthalmic solution in an infant and reversal with naloxone. J Toxicol Clin Toxicol 1997;35:506. Abstract.
10. Bock GW: Skin exposure to cyanoacrylate adhesive. Ann Emerg Med 1984;13:486.
11. Boland ME, Brennand Roper SM, Henry JA: Complications of quinine poisoning. Lancet 1985;1:384–385.
12. Brown VKH, Box VL, Simpson BJ: Decontamination procedures for skin exposed to phenolic substances. Arch Environ Health 1975;30:1–6.
13. Burke J, Kharlamb A, Shan T, et al: Adrenergic and imidazoline receptor-mediated responses to UK–14,304–18 (brimonidine) in rabbits and monkeys. A species difference. Ann NY Acad Sci 1995;763:78–95.
14. Burns FR, Paterson CA: Prompt irrigation of chemical eye injuries may avert severe damage. Occup Health Saf 1989; 58:33–36.
15. Carney LG, Hill RM: Human tear pH: Diurnal variations. Arch Ophthalmol 1976;94:821–824.
16. Chen FS, Maurice DM: The pH in the precorneal tear film and under a contact lens measured with a fluorescent probe. Exp Eye Res 1990;50:251–259.
17. Chung J-H, Fagerholm P, Linstrom B: Hyaluronate in healing of corneal alkali wound in the rabbit. Exp Eye Res 1989;48:569–576.
18. Davson H: Physiology of the Eye, 5th ed. New York, Pergamon Press, 1990.
19. Dean BS, Krenzelok EP: Cyanoacrylates and corneal abrasions. J Toxicol Clin Toxicol 1989;27:169–172.
20. Devine SM, Newman NJ, Siegel JL, et al: Tacrolimus (FK506)-induced cerebral blindness following bone marrow transplantation. Bone Marrow Transplant 1996;18: 569–572.
21. Donshik PC, Berman MB, Dohlman CH, et al: Effect of topical corticosteroids on ulceration in alkali-burned corneas. Arch Ophthalmol 1978;96:2117–2120.
22. Drachman BM, DeNofrio D, Acker MA, et al: Cortical blindness secondary to cyclosporine after orthotopic heart transplantation: A case report and review of the literature. J Heart Lung Transplant 1996;15:1158–1164.
23. Eells JT, Salzman MM, Lewandowski MF, Murray TG: Formate-induced alterations in retinal function in methanol-intoxicated rats. Toxicol Appl Pharmacol 1996;140:58–69.
24. Fraunfelder FT, Bagby GC, Kelly DJ: Fatal aplastic anemia following topical administration of ophthalmic chloramphenicol. Am J Ophthalmol 1982;93:356–360.
25. Fraunfelder FT, Meyer SM, eds: Drug-Induced Ocular Side Effects and Drug Interactions, 3rd ed. Philadelphia, Lea & Febiger, 1989.
26. Friberg TR, Gragoudas ES, Regan CDJ: Talc emboli and macular ischemia in intravenous drug abuse. Arch Ophthalmol 1979;97:1089–1091.
27. Friedman L, Rothkoff L, Zaks U: Clinical observations on quinine toxicity. Ann Ophthalmol 1980;12:640–642.
28. Garner CD, Lee EW, Terzo TS, Louis-Ferdinand RT: Role of retinal metabolism in methanol-induced retinal toxicity. J Toxicol Environ Health 1995;44:43–56.
29. Garner CD, Lee EW, Louis-Ferdinand RT: Muller cell involvement in methanol-induced retinal toxicity. Toxicol Appl Pharmacol 1995;130:101–107.
30. Gottschalk HR, Stone Orville J: Stevens-Johnson syndrome from ophthalmic sulfonamides. Arch Dermatol 1976;112: 513–514.
31. Grant WM: Toxicology of the Eye, 3rd ed. Springfield, IL, Thomas, 1986.
32. Grant WM: The peripheral visual system as a target. In: Spencer PS, Schaumberg HH, eds: Experimental and Clinical Neurotoxicology. Baltimore, Williams & Wilkins, 1980, pp. 77–91.
33. Haddox JL, Pfister RR, Slaughter SE: An excess of topical calcium and magnesium reverses the therapeutic effect of citrate on the development of corneal ulcers after alkali injury. Cornea 1996;15:191–195.
34. Herr RD, White GL, Bernhisel K, et al: Clinical comparison of ocular irrigation fluids following chemical injury. Am J Emerg Med 1991;9:228–231.
35. Hugues FC, Le Jeunne C: Systemic and local tolerability of ophthalmic drug formulations. An update. Drug Saf 1993; 8:365–380.
36. Karp BI, Yang JC, Khorsand M, et al: Multiple cerebral lesions complicating therapy with interleukin-2. Neurology 1996;47:417–424.
37. Lang K: Treatment of phenol burns of the eye with polyethyleneglycol-400. Z Aerztl Fortbild (JENA) 1969;63:705–708.
38. Martin-Amat G, Tephly TR, McMartin KE, et al: Methyl alcohol poisoning: II. Development of a model for ocular toxicity in methyl alcohol poisoning using the Rhesus monkey. Arch Ophthalmol 1977;95:1847–1850.
39. Martinasevic MK, Green MD, Baron J, Tephly TR: Folate and 10-formyltetrahydrofolate dehydrogenase in human and rat retina: Relation to methanol toxicity. Toxicol Appl Pharmacol 1996;141:373–381.
40. McCarron MM, Schulze BW, Thompson GA, et al: Acute phencyclidine toxicity: Incidence of clinical findings in 1,000 cases. Ann Emerg Med 1981;10:237–242.
41. McCulley JP: Ocular hydrofluoric acid burns: Animal model, mechanism of injury and therapy. Trans Am Ophthalmol Soc 1990;88:649–684.
42. McCulley JP, Whiting DW, Petitt MG, Lauber SE: Hydrofluoric acid burns of the eye. J Occup Med 1983;25:447–450.
43. McLane NJ, Carroll DM: Ocular manifestations of drug abuse. Surv Ophthalmol 1986;30:298–311.
44. Murphy SB, Jackson WB, Dare JA: Talc retinopathy. Can J Ophthalmol 1977;95:861–868.
45. Murray TG, Burton TC, Rajani C, et al: Methanol poisoning: A rodent model with structural and functional evidence of retinal involvement. Arch Ophthalmol 1991;109:1012–1016.
46. Nelson JD, Kopietz LA: Chemical injuries to the eyes. Emergency, intermediate, and long-term care. Postgrad Med 1987;81:62–75.

47. Neymeyer VR, Tephly TR: Detection and quantification of 10-formyltetrahydrofolate deydrogenase (10-FTHFDH) in rat retina, optic nerve, and brain. Life Sci 1994;54:PL395–399.
48. Palmer EA: How safe are ocular drugs in pediatrics? Ophthalmology 1986;93:1038–1040.
49. Paterson CA, Pfister RR, Levinson RA: Aqueous humor pH changes after experimental alkali burns. Am J Ophthalmol 1975;79:414–419.
50. Petroutsos G, Pouliquen Y: Effect of ascorbic acid on ulceration in alkali-burned corneas. Ophthalmic Res 1984;16:185–189.
51. Pfister RR: Chemical injuries of the eye. Ophthalmology 1983;90:1246–1253.
52. Pfister RR: The effects of chemical injury on the ocular surface. Ophthalmology 1983;90:601–609.
53. Pfister RR, Haddox JL, Yuille-Barr D: The combined effect of citrate/ascorbate therapy in alkali-injured rabbit eyes. Cornea 1991;10:100–104.
54. Pfister RR, Koski J: Alkali burns of the eye: Pathophysiology and treatment. South Med J 1982;75:417–422.
55. Pfister RR, Paterson CA: Ascorbic acid in the treatment of alkali burns of the eye. Ophthalmology 1980;87:1050–1057.
56. Pfister RR, Paterson CA, Hayes SA: Topical ascorbate decreases the incidence of corneal ulceration after experimental alkali burns. Invest Ophthalmol Vis Sci 1978;17:1019–1024.
57. Pfister RR, Paterson CA, Spiers JW, Hayes SA: The efficacy of ascorbate treatment after severe experimental alkali burns depends on the route of administration. Invest Ophthalmol Vis Sci 1980;19:1526–1529.
58. Rozenbaum D, Baruchin AM, Dafna Z: Chemical burns of the eye with special reference to alkali burns. Burns 1991;17:136–140.
59. Rubenfeld RS, Silbert DI, Arentsen JJ, Laibson PR: Ocular hydrofluoric acid burns. Am J Ophthalmol 1992;114:420–423.
60. Rumack BH, ed: Poisindex Information System, Vol. 91. Denver, Micromedex, edition expires 2/28/97.
61. Saari KM, Leinonen J, Aine E: Management of chemical eye injuries with prolonged irrigation. Acta Ophthalmol 1984;161(suppl 16):52–59.
62. Sachs R, Zagelbaum BM, Hersh PS: Corneal complications associated with the use of crack cocaine. Ophthalmology 1993;100:181–191.
63. Sanghvi A, Basti S: Conjunctival transplantation for corneal surface reconstruction—Case reports and review of the literature. Ind J Ophthalmol 1996;44:33–38.
64. Shell JW: Pharmacokinetics of topically applied ophthalmic drugs. Surv Opthalmol 1982;26:207–217.
65. Singh G, Foster CS: Epidermal growth factor in alkali-burned corneal epithelial wound healing. Am J Ophthalmol 1987;103:802–807.
66. Skrypuch OW, Tokarewicz AC, Willis NR: Effects of dimethyl sulfoxide on a model of corneal alkali injury. Can J Ophthalmol 1987;22:17–20.
67. Smilkstein MJ, Kulig KW, Rumack BH: Acute toxic blindness: Unrecognized quinine poisoning. Ann Emerg Med 1987;16:98–101.
68. Valman HB, White DC: Stellate block for quinine blindness on a child. Br Med J 1977;1:1065.
69. Verschraegen C, Conrad CA, Hong WK: Subacute encephalopathic toxicity of cisplatin. Lung Cancer 1995;13:305–309.
70. Victor M, Adams RD: The effect of alcohol on the nervous system. In: Meritt HH, Hare CC, eds: Metabolic and Toxic Diseases of the Nervous System. Baltimore, Williams & Wilkins, 1953.
71. Walters TR: Development and use of brimonidine in treating acute and chronic elevations of intraocular pressure: A review of safety, efficacy, dose response, and dosing studies. Surv Ophthalmol 1996;41(suppl 1):S19–S26.

CHAPTER 27

Otolaryngologic Principles

William K. Chiang

Many toxins adversely affect the special senses of olfaction and gustation and cochlear-vestibular functions. These toxic effects are not life threatening and frequently not considered critical. Because of the lack of standardized testing techniques and normal parameters, particularly for olfactory and gustatory functions, there is a likelihood that adverse effects will be overlooked and dismissed by healthcare providers, despite significant patient distress and dysfunction. This chapter delineates the effects of toxins on these senses and examines the significant diagnostic information these senses contribute to the detection of toxins. Understanding the effects of toxins on these senses may allow for early detection of certain toxins, which can occasionally be lifesaving.

Olfaction

The sense of smell is an extremely sensitive detector of certain substances. Olfactory receptors can detect a few molecules of certain agents with a sensitivity that is orders of magnitude better than most sophisticated laboratory detection instruments.[62] Olfactory receptors are bipolar neurons located in the superior nasal turbinates and the adjacent septum. There are 10 to 20 million cells per nasal chamber, and the receptor portion of the cell undergoes continuous renewal.[100,103] The axons of these cells form small bundles that traverse the holes of the cribriform plate of the ethmoid bone to the dura. Within the dura, these bundles form connections with the olfactory bulb. Neural projections then connect to the olfactory cortex. There are extensive central interconnections to other parts of the brain, such as the hippocampus, thalamus, hypothalamus, and frontal lobe, suggesting effects on other biologic functions.[100] Although primary odor detection is a function of the olfactory (I) nerve, some irritant odors, such as ammonia and acetone, are transmitted through the trigeminal (V) nerve and its receptors.[41,131]

The actual olfactory receptor sites are structurally similar to taste receptors of the mouth and photoreceptors of the retina. The receptor consists of a single polypeptide chain consisting of approximately 350 amino acids, which folds back and forth on itself to transverse the cellular membrane seven times. The outer end of the polypeptide contains an amine group (*N*-terminal) and the cytosol end contains a COOH group (C-terminal). The transmembranous portions determine the receptor shape and characteristics of the binding site. When a molecule binds to a specific receptor site, the resultant conformational change leads to the activation of the G-protein system, and calcium and/or sodium channel activation and neurotransmission.[68]

What Are the Limitations of the Olfactory Senses?

A number of problems result from the utilization of smell as a toxicologic warning sign. Human olfaction is a variable trait.[5,109,151] Forty to forty-five percent of the population has specific anosmia for cyanide (a bitter almond smell) and androsterone (a woody smell of urine).[42,82,109] There are limited data on the inheritance characteristics or genetic basis of these specific forms of anosmia. While some studies suggest that the ability to detect the odor of cyanide is a sex-linked recessive trait,[53] other studies have yielded conflicting results.[5,20,84] Females have a greater ability to detect androsterone, which is also prominent in human underarm secretion.[62] Human olfaction usually can distinguish a mixture of no more than four substances,[88] and therefore specific odors may be masked by other stimuli.

Olfactory fatigue is the process of olfactory adaptation on exposure to a stimulus for a variable period of time, leading to temporal diminution of the smell. This adaptation may lead to a false sense of security with continued exposure to a toxin. For example, hydrogen sulfide, a toxin that binds to cytochrome oxidase, is readily detectable as a distinct and offensive substance at the very low concentration of 0.025 ppm. At the higher and potentially toxic concentration of 50 ppm, the odor is less offensive, and recognition may disappear after 2 to 15 minutes of exposure.[8,144] At even higher concentration, when toxicity is likely, the onset of olfactory fatigue is more rapid. The combination of the rapid onset of olfactory fatigue and toxicity at high concentrations of hydrogen sulfide exposure has contributed to numerous fatalities.[1,26]

In industrial settings, it is important to be aware of impaired olfactory function in any worker who may be exposed to chemical vapors or gases.[66,137] Such workers are at increased risk for toxic injury. The National Institute for Occupational Safety and Health (NIOSH) requires that an individual using an air-purifying respirator be able to detect a compound's odor at levels below those producing toxicity.[6,137] Sensory perception at this level ensures that the individual can detect filter cartridge "breakthrough" (failure) at a safe level.[137] The odor safety factor refers to the ratio of the time-weighted average threshold limit value (TLV) to the odor threshold for a given compound. A chemical with a high odor safety factor can be detected despite prolonged exposure.[6] Nontoxic agents, such as ethyl mercaptan, with a very high odor safety factor, can be added to agents with lower safety factors or no odor, so that olfactory detection is predictable. This is the premise for the addition of mercaptans to the odorless natural gases used in the home to limit the potential for unrecognized hazardous exposure.

How Can Odor Recognition Be Used Clinically?

The recognition of odors has traditionally been considered an important diagnostic skill in clinical medicine. Diseases can occasionally be diagnosed solely by a recognizable odor. Characteristic odors have been described: diabetic coma has a fruity odor, diphtheria has a sweetish odor, scurvy has a putrid odor, typhoid fever smells like fresh-baked brown bread, and scrofula has the odor of stale beer.[36] More recently, odors have been described for disorders of amino acid and fatty acid metabolism, such as phenylketonuria, maple syrup urine disease, hypermethioninemia, and isovaleric acidemia.[36]

The recognition of odors continues to be an important diagnostic skill for the rapid detection of toxins (Table 27–1). To increase the awareness of odors of toxic products, a simple and inexpensive "sniffing bar" may be prepared (Table 27–2).[57] Toxic odor-producing substances are placed in blood drawing tubes, numbered, and inserted in a test tube rack for circulation among staff. The sniffing bar, along with short descriptions of clinical presentations, and a table of diagnostic odors (Table 27–1), may be used to teach the recognition of odors in medical toxicology.[57]

What Are the Causes of Olfactory Impairment?

There are different types of olfactory dysfunction (Table 27–3). Anosmia, the inability to detect certain odors, and hyposmia, a decrease in the perception of certain odors, are the most common forms of olfactory impairment. The etiology of olfactory impairment may be classified as conductive, from anatomic obstruction of inspired air, or perceptive, from dysfunction of the olfactory receptors or signal transmission. Most conductive olfactory dysfunction results in hyposmia, since the obstruction is usually incomplete.[100,128]

TABLE 27–1. DIAGNOSTIC ODORS

Characteristic Odor	Responsible Toxin
Acetone (sweet, fruity, pearlike)	Lacquer, ethanol, isopropanol, chloroform, trichloroethane, paraldehyde, chloral hydrate, methylbromide
Alcohols	Ethanol, isopropyl alcohol
Automobile exhaust	Carbon monoxide (odorless, but associated with exhaust)
Bitter almond	Cyanide
Carrots	Cicutoxin (water hemlock)
Coal gas (stove gas)	Carbon monoxide (odorless, but associated with coal gas)
Disinfectants	Phenol, creosote
Eggs (rotten)	Hydrogen sulfide, carbon disulfide, mercaptans, disulfiram, *N*-acetylcysteine
Fish or raw liver (musty)	Zinc phosphide, aluminum phosphide
Fruitlike	Nitrites (amyl, butyl, etc), ethanol, isopropanol
Garlic	Phosphorus, tellurium, arsenic, parathion, malathion, selenium, thallium, dimethyl sulfoxide (DMSO)
Hay	Phosgene
Mothballs	Naphthalene, p-dichlorobenzene, camphor
Peanuts	*N*-3-pyridyl-methyl-*N*-p-nitrophenyl urea (Vacor)
Pepperlike	O-chlorobenzylidene malonitrile
Rope (burned)	Marijuana, opium
Shoe polish	Nitrobenzene
Tobacco	Nicotine
Vinegar	Acetic acid
Vinyl-like	Ethchlorvynol (Placidyl)
Violets	Turpentine (metabolites excreted in urine)
Wintergreen	Methyl salicylate

The most common causes of anosmia and hyposmia are viral infections, trauma, toxins, tumors, and congenital and psychiatric disorders (Table 27–3).[41,119,123,128,131] Viral infections may result in olfactory impairment either by obstructing nasal airflow or causing damage to the olfactory epithelium.[69] Trauma to the head or nose can shear fragile olfactory nerves crossing the cribriform plate. Up to 5% of patients with head trauma have some olfactory dysfunction.[131,146]

Following chronic exposure, numerous chemicals or toxins are associated with olfactory dysfunction (Table 27–3). The commonest toxic mechanism related is perceptive olfactory dysfunction. This may be due to a direct injury or structural alteration of the receptor, or components of the receptor such as G-proteins, adenylate cyclase, or receptor kinase.[67,68] Anosmia or hyposmia from hydrocarbons, formaldehyde, heavy metals such as cadmium, and antineoplastic agents such as cytarabine result from direct effects on the receptor sites.[45,68,73] Local effects on the epithelium and the receptors from antibiotic nosedrops may lead to temporary anosmia and hy-

TABLE 27–2. CASE STUDIES FOR "SNIFFING BAR"

Tube 1	
Case history:	A lethargic 28-year-old woman was brought to emergency department with an altered mental status.
Odor:	Vinyl-like smell
Toxin:	Ethchlorvynol
Contents of tube:	Liquid contents of Placidyl capsule
Tube 2	
Case history:	A 34-year-old man in cardiopulmonary arrest found in a chemical plant near several gas cylinders.
Odor:	Bitter almonds
Toxin:	Cyanide
Contents of tube:	Macerated seeds from inside of peach pit
Tube 3	
Case history:	A 5-year-old child ingested unknown rodenticide, presented to emergency department with orthostatic hypotension, hyperglycemia, ketoacidosis. A small sample of rodenticide had this odor.
Odor:	Peanuts
Toxin:	Vacor. (Odor is from a flavoring agent used in commercially available products.)
Contents of tube:	Macerated peanuts
Tube 4	
Case history:	A 27-year-old man was brought to emergency department with necrotic burns on his oral mucosa after gargling with an unknown liquid germicide. The patient thought that it would help his sore throat. The pH of the germicide was 5.
Odor:	White paste
Toxin:	Phenol
Contents of tube:	Phenol (liquefied) (<1% concentration)
Tube 5	
Case history:	A comatose 35-year-old man employed as sanitary engineer was pulled out of sewer by fellow worker. CPR was initiated. When he was brought to emergency department, the patient smelled like rotten eggs.
Odor:	Rotten eggs
Toxin:	Hydrogen sulfide
Contents of tube:	Sulfurated potash
Tube 6	
Case history:	A photographer was brought to the emergency department after unintentionally ingesting a chemical used in developing film.On presentation, patient was drooling and grasping his throat in considerable distress. On examination the patient's mouth and throat were erythematous and he smelled "like a salad."
Odor:	Vinegar
Toxin:	Glacial acetic acid
Contents of tube:	Vinegar
Tube 7	
Case history:	A crop duster was brought to the emergency department in acute respiratory distress. The patient had hypersalivation, miotic pupils (2 mm), a very unpleasant breath odor, and coarse rhonchi in both lung fields.
Odor:	Garlic
Toxin:	Organophosphate insecticide
Contents of tube:	Garlic
Tube 8	
Case history:	A 4-year-old child was brought to the emergency department with a temperature of 39.7°C, a respiratory rate of 32/min, and markedly altered mental status. Laboratory tests on admission showed a high anion gap metabolic - acidosis. The patient smelled like a "wintergreen candy."
Odor:	Oil of wintergreen
Toxin:	Methyl salicylate
Contents of tube:	Oil of wintergreen
Tube 9	
Case history:	A 3-year-old was brought to the emergency department in considerable pain. On examination, the child exhibited dysphagia and dysphonia, the oral mucosa appeared blistered and erythematous. The child's mother stated that he must have gotten into cleaning supplies.
Odor:	Ammonia
Toxin:	Ammonia
Contents of tube:	Ammonia (diluted household)
Tube 10	
Case history:	A 2-year-old was brought to the emergency department after vomiting and having what was described as a grand mal seizure. The child had been playing several minutes earlier in a storage closet.
Odor:	Moth balls
Toxin:	Camphor
Contents of tube:	Camphor

Reprinted, with permission, from Goldfrank LR, Weisman R, Flomenbaum N: Teaching the recognition of odors. Ann Emerg Med 1982;11:685.

TABLE 27–3. DIFFERENTIAL DIAGNOSIS OF DISORDERS OF SMELL

Hyposmia/Anosmia

- Chronic diseases
  - Cirrhosis
  - Renal failure
- Endocrine
  - Cushing's syndrome
  - Diabetes mellitus
  - Hypothyroidism
  - Pseudohypoparathyroidism
  - Gonadal dysgenesis (Turner's syndrome)
  - Hypogonadotropic hypogonadism (Kallmann's syndrome)
    - Primary amenorrhea
- Hereditary
  - Hydrocyanic acid (inability to smell)
- Infection (systemic)
  - Viral hepatitis
  - Influenza
  - Meningitis
- Local
  - Adenoid hypertrophy
  - Allergic rhinitis
  - Asthma
  - Cocaine
  - Cystic fibrosis
  - Gentamicin nose drops
  - Inflammatory—upper respiratory infections
  - Laryngectomy
  - Leprosy
  - Nasal polyposis
  - Sarcoidosis
  - Sinusitis
  - Sjögren's syndrome
  - Tumor of the nasopharynx
- Neurologic
  - Frontal lobe tumors
  - Multiple sclerosis
  - Parkinson's disease
- Nutritional
  - Vitamin B_{12} deficiency
  - Zinc deficiency
- Psychological
  - Hysteria
  - Malingering
- Toxicologic
  - Acrylic acid
  - Antihyperlipidemics: Cholestyramine, clofibrate, gemfibrozil, HMG-CoA reductase inhibitors
- Cadmium
- Chlorhexidine
- Formaldehyde
- Hydrogen sulfide
- Hydrocarbons (volatile)
- Methylbromide
- Pentamidine
- Sulfur dioxide

Dysosmia/Cacosmia/Phantosmia

- Disease states
  - Addison's disease
  - Head trauma
  - Hysteria
  - Hypothyroidism
  - Pregnancy
  - Rhinitis
  - Sinusitis
  - Temporal lobe epilepsy
- Toxicologic
  - Amebicides/antihelminthics: Metronidazole
  - Anesthetic local: Varied
  - Anticonvulsants: Phenytoin, carbamazepine
  - Antihistamines
  - Antihypertensives: ACE inhibitors, diazoxide
  - Antimicrobials
  - Antiinflammatory/antirheumatics: Allopurinol, colchicine, gold, *D*-penicillamine
  - Anti-Parkinsonian agents: Levodopa, bromocriptine
  - Antithyroid agents: Methimazole, methylthiouracil, propylthiouracil
  - Beta-adrenergic antagonists
  - Calcium channel blockers
  - Dental: Tooth pastes
  - DSMO (dimethylsulfoxide)
  - Diuretics: Ethacrynic acid
  - Insecticides
  - Lithium
  - Nicotine
  - Opioids: Varied
  - Sympathomimetics: Varied
  - Vitamin D

Definitions

Anosmia:	The loss of smell
Hyposmia:	A decreased perception of smell
Dysosmia:	A distorted perception of smell
Phantosmia:	Sensation of smell without stimulus
Aliosmia:	Sensation of unpleasant odor from a nominally pleasant stimulus (includes cacosmia and torqosmia)
Cacosmia:	Sensation of a foul smell
Torqosmia:	Sensation of the smell of burnt or metallic materials

posmia.[79,150] Inhaled corticosteroids may have both local effects on the epithelium as well as direct effects on both G proteins and adenylate cyclase.[68] Cocaine insufflation causes direct local effects as well as effects on receptor functions.[60,68]

Most people have selected congenital forms of anosmia to individual molecules, such as hydrogen cyanide, n-butyl mercaptan, trimethylamine, and isovaleric acid.[7,41] Some extreme forms of congenital anosmia are associated with other abnormalities, such as Kallmann's syndrome, a hereditary form of anosmia associated with hypogonadotropic hypogonadism. This form of anosmia is caused by agenesis of the olfactory bulbs and incomplete development of the hypothalamus.[41,131]

Dysosmia (or parosmia) is the distorted perception of smell (Table 27–3). Subclassifications of dysosmia include the perception of foul smell (cacosmia), the sensation of smell without a stimulus (phantosmia), and the sensation of the smell of a burnt or metallic material (torqosmia).[128] The etiologies are classified as peripheral or central. Peripheral etiologies include abnormalities of the nose, sinuses, and upper respiratory tract. Central etiologies may be related to disorders such as Addison's disease, hypothyroidism, temporal lobe epilepsy, and psychosis or conditions such as pregnancy.[41,100,129] How these conditions actually alter the perception of smell is unclear. A number of drugs or toxins with similar effects are listed in Table 27–3. Bromocriptine exerts its effect by affecting dopaminergic transmission and inhibiting adenylate cyclase. Levodopa also affects the dopaminergic transmission and chelates zinc, which is important in the maintenance of normal receptor functions.[68]

What Should Be Done to Evaluate Patients With Olfactory Disorders?

General evaluation of olfactory function should include a detailed history, focusing on types, duration, and progression of symptoms, recent illnesses, head and nose trauma, sinus problems, family history, occupational history, hobbies, medications, and drug history.[37,61] A complete physical examination and detailed examination of the nasopharynx and sinuses should be performed to assess the potential for inflammation or structural abnormality. A simple set of olfactory stimulants, such as ground coffee, almond extract, peppermint extract, and musk, should be used to test each nostril individually with the patient's eyes closed.[61,131] Trigeminal stimulants such as ammonia, acetone, or menthol may be used to identify malingerers denying all odors. Because these agents depend not on olfactory (I) nerve function but on the trigeminal (V) nerve, a patient who has olfactory nerve damage should nevertheless be able to detect these substances. Conversely, a malingerer may deny detection of these substances also.[61,131,150] Radiographs of the sinuses and nose or CT scan of the nose, sinuses, and brain may be required if structural abnormalities are suspected.[131,150] Gas chromatographic analysis of the urine may be useful in patients with fish odor syndrome associated with trimethylaminuria.[89,136] Complicated cases and patients with significant impairment should be referred to an otolaryngologist or neurologist.

Gustation

Taste, the sensory interpretation of orally ingested materials, is determined by taste buds on the tongue, palate, throat, and upper third of the esophagus. The cells in the taste buds are constantly renewed, and have a life span of 10 days.[11,128] The taste buds on the anterior two thirds of the tongue and the palate are innervated by the facial (VII) nerve, those on the posterior one third of the tongue by the glossopharyngeal (IX) nerve, and those on the laryngeal and epiglottal regions by the vagus (X) nerve. There are at least 13 known chemical taste receptors responsible for the four primary taste sensations, sweet, sour, bitter, and salty: two sodium receptor types, two potassium receptor types, one chloride receptor, one adenosine receptor, one ionosine receptor, two sweet receptor types, two bitter receptor types, one glutamate receptor, and one hydrogen ion receptor.[63] The structure of the taste receptors is similar to that of the olfactory receptors mentioned earlier, as they are coupled to G proteins and sodium and calcium channels permitting neural stimulation. The pH of the substance determines sour or acid taste, while sodium or potassium concentrations determine salty taste. Many substances will activate the sweet receptors, such as sugars, glycols, aldehydes, ketones, amides, amino acids, inorganic salts of lead, and bretylium. Bitter taste many be the result of long-chain organic substances containing nitrogen, or alkaloids, including quinine, strychnine, caffeine, and nicotine.[63] Salivary proteins, such as zinc-containing gustin and ebnerin, are important in the regulation of taste sensation.[68,70,72,90,135] These molecules may serve as binding proteins and growth factors for the regeneration of taste receptors. Taste is also affected significantly by the appreciation of aromas or odors and, to a lesser extent, by visual perception.[129]

What Causes Gustatory Impairment?

Types of gustatory dysfunction include ageusia, inability to perceive taste; hypogeusia, diminished sensitivity of taste; and dysgeusia, distortion of normal taste. There are several variations of dysgeusia, such as cacogeusia, which is a perceived foul, perverted, or metallic taste.[63,103] Taste impairment is commonly related to direct damage to the taste receptors, adverse effects on their regeneration, or effects on receptor mechanisms.[68] These effects can result from various pharmacologic and toxicologic agents, diseases, aging, and nutritional disorders (Table 27–4).[56,63,122,128,142] Any abnormality that interferes with either the direct contact of a substance with the gustatory cells of the tongue or cranial nerves VII, IX, or X will dramatically affect taste.[128] Most common forms of toxin or drug-induced dysgeusia are related to direct ef-

TABLE 27–4. DIFFERENTIAL DIAGNOSIS OF DISORDERS OF TASTE

Hypogeusia/Ageusia

Endocrinologic: Cushing's syndrome, cretinism, hypothyroidism, diabetes mellitus, gonadal dysgenesis, pseudohypoparathyroidism

General: Renal failure, cirrhosis, hepatitis, hypertension, hysteria, niacin deficiency, deficiency of copper, nickel, or zinc, alcoholism, aging

Local: Neoplasm of mouth, Sjögren's syndrome, laryngectomy, radiation therapy, glossitis, thermal burn, upper respiratory infections, lichen planus, candidiasis

Neurologic: Ear trauma or surgery, familial dysautonomia, Parkinson's disease, multiple sclerosis, head trauma, nerve injury (lingual nerve, chlorda tympani, or glossopharyngeal), Bell's palsy, migraine headache(?)

Toxicologic: Pyrethrins, carbon monoxide, cocaine, gasoline, penicillamine, spironolactone, hydrochlorothiazide, amiloride, nitroglycerine, DMSO (dimethylsulfoxide), smoking, phenylbutazone, methylthiouracil, amrinone, triazolam, captopril, enalapril, propranolol

Dysgeusia

Hereditary (phenylthiourea)

Pregnancy

Glossitis

CNS disorders (uncinate lesions, Raeder's paratrigeminal syndrome, multiple sclerosis)

Dengue fever

Zinc deficiency

Local: Influenza, radiation therapy, laryngectomy

Botulism (in recovery)

Toxicologic: Griseofulvin, ACE inhibitors, nicotine, DMSO (dimethylsulfoxide), quinine, 5-fluorouracil, adriamycin, levodopa, amphotericin B, nifedipine, carbamazepine, bretylium, ibuprofen, naproxen, isotretinon

Cacogeusia

Local: Gingival disease, dental abscess, lingual disease, sarcoidosis

Gastrointestinal disease: Esophageal diverticulum

Pulmonary disease: Abscess, bronchiectasis

Metallic Taste

Chronic renal failure

Toxicologic

Acetaldehyde	Ethambutol	Metronidazole
Allopurinol	Ferrous salts	Pentamidine
Arsenicals	Flurazepam	Procaine penicillin
Cadmium	Iodine	Propafenone
Ciguatoxin	Lead	Snake envenomation
Copper	Levamisole	Tetracycline
Coprinus spp	Lithium	
Dipyridamole	Mercury (elemental and salts)	
Disulfiram	Methotrexate	
Enalapril	Metoclopramide	

fects on the taste receptor site or effects related to receptor mechanisms such as G proteins, adenylate cyclase, and calcium channels.[87] Other forms of dysgeusia may result from direct stimulation of chemical receptors by drugs or toxins.[63,68]

Angiostensin-converting enzyme (ACE) inhibitors such as captopril, enalapril, and lisinopril commonly cause gustatory impairment, usually hypogeusia and dysgeusia.[19,58,99,152] ACE inhibitors work by inhibiting zinc-dependent ACE, and chelating zinc from taste receptors and salivary proteins resulting in taste dysfunctions. Calcium channel blockers act by inhibiting calcium channels of the taste receptor mechanisms.[63] Many diuretics cause zinc depletion by enhancing zinc elimination in the urine.[68] In addition, furosemide and spironolactone may also chelate zinc as a second mechanism involved in zinc depletion. Numerous other substances also cause gustatory dysfunction through variable degrees of zinc chelation, such as amrinone, ethambutol, hydralazine, methyldopa, the nonsteroidal antiinflammatory drugs (NSAIDs), the antithyroid agents, and penicillamine.[63,68] Heavy metals such as arsenic, mercury, chromium, and lead may either chelate zinc or replace zinc in salivary proteins due to a higher level of affinity. Antineoplastic agents and antimicrotubular agents such as colchicine inhibit cellular division and taste receptor regeneration.[65] The oral antiseptic agent, chlorhexidrine directly alters taste receptor function.[51] Acetazolamide causes cacogeusia when carbonated beverages are consumed. The exact mechanism is unclear, but is postulated to be due to the inhibition of carbonic anhydrase causing carbon dioxide accumulation and an increased tissue bicarbonate.[68,80,101]

What Role Can Taste-Aversive Agents Have in Poison Prevention?

Nontoxic taste-aversive agents are frequently added to products such as shampoo, cosmetics, cleaning and automotive products, and rubbing alcohols to discourage ingestion.[65] Except in the case of rubbing alcohol, this is done primarily to prevent poisoning in children. The most common taste-aversive agents are the denatonium salts, particularly denatonium benzoate (Bitrex), one of the most bitter tasting substances known.[25,40] The bitter taste of denatonium benzoate can be detected at 50 parts per billion (ppb). This agent is used in concentrations of 6 to 50 parts per million (ppm), typically 6 ppm in cosmetic products and ethanol and 30 to 50 ppm in methanol and ethylene glycol.[16,110] Only limited data are available on the utility of taste-aversive agents for prevention of poisoning. Denatonium benzoate added to liquid detergent and orange juice can decrease the amount ingested by children.[13,138] However, the degree of taste aversion is not universal; in one study, some children were noted to take more than one sip of denatonium benzoate-laced orange juice.[138] Taste aversion is partially a learned response; frequently young children do not find bitter taste as offensive as do adults.[14] It seems unlikely that taste-aversive agents will eliminate unintentional ingestions in children, because oral ingestion is required for aversive effects to occur. Taste-aversive agents may be most beneficial in the prevention of poisoning by moderately toxic and nonaversive products, such as ethylene glycol, methanol, paraquat, certain pesticides, acetonitrile, and bromate-containing cosmetics where more than one or two sips of product must be ingested to cause toxicity. Taste aversive agents are not and cannot be substitutes for other poison prevention modalities.

Hearing

Normal hearing begins when sound waves traverse the external auditory canal. They are then conducted to the tympanic membrane, the auditory ossicles of the middle ear, and through the oval window to the perilymph in the scala vestibuli of the cochlea (Figs. 27–1 and 27–2). The wave is then transferred through Reissner's membrane at the roof of the cochlear duct, to the endolymph and the organ of Corti.[48,139] The specialized hair cells of the organ of Corti convert mechanical waves into neurologic signals, which are then transmitted via the cochlear nerve.[39,91] Neurologic transmission is then conducted to the cochlear nucleus of the pons; bilateral projections are sent to the superior olivary nucleus of the midbrain, nuclei of lateral lemnisci, inferior colliculus, medial geniculate body of the thalamus, and then to the auditory cortex of the temporal lobe.[139] Interruption or damage to any part of the hearing mechanism may lead to auditory impairment (Table 27–5).

The anatomy and physiology of the cochlea and its importance in the biomechanics of hearing are reviewed to understand the potential for toxicologic injury. The word "cochlea" is derived from the Greek word "kochlias," meaning snail, and describes its general structure of a 2 1/2-turn spirally wound tube. The cochlea is further divided into 3 inner tubular structures, the upper tube or scala vestibuli, the middle tube or cochlear duct, and the lower tube or scala tympani. The scala vestibuli and the scala tympani contain the perilymph fluid. The cochlear duct contains endolymph fluid, Reissner's membrane at the roof, and the organ of Corti.[139] The cochlear fluids serve multiple functions: to conduct sound waves to the hair cells, to provide nutrients and waste removal for the cells lining the cochlear duct, and to control pressure distribution in the cochlea, and to maintain an electrochemical gradient for the function of the hair cells. The sodium concentration of the perilymph is similar to that of the extracellular fluid, and the potassium concentration of the endolymph is similar to that of the intracellular fluid.[50] Any significant alterations of the sodium or potassium concentrations will depress cochlear potential and function. The stria vascularis controls the production of the cochlear fluids and maintains the electrochemical gradient between the endolymph and the perilymph. The stria vascularis contains a high concentration of the oxidative enzymes, Na-K-ATPase, adenylate cyclase, and carbonic anhydrase, which are highly susceptible to toxins.[21,74,126]

Although human speech is composed of sounds in the frequency of 250 to 3000 Hz, humans can normally detect sounds in the frequency range of 20 to 20,000 Hz.[108] The cochlea is a "tuned" structure with varying width and stiffness, such that different regions can re-

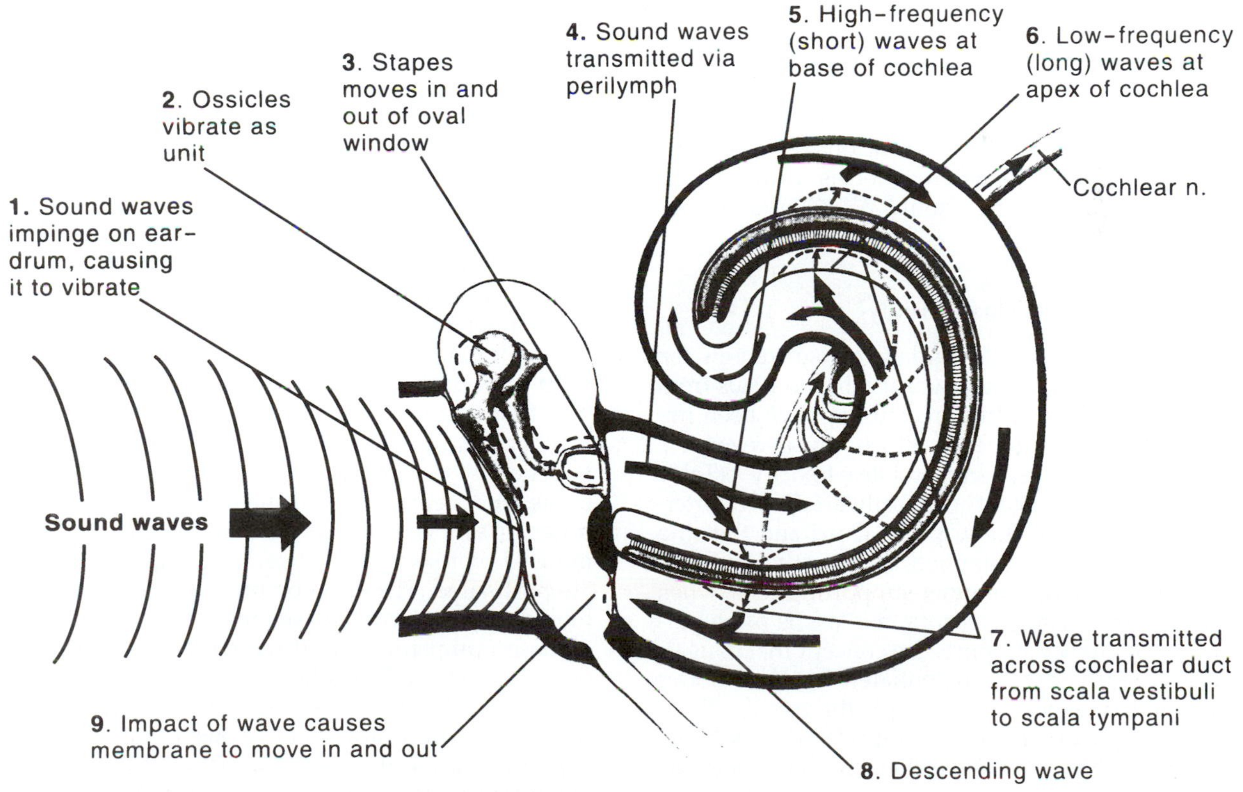

Figure 27–1. Pathways of sound conduction in the ear. *(Reproduced, with permission, from Silverstein H, Wolfson RJ, Rosenberg S: Diagnosis and management of hearing loss. Clin Symposia 1994;44:3.)*

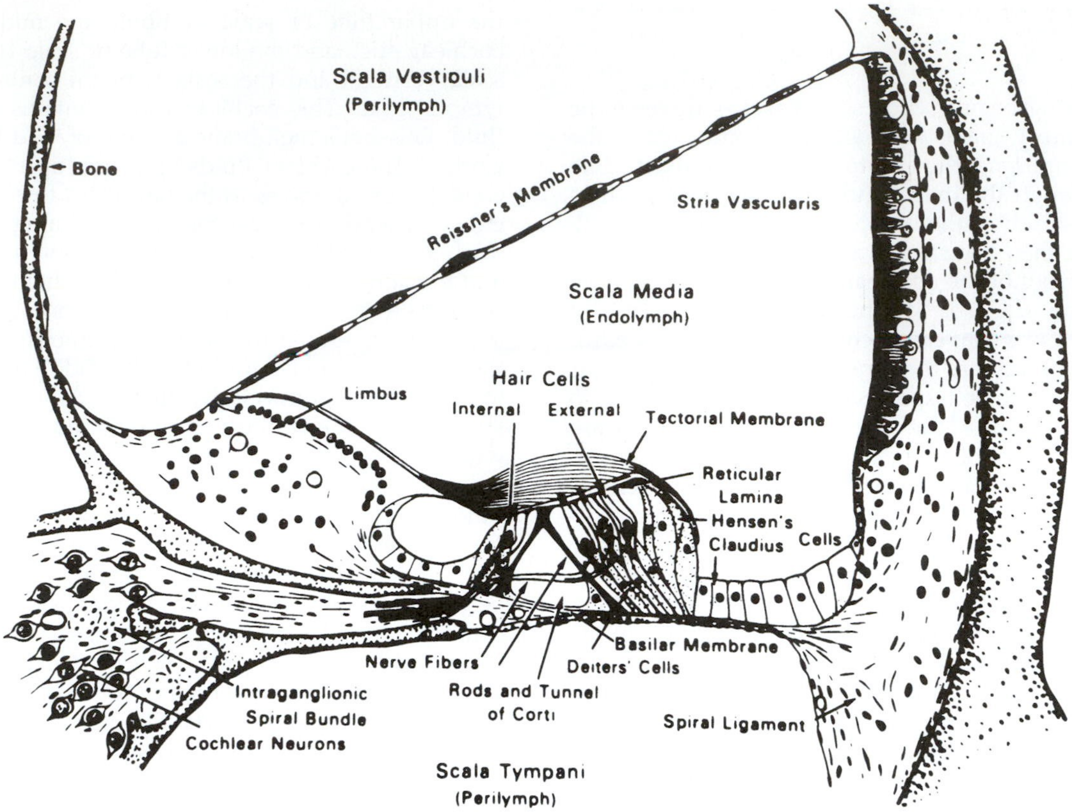

Figure 27–2. Cross-section of the organ of Corti. *(Reproduced, with permission, from Davis H: Advances in the neurophysiology and neuroanatomy of the cochlea. J Acoust Soc Am 1962;34:1379.)*

ceive different sound waves. The stiffer and wider base of the cochlea serves as a receptacle for higher-frequency sounds, whereas the apex is responsible for receiving the lower-frequency sounds.[48] Because various regions of the cochlea are susceptible to different forms of injury, appropriate audiologic testing should be tailored specifically to each patient.[28]

Which Drugs or Toxins Result in Ototoxicity?

Ototoxicity from drugs was widely recognized in the 1800s from quinine and salicylates and in the 1940s from streptomycin.[74,124] Several hundred drugs have been implicated as ototoxins, some of which cause reversible ototoxicity and others, irreversible toxicity (Table 27–5).[24,78,85,105] Ototoxic agents primarily affect two different sites in the cochlea: the organ of Corti and the stria vascularis. Because of the limited regenerative capacity of the sensory hair cells and other supporting cells, when significant cellular damage occurs, the loss is often permanent.[43,48,74] Evidence supports the concept that drug or toxin-related injury can be potentiated by loud noises and other ototoxic agents.[21,24,74,78] While the actual cellular mechanisms for many forms of drug-related toxicity remains unclear, some of the mechanisms have been recently elucidated.

Loop diuretics, such as furosemide, bumetanide, and ethacrynic acid, cause physiologic dysfunction and edema at the stria vascularis, resulting in reversible hearing loss.[74,95] The underlying mechanisms appear to be the inhibition of potassium pumps and G proteins associated with adenyl cyclase.[9] Physiologic studies of loop diuretics demonstrated the decrease in potassium activity in the endolymph and a decreased endocochlear potential.[125] Permanent hearing loss associated with furosemide and ethacrynic acid has been reported, and may be related to direct interference with oxidative metabolism in the outer hair cells.[86,95,125]

Salicylates are well known to cause ototoxicity. Aspirin (acetylsalicylic acid)-induced hearing impairment was first reported in 1877.[81] Salicylate-induced hearing loss is generally mild to moderate (20 to 40 dB loss) and is generally reversible.[18,76] Animal studies demonstrate immediate hearing impairment with the use of high doses of salicylates.[17,97,114] The mechanism of salicylate-induced ototoxicity is unclear, although multiple factors are postulated. The effect on prostaglandin synthesis (inhibition of cyclooxygenase) may interfere with Na-K-ATPase pump function at the stria vascularis, and also decrease cochlear blood flow.[30,46,81] Reversible decrease in outer hair cell turgor secondary to membrane permeability changes may impair otoacoustic emissions.[115,118] In support of these theories, pretreatment of animals with leukotriene antagonists and alpha-adrenergic receptor antagonists attenuates or prevents salicylate-induced ototoxicity.[81]

TABLE 27–5. ETIOLOGY OF HEARING LOSS

Infectious
- Otitis media, mumps, rubella, herpes zoster, syphilis, tuberculosis, cytomegalovirus

Trauma
- Perforated tympanic membrane, temporal bone fracture

Environmental
- Acoustic trauma

Neoplastic
- Acoustic neuroma, meningioma, glomus tumor

Systemic
- Sarcoidosis, giant cell granuloma, histiocytosis, collagen vascular disease, Paget's disease, Behçet's syndrome, Hurler's syndrome

Local
- Obstructed ear canal from cerumen or foreign body, Meniere's disease, otosclerosis, congenital cochlear deformity

Drugs and Toxins:

Primarily reversible
- Antimicrobials
  - Erythromycin, quinine, chloroquine
- Carbon monoxide
- Diuretics
  - Furosemide, bumetanide, ethacrynic acid, acetazolamide, mannitol
- NSAIDs
  - Ibuprofen, indomethacin, piroxicam, naproxen, sulindac, ketoprofen, mefenamic acid
- Salicylates

Primarily irreversible
- Antimicrobials
  - Aminoglycosides (kanamycin, neomycin, gentamicin, tobramycin, streptomycin, netilmicin, amikacin), vancomycin
- Anti-neoplastics
  - Cisplatin, vincristine, vinblastine, nitrogen mustard, bleomycin
- Bromates
- Heavy metals
  - Arsenic, mercury, lead
- Hydrocarbons
  - Toluene, xylene, styrene

Nonsteroidal antiinflammatory drugs (NSAIDs) and the cinchona alkaloid quinine also cause reversible hearing loss, particularly at the higher frequencies.[32,74] Occasionally, quinine-induced hearing loss may be permanent.[74,127] The primary mechanism is related to the prostaglandin inhibition.[81] The NSAIDs inhibit cyclooxygenase, which converts arachidonic acid to prostaglandin G_2 and prostaglandin H_2. Quinine inhibits phospholipase A_2 enzyme, which converts phospholipids to arachidonic acid. Quinine also inhibits calcium channels that interact with prostaglandins.[81]

Antineoplastic agents, such as cisplatin, vinblastine, and vincristine, can cause permanent ototoxicity.[74] Cisplatin is the most toxic of the group, with clinically apparent hearing loss noted in 30 to 70% of the patients receiving doses of 50 to 100 mg/m^2. Children may be even more suspectible to ototoxcity. These agents typically damage the outer hair cells but may also affect the stria vascularis.[74] The underlying mechanisms may be related to the inhibition of adenylate cyclase in the stria vascularis, the inhibition of protein synthesis, and the formation of oxygen free radicals.[9,74,132]

The aminoglycosides are the best known group of drugs associated with irreversible ototoxicity.[113] Neomycin and kanamycin are the most toxic of these agents, although all aminoglycosides are potentially toxic.[86] With the development of newer aminoglycosides and drug monitoring, the incidence of aminoglycoside-related ototoxicity appears to be decreasing. The reported rates of ototoxicity for the more commonly used aminoglycosides gentamicin and tobramycin are between 5 and 8%.[94] In China, where aminoglycosides are readily available over the counter, up to 66% of deaf-mutism may be secondary to aminoglycoside toxicity.[52,92] Aminoglycosides are not concentrated in the cochlear or the renal cells. Few mechanisms of ototoxicity have been postulated. Aminoglycosides antagonize calcium channels of the outer hair cells of the cochlea, blocking transduction of the hair cells and resulting in acute reversible hearing deficits. Aminoglycosides bind to polyphosinositides of cell membranes and alter their functions. Polyphosphoinositides are essential for the generation of second messengers diacylglycerol and inositol trisphosphate and their cellular functions, for the maintenance of lipid membrane structure and permeability, and as a source for arachidonic acid.[147] Aminoglycosides also inhibit ornithine decarboxylase. The inhibition of this enzyme, important for cellular recovery following an injury, makes the cell more susceptible to toxicity.[126] It has been postulated that toxicity is related to the metabolites of aminoglycosides and not the parent compounds, because toxicity can only be reproduced in in vivo models and not in vitro.[126] The other hair cells of the cochlea are increasingly susceptible to aminoglycosides and damage progresses from the inner row of the outer hair cells to the basal turn of the cochlea, and ultimately to the apex.[4,7,86,121] Therefore, high-frequency hearing is most vulnerable, and early or limited impairment may not be noticeable unless audiometry (especially at 8 kHz and above) is performed.[147] Hearing tests in infants can be performed using the nonbehavioral method based on the measurement of auditory brainstem response.[12] The risks of ototoxicity are increased with prolonged duration of therapy (greater than 10 days), concomitant use of other ototoxic agents, and elevated serum levels.[7,49] In animal models, certain free radical scavengers such as glutathione, WR–2721, and deferoxamine decrease aminoglycoside-induced ototoxicity.[54,127,141] Fosfomycin, a phosphonic antibiotic, has also demonstrated limited efficacy in reducing aminoglycoside-induced ototoxicity.[107] Further studies will be required to elucidate the mechanisms of protection and their applicability to humans.

Other antibiotics are also implicated as causing ototoxicity, particularly erythromycin, vancomycin, and their respective analogues. There are a number of human reports of hearing loss following erythromycin therapy and an animal study supporting the otoxic potential. Most human deficits are transient, although several cases of permanent hearing loss are reported.[22,23] The mechanisms of toxicity remain unclear although the proposed effects are on the central auditory pathways. Erythromycin-induced hearing loss occurs at both lower and higher frequencies for speech, allowing for recognition in the early stages of ototoxicity.[22] Ototoxicity from the newer macrolide antibiotics has not been reported.

The evidence for vancomycin-induced ototoxicity is less convincing. Although numerous cases of presumed vancomycin-related ototoxicity are reported, concomitant use of other ototoxic antibiotics was common or audiometric studies were not performed. In limited animal studies, vancomycin alone did not induce ototoxicity, but the agent increases ototoxicity when administered concomitantly with an aminoglycoside. Vancomycin analogues such as teichoplanin and daptomycin probably have similar ototoxic potentials.

Bromates are among the most extensively studied ototoxic agents.[93,116] Bromates are used in hair neutralizers, bread preservatives, and as fuses in explosive devices.[75,116,143] The stria vascularis and hair cells of the organ of Corti can be irreversibly damaged with significant exposure.[116] Bromates may also cause renal failure with substantial exposure, perhaps increasing the ototoxic potential.[75,116] It is intriguing that agents such as the bromates and aminoglycosides primarily affect both the cochlea and the kidneys. One possible explanation is that the stria vascularis and the renal tubules have similar functions in maintaining electrochemical gradients.[116,117] However, renal tubules may regenerate while damage to the hair cells and the stria vascularis of the cochlea is more likely to be permanent.

Other agents also implicated as ototoxins are carbon monoxide, lead, arsenic, mercury, toluene, xylene, and styrene.[71,137] However, both human and animal data are quite limited. A number of chemicals, such as carbon disulfide, carbon tetrachloride, and trichlorethylene, are suspected of being ototoxic, but toxicity has not been demonstrated in humans.[71,137] Since exposures to chemicals and toxins are frequently occupational, they are of great concern as they may potentiate or be additive to other types of occupational hearing impairments.[83,120]

Noise-Induced Hearing Impairment

Noise-induced hearing impairment had been recognized for hundreds of years, but became of great concern and prevalent with the discovery of gunpowder and the industrial revolution.[48] Some of the anatomic changes in the organ of Corti and the audiometric features of noise-induced hearing impairment were well described by 1900.[2,3,98] Few longitudinal studies on noise-induced hearing impairment have been performed.

Although noises of sufficient magnitude may cause hearing impairment with limited exposure, most noise-induced hearing losses result from preventable prolonged cumulative occupational exposure. The National Institute for Occupational Safety and Health has estimated that up to 1.7 million workers in the United States between 50 and 59 years of age have significant occupational hearing loss.[108] Noise can be defined as any unwanted sound, which can be further characterized by duration, time pattern (continuous, intermittent, or impulsive), frequency, and intensity. The intensity is measured in sound pressure levels (SPL) and expressed in a logarithmic scale in decibels (dB). The intensity of a normal conversation is approximately 65 dB (Table 27–6).[108] The risk of noise-induced hearing loss is related to cumulative duration of exposure, intensity, and individual susceptibility.[106,111,149] Much of the risk assessment of noise-induced hearing loss is inexact. Most authorities agree that sounds with maximal intensity below 75 to 80 dB will not cause hearing impairment, regardless of the duration of exposure.[106] At higher intensity, the risk of hearing impairment increases with increased duration of exposure. Continued occupational exposure at 90 to 94 dB will typically cause some high-frequency hearing loss in approximately 10 years.[2,111] Further exposure will result in hearing loss in the lower-frequency range. The Occupational Safety and Health Administration (OSHA) has established guidelines for permissible occupational noise exposure, based on an analysis of the average intensity and duration of exposure (Table 27–7).[2,149]

The pathophysiology of noise-induced hearing impairment is related to an excessive energy impact on the cochlea, but the exact biochemical changes are unclear. Exposure to short duration of excessive noises has been demonstrated to result in a temporary hearing impairment (temporary threshold shift) with a duration of hours to weeks. However, prolonged exposure results in a permanent threshold shift or hearing impairment.[3,48,149] Initially, outer hair cells are lost, but with more significant exposures damage to both inner and outer hair cells and all supporting structures in the organ of Corti results. Cochlear nerve fibers degenerate after hair cell damage.[48,149] The section of the cochlea most at risk from loud noises is at the 9 to 13 mm region (the total length is 32 mm).[98] This region is responsible for hearing at the 3 to 6 kHz range, corresponding to the typical noise-induced hearing loss pattern.

Much of the clinical assessment and monitoring of

TABLE 27–6. TYPICAL SOUND LEVELS ON THE DECIBEL SCALE

Decibels	Sound
10	Weakest sound that humans can detect
20	Quiet bedroom, soft whisper
25–30	Broadcast studio
50	Insulated lounge
65	Normal conversation
70	Television-audio
95	Machine press, subway car (35 mph)
105	Spray painting, snowmobile
110	Power saw
115	Coarse grinding
120	Armored personnel carrier; ear pain begins
145	Jet plane engine
194	Highest sound level that can occur

TABLE 27–7. OSHA STANDARD FOR PERMISSIBLE NOISE EXPOSURE[a]

Duration of Exposure (hr)	dBA[b]
16	85
8	90
6	92
4	95
3	97
2	100
1.5	102
1	105
0.5	110
0.25 or less	115

[a]If daily noise exposure is composed of 2 or more periods at different exposure level, then use the following formula:

Σ Cn/Tn < 1

Cn = time of exposure at the specific noise level

Tn = total time of exposure permissible at that noise level

Σ = summation of the each Cn/Tn

[b]Decibels using the A-scale filter.

noise-induced hearing loss is based on pure tone hearing loss, demonstrating an audiometric deficit at 3 to 6 kHz.[108,149] This typical pattern is seen in other conditions and becomes less typical with aging.[111] Although human speech is composed mainly of low-frequency sounds, the ability to perceive the higher frequency sounds is extremely important in speech recognition. For this reason, the major impairment in patients with noise-induced hearing loss is an inability to discriminate speech, particularly from background noise.[2,38] Currently, the science of the investigation of speech discrimination is limited with extensive areas for research.

Blast injury to the ear is an exposure of extremely short duration, but very high-intensity sound waves (usually greater than 140 dB). Military personnel are particularly at risk.[31,112,145] Hearing loss from blast injury may be related to rupture of the tympanic membrane, disruption of the ossicles, temporary cochlear dysfunction, and permanent cochlear dysfunction from labyrinthine fistulae and basilar membrane rupture.[29] When a large tympanic membrane rupture or disruption of the ossicles occurs, surgical intervention may be required to treat hearing impairment.[29]

Prevention of any type of noise-induced hearing loss remains the best solution. Various hearing protection devices are available if the noise exposure cannot be reduced. Better monitoring and more longitudinal studies are required on noise-induced hearing loss. Exposure to chemicals or toxins that can impair hearing may have synergistic effects with noise-induced hearing loss.[83,85] These factors should be considered when noise exposure is evaluated. Furthermore, noise exposure is not limited to the workplace. Significant noise exposure may occur at home or from leisure activities, such as power tools, stereo, and ambient exposure.[15,35,64,111] The impact of noise exposure outside of the workplace has only recently attracted the attention of investigators.

What Is the Etiology of Tinnitus?

Tinnitus is the sensation of sound not resulting from mechanoacoustic or electrical signals. Virtually all humans will experience tinnitus in their lifetime. The exact mechanism or mechanisms resulting in tinnitus are largely unknown.[130] Several theories have been proposed, but none is completely satisfactory. Tinnitus may result from spontaneous neurologic discharges when the hair cells or cochlear nerve are injured. Altered sound perception may result from local or central effects when feedback mechanisms are interrupted.[44,47,77,96] Severing the cochlear nerve will terminate tinnitus in less than half of affected patients, suggesting important central mechanisms.[10] Furthermore, certain etiologies of tinnitus, such as migraine headache and temporal lobe seizures, do not affect hearing directly. Drugs or toxins including salicylate may cause hair cell dysfunction and may modify neurotransmission centrally in both the cochlear nucleus and the inferior colliculis.[55,148] Although the probable sites involved in tinnitus may be classified as peripheral (external ear, middle ear, cochlear or eighth cranial nerve), central, or extraauditory (vascular, nasopharyngeal), some etiologies may affect peripheral and central sites, and many etiologies remain unknown.[34,47,96]

Tinnitus may result from trauma or disease or as a manifestation of drug toxicity. Tinnitus is most commonly related to any mechanism that affects hearing. Excessive cerumen, fluid, or a foreign body in the external canal, perforated tympanic membrane, acoustic trauma resulting from exposure to excessive noise, otosclerosis, acoustic neuroma, and otitis media may produce tinnitus. However, the only otologic problem that always results in tinnitus is Meniere's disease. Other etiologies for tinnitus include diabetes, hypertension, autoimmune disease, hypothyroidism, and arteriovenous aneurysms.[33,96]

Numerous drugs are associated with tinnitus (Table 27–8), but the incidence is probably low and the implied relationships have usually been supported only by case reports.[33,133,134] Drugs and toxins may produce tinnitus with or without transient or permanent hearing loss. It is probable that these agents also associated with hearing loss affect cochlear function, while those that produce tinnitus without hearing loss probably act on the central nervous system. Drugs that frequently produce tinnitus are streptomycin, neomycin, indomethacin, doxycycline, ethacrynic acid, furosemide, heavy metals, and high doses of caffeine.[59,133,134] Only a few drugs, such as quinine and salicylates, consistently cause tinnitus at toxic doses.[17,47] These two drugs also serve as examples of how the presence of tinnitus may be an indicator of drug toxicity.

Tinnitus associated with salicylates usually begins at the high therapeutic or low toxic level (approximately 20 to 40 mg/dL).[102] Before the wide availability of salicylate serum measurements, physicians treating gout or rheumatoid arthritis often titrated the salicylate dosage until tinnitus developed.[35] Tinnitus and other signs and symptoms of salicylism (Chap. 32) should be sufficient

TABLE 27–8. DRUGS AND TOXINS THAT CAUSE TINNITUS

Antifungal agents	Amphotericin B
Anticonvulsants	Carbamazepine
Antidepressants	Tricyclic antidepressants, amoxapine, lithium, trancylcypromine
Antihistamines	
Antimicrobials	Aminoglycosides (streptomycin, dihydrostreptomycin, neomycin, kanamycin, gentacmicin, tobramycin, paromomycin, capreomycin), vancomycin, dapsone, doxycycline, tetracycline, sulphonamide, sulfasoxazole, sulphamethoxazole, metronidazole, thiabendazole, clindamycin
Antineoplastics	Cisplatin, nitrogen mustard, 6-aminonicotinamide, methotrexate
Antiparasitics	Chloroquine, hydroxychloroquine
Neuroleptics	Haloperidol, molindone
Beta-adrenergic antagonists	
Bromates	
Cinchona alkaloids	Quinine, quinidine, salicylates
Diuretics	Furosemide, ethacrynic acid, bumetanide
Hydrocarbons	Benzene
Local anesthetics	Mepivacaine, bupivacaine, lidocaine
Nonsteroidal antiinflammatory drugs	
Oral contraceptives	
Sympathomimetics	Caffeine, theophylline, metaproterenol, albuterol, methylphenidate

for physicians to diagnose salicylate toxicity before serum salicylate levels are available. However, tinnitus may not be evident in elderly patients with hearing impairment despite significantly elevated salicylate concentrations.[102] The classic constellation of symptoms of quinine and salicylate toxicity, called cinchonism, is nausea, vomiting, tinnitus, and visual disturbances.[4,27,104] Because serum quinine level analysis is not readily available, symptoms of quinine toxicity remain a clinical diagnosis (see Chap. 44).[140]

Summary

The sense of smell, taste, and hearing are commonly affected by numerous drugs and toxins. They may cause significant patient morbidity. Some of the events may be foreseeable and others will require monitoring and appropriate testing. Understanding some of the basic pathophysiology of the otolaryngologic organs as well as a heightened suspicion on the part of healthcare providers may avoid significant patient risk and discomfort. In the future, further understanding of the pathophysiology of toxins and these special organs will spur the development of therapeutic modalities.

References

1. Adelson L, Sunshine I: Fatal hydrogen sulfide poisoning. Report of three cases occurring in a sewer. Arch Pathol 1966;81:375–380.
2. Alberti PW: Noise induced hearing loss. Br Med J 1992; 304:522.
3. Alberti PW: Occupational hearing loss. In: Ballenger JJ, ed: Diseases of the Nose, Throat, Ear, Head, and Neck, 14th ed. Philadelphia, Lea & Febiger, 1991, pp. 1053–1068.
4. Alvan G, Karlsson KK, Villen T: Reversible hearing impairment related to quinine blood concentration in guinea pigs. Life Sci 1989;45:751–755.
5. Amoore JE: Olfactory genetics and anosmia. In: Beidler LM, ed: Handbook of Sensory Physiology, vol 4. Chemical Senses, part I. Berlin, Springer-Verlag, 1971, pp. 145–156.
6. Amoore JE, Hautala E: Odor as an aid to chemical safety: Odor thresholds compared with threshold limit values and volatilities for 214 industrial chemicals in air and water diluted. J Appl Toxicol 1983;3:272–290.
7. Assael BM, Parini R, Rusconi F: Ototoxicity of aminoglycoside antibiotics in infants and children. Pediatr Infect Dis 1982;1:357–365.
8. Audeau FM, Gnanaharan C, Davey K: Hydrogen sulfide poisoning: Associated with pelt processing. NZ Med J 1985;98:145–147.
9. Bagger-Sjoback D, Filipek CS, Schacht J: Characteristics and drug responses of cochlear and vestibular adenylate cyclase. Arch Otorhinolaryngol 1980;228:217–222.
10. Barrs DM, Brackmann DE: Translabyrinthine nerve section: Effect on tinnitus. J Laryngol Otol 1984;98(S9):287–293.
11. Beidler LM: Renewal of cells within taste buds. J Cell Biol 1965;27:263–272.
12. Bergstorm L, Thompson PL: Ototoxicity. In: Brown RD, Daigneault EA, eds: Pharmacology of Hearing: Experimental and Clinical Basis. New York, Wiley, 1981, pp. 119–134.
13. Berning CK, Griffith JF, Wild JE: Research on the effectiveness of denatonium benzoate as a deterrent to liquid detergent ingestion by children. Fundam Appl Toxicol 1982; 2:44–48.
14. Bernstein IL, Webster MM: Learned taste aversions in humans. Physiol Behav 1980;25:363–366.
15. Bess FH, Poynor RE: Noise-induced hearing loss and snowmobiles. Arch Otol 1974;99:45–51.
16. Bitrex Product Information. Edinburgh, Macfarlan Smith, 1989.
17. Boettcher FA, Bancroft BR, Slvi RJ, et al: Effects of sodium salicylate on evoked-response measures of hearing. Hearing Res 1989;42:129–142.
18. Boettcher FA, Salvi RJ: Salicylate ototoxicity: Review and synthesis. Am J Otol 1991;12:33–47.

19. Boyd O: Captopril induced taste disturbance. Lancet 1993; 342:304.
20. Brown KS, Robinette RR: No simple pattern of inheritance in ability to smell solutions of cyanide. Nature 1967;215: 406–408.
21. Brown RD, Penny JE, Henley CM, et al: Ototoxicity drugs and noise. In: Tinnitus, Ciba Foundation Symposium 85. London, Putnam, 1981, pp. 151–171.
22. Brummett RE: Otoxicity of erythromycin and analogues. Otolaryngol Clin North Am 1993;26:811–819.
23. Brummett RE: Otoxicity of vancomycin and analogues. Otolaryngol Clin North Am 1993;26:821–827.
24. Brummett RE, Traynor J, Brown R, et al: Cochlear damage resulting from kanamycin and furosemide. Acta Oto-Laryngol 1975;80:86–92.
25. Budavari S, O'Neil MJ, Smith A, et al, eds: The Merck Index: An Encyclopedia of Chemicals, Drugs, and Biologicals, 11th ed. Rahway, NJ, Merck, 1989, pp. 454–455.
26. Burnett WW, King EG, Grace M, et al: Hydrogen sulfide poisoning: Review of 5 years' experience. Can Med Assoc J 1977;117:1277–1280.
27. Burst JCM, Richter RW: Quinine amblyopia related to heroin addiction. Ann Intern Med 1971;74:84–86.
28. Campbell KCM, Durrant J: Audiologic monitoring for ototoxicity. Otol Clin North Am 1993;26:903–914.
29. Casler JD, Chait RH, Zajtchuk JT: Treatment of blast injury to the ear. Ann Otol Rhinol Laryngol 1989;98:13–22.
30. Cazals Y, Li XQ, Aurousseau C, et al: Acute effects of noradrenaline related vasoactive agents on the otoxicity of aspirin: An experimental study in guinea pigs. Hear Res 1988;36:89–96.
31. Chait R, Casler J, Zajtchuk JT: Blast injury of the ear: Historical perspective. Ann Otol Rhinol Laryngol 1989;98:9–12.
32. Chapman P: Naproxen and sudden hearing loss. J Laryngol Otol 1982;96:163–166.
33. Ciba Foundation Symposium 85: A central or peripheral source of tinnitus. London, Putnam, 1981, pp. 279–294.
34. Ciba Foundation Symposium 85:Appendix I: Definition and classification of tinnitus. London, Putnam, 1981, pp. 300–302.
35. Clark WW: Noise exposure from leisure activities. J Acoust Soc Am 1991;90:175–181.
36. Cone TE Jr: Diagnosis and treatment: Some diseases, syndromes, and conditions associated with an unusual odor. Pediatrics 1968;41:993–995.
37. Davidson TM: The loss of smell. Emerg Med 1988;20: 104–116.
38. Davignon DD, Leshowitz BH: The speech-in-noise test: A new approach to the assessment of communication capability of elderly persons. Int J Aging Hum Dev 1986;23: 149–160.
39. Davis H: Advances in the neurophysiology and neuroanatomy of the cochlea. J Acoust Soc Am 1962;34: 1377–1385.
40. DeCourcy Hinds M: Mother fights to ruin the taste of poison. New York Times, May 20, 1989.
41. Doty RL: A review of olfactory dysfunctions in man. Am J Otol 1979;1:57–79.
42. Drewnowski A: Genetics of taste and smell. World Rev Nutr Diet 1990;63:194–208.
43. Duckert LG, Rubel EW: Current concepts in hair regeneration. Otolaryngol Clin North Am 1993;26:873–901.
44. Eggermont JJ: On the pathophysiology of tinnitus: A review and a peripheral model. Hear Res 1990;48:111–123.
45. Emmett EA: Parosmia and hyposmia induced by solvent exposure. Br J Ind Med 1976;3:196–198.
46. Escoubet B, Amsallem P, Ferrary E, et al: Prostaglandin synthesis by the cochlea or the guinea pig. Influence of aspirin, gentamicin, and acoustic stimulation. Prostaglandins 1985;29:589–599.
47. Evans EF: Chairman's closing remarks. In: Tinnitus, Ciba Foundation Symposium 85. London, Putnam, 1981, pp. 295–302.
48. Falk SA: Pathophysiological responses of the auditory organ to excessive noise. In: Lee DHK, Falk HL, Geiger SR, eds: Handbook of Physiology: Reactions to Environmental Agents. Bethesda, American Physiological Society, 1977, pp. 17–30.
49. Fee WE Jr: Aminoglycoside ototoxicity in the human. Laryngoscope 1980;90(suppl 24):1–19.
50. Feldman AM: Cochlear fluids: Physiology, biochemistry, and pharmacology. In: Brown RD, Daigneault EA, eds: Pharmacology of Hearing. Experimental and Clinical Basis. New York, Wiley, 1981, pp. 81–97.
51. Flotra L, Gjermo P, Rolla G, et al: Side effects of chlorhexidine mouth washes. J Dent Res 1971;79:119–125.
52. Fu DM: Survey of 1583 deaf mutes. Qinghai Med J 1985;1: 105–112.
53. Fukumoto Y, Nakajima H, Uetake M, et al: Smell ability to solution of potassium cyanide and its inheritance. Jpn J Hum Genet 1957;2:7–16.
54. Garetz SL, Altschuler RA, Schacht J: Attenuation of gentamicin ototoxicity by glutathione in the guinea pig in vivo. Hear Res 1994;77:81–87.
55. Gerken GM: Central tinnitus and lateral inhibition: An auditory brainstem model. Hear Res 1996;97:75–83.
56. Glover J, Dibble S, Miaskoski C, et al: Changes in taste associated with intravenous administration pentamidine. J Assoc Nurses AIDS Care 1995;6:43–48.
57. Goldfrank LR, Weisman R, Flomenbaum N: Teaching the recognition of odors. Ann Emerg Med 1982;11:684–686.
58. Gomez HJ, Cirillo VJ, Irvin JD: Enalapril: A review of human pharmacology. Drugs 1985;30S:13–24.
59. Goodey RJ: Drugs in the treatment of tinnitus. In: Tinnitus, Ciba Foundation Symposium 85. London, Putnam, 1981, pp. 263–278.
60. Gordon AS, Moran DT, Jafek BW, et al: The effect of chronic cocaine abuse on human olfaction. Arch Otolaryngol Head Neck Surg 1990;116:1415–1418.
61. Gordon CB: Practical approach to the loss of smell. Am Fam Phys 1982;26:191–193.
62. Gorman W: The sense of smell. Eye Ear Nose Throat 1964;43:54–58.
63. Griffin JP: Drug-induced disorder of taste. Adv Drug React Rev 1992;11:229–239.
64. Grumet GW: Pandemonium in the modern hospital. N Engl J Med 1993;322:433–437.
65. Hansen SR, Janssen C, Beasley VR: Denatonium benzoate as a deterrent to ingestion of toxic substances: Toxicity and efficacy. Vet Hum Toxicol 1993;35:234–236.

66. Hastings L: Sensory neurotoxicology: Use of the olfactory system in the assessment of toxicity. Neurotoxicol Teratol 1990;12:455–459.
67. Henkin RI: Concepts of therapy in taste and smell dysfunction: Repair of sensory receptor functions as primary treatment. In: Kurihara K, Suzuki N, Ogawa H, eds: Olfaction and Taste. Tokyo, Springer Verlag, 1994, pp. 568–570.
68. Henkin RI: Drug-induced taste and smell disorders. Incidence, mechanisms and management related primarily to treatment of sensory receptor dysfunction. Drug Saf 1994; 11:318–377.
69. Henkin RI, Larson AL, Powell RD: Hypogeusia, dysgeusia, hyposmia, and dysosmia following influenza-like infection. Ann Otol Rhinol Laryngol 1975;84:672–682.
70. Henkin RI, Lippoldt RE, Bilstad J, et al: A zinc protein isolated from human parotid saliva. Proc Natl Acad Sci 1975; 72:488–492.
71. Hetu R, Phaneuf R, Marien C: Non-acoustic environmental factor influences on occupational hearing impairment: A preliminary discussion. Paper presented at the second international conference on the combined effects of environmental factors, Kanazama, Japan, 1986, pp. 17–31.
72. Heyneman CA: Zinc deficiency and taste disorders. Ann Pharmacother 1996;30:186–187.
73. Hotz P, Tshchopp A, Soderstrom D, et al: Smell or taste disturbances, neurological symptoms, and hydrocarbon exposure. Int Arch Occup Environ Health 1992;63:525–530.
74. Huang MY, Shacht J: Drug-induced ototoxicity: Pathogenesis and prevention. Med Toxicol 1989;4:452–467.
75. Hymes LC, Bruner BS, Rauber AP: Bromate poisoning from hair permanent preparations. Pediatrics 1985;76: 975–978.
76. Jardini L, Findlay R, Burgi E, et al: Auditory changes associated with moderate blood salicylate levels. Rheumatol Rehab 1978;14:233–236.
77. Jastreboff PJ: Phantom auditory perception (tinnitus): Mechanisms of generation and perception. Neurosci Res 1990;8:221–254.
78. Jobe PC, Brown RD: Auditory pharmacology. Trends Pharmacol Sci 1980;1:202–206.
79. Jojart G: Sense of smell after gentamicin nose-drops. Lancet 1992;339:313.
80. Joyce PW: Taste disturbance with acetazolamide. Lancet 1990;336:1446. Letter.
81. Jung TTK, Rhee CK, Lee CS, et al: Ototoxicity of salicylate, nonsteroidal anti-inflammatory drugs, and quinine. Otolaryngol Clin North Am 1993;26:791–810.
82. Kare MR, Mattes RD: A selective overview of the chemical senses. Nutr Rev 1990;48:39–48.
83. Keeve JP: Ototoxic drugs and the workplace. Am Fam Phys 1988;38:177–181.
84. Kirk RL, Stenhouse NS: Ability to smell solutions of potassium cyanide. Nature 1953;171:698–699.
85. Kisiel DL, Bobbin RP: Miscellaneous ototoxic agents. In: Brown RD, Daigneault EA, eds: Pharmacology of Hearing: Experimental and Clinical Basis. New York, Wiley, 1981, pp. 231–269.
86. Koegel L: Ototoxicity: A contemporary review of aminoglycosides, loop diuretics, acetylsalicylic acid, quinine, erythromycin, and cisplatinum. Am J Otol 1985;6:190–199.
87. Kusakabe Y, Abe K, Tanemura K, et al: GUST27 and closely related G-protein-coupled receptors are localized in taste buds together with Gi-protein alpha-subunit. Chem Senses 1996;21:335–340.
88. Laing DG, Francis GW: The capacity of humans to identify odors in mixtures. Physiol Behav 1989;46:809–814.
89. Leopold DA, Preti G, Mozell MM, et al: Fish-odor syndrome presenting as dysosmia. Arch Otolaryngol Head Neck Surg 1990;116:354–355.
90. Li XJ, Snyder SH: Molecular cloning of ebnerin, a von Ebner's gland protein associated with taste buds. J Biol Chem 1995;270:17674–17679.
91. Lim DJ: Functional structure of the organ of Corti: A review. Hear Res 1986;22:117–146.
92. Lu YF: Cause of 611 deaf mutes in schools for deaf children in Shanghai. Shanghai Med J 1987;10:159.
93. Matsumoto I, Morizona T, Paparella MM: Hearing loss following potassium bromate: Two case reports. Otolaryngol Head Neck Surg 1980;88:625–629.
94. Matz GJ: Aminoglycoside cochlear ototoxicity. Otolaryngol Clin N Am 1993;26:705–736.
95. Matz GJ: The ototoxic effects of ethacrynic acid in man and animals. Laryngoscope 1976;86:1065–1086.
96. McFadden D: Tinnitus: Facts, Theories, and Treatment. Washington, DC, National Academy Press, 1982, pp. 10–24.
97. McFadden D, Plattsmier HS: Aspirin abolishes spontaneous oto-acoustic emissions. J Accoust Soc Am 1984;76: 443–448.
98. McGill TJ, Schuknecht HF: Human cochlear changes in noise induced hearing loss. Laryngoscope 1976;86: 1293–1302.
99. McNeil JJ, Anderson A, Christophidis N, et al: Taste loss associated with oral Captopril treatment. BMJ 1979;15: 1555–1556.
100. Meyerhoff WL: Physiology of the nose and paranasal sinuses. In: Paparella MM, Schumrick DA, eds: Otolaryngology: Basic Sciences and Related Disciplines, Vol. 1. Philadelphia, Saunders, 1980, pp. 308–311.
101. Miller LG, Miller SM: Altered taste secondary to acetazolamide. J Fam Pract 1990;31:199–200.
102. Mongan E, Kelly P, Nies K, et al: Tinnitus as an indication of therapeutic serum salicylate levels. JAMA 1973;226: 142–145.
103. Mott AE, Leopold DA: Disorders of taste and smell. Med Clin North Am 1991;75:1321–1353.
104. Myers EN, Bernstein JM: Salicylate ototoxicity. Arch Otolaryngol 1965;82:483–493.
105. Nadol Jr. JB: Hearing loss. N Engl J Med 1993;329; 1092–1102.
106. National Institute of Health: Noise and hearing loss. Consensus Development Conference Statement. JAMA 1990; 263:3185–3190.
107. Ohtani I, Ohtsuki K, Aikawa T, et al: Mechanism of protective effect of fosfomycin against aminoglycoside ototoxicity. Auris Nasus Larynx 1984;11:119–124.
108. Olishifski JB: Occupational hearing loss, noise, and hearing conservation. In: Zenz C, ed: Occupational Medicine: Principles and Practical Applications. Chicago, Year Book, 1988, pp. 274–323.

109. Patterson PM, Lauder BA: The incidence and probable inheritance of "smell blindness." J Heredity 1948;39:295–297.
110. Payne HAS, Smalley HM, Tracy MJ: Denatonium benzoate as a bitter aversive additive in ethylene glycol and methanol-based automotive products. SAE Technical Paper Series, 1993, pp. 125–131.
111. Phaneur R, Hetu R: An epidemiological perspective of the causes of hearing loss among industrial workers. J Otolaryngol 1990;19:31–40.
112. Phillips YY, Zajtchuk JT: Blast injuries of the ear in military operations. Ann Otol Rhinol Laryngol 1989;98:3–4.
113. Prazma J: Ototoxicity of aminoglycoside antibiotics. In: Brown RD, Daigneault EA, eds: Pharmacology of Hearing: Experimental and Clinical Basis. New York, Wiley, 1981, pp. 155–193.
114. Puel JL, Bobbin RP, Fallon M: Salicylate, meclofenomate, and quinine on cochlear potentials. Otolaryngol Head Neck Surg 1990;102:66–73.
115. Puel JL, Bobbin RP, Fallon M: Salicylate abolishes cochlea potentials through a mechanism that does not involve prostaglandin synthesis and is different than quinine. Otolaryngol Head Neck Surg 1988;99:154.
116. Quick CA, Chole RA, Mauer SM: Deafness and renal failure due to potassium bromate poisoning. Arch Otolaryngol 1975;101:494–495.
117. Quick CA, Fish A, Brown C: The relationship between cochlea and kidney. Laryngoscope 1973;83:1469–1482.
118. Ramsden RT, Latif A, O'Malley S: Electrocochleographic changes in acute salicylate overdosage. J Laryngol Otol 1985;99:1269–1273.
119. Razani J, Murphy C, Davidson TM, et al: Odor sensitivity is impaired in HIV-positive cognitively impaired patients. Physiol Behav 1996;59:877–881.
120. Riggs LC, Brummett RE, Guitjens SK, et al: Ototoxicity resulting from combined adminstration of cisplatin and gentamicin. Laryngoscope 1996;106:401–406.
121. Roche RJ, Silamut K, Pukrittayakamee S, et al: Quinine induces reversible high-tone hearing loss. Br J Clin Pharmacol 1990;29:780–782.
122. Rollin H: Drug-related gustatory disorders. Ann Otol 1978;87:37–42.
123. Rose CS, Heywood PG, Costanzo RM: Olfactory impairment after chronic occupational cadmium exposure. J Occup Med 1992;34:600–605.
124. Rutka J, Alberti PW: Toxic and drug-induced disorders in otolaryngology. Otolaryngol Clin North Am 1984;17:761–774.
125. Rybak LP: Ototoxicity of loop diuretics. Otolaryngol North Am 1993;26:829–844.
126. Schacht J: Biochemical basis of aminoglycoside ototoxicity. Otolaryngol Clin North Am 1993;26:845–856.
127. Schacht J: Molecular mechanisms of drug-induced hearing loss. Hear Res 1986;22:297–304.
128. Schiffman SS: Taste and smell in disease (part 1). N Engl J Med 1983;308:1275–1279.
129. Schiffman SS: Taste and smell in disease (part 2). N Engl J Med 1983;308:1337–1343.
130. Schleuning AJ: Management of the patient with tinnitus. Med Clin North Am 1991;75:1225–1237.
131. Schneider BA: Anosmia: Verification and etiologies. Ann Otol 1972;81:272–277.
132. Schweitzer VG: Ototoxicity of chemotherapeutic agents. Otolaryngol Clin North Am 1993;26:759–789.
133. Seidman MD, Jacobson GP: Update on tinnitus. Otolaryngol Clin North Am 1996;29:455–465.
134. Seligmann H, Podoshin L, Ben-David J, et al: Drug-induced tinnitus and other hearing disorders. Drug Saf 1996;14:198–212.
135. Shatzman AR, Henkin RI: Metal-binding characteristics of the parotid salivary protein gustin. Biochim Biophys Acta 1980;623:107–118.
136. Shelley WB: A diagnosis you can smell. Emerg Med 1992;24:232–235.
137. Shusterman DJ, Sheedy JE: Occupational and environmental disorders of the special senses. Occup Med 1992;7: 515–542.
138. Sibert JR, Frude N: Bittering agents in the prevention of accidental poisoning: Children's reactions to denatonium benzoate (Bitrex). Arch Emerg Med 1991;8:1–7.
139. Silverstein H, Wolfson RJ, Rosenberg S: Diagnosis and management of hearing loss. Clin Symp 1994;44:1–32.
140. Smilkstein MJ, Kulig KW, Rumack BH: Acute toxic blindness: Unrecognized quinine poisoning. Ann Emerg Med 1987;16:98–101.
141. Song BB, Schacht J: Variable efficacy of radical scavengers and iron chelators to attenuate gentamicin ototoxicity in guinea pig in vivo. Hear Res 1996;94:87–93.
142. Stevens JC, Cruz LA, Hoffman JM, et al: Taste sensitivity and aging: High incidence of decline revealed by repeated threshold. Chem Senses 1995;20:451–459.
143. Stewart TH, Sherman Y, Politzer WM: An outbreak of food-poisoning due to a flour improver, potassium bromate. South Afr Med J 1969;200–202.
144. Stine R, Slosberg B, Beacham BE: Hydrogen sulfide intoxication. Ann Intern Med 1976;85:756–758.
145. Sullivan P: MD launches study to determine amount of job-related hearing loss in military. Can Med Assoc J 1992;146:2061–2062.
146. Sumner D: Post-traumatic anosmia. Brain 1964;87:107–120.
147. Tange RA, Dreschler WA, van der Hulst RJ: The importance of high-tone audiometry in monitoring for ototoxicity. Arch Otorhinolaryngol 1985;242:77–81.
148. Wallhauser-Frank E, Braun S, Langner G: Salicylate alters 2-DG uptake in the auditory system: A model for tinnitus? Neuroreport 1996;7:1585–1588.
149. Ward WD: Noise-induced hearing loss. In: Northern JL, ed: Hearing Disorder, 2nd ed. Boston, Little, Brown, 1984, pp. 143–152.
150. Wright HN: Characterization of olfactory dysfunction. Arch Otolaryngol Head Neck Surg 1987;113:163–168.
151. Wysocki CJ, Gilbert AN: The National Geographic Smell Survey: The effects of age are heterogenous. Ann NY Acad Sci 1989;561:12–28.
152. Zazgornick J, Kaiser W, Biesenbach G: Captopril induced dysgeusia. Lancet 1993;341:1542. Letter.

CHAPTER 28

Dermatologic Principles

David E. Cohen and Miguel R. Sanchez

Although vulnerable to chemical injury due to its large surface area and exposed location, human skin effectively shields our bodies from damage by most noxious substances. Some chemical agents, however, are absorbed percutaneously in sufficient quantities to produce local or systemic toxic effects, which result in acute and chronic diseases.[39]

Excluding injuries, 30 to 50% of all reported occupational illnesses involve the skin, and the number may well be higher because many cases are never recorded or diagnosed.[13,88] It is estimated that work-related dermatoses account for 5.7 million physician visits each year and result in an annual financial burden of $222 million to $1 billion.[19] These statistics are not surprising considering that more than 100,000 chemical substances are used by American industries.[87] The Bureau of Labor Statistics Data indicate a case rate of occupational skin disease of 7.9 cases per 10,000 or 61,000 new cases each year. Although the frequency of occupational dermatosis has substantial economic impact, physicians more frequently encounter skin disease caused by household cleansers, detergents, cosmetics, personal hygiene products, medications, and other chemical products.

Anatomy of the Skin

The skin is composed principally of two major anatomic subdivisions: the epidermis and dermis. The epidermis is composed primarily of keratinocytes that form a stratified squamous epithelium. Basal cells, the progenitor cells for squamous cells, reside at the epidermis in direct contact with the basement membrane. Rather than forming a flat interface at the dermal–epidermal junction, the basement membrane and its attached basal cells form an undulating surface, which increases the amount of surface available for exchange of substances through the epidermis.

The keratinocytes derived from basal cell division migrate upward, and undergo a process of terminal differentiation that results in changes in cell surface markers and accumulation of specific proteins called keratins. During the process of differentiation, intracellular organelles and the nucleus are degraded. It takes 14 days for the keratinocyte to undergo differentiation from the basal cell layer to the stratum corneum. Eighty percent of the weight of the differentiated keratinocyte (the corneocyte) in this outermost layer of the skin is keratin. The structure of the stratum corneum allows excretion of certain substances such as sweat, excludes penetration of most infectious agents and toxic substances, and provides flexibility and insulation.

Traversing the epidermis, ducts of the skin appendages ascend from the deeper dermis. These include eccrine and apocrine sweat and sebaceous glands. The distribution of these structures is not uniform throughout the body. Eccrine sweat glands predominate on palms, soles, and axillae, while sebaceous glands with their oil-producing capacity predominate on the face and scalp. Apocrine sweat glands, which perform an incompletely understood function, are present in the axillae and on the areolae, and are responsible for the odor associated with sweat. These glands and ductal structures are sites of percutaneous absorption, and may be reservoirs for delayed transcutaneous absorption.

Although the overwhelming majority of cells present in the epidermis are keratinocytes, other specialized cells reside there as well. The melanocytes are interspersed in the lower epidermal layers and, through their dendritic processes, transfer melanin to keratinocytes. Their primary role is the production of melanin, which is packaged in membrane-bound capsules called melanosomes. Melanin is the skin's main chromophore and absorbs broad spectrums of electromagnetic radiation in its effort to protect vital intracellular structures from damage. Langerhans cells migrate throughout the epidermis and function primarily as immune surveillance cells. These cells continuously sample chemicals that contact the skin and process them for presentation to T lymphocytes. It is through this mechanism that primary sensitization and elicitation of contact dermatitis occurs.

Underlying the epidermis is the dermis, which consists primarily of type I collagen and some elastin and proteoglycans. Its main functions are to provide a supportive structure to the overlying epidermis as well as to house appendegeal and neurovascular structures. Beneath the dermis is the subcutis, a layer of adipose tissue that supplies cushioning from physical trauma, and stores energy in the form of fat. From a toxicologic point of view, the subcutaneous fat may be a reservoir for percutaneously or systemically absorbed hydrophobic substances.

Skin Response to Toxicity

The skin is capable of numerous overt physical responses to diseases produced by internal or external causes. An understanding of these responses can lead the clinician to diagnosis or suspicion of a specific illness. The more common skin lesions are:

- *Vesicle.* A circumscribed, fluid-filled elevation measuring less than 0.5 cm.
- *Macule.* A flat, nonpalpable discoloration, which may be erythematous (red), hyperpigmented (brown or dark), or hypopigmented (lighter in color than the normal skin), and less than 1 cm in diameter.
- *Papule.* A circumscribed, elevated lesion measuring up to 1.0 cm. May be flesh-colored or dyspigmented.
- *Nodule.* Possesses the same morphologic characteristics as a papule, but is greater than 1.0 cm, and the vertical size of the lesion nears that of its width.
- *Tumor.* A circumscribed lesion greater than 1 cm.
- *Patch.* The characteristic findings of the macule with lesions greater than 1 cm in size.
- *Plaque.* An elevated solid lesion that is well circumscribed and measures greater than 1.0 cm. It can be formed by a confluence of papules or nodules.
- *Bulla.* A blister measuring greater than 0.5 cm.
- *Comedone.* The classic acne lesion consisting of open and closed varieties commonly referred as black-heads and white-heads, respectively.
- *Erosion.* Loss of epidermis caused by physical, chemical, or metabolic disorders up to the full thickness of the epidermis, but not through the basement membrane.
- *Ulcer.* Loss of full-thickness epidermis and papillary dermis, reticular dermis, or subcutis.
- *Lichenification.* A compensatory pathologic process marked by accentuation of skin surface markings, usually in the form of a plaque that results from persistent rubbing or scratching.

The overused term "maculopapular" lacks any degree of precision that would assist a clinician to make a proper diagnosis, and is a pattern predominantly associated with some viral or drug eruptions. The overwhelming majority of primary and secondary cutaneous diseases are characterized by the presence of specific skin changes. For example, psoriasis is hallmarked by well-demarcated erythematous plaques with adherent silver scaling, herpes simplex by grouped vesicles on an erythematous base, or an exanthematous drug eruption by a morbilliform lacy pattern of macules and patches.

Percutaneous Absorption

The degree of protection from chemical toxicity provided by the skin varies among individuals and appears to be inherited. The principal barrier to percutaneous absorption is the outermost layer of the skin, the stratum corneum, which is composed of 15 to 25 stacked sheets of keratin-filled cells (keratinocytes) devoid of nuclei and organelles.[29] A thick envelope attached to the inner surface of the keratinocyte's plasma membrane is responsible for the cell's resistance to chemical and mechanical trauma. The spaces between these cells are sealed with stacked layers of lipid. The integrity of the stratum corneum is compromised by regular exposure to soaps and household detergents, which in most individuals produces substantial transepidermal loss of water and variable degrees of dryness, scaling, erythema, and fissuring.[52] The surfactant-induced skin damage leads to increased skin permeability, which may persist for up to 4 weeks.[68]

The toxicologic activity of many chemicals that penetrate the skin surface is modified by enzymes present in the cells below the stratum corneum.[83] The top layer of the skin, the epidermis, undertakes virtually all of the phase I (oxidative, reductive, and hydrolytic) as well as phase II (conjugative) enzymatic reactions.[49] Although the skin possesses only 2% of the metabolizing potential of the liver, its enzymes are strategically located to inactivate noxious substances that challenge its barrier effect.[10]

Among the factors that determine percutaneous absorption (Table 28–1), the most significant is the substance's lipid solubility.[93] Life-threatening poisoning can follow skin contact with a number of chemicals, especially organophosphate insecticides, organochlorines, nitrates, and industrial aromatic hydrocarbons (Table 28–2). Highly lipophilic solvents, such as benzene, toluene, carbon tetrachloride, *n*-hexane, dichloroethane, tetrachloroethane, xylene, trichloroethylene, and vinyl chloride, penetrate the skin within 30 minutes of contact, often without causing a burning sensation. Immediate decontamination with soap and water is essential except in cases of exposure to volatile agents, such as titanium tetrachloride, calcium oxide, and chlorosulfonic acid, which can explode or produce toxic fumes on contact with water.[17] Following absorption of some organic solvents, the skin becomes a reservoir from which these chemicals are gradually released into the circulation.[58] The concentration, extent, and duration of application of a substance are also important factors.[92] Some chemicals used as topical medications, including podophyllin, camphor, phenol, and salicylic acid, can be lethal if higher

TABLE 28–1. FACTORS THAT ENHANCE PERCUTANEOUS ABSORPTION

Body Site

Anatomic parts with thin skin (eg, face and genitalia) or where skin touches skin (eg, body folds)

Chemical Enhancers

Urea

Dimethyl sulfoxide

Propylene glycol

Chemical Factors

Chemical concentration

pH

Lipid solubility

Small molecular size

Skin Integrity

Damage by trauma, inflammation or dehydration

Decreased lipid content

Old age or infancy

Occlusion

Occlusive dressings (eg, plastic film, protective equipment)

Vehicle (eg, petrolatum)

Physical Factors

Frequency of application

Heat

Skin hydration

Surface area exposed

than recommended concentrations are liberally applied to the skin.[73] Lethal intoxication has been reported in infants and young children from enhanced percutaneous absorption after application of ethyl alcohol, benzene hexachloride, malathion, salicylic acid, and other chemicals in concentrations that are safe for adults.[21]

Chemicals can also produce adverse cutaneous effects following absorption through other organ systems. Notable examples of such reactions are drug-induced eruptions. Ingestion or inhalation of a number of organic substances, such as some chlorinated hydrocarbons, can cause skin disease.

Toxicologic Skin Signs

Toxic exposure to certain chemicals is occasionally suspected from the presence of specific cutaneous findings. Cyanosis, diaphoresis, jaundice, pallor, or flushing may be signs of acute poisoning. Pigmentary changes (Table 28–3), skin thickening, acneiform eruptions, and hair loss (Table 28–4) may be due to medications or chronic chemical toxicity. Careful dermatologic examination can also reveal critical evidence about drug or medication usage, systemic conditions, psychiatric illness, and emotional instability. A muscular man with acne, striae, and skin edema is probably taking anabolic steroids.[62] Ethanol abusers may have facial flushing, exacerbation of acne

TABLE 28–2. SELECTED SUBSTANCES THAT CAUSE LIFE-THREATENING SYSTEMIC TOXICITY THROUGH PERCUTANEOUS ABSORPTION

Chemical	Toxicity
Acrylamide	Ataxia, hyporeflexia, peripheral neuropathy, other CNS and PNS toxicity, teratogenicity; local reactions include peeling, redness, or increased sweating on hands and feet
Aniline, related azo dyes and derivatives (chloroaniline, dimethylaniline, nitroaniline, benzidine, etc)	Methemoglobinemia, liver disease, bladder carcinoma
Arsenic	Neurotoxicity, GI inflammation, malaise, cardiac abnormalities, headaches, weight loss
Benzene	Aplastic anemia, acute myelogenous leukemia, myelofibrosis, multiple myeloma
Chlorinated hydrocarbons	Neurotoxicity, GI disease, liver disease, porphyria
Cyanide and its salts	Vomiting, colic, headache, dyspnea, death
Formaldehyde	Metabolic acidosis
Hydrofluoric acid	Irritant dermatitis and necrosis, electrolyte abnormalities, pulmonary edema, eye disease, death
Mercury compounds	GI distress, neurotoxicity, nephrotic syndrome
Nitrates	Methemoglobinemia, headache, nausea, seizures, coma, vasodilation, metabolic acidosis
Organic solvents	CNS toxicity
Pesticides	
Fumigants	
Chlorophenoxyacetic acid	Chloracne, melanosis, porphyria cutanea tarda (chronic exposure)
Dinitrophenol	Facial flushing, sweating, metabolic acidosis
Methyl bromide	Nausea, vomiting, CNS depression, bronchospasm
Paraquat/diquat	Lung damage, renal damage
Fungicides	
Organic mercury compounds	Severe irritant dermatitis with vesiculation may occur without associated systemic illness
Pentachlorophenol	Chloracne, irritant dermatitis with vesiculation
Thiuram	Disulfiram-like reactions
Insecticides	
Carbamates	Cholinergic symptoms, muscle weakness
Halogenated hydrocarbons	DDT and methoxychlor are poorly absorbed and only when in solution, but other compounds are readily absorbed and stored in fat
Organophosphates	Slow absorption, cholinergic symptoms
Thiocyanates	Neurotoxicity
Rodenticides	
Fluoracetamide	Seizures, coma
Phosphorus	Cutaneous burns, cardiac, hepatic, and CNS toxicity
Thallium	Intoxication after depilation with 3 to 7% thallium acetate (see Chap. 82)
Phenols	Cardiovascular collapse, tachypnea, seizures, vomiting, diarrhea, abdominal pain, renal and liver failure, methemoglobinemia
Sulfides	Cardiopulmonary decompensation, CNS toxicity
Sulfites	Vomiting, abdominal pain, diarrhea, GI bleeding, CNS stimulation, seizure, cardiovascular collapse
Toluidine	Anoxia, methemoglobinemia, hematuria, CNS toxicity

TABLE 28–3. SUBSTANCES RESPONSIBLE FOR PIGMENTARY CHANGES

Blue-Black	***Pallor***
Minocycline	Lead
Oxalic acid	
Resorcinol (topical)	***Red***
Tetracycline	Borates
	Mercury
Blue-Gray	Rifampin
Amiodarone	
Bismuth	***Red-Brown***
Gold (sun-exposed areas)	Danthron
Mercury	Clofazimine
Osmium	***Red-Orange***
Phenothiazines	Dihydroxynaphthoquinone
Quinine	Nitric acid
Silver	Tetrylchlorine
Bronze	***Salmon***
Arsenic	Cathaxanthin
Brown	***Yellow***
Alpha-methyldopa	Carotene
BCNU	2–4 dinitrosalicylic acid
Bleomycin (linear)	Hexanitrodiphenylamine (topical)
Busulfan	Lycopene (tomato and beet)
Chromium	Nitrazepam
Cyclophosphamide (exposed areas)	Nitric acid (topical)
Dactinomycin	Picric acid
Dioxin	Quinacrine
Doxorubicin (hands and feet)	Sodium nitrate
Fluorouracil	Tetryl (topical)
Hydroquinone (topical)	Trintrotoluene (topical)
Hydroxyurea	
Imipramine	***Yellow-Brown***
Levodopa	Amiodiquin
Mechlorethamine (topical)	Chloroquine
Nitrates/nitrites	Epoxy resins
Phenacetin	Hydroxychloroquine
Procarbazine	Methylenedianiline
	Yellow-Orange
Green	Dihydroxyacetone
Copper salts (topical)	

TABLE 28–4. SUBSTANCES THAT CAUSE HAIR LOSS

Allopurinol	Cimetidine
Androgens	Cytotoxic agents
Anticoagulants	Gold salts
Antimetabolites	Hexachlorobenzene
Antithyroid drugs	Lead
Arsenic	Mercury
Beta-adrenergic antagonists	Nonsteroidal antiinflammatory agents
Boric acid	Selenium
Captopril	Thallium
Carbamazepine	Thiocyanates
Chemotherapeutic agents	Trimethadione
Chloral hydrate	Valproic acid
Chloroquine	

rosacea, or stigmata of cirrhosis such as spider angiomata, petechiae, jaundice, salivary gland hypertrophy, palmar erythema, gynecomastia, and decreased body hair. The shape and distribution of some skin lesions can be important clues to psychologic dysfunction. Linear nonsurgical scars are usually traumatic and can be a sign of physical abuse. Previous suicide attempts should be suspected in persons with scars over the wrists and antecubital fossae. "Punched-out" excoriations exclusively on body areas readily accessible to the patient's reach suggest a factitial dermatosis. Self-induced panniculitis presenting as painful, deep subcutaneous nodules is reported after injections of acids, alkalis, oils, paraffin, iodine, milk, paint, feces, pentazocine, meperidine, morphine, and other drugs.[70] Trichotillomania, irregular patches of alopecia with broken hair shafts resulting from hair pulling, indicates emotional instability.

Chronic or repeated parenteral drug addiction can be diagnosed by the presence of specific scars, multiple venopuncture marks, and bruises along veins. "Skin tracks" are hyperpigmented, indurated, or atrophic streaks from repeated intravenous injections of opioids or cocaine, mixed with quinine, talc, other potentially sclerosing agents, and protoplasmic poisons.[72] These lesions are found on the hands, forearms, wrists, neck, dorsal surface of the penis, and supraclavicular, popliteal, and antecubital fossae. Scattered atrophic guttate scars from "skin popping" are found on the forearms, abdomen, thighs, and other areas favored for subcutaneous injection. In these patients deep, firm cutaneous nodules develop as a reaction to the inadvertent inoculation of adulterants such as talc or sugar and from particulate material, such as glass or plastic. Drug users who "nod off" while smoking may drop cigarette ashes in an organized "necklace sign" around the neck.

In heroin users, pseudoacanthosis nigricans, cheilitis, thrombophlebitis, leukocytoclastic vasculitis, fixed drug eruptions, and systemic amyloidosis may develop. Skin necrosis can occur due to thrombosis induced by injection of adulterants such as quinine. Impetigo, abscesses, infected skin ulcerations, thrombophlebitis, and localized cellulitis can develop in injected sites (see Color Plate, Fig. 11). These infections may progress to more extensive pyodermas or gangrene. Repeated infection and vascular injury predispose to lymphedema. Intraarterial injection can cause vasospasm and necrosis, which may require amputation.

Irritation of the nasal mucosa, a frequent finding in cocaine snorters, may be so severe as to result in perforation of the nasal septum. Madarosis—the loss of eyebrows and eyelashes—can occur in persons who "freebase" cocaine. Widespread excoriations due to pruritus and delusions of parasitosis, as well as behavioral abnormalities that lead to stereotypical, repetitious skin picking and self-mutilation (Magnan's sign) are occasionally observed in cocaine addicts. Intravenous cocaine use has resulted in skin and muscle infarction due to severe vasoconstriction. Piloerection is a sign of opioid withdrawal.

The diagnosis of chemically induced skin disease requires a detailed history of the patient's habits, chemical exposure, and symptomatology as well as evaluation of the distribution and morphology of cutaneous lesions. The absence of skin lesions, however, by no means excludes poisoning through percutaneous absorption of a substance.

Systemic Toxicity Through Percutaneous Absorption

The agents most frequently implicated in the development of systemic toxicity from skin absorption are listed in Table 28–5. Their systemic effects are discussed in greater depth in other chapters. Adverse effects from contact with agricultural chemicals are reviewed in more detail here due to the frequency of disease from skin contamination with these agents.[42] The Environmental Protection Agency estimated in 1991 that 25,000 pesticide formulations with 750 active ingredients were available, and that 2.7 billion pounds of active ingredients are used each year.

Some pesticides penetrate the skin rather easily. Ironically, although farm workers and amateur gardeners regularly take precautions against inhalation and ingestion of pesticides, avoidance of skin contact is frequently ignored, especially during hot weather or rigorous work periods.[31] In general, agricultural pesticides are more toxic than those pesticides used primarily in the home. All pesticides potentially cause irritant dermatitis. Captafol, sulfur derivatives, organophosphates, organic mercury compounds, and chlorinated hydrocarbons are particularly irritating to the skin; third-degree burns can occur after prolonged skin exposure with some of these agents.[55] Others, such as the thiophthalidamides, phosphothioates, dithiocarbamates, pyrethrin, benzene hexachloride, triazine, and fungicides, also sensitize the skin. When airborne contact with these chemicals occurs during spraying, the dermatitis predominantly involves the face and hands. Allergic contact dermatitis in farm workers is more often due to common sensitizers, such as preservatives, leather tanners, rubber chemicals, formaldehyde, plants, and, occasionally, feed additives. Carbamates and thiuram are related to disulfiram and may cause antabuse-like reactions. Halogenated hydrocarbons are extensively used as insecticides and can be absorbed through the skin in sufficient quantities to cause intoxication and central nervous system disease. Chronic exposure may cause an eczematous dermatitis.

Following contact with most pesticides, immediate washing with soap and water suffices to decontaminate the skin. However, repeated washes are necessary for the more lipophilic agents, such as chlordane.[94] Organophosphates are difficult to remove. The skin should be washed with soap, detergent, and generous volumes of water and then sponged with ethyl alcohol. If available, green soap and dilute hypochloride solutions should be used. All contaminated clothing should be carefully deposited in plastic bags and discarded to avoid reexposure of the patient and staff.

TABLE 28–5. SYSTEMIC TOXICITY OF AGENTS THROUGH PERCUTANEOUS ABSORPTION

Agent	Systemic Disease
Aminoglycosides	Vestibular dysfunction, deafness
Antihistamines	Psychomotor instability
Arsenic	Arsenical keratosis, malignancies
Benzocaine	Methemoglobinemia
Boric acid	Nausea, vomiting, diarrhea
Camphor	Seizures, CNS manifestations
Carmustine	Bone marrow depression
Chloramphenicol	Aplastic anemia after ophthalmic preparations
Clindamycin	Pseudomembranous colitis
Diethyltoluamide (insect repellant)	Fatal toxic encephalopathy
Dimethyl sulfoxide	Oyster breath, rash, nausea
Dinitrochlorobenzene	Mutagenicity
Ethyl alcohol	Hypoglycemia, respiratory depression and death in infants
Fumaric acid (monoethyl ester)	Renal toxicity
Henna dye with paraphenylenediamine	Severe angioneurotic edema, acute renal failure
Hexachlorophene	Neurotoxicity in infants and persons with extensive burns
Hydrofluoric acid	Hypocalcemia, hyperkalemia, hypomagnesemia, death
Lidocaine	Neurotoxicity
Lindane	Neurotoxicity
Monobenzyl ether of hydroquinone	Conjunctival and corneal melanosis
Phenol	Cardiac dysrhythmias, renal failure, death
Podophyllin	Neurotoxicity, convulsions
Povidone-iodine	Toxicity in infants and extensively burned patients
Resorcinol	Edema, hemolysis and methemoglobinemia in infants
Salicylates	Coma and fatal intoxication in young children and infants; death after widespread applications of high concentrations (20%) in adults
Silver nitrate	Argyria, renal disease, electrolyte disturbances, methemoglobinemia in children
Silver sulfadiazine	Leukopenia, nephrotic syndrome (rare)
Sulfamylon	Hyperchloremic acidosis in burned patients, methemoglobinemia, reversible pulmonary disease
Triclocarban	Methemoglobinemia in neonates

Local Reactions

Contact dermatitis comprises approximately 80% of all occupational skin diseases. The term describes two major categories of eczematous processes—allergic and irritant. The first step in the evaluation of occupational dermatosis is identification of the chemical agents to which a per-

TABLE 28–6. COMMON IRRITANTS AND SENSITIZERS IN SELECTED OCCUPATIONS

Occupation	Irritants	Sensitizers
Automobile workers	Cutting oils, paints, solvents, oils, hand cleaners	Nickel, cobalt, beryllium, rubber, epoxy or acrylic resins, chromates, soluble oil preservatives
Bakers	Detergents, citrus fruits	Sodium carboxymethyl cellulose, citrus fruits, spices, nickel, balsam, dyes, BHA, BHT, proprionic acid
Bartenders	Detergents, citrus fruits	Citrus fruits, detergents
Butchers	Detergents, meat products	Nickel, colophony
Canners	Brine, seafood	Vegetables, preservatives, rubber
Carpenters	Solvents, polish, glues, cleansers, glass fiber	Wood, turpentine, paints, polishes, colophony, epoxy and formaldehyde resins, glues, rubber, formaldehyde
Coal miners	Oil, grease, limestone, stone dust, coal dust	Rubber, chromate, cobalt, plastics, explosives
Construction workers	Cement, glass wool, wood preservatives, hydrochloric and hydrofluoric acid	Chromate, cobalt, rubber, urea formaldehyde resins, woods, epoxy resins, polyurethane
Dentists	Detergents, soaps, acrylic monomer, plaster of Paris, fluxes	Rubber, enamel, acrylic monomers, nickel, palladium, cobalt, epoxy resin, balsam of Peru, colophony, eugenol, titanium, impression and sealant materials, anesthetics, methacrylic glues
Electricians	Soldering flux, bitumen	Rubber, nickel, tar, epoxy resins, glues, polyurethanes, soldering flux
Florists	Pesticides, fertilizers, bulbs	Pesticides, plants, lichens
Hairdressers	Soaps, dyes, shampoos, permanent wave solutions	Dyes, perfumes, rubber, nickel, thioglycolates, phenylenediamine
Health care workers (see Chap. 109)	Disinfectants, soaps, detergents, quaternary ammonium compounds, talc	Rubber, antibiotics, hand lotion, phenothiazines, anesthetics, antiseptics
Housekeepers	Soaps, detergents, polishes, vegetables	Nickel, chromate, rubber, polishes, cosmetics and lotions, fruits, vegetables, plants
Jewelers	Fluxes, solvents	Nickel, enamels, cobalt, gold, palladium
Mechanics	Degreasers, solvents, oils, detergents, soldering flux, battery acid, cooling system fluids	Chromate, rubber, epoxy resins, cutting and cooling fluids, soluble oil preservatives
Painters	Turpentine, solvents, paints. plaster	Turpentine, cobalt, chromate, polyurethane, epoxy and acrylic resins, varnish, glues, preservatives
Photographers	Reducing and oxidizing agents, alkalis, solvents	Color developers, chromate, formaldehyde, metals
Plumbers	Oils, hand cleansers, soldering flux	Rubber, chromate, glues, hydrazine
Secretaries	Photocopy paper	Rubber, formaldehyde, glues

son is exposed at work (Table 28–6).[63] Direct skin exposure to exogenous chemicals can produce cutaneous inflammation through irritation or sensitization. Currently, over 3000 chemical agents are known to cause allergic contact dermatitis and over 65,000 chemicals may produce irritant dermatitis.[23]

Irritant Dermatitis

Under specific conditions any chemical agent, including water, can produce irritation.[1] Skin that is eroded, chapped, or damaged is more susceptible to irritation by chemicals. Inflamed skin is more readily sensitized to allergens, and for this reason half of all patients with stasis dermatitis develop hypersensitivity reactions to at least one agent during the course of the disease.

Practically everyone has experienced itching, burning, or pain after touching a chemical substance. In acute primary irritant dermatitis, a reversible inflammatory response is produced by a single application of a chemical agent. Cumulative irritation develops after repeated exposures to chemicals at concentrations too low to cause acute primary irritation. In corrosion, the most severe form of irritant dermatitis, chemicals cause severe irreversible skin alterations that result in blistering, necrosis, ulceration, and scarring. Irritant dermatitis represents the most frequent type, accounting for approximately 75 to 80% of all cases of contact dermatitis.[43]

The characteristic lesions of irritant dermatitis are eczematous, pink to red patches or plaques with fine scale. Edema in the epidermis may be so pronounced that blisters form. In acute cases, burning or intense itching is common. The surface of subacute or chronic lesions is dry and scaly. Prolonged rubbing due to itching results in lichenification. The mechanism of induction of irritant dermatitis is nonimmunologic.

Some substances are potent irritants and can cause damage independent of clinical conditions, but others require the presence of specific factors to exert their effects. First, the agent must be able to diffuse through the skin or damage the stratum corneum.[60] The irritation potential of a substance can vary depending on the integrity of the stratum corneum, the chemical properties and concentration of the substance, the duration of exposure, and a variety of physical factors such as occlusion, overt sweating, excessive dryness, increased body temperature, and friction. The most significant clinical factor in assessing the risk of irritant dermatitis is a history of atopy. Individuals with atopy have a risk as high as 13.5% for developing occupational dermatitis.[76] Irritant dermatitis most commonly develops on the hands, which have the greatest exposure to chemicals. The palms, with their thick stratum corneum, are more resistant to injury from irritating substances than the dorsa of the hands and fingers, but can transport these substances to other parts of the body, especially the face.

Irritants that spill on clothing most often affect the upper back, anterior thighs, axillae, and feet. Dust may collect under the collar or belt, leading to prolonged occluded exposure. Chronic low-grade irritation actually induces a protective "hardening" of the skin. Because the cutaneous changes caused by contact, atopic, nummular, and dyshidrotic dermatitis are indistinguishable histopathologically, the term *eczema* is often used interchangeably to describe these diseases.

TABLE 28–7. COMMON SKIN SENSITIZERS

Balsam of Peru	Mercaptobenzothiazole
Benzocaine	Neomycin
Benzyl alcohol	Nickel sulfate
Black rubber mix	Parabens
Captan	Polyethylene glycol (solvent)
Carba mix	Potassium dichromate
Chloroxylenol (disinfectant)	p-Phenylenediamine
Cinnamic aldehyde	Propylene glycol (solvent)
Colophony	p-Tert-butylphenol formaldehyde resin
Epoxy resin	Quaternium-15
Ethylenediamine dihydrochloride	Sorbic acid
Formaldehyde	Thimerosal
Glutaraldehyde	Thiuram mix
Imidazolidinyl urea	Wood wax alcohol
Mercapto mix	

Allergic Contact Dermatitis

Unlike irritant dermatitis, where overt skin reactivity may occur on initial exposures, allergic contact dermatitis requires an initiating process called sensitization. For this to occur, a purported allergen must link with a host protein to form a complete allergen. Langerhans cells subsequently process the antigen and present them to regional T-helper cells. Through a series of cytokine-driven amplification processes, a clone of now-sensitized cells forms. This process may take up to 7 days to complete. Subsequent challenges with the same or cross-reacting antigens can produce overt dermatitis within 48 to 72 hours. A molecule's antigenic potential is largely determined by its molecular weight and lipid solubility. Implicated chemicals usually have molecular weights less than 500 d. The risk of developing allergic contact dermatitis from a substance increases in direct proportion to both the number of applications and the concentration of the potential allergen.[90] The most common skin sensitizer is nickel. Among topical medications, neomycin most frequently causes allergic contact dermatitis. Allergy to topical corticosteroids is increasingly found. Bacitracin is the topical medication most frequently implicated in cases of anaphylaxis.

Allergic contact dermatitis is diagnosed in approximately 25% of documented cases of occupational skin disease. The disease is more common in women, probably due to greater exposure to allergens associated with jewelry, cosmetics, perfumes, and toiletries. The skin lesions are similar to those of irritant dermatitis, although itching is usually more intense. The mechanism is a cell-mediated (type IV) immunologic reaction (Table 28–7).[57]

Proper diagnosis of allergic versus irritant contact dermatitis can only accurately be performed via patch testing. This test involves the direct application of standardized concentrations of a variety of chemicals to a patient's skin, usually the upper back, under stainless steel occlusive disks. The chemicals remain on for 48 hours and are removed at that time for an initial reading. Approximately 48 hours later, a delayed reading is performed as well. Positive reactions are graded according to the degree of inflammation and induration and most importantly, clinical relevance. Without properly identifying relevant positive reactions, patients are improperly advised about potential allergens that may not be participating in the etiology of their eruption. Testing to specific chemicals must be directed according to known and suspected exposures. Commercial patch testing kits that contain only 20 or 24 allergens are not sufficient in the proper evaluation of patients with allergic contact dermatitis. Supplementary allergens based on occupation must be included.[18]

Immediate Contact Reactions (Contact Urticaria Syndrome)

Within minutes to an hour of contact with skin, certain chemicals can provoke a wheal and flare response that fades away within 24 hours.[51] When the reaction is mediated by an immunologic mechanism, the lesions may be localized or widespread and accompanied by respiratory or GI symptoms and even anaphylaxis.[40] Fortunately, in the more common nonimmunologic contact urticaria, serious systemic reactions have not been reported.

Nonimmunologic contact urticaria is produced without antecedent sensitization, but the immunologic type requires prior exposure and worsens after repeated contact with the allergen. Foods (egg, meat, seafood) are the most common cause of immediate allergic contact urticaria, followed by textiles (silk and wool), animal products, cosmetics (hair spray, nail polish, perfumes), medications (bacitracin, neomycin, ampicillin), and a number of chemicals (Table 28–8).[50] A diagnosis of immediate contact reaction is confirmed by skin testing with the suspected substance. The patient must be observed closely during testing, as anaphylaxis can develop. Rubber-induced contact urticaria has become a serious prob-

TABLE 28–8. SUBSTANCES THAT CAUSE CONTACT URTICARIA

Nonimmunologic Contact Urticaria	Immunologic Contact Uriticaria	
Animals/Plants	***Animals/Animal Products***	***Plant/Plant Products***
Arthropods	Blood	Algae
Corals	Dander	Birch
Jellyfish	Hair	Castor bean
Moths	Liver	Garlic
Nettles	Mealworms	Henna
Seaweed	Mites	Latex
Food	Roaches	Lichens
Cayenne pepper	Saliva	Papain
Fish	Silk	Perfumes
Thyme	Wool	Pickles
Fragrances and Flavorings	***Food***	Rose
Balsalm of Peru	Dairy products	Rubber latex[b]
Cinnamic acid[a]	Egg[b]	Spices
Cinnamic aldehyde[a] (mouthwash, chewing gum)	Flour	Strawberry
Cinnamon oil	Fruits	Teak
Medications	Grains	***Preservatives***
Alcohol	Honey	Balsam of Peru[b]
Benzocaine	Meats	Benzoic acid
Benzoin	Menthol	Benzyl alcohol
Camphor	Nanella	Chloramines
Cantharidine	Nuts	Formaldehyde
Capsaicin	Seafood	Parabens
Chloroform	Vegetables	Polysorbates
Dimethylsulfoxide (DMSO)	***Medications***	Sodium hypochlorite
Methyl salicylate	Acetylsalicylic acid	Sorbitan monolaurate
Nicotinic acid esters[a]	Alcohols	***Others***
Resorcinol	Ampicillin[b]	Acrylic monomers
Tar extracts	Antibiotics	Aliphatic polyamides
Witch hazel	Bacitracin[b]	Ammonia
Metals	Benzoyl peroxide	Benzophenone
Cobalt chloride	Chloramphenicol[b]	Carbonless copy paper
Preservatives	Chlorhexidine	Diethyltoluamide[b]
Benzoic acid[a]	Neomycin[b]	Epoxy resin[b]
Formaldehyde	Penicillin[b]	Formaldehyde
Sodium benzoate[a]	Phenothiazines	Hydroxytoluene
Sorbic acid	Pyrazolones	Lanolin alcohol
Others	Streptomycin[b]	Lindane
Butyric acid	***Metals***	Mechlorethamine[b]
Diethyl fumarate	Copper	Nylon
Pine oil	Nickel	Paraphenylenediamine
Turpentine	Platinum	Patent blue dye
	Rhodium	Plastic
		Polyethylene glycol
		Sodium silicate
		Sodium sulfide

[a]More commonly implicated agents.
[b]Anaphylaxis reported during skin tests.

lem for healthcare workers with the increased use of latex gloves.[41]

Latex Hypersensitivity

Healthcare professionals responding to emergency situations are keenly aware of the need for personal protective equipment. The most prevalently used form of personal protective equipment in the healthcare field is protective gloves.[41] Currently, protective gloves come in a variety of forms and sizes and are made up from pure or hybrid substances. It is estimated that 5.7 million health care workers use 7 billion pairs of latex gloves yearly. Other glove materials such as vinyl, nitrile, and other combination polymers, are available for specific uses. Latex imparts the combination of high barrier function against microbiologic agents, form-fitting flexibility, excellent tactile sensation, and affordability, which continues to make it the premier constituent in the manufacturing of gloves. The same qualities have made it the most preferred material for the use of condoms and diaphragms. In addition to gloves, medical personnel and potential patients are also exposed to natural rubber latex because of its ubiquitous presence in modern society.

In 1991, the Food and Drug Administration was notified about the deaths of 15 patients who had undergone routine barium enemas with latex-tipped catheters. Investigations revealed that the deaths were related to type I hypersensitivity to natural latex rubber proteins. Since then, latex hypersensitivity has been a well-recognized syndrome with clinical characteristics including contact urticaria, coryza, sneezing, asthma, and rarely anaphylaxis and death. This type of hypersensitivity is mediated by immunoglobulin E (IgE) with the subsequent release of histamine and other mast cell products. Proteins derived from latex extracts are not known to cause delayed-type (type IV) hypersensitivity or contact dermatitis.

Patients with inexplicable urticaria, angioedema, or type I hypersensitivity reactions following medical procedures should be suspect for latex hypersensitivity. Such reactions are often erroneously diagnosed as anesthetic reactions or paradoxical reactions to medications.

Evaluation of the Suspected Latex Allergic Patient

The suspected latex-allergic patient should be carefully questioned regarding symptoms of type I hypersensitivity temporally related to exposure to purported latex agents. Often, histories suggestive of allergic contact dermatitis to rubber accelerators, irritant dermatitis from glove constituents and powders, or contact dermatitis to exogenous chemicals will be elicited. Physical examination may show urticaria in direct areas of contact with suspect agents, but more frequently, the lesions have disappeared by the time a patient is evaluated. Repeated exposures on the hands may result in a chronic dermatitis not suggestive of type I hypersensitivity. Under these circumstances, patients should be evaluated for both type I and type IV hypersensitivity to rubber-related products. The evaluation of allergic contact dermatitis is described later in this chapter. For suspected type I hypersensitivity to latex, a radioallergosorbent assay (RAST) for IgE to latex protein should initially be obtained. Those patients with positive latex-RAST tests and histories suggestive of latex hypersensitivity should be counseled accordingly. Patients must be extensively counseled regarding the avoidance of latex products in the home and in the workplace. Depending on the severity of their symptoms, antihistamines, bronchodilators, and an epinephrine autoinjector should be prescribed. Patients with negative latex RAST tests must have a more elaborate evaluation, because RAST testing may miss over 30% of allergic patients.

Patients presenting with known or suspected latex hypersensitivity reaction should be treated as any patient with type I hypersensitivity.

Protein Contact Dermatitis

Within minutes of handling certain food proteins, some persons with chronic hand dermatitis experience itching or burning and may develop erythema, edema, and occasionally vesicles.[86] Some bakers may experience this type of immediate contact reaction after touching wheat flour.

Airborne Dermatitis

Aerosolized chemicals in gases, vapors, and sprayed liquids can produce irritant and allergic contact dermatitis (Table 28–9). Exposed areas, such as the face, hands, and forearms, are characteristically involved.[26] In office workers, irritation of mucous membranes, fatigue, nau-

TABLE 28–9. SELECTED AGENTS THAT CAUSE AIRBORNE CONTACT DERMATITIS

Allergens	Irritants
Acrylates	Acid vapors
Animal feed	Alkaline vapors
Chromates	Alumina
Cobalt	Anhydrous calcium sulfate (anhydrite)
Colophony	Arsenic
Epoxy hardeners	Cellulose
Epoxy resin	Cement
Formaldehyde	Chromate
Fulminate	Fiberglass
Pesticides	Food additives
Phenolformaldehyde resins	Formaldehyde
Sawdust	Mica
Sesquiterpene lactones	Sawdust
Sulfur compounds	Sewage sludge
Turpentine	Slag
	Sodium sesquicarbonate

sea, headaches, laryngeal edema, and airway obstruction, in addition to palmar dermatitis, was associated with the use of carbonless copy paper.

Particulate Dusts

Small particles from cement, plaster, dust, paper, and sawdust accumulate in clothes or around poor-fitting masks and gloves, causing pruritus. Itching is worse in the neck, antecubital and popliteal fossae, forearms, wrists, and frictional sites, such as the belt and sock lines. Wool fiberglass used in housing insulation and less commonly textile fiberglass penetrate clothing. The greater the diameter of the fiber, the worse the symptoms. Fibers less than 4.57×10^{-4} cm in diameter do not cause itching. Under normal circumstances, the concentration of fiberglass in the air is too low to produce irritation.[75]

Although the eruption caused by particulate dust dermatitis is described as resembling widespread miliaria, commonly the dermatitis is limited to pressure points on the forearms and between the fingers, with only few excoriations present in other body areas. To verify the diagnosis of fiberglass dermatitis, the uppermost cells of the stratum corneum are stripped with cellophane tape, which is then applied to a glass slide. Microscopic examination demonstrates the characteristic rodlike fibers. Fiberglass dermatitis can be prevented by wearing loose, long-sleeved clothing and gloves and rinsing exposed areas with water.

Plant Dermatitis

Plants cause many dermatoses that afflict workers in the forestry and agricultural industries, two of the three industries with the highest incidence of occupational disease. Among the sensitizing plants (Table 28–10), the *Compositae*, the largest family of flowering plants, are frequently found in homes and gardens.[64]

The highly sensitizing plants of the genus *Toxicodendron* (poison ivy, poison oak, poison sumac), commonly cause severe eruptions (see Color Plate, Fig. 7). All parts of these plants, including the roots, are allergenic. Erythematous, weeping papules and plaques, vesicles, and bullae characteristically aligned in linear patterns, erupt on exposed skin (see Color Plate, Fig. 8). The dermatitis is further spread by urushiol-containing oleoresin under the fingernails and in clothing. Following initial sensitization, an eruption develops 9 to 14 days after contact. Once initial sensitization has occurred, contact with urushiol causes a rash within hours to days. The eruption can be prevented by washing the skin within 10 minutes of contact. Related species of *Anacardiaciae* (Japanese lacquer tree, ginkgo fruit tree, India marking nut tree, cashew, mango) contain sufficient amounts of urushiol to produce dermatitis in persons who have been previously sensitized.[82]

Plants of the *Urticaceae* family release pharmacologically active substances that cause dermatitis. Over 500 varieties exist worldwide, but in the United States the most common species are the nettles. These plants have hairs that inoculate the skin with histamine, acetylcholine, and serotonin, producing burning, pruritus, and hives at the site of the sting.[30]

Some plants (parsnip, lime, wild carrot, bergamot orange) contain furocoumarins that cause photodermatitis with erythema, blisters, and hyperpigmentation in persons exposed to those agents and ultraviolet A light. This reaction is a significant occupational hazard among those who harvest or grow celery but has also been seen after eating lemon sorbert while sunbathing.[35] Berloque dermatitis, a type of photo-dermatitis with streaks of erythema that become hyperpigmented, is caused by perfumes or colognes containing furocoumarins.[4]

Contact dermatitis from sensitization to hardwoods and timbers occurs in woodcutters, construction workers, joiners, carpenters, furniture makers, sawyers, shipbuilders, and polishers. Many timbers contain sensitizing quinones (dalbergiones).[12] In most cases, the dermatitis affects the dorsa of the hands initially and later the face, neck, and genitalia. In addition, exposure to sawdust may cause mucous membrane irritation, conjunctivitis, and contact urticaria. Woodcutters eczema arises from sensitization to sesquiterpene lactones in liverworts or usnic and attranorin in lichens.

Explosives

Among the chemical agents used in explosives, Tetryl, Amatol, and trinitrotoluene are more frequently responsible for causing dermatitis. The face, collar line, wrists, and hands are chiefly affected, and with Tetryl the skin characteristically develops a yellow hue.

Treatment of Contact Dermatitis

Treatment of contact dermatitis begins with identification and avoidance of the offending agent, although the allergens may not always be immediately identifiable from the patient's history. Topical corticosteroids are the most effective therapeutic agents used in the treatment of contact dermatitis. Since inflamed skin is more easily sensitized to contact allergens and also more susceptible to irritants, corticosteroid ointments with few or no additives are preferred to creams. Optimal frequency for the application of topical corticosteroids is twice a day. If the dermatitis is acute and weeping, saline or aluminum subacetate compresses can be applied two to four times daily to dry the skin. Oral antihistamines and lotions with menthol in concentrations of 0.25% to 0.5% relieve itching. Treatment of "poison ivy" dermatitis consists of high-potency corticosteroid creams for few lesions and tapering oral doses of prednisone for widespread erup-

TABLE 28–10. PLANTS THAT CAUSE DERMATITIS

Plant	Substance	Dermatitis
Elecampane	Alantolactone, isoalantolactone	ACD
Garlic	Allium, diallydisulfide	ACD, ICD
Allium (chives, leek, onion, shallot)	Allyldisulfide	ICD
Tulips	Alpha methylene gamma butyrolactone	ACD
Tansy	Arbusculin A	ACD
Chrysanthemum	Arteglassin A, parthenolide	ACD photoallergic
Ragweed	Artemiscifolin, isabelin	ACD
Field chamomile	Sesquiterpene lactones	Anaphylaxis after ingestion of camomile tea
Myroxolon balsamum	Balsam of Peru (coniferyl benzoate)	ACD
Styrax tonkinensis, styrax benzoin	Benzoin	ACD, ICD
Hyacinth	Calcium oxalate	ICD
Red pepper	Capsaicin	ICD with blistering submucous fibrosis of palate
Mountain tobacco	Carabron, helenalin	ACD
Cashew nut tree	Cardanol	ACD to unroasted cashew nut. Ingestion causes generalized eczematoid dermatitis
Scorpion weed	Cinnamic acid and derivatives	ACD
Cinnamon	Cinnamic aldehyde	ACD
Eucalyptus	Citronellal	Usually ICD, sometimes ACD
Pine tree	Colophony	ACD, ICD
Benzoin	Comferylbenzoate (cinnamate esters)	ACD
Saussurea lappa roots	Costus oil (costunolide, dihydrocostunolactone, dihydrocostunolide)	ACD
Common mugwort	Eudovicins	ACD
Cloves	Eugenol	ACD, ICD, cheilitis
Geranium	Geraniol	Lip dermatitis
Lavender	—	ICD, ACD
Star anise	Geranylhydroquinone	ACD, ICD, hypopigmentation
Gingko tree	Gingkolic acid	ACD to fruit pulp, ingestion of fruit causes cheilitis, stomatitis, proctitis, and pruritus ani
Caper bush, croton	Glucocapparin	ACD, ICD
Dandelion	Glycopyronosid	ACD
Nettles	Histamine (also acetylcholine)	
Hops	Humulone, lupulone, myrcene	Probable irritant
Radish	Isothiocyanates	Allergic hand dermatitis
Jasmine	Jasmine oil	ACD
Endive/chicory	Lactucin	ACD, palmar hyperkeratosis
Lettuce	Lactucopicrin	ACD
Laurel, sweet bay	Laurel oil (costunolide, laurenobiolide)	ACD
Lemongrass	Lemongrass oil	ICD
Citrus	Limonine citral (citrus oil)	Photodermatitis, irritant dermatitis
Mint	Menthol or carvone	ICD
Cajuput tree	Niaouli oil	ACD
Congress grass	Parthenin	ACD
Euphorbs	Phorbol esters	ICD
Primrose	Primrose oil	ACD, conjunctivitis, erythema multiforme
Garden angelica	Psoralen	Phototoxic dermatitis
Rue	—	Photoallergic dermatitis, ACD
Carrots, parsnip, fig	Psoralen	ICD
Celery	Psoralen	Photodermatitis
Pyrethrum	Pyrethrum oil (Pyrethrosin)	ACD
Orchids	Quinone	ACD
Castor bean	Ricinoleic acid	Lip dermatitis, ICD, ACD
Black mustard	Senevols	ICD Punctate keratosis
Sandalwood	Santal oil	Photoallergy
Sesame oil	Sesamol or sesamin	ICD, ACD
Liverwort dahlia, small-headed sneezeweed	Sesquiterpene lactones	ACD

(continued)

TABLE 28–10. PLANTS THAT CAUSE DERMATITIS (continued)

Plant	Substance	Dermatitis
Norway spruce tree	Stilbestrols	ACD
Dandelion	Tarazin acid	ACD
Thyme	Thyme oil (limonene)	Glossitis, cheilitis, ACD
Tulip	Tuliposide	Allergic hand eczema
Pine tree	Turpentine	ACD, ICD, subungual hyperkeratosis
Mango tree	Urushiol (pentadecylcatechol)	ACD to mango pulp
Poison oak	Urushiols (pentadecylcatechol)	Dermatitis, ACD, leukoderma
Poison ivy	Urushiols (pentadecylcatechol)	ACD, leukoderma
Poison sumac	Urushiols (pentadecylcatechol)	ACD
Marking nut tree (Bhilawa)	Urushiols (pentadecylcatechol)	ACD
Ylang Ylang	Urushiols (pentadecylcatechol)	ACD
Japanese lacquer tree	Urushiols (pentadecylcatechol)	ACD
Lichens	Usnic acid	Photosensitivity
Vanilla	Vanillin	ACD, headache, somnolence, facial and hand dermatitis and vertigo ("vanillism")
Narcissus	Unknown	"Tulip rash" contact dermatitis
Jonquil	Unknown	"Tulip rash" contact dermatitis
Daffodil	Unknown	"Tulip rash" contact dermatitis
Diffenbachia	Unknown	ICD, glossitis and edema of oral mucosa if chewed
Philodendron	Unknown	ACD
Asparagus	Unknown	Contact dermatitis
Wandering Jew	Unknown	ICD

ACD = Allergic contact dermatitis; ICD = Irritant contact dermatitis.

tions. Antihistamines, colloidal oatmeal baths, talcum-based shake lotions with menthol, phenol, or calamine, and compresses provide additional relief.

Commercially available hyposensitizers have produced disappointing results. High-potency corticosteroids should be avoided on facial and intertriginous skin since they may quickly result in irreversible atrophy and striae. Corticosteroids will produce atrophy if used for periods exceeding weeks. The greater the potency, the greater the risk of developing atrophy, purpura, folliculitis, striae and telengiectasiae.

Approximately, 30 g of ointment is required to cover the entire body. The quantity prescribed depends on the involved area and the frequency and duration of treatment. If the dermatitis is widespread and very severe, a systemic corticosteroid, such as prednisone, at a dose of 40 to 60 mg/day gradually tapered over 10 to 14 days, is prescribed. Barrier creams have often been touted to reduce the incidence of irritant and allergic contact dermatitis. In vivo laboratory studies using barrier creams for the prevention of rust dermatitis show some promise. Practical uses in industry and in the field have had disappointing results. Frequent applications of these products are necessary, since the creams are easily removed through friction and rubbing.[38]

Photosensitivity Reactions

An ingested or topically applied chemical may not result in adverse cutaneous effects until the skin is exposed to sunlight. Photosensitivity reactions are divided into two groups: phototoxicity and photoallergy. Phototoxicity occurs when the chemical causes direct damage by intensifying the skin's sensitivity to sunlight. The resulting condition simulates a sunburn and predominantly involves areas exposed to sunlight, such as the face, neck, forearms, and dorsa of the hands, but spares the submental portion of the chin, the palms, and usually the flexor region of the extremities. The reaction may be immediate but more commonly is delayed for 48 hours or longer.[3] Some chemicals, such as coal tar and amyl-O-dimethylbenzoic acid, exhibit diphasic reactions with immediate wheals that resolve within hours, followed by raised erythematous plaques 12 to 24 hours later. In dark-colored individuals, symptoms may be minimal or absent, and only hyperpigmentation may be present. Photoallergy occurs when chemicals react with ultraviolet light to induce an allergic reaction. Initially, intensely pruritic, eczematous lesions with sharply demarcated margins appear over areas exposed to sunlight. Later the lesions become widespread and lichenified from rubbing.

Photosensitivity reactions are frequently caused by systemic drugs (Table 28–11), but a variety of environmental substances may also be responsible. Both phototoxicity and photoallergy are generally caused by ultraviolet A (UVA) light (wavelengths of 320 to 400 nm) and less often by ultraviolet B (UVB) light (wavelengths of 280 to 320 nm).[32]

A complication of photoallergy is persistent light reaction, a form of chronic actinic dermatitis. This photosensitivity reaction continues indefinitely and may worsen even after removal of the allergen. The ability to tolerate UVB light and occasionally UVA and visible light is markedly diminished. This incapacitating condition

TABLE 28–11. PHOTOSENSITIZING MEDICATIONS

Phototoxic Reactions	Photoallergic Reactions
Amiodarone	Antihistamines
Captopril	Barbiturates
Dicarbazine	Chlorpropamide
Fluorouracil	Diltiazem
Furosemide[a]	Glyburide
Nalidixic acid	Griseofulvin
Naproxen	NSAIDs
NSAIDs	PABA
Phenothiazines[a]	Phenothiazines[a]
Psoralens[a]	Procaine
Tars	Quinidine
Tetracyclines	Quinine
Tricyclic antidepressants	Sulfonamides
Vinblastine	Thiazides[a]
Warfarin	Tricyclic antidepressants

[a]Most commonly implicated drugs.

may last months to years. The more frequently reported agents associated with persistent light reaction are halogenated salicylanilides, musk ambrette, chlorpromazine, and promethazine.[71] Acute phototoxicity is a rare complication of methylene blue poisoning.[67] The diagnosis of photoallergic contact dermatitis is confirmed with photopatch testing. The suspected substances are applied over two sites. One patch is covered and the other is exposed to a measured dose of ultraviolet light. Both areas are examined 48 hours later. Development of erythema only on the irradiated patch confirms the diagnosis. Treatment of photosensitivity involves identification and removal of the photosensitizing agent. Antihistamines, topical antipruritic agents, and cool compresses relieve symptoms. Topical corticosteroids reduce the inflammatory response and may diminish the pigmentation sequelae. If the reaction is intense, treatment with systemic corticosteroids is usually required. Antimalarials, beta carotene, and PUVA are not very effective in chronic photoallergic dermatitis. Minimal light exposure during the symptomatic period is recommended and topical sunscreen with sun protective factors of 15 or greater is prescribed for UVB protection. Combinations of PABA (para-aminobenzoic acid) and its esters, cinnamates, and salicylates adequately screen UVB light, and benzophenones and parasol protect against UVA. Because UVA light penetrates glass, patients must utilize sunblock even during automobile rides. Opaque agents, such as titanium dioxide, red veterinary petrolatum, and tincture of zinc oxide, are less cosmetically appealing but block longwave light in addition to UVA and UVB light.

Chemical Burns

As a rule, chemical burns produce more extensive tissue destruction than thermal burns. Direct skin contact causes tissue damage that results in inflammation, edema, serum exudation, and necrosis. With some chemicals, such as gaseous fluoride, an almost instantaneous burn results, but with other agents, such as cement, the burn may be delayed for hours after exposure. Depending on the depth of cutaneous damage, the burns are classified as first, second, or third degree.

In first-degree burns, the injury is limited to the epidermis. The skin is tender, dry, and hyperemic and there are no blisters. Healing occurs within a week without scarring. Hypopigmentation may result if the burn is sufficiently deep to destroy melanocytes, but if more superficial, postinflammatory hyperpigmentation will be present.

Superficial second-degree burns involve the epidermis and the upper (papillary) dermis. The painful blistering, suppurative, erythematous plaque heals within 3 weeks with pigmentary changes but little or no scarring. Deep second-degree burns involve the lower dermis. The burned area does not blanch with pressure, and may lack sensation. Even when infection is absent, healing may require more than 1 month, and disfiguring scarring with localized loss of hairs and sebaceous glands can result.

Third-degree burns result from destruction of the entire skin, including the subcutaneous tissue. The skin is firm and gray-white or brown and is anesthetic.

Chemical burns are often caused by acids or alkalis (Table 28–12). Acids coagulate protein and dehydrate tissue. The resulting coagulation necrosis leaves the skin hard and dry. In contrast, alkalis dissolve and damage keratin, saponify fats, and cause liquefaction necrosis, leaving the skin soft and gelatinous.

Common chemicals causing burns that may require hospitalization include hydrofluoric acid, sulfuric acid, black lacquor, lye, potassium permanganate, and phenol. Sequelae of chemical burns include ocular injury, wound infection, tendon exposure, amputations, and systemic reactions from absorption of the chemical.[15]

Hemodialysis and intravenous bicarbonate to correct metabolic acidosis may be needed if systemic toxicity to some chemicals, such as formic acid, develops.[16]

Phenol, in concentrations greater than 5%, causes skin sloughing, denatures proteins, and on prolonged contact causes necrosis.[11] Cement burns develop in construction workers without adequate protective equipment or in inexperienced "weekend builders." The abrasiveness and alkalinity of the calcium hydroxide in wet cement initially causes only mild irritation, but 12 to 24 hours after exposure necrotic ulcers develop. Because cement readily leaks under gloves and boots, the ankles, patellar region, and wrists are most commonly affected.

The most dramatic chemical burns are produced by hydrofluoric acid. Pain may not begin for hours after contact with concentrations below 50%, and there may not be detectable physical findings even when the patient complains of agonizing pain (Chap. 86 and Color Plate, Fig. 12). Early diagnosis and treatment of hydrofluoric acid exposures prevents devastating tissue damage, serious dysrhythmias, and possibly death.[5,27]

For many highly irritating substances, development of a burn depends on the concentration and exposure time. At low concentrations, ammonia produces ery-

TABLE 28–12. SELECTED CAUSES OF CHEMICAL BURNS

Chemical	Cutaneous Reactions	Systemic Reactions	Initial Treatment
Alkyl mercury compounds	Irritant dermatitis, burns	See Chapter 80	Irrigate with water; remove blister to prevent systemic intoxication
Bitumen (hot pitch and tar)[47]	Burns	None	Irrigate with cold water until the bitumen cools and hardens; clean with an antiseptic and apply an adherent hydrocarbon solvent; unroof any bitumen blisters; bitumen that has not been removed initially will become emulsified by the solvent and easily removed in several days
Bromine gas[14]	Burns	Respiratory symptoms, eye irritation, headache, fatigue	Copious aqueous irrigation
Cement	Second-degree burns that may be delayed for hours after exposure	None	Copious aqueous lavage
Chromic acid[84]	Small, often painless skin ulcers	Cough, chest pain, wheezing, headache, fever, weight loss	Copious aqueous lavage and frequent rinsing with 10% ascorbic acid solution to reduce the hexavalent chromate
Ethylene oxide[36]	Burns	Local irritation of eyes and respiratory tract (see Chaps. 53, 109)	Irrigate with soap and water
Hydrofluoric acid[27]	Burns	Pulmonary edema, laryngospasm, hypocalcemia	Superficial burns: following copious water irrigation zephiran (benzalkonium chloride) topically applied is most effective; calcium acetate, magnesium hydroxide antacid, and calcium gluconate gels are not as effective (see Chap. 86)
Monochloracetic acid[34]	Burns	Disorientation, cardiac failure, coma, metabolic acidosis, cerebral edema, renal insufficiency and death if 10% of body area is exposed	Water irrigation. No available antidote
Phenol[45]	Erythema and blistering	Dysrhythmias, cardiopulmonary arrest, convulsions, coma	Decontaminate skin with low molecular weight polyethylene glycol diluted 2:1 with isopropyl alcohol
Selenium oxychloride	Burns	None	Irrigate with water and apply 10% sodium thiosulfate
White phosphorus[28]	Ignites on contact with air causing thermal burns	Dysrhythmias, shock, sudden death	Irrigate with 1 to 2% copper sulfate and debride residue

thema and edema, but first to third-degree burns sometimes resembling deep frostbite injuries have occurred following prolonged contact with concentrated vapors or liquid ammonia, and widespread contact leading to extensive systemic absorption has been fatal. Liquid nitrogen used as a refrigerant and for treatment of cutaneous neoplasms and warts produces rapid freezing of the skin that results in erythema, blistering, and, with prolonged contact, frostbite injuries. Adhesives cause irritant and allergic contact dermatitis, and cyanoacrylate adhesives bond skin instantly, causing burns due to heat release. The skin surface bonded by the adhesive should be immersed in soapy water, or preferably acetone, and the surface then carefully pulled or rolled apart with a blunt edge, such as a spatula or spoon handle. Pulling the bonded surfaces apart with a direct opposing action can result in severe tears. Any glue residue will be shed in time.

The treatment of chemical burns begins with immediate removal of all contaminated clothing, followed by irrigation of the skin with copious volumes of water. After application of a topical antibiotic, the wound is covered with a nonadherent dressing. Analgesics are prescribed as necessary. During the following days, the wound is surgically debrided. For deep burns, grafting may be necessary. In general, hospitalization is required for severe burns of the face, hands, feet, genitals, anus, perineum, and flexor areas; for partial-thickness burns over 10% or more of the body surface area; and for full-thickness burns exceeding 2% of the body surface area.

Solvents and Plasticizers

Solvents are fluids capable of dissolving substances. Plasticizers are nonvolatile chemicals incorporated into plastics to improve flexibility. Almost all solvents are irritants, as they can dissolve the surface lipids of the stratum corneum and cell membranes. The lower the boiling point, the higher the irritating potential of a solvent. Highly volatile solvents (Table 28–13) can produce severe burns after prolonged skin contact. Older, highly viscous diesel oils with high content of aromatic compounds and sulfur cause little irritation compared to lighter, less polluting diesel oils.[34] Death is reported after widespread contact with gasoline for 1 hour. Plasticizers rarely cause allergic contact dermatitis.

TABLE 28–13. IRRITATING SOLVENTS IN ORDER OF DESCENDING SEVERITY

Carbon disulfide
Coal tar solvents (xylol, tuluol)
Petroleum distillates (diesel, gasoline, kerosene, turpentine)
Chlorinated hydrocarbons (methylene chloride, freon, thrichlorethylene)
Alcohols (methyl, ethyl)
Glycols (propylene glycol)
Esters (methyl acetate, butyl acetate)
Ketones (acetone, methylethyl ketone)
Dimethyl sulfoxide

Acneiform Eruptions

The exact mechanism by which acneiform eruptions occur remains unknown. Comedones, inflammatory papules, and pustules develop, predominantly on the face and back. Cysts, abscesses, and scarring can occur. The eruptions can be follicular and pustular and resemble bacterial folliculitis. In one study, 87% of cases of acute generalized exanthematous pustulosis were caused by drugs, usually antibiotics. In some of the cases caused by penicillin, the histologic changes were consistent with a leukocytoclastic vasculitis.

Chloracne

Although chloracne is listed under the subheading of acneiform eruptions, its commonality with classical acne is limited only to its similar-sounding name. Chloracne represents a distinct pathophysiologic entity caused by exposures to classical chloracnegens (Table 28–14).[96] Chloracne represents a rare disease, but it is an occupational and environmental skin disease. Classically, open and closed comedones and straw-colored cysts are present behind the ears, around the eyes, and may be present on the trunk with predilection for the shoulders and back as well as the groin and genitalia. Exposure to chloracnegens is also associated with other integumentary findings such as hypertrichosis, hyperpigmentation, brown discoloration of the nails, conjunctivitis, and eye discharge.[85] The histologic distinctness of chloracne in contrast to folliculitis and classical acne may be useful in diagnosis. In chloracne there is degeneration of sebaceous units with prominent hyperkeratosis around follicular orifices.[61]

TABLE 28–14. CHLORACNEGENS

Hexachlorodibenzo-*p*-dioxin
Polybrominated dibenzofurans
Polybrominated biphenyls
Polychlorinated biphenyls
Polychlorinated dibenzofurans
Polychloronapthalenes
Tetrachloroazobenzene

Despite anecdotal reports of exposure to chloracnegens and illnesses involving the gastrointestinal, reproductive, cardiovascular, central nervous, immune, and other systems, epidemiologic studies of people exposed to these chemicals through their occupational or industrial accidents have failed to demonstrate reproducible organ-specific illnesses. The exception are the changes of chloracne. Relatively high levels of oral or topical exposure are necessary to produce these cutaneous changes.[33]

Chloracne is classically recalcitrant to the use of topical and oral antibiotics, and keralytics. Occasionally, systemic isotretinoin can produce some improvement, but no regimen has consistently provided good success. Chloracne may remain active years after exposure and the routine scarring from these lesions is permanent. Elevated serum levels of high and low chlorinated biphenyls are associated with PCB-induced chloracne. However, the degree of elevation cannot be directly correlated with disease activity. Determinations of serum PCB levels for both low and high chlorinated congeners are useful in evaluating patients with suspect disease. Serum levels of both higher and lower chlorinated PCBs range may remain elevated from several years to decades. Hence, long-term evaluation is needed.

Chlorinated hydrocarbon decontamination should be undertaken with a 10-minute application of mineral oil, which is wiped off with acetone. If these substances are unavailable, the skin should be immediately washed with soap and water. Chlorinated hydrocarbons induce the more severe occupational acneiform eruptions but occupational acne more commonly occurs in machinists, mechanics, and other workers regularly exposed to insoluble cutting oils and semisynthetic metal.[59] In these workers, an inflammatory folliculitis may develop on the hands, arms, and trunk. Coal tar factory laborers, roofers, and construction or road maintenance workers may develop tar acne. Comedones predominate, but hyperpigmentation may develop after phototoxic reactions to tar.

A number of medications can induce or worsen acne. Chronic ingestion of bromides or iodides can lead to acneiform eruptions and granulomatous papules, nodules, and plaques with pustular, crusted, vegetating, papillomatous, or ulcerated surfaces.[79] The condition (bromoderma, iododerma) commonly appears on the face but can involve any area of skin, including the mucous membranes (see Color Plate, Fig. 16). Bromoderma occurs in about 25% of patients with systemic bromism. Skin involvement does not correlate with serum bromide levels, but patients with bromoderma have elevated bromide concentrations in their skin. Lesions that resemble pyoderma gangrenosum including plaques covered with pustules, abscesses, and weeping ulcers are also reported in patients treated with gold salts.

Treatment of chemical- and drug-induced acne consists of oral antibiotics (tetracycline or erythromycin), topical antibiotics (clindamycin, erythromycin, benzoyl peroxide), azelaic acid, and topical retinoids such as tretinoin (Retin-A) and adapalene. If only comedones are present, topical retinoids and comedone extraction suf-

TABLE 28–15. SUBSTANCES THAT CAUSE VESICULAR REACTIONS

Alkyl mercurials
Carbon monoxide
Caustic agents
Diphenoxylate
Dimethyl sulfate
Drugs (see Table 28–18)
Ethylene oxide
Hexachlorobenzene

fices. In recalcitrant cases, oral isotretinoin (Accutane), 1 mg/kg per day for 20 weeks, can be prescribed after careful counseling against pregnancy.

Vesiculobullous Reactions

Vesicular reactions develop after contact with or ingestion of a number of chemical agents (Table 28–15). Blisters may also be present in a number of drug eruptions, including erythema multiforme, fixed drug reactions, vasculitis, and phototoxic eruptions. A number of drugs produce flaccid vesicles and bullae that are clinically and often histopathologically indistinguishable from pemphigus vulgaris or pemphigus foliaceous, as well as tense blisters that are similar to bullous pemphigoid or cicatricial pemphigoid. Immunofluorescence studies may show epidermal intracellular immunoglobulin deposits in the pemphigus and dermal–epidermal junction deposits in the pemphigoid drug eruptions. When widespread blistering occurs, systemic corticosteroids should be used.

Vesicles and bullae resembling epidermolysis bullosa acquisita, another immunologic blistering disease, are reported in patients with sedative-hypnotic overdoses, such as barbiturates and glutethimide, as well as after carbon monoxide exposure (see Color Plate, Fig. 10). Certain drugs, such as alcohol and oral contraceptives, can unmask porphyria cutanea tarda resulting in blisters over sun-exposed areas such as the face and dorsa of hands (Table 28–16). These blisters heal with scars, pigmentary changes, and milia. Hypertrichosis may be evident in the affected areas.

Agents such as sulfur mustard, an agent used in chemical warfare, produce blistering by disruption of the anchoring filaments of basal cell desmosomes at the dermal–epidermal junction, and in high concentrations necrosis of skin and mucous membranes.[20]

TABLE 28–16. SUBSTANCES THAT CAUSE PORPHYRIA CUTANEA TARDA

Estrogens
Chlorinated dibenzofurans
Chlorinated dioxins
Chlorinated hydrocarbons
Chlorinated phenols
Drugs (see Table 28–18)
Hexachlorobenzene

Sclerodermatous Changes

Distinct or confluent papular or sclerodermatous changes of the hands, trunk, face, and forearms, often associated with Raynaud syndrome of the hands and feet—facial telangiectasias, and mottling of the skin of the hands—occur in 1 to 6% of workers in factories where the polyvinyl chloride level in the air is greater than 4 ppm. Through its metabolites, this agent has the potential to stimulate collagen production as well as to induce immunologic alterations, such as hypergammaglobulinemia, cryoglobulinemia, and cryofibrinogenemia. Impotence, dyspnea, dizziness, and irrational laughter as well as hepatosplenomegaly may also be seen. The skin changes do not always improve after exposure ceases.[56] Chlordane, heptachlor, malathion, parathion, DDT, sodium dinitro-orthocresolate, and 7-chlorocyclohexane have been reported to cause sclerodermatous changes, particularly on the hands, occasionally accompanied by Raynaud syndrome. Acrosclerosis and acrocyanosis have also been associated with perchloroethylene, a dry cleaning solvent; trichloroethane; trichloroethylene, a metal cleanser; polyvinyl chloride (see Color Plate, Fig. 15), and after treatment with bleomycin, bromocriptine, vitamin K, sodium valproate, and 5-hydroxytryptophan. Eosinophilic fasciitis has been reported after therapy with phenytoin (Dilantin) and tryptophan.[8] Tryptophan was implicated in numerous cases of eosinophilia-myalgia syndrome (EMS).[77] The acute features of EMS included myalgia, arthralgia, peripheral edema, fever, fatigue, pulmonary symptoms, and dysrhythmias in association with peripheral eosinophilia and a variety of skin manifestations, including morbilliform eruptions, urticaria, angioedema, dermatographism, papular mucinosis, livedo reticularis, and alopecia. Several patients who had ingested high doses of tryptophan developed chronic muscle weakness and sclerodermatous changes or fasciitis preferentially involving the proximal extremities and trunk but sparing the face, hands, and feet. A contaminant of levotryptophan introduced during manufacturing changes appears to have been responsible for this disease. Diffuse cutaneous sclerosis has been observed in workers exposed to organic solvents or the vapors of epoxy resins and in silica coal miners.

In Spain, ingestion of rapeseed oil denatured with aniline caused a cluster of symptoms that became known as the epidemic toxic oil syndrome.[66] The disease, which was caused by a non-necrotizing vasculitis, consisted of pneumonitis, gastrointestinal and neurologic symptoms, and a widespread, pruritic maculopapular eruption that lasted about 5 to 20 days. Some patients developed cutaneous leukocytoclastic vasculitis (palpable purpura) or erythema multiforme. Five to 6 months after ingesting the oil, 10% of patients developed brown or yellow papules over all areas except the palms and soles. Localized or generalized morphea with esophageal dysmotility was observed in several patients, most of them women. Immunoglobulin levels, eosinophil counts, liver function tests, and antinuclear antibody levels often remained elevated 4 months after exposure. Neuromyopathy, sicca syndrome, pulmonary hypertension, and renal disease were observed in some patients with chronic disease, many of whom had expression of HLA-DR3 and -DR4 antigens.

Oil Dermatitis

Insoluble "neat" oils are derived from animals, vegetables, or minerals and may contain sulfur, chlorine, phosphorus, or other additives to enhance performance. Besides follicular eruptions, these oils may cause hyperpigmentation, keratosis, cancer of the scrotum or exposed skin, epitheliomas, and contact dermatitis.

Soluble oils are oil-in-water emulsions and contain emulsifiers (petroleum sulfonates, carboxylic acid soaps), antifoaming agents, corrosion inhibitors, extreme-pressure additives, germicides, and dyes. Aqueous oil solutions do not contain emulsifiers and depend on the effect of surfactants and water. Unlike insoluble neat oils, soluble oils and aqueous solutions do not produce acne and only rarely produce keratoses or epitheliomas, but they frequently cause eczematous dermatitis in mechanics. Usually the etiology is irritation but sensitization to the additives is documented in a number of cases. Characteristically, soluble oil eczema starts in a follicular distribution, but eventually discrete patches and plaques form on the hands and the forearms. Rarely, vesicles on the palms and fingers develop.

Metals and Metallic Salts

Direct subcutaneous injections or extravasation of mercury injected into blood vessels can produce local granuloma and abscesses. Five cases of systemic toxicity were reported after subcutaneous mercury injection without evidence of elemental dissemination.[6]

Metals can cause diverse cutaneous manifestations (Table 28–17). Elements such as nickel can induce dermatitis in solid form but do so more commonly through solutions of metallic salts. Local reactions or systemic poisoning occurs after ingestion, inhalation, and, rarely, percutaneous absorption of metals. Any metal that forms salts can be irritating to the skin, and a number of metal compounds are known to cause irritant and allergic contact dermatitis. Some, such as antimony trioxide, produce an irritant folliculitis. Allergic contact dermatitis to nickel, chromium, cobalt, and mercury is a major form of industrial morbidity. In fact, nickel is the most common sensitizer in the general population.

Chromium exposure can result from a variety of occupational and nonoccupational sources such as cement, leather, pigments, and metal plating chemicals.[24] Potassium dichromate containing hexavalent chromium is the most sensitizing species. Trivalent chromium rarely causes contact dermatitis even in many chromium-sensitive patients. Hand dermatitis resulting from chrome sensitization may be particularly recalcitrant to treatment. Even after discontinuation of exposure, debilitating hand dermatitis may persist for years.

Photocontact dermatitis is reported after applications of compounds containing salts of silver, selenium, gold, arsenic, and cadmium. Beryllium contact dermatitis develops 2 weeks after contact. The lesion becomes verrucous and remains for approximately 1 month.

Zinc-beryllium silicate in fluorescent light tubes, introduced into the skin through lacerations, produces local swelling, induration, tenderness, ulceration, granuloma formation, and necrosis.[54] Deposition of beryllium crystals into the skin produces ulceration that heals only if the ulcer is excised or the beryllium is removed from the ulcer surface through curettage. Soft, red-brown, noncaseating dermal granulomas have also developed after recurrent skin application of deodorants containing zirconium lactate or oxide. Sarcoidal granulomas, which may not appear for up to 5 decades, can develop in wounds contaminated with silicon dioxide (silica). Pruritic photoallergic, sarcoidal granulomatous reactions have been described in red tattoos. The responsible agent was cadmium sulfide, a photosensitizing yellow pigment added to mercury to brighten the red color. Sun-blockers relieve the symptoms. The granulomatous hypersensitivity reaction may be delayed for several decades. Organic compounds, such as silica, silastic, and silicone, are associated with systemic sclerosis, polymyositis, and other connective tissue disorders. These compounds were identified in sclerodermatous skin of patients with silicone breast implants.[78]

Bluish gray discoloration can result from skin inoculation (iron, mercury, silver, or oral administration (gold, silver) of certain metal particles (see Color Plate, Fig. 18). Hyperpigmentation from mercury, lead, silver, or bismuth may involve the oral mucosa due to dermal metal deposits (see Color Plate, Fig. 17) and, in the case of mercury, due to increased melanosis. Arsenic salts appear to stimulate melanin synthesis by enhancing tyrosinase activity. Months to years after exposure to arsenic-containing products, such as Fowler solution, discrete, hard, hyperkeratotic yellow or tan keratosis appear predominantly on the palms, soles, and digits (see Color Plate, Fig. 13). These lesions are precursors of invasive squamous cell carcinomas and should be excised or destroyed by cryotherapy or electrodesiccation and curettage.[81] The skin of patients with previous arsenic exposure should be periodically examined. Arsenic (Chap. 78) and thallium (Chap. 82) toxicities are further discussed elsewhere. In general, cutaneous changes follow the development of systemic manifestations. Some lead compounds, especially tetrabutyl lead and lead naphthanate, can be absorbed through unbroken skin. The absorption of lead acetate and lead oxide, however, is insignificant.[9]

Chelating agents, although beneficial in the management of certain metal intoxications, do not improve

TABLE 28–17. CUTANEOUS MANIFESTATIONS OF METALS

Metal	Topical Application	Ingestion
Aluminum	Irritant dermatitis	—
	Allergic contact dermatitis (rare)	—
Antimony	Irritant dermatitis	—
Arsenic	Irritant dermatitis	—
	Allergic contact dermatitis	
	Irritant folliculitis	
	Bodyfold ulcerations (especially on creases and webs of hands)	
	Cheilitis	
Beryllium	Irritant dermatitis	—
	Allergic contact dermatitis	
	Irritation ulcers	
	Implant granulomas	
Boron	Irritant dermatitis	—
Cadmium	Irritant dermatitis	—
	Photodermatitis	
Chromium	Irritant dermatitis	—
	Skin ulcers	
	Perforation of nasal septum	
	Allergic contact dermatitis	
	Photocontact dermatitis	
Cobalt	Irritant dermatitis	—
	Allergic contact dermatitis	
	Contact urticaria	
Copper	Irritant dermatitis (rare)	Green-black pigmentation of skin, hair and teeth (copper dust)
	Allergic contact dermatitis (rare)	
Gold	Allergic contact dermatitis (rare)	Blue-gray pigmentation (chrysiasis)
	Irritant dermatitis	Maculopapular eruptions
	Allergic contact dermatitis from solutions of gold salts	Lichenoid dermatitis
		Exfoliative dermatitis
	Blue-gray discoloration (hydrargyrosis)	Stomatitis
		Generalized spongiotic dermatitis
Lithium	Irritant to mucous membranes and skin in high concentration	Acneiform eruption
Magnesium	Mild irritant to mucous membranes	—
Mercury	Irritant dermatitis	Tenderness and swelling
	Allergic contact dermatitis	
	Dermatitits is particularly common with mercury fulminate ("fulminate itch") and pigments in cosmetics	
	Blue-gray pigmentation (hydrargyrosis)	
	Implant granulomas	
Molybdenum	—	Hair discoloration
Nickel	Allergic contact dermatitis	—
Palladium	Irritant dermatitis	—
Platinum	Irritant dermatitis	—
	Allergic contact dermatitis	
	Urticaria	
	Exacerbation of atopic dermatitis	
Selenium	Irritant dermatitis	Loss of hair and nails
		Garlic breath
Silica	Irritant dermatitis, granulomas	Scleroderma-like syndrome
Silver	Blue-black discoloration of skin	Slate-gray pigmentation on light-exposed areas (argyria)
	Irritant to skin and mucous membranes	Nail bed pigmentation
Strontium	Contact with water may result in explosion and burn	—
Tellurium	No direct reaction	Dental discoloration
		Garlic breath and smell
Thallium	No direct reaction	Alopecia
		Stomatitis
		Gingivitis
		Purpura
		White transverse lines

(*continued*)

TABLE 28–17. CUTANEOUS MANIFESTATIONS OF METALS (continued)

Metal	Topical Application	Ingestion
Tungsten carbide	Eczematous dermatitis	Green tongue
Vanadium	Eczematous dermatitis Irritation of mucous membranes	Nonspecific dermatitis
Zinc	Irritant dermatitis Irritant ulcerations (zinc chloride) Perforation of nasal septum (zinc chloride) "Zinc pox"—vesicular eruptions of intertriginous areas (zinc oxide dust)	Metallic oral taste
Zirconium	Hypersensitivity cutaneous granulomas	—
Rare Earths and Others		
Dysprosium, holmium, erbium	Subcutaneous nodule if injected	—
Gallium	In situ necrosis when injected subcutaneously	—
Gadolinium and samarium	Ulcers on abraded skin	—
Lead	Gray gingival "lead lines," pallor and lividity	—
Lutetium and europium	Scarring on abraded skin, subcutaneous nodule if injected	—
Manganese	Mask-like facies, excessive sweating	—
Osmium	Mucous membrane changes, petechiae	—
Terbium	Irritant dermatitis	—

metal-induced skin disease. Hypersensitivity granulomas usually respond to systemic corticosteroids or triamcinolone acetonide at a dose of 3 to 5 mg/mL injected into the granuloma. Other local cutaneous manifestations of metal toxicity are treated in the usual manner for the particular disorder.

Pigmentary Disorders

Any chemical agent may produce a change in pigmentation by causing an inflammatory dermatitis. Metals, drugs, and red azo dye (used by Hindu women as a cosmetic) may produce skin discoloration. Ironically, in black persons, hydroquinone, a hypopigmenting agent, can cause disfiguring rebound pigmentation (ochronosis).[44] Both hypopigmentation and hyperpigmentation are more pronounced in black and Asian individuals. Severe injuries, such as hydrofluoric acid or lye burns, damage the melanocytes and produce hypopigmentation.

Depigmentation indistinguishable from vitiligo may develop within 2 weeks of contact with some chemicals derived from phenol, alkyl phenol, and catechol. Industrial leukodermas are caused by monobenzyl ether of hydroquinone, formerly used as an antioxidant to prolong durability of rubber products; hydroquinone, used in photograph development; *p*-tert-butylphenol, a chemical used in adhesives for shoe repair; phenolic compounds used in disinfectants; and catechol derivatives used in auto assembly oils.[80] The hands are most commonly affected in occupational leukoderma, but unexposed sites may also become depigmented. The mechanism by which phenol compounds depigment appears to involve formation of free radicals, which initiate lipid peroxidation and disrupt the lipoprotein membrane of the melanocyte. Some compounds may also inhibit tyrosinase activity.

Epidermal hyperpigmentation is treated with hydroquinone. Treatment is required for weeks to months. It is imperative that the patient shield the pigmented area from sunlight by applying a sunscreen with a protection factor of 15 or higher, or by wearing protective clothing. Mild hypopigmentation usually improves with time, and camouflage cosmetics such as Covermark or Dermablend can be applied during the period of resolution. Cosmeticians can assist the patient in matching skin color. Disfiguring or extensive hypopigmentation and depigmentation can be treated with PUVA (psoralens and UVA light). Due to the risk of serious burning, this therapy should be undertaken only by physicians experienced in this treatment modality.

Drug Reactions

Cutaneous drug reactions are one of the more common and intolerable adverse effects of systemic medications (Table 28–18). Between 2 and 3% of hospitalized adult patients develop drug-induced skin eruptions. When patients are receiving multiple medications, it can be difficult to identify the responsible drug. The frequency of reactions elicited by a drug, the duration of treatment, and the type of cutaneous lesions typically associated with a drug are important considerations in identification of the causative agent. For instance, penicillins are most frequently implicated in maculopapular drug eruptions but rarely cause lichenoid reactions. A recently prescribed drug is more suspect than one that has been administered for weeks, unless the patient has taken the drug intermittently. Penicillins, sulfonamides, and blood products account for approximately two thirds of all drug reactions involving the skin.

Although toxic, photosensitive, and pharmacologic mechanisms may be responsible, drug hypersensitivity accounts for the majority of cutaneous drug reactions.

TABLE 28–18. MEDICATIONS THAT CAUSE CUTANEOUS REACTIONS

Acanthosis Nigricans
Corticosteroids
Diethylstilbestrol
Niacinamide

Acneiform Reactions
Androgens
Anticonvulsants (phenytoin, (carbamazepine, trimethadione, paramethadione)
Antituberculous agents (isoniazid, ethambutol, ethionamide)
Azathioprine
Bromides
Corticosteroids
Danazol
Dantrolene
Hypocholesterolemic agents
Iodides
Isoniazid
Lithium
Oral contraceptives (progesterone dominant)

Annular or Gyrate
Antimalarials
Cimetidine
Estrogens
Penicillin
Piroxicam
Salicylates
Spironolactone
Thiazides
Vitamin K

Eczematous
Aminophylline
Antihistamines
Chloral hydrate
Disulfiram
Ethylenediamine
Gentamicin
Iodides
Kanamycin
PAS
Piperazine
Procaine
Streptomycin
Thiazides
Tolbutamide

Erythema Multiforme
Barbiturates
Carbamazepine
Chlorpropamide
Cimetidine
Codeine
Cyclophosphamide
Furosemide
Gold
Griseofulvin
Hydantoins
Minoxidil
Nonsteroidal antiinflammatory drugs
Penicillins
Pentazocine
Phenolphthalein
Phenothiazines
Progesterone
Rifampin
Sulfonamides[a]
Sulfones
Tetracyclines
Thiazides
Trimethodione
Sulfamethoxazole with trimethoprim[a]

Erythema Nodosum
Amiodarone
Bromides
Iodides
Oral contraceptives
Penicillins
Salicylates
Sulfones
Tetracyclines

Exfoliative Erythroderma
Allopurinol[a]
Barbiturates[a]
Captopril
Carbamazepine
Cefoxitin[a]
Chloroquine
Chlorpromazine
Cimetidine
Diltiazem
D-penicillamine
Gold
Griseofulvin
Hydantoins
Isoniazid
Lithium
Nitrofurantoin
Penicillins[a]
Phenylbutazone
Quinidine
Streptomycin
Sulfonamides[a]
Sulfonylureas

Fixed Drug Reactions
Acetaminophen
Allopurinol[a]
Anthralin
Barbiturates[a]
Captopril
Carbamazepine
Cefoxitin[a]
Chloral hydrate
Chlordiazepoxide
Chloroquine
Chlorpromazine
Cimetidine
Dextromethorphan
Diltiazem
D-penicillamine
Erythromycin
Gold
Griseofulvin
Hydantoins
Hydralazine
Isoniazid
Lithium
Metronidazole
Nitrofurantoin
Nonsteroidal antiinflammatory drugs
Opioids
Oral contraceptives
Penicillins[a]
Phenacetin
Phenolphthalein[a]
Phenylbutazone
Quinidine
Quinine
Salicylates[a]
Streptomycin
Sulfonamides[a]
Sulfonylureas
Sympathomimetics
Tetracyclines[a]
Trimethoprim

Hypertrichosis
Androgens
Corticosteroids
Cyclosporine
Diazoxide
Hydantoin
Minoxidil
Penicillamine
Psoralens
Streptomycin

Lichenoid Reactions
Alpha-methyldopa
Antimalarials[a]
Beta-adrenergic Antagonists
Captopril
Carbamazepine
Chlorpropamide
Furosemide
Gold[a]
Levamisole
Nandrolone
Naproxen
Penicillamine
Phenothiazines
Pyrimethamine
Quinidine
Streptomycin
Sulfonylureas
Tetracyclines
Thiazides

Livedo Reticularis
Acyclovir
Metronidazole
Miconazole
Thrombostatic agents
Vancomycin

Lupus-like Reactions
Alpha-methyldopa
Barbiturates
Griseofulvin
Hydralazine[a]
Ibuprofen
Isoniazid
Penicillamine
Phenothiazines
Phenytoin
Procainamide[a]
Quinidine
Trimethoprim

Maculopapular Reactions (> 5% of patients exposed)
Aclofenac
Amoxicillin[a]
Ampicillin[a]
Atropine
Barbiturates
Bleomycin
Captopril
Carbamazepine
Cephalosporins[a]
Chlorpromazine
Daunorubicin
D-penicillamine
Dipyrone
Gentamicin[a]
Gold[a]
Isoniazid
Meprobamate
Methsuximide
Miconazole
Nalidixic acid
Naproxen
Penicillins[a]
Phenothiazines
Phenylbutazone[a]
Phenytoin[a]
Piroxicam
Quinidine
Streptomycin
Sulfonamides[a]
Sulfamethoxazole with trimethoprim
Thiabendazole
Thiazides

Nail Pigmentation
Azathioprine (pink)
5-Fluorouracil (half-blue, half-brown)
Gold (borwn)
Methotrexate (brown)
Phenothiazines (tan or slate)
Quinacrine (yellow or brown)
Tetracyclines (yellow)
Timolol (brown)
Zidovudine (AZT) (dark brown)

Onycholysis
Adriamycin
5-Fluorouracil
Gold
Phenothiazines
Practolol
Psoralens
Tetracyclines
Thiazides

Pellagra
Chloramphenicol
5-Fluorouracil
Isoniazid[a]
6-Mercaptopurine

Pemphigoid
Furosemide
Penicillins
Penicillamine
Phenacetin
Psoralens
Sulfasalazine

Pemphigus
Captopril
Cephalosporins
D-penicillamine[a]
Gold
Heroin
Hydantoin
Indomethacin
Levodopa
Penicillins
Phenylbutazone
Progesterone
Propranolol
Rifampin

(continued)

TABLE 28–18. MEDICATIONS THAT CAUSE CUTANEOUS REACTIONS (continued)

Pigmentation
Amiodarone (yellow)
Antimalarials (blue-black)
BCNU (brown)
Bleomycin (brown)
Busulfan (brown)
Carotene (orange)
Chlorpromazine (gray or brown)
Clofazimine (red-brown)
Cyclophosphamide (brown)
Daunorubicin (brown)
Fluorouracil (brown)
Gold (blue-gray)
Hydroquinone (ochronosis)
Imipramine (brown)
Methotrexate (brown)
Mithramycin (brown)
Mitomycin (brown)
Minocycline (blue-gray)
Oral contraceptives (chloasma)[a]
Phenothiazines (gray or brown)
Phenytoin (brown)
Quinacrine (yellow)
Thio-TEPA (brown)

Pityriasis Rosea-like Reactions
Arsenicals
Barbiturates
Beta-adrenergic antagonists
Bismuth
Captopril
Clonidine
Gold[a]
Griseofulvin
Isotretinoin
Metronidazole
Penicillin
Pyribenzamine

Porphyria
Barbiturates
Estrogens
Ethanol
Griseofulvin
Rifampin
Sulfonamides

Pseudoporphyria
Furosemide
NSAIDs
Nalidixic acid
Sulfonylureas
Tetracyclines

Psoriasis
Beta-adrenergic antagonists
Captopril
Cimetidine
Clonidine
Interferon
Lithium
NSAIDs
Quinidine

Seborrheic Dermatitis-like Reactions
Cimetidine
Gold

Toxic Epidermal Necrolysis
Allopurinol[a]
Barbiturates
Carbamazepine
Dapsone
Ethambutol
Griseofulvin
Gold
Hydantoin
Isoniazid[a]
NSAIDs
Nitrofurantoin
Penicillins[a]
Pentamidine
Salicylates
Streptomycin
Sulfonamides[a]
Tetracyclines

Urticarial Reactions (1 to 5% of persons exposed)
Amiodarone
Aminoglycosides
Blood products[a]
Cephalosporins[a]
Chemotherapeutic agents
Codeine[a]
Dextran
Fluconazoles
Hydantoin
Hydralazine
Ketoconazole
Methimazole
NSAIDs
Opioids
Penicillin and derivatives
Procainamide
Progesterone
Quinidine
Radiographic contrast material[a]
Salicylates
Streptokinase
Sulfonamides
Thiouracil
Vaccines with egg protein

Vasculitis
Allopurinol[a]
Amiodarone
Amphetamine
Aspirin
Barbiturates
Captopril
Cimetidine
Coumadin
Erythromycin
Fluoroquinolones
Furosemide[a]
Gold
Griseofulvin
Hydantoin
Hydralazine
Iodides
Methotrexate
Penicillins
Penicillamine[a]
Phenothiazines
Phenylbutazone
Phenytoin[a]
Procainamide
Propylthiouracil
Quinidine
Quinine
Radiocontrast material
Streptomycin
Sulfonamides
Tetracyclines
Thalidomide
Thiazides

[a]Most commonly implicated drugs.

Any of the four types of immunologic reactions (IgE-mediated, cytotoxic, immune complex, and cell-mediated) may be involved.[48]

Immediate allergic reactions usually develop within 1 hour of drug administration and constitute a medical emergency, as life-threatening anaphylaxis can occur.

Accelerated reactions are usually urticarial and begin 1 to 72 hours after initiation of therapy. The urticarial reaction is potentially life threatening, as laryngeal edema may develop. Delayed reactions appear during and as long as 3 weeks after discontinuing drug intake and have protean manifestations.

Some drugs produce unusual cutaneous changes.[90] Cholesterol-lowering agents, such as clofibrate, may lead to the development of dry, brittle, ichthyotic skin. Adriamycin, methotrexate, 5-fluorouracil, and vinblastine administration are associated with reactivation of radiodermatitis. Isotretinoin can induce pyogenic granulomas and postsurgical keloids. Ulcerated lichen planus limited to the palms and soles resembling crucifixion stigmata has occurred during treatment with hydroxyurea.[69] Anthroquinones in laxatives have caused weeping nonallergic perianal and gluteal dermatitis from skin contact with feces. Pseudoporphyria, a vesicular phototoxic reaction that resembles porphyria cutanea tarda, can occur during treatment with furosemide, nalidixic acid, naproxen, and tetracyclines. Rapid infusion of vancomycin produces widespread erythema (the red man syndrome). Drug toxicity should always be considered in the evaluation of unusual cutaneous lesions.

Percutaneously absorbed drugs can also cause systemic toxicity (see Tables 28–2 and 28–5). For instance, topical gamma benzene hexachloride (lindane) causes seizures and death in small infants; mercury-containing ointments are implicated as a cause of gingivitis, stomatitis, and nephrotic syndrome; and urticaria and anaphylaxis are reported from use of topical bacitracin, neomycin, penicillin, and benzocaine. Topical medications in preparations for opthalmologic, ottic, nasal, vaginal, and rectal diseases can occasionally cause generalized drug eruptions.

Exanthematous, Morbilliform, and Maculopapular Eruptions

Morbilliform eruptions account for almost 50% of dermatoses induced by systemic drugs. Erythematous, discrete or confluent, symmetrically distributed, and frequently pruritic macules and papules usually appear initially on the trunk and over pressure areas and eventually spread over the entire body.[95] Mucous membranes and palms and soles are occasionally involved. Low-grade fever and, less often, lymphadenopathy may appear. The presence of eosinophilia can be a valuable diagnostic finding in cases where the eruption is clinically indistinguishable from a viral exanthem.

Although the eruption can appear at any time within 3 weeks of initiating drug therapy, the majority develop during the first week. The onset may be delayed for up to 1 week after discontinuation of the drug. Despite withdrawal of the medication, the eruption may become more intense for a few days, but clearing can be expected within 2 weeks. The eruption usually, but not always, reappears if the drug is readministered at the same or higher doses. Although histologic findings are not specific, the presence of a perivascular lymphohistocytic infiltrate with occasional eosinophils, extravasation of erythrocytes, and necrotic epidermal keratinocytes all point to a diagnosis of drug hypersensitivity. Complications may consist of progression to vasculitis, erythema multiforme, and exfoliative erythroderma. Drug eruptions may resolve despite continuation of the medication, but more commonly they become widespread.

Antihistamines, topical corticosteroids, and antipruritic lotions provide relief of symptoms, and the first two may also hasten resolution of the lesions.

Exfoliative Erythrodermic Eruptions

Exfoliative erythroderma may be caused by skin diseases such as psoriasis, atopic dermatitis, and cutaneous T-cell lymphoma in addition to drugs and chemicals. The skin becomes red and desquamates over 80% or more of the body. Patients may complain of pruritus or a burning sensation. Serious complications of exfoliative erythroderma include dehydration, metabolic imbalance, hypoalbuminemia, hypothermia, cardiac failure, and septicemia. Hospitalization for management of complications and topical corticosteroid therapy is recommended. The most striking manifestation of borate toxicity is a bright red, generalized exfoliation (boiled lobster appearance), which develops 1 to 3 days after chronic ingestion of boric acid.

Urticarial Eruptions

Urticarial lesions are pink or red, edematous papules and plaques that blanch with pressure and sometimes have serpiginous borders. When single lesions persist longer than 24 hours, urticarial vasculitis should be considered. In angioedema, swelling of the entire dermis and subcutaneous tissue involves localized areas such as the lips and dorsa of the hands. Edema of the larynx, epiglottis, or surrounding tissues produces upper airway obstruction. Urticarial reactions can become chronic, arbitrarily defined as lasting longer than 6 weeks. The reaction is mediated by histamine and other substances released by cutaneous mast cells. Degranulation of mast cells in the GI tract and lungs produces abdominal cramping and bronchospasm.

Drugs elicit urticarial reactions by several mechanisms. Type I, IgE-dependent, immune reactions are the most serious due to the possible development of anaphylaxis, but more commonly drugs evoke a type III immune reaction that involves activation of the mast cell degranulating complement subunits, $C3_a$ and $C5_a$. In the case of opioids and other drugs, the mechanism involves direct histamine release from mast cells by the pharmaceutical agent. Finally, certain prostaglandin inhibitors, such as salicylates and nonsteroidal antiinflammatory drugs, may stimulate urticarial reactions by impeding the suppressive influence of prostaglandins on mast cells. Notably, in some of these patients hives can also be triggered by chemicals, particularly benzoates, and some azo dyes, such as the popular yellow food colorant, tartrazine. Sulfite preservatives occasionally induce urticarial reactions. The responsible agent is sometimes extremely difficult to identify, as in cases of chronic urticaria caused by exposure to wood preservatives containing pentachlorophenol.[53] H_1 antihistamines are the treatment of choice for urticaria. When high doses of antihistamines from one class are ineffective, an antihistamine from a different class should be prescribed. In recalcitrant cases, an H_2 antihistamine, an oral beta-adrenergic antagonist, or a calcium channel blocker can be added. Subcutaneous epinephrine and systemic corticosteroids may be necessary in severe cases.

Erythema Multiforme

Drugs are responsible for 10 to 20% of cases of erythema multiforme. The causative mechanism is a type III immune complex reaction that involves complement activation. The characteristic "target" lesions consist of concentric rings of different colors: red from vasodilation, purple from erythrocyte extravasation, white from edema, and black from necrosis. Pink or violaceous papules or plaques with or without central urticarial blistering may be the only lesions present. The palms and soles are often involved. Mucosal vesicles and erosions may be accompanied by fever and a toxic appearance (Stevens-Johnson syndrome).

The effect of systemic corticosteroids in the treatment of erythema multiforme is controversial. Advocates of corticosteroids claim that doses of prednisone greater than 60 mg daily must be started early in the illness to be effective.

Toxic Epidermal Necrolysis

With a 30 to 50% mortality rate when diffuse sloughing is present, toxic epidermal necrolysis (TEN) is second only to anaphylaxis as the most serious cutaneous drug reaction. Initially, the skin becomes erythematous and tender over large areas, particularly on the face and extremities. Discrete papules, patches, or plaques with dark centers may be present. Over several hours, severe epidermal detachment occurs. Mucosal lesions and fever are invariably present. Application of moderate pressure can dislodge the epidermis from the dermis (Nikolsky sign). Fever, malaise, and pharyngitis may appear early in the course. If the patient recovers, transient hair loss, nail dystrophy, and cicatricial conjunctivitis frequently occur. Some dermatologists regard drug-induced epidermal necrolysis as the extreme end of a spectrum that comprises erythema multiforme and Stevens-Johnson syndrome. According to revised definitions, the extent of detachment of the epidermis from the underlying dermis must be greater than 10% of the skin surface if target lesions are absent, or at least 30% if target lesions are also present.[2]

The etiology of toxic epidermal necrolysis has remained controversial with immunologic and metabolic mechanisms described in the literature. Recent data indicate that TEN may be the result of metabolic abnormalities in epoxide hydrolase and glutathione transferase, particularly in circulating lymphocytes. In patients with TEN from carbamazepine, an arene oxide intermediate was toxic to the patient's lymphocytes. Free carbamazepine was not similarly toxic.[37]

Patients should be treated in an intensive care or burn unit, with meticulous attention to infection control, metabolic balance, and temperature regulation. Treatment with systemic corticosteroids is highly controversial, and diverse results have been noted. The better studies indicate that corticosteroids do not improve mortality and predispose to septicemia.[2]

Fixed Drug Reactions

Cutaneous drug reactions may be "fixed" in that the lesions recur in the same sites on repeated administration of the medication. The typical lesion is a bright or dusky red, oval, or circular patch or plaque with central pigmentation. Occasionally blisters form in the center of the patch. The lesions may be asymptomatic or may cause burning.

Although any region of the body may be involved, the face, mouth, hands, feet, and genitalia are favored. In addition to drugs, food substitutes and flavors have been implicated as causes of these eruptions.

Erythema Nodosum

Erythema nodosum lesions result from a septal panniculitis in the adipose tissue. Deep, painful, pink, or violaceous nodules or indurated plaques appear in the pretibial area or calves and less frequently on the thighs, buttocks, and upper extremities. Treatment includes discontinuation of the responsible medication, bed rest, and high doses of salicylates or nonsteroidal antiinflammatory agents.

Lichenoid Reactions

As in lichen planus, the lesions of lichenoid reactions are flat-topped (planar), purpuric, polygonal, and intensely pruritic papules that coalesce into plaques. Lichenification from rubbing and postinflammatory hyperpigmentation are common. On histopathologic examination, the main feature that distinguishes lichenoid reactions from lichen planus is the presence of eosinophils in the band-like dermal infiltrate of mononuclear cells. Potent fluorinated corticosteroids, antipruritic lotions, and in severe cases, systemic corticosteroids accelerate resolution. Lichenoid eruptions have occurred after exposure to certain color developers.[7]

Drug-Induced Lupus Erythematosus

Cutaneous lesions are common in lupus erythematosus induced by drugs. Usually erythematous or violaceous papules or plaques or a "butterfly rash" is seen. Systemic symptoms can be present, such as arthritis, pleurisy, fever, and malaise. Although the clinical and histologic findings may be indistinguishable from those of idiopathic lupus erythematosus, the presence of antihistone antibodies is a differentiating factor in drug-induced lupus. Also, serum complement and gamma globulin levels are usually normal.

Some of the implicated drugs are known to bind to DNA on exposure to ultraviolet light. It is postulated that the transformed DNA molecule is more antigenic.

Although improvement occurs after discontinuation of the drug, resolution may require months.

Pityriasis Rosea-Like Eruptions

Some drugs produce eruptions that resemble pityriasis rosea. The lesions are oval, pink patches or flattened plaques that often have fine scaling in the center. The eruptions usually involve the trunk in an "inverted pine tree" pattern, occasionally affecting the extremities, buttocks, and groin. Treatment consists of discontinuation of the drug, oral antihistamines, and topical corticosteroids.

Purpura

Necrotizing vasculitis due to drugs, produce purpuric, nonblanching macules become raised (palpable purpura) on the feet, legs, and occasionally the upper extremities and other body regions. Sometimes the lesions are wheals (urticarial vasculitis), hemorrhagic bullae, or ulcerations.

Histologically, the reaction is characterized by a leukocytoclastic vasculitis with fibrin deposition in the vessel walls and a perivascular infiltrate with intact and fragmented neutrophils (nuclear dust). Involvement of other organs, particularly the kidneys, joints, liver, lungs, and brain should be excluded. The treatment is the withdrawal of the offending agent. When the vasculitis is disabling or affects essential organs, therapy with systemic corticosteroids should be instituted. Milder vasculitis may respond to antihistamines, indomethacin, colchicine, or dapsone alone or in combination. Drugs that interfere with platelet aggregation, such as valproic acid and aspirin, or anticoagulation, such as warfarin and heparin, can cause purpura. Cytotoxic drugs that suppress the bone marrow and depress platelet counts below 30,000/mm^3 also produce bleeding into the skin. Bleomycin causes direct endothelial damage. Pigmented purpura, a benign lymphocytic capillaritis, has been noted during therapy with carbamazepine, meprobamate, phenacetin, thiamine, and chlordiazepoxide.

Coumarin Necrosis

Direct toxic effects on blood vessel walls from warfarin and, less often, heparin, can lead to ecchymosis, hemorrhagic blisters, ulcers, and massive subcutaneous necrosis, usually around day 7 to 10 of treatment.[65] The reaction is associated with vitamin K-related protein C deficiency (see Chap. 42).

Carcinogens

Premalignant keratosis as well as squamous cell and, less often, basal cell carcinomas can develop years after arsenic ingestion. Prolonged contact with dimethylbenzanthracene, 3,4-benzopyrene, and other tar derivatives such as creosote, pitch, asphalt, and mineral oil, result in papillated keratosis (tar warts) and squamous cell carcinomas. These carcinomas also occur in workers exposed to formaldehyde. Vinyl chloride is transformed in the skin and liver to metabolites that induce hepatic angiosarcomas and cutaneous melanomas. Workers repeatedly exposed to benzidine or alpha or beta-naphthylamine have increased rates of bladder neoplasms. A higher incidence of cutaneous T-cell lymphoma is reported in workers with chronic allergic contact dermatitis, particularly those in the construction, manufacturing, and agricultural industries.[89] Mercury salts can sensitize the skin and may be linked to the development of these lymphomas.[46] Other suspected skin carcinogens include acrylamide, acrylonitrile, arsenic, polychlorinated biphenyls, carbon tetrachloride, 3,3-dichlorobenzidine, 1,1-dimethylhydrazine, dimethylsulfate, ethylene dibromide, hexamethyl phosphoramide, hydrazine, phenylhydrazine, methyl hydrazine, methyl iodide, *N*-nitrosodimethylamine, *O*-toluidine, and pharmaceutical agents.[25] Nitrosamines formed from nitrites and amines are implicated in some cases of skin cancer.

Atypical Lymphoid Infiltrates

Oral intake and topical application of volatile oils are reported to cause lymphoreticular hyperplasia in the skin. In some of these cases, lymphocytoma cutis appeared at the site of intradermal injections for desensitization. Rarely, hydantoin derivatives cause lesions that are indistinguishable from cutaneous T-cell lymphomas. They usually rapidly regress after discontinuation of the drug but may progress to death with further drug intake.

Nail Abnormalities

Allergic and irritant contact dermatitis can produce a variety of nail changes.[74] The more common are onycholysis (distal detachment of the nail plate from the nail bed), paronychia (inflammation of the periungual skin), thinning and splitting of the nail plate, leukonychia (white discoloration), nail pigmentation or coloration, pitting, Mee's lines (white transverse bands—see Color Plate, Fig. 14), and Beau's lines (horizontal notches in the nail plate). Onycholysis has developed after contact with rust-removing agents containing hydrofluoric acid, laundry detergents with enzymes, a number of drugs, sodium hypochlorite in swimming pool solutions, and various other irritants.[22]

Solvents, alkalis, acids, and other chemicals—such as formaldehyde, motor oils, diquat, paraquat, and dinitroorthocreosol—can soften and gradually damage the nail plate, producing nail dystrophy, longitudinal striations (onychorrhixis), and horizontal splitting of the nail plate (onychoschizia). Koilonychia, concave, spoon-shaped nail plates, is reported from contact with organic solvents, acids, alkalis, and oils, which soften the nail plate and make it susceptible to reshaping from direct pressure during work.

Several chemicals stain nails, including cupric sulfate (blue); mercury and eosin (red); nail lacquer (red-brown); formaldehyde (gray); silver nitrate (gray-black); iodine and resorcinol (brown); methyl green (green); vioform and fluorescein (yellow); picric acid, nicotine, and photographic developers (yellow-brown); and tars (black/yellow).

Flushing

Flushing may be produced by a number of chemicals and pharmaceutical agents (Table 28–19). Facial flushing and tachycardia following ingestion of ethanol correlate with serum levels of acetaldehyde and are more frequently observed in Asians and Native Americans (55 to 85%) than in whites (5 to 23%). A peculiar reaction occurs in workers exposed to trichloroethylene, a solvent and degreaser. After drinking alcohol, they may develop bright red patches on the face, neck, shoulders, and chest (degreaser's flush). The appearance is most dramatic about 30 minutes after ethanol ingestion and fades in approximately 1 hour. Rubber industry workers develop an identical reaction after exposure to tetramethyl or tetraethylthiuram disulfide (disulfiram), also used to control alcohol addiction. Exposure to *N*-*N*-dimethylformamide or *N*-butyraldoxime can cause flushing after concomitant ethanol ingestion.

TABLE 28–19. MEDICATIONS THAT CAUSE FLUSHING

Medication	Ethanol Interaction
Ergotamine	Disulfiram
Niacinamide	Chloral hydrate
Nitrates	MAO inhibitors
Clonidine	Metronidazole
Reserpine	Sulfonylureas
Sympathomimetic agents	Procarbazine
Calcium channel blockers	Griseofulvin
Theophylline	Trichloroethylene
Ethanol	—

In addition to disulfiram, a number of other drugs cause clinically significant vasodilation after ingestion of ethanol. Patients taking chloral hydrate for at least a week who then drink ethanol may develop flushing with tachycardia and headaches. The reaction seems to be mediated by trichloroethanol, a chloral hydrate metabolite whose production is stimulated by ethanol. The trichloroethanol in turn inhibits ethanol metabolism, leading to pronounced vasodilation. Prominent flushing can also follow coadministration of ethanol and metronidazole, procarbazine, sulfonylureas, or griseofulvin. The metronidazole-ethanol reaction is usually mild and has been described as a "pleasant rush," but symptoms such as confusion and dizziness can frighten patients who are unaware of the interaction. Monoamine-oxidase inhibitors block the metabolism of tyramine, which is present in large concentrations in Chianti wine, aged cheeses, pickled herring, and chicken livers, resulting in increased norepinephrine release and potentially lethal hypertensive crisis. A similar reaction occurs less commonly when patients taking isoniazid eat large portions of Swiss cheese. Vasodilation produced by ethanol or nicotinic acid can be prevented by the prostaglandin-inhibiting effect of NSAIDs.

Summary

The skin is repeatedly exposed to potentially toxic substances. Whether by design or by accident, we breathe and ingest, touch, smear, wear, brush, and gargle chemicals that can induce a variety of cutaneous reactions through diverse mechanisms. Although these skin reactions are rarely lethal, they are invariably disconcerting to the patient, often symptomatic, occasionally disfiguring, and at times disabling.

In certain instances, the diagnosis and even the source of poisoning may become evident from the cutaneous findings. Careful examination of the skin should always be part of the evaluation of a patient presenting with a toxicologic emergency.

References

1. Bason M, Lammintausta K, Howard IM: Irritant dermatitis (irritation). In: Marzulli FN, Maibach HI, eds: Dermatotoxicology, 4th ed. New York, Hemisphere, 1991, pp. 223–253.
2. Bastuji-Garin S, Rzany B, Stern RS, et al: Clinical classification of cases of toxic epidermal necrolysis, Stevens-Johnson syndrome, and erythema multiforme. Arch Dermatol 1993; 129:92–96.
3. Beijersbergen van Henegouwen GM: (Systemic) phototoxicity of drugs and other xenobiotics. J Photochem Photobiol 1991;10:183–210.
4. Benezra C, Ducombs G, Sell Y, Fousserau J: Plant Contact Dermatitis. Toronto, BC Decker, 1985.
5. Bertolini JC: Hydrofluoric acid: A review of toxicity. J Emerg Med 1992;10:163–168.
6. Bradberry SM, Feldman MA, Braithwaite RA, et al: Elemental mercury-induced skin granuloma: A case report and review of the literature. J Toxicol Clin Toxicol 1996;34: 209–216.
7. Brandao FM: Colour developers and lichen planus. Contact Dermatitis 1986;15:253.
8. Breathnack SM, Hintner H: Scleroderma-like reactions. In: Breathnack SM, Hintner H, eds: Adverse Drug Reactions and the Skin. London, Blackwell Scientific, 1992, pp. 118–122.
9. Bress WC, Bidanset JH: Percutaneous in vivo and in vitro absorption of lead. Vet Hum Toxicol 1991;33:212–214.
10. Bronaugh RL, Stewart RF, Storm JE: Extent of cutaneous metabolism during percutaneous absorption of xenobiotics. Toxicol Appl Pharmacol 1989;99:534–543.
11. Bruze M, Almgren G: Occupational dermatoses in workers exposed to resins based on phenol and formaldehyde. Contact Dermatitis 1988;19:272–277.
12. Burrall BA: Plant-related allergic contact dermatitis. Clin Rev Allergy 1989;7:417–439.
13. California Department of Industrial Relations, Division of Labor Statistics and Research: Occupational Skin Disease in California. San Francisco, California Department of Industrial Relations, 1982.
14. Carel RS, Belmaker I, Potashnik G, et al: Delayed health sequelae of accidental exposure to bromine gas. J Toxicol Environ Health 1992;36:273–277.
15. Cartotto RC, Peters WJ, Neligan PC, et al: Chemical burns. Can J Surg 1996:39:205–211.
16. Chan TC, Williams SR, Clark RF: Formic acid skin burns resulting in systemic toxicity. Ann Emerg Med 1995;26: 383–386.
17. Christoph RA: General protocol for dermatologic poisoning. In Noji EK, Kelen GD, eds: Manual of Toxicologic Emergencies. Chicago, Year Book, 1989, pp. 119–121.
18. Cohen DE, Brancaccio R, Andersen D, Belsito DV: Utility of a standard allergen series alone in the evaluation of allergic contact dermatitis: A retrospective study of 732 patients. J Am Acad Dermatol. 1997;36:914–918.
19. Cohen SR, Samitz MH: Occupational skin disease. In: Moschella SL, Hurley HJ, eds: Dermatology. Philadelphia, Saunders, 1992, pp. 1871–1920.
20. Dacre JC, Goldman M: Toxicology and pharmacology of the chemical warfare agent sulfur mustard. Pharm Rev 1996;48: 289–326.
21. Dalt LD, DallAmico R, Laverda AM, et al: Percutaneous ethyl alcohol intoxication in a one-month-old infant. Pediatr Emerg Care 1991;7:343–344.

22. Daniel CR: Onycholysis: An overview. Semin Dermatol 1992;10:34–40.
23. DeGroot AC, Wheeland JW, Nater JP: Unwanted Effects of Cosmetics and Drugs Used in Dermatology, 3rd ed. Amsterdam, Elsevier, 1994.
24. Deng JF, Fleeger AK, Sinks T: An outbreak of chromium ulcer in a manufacturing plant. Vet Hum Toxicol 1990;32: 142–146.
25. Dodson VN, Zenz C: Occupational cancer risks. In: Zenz C, ed: Occupational Medicine: Principles and Practical Applications. Chicago, Year Book, 1988, pp. 815–832.
26. Dooms-Goosens E, Delusschene KM, Gevers DM, et al: Contact dermatitis caused by airborne irritant. J Am Acad Dermatol 1986;15:1–10.
27. Dunn BJ, Mackinnon MA, Knowlden NF, et al: Hydrofluoric acid dermal burns: An assessment of treatment efficacy using an experimental pig model. J Occup Med 1992;34: 902–909.
28. Eldad A, Chaouat M, Weinberg A, et al: Phosphorous pentachloride chemical burn: A slowly healing injury. Burns 1992;18:340–341.
29. Elias JJ: The microscopic structures of the epidermis and its derivatives. In: Bronaugh RL, Maibach HI, eds: Percutaneous Absorption. New York, Dekker, 1989, pp. 1–26.
30. Epstein WL: Plant-induced dermatitis. Ann Emerg Med 1987;16:950–955.
31. Fenske RA, Blacker AM, Hamburger SJ, Simon GS: Worker exposure and protective clothing performance during manual seed treatment with lindane. Arch Environ Contam Toxicol 1990;19:190–196.
32. Ferguson J: Photosensitivity dermatitis and actinic reticuloid syndrome (chronic actinic dermatitis). Semin Dermatol 1990;9:47–54.
33. Fischbein A, Wolff MS, Bernstein J, Selikoff IJ: Dermatologic findings in capacitor manufacturing workers exposed to dielectric fluids containing polychlorinated biphenyls. Arch Environ Health 1982;37:69–74.
34. Fischer T, Bjarnason B: Sensitizing and irritant properties of 3 environmental classes of diesel oil and their indicator dyes. Contact Dermatitis 1996;34:309–315.
35. Fisher AA: Contact Dermatitis, 4th ed. Baltimore, Williams & Wilkins, 1995.
36. Fisher AA: Burns of the hands due to ethylene oxide used to sterilize gloves. Cutis 1988;42:267–268.
37. Friedmann PS, Strickland I, Pirmohamed M, Park BK: Investigation of the mechanisms in toxic epidermal necrolysis induced by carbamazepine. Arch Dermatol 1994;130: 598–604.
38. Grevelink SA, Murrell DF, Olsen EA: Effectiveness of various barrier preparations in preventing and/or ameliorating experimentally produced toxicodendron dermatitis. J Am Acad Dermatol 1992;27:182–188.
39. Hadgraft J, Brain K: Xenobiotic experimentation: Predicting percutaneous penetration. In: Marks R, Plewig G, eds: The Environmental Threat to the Skin. London, Martin Dunitz, 1992, pp. 179–184.
40. Harvell J, Bason M, Maibach HI: Contact urticaria (immediate reaction syndrome). Clin Rev Allergy 1992;10:303–323.
41. Heese A, Van-Hintzenstern J, Peters KP, et al: Allergic and irritant reactions to rubber gloves in medical health services: Spectrum, diagnostic approach, and therapy. J Am Acad Dermatol 1991;25:831–839.
42. Hoffer E, Taitelman U: Exposure to paraquat through skin absorption: Clinical and laboratory observations of accidental splashing on healthy skin of agricultural workers. Hum Toxicol 1989;8:483–485.
43. Hogan DJ: Pesticides and other agricultural chemicals. In: Adams RM, ed: Occupational Skin Disease, 2nd ed. Philadelphia, Saunders, 1990, p. 557.
44. Hull PR, Procter LR: The melanocyte: An essential link in hydroquinone-induced ochronosis. J Am Acad Dermatol 1990;22:529–531.
45. Hunter DM, Timerding BL, Leonard RB, et al: Effects of isopropyl alcohol, ethanol, and polyethylene glycol/industrial methylated spirits in the treatment of acute phenol burns. Ann Emerg Med 1992;21:1303–1307.
46. Hursh JB, Clarkson TW, Miles EF, Goldsmith LA: Percutaneous absorption of mercury vapor by man. Arch Environ Health 1990;44:120–127.
47. James NK, Moss AL: Review of burns caused by bitumen and the problems of its removal. Burns 1990;16:214–216.
48. Kahsh RS: Drug eruptions: A review of clinical and immunological features. Adv Dermatol 1987;6:221–237.
49. Kao J, Carver MP: Skin metabolism. In Marzulli FN, Maibach HI, eds: Dermatotoxicology, 4th ed. New York, Hemisphere, 1991, pp. 143–200.
50. Kenerva L, Estlander T, Jolanki R: Skin testing for immediate hypersensitivity in occupational allergology. In: Menne T, Maibach HI, eds: Exogenous Dermatoses: Environmental Dermatitis. Boca Raton, CRC Press, 1991, pp. 52–63.
51. Keyman AM: The spectrum of contact urticaria: Wheals, erythema and pruritus. Dermatol Clin 1990;8:57–60.
52. Klein G, Grubauer G, Fritsch P: The influence of daily dishwashing with synthetic detergent on human skin. Br J Dermatol 1992;127:131–137.
53. Lambert J, Schepens P, Janssens J, Dockx P: Skin lesions as a sign of subacute pentachlorophenol intoxication. Acta Derm Venereol (Stockh) 1986;66:170–172.
54. Maceira JM, Fukuyama K, Epstein WL: Appearance of T-cell subpopulations during the time course of beryllium-induced granulomas. J Invest Dermatol 1984;83:314–316.
55. Manoguerra AS: Full thickness skin burns secondary to an unusual exposure to diquat dibromide. J Toxicol Clin Toxicol 1990;28:107–110.
56. Markowitz SS, McDonald CJ, Fethiere W, et al: Occupational acroosteolysis. Arch Dermatol 1972;106:219–233.
57. Marks JG, Belsito DV, DeLeo VA, et al: North American Contact Dermatitis Group standard tray patch test results (1992–1994). Am J Contact Derm 1995;6:160–165.
58. McDougal JN, Jepson GW, Clewell HJ III, et al: Dermal absorption of organic chemical vapors in rats and humans. Fundam Appl Toxicol 1990;14:299–308.
59. Mills OH, Kligman AM: Acne mechanica. Arch Dermatol 1975;111:481–484.
60. Moloney SJ, Teal JJ: Alkane-induced edema formation and cutaneous barrier dysfunction. Arch Dermatol Res 1988; 280:375–379.
61. Moses M, Prolieau PG: Cutaneous histologic findings in chemical workers with and without chloracne with past ex-

posure to 2,3,7,9-Tetrachlorodibenzo-p-dioxin. J Am Acad Dermatol 1985;12:497–506.

62. Narducci WA, Wagner JC, Hendrickson TP, Jeffrey TP: Anabolic steroids: A review of the clinical toxicology and diagnostic screening. J Toxicol Clin Toxicol 1990;28:287–310.
63. Occupations commonly associated with contact dermatitis. In: Marks JG, DeLeo VA, eds: Contact and Occupational Dermatology. St. Louis, Mosby-Year Book, 1992, pp. 1–346.
64. Paulsen E: Compositae dermatitis: A survey. Contact Dermatitis 1992;26:76–86.
65. Peterson CE, Kwaan HC: Current concepts of warfarin therapy. Arch Intern Med 1986;146:581–584.
66. Phelps RG, Fleischmajer R: Clinical, pathologic, and immunopathologic manifestations of the toxic oil syndrome: Analysis of fourteen cases. J Am Acad Dermatol 1988;18: 313–324.
67. Porat R, Gilbert S, Malgilner D: Methylene blue-induced phototoxicity: An unrecognized complication. Pediatrics 1996;97:717–721.
68. Priborsky J, Takayama K, Priborska Z, et al: The influence of detergents on skin barrier properties. Pharmacol Toxicol 1992;70:344–346.
69. Renfro L, Kamino H, Raphael B, et al: Ulcerative lichen planus-like dermatitis associated with hydroxyurea. J Am Acad Dermatol 1991;24:143–145.
70. Renfro L, Sanchez MR, Moy JA: Cutaneous ulcers caused by drugs. Wounds 1990;2:236–246.
71. Roelandts R: Chronic actinic dermatitis. J Am Acad Dermatol 1993;28:240–249.
72. Sanchez MR, Moy JA: The cutaneous manifestations of violence and poverty. Arch Dermatol 1992;128:829–839.
73. Sanchez MR, Spielman T, Epstein W, Moy JA: Treatment of oral hairy leukoplakia. Arch Dermatol 1992;128:1659. Letter.
74. Scher RK, Daniel CR: Nails: Therapy, Diagnosis, Surgery. Philadelphia, Saunders, 1990.
75. Sertoli A, Giorgini S, Farli M: Fiberglass dermatitis. Clin Dermatol 1992;10:167–174.
76. Shmunes E: The role of atopy in occupational skin diseases. Occup Med 1986;1:219–228.
77. Silver R, Heyes P, Jaize J,et al: Scleroderma, fasciitis and eosinophilia associated with the ingestion of tryptophan. N Engl J Med 1990;322:874–878.
78. Silver RM, Sahn EE, Allen J, et al: Demonstration of silicon in sites of connective-tissue disease in patients with silicone-gel breast implants. Arch Dermatol 1993;129:63–68.
79. Soria C, Allegue F, Espana A, et al: Vegetating iododerma with underlying systemic diseases: Reports of three cases. J Am Acad Dermatol 1990;22:418–422.
80. Stevenson CJ: Environmentally induced vitiligo (leukoderma) from depigmenting agents and chemical. J Toxicol Cut Ocular Toxicol 1984;3:299–307.
81. Stohrer G: Arsenic: Opportunity for risk assessment. Arch Toxicol 1991;65:525–531.
82. Stoner JG, Rasmussen JE: Plant dermatitis. J Am Acad Dermatol 1983;9:1–15.
83. Storm JE, Collier SW, Stewart RF, Bronaugh RL: Metabolism of xenobiotics during percutaneous penetration: Role of absorption rate and cutaneous enzyme activity. Fundam Appl Toxicol 1990;15:132–141.
84. Terrill PJ, Gowar JP: Chromic acid burns: Beware, be aggressive, be watchful. Br J Plast Surg 1990;43:699–701.
85. Tosti A, Guerra L: Protein contact dermatitis in food handlers. Contact Dermatitis 1988;19:149–150.
86. U.S. Department of Health and Human Services, Agency for Toxic Substance and Disease Registry. Skin lesions and environmental exposures. In: Cases Studies in Environmental Medicine. Atlanta, May 1993, Vol. 28.
87. U.S. Department of Health and Human Services, National Institute for Occupational Safety and Health: Registry of the Toxic Effects of Chemical Substances, 1981–82, DHHS (NIOSH), publ. no. 83-107. Washington, DC: U.S. Government Printing Office, 1983.
88. U.S. Department of Labor, Bureau of Labor Statistics: Occupational Injuries and Illnesses in the United States by Industry. Washington, DC: U.S. Government Printing Office, 1985.
89. Van der Harst-Osstveen CJGR, Van Vloten WA. Delayed-type hypersensitivity in patients with mycosis fungoides. Dermatologica 1978;157:129–135.
90. Venning GR: Rare and serious adverse reaction. Med Toxicol 1987;2:235–241.
91. VonBlomberg BME, Bruynzeel DP, Scheper RJ: Advances in mechanisms of allergic contact dermatitis: In vitro and in vivo research. In: Moschella SL, Hurley HJ, eds: Dermatotoxicology. Philadelphia, Saunders, 1992, pp. 255–362.
92. Webster RC, Maibach HI: Percutaneous absorption of drugs. Clin Pharmacokinet 1992;23:253–266.
93. Webster RC, Maibach HI: In vivo percutaneous absorption: Critical factors in transdermal transport. In: Marzulli FN, Maibach HI, eds: Dermatotoxicology, 4th ed. New York, Hemisphere, 1991, pp. 1–36.
94. Webster RC, Maibach HI, Sedik L, et al: Percutaneous absorption of (14C) chlordane from soil. J Toxicol Environ Health 1992;35:269–277.
95. Wintroub BU, Stern R: Cutaneous drug reactions: Pathogenesis and clinical classification. J Am Acad Dermatol 1985;12:167–179.
96. Zugerman C: Chloracne: Clinical manifestations and etiology. Dermatol Clin 1990;8:209–213.

CHAPTER 29

Genitourinary Principles

Leslie R. Wolf

The genitourinary tract encompasses two major organ systems, both with multifactorial influences. The process of fertility is complicated, and the definition of sexual dysfunction varies. Historically, humans have continued to search for the perfect aphrodisiac, from oysters to toads. Efficacy is variable, and toxic consequences occur commonly. Various treatments have been evaluated for male impotence, but the perfect remedy remains a mystery. While many people search for a cure for impotence or infertility, many others explore drugs and plants that can be used to terminate pregnancy. This chapter examines all of these issues, as well as the causes of priapism, urinary incontinence, and abnormalities detected in urine specimens. Renal (Chap. 23), teratogenic, and carcinogenic (Chap. 16) principles are discussed in further detail elsewhere in this text.

Spermatogenesis/Oogenesis

The process of spermatogenesis begins by secretion of releasing hormones from the hypothalamus, which stimulate the pituitary to release follicle-stimulating hormone (FSH) and luteinizing hormone (LH). Follicle-stimulating hormone stimulates the development of Sertoli cells in the testes, which are responsible for the maturation of spermatids to spermatozoa. Luteinizing hormone promotes production of testosterone by Leydig cells. Testosterone levels must be maintained to ensure the formation of spermatids.[16] Spermatogenesis can be inhibited by decreases in FSH and/or LH or Sertoli cell toxicity. Spermatogenic capacity is evaluated by semen analysis, including sperm count, motility, sperm morphology, and penetrating ability.[16,102] The normal sperm count is above 40 million sperm/mL semen, and a count below 20 million/mL is indicative of infertility.[16,105] Motility below 40% of normal or abnormal morphology of more than 40% of the total number of sperm also indicates infertility.[16,105]

The process of oogenesis also requires secretion of releasing hormones from the hypothalamus resulting in production of LH and FSH from the pituitary, which are required for ovarian follicle maturation.[16] FSH is needed for early maturation, and LH is required for ovulation and for the formation of the corpus luteum. The corpus luteum then produces estrogen and progesterone.

Physiology of Erection

Normal penile erection is a result of both neural and vascular effects on the erectile tissue of the penis. Psychogenic neural stimulation arises from the cerebral cortex and is mediated through the thoracolumbar sympathetic and sacral parasympathetic tracts. Reflex stimulation can also occur from the sacral spinal cord. The afferent limb of the reflex arc is supplied by the pudendal nerves and the efferent limb by the nervi eregentes. The internal pudendal arteries supply blood to the penis via four branches. Multiple emissary veins drain into the dorsal vein of the penis and plexus of Santorini. Within the penis, the corpora cavernosa share vascular supply and drainage due to extensive arteriolar, arteriovenous, and sinusoidal anastomoses.[121]

When penile blood flow is above 20 to 50 mL/minute, erection occurs. Maintenance of tumescence occurs with flow rates of 12 mL/minute. The tunica albuginea limits the absolute size of erection. The ability to increase blood flow and size depends on parasympathetic dominance, either by stimulation of parasympathetic receptors or inhibition of the sympathetic axis. Alpha-adrenergic receptor agonism in the erectile tissues results in detumescence, while alpha-adrenergic antagonism can result in pathologic erection (priapism) as a consequence of parasympathetic dominance.[121]

Bladder Anatomy and Physiology

The bladder is a hollow, muscular reservoir that stores 350 to 450 mL of urine in adults. Nerve supply and neu-

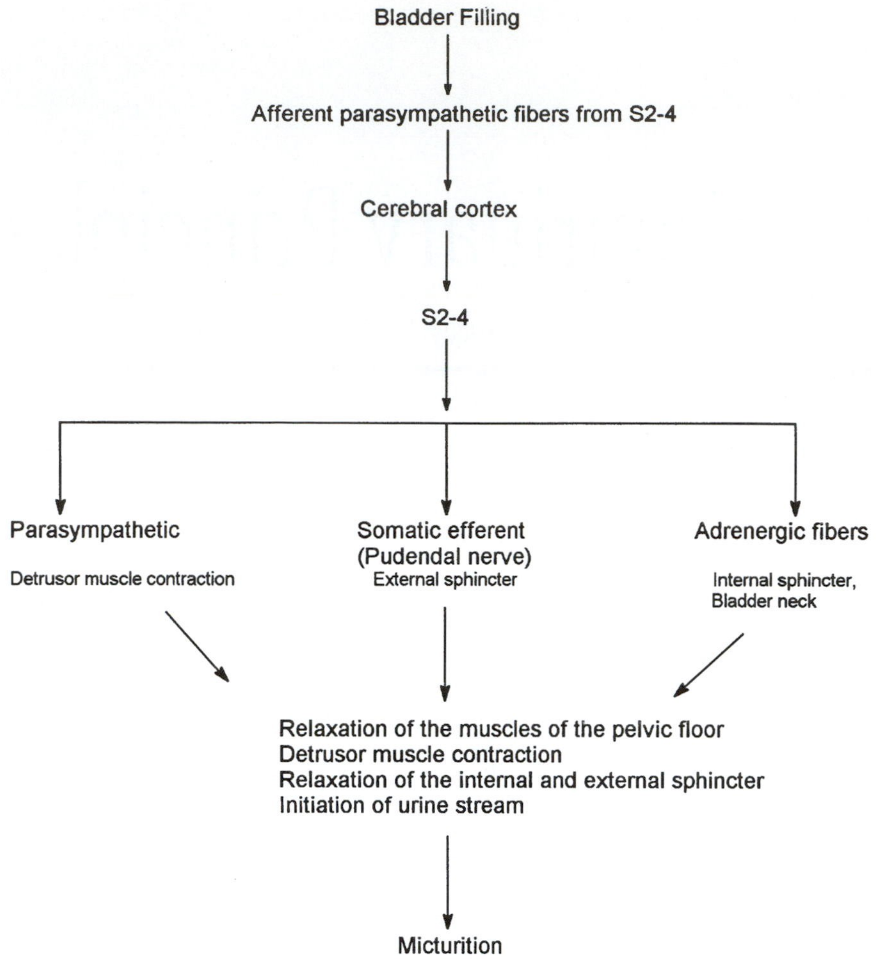

Figure 29–1. A schematic description of the physiology of micturition.

rophysiology involve interplay by the sympathetic and parasympathetic nervous systems arising from the sacral portion of the spinal cord (S2 to S4). Figure 29–1 shows the physiology of micturition. Norepinephrine is released by sympathetic postganglionic fibers, whereas parasympathetic pre- and postganglionic fibers release acetylcholine. Beta-adrenergic receptors supply the bladder wall, and agonism facilitates filling. Alpha-adrenergic receptors predominate in the internal sphincter and the bladder neck. Consequently, stimulation of alpha or beta-adrenergic receptors results in sphincter contraction and bladder outlet resistance, resulting in retention of urine.[24] Stimulation of acetylcholine receptors results in parasympathetic-mediated detrusor muscle contraction and micturition. Conversely, anticholinergic drugs prevent bladder emptying and result in urinary retention.[20,21,22,39,45,79]

Agents Affecting Fertility or Sexual Dysfunction

Fertility is a complex biologic phenomenon. Laboratory tests used to evaluate fertility are relatively unreliable, clinical endpoints are unclear, exposure is difficult to monitor, and indicators of biologic effects are indefinite. Because of these factors, well-designed, conclusive epidemiologic studies are uncommon. Therefore, the role of occupational and environmental exposures in the development of infertility is difficult to define.[6,31,88,92] The negative impact on fertility as an adverse effect of drugs or chemicals is often ignored, but the evaluation of infertility is incomplete without a thorough drug and occupational history. Drug-related, primary infertility may be the result of effects on the hypothalamic–pituitary–gonadal axis or of a direct toxic effect on the gonads.[75] Differences in toxicity of agents in individuals may be sex- and/or age-related. Females usually notice reproductive abnormalities more quickly than males, because menses may be affected, although infertility may occur while normal menses persists. Female infertility may result from changes in hormone levels, direct toxicity to the ovum, interference with the transport of the ovum, or inhibition of implantation of the ovum in the uterus.

Fertility is also affected by exposures that cause abnormal sexual performance. Sexual dysfunction can be a result of decreased libido, impotence, erectile dysfunction, and diminished ejaculation. Categories of drugs known to affect male sexual function include drugs of abuse, CNS depressants, antihypertensive agents, anticholinergics, psychotropic drugs, exogenous hormones, antibiotics,[104] and chemotherapeutic agents.[117] Libido can be decreased by drugs that block dopamine or testosterone production or by those producing dysphoria. Erectile dysfunction is associated with ganglion blockers or any drug that diverts blood flow from the penis. Agents that affect spinal reflexes can cause diminished ejaculation and erectile dysfunction.[117]

Antihypertensive Drugs

Impotence is reported as an adverse effect with all antihypertensive agents and may be due, in part, to a decrease in hypogastric artery pressure, which impairs blood flow to the pelvis.[116] Methyldopa and clonidine both are centrally acting alpha$_2$-adrenergic agonists that inhibit sympathetic outflow from the brain. Sexual dysfunction has been reported in 26% of patients taking methyldopa and in 24% of those receiving clonidine.[8,84] Erectile dysfunction associated with thiazide diuretics may be related to decreased vascular resistance, diverting blood from the penis.[18] Spironolactone acts as an antiandrogen by inhibiting the binding of dihydrotestosterone to its receptors. Impotence related to use of the beta-adrenergic antagonist, propranolol, is well-documented[19,53,76,115] and may be due to unopposed alpha-mediated vasoconstriction resulting in reduced penile blood flow.

Oral Contraceptive Agents

Oral contraceptive agents are toxic to the male and female reproductive systems in different ways. In males, work-related exposure to estrogens and progestins in the oral contraceptive industry may result in decreased libido, impotence, and gynecomastia due to hyperestrogenism.[105] Persistent infertility can occur in women, particularly those who are nulliparous, following the discontinuation of oral contraceptives. Prolonged infertility is more common with the use of the combined preparations as opposed to the use of sequential estrogen/progesterone contraceptives.[16] These agents may affect the hypothalamic–pituitary axis, gonadotropin release, or end-organ sensitivity to hormonal stimulation.

Sulfasalazine

Oligospermia, abnormal sperm motility and morphology, and infertility are reported in males receiving long-term treatment with sulfasalazine for inflammatory bowel disease.[8] Treatment for more than 2 months is commonly associated with depressed spermatogenesis, and the effect is usually reversible when the drug is withdrawn.[8,16] The mechanism for toxicity may be an antifolate effect inhibiting rapidly dividing cells. Sperm motility can also be inhibited by the antiprostaglandin action of the drug.[16]

1,2-Dibromo-3-chloropropane (DBCP)

A soil fumigant used in agriculture to control nematodes, 1,2-dibromo–3-chloropropane (DBCP) provides the clearest example of occupational exposure resulting in testicular toxicity and human reproductive dysfunction. In one series, 7 of 10 patients who were exposed to DBCP had decreased or absent spermatogenic activity on testicular biopsy. This correlated with duration of exposure and was most consistently observed after inhalation exposure. A selective decrease or loss of spermatogenic activity was observed without any other consistent testicular defect, and all stages of differentiation were affected. In the most severe cases, the seminiferous tubules were devoid of germ cells.[9]

The mechanism of toxicity of DBCP is unknown but may be the result of transformation of the parent compound to an alkylating agent. Testosterone levels remain normal, although testicular size is decreased. After removal from exposure, improvement in sperm counts occurred in most oligospermic men, but those who had developed azoospermia showed no recovery of spermatogenic function.[116]

Lead

Painters and artisans are commonly exposed to inorganic lead, which is also a hazard in the smelting and battery industries.[61] Lead is a proven spermicide and abortifacient and can jeopardize the health of a newborn. Lead exposure is also associated with decreased libido, decreased sperm counts, abnormal sperm morphology, and testicular atrophy. An increase in the frequency of stillbirths and spontaneous abortions results when the male partner is a lead worker.[118] Lead levels of 35 to 50 μg/dL are associated with direct spermatogenic toxicity. Indirect effects result from the inhibition of general metabolic processes by lead (see Chaps. 12 and 79).[118]

Other Agents

Many other drugs and chemicals have been implicated in infertility and sexual dysfunction (see Tables 29–1 and 29–2), although substantiation of these effects varies.

Toxicity of Aphrodisiacs and Agents Used to Treat Impotence

An aphrodisiac is defined as a substance that heightens sexual desire, pleasure, and/or performance.[27] The search for an effective aphrodisiac has continued for thousands of years by a variety of societies. Ancient fertility cults used *Datura,* belladonna, and henbane as aphrodisiacs. Yohimbine has been used by African cultures to enhance sexual prowess, and mandrake was used in medieval Europe. Other substances recommended include oysters, vitamin E, and ginseng. Because there are no measurable objective parameters, research in this area is lacking. Most published studies evaluating aphrodisiacs have been conducted in male rodents, and little information is available in humans.

Dopamine, oxytocin, and adrenocorticotrophic hormone all facilitate sexual behavior. Dopamine stimulates

TABLE 29–1. DRUGS AND TOXINS ASSOCIATED WITH INFERTILITY

Agent	Effects
Anabolic steroids	↓LH
Androgens	Suppress testosterone production
Antineoplastic agents	Gonadal toxicity
Chlorambucil	Oligospermia
Busulphan	Amenorrhea
Methotrexate	Oligospermia
Carbon disulfide	↓FSH, ↓LH, ↓spermatogenesis
Cimetidine	Oligospermia
1,2-dibromo-3-chloropropane	Oligospermia, azospermia
Ethanol	↓Testosterone production, Leydig cell damage, ↓Sperm motility, oligospermia, abnormal sperm morphology
Lead	↓Spermatogenesis, abnormal sperm morphology, stillbirths, spontaneous abortions
Opioids	↓LH, ↓testosterone
Oral contraceptives	Affect hypothalamic–pituitary axis, end-organ resistance to hormones
Sulfasalazine	↓Spermatogenesis
Thyroid hormones	↓Ovulation
Tobacco	↓Testosterone

the forebrain and midbrain and leads to an increase in sexual response and arousal. Several dopamine agonists are associated with prosexual effects, but none have proven efficacy in the laboratory. Other preparations tested for the treatment of impotence include bromocriptine,[1,10] glyceryl trinitrate,[81] zinc,[3] oxytocin,[65] and LH.[64] Serotonin, GABA, endogenous opioids, and norepinephrine are all inhibitory. However, various serotonergic drugs, including trazadone, clomipramine, and fluoxetine, appear to have potential prosexual activity in some individuals.[101]

Yohimbine

Yohimbine, an indolealkylamine alkaloid from the West African yohimbe tree (*Corynanthe yohimbe*), is an alpha$_2$-adrenergic antagonist with cholinergic activity used to treat erectile dysfunction and postural hypotension associated with anticholinergic drugs.[66] It is structurally similar to reserpine. Other names for yohimbine include aphrodine, corynine, hydroaergotocin, quebrachine, and the street name "yo-yo."[67] Its use in the treatment of impotence is based on the theory that erection is linked to cholinergic stimulation and alpha$_2$ antagonism, resulting in an increase inflow and decrease outflow of blood to the penis. Although the agent Aphrodex, which contained 5 mg yohimbine, 5 mg methyltestosterone, and 5 mg strychnine, was shown to improve performance in males with erectile failure,[71] its distribution was halted in 1973 due to safety concerns.[101]

TABLE 29–2. DRUGS AND TOXINS ASSOCIATED WITH SEXUAL DYSFUNCTION

Agent	Effects
Anabolic steroids	↓Libido, impotence
Anticholinergics	Erectile failure
Antihypertensives	Impotence
Cimetidine	↓Libido, impotence
Ethanol	Impotence, erectile failure
Lead	↓Libido
Lithium	↓Libido, erectile failure
Monamine oxidase inhibitors	Ejaculatory and erectile dysfunction
Opioids (high dose)	↓Libido, impotence
Oral contraceptives	↓Libido, impotence
Phenothiazines	↓Libido
Tricyclic antidepressants	↓Libido, impotence

Yohimbine can be obtained by prescription, but extracts can be found in "health food" products marketed as "vitalizing agents for men."[29] Yohimbine can also be extracted from the Rauwolfia root.[40] The "therapeutic" dose is 2 to 6 mg three times daily. The drug is rapidly absorbed, with peak serum levels occurring in 45 to 60 minutes. The half-life is 36 minutes, and clearance is by hepatic metabolism without renal excretion.[89] Maximum pharmacologic effects are seen 1 to 2 hours after ingestion and last 3 to 4 hours.[67]

Because the erectile process involves various neurotransmitters, a single agent would be expected to only have a partial effect. In a double-blind study of 100 males with erectile failure treated with 18 mg/day of yohimbine, 42.6% of the treatment group and 27.6% of the placebo group reported some improvement in erectile function, which was not statistically significant.[80] Another study comparing a higher dose of yohimbine and placebo in 82 elderly males showed a statistically significant improvement with treatment.[109]

Adverse effects can occur with relatively low doses of yohimbine. Tachycardia, hypertension, mydriasis, diaphoresis, lacrimation, salivation, nausea, vomiting, and flushing can occur following intravenous administration.[42,54] Ten milligrams can elicit manic symptoms in patients with bipolar disorder,[97] and 15 mg/day is associated with bronchospasm[60] and a lupus-like syndrome.[103] A 16-year-old female who ingested 250 mg of yohimbine powder, purchased for its purported aphrodisiac activity, developed an acute dissociative reaction with weakness, paresthesias, headache, nausea, palpitations, and chest pain. She also developed tachycardia, tachypnea, diaphoresis, tremors, and a rash. Her symptoms resolved without treatment after 36 hours.[67] Another case report describes a 62-year-old male who ingested 200 mg of yohimbine and developed tachycardia, hypertension, and a brief period of anxiety that resolved without treatment.[40] Symptomatic patients who ingest yohimbine should receive activated charcoal and be observed until asymptomatic. Clonidine has been recommended for treatment,[67] but may result in unopposed alpha$_1$-adrenergic activity and worsening of hypertension. Because beta-adrenergic antagonists may also produce unopposed alpha-adrenergic effects, they too should be avoided. Benzodiazepine administration may be sufficient for the treatment of agitation and sympathomimetic effects related to yohimbine.

Spanish Fly

Spanish fly is a cantharidin derived from crushed blister beetles (*Cantharis vesicatoria*), used to enhance sexual potency.[56] A 1% topical solution available for use in wart removal has also been marketed in adult sex shops and by mail order as an aphrodisiac. Adverse effects are a consequence of the vesicant properties of the agent, and gastrointestinal, dermatologic, genitourinary, renal, cardiac, pulmonary, neurologic, and hematologic effects are all described.

After absorption of ingested cantharidin, it is bound to albumin and excreted by the kidney.[96] Symptoms generally occur 2 to 6 hours after ingestion. Gastrointestinal and genitourinary signs include dysuria, oral pain, dysphagia, nausea, hematemesis, and hematuria. Blistering of mucous membranes also occurs, and patients commonly develop hemorrhagic mucositis of the mouth, esophagus, and stomach. Fatal gastrointestinal hemorrhage has been reported, and the lethal dose varies from 10 to 80 mg in adults.[26,85,96] Blister formation in the urinary tract, tubular necrosis, and glomerular damage all result in gross hematuria, which can continue for 2 weeks after ingestion. Proteinuria is common, and death from acute tubular necrosis and renal failure can occur.[111] Dermal exposure can result in blistering, ulceration, and systemic toxicity.

Hemorrhage occurs in the ureters, bladder, and urethra, and hemorrhagic bullae may be noted in the bladder. Priapism, ovarian engorgement, and vaginal bleeding can also occur.[87] Sinus tachycardia is the most common cardiac manifestation of toxicity, but pericardial and subendocardial hemorrhage are also described. Patients may also develop dysrhythmias, ST segment elevation, and T-wave changes.[87] Pulmonary effects are rare and include pulmonary edema and bronchial hemorrhage. Disseminated intravascular coagulation has been reported and may be caused by vesicant-related vascular injury. Neurologic symptoms are rare. No specific antidote is available and treatment is supportive. Cantharidin exposure should be considered in the differential diagnosis of unexplained hematuria or gastrointestinal hemorrhage.

Bufotoxin

"Stone," "love stone," "black stone," and "rock hard" all refer to topical aphrodisiac preparations made from dried toad venom that contains bufalin, cinobufalin, cinobufagin, and other cardioactive steroids in the bufadienolide class. A 90-year-old male presented with bradycardia and a history of syncope after ingesting Yixin Wan, a nonprescription Chinese medication containing toad venom, ginseng, pearl, and musk.[59] Chan Su is a traditional Chinese medication produced from the venom of *Bufo bufo gargarizans*, which contains several cardiac glycosides, a topical anesthetic, and bufotenine.[14] Kyushin is another popular Asian traditional medication that contains dried toad venom. The cardiac glycosides have a similar structure and action to digoxin. Digoxin immunoassay may be positive after exposure to these agents, although the level may not correlate with toxicity. Four deaths were reported between 1993 and 1995 following ingestion of these topical aphrodisiacs. The patients presented with bradycardia and measurable digoxin levels. Hyperkalemia also occurred. One patient was successfully treated with digoxin-specific Fab fragments.[13,15] An animal study evaluating the usefulness of Fab fragments in mice intoxicated with Chan Su demonstrated survival in 8 of 15 mice treated with digoxin-specific Fab fragments, compared with no survivors in the control group.[13] Digoxin Fab fragments (10 vials) should be administered to any patient with a suspected cardioactive steroid overdose with hyperkalemia and/or dysrhythmia (see Chap. 48 and "Antidotes in Depth").

Lead

Some "aphrodisiacs" in Asian countries contain lead and are associated with toxicity after ingestion. In a British report, a 50-year-old male from Pakistan presented with anorexia, abdominal pain, and anemia with basophilic stippling. A whole blood lead level was 96 μg/dL. He reported ingestion of a yellow-white powder provided to him by a traditional Asian practitioner for the treatment of impotence, which contained 84% elemental lead by weight.[32] A 24-year-old male from Bangladesh presented to a London hospital with similar complaints and a whole blood lead level of 102 μg/dL after chronic ingestion of an aphrodisiac containing 46% lead.[12] Traditionally, aphrodisiacs from the Indian subcontinent contain silver and/or gold, but occasionally lead is substituted. The indications for chelation therapy are the same as in other cases of lead poisoning (see Chap. 79).

Nitrites

Alkyl (amyl, butyl, and isobutyl) nitrites are aliphatic esters of nitrous acid and are yellow, highly volatile, sweet-smelling liquids administered by inhalation. Glass capsules typically contain 0.3 mL and are enclosed in a gauze jacket of woven absorbent covering that can be crushed and held to the nostrils. The capsules are called "poppers" due the sound produced when they are broken.[52,69] The vasodilatory effects produced by inhalation of amyl nitrite were first described in 1859, and amyl nitrite was first used for the treatment of angina in 1867. Amyl nitrite was originally marketed as a prescription drug in 1937, but the FDA removed the requirement for a prescription in 1960. After 1960, nitrates replaced nitrites in the treatment of angina. Because the abuse of inhaled nitrites became widespread in the 1960s, particularly by healthy young males, the FDA reinstated the prescription requirement for amyl nitrite in 1968.[52] Since that time, isobutyl and butyl nitrite have been legally marketed as "room deodorizers" in bottles containing 10–30 mL.[46]

Amyl nitrite and other alkyl nitrites are especially popular aphrodisiacs among homosexual males. They are inhaled during foreplay to obtain a "high," to produce anal sphincter relaxation, or just before orgasm to heighten and prolong the climax.[37] Butyl nitrite is also popular among teens who seek a "high." In a 1986 survey by NIDA, 8.6% of 3000 U.S. high school seniors and

9% of teens between 12 and 17 years old reportedly used nitrites, with 0.5% using them daily.[52]

Nitrites are absorbed via the skin, lungs, mucus membranes, and the gastrointestinal tract. They are metabolized in the liver and excreted, partially unchanged, in the urine.[69] In mice, butyl nitrite undergoes rapid hydrolysis to nitrite ion and butyl alcohol. The half-life is 2 to 3 seconds, and metabolism is by first-order kinetics.[52] The relaxation of vascular smooth muscle results in potent vasodilation and hypotension. Blood pressure can decrease significantly within 30 seconds of inhalation. Inhalation of as little as 5 drops can result in hypotension and reflex tachycardia.[69] Cardiovascular collapse can occur, especially if nitrites are injected intravenously. Vasodilation of cerebral blood vessels results in increased intracranial pressure, and cerebral aneurysm rupture has been reported after amyl nitrite inhalation.[86]

A feeling of warmth and palpitations are frequently described after nitrite inhalation.[52] Headache, nausea, and syncope are also common. Nitrite use can be dangerous in patients with glaucoma due to a transient increase in intraocular pressure.[37] Nitrites are a well-known cause of methemoglobinemia[34] (see Chap. 93), which can be fatal. Successful treatment of nitrite-induced methemoglobinemia with methylene blue is well reported. Hemolytic anemia is also reported[11,69] and is probably due to the oxidizing effects of nitrites.

"Popper dermatitis" is a characteristic rash that can be noted around the nose, lips, face, penis, and scrotum and presents as erythematous, edematous, and crusted lesions.[37,68,69] It may have a similar appearance to impetigo and seborrheic dermatitis. The rash usually clears within 10 days, but reappears with repeat nitrite inhalation.[37] A generalized allergic dermatitis can also occur.[28]

The carcinogenic and immunosuppressive effects of amyl nitrite are not adequately tested in animals, although it is mutagenic with the Ames test.[35] There are some data to suggest that nitrites may be immunosuppressive in the setting of repeated viral antigenic stimulation.[46] It is postulated that this may contribute to the high frequency of Kaposi's sarcoma in homosexual males. In one study, amyl nitrite was the only drug that 100% of patients with Kaposi's sarcoma reported using.[73] Concern for carcinogenicity associated with amyl nitrite has resulted in a recent decline in its use by homosexual males.

Agents Associated with Priapism

Priapism is prolonged involuntary erection, which is painful, unassociated with sexual stimulation, and can result in impotence. It most commonly occurs during the third and fourth decades of life and is caused by inflow of blood to the penis in excess of outflow. The corpora cavernosa become firm and the corpus spongiosum flaccid. Intracavernosal pressures can exceed arterial systolic pressure, resulting in cell death. Priapism can occur due to an imbalance in neural stimuli and/or from interference with venous outflow. Priapism can occur as a result of drug-induced inhibition of penile detumescence. Alpha-adrenergic antagonist agents prevent constriction of blood vessels supplying erectile tissue, resulting in priapism.[121] Priapism occurs in one per 10,000 patients taking trazadone and is thought to be related to its alpha-adrenergic antagonist effects.[101] A common cause of priapism is iatrogenic, resulting from the injection of papaverine for the treatment of impotence.[110] Other agents associated with drug-induced priapism include prazosin, labetalol, guanethidine, hydralazine, phenothiazines, androgens, anticoagulants, ethanol, marijuana, and cantharidin.[56,110,121]

The goal in treatment of priapism is detumescence with retention of potency. Initial therapy includes sedation and analgesia with benzodiazepines and opioids. Urology consultation should also be obtained early. Aspiration and normal saline irrigation of the corpora cavernosa may be effective. If priapism occurs secondary to alpha-adrenergic antagonism, an alpha-adrenergic agonist (0.25 mg metaraminol, 10 to 15 μg norepinephrine, or 500 mg phenylephrine) can be instilled by placing a 19-gauge butterfly needle into the corpora cavernosa. If the above measures fail, operative venous shunt placement may be required.[110,121]

Abortifacients

An abortifacient is defined as an agent that induces abortion. These substances may act by flushing the zygote from the fallopian tube, causing uterine horn blockade, inhibiting implantation, causing fetal resorption, or by producing oxytocin-like activity that results in uterine irritation and contraction. Abortifacients may also indirectly affect pregnancy by altering hormonal levels. Inhibition of HCG or progesterone production by the placenta or interference with progesterone receptors can also induce abortion. In a U.S. poison center study, 5 of 43 pregnant patients intentionally overdosed on known abortifacients, including quinine, misoprostol, methylergonovine, and oral contraceptives. Four developed vaginal bleeding and cramping, but no short-term (1 to 3 days) fetal demise was reported.[94] The use of these agents is more common in underdeveloped countries in populations without access to safer methods for termination or prevention of pregnancy. Many abortifacients are derived from plants and their extracts (Table 29–3). Not only are these agents toxic to the mother, but because many are ineffective in producing abortion, the possibility of teratogenicity is a concern.

Trichosanthin is an abortifacient protein extracted from the root of *Trichosanthes kirilowii*, a Chinese medicinal plant. The root is powdered and is used as a folk remedy to induce menstrual bleeding and produce expulsion of the fetus.[112] The active ingredient, trichosanthin, has abortifacient activity in animals and in humans when injected or applied intravaginally.[112] The mechanism is unknown, but may be related to inhibition of protein synthesis by preventing the incorporation of leucine.[112] Trichosanthin's injurious effect on tropho-

TABLE 29–3. DRUGS AND TOXINS USED AS ABORTIFACIENTS

Substance	Source	Country of Origin or Use	Miscellaneous/Toxicity
Acanthospermum hispidum	*Acanthospermum hispidum* (whole plant)	Brazil	Pre-implantation effects
Adhatoda vasica	*Adhatoda vasica*	India	100% abortifacient effect in rats
Alpha-momorcharin	*Momordica charantia*	China	Similar to trichosanthin
Cajanus cajan	*Cajanus cajun* (fresh leaves)	Brazil	Pre-implantation effects
Cinchona alkaloid	Quinine	—	Anti-malarial, oxytocic
Devil's claw	*Ranunculus sp* (root)	South Africa	Similar to pennyroyal oil
Legenaria breviflora Robert	*Legenaria breviflora* Robert (fruit juice)	Nigeria	Anti-implantation, oxytocic
Lysol disinfectant	—	—	Death after intrauterine administration
Moringa oleifera	*Moringa oleifera*	India	100% abortifacient effect in rats
Prostaglandin E analog	Misoprostol	Brazil, U.S.	Marketed as Cytotec for gastric ulcers
Pulegone	*Hedeoma pulegiodes*, pennyroyal oil or tea	—	Hepatotoxicity, NAC may be effective
RU 486	Mifepristone	France	Marketed as abortion pill, administered with prostoglandins
Trichosanthin	*Trichosanthes kirilowii*	China	Inhibits protein synthesis, ↓ HCG, ↓ progesterone

blasts has also been demonstrated, and it may inhibit HCG and progesterone production by the placenta as well.[112] Hypersensitivity occurs in some patients, limiting its clinical usefulness. Alpha-momorcharin is produced by purification of *Momordica charantia* seeds and has biologic activity similar to trichosanthin.[112]

The juice from the fruit of *Legenaria breviflora* Robert, an antifertility plant used by traditional medical practitioners in southern Nigeria,[36] possesses anti-implantation and oxytocin-like activity in rats. After a survey of herbal practices in two Indian districts, 17 plants used as abortifacients were identified and studied in a rat model. Only two of the 17, *Moringa oleifera* and *Adhatoda vasica*, showed 100% abortifacient activity.[83] The toxicity of these agents is unknown.

Extracts of two plants, *Acanthospermum hispidum* and *Cajanus cajan*, are ingested in Brazil to induce abortion.[63] A solution is prepared by adding the fresh leaves of the *C. cajan* plant and the whole *A. hispidum* plant to boiling water. When the mixture reaches room temperature, it is filtered and ingested. The efficacy of these agents has not been scientifically well proven, but their effects probably occur during the preimplantation period.[63]

Misoprostol is a synthetic prostaglandin E methyl analog indicated for the prevention of gastric ulcers caused by nonsteroidal antiinflammatory drugs; it was approved for marketing in Brazil in 1985 and in the US in 1988. The abortifacient properties of prostaglandins are well established,[70] and misoprostol can produce uterine contractions, uterine bleeding, and expulsion of the products of conception.[98] This drug has been extensively misused in Brazil to induce abortion.[23,25,93] In 1991, an estimated 10% of mothers giving birth at public hospitals in Rio de Janeiro were exposed to misoprostol.[25,93] Although the rate of successful pregnancy termination with this agent is 11 to 50%, abortion can occur after amounts just above the recommended therapeutic dose.[58,98]

Mifepristone, or RU 486, an antiprogesterone agent legally used in Europe, is an effective abortifacient, especially when used in conjunction with a prostaglandin.[90,91,100] RU 486 is chemically related to progesterone and competes with progesterone for receptors. The sensitivity of the uterus to prostaglandins is also increased.[7] Adverse effects include excessive blood loss and fatigue, gynecomastia, alopecia, nausea, vomiting, and abdominal pain.[41,50]

Pennyroyal oil is a volatile oil extracted from the leaves of *Mentha pulegium* and *Hedeoma pulegiodes* and contains the ketone, pulegone (see Chap. 76). Preparations also include a tablet, tea, essence of pennyroyal, and leaves. There are several reports of its use as an emmenagogue and illicit abortifacient. Pulegone depletes glutathione stores in the liver and is a direct hepatotoxin. The epoxide metabolite, menthofuran, may also contribute to hepatotoxicity. Fulminant hepatic failure can occur after ingestion of 2 ounces of pennyroyal oil.[2,5] Renal failure is also described.[108] *N*-acetyl cysteine has been successfully used to prevent pulegone-induced hepatotoxicity.[17] Devil's claw root (*Ranunculus spp*), an herb from South Africa, has properties similar to pennyroyal oil and has also been used as an abortifacient.[49]

Due to its oxytocic action, the cinchona alkaloid, quinine, has been used intravenously to induce labor in cases of fetal death.[82] It has also been used as an illicit abortifacient.[119,120] Because it is ineffective when ingested orally for this purpose, it may be taken in repeated doses leading to toxicity (see Chap. 44). Black cohosh root (*Cimicifuga racemosa*) extract is an herbal preparation used to induce abortion and primarily results in gastrointestinal toxicity after ingestion. Intrauterine injection of Lysol (1 to 5% ethanol, 1 to 5% isopropanol, 5.5% ortho-benzyl-*p*-chlorophenol) to induce abortion has also been reported, resulting in coma, shock, and death within 2 hours, secondary to oil embolism.[113]

Urinary Abnormalities

Urinary incontinence is common in the elderly population. As age increases, bladder size decreases, resulting in more frequent emptying. Early detrusor contraction, even with low bladder volumes, occurs more commonly in the elderly causing a sense of urgency. There are many

TABLE 29–4. DRUGS THAT CAUSE INCONTINENCE

Drug	Action
Alpha-adrenergic agonists	Increase internal sphincter tone
Alpha-adrenergic antagonists	Decrease internal sphincter tone
Anticholinergic agents	Impair detrusor contraction
Calcium channel blockers	Decrease detrusor contraction
Diuretics	Overflow of bladder
Opioids	Impair detrusor contraction
Sedatives-hypnotics	Decrease sensorium

Reprinted with permission from Chutka DS, Fleming KC, Evans MP, et al: Urinary incontinence in the elderly population. Mayo Clin Proc 1996;71:93–101.

etiologies for urinary incontinence, including various drug exposures (Table 29–4). General or regional anesthesia, bladder instrumentation, and medications may produce bladder atony leading to incontinence.[22] Functional incontinence can also result from use of any medication that causes impaired cognition or decreased mobility (sedative/hypnotics, opioids, etc.).[22] Urinary retention can occur as a side effect or as with toxicity of various agents, including sympathomimetics, anticholinergics, antidysrhythmics (quinidine, procainamide, disopyramide), and hormonal agents (progesterone, estrogen, testosterone).[22,39]

Abnormalities in Urinalysis

Abnormalities of the urinalysis are often useful in identifying drug or chemical exposures. Color change or the presence of crystals may aid in diagnosis. The urinalysis in patients who ingest ethylene glycol often (but not always) reveals calcium oxalate or hippurate crystals. Calcium oxalate crystals are monohydrates (prism- or needlelike) or dihydrates (envelope shaped). Hippurate crystals are needle shaped.[91] Crystalluria is present in 50% of cases of ethylene glycol poisoning (see Chap. 64). Hexagonal crystals are noted after massive primidone poisoning and result from precipitation of primidone in the urine.[114] Crystalluria is also described after therapeutic doses of salicylate, phenacetin, sulfonamide, and quinolones. After large ingestions, crystals can be seen with methotrexate, amoxicillin, cephalexin, and ampicillin. Urine color is dependent on several factors, including pH, concentration, natural pigments, and length of time exposed to air.[48] Dilute urine secondary to diuretic use, diabetes mellitus, diabetes insipidus, or overhydration can appear colorless, whereas concentrated urine is usually orange. The presence of fluorescein, detected by illumination of the urine with a Wood's lamp, suggests ethylene glycol (commercial antifreeze) ingestion. Other causes of colored urine are noted in Table 29–5.

There are multiple causes of hematuria.[72] It can occur with drug-induced interstitial nephritis, a condition distinguished by fever, rash, eosinophilia, azotemia, and oliguria.[30] Hemorrhagic cystitis is a more frequent cause of hematuria, and is associated with a number of drugs. The clinical presentation of hemorrhagic cystitis includes hematuria, dysuria, and urinary frequency. Criteria for diagnosis include a history of gross hematuria, laboratory findings of gross hematuria (>5 RBC/HPF), platelet count above 50,000/mm^3, and a negative urine culture.[99] When in doubt, the diagnosis may be confirmed by cystoscopy, which reveals an inflamed, hyperemic, and sometimes ulcerated bladder mucosa.

Cyclophosphamide-related hemorrhagic cystitis was first described in 1959,[78] and is the best-documented type of drug-induced hemorrhagic cystitis.[43] Up to 46% of patients receiving cyclophosphamide will develop hemorrhagic cystitis.[33,55,57,62] Acrolein, the causative agent, is a

TABLE 29–5. DRUGS, TOXINS, AND OTHER MATERIALS THAT CAUSE COLORED URINE

Milky		***Black***
Chyle		Alcaptonuria
Lipids		Homogentisic acid
Neutrophils		Melanin
		p-hydroxyphenylpyruvic acid
Reddish-Brown		***Brown-Black***
Anthraquinone	Phenacetin	Cascara
Bilirubin	Phenazopyridine	Iron
Chloroquine	Phenothiazines	Methyldopa
Ibuprofen	Phenytoin	Phenylhydrazine
Levadopa	Porphyrins	Senna
Methyldopa	Trinitrophenol	
Reddish-Orange		***Greenish-Blue***
Aminopyrine	Phenacetin	Amitriptyline
Aniline dyes	Phenazopyridine	Anthraquinones
Antipyrine	Phenothiazines	Biliverdin
Chlorzoxazone	Phenytoin	Chlorophyll breath mints
Doxorubicin	Rifampin	Flavin derivatives
Ibuprofen	Salicylazosulfapyridine	Indicans
Mannose		Indigo blue
		Magnesium salicylate
Red		Methylene blue
Anthraquinones	Erythrocytes	Phenol
Beets	Hemoglobin	Thymol
Blackberries	Myoglobin	
Eosin	Rhubarb	
Yellow-Brown		
Aloe	Nitrofurantoin	
Anthraquinones	Primaquine	
Chloroquine	Rhubarb	
Fava beans	Sulfamethoxazole	
Yellow		
Fluorescein	Riboflavin	
Phenacetin	Santonin	
Quinacrine		
Yellow-Orange		
Aminopyrine	Sulfasalazine	
Anisindione	Vitamin A	
Carrots	Warfarin	

metabolite of cyclophosphamide that damages the urothelium when excreted. There is no sex or age predilection, and symptoms can occur months after exposure. Hemorrhagic cystitis is described after oral doses exceeding 100 g and after a single intravenous dose of cyclophosphamide.[107] Sloughing of the bladder mucosa occurs, and 5% of patients die from intractable hemorrhage.[51,95] Patients at highest risk are those who are dehydrated, receive cyclophosphamide intravenously, or have previous or concomitant exposure to busulfan or radiotherapy.[78] Treatment with cyclophosphamide is also associated with a dose-related increase (9 to 45 fold) in the risk of subsequent bladder cancer (see Chap. 47).[94,107]

Prophylaxis against cyclophosphamide-induced hemorrhagic cystitis includes bladder catheterization and drainage, bladder irrigation, hydration, forced diuresis, and administration of oral sodium 2-mercaptoethanesulfonate (MESNA).[78] MESNA binds to acrolein in the urine to form an inert, nontoxic thioester, reducing the incidence of hemorrhagic cystitis by 85%.[107] Bladder irrigation with alum, silver nitrate, prostaglandins, and formalin[4] has also been used to treat cyclophosphamide-induced hemorrhagic cystitis.[78] In an animal model, pretreatment with hyperbaric oxygen reduces the incidence of hemorrhagic cystitis.[51] In severe cases, hypogastric artery ligation and/or cystectomy may be required to control bleeding.[51]

An outbreak of hemorrhagic cystitis occurred in workers in a packaging plant after exposure to chlordimeform, a formamidine insecticide used to control mites and insects on cotton. Nine workers developed abdominal pain, dysuria, urgency, and hematuria, with biopsy-proven hemorrhagic cystitis.[38] Eight young adults developed painful hematuria after consuming "bootleg" methaqualone. The cause was orthotoluidine, a compound utilized in the synthesis of methaqualone, and the symptoms occurred within 6 hours of ingestion.[47] Cases of hemorrhagic cystitis have also been described with ticarcillin,[74] nafcillin, penicillin G, carbenicillin, piperacillin, isoniazid, indomethacin, tiaprofenic acid, and busulphan.[44,77,106]

Summary

Adverse effects on the genitourinary tract are often overlooked when evaluating the toxicologic potential of various agents. Few physical examination findings, laboratory tests, or ancillary studies will aid in diagnosis. A thorough history including past and present medications, illicit drug use, occupational and environmental exposures, or the use of herbal or alternative therapies is mandatory in the evaluation of patients with genitourinary complaints.

References

1. Ambrosi B, Bara R, Travaglini P, et al: Study of the effects of bromocriptine on sexual impotence. Clin Endocrin 1977; 7:417–421.
2. Anderson IB, Mullen WH, Meeker JE, et al: Pennyroyal toxicity: Measurement of toxic metabolite levels in two cases and review of the literature. Ann Intern Med 1996;124:726–734.
3. Antomiou LD, Shalhoub RJ, Sudbaker T, Smith JC: Reversal of uraemic impotence by zinc. Lancet 1977;2:895–898.
4. Axelsen RA, Leditschke JF, Burke JR: Renal and urinary tract complications following the intravesical instillation of formalin. Pathology 1986;18:453–458.
5. Bakerink JA, Gospe SM, Dimand RJ, et al: Multiple organ failure after ingestion of pennyroyal oil from herbal tea in two infants. Pediatrics 1996;98:944–947.
6. Baranski B: Effects of the workplace on fertility and related reproductive outcomes. Env Health Perspect 1993; 101(suppl 2):81–90.
7. Baulieu EE: RU–486 as an antiprogesterone steroid: From receptor to contragestion and beyond. JAMA 1989;262: 1808–1814.
8. Beeley L: Drug-induced sexual dysfunction and infertility. Adv Drug React Pois Rev 1984;3:23–42.
9. Biava CG, Smuckler EA, Whorton D: The testicular morphology of individuals exposed to dibromochloropropane. Exp Mol Pathol 1978;29:448–458.
10. Bommer J, Ritz E, del Pozo E, Bommer G: Improved sexual function in male hemodialysis patients on bromocriptine. Lancet 1979;2:496–497.
11. Brandes JC, Bufill JA: Amyl nitrite-induced hemolytic anemia. Am J Med 1989;86:252–254.
12. Brearly RL, Forsythe AM: Lead poisoning from aphrodisiacs: Potential hazard in immigrants. Br Med J 1978;2: 1748–1749.
13. Brubacher JR, Lachmanen D, Ravikumar PR, et al: Treatment of toad venom poisoning with digoxin-specific Fab fragments. Chest 1996;110:1282–1288.
14. Brubacher JR, Ravikumar PR, Hoffman RS: Analysis of fatal aphrodisiac known as love stone or rock hard. J Toxicol Clin Toxicol 1995;33:539. Abstract.
15. Brubacher JR, Ravikumar PR, Hoffman RS: Deaths associated with a purported aphrodisiac—New York City, February 1993–May 1995. MMWR 1995;44:853–854.
16. Buchanan JF, Davis LJ: Drug-induced infertility. Drug Intell Clin Pharm 1984;18:122–132.
17. Buechel DW: Pennyroyal oil ingestion: Report of a case. J Am Osteopath Assoc 1983;2:793–794.
18. Buffum J: Pharmacosexology updates: Prescription drugs and sexual function. J Psychoactive Drugs 1986;18:97–102.
19. Burnett WC, Chahine RA: Sexual dysfunction as a complication of propranolol therapy in men. Cardiovasc Med 1979;5:811–815.
20. Castleden CM, Duffin HM, Gulati RS: Double-blind study of imipramine and placebo for incontinence due to bladder instability. Age Ageing 1986;15:299–303.
21. Chapple CR, Parkhouse H, Gardener C, et al: Double-blind, placebo-controlled, crossover study of flavoxate in the treatment of idiopathic detrusor instability. Br J Urol 1990;66:491–494.
22. Chutka DS, Fleming KC, Evans MP, et al: Urinary incontinence in the elderly population. Mayo Clin Proc 1996; 71:93–101.
23. Coelho HLL, Teixeira AC, Santos AP, et al: Misoprostol

and illegal abortion in Fortaleza, Brazil. Lancet 1993;341: 1261–1263.
24. Collste L, Lindskog M: Phenylpropanolamine in treatment of female stress urinary incontinence: Double-blind placebo controlled study in 24 patients. Urology 1987;30: 398–403.
25. Costa SH, Vessey MP: Misoprostol and illegal abortion in Rio de Janerio, Brazil. Lancet 1993;341:1258–1261.
26. Craven JD, Polak A: Cantharidin poisoning. Br Med J 1954;2:1386–1389.
27. Czajka P, Field J, Novak P, Kunnecke J: Accidental aphrodisiac ingestion. J Tenn Med Assoc 1978; 71: 747–750.
28. Dax EM, Lange WR, Jaffe JH: Allergic reactions to amyl nitrite inhalation. Am J Med 1989;86:732.
29. DeSmet PA, Smeets OS: Potential risks of health food products containing yohimbe extracts. Br Med J 1994;309: 958.
30. Ditlove J, Weidmann P, Bernstein M, et al: Methicillin nephritis. Medicine 1977;56:483–491.
31. Dlugosz L, Bracken MB: Reproductive effects of caffeine: A review and theoretical analysis. Epidemiol Rev 1992;14: 83–100.
32. Dolan G, Blumsohn A, Brown MJ, et al: Lead poisoning due to Asian ethnic treatment for impotence. R Soc Med 1991;84:630–631.
33. Droller MJ, Saral R, Santos G: Prevention of cyclophosphamide-induced hemorrhagic cystitis. Urology 1982;20: 256–258.
34. Ducker TE, Fleet WF, Morgan HJ: A case of cyanosis without hypoxemia. J Tenn Med Assoc 1990;83:22.
35. Dunkel VC, Rogers-Back AM, Lawlar TE, et al: Mutagenicity of some alkyl nitrites used as recreational drugs. Environ Mol Mutag 1989;14:115–122.
36. Elujoba AA, Olagbende SO, Adesina SK: Anti-implantation activity of the fruit of *Legenaria Breviflora* Robert. J Ethnopharmacol 1985;13:281–288.
37. Fisher AA: "Poppers" or "Snappers" dermatitis in homosexual men. Cutis 1984;34:120–122.
38. Folland DS, Kimbrough RD, Cline R, et al: Acute hemorrhagic cystitis. JAMA 1978;239:1052–1055.
39. Fontanarosa PB, Roush WR: Acute urinary retention. Emerg Med Clin North Am 1988;6:419–437.
40. Friesen K, Palatnick W, Tenenbein M: Benign course after massive ingestion of yohimbine. J Emerg Med 1993;11: 287–288.
41. Gaillard RC,Herrmann W: Clinical use of RU–486: Control of the menstrual cycle and effect on the hypophyseal-adrenal axis. Ann Endocrinol 1983;44:345–346.
42. Garfield SL, Gershon S, Sletten F, et al: Chemically induced anxiety. Int J Neuropsychiatry 1967;3:426–433.
43. Gellman E, Kissane J, Frech R, et al: Cyclophosphamide cystitis. J Can Assoc Radiol 1969;20:99–101.
44. Ghose K: Cystitis and nonsteroidal antiinflammatory drugs: An incidental association or an adverse effect? NZ Med J 1993;106:501–503.
45. Gilja I, Radej M, Kovacic M, Parazajder J: Conservative treatment of female stress incontinence with imipramine. J Urol 1984;132:909–911.
46. Goedert JJ, Neuland CY, Wallen WC, et al: Amyl nitrite may alter T lymphocytes in homosexual men. Lancet 1982; 1:412–415.
47. Goldfarb M, Finelli: Necrotizing cystitis secondary to "Bootleg" methaqualone. Urology 1974;3:54–55.
48. Goldfrank L, Osborn H: Rainbow urine. Hosp Phys 1978;3: 22–26.
49. Grouse LD: Hidden bias in research design. JAMA 1980;243:1365. Editorial.
50. Grunberg SM, Weiss MH, Spitz JM, et al: Treatment of unresectable meningiomas with the antiprogesterone agent mifepristone. J Neurosurg 1991;74:861–866.
51. Hader JE, Marzella L, Myers RA, et al: Hyperbaric oxygen treatment for experimental cyclophosphamide-induced hemorrhagic cystitis. J Urol 1993;149:1617–1621.
52. Haverkos HW, Dougherty J: Health hazards of nitrite inhalants. Am J Med 1988;84:479–482.
53. Hogan MJ, Wallin JD, Baer RM: Antihypertensive therapy and male sexual dysfunction. Psychosomatics 1980;21: 234–237.
54. Holmberg G, Gershon S: Autonomic and psychic effects of yohimbine hydrochloride. Psychopharmacologia 1961;2: 93–106.
55. Jayalakshmamma B, Pinkel D: Urinary-bladder toxicity following pelvic irradiation and simultaneous cyclophosphamide therapy. Cancer 1976;38:701–707.
56. Karras DJ, Farrell SE, Harrigan RA, et al: Poisoning from "Spanish fly" (Cantharidin). Am J Emerg Med 1996;14: 478–483.
57. Klein FA, Smith MJV: Urinary complications of cyclophosphamide therapy. South Med J 1983;76:1413–1416.
58. Kotsonis FN, Dood DC, Regnier B, et al: Preclinical toxicology profile of misoprostol. Dig Dis Sci 1985;30: 142S–146S.
59. Kwan T, Palusco AD, Kohl L: Digitalis toxicity caused by toad venom. Chest 1992;102:949–950.
60. Landis E, Shore E: Yohimbine-induced bronchospasm. Chest 1989;96:1424.
61. Landrigan PJ: Current issues in the epidemiology and toxicology of occupational exposure to lead. Environ Health Perspect 1990;89:61–66.
62. Lawrence HJ, Simone J, Aur RJA: Cyclophosphamide-induced hemorrhagic cystitis in children with leukemia. Cancer 1975;36:1572–1576.
63. Lemonica IP, Alvarenga CMD: Abortive and teratogenic effect of *Acanthospermum hispidum* DC. and *Cajanus cajan* (L.) Millps. in pregnant rats. J Ethnopharmacol 1994;43:39–44.
64. Levitt NS, Vinik AL, Sive AA, et al: Synthetic leutinizing hormone in impotent male diabetics: A double-blind cross-over trial. S Afr Med J 1980;57:701–704.
65. Lidberg L, Sternthal V: A new approach to the hormonal treatment of impotentia erectonis. Pharmacopsychiatry Neuropsychopharmacol 1977;10:21–25.
66. Lin SC, Hsu T, Fredrickson PA, Richelson E: Yohimbine- and tranylcypromine-induced postural hypotension. Am J Psychiatry 1987;144:119.
67. Linden CH, Vellman WP, Rumack B: Yohimbine: A new street drug. Ann Emerg Med 1985;14:1002–1004.
68. Lycka B: Amyl and butyl nitrites and telangiectasias in homosexual men. Ann Intern Med 1987;106:476.

69. Machabert R, Testud F, Descotes J: Methaemoglobinaemia due to amyl nitrite inhalation: A case report. Human Exp Toxicol 1994;13:313–314.
70. MacKenzie IZ, Davies AJ, Embrey MP, Guillebaud J: Very early abortion by prostaglandins. Lancet 1978;1:1223–1226.
71. Margolis R, Prieto P, Stein L, Chinn S: Statistical summary of 10,000 male cases using aphrodex in treatment of impotence. Curr Ther Res 1971;13:616–621.
72. Marks LB, Carroll PR, Dugan TC, Anscher MS: The response of the urinary bladder, urethra, and ureter to radiation and chemotherapy. Int J Radiat Oncol Biol Phys 1995;31:1257–1280.
73. Marmor M, Friedman-Kein AE, Laubenstein LL, et al: Risk factors for Kaposi's sarcoma in homosexual men. Lancet 1982;1:1083–1087.
74. Marx CM, Alpert SE: Ticarcillin-induced cystitis. AJDC 1984;138:670–672.
75. Mattison DR, Plowchalk DR, Meadows MJ, et al: Reproductive toxicity: Male and female reproductive systems as targets for chemical injury. Med Clin North Am 1990;74: 391–411.
76. Medical Research Council Working Party: Adverse reactions to bendrofluazide and propranolol for the treatment of mild hypertension. Lancet 1981;2:539–543.
77. Millard RJ: Busulphan haemorrhagic cystitis. Br J Urol 1978;50:210.
78. Miller LJ, Chandler SW, Ippoliti CM: Treatment of cyclophosphamide-induced hemorrhagic cystitis with prostaglandins. Ann Pharmacother 1994;28:590–594.
79. Moore KH, Hay DM, Imrie AE, et al: Oxybutynin hydrochloride (3 mg) in the treatment of women with idiopathic detrusor instability. Br J Urol 1990;66:479–485.
80. Morales A, Condra M, Owen JA, et al: Is yohimbine effective in the treatment of organic impotence? Results of a controlled trial. J Urol 1987;137:1168–1172.
81. Mudd JW: Impotence responsive to glyceryl trinitrate. Am J Psychiatry 1977;134:922–925.
82. Mukherjee B, Bhose IN: Induction of labour and abortion with quinine infusion in intrauterine foetal death. Am J Obstet Gynecol 1968;101:853–854.
83. Nath D, Sethi N, Jain S, Jain AK: Commonly used Indian abortifacient plants with special reference to their teratologic effects in rats. J Ethnopharmacol 1992;36:147–154.
84. Newman RJ, Salerno HR: Sexual dysfunction due to methyldopa. Br Med J 1974;4:106.
85. Nickolis LC, Teare D: Poisoning by cantharidin. Br Med J 1954;2:1384–1388.
86. Nudelman RW, Saleman M: The birth of the blues II: Blue movie. JAMA 1987;257:3230.
87. Oaks WW, DiTunno DJ, Magnani T, et al: Cantharidin poisoning. Arch Intern Med 1960;105:574–582.
88. Olsen J: Is human fecundity declining—And does occupational exposure play a role in such a decline if it exists? Scand J Work Environ Health 1994;20:72–77.
89. Owen JA, Nakatsu SL, Fenemore J, et al: The pharmacokinetics of yohimbine in man. Eur J Clin Pharmacol 1987;32: 577–582.
90. Paeyron R, Aubeny E, Targosz V, et al: Early termination of pregnancy with mifepristone (RU 486) and the orally active prostaglandin misoprostol. N Engl J Med 1993;328: 1503–1513.
91. Parry MF, Wallach R: Ethylene glycol poisoning. Am J Med 1974;57:143–150.
92. Paumgartten FJ, Castilla EE, Monteleone-Neto R, et al: Risk assessment in reproductive toxicology as practiced in South America. In: Neubert D, Kavlock RJ, Merker HJ, Klein J, eds: Risk Assessment of Prenatally Induced Adverse Health Effects. Berlin, Springer-Verlag, 1992, pp. 163–179.
93. Paumgartten FJR, Magalhaes-de-Souza CA, de-Carvalho RR, Chahoud I: Embryotoxic effects of misoprostol in the mouse. Braz J Med Biol Res 1995;28:355–361.
94. Perrone J, Hoffman RS: Toxic ingestions in pregnancy: Abortifacient use in a case series of pregnant overdose patients. Acad Emerg Med 1997;4:206–209.
95. Plotz PH, Klippel JH, Decker JL, et al: Bladder complications in patients receiving cyclophosphamide for systemic lupus erythematosus or rheumatoid arthritis. Ann Intern Med 1979;91:221–223.
96. Polettini A, Crippa O, Ravagli A, Saragoni A: A fatal case of poisoning with cantharidin. Forensic Sci Int 1992;56: 37–43.
97. Price LH, Charney DS, Heninger GR: Three cases of manic symptoms following yohimbine administration. Am J Psychiatry 1984;141:1267–1268.
98. Rabe T, Basse H, Thuro H, et al: Wirkung des PGE-1-Methylanalogons Misoprostol auf den schwangeren Uterus im ersten Trimester. Geburtshilfe Frauenheilkol 1987;47:324–331.
99. Relling MV, Schunk JE: Drug-induced hemorrhagic cystitis. Clin Pharm 1986;5:590–597.
100. Reproductive health and mifepristone. Lancet 1990;336: 1480–1481. Editorial.
101. Rosen RC, Ashton AK: Prosexual drugs: Empirical status of the "new aphrodisiacs." Arch Sex Behav 1993;22: 521–543.
102. Rosoff MH, Cohen MV: Profound bradycardia after amyl nitrite in patients with a tendency to vasovagal episodes. Br Heart J 1986;55:97–100.
103. Sandler B, Aronson P: Yohimbine-induced cutaneous drug eruption, progressive renal failure, and lupus-like syndrome. Urology 1993;41:343–345.
104. Schlegel PN, Chang TK, Marshall FF: Antibiotics: Potential hazards to male fertility. Fertil Steril 1991;55:235–242.
105. Schrag SD, Dixon RL: Occupational exposures associated with male reproductive dysfunction. Annu Rev Pharmacol Toxicol 1985;25:567–592.
106. Shieh C, Chen B, Lin K: Late onset hemorrhagic cystitis after allogeneic bone marrow transplantation. Taiwan I Hsuen Hui Tsa Chih 1989;88:508–511.
107. Stillwell TJ, Benson RC: Cyclophosphamide-induced hemorrhagic cystitis. Cancer 1988;61:451–457.
108. Sullivan JB, Rumack BH, Thomas H, et al: Pennyroyal oil poisoning and hepatotoxicity. JAMA 1979;242:2873–2874.
109. Susset JG, Tessier CD, Wincze J, et al: Effect of yohimbine hydrochloride on erectile impotence: A double-blind study. J Urol 1989;141:1360–1363.
110. Tackett RE: Priapism. In: Stine RJ, Chudnofsky CR, eds: A

Practical Approach to Emergency Medicine, 2nd ed. Boston, Little, Brown, 1994, pp. 710–711.

111. Till JS, Majmudar BN: Cantharidin poisoning. South Med J 1981;74:444–447.
112. Tsao SW, Ng TB, Yeung HW: Toxicities of trichosanthin and alpha-momorcharin, abortifacient proteins from Chinese medicinal plants, on cultured tumor cell lines. Toxicon 1990;28:1183–92.
113. Vance BM: Intrauterine injection of lysol as an abortifacient. Report of a fatal case complicated by oil embolism and lysol poisoning. Arch Pathol 1945:40:395–398.
114. Van Jeijst ANP, de Jong W, Seldenrijk R, et al: Coma and crystalluria: A massive primidone intoxication treated with hemoperfusion. J Toxicol Clin Toxicol 1983;20: 307–318.
115. Warren SC, Warren SG: Propranolol and sexual impotence. Ann Intern Med 1977;86:112. Letter.
116. Whorton MD, Foliart DE: Mutagenicity, carcinogenicity, and reproductive effects of dibromochloropropane (DBCP). Mutat Res 1983;123:13–30.
117. Wilson B:The effect of drugs on male sexual function and fertility. Nurse Practitioner 1991;16:12–24.
118. Winder C: Reproductive and chromosomal effects of occupational exposure to lead in the male. Reproduction Toxicology 1989;3:221–233.
119. Winek CL, Davis ER, Collom WD, Shanon SP: Quinine fatality—Case report. Clin Toxicol 1974;7:129–132.
120. Wolf LR, Otten EJ, Spadafora MP: Cinchonism: Two case reports and review of acute quinine toxicity and treatment. J Emerg Med 1992;10:295–301.
121. Yealy DM, Hogya PT: Priapism. Emerg Med Clin North Am 1988;6:509–520.

PART D

The Clinical Basis of Medical Toxicology

CHAPTER 30

Managing the Patient With an Unknown Overdose

Neal E. Flomenbaum, Lewis R. Goldfrank, Neal A. Lewin, Richard S. Weisman, Mary Ann Howland, and Robert S. Hoffman

EMS was asked to respond to the house of an 18-year-old male described by his mother as barely arousable. When the paramedics arrived, the patient was lethargic, seemingly disoriented, hyperventilating, and "intermittently shaking" or shivering. In the patient's bedroom, the paramedics found empty bottles of erythromycin 500 mg, Tylenol and Codeine #3, and Robitussin DM. Upon questioning, the patient told the paramedics that he was trying to kill himself. After obtaining vital signs, consisting of blood pressure, 130/70 mm Hg, pulse rate, 120/min, and respiratory rate, "24 to 36/min," the paramedics started an IV of D_5W, and then transported the patient and the empty medication containers to the ED.

In the ED, the patient was arousable when his name was called and he was able to follow simple commands. Vital signs soon after arrival were BP 120/80 mm Hg, pulse rate, 96 to 108/min, respiratory rate, 20 breaths/min, and temperature, 98.4°F (36.9°C) per rectum. The initial physical evaluation revealed no evidence of head or body trauma; pupils that were equal, round, and reactive to light; a poor gag reflex; a supple neck; clear breath sounds bilaterally; regular rapid heart sounds without murmurs, rubs, or gallops; a soft abdomen without scars or organomegally; and normal extremities without clubbing, cyanosis, or edema.

A bedside glucose determination revealed a blood sugar of 100 mg/dL, and despite the history of codeine ingestion, based on the patient's condition, the staff felt that naloxone was not indicated at that time. Oxygen was administered at 10 L/min by mask. Blood samples were drawn for CBC, BUN, glucose, electrolyte, acetaminophen, and salicylate levels.

A portable chest radiograph was requested and an ECG was obtained, which revealed a supraventricular tachycardia with narrow complexes at a rate of 120 to 140 beats/min and right-axis deviation. Preparations were made for an arterial blood gas determination to be followed by intubation for airway protection, orogastric lavage, and the administration of activated charcoal. However, while the patient was being intubated he began having generalized tonic-clonic convulsions, requiring a total of 20 mg of diazepam IV to achieve control. After the seizure activity ended, the patient was intubated, lavaged, and given activated charcoal. The pink lavage fluid contained white pill fragments. Urine obtained by Foley catherization appeared normal. A portable chest radiograph revealed clear lungs and endotracheal and nasogastric tubes that appeared to be correctly placed. The patient remained comatose throughout the time he spent in the ED prior to transfer to the ICU.

The CBC revealed a WBC of 18,000/mm^3 and a normal hemoglobin. Urinalysis was within normal limits as were the PT and PTT. Blood glucose was 134 mg/dL and K^+ was 3.1 mEq/L. BUN and all other electrolytes tested, including Ca^{2+} and Mg^{2+}, were normal. The blood ethanol level was 75 mg/dL. Salicylate and theophylline levels were negative. The initial acetaminophen level was 40 μg/mL. The ABG specimen drawn immediately after cessation of seizure activity revealed a pH of 7.29, PCO_2 of 45.5 mm Hg, and PO_2 of 570 mm Hg on supplemental oxygen. One hour later, the ABG values were pH 7.49, PCO_2 31.7 mm Hg, and PO_2 307 mm Hg.

The patient was extubated the next morning. He subsequently told the psychiatrist that he was depressed and had tried to commit suicide. He confirmed the ingestion of unknown quantities of erythromycin, Tylenol and Codeine, Robitussin DM, and several other pills that he could not identify from his medicine chest at home. He denied use of any other medications or illicit drugs.

The patient was transferred from the ICU to a "med-psych" floor on the second hospital day and then transferred to a psychiatric facility on day five.

This case is presented here because it illustrates many of the problems clinicians frequently face in managing patients with possible drug overdoses or poisonings. Rarely, if ever, are all of the circumstances of a toxic exposure known: the history may be incomplete, unreliable, or unobtainable; multiple drugs or medications may be involved; and even when a drug etiology is identified, it may not be easy to determine whether we are dealing with an overdose, an allergic or idiosyncratic reaction, or a drug–drug interaction. Similarly, it is sometimes difficult or impossible to differentiate between adverse effects of a correct dose of medication or the consequences of a deliberate or unintentional overdose. The patient's presenting signs and symptoms may force us to intervene at a time when we have almost no information about the etiology of the patient's condition and therefore medications often must be thoughtfully chosen empirically to treat or diagnose a condition without exacerbating the situation. What is the initial management of a patient with an unknown overdose? What constitutes a "primary survey" and primary treatment for a comatose patient suspected of a drug overdose? What is an adequate "secondary survey," and what further interventions are required early on? When should attempts be made to eliminate absorbed toxins from the body, and what methods to do so are available? Which treatments for an unknown overdose are now considered outmoded or dangerous, and what are the management pitfalls to be avoided?

Conscious patients, asymptomatic patients, and pregnant patients with possible overdoses or poisonings pose additional management questions, as do the victims of toxic cutaneous exposures or caustic eye injuries. This chapter represents our efforts to formulate a logical approach to managing the patient with an unknown overdose.

Probably the most frequent toxicologic emergency that clinicians deal with is the patient with an unknown overdose. Considering not only the patient with an altered mental status but those patients who are suicidal, those who are using illicit drugs, and those who are exposed to medications or substances that they are unaware of, the majority of toxicologic emergencies at least partially fall under this category.

To effectively manage the unknown overdose, clinicians must be able to utilize the principles developed in Part A of this text, General Approach to Medical Toxicology. In that section, a basic principle of modern toxicologic management was described, which is that for the vast majority of poisoned or overdosed patients, the clinical condition of the patient, rather than the specific ingredients of the ingestion, dictates the management. In other words, *treat the patient, not the poison.* Such an approach does not preclude identifying and treating specifically for certain toxins and/or toxic syndromes. But even in these situations, basic clinical management techniques must never be neglected.

When the principle of treating the patient, not the poison, is applied to managing the patient with an unknown overdose, the answers to several early management questions become apparent. For example, when an unconscious patient presents, how do we know that we are dealing with an overdose? If the patient has obvious trauma, how do we know the patient has not also overdosed on a medication or drug or been poisoned by a toxic substance? Clearly what is required is an approach that will hopefully identify and treat or exclude toxicologic etiologies of the patient's condition and, in any case, cause no harm to the patient.

What Is the Initial Management of a Patient With an Unknown Overdose?

Similar to the management of any seriously compromised patient, the clinical approach to the poisoned or overdosed patient begins with the recognition and treatment of life-threatening conditions: *a*irway compromise, *b*reathing difficulties, and *c*irculatory problems such as hypotension and serious dysrhythmias. Once the ABCs are addressed, the patient's level of consciousness should be assessed, as this will help determine the techniques to be utilized for further management of the ingestion or exposure.

What Constitutes a "Primary Survey" for the Patient With an Altered Mental Status and Suspected Drug Overdose?

Once the airway itself is clear, and cervical spine trauma excluded or the cervical spine protected, an initial bedside assessment should be made regarding the adequacy of respirations. If a qualitative bedside assessment of depth and rate is not possible, then at least the presence or absence of regular breathing should be determined. In this setting, any irregular breathing pattern should be considered a possible sign of the incipient cessation of breathing requiring hyperventilation with 100% oxygen by bag-valve-mask followed as soon as possible by tracheal intubation. Tracheal intubation is probably indicated for most cases of coma resulting from a poisoning or overdose, not only to insure and maintain control of the airway but also to enable safe performance of procedures to prevent gastrointestinal absorption or eliminate previously absorbed toxins. As soon as practicable, an arterial blood gas determination will more accurately define the adequacy of oxygenation (PO_2, O_2 sat) and ventilation (PCO_2) and may also alert the physician to possible toxic-metabolic etiologies of coma (pH, PCO_2). In addition, when clinically indicated, a carboxyhemoglobin determination will be necessary to diagnose or exclude carbon monoxide poisoning.

Once the patient's respiratory status is assessed and treated, the strength, rate, and regularity of the pulse should be evaluated, the blood pressure determined, and a rectal temperature obtained. Both a 12-lead electrocardiograph (ECG) and continuous ECG monitoring are essential. Monitoring will alert the clinician to dysrhythmias primarily or secondarily (via hypoxemia, electrolyte imbalance) related to drug or toxin ingestions. A 12-lead ECG demonstrating QRS widening and axis deviations may indicate a life-threatening cyclic antidepressant or phenothiazine overdose, enabling the physician to anticipate such serious sequelae as ventricular tachydysrhythmias, seizures, and cardiac arrest, and suggesting both the early use of specific treatment and antidotes and the avoidance of some medications (such as procainamide) that could exacerbate the situation. Other ECG changes such as PR and QTc lengthening or shortening, baseline changes, and T and U-wave abnormalities may point to cardioactive drug toxicity and serious electrolyte abnormalities.

Extremes of core body temperature must be addressed early in the evaluation and treatment of a comatose patient. Life-threatening hyperthermia (temperature ≥ 105°F or ≥ 40.5°C) is usually appreciated when the patient is touched. Regardless of the etiology, such temperatures must be immediately reduced to about 101.5°F (38.7°C) by ice water immersion or fan-mist treatment to prevent catastrophic complications or death. True hypothermia is probably easier to miss than hyperthermia, especially in Northern states during winter months, when most arriving patients feel cold to the touch. Early recognition of hypothermia, however, will help avoid administering a variety of medications that may be ineffective until the patient becomes relatively euthermic, at which time iatrogenic drug toxicity may result.

For the hypotensive patient with clear lungs and an unknown overdose, a fluid challenge with 0.9% NaCl (normal saline) or lactated Ringer's solution may be started. At the time the IV line is secured, blood samples for glucose, electrolytes, BUN, a CBC, and toxicologic analysis should be drawn. *In the vast majority of cases, the blood tests that are most useful in diagnosing toxicologic emergencies are not the toxicologic assays but the nontoxicologic tests such as BUN, glucose, electrolytes, and arterial blood gas.* If the patient remains hypotensive or cannot tolerate fluids, a vasopressor such as norepinephrine may be indicated.

Drug or toxin-related seizures may broadly be divided into three categories: (1) those that respond to standard (typically benzodiazepine) anticonvulsant treatment (eg, ethanol withdrawal); (2) those that either require specific antidotes to control seizure activity or do not respond consistently to standard anticonvulsant treatment (eg, isoniazid-induced seizures requiring pyridoxine administration); and (3) those that may appear to respond—the tonic-clonic activity ceases—but nevertheless leave the patient exposed to the underlying, unidentified toxin or to continued electrical seizure activity in the brain (eg, carbon monoxide or hypoglycemia of any etiology).

What Is the "Primary Treatment" for the Patient With an Altered Mental Status Resulting from a Suspected Drug Overdose?

Early (within the first five minutes) in the management of a patient with altered mental status, four therapeutic modalities should either be administered or considered: (1) *dextrose 0.5 to 1.0 g/kg of $D_{50}W$ for an adult*, or *a more dilute dextrose solution ($D_{10}W$ or $D_{25}W$) for a child* to diagnose and treat or to exclude hypoglycemia; (2) *thiamine 100 mg IV for an adult* (usually unnecessary for a child) to prevent or treat Wernicke-Korsakoff syndrome; (3) *naloxone 2 mg IV for adults and children with respiratory compromise*; and (4) *oxygen, high flow (8 to 10 L/min).*

What Is the "Secondary Survey" for a Patient With an Altered Mental Status and a Suspected Drug Overdose?

While examining a comatose patient for clues to the etiology of a presumably toxic-metabolic form of coma, it is especially important to search for any indication that trauma may have caused, contributed to, or resulted from the patient's altered mental status.

The remainder of the physical examination should be performed rapidly but reasonably thoroughly. In addition to evaluating the level of consciousness, the physician should note abnormal posturing (decorticate or decerebrate), abnormal or unilateral withdrawal responses, and pupil size and reactivity. Pinpoint pupils suggest exposure to opioids or organophosphate insecticides, and widely dilated pupils suggest anticholinergic or sympathomimetic poisoning. The presence or absence of nystagmus, abnormal reflexes, and any other focal neurologic findings may provide important clues to a structural cause of coma. Assigning the patient a Glasgow Coma Score (GCS) (if not already done during the first survey) will provide a useful measure for assessing any changes in neurologic status, but the GCS should never be used for prognostic purposes, because complete recovery from properly managed toxic-metabolic coma despite a low GCS is the rule rather than the exception.

Characteristic breath or skin odors frequently identify the etiology of coma. The fruity odor of ketones on the breath suggests diabetic ketoacidosis, but also the possible ingestion of acetone, or isopropyl alcohol which is metabolized to acetone. The pungent, minty odor of oil of wintergreen on the breath or skin suggests methyl salicylate poisoning. The odors of other substances such as cyanide ("bitter almonds"), hydrogen sulfide ("rotten eggs"), and organophosplates ("garlic") are described in detail in Chapter 27.

What Is the "Secondary Survey" for Patients With a Suspected Drug Overdose?

Reauscultation of respiratory sounds, particularly after a fluid challenge has been initiated, will help diagnose or exclude cardiogenic or noncardiogenic pulmonary edema and aspiration pneumonia. Coupled with an abnormal breath odor of hydrocarbons or organophosphates, for example, rales and rhonchi may point to a *noncardiogenic etiology*. This is of particular consequence as the administration of cardiac medications may be inappropriate or dangerous in these circumstances.

Heart murmurs in an intravenous drug user, especially when accompanied by fever, may point to bacterial endocarditis. Bradydysrhythmias and tachydysrhythmias may suggest overdoses or inappropriate use of cardioactive medications (digoxin, beta-adrenergic antagonists, calcium channel blockers, cyclic antidepressants).

Abdominal examination may reveal signs of trauma or alcohol-related hepatic disease (small or large liver, spider angiomata). The presence or absence of bowel sounds will help exclude or diagnose anticholinergic toxicity, and will be important in considering whether or not to manipulate the gastrointestinal tract in an attempt to remove toxin.

Examination of the extremities may reveal clues to current or former drug use (track marks, skin popping scars), poisoning (Mees lines, arsenical dermatitis), and the presence of cyanosis or edema suggesting preexisting cardiac or renal disease.

Reevalution of the patient suspected of an overdose is essential in identifying new or developing findings or toxidromes and in early identification and treatment of a deteriorating condition. Until the patient is completely recovered or considered no longer at risk for the consequences of a poisoning or overdose, frequent reassessment must be provided even as the procedures described below are carried out.

What Is the Secondary Treatment for the Patient With a Suspected Drug Overdose? What Is the Role for Gastrointestinal Evacuation Techniques?

After stabilizing the patient, completing the primary and secondary surveys, and considering or administering the use of hypertonic dextrose, thiamine, naloxone, and oxygen, the physician must now make a series of individualized treatment decisions. Although many patients may benefit from gastrointestinal evacuation, those patients who have any evidence of possible structural neurologic problems should ordinarily have a CT scan as well as hyperventilation and intubation, *prior* to any stressful procedure such as gastric intubation or lavage that might raise intracranial pressure.

As the discussion in Chapter 4 demonstrates, even the decision to evacuate the GI tract and/or administer activated charcoal can no longer be considered an automatic or generalized form of care. Instead, the decision should be based on the type of ingestion, estimated quantity and size, time since ingestion, concurrent ingestions, ancillary medical conditions, age and size of the patient, and so forth.

The indications, contraindications, and procedures for performing orogastric lavage and for administering whole-bowel irrigation, single or multiple-dose activated charcoal (AC, MDAC), cathartics, and, in the conscious patient, syrup of ipecac to induce emesis, are listed in Tables 30–1 through 30–5 and discussed in detail in Chapter 4.

TABLE 30–1. OROGASTRIC LAVAGE

Indications

1. Life-threatening or serious overdoses when a drug or toxin is still expected to be accessible in the stomach.

Tube Type and Size

Adults/adolescents: 36-40 French
Children: 22-28 French

Procedure

1. If there is potential airway compromise, endotracheal or nasotracheal intubation should precede orogastric lavage. Vomiting commonly follows lavage.
2. The patient should be kept in the left lateral decubitus position.
3. Prior to insertion, the proper length of tubing to be passed should be measured and marked on the tube. Once the tube is introduced, confirmation that the distal end of the tube is in the stomach is essential.
4. Withdraw any material present and consider instillation of AC (Table 30–2).
5. Via a funnel (or lavage syringe), 250 mL aliquots of a saline lavage solution should be instilled in an adult, and 10 to 15 mL/kg aliquots—not to exceed 250 mL—instilled in a child.
6. Lavage should continue for at least several liters in an adult and for 500 mL to 1 L in a child *or* until no particulate matter returns and the effluent lavage solution is clear.
7. Following lavage, the same tube should be used to instill activated charcoal and a cathartic, if indicated (Tables 30–2 and 30–3).

Contraindications

Caustic (strong acid or alkali) ingestions
Sharp material ingestions or coingestions
Drug packet ingestions
Significant hemorrhagic diathesis, esophageal varices, thrombocytopenia (relative contraindication)
Prior significant emesis
Nontoxic ingestions

Adverse Effects

Inadvertent endotracheal intubation and/or airway trauma
Aspiration pneumonitis
Emesis
Gastrointestinal hemorrhage and/or perforation

When Should Attempts Be Made to Eliminate Absorbed Toxins from the Body?

After the decision regarding intervention to prevent absorption of toxic compounds is made, the clinician must next consider the applicability of techniques available to eliminate toxic compounds already absorbed. A detailed discussion of the indications and techniques of manipulating urinary pH (ion trapping), forced diuresis, hemodialysis, hemoperfusion, hemofiltration, and exchange transfusion may be found in Chapter 5. Briefly, patients who may benefit are those who have ingested substances amenable to one of these techniques and whose clinical condition is both serious (or potentially serious) and unresponsive to supportive care, or whose physiologic route of elimination (liver-stools, kidney-urine) is impaired.

TABLE 30–2. ACTIVATED CHARCOAL (SEE P. 527)

Indications

Single-dose (AC)

Ingestions of drugs or toxins that bind to AC when no contraindication exists.

Multiple-dose (MDAC).

Ingestions of drugs or toxins that bind to AC

When a prolonged absorption phase is expected

When potential toxicity is great

When gastrointestinal dialysis is expected to be beneficial

Drugs with a small volume of distribution (<1.0 L/kg), low endogenous clearance, low plasma protein binding, and biliary or gastric secretion of active metabolites that recirculate are most amenable to gastrointestinal dialysis.

Initial Dose (AC, MDAC), Orally or Via Orogastric Tube

Adults and children: 1 g/kg body weight. Following massive ingestions, 2 g/kg may be indicated, if such a large dose can be easily administered.

Repeat Doses (MDAC), Orally or Via Nasogastric Tube

Adults and children: 0.5–1 g/kg body weight q 1–4 h, in accordance with the dose and dosage form of drug ingested (larger doses and shorter dosing intervals may occasionally be indicated).

Procedure

1. Add 8 parts of water to the selected amount of powdered form. All formulations, including prepackaged slurries, should be shaken well for at least one minute to form a transiently stable suspension prior to drinking or instillation via an orogastric tube.
2. AC can be administered as a mixture with a cathartic, for the first dose only.
3. If the patient vomits the dose of AC, it should be repeated. Smaller, more frequent doses, or continuous nasogastric administration, may be better tolerated. An antiemetic may be needed to control nausea or emesis.
4. If a nasogastric or orogastric tube is utilized for MDAC administration, time should be allowed for the last dose to pass through the stomach before suctioning and prior to removing the tube. The suctioning may prevent subsequent charcoal aspiration.

Contraindications

Patients at risk for aspiration who have an unprotected airway.

Caustics: activated charcoal is not only ineffective as an adsorbent, but may accumulate in burned areas, interfering with endoscopy.

Ileus (a contraindication for MDAC).

Adverse Effects

Aspiration

Emesis

Obscuring of gastrointestinal mucosa

Constipation

Obstruction

Alkalinization of the urinary pH for acidic substances, also referred to as *manipulation of the urinary pH,* has limited applicability. Commonly, sodium bicarbonate can be used to enhance salicylate, phenobarbital, chlorpropamide, methotrexate, or myoglobin elimination. Acidification for alkaline substances is difficult to accomplish, probably useless, possibly dangerous, and therefore has no role currently in poison management. *Forced diuresis* has no indication and may endanger the patient by causing pulmonary or cerebral edema. If a form of extracorporeal elimination is contemplated, consider *hemodialysis* for salicylates, methanol, ethylene glycol, lithium, and drugs that are both dialyzable and cause fluid and electrolyte problems; consider *hemoperfusion* for theophylline, phenobarbital, phenytoin and carbamazepine (though rarely for the last three). *Peritoneal dialysis* is too ineffective to be of practical utility, and *hemofiltration* too new to have an established role. At times both *hemodialysis* and *hemoperfusion in series* may be considered for life-threatening overdoses (salicylates). When hemoperfusion is the method of choice (as for a theophylline overdose) but not available, hemodialysis is a logical, effective alternative, and certainly preferable to delaying treatment until hemoperfusion becomes available.

The indications for qualitative and quantitative diagnostic laboratory studies, and the use and interpretation of the ECG and radiologic and imaging procedures in diagnosing and managing the poisoned or overdosed patient are discussed fully in Chapters 6 to 8.

TABLE 30-3. CATHARTICS (SEE P. 535)

Indications

Drugs or toxins that remain in the gastrointestinal tract and may continue to be absorbed (or desorbed from AC) if not rapidly eliminated. Cathartics should be used only with the first dose of AC (or MDAC) and not repeated. Cathartics should not be used routinely in children.

Types and Doses (Adults and Children)

Magnesium citrate (10% Mg citrate)	4 mL/kg, to a maximum of 300 mL
Magnesium sulfate ($MgSO_4$)	250 mg/kg, to a maximum of 30 g
Sorbitol	0.5–1 g/kg (0.5 g/kg in children, with a maximum 50 g of 35% concentrate in children over 5 year of age)

Precautions

Cathartics are not warranted for routine management of trivial ingestions.

Cathartics should not be used more than once for any ingestion—beware of packaging and labeling of AC and cathartic (sorbitol) combinations that appear similar to AC alone.

Sorbitol should be administered cautiously in children if at all, and only with strict attention to fluid and electrolyte status.

Phosphosoda preparations should not be used either in children or adults.

Oil-based cathartics should not be used because of the risks of aspiration and enhanced toxin absorption.

Contraindications

Abdominal trauma

Intestinal obstruction

Adynamic ileus

Renal failure (a contraindication for $MgSO_4$ or Mg citrate cathartics)

Diarrhea

Adverse Effects

Volume depletion

Emesis

Electrolyte imbalance (hypermagnesemia, hypokalemia, hyponatremia)

Diarrhea (excessive)

TABLE 30-4. EMESIS WITH SYRUP OF IPECAC (SEE P. 523)

Indications

Early treatment of a potentially toxic ingestion—particularly for children, at home, when there are no contraindications (see below).

Dose

Adult	30 mL (2 tbsp)
Children	
6–12 months	10 mL (2 tsp)
1–5 years	15 mL (1 tbsp)
Over 5 years	30 mL (2 tbsp)

One additional dose may be given if the patient has not vomited within 30 min.

Contraindications

Caustic acid or alkali ingestions
Sharp solid-material ingestions or coingestions
Easily aspirated substances (eg, a pure petroleum distillate with little systemic toxicity in the amount ingested)
Comatose patients
Seizing patients
Patients expected to deteriorate rapidly
Patients with a compromised gag reflex
Patients with a hemorrhagic diathesis, esophageal varices, thrombocytopenia (relative contraindication)
Children less than 6 months of age
Significant prior vomiting or when vomiting will delay the administration of an oral antidote or AC
Nontoxic ingestions

Adverse Effects

Intractable vomiting (rare)
Mallory-Weiss tears
Pneumothorax and/or pneumomediastinum
Aspiration
Delayed emesis after patient loses consciousness
Diarrhea (unlikely with therapeutic doses)
Electrolyte abnormalities (with chronic use or abuse by patients)

Which Treatments for a Patient With an *Unknown* Overdose Are Now Considered Outmoded or Dangerous?

- Analeptics, including physostigmine (see pp. 17, 614)
- Flumazenil (see p. 1017)
- Forced diuresis (see p. 17)
- Urinary acidification (see p. 18)
- Types IA and IC antidysrhythmics (see pp. 364–373)
- Inappropriate choices of vasopressors (see pp. 357–363)
- Long-acting opioid antagonists such as naltrexone and nalmefene (see p. 996)

How Can the Pitfalls in Managing a Patient With a Suspected Drug Overdose or Alcohol Intoxication Be Avoided?

1. Do not rely solely on the history to predict which patients require naloxone, hypertonic dextrose ($D_{50}W$), thiamine, and oxygen. Instead, consider the use for all patients with altered mental status unless specifically contraindicated. Use the physical examination to guide the use of naloxone. If dextrose or naloxone is indicated, administer sufficient amounts to exclude and/or treat hypoglycemia or opioid toxicity.
2. Do not use vasopressors in the initial management of hypotension in a patient with a suspected or unknown overdose prior to using fluids or inserting a pulmonary artery (Swan-Ganz) catheter.
3. Do not neglect the possibility of concomitant trauma in cases of suspected drug overdose or poisoning. Conversely, do not neglect the possibility of a drug ingestion or toxic-metabolic disorder in the patient with obvious head trauma. In any case, do not use the Glasgow Coma Score as a determinant for therapy.
4. Do not hold a patient with altered mental status in the ED for a prolonged period of time after initial treatment. Make every effort to provide the patient with definitive care in the appropriate intensive care setting as rapidly as possible (see Chap. 103).
5. Do not attribute altered mental status to an alcohol odor on a patient's breath. Small amounts of alcohol and its associated odor emitting congeners generally produce the same breath odor as do intoxicating

TABLE 30-5. WHOLE-BOWEL IRRIGATION (SEE P. 538)

Description

Whole-bowel irrigation with polyethylene glycol electrolyte lavage solution may be helpful in managing poisonings and overdoses when it is desirable or necessary to (1) rapidly clear the entire GI tract without emesis or causing fluid or electrolyte disturbances or (2) prepare the GI tract for visualization. It is not to be substituted for activated charcoal (AC) when the latter is indicated, and its precise role in managing poisonings and overdoses is currently under evaluation.

Indications (Potential)

Sustained-release medications
Slowly dissolving substances (eg, iron tablets, paint chips, bezoars, concretions)
Crack vials
Drug packets prepared for smuggling (eg, heroin, cocaine)
Drugs or toxins not adsorbed by AC (eg, lithium, iron, metals)

Dose Orally or Via Nasogastric Tube

Adults: 2 L/h
Children: 0.5 L/h

Duration of Therapy

For 4–6 hr, or until the rectal effluent is clear
Note: AC should be administered before and during WBI if a charcoal adsorbable drug or toxin is involved

Not Indicated For:

Quickly absorbed drugs or toxins
Liquids
Parenterally administered drugs
Acids or alkalis

Adverse Effects

Rectal itching
Vomiting (especially with rapid administration)
Bloating
Decreased efficacy of AC

amounts. Conversely, even when an extremely high blood ethanol level is *confirmed* by the laboratory, it is dangerous to ignore other possible etiologies of altered mental status: chronic alcoholics may be awake and seemingly alert with ethanol levels in excess of 500 mg/dL, a level that would result in coma and possibly apnea and death in a nonalcoholic.

As a general rule, a supposedly "inebriated" comatose patient still "sleeping it off" 3 to 4 hours after arrival should be considered to have structural CNS damage (head trauma) and/or another toxic-metabolic etiology for the alteration in consciousness, until proven otherwise. Careful neurologic reevaluation supplemented by a head CT scan is always indicated in such a case. The metabolism of ethanol is fairly consistent, at 15 to 30 mg/dL/h, and regardless of the initial level, the patient who is comatose from ethanol alone should be more awake 3 to 4 hours after arrival. This is especially important in dealing with a patient who appears to have a minor bruise and is "intoxicated," as the early treatment of a subdural or epidural hematoma is critical to a successful outcome.

How Does Management of a Patient With Normal Mental Status and a Suspected Overdose Differ from that of the Patient With Altered Consciousness?

As in the case of the patient with altered consciousness, vital signs must be obtained and recorded. Initially, an assumption may have been made that the patient was breathing adequately, and if the patient is alert, talking, and in no respiratory distress, all that remains to document is the respiratory rate and rhythm. Because the patient is alert, additional history should be obtained at this point, keeping in mind that information regarding the number and types of substances ingested, time elapsed, whether or not the patient vomited previously, and other critical information may be unreliable, depending in part on whether the ingestion was deliberate or unintentional.

If possible, another history should be privately and independently obtained from a friend or relative after the patient is initially stabilized. Speaking to the friend or relative may provide an opportunity to learn useful and reliable information regarding the ingestion, the patient's frame of mind, a history of previous ingestions, and the type of support that is available should the patient be discharged from the ED. It is essential to separate the patient from any relatives or friends initially, as the patient may not cooperate in their presence. Also, although friends or relatives may be clinical assets, their anxiety may interfere with therapy. As unreliable as the history taken from a patient with an overdose may be, it may nevertheless provide a clue to an overlooked possibility or a second ingestant, or may reveal the patient's mental and emotional condition. As is often true of the history, physical examination, or laboratory assessment in other clinical situations, the information obtained may confirm but never exclude possible etiologies.

At this point in the management of the conscious patient, a focused physical examination should be performed, concentrating on breath and heart sounds and abdominal examination. A neurologic survey should emphasize reflexes and/or any focal findings.

How Should the Patient With a Deliberate Overdose Be Managed?

Initial efforts at establishing rapport with the patient, such as advising the patient that you are concerned about the problems that led up to the ingestion and that help is available after the drug or poison is removed, will ultimately make management easier. At the same time, the appropriate options for gastrointestinal decontamination must be firmly explained. The patient should be reassured that after the chosen procedure is accomplished there will be time to discuss related problems and obtain additional appropriate care. These considerations are especially important in managing the patient with a deliberate overdose.

Are There Special Considerations for Managing the Pregnant Patient With an Overdose?

In general, a successful outcome for both mother and fetus is dependent on optimum management of the mother. Proven effective treatment of a potentially serious overdose by the mother should never be withheld based on theoretical concerns regarding the fetus.

Physiologic Factors

A pregnant woman's total blood volume and cardiac output are elevated through the second trimester and into the later stages of the third trimester. This means that signs of hypoperfusion and hypotension will manifest later than they would in a woman who is not pregnant, and when they do, uterine blood flow might already be compromised. For these reasons, hypotension must be more aggressively identified and treated in the pregnant woman. Maintaining the patient in the left-lateral decubitus position will prevent supine hypotension resulting from impairment of systemic venous return; this position is also the preferred position for orogastric lavage.

Because the tidal volume is increased in pregnancy, the baseline PCO_2 will normally be lower by approximately 10 mm Hg. Appropriate adjustment should be made for this effect when interpreting arterial blood gas results.

Use of Antidotes

Few data are available on the use of antidotes in pregnancy. In general, antidotes should not be used if the indications for use are equivocal. On the other hand, antidotes should not be withheld if their use might reduce potential morbidity and mortality. Risk-to-benefit ratios should be assessed. For example, reversal of opioid-induced respiratory depression calls for the use of naloxone, but if the woman is opioid dependent, the naloxone may precipate acute withdrawal, including uterine contractions and possible induction of labor. Very slow, careful titration, starting with 0.05 to 0.1 mg naloxone, may therefore be indicated, unless apnea is present, cessation of breathing appears imminent, or the PO_2 or O_2 saturation is already grossly inadequate. In these instances naloxone may have to be administered in the usual manner, or assisted ventilation utilized.

Carbon monoxide (CO) poisoning is particularly threatening to fetal survival. The normal PO_2 of the fetal blood is about 15 to 20 mm Hg. Oxygen delivery to fetal tissues is impaired by the presence of carboxyhemoglobin, which shifts the O_2 hemoglobin dissociation curve to the left, potentially compromising an already tenuous balance. For this reason, many authors recommend aggressive use of hyperbaric oxygen for much lower carboxyhemoglobin levels in pregnancy (see Chap. 96 and Antidotes-in-Depth: Hyperbaric Oxygen). Early notification of the obstetrician and close cooperation between physicians are essential for the best results.

How Should Toxic Cutaneous Exposures Be Managed?

The chemicals that people are commonly exposed to externally include household cleaning materials; organophosphate or carbamate insecticides from crop dusting, gardening, or roach extermination; acids from exploding batteries; alkalies, such as lye; and lacrimating agents, which are used in crowd control. In all cases, the principles of management are as follows:

1. The staff should avoid secondary exposures by wearing protective (rubber or plastic) gowns, gloves, shoe covers, and so on. Many severe cases of secondary poisoning have occurred because emergency personnel were exposed to toxins such as organophosphates merely by touching the victim or the victim's clothing.
2. Remove the patient's clothing and place it in a plastic bag.
3. Wash the patient with soap and copious amounts of water *twice*, no matter how much time has elapsed since the exposure.
4. Never try to neutralize an acid with a base, or vice versa.
5. Avoid using any greases or creams. These will only keep the poison in close contact with the skin and ultimately make removal more difficult.

How Should Toxic or Caustic Eye Injuries Be Managed?

Irrigate the eyes with lids fully retracted for no less than 20 minutes. A drop of anesthetic such as proparacaine in each eye facilitates irrigation. Lids may be held open with a lid retractor or one fashioned from paperclips. An adequate irrigation stream may be obtained by running 1 L of normal saline through regular IV tubing held a few inches from the eye or by using a Morgan lens. Checking the lid fornices with pH paper strips is important to ensure adequate irrigation; the pH should be 6.5 to 7.6 if accurately tested, although when using paper test strips, the measurement is often near 8 (see Chap. 26).

How Can Successful Management of the Patient With an Unknown Overdose Be Assured?

As in the case described at the beginning of this chapter, optimal outcome for the patient suspected of an overdose largely depends on faithfully implementing the principles of basic and advanced life support (BLS and ALS) and a modified version of the "primary" and "secondary" surveys described in Advanced Trauma Life Support (ATLS). Typically, only some of the substances the patient actually ingested will ever be confirmed by the laboratory. In the case at the start of the chapter, the acetaminophen was confirmed whereas the erythromycin and other possible ingestants were either not tested for or remained undetermined throughout the hospitalization. Nevertheless, a successful outcome was possible. In addition to the general management techniques applicable to all overdoses, the careful use of specific treatments or antidotes indicated by the presentation may be reasonable even if not ultimately beneficial.

The thoughtful combination of stabilization, general management, and specific treatment when indicated, will result in successful outcomes in the vast majority of poisoned or overdosed patients.

ANTIDOTES IN DEPTH

Syrup of Ipecac

Mary Ann Howland

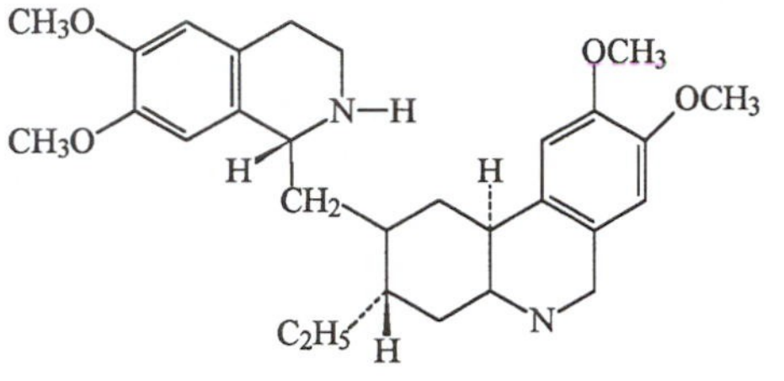

Emetine

Syrup of ipecac is an emetic that has been in use for the management of poisonings since the 1950s and has been available over the counter since the late 1960s. Ipecac comes from the dried rhizome and roots of plants found in Brazil belonging to the family *Rubiaceae*, such as *Cephaelis acuminata* or *Cephaelis ipecacuanha*.[44] Cephaeline and emetine are the two alkaloids believed to be largely responsible for the production of nausea and vomiting, with cephaeline being the more potent.[22] Each 15-mL dose of the syrup of ipecac contains 16 to 21 mg of cephaeline and 6.4 to 21 mg of emetine, giving a cephaeline-to-emetine ratio of between 1:1 and 2.5:1.[44] Syrup of ipecac also contains a small amount of psychotrine, but this is of minor importance. Syrup of ipecac induces vomiting in two ways: local activation of peripheral sensory receptors in the gastrointestinal tract, and central stimulation of the chemoreceptor trigger zone that serves as a sensory area with subsequent activation of the central vomiting center.[40] Recent evidence suggests that $5HT_3$ receptors mediate the nausea and vomiting produced by syrup of ipecac. This was demonstrated when a specific $5HT_3$ antagonist given 30 minutes prior to syrup of ipecac in 40 volunteers prevented or attenuated the nausea and vomiting in a dose-dependent fashion.[13]

In one of the earliest studies evaluating the delay in onset between administration of syrup of ipecac and vomiting, 214 children were given 20 mL of syrup of ipecac and copious amounts of water.[35] Eighty-eight percent of the children vomited within 30 minutes or less, with a mean of 18.7 minutes.[35] Toxicity secondary to syrup of ipecac was not noted. Subsequent studies demonstrate similar findings.[3,8,9,11,15,21,23,41,43]

The onset of emesis does not appear to be affected by fluid administration before or after the administration of syrup of ipecac, by the temperature of the fluids, or by gentle patient motion or walking.[11,12,15,39] Therefore it is not advisable to force fluids. Similarly, milk should not be given with the syrup of ipecac, as the onset of emesis may be delayed, although the actual incidence of vomiting does not appear to be affected.[12] Because the peripheral emetic sensory receptors are located in the proximal small intestine, this delay is consistent with milk's ability to delay gastric emptying.[45] Although traditionally it was thought that activated charcoal inhibited the effectiveness of syrup of ipecac, a study in overdose patients suggests that when activated charcoal is given 10 minutes after syrup of ipecac, vomiting still occurs in the majority of cases, probably because the syrup of ipecac is absorbed so quickly.[14]

The number of episodes of vomiting averages about three, with a range of one to eight.[21] The duration of syrup of ipecac-induced vomiting is reported to average 23 to 60 minutes in the United States,[21,33] although investigators in Finland report longer times (3 to 4 hours).[29] In spite of these data it is probably reasonable to assume that persistent vomiting for more than 2 hours is unrelated to syrup of ipecac and another cause should be sought. This warning is of particular importance when syrup of ipecac is used in the home.

Many studies assessed the effectiveness of syrup of ipecac-induced emesis in decreasing absorption of an ingestion, and compared this to other methods of gastric decontamination, such as gastric lavage or activated charcoal.[29,30,36] There appears to be a wide range of results, largely due to differences in study design, including time to administration of the various techniques and the particular substance or marker used to assess efficacy. Older studies using small lavage tubes and volunteers were further limited due to the quantity of drug that was administered and recovered.

Numerous studies support the concept that the sooner syrup of ipecac is administered after an ingestion, the greater the amount of the ingested substance that will be recovered. In a small, well-quantified study, when 6 adult volunteers were given 20 mL of syrup of ipecac at 5 or 30 minutes after acetaminophen ingestion, absorption was inhibited by 65 and 0%, respectively.[31] In this same volunteer model, absorption was inhibited by 80 and 40% when 50 g of activated charcoal was given at 5 and 30 minutes post ingestion.[31]

A subsequent investigation demonstrated that reduction in the area under the concentration–time curve was equivalent for patients treated with syrup of ipecac-induced emesis and patients treated with activated charcoal plus a cathartic in patients who ingested 40 mg/kg of acetaminophen 60 minutes prior to treatment administration.[26] Comparison of orogastric lavage, syrup of ipecac-induced emesis, and activated charcoal, all given at 60 minutes after ingestion of ampicillin in adult volunteers, showed reductions of 32, 38, and 57%, respectively.[43] Adult volunteers given syrup of ipecac 5 minutes after 30 capsules containing a radionucleotide marker demonstrated a mean 54% removal (range, 21 to 89%) compared to a mean removal of 35.5% (range, 1 to 71%) with orogastric lavage.[48] Other researchers demonstrated recoveries from 0 to 85%.[3,9,10,41] In a study of 13 children given a magnesium hydroxide marker before syrup of ipecac, mean recovery was 28%, but the range was 0 to 78%.[9]

In a study of self-poisoned adults randomized to receive either syrup of ipecac or orogastric lavage with a 33 French lavage tube, all patients had subsequent endoscopy.[37] Thirteen patients were given syrup of ipecac and vomited within 23 minutes (range, 11 to 25 min). Two of these patients had tablets in the vomitus. Upon endoscopy only those 2 patients with tablets in the vomitus had residual tablets in the stomach. Ten of 17 patients who were lavaged had tablets in the lavage fluid. These 10 patients all had tablets in the stomach at the time of endoscopy. Two additional patients also had residual tablets in the stomach. This study suggests that the presence of tablets in the vomitus or lavage fluid supports the presence of additional tablets in the stomach.[37]

This same group of investigators went on to use barium-marked 3-mm^3 pellets to evaluate the effectiveness of gastric emptying.[38] Forty self-poisoned patients were given 20 pellets on admission and randomized immediately to therapy with either orogastric lavage or syrup of ipecac-induced emesis. About 50% of the pellets were removed in both the orogastric lavage and the syrup of ipecac groups. Two patients in the lavage group and one in the syrup of ipecac group had 100% removal of pellets, and 2 patients in the lavage group had no removal.[38]

A large study was designed to address the issue of whether gastric emptying with either syrup of ipecac or orogastric lavage followed by activated charcoal was more effective than activated charcoal alone in overdosed emergency department (ED) patients.[20] Syrup of ipecac did not affect the outcome of patients who arrived in the ED awake and alert.

Three subsequent studies (two adult and one pediatric) have failed to show a benefit for patients who have gastric emptying before activated charcoal[2,28] compared to those who have activated charcoal alone.[18] Furthermore, aspiration was more common in patients who had the combined regimen.[2,28]

Logically, the sooner that syrup of ipecac is administered after an ingestion, the more effective it might be in reducing absorption of the agent. For this reason syrup of ipecac should retain its role in toxicologic management in the home setting.[4] Activated charcoal has a role in the home setting as well, and the increased availability of more appealing products will increase its utility. Syrup of ipecac has lost favor in the ED for the care of adults because the sickest patients are lavaged and given activated charcoal while others receive activated charcoal alone. Administration of syrup of ipecac to children in the ED setting delays time to activated charcoal administration by 100 minutes (2.6 versus 0.9 hours),[18] and therefore is rarely recommended. Although syrup of ipecac may still be useful for toxins not adsorbed to activated charcoal, whole-bowel irrigation is generally preferred.

Syrup of ipecac should *not* be administered to patients who have ingested acids or alkalis, are younger than 6 months of age, are expected to deteriorate rapidly, have a depressed mental status, have a compromised gag reflex, have ingested objects such as batteries or sharps, or have a need for rapid gastrointestinal evacuation to prevent absorption. It should *not* be administered to those in whom the hazard of vomiting and aspiration of the ingested substance outweighs the risk associated with systemic absorption (eg, hydrocarbons), those who have significant prior vomiting or when vomiting will delay administration of an oral antidote, those with hemorrhagic diathesis, or to patients with nontoxic ingestions.

Considering the number of times syrup of ipecac has been administered without incident in this country, it must be considered a relatively safe drug when given in therapeutic doses and when no contraindications exist. Uncommon problems that have occurred after therapeutic doses include a Mallory-Weiss esophageal tear in an adult given 30 mL of syrup of ipecac for a multidrug overdose[42]; herniation of the stomach into the left chest in a child who had a previously unrecognized underlying congenital defect of the diaphragm[34]; and intracerebral hemorrhage[17] and pneumomediastinum.[46] Additional problems include aspiration of stomach contents, aspiration of a volatile hydrocarbon or foreign body, and time delay occurring before it is possible to perform a necessary therapeutic intervention (activated charcoal) or administer an antidote (*N*-acetylcysteine). Another reported problem is the emesis-induced vagal response of bradycardia.[27]

Administration of very large doses of ipecac, such as by giving the fluid extract of ipecac (no longer available), which was 14 times more potent than syrup of ipecac; or repeated and frequent doses of syrup of ipecac (as in patients with anorexia and bulemia), has resulted in substantial morbidity including congestive cardiomyopathy and mortality.[1,5,22,24,32,38,47] When emetine was used for the treatment of amebiasis in the early 1900s, cardiovascular and neuromuscular toxicity ensued. Similarly, inadvertent administration of the fluid extract of ipecac has produced violent and protracted vomiting; diarrhea; seizures; cardiac toxicity (PR prolongation, T-wave abnormalities, QRS abnormalities, atrial dysrhythmias and premature ventricular beats, and ventricular fibrillation); neuromuscular toxicity (weakness and neuropathy); shock; and death.[22]

Surreptitious chronic intentional ipecac poisoning of children (Münchausen's syndrome by proxy) is reported.[6,25] The findings in these children included vomiting, diarrhea, lethargy, irritability, hypothermia, and hypotonia. These children were referred by their parents for atypical patterns of vomiting and had multiple unsuccessful clinical evaluations. When surreptitious use of ipecac is suspected as the cause of chronic vomiting, screening the urine and vomitus for emetine (thin-layer chromatography screen—Toxi-Lab) may be useful.[25] Chronic and prolonged use of syrup of ipecac in patients with eating disorders also results in cardiac and neuromuscular toxicity as well as fatalities.[5,16,24,32,38]

The dose of syrup of ipecac is 15 mL in children 1 to 12 years old and 30 mL in older children and adults. If vomiting does not ensue after the first dose, the same dose may be repeated once in 20 to 30 minutes. For children 6 to 12 months of age, some researchers recommend limitation to a single dose of 10 mL.[7,19] Water can be offered, but is not essential for success. Vomiting will occur in most patients. Home users should be warned that persistent vomiting for more than 2 hours may indicate toxicity from the primary substances ingested and not the antidote, and will necessitate medical evaluation.

Parents should still be encouraged to keep syrup of ipecac at home as a potential first aid measure, but they should be cautioned to use it only on the advice of their regional poison center or physician. In fact, there are very few cases in which syrup of ipecac is indicated and recommended in the home setting because either the ingestion is nontoxic or of such consequence that an imminent deterioration in mental status would be expected to contraindicate its administration. Activated charcoal appears to be gaining acceptance as the first and sometimes only gastric decontamination procedure in the ED, whereas the role of syrup of ipecac is becoming extremely limited. The data seem adequate to consider administering syrup of ipecac to a child who arrives in the ED shortly after the ingestion of a large number of poorly soluble tablets of a size unlikely to be removed by lavage, as well as for the patient who has taken such a large amount of a highly toxic substance that a favorable activated-charcoal-to-drug ratio cannot be attained with certainty. Whole-bowel irrigation is probably a suitable alternative in either case.

References

1. Adler AG, Walinsky P, Krall RA, Cho SY: Death resulting from ipecac syrup poisoning. JAMA 1980;243:1927–1928.
2. Albertson TE, Derlet RW, Foulke GE, et al: Superiority of activated charcoal alone compared with ipecac and activated charcoal in the treatment of acute toxic ingestions. Ann Emerg Med 1989;18:56–59.
3. Auerbach P, Osterloh J, Braun O, et al: Efficacy of gastric emptying: Gastric lavage versus emesis induced with ipecac. Ann Emerg Med 1986;15:692–698.
4. Banner W, Veltri J: The case of ipecac syrup. Am J Dis Child 1988;142:596. Editorial.
5. Bennett H, Spiro A, Pollack M, et al: Ipecac-induced myopathy simulating dermatomyositis. Neurology 1982;32: 91–94.
6. Berkner P, Kaster T, Skolnick L: Chronic ipecac poisoning in infancy: A case report. Pediatrics 1988;82:384–386.
7. Boehnert M, Lewander W, Gaudreault P, et al: Advances in clinical toxicology. Pediatr Clin North Am 1985;32:193–211.
8. Boxer L, Anderson F, Rowe D: Comparison of ipecac-induced emesis with gastric lavage in the treatment of acute salicylate ingestion. J Pediatr 1969;74:800–803.
9. Corby D, Decker W, Moran M, et al: Clinical comparison of pharmacologic emetics in children. Pediatrics 1968;42: 361–364.
10. Curtis R, Barone J, Giacona N: Efficacy of ipecac and activated charcoal and cathartic: Prevention of salicylate absorption in a simulated overdose. Arch Intern Med 1984; 144:48–52.
11. Dean B, Krenzelok E: Syrup of ipecac: 15 mL versus 30 mL in pediatric poisonings. J Toxicol Clin Toxicol 1985;23: 165–170.
12. Eisenga B, Meester W: Evaluation of the effect of motility on syrup of ipecac-induced emesis. Vet Hum Toxicol 1978; 20:462. Abstract.
13. Forster ER, Palmer JL, Bedding AW, et al: Syrup of ipecacuanha-induced nausea and emesis is medicated by $5HT_3$ receptors in man. J Physiol 1994;477:72.
14. Freedman G, Pasternak S, Krenzelok E: A clinical trial using syrup of ipecac and activated charcoal concurrently. Ann Emer Med 1987;16:164–166.
15. Grande G, Ling L: The effect of fluid volume on syrup of ipecac emesis time. J Toxicol Clin Toxicol 1987;25:473–481.
16. Isner JM: Effects of ipecac on the heart. N Engl J Med 1986; 314:1253.
17. Klein-Schwartz W, Gorman R, Oderda G, et al: Ipecac use in the elderly: The unanswered question. Ann Emerg Med 1984;13:1152–1154.
18. Kornberg AE, Dolgen J: Pediatric ingestions: Charcoal alone versus ipecac and charcoal. Ann Emerg Med 1991;20: 648–651.
19. Krenzelok K, Dean B: Syrup of ipecac in children less than one year of age. J Toxicol Clin Toxicol 1985;23:171–176.
20. Kulig K, Bar-Or D, Cantrill SV, et al: Management of acutely poisoned patients without gastric emptying. Ann Emerg Med 1985;14:562–567.
21. MacLean W: A comparison of ipecac syrup and apomorphine in the immediate treatment of ingestion of poisons. J Pediatr 1973;82:121–124.
22. Manno B, Manno J: Toxicology of ipecac. Clin Toxicol 1977; 10:221–242.
23. Manoguerra A, Krenzelok E: Rapid emesis from high dose ipecac syrup in adults and children intoxicated with antiemetics and other drugs. Am J Hosp Pharm 1978;35: 1360–1362.
24. Mateer J, Farrell B, Chou SM, Gutman, L: Reversible ipecac myopathy. Arch Neurol 1985;42:188–190.
25. McClung H, Murray R, Braden N, et al: Intentional ipecac poisoning in children. Am J Dis Child 1988;142:637–639.
26. McNamara R, Aaron C, Gemborys M, Davidheiser S: Efficacy of charcoal versus ipecac in reducing serum acetaminophen in a simulated overdose. Ann Emerg Med 1988; 17:243–246.
27. Meester W: Emesis and lavage. Vet Hum Toxicol 1981;22: 225–234.

28. Merigian KS, Woodard M, Hedges JR, et al: Prospective evaluation of gastric emptying in the self poisoned patient. Am J Emerg Med 1990;8:479–483.
29. Neuvonen P: Clinical pharmacokinetics of oral activated charcoal in acute intoxications. Clin Pharmacokinet 1982;7: 465–489.
30. Neuvonen P, Olkkola K: Activated charcoal and syrup of ipecac in the prevention of cimetidine and pindolol absorption in man after administration of metoclopramide as an antiemetic. J Toxicol Clin Toxicol 1984;22:103–114.
31. Neuvonen P, Vartiainen M, Tokola O: Comparison of activated charcoal and ipecac syrup in prevention of drug absorption. Eur J Clin Pharmacol 1983;24:557–562.
32. Palmer E, Guay A: Reversible myopathy secondary to abuse of ipecac in patients with major eating disorders. N Engl J Med 1985;313:1457–1459.
33. Rauber A, Maroncelli R: The duration of emetic effect of ipecac; duration and frequency of vomiting. Vet Hum Toxicol 1982;24:281. Abstract.
34. Robertson WO: Syrup of ipecac associated fatality: A case report. Vet Hum Toxicol 1979;21:87–89.
35. Robertson WO: Syrup of ipecac: A slow or fast emetic? Am J Dis Child 1962;103:136–139.
36. Saetta JP, March S, Gaunt ME, Quinton DN: Gastric emptying procedures in the self poisoned patient: Are we forcing gastric content beyond the pylorus? J R Soc Med 1991;84: 274–277.
37. Saetta JP, Quinton DN: Residual gastric content after gastric lavage and ipecacuanha induced emesis in self poisoned patients: An endoscopic study. J R Soc Med 1991;84:35–38.
38. Schiff R, Wurzel C, Brunson S, et al: Death due to chronic syrup of ipecac use in a patient with bulimia. Pediatrics 1986;78:412–416.
39. Spiegel R, Addouch I, Munn D: The effect of temperature on concurrently administered fluid on the onset of ipecac-induced emesis. Clin Toxicol 1979;14:281–284.
40. Stewart J: Effects of emetic and cathartic agents on the gastrointestinal tract and the treatment of toxic ingestion. J Toxicol Clin Toxicol 1983;20:199–253.
41. Tandberg D, Diven B, McLeod J: Ipecac-induced emesis versus gastric lavage: A controlled study in normal adults. Am J Emerg Med 1986;4:205–209.
42. Tandberg D, Liechty E, Fishbein D: Mallory-Weiss syndrome: An unusual complication of ipecac-induced emesis. Ann Emerg Med 1981;10:521–523.
43. Tenenbein M, Cohen, Sitar D: Efficacy of ipecac-induced emesis, orogastric lavage, and activated charcoal for acute drug overdose. Ann Emerg Med 1987;16:838–841.
44. United States Pharmacopeia 21 and National Formulary 16: Suppl 2. Rockville, MD, U.S. Pharmacopeial convention, 1985.
45. Varipapa RJ, Oderda GM: Effect of milk on ipecac-induced emesis. J Am Pharm Assoc 1977;17:510.
46. Wolowoduik O, McMicken D, O'Brien P: Pneumomediastinum and pneumoretroperitoneum: An unusual complication of syrup of ipecac induced emesis. Ann Emerg Med 1984;13:1148–1151.
47. Woolf AD, Grew JM: Acute poisonings among adolescents and young adults with anorexia nervosa. AJDC 1990;144: 785–788.
48. Young WF, Bruin SMG: Evaluation of gastric emptying using radionucleotides: Gastric lavage versus ipecac-induced emesis. Ann Emerg Med 1993;22:1423–1427.

ANTIDOTES IN DEPTH

Activated Charcoal

Mary Ann Howland

Activated charcoal, a fine, black, odorless powder has been recognized for almost two centuries as an effective adsorbent of many substances. It was initially observed that colored fluids were decolorized by charcoal.[5] In 1930, the French pharmacist Touery dramatically demonstrated his belief in the powerful adsorbent qualities of activated charcoal by ingesting several times the lethal dose of strychnine mixed with 15 g of activated charcoal in front of colleagues. He suffered no ill effects.[5] An American physician, Holt, first used activated charcoal to save a patient from mercury bichloride poisoning in 1934.[5] It was not until 1940s that Anderson performed research on activated charcoal's adsorbency.[3–5] Today, although more in vitro and in vivo studies are needed, the available evidence clearly supports the use of activated charcoal as an excellent broad-spectrum gastrointestinal adsorbent.

Activated charcoal is produced in a two-step process beginning with the pyrolysis of various carbonaceous materials such as wood, coconut, or peat followed by treatment at high temperatures with a variety of activating (oxidizing) agents such as steam or carbon dioxide to increase the agent's adsorptive capacity through the formation of an internal maze of pores with a huge surface area.[47,94,117] The rate of adsorption depends on external surface area, while the adsorptive capacity is dependent on the far larger internal surface area.[21,84,92] The actual adsorption is believed to rely on hydrogen bonding, ion–ion, dipole, and van der Waals' forces. This suggests that most drugs will be best adsorbed in their dissolved, nonionized form. Therefore strongly ionized and dissociated salts like sodium chloride are not adsorbed, while iodine and mercuric chloride are well adsorbed. Nonpolar, poorly water soluble organic substances are more likely to be adsorbed, and adsorption is enhanced with an increase in size in comparison to small, polar, water-soluble organic substances. Among the organic molecules, aromatics are better adsorbed than aliphatics, branched chains better than straight chains, and the presence of nitro groups rather than hydroxyl, amino, or sulfonic groups also proves advantageous.[21] In vitro studies demonstrate that adsorption begins within about 1 minute of administration, but may not reach equilibrium for about 10 to 25 minutes.[22,81]

Activated charcoal decreases the systemic absorption of a number of drugs, including aspirin, acetaminophen, barbiturates, glutethimide, phenytoin, theophylline, cyclic antidepressants, and most inorganic and organic materials.[36,81,96] Notable exceptions are the alcohols, strong acids and alkalies, iron, and lithium. Efficacy of activated charcoal is inversely related to the time elapsed following ingestion and directly related to the amount of activated charcoal administered. The effect of the activated charcoal-to-drug ratio in vitro and in vivo was demonstrated with para-aminosalicylate (PAS). In vitro the fraction of unadsorbed PAS decreased from 55 to 3% as the activated charcoal-to-PAS ratio increased from 1:1 to 10:1 at pH 1.2.[91] In human volunteers, as the activated charcoal-to-PAS ratio increased from 2.5:1 to 50:1, the total 48-hour urinary excretion decreased from 37 to 4%.[92] These studies demonstrate activated charcoal saturation at low ratios of activated charcoal to drug.

It is clear that the sooner activated charcoal is administered after an ingestion, the more efficacious the intervention. The effect of timing depends largely on the rate of absorption of the drug. Therefore, early administration is even more important with rapidly absorbed drugs. The rate of absorption of a drug depends on many factors. In general, lipid solubility and rapid passage into the intestine speeds absorption and sustained release dosage forms and anticholinergic drugs slow absorption, as may the presence of food.[93] However, the presence of food also decreases the adsorptive capacity of activated charcoal.[3,64]

Drugs are best adsorbed to activated charcoal in their undissociated form. According to the Henderson-Hasselbalch equation, weak bases are best adsorbed at basic pHs and weak acids are best adsorbed at acid pHs. For example, cocaine, a weak base, binds to activated charcoal with a maximum adsorptive capacity of 273 mg of cocaine per gram of activated charcoal at pH 7.00; this capacity is reduced to 212 mg of cocaine per gram of activated charcoal at pH 1.20.[68]

The adsorption of weakly dissociated metallic salts to activated charcoal decreases with decreasing pH because the number of complex ions increases.[4] Accordingly, desorption may occur, especially for weak acids, as the charcoal–drug complex passes from the stomach through the intestine and the pH changes from acidic to basic.[8,37,87,92,115] Desorption may lead to systemic absorption of larger total amounts of drug over several days; in this case, the elimination half-life of the drug appears to increase, but peak levels remain unaffected.[87] Desorption can be minimized by giving a large enough dose of activated charcoal to overcome the decreased affinity of the drug secondary to pH change and by utilizing multiple-dose activated charcoal. An ionic cathartic or sorbitol should reduce gastrointestinal transit time and possibly increase drug elimination. In spite of numerous human volunteer studies[75,85,97,109] this has only been demonstrated in a single study.[53] The importance of these negative results remains in question, as the overdose setting may not be clinically comparable to these study settings.

Although ethanol is minimally adsorbed by activated charcoal, theoretically it and other solvents may decrease the adsorptive capacity of activated charcoal for a given drug by competing for binding with that drug.[87,92]

Activated charcoal is best administered as a water slurry. It may be used following vomiting induced by syrup of ipecac, shortly after ipecac administration but prior to vomiting (reports suggest 50 to 100% incidence of vomiting),[39] following orogastric lavage, or more commonly today as the sole intervention in patients where removal of gastric contents is deemed unnecessary or contraindicated for any reason.

The use of activated charcoal is relatively safe. Vomiting (especially after rapid administration), constipation, and diarrhea are all noted,[84] but constipation and diarrhea probably result from the ingestion rather than the activated charcoal. Serious adverse effects include lethal complications that may result from the simultaneous aspiration of activated charcoal alone or with gastric contents,[6,34,41,44,45,50,76,81,98,108] peritonitis from spillage of activated charcoal in the peritoneum subsequent to perforation following orogastric lavage,[70] and intestinal obstruction and pseudo-obstruction, especially following repeated doses of activated charcoal in the presence of dehydration[12,66,78,103,120] and prior bowel adhesions.[42]

The black and gritty nature of activated charcoal has led to many proposed formulations to increase palatability and patient acceptance. Bentonite, carboxymethyl cellulose, and starch[43,80,107] have been used as thickening agents; and cherry syrup, chocolate syrup, sorbitol, sucrose, saccharin, ice cream, and sherbet[24,63,69,122] have been used as flavoring agents. The thickening agents do not appear to decrease the antidotal efficacy of activated charcoal if the mixtures are fluidlike rather than gelatinous in consistency.[23,71] In fact, a 20% activated charcoal slurry prepared with 70% sorbitol was shown to be more effective than activated charcoal alone.[97] Ice cream and sherbet decreased the activated charcoal's adsorptive capacity in one study,[63] but contradictory results were reported for chocolate syrup.[43,80] The other flavoring agents were free of adverse effects on activated charcoal's adsorptive property. However, improvement in palatability and acceptance was minimal or nonexistent with all of these formulations. A milk chocolate formulation evaluated by a group of children was rated superior in palatability compared to standard activated charcoal preparations,[32] but never marketed.

The acceptance by 50 young children of a dose of activated charcoal given as a water slurry in a paper cup was studied.[14] The children were told to drink the contents, that the substance did not taste bad, and that it would make them feel better and not sick. Eighty-six percent of the children readily accepted the activated charcoal slurry to drink, and 76% of them consumed 95 to 100% of the dose administered.

Other attempts were not as successful. Difficulty was noted in the administration of the standard activated charcoal in 70% of children in the home setting.[30] Similarly, in an emergency department setting, only 30% of children drank the activated charcoal, the remainder required placement of a nasogastric tube.[57]

Adult human volunteers rated a recently newly marketed activated charcoal product with cherry flavoring as preferrable over plain activated charcoal and ingested a statistically significant larger quantity.[20] This novel formulation that calls for the instillation of a very small quantity of cherry flavoring to the straw immediately prior to ingestion, accomplished improved acceptance without loss of adsorptive capacity.[20]

Activated charcoal is supplied as powder in a container to which sufficient water is added to make it watery in consistency (8:1 water-to-charcoal ratio), or it is supplied premixed with water or sorbitol. There are many activated charcoal products available commercially. They differ in source of activated charcoal, amount per container, surface area of the activated charcoal used, presence or absence of sorbitol, and cost. Products used outside the United States may contain other additives, such as sodium bicarbonate.[105] Activated charcoal surface area as it relates to adsorption capacity was studied in vitro and in vivo in animals and in humans. In vitro studies demonstrated significant differences in maximum binding capacities (MBC) and binding affinities. The enhanced MBC of the petroleum-based activated charcoals results from their physical structure, which has been described as a nearly random array of graphite sheets with micropores. When surface area is large, capacity is increased, but affinity is decreased because van der Waals' forces and hydrophobic forces are lessened.[119] The net result in most studies is that activated charcoals with the largest surface area can decrease the absorption of drugs about 2.5 to 3 times that of standard activated charcoals.[25–27,58,119] Superactivated charcoals, which are petroleum-based and have the largest surface areas (approximating 3150 m^2/g), have the greatest maximum binding capacity; binding affinities show an inverse relationship with maximum binding capacity.[119] All of the superactivated charcoal preparations once available in the United States were removed from the market because they contained undesirable impurities. In 1996 a new superactivated charcoal was marketed with a surface area approximately double the current formulations. Both in vitro and in vivo studies indicate a greater MBC.[22,106]

Most of the evidence suggests that activated charcoal plus a single dose of cathartic (sorbitol or magnesium citrate) is about as effective as activated charcoal alone.[2,53,71,72,75,80,84,95] There may, however, be some benefit in combining multiple-dose activated charcoal with whole-bowel irrigation in overdoses with delayed or sustained-release drugs. Repeated doses of cathartics are not recommended due to reports of hypermagnesemia associated with repetitive doses of magnesium-containing cathartics[79,111] as well as severe fluid and electrolyte problems and several deaths related to repeated doses of sorbitol.[35] Whole-bowel irrigation with a nonabsorbable polyethylene glycol electrolyte lavage solution (PEG-ELS) alone or in combination with activated charcoal is not associated with morbidity, and further study may indicate that it is the preferred technique in certain circumstances.

PEG-ELS significantly decreases the in vitro adsorptive capacity of activated charcoal; this effect is most pronounced when the two are premixed (in vitro) together.[46] This capacity is pH dependent and more pronounced at pH 1.20 than pH 7.00.[68] The osmolar characteristics of PEG-ELS do not appear to be affected by the admixture.[55]

The standard treatment of an acetaminophen overdose includes gastric decontamination (in an acute recent ingestion) and *N*-acetylcysteine (NAC). The role of activated charcoal for this ingestion has been questioned due to the concern that it may adsorb substantial quantities of the administered NAC. Two in vitro studies presented evidence that a significant amount of NAC is adsorbed by activated charcoal.[17,56] Subsequent in vitro data suggest that NAC has a limited inhibitory effect on activated charcoal's adsorption of acetaminophen, and that NAC itself is not appreciably adsorbed by activated charcoal.[119] Data from two in vivo studies involving small numbers of healthy volunteers reveal no significant differences in plasma NAC levels when 50- and 60-g doses of activated charcoal were administered immediately prior to, or following, NAC.[89,104] Another study, involving 19 healthy volunteers, compared peak and total absorption of NAC following a loading dose given alone and the same loading dose given with 100 g of activated charcoal. A significant decrease in peak levels and a 40% reduction in total absorption of NAC were demonstrated.[33] When a near double dose of NAC was administered in a subsequent study with activated charcoal, good bioavailability was demonstrated.[16]

The critical issue, which has not been effectively addressed in any study to date, is the minimum amount of NAC necessary to prevent acetaminophen-induced liver damage. Measuring NAC plasma levels is probably not a true representation of AC's ultimate effect on efficacy, since NAC itself is rapidly metabolized due to first-pass metabolism and it is conceivably the NAC metabolites that are not measured that contribute to clinical efficacy.[121] Ultimately, outcome studies are more telling. A multicenter study on the efficacy of NAC suggests that the amount of NAC currently administered far exceeds the amount needed to treat mild to moderate acetaminophen overdoses.[110] A study of 100 patients with acetaminophen (APAP) overdoses from 3 regional poison centers treated with NAC, AC before NAC, or AC before increased NAC, could detect no differences in AST concentrations and concluded that AC before NAC had no significant detrimental effect. Activated charcoal administered within 4 hours of APAP ingestion may decrease absorption sufficiently to transform a potentially toxic acetaminophen ingestion into a nontoxic one.[54,116]

Considering all of the available information, activated charcoal should be administered to all adolescent and adult patients who attempt suicide with APAP, whether indicated for the acetaminophen or for a concurrent ingestion. The dose of NAC administered should be adequate to treat all except the rarest case, of an acetaminophen ingestion so large that it results in an altered mental status and metabolic acidosis (see Chap. 31).[38,65] Although no studies support this hypothesis, an increase in the first and second oral doses of NAC should be considered only in these rare cases.

Multiple-Dose Activated Charcoal

Oral multiple-dose activated charcoal enhanced the total body clearance (nonrenal clearance) of 6 healthy volunteers given 2.85 mg/kg of IV phenobarbital.[9] The serum half-life of phenobarbital decreased from 110 ± 8 to 45 ± 6 hours. An editorial on this study proposed that activated charcoal enhanced the diffusion of phenobarbital from the blood into the gastrointestinal tract and trapped it there, to be excreted later in the stool. In this manner, activated charcoal performs as an "infinite sink" and allows "gastrointestinal dialysis" to take place.[62] This has been confirmed by studies in dogs and rats using IV aminophylline.[29,73] The later study used an elegant isolated vascularly perfused rat small intestine to demonstrate this concept of gastrointestinal dialysis.[73] Activated charcoal dramatically affected the pharmacokinetics of theophylline, producing a constant intestinal clearance that was approximately equivalent to intestinal blood flow. Multiple-dose activated charcoal has been reported to increase the elimination of digitoxin,[99] phenobarbital,[101] carbamazepine,[11] phenylbutazone,[82] dapsone,[83] methotrexate,[40] nadolol,[31] theophylline,[10,67,114] salicylate,[102] cyclosporine,[48] propoxyphene,[52] nortriptyline, and amitriptyline.[51,112] Extensive lists of adsorptive capacities are available.[15,18,21,74]

An analysis of 28 volunteer studies involving 17 drugs was unable to correlate an individual drug's physiochemical properties with the ability of multiple-dose activated charcoal to decrease the drug's plasma half-life.[15] The half-life was not thought to be the best marker of enhanced elimination, but it was the only variable consistently mentioned in all of the studies with their substantially different designs. The drugs with the longest intrinsic plasma half-lives seemed to demonstrate the largest percent reduction in plasma half-life when multiple-dose activated charcoal was utilized. A study utilizing therapeutic doses of four simultaneously administered intravenous drugs in pigs offered clarification of the role that the pharmacokinetics of a drug plays on the effectiveness of activated charcoal.[19] The four drugs utilized were acetaminophen, digoxin, theophylline, and valproic acid. Theophylline, acetaminophen, and valproic acid all have small volumes of distribution. Only valproic acid is highly protein bound at the doses employed, and probably accounted for the inability of activated charcoal to increase its clearance. The three other drugs all responded to MDAC with an increased clearance. Theophylline showed the most dramatic effect, occuring very quickly. Although digoxin has a large volume of distribution, it takes several hours to distribute from the blood to the tissues. MDAC is beneficial before distribution is complete, while the digoxin is still accessible in the blood compartment.

It appears likely that the benefits of multiple-dose activated charcoal depend on a number of patient variables and drug factors. Most importantly, volunteer studies do not accurately reflect the overdose situation[74] in which saturation of plasma protein binding, saturation of liver enzymes, and acid–base disturbances may make more free drug available for an enteroenteric effect.

Multiple-dose activated charcoal may be beneficial to decrease drug absorption when large amounts of drugs are ingested and dissolution is delayed (masses, bezoars), when drugs exhibit a delayed or prolonged release phase (enteric coated, sustained release), or when reabsorption can be prevented (enterohepatic circulation of active drug, active metabolites or conjugated drug hydrolyzed by gut bacteria to active drug). Once drug absorption is complete, multiple-dose activated charcoal is most useful when free drug in the plasma is substantial enough to permit an enteroenteric effect. For this effect to be of clinical importance the drug or metabolite must possess a lengthy elimination phase, as multiple-dose activated charcoal is given every 2 to 6 hours. Drugs with a small volume of distribution and low or saturable plasma protein binding are theoretically most accessible.

Multiple-dose activated charcoal appears to enhance gastrointestinal elimination of many drugs by interfering with enteroenteric circulation, interrupting enterohepatic circulation, and/or minimizing desorption. It is believed that shortening the drug's half-life in overdose benefits the patient clinically by limiting the time of associated CNS depression, risk of aspiration, intensive care, nursing hours, and hospitalization. In a randomized clinical study of this potential benefit, some patients who overdosed with phenobarbital were given a single dose of activated charcoal and some were given multiple doses.[101] Although the half-life of phenobarbital was significantly decreased in the multiple-dose group (36 versus 93 hours), the length of time that each group required intubation did not differ. This study has been criticized as being too small, having unevenly matched groups, and focusing on a single endpoint (extubation) that may be dependent on factors other than the patient condition, such as the time of day to determine potential clinical benefit.

The hazards of multiple-dose activated charcoal include diarrhea (only when sorbitol-containing charcoal preparations are used), constipation, vomiting with a subsequent risk of aspiration, intestinal obstruction, and reduction of serum concentrations of therapeutically employed drugs.[78,81,98]

To prevent aspiration pneumonitis, it is imperative that the patient's airway be protected if necessary. Gastrointestinal motility should be assured by the presence of bowel sounds and lack of abdominal distention. The stomach should be decompressed to decrease the risk of subsequent vomiting and aspiration, if bowel function is lost.

An initial loading dose of activated charcoal in an activated charcoal-to-drug ratio of 10:1 or 1 to 2 g/kg of body weight (if drug dose is unknown) should be administered (to both children and adults). The correct dose of activated charcoal for multiple dosing, when it is indicated, is best tailored to the dose and dosage form of the drug ingested, seriousness of the overdose, potential lethality of the ingestant, and patient's ability to tolerate activated charcoal. Benefit should always be weighed against risk. Doses of activated charcoal for multiple dosing have varied considerably, from 0.25 to 0.5 g/kg every 1 to 6 hours, to 20 to 60 g for adults every 1, 2, 4, or 6 hours. The total dose administered may be more important than frequency of administration.[49,118] In some cases, continuous nasogastric administration of activated charcoal can be employed, especially when vomiting is a problem.[37,90,118]

Activated Charcoal Versus Other Methods of Gastrointestinal Decontamination

The best overall method of gastric decontamination remains a controversial topic. Experimental studies using toxic doses of drugs in animals and therapeutic doses of drugs in volunteers have attempted to address the merits of syrup of ipecac, orogastric lavage, and activated charcoal singly and in a variety of combinations.[7,13,28,86,88,101,113] Due to differences in timing, size of lavage tube, and doses of activated charcoal, these studies are not directly comparable. However, most studies suggest that activated charcoal is at least as effective as syrup of ipecac-induced emesis or lavage and often better, due to the potential for the immediate benefit of activated charcoal. All of these studies involved drugs adsorbable by activated charcoal in the presence of high activated charcoal-to-drug ratios.

The first outcome study that attempted to show whether gastric emptying with syrup of ipecac or orogastric lavage followed by activated charcoal is more effective than activated charcoal alone in overdose found no differences between the two, except when patients arrived within 60 minutes of ingestion and were obtunded.[59] In this case, orogastric lavage was found to lead to a more satisfactory clinical outcome. Three subsequent studies showed no benefit from gastric emptying before activated charcoal administration, and two of them demonstrated a higher incidence of aspiration when gastric emptying was performed first.[1,77,100]

Most critical data suggest that activated charcoal should be the first intervention given to overdosed patients. Patients initially or subsequentially can have an orogastric tube placed for suction of gastric contents if very large amounts of a drug have been ingested and if the time since ingestion has been relatively short. Orogastric lavage may be indicated for life-threatening ingestions when a poor outcome may be expected, or if the substance ingested is not adsorbed by activated charcoal and is still expected to be in the stomach given absorption considerations.

In conclusion, activated charcoal is a very effective nonspecific adsorbent. It should be an integral part of basic poison management. Recent information reveals that oral multiple-dose activated charcoal can decrease the elimination half-lives of a variety of drugs through diverse mechanisms, including gastrointestinal dialysis, making treatment applicable even to some nonoral drug overdoses. Care must be taken to avoid pulmonary aspiration and intestinal obstruction. Home availability of activated charcoal should be encouraged, and as more palatable forms of activated charcoal are developed children may accept this agent more readily.[60,61]

References

1. Albertson TE, Derlet RW, Foulke GE, et al: Superiority of activated charcoal alone compared with ipecac and activated charcoal in the treatment of acute toxic ingestions. Ann Emerg Med 1989;18:56–59.
2. Al-Shareef AM, Buss DC, Allen EM, Routledge PA: The effects of charcoal and sorbitol (alone and in combination) on plasma theophylline concentration after a sustained release formulation. Hum Exp Toxicol 1990;9:179–182.
3. Anderson H: Experimental studies on the pharmacology of activated charcoal. Acta Pharmacol 1948;4:275–284.
4. Anderson H: Experimental studies on the pharmacology of activated charcoal. II. The effect of pH on the adsorption by charcoal from aqueous solutions. Acta Pharmacol 1947;3:199–218.
5. Anderson H: Experimental studies on the pharmacology of activated charcoal. I. Adsorption power of charcoal in aqueous solutions. Acta Pharmacol 1946;2:69–78.
6. Anderson I, Ware C: Syrup of ipecacuanha. Br Med J 1987; 294:578. Letter.
7. Auerbach PS, Osterloh J, Braun O, et al: Efficacy of gastric emptying: Gastric lavage versus emesis induced with ipecac. Ann Emerg Med 1986;15:692–698.
8. Augenstein WL, Kulig KW, Rumack BH: Delayed rise in serum drug levels in overdose patients despite multiple dose charcoal and after charcoal stools. Vet Hum Toxicol 1987;29:491. Abstract.
9. Berg M, Berlinger W, Goldberg M, et al: Acceleration of the body clearance of phenobarbital by oral activated charcoal. N Engl J Med 1982;307:642–644.
10. Berlinger WG, Spector R, Goldberg MJ, et al: Enhancement of theophylline clearance by oral activated charcoal. Clin Pharmacol Ther 1983;33:351–354.
11. Boldy DAR, Heath A, Ruddock C, et al: Activated charcoal for carbamazepine poisoning. Lancet 1987;1:1027. Letter.
12. Brubacher JR, Levine B, Hoffman RS: Intestinal pseudo-obstruction (Ogilvie's syndrome) in the theophylline overdose. Vet Hum Toxicol 1996; 38:368–370.
13. Burton BT, Bayer MJ, Barron L, Aitchison JP: Comparison of activated charcoal and gastric lavage in the prevention of aspirin absorption. J Emerg Med 1984;1:411–416.
14. Calvert W, Corby D, Herbertson L, Decker W: Orally administered activated charcoal: Acceptance by children. JAMA 1971;215:641.
15. Campbell J, Chyka P: Physiochemical characteristics of drugs and response to repeat dose activated charcoal. Am J Emerg Med 1992;10:208–210.
16. Chamberlain JM, Gorman RL, Oderda GM, et al: Use of activated charcoal in a simulated poisoning with acetaminophen: A new loading dose for *N*-acetylcysteine? Ann Emerg Med 1993;22:1398–1402.
17. Chinough R, Czajka P: *N*-acetylcysteine adsorption by activated charcoal. Vet Hum Toxicol 1980;22:392–394.
18. Chyka PA: Multiple dose activated charcoal and enhancement of systemic drug clearance: Summary of studies in animals and human volunteers. J Toxicol Clin Toxicol 1995;33:399–405.
19. Chyka PA, Holley JE, Mandrell TD, Sugathan P: Correlation of drug pharmacokinetics and effectiveness of multiple-dose activated charcoal therapy. Ann Emerg Med 1995;25:356–362.
20. Cohen V, Howland MA, Hoffman RS: Palatability of Insta-Char with cherry flavoring: A human volunteer study. J Toxicol Clin Toxicol 1996;34:635. Abstract.
21. Cooney D, ed: Activated Charcoal in Medical Applications. New York, Marcel Dekker, 1995.
22. Cooney D: In vitro adsorption of phenobarbital, chlorpheniramine maleate, and theophylline by four commercially available activated charcoal suspensions. J Toxicol Clin Toxicol 1995;33:213–217.
23. Cooney D: Effect of type and amount of carboxymethylcellulose on in vitro salicylate adsorption by activated charcoal. Clin Toxicol 1982; 19:367–376.
24. Cooney D: Palatability of sucrose-sorbitol and saccharin sweetened activated charcoal formulations. Am J Hosp Pharm 1980;37:237–239.
25. Cooney D: "Superactive" charcoal adsorbs drugs as fast as standard antidotal charcoal. Clin Toxicol 1980;16:123–125.
26. Cooney D: A "superactive" charcoal for antidotal use in poisonings. Clin Toxicol 1977;11:387–390.
27. Curd-Sneed C, Parks K, Bordelon J, et al: In vitro adsorption of sodium phenobarbital by Superchar, USP, and Darco G-60 activated charcoals. J Toxicol Clin Toxicol 1987;25:1–11.
28. Curtis RA, Barone J, Giacona N: Efficacy of ipecac and activated charcoal/cathartic: Prevention of salicylate absorption in a simulated overdose. Arch Intern Med 1984;144: 48–52.
29. DeVries MH, Rademaker C, et al: Pharmacokinetic modelling of the effect of activated charcoal on the intestinal secretion of theophylline, using the isolated vascularly perfused rat small intestine. J Pharm Pharmacol 1989;41: 528–533.
30. Docksteder LL, Lawrence RA, Bresnick HL: Home administration of activated charcoal: Feasibility and acceptance. Vet Hum Toxicol 1986;28:471. Abstract.
31. DuSoeuch P, Caille G, Larochelle P: Reduction of nadolol plasma half-life by activated charcoal and antibiotics in man. Clin Pharmacol Ther 1982;31:222. Letter.
32. Eisen TF, Grbcich PA, Lacouture PG, Woolf A: The adsorption of salicylates by a milk chocolate–charcoal mixture. Ann Emerg Med 1991;20:143–146.
33. Ekins B, Ford D, Thompson M, et al: The effect of activated charcoal on *N*-acetylcysteine absorption in normal subjects. Am J Emerg Med 1987;5:483–487.

34. Elliot CG, Colby TV, Kelly TM, et al: Charcoal lung: Bronchiolitis obliterans after aspiration of activated charcoal. Chest 1989;96:672–674.
35. Farley T: Severe hypernatremic dehydration after use of an activated charcoal-sorbitol suspension. J Pediatr 1986; 109:719–722.
36. Farrar HC, Herold DA, Reed M: Acute valproic acid intoxication enhanced drug clearance with oral activated charcoal. Crit Care Med 1993;21:299–301.
37. Fillippone G, Fish S, Lacouture P, et al: Reversible adsorption (desorption) of aspirin from activated charcoal. Arch Intern Med 1987;147:1390–1392.
38. Flanagan RJ, Mani TGK: Coma and metabolic acidosis early in severe acute paracetamol poisoning. Hum Toxicol 1986;5:179–182.
39. Freedman G, Pasternak S, Krenzelok E: A clinical trial using syrup of ipecac and activated charcoal concurrently. Ann Emerg Med 1987;16:164–166.
40. Gadgil SD, Damle SR, Advani SH, Vaidya AB: Effect of activated charcoal on the pharmacokinetics of high dose methotrexate. Cancer Treat Rep 1982;66:1169–1171.
41. Givens T, Holloway M, Watson S: Pulmonary aspiration of activated charcoal: A complication of its misuse in overdose management. Pediatr Emerg Care 1992;8:137–140.
42. Goulbourne KB, Cisek JE: Small bowel obstruction secondary to activated charcoal and adhesions. Ann Emerg Med 1994;24:108–110.
43. Gwelt P, Perrier D: Influence of thickening agents on the antidotal efficacy of activated charcoal. Clin Toxicol 1976; 9:89–92.
44. Harris CR, Filandrinos D: Accidental administration of activated charcoal into the lung: Aspiration by proxy. Ann Emerg Med 1993;22:143–146.
45. Harsch H: Aspiration of activated charcoal. N Engl J Med 1986;314:318. Letter.
46. Hoffman RS, Chiang WK, Howland MA, et al: Theophylline desorption from activated charcoal caused by whole bowel irrigation. J Toxicol Clin Toxicol 1991;29:191–202.
47. Holt E, Holz P: The black bottle. J Pediatr 1963;63:306–314.
48. Honcharik N, Anthone S: Activated charcoal in acute cyclosporin overdose. Lancet 1985;1:1051.
49. Ilkhanipour K, Yealy D, Krenzelok E: The comparative efficacy of various multiple dose activated charcoal regimens. Am J Emerg Med 1992;10:298–300.
50. Justiniani F, Hippalgaonkar R, Martinez L: Charcoal-containing empyema complicating treatment for overdose. Chest 1985;87:404–405.
51. Karkkainen S, Neuvonen P: Pharmacokinetics of amitriptyline influenced by oral charcoal and urine pH. Int J Clin Pharmacol Ther 1986;24:326–332.
52. Karkkainen S, Neuvonen PJ: Effect of oral charcoal and urine pH on dextropropoxyphene pharmacokinetics. Int J Clin Pharmacol Ther Toxicol 1985;23:219–225.
53. Keller R, Schwab R, Krenzelok E: Contribution of sorbitol combined with activated charcoal in prevention of salicylate absorption. Ann Emerg Med 1990;19:654–656.
54. Kirk MA, Peterson J, Kulig KW, et al: Acetaminophen overdose in children—A comparison of syrup of ipecac versus activated charcoal versus no gastrointestinal decontamination. Ann Emerg Med 1991;20:472–473.
55. Kirshenbaum LA, Sitar DS, Tenenbein M: Interaction between whole bowel irrigation solution and activated charcoal: Implications for the treatment of toxic ingestions. Ann Emerg Med 1990;19:1129–1132.
56. Klein-Schwartz W, Oderda G: Adsorption of oral antidotes for acetaminophen poisoning (methione and *N*-acetylcysteine) by activated charcoal. Paper presented at the National Poison Center Network annual symposium, Pittsburgh, June 1980.
57. Kornberg AE, Dolgin J: Pediatric ingestions: Charcoal alone versus ipecac and charcoal. Ann Emerg Med 1991; 20:648–651.
58. Krenzelok E, Heller M: Effectiveness of commercially available aqueous activated charcoal products. Ann Emerg Med 1987;16;1340–1343.
59. Kulig KW, Bar-Or D, Cantrill SV, et al: Management of acutely poisoned patients without gastric emptying. Ann Emerg Med 1985;14:562–567.
60. Lamminpaa A, Vilska J, Hoppu K: Medical activated charcoal for a child's poisoning at home: Availability and success of administration in Finland. Hum Exp Toxicol 1993; 12:29–32.
61. Lee RJ: Ancient antidote ignored. Activated charcoal is an underused antidote to a variety of drugs and chemicals, says this author. Am Pharm 1992;32:34–35.
62. Levy G: Gastrointestinal clearance of drugs with activated charcoal. N Engl J Med 1982;307:676–678. Editorial.
63. Levy G, Soda GM, Lampman TA: Inhibition by ice cream of the antidotal efficacy of activated charcoal. Am J Hosp Pharm 1975;32:289–291.
64. Levy G, Tsuchiya T: Effect of activated charcoal on aspirin absorption in man. Clin Pharmacol Ther 1972;13:317–322.
65. Lieh-Lai M, Sarnack A, Newton J, et al: Metabolism and pharmokinetics of acetaminophen in a severely poisoned young child. J Pediatr 1984;105:125–128.
66. Longdson P, Henderson A: Intestinal pseudoobstruction following the use of enteral charcoal and sorbitol with mechanical ventilation with papaverum sedation for theophylline poisoning. Drug Saf 1992;7:74–77.
67. Mahutte CK, True RJ, Michiels TN, et al: Increased serum theophylline clearance with orally administered activated charcoal. Am Rev Resp Dis 1983;128:820–822.
68. Makosiej F, Hoffman RS, Howland MA, et al: An in vitro evaluation of cocaine hydrochloride adsorption by activated charcoal and desorption upon addition of polyethlene glycol electrolyte solution. J Toxicol Clin Toxicol 1993;31:381–386.
69. Manes M, Mann JF: Easily swallowed formulations of antidote charcoals. Clin Toxicol 1974;7:355–364.
70. Mariani PJ, Poole N: Gastrointestinal tract perforation with charcoal peritoneum complicating orogastric intubation and lavage. Ann Emerg Med 1993;22:606–609.
71. Mathur LK, Jaffe JM, Colaizzi JL, Moriarity RW: Activated charcoal-carboxymethylcellulose gel formulation as an antidotal agent for orally ingested aspirin. Am J Hosp Pharm 1976;33:717–729.
72. Mayersohn M, Perrier D, Picchioni A: Evaluation of a charcoal-sorbitol mixture as an antidote for oral aspirin overdose. Clin Toxicol 1977;11:561–567.
73. McKinnon RS, Desmond PV,Harmon PJ, et al: Studies on

the mechanisms of action of activated charcoal on theophylline pharmacokinetics. J Pharm Pharmacol 1987;39: 522–525.
74. McLuckie A, Forbes AM, Ilett KF: Role of repeated doses of oral activated charcoal in the treatment of acute intoxications. Anesth Intens Care 1990;18:375–381.
75. McNamara R, Aaron C, Gemborys M: Sorbitol catharsis does not enhance efficacy of charcoal in simulated acetaminophen overdose. Ann Emerg Med 1988;17:243–246.
76. Menzies DG, Busuttel A, Prescott LF: Fatal pulmonary aspiration of oral activated charcoal. Br Med J 1988;297: 459–466.
77. Merigian KS, Woodard M, Hedges JR, et al: Prospective evaluation of gastric emptying in the self poisoned patient. Am J Emerg Med 1990;8:479–483.
78. Mezutani T, Waits H, Oohashi W: Rectal ulcer with massive hemorrhage due to activated charcoal treatment in oral organophosphate poisoning. Hum Exp Toxicol 1991; 10:385–386.
79. Mofenson H, Caraccio T: Magnesium intoxication in a neonate from oral magnesium hydroxide laxative. J Toxicol Clin Toxicol 1991;29:215–222.
80. Navarro R, Navarro K, Krenzelok E: Relative efficacy and palatability of three activated charcoal mixtures. Vet Hum Toxicol 1980;22:6–9.
81. Neuvonen PJ: Clinical pharmacokinetics of oral activated charcoal in acute intoxications. Clin Pharmacokinet 1982;7: 465–489.
82. Neuvonen PJ, Elonen E: Effect of activated charcoal on absorption and elimination of phenobarbitone, carbamazepine, and phenylbutazone in man. Eur J Clin Pharmacol 1980;17:51–57.
83. Neuvonen PJ, Elonen E, Mattila MJ: Oral activated charcoal and dapsone elimination. Clin Pharmacol Ther 1980; 6:823–827.
84. Neuvonen PJ, Olkkola K: Oral activated charcoal in the treatment of intoxications. Med Toxicol 1988;3:33–58.
85. Neuvonen PJ, Olkkola K: Effect of purgatives on antidotal efficacy of oral activated charcoal. Hum Toxicol 1986;5: 255–263.
86. Neuvonen PJ, Olkkola K: Activated charcoal and syrup of ipecac in prevention of cimetidine and pindolol absorption in man after administration of metoclopramide as an antiemetic agent. J Toxicol Clin Toxicol 1984;22: 103–114.
87. Neuvonen PJ, Olkkola K, Alanen T: Effect of ethanol and pH on the adsorption of drugs to activated charcoal: Studies in vitro and in man. Acta Pharmacol Toxicol 1984;54: 1–7.
88. Neuvonen PJ, Vartiainen M, Tokola O: Comparison of activated charcoal and ipecac syrup in the prevention of drug absorption. Eur J Clin Pharmacol 1983;24:557–562.
89. North D, Peterson R, Krenzelok E: Effect of activated charcoal administration on acetylcysteine serum levels in humans. Am J Hosp Pharm 1981;38:1022–1024.
90. Ohning B, Reed M, Blumer J: Continuous nasogastric administration of activated charcoal for the treatment of theophylline intoxication. Pediatr Pharmacol 1986;5: 241–245.
91. Olkkola K: Effect of charcoal–drug ratio on antidotal efficacy of oral activated charcoal in man. Br J Clin Pharmacol 1985;19:767–773.
92. Olkkola K: Factors affecting the antidotal efficacy of oral activated charcoal. University of Helsinki, 1985. Dissertation.
93. Olkkola K, Neuvonen P: Do gastric contents modify antidotal efficacy of oral activated charcoal? Br J Clin Pharmacol 1984;18:663–669.
94. Osol A, ed: Remington's Practice of Pharmacy, 16th ed. Easton, PA, Mack Publishing, 1980.
95. Park G, Spector R, Goldberg M, et al: Effect of the surface area of activated charcoal on theophylline clearance. J Clin Pharmacol 1984;24:289–292.
96. Picchioni A: Activated charcoal: A neglected antidote. Pediatr Clin North Am 1970;17:535–543.
97. Picchioni A, Chin L, Gillespie T: Evaluation of activated charcoal-sorbitol suspension as an antidote. Clin Toxicol 1982;19:435–444.
98. Pollack M, Dunbar B, Holbrook P, Fields A: Aspiration of activated charcoal and gastric contents. Ann Emerg Med 1981;10;528–529.
99. Pond SM, Jacobs M, Marks J, et al: Treatment of digitoxin overdose with oral activated charcoal. Lancet 1982;2: 1177–1178.
100. Pond SM, Lewis-Driver DJ, Williams G, et al: Gastric emptying in acute overdose: A prospective randomised controlled trial. Med J Austral 1995;163:345–349.
101. Pond SM, Olson KR, Osterloh JD, Tong TG: Randomized study of the treatment of phenobarbital overdose with repeated doses of activated charcoal. JAMA 1984;251: 3104–3108.
102. Prescott L, Hillman R: Treatment of salicylate poisoning with repeated oral charcoal. Br Med J 1985;291:1472.
103. Ray MJ, Padin DR, Condie JD, Halls JM: Charcoal bezoar: Small bowel obstruction secondary to amitriptyline overdose therapy. Dig Dis Sci 1988;33:107.
104. Renzi F, Donovan J, Morgan L, et al: Concomitant use of activated charcoal and *N*-acetylcysteine. Ann Emerg Med 1985;14:568–572.
105. Reynolds JEF, ed: Martindale: The Extra Pharmacopoeia, 29th ed. London, Pharmaceutical Press, 1989, p. 835.
106. Roberts JR, Gracely EJ: High surface area oral activated charcoal has superior clinical properties. Acad Emerg Med 1996;3:419–420.
107. Scholtz E, Jaffe J, Colaizzi J: Evaluation of five activated charcoal formulations for inhibition of aspirin adsorption and palatability in man. Am J Hosp Pharm 1978;35:1355–1359.
108. Siberman H, Davis SM, Lee A: Activated charcoal aspiration. NC Med J 1990;51:79–80.
109. Sketris I, Mowry J, Czajka P, et al: Saline catharsis: Effect on aspirin bioavailability in combination with activated charcoal. J Clin Pharmacol 1982;22:59–64.
110. Smilkstein MJ, Knapp GL, Kulig KW, Rumack BH: Efficacy of oral *N*-acetylcysteine in the treatment of acetaminophen overdose: Analysis of the National Multicenter Study (1976–1985). N Engl J Med 1988;319:1557–1562.
111. Smilkstein MJ, Smolinske S, Kulig KW, et al: Severe hypermagnesemia due to multiple-dose cathartic therapy. West J Med 1988;148:208–211.
112. Swartz C, Sherman A: The treatment of tricyclic antide-

pressant overdose with activated charcoal. J Clin Psychopharmacol 1984;4:336–340.

113. Tenenbein M, Cohen S, Sitar DS: Efficacy of ipecac induced emesis, orogastric lavage and activated charcoal for acute drug overdose. Ann Emerg Med 1987;16: 838–841.
114. True RJ, Berman JN, Mahutte CK: Treatment of theophylline toxicity with oral activated charcoal. Crit Care Med 1984;12:113–114.
115. Tsuchiya T, Levy G: Relationship between effect of activated charcoal on drug adsorption characteristics in vitro. J Pharm Sci 1972;61:586–589.
116. Underhill TJ, Greene MK, Dove AF: A comparison of the efficacy of gastric lavage, ipecacuanha and activated charcoal in the emergency management of paracetamol overdose. Arch Emerg Med 1990;7;148–154.
117. United States Pharmacopoeial Convention: The United States Pharmacopieia, 20th rev. The National Formulary, 15th ed. Easton, PA, Mack Publishing, 1980.
118. Vale JA, Proudfoot AT: How useful is activated charcoal? Br Med J 1993;306:78–79.
119. Van de Graaf W, Thompson WL, Sunshine I, et al: Adsorbent and cathartic inhibition of enteral drug adsorption. J Pharmacol Exp Ther 1982;221:656–663.
120. Watson WA, Cremes KF, Chapman JA: Gastrointestinal obstruction associated with multiple dose activated charcoal. J Emerg Med 1986;4;401–407.
121. Watson WA, McKinney PE: Activated charcoal and acetylcysteine absorption: Issues in interpreting pharmacokinetic data. Ann Pharmacother 1991;25:1081–1084.
122. Yancy RE, O'Barr TP, Corby DG: In vitro and in vivo evaluation of the effect of cherry flavoring on the adsorptive capacity of activated charcoal for salicylic acid. Vet Hum Toxicol 1980;22:163–165.

ANTIDOTES IN DEPTH

Cathartics

Mary Ann Howland

Drugs that promote intestinal evacuation are referred to as *laxatives, cathartics*, or *purgatives*. Laxatives promote a soft formed or semifluid stool within 6 to 8 hours or 1 to 3 days, depending on the agent and the dose employed. Cathartics promote a rapid watery evacuation within 1 to 3 hours.[4] Purgatives imply an even stronger evacuation. The same drug may accomplish any or all of these tasks, depending on the dose.

The traditional classification of laxatives into the five categories of bulk-forming, stimulant or irritant, softeners, saline or osmotic, and lubricant is largely empirical.[3] Additional investigation is needed to determine how laxatives affect gastrointestinal motility and fluid and electrolyte movement.[3]

Traditionally, the effects of saline cathartics, such as magnesium citrate and sulfate salts, were attributed to the fact that they were relatively nonabsorbable anions and cations that established an osmotic gradient and drew water into the gut. The increased water retention led to increased intestinal pressure and a subsequent increase in intestinal motility.[6] This hypothesis, however, is probably overly simplistic.[3] Recent evidence shows that magnesium releases cholecystokinin, a gastrointestinal hormone, from the duodenal mucosa, which stimulates intestinal motor activity and alters fluid movement.[3,36] Magnesium decreases transit time while paradoxically decreasing smooth muscle contractibility in the ileum.[3,36] In animals, saline cathartics may delay gastric emptying, which may affect the rate of absorption but not necessarily the extent of absorption of some drugs.[36] Bisacodyl and phenolphthalein are stimulant cathartics whose action has recently been at least partially linked to the induction of nitric oxide synthase and an increased production of nitric oxide.[10]

Sorbitol (D-glucitol) is naturally found in many ripe fruits and prepared industrially from glucose. Sorbitol is about 60% as sweet as glucose, and upon metabolism yields the same 4 calories per gram as glucose. It is slowly absorbed from the GI tract with some conversion to glucose, but the majority is converted to carbon dioxide. Sorbitol presumably works by an osmotic action, but little is known about the mechanisms of action of this drug. Sorbitol is not even mentioned as a laxative or cathartic in numerous reviews.[3,4,6,36,38,39]

Cathartics have been recommended for basic poison management for many years. Intuitively, the advantages of cathartics appear to be decreasing the potential for constipation or obstruction from activated charcoal, hastening the delivery of activated charcoal to the small intestine, and hastening the elimination of poorly absorbed or sustained-released drugs or toxins before they can be absorbed. A 1981 review of cathartic use in toxic ingestions confirmed frequent utilization, but found little evidence for their efficacy.[32] This analysis remains true today.

Given alone, cathartics such as sorbitol or sodium sulfate may decrease peak and/or total absorption of some drugs, but in no study has this effect achieved the results reported with activated charcoal alone.[2,5,22,30,40] When comparing the efficacy of a single dose of activated charcoal alone with that of activated charcoal plus a single dose of cathartic, studies suggest the combination to be as good as,[2,24,29,30,33] a little better than,[5,14] or even a little worse than activated charcoal alone.[22,40] A study of a sustained-release theophylline preparation (Theo 24) found that a combination of activated charcoal and sorbitol decreased total absorption a little more than activated charcoal alone when given at 6 and 8 hours after ingestion.[11]

In contrast to studying effects on total amount of drug absorbed, some studies have compared cathartic use with respect to time to first stool and number of stools. These studies used a variety of products and doses.[12,17,25,26,37] In general sorbitol produced stools in the shortest amount of time but with the highest incidence of nausea and vomiting. When comparing gram doses of sorbitol, the specific gravity of 1.285 g/mL, the concentration, and the mL amount must be used in the calculation. For example, 70 mL of sorbitol 70% is equivalent to 62.965 g (70 mL × 70% × 1.285 g/mL).[42] The lack of precise calculations has led to inaccurate estimates of g/kg doses of sorbitol in some studies.

In nonpoisoned adult volunteers, four regimens were used each including 50 g activated charcoal administered as a water slurry with 300 mL ginger ale. Given alone it was the first regimen. Other groups had 70% sorbitol (240 mL), 300 mL magnesium citrate (17.45 g), or 30 mL 50% magnesium sulfate (15 g) added. The times to first charcoal stool were 23.5, 0.9, 4.2, and 9.3 hours, respectively.[17] Sorbitol produced 10 to 15 watery stools, the most abdominal cramping before catharsis, and its taste was rated second behind magnesium citrate because of its nauseating sweetness. In a study of 6 adult volunteers, the ingestion of 30 g activated charcoal in 150 mL of 70% sorbitol resulted in severe diarrhea with mild to moderate abdominal cramping and gurgling.[26] The first charcoal stool was noted in 89 min, 12 hours ± 10 hours of diarrhea occurred, and 62 hours of black stools were reported.[26] There were no effects on routinely measured laboratory values.

A study of catharsis in poisoned children 1 to 5 years of age compared 4 mL/kg of sorbitol (50%) (actually 2.48 g/kg, although reported as 2.57g/kg), magnesium citrate (233 mg/kg), magnesium sulfate (250 mg/kg) and water, each added as a slurry with activated charcoal (1 g/kg) and delivered via a nasogastric tube.[12] Sorbitol produced the shortest time to first stool at 8.48 hours compared to magnesium citrate at 12.84 hours, water at 14 hours, and magnesium sulfate at 22.65 hours. Forty-two percent of the patients using sorbitol vomited, while only 17% vomited with the other regimens. The mean number of stools in 24 hours produced with sorbitol was 2.97, with magnesium citrate was 1.79, with water was 1.75, and with magnesium sulfate was 1.65 stools.

The risks associated with cathartics are dehydration, absorption of magnesium or other salts, hypokalemia, and metabolic alkalosis from dehydration and activation of the renin–angiotensin–aldosterone system. In two elderly patients, rectal prolapse occurred.[16] Nausea, vomiting, abdominal cramping, and frequent watery stools are common complaints after sorbitol administration.[14,15,28]

Hypocalcemia, hyperphosphatemia, and hypokalemia were reported following the use of hypertonic phosphate enemas.[7,9,19,20,31,35] In some of these cases, the recommended dose was used.[7] Consequential morbidity and mortality were reported in previously healthy children as well as in those with bowel abnormalities who received phosphosoda. In none of the case reports were the enemas used as part of basic poison management; nonetheless, hypertonic phosphate enemas or oral solutions of phosphosoda should never be used in children as part of poison management.

Because of the demonstrable efficacy of repetitive doses of activated charcoal in certain overdoses, some clinicians mistakenly assume that repetitive doses of cathartics should be given concomitantly.[21] Significant toxicity results from the repetitive administration of either magnesium or sorbitol-containing cathartics. A patient who received 300-mL doses of magnesium citrate every 4 hours for approximately 72 hours developed neuromuscular toxicity and coma and had a magnesium level of 11.4 mEq/L.[13] The patient was treated with intravenous calcium chloride and hemodialysis. A 25-day-old girl was given 8 teaspoons of milk of magnesia each day for 3 days (not in the management of an overdose). She became limp and difficult to arouse and had a serum magnesium level of 7.6 mEq/L.[27] A study investigating the effect of single versus two or three doses of 30 g of magnesium sulfate in suspected overdose patients revealed increasingly elevated serum magnesium levels after the second and third doses, with a resultant mean peak of 2.6 mEq/L.[34] These increases occurred in patients with normal renal function. Clinical signs and symptoms of hypermagnesemia were not reported. Aspiration of magnesium would be expected to lead to consequential hypermagnesemia.

Multiple-dose activated charcoal regimens used to facilitate "gastrointestinal dialysis" have resulted in severe cathartic-related adverse effects in four cases reports.[1,8,18,23] In each instance the charcoal preparations used also contained 70% sorbitol and repeat-dose sorbitol presumably led to severe dehydration and hypernatremia, with neurologic sequelae in one instance.[1,8,23] The retention of sorbitol after repetitive doses in an aperistaltic gut may lead to significant morbidity due to the gas formation and abdominal distention as a result of the digestive action of gut bacteria.[18] Highlighting the potential for toxicity from repetitive activated charcoal dosing was a survey revealing that 16% of those hospitals surveyed only stocked activated charcoal premixed with sorbitol.[41]

Contraindications to the use of cathartics include an adynamic ileus, preexisting or anticipated diarrhea, abdominal trauma, and intestinal obstruction. Renal failure is a contraindication to the use of magnesium-containing cathartics. Oil-based cathartics such as mineral oil should not be used because of the risks associated with aspiration and the possibility for enhancing the absorption of certain lipid-soluble toxins.

Cathartics should no longer be considered part of the routine management of either pediatric or adult overdoses. There is no evidence to indicate that single doses of cathartics alone without activated charcoal are more effective than activated charcoal alone at decreasing absorption or enhancing elimination of substances capable of binding to activated charcoal. Cathartics should never be used as a substitute for activated charcoal when drugs that are adsorbed to activated charcoal are involved. When total drug absorption is evaluated, a single dose of a cathartic given with activated charcoal appears to be as efficacious as activated charcoal given alone. In children given 1 g/kg activated charcoal alone or with 233 mg/kg of magnesium citrate solution, the time to first charcoal stool was 19.5 hours versus 13 hours.[37] This was comparable to 14 hours versus 12.84 hours in another study, and 8.4 hours for 2.48 g/kg of 50% sorbitol.[12] Nonpoisoned adults given 50 g activated charcoal alone versus activated charcoal with 70% sorbitol (130 or 216 g depending on how the calculation was determined) or 300 mL of magnesium citrate produced stools in 23.5, 0.9, or 4.2 hours, respectively. Although in all cases sorbitol produced stool more rapidly, side effects were also more pronounced. In adults, when large amounts of drugs have been ingested or when desorption from charcoal may be an important consideration (such as ASA), a single dose of a cathartic, preferably magnesium citrate or sorbitol, may be given with the activated charcoal. When multiple-dose activated charcoal is used, cathartics should be used only with the first dose. Patients should be administered sufficient fluids orally to avoid inspissation and dehydration. Whole-bowel irrigation, unless contraindicated, is preferable to repetitive dose cathartics for the evacuation of sustained-release or poorly soluble drugs or toxins not adsorbed to activated charcoal.

References

1. Allerton J, Strom J: Hypernatremia due to repeated doses of charcoal-sorbitol. Am J Kidney Dis 1991;7:581–584.

2. Al-Shareef AH, Buss DC, Allen EM, Routledge PA: The effects of charcoal and sorbitol (alone and in combination) on plasma theophylline concentration after a sustained release formulation. Hum Exp Toxicol 1990;9:179–182.
3. Binder H: Pharmacology of laxatives. Annu Rev Pharmacol Toxicol 1977;17:355–367.
4. Brunton LL: Laxatives. In: Goodman LS, Gilman AG, Rall TW, Murad F, eds: The Pharmacological Basis of Therapeutics, 7th ed. New York, Macmillan, 1985, pp. 994–1003.
5. Chin L, Picchioni A, Gillespie T: Saline cathartics and saline cathartics plus activated charcoal as antidotal treatments. Clin Toxicol 1981;18:865–871.
6. Darlington RC: Laxatives. In: Griffenhagen GB, Hawkins LL, eds: Handbook of Nonprescription Drugs. Washington, DC, American Pharmaceutical Association, 1973, pp. 62–76.
7. Davis R, Eichner J, Bleyer W, et al: Hypocalcemia, hyperphosphatemia, and dehydration following a single hypertonic phosphate enema. J Pediatr 1977;90:484–485.
8. Farley T: Severe hypernatremic dehydration after use of an activated charcoal-sorbitol suspension. J Pediatr 1986;109: 719–722.
9. Forman J, Baluarte J, Gruskin A: Hypokalemia after hypertonic phosphate enemas. J Pediatr 1979;94:149–151.
10. Gaginella TS, Mascolo N, Izzo AA, et al: Nitric oxide as a mediator of bisacodyl and phenolphthalein laxative action: Induction of nitric oxide synthase. J Pharm Exp Ther 1994;270:1239–1245.
11. Goldberg M, Spector R, Park G, et al: The effect of sorbitol and activated charcoal on serum theophylline concentrations after slow release theophylline. Clin Pharmacol Ther 1987;41:108–111.
12. James LP, Nichols MH, King WD: A comparison of cathartics in pediatric ingestions. Pediatrics 1995;96:235–238.
13. Jones J, Heiselman D, Dougherty J, et al: Cathartic-induced magnesium toxicity during overdose management. Ann Emerg Med 1986;15:1214–1218.
14. Keller R, Schwab R, Krenzelok E: Contribution of sorbitol combined with activated charcoal in prevention of salicylate absorption. Ann Emerg Med 1990;19:654–656.
15. Kirshenbaum CA, Mathews SC, Sitar DS, Tenenbein M: Whole bowel irrigation versus activated charcoal in sorbitol for the ingestion of modified-release pharmaceuticals. Clin Pharmacol Ther 1989;46:264–271.
16. Korkis A, Miskowitz P, Kurt R, Klein H: Rectal prolapse after oral cathartics. J Clin Gastroenterol 1992;14:339–341.
17. Krenzelok EP, Keller R, Stewart RD: Gastrointestinal transit times of cathartics combined with charcoal. Ann Emerg Med 1985;14:1152–1155.
18. Longdon P, Henderson A: Intestinal pseudo-obstruction following the use of enteral charcoal and sorbitol and mechanical ventilation with papaveretum sedation for theophylline poisoning. Drug Saf 1992;7:74–77.
19. Loughnan P, Mullins G: Brain damage following a hypertonic phosphate enema. Am J Dis Child 1977;131:1032.
20. Martin R, Lisehora G, Braxton M, et al: Fatal poisoning from sodium phosphate enema: A case report and experimental study. JAMA 1987;257:2190–2192.
21. Massanari MJ, Hendeles L, Hill E, et al: The efficacy of sorbitol and activated charcoal in reducing theophylline absorption from a slow release formulation. Drug Int Clin Pharm 1986;20:471.
22. Mayershohn M, Perrier D, Picchioni A: Evaluation of a charcoal-sorbitol mixture as an antidote for oral aspirin overdose. Clin Toxicol 1977;11:561–567.
23. McCord M: Toxicity of sorbitol-charcoal suspension. J Pediatr 1987;110:307–308.
24. McNamara R, Aaron C, Gemborys M: Sorbitol catharsis does not enhance efficacy of charcoal in simulated acetaminophen overdose. Ann Emerg Med 1988;17:243–246.
25. Minocha A, Krenzelok EP, Spyker D: Dosage recommendations for activated charcoal—sorbitol treatment. J Toxicol Clin Toxicol 1985;23:579–587.
26. Minocha A, Merold DA, Bruns DE, et al. Effect of activated charcoal in 70% sorbitol in healthy individuals. J Toxicol Clin Toxicol 1984–85;22:529–536.
27. Mofenson HC, Caraccio TR: Magnesium intoxication in a neonate from oral magnesium hydroxide laxative. J Toxicol Clin Toxicol 1991;29:215–222.
28. Muller-Lissner SA: Adverse effects of laxatives: Fact and fiction. Pharmacol 1993;47:(suppl 1)138–145.
29. Neuvonen P, Olkkola K: Effect of purgatives on antidotal efficacy of oral activated charcoal. Vet Hum Toxicol 1986; 5:255–263.
30. Picchioni A, Chin L, Gillespie T: Evaluation of activated charcoal-sorbitol suspension as an antidote. Clin Toxicol 1982;19:435–444.
31. Reedy J, Zwiren G: Enema-induced hypocalcemia and hyperphosphatemia leading to cardiac arrest during induction of anesthesia in an outpatient surgery center. Anesthesiology 1983;59:578–579.
32. Riegel J, Becker C: Use of cathartics in toxic ingestions. Ann Emerg Med 1981;10:254–258.
33. Sketris I, Mowry J, Czajka P, et al: Saline catharsis: Effect on aspirin bioavailability in combination with activated charcoal. J Clin Pharmacol 1982;22:59–64.
34. Smilkstein MJ, Steedle D, Kulig KW, et al: Magnesium levels after magnesium containing cathartics. J Toxicol Clin Toxicol 1988;26:51–65.
35. Sotos J, Cutler E, Finkel M, et al: Hypocalcemic coma following two pediatric phosphate enemas. Pediatrics 1977;60: 305–307.
36. Stewart J: Effects of emetic and cathartic agents on the gastrointestinal tract and the treatment of toxic ingestions. Clin Toxicol 1983;20:199–253.
37. Sue YJ, Woolf A, Shannon M: Efficacy of magnesium citrate cathartic pediatric toxic ingestions. Ann Emerg Med 1994; 24:709–712.
38. Tedesco F: Laxative use in constipation. Am J Gastroenterol 1985;80:303–309.
39. Thompson WG: Laxatives: Clinical pharmacology and rational use. Drugs 1980;19:49–58.
40. Van de Graff W, Thompson L, Sunshine I, et al: Absorbent and cathartic inhibition of enteral drug absorption. J Pharmacol Exp Ther 1982;221:656–663.
41. Wax PM, Wang RY, Hoffman RS, et al: Prevalence of sorbitol in multiple-dose activated charcoal regimens in emergency departments. Ann Emerg Med 1993;22:1807–1812.
42. Weaver WR: Calculating sorbitol dosage. Ann Emerg Med 1988;17:661–662.

ANTIDOTES IN DEPTH

Whole-Bowel Irrigation

Mary Ann Howland

Rapid ingestion of a large volume of fluid can cause bowel evacuation and achieve the quality of cleansing necessary for bowel surgery. Solutions previously employed for this purpose consisted of normal saline or balanced electrolytes but were absorbable and led to significant sodium and water retention.[7] A nonabsorbable solution is readily available, composed of polyethylene glycol and electrolytes lavage solution (PEG-ELS), which caused only minimal net water and electrolyte shifts.[7] Subsequent studies demonstrated patient acceptance, effectiveness, and safety when used for bowel preparation.[1,3,8,9,24,34,35]

Historically, whole-bowel irrigation with saline and potassium chloride was utilized for two cases of drug overdoses. As expected, fluid and electrolyte abnormalities did occur; nevertheles, the author concluded that the technique was safe in pediatric patients.[24] Whole-bowel irrigation was later applied to a series of 8 patients with toxic ingestions, including 4 patients who swallowed disk batteries.[31] Efficacy was difficult to prove in this series, and one patient who was given lactated Ringer's solution developed peripheral edema. A study was then done with volunteers who ingested 5 g of ampicillin and had whole-bowel irrigation with PEG-ELS.[32] After 234 minutes and 7.71 L of fluid there was a 67% decrease in ampicillin absorption without any significant changes in fluid or electrolytes.

In a dog model involving sustained-release theophylline, and in a volunteer study involving enteric-coated aspirin, whole-bowel irrigation was shown to be as effective as, or slightly more effective than, a single dose or repeated doses of activated charcoal (with a single dose of sorbitol).[6,15] In another volunteer study involving sustained-release lithium preparations, whole-bowel irrigation significantly decreased peak lithium serum concentration and lithium bioavailability.[28] However, whole-bowel irrigation was inferior to activated charcoal when administered following 650 mg of immediate-release aspirin.[26] Once aspirin was absorbed, whole-bowel irrigation was unable to enhance systemic clearance.[21]

There are reports of the use of whole-bowel irrigation in the management of overdoses of iron,[10,20,30,33] sustained-release theophylline,[14] sustained-release verapamil,[4] zinc sulfate,[5] lead,[23,25] sustained-release fenfluramine,[22] and for body packers.[13,37]

As mentioned, whole-bowel irrigation with PEG-ELS flushes out the gastrointestinal tract without causing fluid and electrolyte shifts, and the hope is to reduce bioavailability by decreasing the time available for drug absorption. However, there is some concern that moving drug from the stomach to the small intestine, or increasing the dissolution of a previously saturated solution, may increase absorption. Once absorption has occurred, it is unlikely that whole-bowel irrigation can play a prominent role. Although animal models suggest that it may enhance systemic clearance via gastrointestinal dialysis, much like multiple-dose activated charcoal,[18] low flow rates, the typical delay in administering WBI in actual clinical situations, and the inconvenience of this procedure make it highly unlikely that the effect can be achieved in humans.

Several in vitro studies demonstrated that the addition of PEG-ELS to activated charcoal significantly decreases the adsorptive capacity of activated charcoal.[12,19] The interaction was affected by pH and magnified by high ratios of PEG-ELS to activated charcoal.[2,16,19] The osmolality of the PEG-ELS did not seem to be affected at simulated clinical ratios.[16] Whole-bowel irrigation in an animal model appeared to have an adverse effect by washing the activated charcoal away from the sustained-release theophylline.[6]

Two case reports and one volunteer study question the efficacy of whole-bowel irrigation.[5,27,29] Whole-bowel irrigation for 5 hours following ingestion of 10 fluorescent coffee beans by 7 volunteers led to the removal of an average of only 4 beans (range, 1 to 8), for a 40% efficiency rate.[27] The coffee bean, because of its physical characteristics (density, solubility, size), might not be representative of substances amenable to WBI.

The recommended dose of PEG-ELS is 0.5 L/h for small children and 2 L/h for adolescents and adults. PEG-ELS solution may be administered orally to a patient or administered through a nasogastric tube for 4 to 6 hours or until the rectal effluent becomes clear. Vomiting may occur and appears to be related to the rate of delivery. An antiemetic such as metoclopramide or a serotonin antagonist may be required, particularly if an emetic agent has been ingested or syrup of ipecac was previously given.

Contraindications to WBI include significant gastrointestinal pathology or dysfunction, such as ileus, perforation, and obstruction.[30] Whole-bowel irrigation was used successfully in 2 pregnant women at 38 and 26 weeks of gestation.[36,38] Adverse effects include vomiting (especially with rapid administration). This is of concern in patients with potential airway compromise. Other adverse affects include abdominal bloating and anal itching (from excessive wiping); the patient will need to remain on a commode for 4 to 6 hours. Two unusual adverse effects have also been reported with PEG-ELS, but in the setting of bowel preparation and not overdose. One was the exacerbation of CHF in an extremely clinically unstable patient with cardiac and renal dysfunction.[11] The other is a case of colonic perforation in the setting of severe diverticulitis.[17]

The role of PEG-ELS in the overdosed patient remains to be defined. Theoretically, ingestions of sustained-release drugs (theophylline, verapamil), drugs not adsorbed by charcoal (iron, sustained-release lithium, lead), and drug packets (in body packers) may be amenable to the use of PEG-ELS for whole-bowel irrigation. An added advantage may be that if these patients subsequently require endoscopy, diagnostic radiography, or surgery, after WBI the gastrointestinal tract mucosa may be easily visualized and surgery will be facilitated if necessary. Activated charcoal should be given initially to those patients who have ingested substances adsorbed by activated charcoal, and activated charcoal should probably also be given during WBI and afterwards to prevent or overcome desorption with its potential for further systemic absorption of the drug. The interaction between activated charcoal and PEG-ELS requires further study.

References

1. Ambrose N, Johnson M, Burdon D, et al: A physiologic approach of polyethylene glycol and a balanced electrolyte solution as bowel preparation. Br J Surg 1983;70:428–430.
2. Atta-Politou J, Macheras P, Koupparis M: The effect of polyethylene glycol on the charcoal adsorption of chlorpromazine studied by ion-selective electrode potentiometry. J Toxicol Clin Toxicol 1996;34:307–316.
3. Beck D, Harford F, diPalma J, et al: Bowel cleansing with polyethylene glycol electrolyte lavage solution. South Med J 1985;78:1414–1416.
4. Buckley N, Dawson A, Howarth D, Whyte I: Slow release verapamil poisoning. Med J Aust 1993;158:202–204.
5. Burkhart KK, Kulig KW, Rumack BH: Whole bowel irrigation as adjunctive treatment for zinc sulfate overdose. Ann Emerg Med 1990;19:1167–1170.
6. Burkhart KK, Wuerz R, Donovan JW: Whole bowel irrigation as adjunctive treatment for sustained release theophylline overdose. Ann Emerg Med 1992;21:1316–1320.
7. Davis G, Santa Ana C, Morawsk S, et al: Development of a lavage solution associated with minimal water and electrolyte absorption or secretion. Gastroenterology 1980;78: 991–995.
8. DiPalma J, Brady C, Stewart D, et al: Comparison of colon cleansing methods in preparation for colonoscopy. Gastroenterology 1984;86:856–860.
9. Erstoff J, Howard D, Marshall J, et al: A randomized blinded clinical trial of a rapid colonic lavage solution (Golytely) compared with standard preparation for colonoscopy and barium enema. Gastroenterology 1983;84:1512–1516.
10. Everson G, Bertaccini E, O'Leary J: Use of whole bowel irrigation in an infant following iron overdose. Am J Emerg Med 1991;9:366–369.
11. Granberry MC, et al: Exacerbation of congestive heart failure after administration of polyethylene glycol–electrolyte lavage solution. Ann Pharmacother 1995;29:1232–1235.
12. Hoffman RS, Chiang WK, Howland MA, et al: Theophylline desorption from activated charcoal caused by whole bowel irrigation. J Toxicol Clin Toxicol 1991;29: 191–202.
13. Hoffman RS, Smilkstein MJ, Goldfrank LR: Whole bowel irrigation and the cocaine body packer. Am J Emerg Med 1990;8;523–527.
14. Janss GJ: Acute theophylline overdose treated with whole bowel irrigation. SD J Med 1990;43:7–8.
15. Kirshenbaum L, Mathews SC, Sitar DS, Tenenbein M: Whole bowel irrigation versus activated charcoal in sorbitol for the ingestion of modified release pharmaceuticals. Clin Pharmacol Ther 1989;46:264–271.
16. Kirshenbaum LA, Sitar DS, Tenenbein M: Interaction between whole bowel irrigation solution and activated charcoal: Implications for the treatment of toxic ingestions. Ann Emerg Med 1990;19;1129–1132.
17. Langdon DE: Colonic perforation with volume laxatives. Am J Gastroenterol 1996;91:622–623.
18. Lenz K, Oroz R, Kleinberger G, et al: Effect of gut lavage on phenobarbital elimination in rats. J Toxicol Clin Toxicol 1983;20:147–157.
19. Makoseij F, Hoffman RS, Howland MA, Goldfrank LR: An in vivo evaluation of cocaine hydrochloride adsorption by activated charcoal and desorption upon addition of polyethylene glycol electrolyte lavage solution. J Toxicol Clin Toxicol 1993;31:381–395.
20. Mann K, Picciotti M, Spevack T, Durban D: Management of acute iron overdose. Clin Pharm 1989;8:428–440.
21. Mayer L, Sitar DS, Tenenbein M: Multiple dose charcoal and whole bowel irrigation do not increase clearance of absorbed salicylate. Arch Intern Med 1992;152:393–396.
22. Melandri R, Re G, Morigi A, et al: Whole bowel irrigation after delayed release fenfluramine overdose. J Toxicol Clin Toxicol 1995;33:161–163.
23. Murphy DG, Gerace RV, Peterson RG: The use of whole bowel irrigation in acute lead ingestion. Vet Hum Toxicol 1991;33:353. Abstract.
24. Postuma R: Whole bowel irrigation in pediatric patients. J Pediatr Surg 1982;17:350–352.
25. Roberge RJ, Martin T, Michelson EA, et al: Whole bowel irrigation in acute lead ingestion. Vet Hum Toxicol 1991;33: 353. Abstract.
26. Rosenberg PJ, Livingston DJ, McLellan B: Effect of whole bowel irrigation on the antidotal efficacy of oral activated charcoal. Ann Emerg Med 1988;17:681–683.
27. Scharman EJ, Lembersky R, Krenzelok EP: Efficiency of whole bowel irrigation with and without metoclopramide pretreatment. Vet Hum Toxicol 1992;34:361. Abstract.
28. Smith S, Ling L, Halstenson C: Whole bowel irrigation as a treatment for acute lithium overdose. Ann Emerg Med 1991;20:536–539.
29. Swanson-Brearman B, Dean BS, Krenzelok EP: Failure of whole bowel irrigation to decontaminate the GI tract fol-

lowing massive jequirity bean ingestion. Vet Hum Toxicol 1992;34:352. Abstract.
30. Tenenbein M: Whole bowel irrigation as gastrointestinal decontamination procedure after acute poisoning. Med Toxicol 1988;3:77–84.
31. Tenenbein M: Whole bowel irrigation for toxic ingestions. J Toxicol Clin Toxicol 1985;23:177–184.
32. Tenenbein M, Cohen S, Sitar DS: Whole bowel irrigation as a decontamination procedure after acute drug overdose. Arch Intern Med 1987;147:906–907.
33. Tenenbein M, Wiseman N, Yatscoff RW: Gastrotomy and whole bowel irrigation in iron poisoning. Pediatr Emerg Care 1991;7;286–288.
34. Thomas G, Brozinsky S, Isenberg J: Patient acceptance and effectiveness of a balanced lavage solution (Golytely) versus the standard preparation for colonoscopy. Gastroenterology 1982;82:435–437.
35. Tuggle D, Hoelzer D, Tunell W, et al: Safety and cost-effectiveness of polyethylene glycol electrolyte solution bowel preparation in infants and children. J Pediatr Surg 1987; 22:513–515.
36. Turk J, Aks S, Ampuero F, et al: Successful therapy of iron intoxication in pregnancy with intravenous deferoxamine and whole bowel irrigation. Vet Hum Toxicol 1993;35:441–444.
37. Utecht M, Stone A, McCarron M: Heroin body packers. J Emerg Med 1990;11:33–40.
38. Van Ameyde K, Tenenbein M: Whole bowel irrigation during pregnancy. Am J Obstet Gynecol 1989;160:646–647.

CHAPTER 31

Acetaminophen

Martin J. Smilkstein

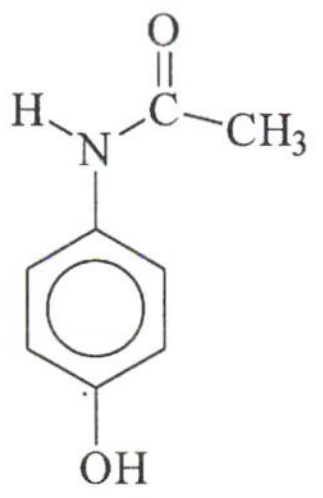

Acetaminophen

Acetaminophen		
MW	=	151 daltons
Therapeutic serum level	=	10–30 μg/mL
	=	66–199 μmol/L
4-hour action level	=	≥150 μg/mL
	=	≥993 μmol/L

Values greater than or equal to the action level necessitate clinical intervention. Values less than this level may necessitate intervention based on the clinical characteristics of the patient.

A 21-year-old woman was brought to the emergency department (ED) by her boyfriend when he learned that she had ingested approximately thirty 325-mg acetaminophen tablets in an attempted suicide. He was unaware of any previous significant medical or psychiatric illness but reported that she had been seen in another ED several days earlier for persistent headaches. He said that she did not abuse alcohol or any other drugs.

The patient was able to provide a history. She admitted to taking about 30 tablets approximately 3 hours before coming to the hospital. She stated that she wanted to kill herself. She said shortly after taking the tablets she developed a bad "stomachache" and felt extremely nauseated, vomiting once. She denied taking any other medications or alcohol in the suicide attempt.

On physical examination the woman was diaphoretic, pale, and suffering from abdominal distress. Her vitals signs were: blood pressure, 95/70 mm Hg; pulse, 100 beats/min; respiratory rate, 20 breaths/min; and oral temperature, 98.6°F (37°C). Examination of the head, eyes, ears, nose, and throat was unremarkable. The neck was supple and the lungs clear, and the cardiac examination was within normal limits. Examination of the abdomen revealed no masses or organomegaly. There was no guarding and only moderate mid-epigastric tenderness. There were no peritoneal signs and bowel sounds were normoactive. Cranial nerves were grossly intact and reflexes were 2+ bilaterally. She was oriented to time, place, and person. Her appearance was consistent with the ingestion of an acute overdose of acetaminophen tablets. She was given 50 g of oral activated charcoal along with 40 mL of 70% sorbitol. A 4-hour serum acetaminophen level was 215 μg/mL, confirming the diagnosis and indicating the need for *N*-acetylcysteine.

Epidemiology and Background

Acetaminophen (*N*-acetyl-*p*-aminophenol [APAP]) is used far more than any other analgesic-antipyretic and as a result, overdosage and toxicity are common considerations. The Toxic Exposure Surveillance System of the American Association of Poison Control Centers reports well over 100,000 calls to United States poison centers each year resulting from APAP exposures, and there are more hospitalizations after APAP overdose than after overdose of any other common pharmaceutical agent.[90–94]

Although first synthesized[111] and used clinically[69] late in the last century, it was only 50 years ago that APAP was rediscovered.[20] As a metabolite of phenacetin, APAP became of interest as an analgesic-antipyretic and was first used clinically in the United States in 1950, but the well-known toxicity of phenacetin led to unfounded concerns about APAP safety that delayed widespread acceptance of APAP until the 1970s. Acetaminophen has since proven to be a remarkably safe drug at appropriate dosage, a fact which, in combination with concerns about salicylate toxicity and association with Reye's syndrome, has resulted in the selection of APAP as the analgesic-antipyretic of choice in most circumstances. Acetaminophen is available alone in myriad single-agent dose formulations and delivery systems, or in combination with opioids, other analgesics, sedatives, decongestants, and antihistamines. The diversity and wide availability of APAP products dictate that APAP toxicity be considered not only after identified APAP exposures, but also after exposure to unknown or multiple drugs in settings of drug overdose, drug abuse, and therapeutic misadventures.

Despite enormous experience with APAP toxicity and long-standing dogma about its management, many controversies and challenges remain unresolved. In order to best understand the continuing evolution in approach to APAP toxicity, it is critical to start with an analysis of certain fundamental principles and then to apply these principles to both typical and atypical presentations in which APAP toxicity must be considered.

APAP Toxicity

How Does APAP Overdose Result in Toxicity?

After the earliest reports,[37,166] a flurry of subsequent case reports, and the first reported series of APAP toxicity,[95,132,133] an intensive research effort clarified the metabolic basis for both the pharmacologic safety and the toxicologic danger of APAP[76,106,107,122] (see Fig. 31–1).

Exact percentages vary among individuals, but approximately 90% of APAP normally undergoes hepatic glucuronide (40–67%) and sulfate (20–46%) conjugation to form inactive, harmless metabolites, which are eliminated in urine. A small fraction of unchanged APAP (<5%) and other minor metabolites reach the urine, but are not thought to be clinically relevant.[124] The remaining fraction, usually ranging from 5 to 15%, is oxidized by the CYP2E1, CYP1A2, CYP3A4 subfamilies of the P450 mixed-function oxidase system, resulting in the formation of a highly reactive electrophile, *N*-acetyl-*p*-benzoquinoneimine (NAPQI).[34] A more exact understanding of P450 metabolism, fundamental to assessing the relationship between ethanol or medication use and APAP toxicity, is still being developed. Experimentally, CYP2E1 and CYP1A2 activation of APAP appears to be prominent at very high dosage,[135] while CYP3A4 oxidation may be most important at low doses.[167]

NAPQI is capable of covalent binding and arylating critical cell proteins, inducing a series of events that may result in cell death.[76] Once thought to be an irreversible process resulting directly from covalent binding of NAPQI, it is now clear that the events leading to cell death are far more complex, and importantly, that the process can be prevented, interrupted, and even reversed after binding has occurred.[21,42,58,120] The potential for intervention after NAPQI binding represents one of the most important advances in understanding of APAP toxicity.

Which, if any, single event is critical and commits the cell to death is still unknown. NAPQI-induced oxidation of enzymes alters normal cell functions and impairs cell defenses against endogenous reactive oxygen species, resulting in further oxidation of vital proteins.[171] Selective arylation of critical cell proteins is likely to be more important than total covalent binding as a determinant of toxicity. Subsequent intracellular calcium dyshomeostasis[110,172] and lipid peroxidation[181] have each been demonstrated, but neither of these processes is consistently required or sufficient to result in cell death.[19,61,64] Recently suggested critical, possibly irreversible, events in cell death include DNA fragmentation[148] and mitochondrial injury,[44] but further work will be required to reliably define the trigger or triggers of APAP-induced cell death. The final pathway of cell death may also vary, with evidence for apoptosis and direct necrosis both demonstrated experimentally.[136]

Macrophages and inflammatory cells infiltrate after necrosis, and destruction due to secondary inflammation[188] and impairment of microcirculation[104] has been demonstrated although, again, neither appears to be necessary for hepatic injury.[72,180]

The safety of appropriate APAP dosing results from the availability of electron donors such as reduced glutathione (GSH) and other thiol-containing compounds. Glutathione quickly combines with NAPQI; the resulting complex is then converted to nontoxic cysteine or mercaptate conjugates, which are then eliminated in urine.[103,108] After appropriate APAP dosing, GSH supply far exceeds that which is required to detoxify NAPQI, and no toxicity occurs. After overdose, the rate and quantity of NAPQI formation may outstrip GSH supply and regeneration, resulting in free NAPQI rapidly binding to hepatocyte constituents. In animal experiments of APAP overdose, hepatic toxicity became evident only when hepatic GSH fell to 30% or less of baseline.[107] This affords APAP a remarkably safe therapeutic index. Although a therapeutic APAP dose is only 10–15 mg/kg, cases of significant toxicity after single acute overdose generally involve doses of 250 mg/kg or higher.[126]

Saturation of the normal, nontoxic routes of metabolism is also important in the development of toxicity.[123]

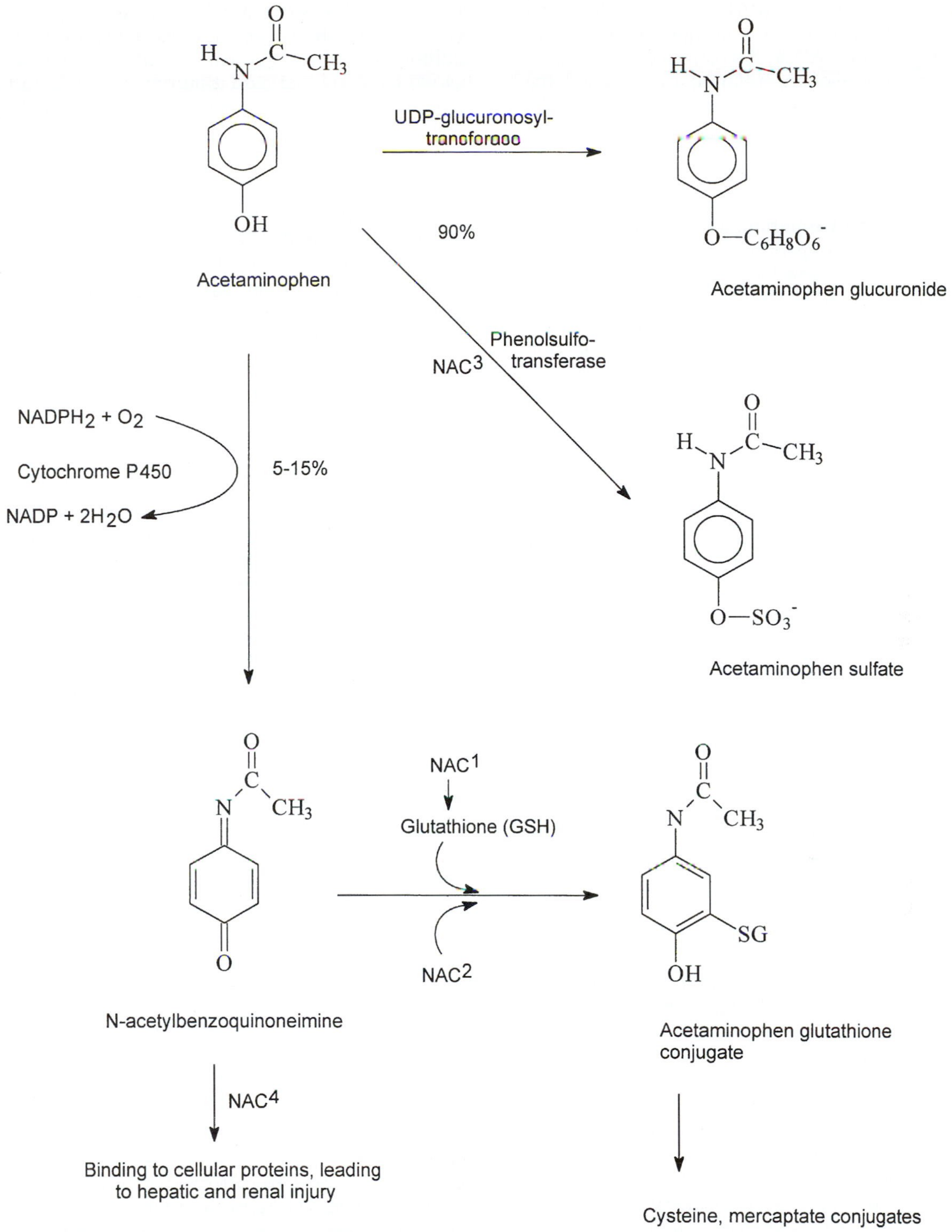

Figure 31–1. Important routes of acetaminophen metabolism in man and mechanisms of *N*-acetylcysteine (NAC) hepatoprotection. NAC[1] is Glutathione (GSH) precursor; NAC[2] is GSH substitute; NAC[3] augments nontoxic sulfation; and, NAC[4] improves multiorgan function during hepatic failure and possibly limits extent of hepatocyte injury.

In experimental or clinical APAP overdose, the total amount of NAPQI increases, but so may the fraction of APAP metabolized to NAPQI. As maximal rates of glucuronidation and, more often, sulfation are exceeded, the fraction of cysteine and mercaptate conjugates in the urine may increase to as high as 39%.[39]

Experimental or clinical conditions that result in increased APAP dose, increased capacity for P450 metabolism, decreased GSH availability, or decreased capacity for glucuronidation and sulfation, all may predispose to hepatotoxicity. Despite experimental evidence for each, clinical consideration of these factors is complex and controversial, and will be discussed under various special categories below.

The pathophysiology of most organ dysfunction resulting directly from APAP is due to the local formation of destructive APAP metabolites. Normally, most oxidative drug metabolism is concentrated in hepatic zone III (centrilobular), and this zone is first and most profoundly affected by APAP toxicity (see Chap. 13). In more severe cases, however, necrosis may extend into zones I and II to destroy the entire liver parenchyma. In perhaps 25% of cases with significant hepatic enzyme elevation, clinically evident renal injury may also occur.[126] Renal P450 formation of NAPQI is the likely cause of acute proximal renal tubular necrosis after acute overdose;[17,52,70] however, several other nephrotoxic mechanisms have been proposed.[67] Conversion of APAP to nephrotoxic *p*-aminophenol[25] and renal conversion of hepatically derived APAP-GSH,[109] both demonstrated in selected animal models, appear unlikely to be significant in toxicity.[51,53,101] NAPQI formation via renal prostaglandin synthetase[177] or prostaglandin-mediated renal medullary ischemia[129] is suspected of contributing to chronic analgesic nephropathy from APAP in combination with other analgesics.[145] In addition, volume depletion and hepatorenal syndrome are often cofactors.

It remains controversial whether local or circulating toxic metabolites cause rare injury to other organs. The mechanism causing myocardial damage, reported in some patients with APAP-induced fulminant hepatic failure, is thought to be part of multisystem organ failure rather than APAP-specific.[18,89] Pancreatic injury from APAP, experimentally produced in mice, appears not to be the result of NAPQI formation,[56] and human cases are too rare to have allowed analysis of the toxic mechanism. Glutathione depletion in rat brain[26] has been suggested as a possible cause of central nervous system effects of APAP, but this finding has been inconsistent[8] and the mechanism of early coma associated with massive APAP doses remains undefined. Similarly, APAP-induced alterations in intermediary metabolism[163] have been presumed to be the cause of lactic acidosis noted to accompany altered mental status in extraordinary cases,[57] but this too is speculative.

The remaining sequelae of severe toxicity are secondary effects of fulminant liver failure, rather than direct APAP effects, and the pathophysiology of these complex multisystem problems is well-described elsewhere.[84] The ability of NAC to ameliorate secondary multiorgan failure via extrahepatic mechanisms (see below) suggests that oxidation of vital thiols and loss of normal microvascular function is an important component of secondary organ failure.[66]

What Are the Clinical Manifestations of APAP Toxicity?

Early recognition and treatment of APAP overdose and toxicity are essential in order to minimize morbidity and mortality. This task is made difficult by the lack of predictive clinical findings early in the course of APAP poisoning, and clinicians should not feel reassured by an asymptomatic patient soon after ingestion. The first symptoms after APAP overdose may be those of hepatic injury, developing many hours after the ingestion, when antidotal therapy is less effective.

The clinical course of APAP toxicity is summarized in Table 31–1. During stage I of toxicity, hepatic injury has not yet occurred and even patients who ultimately develop hepatotoxicity may be asymptomatic at this stage. If clinical findings are present at this stage, they are nonspecific symptoms such as nausea, vomiting, and malaise and signs such as pallor and diaphoresis; laboratory studies are normal. In extremely rare cases of massive overdose, decreased level of consciousness and metabolic acidosis may occur during this stage, in the absence of hepatotoxicity, apparently due directly to the effects of APAP.[57,187] These findings are so uncommon that they should never be attributed to APAP alone without thorough evaluation of other possible causes.

TABLE 31–1. PHASES OF ACETAMINOPHEN POISONING

Phase I (0.5–24 h)

Patients experience anorexia, nausea, pallor, vomiting, and diaphoresis. Malaise may be present. The patient may appear normal.

Phase II (24-72 h)

The symptomatology of phase I becomes less pronounced. Right upper quadrant pain may be present secondary to hepatic damage. Blood chemistries become abnormal, with elevation of liver enzymes and bilirubin. Prothrombin time is prolonged. Renal function may begin to deteriorate, but BUN usually remains low as a result of decreased hepatic urea formation.

Phase III (72–96 h)

Characterized by the sequelae of hepatic necrosis. Coagulation defects, jaundice, renal failure, and myocardial pathology may frequently be present. Hepatic encephalopathy has been observed. Liver biopsy at this time reveals centrilobular necrosis. Nausea and vomiting may reappear. Death is related to hepatic failure and is frequently preceded by anuria and coma.

Phase IV (4 d–2 wk)

If the damage done during phase III is not irreversible, complete resolution of hepatic dysfunction will occur.

Reprinted, with permission, from Linden CH, Rumack BH: Acetaminophen overdose. Emerg Med Clin North Am 1984;2:103–119.

Stage II represents the onset of liver injury, most common approximately 24 hours after ingestion but nearly universal by 36 hours.[149] Symptoms and physical signs during stage II vary with the severity of liver injury but mimic other causes of hepatocellular injury such as infectious hepatitis. Aspartate aminotransferase (AST) is the most sensitive widely available measure to detect the onset of hepatotoxicity, and AST abnormalities always precede evidence of actual liver dysfunction (elevated prothrombin time, elevated bilirubin, hypoglycemia, and metabolic acidosis). Although uncommon, AST elevations may occur as early as 8–12 hours after ingestion in the most severely poisoned patients.

Stage III, defined as the time of maximal hepatotoxicity, is most common between 72 and 96 hours after ingestion. Symptoms and signs vary with the severity of injury, ranging from asymptomatic to fulminant hepatic failure with encephalopathy, coma, and exsanguinating hemorrhage. Laboratory studies are also variable: AST and alanine aminotransferase (ALT) values above 10,000 IU/L are common, even in patients without evidence of liver failure. The highest reported ALT due to APAP toxicity is over 100,000 IU/L.[115] When hepatic failure does occur, dysfunction is evident by abnormalities of prothrombin time, bilirubin, glucose, pH, and other laboratory measures.

Fatalities from fulminant hepatic failure generally occur between 3 and 5 days after overdose but have been reported at other times. Death results from either single or combined complications of multiorgan failure, including hemorrhage, ARDS, sepsis, and most importantly, cerebral edema.[97] Patients who survive this period reach stage IV, defined as the recovery phase. Hepatic regeneration becomes complete in survivors; there are no reported cases of chronic hepatic dysfunction from APAP poisoning. The rate of recovery varies; in most cases laboratory evaluation is normal by 5–7 days after overdose; but recovery may take much longer in severely poisoned patients, and microscopic histologic abnormalities may persist for months.[86,99,121]

Renal function abnormalities are rare overall,[63,126] but occur in as many as 25% of cases with significant hepatotoxicity[36,131] and in more than 50% of those with hepatic failure.[97,184] Overt renal failure necessitating hemodialysis may occur, nearly always among patients with marked hepatic injury.[24] In cases of APAP-induced fulminant liver failure, the incidence of acute renal failure is nearly the same as among patients with hepatic failure of other causes.[184]

Serious clinical manifestations other than hepatic and renal injury are unusual but have been reported. Electrocardiographic and histologic evidence of myocardial injury, first noted in early case reports,[32,118] is often noted in patients with fulminant hepatic and multisystem failure, but never as a consequential isolated problem.[89] Hyperamylasemia and pancreatitis both presumed[46] and proven,[59] have also been attributed to APAP alone or in combination with ethanol abuse.[55] Clinical findings in these rare cases were typical of acute pancreatitis.

Diagnosis

Assessing Risk of Toxicity: What Principles Guide the Diagnostic Approach?

Fatalities from APAP overdose are common, but completely preventable by timely diagnosis and use of a very safe antidote. Therefore, to limit patient risk, a low threshold for treating and erring on the side of overtreatment are advocated. At the same time, the overwhelming majority of APAP exposures result in no toxicity. Therefore, an appropriate approach must avoid the enormous costs of unnecessary overtreatment. In order to balance these seemingly divergent goals, the clinician must understand the basis for and sensitivity of current toxicity screening methods.

When considering risk determination, it is useful to separate different categories of APAP exposure. For acute overdose in typical circumstances, there is an extensive body of experience and literature, permitting a more rigid, defined approach. For issues related to repeated excessive APAP dosing, uncertain circumstances, patients with possible predisposition to toxicity, new APAP formulations, and many other permutations, there is an important conceptual framework for decision making, but little in the way of validated strategies. For these challenges, the central concepts and one approach will be presented, with the understanding that these are dynamic and that more than one approach may have validity. An overview summary of risk determination is presented in Tables 31–2 and 31–3.

The amount and rate of NAPQI formation, the availability of hepatic GSH, and the capacity for nontoxic metabolism are major determinants of toxicity,[105] thus the ideal model for determining risk after APAP overdose would assess each of these. At present, none of these measures is available to clinicians. As noted above, the profile of urinary APAP metabolites may reflect increased NAPQI formation,[39] but there is no indication that measurement would be of any predictive value in any given case. Plasma GSH can be measured, but has an uncertain relationship to hepatic GSH availability.[157] Protein adducts, indicating binding of NAPQI to hepatocyte proteins, can be determined experimentally and are a marker of covalent binding[134,179] but are unlikely to prove useful as a screening measure. Intrahepatic adduct formation should precede APAP-induced liver injury, but some degree of hepatocyte necrosis must precede the appearance of measurable serum adducts, thereby limiting the early warning value of the test. Prior to actual hepatotoxicity, there are no reliable indirect measures of APAP excess. Therefore, the clinician must rely solely upon the ingestion history and measurement of APAP concentration (defined as [APAP]) in the patient to assess

TABLE 31–2. A RISK DETERMINATION STRATEGY AFTER ACUTE APAP INGESTION[a]

A. Assess for risk of APAP toxicity:
   1. If there is a history of APAP overdose and the amount is > 7.5 g in adults, >150 mg/kg in children, unknown, or the history is unreliable
   2. If there is no history of APAP ingestion but another overdose is suspected and there is altered mental status, evidence of oral opioid exposure, nausea and vomiting, or unreliable history
   3. If there are signs or symptoms of hepatic injury
B. Initial laboratory assessment should consist of:
   1. Acetaminophen concentration ([APAP]) 4 h after ingestion or as soon as possible thereafter
   2. AST[b] if [APAP] is above the lower nomogram line or symptoms or physical examination suggest hepatic injury
   3. PT, electrolytes, glucose, BUN, and creatinine if very ill-appearing or marked elevation of AST
C. On the basis of the initial laboratory assessment, consider the patient at risk:
   1. If [APAP] is on or above the lower nomogram line OR
   2. If AST is elevated OR
   3. If [APAP] is > 10 μg/mL and the time of ingestion is completely unknown

[a]The approach described is that of the author, but contains many controversial elements. It is essential that the reader understand the background as discussed in the text, in order to use these guidelines appropriately.

[b]Early in the clinical course of toxicity, and particularly in certain subgroups, the AST may exceed ALT; therefore, AST is listed as the preferred measure. In most circumstances, however, ALT can be substituted for AST in patient assessment, particularly if nonhepatic sources of AST (eg, rhabdomyolysis) are suspected.

the risk for subsequent toxicity and thus the need for treatment.

How Is Risk Assessed After Acute Overdose?

Acute overdose is usually considered to be a single ingestion, although, in fact, many patients consume the overdose in increments over some period. For purposes of this discussion, a single acute overdose is arbitrarily defined as one in which the entire ingestion occurs within a single 4-hour period. Figures of 7.5 g in an adult or 150 mg/kg in a child have been widely disseminated as the lowest acute dose capable of causing toxicity.[1,88] Although these standards have stood the test of time as sensitive markers, they are not based on human data and are quite conservative since historical data suggest that toxicity generally occurs only above 250 mg/kg.[126] Animal data are not reliable in this assessment due to wide interspecies variation in susceptibility to APAP;[125] however, extrapolation of animal data suggests that a single dose of at least 15 g would be required to cause consequential GSH depletion in an adult.[108]

Higher dose cutoffs for consideration of risk would improve specificity; however, the value of improving specificity has not been weighed against the current, sensitive lower cutoff. In the face of an enormous variety of potential outliers, the near-absence of screening failures is almost certainly due to the use of these standards as well as a very sensitive screening nomogram (see below). The adult standard is less controversial than that for children (see below) because massive ingestions, unreliable histories, and factors that might predispose to toxicity occur primarily in adults, justifying continued use of 7.5 g as a screening amount as a "safety net" to avoid missing serious toxicity.

The dose history should be used in the assessment of risk only if there is reliable corroboration or direct evidence of validity. Therefore, dose estimates may be useful in determining risk in many cases of unintentional or therapeutic APAP exposures, but this information is not adequately reliable in most cases of ingestion due to self-harm attempts or drug abuse. If used at all, a credible ingestion history should be used only to exclude toxicity risk and obviate the need for laboratory testing or treatment. When history does suggest possible risk, however, this is not sufficient evidence on which to base treatment decisions, and risk should then be assessed using determination of [APAP].

Interpretation of [APAP] after acute exposures is based on adaptation of the Rumack-Matthew nomogram (see Fig. 31–2),[141] which itself is an adaptation of previous data.[128] The original nomogram was based on the observation that patients who subsequently developed AST or

TABLE 31–3. A RISK DETERMINATION STRATEGY AFTER REPEATED APAP DOSING[a]

A. Assess for risk of APAP toxicity:
   1. If there are signs or symptoms of hepatic injury OR
   2. If the patient is a child with antecedent/concurrent febrile illness who has received >75 mg/kg APAP in any 24-h period
   3. If there is evidence of chronic use of alcohol, anticonvulsants, or isoniazid; or malnourishment in a patient who has received >4 g APAP in any 24-h period
   4. If the patient is not in one of the above groups and has received >7.5–10 g APAP (adults) or >150 mg/kg APAP (children) in any 24-h period
B. Initial laboratory assessment should consist of:
   1. [APAP] immediately if symptomatic or if time of last dose unknown; otherwise, 4 h after last APAP dose or as soon as possible thereafter
   2. AST[b]
   3. PT, electrolytes, glucose, BUN, and creatinine if very ill-appearing or marked elevation of AST
C. On the basis of the initial laboratory assessment, consider the patient at risk (also see below for low-risk subgroup):
   1. If the AST is elevated OR
   2. If the [APAP] is >10 μg/mL
D. Consider the patient at risk, but in a low-risk subgroup:
   1. If [APAP] minimally above 10 μg/mL is the sole abnormality, ie, there are no symptoms and a normal AST OR
   2. If a minimally elevated AST (< 2× normal) is the sole abnormality, ie, there are no symptoms and [APAP] < 10 μg/mL AND
   3. If the patient is reliable and understands the need to return immediately for symptoms or signs consistent with hepatic injury AND
   4. Phone or clinic follow-up is feasible in 24 h

[a]The approach described is that of the author, but contains many controversial elements. It is essential that the reader understand the background as discussed in the text, in order to use these guidelines appropriately.

[b]Early in the clinical course of toxicity, and particularly in certain subgroups, the AST may exceed ALT; therefore, AST is listed as the preferred measure. In most circumstances, however, ALT can be substituted for AST in patient assessment, particularly if nonhepatic sources of AST (eg, rhabdomyolysis) are suspected.

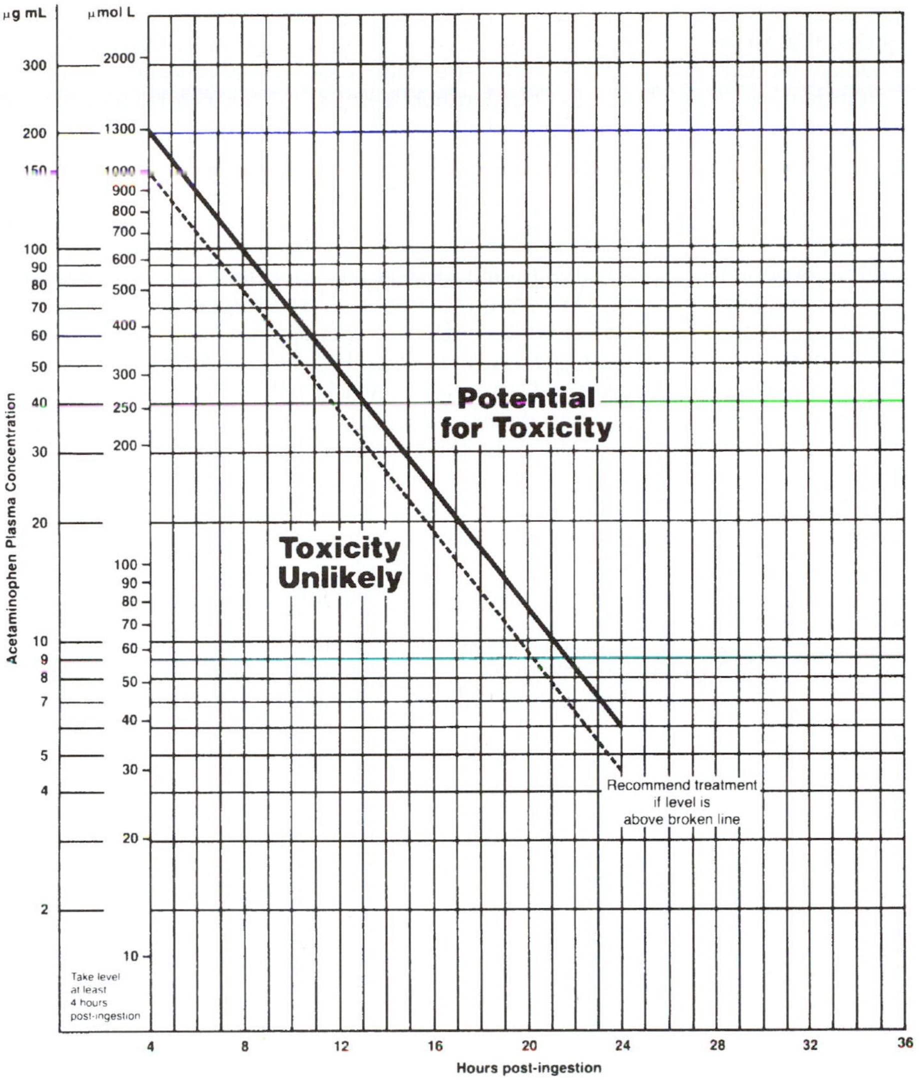

Figure 31–2. Acetaminophen toxicity nomogram: plasma or serum acetaminophen concentration versus time after acetaminophen ingestion. *(Reprinted, with permission, from Management of Acetaminophen Overdose. McNeil Consumer Products Co., 1986.)*

ALT values greater than 1000 IU/L could be separated from those who did not on the basis of initial [APAP]. It was known that APAP elimination followed first-order kinetics, that absorption is generally complete within 4 hours, and that the elimination half-life in those without toxicity is generally less than 4 hours. On the basis of these facts and observations, these authors constructed the nomogram line on a plot of ln[APAP] versus time since ingestion. The line chosen started at an [APAP] of 200 μg/mL, 4 hours postingestion; declined with a 4-hour half-life through 50 μg/mL, 12 hours postingestion; and ended at 6.25 μg/mL, 24 hours after the overdose.

It is important to realize that the line was based on aminotransferase elevation rather than hepatic failure or death and was positioned to be very sensitive, with little regard to specificity. Without antidotal therapy, 60% of those with initial [APAP] above this line will develop aminotransferase values above 1000 IU/L,[127] but the risk is not the same for all such patients. Aminotransferase elevation develops in virtually all patients with [APAP] far above the line, and serious hepatic dysfunction is not uncommon, whereas the incidence of hepatotoxicity among cases with [APAP] values immediately above the line is very low, and the risk of hepatic failure or death far less still.[126,127]

The original line is still used in the United Kingdom and other locations; however, the line used in the United States runs parallel to the original, but has been arbitrarily lowered by 25% in order to add even greater sensitivity.[143] Given the original basis of the nomogram and this subequent change, it is not surprising that the line has proven to be one of the most sensitive screening tools used in medicine. A vanishingly small number of anecdotal cases of nomogram failure involve either special circumstances of increased risk,[29,112] questionable facts, or both. Some authors have suggested that the incidence of nomogram failures may be higher in the United Kingdom, and have recommended that the nomogram in use there is not sensitive enough for high-risk cases.[16,38,174] The validity of this observation has not been adequately studied, but the incidence of nomogram failures in the United States, using the lower line, approaches zero.[152]

On the basis of these observations over 20 years of use, the lower nomogram line is an adequate screening device in nearly all cases and should be rigorously followed. When using the nomogram, it is essential to precisely define the time "window" during which the APAP exposure occurred, and if the time is unknown, to use the earliest possible time as the time of ingestion. Using this approach, patients with [APAP] values below the lower nomogram line, even if only slightly so, do not require further evaluation or treatment for their acute APAP overdose. This applies to most "high-risk" patients, as well. There appears to be adequate experience with acute APAP overdose in the settings of suggested risk factors such as chronic alcohol abuse, chronic medication with anticonvulsants, or inadequate nutrition to recommend that no special approach is required in such cases. Further study will be needed to determine if there are exceptions. Isolated case reports[112] suggest that chronic use of isoniazid, for example, may uniquely predispose[54,186] patients for toxicity after APAP overdose.

The goal should be to determine [APAP] at the earliest point at which it will be meaningful in decision making. To *confirm* risk of toxicity, and thus the need to initiate NAC, that point is 4 hours after ingestion or as soon as possible thereafter. There are no established guidelines for the use of determinations made less than 4 hours after ingestion, and because of variability in absorption such values will have less predictive value. Furthermore, there is no advantage to earlier initiation of therapy because there is no improvement in NAC efficacy when started earlier than 4 hours after the overdose.[154] In light of these facts, there is no advantage to assessing [APAP] earlier in any case in which there is strong suspicion of a significant APAP overdose.

Only if the results of [APAP] determination cannot be obtained within 8 hours of the overdose should history alone be considered adequate to consider the patient at risk and as an indication to start NAC. In such cases, [APAP] should still be determined as soon as possible. When the result becomes available it should be interpreted according to the nomogram, and NAC either continued or discontinued on the basis of this result. In the unusual circumstance that no determination of [APAP] can be obtained, evidence of possible risk by history alone is sufficient to initiate and complete a course of NAC therapy.

Are Determinations of [APAP] Within 4 Hours of Ingestion Useful?

To *exclude* toxicity and the need for antidotal therapy, [APAP] determination less than 4 hours after ingestion may sometimes be useful. This is irrelevant in most cases since the delay to presentation and time required to complete medical clearance usually exceeds 4 hours, but in some circumstances earlier clearance is possible. If there is little evidence to suggest a substantial APAP exposure, and it is feasible and desirable to facilitate more rapid psychiatric evaluation or discharge, determination of [APAP] less than 4 hours after exposure may then be considered. Assays obtained within 1 hour of ingestion are of no value, but between 1 and 4 hours after ingestion, a negligible [APAP] may be sufficient to exclude risk of toxicity without further assessment in many cases. In cases with subsequent [APAP] above the nomogram, values obtained between 1 and 4 hours after ingestion already exceed 100 μg/mL in nearly all cases.[48] These data, studied retrospectively in patients treated with NAC, include several outliers for which early levels were not predictive, however, and thus preclude establishment of firm guidelines. Until further prospective study, it is reasonable to include a safety margin when utilizing early [APAP] determinations. Therefore, when suspicion of consequential APAP overdose is low and there is a compelling reason to consider early [APAP], the author's practice is to consider an [APAP] of 50 μg/mL or less obtained between 1 and 4 hours after exposure adequate to exclude risk of toxicity if there are no extenuating circumstances such as sustained-relief formulation, coingestion of agents that delay gastric emptying and gut motility, or other factors.

How Is Risk Determined if the Time of Ingestion Is Unknown?

Another challenging variation on risk determination is the case in which the time of ingestion simply cannot be determined. Although this is a common initial concern, it is unusual after thoughtful questioning of the patient, family, and others. It is almost always possible to at least establish a time window during which the exposure must have occurred, then to treat the earliest possible time as the time of ingestion for risk-determination purposes. If this time window cannot be established or is so broad that it encompasses a span of more than 24 hours, the following approach is suggested. Determine both the [APAP] and AST. If the AST is elevated, regardless of [APAP], treat with NAC as discussed below. If the [APAP] is <10 μg/mL (or below the lower level of detection) and the AST normal, there is no evidence that subequent consequential hepatic injury is possible, and NAC is unnecessary. Although some have speculated that subsequent liver injury could follow an interval during which [APAP] was negligible and AST was normal, this does not appear to be the case. In all documented cases of serious hepatotoxicity from APAP there has been either delayed elimination of APAP resulting in persistence of measurable levels well beyond 24 hours or early elevation of AST or both.

In the remaining cases, in which there is concern on the basis of the history, the time of ingestion is completely unknown, and [APAP] is above 10 μg/mL (or the lower limit of detection), it is prudent to assume that the patient is at risk. Treatment with NAC should be initiated, but consideration of a shorter course of therapy is appropriate, according to the protocols discussed below.

Is APAP Elimination Half-Life Valuable in Risk Assessment?

There is a clear relationship between the elimination half-life of APAP and hepatotoxicity; therefore, some have advocated determination of half-life as a method of determining risk. A more detailed analysis shows that this is not a valid approach. This concept originated from work showing that among 30 patients with APAP overdose, APAP half-life was > 4 hours in all individuals who developed hepatotoxicity and <4 hours in all those who did not.[132]

There are several features that limit the applicability of these data as justification for use of half-life for screening. Most importantly, these data were serial [APAP] obtained during the 36 hours after overdose, and patients were not treated with NAC. Multiple determinations eliminate errors that are common if half-life is based on only 2 or even 3 values. Measurement over such a long period reflects changes that may take many hours to occur, such as saturation of nontoxic metabolic routes and even slowed metabolism due to incipient liver injury. It is therefore not surprising that half-life is strongly associated with hepatotoxicity. Such data in no way indicate that half-life based on few values obtained early would be at all predictive.

It is also important to realize that this series was reported prior to the availability of an antidote. Certainly observation and serial [APAP] determinations cannot be justified over many hours without initiation of NAC in the interim. Once NAC is initiated, comparison of serial [APAP] with the previous data is impossible, since treatment with NAC alters APAP elimination. After subtoxic APAP doses, clearance of APAP increases slightly while on NAC, but the magnitude of such an effect after APAP overdose is unclear.[150]

Finally, the excellent predictive value of the half-life found in this small study is lost when applied on a large scale. This method, which requires serial venipunctures and many hours, offers no improved predictive value over a single value plotted against the nomogram when the time of ingestion is unknown. In order to equal the sensitivity of the nomogram, a half-life of 2.5 hours, not 4 hours, would need to be used.[156] Even this may not be reliable, as evidenced in a study of cancer patients treated with very high dose APAP followed by NAC rescue.[80] Despite APAP doses from 6 to 20 g/m^2 (200–670 mg/kg) and 4-hour [APAP] as high as 473 μg/mL, the mean elimination half-life of these patients was just under 4 hours with wide variation, indicating that some patients exhibited very short half-life. When time, expense, patient discomfort, and predictive value are considered, there is no reason to consider use of half-life determination when the nomogram can be used instead.

When time of ingestion is unknown and the nomogram cannot be used, use of half-life is tempting but again not of practical value compared to other options. In order to meaningfully determine half-life, at least three [APAP] determinations would be needed, each several hours apart, NAC would need to be started while awaiting final determination of risk, and NAC would be discontinued only in the rare case that the half-life was less than 2.5 hours. Other alternatives, such as consideration of NAC in a short-course protocol (see below), may result in a similar length of stay, less venipuncture, and less risk of errors from inaccurate timing or testing of [APAP] and should be based on patient condition as the final determinant.

How Is Risk Assessed After Overdose of Extended-Relief APAP?

Previously, whether tablets, caplets, capsules, liquids, or suppositories, APAP formulations were all immediate-release preparations (IR APAP) and exposures to these agents formed the basis for the nomogram and a successful diagnostic and therapeutic approach. A new product, Extended Relief Tylenol (ER APAP), consists of an outer 325 mg IR APAP dose of APAP and an inner 325 mg designed for delayed dissolution. These dissolution characteristics have given rise to concern about whether or not the nomogram is an appropriate method to evaluate patients with suspected overdosage of this new agent.

Following discussion with various authorities, the manufacturer has initially recommended measurement of [APAP] with three possible results.[165] If nondetectable, risk of toxicity is excluded. If above the nomogram line, the patient is considered at risk, and NAC initiated. If a detectable value below the nomogram is obtained, the recommendation has been to repeat the [APAP] determination in 4–6 hours, treating with NAC if the second value is above the nomogram, and excluding toxicity if the value is below the line.

This approach, and most analyses that have followed, are based on concern that an initial [APAP] below the line could be followed by a subsequent value above the line, and that failing to recognize a value above the line would place the patient at risk for hepatotoxicity. Critical evaluation of the available information confirms that such nomogram "crossing" is indeed likely; however, despite intuitive concerns, it is not at all clear that this implies risk to the patient.

Whether or not [APAP] is above the nomogram is far less relevant than assessment of the temporal pattern and magnitude of the elevation of [APAP]. The critical threshold for APAP toxicity is dependent on the rate, amount, and duration of NAPQI formation balanced against the supply and regeneration of GSH. The nomogram serves as a marker for risk of reaching that threshold after IR APAP overdoses. In order to compare the risk after ER APAP overdose, it is conceptually useful to separate the first few hours from the subsequent hours in the analysis.

IR APAP results in early, rapid, massive peaks in [APAP], usually within the first 2 hours, which decline steadily thereafter. By the time the [APAP] is plotted on the nomogram after IR APAP overdose, there has already been dramatically increased and sustained NAPQI production and GSH consumption. Volunteer studies clearly show that peak [APAP] and area-under-the-time-versus-concentration-curve (AUC) after ER APAP are far less in the first 4 hours.[47,162] On the basis of time versus concentration curves after actual overdoses of ER APAP, the same appears to be true.[27,175] Therefore, considering for the moment only the NAPQI formation and GSH depletion that occurs in the first few hours, the risk associated with any given 4-hour [APAP] after ER APAP is likely to be far less than for the same [APAP] after IR APAP.

Next, it is important to consider whether subsequent ER APAP metabolism is likely to generate late risk, which might be unanticipated after an initial [APAP] below the nomogram. This would require either delayed massive elevation of [APAP] or delayed sustained moderate elevations of [APAP] sufficient to result in GSH depletion. Neither seems likely to occur. Between 4 and 8 hours, [APAP] declines more slowly after ER APAP than for IR APAP and nomogram "crossings" clearly occur, but subsequent elimination is identical to IR APAP. The duration and magnitude of this *delayed* increased [APAP] after *ER* APAP appears to be quantitatively far less than the duration and magnitude of *early* increased [APAP] after *IR* APAP. Cases of sustained, delayed elimination attributed to ER APAP have been reported,[60] but are no different from what occurs after serious IR APAP overdoses, with delayed elimination resulting from a combination of a very large dose and early APAP-induced liver dysfunction. Thus far, only one reported case fails to fit these reassuring observations.[9] In this case, a dramatic late rise in [APAP] was noted after overdose of ER APAP, IR APAP, NSAIDs, and an anticholinergic agent, suggesting that coingestants may have played a role in the unique [APAP] profile. The actual risk to the patient is difficult to assess since the impressive late rise in [APAP] was brief with rapid decline, and the patient was receiving NAC at the time.

Given the paucity of data regarding ER APAP, it is instructive to look at the IR APAP experience for perspective. First of all, it is important to recognize that the course of [APAP] after IR APAP does not always follow a typical pattern. Not only does nomogram "crossing" occur, but [APAP] occasionally continues to rise more than 4 hours after ingestion.[80,170] When serial levels are obtained, as many as 5% of cases with initial [APAP] below the lower nomogram line may have subsequent determinations above the line (author's unpublished data). Since most patients with an initial [APAP] below the line are medically cleared without a repeat assay, it seems certain that among the thousands of cases screened by this method, many potential nomogram "crossers" have been medically cleared without treatment and without reported subsequent serious toxicity. This is not surprising when the derivation of the nomogram is considered. In almost all cases who "cross" the nomogram after IR APAP or ER APAP overdose, [APAP] is only slightly above the lower line, in a range associated with little or no serious toxicity after IR APAP overdose.[126]

Experience with repeated IR APAP ingestions during a short period may offer further insight. When the formulation of ER APAP is considered, it is evident that its pharmacokinetics closely mimic repeated doses of IR APAP separated by a short interval. Incremental overdoses of IR APAP are not uncommon, although the actual incidence is unknown. Considering the time of the first dose as time zero in order to maximize sensitivity, the nomogram has commonly been used to screen such cases. If ER APAP toxicokinetics are similar to cases of short-term incremental IR APAP overdose, then it is reassuring that the nomogram has proven to be effective in such cases, without reported cases of failure to detect serious risk.

In summary, when considering use of the nomogram as a screening tool for ER APAP overdose, it is unimportant whether reliance upon an initial [APAP] below the line would fail to detect a patient whose subsequent [APAP] would be above the line. What is important is whether reliance upon an initial [APAP] below the line would fail to detect a patient who might develop consequential liver injury. It is evident that a single [APAP] will miss nomogram "crossing," which occurs in a small fraction of ER APAP cases, but because of limited early absorption of APAP and lack of late sustained elevations in [APAP], it is very unlikely that such cases are at risk for toxicity. Therefore, the approach suggested by the manufacturer and described above would certainly be expected to be safe, and it is the view of the author that, unless unusual circumstances are evident, a single [APAP] determination, plotted on the nomogram, is probably adequate to exclude the need for antidotal therapy after ER APAP overdose. This conclusion will require ongoing evaluation, and any new delayed-release APAP formulations will need to be evaluated separately.

How Is Risk Assessed After Repeated or Chronic APAP Overdose?

There are no proven guidelines for risk determination after repeated APAP exposures; nonetheless, there is information that can make these difficult decisions less arbitrary (see Table 31–3). First, it is important to realize that hepatotoxicity from repeated dosing is remarkably rare given the extent of acetaminophen use. Second, despite such patients being only a small fraction of those using APAP, nearly all cases of reported "chronic" APAP toxicity occur within only a few groups: infants with febrile illness who receive excessive dosing,[23,28,31,41,49,68,114,158,164] chronic alcohol users,[3,6,146,189] and patients taking P450-inducing medications chronically.[16] Short-term fasting has also been suggested as a risk factor;[183] however, it is impossible to determine whether fasting is causal, or merely a marker of the severity of other associated conditions. It is striking that outside of these "high-risk" groups, the incidence of serious APAP toxicity after repeated doses is negligible and appears to only follow massive dosing[85,94,100,178] or prolonged excessive dosing.[7,15] Less serious hepatic abnormalities with atypical clinical or histologic features indicating other pathophysiologic mechanisms have been reported at lower doses taken for months to years.[2,11,75]

Thus far, it has been impossible to establish an upper limit for safe repeated dosing. Unlike acute dosing, not only is the total dose important but apparently so are the interval between dosing and the duration of dosing. When interindividual variations such as P450 activity, GSH supply, and regeneration capacity are considered, predicting the dose that will reach the critical threshold for the development of toxicity becomes impossible. Analysis has been further complicated by the likelihood of unreliable information. A substantial proportion of these cases involve parental dosing errors, iatrogenic errors, alcoholics, litigants in product liability cases, and other situations in which those providing the history may be unable or unwilling to accurately describe the dosing. Furthermore, because liver injury often accompanies alcoholism, acute infectious illnesses, and even other medication use, it is unclear in which cases APAP is causative, contributory, or completely unrelated to the hepatotoxicity. Ultimately, resolution of this problem will require development of other laboratory markers of impending toxicity but no such methods are yet available.

When there is concern about toxicity risk after repeated excessive APAP dosing, many approaches have been suggested, but none has been adequately studied. Conceptually, the goal should be to select patients at risk on the basis of dosing history and other risk factors, and then to use limited laboratory testing to determine need for NAC. A logical screening laboratory evaluation consists of determination of [APAP] and AST, with additional testing as indicated by these results and other clinical features. As discussed below (see treatment), the objective is to identify the two conditions that would warrant NAC therapy: remaining APAP yet to be metabolized, or potential serious liver injury. Obviously, since many patients being evaluated for a variety of conditions have detectable [APAP], the predictive value of this approach depends almost entirely on proper selection of patients at risk.

The first consideration when evaluating a patient with a history of repeated excessive APAP dosing is the presence or absence of signs or symptoms of hepatotoxicity. Regardless of risk factors or dosing history, such findings should prompt laboratory evaluation. This is particularly important since most reported cases of serious toxicity after repeated dosing have been symptomatic for more than 24 hours prior to diagnosis, and earlier diagnosis should improve outcome. In the asymptomatic patient, the next consideration should be the presence or absence of risk factors that predispose to toxicity. This is most important because of the near absence of reported toxicity in cases outside these groups. In fact, it is likely that the adult dosing threshold for laboratory evaluation of asymptomatic patients without risk factors should be at least 7.5 g, and perhaps as high as 10–12 g, in any 24-hour period.[96]

Despite the lack of verifiable data, logic and respect for anecdotal reports justify use of a lower threshold in patients with risk factors. Although some retrospective series and some reports from litigation suggest that toxicity can occur after recommended dosing, this has not been supported by other major studies or personal experience. Therefore, it is reasonable to use the recommended upper limit of daily APAP dosing (4 g in adults; 75 mg/kg in children) as a cutoff for considering laboratory evaluation of asymptomatic, high-risk patients. The duration of dosing, any occurrence of large bolus dosing, the presence of multiple risk factors, and other features almost certainly affect risk, but until they can be factored in, the lowest logical risk cutoff seems appropriate. These amounts are almost certainly substantially less than that required to cause toxicity,[96] but it is prudent to start from this sensitive cutoff while better screening strategies are developed. We currently use this approach in alcoholics, patients taking anticonvulsants or isoniazid, and infants and young children with febrile illnesses. Others deserving similar consideration include those with chronic malnutrition, HIV infection, or other conditions that lead to GSH depletion.

Using the strategy described here, patients with elevated AST values are considered at risk, regardless of [APAP]. Therefore, the [APAP] in this setting is useful in patients with normal AST values as a tool to determine only whether there is sufficient remaining APAP to lead to subsequent NAPQI formation and delayed hepatotoxicity. In most cases, this is essentially a qualitative assessment of the presence or absence of APAP, since the numerical value of [APAP] is usually difficult to interpret. In rare cases of repeated dosing, [APAP] will be above the nomogram when plotted as if the case were an acute overdose. If so, obviously NAC is indicated. In other cases, [APAP] will be nondetectable, obviating the need for NAC if the AST is normal.

In most cases of repeated excessive dosing, however, [APAP] is usually intermediate between these two conditions. When this is the case, [APAP] is used only to dichotomize between patients with significant remaining APAP and those who have completed APAP metabolism. Because there is no evidence in the literature or experience that a patient with [APAP]<10 μg/mL and a normal AST has the potential to develop subsequent consequential liver injury, this value is appropriate as a sensitive cutoff to define presence or absence of remaining APAP.

Although the above approach has not been studied, the decision to treat patients who have any remaining APAP or any elevation of AST is likely to prove very conservative (ie, sensitive but not specific), particularly because of recent APAP dosing and comorbidity likely to elevate AST (eg, ethanol use, infectious illness). An alternative strategy in reliable patients after repeated ingestions may be to treat only patients with elevated AST or extraordinarily high [APAP]. For patients without AST elevation and with typical midrange [APAP], risk is likely to be low enough to forgo NAC and instead to arrange for a repeat AST in 24 hours, with careful instructions to return immediately if symptoms arise. These and other possible approaches require thoughtful study.

Unlike the acute overdose setting, patients at risk for toxicity after repeated excessive dosing are more likely to already be symptomatic upon presentation because of time elapsed during the days of their ingestion period. Such cases will not be missed by a thoughtful evaluation. Careful history, physical examination, and the laboratory approach described above should include nearly all patients at risk. The theoretical patient with impending toxicity but without signs or symptoms of toxicity, who might be missed by the above approach, can still be detected in a timely manner by appropriate patient discharge instruction and follow-up.

How Should Risk be Assessed in Children?

Serious hepatotoxicity after acute overdose is clearly less common in children than in adults, but it is unclear whether this reflects relative hepatoprotection or merely results from differences in the characteristics of poisoning in children. Although some data suggest that children are relatively protected from toxicity after acute overdose, closer evaluation shows this to be unresolved. Serious hepatotoxicity or death after acute APAP overdose is reported in children, but is extremely rare. When all cases with initial [APAP] above the lower nomogram are considered, the incidence of hepatotoxicity is lower in children under 5 years of age than in adults.[139] This comparison is valid only if the two groups are comparably stratified by [APAP] and delay to NAC, and this is not the case with pediatric APAP overdose. Despite the enormous number of reported pediatric APAP exposures, there are insufficient documented cases with very high [APAP] and comparable delays to NAC to allow this comparison.

Although limited by methodology, recent studies advocate increasing the threshold APAP dose for screening after pediatric acute overdose to 200 mg/kg.[10] Similarly, because of the paucity of reported toxicity, some have recommended that children be screened using the original, higher, nomogram. Although both of these suggestions are statistically likely to be safe, we advocate continued use of 150 mg/kg as the risk-defining dose and use of the lower nomogram line for [APAP] screening until valid data demonstrate children to be selectively protected, or accumulated experience with 200 mg/kg as a dose threshold for screening proves safe.

If, in fact, children are protected after acute overdose, several theories have been advanced to account for it. In adults, APAP glucuronidation exceeds sulfation (60% to 30%); in young children, sulfation is much greater and the ratio may even be reversed. The relatively greater proportion of sulfate conjugation in young children[103] has been suggested as protective; however, the sulfation/glucuronide ratio itself should not make a difference unless it results in less oxidative metabolism to NAPQI. This has not been shown.[176] A more likely explanation would be the increased glutathione supply and regenerative capacity of children.[82]

Following excessive repeated APAP dosing, there is no evidence that children are relatively protected; in fact, infants and children with acute febrile illnesses comprise one of the few groups in which toxicity after repeated excessive dosing has been described.[23,28,31,41,49,68,114,158,164] Common sources of dosing errors include substitution of adult for pediatric preparations, substitution of drops for elixir, overzealous dosing by amount or frequency in attempts to maximize effect, and failure to read the label and dose carefully. As in all examples of repeated dosing toxicity, the precise dosing pattern required to produce risk is unclear. In nearly all cases, the reported doses associated with toxicity are more than 150 mg/kg/day and generally much higher. Particularly in reports of lesser dosing, confounding factors make dose determination and APAP attribution extremely difficult.

Toxicity after repeated excessive dosing in febrile children may simply reflect that this is the most common setting for pediatric APAP use and that children are at greater relative risk for excessive dosing because of their size. In the absence of pediatric cases outside this group and in light of the paucity of toxicity in normal adults after repeated excessive dosing, it is appropriate to consider whether acute febrile illness predisposes to toxicity. It is logical that oxidative drug metabolism and glutathione supply would be affected by inflammatory oxidant stress and short-term fasting during febrile infectious illnesses, but this relationship is complex and not well-defined. Chronic infectious diseases, particularly HIV-related, have been associated with glutathione depletion, but this has not been evident during acute illness.[125] Among reported cases, it is likely that hepatic injury is the result of the infectious illness in some, the result of APAP in others, and the result of both in still others. The relative contributions of the underlying illness and APAP in these cases is currently difficult to determine and an area of important research.

Although extremely rare, reports of serious hepatoxicity in children necessitate vigilance and the need to develop a reasonable strategy for screening. Because acute febrile illness is an important feature, and because there is no credible evidence that recommended therapeutic dosing of APAP poses a risk, a preliminary strategy can be proposed. Our practice is to consider measurement of [APAP] and AST in any child with acute febrile illness and reported dosing that exceeds 75 mg/kg in any 24-hour period, or if symptoms or signs of hepatotoxicity are evident, regardless of dosing. This suggested cutoff for screening is well below an amount actually expected to produce toxicity in order to provide a sensitive screening strategy. Results of this screening are used as in the case of multiple dosing described above.

How Does Ethanol Use Alter Risk Determination?

The effect of ethanol on APAP toxicity is complex and best described by clearly separating experimental animal data from actual human overdose, acute from chronic ethanol abuse, and acute from repeated excessive APAP dosing. Although not entirely consistent, most animal data indicate that acute ethanol co-administration with APAP may be somewhat hepatoprotective,[169,173] presumably by competitive inhibition of P450 APAP metabolism to NAPQI. Chronic ethanol dosing in animal models, however, increases risk from acute APAP dosing,[87,146,173] on the basis of induced P450 APAP metabolism or decreased GSH supply or regeneration.[83]

After acute APAP overdose, these factors appear to be of little importance.[140,153,168] Although it has been suggested that toxicity may be less after ethanol-containing

APAP formulations,[139] these data lack power and there is no evidence that co-ingestion of ethanol significantly alters the course of human acute APAP overdose. More interestingly, there is also no evidence that chronic ethanol use should alter the approach after acute overdose. Due to failure of the higher original nomogram to adequately screen alcoholics and those chronically taking anticonvulsants, some have suggested that a much lower standard be used.[29,38,174] There is only one reported case of nomogram "failure" in an alcoholic using the lower nomogram line, and the actual events of the case are unclear.[29,152] Furthermore, unpublished data from a large series revealed no difference in incidence of hepatotoxicity among groups identified as chronic, acute, or acute and chronic ethanol users, and ethanol nonusers.[153] These observations indicate that the lower nomogram line is adequately sensitive for screening after acute overdose, regardless of ethanol use.

Chronic ethanol abuse does appear to impact toxicity after repeated excessive APAP dosing.[3,6,146,189] Characterization of this relationship has been complicated by the challenges of obtaining accurate histories in alcoholics, failure to exclude non-APAP causes of hepatotoxicity, and other factors in many cases. These limitations prevent valid definition of the APAP dosing likely to cause toxicity, but the literature and personal experience confirm increased risk in alcoholics after excessive APAP dosing. An approach to screening is discussed above (see repeated or chronic overdose).

Given the prevalence of both ethanol and APAP use, this remains perhaps the most important unresolved issue in risk determination after APAP. Resolution will require innovative methods of risk determination, but also clear case definition and meticulous recording of relevant clinical data. We have observed cases of definite end-stage alcoholic liver disease erroneously attributed to APAP as well as apparent APAP-induced fulminant liver failure erroneously attributed to ethanol use. A public health issue of this importance deserves a much less haphazard approach to study.

A Final Comment Regarding Difficult Risk Determination

Although early NAC is optimum, there is now clear evidence that delayed treatment is beneficial.[77] Therefore, even when a decision not to treat with NAC has been made, careful discharge instructions and appropriate short-term follow-up to detect early signs of hepatotoxicity serve as an additional safety net for patients. This is particularly important in the case of those possibly at higher risk after repeated excessive dosing (eg, alcoholics, those taking P450-inducing medications, fasted or malnourished patients, young children) and when the ingestion involves new delayed-release APAP formulations. While further data are gathered and the approach to atypical presentations is refined and validated, the current lack of proven guidelines dictates the wisdom of assuring close follow-up when admission and treatment are not indicated.

Assessing Actual Toxicity: What are the Critical Components of the Diagnostic Approach?

Earlier protocols and guidelines recommended extensive and ongoing laboratory assessment after APAP overdose.[88,143] On the basis of the pathophysiology and time course of toxicity, a simplified and far more cost-effective approach is logical.

What Initial Testing is Appropriate?

As outlined above, patients with acute APAP overdose and no indication of evident hepatotoxicity should have [APAP] measured, but require no other initial laboratory assessment. Patients found to be at risk by use of the nomogram or by history (in the case of repeated excessive dosing), or those suspected to already have mild hepatotoxicity by history and physical examination should then have AST measured. The first AST determination serves as a screen to detect already established serious liver injury, which may require closer monitoring, and, as mentioned, is also a key component of decision making after repeated excessive dosing and other unusual circumstances.

Unless there is evident serious hepatotoxicity, AST is sufficient, and no additional testing is initially needed. Death of hepatocytes, resulting in release of measurable hepatic enzymes, precedes all cases of serious liver dysfunction. Abnormalities of other markers have been suggested to precede AST elevation, but there is no evidence that their detection benefits the patient.[5] Renal toxicity may occur without significant hepatotoxicity; however, at least minimal AST elevation nearly always precedes evidence of nephrotoxicity.[33] Exceptions[26,78,131] are so rare that routine screening of renal function in the absence of AST elevation is unnecessary.

We have noted many cases in which minor hepatic abnormalities such as elevated bilirubin or prothrombin time (PT) are noted in patients with normal AST after APAP overdose. Preexisting conditions, laboratory error, and possible interference with the PT assay by NAC[73] make it unclear in these sporadic cases whether these abnormalities are related to APAP effects. Even in these cases, if consequential liver injury does develop, AST elevation precedes serious liver dysfunction.

What Testing is Needed for Ongoing Monitoring?

If no AST elevation is noted, repeated AST determination every 24 hours until completion of treatment is sufficient, without other biochemical testing. If AST elevation is noted, then PT should be measured and repeated every 24 hours, or more frequently if clinically indicated. Other liver tests such as GGT, alkaline phosphatase, LDH, and bilirubin, which are useful when determining the etiology of liver abnormalities, will be abnormal in cases of serious APAP-induced hepatotoxicity but provide little additional useful information if the etiology is certain.

If AST exceeds 1000 IU/L or PT elevation is noted, then monitoring BUN and creatinine is warranted. If evidence of actual liver failure is noted, then careful monitoring of blood glucose and acid–base status is important, in addition to meticulous bedside evaluation to detect and document vital signs, neurologic status, and evidence of bleeding. Many additional tests may be useful in the setting of liver failure, on the basis of clinical condition and local protocols. Testing for other rare APAP-associated conditions by electrocardiograph, amylase determination, or other studies should be on a case-by-case basis only.

How Is Prognosis Assessed?

The availability and success of liver transplantation after APAP-induced liver failure has created an important unmet need for early prognostic assessment. Survival without transplantation is certain if AST is normal at the time of NAC initiation,[154] but while this identifies patients at the lowest risk, the converse is of no value in identifying those who will not survive without transplant. Earlier reports described poor prognostic features that are sensitive but inadequately specific, and based on findings too late in the course to be useful.[32] Efforts to determine earlier or more specific markers of poor prognosis have improved our understanding; however, accurate early prediction of need for transplant remains one of the greatest challenges related to APAP toxicity.

One strategy utilizes a combination of clinical features of fulminant hepatic failure. The single criteria of pH < 7.30 after fluid and hemodynamic resuscitation or the combination of PT > 100 seconds (approximately equal to 1.8 × control US standard), creatinine > 3.3 mg/dL, and grade III or IV encephalopathy is extremely predictive of a patient who will die without transplant.[96,116] Any patient meeting these criteria should be considered for transplant. Other prognostic strategies utilize only the coagulation profile, in an attempt to simplify the approach, and more importantly to allow earlier intervention. Using this approach, a markedly abnormal PT that continues to rise on the fourth day after overdose indicates a very poor prognosis.[65] In most cases, other poor prognostic criteria will be evident by that time, but occasionally time will be saved. For earlier screening, others have suggested that any patient whose PT in seconds exceeds the number of hours since ingestion should be considered at extreme risk.[113] Attempts to correlate individual clotting factor levels or ratios have shown promise; however, these correlates appear to offer no benefit over use of PT alone.[14,117]

Interpretation of PT must include awareness of therapy. Use of vitamin K does not confuse interpretation. If it is effective, it implies that transplant is unnecessary since viable liver remains. If vitamin K is ineffective, PT can be used as above. Transfusion of exogenous clotting factors, such as fresh frozen plasma (FFP), obviously alters interpretation because improvement in PT may not indicate any improvement in liver function. Depending on the volume of factors transfused, the subsequent decline in factors must be considered when interpreting PT values. The prognostic importance of monitoring PT in this setting suggests that FFP should be given only for evidence of bleeding, risk of bleeding from known concomitant trauma, or prior to invasive procedures, but not merely on the basis of the PT value.

As mentioned above, survivors regenerate normal liver, and as a result, no long-term laboratory monitoring is indicated, once return to adequate function is demonstrated.

Treatment

What General Treatment Is Appropriate?

Decisions regarding gastrointestinal decontamination are discussed elsewhere (see Chap. 4) and these principles apply to APAP overdose. In cases of very early presentation (< 1 hour), ingestion of delayed-release formulations, or co-ingestion of agents that delay GI absorption, there may be rare patients for whom gastric emptying is appropriate. In general, however, gastric emptying is rarely a consideration for patients with isolated APAP overdose because of the very rapid gastrointestinal absorption of APAP and the availability of an excellent antidote (see Table 31–4).

The role of activated charcoal after APAP overdose has been controversial because of concern that activated charcoal, administered to adsorb APAP, might also adsorb orally administered NAC enough to limit its antidotal effect (see Antidotes in Depth: Activated Charcoal). This led many to recommend that activated charcoal not be used following APAP overdose. Closer examination of the issue suggests that this concern is unfounded for several reasons.

In a large fraction of cases, there should be no potential conflict since the time period after ingestion during which activated charcoal would be used does not overlap with administration of NAC. There is no known value to the use of activated charcoal as a method of speeding APAP elimination, so in this setting its only role is to limit GI absorption, and use of activated charcoal is logical only if ongoing APAP absorption is likely. In nearly all isolated IR APAP overdoses, GI absorption can be considered complete by 4 hours after ingestion; thus there is no value to activated charcoal beyond that point. Because there is no loss of NAC efficacy unless started more than 8 hours after ingestion,[154] there is no difficulty in separating an activated charcoal dose from the initial NAC dose.

If delayed or repeated activated charcoal dosing is indicated because of suspected delayed absorption or co-ingestants, then the strategy of separating any NAC and activated charcoal doses by 1–2 hours is logical, as long as it can be accomplished safely. NAC is quickly well-absorbed high in the GI tract and unlikely to interact with activated charcoal if the doses are not simultaneous.

In unusual cases, due to co-ingestants and timing of presentation, it may be important to administer NAC and activated charoal simultaneously, and it is these cases that pose theoretical concerns. There is clear in vitro evidence of activated charcoal to NAC bind-

TABLE 31–4. SUGGESTED NAC TREATMENT APPROACH[a] AFTER RISK DETERMINATION AS DESCRIBED IN TABLES 31–2 AND 31–3

This approach applies to patients with either acute or repeated APAP dosing.

I. For patients not at risk by any criteria listed in Tables 31–2 and 31–3:
   A. They may be medically cleared relative to APAP toxicity
   B. Advise the patient to return immediately if he/she develops signs or symptoms consistent with hepatic injury

II. For patients in low-risk subgroup after repeated ingestions as described in Table 31–3:
   A. Advise the patient to return immediately if he/she develops signs or symptoms consistent with hepatic injury
   B. Arrange phone or clinic follow-up, as appropriate, in 24 h
   C. If signs or symptoms do subsequently develop, initiate laboratory assessment and reassess for risk as described in Table 31–3

III. For all other patients at risk as described in Tables 31–2 and 31–3:
   A. Initiate oral/enteral NAC
   B. Consider IV NAC:[b]
      1. If the patient exhibits hepatic failure
      2. If the patient is pregnant[b]*
      3. If 8 or more hours have elapsed since the APAP ingestion and the patient is unable to retain oral/enteral NAC
   C. At time of admission and every 24 h: Determine AST. Assess PT and other chemistries as indicated by the clinical condition
   D. If all preceding AST values are normal: Determine AST and [APAP] 36 h after the time of the most recent APAP ingestion[b]

IV. Selection of NAC treatment protocol:
   A. Standard United States protocol: 17 doses (68 h) oral/enteral NAC following the loading dose (see Antidotes in Depth: *N*-Acetylcysteine)
   B. Appropriate circumstances for consideration of alternative protocols:[b]
      1. Short-course NAC: On the basis of assessment done 36 h after most recent APAP ingestion, if the [APAP] < 10 μg/mL, AST is normal, and the patient is not pregnant; discontinue NAC; otherwise continue NAC**
      2. Modified traditional course NAC: On the basis of daily assessment, if, at any time, the AST is elevated but no hepatic failure develops, and the patient is not pregnant; treat with NAC until the AST returns to normal or for 17 doses (68 h)—whichever is first**
      3. Long-course NAC: If the patient develops hepatic failure; treat with IV NAC until the INR is < 2 and encephalopathy, if present, is resolving

[a]The approach described is that of the author, but contains many controversial elements. It is essential that the reader understand the background as discussed in the text, in order to use these guidelines appropriately.

[b]Denotes particularly controversial elements that differ from the traditional approach in the United States. See text for discussion.

*Editors' Note: Currently there is inadequate scientific evidence to justify routine deviation from the use of oral NAC in pregnancy.

**Editors' Note: Currently there is inadequate scientific evidence to justify routine deviation from the use of the 72-hour oral NAC regimen.

ing,[30,79,144] and volunteer data suggest that activated charcoal causes statistically significant decreases in NAC absorption;[50] however, there is no evidence that this interaction is clinically significant.[161] There is no study of patients with serious APAP overdose designed to investigate this issue; however, indirect information is available which suggests that even simultaneous activated charcoal and NAC is unlikely to cause consequential decrease in NAC availability.

Animal data demonstrate that the amount of NAC needed is dependent on the amount of APAP ingested.[119] If the NAC dose given were very close to the threshold of efficacy, then adsorption of a fraction of the NAC to activated charcoal would likely be significant. It appears, however, that the dosing protocol routinely used in the United States far exceeds the NAC dose actually needed, suggesting that partial adsorption of NAC by activated charcoal would still result in an effective dose. This is suggested by the observation that all patients treated with NAC within 8 hours of overdose have similar excellent outcome, with no decrease in efficacy even after massive overdose. In fact the incidence of hepatotoxicity is the same whether the initial [APAP] is below the nomogram or is above 500 μg/mL.[154]

General supportive care consists primarily of control of nausea and vomiting. There are no well-controlled studies to determine choice of optimal antiemetic agent and dose. Because of the time-critical nature of NAC dosing, choice of agent and dose may differ from other circumstances in which a stepwise trial of increasing antiemetic potency and dose might be appropriate. After APAP overdose, patients with very high [APAP] who are approaching or beyond 8 hours from ingestion but still vomiting are placed at greater risk by subsequent delays in NAC administration. These patients should be treated with a potent antiemetic at moderate or high dose if oral NAC is to be tried. If oral NAC is then vomited, a loading dose of IV NAC should be considered, despite the lack of a formulation intended for IV use in the United States (see below). Unless significant liver injury is already evident, vomiting generally resolves within 12–16 hours after ingestion, so that subsequent oral dosing can be accomplished.

The remainder of general treatment issues relate to the management of hepatic injury, renal dysfunction, and the other rare manifestations listed above. Treatment of these problems is based on general principles and is not APAP-dependent. Discussion of the management of liver failure is clearly beyond the scope of this chapter; however, certain aspects deserve mention. Monitoring for and treatment of hypoglycemia due to liver failure is critical and represents one of the most readily treatable of the life-threatening effects of liver failure. If there are adequate viable hepatocytes, vitamin K may produce some improvement in coagulopathy; thus trial dosing is logical as liver injury develops and as it resolves. As mentioned above, administration of FFP should be based on specific indications rather than upon the PT alone.

One of the most important advances in care has been the use of NAC to treat fulminant hepatic failure, discussed in detail below. Parenteral NAC, other advances in supportive care, and successful liver transplantation programs appear to have substantially improved survival.[96]

How Does *N*-Acetylcysteine Work?

Conceptually, it is helpful to think of NAC as serving two separate roles. First, NAC *prevents* toxicity by limiting the formation of NAPQI, but more importantly, by increasing the capacity to detoxify NAPQI that is formed. Second, NAC *treats* toxicity through nonspecific mechanisms that preserve multiorgan function in liver failure. The mechanisms by which NAC prevents and treats toxicity are noted in Figure 31–1 in relation to APAP metabolism.

NAC prevents toxicity by serving as a glutathione precursor, leading to increased GSH availability.[81] NAC can also serve as a GSH substitute, combining with NAPQI and being converted to cysteine and mercaptate conjugates, just as GSH is.[22] NAC may also lead to increased substrate for nontoxic sulfation, allowing increased metabolism by this route and thus less by oxidation to NAPQI.[150] In a mouse model, NAC may actually reverse NAPQI oxidation,[34] but there is no evidence of this process in humans.

Each of these preventive mechanisms must be in place early, and none is of benefit once NAPQI has initiated cell injury. Time is required to saturate nontoxic metabolism, form excessive NAPQI, and deplete GSH; thus there is a window of opportunity after overdose during which NAC can be initiated prior to the onset of liver injury, without any loss of efficacy. Based on large clinical trials, it appears that NAC efficacy is nearly complete as long as it is initiated within 8 hours of the overdose.[154] In fact, there is no evident difference in efficacy between NAC started 0–2 hours, compared to 2–4, 4–6, or 6–8 hours after ingestion.[155] Therefore, delays in NAC initiation that might result from gastrointestinal decontamination or awaiting results of [APAP] determination pose no harm to the patient, as long as NAC can be started within 8 hours of the overdose.

Although no side-by-side comparative studies have been done, historical comparisons indicate that all suggested NAC treatment protocols, as well as earlier methionine or cysteamine protocols appear to be equally effective if started within 8 hours of overdose.[127,130,151,154] Efficacy then decreases in a stepwise fashion with further delays. Compared with historical controls, late methionine and cysteamine were ineffective and possibly harmful, and there was no benefit to the 20-hour IV NAC protocol if started more than 15 hours after the overdose.[127] These findings presumably reflect the time course of events that are preventable by early NAC and led to the conclusion that later treatment was of no value.

Several subsequent observations illustrated that NAC has other mechanisms of action that are effective even after NAPQI formation and binding. In a large clinical trial of the 17-dose oral NAC protocol,[153] it was noted that the severity of hepatotoxicity among high-risk patients first treated with NAC between 16 and 24 hours after overdose was far less than had been observed in untreated historical controls or patients treated with the 20-hour IV NAC protocol.[127] Other experimental work showed that even after cell injury had been initiated, late interventions could diminish hepatocyte injury.[21] Most significantly, in a prospective, randomized trial, British investigators found that even after fulminant hepatic failure was evident, starting IV NAC diminished the need for vasopressors, as well as the incidences of cerebral edema and death.[77]

These dramatic findings were accompanied by a fascinating observation. Despite improved organ function and survival in the NAC-treated group, there was no apparent difference in the degree of hepatic injury. Enzyme elevations and PT were equivalent in the two groups, suggesting that much of the NAC benefit may not have been derived from lessening of hepatic injury. Further investigation supported this hypothesis, showing that oxygen delivery and utilization in extrahepatic organs was enhanced by NAC.[43,66,160]

Whether on the basis of its nonspecific antioxidant effects, enhanced GSH supply, or more likely its role in mediating microvascular tone, NAC results in improved organ function in several organs affected by multisystem failure. Perhaps most importantly, NAC appears to be the agent of choice for cerebral edema after liver failure.[182] With aggressive hemodynamic treatment, hemodialysis and availability of blood products, cerebral edema remains the most feared and most lethal manifestation of liver failure. In this setting, NAC may preserve cerebral blood flow and perfusion better than traditional therapies such as mannitol and hyperventilation, which may actually be detrimental.

How Long Should NAC Be Given?

Known mechanisms of action and the observation that all studied durations of NAC have been effective when started early suggest that shorter courses of treatment are effective when NAC is used for its early, preventive actions (see Table 31–4). In contrast, both the oral NAC data and the liver failure study seem to confirm the importance of longer duration of NAC when treating already established liver injury. In fact, except for duration of treatment, the IV NAC dosing protocol that demonstrated late benefit in liver failure[77] is the same as that previously found to be of no value after 15 hours.[127] In the earlier study, NAC was stopped after 20 hours; in the liver failure study, it was continued until resolution of hepatic failure or death. The above observations suggest that, rather than a single duration of therapy for all patients, it is appropriate to utilize varying treatment protocols, selected on the basis of the clinical course of the patient.

All available information indicates that the conceptual basis for discontinuing NAC should be the completion of APAP metabolism and the absence or resolution of consequential liver injury. The challenge lies in translating these concepts into reliable practical guidelines and in the lack of formal study of such guidelines. In the United States, only the 17-dose oral NAC regimen has been studied or used on a large scale. Results from the traditional use of the 20-hour IV NAC protocol in the United Kingdom,[127] a 48-hour IV NAC protocol studied in the United States,[151] and other "short-course" dosing protocols[185] indicate that NAC therapy of shorter duration than the current United States standard may be safe and effective in many patients.

Currently, the only formally studied standard treatment protocols are those listed above, all of which are based on a standard predetermined duration of NAC. In the United States, only the 17 dose (72-hour) oral NAC protocol is traditionally used (see Table 31–5). The alternative approach described below uses the clinical course of the patient to define the length of NAC therapy. It has been used for several years by the author, ***but it should be clearly understood that it is a departure from routine guidelines and has not been formally studied.*** It is presented here as an alternative in current use and to introduce important conceptual features that should form the basis for future protocol refinement.

The first criterion for discontinuation of NAC should be the completion of APAP metabolism, and measurement of [APAP] is the only widely available method to make this assessment. Although it is theoretically possible that intrahepatic APAP might remain after circulating [APAP] is negligible, there is no evidence that this is consequential. Therefore, [APAP] less than 10 μg/mL is adequate to define the completion of APAP metabolism and exclude risk of subsequent substantial conversion of APAP to NAPQI.

The second criterion for discontinuation of NAC should be the determination that there is no consequential hepatotoxicity and that none will develop, or if it has developed, that it has resolved. As described above, the most practical measure for confirmation or exclusion of liver injury is AST, whereas the measures of liver function such as PT are more appropriate to confirm resolution of serious hepatotoxicity.

Risk of serious hepatic injury can be excluded in patients who show no elevation of AST, if adequate time has passed to exclude the possibility of subsequent significant AST rise. Defining the time point at which subsequent development of liver injury can be excluded is controversial. There are anecdotal descriptions of the time course of AST rise[126,142] and some case series data;[149] however, there are *no comprehensive studies to define the latest point at which liver injury may become evident.* On the basis of these reports and extensive experience, the author has used the conservative figure of 36 hours after ingestion as the time at which all cases of AST elevation should be evident. While it is likely that serious liver injury is always evident sooner than this, a conservative approach seems warranted until further study because of the need to provide a safety net for outliers, errors in history or laboratory timing, and other factors.

Regardless of the acuity or chronicity of the ingestion, the risk characteristics of the patient, the delay to presentation, or other factors that may have impact on outcome, the above criteria should apply. Therefore, in any patient determined to be at risk and treated with NAC, clearance of measurable APAP and continued normal AST values 36 hours after the most recent ingestion seem adequate to exclude risk of serious hepatotoxicity and adequate to justify discontinuation of NAC. Depending on circumstances and the delay to presentation, this may represent a duration of NAC treatment ranging from 0 to 36 hours. Many who use predetermined 20-hour or 24-hour dosing protocols instead recommend reevaluation at the completion of therapy, resulting in a similar net result in most cases. Refinement and validation of these guidelines will be an important area of research.

The aminotransferases of approximately half of all NAC-treated patients with [APAP] above the nomogram line will remain below 100 IU/L.[155] Therefore, the use of a "short-course" of NAC may be appropriate in a large proportion of cases, substantially shortening hospital stays without subjecting the patient to any increased risk.

In contrast, for patients with liver failure IV NAC is recommended (see below) to be continued until the INR is less than 2 and encephalopathy, if present, is nearly resolved.[96] This approach usually results in NAC dosing that continues well beyond other traditional endpoints.

Current information indicates that "short-course" NAC may be appropriate for those with no hepatotoxicity and that very long-course NAC is appropriate for those who develop liver failure. The most difficult approach to define is that for those in between, with increased AST but no liver failure. For these cases, "short-course" therapy seems inappropriate given the superiority of the 17-dose oral protocol over the 20-hour IV protocol for high-risk cases. Among patients without liver failure, there are no reports of deterioration after completion of the 17-dose protocol; thus, there is no indication that such cases benefit from NAC beyond the 17-dose duration. Because of the proven safety and efficacy of the 17-dose duration of NAC, use of this protocol seems the most logical for these patients. In the author's practice, on the basis of daily laboratory testing, NAC is discontinued sooner if all liver abnormalities completely resolve and treatment extended until resolution if liver failure develops.

Given the current understanding of these issues and the extensive experience outside the United States, using a shorter course of NAC for appropriate patients is easily justified. Nonetheless, it must be recognized that definitive comparitive studies have not been done. As a result,

TABLE 31–5. ADMINISTRATION OF ORAL *N*-ACETYLCYSTEINE (MUCOMYST) IN ACETAMINOPHEN OVERDOSE

How supplied

As 10% (10 g/100 mL) or 20% (20 g/100 mL) solution

Dosing

Loading	140 mg/kg
Maintenance	70 mg/kg every 4 h, for 17 doses

Administration

Dilute each dose 1:4 (for 20% concentration) with water, carbonated beverage, or fruit juice to make a 5% concentration (chilled is more palatable).

Repeat dose if patient vomits within 1 h of administration.

Try antiemetic (eg, metoclopramide) if vomiting persists.

Use nasogastric tube if vomiting persists.

a thoughtful, circumspect analysis is always warranted. Use of a longer course of therapy is safe, and it is appropriate in any case in which there is suspicion of unusual circumstances. For example, there are theoretical reasons why pregnancy should be considered a contraindication to short-course therapy. Maternal course may not reflect the condition of the fetus,[62,137] and there is suspicion that NAC may provide limited sulfhydryls to the fetus.[74,147] It seems prudent, therefore, to continue therapy for the full 17-dose duration.

What Is the Ideal Route of Administration for NAC?

As with many issues related to APAP toxicity, the choice of oral versus intravenous NAC is not a simple one. Available information suggests that there are advantages and disadvantages to each, and settings in which each may be preferable. Understanding the risks and benefits of each route is necessary to a rational approach.

Safety is the best understood of these issues; oral NAC is clearly safer. Nausea or vomiting, common prior to NAC, is present in about half of patients treated with oral NAC and diarrhea is also prevalent, but there is no credible evidence of more serious complications.[102] Reports of skin rash and extraordinary complications have occurred but are so rare as to be insignificant. In contrast, intravenous NAC has been clearly associated with anaphylactoid reactions including rash, bronchospasm, hypotension, and death.[4,40,45,98,151] Fortunately, these serious complications are now known to be dose and concentration dependent and eliminated by slow administration of dilute NAC.[45,151] With the rapid 15-minute initial infusion originally recommended in the 20-hour IV protocol, such reactions were common. The same dose, or similar dose, diluted and given slowly appears to be entirely safe. Given in this manner, approximately 15% of patients develop a transient rash during the loading dose, without more serious sequelae unless a dosing or administration error occurs. The rash does not generally require treatment, does not preclude subsequent doses, and rarely recurs during maintenance dosing.[151] Although proper dosing of IV NAC is very safe, it must still be considered more dangerous, due to the risk of dosing errors. For any medication there is an expected incidence of dosing errors; with intravenous NAC this may be life-threatening.

Because there have been no controlled side-by-side studies comparing IV and oral NAC, conclusions about relative benefit of each is more speculative, but nonetheless several observations are relevant. The theoretical, albeit unproven, advantage of oral NAC is that direct delivery via the portal circulation might yield higher intrahepatic concentration of NAC (defined as [NAC]). Because of this first-pass clearance, oral NAC results in circulating [NAC] 20–30-fold lower than after IV dosing;[12,71] higher blood [NAC] and consistent delivery regardless of vomiting represent the theoretical advantages of IV NAC.

Despite theoretical considerations and strong viewpoints of proponents of each, for patients without liver failure there is no evidence of superiority of one route over the other. The advantage of oral delivery is not evident, since each appears equivalent if treatment is started within 8 hours of ingestion and the apparent superiority of oral NAC over IV NAC when started 16–24 hours after overdose is almost certainly related to the duration of NAC rather than the route. Similarly, the concern about delays in oral NAC administration due to vomiting are not borne out by the apparently equivalent outcome. In fact, there was no evidence of any worsening of outcome among patients who required additional NAC doses due to vomiting of NAC doses within an hour of administration (author's unpublished data). This counterintuitive observation may be accounted for by partial NAC absorption prior to vomiting, but this remains speculative.

Lower costs of care have been recently emphasized as an advantage of oral NAC. Avoidance of IV administration costs can reduce inpatient costs, and oral dosing allows the option of outpatient dosing. Whether or not this is appropriate will require further analysis, but it must be considered in any cost-effectiveness evaluation of this issue.

Until a formulation intended for IV use is available in the United States, the above considerations indicate to us that oral NAC should be the treatment of choice for most patients. In other countries where IV NAC is readily available, patient comfort and ease of administration suggest that IV NAC may be preferable, as long as it is carefully administered.

There is no proven advantage to either of the best known IV dosing protocols. One involves dosing identical to oral NAC: 140 mg/kg loading dose followed by 70 mg/kg every 4 hours.[143,154] The other provides a loading dose of 150 mg/kg, followed by 50 mg/kg over 4 hours, followed by a continuous infusion of 6.25 mg/kg/h.[96,127] We use the intermittent-dosing protocol rather than the continuous infusion protocol because of familiarity, lower published incidence of adverse effects, and the substantially higher total dose of NAC given. It must be acknowledged, however, that only the continuous-infusion protocol has been studied in the treatment of liver failure.[77]

In the United States, currently available formulations do not undergo the routine testing and documentation that is required for drugs listed for parenteral use. Thus, the manufacturers do not guarantee that the drug is sterile and pyrogen-free. This does not indicate that the product is not sterile, only that it is not documented to be so. In fact, sterility is expected in light of NAC use for inhalation by patients with a variety of lung diseases. Extensive IV use of these products has indicated that there is no evidence of infectious or febrile consequences of its use.[13] Because these products are not intended for parenteral use, they should never be used IV unless there is good reason to believe that the patient may be harmed by failure to administer IV NAC. In such cases, however, we believe that the potential benefits of IV NAC outweigh the risk of parenteral use of nonparenteral formulations. It has become customary to use an in-line 0.22-μm filter, although there is no evidence that this is necessary.

Are There Circumstances in Which IV NAC Is Currently Indicated?

Despite the lack of an available parenteral form, there are three situations in which the available information suggests that IV NAC is preferable. Each will require further study to validate, but seem well-supported by current information.

Fulminant hepatic failure is an important indication for IV NAC. The choice of IV over oral or enteral NAC is based on several observations. Most importantly, IV is the only route that has been studied in liver failure. Oral NAC may prove effective, but this has not yet been shown. Second, the evidence that the benefit of NAC in liver failure is extrahepatic suggests that IV is preferable. Intravenous NAC results in manyfold higher blood [NAC], which would presumably lead to more NAC delivery to critical organs. Finally, concomitant GI bleeding, use of lactulose, and other factors make IV NAC more practical.

A more common indication for IV NAC is the patient with a very high [APAP] approaching or beyond 8 hours since ingestion who is unable to tolerate oral NAC after a brief, aggressive trial of antiemetic therapy. In order to avoid further delays and resultant loss of NAC efficacy, IV NAC is logical, even without proof that continued vomiting significantly limits NAC absorption.

The most controversial indication for IV NAC is pregnancy. Fetal toxicity is rare, but clearly can occur, with adverse outcomes documented at all stages of pregnancy. Because maternal condition and thiol depletion certainly affect the fetus, the relative contribution to toxicity of fetal NAPQI production at various stages of pregnancy remains hard to define. Fetal oxidation of APAP has been demonstrated and is thought to increase with advancing fetal age, but little else is known.[138] There is every indication that NAC is both safe and effective to treat the mother,[137] but there are inadequate data to evaluate efficacy in the fetus. Fetal outcome has generally been excellent after maternal treatment with oral NAC,[137] but concern exists about those at greatest risk.

Placental transfer of NAC to the fetus is clearly limited, if it occurs at all.[74,147] In order to maximize the maternal-to-fetal gradient for NAC or, perhaps more importantly, other thiol-containing NAC metabolites, IV NAC is logical. In the United States, lacking availability or study of IV NAC in this setting, oral NAC is routinely used; however, it is the author's view that IV NAC is warranted, particularly in the later stages of pregnancy. In addition, since lack of maternal toxicity may or may not exclude fetal toxicity it is logical to continue NAC for 72 hours (the duration of the 17-dose protocol), and not utilize short-course protocols.

Are There Other Specific Antidotes That Can Benefit the Patient?

Other antidotal therapy has been suggested to either enhance thiol supply or decrease NAPQI formation. Prior to the utilization of NAC, both cysteamine and methionine were successfully used to treat APAP poisoning.[130] Both were effective if given early; however, efficacy could not be demonstrated if started more than 10–12 hours after APAP overdose, and both, particularly cysteamine, caused more adverse effects than NAC. There is no evident advantage over NAC in any patient subset, and therefore NAC is preferred. Glutathione and cysteine have each been used experimentally, but have been abandoned. Oral glutathione bioavailability is minimal, intracellular penetration is limited even after parenteral administration, and its efficacy to prevent serious hepatotoxicity is poor. Cysteine has been used intravenously with success equivalent to that of cysteamine or methionine, but without apparent advantage. Dimercaprol and *D*-penicillamine have also been tried and found to be ineffective. In short, no other available glutathione precursor or substitute has matched NAC in safety or efficacy.

Methods to decrease NAPQI formation have focused primarily on inhibition of P450 metabolism, and thus have not demonstrated a logical role in treatment. Such antidotes would be effective only prior to NAPQI covalent binding and arylation of hepatocyte proteins, at a stage when NAC has already proven to be safe and essentially completely effective. Inhibitors of P450 metabolism such as cimetidine have been effective after massive dosing prior to experimental APAP overdose,[159] but there is no evidence or rationale to suggest significant efficacy against serious human APAP overdose,[35] particularly when compared to NAC.

Summary

There have been tremendous advances in our understanding of APAP toxicity, but there are many remaining important challenges. In order to accurately determine risk of toxicity in atypical patients, high-risk patients, after repeated dosing, after sustained-release formulations, and in other settings, it is likely that an entirely new method of toxicity screening will need to be developed. Ongoing study of antidotal therapy dosing protocols is needed to assess the validity of many assumptions. Improved methods to determine need for liver transplantation in a timely manner are very important. These and other issues indicate that further changes are likely. The principles and current strategies presented in this chapter should serve as a strong foundation for these important future advances.

References

1. Anker AL, Smilkstein MJ: Acetaminophen: Concepts and controversies. Emerg Med Clin North Am 1994;12:335–349.
2. Arthurs Y, Fielding, JR: Paracetamol and chronic liver disease. J Irish Med Assoc 1980;73:273–274.
3. Barker JD, deCarle DJ, Anuras S: Chronic excessive acetaminophen use and liver damage. Ann Intern Med 1977;87:299–301.
4. Bateman DN, Woodhouse KW, Rawlins MD: Adverse reactions to *N*-acetylcysteine. Hum Toxicol 1984;3:393–398.
5. Beckett GJ, Donovan JW, Hussey AJ, et al: Intravenous *N*-acetylcysteine, hepatotoxicity and plasma glutathione

S-transferase in patients with paracetamol overdosage. Hum Exp Toxicol 1990;9:183–186.
6. Benson GD: Acetaminophen in chronic liver disease. Clin Pharmacol Ther 1983;33:95–101.
7. Bidault I, Lagier G, Garnier R, et al: Les hepatites par toxicité subaigue du paracetamol existent-elles? Therapie 1987;42:387–388.
8. Bien E, Vick K, Skorka G: Effects of exogenous factors on the cerebral glutathione in rodents. Arch Toxicol 1992; 66:279–285.
9. Bizovi KE, Aks SE, Paloucek F, et al: Late increase in acetaminophen concentration after overdose of Tylenol Extended Relief. Ann Emerg Med 1996;28:549–551.
10. Bond GR, Krenzelok EP, Normann SA, et al: Acetaminophen ingestion in childhood—cost and relative risk of alternative referral strategies. J Toxicol Clin Toxicol 1994;32:513–525.
11. Bonkowsky HL, Mudge GH, McMurtry RJ: Chronic hepatic inflammation: Role of intracellular calcium in paracetamol toxicity. Lancet 1978;1:1016–1018.
12. Borgstrom L, Kagedal B, Paulsen O: Pharmacokinetics of *N*-acetylcysteine in man. Eur J Clin Pharmacol 1986;31: 217–222.
13. Borys DJ, Jackson TW, Jacobs MR, et al: Intravenous *N*-acetylcysteine. Use of an unapproved drug product. A two year retrospective review. Vet Hum Toxicol 1992; 34:350. Abstract.
14. Bradberry SM, Hart M, Bareford D, et al: Factor V and factor VII:V ratio as prognostic indicators in paracetamol poisoning. Lancet 1995;1:646–647.
15. Bravo-Fernandez EF, Reddy KR, Jeffers L, Schiff ER: Hepatotoxicity after prolonged use of acetaminophen: A case report. Bol Asoc Med Puerto Rico 1988;80:417–419.
16. Bray GP, Harrison PM, O'Grady JG, et al: Long-term anticonvulsant therapy worsens outcome in paracetamol-induced fulminant hepatic failure. Hum Exp Toxicol 1992;11:265–270.
17. Breen K, Wandscheer JC, Peignoux M, Pessayre D: In situ formation of the acetaminophen metabolite covalently bound in kidney and lung: Supportive evidence provided by total hepatatectomy. Biochem Pharmacol 1982;31: 115–116.
18. Brent JA: New ways of looking at an old molecule. J Toxicol Clin Toxicol 1996;34:149–153.
19. Brent JA, Rumack BH: Role of free radicals in toxic hepatic injury. II. Are free radicals the cause of toxin-induced liver injury? J Toxicol Clin Toxicol 1993;31:173–196.
20. Brodie BB, Axelrod J: The fate of acetanilide in man. J Pharmacol Exp Ther 1948;94:29–38.
21. Bruno MK, Cohen S, Khairallah EA: Antidotal effectiveness of *N*-acetylcysteine in reversing acetaminophen-induced hepatotoxicity: Enhancement of the proteolysis of arylated proteins. Biochem Pharmacol 1988;37:4319–4325.
22. Buckpitt AR, Rollins DE, Mitchell JR:Varying effects of sulfhydryl nucleophiles on acetaminophen oxidation and sulfhydryl adduct formation. Biochem Pharmacol 1979;28: 2941–2946.
23. Calvert LJ, Linder CW:Acetaminophen poisoning. J Fam Pract 1978;7:953–956.
24. Campbell NR, Baylis B: Renal impairment associated with an acute paracetamol overdose in the absence of hepatotoxicity. Postgrad Med J 1992;68:116–118.
25. Carpenter HM, Mudge GH: Acetaminophen nephrotoxicity: Studies on renal acetylation and deacetylation. J Pharmacol Exp Ther 1981;218:161–167.
26. Cerretani D, Micheli L, Fiaschi AI, et al: MK–801 potentiates the glutathione depletion induced by acetaminophen in rat brain. Curr Ther Res 1994;55:707–717.
27. Cetaruk EW, Dart RC, Horowitz RS, Hurlbut KM: Extended-release acetaminophen overdose. JAMA 1996;275: 686. Letter.
28. Chao TC: Adverse drug reactions: Tales of a forensic pathologist. Ann Acad Med Singapore 1993;22:86–89.
29. Cheung L, Potts RG, Meyer KC: Acetaminophen treatment nomogram. N Engl J Med 1994;330:1907–1908.
30. Chinouth RW, Czajka PA, Peterson, RG: *N*-Acetylcysteine adsorption by activated charcoal. Vet Hum Toxicol 1980; 22:392–394.
31. Clark JH, Russell GJ, Fitzgerald JF: Fatal acetaminophen toxicity in a 2-year-old. J Indiana State Med Assoc 1983; 76:832–835.
32. Clark R, Thompson RPH, Borirakchanyavat V, et al: Hepatic damage and death from overdose of paracetamol. Lancet 1973;1:66–70.
33. Cobden I, Record CO, Ward MK, Derr DNS: Paracetamol-induced acute renal failure in the absence of fulminant liver damage. Br Med J 1982;284:21–22.
34. Corcoran GB, Mitchell JR, Vaishnav YN, Horning EC: Evidence that acetaminophen and *N*-hydroxyacetaminophen form a common arylating intermediate, *N*-acetyl-*p*-benzoquinoneimine. Mol Pharmacol 1980;18:536–542.
35. Critchley JAJH, Dyson EH, Scott AW, et al: Is there a place for cimetidine or ethanol in the treatment of paracetamol poisoning? Lancet 1983;1:1375–1376.
36. Davenport A, Finn R: Paracetamol (acetaminophen) poisoning resulting in acute renal failure without hepatic coma. Nephron 1988;50:55–56.
37. Davidson DGD, Eastham WN: Acute liver necrosis following overdosage of paracetamol. Br Med J 1966;2:497–499.
38. Davie A: Acetaminophen poisoning and liver function. N Engl J Med 1994;331:1311. Letter.
39. Davis M, Simmons CJ, Harrison NG, Williams R: Paracetamol overdose in man: Relationship between pattern of urinary metabolites and severity of liver damage. Q J Med 1976;45:181–191.
40. Dawson AH, Henry DA, McEwan J: Adverse reactions to *N*-acetylcysteine during treatment for paracetamol poisoning. Med J Aust 1989;150:329–331.
41. Day A, Abbott GD: Chronic paracetamol poisoning in children: A warning to health professionals. NZ Med J 1994;107:201.
42. Devalia JL, Ogilvie RC, McLean AEM: Dissociation of cell death from covalent binding of paracetamol by flavones in a hepatocyte system. Biochem Pharmacol 1982;31:3745–3749.
43. Devlin J, Ellis AE, McPeake J, et al: *N*-Acetylcysteine improves indocyanine green extraction and oxygen transport during hepatic dysfunction. Crit Care Med 1997;25: 236–242.
44. Donnelly PJ, Walker RM, Racz WJ: Inhibition of mitochondrial respiration in vivo is an early event in acetamino-

phen-induced hepatotoxicity. Arch Toxicol 1994;68:110–118.

45. Donovan JW, Jarvie DR, Prescott LF, Proudfoot AT: Adverse reactions of *N*-acetylcysteine and their relation to plasma levels. Vet Hum Toxicol 1987;29:470. Abstract.
46. Douglas AP, Hamlyn AN, James O: Controlled trial of cysteamine in treatment of acute paracetamol (acetaminophen) poisoning. Lancet 1976;1:111–115.
47. Douglas DR, Sholar JB, Smilkstein MJ: A pharmacokinetic comparison of acetaminophen products (Tylenol Extended Relief vs regular Tylenol). Acad Emerg Med 1996;3:740–744.
48. Douglas DR, Smilkstein MJ, Rumack BH: APAP levels within 4 hours: Are they useful? Vet Hum Toxicol 1994;36:350. Abstract.
49. Douidar SM, Al-Khalil I, Habersang RW: Severe hepatotoxicity, acute renal failure, and pancytopenia in a young child after repeated acetaminophen overdosing. Clin Pediatr 1994;33:42–45.
50. Ekins BR, Ford DC, Thompson MIB, et al: The effect of activated charcoal on *N*-acetylcysteine absorption in normal subjects. Am J Emerg Med 1987;5:483–487.
51. Emeigh Hart SG, Beierschmitt WP, Bartolone JB, et al: Evidence against deacetylation and for cytochrome P450-mediated activation in acetaminophen-induced nephrotoxicity in the CD-1 mouse. Toxicol Appl Pharmacol 1991;107:1–15.
52. Emeigh Hart SG, Beierschmitt WP, Wyand DS, et al: Acetaminophen nephrotoxicity in CD-1 mice. I. Evidence of a role for in situ activation in selective covalent binding and toxicity. Toxicol Appl Pharmacol 1994;126:267–275.
53. Emeigh Hart SG, Birge RB, Cartun RW, et al: In vivo and in vitro evidence for in situ activation and selective covalent binding of acetaminophen (APAP) in mouse kidney. Adv Exp Med Biol 1991;283:711–716.
54. Epstein MM, Nelson SD Slattery JT, et al: Inhibition of the metabolism of paracetamol by isoniazid. Br J Clin Pharmacol 1991;31:139–142.
55. Erickson RA, Runyon BA: Acetaminophen hepatotoxicity associated with alcoholic pancreatitis. Arch Intern Med 1984;144:1509–1510.
56. Ferguson DV, Roberts DW, Han-Shu H, et al: Acetaminophen-induced alterations in pancreatic B cells and serum insulin concentrations in B6C3F1 mice. Toxicol Appl Pharmacol 1990;104:225–234.
57. Flanagan RJ, Mant TGK: Coma and metabolic acidosis early in severe acute paracetamol poisoning. Hum Toxicol 1986;5:256–259.
58. Gerber JG, MacDonald JS, Harbison RD, et al: Effect of *N*-acetylcysteine on hepatic covalent binding of paracetamol (acetaminophen). Lancet 1977;1:657–658.
59. Gilmore JT, Tourvas E: Paracetamol-induced acute pancreatitis. Br Med J 1977;1:753–754.
60. Graudins A, Aaron CK, Linden CH: Overdose of extended-release acetaminophen. N Engl J Med 1995;333:196. Letter.
61. Grewal KK, Racz WJ: Intracellular calcium disruption as a secondary event in acetaminophen-induced hepatotoxicity. Can J Physiol Pharmacol 1993;71:26–32.
62. Haibach H, Akhter JE, Muscato MS, et al: Acetaminophen overdose with fetal demise. Am J Clin Pathol 1984;82:240–242.
63. Hamlyn AN, Douglas AP, James O: The spectrum of paracetamol (acetaminophen) overdose: Clinical and epidemiological studies. Postgrad Med J 1978;54:400–404.
64. Harman AW, Mahar SO, Burcham PC, Madsen BW: Level of cytosolic free calcium during acetaminophen toxicity in mouse hepatocytes. Mol Pharmacol 1992, 41:665–670.
65. Harrison PM, O'Grady JG, Keays RT, et al: Serial prothrombin time as prognostic indicator in paracetamol induced fulminant hepatic failure. Br Med J 1990;301:964–966.
66. Harrison PM, Wendon JA, Gimson AES, et al: Improvement by acetylcysteine of hemodynamics and oxygen transport in fulminant hepatic failure. N Engl J Med 1991;324:1852–1857.
67. Hart SG, Beierschmitt WP, Wyand DS, et al: Acetaminophen nephrotoxicity in CD-1 mice. I. Evidence of a role for in situ activation in selective covalent binding and toxicity. Toxicol Appl Pharmacol 1994;126:267–275.
68. Henretig FM, Selbst SM, Forrest C, et al: Repeated acetaminophen overdosing: Causing hepatotoxicity in children. Clin Pediatr 1989;28:525–528.
69. Hinsberg O, Treupel G: Ueber die physiologische Wirkung des *p*-Amidophenols und einiger Derivate desselben. Arch Exp Pathol Pharmakol 1894;33:216–250.
70. Hoivik DJ, Manautou JE, Tviet A, et al: Gender-related differences in susceptibility to acetaminophen-induced protein arylation and nephrotoxicity on the CD-1 mouse. Toxicol Appl Pharmacol 1995;130:257–271.
71. Holdiness MR: Clinical pharmacokinetics of *N*-acetylcysteine. Clin Pharmacokinet 1991;20:123–134.
72. Jaeschke H, Smith CW, Farhood A: Role of neutrophils in acetaminophen-induced liver injury. Toxicologist 1991;11:32.
73. Jepsen S, Hansen AB: The influence of *N*-acetylcysteine on the measurement of prothrombin time and activated partial thromboplastin time in healthy subjects. Scand J Clin Lab Invest 1994;54:543–547.
74. Johnson D, Simone C, Koren G: Transfer of *N*-acetylcysteine by the human placenta. Vet Hum Toxicol 1993;35:365. Abstract.
75. Johnson GK, Tolman KG: Chronic liver disease and acetaminophen. Ann Intern Med 1977;87:302–304.
76. Jollow DJ, Mitchell JR, Potter, WZ, et al: Acetaminophen-induced hepatic necrosis. II. Role of covalent binding in vivo. J Pharmacol Exp Ther 1973;187:195–202.
77. Keays R, Harrison PM, Wendon JA, et al: Intravenous acetylcysteine in paracetamol induced fulminant hepatic failure: A prospective controlled trial. Br Med J 1991;303:1026–1029.
78. Kher K, Makker S: Acute renal failure due to acetaminophen ingestion without concurrent hepatotoxicity. Am J Med 1987;82:1280–1281.
79. Klein-Schwartz W, Oderda GM: Adsorption of oral antidotes for acetaminophen poisoning (methionine and *N*-acetylcysteine) by activated charcoal. J Toxicol Clin Toxicol 1981;18:283–290.
80. Kobrinsky NL, Hartfield D, Horner H, et al: Treatment of advanced malignancies with high-dose acetaminophen. Cancer Invest 1996;14:202–210.

81. Lauterburg BH, Corcoran GB, Mitchell JR: Mechanism of action of *N*-acetylcysteine in the protection against hepatotoxicity of acetaminophen in rats in vivo. J Clin Invest 1983;71:980–991.
82. Lauterburg BH, Vaishnav Y, Stillwell WG, Mitchell JR: The effect of age and glutathione depletion on hepatic glutathione turnover in vivo determined by acetaminophen probe analysis. J Pharmacol ExpTher 1980;213:54–58.
83. Lauterburg BH, Velez ME: Glutathione deficiency in alcoholics: Risk factor for paracetamol hepatotoxicity. Gut 1988;29:1153–1157.
84. Lee WM: Acute liver failure. N Engl J Med 1993; 329:1862–1872.
85. Leibowitz H, Kuhn JA: Acetaminophen overdosage: A case presentation and review of current therapy. Del Med J 1980;52:135–138.
86. Lesna M, Watson AJ, Douglas AP, et al: Evaluation of paracetamol-induced damage in liver biopsies. Virchows Arch [Pathol Anat] 1976;370:333–344.
87. Lieber CS, Lasker JM, Alderman J, Leo MA: The microsomal ethanol oxidizing system and its interaction with other drugs, carcinogens, and vitamins. Ann NY Acad Sci 1987;492:11–24.
88. Linden CH, Rumack BH: Acetaminophen overdose. Emerg Med Clin North Am 1984;2:103–119.
89. Lip GYH, Vale JA: Does acetaminophen damage the heart? J Toxicol Clin Toxicol 1996;34:145–147.
90. Litovitz TL, Clark LR, Soloway RA: 1993 Annual Report of the American Association of Poison Control Centers Toxic Exposure Surveillance System. Am J Emerg Med 1994; 12:546–584.
91. Litovitz TL, Felberg L, Soloway RA, et al: 1994 Annual Report of the American Association of Poison Control Centers Toxic Exposure Surveillance System. Am J Emerg Med 1995;13:551–597.
92. Litovitz TL, Felberg L, White S, Klein-Schwartz W: 1995 Annual Report of the American Association of Poison Control Centers Toxic Exposure Surveillance System. Am J Emerg Med 1996;14:487–537.
93. Litovitz TL, Holm KC, Clancy C, et al: 1992 Annual Report of the American Association of Poison Control Centers Toxic Exposure Surveillance System. Am J Emerg Med 1993;11:494–555.
94. Litovitz TL, Smilkstein MJ, Felberg L, et al: 1996 Annual Report of the American Association of Poison Control Centers Toxic Exposure Surveillance System. Am J Emerg Med 1997;15:447–500.
95. MacLean D, Peters TJ, Brown RAG, et al: Treatment of acute paracetamol poisoning. Lancet 1968;2:849–852.
96. Makin AJ, Wendon J, Williams R: A 7-year experience of severe acetaminophen-induced hepatotoxicity (1987–1993). Gastroenterology 1995;109:1907–1916.
97. Makin AJ, Williams R: The current management of paracetamol overdosage. Br J Clin Prac 1994;48:144–148.
98. Mant TGK, Tempowski JH, Volans GN, Talbot JCC: Adverse reactions to acetylcysteine and effects of overdose. Br Med J 1984;289:217–219.
99. Mathew J, Hines JE, James OFW, Burt AD: Non-parenchymal cell responses in paracetamol (acetaminophen)-induced liver injury. J Hepatol 1994;20:537–541.
100. Mathis RD, Walker JS, Kuhns DW: Subacute acetaminophen overdose after incremental dosing. J Emerg Med 1988;6:37–40.
101. McCrae TA, Furuhama K, Roberts DW, et al: Evaluation of 3-(cystein-*S*-yl) acetaminophen in the nephrotoxicity of acetaminophen in rats. Toxicologist 1989;9:47.
102. Miller LF, Rumack BH: Clinical safety of high oral doses of *N*-acetylcysteine. Semin Oncol 1983;10(suppl 1):76–85.
103. Miller RP, Roberts RJ, Fischer LJ: Acetaminophen elimination kinetics in neonates, children, and adults. Clin Pharmacol Ther 1976;19:284–294.
104. Mitchell JR: Acetaminophen toxicity. N Engl J Med 1988;319:1601–1602.
105. Mitchell JR: Host susceptibility and acetaminophen liver injury. Ann Intern Med 1977;87:377–388.
106. Mitchell JR, Jollow DJ, Potter WZ, et al: Acetaminophen-induced hepatic necrosis. I. Role of drug metabolism. J Pharmacol Exp Ther 1973;187:185–194.
107. Mitchell JR, Jollow DJ, Potter WZ, et al: Acetaminophen-induced hepatic necrosis. IV. Protective role of glutathione. J Pharmacol Exp Ther 1973;187:211–217.
108. Mitchell JR, Thorgeirsson SS, Potter WZ, et al: Acetaminophen-induced hepatic injury: Protective role of glutathione in man and rationale for therapy. Clin Pharmacol Ther 1974;16:676–684.
109. Moller-Hartmann W, Siegers CP: Nephrotoxicity of paracetamol in the rat—mechanistic and therapeutic aspects. J Appl Toxicol 1991;11:141–146.
110. Moore M, Thor H, Moore G, et al: The toxicity of acetaminophen and *N*-acetyl-*p*-benzoquinone imine in isolated hepatocytes is associated with thiol depletion and increased cytosolic Ca^{2+}. J Biol Chem 1985;260:13035–13040.
111. Morse HN: Ueber eine neue Darstellungsmethode der Acetylamidophenole. Ber Deutsc Chem Ges 1878;11: 232–233.
112. Murphy R, Swartz R, Watkins PB: Severe acetaminophen toxicity in a patient receiving isoniazid. Ann Intern Med 1990;113:799–800.
113. Mutimer DJ, Ayres RCS, Neuberger JM, et al: Serious paracetamol poisoning and the results of liver transplantation. Gut 1994;35:809–814.
114. Nogen AG, Bremner JE: Fatal acetaminophen overdosage in a young child. J Pediatr 1978;92:832–833.
115. Ohtani N, Matsuzaki M, Anno Y, et al: A case of myocardial damage following acute paracetamol poisoning. Jpn Circ J 1989;53:278–282.
116. O'Grady JG, Alexander GJM, Hayllar KM, Williams R: Early indicators of prognosis in fulminant hepatic failure. Gastroenterology 1989;97:439–445.
117. Pereira LMMB, Langley PG, Hayllar KM, et al: Coagulation factor V and VII/V ratio as predictors of outcome in paracetamol induced fulminant hepatic failure: Relation to other prognostic indicators. Gut 1992;33:98–102.
118. Pimstone BL, Uys CJ: Liver necrosis and myocardiopathy following paracetamol overdosage. South Afr Med J 1968;42:259–262.
119. Piperno E, Berssenbruegge DA: Reversal of experimental paracetamol toxicosis with *N*-acetylcysteine. Lancet 1976; 2:738–739.
120. Piperno E, Mosher AH, Berssenbruegge DA, et al: Patho-

physiology of acetaminophen overdosage toxicity: Implications for management. Pediatrics 1978;62(suppl): 880–889.
121. Portmann B, Talbot IC, Day DW, et al: Histopathological changes in the liver following a paracetamol overdose: Correlation with clinical and biochemical parameters. J Pathol 1975;117:169–181.
122. Potter WZ, Davis DC, Mitchell JR, et al: Acetaminophen induced hepatic necrosis. III: Cytochrome P450 mediated covalent binding in vitro. J Pharmacol Exp Ther 1973; 187:203–210.
123. Prescott LF: Kinetics and metabolism of paracetamol and phenacetin. Br J Clin Pharmacol 1980;10(suppl 2): 291S–298S.
124. Prescott LF: The metabolism of paracetamol. In: Prescott LF, ed: Paracetamol (Acetaminophen). A Critical Bibliographic Review. London, Taylor & Francis, 1996, pp. 67–102.
125. Prescott LF: Factors influencing paracetamol metabolism. In: Prescott LF, ed: Paracetamol (Acetaminophen). A Critical Bibliographic Review. London, Taylor & Francis, 1996, pp. 103–106.
126. Prescott LF: Paracetamol overdosage: Pharmacological considerations and clinical management. Drugs 1983; 25:290–314.
127. Prescott LF, Illingworth RN, Critchley JAJH, et al: Intravenous *N*-acetylcysteine: The treatment of choice for paracetamol poisoning. Br Med J 1979;2:1097–1100.
128. Prescott LF, Newton RW, Swainson CP, et al: Successful treatment of severe paracetamol overdosage with cysteamine. Lancet 1974; 1:588–592.
129. Prescott LF, Mattison P, Menzies DG, Manson LM: The comparative effects of paracetamol and indomethacin on renal function in healthy female volunteers. Br J Clin Pharmacol 1990;29:403–412.
130. Prescott LF, Park J, Sutherland GR, et al: Cysteamine, methionine and penicillamine in the treatment of paracetamol poisoning. Lancet 1976;2:109–114.
131. Prescott LF, Proudfoot AT, Cregeen RJ: Paracetamol-induced acute renal failure in the absence of fulminant liver damage. Br Med J 1982;284:421–422.
132. Prescott LF, Wright N, Roscoe P, Brown SS: Plasma paracetamol half-life and hepatic necrosis in patients with paracetamol overdosage. Lancet 1971;1:519–522.
133. Proudfoot AT, Wright N: Acute paracetamol poisoning. Br Med J 1970;3:557–558.
134. Pumford NR, Hinson JA, Potter WZ, et al: Immunochemical quantitation of 3-(cystein-*S*-yl)acetaminophen adducts in serum and liver proteins of acetaminophen-treated mice. J Pharmacol Exp Ther 1989;248:190–196.
135. Raucy JL, Sker JML, Lieber CS, Black M: Acetaminophen activation by human liver cytochromes P450 IIE1 and P450 IA2. Arch Biochem Biophys 1989;271:270–283.
136. Ray SD, Mumaw VR, Raje RR, Fariss MW: Protection of acetaminophen-induced hepatocellular apoptosis and necrosis by cholesteryl hemisuccinate pretreatment. J Pharmacol Exp Ther 1996;279:1470–1483.
137. Riggs BS, Bronstein AC, Kulig KW, et al: Acute acetaminophen overdose during pregnancy. Obstet Gynecol 1989;74:247–253.
138. Rollins DE, Von Bahr C, Glaumann H, et al: Acetaminophen: Potentially toxic metabolite formed by human fetal and adult liver microsomes and isolated fetal liver cells. Science 1979;205:1414–1416.
139. Rumack BH: Acetaminophen overdose in young children: Treatment and effects of alcohol and other additional ingestants in 417 cases. Am J Dis Child 1984;138:428–433.
140. Rumack BH: Acetaminophen overdose. Am J Med 1983;75(suppl 5A):104–112.
141. Rumack BH, Matthew H: Acetaminophen poisoning and toxicity. Pediatrics 1975;55:871–876.
142. Rumack BH, Peterson RG: Acetaminophen overdose: Incidence, diagnosis and management in 416 patients. Pediatrics 1978;62(suppl):898–903.
143. Rumack BH, Peterson RG, Koch GC, Amara IA: Acetaminophen overdose. 662 cases with evaluation of oral acetylcysteine treatment. Arch Intern Med 1981;141: 380–385.
144. Rybolt TR, Burrell DE, Shults JM, Kelley AK: In vitro coadsorption of acetaminophen and *N*-acetylcysteine onto activated carbon powder. J Pharm Sci 1986;75:904–906.
145. Sandler DP, Smith JC, Weinberg CR, et al: Analgesic use and chronic renal disease. N Engl J Med 1989;320:1238–1243.
146. Seeff LB, Cuccherini BA, Zimmerman HJ, et al: Acetaminophen hepatotoxicity in alcoholics. A therapeutic misadventure. Ann Intern Med 1986;104:399–404.
147. Selden BS, Curry SC, Clark RF, et al: Transplacental transport of *N*-acetylcysteine in an ovine model. Ann Emerg Med 1991;20:1069–1072.
148. Shen W, Kamendulis LM, Ray SD, Corcoran GB: Acetaminophen-induced cytotoxicity in cultured mouse hepatocytes: Effects of Ca^{2+}-endonuclease, DNA repair, and glutathione depletion inhibitors on DNA fragmentation and cell death. Toxicol Appl Pharmacol 1992;112:32–40.
149. Singer AJ, Carracio TR, Mofenson HC: The temporal profile of increased transaminase levels in patients with acetaminophen-induced liver dysfunction. Ann Emerg Med 1995;26:49–53.
150. Slattery JT, Wilson JM, Kalhorn TF, Nelson SD: Dose-dependent pharmacokinetics of acetaminophen: Evidence for glutathione depletion in humans. Clin Pharmacol Ther 1987;41:413–418.
151. Smilkstein MJ, Bronstein AC, Linden C, et al: Acetaminophen overdose: A 48-hour intravenous *N*-acetylcysteine treatment protocol. Ann Emerg Med 1991;20: 1058–1063.
152. Smilkstein MJ, Douglas DR, Daya MR: Acetaminophen poisoning and liver function. N Engl J Med 1994:330: 1310–1311.
153. Smilkstein MJ, Knapp GL, Kulig KW, Rumack BH: *N*-Acetylcysteine in the treatment of acetaminophen overdose. N Engl J Med 1989;320:1418.
154. Smilkstein MJ, Knapp GL, Kulig KW, Rumack BH: Efficacy of oral *N*-acetylcysteine in the treatment of acetaminophen overdose: Analysis of the national multicenter study (1976–1985). N Engl J Med 1988;319:1557–1562.
155. Smilkstein MJ, Knapp GL, Kulig KW, Rumack BH: Acetaminophen overdose: How critical is the delay to *N*-acetylcysteine? Vet Hum Toxicol 1987;29:486. Abstract.
156. Smilkstein MJ, Rumack BH: Elimination half-life as a pre-

dictor of acetaminophen-induced hepatotoxicity. Vet Hum Toxicol 1994;36:377. Abstract.

157. Smith CV, Jones DP, Guenther TM, et al: Compartmentation of glutathione: Implications for the study of toxicity and disease. Toxicol Appl Pharmacol 1996;140:1–12.
158. Smith DW, Isakson G, Frankel LR, Kerner JA: Hepatic failure following ingestion of multiple doses of acetaminophen in a young child. J Pediatr Gastroenterol Nutr 1986; 5:822–825.
159. Speeg KV, Mitchell MC, Maldonado L: Additive protection of cimetidine and *N*-acetylcysteine treatment against acetaminophen-induced hepatonecrosis in the rat. J Pharmacol Exp Ther 1985;234:550–554.
160. Spies CD, Reinhart K, Witt I, et al: Influence of *N*-acetylcysteine on indirect indicators of tissue oxygenation in septic shock patients: Results from a prospective, randomized, double-blind study. Crit Care Med 1994;22: 1738–1746.
161. Spiller HA, Krenzelok EP, Grande GA, et al: A prospective evaluation of the effect of activated charcoal before oral *N*-acetylcysteine in acetaminophen overdose. Ann Emerg Med 1994;23:519–523.
162. Stork CM, Rees S, Howland MA, et al: Pharmacokinetics of extended relief vs regular release Tylenol in simulated human overdose. J Toxicol Clin Toxicol 1996;34:157–162.
163. Strubelt O, Younes M: The toxicological relevance of paracetamol-induced inhibition of hepatic respiration and ATP depletion. Biochem Pharmacol 1992;44:163–170.
164. Swetnam SM, Florman AL: Probable acetaminophen toxicity in an 18-month-old infant due to repeated overdosing. Clin Pediatr 1984;23:104–105.
165. Temple AR: "Dear Doctor" Tylenol ER letter. Fort Washington, PA: McNeil Consumer Products Company. January 3, 1995.
166. Thomson JS, Prescott LF: Liver damage and impaired glucose tolerance after paracetamol overdosage. Br Med J 1966;2:506–507.
167. Thummel KE, Lee CA, Kunze KL, Nelson SD: Oxidation of acetaminophen to *N*-acetyl-*p*-benzoquinone imine by human CYP3A4. Biochem Pharmacol 1993;45:1563–1569.
168. Thummel KE, Slattery JT, Nelson SD, et al: Effect of ethanol on hepatotoxicity of acetaminophen in mice and on reactive metabolite formation by mouse and human liver microsomes. Toxicol Appl Pharmacol 1989;100: 391–397.
169. Thummel KE, Slattery JT, Nelson SD: Mechanism by which ethanol diminishes the hepatotoxicity of acetaminophen. J Pharmacol Exp Ther 1988;245:129–136.
170. Tighe TV, Walter FG: Delayed toxic acetaminophen level after initial four hour nontoxic level. J Toxicol Clin Toxicol 1994;32:431–434.
171. Tirmenstein MA, Nelson SD: Acetaminophen-induced oxidation of protein thiols: Contributions of impaired thiol-metabolising enzymes and the breakdown of adenosine nucleotides. J Biol Chem 1990;265:3059–3065.
172. Tirmenstein MA, Nelson SD: Subcellular binding and effects on calcium homeostasis produced by acetaminophen and a non-hepatotoxic regioisomer, 3-hydroxyacetanilide in mouse liver. J Biol Chem 1989;264:9814–9819.
173. Tredger JM, Smith HM, Read RB, Williams R: Effects of ethanol ingestion on the metabolism of a hepatotoxic dose of paracetamol in mice. Xenobiotica 1986;16:661–670.
174. Vale JA, Proudfoot AT: Paracetamol (acetaminophen) poisoning. Lancet 1995;346:547–552.
175. Vassallo S, Khan AN, Howland MA: Use of the Rumack-Matthew nomogram in cases of extended-release acetaminophen toxicity. Ann Intern Med 1996;125:940. Letter.
176. Volans GN: Antipyretic analgesic overdosage in children. Comparative risks. Br J Clin Pract 1991;(suppl)70:26–29.
177. Walker RJ, Fawcett JP: Drug nephrotoxicity—the significance of cellular mechanisms. Prog Drug Res 1993; 41:51–94.
178. Ware AJ, Upchurch KS, Eigenbrodt EH, Norman DA: Acetaminophen and the liver. Ann Intern Med 1978; 88:267–268.
179. Webster PA, Roberts DW, Benson RW, Kearns, GL: Acetaminophen toxicity in children: Diagnostic confirmation using a specific antigenic biomarker. J Clin Pharmacol 1996;36:397–402.
180. Welty SE, Smith CV, Benzick AE, et al: Investigation of possible mechanisms of hepatic swelling and necrosis caused by acetaminophen in mice. Biochem Pharmacol 1993;45:449–458.
181. Wendel A, Feuerstein S, Konz KH: Acute paracetamol intoxication of starved mice leads to lipid peroxidation in vivo. Biochem Pharmacol 1979;28:2051–2055.
182. Wendon JA, Harrison PM, Keays R, Williams R: Cerebral blood flow and metabolism in fulminant liver failure. Hepatology 1994;19:1407–1413.
183. Whitcomb DC, Block GD: Association of acetaminophen hepatotoxicity with fasting and ethanol use. JAMA 1994;272:1845–1850.
184. Wilkinson SP, Moodie H, Arroyo VA, Williams R: Frequency of renal impairment in paracetamol overdose compared with other causes of acute liver damage. J Clin Pathol 1977;30:220–224.
185. Woo OF, Anderson IB, Kim SY, et al: Shorter duration of *N*-acetylcysteine for acute acetaminophen poisoning. J Toxicol Clin Toxicol 1995;33:508. Abstract.
186. Zand R, Nelson SD, Slattery JT, et al: Inhibition and induction of cytochrome P4502E1-catalyzed oxidation by isoniazid in humans. Clin Pharmacol Ther 1993;54:142–149.
187. Zezulka A, Wright N: Severe metabolic acidosis early in paracetamol poisoning. Br Med J 1982;285:851–852.
188. Zieve L, Anderson WR, Dozeman R, Draves K, Lyftogt C: Acetaminophen liver injury: Sequential changes in two biochemical indices of regeneration and their relationship to histologic alterations. J Lab Clin Med 1985;105:619–624.
189. Zimmerman HJ, Maddrey WC: Acetaminophen (paracetamol) hepatotoxicity with regular intake of alcohol: Analysis of instances of therapeutic misadventure. Hepatology 1995;22:767–773.

ANTIDOTES IN DEPTH

N-Acetylcysteine

Mary Ann Howland

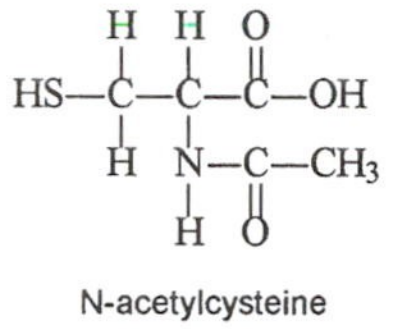

N-acetylcysteine

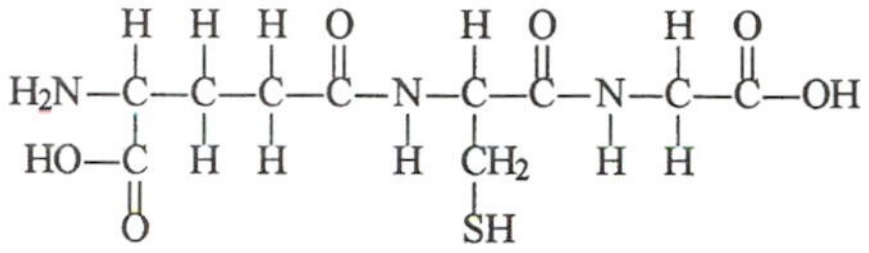

Glutathione

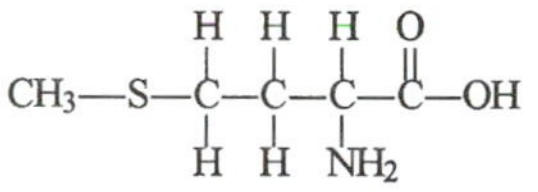

Methionine

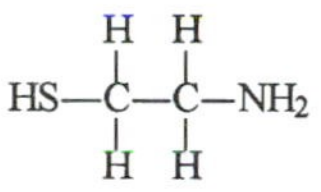

Cysteamine

In 1985, *N*-acetylcysteine (NAC) was approved by the Food and Drug Administration as an antidote for acetaminophen overdose. Since that time, it has become the cornerstone of therapy for the potentially lethal acetaminophen overdose.

In 1974, Mitchell and co-workers described the protective effect that glutathione exerts as acetaminophen is metabolized in the liver.[31] Ninety percent of a therapeutic dose of acetaminophen is metabolized to the nontoxic glucuronide (approximately 60%) and sulfate (approximately 30%) conjugates.[35] Only 4% is metabolized by the cytochrome P450 mixed-function oxidase system (3A4 at low doses; 2E1 and 1A2 at high doses) to a potentially toxic reactive intermediate, *N*-acetyl-*p*-benzoquinoneimine (NAPQI). This intermediate is then conjugated with glutathione to form nontoxic cysteine and mercapturic acid conjugates. After acetaminophen overdose, both the fraction and the total amount of drug undergoing P450 metabolism increases, leading to glutathione depletion, persistence of the highly reactive intermediate, and resultant hepatic centrilobular necrosis.[8]

Cysteamine, methionine, and NAC all have been used successfully to prevent hepatotoxicity, but cysteamine and methionine both produce more adverse effects, and methionine is less effective. Therefore, NAC has emerged as the preferred treatment.[38,44,50]

NAC is a thiol-containing compound that is diacetylated in the body to cysteine. Cysteine is a thiol-containing amino acid that is used intracellularly along with the plentiful amino acids glycine and glutamate to synthesize glutathione.[43] The availability of cysteine becomes the rate-limiting step in the synthesis of glutathione and NAC is effective in replenishing diminished supplies. Glutathione serves as the body's protection against many stressors, including electrophilic compounds, by forming thioether bonds through conjugation, and as a reducing agent and antioxidant.[43] Glutathione reduction to 30% of normal levels sets in motion a cascade of inflammatory events that allows cytoxic damage and possibly cell death to occur. This inflammatory response is presumed secondary to the generation of "oxidants" or "free radicals" (electron acceptors containing an unpaired electron in an orbital) or, more specifically, "reactive oxygen species." These reactive oxygen species deplete thiols including glutathione, endothelium-derived relaxant factor, NAD, and ATP and cause lipid peroxidation, ultimately increasing intracellular calcium and activating proteases and phospholipases and causing more damage.[1,17,45] This inflammatory damage can occur in many tissues including the liver, lung, and heart. Antioxidants function as electron donors. They are oxidized preferentially to a relatively less reactive and destructive species, although antioxidants can have prooxidant action in certain settings.[1] Examples of endogenous antioxidants include vitamins C and E, superoxide dismutase, and reduced glutathione. Glutathione replenishment prior to initiation of the inflammatory cascade is the goal. Glutathione replenishment may protect against further cell damage but is incapable of completely restoring damaged tissues. In this second stage, NAC may act directly as an antioxidant or may act as a reservoir for thiol groups, for the formation of essential endogenous antioxidants (ie, glutathione), and for substances depleted by the oxidant stress (ie, endothelium-derived relaxant factor).[15,19] In this manner NAC can modulate the inflammatory cascade and can improve systemic oxygenation.

The message is clear. For NAC to be most effective it must be administered before glutathione is depleted to 30% of normal, which occurs at approximately 8 hours after a toxic acetaminophen ingestion.[37,42,47] NAC appears to work by preventing the binding of NAPQI to hepatocytes. This is accomplished by enhancing the synthesis of additional glutathione[26] and sulfate,[46] by acting intracellularly as a glutathione substitute by directly binding to NAPQI,[6] and by enhancing the reduction of NAPQI to APAP.[26] Once NAPQI covalently binds to hepatocytes, presumably through the formation of a 3-(cystein-5-yl) APAP protein adduct,[42] NAC appears to modulate the subsequent cascade of inflammatory events as noted above.[19]

NAC is most effective if administered within 8 hours of the ingestion. Therefore, if the history suggests an APAP ingestion of 150 mg/kg close to 8 hours earlier or if plasma APAP concentration falls on or above the nomogram, NAC should be instituted expeditiously. In chronic overdose, adults ingesting more than the recommended maximum daily dose of 4 g/d or children ingesting more than 75 mg/kg/d may be at risk for hepatotoxicity. NAC should be administered when hepatotoxicity is evident either by symptoms or enzymes or when the APAP serum concentration is above 10 μg/mL 4 hours after the last ingestion (see Chap. 31 for details). Interpretation of acetaminophen levels in chronic overdoses is difficult, and the acetaminophen nomogram cannot be applied.

Patients at increased risk of acute or chronic APAP toxicity may need to receive NAC at a lower threshold. Unfortunately, this threshold has not yet been well defined. Glutathione-deficient patients (ie, the malnourished, chronic alcoholic, anorexic, or those with AIDS) and those on cytochrome P450-inducing agents (ie, phenobarbital, phenytoin, carbamazepine) or those on isoniazid should theoretically be at increased risk for APAP toxicity.[4,20,27,47] A recent analysis of a small number of patients who were receiving anticonvulsant therapy or chronically ingesting alcohol did not demonstrate these to be risk factors independent of APAP dose.[29] However, these same authors suggested that genetic factors may have led to hepatotoxicity in patients with ingestions of < 12 g of APAP.[29]

When NAC is administered, the patient should receive a 140 mg/kg loading dose either orally or by enteral tube. Starting 4 hours after the loading dose, 70 mg/kg should be given every 4 hours for an additional 17 doses. The solution should be diluted to 5% with a soft drink to enhance palatability. If any dose is vomited within 1 hour of administration, it should be repeated.[28] Antiemetics (such as metoclopramide or serotonin antagonists) should be used to ensure absorption. If the acetaminophen level is above the nomogram line, the patient should receive a full course of therapy, regardless of subsequent levels. This regimen may need to be continued if hepatic failure intervenes. When fulminant hepatic failure occurs, NAC should be administered until the patient recovers or receives a liver transplant.[5,18,23] However, the route of administration is problematic. Only oral NAC is FDA approved, and only intravenous NAC has been used in these transplantation studies. Currently, oral NAC is preservative free and pyrogen free (communication with manufacturer).

The 20-hour intravenous NAC protocol (150 mg/kg loading dose over 15 minutes, followed by an additional dose of 50 mg/kg over 4 hours and then 100 mg/kg over 16 hours) used in Britain and Canada is effective in preventing hepatic damage when given within 8 hours of acetaminophen ingestion.[37] A 48-hour intravenous regimen (140 mg/kg, then 70 mg/kg every 4 hours) studied in the United States appears to be superior to the 20-hour regimen, but is still experimental.[47] The question of which is better, the IV short (20 hours) or long (48 hours) course or oral course (72 hours) of NAC,[48] will not be settled until additional studies are complete. Perhaps most patients who receive their first dose of NAC within 8 hours will require only the short course since the inflammatory cascade will not be initiated, while those whose treatment is delayed will benefit from a longer course of therapy and the antiinflammatory effects of NAC. Some authors are recommending a 36-hour course in low-risk patients with proper evaluation and follow-up, but this recommendation has not been studied.

Anaphylactoid reactions described after intravenous dosing[2,3,9,10,13,16,21,30,36,40,51,52] of NAC are not noted after oral therapy and may be either rate related or related to high serum NAC levels.[13,36] Iatrogenic overdoses with intravenous NAC have resulted in a number of significant adverse effects and a few deaths.[10,30] It is also unclear whether oral or intravenous dosing results in superior drug delivery to the liver and whether the higher hepatic concentrations enhance the efficacy.[34] All treatment regimens are effective when started within 8 hours of overdose. However, reliable comparative studies of patients treated later than 8 hours of ingestion have not been performed. Based on current data, the 72-hour oral protocol appears to be the most effective for late-treated, high-risk patients with acetaminophen overdose,[48] and this is the only approved protocol in the United States.

Oral NAC is rapidly absorbed, but the bioavailability is low (10–30%) due to significant first-pass metabolism.[15,36] Intact NAC has a relatively small volume of distribution (0.5 L/kg).[52] Serum concentrations after intravenous administration of an initial loading dose of 150 mg/kg over 15 minutes are about 500 mg/L.[36] A steady-state plasma concentration of 35 mg/L (10–90 mg/L) was reached in about 12 hours following the loading dose with a continuous infusion of 50 mg/kg over 4 hours and 100 mg/kg over the next 16 hours.[36] An elimination half-life of 5.7 hours was calculated when this infusion protocol was terminated. Severe liver damage does not appear to affect NAC elimination.[36] Pharmacokinetics and pharmacodynamics of oral NAC were determined in a phase 1 trial in 26 adult volunteers at risk for new onset or recurrent cancer.[33] Oral NAC is being studied as a potential chemopreventive agent. Absorption of NAC is rapid, with a mean time to maximum peak concentration of 1.4 ± 0.7 h and a mean elimination half-life of 2.5 ± 0.6 h that is linear with increasing dose up to 3200 mg/m^2/d given as a single daily dose. Intersubject plasma NAC levels vary 10-fold from a maximum concentration of 1.7 to 20.8 mg/L at a dose of 800 mg/m^2/d. Chronic administration leads to a decrease in plasma concentrations from a C_{max} of 8.9 mg/L at the end of 1 month to 5.1 at the end of 6 months.[33]

N-Acetylcysteine is present in plasma in the reduced or oxidized state and is either free or bound with other thiols (ie, *N*-acetylcysteine-cysteine). *N*-Acetylcysteine is metabolized to many sulfur-containing compounds (eg, cysteine, glutathione, methionine, cystine).[15,33,36] Thus the study of NAC is complicated.

Conflicting in vitro[7,24] and in vivo[32,39] data regarding the concomitant use of activated charcoal have suggested that the resultant bioavailability of NAC is either decreased or unchanged. In vitro studies[7,24] have been conflicting, as have recent in vivo data.[32,39] A study involving 19 healthy volunteers compared peak and total absorption of NAC given alone as a loading dose and when it was followed by 100 g of activated charcoal.[14] The authors demonstrated a statistically significant decrease in peak NAC and a 40% reduction in total absorption of NAC. The issue not addressed by any study, however, is the critical amount of NAC necessary to prevent acetaminophen-induced liver damage. The current dose of NAC used is effective for even the largest acetaminophen overdoses, suggesting that current dosage has a built-in safety margin, and thus a small decrease in available NAC secondary to activated charcoal may not be critical.[48] Given all of the information available, the risk-to-benefit ratio favors using activated charcoal with NAC unless activated charcoal is otherwise contraindicated or unnecessary. It seems prudent to separate NAC and activated charcoal doses by 1–2 hours, if possible.

Although teratogenicity data are unavailable for NAC, it appears that untreated acetaminophen toxicity is a far greater threat to a fetus than NAC treatment.[41] The risk of not treating pregnant women almost certainly far exceeds any potential risk to the developing fetus if a toxic ingestion has occurred.

Intravenous NAC has been shown to decrease clotting factors and increase the prothrombin time in healthy volunteers.[22] This effect occurred rapidly after the first hour, plateaued after 16 hours of continuous IV NAC, with a rapid return to normal noted when the infusion was stopped.[22] Since prothrombin time is used as a marker for severity of intoxication and one of the criteria for transplantation, the effect of NAC should be considered.

N-Acetylcysteine has also been investigated as a treatment for a number of agents where free radicals or reactive metabolites are thought to be responsible for the toxicity. Some of these toxins and chemotherapeutic agents include chloroform, carbon tetrachloride, 1,2-dichloropropane, acrylonitrile, doxorubicin, and cyclophosphamide.[15] A theoretical role for the use of NAC in carbon monoxide poisoning has been suggested, but cannot be recommended until further studies are performed.[15]

NAC is also being studied as a chemopreventive agent against cancer, lung injury, cardiac injury and in a variety of areas where glutathione depletion is believed to play an important protective role.[11,12,43,49] NAC has demonstrated extracellular antimutagenic effects, enhanced repair of nuclear DNA damaged by carcinogens, and inhibition of malignant cell invasion and metastases.[12] NAC rescue is also being used with high-dose acetaminophen (up to 20 g) in patients with advanced malignancies.[25] The use of NAC in these settings may further enhance our understanding of its beneficial effects both in the early and late phases of acetaminophen poisoning.

Acknowledgment

Martin Jay Smilkstein, MD contributed to this Antidotes in Depth in a previous edition.

References

1. Bast A, Haenen G, Doleman C: Oxidants and antioxidants: State of the art. Am J Med 1991;91:2–13.
2. Bateman DN, Woodhouse KW, Rawlins MD: Adverse reactions to *N*-acetylcysteine. Hum Toxicol 1984;3:393–398.
3. Bonfiglio M, Traeger S, Hulisz D, et al: Anaphylactoid reaction to IV acetylcysteine associated with electrocardiographic abnormalities. Pharmacotherapy 1992;26:22–25.
4. Bray G, Harrison P, O'Grady J, et al: Long term anticonvulsant therapy worsens outcome in paracetamol induced fulminant hepatic failure. Hum Exp Toxicol 1992;11:265–272.
5. Bromley PN, Cottam SJ, Hilmi I, et al: Effects of intraoperative *N*-acetylcysteine in orthotopic liver transplantation. Br J Anaesth 1995;75:352–354.
6. Buckpitt AR, Rollins DE, Mitchell JR: Varying effects of sulfhydryl nucleophiles on acetaminophen oxidation and sulfhydryl adduct formation. Biochem Pharmacol 1979;28: 2841–2946.
7. Chinough R, Czajka P: *N*-Acetylcysteine adsorption by activated charcoal. Vet Hum Toxicol 1980;22:392–394.
8. Corcoran GB, Mitchell JR, Vaishnav YN, Horning EC: Evidence that acetaminophen and *N*-hydroxyacetaminophen form a common arylating intermediate, *N*-acetyl-*p*-benzoquinoneimine. Mol Pharmacol 1980;18:536–542.
9. Dawson A, Henry D, McEwen J: Adverse reactions to *N*-acetylcysteine during treatment for paracetamol poisoning. Med J Aust 1989;150:329–331.
10. Death after *N*-acetylcysteine. Lancet 1984;1:1421. Editorial.
11. De Backer WA, Amsel B, Jorens PG, et al: *N*-Acetylcysteine pretreatment of cardiac surgery patients influences plasma neutrophil elastase and neutrophil influx in bronchoalveolar lavage fluid. Intensive Care Med 1996;22:900–908.
12. De Flora S, Cesarone CE, Balansky RM, et al: Chemopreventive properties and mechanisms of *N*-acetylcysteine. The experimental background. J Cell Biochem 1995;(suppl) 22:33–41.
13. Donovan JW, Jarvie DR, Prescott LF, et al: Hypersensitivity reactions to *N*-acetylcysteine: A concentration dependent phenomenon. Presented to European Association of Poison Control Congress, Edinburgh, September 1988.
14. Ekins B, Ford D, Thompson M, et al: The effect of activated charcoal on *N*-acetylcysteine absorption in normal subjects. Am J Emerg Med 1987;5:483–487.
15. Flanagan R, Meredith TJ: Use of *N*-acetylcysteine in clinical toxicology. Am J Med 1991;91:131–139.
16. Gervais S, Lussier-Labelle F, Beaudet G: Anaphylactoid reaction to acetylcysteine. Clin Pharm 1984;3:586–587.
17. Halliwell B: Reactive oxygen species in living systems: Source, biochemistry and role in human disease. Am J Med 1991;91:14–22.

18. Harrison P, Keays R, Bray G, et al: Improved outcome of paracetamol-induced fulminant hepatic failure by late administration of acetylcysteine. Lancet 1990;335:1572–1573.
19. Harrison P, Wendon J, Gimson A, et al: Improvement by acetylcysteine of hemodynamics and oxygen transport in fulminant hepatic failure. N Engl J Med 1991;324:1852–1857.
20. Henry JA: Glutathione and HIV. Lancet 1990;335:235–236.
21. Ho SW, Beilin JJ: Asthma associated with *N*-acetylcysteine infusion and paracetamol poisoning: Report of two cases. Br Med J 1983;287:876–877.
22. Jepsen S, Hansen AB: The influence of *N*-acetylcysteine on the measurement of prothrombin time and activated partial thromboplastin time in healthy subjects. Scand J Clin Lab Invest 1994;54:543–547.
23. Keays R, Harrison P, Wendon J, et al: Intravenous acetylcysteine in paracetamol induced fulminant hepatic failure: A prospective controlled trial. Br Med J 1991;303:1026–1029.
24. Klein Schwartz W, Oderda G: Adsorption of oral antidotes for acetaminophen poisoning (methionine and *N*-acetylcysteine) by activated charcoal. Clin Toxicol 1981;18:283–290.
25. Kobrinsky NL, Hartfield D, Horner H, et al: Treatment of advanced malignancies with high-dose acetaminophen and *N*-acetylcysteine rescue. Cancer Invest 1996;14:202–210.
26. Lauterburg BH, Corcoran GB, Mitchell JR: Mechanism of action of *N*-acetylcysteine in the protection against the hepatotoxicity of acetaminophen in rats. J Clin Invest 1983; 71:980–991.
27. Lauterburg BH, Velez M: Glutathione deficiency in alcoholics: Risk factor for paracetamol hepatotoxicity. Gut 1988;29:1153–1157.
28. Linden CH, Rumack BH: Acetaminophen overdose. Emerg Med Clin North Am 1984;2:103–119.
29. Makin AJ, Wendon J, Williams R: A 7 year experience of severe acetaminophen-induced hepatotoxicity (1987–1993). Gastroenterology 1995;109:1907–1916.
30. Mant TGK, Tompowski JH, Volans GN, Talbot JC: Adverse reactions to acetylcysteine and effects of overdose. Br Med J 1984;289:217–219.
31. Mitchell JR, Thorgeirsson SS, Potter WZ, et al: Acetaminophen induced hepatic injury: Protective role of glutathione in man and rationale for therapy. Clin Pharmacol Ther 1974;16:676–684.
32. North D, Peterson RG, Krenzelok E: Effect of activated charcoal administration on acetylcysteine serum levels in humans. Am J Hosp Pharm 1981;38:1022–1024.
33. Pendyala L, Creaven PJ: Pharmacokinetic and pharmacodynamic studies of *N*-acetylcysteine, a potential chemopreventive agent during a phase 1 trial. Cancer Epidem Biomarkers Prevent 1995;4:245–251.
34. Peterson RG, Rumack BH: Treating acute acetaminophen poisoning with *N*-acetylcysteine. JAMA 1977;237: 2406–2407.
35. Prescott LF: Paracetamol toxicity: Pharmacological considerations and clinical management. Drugs 1983;25: 290–314.
36. Prescott LF, Donovan JW, Jarvie DR, et al: The disposition and kinetics of intravenous *N*-acetylcysteine in patients with paracetamol overdosage. Eur J Clin Pharmacol 1989; 37:501–506.
37. Prescott LF, Illingworth RN, Critchley JAJH, et al: Intravenous *N*-acetylcysteine: The treatment of choice for paracetamol poisoning. Br Med J 1979;2:1097–1100.
38. Prescott LF, Sutherland GR, Park J, et al: Cysteamine, methionine, and penicillamine in the treatment of paracetamol poisoning. Lancet 1976;2:109–113.
39. Renzi F, Donovan J, Morgan L, et al: Concomitant use of activated charcoal and *N*-acetylcysteine. Ann Emerg Med 1985;14:568–572.
40. Reynard K, Riley A, Walker BE: Respiratory arrest after *N*-acetylcysteine for a paracetamol overdose. Lancet 1992;340:675. Letter.
41. Riggs BS, Bronstein AC, Kulig KW, et al: Acute acetaminophen overdose during pregnancy. Obstet Gynecol 1989;74:247–253.
42. Roberts DW, Bucci TJ, Benson RW, et al: Immunohistochemical localization and quantification of the 3 (cystein-5-yl) acetaminophen protein adduct in acetaminophen hepatotoxicity. Am J Pathol 1991;138:359–371.
43. Ruffmann R, Wendel A: GSH rescue by *N*-acetylcysteine. Klin Wochenschr 1991;69:857–862.
44. Shriner K, Goetz M: Severe hepatotoxicity in a patient receiving both acetaminophen and zidovudine. Am J Med 1992;93:94–96.
45. Sies H: Oxidative stress: From basic research to clinical application. Am J Med 1991;91:31–38.
46. Slattery JT, Wilson JM, Kalhorn TF, Nelson SD: Dose dependent pharmacokinetics of acetaminophen: Evidence of glutathione depletion in humans. Clin Pharmacol Ther 1987;41:413–418.
47. Smilkstein MJ, Bronstein AC, Linden CH, et al: Acetaminophen overdose: A 48 hour intravenous *N*-acetylcysteine protocol. Ann Emerg Med 1991;20:1058–1063.
48. Smilkstein MJ, Knapp GL, Kulig KW, et al: Efficacy of oral *N*-acetylcysteine in the treatment of acetaminophen overdose. Analysis of the national multicenter study (1976–1985). N Engl J Med 1988;319:1557–1562.
49. Sochman J, Vrbska J, Musilova B, et al: Infarct size limitation: Acute *N*-acetylcysteine defense (ISLAND) trial. Start of the study. Intl J Cardiol 1995;49:181–182. Letter.
50. Vale JA, Meredith TJ, Goulding R. Treatment of acetaminophen poisoning. The use of oral methionine. Arch Intern Med 1981;141:394–396.
51. Vale JA, Wheeler DC: Anaphylactoid reactions to *N*-acetylcysteine. Lancet 1982;2:988. Letter.
52. Walton NG, Mann TN, Shaw KM: Anaphylactoid reaction to *N*-acetylcysteine. Lancet 1979;2:1298. Letter.

CHAPTER 32

Salicylates

Neal E. Flomenbaum

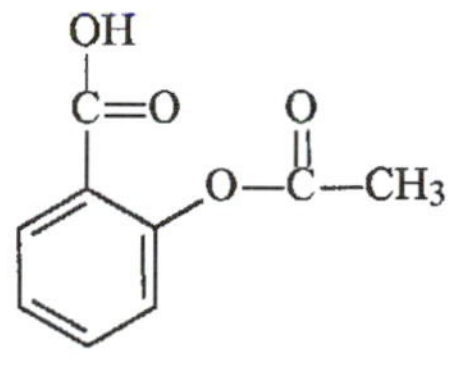

Acetyl salicylic acid

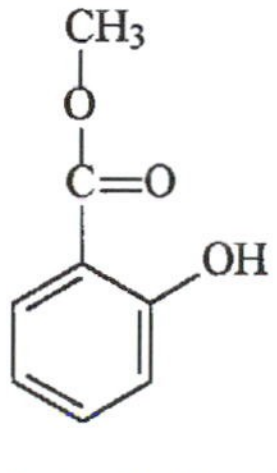

Methyl salicylic acid

Salicylic Acid		
MW	=	138 daltons
Therapeutic serum level	=	15–30 mg/dL
	=	1.1–2.2 mmol/L
Action level	=	100 mg/dL
	=	7.2 mmol/L

Values greater than or equal to the action level necessitate clinical intervention. Values less than this level may necessitate intervention based on the clinical characteristics of the patient.

A 22-year-old woman came to the emergency department (ED) complaining of abdominal pain, nausea, and vomiting. She had a history of depression, but stated that she was not currently seeing a psychiatrist or taking any psychiatric medications. Upon further questioning, the patient said that 6 hours prior to admission she became severely depressed and ingested at least one-half bottle of aspirin tablets in a suicide attempt. A single episode of vomiting occurred shortly afterwards. The patient denied tinnitus but said that she was short of breath. She also denied any other significant past medical or surgical history.

On physical examination, the patient appeared to be well-developed, well-nourished, and diaphoretic. Vital signs were: blood pressure, 120/60 mm Hg; pulse, 110 beats/min; respiratory rate, 30 breaths/min; and rectal temperature, 37.9°C (100.2°F). Examination of the head, eyes, ears, nose, and throat was unremarkable. The neck was supple and without jugular venous distention. The chest was clear to auscultation and percussion. Cardiac examination revealed normal heart sounds and no murmurs, rubs, or gallops. Bowel sounds were normal but the abdomen was diffusely tender, without guarding; stools were negative for occult blood. There was no clubbing, cyanosis, or edema. The patient was alert and fully oriented. No cranial nerve abnormalities were noted; deep tendon reflexes were intact and symmetric with plantar flexion of the toes; and motor and sensory testing was normal.

An intravenous catheter was inserted and blood was drawn and sent for BUN, glucose, electrolytes, a complete blood count, coagulation studies, and salicylate and acetaminophen levels. The patient was placed on a cardiac monitor and an arterial blood gases (ABG) specimen was obtained and sent prior to administering supplemental oxygen. A Foley catheter was inserted and the bedside ferric chloride test of the urine was positive. With the patient in the left lateral decubitus position, orogastric lavage was performed using a 40-French lavage tube. After food and particulate matter were recovered and a total of 2 L of fluid instilled and removed, the lavage fluid was clear. Sixty grams of activated charcoal in a slurry of water and sorbitol (60 g) were administered next and then the lavage tube was removed.

The initial laboratory data revealed a urine pH, 5.5; sp gr, 1.025; 1+ protein; 2+ ketones; no RBCs or WBCs. ABG values on room air were: pH, 7.51; PCO_2, 11 mm Hg; PO_2, 134 mm Hg. Serum electrolytes were Na^+ 144 mEq/L; K^+ 3.8 mEq/L; Cl^- 98 mEq/L; BUN was 23 mg/dL, creatinine 0.9 mg/dL, and glucose 88 mg/dL; calcium was 9.6 mg/dL; and a urine pregnancy test was negative.

A bolus of 88 mEq of sodium bicarbonate was administered and a bicarbonate drip consisting of 132 mEq of $NaHCO_3$ in 1 L of D_5W was started at a rate of 250 mL/h. Potassium replacement was also initiated.

Two and one-half hours later, the patient's pulse had increased to 140 beats/min and her blood pressure dropped to 106/64 mm Hg. Although the salicylate level was not yet available, a nephrology consultation was requested. Fluid rates were increased and a second dose of activated charcoal was administered. A repeat ABG determination revealed a pH, 7.48; PCO_2, 13.9 mm Hg; and PO_2, 116 mm Hg.

About 1 hour later (4 hours after presentation), a third ABG analysis on room air revealed: pH, 7.44; PCO_2, 14 mm Hg; PO_2, 93 mm Hg. At this time the initial salicylate level was reported to be 107 mg/dL and the acetaminophen level was 0. Arrangements for hemodialysis were made.

Another ABG determination on room air 30 minutes later revealed: pH, 7.37; PCO_2, 24 mm Hg; PO_2, 64 mm Hg and at this time rales could be auscultated at both bases. The bicarbonate infusion was reduced to 125 mL/h, and a third dose of activated charcoal was administered.

The patient became agitated shortly thereafter. A fifth ABG determination on 4 L of nasal O_2 revealed pH, 7.20; PCO_2, 46 mm Hg; PO_2, 92 mm Hg. The ABG determination was immediately repeated and the results were: pH, 7.10; PCO_2, 63 mm Hg; PO_2, 80 mm Hg.

Because of her rapidly deteriorating condition, the patient was intubated and hyperventilated, but her systolic blood pressure fell to 80 mm Hg by palpation and did not respond to a fluid bolus of 1 L of normal saline. A post-intubation ABG determination revealed: pH, 6.90; PCO_2, 41 mm Hg; and PO_2, 182 mm Hg. Ventilation was increased, a second bolus of 88 mEq of bicarbonate was administered, and an intravenous dopamine infusion was started. Blood pressure was maintained at approximately 100 mm Hg while hemodialysis was started in the medical intensive care unit.

After 4 hours, the patient's salicylate level was 22 mg/dL and her ABG was pH, 7.42; PCO_2, 36 mm Hg; and PO_2, 190 mm Hg. Eight hours later with hemodialysis completed, the patient appeared to be significantly improved clinically. A psychiatric consultation was obtained the next day; 3 days after that the patient was transferred to the psychiatric service from which she was later discharged home. One week after discharge the patient returned to her job.

What Are the Pathophysiologic Consequences of Salicylate Poisoning?

Acid–Base Patterns of Salicylate Poisoning—Differences between Adult and Pediatric Patients

Salicylates stimulate the respiratory center in the brainstem, leading to hyperventilation and respiratory alkalosis.[83] Salicylates also interfere with the Krebs cycle, limit production of ATP,[40] and increase lactate production,[46] leading to ketosis and a wide anion gap metabolic acidosis (Chaps.15, 64). Although the metabolic acidosis begins with the earliest stages of toxicity, the respiratory alkalosis predominates initially.[27] However, by the time an adult patient presents to the hospital, a mixed respiratory alkalosis and metabolic acidosis is usually discernible on arterial blood gas (ABG) analysis.[27] It is important to understand that the respiratory alkalosis is not merely compensatory for the metabolic acidosis (or vice versa), but that adults acutely poisoned by salicylates characteristically present with a mixed acid–base disturbance initially.[27]

In children, the respiratory alkalosis may be quite transient, and very early in the course the metabolic acidosis becomes significant,[28,80] leading some to incorrectly suggest that pediatric salicylate poisoning is characterized by only a metabolic acidosis. Although some children also may present with a mixed acid–base disturbance and a normal pH, most present with acidemia.[28]

Mixed respiratory alkalosis and metabolic acidosis is found in the majority of adults with serum salicylate levels greater than 40 mg/dL.[27] The initial predominant respiratory alkalosis is characteristic of adult salicylate poisoning. Any adult who is salicylate poisoned who presents early on with a respiratory acidosis has either salicylate-induced pulmonary edema, CNS depression from a mixed overdose, or severe fatigue from the strenuous exercise of hyperventilating for a prolonged period. A study of this issue[27] emphasized how common such mixed drug overdoses are in the adult population by demonstrating that one-third of patients with a presumed primary salicylate overdose had in fact taken other drugs. Benzodiazepines, barbiturates, alcohol, and cyclic antidepressants all appear to blunt the hyperventilatory response to salicylates, resulting in respiratory acidosis or minimizing the centrally induced respiratory alkalosis, and leaving the patient with what appears to be only a metabolic acidosis. The combination of metabolic and respiratory acidosis from salicylate poisoning in an adult indicates an exceedingly grave prognosis and is almost invariably a preterminal event.[69]

Glucose Metabolism

Salicylate poisoning appears to produce a discordance between plasma and CSF glucose levels. Despite normal plasma glucose, CSF glucose fell 33% in salicylate-poisoned mice, compared to controls.[84] In other words, the rate of CSF glucose used exceeded the rate of supply, even in the presence of normal serum glucose. There was also a marked increase in oxygen consumption in mice, even with low salicylate levels.[32] A case report of refractory hypoglycemia secondary to poisoning from topical salicylate absorption underscores the problems of glucose metabolism caused by salicylates.[70]

Hepatic Effects

The effects of salicylates on the liver have been studied in mice.[32] Salicylate-poisoned mice had a marked decrease in glycogen and a dramatic increase in lactate compared to controls. Increased glycolysis apparently compensates for the uncoupling of oxidative phosphorylation.[62] In humans, the increased metabolic demands resulting from salicylate poisoning stimulate peripheral use of glucose and fat with resultant hypoglycemia and ketosis.

Salicylate-induced hepatitis occurs in children being treated with high (average level 30.9 mg/dL) or chronic doses of salicylates for rheumatic fever and rheumatoid arthritis.[29,59,75] Another form of salicylate-induced liver disease, also primarily seen in children, is Reye's syndrome, which is characterized by nausea, vomiting, hypoglycemia, elevated liver enzymes (AST, ALT), fatty infiltration of the liver, and coma following a viral illness.[5] Although the nature of the link between Reye's syndrome and salicylates has never been fully elucidated, the incidence of Reye's syndrome in the United States has fallen steadily concomitantly with decreased use of salicylates in children.[71,87]

Pulmonary Effects

When the patient with a salicylate overdose presents with pulmonary edema, major etiologies to be considered include aspiration pneumonitis, postictal and neurogenic pulmonary edema, and salicylate-induced noncardiogenic pulmonary edema (NCPE)[36,41] (Chap. 20).

Aspiration of acidic material can result in severe chemical pneumonitis with increased pulmonary capillary permeability and subsequent exudation of high-protein edema fluid into the interstitial or alveolar spaces. Frequently referred to as adult respiratory distress syndrome (ARDS) in its severe stages, similar capillary injury has also been associated with pulmonary infections of both viral and bacterial origin. Aspiration pneumonitis can mimic pulmonary edema both clinically and radiographically.

Severe traumatic CNS injuries and elevation of intracranial pressure may be responsible for a form of "central" NCPE.[37] Hypothalamic lesions from trauma, increased intracranial pressure, or salicylate poisoning may be the critical factor, with resultant adrenergic overactivity producing a shift of blood from the systemic to the pulmonary circulation, loss of left ventricular compliance with left atrial and pulmonary capillary hypertension, and subsequent pulmonary edema (Chap. 20).

In 111 consecutive patients with peak salicylate levels > 30 mg/dL, salicylate-induced NCPE occurred in 35% of patients over 30 years of age and none of the 55 patients under 16 years of age. Risk factors for developing NCPE included cigarette smoking, chronic salicylate ingestion, and the presence of neurologic symptoms on admission. The average arterial blood pH was 7.37 ± 0.022 in the 6 adult patients with NCPE and 7.46 ± 0.010 in the 30 adults without it. There was no significant difference in salicylate levels, which were approximately 57 mg/dL in both groups.[88]

Although the exact mechanism for salicylate-induced NCPE is obscure, hypoxia may be an important factor.[35,36] Hypoxia can result in pulmonary arterial hypertension and also a local release of vasoactive substances. Severe salicylate poisoning has also been identified as a distinct cause of NCPE in children as well as adults.[23]

Treatment for salicylate-induced NCPE includes adequate ventilation, oxygenation, and hemodialysis. Close monitoring of the arterial blood gas values is essential and the PO_2 should be maintained at 60–100 mm Hg. If this cannot be done with an FIO_2 of less than 50% by either face mask or mechanically assisted ventilation, then positive end-expiratory pressure (PEEP) or continuous positive airway pressure (CPAP) is indicated together with a pulmonary artery catheter to monitor cardiac output (which may become compromised as a result of PEEP). Potent diuretics to induce hypovolemia have *not* proven useful in managing NCPE which, as noted previously, results from increased capillary permeability (see Chap. 20).

Hematologic Effects

Hematologic effects of salicylate ingestion include hypoprothrombinemia and platelet dysfunction.[26] Anemia in patients who chronically abuse salicylates may be a result of the effects of both platelet dysfunction and gastric mucosal barrier breakdown,[26] particularly in the elderly.[4,13] Hemolysis is unusual and alterations in leukocyte function are of no apparent clinical significance.[74]

Gastrointestinal Effects

Gastrointestinal manifestations include nausea, vomiting, hemorrhagic gastritis, decreased gastric motility, and pylorospasm.[73] Again, the effects appear more pronounced or consequential in the elderly.[42]

Musculoskeletal Effects

Rhabdomyolysis after pure salicylate overdoses has been described and is probably another result of the dissipation of heat and energy from uncoupling oxidative phosphorylation.[49,62,63]

Otolaryngologic Effects

Hearing loss preceded by tinnitus typically occurs with serum salicylate concentrations of 20–45 mg/dL or higher.[11,66] The mechanism of ototoxicity may include the biochemical effects of salicylates on glucose and protein metabolism affecting the endolymph and perilymph, which in turn result in electrophysiologic changes in the inner ear and eighth cranial nerve impulse transmission. Drug accumulation and vasoconstriction in the stria vascularis may also contribute to ototoxicity.[11]

What Are the Pharmacokinetics of Salicylates?

Salicylates are rapidly absorbed from the stomach, as the pK_a of 3.5 leaves approximately 50% of salicylate nonionized in the acid stomach.[14,34,76] Absorption is less efficient in the small bowel, but because of its large surface area, absorption is rapidly effected there as well.[76] The dosage form (effervescent,enteric-coated) often influences the absorption rate.[73,90] Delayed absorption may also be due to salicylate-induced pylorospasm, pyloric stenosis,[30,73] gastric outlet obstruction,[77] or bezoar formation.[9] Protein-binding abnormalities, urine and plasma pH variations, and delayed absorption all influence the maximum salicylate levels and the rates of decline.[64]

After therapeutic doses of salicylates, significant levels are achieved in 30 minutes, and maximum levels are often attained in less than 1 hour.[14] Salicylates are typically prescribed in doses of 15 mg/kg as two regular strength (650 mg) aspirin tablets every 4 hours to achieve an antiinflammatory effect on chronic conditions such as rheumatoid arthritis. The goal of such dosing is to achieve salicylate levels of 15–30 mg/dL, which are considered to be in the therapeutic range.[51]

As levels rise beyond 30 mg/dL, salicylate begins to produce signs and symptoms of toxicity. In overdosage, peak serum levels may not be reached for 4–6 hours or longer. Salicylates also have substantially longer apparent half-lives at toxic levels than at therapeutic levels.[14,52] As the concentration increases, two of the five pathways of elimination—those for salicyluric acid and the salicylic phenolic glucuronide—become saturated and exhibit zero-order kinetics (Fig. 32–1 and see Chap. 11). The result of this saturation changes overall salicylate elimination from the initial first-order kinetics to zero-order kinetics.[50] The half-life of salicylate is 2–4 hours at therapeutic levels but the apparent half-life is as long as 20 hours at toxic levels.[16,52] There is also a decrease in protein binding from 90% at therapeutic levels to less than 75% at toxic levels[1,10,19] and the apparent volume of

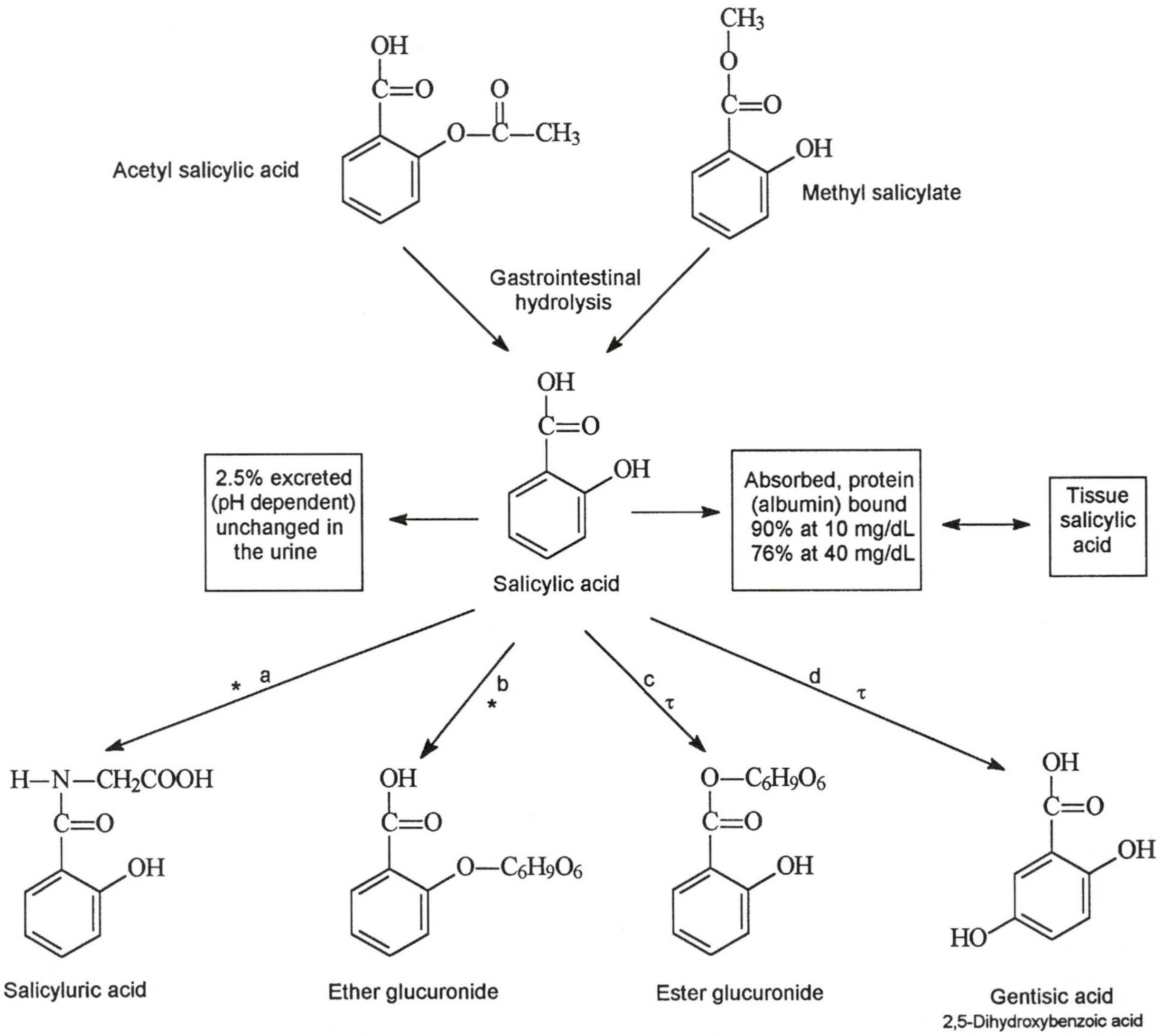

Figure 32–1. Salicylate metabolism. At excessive doses, the a, b, c, and d mechanisms are overloaded, leading to increased tissue binding, decreased protein binding, and increased excretion of unconjugated salicylic acid. * = Michaelis-Menten kinetics; τ = first-order kinetics.

distribution simultaneously increases (from 0.2 L/kg at low levels to more than 0.3 L/kg at higher levels).[53,79] Elimination varies with concentration and is complex, as first-order metabolism is initially substantial but with higher doses certain pathways become saturated.

How Does Salicylate Toxicity Correlate with Serum Levels?

Except in certain narrowly defined situations, the toxicity of salicylates correlates poorly with serum levels. The Done nomogram,[16] first published in 1960, continues to be used despite severely limited applicability: It was based on data from a predominantly pediatric population and intended to be applied only 6 hours or more after a single acute ingestion of non-enteric-coated, orally ingested aspirin. Moreover, the patient's blood pH must be approximately 7.4 or higher. Such conditions rarely apply to serious acute and chronic salicylate overdoses and poisonings. As an example of the shortcomings of the nomogram, a patient who presents with lethargy and/or a coagulation abnormality associated with salicylism can be classified on the nomogram as "mild" or "moderate" although such a patient must be considered severely poisoned. The poor predictive value of the nomogram when applied retrospectively to a group of 55 predominantly adult salicylate intoxications is evident from a 1989 study.[18]

Patients with acute ingestions whose initial serum salicylate determinations are either considered "acceptable," low, or moderate sometimes deteriorate rapidly thereafter. For this reason, careful observation of the patient, correlation of the serum salicylate values with blood pH values, and repeat testing of serum salicylate levels every 2–4 hours are essential until the patient is clinically improving and has a low salicylate level in the presence of a normal or high blood pH. Methyl salicylate exposures have resulted in deaths in less than 6 hours, emphasizing the need for early salicylate determinations in addition to frequent testing after such exposures. In all cases, once a peak salicylate level has been reached, at least one additional level should be obtained in several hours and even more frequent levels obtained in the seriously ill patient, to assess efficacy of treatment and possible need for hemodialysis.

The reason that a concurrent arterial blood pH should be determined when a blood salicylate level is obtained is that in the presence of acidemia, more salicylic acid leaves the blood and enters the CSF and other tissues (Fig. 32–2), increasing the toxicity. Therefore, meaningful interpretation of *serum* salicylate levels must take into account the effect of the blood pH on salicylate distribution, unless the serum salicylate level is so high that hemodialysis is indicated regardless of the pH. A falling serum salicylate concentration may also be difficult to interpret as it can reflect either an increased tissue distribution with increased toxicity or an increased clearance with decreased toxicity: A falling serum salicylate level accompanied by a falling or low blood pH should be presumed to reflect a serious or worsening situation, not a benign or improving one.

When the patient's clinical signs and symptoms are given the highest priority and the serum salicylate level is interpreted in conjunction with a simultaneously obtained arterial blood pH, the severity of toxicity can usu-

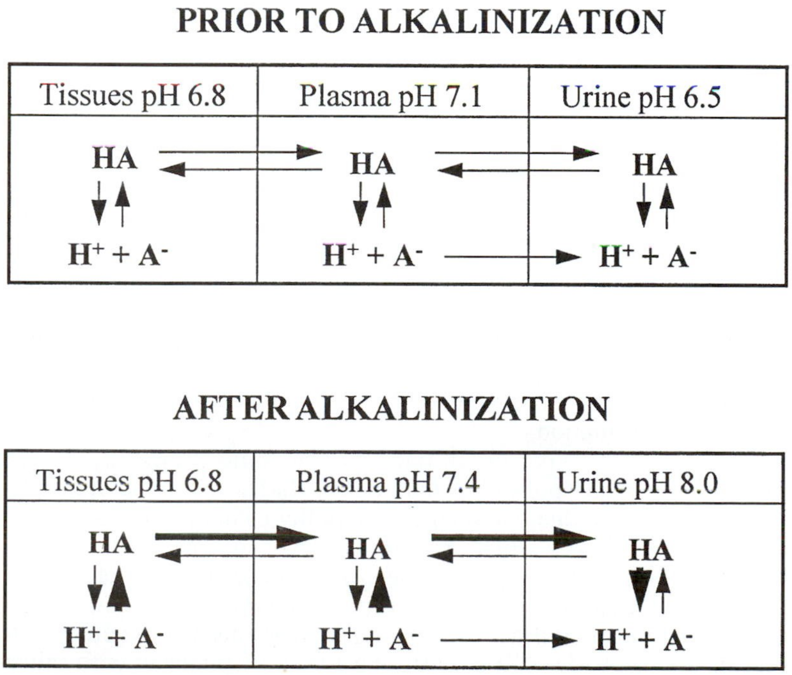

Figure 32–2. Rationale for alkalinization. Alkalinization of the plasma with respect to the tissues and alkalinization of the urine with respect to plasma shifts the equilibrium to the plasma and urine and away from the tissues (including the brain). This equilibrium shift has been called "ion trapping." *(Adapted, with permission, from Temple AR: Acute and chronic effects of aspirin toxicity and their treatment. Arch Intern Med 1981;141:367.)*

ally be predicted and the need for hemodialysis accurately determined.

How Do Serum Salicylate Levels Correlate with CSF Levels?

Although peak serum salicylate levels may provide useful clinical correlations at a normal or high blood pH, serum salicylate determinations not reflecting the peak level may be of limited value. Experimentally, there appears to be a critical CSF salicylate level that correlates well with mortality.[32] In addition, the CSF salicylate level correlates best with the peak serum salicylate level and reequilibrates more slowly than the serum salicylate level. As noted above, a serum salicylate level in the presence of acidemia may have little or no correlation with the CSF salicylate level. However, although more predictive of toxicity, the use of CSF salicylate levels in clinical management is currently not practical.

What Are the Signs and Symptoms of Salicylate Poisoning and How Do Acute and Chronic Cases Differ?

The earliest signs and symptoms of salicylate toxicity include nausea, vomiting, diaphoresis, and tinnitus, which is a subjective sensation of ringing or hissing, with or without hearing loss.[11,26,80] As CNS salicylate levels increase, tinnitus is rapidly followed by diminished auditory acuity sometimes leading to deafness.[11] Other early CNS effects may include vertigo and hyperventilation as well as hyperactivity, agitation, delirium, hallucinations, convulsions, lethargy, and stupor. Coma is rare and generally occurs only after massive ingestions (serum salicylate levels greater than 100 mg/dL) or mixed overdoses (Table 32–1).[26] A marked elevation in temperature resulting from the uncoupling of oxidative phosphorylation caused by salicylate poisoning[62] is an indication of severe toxicity and often a preterminal condition. Many of the signs and symptoms of salicylate toxicity may be mistakenly attributed to the illness for which the salicylates were administered, with disastrous consequences.[80]

Chronic salicylate poisoning most typically occurs in the elderly as a result of unintentional overdosing on salicylates used to treat chronic conditions such as rheumatoid arthritis or osteoarthritis.[3,18,42] Although neither age nor gender appears to affect the absorption rate or plasma clearance of acute therapeutic doses of aspirin (900 mg) administered to healthy adults,[64] when used chronically, a small increase in dosage (eg, in response to increasing pain) or a small decrease in metabolism or renal function can result in substantial increases in serum salicylate levels.[42]

Presenting signs and symptoms of *chronic* salicylate poisoning include hearing loss and tinnitus, nausea, vomiting, dyspnea and hyperventilation, tachycardia, hyperthermia, and neurologic manifestations such as confusion, agitation, hyperactivity, slurred speech, hallucinations, seizures, and coma.[2,26] Although there is considerable overlap with some of the presenting signs and symptoms of *acute* salicylate poisoning, the slow onset and less severe appearance of some of these signs of chronic poisoning in the elderly frequently cause delayed recognition of the true etiology of the patient's presentation.

Typically, ill patients who suffer from chronic salicylate poisoning may be misdiagnosed as having delirium, dementia, encephalopathy of undetermined origin, diseases such as sepsis (fever of unknown origin), alcoholic ketoacidosis, respiratory failure, or cardiopulmonary disease—especially congestive heart failure, acute pulmonary edema, or even unstable angina.[2,6,26] In a study of 73 consecutive adults hospitalized with salicylate intoxication, 27% were not correctly diagnosed for

TABLE 32–1. CLINICAL AND LABORATORY MANIFESTATIONS OF SALICYLATE TOXICITY

Acid–base and electrolyte disturbances	***Hepatic***
Anion gap increased	Abnormal liver enzymes
Metabolic acidosis	Altered glucose metabolism
Metabolic alkalosis (vomiting)	***Metabolic***
Respiratory alkalosis (predominates early)	Hyperthermia
Respiratory acidosis (late grave prognosis)	Hypoglycemia
Hyponatremia or hypernatremia	Hyperglycemia
Hypokalemia	Hypoglycorrhachia
CNS	Ketonemia
Tinnitus	Ketonuria
Diminished auditory acuity	***Pulmonary***
Deafness	Hyperpnea
Vertigo	Tachypnea
Hallucinations	Respiratory alkalosis
Agitation	Noncardiogenic pulmonary edema (NCPE)
Hyperactivity	***Renal***
Delirium	Tubular damage
Stupor	Proteinuria
Coma	NaCl and water retention
Lethargy	Hypouricemia (hyperuricemia)
Convulsions	***Volume status***
Cerebral edema	Nausea
Syndrome of inappropriate secretion of antidiuretic hormone	Vomiting
Coagulation abnormalities	Perspiration
Hypoprothrombinemia	
Inhibition of factors V, VII, X	
Platelet dysfunction	
Gastrointestinal	
Nausea	
Vomiting	
Hemorrhagic gastritis	
Decreased motility	
Pylorospasm	

TABLE 32–2. DIFFERENTIAL CHARACTERISTICS OF ACUTE AND CHRONIC SALICYLATE POISONING

	Acute	Chronic
Age	Younger	Older
Etiology	Overdose, rarely unintentional	Therapeutic misadventures; iatrogenic
Diagnosis	"Classic"	Frequently unrecognized
Other diseases states	None	Underlying disorders (especially chronic pain conditions, etc)
Suicidal ideation	Typical	No
Clinical differences	Rapid progression of signs	Noncardiogenic pulmonary edema (NCPE)[a] CNS abnormalities[a]
Serum concentrations	Marked elevation	Intermediate elevation
Mortality	Uncommon when recognized, unless ingestion massive	Approximately 25%

[a]More common

up to 72 hours after admission.[2] These patients manifested toxicity with standard or excessive therapeutic regimens and had significant associated diseases without a history of previous overdoses. In this group, 60% had had a neurologic consultation before the diagnosis of salicylism was established. When diagnosis is delayed in the elderly, the morbidity and mortality associated with salicylate poisoning is high. Mortality was reported to be as high as 25% in the 1970s,[2] and there is no reason to believe from clinical experience that survival after delayed diagnosis is substantially better today (Table 32–2).

How Can Salicylate Use Be Confirmed Quickly?

Although serum salicylate levels are relatively easy to obtain in most hospital laboratories, salicylate use may be quickly confirmed qualitatively with a simple bedside ferric chloride ($FeCl_3$) test. To perform the test, add several drops of 10% $FeCl_3$ to 1 mL of urine. A purple color indicates the presence of salicylic acid, acetoacetic acid, or phenylpyruvic acid[89] (Fig. 32–3 and see Color Plate 19). This test is extremely sensitive to very small quantities of salicylates, and for this reason a positive test result indicates only salicylate usage and not necessarily poisoning or overdosage. Since the test is only a qualitative test, a positive $FeCl_3$ test must be confirmed with an actual serum salicylate determination. False negative results of $FeCl_3$ testing do not occur or are exceedingly rare: A single (abstract) report noted three false negatives of 187 patients tested.[24] False positive tests may occur when a small quantity of urine that has been used for dipstick analysis with the N-Multistix or Bili Labstix is then used for $FeCl_3$ testing. Presumably, in these cases, some impregnated chemical from the dipstick dissolves in the urine and then causes a false positive reaction.

Another quick bedside urine test for salicylate usage is known as the "urine Trinder spot test."[44] This test utilizes a premixed reagent consisting of mercuric chloride, ferric nitrate, deionized water, and concentrated hydrochloric acid. One milliliter of urine containing salicylates mixed with 1mL of Trinder reagent will turn violet or purple instantly. The sensitivity of the test was 100% when applied to urine collected 2–4 hours after (volunteer) ingestion of 975 mg of salicylate orally.[44]

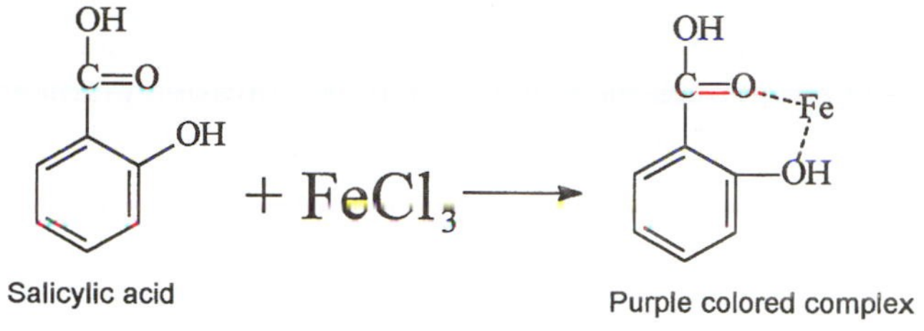

Figure 32–3. The formation of the purple-colored salicylic acid–iron complex is the result of the bedside ferric chloride test.

Yet another bedside test for salicylates utilizes the Ames Phenistix, which was originally created to detect phenylketonuria (PKU). The test is often difficult to interpret and, therefore, only should be used when $FeCl_3$ testing is not available.

A positive bedside urine ketone determination will also help establish the diagnosis of salicylate usage, reflecting the ketogenesis resulting from increased fatty acid metabolism[33] and perhaps the ketone forms of salicylates present.

What Is the Role of Fluid Replacement for Salicylate-Poisoned Patients—Is There a Role for Forced Diuresis?

There is a need to differentiate between restoration of fluid and electrolyte balance in salicylate-poisoned patients as opposed to increasing the fluid load presented to the kidneys with the goal of achieving "forced diuresis": Fluid losses from salicylate poisoning are prominent, especially in children, and can be attributed to tachypnea, vomiting, fever, a hypermetabolic state, hyperpnea, and insensible perspiration.[81] The kidneys also respond to salicylate poisoning by excreting an increased solute load, including large quantities of bicarbonate, sodium, potassium, and organic acids, but renal tubular damage leading to renal failure is rare. Ketoacidosis, hypoglycemia, or hyperglycemia may occur.[3] For all of these reasons the patient's volume status must be adequately assessed and corrected if necessary along with any glucose and electrolyte abnormalities. As in other cases, accurate management of volume status in the poisoned patient may necessitate invasive monitoring with a central venous pressure monitor or, preferably, a pulmonary artery catheter, especially in patients with cardiac disease, noncardiogenic pulmonary edema, or renal compromise.

Increasing fluids *beyond* restoration of fluid balance in order to achieve a forced diuresis is a practice that has been inappropriately emphasized in the past. Although forced diuresis, theoretically, will increase renal tubular flow and reduce the urine tubular cell diffusion gradient for reabsorption, the renal excretion of salicylate depends much more on urine pH than on flow rate, and the use of forced diuresis alone has not been shown to be effective regardless of whether diuretics, osmotic agents, or fluid volumes were used to achieve the diuresis.[68] Although salicylate clearance varies in direct proportion to flow rate, its relation to pH is logarithmic.[47] In summary, although fluid imbalance must be corrected, forced saline diuresis does little more than oral fluids to enhance elimination over a 24-hour period[68] and subjects the patient to the hazards of fluid overload.

What Is the Role of Alkaline Diuresis? How Should Alkalinization Be Achieved?

Alkalinization of both blood *and* urine with $NaHCO_3$ is highly desirable, and alkaline diuresis should be differentiated from forced (saline) diuresis, as the renal excretion of salicylic acid is very dependent on the urinary pH.[68,86] The percentage of a single dose of 1.5 g of sodium salicylate administered to volunteers, excreted unchanged, increased from 2.3 ± 1.5% under acidic conditions to 30.5 ± 9.1% under alkaline conditions. When urine acidity was maintained using ammonium chloride, salicylic acid had a terminal plasma $t_{1/2}$ value of 3.29 ± 0.52 h, which was significantly reduced to 2.50 ± 0.41 h when an alkaline urine was maintained with sodium bicarbonate treatment. The total body clearance of salicylic acid was significantly lower under acidic urine conditions (1.38 ± 0.43) than under alkaline urine conditions (2.27 ± 0.83 L/h).[86]

Because acidemia enhances salicylate transfer into tissue, and particularly into the brain, it must be treated aggressively by raising the blood pH compared to the brain pH, thereby shifting the equilibrium from the tissues to the plasma[31] (Fig. 32–2). To accomplish this, only $NaHCO_3$ and not acetazolamide can be used for alkalinization. Although the administration of acetazolamide, a noncompetitive carbonic anhydrase inhibitor, results in the formation of a bicarbonate-rich alkaline urine, unfortunately, it also causes a systemic metabolic acidosis (acidemia).[21,31] The effect is usually self-limited and mild but results in an increase in the concentration of freely diffusible non-ionized molecules of salicylic acid, thereby increasing the volume of distribution and probably the penetrance of salicylate into the CNS.[52] Because salicylate also appears to inhibit acetazolamide plasma protein binding and renal tubular secretion of acetazolamide, older patients with diminished protein binding and renal function may be at even greater risk for significant metabolic acidosis.[31,78]

Although early endotracheal intubation to maintain hyperventilation may aid in the management of patients whose respiratory efforts may falter after hours of hyperventilating, a respiratory alkalosis sustained by hyperventilation (assisted or unassisted) should never be considered a substitute for either alkalinization with $NaHCO_3$ to achieve alkalemia and an alkaline diuresis or hemodialysis, if necessary.

For all of these reasons, alkalinization with intravenous $NaHCO_3$, should be considered for patients whose salicylate level exceeds 35 mg/dL, and for clinically suspected cases of serious salicylism, until a salicylate level and simultaneously obtained blood pH are available to guide treatment. Patients on therapeutic regimens of salicylates who feel well with salicylate levels of 30–40 mg/dL and who do not manifest toxicity do not require intervention. Oral bicarbonate administration should never be substituted for intravenous bicarbonate to achieve alkalinization, because the oral route may increase salicylate absorption from the GI tract by enhancing dissolution.

Hemodynamically stable adults and children with significant salicylate levels may be alkalinized with a bolus of 1–2 mEq/kg, followed by an intravenous infusion of 3 ampules of $NaHCO_3$ (132 mEq) in 1 L of D_5W, to run at 1.5–2 times maintenance fluid range. Urine pH must be maintained at 7.5–8.0 to achieve maximum ion trapping and maximum excretion. Volume load should remain modest while repleting previous losses. Early hemodialysis must be considered when a patient cannot tolerate the increased solute load that results from alkalinization because of congestive heart failure, renal failure, or cerebral edema.

What Is Meant by "Ion Trapping"?

Because salicylic acid is a weak acid (pK_a 3.5) it will be ionized in an alkaline milieu and, as a result, be "trapped." For this reason, concomitant alkalinization of the blood and the urine will keep salicylates away from the brain and in the blood in addition to enhancing urinary excretion. Alkalinization for salicylate poisoning is the best clinical example of the concept of ion trapping, which in this instance enhances the excretion of the ionized form of salicylate in the alkaline urine, although at least one investigator maintains that ion trapping alone does not account for the increased excretion caused by $NaHCO_3$.[61] When the urine pH increases from 5 to 8, the renal clearance of salicylate increases 10–20 times[65] (Fig. 32–2) (see Antidotes in Depth: Sodium Bicarbonate).

What Problems Associated With Salicylate Poisoning Hinder Alkalinization and Treatment?

Hypokalemia is a common complication of salicylate poisoning and will prevent urinary alkalinization unless corrected. Hypokalemia results from the movement of potassium into cells in exchange for hydrogen ions in the presence of alkalemia, from potassium loss in the urine, and from vomiting, with subsequent metabolic alkalosis and bicarbonaturia.[26] If urinary alkalinization cannot be achieved easily, hypokalemia, excretion of organic acids, and volume depletion should be considered as possible reasons. Calcium should also be monitored, as decreases in both ionized[17] and total serum calcium[25] have also been reported to be complications of bicarbonate therapy.

Frequent blood gas monitoring is necessary for all patients. Although alkalemia is clearly essential, arterial pH should probably not be allowed to rise above 7.55, as alkalemia shifts the oxyhemoglobin dissociation curve to the left and may be otherwise detrimental and difficult to treat. It should be noted, however, that large amounts of bicarbonate may be given to patients with severe salicylism and a blood pH of 7.45–7.50 without necessarily resulting in a further increase in pH. Frequent reassessment of blood pH (and fluid status) almost always allows administration of more $NaHCO_3$ than was initially thought possible.

How Effective Is Activated Charcoal in Managing Salicylate Poisoning and What Are the Roles of Lavage, Catharsis, and Whole-Bowel Irrigation?

In vitro studies suggest that each gram of activated charcoal (AC) can adsorb approximately 550 mg of salicylic acid.[53,67] In vitro, aspirin is adsorbed to AC with moderate efficacy. In humans, AC reduces the absorption of therapeutic aspirin doses by 50–80%, effectively binding enteric-coated and sustained-release preparations in addition to immediate-release tablets.[53] The sooner the AC is given after the salicylate ingestion, the more effective it is in reducing absorption. A 10:1 ratio of AC to salicylate ingested appears to result in maximal efficiency. Although peak serum levels are markedly decreased from predicted concentrations, aspirin desorption from the aspirin–AC complex may diminish the impact on total absorption.[22,60,67] The initial dose of AC is usually given with a cathartic to enhance elimination and, in fact, the benefits of adding sorbitol to AC in achieving salicylate adsorption have been demonstrated.[43]

Repetitive or multiple dosing of activated charcoal (MDAC) probably prevents desorption, which may reduce the level of initially adsorbed salicylate to only 15–20%.[22] Although MDAC increases salicylate elimination in this manner,[7,33] whether MDAC enhances the excretion of salicylates already systematically absorbed is not clear: In one study involving 2800 mg of aspirin followed by 25 g of activated charcoal at 4, 6, 8, and 10 hours after the ingestion, salicylate excretion from the body increased 9–18% but was not considered statistically significant.[45] The authors hypothesized that MDAC might be more effective in enhancing salicylate excretion in the *overdose* situation, when more salicylate is available because of decreased protein binding. However, in another study of the effects of MDAC on the clearance of high-dose intravenous aspirin in a porcine model, MDAC did not enhance the clearance of salicylates under alkaline conditions, ie, when the venous bicarbonate was kept at ≥ 15 mEq/L and urine pH kept at ≥ 7.5.[39] In contrast to the findings of both of these studies, two pediatric patients with salicylate overdoses were successfully treated with MDAC given every 4 hours for 36 hours, and the authors concluded that MDAC is effective in an overdose situation, even after alkalinization.[85] In summary, although its value is controversial in this instance, MDAC is warranted to decrease gastrointestinal absorption (see Antidotes in Depth: Activated Charcoal).

Theoretical support may be found for the use of whole-bowel irrigation (WBI) together with AC to diminish potential desorption, particularly for enteric-coated aspirin preparations.[82] However, the addition of WBI with polyethlyene glycol-electrolyte solution (PEG-ELS) to MDAC did not increase the clearance of absorbed salicylate, even though its effectiveness in preventing absorption of other drugs has been established.[60]

When Should Extracorporeal Removal of Salicylates Be Considered and Which Methods Should Be Used?

Extracorporeal removal of salicylates should be used if the patient is very ill with salicylate poisoning, has a very high salicylate level, has severe fluid or electrolyte disturbances, or is unable to eliminate the salicylates (Table 32–3). In most instances of severe salicylate poisoning, hemodialysis (HD) is the extracorporeal technique of choice, allowing for clearance of the drug as well as rapid correction of fluid, electrolyte and acid–base disorders that are not correctable by hemoperfusion (HP). Apart from this concern, both HP and HD have similar indications. Hemoperfusion has a better clearance (57–116 mL/min) than HD (35–80 mL/min) and is acceptable if (1) HD is unavailable, (2) a mixed overdose might be better treated with HP, or (3) severe hypernatremia is present. Theoretically, the combination of HD and HP in series is both feasible[15] and perhaps more useful for treating severe or mixed overdoses, but is rarely, if ever, employed.

Although peritoneal dialysis (PD) had often been suggested in the past as a simpler extracorporeal procedure for eliminating salicylates in the setting of hemodynamic compromise, a coagulopathy, or the inability to perform HP or HD, PD is only 10–25% as efficient as HP or HD and not even as efficient as renal excretion itself.

TABLE 32–3. INDICATIONS FOR HEMODIALYSIS IN THE SALICYLATE-POISONED PATIENT

Renal failure
Congestive heart failure (relative)
Noncardiogenic pulmonary edema
Persistent CNS disturbances
Progressive deterioration in vital signs
Severe acid–base or electrolyte imbalance, despite appropriate treatment
Hepatic compromise with coagulopathy
Salicylate level (acute) >100 mg/dL

The 24-hour clearance of salicylates with PD is less than the 4-hour clearance of salicylates by HP or HD and for all of these reasons, PD is not recommended. (See Chap. 5 for further discussion.)

What Are the Principles of Immediate Evaluation and Treatment?

Initial assessment of a patient who has ingested an overdose of salicylates includes a determination of the vital signs, particularly the depth and frequency of respiration and temperature. The clinical presentation of a salicylate overdose is characterized by the early onset of nausea, vomiting, abdominal pain, blood-tinged vomitus or gross hematemesis, tinnitus, and lethargy. The presence of hyperventilation, hyperthermia, confusion, coma, seizures, and any other nonspecific neurologic presentation should further heighten the clinician's suspicion of salicylate poisoning (Tables 32–1, 32–2).

If either salicylism or salicylate poisoning is suspected, a bedside ferric chloride ($FeCl_3$) test will confirm salicylate *exposure* (see Fig. 32–3). Using the combination of symptoms, signs, bedside laboratory studies, and characteristic ABG findings, the clinician can rapidly confirm a significant salicylate ingestion, institute immediate alkalinization with $NaHCO_3$, achieve gastric decontamination by orogastric lavage (if indicated), AC, and MDAC, and consider the need for hemodialysis early in the course of management.

For the patient who presents severely ill, maintenance of the airway is essential and requires an extremely careful approach: During initial airway management, death has occurred following sedation.[8] In patients with pulmonary and central nervous system (CNS) manifestations of salicylate toxicity, the possibly protective nature of the hyperpnea or hyperventilation in maintaining alkalemia must be recognized. These patients typically have a significant respiratory alkalosis, and maintaining a high pH (≥ 7.5) at all times is of paramount importance. Urinary alkalinization with $NaHCO_3$ to eliminate salicylates by ion trapping is important, even though the use of $NaHCO_3$ may further complicate electrolyte abnormalities. Fluid and electrolyte replacement (especially potassium) is essential.

How Are People Exposed to Salicylates?

During each year between 1991 and 1995 there were over 181,000 analgesic exposures and 172–235 deaths reported to the American Association of Poison Control Centers Toxic Exposure Surveillance System.[54–58] Among the substances most frequently involved in human exposures, "analgesics" consistently ranked second only to cleaning substances, and among the categories responsible for the largest number of deaths, "analgesics" ranked first (4 out of 5 years) or second (to antidepressants, once). Of the average 200 analgesic-related deaths per year reported, acetaminophen, alone or in combination, accounted for about 46% and aspirin, alone or in combination, accounted for about 24%. If "aspirin, salicylates and salsalate" were listed as a separate category, it would be the seventh most common cause of death from toxic exposures.

Safety packaging, the increasing use of nonsteroidal antiinflammatory drugs (NSAIDs), acetaminophen, or other aspirin substitutes by adults, and the substitution of acetaminophen for aspirin in children to avoid Reye's syndrome[38] all have contributed to decreasing the incidence of unintentional salicylate poisoning. On the other hand, the widespread availability of salicylate preparations without prescription,[48] confusion between product names and brand names, and the ease with which small increments in dosage cause toxicity when salicylates are used chronically, make salicylate poisoning a very common and sometimes fatal occurrence.[42]

In recent years, manufacturers of analgesics have extended popular brand and product names associated with either salicylates or acetaminophen to the other marketed drug or to products containing both. For example, the names "Alka-Seltzer," "Anacin," and "Excedrin," which had once been used exclusively for salicylate-containing products, now are used as brand names for products containing either aspirin, acetaminophen, or both. "Bayer," a company name once exclusively associated with aspirin, now markets, in addition to its aspirin products, a line of products called "Bayer Select" containing ibuprofen or acetaminophen.

Because of the confusion between aspirin and acetaminophen products and the likelihood that either or both may be used in a suicide gesture or attempt, toxicologic analysis for both should always be requested when either one is implicated in a poisoning or exposure. Parents and physicians seeking to use acetaminophen for children with viral illnesses to avoid the possibility of Reye's syndrome should guard against inadvertently selecting a product containing aspirin.

Another common source of patient confusion concerns correct dosage. Terminology such as "grains" and "milligrams" and "baby," "children's," "junior," and "adult" aspirin are often misinterpreted. Both parents and practitioners must remember that a small individual should not receive the maximum dose based on age range; instead, doses should always be based on body weight.

Many patients are unaware that some fixed-dose cold preparations contain aspirin and, therefore, may take aspirin tablets in addition to the fixed-dose preparations, enhancing the likelihood of overdose and toxicity.[48] Others also use preparations such as Pepto Bismol (bismuth subsalicylate), not recognizing that it contains 8.7 mg of salicylic acid/mL.[20] Travelers using large quantities (200–300 mL) of Pepto Bismol may expose themselves to large amounts of salicylate.

Salicylate poisoning (particularly in children) may also result from the extensive application of salicylate-containing ointments,[12] keratolytic agents, or other agents containing methyl salicylate (oil of wintergreen). Due to the high concentration of methyl salicylate (up to 30% in liniments and 100% in pure oil of wintergreen) found in liniments and products used in hot vaporizers, methyl salicylate can be lethal for a young child in the 1–2 teaspoon (5–10 mL) range. Unintentional ingestion of one milliliter of 98% methyl salicylate has the salicylate potency of 1.4 g of acetyl salicylic acid. In a 10-kg child the minimum toxic salicylate dose of approximately 150 mg/kg body weight can almost be achieved with 1 mL, which results in 140 mg/kg of salicylates! (See Chap. 105.)

Overdoses in adolescents and adults usually result from suicide attempts. Rapid diagnosis and appropriate therapy initiated quickly have made mortality uncommon. Salicylism must be considered in all patients with focal and nonfocal neurologic abnormalities, tachypnea, acid–base disorders, and pulmonary edema. As noted previously, older patients and children who develop chronic iatrogenic salicylate intoxication are not usually rapidly diagnosed.

The Food and Drug Administration Advisory Panel on Internal Analgesic and Antirheumatic Products recommends that the maximum adult maintenance dose of aspirin not exceed 3900 mg in 24 hours for more than 10 days in a 70-kg person. No more than 650 mg should be given every 4 hours, except for the initial dose, which should not exceed 1000 mg.

Acknowledgments

Eddy A. Bresnitz, MD and Lorraine Hartnett, MD contributed to this chapter in a previous edition.

References

1. Alvan G, Bergman V, Gustafsson L: High unbound fraction of salicylate in plasma during intoxication. Br J Clin Pharmacol 1981;11:625–626.
2. Anderson RJ, Potts DE, Gabow PA, et al: Unrecognized adult salicylate intoxication. Ann Intern Med 1976;85: 745–748.
3. Arena FP, Dugowson C, Saudek CD: Salicylate-induced hypoglycemia and ketoacidosis in a nondiabetic adult. Arch Intern Med 1978;138:1153–1154.
4. Armstrong CP, Blower AL: Non-steroidal anti-inflammatory drugs and life-threatening complications of peptic ulceration. Gut 1987;28:527–532.
5. Arrowsmith JB, Kennedy DL, Kuritsky JN, et al: National patterns of aspirin use and Reye syndrome reporting. United States 1980 to 1985. Pediatrics 1987;79:858–863.
6. Bailey RB, Jones SR: Chronic salicylate intoxication: A common cause of morbidity in the elderly. J Am Geriatr Soc 1989;37:556–561.
7. Barone J, Raia J, Chain Y: Evaluation of the effects of multiple dose activated charcoal on the absorption of orally administered salicylate in a simulated toxic ingestion model. Ann Emerg Med 1988;17:34–37.
8. Berk WA, Anderson JC: Salicylate associated asystole: Report of two cases. Am J Med 1989;86:505–506.
9. Bogazc K, Caldron P: Enteric coated aspirin bezoar: Elevation of serum salicylate level by barium study. Am J Med 1981;83:783–786.
10. Borga O, Odar-Cederlof I, Ringberger V-A, et al: Protein binding of salicylate in uremic and normal plasma. Clin Pharmacol Ther 1976;20:464–475.
11. Brien J: Ototoxicity associated with salicylates. Drug Safety 1993;9:143–148.
12. Brubacher JR, Hoffman RS: Salicylism from topical salicylates: Review of the literature. J Toxicol Clin Toxicol 1996; 34:431–436.
13. Coggon D, Langman MJS, Spiegelhalter D: Aspirin, paracetamol, hematemesis and melena. Gut 1982;23: 340–344.
14. Davison C: Salicylate metabolism in man. Ann NY Acad Sci 1971;179:249–268.
15. DeBroe ME, Verpooten GA, Christiaens ME, et al: Clinical experience with prolonged combined hemoperfusion-hemodialysis treatment of severe poisoning. Artif Organs 1981;5:59–66.
16. Done AK: Salicylate intoxication: Significance of measurements of salicylate in blood in cases of acute ingestion. Pediatrics 1960;26:800–807.
17. Done AK, Temple AR: Treatment of salicylate poisoning. Mod Treat 1971;8:528–551.
18. Dugandzic RM, Tierney MG, Dickinson GE, et al: Evaluation of the validity of the Done nomogram in the management of acute salicylate intoxication. Ann Emerg Med 1989; 18:1186–1190.
19. Ekstrand R, Alvan A, Borga O: Concentration dependent plasma protein binding of salicylate in rheumatoid patients. Clin Pharmacokinet 1979;4:137–143.
20. Feldman S, Chen SL, Pickering LK: Salicylate absorption from bismuth subsalicylate preparation. Clin Pharmacol Ther 1981;29:788–792.
21. Feuerstein RC, Finberg L, Fleishman BS: The use of acetazolamide in the therapy of salicylate poisoning. Pediatrics 1960;25:215–227.
22. Fillippone G, Fish S, Lacouture P, et al: Reversible adsorption (desorption) of aspirin from activated charcoal. Arch Intern Med 1987;147:1390–1392.
23. Fisher CJ, Albertson TE, Foulke GE: Salicylate induced pulmonary edema. Clinical characteristics in children. Am J Emerg Med 1985;3:33–37.
24. Ford M, Tomaszewski C, Kerns W, et al: Bedside ferric chloride urine test to rule out salicylate intoxication. Vet Hum Toxicol 1994;36:364. Abstract.
25. Fox GN: Hypocalcemia complicating bicarbonate therapy for salicylate poisoning. West J Med 1984;141:108–109.
26. Gabow PA: How to avoid overlooking salicylate intoxication. J Crit Illness 1986;1:77–85.
27. Gabow PA, Anderson RJ, Potts DE, Schrier RW: Acid–base disturbances in the salicylate poisoning in adults. Arch Intern Med 1978;138:1481–1484.
28. Gaudreault P, Temple AR, Lovejoy FH Jr: The relative severity of acute versus chronic salicylate poisoning in children: A clinical comparison. Pediatrics 1982;70:566–569.
29. Hamdan JA, Manasra K, Ahmed M: Salicylate-induced hepatitis in rheumatic fever. Am J Dis Child 1985;139:453–455.
30. Harris FC: Pyloric stenosis: Holdup of enteric-coated aspirin tablets. Br J Surg 1973;60:979–981.
31. Heller I, Halevy J, Cohen S, et al: Significant metabolic acidosis induced by acetazolamide: Not a rare complication. Arch Intern Med 1985;145:1815–1817.

32. Hill JB: Salicylate intoxication. N Engl J Med 1973;288: 1110–1113.
33. Hillman RJ, Prescott LF: Treatment of salicylate poisoning with repeated oral charcoal. Br Med J 1986;291:1472.
34. Hogben CAM, Schanker LS, Jocco DJ, Brodie BB: Absorption of drugs from the stomach. II: The human. J Pharmacol Exp Ther 1957;120:540–545.
35. Hormaechea E, Carlson RW, Rogove H, et al: Hypovolemia, pulmonary edema and protein changes in severe salicylate poisoning. Am J Med 1979;66:1046–1050.
36. Hrnicek G, Skelton J, Miller W: Pulmonary edema and salicylate intoxication. JAMA 1974;230:866–867.
37. Huff RW, Fred HL: Postictal pulmonary edema. Arch Intern Med 1966;117:824–828.
38. Hurwitz ES, Barrett MJ, Bregman D, et al: Public Health Service study on Reye's syndrome and medications: Report of the pilot phase. N Engl J Med 1985;313:849–857.
39. Johnson D, Eppler J, Giesbrecht E, et al: Effect of multiple dose activated charcoal on the clearance of high-dose intravenous aspirin in a porcine model. Ann Emerg Med 1995;26:569–574.
40. Kaplan E, Kennedy J, David J: Effects of salicylate and other benzoates on oxidative enzymes of the tricarboxylic acid cycle in rat tissue homogenates. Arch Biochem Biophys 1954;51:47–61.
41. Karliner J: Noncardiogenic forms of pulmonary edema. Circulation 1972;46:212–215.
42. Karsh J: Adverse reactions and interactions with aspirin—considerations in the treatment of the elderly patient. Drug Safety 1990;5:317–327.
43. Keller RE, Schwab RA, Krenzelok EP: Contribution of sorbitol combined with activated charcoal in prevention of salicylate absorption. Ann Emerg Med 1990;19:654–656.
44. King JA, Storrow AB, Finkelstein JA: Urine Trinder spot test: A rapid salicylate screen for the emergency department. Ann Emerg Med 1995;26: 330–333.
45. Kirshenbaum LA, Mathews SC, Sitar DS, Tenenbein M: Does multiple-dose charcoal therapy enhance salicylate excretion? Arch Intern Med 1990;150:1281–1283.
46. Krebs HG, Woods HG, Alberti KG: Hyperlactatemia and lactic acidosis. Essays Med Biochem 1975;1:81–103.
47. Lawson AAH, Proudfoot AT, Brown SS, et al: Forced diuresis in the treatment of acute salicylate poisoning in adults. Q J Med 1968;149:31–48.
48. Leist ER, Banwell JC: Products containing aspirin. N Engl J Med 1974;291:710–712.
49. Leventhal LJ, Kuritsky L, Ginsburg R, et al: Salicylate induced rhabdomyolysis. Am J Emerg Med 1989;7:409–410.
50. Levy G: Clinical pharmacokinetics of salicylates: A reassessment. Br J Clin Pharmacol 1980;10:285S–290S.
51. Levy G: Clinical pharmacokinetics of aspirin. Pediatrics 1978;62(suppl):867–872.
52. Levy G: Pharmacokinetics of salicylate elimination in man. J Pharm Sci 1965;54:959–967.
53. Levy G, Tsuchiya T: Effect of activated charcoal on aspirin absorption in man. Clin Pharmacol Ther 1972;13:317–322.
54. Litovitz TL, Clark LR, Soloway RA: 1993 Annual Report of the American Association of Poison Control toxic exposure surveillance system. Am J Emerg Med 1994;12:546–599.
55. Litovitz TL, Felberg L, Soloway RA, et al: 1994 Annual Report of the American Association of Poison Control Centers toxic exposure surveillance system. Am J Emerg Med 1995; 13:551–597.
56. Litovitz TL, Felberg L, White S, Klein-Schwartz W: 1995 Annual report of the American Association of Poison Control Centers toxic exposure surveillance system. Am J Emerg Med 1996;14:487–537.
57. Litovitz TL, Holm KL, Bailey KM, et al: 1991 Annual Report of the American Association of Poison Control Centers National Data Collection System. Am J Emerg Med 1992;10: 452–505.
58. Litovitz TL, Holm KC, Clancy C, et al: 1992 Annual Report of the American Association of Poison Control Centers toxic exposure surveillance system. Am J Emerg Med 1993; 11:494–555.
59. Manso C, Taranta A, Nydick I: Effect of aspirin administration on serum glutamic oxaloacetic and glutamic pyruvic transaminases in children. Proc Soc Exp Biol Med 1956;93:84–88.
60. Mayer AL, Sitar DS, Tenenbein M: Multiple-dose charcoal and whole bowel irrigation do not increase clearance of absorbed salicylate. Arch Intern Med 1992;152:393–396.
61. Macpherson CR, Milne MD, Evans BM: The excretion of salicylate. Br J Pharmacol 1955;10:484–489.
62. Miyahara JT, Karler R: Effect of salicylate on oxidative phosphorylation and respiration of mitochondrial fragments. Biochem J 1965;97:194–198.
63. Montgomery H, Porter JC, Bradley RD: Salicylate intoxication causing a severe systemic inflammatory response and rhabdomyolysis. Am J Emerg Med 1994;12:531–532.
64. Montgomery PR, Berger LG, Mitenko PA, Sitar DS: Salicylate metabolism: Effects of age and sex in adults. Clin Pharmacol Ther 1986;39:571–576.
65. Morgan AG, Polak A: The excretion of salicylate in salicylate poisoning. Clin Sci 1971;41:475–484.
66. Myers EN, Bernstein JM, Fostiropolous G: Salicylate ototoxicity. N Engl J Med 1965;273:587–590.
67. Neuvonen PJ, Elfving SM, Elonen E: Reduction of absorption of digoxin, phenytoin and aspirin by activated charcoal in man. Eur J Clin Pharmacol 1978;13:213–218.
68. Prescott LF, Balali-Mood M, Critchley JA, et al: Diuresis or urinary alkalinization for salicylate poisoning. Br Med J 1982;285:1383–1386.
69. Proudfoot AT, Brown SS: Acidaemia and salicylate poisoning in adults. Br Med J 1969;2:547–550.
70. Raschke R, Arnold-Capell P, Richeson R, Curry SC: Refractory hypoglycemia secondary to topical salicylate intoxication. Arch Intern Med 1991;151:591–593.
71. Reye's syndrome surveillance—United States 1989. MMWR 1991;40:88–89.
72. Roberts MS, Cossum PA, Kilpatrick D: Implications of hepatic and extrahepatic metabolism of aspirin in selective inhibition of platelet cyclooxygenase. N Engl J Med 1985;312: 1388–1389.
73. Romankiewicz JA, Reidenberg MM: Factors that modify drug absorption. Ration Drug Ther 1978;12:1–6.
74. Rothschild BM: Hematologic perturbations associated with salicylate. Clin Pharmacol Ther 1979;26:145–150.
75. Schaller JG: Chronic salicylate administration in juvenile rheumatoid arthritis: Aspirin "hepatitis" and its clinical significance. Pediatrics 1978;62(suppl):916–925.

76. Schanker LS, Tocco DJ, Brodie BB, Hogben CAM: Absorption of drugs from the rat's small intestine. J Pharmacol Exp Ther 1958;123:81–88.
77. Sogge MR, Griffith JL, Sinar DR, Mayes GR: Lavage to remove enteric-coated aspirin and gastric outlet obstruction. Ann Intern Med 1977;87:721–722.
78. Sweeney KR, Chapron DJ, Brandt JL, et al: Toxic interaction between acetazolamide and salicylate: Case reports and a pharmacokinetic explanation. Clin Pharmacol Ther 1986;40: 518–524.
79. Swintosky JV: Illustrations and pharmaceutical interpretations of first order drug elimination rate from the bloodstream. J Am Pharm Assoc 1956;45:395–400.
80. Temple AR: Acute and chronic effects of aspirin toxicity and their treatment. Arch Intern Med 1981;141:364–369.
81. Temple AR, George DJ, Done AK, Thompson JA: Salicylate poisoning complicated by fluid retention. Clin Toxicol 1976; 9:61–68.
82. Tenenbein M: Whole bowel irrigation as a gastrointestinal decontamination procedure after acute poisoning. Med Toxicol 1988;3:77–84.
83. Tenney SM, Miller RM: The respiratory and circulatory action of salicylate. Am J Med 1955;19:498–508.
84. Thurston JH, Pollock PG, Warren SK, Jones EM: Reduced brain glucose with normal plasma glucose in salicylate poisoning. Clin Invest 1970;49:2139–2145.
85. Vertrees JE, McWilliams BC, Kelly HW: Repeated oral administration of activated charcoal for treating aspirin overdose in young children. Pediatrics 1990;85: 594–597.
86. Vree TB, Van Ewuk-Beneken Kolmer EWJ, Verwey-Van Wissen CPWGM, Hekster YA. Effect of urinary pH on the pharmacokinetics of salicylate acid, with its glycine and glucuronide conjugates in human. Int J Clin Pharm Ther 1994;32:550–558.
87. Waldman RJ, Hall WN, McGee H, Van Amburg G: Aspirin as a risk factor in Reye's syndrome. JAMA 1982;247: 3089–3094.
88. Walters JS, Woodring JH, Stelling CB, et al: Salicylate-induced pulmonary edema. Radiology 1983;146:289–293.
89. Weisberg HF: Water and electrolytes. In: Davidsohn I, Wells BB, eds: Clinical Diagnosis by Laboratory Methods. Philadelphia, Saunders, 1962, p. 500.
90. Wortzman DJ, Grunfeld A: Delayed absorption following enteric coated aspirin overdose. Ann Emerg Med 1987;16: 434–436.

ANTIDOTES IN DEPTH

Sodium Bicarbonate

Paul M. Wax

Sodium bicarbonate ($NaHCO_3$) is one of the most useful agents available for the treatment of the poisoned patient. Unlike more specific antidotes in which utility is usually limited to antagonizing a single drug or toxin, sodium bicarbonate is a nonspecific antidote effective in the treatment of a number of diverse poisonings. Its most valuable roles are in the treatment of patients with tricyclic antidepressant (TCA) and salicylate overdoses. These two poisonings are among the most frequently encountered and are associated with significant morbidity and mortality. Sodium bicarbonate may also have a role in the treatment of phenobarbital, chlorpropamide, chlorophenoxy herbicide poisonings, and cocaine-induced wide complex tachydysrhythmias. Correcting the life-threatening acidosis generated by methanol and ethylene glycol intoxication and enhancing formate elimination are other important indications for sodium bicarbonate. Alkalinization of the urine for patients with drug- or toxin-associated myoglobinuria may also be useful. The use of sodium bicarbonate in the treatment of common nontoxicologic problems such as lactic acidosis, cardiac resuscitation, and diabetic ketoacidosis is more questionable. Recent studies suggest much less utility for sodium bicarbonate in the treatment of these nontoxicologic disorders than previously thought,[17,52,84] but its use in these situations remains controversial.[81]

The antidotal actions of sodium bicarbonate occur through a number of distinct mechanisms (see Table 32–4). Altering drug ionization, changing sodium gradients, and buffering acidemia are among the most important actions of sodium bicarbonate. A change in the amount of ionized drug may have significant impact on how the drug is distributed to the tissues and how much of the drug is eliminated in the urine. Ionization of weak acids, such as salicylate, phenobarbital, and chlorpropamide, occurs whenever the pH is greater than the pK_a. Since cellular membranes are relatively impermeable to ionized compounds, alkalinization of the blood prevents the movement of ionized drug into the tissues (eg, brain), while alkalinization of the urine increases the amount of ionized drug trapped in the urine. Sodium bicarbonate may also prove beneficial in cases of some cardiotoxic poisonings via a direct sodium effect by increasing the sodium gradient and overcoming sodium channel blockade. This action may be partly responsible for sodium bicarbonate's utility in treating TCA toxicity. Sodium bicarbonate's ability to titrate acid makes it particularly helpful in reversing the life-threatening acidemia generated during methanol or ethylene glycol intoxication. Other mechanisms of sodium bicarbonate in toxicology include increasing drug solubility (eg, methotrexate), preventing myoglobin dissociation (eg, rhabdomyolysis), and neutralization (eg, chlorine gas). Although sodium bicarbonate may work by more than one mechanism in treating a specific poisoning, for the remainder of this section, each drug will be discussed under the most important mechanism.

Sodium bicarbonate is usually administered as a hypertonic solution. The most commonly used preparations are an 8.4% solution (1 M) containing 1 mEq each of sodium and bicarbonate ions per milliliter (calculated osmolarity of 2000 mOsm/L) and a 7.5% solution containing 0.892 mEq each of sodium and bicarbonate ions per milliliter (calculated osmolarity of 1786 mOsm/L). Fifty-milliliter ampules of the 8.4% and 7.5% solutions contain 50 mEq and 44.6 mEq of $NaHCO_3$, respectively.

Altered Drug Ionization Resulting in Altered Drug Distribution

Tricyclic Antidepressants

Sodium bicarbonate's most important role in toxicology appears to be its ability to reverse potentially fatal cardiotoxic effects of the tricyclic antidepressant drugs. The use of sodium bicarbonate for TCA overdose developed as an extension of sodium bicarbonate use in the treatment of other cardiotoxic exposures. Noting similarities in electrocardiographic findings between hyperkalemia and quinidine toxicity (ie, QRS widening), investigators began to use sodium lactate (which is metabolized to sodium bicarbonate by cellular oxidative activity) in the late 1950s for the treatment of quinidine toxicity.[1,5,83] In a dog model, quinidine-induced electrocardiographic changes and hypotension were consistently reversed by the infusion of sodium lactate.[4] Clinical experience confirmed this benefit.[5] Similar efficacy in the treatment of procainamide cardiotoxicity was also reported.[83]

With the introduction of the tricyclic antidepressants during the late 1950s and early 1960s, significant conduction disturbances, dysrhythmias, and hypotension were reported. Extending the use of sodium lactate from the Type I antidysrhythmics to the TCAs, uncontrolled observations in the early 1970s showed a decrease in mortality from 15% to less than 3% when sodium lactate was administered to patients with TCA poisoning.[25] In 1976 the first report of clinical success with the use of sodium bicarbonate in the treatment of a series of TCA-

TABLE 32–4. SODIUM BICARBONATE IN TOXICOLOGY: MECHANISMS, SITE OF ACTION, AND USES

Mechanism	Site of Action	Uses
Altered interaction between drug and sodium channel (also altered sodium gradient)	Heart	Amantadine
		Carbamazepine
		Cocaine
		Encainide
		Flecainide
		Mesoridazine
		Procainamide
		Quinidine
		Quinine
		Thioridazine
		Tricyclic antidepressants
Altered drug ionization leads to altered tissue distribution	Brain	Formic acid
		Phenobarbital
		Salicylates
Altered drug ionization leads to enhanced drug elimination	Kidneys	Chlorophenoxy herbicides
		Chlorpropamide
		Formic acid
		Methotrexate
		Phenobarbital
		Salicylates
Correct acidosis	Metabolic	Cyanide
		Ethylene glycol
		Isoniazid
		Methanol
Increase drug solubility	Kidneys	Methotrexate
Prevent myoglobin dissociation	Kidneys	Rhabdomyolysis
Neutralization	Lungs	Chlorine gas
		Hydrogen chloride
		Phosgene

induced dysrhythmias in children was reported.[12] In this series, 9 out of 12 children who had developed multifocal PVCs, ventricular tachycardia, or heart block reverted to normal sinus rhythm with sodium bicarbonate therapy alone. An early animal experiment at this time in amitriptyline-poisoned dogs demonstrated resolution of dysrhythmias upon alkalinization of the blood to a pH above 7.40.[12] Other methods of alkalinization including hyperventilation and administration of a nonsodium buffer, tris(hydroxymethyl)aminomethane (THAM), also appeared effective in reversing the dysrhythmias.[13,37]

A better understanding of the mechanism and utility of sodium bicarbonate has come about through a series of additional animal experiments during the 1980s. In amitriptyline-poisoned dogs, it was shown that sodium bicarbonate reversed conduction slowing and ventricular dysrhythmias and suppressed ventricular ectopy.[54] When comparing sodium bicarbonate, hyperventilation, hypertonic sodium chloride, and lidocaine, sodium bicarbonate and hyperventilation proved most efficacious in reversing ventricular dysrhythmias and narrowing QRS interval prolongation. Although lidocaine transiently antagonized dysrhythmias, this antagonism was demonstrated only at nearly toxic lidocaine levels and was associated with hypotension. In these studies, hypertonic sodium chloride failed to reverse dysrhythmias. Furthermore, prophylactic alkalinization protected against the development of dysrhythmias in a pH-dependent manner.

In another study, this time in desipramine-poisoned rats, the isolated use of sodium chloride was also effective in decreasing QRS duration as well as the use of sodium bicarbonate.[59] Both sodium bicarbonate and sodium chloride also increased mean arterial pressure but hyperventilation or direct intravascular volume repletion with mannitol did not. In further experimental studies, in vivo, and on isolated cardiac tissue, it was demonstrated that both alkalinization and sodium concentration modulate TCA effects on cardiac conduction.[70,71] Though hypocapnia and sodium chloride each independently improved conduction velocity, this effect was greater when sodium bicarbonate was administered.

Since TCAs are weak bases (high pK_a), alkalinization increases the proportion of nonionized drug. This increase in the proportion of nonionized drug at the sodium channel may decrease drug–receptor binding (possibly due to a redistribution of drug from the central compartment to the periphery because of less ion trapping in the blood), thus diminishing the TCA effect on cardiac conduction. Decreased ionization should not significantly decrease the rate of TCA elimination because of the small contribution of renal pathways to overall TCA elimination (less than 5%).

Sodium bicarbonate seems to work independently of initial blood pH. Animal studies showed that cardiac conduction improved after treatment with sodium bicarbonate or sodium chloride in both normal pH and acidemic animals.[59] Clinically, TCA-poisoned patients who are already alkalemic have also responded to repeat doses of sodium bicarbonate.[49]

Although several authorities have suggested that sodium bicarbonate's efficacy is modulated via a pH-dependent change in protein binding that decreases the proportion of free drug,[13,43] further study failed to support this hypothesis.[61] The administration of large doses of a binding protein alpha-1-acid glycoprotein (AAG) (to which TCAs show great affinity) to desipramine-poisoned rats only minimally decreased cardiotoxicity. Although the addition of AAG increased the concentration of total desipramine and protein-bound desipramine in the serum, the concentration of active free desipramine did not decline significantly. A redistribution of TCA from peripheral sites may have prevented lowering of free desipramine. The persistence of other TCA-associated toxicity such as the anticholinergic effects and seizures also argues against changes in protein binding modulating toxicity. In vitro studies performed in a protein-free bath further support that sodium bicarbonate's efficacy is independent of protein binding.[70]

Hence, sodium bicarbonate appears to have a crucial antidotal role in TCA poisoning by partially reversing the fast sodium channel blockade caused by these drugs. The animal evidence supports two distinct and additive mechanisms for this effect: (1) a pH-dependent effect manifested by the production of an increased fraction of the more freely diffusible nonionized drug that can be liberated from the sodium channel and (2) a sodium-dependent effect manifested by increasing the sodium gradient across the partially closed sodium channels. The actual contribution of each mechanism requires further clarification. Sodium bicarbonate reverses the quinidine-like effects that produce the major, life-threatening cardiovascular manifestations of TCA overdose. Other effects caused by the anticholinergic, alpha-adrenergic antagonism, reuptake inhibition, and direct CNS properties of the TCAs are not affected by the administration of sodium bicarbonate.

Although there are many anecdotal accounts supporting the efficacy of sodium bicarbonate in treating TCA cardiotoxicity in humans,[31] these reports are all uncontrolled observations; controlled studies are not available. In one of the largest retrospective observational studies involving 91 patients who received sodium bicarbonate after TCA overdose, QRS prolongation corrected in 39 of 49 patients who had QRS duration greater than 0.12 seconds, and hypotension corrected within 1 hour in 20 of 21 patients who had systolic BP < 90 mm Hg.[32] The use of sodium bicarbonate was not associated with any complications in this study.

The exact indications for the use of sodium bicarbonate after TCA overdose have not been studied. Since studies have shown that there is a critical QRS duration at which ventricular dysrhythmias may occur (> 0.16 sec),[9] it seems reasonable that narrowing the QRS interval through the use of sodium bicarbonate or hyperventilation may prophylactically prevent the development of dysrhythmias. Controversy exists, however, over the use of sodium bicarbonate in situations in which the QRS interval is less than 0.16 sec. Although sodium bicarbonate has no proven efficacy in either the treatment or prophylaxis of TCA-induced seizures, seizures often cause acidemia, which rapidly increases the risks of conduction disturbances and ventricular dysrhythmias. Administering sodium bicarbonate in situations in which the QRS duration is 0.10 sec or greater may establish a theoretical margin of safety in the event that the patient suddenly deteriorates by lessening the likelihood of subsequent dysrhythmias without adding significant demonstrable risk. In situations in which the QRS duration is less than 0.10 sec (given the negligible risk of seizures or dysrhythmias), prophylactic use of sodium bicarbonate is not indicated.

Since cardiotoxicity may worsen during the first few hours after ingestion, sodium bicarbonate should be started immediately if QRS interval widening to 0.10 sec or greater is noted. Since TCA-induced hypotension also responds to sodium bicarbonate in experimental models, hypotension is another indication for sodium bicarbonate. However, there is no evidence to support a role for sodium bicarbonate in a TCA-poisoned patient who presents with an altered mental status without QRS widening or hypotension.

Since the potential benefits of alkalinization in TCA overdose usually outweigh the risks, sodium bicarbonate should be administered regardless of whether the patient has an acidemic or normal pH. One to two mEq/kg body weight should be administered intravenously as a bolus over a period of 1–2 minutes.[58] Greater amounts may be required to treat unstable ventricular dysrhythmias. Sodium bicarbonate can then be repeated as needed to achieve a blood pH of 7.50–7.55.[60,74] The endpoint of treatment is a narrowing of the QRS interval. Excessive alkalemia (pH > 7.55) and hypernatremia should be avoided. Since sodium bicarbonate has a brief duration of effect, a continuous infusion is usually required after the intravenous bolus. One to three 50-mL ampules may be placed in a liter of fluid and run at maintenance or more than maintenance, depending on the fluid requirements and blood pressure of the patient. If a multiple-ampule infusion is contemplated, the sodium bicarbonate should be placed in a hypotonic solution such as 5% dextrose in water in order to limit the sodium load. Frequent evaluation of fluid status should also be performed to avoid precipitating pulmonary edema. Hyperventilation may be a useful alternative to sodium bicarbonate in reversing the cardiotoxicity of TCAs. Recent experimental evidence suggests that 7.5% hypertonic saline may also prove beneficial in reversing QRS prolongation and hypotension after TCA overdose but significant clinical experience with this approach is lacking.[46]

Other Cardiotoxic Drugs

Sodium bicarbonate may also be useful in treating cardiotoxicity from other drugs with "quinidine-like effects" that impair sodium channel functioning manifested by widened QRS complexes, dysrhythmias, and hypotension. Isolated case reports provide the bulk of the evidence in these situations. Demonstrable utility of sodium bicarbonate in treating Type IA antidysrhythmics such as quinidine and procainamide has already been shown.[5,83] The use of sodium bicarbonate in the successful treatment of conduction disturbances from an overdose of quinine (an optical isomer of quinidine) has also been reported.[8] Studies on dogs poisoned with the Type IC antidysrhythmics, flecainide and encainide, show reversal of the conductance slowing with sodium bicarbonate.[2,68] In a clinical case of encainide overdose, bradycardia, hypotension, and increased QRS duration all resolved after the administration of sodium bicarbonate.[60] Sodium bicarbonate has also proven effective in narrowing the QRS complex in the setting of a propoxyphene-induced wide complex dysrhythmia.[77] The use of sodium bicarbonate in the treatment of an amantadine overdose manifested by prolongation of the QRS and QT_C intervals was associated with a narrowing of the QT_C but not the QRS interval.[21] Sodium bicarbonate may also help in the management of other ingestions associated with Type IA like cardiac conduction abnormalities and dysrhythmias such as the phenothiazines, thioridazine and mesoridazine, and carbamazepine, but documentation of such benefit is lacking.

Cocaine (a local anesthetic with membrane-stabilizing properties resembling other Type I antidysrhythmics) may also cause similar conduction disturbances. In a dog model, sodium bicarbonate successfully reversed cocaine-induced QRS prolongation.[3,57] Similar findings were demonstrated in cocaine-treated guinea pig hearts.[86] Clinical experience with this approach is not well documented.

Altered Drug Ionization Resulting in Enhanced Elimination

Salicylates

Although there is no known specific antidote for salicylate toxicity, judicious use of sodium bicarbonate is an essential treatment modality in moderate and severe salicylism. Sodium bicarbonate, through its ability to change the concentration gradient of the ionized and nonionized fractions of salicylates, has proven utility in decreasing tissue (eg, brain) levels and enhancing urinary elimination of salicylates. This therapy may also limit the need for more invasive treatment modalities such as hemodialysis.

Salicylate is a weak acid with a pK_a of 3.0. According to the Henderson-Hasselbalch equation, at a pH of 3.0, equal concentrations of nonionized and ionized salicylate exist. As pH increases, more of the drug is in the ionized form. This change in ionization occurs in a logarithmic fashion such that 90% of the molecules are ionized at a pH of 4.0 and 99% are ionized at a pH of 5.0. Ionized molecules penetrate lipid-soluble membranes less rapidly than nonionized molecules due to the presence of polar groups on the ionized form. Consequently, weak acids such as salicylates may accumulate in an alkaline milieu such as an alkaline urine when the ionized forms predominate.[47]

Although alkalinizing the urine to increase salicylate elimination is certainly an important intervention in the treatment of salicylate poisoning, increasing the serum pH in patients with severe salicylism may prove even more consequential by protecting the brain from a lethal CNS salicylate burden. Using sodium bicarbonate to "trap" salicylate in the blood (keeping it out of the brain) may prevent clinical deterioration of the salicylate-intoxicated patient. Salicylate lethality is directly related to primary central nervous system dysfunction, which, in turn, corresponds to a "critical brain salicylate level."[29] At physiologic pH where a very small proportion of the salicylate is in the nonionized form, a small change in pH will be associated with a significant change in amount of nonionized molecules (eg, at a pH of 7.4, 0.004% of the salicylate molecules are in the nonionized form, at a pH of 7.2, 0.008% of the salicylate is in the nonionized form). In experimental models, lowering the blood pH by inhaling a mixture of 20% carbon dioxide and 80% oxygen or infusing ammonium chloride produces a shift of salicylate into the tissues.[14] Hence, the metabolic acidemia that is observed in significant salicylate intoxications can be devastating.

Fortunately, in salicylate intoxication, the earliest and most common acid–base disturbance is a respiratory alkalosis. Alkalemia slows the entrance of salicylate into the brain by widening the arterial–cerebral spinal fluid pH difference. In salicylate-poisoned rats, increasing the blood pH with sodium bicarbonate produced a shift in salicylate out of the tissues and into the blood.[30] This change in salicylate distribution did not result from enhanced urinary excretion since occlusion of the renal pedicles failed to alter these results. Acidemia with resultant aciduria, however, will tend to further inhibit elimination of salicylates, thus prolonging toxicity and possibly leading to worsening acidemia.

Trapping the ionized salicylate moiety in the urine may also provide great benefit. Salicylate elimination at low therapeutic concentrations consists predominantly of first-order hepatic metabolism At these low concentrations, without alkalinization, only about 10–20% of salicylate is eliminated unchanged in the urine. With increasing concentrations enzyme saturation occurs (Michaelis-Menten kinetics); thereby, a larger percentage of elimination occurs as unchanged free salicylate. Under these conditions, in an alkaline urine, urinary excretion of free salicylate becomes even more significant, accounting for 60–85% of total elimination.[26,65]

The exact mechanism of pH-dependent salicylate elimination has generated controversy. The pH-dependent increase in urinary elimination was initially ascribed to "ion trapping": the filtering of both ionized and nonionized salicylate while reabsorbing only the nonionized salicylate.[75] Other authorities, however, argue that limiting reabsorption of the ionizable fraction of filtered salicylate cannot be the primary mechanism responsible for enhanced elimination produced by sodium bicarbonate.[44] Since the quantitative difference between the percentage of molecules trapped in the ionized form at a pH of 5.0 (99% ionized) and a pH of 8.0 (99.999% ionized) is small, decreases in tubular reabsorption cannot fully explain the rapid increase in urinary elimination seen above a pH of 7.0.

"Diffusion theory" offers a reasonable alternative explanation. Fick's Law of Diffusion states that the rate of flow of a diffusing substance is proportional to its concentration gradient. A large concentration gradient between the nonionized salicylate in the peritubular fluid (and blood) and the tubular luminal fluid is found in alkaline urine. Since at a higher urinary pH a greater proportion of secreted nonionized molecules quickly become ionized upon entering the alkaline environment, more salicylate (ie, nonionized salicylate) must pass from the peritubular fluid into the urine in an attempt to reach equilibrium with the nonionized fraction. In fact, as long as nonionized molecules are rapidly converted to ionized molecules in the urine, equilibrium in the alkaline milieu will never be achieved. The concentration gradient of peritubular nonionized salicylates to urinary nonionized salicylates continues to increase with rising urinary pH. Hence, increased tubular secretion, not decreased reabsorption, accounts for most of the increase in salicylate elimination observed in the alkaline urine.[44]

Controversies regarding the indications for alkalinization in the treatment of salicylism have persisted. Although urinary alkalinization undoubtedly works to lower serum salicylate levels and enhance urinary elimination, the risks associated with alkalinization in the management of salicylism have generated concern. Questions regarding excessive alkalemia, hypernatremia, fluid overload, hypokalemia, and hypocalcemia, as well as the potential delay in achieving alkalinization with sodium bicarbonate (as opposed to more rapid response achieved with hyperventilation), have all been raised.[23,42,58,65,73] Some authorities have even suggested that the administration of sodium bicarbonate to adolescents and adults with prolonged hyperventilation and hypocapnia who have a pure respiratory alkalosis may result in tetany, encephalopathy, and death.[73] Patients with pure respiratory alkalosis often have alkaluria as well as alkalemia and do not require urinary alkalinization. In the more common scenario in which patients present with a mixed respiratory alkalosis and metabolic acidosis, sodium bicarbonate must be administered cautiously. The young child, who rapidly develops a metabolic acidosis, often requires alkalinization, but should be at less risk for complications of this therapy.[56]

Sodium bicarbonate is indicated in the treatment of salicylate poisoning for most patients with evidence of significant systemic toxicity. Although some authors have suggested alkali therapy for asymptomatic patients with levels above 30 mg/dL,[85] there are few data to support this approach. For patients suffering from a chronic intoxication, levels are not as helpful and may be misleading; clinical criteria remain the best indicators for therapy. A chest radiograph and arterial blood gas analysis to determine the alveolar–arterial oxygen gradient may be helpful in evaluating more subtle cases of acute or chronic intoxications. Patients with contraindications to sodium bicarbonate use, such as renal failure or pulmonary edema, may benefit from hyperventilation; extracorporeal removal may be required in some instances.

Dosing recommendations depend on the acid–base status of the patient. For the patient with acidemia, rapid correction is indicated with intravenous administration of 1–2 mEq/kg body weight of sodium bicarbonate.[78] Once the blood is alkalinized, or if the patient has already presented with an alkalemia, continued titration with sodium bicarbonate over 4–8 hours is recommended until the urine pH reaches 7.5–8.0.[76,78] Alkalinization can be maintained with a continuous sodium bicarbonate infusion of 100–150 mEq in 1 L of 5% dextrose in water at 150–200 mL/h (or about twice the maintenance requirements in a child). Obtaining a urinary pH of 8.0 is difficult but is considered the goal. Fastidious attention to the changing acid–base status is required. Systemic pH should be kept below 7.55 to prevent complications of alkalemia. Acetazolamide (Diamox) should not be used in the treatment of salicylate toxicity.[78] Although recommended in the past because of its ability to alkalinize the urine,[51,65] acetazolamide produces a systemic and possibly CSF acidosis that may potentiate salicylate toxicity.[18,27]

Hypokalemia can make urinary alkalinization particularly problematic.[42,72] In the hypokalemic patient, regardless of total body potassium stores, the kidney will preferentially reabsorb potassium in exchange for hydrogen ions. Alkalinization will be unsuccessful as long as hydrogen ions are excreted into the urine. Thus, appropriate potassium supplementation to achieve normokalemia may be required in order to alkalinize the urine.[87]

In the past, proper urinary alkalinization was thought to require forced diuresis in order to maximize salicylate elimination.[19,42] Suggestions included administering enough fluid (2 L/h) to produce a urine output of 500 mL/h. This method of alkalinization, however, often leads to fluid retention. Excess fluid may be of particular concern in salicylate-poisoned patients who present with or are at high risk of pulmonary edema, cerebral edema, and renal failure.[34,76,79,88] A significantly higher urinary pH was obtained with sodium bicarbonate alone (pH = 8.10) compared to forced alkaline diuresis.[63] Since forced alkaline diuresis appears unnecessary and is potentially harmful due to its unnecessarily large fluid load, alkalinization at a rate of approximately twice maintenance requirements to achieve a urine output of 3–5 mL/kg/h is the goal.

Phenobarbital

Although cardiopulmonary support is the most critical intervention in the treatment of severe phenobarbital overdose, sodium bicarbonate may be a useful adjunct to the general supportive care. The utility of sodium bicarbonate may be particularly important considering the long plasma half-life (about 100 hours) of phenobarbital. Phenobarbital is a weak acid (pK_a of 7.24) that undergoes significant renal elimination. As in the case of salicylates, alkalinization of the blood and urine may reduce the severity and duration of toxicity. In an mouse study, the median anesthetic dose for mice receiving phenobarbital increased by 20% with the addition of 1 g/kg of sodium bicarbonate (raising the blood pH from 7.23 to 7.41), suggesting decreased tissue levels associated with increased pH.[82] Extrapolating the animal evidence to humans, it has been suggested that phenobarbital-intoxicated patients in deep coma might develop a respiratory acidosis secondary to hypoventilation, with the acidemia enhancing the entrance of phenobarbital into the brain, thus worsening central nervous system and respiratory depression. Alternatively, increasing the pH with bicarbonate and/or ventilatory support would enhance the passage of phenobarbital out of the brain, thus lessening toxicity. Given the relatively high pK_a of phenobarbital, significant phenobarbital accumulation in the urine is evident only when urinary pH is raised above 7.5.[7] As the pH approaches 8.0, a threefold increase in urinary elimination occurs. The urine to serum ratio of phenobarbital, while much higher in the alkaline urine than acidic urine, remains less than unity, thereby suggesting less of a role for tubular secretion than in salicylate toxicity.

Unfortunately, clinical studies examining the role of alkalinization in phenobarbital toxicity have been inadequately designed. Many are poorly controlled and fail to examine the effects of alkalinization independent of co-administered diuretic therapy. In one uncontrolled study, a 59–67% decrease in duration of unconsciousness in patients with phenobarbital overdoses occurred in patients administered alkali when compared to nonrandomized controls.[48] In other older studies treatment with sodium lactate and urea reduced mortality and frequency of tracheotomy to 50% of controls, enhanced elimination, and shortened coma.[41,53] In a more recent human volunteer study, urinary alkalinization with sodium bicarbonate was associated with a decrease in phenobarbital elimination half-life from 148 hours to 47 hours. However, this beneficial effect was less than the effect achieved by multiple-dose activated charcoal, which reduced the half-life to 19 hours.[24] Sodium bicarbonate therapy does not appear warranted in the treatment of ingestions of other barbiturates, such as pentobarbital and secobarbital, each of which has a pK_a above 8.0 and is predominantly eliminated by the liver.

Chlorpropamide

Alkalinization has also been shown to enhance the renal elimination of chlorpropamide.[55] Chlorpropamide is a weak acid (pK_a of 4.80) and has a long half-life (30–50 hours). Since patients who ingest this agent in overdose are at risk for prolonged hypoglycemia, enhancing the elimination should shorten the duration of intoxication and lessen the risk of complications. In a human study using therapeutic doses of chlorpropamide, urinary alkalinization with sodium bicarbonate significantly increased renal clearance of the drug.[55] This study showed that nonrenal clearance was the more significant route of elimination at a urinary pH of 5.0–6.0 (only slightly above pK_a), while at a pH of 8.0, renal clearance was 10 times that of nonrenal clearance. Alkalinization reduced the area under the curve almost fourfold and shortened elimination half-life from 50 hours to 13 hours; acidification increased the area under the curve by 41% and increased the half-life to 69 hours. While not a study in overdose patients, this report suggests that sodium bicarbonate may be useful in the management of patients with chlorpropamide overdose. The effect of alkalinization on elimination of other sulfonylureas is unknown.

Chlorophenoxy Herbicides

Alkalinization has also been used in the treatment of poisonings from the weed killers that contain chlorophenoxy compounds such as 2,4-dichlorophenoxyacetic acid (2,4-D) or 2-4-chloro-2-methylphenoxy propionic acid (MCPP).[64] Significant exposure to these herbicides may result in muscle weakness, peripheral neuropathy, coma, hyperthermia, and acidemia. These compounds are weak acids (pK_a 2.6 and 3.8 for 2,4-D and MCPP, respectively) that are excreted largely unchanged in the urine. In an uncontrolled case series of 41 patients poisoned with a variety of chlorophenoxy herbicides, 19 of whom received sodium bicarbonate, alkaline diuresis significantly reduced the half-life of each compound by enhancing renal elimination.[22] In one patient, resolution of hyperthermia and metabolic acidosis and improvement in mental status were associated with a transient elevation of serum levels of these compounds, perhaps reflecting chlorophenoxy compound redistribution from the tissues into the more alkalemic blood. The limited data suggest that the increased ionized fractions of the weak-acid chlorophenoxy compounds produced by alkalinization appear to be trapped in both the blood and the urine (as demonstrated with salicylates and phenobarbital), thus ameliorating toxicity and shortening duration of effect.

Correcting Metabolic Acidosis

Toxic Alcohols

Sodium bicarbonate has two important roles in treating toxic alcohol ingestions. As an immediate temporizing measure, administration of sodium bicarbonate may reverse the life-threatening acidemia associated with methanol and ethylene glycol ingestions. In rats poisoned with ethylene glycol, the administration of sodium bicarbonate alone resulted in a fourfold increase in median lethal dose, perhaps due to decreased calcium excretion.[10] Clinically, titrating the exogenous acid with bicarbonate may be of great assistance in reversing the consequences of the severe acidemia, such as hemodynamic instability and multiorgan dysfunction.

The second role for bicarbonate involves its ability to favorably alter the distribution and elimination of toxic metabolites. This effect has been investigated only in methanol toxicity. Although still not extensively studied, it has been suggested that visual impairment associated with methanol toxicity improved with sodium bicarbonate therapy.[66] Some authorities have suggested that decreased ocular toxicity may result from tissue redistribution of formic acid induced by rising pH.[36,45] The proportion of ionized formic acid can be increased by administering bicarbonate, thereby trapping formate in the blood compartment. Consequently, decreased visual toxicity may result not from a nonspecific correction of the acidosis but from the removal of the toxic metabolite from the optic nerve. In cases of formic acid (pK_a 3.7) ingestion, sodium bicarbonate may also decrease tissue penetration of the formic acid and enhance urinary elimination.[50] Further investigation is required to delineate the beneficial effects of sodium bicarbonate in the treatment of toxic alcohol ingestions.

Early treatment of acidemia with sodium bicarbonate is strongly recommended in cases of methanol and ethylene glycol intoxications.[28] This early use of sodium bicarbonate differs from the management of diabetic ketoacidosis and lactic acidosis where the threshold for bicarbonate use should be high. Sodium bicarbonate should be administrated to toxic alcohol-poisoned patients with an arterial pH below 7.30.[40] More than 400–600 mEq of sodium bicarbonate may be required in the first few hours.[35] In cases of ethylene glycol toxicity, sodium bicarbonate administration may worsen hypocalcemia; therefore serum calcium should be monitored. Combating the acidemia, however, is not the mainstay of therapy, and concurrent administration of intravenous ethanol and preparation for hemodialysis are almost always indicated.

Increasing Drug Solubility

Methotrexate

Urinary alkalinization with sodium bicarbonate is also routinely employed during high-dose methotrexate cancer chemotherapy therapy. Methotrexate is predominantly eliminated unchanged in the urine. Unfortunately, it is poorly water soluble in acidic urine. Under these conditions, tubular precipitation of the methotrexate may occur, leading to nephrotoxicity and decreased elimination, increasing the likelihood of methotrexate toxicity. The administration of sodium bicarbonate (as well as intensive hydration) during high-dose methotrexate infusions increases methotrexate solubility as well as increasing the elimination of methotrexate.[16,69]

Preventing Myoglobin Dissociation

Rhabdomyolysis

Skeletal muscle injury (rhabdomyolysis) is a frequent complication of significant poisoning. This occurs as a direct toxic effect (eg, doxylamine, heroin) or indirect manifestation of muscle ischemia (eg, barbiturates, cocaine, carbon monoxide, ethanol withdrawal). Subsequent myoglobinuria may lead to renal injury and accounts for approximately 10% of cases of acute renal failure.[39] Animal evidence suggests that renal injury from myoglobinuria is dependent on the pH of the urine.[62] At or below urine pH of 5.60, myoglobin dissociates into ferrihemate and globin; ferrihemate is apparently toxic to the renal tubule.

Routine urinary alkalinization in patients with rhabdomyolysis as a means of preventing renal impairment and hyperkalemia has been suggested.[6] In an uncontrolled retrospective study, forced alkaline diuresis (with an intravenous infusion of 25 g of mannitol and 100 mEq of sodium bicarbonate in 1 L of 5% dextrose in water at a rate of 250 mL/h for 4 hours as soon as possible after admission and after obvious volume deficits have been replaced) may prevent development of renal injury in some patients with rhabdomyolysis.[20] Urinary pH, however, was not measured. In a case series of traumatic rhabdomyolysis, a similar protocol appeared to prevent renal damage in patients who achieved a urine pH above 6.5.[67]

Given the lack of strong clinical data, other authorities have questioned the necessity for sodium bicarbonate as long as the urine pH is kept above 6.0.[33,38] Fluid repletion and mannitol may increase the urine flow to 200–300 mL/h, thus creating alkaline urine simply from a dilution effect. Concerns about sodium bicarbonate precipitating tetany in patients already at risk for hypocalcemia have also been raised.[38] If it is not possible to keep the urine pH above 6.0 with fluid resuscitation and mannitol alone, however, alkalinization with sodium bicarbonate is indicated. Large amounts (eg, 300 mEq/d) may be required.

Neutralization

Chlorine Gas

Nebulized sodium bicarbonate has recently been suggested as a useful adjunct in the treatment of pulmonary injuries resulting from chlorine gas inhalation.[15,80] Inhaled sodium bicarbonate is purported to neutralize the hydrochloric acid that is formed when the chlorine gas reacts with the water in the respiratory tree. Although oral sodium bicarbonate is not recommended to neutralize acid ingestions because of the problems associated with the exothermic reaction and production of carbon dioxide in the relatively closed gastrointestinal tract, the rapid exchange of air with the environment should facilitate heat dissipation. In a chlorine-inhalation sheep model, animals treated with 4% nebulized sodium bicarbonate solution demonstrated higher PO_2 and lower PCO_2 than did the normal, saline-treated animals.[15] There was no difference, however, in 24-hour mortality or pulmonary histopathology. Anecdotal experience suggests that nebulized bicarbonate therapy may lead to improvement of symptoms.[80] In a recent retrospective review, 86 cases of chlorine gas inhalation were treated with nebulized sodium bicarbonate.[11] Sixty-nine patients were sent home from the ED, 53 of whom had clearly improved. Such uncontrolled observations do not provide convincing evidence for the efficacy of such an approach, but the nebulized sodium bicarbonate was well tolerated. Further clinical studies are required to further assess the efficacy and safety of this treatment.

Nontoxicologic Uses of Sodium Bicarbonate

Sodium bicarbonate has also been advocated for a variety of other critical care situations not directly pertaining to poisonings, such as hyperkalemia, lactic acidosis, cardiac resuscitation, and diabetic ketoacidosis. For most of these states, other than hyperkalemia, bicarbonate is given in an attempt to correct acidemia. Its use, however, in some of these conditions remains debatable and may actually prove detrimental.

Summary

Despite the increasing tendency to avoid sodium bicarbonate administration in the critically ill acidemic patient, sodium bicarbonate remains an important agent in the treatment of a wide variety of drug and toxin exposures. In fact, its utility in the poisoned patient continues to expand. Not only is sodium bicarbonate effective in the treatment of poisonings by tricyclic antidepressants, salicylates, and phenobarbital, but it also shows promise in the treatment of toxicity from newer antidysrhythmics, cocaine, chlorophenoxy herbicides, and chlorine gas. In the severely poisoned patient such as those manifesting quinidine-like effects, sodium bicarbonate is specific therapy. In the more common causes of metabolic acidosis (eg, lactic acidosis), specific therapy such as antibiotics, volume resuscitation, and inotropic support usually takes precedence over bicarbonate administration.

References

1. Bailey DJ: Cardiotoxic effects of quinidine and their treatment. Arch Intern Med 1960;105:37–46.
2. Bajaj AK, Woosley RL, Roden DM: Acute electrophysiologic effects of sodium administration in dogs treated with O-desmethyl encainide. Circulation 1989;80:994–1002.
3. Beckman KJ, Parker RB, Hariman RJ, et al: Hemodynamic and electrophysiological actions of cocaine. Effects of sodium bicarbonate as an antidote in dogs. Circulation 1991; 83:1799–1807.
4. Bellet S, Hamdan G, Somiyo A, Lara R: The reversal of cardiotoxic effects of quinidine by molar sodium lactate: An experimental study. Am J Med Sci 1959;237:165–176.
5. Bellet S, Wasserman F: The effects of molar sodium lactate in reversing the cardiotoxic effect of hyperpotassemia. Arch Intern Med 1957;100:565–581.
6. Better OS, Stein JH: Early management of shock and prophylaxis of acute renal failure in traumatic rhabdomyolysis. N Engl J Med 1990;322:825–829.
7. Bloomer HA: A critical evaluation of diuresis in the treatment of barbiturate intoxication. J Lab Clin Med 1966;67: 898–905.
8. Bodenhamer JE, Smilkstein MJ: Delayed cardiotoxicity following quinine overdose: A case report. J Emerg Med 1993; 11:279–285.
9. Boehnert MT, Lovejoy FH Jr: Value of the QRS duration versus the serum drug level in predicting seizures and ventricular arrhythmias after an acute overdose of tricyclic antidepressants. N Engl J Med 1985;313:474–479.
10. Borden TA, Bidwell CD: Treatment of acute ethylene glycol poisoning in rats. Invest Urol 1968;6:205–210.
11. Bosse GM: Nebulized sodium bicarbonate in the treatment of chlorine gas inhalation. J Toxicol Clin Toxicol 1994;32: 233–241.
12. Brown TCK: Sodium bicarbonate treatment for tricyclic antidepressant arrhythmias in children. Med J Aust 1976;2: 380–382.
13. Brown TCK, Barker CA, Dunlop ME, Loughnan PM: The use of sodium bicarbonate in the treatment of tricyclic antidepressant-induced arrhythmias. Anaesth Intensive Care 1973;1:203–210.
14. Buchanan N, Kundig H, Eyberg C: Experimental salicylate intoxication in young baboons. J Pediatr 1975;86:225–232.
15. Chisholm CD, Singletary EM, Okerberg CV, Langlinais PC: Inhaled sodium bicarbonate therapy for chlorine inhalation injuries. Ann Emerg Med 1989;18:466. Abstract.
16. Christensen ML, Rivera GK, Crom WR, et al: Effect of hydration on methotrexate plasma concentrations in children with acute lymphocytic leukemia. J Clin Oncol 1988;6: 797–801.
17. Cooper DJ, Walley KR, Wiggs BR, Russell JA: Bicarbonate does not improve hemodynamics in critically ill patients who have lactic acidosis. Ann Intern Med 1990;112:492–498.
18. Cowan RA, Hartnell GG, Lowdell CP, et al: Metabolic acidosis induced by carbonic anhydrase inhibitors and salicylates in patients with normal renal function. Br Med J 1984;289:347–348.
19. Dukes DC, Blainey JD, Cumming G, Widdowson G: The treatment of severe aspirin poisoning. Lancet 1963;2:329–331.
20. Eneas JF, Schoenfeld PY, Humphreys MH: The effect of infusion of mannitol-sodium bicarbonate on the clinical course of myoglobinuria. Arch Intern Med 1979;139:801–805.
21. Farrell S, Lee DC, McNamara RM: Amantadine overdose: Considerations for the treatment of cardiac toxicity. J Toxicol Clin Toxicol 1995;33:516–517. Abstract.
22. Flanagan RJ, Meridith TJ, Ruprah M, et al: Alkaline diuresis for acute poisoning with chlorophenoxy herbicides and ioxynil. Lancet 1990;335:454–458.
23. Fox GN: Hypocalcemia complicating bicarbonate therapy for salicylate poisoning. West J Med 1984;141:108–109.
24. Frenia ML, Schauben JL, Wears RL, et al: Multiple-dose activated charcoal compared to urinary alkalinization for the enhancement of phenobarbital elimination. J Toxicol Clin Toxicol 1996;34:169–175.
25. Gaultier M: Sodium bicarbonate and tricyclic antidepressant poisoning. Lancet 1976;2:1258. Letter.
26. Gutman AB, Sirota JH: A study by simultaneous clearance techniques of salicylate excretion in man: Effect of alkalinization of the urine by bicarbonate administration; effect of probenecid. J Clin Invest 1955;34:711–721.
27. Heller I, Halevy J, Cohen S, et at: Significant metabolic acidosis induced by acetazolamide not a rare complication. Arch Intern Med 1985;145:1815–1817.
28. Herken W, Rietbrock N: The influence of blood-pH on ionization, distribution, and toxicity of formic acid. Naunyn Schmiedebergs Arch Pharmacol 1968;260:142–143.
29. Hill JB: Salicylate intoxication. N Engl J Med 1973;228: 1110–1113.
30. Hill JB: Experimental salicylate poisoning: Observations on the effects of altering blood pH on tissue and plasma salicylate concentrations. Pediatrics 1971;47:658–665.
31. Hoffman JR, McElroy CR: Bicarbonate therapy for dysrhythmia and hypotension in tricyclic antidepressant overdose. West J Med 1981;134:60–64.
32. Hoffman JR, Votey SR, Bayer M, Silver L: Effect of hypertonic sodium bicarbonate in the treatment of moderate-to-severe cyclic antidepressant overdose. Am J Emerg Med 1993;11:336–341.
33. Honda N: Acute renal failure and rhabdomyolysis. Kidney Int 1983;23:888–898.
34. Hormaechea E, Carlson RW, Rogove H, et al: Hypovolemia, pulmonary edema and protein changes in severe salicylate poisoning. Am J Med 1979;66:1046–1050.
35. Jacobsen D, McMartin KE: Methanol and ethylene glycol poisonings: Mechanism of toxicity, clinical course, diagnosis and treatment. Med Toxicol Adverse Drug Exp 1986;1: 309–334.
36. Jacobsen D, Webb R, Collins TD, McMartin KE: Methanol and formate kinetics in late diagnosed methanol intoxication. Med Toxicol Adverse Drug Exp 1988;3:418–423.
37. Kingston ME: Hyperventilation in tricyclic antidepressant poisoning. Crit Care Med 1979;7:550–551.
38. Knochel JP: Rhabdomyolysis and myoglobinuria. Annu Rev Med 1982;33:435–443.
39. Koppel C: Clinical features, pathogenesis and management of drug-induced rhabdomyolysis. Med Toxicol Adverse Drug Exp 1989;4:108–126.
40. Kulig KW, Duffy JP, Linden CH, Rumack BH: Toxic effects of methanol, ethylene glycol, and isopropyl alcohol. Top Emerg Med 1984;6:14–28.

41. Lassen NA: Treatment of severe acute barbiturate poisoning by forced diuresis and alkalinisation of the urine. Lancet 1960;2:338–342.
42. Lawson AAH, Proudfoot AT, Brown SS, et al: Forced diuresis in the treatment of acute salicylate poisoning in adults. Q J Med 1969;149:31–48.
43. Levitt MA, Sullivan JB, Owens SM, et al: Amitriptyline plasma protein binding: Effect of plasma pH and relevance to clinical overdose. Am J Emerg Med 1986;4:121–125.
44. MacPherson CR, Milne MD, Evans BM: The excretion of salicylate. Br J Pharmacol 1955;10:484–489.
45. Martin-Amat C, McMartin KE, Hayreh MS, Tephly TR: Methanol poisoning: Ocular toxicity produced by formate. Toxicol Appl Pharmacol 1978;45:201–208.
46. McCabe J, Menegazzi JJ, Cobaugh DJ, Auble TE: Recovery from severe cyclic antidepressant overdose with hypertonic saline/dextran in a swine model. Acad Emerg Med 1994;1: 111–115.
47. Milne MD, Scribner BH, Crawford MA: Non-ionic diffusion and the excretion of weak acids and bases. Am J Med 1958; 24:709–729.
48. Mollaret P, Rapin M, Pocidalo JJ, Monsallier JF: Treatment of acute barbiturate intoxication through plasmatic and urinary alkalinization. Presse Med 1959;67:1435–1437.
49. Molloy DW, Penner SB, Rabson J, Hall KW: Use of sodium bicarbonate to treat tricyclic antidepressant-induced arrhythmias in a patient with alkalosis. Can Med Assoc J 1984;130:1457–1459.
50. Moore DF, Bentley AM, Dawling S, Henry JA: Folinic acid and enhanced renal elimination in formic acid intoxication. J Toxicol Clin Toxicol 1994;32:199–204.
51. Morgan AG, Polak A: Acetazolamide and sodium bicarbonate in treatment of salicylate poisoning in adults. Br Med J 1969;1:16–19.
52. Morris LR, Murphy MB, Kitabchi AE: Bicarbonate therapy in severe diabetic ketoacidosis. Ann Intern Med 1986; 105:836–840.
53. Myschetzky A, Lassen NA: Urea-induced, osmotic diuresis and alkalization of urine in acute barbiturate intoxication. JAMA 1963;185:936–942.
54. Nattel S, Mittleman M: Treatment of ventricular tachyarrhythmias resulting from amitriptyline toxicity in dogs. J Pharmacol Exp Ther 1984;231:430–435.
55. Neuvonen PJ, Karkkainen S: Effects of charcoal, sodium bicarbonate, and ammonium chloride on chlorpropamide kinetics. Clin Pharmacol Ther 1983;33:386–393.
56. Oliver TK, Dyer ME: The prompt treatment of salicylism with sodium bicarbonate. Am J Dis Child 1960;99:553–564.
57. Parker RB, Beckman KJ, Hariman RJI, et al: The electrophysiologic and arrhythmogenic effects of cocaine. Pharmacotherapy 1989;9:176. Abstract.
58. Pentel PR, Benowitz NL: Tricyclic antidepressant poisoning: Management of arrhythmias. Med Toxicol Adverse Drug Exp 1986;1:101–121.
59. Pentel PR, Benowitz NL: Efficacy and mechanism of action of sodium bicarbonate in the treatment of desipramine toxicity in rats. J Pharmacol Exp Ther 1984;230:12–19.
60. Pentel PR, Goldsmith SR, Salerno DM, et al: Effect of hypertonic sodium bicarbonate on encainide overdose. Am J Cardiol 1986;57:878–880.
61. Pentel PR, Keyler DE: Effects of high dose alpha-1-acid glycoprotein on desipramine toxicity in rats. J Pharmacol Exp Ther 1988;246:1061–1066.
62. Perri GC, Gorini P: Uraemia in the rabbit after injection of crystalline myoglobin. Br J Exp Pathol 1952;33:440–444.
63. Prescott LF, Balali-Mood M, Critchley A, et al: Diuresis or urinary alkalinization for salicylate poisoning. Br Med J 1982;285:1383–1386.
64. Prescott LF, Park J, Darrien I: Treatment of severe 2,4-D and mecoprop intoxication with alkaline diuresis. Br J Clin Pharmacol 1979;7:111–116.
65. Reimold EW, Worthen HG, Reilly TP: Salicylate poisoning: Comparison of acetazolamide administration and alkaline diuresis in the treatment of experimental salicylate intoxication in puppies. Am J Dis Child 1973;125:668–674.
66. Roe O: Methanol poisoning: Its clinical course, pathogenesis and treatment. Acta Med Scand 1946;126(suppl 182):1–253.
67. Ron D, Taitelman U, Michaelson M, et al: Prevention of acute renal failure in traumatic rhabdomyolysis. Arch Intern Med 1984;144:277–280.
68. Salerno DM, Murakami MM, Johnston RB, et al: Reversal of flecainide-induced ventricular arrhythmias by hypertonic sodium bicarbonate in dogs. Am J Emerg Med 1995;13: 285–293.
69. Sand TE, Jacobsen S: Effect of urine pH and flow on renal clearance of methotrexate. Eur J Clin Pharmacol 1981;19: 453–456.
70. Sasyniuk BI, Jhamandas V: Mechanism of reversal of toxic effects of amitriptyline on cardiac Purkinje fibers by sodium bicarbonate. J Pharmacol Exp Ther 1984;231:387–393.
71. Sasyniuk BI, Jhamandas V, Valois M: Experimental amitriptyline intoxication: Treatment of cardiac toxicity with sodium bicarbonate. Ann Emerg Med 1986;15:1052–1059.
72. Savege TM, Ward JD, Simpson BR, Cohen RD: Treatment of severe salicylate poisoning by forced alkaline diuresis. Br Med J 1969;1:35–36.
73. Segar WE: The critically ill child: Salicylate intoxication. Pediatrics 1969;44:440–444.
74. Smilkstein MJ: Reviewing cyclic antidepressant cardiotoxicity: Wheat and chaff. J Emerg Med 1990;8:645–648.
75. Smith PK, Gleason HL, Stoll CC, et al: Studies on the pharmacology of salicylates. J Pharmacol Exp Ther 1946;87: 237–255.
76. Snodgrass W, Rumack BH, Peterson RG, Holbrook ML: Salicylate toxicity following therapeutic doses in children. J Toxicol Clin Toxicol 1981;18:247–259.
77. Stork CM, Redd JT, Fine K, Hoffman RS: Propoxyphene-induced wide QRS complex dysrhythmia responsive to sodium bicarbonate—A case report. J Toxicol Clin Toxicol 1995;33:179–183.
78. Temple AR: Acute and chronic effects of aspirin toxicity and their treatment. Arch Intern Med 1981;141:364–369.
79. Temple AR, George DJ, Done AK, Thompson JA: Salicylate poisoning complicated by fluid retention. J Toxicol Clin Toxicol 1976;9:61–68.
80. Vinsel PJ: Treatment of acute chlorine gas inhalation with nebulized sodium bicarbonate. J Emerg Med 1990;8: 327–329.
81. Vukmir RB, Bircher N, Safar P: Sodium bicarbonate in cardiac arrest: A reappraisal. Am J Emerg Med 1996;14:192–206.

82. Waddell WI, Butler TC: The distribution and excretion of phenobarbital. J Clin Invest 1957;36:1217–1226.
83. Wasserman F, Brodsky L, Dick MM, et al: Successful treatment of quinidine and procaine amide intoxication. N Engl J Med 1958;259:797–802.
84. Weil MH, Ruiz CE, Michaels S, Rackow EC: Acid–base determinants of survival after cardiopulmonary resuscitation. Crit Care Med 1985;13:888–892.
85. Whitten CF, Kesaree NM, Goodwin JF: Managing salicylate poisoning in children. Am J Dis Child 1961;101:178–194.
86. Winecoff AP, Hariman RJ, Grawe JJ: Reversal of the electrocardiographic effects of cocaine by lidocaine Part 1: Comparison with sodium bicarbonate and quinidine. Pharmacotherapy 1994;14:698–703.
87. Yip L, Dart RC, Gabow PA: Concepts and controversies in salicylate toxicity. Emerg Med Clin North Am 1994;12:351–364.
88. Zimmerman GA, Clemmer TP: Acute respiratory failure during therapy for salicylate intoxication. Ann Emerg Med 1981;10:104–106.

CHAPTER 33

Nonsteroidal Antiinflammatory Agents

Mary E. Palmer and Mary Ann Howland

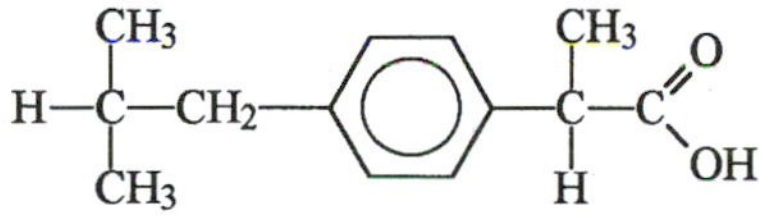

Ibuprofen

Following an argument with his girlfriend, an unresponsive 26-year-old Hispanic male was brought to the hospital by ambulance after ingesting an unknown amount of ibuprofen 800 mg. His girlfriend stated that he may have taken heroin or cocaine as well, and the patient received 0.8 mg naloxone by EMS for pinpoint pupils without improvement in mental status. His vital signs were: blood pressure, 100/70 mm Hg; heart rate, 140 beats/min; respiratory rate, 16 breaths/min; and temperature, 97.5°F (36.4°C). On physical examination, his pupils were both equal and of midrange size with normal response to light. His neck was supple. Skin was of normal turgor and moisture.

Given the severity of his symptoms and the potential for co-ingestants, this patient was lavaged with an orogastric tube and given activated charcoal (1 g/kg). Stool and vomitus were tested for the presence of occult blood. Plasma acetaminophen and salicylate levels were ordered. Urine was tested for ketones and myoglobin and with ferric chloride to assess the possibility of salicylate ingestion. The patient's acetaminophen level was negative.

The patient vomited one half hour after receiving a dose of activated charcoal and was intubated for airway protection. His pre-intubation arterial blood gas on 100% oxygen revealed a respiratory and metabolic acidosis and an increased alveolar–arterial gradient: pH 7.25, PCO_2 44.3 mmHg, and PO_2 162 mmHg. His sodium was 138 mEq/dL; potassium 3.5 mEq/dL; chloride 102 mEq/L; bicarbonate 19.9 mEq/L, with an anion gap of 16. Two hours later, the repeat electrolytes were: sodium, 132 mEq/L; potassium 3.3 mEq/L; chloride 104 mEq/L; and bicarbonate 11.2 mEq/L, with an anion gap of 17. His blood urea nitrogen was 12 mg/dL, creatinine 1.4 mg/dL, and glucose 153 mg/dL. His urine was negative for ketones and myoglobin. His lactic acid level returned at 7.5 mmol/L. An ethanol level was 17 mg/dL. Complete blood count and calcium were normal. Salicylate and acetaminophen levels were negative and opioid urine screen was negative.

During his hospital course, the patient developed acute renal failure; by the second day he had a BUN of 60 mg/dL and creatinine 2.8 mg/dL. His aminotransferases and prothrombin time stayed normal. During his hospital course, repeated stool specimens remained negative for occult blood.

To establish ibuprofen intoxication for academic purposes, an ibuprofen level was sent to a specialty laboratory and was reported as 1220 mg/dL. A typical therapeutic level is 3 mg/dL.

Although a nomogram has been developed for ibuprofen[39,49,64] it is not clinically useful since serum levels do not correlate with clinical symptoms. Testing for ibuprofen plasma concentrations was not indicated for clinical management. It was however, imperative to screen for acetaminophen toxicity since overdose of acetaminophen is potentially fatal and treatable.

How Commonly Do Nonsteroidal Antiinflammatory Agents Result in Overdose?

Nonsteroidal antiinflammatory drugs (NSAIDs) are usually categorized according to their chemical classification. There are six main chemical classes (Table 33–1), two of which tend to cause the most serious and life-threatening consequences: the pyrazolone (phenylbutazone) and the anthranilic acids (mefenamic acid and meclofenamate). Agents in the other four classes, if ingested in large overdose amounts, are capable of causing central nervous system (CNS) depression, respiratory depression, hypotension, hypothermia, gastrointestinal (GI) distress, acute renal failure, mild liver toxicity, elevated prothrombin time, and, rarely, hallucinations and seizures. In general, the remaining agents represent a low order of toxicity, although severe symptoms occasionally do occur. Any patient known to experience an anaphylactoid reaction to any NSAIDs should be considered to be "allergic" to all NSAIDs as well as to aspirin. Fatal and near-fatal reactions have occurred after the first exposure to a newly introduced NSAID.[95]

It is estimated that more than 73 million prescriptions are written annually for NSAIDs, costing over $2.2 billion, in addition to nonprescription NSAIDs.[3] Reported fatalities are 6–7 times greater for salicylates and acetaminophen than for NSAIDs, and the overall morbidity of those who survive is greater as well[99] (Table 33–2).

The popularity of the NSAIDs is demonstrated by their share of the analgesic market and the pervasive nature of the mass advertising campaigns promoting their use. The rarity of toxic reactions has led to increased dosage and the nonprescription availability of ibuprofen, naproxen, and ketoprofen. The effects of increasing availability on the incidence of toxicity remain to be seen.[83]

TABLE 33–1. CHEMICAL CLASSES OF NONSTEROIDAL ANTIINFLAMMATORY AGENTS

Salicylates
Acetyl salicylic acid (aspirin)
Nonacetylated derivatives (metabolized to salicylic acid)
Salicylsalicylic acid (salsalate)
Sodium salicylate
Choline salicylate
Magnesium salicylate
Magnesium choline salicylate
Diflunisal (Dolobid; not metabolized to salicylic acid)
Pyrazolones
Phenylbutazone
Fenamates (anthranilic acids)
Meclofenamate (Meclomen)
Mefenamic acid (Ponstel)
Acetic acids
Diclofenac (Voltaren)
Etodolac (Lodine)
Indomethacin (Indocin)
Ketorolac (Toradol)
Nabumetone (Relafen)
Sulindac (Clinoril)
Tolmetin (Tolectin)
Propionic acids
Carprofen (Rimadyl)[a]
Fenoprofen (Nalfon)
Flurbiprofen (Ansaid)
Ibuprofen (Motrin, Advil, Medipren)[b]
Ketoprofen (Orudis)[b]
Naproxen (Naprosyn, Anaprox)[b]
Oxaprozin (Daypro)
Oxicams
Piroxicam (Feldene)
Meloxicam[a]

[a]Investigational
[b]Nonprescription

What Are the Mechanisms of Action of NSAIDs? How Does This Relate to Adverse Effects and Toxicity?

Understanding the therapeutic and adverse effects of NSAIDs follows from an understanding of their mechanism of action. While steroids block formation of the inflammatory products of both lipooxygenase and cyclooxygenase, the NSAIDs bind only to cyclooxygenase and prevent formation of prostaglandins, prostacyclins, and thromboxane, but not leukotrienes and other eicosanoids[47,98] (Fig. 33–1). Salicylates covalently bind cyclooxygenase 1 and 2 (COX-1 and COX-2), and the irreversibility of this reaction means that the effect persists for the life of the cell. A number of NSAIDs, including diclofenac and indomethacin, inhibit various lipooxygenase enzymes in animals and also decrease the production of leukotrienes.[36,47]

All NSAIDs share the common therapeutic mechanism of inhibiting synthesis of prostaglandins and blocking production of inflammation, pain, or fever. Although the effects of prostacyclins and thromboxanes are complex, with one opposing the other, on balance these effects tend toward decreased platelet aggregation and increased vasoconstriction.

Although death due to overdose is relatively uncommon, the line between adverse effects and toxicity in therapeutic use is not always clear (Table 33–3). NSAIDs are implicated in about a quarter of all adverse drug reactions in the United States.[12,14,92] The most common adverse effects are gastrointestinal (GI). Although NSAIDs cause local irritation in the GI tract, the main mechanism of toxicity is via blockade of cytoprotective prostaglandins, PGI_2 and PGE_2, as demonstrated by the perforation and bleeding that occurs with topical[29,102] as well as parenteral administration. Most notably, NSAIDs cause gastric and duodenal ulceration, and about 3% of these patients suffer hemorrhage or perforation.[32,35,45,61]

TABLE 33–2. TEN YEARS (1986–1995) OF AMERICAN ASSOCIATION OF POISON CONTROL CENTERS (AAPCC) DATA COMPARING OUTCOMES AMONG PATIENTS OVERDOSING ON SALICYLATES, ACETAMINOPHEN, AND NON-SALICYLATE NSAIDS

Analgesic	Moderate Outcomes	Major Outcomes	Fatalities	Total
Salicylates	11,563 (23.5%)	1,197 (1.2%)	377 (0.38%)	49,273
Acetaminophen	13,345 (3.8%)	2,568 (0.73%)	412 (0.12%)	352,067
NSAIDs	9,838 (4.6%)	976 (0.45%)	59 (0.03%)	215,569

The large intestine is also susceptible to increased bleeding tendencies.[9,23,53]

NSAIDs increase the relative risk of a serious gastrointestinal hemorrhage by approximately threefold,[16,34,101,102] although estimations as high as 10-fold have been reported.[44] What is clear is that the risk of GI bleeding increases with advancing age and higher doses of longer duration (as occur in treatment of rheumatoid arthritis).[7,54,62,63] History of previous ulcer or bleeding, alcohol abuse, and use of more than one agent, including steroids,[15,16,31,34,40,101] contribute to this risk as well. Unfortunately, there is no predictable prodrome to the development of serious GI pathology and life-threatening bleeding may not be associated with abdominal pain or other symptoms.[1,26,42,43,80,94]

Finally, transient, asymptomatic elevations in hepatic transaminases are reported in about 25% of NSAID users. Hepatocellular necrosis, particularly associated with diclofenac, and cholestasis are uncommonly reported.[58]

The second most common class of adverse effects of NSAID use is renal. Prostaglandins cause local dilation of renal arterioles in the presence of renal vasoconstrictor substances such as angiotensin.[36,74] In normal patients, NSAIDs have little effect on renal function. However, in the setting of high angiotensin and low intravascular flow such as in congestive heart failure, cirrhosis, intrinsic renal disease or hypovolemia, NSAID-induced decrease in prostaglandins decreases renal blood flow and

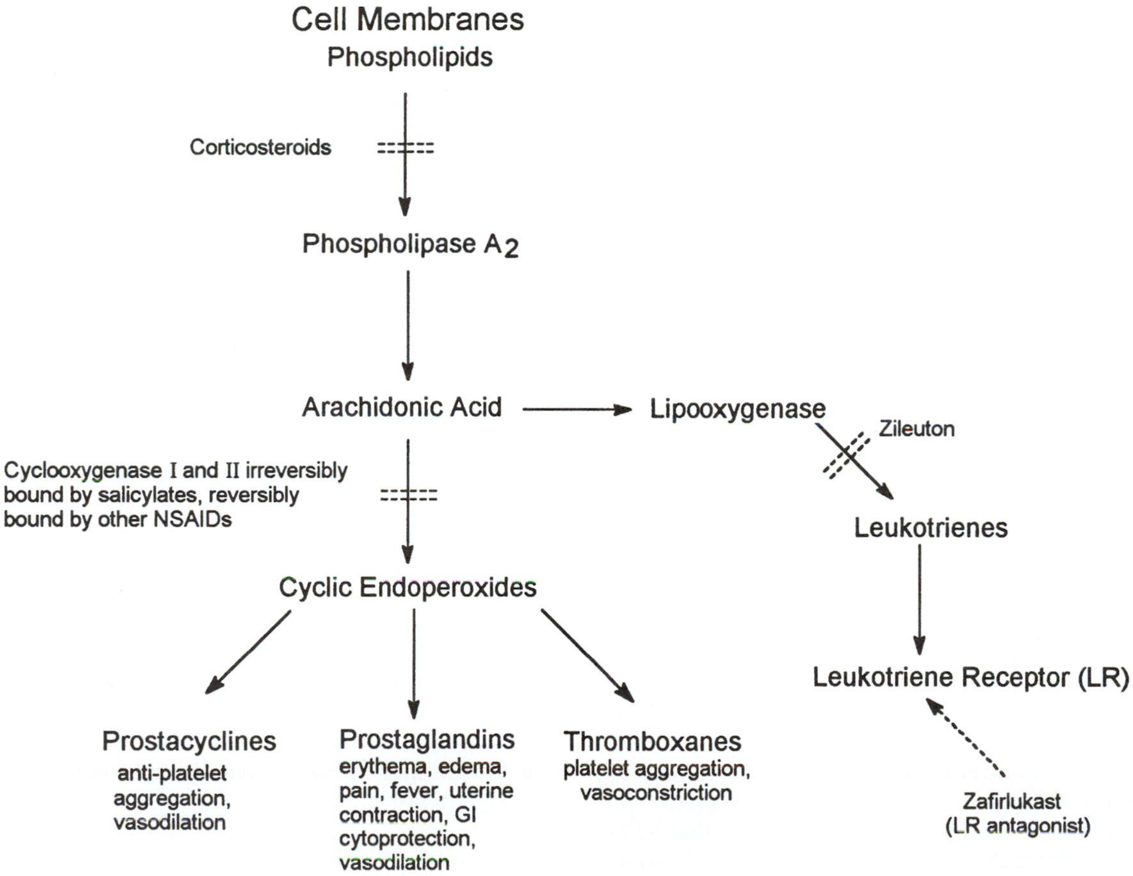

Figure 33–1. Mechanism of action of NSAIDs. Cyclooxygenase-1 (COX-1) is constitutive and always acts in the kidney and GI tract. Cyclooxygenase-2 is induced by inflammatory mediators like cytokines and endotoxin and produces prostaglandins at the site of inflammation. Most NSAIDs block these enzymes nonselectively, with the exception of meloxicam and other experimental agents. Leukotrienes and other products of lipooxygenase are blocked by corticosteroids but not salicylates and other NSAIDs; these may be involved in the allergic or asthmatic reactions produced by NSAIDs but blocked by corticosteroids. Leukotriene receptor antagonists (LTRAs) are designed to alleviate the effects of leukotrienes.

TABLE 33–3. SELECTED ADVERSE EFFECTS OF NONSTEROIDAL ANTIINFLAMMATORY DRUGS

Gastrointestinal
Indigestion
Ulceration
Perforation
Hemorrhage
Elevated hepatic aminotransferases (transient)
Hepatocellular injury (rare)

Renal
Acute renal failure
Fluid and electrolyte retention
Interstitial nephritis
Nephrotic syndrome
Papillary necrosis

Hypersensitivity/pulmonary
Asthma exacerbation
Anaphylactoid reaction
Pneumonitis

Hematologic
Increased bleeding time
Agranulocytosis
Aplastic anemia
Thrombocytopenia
Neutropenia
Hemolytic anemia

Central nervous system
Headache
Aseptic meningitis
Delirium
Cognitive dysfunction, especially in the elderly
Hallucinations

Drug interactions
Anticoagulants: NSAIDs increase risk of GI bleeding
Antihypertensives (especially diuretics, beta-adrenergic antagonists, and ACE inhibitors): NSAIDs reduce antihypertensive effects
Sulfonylureas: NSAIDs increase hypoglycemic effect
Lithium: NSAIDs increase risk of lithium toxicity
Digoxin: NSAIDs increase risk of digoxin toxicity
Aminoglycosides: NSAIDs increase risk of aminoglycoside toxicity

the rate of glomerular filtration. This is also associated with retention of salt and water, and hyperkalemia. Such circumstances may further exacerbate congestive heart failure.[85]

Acute renal failure associated with NSAID use accounts for approximately 15% of drug-induced renal failure.[24] Renal failure among NSAID users may also be associated with the risk factor of binge drinking.[50] Acute and chronic forms of interstitial nephritis and nephrotic syndrome occur in NSAID users.[17,57,73] In heavy analgesic use, the risk for papillary necrosis (69 out of 259 patients) may be higher than previously presumed.[89]

The respiratory system is not spared. Life-threatening anaphylactoid reactions occur and should be treated like anaphylaxis. Up to 25% of adult asthmatics with nasal polyps or chronic urticaria manifest an acute asthmatic attack minutes to hours after NSAID exposure.[96] The asthma is often accompanied by flush of the head and neck, rhinorrhea, conjunctivitis, and/or angioedema. About 2.5% cross-reactivity is noted in patients allergic to tartrazine dyes. The probable mechanism is inhibition of cyclooxygenase, resulting in an increased production of leukotrienes LTC_4, LTD_4, and LTE_4.[88] This is rare in children. It is important to know that there is cross-reactivity among NSAIDs despite their chemical diversity. Blockade of 5-lipooxygenase with zileuton or the use of leukotriene receptor antagonists (LTRAs) such as zafirlukast may prevent symptoms and signs of aspirin intolerance[3,48] (see Fig. 33–1). Zafirlukast and zileuton are now marketed for the treatment of chronic asthma.[3]

Serious hematologic effects can also occur. In addition to decreased platelet aggregation, various NSAIDs have been reported to cause aplastic anemia (especially phenylbutazone but also indomethacin and etodolac), agranulocytosis (eg, naproxen, phenylbutazone), hemolytic anemia (eg, mefenamic acid), neutropenia (eg, indomethacin), and thrombocytopenia (eg, indomethacin, ibuprofen, naproxen).[21,78,79,86,87]

A wide range of CNS signs and symptoms is associated with the use of NSAIDs, including delirium, confusion, and headache.[55] Aseptic meningitis in patients with and without[19] autoimmune disorders is reported with ibuprofen, sulindac and tolmetin use.[19,79] Some agents may cause tinnitus (ibuprofen, naproxen, fenoprofen, sulindac, tolmetin) or transient loss of hearing (ibuprofen, indomethacin, phenylbutazone).[47,79]

Production of prostaglandins E and F increases dramatically in the hours before parturition. This has led to the use of NSAIDs as tocolytics.[72] However, this may be associated with untoward intrauterine closure of the ductus arteriosus and has been associated with renal failure and oligohydramnios in neonates.[51]

Numerous drug interactions can occur with NSAIDs[14] (see Table 33–3), at times producing catastrophic effects.[33] Concurrent use with oral anticoagulants may result in increased NSAID drug levels with competition for protein binding and additive hemostatic effects, resulting in a 13-fold increase of relative risk for GI bleeding, which can be fatal, especially in the elderly.[91] Digoxin, lithium, oral hypoglycemics, and aminoglycosides are among drugs whose levels increase in combination with NSAIDs. Conversely, NSAIDs may reduce the effect of antihypertensives (diuretics, beta-adrenergic antagonists, and ACE inhibitors in particular), resulting in undertreated hypertension or potentiation of nephrotoxicity.[14]

What Toxicity Can Be Expected in a Patient With an Overdose of NSAIDs?

Toxicity is approached by classes of most serious toxicity. Both acetylated and nonacetylated salicylate toxicity is discussed in detail elsewhere (see Chap. 32). Diflunisal

(Dolobid) is not metabolized to salicylate but may demonstrate cross-reactivity with some salicylate assays. It has a prolonged half-life (approximately 13 hours) and in massive overdoses (15–33 g), hyperventilation, tachycardia, sweating, tinnitus, coma, and death are reported.[20,90,97]

Pyrazolones

Historically, phenylbutazone is probably responsible for most of the serious toxicity attributed to NSAIDs. In a review of 99 cases early GI symptoms, acid-base and electrolyte disturbances, pulmonary edema, dizziness, seizures, coma, hypotension, and respiratory and cardiac arrest characterized phenylbutazone overdoses.[20,81] These may be followed by renal, hepatic, and hematologic dysfunction 2–7 days later. At least 50 fatalities have occurred in children.[80] The fatal dose in a 1-year-old is reported to be 2 g, and serious symptoms have occurred in adults after the ingestion of 4–40 g.[20,84,95]

Phenylbutazone is also used in veterinary medicine in high-dosage formulations. For instance, the form used in horses, often referred to as "bute," is available in 1000-mg tablets. An overdose in a race-dog handler resulted in seizure, coma, hemodynamic instability, noncardiogenic pulmonary edema, and acute renal failure with hepatic dysfunction. Recovery took 5 weeks.[76]

Aggressive management is warranted even in the asymptomatic patient with reported phenylbutazone overdose.[76,84] Urine tests positive (color changes to purple or brown) with a qualitative bedside ferric chloride test or Phenistix. Therefore, phenylbutazone should be considered in the differential diagnosis of a positive ferric chloride test along with diflunisal,[77] salicylates, or phenothiazines, whose phenolic metabolites also change the indicator from yellow to purple or brown. Gastric lavage should be considered and multiple dose activated charcoal[75] should be employed. Only 1–5% of phenylbutazone is eliminated unchanged, and forced diuresis is of no value. Hemodialysis is also of no benefit. The value of hemoperfusion is unknown, but may be tried in life-threatening cases.

Therapeutic doses of phenylbutazone can cause aplastic anemia and agranulocytosis. Although the pyrazolones have been withdrawn from the market, phenylbutazone is still available from veterinary sources and from other countries. For instance, it has presented problems in the southwestern United States with its ready availability in Mexican markets (San Diego Poison Control Center, personal comm.).

Anthranilic Acids

Mefenamic acid (Ponstel) and meclofenamate (Meclomen) are the two drugs in this category currently available in the United States. There are no reported cases of meclofenamate overdose, but since its structure is similar to that of mefenamic acid it should be considered in a similar manner.

Muscle twitching and seizures are characteristic of symptomatic overdose, as reported in two case series.[4,20] Muscle twitching may be focal or generalized and in one series lasted 3–10 minutes with 20% of 54 patients progressing to grand mal seizures 2–7 hours postingestion.[4] Gastrointestinal distress (vomiting or diarrhea) was noted in 15% of these patients. Seizures were responsive to benzodiazepines and all patients recovered. Doses as low as 2 g in a child or 6 g over 24 hours in an adult have produced seizures.

Airway management and seizure management should be the primary focus of treatment in patients with anthranilic acid overdoses, where the combination of vomiting and seizures can result in aspiration. In the setting of overdose, aggressive GI decontamination is warranted with activated charcoal and possibly orogastric lavage.

Propionic Acids

Ibuprofen overdoses are well-represented in the literature.[46,56] In a comparative survey of adults who ingested ibuprofen, salicylates, or acetaminophen, fewer adults required hospitalization after ibuprofen ingestion than with either of the other over-the-counter agents.[99] However, toxicity can occur in overdose in adults and children.[37,38,41,65,93,103] In a retrospective case series of 126 patients with ibuprofen overdose, 19% of patients developed symptoms, predominantly CNS depression and GI upset, usually within 4 hours.[37,38] This retrospective analysis was validated in a prospective study of 45 adults and 39 pediatric patients in which all who were to become ill did so within 4 hours. Serious manifestations of coma, apnea, and/or metabolic acidosis developed in 9% of adults and 5% of children. Patients who ingested more than 400 mg/kg (especially children) were at risk for seizures, apnea, hypotension, bradycardia, metabolic acidosis, and renal and hepatic dysfunction.[41,65,93] Atrial fibrillation, probably related to acidemia, was reported as well.[69] Patients with ibuprofen overdose should be evaluated for the following delayed effects: acute renal failure, hepatic toxicity, and thrombocytopenia.[64] Plasma levels are not necessary for patient management,[39] but general poison management with airway support, activated charcoal, and possibly orogastric lavage may be necessary in massive overdoses.

Only a few cases of fenoprofen overdose have been reported. One study reported that 12 out of 16 patients developed symptoms after ingestions of unknown amounts.[20] One adult died of cardiopulmonary arrest after presenting with hypothermia and coma. The others developed drowsiness, ataxia, tinnitus, nausea, hypotension, tachycardia, and/or Kussmaul respirations. Five children exhibited only drowsiness. A few other cases of serious toxicity have been reported as well.[2,59]

Most reported overdoses of naproxen result in mild symptoms: nausea, abdominal pain, or drowsiness.[30] Elimination may be improved in overdose: in 16 healthy volunteers, excretion tended to accelerate as naproxen levels rose.[86] Renal failure is also reported for two cases of overdose with this agent.[60] A 15-year-old who ingested approximately 50 naproxen sodium tablets developed metabolic acidosis and seizures.[67] Similarly, cases have occurred in ketoprofen poisoning with rare reports of seizures[10] and common reports of mild GI symptoms and drowsiness.[20] Little information is available about overdoses of carprofen except that rare but serious photosensitivity reactions may occur as well as transient asymptomatic elevations in liver aminotransferases.[78] Coma and respiratory depression were reported in a single patient who overdosed on flurbiprofen.[20]

Acetic Acids

Intoxication with indomethacin and diclofenac appears to be relatively benign, resulting in nausea, abdominal pain, drowsiness, headache, and tinnitus.[20] However, there is one reported case of seizures after ingestion of "a bottle" of indomethacin by a 6-year-old child.[82] Renal compromise was also reported in a case of diclofenac and in nine cases of sulindac overdose.[60] Little can be said about toxicity from overdoses of the other agents (etodolac, ketorolac, nabumetone, and tolmetin in the acetic acid category), as there are very few reported cases in the literature and almost all of these remained asymptomatic.

Oxicams

The single drug currently available in this category is piroxicam (Feldene). Thirteen of the 16 patients in which piroxicam was the sole agent ingested remained asymptomatic and 2 patients developed dizziness and blurred vision.[20] One patient, who supposedly ingested 600 mg, developed coma with recovery within 24 hours. The safety profile of meloxicam is being developed.[25]

What Clinical and Experimental Modalities Are Being Developed to Limit Adverse Effects and Toxicity?

Several therapeutic efforts have been tried to prevent the gastrointestinal side effects resulting from loss of cytoprotection from prostaglandins. Use of HCl pump inhibitors has shown some success,[22,100] whereas H_2-receptor blockade was unsuccessful in 1920 patients.[92] Concurrent administration of misoprostol, a PGE analog, may also be effective in preventing GI side effects of NSAIDs. Other experimental efforts have involved the co-administration of nitric oxide[27] or substance P inhibitors.[52]

Other efforts focus on enzymatic protection (Fig. 33–1). Since the isoform of cyclooxygenase has been discovered (COX-2), a great deal of research has been focused on the development of COX-2 NSAIDs. While cyclooxygenase-1 (COX-1) is found in blood vessels, stomach, and kidney, COX-2 is induced by cytokines and other inflammatory mediators at the site of inflammation only. COX-2 inhibits prostaglandin only at sites of inflammation, thereby protecting the gastrointestinal tract and kidney.[68,70,71] Other more specific COX-2 inhibitors, such as meloxicam, have been released in France, and the search for other COX isoforms is ongoing.[5,6,18,28,97] In addition, leukotriene-receptor antagonists such as zafirlukast and zileuton, a lipooxygenase inhibitor,[3,48,66] are designed to circumvent the airway constriction in NSAID hypersensitivity and have shown some promise.

Other research focuses in modifying other mediators of inflammation. For instance, tenatap sodium inhibits production or effect of interleukin-1.[13] Another approach to decreasing inflammation focuses on cell-adhesion molecules.[8]

What Are the Pharmacokinetics of NSAIDs in Overdose?

Absorption of NSAIDs is usually rapid, with peak levels achieved within 2 hours for most agents. Sustained-release indomethacin, enteric-coated diclofenac, mefenamic acid, piroxicam, and the two prodrugs sulindac and nabumetone require 2–5 hours to reach peak levels.[11,93] These agents are weakly acidic. Unlike salicylates, these drugs are highly protein-bound (> 90%), with volumes of distribution of approximately 0.1–0.2 L/kg. The high degree of protein binding will make hemodialysis useless in overdose and there is not sufficient experience with hemoperfusion to determine its usefulness.

Liver metabolism is important for the elimination of NSAIDs.[47] Renal elimination of unchanged drug accounts for less than 10% of clearance (except indomethacin at 10–20%). However, in renal failure, conjugated metabolites for some drugs may be transformed to the parent compound, which may then accumulate (ketoprofen, fenoprofen, naproxen, diflunisal). Some agents undergo extensive biliary–fecal elimination (carprofen, indomethacin, piroxicam, sulindac, and to a lesser extent, meclofenamic acid, meclofenamate, and diclofenac), and these agents may theoretically lend themselves to multiple-dose activated charcoal, but toxicity is rarely severe enough to warrant this therapy. Only salicylate is excreted unchanged in the urine in sufficient quantity to benefit from alkalinization of the urine to enhance clearance in overdose. At least two NSAIDs will produce a color change on ferric chloride testing of the urine (phenylbutazone and diflunisal), and these should be considered in the differential diagnosis if this qualitative bedside test is positive[77] (see Chap. 32). In addition, NSAID metabolites in the urine can lead to false positive drug screens, and this would need to be reviewed on a case-by-case basis. For instance, oxaprozin can interfere with the urine drug screen for benzodiazepines (Abbott laboratories).

Half-lives are less than 8 hours for the majority of these agents. Phenylbutazone and piroxicam have very long half-lives (30 hours) and diflunisal, nalbumetone, nalbumetine, naproxen, and sulindac have half-lives of between 8 and 30 hours. Prolonged half-life may contribute to prolonged toxicity in severe overdoses. Multiple-dose activated charcoal may play a role in management of very serious overdoses of NSAIDs, but is rarely required of agents with an extensive enterohepatic elimination. Orogastric lavage may be considered in patients with phenylbutazone and mefenamic acid overdoses, and multiple-dose activated charcoal may be considered for phenylbutazone overdose. All patients require basic poison management including consideration of co-ingestants, evaluation for toxidromes, screening for acid–base disturbances as well as fluid and electrolyte disorders, and psychosocial support. Most NSAID toxicity responds well to supportive care. These patients require further evaluation of gastrointestinal, renal, hepatic, and hematologic injury over their hospital course.

References

1. Agrawal NM: Epidemiology and prevention of nonsteroidal antiinflammatory drug effects in the gastrointestinal tract. Br J Rheumatol 1995;34 (suppl 1):5–10.
2. Appleby D: Fenoprofen overdose. Drug Intell Clin Pharm 1981;15:129–130.
3. Anonymous. Zafirlukast for asthma. Med Lett 1996;38: 111–112.
4. Balali-Mood M, Proudfoot AT, Critchley J, et al: Mefenamic acid overdosage. Lancet 1981;2:1324–1356.
5. Barner A: Review of clinical trials and benefit/risk ratio of meloxicam. Scand J Rheumatol 1996;102 (suppl):29–37.
6. Battistini B, Botting R, Bakhle YS: COX-1 and COX-2: toward the development of more selective NSAIDs. Drug News Perspect 1994;8:501–512.
7. Beard K, Walker AM, Perera DR, Jick H: Nonsteroidal antiinflammatory drugs and hospitalization for gastroesophageal bleeding in the elderly. Arch Intern Med 1987; 147:1621–1623.
8. Bevilacqua MP, Nelson RM: Selectins. J Clin Invest 1993; 91:379–387.
9. Bjarnason I, Zanelli G, Prowse P, et al: Blood and protein loss via small intestinal inflammation induced by nonsteroidal antiinflammatory drugs. Lancet 1987;2:711–714.
10. Bond G, Curry S, Arnold-Cappel P, et al: Generalized seizures and acidosis after ketoprofen overdose. Vet Hum Toxicol 1989;31:369. Abstract.
11. Bond WS: Nonsteroidal antiinflammatory drugs: Are there significant differences? Facts Comp Drug Newsletter 1992;11:81–83.
12. Borda IT: The spectrum of adverse gastrointestinal effects associated with nonsteroidal antiinflammatory drugs. In: Borda I, Koff R, eds: Nonsteroidal Antiinflammatory Drugs: A Profile of Adverse Effects. Philadelphia, Hanley & Belfus, 1992.
13. Brooks PM: Tenidap—a new antiarthritic agent. Agents Actions 1993;44 (suppl):161–163.
14. Brooks PM, Day RO: Nonsteroidal antiinflammatory drugs—differences and similarities. N Engl J Med 1991; 324:1716–1725.
15. Carson JL, Strom BL, Soper KA, et al: The association of nonsteroidal antiinflammatory drugs with upper gastrointestinal tract bleeding. Arch Intern Med 1987;147:85–88.
16. Carson JL, Willett LR: Toxicity of nonsteroidal antiinflammatory drugs. An overview of the epidemiology evidence. Drugs 1993; 46 (suppl 1):243–248.
17. Clive DM, Stoff J: Renal syndromes associated with nonsteroidal antiinflammatory drugs. N Engl J Med 1984;310: 563–572.
18. Chan CC, Boyce S, Brideau C, et al: Pharmacology of a selective cyclooxygenase–2 inhibitor, L–745, 337: A novel nonsteroidal antiinflammatory agent with an ulcerogenic sparing effect in rat and nonhumam primate stomach. J Pharmacol Exp Ther 1995;274:1531–1537.
19. Chez M, Sila CA, Ransohoff RM, et al: Ibuprofen-induced meningitis: Detection of intrathecal IgG synthesis and immune complexes. Neurology 1989;39:1578–1580.
20. Court H, Volans G: Poisoning after overdose with nonsteroidal antiinflammatory drugs. Adv Drug React Ac Pois Rev 1984;3:1–21.
21. Cramer RL Aboko-Cole VC, Gualtieri RJ: Agranulocytosis associated with etodolac. Ann Pharmacother 1994;28: 428–460.
22. Dajani EZ, Agrawal NM: Prevention of ulcers induced by nonsteroidal antiinflammatory drugs: An update. J Physiol Pharmacol 1995;46:3–16.
23. Davies NM: Toxicity of nonsteroidal antiinflammatory drugs in the large intestine. Dis Colon Rectum 1995;38: 1311–1321.
24. Delmas PD: Nonsteroidal antiinflammatory drugs and renal function. Br J Rheumatol 1995;34 (suppl 1):25–28.
25. Distel M, Mueller C, Bluhmki, Fried J: Safety of meloxicam: A global analysis of clinical trials. Br J Rheumatol 1996;35(suppl 1):68–77.
26. Dowd JE, Cimaz R, Fink CW: Nonsteroidal antiinflammatory drug-induced gastroduodenal injury in children. Arthritis Rheum 1995;38:1225–1231.
27. Elliott SN, McKnight W, Cirino G, Wallace JL: A nitric oxide-releasing nonsteroidal antiinflammatory drug accelerates gastric ulcer healing in rats. Gastroenterology 1995;109:524–530.
28. Engelhardt G, Hoffman D, Schlegel K, et al: Antiinflammatory, analgesic, antipyretic and related properties of meloxicam, a new nonsteroidal antiinflammatory agent with favorable gastrointestinal tolerance. Inflamm Res 1995;44:423–433.
29. Evans JM, McMahon AD, McGilchrist MM, et al: Topical nonsteroidal antiinflammatory drugs and admission to hospital for upper gastrointestinal bleeding and perforation: A record linkage case-control study. Br Med J 1995; 311:22–26.
30. Fredell E, Strand L: Naproxen overdose. JAMA 1977;238: 938. Letter.
31. Fries J: Toward an understanding of NSAID-related adverse events: The contribution of longitudinal data. Scand J Rheumatol 1996;102 (suppl):3–8.
32. Fries JF, Miller SR, Spitz PW, et al: Towards an epidemiology of gastropathy associated with nonsteroidal antiinflammatory drug use. Gastroenterology 1989;96: (suppl 2): 647–655.
33. Gabb GM: Fatal outcome of interaction between warfarin and a nonsteroidal antiinflammatory drug. Med J Aust 1996;164:700–701. Letter.
34. Gabriel SE, Jaakimainen L, Bombardier C: Risk for serious gastrointestinal complications related to use of nonsteroidal antiinflammatory drugs: A meta-analysis. Ann Intern Med 1991;115:787–796.
35. Garcia Rodriguez LA, Jick H: Risk of upper gastrointestinal bleeding and perforation associated with individual nonsteroidal antiinflammatory drugs. Lancet 1994;343:769–772.
36. Garella S, Matarese R: Renal effects of prostaglandins and

clinical adverse effects on nonsteroidal antiinflammatory agents. Medicine 1984;63:165–181.
37. Hall AH, Smolinske SC, Conrad FL, et al: Ibuprofen overdose: 126 cases. Ann Emerg Med 1986;15:1308–1312.
38. Hall AH, Smolinske SC, Kulig KW, at al: Ibuprofen overdose: A prospective study. West J Med 1988;48:653–656.
39. Hall AH, Smolinske SC, Stover B, et al: Ibuprofen overdose in adults. J Toxicol Clin Toxicol 1992;30:23–37.
40. Hallas J, Lauritsen J, Villadsen HD, Gran KF: Nonsteroidal antiinflammatory drugs and upper gastrointestinal bleeding, identifying high-risk groups by excess risk estimates. Scand J Gastroenterol 1995;30:438–444.
41. Halpern SM, Fitzpatrick R, Volans GN: Ibuprofen toxicity. A review of adverse reactions and overdose. Adverse Drug React Toxicol Rev 1993;12:107–128.
42. Henry DA: Side effects of nonsteroidal antiinflammatory drugs. Ballieres Clin Rheumatol 1988;2:425–454.
43. Henry D, Lim LL, Garcia Rodriguez LA, et al: Variability in risk of gastrointestinal complications with individual nonsteroidal antiinflammatory drugs: Results of a collaborative meta-analysis. Br Med J 1996;312:1563–1566.
44. Hirschowitz BI: Nonsteroidal antiinflammatory drugs and the gastrointestinal tract. Gastroenterologist 1994; 2:207–223.
45. Hoachain P, Berkelmans I, Czernichow P, et al: Which patients taking non-aspirin non-steroidal anti-inflammatory drugs bleed? A case control study. Eur J Gastroenterol Hepatol 1995;7:419–426.
46. Hunt DP, Leigh RJ: Overdose with ibuprofen causing unconsciousness and hypotension. Br Med J 1980;2: 1458–1459. Letter.
47. Insel PA: Analgesic-antipyretic and antiinflammatory agents and drugs employed in the treatment of gout. In: Hardman JG, Limbard LE, Molinoff PB, et al, eds: Goodman and Gilman's The Pharmacological Basis of Therapeutics. McGraw-Hill, New York, 1996, pp. 617–657.
48. Israel E, Fischer AR, Rosenberg MA, et al: The pivotal role of 5-lipoxygenase products in the reaction of aspirin-sensitive asthmatics to aspirin. Am Rev Respir Dis 1993;148: 1447–1451.
49. Jenkinson ML, Fitzpatrick R, Streete PJ, et al: The relationship between plasma ibuprofen concentrations and toxicity in acute ibuprofen overdose. Hum Toxicol 1988;7: 319–324.
50. Johnson GR, Wen SF: Syndrome of flank pain and acute renal failure after binge drinking and nonsteroidal antiinflammatory drug ingestion. J Am Soc Nephrol 1995;5: 1647–1652.
51. Kaplan BS, Restaino I, Raval DS, et al: Renal failure in the neonate associated with in utero exposure to nonsteroidal antiinflammatory agents. Pediatr Nephrol 1994;8:700–704.
52. Kataeva G, Argo A, Stanisz AM: Substance-P-mediated intestinal inflammation: Inhibitory effects of CP 96,345 and SMS 201–995. Neuroimmunmodulation 1994;1:350–356.
53. Kaufman HL, Fischer AH, Carroll M, Becker JM: Colonic ulceration associated with nonsteroidal antiinflammatory drugs. Report of three cases. Dis Colon Rectum 1996;39: 705–710.
54. Keenan GF, Giammini EH, Athreya BH. Clinically significant gastropathy associated with nonsteroidal antiinflammatory drug use in children with juvenile rheumatoid arthritis. J Rheumatol 1995;22:1149–1151.
55. Kertesz A: Neurological complications of nonsteroidal antiinflammatory agents. In: Borda I, Koff R, eds: Nonsteroidal Antiinflammatory Drugs: A Profile of Adverse Effects. Philadelphia, Hanley & Belfus, 1992.
56. Kim J, Gazarian M, Verjee, Johnson D: Acute renal insufficiency in ibuprofen overdose. Pediatr Emerg Care 1995;11: 107–108.
57. Kincaid-Smith P: Effects of non-narcotic analgesics on the kidney. Drugs 1986;32 (suppl 4):109–128.
58. Koff RS: Liver disease induced by nonsteroidal antiinflammatory drugs. In: Bora I, Koff R, eds: Nonsteroidal Antiinflammatory Drugs: A Profile of Adverse Effects. Philadelphia, Hanley & Belfus, 1992.
59. Kolodzik J, Eilers M, Angelos MG: Nonsteroidal antiinflammatory drugs and coma: A case report of fenoprofen overdose. Ann Emerg Med 1990;19:378–381.
60. Kulling PE, Backman EA, Skagius AS: Renal impairment after acute diclofenac, naproxen and sulindac overdoses. Clin Toxicol J Toxicol 1995;33:173–177.
61. Laine L, Comminelli F, Sloane R, et al: Interaction of NSAIDs and *Helicobacter pylori* on gastrointestinal injury and prostaglandin production: A controlled double-blind trial. Aliment Pharmacol Ther 1995;9:127–135.
62. Langman MJS: Epidemiologic evidence on the association between peptic ulceration and antiinflammatory drug use. Gastroenterology 1989;96 (suppl 2):640–646.
63. Lanza FL: Gastrointestinal toxicity of newer NSAIDs. Am J Gastroenterol 1993;88:1318–1323.
64. Lee CY, Finkler: Acute intoxication due to ibuprofen overdose. Arch Pathol Lab Med 1986;110:747–749.
65. Linden CH, Towsend PL: Metabolic acidosis after acute ibuprofen overdosage. J Pediatr 1987;111:922–925.
66. Malo PE, Bell RL, Shaughnessy TK, et al: The 5-lipoxygenase inhibitory activity of zileuton in in vitro and in vivo models of antigen-induced airway anaphylaxis. Pulmonol Pharmacol 1994;773–779.
67. Martinez R, Smith D, Frankel L: Severe metabolic acidosis after acute naproxen sodium ingestion. Ann Emerg Med 1989;18:1102–1104.
68. Masferrer JL, Zweifel BS, Manning PT, et al: Selective inhibition of inducible cyclooxygenase–2 in vivo is antiinflammatory and nonulcerogenic. Proc Natl Acad Sci USA 1994; 91:3228–3232.
69. McCune KH, O'Brien CJ: Atrial fibrillation induced by ibuprofen overdose. Postgrad Med J 1993;69:325–356.
70. Meade EA, Smith WL, DeWitt DL: Differential inhibition of prostaglandin endoperoxide synthase (cyclooxygenase) isozymes by aspirin and other nonsteroidal antiinflammatory drugs. J Biol Chem 1993;268:6610–6614.
71. Mitchell JA, Akarasereento P, Thiemermann C, et al: Selectivity of nonsteroidal antiinflammatory drugs as inhibitors of constitutive and inducible cyclooxygenase. Proc Natl Acad Sci USA 1993;90:11693–11697.
72. Moise KJ, Huhta JC, Sharif DS, et al: Indomethacin in the treatment of premature labor: Effects on the fetal ductus arteriosus. N Engl J Med 1988;319:327–331.
73. Murray MD, Brater DC: Renal toxicity of the nonsteroidal

antiinflammatory drugs. Annu Rev Pharmacol Toxicol 1993;33:435–465.
74. Murray MD, Brater DC: Adverse effects of nonsteroidal antiinflammatory drugs on renal function. Ann Intern Med 1990;112:559–560.
75. Neuvonen PJ: Clinical pharmacokinetics of oral activated charcoal in acute intoxications. Clin Pharmacokinet 1982;7: 465–489.
76. Newton T, Rose R: Poisoning with equine phenylbutazone in a racetrack worker. Ann Emerg Med 1991;20:204–207.
77. Nordt SP: Diflunisal cross-reactivity with the Trinder method from salicylate determination. Ann Pharmacother 1996;30:1041–1042.
78. O'Brien WM, Bagby GF: Carpofen: A new nonsteroidal antiinflammatory drug. Pharmacology clinical efficacy and adverse effects. Pharmacotherapy 1987;7:16–24.
79. O'Brien WM, Bagby GF: Rare adverse reaction to nonsteroidal antiinflammatory drugs. J Rheumatol 1985;12: 785–790.
80. Okada H, Suzuki H, Awaya N, et al: Serious adverse effects induced by simultaneous administration of two nonsteroidal antiinflammatory drugs. South Med J 1993;86: 1266–1268.
81. Okoneke S: Intoxication with pyrazolones. Br J Clin Pharmacokinet 1982;7:465–489.
82. Physicians Desk Reference, 49th ed. Oradell, NJ, Medical Economics Data, 1995.
83. Polisson R. Nonsteroidal antiinflammatory drugs: The practical and the theoretical considerations in this selection. Am J Med 1996;100:31S–36S.
84. Prescott L, Critchley J, Balali-Mood M: Phenylbutazone overdosage: Abnormal metabolism associated with hepatic and renal damage. Br Med J 1980;281:1106–1107.
85. Riley DJ, Weir M, Balris GL: Renal adaptation to the failing heart. Avoiding a "therapeutic misadventure." Postgrad Med 1994;95:153–156.
86. Runkel R, Chaplin M, Savelium H, et al: Pharmacokinetics of naproxen overdoses. Clin Pharmacol Toxicol. 1976;20: 269–277.
87. Ryback M: Hematologic effects of nonsteroidal antiinflammatory drugs. In: Borda I, Koff R, eds: Nonsteroidal Antiinflammatory Drugs: A Profile of Adverse Effects. Philadelphia, Hanley & Belfus, 1992.
88. Schapowal AG, Simm HU, Schmitz-Schumann M: Phenomenology, pathogenesis, diagnosis and treatment of aspirin-sensitive rhinosinusitis. Acta Otorhinolaryngol Belg 1995;49:235–250.
89. Segasothy M, Samad SA, Zulfigar A, Bennett WM: Chronic renal disease and papillary necrosis associated with the long-term use of nonsteroidal antiinflammatory drugs as the sole or predominant analgesic. Am J Kidney Dis 1994;24:17–24.
90. Settipane G: Adverse reactions to aspirin and related drugs. Arch Intern Med 1981;141:328–332.
91. Shorr RO, Ray WA, Daugherty JR, Griffin MR. Concurrent use of nonsteroidal antiinflammatory drugs and oral anticoagulants places elderly persons at high risk for hemorrhagic peptic ulcer disease. Arch Intern Med 1993;153: 1665–1670.
92. Singh G, Ramey DR, Morfeld D, et al: Gastrointestinal tract complications of nonsteroidal antiinflammatory drug treatment in rheumatoid arthritis. A prospective observational cohort study. Arch Intern Med 1996;156: 1530–1536.
93. Smolinske S, Hall A, Vandenberg S, et al: Toxic effects of nonsteroidal antiinflammatory drugs in overdose. Drug Safety 1990;5:252–274.
94. Somerville K, Faulkner G, Langman M: Nonsteroidal antiinflammatory drugs and bleeding peptic ulcer. Lancet 1986;1:462–464.
95. Strong J, Wilson J, Douglas J, et al: Phenylbutazone self-poisoning treated by charcoal hemoperfusion. Anesthesiology 1979;34:1038–1040.
96. Szczeklik A, Gryglewshi R, Czerniawska-Myski G: Clinical patterns of hypersensitivity to nonsteroidal antiinflammatory drugs and their pathogenesis. J Allergy Clin Immunol 1997;60:276–284.
97. Upadhyay H, Gupta S: Diflunisal overdosage. Br Med J 1978;2:640. Letter.
98. Vane JR, Botting RM: New insights into the mode of action of antiinflammatory drugs. Inflamm Res 1995;44:1–10.
99. Veltri JC, Rollins DE: A comparison of the frequency and severity of poisoning cases for ingestion of acetaminophen, aspirin, and ibuprofen. Am J Emerg Med 1988; 6:104–107.
100. Wilde MI, McTavish D: Omeprazole. An update of its pharmacology and therapeutic use in acid-related disorders. Drugs 1994;48:91–132.
101. Willet LR, Carson JL, Strom BL: Epidemiology of gastrointestinal damage associated with nonsteroidal antiinflammatory drugs. Drug Safety 1994;10:170–181.
102. Zimmerman J, Siguencia J, Tsvang E: Upper gastrointestinal hemorrhage associated with cutaneous application of diclofenac gel. Am J Gastroenterol 1995;90: 2032–2034.
103. Zuckerman GD, Uy CC: Shock, metabolic acidosis and coma following ibuprofen overdose in a child. Ann Pharmacother 1995;29:869–871.

CHAPTER 34

Antihistamines and Decongestants

Richard S. Weisman

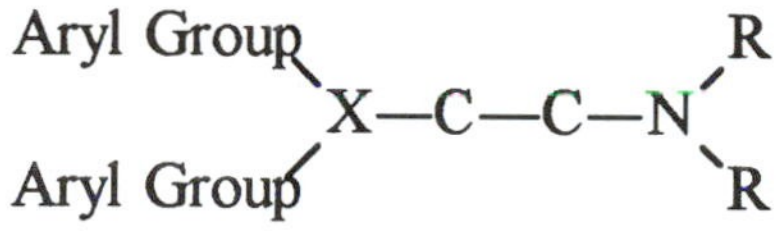

General Structure

An 18-year-old male was brought to the hospital after telling his family that he ingested 100 diphenhydramine capsules in a suicide attempt. An empty bottle was found on the floor. Upon arrival in the emergency department 3 hours later, the patient was lethargic, with garbled speech, and became agitated when aroused. His initial vital signs were: blood pressure, 200/90 mm Hg; pulse, 140/min; respirations, 18 breaths/min; and a rectal temperature of 101.2° F (38.4°C). His skin was dry and flushed. Examination of the head, eyes, ears, nose, and throat was remarkable only for pupils that were 5–6 mm and sluggishly reactive to light. His neck was supple. The chest examination was clear to auscultation and percussion. Heart sounds were normal; no murmurs or gallops were noted. His abdomen was soft, nontender, and without organomegaly. Bowel sounds were absent. There was no clubbing, cyanosis, or edema. Neurologic assessment was notable for periods of lethargy alternating with agitation, disorientation to place and time, and myoclonic jerks. There was no evidence of tremor, asterixis, or meningeal irritation. Deep tendon reflexes were symmetrical, and plantar flexion was noted.

The patient was administered oxygen via nasal cannula at 8 L/min and placed on a cardiac monitor. An intravenous line was established and hydration was initiated with D_5NS at 200 mL/h. Blood was sent for a complete blood count, electrolytes, glucose, and an acetaminophen level. Fifty milliliters of 50% dextrose in water and 100 mg of thiamine were given intravenously without response. An orogastric tube was inserted and 60 g of activated charcoal in a slurry of water and 60 g of sorbitol were administered. A Foley catheter was inserted and 700 mL of clear urine was immediately drained. An ECG was obtained, and demonstrated sinus tachycardia at 140 beats/min with a QRS complex duration of 0.08 seconds and a normal QT_c interval of 0.30 sec.

One milligram of physostigmine was given intravenously over 5 minutes. The patient's mental status did not improve. There were no changes in vital signs. His facial flush faded. There were no signs of salivation, lacrimation, or bronchorrhea. Five minutes later his vital signs were: blood pressure, 180/110 mm Hg; pulse, 130 beats/min; and respirations of 16 breaths/min. Bowel sounds remained absent. A second 1-mg dose of physostigmine was given intravenously over 5 minutes. The patient became alert and oriented over the next 3–5 minutes. His blood pressure and pulse fell to 140/90 mm Hg and 120 beats/min, respectively. Bowel sounds were present.

Laboratory analysis demonstrated normal CBC, electrolytes, and glucose, and a negative acetaminophen level.

Twelve hours later the patient was still alert and oriented, with no facial flushing. Vital signs included a blood pressure of 146/88 mm Hg, a pulse of 110 beats/min, respirations of 16 breaths/min, and a rectal temperature of 100.0°F. His Foley catheter was removed and he was able to void spontaneously.

The patient was admitted to the intensive care unit for monitoring and stabilization and subsequently was referred for psychiatric evaluation.

What Is the Pharmacology of Histamine Receptors?

Stimulation of histamine receptors results in numerous physiologic changes including capillary dilation, increased capillary permeability, increased myocardial contractility, increased gastric acid secretion, and stimulation of epidermal nerve endings causing pain and pruritis.[3] Histamine antagonists or antihistaminergic chemicals exist for three different histamine-modulated receptor sites. All of the receptors allow histamine to interact with G proteins in the plasma membranes.[17] The stimulation of H_1 receptors results in an increased synthesis of inositol-1,4,5-triphosphate and several diacylglycerols from phospholipids located in cell membranes. Inositol-1,4,5-triphosphate causes a release of calcium, which then activates calcium–calmodulin-dependent myosin light chain kinase resulting in enhanced cross-bridging and contraction.[30] The reaction at the H_1 receptors is mediated by phospholipase C.[2] H_2-receptor stimulation is mediated by adenyl cyclase activation of cyclic AMP–dependent protein kinase in smooth muscle and in parietal cells.

This discussion will focus on toxicity, diagnosis, and treatment of patients who have had an excessive exposure to H_1 or H_2 antagonists. The H_1-receptor antagonists are the classical antihistamines, used to lessen histamine-mediated symptoms of allergic reactions. The H_2 antagonists' primary pharmacologic activity is to reduce gastric acidity. The H_3 receptor is located in the central nervous system. The agonists and antagonists at the H_3 receptor do not have therapeutic indications and will not be discussed.

What Are the Pharmacologic Properties of the Specific Histamine H_1 Antihistamines?

Antihistamines are available worldwide and most do not require a prescription. They are often used for the symptomatic relief of cold and allergy symptoms. Several of the H_1 antihistamines with potent central nervous system depressant and anticholinergic properties are available as nonprescription sleep aids.

The importance of establishing the identity of an ingested H_1 antihistamine has increased with the recognition of potentially life-threatening cardiotoxicity with relatively small exposures to terfenadine and astemizole. This identification of the class of antihistamine can often be accomplished by taking a good history, but may on occasion be established by performing a physical examination and by recognizing a specific pattern of toxicity.

All of the histamine H_1 antagonists are reversible, competitive inhibitors of histamine. Terfenadine, cetirizine, fexophenadine, astemizole, and loratadine have a distinct pharmacology in that they bind more selectively to peripheral H_1 receptors and have a lower binding affinity for the cholinergic, alpha- and beta-adrenergic receptor sites than the older antihistamines. Terfenadine, astemizole, cetirizine, fexophenadine, and loratadine are postulated to cause less central nervous system depression than other antihistamines because they do not avidly partition across the blood–brain barrier into the brain.[59] Additionally, this group of antihistamines has become extremely popular because at therapeutic doses their specificity for the peripheral histamine receptor site eliminates many anticholinergic side effects including central nervous system depression, blurred vision, dry mouth, and tachycardia.

Many of the older antihistamines are substituted ethylamine structures with a tertiary amino group linked by a two-to-three carbon chain with two aromatic groups.[17] This differs from histamine by the absence of a primary amino group and the presence of a single aromatic moiety. There are six major classes of antihistamines. These include derivatives of ethylenediamine, ethanolamine, the alkylamines, phenothiazines and piperazines, and the peripherally selective H_1 antagonists. The peripheral selectivity which is defined by the presence of diminished anticholinergic and sedative properties of the H_1 antagonists is shown in Table 34–1. The structures of the various pharmacologic classes of the antihistamines appear in Figure 34–1.

The antihistamines are well absorbed following oral administration and most achieve peak plasma concentrations within 2–3 hours. The duration of action ranges from 3 to more than 24 hours. Hepatic metabolism is the primary route of metabolism for the antihistamines.[45] Asian patients can acetylate diphenhydramine to a nontoxic metabolite twice as rapidly as patients of Caucasian decent, making them much less sensitive to both the effects on psychomotor performance and the sedative effects.[53]

Astemizole is metabolized by the cytochrome P450 enzyme (isoenzyme CYP3A4) to an active metabolite desmethylastemizole, with a half-life of 19 days.[32] Terfenadine is extensively metabolized by the same enzyme to the active metabolite terfenadine carboxylate, which possesses peripheral antihistaminic activity. Further, carboxylate oxidation produces an inactive metabolite, which has a terminal half-life of 17 hours.[15] Drugs such as those listed in Table 34–2, which inhibit the cytochrome P450 isoenzyme CYP3A4, will delay metabolism, causing accumulation of parent astemizole or ter-

TABLE 34–1. ANTIHISTAMINES

Antihistamine	Class	Anticholinergic/ Sedating	Duration of Action	Adult Dose
Acrivastine	Alkylamine (newer)	+	6–8 h	8 mg tid
Astemizole	Piperidine	+	>24 h	10 mg daily
Brompheniramine	Alkylamine	++	4–6 h	4 mg qid
Buclizine	Piperazine	++	4–6 h	50 mg bid
Carbinoxamine	Ethanolamine	++++	3–6 h	4–8 mg qid
Cetirizine	Piperazine (newer)	+	12 h	5–10 mg qd
Chlorpheniramine	Alkylamine	++	4–6 h	4 mg qid
Clemastine	Ethanolamine	++++	12–24 h	2 mg bid
Dexbrompheniramine	Alkylamine	++	12 h	3–12 mg bid
Dexchlorpheniramine	Alkylamine	++	3–6 h	4–6 mg tid
Dimenhydrinate	Ethanolamine	++++	4–6 h	50–100 mg qid
Dimethindene	Alkylamine	++	8 h	1–2 mg tid
Diphenhydramine	Ethanolamine	++++	4–6 h	25–50 mg qid
Doxylamine	Ethanolamine	++++	6 h	7.5–12.5 mg qid
Fexophenadine	Piperidine	+	12 h	60 mg bid
Hydroxyzine	Piperazine	++	6–8 h	25 mg qid
Loratadine	Piperidine	+	8–12 h	10 mg qd
Meclizine	Piperazine	++	6–8 h	25 mg tid
Pheniramine	Alkylamine	++	4–6 h	5–15 mg q4h
Phenyltoloxamine	Ethanolamine	++++	4–8 h	7.5–25 mg tid
Promethazine	Phenothiazine	++++	4–6 h	12.5–25 mg qid
Terfenadine	Piperidine	+	12 h	60 mg bid
Trimeprazine	Phenothiazine	++++	4–6 h	2.5 mg qid
Tripelennamine	Ethylenediamine	+++	4–6 h	25–50 mg qid
Triprolidine	Alkylamine	++	4–6 h	2.5 mg qid

fenadine, which can block potassium efflux, resulting in life-threatening cardiac dysrhythmias.[19] In February 1997, the United States Food and Drug Administration suggested withdrawal of approval of all medications containing terfenadine because safer alternatives were available and in February 1998, the manufacturers voluntarily withdrew these agents.

What Are the Most Common Diagnostic Findings Associated with H_1 Antihistamine Toxicity?

Following exposure to an excessive amount of an antihistamine, most patients will present with central nervous system depression and excessive anticholinergic symptoms. Patients who have ingested cetirizine, fexophenadine, loratadine, terfenadine, or astemizole may not have significant CNS depression or anticholinergic symptoms.

In a review of 136 patients with diphenhydramine overdose, somnolence, lethargy, or coma occured in approximately 55% of patients, while a catatonic stupor occurred in 15% of patients.[31] Several reports suggest that young children will suffer more pulmonary dysfunction,[50] central nervous system stimulation, anticholinergic symptoms, and seizures than adult patients.[63]

Mydriasis is noted with both therapeutic doses and overdose. These patients note blurred vision and/or diplopia. Both vertical and horizontal nystagmus has been reported with diphenhydramine in overdose.[10] Other central nervous system effects may include seizures, hallucinations, acute extrapyramidal movement disorders, and toxic psychoses.[29,35,36,61] A severe anxiety reaction has been reported after the first therapeutic dose of terfenadine.[43] This is considered to be an adverse drug reaction and not a symptom of an acute overdose. Sedation without other anticholinergic effects has been reported with cetirizine, terfenadine, loratadine, and astemizole.

A sinus tachycardia is a consistent finding in any exposure that has anticholinergic effects. The absence of a tachycardia should lead to suspicion that excessive exposure to an anticholinergic substance has not occurred, or the patient has been exposed to another toxin capable of preventing the development of a tachycardia. Both hypotension and hypertension have been reported to occur with tachycardia. This probably relates more to the patient's age, state of hydration, and vascular tone then to a specific class of antihistamines.

Following large diphenhydramine overdoses, prolonged QT intervals and QRS complexes may be observed.[22,47] Overdoses of terfenadine and astemizole have resulted in hypotension, palpitations, and syncope. Torsades de pointes and other ventricular dysrhythmias have been reported in overdoses of terfenadine and

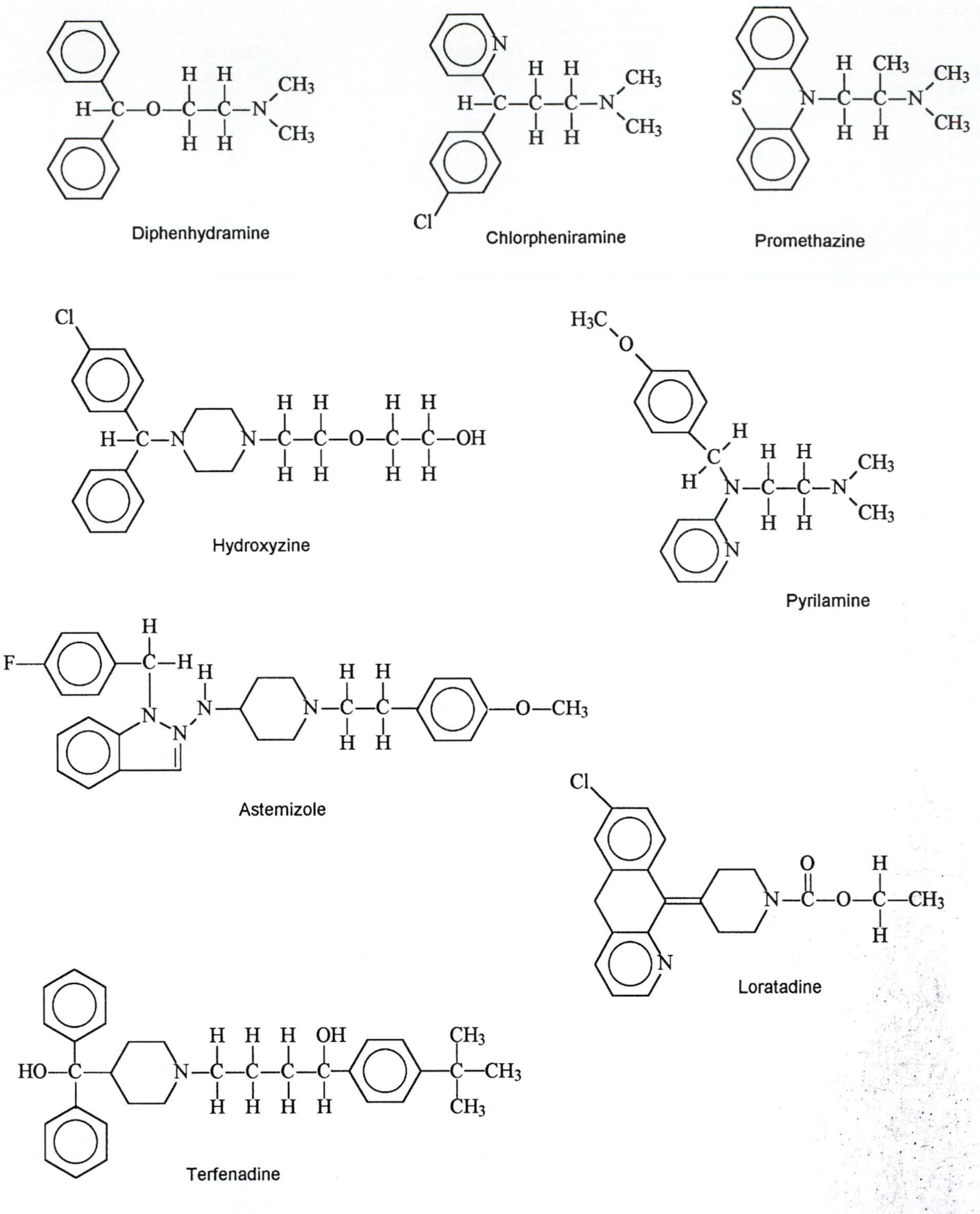

Figure 34–1. Structures of the various pharmacologic classes of antihistamines.

astemizole,[25,39,45] and in patients with significant hepatic dysfunction receiving therapeutic doses of terfenadine and astemizole. Patients with normal hepatic function who concurrently receive an inhibitor of the cytochrome P450 (CYP3A4) oxidative pathway such as erythromycin, troleandomycin, or ketoconazole and as little as 360 mg of terfenadine may manifest QT interval prolongation and ventricular dysrhythmias.[25,42] Cardiac conduction disturbances including atrioventricular dissociation and bundle branch blocks have been reported in a 3-year-old girl who ingested 100 mg of astemizole.[54]

The anticholinergic symptoms commonly seen in both adults and children can be observed at all hollow viscous organs. All mucous membranes and skin sur-

TABLE 34–2. INHIBITORS OF CYTOCHROME P450 ISOENZYME CYP3A4

Cimetidine	Itraconazole
Clarithromycin	Ketoconazole
Danazol	Miconazole
Diltiazem	Nefazodone
Erythromycin	Norfluoxetine
Flavonoids	Omeprazole
Fluconazole (large doses)	Quinidine
Fluoxetine	Troleandomycin

Reprinted, with permission, from Eller MG, Okerholm RA: Effect of cimetidine on terfenadine and terfenadine metabolite pharmacokinetics. Pharm Res 1991;7:206–210.

faces will appear dry. The skin may appear flushed and warm and even if the patient is agitated there will be a notable absence of sweat. Agitation concomitant with the inability to sweat usually results in hyperthermia that can be correlated with the extent of agitation, the ambient temperature and humidity, and the length of time during which the patient has been unable to dissipate heat. Muscle breakdown can occur with extreme agitation. Rhabdomyolysis has been reported in seven patients with doxylamine overdoses with none of the common etiologies such as seizures, shock, or crush injuries.[40] Urinary retention has been associated with all of the antihistamines possessing anticholinergic effects[61] (see Table 34–1). Gastrointestinal symptoms, including nausea, vomiting, diarrhea, and constipation, vary depending upon the specific antihistamine.[52] Various other clinical manifestations such as jaundice[21] and agranulocytosis[20] have been reported.

What Initial Diagnostic and Therapeutic Interventions Are Appropriate for the Patient Who Has Overdosed on an H_1 Antihistamine?

On initial presentation the patient who is likely to develop a severe complication may not be easily distinguished from the patient who will have a benign course. The patient's vital signs must be monitored and corrected when necessary, and the patient must be observed for the development of seizures and dysrhythmias. The patient should be placed on a cardiac monitor, have intravenous access established, and have blood obtained for routine laboratory studies. Early recognition of those at high risk for toxicity can be determined only by performing serial assessments of vital signs and mental status. Particular attention should be given to the patient with a rising temperature or pulse rate as these findings are often prognostic of worsening toxicity. The patient who is going to require more than supportive care will have unstable vital signs or a mental status that fails to improve or deteriorates after several hours. The potential for clinical deterioration necessitates that the patient be managed in a critical care environment where life support is immediately available if stabilization of the airway, cardiovascular, or thermoregulatory systems becomes necessary.

The vast majority of patients with antihistamine ingestions will present with central nervous system depression and tachycardia, which can be managed initially with supportive care and activated charcoal. The most serious complications of an antihistamine ingestion include supraventricular and ventricular dysrhythmias, seizures, hypotension, or hyperthermia.

If the patient is hypotensive, normal saline or lactated Ringer's solution should be administered and the patient should receive oxygen. If the desired increase in blood pressure is not attained, dopamine or norepinephrine may be titrated to achieve an acceptable blood pressure. Cardiogenic shock and myocardial depression that resulted from a 10-g ingestion of pyrilamine maleate could only be reversed with an intraaortic-balloon counterpulsation device.[16]

When Should Physostigmine Be Used to Treat the Anticholinergic Symptoms Associated With an H_1 Antihistamine Overdose?

Physostigmine can be an extremely effective antidote for anticholinergic toxicity. For physostigmine to be used safely the patient should have both peripheral and central anticholinergic effects (see Table 34–3), a narrow QRS complex on ECG, a narrow QRS complex on the currently obtained monitor strip, and no history of exposure to other toxins that may cause intraventricular conduction delays such as the class Ia or Ic antidysrhythmic agents, carbamazepine, cocaine, cyclic antidepressants, mesoridazine, propoxyphene, or thioridazine.

It must always be determined that the benefits of physostigmine outweigh the potential risks prior to use. The patient should be placed on a cardiac monitor and have a secure intravenous access site available. Physostigmine (2 mg adults, 0.5 mg children) should be administered by *slow* intravenous push. Vital signs must be frequently assessed during the administration of physostigmine. This dose may be repeated at 5–10-minute intervals if the reversal of anticholinergic symptoms does not occur and cholinergic symptoms such as salivation, diaphoresis, bradycardia, lacrimation, urination, or defecation do not occur. If improvement occurs it may be

TABLE 34–3. ANTICHOLINERGIC SYMPTOMS

Central	Peripheral
Agitation	Hypertension
Hallucinations	Tachycardia
Confusion	Hyperthermia
Sedation	Mydriasis
Coma	Dry, flushed skin
Seizures	Decreased GI motility
	Urinary retention

necessary to readminister the physostigmine at 30–60-minute intervals. With each readministration the minimum dose to reverse anticholinergic toxicity must be determined. A dose of intravenous atropine equal to one-half of the dose of physostigmine should be available at the patient's bedside if cholinergic toxicity occurs. See Antidotes in Depth, Physostigmine, for more information.

Agitation, hallucinations, and psychosis can often be treated with the administration of either physostigmine or diazepam. If the history is unclear, if the ECG manifests a wide QRS complex, or if the physician is uncertain whether physostigmine is safe, an intravenous benzodiazepine is an efficacious and safe alternative for the management of agitation. The intravenous benzodiazepine may be repeated as necessary until the patient's agitation is controlled and the patient is resting comfortably. Most patients will not require any additional pharmacologic interventions.

The presence of agitation should heighten the awareness that hyperthermia may be present or may develop. If the patient's temperature has reached 40.5°C or the temperature is rising rapidly, the patient should be promptly cooled in an ice bath or with cold water mist and fan.

If the patient has a seizure, an intravenous benzodiazepine such as diazepam 10 mg (0.1–0.2 mg/kg in children) should be given and repeated as necessary. If the seizures are refractory to the benzodiazepine, phenobarbital or general anesthesia with thiopental and paralysis with a neuromuscular blocking agent may be necessary.

What Cardiac Dysrhythmias May Occur With Terfenadine and Astemizole?

Ventricular dysrhythmias from antihistamine ingestions are most commonly associated with astemizole or terfenadine. Torsades de pointes, a variation of polymorphic ventricular tachycardia, is a recognized complication of terfenadine and astemizole overdose. It also occurs with standard dosing in patients with hepatic dysfunction or in patients concurrently receiving an inhibitor of CYP3A4. Terfenadine and astemizole inhibit outward potassium currents along the (hKv1.5) delayed-rectifier potassium channel by entering into the internal mouth of the channel after it opens[48,62] (see Chap. 21). The carboxylic acid metabolite of terfenadine, in contrast, causes only minimal inhibition of this current. Inhibition of the potassium channel prolongs the action potential duration. Excessive action potential duration can cause torsades de pointes.[9,42] Loratadine, cetirizine, and fexophenadine do not inhibit potassium currents along the (hKv1.5) delayed-rectifier potassium channel and therefore are not expected to cause torsades de pointes.[60]

The recommended adult daily dose of astemizole is 10 mg. Astemizole is not approved for use in children less than 12 years of age. As little as 1.7 mg/kg of astemizole in children may be sufficient to cause cardiac toxicity.[57] All children who ingest any amount of astemizole should receive 1 g/kg of body weight of activated charcoal and a prolonged period of cardiac monitoring because of the risk of cardiotoxicity with small ingestions.[57]

Torsades de pointes may initially be treated with cardioversion; however, the success rate for cardioversion of any drug-induced dysrhythmias is limited due to the persistence of the toxin. Magnesium sulfate (2–6 g in adults or 25–50 mg/kg in children) should be administered as a slow intravenous bolus over 10–40 minutes.[55] When magnesium sulfate is administered, the patient should be carefully monitored for changes in blood pressure, rhythm, and reflexes. If the ventricular dysrhythmia remains unresponsive, overdrive pacing may be necessary.

What Methods of Gastrointestinal Decontamination Should Be Used for Patients Who Have Overdosed With an H_1 Antihistamine?

Emesis with syrup of ipecac is reserved solely for the patient who can be treated immediately after the ingestion, outside of the hospital, if activated charcoal is not available. In the emergency department the administration of the syrup of ipecac may delay the administration of activated charcoal, which may be the most beneficial therapeutic intervention for the antihistamine overdose.

Patients who are cooperative, retain a good gag reflex, and can safely take liquids by mouth should receive a slurry of 1 g/kg of body weight of activated charcoal mixed in water to drink. If the patient has significant central nervous system depression, lacks a gag reflex, or is unable to protect his or her airway, endotracheal intubation should be considered and the activated charcoal should be administered through a nasogastric tube. Orogastric lavage is only rarely indicated to decontaminate the GI tract in a massive antihistamine overdose. If the patient with an antihistamine overdose has not developed CNS depression, activated charcoal should be given by mouth. If sufficient time has elapsed since ingestion for the patient to develop CNS depression, a nasogastric tube should be placed for the administration of the activated charcoal. The finding of CNS depression on physical examination indicates that significant absorption of the antihistamine has already occured and orogastric lavage would be unlikely to be beneficial.

What Are the Pharmacologic Properties of the Histamine H_2-specific Antihistamines?

The H_2-receptor antagonists became available shortly after the characterization of the H_2 receptor in 1972.[4] They are presently in widespread use for the treatment of peptic and duodenal ulcer disease, and acid hypersecretory states including Zollinger-Ellison syndrome. Less common uses include systemic mastocytosis and multiple endocrine adenomas.

TABLE 34–4. HISTAMINE H_2-RECEPTOR ANTAGONISTS

Cimetidine
Ranitidine
Nizatidine
Famotidine

Cimetidine is the prototype H_2-receptor antagonist. Table 34–4 lists the other available H_2-receptor antagonists. Cimetidine is rapidly and completely absorbed following oral administration. Cimetidine has a volume of distribution of approximately 2 L/kg with 13–25% protein binding.[1] Seventy percent of cimetidine is eliminated unchanged in the urine, 15% is metabolized by the liver, and 10% is found unchanged in the stool.[43] The elimination half-life in patients with normal renal function is approximately 2 hours.[1] Cimetidine is responsible for numerous drug–drug interactions because it can inhibit cytochrome P450 mixed function oxidase activity and can reduce hepatic blood flow. Cimetidine inhibits P450 isoenzymes CYP1A2, CYP2C9, and CYP3A4.[19] Cimetidine has been implicated in causing significant drug interactions with amitriptyline, the benzodiazepines, carbamazepine, imipramine, lidocaine, nifedipine, phenytoin, quinidine, terfenadine, tolbutamide, theophylline, verapamil, and warfarin.[19,49] All of the other available H_2-receptor antagonists have been shown not to inhibit the cytochrome P450 mixed function oxidase system.[19]

What Are the Toxic Effects of the H_2 Antagonists?

Acute toxic effects appear to be extremely rare following large (20-g) oral ingestions of cimetidine.[26] One patient developed tachycardia, dilated and sluggishly reactive pupils, and slurred speech following a 12-g ingestion.[44]

Bradycardia, hypotension, and cardiac arrest have followed rapid intravenous administration of cimetidine in seriously ill patients.[51]

What Methods of Gastrointestinal Decontamination Should Be Used for Patients Who Have Overdosed With an H_2 Antihistamine?

Patients who have overdosed on an H_2 antihistamine should receive 1 g/kg of body weight of activated charcoal mixed in water to drink as the only gastrointestinal decontamination. These medications rarely result in significant toxicity and do not warrant the risk of complications from orogastric lavage or emesis with syrup of ipecac.

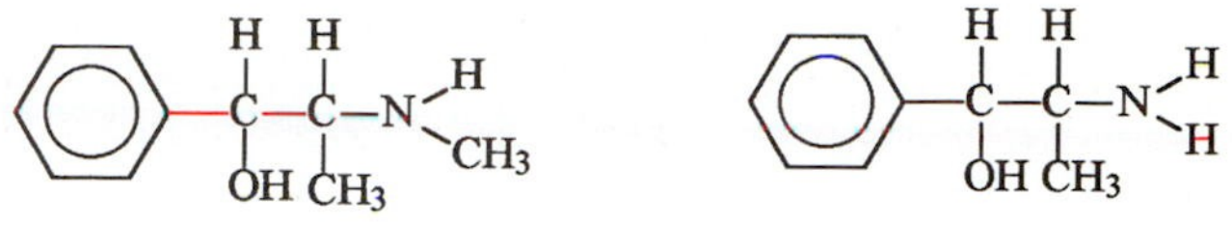

Ephedrine   Phenylpropanolamine

Figure 34–2. Structures of ephedrine and phenylpropanolamine.

What Are the Pharmacologic Properties of the Decongestants?

The decongestants pseudoephedrine, ephedrine, and phenylpropanolamine (see Fig. 34–2) reduce nasal congestion by stimulating the alpha-adrenergic receptor sites on vascular smooth muscles. This results in the constriction of dilated arterioles and reduces blood flow to engorged nasal vascular beds. Pseudoephedrine and ephedrine are direct nonspecific $alpha_{(1, 2)}$- and $beta_{(1, 2)}$-adrenergic receptor stimulants. Pseudoephedrine is the *d*-isomer of ephedrine and has only 25% the adrenergic receptor activity of ephedrine.[12] Phenylpropanolamine is a pure $alpha_{(1, 2)}$-adrenergic receptor stimulant devoid of beta-adrenergic receptor activity. Phenylpropanolamine can directly stimulate $alpha_{(1, 2)}$ receptors and can indirectly stimulate receptors by causing a release of norepinephrine (see Table 34–5). The decongestants are rapidly absorbed from the gastrointestinal tract with peak blood levels occurring within 2–4 hours of ingestion.

Symptoms of toxicity from decongestants will usually resolve within 8–16 hours. Symptoms may persist for greater than 24 hours if a sustained-release product has been ingested.

The imidazoline decongestants naphazoline, oxymetazoline, tetrahydrozoline, and xylometazoline are potent central and peripheral $alpha_2$-adrenergic receptor stimulants and in overdose can cause central nervous system depression, hypotension, bradycardia, and respiratory depression[24] (see Fig. 34–3). These medications are primarily used as nasal decongestants. Tetrahydrozoline is available without prescription as an eye drop to de-

TABLE 34–5. DECONGESTANTS

Decongestant	Class	Duration of Action	Alpha/Beta Activity
Ephedrine	Sympathomimetic	3–5 h	$\alpha_{1,2}$ and $\beta_{1,2}$
Naphazoline	Imidazoline	8 h	α_2
Oxymetazoline	Imidazoline	6–7 h	α_2
Phenylephrine	Sympathomimetic	1 h	$\alpha_{1,2}$
Phenylpropanolamine	Sympathomimetic	12 h (sust. release)	$\alpha_{1,2}$
Pseudoephedrine	Sympathomimetic	3–4 h	$\alpha_{1,2}$ and $\beta_{1,2}$
Tetrahydrozoline	Imidazoline	4–8 h	α_2
Xylometazoline	Imidazoline	5–6 h	α_2

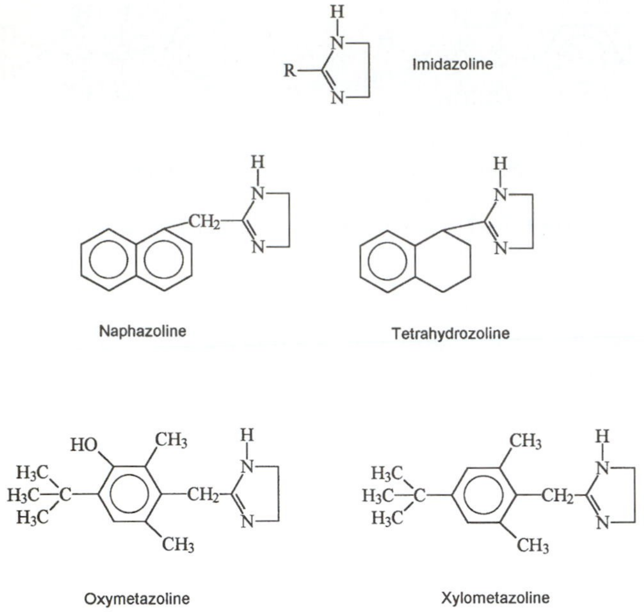

Figure 34–3. Structures of imidazoline decongestants naphazoline, tetrahydrozoline, oxymetazoline, and xylometazoline.

crease eye irritation and redness. Children are particularly sensitive to the effects of the imidazoline decongestants. Oxymetazoline and naphazoline are pure central and peripheral $alpha_2$-adrenergic receptor agonists; tetrahydrozoline stimulates $alpha_2$ receptors and H_2 receptors. The imidazolines are rapidly absorbed from both the gastrointestinal tract and mucous membranes. The elimination half-lives range from 2 to 4 hours.

What Are the Life-Threatening Complications of Decongestant Overdoses? How Should They Be Treated?

Patients who have overdosed on a decongestant will present with central nervous system stimulation, hypertension, and tachycardia if they have ingested ephedrine or pseuoephedrine, or bradycardia if they have ingested phenylpropanolamine.[23] The most serious complications following a decongestant ingestion include hypertension, tachycardia, bradycardia, seizures, and cerebral hemorrhage.[5,7,14,46]

The most serious complications following an ephedrine, pseudoephedrine, or phenylpropanolamine overdose include hypertension, dysrhythmias (tachycardia or bradycardia), seizures, and cerebral hemorrhage.[7,46] In a review of 500 reports of adverse reactions from patients who had ingested ephedrine and associated stimulants as dietary supplements, eight fatalities from myocardial infarction and cerebral hemorrhage were reported.[46] A patient with an abnormal neuropsychiatric examination following the ingestion of a decongestant should be evaluated for cerebral hemorrhage with a CT scan and subsequently a lumbar puncture if indicated.[33]

Extreme agitation, seizures, tachycardia, hypertension, and psychosis should be initially treated with the administration of oxygen and a benzodiazepine. Vital signs must be frequently assessed during the administration of the benzodiazepine. The intravenous benzodiazepine may be repeated as necessary until the patient's agitation is controlled and the patient is resting comfortably. If still hypertensive, the patient may be treated with nifedipine, phentolamine, or nitroprusside.[18]

If seizures are refractory to the intravenous benzodiazepine, phenobarbital, general anesthesia with thiopental, or paralysis with a neuromuscular blocking agent may be necessary.

Ventricular dysrhythmias from decongestant ingestions should be treated with standard doses of lidocaine or bretylium.[56] If the dysrhythmia fails to respond to lidocaine, propranolol can be administered.[38]

Phenylpropanolamine ingestions may cause a reflex bradycardia with an atrioventricular block that will be responsive to standard doses of atropine.[58]

The imidazoline decongestants naphazoline, oxymetazoline, tetrahydrozoline, and xylometazoline are potent central alpha-adrenergic receptor stimulants and in overdose can cause central nervous system depression, hypotension, bradycardia, and respiratory depression.[24] An adolescent male developed sinoatrial node arrest, central nervous system depression, miosis, bradycardia, and hypotension following an inadvertent ingestion of 15 mL of 0.05% tetrahydrozoline.[28]

What Are the Most Common Diagnostic Findings That Have Been Associated With Decongestant Toxicity?

Following overdose of a decongestant most patients will present with central nervous system stimulation, hypertension, tachycardia, or bradycardia. Approximately 4–5 times the recommended dose of pseudoephedrine[12] and 17.5 mg/kg of phenylpropanolamine is required to cause hypertension.[14] Dysrhythmias have been reported in adults with the ingestion of 120 mg of pseudoephedrine and moderate exercise.[5,6,8] Headache was the most common symptom (39%) reported by patients who developed severe toxicity.[33] Approximately 36% of patients with phenylpropanolamine overdoses will present with central nervous system depression.[34] In more severe exposures, seizures,[11] myocardial infarction,[37] atrial and ventricular dysrhythmias, ischemic bowel infarction,[27] and cerebral hemorrhages have been reported.[13,41] In 45 patients who developed hypertensive encephalopathy from the ingestion of phenylpropanolamine, 24 patients developed intracranial hemorrhages, 15 developed seizures, and 6 died.[33]

What Methods of Gastrointestinal Decontamination Should Be Used for Patients Who Have Overdosed With a Decongestant?

Emesis with syrup of ipecac is reserved solely for the patient who can be treated immediately after the ingestion, outside of the hospital, if activated charcoal is not available. In the emergency department the administration of the syrup of ipecac may delay the administration of activated charcoal, which may be the most beneficial therapeutic intervention for the decongestant overdose.

Patients who are cooperative, retain a good gag reflex, and can safely take liquids by mouth, should receive a slurry of 1 g/kg of body weight of activated charcoal mixed in water to drink.

The patient with significant central nervous system toxicity, who lacks a gag reflex, and is unable to protect his or her airway should have a nasogastric tube placed for the instillation of 1 g/kg of body weight of activated charcoal. If the patient already manifests CNS toxicity, orogastric lavage is usually of limited benefit.

What Other Toxins Can Have a Similar Clinical Presentation to H_1 Antihistamine and Decongestant Toxicity and Should Be Considered in the Differential Diagnosis?

Distinguishing between the symptoms of a patient who has overdosed with an antihistamine and a patient who has overdosed with a decongestant (sympathomimetic amines) is often difficult. Both overdoses can cause agitation, tachycardia, mydriasis, urinary retention, a flush, and a low-grade fever. The differences between an antihistamine overdose and a decongestant overdose are that antihistamines more commonly depress mental status, dry mucous membranes, and depress bowel sounds, while the decongestants cause sweating and increase or do not affect bowel sounds.

Other toxins that cause anticholinergic syndromes may include the cyclic antidepressants, phenothiazines, antispasmodics, and the anticholinergic drugs that are used to treat or prevent extrapyramidal symptoms associated with neuroleptic therapy.

Patients who ingest plants containing the belladonna alkaloids such as jimson weed (*Datura stramonium*), angel's trumpet (*Solandra* spp.) and nightshade (*Atropa belladona*) will also present with anticholinergic symptoms. See Chapter 77 for a complete discussion of plants with anticholinergic symptoms.

Other toxins that can cause sympathomimetic symptoms include caffeine, cocaine, the amphetamines, theophylline, thyroid hormones, epinephrine, dopamine, terbutaline, ritodrine, salbutamol, the monoamine oxidase inhibitors, phencyclidine, and phencyclidine congeners.

Can the Toxicology Laboratory Be Helpful in Caring for the Patient With Antihistamine or Decongestant Toxicity?

There appears to be little justification for obtaining either qualitative testing or quantitative screening of the blood or urine for antihistamines or decongestants. Most laboratories are not capable of testing for antihistamines.

Most cough and cold preparations combine antihistamines, decongestants, caffeine, antipyretics, and analgesics. All adults with intentional ingestions of these agents and children with very large ingestions should have blood obtained at 4 hours or as soon thereafter as possible for acetaminophen and salicylate determinations.

Summary

The popularity and availability of antihistamines and decongestants make them readily accessible for overdose in both adults and children. Fortunately, almost all patients will have excellent outcomes with no expected sequelae if they receive activated charcoal soon after ingestion and continuous assessment of and management for abnormalities in their vital signs, electrocardiogram, and mental status during the critical phase. If the clinician is familiar with the more severe sequelae of antihistamine overdoses, early and appropriate interventions will reduce both morbidity and mortality from these exposures.

References

1. Abate MA, Hyneck ML, Cohen IA, et al: Cimetidine pharmacokinetics. Clin Pharm 1982;1:225–233.
2. Arrang JM, Garbarg M, Lacelot JC, et al: Highly potent and selective ligands for histamine H_3 receptors. Nature 1987; 327:117–123.
3. Ash ASF, Schild HO: Receptors mediating some actions of histamine. Br J Pharmacol 1966;27:427–439.
4. Black JW, Duncan WAM, Durant CJ, et al: Definition and antagonism of histamine H_2 receptors. Nature 1972;236: 385–390.
5. Bright TP, Sandage BW Jr, Fletcher HP: Selected cardiac and metabolic responses to pseudoephedrine with exercise. J Clin Pharmacol 1981;21:488–492.
6. Burton BT, Rice M, Schmertzler LE: Atrioventricular block following overdose of decongestant cold medication. J Emerg Med 1985;2:415–419.
7. Cetaruk EW, Aaron CK: Hazards of nonprescription medications. Curr Controv Toxicol 1994;12:483–510.
8. Conway EE, Walsh CA, Palomba AL: Supraventricular tachycardia following the administration of phenylpropanolamine in an infant. Pediatr Emerg Care 1989;5: 173–174.
9. Davies AJ, Harinda V, McEwan A, Ghose RR: Cardiotoxic

effect with convulsions in terfenadine overdose. Br Med J 1989;298:325.
10. Daya L, Spyker DA, Hendin P, et al: Massive diphenhydramine overdose: A case report and comparison of pharmacokinetic models. Vet Hum Toxicol 1991;33:357. Abstract.
11. Dilsaver SC, Votolato NA, Alessi NE: Complications of phenylpropanolamine. Am Fam Physician 1989;39:201–206.
12. Drew CDM, Knight GT, Hughes DTD: Comparison of the effects of D-ephedrine and L-pseudoephedrine on the cardiovascular and respiratory systems in man. Br J Clin Pharmacol 1978;6:221–225.
13. Edwards M, Russo L, Harwood-Nuss A: Cerebral infarction with a single oral dose of phenylpropanolamine. Am J Emerg Med 1987;5:163–164.
14. Ekins BR, Spoerke DG: An estimation of the toxicity of nonprescription diet aids from seventy exposure cases. Vet Hum Toxicol 1983;25:81–85.
15. Eller MG, Okerholm RA: Effect of cimetidine on terfenadine and terfenadine metabolite pharmacokinetics. Pharm Res 1991;7:206–210.
16. Freedberg RS, Friedman GR, Palu RN, Feit F: Cardiogenic shock due to antihistamine overdose: Reversal with intraaortic balloon counterpulsation. JAMA 1987;257:660–661.
17. Ganellin CR, Parsons ME, eds: Pharmacology of Histamine Receptors. Bristol, MA, Wright/PSG, 1982, pp. 1–43.
18. Gibson RG, Oliver JA, Leak D: Nifedipine therapy of phenylpropanolamine-induced hypertension. Am Heart J 1987;113:406–407.
19. Hansten PD. Drug interactions of gastrointestinal drugs. In: Lewis JH, ed: A Pharmacologic Approach to Gastrointestinal Disorders. Baltimore, Williams & Wilkins, 1994, pp. 47–74.
20. Hardin AS, Padilla F: Agranulocytosis during therapy with a brompheniramine-medication. J Arkansas Med Soc 1978; 75:206–208.
21. Henry DA, Lowe JM, Donelly T: Jaundice during cyproheptadine treatment. Br Med J 1978;1:753.
22. Hestand HE, Teske DW: Diphenhydramine hydrochloride intoxication. J Pediatr 1977;90:1017–1018.
23. Heyman SN, Mevorach D, Ghanem J: Hypertensive crisis from chronic intoxication with nasal decongestant and cough medications. Ann Pharmacother 1991;25:1068–1070.
24. Higgins GL, Campbell B, Wallace K, et al: Pediatric poisoning from over-the-counter imidazoline-containing products. Ann Emerg Med 1991;20:655–658.
25. Honig PK, Woosley RL, Zamini K, et al: Changes in the pharmacokinetics and electrocardiographic pharmacodynamics of terfenadine with concomitant administration of erythromycin. Clin Pharmacol Ther 1992;52:231–238.
26. Illingworth RN, Jarvie DR: Absence of toxicity in cimetidine overdosage. Br Med J 1979;1:453–454.
27. Johnson DA, Stafford PW, Volpe RJ: Ischemic bowel infarction and phenylpropanolamine use. West J Med 1985; 142:399–400.
28. Jones DG, Osterhoudt K, Stone M, et al: Sinoatrial node dysfunction following tetrahydrozoline (Visine®) ingestion. J Toxicol Clin Toxicol 1996;34:564. Abstract.
29. Jones IH, Stevenson J, Jordan A, et al: Pheniramine as an hallucinogen. Med J Aust 1973;1:382–386.
30. Kamm KE, Stull JT: The function of myosin and myosin light chain kinase phosphorylation in smooth muscle. Annu Rev Pharmacol Toxicol 1985;25:593–620.
31. Koppel C, Ibe K, Tenczer J: Clinical symptomatology of diphenhydramine overdose: An evaluation of 136 cases, 1982 to 1985. J Toxicol Clin Toxicol 1987;25:53–70.
32. Krestansky PM, Cluxton RJ Jr: Astemizole: A long-acting nonsedating antihistamine. Drug Intell Clin Pharm 1987; 21:947–953.
33. Lake CR, Gallant S, Masson E, et al: Adverse drug effects attributed to phenylpropanolamine: A review of 142 case reports. Am J Med 1990;89:195–208.
34. Larson WL, Rogers A: Overdosage from phenylpropanolamine: Experience of the Hennepin Regional Poison Center. Vet Hum Toxicol 1986;28:546–548.
35. Lavenstein BL, Cantor FK: Acute dystonia: An unusual reaction to diphenhydramine. JAMA 1976;236:291.
36. Leighton KM: Paranoid psychosis after abuse of Actifed. Br Med J 1982;284:789–790.
37. Leo PJ, Hollander JE, Shih RD, Marcus SM: Phenylpropanolamine and associated myocardial infarction. Ann Emerg Med 1996;28:359–362.
38. Liddle GG: Phenylpropanolamine induced dysrhythmias. JAMA 1973;223:324–326.
39. MacConnell TJ, Stanner AJ: Torsades de pointes complicating treatment with terfenadine. Br Med J 1991;302:1469. Letter.
40. Mendoza FS, Atiba JO, Krensky AL, et al: Rhabdomyolysis complicating doxylamine overdose. Clin Pediatr 1987;26: 595–597.
41. Mesnard B, Ginn DR: Excessive phenylpropanolamine ingestion followed by subarachnoid hemorrhage. South Med J 1984;77:939. Letter.
42. Monahan BP, Ferguson CL, Killeavy ES, et al: Torsade de pointes occurring in association with terfenadine use. JAMA 1989;264:2788–2790.
43. Napke E, Biron P: Nervous reactions after first dose of terfenadine in adults. Lancet 1989;2:615–616. Letter.
44. Nelson PG: Cimetidine and mental confusion. Lancet 1977;2:928. Letter.
45. Patan DM, Webster DR: Pharmacokinetics of the H_1 receptor antagonists (the antihistamines). Clin Pharmacokinet 1985;10:477–497.
46. Perrotta DM, Coody G, Culmo C: Adverse events associated with ephedrine-containing products—Texas, December 1993–September 1995. MMWR 1996;45:689–693.
47. Rinder CS, D'Amato SL, Rinder HM: Survival in complicated diphenhydramine overdose. Crit Care Med 1988; 16:1161–1162.
48. Sakeuir H, Vannata B: Torsades de pointes induced by astemizole in a patient with prolongation of the QT interval. Am Heart J 1993;125:1436–1438.
49. Sawyer D, Conner CS, Scalby R: Cimetidine adverse reactions and acute toxicity. Am J Hosp Pharm 1981;38:188–197.
50. Schuller DE: The spectrum of antihistamines adversely affecting pulmonary function in asthmatic children. J Allergy Clin Immunol 1983;71:147.
51. Shaw RG, Mashford MI, Desmond PV: Cardiac arrest after intravenous injection of cimetidine. Med J Aust, 1980; 2:629–630.
52. Simons FER, Simons KG: Pharmacokinetics and antipruritic

effects of hydroxyzine in children with atopic dermatitis. Pediatrics 1984;104:123–127.

53. Spector R, Choudhury AK, Chiang CK, et al: Diphenhydramine in Orientals and Caucasians. Clin Pharmacol Ther 1980;28:229–231.
54. Tobin JR, Doyle TP, Ackerman AD, Brenner JI: Astemizole-induced cardiac conduction disturbances in a child. JAMA 1991;266:2737–2740.
55. Tzivoni D, Banai S, Schuger C, et al: Treatment of torsade de pointes with magnesium sulfate. Circulation 1988;77:392–397.
56. Weesner KM, Denison M, Roberts RJ: Cardiac dysrhythmias in an adolescent following ingestion of an over-the-counter stimulant. Clin Pediatr 1982;21:700–701.
57. Wiley JF, Gelber ML, Henretig FM, et al: Cardiotoxic effects of astemizole overdose in children. J Pediatr 1992;120:799–802.
58. Woo OF, Benowitz NL, Baily FW: Atrioventricular conduction block caused by phenylpropanolamine. JAMA 1985;253:2646–2647.
59. Woodward JK: Pharmacology and toxicology of nonclassical antihistamines. Cutis 1988;42:5–9.
60. Woosley R, Darrow WR: Analysis of potential adverse drug reactions—A case of mistaken identity. Am J Cardiol 1994;74:208–209.
61. Wyngaarden JB, Seevers MH: Toxic effects of antihistamines. JAMA 1951;145:277–288.
62. Yang T, Prakash C, Roden DM, Snyders DJ: Mechanism of block of a human cardiac potassium channel by terfenadine racemate and enantiomers. J Pharmacol 1995;115:267–274.
63. Zavitz M, Lindsay C, McGuigan MA: Acute diphenhydramine ingestion in children. Vet Hum Toxicol 1989;31:349. Abstract.

ANTIDOTES IN DEPTH

Physostigmine

Mary Ann Howland

Physostigmine is a carbamate that reversibly inhibits cholinesterases both in the periphery and in the central nervous system (CNS).[30] This action inhibits the metabolism of acetylcholine, thereby allowing acetylcholine to accumulate. This indirect action of acetylcholine accumulation is used to antagonize the anticholinergic effects of drugs such as atropine, scopolamine,[34] and diphenhydramine. Although past practice was to use physostigmine as an antagonist to the anticholinergic effects of the tricyclic antidepressants and the phenothiazines, this is no longer recommended due to a poor risk–benefit ratio given the potential for exacerbation of life-threatening quinidine-like effects. Physostigmine's tertiary amine structure differentiates it from all other marketed anticholinesterases, which are quaternary amines, and permits CNS penetration.

The history of physostigmine use dates back to the Efik people of Old Calabar in Nigeria on the west coast of Africa.[11,13,15,30] The chiefs used a poisonous concoction made from the beans of an aquatic leguminous perennial plant found in the area to deliver the esere ordeal. Esere was the word used to represent both the bean and the ritual used to test the innocence or guilt of an accused person. It was also believed that the esere had the power to detect and kill those practicing witchcraft. Supposedly the innocent swallowed the poison quickly, causing immediate emesis.[15] Vomiting allowed them to survive on their own or be given an antidote of excrement in water. The guilty, however, hesitated swallowing, leading to speculation that sublingual absorption led to severe systemic symptoms without the benefit of vomiting. They were noted to develop mouth fasiculations and died foaming at the mouth.

Daniell, a British medical officer stationed in Calabar, brought samples of the bean and the plant back to England in 1840.[15] John Balfour, a famous professor of medicine and botany at the Edinburgh Medical School, is credited with characterizing the plant, which became known as *Physostigma venenosum Balfour* (family *Leguminosae*) in 1857. The active alkaloid that was isolated from the Old Calabar or ordeal bean by Jobst and Hesse in 1864 was named physostigmine. Independently a year later Vee and Leven also isolated the active alkaloid and named it eserine.

Christison performed the first toxicologic studies including self-experimentation with increasing doses of the seed. Fraser, Christison's student and later successor, originated the concept of antagonism from his experiments with physostigmine and atropine. Unlike others, he plotted graphs of the dose relationships between the effects of atropine versus physostigmine on various organs such as the eye and the heart.[11] He also demonstrated that, up to a certain dose, atropine acted as an antidote to the lethal effects of physostigmine. Experiments with physostigmine paved the way for Anderson in 1906 to propose the existence of a transmitter through which physostigmine was working. Loewi in the 1920s proposed and then proved the theory of neurohumoral transmission. Stedman and Burger established the chemical structure of physostigmine in 1925. Julian and Pikl synthesized physostigmine in 1935. During this time physostigmine was being employed as a miotic in patients with glaucoma, and in patients with myasthenia gravis, as a reversal agent to the paralytic effects of curare, as an antidote to atropine, and as a prototypical insecticide. In summary, physostigmine was instrumental in the development of a bioassay for acetylcholine, concepts of neurohumoral transmission, mapping of cholinergic nerves, the concept of antagonism, the kinetics of enzyme inhibition, and improved understanding of the blood brain–barrier, as well as being a prototypical carbamate insecticide.[13]

The general formula for carbamate inhibitors is shown in Figure 34–4A. Figures 34–4B and C show the chemical structures of physostigmine ($C_{15}H_{21}O_2N_3$), a tertiary amine, and neostigmine, a quaternary amine agent used therapeutically. Like acetylcholine, physostigmine is a substrate for the cholinesterases: erythrocyte acetylcholinesterase and plasma or pseudocholinesterase. Both acetylcholine and physostigmine bind to the cholinesterase enzymes to form a complex; then a part of the substrate known as the leaving group (ie, choline for acetylcholine) leaves, and the remaining acetylated (for acetylcholine) or carbamyolated (for physostigmine) enzyme is hydrolyzed, regenerating the enzyme and freeing the acetate or carbamate groups, respectively (see Fig. 87–1, Chap. 87). For acetylcholine the process is extremely quick with a turnover time of 150 μsec, whereas the half-life for hydrolysis of the carbamoylated enzyme is 15–30 minutes.[30] This can be compared to several hours for some organophosphates and negligible for others. The I_{50} (molar concentration that inhibits 50% of the enzyme) of physostigmine is 2.3×10^{-7} M for acetylcholinesterase, which is much weaker than other carbamates at 1×10^{-10} M or many organophosphates at 1×10^{-11} M.[16] The mouse LD_{50} for physostigmine is 0.47

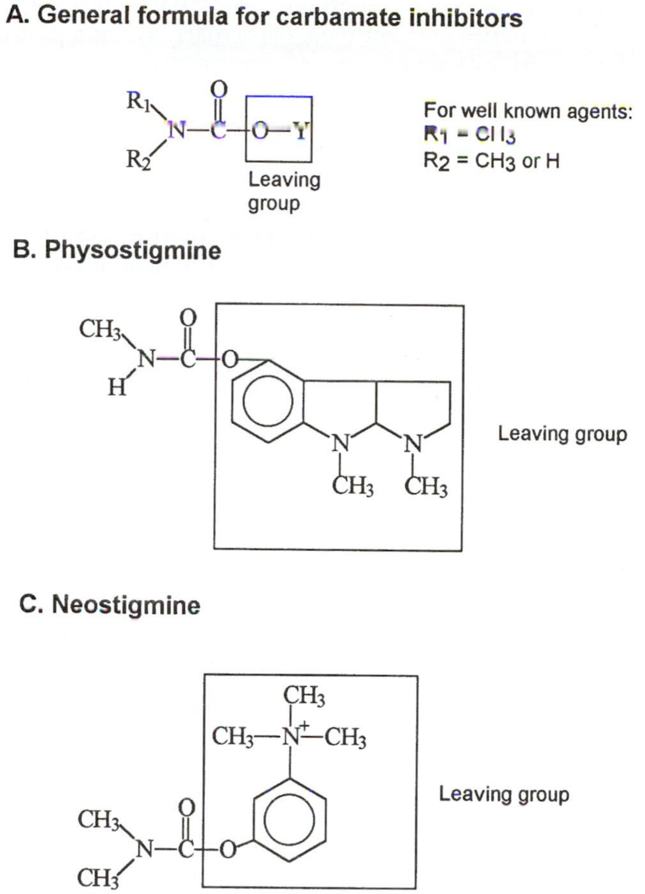

Figure 34–4. A. General formula for carbamate inhibitors. **B.** Structure of physostigmine. **C.** Structure of neostigmine.

mg/kg IV and 2.5 mg/kg po.[16] Only the (–) isomer inhibits cholinesterases, with plasma cholinesterase just a little more sensitive than acetylcholinesterase.[4]

The actions of physostigmine depend on the accumulation of acetylcholine at muscarinic, nicotinic (skeletal muscle, autonomic ganglia, adrenal glands), and the CNS sites.[16] Muscarinic effects produce the stimulation of smooth muscle and glandular secretions (respiratory, GI, GU) and the inhibition of contraction of most vascular smooth muscle. Nicotinic effects are stimulatory at low doses and depressant at high doses. For example, muscle fasiculations are followed by weakness and paralysis. CNS effects produce anxiety, dizziness, tremors, confusion, ataxia, coma, and seizures.[16] The EEG demonstrates desynchronous discharges followed by higher voltage discharges and a pattern similar to tonic-clonic seizures.[16] Terminally, the EEG becomes isoelectric. The cardiac effects are dose dependent and a function of often opposing actions from the muscarinic and nicotinic effects. Small doses produce a rise in blood pressure whereas moderate doses decrease heart rate and produce varying degrees of AV block.[16] At large doses, AV block appears de novo, the P wave is often absent, and the T waves are large and of variable shapes.[16] In addition to its inhibition of cholinesterase, physostigmine has direct actions on the nicotinic acetylcholine-receptor ionic channel, on the neuromuscular junction, and produces a decrease in GABA in the striatum.[29]

Physostigmine is poorly absorbed orally, with a bioavailability of < 5–12%.[1,2] Cholinesterases (choline ester hydrolases) cleave the ester linkage and very little drug is eliminated unchanged in the urine. Pharmacokinetic parameters following IV administration of 1.5 mg over 60 minutes in nine patients with Alzheimer's disease demonstrated the following: V_d 2.4 ± 0.6 L/kg; $t_{1/2}$ 16.4 ± 3.2 min; peak plasma concentration 3 ± 0.5 ng/mL; clearance 0.1 L/min/kg (7.7 L/min). There was a threefold interindividual variability in plasma physostigmine concentrations. Plasma cholinesterase concentrations showed inhibition as early as 2 minutes into the physostigmine infusion; the half time of plasma cholinesterase inhibition was 83.7 ± 5.2 min, with full recovery at 3 hours following the end of the physostigmine infusion. A graph of physostigmine concentration versus either percent plasma or acetylcholinesterase inhibition demonstrated hysteresis.[3,17] The effects on plasma cholinesterase inhibition lasts about 5 times longer than the half-life of physostigmine. In this study memory enhancement by physostigmine was directly related to plasma cholinesterase inhibition. All patients experienced varying degrees of nausea, diaphoresis, vomiting, headache, and generalized fatigue despite pretreatment with 2.5 mg methscopolamine.[3]

Physostigmine was first used as an antidote in 1864 to counteract severe atropine poisoning.[22] Today its role remains primarily in the treatment of antimuscarinic agents. Over 600 anticholinergic agents have been reported to respond to physostigmine.[7]

The past two decades have seen the rise and fall of physostigmine use.[28] Enamored with its ability to cause CNS arousal, physostigmine was used in the 1970s to reverse the CNS effects of a large number of anticholinergic and nonanticholinergic agents.[12,20,21,23,25] The success against anticholinergic agents is easily explained and directly antidotal by virtue of its inhibition of cholinesterase. Effects versus agents like benzodiazepines and opioids[18,26,32] can be attributed to either acetylcholine's direct action on the reticular activating system or as a result of interdependence of central neurotransmitters.[23] Remarkably few serious adverse effects were reported.[31] However, asystole followed the administration of physostigmine in two patients with tricyclic antidepressant overdose.[24] This led to the realization that toxicity from tricyclic antidepressants is complex and consists of more than just anticholinergic effects.[24] Sodium channel blockade causes myocardial depression, QRS and QT interval prolongation, and ventricular dysrhythmias. Physostigmine probably augments vagal effects, thus contributing to a decreased cardiac output and cardiac conduction defects. A reevaluation must conclude that the risks of physostigmine for agents that are not primarily antimuscarinic often outweigh the benefits. Anticholinergic agents fall into the categories of antimuscarinic (atropine, scopolamine, propantheline benztropine, trihexyphenidyl), neuromuscular blockers (eg, curare), and ganglionic blockers (eg, trimethaphan). Other agents have anticholinergic properties that are subordinate to their primary therapeutic action and often considered a side effect (eg, older antihistamines like diphenhydramine, psychotropics like chlorpromazine, tricylic antidepressants like amitriptyline). Physostigmine toxicity, as noted above, causes acetylcholine excess at muscarinic, nicotinic, and CNS sites. This results when physostigmine is given in overdose, when it is used in the absence of an antimuscarinic agent, or when an excess is administered in relation to the antimuscarinic agent. Patients overdosed with physostigmine should be managed with intensive supportive care including mechanical ventilation if needed, intravenous atropine[33] titrated to reverse bronchial secretions, and rarely pralidoxime to reverse the skeletal muscle findings.[6]

Indications for the use of physostigmine include peripheral and central anticholinergic manifestations. Peripheral manifestations include dry mucosa, dry skin, flushed face, mydriasis, hyperthermia, decreased bowel sounds, urinary retention, and tachycardia. Central manifestations include agitation, delirium, hallucinations, seizures, and coma.[10,19] The peripheral and central findings usually occur together. It is uncommon to have just the central findings, although they are often more remarkable.[2,5,8,9,14,27] The central findings may persist longer than the peripheral findings, particularly when a patient is recovering from an antimuscarinic overdose.

The relative contraindications to physostigmine include bronchospastic disease, peripheral vascular disease, intestinal or bladder obstruction, intraventricular conduction defects, and AV block. Little information is available regarding the effects of physostigmine in pregnancy. Transient muscular weakness occurred in 10–20% of neonates whose mothers received anticholinesterases for the treatment of their myasthenia gravis.[1] Drug interactions with cholinergic agonists (eg, pilocarpine), depolarizing neuromuscular blockers, or other anticholinesterase agents (carbamates, organophosphates, pyridostigmine) would be expected to be at least additive. The actions of drugs metabolized by plasma cholinesterase to inactive metabolites (eg, cocaine, succinylcholine, mivacurium) are prolonged.

The dose of physostigmine is 1–2 mg in adults and 0.02 mg/kg (max 0.5 mg) in children intravenously infused over at least 5 minutes. Rapid administration may cause bradycardia, hypersalivation leading to respiratory difficulty, and possible seizures. Additional doses may be required depending on the ingested dose of the antimuscarinic agent, although 4 mg is usually sufficient.[10] The onset of action is usually within minutes.[14] Although the half-life of physostigmine is about 16 minutes, its duration of action is usually much longer (about 5 times) and directly related to the duration of cholinesterase inhibition.[3] However, significant interindividual variability exists.

Physostigmine is available as Antilirium in 2-mL ampules with each milliliter containing 1 mg of physostigmine salicylate. The vehicle contains sodium bisulfite and benzyl alcohol.

References

1. American Hospital Formulary Service (AHFS) 1997. McEvoy CK, ed. American Society of Health-System Pharmacists, Inc, pp. 902–904.
2. Aquilonius S, Hartvig P: Clinical pharmacokinetics of cholinesterase inhibitors. Clin Pharmacokinet 1986;11: 236–249.
3. Asthana S, Greig NH, Hegedus L, et al: Clinical pharmacokinetics of physostigmine in patients with Alzheimer's disease. Clin Pharmacol Ther 1995;58:299–309.
4. Atack JR, Yu Q-S, Soncrant TT, et al: Comparative inhibitory effects of various physostigmine analogs against acetyl and butyrlcholinesterases. J Pharmacol Exp Ther 1989;249:194–202.
5. Crowell EB, Ketchum JS: The treatment of scopolamine—induced delirium with physostigmine. Clin Pharmacol Ther 1967;8:409–414.
6. Cumming G, Harding LK, Prowse K: Treatment and recovery after massive overdose of physostigmine. Lancet 1968;20:147–149.
7. Daunderer M: Physostigmine salicylate as an antidote. Int J Clin Pharmacol Ther Toxicol 1980;18:523–535.
8. Duvoisin R, Katz R: Reversal of central anticholinergic syndrome in man by physostigmine. JAMA 1968;206: 1963–1965.

9. El-Yousef MK, Janowsky D, Davis JM, Sekerke HJ: Reversal of antiparkinsonian drug toxicity by physostigmine: A controlled study. Am J Psychiatry 1973;130:141–145.
10. Forrer GR, Miller JJ: Atropine coma—a somatic therapy in psychiatry. Am J Psychiatry 1958;115:455–458.
11. Fraser TR: On the characters, action and therapeutic uses of the bean of Calabar. Edinburgh Med J 1863;9:36–56; 235–245.
12. Giannini AJ, Castellani S: A case of phenylcyclohexylpyrolidine (PHP) intoxication treated with physostigmine. J Toxicol Clin Toxicol 1982;19:505–508.
13. Holmstedt BO: The ordeal bean of old Calabar: The pageant of *Physostigmine venenosum* in medicine. In: Swain T, ed: Plants in the development of modern medicine. Cambridge, MA, Harvard University Press, 1975, pp. 303–360.
14. Holzgrate RE, Vondrell JJ, Mintz SM: Reversal of postoperative reactions to scopolamine with physostigmine. Anesth Analg 1973;52:921–925.
15. Karczmar AG: History of the research with anticholinesterase agents. In: Karczmar AG, ed: International Encyclopedia of Pharmacology and Therapeutics, Vol. I. Oxford, Pergamon Press, 1970, pp. 1–44.
16. Karczmar AG: Pharmacology of anticholinesterase agents. In: Karczmar AG, ed: International Encyclopedia of Pharmacology and Therapeutics, Vol. I. Oxford, Pergamon Press, 1970, pp. 45, 363.
17. Knapp S, Wardlow ML, Albert K, et al: Correlation between plasma physostigmine concentrations and percentage of acetylcholinesterase inhibition over time after controlled release of physostigmine in volunteer subjects. Drug Metab Dispos 1991;19:400–404.
18. Larson GF, Hurbert BJ, Wingard DW: Physostigmine reversal of diazepam-induced depression. Anesth Analg 1977;56: 348–351.
19. Longo VG: Behavioral and electroencephalographic effects of atropine and related compounds. Pharmacol Rev 1966; 18:965–996.
20. Manoguerra AS: Poisoning with tricyclic antidepressant drugs. Clin Toxicol 1977;10:149–158.
21. Nattel S, Bayne L, Ruedy J: Physostigmine in coma due to drug overdose. Clin Pharmacol Ther 1979;25:96–102.
22. Nickalls RWD, Nickalls EA: The first use of physostigmine in the treatment of atropine poisoning. Anesthesiology 1988;43:776–779.
23. Nilsson E: Physostigmine treatment in various drug-induced intoxications. Ann Clin Res 1982;14:165–172.
24. Pentel P, Peterson CD: Asystole complicating physostigmine treatment of tricyclic antidepressant overdose. Ann Emerg Med 1980;9:588–590.
25. Rumack BH: 707 cases of anticholinergic poisoning treated with physostigmine. Presented at annual meeting of American Academy of Clinical Toxicology, Montreal, Quebec, Canada, 1975. Abstract.
26. Rupreht J, Dworacek B, Oosthoek H, et al: Physostigmine versus naloxone in heroin overdose. J Toxicol Clin Toxicol 1983–84;21:387–397.
27. Smiler BG, Bartholomew EG, Sivak BJ, et al: Physostigmine reversal of scopolamine delirium in obstetric patients. Am J Obstet 1973;116:326–329.
28. Smilkstein MJ: Physostigmine. J Emerg Med 1991;9:275–277. Editorial.
29. Somani SM, Dube SN: Physostigmine—an overview as pretreatment drug for organophosphate intoxication. Int J Clin Pharmacol Ther Toxicol 1989;27:367–387.
30. Taylor P: Anticholinesterase agents. In: Hardman JG, Limbird CE, Molinoff PB, Ruddon RW, eds: Goodman and Gilman's The Pharmacologic Basis of Therapeutics, 9th ed. New York, McGraw-Hill, 1996, pp. 161–176.
31. Walker WE, Levy RC, Hanenson IB: Physostigmine—its use and abuse. JACEP 1976;5:436–439.
32. Weinstock M, Davidson JT, Rosin AJ, et al: Effect of physostigmine on morphine-induced postoperative pain and somnolence. Br J Anesth 1982;54:429–443.
33. Weiss S: Persistence of action of physostigmine and the atropine-physostigmine antagonism in animals and in man. J Pharmacol Exp Ther 1925;27:181–188.
34. Young SE, Ruiz RS, Falletta J: Reversal of systemic toxic effects of scopolamine with physostigmine salicylate. Am J Ophthalmol 1971;72:1136–1138.

CHAPTER 35

Iron

Jeanmarie Perrone

Iron		
MW	=	55.85 daltons
Serum normal	=	80–180 μg/dL
	=	14–32 μmol/L
Action level	>	500 μg/dL
	>	90 μmol/L

Values greater than or equal to the action level necessitate clinical intervention. Values less than this level may necessitate intervention based on the clinical appearance of the patient.

An 18-month-old toddler was found playing with a nearly empty bottle of iron tablets at 11 A.M. He was noted to vomit several times by his mother, who then put him to bed for a nap. At 3 P.M. when he still had not awakened, she became concerned and brought him to the emergency department. He arrived at 5 P.M. with the following vital signs: blood pressure, 130/85 mm Hg; heart rate, 140 beats/min; respiratory rate, 25 breaths/min; and temperature, 99°F (37.2°C). He was markedly lethargic but responded appropriately when intravenous access was obtained. Physical examination was significant for warm, dry pink skin with slightly dry mucous membranes, soft abdomen without tenderness, and guaiac negative stool. An arterial blood gas was obtained and blood samples for CBC, electrolytes, BUN, creatinine, and iron level were sent. A rapid serum glucose was 180 mg/dL. A fluid bolus of 20 mL/kg normal saline was administered.

An abdominal radiograph was obtained and revealed multiple radiopaque pill fragments. Whole-bowel irrigation was initiated at 300 mL/h with polyethylene glycol–electrolyte lavage solution via nasogastric tube.

Laboratory results are reported as: ABG on supplemental oxygen: pH 7.30; PCO_2 30 mmHg; PO_2 287 mm Hg; WBC 28,000/mm^3; Hgb,14.7 g/dL; Hct, 45%; platelet count, 409,000/mm^3. Chemistries revealed sodium, l30 mEq/L; potassium, 3.2 mEq/L; chloride, 98 mEq/L; bicarbonate, 15 mEq/L; BUN, 18 mg/dL; creatinine, 0. 2 mg/dL; and glucose, 302 mg/dL. The anion gap was 17. His serum iron level was 755 μg/dL. A baseline urine sample was obtained. This patient was started on an intravenous deferoxamine infusion beginning at a dose of 5 mg/kg/h. Initially, no urine color change was noted. However, as the patient tolerated increasing the rate of infusion up to 15 mg/kg/h, a subsequent urine color change was reported. The patient was continued on a dose of deferoxamine 15 mg/kg/h for 12 hours. At the time of cessation of therapy, the patient was alert, active, and taking oral liquids and had resolution of his anion gap acidosis.

What Is in Iron Tablets? What Is the Toxic Dose?

Iron supplements are available as iron salts commonly consisting of 325 mg of ferrous gluconate, ferrous sulfate, or ferrous fumarate or can be found in significant quantities in vitamin preparations, especially prenatal vitamins (see Table 35–1). The quantity of elemental iron in each of these formulations varies between 12% and 33% and is the primary determinant of toxicity (eg, see Fig. 35–1). Chewable pediatric multivitamins with iron contain less

TABLE 35–1. ELEMENTAL IRON EQUIVALENTS

	Percentage of Elemental Fe
Ferrous sulfate[a]	20[b]
Ferrous gluconate[a]	12
Ferrous fumarate[a]	33
Ferrous lactate	19
Ferrous chloride	28
Ferrous ferrocholinate	13

[a]Most common
[b]325 mg = 65 mg Fe

iron by comparison (10–18 mg elemental iron/tablet) but toxicity may occur when large quantities are ingested.

Toxic effects occur at doses between 10 and 20 mg/kg elemental iron. A study in human volunteers demonstrated adverse symptoms and elevated iron levels at doses of 10 mg/kg.[42] In another study of human volunteers ingesting 20 mg/kg elemental iron, all developed nausea and voluminous diarrhea within 2 hours as well as serum iron levels above 300 μg/dL in five of six subjects.[10] Previously, recommendations for the hospital referral of ingestions in toddlers ranged from potential exposures > 20 mg/kg up to 60 mg/kg.[5,38] This discrepancy derives from retrospective review of toddlers "exposed" to those doses and who subsequently do not develop toxicity.

Why Is Iron Toxic?

Much of the pathophysiology in iron poisoning is related to the etiologies of metabolic acidosis. Iron toxicity is mediated via both local and systemic effects. Initial toxicity including vomiting, abdominal pain, and diarrhea is the result of direct corrosive effects on the gastric and intestinal mucosa. This may induce intestinal ulceration, edema, and occasionally hematemesis, melena, or hematochezia.[71] Early hypovolemia resulting from GI losses contributes to tissue hypoperfusion and metabolic acidosis.

Absorption of iron also contributes to metabolic acidosis. Following absorption, ferrous iron is converted to ferric iron and an unbuffered hydrogen ion is liberated.[60] Iron concentrated intracellularly in mitochondria disrupts oxidative phosphorylation and results in free radical formation and lipid peroxidation.[60,62] This exacerbates metabolic acidosis and contributes to cell death and tissue injury at the organ level.

10 pills × 325 mg (20% elemental iron/pill)

10 × 65 mg elemental iron/pill

650 mg/10 kg = 65 mg/kg

Figure 35–1. A 10-kg toddler is found playing with 325-mg ferrous sulfate tablets. Ferrous sulfate contains 20% elemental iron. If 10 pills are missing, the potential ingestion consists of 65 mg/kg, a toxic exposure.

Reports of early coagulopathy not related to hepatotoxicity prompted investigations into the effect of iron on clotting.[69] Free iron was shown to inhibit the formation of thrombin and thrombin's effect on fibrinogen in vitro.[63]

Multiple cardiovascular effects can be demonstrated in animals, including decreased cardiac output contributing to shock.[75,80] Although the decreased cardiac output was initially proposed to result from decreased venous filling pressures and decreased preload, a relative bradycardia[75] and a negative inotropic effect of absorbed iron on the myocardium can be demonstrated in animal models.[2]

Early autopsy reports from patients with fatal iron ingestions revealed a hemorrhagic periportal necrosis of the liver.[45] This hepatic injury was experimentally reproduced in rabbits given lethal doses of iron.[45]

How Should a Patient With a Life-Threatening Ingestion of Iron Be Approached?

Iron supplements were previously the leading cause of fatal ingestions in children;[77] fortunately, the incidence of fatal exposures appears to be declining.[44] The FDA recently announced that all packages of iron-containing preparations must have a warning label regarding potential toxicity of accidental overdose in children.[21] A toddler who presents to the emergency department with evidence of gastrointestinal toxicity and lethargy has most certainly ingested a significant amount of iron. Initial stabilization of the patient should focus on an assessment of airway, breathing, and circulation. When a child is lethargic but arousable, the presence of a tachycardia is likely due to relative volume loss, although perfusion may appear adequate.

How Can the Absorption of This Ingested Iron Be Decreased?

Following stabilization including the "ABCs" of basic life support, gastrointestinal decontamination procedures should be considered. Gastric emptying may have added value following ingestion of substances such as iron, which are not bound to activated charcoal. However, little benefit is expected from administration of syrup of ipecac in a child who has already vomited spontaneously several times. Likewise, orogastric lavage may not be effective if the iron tablets are large or if several hours have elapsed since ingestion. The location of the pills on the abdominal radiograph (if radiopaque) may guide the use of lavage. If many pills remain in the stomach, lavage may be able to remove some of them. However, if the pills are further along in the gastrointestinal tract, lavage will be of little benefit and whole-bowel irrigation may be indicated (see Fig. 35–2).

Perhaps because of the lack of efficacy of activated charcoal, many different substances have been investi-

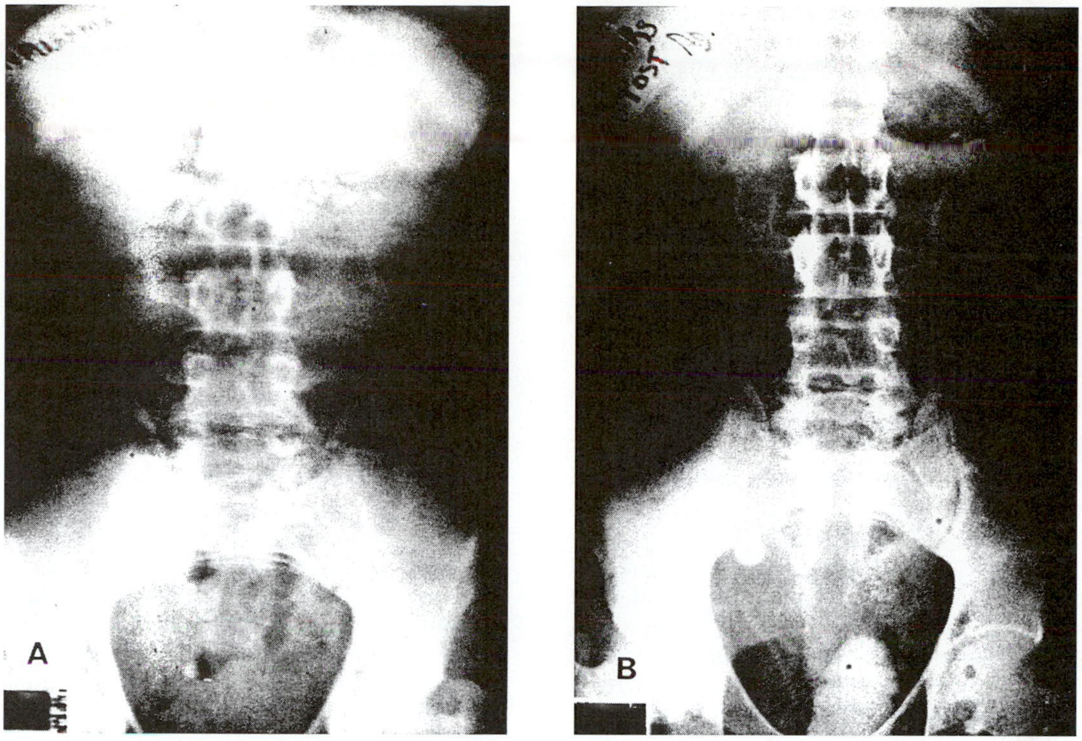

Figure 35–2. (A) Admission abdominal radiograph from a patient who ingested numerous iron tablets shows well-defined radiopaque tablets in the stomach. **(B)** Radiograph taken 5 hours after the patient was admitted and made to vomit shows a large number of pills remaining in the stomach and small bowel. *(Courtesy of Elmhurst City Hospital Emergency Staff).*

gated as lavage solutions. A review of these previous studies on various irrigants is helpful in understanding our current approach. Early studies in the 1960s investigated the usefulness of the iron chelator deferoxamine in the lavage solution in an attempt to chelate iron before it was absorbed. In a canine model of iron poisoning, toxicity secondary to high levels of ferrioxamine was attributed to increased absorption of the iron–deferoxamine complex.[81,82] Thus, while iron was successfully chelated by deferoxamine, forming ferrioxamine, there was an increase in toxicity secondary to increased ferrioxamine absorption.

The previous practice of orogastric lavage with sodium bicarbonate or phosphosoda was based on the belief that these solutions decreased the solubility of iron and prevented its absorption. In an in vitro model, a minimal reduction in iron solubility was demonstrated with the use of sodium bicarbonate.[15] In a rat model of iron poisoning, neither lavage with sodium bicarbonate nor lavage with sodium dihydrogen phosphate had any effect on subsequent serum iron levels compared to control animals lavaged with water.[16] Hyperphosphatemia and other electrolyte imbalances are reported following the use of phosphate lavage.[3,25] Magnesium hydroxide was effective in decreasing serum iron levels in a dog model; however, elevated magnesium levels were also noted.[13] In summary, many solutions have been used for gastric lavage. Despite limited efficacy of some, their potential risks mandate the use of only normal saline or tap water for orogastric lavage.

Whole-bowel irrigation (WBI) has demonstrated efficacy in certain ingestions; its utility in patients with iron poisoning is supported primarily by case reports and one uncontrolled case series.[18,68,73] A recent case report described the safety of using large volumes (44 L) of WBI over 5 days in a child with persistent iron tablets on abdominal radiographs.[35] The usual dose of whole-bowel irrigation is 250–500 mL/h in children and 2 L/h in adults. This rate is best achieved by starting more slowly and increasing as tolerated, often using a nasogastric tube due to the large volumes that must be taken orally. Antiemetics such as metoclopramide can be used to treat nausea and vomiting. Several case reports describe gastrotomy and surgical removal of large numbers of iron tablets adherent to the gastric mucosa and not removable by lavage or syrup of ipecac.[22,55,74] This may no longer be necessary with the increased use of whole-bowel irrigation.

How Reliable Is the Abdominal Radiograph in Iron Ingestions?

Since iron is available in many forms, it must be remembered that iron preparations vary in their radiopacity on abdominal radiography.[65] Factors such as time since ingestion and elemental iron content also play a role.[50,65] Liquid iron formulations and chewable iron tablets are often not radiopaque and yet, due to their pleasant taste, may be ingested by children in significant quantities.[19] In one retrospective review of pediatric iron ingestions, only one of 30 patients ingesting chewable vitamins had a positive abdominal radiograph for iron.[19] In contrast, adult preparations with higher elemental iron content tend to be more persistently radiopaque.[50] Although finding radiopaque pills on an abdominal flat plate may be helpful in guiding and following gastrointestinal decontamination,[31] their absence is not a reliable indicator of the lack of toxic potential.[50,54]

What Is the Expected Clinical Course of the Iron-Poisoned Patient?

Five clinical stages of iron toxicity have been described and correspond to the pathophysiology of iron poisoning.[5,34,58] The first stage of iron toxicity is characterized by the symptoms of nausea, vomiting, abdominal pain, and diarrhea. Iron is corrosive to the gastrointestinal tract and causes gastric mucosal hemorrhage, ulcerations, transmural inflammation, and even necrosis of the bowel wall and small bowel infarction in some extreme cases.[22,61,77] Gastrointestinal symptoms are present in cases of significant overdose. Their absence in the first 6 hours following ingestion essentially excludes serious toxicity. Dehydration may result from volume loss and contributes to the toxic appearance of the iron-poisoned patient. Occasionally, corrosive gastric effects progress to hematemesis, melena, or hematochezia and exacerbate hemodynamic instability. Patients with large ingestions may progress directly from gastrointestinal symptoms (stage 1) to signs of systemic toxicity (stage 3).

The "latent" or "second stage" of iron poisoning refers to the 6–24-hour period following the resolution of gastrointestinal symptoms and before overt systemic toxicity has developed. Controversy exists over whether this is a true quiescent phase or if it represents the failure to recognize ongoing toxicity.[5] While patients who have remained asymptomatic since their ingestion are clearly not in this quiescent stage, clinicians should be cautious in interpreting the absence of ongoing gastrointestinal symptoms in patients who present late. During this time, the hypovolemia and poor tissue perfusion resulting from the gastrointestinal symptoms may result in worsening metabolic acidosis if volume resuscitation has not been adequate. Conversely, many patients with lesser ingestions will have resolution of their toxicity and recover from this point. In summary, patients who appear well with stable vital signs, normal mental status, and toleration of fluids will continue to improve during this period.

Profound toxicity is evident in patients with severe ingestions who progress to the third stage of iron poisoning. Shock results from hypovolemia, vasodilation and poor cardiac output.[75,80] Subsequent poor perfusion and tissue ischemia worsen the metabolic acidosis. Iron may also directly inhibit oxidative metabolism at the cellular level and exaggerate tissue ischemia.[60] An iron induced coagulopathy may worsen bleeding and hypovolemia.[69] Systemic toxicity manifests as lethargy, hyperventilation, seizures, or coma.

A fourth stage consists of hepatic failure, which may occur 2–3 days following severe iron poisoning.[28] It is thought to result from direct uptake of iron by the reticuloendothelial system in the liver.[24,83]

The fifth stage of iron toxicity only rarely occurs. Gastric outlet obstruction secondary to strictures and scarring from the initial corrosive injury can develop 2–8 weeks following ingestion.[27,30,71]

Are Laboratory Measurements Helpful in the Assessment of the Iron-Poisoned Patient?

Many laboratory studies have been examined in the assessment of iron poisoning. Anion gap metabolic acidosis is a common finding in patients with serious iron ingestions. Serial electrolyte measurements can assess progression and response to volume replacement in iron poisoning. Anemia may result from gastrointestinal blood loss, but may not be evident initially due to hemoconcentration secondary to plasma volume loss.

Other tests, such as the WBC and glucose, have been extensively examined for their ability to predict serious iron toxicity. In a retrospective review of a small number of iron-poisoned children, a WBC > 15,000/mm^3 or a glucose > 150 mg/dL were 100% predictive of an iron level > 300 μg/dL.[41] However, WBC < 15,000/mm^3 and glucose < 150 mg/dL were also associated with serum iron > 300 μg/dL in approximately half of the cases. Therefore, these findings in this small study were specific for iron poisoning, but had a limited sensitivity. Three subsequent studies reexamined this issue in a similar manner and were unable to validate the association of elevated WBC and glucose as predictors of elevated (> 300 μg/dL) serum iron levels.[12,39,54] In practice, an elevated WBC or glucose should raise concern about an elevated iron level; however, iron poisoning is a clinical diagnosis, and an assessment of the signs and symptoms of the patient is more reliable than specific laboratory parameters. It is especially important to understand that an elevated serum iron level frequently occurs in the absence of an elevated WBC or glucose.

Although iron poisoning is a clinical diagnosis, serum iron levels have been used to gauge toxicity and treatment.[5] In a study of iron poisoning in six human volunteers who ingested 20 mg/kg elemental iron, all demonstrated significant gastrointestinal toxicity, and four of six required IV fluid resuscitation and had peak serum iron levels in the range of 300 μg/dL between 2 and 4 hours after ingestion.[10] Serum iron levels between 300 and 500 μg/dL usually correlate with significant gastrointestinal toxicity and modest systemic toxicity. When serum levels are between 500 and 1000 μg/dL, pronounced systemic toxicity and shock occur with increased probability.[78] Levels above 1000 μg/dL are associated with significant morbidity.[78] Although elevated levels may reinforce the potential for serious toxicity, lower levels cannot be used to dismiss the possibility of serious toxicity. Any serum iron level may not represent a peak level or may be falsely lowered in the presence of deferoxamine, unless atomic absorption technique is used for measurement.[26,29] Peak levels are thought to occur between 2 and 6 hours after ingestion, depending on the iron preparation.[10,42] In a study of human volunteers ingesting 5–10 mg/kg elemental iron in the form of chewable vitamins, peak serum iron levels occurred between 4.2 and 4.5 hours in all subjects.[42]

Total iron-binding capacity (TIBC) is a measurement of the total amount of iron that can be bound by transferrin in a given volume of serum.[20] It was previously taught that iron toxicity did not occur if the serum iron level was less than the TIBC since there would not be enough circulating "free" iron to cause tissue damage. Further understanding has altered the interpretation of the importance of TIBC values. In patients with hemochromatosis and chronic iron overload, the TIBC remains higher than the serum iron level, yet myocardial and liver injury occur as a result of excess iron. Second, the in vitro measurement of TIBC is spuriously increased as a result of iron poisoning and thus has a tendency to rise above a concurrently measured serum iron level.[72] This occurs as an aberration of the method used to measure TIBC in the laboratory. This false elevation in measuring TIBC can be corrected by adding excess magnesium carbonate reagent during the laboratory process, but this is usually not done. The rise in TIBC above elevated serum iron levels was confirmed in all subjects in a human volunteer study of iron poisoning.[10] A final confounder exists when a patient is treated with deferoxamine, which also may falsely elevate the TIBC.[7] In summary, TIBC has little value in the assessment of the iron-poisoned patient and should not be determined.

How Does Iron Cause an Increased Anion-Gap Metabolic Acidosis?

Serious iron poisoning induces a significant anion-gap metabolic acidosis and should be considered in the differential diagnosis of increased anion-gap metabolic acidosis. The following four mechanisms contribute to the anion-gap acidosis. Absorption of iron and conversion from Fe^{2+} to Fe^{3+} leads to the liberation of an unbuffered proton. Free iron is a vasodilator and contributes to hypotension, poor tissue perfusion, and lactic acidosis. Iron has a negative inotropic effect on the heart, also contributing to hypotension. Iron disrupts oxidative phosphorylation, leading to anaerobic metabolism and lactic acidosis.

What Is Deferoxamine and When Should It Be Used?

Deferoxamine was first used in the 1960s as a specific iron chelator for acute iron overdose as well as for chronic iron toxicity resulting from such diseases as thalassemia major. Deferoxamine is derived from culture of *Streptomyces pilosus* and is very specific for iron with an affinity constant of 10^{31}. In the presence of ferric iron, deferoxamine forms the complex ferrioxamine, which is then excreted by the kidneys[36] and imparts a reddish brown discoloration to the urine (see Color Plate 21). Deferoxamine chelates free iron and iron being transported between transferrin and ferritin,[43,56] but not iron present in hemoglobin, hemosiderin, or ferritin directly.[36] In addition, it appears that deferoxamine cannot remove iron once it is bound to transferrin.[4] There is sufficient evidence to suggest that deferoxamine can access intracytoplasmic and mitochondrial free iron, and thereby limits intracellular toxicity from excess iron.[43] Deferoxamine may work in other ways in addition to binding excess iron, since 100 mg of deferoxamine chelates approximately 9.3 mg of ferric iron. Therapeutic dosing of deferoxamine does not account for a significant amount of chelated iron excretion in the urine.

Deferoxamine is a parenteral iron chelator, although it has also been unsuccessfully used enterally to bind iron in the stomach and as a lavage solution.[30,82] Deferoxamine via IV, IM, and subcutaneous infusion is used extensively in the management of chronic iron overload.[9,57] Intravenous infusions are advantageous in that they result in more constant deferoxamine levels and increased urinary excretion of iron.[57] In patients manifesting serious signs and symptoms of iron poisoning, deferoxamine should be initiated as an intravenous infusion, starting slowly and gradually increasing to a dose of 15 mg/kg/h. Hypotension is the rate-limiting factor in more rapid infusions and occurs commonly.[79,82] Intramuscular administration of deferoxamine, although once a popular method of performing the recommended "deferoxamine challenge" test, is rarely indicated today.

The deferoxamine challenge test consisted of a 1–2-g (90 mg/kg) IM dose of deferoxamine followed by collection of subsequent urine samples to await a "vin rosé" urine color change. This urine color change represented toxic free iron that was being excreted as the colored compound ferrioxamine. Following a "positive" deferoxamine challenge test, a patient would then be treated with either additional IM deferoxamine every 4 hours or an intravenous regimen as described above. Those patients without a urine color change were considered not to be significantly poisoned, and further deferoxamine was withheld. There are several problems with this approach. The use of a single dose of deferoxamine has been shown to be unreliable since cases have been reported with high serum iron levels and no detectable urine color change.[23] Second, intramuscular therapy leads the clinician to manage patients without adequate intravenous access and volume therapy. Overlooking this critical resuscitation measure in a seriously poisoned toddler or adult may lead to hemodynamic instability and potentially devastating outcomes. Patients who appear toxic and/or have serum iron levels above 500 μg/dL should be treated with deferoxamine intravenously. Patients with levels less than 500 μg/dL or who do not appear toxic should be treated supportively without the administration of parenteral deferoxamine (see algorithm, Fig. 35–3).

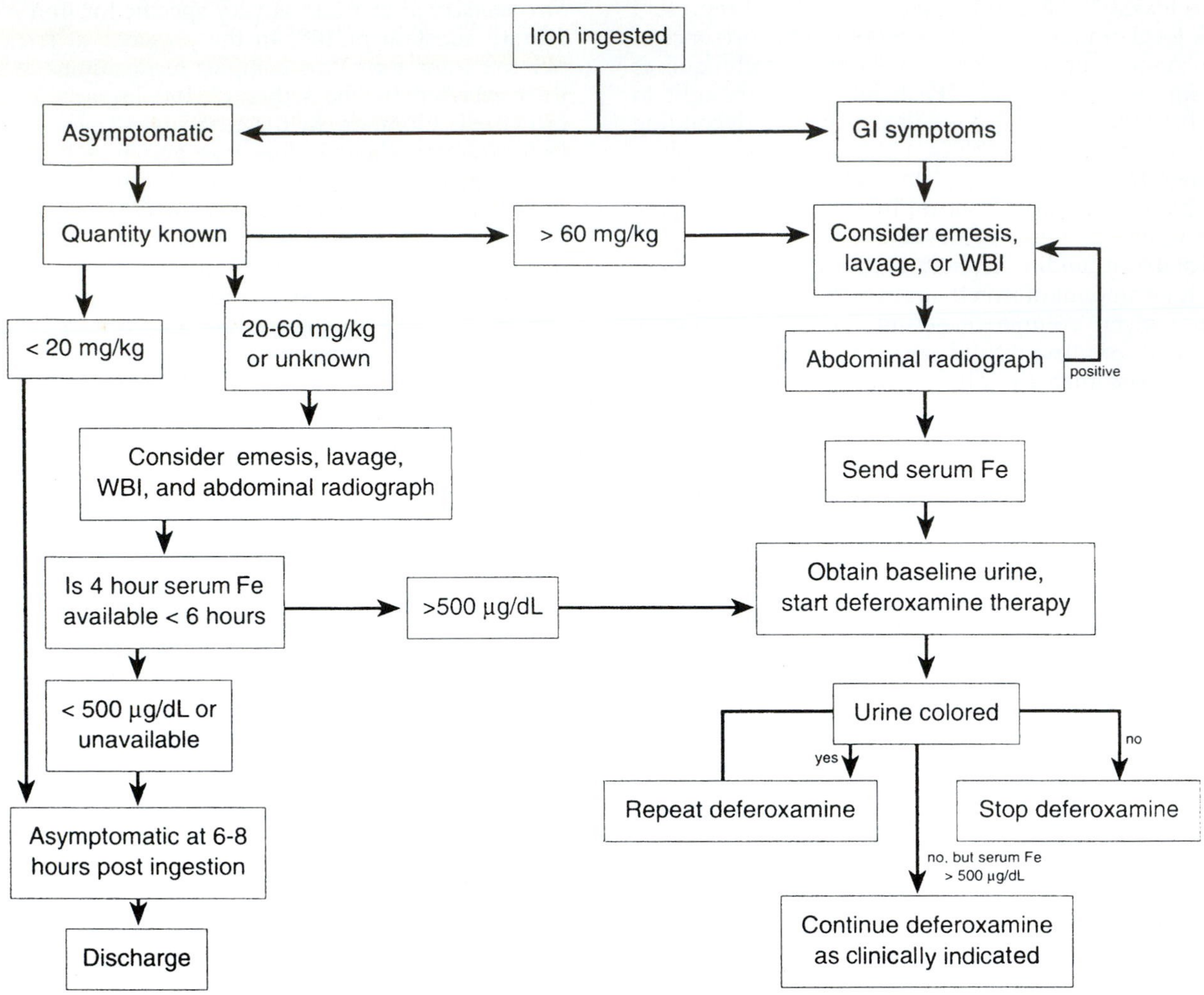

Figure 35–3. Algorithm for decision making following iron ingestion.

What Are the Possible Adverse Effects of Deferoxamine Treatment?

Various toxic effects of deferoxamine are reported in the setting of chronic administration for hemochromatosis,[53,64] however, pulmonary toxicity and ARDS were more recently described in four patients treated for acute iron overdose.[70] These four patients were treated with intravenous deferoxamine for 32–72 hours for serum iron levels ranging from 430 to 620 µg/dL. Although it is not clear whether pulmonary toxicity was the result of iron-induced cardiovascular compromise or deferoxamine effect directly, dose and duration of deferoxamine therapy likely contributed to toxicity. A subsequent animal study revealed significantly increased pulmonary toxicity when high-dose deferoxamine therapy was administered in the presence of high concentrations of oxygen (75–80% FIO_2).[1] The authors proposed that this effect was mediated via an oxygen free radical mechanism. A recent review favored higher doses of deferoxamine during the first 24 hours of serious iron poisoning prior to tissue distribution of iron and subsequently decreasing the dose or limiting the duration of deferoxamine therapy to 24 hours.[32]

When Should Deferoxamine Therapy Be Stopped?

Due to potential deferoxamine toxicity, clinicians have attempted to describe endpoints for deferoxamine therapy. A urine iron-to-creatinine ratio was used to determine whether free iron continued to be excreted in the urine during deferoxamine therapy.[84] This is an objective measure of the presence of ferrioxamine in the urine rather than the less reliable and subjective endpoint of urine color change.[17,38,76] This method, however, must be further studied clinically before it can be advocated. Most authors agree that deferoxamine therapy should be discontinued when the patient appears clinically well, the anion-gap acidosis has resolved, and there is no further urine color change.[48] In patients with signs and symptoms of serious toxicity after 24 hours of intravenous deferoxamine, continuing therapy should be undertaken cautiously and perhaps at a lower dose.

What Other Therapies Are Available for Iron Poisoning?

Many patients with chronic iron overload are dependent on long-term chelation therapy. The use of a new orally active iron chelator 1,2-dimethyl-3-hydroxypyrid-4-one (deferiprone) may prove beneficial. In a small group of patients with thalassemia major, oral deferiprone was effective in decreasing and sustaining lower hepatic iron concentrations.[52] Deferiprone appears to be rapidly absorbed from the stomach, metabolized and excreted as a glucuronide and an iron complex in the urine.[40] Studies are underway to examine the efficacy of deferiprone in a murine model of acute iron poisoning.[33]

One other modality that is described experimentally in the treatment of iron intoxication is continuous arteriovenous hemofiltration (CAVH). In a study of five iron-poisoned dogs, increasing excretion of ferrioxamine in the ultrafiltrate was demonstrated when increasing doses of deferoxamine were infused into the arterial side of the system.[6] This technique has not been described in iron-poisoned patients.

What Special Considerations Are Needed in the Pregnant Patient With Iron Overdose?

The frequent diagnosis of iron deficiency anemia during pregnancy has lead to several reports of serious and even fatal iron ingestions in pregnant women.[8,37,51,59] Although maternal resuscitation is always the primary objective in caring for pregnant women, concerns regarding deferoxamine toxicity in the fetus have delayed appropriate therapy in some cases.[51,67] This theoretical consideration of fetal deferoxamine toxicity has not been supported in human[14] or animal studies.[46] An elaborate study in pregnant ewes near term demonstrated that iron poisoning did not produce elevated fetal serum iron levels, nor could deferoxamine be detected in fetal circulation following maternal administration. It is therefore presumed that fetal demise results from maternal iron toxicity and not from a direct iron toxicity to the fetus. This suggests that appropriate doses of deferoxamine should be used in the treatment of serious maternal iron poisoning.

What Other Complications Have Been Reported in the Setting of Acute Iron Overdose?

Patients with chronic iron overload are known to be at increased risk of *Yersinia enterocolitica* infection. Iron is a required growth factor for *Y. enterocolitica;* however, it lacks the siderophore to solubilize iron and facilitate intracellular entry. Deferoxamine is a siderophore, which thus fosters the growth of *Y. enterocolitica.* Patients with chronic iron overload or acute poisoning have developed *Yersinia* infection or sepsis as a complication of their clinical course.[11,47,49,66] Patients who develop abdominal pain, fever, and diarrhea following resolution of iron toxicity should be suspected of having *Yersinia* infection and should be cultured and treated with appropriate antibiotic therapy.

What Should the Disposition Be for Patients Exposed to Iron?

Fortunately, many patients who are exposed to iron do not develop significant toxic effects. If a toddler remains asymptomatic and develops minimal or no gastrointestinal manifestations and appears well after an observation period of 6 hours in the emergency department, discharge can be considered to an appropriate home situation. Patients who develop gastrointestinal symptoms and signs of mild poisoning (dehydration, minimal anion-gap acidosis) can be observed in a non-ICU hospital setting. Patients who manifest signs and symptoms of significant iron poisoning such as metabolic acidosis, potential hemodynamic instability, and/or lethargy should be treated in an intensive care unit.

References

1. Adamson IY, Sienko A, Tenenbein M: Pulmonary toxicity of deferoxamine in iron poisoned mice. Toxicol Appl Pharmacol 1993;120:13–19.
2. Artman M, Olson RD, Boerth RC: Depression of myocardial contractility in acute iron toxicity in rabbits. Toxicol Appl Pharmacol 1982;66:329–337.
3. Bachrach L, Correa A, Levin R, Grossman M: Iron poisoning: Complications of hypertonic phosphate lavage therapy. J Pediatr 1979;94:147–149.
4. Balcerzak SP, Jensen WN, Pollack S: Mechanism of action of desferrioxamine on iron absorption. Scand J Haematol 1966; 3:205–212.
5. Banner W, Tong TG: Iron poisoning. Pediatr Clin North Am 1986,33:393–409.
6. Banner W, Vernon DD, Ward RM, et al: Continuous arteriovenous hemofiltration in experimental iron intoxication. Crit Care Med 1989;17:1187–1190.
7. Bentur Y, Klein J, Koren G: Misinterpretation of the iron-binding capacity in the presence of deferoxamine. J Pediatr 1991;118:139–142.
8. Blanc P, Hryhorczuk D, Danel L: Deferoxamine treatment of acute iron intoxication in pregnancy. Obstet Gynecol 1984;64:125–145.
9. Brittenham GM, Griffith PM, Nienhuis AW, et al: Efficacy of deferoxamine in preventing complications of iron overload in patients with thalassemia major. N Engl J Med 1994; 331:567–573.
10. Burkhart KK, Kulig KW, Hammond KB, et al: The rise in the total iron binding capacity after iron overdose. Ann Emerg Med 1991;20:532–535.

11. Chiesa C, Pacifico L, Renzulli F, et al: *Yersinia* hepatic abscesses and iron overload. JAMA 1987;257:3230–3231. Letter.
12. Chyka PA, Butler AY: Assessment of acute iron poisoning by laboratory and clinical observations. Am J Emerg Med 1993;11:99–102.
13. Corby DG, McCullen AH: Effect of orally administered magnesium hydroxide in experimental iron intoxication. J Toxicol Clin Toxicol 1985;23:489–499.
14. Curry SC, Bond GR, Raschke R, et al: An ovine model of maternal iron poisoning in pregnancy. Ann Emerg Med 1990;19:632–638.
15. Czajka PA, Konrad JD, Duffy JP: Iron poisoning: An in vitro comparison of bicarbonate and phosphate lavage solutions. J Pediatr 1981;98:491–494.
16. Dean BS, Krenzelok EP: In vivo effectiveness of oral complexation agents in the management of iron poisoning. J Toxicol Clin Toxicol 1987;25:221–230.
17. Eisen TF, Lacouture PG, Woolf A: Visual detection of ferrioxamine color changes in urine. Vet Hum Toxicol 1988;30: 369–370.
18. Everson GW, Bertaccini EJ, O'Leary JO: Use of whole bowel irrigation in an infant following iron overdose. Am J Emerg Med 1991;9:366–369.
19. Everson GW, Oudjhane K, Young LW, Krenzelok EP: Effectiveness of abdominal radiographs in visualizing chewable iron supplements following overdose. Am J Emerg Med 1989;7:459–463.
20. Finch CA, Huebers H: Perspectives in iron metabolism. N Engl J Med 1982;306:1520–1528.
21. Food and Drug Administration: Iron-containing supplements and drugs: Label warning statements and unit-dose packaging requirements. Fed Register 1997;62:2217.
22. Foxford R, Goldfrank L: Gastrotomy: A surgical approach to iron overdose. Ann Emerg Med 1985;14:1223–1226.
23. Freeman DA, Manoguerra AS: Absence of urinary color change in a severely iron poisoned child treated with deferoxamine. Vet Hum Toxicol 1981;23:351. Abstract.
24. Ganote CE, Nahara G: Acute ferrous sulfate hepatotoxicity in rats. Lab Invest 1973;28:426–436.
25. Geffner ME, Opas LM: Phosphate poisoning complicating treatment for iron ingestion. Am J Dis Child 1980;134: 509–510.
26. Gervitz NR, Wasserman LR: The measurement of iron and iron-binding capacity in plasma containing deferoxamine. J Pediatr 1966;68:802–804.
27. Ghandi R, Robarts F: Hourglass stricture of the stomach and pyloric stenosis due to ferrous sulfate poisoning. Br J Surg 1962:49:613–617.
28. Gleason WA, de Mello DE, de Castro FJ, et al: Acute hepatic failure in severe iron poisoning. J Pediatr 1979;95:138–140.
29. Helfer RE, Rodgerson DO: The effect of deferoxamine on the determination of serum iron and iron-binding capacity. J Pediatr 1966;68:804–806.
30. Henretig FM, Karl SR, Weintraub WH: Severe iron poisoning treated with enteral and intravenous deferoxamine. Ann Emerg Med 1983;12:306–309.
31. Hosking CS: Radiology in the management of acute iron poisoning. Med J Aust 1969;1:576–579.
32. Howland MA: Risks of parenteral deferoxamine for acute iron poisoning. J Toxicol Clin Toxicol 1996;34:491–497.
33. Hung O, Manoach S, Howland MA, et al: Deferiprone for acute iron poisoning. J Toxicol Clin Toxicol 1997;35:565.
34. Jacobs J, Greene H, Gendel BR: Acute iron intoxication. N Engl J Med 1965;273:1124–1127.
35. Kaczorowski JM, Wax PM: Five days of whole bowel irrigation in a case of pediatric iron ingestion. Ann Emerg Med 1996:27:258–263.
36. Keberie M: The biochemistry of desferrioxamine and its relation to iron metabolism. Ann NY Acad Sci 1964;119: 758–768.
37. Khoury S, Odeh M, Oettinger M: Deferoxamine treatment for acute iron intoxication in pregnancy. Acta Obstet Gynecol Scand 1995:74:756–757.
38. Klein-Schwartz W, Oderda GM, Gorman RL, et al: Assessment of management guidelines: Acute iron ingestion. Clin Pediatr 1990;29:316–321.
39. Knasel AL, Collins-Barrow NM: Applicability of early indicators of iron toxicity. J Natl Med Assoc 1986;78:1037–1041.
40. Kontoghiorghes GJ, Goddard JG, Bartlett AN, Sheppard L: Pharmacokinetic studies in humans with the oral iron chelator 1,2-dimethyl-3-hydroxypyrid-4-one. Clin Pharmacol Ther 1990;48:255–261.
41. Lacouture PG, Wason S, Temple AR, et al: Emergency assessment of severity in iron overdose by clinical and laboratory methods. J Pediatr 1981;99:89–91.
42. Ling LJ, Hornfeldt CS, Winter JP: Absorption of iron after experimental overdose of chewable vitamins. Am J Emerg Med 1991;9:24–26.
43. Lipschitz D, Dugard J, Simon M, et al: The site of action of desferrioxamine. Br J Haematol 1971;20:395–404.
44. Litovitz TL, Felberg L, White S, Klein-Schwartz W: 1995 Annual Report of the American Association of Poison Control Centers Toxic Exposure Surveillance System. Am J Emerg Med 1996;14:487–537.
45. Luongo MA, Bjornson SS: The liver in ferrous sulfate poisoning: A report of three fatal cases in children and an experimental study. N Engl J Med 1954;251:996–999.
46. McElhatton PR, Roberts JC, Sullivan FM: The consequences of iron overdose and its treatment with desferrioxamine in pregnancy. Hum Exp Toxicol 1991;10:251–259.
47. Melby K, Slordahl S, Gutterberg T, et al: Septicemia due to *Yersinia enterocolitica* after oral overdoses of iron. Br Med J 1982;285:467–468.
48. Mills KC, Curry SC: Acute iron poisoning. Emerg Med Clin North Am 1994;12:397–413.
49. Mofenson HC, Caraccio TR, Sharieff N: Iron sepsis: *Yersinia enterocolitica* septicemia possibly caused by an overdose of iron. N Engl J Med 1987;316:1092–1093.
50. Ng RCW, Perry K, Martin DJ: Iron poisoning: Assessment of radiography in diagnosis and management. Clin Pediatr 1979;18:614–616.
51. Olemnark M, Biber B, Dottori O, Rybo G: Fatal iron intoxication in late pregnancy. J Toxicol Clin Toxicol 1987;25: 347–359.
52. Olivieri NF, Brittenham GM, Matsui D, et al: Iron-chelation therapy with oral deferiprone in patients with thalassemia major. N Engl J Med 1995;332:918–922.
53. Olivieri NF, Buncic JR, Chew E, et al: Visual and auditory neurotoxicity in patients receiving subcutaneous deferoxamine infusions. N Engl J Med 1986;314:869–873.

54. Palatnick W, Tenenbein M: Leukocytosis, hyperglycemia, vomiting, and positive x-rays are not indicators of severity of iron overdose in adults. Am J Emerg Med 1996;14: 454–455.
55. Peterson CD, Fifield GC: Emergency gastrotomy for acute iron poisoning. Ann Emerg Med 1980:9:262–264.
56. Propper R, Nathan D: Clinical removal of iron. Annu Rev Med 1982, 33:509–519.
57. Propper R, Shurn S, Nathan D: Reassessment of the use of desferrioxamine B in iron overload. N Engl J Med 1976;294: 1421–1423.
58. Proudfoot AT, Simpson D, Dyson EH: Management of acute iron poisoning. Med Toxicol 1986;1:83–100.
59. Rayburn WF, Donn SM, Wolf ME: Iron overdose during pregnancy: Successful therapy with deferoxamine. Am J Obstet Gynecol 1983;147:717–718.
60. Reissman KR, Coleman TJ: Acute intestinal iron intoxication. II: Metabolic, respiratory and circulatory effects of absorbed iron salts. Blood 1955;10:46–51.
61. Roberts RJ, Nayfield S, Soper R, et al: Acute iron intoxication with intestinal infarction managed in part by small bowel resection. Clin Toxicol 1975;8:3–12.
62. Robotham JL, Troxler RF, Lietman PS: Iron poisoning: Another energy crisis. Lancet 1974;2:664–665.
63. Rosenmund A, Haeberli A, Struab PW: Blood coagulation and acute iron toxicity. J Lab Clin Med 1984;103:524–533.
64. Scanderbeg AC, Izzi GC, Butturini A, Benaglia G: Pulmonary syndrome and intravenous high-dose desferrioxamine. Lancet 1990;336:1511. Letter.
65. Staple TW, McAlister WH: Roentgenographic visualization of iron preparations in the gastrointestinal tract. Radiology 1964;83:1051–1056.
66. Stein ZL, Barkin RL: *Yersinia* and iron intoxication. Drug Intell Clin Pharmacy 1987;21:661. Letter.
67. Strom RL, Schiller P, Seeds AE, ten Bensel R: Fatal iron poisoning in a pregnant female. Minn Med 1976;99:483–489.
68. Tenenbein M: Whole bowel irrigation in iron poisoning. J Pediatr 1987;111:142–145.
69. Tenenbein M, Israels SJ: Early coagulopathy in severe iron poisoning. J Pediatr 1988;113:695–697.
70. Tenenbein M, Kowalski S, Bowden DH, Adamson IYR: Pulmonary toxic effects of continuous desferrioxamine administration in acute iron poisoning. Lancet 1992;339: 699–701.
71. Tenenbein M, Littman C, Stimpson RE: Gastrointestinal pathology in adult iron overdose. J Toxicol Clin Toxicol 1990;28:311–320.
72. Tenenbein M, Yatscoff RW: The total iron-binding capacity in iron poisoning. Is it useful? Am J Dis Child 1991;45: 437–439.
73. Turk J, Aks S, Ampuero F, Hryhorczuk DO: Successful therapy of iron intoxication in pregnancy with intravenous deferoxamine and whole bowel irrigation. Vet Hum Toxicol 1993;35:441–444.
74. Venturelli J, Kwee Y, Morris N, et al: Gastrotomy in the management of acute iron poisoning. J Pediatr 1982;100: 768–769.
75. Vernon DD, Banner W Jr, Dean JM: Hemodynamic effects of experimental iron poisoning. Ann Emerg Med 1989;18: 863–866.
76. Villalobos D: Reliability of urine color changes after deferoxamine challenge. Vet Hum Toxicol 1992;34:330. Abstract.
77. Weiss B, Alkon E, Weindlar F, et al: Toddler deaths resulting from ingestion of iron supplements—Los Angeles, 1992–1993. MMWR 1993;42:111–113.
78. Westlin WF: Deferoxamine as a chelating agent. Clin Toxicol 1971;4:597–602.
79. Westlin W: Deferoxamine in the treatment of acute iron poisoning: Clinical experiences with 172 children. Clin Pediatr 1966;5:531–535.
80. Whitten CF, Chen YC, Gibson GW: Studies in acute iron poisoning. III. The hemodynamic alterations in acute experimental iron poisoning. Pediatr Res 1968:2:479–485.
81. Whitten CF, Chen YC, Gibson GW: Studies in acute iron poisoning: II. Further observations on desferrioxamine in the treatment of acute experimental iron poisoning. Pediatrics 1966;38:102–110.
82. Whitten CF, Gibson GW, Good MH, et al: Studies in acute iron poisoning. I. Desferrioxamine in the treatment of acute iron poisoning: Clinical observations, experimental studies, and theoretical considerations. Pediatrics 1965;36:322–335.
83. Witzleben CL, Chaffey NJ: Acute ferrous sulphate poisoning: A histochemical study of its effect on the liver. Arch Pathol Lab Med 1966;82:454–460.
84. Yatscoff RW, Wayne EA, Tenenbein M: An objective criterion for the cessation of deferoxamine therapy in the acutely iron poisoned patient. J Toxicol Clin Toxicol 1991; 29:1–10.

ANTIDOTES IN DEPTH

Deferoxamine

Mary Ann Howland

Deferoxamine is the parenteral chelator of choice for iron poisoning. Iron toxicity was recognized as early as the 1800's, forgotten, and subsequently rediscovered.[22] The history of deferoxamine can be traced back to the analysis of the metabolites of actinomycetes. Keberle isolated ferrioxamine B from the organism *Streptomyces pilosus*.[25] It is a brownish red compound containing trivalent iron and three molecules of trihydroxamic acid. Deferoxamine (desferrioxamine B) is the colorless compound that results when the trivalent iron is chemically removed from ferrioxamine B (Fig. 35–4 and 35–5).[25] Deferoxamine (DFO) is a water-soluble compound with a molecular weight of 597 D. The commercial formulation is the mesylate salt with a molecular weight of 693 D. One mole of DFO binds 1 mole of Fe^{3+}; therefore, 100 mg of DFO can bind 9.35 mg of Fe^{3+}. Shortly after DFO was first isolated, it was used as a chelator in patients with iron toxicity. It was shown to have a far greater affinity constant for iron (10^{31}) than for zinc, copper, nickel, magnesium, or calcium (10^{2}–10^{14}).[25] Therefore, at physiologic pH values, deferoxamine complexed almost exclusively with ferric iron.[19]

When DFO comes into contact with ferric ion, it binds the Fe^{3+} at the three N–OH sites, forming an octahedral iron complex (Fig. 35–5). Once bound, the resultant ferrioxamine is very stable, with an affinity constant for iron of $10^{30.7}$, as compared with 10^{29} for transferrin. Theoretically it should therefore be possible to chelate the iron from transferrin.[35] In fact, in vitro experiments demonstrate that DFO removes iron from transferrin and ferritin but can remove only very little from hemosiderin.[35] However, once iron is bound to transferrin in vivo, DFO is unable to remove it.[4] Deferoxamine can, however, chelate iron in transit between transferrin and ferritin in the plasma,[30,42] ultimately decreasing ferritin stores. Deferoxamine chelates and inactivates cytoplasmic and mitochondrial iron, preventing disruption of mitochondrial function and injury.[30] Deferoxamine appears to be of benefit to patients with iron poisoning by chelating free iron and iron in transit between transferrin and ferritin, while not directly affecting the iron of hemoglobin, hemosiderin, or ferritin.[25] Absorbed iron peaks in 2–5 hours and distributes from the blood compartment by 24 hours.[15,28] In vitro studies demonstrate that ferritin can donate iron to deferoxamine and chelation may lead subsequently to biliary excretion and fecal elimination.[34]

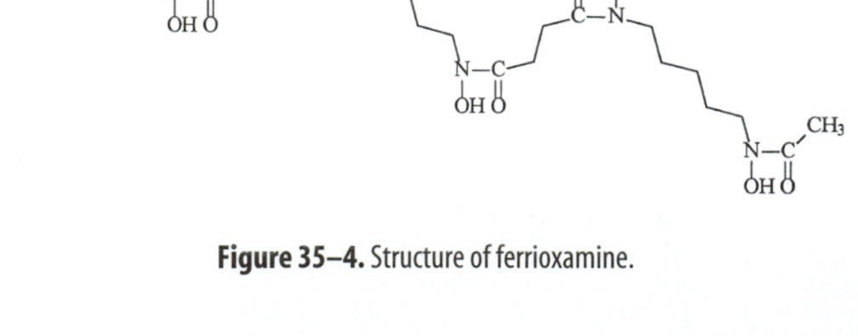

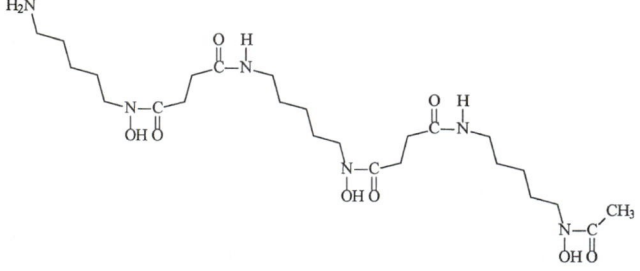

Figure 35–4. Structure of ferrioxamine.

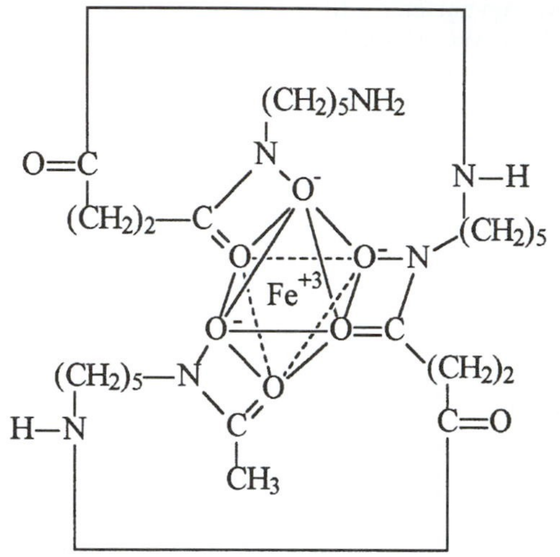

Figure 35–5. Structure of deferoxamine.

Experiments in dogs demonstrate that intravenous (IV) ferrioxamine is entirely eliminated by the kidney within 5 hours, whereas only 70% of the same IV dose of DFO appears in the urine after 72 hours.[25] Even though ferrioxamine is eliminated more quickly than DFO, as unchanged drug and metabolites, ferrioxamine is partially reabsorbed following glomerular filtration, whereas DFO undergoes glomerular filtration and tubular secretion.[34] The remaining DFO is probably metabolized in the plasma to a number of metabolites (A–F), of which metabolite B may be toxic.[25,27,40] In nephrectomized dogs, the volume of distribution of ferrioxamine was calculated to be 19% of body weight, versus about 50% of body weight for DFO,[25] implying that DFO has a wider tissue distribution. This different pharmacokinetic pattern might be explained by comparing the straight chain deferoxamine to the octahedral structure of ferrioxamine.

The initial distribution half-life of DFO is approximately 1 hour in the dog,[40] but is about 5–10 minutes in humans.[27,46] The pharmacokinetics of DFO and ferrioxamine differ in healthy versus iron-overloaded patients. The terminal elimination half-life of DFO is approximately 6 hours in healthy patients,[2] but about 3 hours in patients with thalassemia. Plasma concentrations of DFO in healthy patients are about twice the level noted in patients with thalassemia, while in these patients ferrioxamine concentrations are 5 times greater than those found in healthy patients.[25,46]

It has been suggested that DFO can be continued and hemodialysis performed to remove ferrioxamine in the presence of renal failure.[54] Although both hemodialysis[11,45] and hemoperfusion[11] are effective in ferrioxamine removal, it is unclear whether these interventions are indicated.

Studies in guinea pigs given LD_{50} and LD_{100} oral doses of ferrous sulfate showed dramatic improvement in survival rates after oral DFO was given in a dose calculated to bind most of the iron.[35] Mortality rates in this study and in a similar study in swine[14] were directly correlated with the delay to DFO administration.[35]

Based on experimental work in guinea pigs with acute iron poisoning and in patients with hemochromatosis, early authors suggested giving DFO orally in doses of 10–15 times the ingested amount of elemental iron while simultaneously administering parenteral DFO, either intramuscularly or intravenously, in a dose of 2.5 times the ingested iron dose to be delivered over 24 hours.[35] In more than 1000 injections (mostly in patients with hemochromatosis), DFO had no consequential adverse effects and only one possible allergic reaction was reported.[35]

In the 1960s twelve children who had unintentionally ingested iron were treated with intravenous DFO; nine of these patients also received oral DFO.[53] Significant hypotension was noted in two children when approximately 80–150 mg/kg of DFO was administered intravenously over 15 minutes. In another study, dogs receiving 3–30 mg/kg/min (180–1800 mg/kg/h) of DFO also developed hypotension.[54]

In a canine model, ferrous iron bound to DFO in equimolar quantities when the pH was greater than 6, which promoted the conversion of Fe^{2+} to Fe^{3+}.[53] Studies in four dogs given iron–DFO complex orally suggested that this complex was absorbed and lethal in all animals. Of nine dogs given oral and intravenous DFO, three survived. In a subsequent, similar study there was about a 50% survival rate in dogs given a lethal dose (225 mg/kg) of iron followed by oral DFO (2.6 g) and intravenous DFO (0.75–1.5 mg/kg/min for 8–12 hours). Oral ferrioxamine was absorbed, and two of the five dogs given a complexed lethal dose of iron died.[54] However, this study has limited any substantial interest in the use of oral DFO despite the more favorable results in guinea pigs[33] and mice noted above.[23,49]

In another study, 172 children who were not severely poisoned and were hemodynamically stable were treated with 5–10 g of oral DFO and either 1 or 2 g of DFO IM every 3–12 hours.[52] One gram administered intravenously at no more than 15 mg/kg/h every 4–12 hours was continued for 2–3 days as necessary for those patients in shock or severely ill. Of the 28 patients who developed coma, shock, or both, only 3 died, one of whom received late treatment with DFO. Adverse effects of DFO were noted only when the drug was given rapidly intravenously and included tachycardia, hypotension, shock, dramatic erythema, and urticaria.[52]

The recommended guidelines for DFO dosing are based on the clinical experience developed in a study of 474 patients.[51] The intramuscular dose of DFO was suggested as 1 g initially, followed by 0.5 g 4 and 8 hours later and then every 4–12 hours as necessary, without exceeding 6 g in 24 hours. Intravenous DFO was recommended for patients in shock at a rate not to exceed 15 mg/kg/h, with an initial dose not to exceed 1 g followed by two 0.5-g doses separated by 4 hours and a total dosage not to exceed 6 g in 24 hours. These recommendations for total dosages were not scientifically developed and appear to be based on arbitrary assumptions.

In an attempt to further define the role of DFO, investigators turned to urinary examinations. A vin rosé color of the urine following DFO was indicative of 10–30 mg of urinary iron excretion per 24 hours.[35] In a review of 107 patients with acute iron poisoning who had received 5 g of DFO orally and 90 mg/kg IV at a rate not greater than 15 mg/kg/h,[32] the appearance of a vin rosé color in urine or a serum iron level greater than 500 μg/dL was suggested to require chelation for at least 24 hours. Further studies have tried to establish a framework for how urinary iron concentrations relate to systemic toxicity.[55] Most data suggest that following DFO administration the absence of a urine color change indicates that very little ferrioxamine is being excreted renally.[18] Problems arise when a baseline urine is not obtained prior to DFO administration and comparisons are inadequate post DFO administration. In any case, no relationship between urinary iron excretion, clinical iron toxicity, and the effectiveness of DFO has ever been established.

Prior to 1976, patients were given IM DFO unless they were in shock, when they received IV DFO. At this time, transfusion-induced iron overload was studied, comparing IM with IV DFO administration, demonstrating a significant enhancement of urinary iron elimination with the latter.[43] The study provided the compelling argument against IM dosing, as do the higher peak concentrations and more stable levels achieved with infusions. A single patient was given 425 mg/kg IV over 24 hours without incident, although the increase in urinary iron excretion seen when the DFO dose increased from 4 to 16 g/d appeared to be of limited consequence. No difficulties were reported in using intravenous DFO at 15 mg/kg/h for 52 hours in an adult patient with a serum iron of 915 μg/dL and a TIBC of 515 μg/dL.[38] A limit to the total daily doses of DFO at 8 g has been suggested, although the same author was uncertain about the appropriate length of DFO chelation.[27] An 18-month-old child with an estimated 336 mg/kg ingestion of elemental iron developed GI symptoms, coma, and shock, had an initial serum iron level of 6798 μg/dL, and was lavaged with DFO and given oral and intravenous DFO. The child survived without severe neurologic, hepatic, metabolic, or cardiovascular toxicity, but developed jejunal obstruction at 6 weeks.[21]

There are no controlled studies of the efficacy of DFO in severe iron poisoning nor are there studies of the appropriate dose, route of administration, or duration of therapy.[47] The manufacturer recommends IM administration un-less the patient is in shock, with a maximum daily dose of 6 g and a maximum intravenous infusion rate of 15 mg/kg/h. Severely poisoned patients probably require higher intravenous doses for 24 hours, whereas mildly poisoned patients are often given excessive DFO doses.[24]

The adverse effects of DFO include a rate-related hypotension, pulmonary toxicity, ocular and ototoxicity, and infection.[7,24] Histamine release is probably at least partially responsible for the rate-related hypotension.[54] The recommendations for intravenous administration of not more than 15 mg/kg/h come from early observations.[52,54] Intravascular volume depletion due to iron toxicity no doubt contributes to the hypotension and certainly must be managed appropriately. These suggested intravenous infusion rates are empiric, have never been scientifically determined, and higher rates are administered successfully.[8,12,15]

Pulmonary toxicity (ARDS) has been described in the setting of acute iron overdoses following IV doses of DFO (15 mg/kg/h) therapy for greater than 24 hours.[3,48] Detailed clinical presentations, the severity of the intoxication, and the rationale behind continued administration of DFO in these patients were not reported. Examination of the nontoxicologic literature reveals other instances of ARDS in patients receiving continuous IV DFO for hemosiderosis and refractory malignancies.[10,17,50] Common to all these patients was the administration of continuous IV doses of DFO for prolonged (> 24 hours) periods of time. The mechanism for the development of this pulmonary toxicity is still unknown. The pulmonary toxicity may result from excessive DFO chelation of intracellular iron and the depletion of catalase, resulting in subsequent oxidant damage[20] or the generation of free radicals.[1]

Ocular toxicity as evidenced by decreased visual acuity, night blindness, color blindness, and retinal pigmentary abnormalities has been observed in patients who received continuous IV DFO for thalassemia and other nonacute iron- and aluminum-excess conditions.[6,9,13,37,39] Ototoxicity resulting in abnormal audiograms and deafness has also been reported.[41] To date, neither ocular nor ototoxicity has been reported in the toxicology literature.

Deferoxamine therapy may lead to infection with a number of unusual organisms, including *Yersinia enterocolitica*, *Zygomycetes*, and *Aeromonas hydrophilia*. The virulence of these organisms is facilitated when the DFO–iron complex acts as a siderophore for their growth.[29,33,36] Most cases have occurred when DFO was employed for aluminum toxicity in patients on chronic hemodialysis.[34] But several cases of *Yersinia* sepsis are also reported following acute iron overdose.[33,36]

New iron chelators are being investigated. Pyridoxal isonicotinylhydrase and pyridoxal benzoylhydrazone are potent lipophilic chelators. Lipophilicity increases iron mobilization but may also increase toxicity. Deferiprone is an oral iron chelator used abroad to treat iron overload. Preliminary animal studies in acute toxicity are contradictory.[16,24a,26]

The indications and dosage schedule for DFO are largely empiric since a controlled study has never been performed.[5,44] Systemic toxicity associated with acute iron poisoning as manifested by coma, shock, or metabolic acidosis warrants aggressive intravenous infusion of DFO. The duration of therapy should probably be limited to about 24 hours to maximize effectiveness while minimizing the risk of pulmonary toxicity. There is a suggestion that more than the recommended dose of 15 mg/kg/h should be employed for life-threatening toxicity, but this approach needs validation.[24] Patients with mild toxicity are treated with IM injections of DFO at 90 mg/kg (maximum, 1 g in children or 2 g in adults), but this volume cannot be given intramuscularly with ease in children. The total daily parenteral dose is limited by the infusion rate in children if the manufacturer's recommendations are adhered to, and in adults conservative recommendations limit the dose to 6–8 g/d, although doses as high as 16 g/d and diverse dosing regimens have been administered without incident.[12,15,38,43,47]

Deferoxamine mesylate (Desferal[R]) is available in vials containing 500 mg of sterile, lyophilized powder. Addition of 2 mL of sterile water for injection to each vial results in a solution of 250 mg/mL. The resulting solution can be further diluted with normal saline, glucose in water, or Ringer's lactate solution for intravenous administration.

References

1. Adamson I, Sienko A, Tenenbein M.: Pulmonary toxicity of deferoxamine in iron-poisoned mice. Toxicol Appl Pharmacol 1993;120:13–19.
2. Allain P, Mauras Y, Chaleil D, et al: Pharmacokinetics and renal elimination of desferrioxamine and ferrioxamine in healthy subjects and patients with hemochromatosis. Br J Clin Pharmacol 1987;24:207–212.
3. Anderson KJ, Rivers PRA: Desferrioxamine in acute iron poisoning. Lancet 1992;339:1602. Letter.
4. Balcerzak SP, Jensen WN, Pollack S: Mechanism of action of desferrioxamine on iron absorption. Scand J Haematol 1966;3:205–212.
5. Banner W, Tong T: Iron poisoning. Pediatr Clin North Am 1986;33:393–409.
6. Bene C, Manzler A, Bene D, et al: Irreversible ocular toxicity from a single "challenge" dose of deferoxamine. Clin Nephron 1989;31:45–48.

7. Bentur Y, McGuigan M, Koren G: Deferoxamine (desferrioxamine), new toxicities for an old drug. Drug Safety 1991;6:37–46.
8. Berland Y, Charhon SA, Olmer M, et al: Predictive value of desferrioxamine infusion test for bone aluminum deposit in hemodialyzed patients. Nephron 1985;40:433–435.
9. Blake D, Winyard P, Lunec J, et al: Cerebral and ocular toxicity induced by desferrioxamine. Q J Med 1985;219: 345–355.
10. Castriota Scanderberg A, Izzi G, Butturini A, Benaglia G: Pulmonary syndrome and intravenous high-dose desferrioxamine. Lancet 1990;336:1511. Letter.
11. Chang TMS, Barne P: Effect of desferrioxamine on removal of aluminum and iron by coated charcoal hemoperfusion and hemodialysis. Lancet 1983;2:1051–1053.
12. Cheney K, Gumbiner C, Benson B, et al: Survival after a severe iron poisoning treated with intermittent infusions of deferoxamine. J Toxicol Clin Toxicol 1995;33:61–66.
13. Davies S, Hungerford J, Arden G, et al: Ocular toxicity of high dose intravenous desferrioxamine. Lancet 1983;2: 181–184.
14. Dean B, Oehme FW, Krenzelok E, Hines R: A study of iron complexation in a swine model. Vet Hum Toxicol 1988;30: 313–315.
15. Douglas D, Smilkstein M: Deferoxamine-iron induced pulmonary injury and *N*-acetylcysteine. J Toxicol Clin Toxicol 1995;33:495.
16. Fassos FF, Berkovitch M, Daneman N, et al: Efficacy of deferiprone in the treatment of acute iron intoxication in rats. J Toxicol Clin Toxicol 1996;34:279–287.
17. Freedman M, Grisaru D, Oliveri NF, et al: Pulmonary syndrome in patients with thalassemia major receiving intravenous deferoxamine infusions. Am J Dis Child 1990;144: 565–569.
18. Freeman DA, Manoguerra AS: Absence of urinary color change in severely iron poisoned child treated with deferoxamine. Vet Hum Toxicol 1981;23(suppl 1):49. Abstract.
19. Goodwin JF, Whitten CF: Chelation of ferrous sulfate solution by deferoxamine B. Nature 1965;205:281–283.
20. Helson L, Helson C, Braverman S, et al: Desferrioxamine in acute iron poisoning. Lancet 1992;339:1602–1603. Letter.
21. Henretig F, Karl S, Weintraub W: Severe iron poisoning treated with enteral and intravenous deferoxamine. Ann Emerg Med 1983;12:306–309.
22. Hoppe JO, Marcell GMA, Tainter ML: A review of the toxicity of iron compounds. Am J Med Sci 1955;230:558–571.
23. Hoskin CS: A pharmacologic investigation of acute iron poisoning and its treatment. Aust Paediatr J 1970;6:92–96.
24. Howland MA: Risks of parenteral deferoxamine. J Toxicol Clin Toxicol 1996;34:491–497.
24a. Hung O, Manoach S, Howland MA, et al: Deferipone for acute iron poisoning. J Toxicol Clin Toxicol 1997;35:565.
25. Keberle M: The biochemistry of desferrioxamine and its relation to iron metabolism. Ann NY Acad Sci 1964;119:758–768.
26. Kontoghiorgher GJ: New concepts of iron and aluminum chelation therapy with oral L1 (Deferiprone) and other chelators. Analyst 1995;120:845–851.
27. Lee P, Mohammed N, Marshal L, et al: Intravenous infusion pharmacokinetics of desferrioxamine in thalassemic patients. Drug Met Dispos 1993;21:640–644.
28. Leikin S, Vossough P, Mochiv-Fatemi F: Chelation therapy in acute iron poisoning. J Pediatr 1969;71:425–430.
29. Lin S, Shieh S, Lin Y, et al: Fatal *Aeromonas hydrophilia* bacteremia in a hemodialysis patient treated with deferoxamine. Am J Kidney Dis 1996;27:733–735.
30. Lipschitz D, Dugard J, Simon M, et al: The site of action of desferrioxamine. Br J Haematol 1971;20:395–404.
31. Lovejoy F: Chelation therapy in iron poisoning. J Toxicol Clin Toxicol 1982;19:871–874.
32. McEnery J: Hospital management of acute iron ingestion. Clin Toxicol 1971;4:603–613.
33. Melby K, Slordahal S, Gutteberg TJ, Nordbo SA: Septicemia due to *Yersinia enterocolitica* after oral doses of iron. Br Med J 1982;285:487–488.
34. Mersko C, Hersko C, Weatherall D: Iron chelating therapy. Crit Rev Clin Lab Sci 1988;26:303–340.
35. Moeschlin S, Schnider U: Treatment of primary and secondary hemochromatosis and acute iron poisoning with a new potent iron eliminating agent (desferrioxamine-B). N Engl J Med 1963;269:57–66.
36. Mofenson HC, Caraccio TR, Sharieff N: Iron sepsis: *Yersinia enterocolitica* septicemia possibly caused by an overdose of iron. N Engl J Med 1987;316:1092–1093.
37. Olivieri N, Buncic J, Chew E, et al: Visual and auditory neuro-toxicity in patients receiving subcutaneous deferoxamine infusions. N Engl J Med 1986;314:869–873.
38. Peck M, Rogers J, Riverbach J: Use of high doses of deferoxamine (Desferal) in an adult patient with acute iron overdosage. J Toxicol Clin Toxicol 1982;19:865–869.
39. Pengloan J, Dantal J, Rossazza M, et al: Ocular toxicity after a single dose of desferrioxamine in two hemodialysis patients. Nephron 1987;46:211–212.
40. Peter G, Keberle M, Schmid K: Distribution and renal excretion of desferrioxamine and ferrioxamine in the dog and in the rat. Biochem Pharmacol 1966;15:93–109.
41. Porter J, Jaswon M, Huehns E, et al: Desferrioxamine ototoxicity: Evaluation of risk factors in thalassemic patients and guidelines for safe dosage. Br J Haematol 1989; 73:403–409.
42. Propper R, Nathan D: Clinical removal of iron. Annu Rev Med 1982;33:509–519.
43. Propper R, Shurn S, Nathan D: Reassessment of the use of desferrioxamine B in iron overload. N Engl J Med 1976; 294:1421–1423.
44. Robotham J, Lietman P: Acute iron poisoning. Am J Dis Child 1980;134:875–879.
45. Stivelman J, Schulman G, Fosburg M, et al: Kinetics and efficacy of deferoxamine in iron overloaded hemodialysis patients. Kidney Int 1989;36:1125–1132.
46. Summers MR, Jacobs A, Tudway D, et al: Studies in desferrioxamine and ferrioxamine metabolism in normal and iron loaded subjects. Br J Haematol 1979;42: 547–555.
47. Tenenbein M: Benefits of parenteral deferoxamine for acute iron poisoning. J Toxicol Clin Toxicol 1996;34:485–489.
48. Tenenbein M, Kowalski S, Sienko A, et al: Pulmonary toxic effects of continuous administration in acute iron poisoning. Lancet 1992;339:699–701.
49. Tripod JA: Pharmacologic comparison of the binding of iron and other metals. In: Gross F, ed: Iron Metabolism.

International Symposium on Iron Metabolism. Berlin, Springer-Verlag, 1964, pp. 503–524.
50. Weitman S, Buchanan G, Kamen B: Pulmonary toxicity of deferoxamine in children with advanced cancer. J Natl Cancer Inst 1991;83:1834–1835.
51. Westlin W: Deferoxamine as a chelating agent. Clin Toxicol 1971;4:597–602.
52. Westlin W: Deferoxamine in the treatment of acute iron poisoning: Clinical experiences with 172 children. Clin Pediatr 1966;5:531–535.
53. Whitten C, Gibson G, Good M, et al: Studies in acute iron poisoning: Desferrioxamine in the treatment of acute iron poisoning—clinical observations, experimental studies and theoretical considerations. Pediatrics 1965;36:322–335.
54. Whitten C, You-chen C, Gibson G: Studies in acute iron poisoning: II. Further observations on deferoxamine in the treatment of acute experimental iron poisoning. Pediatrics 1966;38:102–110.
55. Yatscoff RW, Wayne EA, Tenenbein M: An objective criterion for the cessation of deferoxamine therapy in the acutely poisoned patient. J Toxicol Clin Toxicol 1991; 29:1–10.

CHAPTER 36

Vitamins

Richard J. Hamilton and Lewis R. Goldfrank

Vitamin A (Retinol)

MW	=	272.43 daltons
Therapeutic serum level	=	65–275 IU/dL
		16.6–83.3 μg/dL
Action level	=	unknown

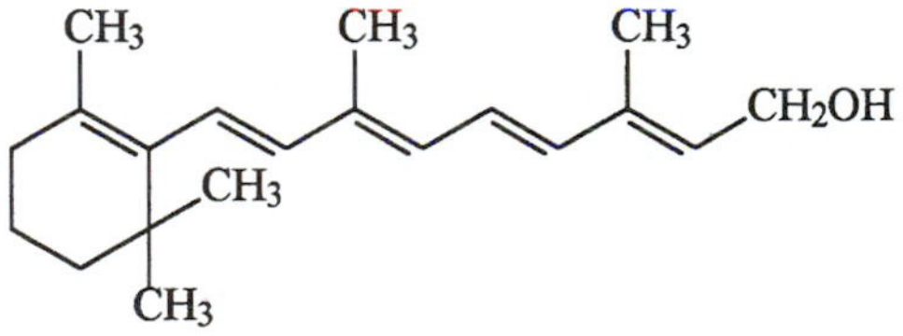

A 19-year-old woman came to the emergency department (ED) complaining of severe headaches and double vision. She had been in relatively good health, with no significant past medical or psychiatric history. For several weeks, however, she had been experiencing generalized headaches that were increasing in severity and duration. In addition, she noted the recent onset of diplopia, which was more marked on lateral gaze. Other complaints included anorexia, arthralgias, dryness and cracking of the lips, muscular stiffness and soreness after prolonged exercise, and a tendency to tire easily. She had had acne vulgaris for several years, for which she was taking vitamins and topical agents prescribed by a local health care clinic. There were no menstrual irregularities, no symptoms of thyroid dysfunction, no history of recent viral syndrome, and no history of head trauma. She was a full-time college student with no exposure to toxins, and had no known drug or alcohol abuse. The family history was unremarkable.

Physical examination revealed a slender, well-nourished young woman in no acute distress. Blood pressure, pulse, respirations, and temperature were within normal limits. Her scalp hair was coarse, with diffuse alopecia. Pubic and axillary hair was scant. Her skin was dry, and there was superficial facial acne vulgaris. Her lips were scaled and cracked, and there were small fissures at the corners of her mouth. Her heart and lungs were unremarkable. Her liver was enlarged to 13 cm, extended 3 cm below the right costal margin, and was smooth and nontender. There was no splenomegaly. Mild to moderate pressure on the long bones elicited moderately severe pain. No other musculoskeletal abnormalities were noted. Neurologic examination revealed bilateral sixth nerve palsies, normal pupillary responses, and blurred and slightly elevated disk margins, with no spontaneous venous pulsations. There were no gross visual field defects. There was no motor weakness, sensory disturbance, abnormal reflexes, or signs of meningeal irritation. Cognitive testing was normal.

We are presented with a previously healthy young woman with a history of a multisystem disorder progressing over several weeks and primarily involving the musculoskeletal, integumentary, and central nervous systems. This multisystem disease process coupled with her use of vitamins to treat acne vulgaris suggests vitamin A intoxication.[27,62,68] After obtaining a CT scan to ensure that the altered mental status is not caused by an intracranial mass or bleeding, a lumbar puncture should be performed.

Laboratory data revealed that complete blood cell count, glucose, BUN, electrolytes, and liver function were all within normal limits. Radiographs of the chest, hands, and legs did not disclose any abnormalities. A lumbar puncture later confirmed the diagnosis of hypervitaminosis A with benign intracranial hypertension. The opening pressure was 320 mm H_2O (normal, 50–180 mm H_2O), the spinal fluid was clear and colorless, with no cells and with normal glucose and protein.

What Is Vitamin A? What Are Normal Needs?

Vitamin A (retinol) is a fat-soluble vitamin. Little is known about its fundamental metabolic action, except in the retina, where it is required for the regeneration of the photosensitive chromoprotein rhodopsin. Vitamin A appears to be necessary for glycoprotein synthesis by mucus-secreting cells and for mucopolysaccharide homeostasis. The vast majority of vitamin A is ingested as retinyl esters, the storage form of retinol. Vitamin A is a significant growth-promoting factor. It is obtained from the diet in two forms: preformed vitamin A from animal sources, particularly liver; and vitamin A precursors, carotenoids, found in vegetables, particularly carrots.[58,70] The average American diet provides about half of its vitamin A activity as carotene and the other half as preformed vitamin A.[20] Several fish-liver oils, such as swordfish and Black Sea bass, may contain more than 180,000 IU of vitamin A per gram of oil. In contrast, vitamin A precursors are converted rather inefficiently to vitamin A in the intestinal wall, where they are absorbed. Massive doses of carotene are not converted rapidly enough to induce vitamin A toxicity. Excess carotene does accumulate in the body, producing a yellow-orange skin discoloration, which can be differentiated from jaundice by the absence of scleral icterus. Absorption depends on the presence of bile and absorbable fat in the intestinal tract. On absorption, retinol-binding protein produced by the liver transports vitamin A to the liver.

Approximately 90% of the total vitamin A content of the mammalian body is stored in the liver, primarily as retinyl ester. The adrenal cortex also concentrates the vitamin. Because vitamin A is insoluble in water but soluble in fats, increased intake does not initially lead to elevated blood levels but rather to hepatic accumulation. When insufficient amounts of vitamin A are consumed, fairly constant blood levels are maintained at the expense of hepatic reserves, which may be sufficient to prevent symptoms of vitamin A deficiency for several months. The normal plasma level of retinol is about 30–70 μg/100 mL.[77] (See Table 36–1 for the Recommended Daily Allowances of vitamin A.)

Transretinoic acid is a metabolite found in tissues or bound to albumin or in blood. Clinical toxicity correlates well with total body vitamin A content and is thus a function of dosage and duration of administration. As little as 25,000–50,000 IU/d for as few as 30 days can induce signs of increased intracranial pressure.[14,68] There is, however, considerable individual variability with respect to the cumulative intake necessary to produce toxicity. As a general guide, acute toxicity requires a single massive ingestion of a medicinal preparation containing in excess of 25,000 IU/kg body weight, and chronic toxicity requires 4000 IU/kg body weight daily for 6–15 months.

TABLE 36–1. RECOMMENDED DAILY ALLOWANCES (RDA) FOR VITAMIN A (REGARDLESS OF FORM) IN INTERNATIONAL UNITS (IU)

Adult men		3300
Adult women		2700
Pregnant women	second and third trimesters	3300
Lactating women		4000
Children	infants to 12 mo	1350
	1–3 y	1350
	4–6 y	1650
	7–10 y	2300
	11–14 y	2700–3300

1 retinol equivalent (μg) = 3.3 IU = 1 μg all transretinols = 6 μg of beta-carotene

Which End Organs Manifest Vitamin A Toxicity and How?

The skin, hair, bones, liver, and brain are each affected by hypervitaminosis A. The exact mechanism of action is unclear, although vitamin A may have hormone-like properties. Some suggest that the retinoids influence gene expression at the level of nuclear DNA, resulting in cell turnover, differentiation, and protein synthesis. Others suggest varied DNA- or RNA-related influences on gene expression.[14,18,63]

In the skin, vitamin A normally assists in epithelial maturation and membrane stability. However, excessive concentrations lead to increased permeability and decreased stability of lipoprotein membranes. These effects may result from unbound retinol and its esters. In excessive dosage, decreased keratinization and sebum production result in extreme thinning of epithelial tissue, manifested as brittle nails, thin rough skin, excessive desquamation, and alopecia.

Asynchronous growth patterns of long bone occurs in children treated with vitamin A for keratinizing disorders. Bone resorption, hypercalcemia, and cartilaginous matrix degradation result in cortical hyperostosis, bony exostoses, metaphyseal flare, and epiphyseal premature closure. Radiographic findings may consist of pericapsular, ligamentous, and subperiosteal calcifications. Areas of new bone formation may be particularly prominent in the shafts of the long bones. Bone demineralization has also been reported. Calcium, phosphorus, and alkaline phosphatase may be abnormal.

Hepatotoxicity results from excessive deposition of vitamin A in the Ito cells of the liver.[56] Ito cells normally function as fat-storage cells and are found in the perisinusoidal space of Disse. They appear responsible, among other things, for maintaining the normal hepatic architecture. Hypertrophy of Ito cells with vitamin A, retinol, and lipids leads to enhanced collagen production and scarring (see Fig. 36–1). Extracellular cholestasis occurs without bile duct proliferation. Liver injury from vitamin A is histiologically defined as cirrhosis. There appears to be a correlation between cirrhotic liver disease and large doses of vitamin A and noncirrhotic liver disease with lower chronic dosing. The disease invariably progresses to portal hypertension, esophageal varices, jaundice, and ascites.[23,32,51] Liver function studies are frequently normal, even in the presence of hepatomegaly, although hepatotoxicity and cirrhosis may be manifested by elevations in bilirubin, aminotransferases, and alkaline phosphatase.

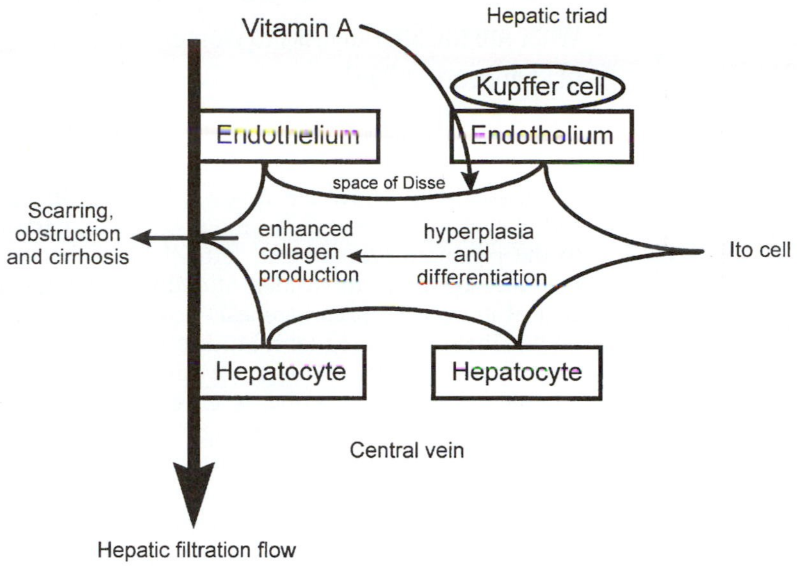

Figure 36–1. A schematic demonstration of hepatotoxicity resulting from excessive deposition of vitamin A in the Ito cells of the liver.

Benign intracranial hypertension (or pseudotumor cerebri) is a syndrome of uncertain etiology found in conjunction with a number of unrelated disorders. The syndrome is defined by the presence of intracranial hypertension without evidence of localizing neurologic findings. In more than 50% of cases no cause can be identified; however, women, usually in their third or fourth decade, represent 75% of these cases.[1,74,88] Benign intracranial hypertension may be seen in patients with altered endocrine function, systemic diseases, impaired venous drainage, or ingestion of various drugs or toxins.[3] Of these ingestions, vitamin A is the most common. Table 36–2 lists the drugs and toxins that have been associated with intracranial hypertension.

TABLE 36–2. DRUGS AND TOXINS ASSOCIATED WITH INTRACRANIAL HYPERTENSION

Drugs
Vitamin A
Oral contraceptives and progestational drugs
Corticosteroid therapy and cessation
Griseofulvin
Phenytoin
Antibiotics: nalidixic acid, tetracycline, ampicillin, minocycline, nitrofurantoin, sulfamethoxazole, metronidazole
Phenothiazines
Lithium
Toxins
Lead
Anesthetics
Halothane
Ketamine
Enflurane
d-Tubocurare

Headaches, blurred vision, and diplopia are the most characteristic initial symptoms of benign intracranial hypertension. The most common ocular complaint is visual blurring, a manifestation of papillitis. Visual loss may be minimal, despite severe chronic papilledema; however, blindness may result from optic atrophy.[57] Visual field assessment may demonstrate blindspot enlargement, scotomata, and peripheral field constriction. A complaint of diplopia may result from sixth nerve palsy secondary to increased intracranial pressure.[73]

How Is the Diagnosis of Hypervitaminosis A Established?

The only consistent laboratory abnormality is the elevation of the serum vitamin A level to a value ranging from 80 to 200 μg/dL. It is important to remember that in chronic intoxication a proportional relationship does not exist between the amount of vitamin A stored in the liver and the serum level. During initial stages of toxicity, much of the vitamin is stored in the liver, and the serum level may remain normal or disproportionately low. Once the capacity for storage is exhausted, the serum level increases rapidly in an apparent nonlinear fashion. Hepatotoxicity may be manifest prior to the elevation of serum vitamin A levels. For this reason, serum levels may be high if a relatively minor excessive amount is given for a sufficiently long time. The serum level may remain low if large amounts are given for a short period of time.

What Treatment, If Any, Is Indicated? What Is the Natural Course of the Disease and What Is the Prognosis?

Treatment consists of withdrawal of vitamin A and appropriate supportive care. Benign intracranial hypertension frequently resolves after treatment of the underlying etiology or withdrawal of the offending agent. Most signs and symptoms begin to resolve within 1 week, although papilledema and skeletal abnormalities may persist for several months after clinical recovery. Visual impairment secondary to optic atrophy is the only major long-term sequela of vitamin A toxicity. Under certain circumstances more aggressive therapy to relieve pressure must be initiated by daily lumbar puncture, an initial dose of 40 mg of IV furosemide, 1 g of mannitol/kg body weight, 250 mg of acetazolamide 4 times a day, and a short course of prednisone, depending on the severity and resistance of the syndrome. The acetazolamide may decrease CSF formation, although there may be a transient increase in CSF pressure. These approaches must be individualized with regard to risk-to-benefit ratio, as remission is usually spontaneous.

Vitamin A-induced hypercalcemia associated with nausea and vomiting may respond to loop diuretics with intravenous fluids, and prednisone (20 mg daily).[9]

The immediate management after an acute overdosage rarely requires more than gastric decontamination. The initial symptoms are usually minor gastrointestinal manifestations and headache. The main manifestations of an acute ingestion include drowsiness or irritability, vomiting, and increased intracranial pressure. These findings are usually followed in 24–72 hours by extensive desquamation. Headache, nausea, and vomiting ensue.[7,30]

Who Is at Risk for Vitamin A Intoxication?

Vitamin A intoxication is uncommon but should be considered in the differential diagnosis of all hepatic and cutaneous diseases. Patients with chronic renal failure requiring dialysis who take even the small amount of vitamin A in multivitamin preparations are at increased risk for hypercalcemia.[25] Hypervitaminosis A usually occurs in adults who have initially been treated with large doses of this vitamin for a variety of dermatologic conditions, such as acne vulgaris, and who subsequently continue using the vitamin without medical supervision.[63,84] Hypervitaminosis A has also been reported in food faddists who ingest large doses of fat-soluble vitamin preparations in their daily dietary regimens, in an adult who had chronically ingested beef liver in large doses, and among Inuits, whose diet may include foods with high vitamin A content, such as polar bear liver.[42]

Vitamin A intoxication may be an occult illness. In fact, several reports demonstrate the unmasking of chronic hypervitaminosis A by intercurrent disease such as hepatitis and protein malnutrition.[36,87] Rat studies demonstrate that modest amounts of vitamin A may become hepatotoxic when associated with ethanol intake.[66] Although prolonged and continuous consumption of doses "theoretically in the therapeutic range" is reported to cause life-threatening hepatotoxicity and cirrhosis, the doses employed were actually 4–80 times the RDA.[18,42]

What Are the Special Risks to Women of Childbearing Age?

Daily doses of 25,000 IU or more should not be used unless severe deficiency of vitamin A exists, as documented by an abnormally low serum level. Doses of this magnitude taken for an extended time pose a risk, particularly to the pregnant woman and fetus.[54] Much lower doses may also be a risk to women of childbearing age. Often critical periods of organogenesis occur before a woman knows that she is pregnant. Studies in pregnant animals have shown that large doses of vitamin A produce CNS anomalies with hydrocephalus, encephalocele, and other teratogenic effects in the offspring.[71]

Isotretinoin (Accutane), a retinoic acid–vitamin A analog, is effective in the management of severe nodulocystic acne. However, since the release of isotretinoin, extremely severe teratogenicity and such complications as spontaneous abortions, mucocutaneous effects, pseudotumor cerebri, corneal opacities, hypercalcemia, hyperuricemia, musculoskeletal symptoms, liver function abnormalities, and elevated triglycerides[28,29] have occurred with alarming frequency.[1,34,35] A major problem arises in that 38% of the users of isotretinoin cited in the National Disease and Therapeutic Index reports are women aged 13–19 years. The risk of pregnancy in this group and the high risk of teratogenicity of this compound further underscore the need to inform all users of the contraindications to the drug's use during pregnancy as well as the need to demonstrate the absence of pregnancy before initiating therapy and the need to have the patient consider the consequences of unintentionally becoming pregnant while taking isotretinoin. The teratogenicity as well as all of the other adverse effects typical of hypervitaminosis A should lead to restraint in the prescription of this drug (see Chaps. 16 and 28).

Megadose Vitamins and the Antioxidants

The megadose school of vitamin therapy has led Americans to spend phenomenal amounts of money for vitamin doses ten to hundreds of times the amount recommended by the National Academy of Science as daily dietary requirements.[65,67] The most frequently promoted health benefit was muscle growth. However, recent evidence has identified ascorbic acid (vitamin C), alphatocopherol (vitamin E), and beta-carotene (a relatively safe precursor of vitamin A) as having potential benefit in prevention of carcinogenic mechanisms via their antioxidant properties.[12]

Nutritional supplements and megadose vitamins often come packaged in tablet form and are labeled to advertise their reported benefits, for example "Energy Pak." Many unusual and unidentifiable ingredients are included; 22.2% of the products advertised had no ingredients listed and no toxicologic data were available on 139 (59%) of the ingredients.[65] Over 90% of these vitamins and supplements are purchased commercially and used without supervision of a physician.[38,72] A 1983 demographic analysis of vitamin use determined that persons older than 65 years of age consumed more supplements than those in younger groups, and people with the highest educational levels had the highest consumption rates.[11,31] A Canadian study determined that the incidence of vitamin overdoses in children was directly related to the number of vitamin preparations used by their families.[43]

Antioxidant vitamins are used to disrupt the peroxidation and epoxidation of DNA that are often essential steps in mutagenesis and to prevent the oxidation of low-density lipoprotein, which is considered an important determinant in atherosclerosis. However, cancer prevention studies have reported mixed benefits of antioxidant vitamins. The Iowa Women's Health Study found no association between dietary antioxidants and breast cancer risk, although a statistically insignificant reduction was noted in those patients who took vitamin supplements.[52] Studies have noted lower antioxidant vitamin levels in cohorts of patients with coronary artery disease when compared to controls matched for age, gender, blood pressure, smoking, alcohol use, serum lipids, and body mass index.[50] The benefits of antioxidants may also include a reduction in markers of severity of myocardial infarction such as creatine kinase fractions and left ventricular dysfunction.[78] A prospective study of a cohort of postmenopausal women demonstrated a protective effect of consumption of vitamin E in the diet but no additional effect was obtained by using vitamin E supplements. Vitamins A or C appeared to have no protective effect.[53] A conclusive discussion of the efficacy of these vitamins in disease prevention is beyond the scope of this chapter. However, sufficient evidence exists to encourage a brisk commerce in vitamin sales and, hence, the potential for toxicity exists. Fortunately, these vitamins are relatively safe at the range of recommended doses (vitamin C: 1000 mg/day; vitamin E: 400 mg/day; beta-carotene: 25 mg/day).[24,29]

Almost every scientific group that has issued a statement on vitamin usage has concluded that healthy adult men and nonpregnant, nonlactating women who eat a normal varied diet do not require supplemental vitamins.[4] Most commercially available preparations contain less than twice the U.S. RDA. These RDAs have long been established at approximately 2 standard deviations above the mean requirement and therefore encompass the needs of 97% of the population.[4,26] While vitamins may have important roles in disease prevention, the question of the efficacy of high-dose supplementation remains to be answered.

Vitamin E (Alpha-Tocopherol)

MW	=	430.69 daltons
Therapeutic serum level	=	0.5–2.0 mg/dL
Action level	=	unknown

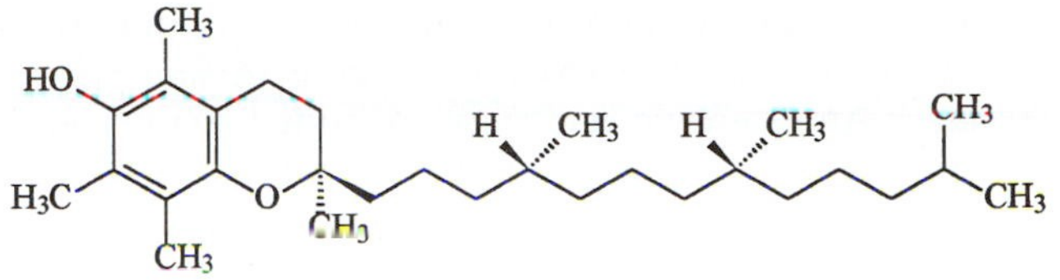

Vitamin E has a wide margin of safety even when taken in doses as high as 400 mg/d (which is ten times the RDA).[6] Reports of adverse symptoms from large doses are anecdotal, with nausea, diarrhea, and flatulence as typical GI manifestations. Numerous other symptoms and toxic effects have been reported. In animals, absorption of vitamins A and K was impaired by large doses of vitamin E.[10,69] In addition, vitamin E appears to enhance the epoxidation of vitamin K to its inactive form (see Fig. 42–2).[6] This can enhance the anticoagulant effect of warfarins, and clinicians should consider vitamin E supplementation as a cause for elevated prothrombin times in patients who are taking coumadin. A severe epidemic of low-birth-weight infants who manifested thrombocytopenia, renal dysfunction, cholestasis, ascites, and death occurred following the intravenous use of E-Ferol (a vitamin E supplement).[13] This product was removed from the market, because questions were raised about the emulsification of lipids and fat-soluble vitamins using polyoxyethylene sorbitan monolaurate and monooleate (polysorbate 20 and polysorbate 80, respectively). It is these agents and not the vitamin E itself that were responsible for this syndrome.

Vitamin C (Ascorbic Acid)

MW	=	176.12 daltons
Therapeutic serum level	=	0.4–2.0 mg/dL
Action level	=	unknown

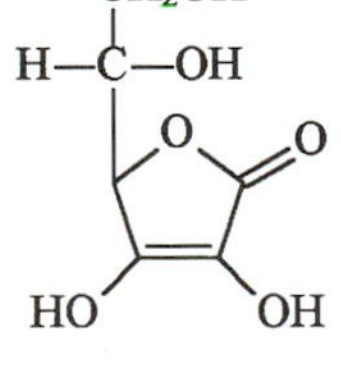

On the basis of its action as a hydrogen donor for the detoxification of peroxy radicals, vitamin C has long been used as a panacea for cancer prevention, to treat or prevent the common cold, to increase mental attentiveness, and to treat minor wounds, cancer, and stress. This belief is so widely held that one study found that 67% of the residents in a California retirement community were using vitamin C, and 6% were taking greater than 2 g/day.[31] An extensive review of 15 studies of the role of ascorbic acid in the treatment of the common cold, however, suggested that only half were truly valid investigations and none demonstrated any therapeutic benefit.[17] Controlled evaluations of the role of vitamin C in cancer therapy also demonstrated no advantage in survival over placebo.[21,61]

Chronic doses in excess of 2 g/day of ascorbic acid may result in diarrhea and urinary cystine or oxalate nephrolithiasis. This results from the metabolism of ascorbic acid to oxalic acid. In addition, ascorbic acid can be oxidized in vitro to oxalate. Subsequently, oxalate crystals precipitate in the renal tubules.[85] Nephropathy and renal failure appear to be associated with single 40–50 g intravenous doses.[55,59]

Vitamin B_6 (Pyridoxine)

MW	=	169 daltons
Therapeutic serum level	=	3.6–18 ng/mL
Action level	=	unknown

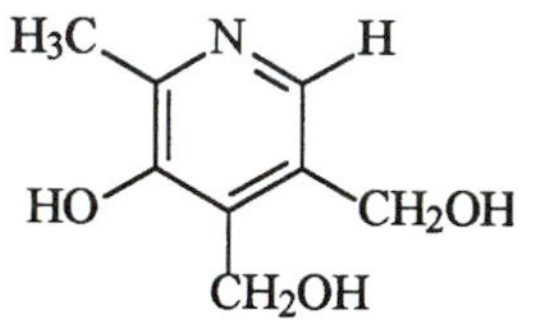

Pyridoxine was thought to be harmless due to its rapid excretion, but a single collection of case reports demonstrated that excessive doses of water-soluble vitamins could be toxic.[75] Seven patients taking pyridoxine at a daily dose of 2–6 g (minimum daily requirement is 2–4 mg) for 2–40 months developed sensory neuropathies. The seven adults studied had normal CNS function but had progressive sensory ataxia and profound distal limb impairment of position and vibration sense. Touch, pain, and temperature sensation were minimally impaired. All tendon reflexes were diminished or absent. Nerve conduction and somatosensory studies showed dysfunction of distal portions of sensory peripheral nerves, and nerve biopsy showed widespread, nonspecific axonal degeneration. This is defined as a toxic sensory neuropathy of the distal axon and neuron. Fortunately, these patients improved over several months with abstinence from pyridoxine.

Since that initial report other cases have been described with lower, but excessive, pyridoxine doses. Pyridoxine is widely available in tablet forms containing 50–500 mg of the drug and is promoted for body building and premenstrual syndrome (PMS). Additionally, use of pyridoxine has been advocated and used for schizophrenia, childhood autism, and attention deficit disorder. Later reports suggest that doses as low as 200–500 mg of pyridoxine per day may prove neurotoxic. In these studies early recognition of symptoms and withdrawal of supplementation has prevented permanent disability in most.[64]

Single doses of pyridoxine can cause acute toxicity but must usually be orders of magnitude above the correct dose. In a case of Gyromitra mushroom poisoning, a husband and wife were inadvertently treated with 183 g and 132 g of pyridoxine, resulting in permanent dorsal root and sensory ganglia deficits.[2]

A prospective study of pyridoxine neurotoxicity in volunteers has characterized the pathophysiology of this syndrome.[8] The investigators administered 1 or 3 g/kg of pyridoxine to five healthy volunteers and closely followed clinical signs and symptoms, serum pyridoxal phosphate levels, quantitative sensory thresholds (QSTs), and sural nerve electrophysiologic determinations. The quantitative sensory threshold is a sensitive measure of toxicity that can be determined prior to changes in nerve conduction studies. Pyridoxine was discontinued at the first sign of either a clinical or laboratory abnormality. In all subjects, sensory symptoms and QST abnormalities occurred simultaneously. Those who received higher doses developed symptoms before those receiving lower doses. Elevation of thermal QSTs preceded or exceeded that for vibration in the low-dose subjects, whereas vibration and thermal QST became abnormal simultaneously in the high-dose subjects. Symptoms continued to progress ("coast") for 2–3 weeks after discontinuation of pyridoxine and the return of serum pyridoxal phosphate to normal levels.

Vitamin D (Cholecalciferol)

MW	=	384.62 daltons
Therapeutic serum level	=	10–50 ng/mL
Action level	=	unknown

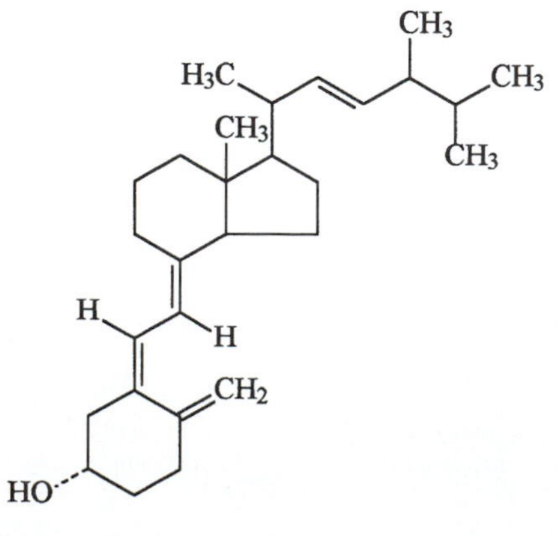

Vitamin D may be more appropriately thought of as a hormone rather than as a dietary nutrient, since it is manufactured in the skin from cholesterol by sunlight. It appears that even casual exposure of cutaneous tissues to ultraviolet light during the summer months produces adequate vitamin D for storage for winter months.[33] A series of British studies[15] of hypercalcemia in the 1950s demonstrated that chronic exposure to relatively small amounts of vitamin D in excess of the RDA can be toxic in children as well as in adults. The manifestations that ensue are directly related to the increased physiologic response to vitamin D, resulting in increased calcium absorption and increased 25-hydroxy vitamin D leading to increased metabolism of calcium (see Fig. 36–2). Children and, especially, infants appear to be susceptible to oversupplementation by vitamin D and will develop cardiovascular, CNS, and renal damage. Symptoms include anorexia, nausea, vomiting, hypertension, and renal compromise associated with hypercalcemia.[76] Consider hypervitaminosis D in children with nephrocalcinosis and hypercalciuria even if the serum calcium and phosphorous are normal.[60] Adults have similar systemic manifestations of anorexia, weakness, malaise, nausea, vomiting, hypertension, renal compromise, and even death. Calcium homeostasis is markedly altered, with hypercalcemia and hyperphosphatemia, resulting in polyuria, polydypsia, nephrolithiasis, renal failure, vascular calcifications, and ectopic calcification.[41]

Recent studies of eight patients who developed hypervitaminosis D associated with drinking milk have led to a reassessment of the appropriate amount of vitamin D necessary to achieve normal skeletal development and mineralization without causing toxicity.[44] This is particularly important in view of the unreliability of fortification of milk and infant formulas. Fortified milk may actually not contain vitamin D_2 (ergocalciferol) but vitamin D_3 (cholecalciferol) and may often be either under- or overfortified, placing the individual at risk.[39]

The elderly and the chronically ill who consume less vitamin D-fortified foods and milk and who have little exposure to sunshine may still benefit from food fortification that is monitored by regulatory agencies for safety. Vitamin D_3 is also currently widely available as a rodenticide (Chap. 89).

Nicotinic Acid (Niacin)

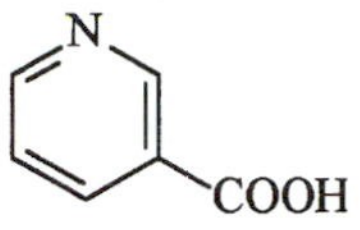

Nicotinic acid is extensively used today as therapy for hyperlipidemias in doses 10–100 times the U.S. RDA. Often the initial therapeutic use results in extensive flushing, vasodilation, headache, and pruritus that appear to be prostaglandin-mediated. The symptoms are usually transient and rarely require therapy. A single aspirin taken 30 minutes before ingestion of nicotinic acid will diminish the flush response.[89] Niacin has been reported to cause amblyopia, hyperglycemia, hyperuricemia, coagulopathy, myopathy, and hyperpigmentation.[37] Excessive doses may result in nausea, diarrhea, and epigastric distress.

Niacin-induced hepatitis appears to be more frequent and more severe among those with hyperlipidemias treated with sustained-release preparations than those receiving crystalline or immediate-release niacin. Hepatotoxicity is consistent with centrilobular cholestasis and parenchymal necrosis. These manifestations appear to be dose related and not a hypersensitivity response.[22,66]

Patients typically develop tolerance to nicotinic acid

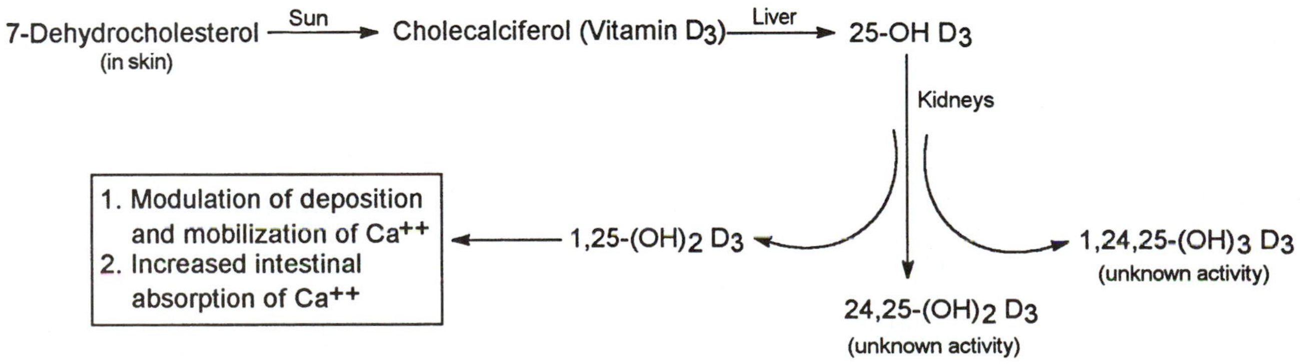

Figure 36–2. A schematic representation of the increased physiologic response to vitamin D resulting in increased calcium absorption and increased 25-hydroxy vitamin D_3.

flushing as plasma levels of 9α–11β prostaglandin F_2, a stable metabolite of prostaglandin D_2, become undetectable in most subjects. Tolerance is not associated with decreased nicotinic acid level nor tolerance to the prostaglandin mediator, but rather to decreased mediator levels. Flushing appears to occur because of the predilection for the skin as a source of prostaglandin D_2 production after niacin ingestion.[82]

Eosinophilia–Myalgia Syndrome

The danger of using "megadoses" of any substance without a sound medical reason was underscored in late 1989 when the CDC began to receive hundreds of reports of illness, and in some cases death, associated with the use of L-tryptophan. Most of the cases involved the use of approximately 150–8400 mg/d of L-tryptophan for 2 weeks to 8 years for its supposed sedative effects.

The illness was named eosinophilia–myalgia syndrome (EMS) and officially defined by the CDC as (1) an eosinophil count greater than 1000 cells/mm^3; (2) generalized myalgias at some time during the illness; and (3) the absence of any infection or neoplasm that could account for (1) or (2).[16] Because of the vast diversity of signs and symptoms reported, a strict case definition will identify only half of those affected.[46] Perimyositis, perivasculitis, or unspecified fasciitis (and no evidence of trichinosis) are demonstrated on muscle biopsy. The manifestations of EMS include pulmonary symptoms and pulmonary infiltrates; cutaneous thickening and edema and a fasciitis resembling scleroderma; neuromuscular manifestations resembling Guillain-Barré syndrome, with an axonal neuropathy; and endarteritis and panarteritis in those with terminal disturbances of cardiac rhythm and conduction.[45]

These clinical manifestations resemble those in patients with intermediate and chronic phases of toxic oil syndrome (TOS), a disease very similar to EMS that occurred as an epidemic in Spain in 1981.[49] Although 50% of TOS patients recovered from the acute illness without apparent sequelae, the remaining patients developed an intermediate or chronic phase or both, manifested by severe myalgia, eosinophilia, peripheral nerve damage, sclerodermiform skin lesions, sicca syndrome, alopecia, and joint contractures (Chap. 117).[47] Toxic oil syndrome resulted from the ingestion of contaminated rapeseed oil denatured with aniline and sold as cooking oil. The clinical manifestations of EMS as with TOS may not regress immediately after the removal of L-tryptophan-containing products. Following the initial case reports about EMS, the FDA sought a nationwide recall of all products containing L-tryptophan. A contaminant introduced in the manufacture of the pure L-tryptophan appears to be the most likely explanation for EMS, rather than the megadoses of L-tryptophan itself. Several epidemiologic studies have demonstrated that the dose of presumably contaminated L-tryptophan is the single most important predictor of toxicity.[46,79] "Peak E," an atypical dimeric form of L-tryptophan (1,1-ethylidene bistryptophan), is also statistically associated with EMS.[5,86] "Peak 5" and "Peak E" appear to enhance the binding of eosinophils to endothelial cells and stimulate eosinophil chemotaxis.[83] This mechanism is consistent with establishment of EMS as a microvascular disease characterized by inflammatory microangiopathy of the dermis, fascia, and muscle. Chronic EMS appears to differ from acute EMS in that the tissue infiltration is largely lymphocytic, rarely eosinophilic.[80]

Recent research has questioned the validity of the epidemiologic studies that originally established the link between the contaminated L-tryptophan and EMS. Animal models do not conclusively reproduce EMS and the original epidemiologic data suffered from recall bias and reporting bias and failed to confirm that the use of tainted product preceded the symptoms.[19,40] Application of the CDC criteria for EMS to populations in Quebec and Ontario uncovered 19 patients who fit the criteria who had not consumed any L-tryptophan.[81] Despite the flaws in the original studies, the incidence of EMS diminished abruptly once L-tryptophan products were recalled; the effect appeared dose related, and no confounding factor or alternative explanation has been produced for the sudden appearance and disappearance of this condition.[48] Further study will be necessary to explain all the facts.

Acknowledgment

Robert A. Kirstein, MD contributed to this chapter in a previous edition.

References

1. Adverse effects with isoretinoin. FDA Drug Bull 1983;13: 1–3.
2. Albin RL, Alpers JW, Greenberg HS, et al: Acute sensory neuropathy-neuronpathy from pyridoxine overdose. Neurology 1987;37:1729–1732.
3. Allain HJ, Weintraub M: Drug induced headache. Ration Drug Ther 1980;14:1–6.
4. AMA Council on Scientific Affairs: Vitamin preparations as dietary supplements and as therapeutic agents. JAMA 1987; 257:1929–1936.
5. Belongia EA, Hedberg CW, Gleich GJ, et al: An investigation of the cause of the eosinophilia myalgia syndrome associated with tryptophan use. N Engl J Med 1990;323: 357–365.
6. Bendich A, Machlin LJ: Safety of oral intake of vitamin E. Am J Clin Nutr 1988;48:612–619.
7. Bergen S, Roels O: Hypervitaminosis A. Am J Clin Nutr 1965;16:265–269.
8. Berger AR, Schaumburg HH, Schroeder C, et al: Dose response, coasting and differential fiber vulnerability in human toxic neuropathy: A prospective study of pyridoxine neurotoxicity. Neurology 1992;42:1367–1370.
9. Bergman SM, O'Mailia J, Krane NK, Wallin JD: Vitamin A in-

duced hypercalcemia: Response to corticosteroids. Nephron 1988;50:362–364.

10. Bieri JG, Corash L, Hubbard VS: Medical uses of vitamin E. N Engl J Med 1983;308:1063–1071.
11. Block G, Cox C, Madans J, et al: Vitamin supplement use by demographic characteristics. Am J Epidemiol 1988;27: 297–309.
12. Block G, Patterson B, Sklar A: Fruit, vegetables, and cancer prevention: A review of the epidemiological evidence. Nutr Cancer 1992;18:1–29.
13. Bove KE, Kosmetatos N, Wedig KE, et al: Vasculopathic hepatotoxicity associated with E-Ferol syndrome in low birth weight infants. JAMA 1985;254:2422–2430.
14. Boyd AS: An overview of the retinoids. Am J Med 1989; 86:568–574.
15. British Pediatric Association: Hypercalcemia in infants and vitamin D. Br Med J 1956;2:149.
16. Centers for Disease Control: Eosinophilia-myalgia syndrome and L-tryptophan-containing products: New Mexico, Minnesota, Oregon, and New York. MMWR 1989;38: 785–788.
17. Chalmers TC: Effect of ascorbic acid in the common cold: An evaluation of the evidence. Am J Med 1975;58:532–536.
18. Chytil F, Sherman DR: How do retinoids work? Dermatologica 1987;175:8–12.
19. Clauw DJ: Animal models of the eosinophilia-myalgia syndrome. J Rheumatol 1996;46(suppl):93–97.
20. Committee on Recommended Dietary Allowances: Report of Food and Nutritional Board, 9th ed. Washington, DC, National Academy of Sciences, National Research Council, 1980, pp. 58–59.
21. Creagan ET, Moertel CG, O'Fallon JR, et al: Failure of high dose vitamin C (ascorbic acid) therapy to benefit patients with advanced cancer: A controlled clinical trial. N Engl J Med 1979;301:687–690.
22. Dalton TA, Berry RS: Hepatotoxicity associated with sustained release niacin. Am J Med 1992;93:102–104.
23. Davis BH, Vucic A: The effect of retinol on Ito cell proliferation in vitro. Hepatology 1988;8:788–793.
24. Diplock A: Safety of antioxidant vitamins and beta-carotene. Am J Clin Nutr 1995;62:1510S–1516S.
25. Farrington K, Miller P, Varghese Z, et al: Vitamin A toxicity and hypercalcemia in chronic renal failure. Br Med J 1981; 282:1999–2002.
26. FDA Consumer Memo: Nutrition Labels and US RDA Publication (FDA) 81-2146, US Department of Health and Human Services, 1981.
27. Feldman M, Schlezinger N: Benign intracranial hypertension associated with hypervitaminosis A. Arch Neurol 1970; 22:1–7.
28. Flynn WJ, Freeman PG, Wickboldt LG: Pancreatitis associated with isotretinoin-induced hypertriglyceridemia. Ann Intern Med 1987;106:63.
29. Garewal HS, Diplock AT: How "safe" are antioxidant vitamins? Drug Safety 1995;13;8–14.
30. Gerber A, Raab A, Sobel A: Vitamin A poisoning in adults. Am J Med 1954;16:729–745.
31. Gray GE, Paganini-Hill A, Ross RK: Dietary intake and nutrition supplement use in a southern California retirement community. Am J Clin Nutr 1983;38:122–128.
32. Guebel AP, de Galocsy C, Alves N, et al: Liver damage caused by therapeutic vitamin A administration: Estimate of dose related toxicity in 41 cases. Gastroenterology 1991; 100:1701–1709.
33. Haddad JG: Vitamin D: Solar rays, the milky way or both? N Engl J Med 1992;326:1213–1215.
34. Hall JG: Vitamin A teratogenicity. N Engl J Med 1984;311: 797–798. Letter.
35. Hall JG: Vitamin A: A newly recognized human teratogen—harbinger of things to come? J Pediatr 1984;105:583–584.
36. Hatoff DE, Gertler SL, Miyai K, et al: Hypervitaminosis A unmasked by acute viral hepatitis. Gastroenterology 1982; 82:124–128.
37. Henkin Y, Oberman A, Hurst DC, Segrest JP: Niacin revisited: Clinical observations on an important but underutilized drug. Am J Med 1991;91:239–246.
38. Herbert V: The vitamin craze. Arch Intern Med 1980;140: 173–176.
39. Holick MF, Shao Q, Liu WW, Chen TC: The vitamin D content of fortified milk and infant formula. N Engl J Med 1992; 326:1178–1181.
40. Horwitz RI, Daniels SR: Bias or biology: Evaluating the epidemiologic studies of L-tryptophan and the eosinophilia myalgia syndrome. J Rheumatol 1996;46(suppl):60–72.
41. Howard JE, Meyer RJ: Intoxication by vitamin D. J Clin Endocrinol Metab 1948;8:895–910.
42. Inkeles SB, Connor WE, Illingworth DR: Hepatic and dermatologic manifestations of chronic hypervitaminosis A in adults: Report of two cases. Am J Med 1986;80:491–496.
43. Issenman RM, Slack R, MacDonald L, Taylor W: Children's multiple vitamins: Overuse leads to overdose. Can Med Assoc J 1985;132:781–784.
44. Jacobus CH, Holick MF, Shao Q, et al: Hypervitaminosis D associated with drinking milk. N Engl J Med 1992;326: 1173–1177.
45. James TN, Kamb ML, Sandberg GA, et al: Postmortem studies of the heart in three fatal cases of the eosinophilia myalgia syndrome. Ann Intern Med 1991;115:102–110.
46. Kamb ML, Murphy JJ, Jones JL, et al: Eosinophilia myalgia syndrome in L-tryptophan exposed patients. JAMA 1992; 267:77–82.
47. Kilbourne EM, de la Paz MP, Borda IA, et al: Toxic oil syndrome: A current clinical and epidemiologic summary including comparisons with the eosinophilia myalgia syndrome. J Am Coll Cardiol 1991;18:711–717.
48. Kilbourne EM, Philen RM, Kamb ML, et al: Tryptophan produced by Showa Denko and epidemic eosinophilia-myalgia syndrome. J Rheumatol 1996;46(suppl):81–88.
49. Kilbourne EM, Rigau-Perez JH, Heath CW, et al: Clinical epidemiology of toxic-oil syndrome: Manifestations of a new illness. N Engl J Med 1983;309:1408–1414.
50. Kim SY, Lee-Kim YC, Kim MK, et al: Serum levels of antioxidant vitamins in relation to coronary disease: A case control study of Koreans. Biomed Environ Sci 1996;9:229–235.
51. Kowalski TE, Falestiny M, Furth E, Malet PF: Vitamin A hepatoxicity: A cautionary note regarding 25,000 IU supplements. Am J Med 1994;97:523–528.
52. Kushi LH, Fee RM, Sellers TA, et al: Intakes of vitamins A, C, and E and postmenopausal breast cancer. The Iowa Women's Health Study. Am J Epidemiol 1996;144:165–174.

53. Kushi LH, Folsom AR, Prineas RJ, et al: Dietary antioxidant vitamins and death from coronary heart disease in postmenopausal women. N Engl J Med 1996;334:1156–1162.
54. Lammer EJ, Chen DT, Hoar RM, et al: Retinoic acid embryopathy. N Engl J Med 1985;313:837–841.
55. Lawton JM, Conway LT, Crosson JT, et al: Acute oxalate nephropathy after massive ascorbic acid administration. Arch Intern Med 1985;145:950–951.
56. Leo MA, Arai M, Sato M, Lieber CS: Hepatotoxicity of moderate vitamin A supplementation in the rat. Gastroenterology 1982;82:194–205.
57. Lysak WR, Svien HJ: Long term follow-up on patients with diagnosis of pseudotumor cerebri. J Neurol Surg 1966;25: 284–287.
58. Marcus R, Coulston AM: Fat-soluble vitamins. In: Gilman AG, Rall TW, Nies AS, Taylor P, eds: The Pharmacological Basis of Therapeutics, 8th ed. New York, Pergamon Press, 1990, pp. 1553–1563.
59. McAllister OJ, Scowden EB, Dewberry FL, et al: Renal failure secondary to massive infusion of vitamin C. JAMA 1984;252:1684. Letter.
60. Misselwitz J, Hesse V, Markestad T: Nephrocalcinosis, hypercalciuria and elevated serum levels of 1,25-dihydrovitamin D in children. Acta Paediatr Scand 1990;79:637–643.
61. Moertel CG, Fleming TR, Creagan ET, et al: High dose vitamin C versus placebo in the treatment of patients who have no prior chemotherapy: A randomized double blind comparison. N Engl J Med 1985;312:137–141.
62. Morrice G, Havener W, Kapetansky F: Vitamin A intoxication as a cause of pseudotumor cerebri. JAMA 1960;173: 1802–1805.
63. Muenter M, Perry H, Ludwig J: Chronic vitamin A intoxication in adults. Am J Med 1971;50:129–136.
64. Parry GJ, Bredesen DE: Sensory neuropathy with low dose pyridoxine. Neurology 1985;35:1466–1468.
65. Philen RM, Ortiz DI, Auerbach SB, Falk H: Survey of advertising for nutritional supplements in health and body building magazines. JAMA 1992;268:1008–1011.
66. Rader JI, Calvert RJ, Hathcock JN: Hepatic toxicity of unmodified and time release preparations of niacin. Am J Med 1992;92:77–81.
67. Read MH, Graney AS: Food supplement usage by the elderly. J Am Diet Assoc 1982;80:250–253.
68. Restak R: Pseudotumor cerebri, psychosis, and hypervitaminosis A. J Nerv Ment Dis 1972;15:572–575.
69. Roberts HJ: Perspective of vitamin E as therapy. JAMA 1981;246:129–131.
70. Roels O: Vitamin A physiology. JAMA 1970;214:1097–1102.
71. Rosa FW, Wilk AL, Kelsey FO: Teratogen update: Vitamin A congeners. Teratology 1986;33:355–364.
72. Rudman D, William PJ: Megadose vitamins: Use and misuse. N Engl J Med 1983;309:488–489.
73. Rush JA: Pseudotumor cerebri: Clinical profile and visual outcome in 63 patients. Mayo Clin Proc 1980;55:541–546.
74. Saul RF, Hamburger HA, Selhorst JB: Pseudotumor cerebri secondary to lithium carbonate. JAMA 1985;253:2869–2870.
75. Schaumburg H, Kaplan J, Windebank A, et al: Sensory neuropathy from pyridoxine abuse: A new megavitamin syndrome. N Engl J Med 1983;309:445–448.
76. Seelig, MS: Vitamin D and cardiovascular, renal and brain damage in infancy and childhood. Ann NY Acad Sci 1969; 147:537–582.
77. Silverman AK, Ellis CN, Vorrhees JJ: Hypervitaminosis A syndrome: A paradigm of retinoid side effects. J Am Acad Dermatol 1987;16:1027–1039.
78. Singh RB, Niaz MA, Rastogi SS, et al: Usefulness of antioxidant vitamins in suspected acute myocardial infarction (the Indian experiment of infarct survival—3). Am J Cardiol 1996;77:232–236.
79. Slutsker L, Hoesly FC, Miller L, et al: Eosinophilia myalgia syndrome associated with exposure to tryptophan from a single manufacture. JAMA 1990;264:213–217.
80. Smith SA: Persistent microvasculopathy in chronic eosinophilia–myalgia syndrome. Adv Exp Med Biol 1996; 398;359–364.
81. Spitzer WO, Haggerty JL, Berkson L, et al: Analysis of Centers for Disease Control and Prevention criteria for the eosinophilia–myalgia syndrome in a geographically defined population. J Rheumatol 1996;46(suppl):73–79.
82. Stern RH, Spence JD, Freeman DJ, Parbtani A: Tolerance to nicotinic acid flushing. Clin Pharmacol Ther 1991;50:66–70.
83. Sternberg EM: Pathogenesis of L-tryptophan eosinophilia myalgia syndrome. Adv Exp Med Biol 1996;398;325–330.
84. Stimson W: Vitamin A intoxication in adults. N Engl J Med 1961;265:369–373.
85. Swartz RD, Wesley JR, Somermeyer MG, et al: Hyperoxaluria and renal insufficiency due to ascorbic acid administration during total parenteral nutrition. Ann Intern Med 1984;100:530–531.
86. Varga J, Vitto J, Jimenez SA: The cause and pathogenesis of eosinophilia myalgia syndrome. Ann Intern Med 1992;116: 140–147.
87. Weber FL, Mitchell GE Jr, Powell DE, et al: Reversible hepatotoxicity associated with hepatic vitamin A accumulation in a protein-deficient patient. Gastroenterology 1982; 82:118–123.
88. Weisberg L: The syndrome of increased intracranial pressure without localizing signs: A reappraisal. Neurology 1975;25:85–88.
89. Whelan AM, Price SO, Fowler SF, Hainer BL: The effect of aspirin on niacin-induced cutaneous reactions. J Fam Pract 1992;34:165–168.

CHAPTER 37

Dieting Agents, Regimens, and Food Supplements

Jeanmarie Perrone

A 34-year-old male bodybuilder was brought to the emergency department by friends on a Friday night after he collapsed in a bar and had a seizure. He was described as initially combative following the seizure and subsequently deeply unresponsive. Vital signs in the emergency department were: blood pressure, 110/60 mm Hg; heart rate, 55 beats/min; respiratory rate, 14 breaths/min; and temperature, 97 °F (36.1°C). A finger stick glucose analysis was 130 mg/dL and no response was noted following 2 mg naloxone intravenously. The patient had a poor gag reflex and was intubated for airway protection and ventilation. The patient underwent orogastric lavage; however, no pill fragments were noted. Activated charcoal (1 g/kg) was administered via the orogastric tube. His blood pressure improved to 130/70 mm Hg following a fluid bolus of 1 L 0.9% NaCl. The heart rate ranged from 55 to 80 beats/min. Physical examination was significant for pupils 3–4 mm and reactive, moist mucous membranes, dry skin, nondistended abdomen with normal bowel sounds, and no palpable bladder. Neurologic examination initially revealed a patient who was sluggishly responsive to deep pain and was otherwise nonfocal. Over 1–2 hours the patient rapidly improved until he was following commands appropriately. Electrolytes were normal. Toxicology testing was negative for salicylates and acetaminophen. He was extubated after 4 hours in the emergency department with a normal mental status. The patient admitted to drinking alcohol with his friends but also using "Somatomax PM," a gamma-hydroxybutyrate supplement that he obtained via a health store mail-order catalog.

Who Uses Diet Aids?

Although obesity is the second leading cause of preventable death in the United States,[56] dieting fads and obsessions influence far more people than the estimated 58 million Americans who are considered obese. A recent search of this topic on the Internet revealed 7873 sites on diets, 39,281 on weight loss, and 9602 on diet medications. Dieting is estimated to be a $33 billion industry annually in the United States.[52] It is easy to anticipate the numerous medical consequences and toxicities of some of these proposed techniques for weight loss. Many dieting regimens of the past resulted in significant toxicity; review of these historical accounts suggests exercising caution before embracing any new diet therapy. Sadly, the extremes of dieting toxicity continue to be manifested in the many people who suffer from anorexia nervosa and bulimia.

Dieting aids are conceptually very simple, yet include an expansive list of modalities to assist in the quest of taking in less energy than needed to produce a net calorie deficit and thus weight loss. Some dieting aids are anorexiants, to decrease appetite and decrease calorie

TABLE 37–1. ANOREXIANTS: PRESCRIPTION AND OTC AGENTS

Serotonergic Agents	Amphetamines and Derivatives
Fenfluramine (Pondimin)	Dextroamphetamine (Dexedrine)
Dexfenfluramine (Redux)	Amphetamine/dextroamphetamine (Biphetamine)
Fluoxetine (Prozac) (not other SSRIs)	Phenmetrazine (Prelu-2)
	Phendimetrazine (Phenazine)
	Diethylpropion (Tenuate)
	Phentermine (Fastin, Ionamin)
	Phenylpropanolamine (Accutrim, Dexatrim, others)

intake. Anorexiants may be amphetamines, serotonergic agents, or both in some of the newer diet aids (Table 37–1). Some anorexiants such as ephedrine are available in "herbal" form, which is neither regulated nor monitored by the Food and Drug Administration. Other agents, such as gelatin or fiber diet pills, act by absorbing large amounts of water and expanding in the stomach and intestinal tract, thus producing the sensation of a large meal. Very-low-calorie diets or those containing high-protein liquid supplements advocate the intake of 300–800 calories per day and are associated with sudden cardiac death.

Another health food supplement, gamma-hydroxybutyrate, was popularized on the premise that it helps "burn fat into muscle" and has led to an epidemic of toxicity. Other techniques previously used and of historical interest include agents that inhibit absorption or prevent energy mobilization from ingested food. The use of both "starch blockers" and dinitrophenol represents attempts to block the caloric yield from an ingested meal.

Which Diet Aids Are Currently Available by Prescription?

Amphetamines and Derivatives

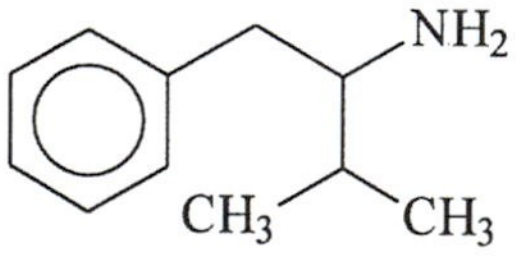

Phentermine

Amphetamines were noted to cause weight loss soon after their introduction in the 1930s. Interestingly, these early observations prompted investigations to characterize whether the weight loss resulted from increased activity (stimulant effects), increased basal metabolic rate, or decreased intake. The net anorexiant effect of amphetamines was well demonstrated in these early studies in animals, although tolerance to the anorectic effects was also noted.[81] Anorectic effects of the amphetamine class are mediated via beta-adrenergic and dopaminergic effects on the hypothalamus.

Despite much controversy within the medical community,[40] amphetamines are still suggested as indicated for short-term weight reduction, according to physician prescribing information.[3] Although many amphetamines and derivatives continue to be available, adverse side effects, dependence, and tolerance to their anorectic effects limit their efficacy and utility. Although the newest anorexiants available affect central serotonergic pathways, one popular combination regimen includes the use of both an amphetamine derivative and serotonergic drug. Known colloquially as "phen-fen," this refers to a combined regimen of phentermine (see above fig., an amphetamine derivative) and fenfluramine (a central serotonin acting agent—see below). This regimen was more popular due to the improved side-effect profile achieved with lower doses of each, and better long-term weight control.[86] Experience with overdose is limited but can be anticipated to reflect amphetamine toxicity (see Chap. 66). As reported with many amphetamines, cardiovascular and cerebrovascular toxicity is described following use of amphetamine derivatives (phentermine, phendimetrazine) for weight loss.[47,67]

Serotonergic Agents

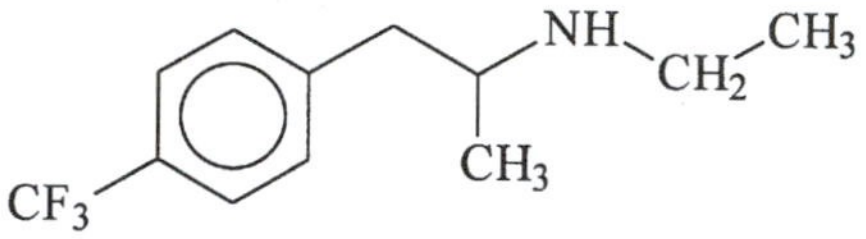

Dexfenfluramine

The use of the newest agents in this category is very controversial. Dexfenfluramine, the *d*-isomer of fenfluramine, was approved in 1995 for treatment of obesity and maintenance of weight loss (see above fig.).[4] Dexfenfluramine stimulates serotonin release and inhibits its reuptake by presynaptic neurons. It is metabolized to *d*-norfenfluramine, which binds to a serotonin receptor on the postsynaptic neuron, increasing activity.[77] Serotonin is believed to mediate satiety and appetite suppression. There is limited experience with overdose of these agents to date.

The well-publicized toxicity associated with therapeutic use of these drugs is an increased incidence of primary pulmonary hypertension. In a multicenter case control study of patients with primary pulmonary hypertension in Europe, an increased risk of the condition was associated with the use of anorectic drugs such as dexfenfluramine and fenfluramine as well as phendimetrazine.[1] The risk of primary pulmonary hypertension was 30 times higher in patients using the drug for more than 3 months compared to obese nonusers.[1] Primary pulmonary hypertension has been reported in association with fenfluramine since 1981.[5,11,15,25,58,66] A similar outbreak of primary pulmonary hypertension in Europe was described with the anorexiant aminorex fumarate in the 1960s.[41]

Several theories have been proposed about the mechanism of pulmonary toxicity of these agents.[15] Serotonin contracts isolated pulmonary arteries in dogs and humans.[10,57] In addition, serotonin-mediated platelet aggregation and vasoconstriction in the lungs appears to be irreversible.[57] This may lead to microembolization, elevated pulmonary vascular resistance, and pulmonary hypertension.

Following a series of case reports of rare cardiovascular manifestations associated with the combined use of fenfluramine and phentermine in 1997 the FDA withdrew its approval of fenfluramine and reiterated that the use of the combination of fenfluramine-phentermine had never been approved for use by the FDA. Of particular importance was the series of cases demonstrating valvular heart disease in 24 women treated with fenfluramine-phentermine who had no history of cardiac disease.[19] These women either presented with cardiovascular symptoms or solely with a heart murmur. They all had either right or left sided valvular abnormalities of morphology or regurgitation. Eight of these women also had newly documented pulmonary hypertension. Several of the patients had cardiovascular surgery which demonstrated plaque-like encasement of the leaflets and chordal structures while preserving intact valve structure. These pathological findings were identical to those seen in patients with the carcinoid syndrome or those with ergotamine induced valvular disease.

Which Anorexiants Are Commonly Available Over the Counter?

Phenylpropanolamine

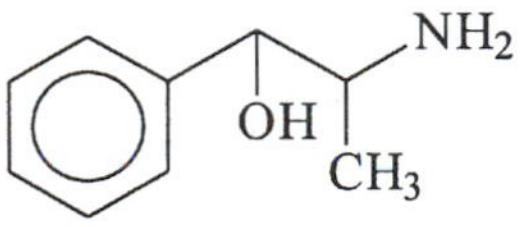

Some amphetamine derivatives, for example phenylpropanolamine (see above fig.), continue to be available in over-the-counter diet preparations. Supplements are available containing 25 to 75 mg phenylpropanolamine in sustained-release preparations. Anorectic effects of the amphetamine class are mediated via beta-adrenergic and dopaminergic effects on the hypothalamus. A second mechanism, involving alpha-adrenergic receptors within the hypothalamus, may account for phenylpropanolamine-mediated anorexia.[87] Phenylpropanolamine is a sympathomimetic amine, similar to ephedrine. It is both a direct-acting agent, via stimulation of alpha-adrenergic receptors, and indirect, through release of norepinephrine. Both actions tend to cause a net increase in blood pressure when given in high doses. Many reports of severe hypertension following "therapeutic" and toxic doses of phenylpropanolamine have been published. Some of the doses resulted in intracranial hemorrhage and death.[31,32,39,42,45,59] Additionally, hypertensive adverse drug interactions between phenylpropanolamine and drugs such as monoamine oxidase inhibitors and nonsteroidal antiinflammatory agents are reported.[51,73] A comprehensive review of over one hundred case reports of adverse drug effects involving phenylpropanolamine described 24 cases of intracranial hemorrhages, 8 with seizures, and 8 fatalities between 1965 and 1990.[49] Many other patients suffered severe hypertension, headaches, and/or encephalopathy. Some of these adverse events occurred following ingestion of diet preparations that contained both phenylpropanolamine and caffeine.[46] The FDA banned PPA–caffeine combination products from the market in 1983. However, patients may continue to experience adverse events from ingesting phenylpropanolamine in combination with caffeine-containing beverages or medications. The toxicologic manifestations of these products may be synergistic, as one author suggested.[50] Cardiac toxicity, although less common, was recently reported in two young patients who suffered myocardial injury following both therapeutic daily dosing and an acute overdose.[53]

What Are the Clinical Findings of Patients With PPA Toxicity? What is the Treatment?

Patients with phenylpropanolamine toxicity may present with anxiety, agitation, psychosis, seizures, palpitations, chest pain, or headache.[63] While hypertension is common following overdose, some patients may also present with confusion and altered mental status as a result of hypertensive encephalopathy. Reflex bradycardia may accompany the hypertension and may be a clue to the diagnosis. Adolescents compose a large group who may be using these agents. Unintentional or intentional overdose in this population may present with seemingly mild elevations in blood pressure. However, this mildly elevated blood pressure may be poorly tolerated by the patient since the individual's baseline blood pressure may be significantly lower. Hypertension should be treated aggressively, either with phentolamine, a rapidly acting alpha-adrenergic antagonist, nifedipine, or nitroprusside. Toddlers with unintentional ingestions may be at especially high risk for hypertensive episodes due to the relatively significant dose ingested on a milligram per kilogram (mg/kg) basis.

Ephedrine

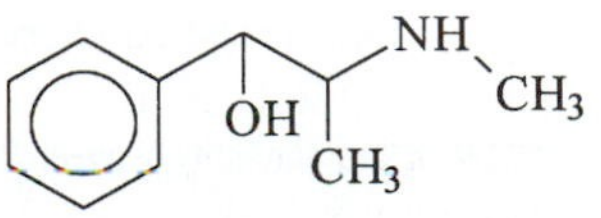

Ephedrine (see above fig.), like gamma-hydroxybutyrate (GHB), has become a popular health food supplement. Known by its Chinese herbal nomenclature, *ma huang*, or simply as Chinese ephedra, it is alleged to have various properties. Ephedrine is advertised as an energy supplement and as a dieting aid. It has become known as "herbal ecstasy," supposedly a safer, plant-derived "herbal" form of ephedrine. Ephedrine is a sympathomimetic amine that has pharmacologic indications in the treatment of asthma, hypotension, and nasal decongestion. It is not indicated or available for treatment of obesity in proprietary form; however, it has been abused for its stimulant and anorectic properties. A recent report described over five hundred adverse events associated with ephedrine-containing dietary supplements over a 2-year period.[64] Adverse effects included palpitations, tachycardia, syncope, hypertension, psychoses, convulsions, coronary vasospasm, chest pain, acute myocardial infarction, and cerebrovascular ischemia.[12,64] There were eight deaths due to cardiovascular or cerebrovascular complications. It has been proposed that most incidents occurred because the public did not perceive the potential for adverse reactions from a "natural" or "herbal" product.[64] Other reports of toxic reactions secondary to "herbal" ephedrine include psychosis and mania.[16,26,44] Abuse by two adolescents of a concentrated ephedrine food supplement led to severe hypertension[61] and life-threatening drug interactions with monoamine oxidase inhibitors.[23] These reports of toxicity underscore the need for regulation of these products. However, the "herbal" industry lobbied successfully in 1993 against FDA regulation of these products, which led to the Health Education Act of 1994. This law created a new category, separate from food and drugs, which includes vitamins, minerals, herbs, and amino acids and is virtually free from FDA regulations.[44] Clinicians should be encouraged to continue reporting adverse events involving these products to poison centers and the FDA in order that appropriate regulations may be sought.

Gamma-Hydroxybutyrate

Gamma-hydroxybutyrate, or GHB, as it is commonly known, is becoming increasingly popular in the United States. GHB emerged as a popular diet fad in bodybuilders in the early 1990s, and was purported to release growth hormone and "burn fat into muscle while you sleep." Although it has no medical indications in the United States, it has been investigated in Europe as an agent to treat alcohol withdrawal and as an anaesthetic.[18] It was initially sold in health food stores; however, reports of toxicity and abuse prompted many states to prohibit sales, and the agent now is largely obtained illicitly and via mail order. Apparently, GHB is synthesized easily by adding sodium hydroxide to gamma-hydroxybutyrolactone, a common industrial solvent.[28] A recent report highlighted the caustic potential of sodium hydroxide in these "homemade" admixtures.[17]

GHB is a catabolite of gamma-aminobutyric acid (GABA), the primary inhibitory neurotransmitter in the central nervous system (see Fig. 37–1). GHB may act by increasing dopamine levels and endogenous opioids in the brain.[55] Potential effects on other neurotransmitters has led to the theory that it may be a direct neuromodulator or a neurotransmitter.[18] GHB is reported to cause seizures[17,29,78] and GHB-induced seizures have been used as a model of absence seizures in monkeys.[75] These seizures do not appear to be mediated via a direct effect of GHB at the $GABA_A$ receptor.[74]

What Are the Clinical Effects of GHB Overdose?

Over one hundred cases of GHB toxicity have been reported to the Centers for Disease Control and Prevention;[17,30] many of these patients manifested CNS and respiratory depression, often following dosing recommendations on the bottle of $\frac{1}{2}$ to 3 teaspoons at bedtime.[30] Of these 114 patients, 15 required intubation, highlighting the potency of the CNS depressant effects of this agent. Concurrent ethanol use, which was common, appears to exacerbate the effects. Additional cases have been reported sporadically, with similar findings.[36,78,79] Two fatalities are described; however, concomitant heroin abuse was suspected in one case.[17,33] Treatment of GHB intoxication is largely supportive, and one of the hallmarks of GHB intoxication is the recovery of consciousness from obtundation relatively rapidly. Although naloxone use has been considered, the lack of response in anecdotal cases does not support its use.[29,78] Because of proposed activity at the GABA receptor, a recent investigation examined the use of flumazenil in an animal model of GHB intoxication. These authors were able to demonstrate efficacy in delaying GHB intoxication in a small number of animals pretreated with flumazenil.[68]

Inadvertent GHB toxicity in two children was re-

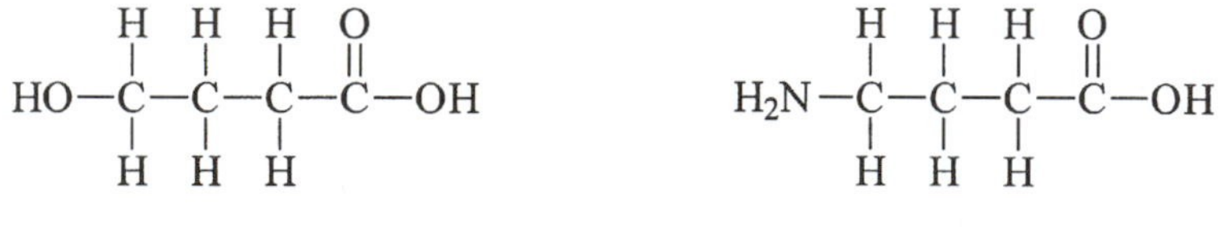

Gamma-hydroxybutyric acid (GHB) Gamma-aminobutyric acid (GABA)

Figure 37–1. Note structural similarity between the inhibitory neurotransmitter gamma-aminobutyric acid (GABA) and gamma-hydroxybutyric acid (GHB).

cently reported, with manifestations consistent with adult presentations.[80] These children became poisoned by unintentionally ingesting an illicit "homemade" GHB preparation synthesized by their parents.

What Other Approaches of Historical Interest Have Been Used for Dieting?

Starch Blockers

Amylase inhibitors, so-called starch blockers, were proposed as diet aids that would prevent the absorption of carbohydrates by blocking their breakdown into sugars. These starch blockers were widely sold over the counter and in health food stores in the early 1980s. However, scientific evidence supporting their efficacy was lacking. In an elegant study in human volunteers, fecal calorie excretion following a high-starch meal of spaghetti and white bread was measured with and without the use of a starch blocker tablet. The authors showed no difference in net calorie excretion, with and without the amylase inhibitor, and proposed that the lack of efficacy was due to the ability of the pancreas to secrete amylase in excess of that which is needed to digest any one particular meal.[8]

Dinitrophenol

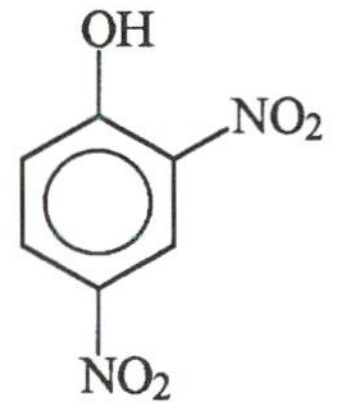

One of the earliest attempts at a pharmaceutical cure for obesity was advanced in the 1930s, when dinitrophenol was popularized as a weight loss adjuvant (see above fig.).[83] Dinitrophenol inhibits metabolism by uncoupling oxidative phosphorylation and thus leads to decreased caloric yield from ingested meals.[22] This net calorie loss is manifested as heat; however, an elevated temperature and occasionally hyperthermia were reported.[82] In addition, yellow skin discoloration, cataracts, hepatotoxicity, and fatalities related to overdose occurred, and eventually DNP use was abandoned.[9,38,48,82] Interestingly, DNP continued to be used in the photochemical industry and a disturbing epidemic occurred in Texas in the 1980s when a chemist processed industrial DNP into tablets and began to distribute them in his weight-loss center. Unfortunately, it was not until the hyperthermic death of a wrestler using this product that authorities became involved and were able to prevent further distribution and sales.[48]

Guar Gum

Guar gum is derived from the bean of the *Cyamopsis psorabides* plant. It was marketed in pill or tablet form as Cal-Ban 3000 (Anderson Pharmaceuticals, Lutz, Florida) until it was banned in 1992. These pills contained the hygroscopic guar gum polysaccharide that expanded 10–20-fold in the stomach, forming a gelatinous mass. This swelling and distention in the stomach led to the sensation of satiety in the dieter and, thus, decreased appetite and intake. However, guar gum was also responsible for many adverse effects, including esophageal and small bowel obstruction.[54,65] Initially, cases of esophageal obstruction were reported in patients with predisposing anatomic lesions such as strictures.[37,70] However, a follow-up report of 26 patients reported to the FDA with obstruction secondary to guar gum ingestion revealed that half had normal gastrointestinal anatomy.[54]

What Is the Relationship Between the Long QT Interval and Hypocaloric Diets?

A variety of extreme calorie-restricted diets resulting in profound weight loss enjoyed great popularity in the late 1970s. Reports followed shortly thereafter of a possible association with sudden death in patients on these diets or during a period of refeeding following profound weight loss and calorie restriction. Several case reports and case series of these patients are reported.[13,60,69,76,84] One case series investigated the circumstances involved in 17 of 58 sudden deaths in patients using these very-low-calorie diets.[76] Several characteristics of these patients emerged that may contribute to an explanation of this association. All of the patients were relatively young (median age 35 years) and morbidly obese (106.5 kg). All had been on the diet for a minimum of 2 months with an average weight loss of 2.1 kg/week. Most (13 of 17) of these patients were taking the "liquid protein" diet as well as vitamin supplement. Daily intake was reported to be 300–400 kcal. A small number of these patients had electrolytes checked while dieting; of note, 6 had hypokalemia ($K < 3.5$ mEq/L, range 2.2–5.2 mEq/L).

The circumstances regarding the deaths of these patients was also of concern. Six patients died while under observation in the hospital after being admitted for syncope and suffered ventricular dysrhythmias refractory to treatment. Although most patients were still dieting, 7 of 17 were refeeding at the time of their death. Electrocardiograms demonstrated low voltage and prolonged QT interval in 10 cases, although some were obtained prior to dieting. Similar electrocardiographic findings were reported in severe calorie restriction, starvation, and refeeding as well as at baseline in 28% percent of obese patients.[34] Three of these patients experienced multiple episodes of torsades de pointes prior to their fatal dysrhythmia.[72] Autopsies were available in 16 cases. Myocardial atrophy was the most common and consistent finding noted. These and other authors have proposed that the cause of death was secondary to the effects of protein–calorie malnutrition on the heart,[27,76] whereas others postulated a diet-induced ECG repolarization abnormality predisposing to these dysrhythmias.[72]

In studies designed to examine possible etiologies for these dysrhythmic events, 11 volunteer patients underwent continuous telemetry in hospital while undergoing complete fasting on a zero-calorie diet.[89] No prolongation of the QT interval or significant dysrhythmia was noted in these patients. However, the study was performed at the initiation of their fasting period, whereas most adverse events have been reported in the setting of prolonged calorie restriction over months. In a second study, six obese subjects were fed a low-calorie diet mixture of proteins as well as minerals, trace elements, vitamins, and essential fatty acids.[2] Holter monitors and EKGs were analyzed over a 40-day period. No dysrhythmias or significant QT prolongation was observed. The authors concluded that dieting with liquid-protein preparations that are adequately supplemented is safe.

Following many of these negative reports and FDA warnings, most enthusiasm for the liquid-protein diets waned until the early 1980s, when a new series of low-calorie diets was popularized. The "Cambridge diet" included a higher grade of protein supplement as well as more calories overall (400–800/day). The proponents of these diets argue that protein wasting is limited and thus the diets may be safer.[88] Some studies support these safety claims,[20,71] but close medical supervision is advocated during dieting.[85] There is one case reported of sudden death in a patient on the Cambridge diet.[21]

Which Medications Have Been Abused by Patients With Eating Disorders?

Although many forms of eating disorders are described, the extent of medication abuse can be remarkable.[14] Starvation, as well as abuse of laxatives, syrup of ipecac, diuretics, and anorexiants, has led to many fatalities, often in young patients.[35,43] Additionally, these agents have been abused by parents or guardians to produce factitious chronic illness in children suffering from Munchausen Syndrome by Proxy. Eating disorders should be considered especially in young women with unexplained dehydration, syncope, or electrolyte disturbances.

Chronic use of syrup of ipecac to induce emesis in patients with anorexia has lead to many cases of cardiomyopathy, subsequent dysrhythmias, and death.[35,62] Emetine, which is toxic to skeletal and cardiac muscle cells, is considered the alkaloid responsible for the severe myopathy in these patients. In addition, chronic administration of syrup of ipecac leads to tolerance of the emetic effects and increased systemic absorption of emetine.[62]

Laxatives are another common modality of abuse in patients with eating disorders. Although not as toxic as syrup of ipecac, chronic laxative abuse results in a vicious cycle of tolerance and increasing doses. There appears to be no net effect of cathartics on decreasing food absorption, and thus these agents do little for weight control chronically.[7] Regardless, chronic laxative abuse results in diarrhea, hypokalemia, metabolic alkalosis, dehydration, and an atonic colon.[6] Various screening methods can be used to detect laxative abuse.[24] Phenolphthalein can be detected in stool following alkalinization. Colonoscopy will reveal the pathognomonic "melanosis coli," dark staining of the colonic mucosa secondary to anthraquinone laxative abuse.

Diuretics are also used to decrease body water and weight. Many diets, especially "herbal" plans, will emphasize the use of some naturally occurring diuretics to "demonstrate efficacy" and bolster encouragement during the first few days of dieting. Like laxatives, diuretics cannot produce a net weight loss when used chronically.

Summary

Although obesity is a major health consideration and a tremendous cause of preventable morbidity and mortality, unproven cures are fraught with failure and toxicity. There is no current substitute for increasing the deficit between calories taken in and those utilized through activity and exercise. The safest approach to weight loss is one that incorporates nutritional counseling, behavioral therapy, and an appropriate exercise regimen to permanently alter lifestyle factors contributing to obesity.

References

1. Abenhaim L, Moride Y, Brenot F, et al: Appetite suppressant drugs and the risk of primary pulmonary hypertension. N Engl J Med 1996;335:609–616.
2. Amatruda JM, Biddle TL, Patton ML, Lockwood DH: Vigorous supplementation of a hypocaloric diet prevents cardiac arrhythmias and mineral depletion. Am J Med 1983;74:1016–1022.
3. Anonymous: Dexedrine. Physician's Desk Reference, 51st ed. Montvale, NJ, Medical Economics, 1997, pp. 2648–2650.
4. Anonymous: Dexfenfluramine for obesity. Medical Lett 1996;38:64–65.
5. Atanassoff PG, Weiss BK, Schmid ER, Tornic M: Pulmonary hypertension and dexfenfluramine. Lancet 1992;339: 436–437.
6. Baker EH, Sandle GI: Complications of laxative abuse. Annu Rev Med 1996;47:127–134.
7. Bo-Linn GW, Santa Ana CA, Morawski SG, Fordtran JS: Purging and calorie absorption in bulimic patients and normal women. Ann Intern Med 1983;99:14–17.
8. Bo-Linn GW, Santa Ana CA, Morawski SG, Fordtran JS: Starch blockers—their effect on calorie absorption from a high-starch meal. N Engl J Med 1982;307:1413–1416.
9. Boardman WW: Rapidly developing cataract after dinitrophenol. JAMA 1935;105:108–110.
10. Boe J, Simonsson BG, Stahl E: Effect of histamine, 5-hydroxytryptamine, and prostaglandins on isolated pulmonary arteries. Eur J Respir Dis 1980;61:12–19.
11. Brenot F, Herve P, Petitprez P, et al: Primary pulmonary

hypertension and fenfluramine use. Br Heart J 1993;70: 537–541.
12. Bruno A, Nolte KB, Chapin J: Stroke associated with ephedrine use. Neurology 1993;43:1313–1316.
13. Brown JM, Yetter JF, Spicer MJ, Jones JD: Cardiac complications of protein-sparing modified fasting. JAMA 1978; 240:120–122.
14. Bulik C: Abuse of drugs associated with eating disorders. J Sub Abuse 1992;4:69–90.
15. Cacoub P, Dorent R, Nataf P, et al: Pulmonary hypertension and dexfenfluramine. Eur J Clin Pharmacol 1995;48:81–83.
16. Capwell RR: Ephedrine induced mania from an herbal diet supplement. Am J Psychiatry 1995;152:647. Letter.
17. Carter J, Mofenson H, Caraccio T, et al: Gamma hydroxy butyrate use—New York and Texas, 1995–1996. MMWR 1997;46:281–283.
18. Cash CD: Gamma-hydroxybutyrate: An overview of the pros and cons for it being a neurotransmitter and/or a useful therapeutic agent. Neurosci Biobehav Rev 1994;18: 291–304.
19. Connolly HM, Crary JL, McGoon MD, et al: Valvular heart disease associated with fenfluramine-phentermine. N Engl J Med 1997;337:581–588.
20. Council on Scientific Affairs: Treatment of obesity in adults. JAMA 1988;260:2547–2551.
21. Coxon A, Kreitzman S: Sudden death and the Cambridge diet. Lancet 1989;2:572. Letter.
22. Cutting WC, Mehrtens HG, Tainter ML: Actions and uses of dinitrophenol. JAMA 1933;101:193–195.
23. Dawson JK, Earnshaw SM, Graham CS: Dangerous monoamine oxidase inhibitor interactions are still occurring in the 1990's. J Accid Emerg Med 1995; 12:49–51.
24. De Wolff FA, Edelbroek PM, De Haas EJM, Vermeij P: Experience with a screening method for laxative abuse. Hum Toxicol 1983;2:385–389.
25. Douglas JG, Munro JF, Kitchin AH, et al: Pulmonary hypertension and fenfluramine. Br Med J 1981;283:881–882.
26. Doyle H, Kargin M: Herbal stimulant containing ephedrine has also caused psychosis. Br Med J 1996;313:756. Letter.
27. Drott C, Lunholm K: Cardiac effects of caloric restriction-mechanisms and potential hazards. Int J Obes Relat Metab Disord 1992:16:481–486.
28. Duchaine D: GHB: A home brew. In: Duchaine D, ed: The Underground Steroid Handbook. Marina Delray, California: Power Distributors 1992, pp. 45–48.
29. Dyer JE: Gamma-hydroxybutyrate: A health food product producing coma and seizurelike activity. Am J Emerg Med 1991;9:321–324.
30. Dyer JE, Kreutzer R, Quattrone A, et al: Multistate outbreak of poisonings associated with illicit use of gammahydroxybutyrate. MMWR 1990;39:861–863.
31. Edwards M, Russo L, Harwood-Nuss A: Cerebral infarction with a single oral dose of phenylpropanolamine. Am J Emerg Med 1987;5:163–164.
32. Fallis RJ, Fisher M: Cerebral vasculitis and hemorrhage associated with phenylpropanolamine. Neurology 1985;35: 405–407.
33. Ferrara SD, Tedeschi L, Frison G, Rossi A: Fatality due to gamma-hydroxybutyric acid (GHB) and heroin intoxication. J Forensic Sci 1995;40:501–504.
34. Frank S, Colliver JA, Frank A: The electrocardiogram in obesity: Statistical analysis of 109 patients. J Am Coll Cardiol 1986;7:295–299.
35. Friedman EJ: Death from ipecac intoxication in a patient with anorexia nervosa. Am J Psychiatry 1984;141;702–703.
36. Friedman J, Westlake R, Furman M: "Grievous bodily harm": Gamma hydroxybutyrate abuse leading to a Wernicke-Korsakoff syndrome. Neurology 1996;46:469–471.
37. Gebhard RL, Albrecht J: The diet pill that worked. N Engl J Med 1990;322:702. Letter.
38. Geiger JC: A death from dinitrophenol poisoning. JAMA 1933;101:1333–1334.
39. Glick R, Hoying J, Cerullo L, Perlman S: Phenylpropanolamine: An over the counter drug causing central nervous system vasculitis and intracerebral hemorrhage. Neurosurgery 1987;20:969–974.
40. Gunby P: Amphetamines may be banned for use in weight control. JAMA 1979;242:1244.
41. Gurtner HP: Aminorex and pulmonary hypertension. Cor Vasa 1985;27:160–171.
42. Horowitz JD, Lang WG, Kowes LG, et al: Hypertensive responses induced by PPA in anorectic and decongestant preparation. Lancet 1980;1:60–61.
43. Isner JM, Roberts WC, Heymsfield SB, Yager J: Anorexia nervosa and sudden death. Ann Intern Med 1985;102:49–52.
44. Jones TL: Dangerously revved. Ephedrine misuse poses health hazards. Tex Med 1996;92:52–53.
45. Kase CS, Foster TE, Reed JE, et al: Intracerebral hemorrhage and phenylpropanolamine use. Neurology 1987;37:399–404.
46. Kikta DG, Devereaux MW, Chandar K: Intracranial hemorrhages due to phenylpropanolamine. Stroke 1985;16: 510–512.
47. Kokkinos J, Levine SR: Possible association of ischemic stroke with phentermine. Stroke 1993;24:310–313.
48. Kurt TL, Anderson R, Petty C, et al: Dinitrophenol in weight loss: The poison center and public safety. Vet Hum Toxicol 1986;28:574–575.
49. Lake CR, Gallant S, Masson E, Miller P: Adverse drug effects attributed to phenylpropanolamine: A review of 142 case reports. Am J Med 1990;89:195–208.
50. Lake CR, Rosenberg DB, Gallant S, et al: Phenylpropanolamine increases plasma caffeine levels. Clin Pharmacol Ther 1990;47:675–685.
51. Lee KY, Vandongen R, Beilin LJ: Severe hypertension after ingestion of an appetite suppressant (phenylpropanolamine with indomethacin). Lancet 1979;2:1110–1111.
52. Lemonick MD: The new miracle drug? Time 1996;148: 61–67.
53. Leo PJ, Hollander JE, Shih RD, Marcus SM: Phenylpropanolamine and associated myocardial injury. Ann Emerg Med 1996;28:359–362.
54. Lewis JH: Esophageal and small bowel obstruction from guar gum-containing "diet pills": Analysis of 26 cases reported to the Food and Drug Administration. Am J Gastroenterol 1992;87:1424–1428.
55. Mamelak M: Gamma-hydroxybutyrate: An endogenous regulator of energy metabolism. Neurosci Biobehav Rev 1989;13:187–198.
56. McGinnis JM, Foege WH: Actual causes of death in the United States. JAMA 1993;270:2207–2212.

57. McGoon MD, Vanhoutte PM: Aggregating platelets contract isolated canine pulmonary arteries by releasing 5-hydroxytryptamine. J Clin Invest 1984;74:828–833.
58. McMurray J, Bloomfield P, Miller HC: Irreversible pulmonary hypertension after treatment with fenfluramine. Br Med J 1986;292:239–240.
59. Mesnard B, Ginn DR: Excessive phenylpropanolamine ingestion followed by subarachnoid hemorrhage. South Med J 1984;77:939. Letter.
60. Michiel RR, Sneider JS, Dickstein RA, et al: Sudden death in a patient on a liquid protein diet. N Engl J Med 1978; 298:1005–1007.
61. Pace S: Ma huang food supplement toxicity in two adolescents. J Toxicol Clin Toxicol 1996;34:598. Abstract.
62. Palmer EP, Guary AT: Reversible myopathy secondary to abuse of ipecac in patients with major eating disorders. N Engl J Med 1985;313:1457–1459.
63. Pentel P: Toxicity of over-the-counter stimulants. JAMA 1984;252:1898–1903.
64. Perrotta DM, Coody G, Culmo C: Adverse events associated with ephedrine-containing products—Texas, December 1993–September 1995. MMWR 1996;45:689–693.
65. Roach J, Martyak T, Benjamin G: Anhydrous pill ingestion: A new cause of esophageal obstruction. Ann Emerg Med 1987;16:913–914.
66. Rosche N, Labrune S, Braun JM, Huchon GJ: Pulmonary hypertension and dexfenfluramine. Lancet 1992;339: 436–437.
67. Rostagno C, Caciolli S, Felici M, et al: Dilated cardiomyopathy associated with chronic consumption of phendimetrazine. Am Heart J 1996;131:407–409.
68. Satz WA, Greene T, Dougherty T, Lee DC: An investigation of flumazenil to antagonize gamma hydroxybutyrate intoxication in a murine model. Acad Emerg Med 1997;4:439. Abstract.
69. Schmidinger H, Weber H, Zwiauer K, et al: Potential life-threatening cardiac arrhythmias associated with a conventional hypocaloric diet. Int J Cardiol 1987;14:55–63.
70. Seidner DL, Roberts IM, Smith MS: Esophageal obstruction after ingestion of a fiber-containing diet pill. Gastroenterology 1990;99:1820–1822.
71. Seim HC, Mitchell JE, Pomeroy C, deZwaan M: Electrocardiographic findings associated with very low calorie dieting. Int J Obesity Rel Metab Dis 1995;19:817–819.
72. Singh BN, Gaarder TD, Kanegae T, et al: Liquid protein diets and torsade de pointes. JAMA 1978;240:115–119.
73. Smookler S, Bermudez AJ: Hypertensive crisis resulting from an MAO-inhibitor and an over-the-counter appetite suppressant. Ann Emerg Med 1982;11:482–484.
74. Snead OC: Gamma hydroxybutyrate in the monkey. Neurology 1978;28:636–642.
75. Snead OC, Liu CC: $GABA_A$ receptor function in the gamma-hydroxybutyrate model of generalized absence seizures. Neuropharmacology 1993;32:401–409.
76. Sours HE, Frattali VP, Brand CD, et al: Sudden death associated with very low calorie weight reduction regimens. Am J Clin Nutr 1981;34:453–461.
77. Spedding M, Ouvry C, Millan M, et al: Neural control of dieting. Nature 1996;380:488. Letter.
78. Steele MT, Watson WA: Acute poisoning from gammahydroxybutyrate (GHB). Mo Med 1995;92:354–357.
79. Stephens BG, Baselt RC: Driving under the influence of GHB? J Anal Toxicol 1994;18:357–358.
80. Suner S, Szlatenyi C, Wang R: Gamma hydroxybutyrate toxicity in children. J Toxicol Clin Toxicol 1996;34:596. Abstract.
81. Tainter ML: Actions of benzedrine and propadrine in control of obesity. J Nutr 1944;27:89–105.
82. Tainter ML, Cutting WC: Febrile, respiratory and some other actions of dinitrophenol. J Pharmacol Exp Ther 1933;48;410–429.
83. Tainter ML, Stockton AB, Cutting WC: Dinitrophenol in the treatment of obesity. JAMA 1935;105:332–337.
84. Thwaites BC, Bose M: Very low calorie diets and pre-fasting prolonged QT interval. A hidden potential danger. West Ind Med J 1992;41:169–171.
85. Wadden TA, Van Itallie TB, Blackburn GL: Responsible and irresponsible use of very low calorie diets in the treatment of obesity. JAMA 1990;263:83–85.
86. Weintraub M, Sundaresan PR, Madan M, et al: Long term weight control study I (weeks 0–34): The enhancement of behavior modification, caloric restriction, and exercise by fenfluramine plus phentermine versus placebo. Clin Pharmacol Ther 1992;51:586–594.
87. Wellman PJ: Overview of adrenergic anorectic agents. Am J Clin Nutr 1992;55:193S–198S.
88. Wilson JHP: Cardiac complications of drastic weight reduction. Neth J Med 1986;29:129–133.
89. Zuckerman E, Yeshurun D, Goldhammer E, Shiran A: 24-hour electrocardiographic monitoring in morbidly obese patients during short-term zero calorie diet. Int J Obes Rel Metab Disord 1993;17:359–361.

CHAPTER 38

Caffeine

Neal A. Lewin

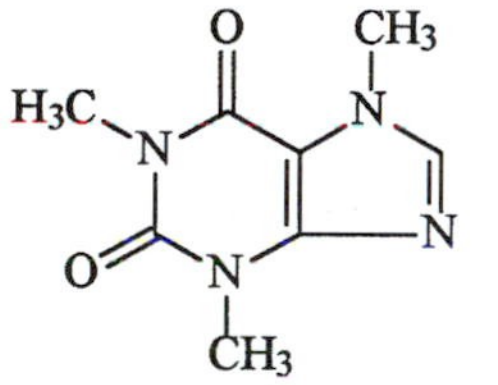

Caffeine
(1,3,7-trimethylxanthine)

Caffeine		
MW	=	194.22 daltons
Therapeutic serum level	=	1–10 μg/mL
Toxic serum level	>	25 μg/mL
	>	129 μmol/L

A 35-year-old woman presented to the emergency department (ED) complaining of a feeling of "impending doom." She stated that her heart was racing and she felt as though she was about to faint. She complained of tingling around her mouth and of her hands and feet. The patient was seen by a physician, blood samples were drawn, and she was given juice with several packets of sugar. A more detailed history revealed that she had recently separated from her husband and had been under tremendous financial strain. She had been getting "viselike" headaches for over a month, for which she was taking at least 10 tablets of Excedrin daily (see Table 38–1). The patient had been upset recently because, despite adhering to a rigid diet, substituting diet soda and black coffee for meals, and taking nonprescription diet pills, she still had been unable to lose weight. She denied use of illicit drugs, specifically cocaine, PCP, and LSD, and denied taking prescription medications such as cyclic antidepressants, amphetamines, asthma medications, thyroid medications, or other sympathomimetic agents.

Physical examination revealed a slender, anxious-appearing woman in no acute distress. Her vital signs were: blood pressure, 140/80 mm Hg; pulse, 120 beats/min with extrasystoles; respirations, 24 breaths/min; and temperature, 99.6°F (37.6°C). She weighed 110 lb and was 67 in. tall. Her skin was warm and diaphoretic and had no lesions. Her head was normocephalic and atraumatic. Pupils were mydriatic (7 mm) and reactive to light; there was no nystagmus, and the fundi were benign. The neck was supple without thyroid enlargement. The chest was clear. Cardiac auscultation revealed a regular tachycardia at a rate of 120 beats/min with four to five extrasystoles per minute; S_1 was normal and S_2 physiologically split. There were no murmurs, gallops, or rubs. The abdomen was scaphoid, without organomegaly; bowel sounds were hyperactive. Extremities showed no cyanosis, clubbing, or edema and no track marks. There were no masses and no occult blood on rectal examination. The neuropsychiatric examination was remarkable only for anxiety and hyperactive reflexes.

The initial arterial blood gas results were: pH 7.58; PCO_2 20 mm Hg; PO_2 95 mm Hg. Complete blood count results were: hematocrit 40%; hemoglobin 13 g/dL; WBC 11,000/mm^3 with a normal differential. Serum glucose (prior to juice and sugar) was 90 mg/dL; electrolytes, BUN, creatinine, and calcium were normal. The electrocardiogram showed a sinus tachycardia, four to five unifocal PVCs/minute, with no abnormalities in the PR, QRS, and QT_c intervals, and no ischemic changes. The salicylate level was 12 mg/dL, consistent with the patient's history of daily Excedrin brand aspirin usage, and acetaminophen level was zero. Thyroid function tests were requested.

Based on the history, physical findings, and laboratory data, the diagnosis was caffeine intoxication and/or phenylpropanolamine toxicity, with resultant anxiety and hyperventilation. Her sources of excessive caffeine intake were diet pills, Excedrin, a decongestant, soda, and coffee. Some physical findings might have been due to phenylpropanolamine, an alpha-adrenergic agonist found in many diet pills. The anxiety as well as the caffeinism resulted in hyperventilation, resulting in an acute respiratory alkalosis, as evidenced by the arterial blood gas (ABG) values.

Once it was determined that the salicylate level was in the low therapeutic range and that the patient was not acidemic, she was reassured that her physical condition was not serious and that she would feel better shortly. She was given 10 mg of diazepam orally, and observed on a cardiac monitor. Within 30 minutes the ectopy ceased and her pulse had slowed to 100 beats/min and respirations to 12 breaths/min. The patient appeared less anxious, and her circumoral paresthesias disappeared. A liaison psychiatrist evaluated the patient and arranged for outpatient psychotherapy; she was instructed to avoid all caffeinated substances.

What Is Caffeine? What Is Caffeinism?

Caffeine, a stimulant and psychoactive drug, is probably the most widely used of all mind-altering substances. The methylxanthines—caffeine (1,3,7-trimethylxanthine), theophylline (1,3-dimethylxanthine), and theobromine (3,7-dimethylxanthine)—are closely related plant-derived structures (Fig. 38–1). Caffeine's structure resembles that of purines such as adenine, guanine, adenosine, xanthine, and uric acid (Fig. 38–2). Pure caffeine is an odorless white powder, bitter in taste, and moderately soluble in water and organic solvents. It is very soluble in boiling water.[11] Beverages are made from the aqueous extracts of *Coffea arabica* (coffee), *Coffea robusta, Thea sinensis* (tea), *Theobroma cacao* (cocoa), and *Cola acuminata* (cola drinks)[5,42] (Table 38–1).

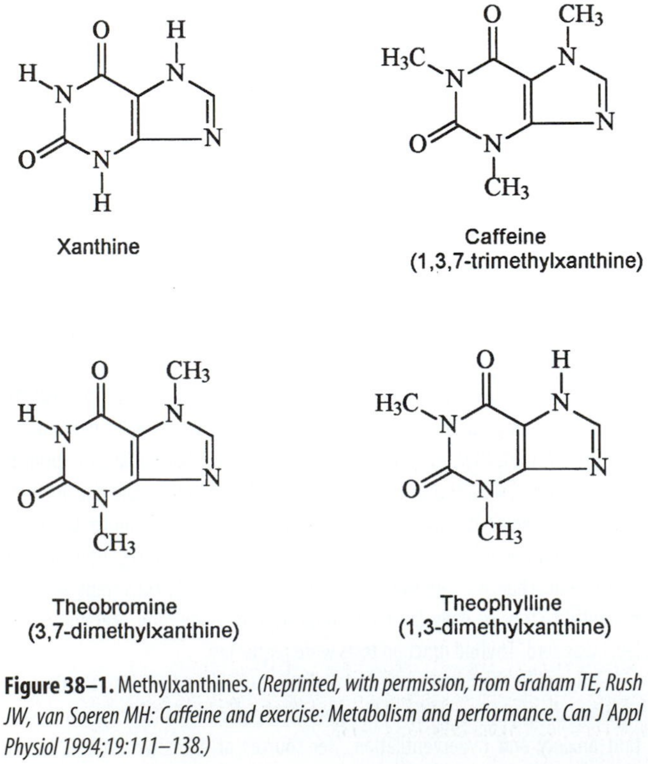

Figure 38–1. Methylxanthines. *(Reprinted, with permission, from Graham TE, Rush JW, van Soeren MH: Caffeine and exercise: Metabolism and performance. Can J Appl Physiol 1994;19:111–138.)*

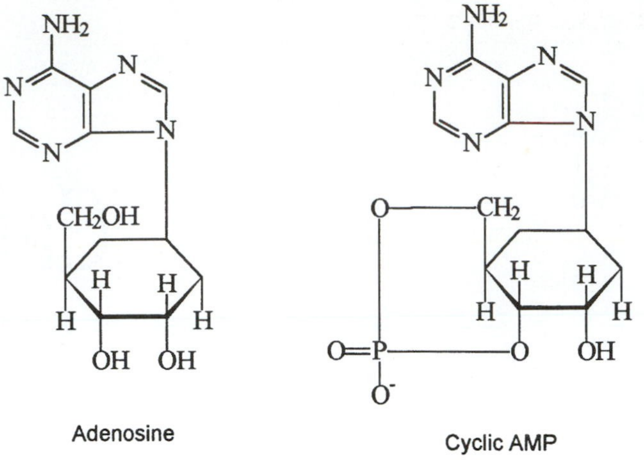

Figure 38–2. Adenosine and cyclic AMP. Note the similarity in the structures with the methylxanthines in Figure 38–1. *(Reprinted, with permission, from Graham TE, Rush JW, van Soeren MH: Caffeine and exercise: Metabolism and performance. Can J Appl Physiol 1994;19:111–138.)*

Caffeine-containing products have been used by both ancient and present societies seeking caffeine's stimulant and antisoporific effects.[47]

Caffeinism, a syndrome related to excessive caffeine use, has typical cardiovascular, gastrointestinal (GI), and neuropsychiatric characteristics. This symptom complex was described by Routh in 1883 and by Kraeplin in 1892. Kraeplin noted headache, delirium, palpitations, and tachycardia in patients with caffeinism.

What Are the Pharmacokinetic and Pharmacologic Properties of Caffeine?

Absorption of caffeine is more rapid after oral than intramuscular administration.[6] After absorption, caffeine, being lipophilic, rapidly diffuses into the total body water and all body tissues.[3,6] Caffeine crosses the placenta and the blood-brain barrier and is in breast milk.[11] Food slows the absorption of caffeine. Peak serum levels are reached in 30–60 minutes (Table 38–2); 36 ± 7% of caffeine is bound in plasma. The major pathway of caffeine catabolism is its demethylation in the liver to 1,7-dimethylxanthine (paraxanthine) via the microsomal cytochrome P450 system, primarily by the isoenzyme CYP1A2 (Fig. 38–3). It is then hydroxylated to 1, 7-dimethyluric acid or demethylated again by CYP1A2 to an *N*-acetylated ring split product or to 1-methylxanthine, which may be hydroxylated to 1-methyluric acid by xanthine oxidase.[22] In preterm infants caffeine is converted to theophylline in significant amounts.[47] Caffeine's urinary excretion is 1.1 ± 0.5%. Its clearance is 1.4 ± 0.5 mL/min/kg. Only 5% of caffeine is recovered in the

TABLE 38–1. THE CONCENTRATION OF CAFFEINE IN COMMON BEVERAGES AND PHARMACEUTICALS

Product	Caffeine Concentration	Quantity per Standard Serving Dose (mg/6 oz)
Beverage and food (mg/100 mL)		
Cocoa	4–10	8–20
Coffee		
Brewed	40–120	72–210
Decaffeinated	1–3	2–5
Cola drinks	10–15	35–55
Chocolate milk	2–7	
Milk chocolate bar (1 oz)	20	
Tea	13–16	25–110
Prescription medication (mg/tablet)		
Cafergot	100	
Darvon compound	32	
Synalgos	30	
Fiorinal	40	
Over-the-counter preparations (mg/tablet)		
Anacin maximum-strength tablets	32	
Bayer Select maximum-strength tablets	65	
Dristan	16.2	
Excedrin analgesic caplets	65	
Midol	32	
No-Doz	100	
Spantrol	150	
Vanquish	33	

TABLE 38–2. CAFFEINE PHARMACOKINETICS

GI Absorption	99–100%
Half-life	4.9 ± 1.8 h
Volume of distribution	0.61 ± 0.2 L/kg
Time to peak blood concentration	30–60 min
Urinary excretion	1.1 ± 0.5%
Bound in plasma	36 ± 7%
Clearance	1.4 ± 0.5 mL/min/kg

Reprinted, with permission, from Busto U, Bendyan R, Sellers EM: Clinical pharmacokinetics of non-opiate abuse drugs. Clin Pharmacokinet 1989;16:1–26.

urine unchanged. The principal urinary metabolites are 1-methylxanthine, 1-methyluric acid, and an acetylated uracil derivative. The half-life is 4.9 ± 1.8 hours.[7] Toxic effects may develop as rapidly as 10 minutes following administration, depending on the dosage and many host variables. For the first 6 months of life, during the late stages of pregnancy,[36] with cirrhosis, and with chronic use of oral contraceptives, the half-life is greatly prolonged. Caffeine's half-life is reduced in smokers,[7,23,42] and serum caffeine levels may double in patients who stop smoking.[11]

The physiologic effects of caffeine are listed in Table 38–3, and the models for its mechanism is depicted in Figure 38–4. The most significant effect of caffeine is mediated through purinoceptors.[18] Caffeine is a nonselective adenosine receptor antagonist, and its structure is similar to cyclic AMP and adenosine[18] (see Fig. 38–2). Adenosine is a naturally occuring nucleoside that acts on receptors A_1 and A_2; these receptors mediate an increase or decrease in cyclic AMP. High-affinity A_1 receptors inhibit adenyl cyclase by a guanyl nucleoside binding protein G_1. Low affinity A_2 receptors stimulate adenyl cyclase via another guanyl nucleoside binding G_2 (see Fig.

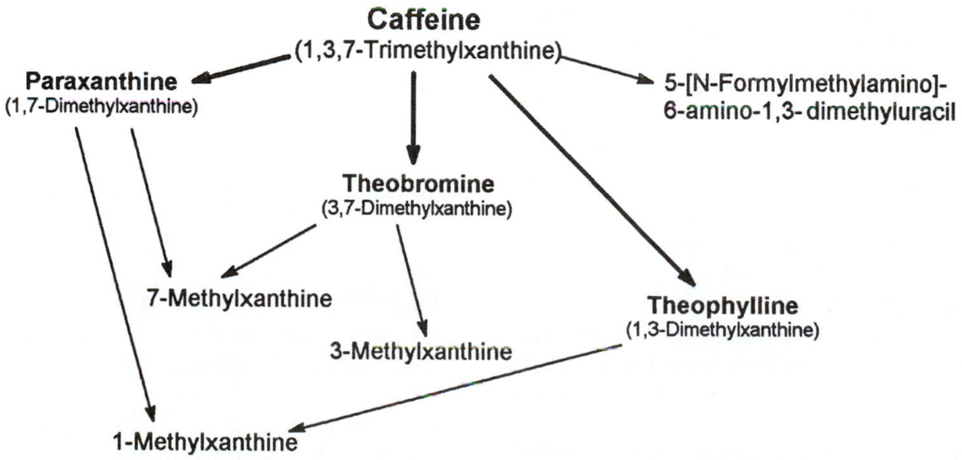

Figure 38–3. Metabolism of caffeine by the liver P450 system. In humans, initial biotransformation (arrows in bold) form the dimethylxanthines, paraxanthine, theobromine, and theophylline. These compounds undergo subsequent metabolism, as shown by lighter arrows. *(Reprinted with permission from Graham TE, Rush JW, van Soeren MH: Caffeine and exercise: Metabolism and performance. Can J Appl Physiol 1994;19:111–138.)*

TABLE 38–3. PHYSIOLOGIC EFFECTS OF CAFFEINE

Metabolic	Gastrointestinal
Increases cAMP concentration	Increases gastric acid and pepsin secretion
Antagonizes adenosine receptors	Increases small intestinal secretions
Increases intracellular calcium concentration	***Cardiovascular***
Hyperpolarizes cell membranes	Atrial and ventricular tachydysrhythmias and ventricular premature contractions
Increases oxygen consumption	Increases stroke volume
Increases basal metabolic rate	Increases cardiac output
Increases plasma renin activity	Increases blood pressure
Increases lactic acid	Increases cerebral arteriolar vasoconstriction
Increases white blood cell count	
Increases urinary catecholamine excretion	
Increases contraction of skeletal muscles (also fasciculations)	
Increases lipolysis, glycogenolysis, and gluconeogenesis	
Decreases serum potassium and calcium	
Increases osteoporosis	
Increases muscle enzymes	
Respiratory alkalosis	

38–4). These purinoceptors are located in the brain, heart, vasculature, respiratory tissue, kidneys, fat, and gastrointestinal tract. Of note is that the withdrawal syndrome described in caffeine-tolerant patients has been ascribed to adenosine receptor upregulation and a shift of A_1 receptors to the high-affinity state and a down regulation of β-adrenergic receptors.[11]

What Are the Cardiovascular Effects of Caffeine?

All of the methylxanthines have a potent effect on the circulatory system (Table 38–4). Large doses of caffeine can stimulate the myocardium directly to produce tachycardia, dysrhythmias, and extrasystoles.[27] The diarrhea, vomiting, and diuresis produced with caffeine toxicity can cause hypocalcemia and hypokalemia, both of which can induce dysrhythmias. In vitro studies show an increase in the duration and amplitude of myocardial action potential, a shortening of cardiac refractory period, and modest increases in blood pressure, force of contraction, and cardiac output. Usually the net effect is an increase in heart rate. The mechanisms by which caffeine causes tachydysrhythmias in overdosage or substantial consumption are thought to include blockade of calcium uptake by the sarcoplasmic reticulum; increases in cytosolic calcium concentrations, adenosine antagonism, phosphodiesterase inhibition, and increased sympathetic activity in the conducting system[4] (see Fig. 38–4 and Table 38–4).

In one prospective study, electrophysiologic testing was done on patients with documented histories of ventricular tachycardia and fibrillation prior to and 1 hour after caffeine ingestion.[9] The conclusion was that caffeine did not significantly alter inducibility or severity of dysrhythmias. An extensive review of both clinical studies and the basic science literature led to the conclusion that moderate ingestion of caffeine did not increase the severity of dysrhythmias in normal patients, patients with ischemic heart disease, or those with preexisting serious ventricular ectopy.[38]

Caffeine causes vasodilation by a direct effect on the media of the vessels (see Table 38–4). At the same time, stimulation of vasomotor centers of the medulla causes vasoconstriction via the sympathetic nervous system. The one exception to this mixed vasoactive response occurs in the cerebral vasculature, which shows a relatively pure vasoconstrictive response to caffeine.

In a recent review of caffeine's pressor effect by the use of a pharmacokinetic and pharmacodynamic model, it was shown that the rapid development and regression of tolerance to caffeine's pressor effect was dependent on how much caffeine is consumed, the schedule of consumption, and the elimination half-life of caffeine.[47,48] Whereas tolerance to the pressor effect of caffeine develops in habitual coffee drinkers, the pressor response is regained after relatively brief periods of abstinence. Positive correlations between plasma levels of caffeine and blood pressure in infrequent coffee drinkers but not in regular coffee drinkers is well defined.[48]

There is no significant relationship between coffee or tea consumption and myocardial infarction, congestive heart failure, cerebrovascular accidents, peripheral vascular disease, hypertension, or sudden death.[26,43] In a recent study assessing the relationship between coffee consumption and risk of coronary heart disease among women in the United States adjusted for age, smoking, and other coronary risk factors, no evidence was found of an increased risk of coronary artery disease.[56]

What Is the Extent of Caffeine Usage? What Are Caffeine Withdrawal and Dependency?

Consumer research indicates that more than half of the coffee produced worldwide is consumed in 98% of American homes each year, or 16 lb per person. Eighty percent of American adults consume an average of 3.5 cups of coffee per day. Caffeine is also consumed by drinking tea, maté, and carbonated beverages, by chewing kola nuts, and from cola and guarana products.[51] Caffeine is widely available not only in these food products but also in medications (see Table 38–1). Unfortunately, many individuals unknowingly ingest toxic dosages of caffeine.[21] Over-the-counter drugs, such as "diet pills," are no longer permitted by FDA regulations to contain the combination of caffeine and phenylpropanolamine, but pure caffeine is still available (Chap. 37). The effects of these drugs in addition to dietary sources place people at greater risk of caffeinism and death.[20] There are preliminary data in rat studies suggesting that when combined with cocaine or *d*-amphetamine, caffeine potentiates toxicity. This toxicity, which increases seizures and death, was felt to be modulated by nonspecific rather than spe-

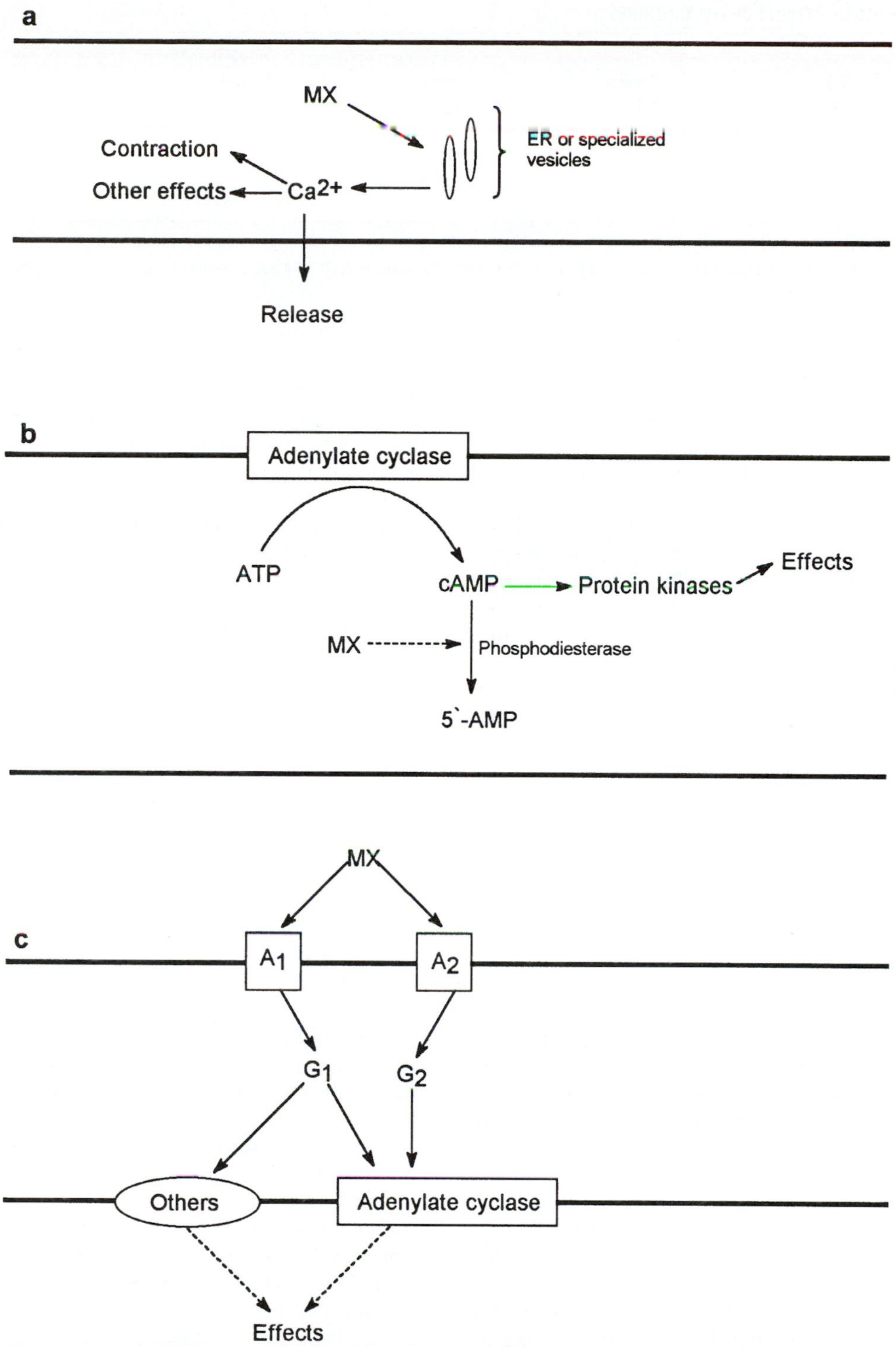

Figure 38–4. Three models for the caffeine mechanism: **(a)** methylxanthines (MX) cause increased mobilization of calcium (Ca^{2+}) from endoplasmic reticulum (ER) and other vesicles. The Ca^{2+} triggers various cellular events. **(b)** MX inhibits phosphodiesterase, causing an elevation in cAMP and greater cellular actions of this second messenger. **(c)** MX binds adenosine receptors (A_1 and A_2) to inhibit adenosine's affects on G_1 and G_2 proteins. *(Reprinted with permission, from Graham TE, Rush JW, van Soeren MH: Caffeine and exercise: Metabolism and performance. Can J Appl Physiol 1994;19:111–138.)*

TABLE 38–4. PHARMACOLOGIC ACTIVITY OF THE XANTHINES

	CNS Stimulation	Cardiac Stimulation	Coronary Vasodilation	Smooth Muscle Relaxation	Diuresis	Skeletal Muscle Stimulation
Caffeine	1	3	3	3	3	1
Theophylline	2	1	3	1	1	2
Theobromine	3	2	2	2	2	3

1 = most active; 3 = least active

Modified, with permission, from Rall TW: Central Nervous System Stimulants: The Xanthines. In: Goodman AG, Goodman LS, Gilman A, eds: Goodman and Gilman's The Pharmacological Basis of Therapeutics, 6th ed. New York, Pergamon Press, 1980, p. 592–604.

cific adenosine- or phosphodiesterase-induced mechanisms. This has important implications since caffeine is easily available to cocaine and amphetamine users.[14]

As is the case with so many other drugs, in addition to its toxicity, sudden abstinence from caffeine by a chronic user may also cause adverse effects. In a study of 62 adults whose usual intake was 2.5 cups of coffee per day (235 mg caffeine) and whose daily consumption was abruptly stopped, 52% of the patients had moderate to severe headaches, 8–10% experienced depression and anxiety, and 13% used analgesics during the placebo period.[50] The patients also described disruption of their normal activities during abstinence. The authors suggested caffeine intake should be reduced gradually rather than abruptly withdrawn.

A syndrome of neonatal caffeine withdrawal has been described in children of women who were substantial users of caffeine during pregnancy.[33] The children had persistently elevated serum caffeine levels from 12 to 120 hours after delivery. They demonstrated irritability, jitteriness, and vomiting that persisted for several days without any other toxicologic or clinical abnormalities.

A recent study examined the extent to which daily caffeine use was associated with a substance-dependence syndrome.[52] The participants were adults who stated they believed they were psychologically or physically dependent on caffeine. Sixteen subjects were identified as being dependent by psychiatrists using structured interviews and as having a diagnosis of caffeine dependence based on generic criteria for DSM IV substance dependency. The median daily caffeine intake was 357 mg. The authors concluded from the study that caffeine dependence existed as a clinical syndrome since some subjects continued to use caffeine despite their desire to stop the drug, and despite recommendations to cease using it, due to their caffeine tolerance and in order to avoid withdrawal effects. This is not surprising since it has been shown in both human and animal studies that caffeine is a reinforcer, maintains self-administration, and is chosen over placebo.[52]

Some issues not evaluated in this study included caffeine blood levels and pharmacokinetic variables that could alter caffeine's elimination, such as liver disease, smoking, and pregnancy. Study subjects were a small group of patients, 57% of whom had a past diagnosis of alcohol abuse or dependence; 7 subjects had a past diagnosis of psychiatric disease, including mood disorder and depression. Though the issues evaluated were not exhaustive, this study was an attempt to recognize that caffeine can cause a dependency syndrome and that there are patients with problematic caffeine dependency who go unrecognized.[52]

What Are the Psychiatric Effects of Caffeine?

The psychiatric manifestations of caffeine dependency vary with plasma levels of caffeine. Doses of 50–200 mg result in increased alertness, decreased drowsiness, and lessened fatigue. Doses in the range of 200–500 mg may produce headache, tremors, nervousness, and irritability.

Five symptom clusters (often confused with other entities) dominate the clinical findings of central nervous system (CNS) involvement from caffeinism. They usually coexist to some degree and may vary in severity.

An *anxiety syndrome* includes diuresis, restlessness, tremulousness, hyperactivity, irritability, dry mouth, dysesthesias, tinnitus, ocular dyskinesias, and scotomata. A biphasic response, manifested initially by anxiety and secondarily by lethargy, is noted.[24] In children and adolescents, the clinical manifestations can mimic hyperactivity. In a study of 62 patients with restless leg syndrome, also seen in chronic renal disease and associated anxiety–depression, caffeine was implicated as a major etiologic factor.[31] It is of interest that the first description of restless leg syndrome was in 17th-century England, when coffee and tea initially were used in that country. The main symptom is discomfort and creeping sensations in the extremities, especially the lower legs, that occurs only at rest, producing an irresistible urge to move the limbs. It may be associated with insomnia, for it generally appears in the evening and early night.

A *hypochondriasis syndrome* includes vague and nonspecific body discomfort, tremor, and myalgias.[15] This is seen most commonly in moderate users (250–750 mg of caffeine, or about 2–6 cups of coffee, per day).

Insomnia and/or headache syndrome is seen in sporadic or moderate users, whereas more frequent drinkers develop a tolerance to this effect.[15] Caffeine delays sleep onset and increases body motility during sleep. Headache can occur simply from excessive use of caffeine; caffeine-containing analgesics, which are used to relieve headache, may establish a vicious cycle of chronic recurring headaches associated with nausea and vomiting.[49]

A *withdrawal syndrome* includes, in addition to headache, yawning, nausea, drowsiness, rhinorrhea, lethargy, irritability, nervousness, a disinclination to work, and a feeling of depression.[15]

Lastly, *a depressive syndrome* may be prevalent among those who consume large amounts of caffeine (750 mg or more daily),[15] but a determination into causality or a secondary relationship needs further evaluation.

Other presentations described include caffeine-induced psychosis in susceptible individuals and exacerbation of symptoms by marked increased consumption of caffeine in patients previously diagnosed as schizophrenic.[35] Symptoms of caffeine intoxication may result in added stress; conversely, caffeine intake may increase considerably during the stressful situation.

In a study of patients with panic disorders, caffeine was shown to increase anxiety, nervousness, fear, nausea, palpitations, restlessness, and tremors more so than in healthy patients.[8] Caffeine also causes a heightened awareness of hypoglycemia at glucose levels not usually considered hypoglycemic, at levels in the "low normal range," and anxiety may result from hypoglycemia.[28]

What Are the Effects of Caffeine on the Musculoskeletal System?

Caffeine increases contractility, thereby decreasing fatigue.[42] Fatigue is also thought to be decreased by the drug's effect on higher cortical centers. The effects of caffeine on muscles are dose-related and complex. Caffeine alters intracellular sequestration of calcium by the sarcoplasmic reticulum, increasing intracytoplasmic calcium concentration. The result is direct cell destruction by toxic doses.[58] Caffeine increases oxygen consumption and the basal metabolic rate by about 10%.[51] Caffeine can enhance performance in short-term intense exercise, which may have implications in competitive situations, such as swimming or cycle sprints.[22]

What Is the Treatment for Caffeine Poisoning?

Serum caffeine levels are rarely available and do not correlate well with outcome and toxicity. Although the more readily available theophylline level may be obtained (since a fraction of caffeine is metabolized to theophylline), it has limited value clinically, except for neonatal overdoses where metabolism to theophylline may be substantial. Caffeine toxicity can induce hypokalemia due to diarrhea, vomiting, and beta-adrenergic agonist effects. Hypocalcemia may occur due to caffeine's effect on calcium metabolism. A leukocytosis due to release of catecholamines is observed. Increased muscle enzymes secondary to increased muscle contractions and ensuing rhabdomyolysis may occur. A respiratory alkalosis can occur secondary to the stimulation of central medullary centers.

There are several case reports of acute caffeine poisoning as a result of both suicide attempts and unintentional overdose.[16,37,39,40,59] General management (Table 38–5), as always, is the primary priority. An airway should be established and circulation maintained. Prevention of absorption can be accomplished by using syrup of ipecac if the patient is seen shortly after ingestion, single and possibly multiple doses of activated charcoal, and a single dose of a cathartic. If the patient is seizing, a benzodiazepine (IV lorazepam or diazepam) should be given or, if the patient fails to respond, a barbiturate such as pentobarbital or phenobarbital.[32] Attempts at diagnosing and treating supraventricular tachycardias should begin with vagal maneuvers. If these fail, sedation with a benzodiazepine or another sedative-hypnotic will usually be adequate. Adenosine in normal doses can be used but may be ineffective in supraventricular tachycardia because of inhibition of adenosine receptors by caffeine. The use of calcium channel blockers, beta-adrenergic antagonists, procainamide, phenytoin, lidocaine, bretylium, defibrillation, cardioversion, and activated charcoal or resin hemoperfusion to lower caffeine levels have all been used to treat caffeine-induced dysrhythmias.[10,39]

Beta-adrenergic receptor antagonists appear to be the drugs of choice in many of the caffeine-induced dys-

TABLE 38–5. TREATMENT OF CAFFEINE TOXICITY

- GI decontamination
  - Syrup of ipecac (early)
  - Activated charcoal (single or MDAC)
  - Cathartic
- Hemoperfusion
- Anticonvulsants
  - Benzodiazepines
  - Barbiturates
- Antidysrhythmics for:
  - Supraventricular tachycardia
    - β-adrenergic antagonists
    - Calcium channel blockers
  - Ventricular tachycardia/fibrillation
    - Cardioversion/defibrillation
    - Bretylium
    - Lidocaine
    - Procainamide
- Antiulcer regimens
  - H_2 antagonists
  - Hydrogen pump inhibitors
  - Sucralfate
- Antiemetics
  - Metoclopramide
  - Ondansetron
- Sedation
  - Benzodiazepines
  - Barbiturates

rhythmias in the normotensive patient due to their cardiac and peripheral antagonism of caffeine's beta-adrenergic stimulatory properties. Beta-adrenergic antagonism in caffeine toxicity may cause hypotension, hypokalemia, and hyperglycemia. Fluids are indicated as the first line of therapy for hypotension. If this fails an alpha-adrenergic receptor agonist should be tried, such as neosynephrine. Gastritis may be treated supportively with antacids; if ulceration is suspected, sucralfate (carafate), H_2 antagonists, or proton pump blockers may be used. Nausea can be treated with metoclopramide, ondansetron or a nasogastric tube. Mild anxiety symptoms usually respond to reassurance, but sedation with benzodiazepines or barbiturates may be indicated (see Table 38–3).

What Are the Gastrointestinal Effects of Caffeine?

Caffeine is a known stimulant of gastric acid and pepsin secretion (see Table 38–4). There is some evidence that individuals with a predisposition to peptic ulcer disease, or with documented ulcer disease in remission, exhibit an abnormal response to caffeine.[12] Large doses of caffeine cause gastric mucosal erosions in animals. Secretions from the small intestine are increased by caffeine, and functional diarrhea may be due to the influx of excess small intestine secretions into the colon.[53,55]

In the evaluation of patients with heartburn in relation to coffee drinking, a reduced tone and dysfunction at the lower esophageal sphincter due to caffeine with resultant acid reflux was found.[13] It is also important to note that coffee, both regular and decaffeinated, may contain other stimulants for acid secretion such as the essential oils and/or possibly a compound that potentiates the action of caffeine.[13]

What Is the Relationship Between Coffee Drinking and Cancer?

The carcinogenic risk of caffeine to humans was evaluated by the International Agency for Research in Cancer Working Group.[51] There is inadequate evidence for the carcinogenicity of caffeine in relationship to the pancreas, ovary, or breast; however a possible correlation with bladder cancer exists. Conversely, there may be an inverse relationship between coffee drinking and colon cancer, although further studies need to be done.

What Effect Does Coffee Have on the Lipid Profile?

Numerous studies have tried to correlate the effect of coffee on serum lipids and its effects on cardiovascular disease. Many are ambiguous, conflicting, and controversial.[29,30,44,51,57,60] A group of researchers evaluated coffee intake in relation to cardiovascular risk and blood lipid profiles. They concluded that coffee had inconsistent effects on lipid profiles and did not have primary or secondary effects on cardiovascular disease.[57] However, boiled, rather than filtered, caffeinated coffee raises serum cholesterol levels. It is postulated that the filter paper adsorbs an active lipid-rich substance and filtered coffee therefore does not raise cholesterol levels[19,60]

In a study that compared filtered decaffeinated coffee, to caffeinated coffee it was shown that neither had cholesterol-elevating effects. This study also compared the different types of coffee beans. Since many decaffeinated beverages contain a higher proportion of *Coffea robusta* rather than *Coffea arabica* (caffeinated), and it is known that the *Coffea robusta* has a much higher phenolic content than *Coffea arabica,* it was postulated that perhaps this could theoretically cause a change in lipid profiles, but no such difference was found due to this chemical difference.[54]

Studies of the effects of coffee consumption on lipid metabolism compared to that of caffeine pills showed that caffeine itself had no effect on serum lipid profiles.[54]

What Is the Relationship Between Caffeinated Coffee and Osteoporosis?

A study of 980 postmenopausal women correlating bone density measurements of their hips and lumbar spine with their lifetime intake of caffeinated coffee found that caffeinated coffee intake of two cups per day was associated with decreased bone density in women who did not drink milk daily, but no bone density diminution in women who drank at least one glass of milk a day.[2] Other studies have confirmed the relationship of low bone densities and caffeine consumption, with hip fractures increasing with increasing caffeine intake. The mechanism invoked in the osteopenia is caffeine's effect of increasing urinary calcium losses.[45]

Does Caffeine Have Any Therapeutic Value?

Historically, caffeine has had a role in the management of headaches, CNS depression associated with alcoholism, and, rarely, neonatal apnea and hyperkinetic children. It is still used in combination with ergot preparations in the treatment of migraine headaches. It may be effective in promoting intestinal absorption of the ergots in the treatment of migraines, and in causing cerebral vascular vasoconstriction or mood elevation.

Caffeine can act as an "analgesic adjuvant" for acetaminophen, aspirin, or ibuprofen in ameliorating headaches, oral surgery pain, episiotomy pain, and sore throat.[25,46] In a study addressing the issue of caffeine as an analgesic adjuvant in outpatients with episodic tension-type headaches, six randomized, double-blind two-period crossover studies concluded that there was a significant analgesic adjuvant effect of caffeine independent of patients' habitual caffeine consumption prior to a headache. The combination of analgesics with caffeine was also found to produce more nervousness and dizziness than resulted from the use of pure analgesics without the addition of caffeine.[34]

In the past, caffeine by mouth and caffeine sodium benzoate IV have been used to manage patients with CNS depression subsequent to drug overdose. This historic application of caffeine is cited only to be condemned (Chap. 1 and Antidotes in Depth: Antiquated Antidotes). When used as an analeptic agent in neonates, caffeine and sodium benzoate have produced fatal complications.[1]

Among the naturopathic therapies used in the United States, a host of questionable therapeutic modalities remain in vogue. A study described a natural food diet with ingredients consisting of potassium salts, Lugol's solution, thyroid extract, niacin, and pancreatin, associated with the use of hypoosmolar caffeine enemas.[17] The two reported patients died, although the hypoosmolarity of the enemas appear to be more responsible for the deaths than the concentration of caffeine.

A potential future use for caffeine may be in the treatment of acetaminophen intoxications. In a study of mice administered toxic and lethal doses of acetaminophen, it was found that caffeine administered after the exposures markedly increased survival and reduced liver damage. The mechanism of caffeine's beneficial effect was postulated to be its prevention of the loss of reduced glutathione.[41]

Summary

In conclusion, caffeine is a ubiquitous substance that can produce multisystem toxicity. The pharmacokinetics and pathophysiology have been well studied. If recognized early, the toxicity of caffeinism can be treated effectively by basic poison management and by the judicious use of pharmacologic agents and extracorporeal techniques.

Acknowledgments

Menachem Melinek, MD and Richard S. Weisman, Pharm D contributed to this chapter in a previous edition.

References

1. Banner W, Czajka PA: Acute caffeine overdose in a neonate. Am J Dis Child 1980;134:495–598.
2. Barrett-Connor E, Chang JC, Edelsltein SL: Coffee-associated osteoporosis offset by daily milk consumption. JAMA 1994;271:280–283.
3. Becker AB, Simons KJ, Gillespie GA, Simons FER: The bronchodilator effects and pharmacokinetics of caffeine in asthma. N Engl J Med 1984;31:743–746.
4. Benowitz N, Osterloh JD, Goldschlager N, et al: Massive catecholamine release from caffeine poisoning. JAMA 1982;248:1097–1098.
5. Blauch JL, Taraka SM: HPLC determination of caffeine and theobromine in coffee, tea and instant hot cocoa mixes. J Food Sci 1983;48:745–750.
6. Bonati M, Latini R, Galletti F, et al: Caffeine disposition after oral doses. Clin Pharmacol Ther 1982;32:98–106.
7. Busto U, Benadyan R, Sellers EM: Clinical pharmacokinetics of non-opiate abuse drugs. Clin Pharmacokinet 1989;16:1–26.
8. Charney DS, Heninger GR, Jatlow PI: Increased anxiogenic effects of caffeine in panic disorders. Arch Gen Psychiatry 1985;42:233–243.
9. Chelsky LB, Cutler JE, Griffith K, et al: Caffeine and ventricular arrhythmias: An electrophysiological approach. JAMA 1990;264:2236–2240.
10. Chopra A, Morrison L: Resolution of caffeine-induced complex dysrhythmia with procainamide therapy. J Emerg Med 1995;13:113–117.
11. Chou TM, Benowitz NL: Caffeine and coffee: Effects on health and cardiovascular disease. Comp Biochem Phys 1994;109:173–189.
12. Cohen S: Pathogenesis of coffee-induced gastrointestinal symptoms. N Engl J Med 1980;303:122–124.
13. Cohen S, Booth G: Gastric acid secretion and lower esophageal sphincter pressure in response to coffee and caffeine. N Engl J Med 1975;293:897–899.
14. Derlet RW, Tseng JC, Albertson TE: Potentiation of cocaine and *d*-amphetamine toxicity with caffeine. Am J Emerg Med 1992;10:211–216.
15. Diagnostic and Statistical Manual of Mental Disorders, 3rd ed. Washington, DC, American Psychiatric Association, 1980, pp. 160–161.
16. Dietrich AM, Mortensen ME: Presentation and management of an acute caffeine overdose. Pediatr Emerg Care 1990;6:296–298.
17. Eisele JW, Reay DT: Deaths related to coffee enemas. JAMA 1980;244:1608–1609.
18. Fredholm BB, Abbrocchio MP, Burnstock G, et al: VI. Nomenclature and classification of purinoceptors. Pharmacol Rev 1994;46:143–156.
19. Fried RE, Levine DM, Kwiterovich MD, et al: The effects of filtered coffee consumption on plasma lipid levels. JAMA 1992;267:811–815.
20. Garriott JC, Simmons LM, Poklis A, Mackell MA: Five cases of fatal overdose from caffeine-containing "look alike" drugs. J Anal Toxicol 1985;9:141–143.
21. Graham DM: Caffeine: Its identity, dietary intake, and biological effects. Nutr Rev 1978;36:97–102.
22. Graham TE, Rush JW, van Soeren MH: Caffeine and exercise: Metabolism and performance. Can J Appl Physiol 1994;19:111–138.
23. Greden JF: Coffee, tea and you. Science 1979;19:6–11.
24. Greden JF, Fontaine P, Lubetsky M, Chamberlain K: Anxiety and depression associated with caffeinism among psychiatric inpatients. Psychiatry 1978;135:963–966.
25. Jain AK, McMahan FG, Ryan JR, Narcisse C: A double blind study of ibuprofen 200 mg in combination with caffeine 100 mg, ibuprofen 400 mg, and placebo in episiotomy pain. Curr Ther Res 1988;43:762–769.
26. Jick H, Miettinen OS, Neff RK, et al: Coffee and myocardial infarction. N Engl J Med 1963;289:63–66.
27. Josephson GW, Etine RJ: Caffeine intoxication: A case of paroxysmal atrial tachycardia. JACEP 1976;5:775–778.
28. Kerr D, Sherwin RS, Pavalkis F, et al: Effect of caffeine on

the recognition of and responses to hypoglycemia in humans. Ann Intern Med 1993;119:799–804.
29. Kokjohn K, Graham M, McGregor M: The effect of coffee consumption on serum cholesterol levels. J Manipulative Physiol Ther 1993;16:327–335.
30. Lewis CE, Caan B, Funkhouser E, et al: Inconsistent associations of caffeine containing beverages with blood pressure and with lipoproteins. Am J Epidemiol 1993;138: 502–507.
31. Lutz EG: Restless legs, anxiety and caffeinism. J Clin Psychiatry 1978;39:693–698.
32. Marangos PJ, Martino AN, Paul SM, et al: The benzodiazepines and inosine antagonize caffeine-induced seizures. Psychopharmacology 1981;72:269–273.
33. McGowan JD, Altman RE, Kant WP: Neonatal withdrawal symptoms after chronic maternal ingestion of caffeine. South Med J 1988;81:1092–1094.
34. Migliardi JR, Armellino JJ, Friedman M, et al: Caffeine as an analgesic adjuvant in tension headache. Clin Pharmacol Ther 1994;56:576–586.
35. Mikkelsen EJ: Caffeine and schizophrenia. J Clin Psychiatry 1978;39:732–736.
36. Mills JL, Holmes LB, Aarons JH, et al: Moderate caffeine use and the risk of spontaneous abortion and intrauterine growth retardation. JAMA 1993;269:593–597.
37. Mrvos RM, Reilly PE, Dean BS, Krenzelok EP: Massive caffeine ingestion resulting in death. Vet Hum Toxicol 1986; 131:571–572.
38. Myers MG, Basinski A: Coffee and coronary heart disease. Arch Intern Med 1992;152:1767–1772.
39. Nagesh RV, Murphy KA: Caffeine poisoning treated by hemoperfusion. Am J Kidney Dis 1988;4:316–318.
40. Price KR, Fligner DJ: Treatment of caffeine toxicity with esmolol. Ann Emerg Med 1990;19:44–46.
41. Rainska T, Juzwiak S, Dulkiewicz T, et al: Caffeine reduces the hepatotoxicity of paracetamol in mice. J Int Med Res 1992;20:331–342.
42. Rall TW: Drugs used in the treatment of asthma: The methylxanthines, cromolyn sodium and other agents. In Goodman AG, Rall TW, Nies AS, Taylor P, eds: Goodman and Gilman's The Pharmacological Basis of Therapeutics, 8th ed. New York, Pergamon Press, 1990 pp. 618–630.
43. Robertson D, Hollister AS, Kincaid D, et al: Caffeine and hypertension. Am J Med 1984;77:54–60.
44. Rosmarin PC, Applegate WB: Coffee consumption and serum lipids: A randomized, crossover clinical trial. Am J Med 1990;88:349–356.
45. Ross PC: Osteoporosis frequency, consequences and risk factors. Arch Intern Med 1996;156:1399–1411.
46. Schaftel BP, Fillman JM, Lane AC, et al: Caffeine as an analgesic adjuvant. Arch Intern Med 1991;151:733–737.
47. Serafin WE: Drugs used in the treatment of asthma. In Hardman JG, Limbird LE, Molinoff PB, Ruddon RW, Gilman AG, eds: Goodman and Gilman's Pharmacological Basics of Therapeutics, 9th ed. New York, McGraw-Hill, 1996 p. 672.
48. Shi J, Benowitz NL, Denaro CP, et al: Pharmacokinetic-pharmacodynamic modeling of caffeine: Tolerance to pressor effects. Clin Pharmacol Ther 1993;53:6–14.
49. Shorolsky MA, Lanh N: Caffeine withdrawal headache and fasting. NY State J Med 1977;77:217–218.
50. Silverman K, Evans SM, Strain EC, Griffiths RR: Withdrawal syndrome after the double blind cessation of caffeine consumption. N Engl J Med 1992;327:1109–1114.
51. Stavric B: An update on research with coffee/caffeine (1989–1990). Fed Chem Toxic 1992;30:533–555.
52. Strain EC, Mumford GK, Silverman K, et al: Caffeine dependence syndrome. JAMA 1994;272:1043–1048.
53. Wagner S, Mekhjian HS, Caldwell JH, Thomas FB: Effects of caffeine and coffee on fluid transport in the small intestine. Gastroenterology 1978;75:379–381.
54. Wahrburg U, Schulte T, Walek T, et al: Effects of two kinds of decaffeinated coffee on serum lipid profiles in healthy young adults. Eur J Clin Nutr 1994;48:172–179.
55. Wald A, Back C, Bayless TH: Effect of caffeine on the human small intestine. Gastroenterology 1976;71:738–742.
56. Willett WC, Stampfer MJ, Manson JE, et al: Coffee consumption and coronary heart disease in women. JAMA 1996;275:458–462.
57. Wilson PWF, Garrison RJ, Kannel WB, et al: Is coffee consumption a contributor to cardiovascular disease? Arch Intern Med 1989;149:1169–1172.
58. Wrenn KD, Oschner I: Rhabdomyolysis induced by caffeine overdose. Ann Emerg Med 1989;18:94–97.
59. Zimmerman PM, Pulliam J, Schwengels J, MacDonald SE: Caffeine intoxication: A near fatality. Ann Emerg Med 1985;14:1227–1229.
60. Zock PL, Katan MB, Merkus MP, et al: Effect of a lipid-rich fraction from boiled coffee on serum cholesterol. Lancet 1990;335:1235–1237.

CHAPTER 39

Theophylline

Richard S. Weisman

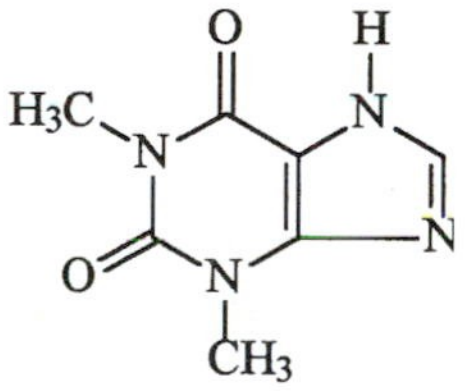

Theophylline
(1,3-dimethylxanthine)

Theophylline	
MW	= 180.17 daltons
Therapeutic serum level	= 5–15 μg/mL
S.I. units	= 10 μg/mL
	= 55.5 μmol/L
Toxic level	> 20 μg/mL
Action levels	
Multiple dose activated charcoal:	>20 μg/mL
Hemoperfusion (acute):	> 90 μg/mL
Hemoperfusion (chronic):	> 40 μg/mL

Values greater than or equal to the action level necessitate clinical intervention. Values less than this level may necessitate intervention based on the clinical characteristics of the patient.

An 18-year-old woman was brought to the emergency department (ED) with her boyfriend, who was in status asthmaticus. After a prolonged resuscitation the boyfriend died. The distraught woman went into the ED bathroom and ingested the deceased patient's entire bottle (60) of sustained-release 300-mg theophylline tablets. Immediately thereafter, she told the triage nurse of her ingestion.

Initially the patient was asymptomatic, with a blood pressure of 130/80 mm Hg, a pulse of 84 beats/min, respirations 14 breaths/min, and a rectal temperature of 98.6°F (37°C). Physical examination was entirely unremarkable. An intravenous line of D_5W was started and blood specimens were sent for electrolytes, glucose, theophylline, and acetaminophen. The patient was given 30 mL of syrup of ipecac and 240 mL of tap water.

Twenty minutes later she vomited large numbers of pills and pill fragments. Her vomiting stopped after three episodes of emesis. The patient was given 60 g of activated charcoal in a slurry of water and 70 mL of 70% sorbitol, which she promptly vomited.

The patient was placed on a monitor in the observation unit until she was able to tolerate another dose of activated charcoal. At $2\frac{1}{2}$ hours post ingestion the results of the initial laboratory studies were available; the glucose was 118 mg/dL, sodium 138 mEq/L, potassium 4.2 mEq/L, chloride 101 mEq/L, bicarbonate 24 mEq/L. The theophylline level was 18 μg/mL and the acetaminophen determination was negative.

Another attempt was made to give oral activated charcoal, and the patient promptly vomited. A nasogastric tube was inserted and 30 g of activated charcoal in a slurry of water were given slowly over 30 minutes.

At about $3\frac{1}{2}$ hours post ingestion, the patient had two episodes of spontaneous emesis. Her pulse was 128 beats/min, and her blood pressure was 120/60 mm Hg. Repeat theophylline level, electrolytes, and glucose were obtained. The patient was admitted to the intensive care unit for continuous observation and monitoring.

The other laboratory studies returned at about 5 hours post ingestion. The glucose was 156 mg/dL, sodium 136 mEq/L, potassium 3.3 mEq/L, chloride 101 mEq/L, bicarbonate 18 mEq/L. The theophylline level was 46 μg/mL.

After two 5-mg doses of intravenous metoclopramide, the patient was able to tolerate activated charcoal. The repeat laboratory studies, drawn about $5\frac{1}{2}$ hours post ingestion and reported at 7 hours post ingestion were: glucose 153 mg/dL, sodium 134 mEq/L, potassium 2.9 mEq/L, chloride 99 mEq/L, and bicarbonate 16 mEq/L. The theophylline level was 83 μg/mL.

An additional dose of 60 g of activated charcoal was given via the nasogastric tube but the patient became tremulous and vomited again. As the nephrologist prepared for charcoal hemoperfusion, the patient had a seizure. Twenty milligrams of intravenous diazepam were administered to treat the seizure. A repeat theophylline level drawn at the initiation of hemoperfusion was 133 μg/mL. The patient underwent $4\frac{1}{4}$ hours of charcoal hemoperfusion. During the procedure she became hypotensive with a blood pressure of 100 mm Hg by palpation. She responded to a 1-L normal saline fluid bolus. Two additional doses of activated charcoal were given after an additional 10 mg of intravenous metoclopramide. Following hemoperfusion the theophylline level was 27 μg/mL.

What Are the Pharmacologic Properties of Theophylline?

For the vast majority of patients the minimum therapeutic response to theophylline occurs with plasma levels of 5–10 μg/mL. The therapeutic range is between 5 and 15 μg/mL. Toxicity usually occurs when levels exceed 20 μg/mL.[19,60] Theophylline, a methylxanthine derivative, exerts its primary pharmacologic effect by antagonizing the activity of adenosine.[9] Adenosine is believed to modulate histamine release and to cause constriction of respiratory smooth muscle. The administration of exogenous adenosine to inhibit theophylline-induced seizure activity has produced conflicting results probably because adenosine fails to cross the blood–brain barrier.[55] The intraventricular and carotid artery administration of adenosine in animal models has been shown to antagonize the neurologic and cardiovascular toxicities of theophylline.[56] In another study, the pretreatment of mice with the adenosine A_1 agonists, cyclohexyladenosine and carbamazepine, failed to inhibit seizures when compared to control mice.[21]

Theophylline is associated with catecholamine release, as demonstrated by very high plasma epinephrine and norepinephrine levels in acute overdoses.[56] In very high concentrations theophylline also inhibits the activity of the enzyme phosphodiesterase, which is responsible for the metabolism of cyclic adenosine monophosphate (cAMP) to 5′-AMP. As the beta-adrenergic receptor is stimulated, levels of cAMP increase intracellularly and persist because metabolism to inactive 5′-AMP is inhibited. Pharmacologically this results in smooth muscle relaxation, peripheral vasodilation, myocardial stimulation, and CNS excitation. The loss of peripheral vascular resistance from excessive $beta_2$-adrenergic receptor stimulation can be antagonized with nonselective beta-adrenergic antagonists such as propranolol.

The volume of distribution for theophylline is 0.5 L/kg, and the drug can be found in all the major body tissues. Approximately 50% of theophylline found in the blood is bound to plasma proteins.[39] Theophylline is me-

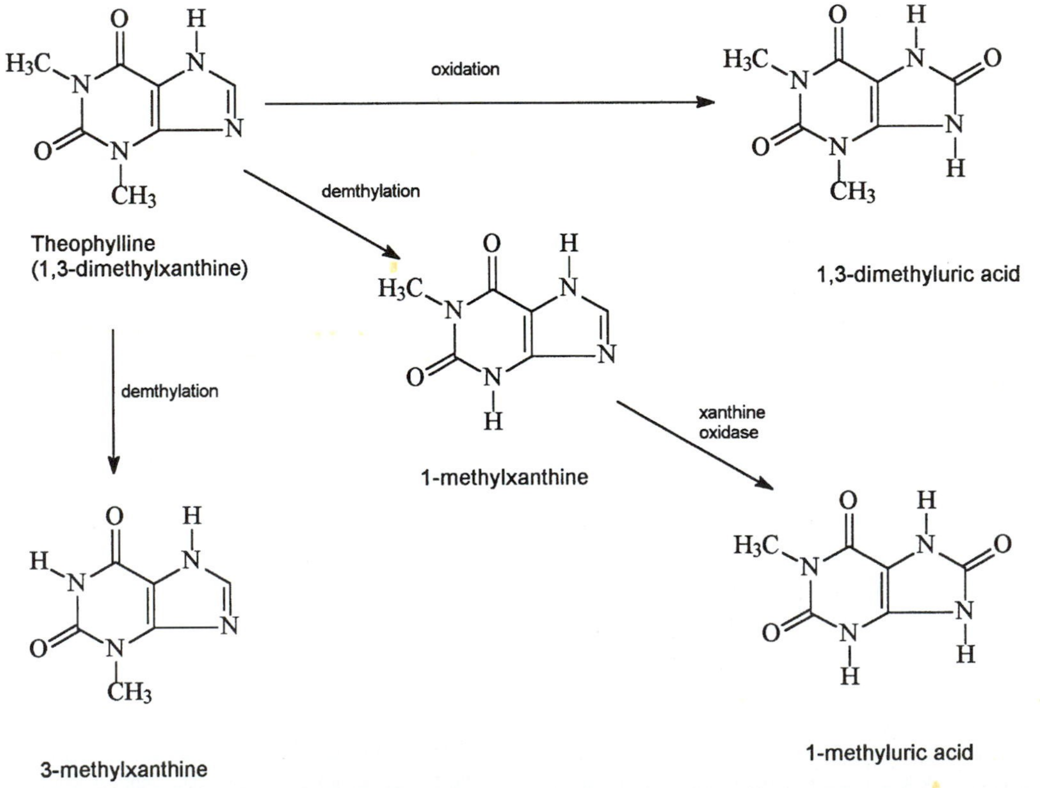

Figure 39–1. The metabolism of theophylline.

tabolized in the liver by the CYP1A2 isozyme of the cytochrome P450 mixed function oxidase enzymes.[17] Theophylline is eliminated primarily as the 3-methylxanthine, 1,3-dimethyluric acid, and 1-methylxanthine, the metabolite which is further broken down to 1-methyluric acid (Fig. 39–1). Only the 3-methylxanthine metabolite is believed to be active; however, it is not usually present in pharmacologically significant concentrations. Cimetidine, ciprofloxacin, diltiazem, enoxacin, erythromycin, fluvoxamine, mexiletine, norfloxacin, and tacrine will inhibit the CYP1A2 isozyme, causing plasma theophylline levels to rise and toxic symptoms to be manifested.[6,17,26,32,33,44] Less than 10% of the absorbed theophylline is eliminated unchanged in the urine.[39] In the geriatric age group, less is eliminated unchanged in the urine and a greater percentage is metabolized to the 1-methyluric acid metabolite.[1] In neonates, unlike older children and adults, theophylline is methylated to form caffeine.[38]

Cigarette smoking, phenobarbital, and phenytoin have been shown to enhance metabolism of theophylline by as much as 50%.[15,35] Congestive heart failure, liver disease, and conditions leading to poor hepatic perfusion decrease the hepatic clearance of theophylline.[18,46,57] These factors are often responsible for the development of chronic toxicity as well as prolonging elimination after an acute ingestion and must be assessed in deciding on the need for hemoperfusion. The factors that are known to alter the metabolic elimination of theophylline can be found in Table 39–1.

TABLE 39–1. FACTORS THAT MODIFY THEOPHYLLINE METABOLISM

Increased Metabolism	*Decreased Metabolism*
Aminoglutethimide	*Drugs and Toxins*
Carbamazepine	Allopurinol
Cigarette smoking	Beta-adrenergic antagonists
Marijuana smoking	Cimetidine
Moricizine	Ciprofloxacin
Phenobarbital	Clarithromycin
Phenytoin	Disulfiram
Primidone	Enoxacin
Rifampin	Erythromycin
Sulfinpyrazone	Estrogen
Other inducers of CYP1A2	Ethanol
	Fluvoxamine
	Interferon
	Methotrexate
	Mexiletine
	Propafenone
	Propranolol
	Tacrine
	Thiobendazole
	Ticlopidine
	Troleandomycin
	Verapamil
	Zileuton
	Pathophysiologic
	Congestive heart failure
	Hepatic failure
	Infections
	Old age

What Are the Toxic Effects of Theophylline?

The most common symptoms of theophylline toxicity include nausea and vomiting, tachydysrhythmias, seizures, hypotension, metabolic acidosis, and hypokalemia. If the patient does not have a tachycardia, the diagnosis of theophylline toxicity must be questioned or a concurrent ingestion with a substance capable of inducing bradycardia must be excluded. The cardiac toxicity that occurs with severe ingestions is due to excessive catecholamine stimulation of the myocardium, aggravated by hypokalemia, hypercalcemia, hypophosphatemia, and a metabolic acidosis.[44,45,50] Beta-adrenergic receptor stimulation is also responsible for the electrolyte and acid–base disturbances.[44] The hypokalemia results largely from a beta$_2$-adrenergic receptor mediated shift of potassium to the intracellular compartment of skeletal muscle, rather than from vomiting and renal losses. Supraventricular tachycardia, atrial fibrillation, multifocal atrial tachycardia (particularly patients with COPD), or, less frequently, ventricular dysrhythmias may result. The blood pressure may initially be mildly elevated or normal, but usually hypotension becomes prominent secondary to beta-adrenergic mediated peripheral vasodilation.[3] Hypotension may be worsened by volume depletion secondary to protracted vomiting and cathartic-induced diarrhea. A widened pulse pressure is commonly observed in patients with severe theophylline toxicity.

The tachydysrhythmias from theophylline toxicity may be worsened by hypoxia or the administration of medications with beta-adrenergic or anticholinergic activity. Antiemetics with anticholinergic activity should be avoided. If a pressor is to be used to raise blood pressure, a drug with pure alpha-adrenergic activity is preferred. Hypoxia lowers the threshold for ventricular fibrillation.[22]

Central nervous system effects include hyperventilation, anxiety, tremor, agitation, and seizures. The exact cause of seizures remains unclear, but loss of central nervous system adenosine anticonvulsant activity appears to be the most probable explanation.[38] Non-type-specific adenosine antagonists have been shown to cause marked prolongation of the ictal phase on the electroencephalogram during theophylline toxicity.[8]

What Are the Initial Therapeutic Interventions for a Patient With Theophylline Toxicity?

Patient Assessment

Upon arrival in the ED the patient's airway and ventilation should be assessed. The vital signs should be evaluated and abnormalities corrected if necessary, and the patient should be placed on a cardiac monitor. A theophylline level along with electrolytes, glucose, BUN, creatinine, a complete blood count, platelets, INR and PTT should be obtained at the time the intravenous line is placed. The baseline INR, PTT, platelets, and calcium should be documented in the event that extracorporeal drug removal becomes necessary.[16]

Gastrointestinal Decontamination

Decisions regarding gastrointestinal decontamination, including orogastric lavage, emesis with syrup of ipecac, activated charcoal, a cathartic or whole-bowel irrigation, will depend on the theophylline dosage form, when the ingestion occurred, and the patient's clinical condition. Emesis with syrup of ipecac should be avoided unless the ingestion has occurred within the hour before arrival at a health care facility, and the patient is asymptomatic. A recent simulated overdose controlled volunteer study with sustained-release theophylline was unable to demonstrate efficacy with the use of syrup of ipecac.[37] The administration of syrup of ipecac may theoretically lead to protracted vomiting, limiting the clinician's ability to utilize activated charcoal which has been shown to be effective in preventing absorption.[37]

Orogastric lavage should be performed in patients with potentially toxic theophylline ingestions, where the administration of activated charcoal requires placement of a tube in the patient's stomach. The efficacy of lavage with even the largest tubes may be limited by the size of the tablets and the dissolution characteristics of the sustained-release product. Orogastric lavage in adult volunteers has not been shown to be effective in removing theophylline tablets.[37] If it becomes apparent that tablets or tablet fragments are not being removed, a slurry of activated charcoal 1–2 g/kg of body weight along with a cathartic should be administered through the lavage tube without delay.[34,48,54] The cathartics that are often administered orally with activated charcoal include either sorbitol (0.5–1 g/kg) or magnesium sulfate (250 mg/kg for children or 30 g for adults).

A 0.5-g/kg dose of activated charcoal without a cathartic can be readministered every hour in patients with rising theophylline levels or significant symptoms but can be readministered every 2 hours in more stable patients. Repeated administration of activated charcoal significantly decreases the half-life and increases the clearance of theophylline.[10] The successful use of two doses of activated charcoal (0.6 g/kg) has been reported in a 2-day-old child with theophylline toxicity.[23] Constipation, diarrhea, and a small bowel obstruction secondary to activated charcoal in an adult patient with adhesions has been described.[14] A more detailed discussion of activated charcoal can be found in Antidotes in Depth: Activated Charcoal.

The administration of a cathartic (sorbitol) along with the first dose of activated charcoal has been shown to be more effective than the administration of activated charcoal alone.[13] If the patient has protracted vomiting and is unable to take the activated charcoal orally, metoclopramide, ondansetron, or a continuous nasogastric instillation of activated charcoal may be helpful.[40] Metoclopramide and ondansetron may theoretically be more beneficial than the phenothiazine antiemetics because they promote gastric motility and do not lower the seizure threshold. Ondansetron, a serotonin (5-HT_3) antagonist, is effective in preventing emesis in patients with theophylline toxicity[53] and in patients unable to tolerate oral *N*-acetylcysteine in acetaminophen overdoses.[5] Ondansetron should be reserved for patients with refractory emesis. Granisetron, a newer and less expensive serotonin antagonist, may also be used for this purpose.

Charcoal hemoperfusion should be considered early for patients with protracted vomiting because the inability to administer multiple doses of activated charcoal may allow theophylline levels to rise rapidly.

Whole-bowel irrigation may be useful to enhance the evacuation of sustained-release theophylline products.[25] The benefit of using whole-bowel irrigation must be weighed against the risk that it may decrease the effectiveness of activated charcoal.[19] The decreased number of available binding sites for theophylline on activated charcoal may be compensated for by increasing the amount of activated charcoal that is administered. In certain situations it may be beneficial to perform whole-bowel irrigation and charcoal hemoperfusion simultaneously.

The delay in absorption of sustained-release products and the potential for bezoar formation make it critical to obtain frequent theophylline levels until the theophylline level falls into the therapeutic range.[36,52] A bezoar consisting of the waxy tablet matrices, activated charcoal, and 29 g of theophylline was recovered at autopsy from the stomach of a patient who had ingested a sustained-release theophylline product.[2]

Health Care Facility Assessment

If the hospital where the patient is being evaluated is unable to provide charcoal hemoperfusion or hemodialysis, arrangements should be initiated to expeditiously transfer the patient to a facility with these capabilities while the patient is still clinically stable enough to be transferred. Because theophylline toxicity can be so effectively treated with extracorporeal techniques, early consideration of a patient's definitive care may necessitate transfer prior to laboratory confirmation when either a massive ingestion is suspected or severe symptoms develop early in the clinical course. Although transfer to another facility is effected, MDAC should be administered.

What Are the Life-Threatening Manifestations That May Be Associated With Theophylline Toxicity?

Agitation and Seizures

Agitation is an extremely common finding in patients with theophylline toxicity and often precedes seizure activity. These patients should have blood obtained for a glucose determination. If the patient is hypoglycemic, intravenous doses of dextrose (0.5 g/kg) and 100 mg of thiamine should be administered. If the patient remains agitated, an intravenous benzodiazepine should be administered. If the patient is agitated and vomiting, extra care must be taken to assure that the patient is able to protect the airway following the administration of the benzodiazepine. The benzodiazepine may be repeated as necessary until the patient is resting comfortably. Vital signs must be frequently assessed during and subsequent to the administration of sedating agents, paying particular attention to respiratory rate and blood pressure.

Initial therapy for seizures should include the administration of an intravenous benzodiazepine followed by phenobarbital or pentobarbital if the seizure fails to respond to the benzodiazepine. Phenytoin has not been found to be an effective anticonvulsant in the mouse or rabbit model of theophylline intoxication.[4,12] It may be necessary to use general anesthesia in addition to a neuromuscular blocking agent and ventilatory support to control the seizures. The patient who has had a seizure as a manifestation of theophylline toxicity requires aggressive management with charcoal hemoperfusion, as status epilepticus may occur if the theophylline level is not rapidly lowered.

Cardiac Dysrhythmias

The patient's electrolytes should be carefully evaluated or reevaluated and rapidly corrected if a dysrhythmia develops. Supraventricular tachycardia rarely requires management; however, low doses of propranolol or diltiazem may be necessary if the patient is unstable or not tolerating the dysrhythmia. These dysrhythmias usually resolve spontaneously as the theophylline level returns to the therapeutic range. Several patients with chronic lung disease, theophylline toxicity, and multifocal atrial tachycardia have been successfully treated using small doses (1–10 mg) of verapamil infused over 2 minutes.[30] Calcium channel blockers or beta-adrenergic antagonists must be administered cautiously to prevent hypotension or high-degree atrioventricular block.

A patient who develops ventricular tachycardia or frequent premature ventricular contractions should be treated with conventional doses of lidocaine. Charcoal hemoperfusion should be initiated for any life-threatening dysrhythmias.

Hypotension

If the patient is hypotensive, intravenous fluids (normal saline or lactated Ringer's) appropriate for the patient's age and weight should be administered and the patient should be placed in the Trendelenburg position. Hypotension unresponsive to intravenous fluid repletion should be considered an immediate indication for charcoal hemoperfusion. If the desired increase in blood pressure is not attained, levarterenol (0.1–0.2 μg/kg/min) or phenylephrine (40–160 μg/min) may be titrated to achieve an acceptable blood pressure. A vasopressor with predominantly alpha-adrenergic receptor activity is preferred because most patients with theophylline activity already have excessive beta-adrenergic receptor stimulation. Hypotension has been reported to be refractory to treatment with vasopressors in some patients.[7] A small number of patients with hypotension associated with a supraventricular tachycardia from theophylline toxicity have been effectively treated with intravenous propranolol.[3] Beta-adrenergic receptor antagonists must be used with extreme caution in patients with asthma or chronic obstructive pulmonary disease. Esmolol has also been used to correct hypotension from theophylline toxicity.[24] If a beta-adrenergic antagonist is used to treat hypotension, the patient should have hemodynamic monitoring of mean arterial pressure, right atrial pressure, pulmonary artery occlusion pressure, cardiac index, systolic index, systemic vascular resistance, and left ventricular stroke work index.

How Can Theophylline Levels Be Used to Predict the Patient's Clinical Course?

The theophylline level can be extremely valuable if it is rapidly available and is evaluated in the context of the ingestion history, therapeutic interventions, and clinical findings. As a general rule theophylline levels should be monitored every 2 hours until two successive levels decline. Thereafter, the levels should be monitored every 4–6 hours until the values are less than 20 μg/mL.

For the level to have the greatest significance the clinician should know if the exposure results from an acute ingestion, chronic toxicity, or an acute ingestion in a patient chronically receiving theophylline. Patients with an acute theophylline exposure and a peak theophylline greater than 90 μg/mL generally are at risk for seizures, hypotension, and dysrhythmias.[41,49] Patients with chronic toxicity may develop life-threatening toxicities with theophylline levels of 40 μg/mL or greater.[49,62] If the patient has concurrently ingested other medications with theophylline, the prognostic value of a level may be altered by the pharmacologic properties of the co-ingestants. Particular consideration should be given to drugs or toxins that alter the seizure threshold, induce dysrhythmias, or lower blood pressure.

A repeat theophylline level 2 hours after the initial determination will significantly improve the prognostic value of both levels. If the second level is higher than the first, more theophylline has been absorbed than has been eliminated and the patient is more likely to develop seizures, dysrhythmias, or hypotension than after the initial level. This situation is particularly serious because clinical deterioration becomes probable until drug absorption is complete.

Conversely, the patient who has a theophylline level that is declining becomes progressively less likely to develop additional toxic effects as the level falls into the therapeutic range of 5–15 μg/mL. The prognosis of a patient with theophylline levels that do not change after several hours depends on how high or how low the unchanged level is. The patient who has an unchanged level at 30 μg/mL is far less likely to develop toxicity than the patient whose level is unchanged at 60 μg/mL. Pharmacokinetically, the unchanged level means that the rate of absorption equals the rate of elimination. As in the case of the patient who has an increasing level, gastrointestinal decontamination has not stopped absorption, and additional decontamination with whole-bowel irrigation may be needed. If the levels fail to decline after the gastrointestinal tract has been theoretically cleared with whole-bowel irrigation and multiple doses of activated charcoal, the presence of a bezoar or retained materials must be considered likely.

What Are the Indications for Charcoal Hemoperfusion in Acute and Chronic Theophylline Toxicity?

Acute Theophylline Toxicity

Many authors[41,43,47] have attempted to identify a specific toxic level that might be predictive of the need for hemoperfusion. Initially it was suggested that if the theophylline level rose above 60 μg/mL or if the patient's clinical status deteriorated, hemoperfusion should be performed while the patient was still hemodynamically stable.[43] Subsequently, others proposed that if the theophylline level approached 90 μg/mL, or if the patient had a seizure or ventricular dysrhythmia, charcoal hemoperfusion should be performed as soon as possible.[41]

In a 5-year, prospective study of more than 270 patients, it was determined that an acute theophylline level greater than 80 μg/mL was predictive of major toxicity and the need for charcoal hemoperfusion.[47] Although the values from these patients range from 60 to 90 μg/mL, the general perspective is quite similar and the indications for hemoperfusion can be defined. Charcoal hemoperfusion is indicated when the theophylline level exceeds 90 μg/mL at any time, or if the patient has a theophylline level greater than 40 μg/mL and seizures, hypotension, ventricular dysrhythmias, or protracted vomiting unresponsive to antiemetics (Table 39–2).

Hemoperfusion and continuous arteriovenous hemoperfusion are more efficient than hemodialysis, which is far better than peritoneal dialysis. Plasmapheresis has also been employed for acute theophylline poisoning, but is less beneficial than either hemodialysis, continuous arteriovenous hemoperfusion, or hemoperfusion and offers little when compared with endogenous clearance.[27] Hemodialysis and hemoperfusion may be used in series for patients with extremely high theophylline levels.[11] The combined use of hemodialysis and hemoperfusion extends the life of the charcoal cartridge, increases the overall extraction fraction and clearance, and allows fluid and electrolyte abnormalities to be corrected.[20] Exchange transfusion may be an option for neonates with severe theophylline poisoning.[42,51]

The estimated clearance for hemoperfusion is 225 mL/min,[28] for hemodialysis 88 mL/min,[29] and for peritoneal dialysis 50 mL/min.[59] Continuous arteriovenous hemoperfusion (nonpump hemoperfusion) has been reported to be 290 mL/min.[31] The normal endogenous clearance of theophylline in an adult patient without enzyme induction is 40 mL/h. The clearance with multiple-dose activated charcoal is approximately 140 mL/min. A comparison of the various clearance rates is found in Figure 39–2.

Patients who are chronically receiving theophylline and then acutely overdose should be treated in the same manner as those with an acute overdose. However, because the total body stores of theophylline will be higher than in patients who are not chronically taking theophylline, the threshold for developing toxicity may be achieved sooner.

TABLE 39–2. INDICATIONS FOR CHARCOAL HEMOPERFUSION

1. Theophylline level >90 μg/mL at any time
2. Theophylline level >40 μg/mL and
   - A. Seizures *or*
   - B. Hypotension, unresponsive to fluids *or*
   - C. Ventricular dysrhythmias *or*
   - D. Protracted vomiting unresponsive to antiemetics

Chronic Theophylline Toxicity

The endogenous clearance of theophylline declines with age and is significantly reduced in patients with congestive heart or liver failure.[18,58] Chronic theophylline toxicity may result from a prescribing error, intentional or unintentional overutilization by the patient, a decrease in hepatic clearance, or a drug interaction. The major distinguishing feature between acute and chronic toxicity is that there is a prolonged period of excessive exposure to theophylline associated with chronic toxicity. Patients often manifest subtle signs such as anorexia, nausea, palpitations, or vomiting; however, the initial presentation in these patients, even with levels in the 40–60 μg/mL range, may be a seizure.[61] In children chronically overdosed with theophylline, the peak theophylline level failed to identify those who would progress to life-threatening toxicity.[49] In the absence of protracted nausea, vomiting, or seizures, the initial electrolytes and blood gases are usually normal in the patient with chronic theophylline toxicity.

The treatment of these patients is often defined by the patient's clinical status and how rapidly the theophylline level can be lowered with multiple-dose activated charcoal. The exact level at which patients with chronic theophylline toxicity should receive charcoal hemoperfusion is controversial. There is no role for either emesis or orogastric lavage in patients with chronic toxicity. If the patient has stable cardiovascular and neurologic function and has not had a seizure or ventricular dysrhythmia, the administration of activated charcoal may be all that is needed. If the patient's theophylline level fails to decline following the administration of activated charcoal or the patient's clinical condition deteriorates, charcoal hemoperfusion is indicated. Charcoal he-

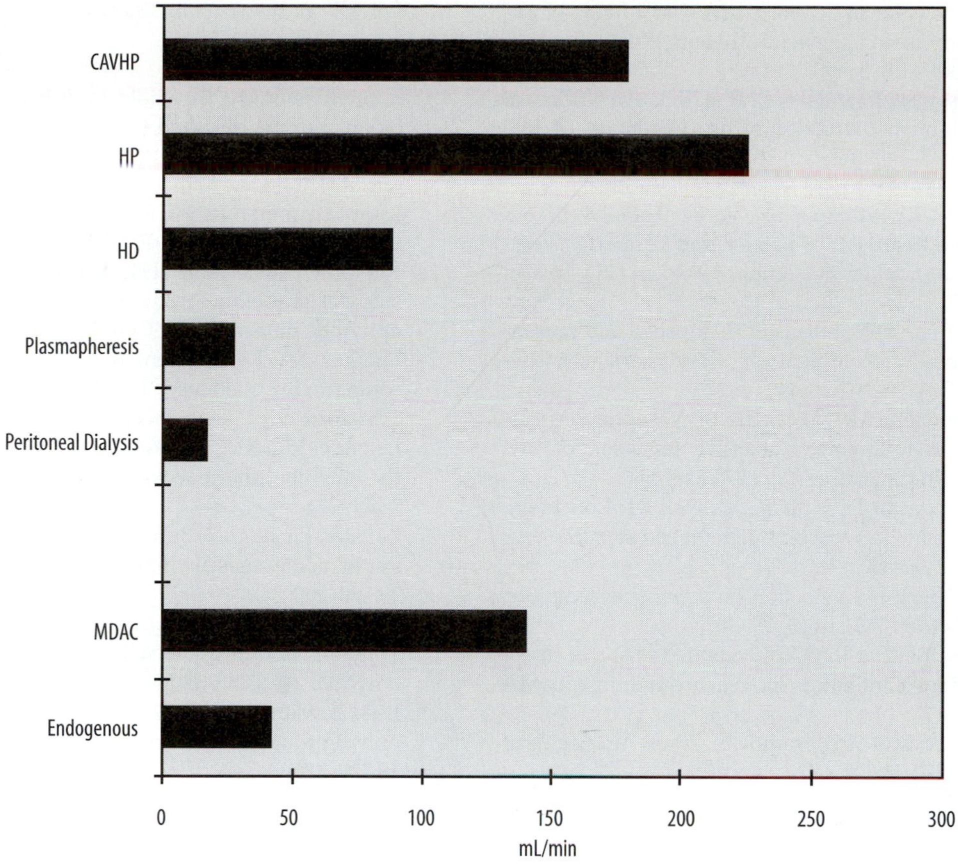

Figure 39–2. Comparative clearance of theophylline via different mechanisms of enhanced removal.

moperfusion is also likely to be needed in patients who have a diminished endogenous clearance. Unfortunately, the patient who is most likely to have diminished clearance is often elderly with congestive heart failure and tachycardia and may not tolerate hemoperfusion very well. Under these circumstances, if congestive heart failure cannot be effectively managed, hemodialysis may be an appropriate alternative to assist in stabilization.

Which Patients Should Be Admitted to a Critical Care Unit?

The decision to admit a patient to a critical care unit should be based on the quantity of theophylline ingested, the patient's present and anticipated clinical condition, the severity of toxic effects since the ingestion, the response to therapy, the laboratory data, and the need for extracoporeal drug removal. Any patient who has had a seizure, ventricular dysrhythmias, or hypotension will require admission to a critical care unit to receive extracorporeal drug removal. Other patients who would benefit from critical care monitoring include those who have significant underlying medical pathology, those who have rising theophylline levels, and those in whom clinical symptoms do not correlate with the theophylline level. In some hospitals admission to the critical care unit may also be necessary if admission elsewhere in the hospital will preclude cardiac monitoring, frequent evaluation of vital signs, the administration of multiple-dose activated charcoal, whole-bowel irrigation, or providing suicide precautions when applicable.

As the frequency with which theophylline is used to treat asthma declines, it is important for today's clinicians to remember the high mortality rate previously associated with sustained-release theophylline overdoses in the 1980s. With experience it was learned that the outcome of these ingestions was usually favorable when the patient was rapidly treated with multiple doses of activated charcoal and when charcoal hemoperfusion was initiated before the patient developed seizures, hypotension, or ventricular dysrhythmias.

References

1. Antal EJ, Kramer PA, Mercik SA, et al: Theophylline pharmacokinetics in advanced age. Br J Clin Pharmacol 1981; 12:637–645.
2. Bernstein G, Jehle D, Bernaski E, Braen GR: Failure of gastric emptying and charcoal administration in fatal sustained-release theophylline overdose: Pharmacobezoar formation. Ann Emerg Med 1992;21:1388–1390.

3. Biberstein MP, Ziegler MG, Ward DM: Use of beta-blockade and hemoperfusion for acute theophylline poisoning. West J Med 1984;141:485–490.
4. Blake KV, Massey KL, Hendeles L, et al: Relative efficacy of phenytoin and phenobarbital for the prevention of theophylline-induced seizures in mice. Ann Emerg Med 1988;17:1024–1028.
5. Clark RF, Chen R, Williams SR, et al: The use of ondansetron in the treatment of nausea and vomiting associated with acetaminophen poisoning. J Toxicol Clin Toxicol 1996;34:163–167.
6. Conrad KA, Nyman DW: Effects of metoprolol and propranolol on theophylline elimination. Clin Pharmacol Ther 1980;28:463–467.
7. Detloff RW, Touchette MA, Zarowitz BJ: Vasopressor-resistant hypotension following a massive ingestion of theophylline. Ann Pharmacother 1993;27:781–784.
8. Eldridge FL, Paydarfar D, Scott SC, Dowell RT: Role of endogenous adenosine in recurrent generalized seizures. Exp Neurol 1989;103:179–185.
9. Fredholm BB: Theophylline action on adenosine receptors. Eur J Respir Dis 1980;180(suppl):29–36.
10. Gal P, Miller A, McCue JD: Oral activated charcoal to enhance theophylline elimination in an acute overdose. JAMA 1984;251:3130–3131.
11. Gibson TP: Kinetics of drug removal. Trans Am Soc Artif Intern Organs 1982;28:672–673.
12. Goldberg MJ, Spector R, Miller G: Phenobarbital improves survival in theophylline-intoxicated rabbits. J Toxicol Clin Toxicol 1986;24:203–211.
13. Goldberg M, Spector R, Park G, et al: The effect of sorbitol and activated charcoal on serum theophylline concentrations after slow release theophylline. Clin Pharmacol Ther 1987;41:108–111.
14. Goulbourne KB, Cisek JE: Small-bowel obstruction secondary to activated charcoal and adhesions. Ann Emerg Med 1994;24:188–190.
15. Grygiel JJ, Birkett DJ: Cigarette smoking and theophylline clearance and metabolism. Clin Pharmacol Ther 1981;4:491–495.
16. Hagstam KE, Larsson LE, Thyssel H: Experimental studies on charcoal hemoperfusion. Acta Med Scand 1966;180:593–603.
17. Hansten PD, Horn JR: Cytochrome P450 Enzyme Drug Interactions. Drug Interactions and Updates Quarterly. Malvern, PA; Lea and Febiger, Vancouver, Washington, Applied Therapeutics, Inc., 1993.
18. Hendeles L, Bighley L, Richardson RH, et al: Frequent toxicity from IV aminophylline infusions in critically ill patients. Drug Intell Clin Pharm 1977;11:12–18.
19. Hoffman RS, Chiang WK, Howland MA, et al: Theophylline desorption from activated charcoal caused by whole bowel irrigation solution. J Toxicol Clin Toxicol 1991;29:191–201.
20. Hootkins R Sr, Lerman MJ, Thompson JR: Sequential and simultaneous "in series" hemodialysis and hemoperfusion in the management of theophylline intoxication. J Am Soc Nephrol 1990;1:923–926.
21. Hornfeldt CS, Larson AA: Adenosine receptors are not involved in theophylline-induced seizures. J Toxicol Clin Toxicol 1994;32:257–265.
22. Horowitz LN, Spear JF, Moore EN, et al: Effects of aminophylline on the threshold for initiating ventricular fibrillation during respiratory failure. Am J Cardiol 1975;35:376–379.
23. Jain R, Tholl DA: Activated charcoal for theophylline toxicity in a premature infant on the second day of life. Dev Pharmacol Ther 1992;19:106–110.
24. Kempf J, Rusterholtz TH, Ber C, et al: Haemodynamic study as guideline for the use of beta blockers in acute theophylline poisoning. Int Care Med 1996;22:585–587.
25. Laggner AN, Kaik G, Lenz K, et al: Treatment of severe poisoning with sustained released theophylline. Br Med J 1984;288:1497.
26. Lalonde RL, McLean WM: The effects of cimetidine on theophylline pharmacokinetics at steady-state. Chest 1983;2:221–224.
27. Laussen P, Shann F, Butt W, Tibballs J: Use of plasmapheresis in acute theophylline toxicity. Crit Care Med 1991;19:288–290.
28. Lawyer C, Aitchison J, Sutton J, et al: Treatment of theophylline neurotoxicity with resin hemoperfusion. Ann Intern Med 1978;38:516–517.
29. Lee CS, Marbury TC, Perrin JH, et al: Hemodialysis of theophylline in uremic patients. J Clin Pharmacol 1979;19:219–226.
30. Levine JH, Michael JR, Guamieri T: Treatment of multifocal atrial tachycardia with verapamil. N Engl J Med 1985;312:21–25.
31. Lin JL, Jeng LB: Critical, acutely poisoned patients treated with continuous arteriovenous hemoperfusion in the emergency department. Ann Emerg Med 1995;25:75–80.
32. Lohmann SM, Miech RP: Theophylline metabolism by the rat microsomal system. J Pharmacol Exp Ther 1976;196:213–225.
33. Maddux MS, Leeds NH, Organek HW, et al: The effect of erythromycin on theophylline pharmacokinetics at steady state. Chest 1982;5:563–565.
34. Mahutte CK, True RJ, Michiels TM, et al: Increased serum theophylline clearance with orally administered activated charcoal. Am Rev Respir Dis 1983;128:820–822.
35. Marquis JF, Carruthers SG, Spence JD, et al: Phenytoin-theophylline interaction. N Engl J Med 1982;307:1189–1190.
36. Minocha A, Spyker DA: Acute overdose with sustained release drug formulations: Perspectives in treatment. Med Toxicol 1986;1:300–307.
37. Minton NA, Glucksman E, Henry JA: Prevention of drug absorption in simulated theophylline overdose. Hum Exp Toxicol 1995;14:170–174.
38. Nahata MC, Powell DA, Franko TG: Some infants receiving theophylline may have caffeine in serum. Ther Drug Monit 1983;5:269–270.
39. Ogilvie RI: Clinical pharmacokinetics of theophylline. Clin Pharmacokinet 1978;3:267–293.
40. Ohning BL, Reed MD, Blumer JL: Continuous nasogastric administration of activated charcoal for the treatment of theophylline intoxication. Pediatr Pharmacol 1986;5:241–245.

41. Olson KR, Benowitz NL, Woo OF, et al: Theophylline overdose: Acute single ingestion versus chronic repeated overmedication. Am J Emerg Med 1985;3:386–394.
42. Osborn HH, Henry G, Wax P, et al: Theophylline toxicity in a premature neonate—elimination kinetics of exchange transfusion. J Toxicol Clin Toxicol 1993;31:639–644.
43. Park GD, Spector R, Roberts RJ, et al: Use of hemoperfusion for the treatment of theophylline toxicity. Am J Med 1983;74:961–966.
44. Renton KW, Gray JD, Hall RJ: Decreased elimination of theophylline after influenza vaccination. Can Med Assoc J 1980;123:288–290.
45. Sawyer WT, Caravati EM, Ellison MJ, Krueger KA: Hypokalemia, hyperglycemia and acidosis after intentional theophylline overdose. Am J Emerg Med 1985;3:408–411.
46. Shammas FV, Deckstein K: Clinical pharmacokinetics in heart failure: An updated review. Clin Pharmacokinet 1988;15:94.
47. Shannon MW: Predictors of major toxicity after theophylline overdose. Ann Intern Med 1993;119:1161–1167.
48. Shannon MW, Amitai Y, Lovejoy FH Jr: Multiple dose activated charcoal for theophylline poisoning in young infants. Pediatrics 1987;80:368–370.
49. Shannon MW, Lovejoy FH Jr: Effect of acute versus chronic intoxication on clinical features of theophylline poisoning in children. J Pediatr 1992;121:125–130.
50. Shannon MW, Lovejoy FH Jr: Hypokalemia after theophylline intoxication. The effects of acute vs chronic poisoning. Arch Intern Med 1989;149:2725–2729.
51. Shannon MW, Wernovsky G, Morris C: Exchange transfusion in the treatment of severe theophylline poisoning. Pediatrics 1992;89:145–147.
52. Sustained release theophyllines. Med Lett Drugs Ther 1984;26:1–3.
53. Roberts JR, Carney S, Boyle SM, Lee DC: Ondansetron quells drug-resistant emesis in theophylline poisoning. Am J Emerg Med 1993;11:609–610.
54. True RT, Berman JM, Mahutte K: Treatment of theophylline toxicity with oral activated charcoal. Crit Care Med 1984; 12:113–114.
55. Ujhelyi MR, Hulula G, Skau KA: Role of exogenous adenosine as a modulator of theophylline toxicity. Crit Care Med 1994;22:1639–1646.
56. Vestal RE, Eiriksson CE Jr, Musser B, et al: Effect of intravenous aminophylline on plasma levels of catecholamines and related cardiovascular and metabolic responses in man. Circulation 1983;67:162–171.
57. Vozeh S, Powell R, Riegelman S, et al: Changes in theophylline clearances during acute illness. JAMA 1978;240: 1882–1884.
58. Weinberger M, Hendeles L: Theophylline in asthma. N Eng J Med 1996;334:1380–1388.
59. Weinberger M, Hendeles L: Role of dialysis in the management and prevention of theophylline toxicity. Dev Pharmacol Ther 1980;1:26–30.
60. Weinberger M, Matthay R, Ginchansky E, et al: Intravenous aminophylline dosage: Use of serum theophylline measurement for guidance. JAMA 1976;235: 2110–2113.
61. Young D, Dragunow M: Status epilepticus may be caused by a loss of adenosine anticonvulsant mechanisms. Neuroscience 1994;58:245–261.
62. Zwillich CW, Sutton FD, Neff TA, et al: Theophylline-induced seizures in adults. Ann Intern Med 1975;82:784–787.

CHAPTER 40

Hypoglycemic Agents

Lewis R. Goldfrank

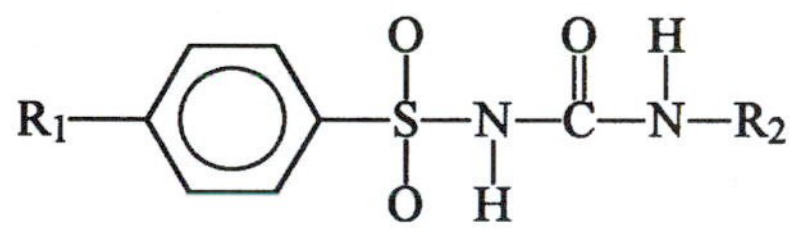

Sulfonylureas

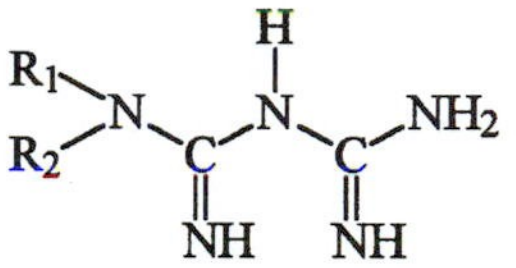

Biguanides

Glucose		
MW	=	180 daltons
Normal range (blood)	=	70–110 mg/dL
	=	3.9–6.1 mmol/L

Five police officers entered the emergency department (ED) with an obese, middle-aged man whose arms were handcuffed behind his back. He was extremely agitated, diffusely diaphoretic, bleeding from the mouth, and had several small lacerations and multiple contusions. His respirations were labored. The police stated that they had been called by the man's family after he had "gone berserk." When they arrived at the apartment, several pieces of furniture had been broken, and it took all five police officers to restrain the man. In a few minutes, the family arrived in the ED. They related that the patient had been despondent recently; they suspected he had been drinking. In addition, they reported, he was taking various unknown medications, "because he's been sick." Shortly after the handcuffs were removed to permit physical examination, the patient developed a focal seizure that began in his right hand and progressed to become a typical generalized tonic-clonic seizure lasting 2 minutes. After the seizure, vital signs were: blood pressure, 120/80 mm Hg; pulse, 120 beats/min; respiration, 24 breaths/ min; temperature, 36.8°C (98.4°F). The patient was lethargic but oriented. The remainder of the neurologic examination revealed a right hemiparesis, right conjugate gaze, right central facial paralysis and right-sided plantar extension. The pupils were equal and reactive to light, and the fundi were unremarkable. He had no evidence of significant head trauma. His chest was clear to percussion and auscultation, and heart sounds were normal except for tachycardia. Abdominal examination revealed no hepatosplenomegaly or palpable mass. The rectal examination was unremarkable, and the stool was negative for occult blood. Multiple contusions were clearly visible on his extremities, but there were no overt fractures and there was no edema.

In this case, the diagnosis was made before the laboratory data returned. Within 5 minutes of administration of IV dextrose and thiamine, the right-sided neurologic findings disappeared, the lethargy cleared, and the patient was sufficiently alert to relate a history. The patient stated that his private physician had placed him on chlorpropamide (Diabinese) for "mild diabetes." Because his mother had died of diabetes, he thought he knew the type of complications he might expect. He became despondent, he said, because of his "inevitable fate" and began to drink. The alcohol, however, only led to more frequent episodes of despondency.

Pretreatment serum glucose was 18 mg/dL. Although the patient's blood sugar remained elevated in the ED, he was admitted to the hospital so that he could be observed for, and if necessary treated for, recurrent hypoglycemia. An IV line was maintained for 24 hours until the patient began to eat regularly. No neurologic sequelae were observed. Diabetic education and alcoholism counseling were initiated during his 2-day hospitalization, which was uneventful. He was discharged to the care of his private physician and the chlorpropamide was discontinued.

Some pharmacologic agents taken in excess produce effects that are exaggerations of the intended therapeutic effects, whereas other drug overdoses produce unique signs of toxicity. An example of the former is an antihypertensive drug overdose, which may result in severe hypotension; examples of the latter are salicylate overdoses resulting in acid–base derangements and hyperthermia, and iron overdoses resulting in gastrointestinal bleeding. For those drug overdoses that result in exaggerated physiologic or pharmacologic effects, it is often difficult to separate out intentional from unintentional overdoses and physiologic conditions from pathophysiologic states.

Nowhere, perhaps, are these issues more relevant than to a discussion of hypoglycemic agents. Hypoglycemic agents are a diverse group of drugs including various types of insulin, sulfonylureas, biguanides and now α-glucosidase inhibitors, all of which—with the possible exception of the biguanides—may produce a nearly identical clinical state of hypoglycemia. In such instances a "unified" therapeutic plan based on the *clinical presentation* (hypoglycemia) is necessary at the same time that a logical diagnostic evaluation is initiated to identify the specific etiology of the hypoglycemia. To discuss the toxicity of sulfonylureas, the biochemistry, physiology, and pharmacology of glucose metabolism must be understood. To be able to diagnose an *exogenous* insulin overdose or poisoning, the production and metabolism of *endogenous* insulin must be understood.

What Are the Etiologies of Hypoglycemia?

Hypoglycemia is the failure to maintain a serum glucose above 60 mg/dL. In healthy individuals neurohormonal control of glucose production maintains a serum glucose level of 70–110 mg/dL. Values less than 60 mg/dL develop when counterregulation becomes impaired or is overwhelmed.[22] Symptoms are usually noted when circulating plasma glucose levels fall below 45 mg/dL or higher when levels fall rapidly. The alcoholic patient is at substantially greater risk than the nonalcoholic for hypoglycemia because as hepatic glycogen is depleted, normal glycemic control is diminished by lack of nutritional intake, and gluconeogenesis is impaired (Chap. 62).

In the alcoholic, carbohydrate intake is typically decreased, and there is a lack of hepatic glycogen stores in the liver; fat is mobilized from adipose tissue as an energy source. The fall in serum glucose that can be induced by sulfonylureas may lead to the release of epinephrine, producing a sense of anxiety and/or malaise, dysesthesias, diaphoresis, and tachycardia. Sulfonylurea agents are also responsible for disulfiram-like reactions (Chap. 63).

The etiologies of hypoglycemia may be divided into three general categories:[3,31] physiologic or pathophysiologic conditions (Table 40–1); direct effects of various hypoglycemic agents (Tables 40–2, 40–3),[40,73] and the potentiation of hypoglycemic agents by interactions with other pharmacologic agents (Table 40–4). The most common cause of severe hypoglycemia resulting in an emergency department visit is actual excessive insulin use or insulin use relatively excessive for the caloric intake or exercise level of the individual at a particular moment. The tightness of glucose control to near normal glucose values, the characteristics of each individual's awareness of hypoglycemia, and the individual counterregulatory mechanisms define the frequency and intensity of hypoglycemia.[74] The Diabetic Control and Complications Trial (DCCT) research group suggested that there are at least 120 episodes of blood glucose < 50 mg/dL with CNS manifestations requiring assistance for every 100 patient years with the current intensive insulin therapy regimens.[23,24] In a review of 1418 medication-related cases of hypoglycemia, sulfonylureas (especially the long-acting agents chlorpropamide and glyburide) alone or with a second agent accounted for the largest percentage of cases: 63%. Conversely, hypoglycemia has been reported in as many as 21% of patients using sulfonylureas.[45] Alcohol, propranolol, and salicylate, either alone or with another hypoglycemic drug, accounted for another 19% of cases of hypoglycemia, and quinine, quinidine, pentamidine, ritodrine, and disopyramide were the most common of the less frequently associated agents.

In overdose, oral sulfonylurea agents produce hypoglycemia by stimulating the release of preformed pancreatic insulin. Extrapancreatic effects may be more important with therapeutic doses. The incidence of sulfonylurea-induced hypoglycemia seems to be directly proportional to the half-life of the agent. It is exceedingly important to realize how commonly hypoglycemia may occur with sulfonylureas, as these agents represent approximately 1% of all U.S. prescriptions.[36] In older studies the mortality rate approached 10% in the sulfonylurea-induced hypoglycemia population.[5]

Drug-induced hypoglycemia is exceedingly dangerous in the elderly, in those with hepatic or renal disease,

TABLE 40–1. CAUSES OF HYPOGLYCEMIA

Endocrine Disorders	***Exogenous***
Addison's disease	Ackee (hypoglycin)
Glucagon deficiency	Alloxan
Panhypopituitarism (Sheehan syndrome)	Beta-adrenergic antagonists
Neoplasms	Cocaine
Carcinomas (diverse extrapancreatic)	Ethanol
Hematologic	Hypoglycemic agents (insulin, sulfonylureas)
Insulinoma	Opioids
Mesenchymal	Pentamidine
Multiple endocrine adenopathy type I (Werner syndrome)	Quinine
	Quinidine
Reactive Hypoglycemia	Ritodrine
	Salicylates
Hepatic Disease	Streptozocin
Acute hepatic atrophy	Sulfonamides
Alcoholism	Vacor
Cirrhosis	Valproic acid
Galactose or fructose intolerance	
Glycogen storage disease	***Artifactual***
Neoplasia	Chronic myelogenous leukemia
	Polycythemia vera
Renal Disease	
Chronic hemodialysis	
Chronic renal insufficiency	
Miscellaneous	
Acquired immunodeficiency syndrome (AIDS)	
Anorexia nervosa	
Autoimmune disorders	
SLE	
Rheumatoid arthritis	
Grave's disease	
Burns	
Diarrhea (childhood)	
Leucine sensitivity	
Muscular activity (excessive)	
Postgastric surgery	
Pregnancy	
Protein calorie malnutrition	
Septicemia	
Shock	
Wasting syndrome	

in the malnourished,[69,84] in alcoholics,[53] and in patients abusing various drugs (Tables 40–1, 40–4). Children are particularly vulnerable to ethanol-induced hypoglycemia. Common medication errors associated with oral hypoglycemic agents attributable to pharmacists, physicians, or patients include the mistaken substitution of Tolinase for Tolectin, Diabinese for Diamox, chlorpropamide for chlorpromazine,[43,75] or acetohexamide for acetazolamide. The last pair are particularly problematic since their corresponding brand names are Dymelor and Diamox, respectively.[77]

An interesting etiology of hypoglycemia observed in Africa and the West Indies for over a hundred years is occasionally seen in this country as well. The ackee tree (*Blighia sapida*), ubiquitous in Jamaica, produces a small fruit, the aril of which is edible. Because this fruit is a staple for the poor, it is often eaten before it is ripe; this practice has resulted in numerous epidemics of a toxic hypoglycemic syndrome.[18] The unripe fruit contains the toxic watersoluble substance hypoglycin, which produces vomiting, seizures, CNS depression, and hypoglycemia.[13] The hypoglycemic activity of hypoglycin results from its inhibition of hepatic gluconeogenesis.[14] Methylenecyclopropane acetic acid, a hypoglycin metabolite, forms nonmetabolizable carnitine and coesters, depressing tissue levels of these cofactors and limiting active gluconeogenesis.[80] Poisoning with ackee has a high fatality rate if unrecognized, partly due to the poor nutritional state of those driven to eat this fruit even though it is widely recognized as toxic when in the unripe state.

What Are the Pharmacologic Characteristics of the Orally Administered Hypoglycemic Agents?

There are two major groups of orally administered hypoglycemic agents (Table 40–1); the sulfonylureas and the biguanides. Recently, the α-glucosidase inhibitors (acarbose) and the thiazolidinedione derivatives (troglitazone) have been introduced.

The sulfonylureas stimulate the β-cells of the pancreas to produce insulin; they are ineffective in type I diabetics who lack the capacity to produce insulin. This stimulatory effect diminishes with chronic therapy. All the hypoglycemic sulfonylureas have molecular mechanisms that involve direct inhibition of potassium channels sensitive to adenosine triphosphate (K_{ATP} channels) in the β-cell membrane.[28,34,36] This inhibition of potassium ion efflux from pancreatic β-cells causes membrane depolarization, calcium influx, and activation of the secretory machinery independent of glucose concentration. High-affinity sulfonylurea receptors are present in pancreatic β-cells, whose binding promotes exocytosis by direct interaction with secretory machinery not involving closure of the plasma membrane K_{ATP} channels.[28,34,36] The first-generation sulfonylureas (acetohexamide, chlorpropamide, tolazamide, and tolbutamide) reduce hepatic clearance of insulin, produce active hepatic metabolites, and are dependent on urinary excretion to maintain euglycemia. The second-generation sulfonylureas (glimepiride, glipizide, and glyburide) have half-lives that approach 24 hours and are associated with substantial fecal excretion of the parent drug and frequent episodes of hypoglycemia (see Fig. 40–1).

Both the sulfonylureas and the biguanides lower the blood glucose in diabetic patients; the biguanides do not lower blood glucose in normal patients, although the sulfonylureas do. The biguanides may stimulate tissue glucose uptake and inhibit gluconeogenesis, but they do not stimulate insulin secretion.[36]

The α-glucosidase inhibitor acarbose competitively inhibits glucoamylase. This effectively reduces intestinal starch and disaccharide absorption by inhibiting intestinal α-glucosidase. Acarbose is completely metabolized in

TABLE 40–2. CHARACTERISTICS OF ORALLY ADMINISTERED HYPOGLYCEMIC AGENTS

Drug	Duration of Action (h)	Active Hepatic Metabolite	Active Urinary Excretory Product (% of dose)	Fecal Excretion (% of dose)	Frequency of Severe Hypoglycemia (other complications)
I. Sulfonylureas					
First generation					
Acetohexamide (Dymelor)	12–18	Hydroxyhexamide (+++) Acetohexamide (2%)	Hydroxyhexamide (65%)	Negligible	~1%
Chlorpropamide (Diabinese)	24–72	2-Hydroxychlorpropamide (+) 3-Hydroxychlorpropamide (+)	Chlorpropamide (20%) 2-Hydroxychlorpropamide (55%) 3-Hydroxychlorpropamide (2%)	Negligible	4–6%
Tolazamide (Tolinase)	16–24	Hydroxytolazamide (++) Tolazamide (7%)	Hydroxytolazamide (35%)	Negligible	~1%
Tolbutamide (Orinase)	6–12	Hydroxytolbutamide (+)	Hydroxytolbutamide (30%) Tolbutamide (2%)	Negligible	<1%
Second generation					
Glimepiride (Amaryl)	24	Cyclohexylhydroxy ethyl derivative (30%)	Cyclohexylhydroxy methyl derivative (63%)	15%	1–2%
Glipizide (Glucotrol, Glucotrol XL)	16–24	None	Glipizide (3%)	12%	2–4%
Glyburide (Micronase, Glynase, DiaBeta)	18–24	4-Hydroxyglyburide (++)	4-Hydroxyglyburide (36%) Glyburide (3%)	50%	4–6%
II. Biguanides					
Metformin (Glucophage)	1.3–4.5	None	Metformin (90%)	Negligible	None (?) (lactic acidosis 0.03 cases/1000 patient years)
Phenformin	6–8	None	Phenformin (66%)	Negligible	Uncommon (lactic acidosis 0.64 cases/1000 patient years)
III. Alpha-Glucosidase Inhibitor					
Acarbose (Precose)	2	None	4-Methyl pyrogallol derivative (<2%)	0%	None (?)
IV. Thiazolidinedione Derivatives					
Troglitazone (Rezulin)	16–34	None	None	Total	None (hepatotoxicity)

+ = Weakly active, ++ = moderately active, +++ = more active than parent drug. The durations of action for the oral agents are cited for therapeutic doses. These values increase for overdoses.
Some of the material is adapted from Gerich JE: Oral hypoglycemic agents. N Engl J Med 1989; 321:1231–1245.

the gastrointestinal tract. Experience with acarbose is limited, but flatulence, abdominal bloating, and malabsorption are common complications.[15] Acarbose does not cause hypoglycemia itself, but may potentiate the action of the sulfonylureas when used concomitantly.

What Are the Characteristics and Risks Associated With the Biguanides: Metformin and Phenformin?

The biguanides metformin and phenformin were developed as derivatives of guanidine, the active components of *Galega officinalis*, the French lilac recognized in medieval Europe as a treatment for diabetes.[6] Metformin, a dimethylbiguanide, improves insulin sensitivity, reduces fasting plasma glucose, increases glycogen formation, and decreases the insulin resistance prevalent in NIDDM.[7] Metformin inhibits gluconeogenesis and reduces hepatic glucose output, thereby reducing fasting blood glucose. In none of the metformin studies was plasma lactate concentration or turnover increased nor metabolism of lactate inhibited.[79] These particular findings differentiate metformin from phenformin, which inhibited mitochondrial lactate utilization.[35] Phenformin was withdrawn from the U.S. market in 1976 due to its unacceptably high risk of refractory lactic acidosis (64 cases/100,000 patient years).[33] Although similar structurally, metformin has a risk of lactic acidosis of only 3 cases/100,000 patient years.[20] However, the risk of adverse reactions from metformin increases with renal impairment, cardiorespiratory insufficiency, a history of lactic acidosis, severe infection, liver disease, or alcohol abuse.

TABLE 40–3. CHARACTERISTICS OF ROUTINELY USED FORMS OF INSULIN

Insulin	Duration of Action (h)	Metabolism
Ultra-short Acting		
Lispro (Humalog)	<5	Renal and hepatic metabolism
Short Acting		
Regular	5–8	Renal and hepatic metabolism
Mixed pork–beef		
Pork		
Human biosynthetic		
Beef		
Semilente	12–16	Renal and hepatic metabolism
Mixed pork–beef		
Beef		
Intermediate Acting		
Lente	18–24	Renal and hepatic metabolism
Mixed		
Beef		
Pork		
Human		
Mixtard		
70% isophane	24	
30% regular		
Pork		
Human		
NPH		
Mixed	18–24	
Beef		
Pork		
Human		
Long Acting		
Protamine zinc insulin (PZI)	24–36	Renal excretion
Ultralente		
Mixed beef–pork	20–36	
Beef		
Human		

Although metformin may be given with insulin, it is generally used in a regimen where a sulfonylurea serves as the hypoglycemic agent while metformin exerts its antihyperglycemic effect.[7] As use of metformin becomes more prevalent, it is extremely important to be clinically vigilant for the occurrence of lactic acidosis.

Even though phenformin was withdrawn from the U.S. market in 1976, cases of phenformin-induced severe lactic acidosis continue to be reported in this country, as phenformin is still available in Canada, Europe, and South America. Travelers and immigrant patients (particularly the elderly) who continue to receive medication from their native countries may present here with metabolic acidosis. This is particularly likely for those with chronic renal failure.

TABLE 40–4. DRUGS OR TOXINS KNOWN TO REACT WITH HYPOGLYCEMIC AGENTS RESULTING IN HYPOGLYCEMIA

ACE inhibitors	Monamine oxidase inhibitors
Allopurinol	Oxytetracycline
Anabolic steroids	Para-aminobenzoic acid
Beta-adrenergic antagonists	Pentamidine
Chloramphenicol	Phenylbutazone
Clofibrate	Probenecid
Dicoumarol	Propoxyphene
Disopyramide	Quinine
Ethanol	Salicylates
Guanethidine	Sulfinpyrazone
Haloperidol	Sulfonamide
Methotrexate	Trimethoprim-sulfamethoxazole

How Do Beta-Adrenergic Antagonists Affect Glucose Metabolism?

The sympathetic nervous system regulates glucagon and insulin secretion, muscle glycogenolysis, adipose lipolysis, and hepatic glucose production. Propranolol and other beta-adrenergic antagonists affect all of these mechanisms and can result in hypoglycemia. In addition, lack of the expected autonomic response to hypoglycemia makes the need for caution with the use of beta-adrenergic antagonists even greater in insulin-dependent diabetics. Although we must still assume this to be true, an adverse effect on hypoglycemic awareness could not be demonstrated in healthy volunteers given metoprolol, atenolol, and propranolol.[49] Renal insufficiency increases insulin half-life and impairs metabolism of insulin. Renal gluconeogenesis is also reduced.[60] For these reasons, in the presence of chronic renal failure, beta-adrenergic antagonist–induced hypoglycemia is a particular risk.[38]

There are now numerous reports[32,72] of neonates with bradycardia and hypoglycemia during the first day of life following delivery from women who had received beta-adrenergic antagonists. Newborn hypoglycemia has also resulted from the use of beta-adrenergic agonists as tocolytics, presumably causing glycogen depletion, hyperinsulinemia, and hypoglycemia.[29]

What Immediate Therapeutic Measures Are Indicated for Hypoglycemia-Induced Seizures?

A patient who presents with generalized seizures should have a patent airway immediately established and maintained. To decrease the chance of aspiration and to facilitate airway suctioning, the patient should be placed left side down on a bed or stretcher (with the side rail up). The patient should be protected from further injury by restraint, if necessary cushioning the head and removing all constricting clothing, and 100% oxygen should be ad-

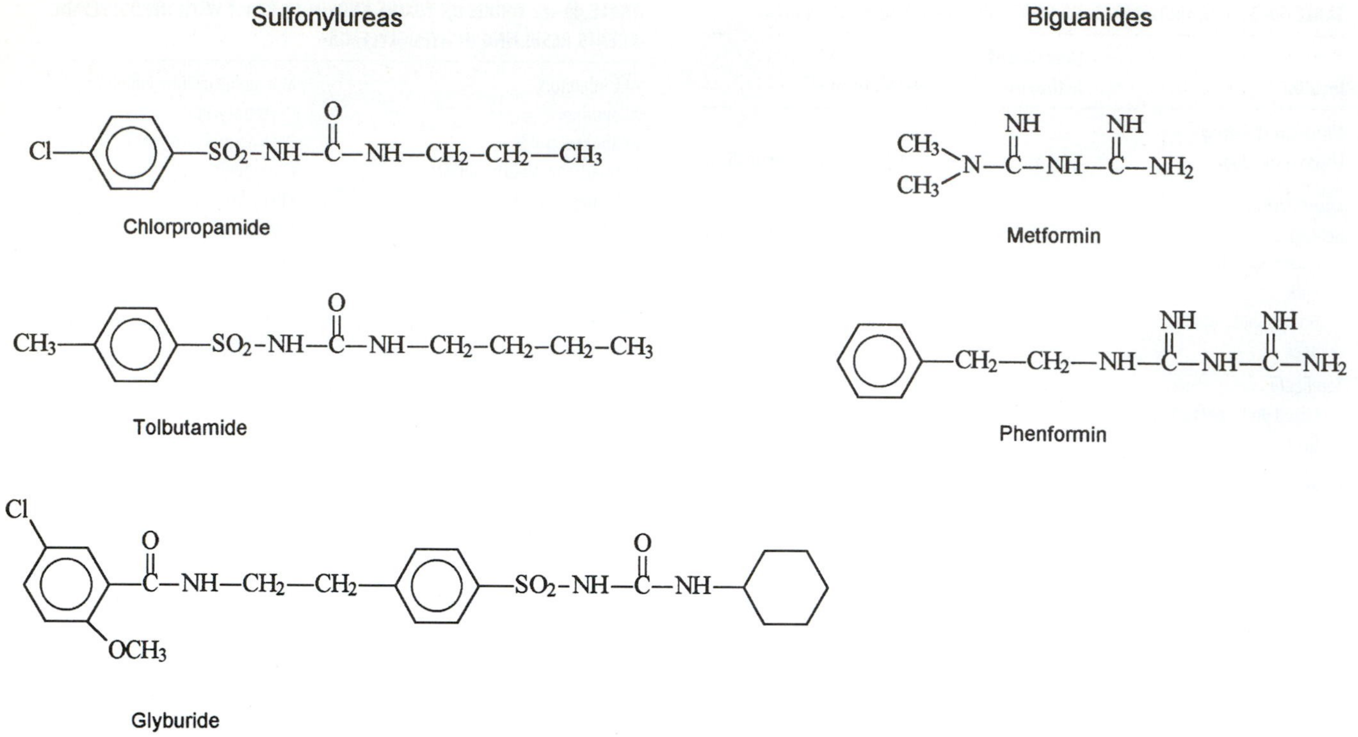

Figure 40–1. The structural formulas of representative first- and second-generation sulfonylureas and the biguanides.

ministered. Cardiac monitoring and pulse oximetry should be utilized. A stable intravenous (IV) line should be established. The nature and duration of any seizures should be observed to assist in localization and determination of possible etiologies.

Blood samples should be drawn for glucose, BUN, electrolytes, calcium, magnesium, CBC, and an ethanol level. Following the use of a bedside glucose determination with a reagent strip or glucometer 1 g/kg body weight dextrose in water and 100 mg of thiamine hydrochloride should be given intravenously as initial therapy. Glucose, not glucagon, should be given to a patient with clinical or laboratory manifestations of hypoglycemia to treat and diagnose or exclude hypoglycemia. Glucagon should not be used for these purposes because many patients are glycogen-depleted (elderly, alcoholic, or cancer patients). Appropriate emergency and toxicologic uses of hypertonic dextrose ($D_{50}W$, $D_{25}W$) as well as glucagon are described in Antidotes in Depth: Dextrose.

Is There a Relationship Between Hypothermia or Hyperthermia and Hypoglycemia?

In a study comparing two groups of comatose and stuporous patients, hypothermia was almost exclusively limited to the hypoglycemic patients; of these, 53% with demonstrated hypoglycemia showed hypothermia.[48] Hypothermia was present in 100% of the hypoglycemic patients presenting between 5:00 A.M. and noon. When mild hypothermia (32.2–35°C; 90–95°F) accompanies hypoglycemia, passive rewarming is usually sufficient treatment, and the temperature usually returns to normal within 2–3 hours. Conversely, in severe and protracted situations, the central hypothalamic response to hypoglycemia stimulated by the sympathetic nervous system may actually "overshoot" normal temperatures, resulting in the hyperthermia found in some hypoglycemic patients[19] (see Chap. 10). Hypoglycemic hypothermic patients who have grand mal seizures may have initially been even more hypothermic since a temperature elevation of several degrees is commonly noted for several hours after a major motor seizure.[82]

What Are the Neurologic Findings of Hypoglycemia?

The presentations of hypoglycemia are extremely variable. Any neuropsychiatric abnormality, whether persistent or transient, focal or generalized, must be considered a possible effect of hypoglycemia (see Table 40–5). The cerebral cortex is usually most severely affected. Categorization of the findings of hypoglycemia have been defined as follows.[64]

1. Delirium with subdued, confused, or manic behavior.
2. Coma with multifocal brainstem abnormalities, including posturing and respiratory abnormalities, with preservation of the oculocephalic (doll's eyes) response, oculovestibular (cold-caloric) response, and pupillary responses.
3. Focal neurologic deficits simulating a CVA with or without the presence of coma.

TABLE 40–5. MANIFESTATIONS OF HYPOGLYCEMIA

Signs due to Catecholamine Release (Neurogenic, Autonomic)	Signs due to Cerebral Glucose Deprivation (Neuroglycopenia)
Tremor, shivering	Blurred vision
Tachycardia, palpitations	Dysesthesias, paresthesias
Diaphoresis	Inability to concentrate
Pallor	Loss of coordination
Piloerection	Weakness
Anxiety	Somnolence, fatigue
Hypertension	Altered behavior pattern
Headache	Hypothermia
Dry mouth	Seizures
Hunger	Hemiplegia
Nausea	Coma
Angina	Death

4. Solitary or multiple seizures, with or without a significant postical phase.

During a 12-month period, three of 125 (2.4%) hypoglycemic patients presented with hemiplegia.[54] There are numerous reports[1] and series[71,83] of patients with focal neurologic deficits. These papers suggest a low but consistent percentage of patients with focal neurologic findings subsequent to hypoglycemia.

Neuropsychiatric symptoms are usually reversible if the hypoglycemia is corrected promptly. The morbidity resulting from missing hypoglycemia is related partly to the etiology and partly to the duration and severity of the hypoglycemia. Because the etiologies of hypoglycemia encompass both severe diseases such as fulminant hepatic failure and some benign problems such as a missed meal by an insulin-requiring diabetic, the literature is confusing with regard to outcome. For example, while an outpatient study reported an 11% mortality in the study group,[54] only one death (0.8%) was attributed to hypoglycemia, whereas four survivors (3.2%), suffered from residual neurologic deficits. In a tertiary care medical center, 1.2% of all admitted patients had hypoglycemia. The overall mortality was 27% for this group of 94 patients.[31] The longer and more profound the hypoglycemic episode, the more likely permanent CNS damage will occur.[4] It cannot be overemphasized that there are no absolute criteria available from the physical examination or history to distinguish one form of metabolic coma from another. Moreover, the findings classically associated with hypoglycemia—tremor, sweating, tachycardia, confusion, coma, and convulsion—may or may not occur (see Table 40–5). This clinical presentation may be further muted when beta-adrenergic antagonists are used concurrently. Typical findings of tachycardia and diaphoresis are not always present and even when both are present cannot be used to conclusively diagnose hypoglycemia.[42] Currently there is a great interest in the concept that patients may be unaware of hypoglycemia, particularly in those with well-controlled insulin-dependent diabetes mellitus. It appears that even in the presence of hypoglycemia, those individuals with near normal glycosylated hemoglobin values maintain near normal glucose uptake by the brain, thereby preserving cerebral metabolism and limiting the response of counterregulatory hormones. The result of this limited response is unawareness of hypoglycemia.[10,12] The authors suggest that a threshold level is achieved below which the glucose concentration is inadequate, but it is a level so close to that which causes serious neuroglycopenia that patients have limited opportunity for corrective action.[12]

Atrial fibrillation and ventricular premature contractions are the most common dysrhythmias associated with hypoglycemia.[50,58] An outpouring of catecholamines, hypoglycemia itself, transient electrolyte abnormalities, and underlying heart disease appear to be the most likely etiologies, as evidenced by the disappearance of these dysrhythmias with glucose repletion. Other cardiovascular manifestations of hypoglycemia include angina and ischemia, which have been reported as the sole manifestations in an individual.[27] Both have been demonstrated to be directly related to hypoglycemia.[9,63]

After Control of the Acute Episode, How Should the Hypoglycemic Patient Be Managed?

The most frequent reasons for missing hypoglycemia and mismanaging hypoglycemic patients are the erroneous conclusions that the patient is not hypoglycemic, but psychotic, epileptic, experiencing a CVA, or intoxicated because of an "odor of alcohol" on the breath (Chap. 62); compounding the problem of misdiagnosis is the erroneous assumption that a single bolus of 0.5–1 g/kg of 50% dextrose in water for an adult will always be sufficient therapy.

Numerous articles have evaluated approaches for treating insulin reactions with carbohydrates in tablets, solutions, or gels in a well-defined diabetic population.[16,76] None of these are appropriate gestures (other than as temporizing measures) for the unknown, possibly hypoglycemic patient. ED patients who have clinical symptoms of hypoglycemia and are unable to care for themselves are almost always glucopenic and run the risk of grave CNS complications unless treated quickly and adequately with glucose.

All patients with hypoglycemic symptoms require intravenous therapy, usually with 10% dextrose, delivering quantities of glucose in the first hour comparable to that delivered in the 1 g/kg IV bolus of $D_{50}W$ in adults. In children 0.5–1.0 g/kg IV should be administered as $D_{25}W$ (a 1:1 dilution with sterile water of $D_{50}W$) and in neonates as $D_{10}W$ (or 1:4 dilution). The hyperosmolarity of these solutions limits their use in peripheral veins. Neonates should not receive more than a 12.5% glucose concentration. One problem that occurs with glucose administration is that individuals who can produce insulin through glucose-stimulated insulin release are at substantial risk of recurrent hypoglycemia. Patients taking oral hypoglycemic agents with prolonged half-lives who are treated with hypertonic glucose solutions can be expected to have a dramatic yet transient increase in glucose concentration, with a subsequent fall in serum glucose possibly to hypoglycemic levels again. A rigorous attempt must be made to avoid recurrent hypoglycemia after successful initial therapy. A state of relative euglycemia may be maintained by delivering large quantities of detrose (50 mL of dextrose is only 100 cal: 25 g at 4 cal/g of dextrose = 100 cal).

Once the patient is awake and alert, 10% dextrose in water should be given intravenously and the rate of infusion adjusted to keep the patient relatively euglycemic (100–250 mg/dL). Some patients may need more concentrated dextrose infusions, such as 20% dextrose in water augmented by repeated doses of 50% dextrose in water. Central venous lines should be used when an infusion of 20% dextrose is instituted, as the solution is a substantial venous irritant. The presence of glycosuria is not an adequate indicator of euglycemia; serial blood glucose, potassium, and phosphate levels must be obtained. The duration of sampling necessary will depend on the stability of the patient, the underlying metabolic disorders, the extent, route, and type of overdose, and the rate of improvement.

As the patient begins to eat an adequate daily diet (at least 300 g of carbohydrates), and if the initial etiology of the hypoglycemia is controlled, the serum glucose will rise and the infusion may then be tapered. At this stage most patients may be switched to D_5W. By the second or third hospital day many patients may actually have significant hyperglycemia.

As noted previously, glucagon should not be used in the ED instead of dextrose. This is true even when glycogen stores are known to be present, because even then there may be a substantial delay in elevating blood sugar and some patients may not respond to this therapy. Only in the known diabetic, when IV access is a problem, should glucagon (1–2 mg IM) be used as emergency therapy. Never under any circumstances should it be assumed that a patient who has no clinical response to glucagon is not hypoglycemic.

The benefits of emesis, lavage, and catharsis should be considered in managing a patient with an overdose of oral hypoglycemic agents. The extensive affinity between carbutamide, chlorpropamide, tolazamide, tolbutamide, glyburide, and glipizide and activated charcoal has been demonstrated in vitro.[47] The affinities ranged from 0.45 to 0.52 g/g activated charcoal at pH 7.5 and were higher at pH 4.9. Single-dose activated charcoal and possibly multiple-dose activated charcoal should theoretically be beneficial in the management of these overdoses. Patients who overdose on glipizide, an agent that has an enterohepatic circulation, may benefit from multiple-dose activated charcoal.

The management of a patient with a sulfonylurea overdose is not always easy. The sulfonylureas have a very prolonged serum half-life and duration of action[36] and may cause refractory hypoglycemia even when 20% dextrose infusion is maintained. Although in this setting glucagon may be effective as an adjunct in the patient who does have hepatic glycogen stores,[61] because it can stimulate glycogenolysis, glucagon may cause further insulin release and is therefore not usually of benefit. The release of insulin may prolong or worsen hypoglycemia after the potential beneficial effect of glucagon has dissipated.[81]

Urinary alkalinization to a pH of 7–8 can reduce the half-life of chlorpropamide from 49 to approximately 13 hours. No advantage from urinary alkalinization has been demonstrated for other oral agents.[57] In patients with chloropropamide overdoses, the plasma insulin levels may remain high for several days, further increasing the risk of recurrent hypoglycemia.

By opening K_{ATP} channels, diazoxide (Hyperstat) directly inhibits insulin secretion in patients who have insulin-secreting tumors, and it is also effective for refractory sulfonylurea-induced hypoglycemia.[46,59] When hypoglycemia is refractory to standard therapeutic measures, the use of an insulin antagonist such as diazoxide may be necessary. Diazoxide can be given by slow IV infusion (300 mg over 30 minutes every 4 hours), thereby producing only a limited hypotensive effect while achieving dextrose regulation. Maintaining an IV infusion of glucose is critical as an additional safeguard when using diazoxide to maintain euglycemia. If diazoxide is used continuously, sodium retention may occur, and therefore a diuretic such as furosemide may need to be employed, particularly when the urine is alkalinized for a chlorpropamide overdose. Oral diazoxide (Proglycem) can also be used at a dose of 200–300 mg every 4 hours, as indicated.

Octreotide, a semisynthetic long-acting analog of somatostatin with an IV half life of 72 minutes, has been shown to inhibit glucose-stimulated β-cell insulin release through receptors coupled to G proteins on β islet cells.[11] Somatostatin present in diverse tissues such as the hypothalamus, pancreas, and GI tract alters the secretion of growth hormone and thyroid-stimulating hormone, gastrointestinal secretions, and the endocrine pancreas (glucagon and insulin).[67,68] In normal subjects brought to hypoglycemia with glipizide, octreotide (30 ng/kg/min IV) was compared to IV hypertonic dextrose and also to diazoxide with dextrose. Insulin concentrations were 4–5 times greater with dextrose alone or in combination with diazoxide than with octreotide. Each of these healthy subjects who had been given 1.43 mg/kg of glipizide developed recurrent hypoglycemia when dextrose or diazoxide therapy was stopped at 13 hours. In contrast, six of eight patients on octreotide had no recurrent hypoglycemia during the next 4 hours of the study, although recurrent episodes of hypoglycemia did occur as long as 30 hours after the overdose. Dextrose requirements were comparable for the dextrose-alone or dextrose-plus-diazoxide groups, whereas only four of eight subjects in the octreotide group required glucose and in these cases only in reduced amounts. The half-life of octreotide and its inhibition of insulin release were responsible for the persistent euglycemia, even in the presence of counterregulatory hormones such as glucagon and growth hormone.[52] Several successful clinical experiences with octreotide use have been reported with quinine-induced hypoglycemia resulting from malaria therapy,[62] with an insulinoma,[41] with nesidioblastosis of infancy,[25] and with a tolbutamide overdose.[11] A successful starting octreotide dosing may be 50 μg every 12 hours.

Successful regimen management of the hypoglycemic patient is defined by maintaining a steady state of euglycemia. This can be done by establishing a glucose infusion rate that avoids peaks or valleys in glucose levels. Success in achieving steady-state euglycemia prevents stimulation of further insulin release and subsequent recurrent hypoglycemia. In addition to maintaining the appropriate glucose infusion, euglycemia is accomplished by preventing further absorption of the oral agent ingested and, in all types of hypoglycemia, feeding the patient as soon as possible. Bolus glucose management should be replaced by an infusion as soon as possible when a steady state is determined. Finally, maintaining a normal potassium level is extremely important in successful management as repetitive glucose bolus and infusion therapy leads to recurrent episodes of hypokalemia.

How Should a Patient With Potential Malicious, Surreptitious, or Unintentional Insulin Overdose Be Evaluated?

Although insulin is used widely, only a limited number of case reports of intentional or unintentional insulin overdosages are reported in the literature.[2,17,39,44] These reviews suggest that diabetics are more likely to overdose with oral preparations than with insulin. Insulin is frequently used surreptitiously for personal abuse or abuse of another by health care professionals, others with medical knowledge, or family members of diabetics. Lethality, duration, and recurrence of hypoglycemia appear to be related in part to amount and type of insulin (or oral agent) used. Delayed release of insulin from fat tissue at the injection site(s) and the presence and efficacy of insulin antibodies may explain a victim's recovery in spite of massive overdoses.[17] Survival cannot be correlated directly with either the dose or type of insulin, as some patients have died with doses estimated in the hundreds of units whereas others have survived doses in the thousands of units.[70] Mortality and morbidity are more likely correlated with delay in recognition of the problem, duration of symptoms, onset of therapy, and type of complications, as opposed to the absolute degree of hypoglycemia or persistence of elevated insulin levels.[55] A significant correlation has been described between the amount of insulin injected and either the total amount of dextrose used for treatment or the duration of dextrose infusion.[78] This same study emphasized that the delay in onset of hypoglycemia was often markedly different from the expected onset with conventional therapy.

Physical examination of the patient with a malicious or surreptitious overdose includes a meticulous search for a potential site of injection. The site may be erythematous, hemorrhagic, atypically boggy in nature, or even painful if the subcutaneous (or intramuscular) injection of insulin was particularly large. The site may provide a clue to the malicious event as well as a depot for ongoing insulin release and subsequent sustained hypoglycemia. Several authors have suggested surgical excision of tissue and insulin from a site of massive insulin injection.[17,56] Although this may assist in a forensic evaluation, there is no documentation in the literature that such an approach is effective or necessary, and we have not employed surgical excision in our clinical management.

The technique of species-specific radioimmunoassay can be employed to elucidate the presence of surreptitious, unintentional, or malicious administration of insulin.[8] An understanding of how the β-cells of the pancreas secrete insulin in response to glucose levels in the blood is essential to understanding the investigation of fasting hypoglycemia.[21] When plasma glucose is less than 45 mg/dL insulin secretion should be almost completely suppressed and therefore plasma insulin concentrations should be minimal or absent.[65] Moreover, insulin is secreted as proinsulin, which is cleaved in vivo to form insulin (a double-stranded peptide) and C peptide, which are released into the blood in equimolar quantities. Only in autoimmune hypoglycemia is proinsulin released in any substantial quantity. Insulin is biologically active, whereas proinsulin has limited activity, and C peptide has no activity. Although insulin is normally cleared during hepatic transit, C peptide is not; therefore C peptide can be utilized as a quantitative marker of endogenous insulin secretion. Commercially available ex-

TABLE 40–6. THE LABORATORY ASSESSMENT OF FASTING HYPOGLYCEMIA

Clinical State	Insulin[a] (Plasma) μU/mL	C Peptide (Plasma) nmol/L	Proinsulin pmol/L	Antiinsulin Antibodies[c]
Normal	<6	<0.2	<5	—
Exogenous insulin	Very high	Low (suppressed)	Absent	Present[d]
Insulinoma	High	High	Present	Absent
Sulfonylurea ingestion[b]	High	High	Present	Absent
Autoimmune	Very high (artifact)	Low (or) high (artifact)	Present	Present
Decreased glucose production	Low	Low	Present	Absent
Neoplasia (non β-cell)	Low	Low	Present	Absent

[a]Insulin levels are determined during fasting hypoglycemia at low levels, preferably <45 mg/dL of blood glucose.
[b]Sulfonylurea ingestion is diagnosed by detection of the drugs or their metabolites in plasma or urine.
[c]The antiinsulin antibodies produced spontaneously differ from those of treated (exposed to exogenous insulin) and those of untreated insulin-dependent diabetics.
[d]The presence of antiinsulin antibodies is noted only after a second dose of insulin has been given and is present less frequently in those exposed only to human insulin.[30]

ogenous human insulin does not contain C-peptide fragments (Table 40–6). When plasma glucose concentration falls to hypoglycemic levels (usually < 60 mg/dL), insulin secretion should fall to less than 6 μU/mL. Therefore, when hypoglycemia is due to exogenous insulin administration, plasma C-peptide levels should be less than 0.2 nmol/L in the presence of insulin levels that are substantially higher than insulin levels resulting from an insulinoma. Animal insulin can also be distinguished from human insulin by high-performance liquid chromatography.[37] Sulfonylurea-stimulated endogenous plasma insulin production will also result in high C-peptide levels, and this combination is not distinguishable from the presence of an insulinoma.

In summary, patients with chronic insulin-induced factitious or surreptitious hypoglycemia will have high insulin levels, the presence of insulin-binding antibodies,[30] and low C-peptide levels. Those who have taken sulfonylureas will have high insulin levels, absent insulin-binding antibodies, high C-peptide levels, and the presence of urinary sulfonylurea metabolites (see Table 40–6). The issues of evidence collection that are appropriate to document malicious or surreptitious use of insulin successfully have been described[51] (Chap. 102).

Which Patients Should Be Admitted to the Hospital?

All patients who present with hypoglycemia due to a sulfonylurea or any etiology other than the use of ultrashort-, short-, or intermediate-acting insulin should be admitted, as should all those who may have delayed, profound, and protracted hypoglycemia resulting from an intentional overdose. The onset of hypoglycemia may be substantially delayed with the use of both oral hypoglycemic agents and insulin. Patients who have recurrent hypoglycemic episodes while using insulin should have their insulin doses adjusted, and a patient who returns to the ED for a second time because of a similar, unexplained episode of hypoglycemia should be admitted for a metabolic evaluation. Although many factors may be responsible for administration of a relative insulin overdose, such as patient error (eg, due to impaired vision), syringe structure, prescription error, and onset of other metabolic derangements, all hypoglycemic patients using oral agents, ethanol, or long-acting insulin, as well as those with hepatic or renal failure or starvation and hypoglycemia of unknown etiology, must be admitted.

Although the etiology for hypoglycemia may not be obvious during the initial evaluation, it is never acceptable to diagnose the etiology as "idiopathic"; to prevent complications while continuing to seek a cause, it must be assumed that the patient has been exposed to a hypoglycemic agent until proven otherwise.

Patients who may be suicidal or victims of attempted homicide and all patients with possible self-induced factitious hypoglycemia should be admitted and evaluated in a hospital setting. Factitious hypoglycemia is particularly prevalent among members of the medical profession. Any patient who has taken a massive insulin overdose should be admitted for observation and psychiatric assessment even if euglycemia is restored in the ED. As noted previously, accurately predicting the time of onset and extent of hypoglycemia is at best extremely limited.[2]

Unindicated insulin administration to a child by a diabetic parent may be a form of child abuse.[26] Children who have accidentally ingested oral preparations or who have been given an inappropriate dose of insulin should be admitted for observation for at least 24 hours—even if they are not hypoglycemic—initially, because there are inadequate data to predict the onset, extent, duration, or potential for hypoglycemia. In a restrospective poison center review of sulfonylurea ingestions by children, hypoglycemia reportedly began from 0.5 to 16 hours after the ingestion. Four of the 25 patients studied became hypoglycemic more than 4 hours after the ingestion.[66] More significantly still, the ingestion of only a single tablet of chlorpropamide (250 mg), glipizide (5 mg), or glyburide (2.5 mg) each produced hypoglycemia in children 1–4 years of age.

Acknowledgment

Robert H. Kirstein, MD contributed to this chapter in a previous edition.

References

1. Andrade R, Mathew V, Morgenstern NJ, et al: Hypoglycemic hemiplegic syndrome. Ann Emerg Med 1984;13:529–531.
2. Arem R, Zoghbi W: Insulin overdosage in eight patients: Insulin pharmacokinetics and review of the literature. Medicine 1985;64:323–332.
3. Arky RA, Arrons DL: Hypoglycemia in diabetes mellitus. Med Clin North Am 1971;55:919–930.
4. Arky RA, Veverbrants E, Abramson EA: Irreversible hypoglycemia. JAMA 1968;206:575–578.
5. Asplund K, Wiholm BE, Lithner F: Glibenclamide-associated hypoglycemia: A report of 57 cases. Diabetologia 1983;24:412–417.
6. Bailey CJ, Day C: Traditional plant medicines in treatments for diabetes. Diabetes Care 1989;12:553–564.
7. Bailey CJ, Turner RC: Metformin. N Engl J Med 1996;334:574–579.
8. Bauman WA, Yalow RS: Hyperinsulinemic hypoglycemia: Differential diagnosis by determination of the species of circulatory insulin. JAMA 1984;252:2730–2734.
9. Bowman CE, MacMahon DG, Mourant AJ: Hypoglycemia and angina. Lancet 1985;1:639–640.
10. Boyle PJ: Plasma glucose concentrations at the onset of hypoglycemic symptoms in patients with poorly controlled diabetes and in non diabetics. N Engl J Med 1988;318:1487–1492.
11. Boyle PJ, Justice K, Krentz AJ, et al: Octreotide reverses hyperinsulinemia and prevents hypoglycemia induced by sulfonylurea overdoses. J Clin Endocrinol Metab 1993;76:752–756.
12. Boyle PJ, Kempers SF, O'Connor AM, Nagy RJ: Brain glu-

cose uptake and unawareness of hypoglycemia in patients with insulin-dependent diabetes mellitus. N Engl J Med 1995;333:1726–1731.

13. Bressler R: The unripe ackee: Forbidden fruit. N Engl J Med 1976;295:500–501.
14. Bressler R, Correder C, Brendel K: Hypoglycin and hypoglycin-like compounds. Pharmacol Rev 1969;21:105–130.
15. Bressler R, Johnson D: New pharmacological approaches to therapy of NIDDM. Diabetes Care 1992;15:792–805.
16. Brodows RG, Williams C, Amatruda JM: Treatment of insulin reactions in diabetics. JAMA 1984;252:3378–3381.
17. Campbell IW, Ratcliffe JG: Suicidal insulin overdose managed by excision of insulin injection site. Br Med J 1982; 285:408–409.
18. CDC: Toxic hypoglycemic syndrome, Jamaica 1989–1991. MMWR 1992;41:53–55.
19. Chochinov R, Daughaday WH: Marked hyperthermia as a manifestation of hypoglycemia in long standing diabetes mellitus. Diabetes 1975;24:859–860.
20. Crofford OB: Metformin. N Engl J Med 1995;333:588–589.
21. Cryer PE: Glucose homeostasis and hypoglycemia. In: Wilson JD, Foster DW, eds: William's Textbook of Endocrinology, 8th ed. Philadelphia, Saunders, 1992, pp. 1223–1253.
22. Cryer PE, Gerich JE: Glucose counterregulation hypoglycemia and intensive insulin therapy in diabetes mellitus. N Engl J Med 1985;313:232–241.
23. DCCT Research Group: Epidemology of severe hypoglycemia in the diabetes control and complications trial. Am J Med 1991;90:450–459.
24. DCCT Research Group: The diabetes control and complications trial: Results of the feasibility study. Diabetes Care 1987;10:1–9.
25. Delemarre-van de waal HA, Veldkamp IJM, Schrander-Stumpel CTRM: Long term treatment of an infant with nesidioblastosis using a somatostatin analogue. N Engl J Med 1987;316:222–223.
26. Dine MS, McGovern ME: Intentional poisoning of children: An overlooked category of child abuse: Report of seven cases and review of the literature. Pediatrics 1982;70:32–35.
27. Duh E, Feinglos M: Hypoglycemia induced angina pectoris in a patient with diabetes mellitus. Ann Intern Med 1994;121:945–946.
28. Eliasson L, Renstrom E, Ammala C, et al: PKC dependent stimulation of exocytosis by sulfonylureas in pancreatic β cells. Science 1996;271:813–815.
29. Epstein MF, Nicholls E, Stubblefield PG: Neonatal hypoglycemia after beta sympathomimetic tocolytic therapy. J Pediatr 1979;94:449–453.
30. Fineberg SE, Galloway JA, Fineberg NS, et al: Immunogenicity of recombinant DNA human insulin. Diabetologia 1983;25:465–469.
31. Fischer KF, Lees JA, Newman JH: Hypoglycemia in hospitalized patients: Causes and outcomes. N Engl J Med 1986;315:1245–1250.
32. Fox RE, Marx C, Stark AR: Neonatal effects of maternal nadolol therapy. Am J Obstet Gynecol 1986;152:1045–1046.
33. Fulop M, Hoberman AD: Phenformin-associated metabolic acidosis. Diabetes 1976;25:292–296.
34. Gaines KL, Hamilton S, Boyd AE III: Characterization of the sulfonylurea receptor on beta cell membranes. J. Biol Chem 1988;263:2589–2592.
35. Gan SC, Barr J, Arieff AI, Pearl RG: Biguanide-associated lactic acidosis. Arch Intern Med 1993;152:2333–2336.
36. Gerich JE: Oral hypoglycemic agents. N Engl J Med 1989;321:1231–1245.
37. Given BD, Ostrega DM, Polonsky KS, et al: Hypoglycemia due to surreptitious injection of insulin: Identification of insulin species by high performance liquid chromatography. Diabetes Care 1991;14:544–547.
38. Grajower M, Walter L, Albin J: Hypoglycemia in chronic hemodialysis patients: Association with propranolol use. Nephron 1980;26:126–129.
39. Grunberger G, Weiner JL, Silverman R, et al: Factitious hypoglycemia due to surreptitious administration of insulin: Diagnosis, treatment and long-term follow up. Ann Intern Med 1988;108:252–257.
40. Hansten PD: Drug Interactions, 3rd ed. Philadelphia, Lea & Febiger, 1976.
41. Hearn PR, Ahmed M, Woodhouse NJY: The use of SMS 201–995 (somatostatin analogue) in insulinomas. Horm Res 1988;29:211–213.
42. Hoffman JR, Schriger DL, Votey SR, Luo JS: The empiric use of hypertonic dextrose in patients with altered mental status: A reappraisal. Ann Emerg Med 1992;21:20–24.
43. Huminer D, Dux S, Rosenfeld JB, Pitlik SD: Inadvertent sulfonylurea-induced hypoglycemia: A dangerous but preventable condition. Arch Intern Med 1989;149: 1890–1892.
44. Jefferys DB, Volans GN: Self-poisoning in diabetic patients. Hum Toxicol 1983;2:345–348.
45. Jennings AM, Wilson RM, Ward JD: Symptomatic hypoglycemia in NIDDM patients treated with oral hypoglycemic agents. Diabetes Care 1989;12:203–208.
46. Johnson SF, Schade DS, Glenn GT: Chlorpropamide induced hypolgycemia: Successful treatment with diazoxide. Am J Med 1977;63:799–804.
47. Kannisto H, Neuvonen PJ: Adsorption of sulfonylureas onto activated charcoal in vitro. J Pharm Sci 1984;73: 253–256.
48. Kedes LH, Field JB: Hypothermia: A clue to hypoglycemia. N Engl J Med 1964;271:785.
49. Kerr D, MacDonald IA, Heller SR, Tattersall RB: β adrenoreceptor blockade and hypoglycemia. A randomized double-blind placebo controlled comparison of metoprolol CR, atenolol and propranolol LA in normal subjects. Br J Clin Pharmacol 1990;29:685–693.
50. Leak D, Starr P: The mechanism of arrhythmias during insulin induced hypoglycemia. Am Heart J 1962;63:688–691.
51. Levy WJ, Gardner D, Moseley J, et al: Unusual problems for the physician in managing a hospital patient who received a malicious insulin overdose. Neurosurgery 1985;17: 992–996.
52. Longnecker SM: Somatostatin and octreotide: Literature review and description of therapeutic activity in pancreatic neoplasia. Drug Intell Clin Pharmacol 1988;22:99–106.
53. Madison LL: Ethanol induced hypoglycemia. In: Levine R, Luft R, eds: Advances in Metabolic Disorders, Vol 3. New York, Academic Press, 1968, pp. 85–109.
54. Malouf R, Brust JCM: Hypoglycemia: Causes, neurologi-

cal manifestations and outcome. Ann Neurol 1985;17: 421–430.
55. Martin FIR, Stocks AE, Pearson MJ: Significance of disappearance of injected insulin. Lancet 1967;1:619–620.
56. McIntyre AS, Woolf VJ, Burnham WR: Local excision of subcutaneous fat in the management of insulin overdose. Br J Surg 1986;73:538.
57. Neuvonen PJ, Karkkainen S: Effects of charcoal, sodium bicarbonate and ammonium chloride on chlorpropamide kinetics. Clin Pharmacol Ther 1983;33:386–393.
58. Odeh M, Oliven A, Bussan H: Transient atrial fibrillation precipitated by hypoglycemia. Ann Emerg Med 1990;19: 565–567.
59. Palatnick W, Meatherall RC, Tennenbein M: Clinical spectrum of sulfonylurea overdose and experience with diazoxide therapy. Arch Intern Med 1991;151:1859–1862.
60. Peitzman SJ, Agarwal BN: Spontaneous hypoglycemia in end-stage renal failure. Nephron 1977;19:131–139.
61. Pfeifer MA, Wolter CF, Samols E: Management of chlorpropamide-induced hypoglycemia with diazoxide. South Med J 1978;71:606–608.
62. Phillips RE, Looareesuwan S, Bloom SR, et al: Effectiveness of SMS 201–995 a synthetic long acting somatostatin analogue in treatment of quinine-induced hyperinsulinaemia. Lancet 1986;1:713–714.
63. Pladziewicz DS, Nesto RW: Hypoglycemia induced silent myocardial ischemia. Am J Cardiol 1989;63:1531–1532.
64. Plum F, Posner JB: The Diagnosis of Stupor and Coma, 3rd ed. Philadelphia, Davis, 1980.
65. Polonsky KS: A practical approach to fasting hypoglycemia. N Engl J Med 1992;326:1020–1021.
66. Quadrani DA, Spiller HA, Widder P: Five year retrospective evaluation of sulfonylurea ingestion in children. J Toxicol Clin Toxicol 1996;34:267–270.
67. Reichlin S: Somatostatin I. N Engl J Med 1983;309: 1495–1501.
68. Reichlin S: Somatostatin II. N Engl J Med 1983;309: 1556–1563.
69. Rich LM, Caine MR, Findling JW, Shaker JL: Hypoglycemic coma in anorexia nervosa: Case report and review of the literature. Arch Intern Med 1990;150:894–895.
70. Samuels MH, Eckel RH: Massive insulin overdose: Detailed studies of free insulin levels and glucose requirements. J Toxicol Clin Toxicol 1989;27:157–168.
71. Seibert DG: Reversible decerebrate posturing secondary to hypoglycemia. Am J Med 1985;78:1036–1037.
72. Seltzer HS: Drug induced hypoglycemia: A review of 1418 cases. Endocrinol Metab Clin North Am 1989;18: 163–183.
73. Seltzer HS: Severe drug induced hypoglycemia: A review. Compr Ther 1979;5:21–29.
74. Service FJ: Hypoglycemic disorders. N Engl J Med 1995;332:1144–1152.
75. Shumak SL, Corenblum B, Steiner G: Recurrent hypoglycemia secondary to drug dispensing error. Arch Intern Med 1991;151:1877–1878.
76. Slama G, Traynard PY, Desplanque N, et al: The search for an optimal treatment of hypoglycemia: Carbohydrates in tablets, solutions or gel for the correction of insulin reactions. Arch Intern Med 1990;150:589–593.
77. Sledge ED, Broadstone VL: Hypoglycemia due to a pharmacy dispensing error. South Med J 1993;86:1272–1273.
78. Stapczynski JS, Haskell RJ: Duration of hypoglycemia and need for intravenous glucose following intentional overdoses of insulin. Ann Emerg Med 1984;13: 505–511.
79. Stumvoll M, Nurjhan N, Perriello G, et al: Metabolic effects of metformin in non-insulin dependent diabetes mellitus. N Engl J Med 1995;333:550–554.
80. Tanaka K, Kean EA, Johnson B: Jamaican vomiting sickness: Biochemical investigation of two cases. N Engl J Med 1976;295:461–467.
81. Thoma ME, Glauser J, Genuth S: Persistent hypoglycemia and hyperinsulinemia caution in using glucagon. Am J Emerg Med 1996;14:99–101.
82. Wachtel TJ, Steele GH, Day JA: Natural history of fever following seizure. Arch Intern Med 1987;147:1153–1155.
83. Wallis WE, Donaldson I, Scott RS, et al: Hypoglycemia masquerading as cerebrovascular disease (hypoglycemic hemiplegia). Ann Neurol 1985;18:510–512.
84. Wharton B: Hypoglycemia in children with kwashiorkor. Lancet 1970;1:171–173.

ANTIDOTES IN DEPTH

Dextrose

Kathleen A. Delaney

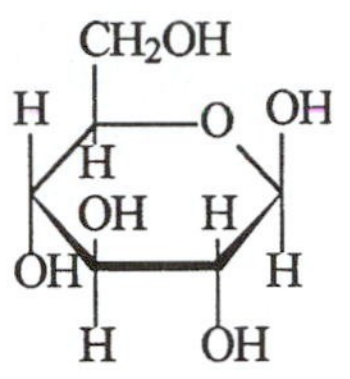

Dextrose

Glucose is the primary energy source for the human brain, although in the mature human alternate substrates such as fatty acids, amino acids, and ketones can also be utilized. Glucose is the obligatory source of metabolic energy for the brain of the fetus and neonate.[61] Hypoglycemia causes neurologic effects that are clinically indistinguishable from those of a variety of toxic-metabolic and structural brain injuries, including focal stroke syndromes, seizures, confusion, delirium, and coma.[3,14,15,21,34,43,46,53,65,71] Hypoglycemia also precipitates myocardial stress and is associated with angina and dysrhythmias.[22,37,44] Prolonged, repeated, or severe episodes of hypoglycemia may result in permanent injury to the central nervous system.[2,6,31]

In most cases where the duration of hypoglycemia is brief, the abnormal clinical effects are immediately reversed by the administration of 0.5–1 g/kg of concentrated intravenous dextrose, given in the form of $D_{50}W$ in adults, $D_{25}W$ in children, or $D_{10}W$ in neonates. Due to the myriad presentations of hypoglycemia, the difficulties inherent in its clinical diagnosis, and the serious consequences of failure to treat it, the empirical administration of hypertonic dextrose to all patients with mental status alteration has been a standard emergency department practice. Only clinically insignificant or very rare complications are attributed to this practice. One theoretical concern is that the osmotic effects of hypertonic dextrose could result in an expanded blood volume and increased myocardial demand, causing pulmonary edema in patients with cardiac insufficiency.[33] The bolus administration of $D_{50}W$ can also precipitate clinically insignificant hypophosphatemia in normal individuals.[40,50,52] Glucose infusion may also increase the hyperkalemia associated with hyporeninemic hypoaldosteronism (type 4 renal tubular acidosis) in insulin-dependent diabetics.[25] The administration of hypertonic dextrose has rarely been associated with lactic acidosis in cancer patients with large tumor loads.[26] Concentrated glucose solutions commonly cause phlebitis, and tissue necrosis is described following soft tissue infiltration of 50% dextrose.[19] Tissue infarction has also followed inadvertent intraarterial injection of 50% dextrose.[4] Seizures, hyperosmolar coma, and death are attributed to the administration of inappropriately large boluses of 50% dextrose to children. In one fatal case, 280 mL of $D_{50}W$ was given to a 15-kg child.[54] Seizures and subdural hemorrhage followed the administration of 100 mL to a 20-kg child.[54] Anecdotal reports of the precipitation of acute Wernicke's encephalopathy by the administration of dextrose have led to the inclusion of thiamine in the "coma cocktail" (see Antidotes in Depth: Thiamine Hydrochloride). Serious problems associated with the administration of hypertonic dextrose are caused by medication errors, such as the inadvertent substitution of a lookalike bolus of concentrated lidocaine or magnesium.[28] These potential or rare complications of dextrose administration are regarded as acceptable in contrast with the risks posed by delay in the recognition and treatment of hypoglycemia.

Concerns Regarding the Administration of Dextrose to the Patient With Cerebral Ischemia

A growing body of laboratory and clinical evidence indicates that in the mature brain, preexisting hyperglycemia is deleterious in the presence of cerebral ischemia.[68] Clinical studies in the previous decade suggested that elevation of blood glucose was associated with more serious neurologic outcomes in patients with head injury or cerebrovascular accidents.[9,48,72] These descriptive clinical studies did not satisfactorily distinguish the primary effects of hyperglycemia from those of obvious associated conditions, such as hyperglycemia secondary to the intense sympathetic response that accompanies more severe brain injury, or hyperglycemia as a marker of diabetes and its attendant severe cerebrovascular disease. However, controlled laboratory investigations of ischemic brain injury in which hyperglycemia was induced prior to the ischemic insult consistently support the clinical observation that higher blood glucose levels are associated with more extensive cerebral injury. Most studies have been conducted in animal models of global cerebral ischemia, using cardiac arrest or four-vessel ligation, and in models of focal ischemia using one- or two-vessel ligation.[45] These animal models of ischemic injury have shown deleterious effects of preischemic hyperglycemia using a variety of outcome endpoints. Infusion of 1.5 g/kg of glucose into cats over 60 minutes prior to 30 minutes of global ischemia resulted in a significantly greater accumulation of lactic acid and severe impairment of recovery of ATP stores in the postreperfusion period.[69] In this study, and in another, similar study of cats that received a dose of 1.5 g/kg, plasma glucose levels were as high as 1000 mg/dL in the infused animals.[24] Monkeys given 0.76 g/kg of glucose followed by 17 minutes of global ischemia had significantly greater neurologic and histopathologic evidence of cerebral injury at 96 hours compared with saline controls. These infusions resulted in increases in the blood glucose levels from a mean of 57 mg/dL to a mean of 244 mg/dL.[35] Infusion of 10% dextrose into cats prior to middle cerebral artery occlusion resulted in a threefold increase in the size of the resultant infarct measured at 2 weeks. Serum glucose levels increased from 90 mg/dL to 360 mg/dL following dextrose infusion in this study.[17] A dog model of cardiac arrest compared six animals pretreated with 500 mL 5% dextrose in lactated Ringers solution (D_5LR) then posttreated with 1 L D_5LR with those treated with LR alone. Glucose levels were 335 mg/dL in the treated animals and 129 mg/dL in the controls. Eleven animals were resuscitated successfully. At 24 hours all of the dextrose-infused animals were dead or had severe neurologic deficits. All of the LR-treated animals walked and ate.[13] Rats subjected to 10 minutes of global ischemia showed no survival in six animals made hyperglycemic prior to ischemia, decreased survival (5 of 8) in animals made hypoglycemic with insulin, and 100% (10 of 10) survival in normoglycemic animals.[55] A comparison of the effects of dextrose infusion with normal saline infusion in a rat four-vessel occlusion model showed a higher incidence of seizures (7 of 10 vs 0 of 5) and higher mortality (5 of 10 vs 0 of 5) in the animals receiving dextrose.[49] The most severe injuries are evident when ischemia is incomplete or focal so that a small amount of blood flow is present.[17,24,29,45,47,49] Comparable clinical situations where lowered perfusion is present would be during CPR, or when collateral circulation is present near an area of focal infarction. The increased severity of injury in these settings has been attributed to the delivery of glucose to ischemic areas.[45] Recently, the administration of insulin to control pre-ischemic hyperglycemia was shown to decrease the extent of ischemic injury.[16,18,27,38,66,68] Hypoglycemia is clearly shown to be deleterious in all models where it has been studied.[17,29,32,55]

The biochemical impact of hyperglycemia in the setting of ischemia has been extensively investigated. In global ischemia there is rapid depletion of brain glucose, ATP, and phosphocreatine, followed by a rapid rise in the intracellular content of lactic acid, disruption of energy-dependent electrolyte gradients, activation of phospholipase by increased intracellular calcium, and generation of destructive free radicals.[56–58,64,67,70] The magnitude of intracellular lactic acid accumulation following the onset of ischemia is proportional to the blood glucose level.[29,51,69] Intracellular lactate levels in models of focal ischemia are significantly elevated in comparison with models of global ischemia. This has been attributed to the availability of a trickle of glucose in the penumbra of ischemia.[45,57] Experimental evidence suggests that hyperglycemia is also associated with increased capillary permeability in ischemic tissue and delay in the resolution of intracellular calcium elevation during recovery from ischemia.[5,20] Hyperglycemia may also interfere with membrane repair systems in injured cells by suppressing the synthesis of "heat shock" proteins.[12,70] Insulin appears to be a promoter of "heat shock" protein synthesis in ischemic cells and may have an independent effect in protecting ischemic tissue, although this remains controversial.[18,27,38,60,62] The induction of normoglycemia (but not hypoglycemia) with insulin appears to offer protection against ischemic injury, but the efficacy of insulin independent of its effect on blood glucose levels is not clear. The deleterious effect of preischemic hyperglycemia appears to be most consistently related to increased intraneuronal production of lactate.[58,64,67] Unlike the case in adult animals, the administration of glucose prolongs survival and is associated with decreased brain damage in fetal and neonatal animal models of anoxia.[61,63]

Clinical Implications of Animal Studies of Hyperglycemia and Cerebral Ischemia

There is no question that the reversal of hypoglycemia is a sound clinical intervention in the patient who is hypoglycemic, regardless of the presence of cerebral ischemia. The failure to administer dextrose in a timely fashion to a patient with significant hypoglycemia may result in permanent neurologic injury. Patients who are hypoglycemic should receive sufficient dextrose to be made euglycemic. There are limited data on the pharmacokinetics of $D_{50}W$. In one study the administration of 25 g (50 mL) of $D_{50}W$ to adults resulted in elevation of the blood glucose from 40 mg/dL to 350 mg/dL above baseline when measured at random times after administration.[1] The significance of the induction of transient hyperglycemia by the empirical administration of a bolus of dextrose in an adult human who was not hypoglycemic at the onset of treatment is unknown. There also remains considerable uncertainty in regard to interpretation of the significance of the animal studies discussed above. The blood glucose levels attained in some of these models were much higher than would be expected following the administration of a 0.5 g/kg dose of hypertonic dextrose to an adult. In addition, they are all pretreatment models in which the blood glucose was persistently elevated prior to the ischemic insult. In a postinfarct scenario, the induction of transient hyperglycemia would not reasonably be expected to affect the area where irreversible infarction had occurred. However, in the situation where a small amount of blood flow is still present, such as during CPR, or in the penumbra of ischemia that surrounds an area of focal infarct, the delivery of prolonged or excessive amounts of glucose would be of greater concern. No studies evaluate the effects of a transient elevation of the blood glucose after the onset of ischemia that might occur during clinical practice. Clearly, for the patient whose neurologic symptoms are due to hypoglycemia, the greatest concern is that the hypoglycemia has not been adequately treated. In these cases consideration should be given to the administration of larger doses (1.0 g/kg) of hypertonic dextrose to the patient who has profound symptoms. On the other hand, the induction of hyperglycemia in the patient who is euglycemic or already hyperglycemic and suffering from ischemia should ideally be avoided.

This dilemma would be easily resolved if bedside blood glucose determinations with reagent strips had the reliability of the chemistry laboratory. Several studies of commonly available reagent strips have failed to demonstrate 100% sensitivity for distinguishing normoglycemia from hypoglycemia.[10,11,23,36,39,41] The best published sensitivities for the detection of hypoglycemia range between 92% and 94%.[30,36] In one study, 2 of 33 hypoglycemic patients (blood glucose < 60 mg/dL) were not detected, but a 90-mg/dL cutoff would have detected 100% of numerically hypoglycemic patients.[36] The "safe" number at which no cases of symptomatic hypoglycemia are missed by reagent strip testing is a subject of debate because poorly controlled diabetics experience hypoglycemic symptoms at blood glucose levels that would normally be regarded as euglycemic. In an important study, the mean blood glucose level for symptomatic hypoglycemia in poorly controlled diabetics was 78 ± 5 mg/dL compared with 53 ± 2 mg/dL in normal controls.[8] Therefore a reasonably conservative cutoff for the assurance of clinical euglycemia in all patients would be a bedside reagent measurement of 120 mg/dL. False positive demonstrations of hypoglycemia are more common than false negatives, especially in patients with shock.[7] A recent study of fingerstick capillary samples in 50 patients with cardiac arrest identified 8 patients as hypoglycemic, while only 3 actually were hypoglycemic when venous blood was analyzed. One true hypoglycemic patient was missed. Tests of venous blood correctly identified all numerically hypoglycemic patients.[59] In another study, 36% of hypotensive patients were incorrectly diagnosed as hypoglycemic.[7] Once again the use of venous blood correctly classified all patients.[7]

A sound clinical solution to this problem would miss no cases of significant symptomatic hypoglycemia and would avoid the administration of dextrose to patients with brain ischemia who have a reasonable expectation of recovery. Infants and neonates should receive glucose when clinically indicated without concern for the presence of associated ischemia or anoxia. The patient with coma or status epilepticus from hypoglycemia will benefit greatly from empiric treatment and will suffer the greatest deterioration if not treated. A patient who is comatose from a major cerebrovascular accident has a very limited chance for recovery and the administration of dextrose is unlikely to impact heavily on the prognosis. It is clinically reasonable to administer $D_{50}W$ to patients in coma who do not have a measured blood glucose of at least 120 mg/dL on bedside reagent strip testing. When a reliable bedside glucose determination cannot be done, all of these patients should receive $D_{50}W$ empirically. Patients with focal deficits constitute a population that would reasonably be expected to have the greatest recovery in the case of a cerebrovascular accident and the greatest theoretical benefit from the withholding of dextrose. Additionally, a focal presentation of hypoglycemia is rare, relative to the numbers of patients with focal presentations who have suffered cerebrovascular accidents. In one study, less than 3% of patients with hypoglycemia presented with focal symptoms.[42] In the patient with a history of diabetes treated with insulin or an oral hypoglycemic agent who presents with focal symptoms, symptomatic hypoglycemia must be strongly considered even when the reagent strip shows a blood glucose level of greater than 90 mg/dL. Confusion and delirium in the absence of focal neurologic findings do occur as a manifestation of structural brain injury; however, toxic-metabolic etiologies are more common in our experience. These patients should receive glucose if the bedside glucose test is not greater than 120 mg/dL. Fingerstick glucose samples are especially unreliable in the patient with hypotension or cardiac arrest; however, bedside reagent strip testing of venous blood appears to be more reliable.[7,59] Hypoglycemia, defined as a serum blood glucose less than 60 mg/dL, was demonstrated in 8% of patients with cardiac arrest in one study.[59] Patients in shock or cardiac arrest should have reagent testing done on a *venous* blood sample (not a fingerstick sample) and should receive glucose if they are numerically hypoglycemic. The administration of glucose to the arrested patient who is euglycemic on reagent strip testing should be considered if the patient is a diabetic. The patient with a clear history and evidence of significant head injury antedated by normal activity (eg, crossing the street, struck by car) should not be treated unless the bedside test indicates hypoglycemia (< 90 mg/dL). Diabetic patients, of course, may suffer unintentional injuries predisposed by hypoglycemic episodes. The treating physician must use his or her best judgment of the mechanism and evidence of injury, witness reports, available medical history, and results of bedside glucose determination to make a decision regarding administration of $D_{50}W$ to the head-injured trauma patient.

References

1. Adler PM: Serum glucose changes after administration of 50% dextrose solution: Pre- and in-hospital calculations. Am J Emerg Med 1986;4:504–506.
2. Agardh CD, Kalimo H, Olsson Y, Siesjo BK: Hypoglycemic brain injury. I. Metabolic and light microscopic findings in rat cerebral cortex during profound insulin-induced hypoglycemia and in the recovery period following glucose administration. Acta Neuropathol 1980;50:31–41.
3. Andrade R, Mathew V, Morgenstern MJ, et al: Hypoglycemic hemiplegic syndrome. Ann Emerg Med 1984;13: 529–531.
4. Arad I, Benady S: Gangrene following intraumbilical injection of hypertonic glucose. J Pediatr 1976;89:327–328.
5. Araki N, Greenberg JH, Sladky JT, et al: The effect of hyperglycemia on intracellular calcium in stroke. J Cereb Blood Flow Metab 1992;12:469–476.

6. Arky RA, Veverbrants E, Abramson EA: Irreversible hypoglycemia. JAMA 1968;206:575–578.
7. Atkin SH, Dasmahapatra A, Jaker MA, et al: Fingerstick glucose determination in shock. Ann Intern Med 1991; 114:1020–1024.
8. Boyle PJ, Schwartz NS, Shah SD, et al: Plasma glucose concentrations at the onset of hypoglycemic symptoms in patients with poorly controlled diabetes and in nondiabetics. N Engl J Med 1988;318:1487–1492.
9. Candelise L, Landi G, Orazio E, et al. Prognostic significance of hyperglycemia in acute stroke. Arch Neurol 1985;42:661–733.
10. Cheeley RD, Joyce SM: A clinical comparison of the performance of four blood glucose reagent strips. Am J Emerg Med 1990;8:11–15.
11. Chernow A, Diaz M, Cruess D, et al: Bedside blood glucose determinations in critical care medicine: A comparative analysis of two techniques. Crit Care Med 1982;10:463–465.
12. Combs DJ, Dempsey RJ, Donaldson D, et al: Hyperglycemia suppresses C-fos mRNA expression following cerebral ischemia in gerbils. J Cereb Blood Flow Metab 1992;12: 169–172.
13. D'Alecy LG: Dextrose containing intravenous fluid impairs outcome and increases death after eight minutes of cardiac arrest and resuscitation in dogs. Surgery 1986;3:505–511.
14. DCCT Research Group: The effect of intensive treatment of diabetes on the development and progression of long-term complications in insulin-dependent diabetes mellitus. N Engl J Med 1993;329:977–986.
15. DCCT Research Group. Epidemiology of severe hypoglycemia in the diabetes control and complications trial. Am J Med 1991;90:450–459.
16. de Courten-Meyers GM, Kleinholz M, Wagner KR, et al: Normoglycemia (not hypoglycemia) optimizes outcome from middle cerebral artery occlusion. J Cereb Blood Flow Metab 1994;14:227–236.
17. de Courten-Myers G, Myers RE, Schoolfield L: Hyperglycemia enlarges infarct size in cerebrovascular occlusion in cats. Stroke 1988;19:623–630.
18. de Courten-Myers GM, Wagner KR, Myers RE: Insulin reduction of cerebral infarction. J Neurosurg 1996;84:146–148.
19. DeLorenzo RA, Vista JP: Another hazard of hypertonic dextrose. Am J Emerg Med 1994;12:262–263.
20. Dietrich WD, Alonso O, Busto R: Moderate hyperglycemia worsens acute blood–brain barrier injury after forebrain ischemia in rats. Stroke 1993;24:111–116.
21. Duarte J, Perez A, Coria F, et al: Hypoglycemia presenting as acute tetraplegia. Stroke 1993;24:143. Letter.
22. Duh E, Feinglos M: Hypoglycemia-induced angina pectoris in a patient with diabetes mellitus. Ann Intern Med 1994; 121:945–946.
23. Frantz ID, Medina G, Taeusch HW: Correlation of Dextrostix values with true glucose in the range less than 50 mg/dL. J Pediatr 1975;87:417–420.
24. Ginsberg MD, Prado R, Deitrich WD, et al: Hyperglycemia reduces the extent of cerebral infarction in rats. Stroke 1987;18:570–574.
25. Goldfarb S, Cox M, Singer I, Goldberg M: Acute hyperkalemia induced by hyperglycemia: Hormonal mechanisms. Ann Intern Med 1976;84:426–432.
26. Goodgame JT, Pizzo P, Brennan MF: Iatrogenic lactic acidosis. Cancer 1978;42:800–803.
27. Hamilton MG, Tranmer BI, Auer RN: Insulin reduction of cerebral infarction due to transient focal ischemia. J Neurosurg 1995;82:262–268.
28. Hoffman RS, Smilkstein MJ, Rubenstein F: An "AMP" by any other name: The hazards of intravenous magnesium dosing. JAMA 1989;261:557. Letter.
29. Ibayashi S: Cerebral blood flow and tissue metabolism in experimental cerebral ischemia of spontaneously hypertensive rats with hyper, normo and hypoglycemia. Stroke 1986;17:261–266.
30. Jones JL, Ray VG, Gough JE, et al: Determination of prehospital blood glucose: A prospective, controlled study. J Emerg Med 1992;10:679–682.
31. Kalimo H, Olsson Y: Effects of severe hypoglycemia on the human brain: Neuropathological case reports. Acta Neurol Scand 1980;62:345–356.
32. Kim YB, Gidday JM, Gonzalez FR, et al: Effect of hypoglycemia on postischemic cortical blood flow, hypercapnic reactivity, and interstitial adenosine concentration. J Neurosurg 1994;81:877–884.
33. Kulling P, Lindholm M, Eklund J: Hemodynamic effects of hyperosmolal glucose infusion in the critically ill patient. Crit Care Med 1981;9:768–771.
34. Lala VR, Vedanarayana VV, Ganesh S, et al: Hypoglycemic hemiplegia in an adolescent with insulin-dependent diabetes mellitus: A case report and a review of the literature. J Emerg Med 1989;7:233–236.
35. Lanier WL, Strangland KJ, Scheithauer BW, et al: The effects of dextrose infusion and head position on neurologic outcome after complete cerebral ischemia in primates: Examination of a model. Anesthesiology 1987;66:39–48.
36. Lavery RF, Allegra JR, Cody RP, et al: A prospective evaluation of glucose reagent test strips in the prehospital setting. Am J Emerg Med 1991;9:304–308.
37. Leak D, Starr P: The mechanism of arrhythmias during insulin-induced hypoglycemia. Am Heart J 1962;63:688–691.
38. LeMay DR, Gehua L, Zelenock GB, D'Alecy LG: Insulin administration protects neurologic function in cerebral ischemia in rats. Stroke 1988;19:1411–1419.
39. MacKay N, Gordon A, Neilson MEJ: Observer error in Dextrostix estimations of blood sugar. Lancet 1965;2:229. Letter.
40. MacLeod DB, Montoya DR, Fick GH, Jessen KR: The effect of 25 grams IV glucose on serum inorganic phosphate levels. Ann Emerg Med 1994;23:524–528.
41. Maisels MJ, Lee CA: Chemstrip glucose test strips: Correlation with true glucose values less than 80 mg/dL. Crit Care Med 1983;11:293–295.
42. Malouf R, Brust JM: Hypoglycemia: Causes, neurological manifestations, and outcome. Ann Neurol 1985;17:421–430.
43. Montgomery BM, Pinner CA: Transient hypoglycemic hemiplegia. Arch Intern Med 1964;114:680–684.
44. Odeh M, Oliven A, Bassan H: Transient atrial fibrillation precipitated by hypoglycemia. Ann Emerg Med 1990; 19:565–567.
45. Plum F: What causes infarction in ischemic brain? The Robert Wartenberg Lecture. Neurology 1983;33:222–226.
46. Plum F, Posner JB: Diagnosis of Stupor and Coma. Philadelphia, Davis, 1978.

47. Prado R, Ginsberg MD, Dietrich WD, et al: Hyperglycemia increases infarct size in collaterally perfused but not end-arterial vascular territories. J Cereb Blood Flow Metab 1988;8:186–191.
48. Pulsinelli WA, Levy DE, Sigsbee B, et al: Increased damage after ischemic stroke in patients with hyperglycemia with or without established diabetes mellitus. Am J Med 1983; 74:540–544.
49. Pulsinelli WA, Waldman S, Rawlinson D, et al: Moderate hyperglycemia augments ischemic brain damage: A neuropathic study in the rat. Neurology 1982;32:1239–1246.
50. Rasmussen A: Hypophosphatemia during postoperative glucose infusion. Acta Chir Scand 1985;151:497–500.
51. Rehncrona S, Rosen I, Siesjo BK: Brain lactic acidosis and ischemic cell damage: 1. Biochemistry and neurophysiology. J Cereb Blood Flow Metabol 1981;1:297–309.
52. Rowlands BJ, Giddings AEB: Postoperative hypophosphataemia. Lancet 1976:3;1077–1078.
53. Seibert DG: Reversible decerebrate posturing secondary to hypoglycemia. Am J Med 1985;78:1036–1037.
54. Shah A, Stanhope R, Matthew D: Hazards of pharmacological tests of growth hormone secretion in childhood. Br Med J 1992;304:173–174.
55. Siemkowicz E, Hansen AJ. Clinical restitution following cerebral ischemia in hypo-, normo-, and hyperglycemic rats. Acta Neurol Scand 1978;58:1–8.
56. Siesjo BK: Basic mechanisms of traumatic brain damage. Ann Emerg Med 1993;22:959–969.
57. Siesjo BK. Cell damage in the brain: A speculative synthesis. J Cereb Blood Flow Metab 1981;1:155–183.
58. Swain JA, Anderson RV, Siegman MG: Low-flow cardiopulmonary bypass and cerebral protection: A summary of investigations. Ann Thorac Surg 1993;56: 1490–1492.
59. Thomas SH, Gough JE, Benson N, et al: Accuracy of finger-stick glucose determination in patients receiving CPR. South Med J 1994;87:1072–1075.
60. Ting LP, Tu CL, Chou CK: Insulin-induced expression of human heat-shock protein hsp-70. J Biol Chem 1989;264: 3404–3408.
61. Vannucci RC, Yager JY: Glucose, lactic acid, and perinatal hypoxic-ischemic brain damage. Pediatr Neurol 1992;8:3–12.
62. Voll CL, Auer RN: Insulin attenuates ischemic brain damage independent of its hypoglycemic effect. J Cereb Blood Flow Metab 1991;11:1006–1014.
63. Voorhies TM, Rawlinson D, Vannucci RC: Glucose and perinatal hypoxic-ischemic brain damage in the rat. Neurology 1986;36:1115–1118.
64. Wagner SR, Lanier WL: Metabolism of glucose, glycogen, and high-energy phosphates during complete cerebral ischemia. Anesthesiology 1994;81:1516–1526.
65. Wallis WE, Donaldson I, Scott RS, Wilson J: Hypoglycemia masquerading as cerebrovascular disease (hypoglycemic hemiplegia). Ann Neurol 1985;18:510–512.
66. Warner DS, Gionet TX, Todd MM, McAllister AM: Insulin-induced normoglycemia improves ischemic outcome in hyperglycemic rats. Stroke 1992;23:1775–1780.
67. Wass CT, Lanier WL: Glucose modulation of ischemic brain injury: Review and clinical recommendations. Mayo Clin Proc 1996;71:801–812.
68. Wass C, Scheithauer BW, Bronk J, et al: Insulin treatment of corticosteroid-associated hyperglycemia and its effect on outcome after forebrain ischemia in rats. Anesthesiology 1996;84:644–651.
69. Welsh FA, Ginsberg MD, Rieder W, et al: Deleterious effect of glucose pretreatment on recovery from diffuse cerebral ischemia in the cat: II. Regional metabolite levels. Stroke 1980;11:355–363.
70. White BC, Krause GS: Brain injury and repair mechanisms: The potential for pharmacologic therapy in closed head trauma. Ann Emerg Med 1993;22:970–979.
71. Winer JB, Fish DR, Sawyers D, Marsden CD: A movement disorder as a presenting feature of recurrent hypoglycemia. Movement Disorders 1990;5:176–177.
72. Woo E, Ma JTC, Robinson JD, et al: Hyperglycemia is a stress response in acute stroke. Stroke 1988;19:1359–1364.

CHAPTER 41

Anticonvulsants

Suzanne Doyon

	Therapeutic serum levels	
Drug	*mg/L*	*μmol/L*
Carbamazepine	4–12	17–51
Ethosuximide	40–100	283–708
Felbamate	N/R	N/R
Gabapentin	N/R	N/R
Lamotrigine	N/R	N/R
Phenobarbital	15–40	65–172
Phenytoin	10–20	40–79
Valproic acid	50–120	347–833
Vigabatrin	N/R	N/R

N/R = Not recommended.

A 28-year-old woman was brought to the Emergency Department (ED) following two generalized seizures. According to her family, she had a 5-year history of generalized tonic-clonic seizures and was well controlled with carbamazepine 1200 mg/day. She had recently become depressed and, according to the family, on the day of presentation had ingested all her remaining carbamazepine tablets and an unknown quantity of phenytoin capsules. Approximately 1 hour following ingestion, as the family was attempting to persuade her to come to the hospital, she began seizing. She had no history of chronic alcohol consumption.

On arrival in the ED, the patient was comatose with a blood pressure of 136/80 mm Hg, pulse of 100 beats/min, respiratory rate of 12 breaths/min, and a temperature of 37°C (98.6° F). The patient responded with withdrawal to deep pain. Her head was atraumatic with dilated pupils (4 mm bilaterally) that responded sluggishly to light. Her gag reflex was depressed. The lungs, heart, and abdomen were unremarkable. There were no signs of track marks, cyanosis, or edema. Deep tendon reflexes were symmetrically brisk and there was bilateral plantar extension.

The patient was intubated and placed on a respirator. An intravenous line was established. A bedside rapid reagent test for blood glucose was 70 mg/dL and the patient was administered 50 mL of 50% dextrose intravenously. A 40 French orogastric tube was placed. The patient was lavaged with 2 L of 0.9% sodium chloride solution, and 60 g of activated charcoal was instilled through the lavage tube. No further seizures were noted.

Laboratory evaluation revealed a normal complete blood count and a serum chemistry profile remarkable only for a serum bicarbonate of 17 mEq/L. An ethanol level was negative. The plasma carbamazepine level was 55 mg/L and phenytoin level was 19 mg/L. A chest radiograph was normal and an ECG revealed a sinus tachycardia with normal axis and intervals.

The patient was admitted to the ICU. Her serum bicarbonate level normalized quickly. Multiple-dose activated charcoal was administered. Hemoperfusion was considered but not instituted. Her ECG remained normal. Twenty-eight hours following presentation, she was stuporous but occasionally arousable and combative. Later, she was noted to exhibit writhing, choreoathetoid movements. Two days later, she was more alert, with horizontal nystagmus and ataxia as her only neurologic abnormalities. Five days after the ingestion, her neurologic examination had returned to normal. She was discharged without permanent sequelae and with psychiatric support.

Toxicity of Anticonvulsants

Due to the diversity of this group of agents, overdose of anticonvulsants can give rise to a wide range of signs and symptoms. The route of administration can determine toxic effects as well. In addition to the amount ingested and the duration of ingestion, age, underlying diseases, concomitant use of other anticonvulsants, and genetic factors all determine individual toxicity. The toxicities of benzodiazepines and barbiturates are discussed in Chapter 61 and will not be reviewed in this chapter.

How Do Anticonvulsants Work?

Extensive research performed over the past decade has served to elucidate the mechanism of action of most of the major anticonvulsants. Table 41–1 summarizes these findings.

TABLE 41–1. MECHANISMS OF ACTION OF VARIOUS ANTICONVULSANTS

Drug	Mechanism of Action
Barbiturates	Enhancement of Cl^- influx at $GABA_A$ receptor
Benzodiazepines	Enhancement of Cl^- influx at $GABA_A$ receptor
Carbamazepine	Prolongation of Na^+ channel inactivation
	Adenosine partial agonist
Ethosuximide	Unknown
Felbamate	Blocks NMDA receptors
	Prolongation of Na^+ channel inactivation
	GABA enhancement
Gabapentin	GABA enhancement
Lamotrigine	Inhibition of release of glutamate and asparate
	Prolongation of Na^+ channel inactivation
	GABA enhancement
Phenytoin	Prolongation of Na^+ channel inactivation
	Inhibits adenosine effect and uptake
Trimethadione	Unknown
Valproic acid	Prolongation of Na^+ channel inactivation
	GABA enhancement
Vigabatrin	GABA enhancement

Data from references 5, 29, 81, and 104.

High-frequency neuronal action potential firing is responsible for seizure development. This pattern of firing is uncommon during normal physiologic neuronal transmission. Suppression of high-frequency firing is related to suppression of voltage-dependent Na^+ channels and inhibition of their rate of recovery. Carbamazepine, felbamate, lamotrigine, phenytoin, and valproic acid all inhibit Na^+ channels by reducing their ability to recover from inactivation. After a depolarization-triggered Na^+ channel opening, the Na^+ channels are prevented from closing spontaneously and are, therefore, unable to evoke another action potential.[66,69,111,113] Low-frequency firing is not affected by these agents. Hypothetically, myocardial Na^+ channels may also be inhibited by these agents, resulting in conduction abnormalities, as illustrated in some cases of carbamazepine overdoses.[6]

Phenytoin and carbamazepine may exert some anticonvulsant effect by acting through adenosine systems. Adenosine, an endogenous anticonvulsant, can suppress seizure continuation.[30] Phenytoin may inhibit adenosine uptake resulting in increased extracellular adenosine.[83] Carbamazepine may act as a partial agonist at the level of the adenosine receptor.[83,96]

Gamma-aminobutyric acid (GABA) is an inhibitory neurotransmitter whose accumulation is protective against seizures. Increased stores of GABA result in increased $GABA_A$ receptors binding and membrane hyperpolarization.[69] This reduces neuronal excitability and raises seizure threshold. GABA stores can be increased by increasing synthesis or decreasing metabolism. Vigabatrin, the first anticonvulsant developed on the basis of a targeted mechanism of action, irreversibly inhibits GABA transaminase, an enzyme responsible for the metabolism of GABA.[29] Valproic acid has similar effects as well.[69] Through a mechanism that remains largely unknown, gabapentin increases threefold the amount of GABA released by presynaptic nerve terminals under certain conditions.[44,69]

Lamotrigine stabilizes presynaptic neuronal membranes by blockade of voltage-dependent Na^+ channels, thus preventing the release of the excitatory amino acid transmitters glutamate and aspartate, resulting in inhibition of excitatory spread.[43,61]

Felbamate prolongs Na^+ channel inactivation, enhances $GABA_A$ receptor Cl^- currents in a barbiturate-like fashion, and, finally, inhibits *N*-methyl-D-aspartate receptors (NMDA).[84]

Phenytoin

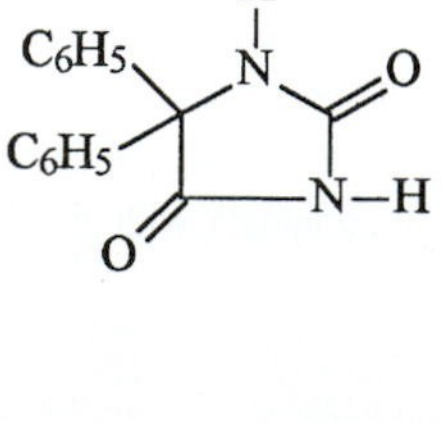

Phenytoin (5,5-diphenyl-2,4-imidazolidinedione), formerly known as diphenylhydantoin, is an effective anticonvulsive agent used in the treatment of most seizure disorders, except absence seizures. Currently available data indicate that it no longer has a role in the treatment of most toxin-induced seizures including the alcohol withdrawal syndrome.[4,16] It is nonsedating in therapeutic doses and is often preferred over the sedative-hypnotic anticonvulsants for the management of epilepsy.

Phenytoin is available parenterally and orally. A loading dose followed by a maintenance dose is usually recommended, whether the medication is administered intravenously or orally.[80] Significant differences in the toxicity of phenytoin exist, depending on the route of administration.[26,87,93,109]

Intravenous phenytoin must be administered with saline, as it precipitates in glucose-containing solutions. The standard loading dose is 15 to 20 mg/kg, to be delivered at a maximal rate of 50 mg per minute in adults and 1 mg/kg per minute in children (up to a maximum of 50 mg/min). Infusion rates should be reduced to 20 to 30 mg/min in the elderly and patients with unstable cardiovascular status.[15,35] Infusion pumps are recommended.[15,92] The medication should be given with established ECG monitoring. Cardiac disturbances are very uncommon when infusion rates are proper. Hypotension, however, is common, and is concentration and dose-related. This side effect has been attributed to the propylene glycol (40%) and ethanol (10%) additives and the adjusted pH of 11 to 12 rather than to the phenytoin itself.[72] Propylene glycol in particular depresses myocardial tissue and decreases peripheral vascular resistance (see Chap. 54).[45,65,107,114] Stopping the infusion for just a few minutes and restarting at a slower rate usually corrects the problem. Occasionally, a saline bolus is necessary.[35] CNS side effects include unusual movement disorders, ataxia, and acute confusion. These symptoms are usually transient and resolve spontaneously in 30 to 60 minutes. Local pain is frequent and has been attributed to the presence of additives. In these cases, stopping the infusion and restarting at a slower rate is also advisable.[35] Extravasation of phenytoin may lead to skin necrosis possibly necessitating surgical intervention.[20,35,58]

Fosphenytoin, a phosphoester prodrug, became available in 1996. It is converted entirely to phenytoin within 6 to 16 minutes of injection. It is diluted with nontoxic, nonirritating additives and has a pH of 8 to 9. Fosphenytoin can be given intramuscularly or intravenously. It is compatible with saline and glucose-containing solutions. The loading dose is the same as phenytoin (and is expressed in phenytoin equivalents). It can be infused at a maximal rate of 150 mg/min. CNS side effects from fosphenytoin infusions are similar to those resulting from phenytoin infusion. Fosphenytoin has no cardiovascular side effects and the risk of skin necrosis from extravasation are minimal. Perineal pruritis has been reported following infusions of fosphenytoin and may last for several hours.[13]

What Are the Pharmacokinetics of Phenytoin?

Table 41–2 details the pharmacokinetic parameters of phenytoin. Phenytoin is rapidly distributed into all tissues. It is extensively bound to albumin. Only the unbound free fraction can cross biologic membranes and exert pharmacologic action.

Individual variations in protein-binding capacity may explain the variance seen in the relationship between serum concentration and clinical intoxication. Pa-

TABLE 41–2. PHARMACOKINETIC PARAMETERS OF MAJOR ANTICONVULSANTS

Drug	Time to Peak Plasma Level (h)	Vd (L/kg)	Plasma Protein Binding (%)	Elimination Unchanged (%)	Active Metabolites	Plasma Half-Life Range (h)	Plasma Half-Life Average (h)
Carbamazepine	3–8	0.8–1.8	75	1	Carbamazepine 10,11-epoxide	6–20[a]	12
Ethosuximide	1–4	0.6	0	25	None	48–72	60[b]
Felbamate	1–4	0.75	25	40	None	20–23	20
Gabapentin	3	0.8	0	100	None	5–7	6
Lamotrigine	2.5	1.2	55	10	None	14–50	25
Phenytoin	5–8	0.6	>90	<5	None	12–36	24
Valproic acid	1–8	0.1–0.22	>90	<5	2-n-valproic acid [2-propyl-2-pentenoic acid] 3-hydroxyvalproic acid 3-ketovalproic	6–18	12
Vigabatrin	2	0.8	0	>80	None	4–8	6

[a]Chronic therapy: 4.9–11.5 h.
[b]Children : 30 h.
Data from references 11, 17, 18, 22, 29, 36, 43, 44, 52, and 60.

tients with decreased protein-binding capacity can theoretically become toxic at total phenytoin levels within the therapeutic range. Examples include neonates; hypoalbuminemic, hyperbilirubinemic, and uremic patients; as well as patients taking phenylbutazone, salicylates, sulfonamides, para-aminosalicylic acid, and chlorothiazide. In such patients, determination of the free phenytoin fraction is essential. The free phenytoin fraction can be measured directly by a number of analytical methods, including serum ultrafiltration followed by gas chromatography or EMIT technology.[8,77] Free phenytoin levels should not exceed 2.1 mg/L.[8,46]

The major metabolite is a parahydroxylphenyl derivative that is conjugated with glucuronide and subsequently excreted in the bile and urine. At plasma concentrations below 10 mg/L, elimination is usually first order. At higher concentrations, zero-order elimination occurs due to saturation of the hydroxylation reaction. Thus the medication's apparent half-life of elimination is progressively prolonged as the plasma concentration increases. This pattern follows the Michaelis-Menten model.

What Are the Manifestations of Phenytoin Toxicity?

Phenytoin toxicity can be extremely variable and symptoms can appear alone or in groups. Acute phenytoin toxicity predominantly produces neurologic signs and symptoms: nystagmus, ophthalmoplegia, ataxia, dysarthria, hyperreflexia, altered mental status, and hallucinations.[71] Toxic phenytoin levels may produce seizures, but this event is extremely rare; when it occurs, it is usually in the setting of overdosage in an epileptic patient.[101] Most patients with phenytoin levels in the toxic range do not have seizures. There is no reported cardiotoxicity resulting from an oral overdose of phenytoin.[112] Young children and the elderly may present with atypical manifestations of toxicity. For example, phenytoin-induced chorea and opisthotonic posturing have been documented after oral overdoses in the pediatric population.[71] Chronic high levels may result in an encephalopathy.

A variety of metabolic, endocrine and hematologic adverse effects are reported with therapeutic phenytoin use: impaired insulin secretion, hypothyroidism, osteomalacia, aplastic anemia, pseudolymphoma, hemorrhagic disease of the newborn, and megaloblastic anemia due to decreased folate absorption and altered folate metabolism that is responsive to folic acid.[85] Gingival hyperplasia occurs in about 20% of patients, especially children and adolescents. The overgrowth of tissue is due to altered collagen metabolism and can be minimized by good oral hygiene.[50] Gastrointestinal disturbances are common and can be reduced by taking the medication with meals.

What Is the Management of Phenytoin Toxicity?

Most cases of phenytoin intoxication, acute or chronic, can be managed conservatively. The use of multiple-dose activated charcoal (MDAC) is shown to reduce the half-life of phenytoin in the overdose setting from 44.5 to 22.3 hours.[68]

Severe ataxia mandates that patients be followed carefully with serial neurologic examinations.

Overdosed patients do not need routine cardiac monitoring.[112] Hemodialysis and hemoperfusion are of little benefit in the management of phenytoin toxicity. No specific antidote is available.

Carbamazepine

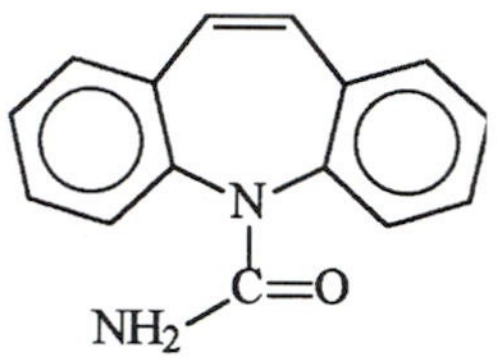

Carbamazepine (5H-dibenzazepine–5-carboxamide) is a potent anticonvulsant used in the treatment of seizures as well as trigeminal neuralgia and bipolar affective disorders.[70] Like phenytoin, it is not effective in the treatment of absence seizures. It has become a first-line therapy for seizures, especially in pregnant patients with epilepsy.[27]

What Are the Pharmacokinetics of Carbamazepine?

Carbamazepine is a carbamylated derivative of iminostilbene and is related structurally to the cyclic antidepressants. Carbamazepine is quite lipophilic with an erratic absorption. Peak levels usually do not occur for 3 to 8 hours following ingestion and may take as long as 24 hours, especially following a large overdose.[19] Like phenytoin, the concentration of carbamazepine in the CNS is correlated with the concentration of free carbamazepine in the plasma. A small amount of the drug is recovered unchanged in the feces, with evidence supporting some enterohepatic circulation.[63] Carbamazepine is largely metabolized to an epoxide and then conjugated with glucuronic acid and excreted in the urine. The metabolite, carbamazepine 10,11-epoxide, is pharmacologically active and its concentration in plasma and blood may reach 50% of that of carbamazepine itself.[36,63] Carbamazepine is also inactivated by conjugation and hydroxylation. The enzymes responsible for the degradation of carbamazepine are not considered saturable.[36,61] Carbamazepine is only available orally. Table 41–2 summarizes the pharmacokinetic properties of carbamazepine.

In managing patients with overdoses of carbamazepine, it is usually only necessary to follow the plasma levels of the parent compound.

The elimination of carbamazepine increases over the first few weeks of therapy due to autoinduction, and the half-life on chronic therapy decreases substantially. Therefore the dose must be increased gradually over a 2 to 4 week period to a final dose of 10 to 20 mg/kg for adults and 20 to 70 mg/kg for children. Children eliminate the drug more rapidly than adults. There is no simple relationship between the dose of carbamazepine and the plasma concentration. Therapeutic levels are 4 to 12 mg/L. Patients on multiple anticonvulsants may not tolerate high levels and should be maintained at 4 to 8 mg/L.

What Are the Manifestations of Carbamazepine Toxicity?

Acute carbamazepine toxicity produces prominent neurologic signs and symptoms occasionally associated with cardiovascular effects. Nystagmus, ataxia, dysarthria, stupor, encephalopathy, myoclonus, dystonia, choreoathetosis, and seizures have been reported.[36] Additional findings associated with acute carbamazepine intoxication include nausea, vomiting, hypothermia, hypotension, tachycardia, and cardiac conduction abnormalities.[93,108] Pancreatitis associated with acute ingestion of carbamazepine is reported.[105]

Some studies have attempted to directly correlate neurologic status to serum levels.[10,108] Many authors, however, have failed to reproduce this correlation on larger groups of patients.[51,94,98,102,103] Periodic fluctuations of level of consciousness followed by sudden relapse or improvement are common.[28,34] Carbamazepine concentrations are not reliable predictors of toxicity, although higher levels, especially levels above 40 mg/L in adults, tend to be associated with increased incidence of coma, seizures, and cardiotoxicity.[51]

Elevated carbamazepine levels can produce paradoxical seizures.[94] Seizures occur independently of a preexistent seizure disorder.[94,103] The mechanism remains largely unknown.

Depression of phase 0, phase 2, and phase 4 of the action potential have been reported in dogs at high doses of carbamazepine.[100] A large case series of patients with carbamazepine overdoses shows a 15% incidence of QRS widening (>100 msec), a 50% incidence of QTc prolongation (>420 msec) and no cases of T40msec axis deviation.[6] Patients with prolonged QTc intervals, congenital or acquired, are at increased risk of developing torsades de pointes or ventricular tachycardia. In comatose patients the onset of ECG abnormalities have been delayed for up to 20 hours postingestion.[32,62,103] They also have been known to occur with chronic carbamazepine therapy.[6,23,56] Severe myocardial dysfunction requiring prolonged support has been reported, but seems to be a rare occurrence.[42,62] Lastly, no correlation between serum concentrations of carbamazepine and ECG abnormalities has been demonstrated.[6,99]

Toxicity of carbamazepine in children differs slightly from that of adults. A higher incidence of dystonic reactions, choreathetosis, and seizures has been described, in contrast to a lower incidence of electrocardiographic abnormalities.[9,10,55,97,102]

Chronic carbamazepine overdose can result in chronic headaches, diplopia, and ataxia. At high concentrations of carbamazepine, vasopressin secretion can be stimulated, leading to hyponatremia and fluid retention (SIADH).[40] This effect is especially detrimental to young children, the elderly, and patients with impaired cardiac function.[12] Another chronic effect is a dose-related leukopenia.[86]

Adverse effects include morbilliform rash, Stevens-Johnson syndrome, lupus like syndrome, aplastic anemia, leukopenia, thrombocytopenia pseudolymphoma,[12,49,85] and fatal eosinophilic myocarditis.[89]

What Is the Management of Carbamazepine Toxicity?

Multiple-dose activated charcoal has a definite therapeutic role in the management of patients with carbamazepine overdose, and is particularly helpful in reducing the enterohepatic circulation.[76,106] Concretions of carbamazepine should be suspected when plasma levels rise or the manifestation of symptoms is delayed. A radiographic contrast study should be performed in order to confirm this diagnosis.

Cardiac monitoring is appropriate. If the QRS duration is longer than 100 msec, it is reasonable to consider the administration of hypertonic sodium bicarbonate at 1–2 mEq/kg IV. Hypertonic sodium bicarbonate reverses some of the electrocardiographic changes induced by cyclic antidepressants, and carbamazepine exhibits cardiotoxicity similar to that of cyclic antidepressants. If the patient is seizing, benzodiazepine administration is recommended.

The lack of water solubility of carbamazepine renders dialysis ineffective. Hemoperfusion has resulted in a modest improvement in elimination in a few cases.[42] It must be emphasized that MDAC is as effective as charcoal hemoperfusion and is much less invasive.[106] No specific antidote is available.

Valproic Acid

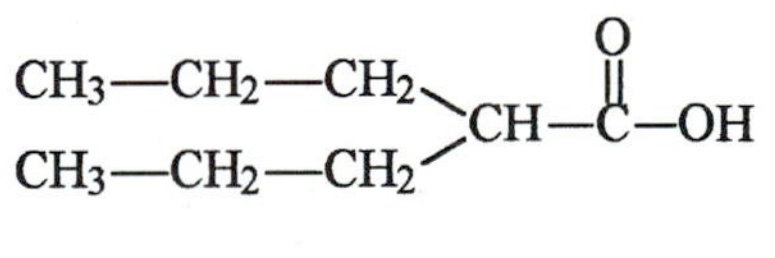

Valproic acid (n-dipropylacetic acid) is a simple branched-chain carboxylic acid. It is used to treat absence seizures, myoclonic seizures, and tonic-clonic seizures. It is also used as a mood stabilizer in the management of many psychiatric illnesses, especially bipolar affective disorder.

What Are the Pharmacokinetics of Valproic Acid?

Valproic acid is extensively metabolized (>95%) in the liver, where it is converted to the conjugate ester of glucuronic acid and oxidized by the mitochondria. Several of the metabolites are biologically active and some are nearly as potent as the parent compound. One in particular, 2-n-valproic acid, accumulates in the plasma and CNS tissue to a significant degree.[47] Table 41–2 summarizes these and other findings.

What Are the Manifestations of Valproic Acid Toxicity?

Acute poisonings with valproic acid may present with neurologic, gastrointestinal, hematologic, metabolic, and respiratory disturbances.[5,33,48,57] Respiratory failure, requiring ventilatory support, frequently complicates the course of patients with severe acute valproic acid overdoses.

CNS toxicity, the most common manifestation of acute valproic acid overdose, ranges from mild lethargy to fatal and delayed cerebral edema.[5,57] The development of cerebral edema may be linked to the production of the metabolite 2-n-valproic acid.[33] There also seems to be an association between valproate-induced encephalopathy and hyperammonemia even in the absence of hepatic dysfunction.[24] This suggests that the hyperammonemia noted with valproate therapy is not always the result of hepatitis, as was previously reported. It now appears that elevated levels of propionate, a valproic acid metabolite, inhibit mitochondrial carbamyl phosphate synthetase activity, which is necessary for the metabolism of ammonia in the urea cycle.[25] In addition to its effect on carbamyl phosphate synthetase, valproic acid combines with carnitine, a nutrient important in long-chain fatty acid and mitochondrial metabolism, and the resulting valproicylcarnitine ester is excreted in the urine. Hypocarnitinemia may be associated with hyperammonemia.[53]

Mild to moderate elevations of liver enzymes are typical in patients with acute valproic acid intoxications.[5] Acute hepatotoxicity has been attributed to the production of intermediate metabolites and to hypocarnitinemia.[31,53,74] Pancreatitis and acute renal failure are rare, possible manifestations of acute toxicity.[5,21,57] Other common metabolic disturbances include metabolic acidosis, hypernatremia, and hypocalcemia.[5,57]

Thrombocytopenia and leukopenia are common manifestations of hematopoietic toxicity.[5,21]

Chronic valproic acid therapy may lead to hepatotoxicity. The clinical findings may vary from asymptomatic elevation of amino transferases to fatal hepatitis. Chronic valproic acid therapy induces steatosis of the liver.

The most frequent adverse effects associated with valproic acid are GI disturbances and ataxia, confusion, sedation, and tremor. Valproic acid has been reported to cause alopecia, pancreatitis, and hematologic disturbances (eg, leukopenia, thrombocytopenia, and inhibition of platelet function). The most important adverse effect however is fulminant hepatitis (Reye's like syndrome) especially in young children receiving multiple anticonvulsants. Unfortunately, fulminant hepatitis, when it occurs, is not consistently preceded by abnormal liver function tests.[85]

What Is the Management of Valproic Acid Toxicity?

Multiple-dose activated charcoal has been shown to reduce the half-life of valproic acid from an average of 12 to 4.8 hours.[37] Although drugs that are extensively protein-bound are usually not amenable to MDAC, it was demonstrated that, in the acute overdose setting, the percentage of bound valproic acid decreases significantly (89 to 29%) as the plasma concentration increases.[37] Whole-bowel irrigation has been suggested as a therapy for intestinal decontamination of enteric-coated preparations of valproic acid.[48]

In vitro, naloxone has been shown to inhibit the effects of valproic acid on GABA transport.[53] Two case reports describe rapid resolution of CNS symptoms in valproate overdosed patients following the administration of naloxone.[3,99] Other reports, however, showed no effect.[21,73]

Carnitine supplementation should be provided to hyperammonemic patients receiving valproic acid.[25] In fact, the administration of carnitine to children on valproate has been shown to normalize ammonia levels.[78] Others have shown that supplemental L-carnitine oral therapy prevented some of the hepatotoxicity of acute valproic acid intoxication.[54]

Valproic acid has a low molecular weight (140 D), a small volume of distribution (0.1 to 0.24 L/kg), and in severe overdose, a large free circulating fraction. Hemodialysis and hemoperfusion result in an increased clearance of valproic acid but resulted in marginal improvement in clinical outcome.[48,73,110] Extracorporeal removal of valproic acid is reserved for patients with rapid deterioration, evidence of hepatic dysfunction, and apparent continued absorption of the drug.

Gabapentin

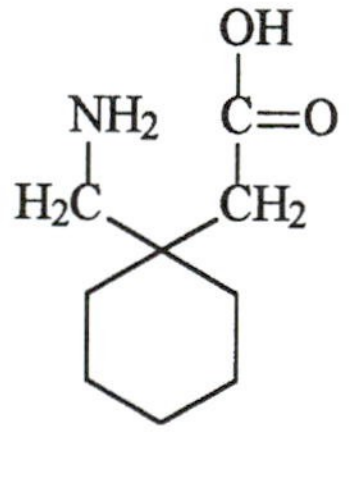

Gabapentin, an anticonvulsant structurally related to gamma-aminobutyric acid (GABA), is an approved adjunct medication in the treatment of partial seizures with and without secondarily generalized seizures in adults.

What Are the Pharmacokinetics of Gabapentin?

Gabapentin possesses quite a few desirable pharmacokinetic characteristics (Table 41–2). Gabapentin is not bound to plasma proteins and is excreted entirely by the kidney. Dosage adjustments must be made in patients with decreased renal function. A definitive therapeutic plasma concentration has not been established, although a range of 2 to 15 mg/mL has been suggested.

What Are the Manifestations of Gabapentin Toxicity?

Toxicity in mice demonstrates ataxia and sedation. In 6 human case reports (largest ingestion, 48.9 g) sedation, ataxia, and slurred speech were observed. The clinical features of acute gabapentin toxicity contrast favorably with the serious neurologic and cardiovascular toxicity of phenytoin and carbamazepine.[38,39,41]

No data exist on the chronic toxicity of gabapentin. The adverse effects associated with gabapentin therapy are somnolence, dizziness, and gastrointestinal distress.

What Is the Management of Gabapentin Toxicity?

The treatment of gabapentin overdose is largely supportive. Activated charcoal may be useful in increasing the clearance of gabapentin.

In all human cases, symptoms resolve within 48 hours without specific therapy. Plasma levels were not documented in these cases. There is no data on hemodialysis or hemoperfusion. No specific antidote exists for gabapentin overdose.

Felbamate

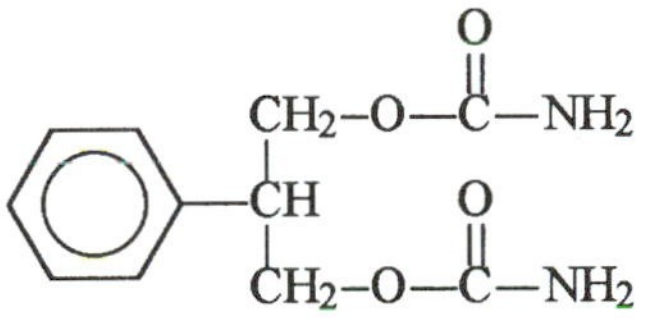

Felbamate was approved in 1993 with indications similar to gabapentin and lamotrigine. Because of the recent occurrence during therapy of cases of hepatic failure and aplastic anemia, the FDA recommends that felbamate be a therapy of last resort.[79]

What Are the Pharmacokinetics of Felbamate?

Felbamate has low plasma protein binding and is eliminated 40% unchanged in the urine with no active metabolites. Felbamate decreases the metabolism of phenytoin and valproic acid and increases the metabolism of carbamazepine.[2]

What Are the Manifestations of Felbamate Toxicity?

Mild gastrointestinal symptoms characterized the single case report of acute felbamate toxicity.[75] Chronic toxicity is not well documented.

Adverse effects from felbamate are frequent. Weight gain or loss, insomnia or somnolence, nausea, vomiting, pancreatitis, and psychosis are documented.[64] Several cases of fulminant hepatic failure with a high mortality rate (20%) were observed. Aplastic anemia, often fatal, developed in another group of patients.[1]

What Is the Management of Felbamate Toxicity?

The treatment of felbamate toxicity is largely supportive. Activated charcoal may be useful. There are no data on hemodialysis and hemoperfusion.

Lamotrigine

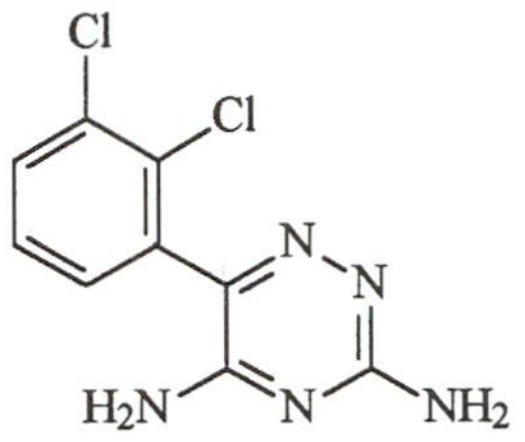

Lamotrigine is an anticonvulsant approved as an adjunctive medication for the treatment of partial seizures or in those with secondarily generalized seizures, in adults. It is not structurally related to other anticonvulsants.

What Are the Pharmacokinetics of Lamotrigine?

Lamotrigine has no active metabolite (Table 41–2). It does not affect the metabolism of other drugs.[17,43] A significantly reduced clearance of lamotrigine occurs in patients with Gilbert's syndrome.[18] No therapeutic serum concentration of lamotrigine is established, nor is there a toxic threshold beyond which intolerable side effects develop.[17,59]

What Are the Manifestations of Lamotrigine Toxicity?

There is only one case report of deliberate lamotrigine overdose. This patient presented with horizontal and vertical nystagmus and ataxia 1 hour after ingestion. His laboratory investigations were all normal except for a potassium level of 3.3 mEq/L. The most important finding was that his admission ECG showed a normal sinus rhythm with QRS width of 112 msec. His ECG 2 months later had a QRS width of less than 100 msec.[14]

The common chronic manifestations are nausea, headache, diplopia, blurred vision, dizziness, and ataxia. Case reports of sudden deaths while on chronic lamotrigine therapy can be found. Most of these patients had a rapidly progressing illness with rhabdomyolysis, disseminated intravascular coagulation, and renal failure secondary to status epilepticus.[67,91]

Adverse effects of lamotrigine include maculopapular rashes, angioedema, Stevens-Johnson syndrome, and, rarely, toxic epidermal necrolysis. The incidence of potentially life-threatening rashes is higher in patients under 16 years of age. Lamotrigine is not approved for use in this particular patient population.

What Is the Management of Lamotrigine Toxicity?

The treatment of patients with lamotrigine toxicity includes close cardiac monitoring and good supportive care. The QRS widening is a newly described phenomenon. Until more is known about the cardiac toxicity of lamotrigine, close ECG monitoring for a period of 24 to 48 hours is recommended if the initial QRS duration is longer than 100 msec. The administration of hypertonic sodium bicarbonate has not been studied but would be recommended.

In the single case report mentioned earlier, signs and symptoms, including ECG changes, gradually resolved over 48 hours.[14] Activated charcoal therapy may be useful. There are no data on hemodialysis and hemoperfusion.

Vigabatrin

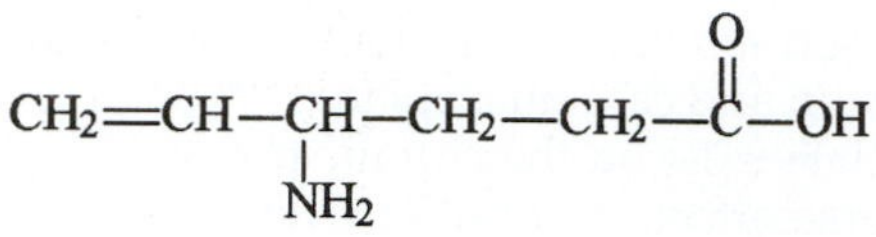

TABLE 41–3. ADVERSE EFFECTS OF ANTICONVULSANTS

Drug	Predictable	Idiosyncratic
Carbamazepine	Diplopia	Agranulocytosis
	Dizziness	Aplastic anemia
	Sedation	Hepatotoxicity
	Headache	Photosensitivity
	Nausea	Stevens-Johnson
	Hyponatremia	Lupus syndrome
	Hypocalcemia	Moribilliform rash
	Orofacial dyskinesia	Thrombocytopenia
	Cardiac dysrhythmias	Pseudolyphoma
		Myocarditis
Ethosuximide	Nausea/vomiting	Rash
	Agitation	Erythema multiforme
	Sedation	Stevens-Johnson
	Headache	Lupus syndrome
	Parkinsonism	Agranulocytosis
	Psychosis	Aplastic anemia
Felbamate	Irritability	Hepatic failure
	Insomnia	Aplastic anemia
	Anorexia	
	Nausea	
	Headache	
Gabapentin	Sedation	None
	Dizziness	
	Diplopia	
	Ataxia	
	Sedation	
Lamotrigine	Dizziness	Rash
	Tremor	Erythema multiforme
	Diplopia	Stevens-Johnson
	Ataxia	Angioedema
	Sedation	
Phenobarbital	Ataxia	Morbilliform rash
	Nystagmus	Exfoliative dermatitis
	Paradoxical excitement	
	Megaloblastic anemia	
	Osteomalacia	
	Neonatal hemorrhage	
Phenytoin	Anorexia	Blood dyscrasias
	Nausea/vomiting	Lupus syndrome
	Aggression	Reduced IgA
	Ataxia	Pseudolymphoma
	Cognitive impairment	Peripheral neuropathy
	Depression	Rash
	Sedation	Stevens-Johnson
	Headache	Dupuytren's contracture
	Nystagmus	Hepatotoxicity
	Neonatal hemorrhage	Teratogenicity
	Gingival hypertrophy	Gingival hyperplasia
	Coarse facies	Aplastic anemia
	Hirsutism	
	Megaloblastic anemia	
	Hyperglycemia	
	Hypocalcemia	
	Osteomalacia	
	Hypothyroidism	
Valproic acid	Anorexia	Pancreatitis
	Nausea/vomiting	Hepatotoxicity
	Alopecia	Thrombocytopenia
	Peripheral edema	Hyperammonemia
	Rash	Stupor
	Sedation	Encephalopathy
	Tremor	Teratogenicity
	Weight gain	
Vigabatrin	Sedation	Psychosis
	Weight gain	
	Behavioral changes	

Currently being investigated in U.S. trials, vigabatrin also has a desirable pharmacokinetic profile (Table 41–2). Vigabatrin, structurally similar to GABA, is a stereospecific inhibitor of GABA-transaminase. The R(−) enantiomer has virtually no effect while S(+) vigabatrin enantiomer inhibits the enzyme.[22] Its short elimination half-life does not indicate a short duration of action. As for gabapentin, dosage adjustments are necessary in the patient with impaired renal function.[52]

What Are the Manifestations of Vigabatrin Toxicity?

An acute psychotic episode lasting 36 hours was documented following deliberate self-poisoning with vigabatrin.[90] Chronic toxicity may result in psychosis.[88,90,95] Several adverse effects have been observed. Neuropathologic studies in rats, mice, and dogs were concerned with the appearance of microvacuoles in the CNS white matter.[82] Studies in humans have not confirmed this finding.

What Is the Management of Vigabatrin Toxicity?

The treatment of vigabatrin toxicity is largely supportive.

Other Anticonvulsant Agents

Trimethadione was the anticonvulsant of choice for absence (petit mal) seizures 50 years ago. It is rapidly demethylated to the active metabolic dimethadione, which is excreted in urine over days. During chronic therapy, the metabolite accumulates and is responsible for the anticonvulsant effects. Acute toxicity presents with gastrointestinal symptoms, sedation, ataxia, hepatitis. Adverse effects include aplastic anemia and a myasthenia gravis-like syndrome.[7]

Ethosuximide has largely replaced trimethadione in the management of absence seizures. Its major metabolite, the hydroxyethyl derivative, is inactive. Acute toxicity presents with sedation and gastrointestinal symptoms. Adverse effects include behavioral disturbances (psychosis, especially in children), Stevens-Johnson syndrome, aplastic anemia, and lupus.

Topiramate, the most recent addition to the anticonvulsant armamentarium is approved as adjunctive therapy for adults with partial seizures. Although the precise

TABLE 41–4. DRUG INTERACTIONS OF COMMON ANTICONVULSANTS

Drug	Increases Levels of	Decreases Levels of	Drug Toxicity Enhanced by	Drug Anticonvulsant Effect Decreased
Carbamazepine	None known	Doxycycline, felbamate, haloperidol, lamotrigine, phenytoin, primidone, valproic acid, warfarin	Danazol, diltiazem, erythromycin, INH, nicotine, propoxyphene, verapamil	Benzodiazepines, carbamazepine, felbamate, phenobarbital, phenytoin, primidone, succinimides, valproic acid
Felbamate	Carbamazepine epoxide (metabolite), phenytoin, valproic acid	Carbamazepine	Valproic acid	Carbamazepine, phenytoin
Gabapentin	None known	None known	None known	None known
Lamotrigine	None known	None known	Valproic acid	Carbamazepine, phenytoin, phenobarbital
Phenobarbital	Valproic acid metabolites	Carbamazepine, corticosteroids, coumadin, doxycycline, estradiol, griseofulvin, lamotrigine, phenytoin, propranolol, quinidine, theophylline, valproic acid	Acetazolamide, chloramphenicol, CNS depressants, dextropropoxyphene, furosemide, methylphenidate, MAOIs, valproic acid	Ammonium chloride, antacids, coumadin, folic acid, pyridoxine
Phenytoin	N-acetyl-P-benzoquinoneimine (NAPQI), oral anticoagulants, primidone	Amiodarone, carbamazepine, contraceptives, corticosteroids, cyclosporine, disopyramide, doxycycline, furosemide, influenza vaccine, levadopa, theophylline, tolbutamide, valproic acid	Amiodarone, chloramphenicol, cimetidine, disulfiram, ethosuximide, felbamate, fluconazole, INH, oral anticoagulants, phenylbutazone, sulfonamides, trimethaprim, valproic acid	Antineoplastic agents, calcium, diazepam, diazoxide, ethanol (chronic), folic acid, phenobarbital, rifampin, sulcrafate, theophylline, vigabatrin
Valproic acid	Felbamate, lamotrigine, phenobarbital, primidone	Carbamazepine	Cimetidine, felbamate, ranitidine	Carbamazepine, phenobarbital, phenytoin, primadone
Vigabatrin	None known	Phenytoin	None known	None known

mechanism of action is unclear, it can block sodium channels, enhance the action of GABA, and diminish the action of Kainate-induced excitatory receptor stimulation.

Therapeutic dosing is 50 to 400 mg daily. Peak plasma levels are reached in about 2 hours. Seventy percent of the drug is eliminated unchanged in the urine. The plasma half-life is about 22 hours. Topiramate can increase phenytoin serum concentrations, while phenytoin, carbamazepine, and valproic acid decrease serum topiramate levels. Topiramate can decrease the effectiveness of oral contraceptives.

Adverse effects noted with therapeutic regimens include lethargy, confusion, somnolence, dizziness, ataxia, diplopia, paresthesias, and weight loss. Nephrolithiasis occurs in about 1 to 2% of patients. Overdose management should include basic GI decontamination with activated charcoal and cardiac monitoring for potential effects on the sodium channel.

Summary

Adverse effects of anticonvulsants and drug interactions with anticonvulsants are often considered in the evaluation of the drug's toxicologic manifestations. Some common adverse effects are considered in Table 41–3, and certain interactions are presented in Table 41–4.

Acknowledgement

Harold Osborn, MD contributed to this chapter in a previous edition.

References

1. Ahmad SR: Felbamate and aplastic anemia. Lancet 1994;344:465.
2. Albani F, Theodore WH, Washington P, et al. Effect of felbamate on plasma levels of carbamazepine and its metabolites. Epilepsia 1991; 32;130–132.
3. Alberto G, Erickson T, Popiel R, et al: Central nervous system manifestations of a valproic acid overdose responsive to naloxone. Ann Emerg Med 1989;18:889–891.
4. Alldredge BK, Lowenstein DH, Simon RP: Placebo-controlled trial of intravenous diphenylhydantoin for short-term treatment of alcohol withdrawal seizures. Am J Med 1989; 87:645–648.
5. Anderson GO, Ritland S: Life threatening intoxication with sodium valproate. J Toxicol Clin Toxicol 1995; 33: 279–284.
6. Apfelbaum JD, Caravati EM, Kerns WP, et al: Cardiovascular effects of carbamazepine toxicity. Ann Emerg Med 1995; 25:631–635.
7. Booker HE, Chun RWM, Sanguino M: Myasthenia gravis syndrome associated with trimethadione. JAMA 1970; 212:2262–2265.
8. Booker HE, Darcey B: Serum concentrations of free diphenylhydantoin and their relationship to clinical intoxication. Epilepsia 1973; 14:177–184.
9. Bradury AJ, Bentick B, Todd PJ: Dystonia associated with carbamazepine toxicity. Postgrad Med J 1982;58:525–526.
10. Bridge TA, Norton RL, Robertson WO: Pediatric carbamazepine overdoses. Pediatr Emerg Care 1994;10: 260–263.
11. Brodie M: Lamotrigine. Lancet 1992;339:1397–1400.
12. Brodie M: Established anticonvulsants and treatment of refractory epilepsy. Lancet 1990;336:350–354.
13. Browne TR, Kugler AR, Eldon MA: Pharmacology and pharmacokinetics of fosphenytoin. Neurology 1996;46: S3–S7.
14. Buckley NA, Whyte IM, Dawson AH: Self-poisoning with lamotrigine. Lancet 1993;342:1552–1553.
15. Carducci B, Hedges JR, Beal JC, et al: Emergency phenytoin loading by constant intravenous infusion. Ann Emerg Med 1984;13:1027–1031.
16. Chance JF: Emergency department treatment of alcohol withdrawal seizures with phenytoin. Ann Emerg Med 1991;20:520–522.
17. Cohen AF, Land GS, Breimer DD, et al: Lamotrigine, a new anticonvulsant: Pharmacokinetics in normal humans. Clin Pharmacol Ther 1987;42:535–541.
18. Cohen AF, Posner J, Moody JP, et al: The pharmacokinetics of lamotrigine (BW 430c), a potential anticonvulsant, in subjects with unconjugated hyperbilirubinemia (Gilbert's Syndrome). Paper presented at Third World Conference on Clinical Pharmacology and Therapeutics, Stockholm, 1986.
19. Cohen H, Howland MA, Luciano DJ, et al: Pharmacokinetic and tolerance study of carbamazepine administered an oral loading dose in tablet or oral suspension. Pharmacotherapy 1992;12:499. Abstract.
20. Comer JB: Extravasation from intravenous phenytoin. Intrav Ther Clin Nutr 1984;11:23–29.
21. Connacher AA, Macnab JP, Jung RT: Fatality due to massive overdose of sodium valproate. Scott Med J 1987; 32:85–86.
22. Connelly JF: Vigabatrin. Ann Pharmacother 1993;27: 197–204.
23. Corday E, Enescu V, Vyden JK, et al: Antiarrhythmic properties of carbamazepine. Geriatrics 1971; 26:78–81.
24. Coulter DL, Allen RJ: Hyperammonemia with valproic acid therapy. J Pediatr 1981;99:317–319.
25. Coulter DL, Allen RJ: Secondary hyperammonemia: A possible mechanism for valproate encephalopathy. Lancet 1980;1:1310–1311.
26. Cranford RE, Leppik IE, Patrick B, et al: Intravenous phenytoin in acute treatment of seizures. Neurology 1979; 29:1474–1479.
27. Dalessio DJ: Seizure disorders and pregnancy. N Engl J Med 1985;312:559–563.
28. De Zeuw R, Westemberg H, Van der Kleijn E: An unusual case of carbamazepine poisoning with a near fatal relapse after two days. J Toxicol Clin Toxicol 1979;14:263–269.
29. Dichter MA, Brodie MJ: New antiepileptic drugs. N Engl J Med 1996;334:1583–1590.

30. Dragunow M, Goddard GV, Laverty R: Is adenosine an endogenous anticonvulsant? Epilepsia 1985;26:480–487.
31. Dreifuss FE, Langer DH, Moline KA, et al: Valproic acid hepatic fatalities. Neurology 1989:39:201–207.
32. Drenck NE, Risbo A: Carbamazepine poisoning, a suprisingly severe case. Anesth Intens Care 1980;8:203–204.
33. Dupuis RE, Lichtman SN, Pollack GM: Acute valproic acid overdose. Clinical course and pharmacokinetic disposition of valproic acid and metabolites. Drug Saf 1990;5: 65–71.
34. Durelli L, Massazza V, Cavallo R: Carbamazepine toxicity and poisoning. Incidence, clinical features and management. Med Toxicol Adv Drug Experience 1989;4:95–107.
35. Earnest MP, Marx JA, Drury LR: Complications of intravenous phenytoin for acute treatment of seizures. JAMA 1983;249:762–765.
36. Eichelbaum M, Ekbom K, Bertilsson L, et al: Plasma kinetics of carbamazepine and its epoxide metabolite in man after single and multiple doses. Eur J Clin Pharmacol 1975;8:337–341.
37. Farrar HC, Harold DA, Reed MD: Acute valproic acid intoxication: Enhanced drug clearance with oral-activated charcoal. Crit Care Med 1993;21:299–301.
38. Fernandez MC, Walter FG, Peterson LR, et al: Gabapentin, valproic acid and ethanol intoxication: Elevated blood levels with mild clinical effects. J Toxicol Clin Toxicol 1996: 34:437–439.
39. Fischer JH, Barr AN, Rogers SL, et al: Lack of serious toxicity following gabapentin overdose. Neurology 1994;44: 982–983.
40. Gandelman MS: Review of carbamazepine-induced hyponatremia. Prog Neuropsychopharmacol Biol Psychiatry 1994;18:211–233.
41. Garofalo E, Koto E, Feuerstein T, Goedecke AG: Experience with gabapentin overdose: Five case studies. Epilepsia 1993;34:157. Abstract.
42. Gary NE, Byra WM, Eisinger RP: Carbamazepine poisoning: Treatment by hemoperfusion. Nephron 1981;27: 202–203.
43. Goa KL, Ross SR, Chrisp P: Lamotrigine. A review of its pharmacological properties and clinical potential in epilepsy. Drugs 1993;46:152–176.
44. Goa KL, Sorkin EM: Gabapentin. A review of its pharmacological properties and clinical potential in epilepsy. Drugs 1993;46:409–427.
45. Goldschlager AW, Karliner JS: Ventricular standstill after intravenous diphenylhydantoin. Am Heart J 1967;74: 410–412.
46. Gordon MF, Gerstenblitt D: The use of free phenytoin levels in averting phenytoin toxicity. NY State J Med 1990; 90:469–470.
47. Gram L, Bentsen KD: Valproate: An updated review. Acta Neurol Scand 1985;72:129–139.
48. Graudins A, Aaron CK: Delayed peak serum valproic acid in massive divalproex overdose: Treatment with charcoal hemoperfusion. J Toxicol Clin Toxicol 1996;34:335–341.
49. Hart RG, Easton JD: Carbamazepine and hematological monitoring. Ann Neurol 1982;11:309–312.
50. Hassell TM, Gilbert GH: Phenytoin sensitivity of fibroblasts as the basis for susceptibility to gingival enlargement. Am J Pathol 1983;112:218–223.
51. Hojer J, Malmlund HO, Berg A: Clinical features in 28 consecutive cases of laboratory confirmed massive poisoning with carbamazepine alone. J Toxicol Clin Toxicol 1993;31: 449–458.
52. Hoke JF, Ruberg ST: Pharmacokinetics and dose proportionality of gamma-vinyl GABA (Vigabatrin) following multiple oral doses. Neurology 1991;41(suppl 1):139.
53. Hyden H, Cupello A, Palm A, et al: Naloxone reverses the inhibition by sodium valproate of GABA transport across the Deiter's neuronal plasma membrane. Ann Neurol 1987;21:416–417.
54. Ishikura H, Matsuo N, Matsubara I, et al: Valproic acid overdose and L-carnitine therapy. J Anal Toxicol 1996; 20:55–58.
55. Jacome D: Carbamazepine-induced dystonia. JAMA 1979;241:2263. Letter.
56. Karsarkis EJ, Kuo CS, Berger R, et al: Carbamazepine-induced cardiac dysfunction. Characterization of two distinct clinical syndromes. Arch Intern Med 1992;152: 186–191.
57. Khoo SH, Layland MJ: Cerebral edema following acute sodium valproate overdose. J Toxicol Clin Toxicol 1992; 30:209–214.
58. Kilarski DJ, Buchanan C, Von Behren L: Soft tissue damage associated with intravenous phenytoin. N Engl J Med 1984;311:1186–1187. Letter.
59. Kilpatrick ES, Forrest G, Brodie MJ: Concentration-effect and concentration-toxicity relations with lamotrigine: A prospective study. Epilepsia 1996;37:534–538.
60. Klotz U, Antonin KH: Pharmacokinetics and bioavailability of sodium valproate. Clin Pharmacol Ther 1977;21: 736–743.
61. Leach MJ, Marden CH, Miller AA: Pharmacological studies on lamotrigine, a novel potential antiepileptic drug, 2. Neurochemical studies on the mechanism of action. Epilepsia 1986;27:490–497.
62. Leslie PJ, Heyworth R, Prescott LF: Cardiac complications of carbamazepine intoxication: Treatment by haemoperfusion. Br Med J 1983;286:1018. Letter.
63. Levy RH, Pitlick WHJ, Troupin AS, et al: Pharmacokinetics of carbamazepine in normal man. Clin Pharmacol Ther 1975;17:657–668.
64. Liporace J, Roberts D: Post-marketing felbamate experience. Epilepsia 1994;35(suppl 8):55. Abstract.
65. Louis S, Kutt H, McDowell F: The cardiocirculatory changes caused by intravenous Dilantin and its solvent. Am Heart J 1967;74:523–529.
66. Macdonald RL. Anticonvulsant drug actions on neurons in cell culture. J Neural Transm 1988;72:173–183.
67. Makin AJ, Fitt S, Williams R: Fulminant hepatic failure induced by lamotrigine. Br Med J 1995;311:292.
68. Mauro LS, Mauro V, Brown D, et al: Enhancement of phenytoin elimination by multiple dose activated charcoal. Ann Emerg Med 1987;16:1132–1135.
69. McNamara JO: Drugs effective in the therapy of the epilepsies. In: Hardman JG, Limbird LE, Molinoff PB, Ruddon RW, eds: Goodman and Gilman's The Pharmaco-

logical Basis of Therapeutics, 9th ed. New York, McGraw-Hill, 1996, pp. 461–486.
70. McQuay H, Carroll D, Jadad AR, et al: Anticonvulsant drugs for management of pain: A systematic review. Br Med J 1995;311:1047–1052.
71. Mellick LB, Morgan JA, Mellick GA: Presentations of acute phenytoin overdose. Ann Emerg Med 1989;7:61–67.
72. Mixter CG, Moran JM, Austen WG: Cardiac and peripheral vascular effects of diphenylhydantoin sodium. Am J Cardiol 1966;17:332–338.
73. Mortensen PB, Hansen HE, Pedersen B, et al: Acute valproate intoxication: Biochemical investigations and hemodialysis treatment. Int J Clin Pharmacol Ther Toxicol 1983;21:64–68.
74. Murakami K, Sugimoto T, Woo M, et al: Effect of *L*-carnitine supplementation on acute valproate intoxication. Epilepsia 1996;37:687–689.
75. Nagel TR, Schunk JE: Felbamate overdose: A case report and discussion of a new antiepileptic drug. Pediatr Emerg Care 1995;11:369–371.
76. Neuvonen PJ, Elonen E: Effect of activated charcoal on absorption and elimination of phenobarbitone, carbamazepine and phenylbutazone in man. Eur J Clin Pharmacol 1980;17:51–57.
77. Oellerich M, Muller-Vahl H: The EMIT free level ultrafiltration technique compared with equilibrium analysis and ultracentrifugation to determine protein binding of phenytoin. Clin Pharmacokinet 1984;9:61–70.
78. Ohtani Y, Endo F, Matsuda I: Carnitine deficiency and hyperammonemia associated with valproic acid therapy. J Pediatr 1982;101:782–785.
79. O'Neil MG, Perdun CS, Wilson MB, et al: Felbamate-associated fatal acute hepatic necrosis. Neurology 1996;46: 1457–1459.
80. Osborn HH, Zistein J, Sparano R: Single-dose oral phenytoin loading. Ann Emerg Med 1987;16:407–412.
81. Pellock JM: The clinical efficacy of lamotrigine as an antiepileptic drug. Neurology 1994;44(suppl 8):S29-S35.
82. Peyster RG, Sussman NM, Hershey BL, et al: Use of ex-vivo magnetic resonance imaging to detect onset of vigabatrin-induced intramyelinic edema in canine brain. Epilepsia 1995;36:93–100.
83. Phillis JW: Interactions of the anticonvulsants diphenylhydantoin and carbamazepine with adenosine on cerebral cortical neurons. Epilepsia 1984;25:765–772.
84. Rho JM, Donovan SD, Rogaushi MA:Mechanism of action of the anticonvulsant felbamate: Opposing effects on *N*-methyl-D-aspartate and gamma-aminobutyric acid A receptors. Ann Neurol 1994;35:229–234.
85. Rogvi-Hansen B, Gram L: Adverse effects of established and new antiepileptic drugs: An attempted comparison. Pharmacol Ther 1993;68:425–434.
86. Rush JA, Beran RG: Leucopenia as an adverse reaction to carbamazepine therapy. Med J Aust 1984; 140:426–428.
87. Russell MA, Bousvaros G: Fatal results from diphenylhydantoin administered intravenously. JAMA 1968;20: 2118–2119.
88. Salke-Kellerman A, Baier H: Acute encephalopathy with vigabatrin. Lancet 1993;342:185. Letter.
89. Salzman MB: Carbamazepine and fatal eosinophilic myocarditis. N Engl J Med 1997;336:878–879. Letter.
90. Sander JW, Hart YM, Trimble MR, et al: Vigabatrin and psychosis. J Neurol Neurosurg Psychiatry 1991;54: 435–439.
91. Schaub JEM, Williamson PJ, Barnes EW, et al: Multisystem adverse reaction to lamotrigine. Lancet 1994;344:481. Letter.
92. Schmidt H, Belleza J, Dougherty JM: Adverse effects with administration of phenytoin: Infusion pump vs manual infusion. Acad Emerg Med 1995;2:758–759.
93. Serrano EE, Roye DB, Hammer RH, et al: Plasma diphenylhydantoin values after oral and intramuscular administration of diphenylhydantoin. Neurology 1973;23: 311–317.
94. Seymour JF: Carbamazepine overdose. Features of 33 cases. Drug Saf 1993;8:81–88.
95. Sharief MK, Sander JWA, Shorvon SD: Acute encephalopathy with vigabatrin. Lancet 1993;342:619. Letter.
96. Skerritt JH, Davies LP, Johnston GAR: Interactions of the anticonvulsant carbamazepine with adenosine receptors. 1. Neurochemical studies. Epilepsia 1983;24:634–642.
97. Soman P, Jain S, Rajsekhar V, et al: Dystonia—A rare manifestation of carbamazepine toxicity. Postgrad Med J 1994;70:54–56.
98. Spiller HA, Krenzelok EP, Cookson E: Carbamazepine overdose: A prospective study of serum levels and toxicity. J Toxicol Clin Toxicol 1990;28:445–458.
99. Steiman GS, Woerpel RW, Sherard ES: Treatment of accidental sodium valproate overdose with an opiate antagonist. Ann Neurol 1979;6:274.
100. Steiner C, Wit AL, Weiss MB, et al: The antiarrhythmic actions of carbamazepine. J Pharmacol Exp Ther 1970;173: 323–335.
101. Stilman N, Masdeu JC: Incidence of seizures with phenytoin toxicity. Neuorolgy 1985;35:1769–1772.
102. Stremski ES, Brady W, Prasad K, et al: Pediatric carbamazepine intoxication. Ann Emerg Med 1995;25:624–630.
103. Sullivan JB, Rumack BH, Peterson RG: Acute carbamazepine toxicity resulting from overdose. Neurology 1981;31:621–624.
104. Swinyard EA, Sofia D, Kupferberg HJ: Comparative anticonvulsant activity and neurotoxicity of felbamate and four prototype antiepileptic drugs in mice and rats. Epilepsia 1986;27:27–34.
105. Tsao CY, Wright FS: Acute chemical pancreatitis associated with carbamazepine intoxication. Epilepsia 1993;34: 174–176.
106. Vale JA: Carbamazepine overdose. J Toxicol Clin Toxicol 1992;30:481–482.
107. Voigt GC: Death following intravenous sodium diphenylhydantoin (Dilantin). Johns Hopkins Med J 1968;123: 153–157.
108. Weaver DF, Camfield P, Fraser A: Massive carbamazepine overdose: Clinical and pharmacologic observation in five episodes. Neurology 1988;38:755–759.
109. Wilensky AJ, Lowden A: Inadequate serum levels after intramuscular administration of diphenylhydantoin. Neurology 1973;23:318–324.

110. William SR, Clark RF: Hemodialysis of a valproic acid poisoning. J Toxicol Clin Toxicol 1995;33:475–486. Abstract.
111. Willow M, Gonoi R, Catterall WA: Voltage clamp analysis of the inhibitory actions of diphenylhydantoin and carbamazepine on voltage-sensitive sodium channels in neuroblastoma cells. Mol Pharmacol 1985;27:549–558.
112. Wyte CD, Berk WA: Severe oral phenytoin overdose does not cause cardiovascular morbidity. Ann Emerg Med 1991;20:508–512.
113. Yoari, Y, Selzer ME, Pincus JH: Phenytoin: Mechanisms of its anticonvulsant action. Ann Neurol 1986;20:171–184.
114. Zoneraich S, Zoneraich O, Seigel J: Sudden death following intraveneous sodium diphenylhydantoin. Am Heart J 1976;91:375–377

CHAPTER 42

Anticoagulants

Robert S. Hoffman

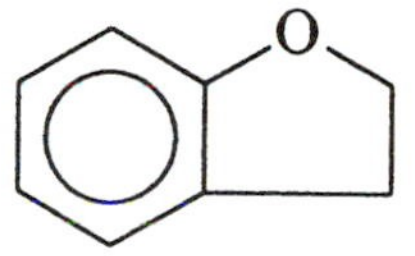

Coumarin

A 30-year-old man presented to the emergency department (ED) complaining of diffuse bruises on his skin and blood in his urine.* Although the patient had no significant past medical history and was on no medication, he reported being depressed and having ingested four packets of rodenticide 8 days prior to presentation. He was well until 4 days after ingestion, when he noted the onset of fatigue, weakness, and blood in his urine. When these symptoms failed to resolve, he came to the ED.

Physical examination revealed a well-developed man in no distress. Vital signs were: blood pressure, 98/50 mm Hg; pulse, 86 beats/min; respiratory rate, 14 breaths/min; and temperature, 98.4°F (36.9°C). There were no orthostatic changes in his vital signs. Although his skin was notable for many ecchymoses of slightly different ages, there were no petechiae. Examination of his head, eyes, ears, nose, and throat was unremarkable except for pallor of the conjunctivae. His chest was clear to auscultation and percussion. His heart and abdomen were unremarkable, and his neurologic evaluation was within normal limits. Rectal examination revealed stool that was brown but tested positive for occult blood.

A large-bore intravenous line was started and lactated Ringer's solution infused at 250 mL/h. Blood specimens were sent for a complete blood count, electrolytes, glucose, coagulation studies, and type and cross-match. Extra specimens of coagulated and anticoagulated blood were drawn and placed aside. The patient was placed on a cardiac monitor and a 12-lead ECG obtained. A urine analysis was obtained and a radiograph of the chest ordered.

Initial laboratory studies revealed a hemoglobin of 9.8 g/dL, a white blood cell count of 9800/mm^3 with a normal differential, and 420,000 platelets/mm^3. The prothrombin time (PT) and the partial thromboplastin time (PTT) were reported as greater than 100 seconds each, with controls of 12 and 32 seconds, respectively. The urine was grossly bloody, with greater than 1000 red blood cells per high-power microscopic field. Electrolytes, glucose, ECG, and chest radiograph were within normal limits.

A fibrinogen level was determined to be 486 mg/dL (within the normal range), which essentially excluded the possibility of disseminated intravascular coagulation. The patient's plasma was then mixed with an equal volume of normal plasma. This resulted in a correction of the PT and PTT to 13.2 and 40 seconds, respectively, which excluded the presence of an inhibitor. Finally, specific factor levels were determined to distinguish between a problem with vitamin K-dependent pathways and liver dysfunction. The vitamin K-dependent factors II, IX, and VII-X complex were determined to be present at levels of 5, 2, and 1%, respectively, of those predicted, whereas factors V (liver) and VIII (endothelium) were present at 94 and 100% of predicted values. This confirmed the diagnosis of anticoagulant poisoning.

*This case was originally reported in Hoffman RS, Smilkstein MJ, Goldfrank LR: Evaluation of coagulation factor abnormalities in long-acting anticoagulant overdose. J Toxicol Clin Toxicol 1988;26:233–248.

How Does the Body Maintain a Balance Between Coagulation and Anticoagulation?

An understanding of the normal function of the coagulation pathways is essential to appreciate the etiology of a coagulopathy. The critical steps of the coagulation cascade will be summarized. For a more detailed discussion, the reader is referred to Chapter 24 and several reviews.[46,95,116]

Coagulation consists of a series of events that prevent excess blood loss and assist in the restoration of blood vessel integrity. Although the traditional impression of the events that occur in the coagulation cascade[34,86] as discussed below adequately describe in vitro events, current comprehension emphasizes some distinct differences that occur in vivo.[46,95,116] Despite these differences, an understanding of the traditional model is most useful for interpreting the results of diagnostic tests of coagulation.

Within the cascade, coagulation factors exist as inert precursors and are transformed into enzymes when activated. Activation of the cascade occurs through one of two distinct pathways, the intrinsic and extrinsic systems (Fig. 42–1).[34,86] Once activated, these enzymes catalyze a series of reactions that ultimately converge and lead to the generation of thrombin and the formation of a fibrin clot.

The intrinsic pathway is activated by the complexation of factor XII (Hageman factor), with high-molecular-weight kininogen (HMWK) and prekallikrein or vascular subendothelial collagen. This results in sequential activation of factor XII, active kallikrein, and active factors IX to XI and prothrombin (Fig. 42–1). Prothrombin is converted to thrombin in the presence of factor V, calcium, and phospholipid. The integrity of this system is usually evaluated by determining the PTT (partial thromboplastin time).

In the extrinsic, or tissue factor-dependent, pathway, a complex is formed between factor VII, calcium,

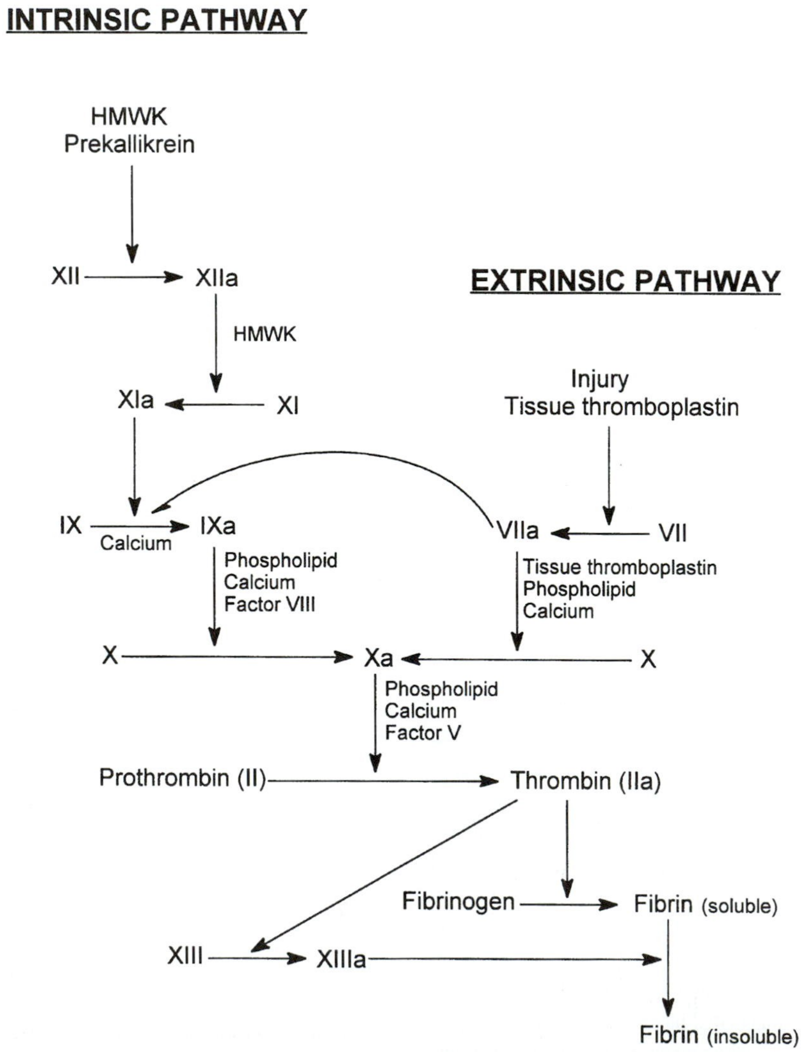

Figure 42–1. The coagulation cascade.

and tissue factor. A calcium and lipid-dependent complex is then created between factors VII and X. Factor VII-X complex subsequently converts prothrombin to thrombin, which promotes the formation of fibrin from fibrinogen (Fig. 42–1). The integrity of this pathway is usually assessed by determining the PT (prothrombin time or INR, described later).

Activation of factors IX and X provides the important link between the traditional intrinsic and extrinsic coagulation pathways. Additional evidence that tissue factor can activate both factors IX and X suggests that the two pathways are more interrelated than originally thought.[105] Furthermore, cell surfaces facilitate the process of clotting. Platelets are also known to interact with proteins of the coagulation cascade through surface receptors for factors V, VIII, IX, and X.[48,128] As a final step, factor XIII assists in the cross-linking of fibrin to form a stable thrombus.

Antithrombin III, protein C, and protein S serve as inhibitors, maintaining the homeostasis that is required to prevent spontaneous clotting and keep blood fluid. Protein C, when aided by protein S, inactivates two plasma factors, V and VIII.[17,29,46] Antithrombin III complexes with all the serine protease coagulation factors except factor VII.[17,46,117]

How Does a Coagulopathy Occur?

Impaired coagulation results from decreased production or enhanced consumption of coagulation factors, the presence of inhibitors of coagulation, activation of the thrombolytic system, or abnormalities in platelet number or function. For the purposes of this chapter a discussion of platelet-related abnormalities is excluded. Some of this information can be found in Chapter 33.

Decreased production of coagulation factors results from congenital and acquired etiologies. Although congenital disorders of factor VIII (hemophilia), factor IX (Christmas factor), factor XI, and factor XII (Hageman factor) have all been reported, their overall incidence is still quite low. Clinical conditions that result in acquired factor deficiencies are much more common and result from either a decrease in synthesis or activation. Factors II, V, VII, and X are entirely synthesized in the liver;[46,95,116] thus hepatic dysfunction is one of the most common causes of acquired coagulopathy. In addition, factors II, VII, IX, and X require postsynthetic activation by vitamin K,[131,135,136] such that vitamin K deficiency (from malnutrition, changes in gut flora, or malabsorption) or inhibition (from warfarin, as will be described) is capable of impairing coagulation.

Excessive consumption of coagulation factors usually results from massive activation of the coagulation cascade. Massive activation occurs during severe hemorrhage or disseminated intravascular coagulation. The latter results from infection (eg, gram-negative sepsis), conditions that introduce tissue factor into the blood (eg, neoplasms, snake envenomations), stagnant blood flow, and diffuse endothelial injury (eg, hyperthermia, aortic aneurysm, or dissection). The hallmark of a consumptive coagulopathy is a depressed level of fibrinogen with an elevation of fibrin degradation products. This combination suggests the rapid turnover of fibrin in the coagulation process. In the other coagulopathic conditions, the failure to activate the coagulation cascade is associated with normal or high fibrin levels and low fibrin degradation products, because of limited clot formation.

Inhibitors of the coagulation cascade (circulating anticoagulants) are of two types: immunoglobulin and nonimmunoglobulin. Immunoglobulins, which are often antibodies to existing coagulation factors, may occur without obvious cause, as part of a systemic autoimmune disorder, or as a result of repeated transfusions with exogenous factors (as occurs in hemophilia).[59,81,126] The clinical syndromes associated with antibody inhibitors are similar to those associated with deficiencies of the particular coagulation factors involved. Antibodies to factors V, VII to XI, and XIII are described.[12,126] Alternatively, nonimmunoglobulin neutralizers of coagulation occur in conditions associated with rapid white cell turnover.[12,57] These neutralizers are positively charged lysosomal proteins that compete with coagulation factors for negatively charged phospholipid membrane surfaces. Although they prolong in vitro coagulation times, they are rarely responsible for clinical coagulopathy because of the excess of phospholipid surface area available in vivo.[59,81]

Thrombolytic agents such as streptokinase, urokinase, anistreplase, and recombinant tissue plasminogen activator (r-TPA) enhance the normal processes that lead to clot degradation.[95] Thrombosis is initiated when exposed endothelium or released tissue factor leads to platelet adherence and aggregation, the formation of thrombin, and cross-linking of fibrinogen to form fibrin strands.[46,95,116] This results in a hemostatic plug or thrombus formation. Thrombus formation, in turn, leads to generation of plasmin from plasminogen, which causes fibrinolysis and eventual dissolution of the hemostatic plug.[30,31] Thus the fibrinolytic system may be thought of as a natural balance against unregulated coagulation. Thrombolytic therapy increases fibrinolytic activity by accelerating the conversion of plasminogen to plasmin, which actively degenerates fibrin.[10,30,31] Following the administration of thrombolytic agents, a consequential coagulopathy results, and fibrin degradation products are elevated secondary to the rapid turnover of clot.

What Initial Therapy Is Indicated for a Patient With Anemia and Coagulopathy?

Blood is required for any patient with a history of blood loss or active bleeding who is hemodynamically unstable, has impaired oxygen transport, or is expected to become unstable. Although a transfusion of packed red blood cells is ideal for replacing lost blood, it cannot correct a coagulopathy, and thus patients will continue to bleed. Whole blood contains not only the cellular elements the patient is losing, but the necessary coagulation factors to reverse the coagulopathy. Although transfusion of whole blood should be considered in severe cases, whole blood contains many components (platelets, white blood cells, and non-vitamin K-dependent factors) that might benefit other patients, and relatively small amounts of vitamin K-dependent factors. Thus selective use of specific blood products is preferred. Packed red blood cells should be given to correct the anemia and fresh frozen plasma (FFP) or other factor concentrates (cryoprecipitate, Konyne) to correct the coagulopathy. Fresh frozen plasma is rich in active vitamin K-dependent coagulation factors and will reverse oral anticoagulant-induced coagulopathy in most patients. Multiple FFP transfusions may be required, however, because of the rapid degradation of coagulation factors in the absence of vitamin K. Although vitamin K administration is required to reverse the blockade of coagulation factor activation, it cannot be relied upon for the patient with acute and consequential hemorrhage (see Antidotes in Depth: Vitamin K). Treatment with vitamin K takes several hours to activate enough factors to reverse the patient's coagulopathy,[89,109] and this delay may potentially be fatal.

When Evaluating a Patient With Prolonged Coagulation Times, How Can the Correct Diagnosis Be Established?

Established screening tests are helpful for diagnosis. Four studies—PT, PTT, thrombin time, and fibrinogen concentration—are usually adequate to determine the diagnosis. Prothrombin time is calculated by adding standardized thromboplastin reagent (phospholipid and tissue factor) to a sample of the patient's citrated plasma (the citrate removes calcium). Calcium is then introduced and the time to clotting measured. The PT is unaffected by factors VIII to XIII, platelets, prekallikrein, and HMWK. The patient's PT is usually expressed as a PT ratio (PT observed/PT control). Because this ratio is related to both laboratory methodology and the source of the thromboplastin reagent used, the results generated suffer from significant variability. The international normalized ratio (INR) was developed in an attempt to limit interlaboratory variability.[61,99] The INR is derived by raising the PT ratio to a power value known as the international sensitivity index (ISI): $(\text{PT ratio})^{\text{ISI}}$. The ISI is a measure of responsiveness of the particular thromboplastin to warfarin. Although the use of the INR does not completely eliminate variability,[62,98] it improves interpretation of values from different institutions.

Partial thromboplastin time is measured by adding kaolin or celite to citrated plasma in order to activate the "contact" components of the intrinsic system. This mixture is then recalcified and the time to clotting observed. Some tests use phospholipids in the reagent to activate the remaining coagulation factors, thereby giving rise to the term activated PTT (aPTT). Since these PTT and aPTT are essentially interchangeable, the term PTT is used hereafter to represent the concept. The PTT is not affected by factors VII, XIII, or platelets.

The thrombin time, determined by adding exogenous thrombin to citrated plasma, evaluates the ability to convert fibrinogen to fibrin, and is thus unaffected by factors II, V, VII to XIII, platelets, prekallikrein, or HMWK. Finally, either a fibrinogen level or a determination of fibrin degradation products will help distinguish between problems with clot formation and consumptive coagulopathy. An evaluation of the combination of normal and abnormal results of these tests will determine the patient's abnormality (Table 42–1).

Inhibitors can be diagnosed by "mixing studies," since only a small percentage of coagulation factors present in normal plasma are necessary to have a normal PTT. If the patient with an abnormal PTT suffers from even a severe factor deficiency, restoration of that factor activity to 50% of normal will completely normalize the PTT. Thus the presence of an abnormal PTT that will not correct by incubation of the patient's plasma with an equal volume of normal plasma is diagnostic of an inhibitor of coagulation. More sophisticated studies can be used to identify specific coagulation factor deficiencies. The reader is referred to one of several standard references for a more detailed discussion of the approach to patients with abnormal coagulation studies.[28,57]

TABLE 42–1. EVALUATION OF ABNORMAL COAGULATION TIMES

PT Normal, PTT Prolonged, Bleeding
Deficiencies of factors VIII, IX, XI
Von Willebrand's disease
Heparin therapy (low dose)
PT Normal, PTT Prolonged, No Bleeding
Deficiencies of factor XII, prekallikrein, high-molecular-weight-kininogen
Inhibitor syndrome
PT Prolonged, PTT Normal
Deficiency of factor VII
Warfarin therapy (early)
Vitamin K deficiency (mild)
Liver disease (mild)
PT and PTT Prolonged, Thrombin Time Normal, Fibrinogen Normal
Deficiencies of factors II, V, IX, vitamin K (severe)
Warfarin therapy (late)
PT and PTT Prolonged, Thrombin Time Abnormal, Fibrinogen Normal
Heparin effect
Dysfibrinogenemia
PT and PTT Prolonged, Thrombin Time Abnormal, Fibrinogen Abnormal
Liver disease
Disseminated intravascular coagulation
Fibrinolytic therapy
Crotalid envenomation

How Do the Warfarin and "Warfarin-Like" Anticoagulants Work?

The oral anticoagulants may be divided into two groups: (1) hydroxycoumarins, including warfarin (coumadin), panwarfarin, warficide, coumachlor, coumafuryl, fumasol, prolin, ethyl biscoumacetate (tromexan), phenprocoumon, di-cumarol bishydroxycoumarin, and acenocoumarin (sintrom); and (2) indandiones, including pindone, pivalyn, diphacinone, diphenadione, phenindione, and anisindione. Regardless of the classification, the mechanism of action involves vitamin K inhibition. Vitamin K is a cofactor in the postribosomal synthesis of clotting factors II, VII, IX, and X (Fig. 42–2). The vitamin K-sensitive step involves the carboxylation in the liver of 10 or more glutamic acid residues at the amino terminal end of the precursor proteins, to form a unique amino acid gamma carboxyglutamate.[36,131,135,136] These amino acids chelate calcium in vivo, which allows the binding of the four vitamin K-dependent clotting factors to phospholipid membranes during activation of the coagulation cascade.[148]

Vitamin K is not active until it is reduced from its quinone form to a quinol (or hydroquinone) form in hepatic microsomes. This reduction of vitamin K must precede the carboxylation of the precursor factors. The carboxylase activity is coupled to an epoxidase activity for vitamin K, whereby vitamin K is oxidized simultaneously to vitamin K 2,3-epoxide (Fig. 42–2).[135,148] This inactive form of the vitamin is converted to the active form by two successive reductions.[36,88,101] In the first step, an epoxide reductase (known as vitamin K 2,3-epoxide reductase) uses reduced nicotinamide adenine dinucleotide (NADH) as a cofactor to convert vitamin K 2,3-epoxide to a quinone form.[101,135] Subsequently, the quinone is reduced to the active vitamin K quinol form (see Antidotes in Depth: Vitamin K).

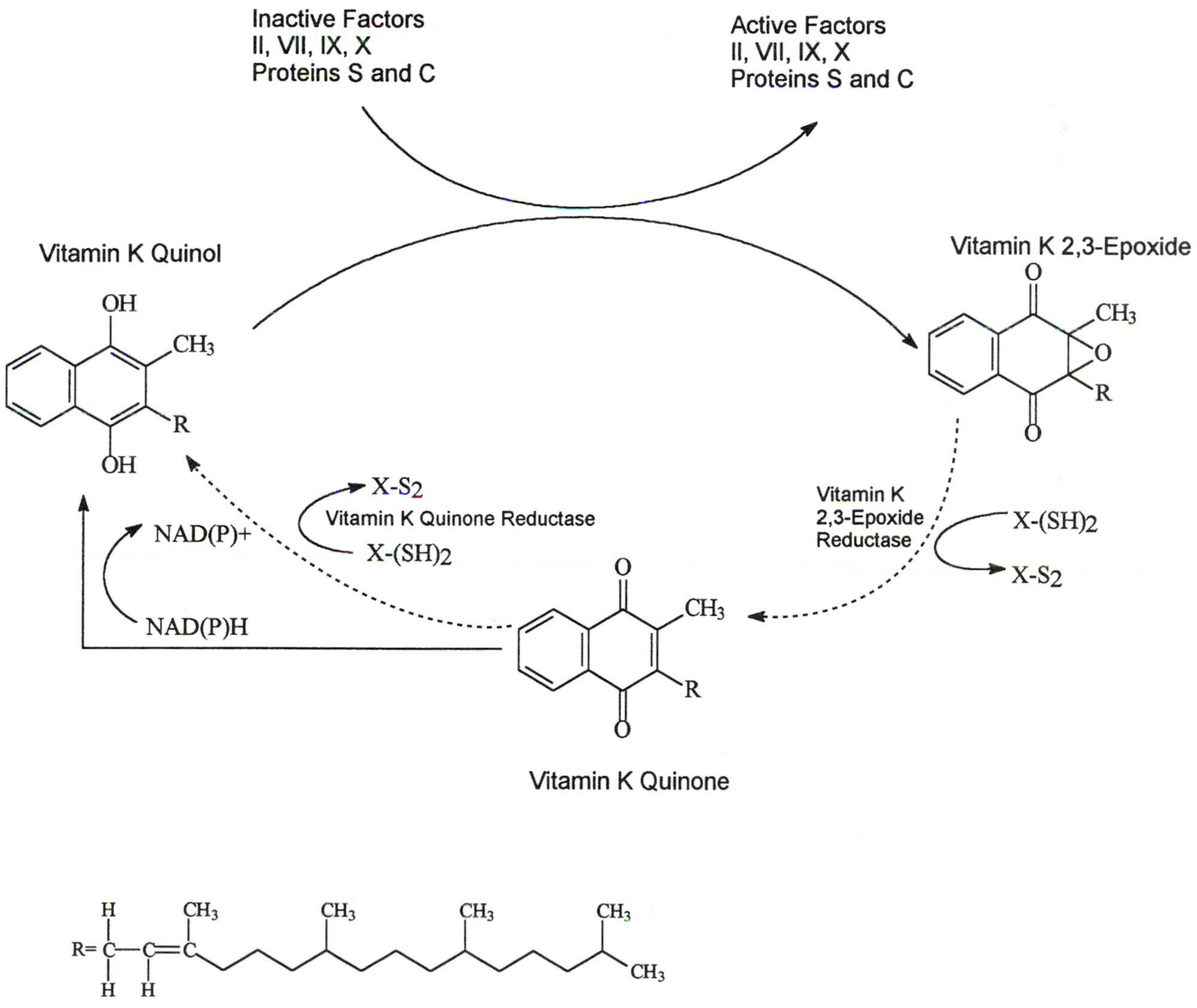

Figure 42–2. The vitamin K cycle. Dotted lines represent pathways that can be blocked with warfarin and warfarin-like anticoagulants. The aliphatic side chain (R) of vitamin K is shown below the metabolic pathway.

Warfarin is a racemic mixture of R warfarin and S warfarin enantiomers. In rodents, S warfarin is three to six times more potent than R warfarin at producing hypoprothrombinemia.[21] In humans, S warfarin may only be about 1.5 times as potent as R warfarin.[20] Warfarin and all warfarin-like compounds inhibit the activity of vitamin K 2,3-epoxide reductase, as can be demonstrated by the observation of elevated levels of vitamin K 2,3-epoxide in anticoagulated subjects.[28,151] Additional evidence suggests that another enzyme system, vitamin K quinone reductase, is also inhibited by warfarin and its related compounds (Fig. 42–2).[36,40] This subsequently inhibits the formation of activated clotting factors.

What Is the Pharmacology of Warfarin?

Orally ingested warfarin is virtually completely absorbed and peak plasma concentrations occur approximately 3 hours after drug administration.[134] Because only the free warfarin is therapeutically active, concurrent administration of drugs that alter the level of free warfarin (eg, by competing for binding to albumin or inhibiting warfarin metabolism) may markedly influence the anticoagulant effect.[8,44,134] Drugs that interfere with or potentiate warfarin's effects are listed in Table 42–2. Although vitamin K regeneration is inhibited almost immediately, the anticoagulant effect of warfarin (and other oral anticoagulant agents) is delayed until the existing stores of vitamin K are depleted and the active coagulation factors are removed from circulation. Because vitamin K turnover is rapid, this effect is dependent on factor half-life ($t_{1/2}$) with factor VII ($t_{1/2}$ = 5 hours) depleted most rapidly.[44] For a prolongation of the PT to occur, factor levels must fall to about 25% of predicted values, suggesting that at least 15 hours (three factor VII half-lives) are required before warfarin's effect is evident.[44]

The half-life of warfarin in humans is 35 hours; thus its duration of action may be up to 5 days.[20,44,134] On average, it takes approximately 6 days of warfarin administration to reach a steady-state anticoagulant effect.

Warfarin is metabolized by isoenzymes CYP1A2 and CYP3A4 of the hepatic microsomal P450 enzyme system. R warfarin is metabolized by side-chain reduction to secondary alcohols that are subsequently excreted by the kidney, whereas S warfarin is metabolized by hydroxylation to 7-hydroxy warfarin, which is excreted into the bile.[44,134] The elimination of R warfarin is more rapid than that of S warfarin.[20]

TABLE 42–2. COMMON DRUG INTERACTIONS WITH WARFARIN

Potentiate Anticoagulation	Antagonize Anticoagulation
Allopurinol	Antacids
Amiodarone	Antihistamines
Anabolic steroids	Barbiturates
Cephalosporins	Carbamazepine
Chloral hydrate	Cholestyramine
Cimetidine	Colestipol
Clofibrate	Corticosteroids
Cyclic antidepressants	Griseofulvin
Erythromycin	Oral contraceptives
Ethanol	Phenytoin
Fluconazole	Rifampin
Ketoconazole	Vitamin K
Metronidazole	
Nonsteroidal antiinflammatory agents	
Omeprazole	
Sulfonylureas	
Thyroxine	
Trimethoprim-sulfamethoxazole	
Vitamin E	

How Should the Patient With an Overdose of a Warfarin-Like Anticoagulant Be Treated?

Several issues influence the decision to treat a patient with a suspected overdose of a warfarin-like anticoagulant. Answers to the following questions should always be considered. Does the ingestion involve a warfarin-containing rodenticide or a pharmaceutical preparation? Is the ingestion unintentional or intentional? Does the patient require maintenance of therapeutic anticoagulation?

The therapeutic dose of warfarin has been established for both adults and children. Typical adult recommendations are to give a loading dose of 5 to 10 mg/day for several days and then maintain the patient on 2 to 10 mg/day as determined by the INR.[88] Therapeutic dosing equivalents for the other oral anticoagulants are available.[88] For children, the suggested loading dose of warfarin is 0.3 to 1.0 mg/kg, followed by a daily maintenance dose that is 15 to 25% of the loading dose.[26] More recently, a 2-year prospective study in children demonstrated that the optimal daily dose of warfarin could be calculated [dose (mg/day) = 0.07 × weight (kg) + 0.54].[138]

Typical warfarin-containing rodenticides contain only small concentrations of anticoagulant, 0.025% (or 25 mg of warfarin per 100 g of product). Using the data just listed, a 10-kg child would require a loading dose of 3 to 10 mg of warfarin (12 to 40 g of rodenticide) and a daily dose of about 1.2 mg of warfarin (5 g of rodenticide) to remain anticoagulated. These quantities are far greater than those seen in typical "tastes." Thus, single unintentional ingestions of warfarin-containing rodenticides pose virtually no threat to either normal or anticoagulated patients.[73] In contrast, intentional and large unintentional ingestions of pharmaceutical-grade anticoagulants have the potential to produce a coagulopathy and consequential bleeding. In one study describing 12 patients with surreptitious ingestion of oral anticoagulants, 9 were healthcare professionals.[102] These patients presented with typical manifestations of impaired coagulation: bruising, hematuria, hematochezia, and menorrhagia. Rare but life-threatening complications such as hemorrhage into the neck with resultant airway compromise are reported.[15] Although warfarin levels may be useful to confirm the diagnosis in unknown cases and study kinetic parameters,[55,100] the routine use of simple and inexpensive measures such as PT determination seems more appropriate.

Although intentional ingestions of warfarin-containing products are uncommon, therapeutic misadventures resulting in excessive anticoagulation and bleeding occur frequently. Older data suggested that the risk for minor bleeding was 20% per year of therapy,[54,112] and that life-threatening hemorrhage occurred in up to 5 to 7% of patients treated per year of therapy.[54,58] More recent data support a modest decline in adverse effects. When 2745 consecutive patients were followed over 2011 patient years, the risks of any bleeding, major bleeding, and fatal bleeding were reported as 7.6, 1.1, and 0.25 per 100 patient-years, respectively.[107] Older patients and those treated for cerebrovascular disease tended to have more adverse events.[107] Another cohort of 1608 patients who were anticoagulated due to their functional mechanical heart valves was followed for 6475 patient years. Major bleeding and CNS bleeding occurred in 2.1 and 0.57 patients per 100 patient years.[25] A similar study in patients anticoagulated as treatment for atrial fibrillation and cerebral ischemia demonstrated a risk of hemorrhage of 3.4 cases per 100 patient years.[38] Other studies give similar results.[43,49] Most studies demonstrate that the incidence of both minor and major bleeding complications increases with increasing INR.[148] Trauma, advanced age, a history of a previous bleeding episode while on therapeutic warfarin, drug interactions, changing liver function, and dietary changes are considered to be additional risk factors for bleeding complications.[43,44,54,58,107,112,150] Clearly, the most serious complication of excessive anticoagulation is intracranial hemorrhage, reported to occur in as many as 2% of patients on long-term therapy.[44] This complication is associated with a fatality rate as high as 77%.[91] Risk factors for intracranial hemorrhage include age, cerebrovascular disease, presence of a prosthetic heart valve, and an increased INR.[66,91]

Life-threatening hemorrhage should immediately be reversed with FFP, followed by vitamin K_1. One recent study characterized events in 32 patients who developed life-threatening hemorrhage while on warfarin therapy.[150] Most patients had multiple risk factors for hemorrhage including excessive anticoagulation, and the gastrointestinal tract was identified as the source of bleeding in two thirds of the patients. Sixty-six percent of patients were given vitamin K_1, 50% were given FFP, and 7% were given both therapies.[150] Repetitive, large doses of vitamin K_1 (on the order of 60 mg/day) may be required in some patients.[15,55,102] If complete reversal of the PT prolongation occurs or is desirable (as in most cases of life-threatening bleeding) and the patient's underlying medical condition still requires some degree of anticoagulation, they can then receive controlled anticoagulation with heparin until the bleeding is controlled and they are otherwise stable. This approach was used in 25% of patients mentioned.[150]

For patients with non-life-threatening hemorrhage, the clinician must consider whether anticoagulation is required for long-term care. In patients not requiring chronic anticoagulation, even small elevations of the PT may be treated (with vitamin K_1 alone) to prevent a deterioration in coagulation status and reduce the risk of bleeding. Because in most cases, coagulopathy persists only for several days, there may be a rationale for prophylactic vitamin K_1 administration in known warfarin-like anticoagulant ingestions in patients not requiring anticoagulation.

Patients requiring chronic anticoagulation can be observed if coagulation studies are only moderately elevated (INRs generally < 50), consequential bleeding is absent, and the patient can be placed in a protected environment (where trauma will be unlikely). For some, especially active children and the elderly, this may still require hospitalization. Patients with greater elevations in the INR or significant bleeding, should receive partial and temporary reversal with periodic administration of FFP. If vitamin K_1 is administered in these circumstances, complete reversal may occur and patients may be difficult to reanticoagulate in the future. One recent study reported on this conservative approach in 51 consecutive patients with INRs greater than 6.[50] Forty-eight patients were treated with observation alone (INRs ranged from 6.1 to 80.9), and only one developed minor bleeding. Three patients where given vitamin K_1 (INRs ranged from 12.8 to 81.8), one of whom required 47 days of heparin therapy before adequate oral anticoagulation was reachieved.[50]

Activated charcoal may be administered as clinically indicated (see Chap. 4). Additionally, oral cholestyramine can also be used to enhance warfarin elimination.[114] No studies are available that compare these two therapies or evaluate the role of combined activated charcoal and cholestyramine therapy. Either of these modalities may be used when complete reversal of the patient's anticoagulation is not desirable and the patient is at risk for significant hemorrhage.

What Is the Difference Between the Long-Acting Anticoagulants and Warfarin?

Within the coumarin group are two 4-hydroxycoumarin derivatives—difenacoum and brodifacoum. These agents differ from warfarin by their longer, higher-molecular weight polycyclic hydrocarbon side chain (Fig. 42–3). Together with a third agent, chlorophacinone, an indandione derivative, they are known as "superwarfarins," or long-acting anticoagulants.

Long-acting anticoagulants were designed to be effective rodenticides in warfarin-resistant rodents.[85] Their mechanism of action is identical to that of the traditional warfarin-like anticoagulants, as demonstrated by the measurement of increased levels of vitamin K 2,3-epoxide after long-acting anticoagulant administration.[18,19,22,82,108] The ability of these agents to perform as superior rodenticides is attributed to their high lipid sol-

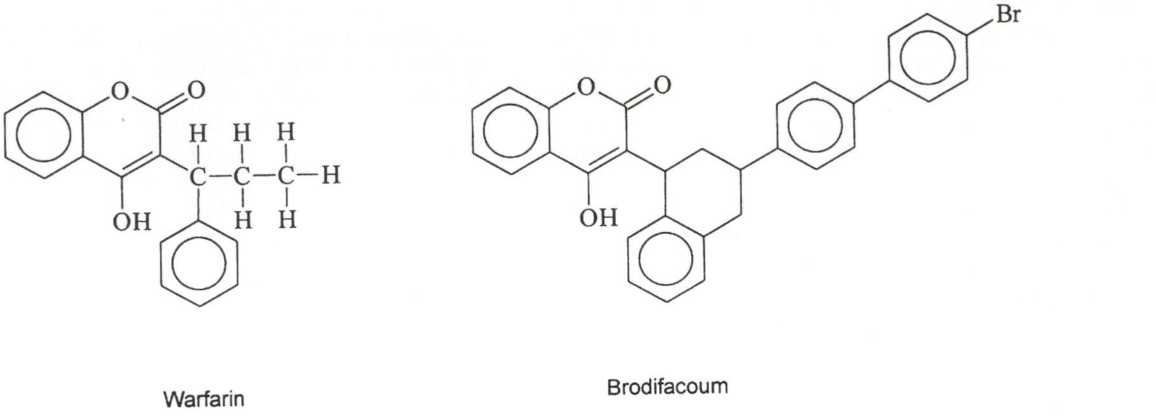

Figure 42–3. Structural comparison of prototypical short-acting (warfarin) and long-acting (brodifacoum) anticoagulants.

ubility and selective concentration in the liver.[82,85,108] They also may saturate hepatic enzymes at very low levels, as demonstrated by zero-order elimination following overdose.[22] These factors make them about 100 times more potent than warfarin on a mole for mole basis.[82,85,108] In addition, they have a longer duration of action than the traditional warfarins.[82,85,108] For example, to obtain 100% lethality in a common house mouse, more than 21 days of feeding with a warfarin-containing rodenticide (0.025% by weight) is required.[85] Similar efficacy can be achieved with a single day's ingestion of brodifacoum (0.005%).[85]

Many animals have been poisoned with long-acting anticoagulants, either secondary to the unintentional ingestion of rodenticides or intentionally for the purposes of investigation. In rats, the half-life of brodifacoum has been reported to be 156 hours.[4] The half-life in dogs has been reported to be between 6 and 120 days.[84,152] Horses intentionally poisoned with brodifacoum showed a half-life of 1.22 days.[14] The veterinary literature is replete with reports of fatalities and animals that remained anticoagulated in excess of 1 month.[96,133]

Many cases of intentional overdose of long-acting anticoagulants in humans are described in the literature. These cases are summarized in Table 42–3. These patients' clinical courses are characterized by a severe coagulopathy that may last weeks to months, often accompanied by consequential blood loss. The most common sites of bleeding include the gastrointestinal and genitourinary tracts. Although initial parenteral vitamin K_1 doses as high as 400 mg have been used,[23] daily vitamin K_1 requirements seem to be in the range of 50 to 100 mg, often administered orally. Recent experience in both animals and humans suggest that parenteral vitamin K_1 therapy may not be required.[22,152] (See Antidotes in Depth: Vitamin K.)

Patients with unintentional ingestions must be distinguished from those with intentional ingestions, because the former demonstrate a low likelihood of producing coagulation abnormalities and rare morbidity or mortality. Actually, with a single, small ingestion of a superwarfarin rodenticide, prolongation of the PT or INR is unlikely. Clinically significant anticoagulation is even rarer. In the combined pediatric case series, prolongation of the PT occurred in only 8 of 142 children (5.6%) reported with single small ingestions of long-acting anticoagulants.[10,72,74,130] Only one child in this group was reported to have "abnormal prolonged bleeding," but this required no medical attention.[130] In a single case report, a 36-month-old child developed epistaxis and hematuria and coagulopathy lasting over 100 days after a presumed, but unwitnessed single unintentional ingestion of brodifacoum.[139] Clinically significant coagulopathy can result, however, following small repeated ingestions. Two children reportedly became unintentionally poisoned by repeated ingestions of a long-acting anticoagulant. One child presented with a neck hematoma that compromised his airway, and the other with a hemarthrosis.[52] Similarly, a 7-year-old girl required multiple hospitalizations over a 20-month period following an unintentional chronic ingestion of brodifacoum.[146]

How Should the Patient With a Suspected Long-Acting Anticoagulant Overdose Be Evaluated?

Once again, the clinician must distinguish an acute unintentional ingestion from chronic or intentional overdose. Following an acute unintentional overdose most patients (usually children) are entirely asymptomatic and have a normal coagulation profile. Knowing the risk of coagulopathy is low and that it will occur over days, most authors recommend nonintervention.[73,130] If the PT is to become abnormal, it will do so within 48 hours of ingestion.[130] This information can be used to plan a rational management strategy. Gastrointestinal decontamination should be performed if more than a few pellets have been ingested (see Chap. 4). Although baseline coagulation studies are not usually helpful, they may provide information about chronic exposure. If the history is reliable and the child is healthy, baseline studies can be

TABLE 42–3. INTENTIONAL LONG-ACTING ANTICOAGULANT OVERDOSES

Reference	Age, Sex	Product	Complications	Initial PT Ratio	Duration of Coagulopathy
Babcock[3]	2	Brodifacoum	Purpura		9 mo
Barlow[6]	17 F	Difenacoum	None	15	5 wk
Reingestion			GI bleeding		42 d
Barnett[7]	27 F	Brodifacoum	Hemoptysis	7	—
Bruno[22]	52 M	Brodifacoum	Hematuria, oral bleeding	6	46 d
Burucoa[23]	20 F	Chlorophacinone	Hematuria	5	49 d
	60 F	Chlorophacinone	Hematuria, menorrhagia	8	25 d
	23 M	Chlorophacinone	Oral bleeding	7	132 d
Butcher[24]	M	Difenacoum	Hematuria	6	10 wk
Chong[27]	20 M	Brodifacoum	Oral bleeding, hematuria	2	8 mo
Exner[39]	25 F	Brodifacoum	Hemoptysis	7	>8 mo
Helmuth[60]	25 M	Brodifacoum	CNS bleed, death	>6	—
Hoffman[63]	30 M	Brodifacoum	Hematuria, GI bleeding	10	64 d
Hollinger[65]	38 M	Brodifacoum	Hematuria	11	114 d
Jones[71]	17 M	Brodifacoum	Hematuria	>10	55 d
Kruse[76]	25 M	Brodifacoum	Upper GI bleeding	4	15 wk
Reingestion			Fatal CNS bleed		
Lipton[84]	31 F	Brodifacoum	Abortion	6	300 d (?Repeat ingestion)
Murdoch[97]	37 F	Chlorophacinone	None	4	59 d
Rauch[113]	26 M	Brodifacoum	Calf hematoma, hematemesis	9	24 mo (?Repeat ingestion)
	37 F	Brodifacoum	Ecchymoses	>8	6 mo
	42 M	Brodifacoum	Hematuria, Epistaxis	>4	>3 mo
Ross[118]	62 M	Brodifacoum	Hematuria	4	3 mo
Routh[119]	29 F	Brodifacoum	Death	9	—
Seidelmann[124]	24 M	Unconfirmed	None	>12	>37 d
Sheen[127]	39 M	Brodifacoum	Hematuria	>12	>152 d
Swigar[137]	52 M	Unconfirmed	Compartment syndrome	—	>82 d
Wallace[144]	36 M	Brodifacoum	Upper GI bleeding	10	—
Weitzel[147]	20 F	Brodifacoum	Melena, menorrhagia, hematuria	>4	>11 mo
	45 M	Brodifacoum	Epistaxis, compartment syndrome	>4	100 d
	37 M	Brodifacoum	Hematuria	>5	>150 d

avoided. Serial PTs at 24 and 48 hours should identify all patients at risk of coagulopathy.[130] These studies can be obtained while the patient remains in the home setting, depending on the social situation. Prophylactic vitamin K_1 should *never* be given to asymptomatic children with accidental ingestions, for several reasons: (1) if the child develops a coagulopathy it will last for weeks, and the one or two doses of vitamin K_1 given will not prevent complications; (2) because a gradual decline in coagulation factors occurs over the first day of anticoagulation, no child would be expected to develop a life-threatening coagulopathy in a single day; (3) after vitamin K_1 is administered, the onset of a prolongation in the PT will be delayed, which could impair the clinician's ability to diagnose any coagulation abnormality or, more likely, require an unnecessarily prolonged observation period.

In contrast, all patients with intentional ingestions of long-acting anticoagulants should be presumed to be at risk for a severe coagulopathy. In fact, most patients do not seek medical care until bruising or bleeding is evident.[6,22,23,27,39,60,63,71,72,74,76,84,97,119,137] These events often occur many days after ingestion, which obviates the need for gastric emptying unless there is a suggestion of repetitive ingestion. These patients should be managed as described below. For patients who present within a few hours of ingestion, gastric decontamination with either orogastric lavage or syrup of ipecac-induced emesis is not indicated (see Chap. 4). Although convincing data on the efficacy of either single- or multiple-dose activated charcoal are lacking, at least a single dose should be administered unless it is contraindicated. The patient should be placed in an environment that will protect him or her against external or self-induced trauma, that has medical and psychiatric support, and permits observation for the onset of coagulopathy. Daily or twice-daily PT evaluations should be adequate to identify most patients at risk for coagulopathy, but early detection (through coagulation factor analysis) may be preferred.[63]

Also, although levels of long-acting anticoagulants can now be measured,[42,77,100] their exact role in determining the onset or duration of effect is unclear. Recent emphasis has been placed on determining a critical superwarfarin level below which anticoagulation does not occur,[23] and using toxicokinetic profiles to predict when levels will be nondetectable or below the given threshold.[22] If these efforts are successful they may prove more reliable than the current empiric endpoints of therapy.

What Specific Treatments Are Indicated for Patients With Long-Acting Anticoagulant Overdoses?

The goal of therapy is to reverse the coagulopathy and replace lost blood. Patients should have large-bore venous access established at the first sign of bleeding and have a blood type and cross-match available for packed red blood cells and FFP. Fresh frozen plasma is the initial treatment of choice for patients with active blood loss. It should be infused as needed, based on clinical symptoms and sequential PT or INR determinations. Vitamin K_1 is required, however, for long-term control of the PT. Vitamin K_1 is preferable over the other forms of vitamin K; the latter have been shown to be ineffective[71,97,101,140] and potentially toxic.[5] Parenteral administration of vitamin K_1 (aquamephyton) is generally preferred as initial therapy by many authors, but success has been achieved with early oral therapy as well.[22] In most cases reviewed, the patient was switched to oral vitamin K_1 preparations for long-term care. Vitamin K_1 can be administered intramuscularly, subcutaneously, intradermally, or intravenously. Although intravenous therapy has the most rapid onset of action, it is still associated with a delay of several hours[89,109] and carries the added risk of anaphylactoid reactions.[115] A slow rate of administration reduces this risk, but we generally prefer that vitamin K_1 be administered by other than the intravenous route (see Antidotes in Depth: Vitamin K).

Finally, long-acting anticoagulants are metabolized by the hepatic mixed-function oxidase system (cytochrome P450).[4,101] In a rat model, the duration of coagulopathy was shortened by administering phenobarbital, CYP3A4 inducer.[4] Although a phenobarbital effect has never been systematically studied in humans, this approach has been employed by several authors in isolated human cases of long-acting anticoagulant toxicity.[23,71,84,139,146] Although these anecdotal reports suggest some improvement with phenobarbital therapy, the risks of producing sedation in a patient who might be prone to bleeding complications appears consequential.[63]

Patients should be followed until their coagulation studies remain normal while off therapy for several days. This usually requires daily or even twice-daily PT determinations while the patient's PT is significantly prolonged, and daily or every-other-day determinations when the optimal vitamin K_1 dose and route have been determined. With standard measures (PT determination) a decreasing vitamin K_1 requirement with time would be expected. Periodic coagulation factor analysis, however, may provide an early clue to the resolution of toxicity.[63] The patient may require weeks to months of close observation (Table 42–3) for both psychiatric and medical reasons.

How Does Heparin Produce Anticoagulation?

Heparin is a heterogeneous group of molecules within the class of glycosaminoglycans.[69] The heparin precursor molecule is composed of long chains of mucopolysaccharides, a polypeptide (sequence of amino acids), and carbohydrates. The main carbohydrate components of heparin molecules include uronic acids and amino sugars in polysaccharide chains. Heparin for pharmaceutical use is extracted from bovine lung tissue and porcine intestines.[123] As a therapeutic agent, heparin inhibits thrombosis by accelerating the binding of the protease inhibitor antithrombin III to thrombin and other serine proteases involved in coagulation.[88,117] Thus, factors IX to XII, kallikrein, and thrombin are inhibited. Heparin also affects plasminogen activator inhibitor, protein C inhibitor, and other components of coagulation. Heparin's therapeutic effect is usually measured through the activated PTT. The activated blood coagulation time (ACT) may be more useful for monitoring large therapeutic doses or in the overdose situation.[78]

Due to heparin's large size and negative charge it is unable to cross cellular membranes. These factors eliminate oral administration as a viable route, and consequently heparin must be administered by either deep subcutaneous injection or continuous intravenous infusion. Following parenteral administration heparin remains in the intravascular compartment, in part bound to globulins, fibrinogen, and low-density lipoproteins, thus resulting in a volume of distribution of 0.06 L/kg in humans.[37,103] Heparin has a short duration of effect, due to its rapid metabolism in the liver by a heparinase.[88] Although the half-life of elimination is dose dependent and ranges from 1 to 2.5 hours,[88,92,103] the duration of anticoagulant effect is usually reported as 1 to 3 hours.[88] Dosing errors or drug interactions with thrombolytic agents, antiplatelet drugs, or nonsteroidal antiinflammatory drugs may increase the risk of hemorrhage.[58]

Although intentional overdoses with heparin are reported,[55,90] most reported cases involve unintentional poisoning in hospitalized infants.[47,51,90,122] One neonate received 8000 U (2666 U/kg) of heparin. Bleeding from injection sites and intrabdominal hemorrhage occurred after 17 hours despite administration of a total of 25.4 mg of protamine sulfate, and the infant died.[47] Similarly, the inadvertent administration of 8620 U/kg of heparin over 4 hours to a neonate via an umbilical catheter resulted in excessive bleeding from all skin puncture sites.[51] Another three cases of infant toxicity related to flushing an indwelling catheter with heparin instead of saline.[122] These infants received 500 to 50,000 U of heparin and presented with respiratory distress, hypotension, bleeding from puncture sites and umbilical stumps, and gross hematuria. Finally, following the unintentional intramuscular administration of 20,000 U of heparin to an 8-month-old girl, a hematoma formed, bleeding from injection sites began within 2 hours, and her hemoglobin fell to 5.5 g/dL. Capillary coagulation times remained abnormal for 31 hours.[106]

How Should a Patient With a Heparin Overdose Be Assessed and Treated?

After stabilization of the airway, breathing, and circulation have been assured, the physician should be prepared to replace blood loss and reverse the coagulopathy, if indicated. Because of the relatively short duration of action of heparin, observation alone may be indicated if significant bleeding has not occurred. For the patient requiring anticoagulation, serial PTT determinations will indicate when it is safe to resume therapy. If significant bleeding occurs, either removal of the heparin or reversal of its anticoagulant effect is indicated. Because heparin has a very small volume of distribution, it can be effectively removed by exchange transfusion.[122] Although this technique has been used successfully in neonates, it is not generally applicable to older children and adults.

When severe bleeding occurs, heparin may be effectively neutralized by protamine sulfate.[1] Protamine is a low-molecular-weight protein found in the sperm and testes of salmon, which forms ionic bonds with heparin and renders it devoid of anticoagulant activity.[88] One milligram of protamine sulfate injected intravenously neutralizes 100 U of heparin.[88] The dose of protamine should be calculated from the dose of heparin administered and heparin's approximate half-life, such that the amount of protamine does not exceed the amount of heparin expected to be found intravascularly at the time of infusion. As with other foreign proteins, protamine administration is associated with numerous adverse effects. Because approximately 0.2% of patients experience anaphylaxis, a complication that carries a 30% mortality rate, authors commonly recommend that protamine be reserved for patients with life-threatening hemorrhage.[64] (See Antidotes in Depth: Protamine.)

Because of the severe adverse effects associated with protamine, current research is focusing on safer methods to reverse heparin anticoagulation. These experimental agents include heparinase,[94] designer protamine variants,[142,143] and platelet factor 4.[35]

What Are Low-Molecular-Weight Heparins and How Do They Differ from Conventional Heparin?

Low-molecular-weight (LMW) heparins are 4000 to 6000-D fractions obtained from conventional (unfractionated) heparin.[45] As such, they share many of the pharmacologic and toxicologic properties of conventional heparin.[16] The major differences between LMW heparins and conventional heparin are greater bioavailability, longer half-life, more predictable anticoagulation with fixed dosing, and targeted activity against activated factor X, but not against activated factor II.[16,45] As a result of this targeted factor X activity, LMW heparins have minimal effect on the activated PTT, thereby eliminating either the need for or the utility of monitoring. As such, they are administered on a fixed-dose schedule.

Low-molecular-weight heparins have been investigated for prevention of thromboembolic disease after hip surgery and trauma, in patients with stroke or deep venous thrombosis, and in other conditions where anticoagulation with heparin would otherwise be indicated. Although most studies demonstrate a lower incidence of embolization, there is a clear trend toward increased bleeding.[11,53,83] If life-threatening bleeding occurs following LMW heparin administration, patients should be treated supportively. The newer (safer) experimental protamine variants appear to be effective against LMW heparins.[142,143]

What Are the Nonbleeding Complications of Anticoagulant Therapy?

Warfarin therapy is associated with three nonhemorrhagic lesions of the skin: urticaria,[121] purple toe syndrome,[41] and warfarin skin necrosis.[32,75,79,93,141] Although skin necrosis was once thought to be a rare and idiosyncratic reaction,[75,79] more recent evidence suggests a link between this disorder and protein C deficiency.[79,141] Protein C is also dependent on vitamin K.[29] Patients who are heterozygotes for protein C deficiency have an increased incidence of thrombosis and embolic events, such that they often require long-term anticoagulant therapy.[29] Because the half-life of protein C is shorter than that of many of the vitamin K-dependent coagulation factors, protein C levels fall rapidly during the first hours of warfarin therapy. In the protein C-deficient patient, protein C reaches a critically low level prior to a reduction in coagulation factors. This results in an imbalance that favors coagulation, and skin necrosis results.[93,141] Although warfarin skin necrosis is more common in patients with protein C deficiency, this disorder has also been described in patients with protein S and antithrombin III deficiencies.[32] Unfortunately, these deficiencies are neither necessary nor sufficient to account for the incidence of warfarin necrosis.[32] A recent review of patients with warfarin skin necrosis suggested that warfarin therapy can be reinitiated, if indicated, without recurrent adverse effects, and provides strategies for doing so.[70] The purple toe syndrome is presumed to result from small atheroemboli that are no longer adherent to their plaques by clot.

The other major nonhemorrhagic complication of warfarin therapy relates to its use in pregnant women. Most warfarin-induced abnormalities occur during weeks 6 to 12 of gestation, but CNS and ocular abnormalities have been reported to develop at any time during gestation.[56,132] Because heparin does not cross the placenta, it is usually recommended for anticoagulation in pregnant women.

Heparin therapy is associated with a transient and mild thrombocytopenia that occurs in about 25% of patients during the first few days of therapy. Although this syndrome results from heparin-induced platelet aggregation, a more severe form of thrombocytopenia occurs in 1 to 5% of patients between days 7 and 14 of therapy.[88] Heparin stimulates platelets to release platelet factor 4, which subsequently complexes with heparin to provoke an IgG response. These antibodies against the heparin–platelet factor 4 complex activate platelets, leading to platelet–fibrin thrombotic events (known as the white clot syndrome).[2,88] Because LMW heparins do not stimulate the release of platelet factor 4, their use is not associated with either severe thrombocytopenia or the white clot syndrome.[145] However, once white clot syndrome occurs, LMWH are not recommended as alternative therapy. When rechallenged with heparin, these events can occur earlier than 7 days. In addition, several authors have described a heparin-induced thrombocytosis–thrombocytopenia syndrome (HITTS) that occurs within 5 to 10 days of initiation of heparin therapy.[87,153] Patients may present with either hemorrhagic or thromboembolic complications. Necrotizing skin lesions[111] and hyperkalemia from aldosterone suppression[104] are rarely reported in patients receiving heparin therapy.

How Do Snake Venins Produce Anticoagulation?

A detailed discussion of snake envenomations is found in Chapter 99; only a few specific issues are discussed here. Envenomation from a member of the *Crotalidae* family of snakes is likely to produce impaired coagulation resulting in either local or systemic hemorrhagic complications. Although venin constituents are complex, several components are capable of producing a coagulopathy.[67,68] Both PT and PTT are elevated, and fibrin levels are decreased with correspondingly elevated levels of fibrin degradation products. These findings are suggestive of a consumptive coagulopathy. Phospholipases, direct lytic factor, and hemolysins directly disrupt red blood cell and platelet membranes, producing cell lysis. Hemorrhagins destroy vascular integrity and contain procoagulants that form intravascular clot. Specific venins have been shown to activate factor X and possess thrombinlike activity (ie, convert fibrinogen to fibrin). In summary, multiple mechanisms create a consumptive coagulopathy that is best treated with antivenin when available.

What Is Hirudin, and What Are Its Uses?

Hirudin, a 65-amino-acid substance originally detected in leech saliva, irreversibly blocks thrombin without the need for antithrombin III.[125] Unlike heparin, the small size of hirudin allows it to enter clots and inhibit clot-bound thrombin, offering the distinct advantage restricting further thrombus formation. Hirudin demonstrates enhanced bioavailability and longer half-life than unfractionated heparin. In addition, there are no known natural inhibitors of hirudin, such as platelet factor 4. Recombinant hirudins have been used in coronary angioplasty and in patients with heparin-induced thrombocytopenia.[13,120,125] These compounds appear to be at least as effective as unfractionated heparin, and to have a lower incidence of bleeding complications. Overdose data are not yet available.

Thrombolytic Agents

The fibrinolytic system is designed to remove unwanted clots and leave those clots protecting sites of vascular injury intact. Plasminogen exists as a proenzyme and is converted to the active form, plasmin, by various plasminogen activators.[30,31] Tissue plasminogen activator (t-PA) is released from the endothelium, and is under the inhibitory control of two inactivators known as tissue plasminogen activator inhibitors 1 and 2 (t-PAI-1 and t-PAI-2).[30,31,88,95] Plasmin's actions are nonspecific in that it degrades not only fibrin clots but also some plasma proteins and coagulation factors.[88] Inhibition at the level of plasmin occurs through α_2-antiplasmin.

With their diverse indications in acute myocardial infarction, unstable angina, arterial and venous thrombosis and embolism, and cerebrovascular disease, the thrombolytic agents (streptokinase, urokinase, alteplase, and anistreplase) are used commonly.[9] The reader is referred to one of a number of reviews for specific indications and dosing regimens.[33,80,88,110,129,149] Although all agents enhance fibrinolysis, they differ in their specific sites of action and durations of effect. Altepase (t-PA) is specific for clot (it does not increase fibrinolysis in the absence of a thrombus), while streptokinase, urokinase, and anistreplase are not clot specific. Altepase has the shortest half-life and duration of effect (5 minutes and 2 hours, respectively), and anistreplase the longest (90 minutes and 18 hours, respectively).[110,129] Streptokinase has the additional risk of severe allergic reaction on rechallenge, limiting its use to once in a lifetime.

Although the incidence of bleeding requiring transfusion may be as high as 7.7% following high-dose (150 mg) altepase and 4.4% following low-dose altepase,[33] the incidence of life-threatening hemorrhage is much lower.[149] The addition of heparin to the thrombolytic regimen increases the risk of bleeding. Reviews of multiple trials suggest that life-threatening events such as intracranial hemorrhage occur in 0.30 to 0.58% of patients receiving anistreplase, 0.42 to 0.73% of patients receiving alteplase, and 0.08 to 0.30% of patients receiving streptokinase.[149] The frequency of bleeding events is essentially equal regardless of the thrombolytic agent used. Currently no agents exist to reverse thrombolysis, and only supportive care is indicated for patients with bleeding complications.

Summary

A complete understanding of the normal mechanisms of coagulation, anticoagulation, and thrombolysis combined with an understanding of the pharmacology of the agent and the patient's clinical needs will allow the clinician to choose from complex therapies that range from observation alone to aggressive reversal with blood products and antidotes.

Acknowledgment

Teresa Kierenia, MD (deceased) contributed to this chapter in a previous edition.

References

1. Andersen MN, Nendelow M, Alfano GA: Experimental studies of heparin-protamine activity with special reference to protamine inhibition of clotting. Surgery 1959; 46:1060–1068.
2. Aster RH: Heparin-induced thrombocytopenia and thrombosis. N Engl J Med 1995;332:1374–1376.
3. Babcock J, Hartman K, Pedersen A, et al: Rodenticide-induced coagulopathy in a young child. A case of Münchausen syndrome by proxy. Am J Pediatr Hematol Oncol 1993;15:126–130.
4. Bachmann KA, Sullivan TJ: Dispositional and pharmacodynamic characteristics of brodifacoum in warfarin-sensitive rats. Pharmacology 1983;27:281–288.
5. Badr M, Yoshihara H, Kauffman F, Thurman RA: Menadione causes selective toxicity to periportal regions of the liver lobule. Toxicol Lett 1987;35:241–246.
6. Barlow AM, Gay AL, Park BK: Difenacoum (Neosorexa) poisoning. Br Med J 1982;285:541.
7. Barnett VT, Bergmann F, Humphrey H, Chediak J: Diffuse alveolar hemorrhage secondary to superwarfarin ingestion. Chest 1992;102:1301–1302.
8. Becker RC: Seminars in thrombosis, thrombolysis, and vascular biology. Cardiology 1991;78:257–266.
9. Benedict CR, Mueller S, Anderson HV, Willerson JT: Thrombolytic therapy: A state of the art review. Hosp Pract 1991;27:61–72.
10. Bennett DL, Caravatti DM, Veltri JC: Long-acting anticoagulant ingestion: A prospective study. Vet Hum Toxicol 1987;29:472. Abstract.
11. Bergqvist D, Benoni G, Bjorgell O, et al: Low-molecular-weight heparin (enoxaprin) as prophylaxis against venous thromboembolism after total hip replacement. N Engl J Med 1996;335:696–700.
12. Bithell TC: Acquired coagulation disorders. In: Lee GR, Bithell TC, Foerster J, et al, eds: Wintrobe's Clinical Hematology, 9th ed. Philadelphia, Lea & Febiger, 1993, pp. 1473–1503.
13. Bittl JA, Strony J, Brinker JA: Treatment with bivalirudin (Hirulog) as compared to heparin during coronary angioplasty for unstable or postinfarction angina. N Engl J Med 1995;333:764–769.
14. Boermans HJ, Johnstone I, Black WD, Murphy M: Clinical signs, laboratory changes and toxicokinetics of brodifacoum in the horse. Can J Vet Res 1991;55:21–27.
15. Boster SR, Bergin JL: Upper airway obstruction complicating warfarin therapy: With a note on reversal of warfarin toxicity. Ann Emerg Med 1983;12:711–715.
16. Bounameaux H, Goldhaber SZ: Uses of low-molecular-weight heparin. Blood Rev 1995;9:213–219.
17. Bowen KJ, Vukeljia SJ: Hypercoagulable states: Their causes and management. Postgrad Med 1992;91:117–132.
18. Braithwaite GB: Vitamin K and brodifacoum. J Am Vet Med Assoc 1982;181:531–534.
19. Breckenridge A, Leck JB, Serlin MJ, Wilson A: Mechanisms of action of the anticoagulants warfarin, 2-chloro-3-phytylnaphthoquinone (CL-K), acenocoumerol, brodifacoum, and difenacoum in the rabbit. Br J Pharmacol 1978;64:339.
20. Breckenridge A, Orme M: Plasma half lives and the pharmacological effect of the enantiomers of warfarin in rats. Life Sci 1972;11:337–345.
21. Breckenridge A, Orme M, Wessling H, et al: Pharmacokinetics and pharmacodynamics of the enantiomers of warfarin in man. Clin Pharmacol Ther 1974;15:424–430.
22. Bruno GR, Howland MA, Hoffman RS: Elimination kinetics of brodifacoum and serum vitamin K_1 concentrations in long-acting anticoagulant overdose. J Toxicol Clin Toxicol 1996;34:568. Abstract.
23. Burucoa C, Mura P, Robert R, et al: Chlorophacinone intoxication a biological and toxicological study. J Toxicol Clin Toxicol 1989;27:79–89.
24. Butcher GP, Shearer MH, MacNicoll AD, et al: Difenacoum poisoning as a cause of hematuria. Hum Exp Toxicol 1992;11:553–554.
25. Cannegieter SC, Rosendaal FR, Wintzen AR, et al: Optimal oral anticoagulant therapy in patients with mechanical heart valves. N Engl J Med 1995;333:11–17.
26. Carpentieri U, Mghiem QX, Harris LC: Clinical experience with an oral anticoagulant in children. Arch Dis Child 1976;51:445–448.
27. Chong L, Chau WK, Ho CH: A case of "superwarfarin" poisoning. Scand J Haematol 1986;36:314–315.
28. Choonara BA, Scott AK, Haynes BP, et al: Vitamin K_1 metabolism in relation to pharmacodynamic response in anticoagulated patients. Br J Clin Pharmacol 1985;20:643–648.
29. Clouse LH, Comp PC: The regulation of hemostasis: The protein C system. N Engl J Med 1986;314:1298–1303.
30. Collen D: On the regulation and control of fibrinolysis. Thromb Haemost 1980;43:77–89.
31. Collen D, Lijnen HR: Basic and clinical aspects of fibrinolysis and thrombosis. Blood 1991;78:3114–3124.
32. Comp PC: Coumarin-induced skin necrosis: Incidence, mechanisms, management and avoidance. Drug Saf 1993; 8:128–135.
33. Conti RC: Brief overview of the endpoints of thrombolytic therapy. Am J Cardiol 1991;67:8E–10E.
34. Davie EW, Ratnoff OD: Waterfall sequence for intrinsic blood clotting. Science 1964;145:1310–1312.
35. Dehmer GJ, Fisher M, Tate DA, Teo S: Reversal of heparin anticoagulation by recombinant platelet factor 4 in humans. Circulation 1995;91:2188–2194.

36. Dowd P, Ham S, Naganathan S, Hershline R: The mechanism of action of vitamin K. Annu Rev Nutr 1995;15:419–440.
37. Estes JW, Poulem PF: Pharmacokinetics of heparin. Thromb Diath Haemorrh 1974;33:26–37.
38. European Atrial Fibrillation Study Group: Optimal oral anticoagulant therapy in patients with nonrheumatic atrial fibrillation and recent cerebral ischemia. N Engl J Med 1995;333:5–10.
39. Exner DV, Brien WF, Murphy MJ: Superwarfarin ingestion. Can Med Assoc J 1992;146:34–35.
40. Fasco MJ, Hildebrandt EF, Suttie JW: Evidence that warfarin anticoagulant action involves two distinct reductase activities. J Biol Chem 1982;257:11210–11212.
41. Feder W, Auerbach R: Purple toes: An uncommon sequela of oral coumarin drug therapy. Ann Intern Med 1961; 55:911–917.
42. Felice LJ, Chalermchaikit T, Murphy MJ: Multicomponent determination of 4-hydroxycoumarin anticoagulant rodenticides in blood serum by liquid chromatography with fluorescence detection. J Anal Toxicol 1991;15:126–129.
43. Fihn SD, Callahan CM, Marin DC, et al: The risk for and severity of bleeding complications in elderly patients treated with warfarin. The National Consortium of Anticoagulation. Ann Intern Med 1996;124:970–979.
44. Freedman MD, Olatidoye AG: Clinically significant drug interactions with the oral anticoagulants. Drug Saf 1994;10:381–394.
45. Frydman A: Low-molecular-weight-heparins: An overview of pharmacodynamics, pharmacokinetics and metabolism in humans. Haemostasis 1996;26(suppl 2):24–38.
46. Furie B, Furie BC: Molecular and cellular biology of blood coagulation. N Engl J Med 1992;326:800–806.
47. Galant SP: Accidental heparinization of a newborn infant. Am J Dis Child 1967;114:313–319.
48. Gilbert GE, Sims PJ, Wiedmer T, et al: Platelet derived microparticles express high affinity receptors for factor VIII. J Biol Chem 1991;266:17261–17268.
49. Gitter MJ, Jaeger TM, Petterson TM, Gersh BJ: Bleeding and thromboembolism during anticoagulant therapy: A population-based study in Rochester, Minnesota. Mayo Clin Proc 1995;70:725–733.
50. Glover JJ: Conservative treatment of over anticoagulated patients. Chest 1995;108:987–990.
51. Glueck HI, Light IJ, Flessa H, et al: Sodium heparin administration to a newborn infant. JAMA 1965;191:159–160.
52. Greeff MC, Mashile O, MacDougall LG: Superwarfarin (bromodialone) poisoning in two children resulting in prolonged anticoagulation. Lancet 1987;2:1269.
53. Green D, Hirsh J, Heit J, et al: Low molecular weight heparin: A critical analysis of clinical trials. Pharmacol Rev 1994;46:89–109.
54. Gurwitz JH, Avron J, Ross-Degnan D, et al: Aging and the anticoagulant response to warfarin therapy. Ann Intern Med 1992;116:901–904.
55. Hackett LP, Ileet KF, Chester A: Plasma warfarin concentrations after a massive overdose. Med J Aust 1985;142: 642–643.
56. Hall JG, Pauli RM, Wilson KM: Maternal and fetal sequelae of anticoagulation during pregnancy. Am J Med 1980;68:122–140.
57. Handin RI, Rosenberg RD: Hemorrhagic disorders. III: Disorders of primary and secondary hemostasis. In: Beck WS, ed: Hematology, 2nd ed. Cambridge, MIT Press, 1977, pp. 547–567.
58. Harrington R, Ansell J: Risk-benefit assessment of anticoagulant therapy. Drug Saf 1991;6:54–69.
59. Harris EN, Gharavi AE, Asherson RA, Hugher GR: Antiphospholipid antibodies: A review. Eur J Rheumatol Inflamm 1984;7:5–8.
60. Helmuth RA, McCloskey OW, Doeden DJ, et al: Fatal ingestion of a brodifacoum-containing rodenticide. Lab Med 1989;20:25–27.
61. Hirsh J: Substandard monitoring of warfarin in North America. Arch Intern Med 1992;152:257–258.
62. Hirsh J, Poller L: The international normalized ratio: A guide to understanding and correcting its problems. Arch Intern Med 1994;154:282–288.
63. Hoffman RS, Smilkstein MJ, Goldfrank LR: Evaluation of coagulation factor abnormalities in long-acting anticoagulant overdose. J Toxicol Clin Toxicol 1988;26: 233–248.
64. Holland CL, Singh AK, McMaster PRB, et al: Adverse reactions to protamine sulfate following cardiac surgery. Clin Cardiol 1984;7:157–162.
65. Hollinger BR, Pastoor TP: Case management and plasma half-life in a case of brodifacoum poisoning. Arch Intern Med 1993;153:1925–1928.
66. Hylek EM, Singer DE: Risk factors for intracranial hemorrhage in outpatients taking Warfarin. Ann Intern Med 1994;120:897–902.
67. Iyaniwura TT: Snake venom constituents: Biochemistry and toxicology, part 1. Vet Hum Toxicol 1991;33:468–474.
68. Iyaniwura TT: Snake venom constituents: Biochemistry and toxicology, part 2. Vet Hum Toxicol 1991;33:475–480.
69. Jacques LB: The discovery of heparin. Semin Thromb Hemost 1978;4:350–353.
70. Jillella AP: Reinstituting warfarin in patients who develop warfarin skin necrosis. Am J Hematol 1996;52:117–119
71. Jones EC, Growe GH, Naiman SC: Prolonged anticoagulation in rat poisoning. JAMA 1984;252:3005–3007.
72. Katona B, Sigell LT, Wason S: Anticoagulant rodenticide poisoning. Vet Hum Toxicol 1986;28:478. Abstract.
73. Katona B, Wason S: Superwarfarin poisoning. J Emerg Med 1989;7:627–631.
74. Katona B, Wason S: Anticoagulant rodenticide poisoning. Clin Toxicol Rev 1986;8:1–2.
75. Koch-Weser J: Coumarin necrosis. Ann Intern Med 1968;68:1365–1367.
76. Kruse JA, Carlson RW: Fatal rodenticide poisoning with brodifacoum. Ann Emerg Med 1992;21:333–336.
77. Kuijpers EA, den Hartigh J, Savelkoul TJ: A method for the simultaneous identification and quantitation of five superwarfarin rodenticides in human serum. J Anal Toxicol 1995;19:557–562.
78. Kunert M, Sorgenicht R, Scheuble L, et al: Value of activated blood coagulation time in monitoring anticoagulation during coronary angioplasty. Z Kardil. 1996;85: 118–124.
79. Lacy JP, Godin RR: Warfarin induced necrosis of the skin. Ann Intern Med 1975;82:381–382.

80. Lawrence PF, Goodman GR: Thrombolytic therapy. Surg Clin North Am 1992;72:899–918.
81. Lechner K, Pabinger-Fasching I: Lupus anticoagulants and thrombosis: A study of 25 cases and review of the literature. Haemostasis 1985;15:254–262.
82. Leck JB, Park BK: A comparative study of the effect of warfarin and brodifacoum on the relationship between vitamin K_1 metabolism and clotting factor activity in warfarin-susceptible and warfarin-resistent rats. Biochem Pharmacol 1981;30:123–128.
83. Levine M, Gent M, Hirsh J, et al: A comparison of low-molecular-weight heparin administered primarily at home with unfractionated heparin administered in the hospital for proximal deep-vein thrombosis. N Engl J Med 1996; 334:677–681.
84. Lipton RA, Klass EM: Human ingestion of a "superwarfarin" rodenticide resulting in a prolonged anticoagulant effect. JAMA 1984;252:3004–3005.
85. Lund M: Comparative effect of the three rodenticides warfarin, difenacoum, and brodifacoum on eight rodent species in short feeding periods. J Hyg 1981;87:101–107.
86. MacFarlane RG: An enzyme cascade in the blood clotting mechanism and its function as a biochemical amplifier. Nature 1964;202:498–499.
87. MacLean JA, Moscicki R, Bloch KJ: Adverse reactions to heparin. Ann Allergy 1990;65:254–259.
88. Majerus PW, Broze GJ, Miletich JP, Tollefsen DM: Anticoagulant, thrombolytic, and antiplatelet drugs. In: Hardman JG, Limbird LE, Molinoff PB, Ruddon RW, eds: Goodman and Gilman's The Pharmacological Basis of Therapeutics, 9th ed. New York, McGraw-Hill, 1996, pp. 1341–1359.
89. Marcus AJ: Hemorrhagic disorders: Abnormalities of platelet and vascular function. In: Wyngaarden JB, Smith LH, eds: Cecil Textbook of Medicine, 18th ed. Philadelphia, Saunders, 1988, pp. 1042–1051.
90. Martin CMM, Engstrom PF, Barrett O: Surreptitious self-administration of heparin. JAMA 1970;212:475–476.
91. Mathiesen T, Benediktsdottir K, Johnsson H, Lindqvist M: Intracranial traumatic and nontraumatic haemorrhagic complications of warfarin treatment. Acta Neurol Scan 1995;91:208–214.
92. McAvoy TJ: Pharmacokinetic modeling of heparin and its clinical implications. J Pharmacokinet Biopharm 1979; 7:331–354.
93. McGhee WG, Klotz TA, Epstein DJ, et al: Coumarin necrosis associated with hereditary protein C deficiency. Ann Intern Med 1984;101:59–60.
94. Michelsen LG, Kikura M, Levy JH, et al: Heparinase I (neutralase) reversal of systemic anticoagulation. Anesthesiology 1996;85:339–346.
95. Mosher DF: Blood coagulation and fibrinolysis: An overview. Clin Cardiol 1990;13:5–11.
96. Mount ME: Diagnosis and therapy of anticoagulant rodenticide intoxications. Vet Clin North Am 1988;18: 115–130.
97. Murdoch DA: Prolonged anticoagulation in chlorophacinone poisoning. Lancet 1983;1:355–356.
98. Ng VL, Lewin J, Corash L, Gottfried EL: Failure of the International Normalized Ratio to generate consistent results within a local medical community. Am J Clin Pathol 1993;99:689–694.
99. Nichols WL, Bowie EJW: Standardization of the prothrombin time for monitoring orally administered anticoagulant therapy with use of the international normalized ratio system. Mayo Clin Proc 1993;68:897–898.
100. O'Bryan SM, Constable DJ: Quantification of brodifacoum in plasma and liver tissue by HPLC. J Anal Toxicol 1991;15:144–147.
101. O'Reilly RA: Vitamin K antagonists. In: Colman RW, Hirsh J, Marder VJ, Salzman EW, eds: Hemostasis and Thrombosis. Philadelphia, Lippincott, 1987, pp. 846–860.
102. O'Reilly RA, Aggeler PM: Surreptitious ingestion of coumarin anticoagulant drugs. Ann Intern Med 1966;64: 1034–1041.
103. Olsson P, Lagergren H, Ek S: The elimination from plasma of intravenous heparin. Acta Med Scand 1963;173:619–630.
104. Oster JR, Singer I, Fishman LM: Heparin-induced aldosterone suppression and hyperkalemia. Am J Med 1995; 98:575–586.
105. Osterud B, Rapaport SI: Activation of factor IX by the reaction product of tissue factor and factor VII: Additional pathway for initiating blood coagulation. Proc Natl Acad Sci USA 1977;74:5260–5264.
106. Pachman DJ: Accidental heparin poisoning in an infant. Am J Dis Child 1965;110:210–212.
107. Palareti G, Leali N, Coccheri S, et al: Bleeding complications of oral anticoagulant treatment: An inception-cohort, prospective collaborative study (ISCOAT). Lancet 1996; 348:423–428.
108. Park BK, Leck JB: A comparison of vitamin K antagonism by warfarin, difenacoum, and brodifacoum in the rabbit. Biochem Pharmacol 1982;31:3535–3639.
109. Park BK, Scott AK, Wilson AC, et al: Plasma disposition of vitamin K_1 in relation to anticoagulant poisoning. Br J Clin Pharmacol 1984;18:655–661.
110. Paspa PA, Movahed A: Thrombolytic therapy in acute myocardial infarction. Am Fam Physician 1992;45: 640–647.
111. Platell CFE, Tan EGC: Hypersensitivity reactions to heparin: Delayed onset thrombocytopenia and necrotizing skin lesions. Aust NZ Surg 1986;56:621–623.
112. Raskob GE, Pineo GF, Hull RD: The technique of administering oral anticoagulant therapy. J Crit Illness 1991;6: 923–930.
113. Rauch AE, Weininger R, Pasquale D, et al: Superwarfarin poisoning: A significant public health problem. J Community Health 1994;19:55–65.
114. Renowden S, Westmoreland D, White JP, Routledge PA: Oral cholestyramine increases the elimination of warfarin after overdose. Br Med J 1985;291:513–514.
115. Rich EC, Prage CW: Severe complications of intravenous phytonadione therapy. Postgrad Med 1982;72:303–306.
116. Roberts HR, Lozier JN: New perspectives on the coagulation cascade. Hosp Pract 1992;27:97–112.
117. Rosenberg RD: Actions and interactions of antithrombin and heparin. N Engl J Med 1975;292:146–151.
118. Ross GS, Zacharski LR, Robert D, Rabin DL: An acquired hemorrhagic disorder from long-acting rodenticide ingestion. Arch Intern Med 1992;151:411–412.

119. Routh CR, Triplett DA, Murphy MJ, et al: Superwarfarin ingestion and detection. Am J Hematol 1991;36:50–54.
120. Schiele F, Vuillemenot A, Mouhat T, et al: Anticoagulant therapy with recombinant hirudin in patients with thrombocytopenia induced by heparin. Presse Med 1996;25: 757–760.
121. Schiff BL, Kern AB: Cutaneous reactions to anticoagulants. Arch Dermatol 1968;98:136–137.
122. Schreiner RL, Wynn RJ, McNulty C: Accidental heparin toxicity in the newborn intensive care unit. J Pediatr 1978;92:115–116.
123. Schwartz BS: Heparin: What is it? How does it work? Clin Cardiol 1990;13:12–15.
124. Seidelmann S, Kubic V, Burton E, Schmitz L: Combined superwarfain and ethylene glycol ingestion: A unique case report with misleading clinical history. Am J Clin Pathol 1995;104:663–666.
125. Serruys PW, Herrman JR, Simon R: A comparison of hirudin with heparin in the prevention of restenosis after coronary angioplasty. N Engl J Med 1995;333:757–763.
126. Shapiro SS: Acquired anticoagulants. In: Williams WJ, Beutler E, Erslev AJ, Rundles RW, eds: Hematology, 2nd ed. New York, McGraw-Hill, 1973, pp. 1447–1454.
127. Sheen SR, Spiller HA, Grossman D: Symptomatic brodifacoum ingestion requiring high-dose phytonadione therapy. Vet Hum Toxicol 1994;36:216–217.
128. Sims PJ, Faioni EM, Wiedmer T, Shattil SJ: Complement proteins CX5b–9 cause release of membrane vesicles from the platelet surface that are enriched in the membrane receptor for coagulation factor Va and express prothrombinase activity. J Biol Chem 1988;263:18205–18212.
129. Smitherman TC: Considerations affecting selection of thrombolytic agents. Mol Biol Med 1991;8:207–218.
130. Smolinske SC, Scherger DL, Kearns PS, et al: Superwarfarin poisoning in children: A prospective study. Pediatrics 1989;84:490–494.
131. Stenflo J, Suttie JW: Vitamin K-dependent formation of the γ-carboxyglutamic acid. Annu Rev Biochem 1977;46: 157–172.
132. Stevenson RE, Burton AM, Ferlauto GJ, et al: Hazards of oral anticoagulants during pregnancy. JAMA 1980; 243:1549–1551.
133. Stowe CM, Metz AL, Arendt TD, Schulman J: Apparent brodifacoum poisoning in a dog. J Am Vet Med Assoc 1983;182:817–818.
134. Sutcliffe FA, MacNicoll AD, Gibson GG: Aspects of anticoagulant action: A review of the pharmacology, metabolism and toxicology of warfarin and congeners. Drug Metabol Drug Interact 1987;5:225–271.
135. Suttie JW: Warfarin and vitamin K. Clin Cardiol 1990;13:16–18.
136. Suttie JW, Jackson CM: Prothrombin structure, activation, and biosynthesis. Physiol Rev 1977;57:1–70.
137. Swigar ME, Clemow LP, Saidi P, Kim HC: Superwarfarin ingestion: A new problem in covert anticoagulant overdose. Gen Hosp Psychiatry 1990;12:309–312.
138. Tait RC: Oral anticoagulation in paediatric patients: Dose requirements and complications. Arch Dis Child 1996; 74:228–231.
139. Travis SF, Warfield W, Breenbaum BH, et al: Spontaneous hemorrhage associated with accidental brodifacoum poisoning in a child. J Pediatr 1993;122:982–984.
140. Udall JA: Don't use the wrong vitamin K. West J Med 1970;112:65–67.
141. Vigano D'Angelo S, Comp PC, Esmon CT, et al: Relationship between protein C antigen and anticoagulant activity during oral anticoagulation and in selected disease states. J Clin Invest 1984;77:416–425.
142. Wakefield TW, Andrews PC, Wrobleski SK, et al: Effective and less toxic reversal of low-molecular weight heparin anticoagulation by a designer variant of protamine. J Vasc Surg 1995;21:839–849.
143. Wakefield TW, Andrews PC, Wrobleski SK, et al: A [+18RGD] protamine variant for nontoxic and effective reversal of conventional heparin and low-molecular-weight heparin anticoagulation. J Surg Res 1995;63:280–286.
144. Wallace S, Paull P, Worsnop C, Mashford ML: Covert self poisoning with brodifacoum, a "superwarfarin." Aust NZ J Med 1990;20:713–715.
145. Warkentin TE, Levine MN, Hirsh J, et al: Heparin-induced thrombocytopenia in patients treated with low-molecular-weight heparin or unfractionated heparin. N Engl J Med 1995;332:1330–1335.
146. Watts RG, Castleberry RP, Sadowski JA: Accidental poisoning with a superwarfarin compound (brodifacoum) in a child. Pediatrics 1990;86:883–887.
147. Weitzel JN, Sadowski JA, Furie BC, et al: Surreptitious ingestion of a long-acting vitamin K antagonist/rodenticide, brodifacoum: Clinical and metabolic studies in three cases. Blood 1990;76:2555–2559.
148. Wessler S, Gitel SN: Warfarin: From bedside to bench. N Engl J Med 1984;311:645–652.
149. White HD: Comparative safety of thrombolytic agents. Am J Cardiol 1991;67:30E–37E.
150. White RH, McKittrick T, Takakuwa J, et al: Management and prognosis of life-threatening bleeding during warfarin therapy. National Consortium of Clinical Anticoagulation. Arch Intern Med 1996;156:1197–1201.
151. Whitlon DS, Sadowski JA, Suttie JW: Mechanisms of coumarin action: Significance of vitamin K epoxide reductase inhibition. Biochemistry 1978;17:1371–1377.
152. Woody BJ, Murphy MJ, Ray AC, Green RA: Coagulopathic effects and therapy of brodifacoum toxicosis in dogs. J Vet Intern Med 1992;6:23–28.
153. Young MA, Ehrenpreis ED, Ehrenpreis M, et al: Heparin-associated thrombocytopenia and thrombosis syndrome in a rehabilitation patient. Arch Phys Med Rehabil 1989; 70:468–470.

ANTIDOTES IN DEPTH

Vitamin K

Mary Ann Howland

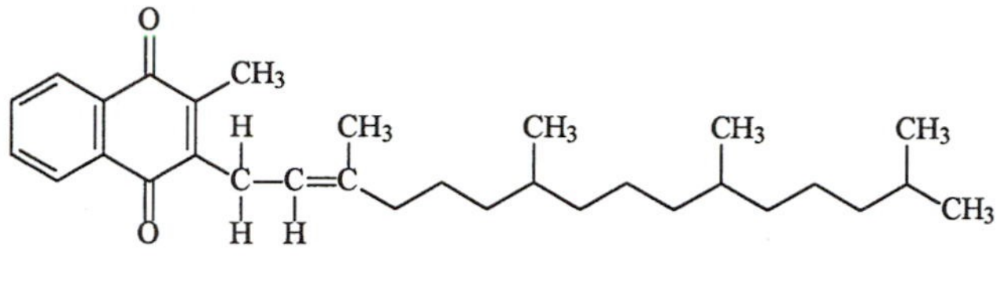

Vitamin K_1

It was noted in 1929 that chickens fed a poor diet developed spontaneous bleeding. In 1935, Dam and coworkers discovered that incorporating a fat-soluble substance in the chickens' diet could correct the bleeding. They named this substance a "koagulation factor," vitamin K.[7,11] Vitamin K, an essential fat-soluble vitamin, is actually a broad term encompassing at least two distinct natural forms. Vitamin K_1 (phytonadione, phylloquinone) is the only form synthesized by plants and algae. Vitamin K_2 (menaquinones) is a series of compounds with the same 2-methyl-1,4-naphthoquinone ring structure as phylloquinone but with a variable number (1 to 13) of repeating 5 carbon units on the side chain (Table 42–4). The menaquinones are synthesized by bacteria. Most of the vitamin K ingested in the diet is phylloquinone.

Activation of the coagulation factors II, VII, IX, and X requires gamma carboxylation of the glutamate residues, a vitamin K-dependent process. Only the reduced (quinol) form of vitamin K manifests biologic activity (see Fig. 42–2). The quinone form of vitamin K can be activated to the quinol form directly by an NADPH-dependent pathway that is relatively insensitive to warfarin.[11,14] During the carboxylation step, the K quinol form is converted to an epoxide. This 2,3-epoxide is reduced and recycled to the active K quinol in a two-step process that is inhibited by warfarin. An in-depth model of the chemical basis of this reaction has recently been proposed.[4]

The human daily requirement for vitamin K is small; the Food and Nutrition Board set the recommended daily allowance at 1 μg/kg per day of phylloquinone for adults, although 10 times that amount is required by infants to maintain normal hemostasis. Other vitamin K-dependent extrahepatic enzymatic reactions include the synthesis of osteocalcin, matrix G_{la} protein, plaque G_{la} protein, and one or more renal G_{la} proteins.[11,14]

Vitamin K deficiency can result from inadequate intake, malabsorption, or interference with the vitamin K cycle. Malnourishment and any condition in which bile salts or fatty acids are inadequate, such as extrahepatic cholestasis or severe pancreatic insufficiency, can lead to vitamin K deficiency. Newborns are at risk for hemor-

TABLE 42–4. VITAMIN K PRODUCTS

	Commercial Preparation	Route of Administration	Strength	Comments
Vitamin K_1 (phylloquinone, phytonadione)	Mephyton	Oral	5 mg	Best for anticoagulant-induced prolonged prothrombin time.
	Aqua Mephyton	SQ, IM, IV	2 mg/mL 10 mg/mL	Oral route preferred; divided doses may be necessary for large requirements; IV reserved for life-threatening situations.
	Konakion	IM	2 mg/mL 10 mg/mL	Must be carefully diluted and slowly infused (IV) to avoid anaphylactoid reactions; SQ for small doses; IM should be avoided; may be used for infants, pregnant women, G-6-PD deficiency; oral absorption requires presence of bile salts.
Vitamin K_3 (precursor to vitamin K_2, menaquinone)	Menadione	Oral	5 mg	Inferior to K_1 for anticoagulant-induced bleeding or prolonged prothrombin time; not used for neonates, pregnant women, G-6-PD deficient patients; absorbed in absence of bile salts.
Vitamin K_4	Menadiol sodium diphosphate	Oral SQ, IM, IV	5 mg 5 mg/mL 10 mg/mL 37.5 mg/mL	See Vitamin K_3. 50% of vitamin K_3 potency.

rhage for the following reasons: (1) phylloquinone does not readily cross the placenta; (2) breast milk contains less phylloquinone than vitamin K-fortified formula; (3) fetal hepatic stores of phylloquinone are low; and (4) maternal anticonvulsant therapy leads to increased vitamin K metabolism and may be contributory.[11,14] Although menaquinones are produced in the colon by bacteria, it is unlikely that enteric production contributes significantly to vitamin K stores or that eradication of the bacteria with antibiotics, without a coexistent dietary deficiency of vitamin K, results in deficiency.[11] Determination of vitamin K deficiency is usually established on the basis of a prolonged prothrombin time (PT) or INR, an indirect measure. Direct measurement of serum vitamin K levels has been technically difficult and probably does not adequately reflect hepatic stores.[11,14]

Oral anticoagulants are vitamin K antagonists that interfere with the vitamin K cycle, causing the accumulation of vitamin K 2,3-epoxide, an inactive metabolite. Warfarin is a strong inhibitor of the dithiol-dependent vitamin K reductases, which maintain vitamin K in its active (quinol) form. The superwarfarins are even more potent vitamin K reductase inhibitors. Other compounds have varying degrees of vitamin K antagonistic activity and include the *N*-methyl-thiotetrazole side chain containing antibiotics (moxalactam, cefamandole) and salicylates (weak).[11]

Dietary vitamin K in the form of phylloquinone and menaquinones are solubilized with the bile salts, free fatty acids, and monoglycerides to enhance absorption. Vitamin K, bound to chylomicrons, enters the circulation via the lymphatic system and then is taken up by the liver.[11] Plasma vitamin K is primarily in the form of phylloquinone, whereas liver stores are 90% menaquinones and 10% phylloquinone.[11] Following 3 days of low vitamin K intake, a group of surgical patients showed a fourfold lowering of liver vitamin K concentrations.[13] Rats given a vitamin K-deficient diet developed severe bleeding within 2 to 3 weeks.

Vitamin K products that are marketed are listed in Table 42–4. Vitamin K_1 (phylloquinone, phytonadione) is the only vitamin K preparation that should be used to reverse anticoagulant-induced vitamin K deficiency or to treat infants, pregnant women, or patients with glucose 6-phosphate dehydrogenase (G-6-PD) deficiency. Vitamin K_1 is superior to other commercially available vitamin K preparations not only because it is more active, thus requiring comparatively smaller doses, but because it works more rapidly (6 versus 12 hours).[6,12] Vitamin K_3 (menadione) and K_4 (menadiol sodium diphosphate) may produce hemolysis, hyperbilirubinemia, and kernicterus in neonates and hemolysis in G-6-PD-deficient patients. The only advantage of menadione and menadiol sodium diphosphate is that they are absorbed directly from the intestine by a passive process that does not require the presence of bile salts. Therefore, in patients with cholestasis or severe pancreatic insufficiency, these agents may be advantageous. They are neither interchangeable with vitamin K_1 nor a substitute for vitamin K_1 when anticoagulants such as warfarin or the superwarfarins are responsible for coagulation deficits.

The pharmacokinetics of vitamin K have been studied in healthy volunteers, brodifacoum-anticoagulated rabbits, and a patient poisoned with brodifacoum.[9] In the volunteers and a poisoned patient, a 10-mg IV dose of vitamin K_1 had a half-life of 1.7 hours. After oral administration of doses of 10 and 50 mg of vitamin K_1, peaks of 100 to 400 ng/mL and 200 to 2000 ng/mL, respectively, occurred at 3 to 5 hours. Bioavailability varied significantly between patients (10 to 65%) for both doses and in individual patients with the 50-mg dose. In maximally brodifacoum-anticoagulated rabbits, IV vitamin K_1 (10 mg/kg) increased prothrombin complex activity (PCA) from 14 to 50% by 4 hours and to 100% at 9 hours, after which it declined with a half-life of 6 hours. The minimum effective concentration of vitamin K_1 was approximately 1 μg/mL. High doses of oral vitamin K_1 were used to treat a patient anticoagulated with brodifacoum.[2] In this patient, a serum vitamin K_1 concentration as low as 200 ng/mL (0.2 μg/mL) was effective in maintaining a normal coagulation profile. This corresponded to 150 mg of vitamin K_1 every 6 hours. Lower doses were not initially evaluated.

Vitamin K_1 may be administered orally, subcutaneously, intramuscularly, or intravenously. The oral route is preferred when possible. Subcutaneous administration is limited to about 5 mL, the amount that can be physically injected at any one administration site. The intramuscular route is best avoided in patients who are anticoagulated and at risk for hematoma formation. The only preparation available for intravenous administration is Aqua Mephyton. This is not available in solution but as an aqueous colloidal suspension of a polyoxyethylated fatty acid derivative dextrose, and benzyl alcohol. Aqua Mephyton is specially formulated as a colloidal suspension due to the vitamin's lipid solubility. Intravenous administration has resulted in death secondary to anaphylactoid reactions, probably as a result of the preparation's colloidal formulation.[1,3,8] The time necessary for PT or INR to return to a safe or normal range depends on the rate of absorption of the vitamin K_1, the plasma concentration achieved, and the time necessary for the synthesis of activated clotting factors. Maintenance of a normal PT or INR depends on the half-life of the vitamin K_1, maintenance of an effective plasma concentration, and the half-life of the anticoagulant involved. The IV route is only slightly faster than the oral route in restoring PT to a safe range because oral absorption takes approximately 2 to 3 hours. If the oral route is not feasible and the dose requirements exceed the 5 mL of subcutaneous administration (ie, > 50 mg) then the intravenous route may be used for an initial dose. To minimize the risk of an anaphylactoid reaction, the preparation should be diluted with preservative-free 5% dextrose, 0.9% sodium chloride, or 5% dextrose in 0.9% sodium chloride, and administered slowly, at a rate not to exceed 1 mg/min in adults.

Oral vitamin K_1 (phytonadione, phylloquinone) is absorbed in an energy-dependent saturable process in the proximal small intestine.[9] Because of this mechanism and its short half-life, divided daily doses should be more effective than single daily doses, especially where requirements are very large. These absorptive and kinetic variables probably explain why it is frequently suggested that patients cannot be adequately managed with oral vitamin K_1 therapy.

The dose and duration of vitamin K_1 necessary to restore and maintain a normal PT or INR varies, depending on vitamin K_1 pharmacokinetics as well as the amount of anticoagulant ingested and whether the patient ingested a warfarin or superwarfin anticoagulant.[10] Reported cases have required as much as 125 mg daily for weeks to months.[5]

A reasonable starting approach in an adult is 50 to 100 mg of vitamin K_1, orally 3 to 4 times a day for 1 to 2 days. The PT or INR should be monitored and the vitamin K_1 dose modified accordingly. If the oral route is impractical, then either a subcutaneous dose of 25 to 50 mg should be given or an intravenous dose of 25 to 50 mg should be diluted and administered slowly as described; preparations should be made for treating an anaphylactoid reaction. Because the duration of action of vitamin K_1 is short-lived, this dose must be repeated 2 to 4 times daily. The onset of the effect of vitamin K_1 is not immediate, regardless of the route of administration; therefore, significant bleeding should be managed acutely with fresh frozen plasma. The risks of anaphylactoid reaction from the IV administration of vitamin K_1 and hematoma formation from IM administration are substantial concerns.

From a practical perspective, vitamin K_1 is available orally as a 5-mg tablet, requiring the adult patient to consume 10 to 30 tablets every 6 to 8 hours.

References

1. Barash P, Kitahata LM, Mandel S: Acute cardiovascular collapse after intravenous phytonadione. Anesth Analg 1976; 55:304–306.
2. Bruno GR, Hoffman RS, Howland MA: Elimination kinetics of brodifacoum and serum vitamin K_1 concentrations in long-acting anticoagulant (LAA) overdose. J Toxicol Clin Toxicol 1996;34:568. Abstract.
3. De la Rubia J, Grau E, Montserrat I, et al: Anaphylactic shock and vitamin K_1. Ann Intern Med 1989;110:943.
4. Dowd P, Ham SW, Naganathan S, et al: The mechanism of action of Vitamin K. Annu Rev Nutr 1995;15:419–440.
5. Exner DV, Brien WF, Murphy MJ: Superwarfarin ingestion. Can Med J 1992;146:34–35.
6. Gamble JR, Dennis EW, Coon WW, et al: Clinical comparison of vitamin K_1 and water-soluble vitamin K. Arch Intern Med 1955;5:52–58.
7. Marcus R, Coulston AM: Water-soluble vitamins: The vitamin B complex and ascorbic acid. In: Gilman AG, Rall TW, Nies AS, Taylor P, eds: Goodman and Gilman's The Pharmacological Basis of Therapeutics, 8th ed. New York, Pergamon, 1990, pp. 1563–1566.
8. Mattea E, Quinn K: Adverse reactions after intravenous phytonadione administration. Hosp Pharm 1981;16: 230–235.
9. Park BK, Scott AK, Wilson AC, et al: Plasma disposition of Vitamin K_1 in relation to anticoagulant poisoning. Br J Clin Pharmacol 1984;18:655–662.
10. Routh CR, Triplett DA, Murphy MJ, et al: Superwarfarin ingestion and detection. Am J Hematol 1991;36:50–54.
11. Shearer MJ: Vitamin K metabolism and nutrition. Blood Rev 1992;6:92–104.
12. Udall JA: Don't use the wrong vitamin K. West J Med 1970; 112:65–67.
13. Usuri Y, Taminura M, Nishimura, N, et al: Vitamin K concentrations in the plasma and liver of surgical patients. Am J Clin Nutr 1990;51:846–852.
14. Vermeer C, Hamulyak K: Pathophysiology of vitamin K deficiency and oral anticoagulants. Thromb Haemost 1991; 66:153–159.

ANTIDOTES IN DEPTH

Protamine

Mary Ann Howland

Although protamine was approved for use as an antidote for heparin in 1968, its characteristics were recognized 30 years earlier.[35] The protamines are a group of simple basic proteins found in fish sperm. Commercially available protamine sulfate is derived from the sperm of mature testes of salmon and related species. On hydrolysis it yields basic amino acids, particularly arginine, proline, serine, and valine, but not tyrosine and tryptophan.

Heparin is a large electronegative substance that is rapidly complexed by the electropositive protamine, forming an inactive salt. Heparin binds to antithrombin III (AT III), altering its stereochemistry and thereby catalyzing the subsequent inactivation of thrombin and other clotting factors. Immunoelectrophoresis demonstrates that due to its net positive charge, protamine has a greater affinity for heparin than AT III, thereby producing a dissociation of the heparin–AT III complex in favor of a protamine–heparin complex.[36]

Since the advent of cardiopulmonary bypass surgery, protamine has been routinely employed in the neutralization of heparin at the completion of the procedure. It is largely in this setting that the adverse effects of protamine are also documented and studied.[17,18,30] Nearly 100 deaths have been attributed to the use of protamine under these circumstances. These adverse effects include both rate-related and non-rate-related hypotension,[8–11,13,21,24,39,40] anaphylactic[20] and anaphylactoid reactions,[23,32,34] bradycardia,[1] thrombocytopenia,[46] leukopenia, decreased oxygen consumption,[43,45] and anticoagulant effects.[2]

The mechanisms for these adverse effects are multifactorial: the strong net positive charge of protamine may be responsible for some of the adverse effects and probably directly injures a variety of organelles, including platelets.[5,47] It is believed that activation of the arachidonic acid pathway is responsible for some of the hemodynamic changes, because pretreatment with indomethacin limits these effects.[7,16,33,47] Free protamine or protamine complexed with heparin can convert *L*-arginine to endothelium-derived relaxing factor (nitric oxide), which in turn causes vasodilation and inhibits platelet aggregation and adhesion.[37] Protamine administered in the absence of heparin or in an amount exceeding that necessary for heparin neutralization, can act as an anticoagulant and may inhibit platelet function with a resultant weaker clot.[3,22] This anticoagulant effect may result from effects on factor VII and/or AT III.

Risk factors for protamine-induced adverse reactions include prior exposure (eg, during a previous surgery), vasectomy, or a history of allergy to fish. Diabetic patients receiving daily subcutaneous injections of a protamine-containing insulin (NPH) have a 40 to 50% increased risk of adverse reactions.[12,15,20,41] The resultant elevation of histamine levels, the activation of complement, and elevated IgE, IgA, and IgG levels are also suggested as mechanisms for the adverse effects.[29,42,48,49] Occasionally patients manifesting a protamine allergy are presumed to have insulin allergy.[27] In diabetic patients receiving protamine insulin injections, the presence of serum antiprotamine IgE antibody is a significant risk factor for acute protamine reactions. Only patients with previous exposure to protamine insulin injections had serum antiprotamine IgE antibodies. However, in the group without previous protamine insulin exposure, antiprotamine IgG antibody was noted as a risk factor for protamine reactions.[49] Either naturally occurring cross-reacting antibodies or more likely previous unrecognized protamine exposure was responsible for the generation of these IgG antibodies.

There are limited options for the reversal of heparin in patients who have previously experienced anaphylaxis following protamine therapy or those who are expected to be at high risk for a protamine reaction. Clotting factors may be replaced and protamine avoided, or protamine may be used while preparing to treat anaphylaxis expectantly. Several alternatives are being investigated and include the placement of heparin removal devices in the extracorporeal circuit, as well as the use of hexadimethrine, methylene blue (incomplete reversal in vitro), platelet factor 4, and heparinase as antidotes.[26] Pretreatment with antihistamines and corticosteroids may be sufficient for immune mediated mechanisms, but will probably not be beneficial for pulmonary vasoconstriction and nonimmune-mediated anaphylactoid reactions.[19]

A heparin rebound effect has been noted after cardiopulmonary bypass. This is an anticoagulant effect that recurs, and is attributed to the presence of detectable circulating heparin several hours after apparently adequate heparin neutralization with protamine. The incidence of heparin rebound and the need for additional protamine (range, 4 to 42%) vary, depending on the neutralization protocol.[14,31,38] The effects of protamine sulfate appear to be comparable to those of protamine chloride.[28] It is likely that larger heparin doses may prolong the clearance of heparin, contributing to higher than expected heparin levels.[38] When 300 U/kg body weight doses of heparin were reversed at the end of cardiopulmonary bypass with 3 mg/kg of protamine, a 14% incidence of small but detectable concentrations of circulating heparin were noted at 2 hours, which lasted less than 1 hour in all but one case.[31] The prothrombin time was prolonged and thrombocytopenia was noted, but there was no increase in blood loss.

Protamine is most frequently used at the end of cardiopulmonary bypass operations to reverse the effects of heparin. There are many regimens used for protamine dosing, and they include (1) giving an arbitrary amount of protamine (eg, > 2mg/kg); (2) giving protamine in a ratio of 0.6 to 1.5:1 times the initial heparin dose, resulting in an activated coagulation time (ACT) of about 480 sec; and (3) giving protamine in a ratio of 0.75 to 2.1:1 times the total operative heparin dose.[50] Two new methods of calculating the protamine dose to improve accuracy and avoid excess protamine have been proposed.[22,50] One advocates an initial protamine dose based upon ACT with subsequent doses based on the ratio of the change in thrombin time to the heparin-neutralized thrombin time. If this ratio is greater than 12 seconds, 10-mg incremental protamine doses should be administered.[22] The other uses a nomogram based on heparin activity in mg/kg versus ACT.[50] Both methods ultimately demonstrated efficacy with 2 mg/kg doses of protamine, about one-half of the dose previously used. With these approaches, the ACT responded to protamine within 5 minutes, decreasing in value from 550 to 700 seconds to a control of 150 seconds.

Approximately 1 mg of protamine will neutralize about 100 U (1 mg) of heparin. A number of tests can directly measure heparin levels or indirectly measure heparin's effect on the clotting cascade.[4,6] These tests may be helpful in determining the appropriate dose of protamine. Because excessive protamine can act as an anticoagulant, the dose chosen should always be an underestimation of that which is needed. In case of unintentional overdose, the half-life of heparin should be considered, because half of the administered dose of heparin will be eliminated within 60 to 90 minutes. In the case of an unintentional overdose without bleeding, the short half-life of heparin and the potential risks of protamine administration usually argue for patient observation, rather than protamine reversal of anticoagulation. If protamine use is necessary to treat active bleeding, the dose must be administered intravenously over 15 minutes to limit rate-related hypotension.[25,44]

When faced with a patient believed to have received an overdose of an unknown quantity of heparin, the decision to use protamine should be made when the setting is correct, and a prolonged PTT and persistent bleeding are present. In each circumstance, evaluate the potential risks of protamine use (especially in those who have had a prior life-threatening reaction to protamine as well as in a diabetic receiving a protamine-containing insulin) and the risks of continued heparin anticoagulation. A baseline ACT, thrombin time, heparin-neutralized thrombin time, heparin activity, platelets, PT/PTT, and Hb/HCT should be obtained. Because of the routine nature of heparin reversal following cardiopulmonary bypass, consultation with members of the bypass team may be helpful. An empiric dose of protamine may be determined by the baseline ACT: (1) an ACT of 150 seconds necessitates no protamine; (2) an ACT of 200–300 seconds necessitates 0.6 mg/kg; and (3) an ACT of 300–400 seconds necessitates 1.2 mg/kg. These doses have not been tested outside the operating room. The ACT should be repeated 5 to 15 minutes following the protamine dose and further dosing based on this value. When the ACT is not available, 25 to 50 mg of protamine can be administered and adjusted accordingly.

Protamine is available either as a parenteral solution ready for injection or as a powder to be reconstituted with 5 mL of sterile or bacteriostatic water for injection. When the vials containing 50 mg of protamine are used, they should be shaken vigorously after the water is added. The final solution of either preparation contains 10 mg of protamine per mL. The dose should be administered intravenously slowly over 15 minutes with resuscitative equipment nearby.

References

1. Alvarez J, Alvarez L, Escudero C, Olivares JLC: Sinus node function and protamine sulfate. J Cardiothorac Anesth 1989;3:44–51.
2. Andersen MN, Mendelow M, Alfano GA: Experimental studies of heparin-protamine activity with special reference to protamine inhibition of clotting. Surgery 1959;46: 1060–1068.
3. Carr ME, Carr, SL: At high heparin concentrations, protamine concentrations which reverse heparin anticoagulant effects are insufficient to reverse heparin antiplatelet effects. Thromb Res 1994;75:617–630.
4. Castellani WJ, Hodges ED, Bode AP: Effect of protamine sulfate on the ACA heparin assay. Clin Chem 1991;37: 1119–1120.
5. Chang SW, Westcott JY, Henson JE, Voelkel NF: Pulmonary vascular injury by polycations in perfused rat lungs. J Appl Physiol 1987;62:1932–1943.
6. Chen W, Yang V: Versatile non-clotting based heparin assay requiring no instrumentation. Clin Chem 1991;37: 832–837.
7. Conzen PF, Habazettl H, Gutmann R, et al: Thromboxane mediation of pulmonary hemodynamic responses after neutralization of heparin by protamine in pigs. Anesth Analg 1989;68:25–31.
8. Fadali MA, Ledbetter M, Papacostas CA, et al: Mechanism responsible for the cardiovascular depressant effect of protamine sulfate. Ann Surg 1974;180:232–235.
9. Fadali MA, Papacostas CA, Duke JJ, et al: Cardiovascular depressant effect of protamine sulfate. Thorax 1976;31: 320–323.
10. Frater RMW, Oka Y, Hong Y, et al: Protamine-induced

circulatory changes. J Thorac Cardiovasc Surg 1984;87: 687–692.
11. Goldman BS, Joison J, Austen WG: Cardiovascular effects of protamine sulfate. Ann Thorac Cardiovasc Surg 1969; 7:459–471.
12. Gottschlich GM, Gravlee GP, Georgitis JW: Adverse reactions to protamine sulfate during cardiac surgery in diabetic and nondiabetic patients. Ann Allergy 1988;61: 277–281.
13. Gourin A, Streisand RL, Greineder JK, Stuckey JH: Protamine sulfate administration and the cardiovascular system. J Thorac Cardiovasc Surg 1971;62:193–204.
14. Gundry SR, Drongowski RA, Klein MD, et al: Postoperative bleeding in cardiovascular surgery: Does heparin rebound really exist? Am Surg 1989;55:162–165.
15. Gupta SK, Veith FJ, Wengerter KR, et al: Anaphylactoid reactions to protamine: An often lethal complication in insulin-dependent diabetic patients undergoing vascular surgery. J Vasc Surg 1989;9:342–350.
16. Hobbhahn J, Conzen PF, Zenker B, et al: Beneficial effect of cyclooxygenase inhibition on adverse hemodynamic responses after protamine. Anesth Analg 1988;67:253–260.
17. Holland CL, Singh AK, McMaster PRB, Fang W: Adverse reactions to protamine sulfate following cardiac surgery. Clin Cardiol 1984;7:157–162.
18. Horrow JC: Protamine: A review of its toxicity. Anesth Analg 1985;64:348–361.
19. Hughes C, Haddock M: Protamine reaction in a patient undergoing coronary artery bypass grafting. Clin Forum Nurse Anesth 1995;6:172–176.
20. Jackson DR: Sustained hypotension secondary to protamine sulfate. Angiology 1970;21:295–298.
21. Jastrebski MK, Sykes MK, Woods DG: Cardiorespiratory effects of protamine after cardiopulmonary bypass in man. Thorax 1974;20:534–538.
22. Jobes DR, Aitken GL, Shaffer GW: Increased accuracy and precision of heparin and protamine dosing reduces blood loss and transfusion in patients undergoing primary cardiac operations. J Thorac Cardiovasc Surg 1995;110:36–45.
23. Kambam JR, Merrill WH, Smith BE: $Histamine_2$ receptor blocker in the treatment of protamine related anaphylactoid reactions: Two case reports. Can J Anaesth 1989;36:463–465.
24. Katz NM, Kim YD, Siegelman R, et al: Hemodynamics of protamine administration. J Thorac Cardiovasc Surg 1987; 94:881–886.
25. Kien ND, Quam DD, Reitan JA, White DA: Mechanism of hypotension following rapid infusion of protamine sulfate in anesthetized dogs. J Cardiothorac Vasc Anesth 1992; 6:143–147.
26. Kikura M, Lee MK, Levy JH: Heparin neutralization with methylene blue, hexadimethrine, or vancomycin after cardiopulmonary bypass. Anesth Analg 1996;83:223–227.
27. Kim R: Anaphylaxis to protamine masquerading as an insulin allergy. Del Med J 1993;65:17–23.
28. Kuitunen AH, Salmenpera MT, Heinonen J, et al: Heparin rebound: A comparative study of protamine chloride and protamine sulfate in patients undergoing coronary artery bypass surgery. J Cardiothorac Vasc Anesth 1991;5:221–226.
29. Lakin JD, Blocker TJ, Strong DM, Yocum MW: Anaphylaxis to protamine sulfate mediated by a complement dependent IgG antibody. J Allergy Clin Immunol 1978;61:102–107.
30. Lindblad B: Protamine sulphate: A review of its effects—Hypersensitivity and toxicity. Eur J Vasc Surg 1989;3: 195–201.
31. Martin P, Horkay F, Gupta NK, et al: Heparin rebound phenomenon: Much ado about nothing. Blood Coagul Fibrinolysis 1992;3:187–191.
32. Moorthy SS, Pond W, Rowland RG: Severe circulatory shock following protamine (an anaphylactoid reaction). Anesth Analg 1980;59:77–78.
33. Morel DR, Zapol WM, Thomas SJ, et al: C5a and thromboxane generation associated with pulmonary vaso- and broncho-constriction during protamine reversal of heparin. Anesthesiology 1987;66:597–604.
34. Neidhart PP, Meier B, Polla BS, et al: Fatal anaphylactoid response to protamine after percutaneous transluminal coronary angioplasty. Eur Heart J 1992;13:856–858.
35. New Drug Application. Washington D.C., Food and Drug Administration, 1968; 6460, log 775.
36. Okajirna Y, Kanayama S, Maeda Y, et al: Studies on the neutralizing mechanism of antithrombin activity of heparin by protamine. Thromb Res 1981;24:21–29.
37. Pearson PJ, Evora PRB, Ayrancioglu K, Schaff HV: Protamine releases endothelium-derived relaxing factor from systemic arteries. Anesth Prog 1991;38:99–100.
38. Raul TK, Crow MJ, Rajah SM, et al: Heparin administration during extracorporeal circulation: Heparin rebound and postoperative bleeding. J Thorac Cardiovasc Surg 1979; 78:95–102.
39. Shapira N, Schaff HV, Piehler JM, et al: Cardiovascular effects of protamine sulfate in man. J Thorac Cardiovasc Surg 1982;84:505–514.
40. Stefaniszyn HJ, Novick RJ, Salerno TA: Toward a better understanding of the hemodynamic effects of protamine and heparin interaction. J Thorac Cardiovasc Surg 1984;87: 678–686.
41. Stewart WJ, McSweeney SM, Kellett MA, et al: Increased risk of severe protamine reactions in NPH insulin-dependent diabetics undergoing cardiac catheterization. Circulation 1984;70:788–792.
42. Stoelting RK, Henry DD, Verburg KM: Hemodynamic changes and circulating histamine concentrations following protamine administration to patients and dogs. Can Anaesth Soc J 1984;31:534–540.
43. Wakefield TW, Bies LE, Wrobleski SK, et al: Impaired myocardial function and oxygen utilization due to protamine sulfate in an isolated rabbit heart preparation. Ann Surg 1990;212:387–393.
44. Wakefield TW, Mantler CB, Wrobleski SK, et al: Effects of differing rates of protamine reversal of heparin anticoagulation. Surgery 1996;119:123–128.
45. Wakefield TW, Ucros I, Kresowik TF, et al: Decreased oxygen consumption as a toxic manifestation of protamine sulfate reversal of heparin anticoagulation. J Vasc Surg 1989;9:772–777.
46. Wakefield TW, Wrobleski SK, Nichol BJ, et al: Heparin-mediated reduction of the toxic effects of protamine sulfate on rabbit myocardium. J Vasc Surg 1992;16:47–53.

47. Wakefield TW, Wrobleski BS, Wirthlin DJ, et al: Increased prostacyclin and adverse hemodynamic responses to protamine sulfate in an experimental canine model. J Surg Res 1991;50:449–456.
48. Weiss ME, Chatham F, Kagey Sobotka A, Adkinson NF: Serial immunological investigations in a patient who had a life threatening reaction to intravenous protamine. Clin Exp Allergy 1990;20:713–720.
49. Weiss ME, Nyhan D, Zhikang P, et al: Association of protamine IgE and IgG antibodies with life-threatening reactions to intravenous protamine. N Engl J Med 1989;320: 886–892.
50. Wright SJ, Murray WB, Hampton WA, et al: Calculating the protamine-heparin reversal ratio. A pilot study investigating a new method. J Cardiothorac Vasc Anesth 1993;7: 416–421.

CHAPTER 43

Antituberculous Agents

Harold H. Osborn

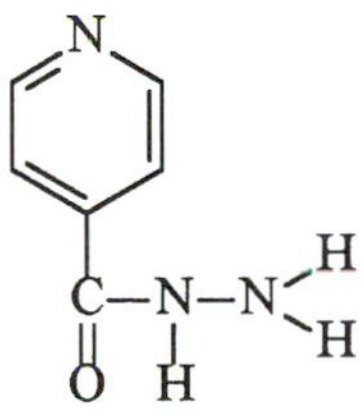

Isoniazid

A 24-year-old woman was found unconscious in her apartment by her brother. She had been despondent for several weeks. An ambulance was called and the patient was transported. On the way to the hospital the patient had a tonic-clonic seizure and became cyanotic. The ambulance personnel administered oxygen and inserted an oropharyngeal airway into her mouth.

On arrival in the emergency department (ED), the patient had a blood pressure of 130/90 mm Hg, a pulse of 100 beats/min, respiratory rate of 12 breaths/min, and a temperature of 101.1°F (38.4°C). The skin was warm, moist, and neither cyanotic nor jaundiced. The head was atraumatic and there were no marks on her body. The pupils were 3 mm bilaterally and reacted to light. The fundi were benign. Her neck was supple and she responded to deep pain. Oculocephalic reflexes were present. Reflexes were diffusely hyperactive, and bilateral plantar extension was present. The remainder of the physical examination was unremarkable.

An intravenous line was inserted and blood was sent for a complete blood count (CBC), electrolytes, glucose, BUN, and prothrombin time. Fifty mL of 50% dextrose in water, 2 mg of naloxone, and 100 mg of thiamine were administered intravenously without response. Because her gag reflex was absent, a cuffed endotracheal tube was inserted before orogastric lavage was performed. A 40 French orogastric tube was passed and the stomach was lavaged with several liters of 0.9% sodium chloride solution. A slurry containing 60 g of activated charcoal and 50 mL of 70% sorbitol was then instilled in the stomach and the orogastric tube removed.

Shortly after the initial treatment, the patient had another generalized seizure, which lasted for 5 minutes after the administration of 10 mg of diazepam IV. Without regaining consciousness she had several more seizures. A total of 500 mg of phenobarbital was given intravenously, but the seizures persisted. The CBC, urinalysis, and prothrombin time were all within normal limits. She had a glucose of 97 mg/dL; BUN, 9 mg/dL; sodium, 145 mEq/L; potassium, 4.4 mEq/L; chloride, 97 mEq/L; and HCO_3, 18 mEq/L (anion gap 30). An arterial blood gas analysis showed pH, 7.32; PCO_2, 32 mm Hg; and PO_2, 90 mm Hg. An acetaminophen level was negative. The ECG revealed a sinus tachycardia.

As soon as the patient's brother arrived in the ED, he stated the patient was taking isoniazid (INH). The patient was then given 5 g of pyridoxine hydrochloride and an additional 10 mg of diazepam IV. The seizures abruptly terminated and the patient was admitted to the intensive care unit. She awoke several hours after admission and stated she wanted to die and had purposely ingested a full bottle of tablets (30 300-mg tablets, or 9 g of INH). The patient did well and had no further seizures. Because she was judged to be severely depressed and still suicidal, arrangements were made to transfer her to a psychiatric unit.

Epidemiology

Because of the recent epidemic of tuberculosis (TB) there has been an increase in isoniazid (INH) use, with consequent overdoses and accidental toxicity. Isoniazid is among the most common causes of drug-induced seizures in the United States.[46] An estimated 1.8 billion people worldwide are infected with tuberculosis, with 10 million new cases and 1 million deaths reported each year.[6,70] In the United States, where the TB rate had been declining for 30 years, it began to increase in 1984. This increase was halted by 1994 in some cities such as New York due to better completion of treatment and the expansion of directly observed therapy.[25] In some communities the incidence is increasing at an alarming rate, especially among children,[34] adults aged 25 to 44 years, and minorities.[6] The acquired immunodeficiency syndrome (AIDS) epidemic has contributed to the increase in TB and to the emergence of multiple drug resistant strains of mycobacteria.[50] Populations at risk for TB and presumably INH toxicity include immigrants from Southeast Asia, Inuits, Native Americans, alcoholics, intravenous drug users, the homeless, people living in overcrowded conditions, and HIV-positive patients. Physicians must be aware of the potential for INH toxicity in these groups. Whenever a patient, especially from one of the high-risk groups, presents to the ED with altered consciousness, agitation, seizures, or coma, INH overdose must be considered. As INH is more frequently prescribed, chronic toxicity also becomes more common, and the practitioner must be able to recognize the adverse effects of this medication.

What Are the Pharmacokinetics of Isoniazid?

Isoniazid is the hydrazide of isonicotinic acid. Following the discovery, in 1945, that nicotinamide possessed tuberculostatic action, other biologically active derivatives of nicotinamide were sought. One of the first intermediates synthesized was isonicotinyl hydrazide (INH). Isoniazid is rapidly absorbed from the GI tract, with peak levels developing within 1 to 2 hours. Following absorption, INH distributes into all body fluids and cells with an apparent volume of distribution of 0.6 L/kg. Isoniazid has little protein binding (10%), and 75 to 95% of a dose of INH is excreted in the urine within 24 hours, mostly as metabolites.

Isoniazid undergoes enzymatic transformation in the liver. The main metabolic pathway involves acetylation followed by hydrolysis (Fig. 43–1). The principal

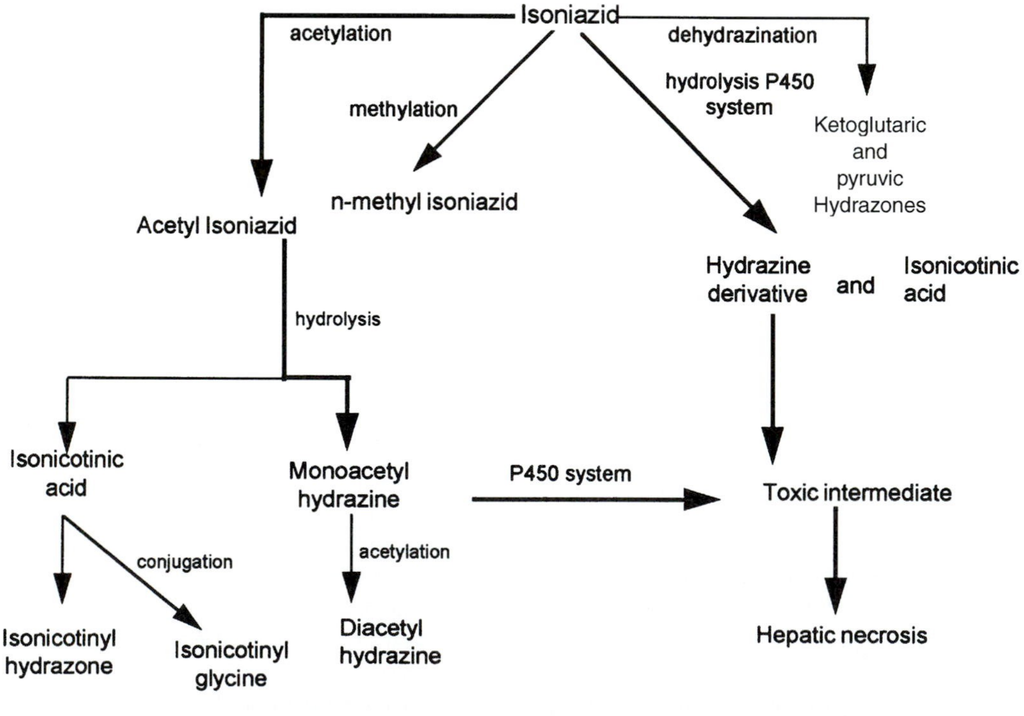

Figure 43–1. Isoniazid metabolism in detail. Bold arrows demonstrate the roles of acetylation and cytochrome P450 in the generation of hepatotoxicity. *(Adapted, with permission, from Ellenhorn MJ, Barceloux DG: Medical Toxicology: Diagnosis and Treatment of Human Poisoning. New York, Elsevier, 1988, p. 366; and Hitchings GH, Burchall JJ: Inhibition of folate biosynthesis and function as a basis for chemotherapy. Adv Enzymol 27:419, 1965.)*

metabolites, acetyl isoniazid and isonicotinic acid, are renally excreted along with small quantities of an isonicotinic acid conjugate (isonicotinyl glycine), isonicotinyl hydrazones, and traces of methylisoniazid.

Humans show a genetically determined heterogeneity with regard to the rate of acetylation of isoniazid based on the activity of the enzyme acetyltransferase.[23] The acetylation rate varies with race but is not influenced by sex or age. This rate determines the half-life of the parent compound in the circulation, and the half-life is also prolonged with hepatic dysfunction. The plasma half-life is 0.7 hours in rapid acetylators and 2 to 4 hours in slow acetylators.[32] Fast acetylation is found in up to 95% of Inuits, Japanese, Chinese, and blacks, while slow acetylation is the predominant phenotype in most Scandinavians and North African Caucasians. The incidence of slow acetylation in the general U.S. population is estimated to be approximately 50%.[37] Fast acetylation, which is inherited as an autosomal dominant trait, permits "fast acetylators" or "rapid inactivators" to have, on average, 30 to 50% of the plasma concentration of INH found in "slow acetylators" or "slow inactivators." Slow acetylators may accumulate substantial amounts of the drug if they have concomitant renal dysfunction, but even azotemic patients with serum creatinine levels in the range of 12 mg/dL tolerate the 300 mg/day of INH normally prescribed for adult patients without consequential manifestations.[9]

What Are the Mechanisms of Action and Toxicity of Isoniazid?

The mechanism of action of INH has not yet been fully elucidated. Hypotheses center on its ability to affect lipid metabolism, nucleic acid biosynthesis, and glycolysis. Its primary action may be to inhibit the synthesis of mycolic acids, which are unique to mycobacteria and are important constituents of their cell walls. Only tubercle bacilli take up the drug, and this uptake is an active process. Isoniazid has a variety of both acute and chronic toxic effects. Much of INH's toxicity, especially the neurotoxicity, is mediated by an INH-induced reduction in the activity of pyridoxine, a cofactor in the synthesis and metabolism of important amino acids. Other toxic effects, such as the hepatotoxic effects, are mediated directly by the products of INH metabolism.

The toxic effects of INH on the human nervous system were recognized almost as soon as the drug became available. In the mid-1950s, evidence began to accumulate to suggest that the neurotoxicity of INH was due to vitamin B_6 (pyridoxine) depletion.[69] Pyridoxine is vital to cellular metabolism and the utilization of amino acids and serves as a cofactor in more than 40 enzyme systems.[68] The frequent occurrence of seizures in infants suffering from a dietary deficiency of pyridoxine is a well-known phenomenon. Because INH seizures were also

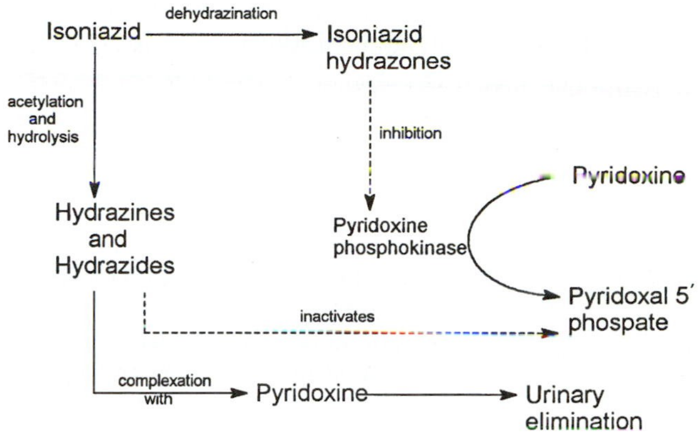

Figure 43–2. The effect of isoniazid on pyridoxine leading to reduced activation and diminished supply of pyridoxine.

noted to be responsive to pyridoxine, vitamin B_6 antagonism was implicated.

In the liver, pyridoxine is phosphorylated by a specific kinase and then oxidized to pyridoxal phosphate, the active form, by a flavoprotein. Isoniazid affects the availability of pyridoxine in a variety of ways. It combines directly with pyridoxine and forms an isonicotinylhydrazide complex that is excreted in the urine (Fig. 43–2).[52] It also forms hydrazones that inhibit pyridoxine phosphokinase, the enzyme that converts pyridoxine to its active form.[4] Finally, INH hydrazides inactivate pyridoxal 5′-phosphate, rendering it ineffective. This interference with the activation and supply of pyridoxine results in a reduction in the synthesis of GABA, which requires pyridoxal phosphate as a cofactor (Fig. 43–3). In addition, INH causes an increase in the transamination of existing GABA to alpha-ketoglutaric acid. Gamma-aminobutyric acid is the main inhibitory neurotransmitter of the central nervous system, and a decrease in the availability of GABA, with resultant loss of its vital inhibitory influence, is the presumed etiology of INH-induced seizures.[67]

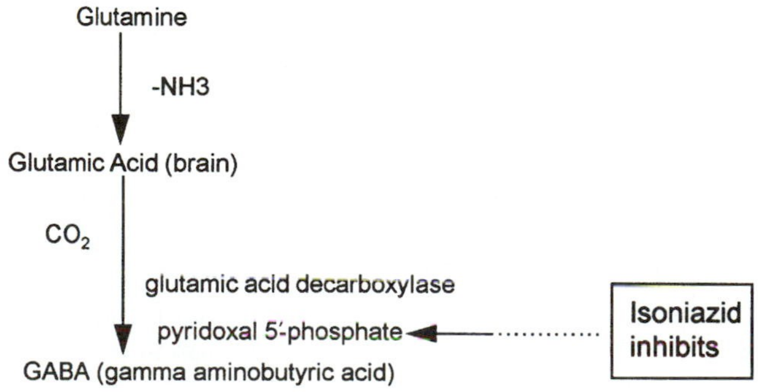

Figure 43–3. The mechanism of the inactivation of pyridoxal 5′-phosphate resulting in the reduction of the synthesis of GABA.

What Are the Clinical Manifestations of Acute INH Toxicity?

Acute INH overdose is characterized by the clinical triad of seizures refractory to conventional therapy, metabolic acidosis, and persistent coma.[11,18,33,62] Following an acute overdose, nausea, vomiting, dizziness, hyperthermia, and hypotension may also be seen. (Table 43–1)[57] Hyperglycemia, glycosuria, ketonemia, and ketonuria are reported and can mimic diabetic ketoacidosis.[59] Patients are usually symptomatic within 30 to 45 minutes of ingestion; however, symptoms may be delayed for up to 2 hours when peak absorption occurs.

TABLE 43–1. TOXICITY OF ISONIAZID

	Acute	Chronic
Cardiovascular	Cyanosis Hypotension Shock Tachycardia	
Gastrointestinal	Nausea Vomiting	Anorexia Constipation Hepatitis Liver failure Nausea Vomiting
Hematologic	Leukocytosis	ANA (positive) Anemia Hemolysis Agranulocytosis Eosinophilia Methemoglobinemia
Metabolic	Hyperthermia Lactic acidosis Hyperglycemia, ketonemia Elevated beta-hydroxybutyrate	
Musculoskeletal		Arthralgias Arthritis Backache
Neurologic	Altered mental status Ataxia Coma Dizziness Hallucinations Hyperreflexia Psychosis Seizures Slurred speech	Vertigo Insomnia Psychosis Pellagra Peripheral neuropathy
Ophthalmic	Keratitis Nystagmus Mydriasis Blurred vision Photophobia	Optic neuritis Optic atrophy
Renal	Oliguria Anuria	Urinary retention

Usually INH-induced seizures are generalized tonic-clonic but may be focal. Seizures frequently occur within the first 2 hours and often develop into status epilepticus that is refractory to anticonvulsants.[11,14,68] The metabolic acidosis is often quite severe, is associated with a high anion gap, and the major component of this acidosis is the accumulation of lactate secondary to seizure activity.[3,14,68] INH may also block the conversion of lactate to pyruvate by interfering with nicotinamide-adenine dinucleotide (NAD), which is a cofactor for the enzyme lactate dehydrogenase that catalyzes this reaction. Although this effect may occur in vitro, the evidence is weak for a significant in vivo effect. Isoniazid has also been linked to an increase in production of beta-hydroxybutyric acid.[47]

Ingestions of less than 1.5 g of INH in adults are usually associated with mild toxicity, while those of 10 g or more are often fatal.[59] Toxic doses of INH are variable. In general, toxicity occurs with doses as low as 10 to 30 mg/kg, seizures occur with doses greater than 20 mg/kg, and death may occur at doses in excess of 50 mg/kg.[45] The LD_{50} of INH in humans is estimated to be 80 to 150 mg/kg.[45] Patients with underlying seizure disorders are at greater risk and have been reported to manifest seizures at doses as low as 14 mg/kg.[45] Mortality rates in the overdose setting are also variable but have been reported to be as high as 20% with significant ingestions[11]; permanent brain damage has been described in survivors.[66]

What Is the Management of Patients With Isoniazid Overdoses?

Patients with massive INH ingestions should be treated with vigorous life support techniques. Airway protection in the setting of seizures or coma is essential. In the actively seizing patient the next priority is seizure control. When the airway is secured and the seizures are controlled, orogastric lavage and treatment with activated charcoal are indicated. Syrup of ipecac is contraindicated, due to the possibility of seizures and aspiration. Since INH is absorbed rapidly, gastrointestinal (GI) evacuation and activated charcoal administration must not be delayed. Activated charcoal has been shown to block the absorption of INH in normal volunteers.[58] The use of multiple-dose activated charcoal (MDAC) has never been studied but would be a reasonable therapeutic modality for the severely ill patient.

Seizing patients should immediately be given 1 g of pyridoxine IV for each gram of INH ingested to a maximum of 5 g, at a rate of 1 g every 2 to 3 minutes. If seizures are controlled before the full amount has been given, the remainder may be mixed with D_5W and infused more slowly. Because pyridoxine is rapidly excreted, it may be beneficial to administer the drug by slow infusion. If the amount of INH ingested is unknown, a dose of 5 g may be administered to an adult or 70 mg/kg to a maximum of 5 g in a child.[11,33] This dose may be repeated if seizures recur. In a classic study of massive INH overdoses among Inuits in Alaska, all patients given large doses of pyridoxine survived.[11] If no parenteral form of pyridoxine is available, pyridoxine tablets may be crushed and administered orally as a slurry in the same dose. Patients who have taken an overdose of INH and who are asymptomatic should be observed for 6 hours, since toxicity usually develops in this time.

Theoretically, gamma-aminobutyric acid (GABA)-enhancing anticonvulsants should be beneficial in the management of INH-induced seizures. In practice, these agents, especially diazepam, have proven utility, but often they are not completely effective and numerous cases of INH seizures refractory to anticonvulsant therapy are described.[18] In animal studies of INH-induced seizures, diazepam alone is not completely protective.[15] However, the combination of diazepam and pyridoxine is both synergistic and protective.[13,15] The administration of pyridoxine to an INH-poisoned patient restores the deficiency in GABA. GABA increases the benzodiazepine affinity on the BZD binding site of the GABA receptor complex. Benzodiazepines increase the affinity of GABA for the GABA binding site of the GABA receptor and increase the frequency of opening of the chloride ionophore. Thus, the effects of pyridoxine and a benzodiazepine are synergistic.

Phenytoin, which works mainly by blocking rate and frequency-dependent sodium channels, is ineffective in the treatment of INH seizures and is therefore not recommended in this setting.[51] The clinician should suspect the possibility of an INH overdose whenever a patient presents with seizures that are resistant to treatment. Hospitals and EDs should be well stocked with sufficient amounts of pyridoxine to treat these patients. The empiric administration of pyridoxine to a patient with refractory seizures or coma of unknown cause is justified if an overdose of isoniazid is considered likely.

Three patients with INH overdose who were obtunded or comatose awoke immediately upon the administration of pyridoxine.[10] In two of these patients, seizures were terminated with IV pyridoxine but the patients remained comatose for prolonged periods until additional pyridoxine was administered. The authors concluded that pyridoxine is effective not only for treating INH induced seizures but also for alleviating the mental status changes that may persist. This issue raises the question of the optimal dosing of pyridoxine (see Antidotes in Depth: Pyridoxine). Patients with INH overdose with persistent mental status changes despite adequate seizure control, should receive additional doses of pyridoxine.

Although pyridoxine is very effective in this setting, it is not totally innocuous. A peripheral neuropathy is described following its chronic use,[55] and a severe sensory neuropathy occurred in an iatrogenic overdose.[1]

In general, good supportive care—coupled with the administration of pyridoxine, GABA-enhancing anticonvulsants, and sodium bicarbonate, if necessary to treat severe acidosis—should suffice. Extracorporeal elimination with hemodialysis or hemoperfusion should be reserved for cases of INH overdose with persistent symptoms despite adequate therapy and for symptomatic patients with renal insufficiency.[35,58] Peritoneal dialysis has been utilized to enhance the elimination of isoniazid but is no longer considered an acceptable alternative.[16]

What Are the Clinical Effects of Chronic INH Toxicity?

Chronic ingestion of therapeutic doses of INH is associated with a number of adverse effects including hepatitis, peripheral neuropathy, optic neuritis, encephalopathy, numerous psychological complaints, and a syndrome indistinguishable from pellagra (Table 43–1).

The incidence of adverse reactions to INH is estimated to be 5.4% in a large series.[48] The most common of these effects are rash, fever, jaundice, and neuritis. Back pain, urinary retention, and dry mouth also occurred. Hypersensitivity is rare but may result in fever, lingual edema, urticaria, and arthritis. Hematologic reactions are reported, and include agranulocytosis, thrombocytopenia, and anemia. A vasculitis associated with antinuclear antibodies is described but disappears when treatment is stopped. The prophylactic administration of pyridoxine usually prevents the development of the peripheral neuropathy and the other nervous system disorders, even when INH therapy is prolonged more than 2 years. Isoniazid has been reported to be embryocidal when administered to pregnant rats, although no INH-related congenital abnormalities have been found in reproductive studies in mammalian species. Isoniazid can be prescribed in pregnancy if it is clinically indicated for active tuberculosis (FDA pregnancy category C).

What Are the Epidemiology and Other Characteristics of Isoniazid Hepatitis?

The most dreaded complication of chronic INH therapy is hepatitis. A 1969 study noted that 10% of patients receiving INH developed elevations of ALT (alanine aminotransferase) and AST (aspartate aminotransferase).[54] It was originally believed that these elevations were only transient and occurred exclusively within the first 2 months of treatment. In the same year, because several cases of TB were discovered among government employees in Washington, DC, a large-scale program of INH prophylaxis was initiated for more than 2000 government workers. After 1 year, 19 cases of hepatitis and 2 deaths from liver failure had occurred.

An ad hoc committee on INH and liver diseases, established by the Centers for Disease Control, conducted a prospective study of 358 patients that revealed that 13% of patients on INH therapy developed AST elevations.[12] Although many of these elevations occurred within the first 8 weeks of therapy, others occurred throughout the study. In two cases, enzyme elevations occurred as late as 52 weeks after INH was started. This challenged the "transitory early occurrence" hypothesis. A 14,000-patient study by the Public Health Service showed that approximately 10% of all patients maintained on INH developed enzyme elevations.[36] Ten percent of this group (1% overall) went on to develop clinical liver disease, and 10% of those who developed hepatitis (0.1% overall) died. More recent studies confirm that 10 to 20% of all patients taking INH develop asymptomatic elevations in liver enzymes (usually 2 to 3 times normal), which usually resolve despite continued therapy.[24,41]

INH hepatitis is characterized by nausea, vomiting, fatigue, fever, abdominal pain, pruritis, and elevated liver enzymes. Most studies emphasize the increasing risk of INH-induced hepatitis as older patients are exposed to the drug.[17] Hepatitis associated with INH is more common in the elderly, the malnourished, alcoholics, those with pre-existent liver disease, and those who also receive rifampin or pyrazinamide.[60] Mortality is higher in patients who develop marked hyperbilirubinemia (> 20 mg/dL), become symptomatic late in the course of INH therapy, and have grade III encephalopathy and factor V levels below 20%.[21,63] Cases of fulminant hepatic failure secondary to INH toxicity requiring liver transplantation are reported.[44] The prophylactic use of INH is controversial but is still widely practiced. Cost-effectiveness and risk-benefit studies have come to conflicting conclusions about the relative merits of INH for TB prevention. Recommendations based on different assumptions of the rates of hepatitis, hepatic failure, and risk of tuberculosis have varied. Some authors have advocated a reevaluation of the management strategy in view of the significant toxicity of INH.[31]

In order to reduce potential hepatotoxicity if INH is prescribed, the liver enzymes should be monitored closely, especially in the first 4 months of therapy; if they exceed two times the normal value, INH should be discontinued. Patients on combination regimens that include rifampin or pyrazinamide should be monitored even more carefully.

The mechanism of INH hepatitis is well described.[5,42,43] The INH metabolite, monoacetylhydrazine, can be converted by hepatic P450 isoenzymes to a hepatotoxic intermediate that binds covalently to hepatocytes, causing hepatic necrosis. This hepatotoxic mechanism is reminiscent of that associated with acetaminophen. Because monoacetylhydrazine is a product of the acetylation reaction, it was postulated that rapid acetylators were at greater risk for hepatotoxicity.[42,43] However, monoacetylhydrazine is in turn acetylated to diacetylhydrazine, which is not toxic to the liver (see Fig. 43–1). Presumably rapid acetylators also perform this conversion more rapidly than slow acetylators, thus reducing the risk of hepatotoxicity. Detailed studies have revealed that both slow and fast acetylators excrete similar proportions of monacetylhydrazine, suggesting that exposure to this hepatotoxic compound is the same for both groups.[22] The current view is that acetylation status does not constitute an independent risk factor for INH hepatitis.[19,29]

Researchers studying patients who received the combination of rifampin and INH have demonstrated an additional mechanism of hepatotoxicity. Among patients on combination therapy, the slow acetylators develop hepatitis more commonly than the rapid acetylators.[53] Apparently, INH can be directly hydrolyzed to a hepatotoxic hydrazine via INH hydroxylase (see Fig. 43–1). This pathway is more prominent in slow acetylators, and because it is mediated by the P450 system, is inducible by rifampin. This would explain the increased incidence of INH hepatitis among slow acetylators taking rifampin and INH.

What Other Chronic Effects Are Associated With Isoniazid?

Isoniazid interferes with a number of other metabolic pathways. Isoniazid blocks the conversion of lactate back to pyruvate by interfering with the cofactor for this reaction, nicotine adenine dinucleotide (NAD).[45] Isoniazid is closely related to the monoamine oxidase inhibitors (a derivative, iproniazide, was historically used as an MAOI). The administration of INH is associated with a typical tyramine syndrome: palpitations, flushing, conjunctival injection, headache, dyspnea, chest tightness, and sweating.

Chronic INH therapy can lead to optic neuritis and optic atrophy.[28] An encephalopathy characterized by dysarthria, euphoria, confusion, and lethargy is reported in dialysis patients maintained on INH.[61] Reduced metabolism of pyridoxine to its active form, and increased dialysis clearance of pyridoxal phosphate, are the presumed etiology of this effect. In a study of 172 patients receiving INH prophylactically, 6 patients had to discontinue treatment due to depression and/or aggressive behavior while an additional 53 patients had a variety of psychological reactions.[64] INH can cause a peripheral neuropathy, which is seen in approximately 20% of patients receiving 6 mg/kg per day without pyridoxine supplementation. This peripheral neuropathy is classically a distal sensory-motor axonopathy, is dose related, and seen more often in slow acetylators and those who are malnourished, alcoholic, uremic, and diabetic.[27]

Finally, chronic INH therapy can lead to a syndrome indistinguishable from pellagra characterized by dermatitis, diarrhea, and dementia. Pyridoxal phosphate is an essential cofactor in the synthesis of niacin (nicotinic acid) from tryptophan, and an INH-mediated decrease in pyridoxal phosphate results in this deficiency.

What Other Antituberculous Agents Are in Use?

Rifampin

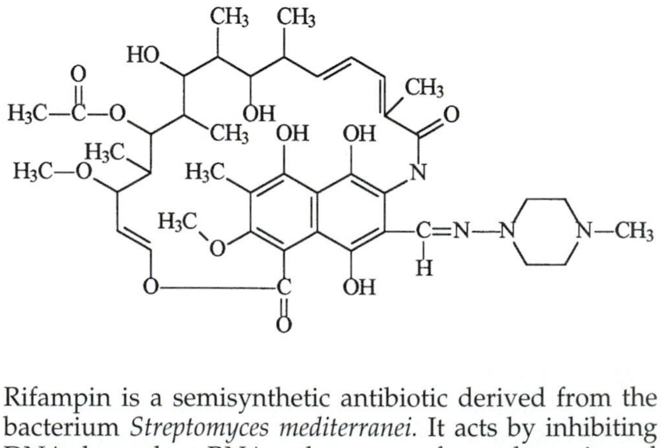

Rifampin is a semisynthetic antibiotic derived from the bacterium *Streptomyces mediterranei.* It acts by inhibiting DNA-dependent RNA polymerase of mycobacteria and other organisms, thereby suppressing the initiation of chain formation in RNA synthesis. It is well absorbed orally, with peak levels occurring within 2 to 4 hours. Rifampin is distributed throughout the body, with an apparent volume of distribution of 1.6 L/kg, and is 75% protein bound. It is deacetylated in the liver to desacetyl rifampin and undergoes an enterohepatic circulation, with eventual GI elimination. Approximately 30% of the drug is excreted in the urine. The half-life varies from 1 to 5 hours. It may be prolonged in patients with liver disease and decreased in slow acetylators who are receiving INH. Rifampin is a potent inducer of the hepatic microsomal (P450) enzyme system. This effect is responsible for many of its well-known drug interactions as well as its ability to induce its own metabolism.[8] The administration of rifampin decreases the half-life of a variety of agents (Table 43–2).

Adverse effects are seen in approximately 6% of patients maintained on rifampin and are more common after intermittent therapy.[26] Gastrointestinal disturbances (nausea, vomiting, and abdominal pain) and cutaneous reactions (rash, pruritis, and facial flushing) are commonly observed. Other reactions include an influenza-like syndrome, thrombocytopenia, hemolytic anemia, eosinophilia, and pseudomembranous colitis.

Like INH, rifampin can cause hepatitis.[38,39,53] Liver damage is more common in persons with a history of liver disease, slow inactivators of rifampin, and those on concomitant therapy with INH (especially slow acetylators). Approximately one third of patients also taking INH exhibit increases in liver enzymes and bilirubin levels during the first few months of rifampin use. Often these abnormalities disappear after approximately 2 weeks, whether or not the drug is stopped.[53] Patients must be closely observed for a substantial increase in LFTs and jaundice, which occurs in 0.6% of those who take rifampin.[65] Total bilirubin levels may be falsely elevated due to interference by rifampin with the bilirubin assay. High-dose intermittent therapy or reinstitution of rifampin after a drug-free interval has resulted in serious adverse effects, such as antibody-mediated immune reactions (autoimmune anemia, thrombocytopenia, and renal failure). Acute renal failure may occur in association with eosinophilia, skin rash, and a hepatorenal syndrome.

Rifampin is teratogenic in mice, and isolated cases of fetal malformations have been described. There are, however, no well-controlled studies of its effect on the human fetus, and it is currently classified as a category C drug for pregnancy by the FDA.

Rifampin and its metabolites are red, and overdose with the drug can produce a characteristic orange-red staining of the tissues and urine ("red man syndrome").[30] This color may be partially removed by washing or scrubbing, a property unique to rifampin ingestion. Rifampin overdose may also be associated with GI effects, flushing, angioedema, and obtundation. Periorbital or facial edema was observed in 18 of 19 children who received an inadvertent overdose of 100 mg/kg.[7] The diagnosis should be suspected in any patient who presents with nausea and vomiting, mental status changes, and reddish discoloration of the skin. Overdosage can result in pulmonary edema and death.[49] Doses over 14 g are potentially fatal. Death is more likely in patients who have underlying liver abnormalities, a history of alcohol abuse, and those not previously on rifampin therapy. Because rifampin undergoes enterohepatic circulation, MDAC may result in additional total clearance of the drug from the body. In light of its extensive volume of distribution and protein binding, rifampin does not lend itself well to elimination by hemodialysis or hemoperfusion.

Ethambutol

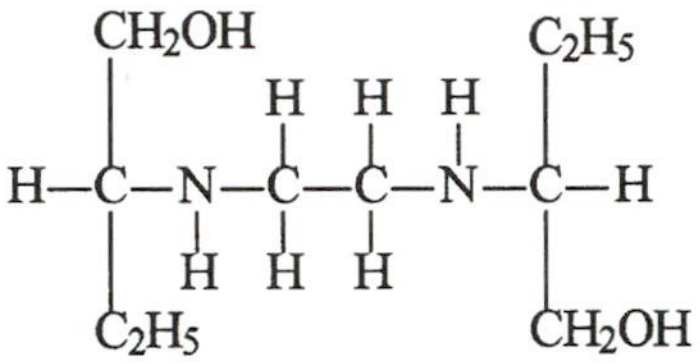

Ethambutol is a synthetic bacteriostatic antituberculous agent that has essentially replaced p-aminosalicylic acid in multidrug regimens. The drug is effective only in actively growing cells and probably acts as an antimetabolite to inhibit the synthesis of RNA. It is well absorbed from the GI tract, with peak levels within 2 to 4 hours. Approximately 50% of an oral dose is excreted in the urine unchanged, 10 to 20% is metabolized in the liver to an aldehyde and a dicarboxylic acid derivative, and 20% is excreted in the feces.

Ethambutol is generally well tolerated. Adverse effects include GI symptoms, pruritis, joint pain, dizziness, confusion, and disorientation. A peripheral neuritis is described. The most important adverse effect is optic neuritis, manifested by decreased visual acuity, loss of red-green color perception, central scotomata, and peripheral visual field defects. The optic neuritis is a dose-related phenomenon and is often reversible. Two types of retrobulbar neuritis are identified. One involves the central fibers of the optic nerve leading to blurred vision, decreased visual acuity, central scotomata, and color blindness. The other, less common, variety involves peripheral fibers and results in constriction of the visual fields.[56] Ocular toxicity may be unilateral or bilateral and is observed in 15% of patients receiving 50 mg/kg per day, 5% of those receiving 25 mg/kg per day, and less than 1% of those receiving 15 mg/kg per day.[40] The degree of visual impairment is related to the duration of therapy after the problem with visual acuity first becomes apparent. Testing of visual acuity and red-green discrimination prior to the start of therapy and periodically thereafter is strongly recommended. The use of ethambutol is associated with increased uric acid in 66% of patients taking doses of 20 mg/kg per day due to decreased renal excretion. Overdosage with ethambutol is associated with nausea, abdominal pain, confusion, hal-

TABLE 43–2. ANTITUBERCULOUS AGENTS

Drug	Major Adverse Reactions	Drug Interactions	Monitoring	Comments
First-Line Agents				
Isoniazid	Elevation of LFTs, hepatitis, CNS effects including seizures, peripheral neuropathy, pellagra	Rifampin, pyrazinamide and ethanol: Increased hepatic toxicity Disulfiram: Psychotic episodes and ataxia Phenytoin metabolism is inhibited	Liver enzymes	Use of pyridoxine can decrease neurologic toxicity
Rifampin	Hepatitis, red-orange discoloration of secretions, urine, contact lenses	INH: Increased toxicity Methadone: Increased metabolism leading to withdrawal Other drugs: Increased metabolism of anticoagulants (↓ PT), barbiturates, beta-adrenergic antagonists, clofibrate, contraceptives, dapsone, digoxin, ketoconazole, sulfonylureas, quinidine, steroids, theophylline, verapamil	Liver enzymes	
Ethambutol	GI effects, optic neuritis, loss of visual acuity, decreased red-green color perception, decreased urate excretion	—	Color vision and visual acuity	Contraindicated in children too young for visual testing
Pyrazinamide	GI effects, hepatitis, decreased urate excretion	INH: Increased hepatotoxicity	Liver enzymes	
Streptomycin	Ototoxicity, nephrotoxicity, neuromuscular paralysis	Neuromuscular blocking agents: Increased potency Capreomycin: Increased ototoxicity and nephrotoxicity Warfarin: Increased PT	Renal function tests, audiometry	Contraindicated in pregnancy
Second-Line Agents				
Capreomycin	Electrolyte disturbances, renal damage, hepatotoxicity, ototoxicity	Neuromuscular blockers: Increased activity Aminoglycosides: Increased ototoxicity and nephrotoxicity	LIver function tests	
Ethionamide	GI effects, thrombocytopenia, hepatitis, CNS effects including seizures, peripheral neuropathy, porphyria, pellagra	Cycloserine: Increased CNS effects, including seizures INH: Increased incidence of pellagra		Contraindicated in patients with porphyria. Pyridoxine can decrease neurologic toxicity
Cycloserine	Megaloblastic anemia, CNS effects including seizures, porphyria, pellagra	INH, ethionamide: Increased CNS effects, including seizures Phenytoin: Increased blood levels	CBC	Pyridoxine can decrease neurologic toxicity
Rifabutin	GI effects, thrombocytopenia, ageusia, elevated LFTs, orange-brown discoloration of secretions and urine	—	Liver enzymes, CBC	
Para-aminosalicylic acid	GI effects, elevated LFTs	Digoxin: Decreased absorption of digoxin Warfarin: Increased PT	Liver enzymes	
Clofazimine	GI effects including bowel obstruction and infarction, leukopenia; CNS effects, corneal and skin pigmentation		CBC	

lucinations, and optic neuropathy (retrobulbar neuritis), particularly with doses greater than 10 g.[20] Acute overdose involving both ethambutol and isoniazid may result in synergistic central nervous system toxicity. Ethambutol has been given to pregnant women without adverse effects on the fetus and is listed as a category B drug.

Pyrazinamide

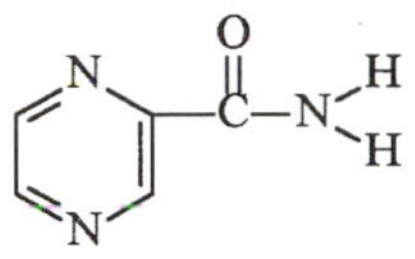

Pyrazinamide is an analog of nicotinamide and is considered to be bactericidal to actively dividing tubercle bacilli. It is well absorbed from the GI tract, with peak levels usually achieved within 2 hours. It is excreted primarily by renal filtration. Pyrazinamide is partly hydrolyzed to pyrazinoic acid and then hydroxylated to 5-hydroxypyrazinoic acid and excreted. Hepatic abnormalities are the most consistent and serious adverse effect of pyrazinamide therapy. In doses of 3 g/d and greater, approximately 15% of patients will develop hepatitis and 2 to 3% will succumb with acute hepatic necrosis. In recent studies, pyrazinamide hepatotoxicity developed in only 1 to 5% of patients taking INH, rifampin, and pyrazinamide.[65] Patients about to receive pyrazinamide therapy should have hepatic function tested first, and these tests should be repeated at frequent intervals throughout therapy. In the presence of a significant elevation of LFTs, pyrazinamide should be immediately stopped. Like ethambutol, pyrazinamide inhibits the excretion of uric acid, resulting in hyperuricemia and, occasionally, acute gouty attacks. Toxic effects from an acute overdose have not been reported. No studies of its effect on the developing fetus have been performed in animals or humans. Pyrazinamide is currently classified as a category C drug.

Streptomycin

Streptomycin is an aminoglycoside antibiotic and was the first effective chemotherapeutic agent for the treatment of tuberculosis. It acts by binding to a protein on the 30s subunit of the bacterial ribosome leading to faulty alignment with messenger RNA. The accumulation of nonfunctional peptide chains leads to bacterial cell death.

Streptomycin can only be given parenterally, and peak serum levels occur 1 hour after IM administration. It is 34% protein bound and has an elimination half-life of 2 to 5 hours. Up to 89% of a given dose is excreted unchanged in the urine.

Streptomycin can cause a hemolytic anemia and is associated with hemorrhage due to an IgG-mediated factor V inhibition. Like other aminoglycosides it can cause a dose-related neuromuscular blockade, which can be reversed by calcium but not neostigmine. Nephrotoxicity does occur following the therapeutic use of streptomycin, although it is much less common than with other aminoglycosides.

Ototoxicity is common following streptomycin therapy and epidemiologic data indicate that the elderly are the most susceptible. Patients typically present with tinnitus, vertigo, dizziness, ataxia, and hearing loss. Severity appears to be dose related and deficits can persist despite discontinuation of the drug. Periodic auditory testing is recommended in patients with renal insufficiency and those receiving high doses. Finally, the use of streptomycin during pregnancy is linked to a non-dose-related hearing impairment and eighth nerve damage in neonates. It is the only antituberculosis agent known to produce harmful effects in the fetus (FDA category D) and is therefore contraindicated during pregnancy.

What Are The Second-Line Antituberculosis Medications?

A variety of second-line antituberculosis agents are in use and include the following: ciprofloxacin, ofloxacin, kanamycin, amikacin, capreomycin, ethionamide, cycloserine, para-aminosalicylic acid, rifabutin, and clofazimine (see Table 43–2).

Capreomycin, a cyclic polypeptide antimicrobial, causes renal tubular damage in a significant percentage of patients. It has also been linked to Bartter's syndrome and to a variety of electrolyte disturbances. Capreomycin may cause pain and sterile abscesses at the site of injections and can cause ototoxicity similar to that seen with streptomycin.

Ethionamide is a bacteriostatic agent that can cause GI upset and neurotoxicity: sensory neuropathy, depression, drowsiness, toxic psychosis, tremors, seizures, and a pellagra-like encephalopathy. Concomitant administration of pyridoxine to prevent these effects is advised. Ethionamide is reported to cause hypoglycemia, hepatitis, optic neuritis, and a rheumatic syndrome. It is contraindicated in patients with porphyria.

Cycloserine interferes with bacterial cell wall synthesis. It is reported to cause a megaloblastic anemia, CHF, and a polyarthritis. Its main toxic effects are manifested neurologically. Confusion, coma, tremors, vertigo, seizures, and a pellagra-like syndrome are described. Neurologic side effects often appear in the first 2 weeks of therapy, and are more common at higher doses and in patients with previous psychiatric problems.[2] Concomitant use of INH and cycloserine can cause increased CNS toxicity, because both affect the metabolism of pyridoxine; prophylactic administration of pyridoxine is recommended.

Rifabutin is an antibacterial agent related to rifampin. The use of rifabutin has resulted in elevation of liver enzymes, thrombocytopenia, neutropenia, uveitis, and loss of taste (ageusia). Like rifampin, rifabutin can cause an orange discoloration of bodily fluids, and as an inducer of microsomal enzymes, can affect the metabolism of a number of drugs when administered concomitantly.

Clofazimine is a phendimetrazine tartrate derivative that binds to mycobacterial DNA and inhibits growth. GI effects and a dose-related, reversible, red-brown discoloration of the skin and eyes are common side effects. Clofazimine can cause CNS dysfunction, depression, and hyperglycemia. Clofazimine deposits on the wall of the small bowel and can cause an enteropathy that can lead to bowel obstruction and infarction.

References

1. Albin RL, Albers JW, Greenberg HS: Acute sensory neuropathy from pyridoxine overdose. Neurology 1987;37: 1729–1732.
2. Anonymous: Treatment of tuberculosis and tuberculosis infection in adults and children. Am J Respir Crit Care Med 1994;149:1359–1374.
3. Bear ES, Hoffman PF, Siegel SR: Suicidal ingestion of isoniazid: An uncommon cause of metabolic acidosis and seizures. South Med J 1976;69:31–32.
4. Biehl JP, Vilter RW: Effects of isoniazid on pyridoxine metabolism. JAMA 1954;165:1549–1552.
5. Black M, Mitchell JR, Zimmerman HJ: Isoniazid associated hepatitis in 114 patients. Gastroenterology 1975;69:289–301.
6. Bloch AB, Reider HL, Kelly GD: The epidemiology of TB in the U.S.: Implications for diagnosis and treatment. Clin Chest Med 1989;10:297–313.
7. Bolan G, Laurie RE, Broone CV: Red man syndrome: Inadvertent administration of an excessive dose of rifampin to children in a daycare center. Pediatrics 1986;77:633–635.
8. Borcherding SM, Baciewicz AM, Self TH: Update on rifampin drug interactions, II. Arch Intern Med 1992;152: 711–716.
9. Bowersox DW, Winterbauer RH, Steward GL: Isoniazid dosage in patients with renal failure. N Engl J Med 1973; 289:84–87.
10. Brent J, Nguyen VO, Kulig K: Reversal of prolonged isoniazid-induced coma by pyridoxine. Arch Intern Med 1990; 150:1751–1753.
11. Brown CV: Acute isoniazid poisoning. Am Rev Respir Dis 1972;105:206–216.
12. Byrd RB, Nelson R, Elliott RC: Isoniazid toxicity: A prospective study in secondary complications. JAMA 1972;220:1471–1473.
13. Chin L, Seivers ML, Herrier RN: Potentiation of pyridoxine by depressants and anticonvulsants in the treatment of acute isoniazid intoxication in dogs. Toxicol Appl Pharmacol 1981;58:504–509.
14. Chin L, Sievers ML, Herrier RN: Convulsions as the etiology of lactic acidosis in acute isoniazid toxicity in dogs. Toxicol Appl Pharmacol 1979;40:377–384.
15. Chin L, Sievers ML, Laird HE: Evaluation of diazepam and pyridoxine as antidotes to isoniazid intoxication in rats. Toxicol Appl Pharmacol 1978;45:713–722.
16. Cocco AE, Pazourek LJ: Acute isoniazid intoxication management by peritoneal dialysis. N Engl J Med 1963;269: 852–853.
17. Comstock GW: New data on preventive treatment with isoniazid. Ann Intern Med 1983;98:663–665.
18. Coyer, JR, Nicholson DP: Isoniazid-induced convulsions. South Med J 1976;69:294–297.
19. Dickinson DS, Bailey WC, Hirschowitz BI: Risk factors for INH-induced liver dysfunction. J Clin Gastroenterol 1981;3: 271–279.
20. Ducobu J, Dupont P, Laurent M: Acute isoniazid/ethambutol/rifampin overdosage. Lancet 1982;1:632. Letter.
21. Durand F, Bernicau J, Pessayre D: Deleterious influence of pyrazinamide on the outcome of patients with fulminant or subfulminant liver failure during antituberculosis treatment including isoniazid. Hepatology 1995;21:929–932.
22. Ellard GA, Mitchison DA, Girling DJ: The hepatic toxicity of isoniazid among rapid and slow acetylators of the drug. Am Rev Respir Dis 1978;118:628–629.
23. Evans DAP, Manley KA, McKusick VA: Genetic control of isoniazid metabolism in man. Br Med J 1960;2:485–491.
24. Farrell FJ, Keefe EB, Man KM: Treatment of hepatic failure secondary to isoniazid hepatitis with liver transplantation. Dig Dis Sci 1994;39: 2255–2259.
25. Frieden TR, Fujiwara PI, Washko RM, Hamburg MA: Tuberculosis in New York City—Turning the tide. N Engl J Med 1995;334:229–233.
26. Girling DJ, Hitze KL: Adverse reactions to rifampin. Bull WHO 1979;57:47–49.
27. Goel UC, Bajaj S, Gupta OP, et al: Isoniazid-induced neuropathy in slow versus rapid acetylators: An electrophysiological study. J Assoc Physicians India 1992;40:671–672.
28. Gonzalez-Gay MA, Sanchez-Andrade A, Aguero JJ: Optic neuritis following treatment with isoniazid in a hemodialyzed patient. Nephron 1993;63: 360. Letter.
29. Gurumurthy P, Krishnamurthy MS, Nazareth O: Lack of relationship between hepatic toxicity and acetylator phenotype in 3,000 South Indian patients during treatment with isoniazid. Am Rev Respir Dis 1984;129:58–61.
30. Holdiness MR: A review of the redman syndrome and rifampin overdosage. Med Toxicol Adverse Drug Exp 1989;4: 444–451.
31. Israel HL, Gotlieb JE, Maddrey WC: Perspective: Preventive isoniazid therapy and the liver. Chest 1992;101:1298–1301.
32. Jeanses CWL, Schaefer O, Eidus L: Inactivation of isoniazid by Canadian Eskimos and Indians. Can Med Assoc J 1972;106:331–335.
33. Katz GA, Jobin EC: Large doses of pyridoxine in the treatment of massive isoniazid ingestion. Am Rev Respir Dis 1970;101:991–992.
34. Kendig EL, Inselman LS: Tuberculosis in children. Adv Pediatr 1991;38:233–255.
35. Konigshansen T, Altrogge G, Hein D: Hemodialysis and hemoperfusion in the treatment of most severe INH poisoning. Vet Hum Toxicol 1979;21:12–15.
36. Kozanoff DE, Snider DE, Caras GJ: Isoniazid hepatitis: A U.S. Public Health Service cooperative surveillance study. Am Rev Respir Dis 1978;117:991–1001.
37. La Du BN: Isoniazid and pseudocholinesterase polymorphisms. Fed Proc 1972;31:1276–1285.

38. Lal S, Singhal SN, Burley DM: Effect of rifampin and isoniazid on liver function. Br Med J 1972;1:148–150.
39. Lees AW, Alan EW, Smith J: Toxicity from rifampin plus isoniazid and rifampin plus ethambutol therapy. Tubercle 1971;52:182–189.
40. Mandell EL, Sande MA: Antimicrobial agents: Drugs used in the chemotherapy of tuberculosis and leprosy. In: Gilman AG, Rall TW, Nies AS, Taylor P, eds: Goodman and Gilman's The Pharmacological Basis of Therapeutics, 8th ed. New York, Pergamon Press, 1990, pp. 1146–1164.
41. Meyers BR, Halpern M, Sheiner P: Acute hepatic failure in seven patients after prophylaxis and therapy with antituberculosis agents. Transplantation 1994;58:372–376.
42. Mitchell JR, Thorgeirsson UP, Black M: Increased incidence of isoniazid hepatitis in rapid acetylators: Possible relation to hydrazine metabolites. Clin Pharmacol Ther 1975;18: 70–79.
43. Mitchell JR, Zimmerman JH, Ishak KG: Isoniazid liver injury. Ann Intern Med 1976;84:181–192.
44. MMWR Weekly Report: Severe isoniazid-associated hepatitis; 1991–1993. MMWR 1993;42:28.
45. Nelson MV, Bailie ER, Krenzelok EP: Central nervous system stimulation from isoniazid therapy. Vet Hum Toxicol 1983;25:90–91.
46. Olson KR, Kearney TE, Dyer JE, et al: Seizures associated with poisoning and drug overdose. Am J Emerg Med 1993;6:565–568.
47. Pahl MV, Jaziri ND, Ness R: Association of beta hydroxybutyric acidosis with isoniazid intoxication. J Toxicol Clin Toxicol 1984;22:167–176.
48. Pitts FW: Tuberculosis: Prevention and therapy. In: Hook EW, Mandell GL, Gwaltney JM, et al, eds: Current Concepts of Infectious Diseases. New York, Wiley, 1977, pp. 181–194.
49. Plomp TA, Battista HJ, Unterdorfer H: A case of fatal poisoning by rifampin. Arch Toxicol 1981;48:245–252.
50. Rieder HL, Cauthen GM, Kelly GD: Tuberculosis in the U.S. JAMA 1989;262: 385–389.
51. Saad SF, el Masry AM, Scott PM: Influence of certain anticonvulsants on the concentration of GABA in the cerebral hemispheres of mice. Eur J Pharmacol 1972;17:386–392.
52. Sah P: Nicotinyl and isonicotinyl hydrazones of pyridoxal. J Am Chem Soc 1954;76:300–304.
53. Sarma GR, Immanuel C, Kailasam S: Rifampin-induced release of hydrazine from isoniazid. A possible cause of hepatitis during treatment. Am Rev Respir Dis 1986;133:1072–1075.
54. Scharer L, Smith JP: Serum transaminase elevations and other hepatic abnormalities in patients receiving isoniazid. Ann Intern Med 1969;71:1113–1120.
55. Schaumberg H, Kaplan J, Windebank A: Sensory neuropathy from pyridoxine overdose. N Engl J Med 1983;309: 445–448.
56. Schild HS, Fox BC: Rapid-onset reversible ocular toxicity from ethambutol therapy. Am J Med 1991;90:404–406.
57. Shah BR, Santucci K, Sinert R, Steiner P: Acute isoniazid neurotoxicity in an urban hospital. Pediatrics 1995;95: 700–704.
58. Siefkin AD, Albertson TE, Corbett MG: Isoniazid overdose: Pharmacokinetics and effects of oral charcoal in treatment. Hum Toxicol 1987;6:497–501.
59. Sievers ML, Herrier RN: Treatment of acute isoniazid toxicity. Hosp Pharm 1975;32:202–207.
60. Singh J, Arrora A, Garg PK: Antituberculosis treatment induced hepatotoxicity in an urban hospital. Pediatrics 1995; 95:700–704.
61. Siskind MS, Thienemann D, Kirlin L: Isoniazid-induced neurotoxicity in chronic dialysis patients: Report of three cases and a review of the literature. Nephron 1993;64: 303–306.
62. Starke H, William S: Acute poisoning from overdose of isoniziad. Lancet 1976;83:406–408.
63. Summary of the report of the tuberculosis advisory committee of isoniazid-associated hepatitis. MMWR 1974;23: 97–98.
64. Van Der Have JJ: Disturbance of the psychological balance during isoniazid preventive chemotherapy. Tubercle 1991; 72: 232. Letter.
65. Van Scoy RE, Wilkowske CL: Anti-tuberculous agents. Mayo Clin Proc 1992;67:179–187.
66. Vysniauskas C, Breuckner HH: Severe reactions of the central nervous system following isoniazid therapy. Annu Rev Tuberc 1954;69:759–765.
67. Wason S, LaCouture PG, Lovejoy FH: Single high-dose pyridoxine treatment for isoniazid overdose. JAMA 1981; 246:1102–1104.
68. Whitefield CL, Klein RG: Isoniazid overdose: Report of 40 patients with a critical analysis of treatment and suggestions for prevention. Am Rev Respir Dis 1971;103: 887–893.
69. Williams HL, Killah MS, Jenny EH: Convulsant effects of isoniazid. JAMA 1953;152:1317–1321.
70. World Health Organization: Statement on AIDS and tuberculosis. Bull Int Union Tuberc Lung Dis 1989;64: 8–11.

ANTIDOTES IN DEPTH

Pyridoxine

Mary Ann Howland

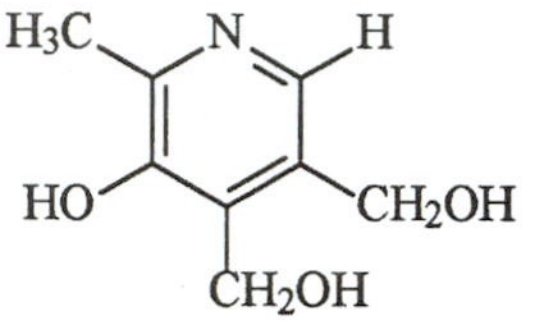

Vitamin B6
(pyridoxine)

The phosphate ester of pyridoxine (vitamin B_6) (pyridoxal-5′-phosphate) is the active form of vitamin B_6.[18] Pyridoxine, an alcohol; pyridoxal, an aldehyde; and pyridoxamine, an aminomethyl form; are all naturally occurring related compounds that are converted to the active pyridoxal-5′-phosphate in the body.[18] Pyridoxine hydrochloride was chosen as the commercial preparation because of its stability.[32] Pyridoxal-5′-phosphate (PLP) is an important cofactor in many enzymatic reactions including decarboxylation and transamination of amino acids, and the metabolism of tryptophan to-5′-hydroxytryptamine and methionine to cysteine.[15,18]

Pyridoxine is not protein bound, has a volume of distribution of 0.6 L/kg, and easily crosses cell membranes, while PLP is nearly entirely plasma protein bound.[32] Pyridoxine is rapidly metabolized at extrahepatic sites to pyridoxal, PLP and 4-pyridoxic acid with only 7% excreted unchanged in the urine.[32] After intravenous infusion of 100 mg of pyridoxine over 6 hours, PLP increases in plasma from a baseline of 183 nmol/L to a peak of 892 nmol/L at 3 hours after the end of the infusion, and in erythrocytes from 88 nmol/L to a peak of 1646 nmol/L at 4 hours into the infusion.[32] Pyridoxal (PL) rose from 37 nmol/L to 2183 nmol/L in plasma and 5593 nmol/L in erythrocytes, with peaks reached at the end of the infusion.[32] Oral pyridoxine in doses of 600 mg is 50% absorbed within 20 minutes, by a first-order process.[31] Peak plasma concentrations of pyridoxine, PLP, and PL were 25,053, 945, and 8682 nmol/L at 1.3, 2.3, and 3.3 hours postingestion of 600 mg.[31] The concentration of PLP appears to be tightly controlled in the plasma and related to alkaline phosphatases. Oral doses of pyridoxine from 10 to 800 mg result in PLP concentrations of 518 to 732 nmol/L 4 hours after ingestion.[31] Chronic alcoholics have lower baseline PLP plasma levels, as acetaldehyde enhances the degradation of PLP in erythrocytes through stimulation of an erythrocyte membrane-bound phosphatase that hydrolyzes phosphate-containing B_6 compounds.[17]

Pyridoxine is used as an antidote for isoniazid, monomethylhydrazine, and ethylene glycol overdoses. The first two overdoses result in seizures due to the competitive inhibition of PLP and the administration of pyridoxine overcomes the inhibition. The administration of pyridoxine may enhance a less toxic pathway of ethylene glycol metabolism.[3]

Pyridoxine's antidotal role in the management of isonicotinic acid hydrazide (isoniazid; INH) and monomethylhydrazine (MMH) poisoning is based on an understanding of the sites of toxicity of these substances. Isoniazid and MMH interfere with the normal utilization and function of pyridoxine as a coenzyme. INH produces a syndrome resembling cerebral vitamin B_6 deficiency, resulting in convulsions. Hydrazides and hydrazines inhibit the enzyme pyridoxine phosphokinase that converts pyridoxine to its active form, PLP.[15] In addition, hydrazides directly combine with PLP, causing inactivation through the production of hydrazones that are then rapidly excreted by the kidney.[15] Gamma-aminobutyric acid (GABA) is synthesized from L-glutamic acid by the enzyme L-glutamic acid decarboxylase and the coenzyme PLP. Animal studies suggest that the interference with PLP by INH disrupts the formation of GABA, an inhibitory neurotransmitter.[15] The decreased GABA formation may decrease the inhibitory tone of the brain, which contributes at least in part to the seizures produced by INH and MMH.[30]

The efficacy of pyridoxine in controlling INH-induced seizures was demonstrated in dogs but not in rats.[10] With regard to INH-induced seizures in dogs, diazepam proved ineffective, but a synergistic effect was noted when diazepam was added to pyridoxine. Pyridoxine thereby resulted in a reduction in the severity of seizures and prevented the mortality in dogs given a lethal dose of INH.[9] Phenobarbital, pentobarbital, phenytoin, ethanol, and diazepam as single agents were ineffective in controlling seizures and mortality, but when combined with pyridoxine each agent protected the animals from seizures and death. It is noteworthy that diazepam and phenobarbital enhance the efficacy of GABA; therefore some degree of synergism may be expected. Clinical experience with pyridoxine for INH overdose in humans has demonstrated generally favorable results. Seizures were controlled in a 22-month-old boy given 100 mg of IV pyridoxine, after an estimated INH ingestion of 5 g.[25] Convulsive activity has been reported in 2 patients following the ingestion of INH-pyridoxine combination tablets, although the actual amount of pyridoxine ingested was not noted.[27] Variable results in control of INH-induced seizures in children have occurred when relatively small doses of pyridoxine were used.[19] In a comprehensive review of the literature, "massive" amounts of IV pyridoxine have been given successfully.[2,8] Rapid seizure control with no fatalities has resulted when the ratio of grams of pyridoxine administered to grams of INH ingested ranged from 0.14 to 1.3, although most patients receive approximately gram-for-gram amounts. In 5 patients the use of gram-for-gram amounts of pyridoxine resulted in the complete control of seizures and a resolution of the metabolic acidosis.[29] In 8 patients with intentional INH overdoses, basic poison management, intensive supportive care, and a mean dose of 5 g of pyridoxine IV resulted in no fatalities.[5]

Two patients with INH overdoses and seizures, who were obtunded for up to 36 to 72 hours after the seizures were reported to awaken immediately after 3 to 10 g of IV pyridoxine was administered.[7] A third patient was treated for lethargy with IV pyridoxine on presentation and awakened. This work suggests that mental status abnormalities associated with INH and hydrazine overdoses may be responsive to pyridoxine and may necessitate repetitive dosing. These papers support the suggestions[8,29] that patients treated with large doses of pyridoxine awakened more rapidly even following status epilepticus.

Monomethylhydrazine poisoning may be encountered in a variety of clinical situations. In the aerospace industry, where MMH is used as a rocket propellant, intoxication through the percutaneous or inhalational route may occur. Ingestion of the false morel mushroom, *Gyromitra esculenta*, can also produce toxicity when its major toxic compound, known as gyromitrin, is metabolized to MMH. Although its name implies edibility, *G. esculenta* is usually toxic if eaten raw. Boiling and rinsing can remove much of the volatile water-soluble toxin, and when so prepared the mushroom has been eaten safely by many. Inhalation of the vapors while boiling, however, can lead to significant absorption of toxin (see Chap. 75).[16]

Poisoning by MMH has many neurologic similarities to INH toxicity (seizures, respiratory failure); even severe liver damage has been described.[11] There is no evidence that the acute liver toxicity may be treated by administration of pyridoxine.[6] Small animal experiments have documented the effectiveness of vitamin B_6 against MMH-induced seizures when used alone[15] or in combination with diazepam.[12] Anticonvulsant efficacy has also been noted in cat[24] and monkey[26] models.

A 10-g dose of pyridoxine improved the mental status and liver function tests of a confused, lethargic, and restless man who had ingested a mouthful of hydrazine.[14] This improvement developed over 24 hours and may have been unrelated to pyridoxine therapy. A severe sensory peripheral neuropathy lasting for 6 months developed 1 week following therapy.

PLP is a cofactor in the conversion of glycolic acid to nonoxalate compounds (see Chap. 64). Patients poisoned with ethylene glycol should receive 100 mg/day of pyridoxine IV to attempt to shunt metabolism preferentially away from the production of oxalic acid. This approach was suggested in an animal model[3] and in the study of primary hyperoxaluria,[13] but has not been conclusively demonstrated in cases of human ethylene glycol poisoning.[21]

Unfortunately, pyridoxine itself has toxic effects, and inadequate information is available to determine the maximal single acute nontoxic dose in humans. Doses of pyridoxine ranging from 70 to 375 mg/kg, or doses equivalent to the milligram-per-kilogram historical dose of ingested INH, were administered without adverse effects.[29] Nevertheless, ataxia has occurred (but resolved) in dogs receiving 1 g/kg of pyridoxine. With larger doses of pyridoxine, incoordination, ataxia, seizures, and death have occurred. Death was sometimes delayed for 2 to 3 days.[28] Delayed peripheral neurotoxicity occurred in patients taking large daily doses of 200 mg to 6 g of pyridoxine for 1 month,[20,22,23] and may also occur after very large single doses.[1] Healthy volunteers administered 1 or 3 g/d developed a small and large-fiber distal axonopathy with sensory findings and quantitative sensory threshold abnormalities occurring after 1.5 months in the high-dose and 4.5 months in the low-dose patients. Once symptoms occurred, the pyridoxine was immediately stopped, but symptoms progressed for 2 to 3 weeks leading to speculation that it took time for neuronal metabolic changes to reverse.[4] Two patients who were treated with 132 and 183 g, respectively, of IV pyridoxine (2 g/kg) over 3 days developed a severe and crippling sensory neuropathy over several days.[1] At 1-year follow-up, both patients were unable to walk.

Considering all of the available data, a safe and effective regimen for INH overdoses in adults is to give 1 g of pyridoxine for each gram of INH ingested, to a maximum of 5 g or 70 mg/kg when the history is uncertain. Initial doses in children should not exceed 70 mg/kg.[29] The best way to administer pyridoxine in an INH overdose has not been established. In a patient who is actively seizing, the pyridoxine may be given by slow IV infusion at approximately 0.5 g/min until the seizures stop or the maximum dose has been reached. Once the seizures stop, the remainder of the dose should be infused over 4 to 6 hours to maintain pyridoxine availability while the INH is being eliminated. The dose should be repeated if seizures persist or recur or if the patient exhibits mental status depression. In cases of MMH poisoning, the dose of pyridoxine is 25 mg/kg.[16] Pyridoxine should not be the sole agent used for INH or MMH poisoning. A benzodiazepine should be used with pyridoxine to control seizures. If the seizures do not respond to both of these measures, they can be repeated, followed by intravenous pentobarbital or phenobarbital and, if necessary, neuromuscular blockade and general anesthesia. Neuromuscular blockade without extinguishing of the CNS seizure activity may lead to irreversible neuronal damage. Although metabolic acidosis is probably a result of the seizures and should therefore resolve once the underlying condition is controlled, severe or refractory metabolic acidosis may require appropriate quantities of sodium bicarbonate.

Pyridoxine HCl is available parenterally at a concentration of 100 mg/mL in 10 and 30-mL vials from various manufacturers.

References

1. Albin R, Albers J, Greenberg H, et al: Acute sensory neuropathy-neuronopathy from pyridoxine overdose. Neurology 1987;37:1729–1732.
2. Alvarez EG, Guntupalli KK: Isoniazid overdose: Four case reports and review of the literature. Intens Care Med 1995;21:641–644.
3. Beasley UR, Buck WB: Acute ethylene glycol toxicosis: A review. Vet Hum Toxicol 1980;22:255–263.
4. Berger AR, Schaumberg HH, Schroeder C, et al: Dose response, coasting, and differential fiber vulnerability in human toxic neuropathy: A prospective study of pyridoxine neurotoxicity. Neurology 1992;42:1367–1370.
5. Blanchard P, Yao J, McAlpine D, et al: Isoniazid overdose in the Cambodian population of Olmsted County, Minnesota. JAMA 1986;256:3131–3133.
6. Braun R, Greeff U, Netter KJ: Liver injury by the false morel poison gyromitrin. Toxicology 1979;12:155–163.
7. Brent J, Vo N, Kulig K, Rumack BH: Reversal of prolonged isoniazid-induced coma by pyridoxine. Arch Intern Med 1990;150:1751–1753.
8. Brown CV: Acute isoniazid poisoning. Am Rev Respir Dis 1972;105:206–216.
9. Chin L, Sievers ML, Herrier RN, et al: Potentiation of pyridoxine by depressants and anticonvulsants in the treatment of acute isoniazid intoxication in dogs. Toxicol Appl Pharmacol 1981;58:504–509.
10. Chin L, Sievers ML, Laird HE, et al: Evaluation of diazepam and pyridoxine as antidotes to isoniazid intoxication in rats and dogs. Toxicol Appl Pharmacol 1978;45:713–722.
11. Franke S, Freimuth U, List PH: Uber die Giftigkeit der fruhjahrslorchel Gyromitra (Helvella) esculenta. Fr Arch Toxicol 1967;22:293–332.
12. George ME, Pinkerton MK, Bach KC: Therapeutics of monomethylhydrazine intoxication. Toxicol Appl Pharmacol 1982;63:201–208.
13. Gibbs DA, Watts RWE: The action of pyridoxine in primary hyperoxaluria. Clin Sci 1970;38:277–286.
14. Harati Y, Niakan E: Hydrazine toxicity, pyridoxine therapy and peripheral neuropathy. Ann Intern Med 1986;104: 728–729.
15. Holtz P, Palm D: Pharmacological aspects of vitamin B_6. Pharmacol Rev 1964;16:113–178.
16. Lincoff G, Mitchell DH: Toxic and Hallucinogenic Mushroom Poisoning. New York, Van Nostrand Reinhold, 1977, pp. 49–61.
17. Lumeng L, Li T: Vitamin B_6 metabolism in chronic alcohol abuse. J Clin Invest 1974; 53:693–704.
18. Marcus R, Coulston AM: Water-soluble vitamins. In: Hardman JG, Limbird LE, Molinoff PB, Ruddon RW, eds: Goodman and Gilman's The Pharmacological Basis of Therapeutics, 9th ed. New York, McGraw-Hill, 1996, pp. 1561–1563.
19. Miller J, Robinson A, Percy AK: Acute isoniazid poisoning in childhood. Am J Dis Child 1980;134:290–292.
20. Parry G, Bredesen D: Sensory neuropathy with low dose pyridoxine. Neurology 1985;35:1466–1468.
21. Parry MF, Wallach R: Ethylene glycol poisoning. Am J Med 1974;57:143–150.
22. Schaumburg H: Sensory neuropathy from pyridoxine abuse. N Engl J Med 1984;310:198.
23. Schaumburg H, Kaplan J, Windebank A, et al: Sensory neuropathy from pyridoxine abuse: A new megavitamin syndrome. N Engl J Med 1983;309:445–448.
24. Shouse MN: Acute effects of pyridoxine hydrochloride on monomethylhydrazine seizure latency and amygdaloid kindled seizure thresholds in cats. Exp Neurol 1982;75: 79–88.
25. Starke H, Williams S: Acute poisoning from overdose of isoniazid: A case report. Lancet 1963;83:406–408.
26. Sterman MB, Kovalesky RA: Anticonvulsant effects of restraint and pyridoxine on hydrazine seizures in the monkey. Exp Neurol 1979;65:78–86.
27. Terman DS, Teitelbaum DT: Isoniazid self-poisoning. Neurology 1970;20:299–304.
28. Unna IC: Studies of the toxicity and pharmacology of vitamin B_6 (2-methyl, 3-hydroxy-4, 5-*bis*- pyridine). Pharmacol Exp Ther 1940;70:400–407.
29. Wason S, Lacouture PG, Lovejoy FH: Single high-dose pyridoxine treatment for isoniazid overdose. JAMA 1981;246: 1102–1104.
30. Wood JD, Peesker SJ: A correlation between changes in GABA metabolism and isonicotinic acid. Hydrazide induced seizures. Brain Res 1972;45:489–498.
31. Zempleni J: Pharmacokinetics of vitamin B_6 supplements in humans. J Am Coll Nutr 1995;14:579–586.
32. Zempleni J, Kubler W: The utilization of intravenously infused pyridoxine in humans. Clin Chim Acta 1994;229: 27–36.

CHAPTER 44

Antimalarial Agents

Lewis R. Goldfrank and Harold H. Osborn

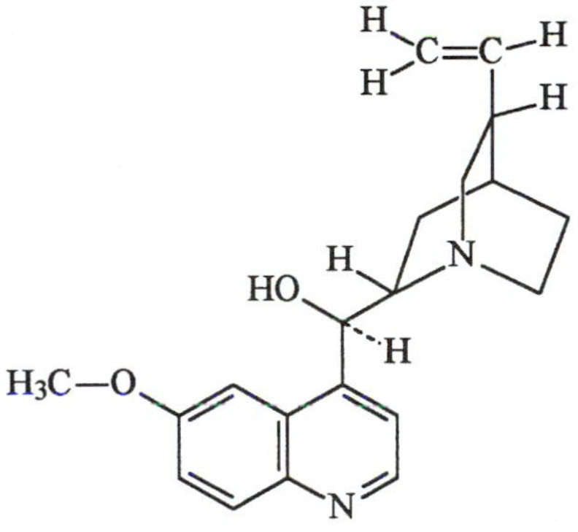

Quinine

Quinine		
MW	=	324.41 D
Cinchonism	=	8–15 μg/mL
(serum levels)	=	24.7–46.02 μmol/L
Visual Toxicity		
Early	=	> 15 μg/mL
		> 46.2 μmol/L
Late	=	> 10 μg/mL
		> 30.8 μmol/L

Values greater than or equal to the action level necessitate clinical intervention. Values less than this level may necessitate intervention based on the clinical condition of the patient.

A 30-year-old man stumbled into the emergency department (ED) appearing to be intoxicated and agitated. However, he was quite coherent. He complained of inability to see, difficulty in hearing, with a continuous ringing in his ears, and the sensation of "a train rushing through his head."

He stated that he had taken "a bunch of pills," drunk some wine, and went off to sleep about 7 hours before coming to the ED. On awakening approximately 6 hours later, he was unable to keep his balance. His mother, hearing his cries for help, accompanied him to the hospital.

The mother related an extensive family, medical, and social history: The patient was an asthmatic taking many drugs. In addition, he took "water pills," later identified as furosemide, to control hypertension. The patient, she said, took aspirin "for arthritis," and "some other pills for malaria." She insisted that he used no illicit drugs and seldom drank, but did smoke two packs of cigarettes per day. She further noted that he had been extremely depressed recently, after his loss of unemployment benefits. In addition, he had had a quarrel on the day of admission.

Physical examination showed a well-developed, talkative, anxious man, with blood pressure, 100/40 mm Hg; pulse, 100 beats/min; respiration, 18 breaths/min; and temperature, 97.2°F (36.2°C). The skin was warm, dry, anicteric, and without pallor or cyanosis.

Ophthalmologic examination revealed fixed, widely dilated pupils (OD 7 mm, OS 8 mm) unresponsive to light and accommodation. Assessment of visual acuity demonstrated some perception of distant shadows but no perception of close objects. The fundi were easily visualized. The optic discs were pale and flat. There was severe arteriolar constriction starting at the disc border with threadlike vessels. The veins appeared normal in diameter. The arteriovenous ratio was 1:7. Extraocular movements were intact.

Examination of the ears revealed normal tympanic membranes. The patient was able to hear a tuning fork on each side, but could not hear the ticking of a watch. Bone versus air conduction (Rinne's test) was difficult to assess, and when the tuning fork handle was placed midline on the patient's forehead the sound was equal in both ears (normal Weber's test). The remainder of the examination was normal except for a systolic ejection murmur.

Blood samples were drawn for complete blood cell count (CBC), blood urea nitrogen (BUN), glucose, calcium, electrolytes, liver function tests, thyroid function tests, arterial blood gas (ABG), prothrombin time (PT), and ethanol level. An ECG was obtained. An IV line was established with 5% dextrose in water (D_5W), and 1 g/kg body weight of activated charcoal and 50 g of sorbitol were given orally.

The initial laboratory data revealed a hematocrit of 37.6%; hemoglobin, 12.1 g/dL; WBCs, 8600/mm^3 with 80% polymorphonuclear cells, 18% lymphocytes, 1% monocytes, and 1% eosinophils. The platelet count and PT were normal.

The electrolyte analysis revealed sodium, 143 mEq/L; potassium, 4.4 mEq/L; chloride, 106 mEq/L; bicarbonate, 29 mEq/L; BUN, 9 mg/dL; and glucose, 65 mg/dL. The creatine phosphokinase of 10,250 IU, lactic dehydrogenase of 700 IU/L, and aspartate aminotransferase of 75 IU/L were all elevated. The urinalysis was normal with a negative urine ferric chloride test for salicylates. The ECG showed a normal sinus rhythm at 96 beats/min, an axis of 90°, and inverted T waves in leads II, III, and aVF. Peaked T waves were present in V_2 to V_4. The chest radiograph was normal. The patient was admitted to the intensive care unit.

Without any additional specific therapy the ophthalmologic and auditory symptoms rapidly abated. Ophthalmologic findings returned to normal. The fundi showed normal vasculature and color within 24 hours. Blood pressure returned to normal by the second day. The abnormal auditory and visual findings entirely resolved within 48 hours.

The patient's mother subsequently revealed that he had taken ten 300-mg quinine tablets, originally intended for the treatment of the *Plasmodium falciparum* malaria he had previously contracted.

What Are the Pharmacologic Features of Quinine?

Quinine and quinidine are extracted from the South American cinchona tree. They are optical isomers. Both drugs are highly protein bound.[45] The average oral lethal dose of quinine is 8 g, although a dose as small as 1.5 g has been reported to cause death.[18,24] Quinine is rapidly and relatively completely absorbed orally. It cannot be injected subcutaneously or intramuscularly for therapeutic purposes because it leads to local tissue necrosis. Peak plasma levels are achieved within 3 hours, and 85 to 95% of quinine is protein bound.[44] The apparent volume of distribution is approximately 1.8 L/kg. Peak myocardial concentrations are achieved at 3 to 6 hours. At a delayed phase of exposure, plasma quinine levels greater than 10 μg/mL are associated with temporary blindness, and levels of 15 μg/mL are associated with increased risk of permanent visual damage,[4] dysrhythmias, and death.[18,24] Similar levels in individuals who are severely ill with malaria do not result in toxicity due to the reduced free fraction of quinine present. This is probably due to the very high levels of α_1-glycoproteins present in severe malaria.[42] The average therapeutic plasma half-life of quinine is 6 to 8 hours. In overdose the elimination half-life is approximately 25 to 26 hours.[3] The liver, kidneys, and muscles metabolize 80% of the ingested dose. Approximately 20% is excreted unaltered in urine. Quinine passes transplacentally as well as via breast milk. The urine assay for quinine is sensitive enough to record the presence of quinine following the ingestion of tonic water. Immunoassay techniques are reliable.

What Is Cinchonism and How Does It Present?

Cinchonism is a syndrome that occurs after the ingestion of cinchona bark or quinine. As in the case of this patient, quinine may rarely be used when *P. falciparum* is resistant to chloroquine and quinacrine.[45] Quinine is also available in small quantities in tonic water (about 2.2 mg/fluid oz) and has been used to adulterate or "cut" heroin.[9,13] Cinchonism is characterized by numerous central nervous system, cardiovascular, gastrointestinal, dermatologic, hematologic, and renal manifestations (Table 44–1).

TABLE 44–1. CLINICAL FINDINGS IN CINCHONISM

System	Signs and Symptoms
Auditory	Hearing loss Tinnitus
Cardiovascular	AV conduction disturbances Hypotension Ventricular dysrhythmias
Central nervous	Coma, confusion, delirium Encephalopathy, headache Seizures, vertigo Syncope
Dermatologic	Diaphoresis Flushing Rashes Angioedema
Endocrinologic	Hypoglycemia
Gastrointestinal	Abdominal pain Nausea, vomiting, diarrhea
Gynecologic	Premature labor Oxytocic effect
Hematologic	Hemolysis Thrombocytopenia Agranulocytosis
Ophthalmic	Altered color perception Blurred vision, blindness Mydriasis, diplopia Optic disc edema Photophobia Retinal artery spasm Scotomata Tunnel vision
Renal	Acute renal failure Hemoglobinuria

The CNS manifestations include headache, vertigo, syncope, and confusion. Delirium, coma, and seizures are uncommon and usually occur only after severe overdoses and may be associated with myocardial depression.[5] Ophthalmologic presentations include blurred vision, visual field constriction, tunnel vision, diplopia, altered color perception, mydriasis, photophobia, scotomata, and sometimes complete blindness due to the direct toxicity.[2,5,8,18,19] Onset of blindness is invariably delayed and usually follows the onset of other manifestations of cinchonism by at least 6 hours.

The pupillary dilation that occurs is usually nonreactive and correlates with the severity of visual loss. Verminform motion[12] or tonic pupil with denervation supersensitivity has been reported.[20] Funduscopic examination may be normal, but usually extreme arteriolar constriction associated with optic disc and retinal edema are seen. Normal arteriolar caliber may be present, but funduscopic manifestations such as vessel attenuation and disc pallor may develop as clinical improvement occurs.[7,12] Electroretinographic studies have shown a well-documented rapid and direct effect on the retina within minutes after doses of quinine.[7,14] Early retinographic changes as well as histologic lesions in photoreceptor and ganglion cell layers of the retina have also been noted.[7] Plasma quinine concentrations are higher in individuals who develop blindness and can be used as a predictor of blindness.[3]

Eighth-nerve dysfunction results in tinnitus and deafness. Quinine inhibits hearing, acting on the transducing function of the cochlea. This effect is a result of micromechanical changes on the contractile structure in the outer hair cells of the organ of Corti.[1,25] This causes a rapid decrease in auditory acuity with a flattening of audiograms. The decreased acuity is not usually clinically apparent, although the patient recognizes tinnitus.[38] These findings usually resolve within 48 to 72 hours, and permanent hearing impairment is unlikely.

Cardiovascular manifestations of cinchonism are related to myocardial drug levels and are similar to those of quinidine. Quinine has a negative inotropic action, slows depolarization and conduction rates, and increases both the action potential duration and the effective refractory period much like class IA antidysrhythmic agents such as quinidine. Prolonged AV conduction and intraventricular conduction occur. A prolonged PR interval, QRS complex, QT interval, and ST depression with or without T wave inversion may be seen. Patients on high doses of quinine must be monitored for torsades de pointes, ventricular tachycardia, and fibrillation. Patients may develop complete heart block, markedly prolonged QRS complexes, or dysrhythmias. Quinine intoxication can also result in significant hypotension, due to vasodilation and probably a concomitant decrease in myocardial contractility.

Quinine formerly was used for muscle cramps, decreases excitability of the motor endplate to nerve stimulation, and increases the muscle refractory period.[31] Chloroquine, a synthetic aminoquinidine derivative, has been associated with a myasthenic syndrome secondary to the failure of the neuromuscular junction.[37]

Hypoglycemia with elevated plasma insulin levels has been noted in severely malnourished patients, with malaria,[33] a patient with severe congestive heart failure,[27] and in a healthy individual[46] all of whom took quinine. The first two patients took therapeutic doses while the third had overdosed on quinine. In vitro experiments demonstrated that the mechanism for quinine's stimulation of insulin release by beta cells of the pancreas is similar to that of sulfonylureas.[23]

Nausea and vomiting due to both central stimulation of the emesis center and local irritation frequently occur, while diarrhea and abdominal pain are also sometimes seen. Dermatologic manifestations include rashes and angioedema. The skin may also be hot, flushed, and diaphoretic. Oliguria and acute renal failure have been reported.[26] Asthma, due to hypersensitivity reactions, sometimes occurs.

Although hematologic manifestions are rare, when they occur they include thrombocytopenia, agranulocytosis, and hemolysis, which may lead to jaundice and hemoglobinuria. Hemolysis occurs most frequently in those with glucose-6-phosphate dehydrogenase deficiency. Thrombocytopenic purpura may develop through an antibody complement-dependent hypersensitivity response (see Chap. 24).

In pregnant women, high doses of cinchona alkaloids exhibit oxytocic activity that may induce abortion or premature labor. For this reason, despite its known dangers, quinine was once used commonly as an abortifacient (see Chap. 29).

How Should Quinine Overdose Be Treated?

Even with low doses of quinine, nausea and vomiting are noted.[24] However, when quinine is ingested in substantial amounts, emesis almost invariably ensues. Even if the patient has not already vomited on his or her own, emetic agents should not be used, as seizures, dysrhythmias, and hypotension may also develop rapidly. Because activated charcoal is so effective at adsorbing quinine, orogastric lavage should only be performed for patients evaluated within one hour of ingestion or those with large ingestions. Otherwise, standard overdose management is indicated and includes activated charcoal (1 g/kg), catharsis, and supportive techniques such as nasal O_2, cardiac monitoring, and an IV line with 0.9% sodium chloride.

Activated Charcoal

The effect of multiple-dose activated charcoal (MDAC) on quinine elimination has been studied in a human experimental model[27] as well as in symptomatic patients.[36] In these patients, MDAC decreased quinine half-life from 8.23 ± 0.57 hours to 4.55 ± 0.15 hours, and increased clearance by 56%.[36]

Numerous authors[3,28,36] have shown that activated charcoal decreases quinine half-life. Although it is unclear whether the reduction in half-life improves clinical outcome, administration of activated charcoal every 2 to 4 hours is prudent.

Manipulation of pH

Quinine has two pK_a values, of 8.0 and 4.11, thereby accounting for confusion in results and analysis of data associated with pH manipulation. It is true that acidification to a urine pH of 4.5 to 5.5 effectively blocks reabsorption of the alkaloidal base and has been shown to produce a two to threefold increase in quinine clearance in dogs[34] and humans (see Chap. 5).[41] However, due to the increased potential for cardiotoxicity associated with acidification, this technique is not recommended. On the contrary, serum alkalinization may be indicated. In the case of quinine, pH manipulation would be utilized primarily to treat cardiac toxicity and not to alter excretion.

It has been shown that the renal clearance of quinine correlates with neither urine flow nor pH,[3] suggesting that neither diuresis nor acidification are justified. In this study, the mean half-life of quinine in the forced acid diuresis group was 25.1 hours, compared with 26.5 hours in the control group.

The cardiotoxic manifestations of quinine make the choice of serum alkalinization a logical therapeutic intervention. In a human quinine overdose, alkalinization with sodium bicarbonate was dramatically effective in narrowing the QRS complex, but torsades de pointes nevertheless ensued and was responsive only to an overdrive pacemaker.[4] Quinine blocks cardiac sodium channels, which results in prolongation of the P-R interval, and QRS complex, myocardial depression, hypotension, and ventricular tachycardia or fibrillation. All of these manifestations of cardiac toxicity should be treated with alkalinization to achieve a serum pH of 7.45 to 7.50 and to alter sodium channel conduction as would be done in the presence of a patient with a serious cyclic antidepressant overdose (see Antidotes in Depth: Sodium Bicarbonate). In addition, quinine inhibits potassium channels. Hypertonic sodium bicarbonate, which may result in hypokalemia, can exacerbate potassium channel blockade. These patients should be treated like other patients with torsades de pointes (see Chap. 21).

Cardiac Dysrhythmias and Conduction Abnormalities

Alkalinization of serum may be effective in preventing further conduction abnormalities and lethal dysrhythmias. If the management of chloroquinine offers a comparable model, diazepam and epinephrine may also have a cardioprotective effect.[39,40] In the chloroquine management model, rapid control of acidemia, hypoxia (early intubation), electrolyte abnormalities, and hypotension (intravenous fluid and epinephrine) are essential for success. However, currently there are no studies to support this approach in quinine-poisoned patients.

Obviously, no class IA and IC antidysrhythmic agents should be used to treat a quinine, quinidine, or chloroquine overdosed patient, as they may exacerbate the toxin-related conduction disturbances or dysrhythmias (see Chap. 21).

Extracorporeal Techniques

Peritoneal dialysis,[29] hemoperfusion,[32] hemodialysis, and exchange transfusion[3,42] have a limited effect on drug removal. Although the blood compartment can be cleared with the last three of these techniques, total body clearance is only marginally altered. Once the rapid tissue distribution has occurred there is little impact on the total body burden because of the relatively large volume of distribution (1.5 L/kg) and the very extensive protein binding ($\geq$ 85%)

How Should the Ophthalmologic Manifestations of Quinine Intoxication Be Evaluated?

The occurrence of blindness and any recovery from blindness depend on the dose of quinine ingested. There is no evidence to support the theories that quinine-induced blindness results from ischemia, nor is there any evidence to support therapeutic gestures directed toward reversal of ischemia such as stellate ganglion block. The electrophysiologic changes noted following quinine administration in a cat model include retinal ganglion, bipolar, and photoreceptor cell dysfunction.[10] In contrast no electrophysiologic, angiographic, or morphologic experimental evidence for retinal ischemia has been found.[10] Quinine may antagonize cholinergic neurotransmission in the inner synaptic layer.[12]

Initial and follow-up funduscopic and visual field examination, electroretinography, electro-oculogram, visual evoked potentials evaluation, and dark adaptation and color testing may be appropriate diagnostic studies. Improvement in symptomatology is expected to be slow, occuring over a period of months after a severe exposure. Initially, improvement occurs centrally and is followed later by improvement in peripheral vision. The pupils may remain dilated even after return to normal vision.[20] Those with the greatest exposure may develop optic atrophy. There is no specific effective treatment for quinine retinal toxicity.[21]

What Are the Pharmacologic Principles of Chloroquine?

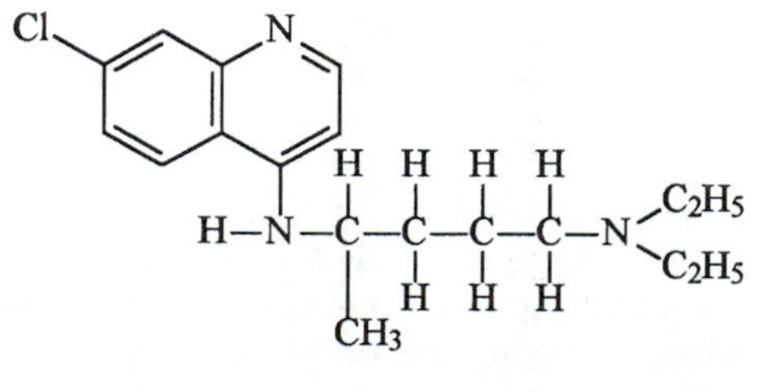

Chloroquine remains a common agent for prophylaxis and treatment of malaria. Chloroquine has the highest fatality rate of all the antimalarial agents; deaths have been frequently reported in the French literature.[39] It has a small toxic to therapeutic margin, making this agent a particularly high-risk in overdose. For this reason extreme care must be used in prescribing chloroquine to prevent unintentional or intentional overdose.

Chloroquine is rapidly absorbed from the GI tract. Toxic symptoms are usually noted within 1 to 3 hours and death may occur as rapidly. Severe chloroquine poisoning is usually associated with serum concentrations exceeding 5 μg/mL. Serum values reflect a small part of total chloroquine load, as the mean apparent volume of distribution is 61 ± 9 L/kg.[45] Chloroquine is highly bound to many different tissues, particularly kidney, liver, and lung.[22]

Chloroquine is eliminated in the urine, 70% as the parent molecule and the remainder as metabolites. An exceedingly long half-life of 41 ± 14 days has been reported.[45] In view of the nature and degree of chloroquine tissue distribution, its high protein binding of 61 ± 9%, and long terminal half-life elimination, it is easy to understand why enhanced elimination procedures have not been beneficial.

What Are the Toxicologic Manifestations and Treatment of Chloroquine Intoxication?

Toxic manifestations of chloroquine are often grave. Although the extent and frequency of the clinical manifestations differ, the mechanisms are presumed to be similar to those of quinine and quinidine. The ophthalmologic manifestations are usually less consequential and are transient in nature.[8] The neurologic manifestations include CNS depression, dizziness, headache, and convulsions. Respiratory compromise and sudden apnea have been noted. Hypotension and cardiovascular compromise can be precipitous. Electrocardiographic abnormalities include QRS prolongation, ST-T depression, increased U waves, and QT interval prolongation. Significant hypokalemia is invariably associated with the cardiac manifestations and may be causal.[24]

Animal[15] and human[40] work suggests that early management of severe chloroquine intoxication may have a cardioprotective effect and decrease the fatality rate. A retrospective historical analysis was used to determine that the ingestion of 5 g (or more) of chloroquine is the most accurate predictor of a fatal outcome. Data from several studies[17,40,44] demonstrate that epinephrine and diazepam counteract the cardiovascular effects of chloroquine and decrease its toxic manifestations.

The protective effects of diazepam in chloroquine poisoning have also been demonstrated experimentally in rats[15] and in pigs.[40] In the rat model,[15] intraperitoneal diazepam was administered after an oral LD_{50} dose of chloroquine. This study demonstrated a decreased mortality rate. In the pig model,[40] a pentobarbital anesthetized animal poisoned with chloroquine was given intravenous diazepam. In the diazepam-treated animals, systolic and diastolic pressures, heart rate, urine volume, urinary chloroquine levels, and plasma and red blood cell chloroquine levels all were higher, and QRS duration was shorter. The authors concluded that diazepam counteracted both hemodynamic and electrocardiographic manifestations of chloroquine intoxication. When this approach was studied in a chloroquine poisoned rat model, the QRS complex narrowed rapidly, although the mean rate of narrowing was quite modest.[16] A small study in a chloroquine-poisoned rat model suggested that barbiturate anesthesia with thiobutobarbitone and isoprenaline was more consequential and efficacious than diazepam and epinephine.[11] The study design, number of animals, and consistency of the data necessitate further investigation to achieve adequate understanding.

In a group of treated patients who had ingested more than 5 g of chloroquine and had exceedingly high blood levels (40 to 80 μmol/L, or 12 to 24 μg/mL), diazepam and epinephrine were used.[39] There were no controls and all patients received early orotracheal intubation initiated by a nurse or physician in the home. Early mechanical ventilation was instituted with an FIO_2 of 40%, a tidal volume of 10 mL/kg, and a ventilatory rate of 14 breaths/min. Epinephrine (0.25 μg/kg/min) was given IV with D_5W, incrementally until a systolic blood pressure over 100 mm Hg was achieved. After intubation, 2 mg/kg of IV diazepam was given over 30 minutes and then 1 to 2 mg/kg per day was administered for 2 to 4 days. These patients also had orogastric lavage performed. Even after this initial therapy, 5 patients manifested transient cardiovascular compromise and required additional epinephrine and other catecholamines. Of the 11 patients in the study, 10 survived, compared with only 1 patient in the historical control group.[39] A single case report is available of a child who ingested chloroquine, developed cardiac arrest, was given CPR, and 40 minutes after collapse was given epinephrine and diazepam with return of heart rate and a sustained pulse.[30] Although the authors suggest the potential benefit of diazepam in this child receiving CPR at an arterial pH of 6.86, epinephrine might have taken 5 minutes to result in a response as opposed to suggesting that the 12 mg (1 mg/kg) of diazepam was responsible for immediate resuscitation in this pulseless child. This child ultimately died of grave posthypoxic central nervous system injury.

The role of epinephrine in the management of chloroquine-related vasodilation and myocardial depression is more easily understandable. The benefit of early intervention for neurologic or cardiorespiratory compromise in patients with chloroquine overdose is evident by the transformation of patients with potentially lethal ingestions into patients who survive the acute toxicity.

Continuous and aggressive cardiorespiratory and neurologic support of these patients appears to be the most critical factor in survival. The precise manner by which diazepam improves hemodynamic function and ECG abnormalities remains to be elucidated.

What Other Antimalarials Are Used?

The chemotherapeutic agents used for malaria are exceedingly diverse and combination regimens have been developed for both prophylaxis and the treatment of resistant strains (Table 44–2). The quinoline agents discussed in this chapter have very narrow toxic to therapeutic ratios and present a substantial risk of toxicity. Three agents that are frequently used are mefloquine and amodiaquine for *P. falciparum*, and primaquine for *P. vivax* or *P. ovale*.

In the last decade, there have been several case reports of mefloquine toxicity.[6,41] Mefloquine has a long half-life and is effective for chloroquine-resistant *P. falciparum* malaria. Most of the cases of toxicity occurred 2 to 3 weeks after a single therapeutic dose. Although the main carboxylic acid metabolite of mefloquine does not traverse the blood–brain barrier, very high plasma and cerebrospinal fluid levels of mefloquine were reported. In each case the clinician's initial assumption was that the patient had cerebral malaria; however, the diffuse encephalopathy and seizures resolved spontaneously with cessation of the mefloquine over several days. The duration of the neuropsychiatric manifestations seems directly correlated with the very long half-life of 20 ± 4 days (Table 44–3). Hypotension, dysrhythmias, and hepatic abnormalities have also been reported. Amodiaquine has limited gastrointestinal toxicity but has been associated with headache, dizziness, visual impairment, and extrapyramidal manifestations.[35] Primaquine may cause methemoglobinemia. No cases of piperaquine overdoses have been reported.

TABLE 44–2. CURRENT ANTIMALARIAL AGENTS FOR PROPHYLAXIS AND TREATMENT[a]

Quinoline Derivatives
- Quinine
- Chloroquine
- Mefloquine
- Piperaquine
- Primaquine
- Amodiaquine

Dihydrofolate Reductase Inhibitors
- Proguanil
- Chlorproguanil
- Pyrimethamine
- (Pyrimethamine/Dapsone = Maloprim)
- (Pyrimethamine/sulfadoxine = Fansidar)

Sulfonamides and Sulfones
- Sulfonamides
- Dapsone
- Sulfonamide and sulfone combinations

Antibacterials
- Tetracycline
- Doxycycline

Others
- Halofantrine
- Artemisinin and derivatives

[a]Only the quinoline derivatives are discussed in this chapter. Discussions of other agents are found in Chapters 24, 28, and 46.

TABLE 44–3. QUINOLINE DERIVATIVES

	Quinine	Chloroquine	Mefloquine
Plasma bound (%)	93 ± 3	61 ± 9	98.2
Volume distribution (L/kg)	1.8 ± 0.4	115 ± 61	19 ± 6
Half-life	11 ± 2 h	41 ± 14 d	20 ± 4 d
Toxic concentration	> 2 μg/mL	0.25 μg/mL	—
Urinary excretion (%)	12	61 ± 4	< 1

Reprinted, with permission, from Silamut K, Molunto P, Ho M, et al: α-1-Acid glycoprotein (orosomucoid) and plasma protein binding of quinine in Falciparum *malaria. Br J Clin Pharmacol 1991;32:311–315.*

References

1. Alvan G, Karlsson KK, Villen T: Reversible hearing impairment related to quinine blood concentrations in guinea pigs. Life Sci 1989;45:751–755.
2. Bankes JLK, Hayward JA, Jones MBS: Quinine amblyopia treated with stellate ganglion block. Br Med J 1972;4:85–86.
3. Bateman DN, Blain PG, Woodhouse KW, et al: Pharmacokinetics and clinical toxicity of quinine overdosage: Lack of efficacy of techniques intended to enhance elimination. Q J Med 1985;54:125–131.
4. Bodenhamer JE, Smilkstein MJ: Delayed cardiotoxicity following quinine overdose: A Case Report. J Emerg Med 1993;11:279–285.
5. Boland ME, Roper SMB, Henry JA: Complications of quinine poisoning. Lancet 1985;384–385.
6. Bourgeade A, Tonin V, Keudjian F, et al: Intoxication accidentelle à la mefloquine. Presse Med 1990;19:1903.
7. Brinton GS, Norton EWD, Zahn JR, Knighton RW: Ocular quinine toxicity. Am J Ophthalmol 1980;90:403–410.
8. Britton WJ, Kevau JH: Intentional chloroquinine overdosage. Med J Aus 1978;21:407–410.
9. Brust JCM, Richter RW: Quinine amblyopia related to heroin addiction. Ann Intern Med 1971;74:84–86.
10. Buchanan TAS, Lyness RW, Collins AD, et al: An experimental study of quinine blindness. Eye 1987;1:522–524.
11. Buckley NA, Smith AJ, Dosen P, O'Connell DL: Effects of catecholamines and diazepam in chloroquine poisoning in barbiturate anaesthetised rats. Hum Exp Tox 1996;15: 909–914.
12. Canning CR, Hague S: Ocular quinine toxicity. Br J Ophthalmol 1988;72:23–26.
13. Christie DJ, Walker RH, Kolins MD, et al: Quinine-induced thrombocytopenia following intravenous use of heroin. Arch Intern Med 1983;143:1174–1175.
14. Cibis GW, Burian HM, Blod FC: Electroretinogram in acute quinine poisoning. Arch Ophthalmol 1973;90:307–309.
15. Crouzette J, Vicaut E, Palombo S, et al: Experimental assess-

ment of the prospective activity of diazepam on the acute toxicity of chloroquine. J Toxicol Clin Toxicol 1983;20: 271–280.

16. Curry SC, Conner DA, Clark RF, et al: The effect of hypertonic sodium bicarbonate on QRS duration in rats poisoned with chloroquine. J Toxicol Clin Toxicol 1996;34:73–76.
17. Don Michael TA, Aiwazzadeh S: The effects of acute chloroquine poisoning with special reference to the heart. Am Heart J 1970;79:831–842.
18. Dyson EH, Proudfoot AT, Bateman DN: Quinine amblyopia: Is current management appropriate? J Toxicol Clin Toxicol 1985–1986;23:571–578.
19. Dyson EH, Proudfoot AT, Prescott LF, Heyworth R: Death and blindness due to overdose of quinine. Br Med J 1985;291:31–33.
20. Gangitano JL, Keltner JL: Abnormalities of the pupil and visual evoked potential in quinine amblyopia. Am J Ophthalmol 1980;89:425–430.
21. Guly U, Driscoll P: The management of quinine induced blindness. Arch Emerg Med 1992;9:317–322.
22. Gustafsson LI, Walker O, Alvan G, et al: Disposition of chloroquine in man after single intravenous and oral doses. Br J Clin Pharmacol 1983;15:471–479.
23. Henquin J: Quinine and the stimulus secretion coupling in pancreatic β cells: Glucose like effects on potassium permeability and insulin release. Endocrinology 1982;110: 1325–1332.
24. Jaeger A, Sauder P, Kopferschmitt J, Flesch F: Clinical features and management of poisoning due to antimalarial drugs. Med Toxicol 1987;2:242–273.
25. Karlsson KK, Flock A: Quinine causes isolated outer hair cells to change length. Neurosci Lett 1990;116:101–105.
26. Lang PA, Jones CC: Acute renal failure precipitated by quinine sulfate in early pregnancy. JAMA 1964;188:464–466.
27. Limburg PJ. Katz H, Grant CS, Service FJ: Quinine induced hypoglycemia. Ann Intern Med 1993;119:218–219.
28. Lockey D, Bateman DN: Effect of oral activated charcoal on quinine elimination. Br J Clin Pharmacol 1989;27:92–94.
29. Markham TN, Dodson VN, Eckberg DL: Peritoneal dialysis in quinine sulfate intoxication. JAMA 1967;202:1102–1103.
30. McCarthy VP, Swabe GL: Chloroquine poisoning in a child. Pediatr Emerg Care 1996;12:207–209.
31. McGee SR: Muscle cramps. Arch Intern Med 1990;150: 511–518.
32. Morgan MD, Rainford DJ, Pusey CD, et al: The treatment of quinine poisoning with charcoal hemoperfusion. Postgrad Med J 1983;59:365–367.
33. Okitolonda W, Delacollette C, Malengreau M, Henquin JC: High incidence of hypoglycemia in African patients treated with intravenous quinine for severe malaria. Br Med J 1987;295:716–718.
34. Orloff J, Berliner RW: The mechanism of the excretion of ammonia in the dog. J Clin Invest 1956;35:233–235.
35. Phillips-Howard PA, Terkville FO:CNS adverse events associated with antimalarial agents. Fact or fiction? Drug Saf 1995;12:370–383.
36. Prescott LF, Hamilton AR, Heyworth R: Treatment of quinine overdose with repeated oral charcoal. Br J Clin Pharmacol 1989;27:95–97.
37. Robberecht W, Bednarik J, Bourgeois P, et al: Myasthenic syndrome caused by direct effect of chloroquine on neuromuscular junction. Arch Neurol 1989;46:464–468.
38. Roche RJ, Silamut K, Pukrittayakamee S, et al: Quinine induces reversible high tone hearing loss. Br J Clin Pharmacol 1990;29:780–782.
39. Riou B, Barriot P, Rimailho A, Baud FJ: Treatment of severe chloroquine poisoning. N Engl J Med 1988;318:1–7.
40. Riou B, Rimailho A, Galliot M, et al: Protective cardiovascular effects of diazepam in experimental acute chloroquine poisoning. Intens Care Med 1988;14:610–616.
41. Rouviex B, Bricaire F, Michon C, et al: Mefloquine and an acute brain syndrome. Ann Intern Med 1989;110:577–578.
42. Sabto J, Pierce RM, West RH, Gurr FW: Haemodialysis, peritoneal dialysis, plasmapheresis and forced diuresis for the treatment of quinine overdose. Clin Nephrol 1981;16: 264–268.
43. Silamut K, Molunto P, Ho M, et al: α-1-Acid glycoprotein (orosomucoid) and plasma protein binding of quinine in *Falciparum* malaria. Br J Clin Pharmacol 1991;32:311–315.
44. Sofola OA: The effects of chloroquine on the electrocardiogram and heart rate in anesthetized dogs. Clin Physiol 1983;3:75–82.
45. Tracy JW, Webster LT: Drugs used in the chemotherapy of protozoal infection: Malaria. In: Hardman JG, Limbird LE, Molinoff PB, et al, eds: Goodman and Gilman's The Pharmacological Basis of Therapeutics, 9th ed. New York, McGraw-Hill, 1996, pp. 965–985.
46. Wenstone R, Bell M, Mostafa SM: Fatal adult respiratory distress syndrome after quinine overdose. Lancet 1989;1: 1143–1144. Letter.

CHAPTER 45

Ergotamines

Neal A. Lewin

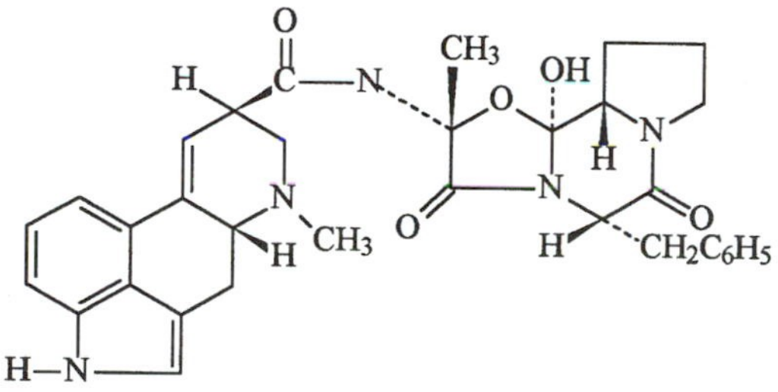

Ergotamine

A 33-year-old man presented to the emergency department (ED) with substernal chest pain. His past medical history was remarkable for 2 weeks of daily headaches. He had visited his personal physician, who prescribed Fiorinal (caffeine 50 mg, aspirin 300 mg, and butalbital 50 mg) for migraine headaches. After failing a trial of Fiorinal, the patient was started on Cafergot (ergotamine tartrate 1 mg and caffeine 100 mg). He was specifically instructed to take no more than 6 Cafergot tablets per day and no more than 10 tablets per week. For the first 5 days he took 4 tablets each day, which relieved his headache. On day 6 he took 4 tablets in the morning, but the headache returned in the afternoon and he took an additional 10 tablets. A total of 34 tablets (34 mg of ergotamine) were consumed within 6 days. Within 10 minutes of taking the 10 tablets he noted tingling in his forehead and the onset of substernal pressure.

The emergency medical service was called within half an hour of the onset of his chest pain. The patient vomited once in the ambulance. On arrival in the ED he still had substernal pressure. His vital signs were: blood pressure, 150/90 mm Hg; pulse, 100 beats/min; respirations, 20 breaths/min; rectal temperature, 98.6°F (37°C). His head was without signs of trauma. The pupils were equal, round (at 3 to 4 mm), and reactive to light, and extraocular movements were intact. Funduscopic examination showed no evidence of increased intracranial pressure or hemorrhage. The neck was supple and there was no thyromegaly or carotid bruits. The chest was clear to auscultation and percussion. Heart sounds were normal. The abdomen was soft, nontender, and without organomegaly. Stool was negative for occult blood. Pulses were strong and symmetric, and there were no signs of clubbing, cyanosis, edema, or ulcerations on the extremities. There were no focal neurologic findings. One inch of 2% nitropaste (nitroglycerin paste) was immediately applied to the chest and an ECG was performed, which showed ST segment elevations in precordial leads V_2 to V_5 interpreted as early repolarization abnormalities, with biphasic T waves in leads III and aVF (Fig. 45–1). Intravenous nitroglycerin was started and the pain resolved. Subsequent ECGs showed inversion of the T waves in leads III and aVF, consistent with inferior myocardial injury (Fig. 45–2). Cardiac isoenzymes were nondiagnostic. A cardiac pyrophosphate scan was consistent with anteroseptal and inferior myocardial infarction.

What Is Ergotism? What Is the Source and History of Ergotism?

Ergotism, a toxicologic syndrome resulting from excessive use of ergot preparations, is characterized by intense

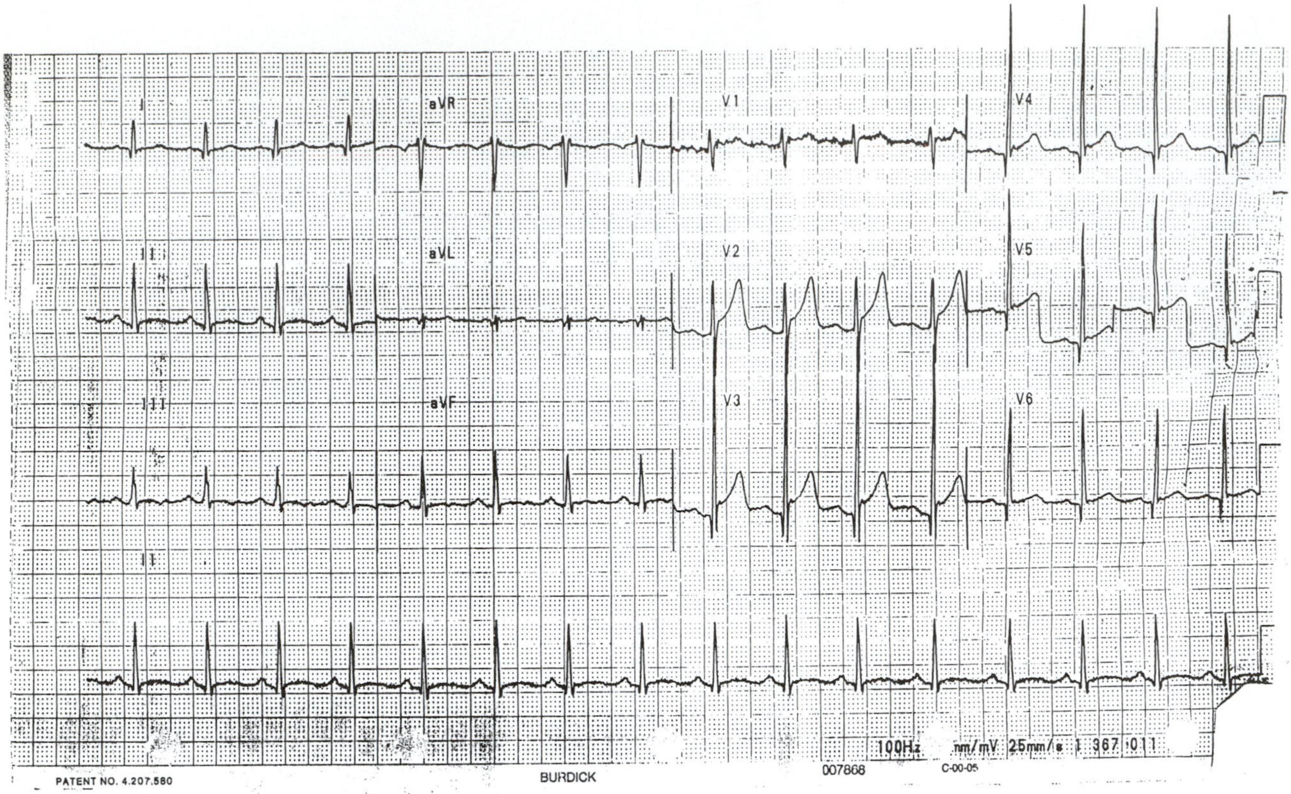

Figure 45–1. This 12-lead electrocardiogram (ECG) was obtained in the patient after the application of 2% nitropaste. The ECG shows ST segment elevation in the precordial leads (V_2 to V_5) interpreted as early repolarization, and biphasic T waves in leads III and aVF.

burning of the extremities, hemorrhagic vesiculations, pruritis, formications, nausea, vomiting, and gangrene (Table 45–1). Headache, fixed miosis, hallucinations, delirium, cerebrovascular ischemia, and convulsions are also associated with this condition.[8] Acute overdose is uncommon. Many published cases describe ingestions of combination preparations containing an ergot alkaloid and caffeine. In an acute overdose—although restlessness, nausea, vomiting, or agitation develop within 4 hours—peripheral vasospasm may not be obvious for 24 hours. Chronic ergotism usually presents with peripheral ischemia of the lower extremities, although ischemia of cerebral, mesenteric, coronary, and renal vascular beds is well documented.[1,5,6,17,18]

Ergot is the product of *Claviceps purpurea*, a fungus that contaminates rye and other grains. The spores of the fungus are both windborn and transported by insects to young rye, where they germinate into hyphal filaments. When these spores germinate they destroy the grain and harden into a curved body called the sclerotium, which is a major commercial source of ergot alkaloids.[15] This fungus can elaborate diverse substances, including ergotamine, histamine, tyramine, isomylamine, acetylcholine, and acetaldehyde.

In 600 B.C., an Assyrian tablet made mention of contamination of grain believed to be *Claviceps purpurea*. In approximately 400 B.C., contaminated grass that killed pregnant women was described. In the Middle Ages epidemics causing gangrene of the extremities, with mummification of limbs, were depicted in the literature. The disease was called holy fire or St. Anthony's fire, due to the blackened limbs resembling the charring from fire and the burning sensation expressed by its victims. It has been postulated that improvement occurred when victims went to visit the shrine of St. Anthony due to a diet free of contaminated grain. Abortion and seizures were also reported with this poisoning. As early as 1582, ergot was used by midwives to assist in the childbirth process. Desgranges was the first physician to use ergot for obstetrical care in 1818. In 1824, Hosack reported that the ergot could be used for the control of postpartum hemorrhage, but that its routine use during labor was to be avoided due to the drug's toxicity.[15] Ergot's clinical use since 1950 has been almost entirely limited to the treatment of vascular headaches. Ergonovine, another ergot derivative, is used in obstetric care for its stimulant effect on uterine smooth muscle. It is also employed during cardiac catheterizations to induce coronary artery spasm

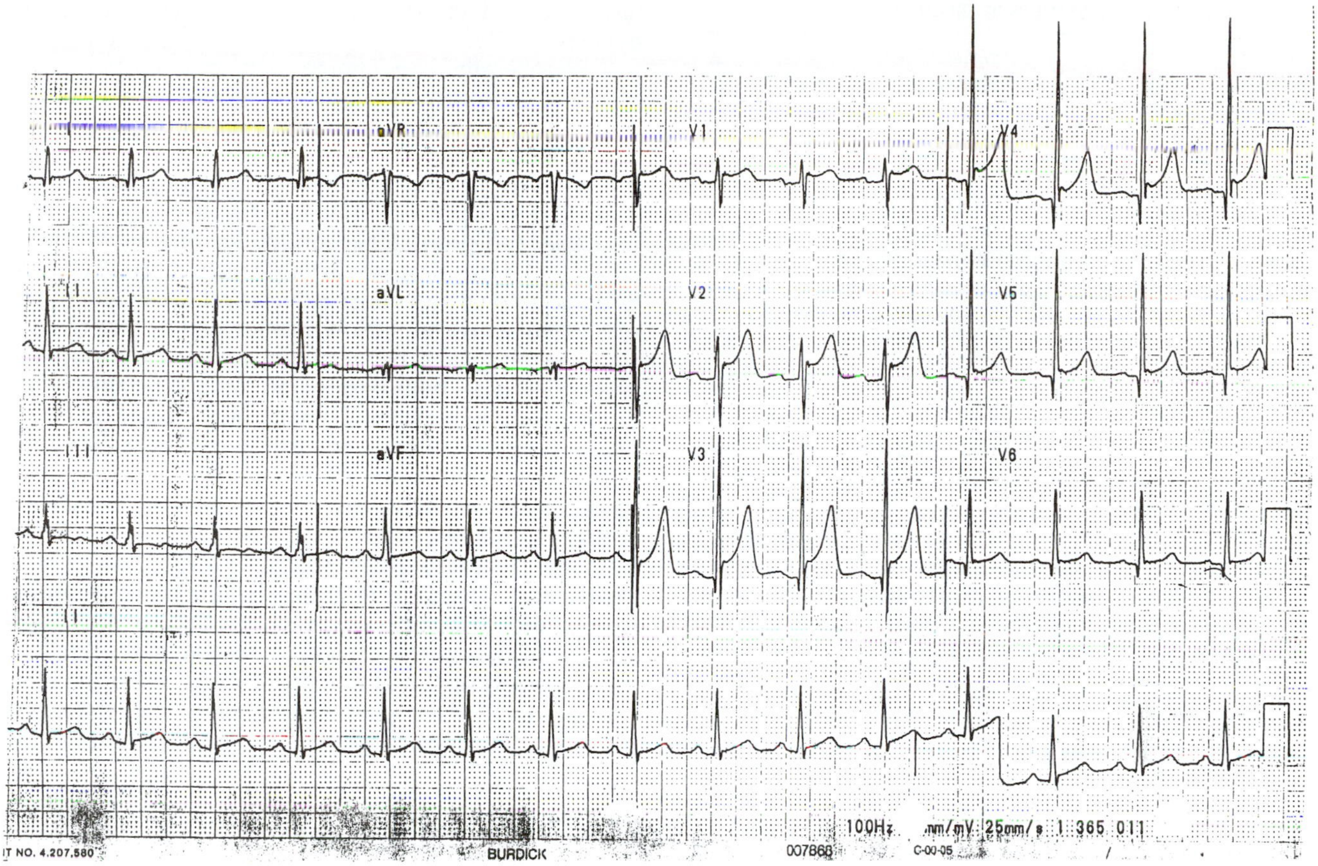

Figure 45–2. A subsequent 12-lead electrocardiogram (ECG) from the patient taken after the initiation of IV nitroglycerin therapy. The ECG now demonstrates inversion of the T wave in lead III and normalization of the T wave in aVF.

and assist in the diagnosis of Prinzmetal's angina. Ergots have also been used as a putative cognition enhancer,[23] in the management of orthostatic hypotension,[22] and to prevent the secretion of prolactin.[16]

Presently, epidemics of ergotism in the United States are prevented by government inspections of grain fields. If a grain field contains more than 0.3% infected grain, it is rejected for commercial sale; there have been years where as much as 36% of the grain was rejected.[15]

What Are the Pharmacologic and Pathophysiologic Features of the Ergot Alkaloids?

The ergot alkaloids can be divided into three groups: amino acid alkaloids, dihydrogenated amino acid alkaloids, and amine alkaloids. All ergot alkaloids are derivatives of the tetracyclic compound 6-methylergoline (Fig. 45–3, Table 45–2).

The amino acid alkaloid group, or ergopeptines, includes ergotamine, ergocristine, ergosine, ergocornine, and bromocriptine. The dihydrogenated group include dihydroergotamine, dihydroergocristine, dihydroergosine, and dihydroergocornine. The amine alkaloids include ergonovine, ergometrine, ergobasine, and methysergide. The pharmacokinetics of the ergot alkaloids are well defined from controlled human volunteer studies, whereas the toxicokinetics are unknown. Almost all of the ergots are poorly absorbed orally and there is considerable first-pass hepatic metabolism, resulting in highly variable bioavailability. Intramuscular absorption is unpredictable and actions are often delayed.[14] The effective oral dose is approximately 10 times the intramuscular dose.[14] Ergotamine suppositories increase bioavailability 20 times compared to orally administered doses.[10,20] Peak plasma levels with most ergots occur within 30 to 120 minutes.[14] The volume of distribution is approximately 2 L/kg, and the half-life varies from 1.4 to 6.2 hours.

The pharmacologic effects of the ergot alkaloids are complex and can be mutually antagonistic.[15] The actions of the ergot alkaloids can be subdivided into central and peripheral effects. In the CNS, ergotamine is believed to

TABLE 45–1. CLINICAL MANIFESTATIONS OF ERGOTISM

Central Effects	Peripheral Effects
Agitation	Bradycardia
Cerebrovascular ischemia	
Hallucinations	***Ischemic Effects***
Headaches	Angina
Miosis (fixed)	Gangrene
Nausea	Hemorrhagic vesiculations and bullae
Seizures	Mesenteric infarction
Twitching (facial)	Myocardial infarction
Vomiting	Renal infarction

have a sympatholytic effect, stimulating and potentiating serotonergic (tryptaminergic) receptors and interfering with neuronal serotonin reuptake (Table 45–2).[16] The ergots interact with all known 5-HT_1 and 5-HT_2 receptors.[15] The result is increased intrasynaptic serotonin activity in the median raphe neurons of the brainstem.[17] Because serotonin is an inhibitory CNS neurotransmitter, ergotamine is thought to decrease the neuronal firing rate and stabilize the cerebrovascular smooth musculature. The stabilization of the cerebrovascular beds by the ergots makes them useful drugs for the treatment of migraine headaches, which are characterized by cerebrovascular hyperreactivity.

Peripherally, ergotamine acts as a partial alpha-adrenergic agonist or as an antagonist at adrenergic, dopaminergic, and serotonergic (tryptaminergic) receptors.[15] Table 45–2 summarizes the pharmacologic actions of selected ergot alkaloids currently used in clinical medicine. The spectrum of effects depends on dosage, host response, and physiologic conditions. The usual clinical effect at therapeutic doses is vasoconstriction. There may be an additional vasoconstrictive effect caused by the direct action of ergotamine on the media of the arterioles.[16]

The difference between the effects of therapeutic and toxic doses, both peripherally and centrally, is that in the peripheral vessels, therapeutic doses of ergotamine produce mild vasoconstriction. The effect is directly dose related; therefore, at toxic doses, extreme vasoconstriction produces the characteristic ischemic changes seen in ergotism.

The cerebrovascular effects of ergots are not as clearly understood. In migraine treatment, for example, therapeutic doses of ergotamine produce a mild vasoconstriction via alpha-adrenergic receptors, especially in intracranial vessels that are already dilated during a migraine attack. This vasoconstriction is considered the basis for the ergot's ability to terminate a migraine

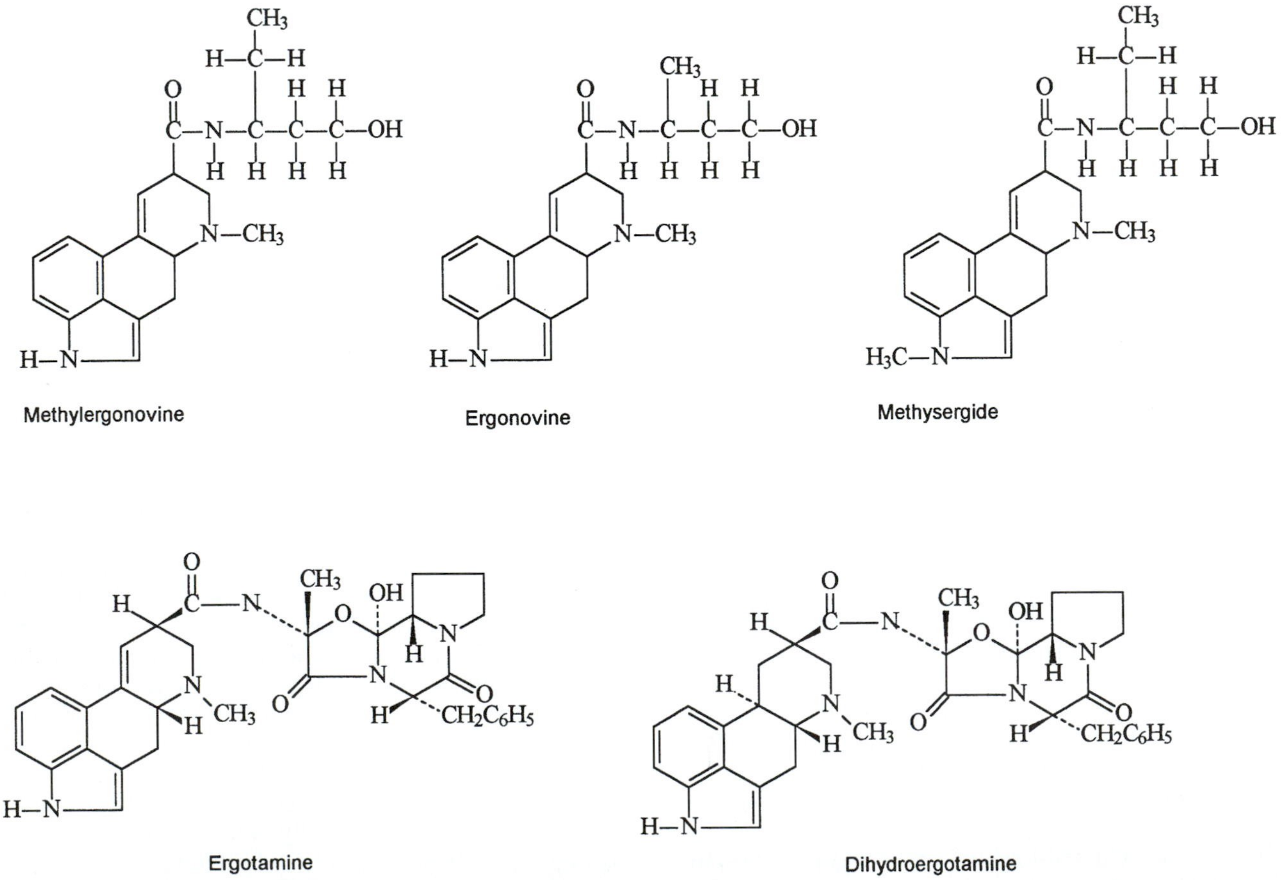

Figure 45–3. Chemical structures of ergot derivatives.

TABLE 45–2. ERGOTAMINE COMPOUNDS

Compound	Interactions With Tryptaminergic (Serotonergic) Receptors	Interactions With Dopaminergic Receptors	Interactions With α-Adrenergic Receptors
Ergotamine (amino acid alkaloid)	Vasculature: Partial agonist Smooth muscles: Nonselective antagonist CNS: Poor agonist/antagonist	CNS: Emetic (potent)	Vasculature: Partial agonist/ antagonist Smooth muscles: Partial agonist/ antagonist CNS: Antagonist PNS: Antagonist
Bromocriptine (amino acid alkaloid)	Weak antagonist	CNS: Partial agonist/antagonist; inhibits prolactin secretion; emetic (mild)	Vasculature: Antagonist
Dihydroergotamine (dihydrogenated group)	Smooth muscles: Partial agonist/antagonist CNS: Agonist lateral geniculate nucleus	CNS: emetic (mild) Sympathetic ganglia: antagonism	Vasculature: partial agonist: veins; antagonist: arteries Smooth muscles: Antagonism CNS/PNS: Antagonism
Ergonovine and methyl ergonovine (amine alkaloid)	Smooth muscles: Potent antagonist Vasculature: Agonist in umbilical and placental vessels CNS: Partial antagonist/agonist	CNS: Emesis (mild); inhibits prolactin (weak); partial agonist/antagonist Vasculature: Weak antagonist	Vasculature: Partial agonists
Methysergide (amine alkaloid)	Vasculature: Partial agonist CNS: Potent antagonist	None	None

Adapted, with permission, from Peroutka SJ: Drugs effective in the therapy of migraine. In: Hardman JG, Limbird LE, Molinoff PB, et al, eds: Goodman and Gilman's The Pharmacological Basis of Therapeutics, 9th ed. New York, McGraw-Hill, 1996, pp. 491–496.

headache. There is very little definitive information, however, regarding toxic doses of the ergots on the cerebrovasculature. Cephalic vasodilation may occur, but the mechanism for this effect is unknown. One hypothesis is that toxic doses of the drug initially produce vasoconstriction and ischemia, just as in the periphery, but as the cerebrovasculature cannot tolerate hypoxia and hypercapnea, rapid vasodilation then ensues to improve local perfusion. Alpha-adrenergic receptors in the CNS function differently from those in the periphery, and it may be that CNS vascular tone cannot be maintained in the setting of local tissue hypoxia.

The toxic vascular effects ascribed to ergot alkaloids are complex and sometimes conflicting (see Table 45–2). Subintimal and medial fibrosis, vasospasm, and arteriolar and venous thrombi (in general, stasis related) are all reported.[11] Angiography can demonstrate distal, segmental vessel spasm with increased collateralization in patients with chronic ergotism. The coronary, renal, cerebral, ophthalmic, and mesenteric vasculature,[19] as well as the vessels of the extremities, may also be affected.[21] Neuropathic changes may be secondary to ischemia of the vasa nervorum injury.

Bradycardia is a characteristic effect of the ergot alkaloids. Bradycardia is believed to be a reflex baroreceptor-mediated phenomenon associated with vasoconstriction, but a reduction in sympathetic tone, direct myocardial depression, and increased vagal activity may also be factors.[15]

Methysergide, an amine alkaloid, has potent vasoconstrictive characteristics and is a serotonin antagonist used to prevent migraine headaches.[7] Methysergide's use is limited due to its well-described adverse effects of retroperitoneal fibrosis[18] as well as pleuropericardial, endocardial, and endovascular fibrosis.[13,18]

What Is the Treatment for Ergotism?

The treatment for ergot toxicity depends on the severity of the clinical findings (Table 45–3). Shortly after an acute oral overdose, if vomiting is not present, basic management should include multiple-dose activated charcoal

TABLE 45–3. TREATMENT OF ERGOTISM

Acute

Basic Management
- Syrup of ipecac or orogastric lavage—often will not be necessary due to spontaneous emesis
- Multiple-dose activated charcoal and sorbitol or magnesium sulfate cathartic

Advanced Management
- Hypertension or cerebral, mesenteric, or cardiac ischemia: IV nitroglycerin, nitroprusside, or phentolamine titrated to adequate blood pressure and perfusion
- Mild peripheral vascular ischemia with adequate perfusion: Oral prazosin, captopril, or nifedipine titrated to adequate perfusion
- Seizures and hallucinations: Diazepam, lorazepam titrated until seizures and hallucinations cease
- Hypercoagulable conditions: Heparin or dextran titrated until anticoagulated; thrombolytic therapy?

Chronic

Withdraw drug

Surgery if gangrene is advanced or to remove a clot

and sorbitol. If emesis is present, metoclopramide can be used as an antiemetic to facilitate the administration of activated charcoal. The use of ipecac or an orogastric tube should be used rarely, if at all, since vomiting is a common early occurrence of acute ergot toxicity. In mild cases, characterized by minimal pain of the extremities, supportive measures such as hydration and analgesia are all that is needed. In more serious cases, severe peripheral vasoconstriction may produce ischemic changes including angina, myocardial infarction, cerebral ischemia, and mesenteric ischemia. Intravenous vasodilators, such as nitroprusside,[1,2,12] nitroglycerin,[9] or phentolamine, are indicated to reverse the ischemia. Prazosin,[3] captopril,[24] and nifedipine[4] have also been used to achieve peripheral vasodilation, and may be appropriate with less severe vasospasm, manifested by dysesthesias and minimal ischemic pain of the digits, where immediate reversal may not yet be imperative.

Although sympathetic block, epidural block, or sympathectomy—all of which have been used in past—may relieve vasoconstriction mediated via the central nervous system (CNS), these modalities would not be expected to antagonize the direct action of ergotamine on arteriolar smooth muscle.[1] Heparinization, corticosteroids, or low-molecular-weight dextran may be used to prevent sludging and subsequent clot formation. The use of thrombolytic agents in this setting has not been evaluated. Arteriotomy may be necessary to remove large clots. Hyperbaric oxygen may correct local tissue hypoxia.

In conclusion, although epidemic ergotism is no longer a concern in this country since testing of grain by the government exists, ergot poisoning both by unintentional and intentional ingestions continues to be reported. Knowledge of these agents' complex pharmacologic and physiologic actions, and use of appropriate pharmacologic agents, allow the clinician to minimize its morbidity and mortality of the past.

Acknowledgment

Richard S. Weisman, PharmD contributed to this chapter in a previous edition.

References

1. Anderson PK, Christensen KN, Hole P, et al: Sodium nitroprusside and epidural blockage in treatment of ergotism. N Engl J Med 1977;296:1271–1273.
2. Carliner NH, Denune DP, Finch CS, Goldberg LI: Sodium nitroprusside treatment of ergotamine-induced peripheral ischemia. JAMA 1974;227:308–309.
3. Cobaugh DS: Prazosin treatment of ergotamine induced peripheral ischemia. JAMA 1980;244:1360.
4. Dagher FJ, Paris SO: Severe unilateral ischemia of the lower extremity caused by ergotamine. Surgery 1985;97:369–373.
5. Finchan RW, Perdue Z, Dunn VD: Bilateral focal cortical atrophy and chronic ergotamine abuse. Neurology 1985;35:720–722.
6. Fisher PE, Silk DBA, Menzies-Gow N, Dingle M: Ergotamine abuse and extra-hepatic portal hypertension. Postgrad Med J 1988;61:461–463.
7. Graham JR: Methysergide for prevention of headache. N Engl J Med 1964;270:67–72.
8. Harrison TS: Ergotaminism. JACEP 1978;7:162–169.
9. Husum B, Metz P, Rasmussen JP, et al: Nitroglycerin infusion for ergotism. Lancet 1979;2:794–795.
10. Ibraheem JJ, Paalzow L, Tfelt-Hansen P: Kinetics of ergotamine after intravenous and intramuscular administration of migraine sufferers. Eur J Clin Pharmacol 1982;23:235–240.
11. Merhoff GC, Porter JM: Ergot intoxication: Historical review and description of unusual clinical manifestations. Ann Surg 1974;180:733–779.
12. O'Dell CW, Davis GB, Johnson AD, et al: Sodium nitroprusside in the treatment of ergotism. Radiology 1977;124:73–74.
13. Orlando RC, Moyer P, Barnett TB: Methysergide therapy and constrictive pericarditis. Ann Intern Med 1978;88:213–214.
14. Orton DA, Richardson RJ: Ergotamine absorption and toxicity. Postgrad Med J 1982;58:6–11.
15. Peroutka SJ: Drugs effective in the therapy of migraine. In: Hardman JG, Limbird LE, Molinoff PB, et al, eds: Goodman and Gilman's The Pharmacological Basis of Therapeutics, 9th ed. New York, McGraw-Hill, 1996, pp. 491–496.
16. Rall TW, Schleifer LS: Oxytocin, prostaglandins, ergot alkaloids and other tocolytic agents. In: Gilman AG, Rall TW, Nies AS, Taylor P, eds: Goodman and Gilman's The Pharmacological Basis of Therapeutics, 8th ed. New York, Pergamon, 1990, pp. 933–953.
17. Raskin N, Appenzeller O: Migraine pathogenesis. In: Raskin N, Appenzeller, O, eds: Major Problems in Internal Medicine. Vol. 19. Philadelphia, Saunders, 1980, pp. 84–104.
18. Redfield MM, Nicholson WJ, Edwards WD, Tajik AJ: Valve disease associated with ergot alkaloid use: Echocardiographic and pathologic correlations. Ann Intern Med 1992;117:50–52.
19. Rogers PA, Mansberger JA: Gastrointestinal vascular ischemia caused by ergotamine. South Med J 1989;82:1058–1059.
20. Sanders SW, Haering N, Mosberg H, Jaegger H: Pharmacokinetics of ergotamine in healthy volunteers following oral and rectal dosing. Eur J Clin Pharmacol 1986;30:331–334.
21. Senta HJ, Lieberman AN, Pinto R: Cerebral manifestations of ergotism: Report of a case and review of the literature. Stroke 1976;7:88–92.
22. Stumpf JL, Mitrzyk B: Management of orthostatic hypotension. Am J Hosp Pharm 1994;51:618–660.
23. Wadsworth AN, Chrisp P: Co-dergocrine mesylate. A review of its pharmacodynamic and pharmacokinetic properties and therapeutic use in age-related cognitive decline. Drugs Aging 1992;2:153–173.
24. Zimran A, Ofek B, Hershko C, et al: Treatment with captopril for peripheral ischemia induced by ergotamine. Br Med J 1984;288:364.

CHAPTER 46

Antibiotics

Christine M. Stork

A 6-day-old girl was given gentamicin as part of treatment for sepsis in the neonatal intensive care unit. Two hours after the initial dose the gentamicin level was reported as 50 mg/L. Upon further examination, it was apparent that the patient received 25 mg/kg instead of an expected 2.5 mg/kg of gentamicin as a loading dose. Twelve hours after the initial dose the gentamicin level was 1.5 mg/L. Renal function remained stable over the next few days.

What Are the Causes of Antibiotic-Related Adverse Events?

The adverse events related to antibiotics often occur as a result of iatrogenic complications rather than intentional overdose. The origin of these complications are diverse and include dosing errors, allergic reactions, idiosyncratic drug reactions, and drug interactions. This chapter will focus on each of these adverse drug effects as they specifically relate to the chosen antibiotic. Overdose data will also be presented, if available.

Prevention and continued vigilance are required to minimize adverse effects. As dosing errors are commonly noted in neonates and infants treated with intravenous antibiotics, careful and constant diligence on the part of all healthcare providers is required to minimize such errors. Antibiotics carry a higher risk for anaphylactic reactions than other medications. A complete and clear allergy history is essential to minimize these reactions in patients being considered for antibiotic therapy.

Many of the adverse effects of antibiotics are difficult to predict even when given patient and populations specific parameters. In some cases, a diluent or additional drug given concurrently with an antibiotic as part of the drug's chemical or physiologic makeup is responsible for the adverse effect, as seen in the case of the procaine component of penicillin G.

Lastly, antibiotics have been involved in many of the common and severe drug interactions primarily through the inhibition of metabolic enzyme systems. Patients being considered for antibiotic therapy should be carefully assessed for the existence of concomitant drug therapy that will interact with the chosen antibiotic.

Penicillins

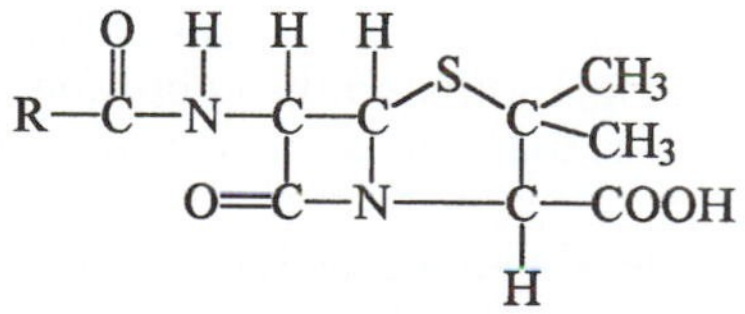

Penicillin nucleus

There are several penicillins available in the United States. Penicillins act to erode bacterial cell walls by interfering with mucopeptide synthesis. Acute oral overdoses of penicillin-containing drugs are usually not life threatening, and most patients can be safely and effectively managed in the home by poison center staff unless psychological or social reasons necessitate transport to a hospital. The most frequent complaints are gastrointestinal and include nausea, vomiting, and diarrhea. Rarely, electrolyte abnormalities resulting in electrocardiographic abnormalities are seen after rapid intravenous doses of potassium penicillin G in patients with renal failure.

Seizures occur in humans given large intravenous or intraventricular doses of penicillins.[20,96,165] Doses of penicillin required to produce seizures are high, usually greater than 50 million units intravenously.[163] In animals, seizures develop when penicillin is administered by parenteral, intraventricular, or intracisternal injection.[71,73] The mechanism for penicillin-induced seizures appears to be through an interaction with the picrotoxin-binding site on gamma amino butyric acid (GABA; see Chap. 10). When this binding site is activated, it inhibits GABA from binding to its receptor, resulting in a relative lack of inhibitory tone.[46] Penicillin analogs (such as imipenem) also cause seizures in animal models and some human case reports, presumably through a similar mechanism.[71,165] Treatment for patients who develop seizures following penicillin exposure should be aimed at increasing central GABA activity using benzodiazepines and barbiturates if needed.

Penicillin G

The most common adverse effects occurring after administration of intramuscular procaine penicillin G are the Hoigne syndrome and the Jarisch-Herxheimer reaction.[7,43,84,94,116,140,168,196] Both occur after the administration of large intramuscular or intravenous doses of penicillin G.[60,70] Hoigne syndrome is characterized by extreme apprehension and fear, illusions or hallucinations, changes in auditory and visual perception, tachycardia, systolic hypertension, and occasionally seizures that begin within minutes of injection.[183] These effects occur in the absence of signs or symptoms of anaphylaxis. The cause of this syndrome is unknown. Procaine is implicated as the causative agent because of this syndrome's similarity to events seen after the administration of other pharmacologically similar local anesthetics.[156,164,181]

Hoigne syndrome is six times more common in males than females.[167] The reason for this increased prevalence is unclear, but autosomal dominance and influences of prostaglandin and thromboxane A_2 activity in this population may account for the differences seen.[7]

The Jarisch-Herxheimer reaction is a self-limited reaction that develops within a few hours of treatment of early syphillis. Symptoms include myalgias, chills, headache, rash, and fever. Symptoms spontanously resolve within 18 to 24 hours even with continued antibiotic therapy.[120,152] The pathogenesis of this reaction is unclear, but some authors hypothesize that the reaction is caused by an acute antigen response to lysed bacteria. Similar reactions have been reported after teatment of other spirochetal and bacterial infections.[24]

Chronic Effects

Penicillin antibiotics are associated with a myriad of chronic toxic effects. They have been implicated in causing immune-related reactions such as bone marrow suppression,[61] intrahepatic cholestatic hepatitis,[169,189] interstitial nephritis,[126,127] and vasculitis.[172] Rare effects include pemphigus after penicillin use and corneal damage after the use of methicillin.[13,191]

Acute Allergy

Penicillins are the most common agents implicated in the development of acute allergy including anaphylactic reactions (see Chap. 14). The incidence of hypersensitivity after penicillin use is 5% overall, with 1% of penicillin reactions resulting in anaphylaxis. The risk for a fatal reaction after penicillin administration is 2/100,000 (0.002%).[184] All routes of penicillin administration can result in anaphylaxis; however, it most commonly results after intravenous administration. The anaphylactic syndrome is caused by local and systemic release of endogenous vasoactive substances including leukotrienes C_4 and D_4, histamine, eosinophilic chemotactic factor, and other vasoactive substances such as bradykinin, kallikrein, prostaglandin D_2, and platelet-activating factor (Table 46–1). (See also Chap. 14.) Type-1 anaphylaxis results after prior exposure to the antigen. IgE is manufactured by plasma cells after initial exposure and is bound to mast cell and basophil surfaces. With secondary exposure, the antigen combines with the antibody and results in mast cell and basophil degranulization. Treatment is supportive with careful attention to airway, breathing, and circulation. Specific therapy is listed in Table 46–2. In addition to supportive care, patients experiencing anaphylaxis after exposure to oral penicillin may benefit from a dose of activated charcoal, 1 g/kg.

TABLE 46–1. CLASSIFICATION OF ANAPHYLACTIC REACTIONS

Grade	Classification Description
I	Large local contiguous cutaneous reaction (> 15 cm)
II	Pruritis (urticaria) generalized
III	Asthma, angioedema, nausea, vomiting
IV	Airway (asthma, tongue swelling, dysphagia, respiratory distress, laryngeal edema)
	Cardiovascular (hypotension, may progress to cardiovascular collapse)

TABLE 46–2. GUIDELINES FOR TREATMENT OF ANAPHYLAXIS

Agent	Indications: Grade	Dose	Complications
Airway Reactions: Goal: Maintain Airway Patency			
Initial Therapy			
Epinephrine	Consider for II, III, IV	0.01 mL/kg (up to 0.5 mL) of 1:1000 dilution SQ every 10–20 min	Dysrhythmias, hypertension
Oxygen	III, IV	40–100%	None
Inhaled β_2-adrenergic agonists	III, IV	Through nebulizer, 0.3–0.5 mL in 2.5 mL of 0.9% NaCl	Dysrhythmias, hypertension
Secondary Therapy			
Corticosteroids	III, IV	125–250 mg of methylprednisolone or equivalent Q 6 hr for 2–4 doses	Hyperglycemia, fluid retention
H_1 and H_2 antagonists	II, III, IV	1 mg/kg of diphenhydramine or equivalent; 300 mg of cimetidine or equivalent	Anticholinergic effects
Aminophylline	Consider for III, IV	6 mg/kg IV infusion; maintenance dose as needed	Nausea/vomiting, dysrhythmias, seizures
Cardiovascular Reactions: Goal: Maintain Hemodynamic Stability			
Initial Therapy			
Intravenous fluids	IV	10–30 mL/kg, titrated to effect	Congestive heart failure, pulmonary edema
Epinephrine	Consider for II, III, IV	See Airway Reactions 1 mL of a 1:10,000 solution IV added to 9 mL of 0.9% NaCl to create a 1:100,000 solution infused slowly	See Airway Reactions
Secondary Therapy			
Norepinephrine	IV	2–12 µg/min IV in adults	Same as epinephrine
H_1 and H_2 antagonists	II, III, IV	See Airway Reactions	See Airway Reactions
Glucagon	IV	5–15 µg/min	Nausea, vomiting, hyperglycemia

Cephalosporins

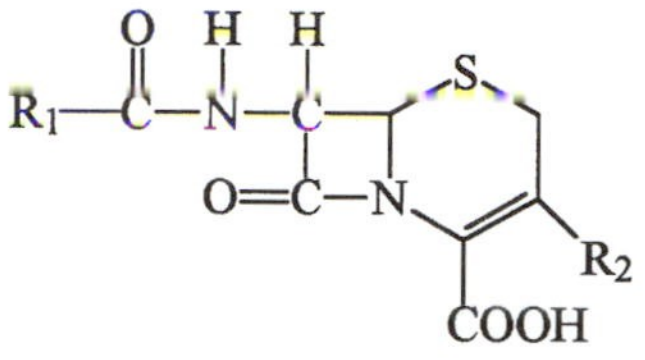

Cephem nucleus

Cephalosporins are similar to penicillin in that they are also beta-lactam antibiotics that interfere with bacterial cell wall function. They are generally divided into first, second, and third generations based upon their antimicrobial spectrum.

Cross Hypersensitivity

The cephalosporins contain a 6-membered dihydrithiazine ring instead of the 5-membered thiazolidine penicillin ring. The incidence of allergy after cephalosporin use is approximately 4% in the general population and 8% in those with prior penicillin allergy. The incidence of anaphylaxis to cephalosporins is less than 0.02%, with an increase to less than 0.04% in those patients with previous penicillin allergy. Cross-reactivity may be greater with agents that are structurally similar to penicillin or are contaminated by penicillin.[3] Antibody binding after cephalosporin exposure occurs at the determinants located on the side chain groups of the cephalosporin.[9] These determinants are quite distinct between cephalosporins, which causes the pattern of cross-hypersensitivity between cephalosporins to be much less well defined than between the penicillins. Caution should be used when considering cephalosporins in penicillin or cephalosporin-allergic patients; however, if a risk-benefit analysis demonstrates a clear benefit to the patient without equivalent alternatives, the cephalosporin should be given.

Acute Overdose

Effects occurring after acute overdose of cephalosporins resemble those occurring after penicillin exposure. Some cephalosporins have similar epileptogenic potential to penicillin in the animal model.[63] Management guidelines for cephalosporin overdose are similar to those of penicillin overdose.

Chronic Toxicity

Cephalosporins are also capable of causing an immune-mediated acute hemolytic crisis.[15,51] Cefaclor is the most common cephalosporin reported to cause serum sickness, although it can occur with other cephalosporins.[100,113] Also, like penicillins, cephalosporins are associated with chronic toxicity including interstitial nephritis and hepatitis with first-generation agents.[126,127,189]

nMTT Side Chain Effects

Cephalothin (without side chain)

Cephamandole (with side chain)

nMTT Side chain

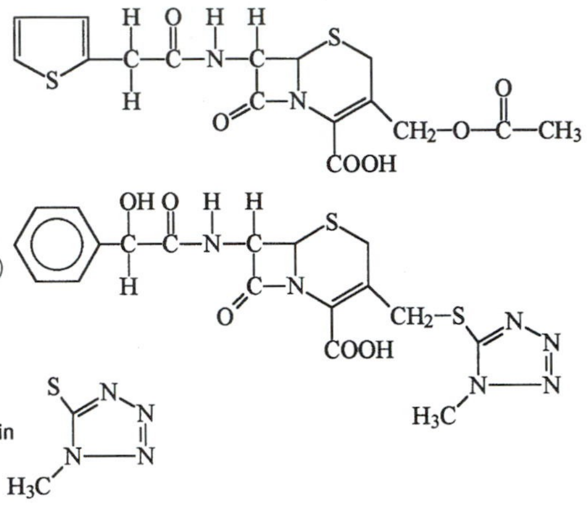

Cephalosporins containing a *N*-methylthiotetrazole (nMTT) side chain (moxalactam, cefazolin, cefperazone, cefmetazole, cefamandole, cefotetan) have toxicity unique to their structure among the cephalosporins. These cephalosporins dissociate and release free nMTT, which results in acute toxicity.[117]

Free nMTT inhibits the enzyme aldehyde dehydrogenase similar to disulfiram, and in conjunction with ethanol can cause a disulfiram-like reaction (see Chap. 63).[25] Patients report flushing, nausea, and vomiting after even small doses of ethanol. Those experiencing more severe manifestations may present with hypotension and shock. Treatment is supportive, with careful attention to hemodynamic status. Activated charcoal may be useful if the cephalosporin has been recently ingested or has enterohepatic recirculation.

The nMTT side chain is also implicated in causing hypoprothrombinemia, although a causal relationship is controversial.[69] It is thought that nMTT depletes vitamin K-dependent clotting factors by inhibition of vitamin K epoxide reductase (see Chap. 42).[132] Treatment of patients suspected of hypoprothrombinemia due to these cephalosporins consists of fresh frozen plasma if bleeding is evident and vitamin K_1 in doses required to resynthesize vitamin K cofactors.

The amount of nMTT formed per dose of cephalosporin is variable among the cephalosporins. In a study involving healthy humans, cefoperazone produced the greatest amount of nMTT, followed by cefotetan and cefmetazole.[188]

Other Beta-Lactam Antibiotics

Acute toxicity

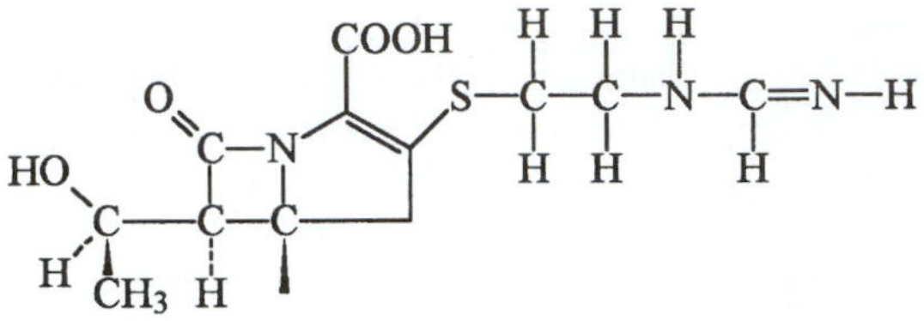

Imipenem

Carbapenem compounds such as imipenem cause seizures in therapeutic doses.[32,99,108,137,171] In a prospective surveillance study, researchers found that risk factors for seizure activity included central nervous system disease, prior seizure disorders, or abnormal renal function.[139] The mechanism for seizures appears to be GABA antagonism (similar to penicillins) in conjunction with enhanced activity excitatory amino acids. In mice, the addition of both excitatory amino acid antagonists and GABA agonists was able to increase the threshold required to provoke carbapenem-induced seizure activity.[47] There appears to be a structural relationship between imipenem and the development of seizures. In the animal model the C–2 side chain of imipenem was required to provoke seizure activity.[175] Treatment for patients with seizures after imipenem use is largely supportive with attention to basic life-support measures and withdrawal of imipenem use. GABA agonists such as benzodiazepines or barbiturates should be used if pharmacologic therapy is required for termination of seizure activity.

Cross-Allergenicity

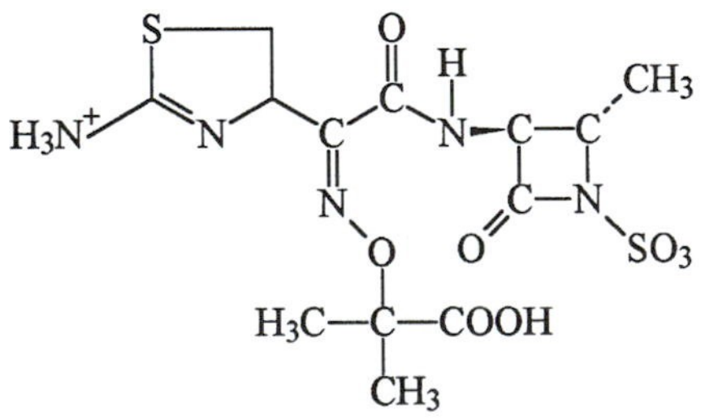

Aztreonam

Aztreonam is a monobactam that does not contain the antigenic components required for cross-allergy with penicillins. Therefore cross-allergenicity is not expected. However, cross-allergenicity is noted between imipenem and penicillins, although the incidence has yet to be determined.

Aminoglycosides

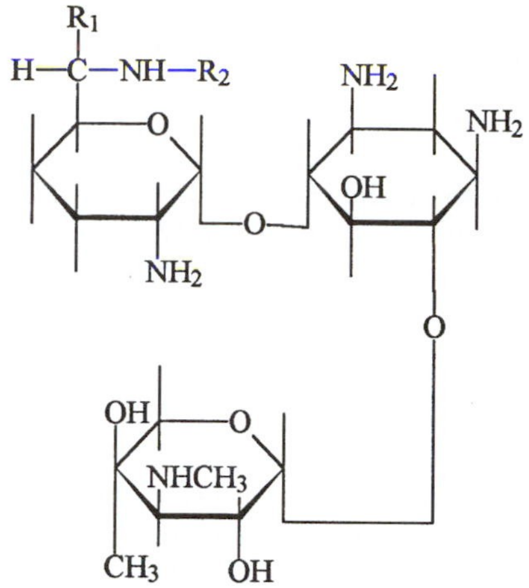

Gentamicin C: $R_1 = R_2 = CH_3$
Gentamicin C_2: $R_1 = CH_3$, $R_2 = H$
Gentamicin C_{1a}: $R_1 = R_2 = H$

Aminoglycosides provide antimicrobial activity by interfering with the 30s ribosomal subunit of RNA. Acute overdoses of aminoglycoside antibiotics (kanamycin, netilmicin, streptomycin, neomycin, gentamicin, tobramycin, amikacin) are almost exclusively the result of dosing error mistakes, especially in neonates. Fortunately these overdoses are rarely life threatening, and most patients can be safely managed with minimal intervention.[59a,86,104] In fact, the role of single daily-dose aminoglycoside administration has been studied extensively. A meta-analysis evaluating the once-daily aminoglycoside dosing studies failed to find an increase in adverse effects from these relatively large doses of aminoglycosides.[78] In rare instances, patients may develop neuromuscular blockade corresponding with high peak serum aminoglycoside levels (see Chap. 53).[135,186] Aminoglycosides inhibit the release of acetycholine from presynaptic nerve terminals and block acetycholine receptors.[2,76] Risk factors for enhanced neuromuscular blockade include patients with abnormal neuromuscular junction function such as those with myasthenia gravis, botulism, and patients receiving concomitant neuromuscular blocking drugs.[2]

Although aminoglycoside antibiotics attain optimum effectiveness through the peak serum concentrations, chronic therapy that results in nephrotoxicity and ototoxicity correlates more closely with trough serum concentrations.[2,56,92,118,121]

The incidence of nephrotoxicity after treatment with aminoglycoside antibiotics is estimated at 5 to 10%.[4] Although the aminoglycosides are almost completely excreted prior to biotransformation in the kidney, a small fraction of filtered aminoglycoside is transported by absorptive endocytosis across the apical membrane of proximal tubular cells and becomes sequestered within lysosomes. Toxicity results as the aminoglycoside binds to phospholipids contained on brush border membranes in the proximal renal tubule, causing cellular dysfunction.[4] Clinically, acute tubular necrosis develops, typically after 7 to 10 days of therapy. Laboratory abnormalities include granular casts, proteinuria, elevated urinary sodium, and increased fractional excretion of sodium. Usually the renal dysfunction is reversible; however, irreversible toxicity has been reported.[5] Renal injury may be manifest days prior to elevations in serum creatinine often causing a delay in diagnosis.[159] Risk factors for the development of nephrotoxicity include genetic predisposition, increased age, renal dysfunction, female sex, previous aminoglycoside therapy, liver dysfunction, large total dose, long duration of therapy, frequent doses, high trough levels, presence of other nephrotoxic drugs, and the presence of shock.[4,123,143]

The antibiotic ticarcillin forms a complex with aminoglycosides to inactivate both antimicrobial efficacy and toxicity. In animals given tobramycin with and without concurrent ticarcillin, ticarcillin provided renal protection against tobramycin-induced renal toxicity.[52] Seven patients with acute elevations in their serum aminoglycoside concentrations underwent a study to determine the relative efficacy of hemodialysis versus ticarcillin or carbenicillin for the removal of aminoglycosides from the serum.[159] During a 48-hour complexation period, ticarcillin removed 50% more aminoglycoside than two 4-hour hemodialysis sessions. Because of the limited toxicity associated with large overdoses of aminoglycosides, this therapy is rarely warranted in clinical settings. In addition, in most instances the aminoglycoside has decreased to a much lower serum concentration before any therapeutic measures can be employed. The use of ticarcillin should be considered in patients with either chronic overdoses or renal failure in which the risks of toxicity are significant.

Ototoxicity can occur after prolonged exposure to aminoglycosides. Both cochlear and vestibular dysfunction is correlated with high aminoglycoside trough concentrations.[27,122] Because aminoglycosides bioaccumulate in the endolymph and perilymph spaces, they have prolonged contact time with sensory hair cells. Aminoglycosides interfere with cell membrane lipids by binding to the plasma membranes and by an energy-dependent uptake that interferes with necessary intracellular processes.[158,190] In animals, a metabolite, but not the parent aminoglycoside, was capable of damaging hair cells.[89] Also, type I hair cells were more susceptible than type II hair cells, although both were affected.[103] The delay in onset of ototoxicity may be related to induction of oxidative metabolism and formation of the highly toxic metabolite (see Chap. 27). Cochlear dysfunction is reported to result in hearing loss in 0.5 to 5% of patients and is caused by the degeneration of hair cells in the organ of Corti.

Vestibular toxicity caused by destruction of sensory receptor portions of the inner ear or distruction of hair cells in the utricle and saccule occurs in 0.4 to 6% of patients.[122] Symptoms may include vertigo or tinnitus. Kanamycin, neomycin, and amikacin are predominantly cochlear toxic, whereas gentamycin and tobramycin have cochlear and vestibulotoxic properties. Streptomycin is the only aminoglycoside that is predominantly vestibulotoxic.

Full-tone audiometric testing may first show high-frequency hearing loss, which may subsequently progress. All hearing loss that develops is permanent due to the inability of hair cells to regenerate. Electronystagmography is the diagnostic tool of choice for vestibular dysfunction, and up to 50% of patients with early findings of vestibular dysfunction may have improvement after discontinuation of the drug.[54] Otoxicity of aminoglycoside antibiotics is enhanced by simultaneous administration of other drugs capable of causing ototoxicity (see Chap. 27).[22,103,174]

Less common adverse effects associated with chronic aminoglycoside use include electrolyte abnormalities, allergic reactions, hepatotoxicity, anemia, granulocytopenia, thrombocytopenia, eosinophilia, reproductive dysfunction, and toxic psychosis.[35,42,179]

Chloramphenicol

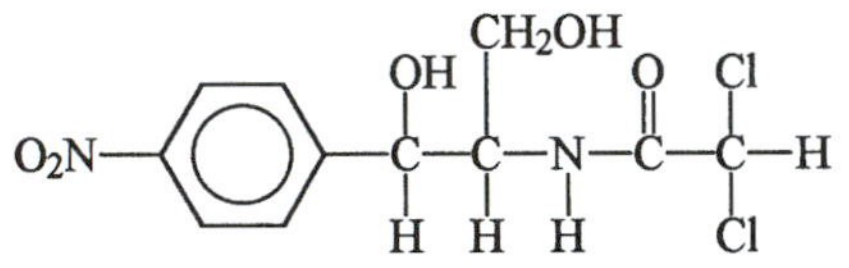

Acute overdose of chloramphenicol is commonly associated with nausea and vomiting. Chloramphenicol works by inhibiting the 50s ribosomal subunit and by inhibition of protein synthesis in rapidly proliferating cells. Metabolic acidosis occurs due to the inhibition of mitochondrial enzymes, oxidative phosphorylation, and mitochondrial biogenesis.[58] Sudden cardiovascular collapse is reported 5 to 12 hours after acute overdoses.[58,101,124,178] All poisoned patients should receive close observation for at least 12 hours after exposure. Orogastric lavage may be useful for recent ingestions in which the patient has not vomited, and activated charcoal 1 g/kg should be given orally. Charcoal hemoperfusion should be considered in large ingestions (> 10 times the normal daily dose) because it has shown to significantly decrease elevated plasma chloramphenicol levels.[57,119] Exchange transfusion successfully lowers chloramphenicol serum concentrations in neonates.[101,173] Surviving patients should be closely monitored for signs of bone marrow suppression.

Chronic overdoses of chloramphenicol cause toxicity similar to that seen after acute poisoning. Several cases of cardiovascular collapse are reported with elevated serum concentrations (> 50 μg/mL).[58,141] Hypotension and cardiovascular collapse are hallmarks of the "gray baby syndrome."[57,58,119,173] Other findings in children with "gray baby syndrome" include vomiting, anorexia, respiratory distress, abdominal distention, green stools, lethargy, cyanosis, ashen color, and metabolic acidosis. Infants, in particular, are predisposed to the gray baby syndrome because they are unable to conjugate chloramphenicol or to excrete unconjugated chloramphenicol in the urine.[66,187]

Dose-dependent bone marrow depression is seen with high serum concentrations of chloramphenicol.[90,91,162] Clinical manifestations usually occur after several weeks of therapy and include anemia, thrombocytopenia, and leukopenia. Bone marrow suppression is reversible with discontinuation of therapy. Chloramphenicol causes bone marrow suppression by causing ultrastructural microsomal changes, thereby decreasing the production of essential proteins and enzymes.[128,129] Rarely, aplastic anemia is seen after topical application.[1]

The development of aplastic anemia after chloramphenicol use is not dose related and generally occurs in susceptible patients within 5 months of treatment (see Chap. 24).[49,194] Although the exact mechanism is unknown, it is theorized that the p-nitrosulfathiazole group on chloramphenicol inhibits DNA synthesis in marrow stem cells.[193]

Other adverse effects associated with chloramphenicol include peripheral neuropathy,[98,145] neurologic abnormalities including confusion and delirium,[110] optic neuritis,[39,98] and contact dermatitis.[106] One case-controlled interview study has linked chloramphenicol use to the development of acute nonlymphocytic leukemia.[166] However, a true association has not been defined.

Fluoroquinolones

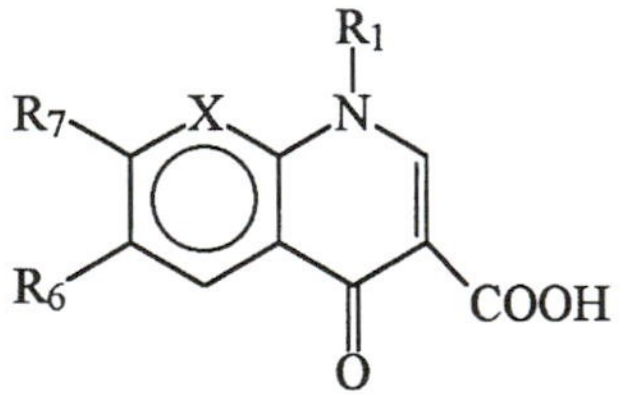

Quinolone nucleus

The fluoroquinolones include levofloxacin, ciprofloxacin, norfloxacin, ofloxacin, nalidixic acid, pefloxacin, lomefloxacin, and enoxacin. The fluoroquinolones act by inhibiting DNA topoisomerase and DNA gyrase in susceptible cells. Like other antimicrobials, the fluoroquinolones are rarely life threatening after acute overdose, and most patients can be safely managed with minimal intervention.[6] Rarely, acute overdoses of fluoroquinolones result in renal failure[41] or seizures. The mechanism of renal failure after fluoroquinolone exposure is controversial. In animals, ciprofloxacin and norfloxacin cause pathologic changes in the kidney, especially with neutral or alkaline urine.[160] In humans, renal failure is reported after both acute and chronic exposure to fluoroquinolones. A hypersensitivity reaction has been postulated to explain pathologic changes consistent with interstitial nephritis.[88,126,127,148,192] Treatment is supportive with discontinuation of the fluoroquinolone. Improvement in renal function is usually noticed within several days.

Seizures are reported with ciprofloxacin.[170] Some investigators suggest inhibition of GABA as the etiology.[180] Other risk factors for the development of seizures include concomitant use of theophylline.[170] Treatment is supportive using benzodiazepines and, if necessary, barbiturates in order to increase GABAergic activity.

Ciprofloxacin inhibits CYP3A4 enzyme system, which is responsible for the metabolism of many drugs (Table 46–3).

Fluoroquinolones should be used with caution in children and pregnant women due to their potential adverse effects on developing cartilage and bone. Damage to articular cartilage is demonstrated in young dogs and rats.[28,177] There are very limited data in humans; however, children given ciprofloxacin on a compassionate basis for cystic fibrosis developed complaints of swollen, painful, and stiff joints after 3 weeks of therapy.[97] All signs and symptoms abated within 2 weeks of discontinuation of therapy. However, 29 children with cystic fibrosis studied with magnetic resonance imaging (MRI) before and after placebo-controlled quinolone (ofloxacin or ciprofloxacin) therapy showed no differences with respect to cartilage thickness, cartilage structure, edema, cartilage-bone borderline, or synovial fluid.[45] In a study of 38 women who received quinolones during pregnancy, these women were shown to have more cesarean deliveries due to fetal distress than the controls. Their infants were heavier than controls, but no congenital malformations, delay to developmental milestones, or musculoskeletal abnormalities were found, while a congenital abnormality was noted in the control group.[12]

Other adverse effects include acute psychosis, transient elevations in liver function tests, hepatic failure, rash, tinnitus, eosinophilia, serum sickness, and photosensitivity.[26,59,72,75,79,102,125,138]

TABLE 46–3. DRUGS METABOLIZED THROUGH CYP3A4

Alprazolam	Lidocaine
Astemizole	Lovastatin
Carbamazepine	Midazolam
Cisapride	Nifedipine
Corticosteroids	Quinidine
Cyclosporine	Simvastatin
Diazepam	Terfenadine
Diltiazem	Triazolam
Erythromycin	Verapamil
Felodipine	

Data from references 77 and 149.

Macrolides

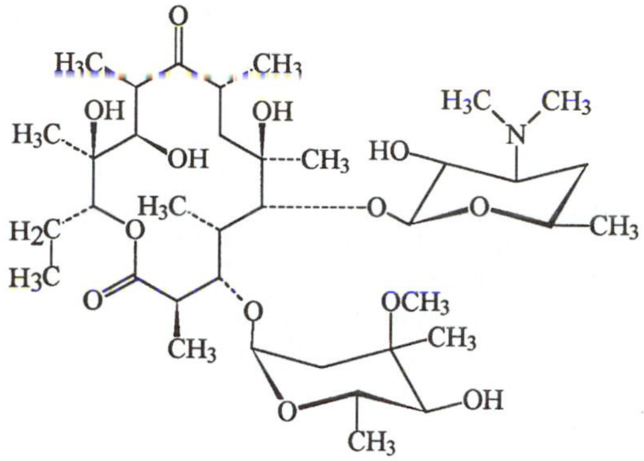

Erythromycin

The macrolide antibiotics include various forms of erythromycin (base, estolate, ethylsuccinate, gluceptate, lactobionate, stearate), clarithromycin, azithromycin, and troleandomycin (see Chap. 107). The macrolides inhibit the 50s ribosomal subunit of RNA in multiplying cells. Acute oral overdoses of macrolide antibiotics are usually not life threatening and symptoms are generally confined to the gastrointestinal tract. Treatment is similar to acute oral penicillin overdoses. Seizures can be produced by erythromycin in animal models, but have not been reported in humans.[71] Erythromycin lactobionate causes QT prolongation and torsades de pointes after intravenous use.[133] In vitro models demonstrate erythromycin's ability to slow repolarization in a concentration-dependent manner.[130] The cause for widened QT was once thought to result from hypokalemia-induced promotion of intracellular efflux of potassium.[146] Current data, however, demonstrate that the QT prolongation results from blockade of delayed rectifier potassium currents (see Chap. 8).[151] In a prospective study designed to determine the incidence of QT prolongation and torsades de pointes after intravenous erythromycin lactobionate, a statistically significant increase in the QT interval was found after therapeutic doses.[133] More pronounced widening occurred in patients with underlying heart disease. One patient of the 278 studied developed torsades de pointes. Another consecutive series of 7 patients demonstrated that 12 of 13 intravenous administrations of erythromycin resulted in widening of the QT interval, the extent of which was significantly correlated with the infusion rate.[74]

Drug Interactions

Erythromycin is the prototypical macrolide and as such has received the most attention with respect to potential and documented drug interactions. Erythromycin and troleandomycin are potent inhibitors of the cytochrome CYP3A4 enzyme system.[44] Erythromycin inhibits P450 after metabolism to a nitroso intermediate, which then forms an inactive complex with the iron (II) of cytochrome P450. Some substrates for the CYP3A4 system are listed in Table 46–3. Clinically significant interactions occur with erythromycin and astemizole, carbamazepine, cisapride, and terfenadine.[29,68,82,87,144] Inhibition of terfenadine, astemizole, and cisapride metabolism has resulted in increased concentrations of the parent drug, all of which are capable of causing a widening of the QT interval. Cases of torsades de pointes are reported as a result of this interaction.[18,136] Cases of carbamazepine toxicity are documented with erythromycin use.[82] Erythromycin also inhibits CYP1A2, producing clinically significant interactions with clozapine, theophylline,[149] and warfarin. Clarithromycin has also demonstrated the ability to inhibit the CYP3A4 in healthy human studies concomitantly using theophylline or carbamazepine.[77] Azithromycin does not appear to influence this enzyme system.

Chronic Toxicity

The macrolides have potential toxicity at therapeutic doses. The most common toxic effect is hepatitis, which may be immune mediated.[33] Erythromycin estolate is the most commonly implicated agent in causing cholestatic hepatitis in adults on prolonged therapy.[65,95]

Large doses of macrolide antibiotics are also associated with high-frequency sensorineural hearing loss.[21,161] A review of 11 patients who experienced hearing loss after erythromycin use demonstrated an erythromycin dose greater than 4 g/day and prior renal impairment as potential risk factors.[155] The hearing loss was reversible in all 11 cases after dosage reduction or discontinuation. A similar case-control study found that 5 of 30 patients treated with erythromycin therapy experienced ototoxicity while none of the 15 controls had any manifestations.[176] Ototoxicity occurred only with doses of 4 g/day or more and was found to correlate with higher serum concentrations. Ototoxicity resolved in all patients 6 to 14 days after discontinuation of therapy. There are rare case reports in which ototoxicity did not resolve following discontinuation of therapy.[50,109] There are insufficient data concerning the ototoxic potential of the other macrolide antibiotics. Macrolides are rarely reported to cause acute pancreatitis.[53]

Sulfonamides

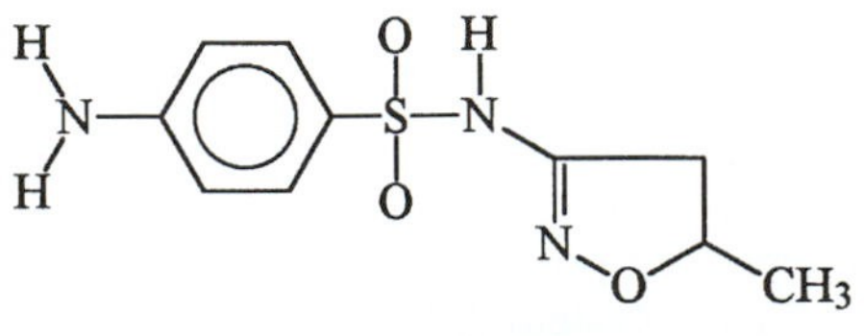

Sulfamethoxazole

Sulfonamides act therapeutically by inhibiting para-aminobenzoic acid or para-aminoglutamic acid required for the biosynthesis of folic acid. The most common adverse effect associated with chronic therapy with sulfonamides include nausea and cutaneous hypersensitivity reactions. Nausea is also common following overdose. The sulfonamides are associated with many chronic adverse effects. Bone marrow suppression is rare, but an increased incidence is seen in folic acid or vitamin B_{12} deficiency, children, pregnant women, alcoholics, dialysis patients, immunocompromised patients, and those receiving folate antagonists. Other adverse effects include hypersensitivity reactions, hypersensitivity pneumonitis, stomatitis, aseptic meningitis, hepatotoxicity, renal toxicity, and central nervous system toxicity.[16]

Tetracyclines

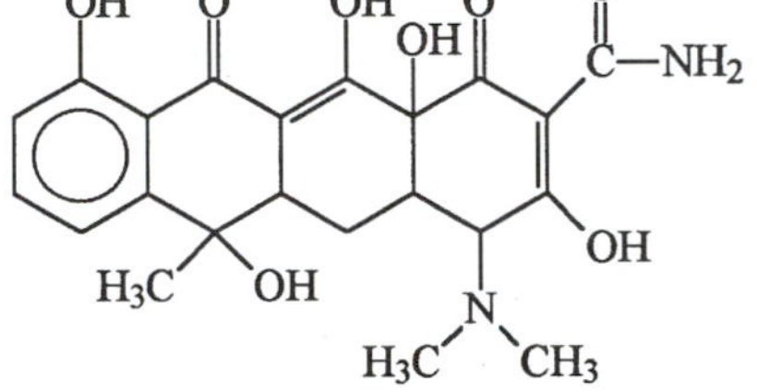

Tetracycline

Tetracyclines act as antimicrobials by inhibiting protein synthesis, the 30s ribosomal subunit, binding to aminoacyl transfer RNA, and binding to the 50s ribosomal subunit. Significant toxicity after acute overdose of tetracyclines including demeclocycline, doxycycline, methacycline, minocycline, oxytetracycline, and tetracycline is unlikely. Gastrointestinal effects consisting of nausea, vomiting, and epigastric pain are reported.[23]

Tetracycline should not be used in children during the first 6 to 8 years of life or in pregnant women after the 12th week of pregnancy because of the risk of development of tooth discoloration in the child or in the offspring.

Other chronic effects associated with the tetracyclines include nephrotoxicity, hepatotoxicity, and skin hyperpigmentation in sun-exposed areas and hypersensitivity reactions.[33,67,93] Demeclocycline has been reported to cause nephrogenic diabetes insipidus.[34] Outdated older formulations of tetracycline are reported to cause hypouricemia, hypokalemia, and a proximal and distal renal tubular acidosis.[37]

Vancomycin

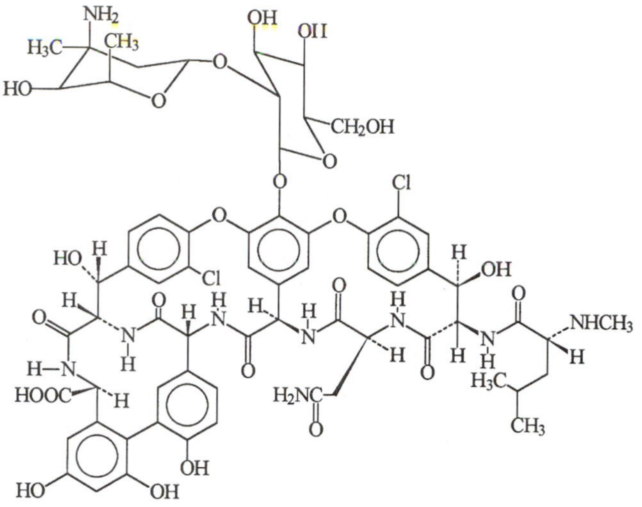

Vancomycin acts therapeutically through inhibition of glycopeptide polymerization, which is required for bacterial cell wall synthesis. Acute oral overdoses of vancomycin rarely cause significant toxicity and most cases can be treated with supportive care alone. Multiple-dose activated charcoal therapy decreases the half-life of vancomycin and can be considered in patients expected to have long clearance times.[107]

Patients exposed to vancomycin develop the "red man syndrome," a glycopeptide-induced anaphylactoid reaction.[62] Symptoms included chest pain, dyspnea, pruritis, urticaria, and angioedema.[150] Signs and symptoms spontaneously resolved within 15 minutes. Other symptoms attributed to "red man syndrome" may include hypotension, cardiovascular collapse, and seizures.[8,131]

The incidence, signs, and symptoms of red man syndrome are variable. In a retrospective evaluation of 76 patients receiving 1 g of vancomycin over 10 minutes, 11 patients experienced marked hypotension.[131] In a prospective study of patients receiving vancomycin over 60 minutes, 3.4% developed red man syndrome.[134] A trial in healthy humans studied the relationship between intradermal skin hypersensitivity and the development of red man syndrome. Each of the 11 subjects underwent skin testing followed 1 week later by an intravenous dose of vancomycin 15 mg/kg over 60 minutes. Following intravenous vancomycin, all subjects developed dermal flare responses and erythema, and 10 of 11 subjects developed pruritis within 20 to 45 minutes. Once the infusion was terminated, symptoms resolved within 60 minutes.[142] A placebo-controlled trial in adult patients studied the incidence of these symptoms in patients given 1 g of vancomycin over 1 hour as well as the effect of diphenhydramine in the prevention of the syndrome.[185] There was a 47% incidence of reaction without diphenhydramine and a 0% incidence with diphenhydramine.

Reports demonstrate that the signs and symptoms of the red man syndrome are related to the rise and fall of histamine concentrations.[81,111] Tachyphylaxis occurs in patients given multiple doses.[80,185] Work in animals demonstrated a direct myocardial depressant effect of vancomycin and a direct ability to produce peripheral vasodilation.[40] More serious reactions result when vancomycin is given via intravenous bolus, supporting a rate-related anaphylactoid mechanism for the development of this reaction.[14]

Patients most often experience red man syndrome after vancomycin is administered intravenously. In rare cases, oral administration of vancomycin can also result in the syndrome.[11] Treatment includes increasing the dilution of vancomycin and a slower intravenous administration. Antihistamines may be useful as pretreatment, especially prior to the first dose.

Chronic use of vancomycin is reported to cause nephrotoxicity. Nephrotoxicity is associated with prolonged excessive serum levels and is usually reversible after discontinuation of the drug.[5,147] Concomitant administration of aminoglycoside antibiotics may increase the risk of nephrotoxicity.[153] Vancomycin also rarely causes thrombocytopenia and neutropenia.[36,48]

Antifungals

Amphotericin B

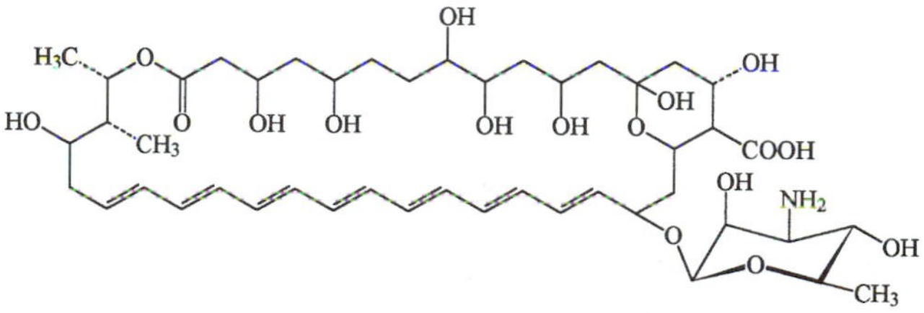

Amphotericin B is a polyene macrolide antifungal agent structurally similar to nystatin. Amphotericin B acts by combining with the ergosterol of the cytoplasmic membrane of the fungus, thereby creating porous cell membranes. This is followed by leakage of cellular organelles and cell lysis. Adverse reactions related to the administration of amphotericin B are common.

There are several case reports of amphotericin B overdose in infants and children. An infant receiving 50 times a normal dose (15 mg/kg) over 3 days experienced hypokalemia and mild increases in aspartate aminotransferase, which spontaneously resolved. Bone marrow depression and renal dysfunction did not occur.[105] Another infant received 31 mg instead of an intended 2.5 mg. The patient underwent a prophylactic exchange transfusion. No adverse clinical effects or laboratory abnormalities were noted.[19] Five pediatric patients (ages: 4.5 and 7 weeks; 2, 3.5, and 7 years) experienced cardiac complications including dysrhythmias and cardiac arrest after being given 5 to 15 mg/kg of amphotericin B. Four

TABLE 46–4. ORGAN SYSTEM MANIFESTATIONS ASSOCIATED WITH ANTIFUNGAL AGENTS AND OTHER ANTIBIOTICS

Drug	Organ System Toxicity	Signs, Symptoms, Laboratory
Bacitracin	Immune	Hypersensitivity reactions
Clindamycin	Immune	Hypersensitivity reactions
	Gastrointestinal	Nausea/vomiting/diarrhea
	Nervous	Dizziness, headache, vertigo
Colistimethate (colistin sulfate)	Renal	Decreased function, acute tubular necrosis
	Nervous	Paresthesias, confusion, coma, seizures, neuromuscular blockade
Griseofulvin	Renal	Proteinuria, nephrosis
	Hepatic	Increased liver enzymes
	Gastrointestinal	Nausea/vomiting/diarrhea
	Immune	Granulocytopenia
	Other	Disulfiram reactions, increased porphyrins
Lincomycin	Gastrointestinal	Nausea/vomiting/diarrhea
	Immune	Hypersensitivity reactions
Metronidazole	Neurologic	Peripheral neuropathy, seizures
	Gastrointestinal	Nausea, vomiting
	Other	Disulfiram reactions
Nitrofurazone	Immune	Hypersensitivity reactions
	Other	Ointment contains polyethylene glycols (renal dysfunction)
Nitrofurantoin	Gastrointestinal	Nausea, vomiting, diarrhea
	Hepatic	Jaundice
	Immune	Rash, acute and chronic pulmonary hypersensitivity
	Neurologic	Peripheral neuropathy
Novobiocin	Immune	Skin rash
	Gastrointestinal	Nausea, vomiting, diarrhea
	Hematologic	Pancytopenia, hemolytic anemia
Polymyxin B sulfate	Neurologic	Muscle weakness, seizures
	Renal	Azotemia, proteinuria
Selenium sulfide	Cutaneous	Contact dermatitis
	Other	Selenium: hair loss (rare)
Silver sulfadiazine	Cutaneous	Contact dermatitis
	Hematologic	Anemia, aplastic anemia
Spectinomycin	Immune	Rash (rare)
Antifungals		
Benzoic acid	Gastrointestinal	Nausea, vomiting, diarrhea
Carbol–fuchsin solution (Phenol/resorcinol/fuchsin)	Gastrointestinal	Nausea, vomiting, diarrhea
Gentian violet	Gastrointestinal	Nausea, vomiting, diarrhea
	Immune	Rash (rare)
Nystatin	Gastrointestinal	Nausea, vomiting, diarrhea
Salicylic acid	Gastrointestinal, dermal	Higher concentrations are caustic
Undecylenic acid and undecylenate salt	Gastrointestinal	Nausea, vomiting, diarrhea

of these five patients died.[38] In animals, the administration of hydrocortisone increased the LD_{50} of amphotericin B; however, this has not been studied in the human model of acute poisoning.[30]

Infusion of amphotericin B results in fever, rigors, headache, nausea, vomiting, hypotension, tachycardia, and dyspnea.[115] Pretreatment with acetaminophen, diphenhydramine, ibuprofen, and hydrocortisone are helpful in alleviating the febrile symptoms along with slower rates of infusion and lower total daily doses.[64,182] Concentrations of amphotericin B greater than 0.1 mg/mL result in phlebitis. Slower infusion rates, hot packs, and frequent line flushing with dextrose in water may also help to alleviate symptoms.

Eighty percent of those patient exposed to amphotericin B will sustain some degree of renal insufficiency (see Chap. 23).[31] Azotemia is caused by distal renal tubule damage, which then causes renal artery vasoconstriction. Studies in animals show depressed renal blood flow and glomerular filtration rate and increased renal vascular resistance. This occurs by a mechanism that does not include the renal nerves, angiotensin II, endothelium-derived relaxing factor, or tubuloglomerular feedback.[154,157] In an in-vitro trial, 40% of amphotericin B's toxic effects were due to the vehicle, deoxycholate.[195] After large total doses of amphotericin B, residual decreases in glomerular filtration rate may occur even after discontinuation of therapy. This is hypothesized to be due to nephrocalcinosis. Potassium and magnesium wasting, proteinuria, decreased renal concentrating ability, renal tubular acidosis, and hematuria also occur.[10,115] Strategies to reduce renal toxicity after amphotericin B include intravenous saline or magnesium and potassium supplementation.[17,55,83] Lipid formulation of amphotericin B may also attenuate the adverse effects associated with amphotericin B. These formulations of amphotericin B are complexed with a lipid until contact is made with a fungus. The fungus produces lipases to free the complexed amphotericin B, resulting in focused cell death.[85]

Other adverse effects reported after treatment with amphotericin B include normochromic, normocytic anemia; decreased erythropoietin release; respiratory insufficiency with infiltrates; and, rarely, dysrhythmias, tinnitus, thrombocytopenia, peripheral neuropathy, and leukopenia.[112,114,115]

Triazole and Imidazoles

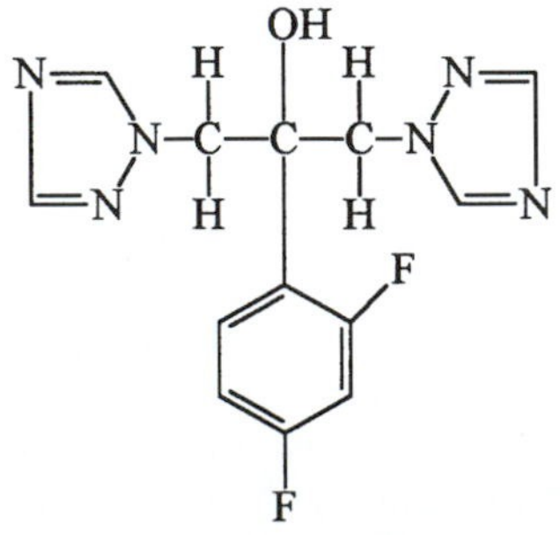

Fluconazole

Common triazole antifungals include fluconazole and itraconazole. Common imidazoles include clotrimazole, econazole, ketoconazole, and miconazole. These drugs act by altering cell membranes to increase their permeability. Severe toxicity is not expected in the overdose setting. The majority of toxic effects seen after the use of these drugs result from their drug interactions. Fluconazole, itraconazole, ketoconazole, and miconazole have the ability to competitively inhibit CYP3A4. This enzyme system is responsible for the metabolism of many drugs. Clinically significant interactions are reported with many of the drugs listed in Table 46–3. Other organ system manifestations to antifungal agents and other antibiotics are shown in Table 46–4.

References

1. Abrams SM, Degnan TJ, Vinciguerra V: Marrow aplasia following topical application of chloramphenicol eye ointment. Arch Intern Med 1980;140:576–577.
2. Adams SL, Mathews J, Grammer LC: Drugs that may exacerbate myasthenia gravis. Ann Emerg Med 1984; 13:532–538.
3. Anne S, Reisman RE: Risk of administering cephalosporin antibiotics to patients with history of penicillin allergy. Ann Allergy Asthma Immunol 1995;74:167–170.
4. Appel GB: Aminoglycoside nephrotoxicity. Am J Med 1990;88(suppl 3C):16S–20S.
5. Appel GB, Given DB, Levine LR, et al: Vancomycin and the kidney. Am J Kidney Dis 1986;8:75–80.
6. Arcieri GM, Becker N, Esposito B, et al: Safety of intravenous ciprofloxacin. Am J Med 1989;87(suppl 5A): 92S–97S.
7. Backon J: Hoigne's syndrome: Relevance of anomalous dominance and prostaglandins. Am J Dis Child 1986; 140:1091–1092. Letter.
8. Bailie GR, Yu R, Morton R, Waldek S: Vancomycin, red neck syndrome and fits. Lancet 1985;2:279–280.
9. Balso BA, Pham NH: Invited review: Structure–activity studies on drug-induced anaphylactic reactions. Chem Res Toxicol 1994;7:703–721.
10. Barton CH, Pahl M, Vaziri ND: Renal magnesium wasting associated with amphotericin B therapy. Am J Med 1984;77:471–474.
11. Bergeron L, Boucher FD: Possible red-man syndrome associated with systemic absorption of oral vancomycin in a child with normal renal function. Ann Pharmacother 1994;28:581–584.
12. Berkovitch M, Pastuszak A, Gazarian M, et al: Safety of the new quinolones in pregnancy. Obstet Gynecol 1994;84: 535–538.
13. Berry M, Gurung A, Easty DL: Toxicity of antibiotics and antifungals on cultured human corneal cells: Effect of mixing, exposure and concentration. Eye 1995;9:110–115.
14. Best CJ, Ewart M, Sumner E: Perioperative complications following the use of vancomycin during anaesthesia: Two clinical reports. Br J Anaesth 1989;62:567–577.
15. Borgna-Pignatti C: Fatal ceftriaxone-induced hemolysis in a child with acquired immunodeficiency syndrome. Pediatr Infect Dis J 1995;14:1116–1117.
16. Bovino JA, Marcus DF: The mechanism of transient myopia induced by sulfonamide therapy. Am J Ophthamol 1982;94:99–102.
17. Branch RA: Prevention of amphotericin B-induced renal impairment. Arch Intern Med 1988;148:2389–2394.
18. Brandriss MW, Richardson WS, Barold SS: Erythromycin-induced QT prolongation and polymorphic ventricular tachycardia (torsades de pointes): Case report and review. Clin Infect Dis 1994;18:995–998.
19. Brent J, Hunt M, Kulig K, Rumack B: Amphotericin B overdoses in infants: Is there a role for exchange transfusion? Vet Hum Toxicol 1990;32:124–125.
20. Brozanski BS, Scher MS, Albright AL: Intraventricular nafcillin-induced seizures in a neonate. Pediatr Neurol 1988;4:188–190.
21. Brummett RE: Ototoxic liability of erythromycin and analogues. Otolaryngol Clin North Am 1993;26:811–819.
22. Brummett RE, Traynor J, Brown R, Himes D: Cochlear damage resulting from kanamycin and furosemide. Acta Otolaryngol (Stockh) 1975;80:86–92.
23. Bryant SG, Fisher S, Kluge RM: Increased frequency of doxycycline side effects. Pharmacotherapy 1987;7:125–129.
24. Bryceson ADM: Clinical pathology of the Jarisch-Herxheimer reaction. J Infect Dis 1976;133:696–704.
25. Buening MK, Wold JS, Israel KS, Kammer RB: Disulfiram-like reaction to beta-lactams. JAMA 1980;245:2027–2028.
26. Burdge DR, Nakielna EM, Rabin HR: Photosensitivity associated with ciprofloxacin use in adult patients with cystic fibrosis. Antimicrob Agents Chemother 1995;39:793. Letter.
27. Buring JE, Evans DA, Mayrent SL, et al: Randomized trials of aminoglycoside antibiotics: Quantitative overview. Rev Infect Dis 1988;10:951–957.
28. Burkhardt JE, Hill MA, Lamar CH, et al: Effects of difloxacin on the metabolism of glycosaminoglycans and collagen in organ cultures of articular cartilage. Fundam Appl Toxicol 1993;20:257–263.
29. Bussey HI, Knodel LC, Boyle DA. Warfarin–erythromycin interaction. Arch Intern Med 1985;145:1736–1737.
30. Butler WT, Bennett JE, Alling DW, et al: Nephrotoxicity of amphotericin B. Ann Intern Med 1964;61:175–187.
31. Butler WT, Bennett JE, Hill GJ, et al: Electrocardiographic and electrolyte abnormalities caused by amphotericin B in dog and man. Proc Soc Exp Biol Med 1964;116:857–863.
32. Calandra GB, Wang C, Aziz M, Brown KR: The safety profile of imipenim/cilastatin: Worldwide experience base on 3,470 patients. J Antimicrob Chemother 1986;18(suppl E):193–202.
33. Carson JL, Strom BL, Duff A, et al: Acute liver disease associated with erythromycins, sulfonamides, and tetracyclines. Ann Intern Med 1993;119:576–583.
34. Castell DO, Sparks HA: Nephrogenic diabetes insipidus due to demethylchlortetracycline hydrochloride. JAMA 1965;193:237.
35. Chen JH, Wiener L, Distenfeld A: Immunologic thrombocytopenia. NY State J Med 1980;80:1134–1135.
36. Christie DJ, Van Buren N, Lennon SS, et al: Vancomycin-dependent antibodies associated with thrombocytopenia and refractoriness to platelet transfusion in patients with leukemia. Blood 1990;75:518–525.

37. Chusil S, Tungsanga K, Wathanavaha A, Pansin P: Hypouricemia, hypokalemia, proximal and distal tubular acidification defect following administration of outdated tetracycline: A case report. J Med Assoc Thailand 1994;77:98–102.
38. Cleary JD, Hayman J, Sherwood J, et al: Amphotericin B overdose in pediatric patients with associated cardiac arrest. Ann Pharmacother 1993;27:715–719.
39. Cocke JG, Brown RE, Geppert LJ: Optic neuritis with prolonged use of chlormaphenicol. J Pediatr 1966;68:27–31.
40. Cohen LS, Wechsler AS, Mitchell JH, Glick G: Depression of cardiac function by streptomycin and other antimicrobial agents. Am J Cardiol 1970;26:505–511.
41. Connor JP, Curry JM, Selby TL, Perlmutter AD: Acute renal failure secondary to ciprofloxacin use. J Urol 1994;154:975–976.
42. Covinsky JO: Aminoglycoside-induced electrolyte imbalance. Hosp Ther 1986;5:17–29.
43. Cummings JL, Barritt CF, Horan M: Delusions induced by procaine penicillin: Case report and review of the syndrome. Int J Psychiatry Medicine 1986–7;16:163–168.
44. Danan G, Descatoire V, Pessayre D: Self-induction of erythromycin by its own transformation into a metabolite forming an inactive complex with reduced cytochrome P-450. J Pharmacol Exp Ther 1989;250:746–751.
45. Danisovicova A, Brezina M, Belan S, et al: Magnetic resonance imaging in children receiving quinolones: No evidence of quinolone-induced arthrophy. A multicenter survey. Chemotherapy 1994;40:209–214.
46. De Boer T, Stoof JC, Van Duyn H: Effect of penicillin on neurotransmitter release from rat cortical tissue. Brain Res 1980;192:296–300.
47. De Sarro A, Ammendola D, De Sarro G: Effects of some quinolones on imipenem-induced seizures in DBA/2 mice. Gen Pharmacol 1994;25:369–379.
48. Domen RE, Horowitz S: Vancomycin-induced neutropenia associated with anti-granulocyte antibodies. Immunohematology 1990;6:41–43.
49. Durosinmi MA, Ajayi AA: A prospective study of chloramphenicol induced aplastic anaemia in Nigerians. Trop Geographic Med 1993;45:159–161.
50. Dylewski J: Irreversible sensorineural hearing loss due to erythromycin. Can Med Assoc J 1988;139:230–231.
51. Ehmann WC: Cephalosporin-induced hemolysis: A case report and review of the literature. Am J Hematol 1992;40:121–125.
52. English J, Gilbert DN, Kohlhepp S, et al: Attenuation of experimental tobramycin nephrotoxicity by ticarcillin. Antimicrob Agents Chemother 1985;27:897–902.
53. Fang CC, Wang HP, Lin JT: Erythromycin-induced acute pancreatitis. J Toxicol Clin Toxicol 1996;34:93–95.
54. Fee WE: Aminoglycoside ototoxicity in the human. Laryngoscope 1980;90(suppl 24):1–19.
55. Fisher MA, Talbot GH, Maislin G, et al: Risk factors for amphotericin B associated nephrotoxicity. Am J Med 1989;87:547–552.
56. French MA, Cerra FB, Plaut ME, Schentag JJ: Amikacin and gentamicin accumulation pharmacokinetics and nephrotoxicity in critically ill patients. Antimicrob Agents Chemother 1981;19:147–152.
57. Freundlich M, Cynamon H, Tames A, et al: Management of chloramphenicol intoxication in infancy by charcoal hemoperfusion. J Pediatr 1983;103:485–487.
58. Fripp RR, Carter MC, Werner JC: Cardiac function and acute chloramphenicol toxicity. J Pediatr 1983;103:487–490.
59. Fuchs S, Simon Z, Brezis M: Fatal hepatic failure associated with ciprofloxacin. Lancet 1994;343:738–739. Letter.
59a. Fuguay D, Koup J, Smith AL: Management of neonatal gentamicin overdose. J Pediatr 1981;99:473–476.
60. Galpin JE, Chow AW, Yoshikawa TT, Guze LB: Pseudoanaphylactic reactions for inadvertent infusion of procaine penicillin G. Ann Intern Med 1974;81:358–359.
61. Garratty G: Immune cytopenia associated with antibiotics. Transfus Med Rev 1993;7:255–267.
62. Garrelts JC, Peterie JD: Vancomycin and the "red man's syndrome." N Engl J Med 1985;312:245. Letter.
63. Gerald MD, Massey J, Spadoro DC: Comparative convulsant activity of various penicillins after intracerebral injection in mice. Pharmacology 1973;25:104–106.
64. Gigliotti F, Shenep JL, Lott L, et al: Induction of prostaglandin synthesis as the mechanism responsible for the chills and fever produced by infusing amphotericin B. J Infect Dis 1987;156:784–789.
65. Gilbert FI Jr.: Cholestatic hepatitis caused by esters of erythromycin and oleandomycin 1962 (classical article). Hawaii Med J 1995;54:603–605.
66. Glazko AJ: Identification of chloramphenicol metabolites and some factors affecting metabolic disposition. Antimicrob Agents Chemother 1966;6:655–665.
67. Gordon G, Sparano BM, Iatripoulos MJ: Hyperpigmentation of the skin associated with minocycline therapy. Arch Dermatol 1985;121:618–623.
68. Goss JE, Ramo BW, Blake K: Torsades de pointes associated with astemizole (hismanal) therapy. Arch Intern Med 1993;153:2705. Letter.
69. Goss TF, Walawander CA, Grasela TH, et al: Prospective evaluation of risk factors for antibiotic-associated bleeding in critically ill patients. Pharmacotherapy 1992;12:283–291.
70. Green RL, Lewis JE, Kraus ST, et al: Elevated plasma procaine concentration after administration of procaine penicillin G. N Engl J Med 1979;291:223–226.
71. Grondahl TO, Langmoen IA: Epileptogenic effect of antibiotic drugs. J Neurosurg 1993;78:938–943.
72. Guharoy SR: Serum sickness secondary to ciprofloxacin use. Vet Hum Toxicol 1994;36:540–541.
73. Gutnick MJ, Van Duijn H, Citri N: Relative convulsant potencies of structural analogs of penicillin. Brain Res 1976;114:139–143.
74. Haefeli WE, Schoenberger RA, Weiss PH, Ritz R: Possible risk for cardiac arrhythmias related to intravenous erythromycin. Intensive Care Med 1992;18:469–473.
75. Halkin H: Adverse effects of the fluoroquinolones. Rev Infect Dis 1988;10(suppl 1):S258–S261.
76. Hall DR, McGibbin DH, Evans CC, et al: Gentamycin, tubocurarine, lignocaine, and neuromuscular blockade. Br J Anaesth 1972;44:1329–1331.
77. Hansten PD, Horn JR, Koda-Kimble MA, Young LY. A clinical perspective and analysis of current developments. Drug Interact Updates Q 1996;16:905.
78. Hatala R, Dinh T, Cook DJ: Once daily aminoglycoside

dosing in immunocompetent adults: A meta-analysis. Ann Intern Med 1996;124:717–725.
79. Hautekeete ML, Kockx MM, Naegels S, et al: Cholestatic hepatitis related to quinolones: A report of two cases. J Hepatol 1995;23:759–760.
80. Healy DP, Polk RE, Garson ML, et al: Comparison of steady-state pharmacokinetics of two dosage regimens of vancomycin in normal volunteers. Antimicrob Agents Chemother 1987;31:393–397.
81. Healy DP, Sahai JV, Fuller SH, Polk RE. Vancomycin-induced histamine release and "red mans syndrome": Comparison of 1- and 2-hour infusions. Antimicrob Agents Chemother 1990;34:550–554.
82. Hedrick R, Williams F, Morin R, et al: Carbamazepine–erythromycin interaction leading to carbamazepine toxicity in four epileptic children. Ther Drug Monit 1983;5:405–407.
83. Heidemann HT, Gerkens JF, Spickard WA, et al: Amphotericin B nephrotoxicity in humans decreased by salt repletion. Am J Med 1983;75:476–481.
84. Heye N, Dunne JW: Jarisch-Herxheimer reaction in a patient with neurosyphilis: Non-convulsive status epilepticus? J Neurol Neurosurg Psychiatry 1995;58:521. Letter.
85. Hiemenz JW, Walsh TJ: Lipid formulation of amphotericin B: Recent progress and future directions. Clin Infect Dis 1996;22:S133–S144.
86. Ho PW, Pien FD, Koninami N: Massive amikacin overdose. Ann Intern Med 1979;91:227–228.
87. Honig PK, Woolsley RL, Zamani K, et al: Changes in the pharmacokinetics and electrocardiographic pharmacodynamics of terfenidine with concomitant administration of erythromycin. Clin Pharmacol Ther 1992;52:231–238.
88. Hootkins R, Fenves AZ, Stephens MK: Acute renal failure secondary to oral ciprofloxacin therapy: A presentation of three cases and a review of the literature. Clin Nephrol 1989;32:75–78.
89. Huang MY, Schacht J: Formation of cytotoxic metabolite from gentamycin by liver. Biochem Pharmacol 1990;40: R11-R14.
90. Hughes DW: Studies on chloramphenicol II. Possible determinants and progress of hemopoietic toxicity during chloramphenicol therapy. Med J Aust 1973;2:1142–1146.
91. Hughes DW: Studies on chloramphenicol I. Assessment of hemopoietic toxicity. Med J Aust 1968;2:436–438.
92. Humes HD: Aminoglycoside nephrotoxicity. Kidney Int 1988;33:900–901.
93. Hunt CM, Washington K: Tetracycline-induced bile duct paucity and prolonged cholestasis. Gastroenterology 1994;107:1844–1847.
94. Ilechukwu STC: Acute psychotic reactions and stress response syndromes following intramuscular aqueous procaine penicillin. Br J Psychiatry 1990;156:554–559.
95. Inman WH, Rawson NS: Erythromycin estolate and jaundice. Br Med J 1983;286:1954–1955.
96. Jalbert EO: Seizures after penicillin administration. Am J Dis Child 1985;139:1075. Letter.
97. Jawad ASM: Cystic fibrosis and drug induced arthropathy. Br J Rheumatol 1989;28:179–180.
98. Joy RJT, Scalettar R, Sodee DB: Optic and peripheral neuritis. Probable effect of prolonged chloramphenicol therapy. JAMA 1960;173:1731–1734.
99. Kaloyanides GJ: Renal pharmacology of aminoglycoside antibiotics. In: Bianchi C, Bertelli A, Duarte CG, eds. Contributions to Nephrology 42, Drug-Induced Nephrotoxicity. Basel, Karger, 1984, pp. 148–167.
100. Kearns OL, Wheeler JO, Childress SH, Letzig LU: Serum sickness-like reactions to cefaclor: Role of hepatic metabolism and individual susceptibility. J Pediatr 1994;125: 805–811.
101. Kessler DL, Smith AL, Woodrum DE: Chloramphenicol toxicity in a neonate treated with exchange transfusion. J Pediatr 1980;96:140–141.
102. Kimura M, Kawada A, Kobayashi T, et al: Photosensitivity induced by fleroxacin. Clin Exp Dermatol 1996;21:56–57.
103. Koegel L: Ototoxicity: A contemporary review of aminoglycosides, loop diuretics, acetysalicylic acid, quinine, erythromycin, and cisplatinum. Am J Otol 1985;6:190–199.
104. Koren G, Barzilay Z, Greenwald M: Tenfold errors in administration of drug doses: A neglected iatrogenic disease in pediatrics. Pediatrics 1986;77:848–849.
105. Koren G, Lau A, Kenyon CF, et al: Clinical course and pharmacokinetics following a massive overdose of amphotericin B in a neonate. J Toxicol Clin Toxicol 1990; 28:371–378.
106. Kubo Y, Nonaka S, Yoshida H: Contact sensitivity to chloramphenicol. Contact Dermatitis 1987;17:245–247.
107. Kucukguclu S, Tuncok Y, Ozkan H, et al: Multiple-dose activated charcoal in an accidental vancomycin overdose. J Toxicol Clin Toxicol 1996;34:83–87.
108. Leo RJ, Ballow CH: Seizure activity associated with imipenem use: Clinical case reports and review of the literature. Ann Pharmacother 1991;25:351–354.
109. Levin G, Behrenth E: Irreversible ototoxic effect of erythromycin. Scand Audiol 1986;15:41–42.
110. Levine PH, Regelson W, Holland JF: Chloramphenicol-associated encephalopathy. Clin Pharmacol Ther 1970;11: 194–199.
111. Levy JH, Kettlekamp N, Goertz P, et al: Histamine release by vancomycin: A mechanism for hypotension in man. Anaesthesia 1987;67:122–125.
112. Lin AC, Goldwasser E, Bernard EM, et al: Amphotericin B blunts erythropoietin response to anemia. J Infect Dis 1990;161:348–351.
113. Lowery N, Kearns GL, Young RA, Wheeler JG: Serum sickness-like reactions associated with cefprozil therapy. J Pediatr 1994;125:325–328.
114. MacGregor RR, Bennett JE, Erslev AJ: Erythropoietin concentration in amphotericin B induced anemia. Antimicrob Agents Chemother 1978;14:270–273.
115. Maddux MS, Barriere SL: A review of complications of amphotericin therapy: Recommendations for prevention and management. DICP Ann Pharmacother 1980;14: 177–180.
116. Malone JD, Lebar RD, Hilder R: Procaine-induced seizures after intramuscular procaine penicillin G. Military Med 1988;153:191–192.
117. Matsubara T, Otsubo S, Ogawa A, et al: Effects of beta-lactam antibiotics and *N*-methyltetrazolethiol on the alcohol-metabolizing system in rats. Japan J Pharmacol 1987;45: 303–315.
118. Mattle H, Craig WA, Pechere PC: Determinants of efficacy

and toxicity of aminoglycosides. J Antimicrob Chemother 1989;24:281–293.

119. Mauer SM, Chavers BM, Kjellstrand CM: Treatment of an infant with severe chloramphenicol intoxication using charcoal-column hemoperfusion. J Pediatr 1980;96: 136–139.
120. Meislin HW, Bremer JC: Jarisch-Herxheimer reaction case report. JACEP 1976;5:779–781.
121. Moore RD, Lietman PS, Smith CR: Clinical response to aminoglycoside therapy: Importance of the ratio of peak concentration to minimal inhibitory concentration. J Infect Dis 1987;155:93–99.
122. Moore RD, Smith CR, Lietman PS: Risk factors for the development of auditory toxicity in patients receiving aminoglycosides. J Infect Dis 1984;149:23–30.
123. Moore RD, Smith CR, Lipsky JJ, et al: Risk factors for nephrotoxicity in patients treated with aminoglycosides. Ann Intern Med 1984;100:352–357.
124. Mulhall A, deLouvois J, Hurley R: Chloramphenicol toxicity in neonates: Its incidence and prevention. Br Med J 1983;287:1424–1427.
125. Mulhall JP, Bergmann LS: Ciprofloxacin-induced acute psychosis. Urology 1995;46:102–103.
126. Murray KM, Keane WR: Review of drug-induced acute interstitial nephritis. Pharmacotherapy 1992;12:462–467.
127. Murray KM, Wilson MG: Suspected ciprofloxacin-induced interstitial nephritis. DICP Ann Pharmacother 1990;24: 379–380.
128. Nahtha MC: Lack of predictability of chloramphenicol toxicity in pediatric patients. J Clin Pharmacol Ther 1989;14:297–303.
129. Nahtha MC: Serum concentrations and adverse effects of chloramphenicol in pediatric patients. Chemotherapy 1987;33:322–327.
130. Nattel S, Ranger S, Talajic M, et al: Erythromycin-induced prolonged QT syndrome: Concordance with quinidine and underlying cellular electrophysiologic mechanism. Am J Med 1990;89:235–238.
131. Newfield P, Roizen MF: Hazards of rapid administration of vancomycin. Ann Intern Med 1979;91:581.
132. Obata H, Lizuka B, Uchida K: Pathogenesis of hypoprothrombinemia induced by antibiotics. J Nutr Sci Vitaminol (Tokyo) 1992;S13–S15:421–424.
133. Oberg KC, Bauman JL: QT prolongation and torsades de pointes due to erythromycin lactobionate. Pharmacotherapy 1995;15:687–692.
134. O'Sullivan TL, Ruffing MJ, Lamp KC, et al: Prospective evaluation of red man syndrome in patients receiving vancomycin. J Infect Dis 1993;168:773–776.
135. Paradelis AG: Aminoglycoside antibiotics and neuromuscular blockade. J Antimicrob Chemother 1979;5:737–738.
136. Paris DG, Parente TF, Bruschetta HR, et al: Torsades de pointes induced by erythromycin and terfenadine. Am J Emerg Med 1994;12:636–638.
137. Park SY, Parker RH: Review of imipenem. Infect Control 1986;7:333–337.
138. Paul J, Brown NM: Tinnitus and ciprofloxacin. BMJ 1995;311:232.
139. Pestotnik SL, Classen DC, Evans RS, et al: Prospective surveillance of imipenem/cilastatin use and associated seizures using a hospital information system. Ann Pharmacother 1993;27:497–501.
140. Phelps G, Nixon M: A case of pseudoanaphylactic reaction to intramuscular procaine penicillin G (Hoigne's syndrome) PNG Med J 1990;33:159–160.
141. Phelps SJ, Tsiu W, Barrett FF, et al: Chloramphenicol-induced cardiovascular collapse in an anephric patient. Pediatr Infect Dis J 1987;6:285–288.
142. Polk RE, Israel D, Wang J, et al: Vancomycin skin tests and prediction of "red man syndrome" in healthy volunteers. Antimicrob Agents Chemother 1993;37:2139–2143.
143. Prazic M, Salaj B, Sunotic R: Familial sensitivity to streptomycin. J Laryngol Otol 1964;78:1037–1043.
144. Ptachainski RJ, Carpenter BJ, Burckart GJ, et al: Effect of erythromycin on cyclosporine levels. N Engl J Med 1985; 313:1416–1417. Letter.
145. Ramilo O, Kinane BT, McCracken GH: Chloramphenicol neurotoxicity. Pediatr Infect Dis J 1988;7:358–359.
146. Regan TJ, Khan MI, Olde IHA, Passannant AJ: Antibiotic effect on myocardial K^+ transport and the production of ventricular tachycardia. J Clin Invest 1969;48:66A. Abstract.
147. Riley HD Jr: Vancomycin and novobiocin. Med Clin North Am 1970;54:1277–1289.
148. Rippelmeyer DJ, Synhavsky A: Ciprofloxacin and allergic interstitial nephritis. Ann Intern Med 1988;109:170. Letter.
149. Rockwood RP, Embardo LS: Theophylline, ciprofloxacin, erythromycin: A potentially harmful regimen. Ann Pharmacother 1993;27:651–652. Letter.
150. Rothenberg HJ: Anaphylactoid reaction to vancomycin. J Am Med Assoc 1959;171:1101–1102.
151. Rubart M, Pressler ML, Pride HP, Zipes DP: Electrophysiological mechanisms in a canine model of erythromycin-associated long QT syndrome. Circulation 1993;88(pt 1): 1832–1844.
152. Rudolph AH, Prince EV: Penicillin reactions among patients in venereal disease clinics: A national survey. JAMA 1973;223:499–501.
153. Rybak MJ, Boike SC: Additive toxicity in patients receiving vancomycin and aminoglycosides. Clin Pharm 1983;2: 508. Letter.
154. Sabra R, Takahashi K, Branch RA, Badr KF: Mechanisms of amphotericin B-induced reduction of glomerular filtration rate: A micropuncture study. J Pharmacol Exp Ther 1990;253:34–37.
155. Sacristan JA, Soto JA, deCos MA: Erythromycin-induced hypoacusis: 11 new cases and literature review. Ann Pharmacother 1993;27:950–955.
156. Saraway SM, Marke J, Steinberg M, et al: Doom anxiety and delirium in lidocaine toxicity. Am J Psychiatry 1987;144:159–163.
157. Sayawa BP, Weihprecht H, Cambell WR, et al: Direct vasoconstriction as a possible cause for amphotericin B-induced nephrotoxicity in rats. J Clin Invest 1991;87: 2079–2107.
158. Schacht J: Molecular mechanisms of drug-induced hearing loss. Hear Res 1986;48:297.
159. Schentag JJ, Plaut ME: Patterns of beta-2-microglobulin excretion in patients treated with aminoglycosides. Kidney Int 1980;16:654–661.

160. Schluter G: Ciprofloxacin: review of potential toxicologic effects. Am J Med 1987;82(suppl 4A):91–93.
161. Schweitzer VG, Olson NR: Ototoxic effect of erythromycin therapy. Arch Otolaryngol 1984;110:258–260.
162. Scott JL, Finegold SM, Belkins GA, et al: A controlled double-blind study of the hematologic toxicity of chloramphenicol. N Engl J Med 1965;272:1137.
163. Seamans KB, Gloor P, Dobell RAR, Wyant JD: Penicillin-induced seizures during cardiopulmonary bypass: A clinical and electroencephalographic study. N Engl J Med 1968;278:861–868.
164. Seldon R, Sasahara AA: Central nervous system toxicity induced by lidocaine. JAMA 1967;202:908–909.
165. Serdaru M, Diquet B, Lhermitte F: Generalized seizures after ampicillin. Lancet 1982;2:617–618. Letter.
166. Shu XO, Gao YT, Linet MS, et al: Chloramphenicol use and childhood leukaemia in Shanghai. Lancet 1987;2: 934–937.
167. Silber T, D'Angelio L: Doom, anxiety, and Hoigne's syndrome. Am J Psychiatry 1987;144:1365. Letter.
168. Silber TJ, D'Angelio LJ: Panic attack following injection of aqueous procaine penicillin G (Hoigne's syndrome). J Pediatr 1985;107:314–315.
169. Silvian C, Levillain P, Labat-Labourdette J, Beauchant M: Granulomatous hepatitis due to a combination of amoxacillin and clavulanic acid. Digestive Dis Sci 1992;37: 150–152.
170. Slavich IL, Gleffe RF, Haas EJ: Grand mal epileptic seizures during ciprofloxacin therapy. JAMA 1989:261: 558–559.
171. Solomkin JS, Fant WK, Rivera JU, Alexander JW: Randomized clinical trial of imipenem/cilastatin versus gentamycin and clindamycin in mixed flora infections. Am J Med 1985;78(suppl 6A):85–91.
172. Somer T, Finegold SM: Vasculitis associated with infections, immunization, and antimicrobial drugs. Clin Infect Dis 1995;20:1010–1036.
173. Stevens DC, Kleiman MB, Lietman PS, et al: Exchange transfusion in acute chloramphenicol toxicity. J Pediatr 1981;99:651–653.
174. Stupp H, Kupper K, Lagler F, et al: Inner ear concentrations and ototoxicity of different antibiotics in local and systemic application. Audiology 1973;12:350–363.
175. Sunagawa M, Matsumura H, Sumita Y, Nouda H: Structural features resulting in convulsive activity of carbapenem compounds: Effect of C-2 side chain. J Antibiot (Tokyo) 1995;48:408–416.
176. Swanson DJ, Sung RJ, Fine MJ, et al: Erythromycin ototoxicity: Prospective assessment with serum concentrations and audiograms in a study of patients with pneunomia. Am J Med 1992;92:61–68.
177. Takada S, Kato M, Takayama S: Comparison of lesions induced by intra-articular injections of quinolones and compounds damaging cartilage components in rat femoral condyles. J Toxicol Environ Health 1994;42:73–88.
178. Thompson WL, Anderson SE Jr, Lipsky JJ, et al: Overdose of chloramphenicol. JAMA 1975;234:149–150.
179. Timmermans L: Influence of antibiotics on spermatogenesis. J Urol 1974;112: 348–349.
180. Tsuji A, Sato H, Kume Y, et al: Inhibitory effects of quinolone antibacterial agents on gamma-aminobutyric acid binding to receptor sites in rat brain membranes. Antimicrob Agents Chemother 1988;32:190–194.
181. Turner WM: Lidocaine and psychotic reactions. Ann Intern Med 1982;97:149–150.
182. Tynes BS, Utz JP, Bennett JE, et al: Reducing amphotericin B reactions. Am Rev Resp Dis 1963;87:264–268.
183. Utley PM, Lucas JB, Billings TE. Acute psychotic reactions to aqueous procaine penicillin. South Med J 1966;59: 1271–1274.
184. Van Arsdel PP Jr: The risk of penicillin reactions. Ann Intern Med 1968;69:1071–1073.
185. Wallace MR, Mascola JR, Oldfield EC 3rd: Red man syndrome: Incidence, etiology and prophylaxis. J Infect Dis 1991;164:1180–1185.
186. Warner WA, Sanders E: Neuromuscular blockade associated with gentamycin therapy. JAMA 1971;215:1153–1154.
187. Weisberger AS, Wessler S, Avioli LV: Mechanisms of action of chloramphenicol. JAMA 1969;209:97–103.
188. Welage LS, Borin MT, Wilton JH, et al: Comparative evaluation of the pharmacokinetics of *N*-methylthiotetrazole following administration of cefoperazone, cefotetan and cefmetazole. Antimicrob Agents Chemother 1990;34: 2369–2374.
189. Westphal JF, Vetter D, Brogard JM: Hepatic side-effects of antibiotics. J Antimicrob Chemother 1994;33:387–401.
190. Williams SE, Zenner HP, Schacht J: Three molecular steps of aminoglycoside ototoxicity demonstrated in outer hair cells. Hear Res 1987;30:11–18.
191. Wolf R, Brenner DS: An active amide group in the molecule of drugs that induce pemphigus: A casual or causal relationship? Dermatology 1994;189:1–4.
192. Ying LS, Johnson CA: Ciprofloxacin-induced interstitial nephritis. Clin Pharm 1989;8:518–521.
193. Yunis AA: Chloramphenicol toxicity: 25 years of research. Am J Med 1989;87:3-44N–3-48N.
194. Yunis AA: Chloramphenicol-induced bone marrow suppression. Semin Hematol 1973;10:255–234.
195. Zager RA, Bredl CR, Schimpf BA: Direct amphotericin B-mediated tubular toxicity: Assessments of selected cytoprotective agents. Kidney Int 1992;42:1588–1594.
196. Zifko U, Wimberger D, Volc B, Grisold W: Jarisch-Herxheimer reaction in a patient with neurosyphilis. J Neurol Neurosurg Psychiatry 1994;57:865–867.

CHAPTER 47

Antineoplastic Agents

Richard Y. Wang and Paul Calabresi

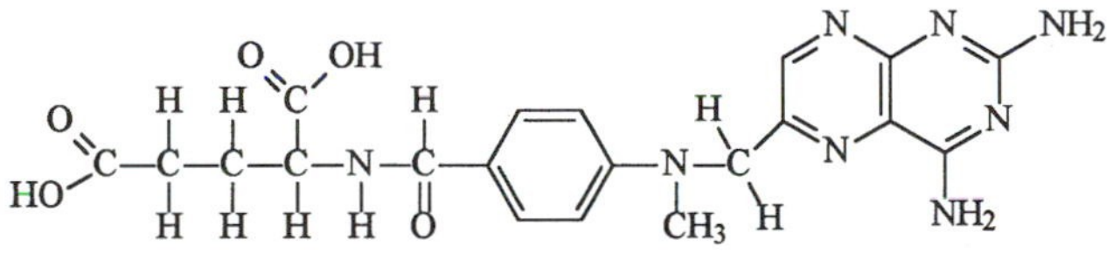

Methotrexate

A 70-year-old female was brought to the emergency department from an extended-care facility due to sudden-onset epistaxis. Vital signs were: blood pressure, 120/70 mm Hg; pulse, 100 beats/min; and respiratory rate, 18 breaths/min. The patient stated that for the last 2 days she had dysphagia, progressive weakness, and intermittent shakes. The patient had a past medical history of rheumatoid arthritis and pulmonary emboli. The patient's medications include methotrexate (MTX) and coumadin, which were both started in the last month for her underlying disorders. An anterior nasal packing was placed to stop the bleeding. Further examination of the oropharynx demonstrated several sores. The skin showed ecchymoses. Chest and abdominal findings were unremarkable. A large-bore IV line was established, and blood was drawn for CBC with platelets, PT, PTT, electrolytes, BUN, and creatinine tests. A MTX level and a type and cross were sent. The CBC showed hemoglobin, 8 g/dL; white cell count, 2000/mm^3 (81% neutrophils, 13% lymphocytes, 1% monocytes, 5% eosinophils); platelet count, 3000/mm^3; prothrombin time, 16.5 seconds; and INR, 2.0 (PTT was normal). Renal function was normal. The extended-care facility was contacted, and it was discovered that the patient was inadvertently administered methotrexate 2.5 mg QD instead of once a week for 1 month.

The patient was transfused with packed red blood cells, platelets, and fresh frozen plasma. Prophylactic broad-spectrum antibiotics were initiated. Leucovorin 10 mg/m^2 was started and administered every 4 hours IV. The serum MTX was determined later to be zero, and leucovorin therapy was discontinued. The WBC was lowest on day 3 of hospitalization and rose thereafter.

Why Do Antineoplastic Overdoses Occur?

Overdoses of antineoplastic medications are infrequent; however, they are of more consequence than many other medications because of their narrow therapeutic margin.[131,186] From 1987 to 1995, 90% of the annual exposures to these agents reported to the American Association of Poison Control Centers Toxic Surveillance Systems (AAPCC TESS) were unintentional.[133–141] Twenty percent of all annual exposures resulted in moderate or severe symptoms.

A review of the 2819 orders for cytotoxic agents at a pharmacy satellite showed that 93 orders (3%) contained at least one error in the dosage regimen and 442 (16%) contained at least one error in the instructions for drug preparation.[72] Three of the errors in dosage regimen were classified as potentially lethal, 13 as serious, 5 as significant, and 72 as minor. Two of the potentially lethal overdoses of cisplatin were due to errors in duration of administration (100 mg/m^2 for 3 to 4 consecutive days instead of for a single day). Lack of healthcare provider familiarity with the agent and its dosing was a major cause of these events. In another study evaluating drug errors, 49% occurred at the ordering/prescribing stage. This was most commonly caused by physicians who lacked knowledge of the drug and the intended patient.[128] Other areas where errors occurred were during transcription and nurse administration (Table 47–1). As more antineoplastic agents become available and their indications broaden, exposures will increase in number and frequency. In the last 9 years, the annual number of exposures reported to the AAPCC TESS increased threefold.[133–141]

TABLE 47–1. REASONS FOR MEDICAL PRESCRIBING ERRORS

Reason for error	Example
Wrong dose	Decimal point
	Calculation
	Rate of administration
	Unit of measure
	Patient pathophysiologic status
	Route of administration
	History taking
	Transcription
Wrong duration	Treatment duration: therapeutic
	Treatment duration: toxic
Wrong drug	Drug interaction
	Duplicative therapy
	No indication
	Combination products
	Wrong drug: same class
	Wrong drug: linked therapies
	Contraindication
Wrong frequency	Product dose/form
	Therapeutics/toxicity
	Abbreviated
Wrong route	Unusual drug use
	Abbreviation
	Dosage form
Wrong dose form	
Wrong patient history/information/identification	Allergy
	Wrong patient
Nomenclature	Sound-alikes
	Failure to specify specific dose
	Brand name lacking suffix

Reprinted, with permission, from Legha SS: Vincristine neurotoxicity, pathophysiology, and management. Med Toxicol 1986;1:421–427.

Most antineoplastic agents can be grouped into one of the following four categories: alkylating agents, antimetabolites, antimitotics, and antibiotics (Table 47–2). The antimetabolites are considered cell-cycle specific and are classified by their mechanism of action. They include pyrimidine, purine, and folic acid antagonists. Methotrexate is a folate antagonist, and other agents with similar but lesser toxicity include trimethoprim and pyrimethamine. Because the majority of the cases of antineoplastic agent overdoses involve the mustards, cisplatin, methotrexate, vincristine, and mitoxantrone, this discussion will focus on these agents.

What Is the Mechanism of Action of Methotrexate?

Methotrexate (MTX) is an important therapy for a variety of cancers, such as lymphoma, lymphocytic leukemia, breast cancer, and small-cell carcinoma. Its immunosuppressive activity allows it to also be used for rheumatoid arthritis, organ transplantation, and trophoblastic diseases.[41,110] Methotrexate's therapeutic and toxic effects are based on its ability to limit DNA and RNA synthesis by inhibiting dihydrofolate reductase (DHFR) and thymidine synthetase (Fig. 47–1). Dihydrofolate reductase reduces folic acid to tetrahydrofolate (FH_4), which serves as an essential cofactor in the synthesis of purine nucleotides. These reduced folates are required by thymidylate synthetase to serve as methyl donors in the formation of thymidylate as well. Thymidylate is then used for DNA synthesis. Methotrexate is a structural analogue of folate and competitively inhibits DHFR by binding to this substrate's site of action. This stops reduced folate production, which is necessary for nucleotide formation and DNA/RNA synthesis. Administration of the reduced folate (folinic acid or leucovorin) will allow for continual purine synthesis despite a blocked DHFR. Leucovorin is used as an antidote or rescue agent to limit the toxic effects of high-dose methotrexate therapy.

The bioavailability of methotrexate appears to be limited by a saturable intestinal absorption mechanism. At doses less than 30 mg/m^2, the absorption is 90%; and at doses greater than 80 mg/m^2, the absorption is less than 10 to 20%.[29] Methotrexate dosing regimens are variable, but can be generally classified as low dose, 30 to 40 mg/m^2 IV every 1 to 3 weeks; moderate dose, 250 to 500 mg/m^2 IV infusion every 2 to 3 weeks; and high dose, greater than 1000 mg/m^2 infusion every 2 to 3 weeks. Conventional doses of up to 100 mg/m^2 can be administered without special precautions. Doses of 1000 mg/m^2 are considered potentially lethal. Much higher doses (eg, 2 to 3 g/m^2) can be given when MTX is followed by leucovorin in order to prevent life-threatening toxicity. Mortality from high-dose methotrexate is about 6%, and occurs primarily when patients are not monitored with methotrexate levels.[70,206,221] Neurotoxicity may occur with high-dose therapy; however, the process reverses upon discontinuation of MTX treatment. The mechanisms re-

TABLE 47–2. CLASSIFICATION OF ANTINEOPLASTIC AGENTS AND THEIR EFFECTS

Class	Agent	Adverse Effects	Overdose
Alkylating	Busulphan	Hyperpigmentation, pulmonary fibrosis, hyperuricemia	Bone marrow suppression
	Dacarbazine	Hypotension, ↑AST, ALT, flu-like syndrome	
	Melphalan	Pulmonary fibrosis	
	Mustards		GI symptoms, seizures, CNS depression, myocardial necrosis
	Chlorambucil, cyclophosphamide, ifosfamide, mechlorethamine	Hemorrhagic cystitis, encephalopathy, pulmonary fibrosis	
	Nitrosourea		
	Carmustine, lomustine, semustine	Pulmonary fibrosis, ↑AST, ↑ALT, renal insufficiency	
	Platinoids		
	Cisplatin	Renal failure, peripheral neuropathy, hypomagnesemia, hypocalcemia, hyponatremia, ototoxicity	Seizures, encephalopathy, ototoxicity, retinal toxicity
	Carboplatin, iproplatin	Myelosuppression, hypomagnesemia, hypocalcemia, hyponatremia	Hepatic and renal compromise
	Procarbazine	MAOI activity	
	Thiotepa		Bone marrow suppression
Antimetabolite	Hydroxyurea		
	Methotrexate	Mucositis, nausea, diarrhea, ↑AST, ↑ALT	Mucositis, myelosuppression, renal failure
	Purine analogues		
	Chlordeoxyadenosine		
	Fludarabine	Encephalopathy, muscle weakness	Coma, seizures, blindness
	Mercaptopurine	Hyperuricemia, pancreatitis, cholestasis	GI symptoms, bone marrow suppression
	Pentostatin	↑AST, ↑ALT	Renal, CNS, and pulmonary toxicity
	Thioguanine	Hyperuricemia	
	Pyrimidine analogues		
	Cytarabine	Noncardiogenic pulmonary edema, neuropathy, cerebellar ataxia	
	Fluorouracil	Cardiogenic shock, cardiomyopathy, neuropathy, cerebellar ataxia	Paralytic ileus
Antimitotic	Epipodophyllotoxin		
	Etoposide, teniposide	CHF, hypotension	Bone marrow suppression
	Paclitaxel	GI perforation, peripheral neuropathy, dysrhythmias	
	Vinca alkaloids		
	Vinblastine, vincristine, vindesine	Peripheral neuropathy	Encephalopathy, seizures, autonomic instability, SIADH, paralytic ileus, myelosuppression
Antibiotics	Anthracycline		
	Daunorubicin, doxorubicin, epirubicin, idarubicin	Congestive cardiomyopathy	Dysrhythmias, CHF
	Bleomycin	Pulmonary fibrosis	
	Dactinomycin	↑AST, ↑ALT	Mucocutaneous toxicity
	Mithramycin	Skin flushing	GI toxicity
	Mitomycin C	Hemolytic uremic syndrome	GI toxicity, thrombocytopenia
	Mitoxantrone	Congestive cardiomyopathy	Pulmonary, CNS, and renal toxicity
Enzyme	L-Asparaginase	Hypersensitivity, pancreatitis	

main unclear, but may be due to direct toxicity to neuronal glial and endothelial cells and decreased neurotransmitter synthesis.[1]

Toxicity of MTX is dependent more on the duration of concentration than the dose itself. Thus, greater toxicity is expected from a 7-g IV dose for 48 hours than a 20-g dose over 24 hours.[81] Patients with a plasma MTX concentration greater than 1.0 μM at 48 hours posttreatment are considered at risk for bone marrow and gastrointestinal mucosal toxicity.[206] Risk factors for MTX toxicity are impaired renal function (primary route of drug elimination), third compartment spacing (eg, ascites, pleural effusions), use of NSAIDs, age, folate deficiency, and concurrent infection.[206]

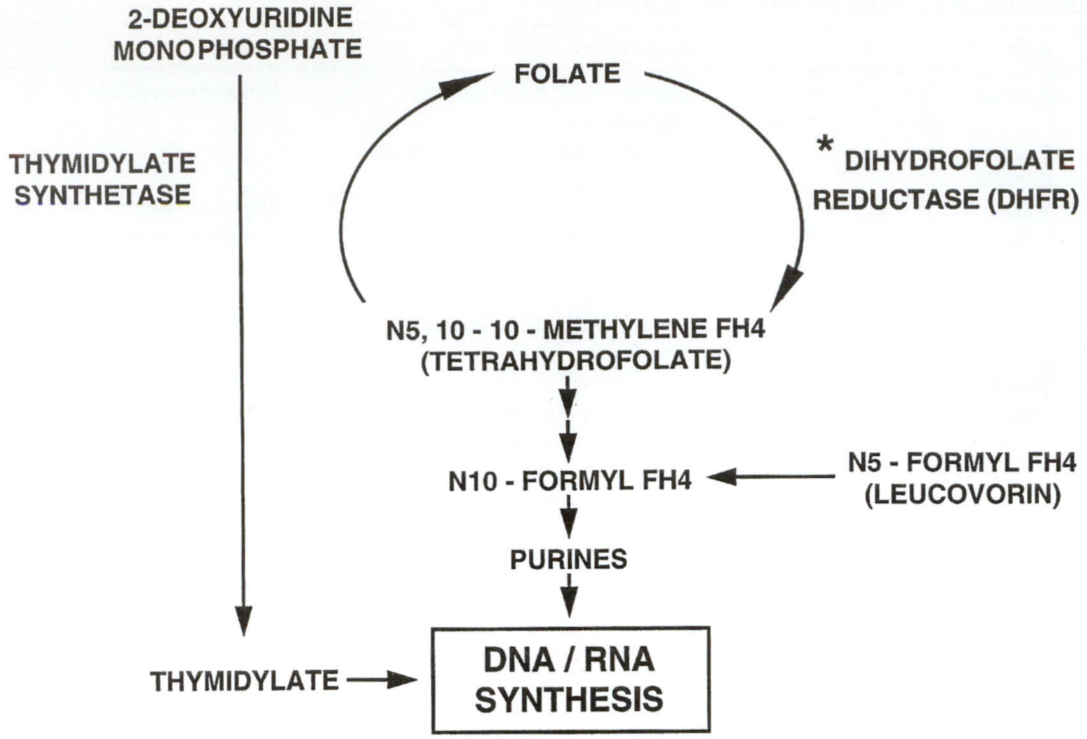

Figure 47–1. Mechanism of methotrexate toxicity. MTX inhibits DHFR activity, which is necessary for DNA and RNA synthesis. Leucovorin bypasses blockade to allow for continued synthesis.

Methotrexate is primarily eliminated by the kidneys. At high doses, drug and insoluble drug metabolites, 7-hydroxy methotrexate and 2,4-diamino-10-methyl pteroic acid, accumulate and may precipitate in the renal tubules, causing reversible acute tubular necrosis. Methotrexate is one tenth as soluble at a pH of 5.5 than at a pH of 7.5.[29,188] The serum concentration threshold for nephrotoxicity is 2.2 mM at a urine pH of 5.5, and 22 mM at a urine pH of 6.9. Acute renal failure may result from drug precipitation in the renal tubule, and is most common in patients who are inadequately hydrated or not alkalinized.[2,75,112] The majority (90%) of methotrexate is excreted unchanged in the urine, within 48 hours, by both glomerular filtration and active tubular secretion. Folic acid blocks MTX renal reabsorption and can enhance drug elimination during leucovorin rescue.[97]

What Are the Clinical Manifestations of MTX Toxicity?

In the course of methotrexate therapy, a variety of disorders may occur resulting from either an adverse reaction or an excessive administration. Some of these clinical manifestations may include hepatic, pulmonary, and neurologic findings.

The clinical manifestations of methotrexate toxicity include stomatitis, esophagitis, renal failure, and myelosuppression. In a group of 23 patients who received 45 courses of high-dose methotrexate therapy, some of the toxic signs that were observed included increased AST/ALT (81%), nausea and vomiting (66%), mucositis (33%), dermatitis (18%), leukopenia (11%), thrombocytopenia (9%), and creatinine elevation (7%).[175]

Nausea and vomiting, considered rare after low-dose therapy, typically begin 2 to 4 hours after high-dose therapy and last for about 6 to 12 hours. Mucositis, characterized by mouth soreness, stomatitis, or diarrhea, usually occurs 1 to 2 weeks after therapy and can last for 4 to 7 days. Other gastrointestinal symptoms resulting from methotrexate therapy include pharyngitis, anorexia, gastrointestinal hemorrhage, and toxic megacolon.[12] Hepatotoxicity, as described by increased AST/ALT and hyperbilirubinemia, can be observed with both acute and chronic therapy.[147,157] It is usually associated with high dosage regimens. Laboratory abnormalities improve within 1 to 2 weeks of discontinuation of MTX. The mechanism is not completely understood, but toxicity is attributed to reduced liver folate stores.[15] Factors associated with toxicity are sustained high plasma levels, cumulative dosages, chronic therapy, and host factors such as increase in age, obesity, diabetes, and alcoholism.[224]

Pancytopenia usually occurs within the first 2 weeks after an acute exposure. The complete blood count should be monitored on days 7, 10, and 14 because life-threatening complications such as bleeding disorders and overwhelming sepsis may occur.[125] There are several reports demonstrating the occurrence of pancytopenia in individuals receiving chronic low-dose methotrexate therapy for rheumatoid arthritis and psoriasis.[59,120,147,179] Leucovorin therapy may be beneficial in these instances, and has been recommended for treatment until the pancytopenia resolves and methotrexate is no longer detected in the serum.[142]

When used in small IV doses of 40 to 60 mg/m^2, methotrexate is not associated with appreciable nephrotoxicity. However, at doses greater than 100 mg/kg, several investigators have reported severe kidney damage, with oliguria, azotemia, and fatal renal failure.[28] Patients at risk for nephrotoxicity include the elderly, those with underlying renal disease (GFR less than 50 mL/min), and those who receive concurrent drug therapy that can delay MTX excretion. This would include agents that reduce renal blood flow (eg, NSAIDs), are nephrotoxic (eg, cisplatin, aminoglycoside), or are weak organic acids (eg, salicylate, piperacillin).[104,206] Some of the acute pulmonary disorders associated with MTX therapy are alveolar infiltrates and hypersensitivity reactions.[117] Symptoms begin from 12 to 17 years after initiation of therapy.[132,200] Host risk factors associated with methotrexate pneumonitis include middle aged males, tobacco use, and preexisting pulmonary disease.[192] Mortality from high-dose methotrexate is about 6%, and occurs primarily when patients are not monitored with methotrexate levels.[70,206,221]

The neurologic complications associated with either high-dose systemic MTX therapy or intrathecal administration are the most consequential manifestations. The incidence of neurologic toxicity from high-dose MTX therapy is about 5 to 15%.[113] The manifestations usually occur days after the initiation of therapy and include hemiparesis, behavioral abnormalities, seizures, and dysreflexia.[68,223] Cerebrospinal fluid analysis and computerized tomography of the brain may be normal or show demyelination of white matter (especially in the anterior and frontal lobes).[5] Leucovorin does not appear to limit or prevent MTX-induced neuropathy.

How Should a Patient With an MTX Overdose Be Managed?

In the event of an oral overdose of methotrexate, the initial concern should be gastric decontamination. If the patient presents soon after ingestion, then syrup of ipecac is an appropriate method. If there are contraindications to emesis, orogastric lavage should be performed. Activated charcoal binds methotrexate and should be administered as soon as possible so as to limit further drug absorption.[76] The administration of multiple-dose activated charcoal and cholestyramine[68] can significantly decrease the elimination half-life of methotrexate by interrupting enterohepatic circulation.[76,85]

Adequate hydration is also important to prevent renal failure in patients who receive inadvertent high doses. Therefore, a good urinary output (1 to 3 mL/kg per hour) and urinary alkalinization with sodium bicarbonate (to pH 7 to 8), should be initiated to prevent renal toxicity.

What Antidotes Are Available for MTX?

Folinic acid (leucovorin, N5-formyl-tetrahydrofolate) rescue therapy has allowed higher doses of methotrexate to be administered therapeutically, as leucovorin limits bone marrow and gastrointestinal toxicity. Leucovorin is most beneficial when administered within 1 hour of exposure, but should still be given to patients as soon as possible after an excessive exposure, because the only complications associated with leucovorin administration are drug interactions[177] and hypersensitivity reactions.[99] Routine doses of leucovorin used for rescue therapy are inadequate for overdose situations. (See Antidotes in Depth: Folinic acid.)

The initial leucovorin dose to be administered should achieve a plasma concentration equal to or greater than that of the methotrexate. In this manner, the reduced folate antidote can successfully compete with MTX for active transport sites on the cell membrane, displace MTX from its intracellular binding site, and most importantly, restore reduced folate stores.[111,171] The lower doses of leucovorin used during methotrexate therapy are an attempt to protect normal body cells but not tumor cells. Under therapeutic circumstances it is recommended to delay leucovorin rescue as long as possible, administer the minimal effective dose, and discontinue therapy as soon as it is no longer necessary.[28]

Serum methotrexate levels should be monitored at 12, 24, and 48 hours postexposure so that leucovorin therapy can be adjusted accordingly (Fig. 47–2). Generally, leucovorin therapy should be continued if the plasma MTX level is above 1.0 μM at 48 hours postexposure,[206] and maintained until the level is below 0.01 μM.[213] In severe cases, leucovorin therapy should be considered until marrow recovery, even if serum MTX is no longer detectable. This is because intracellular MTX activity may still be ongoing and folinic acid would be of benefit. It should be noted that trimethoprim, a folate antagonist, can interfere with certain MTX assays (radioenzymatic, enzyme inhibition).[18] Spectrophotofluorimetric analysis may misinterpret folinic acid for MTX and should not be used as the analytic method during leucovorin therapy.[121]

Thymidine has also been used to rescue cells from the cytotoxic effects of methotrexate by what is called "thymidylate salvage."[67,209] Thymidine can be converted to thymidine synthetase by thymidine kinase, which is not inhibited by MTX, thus allowing for the formation of thymidylate for DNA synthesis (see Fig. 47–1). Thymidine rescue is investigational, but has limited application as it does not appear to be as effective as leucovorin.[152,209]

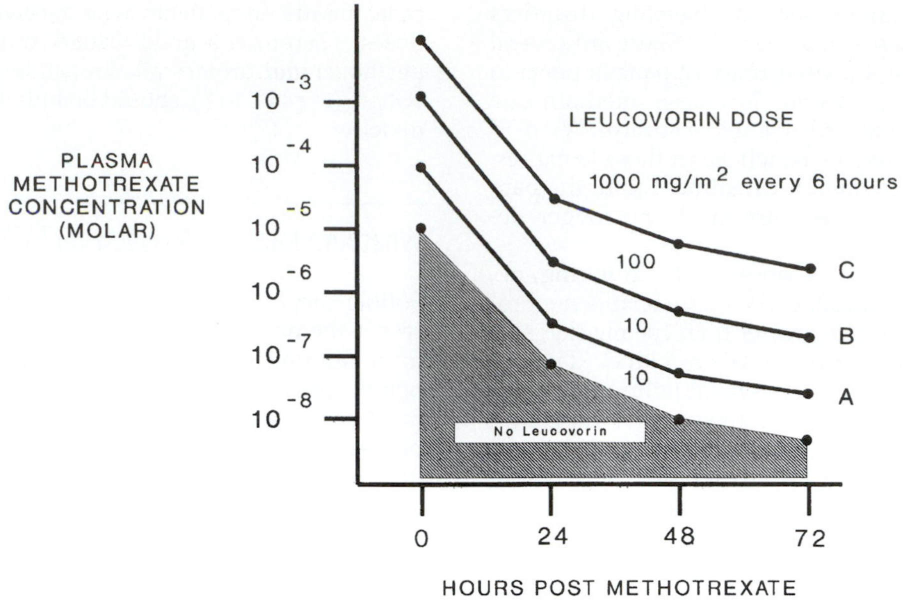

Figure 47–2. Leucovorin rescue nomogram for methotrexate toxicity. Shaded area = MTX levels observed after doses < 60 mg/m^2; leucovorin is usually not required. Up to curve B requires 10 mg/m^2 of leucovorin per dose every 6 hours until the MTX level is $< 1 \times 10^{-7}$ M. Up to curve C requires 100 mg/m^2 per dose. *(Reprinted, with permission, from Young LY, Koda-Kimble MA (eds): Applied Therapeutics: The Clinical Use of Drugs, 4th edition. Vancouver, Washington, Applied Therapeutics, Inc., 1988.)*

What Other Approaches Are Available for Patients With Methotrexate Overdose?

There are several reports of the use of hemodialysis and/or hemoperfusion for patients with methotrexate toxicity. Although the volume of distribution and protein binding suggest that methotrexate is dialyzable, clinical evidence suggests otherwise.[203] In one report, less than 10% of an initial 0.7 g of methotrexate was cleared in 12 sessions of hemodialysis.[211] The measured clearance was only 38 mL/min.

Charcoal hemoperfusion removed more than 50% of methotrexate in 4 patients with delayed renal MTX clearance during high-dose MTX therapy.[58] This was felt to have prevented severe skin and mucosal toxicity. Sequential hemodialysis and hemoperfusion were used for a patient with substantial methotrexate toxicity.[85] These procedures decreased the half-life of elimination from 45 to 7.6 hours. In experimental animals, hemoperfusion significantly reduced both the terminal half-life and the blood concentration of methotrexate. In anephric dogs, hemoperfusion decreased the half-life from greater than 20 hours to 1.3 hours.[103] Thus, hemoperfusion is recommended over hemodialysis.

In vitro studies indicate that the toxic effects of 100 μmol MTX cannot be reversed by 1000 μmol of leucovorin.[171] The efficacy of leucovorin rescue appears limited when the plasma MTX levels exceed 10 μmol. This suggests the potential need for hemoperfusion to lower persistent MTX plasma concentrations of greater than 100 μmol.[176] It is important to perform hemoperfusion early, prior to distribution into tissues. Inline hemoperfusion and hemodialysis may remove more MTX than hemoperfusion alone and should be considered. Rebound in MTX levels may be expected after hemodialysis.[80,90] Folic acid is water soluble and can also be removed by hemodialysis. Thus, replacement therapy may be necessary postdialysis.[50,194,197] This is probably also applicable for leucovorin, and postdialysis doses of leucovorin should be considered.

Enzymatic cleavage is another method of inactivating antineoplastic agents. Carboxypeptidase G2 is a new rescue agent able to inactivate MTX by cleaving its terminal glutamate group.[234] Its use in high-dose MTX therapy in humans has been tolerated, but it is associated with hypersensitivity reactions because of its bacterial origin. To avoid systemic sensitization, this enzyme has been attached to extracorporeal filters used to enhance drug detoxification.[24] Further clinical investigation is needed to better define the role of this enzyme in therapy.

Granulocyte colony stimulating factor (G-CSF) was used in a patient with a chronic MTX overdose and pancytopenia.[203] The patient had a serum MTX concentration of 1.25 μmol upon admission and was in renal failure. Bone marrow biopsy showed promyelocytes but no mature white cells and a marked reduction of megakaryocytes. Due to deteriorating conditions, granulocyte-macrophage G-CSF (125 μg/m^2 per day) was administered when the

MTX level fell below the reference limit for toxicity. Seven days after the initiation of G-CSF, the WBC count rose and reached normal values within 10 days.

The decision for using G-CSF in patients with agranulocytosis depends on the severity of neutropenia and anticipated speed of recovery. If promyelocytes and myelocytes are present in the bone marrow, neutrophil recovery will occur spontaneously in 4 to 7 days following the withdrawal of the offending agent.[74] However, when granulopoiesis is completely absent, neutrophil recovery can not be expected for at least 14 days. This latter situation can be accelerated by using granulocyte or granulocyte-macrophage G-CSF. When myeloid precursors are present in the bone marrow, G-CSF can accelerate neutrophil recovery in 1 to 4 days. If myeloid precursors are absent, neutrophil recovery with G-CSF would take longer, but would still occur sooner than without G-CSF therapy.

Rapid neutrophil recovery following G-CSF use was also demonstrated with several drug-induced disorders,[14,42] but without a clear advantage. When consideration is given to these findings and the high mortality associated with agranulocytosis, it is only rational to use these agents. Indications for G-CSF use are severe neutropenia with proven infection or when bone marrow recovery is expected to be delayed. Serum levels of the antineoplastic agent should be below detection before institution of G-CSF; otherwise, no benefit may be expected.

What Are the Clinical Manifestations of Vincristine Toxicity?

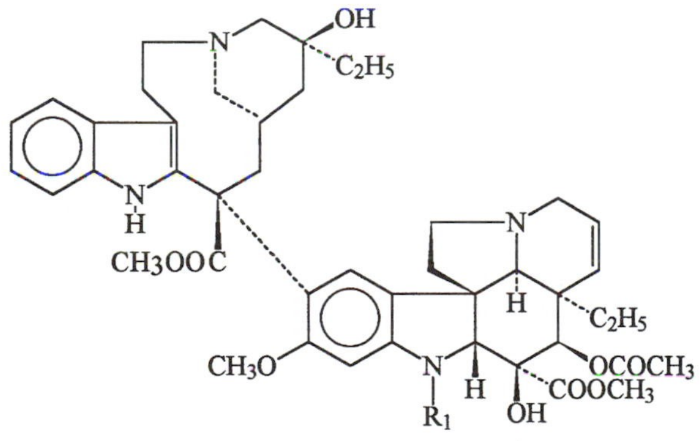

Vinblastine: $R_1 = CH_3$
Vincristine: $R_1 = CHO$

Vincristine and vinblastine are derived from the periwinkle plant and used for the treatment of leukemias, lymphomas, and certain solid tumors. Their mechanism of activity is similar to that of colchicine and podophyllotoxin. These agents bind to tubulin at different sites, and prevent its polymerization into microtubules.[54,63] Microtubules are responsible for several basic cellular functions including reproduction, axonal transport of organelles, and cellular movement. Metaphase arrest is commonly observed due to the inability to form spindle fibers from the microtubules. Cell death quickly ensues as a result of the interruption of these homeostatic functions, accounting for the clinical manifestations.

Despite their similarity in structure, vincristine and vinblastine differ in clinical toxicity. Vincristine has less bone marrow suppression and more neurotoxicity than vinblastine. In the therapeutic use of vincristine, the occurrence of myelosuppression is only 5 to 10%.[94] However, this is common in the overdose setting and the need for replacement blood products and concern for overwhelming infection is apparent. The fall in cell counts begins within the first week and may last for up to 3 weeks. Other manifestations of acute vincristine toxicity are mucositis, CNS disorders, and syndrome of inappropriate antidiuretic hormone (SIADH).

Central nervous system disorders are varied and unusual during therapeutic vincristine therapy because of the agent's poor penetrance of the blood–brain barrier.[108] They are, however, common when there is delayed drug elimination, damage to the blood brain–barrier, and overdose of the patient. Generalized seizures from toxicity or secondary effects may occur from 1 to 7 days after drug exposure.[100,115,119] Treatment is with benzodiazepines and phenobarbital, although phenytoin was used successfully in a patient with barbiturate hypersensitivity.[119] Other manifestations are depression, agitation, insomnia, and hallucinations.

Autonomic dysfunction is observed, and it commonly includes bowel ileus, constipation, and abdominal pain. Atony of the bladder, hypertension, and hypotension can occur as well.[119] Vincristine stimulation of the hypothalamus may be responsible for the fevers and SIADH noted in overdosed patients.[181] The fevers begin 24 hours after exposure and last 6 to 96 hours. Serum electrolytes need to be monitored typically for 10 days.

Ascending peripheral neuropathies occur during vincristine therapy and can be limited by keeping the total for a single dose below 2 mg.[198] Neuropathy may appear after an overdose, starting at about 2 weeks and lasting for 6 to 7 weeks. Paresthesias, ataxia, bone pain, wrist drop, foot drop, cranial nerve involvement (III to VII and X), and diminished reflexes can be observed.[225] The loss of reflexes, the earliest and most consistent sign of vincristine neuropathy, is maximal at 17 days after a single dose. Muscular weakness is a limiting point in therapy, and typically involves the distal dorsiflexors of the extremities, although laryngeal involvement has also been reported.[130,187] These severe neurologic symptoms may be reversed by either withholding therapy or reducing dosage upon manifestation of these findings.[130] The mechanism of toxicity is not well understood, but appears to be related to inhibition of microtubular synthesis, which leads to axonal degeneration.[84,158] A brain biopsy of a vincristine-related death showed neurotubular dissociation, which is characteristic of vincristine damage in experimental animals.[32,44] Nerve conduction studies and the Achilles tendon reflex are useful in monitoring patients for toxicity after exposure.

Vincristine-induced myocardial infarctions are reported but not understood.[144,199,207,231] The mechanism of the effect may be related to vinca alkaloid-induced platelet aggregation, coronary artery spasm, or increased sensitivity of myocardium to hypoxia.

How Is a Patient With a Vincristine Overdose Managed?

Vincristine overdose is the most frequently reported antineoplastic overdose in the literature. This is because there are three different ways to misdose this agent, including confusing it with vinblastine, misinterpreting the dose, and confusing two different-strength vials. The normal dose for vincristine is 0.06 mg/kg, and a single dose is not to exceed 2.0 mg for an adult or child. Patients receiving an inadvertent amount of an IV dose of vincristine are to be admitted to a cardiac-monitored bed and observed for 24 to 72 hours.[143] Seizures, dysrhythmias, and alterations in blood pressure can be expectantly managed, although prophylactic phenobarbital was used to prevent seizures in one report.[122]

If patients remain asymptomatic, they can be discharged with follow-up for bone marrow suppression and SIADH; otherwise, depending upon the patient's clinical condition, continual observation for progression of neurologic symptoms is warranted.[21] The symptoms of acute toxicity usually last for 3 to 7 days, and the neurologic sequelae may last for months with some resolution.

In the early 1960s, some investigations suggested that glutamic acid might reduce the incidence of vinblastine-induced myelosuppression.[11,52,116,216] Further investigations led to a controlled study, where patients receiving vincristine therapy were given glutamic acid as 500 mg orally three times a day.[109] It was observed that there was a decreased incidence in loss of Achilles tendon reflex and delayed onset of paresthesias in the glutamic acid-treated group. However, the frequency of hematologic and gastrointestinal effects from vincristine were not significantly different between the two treatment groups. There were no reported adverse effects with glutamic acid in this study. Animal studies involving the administration of glutamic and aspartic acid to mice poisoned with either vinblastine or vincristine, demonstrate increased survival.[52,107] The mechanisms of these observed effects with glutamic acid are not clear. One possibility is that glutamic acid may competitively inhibit a common cellular transport mechanism for vincristine.[30,49] Another possibility would be that glutamic acid may assist in the stabilization of tubulin and promote its polymerization into microtubules, thus improving peripheral neuropathy.[33,89] Finally, exogenous glutamic acid may improve cellular metabolism by overcoming its inhibition by vinblastine in the Kreb's cycle.[62,178] Although the role of glutamic acid for acute toxicity needs further study, it is probably not harmful and should be considered.

Leucovorin may shorten the course of vincristine-induced peripheral neuropathy[87] and myelosuppression.[122] The mechanism is attributed to leucovorin's ability to overcome a vincristine-mediated block of dihydrofolate reductase and thymidine synthetase.[87] However, neither leucovorin,[19,105,212] nor pyridoxine[106] have been shown to be definitely effective.

What Is the Role of Enhanced Elimination in Vincristine Overdoses?

Vincristine is rapidly distributed to tissue stores and highly bound to proteins and red cells.[40] Elimination is via the hepatobiliary system.[40] In more than 50% of children given this agent IV, their plasma levels were not detected 4 hours after administration.[154] Such characteristics favor early intervention and methods other than hemodialysis. Double-volume exchange transfusion was performed at 6 hours postexposure in 3 children who were overdosed with 7.5 mg/m^2 of vincristine IV.[122] Of the two survivors, their respective postexchange serum vincristine concentrations were 57 and 71% lower than their pre-exchange concentrations. The amount of vincristine removed was not determined. Although these patients developed peripheral neuropathies, myelosuppression, and autonomic instability, the author noted that the duration of illness was shorter than previously reported. The pre- and post-serum vincristine concentrations were unchanged in the nonsurvivor. Plasmapheresis was attempted in an 18-year-old patient who received two 8-mg IV doses of vincristine, 12 hours apart. The procedure was performed 6 hours after the second dose and 1.5 times the plasma volume was pheresed.[169] Postserum vincristine concentration was only 23% lower than the preconcentration. The patient survived with myelosuppression, neurotoxicity, and SIADH. Thus, based on the pharmacodynamic profile of vincristine and these two reports, exchange transfusion in the child would be the preferred method of enhanced elimination upon early arrival.

What Are the Manifestations of Anthracycline Toxicity?

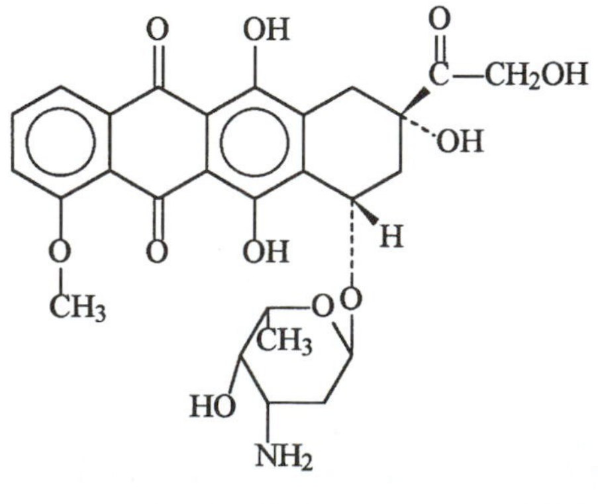

Doxorubicin

The antineoplastic agents derived from the bacterium *Streptomyces* are dactinomycin, daunorubicin, doxorubicin, bleomycin, mitomycin, and plicamycin. All except the latter are known not to cross the blood–brain barrier. The red anthracycline antibiotics, dactinomycin and doxorubicin, are best known for their associated cardiotoxicity, which limits their therapeutic use. The mechanism responsible for their therapeutic effects is different from that which causes cardiotoxicity.[210] The latter is believed to result from the formation of free radicals.[155] Doxorubicin and dactinomycin are quinone derivatives and can be reduced to free radicals. These metabolites are extremely cytotoxic through the promotion of lipid peroxidation. Paraquat and bleomycin have similar mechanisms of toxicity. The limited efficacy of free radical scavengers (alpha-tocopherol, *N*-acetylcysteine) for anthracycline cardiotoxicity have led to the evaluation of other toxic mechanisms.[156] From this, the importance of iron as a cofactor for these radical-producing reactions was realized. The anthracyclines have a high affinity for metal ions. Doxorubicin has an iron (Fe^{3+}) binding constant of 10^{33}, which is comparable to deferoxamine.[78]

The heart's increased susceptibility to free radicals is attributed to its lack of sufficient enzyme activity responsible for free radical scavenging.[60] The cardiotoxicity can be divided into acute and chronic manifestations. The acute form of toxicity consists of dysrhythmias, ST and T-wave changes on the electrocardiograph, diminished ejection fraction that usually resolves over 24 hours, and sudden death.[34,204,230] Abnormal findings on the ECG are present in 41% of patients receiving doxorubicin.[9,91,129,204,222,233,236] These are neither dose related nor associated with the development of cardiomyopathy. Acute pericarditis and myocarditis resulting in conduction defects and congestive heart failure are also reported.[34] Animal studies with doxorubicin demonstrate beneficial effects of adrenergic antagonists for toxicity due to elevated levels of catecholamines,[35] although the use of beta-adrenergic antagonists in the potential setting of diminished cardiac output needs to be considered.

Significant cardiotoxicity results from elevated peak serum drug levels and accounts for the continuous and periodic infusions practiced in therapy. In cumulative doses, the anthracycline antibiotics cause a cardiomyopathy that results in congestive heart failure. The condition is irreversible and is associated with a 48% mortality.[172] This drug-induced CHF is associated with pathognomonic changes on electron microscopy that can distinguish it from infectious and ischemic etiologies. These histologic changes include reduced number of myocardial fibrils, and mitochondrial and cellular degeneration.[26] The incidence of chronic cardiotoxicity for doxorubicin is between 1 and 10% when the cumulative dose is less than 450 mg/m^2, and becomes greater than 20% when more than 550 mg/m^2 (comparable to dactinomycin, 950 mg/m^2) is administered.[220] The best way of monitoring cardiac function during therapy is by measuring left ventricular ejection fraction by radionuclide cineography.[4] Therapy should be discontinued when the ejection fraction falls below 50%. Some of the factors associated with an increased risk for cardiotoxicity include mediastinal irradiation, preexisting cardiac disease, the pediatric age group, and the concomitant use of cyclophosphamide and other anthracycline agents.[34] Fatalities are been reported with minimum doses of 150 to 333 mg/m^2, and occur within 1 to 16 days after exposure.[51]

Myelosuppression and mucositis are other effects associated with the use of the anthracycline agents. They typically occur in 1 to 2 weeks and recover.[20] The white cells are affected more than either the red cells or platelets. Patients with diminished drug clearance (eg, liver failure) are at risk for the development of these findings.

Newer agents with less cardiotoxicity are epirubicin, idarubicin, and mitoxantrone. The potential therapeutic benefits and questionable degree of lesser toxicity of the former two agents limit their current use. Mitoxantrone is an anthraquinone and is recognized to be less toxic than doxorubicin and daunorubicin. Major organs of toxicity remain the heart, bone marrow, and gut. Gastrointestinal effects are less severe and frequent with mitoxantrone than doxorubicin.[196] There are four cases of mitoxantrone overdoses reported in the literature.[88,196] Common to these events was a tenfold error in dosing (100 mg/m^2 instead of 10 mg/m^2), early onset of nausea with vomiting, and myelosuppression with fever. Acute decreased cardiac contractility was observed by echocardiography in one patient who was asymptomatic.[88] Otherwise, no patient developed dysrhythmias, congestive failure, ECG changes, or elevated creatine phosphokinase levels early after exposure. Three patients developed fatal congestive heart failure from 1 to 4 months later.[196]

How Should Patients With an Anthracycline Overdose Be Managed?

There are no specific antidotes for this class of agents; thus, management is largely supportive. Monitoring for cardiotoxicity and pancytopenia is necessary. Left ventricular function is the best predictor for cardiomyopathy.[71,190] When there is more than a 10% absolute decrease in the left ventricular ejection fraction (LVEF) and a drop in LVEF of 50% from baseline, doxorubicin therapy is discontinued.[190] Acute congestive failure was successfully managed with digoxin and furosemide.[196]

A variety of cardioprotectants have been evaluated for doxorubicin; however, only a few were used in clinical trials. Digoxin and low-dose verapamil were shown to benefit patients treated with doxorubicin.[77,226] At higher doses of verapamil, hypotension and heart block were observed and limited further use.[164,205] Dexrazoxane (ICRF–187), an iron chelator, limited the cardiotoxic effects of doxorubicin in a randomly controlled human trial.[201] In comparison with the controls, the treatment group had smaller decreases in the left ejection fraction per dose of doxorubicin, fewer histologic changes on cardiac biopsy, and more patients tolerated doses greater than 600 mg/m^2. The use of dexrazoxane in this study also had a slight increase in myelosuppression. The current role of this chelator is in limiting cardiotoxicity during therapeutic use. It is administered 30 minutes before doxorubicin in a 10:1 ratio. Further investigations are required to determine the use of dexrazoxane in overdose exposures.

The anthracycline agents are highly protein bound and have a large volume of distribution, thus making them unlikely candidates for hemodialysis. However, the early institution of hemoperfusion may enhance elimination. In an animal model, plasma doxorubicin clearance could be enhanced up to 20-fold with hemoperfusion.[228] Factors determining this were duration of therapy, rate of flow, and type of cartridge. The recommended cartridge was 2% acrylic hydrogel-coated. Three patients with an doxorubicin overdose were treated with hemoperfusion, one with an Amberlite cartridge, and all had a rapid reduction in their serum levels.[51] One survived a tenfold error in dosing. In a patient with a mitoxantrone overdose of 98 mg IV, hemoperfusion was begun within hours and only 0.287 and 0.236 mg of drug was removed in two trials.[88]

What Is the Management for a Patient With Nitrogen Mustard Overdose?

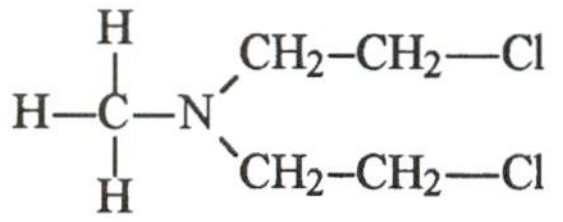

Mechlorethamine

The nitrogen mustard agents are cyclophosphamide, ifosfamide, chlorambucil, mechlorethamine, and melphalan. The tumoricidal activity of these agents is the result of the formation of reactive intermediates that bind to nucleophilic moieties on the DNA chain. Mechlorethamine is the original compound from which all of the others were derived. It is highly reactive when it comes in contact with water and undergoes rapid chemical transformation. Local reactions due to mechlorethamine include extravasation-induced tissue injury and thrombophlebitis. Spillage onto skin should be thoroughly washed with soap and water, and then irrigated with a 2 to 4% sodium thiosulfate solution. Extravasations can cause significant injury and should be managed by infiltrating the area with isotonic sodium thiosulfate (see the section on extravasations later in the chapter). Ingestions of mechlorethamine should be managed as caustic exposures.

Chlorambucil and ifosfamide can produce CNS toxicity from therapeutic use or an overdose.[38] Both compounds undergo *N*-dechloroethylation to produce chloroacetaladehyde, which is believed to be toxic to the nervous system.[83] Encephalopathy occurs in 9% of patients receiving 5 g/m^2 of ifosfamide, and is more frequent with oral versus IV administration because of the first-pass effect and increased chloroacetaldehyde production.[148] The encephalopathy can be managed with methylene blue (50 mg IV as a 1% solution), although the mechanism is unknown.[124,235] Seizures are more commonly associated with chlorambucil. Acute overdoses reported in the literature are all from the oral route, and range in dosing from 1.5 to 6.8 mg/kg (therapeutic is 0.1 to 0.2 mg/kg).[7,39] The seizures occur within 6 hours, may appear as generalized tonic clonic activity or staring spells, and can last for 24 hours. However, in one instance where therapeutic dosing was increased, seizures occurred 17 hours later. This delay may be attributed to a lower serum concentration or a slower time to peak than in the overdose setting. A similar reasoning would explain why a patient with a chronic overdose of 4.1 mg/kg over 5 days did not sustain CNS toxicity.[66] EEGs demonstrated multiple paroxysms of bilaterally symmetrical 2 to 3-Hz spikes and slow high-voltage rhythmic slowing that progressed to slower bursts of rhythmic spike and wave discharge in a child with an acute overdose.[39] Barbiturates and benzodiazepines are more effective than phenytoin in seizure management.[7,27,229] Myelosuppression occurs in patients with both acute and chronic overdoses, and can present as late as 41 days postexposure. Recovery is expected within 1 week of the nadir. Recommendations for an acute chlorambucil exposure are routine gastrointestinal decontamination, a 6-hour observation, a baseline CBC and LFT, and a follow-up CBC weekly for 4 weeks.[217]

Cyclophosphamide is a commonly used agent that is known for inducing hemorrhagic cystitis from its irritating metabolite acrolein. This occurs in about 5 to 10% of patients who receive therapy.[37,48] The incidence of cystitis does not appear to be related to the total dose and route administered, age, or gender. The course is usually self-limiting, although blood transfusions may be required. In refractory cases electrocauterization, systemic vasopressin,[173] and intravesical administration of silver nitrate,[123] formalin,[73,193] prostaglandin F_2 alpha,[195] and hydrostatic pressure[95] have been tried. Some of the preventive therapies that seem to reduce this occurrence include adequate hydration for dilution effect, IV administration of sodium 2-mercaptoethanesulfonate (MENSA), and intravesical *N*-acetylcysteine.[37] MENSA is believed to work by inactivating acrolein to an inert thioether.[96]

In the overdose setting, cyclophosphamide can cause dysrhythmias, myocardial necrosis, and death. ECG changes are noted at doses of 120 mg/kg and heart failure and myocarditis at doses greater than 150 mg/kg.[8,153] An error in writing an order led to the death of one patient and irreversible cardiac damage in another from cyclophosphamide overdose. These two patients received 6520 mg of the agent daily for 4 consecutive days, when the amount was to be given over 4 days.[183]

What Are the Manifestations of a Platinoid Agent Overdose?

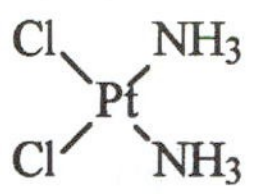

Cisplatin

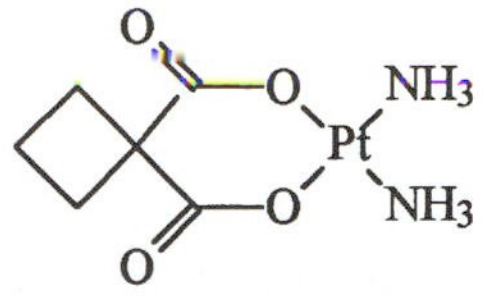

Carboplatin

The cytotoxic effects of the platinum-containing compounds were first recognized in 1965, and since then many types have been derived. The ones of clinical significance are cisplatin, carboplatin, and iproplatin. The latter two were designed to reduce the incidence of nephrotoxicity. Differences in chemical structure exist among these agents as well. Most notably, cisplatin is an inorganic and carboplatin an organic compound. When these agents enter an environment with a low chloride concentration (eg, intracellular), they are activated by hydrolysis and promote intra and interstrand crosslinks with DNA molecules.[180] The more common manifestations of toxicity with cisplatin during therapy are renal dysfunction, auditory impairment, and peripheral neuropathy. Myelosuppression is a dose-limiting factor for carboplatin and iproplatin. At a carboplatin dose of 800 mg/m^2, 25% of patients will develop marrow toxicity.[165] The marrow effects are delayed, with nadir occurring 3 to 5 weeks after the start of therapy. Thrombocytopenia can be life threatening. Patients developing an anemia within the first week of cisplatin therapy should be evaluated for hemolytic anemia.[46]

The sources of error associated with cisplatin overdoses are frequency of administration (total dose versus over a period of time), mistaking it for carboplatin, and writing the wrong dose.[170] Manifestations in the overdose setting involve neurologic, visual, hearing, bone marrow, and renal disorders. The most common renal disorder is renal failure, which is dose-related and begins at 50 mg/m^2. The result is irreversible distal tubular necrosis.[182,189] Cell death may be from intracellular glutathione depletion.[53,57,82] The presence of urinary alanine aminopeptidase and *N*-acetyl-beta-D-glucosamidase may be used as early indicators of renal tubular damage.[53,57,82] At doses greater than 200 mg/m^2, the development of seizures, encephalopathy, and peripheral neuropathy are of concern.[22,47,93,165,167] The pathology is axonal degeneration, which is similar to that of other heavy metals. At this dose, visual impairment may occur within the first week of exposure.[45,146,227] This can include temporary visual loss with permanent loss of color discrimination. Physical examination of the anterior chamber and fundus of the eye will be normal; however, an electroretinogram will be abnormal with a negative-type response. High-frequency hearing loss is evident 2 to 3 days after exposure to doses greater than 500 mg/m^2.[43]

What Is the Management of a Patient With Platinoid Overdose?

Renal protection and enhanced elimination of platinum are the two primary goals in the management of a cisplatin overdose. Expectant management for myelosuppression and neurotoxicity can follow. Chloride diuresis both promotes the inactive anionic state of cisplatin and decreases the urine platinum concentration to limit nephrotoxicity during therapy.[6,219] Hydration with 0.9% NaCl and an osmotic diuretic (eg, mannitol) should be administered to achieve a high urine output (eg, 1 to 3 mL/kg per hour) for 6 to 24 hours postexposure. In the setting of nonoliguric renal failure, careful hydration is recommended to maintain urinary output, because platinum renal excretion is directly related to urinary flow and independent of creatinine clearance.[45] Aside from the serum BUN and creatinine, assessment of renal function can include the glomerular filtration, filtration fraction, and renal plasma flow.[86,150,151,159]

Nephroprotectants found to be effective postexposure are sodium thiosulfate and diethyldithiocarbamate (DDTC). Thiosulfate binds to free platinum to prevent cellular damage. Little or no renal toxicity was seen in patients receiving up to 270 mg/m^2 of cisplatin when thiosulfate was given as an IV bolus of 4 g/m^2 with an infusion of 12 g/m^2 over 6 hours.[92,168] Thiosulfate may offer the additional benefit of limiting neurotoxicity.[145] DDTC affects platinum binding after coupling to protein adducts and can enhance biliary excretion by 30-fold. Clinical trials with DDTC (4 g/m^2) as a 1.5 to 3.5-hour infusion, 45 minutes after cisplatin, limited renal toxicity.[55] Disulfiram is metabolized to DDTC and may be used if DDTC is not readily available. Disulfiram was shown to be nephroprotectant when administered as 75 or 150 mg/m^2 over 90 minutes, 30 minutes after cisplatin (50 to 120 mg/m^2).[174] The use of thiosulfate and DDTC is limited by the time in which it needs to be administered after exposure (ie, 1 to 2 hours).

Plasmapheresis and hemodialysis have been attempted in patients with cisplatin overdoses and owing to this agent's high protein binding, hemodialysis was found not to be effective.[36] However, in patients with renal failure, dialysis may benefit. Plasmapheresis was performed in 2 adults and there was a fall in blood platinum levels with clinical improvement. The first patient received an overdose of 280 mg/m^2 and was plasmapheresed on day 12 of exposure.[45] After 3 daily treatments, the serum platinum level decreased from 2900 to 200 ng/mL and the patient had noticable improvement in gastrointestinal and visual symptoms. On day 20, the serum platinum level rebounded to 700 ng/mL and the symptoms worsened. Further plasmapheresis lowered the level to 290 ng/mL by day 27 and symptoms improved. The other patient received 300 mg/m^2 of cisplatin and received 4 daily treatments of plasmapheresis starting on day 6 postexposure.[118] The plasma platinum level declined from 2979 to 430 ng/mL and the patient became more awake and less nauseous. On day 11, platinum levels rebounded to 834 ng/mL and fell to 279 ng/mL upon reinstitution of plasmapheresis. The amount of platinum removed by three trials was 4622 μg. The author of the paper contends that plasmapheresis prevented the need for hemodialysis for renal failure. Thus, plasmapheresis appears to be effective in cisplatin overdose and should be instituted immediately after exposure. Patients who remain symptomatic days later may benefit as well.

How Should a Patient With an Intrathecal Overdose Be Managed?

Intrathecal (IT) overdoses with vincristine, methotrexate, doxorubicin, and daunorubicin are reported in the literature. Common sources of error are confusing the IV for the IT agent and misidentifying the strength of the solution vial in the preparation of the medication. These events are stressful because of the disastrous consequences they bring and the immediacy with which the agent must be removed from the thecal space. Removal of as much of the agent as possible is the patient's only chance of having an acceptable prognosis.

Upon recognition of the occurrence, the patient needs to be placed in a gravity-dependent position to prevent upward flow of the agent towards the cisterna magnum. The upright position significantly delays the flow of an intralumbar administered agent to the cerebral ventricles when compared to lying flat or being in the Trendelenberg position.[65] The lumbar puncture site needs to be maintained or reestablished so that as much of the CSF can be drained as possible. With an IT MTX model, if 20 mL of CSF were removed within 30 minutes of administration, 94% of the agent given was retrieved.[3] However, by removing the same volume at 3 hours, only 10% of the agent was recovered. Cerebrospinal fluid drainage can be accomplished in short time intervals while considering CSF production is 30 mL/h. CSF exchange should then be accomplished by lavaging the intrathecal space with lactated Ringer's solution. An equal volume of the CSF space should be used in each pass, and two to three passes should be performed. The volume of CSF in a child older than 3 years approaches that of an adult (ie, 120 mL). For large and significant exposures, CSF perfusion must follow. This is performed by passing solution through a ventriculostomy and out a lumbar drainage catheter. Lactated Ringer's with 15 to 25 mL of fresh frozen plasma added per liter of crystalloid is infused at 150 mL/h for 18 to 24 hours.[64,232] The ventriculostomy and lumbar drain can then be removed. The thecal effluent can be collected to determine the amount of agent recovered. Depending on the antineoplastic agent involved, additional measures may be necessary.

Vincristine IT overdoses are devastating because of the 13 patients reported in the literature, only 2 survived.[64,232] There is no indication for the intrathecal administration of vincristine or vinblastine. This mishap is usually the result of confusing vincristine with the other medications (eg, cytarabine, MTX) that are commonly dispensed for intrathecal use. Death follows a characteristic course, consisting of back pain, meningismus, lower limb weakness, urinary difficulty, loss of deep tendon reflexes, encephalopathy, and then respiratory failure. Alteration in mental status appeared earlier when VCR was administered intraventricularly.[149] Pathologic changes are most notable in the cerebellum, brainstem, and the anterior horns of the spinal cord.[13] There are only two reported survivors from IT VCR, and is believed that their success was because CSF evacuation of the agent was instituted within minutes as described above.[64,232] The amount of VCR recovered in one case was 95% of the 2 mg VCR that had been administered.[64] Additional therapies provided in these cases were glutamic acid (10 g IV over 24 hours, then 500 mg po tid),[109] folinic acid (25 mg IV every 6 hours) and pyridoxine (50 mg IV every 8 hours). These agents were continued for 1 week or until the neurologic symptoms stabilized. Dexamethasone (4 mg/m^2 IV every 6 hours) may be given for meningeal inflammation. The role for these agents is unclear, but because of the seriousness of the situation, aggressive therapy should be offered.

Intrathecal overdoses of MTX commonly occur because a more concentrated solution vial is mistaken for one that is less concentrated.[202] Overdoses reported in the literature range as high as 650 mg—death is associated with amounts greater than 500 mg.[202] The therapeutic intralumbar MTX dose according to age is as follows: 6 mg for a patient less than 1 year old, 8 mg for between the ages of 1 and 2 years, 10 mg for between the ages of 2 and 3 years, and 12 mg for greater than 3 years of age.[29] The neurotoxicity associated with these events includes chemical arachnoiditis, ascending neuropathy, encephalopathy, and seizures. The most common form of toxicity is chemical arachnoiditis, which is associated with the acute onset of fever, back pain, dizziness, neck stiffness, vomiting, and headaches that can last for hours.[98] The cerebrospinal fluid in these cases demonstrated elevated intracranial pressure, pleocytosis, and elevated protein levels.

Unlike IT VCR overdoses, the prognosis for a IT MTX exposure is more favorable because of the agent's different mechanism of action and the availability of rescue therapy. Two deaths have been reported with IT MTX overdose and they received amounts greater than 500 mg.[69,202] CSF removal of MTX is still crucial, and for amounts less than 100 mg CSF, drainage may be adequate if performed within 30 to 60 minutes of administration.[114,162] When a longer period of time has elapsed, or a larger amount is involved, CSF exchange is necessary, and possibly CSF perfusion as well. At amounts greater than 500 mg, CSF perfusion must follow because drainage and exchange cannot remove enough MTX to prevent significant toxicity. CSF decontamination should continue until the final MTX concentration is about 100 μmol, which is a peak therapeutic level for a 12 mg IT MTX dose.[162] Large amounts of MTX administered IT will pass into the systemic circulation, which poses a threat to the bone marrow. Although there are no reports of myelosuppression resulting from such an event, IV leucovorin is indicated. High-dose leucovorin rescue is to be started upon recognition of the overdose. The following IV regimen was used in a patient who received 600 mg and survived: 1000 mg/m^2, followed by 100 mg/m^2 every 3 hours until the plasma MTX was less than 0.1 μmol.[162] Leucovorin is not to be administered IT because seizures with resultant death can occur, and the etiology of MTX-induced neurotoxicity is chemical irritation, not folate inhibition.[114] Additional therapies are hydration and urinary alkalinization to prevent renal toxicity, and IV dexamethasone to lessen meningeal inflammation. Enzymatic agents that inactivate MTX are a new and promising form of rescue therapy for IT overdoses. Carboxypeptidase G2 was shown to dramatically shorten the MTX CSF half-life in a patient with a 600 mg IT overdose.[162] The patient received the carboxypeptidase agent IT, following CSF decontamination, and survived. Information regarding the availability of carboxypeptidase G-class agents can be obtained from the Cancer Therapy Evaluation Program at the National Cancer Institute (telephone 301/496-5725). Enzymatic cleavage may obviate the future need for CSF perfusion in large overdoses.

What Should Be Done When Extravasations Occur?

Extravasational injuries are one of the most consequential local toxic events. Another is arterial vasospasm resulting in limb ischemia. When an antineoplastic agent leaks from the blood vessel into the surrounding tissue, significant necrosis of skin, muscles, and tendons can occur with resultant loss of function. The initial manifestations may include swelling, pain, and a burning sensation that can last for hours. Days later, the area becomes erythematous and indurated and can either resolve or proceed to ulceration and necrosis.[184] Sometimes, these early findings may be difficult to distinguish from other forms of local drug toxicity, such as irritation and hypersensitivity. Local irritation may be due to either the agent or its vehicle (ethanol, propylene glycol). The agents associated with local irritation include fluorouracil, carmustine, bisantrene, cisplatin, and dacarbazine. The local irritation and hypersensitivity manifestations are self-limiting and typified by an immediate onset of a burning sensation, pruritis, erythema, and a flare reaction of the vein in which the agent is being infused. Pretreatment with an antihistamine will usually prevent some of the hypersensitivity manifestations upon subsequent administrations.[218] Agents reported to cause hypersensitivity reactions include daunorubicin, doxorubicin, idarubicin, and mitoxantrone. This event is typified by the presence of pruritis. Nevertheless, when local reactions cannot be differentiated, it is always best to presume extravasation and manage the situation accordingly.

The occurrence of these inadvertent events appears to be about 50 times more frequent in the hands of the inexperienced clinician.[101] There are several factors that have been associated with extravasational injuries. They include (1) patients with poor vessel integrity and blood flow, such as the elderly, those who have undergone numerous venipunctures, and radiation therapy to the site; (2) limited venous and lymphatic drainage due to either obstruction or surgical resection; and (3) use of sites over joints, which increases the risk of dislodgments due to movement.[102,184] The factors that are associated with a poor outcome include (1) areas of the body with little subcutaneous tissue, such as the dorsum of the hand, volar surface of the wrist, and antecubital fossa, where healing is poor and vital structures are more likely to be involved; (2) concentration of extravasant; (3) increased volume and duration of contact with tissue; and (4) the type of agent.[184,185] The vesicant agents appear to result in more significant local tissue destruction. These include doxorubicin, daunorubicin, dactinomycin, epirubicin, idarubicin, mechlorethamine, mitomycin, and the vinca alkaloids. The anthracycline antibiotics are associated with a higher incidence of significant injuries and delayed healing, which may be due to their slow release from bound tissue into surrounding viable tissue. Doxorubicin extravasation is associated with local tissue necrosis in approximately 25% of cases. The best form of therapy for these injuries is one of prevention. Specialized nursing care and the use of indwelling central venous catheters have limited the extent of these injuries.

Management

The treatment for extravasational injuries is somewhat controversial; varying from conservative care to early surgical debridement and the use of selective antidotes.[191] This uncertainty is because of the limited number of clinical cases available for study, and the discordance between animal studies and clinical findings. However, there are some recommended general management guidelines for an extravasation (Table 47–3).[23,31]

Once extravasation of an agent is suspected, the infusion should be immediately halted. A physician should be notified and the agent, its concentration, and the approximate amount infused be noted. The venous access should be maintained so that aspiration of as much of the infusate can be performed and antidote can be administered, if indicated. Injection of normal saline into the catheter to dilute the extravasant may be beneficial.[191] The intermittent local application of ice (20 minutes four times a day) and elevation of the extremity should be done for 24 to 48 hours, so as to limit further progression of the agent. Cooling the area is believed to prevent cell injury by reducing the amount of drug absorbed by the tissue and lowering the cellular metabolic rate. It was demonstrated that with just cold application and strict elevation, only 11% of 119 patients required surgical intervention for their injuries.[126] In the past, heat was recommended to disperse the agent, but investigations with mice demonstrated that this practice increases the area of skin ulceration.[61,126] However, dry warm compresses are

TABLE 47–3. MANAGEMENT OF EXTRAVASATIONAL INJURIES

Agent	Therapy	Mechanism
Anthracyclines Doxorubicin Daunorubicin Dactinomycin Epirubicin Idarubicin	Dimethyl sulfoxide—Applied topically and allowed to dry. Every 6 to 8 hours for 3 to 10 days Cool compresses	Free radical scavenger Localizes area of involvement
Mechlorethamine	Sodium thiosulfate—Prepare a sterile 0.17-mol solution by mixing 4 mL thiosulfate 10% weight/volume with 6 mL water for injection. Infiltrate the site of extravasation	Inhibits tissue alkylation
Mitomycin	DMSO	
Vinca alkaloids and epipodophyllotoxins	Hyaluronidase—Reconstitute with normal saline (15 U/mL) and inject, intradermally or subcutaneously, 150 to 900 U into the site	Degrades hyaluronic acid to enhance systemic absorption
	Dry warm compresses only	To promote systemic absorption

Adapted, with permission, from Bertelli G: Prevention and management of extravasation of cytotoxic drugs. Drug Saf 1995;12:245–255.

still recommended for the vinca alkaloids and etoposide to promote systemic uptake.[23] This is combined with the local infiltration with hyaluronidase to enhance absorption. The wound should be observed closely for the first 7 days, and a surgeon consulted if either pain persists or evidence of ulceration appears.[184] However, in severe extravasations—where there is a high incidence of necrosis due to the type of drug (doxorubicin), the volume or concentration, and any area where there may be significant long-term morbidity (over joints)—early surgical consultation would be warranted. If tissue ulceration occurs, initial management can be with antiseptic dressings. After the area of necrotic skin has evolved to the point where it can be clearly delineated from surviving tissue, surgical debridement may be beneficial to limit secondary infection. The use of intravenous fluorescein can aid in identifying viable tissue.[10]

Antidotal therapy should be considered when the extravasant is known to respond poorly to conservative care. The vesicant type agents are associated with a significantly worse outcome, and when the exposure is large, a more aggressive approach should be initiated. Otherwise, conservative management may be the accepted form of care. The specific antidotal treatments can be divided into several categories based upon their mechanism of action, one of which is the reduction of the inflammatory response through the application of steroids. Hydrocortisone has been used in varying concentrations (50 to 200 mg) as either subcutaneous or intradermal injections for doxorubicin and the vinca alkaloids.[16,101,127,215] Steroids may have only a limited role in doxorubicin-induced lesions because inflammatory cells are not found in predominance at the wound site.[25] The addition of steroids to doxorubicin infusions, so as to limit morbidity if extravasation should occur, is not recommended because the drugs are chemically incompatible.[214] Another approach is to inactivate the agents by affecting the pH of the environment. The administration of 5 mL of 8.4% sodium bicarbonate through the same IV line has been advocated to decrease the DNA binding of doxorubicin.[17] The use of bicarbonate should be cautioned because its hyperosmolarity can cause tissue necrosis.[79] Sodium thiosulfate is recommended for mechlorethamine extravasations, and is believed to work by inactivating the agent by reacting with the active ethylenimmonium ring.[102,163] The site is infiltrated with sterile sodium thiosulfate solution and then ice compresses are applied intermittently for 6 to 12 hours.[23] Finally, there are agents, like dimethyl sulfoxide (DMSO), that scavenge the free radicals that are believed to cause tissue damage from doxorubicin. Dimethyl sulfoxide is beneficial for anthracycline extravasations in both animal and human clinical trials.[56,127,161,163,208] The concentration of DMSO used ranged from 55 to 99% and was applied topically.[127,160] Some of the other beneficial properties of DMSO include its antiinflammatory, analgesic, and vasodilatory effects. In conclusion, although the overall incidence of extravasations with antineoplastic agents is small, the associated morbidity from any one event may be significant. The best form of therapy is one of prevention.

References

1. Abelson HT: Methotrexate and central nervous system toxicity. Cancer Treat Rep 1978;62:1999–2001.
2. Abelson HT, Fosburg MT, Beardsley P, et al: Methotrexate induced renal impairment: Clinical studies and rescue from systemic toxicity with high dose leucovorin and thymidine. J Clin Oncol 1983;1:208–216.
3. Addiego JE, Ridgway D, Bleyer WA: The acute management of intrathecal methotrexate overdose: Pharmacologic rationale and guidelines. J Pediatr 1981;98:825–828.
4. Alexander J, Dainiak N, Berger HJ, et al: Serial assessment of doxorubicin cardiotoxicity with quantitative radionuclide angiocardiography. N Engl J Med 1979;300:278–283.
5. Allen JC, Rosen G, Mehta BM, Horten B: Leukoencephalopathy following high dose IV methotrexate chemother-

apy with leucovorin rescue. Cancer Treat Rep 1980;64: 1261–1273.
6. Al-Sarraf M, Fletcher W, Oishi N, et al: Cisplatin hydration with and without mannitol diuresis in refractory disseminated malignant melanoma. Cancer Treat Rep 1982; 66:31–35.
7. Ammenti A, Reitter B, Muller-Wiefel DE: Chlorambucil neurotoxicity: Report of two cases. Helvetic Paediatr Acta 1980;35:281–287.
8. Appelbaum FR, Strauchen JA, Gram RG: Acute lethal carditis caused by high-dose combination chemotherapy. Lancet 1976;31:58–62.
9. Arena E, D'Alessandro N, Dusonchet L, et al: Influence of pharmacokinetic variations on the pharmacologic properties of adriamycin. In: Carter SK, DiMarco A, Ghione M, Krakoff IH, et al (eds): International Symposium on Adriamycin. Berlin, Springer-Verlag, 1972, pp. 96–116.
10. Argenta LC, Manders EK: Mitomycin C extravasation injuries. Cancer 1983;51:1080–1082.
11. Armstrong JG, Dyke RW, Forts PJ, et al: Hodgkin's disease, carcinoma of the breast, and other tumors treated with vinblastine sulfate. Cancer Chemother Rep 1962;18: 49–51.
12. Atherton LD, Leib ES, Kaye MD: Toxic megacolon associated with methotrexate therapy. Gastroenterology 1984; 86:1583–1585.
13. Bain PG, Lantos PL, Djurovic V, West I: Intrathecal vincristine: A fatal chemotherapeutic error with devastating central nervous system effects. J Neurol 1991;238:230–234.
14. Balfour HH, Bean B, Laskin OL, et al: Acyclovir halts progression of herpes zoster in immunocompromised patients. N Engl J Med 1983;308:1448–1453.
15. Barak AJ, Tuma DJ, Beckenhauer HC: Methotrexate hepatotoxicity. J Am Coll Nutr 1984;3:93–96.
16. Barlock AL. Howsen DM, Hubbard SM: Nursing management of adriamycin extravasation. Am J Nurs 1979;79: 94–96.
17. Bartowski-Dodds L, Daniels JR: Use of sodium bicarbonate as a means of ameliorating doxorubicin induced dermal necrosis in rats. Cancer Chemother Pharmacol 1980;4: 179–181.
18. Baselt RC: Disposition of Toxic Drugs and Chemicals in Man. Davis, CA, Biomedical Publications, 1982.
19. Beer M, Cavalli F, Martz G: Vincristine overdose: Treatment with and without leucovorin rescue. Cancer Treat Rep 1983;67:746–747.
20. Benjamin RS, Wiernik PH, Bachur NR: Adriamycin chemotherapy—Efficacy, safety, and pharmacologic basis of an intermittent single high-dosage schedule. Cancer 1974;33:19–27.
21. Berenson MP: Recovery after inadvertent massive overdosage of vincristine. Cancer Chemother Rep 1971;55: 525–526.
22. Berman IF, Mann MP: Seizures and transient cortical blindness associated with cisplatinum diamminedichloride therapy in a thirty year old man. Cancer 1980;45: 764–766.
23. Bertelli G: Prevention and management of extravasation of cytotoxic drugs. Drug Saf 1995;12:245–255.
24. Bertino JR, Condos S, Horvath C, et al: Immobilized carboxypeptidase G1 in methotrexate removal. Cancer Res 1978;38:1936–1941.
25. Bhawan J, Petry J, Pybak ME: Histologic changes induced in skin by extravasation of doxorubicin. J Cutan Pathol 1989;16:158–163.
26. Billingham ME, Mason GW, Bristow MT, Daniels JR:Anthracycline cardiomyopathy monitored by morphologic changes. Cancer Treat Rep 1978;62:865–872.
27. Blank DQ, Nanji AA, Schreiber DH: Acute renal failure and seizures associated with chlorambucil overdose. J Toxicol Clin Toxicol 1983; 20:361–365.
28. Bleyer WA: New vistas for leucovorin in cancer chemotherapy. Cancer 1989; 63:995–1007.
29. Bleyer WA: The clinical pharmacology of methotrexate. Cancer 1978;41:36–51.
30. Bleyer WA, Frisby SA, Oliverio VT: Uptake and binding of vincristine by murine leukemia cells. Biochem Pharmacol 1975; 24:633–639.
31. Boyle D, Engelking C: Vesicant extravasation: Myths and realities. Oncol Nurs Forum 1995; 22:57–67.
32. Bradley WG, Lassman LP, Pearce GW, Walton JN: The neuromyopathy of vincristine in man: Clinical electrophysiological and pathological studies. J Neurol Sci 1970;10:107–131.
33. Brady ST: Basic properties of fast axonal transport and the role of fast axonal transport in axonal growth. In: Elam JS, ed: Axonal Transport in Neuronal Growth and Regeneration. New York, Plenum, 1984, pp.13–27.
34. Bristow MR: Toxic cardiomyopathy due to doxorubicin. Hosp Pract 1982;17:101–111.
35. Bristow MR, Minobe WA, Billingham BE, et al: Anthracycline associated cardiac and renal damage in rabbits. Lab Invest 1981;45:1579–1681.
36. Brivet F, Pavlovitch JM, Gouyette A, et al: Inefficiency of early prophylactic hemodialysis in cis-platinum overdose. Cancer Chemother Pharmacol 1986;18:183–184.
37. Brock N, Pohl J: Prevention of urotoxic side effects by regional detoxification with increased selectivity of oxazophosphorine cytostatics. IARC Sci Publ 1986;78: 269–279.
38. Brock N, Stekar J, Pohl J, et al: Acrolein, the causative factor of nontoxic side effects of cyclophosphamide, ifosfamide, trofosfamide and sufosfamide. Arzneimittelforschung 1979;29:659–661.
39. Byrne TN, Moseley TA, Finer MA: Myoclonic seizures following chlorambucil overdose. Ann Neurol 1981;9: 191–194.
40. Calabresi P, Chabner BA: Antineoplastic agents. In: Gilman AG, Rall TW, Nies AS, Taylor P, eds: The Pharmacological Basis of Therapeutics. New York, McGraw-Hill, 1990, p. 1238.
41. Chabner BA, Allegre CG, Curt GA, et al: Polyglutamation of methotrexate. Is methotrexate a pro-drug? J Clin Invest 1985;76:907–912.
42. Chia HM, Kalra L, Lakhani AK: Filgrastim for low-dose captopril-induced agranulocytosis. Lancet 1993;342:304.
43. Chiuten D, Vogl SE, Kaplan BH, Greenwald R: Is there a cumulative or delayed toxicity from cis-diamminedichloroplatinum? Proc Am Assoc Cancer Res 1981;22: 163–164.

44. Cho ED, Lowndes HE, Goldstein BD: Neurotoxicology of vincristine in the cat. Arch Toxicol 1983;52:83–90.
45. Chu G, Mantin R, Shen YM: Massive cisplatin overdose by accidental substitution for carboplatin. Cancer 1993;73: 3707–3714.
46. Cinollo G, Dini G, Lanino E, et al: Positive direct antiglobulin test in a pediatric patient following high dose cisplatin. Cancer Chemother Pharmacol 1988;21: 85–86.
47. Cohen RJ, Cuneo RA: Transient left homonymous hemianopsia and encephalopathy following treatment of testicular carcinoma with cisplatin, vinblastine and bleomycin. J Clin Oncol 1983;1:392–393.
48. Cox PJ: Cyclophosphamide cystitis—Identification of acrolein as the causative agent. Biochem Pharmacol 1979; 28:2045–2049.
49. Creasey WA, Bensch KB, Malawista SE: Colchicine, vinblastine and griseofulvin pharmacological studies with human leukocytes. Biochem Pharmacol 1971;20:1579–1588.
50. Cunningham J, Sharman BL, Goodwin FJ, et al: Do patients receiving hemodialysis need folic acid supplements? Br Med J 1981;282:1582–1585.
51. Curran CF: Acute doxorubicin overdoses. Ann Intern Med 1991;115:913. Letter.
52. Cutts HJ: Effects of other agents on the biologic responses to vincaleukoblastine. Biochem Pharmacol 1964;13: 421–430.
53. Daugaard G, Abildgarrd U, Holstein-Rathlou N, et al: Renal tubular function in patients treated with high-dose cisplatin. Clin Pharmacol Ther 1988;44:164–172.
54. Deconti RC, Creasey WA: Clinical aspects of the dimeric Cantharanthus alkaloids. In Taylor WI, Farnsworth NR, eds: The Cantharanthus Alkaloids: Botany, Chemistry, Pharmacology and Clinical Use. New York, Dekker, 1975, pp. 237–278.
55. De Gregorio MW, Gandara DR, Hollerman WM, et al: High-dose cisplatin with diethyldithiocarbamate (DDTC) rescue therapy: Preliminary pharmacologic observations. Cancer Chemother Pharmacol 1989;23:276–278.
56. Desao MH, Teres D: Prevention of doxorubicin induced skin ulcers in the rat and pig with dimethyl sulfoxide. Cancer Treat Rep 1982;66:1371–1374.
57. Diener U, Knoll E, Langer G, et al: Urinary excretion of *N*-acetyl-beta-D-glucosaminidase and alanine aminopeptidase in patients receiving amikacin or cisplatin. Clin Chim Acta 1981;112:149–157.
58. Djerassi I, Ciesielka W, Kim JS: Removal of methotrexate by filtration adsorption using charcoal filters or by hemodialysis. Cancer Treat Rep 1977;61:751–752.
59. Doolittle GC, Simpson KM, Lindsley HB: Methotrexate associated, early onset pancytopenia in rheumatoid arthritis. Arch Intern Med 1989;149:1430–1431.
60. Doroshow JH, Locker GY, Myers CE: The enzymatic defenses of the heart against reactive oxygen metabolites. J Clin Invest 1980;65:128–135.
61. Dorr RT, Alberts DS, Stone A: Cold protection and heat enhancement of doxorubicin skin toxicity in the mouse. Cancer Treat Rep 1985;69:431–437.
62. Dorr RT, Fritz WL: Cancer Chemotherapy Handbook. New York, Elsevier, 1980, pp. 677–684.
63. Dustin P: Micorotubule poisons. In: Justin P, ed: Microtubules. Berlin, Springer-Verlag, 1984, pp. 167–225.
64. Dyke RW: Vincristine must not be administered intrathecally. JAMA 1982;248:171. Letter.
65. Echelberger CK, Ricccardi R, Bleyer A, et al: Influence of body position on ventricular cerebrospinal fluid methotrexate concentration following intralumbar administration. Proc Am Assoc Cancer Res Am Soc Clin Oncol, March 1981, p. 365. Abstract C-131.
66. Enck RE, Bennett JM: Inadvertent chlorambucil overdose in adult. NY State J Med 1977;77:1480–1485.
67. Ensminger WD, Frei E: The prevention of methotrexate toxicity thymidine infusions in humans. Cancer Res 1977; 37:1857–1863.
68. Erttmann R, Landbeck G: Effect of oral cholestyramine on the elimination of high dose methotrexate. J Cancer Res Clin Oncol 1985;110:48–50.
69. Ettinger LJ: Pharmacokinetics and biochemical effects of a fatal intrathecal methotrexate overdose. Cancer 1982;50: 444–450.
70. Evans WE, Pratt CB, Taylor RH, et al: Pharmacokinetic monitoring of high dose methotrexate: Early recognition of high risk patients. Cancer Chemother Pharmacol 1979; 3:161–166.
71. Fantine EO, Garnier-Suillerot G: Interaction of 5-amino daunorubicin with Fe II and with cardiolipin-containing vesicles. Biochim Biophys Acta 1986;856:130–136.
72. Favier M, de Carzanove F, Saint-Martin F, et al: Preventing medication errors in antineoplastic therapy. Am J Hosp Pharm 1984;51:832–833. Letter.
73. Firlit CF: Intractable hemorrhagic cystitis secondary to extensive carcinomatosis: Management with formalin solution. J Urol 1973;110:57–58.
74. Fleischman RA: Clinical use of hematopoietic growth factors. Am J Med Sci 1993;11:248–273.
75. Fox RM: Methotrexate nephrotoxicity. Clin Exp Pharmacol Physiol 1977;5:43–45.
76. Gadgil SD, Damle SR, Advani SH, Vaidya AB: Effect of activated charcoal on the pharmacokinetics of high dose methotrexate. Cancer Treat Rep 1982;66:1169–1171.
77. Garbrecht M, Mullerlie U: Verapamil in the prevention of adriamycin-induced cardiomyopathy. Klin Wochenschr 1986;64:132–134.
78. Garnier-Suillerot A: Metal anthracycline and anthracene dione complexes as a new class of anticancer agents. In: Lown JW, ed: Anthracycline and Anthracenedione-Based Anticancer Agents. Amsterdam, Elsevier, 1988, pp. 129–157.
79. Gaze NR: Tissue necrosis caused by commonly used intravenous infusions. Lancet 1978;2:417–419.
80. Gibson TP, Reisch SD, Krumlousky FA, et al: Hemoperfusion for methotrexate removal. Clin Pharmacol Ther 1978;23:351–355.
81. Goldie JH, Price LA, Harrap KR: Methotrexate toxicity: Correlation with duration of administration, plasma levels, dose and excretion pattern. Eur J Cancer 1072;8: 409–414.
82. Goren MP, Wright RK, Horowitz ME: Cumulative renal tubular damage associated with cisplatin nephrotoxicity. Cancer Chemother Pharmacol 1986;18:69–73.

83. Goren MP, Wright RK, Pratt CP, Pell FE: Dechlorethylation of ifosfamide and neurotoxicity. Lancet 1986;2: 1219–1220.
84. Green LS, Donoso JA, Heller-Bettinger IE, Samson FE: Axonal transport of disturbances in vincristine-induced peripheral neuropathy. Ann Neurol 1977;12:255–262.
85. Grimes DJ, Bowles MR, Buttsworth JA, et al: Survival after unexpected high serum methotrexate concentrations in a patient with osteogenic sarcoma. Drug Saf 1990;5:447–454.
86. Groth S, Nielsen H, Sorensen JB, et al: Acute and long-term nephrotoxicity of cisplatinum in man. Cancer Chemother Pharmacol 1986;17:191–196.
87. Grush OC, Morgan SK: Folinic acid rescue for vincristine toxicity. Clin Toxicol 1979;14:71–78.
88. Hachimi-Idrissi S, Schots R, DeWolf D, et al: Reversible cardiopathy after accidental overdose of mitoxantrone. Pediatr Hematol Oncol 1993;10:35–40.
89. Hamel E, Lin CM: Glutamate induced polymerization of tubulin: Characteristics of the reaction and application to the large scale purification of tubulin. Arch Biochem Biophys 1981;209:29–40.
90. Hande KR, Balow JE, Drake JC, et al: Methotrexate and hemodialysis. Ann Intern Med 1977;87:495–596.
91. Herman EH, Matre RM, Lee IP, et al: A comparison of the cardiovascular actions of daunomycin, adriamycin and *N*-acetyl-daunomycin in hamsters and monkeys. Pharmacology 1971;6:230–241.
92. Hirosawa A, Niitani H, Hayashibara K, Tsuboi E: Effects of sodium thiosulfate in combination therapy of cis-dichlorodiammineplatinum and vindesine. Cancer Chemother Pharmacol 1989;23:255–258.
93. Hitchings RN, Thompson DB: Encephalopathy following cisplatin, bleomycin and vinblastine therapy for non-seminomatous germ cell tumor of testis. Aust NZ J Med 1988;18:67–68.
94. Holland JF: Vincristine treatment of advanced cancer: A cooperative study of 392 cases. Cancer Res 1973;33: 1258–1265.
95. Holstein P, Jacobsen K, Pedersen JF, Sorensen JS: Intravesical hydrostatic pressure treatment: New method for control of bleeding from the bladder mucosa. J Urol 1973; 109:234–236.
96. Hows JM, Mehta AM, Ward L, et al: Comparison of MENSA with forced diuresis to prevent cyclophosphamide induced hemorrhage cystitis in marrow transplantation: A prospective randomized study. Br J Cancer 1984;50:753–756.
97. Huang KC, Wenczak BA, Liu YK: Renal tubular transport of methotrexate in the rhesus monkey and dog. Cancer Res 1979;39:4843–4848.
98. Hughes PJ, Lane RJM: Acute cerebral edema induced by methotrexate. Br Med J 1989;289:1315.
99. Hunter R, Barnes J, Oakeley JF, Mattews DM: Toxicity of folic acid given in pharmacological doses to healthy volunteers. Lancet 1970;1:61–63.
100. Hurwitz RL, Mahoney DH, Armstrong DL, Browder TM: Reversible encephalopathy and seizures as a result of conventional vincristine administration. Med Pediatr Oncol 1988;16:216–219.
101. Ignoffo RJ: Neoplastic disorders. In: Young LY, Koda Kimble MA, eds: Applied Therapeutics: The Clinical Use of Drugs. Vancouver, Applied Therapeutics, 1988, pp. 1197–1201.
102. Ignoffo RJ, Friedman MA: Therapy of local toxicities caused by extravasation of cancer chemotherapeutic drugs. Cancer Treat Rev 1980;7:17–27.
103. Isacoff WH: Effects of extracorporeal charcoal hemoperfusion on plasma methotrexate. Proc Am Assoc Cancer Res 1977;18:145. Abstract.
104. Iven H, Brasch H: The effects of antibiotics and uricosuric drugs on the renal elimination of methotrexate and 7-hydroxy methotrexate in rabbits. Cancer Chemother Pharmacol 1988;21:337–342.
105. Jackson DV, McMahan RA, Pope EK, et al: Clinical trial of folinic acid to reduce vincristine neurotoxicity. Cancer Chemother Pharmacol 1986;17:281–284.
106. Jackson DV, Pope EK, McMahan RA, et al: Clinical trial of pyridoxine to reduce vincristine neurotoxicity. J Neurol Oncol 1986;4:37–41.
107. Jackson DV, Pope EK, Case LD, et al: Improved tolerance of vincristine by glutamic acid. A preliminary report. J Neurooncol 1984;2:219–222.
108. Jackson DV, Rosenbaum DL, Carlisle LJ, et al: Glutamic acid modification of vincristine toxicity. Cancer Biochem Biophys 1984;7:245–252.
109. Jackson DV, Wells HB, Atkins JN, et al: Amelioration of vincristine neurotoxicity by glutamic acid. Am J Med 1988;84:1016–1022.
110. Jackson RC: Biological effects of folic acid antagonists with antineoplastic activity. Pharmacol Ther 1984;25:61–82.
111. Jackson RC, Grindey GB: The biochemical basis for methotrexate cytotoxicity. In: Sirotnak FM, ed: Folate Antagonists as Therapeutic Agents, Vol. 1. Orlando, Florida, Academic Press, 1984, pp. 289–315.
112. Jacobs SA, Stoller RG, Chabner BA, Johns DG: 7 Hydroxy methotrexate as a urinary metabolite in human subjects and rhesus monkeys receiving high dose methotrexate. J Clin Invest 1978;57:534–538.
113. Jaffe N, Takaue Y, Anzai T, Robertson RR: Transient neurologic disturbances induced by high-dose methotrexate treatment. Cancer 1985;56:1356–1360.
114. Jardine LF, Ingram LC, Bleyer WA: Intrathecal leucovorin after intrathecal methotrexate overdose. J Pediatr Hematol Oncol 1996;18:302–304.
115. Johnson FL, Bernstein ID, Hartman JR: Seizures associated with vincristine sulfate therapy. J Pediatr 1973;82:699–702.
116. Johnson IS, Wright HF, Svoboda GH, et al: Antitumor principles derived from vinca rosea linn, I. Vincaleukoblastine and leurosine. Cancer Res 1960;20:1016–1022.
117. Jones G, Mierins E, Karsh J: Methotrexate induced asthma. Am Rev Respir Dis 1991;143:179–181.
118. Jung HK, Lee J, Lee SN: A case of massive cisplatin overdose managed by plasmapheresis. Korean J Intern Med 1995;10:150–154.
119. Kaufman IA, Kung FH, Koenig HM, Giammona ST: Overdosage with vincristine. J Pediatr 1976;89:671–674.
120. Kevat SG, McCarthy PJ, Hill WR, Ahern MJ: Pancytopenia induced by low dose methotrexate for rheumatoid arthritis. Aust NZ J Med 1988;18:697–700.
121. Kinkade JM, Volger WR, Dayton PG: Plasma levels of

methotrexate in cancer patients as studied by an improved spectrophotofluoromitric method. Biochem Med 1974; 10:337–350.

122. Kosmidos HV, Bouhoutsou DO, Varvoutsi MC, et al: Vincristine overdose: Experience with 3 patients. Pediatr Hematol Oncol 1991;8:171–178.
123. Kumar APN, Wrenn EL, Conrad L, et al: Silver nitrate irrigation to control bladder hemorrhage in children receiving cancer therapy. J Urol 1976;166:85–86.
124. Kupfer A, Aeschlimann C, Wermuth B, Cerny T: Prophylaxis and reversal of ifosfamide encephalopathy with methylene-blue. Lancet 1994;26:763–764.
125. Langlsow A: Nursing and the law. Deadly doses of methotrexate. Aust Nurs J 1995;2:32–34.
126. Larson DL: Treatment of tissue extravasation by antitumor agents. Cancer 1982;49:1796–1799.
127. Lawrence HJ, Goodnight SH: Dimethyl sulfoxide and extravasation of anthracycline agents. Ann Intern Med 1983;98:1026. Letter.
128. Leape LL, Bates DW, Culler DJ, et al: Systems analysis of adverse drug events. JAMA 1995;274:35–43.
129. LeFrak EA, Pitha J, Rosentheim S, Gottlieb JA: A clinicopathologic analysis of adriamycin cardiotoxicity. Cancer 1973;32:302–314.
130. Legha SS: Vincristine neurotoxicity, pathophysiology and management. Med Toxicol 1986;1:421–427.
131. Lesar TS, Briceland L, Stein D: Factors related to errors in medication prescribing. JAMA 1997;227:312–317.
132. Lewis JH, Walter JF: Methotrexate-induced pulmonary fibrosis. Arch Dermatol 1979;115:1169–1170.
133. Litovitz T, Bailey KM, Schmitz B: 1990 Annual report of the American Association of Poison Control Centers Toxic Exposure Surveillance System. Am J Emerg Med 1991; 9:461–509.
134. Litovitz T, Clark L, Soloway R: 1993 Annual report of the American Association of Poison Control Centers Toxic Exposure Surveillance System. Am J Emerg Med 1994; 12:546–584.
135. Litovitz T, Felberg L, Soloway R, et al: 1994 Annual report of the American Association of Poison Control Centers Toxic Exposure Surveillance System. Am J Emerg Med 1995;13:551–598.
136. Litovitz T, Felberg L, White S, Klein-Schwartz W: 1995 Annual report of the American Association of Poison Control Centers Toxic Exposure Surveillance System. Am J Emerg Med 1996;14:487–538.
137. Litovitz T, Holm K, Bailey KM, Schmitz F: 1991 Annual report of the American Association of Poison Control Centers Toxic Exposure Surveillance System. Am J Emerg Med 1992;10:452–490.
138. Litovitz T, Holm KC, Clancy C, et al: 1992 Annual report of the American Association of Poison Control Centers Toxic Exposure Surveillance System. Am J Emerg Med 1993;11:494–529.
139. Litovitz T, Schmitz B, Bailey KM: 1989 Annual report of the American Association of Poison Control Centers Toxic Exposure Surveillance System. Am J Emerg Med 1990; 8:394–442.
140. Litovitz T, Schmitz B, Holm K: 1988 Annual report of the American Association of Poison Control Centers Toxic Exposure Surveillance System. Am J Emerg Med 1989;7: 495–521.
141. Litovitz T, Schmitz B, Matyunas N, Martin TG: 1987 Annual report of the American Association of Poison Control Centers Toxic Exposure Surveillance System. Am J Emerg Med 1989;6:479–515.
142. MacKinnon SK, Starkebaum G, Wilkens RF: Pancytopenia associated with low dose pulse methotrexate in the treatment of rheumatoid arthritis. Semin Arthritis Rheum 1985;15:119–126.
143. Maeda K, Ueda M, Ohtaka H, et al: A massive dose of vincristine. Jpn J Clin Oncol 1987;7:247–253.
144. Mandel EM, Lewinski U, Djaldetti M: Vincristine induced myocardial infarction. Cancer 1975; 36:1979–1982.
145. Markman M, Cleary S: High-dose intracavitary cisplatin with intravenous thiosulfate. Low incidence of serious neurotoxicity. Cancer 1985;56:2364–2368.
146. Marmor MF: Negative type electroretinogram from cisplatin toxicity. Doc Ophthalmol 1993;84:237–246.
147. McIntosh S, Davis DL, O'Brian RT, Pearson HA: Methotrexate hepatotoxicity in children with leukemia. J Pediatr 1977;90:1019–1021.
148. Meanwell CA, Blake AE, Kelly KA, et al: Prediction of ifosfamide mesna associated encephalopathy. Eur J Cancer Clin Oncol 1986;22:815–819.
149. Meggs WJ, Hoffman RS: Intraventricular vincristine fatality. J Toxicol Clin Toxicol 1996;34:575. Abstract.
150. Meijer S, Mulder NH, Sleiffer DD, et al: Influence of combination chemotherapy with cis-diamminedichloroplatinum on renal function: Long term effects. Oncology 1983;40:170–173.
151. Meijer S, Sleijfer DT, Mulder NH, et al: Some effects of combination chemotherapy with cisplatinum on renal function in patients with nonseminomatous testicular carcinoma. Cancer 1983;51:2035–2040.
152. Meyer WH, Houghton JA, Houghton PJ: Hypoxanthine: Guanine phosphoribosyltransferase activity in primary human osteosarcomas. A rationale for therapy with methotrexate-thymidine rescue? J Clin Oncol 1987;5:657–661.
153. Mills BA, Roberts RW: Cyclophosphamide-induced cardiomyopathy: A report of two cases and review of the English literature. Cancer 1979;43:2223–2226.
154. Moraska L, Rainisio C, Masera G: Duration of cytotoxicity activity of vincristine in the blood of leukemia in children. Rur J Cancer 1969;5:79–84.
155. Myers CE: Role of iron in anthracycline action. In: Hacker MP, Lazo JS, Tritton TR, eds: Organ Directed Toxicities of Anticancer Drugs. Boston, Marinus Nijhoff, 1988, pp. 17–30.
156. Myers CE, Bonow R, Palmeri S, et al: Prevention of doxorubicin cardiomyopathy by *N*-acetylcysteine. Semin Oncol 1983;10:53–55.
157. Nesbit M, Kririt W, Heyn R, Sharp H: Acute and chronic methotrexate on hepatic, pulmonary, and skeletal systems. Cancer 1976;27:1048–1057.
158. Ochs S, Worth R: Comparison of the block of fast axoplasmic transport in mammalian nerve by vincristine, vinblastine, and desacetyl vinblastine amide sulfate (DVA). Proc Am Assoc Cancer Res 1975;16:70–75.
159. Offerman JJ, Meijer S, Sleijfer DT, Mulder NH, et al: Acute

effects of cis-diamminedichloroplatinum on renal function. Cancer Chemother Pharmacol 1984;12:36–38.

160. Olver IN, Aisner J, Hament A, et al: A prospective study of topical dimethyl sulfoxide for treating anthracycline extravasation. J Clin Oncol 1988;6:1732–1735.
161. Olver IN, Schwartz MA. The use of dimethyl sulfoxide in limiting tissue damage caused by extravasation of doxorubicin. Cancer Treat Rep 1983;67:407–408.
162. O'Marcaigh AS, Johnson MC, Smithson WA, et al: Successful treatment of intrathecal methotrexate overdose by using ventriculolumbar perfusion and intrathecal instillation of carboxypeptidase G2. Mayo Clin Proc 1996;71: 161–165.
163. Owen OE, Dellatorre DL, Van Scott EJ, Cohen MR: Accidental intramuscular injection of mechlorethamine. Cancer 1980;45:2225–2226.
164. Ozols RF, Cunnion RE, Klecker RW, et al: Verapamil and adriamycin in the treatment of drug-resistant ovarian cancer patients. J Clin Oncol 1987;5:641–664.
165. Ozols RF, Ostchega Y, Curt G, Young RC: High dose carboplatin in refractory ovarian cancer patients. J Clin Oncol 1987;5:197–201.
166. Ozols RF, Young RC: High dose cisplatin therapy in ovarian cancer. Semin Oncol 1985;12:21–30.
167. Panici PB, Greggi S, Scambia G, et al: High dose cisplatin induced neurotoxicity in primary advanced ovarian cancer patients. Cancer Treat Rep 1987;71:669–670.
168. Pfeifle CE, Howell SB, Felthouse RD, et al: High dose cisplatin with sodium thiosulfate protection. J Clin Oncol 1985;3:237–244.
169. Pierga JY, Beuzeboc P, Dorval T, et al: Favorable outcome after plasmapheresis for vincristine overdose. Lancet 1992; 640:185. Letter.
170. Pike IM, Arbus MH: Cisplatin overdosage. J Clin Oncol 1992;10:1503–1504. Letter.
171. Pinedo HM, Zaharko DS, Bull JM: The reversal of methotrexate cytotoxicity to mouse bone marrow cells by leucovorin and nucleoside. Cancer Res 1976;336: 4418–4424.
172. Pratt CB, Ransom JL, Evans WE: Age related adriamycin cardiotoxicity in children. Cancer Treat Rep 1978;62: 1381–1385.
173. Pyeritz RE, Droller MJ, Bender WL, Saral R: An approach to the control of massive hemorrhage in cyclophosphamide induced cystitis by intravenous vasopressin: A case report. J Urol 1978;120:253–254.
174. Qazi R, Chang AY, Borch RF, et al: Phase I clinical and pharmacokinetic study of diethyldithiocarbamate as a chemoprotector for toxic effects of cisplatin. J Natl Cancer Inst 1988;80:1486–1488.
175. Reggev A, Djerassi I: The safety of administration of massive doses of methotrexate (50 gm) with equimolar citrovorum factor rescue in adult patients. Cancer 1988;61: 2423–2428.
176. Relling MV, Srapleton FB, Ochs J, et al: Removal of methotrexate, leucovorin, and their metabolites by combined hemodialysis and hemoperfusion. Cancer 1988;62: 884–888.
177. Reynolds EH: Mental effects of anticonvulsants and folic acid metabolism. Brain 1968;91:197–214.
178. Reynolds JEF: Vinblastine. In: Reynolds JEF, ed: Martindale: The Extra Pharmacopoeia. England, The Pharmaceutical Press, 1990.
179. Roenigk H, Maibach HI, Weinstein GP: Methotrexate therapy for psoriasis. Guidelines revisions. Arch Dermatol 1973;108:3535
180. Rosenberg B: Anticancer activity of cis-dichlorodiammineplatinum and some relevant chemistry. Cancer Treat Rep 1979;63:1433–1438.
181. Rosenthal S, Kaufman S: Vincristine neuropathy. Ann Intern Med 1974;81:733–737.
182. Rossof RH, Slayton RE, Perlia CP: Preliminary clinical experience with cis-diamminedichloroplatinum. Cancer 1972;30:1451–1456.
183. Roush W: Dana-Farber death sends a warning to research hospitals. Science 1995;269:295–306.
184. Rudolph R, Larson DL: Etiology and treatment of chemotherapeutic agent extravasation injuries: A review. J Clin Oncol 1987;5:1116–1126.
185. Rudolph R, Suzuki M, Luca JK: Experimental skin necrosis produced by adriamycin. Cancer Treat Rep 1979;63: 529–537.
186. San Angel F: Current controversies in chemotherapy administration. J Intraven Nur 1995;18:16–22.
187. Sandler SG, Tobin W, Henderson ES: Vincristine induced neuropathy: A clinical study of fifty leukemic patients. Neurology 1969;19:367–374.
188. Sasaki K, Tanaka J, Fujimoto T: Theoretically required urinary flow during high dose methotrexate infusion. Cancer Chemother Pharmacol 1984;13:9–14.
189. Schilsky RL: Renal and metabolic toxicities of cancer chemotherapy. Semin Oncol 1982;9:75–83.
190. Schwartz RG, McKenzie WB, Alexander J, et al: Congestive heart failure and left ventricular dysfunction complication doxorubicin therapy. Am J Med 1987;82:1110–1118.
191. Scuderi N, Onesti MG: Antitumor agents: Extravasation, management, and surgical treatment. Ann Plast Surg 1994;32:39–44.
192. Searles G, McKendry RJR: Methotrexate pneumonitis in rheumatoid arthritis: Potential risk factors. Four case reports and a review of the literature. J Rheumatol 1987;14: 1164–1171.
193. Shah BC, Albert DJ: Intravesical instillation of formalin for the management of intractable hematuria. J Urol 1973; 110:519–520.
194. Sharman VL, Cunningham J, Goodwin JF, et al: Do patients receiving regular hemodialysis need folic acid supplements? Br Med J 1982;285:96–97.
195. Shurafa M, Shumaker E, Cronin S: Prostaglandin F_2-alpha bladder irritation for control of intractable cyclophosphamide induced hemorrhagic cystitis. J Urol 1987;137: 1230–1231.
196. Siegert W, Hiddemann W, Koppensteiner R, et al: Accidental overdose of mitoxantrone in three patients. Med Oncol Tumor Pharmacother 1989;6:275–278.
197. Skoutakis VA, Acchiardo DR, Meyer MC, Hatch FE: Folic acid dosage for chronic hemodialysis patients. Clin Pharmacol Ther 1975;18:200–204.
198. Slimowitz R: Thoughts on a medical disaster. Am J Health Syst Pharm 1995;52:1464–1465.

199. Somers G, Abramow M, Witter M, Naets JP: Myocardial infarction: A complication of vincristine treatment? Lancet 1976;2:690. Letter.
200. Sostman HD, Matthay RA, Putman CE, Smith GJ: Methotrexate-induced pneumonitis. Medicine 1976;55: 371–388.
201. Speyer J, Green MD, Kramer E, et al: Protective effect of the bispiperazinedione ICRF–187 against doxorubicin induced cardiac toxicity in women with advanced breast cancer. N Engl J Med 1988;319:745–752.
202. Spiegel RJ, Cooper PR, Blum RH, et al: Treatment of massive intrathecal methotrexate overdose by ventriculolumbar perfusion. N Engl J Med 1984;311:386–388.
203. Steger GG, Mader RM, Gnant MFX, et al: GM-CSF in the treatment of a patient with severe methotrexate intoxication. J Intern Med 1993;233:499–502.
204. Steinberg JS, Cohen AJ, Wasserman AG, et al: Acute arrhythmogenicity of doxorubicin administration. Cancer 1987;60:1213–1218.
205. Stephens LC, Wang YM, Schultheiss TE, Jarkdine JN: Enhanced cardiotoxicity in rabbits treated with verapamil and adriamycin. Oncology 1987;44:302–306.
206. Stoller RG, Hande KR, Jacobs SA, et al: Use of plasma pharmacokinetics to predict and prevent methotrexate toxicity. N Engl J Med 1977;297:630–633.
207. Subar M, Muggia FM: Apparent myocardial ischemia associated with vinblastine administration. Cancer Treat Rep 1986;70:690–691.
208. Svingen BA, Powis G, Appel PL, Scott M: Protection against adriamycin induced skin necrosis in the rat by dimethyl sulfoxide and alpha tocopherol. Cancer Res 1979; 41:3395–3399.
209. Tattersall MHN, Brown B, Frei E: The reversal of methotrexate toxicity by thymidine with maintenance of antitumor effects. Nature 1981;253:198–200.
210. Tewey KM, Chen GL, Nelson EM, Liu IF: Interactive anticancer drugs interfere with the breakage reunion reaction of mammalian DNA topoisomerase II. J Biol Chem 1984;259:9182–9187.
211. Thierry FX, Vernier I, Dueymes HM, et al: Acute renal failure after high dose methotrexate therapy. Nephron 1989; 51:416–417.
212. Thomas LL, Brasst PC, Somers R, Goudsmit R: Massive vincristine overdose: Failure of leucovorin to reduce toxicity. Cancer Treat Rep 1982;66:1967–1969.
213. Treon SP, Chabner BA: Concepts in use of high dose methotrexate therapy. Clin Chem 1996;42:1322–1329.
214. Trissel LA: Handbook of Injectable Drugs. Bethesda, American Society of Hospital Pharmacists, 1988.
215. Tsavaris NB, Karagiaouris P, Tzannou I: Conservative approach to the treatment of chemotherapy induced extravasation. J Dermatol Surg Oncol 1990;16:519–522.
216. Vaitkevicius VK, Talley RW, Tucker JL, et al: Cytological and clinical observations during vincaleukoblastine therapy of disseminated cancer. Cancer 1962;15: 294–297.
217. Vandenberg SA, Julig K, Spoerke DG, et al: Chlorambucil overdose: Accidental ingestion of an antineoplastic drug. J Emerg Med 1988;6:495–508.
218. Vogelzang NJ: "Adriamycin flare": A skin reaction resembling extravasation. Cancer Treat Rep 1979;63:2067–2069.
219. Vogl SE, Zaravinos T, Kaplan BH: Toxicity of cis-diamminedichloroplatinum given in a two hour outpatient regimen of diuresis and hydration. Cancer 1980;45:11–15.
220. Von Hoff DD, Layard MY, Basa P, et al: Risk factors for doxorubicin induced congestive heart failure. Ann Intern Med 1979;91:710–717.
221. Von Hoff DD, Penta JS, Helman LG, Slavik M: Incidence of drug related deaths secondary to high dose methotrexate and citrovorum factor administration. Cancer Treat Rep 1977;61:745–748.
222. Von Hoff DD, Rozencweig M, Picat M: The cardiotoxicity of anticancer agents. Semin Oncol 1982;9:23–33.
223. Walker RW, Allen JC, Rosen G, Caparros B: Transient cerebral dysfunction secondary to high dose methotrexate. J Clin Oncol 1986;4:1845–1850.
224. Weinstein GO: Methotrexate. Ann Int Med 1988;86: 199–204.
225. Weiss HD, Walker MD, Wiernick PH: Neurotoxicity of commonly used antineoplastic agents. N Engl J Med 1974;29:75–81.
226. Whittaker JA, Al-Ismail SA: Effect of digoxin and vitamin E in preventing cardiac damage caused by doxorubicin in acute myeloid leukemia. Br Med J 1984;288:283–284.
227. Wilding G, Caruso R, Lawrence TS, et al: Retinal toxicity after high dose cisplatin therapy. J Clin Oncol 1985; 3:1683–1689.
228. Winchester JF, Rahman A, Tilstone WJ, et al: Will hemoperfusion be useful for cancer chemotherapeutic drug removal? Clin Toxicol 1980;17:557–569.
229. Wolfson S, Olney MB: Accidental ingestion of a toxic dose of chlorambucil. Report of a case in a child. JAMA 1957; 165:239–240.
230. Wortman JR, Lucas VS, Schuster E, et al: Sudden death during doxorubicin administration. Cancer 1979;44: 1588–1590.
231. Yancey RS, Talpaz M: Vindesine-associated angina and ECG changes. Cancer Treat Rep 1982;66:587–589.
232. Zaragoza MR, Ritchey ML, Walter A: Neurologic consequences of accidental intrathecal vincristine: A case report. Med Pediatr Oncol 1995;24:61–62.
233. Zbinden G, Brandle E: Toxicologic screening of daunorubicin NSC–82151, adriamycin, NSC-123127 and their derivatives in rats. Cancer Chemother Rep 1975;59:707–715.
234. Zoubek A, Zaunschirm HA, Lion T, et al: Successful carboxypeptidase G2 rescue in delayed methotrexate elimination due to renal failure. Pediatr Hematol Oncol 1995;12:471–477.
235. Zulian GB, Tullen E, Maton B: Methylene blue for ifosfamide associated encephalopathy. N Engl J Med 1996; 332:1239–1240.
236. Zweier JL: Iron mediated formation of an oxidized adriamycin free radical. Biochim Biophys Acta 1985;839: 209–213.

CHAPTER 48

Cardiac Glycosides

Neal A. Lewin

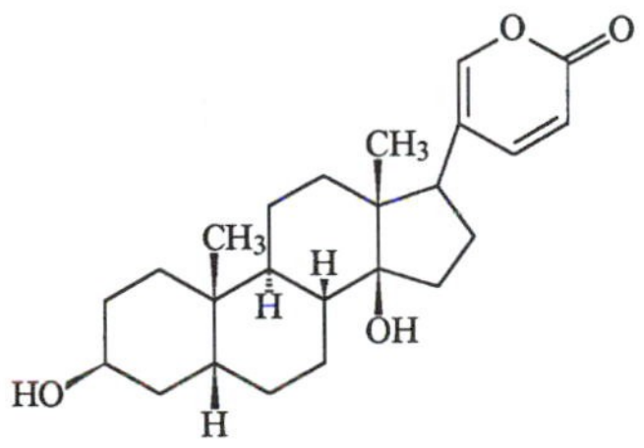

Bufalin

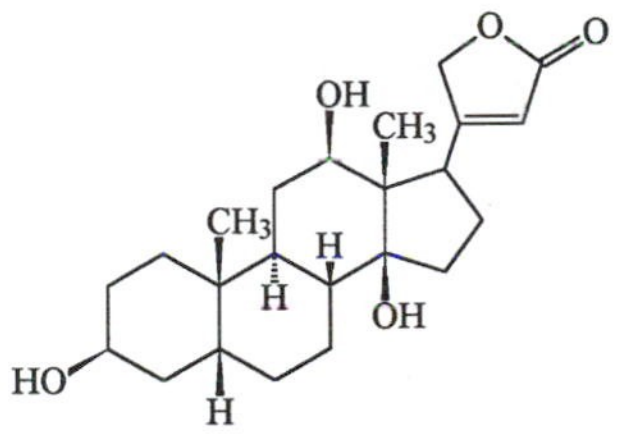

Digoxigenin

Digoxin	
MW: 780 daltons	
Action Levels	
Serum Digoxin	> 2 ng/mL
	> 10–15 ng/mL (serious)
Serum Digitoxin	> 4 ng/mL
	> 150 ng/mL (serious)
Ingestion	> 4 mg digoxin in child
	> 10 mg digoxin in adult
Serum K+ Level	≥ 5.0 mEq/L (acute)

Values greater than or equal to the action level necessitate clinical intervention. Values less than this level may necessitate intervention based on the clinical condition of the patient.

A 72-year-old retired nurse presented to the hospital about 5 hours after taking 20 digoxin pills of unknown strength in a suicide attempt. She complained of nausea and one episode of vomiting. She stated that her husband died 2 months earlier of a heart attack and that she no longer wanted to live. Her past medical history was remarkable for hypothyroidism, congestive heart failure, hypertension, and Familial Mediterranean Fever. Her current medicines included colchicine, digoxin, diltiazem, isordil, and dipyridamole. She denied ingestion of any of her other medications.

On presentation to the emergency department she was described as an elderly woman in no distress. Her vital signs were: blood pressure, 120/80 mm Hg; pulse, 80 beats/min and regular; respiratory rate, 20 breaths/min; and rectal temperature, 98.8°F (37.1°C). Her weight was estimated at 70 kg. The skin was moist. Examination of the head, eyes, ears, nose, and throat was unremarkable. Her neck was supple and without jugular venous distention or hepatojugular reflux. Chest was clear to auscultation and percussion. Heart examination revealed a normal S_1 and S_2 and an S_3 gallop. The abdomen was nontender with active bowel sounds and no hepatosplenomegaly. The extremities were without clubbing or cyanosis but had a trace amount of pedal edema. Neurologic assessment demonstrated intact orientation, concentration, and memory. No cranial nerve abnormalities were noted, and deep tendon reflexes were intact and symmetric. Plantar flexion was noted. Motor and sensory testing were grossly normal. The patient's mood was described as angry, uncooperative, and depressed.

An intravenous line was started and blood samples were sent for BUN, creatinine, electrolytes including calcium and magnesium, glucose, serum digoxin level, complete blood count, and acetaminophen level. She was placed

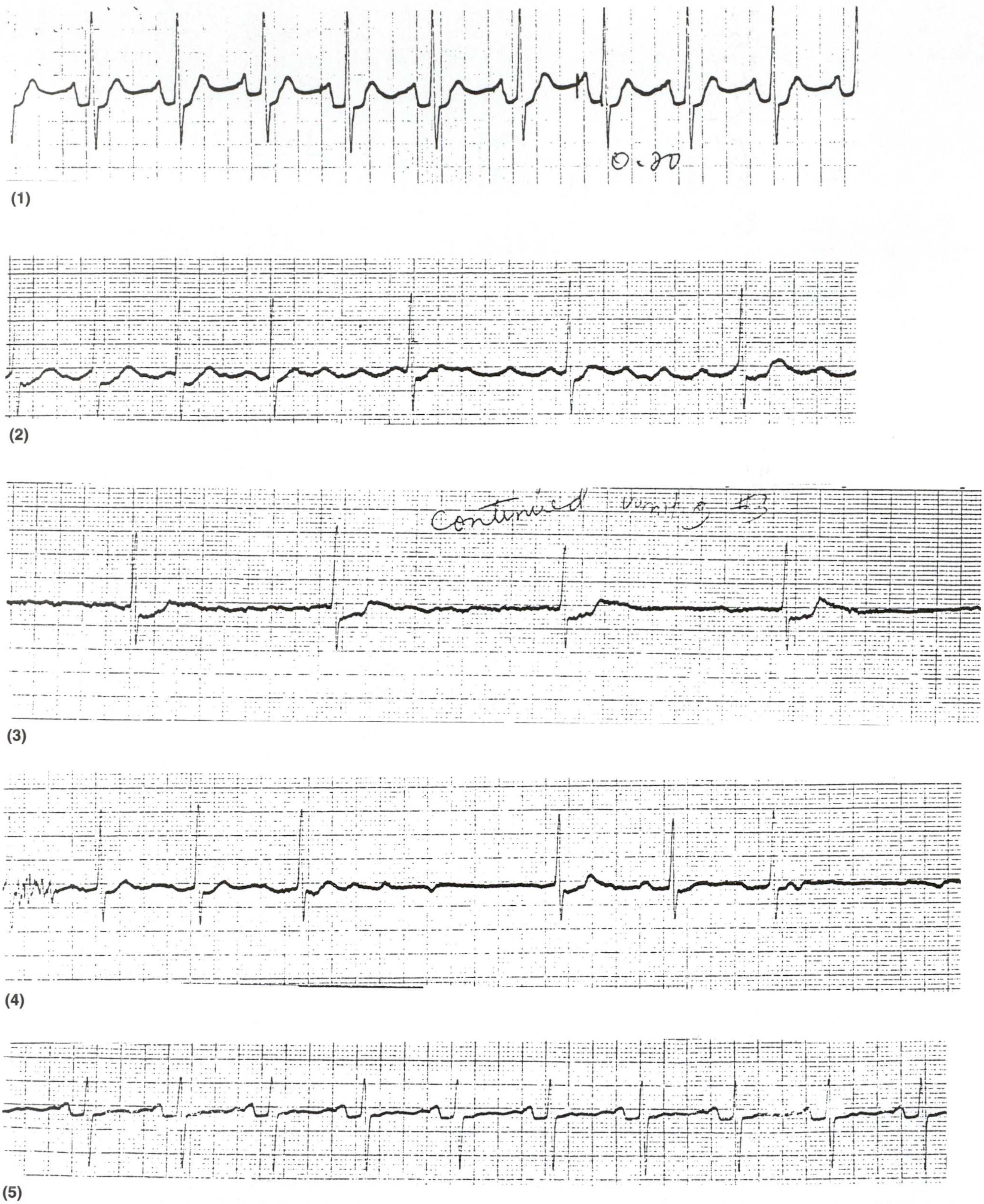

Figure 48–1. Serial ECG rhythm strips in a patient with acute digoxin intoxication. (1) Presentation ECG demonstrates normal sinus rhythm with a ventricular rate of about 80 beats/min. (2) Second rhythm strip demonstrates atrial fibrillation (or flutter) that occurred during emesis. (3) With further emesis, the ventricular response to the patient's atrial fibrillation slowed significantly and her blood pressure fell. (4) A rhythm strip, taken 1 hour after the IV administration of 400 mg (10 vials) of digoxin-specific antibody fragments and 1 mg of atropine, demonstrates occasional sinus rhythm with an increased ventricular response. (5) A rhythm strip taken 3.5 hours after therapy demonstrates restoration of normal sinus rhythm.

on a cardiac monitor (Fig. 48–1, rhythm strip 1), which revealed a normal sinus rhythm at 80 beats/min. Sixty grams of activated charcoal and 70 mL of 70% sorbitol were given orally. The patient immediately vomited. Metoclopramide, 10 mg IV, was given but vomiting persisted. The poison center was contacted and the hospital was advised to admit the patient to an intensive care unit and to have at least 10 vials of Digibind (digoxin-specific Fab) at her bedside. The following stat laboratory results returned: serum sodium, 134 mEq/L; chloride, 110 mEq/L; potassium, 6.7 mEq/L; bicarbonate, 24 mEq/L; BUN, 14 mg/dL; creatinine, 1.0 mg/dL; glucose, 101 mg/dL; calcium, 9.8 mg/dL; acetaminophen, negative; hematocrit, 40.3%; digoxin level and magnesium level, pending.

Within 5 minutes the serum potassium was repeated and reported as 4.8 mEq/L. Repeat ECG was consistent with atrial fibrillation or flutter (Fig. 48–1, rhythm strip 2). The patient vomited again, was noted to become more bradycardic (Fig. 48–1, rhythm strip 3), and her blood pressure fell to 90/40 mg Hg. A repeat potassium concentration was reported as 5.4 mEq/L and a second digoxin concentration was sent. Ten vials of Digibind were given intravenously, as well as 1 mg of atropine and a fluid challenge of 500 mL of 0.9% sodium chloride solution. Atropine raised the heart rate transiently to 46 beats/min and the blood pressure increased to 100/50 mm Hg. An external pacemaker was placed on standby. About 1 hour later the patient's rhythm began to improve. (Fig. 48–1, rhythm strip 4). Three and one-half hours after Digibind administration a normal sinus rhythm was restored (Fig. 48–1, rhythm strip 5). The initial serum digoxin concentration was reported as 14.6 ng/mL and the second concentration as 12.3 ng/mL. After Digibind therapy, the potassium concentration fell to 4.2 mEq/L. The patient had an uneventful recovery and was ultimately referred for psychiatric counseling.

Overview

Since Withering wrote the classic treatise on digitalis in the 18th century, both acute and chronic digitalis toxicity have remained an important problem.[78] Acute digitalis toxicity occurs with intentional overdoses and quite commonly unintentionally in young children. Acute digitalis toxicity is frequently superimposed on chronic use, for example, as may result from a dosing error in the elderly, or due to drug–drug interactions that cause changes in digitalis clearance. The most commonly prescribed cardiac glycoside in the United States is digoxin; other preparations rarely if ever used include digitoxin, ouabain, lanatoside C, deslanoside, and gitalin. Cardiac glycoside toxicity also accounts for a small percentage of the reported toxicity from plant ingestions (see Chap. 77), with most instances occurring in children 6 years old or younger. Herbal exposure to cardiac glycosides can occur from drinking contaminated water, eating meat cooked with or stirred by stems, inhaling smoke from burning plants, or ingesting sap, leaves, blossoms, seeds, or tea from cardiac glycoside-containing plants. Some of these plants include oleander, foxglove, yew berry, lily of the valley, dogbane, siberian ginseng, and red squill (see Chap. 77).[12,33,51,56,60,71] Cases of toad venom poisoning following ingestion of a topical aphrodisiac containing a cardioactive steroid of the bufadienolide class have been reported.[8,9,11] It is postulated that plants and some toad species contain these cardiac glycosides to serve as protection against their natural predators.[6,37]

What Are the Mechanisms of Action and Pathophysiology of the Cardiac Glycosides?

The cardiac glycosides inhibit active transport of Na^+ and K^+ across cell membranes by binding onto a specific site on the extracytoplasmic face of the α subunit of Na^+-K^+-ATPase. The binding of the glycosides to the Na^+-K^+-ATPase as well as the inhibition of the cellular Na^+ pump is reversible and entropically driven.[17]

The glycosides increase the force of contraction of the heart (positive inotropic effect) due to an increase of cytosolic Ca^{2+} during systole. Both Na^+ and Ca^{2+} ions enter cardiac muscle cells during each cycle of depolarization, contraction, and repolarization. The calcium enters the cardiac myocyte through L-type calcium channels during depolarization which subsequently triggers the release of more calcium into the cytosol from the sarcoplasmic reticulum. During repolarization and relaxation, calcium is pumped back into the sarcoplasmic reticulum by a Ca^{2+}-ATPase and is removed intracellularly by a Na^+-Ca^{2+} exchanger and a sarcolemmal Ca^{2+}-ATPase.[50]

The amount of intracellular Na^+ will determine how much Ca^{2+} will be extruded from the cell. The cardiac glycosides bind to sarcolemmal Na^+-K^+-ATPase, and inhibit cellular Na^+ pump activity, which decreases Na^+ extrusion and increases Na^+ in the cytosol, thereby decreasing transmembrane Na^+ gradient preventing extrusion of intracellular Ca^{2+} during repolarization. Small changes in intracellular Na^+ concentration yield large increases in cardiac muscle shortening. Excessive increases in intracellular Ca^{2+} caused by excessive cardiac glycoside levels results in a transient late depolarization (delayed afterdepolarization) that may be accompanied by an aftercontraction often seen with digitalis toxicity.[16,38]

The alterations in cardiac rate and rhythm occurring in digitalis toxicity may simulate almost every known type of dysrhythmia. Although no dysrhythmia is diagnostic of digoxin toxicity, toxicity should be suspected when there is evidence of increased automaticity and depressed conduction.[38] Underlying these dysrhythmias is the complex influence of digitalis on the electrophysiologic properties of the heart as discussed, as well as via the cumulative result of the direct, vagotonic, and antiadrenergic actions of digitalis. The effects of digoxin vary with the dose and differ depending on the type of cardiac tissue involved. The atria and ventricles exhibit increased automaticity and excitability, resulting in extrasystoles and tachydysrhythmias. Conduction velocity is reduced in both myocardial and nodal tissue, resulting in an increased PR interval and AV block accompanied by a decrease in the QT interval. These phenomena are summarized in Table 48–1.

In addition to the effects described above, the direct effect of digitalis on repolarization is often reflected in

TABLE 48–1. EFFECTS OF DIGITALIS GLYCOSIDES

	Atria and Ventricles	AV Node	ECG
Excitability	↑	—	Extrasystoles, tachydysrhythmias
Automaticity	↑	—	Extrasystoles, tachydysrhythmias
Conduction velocity	↓	↓	Increased PR interval, AV block
Refractoriness	↓	↑	Increased PR interval, AV block, decreased QTc interval

↑ = Increase; ↓ = Decrease.

the ECG by ST segment and T-wave forces opposite in direction to the major QRS forces. The initial electrophysiologic manifestations of digitalis effects and toxicity are usually mediated indirectly by increased vagal tone. Early in acute intoxication, depression of SA or AV nodal function may be reversed by atropine. Subsequent manifestations are the result of direct and vagomimetic actions of the drug on the heart and are not reversed by atropine. In 10 to 15% of cases, ectopic rhythms appear as the first sign of intoxication.[58]

Ectopic rhythms—such as nonparoxysmal junctional tachycardia, ventricular premature extrasystoles, ventricular flutter and fibrillation, atrial flutter and fibrillation, and bidirectional ventricular tachycardia—are due to enhanced automaticity, reentry, or both (Tables 48–2 and 48–3).[58]

Bidirectional ventricular tachycardia (see Fig. 8–15) is particularly characteristic of severe digitalis toxicity and results from alterations of intraventricular conduction, junctional tachycardia with aberrant intraventricular conduction, or on rare occasions, alternating ventricular pacemakers. Depression of the atrial pacemakers resulting in SA arrest may also be seen. Other features are SA block, AV block, and sinus exit block resulting from depression of normal conduction. Nonparoxysmal atrial tachycardia with block is associated with digitalis toxicity.[47] When conduction and the normal pacemaker are both depressed, ectopic pacemakers may take over, producing atrial tachycardia with AV block and nonparoxysmal automatic AV junctional tachycardia.[38] Indeed, AV junctional block of varying degrees, along with increased ventricular automaticity, are the most common manifestations of digoxin toxicity, occurring in 30 to 40% of patients with recognized digoxin toxicity.[48] Atrioventricular dissociation may occur due to suppression of the dominant pacemaker with escape of a subsidiary pacemaker or to an inappropriate acceleration of a ventricular pacemaker. Hypotension, shock, and cardiovascular collapse can ensue.

Elevated serum potassium levels occur in a significant number of cases of acute digitalis poisoning.[38,40] Hyperkalemia in the initial stage of digitalis intoxication has important prognostic implications, in that serum potassium concentration has a better prognostic correlation than either the initial ECG changes or the serum digoxin concentration.[4,5] In a study of acutely digoxin-poisoned patients, approximately 50% of the patients with serum potassium levels of 5.0 to 5.5 mEq/L died. Serum potassium levels of 5.5 to 6.4 mEq/L were associated with death in 4 out of 7 patients. All of the 10 patients with serum potassium levels above 6.4 mEq died.[4] Hyperkalemia causes further depolarization of myocardial conduction tissue, particularly the AV node, leading to an exacerbation of digitalis-induced conduction delays.[38] The elevation of the serum potassium concentration after therapeutic as well as toxic administration of digitalis is due to (1) the release of potassium from many tissues, including the liver; (2) inhibition of potassium uptake by skeletal muscle; and (3) inhibition of the Na^+-K^+-ATPase pump (as discussed earlier). The interrelationships be-

TABLE 48–2. ADULT DIGITALIS INTOXICATION

Common Cardiac Abnormalities
- High degrees of AV block
- Ventricular ectopic activity, bigeminy, salvoes
- Ventricular fibrillation
- Ventricular tachycardia
- Nonparoxysmal atrial tachycardia with block
- Sinus bradycardia

Noncardiac Abnormalities
- Anorexia
- Confusion
- Nausea
- Vomiting
- High digoxin serum concentrations
- Rising potassium concentrations

TABLE 48–3. PEDIATRIC DIGITALIS INTOXICATION[a]

Common Cardiac Abnormalities
- Often not life threatening
  - Bradycardia
  - First or second-degree AV block
  - ST segment depression
  - Junctional rhythm with SA block or arrest
- In most severe cases
  - AV junctional tachycardia alternating with slow ventricular rate
  - Ventricular fibrillation

Noncardiac Abnormalities
- Vomiting and lethargy common

[a]Children appear more resistant to life-threatening toxicity than adults (appear to require a higher μg/kg dose to induce toxicity). In neonates, lethargy and feeding difficulties may be manifestations of chronic intoxication.

tween intracellular and extracellular potassium and digitalis therapy are complex and not clearly understood.

Hypokalemia probably results from the kaliuresis induced by potent loop diuretics that are frequently used concomitantly with digitalis in patients with congestive heart failure. Severe hypokalemia (<2.5 mEq/L) reduces the rate of sodium pump turnover, slowing the pump and exacerbating concomitant sodium pump inhibition due to cardiac glycosides.[38] Chronic hypokalemia reduces the number of Na^+-K^+-ATPase units in skeletal muscle, thereby potentially decreasing the volume of drug distribution.[2,40]

What Are the Pharmacologic Features of Digitalis Glycosides?

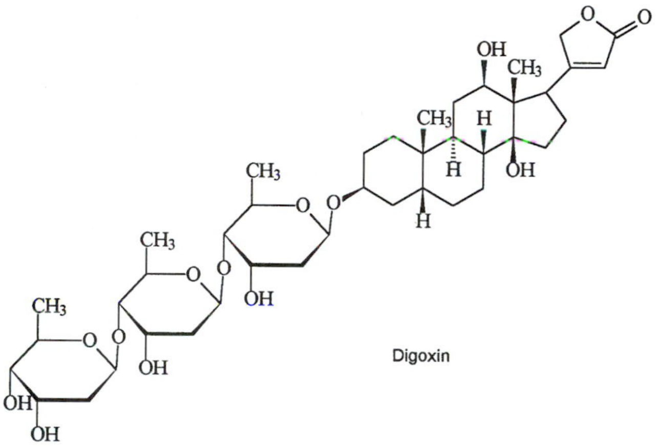

Digoxin

Cardiac glycosides are composed of a steroid nucleus containing an unsaturated lactone ring at the C–7 position and one or more glycoside residues at C–3. The effects of digoxin depend upon the preparation, mode of administration, absorption, protein binding, volume of distribution, route of administration, route of elimination, drug–drug interactions, and pathophysiologic characteristics of the host (Table 48–4). Factors such as age, hypothyroidism, hepatic and renal disease, hypokalemia, hypernatremia, alkalosis, hypercalcemia, hypomagnesemia, hypoxemia, myocardial disease, and cor pulmonale can all result in digitalis toxicity unless therapeutic regimens of digoxin are appropriately adjusted. Drug interactions are reported with digitalis and quinidine, verapamil, diltiazem, amiodarone, and spironolactone.[13,29,43,57] The inactivation of digoxin in the gut, in particular by the enteric bacterium *Eubacterium lentum*, present in approximately 10% of the population, and the reversal of the inactivation by erythromycin or tetracycline is well demonstrated.[46] Indeed, antibiotics may produce as much as a twofold increase in serum digoxin concentration, potentially leading to digitalis toxicity.[43]

TABLE 48–4. PHARMACOLOGY OF DIGOXIN

Onset of action	
Oral	1.5–6 h
IV	5–30 min
Maximal effect	
Oral	4–6 h
IV	1.5–3 h
Intestinal absorption[a]	40–90% (mean, 75%)
Plasma protein binding	25%
Volume of distribution	6–7 L/kg (adults)
	16 L/kg (infants)
	10 L/kg (neonates)
	4–5 L/kg (adults with renal failure)
Elimination half-life	1.6 days
Route of elimination	Renal excretion (60–80%) of unchanged drug, limited hepatic metabolism
Enterohepatic circulation	Small
"Therapeutic" plasma concentration	0.5–2.0 ng/mL

[a]Dependent on tablet dissolution, coadministered food, antacids, malabsorption, and motility disorders.

What Are the Most Frequently Encountered Noncardiac Toxic Effects of Digitalis?

An asymptomatic period of several minutes to several hours follows a single orally administered toxic dose. The first symptom of digitalis toxicity may be anorexia, and is often followed by nausea, vomiting, and abdominal pain. Neuropsychiatric disorders include confusion, disorientation, drowsiness, headache, hallucinations, and, rarely, convulsions.[24,26] Digitalis-induced central nervous system symptoms can play a role in the early detection of digitalis toxicity.[12] Visual disturbances include transient amblyopia, photophobia, blurring, scotomata, photopsia, decreased visual activity, and aberrations of color vision (chromatopsia), such as yellow halos (xanthopsia) around light.[44]

What Does a Serum Digoxin Concentration Mean?

Properly obtained and interpreted serum digoxin concentrations significantly aid in management. After massive digoxin ingestions, the plasma elimination half-life may be shortened to as little as 13 to 15 hours from the usual 36 hours. Although digitalis toxicity is the result of the interaction of the diverse factors previously mentioned, there is a significant correlation between the clinical condition and the serum digoxin or digitoxin concentration. In general, toxic patients have mean serum concentrations (as determined by radioimmunoassay) above 2 ng/mL for digoxin and above 40 ng/mL for digitoxin.[36] The significance of these concentrations depends on when the value is obtained in relation to an acute ingestion and the distribution phase of the drug. A value of 15 ng/mL of digoxin is, therefore, more ominous 6 hours after an ingestion than 1 hour after an ingestion. Because there are multiple determinants of digitalis intoxication and there is an overlap in serum digitalis concentrations between toxic and nontoxic patients, it may be inaccurate to use the therapeutic range of digoxin of 0.5 to 2.0 ng/mL as the sole indicator of toxicity.[62]

The use of digoxin-specific Fab can cause a false elevation in serum digoxin concentrations as measured by standard immunoassay techniques. Most assay systems involve a complex balance between reagent digoxin, serum digoxin, and solid-phase digoxin antibodies. Any excess digoxin antibody results in less reagent digoxin binding to the solid-phase antibody, which causes a further false elevation in concentration (Table 48–5).[22]

Endogenous Digoxin-like Immunoreactive Factors (DLIS)

Patients not receiving digoxin therapy may also have a false positive digoxin assay.[29] Patients with renal insufficiency,[8,10,27,34] pregnancy,[19,28,32] liver disease,[52] subarachnoid hemorrhage,[77] congestive heart failure,[25,63] insulin-dependent diabetes,[21] stress,[26,73] acromegaly,[15] and neonates[72] may have an endogenous cross-reacting substance. Spironolactone and hyperbilirubinemia cross-react with the digoxin assay and cause a false-positive result.[64] In a recent report an inhibitor of the sodium pump obtained from human placenta was identified as a dihydropyrone-substituted steroid. This substance, described as a bufenolide, is believed to be of endogenous origin, with a mass of 370 D and an empirical formula $C_{24}H_{34}O_3$. It differs from the toad bufadenolides solely by a single double-bond pyrone ring. The authors speculate that because bufenolides are not found in plant or animal kingdoms, a synthetic pathway to dihydropyrone-substituted steroids in humans may be responsible for this endogenous digoxin-like immuoreactive factor. Further research is necessary to confirm this pathway.[32] The use of ultrafiltration techniques while altering incubation time and temperature at which the digoxin assay is performed can eliminate the contribution of DLIS.[20] The clinician suspecting this problem should consult the laboratory. Clinical observations indicate that the serum digoxin level contributed by endogenous digoxin-like immunoreactive substances is usually less than 2 ng/mL.

TABLE 48–5. PITFALLS IN USING SERUM DIGOXIN LEVELS

1. Serum levels must be interpreted in relation to other metabolic abnormalities and medications: hypokalemia, hypomagnesemia, hypercalcemia, hypernatremia, alkalosis, hypothyroidism, hypoxemia, catecholamines, calcium channel blockers, quinidine, amiodarone, diuretics.
2. Correlation between clinical effects and toxic serum levels are based on steady-state levels; measurements of level before 6 hours after ingestion gives high levels, which reflect biphasic distribution.
3. Endogenous-like immunoreactive factors (substances) can cause a false-positive assay (<2 ng/mL).
4. After Fab administration, the total serum digoxin level is no longer clinically useful, as it is exceedingly high. Solution: request free serum digoxin level (rarely available).
5. Cardioactive steroids other than digitalis preparations may not be detected by *monoclonal* digoxin immunoassay. Solution: request polyclonal digoxin immunoassay from laboratory.

What Therapeutic Measures Are Indicated?

Basic Management

Initial treatment of a patient with acute digitalis poisoning is comparable to that of any toxicologic emergency. Therapy includes providing general supportive care, preventing further exposure, preventing further GI absorption, increasing excretion, administering digoxin-specific antibodies, and treating specific complications such as dysrhythmias and electrolyte abnormalities (Table 48–6).

Initial therapy should be directed toward prevention of further GI absorption by either emesis or lavage, followed by the administration of multiple-dose activated charcoal and a cathartic (Table 48–6). The optimal effectiveness of activated charcoal depends on the time elapsed since ingestion. Because digitoxin and digoxin are recirculated enterohepatically and enteroenterically, late as well as repeated activated charcoal administration (1 g/kg body weight every 2 to 4 hours) may be beneficial.[42,45,53,75] Steroid-binding resins, such as cholestyramine and colestipol,[31] like activated charcoal, can prevent further absorption of digoxin and digitoxin from the GI tract and reduce serum half-life by interrupting both enteroenteric and enterohepatic circulation. This effect is especially important when digitoxin, a less polar compound, has been ingested or when digoxin has been ingested by a patient with significant renal insufficiency (Table 48–6).

TABLE 48–6. MANAGEMENT OF DIGITALIS TOXICITY

General Therapy

Discontinue digitalis
Monitor for dysrhythmias
Determine electrolytes and serum digoxin concentration
Observe for hemodynamic compromise
Multiple-dose activated charcoal
Steroid-binding resins for digitoxin and for patients with renal insufficiency

Management of Dysrhythmias

Electrolyte abnormalities:
- Hyperkalemia ≥5.0 mEq/L—digoxin-Fab therapy. If Digibind not available: insulin and glucose, sodium bicarbonate, sodium polystyrene sulfonate
- Hypokalemia—Replete with IV KCl until eukalemic
- Hypomagnesemia—Replete with IV $MgSO_4$

Supraventricular tachydysrhythmia—β-adrenergic antagonists, digoxin-Fab
Supraventricular bradydysrhythmia—Atropine, digoxin-Fab
High-degree A-V block—digoxin-Fab
Ventricular tachycardia/fibrillation—Cardioversion/defibrillation, digoxin-Fab, lidocaine, phenytoin, $MgSO_4$

Forced diuresis,[41] hemoperfusion,[49] and hemodialysis[74] are not effective in hastening the elimination of digoxin due to its large volume of distribution (4 to 10 L/kg), making it relatively inaccessible to these techniques (see Table 48–4). Only 1% of the total body digoxin is in the serum, and of that amount approximately 25% is protein-bound.

Advanced Management

The standard of care for patients with life-threatening digitalis toxicity is the use of digoxin-specific antibodies.[1,20,22,54,56,60,67,69,79] Purified digoxin-specific Fab has been successfully administered to severely poisoned patients with a subsequent sharp decrease in free digoxin levels, a concomitant massive increase in total serum digoxin, an increase in renal excretion of digoxin bound to digoxin Fab, and a decrease of serum potassium toward normal.[1] Digoxin-specific Fab represents a significant advance when life-threatening digoxin or digitoxin toxicity is present. Indications are listed in Table 48–7. Extensive discussion is found in Antidotes in Depth: Digoxin-Specific Antibody Fragments.

With life-threatening digitalis toxicity the patient should be monitored continuously in an intensive care setting, with frequent ECGs and electrolyte determinations. Specific therapy depends on the pattern of cardiotoxicity. Rhythm disturbances that impair cardiac output because of significant bradycardia or tachycardia, or that portend ventricular fibrillation, require active intervention. Patients with preexisting heart disease tend to develop ectopic ventricular dysrhythmias that are more prominent than conduction disturbances.[38]

In the event that digoxin-specific fragments are not immediately available, the drugs of choice for the management of ventricular irritability include phenytoin and lidocaine, because they depress the enhanced ventricular automaticity without significantly slowing AV nodal conduction.[59] In fact, phenytoin may reverse digitalis-induced prolongation of AV nodal conduction. Phenytoin dissociates the inotropic and dysrhythmic actions of digitalis, thus suppressing digitalis-induced tachydysrhythmia without diminishing the contractile effects. In addition, phenytoin can terminate supraventricular dysrhythmias induced by digitalis, whereas lidocaine is not as effective.[59] Atrial fibrillation and flutter typically do not respond to phenytoin or lidocaine. Phenytoin should be infused slowly intravenously (up to 50 mg/min) until control of the dysrhythmias is achieved, phenytoin toxicity occurs, or a maximum of 1000 mg has been given in an adult or 15 to 20 mg/kg in a child. The role of fosphenytoin has not been evaluated in this setting. Maintenance oral doses of phenytoin 300 to 400 mg/d in an adult and 6 to 10 mg/kg per day in a child should be continued until digoxin toxicity is resolved. Lidocaine is given as a 1-mg/kg IV bolus followed by continuous infusion at 1 to 4 mg/min in an adult, or given as a 1-mg/kg IV bolus followed by 20 to 50 μg/kg per minute in a child, as required to control the rhythm disturbance. Fifteen minutes after the initial bolus, an additional 1 mg/kg IV bolus should be administered in an adult and child (see Chap. 50). As noted, the use of lidocaine or phenytoin should be rare with the availability of Digibind.

Beta-adrenergic receptor antagonists may be useful in the treatment of both supraventricular and ventricular tachydysrhythmias. In the presence of SA node or AV node depression, however, these drugs may further depress activity. All class IA antidysrhythmic agents are contraindicated because they may induce or worsen AV nodal block and decrease His–Purkinje conduction. These agents may also induce ventricular dysrhythmias (prodysrhythmogenic effects).

In patients with severe supraventricular bradydysrhythmias or varying high degrees of AV block, 0.5 mg of atropine IV should be administered in an adult or 0.02 mg/kg with a minimum of 0.1 mg in a child, with a maximum of 1.5 mg, to block the vagotonic effects of digitalis. The dose may be repeated at 5-minute intervals if necessary. Therapeutic success is unpredictable because the depressant actions of digitalis are mediated only in part through the vagus nerve. When effective, additional doses of atropine may be given as indicated. At high serum levels of digitalis, the direct effects of digitalis may predominate, making management more difficult. *The use of isoproterenol should be avoided in digitalis-induced conduction disturbances, as there may be an increased incidence of ventricular ectopic activity in the presence of toxic levels of digitalis.*

External or transvenous pacemakers have limited value with the availability of digoxin-specific Fab. In one retrospective study over a 6-year period, 92 digitalis-intoxicated patients were studied.[70] Fifty-one patients were treated with cardiac pacing and/or digoxin-specific Fab, and the overall mortality rate was 13%. Prevention of life-threatening dysrhythmias failed in 8% of patients treated with immunotherapy and 23% of patients treated with pacemakers. The main reason for failure of digoxin-specific Fab was pacing-induced dysrhythmias and delayed or insufficient administration of digoxin-specific Fab. Iatrogenic complications of pacing occurred in 36% of patients and proved fatal in 13%. The authors concluded that the pacemaker has limited utility in digitalis toxicity and encouraged early use of digoxin-specific Fab as first-line therapy.[70]

Hypokalemia, hyperkalemia, and hypomagnesemia

TABLE 48–7. INDICATIONS FOR ADMINISTRATION OF DIGOXIN-SPECIFIC ANTIBODY FRAGMENTS

Severe ventricular dysrhythmias
Progressive bradydysrhythmias unresponsive to atropine
Potassium concentration ≥5 mEq/L in setting of suspected digoxin toxicity
Rapidly progressive cardiac or gastrointestinal symptoms, or a rising potassium concentration
Serum digoxin concentration ≥15 ng/mL at any time or ≥10 ng/mL at steady state
Ingestion of ≥10 mg or ≥4 mg in a previously healthy adult or child, respectively
To establish the diagnosis

can exacerbate digitalis cardiotoxicity. Hypokalemia inhibits Na^+-K^+-ATPase activity and increases the pump inhibition induced by toxic levels of digitalis, enhances myocardial automaticity, and therefore exacerbates digitalis-related dysrhythmias. Hyperkalemia increases AV nodal block, exacerbating digitalis-induced bradydysrhythmias and conduction delays. When hypokalemia is noted in conjunction with tachydysrhythmias or bradydysrhythmias, potassium replacement should be given cautiously, with close monitoring of serum potassium, as hyperkalemia is detrimental. Intravenous potassium chloride in 0.9 or 0.45% sodium chloride solution should be infused at rates of 0.5 to 1.0 mEq/min in an adult, and a maximum of 1 mEq/kg per hour in a child, to achieve eukalemia. Rarely should overdrive suppression with a temporary transvenous pacemaker be used to abolish ventricular tachydysrhythmias.[5,70]

Hypomagnesemia may also occur in digitalis-poisoned patients, and concomitant hypomagnesemia and hypokalemia may result in refractory hypokalemia despite potassium replacement. Transient inward calcium current blockade, antagonism of calcium at intracellular binding sites, decreased digitalis-related ventricular irritability, and blockade of potassium egress from digitalis-poisoned cells have been hypothesized as the causes of hypomagnesemia.[3,18,35,55,61,68,76]

Hypomagnesemia increases myocardial digoxin uptake and decreases cellular NA^+-K^+-ATPase activity. Patients with hypomagnesemia, hypokalemia, or both may become cardiotoxic even with therapeutic digitalis levels.[76]

The successful use of intravenous magnesium sulfate in the treatment of ventricular dysrhythmias due to digoxin toxicity even in the presence of elevated serum magnesium levels was reported.[39] The mechanism of magnesium's efficacy may be its ability to suppress early afterdepolarizations and its indirect antagonism of digoxin at the sarcolemma Na^+-K^+-ATPase pump. However, this treatment would only be temporizing until digoxin-specific Fab was available for definitive therapy, and is not advocated as first-line therapy. The precise dosing of magnesium sulfate in digitalis-poisoned patients is not established.[3,18,35,39,55,61,76] A common regimen is the use of 2 g of magnesium sulfate (10%) IV over 20 minutes in an adult, or 25 to 50 mg/kg/dose to a maximum of 2 g in a child. Following stabilization an infusion of 1 to 2 g/h in an adult or 25 to 50 mg/kg/ per hour to a maximum of 2 gm in a child with serial monitoring of serum magnesium levels, telemetry, respiratory rate (observing for bradypnea), deep tendon reflexes (observing for hyporeflexia), and monitoring of blood pressure. Magnesium is contraindicated in the setting of bradycardia or atrioventricular block.

In the presence of digitalis toxicity when hyperkalemia exceeds 5.0 mEq/L, many believe digoxin-specific antibodies are indicated. Most investigators agree that when marked hyperkalemia develops in conjunction with ECG evidence of potassium toxicity, an attempt should be made to lower the serum potassium with IV insulin, dextrose, sodium bicarbonate, and oral administration of ion-exchange resins such as sodium polystyrene sulfonate if digoxin-specific Fab is not available immediately. *Whereas in most hyperkalemic patients calcium chloride is beneficial, in the presence of digitalis intoxication it could theoretically be disastrous, as intracellular hypercalcemia already exists.* Intractable ventricular fibrillation or tachycardia could ensue if additional calcium is administered, although the literature is unclear if this effect is additive or synergistic.[7,23,65] In digitalis toxic patients with unstable rhythms such as ventricular tachycardia or ventricular fibrillation, cardioversion and defibrillation, respectively, are indicated.

In conclusion, the cardiac glycosides have a narrow therapeutic to toxic index, and both unintentional and intentional overdoses can have profound cardiac and noncardiac effects. The use of basic management and advanced techniques such as immunotherapy can reduce morbidity and mortality in these high-risk patients.

Acknowledgments

Mary Ann Howland, PharmD and Robert H. Kirstein, MD contributed to this chapter in a previous edition.

References

1. Banner W, Bach P, Burk B, et al: Influence of assay methods on serum concentrations of digoxin during Fab fragment treatments. J Toxicol Clin Toxicol 1992;30:259–267.
2. Bayer MJ: Recognition and management of digitalis intoxication: Implications for emergency medicine. Am J Emerg Med 1991; 9 (suppl 1):29–32.
3. Beller GA, Hood WB, Smith TW, et al: Correlation of serum magnesium level and cardiac digitalis intoxication. Am J Cardiol 1974;33:225–229.
4. Bismuth C, Gaultier M, Conso F, Efthymiou ML: Hyperkalemia in acute digitalis poisoning: Prognostic significance and therapeutic implications. Clin Toxicol 1973;6:153–162.
5. Bismuth C, Motte G, Conso F, Chauvin M: Acute digitoxin intoxication treated by intracardiac pacemaker: Experience in sixty-eight patients. Clin Toxicol 1977;10:443–456.
6. Blaustein MP: Physiologic effects of endogenous ouabain: Control of intracellular Ca^{2+} stores and cell responsiveness. Am J Physiol 1993;264: C1367-C1387.
7. Bower JO, Mengle HAK: The additive effect of calcium and digitalis. JAMA 1936;106:1151–1153.
8. Brubacher JR, Hoffman RS, Bania T, et al: Deaths associated with a purported aphrodisiac. New York City, February 1993–May 1995. MMWR 1995;44:853–855.
9. Brubacher JR, Ravikumar PR, Bania T, et al: Treatment of toad venom poisoning with digoxin-specific Fab fragments. Chest 1996;110:1282–1288.
10. Carver JL, Valdes R. Anomalous serum digoxin concentrations in uremia. Ann Intern Med 1983;98:483–484.
11. Chern MS, Ray CY, Wu DL: Biological intoxication due to digitalis-like substance after ingestion of cooked toad soup. Am J Cardiol 1991;67:443–444.
12. Cooke D: The use of central nervous system manifestations in the early detection of digitalis toxicity. Heart Lung 1993;22:477–481.
13. Cummins RO, Haulman J, Quan L. Near-fatal yew berry in-

toxication treated with external cardiac pacing and digoxin-specific Fab antibody fragments. Ann Emerg Med 1990; 19:38–43.
14. Doering W: Quinidine-digoxin interaction: Pharmacokinetics, underlying mechanism and clinical implications. N Engl J Med 1979;301:400–404.
15. Doolittle MH, Lincoln K, Graves SW. Unexplained increase in serum digoxin: A case report. Clin Chem 1994;40:487–492.
16. Eisner DA, Lederer WJ, Vaughan-Jones RD: The quantitative relationship between twitch tension and intracellular sodium activity in sheep cardiac Purkinje fibres. J Physiol 1984; 355:251–266.
17. Eisner DA, Smith TW: The Na-K pump and its effect in cardiac muscle. In: Fozzard HA, ed: The Heart and Cardiovascular System, 2nd ed. New York, Raven, 1991, pp. 863–902.
18. French JH, Thomas RG, Siskind AP, et al: Magnesium therapy in massive digoxin intoxication. Ann Emerg Med 1984;13:562–566.
19. Friedman HS, Abramowitz I, Nguyen T, et al: Urinary digoxin-like immunoreactive substance in pregnancy. Am J Med 1987;83:261–264.
20. George S, Brathwaite RA, Hughes EA. Digoxin measurements following plasma ultrafiltration in two patients with digoxin toxicity treated with specific Fab fragments. Ann Clin Biochem 1994;31:380–381.
21. Giampietro O, Clerico A, Gregori G, et al: Increased urinary excretion of digoxin-like immunoreactive substance by insulin-dependent diabetic patients: A linkage with hypertension? Clin Chem 1988;34:2418–2422.
22. Gibb T, Adams PC, Parnham AJ, Jennings K: Plasma digoxin: Assay anomalies in Fab-treated patients. Br J Clin Pharmacol 1983;16:445–447.
23. Gold H, Edwards DJ: The effects of ouabain on heart in the presence of hypercalcemia. Am Heart J 1927;3:45–50.
24. Gorelick DA, Kussin SZ, Kahn I: Paranoid delusions and auditory hallucinations associated with digoxin intoxication. J Nerv Ment Dis 1978;166:817–819.
25. Graves SW: Endogenous digitalis-like factors. Crit Rev Clin Lab Sci 1986;23:177–200.
26. Graves SW, Adler G, Stuenkel C, et al: Increases in plasma digitalis-induced hypoglycemia. Neuroendocrinology 1989; 49:586–591.
27. Graves SW, Brown BA, Valdes R: Digoxin-like substances measured in patients with renal impairment. Ann Intern Med 1983;99:604–608.
28. Graves SW, Valdes R, Brown BA, et al: Endogenous immunoreactive digoxin-like substance in human pregnancies. J Clin Endocrinol Metab 1984;58:748–751.
29. Haddy FJ: Endogenous digitalis-like factor or factors. N Engl J Med 1987;316:621–622. Letter.
30. Hager WD, Fenster P, Mayersohn M, et al: Digoxin-quinidine interaction: Pharmacokinetic evaluation. N Engl J Med 1979;300:1238–1241.
31. Henderson RP, Solomon CP: Use of cholestyramine in the treatment of digoxin intoxication. Arch Intern Med 1988; 148:745–746.
32. Hilton PJ, White G, Lord A, et al: An inhibitor of the sodium pump obtained from human placenta. Lancet 1996; 348:303–305.
33. Hollman A: Plants and cardiac glycosides. Br Heart J 1985;54:258–261.
34. Isensee L, Solomon RJ, Weinberg MS, et al: Digoxin levels in dialysis patients. Hosp Physician 1988;24:50–52.
35. Karkal SS, Ordog G, Wasserberg J: Digitalis intoxication: Dealing rapidly and effectively with a complex cardiac toxidrome. Emerg Med Rep 1991;12:29–44.
36. Kelly RA, Smith TW: Pharmacological treatment of heart failure. In: Hardman JG, Limbird LE, Molinoff PB, Ruddon RW, eds: Goodman and Gilman's The Pharmacological Basis of Therapeutics, 9th ed. New York, McGraw-Hill, 1996, pp. 809–838.
37. Kelly RA, Smith TW: Endogenous cardiac glycosides. Adv Pharmacol 1994 25:263–288.
38. Kelly RA, Smith TW: Recognition and management of digitalis toxicity. Am J Cardiol 1992;69:108G–109G.
39. Kinlay S, Buckley N: Magnesium sulfate in the treatment of ventricular arrhythmias due to digoxin toxicity. J Toxicol Clin Toxicol 1995;33:55–59.
40. Klausen T, Kjeldsen K, Norgaard A: Effects of denervation on sodium, potassium and [3H] ouabain binding in muscles of normal and potassium depleted rats. J Physiol 1983: 345:123–124.
41. Koren G, Klein J: Enhancement of digoxin clearance by mannitol diuresis: In vivo studies and their clinical implications. Vet Hum Toxicol 1988;30:25–27.
42. Lalonde RL, Deshpande R, Hamilton PP, et al: Acceleration of digoxin clearance by activated charcoal. Clin Pharmacol Ther 1985;37: 367–371.
43. Leahy EB Jr, Reiffel JA, Drusin RE, et al: Interaction between quinidine and digoxin. JAMA 1978;240:533–534.
44. Lee TC: Van Gogh's vision. JAMA 1981;245: 727–729.
45. Levy G: Gastrointestinal clearance of drugs with activated charcoal. N Engl J Med 1982;307:676–678.
46. Lindenbaum J, Rund DG, Butler VP: Inactivation of digoxin by the gut flora: Reversal by antibiotic therapy. N Engl J Med 1981;305:789–794.
47. Lown B, Byatt NF, Levine HD: Paroxysmal atrial tachycardia with block. Circulation 1960; 21:129–143.
48. Mahdyoon H, Battilana G, Rosman H, et al: The evolving pattern of digoxin intoxication: Observations at a large urban hospital from 1980 to 1988. Am Heart J 1990; 120: 1189–1194.
49. Marbury T, Mahoney J, Juncos L, et al: Advanced digoxin toxicity in renal failure: Treatment with charcoal hemoperfusion. South Med J 1979;72:279–282.
50. McGary SJ, Williams AJ: Digoxin activates sarcoplasmic reticulum Ca^{2+} release channels: A possible role in cardiac inotropy. Br J Pharmacol 1993;108:1043–1050.
51. McRae S: Elevated serum digoxin levels in a patient taking digoxin and siberian ginseng. Can Med Assoc J 1996; 155:292–295.
52. Nanji AA, Greenway DC: Falsely raised plasma digoxin concentrations in liver disease. Br Med J 1985;290:432–433.
53. Pond S, Jacos M, Marks J, et al: Treatment of digitoxin overdose with oral activated charcoal. Lancet 1981;2:1177–1178.
54. Rabetory GM, Price CA, Findlay JWA, et al: Treatment of digoxin intoxication in a renal failure patient with digoxin-specific antibody fragments and plasmapheresis. Am J Nephrol 1990;10:518–521.

55. Reisdorff EJ, Clark MR, Walter BL: Acute digitalis poisoning: The role of intravenous magnesium sulfate. J Emerg Med 1986;4:463–469.
56. Rich SA, Libera JM, Locke RJ: Treatment of foxglove extract poisoning with digoxin-specific Fab fragments. Ann Emerg Med 1993;22:1904–1907.
57. Rodin SM, Johnson BF: Pharmacokinetic interactions with digoxin. Clin Pharmacokinetic 1988;15:227–244.
58. Rosen MR, Wit AL, Hoffman BF: Cardiac antiarrhythmic and toxic effects of digitalis. Am Heart J 1975;89:391–399.
59. Rumack BH, Wolfe RR, Gilfinch H: Diphenylhydantoin treatment of massive digoxin overdose. Br Heart J 1974; 36:405–408.
60. Safadi R, Levy T, Amitai Y, et al: Beneficial effect of digoxin-specific Fab antibody fragments in oleander intoxication. Arch Intern Med 1995;155:2121–2125.
61. Seller RH: The role of magnesium in digitalis toxicity. Am Heart J 1971;82:551–556.
62. Selzer A: Role of serum digoxin assay in patient management. J Am Coll Cardiol 1985, 5:106A–110A.
63. Shilo LM, Adawi A, Solomon G, Shenkman L: Endogenous digoxin-like immunoreactivity in congestive heart failure. Br Med J 1987;295:415–416.
64. Silber B, Sheiner LB, Powers JL, et al: Spironolactone-associated digoxin radioimmunoassay interference. Clin Chem 1979;25:48–54.
65. Smith PK, Winkler AW, Hoff HE: Calcium and digitalis synergism: The toxicity of calcium salts injected intravenously into digitalized animals. Arch Intern Med 1939; 64:322–328.
66. Smith TW: Digitalis. N Engl J Med 1988;318:358–365.
67. Smith TW, Haber E, Yeatman L, et al: Reversal of advanced digoxin intoxication with Fab fragments of digoxin-specific antibodies. N Engl J Med 1976;294:797–800.
68. Spechter MJ, Schweizer E, Goldman RH: Studies on magnesium's mechanism of action in digitalis induced arrhythmias. Circulation 1975;52:1001–1005.
69. Sullivan JB: Immunotherapy in the poisoned patient. Med Toxicol 1986;1:47–60.
70. Taboulet P, Baud FJ, Bismuth C, et al: Acute digitalis intoxication: Is pacing still appropriate? J Toxicol Clin Toxicol 1993;31:261–273.
71. Tuncok Y, Kozan O, Cavdar C, et al: Urginea maritima (squill) toxicity. J Toxicol Clin Toxicol 1995;33:83–86.
72. Valdes R, Graves SW, Brown BA, et al: Endogenous substances in newborn infants causing false-positive digoxin measurements. J Pediatr 1983;102:947–950.
73. Valdes R, Hagberg JM, Vaughn TE, et al: Endogenous digoxin-like immunoreactivity in blood is increased during prolonged strenuous exercise. Life Sci 1988;42:103–110.
74. Warren SE, Fanestil DD: Digoxin overdose: Limitations of hemoperfusion-hemodialysis treatment. JAMA 1979;242: 2100–2101.
75. Watson WA: Factors influencing the clinical efficacy of activated charcoal. Drug Intell Clin Pharm 1987,21:160–166.
76. Whang R, Aikawa J: Magnesium deficiency and refractoriness to potassium repletion. J Chron Dis 1977;30: 65–68.
77. Wildicks EFM, Vermeulen M, van Brummelen P, et al: Digoxin-like immunoreactive substance in patients with aneurysmal subarachnoid hemorrhage. Br Med J 1987;294: 729–732.
78. Withering W: An account of the fox glove and some of its medical uses: With practical remarks on dropsy and other diseases. Med Classics 1937;2:295–443.
79. Woolf AD, Wenger T, Smith TW, et al: The use of digoxin-specific Fab fragments for severe digitalis intoxication in children. N Engl J Med 1992;326:1739–1744.

ANTIDOTES IN DEPTH

Digoxin-Specific Antibody Fragments (Fab)

Mary Ann Howland

The production of digoxin antibody fragments to treat patients intoxicated with digoxin began with the development of digoxin antibodies for measuring serum digoxin concentrations by radioimmunoassay (RIA).[8] The RIA technique permitted the correlation between serum digoxin concentrations and clinical digoxin toxicity. One of the earliest prospective studies of patients receiving therapeutic digoxin demonstrated that toxic patients had statistically significantly higher mean serum digoxin concentrations (2.3 ± 1.6 ng/mL) than nontoxic patients (1.0 ± 0.5 ng/mL), although considerable overlap was present (29% of the toxic group had levels less than 1.7 ng/mL and 15% of the nontoxic group had levels greater than 1.7 ng/mL).[3] Subsequent studies have reaffirmed the benefits of appropriate monitoring of serum digoxin concentrations.[14,15,41]

Butler and Chen suggested that purified digoxin antibodies with a high affinity and specificity should be developed to treat digoxin toxicity in humans.[8] The digoxin molecule alone, with a molecular weight of 780 D, would be too small to be immunogenic. But digoxin could function as a hapten when joined to an immunogenic protein carrier such as serum albumin. These investigators immunized sheep with this conjugate to generate antibodies. The immunized sheep subsequently produced a mixture of antibodies that included antialbumin antibodies and antidigoxin antibodies. The antibodies were separated and highly purified to retain the digoxin antibodies while removing the antibodies to the albumin and all other extraneous proteins. The antibodies developed have a high affinity for digoxin and sufficient cross-reactivity with digitoxin to be clinically useful for the treatment of intoxication from either agent. Moreover, the specificity is so significant that endogenous steroids, which resemble digoxin structurally, are not affected by antibody administration.

In vitro studies followed by in vivo studies in animals demonstrated biologic activity of these antibodies.[10,13,49,50] Investigations proceeded and contributed significantly to understanding of the pharmacodynamics and pharmacokinetics of the antibodies.[9,35,57] Intact IgG antidigoxin antibodies reversed digoxin toxicity in dogs. Unfortunately the urinary excretion of digoxin was delayed, and free digoxin was released later after antibody degradation occurred. Furthermore, concern for hypersensitivity reactions also existed. To make these antibodies safe and effective in humans the whole IgG antidigoxin antibodies were then cleaved with papain, yielding two antigen-binding Fab with a molecular weight of 50,000 D each and one Fc.[9] Because the Fc does not bind antigen, and it increases the potential for hypersensitivity reactions, it was eliminated. The advantages of the digoxin-specific Fab when compared to the whole IgG antibodies include larger volume of distribution, more rapid onset of action, smaller risk of adverse immunologic effects, and more rapid elimination.[9,35,37] Ultimately, the commercial product (Digibind) is a relatively pure Fab product that is very safe and extremely effective.

Mechanism of Action of Digoxin-Specific Antibodies

Immediately following IV administration, Fab digoxin-specific antibodies bind intravascular free digoxin. They then diffuse into the interstitial space, binding free digoxin there. This accounts for the threefold larger V_d at steady state.[60] A concentration gradient is then established, which facilitates movement of the free intracellular digoxin and digoxin that is dissociated from its binding sites (the external surface of Na-K-ATPase enzyme) in the heart into the interstitial or intravascular spaces. The binding affinity of Digibind for digoxin is about 10^9 to 10^{11}, which is greater than the affinity of digoxin for the Na-K-ATPase pump receptor. Intravascular concentrations of inactive, antibody-bound digoxin rise substantially. The elimination kinetics of the Fab antibody-bound digoxin then depends on the patient's renal function and capacity for renal and nonrenal elimination.

Efficacy of Digoxin-Specific Antibodies

One hundred twenty-five patients with a median age of 65 years (all 16 years or older) and 25 patients with a median age of 3 years were treated.[1] Forty-nine percent of cases involved a single unintentional or suicidal overdose, and the remainder involved patients on chronic digitalis therapy. Of the 150 patients treated, 148 were evaluated for cardiovascular manifestations of toxicity; 79 patients (55%) had high-grade AV block, 68 (46%) had refractory ventricular tachycardia, 56 (37%) had hyperkalemia, and 49 (33%) had ventricular fibrillation. Ninety percent of patients have a response to digoxin-specific Fab within minutes to several hours of Digibind administration. Complete resolution of all signs and symptoms of digoxin toxicity occurred in 80% of cases. A partial response was observed in 10% of patients, and of the 15 patients who did not respond, 14 were moribund or actually found not to be digoxin toxic. The spectacular success of digoxin-specific Fab antibodies for patients with digoxin toxicity is demonstrated by the fact that of the 56 patients who had cardiac arrest due to digoxin, 54% survived hospitalization, compared with 100% mortality before the advent of these fragments.[1,5] Newborns, infants, and children have all been successfully treated with Digibind.[4,28,51] Pediatric patients with cardiac abnormalities who develop chronic digoxin toxicity will require small doses of Fab because the total body burden of digoxin will be small, while acute overdoses require Fab doses based on the amount of digoxin ingested, similar to adults.

Safety of Digoxin-Specific Antibody Fragments

Digoxin-specific antibody fragments are not only effective, they are also very safe. In the multicenter study of 150 patients, the only acute clinical manifestations were hypokalemia in 6 patients (4%), worsening of congestive heart failure in 4 patients (3%), and transient apnea in a several-hour old neonate.[1] There were no other reactions reported in any of the patients in this series, although concern for allergic reactions and/or serum sickness remains. In a postmarketing surveillance study of Digibind that included 451 patients, however, 2 patients with a prior history of allergy to antibiotics reportedly developed rashes.[44] One of these patients developed a total body rash, facial swelling, and a flush during the infusion. The other experienced a pruritic rash. Two other adverse reactions (thrombocytopenia and shaking chills) were probably unrelated to the use of Digibind.[44] One patient received Digibind three separate times over the course of 1 year for multiple suicide attempts with no evidence of adverse effects.[6]

Indications for Digoxin-Specific Fab Antibodies

To define the indications for digoxin-specific Fab antibodies, the signs and symptoms of digoxin toxicity must be recognized.[17,55] In general, the manifestations of digoxin toxicity are exaggerations of the pharmacologic effects or alterations of these effects due to ingestion of a single large dose (suicidal or unintentional) or accumulation from chronic dosing, the presence or absence of cardiac pathology, or the patient's age.[17,55] Although there are no absolutes, pediatric patients with normal hearts generally tolerate higher μg/kg dosages of digoxin than do adults. Potassium concentrations in these children tend to remain in the therapeutic range. Serum potassium concentrations result from a balance between the degree and extent of inhibition of the Na-K-ATPase pump and the renal capacity to excrete potassium.[17,55] Healthy children typically maintain renal excretion of potassium except in extreme circumstances. Both adults and children with diseased hearts become digoxin toxic at lower total body loads than their respective healthy counterparts. In the chronically exposed patient, the magnitude of Na-K-ATPase enzyme inhibition in the heart and throughout the body is less extensive prior to the development of symptoms. Many patients who chronically receive digoxin also receive diuretics, which may contribute to smaller rises in serum potassium levels in these patients. Adult patients who ingest a large single dose of digoxin or digitoxin have extensive Na-K-ATPase inhibition and consequently have significant elevations in potassium. When hyperkalemia occurred, before the advent of digoxin-specific Fab, rises in potassium above 5.0 or 5.5 mEq/L indicated a 50 or 100% probability of death, respectively.[5]

Digoxin-specific antibody fragments are indicated for potentially life-threatening digoxin or digitoxin toxicity.[43] Patients with progressive bradydysrhythmias, including severe sinus bradycardia or second or third-degree heart block unresponsive to atropine; and those patients with severe ventricular dysrhythmias, including ventricular tachycardia or ventricular fibrillation, should be treated with digoxin-specific antibody fragments. A ventricular tachycardia with a fascicular block is likely to be a digoxin toxic rhythm.[36] Any patient with a potassium concentration exceeding 5 mEq/L should also be treated. Acute ingestions greater than 4 mg in a healthy child or 10 mg in a healthy adult will probably require antibody treatment. Serum digoxin concentrations do not correlate with myocardial concentrations and are not stable until tissue distribution occurs within about 4 to 6 hours. This time delay is required for digoxin to distribute from the serum to the heart. Serum concentrations of ≥ 15 ng/mL in an acute ingestion will probably require digoxin-specific antibody fragments and are an indication for treatment. A rapid progression of clinical signs and symptoms, such as cardiac and gastrointestinal effects and a rising potassium level in the presence of an acute overdose, suggests a potentially life-threatening ingestion and the need for digoxin antibodies.

In a patient with an unknown ingestion who is clinically ill with characteristics suggestive of intoxication by digoxin, a calcium channel blocking agent, or a beta-adrenergic antagonist, digoxin antibodies should be administered early in management and always prior to calcium use. If digoxin is involved, its effects can be reversed, obviating the need to administer calcium and avoiding the danger of giving calcium to a digoxin-toxic patient. Digoxin toxicity causes intracellular myocardial hypercalcemia, and the administration of exogenous calcium may further exacerbate conduction abnormalities.

When it is difficult to distinguish clinically between digoxin intoxication and intrinsic cardiac disease, the administration of digoxin antibodies can help establish the diagnosis (see Table 48–7).

Time of Onset of Response to Digoxin-Specific Fab

In the multicenter study of 150 patients, the mean time to initial response from the completion of the digoxin antibody infusion (accomplished over 15 minutes to 2 hours) was 19 minutes (range, 0 to 60 minutes), and the time to complete response was 88 minutes (range, 30 to 360 minutes).[13] Time to response was not affected by age, concurrent cardiac disease, or presence of chronic or acute ingestion.[1]

TABLE 48–8. SAMPLE CALCULATION BASED ON HISTORY OF DIGOXIN INGESTION

Adult

Weight: 70 kg

Ingestion: Fifty 0.25-mg digoxin tablets

Calculation:

0.25 mg × 50 = 12.5 mg ingested dose

12.5 mg × 0.80 (80% bioavailability) = 10.0 mg (absorbed dose)

$$\frac{10.0\ \text{mg}}{0.5\ \text{mg}} = 20\ \text{vials}$$

Child

Weight: 10 kg

Ingestion: Fifty 0.25-mg digoxin tablets

Calculation: Same as for adult. Child will require 20 vials

Dosing of Digoxin-Specific Fab

The dose of antibodies depends on the total body load (TBL) of digoxin. Estimates of TBL can be made in three ways: (1) estimate the quantity of digoxin ingested in the acute ingestion and assume 80% bioavailability (X mg ingested × 0.8 = TBL); (2) obtain a serum digoxin concentration, and using a pharmacokinetic formula, incorporate the volume of distribution (V_d) of digoxin and the patient's body weight (in kg); or (3) use an empiric dose based on average requirements for an acute or chronic overdose in an adult or child. Sample calculations for each of these methods are shown in Tables 48–8 to 48–10. Each vial of Digibind contains 38 mg of purified digoxin-specific antibody fragments, which will bind approximately 0.5 mg of digoxin or digitoxin. If the quantity of ingestion cannot be reliably estimated, it may be safest to use the largest calculated estimate. Alternatively, the clinician should be prepared to increase dosing should resolution be incomplete. Inaccurate estimations can occur if the history is faulty; if serum digoxin concentration is determined during the acute phase of distribution—overestimating requirements; and because the volume of distribution figure of 5 L/kg is merely a population estimate that varies considerably in individuals and in certain disease states (decreased in patients with renal disease, hypothyroid, on quinidine).[66]

Administration and Pharmacokinetics

According to the manufacturer, Digibind should be administered IV over 30 minutes via a 0.22-μm membrane filter.[43] The 38-mg vial must be reconstituted with 4 mL of sterile water for IV injection, furnishing an isoosmotic solution. This preparation can be further diluted with sterile isotonic saline (for small infants, addition of 34 mL achieves 1 mg/mL). Once reconstituted it should be used immediately or, if refrigerated, used within 4 hours.[43] In an unstable clinical situation Digibind is given by IV bolus.

In 1976, Smith and associates described the first clinical use of digoxin-specific antibody fragments in a human.[56] Within 1 hour of administration, free (unbound and active) digoxin dropped to an undetectable level. It did not rise until 9 hours later, and the free digoxin reached a peak of only 2 ng/mL at 16 hours and remained at approximately 1.5 ng/mL for the next 40 hours.[56] Total (free plus bound) digoxin, which was 17.6 ng/mL before digoxin-specific antibody fragments were given, rose to 226 ng/mL 1 hour after the start of the infusion, remained there for 11 hours, and then fell over

TABLE 48–9. SAMPLE CALCULATIONS BASED ON THE SERUM DIGOXIN CONCENTRATION

Adult

Weight: 70 kg

Serum digoxin concentration = 10 ng/mL

Volume of distribution = 5 L/kg

Calculation[a]:

$$\frac{\text{Total body load}}{0.5\ \text{mg/vial}} = \text{no. of vials} = \frac{\text{Digoxin serum concentration} \times V_d \times \text{Pt Wt (kg)}}{1000 \times 0.5\ \text{mg/vial}}$$

$$\text{No. of vials} = \frac{10\ \text{ng/mL} \times 5\ \text{L/kg} \times 70\ \text{kg}}{1000 \times 0.5\ \text{mg/vial}}$$

No. of vials = 7

Child

Weight: 10 kg

Serum digoxin concentration: 10 ng/mL

Volume of distribution: 5 L/kg

Calculation[a]:

$$\text{No. of vials} = \frac{10\ \text{ng/mL} \times 5\ \text{L/kg} \times 10\ \text{kg}}{1000 \times 0.5\ \text{mg/vial}}$$

No. of vials = 1

Quick Estimation (for Adults and Children)

$$\text{No. of vials} = \frac{\text{Digoxin serum concentration} \times \text{Pt Wt}}{100}$$

[a]1000 is a conversion factor to change ng/mL and L to mg.

TABLE 48–10. EMPIRIC DOSING RECOMMENDATIONS

Acute Ingestion
Adult: 10–20 vials
Child[a]: 10–20 vials
Chronic Toxicity
Adult: 3–6 vials
Child[b]: 1/4–1/2 vial

[a]Monitor for volume overload in children.

[b]Package insert contains table for infants and children, with corresponding serum concentrations.

the next 44 hours, with a half-life of 20 hours.[56] Fab concentrations peaked at the end of the infusion and then apparently exhibited a biphasic or triphasic decline, probably reflecting distribution into different compartments as well as excretion and catabolism. An analysis of renal elimination based on an incomplete collection suggested that digoxin was excreted only in the bound form during the first 6 hours, but by 30 hours after Fab administration all digoxin was free digoxin. However, this value is very dependent on the dose of Fab in relation to the total body load of digoxin.

Schaumann and associates studied the pharmacokinetics of Fab in 17 patients with acute suicidal ingestions of digoxin.[48] Data from 11 of those patients were used to calculate a median total body digoxin-specific Fab clearance of 24.5 mL/min, of which 13.6 mL/min was renal clearance. The apparent distribution volume for the Fab varied from 25.4 to 54 L, depending on when the calculation was made. In the first 11 patients the dose was 400 to 480 mg (10 to 12 vials), infused over 0.5 to 5 hours. In the last 6 patients, 160 mg (4 vials) was given as a loading dose over 15 minutes, followed by an additional 160 mg given over 7 hours. If the Fab is given so rapidly that elimination occurs before redistribution of digoxin from the binding sites, the total amount of Fab actually bound to digoxin will be less than the predicted or the optimal amount, and digoxin levels may once again increase. In the first 11 patients, the amount of bound to unbound digoxin-specific Fab was about 50%, free digoxin concentrations appeared earlier, and maximum levels were higher than in the last 6 patients. In those 6 patients who received a loading dose followed by a maintenance infusion, the amount of bound Fab was 70%, indicating a better interaction between Fab and digoxin. Free digoxin levels reappeared at 12 to 24 hours and maximum levels averaged only 2.2 ng/mL (0 to 4.4 ng/mL).[48]

These findings[48] suggest some important points. First, it makes more sense to give a loading dose of Fab followed by a maintenance infusion to optimize the binding of digoxin to Fab. The loading dose immediately captures digoxin already in the vascular space and that which can be rapidly redistributed to the vascular space. The maintenance dose provides enough Fab to continue to draw digoxin from the tissues into the serum to be bound. It appears that in acute intentional overdose, 4 to 6 vials given as a loading dose, followed by 0.5 mg/min for 8 hours and then 0.1 mg/min for about 6 hours, should be safe, effective, and efficient.[48] More patients should be studied and the protocol validated before this approach can be generally adopted or recommended. The other important issue raised by Schaumann's study is that the distribution volumes of Fab suggest that they may enter the cells in spite of a molecular weight of 50,000 D.[48]

Additional pharmacokinetic studies indicate that in renal failure the half-life of Fab is prolonged 10-fold with no change in the Vd.[60] Fab serum concentrations remain detectable for 2 to 3 weeks. Total digoxin serum concentrations generally follow Fab. There is no evidence for dissociation of digoxin–Fab over time.[65] However, there is a rebound in free digoxin levels that appears at 12 to 130 hours in patients with renal dysfunction as compared to 12 to 24 hours in patients with normal renal function.[12,16,18,30,39,40,52,54,61,62,65] This rebound is presumed secondary to changes in distribution, with Fab leaving the vascular space and digoxin leaving the tissues. The rebound is delayed in patients with renal dysfunction presumably secondary to a prolonged distribution phase.

Measurement of Digoxin Serum Concentration After Fab Administration

Many laboratories are not equipped to determine free serum digoxin concentrations. Therefore, once digoxin-specific antibody fragments are administered, serum digoxin concentrations are no longer clinically useful, since they represent free plus bound digoxin.[2,21,26,33,58] The type of test employed can either result in falsely high or falsely low serum concentrations depending on which phase (solid or supernatant) is sampled.[25] If the correct dose of Fab is administered, the free serum digoxin concentrations should be near zero. Free digoxin concentrations begin to reappear 5 to 24 hours or longer after Fab administration, depending on the antibody dose, infusion technique, and the patient's renal function. Newer commercial methods employing ultrafiltration make free digoxin measurements easier to perform and therefore more clinically useful.[20,59] Free digoxin concentrations are particularly useful in patients with severe renal dysfunction. Regardless, the patient's cardiac status must be carefully monitored for signs of recurrent toxicity.

Other pitfalls in the measurement and utility of serum digoxin concentrations include endogenous and exogenous factors. Endogenous digoxinlike immunoreactive substances (DLIS) have been described in infants, in women in the third trimester of pregnancy, and in patients with renal and hepatic failure.[19,22,23,27,29,38,63,64] When endogenous DLIS are free or weakly bound, as in these circumstances, they are measurable by the typical RIA assay and can account for factitiously high reported serum digoxin concentrations when the patient is not being treated with digoxin. The role of endogenous DLIS in the body has not been fully elucidated, but it does have an effect on both the sodium potassium ATPase pump and the digoxin glycoside receptor site.[23] Endogenous DLIS have been implicated as a causative factor in hypertension and renal disease. Exogenous factors relate primarily to measurement techniques and interpretation.[31] Digoxin is metabolized to compounds with varying levels of cardioactivity.[34] Some metabolites cross-react and are measured by RIA, while others are not. The in vivo production of these metabolites varies in patients, and may depend on intestinal metabolism by gut flora as well as renal and liver clearance.

Hemodialysis and activated charcoal hemoperfusion have no role in the management of digoxin intoxication. Without the use of Fab, these procedures are not indicated because the molecular weight of digoxin is too large for hemodialysis to be successful. In addition, digoxin's volume of distribution is too large to make either approach feasible. Digoxin-specific antibody fragments are effective even in anephric patients, although symptoms may recur 7 to 14 days later, possibly indicating the need for another dose of Fab. Hemoperfusion through columns with antidigoxin antibodies bound to agarose polyacrolein microsphere beads has been accomplished, but the availability of Fab in the United States makes this modality outmoded.[37,47] The principles that make activated charcoal hemoperfusion less than ideal (V_d of digoxin, extracorporeal access, anticoagulation) also apply to this technique. Continuous arteriovenous hemofiltration in an experimental model has failed to remove the digoxin–Fab complex.[45]

Future research in digoxin-specific antibody fragments hopefully will lead to developing an even smaller antigen-binding fragment, and then manufacturing a consistent product through the use of monoclonal antibody techniques. Experimental studies using monoclonal antibodies in animals have already met with great success.[32]

Role of Digoxin-Specific Antibody Fragments in Poisoning With Other Cardiac Glycosides

Digoxin-specific antibody fragments were designed to have high-affinity binding for digoxin and digitoxin. There are structural similarities, however, between all cardiac glycosides. In fact, radioimmunoassay-determined digoxin levels have been reported in patients following intoxication with nondigoxin cardiac glycosides,[24,42,53] suggesting that cross-reactivity exists between digoxin-specific antibodies and other cardiac glycosides. Thus Digibind may have some efficacy in all natural cardiac glycoside poisonings including oleander, squill, and toad venom.[7,11,46] The successful reversal by Digibind of cardiotoxicity resulting from ingestion of *Nerium oleander* was reported.[53] This patient responded to 5 vials (200 mg) of Fab, but larger doses may be required in other cardiac glycoside poisonings because of the lower-affinity binding of Digibind for these toxins. Treatment decisions should be based on empirical grounds, with initial therapy consisting of 10 to 20 vials. Subsequent doses can be based on clinical response.

References

1. Antman EM, Wenger TL, Butler VP, et al: Treatment of 150 cases of life threatening digitalis intoxication with digoxin specific Fab antibody fragments: Final report of multicenter study. Circulation 1990;81:1744–1752.
2. Argyle JC: Effect of digoxin antibodies on TDX digoxin assay. Clin Chem 1986;32:1616–1617.
3. Beller GA, Smith TW, Abelmann WH, et al: Digitalis intoxication: A prospective clinical study with serum level correlations. N Engl J Med 1971;284:989–997.
4. Berkovitch M, Akilesh MR, Gerace R, et al: Acute digoxin overdose in a newborn with renal failure: Use of digoxin immune Fab and peritoneal dialysis. Ther Drug Monit 1994;16:531–533.
5. Bismuth C, Gaultier M, Conso F, et al: Hyperkalemia in acute digitalis poisoning: Prognostic significance and therapeutic implications. Clin Toxicol 1973;6:153–162.
6. Bosse GM, Pope TM: Recurrent digoxin overdose and treatment with digoxin-specific Fab antibody fragments. J Emerg Med 1994;12:179–185.
7. Brubacher J, Ravikumar P, Bania T, et al: Treatment of toad venom poisoning with digoxin-specific Fab fragments. Chest 1996;110:1282–1288.
8. Butler VP, Chen J: Digoxin specific antibodies. Proc Natl Acad Sci USA 1967;57:71–78.
9. Butler VP, Schmidt DH, Smith TW, et al: Effects of sheep digoxin: Specific antibodies and their Fab fragments on digoxin pharmacokinetics in dogs. J Clin Invest 1977;59: 345–359.
10. Butler VP, Smith TW, Schmidt DH, et al: Immunological reversal of the effects of digoxin. Fed Proc 1977;36: 2235–2241.
11. Cheung K, Urech R, Taylor L, et al: Plant cardiac glycosides and digoxin Fab antibody. J Pediatr Child Health 1991; 27:312–313.
12. Colucci R, Choses M, Kluger J, et al: The pharmacokinetics of digoxin immune Fab, total digoxin and free digoxin in patients with renal impairment. Pharmacotherapy 1989;9: 175. Abstract.
13. Curd J, Smith TW, Jaton J, et al: The isolation of digoxin specific antibody and its use in reversing the effects of digoxin. Proc Natl Acad Sci 1971;68:2401–2406.
14. D'Angio RG, Stevenson JG, Lively BT, et al: Therapeutic drug monitoring: Improved performance through educational intervention. Ther Drug Monit 1990;12:173–181.
15. Duhme DW, Greenblatt DJ, Kock-Weser J: Reduction of digoxin toxicity associated with measurement of serum levels: A report from the Boston Collaborative Drug Surveillance Program. Ann Intern Med 1974;80:516–519.
16. Durham G, Califf RM: Digoxin toxicity in renal insufficiency treated with digoxin immune Fab. Prim Cardiol 1988;1:31–34.
17. Eagle KA, Haber E, DeSanctis RW, et al, eds: The Practice of Cardiology, 2nd ed. Boston, Little, Brown, 1989.
18. Erdmann E, Mair W, Knedel M, et al: Digitalis intoxication and treatment with digoxin antibody fragments in renal failure. Klin Wochenschr 1989;67:16–19.
19. Frisolone J, Sylvia LM, Gelwan J, et al: False positive serum digoxin concentrations determined by three digoxin assays on patients with liver disease. Clin Pharm 1988;7: 444–449.
20. George S, Braithwaite RA, Hughes EA: Digoxin measurements following plasma ultrafiltration in two patients with

digoxin toxicity treated with specific Fab fragments. Ann Clin Biochem 1994;31:380–381.

21. Gibb I, Adams PC, Parnham AJ, et al: Plasma digoxin: Assay anomalies in Fab treated patients. Br J Clin Pharmacol 1983;16:445–447.
22. Graves SW, Brown B, Valdes R: An endogenous digoxin like substance in patients with renal impairment. Ann Intern Med 1983;99:604–608.
23. Hastreiter AR, John EG, Nander Hoist RL: Digitalis, digitalis antibodies, digitalis like immunoreactive substances, and sodium homeostasis: A review. Clin Perinatol 1988;15: 491–522.
24. Haynes BE, Bessen HA, Wightman WD, et al: Oleander tea: Herbal draught of death. Ann Emerg Med 1985;14:350–353.
25. Honda SAA, Rios CN, Murakami L, et al: Problems in determining levels of free digoxin in patients treated with digoxin immune Fab. J Clin Lab Anal 1995;9:407–412.
26. Hursting MJ, Raisys VA, Opheim KE, et al: Determination of free digoxin concentrations in serum for monitoring Fab treatment of digoxin overdose. Clin Chem 1987;33: 1652–1655.
27. Karboski JA, Godley PJ, Frohna PA, et al: Marked digoxin like immunoreactive factor interference with an enzyme immunoassay. Drug Intell Clin Pharm 1988;2:703–705.
28. Kaufman J, Leikin J, Kendzierski D, Polin K: Use of digoxin Fab immune fragments in a seven-day-old infant. Pediatr Emerg Care 1990;6:118–121.
29. Kelly RA, O'Hara DS, Canessa MG, et al: Characterization of digitalis like factors in human plasma. J Biol Chem 1905;260:11396–11405.
30. Koren G, Deatie D, Soldin S: Agonal elevation in serum digoxin concentrations in infants and children long after cessation of therapy. Crit Care Med 1988;16:793–795.
31. Koren G, Parker R: Interpretation of excessive serum concentrations of digoxin in children. Am J Cardiol 1985; 55:1210–1214.
32. Lechat P, Mudgett-Hunter M, Margolies M, et al: Reversal of lethal digoxin toxicity in guinea pigs using monoclonal antibodies and Fab fragments. J Pharmacol Exp Ther 1984; 229:210–215.
33. Lemon M, Andrews DJ, Binks AM, et al: Concentrations of free serum digoxin after treatment with antibody fragments. Br Med J 1987;295:1520–1521.
34. Lindenbaum J, Rund D, Butler VP, et al: Inactivation of digoxin by the gut flora: Reversal by antibiotic therapy. N Engl J Med 1981;305:789–794.
35. Lloyd BL, Smith TW: Contrasting rates of reversal of digoxin toxicity by digoxin: Specific IgG and Fab fragments. Circulation 1978;58:280–283.
36. Marchlinski FE, Hook BG, Callans DJ: Which cardiac disturbances should be treated with digoxin immune Fab (ovine) antibody? Am J Emerg Med 1991;9:24–34.
37. Marcus L, Margel S, Savin H, et al: Therapy of digoxin intoxication in dogs by specific hemoperfusion through agarose polyacrolein microsphere beads: Antidigoxin antibodies. Am Heart J 1985;110:30–39.
38. Naomi S, Graves S, Lazarus M, et al: Variation in apparent serum digitalis-like factor levels with different digoxin antibodies: The "immunochemical fingerprint." Am J Hypertens 1991;4:795–800.
39. Nollet H, Verhaaren H, Stroobandt R, et al: Delayed elimination of digoxin antidolum determined by RIA. J Clin Pharmacol 1989;29:41–45.
40. Nuwayhid N, Johnson G: Digoxin elimination in a functionally anephric patient after digoxin specific Fab fragment therapy. Ther Drug Monit 1989;11:680–685.
41. Ordog GJ, Benaron S, Bhasin V: Serum digoxin levels and mortality in 5100 patients. Ann Emerg Med 1987;16:32–39.
42. Osterloh J, Herold S, Pond S: Oleander interference in the digoxin radioimmunoassay in a fatal ingestion. JAMA 1982;247:1596–1597.
43. Physicians Desk Reference, 45th ed. Oradell, NJ, Medical Economics, 1991, pp. 755–756.
44. Postmarketing Surveillance Study of Digibind: Interim Report to Contributors. Research Triangle Park, NC, Burroughs Wellcome, July 1986–July 1987.
45. Quaife EJ, Banner W, Vernon D, et al: Failure of CAVH to remove digoxin Fab complex in piglets. J Toxicol Clin Toxicol 1990;28:61–68.
46. Safadi R, Levy I, Amitai Y, Caraco Y: Beneficial effect of digoxin-specific Fab antibody fragments in oleander intoxication. Arch Inter Med 1995:155:2121–2125.
47. Savin H, Marcus L, Margel S, et al: Treatment of adverse digitalis effect by hemoperfusion through columns with antidigoxin antibodies bound to agarose polyacrolein microsphere beads. Am Heart J 1987;113:1078–1084.
48. Schaumann W, Kaufmann B, Neubert P, et al: Kinetics of the Fab fragments of digoxin antibodies and of bound digoxin in patients with severe digoxin intoxication. Eur J Clin Pharmacol 1986;30:527–533.
49. Schmidt DH, Butler VP: Immunological protection against digoxin toxicity. J Clin Invest 1971;50:866–871.
50. Schmidt DH, Butler VP: Reversal of digoxin toxicity with specific antibodies. J Clin Invest 1971;50:1738–1744.
51. Schmitt K, Tulzer G, Hackel F, et al: Massive digitoxin intoxication treated with digoxin-specific antibodies in a child. Pediatr Cardiol 1994;15:48–49.
52. Sherron PA, Gelband H: Reversal of digoxin toxicity with Fab fragments in a pediatric patient with acute renal failure. Paper presented at Management of Digitalis Toxicity: The Role of Digibind, San Francisco, July 26–28, 1985. Burroughs Wellcome, sponsor.
53. Shumaik GM, Wu AU, Ping AC: Oleander poisoning: Treatment with digoxin-specific Fab antibody fragments. Ann Emerg Med 1988;17:732–735.
54. Sinclair AJ, Hewick DS, Johnston PC, et al: Kinetics of digoxin and anti-digoxin antibody fragments during treatment of digoxin toxicity. Br J Clin Pharmacol 1989;28: 352–356.
55. Smith TW: New advances in the assessment and treatment of digitalis toxicity. J Clin Pharmacol 1985;25:522–528.
56. Smith TW, Haber E, Yeatman L, et al: Reversal of advanced digoxin intoxication with Fab fragments of digoxin specific antibodies. N Engl J Med 1976;294:797–800.
57. Smith TW, Lloyd BL, Spicer N, et al: Immunogenicity and kinetics of distribution and elimination of sheep digoxin specific IgG and Fab fragments in the rabbit and baboon. Clin Exp Immunol 1979;36:384–396.
58. Soldin S: Digoxin: Issues and Controversies. Clin Chem 1986;32:5–12.

59. Ujhelyi MR, Colucci RD, Cummings DM, et al: Monitoring serum digoxin concentrations during digoxin immune Fab therapy. Ann Pharmacother 1991;25:1047–1049.
60. Ujhelyi MR, Robert S: Pharmacokinetic aspects of digoxin-specific Fab therapy in the management of digitalis toxicity. Clin Pharmacokinet 1995;28:483–493.
61. Ujhelyi MR, Robert S, Cummings DM, et al: Disposition of digoxin immune Fab in patients with kidney failure. Clin Pharmacol Ther 1993;54:388–394.
62. Ujhelyi MR, Robert S, Cummings DM, et al: Influence of digoxin immune Fab therapy and renal dysfunction on the disposition of total and free digoxin. Ann Intern Med 1993;119:273–277.
63. Vasdev S, Johnson E, Longerich L, et al: Plasma endogenous digitalis like factors in healthy individuals and in dialysis dependent and kidney transplant patients. Clin Nephrol 1987;27:169–174.
64. Vinge E, Ekman R: Partial characterization of endogenous digoxin like substance in human urine. Ther Drug Monit 1988;10:8–15.
65. Wenger TL: Experience with digoxin immune Fab (ovine) in patients with renal impairment. Am J Emerg Med 1991;9:21–23.
66. Winter ME: Digoxin. In: Koda-Kimble MA, Young LY, eds: Basic Clinical Pharmacokinetics, 3rd ed. Vancouver, Applied Therapeutics, 1994, p. 200.

CHAPTER 49

Beta-Adrenergic Antagonists

Jeffrey R. Brubacher

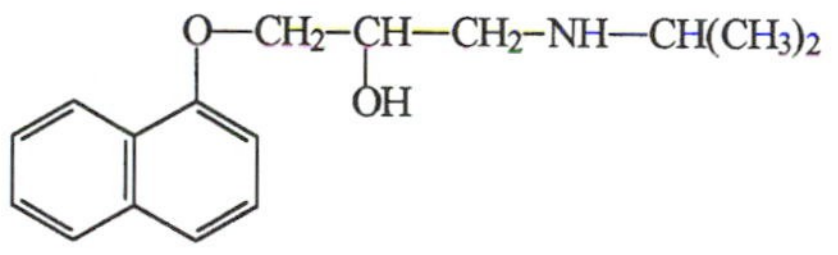

Propranolol

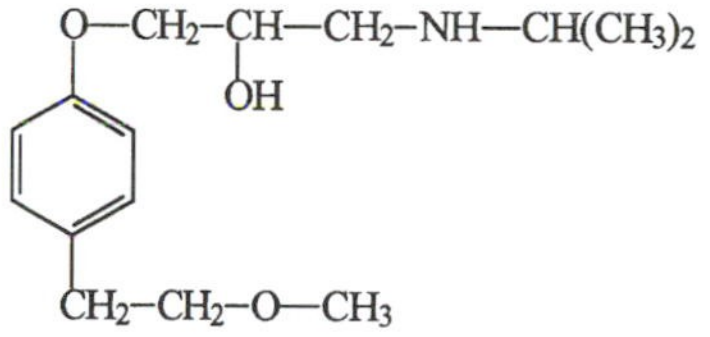

Metoprolol

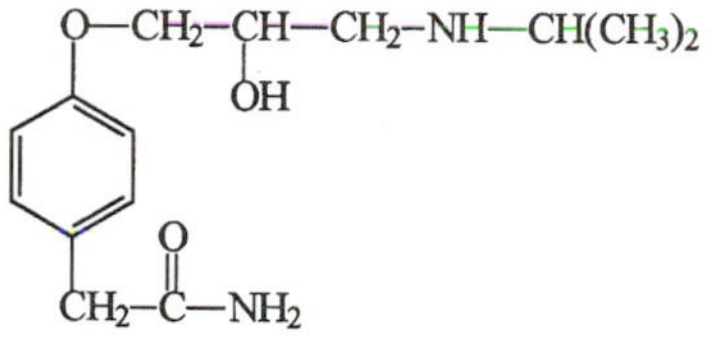

Atenolol

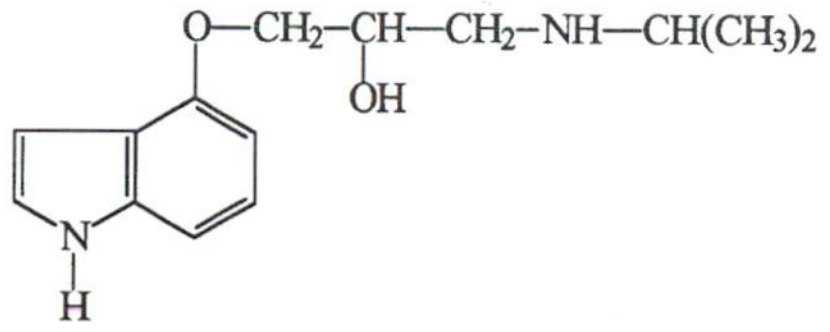

Pindolol

A 64 year-old-man was brought to the emergency department by ambulance after being found comatose by his family. The paramedics had found him to be hypoventilating with respirations of 10 breaths/minute, a pulse of 45 beats/minute, and a blood pressure of 80 mm Hg by palpation. He was intubated and received 2 mg naloxone IV, 1 mg atropine IV, and a 500-mL bolus of normal saline. During transport to hospital, the patient had a generalized seizure that responded to 5 mg of intravenous diazepam. On arrival in the emergency department, the patient was intubated and ventilated with the following vital signs: blood pressure, 85 mm Hg by palpation; pulse, 50 beats/minute; temperature 96.8°F (36°C). On 100% oxygen the patient's oxygen saturation by pulse oximetry was 99% and his fingerstick glucose level was 80 mg/dL. Physical examination was otherwise unremarkable except for occasional scattered basilar crackles. Heart sounds were normal with no murmurs. Pupils were 6 mm and reactive, skin was cool, and bowel sounds were decreased. The patient was given 100 mg thiamine IV, 50 mL 50% dextrose IV, and 2 mg naloxone IV with no response. One of the medical staff was sent to interview the family.

Blood specimens were sent for a complete blood count, electrolytes, glucose, renal function, and creatine phosphokinase. Arterial blood was sent for blood gas analysis. A 12-lead electrocardiogram showed sinus bradycardia with a PR interval of 280 msec and a QRS width of 140 msec. During the next several minutes the patient's vital signs deteriorated. His blood pressure decreased to 75 mm Hg and his pulse decreased to 40 beats per minute. He was given an additional 2 mg of atropine IV and another 500 mL of normal saline, with little change in blood pressure or heart rate. External cardiac pacing was instituted and increased the pulse to 70 per minute. Unfortunately, the blood pressure fell to 60 mm Hg with pacing, and this intervention was discontinued. A central venous line was placed and a dopamine infusion was started. There was no response to a dopamine infusion at 20 μg/kg per minute.

Further history was obtained from the patient's son. The patient had previously been healthy except for a history of depression and hypertension. He had been taking antidepressants, but his son believed that these had been stopped for several months. He was currently taking only an antihypertensive medication that had been prescribed recently. No one else in the family took any pills. The family stated that the patient had been more depressed in the last 2 weeks, with apathy, decreased appetite, and inability to sleep. On the day of admission, however, he had seemed better. He had eaten breakfast, taken a shower, and went for a walk before he returned home to take a nap. The patient was well prior to his nap, but 2 hours later the family could not arouse him for lunch and they called the ambulance. A family member was requested to return home and bring all medication bottles to the emergency department. A call was placed to the patient's family physician.

Given the possibility of an overdose, analysis of acetaminophen and salicylate was added to the bloodwork. Because the history of depression, seizures, hypotension, and widened QRS interval suggested a tricyclic antidepressant overdose, the patient was given 2 ampules (50 mL each) of hypertonic sodium bicarbonate. There was no change in the patient's vital signs afterwards, and a repeat electrocardiogram was essentially unchanged except that the QRS interval had narrowed to 130 msec. A bicarbonate infusion was started. Because of the possibility that a calcium channel blocking medication had been ingested, the patient was given 1 g of calcium chloride intravenously. Following this the blood pressure increased to 75 mm Hg while the pulse remained at 40 per minute.

The family physician called and stated that he had given the patient an immediate release form of propranolol for hypertension 2 weeks earlier. One of the patient's daughters returned with all the medication bottles that she could find. Several bottles of vitamins and over-the-counter analgesics were almost full but the propranolol bottle was empty. About 5 g of propranolol were missing from the bottle.

As a result of obtaining this additional information, the patient was given intravenous glucagon. After a total of 5 mg of glucagon was administered over a 10-minute period the patient's blood pressure increased to 105/60 mm Hg and his pulse increased to 55 beats per minute. A glucagon infusion at 5 mg/h was started and the patient was admitted to the intensive care unit. Laboratory analysis was negative for salicylates and acetaminophen. The electrolytes, glucose, renal function, complete blood count, and arterial blood gas were all within normal limits except for a mild anion gap metabolic acidosis, which resolved when the analysis was repeated after the patient's vital signs had normalized.

By the next day, the patient had regained consciousness and his blood pressure remained normal after the glucagon infusion was stopped. He was extubated and later admitted to taking an overdose of propranolol in a suicide attempt. The patient was assessed by a psychiatrist, who felt that his depression had been exacerbated by propranolol. Propranolol was discontinued, and his antidepressants were restarted. The patient was started on a calcium channel blocker for hypertension and briefly admitted to psychiatry. On follow-up one month after discharge he was doing well with no complaints. He no longer felt depressed and his blood pressure was well controlled.

What Is the Epidemiology of Beta-Adrenergic Antagonist Overdose?

Intentional beta-adrenergic antagonist overdose is relatively uncommon but continues to account for a small number of deaths annually. During the 7-year period from 1989 to 1995, there were over 5000 beta-adrenergic antagonist exposures per year reported by the Toxic Exposure Surveillance System of the American Association of Poison Control Centers. These exposures accounted for an average of 15 deaths and 90 "major outcomes" annually. Children under the age of 6 accounted for about one third of the exposures, but no deaths were reported in this age group.[59–65] In England and Wales, beta-adrenergic antagonist toxicity accounted for just over 20 deaths annually during the period from 1975 to 1984. In comparison, carbon monoxide annually causes over 5000 deaths in the United States and over 1000 deaths in England and Wales.[32]

Several authors report that, compared to the other beta-adrenergic antagonists, propranolol accounts for a disproportionate number of cases of self-poisoning[17,89] and deaths.[51] This may be explained by the fact that propranolol is frequently prescribed to patients with diagnoses such as anxiety, stress, and migraine who may be more prone to suicide attempts.[89] Propranolol may also be more toxic due to its lipophilic and membrane-stabilizing properties.[33,89]

How Does Myocyte Calcium Flow Relate to Contractility?

Striated muscle contraction is an energy-dependent process that involves the calcium dependent interaction of actin and myosin. At rest this is prevented by the troponin–tropomyosin complex, which is in intimate contact with actin. Myocyte excitation triggers a series of events that increase cytoplasmic calcium concentrations from approximately 10^{-7} M during diastole to 10^{-5} M during systole. Calcium binds to troponin C, causing a conformational change in the troponin–tropomyosin complex that permits actin–myosin cross-linkage. Actin activates the myosin ATPase, which links ATP hydrolysis to conformational changes in the globular ends of myosin heavy chains, resulting in sliding of myosin and actin chains relative to each other and ultimately in muscle contraction.[1,6]

Extracellular calcium concentrations are 5000 to 10,000 times greater than intracellular concentrations. This gradient is maintained by ion pumps that actively remove calcium from the cytoplasm.[87,88] Voltage-sensitive slow calcium channels open in response to cell depolarization and calcium flows into the myocyte. This calcium current opens calcium-release channels in the sarcoplasmic reticulum, which releases large amounts of calcium from sarcoplasmic stores. The strength of contraction is proportional to the amount of calcium released from the sarcoplasmic reticulum, which in turn is proportional to the amount of calcium entering the cell through slow calcium channels and to the amount of calcium stored in the sarcoplasmic reticulum. The actin–myosin interaction is also modulated by other factors including troponin phosphorylation and intracellular pH (Fig. 49–1).[6]

Following contraction, calcium must be removed from the cytoplasm to allow muscle relaxation. Unlike calcium entry, calcium removal occurs against a concentration gradient and requires the expenditure of energy. The most rapid mechanism for calcium removal is the calcium–sodium transporter, which exchanges 1 molecule of calcium for 3 molecules of sodium. Under most conditions, electrochemical gradients favor the extrusion of calcium from the cell coupled to the entry of sodium. Increased intracellular sodium concentration and cell depolarization decrease this gradient, and under these conditions the pump may actually "run in reverse" and allow entry of calcium coupled with extrusion of sodium. A second mechanism for calcium removal is the cytoplasmic membrane calcium pump, which uses energy from the hydrolysis of ATP to pump calcium out of the cell. A similar calcium ATPase located on the sarcoplasmic membrane pumps calcium into the sarcoplasmic reticulum, where it is bound to calsequestrin. The sarcoplasmic calcium pump is inhibited by the binding of phospholamban. Phosphorylation of phospholamban removes this inhibition, resulting in greater calcium stores in the sarcoplasmic reticulum and hence greater calcium release with subsequent cell depolarizations.[6]

What Are the Different Subtypes of Beta-Adrenergic Receptors?

All beta-adrenergic receptors are coupled to G_s proteins, which activate adenylate cyclase when the receptor is stimulated by catecholamines such as epinephrine or norepinephrine. This activation increases intracellular cyclic AMP (cAMP), which in turn activates protein kinase A and other cAMP-dependent protein kinases.[58] These activated protein kinases mediate the ultimate cellular effects of β-stimulation by phosphorylation of key intracellular enzymes, ion channels, and other proteins (Fig. 49–2).

Beta-adrenergic stimulation modulates the function of the heart, vasculature, lungs, and numerous other organs and causes complex metabolic effects. Beta-adrenergic receptors are divided into β_1, β_2, and β_3 subtypes. The most prevalent subtype in the heart is the β_1-adrenergic receptor, although cardiac β_2-adrenergic receptors also exist. Beta-adrenergic stimulation of the heart results in increased contractility, increased conduction velocity,

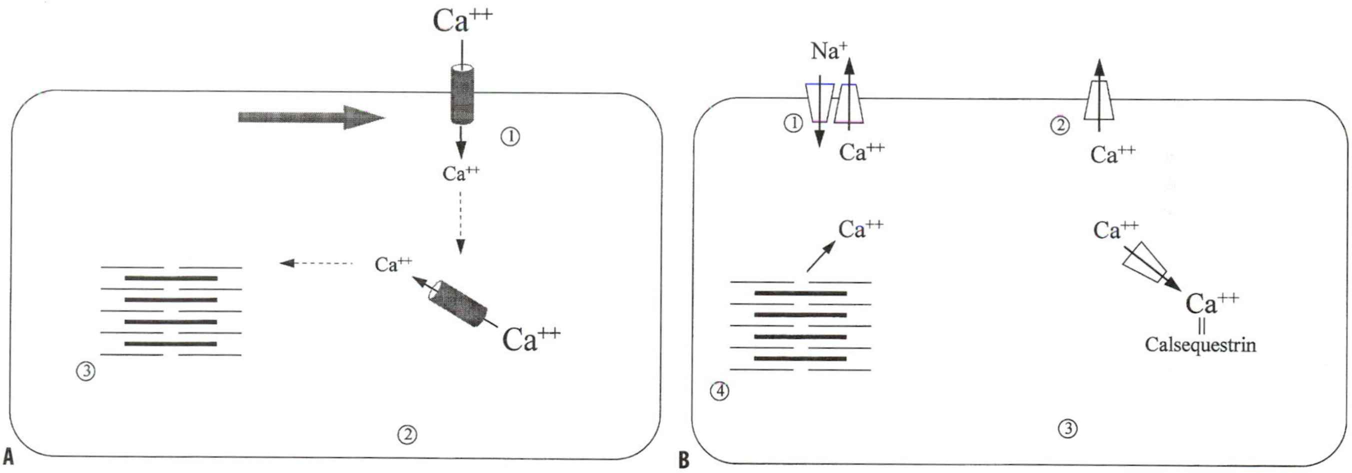

Figure 49–1. A. Fluctuations in calcium levels couple myocyte depolarization with contraction and myocyte repolarization with relaxation. 1. Depolarization causes voltage-sensitive calcium channels to open and calcium to flow down its concentration gradient into the myocyte. 2. This triggers the opening of calcium release channels in the sarcoplasmic reticulum (SR), and calcium pours out of the SR. The amount of calcium released from the SR is proportional to the initial inward calcium current and to the amount of calcium stored in the SR. 3. At rest, actin–myosin interaction is prevented by troponin. When calcium binds to troponin, this inhibition is removed and actin and myosin slide relative to each other and the cell contracts. **B.** Following contraction, calcium is actively removed from the myocyte to allow relaxation. 1. The calcium sodium transporter couples the flow of three molecules of sodium flow in one direction to that of a single molecule of calcium in the opposite direction. This transporter is passively driven by electrochemical gradients that usually favor the inward flow of sodium coupled to the extrusion of calcium. Extrusion of calcium is inhibited by higher intracellular sodium concentrations and by cell depolarization, and under these conditions the pump may actually "run in reverse." 2. Calcium is actively pumped from the cell by a calcium ATPase. 3. Another similar calcium ATPase pumps calcium into the SR, where it is bound to calsequestrin. Calcium stored in the SR is available for release during subsequent depolarizations. The sarcoplasmic calcium ATPase is inhibited by phospholamban (see Fig. 49–2). 4. As myocyte calcium concentrations fall, calcium is released from troponin and the myocyte relaxes.

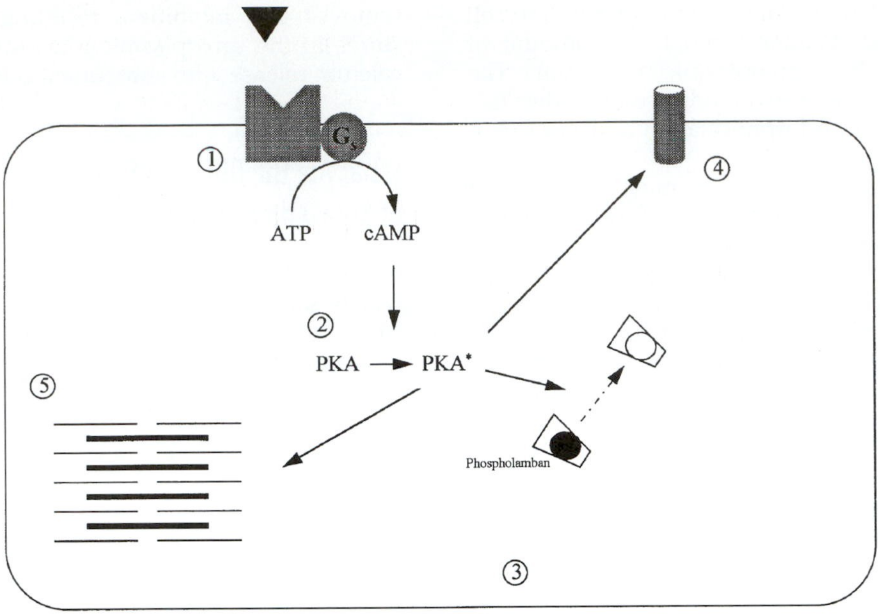

Figure 49–2. Beta-adrenergic agonists are positive inotropes by virtue of their ability to activate protein kinase A (PKA). 1. Beta-adrenergic receptors are coupled to G_S proteins, which activate adenyl cyclase when catecholamines bind to the receptor. Adenyl cyclase increases formation of cAMP from ATP. 2. Increased cAMP levels activate PKA, which mediates the ultimate effects of beta-adrenergic receptor stimulation by phosphorylating key intracellular proteins. 3. Phosphorylation of phospholamban disinhibits the sarcoplasmic reticulum (SR) calcium ATPase, resulting in increased SR calcium stores available for release during subsequent depolarizations. 4. Phosphorylation of voltage-sensitive calcium channels increases calcium influx through these channels during systole. 5. The phosphorylation of troponin improves cardiac performance by facilitating calcium liberation during diastole.

and increased automaticity. Peripheral vascular resistance is largely controlled by arteriolar muscle tone. Alpha-adrenergic stimulation causes arteriolar constriction in contrast to β_2 receptor stimulation which causes arteriolar dilation. In the lungs, β_2-adrenergic receptor stimulation results in bronchodilation and also increases respiratory secretions. Beta-adrenergic agonists have important endocrine and metabolic effects. Renin secretion is increased by β_1 stimulation and insulin secretion is increased by β_2 stimulation. In spite of increased insulin, β_2-adrenergic receptor stimulation increases glucose by increasing hepatic gluconeogenesis, and skeletal muscle and hepatic glycogenolysis. Skeletal muscle potassium uptake is increased by β_2 stimulation, resulting in hypokalemia. Gut motility is decreased by both β_1 and β_2 stimulation. Beta agonists act at fat cells to cause lipolysis and thermogenesis.[39]

Recently a new beta-adrenergic receptor, referred to as the β_3 receptor, has been discovered. The pharmacology of this receptor differs substantially from that of the other beta receptors. In fact, the classic beta-adrenergic antagonists actually act as agonists at this receptor. Isoproterenol is an agonist at all three beta receptors.[109] The role of the β_3-adrenergic receptor in humans is incompletely understood. This receptor is found on human adipocytes, where it plays a role in mediating thermogenesis and lipolysis.[22] Some investigators have shown that β_3 receptors in the human heart increase cardiac contractility.[127]

What Are the Mechanisms of Action of Beta-Adrenergic Receptor Agonists and Other Inotropic Agents?

Cardiac contractility can be increased by several mechanisms. As discussed, any agent that increases sarcoplasmic calcium stores will enhance contractility by increasing the pool of calcium available for release during depolarization. This is the ultimate mechanism of action of most inotropic agents and may be achieved by increasing the activity of the sarcoplasmic calcium pump, increasing calcium influx during depolarization or decreasing calcium efflux during repolarization. Agents that decrease or reverse the activity of the calcium–sodium exchange pump will increase contractility by slowing calcium efflux. This provides higher calcium concentrations throughout the cardiac cycle, and allows greater time for the sarcoplasmic pump to move calcium into the sarcoplasmic reticulum, translating into greater sarcoplasmic calcium stores. Digoxin and similar compounds achieve this effect by increasing intracellular sodium concentrations. Similarly, a prolonged action potential duration (APD) will inhibit the calcium–sodium exchange pump by increasing the time when the cell is depolarized. Increased APD will further increase intracellular calcium concentrations by prolonging the time that voltage-sensitive calcium channels are open. Agents such as 4-aminopyridine, which prolong APD by blocking outward potassium channels, may increase contractility by these mechanisms.[6,7,36,112]

Cyclic AMP mediates the inotropic effect of beta-adrenergic agonists, glucagon, forskolin, and the phosphodiesterase inhibitors by activating protein kinase A, which in turn phosphorylates important myocyte proteins including phospholamban, the voltage-sensitive calcium channels, and troponin.[31,111] Calcium channel phosphorylation increases contractility by increasing the influx of calcium during each cell depolarization.[91,107] Phosphorylation of phospholamban increases the activity of the sarcoplasmic calcium ATPase and thus enhances contractility by increasing sarcoplasmic calcium stores.[18,111] Dephosphorylation of phospholamban probably also plays an important role in intracellular calcium handling, but the mechanisms controlling this event are poorly understood. Troponin phosphorylation facilitates calcium unbinding and improves cardiac performance by enhancing actin–myosin relaxation (Fig. 49–3).[1,6,111]

Glucagon receptors, like beta-adrenergic receptors, are coupled to G_S proteins. Glucagon binding increases adenyl cyclase activity independent of beta-adrenergic stimulation.[128] It has recently been shown that humans have cardiac glucagon receptors identical to those found in the pancreas,[124] and it is probable that glucagon's positive inotropic action is due to increased adenyl cyclase activity causing increased myocyte cAMP levels. The inotropic effect of glucagon is enhanced by its ability to inhibit phosphodiesterase and thereby prevent cAMP breakdown.[72] The experimental agent forskolin also increases cAMP levels by a non-beta-adrenergic mechanism.[15] Phosphodiesterase inhibitors such as amrinone, milrinone, and enoximone are also positive inotropes by virtue of their ability to increase cAMP levels.

The actions of alpha$_1$-adrenergic stimulation are ultimately mediated by protein kinase C (PKC), which like protein kinase A, phosphorylates intracellular proteins and modifies their function. Protein kinase C is actually a heterogenous group of proteins that is activated by other signals in addition to alpha$_1$ stimulation. Compared with protein kinase A, the consequences of PKC stimulation are not well understood. In many tissues, PKC modifies long-term functions such as gene expression, receptor downregulation, and immune and inflammatory responses.[77,85] In the heart, PKC does not phosphorylate phospholamban but appears to phosphorylate slow calcium channels, and this may play a role in the positive contractile response to alpha$_1$ simulation.[114] Nevertheless, some studies have demonstrated decreased contractility following PKC activation.[13]

Intracellular pH also modifies contractility. Alkalosis augments the sensitivity of the contractile proteins to calcium. Agents such as angiotensin II and endothelin are believed to exert their inotropic effect by increasing intracellular pH,[6] and the positive inotropic action of 4-aminopyridine may be caused in part by this mechanism.[102]

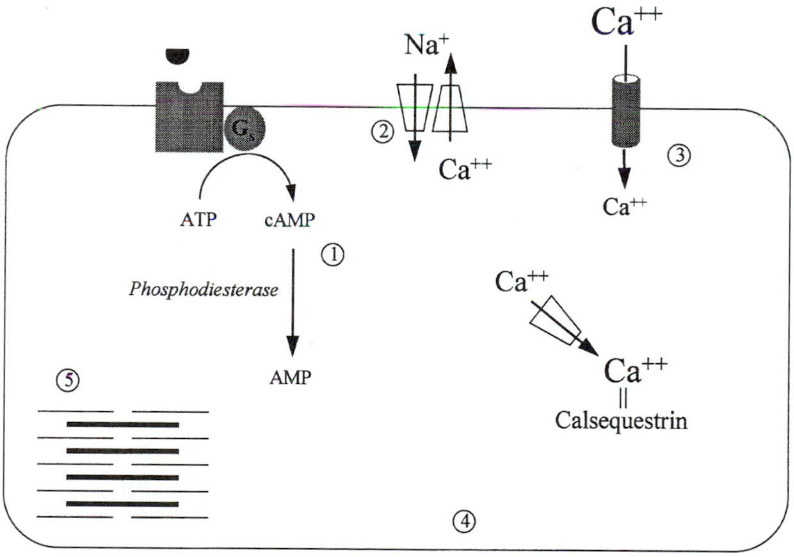

Figure 49–3. Inotropic agents act by several mechanisms. 1. Agents that increase cAMP increase contractility, as outlined in Fig. 49–2. Glucagon receptors and beta-adrenergic receptors are coupled to G_S proteins so that receptor binding increases cAMP by activation of adenyl cyclase. Phosphodiesterase inhibitors such as amrinone, milrinone, and enoxime increase cAMP by preventing its breakdown. The experimental inotropic agent, forskolin, also increases cAMP. 2. Agents such as digoxin that increase intracellular sodium concentrations, or agents such as 4-aminopyridine that prolong the time that the myocyte is depolarized, will decrease or reverse the electrochemical gradient favoring calcium extrusion by the sodium–calcium transporter. This increases intracellular calcium levels, resulting in increased contractility. 3. The activity of the voltage-sensitive calcium channels is increased by protein kinase A-mediated phosphorylation. Agents that prolong the action potential duration also allow greater calcium influx through these channels by allowing them to remain open for longer. 5. Intracellular alkalosis increases sensitivity of the contractile elements to calcium. Angiotensin II and endothelin are inotropes by virtue of their ability to induce intracellular alkalosis. Cardiac performance is also increased by troponin phosphorylation as described in Fig. 49–2.

What Are the Clinical Uses of Beta-Adrenergic Antagonists?

Beta-adrenergic antagonists are used in the treatment of hypertension, angina, tachydysrhythmias, and theophylline overdoses and have been shown to decrease mortality following myocardial infarction. Additional indications of beta-adrenergic antagonists include migraine headaches, tremor, panic attack, and hyperthyroidism. Ophthalmic preparations containing beta-adrenergic antagonists are used in the treatment of glaucoma.[39]

Beta-adrenergic antagonists competitively antagonize the effects of catecholamines at the beta-adrenergic receptor resulting in decreased chronotropy and contractility, which are manifested clinically as lowered heart rate and blood pressure. These effects are more important in times of exertion or stress, when sympathetic tone is increased. The antihypertensive effect of beta-adrenergic antagonists is counteracted by a reflex increase in peripheral vascular resistance. This effect is augmented by the β_2 antagonism seen with nonselective beta-adrenergic antagonists. Long-term use of beta-adrenergic antagonists causes decreased peripheral vascular resistance. The mechanism for this effect is poorly understood.[39]

Patients with reactive airways disease may suffer severe bronchospasm after using beta-adrenergic antagonists. This effect is caused by loss of β_2-mediated bronchodilation and is more likely to be a problem following the use of nonselective beta-adrenergic antagonists. Catecholamines inhibit mast cell degranulation through a β_2-adrenergic mechanism. Interference with this effect by beta-adrenergic antagonism may predispose to life-threatening anaphylactic reactions in atopic individuals. Patients taking beta-adrenergic antagonists who develop allergic reactions should therefore be monitored more closely than other patients, and allergy testing should be avoided in these patients. Beta-adrenergic antagonists interfere with glycogenolysis and gluconeogenesis, resulting in impaired ability to recover from hypoglycemia. Furthermore, beta-adrenergic antagonism may mask the sympathetic discharge that serves to warn of hypoglycemia. This combination frequently proves dangerous for diabetic patients at risk for hypoglycemic episodes.[39]

What Are the Pharmacologic Properties of Beta-Adrenergic Antagonists?

Beta-adrenergic antagonists differ in their lipid solubility, oral availability, first-pass effect, protein binding, metabolism, β_1 selectivity, and intrinsic sympathomimetic activity. Certain beta-adrenergic antagonists possess additional properties such as the ability to block sodium channels (membrane-stabilizing activity), potassium channels (delayed repolarization), and to act as an α-adrenergic agonist. Table 49–1 summarizes the pharmacologic properties of individual beta-adrenergic antagonists.[26,39,80,113]

The important nonselective beta-adrenergic antagonists are labetolol, nadolol, oxprenolol, pindolol, propranolol, sotalol, and timolol. The nonselective agents are theoretically less effective antihypertensive agents than the selective agents because they prevent β_2-mediated vasodilation. The important β_1-selective agents are acebutolol, atenolol, esmolol, and metoprolol. These agents are, in theory, safer to use for patients with reactive airways or diabetes mellitus. It is important to realize that β_1 selectivity is incomplete, and adverse reactions sec-

TABLE 49–1. PHARMACOLOGIC PROPERTIES OF THE BETA-ADRENERGIC ANTAGONISTS

	Adrenergic Agonist Activity	Partial Agonist Activity (ISA)	Membrane-Stabilizing Activity	Lipid Solubility	Protein Binding (%)	Oral Bio-availability (%)	Half-Life	Metabolism	Volume of Distribution (L/kg)
Acebutolol	β_1	Yes	Yes	Low	25	40	2–4 h	Hepatic/ renal	1.2
Atenolol	β_1	No	No	Low	<5	50	5–8 h	1° Renal	1
Esmolol	β_1	No	No	Low	50	0	~8 min	RBC esterases	2
Labetalol	$\alpha_1, \beta_1, \beta_2$	No	Low	Moderate	50	20	4–6 h	1° Hepatic	9
Metoprolol	β_1	No	Low	Moderate	10	40	3–4 h	1° Hepatic	4
Nadolol	β_1, β_2	No	No	Low	20	35	10–20 h	1° Renal	2
Oxprenolol	β_1, β_2	Yes	Yes	High ??	80	20–70	1–2 h	1° Hepatic	1.3
Pindolol	β_1, β_2	Yes	Low	Moderate	50	75	3–4 h	Hepatic/ renal	2
Propranolol	β_1, β_2	No	Yes	High	90	25	3–5 h	1° Hepatic	4
Sotalol	β_1, β_2	No	No	Low	0	90	~12 h	1° Renal	2
Timolol	β_1, β_2	No	No	Moderate	60	75	3–5 h	Hepatic/ renal	2

Data from references 16, 32, and 39.

ondary to β_2 antagonism may occur even with the β_1-selective agents. This is especially likely to be the case when higher doses are used.[8,66,104]

Intrinsic sympathomimetic activity (ISA) describes beta-adrenergic antagonists that are also partial agonists at the beta-adrenergic receptors. This property is unrelated to β_1 selectivity. Like other beta-adrenergic antagonists, these agents are antihypertensives and prevent exercise-induced tachycardia. The clinical benefit of agents with ISA has not been shown in controlled trials, but these agents may avoid the severe decrease in resting heart rate that occurs with beta-adrenergic antagonism in susceptible patients.[23] The important agents with ISA are oxprenolol, pindolol, and acebutolol.[26,39,81]

Lipid solubility is a measure of the ability of a drug to partition into fat. Highly lipid-soluble agents cross lipid membranes rapidly and concentrate into adipose tissue. These properties allow rapid entry into the central nervous system, and result in large volumes of distribution. Lipid solubility tends to enhance intestinal absorption by allowing rapid transit across lipid membranes, but because compounds must enter an aqueous phase in the intestines before being absorbed, excessive lipid solubility may actually impede absorption. Highly lipid-soluble agents are poorly excreted by the kidneys and require hepatic biotransformation before they can be eliminated. These agents also tend to be highly protein bound. Propranolol is the most lipid soluble of the beta-adrenergic antagonists. Other important moderately to highly lipid-soluble beta-adrenergic antagonists are acebutolol, metoprolol, oxprenolol, and timolol. These drugs tend to accumulate in liver failure and have greater CNS toxicity in overdose.[39,80,113]

Highly water-soluble compounds cross lipid membranes slowly and distribute in total body water. These compounds are generally slowly absorbed, poorly protein bound, renally eliminated, and slow to enter the CNS. Atenolol is the most water-soluble beta-adrenergic antagonist. Acebutolol, esmolol, nadolol, and sotalol are the other important highly water-soluble beta-adrenergic antagonists. These drugs tend to accumulate in renal failure and generally have less CNS toxicity. Esmolol, although water soluble, is rapidly eliminated by red blood cell esterases and does not accumulate in renal failure.[92]

Bioavailability reflects both the degree of absorption and the amount of first-pass metabolism. Compounds with extensive first-pass hepatic metabolism or poor absorption will have low bioavailability. Beta-adrenergic antagonist bioavailability ranges from approximately 25% for propranolol to almost 100% for pindolol. Propranolol and other lipophilic agents with extensive first-pass hepatic metabolism have greater bioavailability in overdose when hepatic enzymes become saturated. The half-life of beta-adrenergic antagonists is generally in the range of 3 to 5 hours. Sotalol and nadolol have longer half-lives, approximately 10 to 20 hours for nadolol and 12 hours for sotalol. Because of its rapid metabolism by erythrocyte esterases, esmolol's half-life is only 8 minutes. The duration of action of beta-adrenergic antagonists is greater than the measured half-life. The protein binding of beta-adrenergic antagonists ranges from essentially none with sotalol to 90% with propranolol. The volume of distribution of most beta-adrenergic antagonists is in the range of 2 to 4 L/kg. Atenolol, being the most water soluble, has the lowest volume of distribution (approximately 1 L/kg), and labetolol has the largest volume of distribution (~ 9 L/kg).[39]

In addition to competitive inhibition of catecholamine binding to beta-adrenergic receptors, several beta-adrenergic antagonists have unique properties that modify their clinical action and toxicity. From a toxicologic point of view, the most important of these properties is the ability of certain beta-adrenergic antagonists to block fast sodium channels, the so-called "membrane stabilizing action." This plays little role in therapeutic doses but is an important cause of morbidity and mortality in the overdose situation, which will be described. Propranolol, and to a lesser extent acebutolol and oxprenolol, are the beta-adrenergic antagonists with significant membrane-stabilizing activity. Sotalol is unique in that it prolongs action potential duration and decreases automaticity by blocking delayed rectifier potassium channels.[40] These actions make sotalol an effective antidysrhythmic agent but unfortunately also cause polymorphic ventricular tachycardia (torsades de pointes) in patients with sotalol toxicity. Labetolol is a nonselective beta-adrenergic antagonist that also blocks alpha$_1$-adrenergic receptors. Labetolol is five to ten times more potent as a beta-adrenergic antagonist than as an alpha-adrenergic antagonist, and so is contraindicated in situations such as pheochromocytoma or cocaine toxicity where beta antagonism could result in an "unopposed alpha" effect. In addition, labetolol has some β_2 agonist activity and inhibits neuronal reuptake of norepinephrine.[30,39]

What Is the Clinical Presentation of a Patient With Beta-Adrenergic Antagonist Overdose?

Beta-adrenergic antagonist overdoses are often quite benign, with about one third of patients remaining asymptomatic.[21,113] This is explained by the fact that beta-adrenergic antagonists act by inhibiting sympathetic stimulation to the heart, resulting in the equivalent of a denervated heart. Thus, in healthy persons who do not rely on sympathetic stimulation to maintain cardiac output, beta-adrenergic antagonism is well tolerated. There are, of course, important exceptions to this rule. Persons with congestive heart failure, sick sinus syndrome, or impaired AV conduction may rely on sympathetic stimulation to maintain heart rate or cardiac output. Even therapeutic doses of beta-adrenergic antagonists may be harmful for such persons. Secondly, beta-adrenergic antagonists severely impair the heart's ability to respond to peripheral vasodilation, bradycardia, or decreased contractility caused by other toxins. Therefore even relatively benign toxins, such as alcohol, may cause catastrophic toxicity when coingested with beta-adrenergic antagonists.[27] Furthermore, severe toxicity and death have occurred in healthy persons who have ingested beta-adrenergic antagonists alone.[26,89,108] This may be explained by an increased susceptibility of certain persons to beta-adrenergic antagonism or by special properties that increase the toxicity of certain beta-adrenergic antagonists.

Patients with symptomatic beta-adrenergic antagonist overdose will be hypotensive and bradycardic. Decreased SA node function results in sinus bradycardia, sinus pauses, or sinus arrest. Impaired atrioventricular conduction is manifested as prolonged PR interval or high-grade AV block. Prolonged QRS interval may occur, and severe poisonings may result in asystole. Congestive heart failure often complicates beta-adrenergic antagonist overdose. Delirium, coma, and seizures occur most commonly in the setting of severe hypotension, but may also occur with normal blood pressure, especially with the more lipophilic agents.[26,89] Respiratory depression and apnea appear to be important determinants of morbidity and mortality in animal models of beta-adrenergic antagonist toxicity,[53–55] and may play a role in human overdoses as well.[4] In fact, in a review of reported cases, 18% of patients with propranolol toxicity and 6% of those with atenolol toxicity had a respiratory rate less than 12 breaths/min.[89] Respiratory depression in this setting typically occurs in patients who are hypotensive and comatose but may also occur in awake patients.[74] Hypoglycemia is relatively common after beta-adrenergic antagonist poisoning in children[34] but is an uncommon result of acute toxicity in adults. In a series of 15 cases of beta-adrenergic antagonist overdose, none of the 13 adults were hypoglycemic but both of the 2 children had hypoglycemia requiring treatment.[26] Bronchospasm is relatively uncommon following beta-adrenergic antagonist overdose and appears to occur only in susceptible patients. In the series mentioned, only 2 of the 15 patients developed bronchospasm,[26] and in a review of 39 cases of symptomatic adult beta-adrenergic antagonist overdose, only one patient developed bronchospasm.[67] Clinical use of beta-adrenergic antagonists slightly increases serum potassium[70] but significant hyperkalemia rarely complicates acute overdose.

Toxicity generally occurs early following beta-adrenergic antagonist ingestion. Propranolol overdose, in particular, may be complicated by the rapid development of seizures, coma, and dysrhythmias. All reported cases of adult beta-adrenergic antagonist overdoses with well-documented times from ingestion to symptom onset were reviewed. All 39 patients who eventually became symptomatic did so within the first 6 hours. In fact, 31 patients were symptomatic at 2 hours, and all but one developed symptoms at 4 hours. The authors conclude that there have been no well-documented cases of beta-adrenergic antagonist overdose resulting in toxicity delayed more than 6 hours after ingestion. Sotalol overdoses, which are well known to cause delayed toxicity, were excluded from this series, and the authors also caution against applying their observations to sustained-release products.[67] The authors of a recent Australian series also noted that in their 58 patients with beta-adrenergic antagonist overdose, all major symptoms began within 6 hours of ingestion.[89]

What Special Properties of Beta-Adrenergic Antagonists May Modify Their Toxicity?

Beta-adrenergic antagonists that inhibit fast sodium channels are said to possess membrane-stabilizing activity. Propranolol posseses the most membrane-stabilizing activity, and the clinical presentation of patients with propranolol overdoses is characterized by coma, seizures, hypotension, and bradycardia associated with impaired atrioventricular conduction and widened QRS interval.[14] Hypotension may be out of proportion to bradycardia, and deaths from propranolol overdose are well reported.[26,32] Acebutolol and oxprenolol also possess significant membrane-stabilizing activity and have caused fatalities.[32,45,80] Several other beta-adrenergic antagonists, including labetolol, metoprolol, and pindolol, have weak membrane-stabilizing activity, which plays little role in their toxicity.[81]

Lipid solubility is another important modifier of beta-adrenergic antagonist toxicity. In overdose, the more lipophilic beta-adrenergic antagonists cause delirium, coma, and seizures even in the absence of hypotension.[26,89] Atenolol is the least lipid soluble of the beta-adrenergic antagonists and also appears to be one of the safest in overdose.[33] In fact, in one series of beta-adrenergic antagonist overdoses none of the 18 patients with atenolol overdose had seizures compared with 8 out of 28 patients with propranolol overdoses.[89]

There is little experience with overdoses of the agents with ISA. In theory these agents should be safer than the other beta-adrenergic antagonists. Sympathetic stimulation with tachycardia or hypertension often predominates in pindolol overdose, and this agent does appear to be relatively safe after overdose.[26,51,81] The other agents with ISA—acebutolol and oxprenolol—have significant membrane-stabilizing activity, making them dangerous in overdose; deaths due to acute toxicity from these agents are reported.[26,32,80,99]

Cardioselective agents are safer in clinical practice because they are less likely to cause bronchospasm and the other undesirable effects of β_2 antagonism. In overdose, cardioselectivity is largely lost and deaths due to the β_1-selective agents including metoprolol[95,108] and acebutolol[32] are reported. Some authors, nevertheless, believe that β_1-selectivity is partially maintained following overdose with these agents.[17]

Sotalol is a nonselective beta-adrenergic antagonist with low lipid solubility, no membrane-stabilizing effect, and no ISA. Sotalol is unique because of its ability to block the delayed rectifier potassium current responsible for repolarization. This prolongs the action potential duration and is manifested on the electrocardiogram by a prolonged QT interval.[40] Prolonged QT intervals predispose to torsades de pointes, and ventricular dysrhythmias may complicate the therapeutic use of sotalol.[50] Torsades de pointes is most common in patients taking sotalol therapeutically who have predisposing factors such as hypokalemia, hypomagnesemia, or bradycardia, or are taking other agents that prolong the QT interval.[40] Sotalol overdoses are also frequently complicated by QT prolongation and ventricular dysrhythmias, especially torsades de pointes.[9] In 6 patients with sotalol overdoses, the average QT interval was 172% of normal, and 5 patients had ventricular dysrhythmias including multifocal ventricular extrasystoles, ventricular tachycardia, and ventricular fibrillation.[76] Sotalol overdoses may also be complicated by hypotension, bradycardia, and asystole,[3,76] and fatalities are well documented.[73,78] Lidocaine is ineffective for sotalol-induced ventricular dysrhythmias but overdrive pacing and magnesium infusions may be effective.[5,115] Hypokalemia should also be corrected. Sotalol overdoses may cause delayed and prolonged toxicity, although electrocardiographic changes occur early. In a series of 6 patients with sotalol overdoses, all had prolonged QT interval noted on the initial electrocardiogram taken 30 minutes to $4\frac{1}{2}$ hours after ingestion. The greatest QT prolongation occured 4 to 15 hours after ingestion and the risk of ventricular dysrhythmias was highest between 4 and 20 hours. All 4 patients who developed ventricular tachycardia did so after 4 hours, and in 2 patients ventricular dysrhythmias first occurred 9 hours after ingestion. One patient continued to have ventricular dysrhythmias at 48 hours and abnormally prolonged QT intervals were noted as long as 100 hours after ingestion. In this series, average sotalol half-life was 13 hours and the average time until normalization of the QT interval was 82 hours.[76]

Labetalol overdoses are rare but appear to be similar to those of other beta-adrenergic antagonists with hypotension and bradycardia as prominent features. Labetalol's $alpha_1$-adrenergic antagonism would theoretically act in synergy with its beta-adrenergic antagonism to increase toxicity. Conversely, labetalol's low-membrane stabilizing effect may make it relatively safe in overdose. Treatment of a patient with labetalol overdose is similar to that for other beta-adrenergic antagonists. If vasodilation from $alpha_1$ antagonism is a prominent feature, then high doses of pressors with alpha agonist properties may be required. Conversely, if beta-adrenergic antagonism is prominent, then agents that act to increase intracellular cAMP may be needed. One patient with labetalol poisoning required large doses of epinephrine to maintain blood pressure[35] and a second patient responded to amrinone after other therapy including glucagon and pressors failed.[46] Renal failure has complicated 2 of the 5 reported cases of labetalol overdose.[47,105]

There has been very little experience with overdoses of the sustained-release beta-adrenergic antagonists, but it is reasonable to expect that an overdose with these agents will result in delayed onset and prolonged duration of toxicity. Therapeutic use of ophthalmic solutions containing beta-adrenergic antagonists may cause adverse effects such as bradycardia, heart failure, bronchospasm, and depression,[11,118] but acute overdose of these agents has not been reported. Combined overdoses with calcium channel blockers and beta-adrenergic antagonists are likely to be very difficult to manage because of synergistic toxicity. An extended-release tablet containing a combination of the calcium channel blocker, felodipine, and metoprolol is being studied as an antihypertensive medication.[41] This medication would be expected to be quite dangerous in overdose.

How Can Beta-Adrenergic Antagonist Toxicity Be Differentiated from Other Causes of Bradycardia?

Bradycardia may result from numerous toxic exposures and medical conditions. The three most common causes of drug-induced bradycardia are calcium channel blockers (see Chap. 50), beta-adrenergic antagonists, and digoxin and other cardioactive steroids (see Chap. 48). Other important toxic causes of bradycardia include $alpha_1$ agonists such as phenylpropanolamine (Chap. 34), $alpha_2$ agonists such as clonidine and other imidazolines (see Chap. 51), cholinergic agents such as carbamates and organophosphates (Chap. 87), sodium channel blockers, opioids, and some sedative hypnotics such as the barbiturates (Chap. 61). Many patients with toxic causes of bradycardia will present with a recognizable toxidrome. A directed history and physical examination together with electrocardiogram and basic laboratory tests can determine the correct diagnosis in most cases of drug-induced bradycardia. Medical causes of bradycardia include hyperkalemia, hypothermia, myocardial infarction, sick sinus syndrome, vasovagal episodes, intracranial hypertension, and benign physiologic bradycardia in resting athletes. The differential diagnosis of bradycardia is summarized in Table 49–2 and discussed in detail in Chapters 17 and 21.

Beta-adrenergic antagonist toxicity typically results in bradycardia and hypotension, although these findings may not occur in all patients.[21] In fact, patients who have ingested agents with intrinsic sympathomimetic activity may actually present with tachycardia and hypertension.[81] Patients will often have a depressed mental status and coma, seizures, and apnea may occur. The electrocardiogram will demonstrate sinus bradycardia and prolonged PR interval. Propranolol and other beta-adrenergic antagonists with membrane-depressant effects prolong the QRS interval. Patients who overdose on beta-adrenergic antagonists may be hypoglycemic and slightly hyperkalemic.

Calcium channel blocker toxicity invariably causes hypotension but may result in bradycardia, normal heart rate, or even reactive tachycardia depending on which agent is ingested. Calcium channel blocker overdose is often characterized by preservation of mental status in

TABLE 49–2. DRUG-INDUCED BRADYCARDIA

Drug	Clinical Characteristics of Overdose	Electrocardiogram
Beta-adrenergic antagonists	Depressed mental status, hypotension, slight hyperkalemia	Prolonged PR interval, QRS narrow or wide
Calcium channel blockers	Preservation of mental status, hypotension	Prolonged PR interval, QRS narrow or wide
Digoxin/cardiac glycosides	Vomiting, hyperkalemia, BP and mental status preserved	Prolonged PR interval, ST segment changes, atrial and ventricular dysrhythmias
Sodium channel blockers	Altered mental status, seizures, hypotension	Wide QRS interval
Cholinergics	Cholinergic toxidrome: SLUDGE (see Chap. 87)	Sinus bradycardia
α-Agonists (phenylpropanolamine)	Hypertension, intracranial hemorrhage	Sinus bradycardia
α_2 Agonists (clonidine)	Opioid toxidrome: miosis, respiratory depression, sedation	Sinus bradycardia
Opioids	Opioid toxidrome: miosis, respiratory depression, sedation	Sinus bradycardia
Sedative-hypnotics	Sedation, +/− miosis, +/− respiratory depression	Sinus bradycardia or tachycardia

the face of marked hypotension. The ECG may show a prolonged PR with normal QRS interval. In contrast to the case with beta-adrenergic antagonists, patients with calcium channel blocker overdose may be hyperglycemic.[38,83] The presence of profound hypotension with preserved mental status and hyperglycemia may differentiate a patient with calcium channel blocker toxicity from one with beta-adrenergic antagonist toxicity, however the two conditions are easily confused clinically. Fortunately, the therapy for these two poisonings is similar.

Acute digoxin toxicity is invariably associated with vomiting. Patients may be bradycardic secondary to increased vagal tone but may also develop ventricular tachydysrhythmias. Blood pressure will typically be preserved despite significant bradycardia. Patients with digoxin toxicity usually have normal mental status. Hyperkalemia is an important marker of digoxin toxicity. Digoxin results in typical electrocardiographic findings, which reflect impaired AV conduction, repolarization changes ("digoxin effect"), and ventricular irritability. Digoxin toxicity is differentiated from beta-adrenergic antagonist toxicity by the presence of vomiting, bradycardia with preserved blood pressure, characteristic ECG changes, and prominent hyperkalemia.

Sodium channel blocker toxicity results in hypotension, seizures, and depressed mental status. Most cases of sodium channel blocker toxicity are associated with tachycardia, but bradycardia may occur. The electrocardiogram will be characterized by a markedly widened QRS interval which narrows with administration of hypertonic sodium bicarbonate. Beta-adrenergic antagonists with membrane-stabilizing effect such as propranolol may also prolong the QRS interval.

Alpha agonists cause marked hypertension and a reactive bradycardia. Patients often complain of headaches, and the clinical course may be complicated by intracranial hemorrhage. Cholinergic toxicity causes an easily recognized symptom complex characterized by vomiting, diarrhea, salivation, lacrimation, urinary incontinence, fasciculations, muscle paralysis, seizures, coma, and hypoxia. Patients are usually bradycardic but may be tachycardic secondary to hypoxia and nicotinic stimulation. Opioids, alpha_2 agonists, and certain sedative hypnotics result in marked sedation, respiratory depression, miosis, and only moderate bradycardia. Toxicity from these agents is usually easily differentiated from that due to beta-adrenergic antagonists. The medical causes of bradycardia are distinguished from beta-adrenergic antagonist toxicity by history, physical examination, and simple laboratory tests (see Chap. 21).

How Should a Patient With Beta-Adrenergic Antagonist Overdose Be Treated?

The initial management of the critically ill patient who has ingested beta-adrenergic antagonists is similar to that of other acutely ill patients. Airway and ventilation should be maintained with endotracheal intubation if necessary. Because laryngoscopy may induce a vagal response, it is reasonable to give atropine prior to intubation of the bradycardic patient. The initial treatment of bradycardia and hypotension consists of atropine and fluids. If these measures fail, then the specific therapy discussed next is indicated. Seizures associated with cardiovascular collapse are treated by attempting to restore circulation. Seizures in the patient with relatively normal vital signs should be treated with benzodiazepines followed by barbiturates if benzodiazepines fail. Refractory seizures are rare in beta-adrenergic antagonist overdose. Consideration should be given to the administration of glucose, thiamine, and naloxone to the lethargic or comatose patient. Hypoglycemia is rare in adults but is common in children who ingest beta-adrenergic antagonists. Naloxone may be effective for patients who are comatose following a mixed drug overdose, but will not reverse coma in a pure beta-adrenergic antagonist overdose.

Gastrointestinal decontamination is warranted for all persons who have ingested significant amounts of a beta-adrenergic antagonist. Because beta-adrenergic antagonist ingestion may be followed by a catastrophic deterioration of mental status and vital signs, induction of emesis is contraindicated. In fact, ipecac may be particularly dangerous in this situation, because it increases vagal stimulation and may worsen bradycardia.[106] Orogastric lavage also causes vagal stimulation, so some clinicians recommend giving atropine prior to lavage.[113] Activated charcoal alone may be effective and avoids some of the potential complications of gastric lavage. Activated charcoal alone is recommended for persons with minor symptoms following an overdose with one of the more water-soluble beta-adrenergic antagonists such as atenolol. Persons who develop severe symptoms such as seizures, significant hypotension, or bradycardia probably warrant orogastric lavage. Lavage is also recommended for patients with large (gram amount) ingestions of propranolol or one of the other more toxic beta-adrenergic antagonists (acebutolol, metoprolol, oxprenolol, and sotalol) who present within the first hour of ingestion even if they have not yet developed symptoms. Because lavage carries the risk of worsening bradycardia, it is reasonable to give atropine prior to lavage for patients who are already bradycardic and to have it available at the bedside for all other persons. Whole-bowel irrigation with polyethylene glycol should be considered for patients who have ingested sustained release preparations (see Antidotes in Depth: Whole-Bowel Irrigation).

Hypotension and bradycardia from beta adrenergic-antagonist poisoning is often refractory to atropine and fluids, and it is important to have an approach to the care of these patients. When time permits, it is preferable to introduce new medications sequentially, so that the effects of each may be assessed. In the critically ill patient there may not be enough time for this approach, and multiple treatments may be started simultaneously. It is often difficult to differentiate clinically between beta-adrenergic antagonist and calcium channel blocker toxicity, and it is fortunate that the therapies for these ingestions are similar. The following recommendations take into consideration the clinical similarities and are broad enough to apply to both overdoses.

Several animal models show the effectiveness of glucagon in treating beta-adrenergic antagonist toxicity.[29,48] Glucagon has been used clinically to treat beta-adrenergic antagonist poisoning for over 20 years,[49,123] and has become recognized as the treatment of choice after atropine and fluids.[79,113,126] Glucagon acts to increase cAMP by pathways that do not involve the beta receptors. The initial adult dose of glucagon for beta-adrenergic antagonist toxicity is 2 to 5 mg given over 30 to 60 seconds. The initial pediatric dose is 50 μg/kg. Normal saline or 5% dextrose are recommended as diluents for doses of glucagon exceeding 2 mg, because the packaged diluent contains 0.2% (2 mg/mL) phenol. If there is no response to the initial dose, higher doses up to a total of 10 mg may be used. Once a response has occurred, a glucagon infusion should be started. Most authors recommend an infusion of 2 to 5 mg/h, although some recommend glucagon infusions as high as 10 mg/h. We suggest that the glucagon infusion be started at the "response dose" per hour. Thus, for example, if the patient receives 7 mg of glucagon before a response occurs, the glucagon infusion should be started at 7 mg/h. When a "full dose" of glucagon fails to restore blood pressure and heart rate and when beta-adrenergic antagonist toxicity remains the likely etiology, we would still recommend starting an infusion of glucagon at 10 mg/h. Adverse effects of glucagon in this setting have included vomiting, hyperglycemia, and mild hypocalcemia,[42] and these should be treated appropriately if they develop (see Antidotes in Depth: Glucagon).

Once cardiac glycolosides have been excluded as the etiology, calcium salts can effectively be used to treat hypotension from calcium channel blocker overdose and are also effective in animal models of beta-adrenergic antagonist toxicity.[53] Calcium chloride has successfully reversed hypotension in patients with beta-adrenergic antagonist overdose[12] and in combined calcium channel blocker and beta-adrenergic antagonist toxicity.[33] The adult starting dose of calcium chloride is 1 g of the 10% solution given as a slow intravenous push. Using up to 3 g of calcium chloride is recommended. The initial pediatric dose of calcium chloride is 20 mg/kg up to 1 g, and up to 60 mg/kg may be given (see Antidotes in Depth: Calcium). Ventricular pacing has been used to increase the heart rate in patients with beta-adrenergic antagonist toxicity.[44] Unfortunately, ventricular pacing typically increases the heart rate with no increase in cardiac output or blood pressure.[2,51,52,113] In fact, some authors have noticed that ventricular pacing frequently results in a decreased blood pressure, presumably secondary to loss of atrial contraction.[113]

When the preceeding measures fail, the next step is usually to begin a catecholamine infusion. The choice of catecholamine is somewhat controversial. Theoretically, the beta agonist isoproterenol would seem to be the ideal agent. Unfortunately, this therapy has several potential drawbacks that limit efficacy. In the presence of beta antagonism, extraordinarily high doses of isoproterenol and other catecholamines are frequently required.[80,94,113,117] In fact, one author suggests that catecholamine infusion rates up to 10,000 times the usual effective rate may be required.[17] Case reports document isoproterenol infusions of 800 μg/min, dobutamine infusions of 500 μg/min, 6 mg of epinephrine given over an hour, and dopamine infusions of 4800 μg/min.[80] At these high doses the $beta_2$ effects of isoproterenol cause peripheral vasodilation and may cause consequential hypotension.[93] Furthermore, isoproterenol is very dysrhythmogenic and is thus potentially harmful for calcium channel blocker overdoses and other causes of hypotension and bradycardia. Nevertheless, in animal models, isoproterenol was the most effective catecholamine and was even more effective than glucagon in reversing beta-adrenergic antagonist toxicity.[110,125] Clinical experience in humans, however, has not shown this to be the case. In a review of reported cases, glucagon increased heart rate 67% of the time and blood pressure 50% of the time. In contrast, isoproterenol was effective in increasing heart rate only 11% of the time and blood pressure only 22% of the time, and epinephrine was more effective than isoproterenol.[126] The selective $beta_1$-agonist prenalterol may avoid some of the problems associated with isoproterenol and has been used successfully to treat beta-adrenergic antagonist overdoses.[24,51] This agent would be expected to be especially effective following overdose of the cardioselective beta-adrenergic antagonists.[24] Prenalterol is not readily available for clinical use, and prenalterol therapy is limited by its half life of approximately 2 hours, which makes dose titration difficult.[96] Dobutamine is a selective $beta_1$ agonist and may be useful in this setting. However, experience is limited, and dobutamine has not always proven effective in beta-adrenergic antagonist overdose, perhaps because inadequate doses were used.[80,103] In the setting of beta-adrenergic antagonism, catecholamines with substantial alpha agonist properties may increase peripheral vascular resistance without improving contractility. This could result in acute cardiac failure. Severe hypertension due to lack of $beta_2$-mediated vasodilation is another potential adverse reaction from this so-called "unopposed alpha" effect.[28] Because of these potential problems, the use of catecholamines should be guided by invasive monitoring whenever possible. Catecholamine infusions should be started at the usual rates and then increased rapidly until a clinical effect is obtained. If invasive monitoring is impossible and the diagnosis of beta-adrenergic antagonist overdose is fairly certain, it is reasonable to begin an isoproterenol or epinephrine infusion with careful monitoring of the patient's blood pressure. The infusion should be stopped immediately if the patient's blood pressure falls further. Recommendations for the treatment of beta-adrenergic antagonist toxicity are summarized in Table 49–3.

All patients who have bradycardia, hypotension, abnormal ECGs, or CNS toxicity following a beta-adrenergic antagonist overdose should be observed in intensive care until these findings have resolved. Toxicity from regular-release beta-adrenergic antagonist poisoning almost always occurs within the first 6 hours.[67] Therefore patients without any findings of toxicity following an overdose of a regular-release beta-adrenergic antagonist may be discharged from medical care if they remain asymptomatic with normal vital signs and a normal electrocardiogram after an observation time of 6 to 8 hours. Ingestion of extended-release preparations may cause delayed toxicity, and these patients should be observed for 24 hours. Patients who may have delayed absorption because of a mixed overdose or underlying gastrointestinal disease may also require longer observation. As discussed, sotalol overdose may also present in a delayed fashion. All patients who ingest medications with suicidal intent should have a psychiatric assessement prior to discharge.

TABLE 49–3. TREATMENT OF BETA-ADRENERGIC ANTAGONIST OVERDOSE IN ADULTS

Asymptomatic

1. Activated charcoal.
2. Consider orogastric lavage early after a large overdose of one of the more toxic beta-adrenergic antagonists (acebutolol, oxprenolol, propranolol, sotalol).
3. Consider whole-bowel irrigation with polyethylene glycol for sustained-release preparations.

Mild Toxicity

1. All of the above plus:
2. Atropine 1 mg IV for bradycardia.
3. Fluid boluses for hypotension (monitor closely to avoid pulmonary edema).

Moderate Toxicity

1. All of the above plus:
2. Monitor ventilation and intubate if necessary.
3. Glucagon: 2–5 mg IV push (may give up to 10-mg IV push), then 2–5 mg/h (up to 10 mg/h).
4. More atropine up to 3 mg IV for bradycardia.

Severe Toxicity

1. All of the above plus:
2. Intraarterial and pulmonary artery pressure monitoring and frequent reassessment.
3. Catecholamine infusion: *Very high doses of the following are typically required.*
   Isoproterenol (β_1, β_2 agonist: Caution with β_2-mediated vasodilation):
   Start at 0.1 μg/kg/min. Titrate rapidly to effect.
   Dobutamine (β_1 agonist: Theoretically useful but limited experience):
   Start at 2.5 μg/kg/min. Titrate rapidly to effect.
   Norepinephrine (α, β_1 agonist: Caution with "unopposed alpha" effects):
   Start at 0.1 μg/kg/min. Titrate rapidly to effect.
   Epinephrine (α, β agonist: Caution with "unopposed alpha" effects):
   Start at 0.02 μg/kg/min. Titrate rapidly to effect.
4. Phosphodiesterase inhibitors:
   Milrinone: 50 μg/kg IV bolus over 2 min, then 0.25–1.0 μg/kg/min.
   Amrinone: 0.75 mg/kg IV bolus over 2 min (may repeat in 30 min), then 2–20 μg/kg/min.
5. Ventricular pacing: *This often increases heart rate without improving cardiac output.*
6. Intra-aortic balloon pump or extracorporeal circulation.

Which Other Modalities May Prove Useful in Treating Beta-Adrenergic Antagonist Overdoses?

The therapy outlined above may fail in the critically ill patient with beta-adrenergic antagonist toxicity. In this case there are several invasive or experimental treatment modalities that may prove to be life saving. The phosphodiesterase inhibitors (PDIs) amrinone, milrinone, and enoximone are theoretically beneficial in beta-adrenergic antagonist overdose because they increase cAMP independently of beta receptor stimulation. Phosphodiesterase inhibitors are able to increase inotropy in the presence of beta-adrenergic antagonism both in animal models[57] and in humans.[116] In fact, these agents appear to be as effective as glucagon in animal models of beta-adrenergic antagonist toxicity,[69,101] but controlled dog models have been unable to demonstrate an additional benefit of these agents over glucagon.[68,100] Phosphodiesterase inhibitors might be useful in selected patients who fail glucagon therapy, and in fact have been used clinically to treat beta-adrenergic antagonist poisonings.[37,46] Therapy with PDIs is often limited by hypotension secondary to peripheral vasodilation. Furthermore, these agents are difficult to titrate because of relatively long half-lives (30 to 60 minutes for milrinone, 2 to 4 hours for amrinone, and approximately 2 hours for enoximone).[43,75] For these reasons, the PDIs should only be considered for patients who have arterial and pulmonary artery pressure monitoring.

High doses of insulin with sufficient glucose to maintain euglycemia have recently been shown to improve cardiac performance and increase survival in a canine model of propranolol toxicity.[44a] The same investigators had previously demonstrated that this therapy was effective in verapamil toxicity in dogs.[45a] High-dose insulin has not yet been evaluated in humans with beta-adrenergic antagonist toxicity. This therapy has, however, been evaluated in postoperative cardiac patients and shown to improve cardiac performance without increasing myocardial oxygen demand.[35a] The physiologic basis for the beneficial effects of insulin are incompletely understood but appear to be at least in part due to its metabolic effects of decreasing cardiac uptake of free fatty acids and increasing carbohydrate use.[44a] Selected patients with beta-adrenergic antagonist toxicity may benefit from high-dose insulin infusions. This treatment would mandate glucose infusions to maintain euglycemia and careful monitoring of glucose and potassium levels.

Extracorporeal removal is ineffective for the lipid-soluble beta-adrenergic antagonists due to their large volumes of distribution. Hemodialysis was used successfully to remove the water-soluble beta-adrenergic antagonist, atenolol.[98] Hemodialysis is rarely indicated in patients with beta-adrenergic antagonist overdose, but may be considered in selected cases.

It is important to remember that the patient with severe hypotension from an acute overdose will typically recover without sequelae if ventilation and circulation are maintained until the toxin is metabolized. When the medical treatment described fails in patients with severe beta-adrenergic antagonist overdose, it is appropriate to consider the use of an intra-aortic balloon pump or extracorporeal circulation. Several case reports describe remarkable recoveries following the use of these therapies for refractory beta-adrenergic antagonist toxicity[52,71] or combined beta-adrenergic antagonist and calcium channel blocker overdose.[25]

In the future, novel new medications may prove beneficial in beta-adrenergic antagonist overdose. Potential new therapeutic agents include forskolin, another drug that increases cAMP independently of the beta-adrenergic receptor, and the potassium channel blocker, 4-aminopyridine. The mechanism of action of these drugs was discussed earlier. These medications have not been studied in beta-adrenergic antagonist overdose and should be considered experimental at this time.

What Is Beta-Antagonist Withdrawal?

Patients with angina who abruptly stop taking beta-adrenergic antagonists after chronic use have an increased incidence of angina, silent myocardial ischemia, and myocardial infarction in the first weeks following discontinuation of therapy.[19,84,119] This is associated with a rebound increase in exertional heart rate to greater than pretreatment values, and with increased sensitivity to isoproterenol infusions. These phenomena are believed to represent adrenergic hypersensitivity secondary to an increased number of beta-adrenergic receptors.[90] This phenomenon can be seen after as little as 2 weeks of beta-adrenergic antagonist therapy.[86,97] Patients may complain of malaise, headache, tremor, palpitations, and diaphoresis associated with increased blood pressure and heart rate.[56] Withdrawal effects are reported for most beta-adrenergic antagonists including atenolol, metoprolol, and propranolol.[86,120] The beta-adrenergic antagonists with intrinsic sympathomimetic activity, however, do not cause adrenergic hypersensitivity.[10,86,119] In fact, these agents may actually cause decreased sensitivity to adrenergic stimulation.[121,122]

Beta-adrenergic antagonist withdrawal is unpredictable, and many patients will not develop withdrawal symptoms. Close clinical monitoring appears to minimize the associated risks, and patients who develop symptoms may be simply treated by restarting beta-adrenergic antagonist therapy.[20] Because heart rate and blood pressure overshoot occurs during periods of adrenergic stimulation, patients withdrawn from beta-adrenergic antagonist therapy should be counseled to avoid exertion during the first several weeks. Gradual reduction in beta-adrenergic antagonist dosage may also minimize the risk of complications.[82]

Summary

Beta-adrenergic antagonists are commonly used to treat hypertension, angina, tachydysrhythmias, tremor, migraines, and panic attack. Although overdoses are relatively uncommon, beta-adrenergic antagonists continue to cause deaths in the United States and around the world. Patients who develop symptoms after ingesting regular-release beta-adrenergic antagonists except for sotalol do so within the first 6 hours. Sotalol may cause delayed and prolonged toxicity. Beta-adrenergic antagonist overdose, when symptomatic, typically causes bradycardia and hypotension. Propranolol and other beta-adrenergic antagonists with membrane stabilizing properties and high lipid solubility are the most toxic in overdose. These drugs cause prolonged QRS intervals, severe hypotension, coma, seizures, and apnea. Hypoglycemia is rare following adult beta-adrenergic antagonist ingestions, but may complicate pediatric ingestions. Bronchospasm may occur in acute beta-adrenergic antagonist toxicity in susceptible persons. Sotalol is unique in its ability to cause extreme prolongation of the QRS interval, and sotalol toxicity results in refractory ventricular dysrhythmias that may respond to overdrive pacing or to magnesium infusions. In addition to supportive care, the most important therapy for beta-adrenergic antagonist toxicity is glucagon. Catecholamine infusions may also be helpful, but should be given in a closely monitored setting, and large doses are typically required. Persons who fail treatment with glucagon and catecholamines are typically critically ill and such patients may respond to phosphodiesterase inhibitors or mechanical support of circulation. Fortunately, most patients respond to simpler measures and this aggressive therapy is rarely required.

References

1. Adelstein RS, Eisenberg E: Regulation and kinetics of the actin–myosin–ATP interaction. Annu Rev Biochem 1980; 49:921–956.
2. Agura ED, Wexler LF: Massive propranolol overdose. Am J Med 1986;80:755–757.
3. Alderfliegel F, Leeman M, Demaeyer P, Kahn RJ: Sotalol poisoning associated with asystole. Intensive Care Med 1993;19:57–58.
4. Annane D: Beta-adrenergic mediation of the central control of respiration: Myth or reality? J Toxicol Clin Exp 1991;11:325–336.
5. Arstall MA, Hii JT, Lehman RG, Horowitz JD: Sotalol induced torsade de pointes: Management with magnesium infusion. Postgrad Med J 1992;68:289–290.
6. Barry WH, Bridge JHB: Intracellular calcium homeostasis in cardiac myocytes. Circulation 1993;87:1806–1815.
7. Basavappa S, Romano-Silva MA, Mangel AW, et al: Inhibition of K^+ channel activity by 4-AP stimulates N-type Ca^+ channels in CHP-100 cells. Neuroreport 1994;5: 1256–1258.
8. Bauer K, Kaik G, Kaik B: Osmotic release drug delivery system of metoprolol in hypertensive asthmatic patients. Pharmacodynamic effects on $beta_2$-adrenoreceptors. Hypertension 1994;24:339–346.
9. Beattie JM: Sotalol induced torsade de pointes. Scott Med J 1984;29:240–244.
10. Bolli P, Buhler FR, Raeder EA, et al: Lack of beta-adrenoreceptor hypersensitivity after abrupt withdrawal of long term therapy with oxprenolol. Circulation 1981;64: 1130–1134.
11. Bourgeois JA: Depression and topical ophthalmic beta adrenergic blockade. J Am Optom Assoc 1991;62:403–406.
12. Brimacombe JR, Scully M, Swainston R: Propranolol overdose—A dramatic response to calcium chloride. Med J Aust 1991;155:267–268.
13. Buenaventura P, Cao-Danh H, Glynn P, et al: Protein kinase C activation in the heart: Effects on calcium and contractile proteins. Ann Thorac Surg 1995;60:S505–S508.
14. Buiumsohn A, Eisenberg ES, Jacob H, et al: Seizures and intraventricular conduction defect in propranolol poisoning: A report of two cases. Ann Int Med 1979;91:860–862.
15. Buschmans E, Hearse DJ, Manning AS: Forskolin: Effects on cyclic AMP and contractile function in the isolated rat and guinea pig heart. Can J Cardiol 1985;1:385–394.
16. Cada DJ, Covington TR, Hussar DA, et al, eds: Diuretics and cardiovasculars. In: Drug Facts and Comparisons, St. Louis, 1995, pp. 593–599.
17. Critchley JA, Ungar A: The management of acute poisoning due to beta adrenoreceptor antagonists. Med Toxicol 1989;4:32–45.
18. Davis BA, Edes I, Gupta RC, et al: The role of phospholamban in the regulation of calcium transport by cardiac sarcoplasmic reticulum. Mol Cell Pharmacol 1990;99: 83–88.
19. Egstrup K: Transient myocardial ischemia after abrupt withdrawal of antianginal therapy in chronic stable angina. Am J Cardiol 1988;61:1219–1222.
20. Eisele G, Gilmore LL, Blanchard EB: Close clinical observation minimizes the complications of beta blocker withdrawal. Ann Pharmacother 1994;28:849–851.
21. Elkharrat D, Bismuth C, Davy JM: Le blocage des beta-recepteurs: Phenomene auto-limite exploquant la benignite des intoxicationa aigues par les beta-bloquantes. Mortalite nulle a la clinique toxicologique de Fernand-Widal sur quarante cas. Semaine Hospitaux 1982;58:1073–1076.
22. Enocksson S, Shimizu M, Lonnqvist F, et al: Demonstration of an in vivo functional beta 3-adrenoceptor in man. J Clin Invest 1995;95:2239–2245.
23. Fitzgerald JD: Do partial agonist beta-blockers have improved clinical utility? Cardiovasc Drugs Ther 1993;7: 303–310.
24. Freestone S, Thomas HM, Bharma RK, et al: Severe atenolol poisoning: Treatment with prenalterol. Hum Toxicol 1986;5:343–345.
25. Frierson J, Bailly D, Shultz T, et al: Refractory cardiogenic shock and complete heart block after unsuspected verapamil-SR and atenolol overdose. Clin Cardiol 1991;14: 933–935.
26. Frishman W, Jacob H, Eisenberg E, et al: Clinical pharmacology of the new beta-adrenergic blocking drugs. Part 8: Self poisoning with beta-adrenoreceptor blocking agents: Recognition and management. Am Heart J 1979;98: 798–811.
27. Frithz G. Toxic effects of propranolol on the heart. Br Med J 1976;1:769–770.
28. Gandy W: Severe epinephrine-propranolol interaction. Ann Emerg Med 1989;18:98–99.
29. Glick G, Parmley W, Weschler A, et al: Glucagon: Its enhancement of cardiac performance in the cat and dog and persistence of its inotropic action despite beta receptor blockade with propranolol. Circ Res 1968;22:789–799.
30. Gold EH, Chang W, Cohen M, et al: Synthesis and comparison of some cardiovascular properties of the sterioisomers of labetalol. J Med Chem 1982;25:1363–1370.
31. Hartzell HC, Hirayama Y, Petit-Jacques J: Effects of protein phosphatase and kinase inhibitors on the cardiac L-type calcium current suggests two sites are phosphorylated by protein kinase A and another protein kinase. J Gen Physiol 1995;106:393–414.
32. Henry JA, Cassidy SL: Membrane stabilizing activity: A major cause of fatal poisoning. Lancet 1986;8495: 1414–1417.
33. Henry M, Kay MM, Viccellio P: Cardiogenic shock associated with calcium channel blockers and beta blockers: Reversal with calcium chloride. Am J Emerg Med 1985; 3:334–336.
34. Hesse B, Pederson JT: Hypoglycemia after propranolol in children. Acta Med Scand 1973;193:551–552.
35. Hicks PR, Rankin AP: Massive adrenaline doses in labetalol poisoning. Anaesth Intens Care 1991;19:447–449.

35a. Hiesmayr M, Haider WJ, Grubhofer G, et al: Effects of dobutamine versus insulin on cardiac performance, myocardial oxygen demand, and total body metabolism after coronary artery bypass grafting. J Cardiothorac Vasc Anesth 1995;9:653–658.
36. Hilgemann DW: Extracellular calcium transients and action potential configuration changes related to post-stimulatory potentiation in rabbit atrium. J Gen Physiol 1986; 87:675–706.
37. Hoeper MM, Boeker KH: Overdose of metoprolol treated with enoximone. N Engl J Med. 1996;335:1538. Letter.
38. Hofer CA, Smith JK, Tenholder MF: Verapamil intoxication: A literature review of overdoses and discussion of therapeutic options. Am J Med 1993;95:431–438.
39. Hoffman BB, Lefkowitz RJ: Catecholamines, sympathomimetic drugs, and adrenergic receptor antagonists. In: Hardman JG, Limbird LE, Molinoff PB, et al, eds: Goodman and Gilman's The Pharmacological Basis of Therapeutics, 9th ed. New York, McGraw-Hill, 1996, pp. 199–248.
40. Hohnloser SH, Woosley RL: Sotalol. N Engl J Med 1994;331:31–38.
41. Hosie J, Dahlof B, Klein G: The long term antihypertensive efficacy and safety of a new felodipine–metoprolol combination tablet. Blood Pressure 1993;(suppl)1:46–50.
42. Illingworth R: Glucagon for beta blocker poisoning. Lancet 1980;2:86.
43. Kelly RA, Smith TW: Pharmacologic treatment of heart failure. In: Hardman JG, Limbird LE, Molinoff PB, et al, eds: Goodman and Gilman's The Pharmacological Basis of Therapeutics, 9th ed. New York, McGraw-Hill, 1996, pp. 809–838.
44. Kenyon CJ, Aldonger GE, Joshipura P, Zaid GJ: Successful resuscitation using external cardiac pacing in beta adrenergic antagonist-induced bradyasystolic arrest. Ann Emerg Med 1988;17:711–713.
44a. Kerns W, Schroeder D, Williams C, et al: Insulin improves survival in a canine model of acute β-blocker toxicity. Ann Emerg Med 1997;29:748–757.
45. Khan A, Muscat-Baron JM: Fatal oxprenolol poisoning. Br Med J 1977;1:552.
45a. Kline JA, Leonova E, Raymond RM: Beneficial myocardial metabolic effects of insulin during verapamil toxicity in the anesthetized canine. Crit Care Med 1995;23:1251–1263.
46. Kollef MH: Labetalol overdose successfully treated with amrinone and alpha receptor agonists. Chest 1994;105: 626–627.
47. Korzets A, Danby P, Edmunds ME, et al: Acute renal failure associated with a labetalol overdose. Postgrad Med J 1990;66:66–67.
48. Kosinski E, Malindzak G: Glucagon and isoproterenol in reversing propranolol toxicity. Arch Intern Med 1973; 132:840–843.
49. Kosinski EJ, Stein N, Malindzak GS, et al: Glucagon and propranolol (Inderal) toxicity. N Engl J Med 1971;285:1325.
50. Krapf R, Gertsch M: Torsade de pointes induced by sotalol despite therapeutic plasma sotalol concentrations. Br Med J 1985;290:1784–1785.
51. Kulling P, Eleborg L, Persson H: β-adrenoreceptor blocker intoxication: Epidemiological data. Prenalterol as an alternative in the treatment of cardiac dysfunction. Hum Toxicol 1983;2:175–181.
52. Lane AS, Woodward AC, Goldman MR: Massive propranolol overdose poorly responsive to pharmacologic therapy: Use of the intra-aortic balloon pump. Ann Emerg Med 1987;16:1381–1383.
53. Langemeijer J, De Wildt D, De Groot G, et al: Calcium interferes with the cardiodepressive effects of beta-blocker overdose in isolated rat hearts. J Toxicol Clin Toxicol 1986;24:111–133.
54. Langemeijer JJM, De Wildt D, De Groot G, et al: Centrally induced respiratory arrest: Main cause of death in β-adrenoreceptor antagonist intoxication. Hum Toxicol 1986;5:65. Letter.
55. Langemeijer J, De Wildt D, De Groot G, et al: Respiratory arrest as main determinant of toxicity due to overdose with different β-blockers in rats. Acta Pharmacol Toxicol 1985;57:352–356.
56. Lederballe Pederson O, Mikkelsen E, Lanng Nielsen J, Christensen NJ: Abrupt withdrawal of beta blocking agents in patients with arterial hypertension. Effect on blood pressure, heart rate and plasma catecholamines and prolactin. Eur J Clin Pharmacol 1979;15: 215–217.
57. Lee KC, Canniff PC, Hamel DW, et al: Cardiovascular and renal effects of milrinone in β-adrenoreceptor blocked and non-blocked anaesthetized dogs. Drugs Exp Clin Res 1991;18:145–158.
58. Levitzki A, Marbach I, Bar-Sinai A: The signal transduction between beta receptors and adenyl cyclase. Life Sci 1993;52:2093–2100.
59. Litovitz TL, Bailey KM, Schmitz BF, Holm KC: 1990 Annual report of the American association of poison control centers national data collecting system. Am J Emerg Med 1991;9:461–509.
60. Litovitz TL, Clark LR, Soloway RA: 1993 Annual report of the American Association of Poison Control Centers National Data Collecting System. Am J Emerg Med 1994; 12:546–584.
61. Litovitz TL, Felberg L, Soloway RA, et al: 1994 Annual report of the American Association of Poison Control Centers National Data Collecting System. Am J Emerg Med 1995;13:551–596.
62. Litovitz TL, Felberg L, White S, Klein-Schwartz W: 1995 Annual report of the American Association of Poison Control Centers National Data Collecting System. Am J Emerg Med 1996;14:487–537.
63. Litovitz TL, Holm KC, Bailey KM, et al: 1991 Annual report of the American Association of Poison Control Centers National Data Collecting System. Am J Emerg Med 1992;10:452–505.
64. Litovitz TL, Holm KC, Clancy C, Schmitz BF: 1992 Annual report of the American Association of Poison Control Centers National Data Collecting System. Am J Emerg Med 1993;11:494–555.
65. Litovitz TL, Schmitz BF, Bailey KM: 1989 Annual report of the American Association of Poison Control Centers National Data Collecting System. Am J Emerg Med 1990; 8:394–442.
66. Lofdahl CG, Svedmyr N: Cardioselectivity of atenolol and

metoprolol. A study in asthmatic patients. Eur J Resp Dis 1981;62:396–404.
67. Love JN: Beta blocker toxicity after overdose: When do symptoms develop in adults? J Emerg Med 1994;12: 799–802.
68. Love JN, Leasure JA, Mundt DJ: A comparison of combined amrinone and glucagon therapy to glucagon alone for cardiovascular depression associated with propranolol toxicity in a canine model. Am J Emerg Med 1993; 11:360–363.
69. Love JN, Leasure JA, Mundt DJ, et al: A comparison of amrinone and glucagon therapy for cardiovascular depression associated with propranolol toxicity in a canine model. J Toxicol Clin Toxicol 1992;30:399–412.
70. Lundborg P: The effect of adrenergic blockade on potassium concentrations in different conditions. Acta Med Scand 1983;672:121–126.
71. Mcvey FK, Corke CF: Extracorporeal circulation in the management of massive propranolol overdose. Anesthesiology 1991;46:744–746.
72. Mery PF, Brechler V, Pavoine C, et al: Glucagon stimulates the cardiac Ca^{2+} current by activation of adenyl cyclase and inhibition of phosphodiesterase. Nature 1990;345: 158–161.
73. Montagna M, Groppi A: Fatal sotalol poisoning. Arch Toxicol 1980;43:221–226.
74. Montgomery AB, Stager MA, Schoene RB: Marked suppression of respiration while awake following massive ingestion of atenolol. Chest 1985;88:920–921.
75. Morita S, Sawai Y, Heeg JF, Koike Y: Pharmacokinetics of enoximone after various intravenous administrations to healthy volunteers. J Pharmaceut Sci 1995;84:152–157.
76. Neuvonen PJ, Elonen E, Vuorenmaa T, et al: Prolonged QT interval and severe tachyarrhythmias, common features of sotalol intoxication. Eur J Clin Pharmacol 1981; 20:85–89.
77. Nishizuka Y: Intracellular signalling by hydrolysis of phospholipids and activation of protein kinase C. Science 1992;258:607–614.
78. Perrot D, Bui-xuan B, Lang J, et al: A case of sotalol poisoning with fatal outcome. J Toxicol Clin Toxicol 1988;26: 389–396.
79. Pollack CV: Utility of glucagon in the emergency department. J Emerg Med 1993;11:195–205.
80. Pritchard BN, Battersby LA, Cruikshank JM: Overdosage with β-adrenergic blocking agents. Adv Drug React Poison Rev 1984;3:91–111.
81. Pritchard BN, Thorpe P: Pindolol in hypertension. Med J Aust 1971;58:1242.
82. Pritchard BN, Tomlinson B, Walden RJ, Bhattacherjee P: The beta-adrenergic blockade withdrawal phenomenon. J Cardiovasc Pharmacol 1983;5(suppl 1):56S–62S.
83. Proano L, Chiang WK, Wang RY: Calcium channel blocker overdose. Am J Emerg Med 1995;13:444–450.
84. Psaty BM, Koepsell TD, Wagner EH, et al: The relative risk of incident coronary heart disease associated with recently stopping the use of beta blockers. JAMA 1990;263: 1653–1657.
85. Puceat M, Vassort G: Signalling by protein kinase C isoforms in the heart. Mol Cell Biochem 1996;157:65–72
86. Ragno RE, Langlois S: Comparison of withdrawal phenomena after propranolol, metoprolol and pindolol. Br J Clin Pharmacol 1982;13(suppl 2):345S–351S.
87. Rasmussen H: The calcium messenger system. N Engl J Med 1986;314:1094–1102.
88. Reiter M: Calcium mobilization and cardiac inotropic mechanisms. Pharmacol Rev 1988;40:189–217.
89. Reith DM, Dawson AH, Epid D, et al: Relative toxicity of beta blockers in overdose. J Toxicol Clin Toxicol 1996;34: 273–278.
90. Reithman C, Thomschke A, Werdan K: The role of endogenous noradrenaline in the beta blocker withdrawal phenomenon—studies with cultured heart cells. Klin Wochenschr 1987;65:308–316.
91. Reuter H, Porzig H: Beta-adrenergic actions on cardiac cell membranes. Adv Myocardiol 1982;3:87–93.
92. Reynolds RD, Gorczynske RJ, Quon CY: Pharmacology and pharmacokinetics of esmolol. J Clin Pharmacol 1986;26:A3–A14.
93. Richards DA, Prichard BN: Self poisoning with β-blockers. Br Med J 1978;1:1623–1624.
94. Richards DA, Pritchard BN, Boakes AJ, et al: Pharmacologic basis for antihypertensive effects of intravenous labetalol. Br Heart J 1977;39:99–106.
95. Riker CD, Wright RK, Matusiak W, et al: Massive metoprolol ingestion associated with a fatality—A case report. J Forensic Sci 1987;32:1447–1452.
96. Ronn O, Graffner C, Johnsson G, et al: Heamodynamic effects and pharmacokinetics of a new selective beta 1-adrenoreceptor agonist, prenalterol, and its interaction with metoprolol in man. Eur J Clin Pharmacol 1979;15: 9–13.
97. Ross PJ, Lewis MJ, Sheridan DJ, Henderson AH: Adrenergic hypersensitivity after beta blocker withdrawal. Br Heart J 1981;45:637–642.
98. Saitz R, Williams BW, Farber HW: Atenolol induced cardiovascular collapse treated with hemodialysis. Crit Care Med 1991;19:116–119.
99. Sangster B, De Wildt D, Van Dijk A: A case of acebutolol intoxication. J Toxicol Clin Toxicol 1983;20:69–77.
100. Sato S, Tsuji MH, Okubo N, et al: Combined use of glucagon and milrinone may not be preferable for severe propranolol poisoning in the canine model. J Toxicol Clin Toxicol 1995;33:337–343.
101. Sato S, Tsuji MH, Okubo N, et al: Milrinone versus glucagon: Comparative hemodynamic effects in canine propranolol poisoning. J Toxicol Clin Toxicol 1994;32: 277–289.
102. Shahid M, Rogers IW: The inotropic effect of 4-aminopyridine and pH changes in rabbit papillary muscle. J Pharm Pharmacol 1989;49:601–606.
103. Shore ET, Cepin D, Davidson MJ: Metoprolol overdose. Ann Emerg Med 1981;10:524–527.
104. Singh BN, Nisbet HD, Harris EA, et al: A comparison of the actions of ICI66082 and propranolol on cardiac and peripheral beta receptors. Eur J Pharmacol 1975;34:75–86.
105. Smit AJ, Mulder PO, de Jong PE, et al: Acute renal failure after overdose of labetalol. BMJ 1986;293:1142–1143.
106. Soni N, Baines D, Pearson IY: Cardiovascular collapse and propranolol overdose. Med J Aust 1983;2:629–630.

107. Sperelakis N, Xiong Z, Haddad G, et al: Regulation of slow calcium channels of myocardial cells and vascular smooth muscle by cyclic nucleotides and phosphorylation. Mol Cell Biochem 1994;140:103–117.
108. Stajic M, Granger RH, Beyer JC: Fatal metoprolol overdose. J Anal Toxicol 1984;8:228–230.
109. Strosberg AD: Structure, function, and regulation of the three beta-adrenergic receptors. Obesity Res 1995;3(suppl 4):501S–505S.
110. Strubelt O: Evaluation of antidotes against the acute cardiovascular toxicity of propranolol. Toxicology 1984;31: 261–270.
111. Sulakhe PV, Vo XT: Regulation of phospholamban and troponin-I phosphorylation in the intact rat cardiomyocytes by adrenergic and cholinergic stimuli: Roles of cyclic nucleotides, calcium, protein kinases and phosphatases and depolarization. Mol Cell Biochem 1995;149/150: 103–126.
112. Szigligeti P, Pankucsi C, Banyasz T, et al: Action potential duration and force–frequency relationship in isolated rabbit, guinea pig and rat cardiac muscle. J Comp Physiol 1996;166:150–155.
113. Taboulet P, Cariou A, Berdeaux A, et al: Pathophysiology and management of self-poisoning with β-blockers. J Toxicol Clin Toxicol 1993;31:531–551.
114. Talosi L, Kranias EG: Effect of α-adrenergic stimulation on activation of protein kinase C and phosphorylation of proteins in intact rabbit hearts. Circ Res 1992;70: 670–678.
115. Totterman KJ, Turto H, Pellinen T: Overdrive pacing as treatment of sotalol induced ventricular tachydysrhythmias (torsades de pointes). Acta Med Scand 1982;668: 28–33.
116. Travill CM, Pugh S, Noble MIM: The inotropic and hemodynamic effects of intravenous milrinone when reflex adrenergic stimulation is suppressed by beta-adrenergic blockade. Clin Ther 1994;16:783–792.
117. Tynan RF, Fisher M, Ibels LS: Self-poisoning with propranolol. Med J Aust 1981;1:82–83.
118. Vinti H, Chichmanian RM, Fournier JP, et al: Systemic complications of beta-blocking eyedrops. Apropos of 6 cases. Rev Med Interne 1989;10:41–44.
119. Walden RJ, Bhattacherjee P, Tomlinson B, et al: The effect of intrinsic sympathomimetic activity on beta-receptor responsiveness after beta-adrenergic blockade withdrawal. Br J Clin Pharmacol 1982;13(suppl):359S–364S.
120. Walden RJ, Hernandez J, Yu Y, et al: Withdrawal of beta-blocking drugs. Am Heart J 1982;104:515–520.
121. Walden RJ, Tomlinson B, Graham B, et al: Withdrawal phenomena after atenolol and bopindolol: Heamodynamic responses in healthy volunteers. Br J Clin Pharmacol 1990;30:557–565.
122. Walden RJ, Tomlinson B, Graham B, et al: Withdrawal phenomena after atenolol and bopindolol: Hormonal changes in normal volunteers . Br J Clin Pharmacol 1990; 30:547–556.
123. Ward DE, Jones B: Glucagon and beta blocker toxicity. Br Med J 1976;6028:151.
124. Wei J, Mojsoc S: Tissue specific expression of the human receptor for glucagon like peptide, 1. Brain, heart and pancreatic forms have the same deduced amino acid sequences. FEBS Lett 1995;358:219–224.
125. Wei J, Spotnitz H, Spotnitz W, et al: Pharmacologic antagonism of propranolol in dogs. J Thorac Cardiovasc Surg 1984;87:732–742.
126. Weinstein RS: Recognition and management of poisoning with beta adrenergic blocking agents. Ann Emerg Med 1984;13:1123–1131.
127. Wheeldon NM, McDevitt DG, Lipworth BJ: Investigation of putative cardiac beta 3-adrenoceptors in man. Q J Med 1993;86:255–261.
128. Yagami T: Differential coupling of glucagon and beta-adrenergic receptors with the small and large forms of the stimulatory G protein. Mol Pharmacol 1995;48:849–854.

ANTIDOTES IN DEPTH

Glucagon

Mary Ann Howland

Glucagon is a polypeptide hormone with a molecular weight of 3500 D that is secreted by pancreatic alpha cells in response to food products and often gastrointestinal hormones. Whereas fuel storage is promoted by insulin, fuel mobilization is stimulated by glucagon.[19] Hypoglycemia causes the release of glucagon and the suppression of insulin. Intracellular food stores are then mobilized to meet the energy demands of the body.[19] This response is probably mediated through stimulation of cyclic AMP (cAMP) synthesis, especially in liver and adipose tissue.[21] This same stimulation of cAMP synthesis in the heart may account for glucagon's inotropic effect in high concentrations.[19,30] In addition, glucagon relaxes smooth muscle in the lower esophageal sphincter, stomach, small and large intestines, common bile duct, and ureters.[13,15]

Glucagon was formerly proposed as part of the initial treatment for all comatose patients.[33] The theoretical rationale for this approach is only partially sound. Hypoglycemic patients may present in coma or with an altered mental status and hypoglycemia can exist concomitantly with a drug overdose. Immediately restoring the patient's blood glucose level may be lifesaving. Glucagon, however, requires time to act and may be ineffective in a patient with depleted glycogen stores. The intravenous administration of 0.5–1.0 g/kg of 50% dextrose in adults rapidly reverses hypoglycemia and does not rely on glycogen stores for its effect. Intravenous dextrose, therefore, is preferred over glucagon as the initial substrate to be given to all patients with an altered mental status presumed to be related to hypoglycemia (see Antidotes in Depth: Dextrose).

The cardiovascular effects of glucagon were extensively studied in 21 patients who were given varied doses and durations of infusion. In 11 patients who received 3–5 mg via IV bolus, increases in the force of contraction as measured by maximum dP/dT, heart rate, cardiac index, blood pressure, and stroke work were all demonstrated. There was no change in systemic vascular resistance, LVEDP, or stroke index. Additionally, glucose increased by 50% and the potassium level fell. Patients who received 1 mg via IV bolus also had an increase in cardiac index but systemic vascular resistance fell, probably secondary to splanchnic and hepatic vascular smooth muscle relaxation. Patients who received an infusion of 2–3 mg/min for 10–15 min responded similarly to the patients who received the 3–5 mg IV boluses, but experienced significant dose-limiting nausea and vomiting. Glucagon's effects began within 1–3 minutes, were maximal within 5–7 minutes, and lasted up to 10–15 minutes.[30] These cardiovascular manifestations demonstrate the positive inotropic and chronotropic effects of glucagon on the intact human heart.[31]

Investigations into the mechanism of action of glucagon on the heart have been performed on cardiac tissue obtained from patients during surgical procedures and in a variety of in vivo and ex vivo animal studies. The results are species specific and dependent on the presence or absence of congestive heart failure. The inotropic action of glucagon appears to be related to an increase in cardiac cAMP levels.[7] The positive inotropic and chronotropic actions of glucagon are very similar to those of the beta-adrenergic agonists except that they are not blocked by beta-adrenergic antagonists. In addition, whereas the beta-adrenergic agonists are dysrhythmogenic, glucagon is not. The effects of glucagon are markedly diminished as the severity and chronicity of congestive heart failure increases.

Administration of ^{125}I-labeled glucagon in the cat demonstrated the presence of a specific glucagon receptor.[21] Binding was closely correlated with activation of cardiac adenylate cyclase. This experiment demonstrated a large number of glucagon binding sites, with as few as 10% of the binding sites occupied at near maximal stimulation of adenylate cyclase. It is currently believed that the binding of glucagon to its receptor results in the combination coupling with the G_s protein, catalyzing the exchange of guanosine triphosphate (GTP) for guanosine diphosphate (GDP) on the alpha subunit of G_s.[15,34] The GTP–G_s unit then stimulates adenylate cylase to convert ATP to cAMP. In the rat ventricular myocyte, stimulation of adenylate cylase enhances cAMP phosphorylation of L-type Ca^{2+} channels.[28] These effects are antagonized by acetylcholine.[28]

Strategies for enhancing the beneficial effects of glucagon have involved combination with the phosphodiesterase inhibitors amrinone and its derivative milrinone. In a canine model, both amrinone and milrinone alone were comparable to glucagon,[23,38] but the combinations caused a decrease in mean arterial pressure in the presence of amrinone and an excessive tachycardia when milrinone was used.[22,37]

Overdoses with beta-adrenergic antagonists are particularly dangerous and are manifested by hypotension, bradycardia, prolonged atrioventricular conduction times, depressed cardiac output, and cardiac failure, in addition to alterations in consciousness, seizures, and, rarely, hypoglycemia.[1,6,8,10] Bradycardia and hypotension may respond to atropine, isoproterenol, epinephrine, norepinephrine, dopamine, dobutamine, or combinations.[9] Glucagon has successfully reversed bradydysrhythmias and hypotension in patients unresponsive to these drugs and should be administered early in the management of patients with severe overdoses.[6,8,18,41] Glucagon, by increasing myocardial cAMP levels,[20,27] is able to increase the inotropic[2,11,25,30] and the chronotropic[2,11,18,25,30,43] activity of the heart and circumvent the beta-adrenergic antagonist effect on the heart.

The relationship between calcium and the chronotropic effects of glucagon was demonstrated in rats.[5] Glucagon's maximal chronotropic effects are dependent on a normal circulating ionized calcium. Both hypocalcemia and hypercalcemia blunt the maximal chronotropic response.[4,5]

Calcium channel blocker overdoses produce a constellation of clinical findings similar to those recognized with beta-adrenergic antagonist overdoses, including hypotension, bradycardia, heart block, and myocardial depression. Animal studies[17,35,39,40,45,46] demonstrate the ability of glucagon to reverse the myocardial depression produced by nifedipine, diltiazem, and verapamil. Several human case reports,[29] including one where amrinone was used in addition to glucagon therapy, also show this benefit.[44]

A single IV dose of glucagon has its onset within minutes, peak level in 5–7 minutes, with a duration of action of 10–15 minutes.[30] An initial IV bolus of 50 μg/kg infused over 1 minute has been recommended (3.5 mg in a 70-kg person).[10] Higher doses may be necessary if the initial bolus is ineffective, and up to 10 mg may be tried in an adult.[16] In many cases the bolus dose should be followed by a continuous infusion of 2–5 mg/h, in 5% dextrose in water, which can then be tapered as the patient improves.[1,14,16,32,36,42]

Glucagon is available as a 1-unit (1-mg) or 10-unit (10-mg) lyophilized powder for injection with an accompanying 1 mL or 10 mL of the diluent, respectively. The diluent contains 2 mg of phenol/mL as a preservative. As a precaution against phenol toxicity, it is recommended that the body burden of phenol should not exceed 50 mg in a 10-hour period.[3] Although systemic adverse effects from the use of parenteral phenol-containing pharmaceuticals have not been reported,[12] the manufacturer recommends reconstituting the glucagon with sterile water for injection, rather than the accompanying diluent, when glucagon doses will exceed 2 mg.

Side effects from glucagon include a dose-dependent nausea and vomiting,[26] hyperglycemia, hypokalemia, and generalized allergic reactions. Commercial glucagon is derived from beef or pork pancreas and therefore the potential for allergic reactions exists.

Glucagon produces positive inotropic and chronotropic effects despite beta-adrenergic antagonism. Glucagon has proved to be beneficial in the treatment of patients with severe overdoses of beta-adrenergic antagonists and calcium channel blockers. The benignity of an IV bolus of glucagon in the patient with a serious overdose of a beta-adrenergic antagonist or calcium channel blocker should lead the clinician to use glucagon early in patient management. The availability of an adequate supply of glucagon in the ED (at least three 10-mg vials) with another 100 mg in the pharmacy should be ensured.[24]

References

1. Agura E, Wexler L, Witzburg R: Massive propranolol overdose. Am J Med 1986;80:755–757.
2. Benvenisty A, Spotnitz H, Rose E, et al: Antagonism of chronic canine beta adrenergic blockage with dopamine, isoproterenol, dobutamine, and glucagon. Surg Forum 1979; 30:187–188.
3. Brancato DJ: Recognizing potential toxicity of phenol. Vet Hum Toxicol 1982;24:29–30.
4. Chernow B, Reed L, Geelhoed G, et al: Endocrine effects and calcium involvement in cardiovascular actions in dogs. Circ Shock 1986;19:393–407.
5. Chernow B, Zaloga G, Malcolm D, et al: Glucagon's chronotropic action is calcium dependent. J Pharm Exp Ther 1987;241:833–837.
6. Ehgartner GR, Zelinka MA: Hemodynamic instability following intentional nadolol overdose. Arch Intern Med 1988;148:801–802.
7. Farah A: Glucagon and the circulation. Pharm Rev 1983; 35:181–217.
8. Fernandes CMB, Daya MR: Sotalol-induced bradycardia reversed by glucagon. Can Fam Physician 1995;41:659–665.
9. Frishman W: Beta-adrenoceptor antagonists: New drugs and new indications. N Engl J Med 1980;305:500–506.
10. Frishman W, Jacob H, Eisenberg E, Ribner H: Clinical pharmacology of the new beta-adrenergic blocking drugs. Part 8. Self poisoning with beta-adrenoceptor blocking agents: Recognition and management. Am Heart J 1979;98:798–811.
11. Glick G, Parmley W, Wechsler AS, Sonnenblick EH: Glucagon. Circ Res 1968;22:798–799.
12. Golightly L, Smolinske S, Bennett M, et al: Pharmaceutical excipients. Med Toxicol 1988;3:128–165.
13. Hall-Boyer K, Zaloga G, Chernow B: Glucagon: Hormone or therapeutic agent. Crit Care Med 1984;12:584–589.
14. Heath A: β-Adrenoreceptor blocker toxicity: Clinical features and therapy. Am J Emerg Med 1984;2:518–526.
15. Homcy CJ: The β-adrenergic signaling pathway in the heart. Hosp Pract 1991;26:43–50.
16. Illingworth RN: Glucagon for beta-blocker poisoning. Practitioner 1979;223:683–685.
17. Jolly S, Kipnis J, Lucchesi B: Cardiovascular depression by verapamil: Reversal by glucagon and interactions with propanolol. Pharmacology 1987;35:249–255.
18. Kosinski EJ, Malidzak GS: Glucagon and isoproterenol in reversing propanolol toxicity. Arch Intern Med 1973; 132:840–843.
19. Larner J: Insulin and oral hypoglycemic drugs: Glucagon. In: Gilman AG, Goodman LS, Gilman A, eds: The Pharmacologic Basis of Therapeutics, 6th ed. New York, Macmillan, 1980, pp. 1497–1523.

20. Levey G, Epstein S: Activation of adenyl cyclase by glucagon in cat and human heart. Circ Res 1969;24:151–156.
21. Levey GS, Fletcher MA, Klein I, et al: Characterisation of I-glucagon binding in a solubilized preparation of cat myocardial adenylate cyclase. J Biol Chem 1974;249: 2665–2673.
22. Love JN, Leasure JA, Mundt DJ: A comparison of combined amrinone and glucagon therapy to glucagon alone for cardiovascular depression associated with propranolol toxicity in a canine model. Am J Emerg Med 1993;11:360–363.
23. Love JN, Leasure JA, Mundt DJ, Janz TG: A comparison of amrinone and glucagon therapy for cardiovascular depression associated with propanolol toxicity in a canine model. J Toxicol Clin Toxicol 1992;30:399–412.
24. Love JN, Tandy TK: β-Adrenoreceptor antagonist toxicity: A survey of glucagon availability. Ann Emerg Med 1993;22: 151–152. Letter.
25. Lucchesi B: Cardiac actions of glucagon. Circ Res 1968;22: 777–787.
26. Lvoff R, Wilcken D: Glucagon in heart failure and in cardiogenic shock—Experience in 50 patients. Circulation 1972;45: 534–542.
27. MacLeod K, Rodgers R, McNeil J: Characterization of glucagon-induced changes in rate, contractility, and cyclic AMP levels in isolated cardiac preparations of the rat and guinea pig. J Pharmacol Exp Ther 1981;217:798–804.
28. Méry PF, Brechler V, Pavoine C, et al: Glucagon stimulates the cardiac Ca^{2+} current by activation of adenyl cyclase and inhibition of phosphodiesterase. Nature 1990;345:158–161. Letter.
29. Mullen JT, Walter FG, Ekins BR, Khasigian PA: Amelioration of nifedipine poisoning associated with glucagon therapy. Vet Hum Toxicol 1991;33:358.
30. Parmley WW: The role of glucagon in cardiac therapy. N Engl J Med 1971;285:801–802.
31. Parmley W, Glick G, Sonnenblick E: Cardiovascular effects of glucagon in man. N Engl J Med 1968;279:12–17.
32. Peterson C, Leeder S, Sterner S: Glucagon therapy for beta-blocker overdose. Drug Intell Clin Pharm 1984;18:394–398.
33. Rappolt R, Inaba D, Gay G: NAGD regime (Naloxone [Narcan], activated charcoal, glucagon, doxapram [Dopram]) for the coma of drug related overdoses. Clin Toxicol 1980; 16:395–396.
34. Rodell M: The role of hormone receptors and GTP-regulatory proteins in membrane transduction. Nature 1980;284: 17–22.
35. Sabatier J, Pouyet T, Shelvey G, Cavero I: Antagonistic effects of epinephrine, glucagon and methylatropine but not calcium chloride against atrio-ventricular conduction of disturbances produced by high doses of diltiazem, in conscious dogs. Fundam Clin Pharmacol 1991;5:93–106.
36. Salzberg M, Gallagher EJ: Propranolol overdose. Ann Emerg Med 1980;9:26–27.
37. Sato S, Tsuhi MH, Okubo N, et al: Combined use of glucagon and milrinone may not be preferable for severe propanolol poisoning in the canine model. J Toxicol Clin Toxicol 1995;33:337–342.
38. Sato S, Tsuhi MH, Okubo N, et al: Milrinone versus glucagon: Comparative effects in canine propranolol poisoning. J Toxicol Clin Toxicol 1994;32:277–289.
39. Stone CK, May WA, Carroll R: Treatment of verapamil overdose with glucagon. Ann Emerg Med 1995;25:369–374.
40. Stone CK, Thomas SH, Koury SI, Low RB: Glucagon and phenylephrine combination vs glucagon alone in experimental verapamil overdose. Acad Emerg Med 1996;3: 120–125.
41. Ward DE, Jones B: Glucagon and beta-blocker toxicity. Br Med J 1976;2:151.
42. Weinstein R: Recognition and management of poisoning with beta-blocking agents. Ann Emerg Med 1984;13: 1123–1131.
43. Whitehouse F, James T: Chronotropic action of glucagon on the sinus node. Proc Soc Exp Biol Med 1966;122:823–826.
44. Wolf LR, Spadafora MP, Otten EJ: Use of amrinone and glucagon in a case of calcium channel blocker overdose. Ann Emerg Med 1993;22:1225–1228.
45. Zaloga G, Malcolm D, Holaday J, et al: Glucagon reverses the hypotension and bradycardia of verapamil overdose in rats. Crit Care Med 1985;13:273.
46. Zaritsky A, Morowitz M, Chernow B: Glucagon antagonism of calcium blocker-induced myocardial dysfunction. Crit Care Med 1988;16:246–251.

CHAPTER 50

Calcium Channel Blockers

Francis DeRoos

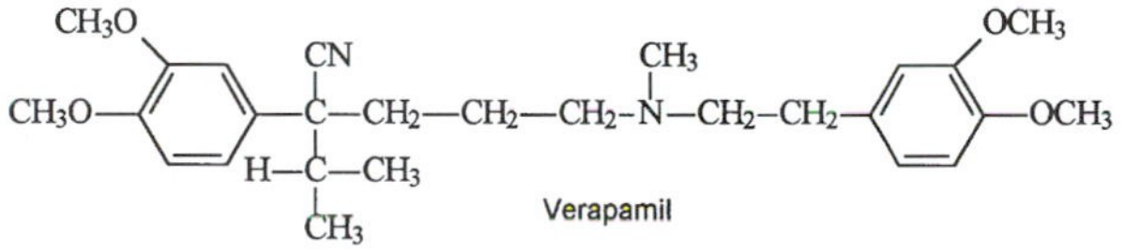

Verapamil

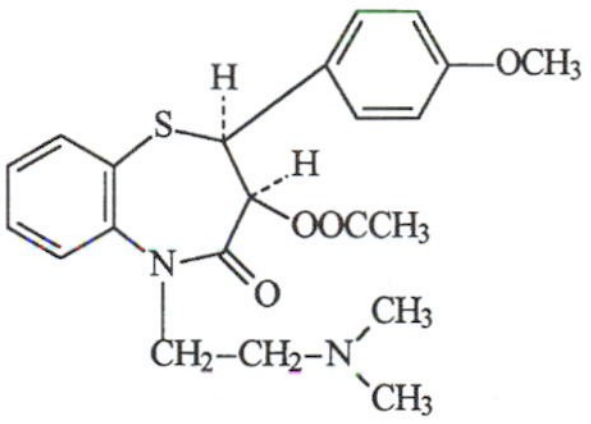

Diltiazem

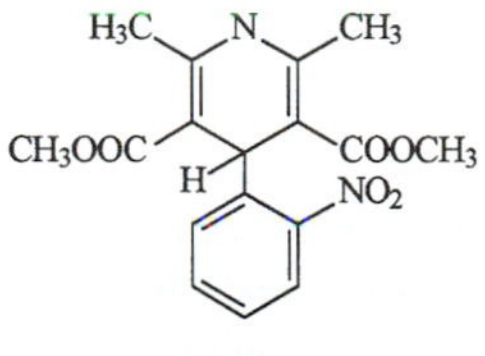

Nifedipine

A 47-year-old female with a history of insulin-dependent diabetes, coronary artery disease, and depression presented to the hospital with multiple nonspecific complaints including "not feeling well," dyspnea, weakness in the legs, and lightheadedness. Physical examination revealed a morbidly obese female in no distress. The initial vital signs were a blood pressure of 120/70 mm Hg, heart rate of 100 beats/min, respiratory rate of 18 breaths/min, and temperature of 98.9°F (37.2°C). The lung fields were clear to auscultation and cardiac examination revealed no murmurs or rubs, but an S_4 gallop was present. Her abdomen was obese with active bowel sounds and no tenderness. Neurologic assessment revealed an alert and oriented female with no gross focal deficits.

Due to the nonspecific complaints in a patient with significant medical conditions, a broad diagnostic evaluation was begun including a rapid blood glucose check, a urinalysis, electrolytes, renal function testing, liver function tests, complete blood count, and an ECG. The ECG demonstrated a sinus rhythm at 100 beats/min with normal PR, QRS and QT_C intervals, left atrial enlargement, and evidence of an old anterior wall infarction (Fig. 50–1). There was no change from previous ECGs.

Following her initial evaluation, the patient confided in the physician that the true reason for her visit was that she was suicidal and that she ingested 20 diltiazem (90 mg) tablets just prior to coming to the hospital. She complained of lightheadedness and weakness. Repeat physical examination revealed a slightly lethargic but arousable and cooperative female. Blood pressure was now 70/30 mm Hg, and heart rate 90 beats/min and regular. A repeat ECG revealed normal sinus rhythm but with first-degree heart block with a PR interval of 24 msec (Fig. 50–2). Initial therapy included normal saline bo-

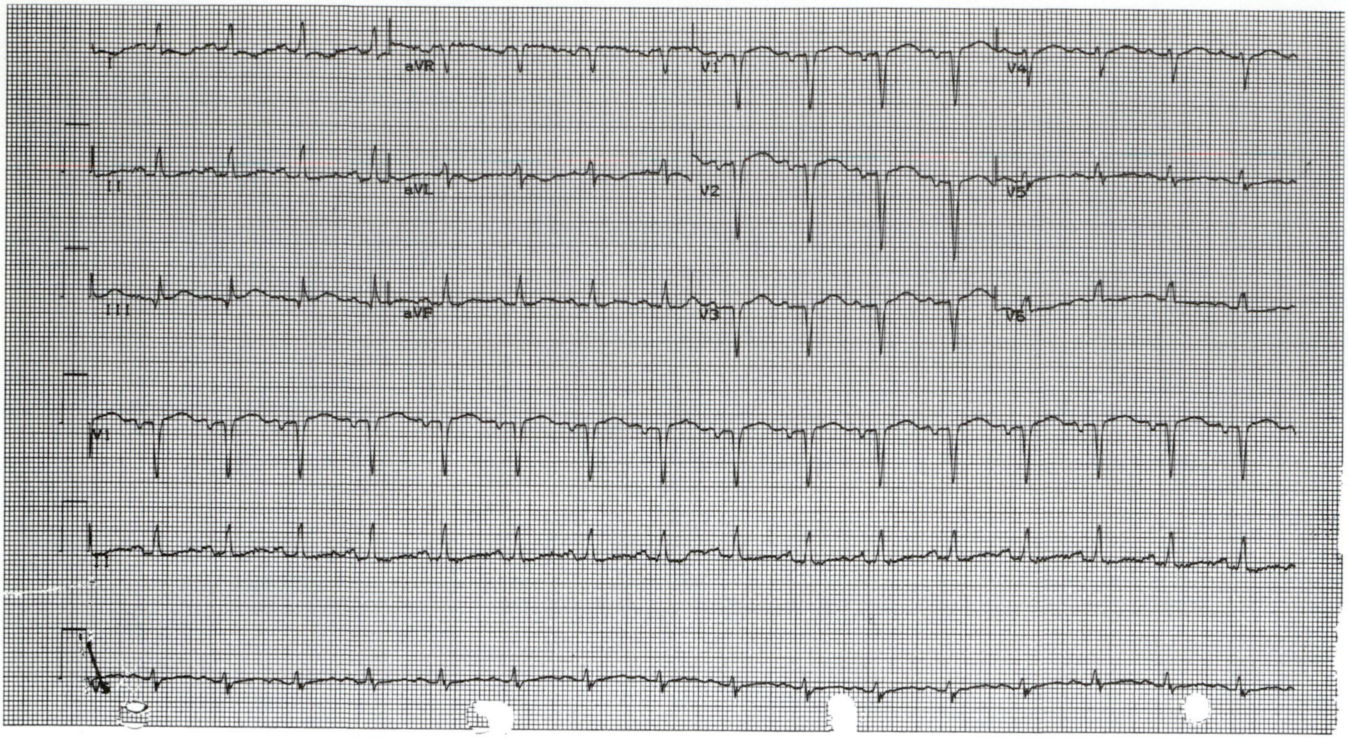

Figure 50–1. This 12-lead electrocardiogram taken 2 hours postingestion of 1800 mg of sustained-release diltiazem demonstrates a sinus tachycardia at 100 beats/min with a normal QRS axis, normal intervals, left atrial enlargement, and an old anterior wall myocardial infarction.

luses, calcium chloride (2 g), glucagon (1 mg), and infusions of dopamine and isoproterenol which resulted in transient improvement in systolic blood pressure from 70 to 98 mm Hg. One hour after she initially became hypotensive, the patient suffered a cardiac arrest with a junctional bradycardia of 65 beats/min and no measurable blood pressure (Fig. 50–3). With aggressive therapy including CPR, endotracheal intubation, atropine (3 mg), large infusions of dopamine and isoproterenol, and a glucagon bolus (5 mg), the systolic blood pressure returned to between 40 to 65 mm Hg with a heart rate of 50 to 60 beats/min. Over the next 3 hours multiple pharmacologic agents including repeat boluses of calcium chloride and continuous infusions of glucagon (5 mg/h) , amrinone (200 mg bolus then 800 mg/h), and phenylephrine were initiated without improvement in blood pressure. During this period the patient's serum glucose had risen from 250 to 800 mg/dL and an insulin infusion was begun.

Because of only limited success after multiple pharmacologic agents, a transthoracic pacer was applied but was unable to capture and a transvenous right ventricular pacemaker was placed with intermittent capture at 70 beats/min but the systolic blood pressure remained below 80 mm Hg. An intraaortic balloon pump (IABP) was placed and within 15 minutes the blood pressure improved to 100/50 mm Hg. The patient was maintained on the IABP and transvenous pacemaker, and slowly weaned off the multiple inotropic agents and vasopressors over the next 24 hours. After a complicated 3-week hospitalization, the patient was discharged to an inpatient psychiatric facility with complete neurologic recovery.

What Is the Physiologic Role of Calcium Channels?

In order to understand the physiologic effects of calcium channel blockers and develop a rational pharmacologic approach to overdose therapy, it is important to understand the role of calcium in normal muscle function. Calcium plays an integral part in excitation–contraction coupling and myocardial conduction. Initially, calcium is driven intracellularly down a large concentration and electrical gradient through calcium-specific, voltage-sensitive channels. These channels, specifically identified as L-type calcium channels, are located in the plasma membrane of all types of muscle cells[70] and are composed of homologous protein subunits also found in some sodium and potassium channels.[69] There are many other types of calcium channels, including the T, N, P, Q, and R types, which can be found either intracellularly on the sarcoplasmic reticulum or on cell plasma membranes, particularly in neuronal and secretory tissue.[132] They may be stimulated by cellular stretch (stretch operated), specific neurohormonal binding (receptor operated), or voltage changes (voltage sensitive).[123] Skeletal muscle depends exclusively upon intracellular calcium stores for excitation contraction coupling, so intracellular influx of calcium has little physiologic consequence. In

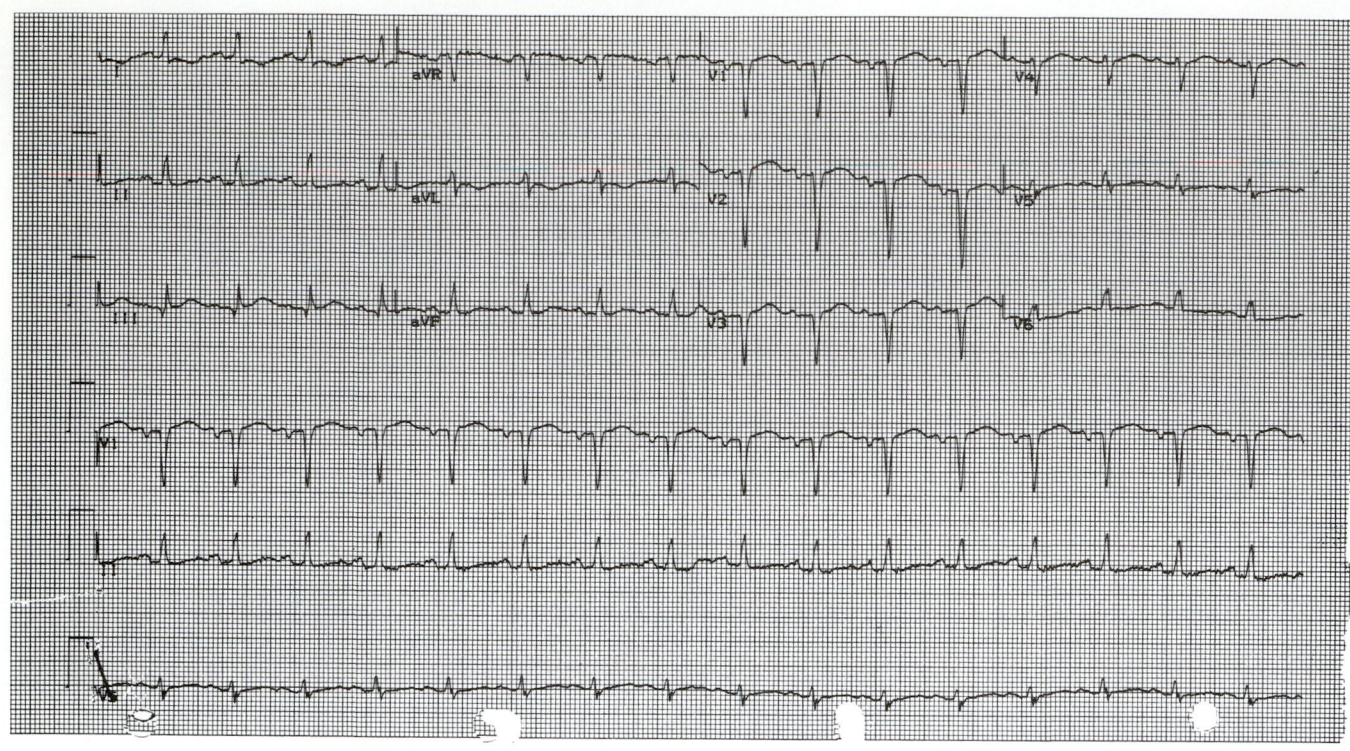

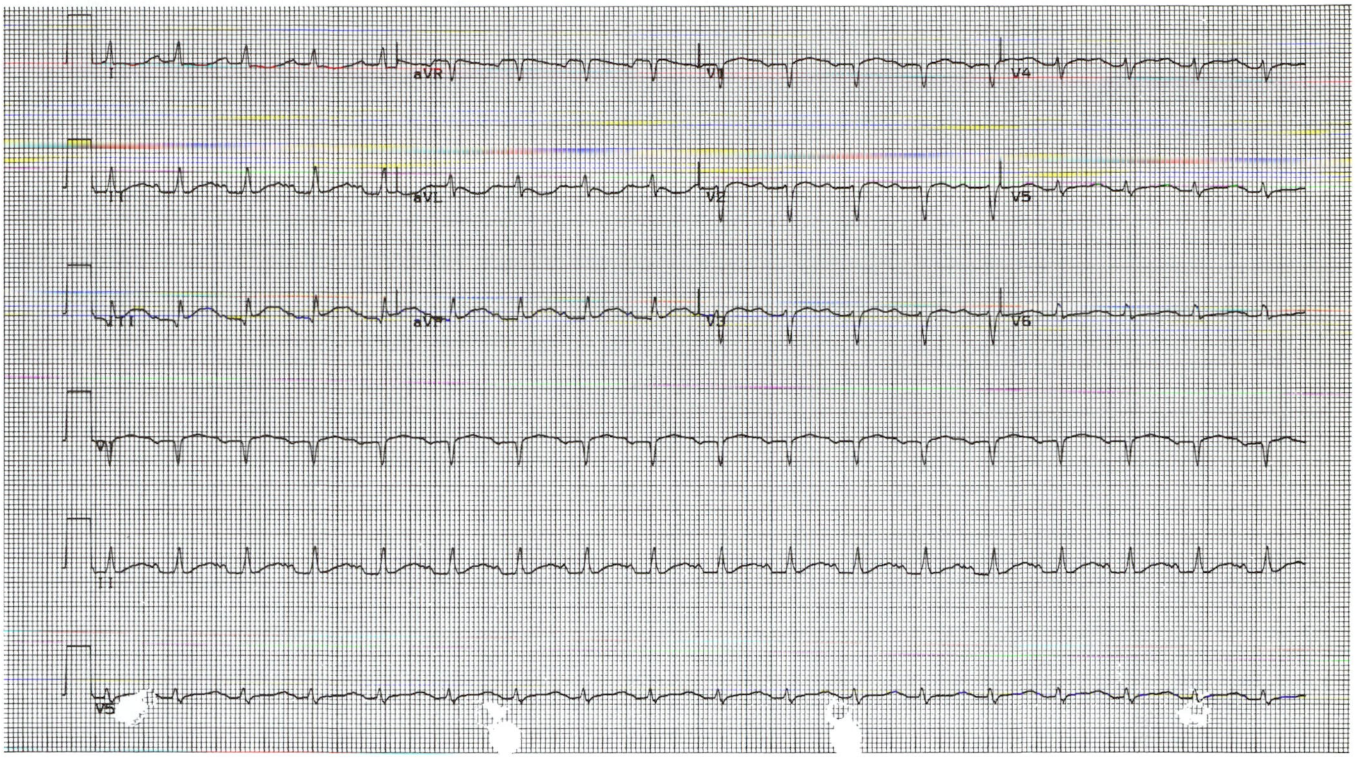

Figure 50–2. This 12-lead electrocardiogram taken 6 hours postingestion of 1800 mg of sustained-release diltiazem now demonstrates first-degree heart block with a PR interval of 0.26 msec and no other changes compared to the patient's previous electocardiogram.

cardiac and smooth muscle cells, however, this influx is critical.

In smooth muscle, the rapid influx of calcium binds calmodulin, and the resulting complex stimulates myosin light-chain kinase activity.[1] The myosin light-chain kinase phosphorylates, and thus activates, myosin, which subsequently binds actin and a contraction occurs.[71,111] In myocardial cells, this slow calcium influx creates the plateau phase (phase 2) of the action potential.[108] The calcium then acts as a second messenger by binding to and opening a receptor-operated calcium channel on the sarcoplasmic reticulum, which releases calcium from the vast stores of the sarcoplasmic reticulum into the cytosol.[62,66] This is often termed calcium-induced calcium release.[33,158] Calcium then binds troponin C, which causes a conformational change that displaces troponin and tropomyosin from the actin. This allows actin and myosin to bind, resulting in a contraction.[72]

In addition to its role in myocardial contractility, calcium influx is also important in myocardial conduction. Calcium influx plays an important role in the spontaneous depolarization (phase 4) of the action potential in the sinoatrial (SA) node.[108] In addition, slow calcium influx allows normal propagation of electrical impulses via the specialized myocardial conduction tissues, particularly the atrioventricular (AV) node.[126]

What Are Calcium Channel Blockers and What Is Their Mechanism of Action?

All commercially available calcium channel blockers (CCBs) exert their physiologic effects by antagonizing L-type voltage-sensitive slow calcium channels, except mibefradil which blocks T channels.[73,150] L channel blockade impairs the calcium influx into muscle cells, particularly the myocardial and smooth muscle, which are dependent upon this influx for normal function. In the vascular smooth muscle, the cytosolic calcium concentration maintains basal tone, and any influx of calcium results in relaxation and arterial vasodilation.[66] In the myocardium this impaired calcium flow results in a decreased force of contraction and negative inotropy. In addition, the sinoatrial (SA) and atrioventricular (AV) nodal tissues are inhibited, producing a reduction in heart rate and intracardiac conduction.[104]

Eleven CCBs are currently available in the United States. These are classified into four structural groups and one functional group (Table 50–1). Each group has a different affinity for the calcium channels in the myocardium and the vascular smooth muscle.[95,106,107,143,150] Verapamil, a phenylalkylamine, has the most profound

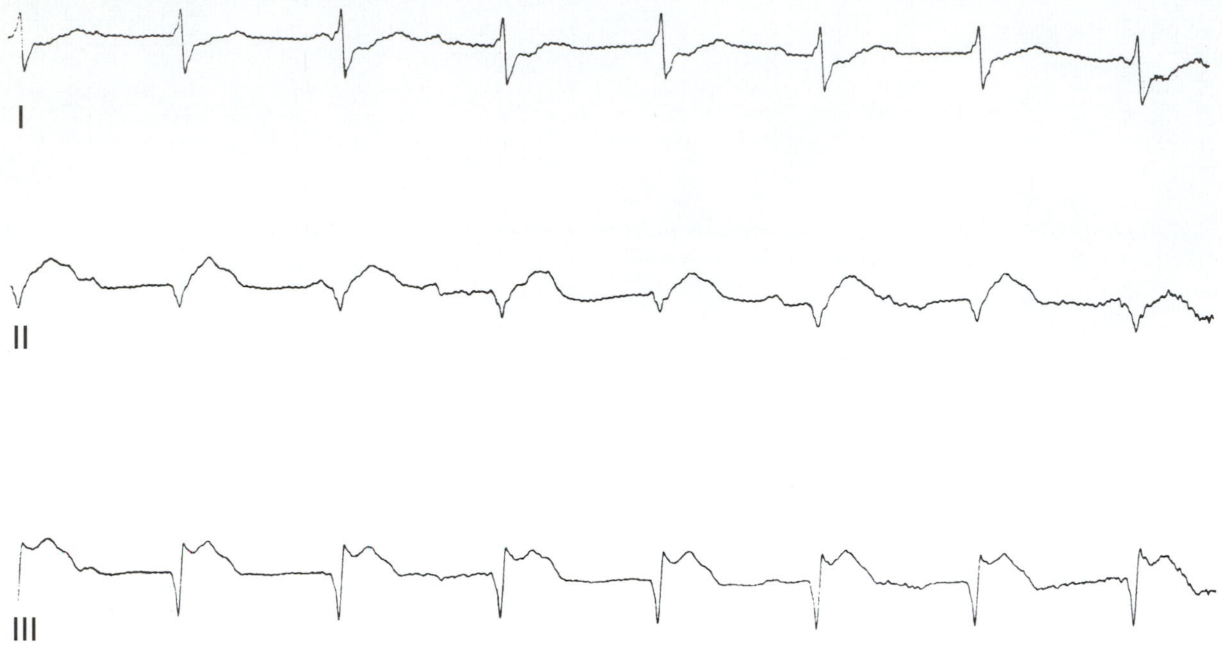

Figure 50–3. This 3-lead rhythm strip was obtained 9 hours postingestion of 1800 mg of sustained-relase diltiazem shortly after the patient became obtunded, hypotensive, and bradycardic. The electrocardiogram now demonstrates a junctional bradycardia at 65 beats/min with widened QRS interval of 0.13 msec and possible inferior ischemia.

inhibitory effects on the SA and AV nodal tissue, while diltiazem has only moderate myocardial depressant effects.[74,106,107] In contrast, nifedipine, the prototypical dihydropyridine, has very little affinity for myocardial calcium channels but has the greatest pharmacologic effect upon the peripheral vascular smooth muscle.[74,106,143] Diltiazem has significant cardiovasular effects although it is not as potent as verapamil. Both verapamil and diltiazem have similar effects on vascular smooth muscle calcium channels.[95] Therefore verapamil is the most potent at decreasing heart rate, cardiac output, and blood pressure, while nifedipine produces the greatest decrease in systemic vascular resistance. However, because dihydropyridines have little myocardial effects at therapeutic levels, the baroreceptor reflex remains intact and an actual slight increase in heart rate and cardiac output may occur.[143] Isradipine is the only dihydropyridine that has a significant enough inhibitory effect on the SA node to blunt any reflex tachycardia.[39]

TABLE 50–1. CLASSIFICATION OF CALCIUM CHANNEL BLOCKERS AVAILABLE IN THE UNITED STATES

Class	Specific Compounds
Phenylalkylamine	Verapamil (Calan, Isoptin, Verelan)
Benzothiazepine	Diltiazem (Cardizem, Dilacor, Tiazac)
Dihydropyridines	Nifedipine (Adalat, Procardia)
	Isradipine (DynaCirc)
	Amlodipine (Norvasc)
	Felodipine (Plendil)
	Nimodipine (Nimotop)
	Nisoldipine (Sular)
	Nicardipine (Cardene)
Diarylaminopropylamine ether	Bepridil (Vascor)
T channel blocker	Mibefradil (Posicor)

Currently bepridil is the only available CCB from the fourth group of agents. Bepridil is unique because in addition to its calcium channel blocking effects, it is a potent fast sodium channel and potassium channel antagonist.[57] This impairs both myocardial contractility and conduction, and results in prolongation of the AV nodal effective refractory period, the action potential itself, and myocardial repolarization.[57] Bepridil induces a prolongation of the QTc interval and has precipitated malignant ventricular dysrhythmias including torsades de pointes.[5,57] This dysrythmogenic effect is potentiated in the setting of hypokalemia.

These receptor-binding differences among the CCB

classes determine the potential therapeutic role of each. Verapamil and diltiazem are used in the management of hypertension, to reduce myocardial oxygen demand, rate control in atrial flutter or fibrillation, and supraventricular reentry tachycardias.[14] Dihydropyridines are typically used to treat diseases with increased peripheral vascular tone such as hypertension, Raynaud's phenomenon, Prinzmetal's angina, esophageal spasm, vascular headaches, and postsubarachnoid hemorrhage vasospasm.[3,14,19,43] Due to its potassium channel blocking effects, bepridil is classified and used exclusively as a class I antidysrhythmic, but due to its dysrythmogenic potential its use is limited to patients who are refractory to all other therapy.[57]

What Are the Pharmacokinetics of Calcium Channel Blockers?

All calcium channel blockers are well absorbed orally. Verapamil undergoes extensive hepatic metabolism and is renally eliminated as inactive metabolites.[102] Norverapamil, formed by *N*-demethylation, is the only active metabolite and retains 20% of the parent compound's activity.[67] Diltiazem also undergoes an extensive first-pass effect and is predominantly deacetylated into deacetyldiltiazem, which has limited activity. This is then eliminated via the biliary tract.[53] Nifedipine also undergoes extensive hepatic metabolism without the production of active metabolites.[38] In overdose, these hepatic enzymes become saturated, reducing the first-pass effect and increasing the quantity of active drug absorbed systemically. This impaired drug metabolism contributes to the prolongation of drug half-lives that has been reported.[15,36,37,125] All CCBs are highly protein bound.[75,102] Volumes of distribution are large for verapamil (5.5 L/kg)[103] and diltiazem (5.3 L/kg),[102] and substantially smaller for nifedipine (0.8 L/kg).[81] Although not well studied, the substantial protein binding and large volume of distribution make it unlikely that extracorporeal drug removal with hemodialysis or hemoperfusion would be of any value in overdose. Several case reports offer clinical support for this conclusion.[128,130,146]

How Common Is Poisoning With Calcium Channel Blockers?

As the utility of calcium channel blockers expands, more and more poisonings are occurring. In 1986, there were just over 1200 exposures and 7 deaths associated with CCB exposures reported to the American Association of Poison Control Centers. In 1995, those figures increased to over 8300 exposures, including over 1000 characterized by moderate to major toxicity, and 69 deaths.[93,94] As a class of drugs, only cyclic antidepressants and opioids were associated with more deaths.[94] These figures partly reflect the increasing popularity and utility of these drugs. A 1989 survey found that verapamil, diltiazem, and nifedipine were among the top 20 prescription drugs dispensed by pharmacies.[122] However, the significant rise in fatalities may also, in part, be due to the introduction of sustained-release preparations in 1988. These dramatic statistics underscore the seriousness of all CCB exposures and the need for thorough gastrointestinal decontamination and critical care monitoring.

What Are the Physiologic Manifestations of Calcium Channel Blocker Poisoning?

The life-threatening toxicity of CCBs is manifested largely within the cardiovascular system and is an extension of their therapeutic effects. Myocardial depression and peripheral vasodilation occur, producing bradycardia and hypotension.[131] Myocardial conduction may be impaired, producing AV conduction abnormalities, idioventricular rhythms, and complete heart block.[9,35,58,64,89,97,112,119] Junctional escape rhythms are frequently noted in patients with significant ingestions.[24] The negative inotropic effects may be so profound, particularly with verapamil, that ventricular contraction may be completely inhibited.[10,49] Patients may present initially asymptomatic but deteriorate rapidly into severe cardiogenic shock.[55,136,152]

Hypotension is the most common physical finding following an overdose.[121,122] The signs and symptoms represent the degree of cardiovascular compromise and hypoperfusion of the patient's central nervous system. Early or mild symptoms include dizziness, fatigue, and lightheadedness, while more severely poisoned patients may manifest lethargy, syncope, altered mental status, coma, and death.[25,51,55,58,84,112,127] Cases of seizures,[51,58,100,114,140] strokes,[129,134,156] ischemic bowel,[46,47,139,153] and renal failure[97,119] occurring in the setting of cardiogenic shock from CCB poisonings are also reported. Severe CNS depression is distinctly uncommon, and if respiratory depression or coma is present without severe hypotension, coingestants or other causes of altered mental status must be considered. Gastrointestinal symptoms of nausea and vomiting are also uncommon.[60]

Although receptor selectivity is lost in overdose and all CCBs can produce severe bradycardia, hypotension, and death,[131] there are some subtle variations in presentation depending upon the agent. The CCBs with the most significant myocardial effects—verapamil and to a lesser extent diltiazem—are associated with more negative inotropic and chronotropic effects.[115,118] In a prospective, poison control center-based study, AV nodal block occurred much more frequently in the setting of verapamil poisoning.[122] In contrast, nifedipine, due to its limited myocardial binding, may produce tachycardia or a "normal" heart rate initially and develop true bradycardia only in patients with more substantial ingestions.[22,54,153,157] Deaths associated with dihydropyridines are distinctly uncommon.[84,115]

Numerous reports document hyperglycemia in severe CCB poisoning.[13,25,31,44,51,58,97,105,119,140,152] Insulin release from the beta islet cells in the pancreas is dependent upon calcium influx via slow calcium channels.[90,99] In CCB overdose, selectivity is lost and this channel is also antagonized. This impairs normal calcium influx and insulin release is reduced.[26] The hyperglycemic effect may be exacerbated in a diabetic patient or if glucagon is used as inotropic therapy.[147]

Noncardiogenic pulmonary edema is also associated with CCB poisoning.[13,17,42,54,60,91] While the mechanism is unknown, it is postulated that there is precapillary vasodilation, causing an increase in transcapillary hydrostatic pressure.[61] The elevated pressure gradient results in increased pulmonary capillary transudates and ultimately interstitial edema.

What Factors Determine the Severity of the Poisoning?

Several factors may affect severity of poisoning, including the agent involved, dose ingested, product formulation, and the patient's underlying cardiovascular health. Coingestion of other agents with cardiovascular activity such as beta-adrenergic antagonists or digoxin will potentiate conduction abnormalities.[18,40,68,85,162]

The product formulation ("immediate" versus sustained release) affects the onset of symptoms and duration of toxicity. With "regular-release" formulations, toxicity is often present within 2 to 3 hours of ingestion.[121] With sustained-release products, however, initial signs or symptoms may be delayed for 6 to 8 hours, and delays of up to 15 hours have been reported.[121,138,148] In addition, with sustained-release ingestions, the drug's apparent half-life is prolonged and toxicity may last longer than 48 hours.[7,9,88]

Comorbidity and age are two factors that negatively impact on both morbidity and mortality in CCB poisonings. Elderly patients and those with underlying cardiovascular disease, such as congestive heart failure, are much more sensitive to the myocardial depressive effects of CCBs.[22,101] Even at therapeutic doses these individuals may develop symptoms of mild hypoperfusion, such as dizziness and fatigue, much more frequently.[50,59,64,110]

What Is the Initial Approach to Patients With Calcium Channel Blocker Ingestions?

Any patient with a suspected calcium channel blocker (CCB) ingestion should be immediately evaluated even if initial vital signs are normal and there are no symptoms. Intravenous access and continuous electrocardiographic monitoring should be initiated. A 12-lead ECG demonstrating the rhythm and intervals should be obtained and repeated every 1 to 2 hours for the first 8 hours and at longer intervals subsequently if the patient's clinical condition normalizes. Initial evaluation should begin with adequate oxygenation and airway protection, intravenous access, continuous cardiac monitoring, and aggressive gastrointestinal decontamination. If the patient is hypotensive and there is no evidence of pulmonary edema, an initial fluid bolus of 10 to 20 mL/kg of crystalloid should be given.

Gastrointestinal decontamination is a critical intervention. Syrup of ipecac should be avoided because CCB-poisoned patients can rapidly deteriorate and become severely hypotensive. Orogastric lavage should be considered for all patients who present early (1 to 2 hours postingestion) after large ingestions, particularly ingestions of sustained-release products, and for patients who are critically ill. All patients with CCB ingestions should receive 1 g/kg of activated charcoal orally. Multiple doses (0.5 g/kg) of activated charcoal (MDAC) without a cathartic should be administered to all patients with sustained-release ingestions or signs of toxicity. Although data are limited, there is no evidence that MDAC increases CCB clearance from the serum.[125,145] Rather, its efficacy may be due to the continuous presence of activated charcoal throughout the gastrointestinal tract in order to adsorb any active drug from its slow-release formulation. Whole-bowel irrigation (WBI) with polyethylene glycol solution (1 to 2 L/h via nasogastric tube in adults, up to 500 mL/h in children) should be initiated for ingestions involving sustained-release products.[16,144] Whole-bowel irrigation may be the most effective means of gastrointestinal decontamination for sustained release products.[79] Dosing should be continued until the rectal effluent is clear.

The importance of early initiation of MDAC and WBI, even in well-appearing patients and particularly in children with a history of sustained-release CCB ingestion, cannot be overemphasized. It is imperative to minimize any absorption and prevent delayed cardiovascular toxicity, which can be profound and difficult to reverse. Several reports describe patients who presented with mild signs of poisoning, in whom gastrointestinal decontamination was not performed aggressively and who subsequently displayed severe toxicity.[138,148]

What Are the Pharmacologic Treatment Options for Patients With Calcium Channel Blocker Poisoning?

Pharmacotherapy should focus upon maintenance or improvement of both cardiac output and peripheral vascular tone.[77] Although many agents—including atropine, calcium, glucagon, isoproterenol, dopamine, epinephrine, norepinephrine, and amrinone—have been used with reported success in the CCB-poisoned patients, no single agent has consistently demonstrated efficacy.[58,115,118,121,122] Little prospective or basic research has been done to evaluate effective treatment modalities.

Atropine

Atropine is considered the drug of choice for all patients with symptomatic bradycardia. In an early dog model of verapamil poisoning, atropine improved heart rate and cardiac output.[41] In one recent prospective study, only 2 of 8 bradycardic CCB-poisoned patients had an improvement in heart rate following the use of atropine.[122] Clinical experience has also demonstrated atropine to be largely ineffective in improving bradycardias in severe CCB-poisoned patients.[25,31,63,118,127,136,156] Initial treatment with calcium may improve the efficacy of atropine.[30,60,65] Given its availability, efficacy in mild poisonings, and safety profile, atropine should still be considered initial therapy in patients with symptomatic bradycardia. Dosing should begin with 0.5 to 1.0 mg (0.02 mg/kg in children) IV every 2 or 3 minutes to a maximum dose of 3 mg in all patients with symptomatic bradycardia. However, due to its limited efficacy in severely poisoned patients, treatment failures with this agent should be anticipated.

Calcium

Pharmacologically, calcium appears to be a logical agent to treat patients with CCB poisoning. Pretreatment with intravenous calcium prior to verapamil use for supraventricular tachydysrhythmias prevents hypotension without diminishing the antidysrhythmic effects.[28,135,154] This is also observed in the overdose setting, where calcium tends to improve blood pressure more than it does the heart rate. Although the mechanism is unclear, boluses of calcium increase the extracellular calcium concentration and increase the intracellular concentration gradient. This may drive calcium through unblocked calcium channels intracellularly. Calcium salts are beneficial in experimental models of CCB poisoning.[30,41,49] Improvement in inotropy and blood pressure in verapamil-poisoned dogs was demonstrated after increasing the serum calcium by 2 mEq/L with an intravenous infusion of 10% calcium chloride at 3 mg/kg per minute.[49]

Calcium has reversed the negative inotropy, impaired conduction, and hypotension in many humans poisoned with CCBs.[16,23,32,48,52,54,89,92,96,109,110,116,122,155,159] Unfortunately, this effect is often short-lived, and more significantly poisoned patients have had no improvement with calcium salt administration.[21,25,31,37,42,45,55,63,125,130] Some authors feel these failures may represent inadequate dosing.[17,60] Unfortunately, the exact dosing of calcium salts is unclear. Reasonable recommendations for poisoned adults include an initial intravenous bolus of approximately 13 to 25 mEq of calcium (10 to 20 mL of 10% calcium chloride or 30 to 60 mL of 10% calcium gluconate), followed by either repeat boluses every 15 to 20 minutes up to 3 or 4 doses or a continuous infusion of 0.5 mEq/kg per hour of calcium (0.2 to 0.4 mL/kg per hour of 10% calcium chloride or 0.6 to 1.2 mL/kg of 10% calcium gluconate).[77,78,115] Careful selection of the calcium salt used is critical for dosing. Although there is no difference in efficacy of calcium chloride or calcium gluconate, 1 g of calcium chloride contains 13.4 mEq of calcium, which is over 3 times the 4.3 mEq found in 1 g of calcium gluconate. Therefore, in order to administer equal doses of calcium, one must administer 3 times the amount of calcium gluconate. If repeat dosing or continuous infusions are used, the serum calcium should be closely monitored to prevent hypercalcemia. This concern is consequential and may significantly limit calcium therapy, particularly the use of a continuous infusion.[84] Other adverse effects of intravenous calcium include nausea, vomiting, flushing, confusion, and angina.[78] *If there is any suspicion that a cardiac glycoside such as digoxin is involved in an overdose, calcium should be avoided because it may further elevate the intracellular calcium and worsen digoxin toxicity unless digoxin-specific Fab has already been utilized* (see Chap. 48).[12]

Catecholamines

Catecholamines and sympathomimetics are the next line of therapy in the treatment CCB poisoning. Numerous case reports describe the success or failure of a wide variety of vasopressors including epinephrine (success,[6,21] failure[51,97]), norepinephrine (success,[58,105] failure[97,100]), dopamine (success,[7,32,156] failure[6,21,29,44,51,97,105,152]), isoproterenol (success,[44,97,112,119,146] failure[6,21,51,152]), and dobutamine (success,[119] failure[25,29,97]). Experimentally, no single agent has been consistently effective.[41] This is not surprising given the significant variability in both the CCBs and the patients involved. Mechanistically, however, stimulation of either β_1-adrenergic receptors on the myocardium or α_1-adrenergic receptors on the peripheral vascular smooth muscle would appear to be the most beneficial depending upon the etiology of the hypotension.

Beta-adrenergic receptor agonists activate adenylate cyclase via G_s protein.[133] This results in formation of cyclic adenosine monophosphate (cAMP), which then stimulates a protein kinase A to phosphorylate the α_1 subunit of various calcium channels (Fig. 50–4).[137] It is unclear whether this phosphorylation allows calcium channels to remain open longer,[22,124] or if it opens dormant channels within the plasma membrane.[14,78] In addition, protein kinase A also phosphorylates phospholamban, which increases intrasarcolemmal calcium, and troponin, which improves calcium release from troponin after contraction.[142] In the myocardium this multifactorial increase in intracellular calcium results in improved chronotropy, dromotropy, and inotropy (see Chap. 49).

In the peripheral vascular smooth muscle, α_1-adrenergic receptor agonists activate receptor-operated calcium channels. This opening of nonpoisoned calcium channels allows calcium influx (Fig. 50–5).[124] Alpha$_1$-adrenergic agonists such as epinephrine, norepinephrine, and phenylephrine are therefore logical choices if the hypotension is primarily the result of peripheral vasodilation.

Based upon these pharmacologic mechanisms, epinephrine appears to be an appropriate initial catecholamine to use in hypotensive CCB-poisoned patients. Its significant β_1-adrenergic activity reverses the myocar-

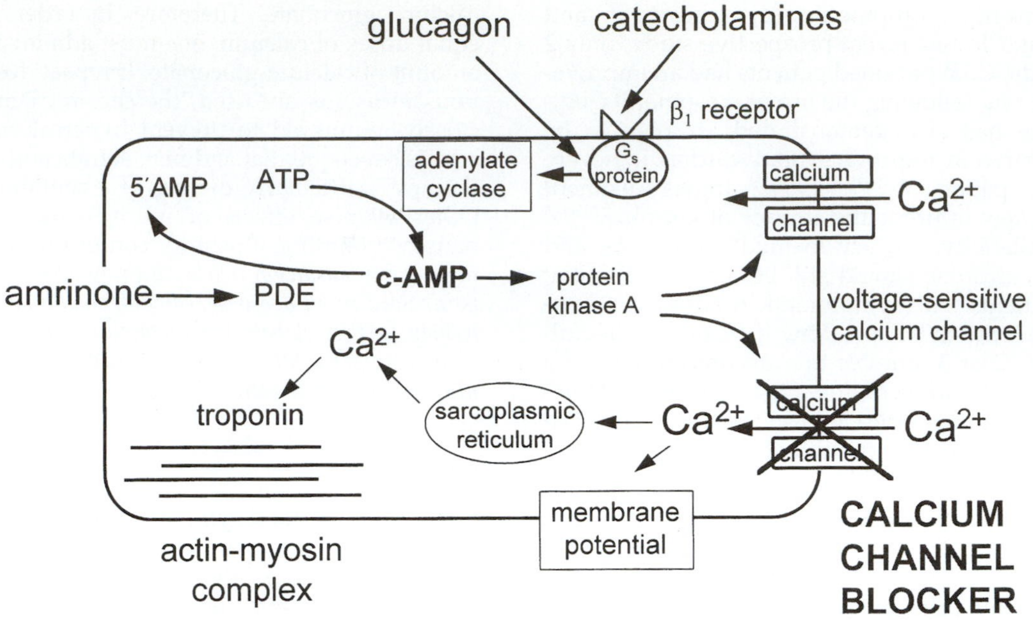

Figure 50–4. Schematic diagram of calcium's role in contractile function of myocardial cells and potential therapeutic options in severe calcium channel blocker toxicity. Mechanisms to increase intracellular calcium include recruitment of new or dormant calcium channels by increasing intracellular cyclic AMP, either by stimulating its formation with catecholamines or glucagon, or inhibiting its degradation with amrinone. In addition, increasing calcium's concentration gradient across the cellular membrane to further its influx may improve contractility.

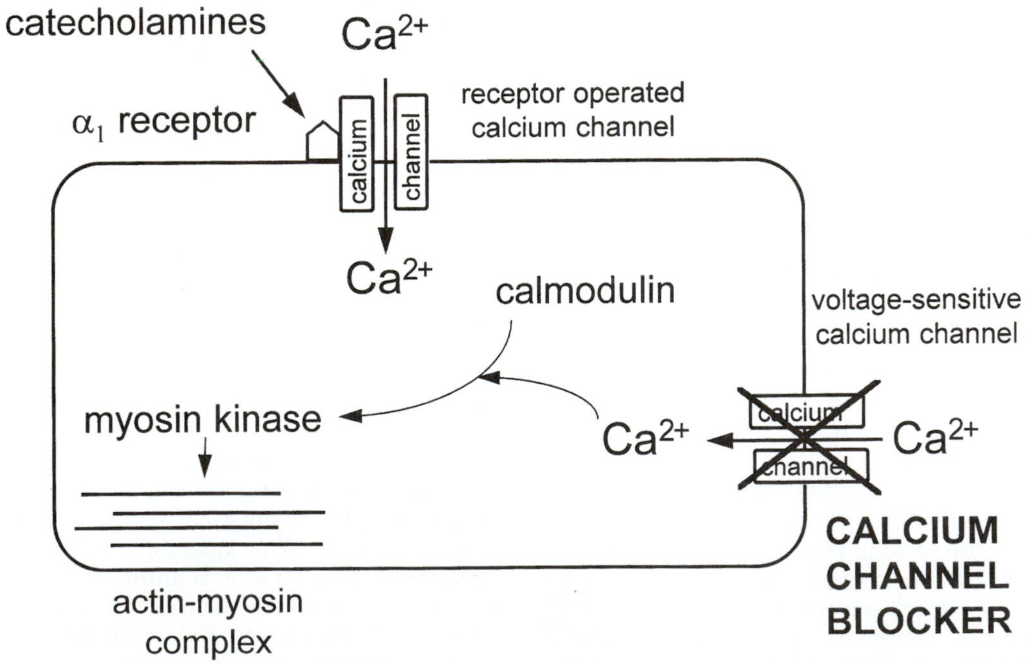

Figure 50–5. Schematic diagram of calcium's role in contractile function of vascular smooth muscle cells and potential therapeutic options in severe calcium channel blocker toxicity. Calcium's entry via voltage-sensitive channels initiates a cascade of events resulting in actin–myosin coupling and contraction. Severe calcium channel blocker poisoning inhibits this influx. Mechanisms to increase intracellular calcium include activation of receptor operator calcium channels with α_1-adrenergic agonists or increasing calcium's concentration gradient across the cellular membrane to further its influx.

dial depressant effects, while its α_1-adrenergic effects increase peripheral vascular resistance. There is some theoretical concern about using pure β-adrenergic receptor agonists, such as isoproterenol and to a lesser extent dobutamine, because β_2-induced peripheral vasodilation may worsen hypotension, particularly at high doses.

Dopamine is predominantly an indirect acting pressor, which acts by stimulating the release of norepinephrine from the distal nerve terminal and not by direct α- and β-adrenergic receptor stimulation.[56] This may limit its effectiveness in severely stressed patients who may have mild catecholamine depletion.[152] Published clinical experience of severe CCB poisonings support these concerns.[6,21,29,44,51,97,105,152] Improvement in blood pressure may be noted with dopamine at high dosing when the drug has additional direct α- and β-adrenergic effects.[56]

The choice of a sympathomimetic agent is based upon numerous factors including the pharmacologic profile of each drug, the patient's underlying physiologic condition, and the physician's familiarity and comfort with the agent. If one sympathomimetic agent is unsuccessful, invasive cardiovascular monitoring, such as a pulmonary artery catheterization, may be helpful in assessing whether the myocardial depressant or peripheral vasodilatory effects are responsible for the hypotension.[118]

Glucagon

Glucagon is an endogenous polypeptide hormone secreted by the pancreatic alpha cells in response to hypoglycemia and catecholamines. In addition, it has significant inotropic and chronotropic effects.[20,113] Glucagon is the drug of choice for beta-adrenergic antagonist poisoning (see Chap. 49 and Antidotes in Depth: Glucagon) because of its ability to bypass the beta-adrenergic receptor and activate adenylate cyclase, probably via a G_s protein.[133] However, in CCB poisoning, this offers no advantage pharmacologically over more traditional vasopressors (see Fig. 50–4).

Cases of CCB-poisoned patients who failed to respond to fluids, calcium, or dopamine and dobutamine but had significant increases in both heart rate and blood pressure after glucagon adminstration have been reported.[29,151] Many other much more severely poisoned patients demonstrated no hemodynamic benefit with glucagon therapy.[6,21,51] Several animal models demonstrate glucagon's efficacy at improving CCB-induced myocardial depression.[68,141,163,164] Unfortunately, none of these studies compared other therapies, including calcium or catecholamines, with glucagon. Although these data are limited, given its experimental and anecdotal efficacy, glucagon should be considered early in the management of refractory hypotension in patients with CCB poisoning. Dosing for glucagon has not been well established. An initial dose of 2 to 5 mg intravenously over 30 to 60 seconds is reasonable in adults followed by 4 to 10 mg over 5 minutes if there is no response. Initial pediatric dose is 50 μg/kg. Due to the short half-life of glucagon, a maintenance infusion must be initiated once a desired effect is achieved. Maintenance infusion dosing must begin at the "response dose" of glucagon per hour. For example, if an initial dose of 4 mg of glucagon effectively improved blood pressure, then the infusion should be started at 4 mg/h (see Antidotes in Depth: Glucagon). Adverse effects include vomiting and hyperglycemia particularly in diabetics or during continuous infusion.[147] It is important to remember to reconstitute the glucagon in normal saline or sterile water and not the 0.2% phenol provided by the manufacturer as a diluent for intramuscular administration.

Amrinone

Another agent that has demonstrated utility in CCB poisoning is amrinone. Amrinone is a noncatecholamine inotropic agent that does not increase myocardial oxygen demand and has been traditionally used for congestive heart failure.[8,11] It specifically inhibits phosphodiesterase III, which is the enzyme responsible for cAMP breakdown and is found in cardiac and vascular tissue (see Fig. 50–4).[27] This inhibition results in increased cAMP and increased intracellular calcium, which improves inotropy. Other phosphodiesterase inhibitors include milrinone and enoximone. Amrinone improved myocardial contractility in two canine models of verapamil poisoning.[4,98] In addition, amrinone has been clinically successful in patients with CCB poisoning.[44,160] In both these cases, amrinone was used in combination with another inotropic agent such as isoproterenol or glucagon. This "two-pronged" approach to increase myocardial cAMP levels, both by stimulating its formation and inhibiting its breakdown, makes pharmacologic sense. However, due to amrinone's nonselective inhibition of phosphodiesterase III, cAMP is also increased in the vascular smooth muscle. This causes smooth muscle relaxation, peripheral vasodilation and, potentially, hypotension.[80] Therefore, amrinone should be used only as a second-line agent and in combination with another inotropic agent. Dosing of amrinone in CCB poisoning is not well defined. Based on traditional dosing for congestive heart failure, the experimental data, and the case reports, an initial bolus of 1 mg/kg over 2 minutes followed by a continuous infusion of 5 to 20 μg/kg per minute is appropriate.[4,27,44,45,160]

Are There Other Treatment Options If Pharmacologic Agents Fail?

Many of the most severely poisoned patients may not respond to any pharmacologic intervention.[51] Transthoracic or intravenous cardiac pacing may be required to improve heart rate, as demonstrated by several case reports.[32,136,152] However, in a prospective cohort of CCB poisonings, 2 of the 4 patients with significant bradycardias treated with electrical pacing had no electrical capture.[122] In addition, even if electrical pacing is effective in increasing the heart rate, often blood pressure remains unchanged.[15,55,58,112]

Intra-aortic balloon counterpulsation is another invasive supportive option. A large balloon is inserted in the femoral artery, which expands during diastole and deflates just before systole. This supports the diastolic pressure to the coronary and carotid arteries during inflation and acts as a vacuum that effectively reduces afterload when the balloon collapses.[149] Intra-aortic balloon counterpulsation has been used successfully to improve cardiac output and blood pressure in a patient with a mixed verapamil and atenolol overdose.[40] The synchronized inflation and deflation is dependent upon regular cardiac electrical activity, so cardiac pacing is often required as well. It is important to understand that overdosed patients who may be candidates for intra-aortic balloon counterpulsation support have a much better prognosis than patients with severe left ventricular failure from ischemic heart disease in whom this technology is traditionally used. Twenty-four to 48 hours of assisted cardiac output allows metabolism and elimination of the CCBs and a return of baseline myocardial function.

Although much more invasive and technologically demanding, emergent cardiopulmonary bypass has also been used to support patients with severe CCB poisoning.[51] Unfortunately, the limited amount of time a patient can be maintained on bypass may not allow for sufficient drug to be metabolized. Extracorporeal membrane oxygenation (ECMO) is a new technology that may be more efficacious than cardiopulmonary bypass. The major limitation of all these technologies is that they are available only at tertiary care facilities. Fortunately they are rarely required.

What Experimental Therapies Are Available for Calcium Channel Blocker Poisoning?

There are several drugs currently being tested as experimental agents that may be effective in treatment of severe hypotension and bradycardia in CCB poisoning. For many years 4-aminopyridine has been used as an antagonist to nondepolarizing neuromuscular blocking agents in Bulgaria.[2] It indirectly increases the calcium influx by blocking voltage-sensitive potassium channels in excitable membranes. This blockade of the outward potassium rectifying current causes a prolonged depolarization at the nerve terminal, allowing for greater calcium influx, and ultimately increasing neurotransmitter release.[41,161] In addition, 4-aminopyridine directly increases both skeletal as well as cardiac muscle contractility.[2] The net effect on the cardiovascular system is an increase in myocardial contractility and in peripheral vascular resistence. Several animal models of severe verapamil poisoning have reported improvements in hemodynamic status as well as survival in animals receiving 4-aminopyridine.[2,41] Two closely related and much more potent dihydropyridines, 3,4-diaminopyridine and Bay K 8664, have had similar experimental success at improving the hemodynamics in verapamil poisoning models but are limited by their significant toxicity, which includes muscle fasciculations, severe hypertension, and coronary artery vasospasm.[55,87,117] In one patient who was verapamil poisoned due to a therapeutic error, 4-aminopyridine was used although other interventions including calcium and isoproterenol infusions were also administered.[146] Although 4-aminopyridine appears safe for human use, its efficacy and possible role in CCB poisoning has yet to be determined.

Insulin has also been evaluated as a potential therapeutic agent in patients with CCB overdose. This is particularly appealing because pancreatic insulin secretion is inhibited in CCB poisoning and many patients already require insulin therapy to correct severe hyperglycemia.[31,140] Insulin has positive inotropic effects, and indirect evidence suggests that increased calcium entry may be responsible.[34,86] In a canine model of verapamil toxicity, high-dose insulin, while maintaining euglycemia with continuous dextrose infusion, improved survival when compared to calcium, epinephrine, or glucagon.[82,83] It appears that verapamil poisoning may alter normal cardiac metabolism primarily of fatty acids and force myocardial cells to become carbohydrate-dependent.[82] Thus, insulin and glucose administration may improve intracellular calcium and improve basic cellular metabolism.

Another drug used experimentally in CCB poisoning is digoxin. Cardiac glycosides inhibit sodium/potassium/ATPase, which increases the intracellular sodium concentration and decreases the transmembrane sodium concentration gradient. This concentration gradient is the driving force for the sodium/calcium exchanger in the cell membrane. When it is decreased, less calcium can exit the cell in exchange for sodium during cellular repolarization.[76] In a canine model of mild to moderate verapamil poisoning, digoxin in conjunction with atropine to block vagally mediated inhibitory effects of digoxin on the heart rate and AV nodal conduction, improved both myocardial dromatropy and inotropy and increased peripheral vascular resistance.[120] Further work is needed before digoxin can be safely administered to any patient with CCB poisoning.

What Is the Appropriate Disposition for Patients Exposed to CCBs?

Any patient who manifests any signs or symptoms of toxicity should be admitted to an intensive care setting. Due to the potential for delayed toxicity, any patient ingesting sustained-release products should be admitted for 24 hours to a monitored setting even if asymptomatic. This is particularly important for small children, in whom even a few tablets may produce significant toxicity.[51,114] All admitted patients should be treated with multiple doses of activated charcoal, and whole-bowel irrigation should be strongly considered for any ingestion involving sustained-release products. Only patients with a precise history of an "immediate-release" preparation who have received adequate gastrointestinal decontamination, who had serial ECGs over 6 to 8 hours that have remained unchanged, and who are asymptomatic, can be medically cleared without hospitalization.

References

1. Adelstein RS, Sellers JR, Conti MA, et al: Regulation of smooth muscle contractile proteins by calmodulin and cyclic AMP. Fed Proc 1982;41:2873–2878.
2. Agoston S, Maestrone E, van Hezik EJ, et al: Effective treatment of verapamil intoxication with 4-aminopyridine in the cat. J Clin Invest 1984;73:1291–1296.
3. Allen GS: Role of calcium antagonists in cerebral arterial spasm. Am J Cardiol 1985;55:149B–153B.
4. Alousi AA, Canter JM, Fort DJ: The beneficial effect of amrinone on acute drug-induced heart failure in the anaesthetised dog. Cardiovasc Res 1985;19:483–494.
5. Anonymous: Studies of bepridil in use against arrhythmias halted. Clin Pharm 1985;4:614.
6. Anthony T, Jastremski M, Elliot W, et al: Charcoal hemoperfusion for the treatment of a combined diltiazem and metoprolol overdose. Ann Emerg Med 1986;15:1344–1348.
7. Ashraf M, Chaudhary K, Nelson J, Thompson W: Massive overdose of sustained-release verapamil: A case report and review of literature. Am J Med Sci 1995;310: 258–263.
8. Baim DS: Effect of phosphodiesterase inhibition on myocardial oxygen consumption and coronary blood flow. Am J Cardiol 1989;63:23A–26A.
9. Barrow PM, Houston PL, Wong DT: Overdose of sustained-release verapamil. Br J Anaesth 1994;72:361–365.
10. Beniam ME: Asystole after verapamil. BMJ 1972;2:169–170.
11. Benotti JR, Grossman W, Braunwald E, Carabello BA: Effect of amrinone on myocardial energy metabolism and hemodynamics in patients with severe congestive heart failure due to coronary artery disease. Circulation 1980; 62:28–35.
12. Bower JO, Mengle HAK: The additive effects of calcium and digitalis: A warning with a report of two deaths. JAMA 1936;106:1151–1153.
13. Brass BJ, Winchester-Penny S, Lipper BL: Massive verapamil overdose complicated by noncardiogenic pulmonary edema. Am J Emerg Med 1996;14:459–461.
14. Braunwald E: Mechanism of action of calcium channel-blocking agents. N Engl J Med 1982;307:1618–1627.
15. Buckley CD, Aronson JK: Prolonged half-life of verapamil in a case of overdose: Implications for therapy. Br J Clin Pharmacol 1995;39:680–683.
16. Buckley N, Dawson AH, Howarth D, Whyte IM: Slow-release verapamil poisoning. Use of polyethylene glycol whole-bowel lavage and high-dose calcium. Med J Aust 1993;158:202–204.
17. Buckley NA, Whyte IM, Dawson AH: Overdose with calcium channel blockers. BMJ 1994;308:1639. Letter.
18. Carruthers SG, Freeman DJ, Gailey DG: Synergistic adverse hemodynamic interaction between oral verapamil and propranolol. Clin Pharmacol Ther 1989;46:469–477.
19. Castell DO: Calcium-channel blocking agents for gastrointestinal disorders. Am J Cardiol 1985;55:210B–213B.
20. Chernow B, Zagola GP, Malcolm D, et al: Glucagon's chronotropic action is calcium dependent. J Pharmacol Exp Ther 1987;241:833–837.
21. Chimienti M, Previtali M, Medici A, Piccinini M: Acute verapamil poisoning: Successful treatment with epinephrine. Clin Cardiol 1982;5:219–222.
22. Clifton DG, Booth DC, Hobbs S, et al: Negative inotropic effect of intravenous nifedipine in coronary artery disease. Relation to plasma levels. Am Heart J 1990; 119:283–290.
23. Coaldrake LA: Verapamil overdose. Anaesth Intensive Care 1984;12:174–175.
24. Connolly DL, Nettleton MA, Bastow MD: Massive diltiazem overdose. Am J Cardiol 1993;72:742–743.
25. Crump BJ, Holt DW, Vale JA: Lack of response to intravenous calcium in severe verapamil poisoning. Lancet 1982;2:939–940.
26. Devis G, Somers G, Van Obberghen E, Malaisse WJ: Calcium antagonists and islet function. I. Inhibition of insulin release by verapamil. Diabetes 1975;24:547–551.
27. DiBianco R: Acute positive inotropic interventions: The phosphodiesterase inhibitors. Am Heart J 1991;121: 1871–1876.
28. Dolan DL: Intravenous calcium before verapamil to prevent hypotension. Ann Emerg Med 1991;20:588–589.
29. Doyon S, Roberts JR: The use of glucagon in a case of calcium channel blocker overdose. Ann Emerg Med 1993; 22:1229–1233.
30. Eccleston DS, Dosen P, Smith AJ: A rat model for calcium channel antagonist toxctiy in man. Clin Exp Pharmacol Physiol 1991;18(suppl):15.
31. Enyeart JJ, Price WA, Hoffman DA, Woods L: Profound hyperglycemia and metabolic acidosis after verapamil overdose. J Am Coll Cardiol 1983;2:1228–1231.
32. Erickson FC, Ling LJ, Grande GA, Anderson DL: Diltiazem overdose: Case report and review. J Emerg Med 1991;9:357–366.
33. Fabiato A: Calcium-induced release of calcium from the cardiac sarcoplamic reticulum. Am J Physiol 1983;245: C1–C14.
34. Farah AE, Alousi AA: The actions of insulin on cardiac contractility. Life Sci 1981;29:975–1000.
35. Fauville JP, Hantson P, Honore P, et al: Severe diltiazem poisoning with intestinal pseudo-obstruction: Case report and toxicological data. J Toxicol Clin Toxicol 1995;33: 273–277.
36. Ferner RE, Monkman S, Riley J, et al: Pharmacokinetic and toxic effects of nifedipine in massive overdose. Hum Exp Toxicol 1990;9:309–311.
37. Ferner RE, Odemuyiwa O, Field AB, et al: Pharmacokinetics and toxic effects of diltiazem in massive overdose. Hum Toxicol 1989;8:497–499.
38. Foster TS, Hamann SR, Richards VR, et al: Nifedipine kinetics and bioavailability after single intravenous and oral doses in normal subjects. J Clin Pharm 1983;23:161–170.

39. Freedman DD, Waters DD: "Second generation" dihydropyridine calcium antagonists. Greater vascular selectivity and some unique applications. Drugs 1987;34: 578–598.
40. Frierson J, Bailly D, Shultz T, et al: Refractory cardiogenic shock and complete heart block after unsuspected verapamil-SR and atenolol overdose. Clin Cardiol 1991;14: 933–935.
41. Gay R, Angeo S, Lee R, et al: Treatment of verapamil toxicity in intact dogs. J Clin Invest 1986;77:1805–1811.
42. Gelbke HP, Schlicht HG, Schmidt G: Fatal poisoning with verapamil. Arch Toxicol 1980;37:89–94.
43. Gelmers HJ: Calcium-channel blockers in the treatment of migraine. Am J Cardiol 1985;55:139B–143B.
44. Goenen M, Col J, Compere A, Bonte J: Treatment of severe verapamil poisoning with combined amrinone-isoproterenol therapy. Am J Cardiol 1986;58:1142–1143.
45. Goenen M, Pedemonte O,Baele P, Col J: Amrinone in the management of low cardiac output after open heart surgery. Am J Cardiol 1985;56:33B–38B.
46. Goglin WK, Elliott BM, Deppe SA: Nifedipine-induced hypotension and mesenteric ischemia. South Med J 1989; 82:274–275.
47. Gutierrez H, Jorgensen M: Colonic ischemia after verapamil overdose. Ann Int Med 1996;124:535.
48. Haddad LM: Resuscitation after nifedipine overdose exclusively with intravenous calcium chloride. Am J Emerg Med 1996;14:602–603.
49. Hariman RJ, Mangiardi LM, McAllister RG, et al: Reversal of the cardiovascular effects of verapamil by calcium and sodium: Differences between electrophysiologic and hemodynamic responses. Circulation 1979;59:797–804.
50. Hattori VT, Mandel WJ, Peter T: Calcium for myocardial depression from verapamil. N Engl J Med 1982;306:238.
51. Hendren WC, Schreiber RS, Garretson LK: Extracorporeal bypass for the treatment of verapamil poisoning. Ann Emerg Med 1989;18:984–987.
52. Henry M, Kay MM, Viccellio P: Cardiogenic shock associated with calcium channel and beta blockers. Reversal with intravenous calcium chloride. Am J Emerg Med 1985;3:334–336.
53. Hermann PH, Rodger SD, Remones G, et al: Pharmacokinetics of diltiazem after intravenous and oral administration. Eur J Clin Pharmacol 1983;24:349–352.
54. Herrington DM, Insley BM, Weinman GG: Nifedipine overdose. Am J Med 1986;81:344–346.
55. Hofer CA, Smith JK, Tenholder MF: Verapamil intoxication: A literature review of overdoses and discussion of therapeutic options. Am J Med 1993;95:431–438.
56. Hoffman BB, Lefkowitz RJ: Catecholamines, sympathomimetic drugs, and adrenergic receptor antagonists. In: Hardman JG, Limbird LE, Molinoff PB, Ruddon RW, eds: Goodman and Gilman's The Pharmacological Basis of Therapeutics, 9th ed. New York, McGraw-Hill, 1996, pp. 199–248.
57. Hollingshead LM, Faulds D, Fitton A: Bepridil. A review of its pharmacological properties and therapeutic use in stable angina pectoris. Drugs 1992;44:835–837.
58. Horowitz BZ, Rhee KJ: Massive verapamil ingestion: A report of two cases and a review of the literature. Am J Emerg Med 1989;7:624–631.
59. Hossack KF: Conduction abnormalities due to diltiazem. N Engl J Med 1982;307:953–954.
60. Howarth DM, Dawson AH, Smith AJ, et al: Calcium channel blocking drug overdose: An Australian series. Hum Exp Toxicol 1994;13:161–166.
61. Humbert VH, Munn NJ, Hawkins RF: Noncardiogenic pulmonary edema complicating massive diltiazem overdose. Chest 1991;99:258–260.
62. Ikemoto N: Structure and function of the calcium pump protein of sarcoplasmic reticulum. Annu Rev Physiol 1982;44:297–317.
63. Immonen P, Linkola A, Waris E: Three cases of severe verapamil poisoning. Int J Cardiol 1981;1:101–105.
64. Ishikawa T, Imamura T, Koiwaya Y, Tanaka K: Atrioventricular dissociation and sinus arrest induced by oral diltiazem. N Engl J Med 1983;309:1124–1125.
65. Jakubowski AT, Mizgala HF: Effect of diltiazem overdose. Am J Cardiol 1987;60:932–933.
66. Johns A, Leijten P, Yamamoto H, et al: Calcium regulation in vascular smooth muscle contractility. Am J Cardiol 1987;59:18A–23A.
67. Johnson KE, Balderston SM, Pieper JA, et al: Electrophysiologic effects of verapamil metabolites in the isolated heart. J Cardiovasc Pharmacol 1991;17:830–837.
68. Jolly SR, Kipnis JN, Lucchesi BR: Cardiovascular depression by verapamil: Reversal by glucagon and interactions with propranolol. Pharmacology 1987;35:249–255.
69. Katz AM: Calcium channel diversity in the cardiovascular system. J Am Coll Cardiol 1996;28:522–529.
70. Katz AM: Cardiac ion channels. N Engl J Med 1993; 328:1244–1251.
71. Katz AM: Basic cellular mechanisms of action of the calcium-channel blockers. Am J Cardiol 1985;55:2B–9B.
72. Katz A: Contractile proteins of the heart. Physiol Rev 1970;50:63–167.
73. Katz AM, Hager DW, Messineo FC, Pappano AJ: Cellular actions and pharmacology of calcium-channel blockers. Am J Emerg Med 1985;3:1–9.
74. Kawai C, Konishi T, Matsuyama E, Okazaki H: Comparative effects of three calcium antagonist, diltiazem, verapamil, and nifedipine, on the sinoatrial and atrioventricular nodes. Circulation 1981;63:1035–1042.
75. Keefe DL, Yee YG, Kates RE: Verapamil protein binding in patients and normal subjects. Clin Pharmacol Ther 1981; 29:21–26.
76. Kelly RA, Smith TW: Pharmacological treatment of heart failure. In: Hardman JG, Limbird LE, Molinoff PB, Ruddon RW, eds: Goodman and Gilman's The Pharmacological Basis of Therapeutics, 9th ed. New York, McGraw-Hill, 1996, pp. 809–838.
77. Kenny J: Treating overdose with calcium channel blockers. BMJ 1994;308:992–993.
78. Kerns W, Kline J, Ford MD: β-blocker and calcium channel blocker toxicity. Emerg Med Clin North Am 1994;12: 365–390.
79. Kirshenbaum LA, Mathews SC, Sitar DS, Tenenbein M: Whole bowel irrigation versus activated charcoal in sor-

bitol for the ingestion of modified-release pharmaceuticals. Clin Pharmacol Ther 1989;46:264–271.

80. Kissling G, Brilla C, Vagt M, et al: Haemodynamic effects of amrinone in the anaesthetized pig. Eur Heart J 1991;9: 800–810.
81. Kleinbloesem CH, van Brummelen P, van de Linde JA, et al: Nifedipine: Kinetics and dynamics in healthy subjects. Clin Pharmacol Ther 1984;35:742–749.
82. Kline JA, Leonova E, Raymond RM: Beneficial myocardial metabolic effects of insulin during verapamil toxicity in the anesthetized canine. Crit Care Med 1995;23: 1251–1263.
83. Kline JA, Tomaszewski CA, Schroeder JD, Raymond RM: Insulin is a superior antidote for cardiovascular toxicity induced by verapamil in the anesthetized canine. J Pharm Exp Ther 1993;267:744–750.
84. Koch AR, Vogelaers DP, Decruyenaere JM, et al: Fatal intoxication with amlodipine. J Toxicol Clin Toxicol 1995;33: 253–256.
85. Kones RJ, Phillips JH: Insulin: Fundamental mechanism of action and the heart. Cardiology 1973;60:280–303.
86. Korstanje C, Honkman FAM, van Kemenade JE: Bay K 8644, a calcium entry promoter as an antidote in verapamil intoxication in rabbits. Arch Int Pharmacodyn Ther 1987;287:109–119.
87. Kounis N: Asystole after verapamil and digoxin. J Clin Pract 1980;43:57–58.
88. Kozlowski JH, Kozlowski JA, Schuller D: Poisoning with sustained-release verapamil. Am J Med 1988;85:127.
89. Kuo MJ, Tseng YZ, Chen TF, Fong DE: Verapamil overdose and severe hypocalcemia. J Toxicol Clin Toxicol 1992;30:309–311.
90. Lebrun P, Malaisse WJ, Herchuelz A: Nutrient induced intracellular calcium movement in rat pancreatic β-cell. Am J Physiol 1982; 243:E196–E205.
91. Leesar MA, Martyn R, Talley JD, Frumin H: Noncardiogenic pulmonary edema complicating massive verapamil overdose. Chest 1994;105:606–607.
92. Lipman J, Jardin I, Roos C, et al: Intravenous calcium chloride as an antidote to verapamil induced hypotension. Intensive Care Med 1982;8:55–57.
93. Litovitz TL, Felberg L, White S, Klein-Schwartz W: 1995 Annual report of the American Association of Poison Control Centers national data collection system. Am J Emerg Med 1996;14:485–537.
94. Litovitz TL, Martin TG, Schmitz B: 1986 Annual report of the American Association of Poison Control Centers National Data Collection System. Am J Emerg Med 1987; 5:405–445.
95. Low R, Takeda P, Mason DT, DeMaria AN: The effects of calcium channel blocking agents on cardiovascular function. Am J Cardiol 1982;49:547–553.
96. Luscher TF, Noll G, Sturmer T, et al: Calcium gluconate in severe verapamil intoxication. N Engl J Med 1994;330: 718–720.
97. MacDonald D, Alguire PC: Case report: Fatal overdose with sustained-release verapamil. Am J Med Sci 1992;303: 115–117.
98. Makela HMV, Kapur PA: Amrinone and verapamil-propranolol induced cardiac depression during isoflurane anesthesia in dogs. Anesthesiology 1987;66:792–797.
99. Malaisse WJ: Role of calcium in insulin secretion. Isr J Med Sci 1972;8:224–251.
100. Malcolm N, Callegari P, Goldberg P, et al: Massive diltiazem overdosage: Clinical and pharmacokinetic observations. Drug Intell Clin Pharmacol 1993;20:888.
101. Materne P, Legrand V, Vandormael M, et al: Hemodynamic effects of intravenous diltiazem with impaired left ventricular function. Am J Cardiol 1984;54:733–737.
102. McAllister RG, Hamann SR, Blouin RA: Pharmacokinetics of calcium-entry blockers. Am J Cardiol 1985;55:30B–40B.
103. McAllister RG, Kirsten EB: The pharmacology of verapamil: IV. Kinetic and dynamic effects after single intravenous and oral doses. Clin Pharmacol Ther 1982;31: 418–426.
104. McCall D: Excitation–contraction coupling in cardiac and vascular smooth muscle. Modification by calcium-entry blockade. Circulation 1987;75(suppl V):V3–V64.
105. McMillan R: Management of acute severe verapamil intoxication. J Emerg Med 1988;6:193–196.
106. Millard RW, Lathrop DA, Grupp G, et al: Differential cardiovascular effects of calcium channel blocking agents: Potential mechanisms. Am J Cardiol 1982;49:246–251.
107. Mitchell BL, Schroeder JS, Mason JW: Comparative clinical electrophysiologic effects of diltiazem, verapamil, and nifedipine: A review. Am J Cardiol 1982;49:629–635.
108. Morad M, Tung L: Ionic events responsible for the cardiac resting and action potential. Am J Cardiol 1982;49: 584–594.
109. Moroni F, Mannaioni PF, Dolara A, Ciaccheri M: Calcium gluconate and hypertonic sodium chloride in a case of massive verapamil poisoning. Clin Toxicol 1980;17: 395–400.
110. Morris DL, Goldschlager N: Calcium infusion for reversal of adverse effects of intravenous verapamil. JAMA 1981;249:3212–3213.
111. Murphy RA, Askoy MO, Dillon PF, et al: Myosin phosphorylation and the crossbridge cycle in arterial smooth muscle. Fed Proc 1983;42:51–56.
112. Orr GM, Bodansky HJ, Dymond DS, Taylor M: Fatal verapamil overdose. Lancet 1982;2:1218–1219.
113. Parmley WW: The role of glucagon in cardiac therapy. N Engl J Med 1971;285:801–802.
114. Passal DB, Crespin FH: Verapamil poisoning in an infant. Pediatrics 1984;73:543–545.
115. Pearigen PD, Benowitz NL: Poisoning due to calcium antagonists. Drug Saf 1991;6:408–430.
116. Perkins CM: Serious verapamil poisoning: Treatment with intravenous calcium gluconate. BMJ 1978;21:1127.
117. Plewa MC, Martin TG, Menegazzi JJ, et al: Hemodynamic effects of 3,4-diaminopyridine in a swine model of verapamil toxicity. Ann Emerg Med 1994;23:499–507.
118. Proano L, Chiang WK, Wang RY: Calcium channel blocker overdose. Am J Emerg Med 1995;13:444–450.
119. Quezado Z, Lippmann M, Wertheimer J: Severe cardiac, respiratory, and metabolic complications of massive verapamil overdose. Crit Care Med 1991;19:436–438.
120. Ramo MP, Grupp I, Pesola MK, et al: Cardiac glycosides

in the treatment of experimental overdose with calcium-blocking agents. Res Exp Med 1992;192:335–343.
121. Ramoska EA, Spiller HA, Winter M, Borys D: A one-year evaluation of calcium channel blocker overdoses: Toxicity and treatment. Ann Emerg Med 1993;22:196–200.
122. Ramoska EA, Spiller HA, Myers A: Calcium channel blocker toxicity. Ann Emerg Med 1990;19:649–653.
123. Rasmussen H: The calcium messenger system. N Engl J Med 1986;314:1094–1102.
124. Reuter H, Stevens CF, Tsien RW, Yellen G: Properties of single calcium channels in cardiac cell culture. Nature 1982;297:501–504.
125. Roberts D, Honcharik N, Sitar DS, Tenenbein M: Diltiazem overdose: Pharmacokinetics of diltiazem and its metabolites and effect of multiple dose charcoal therapy. J Toxicol Clin Toxicol 1991;29:45–52.
126. Roden DM, George AL: The cardiac ion channels: Relevance to management of arrhythmias. Annu Rev Med 1996;47:135–148.
127. Roper TA, Sykes R, Gray C: Fatal diltiazem overdose: Report of four cases and review of the literature. Postgrad Med J 1993;69:474–476.
128. Rosansky SJ: Verapamil toxicity—Treatment with hemoperfusion. Ann Intern Med 1991;114:340.
129. Samniah N, Schlaeffer F: Cerebral infarction associated with oral verapamil overdose. J Toxicol Clin Toxicol 1988; 26:365–369.
130. Schiffl H, Ziupa J, Schollmeyer P: Clinical features and management of nifedipine overdosage in a patient with renal insufficiency. J Toxicol Clin Toxicol 1984;22:387–395.
131. Schoffstall JM, Spivey WH, Gambone LM, et al: Effects of calcium channel blocker overdose-induced toxicity in the conscious dog. Ann Emerg Med 1991;20:1104–1108.
132. Schwartz A: Molecular and cellular aspects of calcium channel antagonism. Am J Cardiol 1992;70:6F–8F.
133. Scott RH, Dolphin AC: Activation of a G protein promotes against responses to calcium channel ligands. Nature 1987;330:760–762.
134. Shah AR, Passalacqua BR: Case report: Sustained-released verapamil overdose causing stroke: An unusual complication. Am J Med Sci 1992;304:257–359.
135. Singh NA: Intravenous calcium and verapamil—When the combination may be indicated. Int J Cardiol 1983;4: 281–284.
136. Snover SW, Bocchino V: Massive diltiazem overdose. Ann Emerg Med 1986;15:1221–1224.
137. Sperelakis N: Cyclic AMP and phosphorylation in regulation of calcium influx into myocardial cells and blockade by calcium antagonist drugs. Am Heart J 1984;107: 347–357.
138. Spiller HA, Meyers A, Ziemba T, Riley M: Delayed onset of cardiac arrhythmias from sustained-release verapamil. Ann Emerg Med 1991;20:201–203.
139. Sporer KA, Manning JJ: Massive ingestion of sustained-release verapamil with a concretion and bowel infarction. Ann Emerg Med 1993;22:603–605.
140. Spurlock BW, Virani NA, Henry CA: Verapamil overdose. West J Med 1991;154:208–211.
141. Stone CK, May WA, Carroll R: Treatment of verapamil overdose with glucagon in dogs. Ann Emerg Med 1995; 25:369–374.
142. Sulakhe MV, Vox T: Regulation of phospholamban and troponin 1 phosphorylation in the intact rat cardiomyocytes by adrenergic and cholinergic stumuli: Roles of cyclic nucleotides, calcium, protein kinases, and phosphatases and depolarization. Mol Cell Biochem 1995; 149/150:103–126.
143. Taira N: Differences in cardiovascular profile among calcium antagonists. Am J Cardiol 1987;59:24B–29B.
144. Tenenbein M, Cohen S, Sitar DS: Whole bowel irrigation as a decontamination procedure after acute drug overdose. Arch Intern Med 1987;147:905–907.
145. Tenenbein M, Honcharik N, Roberts D, Sitar DS: Pharmacokinetics of massive diltiazem overdose and effects of multiple dose charcoal therapy. Vet Hum Toxicol 1989;31: 335. Abstract.
146. Ter Wee PM, Kremer Hovinga TK, Uges DRA, van der Geest S: 4-Aminopyridine and haemodialysis in the treatment of verapamil intoxication. Hum Toxicol 1985;4: 327–329.
147. Thomas SH, Stone K, May WA: Exacerbation of verapamil-induced hyperglycemia with glucagon. Am J Emerg Med 1995;13:27–29.
148. Tom PA, Morrow CT, Kelen GD: Delayed hypotension after overdose of sustained release verapamil. J Emerg Med 1994;12:621–625.
149. Underwood MJ, Firmin RK, Graham TR: Current concepts in the use of intra-aortic balloon counterpulsation. Br J Hosp Med 1993;50:391–397.
150. Vaghy PL, Williams JS, Schwartz A: Receptor pharmacology of calcium entry blocking agents. Am J Cardiol 1987;59:9A–17A.
151. Walter FG, Frye G, Mullen JT, et al: Amelioration of nifedipine poisoning associated with glucagon therapy. Ann Emerg Med 1993;22:1234–1237.
152. Watling SM, Crain JL, Edwards TD, Stiller RA: Verapamil overdose: Case report and review of the literature. Ann Pharmacother 1992;26:1373–1377.
153. Wax P: Intestinal infarction due to nifedipine overdose. J Toxicol Clin Toxicol 1995;33:725–728.
154. Weiss AT, Lewis BS, Halon DA, et al: The use of calcium with verapamil in the management of supraventricular tachyarrhythmias. Int J Cardiol 1983;4:275–280.
155. Welch RD, Todd K: Nifedipine overdose accompanied by ethanol intoxication in a patient with congenital heart disease. J Emerg Med 1990;8:169–172.
156. Wells TG, Graham CJ, Moss MM, Kearns GL: Nifedipine poisoning in a child. Pediatrics 1990;86:91–94.
157. Whitebloom D, Fitzharris J: Nifedipine overdose. Clin Cardiol 1988;11:505–506.
158. Winegrad S: Calcium release from cardiac sarcoplasmic reticulum. Annu Rev Physiol 1982;44:451–462.
159. Woie L, Storstein L: Successful treatment of suicidal verapamil poisoning with calcium gluconate. Eur Heart J 1981;2:239–242.
160. Wolf LR, Spadafora MP, Otten EJ: Use of amrinone and glucagon in a case of calcium channel blocker overdose. Ann Emerg Med 1993;22:1225–1228.

161. Yeh JZ, Oxford GS, Wu CH: Interactions of aminopyridines with potassium channels of squid axon membranes. Biophys J 1976;16:77–81.
162. Yust I, Hoffman M, Aronson RJ: Life-threatening bradycardic reactions due to beta blocker–diltiazem interactions. Isr J Med Sci 1992;28:292–294.
163. Zaloga GP, Malcolm D, Holaday J, Chernow B: Glucagon reverses the hypotension and bradycardia of verapamil overdose in rats. Vet Hum Toxicol 1985;13:273. Abstract.
164. Zaritsky AL, Horowitz M, Chernow B: Glucagon antagonism of calcium channel blocker-induced myocardial dysfunction. Crit Care Med 1988;16:246–251.

CHAPTER 51

Miscellaneous Antihypertensive Agents

Francis DeRoos

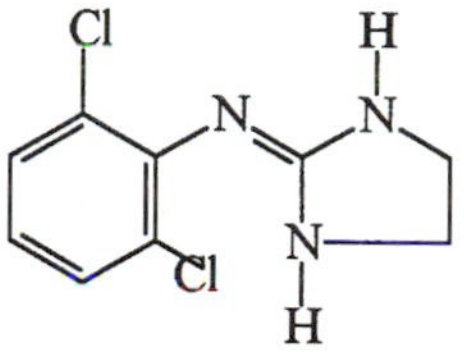

Clonidine

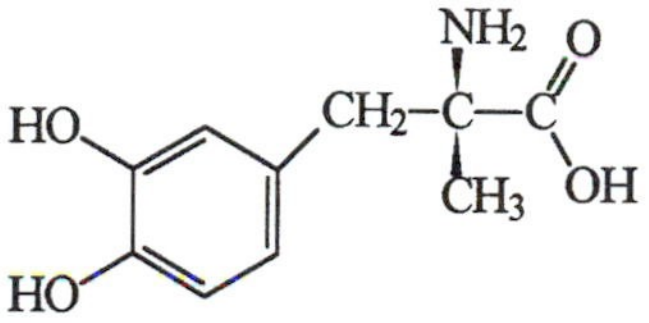

Methyldopa

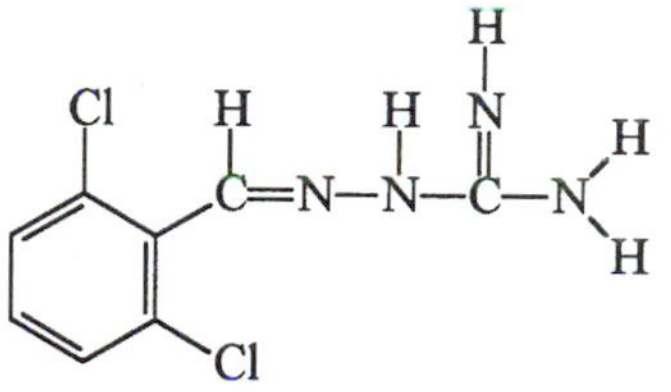

Guanabenz

CASE 1. A 2-year-old male was brought into the emergency department after he became lethargic and difficult to arouse. The patient has no medical history. Earlier in the afternoon he was found playing with a bottle of clonidine tablets. Initial vital signs were a blood pressure of 110/70 mm Hg; a heart rate of 55 beats/min at rest and 80 beats/min with stimulation; a respiratory rate of 16–20 breaths/min with intermittent deep, sighing respirations; and a temperature of 97.8°F (36.6°C). The head and neck examination was significant for 2-mm pupils that were slightly reactive to light. Lung and abdominal examinations were normal. Heart examination was notable for a regular bradycardia. Neurologic evaluation revealed a somnolent male with poor muscle tone and slight hyporeflexia. The gag reflex was intact. Of note, the patient became much more active and at times agitated with tactile stimulation, and he had strong purposeful movements when intravenous access was initiated. Supplemental oxygen was administered and naloxone 0.5 mg was given intravenously and a repeat dose of 1.5 mg was given without clinical response. Activated charcoal (12.5 g) was administered via nasogastric tube. Laboratory tests included an ECG, which revealed normal sinus rhythm with a rate of 60 beats/min with no conduction abnormalities and an arterial blood gas with pH, 7.36; PCO_2, 42 mm Hg; PO_2, 113 mm Hg. The patient was admitted to the pediatric intensive care unit for close observation and cardiac monitoring. Over the next 16 hours the patient's blood pressure remained stable, his heart rate increased to 90 beats/min and his mental status returned to normal.

What is Clonidine?

Clonidine is an imidazoline compound that was synthesized in the early 1960s. Due to its potent α_2-adrenergic agonist effects, it was initially tested as a topical nasal decongestant. However, since hypotension was a common side effect, the search for therapeutic applications was redirected.[66] Clonidine is the best studied and most commonly used of all the centrally acting antihypertensive agents. The other agents include methyldopa, guanfacine, and guanabenz. Though these drugs differ chemically and structurally, they all decrease blood pressure in a similar manner by reducing the sympathetic outflow from the central nervous system.

Over the past 15 years, the increased efficacy and improved side-effect profiles of the newer antihypertensives have diminished the use of the α_2-adrenergic agonists in hypertension management. However, a wide variety of new applications for clonidine have been promoted, including migraine headache prophylaxis, attention deficit/hyperactivity disorder, and the management of opioid, ethanol, and nicotine withdrawal.[50,51,69,70,77] Although unintentional exposure to clonidine is relatively uncommon, it can cause significant toxicity, particularly in children. One report from two large pediatric hospitals identified 47 children requiring hospitalization for clonidine ingestions over a 5-year period.[168]

What Is the Mechanism of Action of Centrally Acting Antihypertensives?

Clonidine and the other centrally acting antihypertensives exert their hypotensive effects primarily via stimulation of α_2-adrenergic receptors in the brain.[80,123] This central α_2-adrenergic receptor agonism enhances the activity of inhibitory neurons in the vasoregulatory regions of the CNS, notably the nucleus tractus solitarius in the medulla, resulting in decreased sympathetic outflow from the intermediolateral cell columns of the thoracolumbar spinal tracts into the periphery.[1,161] This sympathetic attenuation reduces heart rate, vascular tone, and ultimately arterial blood pressure.[122,171]

One area of controversy is the precise cellular location of the α-adrenergic receptors that are activated by clonidine. While compelling arguments are published for both presynaptic and postsynaptic effects, it appears that the effects are postsynaptic.[94,160] When the central presynaptic pathways and receptors are destroyed or inactivated with various compounds, there is little alteration in the hypotensive response to clonidine.[80] Therefore it appears that these α_2-adrenergic receptors are located postsynaptically.

In therapeutic oral dosing, clonidine and the other centrally acting antihypertensives have little effect on the peripheral α-adrenergic receptors, the peripheral sympathetic nervous system, or the normal circulatory responses seen with exercise or with the Valsalva maneuver.[106,115] In overdose or with intravenous administration, peripheral α-adrenergic stimulation can occur, causing norepinephrine release, which produces vasoconstriction and hypertension.[24,108] This hypertension is short-lived, however, as clonidine's potent centrally mediated sympathetic inhibition becomes overwhelming and hypotension ensues.[4,34,88,98]

Recently imidazoline-specific binding sites have been identified in both the brain and periphery.[154] Although their significance has not been identified, they may become targets of new antihypertensive drug therapy.[66]

What Is the Pharmacology of These Agents?

Clonidine is well absorbed from the gastrointestinal tract (approximately 75%) with an onset of action within 30–60 minutes and demonstrates a peak effect at 2–3 hours, lasting up to 8 hours.[36] It is widely distributed to all tissues including the brain, with 20–40% protein binding and an apparent volume of distribution of 3.2–5.6 L/kg.[95] Clonidine is predominantly eliminated unchanged via the kidneys.[95]

Guanfacine and guanabenz are structurally and pharmacologically very similar. They are well absorbed orally, acheiving peak levels within 3–5 hours, and have large volumes of distribution (4–6 L/kg for guanfacine, 7–17 L/kg for guanabenz).[68,147] Guanabenz is metabolized predominantly in the liver and undergoes extensive first-pass effect, whereas guanfacine is eliminated equally by the liver and kidney.[68,147] Neither drug has significant active metabolites.

Whereas clonidine, guanabenz, and guanfacine are all active agents with direct α_2-adrenergic agonist effects, methyldopa is a prodrug. It enters the CNS, probably by an active transport mechanism, before it is converted into its pharmacologically active degradation products.[14] Alpha-methylnorepinephrine is the most significant of the metabolites, although α-methyldopamine and α-methylepinephrine may also be important.[43,62,132] These metabolites are direct α_2-adrenergic agonists and impart their hypotensive effect just like the other centrally acting antihypertensives. Approximately 50% of an oral dose of methyldopa is absorbed and peak serum levels are achieved in 2–3 hours.[107] However, because methyldopa requires metabolism into its active form, these serum levels have little correlation to clinical effects. It has a small volume of distribution (0.24 L/kg) with little protein binding (15%).[107] It is eliminated in the urine both as parent compound and after hepatic sulfation.[112]

Clonidine is available in both oral and patch form. The patch, referred to as the clonidine transdermal therapeutic system (TTS), allows slow, continuous delivery of drug over a prolonged period of time, typically 1 week. Similar delivery systems have been effective in management of chronic pain with fentanyl and in the cessation of smoking tobacco with nicotine. This formulation, however, offers new challenges to the medical toxicologist. Each patch contains significantly more drug than is delivered. One that delivers 0.1 mg/day of clonidine contains 2.5 mg total while the 0.3 mg/day product contains 7.5 mg.[20] Even after 1 week of use between 35 and 50% and, in some instances, possibly as high as 70%, of the drug remains in the patch.[20,60] Puncturing the outer membrane layer or backing opens the drug reservoir and allows significant drug to be released rapidly. In addition, patients who do not perceive this TTS as a medication may discard the vehicle in open wastebaskets. This is an invitation for toddlers, who often are fascinated with stickers and other adhesive objects and who may remove an improperly disposed of patch and apply, taste, or ingest it. Numerous reports of significant toxicity from dermal exposure, mouthing, or ingesting a single clonidine patch emphasize this concern.[20,26,58,60,64,79,128]

What Are the Clinical Manifestations of Patients With Centrally Acting Antihypertensive Poisoning?

The signs and symptoms of poisoning with any centrally acting antihypertensive are variable but reflect an exaggeration of their pharmacologic action. Although the majority of the published cases involve clonidine, it appears that all these agents produce similar toxicity, especially to the central nervous system (CNS) and cardiovascular system. Common signs include CNS depression, bradycardia, hypotension, and occasionally hypothermia.[6,121,141,158] Most patients who ingest clonidine and the other similarly acting agents will manifest symptoms rapidly, typically within 30–90 minutes.[168] The exception may be with methyldopa, which requires metabolism before it is active. This may delay toxicity until several hours postingestion.[141,173]

Central nervous system depression is the most frequent complication and can vary from mild lethargy to somnolence, stupor, or coma.[26,56,57,96,98,103,105,110,114,127] In addition, severely obtunded patients may suffer from decreased ventilatory effort and hypoxia.[4] Respirations may be slow and shallow with intermittent deep sighing breaths. Various terms have been used to describe this phenomenon including shallow, gasping, or Cheyne-Stokes respirations or periodic apnea.[6,9,79,98,99] This hypoventilation is typically responsive to tactile stimuli alone, although endotracheal intubation may be required in rare instances.[4,6,63,79,103] This CNS depression typically resolves over 12–36 hours,[9,61,114] although prolonged coma has been reported.[120] Other manifestations of this CNS depression include hypotonia, hyporeflexia, and irritability.[24,98,149] The cranial nerve examination often demonstrates miotic pupils that may remain reactive to light.[4,6,117,152] Two unusual case reports describe seizures in the setting of clonidine poisoning.[71,97] The mechanism for producing these seizures is unclear.

Hypothermia has also been associated with overdoses involving centrally acting antihypertensives.[6,98,99,121] This is thought to be due to α-adrenergic effects within the thermoregulatory center, although others suggest that these agents activate central serotonergic pathways that alter normal heat production and/or loss.[89,102] Though this phenomenon may last several hours, it rarely requires treatment and responds well to passive rewarming.[24,121]

Sinus bradycardia may be seen in up to 50% of ingestions.[149,168] Though usually associated with hypotension, it may be an isolated finding. The exact mechanism resposible for this is not clearly defined, but plausible explanations include an exaggerated centrally mediated sympatholytic effect, a centrally mediated increase in vagal tone, or a direct stimulation of α_2-adrenergic receptors on the myocardium.[31,85,162] All these mechanisms may play a role in various patients.

Conduction abnormalities, including first-degree heart block, second-degree atrioventricular block, and complete heart block, are described both in overdose and after therapeutic dosing.[53,78,114,137,139,159,169] It appears that patients who have underlying sinus node dysfunction, concurrent sympatholytic drug therapy, or renal insufficiency and the very young are at greatest risk of developing sinus bradycardia and conduction delays.[18,149,155]

Hypotension is another hemodynamic manifestation of central antihypertensive toxicity.[6,20103,114,149,168] This typically occurs within the first few hours after the exposure and represents profound inhibition of central sympathetic outflow.[45] Paradoxically, severe hypertension may be noted early in dosing or in massive overdoses.[4,34,71,88,98] This is the result of nonspecific peripheral α-adrenergic agonism resulting in norepinephrine release and vasoconstriction. Typically this hypertensive effect is short-lived as the central sympatholytic effects become more prominent.[71] However, in massive ingestions hypertension can be protracted, requiring pharmacologic intervention.[4,34,98,149]

There is no clear association between the amount of any centrally acting antihypertensive ingested and the clinical manifestations. In children, clonidine ingestions as small as 0.2 mg have resulted in severe poisoning.[114] Fatalities from any of these agents is extremely rare, with few published reports.[92,141]

In addition to the common clinical findings in overdose, these centrally acting antihypertensive agents also produce similar adverse effects with therapeutic dosing. Symptoms include drowsiness, depression, lightheadedness, dry mucous membranes, constipation, and sexual dysfunction.[41] In rare instances hallucinations are reported,[16] and transdermal clonidine patch therapy may result in skin depigmentation.[35]

Methyldopa has the highest incidence of these adverse effects—thus its limited therapeutic use.[173] It is associated with a 10% incidence of a positive direct Coombs test, and fatal hemolytic anemia is also reported.[21,170] Methyldopa therapy is associated with elevation in hepatic aminotransferases and hepatitis.[40,133]

Abrupt cessation of central antihypertensive therapy may result in withdrawal, characterized by excessive sympathetic activity. Symptoms include agitation, insomnia, tremor, palpitations, and hypertension and present between 16 and 48 hours of cessation of therapy.[59,129,151] The frequency and severity of symptoms appear to be greater in patients treated with higher doses for several months and in those with the most consequential underlying hypertension.[129] However, withdrawl occurs even when the drug dosing is gradually reduced.[19,163] While this phenomenon is associated with all centrally acting α_2–adrenergic-agonists, it appears to be most prominent following use of the shorter acting agents such as clonidine and guanabenz.[1,17,48,126,172]

What Is the Treatment for Patients With Centrally Acting Antihypertensive Poisoning?

Appropriate therapy begins with particular focus on the respiratory and hemodynamic status. Administration of activated charcoal is the primary mode of gastrointestinal decontamination. Emesis induced by syrup of ipecac is contraindicated due to the possibility for rapid deterioration in mental status. Orogastric lavage has limited utility because these agents are rapidly absorbed and patients often present following the onset of symptoms and respond well to supportive care. In cases involving clonidine patch ingestions, whole-bowel irrigation appears to be an effective intervention.[64]

All patients with CNS depression should be routinely evaluated for hypoxia and hypoglycemia. Respiratory compromise including apnea often responds well to simple auditory or tactile stimulation.[4,6,63,79] Significant arousal during preparation for intubation precluding any need for mechanical ventilation has been reported.[4] Endotracheal intubation may be required, however, in the most severely poisoned patients.

Naloxone was probably first used in clonidine poisoning due to the similarity in clinical findings with opioid toxicity, namely CNS and respiratory depression and miosis. Although the interaction between clonidine and opioid receptors is poorly understood, several clonidine-poisoned patients have had significant arousal after naloxone administration, demonstrating increased respiratory effort, heart rate, and blood pressure.[9,83,109,111,152] Due to naloxone's short duration of effect, 20–60 minutes, redosing or continuous infusion may be required. As with some synthetic opioids, such as propoxyphene and fentanyl, clinical improvement may occur only after high doses of naloxone, 4–10 mg,[79] and some patients may have no response regardless of dosing.[10,96,168] Due to the paucity of clinical experience, it is unclear how efficacious naloxone may be in overdoses involving other α-adrenergic agents. In one adult with severe guanabenz poisoning, 7 mg of naloxone failed to improve her clinical status.[121] Rarely, naloxone administration in the setting of clonidine overdose may result in significant hypertension, necessitating the use of continuous hemodynamic monitoring.[79,168]

Bradycardia following overdose with a centrally acting α-adrenergic agonist may be mild and does not require any therapy if adequate peripheral perfusion exists. If the bradycardia is severe, however, standard doses of atropine are effective, but redosing may be required.[4,6,96,149] If bradycardia is associated with severe hypotension, dopamine may increase both heart rate and blood pressure.[6,54,96] Isolated hypotension should initially be treated with intravenous boluses of crystalloid. If ineffective, pressor support with a dopamine infusion is typically beneficial.[4,6,20]

Some investigators have recommended the use of central α-adrenergic antagonists such as tolazoline as a specific antidote for patients with α-adrenergic agonist overdoses. Although some patients have had significant hemodynamic improvements,[103,114,138] tolazoline administration was ineffective in others.[4,149] An adult dose of tolazoline is 5–10 mg by intravenous infusion every 15 minutes up to a total maximum of 40 mg.[24] Given that this agent is variably successful and that most physicians are unfamiliar with this agent, tolazoline cannot be recommended in the primary management strategy for centrally acting antihypertensive poisoning. It should be considered only after tactile stimulation, naloxone, atropine, intravenous fluids, and dopamine have failed.

If the patient presents early or after a massive overdose, paradoxical hypertension may be seen. This hypertension is typically self-limited and routinely followed by profound hypotension. If severe or prolonged, then treatment with a short-acting antihypertensive such as sodium nitroprusside is appropriate.[98] Oral nifedipine has been used,[34] but its lack of titratability and its unpredictable efficacy make its use inappropriate.

Are There Any Other Sympatholytic Antihypertensive Agents?

In addition to the centrally acting α_2-adrenergic agonists such as clonidine, there are several other agents that exert their antihypertensive effect by decreasing the effects of the sympathetic nervous system. Often termed sympatholytics, they can be classified as either ganglionic blocking agents, peripheral neuron blocking agents, or α_1-adrenergic antagonists, depending upon their mechanism of action. All these agents are rarely used clinically and little is known about their toxicologic effects.

Ganglionic Blocking Agents

Ganglionic blocking agents, such as trimethaphan, are extremely potent antihypertensive agents. They inhibit impulse transmission down the postganglionic sympathetic, as well as parasympathetic, nerves and thus decrease vascular tone, cardiac output, and blood pressure. These agents were used more frequently in the 1950s and 1960s in Europe, but because of their significant side effects, they were quickly replaced with other agents. These side effects stem from the unpredictable degree of sympathetic, as well as additional parasympathetic, blockade and include paralytic ileus, constipation, urinary retention, impotence, dry mouth, and blurred vision.[112] Trimethaphan is the only ganglionic blocker available in the United States and it is administered intravenously. While there are no reported cases of intentional overdose reported, there are several cases of cardiopulmonary arrest associated with administration of continuous doses of trimethaphan in the treatment of a severe hypertensive crisis.[29] In overdose, the exaggerated hypotensive response should respond well to intravenous crystalloid boluses and a direct-acting vasopressor such as norepinephrine.

Peripheral Adrenergic Neuron Blocking Agents

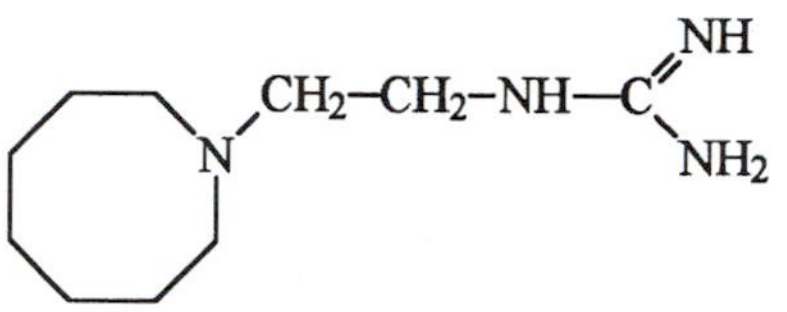

Guanethidine

These agents exert their sympatholytic action by decreasing norepinephrine release from the distal nerve terminals. Guanethidine and guanadrel interfere with the action potential that triggers the release of norepinephrine, whereas reserpine depletes norepinephrine and other catecholamines from the nerve end terminals. Adverse effects of these agents again limit their clinical utility. These include a high incidence of orthostatic and exercise-induced hypotension, diarrhea, increased gastric secretions, and impotence.[112] Reserpine, due to its ability to cross the blood–brain barrier, may also deplete central catecholamines and produce drowsiness, extrapyramidal symptoms, hallucinations, or depression.[93] An exaggeration of their pharmacologic effects would be expected in overdose. Severe orthostatic hypotension should be anticipated and treatment should consist of intravenous crystalloid boluses and a direct-acting vasopressor. If reserpine is involved, significant CNS depression should be anticipated.[93]

Peripheral α_1-Adrenergic Antagonists

The fourth group of sympatholytic agents are the selective α_1-adrenergic antagonists, which include prazosin, terazosin, and doxazosin. The α_1-adrenergic receptor is a postsynaptic receptor primarily located on vascular smooth muscle, although these receptors are also found in the eye and gastrointestinal and genitourinary tracts.[27] The adrenergic antagonism of these drugs results in arterial smooth muscle relaxation, vasodilation, and lowering of the blood pressure. Although better tolerated than ganglionic blockers and peripheral adrenergic neuron blockers, these agents may still produce significant symptoms of postural hypotension, including lightheadedness, near syncope, and palpitations, particularly after the first dose or if the dosing is rapidly increased.[12] In overdose, hypotension and CNS depression ranging from lethargy to coma are reported.[87,100] In addition, priapism may occur.[130] Treatment with supportive care including intravenous fluid boluses and vasopressors such as dopamine were effective in the few overdose cases reported.[87,100]

Which Agents Are Direct Vasodilators?

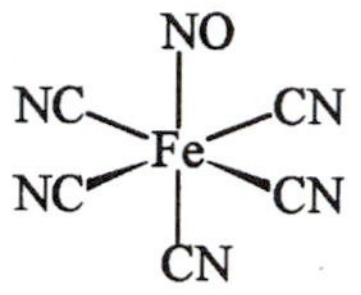

Nitroprusside

The direct vasodilators, including hydralazine, minoxidil, diazoxide, and sodium nitroprusside represent another class of antihypertensive drugs. These drugs produce vascular smooth muscle relaxation independent of innervation or known pharmacologic receptors.[37,81,82] This direct vasodilatory effect appears to be related to alterations in smooth muscle intracellular calcium ion homeostasis. As this vasodilation occurs, the baroreceptor reflexes, which remain intact, produce an increased sympathetic outflow to the myocardium, resulting in an increase in heart rate and contractile force. Typically these agents are utilized in patients with severe, refractory hypertension and in conjunction with a β-adrenergic antagonist to diminish the reflex tachycardia. Hydralazine and minoxidil are effective orally, whereas diazoxide and sodium nitroprusside are used only intravenously. Minoxidil is also used topically to promote hair growth in patients with male pattern baldness, and significant overdoses have occurred with this formulation.[101] Diazoxide, although previously used to rapidly reduce blood pressure in hypertensive emergencies, is rarely used for this indication due to its poor titratability and its variable hypotensive effect. It is currently used to treat refractory hypoglycemia in patients who have overdosed with insulin or oral hyperglycemic agents (see Chap. 40).

Adverse effects associated with hydralazine use include several immunologic phenomena, including hemolytic anemia, vasculitis, acute glomerulonephritis, and, most notably, a lupus-like syndrome.[124] Minoxidil may cause electrocardiographic changes, both in therapeutic doses and in overdose, including sinus tachycardia, ST segment depressions, and T-wave inversions.[57,125,145] The significance of these changes is unknown, and they typically resolve with either continued therapy or as other toxic manifestations resolve.[57,145]

The toxic manifestations of these agents are an exaggeration of their pharmacologic action. Symptoms may include lightheadedness, syncope, palpitations, and nausea.[3] Signs may be isolated to tachycardia alone [72,125,145] or include flushing or alterations in mental status, depending on the degree of hypotension.[101] After appropriate gastrointestinal decontamination, routine supportive care with special consideration to maintaining adequate mean arterial pressure should be performed. If intravenous fluid boluses are insufficient to restore blood pressure, a peripherally acting vasopressors such as norepinephrine or neosynephrine would be an appropriate next therapy. Catecholamines such as dopamine and epinephrine should be avoided to prevent an exaggerated myocardial response and tachycardia.

Sodium nitroprusside, which exerts its vasodilatory effects after being metabolized in the erythrocyte and releasing the vasodilator nitric oxide, also releases five atoms of cyanide. If the patient has renal insufficiency or low thiosulfate stores (eg, infancy, the malnourished, or the critically ill) or is maintained on an infusion rate of greater than 3–4 μg/kg/min, then the individual is at risk of developing cyanide toxicity.[28] Signs and symptoms include an alteration in mental status, anion gap metabolic acidosis, and in late stages, hemodynamic instablility. (For a complete discussion of Cyanide, see Chap. 97.)

What Is the Toxicity of Diuretics?

Antihypertensive diuretic agents can be divided into three main groups: (1) the thiazides, and related compounds including hydrochlorothiazide and chlorthalidone; (2) the loop diuretics, including furosemide, bumetanide, and ethacrynic acid; and (3) the potassium-sparing diuretics, including amiloride, triamterene, and spironolactone. Two other groups of diuretics include carbonic anhydrase inhibitors, such as acetazolamide, and osmotic diruretics, such as mannitol, but are not used as antihypertensive agents.

The thiazides are a broad class of diuretics that share both a core benzothiadiazine structure and a function. Their diuretic effect involves inhibition of sodium and chloride reabsorption in the distal convoluted tubule. Loop diuretics, in contrast, inhibit the coupled transport of sodium, potassium, and chloride in the thick ascending limb of the loop of Henle. Although their exact antihypertensive mechanism is unclear, an increased urinary excretion of sodium, potassium, and magnesium results from their use.[167] Potassium-sparing diuretics act either as aldosterone antagonists, such as spironolactone, or as renal epithelial sodium channel antagonists in the late distal tubule and collecting duct, such as triamterene.[74]

Most toxic effects associated with these agents are metabolic and seen during chronic therapy or overuse. Hyponatremia occurs within the first 2 weeks of initiation of therapy in over two thirds of susceptible patients.[146] Patients who are elderly, female, malnourished, or taking thiazides are at greatest risk.[8] With severe hyponatremia (< 120 mmol/L) symptoms may include headache, nausea, vomiting, confusion, seizures, or coma. Pontine demyelination has been reported during correction of severe hyponatremia secondary to diuretic abuse.[25]

Other electrolyte abnormalities associated with diuretic use include hypokalemia and hypomagnesemia, which increase the risk of precipitating ventricular dysrhythmias and sudden death. This is an extremely controversial topic, with several excellent studies providing conflicting results.[13,44,118,142,143] Although it is unclear how great a risk, if any, diuretic use may be, it remains prudent to monitor and correct the patient's potassium levels.[67,142,166] This is particularly critical in elderly patients and in those concomitantly taking digoxin, where hypokalemia is clearly associated with dysrhythmias.[15,150] Potassium-sparing diuretics may cause hyperkalemia, particularly in the setting of renal insufficiency.

Several unusual reactions are associated with diuretic use, including pancreatitis, cholecystitis, and hematologic abnormalities such as hypercoagulability, thrombocytopenia, and hemolytic anemia.[38,39,134,136,157,165] Impotence remains an underappreciated adverse effect of these agents.

Despite the widespread use of these agents, acute overdoses are rare.[91] Major signs and symptoms include gastrointestinal distress, brisk diuresis, hypovolemia, electrolyte abnormalities, and altered mental status.[91] Typically the diuresis is short-lived due to the limited duration of effect and rapid clearance of the majority of diuretics. Assessment should focus on fluid and electrolyte status and be corrected as needed. If hyperkalemia is unexpectedly discovered, consider an ingestion of a potassium-sparing agent, or more likely an overdose of potassium supplements, which are frequently prescribed in conjuction with thiazides. Altered mental status including coma may result from diuretic overdosage without evidence of any fluid or electrolyte abnormalities.[11,91,135] Postulated mechanisms include a direct drug effect or induction of transient cerebral ischemia.[113]

CASE 2. A 56-year-old male presents complaining of progressive lip and tongue swelling. The patient has a history of non-insulin-dependent diabetes and hypertension. His medications include aspirin, glyburide, and hydrochlorothiazide, and 3 weeks earlier he began a second antihypertensive agent. Physical examination revealed a well-appearing male in mild distress with obvious swelling of lips, face, and tongue. Initial vital signs were a blood pressure of 154/88 mm Hg; a heart rate of 90 beats/min; a respiratory rate of 18 breaths/min; and a temperature of 97.8°F (36.6°C). Head and neck examination was remarkable for marked swelling of lips, slight protrusion of tongue forcing the mouth open at rest, and left cheek swelling. Lung examination revealed no wheezes or rhonchi, with good air movement. No stridor was noted, although his voice was muffled. Cardiac, abdominal, and neurologic examinations were unremarkable. A diagnosis of angiotensin converting enzyme inhibitor–induced angioedema was made and a nasopharyngeal airway was immediately placed. Diphenhydramine (50 mg IV) and methylprednisolone (125 mg IV) were administered without significant improvement. Epinephrine was not administered due to concerns about possible atherosclerotic heart disease and the precipitation of myocardial ischemia. Although the patient's upper airway was patent, the rapidity of the onset of such significant oropharyngeal swelling threatened his respiratory status. Direct fiberoptic nasopharyngeal intubation was performed using topical anesthetics and a benzodiazepine. The patient remained intubated for 36 hours. After the swelling had decreased, the patient tolerated extubation without difficulty. He was discharged from the hospital with specific instructions to discontinue his new antihypertensive, enalapril, and a replacement antihypertensive, verapamil, was prescribed.

What Are Angiotensin Converting Enzyme Inhibitors?

Angiotensin converting enzyme (ACE) inhibitors are among the most widely prescribed antihypertensive drugs. There are currently nine ACE inhibitors approved by the U.S. Food and Drug Administration for the treatment of hypertension (Table 51–1). They exert their antihypertensive effect by inhibiting the conversion of angiotension I to angiotensin II in the lung and vascular endothelium. This reduction in angiotensin II, which is a potent vasoconstrictor and stimulant of aldosterone secretion, results in vasodilation, decreased peripheral vascular resistance, decreased blood pressure, increased cardiac output, and a relative increase in renal, cerebral, and coronary blood flow.[47] This hypotensive response may be severe in select patients after their initial dose, resulting in syncope and cardiac ischemia.[23,65] Patients with renovascular-induced hypertension and those who are mildly hypovolemic from concomitant diuretic use appear to be at greatest risk.[65] Overall, however, these agents are well tolerated and have a very low incidence of side effects. Some reported adverse effects include rash, dysgeusia, neutropenia, hyperkalemia, chronic cough, and angioedema.[32,47,153]

How Are ACE Inhibitors Associated With Angioedema?

Angioedema is an inflammatory reaction in which there is increased capillary blood flow and permeability, resulting in an increase in interstitial fluid. If this process is confined to the superficial dermis, urticaria is seen, while if the deeper layers of the dermis or subcutaneous tissue are involved, angioedema results. Angioedema most commonly involves the periorbital, perioral, or oropharyngeal tissues.[131] This swelling may progress rapidly over minutes and result in complete airway obstruction and death.[46,49,140] The pathogenesis of acquired angioedema in-

TABLE 51–1. CLASSIFICATION OF ANTIHYPERTENSIVE AGENTS

Beta-adrenergic antagonists (see Chap. 49)

Calcium channel blockers (see Chap. 50)

Sympatholytics

a. Central acting agents: α_2-adrenergic agonists
  - methyldopa (Aldomet)
  - clonidine (Catapres)
  - guanabenz (Wytensin),
  - guanfacine (Tenex)

b. Ganglionic blocking agents
  - trimethaphan (Arfonad)

c. Peripheral adrenergic neuron blocking agents
  - guanethidine (Ismelin)
  - guanadrel (Hycorel)
  - metyrosine (Demser)
  - reserpine

d. Peripheral α_1-adrenergic antagonists
  - prazosin (Minipress)
  - terazosin (Hytrin)
  - doxazosin (Cardura)

Diuretics

a. Thiazide
  - hydrochlorothiazide (Hydrodiuril)
  - metolazone (Zaroxolyn)
  - chlorthalidone (Hygroton)

b. Loop diuretics
  - furosemide (Lasix)
  - bumetanide (Bumex)
  - ethacrynic acid (Edecrin)

c. Potassium sparing
  - amiloride (Midamor)
  - triamterene (Maxzide)
  - spironolactone (Aldactone)

Vasodilators

- hydralazine (Apresoline)
- minoxidil (Loniten, Rogaine)
- diazoxide (Hyperstat IV)
- sodium nitroprusside (Nipride)

ACE inhibitors

- captopril (Capoten)
- enalapril (Vasotec)
- lisinopril (Prinivil, Zestril)
- quinapril (Accupril)
- ramipril (Altace)
- benazepril (Lotensin)
- moexipril (Univasc)
- fosinopril (Monopril),
- trandolapril (Mavik)

Angiotensin II receptor antagonists

- losartan (Cozaar)
- Valsartan

volves multiple vasoactive substances, including histamine, protaglandin D_2, leukotrienes, and bradykinin. Angiotension converting enzyme not only converts angiotensin I to angiotensin II, but also metabolizes bradykinin into inactive products (Fig. 51–1). Thus ACE inhibition results in elevations in bradykinin levels, and these elevations appear to be the primary cause of ACE inhibitor–induced angioedema as well as cough.[5,73] There is no evidence that this is an allergic phenomenon.[5]

Although the literature is replete with ACE inhibitor–induced angioedema, the overall incidence is only approximately 0.1%.[42,73,76,144] One third of these reactions occur within hours of the first dose and another third within the first week.[144] It is important to remember that the additional one third of cases may occur at any time during therapy, even after years.[22] Patients with a history of idiopathic angioedema and possibly atopy may be at greater risk.[116] There does not appear to be any dose–response relationship.

Treatment varies depending on the severity and rapidity of the swelling. Due to the propensity to involve the tongue, face, and oropharynx, the airway must remain the primary focus of management. A nasopharygeal airway is often helpful. If there is any potential for or suggestion of airway compromise, endotracheal intubation should be performed. Severe tongue and oropharyngeal swelling may make orotracheal or nasotracheal intubation extremely difficult if not impossible. If this occurs, fiberoptic nasal intubation may be an attractive option provided the resources are available. Other techniques including retrograde intubation over a guidewire that was passed through the cricothyroid membrane and emergent cricothyrotomy should also be considered.[131]

Pharmacologic therapy for ACE inhibitor–induced angioedema should include standard agents used for anaphylaxis such as epinephrine, intravenous diphenhydramine, and corticosteroids. However, this is not an antibody-mediated allergic phenomenon and these interventions may be ineffective. In addition, epinephrine may be harmful by inducing vasospasm and myocardial ischemia in elderly patients, particularly those with known atherosclerotic heart disease.

All patients with mild or quickly resolving angioedema should be observed for several hours to assure that the swelling does not progress or return. Outpatient therapy with a short course of oral antihistamines and corticosteroids is appropriate. These patients should be instructed to discontinue ACE inhibitor therapy permanently and to consult their primary physician about other antihypertensive options. Because this is a mechanistic and not allergic adverse effect, the use of any other ACE inhibitors is contraindicated.

What Are the Consequences of an ACE Inhibitor Overdose?

The toxicity of ACE inhibitors in overdose appears to be limited.[90,148] While there have been several case reports of overdoses involving ACE inhibitors published, the majority demonstrated toxicity of a co-ingestant.[30,55,75,166] Pa-

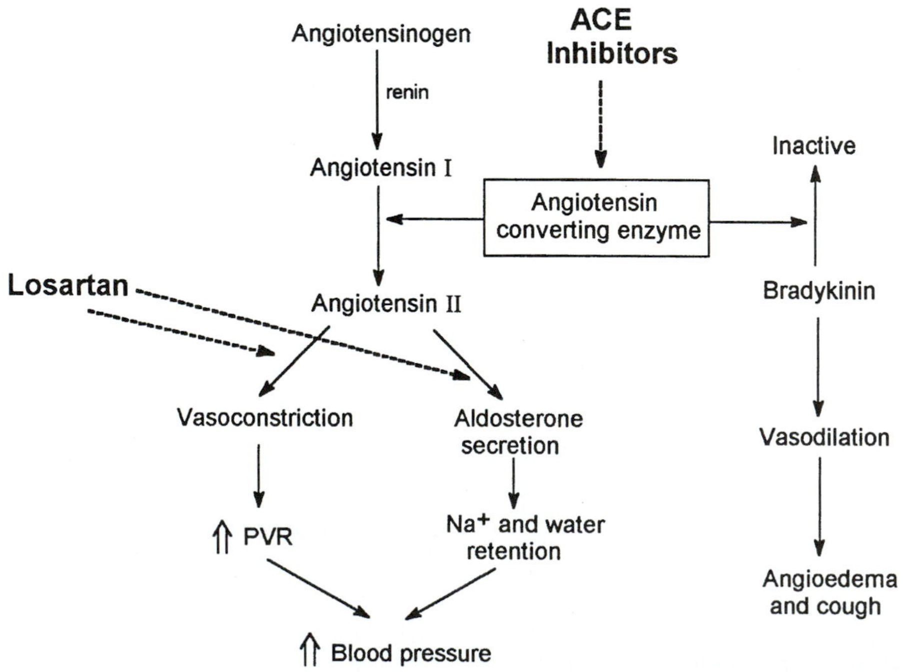

Figure 51–1. An overview of the normal function of angiotensin II and the mechanisms of action of angiotensin-converting enzyme inhibitors and the angiotensin II receptor antagonist, losartan (PVR = peripheral vascular resistance). The inhibitory effects of losartan and valsartan are shown with dotted lines.

tients may remain asymptomatic despite high serum ACE inhibitor drug levels, particularly in isolated ingestions.[86] Hypotension may occur in select patients and is typically responsive to intravenous fluids.[84] One report of death associated with captopril overdose has been reported.[119]

Treatment should focus on supportive care and identifying any co-ingestants that may be more toxic, particularly other antihypertensives such as β-adrenergic antagonists and calcium channel blockers. Activated charcoal alone is sufficient gastrointestinal decontamination in most cases. Intravenous crystalloid boluses are often effective in correcting hypotension, although in rare cases catecholamines may be required.[7]

Naloxone may also be effective in reversing the hypotensive effects of ACE inhibitors. ACE inhibitors may inhibit the metabolism of enkephalins and potentiate their opioid effects, which include lowering blood pressure.[33,104] In a controlled human volunteer study, continuous naloxone infusion effectively blunted the hypotensive response of captopril.[2] In one case report naloxone also appears effective in reversing symptomatic hypotension secondary to a captopril overdose.[164] Although its role in the setting of ACE inhibitor overdose remains unclear, naloxone may obviate the need for large quantities of crystalloid or vasopressors, and it should be utilized.

Are There Any New Antihypertensive Agents Available?

Two new antihypertensive agents became available in the United States called losartan and valsartan. They are similar to ACE inhibitors in that they decrease the effects of angiotensin II. However, ACE inhibitors decrease the formation of angiotensin II, whereas these drugs antagonize angiotensin II at its receptors[156] (see Fig. 51–1). A predicted benefit of this mechanism of action is that the bradykinin system is unaffected and adverse effects, including chronic cough and angioedema, would not be expected. Similar to ACE inhibitors approximately 0.5–1% of patients developed orthostatic hypotension associated with the first dose.[52] There are no reported overdoses, although hypotension should be anticipated.

References

1. Abrams WB: In summary: Satellite symposium on central α-adrenergic blood pressure regulating mechanisms. Hypertension 1984;6(suppl II):87–93.
2. Ajayi AA, Campbell BC, Rubin PC, Reid JL: Effect of naloxone on the actions of captopril. Clin Pharmacol Ther 1985;38:560–565.
3. Allon M, Hall WD, Macon EJ: Prolonged hypotension after initial minoxidil dose. Arch Intern Med 1986;146: 2075–2076.
4. Anderson FJ, Hart GR, Crumpler CP, Lerman MJ: Clonidine overdose: Report of six cases and review of the literature. Ann Emerg Med 1981;10:107–112.
5. Anderson MW, deShazo RD: Studies of the mechanism of ACE inhibitor-associated angioedema: The effect of an ACE inhibitor on cutaneous responses to bradykinin, codeine, and histamine. J Aller Clin Immunol 1990;85: 856–858.
6. Artman M, Boerth RC: Clonidine poisoning. Am J Dis Child 1983;137:171–174.
7. Augenstein WL, Kulig KW, Rumack BH: Captopril overdose resulting in hypotension. JAMA 1988;259:3302–3305.
8. Baglin A, Boulard JC, Hanslink T, Prinseau J: Metabolic adverse reactions to diuretics. Drug Safety 1995;12: 161–167.
9. Bamshad MJ, Wasserman GS. Pediatric clonidine intoxications. Vet Hum Toxicol 1990;32:220–223.
10. Banner WJR, Lund ME, Clawson L: Failure of naloxone to reverse clonidine toxic effect. Am J Dis Child 1983;137: 1170–1171.
11. Bass JW, Beisel WR: Coma due to acute chlorothiazide intoxication. Am J Dis Child 1973;106:620–623.
12. Bendall MJ, Baloch KH, Wilson PB: Side effects due to treatment of hypertension with prazosin. Br Med J 1975; 2:727–729.
13. Bigger TJ: Diuretic therapy, hypertension, and cardiac arrest. N Engl J Med 1994;330:1899–1900.
14. Bobik A, Jennings G, Jackman G, et al: Evidence for a predominantly central hypotensive effect of alpha-methyldopa in humans. Hypertension 1986;8:16–23.
15. Brater DC, Morrelli HF: Digoxin toxicity in patients with normokalemic potassium depletion. Clin Pharmacol Ther 1978;22:21–33.
16. Brown MJ: Clonidine hallucinations. Ann Intern Med 1980;93:456–457.
17. Burden AC, Alexander CPT: Rebound hypertension after acute methyldopa withdrawal. Br Med J 1976;2:1056–1057.
18. Byrd BF III, Collins HW, Primm RK: Risk factors for severe bradycardia during oral clonidine therapy for hypertension. Arch Intern Med 1988;148:729–733.
19. Cairns SA, Marshall AJ: Clonidine withdrawal. Lancet 1976;1:268. Letter.
20. Caravati EM, Bennett DL: Clonidine transdermal patch poisoning. Ann Emerg Med 1988;17:175–176.
21. Carstairs KC, Brechenridge A, Dollery CT, Worlledge SM: Incidence of a positive direct Coombs test in patients on alpha-methyldopa. Lancet 1966;2:133–135.
22. Chin HL, Buchan DA: Severe angioedema after long term use of an angiotensin-converting enzyme inhibitor. Ann Intern Med 1990;112:312–313.
23. Cleland JGF, Dargie HJ, McAlpine, et al: Severe hypotension after first dose of enalapril in heart failure. Br Med J 1985;291:1309–1312.
24. Conner CS, Watanabe AS: Clonidine overdose: A review. Am J Hosp Pharm 1979;36:906–911.
25. Copeland PM: Diuretic abuse and central pontine myelinolysis. Psychother Psychosom 1989;52:101–105.
26. Corneli HM, Banner WW, Vernon DD, Swenson PH: Toddler eats clonidine patch and nearly quits smoking for life. JAMA 1989;261:42. Letter.
27. Cubeddu LX: New $alpha_1$-adrenergic receptor antagonists for the treatment of hypertension: Role of vascular alpha receptors in the control of peripheral resistance. Am Heart J 1988;116:133–162.
28. Curry SC, Arnold-Capell P: Nitroprusside, nitroglycerin,

and angiotensin-converting enzyme inhibitors. Crit Care Clin 1991;7:555–581.

29. Dale RC, Schroeder ET: Respiratory paralysis during treatment of hypertension with trimethaphan camsylate. Arch Intern Med 1976;126:816–818.
30. Dawson AH, Harvey D, Smith AJ, et al: Lisinopril overdose. Lancet 1990;335:487–488.
31. De Jonge A, Timmermans PB, van Zwieten PA: Qualitative aspects of α-adrenergic effects induced by clonidine-like imidazolidines: II. Central and peripheral bradycardia activities. J Pharmacol Exp Ther 1982;222:712–719.
32. DiBianco R: Adverse reactions with angiotensin converting enzyme (ACE) inhibitors. Med Toxicol 1986;1:122–141.
33. Di Nicolantonia R, Hutchinson JS, Takata Y, Veroni M: Captopril potentiates the vasodepressor action of met-enkephalin in anaesthetised dogs. Br J Pharmacol 1983;80: 405–408.
34. Dire DJ, Kuhns DW: The use of sublingual nifedipine in a patient with a clonidine overdose. J Emerg Med 1988; 6:125–128.
35. Doe N, Seth S, Hebert LA: Skin depigmentation related to transdermal clonidine therapy. Arch Intern Med 1995; 155:2120. Letter.
36. Dollery CT, Davies DS, Draffan GH, et al: Clinical pharmacology and pharmacokinetics of clonidine. Clin Pharmacol Ther 1976;19:11–17.
37. DuCharme DW, Freyburger WA, Graham BE, Carlson RG: Pharmacologic properties of minoxidil: A new hypertensive agent. J Pharmacol Exp Ther 1973;184:662–670.
38. Eckhauser ML, Dokler MA, Imbembo AL: Diuretic-associated pancreatitis: A collective review and illustrative cases. Am J Gastroenterol 1987;82:865–870.
39. Eisner EV, Crowell EB: Hydrochlorothiazide-dependent thrombocytopenia due to IgM antibodies. JAMA 1971; 215:480–482.
40. Elkington SG, Schreiber WM, Conn HO: Hepatic injury caused by L-alpha-methyldopa. Circulation 1969;40:589–590.
41. Engelman K: Side effects of sympatholytic antihypertensive drugs. Hypertension 1988;11(suppl II):30–33.
42. Finley CJ, Silverman MA, Nunez AE: Angiotensin converting enzyme inhibitor–induced angioedema: Still unrecognized. Am J Emerg Med 1992;10:550–552.
43. Freed CR, Quintero E, Murphy RC: Hypotension and hypothalamic amine metabolism after long-term alpha-methyldopa infusions. Life Sci 1978;23:313–322.
44. Freis ED: Adverse effects of diuretics. Drug Safety 1992;7:364–373.
45. Frohlich ED, Messerli FH, Pegram BL, Kardon MB: Hemodynamic and cardiac effects of centrally acting antihypertensive drugs. Hypertension 1984;6(suppl II):76–81.
46. Gannon TH, Eby TI: Angioedema for angiotensin-converting enzyme inhibitors: A cause of upper airway obstruction. Laryngoscope. 1990;100:1156–1160.
47. Gavras H, Gavras I: Angiotensin converting enzyme inhibitors. Properties and side effects. Hypertension 1988;11 (suppl II):37–41.
48. Geyskes GG, Boer P, Dorhout MEJ: Clonidine withdrawal: Mechanism and frequency of rebound hypertension. Br J Clin Pharmacol 1979;7:55–62.
49. Giannoccaro PJ, Wallace GJ, Higginson LAJ, et al: Fatal angioedema associated with enalapril. Can J Cardiol 1989;5: 335–336.
50. Glassman AH, Steiner F, Walsh BT, et al: Heavy smokers, smoking cessation, and clonidine. JAMA 1988;259: 2863–2866.
51. Gold MS, Pottash AC, Sweeney DR, Kleber HD: Opiate withdrawal using clonidine. A safe, effective and rapid nonopiate treatment. JAMA 1980;243:343–346.
52. Goldberg AJ, Dunlay MC, Sweet CS: Safety and tolerability of losartan potassium, an angiotensin II receptor antagonist, compared with hydrochlorothiazide, atenolol, felodipine ER, and angiotensin converting enzyme inhibitors for the treatment of systemic hypertension. Am J Cardiol 1995;75:793–795.
53. Golusinski CL, Blount BW: Clonidine-induced bradycardia. J Fam Pract 1995;41:399–401.
54. Grabert B: Clonidine: Recurrent apnea following overdose. DICP Ann Pharmacother 1979;13:1778–1780.
55. Graham SR, Day RO, Hardy M: Captorpril overdose. Med J Aust 1989;151:111. Letter.
56. Hall AH, Smolinske SC, Kulig KW, Rumack BH: Guanabenz overdose. Ann Intern Med 1985;102:787–788.
57. Hall D, Charocopos F, Froer K-L, Rudolph W: ECG changes during long term minoxidil therapy for severe hypertension. Arch Intern Med. 1979;139:790–794.
58. Hamblin JE, Martin CA: Transdermal patch poisoning. Pediatrics 1987;79:161. Letter.
59. Hansson L: Clinical aspects of blood pressure crisis due to withdrawal of centrally acting antihypertensive drugs. Br J Clin Pharmacol 1983;15:485–490.
60. Harris JM: Clonidine patch toxicity. DICP Ann Pharmacother 1990;24:1191–1194.
61. Heidemann SM, Sarnaik AP: Clonidine poisoning in children. Crit Care Med 1990;18:618–620.
62. Henning M, Rubenson A: Evidence that the hypotensive action of alpha-methyldopa is mediated by central actions of methylnoradrenaline. J Pharm Pharmacol 1971;23: 407–411.
63. Henretig F: Clonidine and central acting antihypertensives. In: Ford M, Delaney DA, Ling L, Rose SR, eds: Clinical Toxicology. Philadelphia, Saunders, in press.
64. Henretig F, Wiley J, Brown L: Clonidine patch toxicity: The proof is in the poop. J Toxicol Clin Toxicol 1995; 33:520. Abstract.
65. Hodsman GP, Isles CG, Murray GD, et al: Factors related to first dose hypotensive effect of captopril: Prediction and treatment. Br Med J 1993;286:832–834.
66. Hoffman BB, Lefkowitz RJ: Catecholamines, sympathomimetic drugs, and adrenoreceptor antagonists. In: Hardman JG, Limbird LE, Molinoff PB, Ruddon RW, eds: Goodman and Gilman's The Pharmacological Basis of Therapeutics, 9th ed. New York, McGraw-Hill, 1996, pp. 199–248.
67. Holland OB, Nixon JV, Kuhnet L: Diuretic induced ventricular ectopic activity. Am J Med 1981;70:762–765.
68. Holmes B, Brogden RN, Heel RC: Guanabenz. A review of its pharmacodynamic properties and therapeutic efficacy in hypertension. Drugs 1983;26:212–229.
69. Hughes PL, Morse RM: Use of clonidine in a mixed drug detoxification regimen: Possibility of masking of clinical

signs of sedative withdrawal. Mayo Clin Proc 1985;60: 47–49.
70. Hunt RD, Minderaa RB, Cohen DJ: Clonidine benefits children with attention deficit disorder and hyperactivity: Report of a double-blind placebo-crossover therapeutic trial. J Am Acad Child Psychiatry 1985;24:617–629.
71. Hunyor SN, Bradstock K, Somerville PJ, Lucas N: Clonidine overdose. Br Med J 1975;4:23.
72. Isles C, Mackay A, Barton PJM, Mitchell I: Accidental overdose of minoxidil in a child. Lancet 1981;1:97. Letter.
73. Israili ZH, Hall WD: Cough and angioneurotic edema associated with angiotensin-converting enzyme inhibitor therapy. Ann Intern Med 1992;117:234–242.
74. Jackson EK: Diuretics. In: Hardman JG, Limbird LE, Molinoff PB, Ruddon RW, eds: Goodman and Gilman's The Pharmacological Basis of Therapeutics, 9th ed. New York, McGraw-Hill, 1996, pp. 685–713.
75. Jackson T, Corke C, Agar J: Enalapril overdosage treatment with angiotensin infusion. Lancet 1993;341:703.
76. Jett KG: Captopril-induced angioedema. Ann Emerg Med 1984;13;489–490.
77. Kallanranta T, Hakkarainen H, Kokkanen E, et al: Clonidine in migraine prophylaxis. Headache 1977;17:169–172.
78. Kibler LE, Gazes PC: Effect of clonidine on atrioventricular conduction. JAMA 1977;238:1930–1932.
79. Knapp JF, Fowler MA, Wheeler CA, Wasserman GS: Case 01–1995: A two-year-old female with alteration of consciousness. Pediatr Emerg Care 1995;11:62–65.
80. Kobinger W: Central α-adrenergic systems as target for hypotensive drugs. Rev Physiol Biochem Pharmacol 1978; 81:39–75.
81. Koch-Weser J: Diazoxide. N Engl J Med 1976;294: 1271–1274.
82. Koch-Weser J: Hydralazine. N Engl J Med 1976;295: 320–323.
83. Kulig K, Duffy J, Rumack BH, et al: Naloxone for treatment of clonidine overdose. JAMA 1982;247:1697. Letter.
84. Lau CP: Attempted suicide with enalapril. N Engl J Med 1986;315:197. Letter.
85. Laubie M, Schmitt H, Drouillat M: Action of clonidine on the baroreceptor pathway and medullary sites mediating vagal bradycardia. Eur J Pharmacol 1976;38:293–303.
86. Lechleitner P: Uneventful self-poisoning with a very high dose of captopril. Toxicology 1990;64:325–329.
87. Lenz K, Druml W, Kleinbergeer G, et al: Acute intoxication with prazosin. A case report. Hum Toxicol 1985;4: 53–56.
88. Levine RH, Stauch BS: Hypertensive responses to methyldopa. N Engl J Med 1966;257:946–948.
89. Lin MT, Chandra A, Ko WC, Chen YM: Serotonergic mechanisms of clonidine-induced hypothermia in rats. Neuropharmacology 1981;20:15–21.
90. Lip GYH, Ferner RE: Poisoning with anti-hypertensive drugs: Angiotensin converting enzme inhibitors. J Hum Hyperten 1995;9:711–715.
91. Lip GYH, Ferner RE: Poisoning with anti-hypertensive drugs: Diuretics and potassium supplements. J Hum Hyperten 1995;9:295–301.
92. Litovitz TL, Schmitz BF, Holm KC: 1988 Annual Report of the American Association of Poison Control Centers National Data Collection System. Am J Emerg Med 1989; 7:495–545.
93. Loggie JMH, Saito H, Kahn I, Femmer A, Gaffmeu TE: Accidental reserpine poisoning: Clinical and metabolic effects. Clin Pharmacol Ther 1967;8:692–695.
94. Lowenstein JS: Clonidine. Ann Intern Med 1980,92.74–77.
95. Lowenthal DT: Pharmacokinetics of clonidine. J Cardiovasc Pharmacol 1980;2(suppl):529–537.
96. Maggi JC, Iskra MK, Nussbaum E: Severe clonidine overdose in children requiring critical care. Clin Paediatr 1986;25:453–455.
97. MacFaul R, Miller G: Clonidine poisoning in children. Lancet 1979;1:1266–1267.
98. Marruecos L, Roglan A, Frati ME, Artigas A: Clonidine overdose. Crit Care Med 1983;11:959–960.
99. Mathew PM, Addy DP, Wright N: Clonidine overdose in children. Clin Toxicol 1981;18:169–173.
100. McClean WJ: Prazosin overdose. Med J Aust 1976;1:592.
101. McCormick MA, Forman MH, Manoguerra AS: Severe toxicity from ingestion of a topical minoxidil preparation. Am J Emerg Med 1989;7:419–421.
102. McLennan PL: The hypothermic effect of clonidine and other imidazolidines in relation to their ability to enter the central nervous system in mice. Eur J Pharmacol 1981; 69:477–482.
103. Mendoza JE, Medalie M: Clonidine poisoning with marked hypotension in a 2½ year old child. Clin Pediatr 1079;18:123–127.
104. Millar JA, Sturani A, Rubin PC, Reid JL: Attenuation of the antihypertensive effect of captopril by the opioid receptor antagonist naloxone. Clin Exp Pharmacol Physiol 1983;10: 253–259.
105. Moore MA, Philips P: Clonidine overdose. Lancet 1976; 2:694. Letter.
106. Muir AL, Burton JL, Lawrie DM: Circulatory effects at rest and exercise of clonidine, an imidazoline derivative with hypotensive properties. Lancet 1969;2:181–185.
107. Myhre E, Rugstad HE, Hansen T: Clinical pharmacokinetics of methyldopa. Clin Pharmacokinet 1982;7:221–223.
108. Nayler WG, Price JM, Swann JB, et al: Effect of the hypotensive drug ST 155 (Catapres) on the heart and peripheral circulation. J Pharmacol Exp Ther 1968;164:45–59.
109. Neimann JT, Getzug T, Mruphy W: Reversal of clonidine toxicity by naloxone. Ann Emerg Med 1986;15:1229–1231.
110. Neuvonen PJ, Vilska J, Keranen A: Severe poisoning in a child caused by small dose of clonidine. Clin Toxicol 1978;14:369–374.
111. North DS, Wieland MJ, Peterson CD, Krenzelok EP: Naloxone administration in clonidine overdose. Ann Emerg Med 1981;10:397. Letter.
112. Oates JA: Antihypertensive agents and the drug therapy of hypertension. In: Hardman JG, Limbird LE, Molinoff PB, Ruddon RW, eds: Goodman and Gilman's The Pharmacological Basis of Therapeutics, 9th ed. New York, McGraw-Hill, 1996, pp. 780–808.
113. O'Doherty NJ: Thiazides and cerebral ischaemia. Lancet 1965;2:1297.
114. Olsson JM, Pruitt AW: Mangement of clonidine ingestion in children. J Pediatr 1983;103:646–650.
115. Onesti G, Schwartz AB, Kim KE, et al: Pharmacodynamic

effects of a new antihypertensive drug. Catapres (ST–155). Circulation 1969;34:219–228.
116. Orfan N, Patterson R, Dykewicz MS: Severe angioedema related to ACE inhibitor in patients with a history of idiopathic angioedema. JAMA 1990;264:1287–1290.
117. Pai GS, Lipsitz DJ. Clonidine poisoning. Pediatrics 1976; 58:749–750.
118. Papademetriou V, Burris JF, Notargiacomo A, et al: Thiazide therapy is not a cause of arrhythmia in patients with systemic hypertension. Arch Intern Med 1988;148: 1272–1276.
119. Park H, Purnell GV, Mirchandani HG: Suicide by captopril overdose. J Toxicol Clin Toxicol 1990;28:379–382.
120. Patnode RE, Brouhard BH, Travis LB, et al: Prolonged clonidine overdosage in a child. J Pediatr 1977;90:849–850.
121. Perrone J, Hoffman RS, Jones B, Hollander JE: Guanabenz induced hypothermia in a poisoned elderly female. J Toxicol Clin Toxicol 1994;32:445–449.
122. Pettinger WA: Pharmacology of clonidine. J Cardiovasc Phamacol 1980;2:521–528.
123. Pettinger WA: Clonidine, a new antihypertensive drug. N Engl J Med 1975;293:1179–1180.
124. Pettinger WA, Mitchell HC: Side effects of vasodilator therapy. Hypertension 1988;11(suppl II):34–36.
125. Poff SW, Rose SR: Minoxidil overdose with ECG changes: Case report and review. Am J Emerg Med 1992;10:53–57.
126. Ram VCS, Holland B, Fairchild C, Gomez-Sanchez CE: Withdrawal syndrome following cessation of guanabenz therapy. J Clin Pharmacol 1979;19:148–150.
127. Raper JH, Shinar C, Finkelstein S: Clonidine patch ingestion in an adult. DICP Ann Pharmacother 1993;27:719–722.
128. Reed MT, Hamburg EL: Person to person transfer of transdermal drug-delivery systems: A case report. N Engl J Med 1986;314:1120–1121.
129. Reid JL, Campbell BC, Hamilton CA: Withdrawal reactions following cessation of central α-adrenergic receptor agonists. Hypertension 1984;6(suppl II):71–75.
130. Robbins DN, Crawford ED, Lackner LH: Priapism secondary to prazosin overdose. J Urol 1983;130:975.
131. Roberts JR, Wuerz RC: Clinical characteristics of angiotensin-converting enzyme inhibitor–induced angioedema. Ann Emerg Med 1991;20:555–558.
132. Robertson D, Tung C, Goldberg MR, et al: Antihypertensive metabolites of α-methyldopa. Hypertension 1984;6 (suppl II);45–50.
133. Rodman JS, Deutsch DJ, Gutman SI: Methyldopa hepatitis. A report of six cases and review of the literature. Am J Med 1976;60:941–948.
134. Rosenberg L, Shapiro S, Slone D, et al: Thiazides and acute cholecystitis. N Engl J Med 1980;303:546–548.
135. Rougraff ME: Chlorothiazide overdosage effects in two year old child. Penn Med J 1959;62:694.
136. Rubinstein I: Fatal thrombosis of left internal carotid artery following diuretic abuse. Ann Emerg Med 1985; 14:275. Letter.
137. Scheinman MM, Strauss HC, Evans GT, et al: Adverse effects of sympatholytic agents in patients with hypertension and sinus node dysfunction. Am J Med 1978;64: 1013–1020.
138. Schieber RA, Kaufman ND: Use of tolazoline in massive clonidine poisoning. Am J Dis Child 1981;135:77–78.
139. Schwartz E, Friedman E, Mouallem M, Farfel Z: Sinus arrest associated with clonidine therapy. Clin Cardiol 1987; 11:53–54.
140. Self F, Bates GHEM, Drake-Lee A: Severe angioneurotic oedema causing acute airway obstruction. J R Soc Med 81;1988;544–545.
141. Shnaps Y, Almog S, Halkin H, Tirosh M: Methyldopa poisoning. Clin Toxicol 1982;19:501–503.
142. Siegel D, Hulley SB, Black DM, et al: Diruetics, serum and intracellular electrolyte levels, and ventricular arrhythias in hypertensive men. JAMA 1992;267:1083–1089.
143. Si^covick DS, Raghunathan TE, Psaty BM, et al: Diuretic therapy for hypertension and the risk of primary cardiac arrest. N Engl J Med 1994;330:1852–1857.
144. Slater EE, Merril DD, Guess HA, et al: Clinical profile of angioedema associated with angiotensin converting enzyme inhibition JAMA 1988;260:967–970.
145. Smith BA, Ferguson DB: Acute hydralazine overdose: Marked ECG abnormalities in a young adult. Ann Emerg Med 1992;21:326–330.
146. Sonnenblick M, Friedlander Y, Rosin AJ: Diuretic-induced hyponatremia. Reproducibility by single dose rechallenge and an analysis of pathogenesis. Chest 1993; 103:601–606.
147. Sorkin EM, Heel RC: Guanfacine. A review of its pharmacodynamic and pharmacokinetic properties and therapeutic efficacy in the treatment of hypertension. Drugs 1986;31:301–336.
148. Spiller HA, Udicious TM, Muir S: Angiotensin converting enzyme inhibitor ingestion in children. J Toxicol Clin Toxicol 1989;27:345–353.
149. Stein B, Volans GN: Dixarit overdose: The problem of attractive tablets. Br Med J 1978;2:667–668.
150. Steiners E: Diuretics, digitalis, and arrhythmias. Acta Med Scand 1981;647(suppl):75–78.
151. Stelzer FP, Stubenbord JJ, Sreenivasan V, Venuto RC: Late toxicity of clonidine withdrawal. N Engl J Med 1976; 294:1182. Letter.
152. Tenenbein M: Naloxone in clonidine toxicity. Am J Dis Child 1984;138:1084–1085.
153. Textor SC, Bravo EL, Fouad FM, Tarazi RC: Hyperkalemia in azotemic patients during angiotensin-converting enzyme inhibition and aldosterone reduction with captopril. Am J Med 1982;73:719–725.
154. Tibirica E, Feldman J, Mermet C, et al: An imidazoline-specific mechanism for the hypotensive effect of clonidine: A study with yohimbine and idazoxan. J Pharmacol Exp Ther 1991;256:606–613.
155. Thormann J, Neuss H, Schlepper M, Mitrovic V: Effects of clonidine on sinus node function in man. Chest 1981;80: 201–206.
156. Triggle DJ: Angiotensin II receptor antagonism: Losartan—sites and mechanism of action. Clin Ther 1995;17: 1005–1030.
157. Van der Linden W, Ritter B, Edlund G: Acute cholecystitis and thiazides. Br Med J 1984;289:654–655.
158. Van Dyke MW, Bonace AL, Ellenhorn MJ: Guanfacine

overdose in a pediatric patient. Vet Hum Toxicol 1990;32: 46–47.

159. van Etta L, Burchell H: Severe bradycardia with clonidine. JAMA 1978;240:2047. Letter.

160. van Zwieten PA: The pharmacology of centrally acting hypotensive drugs. Br J Clin Pharmacol 1980;10:135S–138S.

161. van Zweiten PA: Antihypertensive drugs with a central action. Prog Pharmacol 1975;1:1–66.

162. van Zwieten PA, Thoolen MJMC, Timmermans PBMWM: The hypotensive activity and side effects of methyldopa, clonidine, and guanfacine. Hypertension 1984;6(suppl II):28–33.

163. Vanholder R, Carpentier J, Schurgers M, Clement DL: Rebound phenomenon during gradual withdrawal of clonidine. Br Med J 1977;1:1138.

164. Varon J, Duncan SR: Naloxone reversal of hypotension due to captopril overdose. Ann Emerg Med 1991;20: 1125–1127.

165. Vila JM, Blum L, Dosik H: Thiazide-induced immune hemolytic anemia. JAMA 1976;236:1723–1724.

166. Waeber B, Nussberger J, Brunner HR. Self-poisoning with enalapril. Br Med J 1984;288:287–288.

167. Weinberger MH: Diuretics and their side effects. Hypertension 1988;11(suppl II):16–20.

168. Wiley JF, Wiley CC, Torrey SB, Henretig FM: Clonidine poisoning in young children. J Pediatr 1990;116: 654–658.

169. Williams PL, Krafcik JM, Potter BB, et al: Cardiac toxicity of clonidine. Chest 1977;72:784–785.

170. Worlledge SM, Carstairs KC, Dacie JV: Autoimmune hemolytic anaemia associated with α-methyldopa therapy. Lancet 1966;2:135–139.

171. Yeh BK, Natel A, Goldberg LI: Antihypertensive effect of clonidine. Arch Intern Med 1971;127:233–237.

172. Zamboulis C, Reid JL: Withdrawal of guanfacine after long term treatment in essential hypertension. Eur J Clin Phamacol 1981;19:19–24.

173. Zarifis J, Lip GYH, Ferner RE: Poisoning with anti-hypertensive drugs: Methyldopa and clonidine. J Hum Hypertension 1995;9:787–790.

CHAPTER 52

Antidysrhythmic Agents

Neal A. Lewin

A 78-year-old woman was brought to the emergency department (ED) complaining of nausea. She had a history of "heart trouble" and reported taking a "water pill" for high blood pressure. On closer questioning she admitted to four episodes of syncope over the previous 9 days.

Her vital signs were: blood pressure, 130/90 mm Hg; irregular pulse at 100 beats/min; respirations, 20 breaths/min; and temperature, 37°C (98.6°F). The patient was moderately obese, slightly diaphoretic, and in moderate distress. There was no cyanosis or peripheral edema. Her lungs were clear. The PMI was in the sixth intercostal space, midway between the midclavicular and anterior axillary line. Auscultation of the heart revealed an irregular rhythm without murmurs. The abdomen was soft, nontender, and without organomegaly. The neurologic examination was within normal limits.

An ECG revealed a sinus rhythm of 70 beats/min with runs of a wide complex dysrhythmia at a rate of 160 beats/min. Blood was drawn for complete blood count, glucose, BUN, and electrolytes, including calcium and magnesium. An intravenous (IV) line was inserted. The patient was given a 100-mg bolus of lidocaine. A lidocaine infusion was started at a rate of 2 mg/min by gravity drip. A second IV line with 0.9% NaCl was placed in the other arm for the administration of fluids. A subsequent ECG showed sinus rhythm without evidence of ectopy.

As the patient could not void, a Foley catheter was inserted. Over the next hour, the urine output was noted to be only 10 mL. It was therefore decided to increase the rate of fluids. Inadvertently, the lidocaine infusion, rather than the 0.9% NaCl line, was run "wide open" and the patient received 600 mg of lidocaine (150 mL of solution) over a 10-minute period. She rapidly became hypotensive with a palpable blood pressure of 70 mm Hg. The patient then developed status epilepticus, followed shortly thereafter by cardiorespiratory arrest. Cardiopulmonary resuscitation (CPR) was initiated. The patient was given 1.0 mg of epinephrine (1:10,000), and 1 amp (44 mEq) of sodium bicarbonate IV, without effect. While a transvenous pacemaker was being inserted, a sinus rhythm of 70 beats/min returned spontaneously. The patient was admitted to the intensive care unit (ICU) with a blood pressure of 124/80 mm Hg.

The initial laboratory data were: hemoglobin, 13 g/dL; hematocrit, 38%; WBC, 6800/mm^3 with a normal differential; creatinine, 1.0 mg/dL; sodium, 143 mEq/L; potassium, 4.0 mEq/L; chloride, 105 mEq/L; bicarbonate, 25 mEq/L; BUN, 10 mg/dL; and glucose, 110 mg/dL.

The patient's mental status returned to normal 7 hours after her cardiac arrest. As she continued to have intermittent multifocal ventricular extrasystoles, a lidocaine infusion was reinstituted using an infusion pump. Despite an infusion rate of 4 mg/min, the lidocaine failed to control the dysrhythmia. Four hundred milligrams of procainamide was slowly administered IV and abolished the ectopy. Serial ECGs and cardiac enzyme studies failed to show any evidence of a myocardial infarction. The patient was placed on oral doses of procainamide and subsequently discharged from the hospital.

Overview of Antidysrhythmic Agents

Dysrhythmias can be benign or malignant, and the mechanisms of these electrophysiologic events are complex and sometimes unknown. There are a plethora of antidysrhythmic agents currently being used, and as a result there exists the potential for both intentional and unintentional overdoses and a multitude of adverse effects. Although there are potential benefits from these agents, such as a reduction in mortality, there is also a risk of inducing dysrhythmias and increasing mortality during long-term treatment.[2,26,27,43,47,63,94,96,128]

The classification of antidysrhythmics is complex and controversial. This chapter will discuss the toxicity of the different classes of antidysrhythmics and the management of their toxicities. A detailed discussion of dysrhythmias and their mechanisms appears in Chapter 21 (Cardiovascular Principles). Toxicity from beta-adrenergic antagonists and calcium channel blockers is discussed in Chapters 49 and 50.

What Classification System Is Currently Used for the Antidysrhythmics?

Classifying antidysrhythmics by electrophysiologic properties emphasizes the connection between the basic electrophysiologic actions and the antidysrhythmic effects. This is the basis of the Vaughan Williams classification[158,159] (Table 52–1). Another approach to classification is to classify dysrhythmia mechanisms and target drug therapy to the electrophysiologic mechanism that it is hoped will terminate the dysrhythmia. The chapter will discuss the antidysrhythmics using the latter classification, recognizing that there remains some criticism of this classification.[157–159,167]

Class I Antidysrhythmics: IA, IB, IC

Antidysrhythmics in this group are sodium channel blockers.[25] The original subdivision of class I drugs was based on clinical observations, before kinetics were examined.[158] The IA class (cibenzoline, disopyramide, pirmenol, procainamide, quinidine) widens the QRS interval and lengthens His-ventricle (H-V) intervals at high drug concentrations, increases effective refractory period (ERP), and delays repolarization. These drugs block sodium channels and multiple cardiac potassium currents. They are open-state blockers of sodium channels with a recovery time in the intermediate range.[128,158,159]

IB compounds (lidocaine, mexiletine, moricizine, phenytoin, tocainide) have little effect on the QRS interval or H-V intervals but prolong the effective refractory period (ERP). The reason for this is that they attach rapidly to sodium channels following depolarization; by the end of a single action potential a substantial proportion of channels are blocked, and at the beginning of diastole less sodium current is available and ERP is prolonged. After repolarization IB drugs dissociate rapidly, and by the end of normal diastole most channels are drug free. Sodium channels are fully available and QRS and H-V intervals are unaffected.[158]

The IC drugs (encainide, flecainide, lorcainide, propafenone) detach very slowly from Na-channels following repolarization so that a steady-state block develops, eliminating a proportion of channels permanently. Sodium current is reduced and conduction velocity is depressed, thereby widening of QRS and H-V intervals.[159]

Class IA Antidysrhythmics: Procainamide, Quindine, Disopyramide

Procainamide. Procainamide (Fig. 52–1) is used predominantly to suppress ventricular ectopy and atrial and ventricular tachydysrhythmias. Although absorption from the GI tract is rapid and relatively complete following a therapeutic dose (75–95%), it may be delayed in overdose situations.[34,130,131] The apparent volume of distribution is 1.7–2.22 L/kg.[131] Elimination follows first-order kinetics. It is metabolized by the liver and undergoes biotransformation by acetylation to *N*-acetylprocainamide (NAPA), which is pharmacologically active.[34,41,131] Its rate of acetylation is genetically determined.[130] Both procainamide and NAPA are renally excreted. In patients with renal failure, procainamide and *N*-acetylprocainamide can reach toxic plasma concentrations.[39] Intravenous dosing is potentially dangerous if done rapidly. Procainamide distributes into an initial volume of distribution that is smaller than the final volume of distribution. The heart is located in this initial volume; therefore, the loading dose should be given in divided doses every 5 minutes.

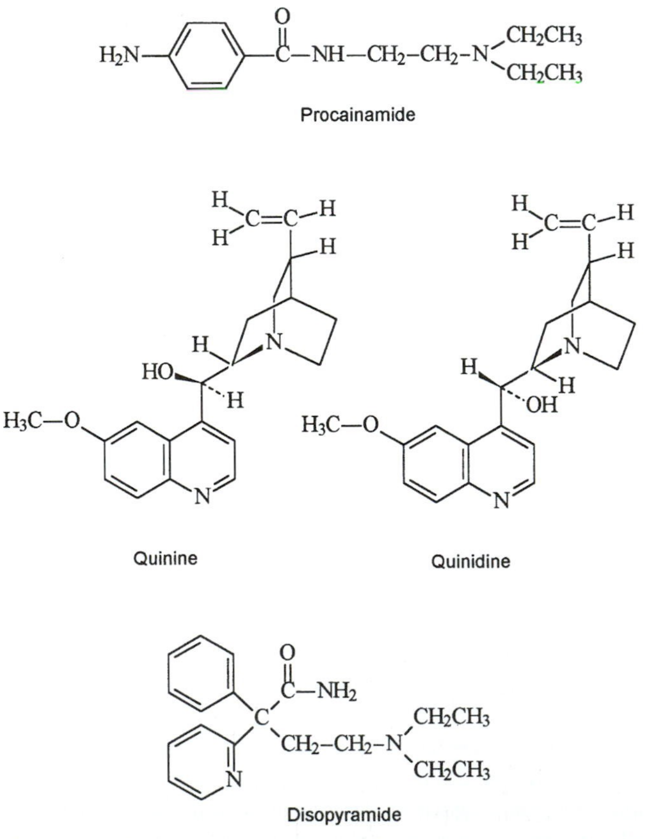

Figure 52–1. Structures of class IA antidysrhythmics and quinine.

TABLE 52–1. ANTIDYSRHYTHMIC DRUGS

Drug	Route	Primary Route of Elimination	Classification	Channel Block	Effect on ECG	Side Effects and Complicating Factors
Disopyramide	PO	Liver, kidney	Class IA	Na^+, K^+	↑QRS, ↑QT, ±PR	Congestive heart failure, negative inotropic effects, anticholinergic, torsades de pointes, heart block, hypoglycemia
Procainamide	IV, PO	50–60% unchanged in kidney, liver active metabolite	Class IA	Na^+, K^+	↑QRS, ↑QT, ±PR	Hypotension, QRS widening, fever, systemic lupus erythematosis like syndrome, torsades de pointes
Quinidine	PO	Liver, kidney, 10–20% unchanged	Class IA	Na^+, K^+, Ca^{2+}	↑QRS, ↑QT, ±PR	Heart block, severe sinus node dysfunction, prolonged QT syndrome, hypotension, cinchonism, torsades de pointes, thrombocytopenia, ↑ digoxin levels
Lidocaine	IV	Liver, active metabolite	Class IB	Na^+	None	Fatigue, agitation, paresthesias, seizures, hallucinations, rarely bundle branch block
Mexiletine	IV, PO	Liver	Class IB	Na^+	None	See lidocaine
Phenytoin	IV, PO	Liver	Class IB	Na^+	None	Hypotension and asystole related to IV infusion, nystagmus, ataxia
Tocainide	IV, PO	Kidney, liver	Class IB	Na^+	None	See lidocaine, aplastic anemia, interstitial pneumonia
Encainide	PO	Liver, active metabolites	Class IC	Na^+, Ca^{2+}, K^+	↑QRS, ↑PR	Negative inotropic effects
Flecainide	IV, PO	Liver 75% Kidney 25%	Class IC	Na^+, Ca^{2+}, K^+	↑PR ↑QRS	Negative inotropic effects, bradycardia, heart block, ventricular fibrillation, ventricular tachycardia, neutropenia
Propafenone	IV, PO	Liver	Class IC	Na^+, K^+	↑PR, ↑QRS	Asthma, congestive heart failure, hypoglycemia, AV block, QRS prolongation, bradycardia, ventricular fibrillation, ventricular tachycardia
Moricizine	PO	Liver	Class I	Na^+	↑QRS, ↓QT_c	↑Mortality after myocardial infarction, bradycardia, CHF, ventricular fibrillation, ventricular tachycardia
Beta-adrenergic antagonist	IV, PO	Liver	Class II		↑PR, ↑QT	Congestive heart failure, asthma, hypoglycemia, Raynaud's disease
Amiodarone	IV, PO	Liver	Class III	Na^+, Ca^{2+}	↑PR, ↑QRS, AV Block, ↑QT	Negative inotropic effects, pulmonary fibrosis, corneal microdeposits, thyroid abnormalities, photosensitivity, ↑diltiazem, quinidine, procainamide, flecainide, digoxin levels
Bretylium	IV, IM	Kidney	Class III	K^+ channel block	None	Hypertension followed by hypotension, nausea, and vomiting
Calcium channel blockers	IV, PO	Liver	Class IV	Ca^{2+}	↑PR	Asystole (if used IV with IV beta-adrenergic receptor antagonists), AV block, hypotension, congestive heart failure, constipation, ↑ digoxin levels
Adenosine	IV	All cells (Adenosine deaminase)	None	Nucleoside-specific G protein coupled adenosine receptors, ↓Ca^{2+} currents activates ACH-sensitive K^+ current	↑PR, heart block	Transient asystole < 5 sec, chest pain, dyspnea, atrial fibrillation, ↓BP, effects potentiated by dipyridamole and in heart transplant patients, ↑ dose needed with methylxanthine use

Procainamide and NAPA concentrations should be determined. Total procainamide and NAPA therapeutic concentrations range from 5 to 30 μg/mL. Some authors report severe toxicity at concentrations greater than 60 μg/mL.[7] Clinically, the QT_c intervals and blood pressure seem to correlate with degree of toxicity.

Cardiac toxicity may include cardiac dysrhythmias due to the drug's prodysrhythmic effect, resultant conduction abnormalities, such as increased QT_c and QRS intervals, torsades de pointes,[127,129,131] and hypotension. Gastrointestinal distress, obtundation, and renal insufficiency may also develop.[13,79]

Treatment should include continuous ECG monitoring and attention to basic management: airway and circulatory support and IV access. Gastrointestinal decontamination, activated charcoal, and a cathartic are indicated following an oral overdose. The use of sodium bicarbonate and sodium lactate may be beneficial in reversing Na^+ blockade with IA and IC overdoses.[118,160]

If renal failure is present, hemodialysis,[7,74] which can increase the clearance of both parent drug and metabolite, may be indicated. The roles of charcoal hemoperfusion, hemofiltration, and continuous arteriovenous hemodiafiltration are inadequately defined, but may be beneficial for removing NAPA.[21,74] Drugs to avoid in treating patients with procainamide-induced dysrhythmias are quinidine, disopyramide, and beta-adrenergic receptor antagonists, all of which may exacerbate conduction abnormalities.

Quinidine. Quinidine (see Fig. 52–1), the *d*-isomer of quinine, is found in cinchona bark.[91] Quinidine shares many pharmacologic properties of quinine (see Chap. 44) but is more toxic, especially in cardiac tissue. It is considered a myocardial depressant, decreasing excitability, conduction velocity, and contractility.[158,159] It also alters cardiac action by its anticholinergic effect.[132] Quinidine's Na^+ channel blocking properties result in an increased threshold for excitability and decreased automaticity. Its K^+ channel blocking actions cause increased action potentials and elicit early afterdepolarizations (EADs) at slow heart rates.[130]

Quinidine is a weak base. It is available clinically as a sulfate, gluconate, and other salts. After oral ingestion, it is 70–80% bioavailable. The sulfate form is absorbed rapidly, within 1–1.5 hours. Its volume of distribution is approximately 3.0–4.0 L/kg and its half-life is approximately 6–8 hours.[130] Liver disease extends the half-life to as long as 50 hours, and in renal failure the half-life is approximately 9–12 hours. It is protein bound (80%) and is hydroxylated in the liver to active and inactive metabolites, with 10–30% of the parent drug excreted unchanged in the urine. Quinidine has substantial acute cardiotoxicity after ingestion, including decreased AV conduction, intraventricular conduction abnormalities, increased QT_c, T-wave inversions, and ST depression.[127] With widening of QT and QRS intervals, ventricular tachycardia, ventricular fibrillation, or torsades de pointes may ensue.[70,72,127,130,136,162] "Quinidine syncope" is believed to be caused by a ventricular dysrhythmia, most commonly torsades de pointes.[127,153] Many of the ECG changes mimic those of hyperkalemia. In contradistinction to procainamide, quinidine is associated with an increased QT_c at therapeutic concentrations.[132] Other acute manifestations of quinidine toxicity include hypotension, seizures, coma, and noncardiogenic pulmonary edema.

Management of a patient with quinidine toxicity is similar to that for procainaimide toxicity. Generally, concentrations greater than 14 μg/mL are associated with cardiotoxicity.[79] Continuous ECG monitoring for evidence of QRS or QT changes is critical. A 50% increase in QT_c or QRS intervals indicates toxicity. Intravenous access, airway and circulatory support, and electrolyte balance are all important. Gastrointestinal decontamination is also indicated. Although acidification of urine may theoretically increase urinary excretion, it is potentially harmful due to presumed benefit of serum alkalinization with sodium bicarbonate[145,160] (see Antidotes in Depth: Sodium Bicarbonate) as the treatment for lengthened QRS complex, and acidification is therefore not recommended. Hemodialysis is not helpful due to the substantial protein binding. The use of glucagon and bretylium to reverse myocardial depression has been studied in canine models, but human studies are lacking. Hypotension can be treated with fluids, dopamine, dobutamine, isoproterenol, norepinephrine, and intraaortic balloon pump.[13,145] Ventricular dysrhythmias can be treated with lidocaine and phenytoin. Magnesium sulfate[155] and overdrive with a pacemaker may be helpful in treating torsades de pointes.[79]

Disopyramide. Disopyramide (see Fig. 52–1) has greater myocardial depressant and anticholinergic effects than other class IA antidysrhythmic agents.[107,158] Disopyramide is 85% bioavailable, but absorption can be delayed due to the decreased GI motility associated with its anticholinergic effects. Its volume of distribution is 40–80 L/kg. The kidney excretes 40–60% of the drug, whereas the liver metabolizes the drug and its metabolite, mono-*N*-dealkylated disopyramide.[93] This metabolite is responsible for most of the anticholinergic effects commonly observed.[107,130] The half-life of disopyramide is 6–8 hours and that of mono-*N*-dealkylated disopyramide is 3–4 hours. Electrocardiographic findings comparable to those associated with toxicity from other class IA drugs can occur.[79] Atrioventricular and intraventricular conduction abnormalities, torsades de pointes, other ventricular dysrhythmias, and congestive heart failure and cardiopulmonary arrest have occurred early in these overdoses.[107,120]

Management of a patient with a disopyramide overdose is similar to that of patients with procainamide and quinidine overdoses. Airway, circulatory support, IV access, and ECG monitoring are of paramount importance. One case report discusses the successful resuscitation of a 16-year-old girl who acutely overdosed on 20 capsules of 100-mg disopyramide.[1] Asystole followed by an idioventricular rhythm was present with electromechanical dissociation. The patient was resuscitated with 75 minutes of cardiopulmonary resuscitation, calcium chloride, isoproterenol, mannitol, dopamine, and a temporary pacemaker. Since disopyramide blocks calcium channels, it has been postulated that the high dosage of calcium may be beneficial, although evidence to support this effect is lacking.

Gastrointestinal decontamination is warranted. There is no clinical evidence to support the use of hemodialysis or hemoperfusion.

Class IB Antidysrhythmics: Lidocaine, Tocainide, Mexilitine, Moricizine

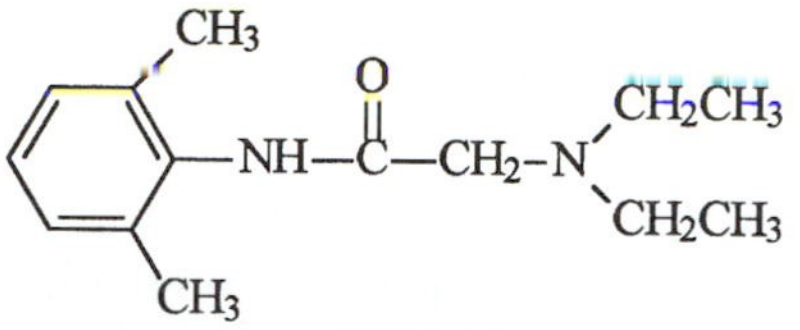

Lidocaine

Lidocaine. Lidocaine is an aminoacyl amide that is a synthetic derivative of cocaine.[3] It is used clinically as both an antidysrhythmic and an anesthetic agent.[9,19,37,62,106,121,137]

Lidocaine inhibits sodium and potassium conductance and decreases the excitability of cells.[25] In peripheral nerves it decreases the rate and degree of depolarization and blocks conduction, thereby causing anesthesia.

Lidocaine is effective in controlling ventricular dysrhythmias resulting from increased automaticity and reentry. Like many other antidysrhythmic agents (including quinidine, disopyramide, bretylium, procainamide, propranolol, and phenytoin), lidocaine decreases cardiac automaticity and membrane responsiveness by depressing the slope of phase 4 depolarization. Lidocaine has been postulated to prevent reentry by preferentially suppressing conduction in compromised tissue.[3,25,40,89,92,131]

Lidocaine is generally used parenterally due to its extensive first-pass hepatic metabolism when it is ingested orally.[20,62] Transtracheal absorption can be significant, as can unintentional or intentional oral ingestion of viscous lidocaine.[9,19,20,62,106,121,131] Lidocaine is a weak base with a of pK_a 7.8. It is 50% bound to protein, with an apparent volume of distribution (V_d) of 1.3 L/kg in adults. Congestive heart failure reduces the V_d by approximately 30% and chronic liver disease increases the V_d by approximately 40%.[12,20]

Lidocaine is 95% metabolized by mixed-function oxidases in the liver by dealkylation to an active metabolite, mono-ethylglycylxylide (MEGX) (half-life, 120 minutes) and subsequently to the inactive glycine xylidide (GX) (half-life, 1 hour) which can be further broken down to monoethylglycine and xylidide.[15,151] The active metabolite (MEGX) may also produce toxicity, but has less Na^+ channel blocking than the parent drug. The rate of degradation is influenced by hepatic blood flow and hepatic function.[154] Only a small percentage of lidocaine is excreted unchanged by the kidney, and about 75% of xylidide is excreted in the urine as the metabolite 4-hydroxy-2,6-dimethylaniline. Toxic reactions to therapeutic doses are most likely to occur in patients with congestive heart failure, shock, liver disease, or concomitant drug therapy with cimetidine or propranolol.[33,58,71,152,154]

Adverse reactions to lidocaine appear to increase with advancing age and decreasing body weight.[33,37,119] Toxic reactions to lidocaine and its metabolites MEGX and GX occur in 6–15% of patients placed on infusions at 3 mg/min.[11,37,57,123,141] The most common toxicity of lidocaine is its effect on the central nervous system (CNS). The typical CNS manifestations of lidocaine toxicity include drowsiness, weakness, a sensation of "drifting away," euphoria, dysphoria, diplopia, decreased hearing, paresthesias, muscular fasciculations, and convulsions.[14] The more severe CNS reactions are commonly seen with blood concentrations greater than 5 μg/mL and are often preceded by somnolence and paresthesias. These symptoms should therefore alert the clinician to reduce the dosage promptly. In neonates apnea, hypotonia and seizures are reported to result from lidocaine toxicity.[80] If seizures develop, an intravenous benzodiazepine or a barbiturate should be administered. Seizures that are induced by lidocaine are generally brief in nature, albeit status epilepticus can occur.[14]

Severe cardiovascular reactions also occur. Massive overdoses resulting from uncontrolled IV infusions can lead to immediate hypotension, convulsions, and cardiopulmonary arrest.[8,44,48,76,119,121] At therapeutic doses, lidocaine suppresses phase 4 automaticity, decreases the refractory period, and increases conduction velocity in diseased tissue. When toxicity develops, however, there is depression in the intrinsic pacemakers, leading to sinus arrest, AV block, hypotension, ventricular tachycardia, ventricular fibrillation, and/or cardiac arrest. Many of these reactions have also been reported at therapeutic doses. Management includes fluid replacement if hypotension exists. If the patient does not respond to fluids, norepinephrine, dopamine, dobutamine, and intraaortic balloon assist can be used.[52,114] Bradydysrhythmias can be treated with atropine, isoproterenol, or a pacemaker.[114] Cardiopulmonary bypass, which maintains hepatic perfusion, allowing lidocaine to be metabolized, has been used.[52,114] Hemoperfusion may be warranted if liver failure or circulatory collapse does not allow for other treatment modalities to be used.[52]

A number of case reports demonstrate the toxicity associated with oral lidocaine.[9,19,37,62,106,121,137] Lidocaine is absorbed from both the oral mucosa and the gastrointestinal (GI) tract. When mucosal absorption occurs, the liver is bypassed; when intestinal absorption occurs, extensive first-pass hepatic extraction and metabolism result and only one third of the drug is bioavailable. Since the primary metabolite, MEGX, is almost as toxic as lidocaine itself,[116] this may explain why toxicity still occurs with oral ingestions. A case report of $3\frac{1}{2}$-year-old, 14-kg child who became toxic when given 15 mL of 2% viscous lidocaine (estimate, 300 mg or 21.4 mg/kg/dose) demonstrated the potential for toxicity of an oral ingestion.[137] The child received two doses 4 hours apart. Ten minutes after the second dose the child developed tonic-clonic seizures. The lidocaine concentration 60 minutes after the second dose was 10 μg/mL. Another child had received multiple doses of 2.5 mL each and developed seizures. Both children were treated supportively and fully recovered.[62]

Another hazard associated with lidocaine is paralysis of the gag reflex with the potential of aspiration.

Drink or food should not be ingested within 60 minutes after oral lidocaine use. The risk associated with oral lidocaine probably outweighs the benefit. If it is used, single doses should be less than 5 mg/kg.

Tocainide. Tocainide is indicated for the treatment of ventricular dysrhythmias. It is a lidocaine analog, but unlike lidocaine it does not undergo first-pass metabolism and is almost 100% bioavailable when administered orally. Its half-life is 9–20 hours; 60% is metabolized hepatically and 40% excreted renally. Its glucuronide metabolites are not pharmacologically active. Ten to 50% of the drug is protein bound. Its therapeutic range is 5–12 μg/mL, and it does not prolong the QT interval.[55,84,85,105,135,142] Tocainide has membrane-stabilizing effects that reduce sodium and potassium conductance and decrease the myocardial cell excitability. It slows the rate of rise of phase 0 of the action potential. It increases ventricular fibrillation threshold in normal and ischemic tissues.[105] Both renal failure and congestive heart failure can prolong the half-life considerably.[85]

The few overdoses reported with tocainide are associated with CNS and cardiovascular complications similar to those that occur with lidocaine overdose (Table 52–1).[10,30] Treatment of a patient with tocainide toxicity therefore should be similar to that of a patient with lidocaine toxicity. Because seizures can develop rapidly, orogastric lavage is warranted, and emesis is contraindicated. Tocainide is significantly removed by hemodialysis and hemoperfusion. The intrinsic clearance of tocainide is low, 200 mL/min; adding hemoperfusion or hemodialysis clearance of 200–300 mL/min should increase clearance.[163]

Mexiletine. Mexiletine was originally developed as an anorectic agent but was found to have antidysrhythmic, local anesthetic, and anticonvulsant activity.[23,24] It is used for ventricular dysrhythmias and is ineffective in treating supraventricular dysrhythmias. Its chemical structure and electrophysiologic properties are similar to lidocaine except it is a primary amine. Mexiletine depresses the rise of phase 0 of the action potential and shortens the effective refractory period similar to other class IB antidysrhythmic agents, and it blocks the fast inward sodium channel.[159] It is a base, with absorption usually occurring in the small intestine. Absorption is increased, however, when the gastric contents are alkalinized. Its therapeutic range is 1–2 μg/mL, with a half-life of 12–13 hours. It is 100% hepatically metabolized. Seventy percent of mexiletine is protein bound. It has a very large volume of distribution (5.5–12 L/kg), is highly lipophilic, is eliminated predominantly as inactive metabolites, and has a long elimination half-life (8–10 hours).[127] Renal disease, CHF, and cirrhosis decrease the clearance of mexiletine. Metabolism of mexiletine is accelerated by phenobarbital, rifampin, and phenytoin and is slowed by cimetidine, INH, and disulfiram.[83]

In the few cases of reported mexiletine overdoses, most patients have cardiovascular toxicity such as complete heart block, torsades de pointes, and asystole.[31,37,51,73] The use of other IB antidysrhythmics such as lidocaine or tocainide can potentiate the neurotoxicity of mexiletine. Neurotoxicity has also been reported with this overdose, including status epilepticus, which can be treated with intravenous benzodiazepines.

One case report described a patient with status epilepticus secondary to mexiletine toxicity but without any hemodynamic or electrocardiographic abnormalities.[6,113] Basic management of this overdose includes activated charcoal possibly with whole-bowel irrigation.[6,113] Mexiletine's extensive distribution and its rapid metabolism make it a poor candidate for extracorporeal drug removal.

Moricizine. Moricizine, previously known as ethmozin (or ethmozine), is a phenothiazine derivative that depresses Na^+ current. In isolated nonischemic canine Purkinje fibers, it reduces maximal upstroke velocity (V_{max}) of both phase 0 depolarization and action potential duration.[157] This action is similar to lidocaine; however, unlike lidocaine it does not affect the slope of spontaneous phase 4 depolarization.

After oral dosing, peak levels are obtained at 1 hour. The drug undergoes extensive and rapid metabolism. Elimination half-life is approximately 10 ± 3 hours with a range of 6.4–13.1 hours with normal renal function and as long as 47.5 hours in patients with renal insufficiency.[105]

Dose-related increases in PR, QRS, H–V intervals as well as hemiblocks, bundle brunch blocks, and sustained ventricular tachydysrhythmias can occur.[105]

Overdose with this drug has not been reported, and management would be similar to that with IB antidysrhythmics mentioned above.

Class IC Antidysrhythmics: Flecainide, Encainide, Propafenone

Flecainide. Flecainide, a fluorobenzamide, is a derivative of procainamide. It is used in treating both supraventricular and ventricular dysrhythmias, although it is approved only for ventricular dysrhythmias.[4] Sodium channel blockade is the major electrophysiologic action of this drug. Flecainide increases QRS, PR, and, to a lesser extent, QT_c intervals.[29,43,60,61,64,69,82,138,144] Flecainide depresses phase 0 of the action potential and slows conduction. It delays repolarization in canine ventricular muscle and prolongs intracardiac monophasic potentials.[114] It is used in the treatment of atrial fibrillation, atrial flutter, and dysrhythmias associated with Wolff-Parkinson-White syndrome.[4,49,50,65,122,134,149,150] Its therapeutic range is 0.2–1.0 μg/mL, with a half-life of 12–27 hours. Its peak plasma concentrations range from 1 to 6 hours after oral dosing. Seventy percent is metabolized hepatically to two major metabolites, one active and the other inactive, and 30% is excreted renally.[105] Ninety to ninety-five percent of the drug is bioavailable and 40% is protein bound. Alkalinization of the urine increases its elimination, and renal insufficiency and congestive heart failure decrease its clearance. In therapeutic dosages, the QRS, QT_c, and PR intervals may be prolonged, and left ventricular dysfunction, increasing CHF, and sudden death may occur.

One case report describes an acute overdose of an adult with flecainide, diazepam, imodium, and alcohol.[166] The patient developed polymorphous ventricular tachycardia and was treated with a variety of agents including dopamine, sodium bicarbonate and sodium chloride, physostigmine, and neostigmine as well as GI decontamination and activated charcoal. It is unclear whether these interventions were appropriate or successful. These authors and others suggest that a 50% increase in QRS duration, a 30% prolongation of the PR interval, or a 15% increase in the QT_c interval indicates flecainide toxicity.[108,115] The marked QRS and PR interval changes associated with minimal QT_c prolongation are noted with flecainide toxicity, in contrast to the toxic findings from the other antidysrhythmics, such as procainamide, tocainide, or quinidine.

Although a recent animal study concludes that the use of hypertonic sodium bicarbonate reverses flecainide-induced ventricular dysrhythmias, human studies have yet to be done.[78] Treatment of flecainide toxicity may include GI decontamination with activated charcoal and a cathartic. Hypertonic sodium bicarbonate has been used to decrease QRS, QT, and PR intervals.[78] The use of hemodialysis is not recommended due to flecanide's lipophilicity. Hemoperfusion may be of minimal efficacy but has not been studied in humans. The use of other class IC or IA antidysrhythmic agents is contraindicated in the treatment of flecainide toxicity due to their potential to exacerbate Na^+ channel blockade. Flecainide increases the threshold for electrical pacing of the ventricle,[61,144] which could decrease the efficacy of a pacemaker used to treat dysrhythmias due to flecainide toxicity.

Encainide. Encainide, a benzanilide compound analog of lysergic acid, with 5–10 times the antidysrhythmic potency of procainamide, was removed from the market in the United States in 1991 due to its prodysrhythmic effects and risk of sudden cardiac death.[26,27] Its electrophysiologic properties are similar to those of flecainide.[98] Absorption of encainide is rapid. Within 30 minutes to 4 hours it is metabolized in the liver to *O*-desmethylencainide (ODE and 3-methoxy–*O*-desmethylencainide (MODE), both active antidysrhythmics. Metabolism of encainide is under genetic control with populations of fast and slow metabolizers. In fast metabolizers (90% of the populace) the half-life of ODE is much longer than encainide. *O*-Desmethylencainide (ODE) is 5–50 times as potent as encainide. 3-Methoxy–*O*-desmethylencainide (MODE) is also active but its therapeutic and toxic effects are less clear.[36,42,59,98,101,128,129,133,164,165] The few overdoses reported with encainide involved its cardiotoxicity.[164] One case of an acute overdose of 3–3.5 g in an otherwise healthy person manifested marked QRS prolongation, hypotension, bradycardia, seizures, and coma. The seizures were treated with diazepam, and 100 mEq of hypertonic sodium bicarbonate was found to improve blood pressure and heart rate. More bicarbonate was administered with a brief improvement of the QRS interval.[118] In one case report a 6-month-old child developed a wide complex sinus tachycardia and then ventricular tachycardia with a single 25-mg tablet ingestion.[109] Fluids, sodium bicarbonate, phenytoin, and defibrillation were performed, resulting in normalization of the ECG within 72 hours.

The use of sodium bicarbonate may be of benefit in encainide overdoses.[54,118] The use of other class IA or IC antidysrhythmic agents is contraindicated. The use of hemoperfusion raises complex questions. In acute overdose, fast metabolizers may achieve high encainide levels and produce toxicity, whereas in chronic use encainide levels would be low and hemoperfusion would add little. The efficacy of removing the active metabolite is unclear. For slow metabolizers high encainide levels may allow hemoperfusion to be helpful, but this is not known.[118]

Propafenone. Propafenone has some structural resemblance to propranolol.[54,139,140] Propafenone blocks fast sodium channels and slows conduction through the AV node and the ventricular conduction system. It has quinidine-like activity, weak beta-adrenergic receptor antagonist activity,[87,88,103,104,110] and calcium channel blocking activity in vitro.[146,147] Propafenone depresses the rate of rise of phase 0 of the action potential by blocking the fast inward sodium channel.[81] It also depresses delayed afterdepolarizations in ischemic Purkinje fibers. In patients with ventricular tachycardia, prolongation of PR and H–V intervals and increase in effective refractory periods are reported.[112,124,125] Endocardial pacing thresholds are increased.[75] It is 95% absorbed after oral dosing and peaks in 2–3 hours; less than 1% of an oral dose is excreted unchanged in the urine.[66,75,147] The plasma half-life is 2–32 hours.[32] Bioavailability is low due to first-pass metabolism. Its principle metabolite, 5-OH-propafenone, may be more active than the parent compound. The activity of a second metabolite, *N*-depropylpropafenone, is not known.[146]

In one case report a 2-year-old child who ingested 1800 mg of propafenone developed a wide complex tachycardia, right bundle branch block, first-degree AV block, and prolongation of the QT interval as well as a generalized seizure.[77,103] Two hours after ingestion, the patient received 135 mg of phenytoin IV, and 0.5 hour later had an irregular bradycardia, widening of QRS and QT intervals, and a cardiopulmonary arrest. Atropine, sodium bicarbonate, and dopamine were administered, and within several hours the ECG normalized. In another case report[77] a 28-year-old man ingested 8.1 g of propafenone in a suicide attempt. The patient had seizures, widened QRS complex, bradycradia, and hypotension. The patient required sodium bicarbonate, glucagon, calcium, atropine, and vasopressors. The authors also report the use of an internal pacemaker and continuous epinephrine infusion. Of note is that 4 months after acute ingestion, the patient had a mild cardiomoypathy and a left bundle branch block, perhaps a result of the overdose. Hemodialysis has been used in a propafenone overdose but studies need to be done to determine its benefit.[22]

Class III Antidysrhythmics: Amiodarone, Bretylium

Amiodarone

Amiodarone is a benzofuran derivative that is iodinated and structurally similar to thyroxine. Nearly 40% of the molecular weight of the drug is iodine.[95] It has weak alpha- and beta-adrenergic receptor antagonist activity. As a class III agent it prolongs repolarization of myocardial tissue.[148] It also prolongs depolarization, thus adding to its antidysrhythmic action.[68,131] Due to its substantial pulmonary, hepatic, corneal, and cutaneous toxicity, it is used only in the treatment of life-threatening ventricular dysrhythmias resistant to less toxic drugs.

Common effects of therapeutic doses are prolongation of the PR and QT_c intervals and abnormal T and U waves. Oral absorption is variable, and the bioavailability is low (28–50%) due to incomplete absorption.[67] First-pass metabolism is low. The parent compound and its metabolite desethylamiodarone[46,56] have large volumes of distribution (10–70 L/kg). Their major route of elimination is by hepatic excretion into the bile where it is concentrated up to 50 times that of the serum.[5] The half-life may be up to 2 months. When used with other antidysrhythmic agents, such as digoxin, quinidine, procainamide, phenytoin, and flecainide, serum levels of these drugs are dramatically increased. Hemodynamic interactions with beta-adrenergic receptor antagonists and calcium channel blockers are also reported.[99]

Ventricular dysrhythmias and sinus bradycardia are the most serious complications of therapeutic doses of amiodarone.[102,143] Monomorphic and polymorphic ventricular tachycardia resistant to cardioversion and pharmacologic interventions are reported.[18,86,97,102,168]

Treatment of amiodarone overdose is limited. Torsades de pointes induced by amiodarone has been treated with isoproterenol and overdrive pacing.[143] Monomorphic ventricular tachycardia has been treated with class IB antidysrhythmics or propranolol.[168] Hemodialysis would not be beneficial since amiodarone is highly protein bound. Hemoperfusion and multiple-dose activated charcoal may be of help if used early in the course, but these approaches have not been studied in human trials.[117]

Bretylium

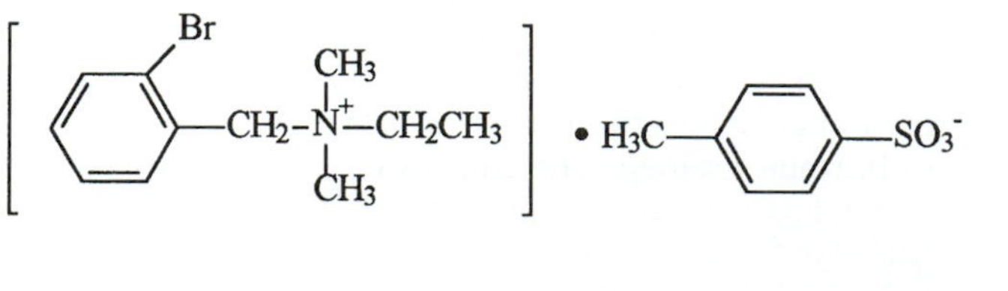

Bretylium tosylate is frequently used to treat resistant ventricular dysrhythmias, including those that occur post-MI. It is a quaternary benzylammonium compound that is concentrated in adrenergic neurons, where it initially releases and later inhibits the release of norepinephrine by adrenergic nerve endings.[129]

It prolongs action potentials in normal Purkinje cells and reduces heterogeneity of repolarization times, and therefore suppresses reentry. It blocks K^+ channels and has no effect on Na^+ channels, and no direct effect on automaticity. Bretylium is excreted unchanged by the kidneys without significant hepatic metabolism. Transient hypertension may be noted initially and hypotension later with administration of bretylium.

A case report of an unintentional 2-g IV bolus of bretylium being administered for treatment of recurrent ventricular tachycardia and fibrillation is reported.[17] This dose of 30 mg/kg of bretylium was 3 times the intended dose. Prior to the administration of the bretylium, the patient had a cardiac arrest and was treated with epinephrine, atropine, sodium bicarbonate, calcium chloride, and lidocaine. Approximately 25 minutes after the massive bretylium bolus, the patient's blood pressure was 310/90 mm Hg and then dropped to 90/40 mm Hg over the next 90 minutes. Despite vasopressors, fluids, and colloids, the patient developed renal failure and cardiac arrest and died within 3 hours. Theoretically, since the hypotension seen with bretylium is due to inhibition of norepinephrine reuptake and not myocardial depression, fluids should be adequate to raise blood pressure in hypotensive patients. Use of vasopressors such as dopamine should be avoided because they may cause hypertension.

Unclassified: Adenosine

Adenosine, a biologic compound, is a nucleoside found in all cells. It is released from myocardial cells under physiologic and pathophysiologic conditions.[16,38,105,111,126] It is used as a rapid IV bolus for terminating reentrant supraventricular tachycardia. The effects of adenosine are mediated by its interaction with specific G protein-coupled adenosine receptors. It activates acetylcholine-sensitive K^+ current in the atrium, sinus nodes, and AV nodes, producing a shortenting of action potential duration, causing hyperpolarization and slowing of normal automaticity; it reduces the Ca^{2+} currents and is antidysrhythmic by increasing AV nodal refractoriness and by inhibiting delayed afterdepolarizations (DADs) elicited by sympathetic stimulation.[90,127]

Adenosine has a half-life of seconds. It is metabolized by extracellular deaminases as well as intracellularly to inosine. Overdoses have not been reported but its adverse effects, include asystole, bronchospasm, hypotension, and atrial fibrillation,[38,111] can be potentiated in patients receiving dipyridamole (adenosine uptake inhibitor) and in cardiac transplant recipients (denervation hypersensitivity). With adenosine receptor blockade produced by methylxanthines (see Chap. 38), larger than usual doses are required to produce an antidysrhythmic effect.

In summary, understanding the electrophysiologic properties of the various antidysrhythmics enables the clinician to effectively treat and manage complex toxicologic emergencies created by intentional and unintentional overdoses.

Acknowledgments

Mary Ann Howland, PharmD and Harold Osborn, MD contributed to this chapter in a previous edition.

References

1. Accornero F, Pellanda A, Ruffini C, et al: Prolonged cardiopulmonary resuscitation during acute disopyramide poisoning. Vet Hum Toxicol 1993;35:231–232.
2. Akiyama T, Pawitan Y, Greenberg H, et al: Increased risk of death and cardiac arrest from encainide and flecainide in patients after non-Q-wave acute myocardial infarction in the Cardiac Arrhythmia Suppression Trial. Am J Cardiol 1991;68:1551–1555.
3. Amitai Y: Lidocaine. Clin Toxicol Rev 1985;8:1–2.
4. Anderson JL, Stewart JR, Perry BA, et al: Oral flecainide acetate for the treatment of ventricular arrhythmias. N Engl J Med 1981;305:473–477.
5. Andreasen F, Agerbaek H, Bjerrgaard P, Gotzsche H: Pharmacokinetics of amiodarone after intravenous and oral administration. Am J Clin Pharm 1981;19:293–299.
6. Arimori K, Deshimaru M, Furukawa E, Nakano M: Adsorption of mexiletine on to activated charcoal in macrogel-electrolyte solution. Chem Pharm Bull (Tokyo) 1993; 41:766–782.
7. Atkinson AJ, Krumlovsky FA, Huang CM, et al: Hemodialysis for severe procainamide toxicity: Clinical and pharmacokinetic observations. Clin Pharmacol Ther 1976; 20:585–592.
8. Badui E, Garcia-Rubi D, Estand B: Inadvertent massive lidocaine overdose causing temporary complete heart block in myocardial infarction. Am Heart J 1981;102:801–803.
9. Bailey DN: Percutaneous absorption of lidocaine hydrochloride in vivo. J Toxicol Cut Ocular Toxicol 1987;6: 233–236.
10. Barnfield C, Kemmenoe AV: A sudden death due to tocainide overdose. Hum Toxicol 1986;5:337–340.
11. Bennett PB, Woolsey RL, Hondeghem LM: Competition between lidocaine and one of its metabolites, glycylxylidide, for cardiac sodium channels. Circulation 1988;78: 692–700.
12. Benowitz NL, Forsyth RP, Melmon KL, Rowland M: Lidocaine disposition kinetics in monkey and man. 1. Prediction by a perfusion model. Clin Pharmacol Ther 1974;16: 87–98.
13. Benowitz NL: Quinidine, procainamide and disopyramide. In: Haddad LM, Winchester JF, eds: Clinical Management of Poisoning and Drug Overdose, 2nd ed. Philadelphia, Saunders, 1990, pp. 1360–1371.
14. Benowitz NL: Lidocaine, mexiletine and tocainide. In: Haddad LM, Winchester JF, eds: Clinical Management of Poisoning and Drug Overdose, 2nd ed. Philadelphia, Saunders, 1990, pp. 1371–1379.
15. Blumer J, Strong JM, Atkinson AJ Jr: The convulsant potency of lidocaine and its *N*-dealkylated metabolites. J Pharmacol Exp Ther 1973;186:31–36.
16. Biaggioni I, Killian TJ, Mosqueda Garcia R, Robertson RM: Adenosine increases sympathetic nerve traffic in humans. Circulation 1991;83:1668–1675.
17. Bodner T, Nowak R, Tomlanovich MC: Massive intravenous bolus bretylium tosylate. Ann Emerg Med 1980; 9:630–633.
18. Bonati M, D'Arranno V, Galletti F: Acute overdose of amiodarone in a suicide attempt. J Toxicol Clin Toxicol 1983;20:181–186.
19. Boster SR, Danzl DF: Translaryngeal absorption of lidocaine. Ann Emerg Med 1982;11:461–465.
20. Boyes RN, Scott DB, Jebson PJ, et al: Pharmacokinetics of lidocaine in man. Clin Pharmacol Ther 1971;12:105–116.
21. Braden G, Fitzgibbons JP, Germain MJ, et al: Hemoperfusion for treatment of *N*-acetylprocainamide intoxication. Ann Intern Med 1986;105:64–65.
22. Burgess ED, Duff HJ: Brief reports: Hemodialysis removal of propafenone. Pharmacotherapy 1989;9:331–333.
23. Campbell NPS, Zaidi SA, Adgey AAJ, et al: Observations on hemodynamic effects of mexiletine. Br Heart J 1979; 41:182.
24. Campbell RW: Mexiletine. N Engl J Med 1987;316:29–34.
25. Campbell TJ: Subclassification of class 1 antiarrhythmic drugs. In: Vaughan Williams EM, ed: Handbook of Experimental Pharmacology. Antiarrhythmic Drugs. Heidelberg, Springer Verlag, 1989, pp. 135–156.
26. The CAST Investigators: Preliminary report: effect of encainide and flecainide on mortality in a randomized trial of arrhythmia suppression after myocardial infarction. N Engl J Med 1989;321:406–412.
27. The CAST Investigators: The cardiac arrhythmia suppression trial: First CAST . . . then CAST 2. J Am Coll Cardiol 1992;19:894–898.
28. Chouty F, Funck-Bretano C, Leenhardt A, et al: Intravenous sodium lactate as a treatment of class I antiarrhythmic agents overdose (ABST). Circulation 1989;80 (suppl II): 114–120.
29. Chung PKC, Tuso P: The electrocardiographic changes in a case of flecainide overdose. Conn Med 1990;54:183–185.
30. Clark CWF, El-Mahdi EO: Fatal oral tocainide overdosage. Br Med J 1984;288:760.
31. Cocco G, Strozzi C, Chu D, Pansini R: Torsade de pointes as a manifestation of mexiletine toxicity. Am Heart J 1980; 100:878–880.
32. Connolly SJ, Kates RE, Lebsack CS, et al: Clinical pharmacology of propafenone. Circulation 1983;68:589–596.
33. Cusson J, Rattel S, Matthew C, et al: Age dependent lidocaine disposition in patients with acute myocardial infarction. Clin Pharmacol Ther 1985;37:381–386.
34. Dangman KH, Hoffman BF: In vivo and in vitro antiarrhythmic and arrhythmogenic effects of *N*-acetylprocainamide. J Pharmacol Exp Ther 1981;217:851–862.
35. Davison R, Parker M, Atkinson AJ Jr: Excessive serum lidocaine levels during maintenance infusions: Mechanisms and prevention. Am Heart J 1982;104:203–207.

36. Dawson AK, Roden DM, Duff HJ, et al: Differential effects of *O*-demethyl encainide on induced and spontaneous arrhythmias in the conscious dog. Am J Cardiol 1984;54: 654–658.
37. Denaro CP, Benowitz NL: Poisoning due to class 1b antiarrhythmic drugs: Lignocaine, mexiletine and tocainide. Med Toxicol Adverse Drug Exp 1989;4:412–428.
38. DiMarco JP, Sellers TD, Lerman BB, et al: Diagnostic and therapeutic use of adenosine in patients with supraventricular tachyarrhythmias. J Am Coll Cardiol 1985;6: 417–425.
39. Domoto D, Brown WW, Briggensmith P: Removal of toxic levels of *N*-acetylprocainamide with continuous arteriovenous hemofiltration or continuous arteriovenous hemodiafiltration. Ann Intern Med 1987;50–552.
40. Dorian P, Fain ES, Davy JM, Winkle RA: Lidocaine causes a reversible, concentration-dependent increase in defibrillation energy requirements. J Am Coll Cardiol 1986;8: 327–332.
41. Drayer DE, Lowenthal DT, Woosley RL, et al: Cumulation of *N*-acetylprocainamide, a metabolite of procainamide, in patients with impaired renal function. Clin Pharmacol Ther 1977;22:63–69.
42. Duff HJ, Dawson AK, Roden DM, et al: Electrophysiologic actions of *O*-demethyl encainide: An active metabolite. Circulation 1983;68:385–391.
43. Echt DS, Liebson PR, Mitchell LB, et al: Mortality and morbidity in patients receiving encainide, flecainide, or placebo: The Cardiac Arrhythmia Suppression Trial. N Engl J Med 1991;324:781–788.
44. Edgren B, Tilelli J, Gehrz R: Intravenous lidocaine overdosage in a child. J Toxicol Clin Toxicol 1986;24:51–58.
45. Engler RL, Le Winter M: Tocainide-induced ventricular fibrillation. Am Heart J 1981;101:494–496.
46. Falik R, Flores BT, Shaw L, et al: Relationship of steady-state serum concentrations of amiodarone and desethylamiodarone to therapeutic efficacy and adverse effects. Am J Med 1987;82:1102–1108.
47. Feld GK, Chen PS, Nocod P, et al: Possible atrial proarrhythmic effects of class 1C antiarrhythmic drugs. Am J Cardiol 1990;66:378–383.
48. Finkelstein F, Kreeft J: Massive lidocaine poisoning. N Engl J Med 1979;301:50.
49. Flecainide-Quinidine Research Group: Flecainide versus quinidine for treatment of chronic ventricular arrhythmias, a multicenter clinical trial. Circulation 1983;67:1117–1123.
50. Flecainide Ventricular Tachycardia Study Group: Treatment of resistant ventricular tachycardia with flecainide acetate. Am J Cardiol 1986;57:1299–1304.
51. Frank SE, Snyder JT: Survival following severe overdose with mexiletine, nifedipine and nitroglycerine. Am J Emerg Med 1991;9:43–46.
52. Freedman MD, Gal J, Freed CR: Extracorporeal pump assistance: Novel treatment or acute lidocaine poisoning. Eur J Clin Pharmacol 1982;22:129–135.
53. Funk-Brentano C, Kroemer HK, Lee JT: Drug therapy: Propafenone. N Engl J Med 1990;322:518–525.
54. Gardner ML, Brett-Smith H, Batsford WP: Treatment of encainide proarrhythmia with hypertonic saline. Pacing Clin Electrophysiol 1990;13:1232–1235.
55. Graffner C, Conradson TB, Hofvendahl S, et al: Tocainide kinetics after intravenous and oral administration in healthy subjects and inpatients with acute myocardial infarction. Clin Pharmacol Ther 1980;27:64–71.
56. Greenberg ML, Lerman BB, Shipe JR, et al: Relationship between amiodarone and desethylamiodarone plasma concentrations and electrophysiologic effects, efficacy and toxicity. J Am Coll Cardiol 1987;9:1148–1155.
57. Greenblatt DJ, Bolognini V, Koch-Weser J, et al: Pharmacokinetic approach to the clinical use of lidocaine intravenously. JAMA 1976;236:273–277.
58. Halkin H, Meffin P, Melmom KL, et al: Influence of congestive heart failure on blood levels of lidocaine and its active monoethylated metabolite. Clin Pharmacol Ther 1975;17:669–676.
59. Harrison DC, Kates RE, Quart BD: Relation of blood level and metabolites to the antiarrhythmic effectiveness of encainide. Am J Cardiol 1986;58:66C–73C.
60. Hellestrand KJ, Bexton RS, Nathan AW, et al: Acute electrophysiologic effects of flecainide acetate on cardiac conduction and refractoriness in man. Br Heart J 1982;48: 140–148.
61. Hellestrand KJ, Nathan AW, Bexton RS, Camm AJ: Electrophysiologic effects of flecainide acetate on sinus node function, anomalous atrioventricular connections, and pacemaker thresholds. Am J Cardiol 1984;53:30B–38B.
62. Hess GP, Walson PD: Seizures secondary to oral viscous lidocaine. Ann Emerg Med 1988;17:725–727.
63. Hine LK, Laird N, Hewitt P, Chalmers TC: Meta-analytic evidence against prophylactic use of lidocaine in acute myocardial infarction. Arch Intern Med 1989;149: 2694–2698.
64. Hodess AB, Follansbee WP, Spear JF, et al: Electrophysiologic effects of a new antiarrhythmic agent, flecainide, in the intact canine heart. J Cardiovasc Pharmacol 1979; 1:427–439.
65. Hodges M, Haugland JM, Granrud G, et al: Suppression of ventricular ectopic depolarization by flecainide acetate, a new antiarrhythmic agent. Circulation 1982; 65:879–885.
66. Hollmann M, Brode E, Holtz D, et al: Investigations on the pharmacokinetics of propafenone in man. Arzneimittel-Forschung 1983;33:763.
67. Holt DW, Tucker GT, Jackson PR, et al: Amiodarone pharmacokinetics. Am Heart J 1985;106:840–846.
68. Hondeghen LM, Mason JW, Katzung BG: Block of inactivated sodium channels and of depolarization-induced automaticity in guinea pig papillary muscle by amiodarone. Circ Res 1984;55:277–285.
69. Ikeda N, Singh BN, Davis LD, Hauswirth O: Effect of flecainide on the electrophysiologic properties of isolated canine and rabbit myocardial fibers. J Am Coll Cardiol 1985;5:303–310.
70. Jackman WM, Friday KJ, Anderson JL, et al: The long QT syndromes: A critical review, new clinical observations and a unifying hypothesis. Prog Cardiovasc Dis 1988;31: 115–172.
71. Jackson JE, Bentley JB, Glass SJ, et al: Effects of histamine-2 receptor blockade on lidocaine kinetics. Clin Pharmacol Ther 1985;37:544–548.

72. Jenzer HJ, Hagemeijer F: Quinidine syncope: Torsades de pointes with low quinidine plasma concentrations. Eur J Cardiol 1976;4:447–451.
73. Jequier P, Jones R, Mackintosh A: Fatal mexiletine overdose. Lancet 1976;1:429. Letter.
74. Kar PM, Kellner K, Ing T, et al: Combined high efficiency hemodialysis and charcoal hemoperfusion in severe *N*-acetylprocainamide intoxication. Am J Kidney Dis 1992;4:403–406.
75. Karagueuzian HA, Katoh T, McCullen A, et al: Electrophysiologic and hemodynamic effects of propafenone, a new antiarrhythmic agent on the anesthetized, closed-chest dog. Comparative study with lidocaine. Am Heart J 1984;107:418.
76. Kempden PM: Lethal/toxic injection of 20% lidocaine: A well known complication of an unnecessary preparation? Anesthesiology 1986:65;564–565.
77. Kerns W, English B, Ford M: Propafenone overdose. Ann Emerg Med 1994;24:98–103.
78. Keyler DE, Pentel PR: Hypertonic sodium bicarbonate partially reverses QRS prolongation due to flecainide in rats. Life Sci 1989;45:101–107.
79. Kim SY, Benowitz, NL: Poisoning due to class Ia antiarrhythmic drugs, quinidine, procainamide and disopyramide. Drug Safety 1990;5:393–420.
80. Kim WY, Pomerance JJ, Miller AA: Lidocaine intoxication in a newborn following local anesthesia for episiotomy. Pediatrics 1979;64:643–645.
81. Kohlhardt M: Basic electrophysiologic actions of propafenone in heart muscle. In: Schlepper M, Olsson B, eds: Cardiac Arrhythmias: Proceedings of the First International Rhythmonorm Congress. New York, Springer-Verlag, 1983, p. 91.
82. Kroemer HK, Turgeon J, Parker RA, Roden DM: Flecainide enantiomers: Disposition in human subjects and electrophysiologic actions in vitro. Clin Pharmacol Ther 1989;46:584–590.
83. Kuhn P, Klicpera M, Kroiss A, et al: Antiarrhythmic and hemodynamic effects of mexiletine. Postgrad Med J 1977; 53:81.
84. Kutalek SP, Morganroth J, Horowitz LN: Tocainide: A new oral antiarrhythmic agent. Ann Intern Med 1985;103: 387–391.
85. Lalka D, Meyer MB, Duce BR, et al: Kinetics of the oral antiarrhythmic lidocaine congener, tocainide. Clin Pharmacol Ther 1976;19:757–766.
86. Lazzara R: Amiodarone and torsade de pointes. Ann Intern Med 1989;549–551.
87. Lee JT, Kroemer HK, Silberstein DJ, et al: The role of genetically determined polymorphic drug metabolism in the beta-blockade produced by propafenone. N Engl J Med 1990;322:1764–1768.
88. Lee JT, Lineberry MD, Funck-Brentano C, et al: Propafenone-induced β-blockade in extensive and poor metabolizer subjects. Circulation 1988;78(suppl II):499.
89. Le Lorier J, Grenon D, Latour Y, et al: Pharmacokinetics of lidocaine after prolonged intravenous infusions in uncomplicated myocardial infarction. Ann Intern Med 1977; 87:700–702.
90. Lerman BB, Belardinelli L: Cardiac electrophysiology of adenosine; basic and clinical concepts. Circulation 1991; 83:1499–1509.
91. Levy S, Azoulay S: Stories about the origin of quinine and quinidine. J Cardiovasc Electrophysiol 1994;5:635–636.
92. Lie KI, Wellens HJ, van Capelle FJ, Durrer D: Lidocaine in the prevention of primary ventricular fibrillation: A double-blind, randomized study of 212 consecutive patients. N Engl J Med 1974;29:1324–1326.
93. Lima JJ, Boudoulas H, Blanford M: Concentration-dependence of disopyramide binding to plasma protein and its influence on kinetics and dynamics. J Pharmacol Exp Ther 1981;219:741–747.
94. Makkar RR, Fromm BS, Steinman RT, et al: Female gender as a risk factor for torsades de pointes associated with cardiovascular drugs. JAMA 1993;270:2590–2597.
95. Marcus F, Fontaine GH, Frank R, et al: Clinical pharmacology and therapeutic applications of the antiarrhythmic agent, amiodarone. Am Heart J 1981;101:480–493.
96. Marcus FI: The hazards of using type IC antiarrhythmic drugs for the treatment of paroxysmal atrial fibrillation. Am J Cardiol 1990;66:366–367.
97. Mattioni TA, Zheutlin TA, Sarmiento JJ, et al: Amiodarone in patients with previous drug-mediated torsade de pointes. Ann Intern Med 1989;549–551.
98. Mason JW: Basic and clinical cardiac electrophysiology of encainide. Am J Cardiol 1986;58:18C–24C.
99. Mason JW: Amiodarone. N Engl J Med 1987;316:455–466.
100. Mason JW, Hondeghen LM, Katzung BG: Amiodarone blocks inactivated cardiac sodium channels. Pflugers Arch 1983;396:79–81.
101. Mason JW, Peters FA: Antiarrhythmic efficacy of encainide in patients with refractory recurrent ventricular tachycardia. Circulation 1981;63:670.
102. McGovern B. Garan H, Kelly E, Ruskin J: Adverse reactions during treatment with amiodarone hydrochloride. Br Med J 1983;287:175–180.
103. McHugh TP, Perina DG: Propafenone ingestion. Ann Emerg Med 1987;16:437–440.
104. McLeod AA, Stiles GL, Spand DG: Demonstration of beta adrenoreceptor blockade by propafenone hydrochloride. Clinical, pharmacologic, radioligand binding and adenyl cyclase activation studies. J Pharmacol Exp Ther 1983; 228:461–466.
105. Michelson EL, Dreifus LS: New antiarrhythmics. Med Clin North Am 1988;72:275–319.
106. Mofenson HC, Caraccio TR, Miller H, et al: Lidocaine toxicity from topical mucosal application. Clin Pediatr 1983; 22:190–192.
107. Morady F, Scheinman MM, Desai J: Disopyramide. Ann Intern Med 1982;96:337–343.
108. Morganroth J, Horowitz LN: Flecainide: Its proarrhythmic effect and expected changes on the surface electrocardiogram. J Am Coll Cardiol 1984;53:89B–94B.
109. Mortenson M, Bolon C, Kelley M, et al: Encainide overdose in an infant. Ann Emerg Med 1992;21:998–1001.
110. Muller-Peltzer H, Greger G, Neugebauer G, et al: Beta-blocking and electrophysiological effects of propafenone in volunteers. Eur J Clin Pharmacol 1983;25: 831–833.
111. Munoz A, Leenhardt A, Sassine A, et al: Therapeutic use

of adenosine for terminating spontaneous paroxysmal supraventricular tachycardia. Eur Heart J 1984;5:735.

112. Nathan AW, Bexton RS, Hellestrand KJ, et al: Fatal ventricular tachycardia in association with propafenone, a new class Ic antiarrhythmic agent. Postgrad Med J 1984; 60:155–156.
113. Nelson L, Hoffman R: Mexiletine overdose producing status epilepticus without cardiovascular abnormalities. J Toxicol Clin Toxicol 1994;32:731–736.
114. Noble J, Kennedy DJ, Lattimer RD, et al: Massive lignocaine overdose during cardiopulmonary bypass, successful treatment with cardiac pacing. Br J Anesthesia 1984; 56:1439–1441.
115. Olsson SB, Edvardsson N: Clinical electrophysiologic study of antiarrhythmic properties of flecainide: Acute intraventricular delayed conduction and prolonged repolarization with programmed stimulation. Am Heart J 1981; 102:864–871.
116. Peat MA, Deyman ME, Crouch DJ, et al: Concentrations of lidocaine and monoethylglycylxylidide (MEGX) in lidocaine-associated deaths. J Forensic Sci 1985;30:1048–1057.
117. Pentel PR, Dunbar DN: New Cardiac Antiarrhythmic Agents. In: Haddad LM, Winchester JF, Clinical Management of Poisoning and Drug Overdose, 2nd ed. Philadelphia, Saunders, 1990, pp. 1380–1392.
118. Pentel PR, Goldsmith SR, Salerno DM, et al: Effects of hypertonic sodium bicarbonate on encainide overdose. Am J Cardiol 1986;57:878–880.
119. Pfeifer HJ, Greenblatt DJ, Koch-Weser J: Clinical use and toxicity of intravenous lidocaine. A report from the Boston Collaborative Drug Surveillance Program. Am Heart J 1976;92:168–173.
120. Podrid PJ, Schoeneberger A, Lown B: Congestive heart failure caused by oral disopyramide. N Engl J Med 1980;302:614–618.
121. Polkis A, Mackell MA, Tucker EF: Tissue distribution of lidocaine after fatal accidental injection. J Forensic Sci 1984;29:1129–1236.
122. Pottage A: Clinical profile of newer class I antiarrhythmic agents: Tocainide, mexiletine, encainide, flecainide and lorcainide. Am J Cardiol 1983;52:240–244.
123. Prescott LF, Adjepon-Yamoah KK, Talbot RG: Impaired lidocaine metabolism in patients with myocardial infarction and cardiac failure. Br Med J 1976;1:939–941.
124. Prystowsky EN, Heger JJ, Chilson DA, et al: Antiarrhythmic and electrophysiologic effects of oral propafenone. Am J Cardiol 1984;54:26D.
125. Prystowsky EN, Heger JJ, Lloyd EA, et al: Clinical electrophysiology of ventricular tachycardia. Cardiol Clin 1983; 1:253.
126. Puech P, Munoz A, Sassine A, Brugada J: Use of adenosine as an antiarrhythmic agent. In: Vaughan Williams EM, ed: Handbook of Experimental Pharmacology. Antiarrhythmic Drugs. Heidelberg, Springer Verlag, 1989, pp. 453–460.
127. Roden DM: Antiarrhythmic drugs. In: Hardman JG, Limbird LE, Molinoff PB, Ruddon RW, eds. Goodman and Gilman's The Pharmacological Basis of Therapeutics, 9th ed. New York, McGraw-Hill, 1996, pp. 839–874.
128. Roden DM: Risks and benefits of antiarrhythmic drug therapy. N Engl J Med 1994;331:785–791.
129. Roden DM: Current status of class III antiarrhythmic drug therapy. Am J Cardiol 1993;72:44B–49B.
130. Roden DM: The long QT syndrome and torsades de pointes: Basic and clinical aspects. In: El-Cherif N, Samet P, eds: Cardiac Pacing and Electrophysiology, 3rd ed. Philadelphia, Saunders, 1991, pp. 265–284.
131. Roden DM, Echt DS, Lee JT, Murray KT: Clinical pharmacology of antiarrhythmic agents. In: Josephson ME, ed: Sudden Cardiac Death. Boston Blackwell Scientific, 1993, pp. 182–185.
132. Roden DM, Hoffman BF: Action potential prolongation and induction of abnormal automaticity by low quinidine concentrations in canine Purkinje fibers. Relationship to potassium and cycle length. Circ Res 1985;56:857–867.
133. Roden DM, Wood AJJ, Wilkinson GR, et al: Disposition kinetics of encainide and metabolites. Am J Cardiol 1986; 58:4C–9C.
134. Roden DM, Woosley RL: Flecainide. N Engl J Med 1986; 315:36–41.
135. Roden DM, Woolsey RL: Tocainide. N Engl J Med 1986; 315:41–45.
136. Roden DM, Woosley RL, Primm RK: Incidence and clinical features of the quinidine-associated long QT syndrome: Implications for patient care. Am Heart J 1986; 111:1088–1093.
137. Rothstein P, Dornbusch J, Shaywitz B: Prolonged seizures associated with the use of viscous lidocaine. J Pediatr 1982;101:461–463.
138. Salerno DM, Granrud G, Sharkey P, et al: Pharmacodynamics and side effects of flecainide acetate. Clin Pharmacol Ther 1986;40:101–107.
139. Salerno DM, Granrud G, Sharkey P, et al: A controlled trial of propafenone for treatment of frequent and repetitive ventricular premature complexes. Am J Cardiol 1984; 53:77–83.
140. Salerno DM, Hodges M: New therapy focus: Propafenone. Cardiovasc Rev Rep 1985;6:924–931.
141. Sawyer DR, Ludden TM, Crawford MH: Lidocaine infusions with cardiac arrhythmias: Unpredictability of plasma concentrations. Arch Intern Med 1981;141:43–45.
142. Schnittger I, Griffith JC, Hill RJ, et al: Effects of tocainide on ventricular fibrillation threshold: Comparison with lidocaine. Am J Cardiol 1978;42:76–81.
143. Sclarovsky S, Lewin RF, Kracoff O, et al: Amiodarone-induced polymorphous ventricular tachycardia. Am Heart J 1983;105:6–12.
144. Sellers TD, DiMarco JP: Sinusoidal ventricular tachycardia associated with flecainide acetate. Chest 1984;85:647–649.
145. Shub G, Gan GT: Management of acute quinidine intoxication. Chest 1978;73:173–178.
146. Siddoway LA, Roden DM, Woosley RE: Clinical pharmacology of propafenone: Pharmacokinetics, metabolism and concentration-response relations. Am J Cardiol 1984; 54:9D–12D.
147. Siddoway LA, Thompson KA, McAllister CB, et al: Polymorphism of propafenone metabolism and disposition in man: Clinical and pharmacokinetic consequences. Circulation 1987;75:785–791.
148. Singh BN, Williams EMV: The effects of amiodarone, a new anti-anginal drug, on cardiac muscle. Br J Pharmacol 1970;39:657–667.

149. Somani P: Antiarrhythmic effects of flecainide. Clin Pharmacol Ther 1980;27:464–470.
150. Soon S, Lal R, Ruffy R: Treatment of paroxysmal reentrant supraventricular tachycardia with flecainide acetate. Am J Cardiol 1986;58:80–85.
151. Strong JM, Mayfield DE, Atkinson AJ Jr, et al: Pharmacological activity, metabolism and pharmacokinetics of glycinexylidide. Clin Pharmacol Ther 1975;17:184–194.
152. Svendsen TL, Tango M, Waldorff S, et al: Effects of propranolol and pindolol on plasma lignocaine clearance in man. Br J Clin Pharmacol 1982;13:223S–226S.
153. Swiryn S, Kim SS: Quinidine induced syncope. Arch Intern Med 1983;143:314–316.
154. Thomson PD, Rowland M, Melmon KL: The influence of heart failure, liver disease, and renal failure on the disposition of lidocaine in man. Am Heart J 1971;82:417–421.
155. Tzivoni D, Banai S, Schuger C, et al: Treatment of torsades de pointes with magnesium sulfate. Circulation 1988;77:392–397.
156. Vaughan Williams EM: Classifying antiarrhythmic actions: By facts or speculation. J Clin Pharmacol 1992;32:964–977.
157. Vaughan Williams EM: Classification of the antiarrhythmic action of moricizine. J Clin Pharmacol 1991;31:216–221.
158. Vaughan Williams EM: Significance of classifying antiarrhythmic actions since the Cardiac Arrythmia Suppression Trial. J Clin Pharmacol 1991;31:123–135.
159. Vaughan Williams EM: Classification of antidysrhythmic drugs. Pharmacol Ther B 1975;1:115.
160. Wasserman F, Brodsky L, Dick MM, et al: Successful treatment of quinidine and procainamide intoxication. N Engl J Med 1958;259:797–802.
161. Webb CR, Morganroth J, Senior S, et al: Flecainide: Steady state electrophysiologic effects in patients with remote myocardial infarction and inducible sustained ventricular arrhythmia. J Am Coll Cardiol 1986;8:214–220.
162. Wetherbee DG, Holzman D, Brown MG: Ventricular tachycardia following the administration of quinidine. Am Heart J 1951;42:89–96.
163. Wieger U, Hanrath P, Kuck KH: Pharmacokinetics of tocainide in patients with renal dysfunction and during hemodialysis. Eur J Clin Pharmacol 1983;24:503–507.
164. Winkle RA, Peters F, Kates RE, et al: Possible contribution of encainide metabolites to the long term antiarrhythmic efficacy of encainide. Am J Cardiol 1983;51:1182–1188.
165. Winkle RA, Mason JW, Griffin JC, et al: Malignant ventricular tachyarrhythmias associated with the use of encainide. Am Heart J 1981;102:857–864.
166. Winkelmann BR, Leinberger H: Life-threatening flecainide toxicity: A pharmacodynamic approach. Ann Intern Med 1987;106:807–814.
167. Working Group on Arrhythmias of the European Society of Cardiology: The Sicilian Gambit. Circulation 1991;84:1831–1851.
168. Zipes DP, Prystowsky EN, Heger JJ: Amiodarone: electrophysiologic actions, pharmacokinetics and clinical effects. J Am Coll Cardiol 1984;3:1059–1071.

CHAPTER 53

Anesthetics and Neuromuscular Blocking Agents

Brian Kaufman, Kenneth M. Sutin, Staffan Wåhlander, and Sanford M. Miller

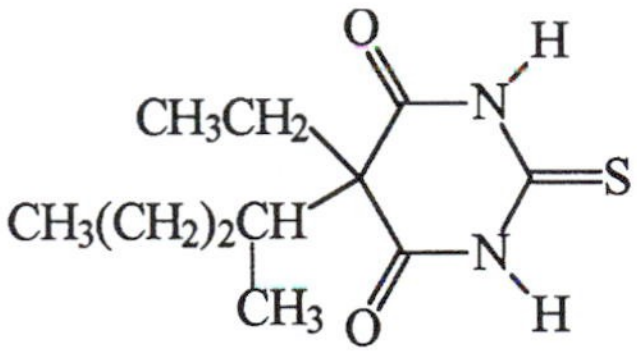

Thiopental

Inhalational Anesthetics

CASE 1. A 40-year-old dentist is found unresponsive in his procedure room by his office staff, who report that he had a mask on his face. The paramedics note that the mask is attached to a supply of nitrous oxide and oxygen. The oxygen tank is empty. Physical examination in the emergency department is normal except for his neurologic examination, which demonstrates that he is in coma and unresponsive to painful stimulation. A CT scan of the head is normal.

What Are the Acute Toxic Effects of Nitrous Oxide?

Nitrous oxide is the most commonly used inhalational anesthetic in the world. Its advantages include a mild odor, absence of airway irritation, rapid induction and emergence from anesthesia, potent analgesia, and minimal respiratory and circulatory effects.

When administered in a modern operating room using current standards of monitoring to prevent unintentional hypoxia, it is a remarkably safe agent. Unfortunately, nitrous oxide also has a potential for abuse, particularly among hospital and dental personnel.[197] Death and permanent brain damage are described; however, these do not result from direct toxic effects, but rather are secondary to asphyxia, either from inhalation of insufficient oxygen, or from use of high concentrations of the gas in a poorly ventilated room.[89] If a patient who has been exposed to nitrous oxide fails to regain consciousness within several minutes after breathing fresh air or oxygen, other etiologies for the altered mental status such as hypoxic encephalopathy or concomitant ingestion of a central nervous system (CNS) depressant drug should be suspected.

Deaths have occurred when patients receive commercially prepared nitrous oxide from tanks contaminated with impurities such as nitric oxide or nitrogen dioxide, and pulmonary toxicity was described when similar contaminants were produced by individual preparation of nitrous oxide by the combustion of ammonium nitrate fertilizer.[233]

Injury can also result from the physical properties of this agent. Nitrous oxide is 35 times more soluble in blood than nitrogen. When it is inhaled, any compliant air-containing space (eg, bowel) will increase in size, while noncompliant spaces will exhibit an increase in pressure (eg, the eustachian tubes). These effects occur because nitrous oxide diffuses along the concentration gradient from the blood into a closed space much more rapidly than nitrogen can be transferred in the opposite direction. Clinical consequences include rapid progression of a pneumothorax to tension pneumothorax, tympanic membrane rupture with hearing loss, bowel distension, and tracheal or laryngeal trauma due to increased endotracheal cuff pressure.

What Are the Toxic Effects of Nitrous Oxide on the Bone Marrow?

Bone marrow depression was first recognized as a complication of long-term nitrous oxide exposure in the 1950s, when the gas was used to sedate intubated patients with severe tetanus.[193] Leukopenia with hypoplastic bone marrow and megaloblastic erythropoiesis developed 3–5 days after initial exposure, followed by thrombocytopenia. Bone marrow recovery usually occurred within 4 days after the agent was discontinued. Healthy patients undergoing routine surgical procedures demonstrate mild megaloblastic bone marrow changes after 12 hours of exposure to 50% nitrous oxide and marked changes after 24 hours.[267] Critically ill patients may be more sensitive to the effects of nitrous oxide on the bone marrow, since megaloblastic changes are described after as little as 1 hour of exposure.[13]

The hematologic effects of exposure to nitrous oxide strongly resemble those characteristic of pernicious anemia. These similarities have a biochemical basis.[12,262] Vitamin B_{12} is a bound coenzyme of methionine synthase. The cobalt in the molecule functions as a methyl carrier in the cytoplasmic reaction in which a methyl group is transferred from 5-methyltetrahydrofolate to homocysteine to form methionine (Fig. 53–1). Nitrous oxide oxi-

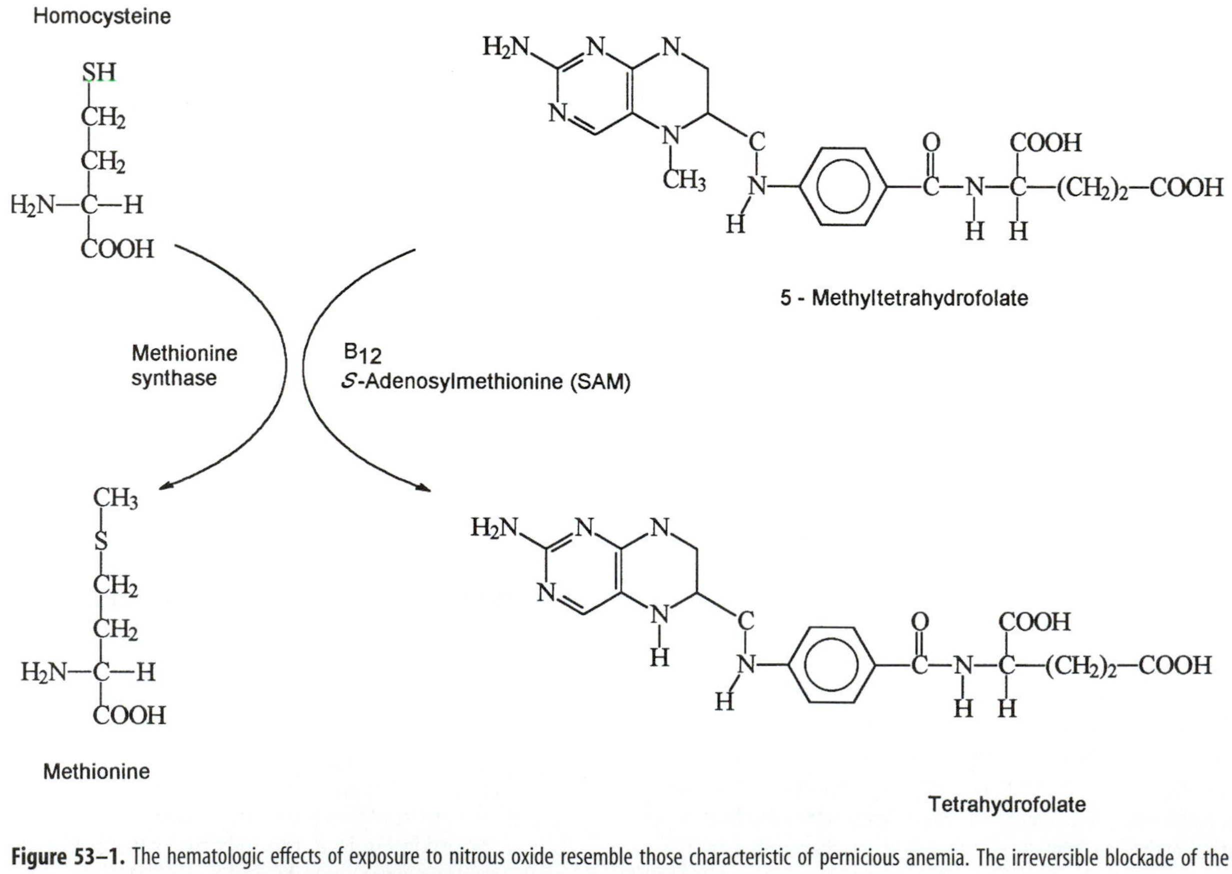

Figure 53–1. The hematologic effects of exposure to nitrous oxide resemble those characteristic of pernicious anemia. The irreversible blockade of the methionine synthase is consequential with regard to DNA synthesis and myelin production.

dizes the cobalt, converting vitamin B_{12} from the active monovalent form (cob(I)alamin) to an inactive bivalent form (cob(II)alamin). Methionine synthase activity thereby becomes irreversibly inhibited.[262] It appears that the sole biochemical effect of nitrous oxide is to block this transmethylation reaction. The metabolic consequences of this block are quite significant, since methionine and tetrahydrofolate are required for DNA synthesis and production of myelin. Interference with these reactions is responsible for the development of bone marrow depression and polyneuropathy resembling those seen in pernicious anemia.[262]

What Are the Toxic Effects of Nitrous Oxide on the Nervous System?

Disabling polyneuropathy in health care workers who habitually abused nitrous oxide was first described in 1978.[197] The neurologic disorder improved slowly when the patients abstained from further nitrous oxide abuse. As discussed, this neuropathy is clinically indistinguishable from subacute combined degeneration of the spinal cord, as associated with pernicious anemia. The syndrome of nitrous oxide neuropathy is characterized by sensorimotor polyneuropathy, often combined with signs of posterior and lateral spinal cord involvement.

Neurologic changes develop only after several months of frequent exposure to nitrous oxide. Those at risk include individuals who chronically abuse the gas and those who are occupationally exposed for prolonged periods to grossly contaminated environments.[22] This is a very unlikely scenario in the modern operating room, where inhalational anesthetics are scavenged, but it may occur in poorly ventilated dental offices, where personnel are exposed to greater than 1000 parts per million (ppm) of nitrous oxide. This problem is probably markedly underdiagnosed, since the neurologic changes seen in mild cases mimic other more common neurologic conditions.[51]

What Are the Effects of Chronic Exposure to Trace Levels of Nitrous Oxide?

Dentists and dental assistants are often exposed to greater concentrations of waste anesthetic gases than individuals working in well-vented operating rooms. Animal studies demonstrate that methionine synthase may be inactivated by exposure to greater than 1000 ppm of nitrous oxide, a level often exceeded in dental procedure rooms. An epidemiologic survey of dentists compared 15,000 who used and 15,000 who did not use nitrous oxide in their practices.[51] A 1.2–1.8-fold increase in liver, kidney, and neurologic disease was found in the dentists and their chair-side assistants who were chronically exposed to trace levels of nitrous oxide. For those with heavy office use of nitrous oxide, there was a fourfold increase in the incidence of neurologic complaints compared to the nonexposed group. Female dental assistants who were exposed to nitrous oxide also had a two- to threefold increase in spontaneous abortion rates, reduced fertility, and a higher rate of congenital abnormalities in their offspring.

How Can Nitrous Oxide Toxicity Be Reversed?

Removal of the affected person from the toxic environment should be the initial intervention. Individuals who have developed toxicity from abuse of the gas should be educated about the relationship between their recreational activities and their clinical findings.

Vitamin B_{12} may help patients with a masked vitamin B_{12} deficiency who develop megaloblastic anemia and neurologic dysfunction after brief exposure to nitrous oxide, but it is not beneficial in patients who have toxicity resulting from more chronic exposure.[308] The reason for the ineffectiveness of vitamin B_{12} in this situation is uncertain.

The bone marrow abnormalities associated with nitrous oxide toxicity may be reversed by the administration of folate. A single intravenous dose of folinic acid, 30 mg, has been effective.[263] A methionine-supplemented diet also greatly reduced the demyelination and neurologic damage induced in monkeys by chronic exposure to 15% nitrous oxide.[312]

CASE 2. A 52-year-old morbidly obese woman was admitted to the hospital because of fever, fatigue, and jaundice. She had undergone an uneventful open cholecystectomy 6 weeks prior to this admission and an incisional hernia repair 2 weeks previously, both under general anesthesia using nitrous oxide, halothane, pancuronium, and fentanyl. She had no history of liver disease, had never received blood products, and was not taking any medication. She had not been exposed to family members with hepatitis. Physical examination was remarkable for her obesity, scleral icterus, and jaundice. The liver was not palpable and there was mild right upper quadrant tenderness. Admission laboratory results were normal except for her liver function tests. The aminotransferases and serum bilirubin were markedly elevated and the prothrombin time was prolonged. A viral hepatitis panel was negative. A presumptive diagnosis of halothane hepatitis was made and supportive care for liver failure was provided. She rapidly deteriorated over the next 48 hours with a clinical course consistent with fulminant hepatic failure, and died 72 hours after admission.

What Are the Clinical Features of Halothane Hepatitis?

Two distinct types of hepatotoxicity are associated with the use of halothane. The first is a mild dysfunction that develops in approximately 20% of exposed patients. Patients are often asymptomatic, but exhibit modest elevations of serum aminotransferase levels that develop within a few days of anesthetic exposure, and recover completely.[256] The second is a life-threatening hepatitis that occurs in approximately 1 in 10,000 exposed patients and produces a fatal outcome from massive hepatic necrosis in 1 of 35,000 patients.[335] The histologic findings of massive hepatocellular necrosis are indistinguishable from those of viral hepatitis.[351] Differentiating halothane hepatitis from viral hepatitis that becomes clinically evident in the postoperative period is difficult without positive serologic studies. Jaundice, common following anesthesia and surgery, is usually due to factors such as preexisting liver disease, blood transfusion, sepsis, or other causes of hepatitis. Halothane hepatitis is thus a diagnosis of exclusion.

What Factors May Increase the Risk of Halothane Hepatitis?

Factors that may increase the risk of developing hepatotoxicity from halothane include: (1) multiple exposures, (2) obesity, (3) female gender, (4) age, and (5) ethnic origin.

Several studies report an association between multiple exposures to halothane and subsequent development of hepatitis.[348,363] In one study, 95% of cases of halothane hepatitis followed multiple exposures, while 55% followed reexposure within 4 weeks.[363] Under these circumstances, the liver dysfunction is usually more severe and the latency before clinical presentation is usually shorter than when the syndrome develops following initial exposure to halothane.[348]

Obesity is implicated in several reports as a risk factor for hepatotoxicity following halothane.[3,358] Increased fat stores may act as a "reservoir" for this agent, with slow and prolonged release into the circulation and subsequent increase in production of potentially hepatotoxic metabolites.

Most cases of halothane hepatitis have occurred in middle-aged patients. Females reportedly have a twofold increase in risk of developing the syndrome.[170] Genetic factors may also play a role in some patients, as there is a report of this syndrome in three pairs of related women of Mexican-Indian or Mexican-Spanish ancestry.[163]

What Is the Mechanism of Toxicity?

The inhaled anesthetics were originally considered to be biologically inert, but it was subsequently recognized that these drugs are metabolized and that their metabolites may be toxic. Halothane is the most extensively metabolized inhalational anesthetic. Approximately 20% of the absorbed drug is metabolized, principally by mixed-function oxidases in the liver. This oxidative reaction produces trifluoroacetic acid. An alternate and usually minor route of halothane metabolism exists (reductive pathway) that requires absence of oxygen and the presence of an electron donor. Reductive metabolism results in the formation of trifluorochloroethane and difluorochloroethylene (Fig. 53–2). These volatile metabolites act as free radicals, which may produce acute hepatic toxicity directly by irreversibly binding to and destroying intracellular structures in the hepatocyte, or by acting as haptens and triggering an immune-mediated hypersensitivity response.[281,359] The high percentage of patients with halothane hepatitis who had prior recent exposure to the drug is consistent with the latter mechanism.[170]

Are the Other Inhalational Anesthetics Hepatotoxic?

Enflurane has been used extensively in North America since 1966, and only a few scattered reports of liver damage have appeared. Some authorities believe that the evidence does not support the existence of enflurane-induced hepatic necrosis.[103,112,329] Isoflurane, desflurane, and sevoflurane all appear to have low hepatotoxic potential.

What Other Visceral Organ Toxicities Are Associated With Use of Inhalational Anesthetics?

The kidneys are the only other organ at risk of toxicity from modern inhalational anesthetics. Methoxyflurane is an anesthetic introduced in 1962. In 1966 it was linked to the development of vasopressin-resistant polyuric renal insufficiency (nephrogenic diabetes insipidus) in 16 of 94 patients receiving prolonged methoxyflurane anesthesia for abdominal surgery.[75] Polyuria was associated with a negative fluid balance; dehydration; elevation of serum sodium, osmolality, and urea nitrogen concentrations;

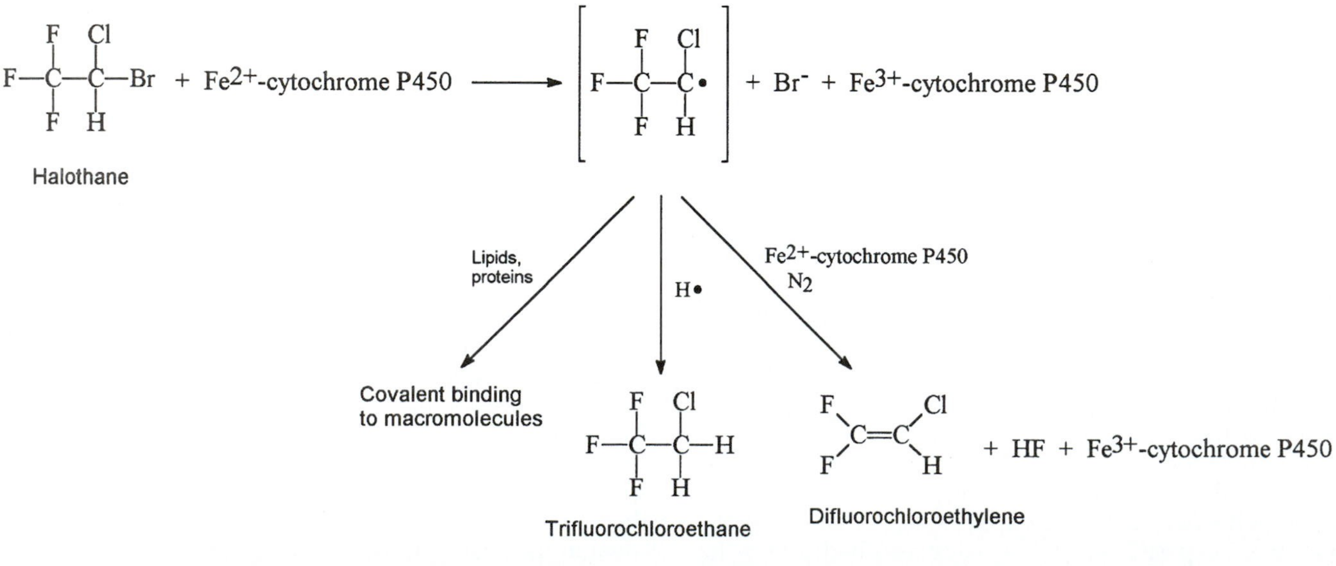

Figure 53–2. The reductive metabolism of halothane results in the formation of trifluorochloroethane and difluorochloroethylene.

and a fixed urinary osmolality close to that of serum. Renal abnormalities lasted from 10 to 20 days in most patients but persisted in three patients for more than 1 year. Subsequent studies demonstrated that the renal toxicity was caused by inorganic fluoride (F^-) released during biotransformation of methoxyflurane.[340] The risk of toxicity was highly correlated with both the total dose of methoxyflurane (concentration × duration) and the peak serum F^- concentration.[74,228] The nephrotoxic serum F^- concentration is 50–60 μmol/L.[74] Factors that enhance biotransformation (obesity, enzyme induction) increased the toxic risk. Although the precise mechanism by which F^- produces its toxic effect on the kidney is not clear, one hypothesis is that F^- induces inhibition of adenylate cyclase activity, and thereby interferes with the normal action of antidiuretic hormone on the distal convoluted tubules.

Although methoxyflurane is no longer used, lessons learned regarding its toxicity have been applied to evaluating the nephrotoxic potential of other fluorinated anesthetics. Of the currently used agents (halothane, isoflurane, enflurane, desflurane, sevoflurane), only enflurane and sevoflurane undergo biotransformation by defluorination to result occasionally in serum concentrations high enough to produce transient decreases in urine-concentrating ability. However, clinically evident renal impairment almost never occurs in surgical patients anesthetized with either agent.[185]

Chronic use of isoniazid induces CYP2E1, which increases metabolism of enflurane, producing higher than usual serum F^- levels in approximately 50% of treated surgical patients who receive an enflurane anesthetic.[228] The F^- concentrations, however, were neither high enough nor sustained long enough to produce clinically significant renal dysfunction. Nonetheless, it would seem prudent to avoid prolonged use of enflurane in patients taking isoniazid or other agents, such as ethanol, phenobarbital, and phenytoin, which elevate the hepatic level of cytochrome CYP2E1.

Unusually high serum F^- concentrations are also reported in morbidly obese patients anesthetized with enflurane.[73] This finding may be related to the large storage capacity of the obese for fat-soluble drugs, which may permit prolonged postoperative release and metabolism of enflurane. Renal dysfunction, however, has not been reported with the use of enflurane in this patient population.

What Is the Clinical Presentation of Patients Who Have Toxicity From Abuse of Halogenated Volatile Anesthetics?

Fatal or life-threatening complications have been described when halogenated inhalational anesthetics are used for nonanesthetic purposes (suicide attempts, mood elevation, topical treatment of herpes simplex labialis). When ingested, halothane usually produces a gastroenteritis with vomiting, followed by depression of consciousness, hypotension, shallow breathing, bradycardia with extrasystoles, and pulmonary edema. Coma usually resolves within 72 hours.[79,373] The diagnosis should be suspected when these features are seen in a patient with the odor (sweet/fruity) of halothane on his or her breath. Supportive care, including endotracheal intubation and orogastric lavage, should be provided. Full recovery can occur without permanent organ injury.

Intravenous injections of halothane are described in both a suicide attempt and unintentionally, during induction of anesthesia. A 19-year-old male self-administered 9 mL of halothane IV in a fatal poisoning.[35] On arrival at the emergency department within 1 hour of the injection, the patient was unconscious and hypotensive and showed minimal respiratory effort. Pulmonary edema fluid was present in the endotracheal tube following intubation. Asystole developed 3 hours later; the patient could not be resuscitated. Pulmonary edema was confirmed on autopsy and was believed to be the cause of death. In another incident, a 16-year-old girl received an unintentional IV injection of 2.5 mL of halothane during induction of anesthesia.[336] She became unconscious and apneic within 30 seconds but began to awaken within 2–3 minutes. Four hours later she developed respiratory distress from pulmonary edema but subsequently made a full recovery.

Transient coma and apnea are probably secondary to a bolus of halothane reaching the brain on its first pass through the bloodstream. Redistribution then occurs, explaining the rapid awakening. The pulmonary edema that develops following injection of halothane may result from a direct toxic effect of high concentrations of this drug on the pulmonary vascular bed. Following injection, the agent likely travels as a bolus during the first passage through the pulmonary circulation because of its poor solubility in blood.

Hospital personnel have been involved in most reported cases of halothane abuse by inhalation.[323] Inhalation of halothane produces a pleasurable sensation similar to that described with glue-sniffing. Death may result from upper airway obstruction following loss of consciousness or from dysrhythmias. Death also occurred in a student nurse anesthetist who applied a full 250-mL bottle of enflurane over 3 hours to "cold sores" on her lower lip.[211]

Intravenous Anesthetics

Nonopioid Intravenous Anesthetics

Intravenous anesthetics were introduced into clinical practice in the 1930s when short-acting barbiturates became available. The first significant adverse effect to be reported following administration of these drugs was profound systemic hypotension. When thiopental was used as a sole anesthetic for management of battle injuries at Pearl Harbor in 1941, it was reported to cause a "cyanosis decolletage" which was "the inevitable and irremedial predecessor of death." The drug was thus named "the ideal form of euthanasia."[151] Since then, other intravenous agents have been introduced to produce hypnosis and we have learned more about their adverse effects. The clinical importance of these effects differs depending on whether the drug is administered as a single dose for induction of anesthesia or as repeated doses or continuous infusions for maintenance of anesthesia or sedation. When used in a single dose, the concerns are not only the inherent ability of the drug itself to produce hemodynamic instability, respiratory depression, and acute effects on CNS blood flow and metabolism, but also unwanted interactions with other drugs and allergic reactions. When repeated doses or continuous infusions are administered, there may be adverse effects on metabolism and hormonal homeostasis in addition to prolonged effects on the cardiovascular, respiratory, and central nervous systems as well as pharmacokinetic interactions with other drugs. This discussion will be limited to the following commonly used nonopioid agents: (1) ultra-short-acting barbiturates (thiopental, methohexital), (2) propofol, (3) etomidate, and (4) ketamine.

What Are the Effects of the Ultra-Short-Acting Barbiturates on Organ Function?

Although there are two main classes of barbiturates in clinical use—oxybarbiturates and thiobarbiturates—they have similar effects. The two most commonly used barbiturates in anesthetic practice are thiopental [5-ethyl-5-(1-methylbutyl)-2-thiobarbituric acid], a thiobarbiturate, and methohexital [1-methyl-5 allyl-5-(1-methyl-2-pentynyl)barbituric acid], an oxybarbiturate (Fig. 53–3).

The anesthetic effect of barbiturates is closely correlated with their ability to potentiate gamma-aminobutyric acid type A ($GABA_A$) receptor-mediated inhibitory synaptic transmission,[311,382] but the drugs affect a variety of other neurotransmitter receptors and ion channels.

Cardiovascular Effects. Barbiturates decrease systemic blood pressure and increase heart rate.[30,346,347] This effect is particularly pronounced in hypovolemic patients in whom the usual anesthetic induction dose of thiopental can cause fatal cardiovascular collapse. The effect on cardiac contractility, however, is somewhat controversial. Most investigators have found reduced stroke volume, increased heart rate, and moderately reduced cardiac output following barbiturate administration. It is thus generally assumed that these drugs are myocardial depressants. Others, however, have questioned whether this effect is clinically significant. They propose instead that the reduced cardiac output observed following barbiturate administration is secondary to venodilation and peripheral pooling of blood with resultant baroreflex-mediated increase in heart rate.[58,116,345] Apart from tachycardia, significant barbiturate-induced dysrhythmias are uncommon. Thiobarbiturates have, however, a dose-dependent biphasic effect on the duration of the action potential[301] and potentiate halothane-epinephrine–induced dysrhythmias, particularly AV dissociation and ventricular dysrhythmias.[18] Some of the cardiovascular effects of these agents are likely related to their activity on both calcium and potassium ion channels.[129,139,301]

Cerebral and Neurophysiologic Effects. Barbiturates inhibit synaptic transmission in the brain, resulting in a reduction of the cerebral metabolic rate for oxygen ($CMRO_2$) of up to 50%.[176,236] This mechanism is coupled with a decrease in global cerebral blood flow (CBF), cerebral blood

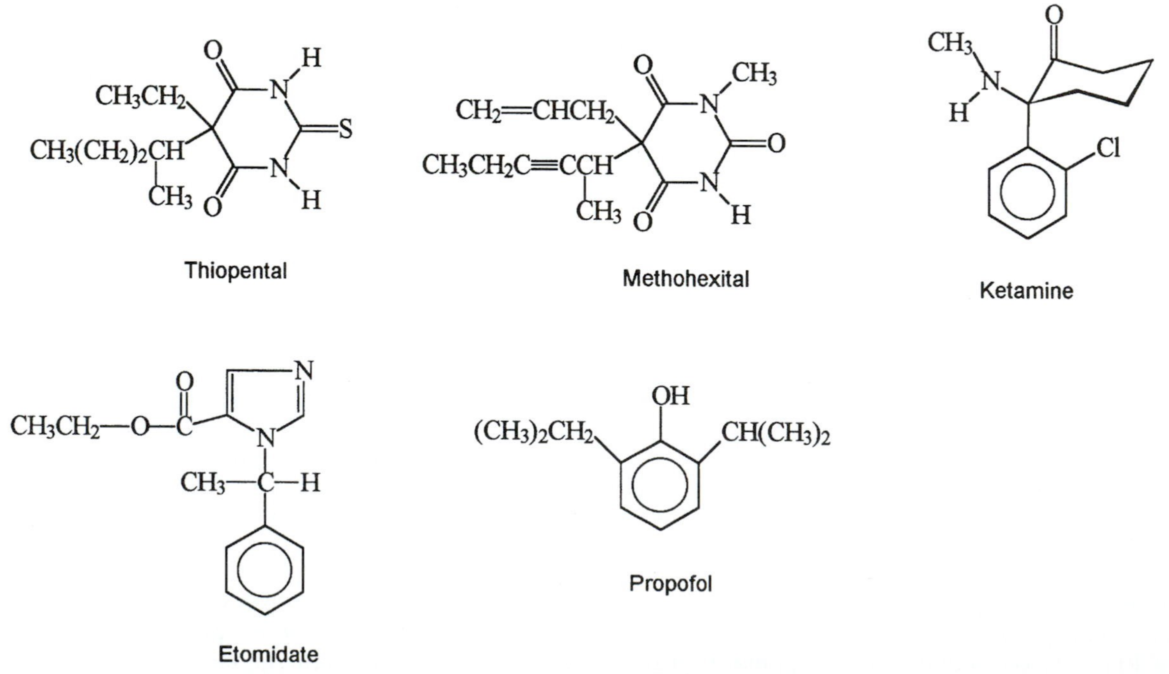

Figure 53–3. Chemical structures of common intravenous anesthetics.

volume (CBV), and intracranial pressure (ICP), when cerebral vasoreactivity to CO_2 is maintained. The effect of the barbiturates on CBF, CBV, and ICP is much more complicated and poorly understood in patients with impaired cerebral autoregulation.[232,260] Barbiturates depress EEG activity in a dose-related fashion parallel to the decrease in cerebral metabolic rate.[176] Suppression of EEG to burst-suppression correlates with the maximal effect on CBF, making it possible to adjust barbiturate infusion by continuous EEG monitoring in order to maximize its effect on cerebral metabolism while minimizing untoward hemodynamic effects.[176] Barbiturates have anticonvulsant activity.[240] Low doses, however, may produce a net excitatory effect on the CNS, as demonstrated by increased sensitivity to painful stimuli after subanesthetic doses of barbiturates[127] and the ability of low-dose methohexital[150,354] and thiopental[240] to provoke seizures in patients with temporal lobe epilepsy. Epileptiform seizures can occur during emergence from high-dose methohexital administration, suggesting the possibility of acute barbiturate withdrawal.[346]

Porphyria. Barbiturates can precipitate a crisis of porphyria and are contraindicated in patients with acute intermittent porphyria.[354]

What Are the Effects of Propofol on Organ Function?

Propofol (2,6-diisopropylphenol) is a hypnotic agent that is chemically unrelated to other intravenous anesthetics (Fig. 53–3). The mechanism of action is not known, but may be related to the ability of propofol to enhance GABA-mediated synaptic inhibition.[25,276] Propofol exists as an oil at room temperature and is available for administration in a 1% solution in 10% soybean oil, 2.25% glycerol, and 1.2% purified egg phosphatide. The solution does not contain preservatives.

Cardiovascular Effects. Propofol consistently decreases systemic blood pressure.[313,326] Factors contributing to this effect include: (1) reduction of systemic vascular resistance[61,117,149] and increased arterial compliance[215] due to decreased sympathetic tone;[105] (2) resetting of the baroreflex, blunting the tachycardic response to hypotension;[19,78,105,303] (3) decreased preload;[205] and (4) a possible negative inotropic effect. Propofol interferes with transsarcolemmal Ca^{2+} flux,[283,337,379] but reports of its effect on isolated cardiac muscle contractility are contradictory.[137,331] Studies of the effect of propofol on inotropy in vivo are inconsistent as well. Whereas some studies demonstrate a significant negative inotropic effect of propofol in humans[63,252,352] and in animals,[52,64] other studies fail to confirm this finding.[61,117,149] The ability to depress cardiovascular function significantly when it is combined with other anesthetics is more pronounced for propofol than for thiopental[252] or etomidate.[52] Propofol has been used for cardiovascular surgery,[146] but the possibility that the drug may have a significant myocardial depressant effect in the presence of heart disease must be borne in mind. Elderly patients may respond to propofol administration with a pronounced depression of cardiac output, apart from the fact that these patients require lower induction doses under these circumstances.[96,192]

Induction of anesthesia with propofol is usually not associated with dysrhythmias.[63,242] There are, however, case reports of propofol-associated significant[26] and persistent[343] bradycardias as well as Mobitz type I atrioventricular block.[134] All cases responded to atropine. Cardiac arrest has been reported following propofol-induced bradycardia.[93,111] The combination of propofol with other drugs that can induce bradycardia, such as fentanyl, succinylcholine, vecuronium, and neostigmine, increases the risk of clinically significant bradydysrhythmias.[26,93,111,134] These problems may result from a reduction of sympathetic tone that occurs prior to decreased vagal tone, resulting in a period of predominantly vagal activity.[104] A recent study in rats in which both pretreatment with atropine and bilateral vagotomy abolished the bradycardic response to propofol supports the theory that propofol-induced bradydysrhythmias are cholinergic and neurally mediated.[39] There is, however, also evidence from animal models of a direct effect of propofol on cardiac conduction tissues.[11,69,331] Frequency-dependent depression of AV nodal conduction by propofol can be demonstrated in isolated guinea pig hearts.[11] When used as a continuous infusion for sedation, the cardiovascular effects can be minimized by slowly titrating the rate.[32,100,118] In this situation there may be no significant hemodynamic difference between propofol and other sedatives.[5,56] Significant decreases in arterial blood pressure, however, have been reported during propofol infusion for sedation of intensive care patients aged 58–77.[257]

Cerebral and Neurophysiologic Effects. Propofol reduces $CMRO_2$, CBF, and ICP.[327] However, since the drug also reduces mean arterial blood pressure, CPP can actually decrease.[252,280] Several case reports of neurologic sequelae have raised concerns about the safety of prolonged infusions in children.[100] Twitching movements of the face, head, and shoulders; choreiform movements and cogwheel rigidity of the arms; and ataxia have been reported in children following doses of propofol that exceeded the recommended dose for adults.[349] These findings have never been correlated with the EEG changes or pathologic eye movements that indicate seizures.

What Other Toxic Effects Are Associated With the Use of Propofol?

Propofol infusions are being used increasingly for long-term sedation in adults, and the safety of this practice is well documented.[100,154] Experience in the pediatric population is more limited.[221,261,287] Metabolic acidosis with fatal myocardial failure has been reported after propofol infusions in children with significant upper airway infections[271] and increased ICP.[333] There are two case reports of children who survived. A 20-month-old girl with epiglottitis was sedated with propofol (5–10 mg/kg/h) for 56 hours and then developed hyperthermia, lactic acidosis, bradycardia, hypotension, oliguria, myoglobinuria, and fixed and dilated pupils, while her serum was lipemic. Echocardiography and head CT were normal, and blood and spinal fluid cultures were negative. The patient gradually improved with hemodiafiltration. She later received propofol anesthesia for a short surgical procedure without complication.[27] A recent report described a 4-year-old boy with laryngitis who received propofol infusion (8.6 mg/kg/h) for 3 days and developed lipemic serum, pulmonary hypertension, rhabdomyolysis, myoglobinuria, and elevated transaminases. Hemodiafiltration was instituted and this patient also had a favorable outcome.[355] Although it is not clear if any relationship exists between propofol administration and the severe morbidity described,[286] the manufacturer warns against the prolonged use of propofol in children.[287] If indeed propofol is responsible for this complication, the question remains whether these effects are caused by the drug itself or by its lipid carrier. There are no data supporting a role of fat emulsions in the serious conditions described in these case reports,[286] and the clinical findings differ from fat overload syndrome, which may occur in children.[31,160] There is, however, an association between high levels of inflammatory cytokines, which strongly suppress lipoprotein lipase activity, and lipid abnormalities, such as increased levels of very-low-density lipoproteins and triglycerides.[157,304] This is supported by another report, which describes a 21-year-old woman with traumatic head injury who received small amounts of 20% fat emulsion for nutrition and developed hemophagocytosis accompanied by high fever, hypertension, multiple organ failure, and high levels of serum triglycerides and C-reactive protein.[297] Increased plasma levels of inflammatory cytokines occur in both serious infections and head injury[229] and, interestingly, all of the children described above suffered from severe infections or significant intracranial pathology. A possible relationship between infusion of fat emulsions and increased levels of inflammatory mediators in the development of these complications is, however, speculative, and serious complications of hyperlipidemia following propofol infusion have not been described in adults. Clinicians should be aware of this possibility and closely monitor for any of the metabolic abnormalities described above when administering lipid emulsions, such as propofol, to patients with increased levels of cytokines, reflected by an increase in C-reactive protein.[297]

Prolonged hypertriglyceridemia without any other significant findings can result from propofol administration.[109] This is an unusual finding in adult patients and the effect of prolonged propofol administration on blood lipids is usually confined to this temporary rise in triglycerides.[56,70]

Early studies of the allergenic properties of propofol indicated that in contrast to the original cremophor formulation, the present soybean emulsion formulation is less likely to produce histamine release or anaphylactoid reactions.[142] Histamine release is minimal with normal anesthetic doses of propofol, but with higher blood levels, which may result from rapid bolus injection in patients with low cardiac output, this may occur.[195] This effect may be of clinical significance, especially if the agent is administered with other histamine-releasing drugs, such as atracurium or thiopental.[196] True anaphylactic reactions to propofol in emulsion also occur.[194] One study described 14 patients with life-threatening reactions that developed within a few minutes of receiving propofol. Thirteen of these patients were positive for at least one of the following: skin test, IgE-dependent leucocyte histamine release, or radioimmunoassay of IgE against propofol.[196]

Blood coagulability and platelet function may also be affected by the fat emulsion in the propofol preparation.[14,54,289] Prolongation of the prothrombin time was reported in ICU patients sedated with a continuous infusion of propofol over 8 hours.[148] No other changes in hemostatic values were noted and no patient displayed any bleeding tendency. The consequences of this effect on hemostasis during longer periods of infusion are not fully known, however, and careful monitoring of blood coagulation is mandatory in this situation.

Why Is Propofol Use Associated With Sepsis?

The Centers for Disease Control and Prevention published a report in 1990 on bacteremia and wound infections caused by *Staphylococcus aureus* associated with the use of contaminated propofol.[1] This was followed by another report in 1995 of seven outbreaks of perioperative infectious complications where extrinsically contaminated propofol was identified as the cause.[34] Propofol emulsion is a fertile medium for growth of *E. coli*, *P. aeruginosa*, and *S. aureus*,[341] whereas thiopental, methohexital, etomidate, and saline are not.[321] Propofol also supports the growth of *C. albicans*,[322] *S. aureus*, and *S. epidermidis* after external contamination.[231] Interestingly, a 1:1 mixture of propofol and thiopental has marked bactericidal properties, indicating that the pH of the solution may be a major factor in the ability to sustain bacterial growth.[76] The packaging has been implicated since it is almost impossible to open the ampules without touching their necks. One study has demonstrated that glass particles from broken ampules can contaminate the contents as it is opened.[322] Routine wiping of the ampule with alcohol is recommended[98] as well as aseptic technique when preparing propofol infusions.[1,2] Propofol should be used immediately after it has been drawn up, and the contents of an opened ampule must be discarded within 6 hours.

What Are the Effects of Etomidate on Organ Function?

Etomidate [R-(+)ethyl-1-(1-phenylethyl)-1-H-imidazole-5-carboxylate] is a short-acting nonbarbiturate induction agent (Fig. 53–3). Etomidate is prepared as a 2% solution in 35% propylene glycol. Although the mechanism by which etomidate produces hypnosis is unknown, it probably modulates GABAminergic neurotransmission.

Cardiovascular Effects. Etomidate has fewer hemodynamic side effects than the other commonly used intravenous anesthetic induction agents.[292,354] There is minimal alteration of cardiac output[144] and systemic blood pressure,[65,144] and the myocardial oxygen supply/demand ratio is maintained.[181,192] The drug has little direct depressant activity on myocardial contractility in clinical doses[137,331] and also preserves sympathetic tone,[105] the baroreflex,[105] and coronary vascular autoregulation.[331] This hemodynamic stability is less reliable in elderly patients and those with heart disease.[145] Etomidate can also produce hypotension in the presence of hypovolemia.[65]

Etomidate does not seem to have any significant intrinsic effect on cardiac rhythm, although both moderate decrease[128] and increase in heart rate immediately after an induction dose are reported.[144]

Cerebral and Neurophysiologic Effects. Etomidate decreases $CMRO_2$, CBF, and ICP[66,291] in the presence of intracranial hypertension.[65,250,291,310] These effects are similar to those of the barbiturates. In contrast to the barbiturates, however, etomidate has minimal effect on systemic blood pressure and cardiac output; thus the CPP is usually preserved or increased.[239,250]

Etomidate can induce convulsion-like EEG patterns in patients with[106,135,190] and without[65,147,190] seizure disorders, but has also been used to treat seizures.[162,240,367] It appears that etomidate possesses both pro- and anticonvulsant properties and it is possible that the dose and rate of administration of the drug determine which of these effects predominates.[240] Myoclonic movements during induction are common.[174,292] This is believed to be caused by disinhibition of the spinal cord.[21,240] Two reports of patients without a history of epilepsy, who were monitored with EEG during induction of anesthesia with etomidate, failed to demonstrate an epileptiform EEG pattern during myoclonic movements.[91,138] Premedication with diazepam and opioids decreases the intensity and frequency of this phenomenon.[165] Even though myoclonus during induction is generally considered to be of little clinical importance, in view of the previously described epileptiform EEG patterns that can be induced by etomidate, it is not possible to exclude subcortical seizure activity as a cause for convulsive movements.[240]

Effects on the Adrenal Gland. Etomidate suppresses adrenal synthesis of both cortisol and aldosterone via a concentration-dependent block of a cholesterol side-chain cleavage enzyme and 11-β-hydroxylase, in a fashion analogous to that of ketoconazole.[361,362] This effect is implicated in the increased mortality of intensive care patients who received etomidate for continuous sedation.[200] One patient received long-term etomidate infusion and developed hypotension unresponsive to vasopressor drugs. The patient's cardiovascular status improved after glucocorticoid administration.[10] Etomidate is therefore no longer recommended for this purpose in spite of its favorable pharmacokinetic profile.[353] Short-term infusions of etomidate (90–170 min) completely block the adrenocortical response to corticotropin stimulation for 24 hours,[364] and even a single dose of etomidate blunts the response to ACTH.[102,130,257] The clinical significance of this decrease in adrenocortical function after a single dose of etomidate is uncertain. Only insignificant changes in plasma cortisol and ACTH levels occur in healthy patients during and after minor surgery following a single induction dose of etomidate. Inhibition of adrenal response to ACTH does occur in these patients, but it was concluded that a single bolus dose of the agent does not cause clinically significant adrenocortical depression.[102] However, we have at present too little knowledge about the clinical consequences of a single dose of etomidate in high-risk patients who may already have adrenal suppression.

What Are the Effects of Ketamine on Organ Function?

Ketamine [2-(*ortho*-chlorophenyl)-2-methylamino cyclohexanone] is an intravenous agent that combines sedative, anesthetic, amnestic, and analgesic properties, making it the only available intravenous agent that can function as a sole anesthetic (Fig. 53–3). It is structurally similar to phencyclidine (PCP) and cyclohexamine, both of which produce anesthesia, but with long-lasting postanesthetic psychotomimetic symptoms. Ketamine also produces disturbing psychic sensations following its use, but significantly less than the other drugs.[92,372] These effects, which include auditory, visual, and sensory hallucinations as well as frank delirium,[371] may recur several weeks after ketamine administration in both adults and children[122,235,277] and is a serious problem when the drug is used as a sole anesthetic. These effects can be overcome by concomitant administration of a benzodiazepine[96,209] or an α_2-adrenergic antagonist.[207] Patients who have developed tolerance to alcohol may react with severe agitation after ketamine administra-tion; the drug should perhaps be avoided in these patients.[208]

The mechanism by which ketamine produces anesthesia remains unknown. It may be complex and probably differs from the actions of the other commonly used intravenous anesthetics. The condition induced by ketamine was initially described as "dissociative anesthesia" and thought to be produced by a functional and electrophysiologic dissociation between the thalamoneocortical and limbic systems.[71] This theory was later challenged by EEG studies showing that ketamine produces excitatory activity in both of these regions.[179] Based on these findings, an alternative mechanism of the anesthetic action of ketamine was proposed: a sustained cataleptoid, or stage II, CNS excitation.[374] More recent studies have demonstrated effects that could explain or contribute to the anesthetic action of the drug, such as blockade of the *N*-methyl-*d*-aspartate (NMDA) receptor[15,342] as well as activity on opioid, noradrenaline, and serotonin receptors.[288]

Cardiovascular Effects. Ketamine has a slight direct myocardial depressant effect in various animal preparations as well as in isolated human atrial muscle.[137] One recent study demonstrates attenuation of baroreceptor function produced by NMDA receptor blockade in the nucleus tractus solitarius of the rat.[264] By themselves these properties would result in cardiovascular effects similar to those of the barbiturates and propofol. However, in vivo administration of the drug usually results in increases in heart rate, systemic and pulmonary blood pressures, and cardiac index.[288,292,354,372,375] This effect is similar in healthy individuals and in those with heart disease, with the possible exception of the rise in pulmonary artery pressure, which seems to be more pronounced in patients with chronic pulmonary hypertension.[292] The mechanism of this effect is most likely centrally mediated release of endogenous catecholamines, possibly augmented by the ability of the agent to enhance peripheral catecholamine activity.[217] In clinical practice it is important to remember that, since the ability of ketamine to preserve or increase systemic blood pressure, heart rate, and cardiac output is dependent on sympathetic stimulation, this effect cannot be relied on in situations in which the sympathetic modulation of the heart and circulation is impaired,[38,368] such as septic shock.[279] Other effects of ketamine on cardiac rhythm are controversial.[288,372] Even though the drug does not have any direct effect on peripheral α- and β-adrenergic receptors,[217,378] it seems to enhance the effect of epinephrine on smooth muscle receptors[217] and to sensitize the myocardium to the dysrhythmogenic effects of catecholamines.[186] It is also possible that ketamine can induce dysrhythmias by promoting atrial reentry.[255] These direct effects may become clinically significant if ketamine is used in combination with other agents with positive chronotropic and bathmotropic properties.

The cardiovascular effects of ketamine may be undesirable in the presence of cardiovascular disease, especially pulmonary hypertension; the drug is probably best avoided in these patients. Cardiostimulatory effects can be attenuated to some degree by premedication with benzodiazepines,[96,372] α_2-adrenergic antagonists,[207] α- and β-adrenergic antagonists,[24,143,288] and/or combination with general anesthetics.[38,325,372] The benzodiazepines seem to be the most reliable agents for blunting the cardiovascular effects of ketamine,[288,292] whereas the response to labetalol, an α- and β-adrenergic antagonist, is much more variable.[97]

Cerebral and Neurophysiologic Effects. The major difference between ketamine and the other commonly used intravenous anesthetics is that anesthesia induced by ketamine is associated with increased regional metabolic activity in the brain, whereas other drugs produce generalized cerebral metabolic depression. As expected, the effects of ketamine administration on cerebral hemodynamics and metabolism are much more complex than those observed after administration of barbiturates, etomidate, and propofol. Early research in both humans and animals demonstrated that ketamine, as opposed to the other intravenous anesthetics in clinical use, could increase ICP and CBF.[136,338] Other reports demonstrate only minor or no effect on ICP and CBF when normocapnia is maintained[6,158,159,278,344] or when ketamine is combined with other anesthetic drugs.[83,344] Questions about the safe use of ketamine in patients with intracranial pathology remain, however. Ketamine may increase neuronal vulnerability to cerebral ischemia,[8,293,318] and one study demonstrated increase in hippocampal neuronal loss after short-term ischemia during ketamine anesthesia.[60]

Myoclonic movements have been reported in children following both induction and maintenance doses of ketamine.[113,268,284] No EEG tracings were available. Absence of cortical EEG changes does not exclude subcortical seizure activity, however.[240] Seizure activity was recorded from the limbic system following ketamine administration to cats[179] and in the limbic and thalamic system in epileptic patients.[121] This activity is associated with excitation, muscle twitching, and posturing.[240] In epileptic patients, this subcortical activity can lead to tonic and clonic motor activity with or without cortical EEG changes, after relatively high doses (> 2 mg/kg).[57,72,121,240] Even though ketamine has occasionally been used to terminate clinical seizures, and may be safe in epileptic patients,[72] most evidence indicates a predominantly cerebral stimulatory effect.

Long-term Ketamine Infusions. Ketamine is infrequently utilized in the ICU, since reliable, safe, long-term sedation and analgesia can usually be achieved with a combination of benzodiazepines and opioids. An exception is the treatment of refractory status asthmaticus in which several case reports indicate a possible role for ketamine infusions.[71,270,295,334] The safe use of ketamine for this purpose is a complicated issue. The well-known adverse effects of the drug must be ameliorated; neuropsychiatric phenomena should be attenuated by concomitant administration of benzodiazepines, and salivary and tracheobronchial hypersecretion often requires treatment with antisialogogues.[241,288] Repeated administration of atropine or glycopyrrolate, however, must be carefully titrated to avoid accumulation of dry secretions in the airways, a potentially dangerous situation, especially in the asthmatic. The adverse cardiovascular interactions between ketamine and other drugs with dysrhythmogenic and sympathomimetic properties must be carefully monitored and treated. There are also theoretical concerns about possible lasting disturbance of N-methyl-*d*-aspartate (NMDA) receptor function after long-term pharmacologic receptor blockade, which may affect learning and memory.[7,68] Activation of NMDA receptors is also necessary for normal visual development in some animals; the safe use of long-term ketamine infusions in human neonates and children has not been studied.[7]

What Are the Toxic Manifestations of Ketamine When Used as a Substance of Abuse?

Abuse of ketamine administered intranasally, intramuscularly, intravenously, and by inhalation in social settings was first reported on the West Coast of the United States in the early 1970s.[120,319] Since the early 1990s, there has been a renewed popularity of ketamine abuse at social gatherings such as "rave" parties and at certain night clubs, particularly in the United States, but also in Europe and Australia. Currently, the most common routes of administration are the nose and mouth.[172] The popularity of the drug for abuse is related to the ability of ketamine to induce a dissociative state, which in subanesthetic doses can produce an "out of body" or "separate reality" experience, with a marked reduction in sensory input, including pain.[4,17,67,172,173] This dissociation is similar to, if not the same as, the psychic sensations commonly experienced during emergence from ketamine anesthesia. This experience, which is extremely frightening to some individuals, is described as "near death," with perceptions of separation from the body, and can in some situations produce an exhilarating sensation of being lost in or transported through space, accompanied by colorful hallucinations, sensations of immobility, and a feeling of disregard for death.[4,67,172,173] Ketamine and its congener phencyclidine block the receptor for NMDA, an excitatory amine in the mammalian brain.[15,180,288] An association between blockade of this receptor and "near death" experiences has been suggested.[173] The sensation of immobility is often accompanied by a real loss of motor coordination and even severe dystonia,[120,172] which may represent a ketamine-induced dopaminergic/noradrenergic imbalance in the basal ganglia.[120] Both voluntary muscle exertion and involuntary myoclonic or dystonic muscle contractions are implicated in rhabdomyolysis following PCP intoxication.[274] This could also be of concern in patients with ketamine intoxication, especially if physical restraints are used.[23] Routine monitoring of, and prophylactic treatment for, myoglobinuria should always be considered when managing these patients. Otherwise, the care of patients under self-administered ketamine influence depends on whether the drug has been taken together with other drugs that can potentiate its respiratory side effects, such as benzodiazepines and alcohol, or cardiovascular complications, such as cocaine.[140,253] Panic attacks are best treated with benzodiazepines,[172] and acute dystonias have been successfully managed with diphenhydramine.[120]

Neuromuscular Blocking Drugs

CASE 3. A 25-year-old, 80-kg man with a 5-year history of steroid-dependent asthma presented to the emergency department complaining of acute shortness of breath. Physical examination revealed a pulse 120 beats per minute; blood pressure, 130/80 mm Hg; tachypnea at RR 40 breaths/min; temperature, 99.7°F (37.6°C); and diffuse wheezing. He was treated with intravenous fluids, nebulized albuterol, and theophylline and methylprednisolone IV. Despite therapy, he remained in respiratory distress. An arterial blood gas performed while he was receiving 60% O_2 by face mask revealed a pH of 7.25, a PCO_2 of 65 mm Hg, and a PO_2 of 70 mm Hg.

He was intubated and mechanical ventilatory support was initiated. Initial pharmacologic therapy consisted of methylprednisolone 100 mg IV every 6 hours, terbutaline 0.1 μg/kg/min IV, and aminophylline 1 mg/kg/h IV. Chest auscultation revealed equal but distant breath sounds bilaterally. A chest roentgenogram was normal except for diffuse hyperinflation. The patient's blood pressure decreased from 120/90 to 80/40 mm Hg. His respiratory rate was 35 breaths/min on synchronous intermittent mandatory ventilation at a rate of 20. The peak airway pressure was 65 cm H_2O. Evaluation of the expiratory flow waveform revealed the presence of auto-PEEP (air trapping). Attempts to relieve this by prolonging the expiratory time were unsuccessful. Fentanyl and then lorazepam were infused to decrease the patient's dyspnea and allow for more complete exhalation. Although the patient's respiratory rate decreased to 15 breaths/min, the measured auto-PEEP was 15 cm H_2O. A 6-mg bolus of vecuronium was given, followed by continuous infusion at 3 mg/h, adjusted to suppress spontaneous ventilatory efforts. The respiratory rate was decreased to 10 breaths/min and the I:E ratio was reset to 1:3; with this treatment the level of auto-PEEP fell to 3 cm H_2O and the peak airway pressure decreased to 45 cm H_2O.

Sedation, paralysis, and antibronchospastic therapy were maintained for 10 days. Before attempting to wean him from mechanical ventilation, residual muscle relaxation was allowed to wear off. Reversal agents were not given because of concern that an anticholinesterase might exacerbate his bronchospasm.

Twenty-four hours after vecuronium was discontinued, the patient was awake and alert and able to move his eyes, tongue, and head; however, he was unable to sustain a voluntary 5-second head lift. Train-of-four stimulation demonstrated four equal twitches without evidence of fade, nor was post-tetanic potentiation evident. Physical examination revealed flaccid quadriparesis with absent deep tendon reflexes. Sensory examination was normal. The maximum negative inspiratory force was −10 cm H_2O (normal −60 to −90), and during brief weaning trials with pressure support of 15 cm H_2O, he rapidly became dyspneic. The blood urea nitrogen, creatinine, and liver chemistry concentrations remained normal. The plasma creatine kinase peaked at 2172 U/L.

Over the next few days, attempts at weaning proved unsuccessful because of profound respiratory muscle weakness. Electromyography demonstrated a markedly decreased compound motor action potential with no evidence of neuromuscular block. Nerve conduction studies were normal. A quadriceps femoris muscle biopsy revealed atrophy and degeneration with vacuolation of type II fibers and extensive loss of thick (myosin) filaments. There was a slow but complete recovery of muscle strength over the subsequent 3 months.

Because of the pattern of respiratory muscle weakness, diffuse motor weakness, preserved sensory function, increased creatine kinase, and the biopsy results, a diagnosis of thick filament (myosin) myopathy following the use of a neuromuscular blocking agent (NMB) was made.

How Do Neuromuscular Blockers Work?*

There are two classes of drugs that inhibit the effects of acetylcholine (ACH) on nicotinic receptors at the neuromuscular junction (NMJ) (Table 53–1). Succinylcholine is the only currently used depolarizing neuromuscular blocker (DNMB), so called because it produces muscle

TABLE 53–1. CLASSIFICATION OF NEUROMUSCULAR BLOCKING DRUGS

	Short-acting	Intermediate-acting	Long-acting
Depolarizers	Succinylcholine		
Nondepolarizers			
Benzylisoquinolinium		Atracurium	Tubocurarine
		cis-Atracurium	Metocurine
		Mivacurium	Doxacurium
Aminosteroid		Vecuronium	Pancuronium
		Rocuronium	Pipecuronium

*The term "neuromuscular blocking drug" (NMB) is used instead of "muscle relaxant" to avoid confusion with drugs that decrease muscle spasms, such as baclofen or diazepam.

depolarization in the same way as ACH. Its effect is of longer duration because it is relatively resistant to hydrolysis by true (junctional) acetylcholinesterase. Succinylcholine produces prolonged depolarization of the junctional muscle membrane, rendering the NMJ insensitive to subsequent cycles of ACH release from the nerve terminal. In contrast, the nondepolarizing neuromuscular blockers (NDNMB) cause skeletal muscle paralysis by competitive inhibition of ACH at the nicotinic receptor.

All NMBs possess at least one positively charged quaternary ammonium group that binds to the negatively charged alpha subunit of the nicotinic receptor. The NMBs are highly water soluble; they do not easily cross lipid membranes (eg, blood–brain barrier, placenta) and are distributed mostly in the extracellular space.

There are different ACH receptors on the pre- and postjunctional membranes. It is commonly believed that the muscle paralysis produced by NMBs is due to inhibition of the muscle end plate. However, these agents also block prejunctional nicotinic receptors, inhibiting ACH-stimulated ACH production and release.[294] This effect reduces the available pool of ACH and enhances the postjunctional block, and also accounts for the decrease in tension ("fade") observed following train-of-four or tetanic stimulation during partial NDNMB block.

The fast onset of NMB effect following IV administration is due to rapid drug uptake at the NMJ, which is a result of its abundant blood supply. In general, the onset of NDNMB is inversely related to the potency of the agent.[48] During induction, paralysis of the diaphragm precedes that of the hand muscles because of the greater perfusion of the former. Termination of NMB effect is primarily the result of drug elimination.

How Is Muscle Blockade Monitored?

A portable nerve stimulator or visual evaluation of limb motion or respiratory efforts are the usual means of evaluating neuromuscular function; however, the nerve stimulator is considerably more reliable and should be used routinely when caring for any patient receiving a NMB.[360] Hand-held units are readily available, cost less than $200, and are simple to use. Surprisingly, in a survey of medical ICUs, neuromuscular monitoring was employed in only 21% and was used routinely only 4% of the time.[152]

The most common test of the degree of neuromuscular blockade is to deliver four supramaximal electrical impulses at 2 Hz train-of-four (TOF) to the ulnar nerve at the wrist and to assess the resultant movement of the adductor pollicis muscle by manual or visual inspection (typically) or by transduction of the electromyogram or twitch force. Adequate recovery of muscular function is usually present when the ratio of the force generated by the fourth twitch is > 70% of the first (ie, TOF ratio < 0.7).[49] With a TOF ratio < 0.7, subjects may experience weakness, negative inspiratory force and vital capacity are diminished, and weakness of upper airway muscles may cause airway obstruction. When TOF > 0.7, respiratory parameters are relatively normal and upper airway muscle tone is usually adequate to permit extubation. This, however, does not indicate that the patient has returned to normal. At a TOF ratio of < 0.90, normal volunteers complained of diplopia and difficulty in tracking moving objects,[187] while at a TOF ratio of < 0.75, normal volunteers reported feeling uncomfortable, had difficulty talking, swallowing, and sipping through a straw, and displayed a "flat" facial expression.[187]

In a prospective, randomized study of ICU patients, vecuronium dosing was titrated by peripheral nerve stimulation (TOF of 1 of 4 or 90% blockade) or clinical criteria (no movement or spontaneous ventilation).[300] When compared to controls, the peripheral nerve stimulator group required less vecuronium (0.040 ± 0.028 vs 0.070 ± 0.030 mg/kg/h, respectively, $p = 0.001$), and more quickly recovered neuromuscular function and spontaneous ventilation. Although the nerve stimulator helps prevent drug overdose and hastens recovery of muscle strength following termination of NMB, it cannot guarantee that pathologic weakness will not occur as a result of the patient's disease or the use of these agents.

What Are the Complications of NMB Administration?

In the presence of adequate oxygenation and ventilation, short-term use of NMB is only rarely a cause of mortality (eg, succinylcholine-related hyperkalemia, malignant hyperthermia, or anaphylactic reaction). However, these drugs are increasingly being used outside the operating room and for prolonged periods. This alteration in use has produced newly recognized side effects. The complications associated with NMB agents can be divided into those due to inadequate or inappropriate supportive care of the paralyzed patient and those due to specific untoward effects.

Complications of Inappropriate Care. Use of NMB drugs to facilitate intubation requires careful planning and a thorough understanding of their effects. Failure to oxygenate and ventilate the paralyzed patient can rapidly lead to cardiac arrest, anoxic encephalopathy, or death.

One of the most terrifying experiences that a patient can endure is to be awake and paralyzed.[273] These concerns are magnified in the critically ill patient, who may be paralyzed for an extended period of time. It is unfortunate that there is no simple, accurate, and continuous monitor to assure the adequacy of analgesia and sedation in the paralyzed ICU patient, although processed EEG may be helpful. The paralyzed patient is unable to communicate feelings of pain, anxiety, or distress, and the vital signs may be the only index of the adequacy of sedation and analgesia.

Misconceptions about the effects of NMB drugs are also an important issue. In a survey, 10% of ICU nurses and 5% of physician house staff believed that pancuronium relieved pain, while 70% of ICU nurses and 50% of house staff believed that this agent relieved anxiety.[213] Pain is common in the ICU; it may be caused by surgery or routine activities, such as insertion of tubes, lines, and catheters. Anxiety may result from interventions (mechanical ventilation, tracheal suction, application of a hypothermia blanket), or when the patient hears an alarm or discussions about his or her care. Opioids should be given to any patient who may have pain, since pain is not diminished by NMB drugs or sedative/hypnotic agents. On the other hand, opioids do not produce hypnosis or amnesia. For this reason, a sedative such as a benzodiazepine, a barbiturate, or propofol should be administered whenever possible to all patients who receive NMBs. Since these patients are unable to communicate their feelings, these agents should be given by continuous infusion or on a regular schedule, rather than as needed. It is best always to assume that the patient is awake and can perceive pain, touch, and the voices of others.[273] It is always a good idea to explain all procedures to any patient who is receiving NMBs, opioids, and/or sedatives. Whenever possible, the patient should be permitted to wake up once each day in order to monitor analgesia, sedation, and mental status and to evaluate his or her neurologic condition.

Agitation in the critically ill patient is a valuable sign; it may indicate pain, ventilatory difficulty, hypoxemia, shock, or metabolic derangement. Obviously, use of NMBs renders the patient unable to communicate serious problems to the caretaker. In this situation, unrecognized mechanical ventilator failure or disconnection, or endotracheal tube obstruction, may result in hypoxemia, hypercapnia, and death. Therefore, all patients who receive NMBs must be vigilantly attended. The caretaker assumes total responsibility for maintenance of both the airway and adequate ventilation.

Immobility from NMB use is associated with other problems: (1) muscular atrophy; (2) an increased risk of deep venous thrombosis and pulmonary embolism; (3) inhibition of the blink reflex with possible drying of the cornea; (4) decubitus ulcers; (5) pressure neuropathy; (6) muscle contractures (especially of the triceps surae); (7) joint stiffening, and (8) diminished range of motion. Furthermore, the only evidence of a seizure may be twitching of the eyes and abnormal EEG activity.

Complications Due to Specific Untoward Drug Effects

Histamine Release. The nonsteroidal NMBs may produce direct, nonimmunologic histamine release from connective tissue mast cells, with dose- and rate-related venous and arterial dilatation, hypotension, tachycardia, bronchospasm, upper body erythema, and increased bronchial secretions. This reaction is usually mild and clinically insignificant.[28] The approximate rank order for histamine release is tubocurarine > metocurine > atracurium, gallamine and mivacurium > succinylcholine.[115] Pancuronium, rocuronium, and vecuronium do not increase plasma histamine. Succinylcholine may also cause a mild increase in whole blood and plasma histamine.[115] Hypersensitivity to NMB drugs may be more common and more severe in patients with asthma or other allergic diseases, possibly as a result of hypersensitivity to histamine.[115] Prophylaxis with both H_1 and H_2 blockers may be needed to inhibit the systemic effects of histamine release, since antagonism of only one receptor population may be insufficient.[214] Although the steroidal relaxants do not typically cause histamine release, unexplained episodes of hypotension and flushing are reported; these are likely caused by noncompetitive inhibition of histamine *N*-methyl transferase (HNMT), which is the primary enzyme responsible for histamine degradation in humans.[133]

Autonomic Side Effects. In clinical doses, some NMBs have potentially serious dose- and rate-related effects on nicotinic and muscarinic receptors. Gallamine is now infrequently used because it produces substantial vagal blockade and tachycardia. Pancuronium causes tachycardia and an increase in blood pressure due to vagal blockade[307] and sympathetic stimulation.[314] These effects may be beneficial, since they may counteract the bradycardia and mild hypotension caused by high doses of opioids. However, this sympathetic stimulation may be hazardous when pancuronium is combined with halothane (which sensitizes the myocardium to catecholamine-induced dysrhythmias) or a tricyclic antidepressant.[110] Vecuronium has no chronotropic effect. This may be partly responsible for the rare bradydysrhythmias and cardiac arrest that have been observed after concurrent administration of high-dose opioids.[171] Succinylcholine stimulates cardiac muscarinic receptors and may produce cardiac dysrhythmias, including bradycardia, junctional rhythm, ventricular dysrhythmias, and cardiac arrest. Tubocurarine, and to a lesser extent metocurine, produces autonomic blockade at clinical doses, which may impair the sympathetic response to surgical stress or hypotension.[47]

Immunosuppression. General anesthetics and sedatives may be associated with an increased incidence of infection or pneumonia, and it is difficult to determine what effect, if any, is attributable to NMB. In patients with severe head injury treated with early routine paralysis, there was an increased incidence of pneumonia (29% vs 15%, $p < 0.001$) when compared to patients who did not receive paralysis.[167] The authors suggested a possible deleterious effect of NMB on polymorphonuclear leukocyte function.

Interactions of NMBs. Many medications and normal or pathologic physiologic conditions may alter the effects of NMBs (Tables 53–2 and 53–3). It is especially important to be aware of conditions associated with an increased risk for hyperkalemia, rhabdomyolysis, and malignant hyperthermia. Medications or diseases may affect the neuromuscular system at any level from the central nervous system (CNS) to the muscle itself. For example, potent inhalation anesthetics depress CNS activity, lithium can inhibit presynaptic synthesis of ACH, local anesthetics inhibit action potential propagation at the nerve terminal, and dantrolene inhibits calcium release from muscle sarcoplasmic reticulum. All of these drugs augment the effects of NMBs.

TABLE 53–2. POSSIBLE INTERACTIONS OF NEUROMUSCULAR BLOCKERS IN CERTAIN PHYSIOLOGIC CONDITIONS

Physiologic or Metabolic State	Response to Depolarizing NMB	Response to Nondepolarizing NMB
Acidosis	Probably best to avoid in patients with hyperkalemia and acidosis.	Respiratory but not metabolic acidosis potentiates tubocurarine and vecuronium block and either produces no effect or antagonizes pancuronium and metocurine. Slowed nonenzymatic elimination of atracurium. Respiratory acidosis inhibits reversal of tubocurarine and pancuronium by neostigmine.
Alkalosis		No effect or potentiates pancuronium and metocurine and antagonizes tubocurarine and vecuronium.
Burns	Avoid succinylcholine because of hyperkalemia.	Following injury, resistance to block.
Cirrhosis		Increased volume of distribution may require increased initial bolus. Drugs with extensive hepatic elimination may have prolonged effect (rocuronium, vecuronium, pancuronium, and pipecuronium).
Elderly age		Reduced cardiac output and muscle blood flow slows drug onset. Diminished renal and hepatic function slows elimination and prolongs drug effect (pancuronium, vecuronium, tubocurarine). Atracurium pharmacokinetics unaffected.
Hepatobiliary disease		Delayed elimination of drugs dependent on hepatic elimination (rocuronium, vecuronium, pancuronium, and pipecuronium).
Hypercalcemia		Resistance to block.
Hyperkalemia	Avoid succinylcholine.	May potentiate block.
Hypermagnesemia		Potentiates block.
Hypernatremia		If associated with hypovolemia, decreases volume of distribution.
Hyperthyroidism		Accelerated drug metabolism. Possible potentiation due to association with myopathy and myasthenia.
Hypocalcemia		Potentiates block. May cause muscle weakness.
Hypokalemia		Potentiates block.
Hyponatremia		If associated with volume overload, increases drug volume of distribution.
Hypophosphatemia	Associated with rhabdomyolysis.	Potentiates block.
Hypothermia		Potentiates block. Reduces muscle blood flow, slowing renal and hepatic drug elimination, and directly depresses muscle response. Altered drug sensitivity and slowed elimination. Slowed nonenzymatic elimination of atracurium.
Hypothyroidism		Delayed drug metabolism may prolong block. May have preexisting weakness.
Infants	Increased volume of distribution requires higher initial dose. Increased cardiac side effects. Increased incidence of MH, myoglobinuria, and hyperkalemia.	Increased volume of distribution and increased sensitivity of neuromuscular junction tend to balance; drug requirement usually same as adult but may be longer lasting (tubocurarine, vecuronium). Reversal of block occurs as fast as in adults.
Protein binding abnormality		Hypoproteinemia may increase free drug fraction and thus drug effect. Overall, effect difficult to predict, and though probably of importance, influence is not well studied.
Renal insufficiency	Cannot be used if plasma potassium is high.	Prolonged elimination of drugs dependent on renal elimination (pancuronium, tubocurarine, pipecuronium, doxacurium, metocurine, gallamine). Accumulation of certain drug metabolites, eg, laudanosine. Neostigmine, pyridostigmine, and edrophonium are primarily eliminated by the kidney and their elimination half-lives are prolonged at least to the same extent as the NDNMBs they antagonize.
Sepsis		Following injury, resistance to block.
Shock (low cardiac output)		Delayed onset and metabolism of drugs.
Trauma	Possible hyperkalemia	During acute trauma, prolonged drug effect due to decreased cardiac output and hypothermia. Following injury, resistance to block.

Adapted, with permission, from Buck ML, Reed MD: Use of nondepolarizing neuromuscular blocking agents in mechanically ventilated patients. Clin Pharm 1991;10:32–48.

TABLE 53–3. DRUGS THAT MAY INTERACT WITH SUCCINYLCHOLINE OR NONDEPOLARIZING NEUROMUSCULAR BLOCKERS (NDNMBs)

Drug	Response to Succinylcholine	Response to Nondepolarizers	Comments
Antibiotics			
Aminoglycosides Amikacin, gentamicin, kanamycin, neomycin, streptomycin, tobramycin	Potentiate	Potentiate	Decrease ACH release and postjunctional response to ACH. Some intrinsic neuromuscular blocking effects.
Polymyxins			
Polymyxin B	Potentiate	Potentiate	Local anesthetic–like action; decreases ACH release and postjunctional response to ACH. Some intrinsic neuromuscular blocking property. Anticholinesterases paradoxically enhance block.
Tetracyclines	Potentiate	Potentiate	
Other Clindamycin, colistin, lincomycin, metronidazole	Potentiate	Potentiate	Lincomycin and clindamycin cause prejunctional muscle inhibition.
Anticonvulsants			
Phenytoin	?	Inhibits	May cause resistance to nondepolarizers (metocurine, pancuronium, and vecuronium) but not to atracurium.
Carbamazepine	?	Inhibits	May cause resistance to nondepolarizers.
Azathioprine	Potentiates in cat, effect in humans uncertain	Inhibits	Mild effect on NDNMB
Aprotinin (trasylol)	? Mild prolongation		Weak inhibitor of plasma acetylcholinesterase.
Cardiac Medications and Antidysrhythmics			
Calcium channel blockers: nifedipine and verapamil	Potentiate	Potentiate	Causes pre- and postjunctional calcium channel block. Verapamil has local anesthetic–like effect on nerve. May inhibit block reversal by cholinesterase inhibitor.
Digitalis	More prone to cardiac dysrhythmias	Pancuronium increases catecholamines and may cause dysrhythmias.	
Nitroglycerin		Prolongs pancuronium in cats, effect in humans uncertain.	
Propranolol	Potentiates in cat, effect in humans uncertain	Potentiates	Given alone may unmask myasthenic syndrome. Blocks ACH binding at postsynaptic membrane. Block reversal with cholinesterase inhibitor may cause bradydysrhthmias in patient on high-dose beta-adrenergic antagonist.
Procainamide	Potentiates in cat, effect in humans uncertain	Potentiates	Decreases presynaptic ACH release and sensitivity of postjunctional membrane.
Quinidine	Potentiates, may get prolonged block	Potentiates	Pre- and postjunctional effects unclear mechanism.
Trimethaphan	Potentiates	Potentiates	Inhibits plasma cholinesterase and acts like NDNMB.
Cholinesterase Inhibitors			
Edrophonium, neostigmine, physostigmine, pyridostigmine	Prolong effect of succinylcholine, especially if patient heterozygous for atypical plasma cholinesterase. May inhibit or potentiate a preexistent phase II block.	Inhibit	Inhibit plasma cholinesterase in dose-dependent manner. Succinylcholine 1–1.5 mg/kg lasts 35–180 min when given within 90 min after neostigmine.
Echothiophate	Potentiates		Irreversible plasma cholinesterase inhibitor. May decrease enzyme activity 70–100%.
Organophosphates	Potentiate; succinylcholine may last 30 min		Irreversible plasma cholinesterase inhibitor. May decrease enzyme activity 100%.
Cimetidine	Potentiates	Prolongs duration	

(*continued*)

TABLE 53–3 DRUGS THAT MAY INTERACT WITH SUCCINYLCHOLINE OR NONDEPOLARIZING NEUROMUSCULAR BLOCKERS (NDNMBs) (continued)

Drug	Response to Succinylcholine	Response to Nondepolarizers	Comments
Contraceptive pills	? Mild prolongation		Decrease plasma cholinesterase activity 20–30%.
Cyclophosphamide	Prolongs	Potentiates	Irreversible plasma cholinesterase inhibitor. May decrease enzyme activity 35–70%.
Cyclosporine	Potentiates	Potentiates	Cyclosporine in solvent or its solvent alone prolongs NDNMB; and especially vecuronium.
Dantrolene	?	Potentiates	Blocks excitation–contraction coupling by blocking ryanodine calcium channel in sarcoplasmic reticulum of skeletal muscle.
Furosemide			Biphasic dose–response in cats; protein kinase inhibition at low doses and phosphodiesterase inhibition at high doses. Diuretic-related hypokalemia potentiates pancuronium in cats.
< 10 μg/kg	Potentiates	Potentiates	
1–4 mg/kg	Inhibits	Inhibits	
Glucocorticoids	Complex effects, ? mild prolongation.	Inhibits	Chronic steroids antagonize pancuronium and decrease plasma cholinesterase activity by 50%. Steroids with or without NDNMB are associated with myopathies.
Hexafluorinium	Prolongation		Inhibits plasma cholinesterase and has weak effect like NDNMB.
Inhalation anesthetics Isoflurane, enflurane, halothane, desflurane, sevoflurane	Potentiate	Potentiate	Decrease CNS neural activity and potentiates NMB in dose-dependent fashion (postsynaptic and muscle effects). Halothane and enflurane facilitate establishment of succinylcholine phase II block.
Intravenous anesthetics Barbiturates (eg, thiopental), etomidate, fentanyl	None	Slight potentiation	Most IV agents increase ACH release and decrease sensitivity of postsynaptic membrane; effects usually balance out. Effects generally clinically insignificant.
Benzodiazepines (diazepam, midazolam)	Diazepam may accelerate block onset.	Midazolam potentiates vecuronium effect.	Clinically insignificant effects.
Ketamine	Variable	Potentiates	Potentiates tubocurarine but not pancuronium.
Local anesthetics			
Lidocaine	Potentiates	Low-dose lidocaine potentiates block. High-dose lidocaine inhibits nerve terminals and blocks ACH binding site at postsynaptic membrane.	The fast Na^+ channel blockers decrease action potential propagation, ACH release, postsynaptic membrane sensitivity, and muscle excitability. Weak inhibitor of plasma cholinesterase.
Procaine	Potentiates	Potentiates	Ester local anesthetics compete with succinylcholine for plasma protein binding sites and for metabolism by plasma cholinesterase. Weak inhibitor of plasma cholinesterase.
Magnesium	Potentiates, may block fasciculations	Potentiates	Decreases prejunctional ACH release, sensitivity of postjunctional membrane and muscle excitability.
Nondepolarizing NMB			
Pancuronium	"Precurarization" with NDNMB prolongs the onset and decreases side effects of succinylcholine. Tubocurarine decreases and pancuronium increases block duration.	Chronic NDNMB use induces resistance to their effects. Mixing different NDNMB may cause greater than additive effects; especially combining pancuronium with either tubocurarine or metocurine.	Pancuronium, and to a lesser extent vecuronium, inhibit plasma cholinesterase. Heterozygotes for atypical cholinesterase may develop phase II block.
Psychotropic medications Lithium carbonate	Prolong onset and duration (especially if heterozygote for atypical cholinesterase)	May cause resistance to, or prolong effect of pancuronium.	Inhibit synthesis and release of ACH. Lithium alone may cause myasthenic reaction.
MAO inhibitors, (eg, Phenelzine)	Prolong		Decrease plasma cholinesterase activity.

(continued)

TABLE 53–3 DRUGS THAT MAY INTERACT WITH SUCCINYLCHOLINE OR NONDEPOLARIZING NEUROMUSCULAR BLOCKERS (NDNMBs) (continued)

Drug	Response to Succinylcholine	Response to Nondepolarizers	Comments
Tricyclic antidepressants (TCA)		Pancuronium and TCA may cause cardiac dysrhythmias due to sympathetic effects.	
Succinylcholine	Self-taming dose may be used to prevent fasciculations.	NDNMB often used following succinylcholine induction. Tubocurarine, pancuronium, and vecuronium block slightly prolonged by prior administration of succinylcholine.	
Theophylline		Inhibits	Pancuronium and theophylline may increase incidence of cardiac dysrhythmias.

Adapted, with permission, from Viby-Mogensen J: Interaction of other drugs with muscle relaxants. In: Katz R, ed: Muscle Relaxants: Basic and Clinical Aspects. New York: Grune & Stratton, 1985; and Ostergaard D, Engbaek J, Viby-Mogensen J: Adverse reactions and interactions of the neuromuscular blocking drugs. Med Toxicol Adverse Drug Exp 1989;4:351–368.

How Do Neuromuscular Blockers Produce Persistent Weakness in the Critically Ill Patient?

Weakness in critically ill patients is a common occurrence. Reports of this problem following use of NDNMB first appeared in 1985: severe, reversible quadriplegia, muscular atrophy, and areflexia were described in 12 of 60 patients who received 4 mg of pancuronium every 3–4 hours for >6 days.[265] In all patients, biopsy revealed myopathic changes, while electromyography was consistent with axonal degeneration. In a prospective study of 25 severe asthmatics who received corticosteroids, 22 of whom also received vecuronium, an elevation of creatine kinase was observed in 76% and clinical myopathy was observed in 36%.[94] Patients with either abnormality had received a significantly higher dose of vecuronium and required more prolonged mechanical ventilation. There are other reports of weakness in 20–30% of patients receiving NMB for as little as 48–72 hours, in 58% of critically ill patients ventilated for >7 days,[204] and in 70% of patients with sepsis and multiple organ failure.[43,44] In the ICU setting, weakness associated with NDNMB toxicity usually presents as failure to wean from mechanical ventilation. In one study, prolonged motor weakness increased hospital charges by $66,000 per patient, not including the cost of rehabilitation.[299] In general, prolonged motor weakness following NDNMB is multifactorial (reflected in the confusing nomenclature: NMB-induced protracted paralysis, postparalytic syndrome, ICU neuromuscular syndrome) and occurs more often in women. Recovery in survivors is usually complete after 6 months.

The differential diagnosis of weakness in the ICU patient includes (1) residual NMB effect due to inadequate reversal; (2) accumulation of the parent drug or an active metabolite (3-OH-pancuronium, 3-desacetylvecuronium), especially in the presence of renal or hepatic dysfunction; (3) other correctable or preexistent causes of muscular weakness (eg, hypothermia, hypophosphatemia, hypokalemia, hypermagnesemia, burn injury, or malnutrition); (4) neuromuscular disorders such as stroke and peripheral neuropathy; and (5) disorders unique to critically ill patients (critical illness polyneuropathy, motor neuropathy, disuse muscular atrophy, corticosteroid myopathy, thick filament myopathy, necrotizing myopathy of critical illness, and rhabdomyolysis).

Basal motor neuron activity exerts a trophic influence at the NMJ. Under normal circumstances, mature ACH receptors are localized at the endplate. The protein ARIA (for acetylcholine receptor-inducing activity), a member of the neureglin family, is most likely responsible for maintaining the population of ACH receptors at the motor endplate.[305] The normal trophic neural activity can be blocked by prolonged pharmacologic paralysis or nerve injury; and, in response, the muscle synthesizes immature ACH receptors, which disperse over the entire muscle membrane. In addition, there is muscle atrophy, subjective weakness, resistance to NDNMB,[164] and hypersensitivity to DNMB.[148] Resistance to the effect of NDNMB drugs may occur as early as 72 hours after initiation of a drug infusion, necessitating an increase in the rate of administration.[380] It has been observed in ICU patients who required ventilation for more than 3 days that those with a high vecuronium requirement had more ACH receptors than patients who had a lower drug requirement.[90] These alterations have been assumed to be a result of muscle inactivity; however, this phenomenon may also be observed when subparalyzing doses of NMBs are used, suggesting that upregulation may in fact be a primary effect of the agent itself.[201] In addition, weakness may result from a compound injury to the neuromuscular system caused by neuropathy, NMB and corticosteroid administration, sepsis, burn injury, and drug or electrolyte disorders. In animal models, denervated skeletal muscle has an increased number of cytosolic glucocorticoid receptors,[95] and glucocorticoids promote muscular atrophy (especially in type II fibers) and induce selective myosin loss.[298] The association between corticosteroids and NDNMB with severe myopathy has been observed for several years.[153]

Prolonged weakness due to NDNMB must be distinguished from the much more common critical illness polyneuropathy (CIP). Critical illness polyneuropathy occurs in 58–82% of critically ill patients with systemic inflammatory response (SIRS) or sepsis and multiple organ dysfunction syndrome (MODS)[204] and is not related to use of NMB agents. Furthermore, the incidence of CIP is related to the severity of MODS.[203] Critical illness polyneuropathy (Table 53–4) is associated with an increase in ICU mortality (19% without CIP vs 48% with CIP, $p < 0.05$)[204] yet ultimately 50% of patients with CIP make a complete recovery.[202]

Thick filament (myosin) myopathy and necrotizing myopathy of intensive care are myopathic disorders that appear to be related to chronic use of NDNMB and high-dose corticosteroids in critically ill asthmatic patients.[80,182] Nerve conduction is relatively preserved; however, electromyography reveals low-amplitude motor-unit potentials, which are of short duration and may be polyphasic.[49] Superimposed CIP can lead to concurrent nerve conduction abnormalities, which often complicate this picture. Thick filament myopathy occurs relatively infrequently and is characterized by loss of myosin filaments, while thin actin filaments are relatively preserved.

A rare finding in patients receiving NDNMB is necrotizing myopathy of intensive care. This syndrome is associated with severe myonecrosis, myoglobinuric renal failure, and death due to multiple organ failure. The electrophysiologic signs of myopathy include low-amplitude motor M response and normal to slightly abnormal spontaneous muscle activity.[383] It has been proposed that this syndrome may be caused when a "priming" factor (high dose of systemic glucocorticoids, myotropic infection, or sepsis) is combined with a "triggering" agent (a NDNMB).[285] Infection with certain myotropic pathogens (eg, influenza A or B, *S. aureus* with toxic shock syndrome, *E. coli*, or Legionellosis) may function as a priming factor and predispose to myonecrosis. The early recognition of myonecrosis should prompt immediate discontinuation of the NDNMB triggering agent; this may improve chances of survival.[285] Certainly, creatine kinase should be monitored routinely in all patients receiving NMBs, and these agents should be avoided whenever possible in severe asthmatics[317] and perhaps in other patients who require systemic glucocorticoids.

Evaluation of weakness in the ICU patient should begin with a detailed neurologic examination including pupillary response; pulmonary function tests (negative inspiratory force, positive expiratory force, and forced vital capacity); and exclusion of cardiac, pulmonary, electrolyte, and endocrine disorders.[191] Other tests may be required[42]: (1) nerve stimulation to exclude residual block; (2) plasma creatine kinase; (3) radiologic examination (computerized tomography or magnetic resonance imaging) to evaluate diseases of the brain, spinal cord, or nerve roots; (4) sensory and motor nerve conduction studies; (5) electromyography (EMG) of the extremities and respiratory system; (6) lumbar puncture; and (7) muscle biopsy. When weakness is the suspected cause of failure to wean from mechanical ventilation, the most specific method to identify a neuromuscular disorder is phrenic nerve conduction and needle EMG of the diaphragm.[223]

Is It Possible to Prevent Persistent Paralysis in Patients Who Receive Nondepolarizing Neuromuscular Blocking Drugs?

The following recommendations should minimize the risk of serious problems following prolonged NMB administration:

1. Optimize analgesia and sedation before administering a NMB. Use a NMB only in circumstances when it is absolutely required.
2. Minimize dose and duration of NMB treatment (preferably < 48 hours).
3. Avoid NMB in patients receiving systemic corticosteroids.
4. Monitor NMB response with a peripheral nerve stimulator and titrate the infusion based on the train-of-four response to maintain at least one or two twitches of the TOF.
5. Allow the patient to wake up every 24 hours (a "drug holiday") to allow assessment of neurologic status and possibly prevent NMB overdosing.
6. Monitor creatine kinase (CK) routinely, and stop the NMB if CK increases.

Absence of diaphragmatic or chest wall motion is an indicator of an adequate degree of paralysis, but this obviously cannot demonstrate drug overdose, accumulation of toxic metabolites, or myopathy. Prolonged muscle weakness may be more common following use of a steroidal NMB (eg, pancuronium or vecuronium), especially when organ dysfunction is likely to cause accumulation of active metabolite. It has been recommended that in all critically ill patients maintained on NMBs, the degree of muscle blockade should be monitored by TOF q4–6h, and the dose of the agent adjusted to maintain one or two twitches at all times.[316] Although TOF monitoring cannot prevent persistent paralysis, it may decrease the incidence of overdosage,[254] shorten the time to full recovery of muscle function,[81] and perhaps reduce the incidence of prolonged paralysis.[166] Even when a nerve stimulator is used to titrate the rate of NMB infusion, this does not guarantee that prolonged paralysis will not occur, as indicated by several reports that describe this complication.[224,234] In addition, adherence to these guidelines will not prevent most instances of weakness in critically ill patients with multiple organ dysfunction syndrome, since the most common cause of weakness in this setting is critical illness polyneuropathy—which is not associated with the use of NDNMB.

What Are the Clinical Effects and Toxicities of Specific Neuromuscular Blocking Agents?

Succinylcholine. Succinylcholine[99] (succinic acid-bis-choline chloride, succinyldicholine, diacetylcholine, suxametho-

TABLE 53–4. NEUROMUSCULAR PATHOLOGY ASSOCIATED WITH CRITICAL ILLNESS AND NMBs

Condition	Incidence	Clinical Feature	Electromyography	Creatine Kinase	Muscle Biopsy
Polyneuropathy					
Critical illness polyneuropathy (CIP)[202]	Common, especially with SIRS/MODS, sepsis, and aminoglycosides	1. Ventilator dependence (100%) 2. Symmetric paralysis LE > UE > face 3. Muscle wasting (21–100%) 4. Absent myotatic reflex (32–100%) 5. Distal sensory neuropathy (0–75%) 6. Absence of pain	Primary axonal sensorimotor polyneuropathy	Near normal	Denervation atrophy, absence of inflammation, normal CSF
Motor neuropathy	Common with NMB	Flaccid tetraplegia and respiratory weakness	Axonal degeneration of motor fibers	Near normal	Denervation atrophy
Neuromuscular Transmission Defect					
Transient neuromuscular blockade, accumulation of drug or its by-product	Common with NMB (especially when combined with other drugs that cause weakness)	Flaccid tetraplegia and respiratory weakness	Abnormal response to repetitive nerve stimulation	Normal	Normal
Myopathy					
Steroid myopathy[182]	Uncommon	Proximal symmetric weakness lower > upper extremity, systemic steroid sequelae	Myopathic changes	Low normal	Atrophy of type IIB fibers
Thick filament (myosin) myopathy[43,80]	Common (associated with glucocorticoids and NDNMBs, also asthma and SIRS)	Severe flaccid tetraplegia and respiratory weakness, intact sensation	Myopathic changes	Increased	Diffuse atrophy, myofibrilar disorganization, selective loss of thick type II filaments, preservation of thin (actin) filaments
Disuse (cachectic) myopathy[191]	Common (?)	Diffuse muscle wasting, reduced muscle mass	Normal	Normal	Normal or type II fiber atrophy
Necrotizing myopathy of intensive care[285,383]	Rare (associated with glucocorticoids and NDNMBs, also severe asthma or sepsis)	Flaccid tetraplegia and myoglobinuria, preserved sensation	Myopathic changes	Severely increased	Panfascicular necrotizing myopathy affecting both fiber types, vacuolation and macrophage invasion, myosin loss, normal mitochondria

LE = lower extremity; MODS = multiple organ dysfunction syndrome; SIRS = systemic inflammatory response; UE = upper extremity.
Adapted, with permission, from Bolton C: Sepsis and the systemic inflammatory response syndrome: neuromuscular manifestations. Crit Care Med 1996;24:1408–1415.

nium) is a bis-quaternary ammonium ion, composed of two ACH molecules attached by their acetate groups. Following a typical IV induction dose (1 mg/kg), intubating conditions are obtained in less than 60 seconds; paralysis usually lasts 3–5 minutes.

Following IV administration, plasma levels of succinylcholine rapidly decline as a result of distribution into the extracellular fluid and neuromuscular junctions; later, the concentration gradient reverses due to rapid enzymatic hydrolysis, and the agent shifts from the NMJ into the plasma.[125] Succinylcholine is metabolized mostly by plasma cholinesterase hydrolysis (true or junctional cholinesterase does not catalyze this reaction), and to a slight extent by alkaline hydrolysis. Succinylcholine is hydrolyzed in a two-step reaction to succinylmonocholine and choline, and then to succinic acid and choline (both of which are products of intermediary metabolism).

Succinylcholine in body fluids or tissues can be detected by gas chromatography or mass spectrometry.[320] Rapid hydrolysis of the parent compound in the plasma may make it difficult to detect the parent compound.[328]

Plasma cholinesterase (MW 300,000) is manufactured in the liver; its half-life is about 11 days.[266] This enzyme is also involved in the metabolism of other drugs including mivacurium, heroin, and ester local anesthetics (cocaine, tetracaine, chloroprocaine, and procaine). The effect of succinylcholine may last for several hours if it cannot be degraded because of the presence of an atypical plasma cholinesterase (incidence 1:2500) or enzyme deficiency or inhibition (eg, from organophosphate intoxication) (Table 53–5). A history of a previously uneventful exposure to succinylcholine excludes the possibility of atypical pseudocholinesterase. The most common atypical plasma cholinesterase (E_1^a) can be assayed by its resistance to inhibition by the local anesthetic dibucaine, although there are different types of atypical cholinesterases.[269] Dibucaine inhibits the ability of normal plasma cholinesterase to hydrolyze benzoylcholine by > 70%, heterozygous atypical by 40–60%, and homozygous atypical enzyme by < 30%. Fresh plasma or pseudocholinesterase concentrate can be infused to hasten recovery in the case of enzyme deficiency, but the simplest treatment is to keep the patient sedated, intubated, and ventilated until the block spontaneously reverses. If enzyme is deficient, inhibited, or unable to hydrolyze substrate, succinylcholine elimination will occur by alkaline hydrolysis, which is a relatively fast process at pH 7.4.[126]

Adverse effects associated with succinylcholine are summarized (Table 53–6). Potentially life-threatening complications are anaphylaxis; hyperkalemia in patients with neuropathy or myopathy; malignant hyperthermia in susceptible patients; and bradycardia from muscarinic stimulation, which is occasionally seen in children during anesthetic induction, especially following large or repeated doses in patients who have not been premedicated with atropine. Severe hyperkalemia may occur in patients with nerve or muscle disease, and rarely in persons without an obvious history of predisposing factors. Because of several reports of acute rhabdomyolysis, hyperkalemic cardiac arrest, and death in apparently healthy children who were subsequently diagnosed with myopathy, a warning now appears in the package insert:

> There have been rare reports of acute rhabdomyolysis with hyperkalemia followed by ventricular dysrhythmias, cardiac arrest and death after the administration of succinylcholine to apparently healthy children who were subsequently found to have undiagnosed skeletal muscle myopathy, most frequently Duchenne's muscular atrophy.
>
> This syndrome often presents as peaked T-waves and sudden cardiac arrest within minutes after the administration of the drug in healthy appearing children (usually, but not exclusively, males, and most frequently 8 years of age or younger). There have also been reports in adolescents.
>
> Therefore, when a healthy appearing infant or child develops cardiac arrest soon after administration of succinylcholine, not felt to be due to inadequate ventilation, oxygenation or anesthetic overdose, immediate treatment for hyperkalemia should be instituted. Due to the abrupt onset of this syndrome, routine resuscitative measures are likely to be unsuccessful. However, extraordinary and prolonged resuscitative efforts have resulted in successful resuscitation in some reported cases. In addition, in the presence of signs of malignant hyperthermia, appropriate treatment should be instituted concurrently.
>
> Since there may be no signs or symptoms to alert the practitioner as to which patients are at risk, it is recommended that the use of succinylcholine in children should be reserved for emergency intubation or instances where immediate securing of the airway is necessary, e.g., laryngospasm, difficult airway, full stomach, or for intramuscular use when a suitable vein is inaccessible.

Succinylcholine is the agent most often implicated as the cause of anaphylaxis during general anesthesia[251] and as the neuromuscular blocker most likely to produce adverse reaction.[366] In 20 of 28 patients with succinylcholine anaphylaxis, immediate circulatory collapse was the *only* manifestation; other more obvious signs such as wheezing and skin rash were notably absent.[381] In addition, more than 50% of these patients had sensitivities to other neuromuscular blockers. Succinylcholine anaphylaxis is 8 times more common in women than in men.

Under light anesthesia, succinylcholine (1 mg/kg IV) may produce an increase in cerebral blood flow, cortical electrical activity, and ICP.[188] When it occurs, these effects are usually modest and can be blunted by deep

TABLE 53–5. ABNORMAL PLASMA CHOLINESTERASE ACTIVITY

Reduced Plasma Cholinesterase Activity
- Decreased quantity of plasma cholinesterase
  - female gender
  - pregnancy, extremes of age
  - liver disease, malignancy, burns, uremia
  - glucocorticoids, estrogens, oral contraceptives
  - alkylating antineoplastic drugs, cyclophosphamide, mechlorethamine
  - plasmapheresis, extracorporeal circulation
- Inhibition of plasma cholinesterase function
  - Irreversible inhibition
    - organophosphates, eg, echothiophate
    - cyclophosphamide, triethylenthiophosphoramine (Thiotepa)
  - Reversible inhibition
    - edrophonium, neostigmine, pyridostigmine, hexafluorinium
    - propranolol, pancuronium, trimethapan, local anesthetics, aprotinin, MAO inhibitors, metoclopramide
    - fluoride, eg, following enflurane or sevoflurane anesthesia
- Atypical plasma cholinesterase
  - E_1^a: able to hydrolyze benzoylcholine, resistant to dibucaine inhibition
  - E_1^f: resistant to fluoride inhibition
  - E_1^s: silent types, little hydrolysis of any substrates

Enhanced Plasma Cholinesterase Activity
- chronic hemodialysis, obesity, hyperlipidemia
- atypical (hyperactive) plasma cholinesterase

Adapted, with permission, from Lee C: Succinylcholine: its past, present, and future. In: Katz R, ed: Muscle Relaxants: Basic and Clinical Aspects. New York: Grune & Stratton, 1984, pp. 69–85.

TABLE 53–6. ADVERSE EFFECTS AND COMPLICATIONS ASSOCIATED WITH SUCCINYLCHOLINE

Complication	Mechanisms and Explanation
Prolonged drug effect	• Homozygous recessive atypical plasma cholinesterase (1:2500)—paralysis may last up to 6 h.[269] • Inadequate production of plasma pseudocholinesterase due to severe liver disease (rare). • Inhibition of normal plasma pseudocholinesterase, eg, anticholinesterases or organophosphates • Phase II block, may occur when 2–8 mg/kg IV succinylcholine given over short time.
Cardiac dysrhythmias due to stimulation of autonomic receptors	• Stimulation of cardiac muscarinic receptors may cause bradycardia, junctional rhythm, and ventricular dysrhythmias. Dysrhythmias more likely when succinylcholine given rapidly, in high dose to nonatropinized pediatric patient. Pretreatment with atropine 15–20 μg/kg inhibits bradycardia.
Hyperkalemia	• Succinylcholine 1 mg/kg IV increases K^+ 0.5 mEq/L in normal patients and in those with renal failure. • Severe hyperkalemia associated with increased extrajunctional muscle acetylcholine receptors due to disease of neuromuscular system (eg, head or spinal cord injury or stroke, neuropathy, muscular dystrophy, thermal burn or cold injury, crush injury, prolonged immobility after prolonged use of a NDNMB, or malignant hyperthermia. Susceptibility to hyperkalemia begins 4–7 days after injury, and may persist indefinitely. Severe hyperkalemia is not prevented by a defasciculating dose of NDNMB.
Increased intracranial pressure (ICP)	• Associated with skeletal muscle fasciculations, there is a volley of skeletal muscle afferent activity, and EEG burst, and ICP may increase. ICP increase blunted by defasciculating dose of NDNMB.
Increased intraocular pressure (IOP)	• The IOP usually increases 5–15 mm Hg after succinylcholine. This is blunted by ensuring deep anesthesia, which prevents coughing and bucking, and by sublingual nifedipine or intravenous opioid. It may also be blunted by defasciculating dose of NDNMB.
Increased intragastric pressure	• Since lower esophageal sphincter pressure is also increased, the gastric barrier pressure gradient (high pressure zone—intragastric pressure) actually increases following succinylcholine.
Myalgias	• May be due to muscle fasciculations. The frequency of myalgias is decreased 30% by prior administration of defasciculating dose of NDNMB.
Rhabdomyolysis and myoglobinuria	• May be caused by muscle fasciculations, sustained muscle contractions, muscular dystrophy, or malignant hyperthermia.
Muscle fasciculations, masseter muscle rigidity, and sustained muscle contractions	• Succinylcholine (1 mg/kg) causes muscle fasciculations, which can be inhibited by giving tubocurarine 3 mg or a small dose of other NDNMB 3–4 min before succinylcholine. • Masseter muscle spasm: may occur in up to 1% of pediatric patients induced with halothane and succinylcholine. It may precede malignant hyperthermia, especially if generalized muscle spasms occur. • With myotonic dystrophy or myotonia congenita, myoclonic spasms after succinylcholine may be severe and make ventilation and/or intubation impossible.
Malignant hyperthermia (MH)	Succinylcholine can trigger MH, especially when combined with a potent fluorinated hydrocarbon (eg, halothane). History of a previous uneventful exposure does not exclude subsequent development of MH. Therapeutic principles include removal of triggering agent, dantrolene sodium (1–10 mg/kg), and treatment of hypoxemia, hypercarbia, hyperthermia, hyperkalemia, and rhabdomyolysis.

Adapted, with permission, from Durant N, Katz R: Suxamethonium. Br J Anaesth 1982;54:195–208.

anesthesia, a small dose of NDNMB, or lidocaine (1.5 mg/kg IV); they were not observed in severely head injured patients more than 3 days following injury.[188]

Nondepolarizing Neuromuscular Blocking Drugs. *Tubocurarine* (see Table 53–7) has an exotic history. Curare is a South American arrow poison derived from the strychnos plant; it was used to paralyze hunted animals. It is unknown why the plant produces this alkaloid. Fortunately for the people who used this toxin, oral ingestion does not cause paralysis. Curare was first used medically by Hunter in 1878 to treat tetanus, and later by West[370] to reduce the muscular rigidity of hemiplegia. The most potent of the curare alkaloids, the toxiferenes, are derived from the bark of the ligneous vine, *Strychnos toxifera*. Tubocurarine is a monoquaternary ammonium with a bulky structure that permits receptor binding but prevents receptor activation.

Tubocurarine does not undergo significant metabolism and is eliminated primarily in the urine. Renal failure thus slows its elimination and prolongs neuromuscular blockade.[238] Poisoning by curariform drugs produces complete skeletal muscle paralysis but does not affect consciousness. Initially there is weakness of the small muscles of the hands, toes, and eyes; then of the face and neck; followed by the extremities; and finally of the intercostals and the diaphragm. In humans, tubocurarine is associated with dose- and rate-dependent histamine release and is best avoided in patients with bronchial asthma. Tubocurarine produces autonomic blockade at clinical doses; this can impair the sympathetic response to surgical stress or hypotension.[47]

Metocurine, produced by methylation of tubocurarine, is twice as potent. Like tubocurarine, it is minimally metabolized and is excreted primarily in the urine.[226] Elimination is thus also impaired in patients with renal insufficiency. Histamine release is half that of tubocurarine, and it produces mild autonomic blockade at clinical doses. The drug, prepared as the iodide, may cause hypersensitivity in patients with seafood or shellfish allergy.

Doxacurium is a highly potent, long-acting NMB devoid of histamine-releasing effects and thus does not

TABLE 53–7. PHARMACOLOGY OF SELECTED NONDEPOLARIZING NMB DRUGS

	Benzylisoquinolinium Derivatives					
	Tubocurarine (Curare)	*Metocurine (Metubine)*	*Atracurium (Tracrium)*	*Doxacurium (Nuromax)*	*Mivacurium (Mivacron)*	*cis-Atracurium (Nimbex)*
Introduced	1942	1952	1983	1991	1992	1996
ED_{95} dose (mg/kg)	0.51	0.3	0.25	0.025–0.030	0.075	0.050
"Initial" dose (mg/kg)	0.2–0.3	0.3–0.35	0.4–0.5	up to 0.1	0.15–0.25	0.1–0.2
Duration (min)	80	70–90	25–35	120–150	10–20	22–30
Infusion dose (μg/kg/min)			4–12		9–10	
Recovery (min)	80–180	90–180	40–60	120–180	10–20	
% renal excretion	40–45	45–55	5–10	70		
Effect in renal failure	↑	↑	No change	↑ to ↑↑	↑ duration	
% biliary excretion	10–40	2	Minimal	Unclear		
Effect in hepatic failure	Minimal to mild ↑	No effect	Minimal to none	?	↑ duration	
Active metabolites	None	None	None, but laudanosine	?	Minimal	None, but laudanosine
Histamine release hypotension	Marked	Moderate	Minimal	None	None	None
Vagal block tachycardia	Minimal	Minimal	None	None	None	None
Ganglionic block hypotension	Marked	Modest	Minimal to none	None	None	None
Prolonged block reported	None	Yes	Yes	Yes	None	None

	Aminosteroid Derivatives			
	Pancuronium (Pavulon)	*Vecuronium (Norcuron)*	*Pipecuronium (Arduan)*	*Rocuronium (Zemuron)*
Introduced	1972	1984	1991	1994
ED_{95} dose (mg/kg)	0.07	0.05	0.05	0.3
"Initial" dose (mg/kg)	0.1	0.1	0.085–0.1	0.6–1.0
Duration (min)	90–100	35–45	90–100	30
Infusion dose (μg/kg/min)	1–2	1–2	0.5–2.0	10–12
Recovery (min)	120–180	45–60	55–160	20–30
% renal excretion	45–70	50	50+	33
Effect in renal failure	↑ to ↑↑, especially metabolites	↑, especially metabolites	↑ duration	Minimal effect
% biliary excretion	10–15	35–50	Minimal	<75%
Effect in hepatic failure	Mild ↑	Mild ↑	Minimal	Moderate ↑
Active metabolites	3-OH- and 17-OH-pancuronium	3-desacetyl-vecuronium	None reported	None reported
Histamine release hypotension	None	None	None	None
Vagal block tachycardia	Modest to marked	None	None	Some at high doses
Ganglionic block hypotension	None	None	None	None
Prolonged block reported	Yes	Yes	None	None

Adapted, with permission, from Coursin DB, Prielipp RC: Use of neuromuscular blocking drugs in the critically ill patient. Crit Care Clin North Am, 1995;11:957–981.

alter heart rate or blood pressure.[29] It is minimally hydrolyzed by plasma cholinesterase and is eliminated mostly in the urine. Drug elimination and pharmacologic effect are prolonged in renal insufficiency.

Atracurium is a mixture of 10 stereoisomers that possess different pharmacokinetic behaviors. Atracurium is rapidly metabolized by spontaneous nonenzymatic elimination at a rate determined by temperature and pH, and by ester hydrolysis. The latter is catalyzed by nonspecific plasma esterases, distinct from the plasma cholinesterases that hydrolyse succinylcholine. Drug elimination is independent of renal and hepatic function; however, it is prolonged during hypothermia or acidemia. Less than 10% of an administered dose of atracurium is eliminated unchanged in the urine or bile.

When metabolized, each atracurium molecule generates two molecules of laudanosine and an acrylate moiety, neither of which possesses neuromuscular blocking activity.[258] Laudanosine is excreted in the urine and bile; its elimination is prolonged in renal insufficiency, biliary obstruction, or cirrhosis.[272] Laudanosine crosses the blood–brain barrier[107] and, at high plasma concentrations, causes neuroexcitation and seizures in mice, rats, and dogs.[59] In humans, the toxic plasma laudanosine concentration is unknown and seizures directly attributable to atracurium have not been observed, even following prolonged drug infusion in the ICU.[380] Atracurium produces dose- and rate-related histamine release. Unintentional overdose in a neonate was associated with flushing, hypotension, bronchospasm, and tachycardia, presumably due to histamine release.[101]

cis-Atracurium is a purified atracurium isomer that retains the advantage of organ-independent elimination. It is degraded in the plasma by pH- and temperature-dependent Hofmann elimination but is not hydrolyzed by plasma esterases. *cis*-Atracurium is an improvement on the parent drug; it is three times more potent and does not produce histamine release or any significant cardiovascular effects.[206,309] *cis*-Atracurium degrades to form laudanosine and a monoquaternary acrylate, and the latter product is metabolized further in the plasma. *cis*-Atracurium is associated with lower plasma laudanosine levels than the parent compound.[108] At clinically relevant doses, *cis*-atracurium does not cause release of histamine and does not produce any significant cardiovascular effects.[206] Drug elimination is not altered by liver or kidney failure, or following prolonged infusions in ICU patients.[169]

Mivacurium is composed of an unequal mixture of three stereoisomers; the two more abundant are also the most potent, and they are rapidly hydrolyzed by plasma cholinesterase.[306] Mivacurium is a short-acting drug, and recovery is twice as fast as that observed following atracurium. Prolonged block has been observed in persons with pseudocholinesterase deficiency. In patients with atypical cholinesterase, the duration of effect is increased to 10–40 minutes in heterozygotes and up to 3–4 hours in homozygotes.[306] Pancuronium given before mivacurium speeds the onset of activity and markedly prolongs its duration of action, probably as a result of inhibition of plasma cholinesterase by pancuronium (see below) or synergistic effects of the two agents.[50]

Pancuronium is a synthetic bis-quaternary aminosteroid drug that is the prototype agent in its class. About 60% of the drug is excreted unchanged in the urine and about 20% is metabolized. Since all aminosteroid drugs undergo some degree of deacetylation in the liver (especially pancuronium and vecuronium), clearance may be slowed and its effect prolonged in hepatic insufficiency. Some of its metabolites are excreted in the urine and bile. The 3-OH-pancuronium metabolite retains 50% of the NMB activity of the parent drug[237] and accumulates in patients with renal failure.[357] Because the aminosteroid drugs undergo substantial biliary excretion (rocuronium > vecuronium > pancuronium > pipecuronium), their clearance is prolonged when this function is impaired.[168] Pancuronium is the only commonly used NMB drug that increases heart rate and arterial blood pressure; this is attributed to a selective cardiac antimuscarinic (atropine-like) action,[307] to an indirect norepinephrine-releasing effect on postganglionic fibers, and perhaps to block of presynaptic muscarinic receptors at the sympathetic nerve terminals.[314] In patients under general anesthesia, pancuronium 0.08–0.1 mg/kg IV caused an increase in heart rate, blood pressure, and cardiac output.[330] Combining pancuronium with halothane in patients receiving chronic tricyclic antidepressant therapy is associated with tachycardia and ventricular dysrhythmias.[110] At clinically relevant doses, pancuronium inhibits normal plasma cholinesterase and, to a lesser extent, atypical plasma cholinesterase, and slows the metabolism of drugs inactivated by this enzyme: succinylcholine, mivacurium, and procaine.[47]

Vecuronium is derived from pancuronium (it lacks one methyl group) and its potency is similar. The structural alteration eliminates the tachycardia and hypertension observed following pancuronium. Vecuronium does not cause clinically significant histamine release or cardiovascular or autonomic side effects.[249] About 10–25% of the agent is excreted in the urine within 24 hours. The drug is rapidly taken up by the liver and excreted in the bile.[33] Vecuronium elimination follows zero-order kinetics.[141] In patients with cholestasis[199] or cirrhosis,[198] slowed elimination may prolong the effect of vecuronium. One third of vecuronium is desacetylated in the liver to 3-desacetyl-, 17-desacetyl-, and 3,17-desacetylvecuronium. These metabolites are renally excreted. The 3-desacetylvecuronium metabolite has 80% of the neuromuscular blocking potency of the parent compound,[55] and it may accumulate in the presence of renal impairment, especially after repeated dosing.[376] In another study, persistent paralysis was observed in 7 of 16 critically ill patients paralyzed with vecuronium for at least 2 days.[315] Paralysis lasted for 6 hours to > 7 days, and was associated with elevated levels of 3-desacetylvecuronium, creatinine clearance < 30 mL/min, metabolic acidosis, female gender, and elevated plasma magnesium.[315] Because vecuronium is devoid of cardiovascular side effects, it is usually ideal for patients with cardiac disease. However, the agent has been associated with significant bradydysrhythmias and even asystole[184] when associated with vagal stimulation, absence of painful stimulation, and concurrent use of fentanyl, sufentanil, etomidate, or propofol.[171]

Pipecuronium is a long-acting analog of pancuronium with minimal hemodynamic and autonomic effects. It produces a block of long duration. The hepatic 3-desacetyl metabolites are excreted in the urine.

Rocuronium is an aminosteroid drug that produces the fastest intubating conditions of all the NDNMBs, approaching those of succinylcholine. In fact, rocuronium may be substituted for succinylcholine when rapid onset is required, for instance, in rapid-sequence inductions when succinylcholine is contraindicated. Rocuronium is eliminated mostly in the liver and bile, and to a lesser extent by the kidneys. The drug is minimally metabolized by the liver and has no active metabolites. Hepatic dysfunction increases the volume of distribution and elimination half-life, but does not affect plasma clearance.[222] This may result in prolonged drug effect in patients with liver disease, especially following prolonged administration. Its effect is not prolonged by renal insufficiency. Rocuronium is associated with a slight increase in heart rate and stroke volume but does not produce histamine release.[230]

What Are the Complications of Reversal of Nondepolarizing Neuromuscular Blocking Agents?

Reversal of NMB block depends on drug redistribution, degradation, metabolism, and/or elimination. Neuromuscular block by NDNMB can be pharmacologically reversed by acetylcholinesterase inhibitors (anticholinesterases), which inhibit both plasma and junctional cholinesterase at nicotinic and muscarinic receptors. The resultant increase in ACH concentration at the NMJ competitively reverses the effects of an NDNMB.

The goal of NMB reversal is to maximize the nicotinic (neuromuscular junctional) effect while minimizing muscarinic (ganglionic) side effects. This is accomplished by administering an antimuscarinic agent. The commonly used acetylcholinesterase inhibitors are neostigmine, pyridostigmine, and edrophonium; these are given in combination with the antimuscarinic agents glycopyrrolate or atropine. Since an increase or decrease in muscarinic effect leads to bradycardia or tachycardia, it is best to combine drugs with similar rates of onset. The rapid-acting agents edrophonium and atropine are generally administered together, as are the slower acting neostigmine or pyridostigmine and glycopyrrolate (Table 53–8). Reversal of neuromuscular blockade should be attempted only when at least one twitch is present on TOF testing.

In addition to their effects at the NMJ, cholinesterase inhibitors inhibit plasma acetylcholinesterase, and for this reason prolong the effects of drugs metabolized by this enzyme, such as succinylcholine and ester local anesthetics. Acetylcholinesterase inhibitors are primarily eliminated by the kidneys; in renal failure, their elimination is slowed more than that of most NDNMBs, so that delayed "recurarization" is unlikely.

Residual neuromuscular blocking effect is an important cause of weakness in the postanesthesia care unit; the reported incidence is 30–42% following long-acting muscle NMBs, but less than 10% when atracurium or vecuronium had been used to maintain muscle paralysis.[37] Postanesthetic death is a rare event; however, postoperative respiratory insufficiency is an important cause, and residual paralysis often plays a significant role in these events.

It should be possible in most situations to limit the incidence of postextubation complications in patients who have received muscle relaxants, if standard criteria for extubation are rigidly adhered to. It should be noted that an overdose of acetylcholinesterase inhibitors may actually cause muscular weakness.[16] Administration of

TABLE 53–8. PHARMACOLOGY OF INTRAVENOUS NEUROMUSCULAR BLOCK REVERSAL AGENTS

	Acetylcholinesterase Inhibitors		
	Neostigmine	*Pyridostigmine*	*Edrophonium*
Structure	Quaternary ammonium	Quaternary ammonium	Quaternary ammonium
"Initial" dose (mg/kg)	0.040–0.080	0.2–0.4	0.5–1.0
Onset (min)	7–11	10–16	1–2
Duration (min)	60–120	60–120	60–120
Recommended antimuscarinic	Glycopyrrolate	Glycopyrrolate	Atropine
% renal excretion	50	75	70
% metabolism in renal failure	50	25	30

	Antimuscarinics	
	Glycopyrrolate	*Atropine*
Structure	Quaternary ammonium	Tertiary amine
"Initial" dose (mg/kg)	0.01–0.02	0.02–0.03
Onset (min)	2–3	1
Duration (min)	30–60	30–60
Elimination	Renal	Renal
Other	Does not cross BBB,[a] minimal CNS effects	Can cross BBB and cause CNS excitation

[a]BBB = blood–brain barrier

Reprinted, with permission, from Bevan D, Donati F, Kopman A: Reversal of neuromuscular blockade. Anesthesiology 1992;77:785–805.

neostigmine in the presence of preexisting respiratory acidosis inhibits its effects; acidosis should be corrected by improving ventilation before administering the reversal agent.

The most common and troublesome clinical side effect of acetylcholinesterase inhibition is bradycardia, which is usually prevented by co-administration of an antimuscarinic drug.[77] Bradydysrhythmias may be severe and lead to nodal or ventricular rhythms, or even asystole. These problems may be more common in patients with preexisting bradycardias or those receiving chronic beta-adrenergic antagonist therapy and are not necessarily prevented by prior administration of atropine.[324] Other side effects may result from excess acetylcholinesterase inhibition (salivation, bronchospasm, increased bronchial secretions and intestinal peristaltic activity, miosis, tearing, and increased bladder tone) or excess antimuscarinic effect (tachycardia, bronchodilation, pupillary dilatation, and increased intraocular pressure). Following general anesthesia, use of anticholinesterases may increase the incidence of nausea, vomiting, and abdominal cramps.[183]

Since atropine crosses the blood–brain barrier, it can produce a central anticholinergic syndrome: dry mouth, fever, tachycardia, pupillary dilatation, increased peristaltic activity, and CNS excitation ranging from agitation and hallucinations to coma. This is treated by withdrawal of the agent, hydration, and physostigmine. Physostigmine is a cholinesterase inhibitor that readily crosses the blood–brain barrier (see Antidotes in Depth: Physostigmine).

Local Anesthetics

Clinically useful local anesthetic agents fall into one of two chemically distinct groups: (1) amino esters, which possess an ester link between the aromatic portion and the intermediate chain, and (2) amino amides, which possess an amide link (Table 53–9). In general, if a local anesthetic has the letter "i" within the first four letters of its name, the agent is an amide, and if not, it is an ester. The amino esters are primarily metabolized by plasma cholinesterase, and the amino amides are metabolized in the liver. Factors that decrease hepatic blood flow or hepatic function increase the risk of toxic reactions to the amino amides and make management of serious reactions more difficult.

TABLE 53–9. CLASSIFICATION OF LOCAL ANESTHETICS

Amino Esters	Amino Amides
Procaine	Lidocaine
Chloroprocaine	Mepivacaine
Tetracaine	Prilocaine
Cocaine	Etidocaine
Benzocaine	Ropivacaine

TABLE 53–10. DIFFERENTIAL DIAGNOSIS OF LOCAL ANESTHETIC REACTIONS

Etiology	Major Clinical Feature
Local anesthetic toxicity	
Intravascular injection	Immediate seizure and/or cardiac toxicity
Relative overdose	Delayed onset (5–15 min), neurologic toxicity
Reaction to catecholamine	Tachycardia, hypertension, headache
Vasovagal reaction	Rapid onset, bradycardia, hypotension, pallor
Allergic reaction	Anaphylaxis, urticaria
High spinal or epidural block	Bradycardia, hypotension, respiratory distress, respiratory arrest

The various local anesthetic agents differ in their potency, duration of action, and degree of effects on sensory and motor fibers. The discussion will be limited primarily to the toxic effects of lidocaine and bupivacaine, which can serve as models for the systemic toxic effects of all of the local anesthetics except cocaine, which is discussed in Chapter 65.

What Is the Differential Diagnosis of a Systemic Toxic Reaction to a Local Anesthetic?

The differential diagnosis of local anesthetic toxic reactions include the effects of catecholamines, which are often added to the anesthetic to delay absorption (usually epinephrine), vasovagal or allergic reactions, high spinal or epidural block, or a CNS or cardiovascular event related to the patient's underlying medical condition (eg, acute myocardial infarction). The clinical features that can help differentiate these possible etiologies are summarized in Table 53–10.

What Are the Systemic Manifestations of Local Anesthetic Toxicity?

Local anesthetics are relatively free of side effects if administered in an appropriate dose and anatomic location. The toxic effects of local anesthetic agents include systemic complications, allergic reactions, and miscellaneous effects of specific drugs, such as the development of methemoglobinemia after the use of prilocaine.[216]

Local anesthetics act by inhibiting membrane conductance of sodium ions and thereby blocking impulse conduction in nerves. Similar effects are seen in other conductive tissues, especially the heart and brain; thus, systemic toxicity usually affects the central nervous and cardiovascular systems. The most common causes of adverse reactions to local anesthetics are unintentional direct intravascular injection (either intravenous or intra-arterial), relative overdose, and inadvertent spinal or epidural administration.

Intravascular injection leads to immediate seizures and/or cardiac dysrhythmias. Seizures may follow even a small dose injected into the vertebral or carotid artery (as may occur during stellate ganglion block).[189] A relative overdose produces a slower onset of symptoms (usually within 5–15 minutes of drug injection), with irritability progressing to seizures.

Systemic toxicity in humans usually involves the CNS. Local anesthetic–induced cardiac toxicity occurs less frequently, but is usually more serious and more difficult to manage. Toxic effects correlate with plasma concentrations. Animal studies and clinical observations demonstrate that CNS toxicity develops at a lower plasma concentration of local anesthetic than is needed to produce cardiac toxicity.[85]

Considering the large number of local anesthetics administered, the frequency of clinically significant toxic reactions is quite low. In a large series of patients receiving bupivacaine, systemic toxicity occurred in only 15 of 11,080 nerve blocks.[245] Of these patients 80% convulsed, whereas 20% had milder symptoms. Although no cardiovascular toxicity was reported in this series, other studies document the potential cardiac toxicity of bupivacaine.[82,212]

What Are the Toxic Effects of Lidocaine on the CNS?

A gradually increasing blood level of lidocaine produces a common pattern of symptoms and signs. In the awake patient, the initial symptoms are subjective and include tinnitus, lightheadedness, circumoral numbness, disorientation, confusion, auditory and visual disturbances, and lethargy. Objective signs then develop, which are usually excitatory, and include shivering, tremors, and ultimately general tonic-clonic seizures. At even higher blood levels depression develops, associated with coma, apnea, and cardiovascular depression. Rapid intravascular injection of lidocaine may produce a brief excitatory phase followed by generalized CNS depression with respiratory arrest.

The mechanism of the initial CNS excitation involves a selective block of cortical cerebral inhibitory pathways.[339] The resulting increase in unopposed excitatory activity leads to seizures. As the blood level rises further, both inhibitory and excitatory neurons are blocked and generalized CNS depression ensues.

There is a linear relationship between local anesthetic potency and CNS toxicity; however, several other factors influence the CNS effects, including the rate of injection (rapid infusion results in a higher blood level and a smaller dose necessary to produce toxicity), drug interactions (sedatives may be protective), and acid–base status. The convulsive threshold of various local anesthetics is inversely related to the arterial PCO_2.[114] Hypercarbia may lower seizure threshold by several mechanisms: (1) increased cerebral blood flow, which increases drug delivery to the CNS; (2) increased conversion of the drug base to the active cation in the presence of decreased intracellular pH; and (3) decreased plasma protein binding, which increases the amount of free drug available for diffusion into the brain.[53,86]

These factors make it difficult to establish maximal safe doses of local anesthetics. Estimates of the toxic doses of various local anesthetics are summarized in Table 53–11.

TABLE 53–11. TOXIC DOSES OF LOCAL ANESTHETICS

Local Anesthetic	Minimum IV Toxic Dose of Local Anesthetic in Humans (mg/kg)
Procaine	19.2
Chloroprocaine	22.8
Tetracaine	2.5
Lidocaine	6.4
Mepivacaine	9.8
Bupivacaine	1.6
Etidocaine	3.4

Adapted, with permission, from Durrani Z, Winnie AP: Brainstem toxicity with reversible locked-in syndrome after intrascalene brachial plexus block. Anesth Analg 1991;72:249–252.

Another factor that creates difficulty in specifying the minimal toxic plasma level of lidocaine results from the fact that its *N*-dealkylated metabolites are pharmacologically active. Subjective side effects are seen at plasma levels between 3 and 6 μg/mL, objective CNS toxicity is usually evident at levels between 5 and 9 μg/mL, seizures may occur at levels above 10 μg/mL, while higher levels produce coma and cardiovascular collapse (see Chap. 52).

How Should Local Anesthetic CNS Toxicity Be Treated?

The treatment of CNS complications is controversial since there are no specific antidotes. At the first sign of possible CNS toxicity, administration of the agent should be stopped. One hundred percent oxygen should be supplied immediately and ventilation should be supported if necessary. Minor symptoms usually do not require treatment provided that adequate respiratory and cardiovascular function are maintained. The patient must be followed closely so that progression to more severe effects can be detected quickly.

Although most seizures caused by local anesthetics are self-limited, they should be treated quickly since the hypoxia and respiratory and metabolic acidosis produced by prolonged convulsions may increase both CNS and cardiovascular toxicity.[246,248] Barbiturates and benzodiazepines have been used for treatment of local anesthetic–induced seizures. Thiopental can rapidly terminate a seizure and acts more quickly than any benzodiazepine, but any of these agents can exacerbate circulatory and respiratory depression.[84,243] Propofol, 1 mg/kg IV, was as effective as thiopental, 2 mg/kg IV, in stopping bupivacaine-induced seizures in rats and has been used successfully in a patient with uncontrolled muscle twitching secondary to local aesthetic toxicity.[40,155]

Succinylcholine may also have an adjunctive role in the treatment of local anesthetic seizures. Although it does not suppress seizure activity in the brain, it rapidly blocks muscular activity and thereby decreases lactic acid production. Succinylcholine also permits intubation and artificial ventilation, which are essential for treating hypoxia and acidosis.[244]

The cardiovascular system must be monitored closely, because cardiovascular depression may go unnoticed while the seizures are being treated. Since local anesthetic–induced hypotension results from both peripheral vasodilation and myocardial depression, alpha- and beta-adrenergic agonists should be used to treat hypotension. Atropine should be used to treat bradycardia.

What Are the Toxic Effects of Local Anesthetics on the Cardiovascular System?

Cardiovascular toxicity is the most feared complication of bupivacaine administration and is usually seen following a sudden increase in the plasma concentration, as in unintentional intravascular injection. Cardiovascular toxicity is rare in other circumstances, since a large dose of the drug is necessary to produce this effect, and also because CNS toxicity precedes cardiovascular events and thus provides a warning. Animal studies have compared the dosage or plasma levels of local anesthetics required to produce irreversible circulatory collapse to those necessary to produce seizures.[247,248] This cardiovascular collapse/central nervous system toxicity ratio (CC/CNS) is approximately 7 for lidocaine; therefore, CNS toxicity should become evident well before potentially cardiotoxic levels are reached. In contrast, the CC/CNS ratio for bupivacaine is 3.7. The electrophysiologic toxicity of bupivacaine is approximately 16 times greater than that of lidocaine.[290] Cardiac events induced by this agent include cardiovascular collapse, bradycardia, atrioventricular and intraventricular blocks, and ventricular dysrhythmias that are often refractory to treatment and may be fatal.

During the late 1970s and early 1980s a series of cases was described in which the use of bupivacaine, particularly in 0.75% concentration, was associated with the development of severe cardiovascular depression, ventricular dysrhythmias, and even death. Pregnant women were disproportionately affected. Some of these cases required prolonged and difficult resuscitation.[290] In 1983, 49 incidents of cardiac arrest or ventricular tachycardia occurring over a 10-year period were presented to the U.S. Food and Drug Administration's Anesthetic and Life Support Advisory Committee. Of these cases, 0.75% bupivacaine was used in 27 obstetric patients with 10 deaths, and 8 followed the use of 0.5% bupivacaine in obstetric patients, with 6 deaths. In nonobstetric patients there were only 14 cases, of whom 5 died. The overall mortality was 21/49 (43%). Partly as a result of these reports, in 1984 the U.S. Food and Drug Administration withdrew approval of bupivacaine 0.75% for obstetric anesthesia.[290]

In vivo and in vitro studies indicate that bupivacaine is more cardiotoxic than other local anesthetics such as lidocaine, and that the toxic blood concentration is lower in pregnant animals than in nonpregnant animals.[247] Both drugs depress the maximum rate of increase of the cardiac action potential (V_{max}) by blocking cardiac sodium channels. Lidocaine binds to both open and inactive channels and dissociates from the channels rapidly after an action potential. Bupivacaine, on the other hand, binds only to inactivated channels and dissociates much more slowly (fast in, slow out).[62] These differences may be fundamental to the relative cardiotoxicity of bupivacaine compared to lidocaine.

The slowing of the action potential in the cardiac conduction system prolongs the PR, QRS, and QT intervals and thereby increases the likelihood of reentrant tachycardia, which may be either ventricular or supraventricular with aberrant conduction. Bupivacaine may also produce dysrhythmias by blockade of GABAergic neurons that tonically inhibit the autonomic nervous system.[36]

In addition to its other effects on the heart, bupivacaine may induce a marked decrease in cardiac contractility by alteration of Ca^{2+} release from sarcoplasmic reticulum.[218] This negative inotropic effect may contribute to the cardiovascular collapse seen in bupivacaine cardiac toxicity.

Ropivacaine is a recently available long-acting amide-type local anesthetic that appears to produce less depression of cardiac conductivity in animal models than equipotent amounts of bupivacaine. Whether this new agent will replace bupivacaine in popularity remains to be seen.[119]

Lidocaine at high plasma levels also produces cardiac toxicity. Blockade of fast sodium channels depresses myocardial automaticity, slows cardiac conduction, decreases the rate of spontaneous depolarization, and thereby increases both PR interval and QRS duration. At progressively higher levels, hypotension, sinus arrest with junctional rhythm, and eventually cardiac arrest occur.[20] Asystole has been described in patients who received unintentional intravenous bolus injections of 800–1000 mg of lidocaine.[20,123] Cardiac toxicity is not usually observed in humans until the plasma lidocaine level greatly exceeds 10 μg/mL unless the patient is also receiving medications that depress sinus and AV nodal conduction (calcium channel or beta-adrenergic antagonists).[377]

How Should Local Anesthetic–Induced Cardiac Toxicity Be Treated?

The treatment of the cardiovascular complications of local anesthetics is controversial. The ACLS protocol should be followed initially, as prompt support of ventilation and circulation will limit hypoxia and acidosis, both of which enhance the cardiac toxicity of local anesthetics.[45,296] The effectiveness of epinephrine in reversing local anesthetic–induced cardiac depression has been inconsistent in various animal models. The dysrhythmic effects of epinephrine are of particular concern. Amrinone, a phosphodiesterase fraction III inhibitor, has been evaluated for the treatment of bupivacaine-induced cardiac toxicity.[132,210] Amrinone reduces cAMP degradation and permits increased concentrations of this second messenger to increase intracellular Ca^{2+} availability and thus reverse the cardiodepressant effects of bupivacaine. Amrinone also opens cellular Ca^{2+} channels and thus compensates in part for the local anesthetic blockade of Na^+ channels.[210] Anesthetized pigs with cardiovascular collapse induced by bupivacaine infusion survived when treated with amrinone; all of the control animals died of irreversible cardiac arrest.[210]

Bupivacaine-induced dysrhythmias are often refractory to cardioversion, defibrillation, and pharmacologic treatment. Lidocaine, phenytoin, magnesium, bretylium, amiodarone, calcium channel blockers, and combined therapy with clonidine and dobutamine have all been used in animal models, with variable results.[87,225,227] Therapy for bupivacaine toxicity should be directed toward dissociating bupivacaine from the myocardial sodium channel, reversing the effects of the drug on cardiac conduction. Lidocaine competes with bupivacaine for cardiac sodium channels, and at high doses may displace it. Anecdotal reports suggest that lidocaine on occasion has helped in this application.[82] However, concern persists about additive CNS effects when lidocaine is used to treat bupivacaine cardiac toxicity.

Bretylium has been used successfully in some, but not all, animal models of bupivacaine cardiac toxicity.[177,178] The use of bretylium has several theoretical advantages for the treatment of this complication: (1) it does not slow conduction; (2) it does not exhibit CNS toxicity, unlike lidocaine, whose CNS affects are additive to those of bupivacaine; and (3) it produces norepinephrine release, which can help overcome some of the depressant effects of bupivacaine on cardiac output, stroke volume, and heart rate.[177] The benefits of this drug need to be established in humans.

The successful treatment of bupivacaine-induced cardiac dysrhythmias with phenytoin has been described in two full-term newborns after other therapies, including bretylium, had failed.[227] Phenytoin has direct cardiac effects similar to lidocaine, but it also blocks cardiac calcium channels and modulates the autonomic control centers in the brain.

Cardiac resuscitation would be expected to be difficult and prolonged (often for greater than 45 minutes) to allow for redistribution and metabolism of bupivacaine or etidocaine, another potent, highly lipid-soluble, protein-bound amide local anesthetic.[9,282] Vital organ perfusion is often seriously compromised despite optimal chest compression. Rapid initiation of cardiopulmonary bypass should be considered if practical; its use has resulted in a successful outcome in some cases of lidocaine overdose.[131,212] Cardiopulmonary bypass provides circulatory support that is far superior to closed chest cardiac massage. The improved perfusion prevents tissue hypoxia and the development of metabolic acidosis and, in turn, decreases the binding of local anesthetics to myocardial sodium channel receptors. Hepatic blood flow is also better maintained, enhancing local anesthetic metabolism, and increased myocardial blood flow helps redistribute local anesthetics out of the myocardium.[212]

Cardiac pacing was used successfully for treatment of cardiac arrest following unintentional administration of a 2-g bolus of lidocaine into a cardiopulmonary bypass circuit as the patient was being removed from bypass.[259] Pharmacologic therapy was unsuccessful and bypass had to be resumed. Forty-five minutes after the injection, atrioventricular pacing restored the cardiac output and permitted discontinuation of support.

What Local Anesthetics Can Be Used in Patients With Local Anesthetic Allergy?

Allergic reactions to local anesthetics are extremely rare. When hydrolyzed, the amino ester local anesthetics produce para-aminobenzoic acid (PABA), a known allergen. Allergic reactions to this group of agents occur more frequently than to amino amides such as lidocaine or bupivacaine. Cross-sensitivity to amino ester anesthetics is common. Some commercial preparations of amino amides contain the preservative methylparaben, which is chemically related to PABA and is the most likely cause of allergic reactions to amino amides. Thus preservative-free amino amides including lidocaine can be used safely in patients who have had reactions to drug preparations containing methylparaben, unless the patient is specifically sensitive to lidocaine.

How Does Prilocaine Produce Methemoglobinemia?

Prilocaine is an amino ester local anesthetic primarily used in obstetric anesthesia because of its rapid onset of action and low systemic toxicity in both mother and fetus. Use of large doses of prilocaine can lead to the development of methemoglobinemia.[216] Prilocaine is an aniline derivative that, when metabolized in the liver, produces *ortho*-toluidine, which may oxidize hemoglobin to methemoglobin.[161] A direct relationship exists between the amount of epidural prilocaine administered and the incidence of methemoglobinemia. A dose greater than approximately 8 mg/kg is generally necessary to produce symptoms, which may not become apparent until several hours after epidural administration of the drug. If necessary, the patient should be treated with intravenous methylene blue (see Chap. 93 and Antidotes in Depth: Methylene Blue). Lidocaine is also a known precipitant of methemoglobin formation.

Topical local anesthetics such as benzocaine can precipitate methemoglobinemia but will not be discussed here.

Malignant Hyperthermia

Malignant hyperthermia (MH) is a genetic disease with autosomal-dominant inheritance involving muscle hypermetabolism associated with an increase in myoplasmic calcium triggered by exposure to certain anesthetic agents.[220] The incidence of MH is about 1:15,000 in children and 1:50,000 in adults. In humans, a defective protein associated with MH was found in the sarcoplasmic calcium release channel (ryanodine-1 receptor, RYR1) in fast- and slow-twitch skeletal muscle.[219] A different gene on chromosome 1, RYR2, codes for the same receptor in cardiac muscle and brain. Several different mutations of RYR1 have been associated with MH. Prior to receiving general anesthesia, patients should be asked about any family history of MH, muscle disease (Duchenne dystrophy, central core disease, or myotonia), or previous problems with anesthesia (eg, perioperative high fever or unexplained death of a family member). However, in a review of MH, it was found that 75.9% of patients had no family history and 20.9% had an uneventful previous anesthetic.[332]

In all anesthetizing locations, staff should be familiar with the treatment of acute MH (Table 53–12), and dantrolene should be immediately available. Before the discovery of dantrolene, the mortality rate from MH was 80%. It resulted from cardiac arrest, dysrhythmias, brain damage, hemorrhage, or multiple organ failure. When patients are treated immediately with dantrolene, volume resuscitation, active cooling, control of hyperkalemia, and supportive care, the mortality from acute MH is under 7%. Therefore, the most important aspects of therapy are rapid initial diagnosis and immediate therapy (within minutes) with dantrolene. Even if delayed for hours or days, dantrolene may still improve survival following acute MH.

The agents that most commonly trigger MH are succinylcholine and all of the potent volatile inhalation anesthetics. NMBs, propofol, ketamine, etomidate, nitrous oxide, benzodiazepines, opioids, barbiturates, and local anesthetics may be safely administered. The manifestations of MH result from hypermetabolism following uncontrolled calcium release from the sarcoplasmic reticulum. This produces muscle contractures, while continuous calcium reuptake by sarcoplasmic Ca-ATPase causes depletion of cellular ATP, excess oxygen consumption and CO_2 production, venous oxygen desaturation and hypercarbia, anaerobic metabolism, generation of lactic acid, and excess heat production.[156] In addition, potassium release from muscle cells may cause life-threatening hyperkalemia, while skeletal myonecrosis causes myoglobin release and renal damage. An abrupt and otherwise unexplained increase in the end-tidal CO_2 is the most sensitive clinical sign of MH. Signs of MH include fever, total-body rigidity, tachycardia, tachypnea, and jaw-muscle rigidity. In contrast to what its name suggests, hyperthermia is actually a late sign of MH. Sudden cardiac arrest, especially immediately following succinylcholine, should be treated as hyperkalemia; and if there is fever, muscle rigidity, or acidosis, dantrolene should also be given.

By partially blocking the release of sarcoplasmic calcium, dantrolene rapidly reverses the signs and symptoms of hypermetabolism: fever, mottled skin, dysrhythmias, muscle rigidity, tachycardia, metabolic acidosis, and hypercapnia. In acute MH, significant dysrhythmias may be treated with standard antidysrhythmic agents; however, calcium entry blockers should *not* be given with dantrolene as they may cause hyperkalemia and severe cardiac depression.[302]

What Are the Indications and Pharmacology of Dantrolene Sodium?

Dantrolene is a hydantoin derivative. It is structurally similar to local anesthetics and anticonvulsants but possesses none of their properties.[365] It inhibits release of calcium from skeletal muscle sarcoplasmic reticulum, dissociating excitation–contraction coupling. Dantrolene has little effect on cardiac and smooth muscle.[356] Its most important use is as therapy for acute malignant hyperthermia.

Indications. Dantrolene has been used to treat the two hyperthermia syndromes believed to be of peripheral etiology, malignant hyperthermia (MH) and thyrotoxicosis. It may be used prophylactically prior to general anesthesia in patients with known MH susceptibility—those with a previous episode of MH after general anesthetic. Dantrolene administration may be considered in the patient with severe hyperthermia, when the diagnosis of MH cannot be excluded with certainty, eg, when it is associated with metabolic acidosis, coagulopathy, or rhabdomyolysis.[88] Unproven uses for dantrolene include other syndromes associated with muscle rigidity and/or hyperthermia, including heat stroke, neuroleptic malignant syndrome (NMS),[41] monoamine oxidase overdose,[175] amphetamine overdose, and organophosphate toxicity. In a prospective study, dantrolene has not been found to be useful in the treatment of heat stroke.[46] In NMS, dantrolene is unlikely to be beneficial unless there is severe muscle rigidity, which can cause uncoupling of excitation–contraction.[275] Finally, dantrolene has been used to treat muscular spasticity; however, long-term administration is associated with hepatic and other toxicities.[365]

Pharmacology of Dantrolene. Dantrolene is supplied as a sterile lyophilized solution in a 70-mL vial that contains 20 mg of dantrolene sodium and 3000 mg of mannitol and, following reconstitution with 60 mL of sterile water for injection USP (without a bacteriostatic agent), it has a pH of about 9.5. Dantrolene is lipophilic and relatively insoluble in water. About 70% of an oral dose of dantrolene is absorbed. In plasma, it is reversibly bound to plasma proteins, especially albumin. Dantrolene is metabolized in the liver to 5-hydroxydantrolene, and up to 25% is excreted in the urine as the hydroxy metabolite. The elimination half-life is 6–9 hours for dantrolene and 15.5 hours for the metabolite.

Dosage. The initial dose of dantrolene for treatment of acute MH is 2–3 mg/kg IV as a bolus. This dose should be repeated approximately every 15 minutes until the signs of hypermetabolism are reversed or until a total dose of about 10 mg/kg has been administered. Following initial treatment, at least 1 mg/kg should be given every 4 hours for 48 hours to prevent recrudescence of the syndrome. For prophylaxis of MH, 2.5 mg/kg of dantrolene is given IV 30 minutes prior to anesthesia or planned exposure. Oral prophylaxis can be given, but its absorption is less predictable.[124]

Adverse Effects and Toxicity. Because of its alkaline pH, dantrolene can cause venous irritation and thrombophlebitis; it should be administered through a well-functioning venous cannula. One case of anaphylaxis has been reported. In therapeutic doses, dantrolene causes

TABLE 53–12. SUGGESTED THERAPY FOR MALIGNANT HYPERTHERMIA

What to Look for:

Tachycardia
Hypercarbia (end-tidal CO_2 and arterial CO_2)
Muscle rigidity
Tachypnea
Central venous desaturation
Respiratory and metabolic acidosis
Fever
Myoglobinuria
Unstable or rising blood pressure
Cyanosis or mottling

Acute Phase Treatment of Malignant Hyperthermia (MH)

Stop volatile anesthetics and succinylcholine.

Hyperventilate with 100% O_2.

Administer dantrolene sodium 2–3 mg/kg initial bolus rapidly with increments up to 10 mg/kg total. Continue to administer dantrolene until signs of MH (eg, tachycardia, rigidity, increased end-tidal CO_2, and temperature elevation) are controlled. Occasionally, a total dose greater than 10 mg/kg may be needed. Each vial of dantrolene contains 20 mg of dantrolene and 3 g mannitol. Each vial should be mixed with 60 mL of sterile water for injection USP without a bacteriostatic agent. Dissolution of the lyophilized solution in water is slow and requires thorough mixing.

Administer sodium bicarbonate to correct metabolic acidosis as guided by blood gas analysis. In the absence of blood gas analysis, 1–2 mEq/kg should be administered only when serious cardiac decompensation has occurred.

Simultaneous with the above, actively cool the hyperthermic patient. Use IV cold saline (not Ringer's lactate) 15 mL/kg q 15 min × 3.

Lavage stomach, bladder, rectum, and open cavities with iced saline as appropriate.

Cool surface with ice and hypothermia blanket.

Monitor core temperature closely since overvigorous treatment may lead to hypothermia.

Dysrhythmias will usually respond to treatment of acidosis and hyperkalemia. If they persist or are life threatening, standard antidysrhythmic agents may be used.

Dysrhythmias should not be treated with calcium channel blockers because they may cause hyperkalemia and cardiovascular collapse.

Determine and monitor end-tidal CO_2, arterial, mixed venous blood gases, serum potassium, calcium, clotting studies, and urine output.

Hyperkalemia is common and should be treated with hyperventilation, sodium bicarbonate, intravenous dextrose, and insulin. Life-threatening hyperkalemia may also be treated with calcium administration.

Ensure urine output of greater than 2 mL/kg/h by hydration and/or administration of mannitol or furosemide. Consider central venous or PA monitoring because of fluid shifts and hemodynamic instability that may occur.

Sudden unexpected cardiac arrest in children: Children less than about 10 y of age who experience sudden cardiac arrest after succinylcholine in the absence of hypoxemia and anesthetic overdose should be treated for acute hyperkalemia first. In this situation calcium chloride, sodium bicarbonate, insulin, and dextrose should be administered to reduce serum potassium. They should be presumed to have subclinical muscular dystrophy and a neurologist should be consulted.

Post-Acute Phase Treatment of Malignant Hyperthermia

Observe the patient in an ICU setting for at least 24 h since recrudescence of MH may occur, particularly following a fulminant case resistant to treatment.

Administer dantrolene 1 mg/kg IV q6h for 24–48 h post episode. After that, oral dantrolene 1 mg/kg q6h may be used for 24 h as necessary.

Follow ABG, CK, potassium, calcium, urine and serum myoglobin, clotting studies, and core body temperature until such time as they return to normal values (eg, q6h). Central temperature (eg, rectal, esophageal) should be continuously monitored until stable.

Counsel patient and family regarding MH and further precautions.

Refer patient to MHAUS:

Malignant Hyperthermia Association of the United States
32 South Main Street
P.O. Box 1069
Sherburne, NY 13460-1069
Phone: (800) 98-MHAUS or (607) 674-7901
Fax: (607) 674-7910
E-mail: mhaus@norwich.net
Website: http://www.mhaus.org/
Fax-on-demand: (800) 440-9990

Fill out an Adverse Metabolic Reaction to Anesthesia (AMRA); this form is available from MHAUS.

Register all patients with the North American MH Registry. Forms can be obtained from MHAUS.

Alert family members to the possible dangers of MH and anesthesia.

Notes:

For help with an MH emergency, call the MH Emergency Hotline:

Inside US Call: (800) MH HYPER (800) 644-9737
Outside US Call: (315) 428-7924

CAUTION: This protocol may not apply to every patient and must of necessity be altered according to specific patient needs.

Also see suggestions at:
http://gasnet.med.yale.edu/gta/suggested_mh_therapy.html

muscle weakness, but not muscle paralysis,[369] nor does it depress pulmonary function.[124] It may, however, cause visual problems, lethargy, nausea, and dizziness. Pulmonary edema has been observed rarely when the agent has been given in large doses to treat acute MH. Vomiting and diarrhea may follow oral administration. Rare complications in patients receiving oral dantrolene include hepatotoxicity, seizures, pleural effusion, visual hallucinations, aplastic anemia, heart failure, lymphocytic lymphoma, and leukopenia. Hepatic dysfunction may present as elevated aminotransferases (incidence 1.8%), symptomatic hepatitis (0.6%), or fatal hepatitis (0.3%).[350] Pathologic findings may include subacute hepatic necrosis, chronic active hepatitis, and cholestasis. Risk factors for hepatitis include female gender, dose over 300 mg/day, and duration of therapy over 60 days.

References

1. Postsurgical infections associated with an extrinsically contaminated intravenous anesthetic agent. California, Illinois, Maine, and Michigan, 1990. MMWR 1990;39: 426–427.
2. Recommendations for Infection Control for the Practice of Anesthesiology. Park Ridge, IL, American Society of Anesthesiologists, 1994.
3. Abernathy D, Greenblatt D: Pharmacokinetics of drugs in obesity. Clin Pharmacokinet 1982;7:108–124.
4. Ahmed S, Petchkovsky L: Abuse of ketamine. Br J Psychiatry 1980;137:303. Letter.
5. Aitkinhead A, Willats S, Park G, et al: Comparison of propofol and midazolam for sedation in critically ill patients. Lancet 1989;2:704–709.
6. Åkesson J, Björkman S, Messeter K, et al: Cerebral pharmacodynamics of anaesthetic and subanaesthetic doses of ketamine in the normoventilated pig. Acta Anaesth Scand 1993;37:211–218.
7. Albers G, Goldberg M, Choi D: *N*-methyl-*d*-aspartate antagonists: Ready for clinical trial in brain ischemia? Ann Neurol 1989;25:398–403.
8. Albin M, Bunegin L, Rasch J, et al: Ketamine hydrochloride (KH) fails to protect against global hypoxia in the rat. Anesth Analg 1989;68:S8. Abstract.
9. Albright G: Cardiac arrest following regional anesthesia with etidocaine or bupivaciane. Anesthesiology 1979;51: 285–287. Editorial.
10. Allolio B, Stuttman R, Fischer H, et al: Long-term etomidate and adrenocortical suppression. Lancet 1983;2:626. Letter.
11. Alphin R, Martens J, Dennis D: Frequency-dependent effects of propofol on atrioventricular nodal conduction in guinea pig isolated heart: Mechanisms and potential antidysrhythmic properties. Anesthesiology 1995;83:382–394.
12. Amess J, Burman J, Rees G, et al: Megaloblastic haemopoieses in patients receiving nitrous oxide. Lancet 1978;2: 339–342.
13. Amos R, Amess J, Hinds C, Mollin D: Incidence and pathogenesis of acute megaloblastic bone marrow change in patients receiving intensive care. Lancet 1982;2:835–839.
14. Amris C, Brockner J, Larsen V: Changes in the coagulability of blood during the infusion of intralipid. Acta Chir Scand 1964;325:70–74.
15. Anis A, Berry S, Burton N, Lodge D: The dissociative anaesthetics, ketamine and phencyclidine, selectively reduce excitation of central mammalian neurons by *N*-methyl-aspartate. Br J Pharmacol 1983;79:565–575.
16. Aracava Y, Deshpande S, Rickett D, et al: The molecular basis of anticholinesterase actions on nicotinic and glutamanergic synapses. Ann NY Acad Sci 1987;505:226–255.
17. Arendt-Nielsen L, Petersen-Felix S, Fischer M, et al: The effect of *N*-methyl-*d*-aspartate antagonist (ketamine) on single and repeated nociceptive stimuli: A placebo controlled experimental human study. Anesth Analg 1995; 81:63–68.
18. Atlee JI, Malkinson B: Potentiation by thiopental of halothane-epinephrine-induced arrhythmias in dogs. Anesthesiology 1982;57:285–288.
19. Aun C, Major E: The cardiorespiratory effects of ICI 35,868 in patients with valvular heart disease. Anaesthesia 1984; 39:1096–1100.
20. Babui E, Garcia-Rubi D, Estanol B: Inadvertent massive lidocaine overdose causing temporary complete heart block in myocardial infarction. Am Heart J 1981;102:801–803.
21. Baiker-Heberlein M, Kennis P, Kikillus H, et al: Investigations on the site of central nervous action of the short-acting hypnotic agent R-(+)-ethyl-1-(alpha-methyl-benzyl)-imidazole-5-carboxylate (etomidate) in cats. Anaesthesia 1979;28:78–84.
22. Baird P: Occupational exposure to nitrous oxide—not a laughing matter. N Engl J Med 1992;327:1026–1027.
23. Baldridge E, Bessen H: Phencyclidine. Emerg Med Clin North Am 1990;8:541–550.
24. Balfors E, Häggmark S, Nyhman H: Droperidol inhibits the effects of intravenous ketamine on central hemodynamics and myocardial oxygen consumption in patients with generalized atherosclerotic disease. Anesth Analg 1983;62:193–197.
25. Bansinath M, Shukla V, Turndorf H: Propofol modulates the effects of chemoconvulsants acting at GABAergic, glycinergic, and glutamate receptor subtypes. Anesthesiology 1995;83:809–815.
26. Baraka A: Severe bradycardia following propofol-suxamethonium sequence. Br J Anaesth 1988;61:482–483.
27. Barclay K, Williams A, Major E: Propofol infusion in children. Br Med J 1992;305:953. Letter.
28. Basta S: Modulation of histamine release by neuromuscular blocking drugs. Curr Opin Anaesth 1992;5:572–576.
29. Basta S, Savarese J, Ali H, et al: Clinical pharmacology of doxacurium chloride: A new long-acting non-depolarizing muscle relaxant. Anesthesiology 1988;69:478–486.
30. Becker KJ, Tonnesen A: Cardiovascular effects of plasma levels of thiopental necessary for anesthesia. Anesthesiology 1978;49:197–200.
31. Belin R, Bivins B, Jona J, Young V: Fat overload with a 10% soybean oil solution. Arch Surg 1976;111:1391–1393.
32. Beller J, Pottecher T, Lugnier A, et al: Prolonged sedation with propofol in ICU patients: Recovery and blood concentration changes during periodic interruptions in infusion. Br J Anaesth 1988;61:583–588.
33. Bencini A, Scaf A, Sohn Y, et al: Hepatobiliary disposition

of vecuronium bromide in man. Br J Anaesth 1986;58: 988–995.
34. Bennet S, McNeil M, Bland L, et al: Postoperative infections traced to contamination of an intravenous anesthetic, propofol. N Engl J Med 1995;333:147–154.
35. Berman P, Tattersall M: Self-poisoning with intravenous halothane. Lancet 1982;I:340. Letter.
36. Bernards C, Artru A: Hexamethonium and midazolam terminate dysrhythmias and hypertension caused by intracerebroventricular bupivacaine in rabbits. Anesthesiology 1991;74:89–96.
37. Bevan D, Donati F, Kopman A: Reversal of neuromuscular blockade. Anesthesiology 1992;77:785–805.
38. Bidwai A, Stanley T, Graves C, et al: The effects of ketamine on cardiovascular dynamics during halothane and enflurane anesthesia. Anesth Analg 1975;54:588–592.
39. Bielen S, Lysko G, Gough W: The effect of a cyclodextrine vehicle on the cardiovascular profile of propofol in rats. Anesth Analg 1996;82:920–924.
40. Bishop D, Johnstone R: Lidocaine toxicity treated with low-dose propofol. Anesthesiology 1993;78:788–789.
41. Bismuth C, Rohan-Chabot PD, Goulon M, Raphael J: Dantrolene—a new therapeutic approach to the neuroleptic malignant syndrome. Acta Neurol Scand 1984;70(suppl 100):193–198.
42. Bolton C: Neuromuscular conditions in the intensive care unit. Intensive Care Med 1996;22:841–843.
43. Bolton C: Sepsis and the systemic inflammatory response syndrome: Neuromuscular manifestations. Crit Care Med 1996;24:1408–1415.
44. Bolton CF: Neuromuscular complications of sepsis. Intensive Care Med 1993;19:S58–S63.
45. Bosnjak Z, Stowe D, Kampine J: Comparison of lidocaine and bupivacaine depression of sinoatrial nodal activity during hypoxia and acidosis in adult and neonatal guinea pigs. Anesth Analg 1986;65:911–917.
46. Bouchama A, Cafege A, Devol E, et al: Ineffectiveness of dantrolene sodium in the treatment of heatstroke. Crit Care Med 1991;19:176–180.
47. Bowman W: Nonrelaxant properties of neuromuscular blocking drugs. Br J Anaesth 1982;54:147–160.
48. Bowman W, Rodger J, Houston J: Structure: Action relationships among some desacetoxy analogues of pancuronium and vecuronium in the anesthetized cat. Anesthesiology 1988;69:57–62.
49. Brand J, Cullen D, Wilson N, Ali H: Spontaneous recovery from nondepolarizing neuromuscular blockade: Correlation between clinical and evoked responses. Anesth Analg 1977;56:55–58.
50. Brandom B, Meretoja O, Taivainem T, Wirtavuori K: Accelerated onset and delayed recovery of neuromuscular block induced by mivacurium preceded by pancuronium in children. Anesth Analg 1993;76:998–1003.
51. Brodsky J, Cohen E, Brown B, et al: Exposure to nitrous oxide and neurologic disease among dental professionals. Anesth Analg 1981;60:297–301.
52. Brüssel T, Theissen J, Vigfusson G, et al: Hemodynamic and cardiodynamic effects of propofol and etomidate: Negative inotropic properties of propofol. Anesth Analg 1989;69:35–40.
53. Burney R, DiFazio C, Foster J: Effects of pH on protein binding of lidocaine. Anesth Analg 1978;57:478–480.
54. Burnham W, Hepinstall S, Cockbill S, Harrison S: Blood platelet behaviour during infusion of an Intralipid-based intravenous feeding mixture. Postgrad Med J 1982;58: 152–155.
55. Caldwell J, Szenohradszky J, Segredo V, et al: The pharmacodynamics and pharmacokinetics of the metabolite 3-desacetylvecuronium (ORG 7268) and its parent compound, vecuronium, in human volunteers. J Pharmacol Exp Ther 1994;270:1216–1222.
56. Carrasco G, Molina R, Costa J, et al: Propofol vs midazolam in short-, medium-, and long-term sedation of critically ill patients. Chest 1993;103:557–564.
57. Celesia G, Chen R, Bamforth B: Effects of ketamine in epilepsy. Neurology 1975;25:169–172.
58. Chamberlain J, Seed R, Chung D: Effect of thiopentone on myocardial function. Br J Anaesth 1977;49:865–870.
59. Chapple D, Miller A, Ward J, Wheatley P: Cardiovascular and neurological effects of laudanosine: Studies in mice and rats, and in conscious and anaesthetized dogs. Br J Anaesth 1987;59:218–225.
60. Church J, Zeman S: Ketamine promotes hippocampal CA1 pyramidal neuron loss after a short duration ischemic insult in the rat. Neurosci Lett 1991;123:65–68.
61. Claeys M, Gepts E, Camu F: Haemodynamic changes during anaesthesia induced and maintained with propofol. Br J Anaesth 1988;60:3–9.
62. Clarkson C, Hondeghem L: Mechanism for bupivacaine depression of cardiac conduction: Fast block of sodium channels during the action potential with slow recovery from block during diastole. Anesthesiology 1985;62: 396–405.
63. Coates D, Monk C, Prys-Roberts C, Turtle M: Hemodynamic effects of infusions of the emulsion formulation of propofol during nitrous oxide anesthesia in humans. Anesth Analg 1987;66:64–70.
64. Coetzee A, Fourie P, Coetzee J, et al: Effect of various propofol plasma concentrations on regional myocardial contractility and left ventricular afterload. Anesth Analg 1989;69:473–483.
65. Cohn B, Reiger V, Hagenouw-Taal J, Voormolen J: Results of a feasibility trial to achieve total immobilization of patients in a neurosurgical intensive care unit with etomidate. Anaesthesia 1983;38(suppl):47–50.
66. Cold G, Eskesen V, Eriksen H, Blatt LB: Changes in $CMRO_2$, EEG and concentration of etomidate in serum and brain tissue during craniotomy with continuous etomidate supplemented with N_2O and fentanyl. Acta Anaesth Scand 1986;30:159–163.
67. Collier B: Long-term dangers of ketamine anaesthesia. Br J Anaesth 1981;53:552. Letter.
68. Collingridge G, Bliss T: NMDA receptors—their role in long-term potentiation. Trends Neurosci 1987;10:288–293.
69. Colson P, Eledjam J: Mechanism of propofol bradycardia. Anesth Analg 1988;67:906–907. Letter.
70. Cook S, Palma O: Propofol as a sole agent for prolonged infusion in intensive care. J Drug Dev 1989;2(suppl 2): 65–67.
71. Corssen G, Gutierrez J, Reves J, Huber F: Ketamine in the

anesthetic management of asthmatic patients. Anesth Analg 1972;51:588–596.

72. Corssen G, Little S, Tavakoli M: Ketamine and epilepsy. Curr Res 1974;53:319–335.
73. Cousins M, Greenstein L, Hitt B, Mazze R: Metabolism and renal effects of enflurane in man. Anesthesiology 1976;44:44–53.
74. Cousins M, Mazze R: Methoxyflurane nephrotoxicity: A study of dose-response in man. JAMA 1973;225:1611–1616.
75. Crandell W, Pappas S, MacDonald A: Nephrotoxicity associated with methoxyflurane anesthesia. Anesthesiology 1966;27:591–607.
76. Croether J, Hrazdil J, Jolly D, et al: Growth of microorganisms in propofol, thiopental, and a 1:1 mixture of propofol and thiopental. Anesth Analg 1996;82:475–478.
77. Cronnelly R, Morris R: Antagonism of neuromuscular blockade. Br J Anaesth 1982;54:183–194.
78. Cullen P, Turtle M, Prys-Roberts C, et al: Effect of propofol anesthesia on baroreflex activity in humans. Anesth Analg 1987;66:1115–1120.
79. Curelaru I, Stanciu S, Nicolau V, et al: A case of recovery from coma produced by the ingestion of 250 ml of halothane. Br J Anaesth 1968;40:283–288.
80. Danon M, Carpenter S: Myopathy with thick filament (myosin) loss following prolonged paralysis with vecuronium during steroid treatment. Muscle Nerve 1991;14: 1131–1139.
81. Darrah W, Johnston J, Mirakhur R: Vecuronium infusions for prolonged muscle relaxation in the intensive care unit. Crit Care Med 1989;17:1297–1300.
82. Davis N, de Jong R: Successful resuscitation following massive bupivacaine overdose. Anesth Analg 1982;61: 62–64.
83. Dawson B, Michenfelder J, Theye R: Effect of ketamine on canine cerebral blood flow and metabolism: Modification by prior administration of thiopental. Anesth Analg 1971;50:443–447.
84. de Jong R, Heavner J: Local anesthetic seizure prevention: Diazepam versus pentobarbital. Anesthesiology 1972;36: 449–457.
85. de Jong R, Ronfeld R, DeRosa R: Cardiovascular effects of convulsant and supraconvulsant doses of amide local anesthetics. Anesth Analg 1982;61:3–9.
86. de Jong R, Wagman I, Prince D: Effect of carbon dioxide on the cortical seizure threshold to lidocaine. Exp Neurol 1967;17:221–232.
87. de la Coussaye J, Bassoul B, Brugada J, et al: Reversal of electrophysiologic and hemodynamic effects induced by high-dose of bupivacaine by the combination of clonidine and dobutamine in anesthetized dogs. Anesth Analg 1992;74:703–711.
88. Denborough M: Heat stroke and malignant hyperpyrexia. Med J Aust 1982;1:204–205.
89. Di Maio V, Garriott J: Four deaths resulting from abuse of nitrous oxide. J Forensic Sci 1978;23:169–172.
90. Dodson B, Kelly B, Braswell L, Cohen N: Changes in acetylcholine receptor number in muscle from critically ill patients receiving muscle relaxants: An investigation of the molecular mechanism of prolonged paralysis. Crit Care Med 1995;23:815–821.
91. Doenicke A, Löffler B, Kugler J, et al: Plasma concentration and EEG after various regimens of etomidate. Br J Anaesth 1982;54:393–400.
92. Domino E, Chodoff P, Corssen G: Pharmacologic effects of CI–581, a new dissociative anesthetic in man. Clin Pharmacol Ther 1965;6:279–291.
93. Dorrington K: Asystole with convulsion following a subanaesthetic dose of propofol plus fentanyl. Anaesthesia 1989;44:658–659.
94. Douglass J, Tuxen D, Horne M, et al: Myopathy in severe asthma. Am Rev Respir Dis 1992;146:517–519.
95. Dubois D, Almon R: A possible role for glucocorticoids in denervation atrophy. Muscle Nerve 1981;4:370–373.
96. Dundee J, Lilburn J: Ketamine-lorazepam. Anaesthesia 1978;33:312–314.
97. Dundee J, Lilburn J, Morre J: Attempted reduction of the cardiostimulatory effects of ketamine by labetalol. Anaesthesia 1978;33:506–511.
98. Dunn S: Contamination of propofol. Anesthesiology 1992; 77:833. Letter.
99. Durant N, Katz R: Suxamethonium. Br J Anaesth 1982; 54:195–208.
100. Durbin C: Sedation in the critically ill patient. New Horizons 1994;2:64–74.
101. Durcan J, Carter J: Overdose of atracurium. Anaesthesia 1986;41:767. Letter.
102. Duthie D, Fraser R, Nimmo W: Effect of induction of anesthesia with etomidate on corticosteroid synthesis in man. Br J Anaesth 1985;57:156–159.
103. Dykes M: Is enflurane hepatotoxic? Anesthesiology 1984; 61:235–237.
104. Ebert T, Muzi M: Propofol and autonomic reflex function in humans. Anesth Analg 1994;78:369–375.
105. Ebert T, Muzi M, Berens R, et al: Sympathetic responses to induction of anesthesia in humans with propofol or etomidate. Anesthesiology 1992;76:725–733.
106. Ebrahim Z, DeBoer G, Luders H, et al: Effect of etomidate on the electroencephalogram of patients with epilepsy. Anesth Analg 1986;65:1004–1006.
107. Eddleston J, Harper N, Pollard B, et al: Concentrations of atracurium and laudanosine in cerebrospinal fluid and plasma during intracranial surgery. Br J Anaesth 1989;63: 525–530.
108. Eddleston J, Harper N, Ward J, Weatley P: Cardiovascular and neurological effects of laudanosine. Br J Anaesth 1987; 59:218–225.
109. Eddelston J, Shelly M: The effect on serum lipid concentration of a prolonged infusion of propofol-hypertriglyceridemia associated with propofol administration. Intensive Care Med 1991;17:424–426.
110. Edwards R, Miller R, Roizen M, et al: Cardiac responses to imipramine and pancuronium during anesthesia with halothane and enflurane. Anesthesiology 1979;50: 421–425.
111. Egan T, Brock-Utne J: Asystole after anesthesia induction with a fentanyl, propofol, and succinylcholine sequence. Anesth Analg 1991;73:818–820.
112. Eger E, Smuckler E, Ferrell L, et al: Is enflurane hepatotoxic? Anesth Analg 1986;65:21–30.
113. Elliot E, Hanid T, Arthur L, Kay B: Ketamine anesthesia

for medical procedures in children. Arch Dis Child 1976; 51:56–59.
114. Englesson S: The influence of acid–base changes on central nervous system toxicity of local anesthetic agents. I. An experimental study in cats. Acta Anaesthesiol Scand 1974; 18:79–87.
115. Ertama P: Histamine liberation in surgical patients following administration of neuromuscular blocking drugs. Ann Clin Res 1982;14:15–26.
116. Etsten B, Li T: Hemodynamic changes during thiopental anesthesia in humans: Cardiac output, stroke volume, total peripheral resistance, and intrathoracic blood volume. J Clin Invest 1955;34:500–510.
117. Fahmy N, Alkhouli H, Sunder M, et al: Diprivan: A new intravenous induction agent. A comparison with thiopental. Anesthesiology 1985;63:A363. Abstract.
118. Farling P, Johnston J, Coppel D: Propofol infusion for sedation of patients with head injury in intensive care. Anaesthesia 1989;44:222–226.
119. Feldman H, Arthur R, Covino B: Comparative systemic toxicity of convulsant and supraconvulsant doses of intravenous ropivacaine, bupivacaine, and lidocaine in the conscious dog. Anesth Analg 1989;69:794–801.
120. Felser J, Orban D: Dystonic reaction after ketamine abuse. Ann Emerg Med 1982;11:673–675.
121. Ferrer-Allado T, Brechner V, Dymond A, et al: Ketamine-induced electroconvulsive phenomena in the human limbic and thalamic regions. Anesthesiology 1973;38:333–344.
122. Fine J, Finestone S: Sensory disturbances following ketamine anesthesia: Recurrent hallucinations. Anesth Analg 1973;52:428–430.
123. Finkelstein F, Kreeft J: Massive lidocaine poisoning. N Engl J Med 1979;301:50.
124. Flewellen E, Nelson T, Jones W, et al: Dantrolene dose response in awake man: Implications for management of malignant hyperthermia. Anesthesiology 1983;59:275–280.
125. Foldes F: Distribution and biotransformation of succinylcholine. Int Anesth Clin 1975;13:101–115.
126. Foldes F, Rendell-Baker L, Birch J: Causes and prevention of prolonged apnea with succinylcholine. Anesth Analg 1956;35:609–615.
127. Fragen R, Avram M: Barbiturates. In: Miller R, ed: Anesthesia, 4th ed. New York, Churchill Livingstone, 1994, pp. 229–246.
128. Fragen R, Avram M: Nonopioid intravenous anesthetics. In: Barash P, Cullen B, Stoelting R, eds: Clinical Anesthesia, 2nd ed. Philadelphia, Lippincott, 1992, pp. 385–412.
129. Fragen R, Caldwell N, Brunner E: Clinical use of etomidate for anesthesia induction: A preliminary report. Anesth Analg 1976;55:730–733.
130. Fragen R, Shanks C, Molteni A, Avram M: Effects of etomidate on hormonal responses to surgical stress. Anesthesiology 1984;61:652–656.
131. Freedman M, Gal J, Freed C: Extracorporeal pump assistance—novel treatment for acute lidocaine poisoning. Eur J Clin Pharmacol 1982;22:129–135.
132. Fujita Y: Amrinone reverses bupivacaine-induced regional myocardial dysfunction. Acta Anaesthesiol Scand 1996;40: 47–52.
133. Futo J, Kupferberg J, Moss J: Inhibition of histamine *N*-methyltransferase (HNMT) in vitro by neuromuscular relaxants. Biochem Pharmacol 1990;39:415–420.
134. Ganansia M-F, Francois T, Ormezzano X, et al: Atrioventricular mobitz I block during propofol anesthesia for laparoscopic tubal ligation. Anesth Analg 1989;69:524–525.
135. Gancher S, Laxer K, Krieger W: Activation of epileptogenic foci by etomidate. Anesthesiology 1984;61:616–618.
136. Gardner A, Olson B, Lichtiger M: Cerebrospinal-fluid pressure during dissociative anesthesia with ketamine. Anesthesiology 1971;35:226–228.
137. Gelissen H, Epema A, Henning R, et al: Inotropic effects of propofol, thiopental, midazolam, and ketamine on isolated human atrial muscle. Anesthesiology 1996;84: 397–403.
138. Ghoneim M, Yamada T: Etomidate: A clinical and electroencephalographic comparison with thiopental. Anesth Analg 1977;56:479–485.
139. Gibbons S, Núñez-Hernández R, Mazé G, Harrison N: Inhibition of a fast inwardly rectifying potassium conductance by barbiturates. Anesth Analg 1996;82:1242–1246.
140. Gill P: Non-medical use of ketamine. Br Med J 1993; 306:1340. Letter.
141. Ginsberg B, Glass P, Quill T, et al: Onset and duration of neuromuscular blockade following high-dose vecuronium administration. Anesthesiology 1989;71:201–205.
142. Glen J, Hunter S: Pharmacology of an emulsion formulation of ICI 36 868. Br J Anaesth 1984;56:617–625.
143. Gold M, Brown M, Coverman S, Herrington C: Heart rate and blood pressure effects of esmolol after ketamine induction and intubation. Anesthesiology 1986;64:718–723.
144. Gooding J, Corssen G: Effect of etomidate on the cardiovascular system. Anesth Analg 1977;56:717–719.
145. Gooding J, Weng J, Smith R, et al: Cardiovascular and pulmonary response following etomidate induction of anesthesia in patients with demonstrated cardiac disease. Anesth Analg 1979;58:40–41.
146. Gordon P, Morrell D, Pamm J: Total intravenous anesthesia using propofol and alfentanil for coronary artery bypass surgery. J Cariothorac Vasc Anesth 1994;8:284–288.
147. Grant I, Hutchison G: Epileptiform seizures during prolonged etomidate sedation. Lancet 1983;2:511–512. Letter.
148. Gronert G: Disuse atrophy with resistance to pancuronium. Anesthesiology 1981;55:547–549.
149. Grounds R, Twigley A, Carli F, et al: The hemodynamic effects of intravenous induction. Anaesthesia 1985;40: 735–740.
150. Gumpert J, Paul R: Activation of the electroencephalogram with intravenous brevital (methohexitone): The findings in 100 cases. J Neurol Neurosurg Psychiatry 1971; 34:646.
151. Halford F: A critique of intravenous anesthesia in war surgery. Anesthesiology 1943;4:67–69.
152. Hansen-Flaschen J, Brazinsky S, Basile C, Lanken P: Use of sedating drugs and neuromuscular blocking agents in patients requiring mechanical ventilation for respiratory failure: A national survey. JAMA 1991;266:2870–2875.
153. Hansen-Flaschen J, Cowen J, Raps E: Neuromuscular blockade in the intensive care unit: More than we bargained for. Am Rev Respir Dis 1993;147:234–236.
154. Harris C, Grounds R, Murray A, et al: Propofol for long-

term sedation in the intensive care unit. Anaesthesia 1990; 45:366–372.
155. Heavner J, Arthur J, Zou J, et al: Propofol vs thiopental for treating bupivacaine-induced seizures in rats. Anesthesiology 1992;77:A801.
156. Heffron J: Malignant hyperthermia: Biochemical aspects of the acute episode. Br J Anaesth 1988;60:274–278.
157. Henter J-I, Carlson L, Söder O, et al: Lipoprotein alterations and plasma lipoprotein lipase reduction in familial hemophagocytic lymphohistiocytosis. Acta Paediatr Scand 1991;80:675–681.
158. Herrschaft H, Schmidt H, Duus P: Cerebral blood flow in man under general anaesthesia with regard to several narcotics. Eur Neurol 1971;6:373–382.
159. Herrschaft H, Schmidt H, Gleim F, Albus G: The response of human cerebral blood flow to anesthesia with thiopentone, methohexitone, propranidid, ketamine, and etomidate. Adv Neurosurg 1975;3:120–133.
160. Heyman M, Storch S, Ament M: The fat overload syndrome. Report of a case and literature review. Am J Dis Child 1981;135:628–630.
161. Hjelm M, Holmdahl M: Biochemical effects of aromatic amines. Acta Anaesthesiol Scand 1965;2:99–120.
162. Hoffmann P, Schockenhoff B: Etomidate as an anticonvulsant agent. Anaesthesist 1984;33:142–144.
163. Hoft R, Bunker J, Goodman H: Halothane hepatitis in three pairs of closely related women. N Engl J Med 1981;304:1023–1024.
164. Hogue C, Ward J, Itani M, Martyn J: Tolerance and upregulation of acetylcholine receptors follow chronic infusion of *d*-tubocurarine. J Appl Physiol 1992;72:1326–1331.
165. Holdcroft A, Morgan M, Whitwam J, Lumley J: Effect of dose and premedication on induction complications with etomidate. Br J Anaesth 1976;48:199–205.
166. Hoyt J: Persistent paralysis in critically ill patients after the use of neuromuscular blocking agents. New Horizons 1994;2:48–55.
167. Hsiang J, Chestnut R, Crisp C, et al: Early, routine paralysis for intracranial pressure control in severe head injury: Is it necessary? Crit Care Med 1994;22:1471–1476.
168. Hunter J: New neuromuscular blocking drugs. New Engl J Med 1995;332:1691–1699.
169. Hunter J, De Wolf A: The pharmacodynamics and pharmacokinetics of cis-atracurium in patients with renal or hepatic failure. Curr Opin Anesthesiol 1996;9(suppl 1): S40–S44.
170. Inman W, Mushlin W: Jaundice after repeat exposure to halothane: A further analysis of reports to the committee on safety of medicines. Br Med J 1978;2:1455–1456.
171. Inoue K, El-Banayosy A, Stolarski L, Reichelt W: Vecuronium induced bradycardia following induction of anaesthesia with etomidate or thiopentone, with or without fentanyl. Br J Anaesth 1988;60:10–17.
172. Jansen K: Non-medical use of ketamine. Br Med J 1993; 306:601–602.
173. Jansen K: Near death experience and the NMDA receptor. Br Med J 1989;298:1708. Letter.
174. Jones D, Laurence A, Thornton J: Total intravenous anaesthesia with etomidate-fentanyl. Use in general and gynaecological surgery. Anaesthesia 1983;38:29–34.
175. Kaplan R, Feinglass N, Webster W, Mudra S: Phenelzine overdose treated with dantrolene sodium. JAMA 1986; 255:642–644.
176. Kassell N, Hitchon M, Gerk M, et al: Alterations in cerebral blood flow, oxygen metabolism and electrical activity produced by high dose sodium thiopental. Neurosurgery 1980;7:598–603.
177. Kasten G, Martin S: Bupivacaine cardiovascular toxicity: Comparison of treatment with bretylium and lidocaine. Anesth Analg 1985;64:911–916.
178. Kasten G, Martin S: Successful cardiovascular resuscitation after massive intravenous bupivacaine overdosage in anesthetized dogs. Anesth Analg 1985;64:491–497.
179. Kayama Y, Iwama K: The EEG, evoked potentials, and single-unit activity during ketamine anesthesia in cats. Anesthesiology 1972;36:316–328.
180. Kemp J, Foster A, Wong E: Non-competitive antagonists of excitatory amino acid receptors. Trends Neurosci 1987; 10:294–298.
181. Kettler D, Sonntag H, Donath U, et al: Hemodynamics, myocardial mechanics, oxygen requirements and oxygen consumption of the human heart during etomidate induction into anaesthesia. Anaesthesist 1974;23:116–121.
182. Khaleeli A, Edwards R, Gohil K, et al: Corticosteroid myopathy: A clinical and pathological study. Clin Endocrinol 1983;18:155–166.
183. King M, Milazkiewicz R, Carli F, Deacock A: Influence of neostigmine on postoperative vomiting. Br J Anaesth 1988;61:403–406.
184. Kirkwood I, Duckworth R: An unusual case of sinus arrest. Br J Anaesth 1983;55:1273.
185. Kobayashi Y, Ochiai R, Takeda J, et al: Serum and urinary inorganic fluoride concentrations after prolonged inhalation of sevoflurane in man. Anesth Analg 1992;74:753–757.
186. Koehntop D, Liao J-C, Van Bergen F: Effects of pharmacologic alterations of adrenergic mechanisms by cocaine, tropolone, and ketamine on epinephrine-induced arrhythmias during halothane-nitrous oxide anesthesia. Anesthesiology 1977;46:83–93.
187. Kopman A, Yee P, Neuman G: Relationship of the train-of-four fade ratio to clinical signs and symptoms of residual paralysis in awake volunteers. Anesthesiology 1997; 86:765–771.
188. Kovarik W, Mayberg T, Lam A, et al: Succinylcholine does not change intracranial pressure, cerebral blood flow velocity, or the electroencephalogram in patients with head injury. Anesth Analg 1994;78:469–473.
189. Kozody R, Ready L, Barsa J, Murphy T: Dose requirements of local anaesthetic to produce grand mal seizure during stellate ganglion block. Can Anaesth Soc J 1982; 29:489–491.
190. Krieger W, Copperman J, Laxer K: Seizures with etomidate anesthesia. Anesth Analg 1985;64:1226–1227. Letter.
191. Kupfer Y, Okrent D, Twersky R, Tessler S: Disuse atrophy in a ventilated patient with status asthmaticus receiving neuromuscular blockade. Crit Care Med 1987;15:795–796.
192. Larsen R, Rathgeber J, Bagdahn A, et al: Effects of propofol on cardiovascular dynamics and coronary blood flow in geriatric patients. A comparison with etomidate. Anaesthesia 1988;43(suppl):25–31.

193. Lassen H, Henriksen E, Neukirch F, Kristensen H: Treatment of tetanus: Severe bone marrow depression after prolonged nitrous-oxide anaesthesia. Lancet 1956;1:527–530.
194. Laxenaire M, Gueant J, Bermejo E, et al: Anaphylactic shock due to propofol. Lancet 1988;2:739–740.
195. Laxenaire M, Mata E, Guéant JL, et al: Basophil histamine release in atopic patients after in vitro provocation thiopental, Diprivan® and chlormethiazole. Acta Anaesth Scand 1991;35:706–710.
196. Laxenaire M-C, Mata-Bermejo E, Moneret-Vautrin D, Guéant J-L: Life-threatening anaphylactoid reactions to propofol (Diprivan®). Anesthesiology 1992;77:275–280.
197. Layzer R, Fishman R, Schafer J: Neuropathy following abuse of nitrous oxide. Neurology 1978;28:504–506.
198. Lebrault C, Berger J, D'Hollander A, et al: Pharmacokinetics and pharmacodynamics of vecuronium (ORG NC 45) in patients with cirrhosis. Anesthesiology 1985;62:601–605.
199. Lebrault C, Duvaldestin P, Henzel D, et al: Pharmacokinetics and pharmacodynamics of vecuronium in patients with cholestasis. Br J Anaesth 1986;58:983–987.
200. Ledingham I, Watt I: Influence of sedation on mortality in critically ill multiple trauma patients. Lancet 1983;1:1270. Letter.
201. Lee C: Intensive care unit neuromuscular syndrome? Anesthesiology 1995;83:237–240.
202. Leijten F, De Weerd A: Critical illness polyneuropathy: A review of the literature, definition and pathophysiology. Clin Neurol Neurosurg 1994;96:10–19.
203. Leijten F, De Weered A, De Ridder V, et al: Critical illness polyneuropathy in multiple organ dysfunction syndrome and weaning from the ventilator. Intensive Care Med 1996;22:856–861.
204. Leijten F, Harinck-de Weerd J, Poortvliet D, de Weerd A: The role of polyneuropathy in motor convalescence after prolonged mechanical ventilation. JAMA 1995;274: 1221–1225.
205. Lepage J, Pinaud M, Helias J, et al: Left ventricular function during propofol and fentanyl anesthesia in patients with coronary artery disease: assessment with a radionuclide approach. Anesth Analg 1988;67:949–955.
206. Lepage J-Y, Malinovsky J-M, Malinge M, et al: Pharmacodynamic dose-response and safety study of cisatracurium (51W89) in adult surgical patients during N_2O-O_2-opioid anesthesia. Anesth Analg 1996;83:823–829.
207. Levänen J, Mäkelä M-L, Scheinin H: Dexmedetomidine premedication attenuates ketamine-induced cardiostimulatory effects and postanesthetic delirium. Anesthesiology 1995;82:1117–1125.
208. Lilburn J, Dundee J, Moore J: Ketamine infusions. Anaesthesia 1978;33:315–321.
209. Lilburn J, Dundee J, Nair S, et al: Ketamine sequelae. Anaesthesia 1978;33:307–311.
210. Lindgren L, Randell T, Suzuki N, et al: The effect of amrinone on recovery from severe bupivacaine intoxication in pigs. Anesthesiology 1992;77:309–315.
211. Lingenfelter R: Fatal misuse of enflurane. Anesthesiology 1981;55:603.
212. Long W, Rosenblum S, Grady I: Successful resuscitation of bupivacaine-induced cardiac arrest using cardiopulmonary bypass. Anesth Analg 1989;69:403–406.
213. Loper K, Butler S, Nessly M, Wild L: Paralyzed with pain: The need for education. Pain 1989;37:315–316.
214. Lorenz W, Ennis M, Doenicke A, Dick W: Perioperative uses of histamine antagonists. J Clin Anesth 1990;2: 345–360.
215. Lowe D, Hettrick D, Pagel P, Warltier D: Propofol alters left ventricular afterload as evaluated by aortic input impedance in dogs. Anesthesiology 1996;84:368–376.
216. Lund P, Cwik J: Propitocaine (eitanest) and methemoglobinemia. Anesthesiology 1965;26:569–571.
217. Lundy P, Gowdey C, Colhoun E: Tracheal smooth muscle relaxant effect of ketamine. Br J Anaesth 1974;46: 333–336.
218. Lynch C: Depression of myocardial contractility in vitro by bupivacaine, etidocaine and lidocaine. Anesth Analg 1986;65:551–559.
219. MacLennan D, Duff C, Zorzato F, et al: Ryanodine receptor gene is a candidate for predisposition to malignant hyperthermia. Nature 1990;343:559–561.
220. MacLennan D, Phillips M: Malignant hyperthermia. Science 1992;257:789–794.
221. Macrae D, James I: Propofol sedation of children. Anaesthesia 1992;47:811. Letter.
222. Magorian T, Wood P, Caldwell J, et al: The pharmacokinetics and neuromuscular effects of rocuronium bromide in patients with liver disease. Anesth Analg 1995;80: 754–759.
223. Maher J, Rutledge F, Remtulla H, et al: Neuromuscular disorders associated with failure to wean from the ventilator. Intensive Care Med 1995;21:737–743.
224. Marik P: Doxacurium-corticosteroid acute myopathy: Another piece to the puzzle. Crit Care Med 1996;24: 1266–1267.
225. Matsuda F, Kinney W, Wright W, Kambam J: Nicardipine reduces the cardio-respiratory toxicity of intravenously administered bupivacaine in rats. Can J Anaesth 1990;37: 920–923.
226. Matteo R, Brotherton W, Nishitateno K: Pharmacodynamics and pharmacokinetics of metocurine in humans: Comparison to *d*-tubocurarine. Anesthesiology 1982;57: 183–190.
227. Maxwell L, Martin L, Yaster M: Bupivacaine-induced cardiac toxicity in neonates: successful treatment with intravenous phenytoin. Anesthesiology 1994;80:682–686.
228. Mazze R, Woodruff R, Heerdt M: Isoniazid-induced enflurane defluorination in humans. Anesthesiology 1982;57: 5–8.
229. McClain C, Cohen D, Phillips R, et al: Increased plasma and ventricular fluid interleukin–6 levels in patients with head injury. J Lab Clin Med 1991;118:225–231.
230. McCoy E, Maddineni V, Elliott P, et al: Hemodynamic effects of rocuronium during fentanyl anaesthesia: Comparison with vecuronium. Can J Anaesth 1993;40:703–708.
231. McLeod G, Pace N, Inglis M: Bacterial growth in propofol. Br J Anaesth 1991;67:665–666.
232. Messeter K, Nordström C-H, Sundbärg G, et al: Cerebral hemodynamics in patients with acute severe head trauma. J Neurosurg 1986;64:231–237.
233. Messina F, Wynne J: Homemade nitrous oxide: No laughing matter. Ann Intern Med 1982;96:333–334.

234. Meyer K, Prielipp R, Grossman J, Coursin D: Prolonged weakness after infusion of atracurium in two intensive care unit patients. Anesth Analg 1994;78:772–774.
235. Meyers E, Charles P: Prolonged adverse reactions to ketamine in children. Anesthesiology 1978;49:39–40.
236. Michenfelder J: The interdependency of cerebral functional and metabolic effects following massive doses of thiopental in the dog. Anesthesiology 1974;41:231–236.
237. Miller R, Agoston S, Booij L, et al: The comparative potency and pharmacokinetics of pancuronium, and its metabolites in anesthetized man. J Pharmacol Exp Ther 1978;207:539–543.
238. Miller R, Matteo R, Benet L, Sohn Y: The pharmacokinetics of *d*-tubocurarine in man with and without renal failure. J Pharmacol Exp Ther 1977;202:1–7.
239. Modica P, Tempelhoff R: Intracranial pressure during induction of anaesthesia and tracheal intubation with etomidate-induced EEG burst suppression. Can J Anaesth 1992; 39:236–241.
240. Modica P, Tempelhoff R, White P: Pro- and anticonvulsant effects of anesthetics (Part II). Anesth Analg 1990;70: 433–444.
241. Mogensen H, Mueller D, Valentin N: Glycopyrrolate during ketamine/diazepam anaesthesia. Acta Anaesth Scand 1986;30:332–336.
242. Monk C, Coates D, Prys-Roberts C, et al: Haemodynamic effects of a prolonged infusion of propofol as a supplement to nitrous oxide anaesthesia. Br J Anaesth 1987;59: 954–960.
243. Moore D, Balfour R, Fitzgibbons D: Convulsive arterial plasma levels of bupivacaine and the response to diazepam therapy. Anesthesiology 1979;50:454–456.
244. Moore D, Bridenbaugh L: Oxygen: The antidote for systemic toxic reactions from local anesthetic drugs. JAMA 1960;174:102–107.
245. Moore D, Bridenbaugh L, Thompson G, et al: Bupivacaine: A review of 11,080 cases. Anesth Analg 1978;57:42–53.
246. Morishima H, Corvino B: Toxicity and distribution of lidocaine in nonasphyxiated and asphyxiated baboon fetuses. Anesthesiology 1981;54:182–186.
247. Morishima H, Pederson H, Finster M, et al: Bupavicaine toxicity in pregnant and nonpregnant ewes. Anesthesiology 1985;63:134–139.
248. Morishima H, Pederson H, Finster M, et al: Toxicity of lidocaine in adult, newborn, and fetal sheep. Anesthesiology 1981;55:57–61.
249. Morris R, Cahalan M, Miller R, et al: The cardiovascular effects of vecuronium (ORG NC45) and pancuronium in patients undergoing coronary artery bypass grafting. Anesthesiology 1983;58:438–440.
250. Moss E, Powell D, Gibson R, McDowall D: Effect of etomidate on intracranial pressure and cerebral perfusion pressure. Br J Anaesth 1979;51:347–351.
251. Moss J: Muscle relaxants and histamine release. Acta Anaesthesiol Scand 1995;39(suppl 106):7–12.
252. Mulier J, Wouters P, Van Aken H, et al: Cardiodynamic effects of propofol in comparison with thiopental: Assessment with a transesophageal echocardiographic approach. Anesth Analg 1991;72:28–35.
253. Murphy J: Hypertension and pulmonary oedema associated with ketamine administration in a patient with a history of substance abuse. Can J Anaesth 1993;40:160–164.
254. Murray M, Coursin D, Scuderi P, et al: Double-blind, randomized, multicenter study of doxacurium vs pancuronium in intensive care unit patients who require neuromuscular-blocking agents. Crit Care Med 1995;23:450–458.
255. Napolitano C, Raatikainen M, Martens J, Dennis D: Effects of intravenous anesthetics on atrial wavelength and atrioventricular nodal conduction in guinea pig heart. Anesthesiology 1996;85:393–402.
256. Neuberger J, Williams R: Halothane hepatitis. Digest Dis 1988;6:52–64.
257. Newman L, McDonald J, Wallace P, Ledingham I: Propofol infusion for sedation in intensive care. Anaesthesia 1987;42:929–937.
258. Nigrovic V, Fox J: Atracurium decay and the formation of laudanosine in humans. Anesthesiology 1991;74:446–454.
259. Noble J, Kennedy D, Latimer R, et al: Massive lignocaine overdose during cardiopulmonary bypass: Successful treatment with cardiac pacing. Br J Anaesth 1984;56: 1439–1441.
260. Nordström C, Messeter K, Sundbärg G: Cerebral blood flow, vasoreactivity, and oxygen consumption during barbiturate therapy in severe traumatic brain lesions. J Neurosurg 1988;68:424–431.
261. Nørreslet J, Wahlgreen C: Propofol infusion for sedation of children. Crit Care Med 1990;18:890–892.
262. Nunn J: Clinical aspects of the interaction between nitrous oxide and vitamin B_{12}. Br J Anaesth 1987;59:3–13.
263. Nunn J, Chanarin I, Tanner A, Owen E: Megaloblastic bone marrow changes after repeated nitrous oxide anaesthesia. Br J Anaesth 1986;58:1469–1470.
264. Ogawa A, Uemura M, Kataoka Y, et al: Effects of ketamine on cardiovascular responses mediated by *N*-methyl-*d*-aspartate receptor in the rat nucleus tractus solitarius. Anesthesiology 1993;78:163–167.
265. Op De Coul A, Lambregts P, Koeman J, et al: Neuromuscular complications in patients given Pavulon (pancuronium bromide) during artificial ventilation. Clin Neurol Neurosurg 1985;87:17–22.
266. Ostergaard D, Viby-Mogensen J, Hanel H, Skovgaard L: Half-life of plasma cholinesterase. Acta Anaesthesiol Scand 1988;32:266–269.
267. O'Sullivan H, Jennings F, Ward K, et al: Human bone marrow biochemical function and megaloblastic hematopoiesis after nitrous oxide anesthesia. Anesthesiology 1981; 55:645–649.
268. Page P, Morgan H, Loh L: Ketamine anesthesia in pediatric procedures. Acta Anaesth Scand 1972;16:155–160.
269. Pantuck E: Plasma cholinesterase: Gene and variations. Anesth Analg 1993;77:380–386.
270. Park W, Lynch C III: Propofol and thiopental depression of myocardial contractility. A comparative study of mechanical and electrophysiologic effects in isolated guinea pig ventricular muscle. Anesth Analg 1992;74:395–405.
271. Parke T, Stevens J, Rice A, et al: Metabolic acidosis and fatal myocardial failure after propofol infusions in children: Five case reports. Br Med J 1992;305:613–616.
272. Parker C, Jones J, Hunter J: Disposition of infusions of atracurium and its metabolite, laudanosine, in patients in

renal and respiratory failure in an ITU. Br J Anaesth 1988;61:531–540.
273. Parker M, Schubert W, Shelhamer J, Parrillo J: Perceptions of a critically ill patient experiencing therapeutic paralysis in an ICU. Crit Care Med 1984;12:69–71.
274. Patel R, Connor G: A review of thirty cases of rhabdomyolysis-associated acute renal failure among phencyclidine users. Clin Toxicol 1985–1986;23:547–556.
275. Pearlman C: Neuroleptic malignant syndrome: A review of the literature. J Clin Psychopharmacol 1986;6:257–273.
276. Peduto V, Concas A, Santoro G, et al: Biochemical and electrophysiologic evidence that propofol enhances GABAergic transmission in the rat brain. Anesthesiology 1991;75:1000–1009.
277. Perel A, Davidson J: Recurrent hallucinations following ketamine. Anaesthesia 1976;31:1081–1083.
278. Pfenninger E, Reith A: Ketamine and intracranial pressure. In: Domino E, ed: Status of Ketamine in Anesthesiology. Ann Arbor, MI, NPP Books, 1990, pp. 109–118.
279. Piepoli M, Garrard C, Kontoyannis D, Bernardi L: Autonomic control of the heart and peripheral vessels in human septic shock. Intensive Care Med 1995;21:112–119.
280. Pinaud M, Lelausque J-N, Chetanneau A, et al: Effects of propofol on cerebral hemodynamics and metabolism in patients with brain trauma. Anesthesiology 1990;73: 404–409.
281. Pohl L, Gillette JR: A perspective on halothane-induced hepatotoxicity. Anesth Analg 1982;61:809–811.
282. Prentiss J: Cardiac arrest following caudal anesthesia. Anesthesiology 1979;50:51–53.
283. Puttick R, Terrar D: Differential effects of propofol and enflurane on contractions dependent on calcium derived from the sarcoplasmic reticulum of guinea pig isolated papillary muscle. Anesth Analg 1993;77:55–60.
284. Radnay P, Badola R: Generalized extensor spasm in infants following ketamine anesthesia. Anesthesiology 1973; 39:459–460.
285. Ramsay D, Zochodne D, Robertson D, et al: A syndrome of acute severe muscle necrosis in intensive care unit patients. J Neuropathol Exp Neurol 1993;52:387–398.
286. Reed M, Blumer J: Propofol bashing: The time to stop is now. Crit Care Med 1996;24:175–176.
287. Reed M, Yamashita T, Marx C, et al: A pharmacokinetically based propofol dosing strategy for sedation of the critically ill, mechanically ventilated pediatric patient. Crit Care Med 1996;29:1473–1481.
288. Reich D, Silvay G: Ketamine: An update on the first twenty-five years of experience. Can J Anaesth 1989;36: 186–197.
289. Reid D, Ingram G: Changes in blood coagulation during infusion of Intralipid. Clin Sci 1967;33:399–407.
290. Reiz S, Nath S: Cardiotoxicity of local anaesthetic agents. Br J Anaesth 1986;58:736–746.
291. Renou A, Vernhiet J, Macrez P, et al: Cerebral blood flow and metabolism during etomidate anesthesia in man. Br J Anaesth 1978;50:1047–1051.
292. Reves J, Glass P, Lubarsky D: Nonbarbiturate intravenous anesthetics. In: Miller R, ed: Anesthesia, 4th ed. New York, Churchill Livingstone, 1994, pp. 247–289.
293. Ridenour T, Warner D, Todd M, Baker M: Effects of ketamine on outcome from temporary middle cerebral artery occlusion in the spontaneously hypertensive rat. Brain Res 1991;565:116–122.
294. Riker W: Pre-junctional effects of neuromuscular blocking and facilitatory drugs. In: Katz R, ed: Muscle Relaxants. Amsterdam, North-Holland, 1975, pp. 59–102.
295. Rock M, Reyes de la Rocha S, L'Hommedieu C, Truemper E: Use of ketamine in asthmatic children to treat respiratory failure refractory to conventional therapy. Crit Care Med 1986;14:514–516.
296. Rosen M, Thigpen J, Shnider S, et al: Bupivacaine-induced cardiotoxicity in hypoxic and acidotic sheep. Anesth Analg 1985;64:1089–1096.
297. Roth B, Grände P, Nilsson-Ehle P, Eliasson I: Possible role of short-term parenteral nutrition with fat emulsions for development of haemophagocytosis with multiple organ failure in a patient with traumatic brain injury. Intensive Care Med 1993;19:111–114.
298. Rouleau G, Karpati G, Carpenter S, et al: Glucocorticoid excess induces preferential depletion of myosin in denervated skeletal muscle fibers. Muscle Nerve 1987;10: 428–438.
299. Rudis M, Guslits B, Peterson E, et al: Economic impact of prolonged motor weakness complicating neuromuscular blockade in the intensive care unit. Crit Care Med 1996; 24:1749–1756.
300. Rudis M, Sikora C, Angus E, et al: A prospective, randomized, controlled evaluation of peripheral nerve stimulation versus standard clinical dosing of neuromuscular blocking agents in critically ill patients. Crit Care Med 1997;25: 575–583.
301. Sakai F, Hiraoka M, Amaha K: Comparative actions of propofol and thiopentone on cell membranes of isolated guinea pig ventricular myocytes. Br J Anaesth 1996;77: 508–516.
302. Saltzman L, Kates R, Corke B, et al: Hyperkalemia and cardiovascular collapse after verapamil and dantrolene administration in swine. Anesth Analg 1984;63:473–478.
303. Samain E, Marty J, Gauzit R, et al: Effects of propofol on baroreflex control of heart rate and on plasma noradrenaline levels. Eur J Anaesthesiol 1989;6:321–326.
304. Sammalkorpi K, Valtonen V, Maury C: Lipoproteins and acute phase response during acute infection. Interrelationships between C-reactive protein and serum amyloid-A protein and lipoproteins. Ann Med 1990;22:397–401.
305. Sandrock AJ, Dryer S, Rosen K, et al: Maintenance of acetylcholine receptor number by neureglins at the neuromuscular junction in vivo. Science 1997;276:599–603.
306. Savarese J, Lien C, Belmont M, Rubin L: The clinical and basic pharmacology of mivacurium: A short-acting nondepolarizing benzylisoquinolinium diester neuromuscular blocking drug. Acta Anaesthesiol Scand 1995;39(suppl 106): 18–22.
307. Saxena P, Bonta I: Mechanism of selective cardiac vagolytic action of pancuronium bromide. Specific blockade of cardiac muscarinic receptors. Eur J Pharmacol 1970;3:332–341.
308. Schilling R: Is nitrous oxide a dangerous anesthetic for vitamin B_{12}-deficient subjects? JAMA 1986;255:1605–1606.
309. Schmith V, Phillips L, Kisor D, et al: Pharmacoki-

netics/pharmacodynamics of cis-atracurium in healthy adult patients. Curr Opin Anesthesiol 1996;9(suppl 1): S9–S15.

310. Schulte A, Esch J, Pfeifer G, Thiemig F: Der Einfluss von Etomidate und Thiopental auf den gesteigerten intracraniellen Druck. Anaesthesist 1978;27:71–75.
311. Schulz D, Macdonald R: Barbiturate enhancement of GABA-mediated inhibition and activation of chloride ion conductance: Correlation with anticonvulsants and anesthetic agents. Brain Res 1981;209:177–188.
312. Scott J, Dinn J, Wilson P, Weir D: Pathogenesis of subacute combined degeneration: A result of methyl group deficiency. Lancet 1981;2:334–337.
313. Sebel P, Lowdon J: Propofol: A new intravenous anesthetic. Anesthesiology 1989;71:260–277.
314. Segarra Domenech J, Carlos Garcia R, Rodrigues Sasiain J, et al: Pancuronium bromide: An indirect sympathomimetic agent. Br J Anaesth 1976;48:1143–1148.
315. Segredo V, Caldwell J, Matthay M, et al: Persistent paralysis in critically ill patients after long-term administration of vecuronium. N Engl J Med 1992;327:524–528.
316. Shapiro B, Warren J, Egol A, et al: Practice parameters for sustained neuromuscular blockade in the adult critically ill patient: An executive summary. Crit Care Med 1995; 23:1601–1605.
317. Shapiro J, Condos R, Cole R: Myopathy in status asthmaticus: Relation to neuromuscular blockade and corticosteroid administration. J Intensive Care Med 1993;8: 144–152.
318. Shimoji K, Takahata Y, Fujiwara N, et al: Effects of pentobarbital and ketamine on brain injury-induced antiischemic activity. Brain Res 1987;408:385–388.
319. Siegel R: Phencyclidine and ketamine intoxication: A study of four populations of recreational users. Natl Inst Drug Abuse Res Monogr Ser 1978;21:119–147.
320. Somogyi G, Varga M, Prokai L, et al: Drug identification problems in two suicides with neuromuscular blocking agents. Forensic Sci Int 1989;43:257–266.
321. Sosis M, Braverman B: Growth of *Staphylococcus aureus* in four intravenous anesthetics. Anesth Analg 1993;77: 766–768.
322. Sosis M, Braverman B, Villaflor E: Propofol but not thiopental supports the growth of *Candida albicans*. Anesth Analg 1995;81:132–134.
323. Spencer J, Raasch F, Trefny F: Halothane abuse in hospital personnel. JAMA 1976;235:1034–1035.
324. Sprague D: Severe bradycardia after neostigmine in a patient taking neostigmine to control paroxysmal atrial tachycardia. Anesthesiology 1975;42:208–210.
325. Stanley T: Blood-pressure and pulse-rate responses to ketamine during general anesthesia. Anesthesiology 1973; 39:648–649.
326. Stephan H, Sonntag H, Schenk H, et al: Effects of propofol on cardiovascular dynamics, myocardial blood flow and myocardial metabolism in patients with coronary artery disease. Br J Anaesth 1986;58:969–975.
327. Stephan S, Sonntag H, Schenk H, Kohlhausen S: Effect of Disoprivan (propofol) on the circulation and oxygen consumption of the brain and CO_2 reactivity of the brain vessels in the human. Anaesthetist 1987;36:60–65.
328. Stevens H, Moffat A: A rapid screening procedure for quaternary ammonium compounds in fluids and tissues with special reference to suxamethonium (succinylcholine). J Forensic Sci Soc 1974;14:141–148.
329. Stock J, Strunin L: Unexplained hepatitis following halothane. Anesthesiology 1985;63:424–439.
330. Stoelting R: The hemodynamic effects of pancuronium and *d*-tubocurarine in anesthetized patients. Anesthesiology 1976;36:612–615.
331. Stowe D, Bosnjak Z, Kampine J: Comparison of etomidate, ketamine, midazolam, propofol and thiopental of function and metabolism of isolated hearts. Anesth Analg 1992; 74:547–558.
332. Strazis K, Fox A: Malignant hyperthermia: A review of published cases. Anesth Analg 1993;77:297–304.
333. Strickland R, Murray M: Fatal metabolic acidosis in a pediatric patient receiving an infusion of propofol in the intensive care unit: Is there a relationship? Crit Care Med 1995;23:405–409.
334. Strube P, Hallam P: Ketamine by continuous infusion in status asthmaticus. Anesthesiology 1986;41:1017–1019.
335. Subcommittee on the National Halothane Study of the Committee on Anesthesia National Academy of Sciences—National Research Council: Summary of the national halothane study: Possible association between halothane anesthesia and postoperative hepatic necrosis. JAMA 1966;197:121–134.
336. Suton J, Harrison G, Hickie J: Accidental intravenous injection of halothane: Case report. Br J Anaesth 1971;43: 513–520.
337. Takahashi H, Puttick R, Terrar D: The effects of propofol and enflurane on single calcium channel currents of guinea-pig isolated myocytes. Br J Pharmacol 1994;111: 1147–1153.
338. Takeshita H, Okuda Y, Sari A: The effects of ketamine on cerebral circulation and metabolism in man. Anesthesiology 1972;36:69–74.
339. Tanaka K, Yamasaki M: Blocking of cortical inhibitory synapses by intravenous lidocaine. Nature 1966;209: 207–208.
340. Taves D, Fry B, Freeman R, Gillies A: Toxicity following methoxyflurane anesthesia. II. Fluoride concentrations and nephrotoxicity. JAMA 1970;214:91–95.
341. Thomas D: Propofol supports bacterial growth. Br J Anaesth 1991;66:274. Letter.
342. Thomson A, West D, Lodge D: An *N*-methylaspartate receptor-mediated synapse in rat cerebral cortex: A site of action of ketamine? Nature 1985;313:479–481.
343. Thomson S, Yate P: Bradycardia after propofol infusion. Anaesthesia 1987;42:430.
344. Thorsen T, Gran L: Ketamine/diazepam infusion anaesthesia with special attention to the effect on cerebrospinal fluid pressure and arterial blood pressure. Acta Anaesth Scand 1980;24:1–4.
345. Todd M, Drummond J, U HS: The hemodynamic consequences of high-dose thiopental anesthesia. Anesth Analg 1985;65:681–687.
346. Todd M, Drummond J, Sang H: The hemodynamic consequences of high-dose methohexital anesthesia in humans. Anesthesiology 1984;61:495–501.

347. Todd M, Drummond J, U HS: The hemodynamic consequences of high-dose thiopental anesthesia. Anesth Analg 1985;64:681–687.
348. Touloukian J, Kaplowitz N: Halothane-induced hepatic disease. Semin Liver Dis 1981;1:134–142.
349. Trotter C, Serpell M: Neurological sequelae in children after prolonged propofol infusion. Anaesthesia 1992;47: 340–342.
350. Utili R, Boitnott J, Zimmerman H: Dantrolene-associated hepatic injury: Incidence and character. Gastroenterology 1977;72:610–616.
351. Uzunalimoglu B, Yardley J, Boitnott J: The liver in mild halothane hepatitis: Light and electron microscopic findings with special reference to the mononuclear cell infiltrate. Am J Pathol 1970;61:457–478.
352. Van Aken H, Meinshausen E, Prien T, et al: The influence of fentanyl and tracheal intubation on the hemodynamic effects of anesthesia induction with propofol/N_2O in humans. Anesthesiology 1988;68:157–163.
353. Van Hamme M, Ghoneim M, Ambre J: Pharmacokinetics of etomidate, a new intravenous anesthetic. Anesthesiology 1978;49:274–277.
354. van Hemelrijk J, White P: Nonopioid intravenous anesthesia. In: Barash P, Cullen B, Stoelting R, eds: Clinical Anesthesia, 3rd ed. Philadelphia, Lippincott–Raven, 1997, pp. 311–328.
355. van Straaten E, Hendriks J, Ramsey G, Vos G: Rhabdomyolysis and pulmonary hypertension in a child, possibly due to long-term high-dose propofol infusion. Intensive Care Med 1996;22:997. Letter.
356. Van Winkle W: Calcium release from skeletal muscle sarcoplasmic reticulum: Site of action of dantrolene sodium? Science 1976;193:1130–1131.
357. Vandenbrom R, Wierda J: Pancuronium bromide in the intensive care unit. A case of overdose. Anesthesiology 1988; 69:996–997.
358. Vaughn R: Biochemical and biotransformation alterations in obesity. Contemp Anesth Pract 1982;5:55–70.
359. Vergani D, Tsantoulas D, Eddleston A, et al: Sensitization to halothane-altered liver components in severe hepatic necrosis after halothane anesthesia. Lancet 1978;2:801–803.
360. Viby-Mogensen J: Clinical assessment of neuromuscular transmission. Br J Anaesth 1982;54:209–223.
361. Wagner R, White P: Etomidate inhibits adrenocortical function in surgical patients. Anesthesiology 1984;61: 647–651.
362. Wagner R, White P, Kan P, et al: Inhibition of adrenal steroidogenesis by the anesthetic etomidate. N Engl J Med 1984;310:1415–1421.
363. Walton B, Simpson B, Strunin L, et al: Unexplained hepatitis following halothane. Br Med J 1976;1:1171–1176.
364. Wanscher M, Tønnesen E, Hüttel M, Larsen K: Etomidate infusion and adrenocortical function: A study in elective surgery. Acta Anaesth Scand 1985;29:483–485.
365. Ward A, Chaffman M, Sorkin E: Dantrolene: A review of its pharmacodynamic and pharmacokinetic properties and therapeutic use in malignant hyperthermia, and neuroleptic malignant syndrome and an update of its use in muscle spasticity. Drugs 1986;32:130–168.
366. Watkins J: Adverse reaction to neuromuscular blockers: Frequency, investigation, and epidemiology. Acta Anaesthesiol Scand 1994;38(suppl 102):6–10.
367. Wauquier A: Profile of etomidate. Anaesthesia 1983;38 (suppl):26–33.
368. Waxman K, Shoemaker W, Lippman M: Cardiovascular effects of anesthetic induction with ketamine. Anesth Analg 1980;59:355–358.
369. Wedel D, Quilan J, Iaizzo P: Clinical effects of intravenously administered dantrolene. Mayo Clin Proc 1995; 70:241–246.
370. West R: Curare in man. Proc R Soc Med 1932;25: 1107–1116.
371. White P, Ham J, Way W, Trevor A: Pharmacology of ketamine isomers in surgical patients. Anesthesiology 1980; 52:231–239.
372. White P, Way W, Trevor A: Ketamine—its pharmacology and therapeutic uses. Anesthesiology 1982;56:119–136.
373. Wig J, Chakravarty S, Krishnamurthy K, Mehta D: Coma following ingestion of halothane: Its successful management. Anaesthesia 1983;38:552–555.
374. Winters W: Epilepsy or anesthesia with ketamine. Anesthesiology 1972;36:309–311.
375. Wood M: Intravenous anesthetic agents. In: Wood M, Wood A, eds: Drugs and Anesthesia. Pharmacology for Anesthesiologists. Baltimore, Williams & Wilkins, 1990, pp. 179–223.
376. Wright P, Hart P, Lau M, et al: Cumulative characteristics of atracurium and vecuronium: A simultaneous clinical and pharmacokinetic study. Anesthesiology 1994;81: 59–68.
377. Wyse D, Kellen J, Tam Y, Rademaker A: Increased efficacy and toxicity of lidocaine in patients on beta-blockers. Int J Cardiol 1988;21:59–70.
378. Yamanaka I, Dowdy E: The effects of ketamine on spiral-cut strips of rabbit aorta. Anesthesiology 1974;40:222–227.
379. Yang C, Wong C, Yu C, et al: Propofol inhibits cardiac L-type calcium current in guinea pig ventricular myocytes. Anesthesiology 1996;84:626–635.
380. Yate P, Flynn P, Arnold R, et al: Clinical experience and plasma laudanosine concentrations during the infusion of atracurium in the intensive therapy unit. Br J Anaesth 1987;59:211–217.
381. Youngman P, Taylor K, Wilson J: Anaphylactoid reactions to neuromuscular blocking agents: A commonly undiagnosed condition? Lancet 1983;2:597–599.
382. Zimmerman S, Jones M, Harrison N: Potentiation of γ-aminobutyric acid A receptor Cl^- current correlates with *in vivo* anesthetic potency. J Pharmacol Exp Ther 1994; 270:987–991.
383. Zochodne D, Ramsay D, Saly V: Acute necrotizing myopathy of intensive care: Electrophysiologic studies. Muscle Nerve 1994;17:285–292.

CHAPTER 54

Pharmaceutical Additives

Sean Patrick Nordt

A 32-year-old man presented to the emergency department (ED) after being found at a local motel. The patient was confused and nonconversive when paramedics arrived on the scene. The patient's tongue was bleeding, and he had urinary incontinence, suggestive of a seizure. In the ED the patient had a blood pressure of 152/80 mm Hg, a pulse of 101 beats/min, respirations of 20 breaths/min, and temperature of 97.4° F (36.3° C). On physical examination the patient was noted to have several abrasions on the left side of his face; his pupils were 6 mm, equal and reactive to light; his tongue was bitten and bleeding; he was tachycardiac with a regular rhythm; his lungs were clear to auscultation; and his abdomen was soft and nontender. A 12-lead electrocardiogram showed sinus tachycardia with a rate of 102 beats/min, a PR interval of 200 msec, a QRS interval of 108 msec, and a corrected QT interval of 450 msec. An old ED chart revealed the patient had suffered a gun shot wound to the head with a subsequent seizure disorder. A loading dose of 1 g of fosphenytoin was ordered to be given intravenously over 5 minutes. Immediately following the fosphenytoin, the patient became hypotensive with a blood pressure of 85/50 mm Hg. His heart rate decreased to 52 beats/min, and his QRS interval widened to 140 msec. Atropine was given, resulting in an increase in heart rate to 82 beats/min. Wide open intravenous 0.9% sodium chloride was administered and restored his blood pressure. The patient's QRS narrowed to 100 msec without intervention several minutes later. Later it was realized the nurse had inadvertently drawn up phenytoin instead of fosphenytoin. Fosphenytoin, a prodrug of phenytoin, can be given more rapidly intravenously than phenytoin, or can be given intramuscularly. The patient had an adverse reaction to the rapid infusion of phenytoin, which contained 400 mg/mL of propylene glycol.

Pharmaceutical agents are labeled to reflect the active ingredient(s) of the product. However, these products often contain additives to improve the consistency, stability, color, or taste or to provide antibacterial and antifungal properties to medications, particularly those intended for multiple dose use (eg, ophthalmic drops). Although these additives or excipients are often termed "inert," implying that they possess no inherent pharmacologic properties of their own, this is not entirely true.

The most commonly used additives and nonimmunologic toxicities associated with their use are discussed. Many of these agents are also associated with hypersensitivity reactions, including anaphylaxis. Although these allergic hypersensitivity reactions are not discussed in this chapter, these additives should all be considered as possible causative agents in any patient developing hypersensitivity reactions.

Propylene Glycol

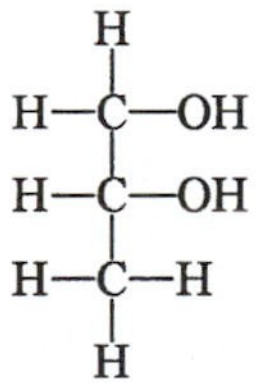

Propylene glycol (PG) or 1,2-propanediol is a clear, colorless, odorless, viscous liquid that is sweet to the taste. Propylene glycol is widely employed as a preservative and solvent in numerous pharmaceuticals (see Table 54–1).

TABLE 54–1. MEDICATIONS CONTAINING PROPYLENE GLYCOL

Medication	Percent Propylene Glycol
Apresoline (hydralazine)	40
Ativan (lorazepam)	80
Bactrim/Septra (trimethoprim/sulfamethoxazole)	40
Brevibloc (esmolol)	25
Dilantin (phenytoin)	40
Lanoxin (digoxin)	40
Librium (chlordiazepoxide)	20
MVI-12 (multivitamins)	30
Phenobarbital sodium	70
Tridil (nitroglycerin)	30
Valium (diazepam)	40

Pharmacokinetics

Propylene glycol is rapidly absorbed from the GI tract following oral administration and has a volume of distribution of approximately 0.6 L/kg.[61,83] When applied to intact epidermis, the absorption of PG is minimal. Percutaneous absorption may occur following application to damaged skin (eg, extensive burn surface areas). Propylene glycol is hepatically metabolized to lactic and pyruvic acid by alcohol dehydrogenase and is then further broken down to carbon dioxide and water.[68] The terminal half-life is reported to be between 1.4 and 5.6 hours in adults and as long as 16.9 hours in neonates.[27,83] Twelve to forty-five percent of propylene glycol is excreted unchanged in the urine.[27]

Cardiovascular

Intravenous preparations of phenytoin contain 40% propylene glycol to facilitate the solubility of phenytoin. Nine years after intravenous phenytoin became available, three deaths were attributed to the rapid administration of phenytoin used for the treatment of cardiac dysrhythmias.[38,88] Several years later, PG was identified as the cardiotoxin. Rapidly infusing PG results in hypotension, apnea, bradycardia, widening of the QRS interval, increased T waves with occasional inversions, and transient ST elevations. Conversely, when PG is infused slowly only minimal hypotension and moderate ECG changes result. Bradycardia and depression of atrial conduction were not observed in cats pretreated with atropine or vagotomy following rapid intravenous infusion of PG, suggesting these effects are vagally mediated. QRS widening was noted in these same pretreated cats, suggesting an additive direct cardiotoxic effect of propylene glycol.[59] Similar results were reported in calves pretreated with atropine that received oxytetracycline in a propylene glycol vehicle.[41]

Serum Osmolarity

There are numerous reports of propylene glycol–induced serum hyperosmolarity following the topical administration of silver sulfadiazine.[6,35,53] Hyperosmolarity was reported in 15 burn patients treated with topical silver sulfadiazine cream.[53] All of these patients had burn areas greater than 35% body surface area, facilitating the systemic absorption of PG. Hyperosmolarity also occurred in four infants receiving parenteral multivitamins dissolved in propylene glycol.[40] A correlation between decreased renal function and serum hyperosmolarity was found in patients receiving nitroglycerin dissolved in a propylene glycol–containing vehicle. A statistically significant increase in osmolar gap was reported in patients who had a calculated creatinine clearance of less than 30 mL/min.[27] Since propylene glycol is a volatile alcohol, the freezing point method of osmolarity determination is recommended for screening for PG overdosage (see Chap. 15). A 20–30 mOsm/kg discrepancy between values reported by freezing point and the vapor pressure was described in two patients being treated with silver sulfadiazine.[6]

Serum pH

Metabolic acidosis is also reported in patients receiving PG. The metabolic acidosis probably results from increased production of lactate, a metabolic by-product of PG metabolism.[20] Nephrotoxicity was associated with PG in an in vitro experiment that assessed the acute toxicity of propylene glycol in a human proximal tubule cell model. Lactate dehydrogenase and creatinine release were measured as indicators of tubular toxicity. The authors reported a concentration and time-dependent effect associated with propylene glycol, suggesting a direct toxic effect on proximal tubule cells.[68]

Neurotoxicity

Smaller infants appear to have a decreased ability to clear propylene glycol when compared to older children and adults.[60] An increased frequency of seizures was reported in low-birthweight infants who received greater than 10 mL a day of a parenteral multivitamin preparation containing 300 mg of PG/mL.[60] Seizures developed in an 11-year-old boy receiving long-term therapy with vitamin D dissolved in PG. Seizures abated after the product was discontinued.[2] Propylene glycol is an alcohol and may possess some inebriating properties similar to ethanol.[61] Central nervous system depression was reported following oral ingestions of propylene glycol–containing products.[20,61]

Ototoxicity

Many otic solutions and suspensions contain PG in their vehicles. Concentrations of PG greater than 10% were reported to result in cochlear hair cell loss and irreversible deafness when instilled into the middle ears of guinea pigs.[67] When this experiment was repeated by another author, 10% propylene glycol produced no negative effects. While 90% PG did impair cochlear function, there was no greater increase in hair cell loss than in controls.[89]

Thrombophlebitis

An increased frequency of thrombophlebitis occurred in patients who received intravenous diazepam in a propylene glycol solvent compared with diazepam suspended in another solvent, cremophor-EL (polyethoxylated castor oil). Sixty-two percent of the propylene glycol–treated patients had evidence of thrombophlebitis 14 days after administration compared to only 3.4% of the cremophor-EL patients. Pain on injection was also greater in intensity in the propylene glycol patients than in those receiving the other preparation, 65% and 8.5% respectively.[63] However, since cremophor-EL was associated with several cases of anaphylaxis, its widespread use is precluded.[28,29]

Drug Interactions

Propylene glycol may cause a transient neutralization of heparin by a mechanism similar to protamine.[21] Higher doses of heparin are sometimes required when used concomitantly with nitroglycerin containing propylene glycol as a diluent. However, heparin resistance seems to occur in patients receiving nitroglycerin whether or not the product contains propylene glycol.[42]

Polyethylene Glycol

Polyethylene glycols (Carbowaxes) include several compounds with varying molecular weights ranging from 150 to 10,000.[8] Polyethylene glycols (PEG) are mixtures that usually have a corresponding number denoting their average molecular weight. Polyethylene glycols possess a wide range of solubilities and compatibilities, making them useful as additives in pharmaceuticals (Table 54–2) and cosmetics. At room temperature, polyethylene glycols with molecular weights less than 600 are liquids, whereas those with molecular weights greater than 1000 are solids.[8] Polyethylene glycols with molecular weights greater than 6000 appear much less toxic than those of lower molecular weights when orally ingested.[80] There appears to be a decrease in toxicity as the molecular weights increase, similar to that of diethylene glycol and triethylene glycol.[79]

Commercially available products such as GoLytely and CoLyte are solutions of PEG 3350 combined with electrolytes (PEG-ELS). They are routinely employed to cleanse the bowel prior to surgery with minimal net water and electrolyte shifts. In addition, they are also used to decontaminate the gut following poisonings with sustained-release products or iron. Polyethylene glycols combined with electrolytes are considered relatively nontoxic even after massive quantities have been ingested. A 33-month-old child received a total of 44.3 L PEG-ELS over 5 days following iron poisoning without any adverse effects.[52]

TABLE 54–2. DRUGS CONTAINING POLYETHYLENE GLYCOL

Chloroptic (chloramphenicol) ointment
CoLyte
Decadron ophthalmic ointment
DepoProvera (progesterone)
GoLytely
Monistat I.V. (miconazole)
Nulytely
Vepesid (etoposide)

Nephrotoxicity

When rats fed various polyethylene glycols (200, 300, and 400) in their drinking water for 90 days were studied, an 8% solution of PEG 200 produced renal tubular necrosis in all the animals, followed by death within 15 days, while a 4% solution of PEG 200 resulted in only two of nine rats dying within 80 days. A 16% solution of polyethylene glycol 400 killed all animals within 13 days; however, both 8% and 4% solutions had no observable effect except for lighter kidney weights than controls.[81]

In a suicide attempt, a 65-year-old male ingested the contents of a lava lamp that contained 13% PEG 200 in addition to water, paraffin, kerosene, and wax. Forty-eight hours after admission, the patient became oliguric with a corresponding BUN of 30 mg/dL and a serum creatinine of 7.9 mg/dL. The patient also had an anion gap metabolic acidosis.[32] He was discharged 3 months later with residual kidney dysfunction attributed to the PEG component of the lamp.

Serum Osmolarity

Serum hyperosmolarity was reported in patients with burn surface areas ranging from 20 to 56%, following the application of Furacin, a topical dressing containing 63% PEG 300 and 32% PEG 1000.[18] Polyethylene glycol produces a greater osmotic effect than can be accounted for by the number of PEG molecules in solution. In addition, the measured serum osmolarity is greater when the freezing point depression method is used than with the vapor pressure method.[77] Renal tubular necrosis and severe hydropic degeneration was seen on autopsy of nine burn patients treated with a topical antibiotic cream in a PEG base. These effects were reproduced with the topical application of PEG for 7 days to rabbits with full thickness skin defects.[84]

Serum pH

Polyethylene glycol is oxidized by alcohol dehydrogenase to hydroxyacid and diacid metabolites, possibly contributing to metabolic acidosis.[47] Two severe cases of metabolic acidosis were reported following intravenous administration of nitrofurantoin mixed with polyethylene glycol.[85] Similarly, an increased anion gap was reported in three patients being treated with a topical polyethylene glycol–based burn cream.[18]

Neurotoxicity

Neurologic complications following intrathecal steroidal injections containing 3% polyethylene glycol as a vehicle are reported.[10] An in vitro experiment exposed sheathed and desheathed rabbit nerves to concentrations of PEG 3350 ranging from 3 to 40% for 1 hour. Three and ten percent PEG had no effect on either nerve conduction or the amplitude of action potentials. Twenty and thirty percent PEG markedly slowed nerve conduction and had varying effects on amplitudes of action potentials. Forty percent PEG completely abolished action potentials.[8] This impairment of nerve conduction may be related to the osmotic effects of polyethylene glycol.[8]

Benzyl Alcohol

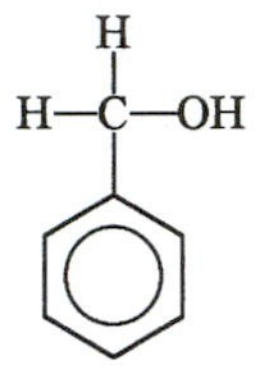

Benzyl alcohol (benzene methanol) is a colorless liquid with a faint aromatic odor that is most commonly added to pharmaceuticals as a bacteriostatic agent (Table 54–3). In 1982 a "gasping" syndrome was first described in low-birth-weight neonates in intensive care units.[17,39] The syndrome manifested with hypotonia, progressive metabolic acidosis, bradycardia, gasping respirations, seizures, hypotension, and cardiovascular collapse and resulted in death.[17,39] The onset of symptoms typically occurred within the first 2 weeks of life.[50] All the infants had received either bacteriostatic water or sodium chloride containing 0.9% benzyl alcohol to flush intravenous catheters or in parenteral medications reconstituted with bacteriostatic water or saline.[17,39] The syndrome only occurred in infants who had received greater than 99 mg/kg of benzyl alcohol (range from 99 to 234 mg/kg) while infants who received less than 99 mg/kg did not develop any symptoms.[39]

TABLE 54–3. DRUGS CONTAINING BENZYL ALCOHOL

Parenteral Medication	Percent Benzyl Alcohol
Bactrim/Septra (trimethoprim/ sulfamethoxazole)	1
Bumex (bumetanide)	1
Compazine (prochlorperazine)	0.75
Cordarone (amiodarone)	2.2
Valium (diazepam)	1.5
Lasix (furosemide)	0.9
Methotrexate	0.9
Norcuron (vecuronium)	0.9
Pronestyl (procainamide)	0.9
Tracurium (atracurium)	0.9
Vasotec (enalapril)	0.9
Vepesid (etoposide)	3
Versed (midazolam)	1
Vistaril (hydroxyzine)	0.9

Pharmacokinetics

In adults, benzyl alcohol is oxidized to benzoic acid, conjugated in the liver with glycine, and then excreted in the urine as hippuric acid. The immature metabolic capacities of the infants diminished their ability to metabolize and excrete benzyl alcohol.[39] Preterm babies actually have an increased ability to metabolize benzyl alcohol to benzoic acid compared to term babies. However, preterm infants are unable to convert benzoic acid to hippuric acid, possibly from glycine deficiency, resulting in the accumulation of benzoic acid[54] (Fig. 54–1). A fatal case of metabolic acidosis was reported in a 5-year-old girl who had received 2.4 mg/kg/h diazepam preserved with benzyl alcohol for 36 hours to control status epilepticus. Elevated benzoic acid levels were identified in serum and urine samples. The estimated daily dosing of benzyl alcohol was 180 mg/kg, which was much higher than the recommended maximum single dosage of 4 mg/kg in adults.[39,56]

Hematologic

An in vitro hemolytic effect was reported in red blood cells preserved with 1.5% benzyl alcohol.[64] Although the consequence of this in vitro phenomenon has not been elucidated in humans, it may have a role in the increased frequency of intraventricular hemorrhages and mortality reported in low-birth-weight infants (< 1000 g) who received flush solutions preserved with benzyl alcohol.[50] An increased incidence of developmental delay and cerebral palsy was also seen in the same patient population.[7]

Neurotoxicity

Amplitudes of action potentials were measured in rats exposed to 0.9% or 1.5% benzyl alcohol in either 0.9% sodium chloride or distilled water. Rats were exposed to benzyl alcohol either acutely (less than 1 minute) or chronically (for 7 days). Acutely, action potentials were 95–100% blocked by benzyl alcohol; however, nerve function was somewhat restored after rinsing the nerves with 0.9% sodium chloride. Chronic exposure to benzyl alcohol 0.9% showed scattered demyelinization and early remyelinization, whereas nerve roots exposed to 1.5% benzyl alcohol showed widespread demyelinization and fatty degeneration of nerve fibers.[45] These results suggest that in cases of inadvertent intrathecal administration of benzyl alcohol–containing products, cerebrospinal fluid exchanges with 0.9% sodium chloride may attenuate nerve dysfunction. There are several reports of transient paraplegia following the intrathecal or epidural administration of antineoplastics or analgesics containing benzyl alcohol as the preservative.[4,22,45,75]

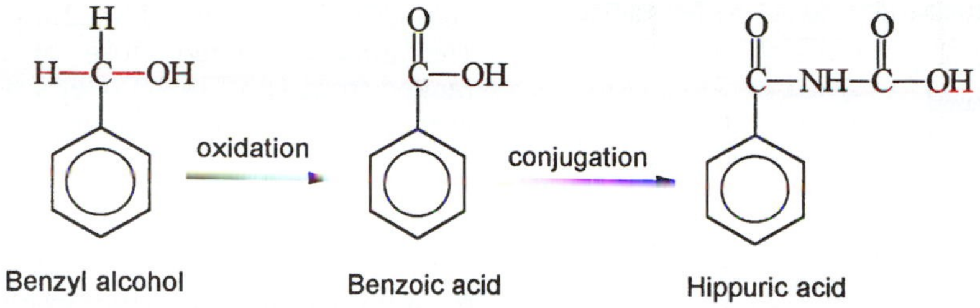

Figure 54–1. The oxidative metabolism of benzyl alcohol.

Chlorobutanol

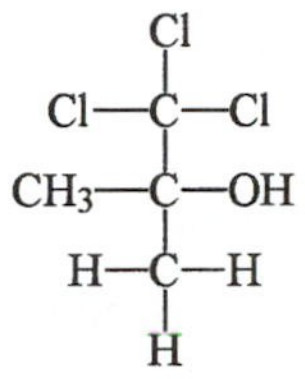

Chlorobutanol or chlorbutol (1,1,1,-trichloro-2-methyl-2-propranol) is widely used as a preservative in pharmaceutical preparations (Table 54–4). It has antibacterial and antifungal properties, in a concentration of 0.5% in injectables, ophthalmics, otics, and cosmetics. Because of its sedative-hypnotic and anxiolytic effects, small doses of chlorobutanol have been used to improve the performance of racing greyhounds.[72]

Central Nervous System Depression

Chlorobutanol has a chemical structure similar to trichloroethanol (see Fig. 61–5), the active metabolite of chloral hydrate. It has therefore been suggested that chlorobutanol has pharmacologic properties similar to those of chloral hydrate, although data to support this are lacking. A 40-year-old alcoholic male chronically abused chlorobutanol in Seducaps, a nonprescription hypnotic available in Australia and other countries. He was noted to have dysarthria, slurred speech, and occasional episodes of irregular clonic jerks. The speech abnormality resolved over 4 weeks as plasma chlorobutanol levels declined. No drugs other than chlorobutanol were detected in the patient's urine or plasma.[11]

TABLE 54–4. DRUGS CONTAINING CHLOROBUTANOL

Adrenalin (epinephrine)
Chloroptic (chloramphenicol)
Epiphrine (epinephrine) opththalmic solution
Methadone injectable
Novocain (procaine)
Phospholine iodide (echothiophate iodide)
Tobrex (tobramycin)

An additive somnolent effect from chlorobutanol was suggested in a 19-year-old woman treated with high doses of morphine preserved with chlorobutanol. It was calculated she received 90 mg/h of chlorobutanol for several days, far in excess of the recommended dosage of 150 mg/d. Her peak plasma chlorobutanol concentration was 83 μg/mL, similar to previously reported concentrations.[11,26]

Cardiovascular

In patients undergoing elective coronary artery bypass graft surgery, a clinically important decrease in arterial blood pressure (15.4 vs 1.3 mm Hg, $p = 0.01$) was reported when heparin preserved with 0.5% chlorobutanol was compared to preservative-free heparin. No effect on heart rate or central venous pressure was noted in this study.[14] Chlorobutanol is a halogenated hydrocarbon and therefore may theoretically sensitize the myocardium to catecholamines in acute poisonings, although no cases of ventricular dysrhythmias have been described in the literature to date.

Ophthalmologic

Chlorobutanol increases the permeability of cells by interrupting the structure of cell membranes.[87] Chlorobutanol has been reported to arrest mitotic activity in human cadaver corneal epithelial cells.[87] However, in another study, although chlorobutanol was shown to be cytotoxic, it had a lesser toxicity than other commonly used ophthalmic preservatives such as benzalkonium chloride.[69]

Thimerosal

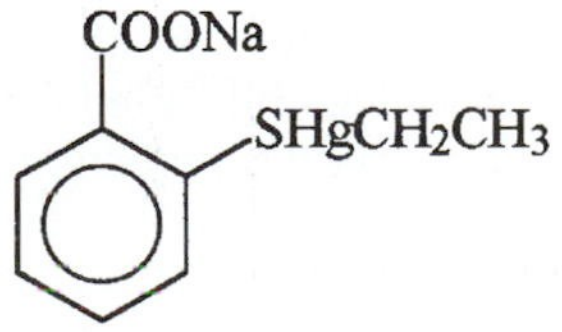

Thimerosal (Merthiolate, Mercurothiolate) or sodium ethylmercuric thiosalicylate is an organic mercury compound that is widely employed as a contact lens disinfectant and as a preservative in numerous pharmaceuti-

TABLE 54–5. DRUGS AND OTHER PREPARATIONS CONTAINING THIMEROSAL

Crotalidae (Wyeth) antivenin
Diphtheria–tetanus toxoid
Gammar (gamma immune globulin)
Lactrodectus mactans antivenin
Micrurus fulvius antivenin
Neosporin (triple antibiotic) ophthalmic solution
Ocufren (flurbiprofen) ophthalmic solution
Pneumovax-23 (pneumococcal) vaccine
Rabies immune globulin

cals[24,66] (Table 54–5). Thimerosal has a wide spectrum of antibacterial activity when used in concentrations of 0.02–0.1%; however, higher concentrations are sometimes used.[66] Thimerosal contains approximately 49% mercury by weight.[74]

Oral Ingestion

In a suicide attempt a 44-year-old man ingested 5 g (83 mg/kg) of thimerosal; within 15 minutes he began vomiting spontaneously. Gastric lavage was performed and chelation therapy begun with 300 mg of dimercaptopropane sulfonate (DMPS) instilled through a nasogastric tube into the stomach. Gastroscopy revealed a grade 2 hemorrhagic gastritis. Polyuric acute renal failure was noted on the day of admission and persisted for 40 days. Four days after admission the patient developed a fever and a maculopapular exanthem not attributed to an allergic reaction to the DMPS. The patient also developed an autonomic and ascending peripheral polyneuropathy that persisted for 13 days. Chelation therapy was continued for a total of 50 days with DMPS followed by dimercaptosuccinic acid (DMSA). Elevated blood and urine mercury levels persisted for more than 140 days. The patient was discharged 148 days following the ingestion with only sensory defects in his toes. No other neurologic sequelae were noted.[71]

Otolaryngologic

An 18-month-old girl died of mercury poisoning following irrigations with an otic solution containing 0.1% thimerosal and 0.14% sodium borate. A total of 1.2 L of solution (500 mg mercury) had been instilled over a 4-week period. Tympanostomy tubes, placed 1 year previously, allowed for the majority of the irrigation solution to be swallowed and subsequently absorbed through the gastrointestinal tract. The child died 3 months later, despite chelation therapy with D-penicillamine.[74]

Intramuscular Administration

Urine mercury levels were studied in 26 patients with hypogammaglobulinemia who received intramuscular weekly IgG replacement therapy preserved with 0.01% thimerosal. The dosage of IgG ranged from 25 mg/kg to 50 mg/kg, containing 0.6–1.2 mg of mercury per dose.[43] The total estimated dose of mercury administered ranged from 4 to 734 mg over a period of 6 months to 17 years. Elevated urine mercury levels were determined in 19 patients; however, no patients had clinical evidence of chronic mercury toxicity.[43]

Six cases of severe mercury poisoning resulting in four deaths were reported following the intramuscular administration of chloramphenicol preserved with thimerosal. A manufacturing error resulted in each vial containing 510 mg of thimerosal instead of 0.51 mg per vial. Extensive tissue necrosis was noted at the site of injection in all patients. Fever, altered mental status, slurred speech, and ataxia were noted. On autopsy there was evidence of widespread degeneration and necrosis of the renal tubules. Elevated mercury concentrations were found in kidneys, livers, brain, and injection site tissues.[3]

Ophthalmologic Administration

Mercury concentrations were measured in the aqueous humor and excised corneal buttons of nine patients undergoing keratoplasty. A contact lens stored for several weeks in a solution containing thimerosal was applied to one eye for 4 hours. After 4 hours the lens was removed and mercury concentrations were determined in aqueous humor, corneal buttons, and the contact lens itself. Markedly elevated levels of mercury were determined in both aqueous humor and corneal buttons of subjects as compared to controls; however, there was little residual mercury on the contact lens after 4 hours. The mercury content in the corneal buttons of subjects ranged from 0.6 to 14 ng per tissue. The mercury content in samples of aqueous humor from subjects ranged from 20 to 46 ng/mL. Untoward effects from the accumulation of mercury in the eye have not been identified, although the authors noted that the aqueous humor concentrations were in the same range as those seen in 10 patients (11–104 ng/mL) with symptomatic mercury poisoning.[91]

Topical Administration

Ten of 13 infants exposed to topical applications of a thimerosal tincture 0.1% for the treatment of exomphalos died. The total number of applications ranged from 9 to 48. Mercury concentrations were determined in various tissues from 6 of the infants. Mean tissue concentrations in fresh samples of liver, kidney, spleen, and heart ranged from 5152 to 11,330 ppb, suggesting percutaneous absorption from repeated topical applications.[33]

A chemical interaction between thimerosal and aluminum electrodes caused skin burns in a woman following a surgical procedure. Thimerosal acted as a catalyst that rapidly oxidized the aluminum electrode, generating heat and causing a subsequent thermal injury.[51]

Benzalkonium Chloride

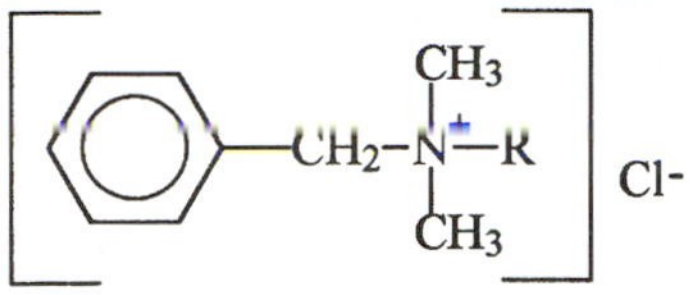

Benzalkonium chloride (BAK) is a quaternary ammonium cationic surfactant composed of a mixture of alkyl benzyl dimethyl ammonium chlorides. It is the most widely used ophthalmic preservative in the United States and is also considered the most cytotoxic[55] (Table 54–6). Benzalkonium chloride possesses activity against gram-positive and gram-negative bacteria as well as some viruses, fungi, and protozoa. Benzalkonium chloride is preferred to other preservatives due to its rapid onset of action, good tissue penetration, and long duration of action. The concentration of BAK in ophthalmic medications usually ranges from 0.004 to 0.01%.[55]

Ophthalmologic Toxicity

A 36-year-old woman complained of decreased vision when she inadvertently switched from Lensrins, a contact lens cleaning solution, to Dacriose, an isotonic boric acid solution preserved with BAK. After 3 days, she was noted to have inflammation, pain, and decreased visual acuity. Examination of the cornea revealed many superficial punctate erosions of the epithelium. An in vitro experiment identified significant binding of BAK to soft contact lenses.[36]

A 56-year-old man diagnosed with keratoconjunctivitis sicca was treated with topical antibiotics and artificial tears containing BAK. Following 1 year of continual use, the patient developed intractable pain, photophobia, and extensive breakdown of the corneal epithelium; however, neither of the BAK-containing products was suspected. The patient continued to use the artificial tear solution for an additional 9 years despite continued pain and decreasing visual acuity. The artificial tear solution was then replaced with a preservative-free saline solution with a dramatic resolution of pain, photophobia, and corneal changes.[55]

In an in vitro experiment, human cadaver corneal cells were exposed to a medium containing 0.01% BAK. Immediate halting of mitotic activity was reported following exposure to the medium. Within 2 hours, degenerative changes to the corneal epithelium were noted. No recovery of cytokinesis or mitosis was seen 24 hours after exposure to BAK.[87] Benzalkonium chloride was shown to possess surfactant properties resulting in the dissolution of the intercellular matrix and the loss of superficial layers of epithelial tissue. Patients with a compromised corneal epithelium may be at an increased risk to the adverse corneal effects of BAK.[87]

In another in vitro experiment, human adenoidal tissue was exposed to oxymetalozine preserved with BAK at various concentrations. A dose- and time-dependent effect was demonstrated on epithelial cell morphology, with the highest concentrations resulting in irregular and broken epithelial cells within 36 hours. Similarly, the number of beating ciliary bodies decreased as the duration and the concentrations increased. Benzalkonium chloride may actually decrease the viscosity of the normal protective mucus blanket, thereby increasing the risk of cytotoxicity.[9] One or two applications of BAK 0.01% irreversibly halted the transport of ciliated epithelial cells in a frog model.[5]

Phenol

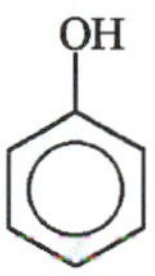

Phenol (carbolic acid) is a commonly used preservative in injectable medications (Table 54–7). Commercially available glucagon is a lyophilized powder containing either 1 mg or 10 mg of glucagon. A diluent containing 1 mL or 10 mL sterile water preserved with 0.2% phenol and 1.6% glycerin is included. Reconstituted glucagon contains 2 mg of phenol per mL. Glucagon in doses of 0.5–1 mg are employed in the treatment of hypoglycemia. High doses

TABLE 54–6. OPHTHALMIC PREPARATIONS CONTAINING BENZALKONIUM CHLORIDE

Acular (ketorolac)	Mydriacil (tropicamide)
Betagan (levobunolol)	Neosynephrine (phenylephrine)
Betoptic (betaxolol)	Ocuflox (ofloxacin)
Ciloxan (ciprofloxacin)	Ocupres (cartelol)
Cyclogyl (cyclopentolate)	Polytrim (trimethoprim)
Decadron (dexamethasone)	Timoptic (timolol)
Garamycin (gentamicin)	Tobrex (tobramycin)
Glaucon (epinephrine)	Various artificial tears
Isoptocarpine (pilocarpine)	Visine (tetrahydrolozine)

TABLE 54–7. DRUGS OR PREPARATIONS CONTAINING PHENOL

Antivenin (*Crotalidae*)
Antivenin (*Micrurus fulvius*)
Glucagon
Meperidine (demerol)
Pneumovax 23 (pneumococcal) vaccine
Prostigmin (neostigmine)
Quinidine gluconate
SusPhrine (epinephrine)

of glucagon (up to 5 mg/h) are advocated in the treatment of severe beta-adrenergic antagonist and calcium channel blockade poisonings. There is a concern of systemic phenol toxicity following the administration of high doses of glucagon reconstituted with the enclosed diluent.[23,65] It is recommended that the total dose of phenol in humans not exceed 50 mg in a 10-hour period.[15] Therefore, glucagon should be reconstituted with either 0.9% sodium chloride, 5% dextrose in water, or sterile water for injection when the dose exceeds 10 mg.[23,65] The diluent is enclosed for reconstitution for intramuscular administration when intravenous access is unavailable. The diluent contains phenol to prolong the shelf life of the glucagon, according to the manufacturer (personal communication Lily Pharmaceuticals).

Topical Administration

Drowsiness, respiratory depression, and blue-colored urine were reported in a 6-month-old child after repeated applications of magenta paint (also known as Castellani's Paint). Magenta paint, which contains 4% phenol, magenta, boric acid, resorcinol, acetone, and methylated spirit, was previously widely employed in the treatment of seborrheic eczema in infants. Due to the suspicion of systemic phenol toxicity, the urines of 16 children treated with topical magenta paint were evaluated for the presence of phenol. Phenol was detected in the urine of four children who had approximately 11–15% of their body surface area painted twice daily for 48 hours.[73] Following the application of a chemical peeling solution, multifocal premature ventricular complexes were observed in a 10-year-old boy. This solution contained 40% phenol; however, no phenol levels were obtained to confirm systemic absorption of phenol.[90]

Parabens

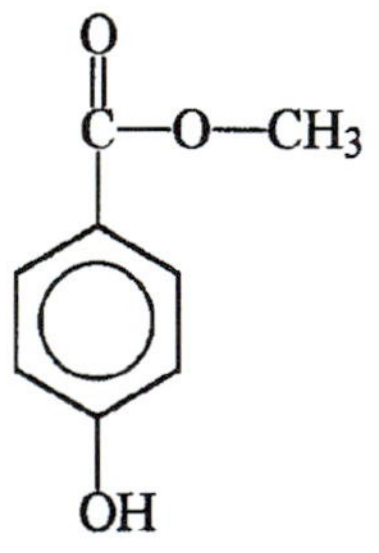

Methylparaben

The parabens or parahydroxybenzoic acids are widely employed as preservatives due to their bacteriostatic, fungistatic, and antioxidant properties[76] (Table 54–8). Parabens are often used in combination, because the presence of two or more parabens results in synergistic action.[57] The two most commonly employed parabens are the methyl and propyl esters.[76] A survey conducted by the Food and Drug Administration identified the parabens as the second most commonly found ingredients in cosmetic formulations, with water being the most common.[57] Therefore, due to the widespread exposure to these agents, it is felt that the parabens have a relatively low order of toxicity, although they are associated with a higher incidence of allergic reactions as compared to other pharmaceutical additives.[76] Food and prescription medications containing greater than 0.1% parabens must be labeled as such, whereas OTCs and cosmetics do not have to list the presence of parabens.[76] In the United States, the concentration of parabens usually ranges from 0.1 to 0.3%; however, Aureomycin and Achromycin each contain methyl paraben 2.4% and propyl paraben 0.6%. In Europe, parabens are used topically in a concentration of 5% as antifungal agents.

TABLE 54–8. DRUGS CONTAINING PARABENS

Bleph-10 (sulfacetamide) ophthalmic solution	Narcan (naloxone)
Dilaudid (hydromorphone)	Oncovin (vincristine)
Haldol (haloperidol)	Prolixin (fluphenazine)
Inapsine (droperidol/fentanyl)	Romazicon (flumazenil)
Marcaine (bupivicaine)	Trandate (labetalol)
Mestinon (neostigmine)	Xylocaine (lidocaine)
Methyldopate	Zofran (ondansetron)

Bilirubin Displacement

Gentamicin injection preserved with methyl and propyl paraben displaces bilirubin from albumin binding sites at serum concentrations ranging from 3 to 15 μg/mL.[25] An in vitro experiment demonstrated bilirubin displacement by methyl paraben 0.2 mg/mL in serum obtained from 28 hyperbilirubinemic newborns, while gentamicin alone had no effect on bilirubin displacement.[58]

Spermicidal Activity

The in vitro spermicidal activity of methyl, ethyl, propyl, and butyl paraben was studied in human semen specimens. All the parabens possessed significant spermicidal activity in concentrations ranging from 1 to 8 mg/mL. The authors suggested the parabens be further investigated as vaginal contraceptives.[82] The impact of routine topical application of cosmetics and medications, particularly to women, as well as the ingestion of foods containing parabens has not been fully elucidated although they are generally considered nontoxic.[57]

Other Pharmaceutical Tragedies

E-Ferol

In December 1983 a new parenteral vitamin E formulation became available marketed as E-Ferol. Each 2-mL unit dose vial contained 25 U/mL of α-tocopherol acetate, 9% polysorbate 80, 1% polysorbate 20, and water for injection. By early 1984 a fatal syndrome was described in low-birth-weight infants characterized by thrombocytopenia, renal dysfunction, cholestasis, hepatomegaly, and ascites.[1,62] The syndrome was seen in infants who received greater than 20 U/kg/d of E-Ferol.[62] Exposure to E-Ferol was associated with progressive intralobular cholestasis, inflammation of hepatic venules, and extensive sinusoidal veno-occlusion by fibrosis. In addition, acute tubular necrosis and substantial deposition of oxalate-type crystals in the distal renal tubules and collecting ducts was reported.[12,16]

Vitamin E was implicated as the offending agent, although it is now believed the polysorbate emulsifiers are responsible. Polysorbates are a mixture of oleate esters of sorbitol and sorbitol anhydrides condensed with ethylene oxide.[1] Polysorbates are used extensively as hydrophilic and nonionic surfactants.

Polysorbate 80 is associated with impaired uptake and secretion of bile acids and loss of microvilli in rabbits.[1] Chronic oral administration of polysorbate 80 in rats results in congestion and dilatation of central veins and sinusoids in liver and possibly capillary wall damage. Polysorbate 20 causes hypotension due to histamine release, increasing capillary permeability. The renal lesions resemble those occurring with arterial hypotension. The presence of oxylate-type crystals may have resulted from ethylene oxide being converted to ethylene glycol in vivo.

Four months after its release, E-Ferol was recalled by the manufacturer. There were 38 deaths and 43 cases of severe symptoms associated with the use of E-Ferol. No premarketing testing was required as E-Ferol was a new formulation of vitamin E. There is a concern that the long-term use of other medications containing polysorbates such as Poly-Vi-Sol and Tri-Vi-Sol may be dangerous, although these data are lacking.

Diethylene Glycol

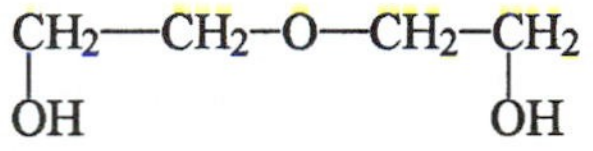

Diethylene glycol (DEG) has been associated with a number of outbreaks following its use as a pharmaceutical adulterant in numerous countries. Diethylene glycol is an excellent solvent, which has been substituted for propylene glycol and glycerin due to its lower cost. The most famous outbreak of mass DEG poisoning was the Massengill sulfanilamide disaster in 1937.[19,37,44] One-hundred-five people died of acute renal failure when a new liquid antibiotic was formulated with DEG to facilitate the solubility of sulfanilamide.[19] More recently there have been a number of outbreaks of acute renal failure when DEG was used to solubilize acetaminophen in South Africa, Bangladesh, Nigeria, and Haiti.[13,34,46,70] One study identified DEG as the sole diluent in 19 of 69 foreign acetaminophen elixirs tested.[46]

The mechanism of toxicity of diethylene glycol is unknown. Diethylene glycol, unlike ethylene glycol, does not produce a profound metabolic acidosis or calcium oxalate deposition in renal tubules. Initially diethylene glycol causes nausea, vomiting, and severe abdominal pain.[13,19] Within 24 hours of ingestion, polyuria is seen followed by oliguria and anuria.[19,37] Renal damage has been suggested to be due to hygroscopic swelling of the renal parenchyma, which obstructs the tubular lumen.[37] Unlike ethylene glycol, DEG causes central hydropic degeneration of hepatic cells, hepatomegaly, and jaundice.[37]

Diethylene glycol does not have a high affinity for alcohol dehydrogenase; therefore, treatment with ethanol or 4-methylpyrazole has a limited role if any. The treatment of DEG poisoning is supportive, and patients often require hemodialysis as a result of renal failure.

Eosinophilia-Myalgia Syndrome

In October 1989 a debilitating syndrome was described in three women chronically ingesting oral preparations of L-tryptophan.[30] All the patients had severe muscle pain, mouth ulcers, and elevated eosinophil counts.[30,48] By late November 1989 the CDC had identified 360 cases of "eosinophilia-myalgia syndrome" (EMS) and one fatality, prompting a recall of all L-tryptophan-containing products.[31] Other common symptoms include arthralgia, rash, dyspnea, cough, peripheral edema, elevated aldolose levels, and increased liver function tests.[86]

L-Tryptophan is an essential amino acid formerly available as a dietary supplement. L-Tryptophan was a popular over-the-counter remedy for insomnia, premenstrual syndrome, and depression and an aid to weight loss.[48] All the L-tryptophan available in the United States was manufactured by six Japanese pharmaceutical companies.[78] Over 98% of patients with EMS had received L-tryptophan manufactured by a single Japanese company, Showa Denko.[49,78] Over 60 contaminants were identified in the Showa Denko L-tryptophan, six of which have been associated with EMS.[49] There have been several thousand cases of EMS and 36 deaths attributed to contaminated L-tryptophan.[49]

Summary

Pharmaceutical additives are often termed "inert," implying they possess no pharmacologic or toxicologic properties of their own. Although these agents are very necessary and very useful, they may also be responsible for severe and sometimes fatal adverse effects. The FDA now requires all new pharmacologic agents to list all ingredients in the package insert. However, package inserts of older agents may not list all the inert ingredients. When assessing whether an agent is responsible for an adverse effect or not, the other additives should be included as well. Many of these additives may be responsible for allergic reactions. They are found in numerous pharmaceuticals, cosmetics, and foods, thus allowing for sensitization. For the most part pharmaceutical agents are safe and effective and allow long-term storage and multiple-dose containers, as well as improving the solubility, stability, and taste of medications.

References

1. Alade SL, Brown RE, Paquet A: Polysorbate 80 and E-Ferol toxicity. Pediatrics 1986;77:593–597.
2. Arulanantham K, Genel M: Central nervous system toxicity associated with ingestion of propylene glycol. J Pediatr 1978;93:515–516.
3. Axton JH: Six cases of poisoning after parenteral organic mercurial compound (merthiolate). Postgrad Med J 1972;48: 417–421.
4. Bagshawe KD, Magrath IT, Golding PR: Intrathecal methotrexate. Lancet 1969;2:1258.
5. Batts AH, Marriott C, Martin GP, et al: The effect of some preservatives used in nasal preparations on mucociliary clearance. J Pharm Pharmacol 1989;41:156–159.
6. Bekeris L, Baker C, Fenton J, et al: Propylene glycol as a cause of an elevated serum osmolality. Am J Clin Pathol 1979;72:633–636.
7. Benda GI, Hiller JL, Reynolds JW: Benzyl alcohol toxicity: Impact on neurologic handicaps among surviving very low birth weight infants. Pediatrics 1986;77:507–512.
8. Benzon HT, Gissen AJ, Strichartz GR, et al: The effect of polyethylene glycol on mammalian nerve impulses. Anesth Analg 1987;66:553–559.
9. Berg ØH, Henriksen RN, Steisvåg SK: The effect of a benzalkonium chloride-containing nasal spray on human respiratory mucosa in vitro as a function of concentration and time of action. Pharmacol Toxicol 1995;76:245–249.
10. Bernat JL: Intraspinal steroid therapy. Neurology 1981;31: 168–171.
11. Borody T, Chinweah PM, Graham GG, et al: Chlorobutanol toxicity and dependence. Med J Aust 1979;1:288.
12. Bove KE, Kosmetatos N, Wedig KE, et al: Vaculopathic hepatotoxicity associated with E-Ferol syndrome in low-birth-weight infants. JAMA 1985;254:2422–2430.
13. Bowie MD, McKenzie D: Diethylene glycol poisoning in children. South Afr Med J 1972;46:931–934.
14. Bowler GM, Galloway DW, Mieklejohn BH: Sharp fall in blood pressure after injection of heparin containing chlorbutol. Lancet 1986;1:848–849.
15. Brancato DJ: Recognizing potential toxicity of phenol. Vet Hum Toxicol 1982;24:29–30.
16. Brown RE, Krouse MA: Polysorbates and renal oxylate crystals in the E-Ferol syndrome. JAMA 1986;255:2445.
17. Brown WJ, Buist WJ, Cory Gipson HT, et al: Fatal benzyl alcohol poisoning in an neonatal intensive care unit. Lancet 1982;1:1250. Letter.
18. Bruns DE, Herold DA, Rodheaver GT, et al: Polyethylene glycol intoxication in burn patients. Burns 1982;9:49–52.
19. Calvery HO, Klumpp TG: The toxicity for human beings of diethylene glycol with sulfanilamide. South Med J 1939; 32:1105–1109.
20. Cate JC, Hedrick R: Propylene glycol intoxication and lactic acidosis. N Engl J Med 1980;303:1237. Letter.
21. Col J, Col-Debeys C, Lavenne-Pardogne E, et al: Propylene glycol-induced heparin resistance during nitroglycerin infusion. Am Heart J 1985;110:171–173.
22. Craig DB, Habib GG: Flaccid parapareis folowing obstetrical epidural anesthesia: Possible role of benzyl alcohol. Anesth Analg 1977;56:219–221.
23. Cronk JD: Phenol with glucagon in cardiotherapy. N Engl J Med 1971;284:219–220.
24. Crook TG, Freeman JJ: Reactions induced by the concurrent use of thimerosal and tetracycline. Am J Optom Physiol Optics 1983;60:759–761.
25. Cukier JO, Seungdamrong S, Odell JL, et al: The displacement of albumin bound bilirubin by gentamicin. Pediatr Res 1974;8:399.
26. DeChristoforro R, Corden BJ, Hood JC, et al: High dose morphine complicated by chlorobutanol-somnolence. Ann Intern Med 1983;98:335–336.
27. Demey HE, Daelemans RA, Verpooten GA, et al: Propylene glycol-induced side effects during intravenous nitroglycerin therapy. Intensive Care Med 1988;14:221–226
28. Doenicke A, Lorenz W, Beigl R, et al: Histamine release after intravenous application of shortacting hypnotics. Br J Anaesth 1973;45:1097–1104.
29. Dundee JW: Hypersensitivity to intravenous anaesthetic agents. Br J Anaesth 1976;48:57–58.
30. Eosinophilia-myalgia syndrome—New Mexico. MMWR 1989;38:765–767.
31. Eosinophilia-myalgia syndrome and L-tryptophan-containing products—New Mexico, Minnesota, Oregon, and New York, 1989. MMWR 1989;38:785–788.
32. Erickson TB, Aks SE, Zabaneh R, et al: Acute renal toxicity after ingestion of lava light liquid. Ann Emerg Med 1996; 27:781–784.
33. Fagan DG, Pritchard JS, Clarkson TW, et al: Organ mercury levels in infant with omphaloceles treated with organic mercurial antiseptic. Arch Dis Child 197;52:962–964.
34. Fatalities associated with ingestion of diethylene glycol-contaminated glycerin used to manufacture acetaminophen syrup—Haiti, November 1995–June 1996. MMWR 1996; 45:649–650.
35. Fligner CL, Jack R, Twiggs GA, et al: Hyperosmolality induced by propylene glycol, a complication of silver sulfadiazine therapy. JAMA 1985;253:1606–1609.
36. Gassett AR: Benzalkonium chloride toxicity to the human cornea. Am J Ophthamol 1977;84:169–171.
37. Geiling EM, Cannon PR: Pathologic effects of elixir of sulfanilamide (diethylene glycol) poisoning. JAMA 1938;111:919–926.
38. Gellerman GL, Martinez C: Fatal ventricular fibrillation following intravenous sodium diphenylhydantoin therapy. JAMA 1967;200:337–338.
39. Gershanik J, Boecler B, Ensley H, et al: The gasping syndrome and benzyl alcohol poisoning. N Engl J Med 1982: 1384–1388.
40. Glasgow AM, Boeckx RL, Miller MK, et al: Hyperosmolality in small infants due to propylene glycol. Pediatrics 1983; 72:353–355.
41. Gross DR, Kitzman JV, Adams HR: Cardiovascular effects of intravenous administration of propylene glycol and oxytetracycline in propylene glycol in calves. Am J Vet Res 1979;40:783–791.
42. Habbab MA, Haft JI: Heparin resistance induced by intravenous nitroglycerin. Arch Intern Med 1987;147:857–860.

43. Haeney MR, Carter GF, Yeoman WB, et al: Long-term parenteral exposure to mercury in patients with hypogammaglobulinaemia. Br Med J 1979;2:12–14.
44. Hagebusch OE: Necropsies of four patients following administration of elixir sulfanilamide—Massengill. JAMA 1937;109:1537–1539.
45. Hahn AF, Feasby TE, Gilbert JJ: Paraparesis following intrathecal chemotherapy. Neurology 1983;33:1032–1038.
46. Hanif M, Mobarak MR, Ronan A: Fatal renal failure by diethylene glycol in paracetamol elixir: The Bangladesh epidemic. Br Med J 1995;311:88–91.
47. Herold DA, Keil K, Bruns DE: Oxidation of polyethylene glycols by alcohol dehydrogenase. Biochem Pharmacol 1989;38:73–76.
48. Hertzman PA, Blevins WL, Mayer J, et al: Association of the eosinophilia-myalgia syndrome with the ingestion of tryptophan. N Engl J Med 1990;322:869–873.
49. Hill RH, Caudill SP, Philen RM, et al: Contaminants in L-tryptophan associated with eosinophilia myalgia syndrome. Arch Environ Contam Toxicol 1993;25:134–142.
50. Hiller JL, Benda GI, Rahatzad M, et al: Benzyl alcohol toxicity: Impact on mortality and intraventricular hemmorrhage among very low birth weight infants. Pediatrics 1986;77:500–506.
51. Jones HT: Danger of skin burns from thiomersal. Br Med J 1972;2:504–505.
52. Kaczorowski JM, Wax PM: Five days of whole-bowel irrigation in a case of pediatric iron ingestion. Ann Emerg Med 1996;27:258–263.
53. Kulick MI, Lewis NS, Bansal V, et al: Hyperosmolality in the burn patient: Analysis of an osmolal discrepancy. J Trauma 1980;20:223–228.
54. LeBel M, Ferron L, Masson M, et al: Benzyl alcohol metabolism and elimination in neonates. Dev Pharmacol Ther 1988;11:347–356.
55. Lemp MA, Zimmerman LE: Toxic endothelial degeneration in ocular surface disease treated with topical medications containing benzalkonium chloride. Am J Ophthamol 1988;105:670–673.
56. Lopez-Herce J, Bonet C, Meana A, Albajara L: Benzyl alcohol poisoning following diazepam intravenous infusion. Ann Pharmacother 1995;29:632. Letter.
57. Lorenzetti OJ, Wernet TC: Topical parabens: Benefits and risks. Dermatologica 1977;154:244–250.
58. Loria CJ, Echeverria P, Smith AL: Effect of antibiotic formulations in serum protein: Bilirubin interaction of newborn infants. J Pediatr 1976;89:479–482.
59. Louis S, Kutt H, McDowell F: The cardiovascular changes caused by intravenous Dilantin and its solvent. Am Heart J 1967;74:523–529.
60. MacDonald MG, Getson PR, Glasgow AM, et al: Propylene glycol: Increased incidence of seizures in low birth weight infants. Pediatrics 1987;79:622–625.
61. Martin G, Finberg L: Propylene glycol: A potentially toxic vehicle in liquid dosage form. J Pediatr 1970;77:877–878.
62. Martone WJ, Williams WW, Mortensen ML, et al: Illness with fatalaties in premature infants: Association with intravenous vitamin E preparation, E-Ferol. Pediatrics 1986;78:591–600.
63. Mattila MA, Ruoppi M, Korhonen HM, et al: Prevention of diazepam-induced thrombophlebitis with cremophor as a solvent. Br J Anaesth 1979;51:891–894.
64. McOrmond P, Gulck B, Duggan HE, et al: Hemolytic effect of benzyl alcohol. Drug Intell Clin Pharm 1980;14:549.
65. Mofenson HC, Caraccio TR, Laudano J: Glucagon for propranolol overdose. JAMA 1986;255:2025–2026.
66. Möller H: Merthiolate allergy: A nationwide iatrogenic sensitization. Acta Demat Venerol 1977;57:509–517.
67. Morizono T, Johnstomne BM: Ototoxicity of chloramphenicol ear drops with propylene glycol as solvent. Med J Aust 1975;2:634–638.
68. Morshed KM, Jain SK, McMartin KE: Acute toxicity of propylene glycol: An assessment using cultured proximal tubule cells of human origin. Fundam Appl Toxicol 1994;23:38–43.
69. Neville R, Dennis, P, Sens D, et al: Preservative cytotoxicity to cultured corneal epithelial cells. Curr Eye Res 1986;5:367–372.
70. Okuonghae HO, Ighogboja IS, Lawson JO, et al: Diethylene glycol poisoning in Nigerian children. Ann Trop Paediatr 1992;12:235–238.
71. Pfab R, Mückter H, Roider G, et al: Clinical course of severe poisoning with thiomersal. J Toxicol Clin Toxicol 1996;34:453–460.
72. Prole JH: Use of chlorobutanol in greyhounds. Vet Record 1986;119:436.
73. Rogers SC, Burrows D, Neill D: Percutaneous absorption of phenol and methyl alcohol in magenta paint BPC. Br J Dermatol 1978;98:559–560.
74. Rohyans J, Walson PD, Wood GA, et al: Mercury toxicity following merthiolate ear irrigations. J Pediatr 1984;104:311–313.
75. Saiki JH, Thompson S, Smith F, et al: Paraplegia following intrathecal chemotherapy. Cancer 1972;29:370–374.
76. Schamberg IL: Allergic contact dermatitis to methyl and propyl paraben. Arch Dermatol 1967;95:626–328.
77. Schiller LR, Emmett M, Santa CA, et al: Osmotic effects of polyethylene glycol. Gastroenterology 1988;94:933–941.
78. Slutsker L, Hoesly FC, Miller L, et al: Eosinophilia-myalgia syndrome associated with exposure to tryptophan from a single manufacturer. JAMA 1990;264:213–217.
79. Smyth HF, Carpenter CP, Shaffer CB: The toxicity of high molecular weight polyethylene glycols; chronic oral and parenteral administration. J Am Pharmaceut Assoc 1947;36:157–160.
80. Smyth HF, Carpenter CP, Weil CS: The chronic oral toxicity of the polyethylene glycols. J Am Pharmaceut Assoc 1955;44;27–30.
81. Smyth HF, Carpenter CP, Weil CS: The toxicology of the polyethylene glycols. J Am Pharmaceut Assoc 1950;39:349–354.
82. Song BL, Li HY, Peng DR: In vitro spermicidal activity of parabens against human spermatozoa. Contraception 1989;39:331–335.
83. Speth PA, Vree TB, Neilen NF, et al: Propylene glycol pharmacokinetics and effect after intravenous infusion in humans. Therapeutic Drug Monitoring 1987;9:255–258.
84. Sturgill BC, Herold DA, Bruns DE: Renal tubular necrosis in

burn patients treated with topical polyethylene glycol. Lab Invest 1982;46:81A.

85. Sweet AY: Fatality from intravenous nitrofurantoin. Pediatrics 1958;22:1204.
86. Swygert LA, Maes EF, Sewell LE, et al: Eosinophilia-myalgia syndrome. Results of a national surveillance. JAMA 1990;264:1698–1703.
87. Tripathi BJ, Tripathi RC: Cytotoxic effects of benzalkonium chloride and chlorobutanol on human corneal epithelial cells in vitro. Lens Eye Toxicity Res 1989;6:395–403.
88. Unger AH, Sklaroff HJ: Fatalities following intravenous use of sodium diphenylhydantoin for cardiac arrhythmias. JAMA 1967;200:35–36.
89. Vernon J, Brummett R, Walsh T: The ototoxic potential of propylene glycol in guinea pigs. Arch Otolaryngol 1978; 104:726–729.
90. Warner MA, Harper JV: Cardiac dysrhythmias associated with chemical peeling with phenol. Anesthesiology 1985;62: 366–367.
91. Winder AF, Astbury NJ, Sheraidah GA, et al: Penetration of mercury from ophthalmologic preservatives into the human eye. Lancet 1980;2:237–239.

CHAPTER 55

Cyclic Antidepressants

Richard S. Weisman

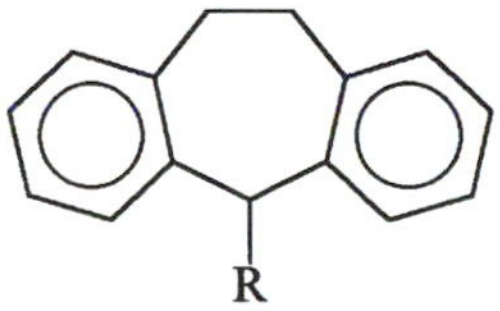

General Structure of Tricyclic Antidepressants

A 15-year-old girl was found awake by her parents after she had ingested the contents of a bottle of amitriptyline 50-mg tablets. She had no medical or surgical problems. She recently had a fight with her boyfriend. A suicide note was at her side. An ambulance was summoned.

When the paramedics arrived 30 minutes later, the patient was lethargic, with a blood pressure of 60/40 mm Hg, a pulse of 160 beats/min, and a respiratory rate of 4 breaths/min. Her pupils were dilated to 7 mm bilaterally. An endotracheal tube was inserted and she was ventilated with 100% oxygen. While on route to the hospital, an intravenous infusion of lactated Ringer's solution was started and the patient was given dextrose (50 g) and thiamine (100 mg) intravenously without response.

By the time the patient reached the hospital 750 mL of lactated Ringer's solution had been infused. Her vital signs were: blood pressure, 84/52 mm Hg; pulse, 150 beats/min; respiratory rate, 20 breaths/min assisted; and a rectal temperature of 98.8°F (37.1°C). The patient was placed on a cardiac monitor, which showed a wide complex rhythm at about 150 beats/min. Her skin was dry, flushed, without track marks, and anicteric. The pupils were 7 mm wide and unresponsive to light. Auscultation of the chest and heart were normal. The abdomen was remarkable for the absence of bowel sounds, and neurologic assessment revealed coma without any focal motor abnormalities.

Blood was obtained for an arterial blood gas, electrolytes, BUN, creatinine, glucose, complete blood count, and a serum acetaminophen determination. A Foley catheter was inserted and 800 mL of urine was obtained.

Several minutes after arrival in the ED, the patient had a brief seizure; her blood pressure fell to 70/46 mm Hg and her QRS complex was noted to be 120 msec. Her lungs were hyperventilated at a rate of 30 breaths/min and she was given a bolus of 44 mEq of sodium bicarbonate. The QRS complex narrowed.

A total of 2 L of lactated Ringer's solution was rapidly infused without a change in heart rate or blood pressure. A norepinephrine drip was initiated at 2 μg/min, which increased the blood pressure to 94/68 mm Hg. Two ampules (88 mEq) of sodium bicarbonate were administered by IV bolus. A sodium bicarbonate infusion was made by adding 132 mEq (3 ampules of 44 mEq/50 mL) to 1 liter of D_5W and infused at 250 mL/h. Simultaneously, a 40 French orogastric lavage tube was inserted and the patient was lavaged until the return was clear. Sixty grams of activated charcoal in a slurry of water and 60 g of sorbitol were then instilled via the tube.

Initial electrolytes were a sodium 139 mEq/L; potassium 3.6 mEq/L; chloride 97 mEq/L; bicarbonate 18 mEq/L; BUN 18 mg/dL; creatinine 1.0 mg/dL; and glucose 120 mg/dL. An arterial blood gas obtained on 100% oxygen showed: pH 7.34; PCO_2 34 mm Hg; and PO_2 252 mm Hg.

Two hours later the patient's blood pressure had increased to 110/80 mm Hg, and the norepinephrine drip was discontinued. A second dose of activated charcoal (0.5 g/kg) was administered through a nasogastric tube 6 hours after admission. Over the next 6 hours the patient began to have spontaneous respirations. By 12 hours after admission the patient withdrew from pain, and by 18 hours she was awake and following commands. The patient was extubated the next day and seen by a psychiatrist, who felt that she remained suicidal. The patient was ultimately transferred to the psychiatry service for long-term care.

What Is the Incidence of Overdose With Cyclic Antidepressants?

In 1987 an epidemiologic study reported that the annual incidence of overdose with cyclic antidepressants was approximately 500,000 each year in the United States.[35] In the United Kingdom in 1992, it was estimated that approximately 50 successful suicides would occur for every million prescriptions written for the first-generation tricyclic antidepressants.[45] In a 1995 retrospective study of 200 consecutive patients who were treated in a critical care unit of a general hospital, 12% were for antidepressant overdoses.[32] The cyclic antidepressants were reported to be the leading cause of life-threatening prescription drug overdose. Typical victims of these overdoses were women, 20–29 years of age, who were living alone, were employed, and did not have a history of drug abuse or prior suicide attempts. Approximately 70% of these earlier cyclic antidepressant suicide attempts never reach medical care.[35]

What Are the Pharmacologic Properties of the Cyclic Antidepressants?

The cyclic antidepressants can be divided into first- and second-generation antidepressants[24] (Table 55–1). The first-generation antidepressants or tricyclic antidepressants were initially marketed in the 1960s. The second generation cyclic antidepressants were developed and released during the 1980s and 1990s to improve the therapeutic index, decrease bothersome side effects and adverse reactions, and reduce the incidence of serious toxicity. As the pharmacologic mechanisms of action became more selective for the inhibition of serotonin and dopamine, the incidence of cardiac and neurologic toxicity has generally decreased.

The first-generation cyclic antidepressants have numerous pharmacologic actions that are well described, yet their exact mechanism for treating depression is still not elucidated.[5] Cyclic antidepressants inhibit voltage-gated sodium channels in myocardial cells (quinidine like effect), block H_1, H_2 and D_2 receptors, block muscarinic receptors, inhibit alpha-adrenergic receptors and potassium efflux, interact with GABA receptors, and inhibit the transport and reuptake of biogenic amines at nerve terminals.[30] Although most of the pharmacologic effects of the cyclic antidepressants occur within minutes of drug administration, clinically most patients will not have an improvement in their depression until they have been treated for 1–3 weeks. The potentiation of biogenic amine activity in the brain may be only the first step of a complex series of actions needed to resolve depression.[6] The inhibition of firing rates in neurons within the *locus coeruleus* and *median raphe,* respectively containing norepinephrine and serotonin (5-HT), are probably mediated by presynaptic D_2 and 5-$HT_{1A/1D}$ autoreceptors. After several weeks of cyclic antidepressant therapy, firing rates return to normal as down regulation of α_2-adrenergic receptors decreases.[44] The α_1-adrenergic receptors do not appear to down-regulate following antidepressant administration and may actually increase functionality. This may be responsible for at least some of the mood elevating effects of these drugs.[44]

Within the class of cyclic antidepressants there are differences in the reuptake inhibition of the biogenic amines that can be related to structure. Imipramine as a parent compound is a potent inhibitor of norepinephrine reuptake. The presence of a tertiary-amine side chain on imipramine (and related compounds) inhibits the reuptake of serotonin. Except for bupropion, most of the cyclic antidepressants do not effectively inhibit dopamine reuptake.[83]

What Are the Pharmacokinetic Properties of the Cyclic Antidepressants?

The cyclic antidepressants are initially rapidly absorbed from the gastrointestinal tract unless anticholinergic effects decrease the rate of absorption by slowing gastrointestinal motility. These drugs have large volumes of distribution (10–50 L/kg). Many of these drugs and their metabolites bind to the plasma protein α_1-glycoprotein, although binding affinities are different.[3,80] Amitriptyline has a higher binding affinity for α_1-glycoprotein than its demethylated metabolite, nortriptyline. Acidemia may increase the percentage of unbound (free) tricyclic antidepressant in the plasma.[35,58] The compounds are all highly lipophilic, sparingly water soluble, and extensively metabolized on their first pass through the liver.[80] The cyclic antidepressants are metabolized by the phase I processes of demethylated and hydroxylation. Both parent and the demethylated metabolites retain pharmacologic activity until hydroxylation occurs by the microsomal enzyme system.[35,80] Several of the metabolites are further solubilized by a phase II complexation reaction with glucuronide. The half-lives of the various cyclic antidepressants range from 4 hours for trazodone to greater than 93 hours for nortriptyline. The complexity of pH-dependent protein binding, the large volumes of distribution, and the wide intrapatient variability of the terminal elimination half-life limit the clinical value of plasma antidepressant levels in overdose. See Table 55–2 for additional pharmacokinetic data.

TABLE 55–1. PHARMACOLOGIC PROPERTIES OF CYCLIC ANTIDEPRESSANTS

	Amine Reuptake Activity						
Drug	***Norepinephrine***	***Serotonin***	***Dopamine***	**Anticholinergic**	**Prolonged QRS Complex**	**Hypotension**	**Seizures**
First generation							
Amitriptyline	++	++++	0	++++	++++	++++	++++
Clomipramine	++	++++	+	++++	++++	++++	++++
Doxepin	+	++	0	+++	++++	++++	++++
Trimipramine	+	+	0	++++	++++	++++	++++
Desipramine	++++	0	0	++	++++	+++	++++
Nortriptyline	+++	0	0	+++	++++	+++	++++
Protriptyline	+++	0	0	+++	++++	+++	++++
Imipramine	+++	+++	0	+++	++++	++++	++++
Second generation							
Amoxapine	+++	0	1,+	+++	+	+	++++
Bupropion	+	0	+	0	0	+	+++
Fluoxetine	0	++++	0	0	0	0	0
Maprotiline	+++	+	0	+++	++++	++++	++++
Trazodone	0	+++	0	0	0	+	0
Sertraline	+	++++	0	+	0	0	0
Fluvoxamine	0	++++	0	0	0	0	0
Paroxetine	0	++++	0	0	0	0	0
Venlafaxine	+	++	++	0	+	0	+++

0 = none; + = very low; ++= low; +++ = moderate; ++++ = high; 1 = blocks dopamine receptors

The ultimate disposition of the cyclic antidepressants is not well characterized. Although approximately 30% of the absorbed dose is eliminated by gastric and biliary secretion, little of the parent compound is found in the stool because of reabsorption.[38,63] Renal clearance of the parent compounds range between 3 and 10%.[21,35,80]

TABLE 55–2. PHARMACOKINETIC PROPERTIES OF THE CYCLIC ANTIDEPRESSANTS

Drug	**Plasma Half-life (h)**	**V_d (L/kg)**	**Plasma Protein Binding (%)**
First generation:			
Amitriptyline	14–40	18–22	93–96
Clomipramine	19–37	12	97
Desipramine	14–76	22–59	73–92
Doxepin	8–24	9–33	80–85
Imipramine	9–24	11–16	76–96
Nortriptyline	18–93	11–27	88–94
Protriptyline	53–90	15–31	?
Trimipramine	20–26	26–35	95
Second generation			
Amoxapine	7.7	60–65	90
Bupropion	10–21	20	82–88
Fluvoxamine	23	25	75
Fluoxetine	90	20–45	95
Maprotiline	30–50	22	88
Paroxetine	7–37	8–28	95
Sertraline	24	20	99
Trazodone	4.6	0.5–1.0	89–95
Venlafaxine	3–10	6–7	30

What Are the Toxicologic Properties of the Cyclic Antidepressants?

The toxicity of the cyclic antidepressants is primarily due to its effects on the myocardium, central nervous system, and peripheral vasculature. The cyclic antidepressants exert a membrane depressant effect on the myocardium by inhibiting voltage-gated sodium channels, known as a quinidine like effect.[1,39,64,97] This results in decreased conduction velocities and in an increased threshold for excitability. As a result of potassium channel blocking actions, the cyclic antidepressants further prolong action potential durations in most cardiac cells. Most of the cyclic antidepressants have anticholinergic effects, which increase heart rate and predispose the patient to tachydysrhythmias. The cyclic antidepressants are also potent α-adrenergic antagonists, which result in a decreased peripheral vascular resistance. This effect, coupled with the myocardial depressant effects from sodium and potassium channel inhibition, result in hypotension.

The seizures resulting from cyclic antidepressant overdoses occur shortly after the ingestion, are usually brief in duration, and often resolve without the necessity of administering an anticonvulsant.[81] Nortriptyline-induced seizures are often accompanied by hypotension.[60] Seizures resulting from cyclic antidepressant overdose are caused by complex interactions within the brain due to altered concentrations of GABA, dopamine, norepinephrine, and acetylcholine.[19,62,88] The cyclic antidepressants that block neuronal reuptake of norepinephrine and dopamine are those drugs most frequently associated with seizure activity.[88] The cyclic antidepressants inhibit the chloride ionophore on the GABA-receptor complex by binding at the picrotoxin receptor site. The degree of chloride inhibition at this location correlates with seizure frequency.[62]

Depending on the dose, the neurotransmitters most affected, and the anticholinergic potency of the specific cyclic antidepressant, patients may present with a variety of different signs and symptoms involving the cardiovascular and neurologic systems.

Many of the signs and symptoms observed in patients with cyclic antidepressant toxicity are due to the anticholinergic effects of these drugs (Table 55–3).[41] Central nervous system anticholinergic toxic effects may include respiratory depression, agitation, lethargy, hallucinations, hyperthermia, ataxia, choreoathetoid movements, seizures, and coma. Peripheral anticholinergic effects may include hypotension, decreased gastrointestinal motility, dry flushed skin, urinary retention, sinus tachycardia, and rarely AV block.[17,18,46,70,93]

Amitriptyline, imipramine, clomipramine, and doxepin are representative of the first-generation, tertiary-amine tricyclic antidepressants that first became available in the 1960s (Fig 55–1). As a group, they are both pharmacologically active and have active metabolites that are formed by demethylation. The presence of the tertiary-amine side chain inhibits the reuptake of serotonin. They are potent inhibitors of both norepinephrine and serotonin. As a class this group has potent anticholinergic effects, are very sedating, and in overdose are likely to cause seizures, hypotension, and cardiac dysrhythmias. Clomipramine is additionally capable of inhibiting the D_2 receptor.[82]

Desipramine, nortriptyline, and protriptyline are the first-generation, secondary-amine tricyclics. They are potent inhibitors of norepinephrine reuptake, but are incapable of inhibiting the reuptake of serotonin. They

TABLE 55–3. ANTICHOLINERGIC EFFECTS OBSERVED WITH SOME CYCLIC ANTIDEPRESSANTS

Central	Peripheral
Agitation	Hypertension
Hallucinations	Tachycardia
Confusion	Hyperthermia
Sedation	Mydriasis
Coma	Dry, flushed skin
Seizures	Decreased GI motility
	Urinary retention

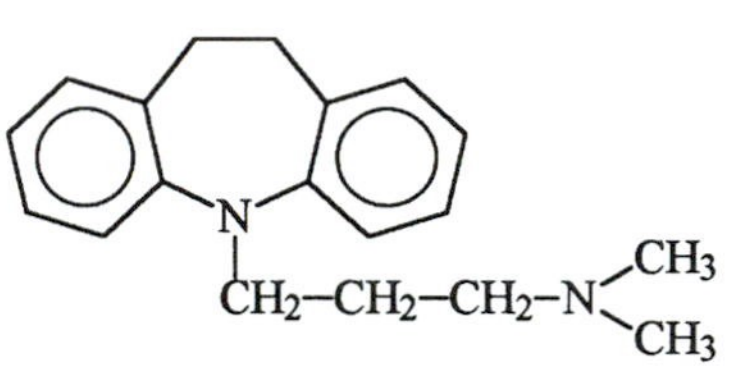

Imipramine

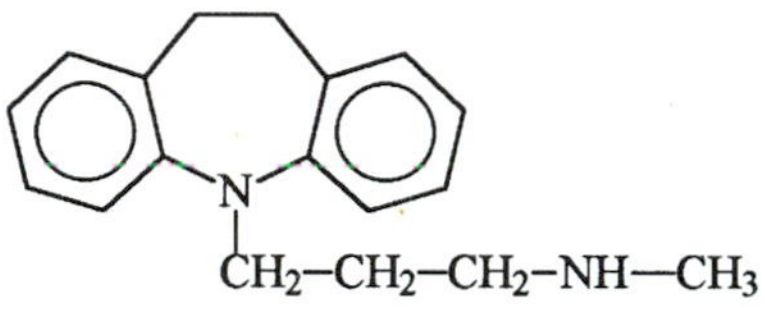

Desipramine

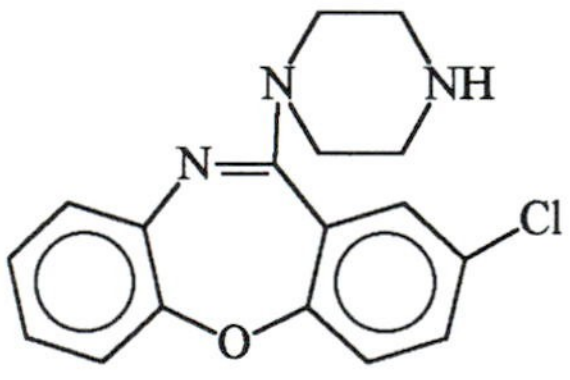

Amoxapine

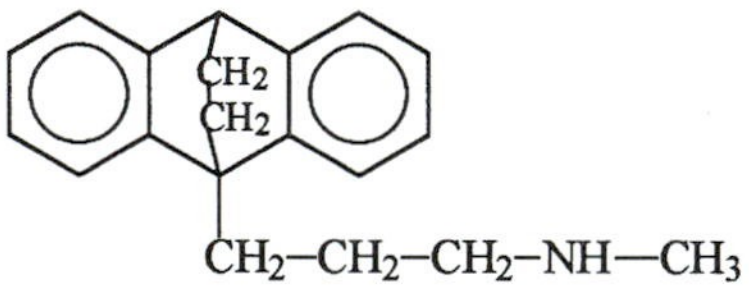

Maprotiline

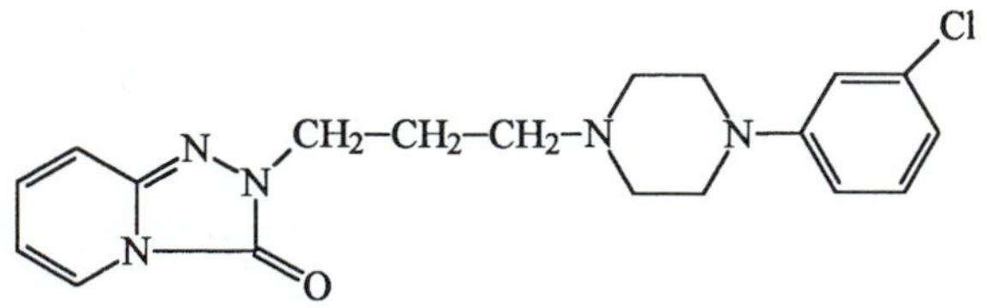

Trazodone

Figure 55–1. Examples of the secondary and tertiary-amine cyclic antidepressants and the atypical antidepressant trazodone.

have fewer anticholinergic effects, are less sedating, and in overdose cause less hypotension and fewer cardiac dysrhythmias. Amoxapine is a dibenzoxapine cyclic antidepressant structurally similar to the secondary-amine tricyclic antidepressants. It inhibits the reuptake of norepinephrine, blocks dopamine (D_2) receptors, but does not inhibit the reuptake of serotonin.[82] Although the incidence of cardiac toxicity is less with amoxapine, the incidence of seizures is almost 9 times greater than with the first-generation antidepressants.[53,61,98]

Maprotiline is the only tetracyclic antidepressant available in the United States. In addition to a four-ring structure, it has a secondary amine side group. It predominantly blocks the reuptake of norepinephrine. Although it was initially suggested to have an excellent safety profile, the incidences of seizures, cardiac dysrhythmias, and duration of coma in overdose are at least 4 times greater than the other first-generation cyclic antidepressants.[28,51,98]

Fluoxetine, fluvoxamine, paroxetine, and sertraline comprise the currently available selective serotonin reuptake inhibitors. As their name suggests, they selectively inhibit the reuptake of serotonin without inhibiting the reuptake of norepinephrine or dopamine. They are devoid of anticholinergic effects, cause minimal sedation, and in overdose do not cause seizures, hypotension, or cardiac dysrhythmias.[82] An extensive discussion of this group of antidepressants can be found in Chapter 56.

Venlafaxine is a heterocyclic antidepressant that is categorized as a selective serotonin reuptake inhibitor, although it also inhibits the reuptake of norepinephrine and to some extent dopamine.[33] In comparison to other antidepressants, venlafaxine is a weaker inhibitor of serotonin reuptake than the selective serotonin reuptake inhibitors, is a weaker inhibitor of norepinephrine reuptake than the first-generation tricyclic antidepressants, but is a more potent inhibitor of dopamine reuptake than either of these other two classes of antidepressants.[12] Venlafaxine causes a dose-dependent increase in systolic blood pressure.[29] There are numerous reports of seizures[34,52,73,100] and several fatalities from venlafaxine ingestions.[22,72]

The atypical antidepressants include trazodone, nefazodone, and bupropion. Trazodone and nefazodone are potent presynaptic serotonin reuptake inhibitors and postsynaptic type 2 serotonin antagonists. They are very sedating, are devoid of anticholinergic effects, and have not been reported to cause seizures or cardiac dysrhythmias. In a multicenter study of 32 exposures, there were no life-threatening toxicities reported.[8]

Buproprion is a unicyclic antidepressant with weak presynaptic dopamine uptake inhibition and some inhibition of norepinephrine reuptake.[82] It does not inhibit the reuptake of serotonin and does not have anticholinergic effects.[13] Seizures are associated with the chronic ingestion of bupropion in doses exceeding 450 mg/day.[31] In a retrospective review of 58 patients with acute bupropion overdoses, and nine additional ingestions of bupropion and a benzodiazepine, neurologic toxicity was commonly encountered and included lethargy, tremor, and seizures.[90] One patient reportedly developed hypotension. Sinus tachycardia was the only cardiac dysrhythmia reported in this case series.

What Are the Immediate Diagnostic and Therapeutic Interventions for a Patient With a Cyclic Antidepressant Overdose?

Patients with a cyclic antidepressant overdose often develop wide complex tachydysrhythmias, hypotension, and seizures within minutes of the ingestion.[96] The initial therapeutic interventions for a patient with a cyclic antidepressant overdose are to secure an airway, to place the patient on a cardiac monitor, and to evaluate, stabilize, and maintain vital signs. A retrospective review of cyclic antidepressant fatalities found that half of the patients who presented to the emergency department with trivial signs of poisoning had a catastrophic deterioration within 1 hour.[19] Life-threatening events occur within the first 6 hours of an ingestion, and most often within the first 2 hours.[11] A low risk for a patient who overdoses on a first-generation tricyclic antidepressant who does not develop a QRS > 100 msec, cardiac dysrhythmias, conduction defects, an altered mental status, seizures, respiratory depression, or hypotension within 6 hours, can be predicted with 100% sensitivity.[36]

In a prospective analysis of ECGs from cases reported to a poison center, the maximal limb lead QRS duration was prognostic of seizures and cardiac dysrhythmias following acute first-generation tricyclic antidepressant ingestions.[11] Seizures occurred in 30% of patients with QRS complexes > 100 msec, and cardiac dysrhythmias occurred in 50% of patients with QRS complexes > 160 msec. None of the 49 patients studied had a seizure with a QRS complex < 100 msec, or cardiac dysrhythmias with a QRS complex < 160 msec.

The finding of a rightward axis shift in the terminal 40 msec of the QRS complex (an R wave in lead aVR and an S wave in aVL) (see Fig. 8–10), together with a prolonged QT_c and a sinus tachycardia, is highly specific and sensitive for first-generation tricyclic antidepressant poisoning,[69] but the absence of all or some of these findings is not exclusionary.[41,69,99]

Several studies with limited clinical data found that the ECGs from first-generation tricyclic antidepressant overdosed patients were 8.6 times more likely to have a terminal 40 msec axis of more than 120 degrees than ECGs from a cohort of patients without a tricyclic antidepressant overdose,[99] and that an R wave in aVR greater of 3 mm or greater was the only ECG variable to reliably predict seizures and dysrhythmias with statistical significance.[59]

Blood should be sent to the laboratory for electrolytes, glucose, BUN, creatinine, a complete blood count, and an acetaminophen level if the ingestion was intentional. While standard cyclic antidepressant blood levels exceeding 1000 ng/mL are often found in patients with cardiac dysrhythmias, seizures, or coma,[40,77,89] life-threatening toxicities are often found in patients with levels below 1000 ng/mL.[10,11,57,99] If the concentration of red blood cell and plasma cyclic antidepressant metabolites can be assayed, these determinations may be more likely to correlate with the risk of developing an intraventricular conduction abnormality[2] than the plasma concentration of the parent drug alone.

Wide Complex Dysrhythmias

The cyclic antidepressants exert a membrane-depressant, local-anesthetic effect on the myocardium by slowing sodium influx into cells during phase 0 of the action potential.[39,64,97] This quinidine like effect causes intraventricular conduction delays, ventricular dysrhythmias, and negative inotropy which decreases cardiac output, decreases coronary perfusion, and causes hypotension.

The effects of the cyclic antidepressants on the voltage-gated sodium channels can be attenuated with the administration of sodium bicarbonate[15,67,75,78,84,85] and/or hyperventilation.[9,50] A similar effect can be achieved by increasing the concentration of extracellular sodium and improving the gradient across the sodium channel.[67] Achieving a blood pH between 7.50 and 7.55 appears to reduce the binding of the cyclic antidepressants to the sodium channel. The contribution that alkalinization may have on expanding the intravascular volume or lowering the extracellular potassium concentration is less clear.[15,75,78]

In amitriptyline-poisoned dogs, sodium bicarbonate restored conduction velocity and suppressed ventricular dysrhythmias.[67] In a comparison of sodium bicarbonate, hyperventilation, hypertonic sodium chloride, and lidocaine, sodium bicarbonate and hyperventilation proved most effective in correcting intraventricular conduction delays.[67] Hypertonic sodium chloride failed to reverse dysrhythmias. Although lidocaine was transiently beneficial, antagonism of myocardial voltage-gated sodium channel depression was demonstrated only at near toxic doses and was associated with hypotension.[67]

In subsequent studies, alkalinization with sodium bicarbonate appeared to be superior to either the administration of hypertonic saline or hyperventilation in animal models.[9,50,75] Hyperventilation without the administration of sodium bicarbonate should be reserved for patients with pulmonary or cerebral edema, head trauma, or poorly controlled congestive heart failure in whom the administration of large quantities of sodium may be contraindicated.[9,50]

Sodium bicarbonate should be administered as an initial bolus of 1–2 mEq/kg. This can be followed with an infusion of 100–150 mEq of sodium bicarbonate in 1 L of 5% dextrose in water, titrated over 4–6 hours to maintain the blood pH between 7.50 and 7.55. During the administration of sodium bicarbonate the patient's potassium must be carefully monitored to prevent the development of hypokalemia. After 4–6 hours, the infusion can be discontinued if the width of the QRS complex remains less than 100 msec without the administration of sodium bicarbonate. For additional discussion of the use of sodium bicarbonate for treating cyclic antidepressant overdoses, see Antidotes in Depth: Sodium Bicarbonate.

Although the use of lidocaine has been suggested by some authors,[4,54,56] animal data have not demonstrated efficacy in the treatment of dysrhythmias. Further studies are needed to evaluate both efficacy and the possibility that lidocaine may exacerbate hypotension.[67]

Both beta-adrenergic antagonists and calcium channel blockers may be dangerous for any patient who has a wide complex dysrhythmia. Both groups slow conduction velocity and heart rate and lower blood pressure. In a canine tricyclic antidepressant toxicity model,[85] propranolol may have assisted in the restoration of a sinus rhythm, although all of the dogs expired from intractable hypotension.

All of the type IA and IC antidysrhythmics exert quinidine-like effects on the voltage-gated sodium channel and produce negative inotropic effects. They worsen both cardiac toxicity and hypotension. The administration of quinidine, procainamide, disopyramide, flecainide, encainide, and propafanone is therefore contraindicated for patients with tricyclic antidepressant overdoses.[42,92] In addition there is no role for physostigmine in tricyclic antidepressant overdose (see Antidotes in Depth: Physostigmine).[68,74]

Seizures

Seizures from cyclic antidepressants usually are brief and respond to intravenous benzodiazepines.[14] Seizures must be promptly treated to prevent hypoxia and lactic acidosis. Both hypoxia and acidemia may predispose to the development of life-threatening ventricular dysrhythmias. Benzodiazepines such as diazepam, lorazepam, or midazolam are effective in controlling seizure activity from the cyclic antidepressants.

Several reports have suggested that seizures refractory to other benzodiazepines are responsive to a bolus of midazolam followed by a continuous infusion.[25,37,55]

If the patient fails to respond to benzodiazepines, barbiturates or propofol can be administered. A patient with an amoxapine overdose and refractory seizures responded to a loading dose of propofol 2.5 mg/kg followed by a continuous infusion of 0.2 mg/kg/min.[66] If seizures persist, neuromuscular blockade and general anesthesia should be promptly administered.

Phenytoin is no longer recommended for the treatment of tricyclic antidepressant seizures due to its limited efficacy[7] as well as animal data suggesting that the drug may have prodysrhythmic effects. In the canine model, pretreatment with phenytoin increased the incidence of ventricular tachycardia following an infusion of amitriptyline.[20]

Patients who have had multiple or protracted seizures are at risk for developing rhabdomyolysis and acute renal failure.[48] These patients should be kept well hydrated and their renal function should be carefully monitored.

Flumazenil is contraindicated in patients who have overdosed on a cyclic antidepressant because it inhibits the benzodiazepine binding site on the chloride ionophore of the GABA-receptor complex. There are several case reports of patients with cyclic antidepressant overdoses who had seizures following the administration of flumazenil.[43,65] For a more in-depth discussion, see Antidotes in Depth: Flumazenil.

Hypotension

Hypotension must be rapidly corrected. Any impairment in coronary perfusion or tissue perfusion may result in the production of lactic acid. Acidemia will increase the binding of cyclic antidepressants to the sodium channel, slow intraventricular conduction, and predispose the patient to life-threatening dysrhythmias.[86]

The hypotensive patient should be given 10–30 mL/kg of lactated Ringer's solution or normal saline in aliquots.[75] If hypotension or hypoperfusion fails to respond to fluids, pulmonary artery catheterization may be necessary to distinguish between myocardial depression with high filling pressures, or peripheral vasodilation with low filling pressures. The risk of precipitating a ventricular dysrhythmia from catheterization must be weighed against the benefit of the data obtained from the pulmonary catheter.

If the cause of the hypotension is a loss of vascular tone, a direct-acting adrenergic receptor agonist such as norepinephrine will increase peripheral vascular resistance with a limited risk of increased myocardial irritability. If hypotension is due to a loss of inotropy characterized by low cardiac output and elevated pulmonary artery wedge pressure, a direct acting β_1-adrenergic agonist such as dobutamine should be selected. Dobutamine will increase the force of contraction without increasing the peripheral vascular resistance or significantly increasing heart rate.

Dopamine should be avoided in treating cyclic antidepressant–induced hypotension because the drug's β_2-adrenergic receptor stimulatory effects may exacerbate vasodilation, worsening the hypotension. Because dopamine works indirectly through the release of norepinephrine, if catecholamine stores have been depleted by the cyclic antidepressant, the response may be less than expected.[16] If hypotension remains refractory to fluids and vasopressors, the use of an intraaortic balloon assist pump should be considered as a temporizing technique.[16,26,33,64]

Which Gastrointestinal Decontamination Techniques Should Be Used for the Patient Who Has Ingested a Cyclic Antidepressant?

Once the patient is stabilized, gastric decontamination should be performed to limit further absorption. Orogastric lavage should be reserved for patients in whom there is a high probability that an absorbed medication still remains in the stomach. The first landmark study to evaluate the benefit of gastric emptying in overdose patients demonstrated a benefit for those patients presenting early after the ingestion. A later study failed to show a difference.[79] Our position is to recommend gastric lavage in those patients who are seriously ill and in whom we believe the drug is still accessible in the stomach. A risk benefit analysis as described in Chapter 4 should be applied. Activated charcoal should be administered in a dose of 1 g/kg body weight, mixed as a water slurry with a cathartic, either after gastric lavage or in place of gastric lavage in those patients in whom lavage is not indicated or where risk outweighs benefit. A second dose of activated charcoal, at 0.5 g/kg without a cathartic, may be administered several hours later if it seems plausible that the unabsorbed drug may still be in the gastrointestinal tract secondary to a massive ingestion or hypotension. Administering multiple dose activated charcoal for the purposes of enhancing systemic elimination is probably not warranted.[94] The marginal[23,27,71,91] enhancement gained through interruption of the enterohepatic circulation is more than offset by these agents' high plasma protein binding and large volumes of distribution making multiple dose activated charcoal ineffective and unnecessary.

The use of syrup of ipecac is contraindicated in all cyclic antidepressant overdoses because of the potential for seizures, coma, hypotension, and cardiac dysrhythmias.

How Long Should the Patient With a Cyclic Antidepressant Overdose Require Monitoring in an ICU?

If the patient with a cyclic antidepressant overdose remains asymptomatic with a normal ECG for 6 hours of observation and has received only gastrointestinal decontamination and no serum alkalinization, the likelihood that the patient will develop late toxic effects from a cyclic antidepressant is extremely small.[11,36] The asymptomatic patient can be discharged from the telemetry unit for psychiatric evaluation.[95]

If the patient has had an altered mental status, seizure, or cardiac dysrhythmia, the patient should remain in an intensive care unit for 12 hours after all supportive therapeutic interventions have been discontinued. If the patient remains asymptomatic with a normal ECG and a normal pH during this phase of observation, the patient can then undergo psychiatric evaluation.

Although specific antibodies[47,49,76,87] may one day be available as an effective antidote for patients with cyclic antidepressant overdose who survive long enough to reach medical care, it is likely that newer, more effective, and less toxic antidepressants will ultimately replace many of the current antidepressants that have low therapeutic indices.

Acknowledgments

Mary Ann Howland, PharmD, Robert S. Hoffman, MD, and Henry Cohen, PharmD, contributed to this chapter in a previous edition.

References

1. Ahmad S: Management of cardiac complications in tricyclic antidepressant poisoning. (Letter) J Soc Med 1980;73:79.
2. Amitai Y, Erickson T, Kennedy EJ, et al: Tricyclic antidepressants in red cells and plasma: Correlation with impaired intraventricular conduction in acute overdose. Clin Pharmacother 1993;54:219–227.
3. Amitai Y, Kennedy EJ, De Sandre P, Frischer H: Distribution of amitriptyline and nortriptyline in blood: Role of α_1-glycoprotein. Ther Drug Monit 1993;15:267–273.
4. Bain DJG, Turner T: Imipramine poisoning. Arch Dis Child 1971;46:887.
5. Baldessarini RJ: Current status of antidepressants: Clinical pharmacology and therapy. J Clin Psychiatry 1989;50:117–126.
6. Baldessarini RJ: Treatment of depression by altering monoamine metabolism: Precursors and metabolic inhibitors. Psychopharmacol Bull 1984;20:224–239.
7. Beaubein AR, Carpenter DC, Mathieu LF, et al: Antagonism of imipramine poisoning by anticonvulsants in the rat. Toxicol Appl Pharmacol 1976;38:1–6.
8. Benson B, Mathiason M, Foley M, et al: Prospective multicenter evaluation of nefazodone exposures. J Toxicol Clin Toxicol 1996;34:565. Abstract.
9. Bessen HA, Niemann JT, Haskell RJ, et al: Effect of respiratory alkalosis in tricyclic antidepressant overdose. West J Med 1983;139;373–376.
10. Biggs JT, Spiker DG, Petit JM, et al: Tricyclic antidepressant overdose—Incidence of symptoms. JAMA 1977;238: 135–138.
11. Boehnert M, Lovejoy FH Jr: Value of the QRS duration versus the serum drug level in predicting seizures and ventricular arrhythmias after an acute overdose of tricyclic antidepressants. N Engl J Med 1985;313:474–479.
12. Bolden-Watson C, Michelson E: Blockade by newly-developed antidepressants of biogenic amine uptake into rat brain synaptosomes. Life Sci 1993;52:1023–1029.
13. Boryant SG, Guernsey BG, Ingrim NB: Review of bupropion. Clin Pharm 1983;2:525–537.
14. Braden NJ, Jackson JE, Walson PD: Tricyclic antidepressant overdose. Ped Clin North Am 1986;33:287–297.
15. Brown TCK, Barker GA, Dunlop ME, et al: The use of sodium bicarbonate in the treatment of tricyclic antidepressant induced arrhythmias. Anesth Intensive Care 1973;1:203–210.
16. Buchman AL, Dauer J, Geiderman J: The use of vasoactive agents in the treatment of refractory hypotension seen in tricyclic antidepressant overdose. J Clin Psychopharmacol 1990;10:409–413.
17. Burks JS, Walker JE, Rumack BH, et al: Tricyclic antidepressant poisoning—Reversal of coma, choreoathetosis and myoclonus by physostigmine. JAMA 1974;230: 1405–1407.
18. Callaham M: Tricyclic antidepressant overdose. JACEP 1979;8:413–423.
19. Callaham M, Kassel D: Epidemiology of fatal tricyclic antidepressant ingestion: Implications for management. Ann Emerg Med 1985;14:1–9.
20. Callaham M, Schumaker H, Pentel P: Phenytoin prophylaxis of cardiotoxicity in experimental amitriptyline poisoning. J Pharmacol Exp Ther 1988; 245:216–220.
21. Caraccio TR, Mofenson HC, Sturman K: Clinical toxicology of tricyclic antidepressants and cyclic antidepressants. NY State J Pharm 1984;4:105–111.
22. Chen NBW, Donahue ER, An TL: Venlafaxine related deaths, postmortem tissue distribution. American Academy of Forensic Sciences: Annual Meeting, Nashville, TN, February 19–24, 1996, p. 209.
23. Chyka P: Multiple-dose activated charcoal and enhancement of systemic drug clearance: Summaries of studies in animals and human volunteers. J Toxicol Clin Toxicol 1995;33:399–405.
24. Cohen H, Hoffman RS, Howland MA: Cyclic antidepressant poisoning: A review and case report. J Pharm Pract 1993;6:89–102.
25. Crisp CB, Gannon R, Knauft F: Continuous infusion of midazolam hydrochloride to control status epilepticus. Clin Pharm 1988;7:322–324.
26. Crome P: Poisoning due to tricyclic antidepressant overdosage: Clinical presentation and treatment. Med Toxicol 1986;1:261–285.
27. Crome P, Dawling S, Braithwaite RA: Effect of activated charcoal on absorption of nortriptyline. Lancet 1977;1: 1203–1205.
28. Crome P, Newman B: Poisoning with maprotiline and mianserin. Br Med J 1977;2:260. Letter.
29. Cunningham LA, Borison RL, Carman JS: A comparison of venlafaxine, trazodone, and placebo in major depression. J Clin Psychopharmacol 1994;14:99–106.
30. Cusack B, Nelson A, Richelson E: Binding of antidepressants to human brain receptors: Focus on newer generation compounds. Psychopharmacology 1994;114:559–565.
31. Davidson J: Seizures and bupropion: A review. J Clin Psychiatry 1989;50:256–261.
32. D'Mello DA, Finkbeiner DS, Kocher KN: The cost of antidepressant overdose. Gen Hosp Psychiatr 1995;17: 454–455.
33. Ellinrod VL, Perry PJ: Venlafaxine: A heterocyclic antidepressant. Am J Hosp Pharm 1994;51:3033–3046.
34. Fantaskey A, Burkhart KK: A case report of venlafaxine toxicity. J Toxicol Clin Toxicol 1995;33:359–361.
35. Frommer DA, Kulig KW, Marx JA, et al: Tricyclic antidepressant overdose: A review. JAMA 1987;257:521–526.
36. Foulke GE: Identifying toxicity risk early after antidepressant overdose. Am J Emerg Med 1995;13:123–126.
37. Galvin GM, Jelinek GA: Midazolam: An effective agent for seizure control. Arch Emerg Med 1987;4:169–172.
38. Gard H, Knapp D, Walle T, et al: Qualitative and quantitative studies on the disposition of amitriptyline and other tricyclic antidepressant drugs in man as it relates to the management of the overdosed patient. Clin Toxicol 1973; 6:571–584.

39. Glassman AH: Cardiovascular effects of tricyclic antidepressants. Ann Rev Med 1984;35:503–511.
40. Goldberg RJ, Capone RJ, Hunt JD: Cardiac complications following tricyclic antidepressant overdose—Issues for monitoring policy. JAMA 1985;254:1772–1775.
41. Guy S, Silke B: The electrocardiogram as a tool for therapeutic monitoring: A critical analysis. J Clin Psychiatry 1990;51(12 suppl B):37–39.
42. Hansten PD, Horn JR: Drug Interactions and Updates. Malvern, PA, Lea & Febiger, 1990.
43. Haverkos GP, DiSalvo RP, Imhoff TE: Fatal seizures after flumazenil administration in a patient with mixed overdose. Ann Pharmacother 1994;28:1347–1349.
44. Henninger GR, Charney DS: Mechanisms of action of antidepressant treatments: Implications for the etiology and treatment of depressive disorders. In: Meltzer HY, ed: Psychopharmacology: The Third Generation of Progress. New York, Raven Press, 1987, pp. 535–544.
45. Henry J: The safety of antidepressants. Br J Psychiatry 1992;160:439–441.
46. Hurst HE, Jarboe CH: Clinical findings, elimination pharmacokinetics, and tissue drug concentrations following a fatal amitriptyline intoxication. Clin Toxicol 1981;18: 119–125.
47. Hursting MJ, Opheim KE, Raisys VA, et al: Tricyclic antidepressant-specific Fab fragments alter the distribution and elimination of desipramine in the rabbit: A model for overdose treatment. J Toxicol Clin Toxicol 1989;27:53–66.
48. Jennings AE, Levey AS, Harrington JT: Amoxapine associated with acute renal failure. Arch Intern Med 1983;143 1525–1527.
49. Keyler DE, Le Couteur DG, Pond SM, et al: Effects of specific antibody Fab fragments on desipramine pharmacokinetics in the rat in vivo and in the isolated, perfused liver. J Pharmacol Exp Ther 1995;272:1117–1123.
50. Kingston ME: Hyperventilation in tricyclic antidepressant poisoning. Crit Care Med 1979;7:550–551.
51. Knudsen K, Heath A: Effects of self poisoning with maprotiline. Br Med J 1984;288:601–603.
52. Kokan L, Dart RC: Life-threatening hypotension from venlafaxine overdose. J Toxicol Clin Toxicol 1996;34:559. Abstract.
53. Kulig K, Rumack BH, Sullivan JB, et al: Amoxapine overdose: Coma and seizures without cardiotoxic effects. JAMA 1982;248:1092–1094.
54. Knudsen K, Abrahamsson J: Effects of magnesium sulfate and lidocaine in the treatment of ventricular arrhythmias in experimental amitryptyline poisoning in the rat. Crit Care Med 1994;22:494–498.
55. Kumar A, Bleck TS: Intravenous midazolam for the treatment of refractory status epilepticus. Crit Care Med 1992; 20:483–488.
56. Langou RA, Van Dyke C, Tahan SR, et al: Cardiovascular manifestations of tricyclic antidepressant overdose. Am Heart J 1980;100:458–464
57. Lavoie FW, Gansert GG, Weiss RE: Value of initial ECG findings and plasma drug levels in cyclic antidepressant overdose. Ann Emerg Med 1990;19:696–700.
58. Levitt MA, Sullivan JB Jr, Owens SM, et al: Amitriptyline plasma protein building: Effect of plasma pH and relevance to clinical overdose. Am J Emerg Med 1986;4: 121–125.
59. Liebelt EI, Francis PD, Woolf AD: ECG lead AVR versus QRS interval in predicting seizures and arrhythmias in acute tricyclic antidepressant toxicity. Ann Emerg Med 1995;26:195–201.
60. Lipper B, Bell A, Gaynor B: Recurrent hypotension immediately after seizures in nortriptyline overdose. Am J Emerg Med 1994;12:451–457.
61. Litovitz TL, Troutman WG: Amoxapine overdose: Seizures and fatalities. JAMA 1983;250:1069–1071.
62. Malatynska E, Knapp RJ, Ikeda M, et al: Antidepressants and seizure-interactions at the GABA-receptor chloride-ionophore complex. Life Sci 1988;43:303–307.
63. Manoguerra AS, Weaver LC: Poisoning with tricyclic antidepressant drugs. Clin Toxicol 1977;10:149–158.
64. Marshall JB, Forker AD: Cardiovascular effects of tricyclic antidepressant drugs: Therapeutic usage, overdose, and management of complications. Am Heart J 1982;103: 401–414.
65. McDuffee AT, Tobias JD: Seizure after flumazenil administration in a pediatric patient. Pediatr Emerg Care 1995; 11:186–187.
66. Merigian KS, Browning RG, Leeper KV: Successful treatment of amoxapine induced refractory status epilepticus with propofol (Diprivan). Acad Emerg Med 1995;2: 128–133.
67. Nattel S, Mittleman M: Treatment of ventricular tachyarrhythmias resulting from amitriptyline toxicity in dogs. J Pharmacol Exp Ther 1984;231:430–435.
68. Newton RW: Physostigmine salicylate in the treatment of tricyclic antidepressant overdosage. JAMA 1975;231: 941–943.
69. Niemann JT, Besssen HA, Rothstein RJ, et al: Electrocardiographic criteria for tricyclic antidepressant cardiotoxicity. Am J Cardiol 1986;57:1154–1159.
70. Noble J, Mathew H: Acute poisoning by tricyclic antidepressants: Clinical features and management of 100 patients. Clin Toxicol 1969;2:403–421.
71. Oppenheim RC, Stewart NF: Adsorption of tricyclic antidepressants by activated charcoal. I. Adsorption in low pH conditions. Aust J Pharm Sci 1975;4:79–84.
72. Parsons AT, Anthony RM, Meeker JE: Two fatal cases of venlafaxine poisoning. J Anal Toxicol 1996;20:266–268.
73. Peano C, Leikin JB, Hanashiro PK: Seizures, ventricular tachycardia, and rhabdomyolysis as a result of ingestion of venlafaxine and lamotrigine. Ann Emerg Med 1997; 30:704–708.
74. Pentel P, Peterson CD: Asystole complicating physostigmine treatment of tricyclic antidepressant overdose. Ann Emerg Med 1980;9:588–590.
75. Pentel PR, Benowitz NL: Tricyclic antidepressant poisoning—Management of arrhythmias. Med Toxicol 1986;1: 101–121.
76. Pentel PR, Keyler DE, Brunn GJ, et al: Redistribution of tricyclic antidepressants in rats using a drug-specific monoclonal antibody: Dose-response relationship. Drug Metab Dispos 1991;19:24–28.

77. Petit JM, Spiker DG, Ruwitch JF, et al: Tricyclic antidepressant plasma levels and adverse effect after overdose. Clin Pharmacol Ther 1977;21:47–51.
78. Pollack BG, Perel GM: Sodium bicarbonate in tricyclic antidepressant—Induced arrhythmias. Can Med Assoc J 1984;131:717. Letter.
79. Pond SM, Lewis-Driver DJ, William GM, et al: Gastric emptying in acute overdose: A prospective randomised controlled trial. Med J Aust 1995;163: 345–349.
80. Preskorn SH, Irwin HA: Toxicity of tricyclic antidepressants—Kinetics, mechanism, intervention: A review. J Clin Psychiatry 1982;43:151–156.
81. Rosenstein DL, Nelson JC, Jacobs SC: Seizures associated with antidepressants: A review. J Clin Psychiatry 1993;54: 289–299.
82. Rudorfer MV, Manji HE, Potter WZ: Comparative tolerability profiles of the newer versus the older antidepressants. Drug Safety 1994;10:18–42.
83. Rudorfer MV, Potter WZ: Antidepressants: A comparative review of the clinical pharmacology and therapeutic use of the "newer" versus the "older" drugs. Drugs 1989;37: 713–738.
84. Sasyniuk BI, Jhamandas V: Mechanism of reversal of toxic effects of amitriptyline on cardiac Purkinje fibers by sodium bicarbonate. J Pharmacol Exp Ther 1984;231: 387–394.
85. Sasyniuk BI, Jhamandas V, Valois M: Experimental amitriptyline intoxication: Treatment of cardiac toxicity with sodium bicarbonate. Ann Emerg Med 1986;15: 1052–1059.
86. Shannon MW, Merola J, Lovejoy FH Jr: Hypotension in severe tricyclic antidepressant overdose. Am J Emerg Med 1988;6:439–442.
87. Shelver WL, Keyler DE, Lin G, et al: Effects of recombinant drug-specific single chain antibody Fv fragment on [^{3}H]-desipramine distribution in rats. Biochem Pharmacol 1996;51:531–537.
88. Skowron DM, Stimmel GL: Antidepressants and the risk of seizures. Pharmacotherapy 1992;2:8–22.
89. Spiker DG, Weiss AN, Chang SS, et al: Tricyclic antidepressant overdose: Clinical presentation and plasma levels. Clin Pharmacol Ther 1975;18:539–546.
90. Spiller HA, Ramoska EA, Krenzelok EP, et al: Bupropion overdose: A 3 year multi-center retrospective analysis. Am J Emerg Med 1994;12:43–45.
91. Swartz CM, Sherman A: The treatment of tricyclic antidepressant overdose with repeated charcoal. J Clin Psychopharmacol 1984;4:336–340.
92. Tatro DS, Olin BR: Drug Interaction Facts and Updates. St. Louis, Lippincott, 1990, p. 623.
93. Taylor P: Anticholinesterase agents. In: Gilman AG, Rall TW, Nies AS, Taylor, P, eds: Goodman and Gilman's The Pharmacological Basis of Therapeutics, 8th ed. Elmsford, NY, Pergamon, 1990, pp. 131–149.
94. Tennenbein M: Multiple doses of activated charcoal: Time for reappraisal. Ann Emerg Med 1991;20:529–531.
95. Tokarski GF, Young MJ: Criteria for admitting patients with tricyclic antidepressant overdose. J Emerg Med 1988; 6:121–124.
96. Tong TG, Benowitz NL, Becker CE, et al: Tricyclic antidepressant overdose. Drug Int Clin Pharm 1976;10: 711–712.
97. Vohra J, Burrows G, Hunt D, et al: The effect of toxic and therapeutic doses of tricyclic antidepressant drugs on intracardiac conduction. Eur J Cardiol 1975;3:219–227.
98. Wedin GP, Oderda GM, Klein-Schwartz W: Relative toxicity of cyclic antidepressants. Ann Emerg Med 1986;15: 797–804.
99. Wolfe TR, Caravati EM, Rollins DE, et al: Terminal 40-ms frontal plane QRS axis as a marker for tricyclic antidepressant overdose. Ann Emerg Med 1989;18:348–351.
100. Woo OF, Vrendenbury M, Freitas P, Olson KR: Seizures after venlafaxine overdose: A case report. J Toxicol Clin Toxicol 1995;33:549–550.

CHAPTER 56

Selective Serotonin Reuptake Inhibitors and Other Antidepressants

Christine M. Stork

A 26-year-old female ingested an unknown amount of fluoxetine (20 mg) capsules in a suicide attempt. The patient vomited once while on route to the hospital. In the emergency department, the patient was noted to be drowsy but awoke to voice and was orientated to person, place, and time. Vital signs were: blood pressure, 110/70 mm Hg; heart rate, 100 beats/min; respiratory rate, 14 breaths/min; and temperature, 98.6°F (37°C). Physical examination was remarkable for a slight hand tremor, but otherwise was noncontributory. The patient's ECG revealed sinus tachycardia with a QRS duration of 0.08 seconds. The patient was given one dose of oral activated charcoal with sorbitol. A 4-four hour acetaminophen level was reported as negative. Over the next several hours the patient's vital signs and mental status normalized.

What Is Fluoxetine?

Fluoxetine (Prozac) (Fig. 56–1) is the first of the class of antidepressants known as selective serotonin reuptake inhibitors (SSRI). Other drugs that belong to the class of SSRIs include paroxetine (Paxil), fluvoxamine (Luvox), sertraline (Zoloft), and citalopram (Nitalpram). Other drugs that also exhibit some SSRI activity include clomipramine, nefazodone, trazodone, venlafaxine, and mirtazapine. Therapeutic doses and pharmacology of the SSRIs and related antidepressants are listed in Table 56–1.

How Do SSRIs Work?

The SSRI's are distinct psychopharmaceutical agents capable of specifically inhibiting the reuptake of serotonin.[3] The selectivity for serotonin receptors may be structurally related to the *p*-trifluoromethyl substitution in some of these agents[90] (Fig. 56–1). By inhibiting serotonin reuptake, these drugs potentiate the activity of neuronally released serotonin and may additionally influence depressive illness by altering the sensitivity of serotonin subtype $5HT_{1A}$ or $5HT_{1C}$ receptors. Unlike tricyclic antidepressants and other atypical antidepressants, SSRIs have little interaction with other receptors such as adrenergic, cholinergic, and GABA receptors and with sodium channels.

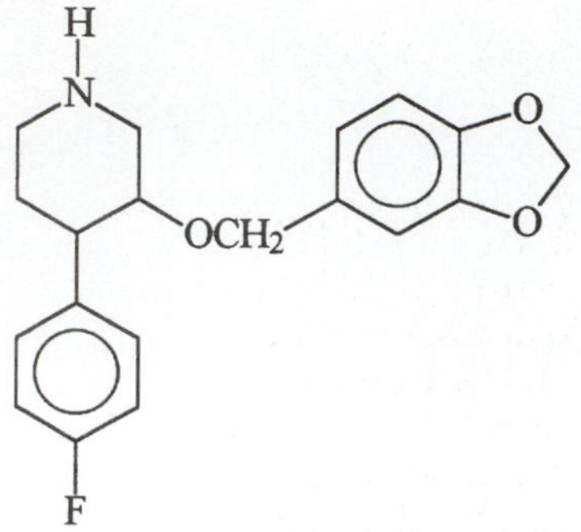
Paroxetine

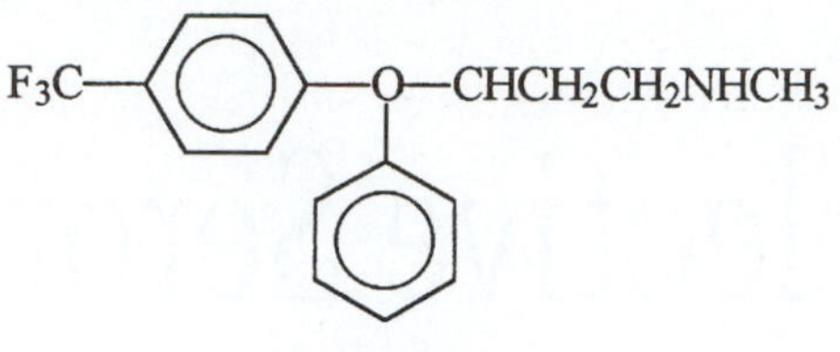
Fluoxetine

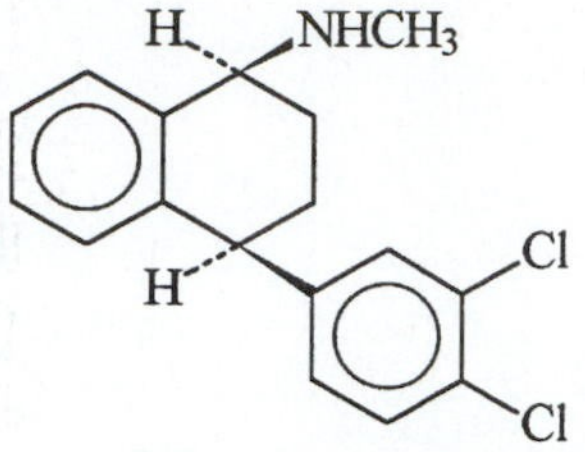
Sertraline

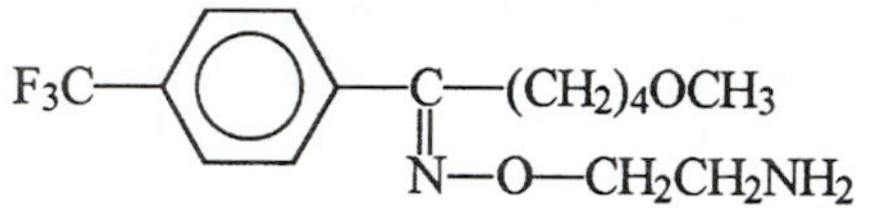
Fluvoxamine

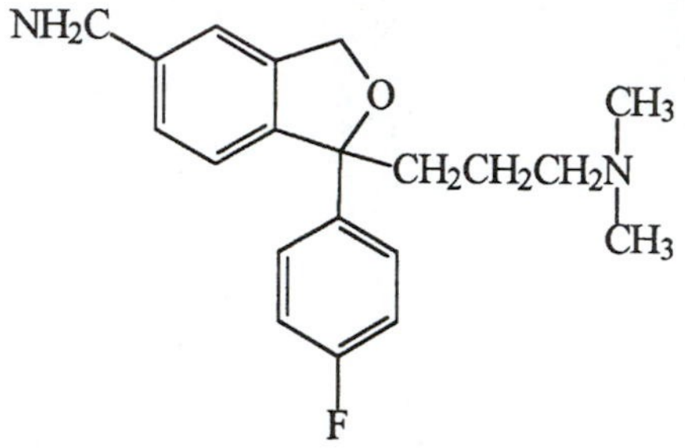
Citalopram

Figure 56–1. The structures of common selective serotonin reuptake inhibitors.

TABLE 56–1. THERAPEUTIC DOSES AND PHARMACOLOGY OF SSRIs AND RELATED ANTIDEPRESSANTS

Drug Mechanism and Drug	Therapeutic Dose Range (mg/d)	V_d (L/kg)	$T_{1/2}$	Active Metabolite(s)
Selective serotonin reuptake inhibitors (SSRI)				
Fluoxetine	10–80	20–45	1–6 d	Yes
Fluvoxamine	100–300	25	15–23 h	No
Paroxetine	10–50	8–28	2.9–44 h	No
Sertraline	50–200	20	24 h	No
SSRI + alpha-adrenergic antagonist				
Trazodone	50–600	0.5–1	3–9 h	No
Nefazodone	300–600	0.22–0.87	3.5 h	Yes
SSRI + inhibition of reuptake of norepinephrine and dopamine				
Venlafaxine	75–375	6–7	3–4 h	Yes
Alpha$_2$-adrenergic antagonist				
Mirtazapine	15–45	?	20–40 h	?
Inhibition of reuptake of biogenic amines or dopamine				
Bupropion	300–450	20	9.6–20.9 h	Yes

How Common Is the Use of SSRIs for the Treatment of Major Depression?

In the treatment of major depression, SSRIs are about as efficacious as the tricyclic antidepressants.[65] Initially marketed in the early 1980s, the SSRIs have become first line therapy for the treatment of depressive disorders.[55] In fact, according to a 1994 report of prescription drug use, SSRIs have become the largest prescribed class of medication used for the treatment of major depression.[78] Selective serotonin reuptake inhibitors differ from older antidepressants in that they have a relative lack of adverse effects, particularly with respect to those characteristics that limit patient compliance[20] (Chap. 55). SSRIs are also useful in the treatment of obsessive/compulsive disorders, alcoholism, obesity, and various other medical and psychologic disorders.[19,57]

What Are the Typical Clinical Manifestations of an SSRI Overdose?

The acute manifestations of SSRI overdose may include nausea, vomiting, dizziness, blurred vision, and, less commonly, central nervous system depression and sinus tachycardia.[6,7] Rarely, cases of seizures are reported after large overdoses.[7]

Citalopram reportedly causes wide QRS complexes and seizures in patients exposed to more than 600 mg. In one case series, seizures occurred early, whereas ECG abnormalities were delayed for as long as 24 hours. Although concurrent exposure to other drugs capable of producing these effects was not excluded by laboratory studies, the high incidence of adverse effects (6 of 18 cases) warrants further investigation. Until more information is available, all patients exposed to citalopram should be carefully monitored for ECG abnormalities and the development of seizures.[62]

How Should Patients with SSRI Overdoses Be Treated?

Treatment of patients with SSRI overdose is largely supportive with careful attention to airway, breathing, and circulation. Dextrose and thiamine (in adults) should be given to patients presenting with an alteration in mental status as indicated. Although cardiac manifestations after SSRI overdose are rare, a 12-lead ECG should be obtained to screen and monitor for other, more life-threatening antidepressants, which may have been co-ingested (Chap. 55). Serum electrolytes and an acetaminophen level are also useful screens for co-ingestants.

Once the patient is stabilized, oral activated charcoal (1 g/kg) in a slurry with a cathartic may be useful to bind drug remaining in the gastrointestinal tract. Syrup of ipecac is too dangerous to use in the management of these patients due to expected changes in mental status. Pure SSRI overdose is rarely life-threatening, obviating the need for orogastric lavage. Multiple doses of activated charcoal without a cathartic may be useful for co-ingestants. Patients with small unintentional overdoses of SSRIs are not expected to develop significant signs and symptoms of poisoning. These patients, particularly children, can be safely and effectively managed in the home with close observation.

What Are the Adverse Effects Associated With Therapeutic Doses of SSRIs?

Therapeutic doses of SSRIs are commonly associated with anorexia, jitteriness, dizziness, and blurred vision. In addition, endocrine alterations are reported after SSRI administration.[22,41] These effects appear to be serotonin mediated. A dose-related increase in serum cortisol concentration, potentiation of oxitriptan-induced elevations in serum cortisol concentrations, and increased corticotrophin (ACTH) and vasopressin concentrations occur in animals.[25] Post-marketing surveillance and case reports have identified instances of hyponatremia resulting from SIADH in humans.[22,41] Hyperglycemia, which resolves with discontinuation of therapy, is also reported after SSRI use. Additionally, platelet dysfunction occurs and is thought to be due to serotoninergic effects on platelets.[40]

What Is the Relationship Between SSRIs and Serotonin Syndrome?

The SSRIs are associated with the development of serotonin syndrome when used alone[21] or in combination with other serotoninergic agents. This syndrome is also referred to as serotonin behavioral or hyperreactivity syndrome.[32] First described in animals, serotonin excess caused hyperactivity and reactivity, forepaw-treading, head-weaving, hind-limb abduction, and an arched tail along with tremor, rigidity, salivation, flushing, myoclonus, and seizures. In humans, the serotonin syndrome was first described in patients treated with monoamine oxidase inhibitors in conjunction with other drugs that enhance serotonergic activity.[12,60,81] This rare, idiosyncratic reaction is characterized by alterations in mental status, autonomic instability, and neuromuscular abnormalities.[5,51,58]

The incidence of serotonin syndrome is unknown; however, a prospective study in depressed inpatients given clomipramine demonstrated that 16 of 38 patients experienced symptoms consistent with serotonin syndrome.[49] Monitored symptoms included confusion, agitation, myoclonus, diaphoresis, tremor, and diarrhea. Fourteen of the 16 patients experienced tremor and myoclonus and 10 developed myoclonus, diaphoresis, and shivering. All except two of the cases spontaneously resolved within 1 week without discontinuation of therapy. Other manifestations of serotonin syndrome may include agitation, delirium, coma, mydriasis, diaphoresis, hyperthermia, tachycardia, unstable blood pressure, tremor, rigidity, myoclonus, and seizures. Untreated patients may develop lactic acidosis, rhabdomyolysis, myoglobinuria, renal and hepatic dysfunction, disseminated intravascular coagulation, or adult respiratory distress syndrome.[52,86] A 1991 study of 38 cases led to the description of the clinical characteristics of the serotonin syndrome.[86] Suggested diagnostic criteria for serotonin syndrome include three out of the following: mental status changes, agitation, myoclonus, hyperreflexia, diaphoresis, tremor, diarrhea, incoordination, and fever when other etiologies are excluded and a neuroleptic is not present. These criteria, although not validated in human trials, can serve as a guide when evaluating potential cases of serotonin syndrome.

The pathophysiologic mechanism of the serotonin syndrome is not completely understood, but may involve excessive stimulation of serotonin $5HT_{1A}$ receptors.[91] Cases of serotonin syndrome have been associated with many agents that can increase synaptic serotonin (Table 56–2). A review of these case reports demonstrates that ingestion of an MAOI is not required for this interaction to exist, and that initiation is unpredictable. It is unclear whether certain combinations of serotoninergic agents place patients at greater risk than others. Although serotonin syndrome is considered an idiosyncratic reaction, genetic polymorphism may be used in the future to predict which patients may be at increased risk.[23,75]

TABLE 56–2. POTENTIAL CAUSES OF THE SEROTONIN SYNDROME

Drugs that inhibit the breakdown of serotonin
Monamine oxidase inhibitors (MAO-A)
phenelzine, moclobemide, corgyline, isocarboxyzid[8,12,29,31,36,64,70,82,89]
cocaine[70]
Drugs that block reuptake of serotonin
SSRIs (fluoxetine, citalopram, paroxetine, fluvoxamine, sertraline)[1,4,8,17,27,31,34,43,56,64,68,79,85]
Venlafaxine[36]
Clomipramine[10,47,64,82]
Doxepin[33]
Trazodone[27,30,68]
Nefazodone[43]
Dextromethorphan[70,79]
Meperidine[29]
Pentazocine[35]
Cocaine[89]
Drugs that act as serotonin precursors or agonists
Lithium[33,47,56]
L-Tryptophan[66,85]
Buspirone[1,30]
Lysergic acid diethylamine (LSD)[77]
Psilocybin[a]
Drugs that enhance serotonin release
MDMA (ecstasy)[45,80]

[a]Theoretical

Serotonin syndrome is reported after a single dose, high therapeutic doses, or overdoses of the precipitant agent.[44,50] Cases are also reported after discontinuation of therapy of one serotoninergic agent in which an insufficient lag time had occurred between initiating alternative therapy.[72,73] Some reasons for the development of serotonin syndrome after the discontinuation of concurrent therapy include residual pharmacologic effect, receptor down- or up-regulation, or the presence of active metabolites. Fluoxetine contains an active metabolite, norfluoxetine, that has a half-life longer than that of the parent drug. Levels of norfluoxetine are still present when the serotonin syndrome develops, weeks after discontinuation of therapy.[13]

Treatment for serotonin syndrome is supportive and is aimed at decreasing muscle rigidity, which is thought to be the major contributor to hyperthermia and death. Rapid external cooling in conjunction with the aggressive use of benzodiazepines should limit the negative effects resulting from sustained hyperthermia. In severe cases, neuromuscular blockade should be considered to achieve rapid muscle relaxation. The serotonin syndrome will resolve in most patients within 24 hours of removal of the offending drug.

Pretreatment with nonselective serotonin antagonists and serotonin $5HT_{1A}$-receptor antagonists prevents the development of serotonin syndrome in animals.[28,38,84] There are also anecdotal reports of the successful use of cyproheptadine (4 mg/h), methysergide (2 mg twice daily), and propranolol in humans.[30,33,48,74] Because of the potential lethality of hyperthermia and the unproven utility of these agents, they should be considered only after aggressive cooling and sedation have been initiated.

What Are the Features That Distinguish Serotonin Syndrome from Neuroleptic Malignant Syndrome?

There are many overlapping features between serotonin syndrome and neuroleptic malignant syndrome (NMS) (Chap. 57). In fact, some authors have called these disorders "spectrum disorders" that can be caused by drugs with both antidopaminergic and/or serotonergic effects.[53] Both syndromes are characterized by changes in mental status, autonomic instability, and changes in neuromuscular tone that may result in hyperthermia; however, the mechanisms are distinct. The development of NMS involves rapid blockade of dopaminergic neurons in the central nervous system, whereas serotonin syndrome appears to result from acute overstimulation of serotonin receptors. Some authors have described NMS after serotonin-enhancing drugs; however, studies determining the levels of dopamine and serotonin metabolites in patients experiencing NMS have supported the hypothesis that central dopaminergic hypoactivity is the main pathophysiologic effect seen in NMS.[2,59]

One of the major clinical differences between the two syndromes appears to be time of onset. Signs and symptoms of serotonin syndrome develop within minutes to hours after exposure to the offending agent, whereas NMS typically develops 3–9 days after exposure. [5,31] Serotonin syndrome is also more likely to present with hyperreflexia and myoclonus rather than acute muscular rigidity as seen in NMS, although rigidity is also reported with serotonin syndrome.[31,46]

What Other Drug Interactions Occur With SSRIs?

Drug interactions reported after therapeutic doses of SSRIs are both pharmacokinetically related and idiosyncratic (serotonin syndrome as described). The SSRIs are both substrates for and potent inhibitors of some cytochrome P450 isoenzymes.[69] Specifically, paroxetine and sertraline are substrates for the CYP2D6 isoenzyme and fluoxetine and paroxetine are potent inhibitors of this same CYP isoenzyme. The consequences of these interactions can be seen with drugs and toxins that either rely on this isoenzyme for metabolic transformation or influence the metabolism of the SSRIs that are substrates for this system. The ability to block CYP2D6 is greatest with paroxetine, and progressively lower with norfluoxetine, fluoxetine, and sertraline.[14] In addition, fluoxetine is a

TABLE 56–3. THE PHARMACODYNAMICS OF SSRIs AND CYP2D6

Substrates for CYP2D6
SSRIs: paroxetine, sertraline
Tricyclic antidepressants: desipramine, nortriptyline, clomipramine, imipramine
Other antidepressants/neuroleptics: venlafaxine, clozapine, risperidone, haloperidol, thioridazine, perphenazine
Beta-adrenergic antagonists: propranolol, metoprolol, timolol
Other: encainide, flecainide, propafenone, codeine/morphine, dextromethorphan
SSRI inhibitory metabolic effects[a]
Fluoxetine: alprazolam, diazepam, metoprolol, desipramine, nortriptyline, imipramine, doxepin, trazodone
Fluvoxamine: imipramine, amitryptiline, clomipramine, theophylline (inhibition of CYP1A2)
Paroxetine: desipramine, amitryptiline
Sertraline: diazepam

[a]Only those drugs demonstrated to have these effects are cited.

Abstracted, with permission, from: Hansten PD, Horn JR, Koda-Kimple MA, Young LY: Drug Interactions and Updates Quarterly. Drug Interactions Newsletter. A clinical perspective and analysis of current developments. Philadelphia, Lea & Febiger, 1992, pp. 713–716.

potent inhibitor of CYP2C19.[23] There is some evidence to suggest that genetic polymorphism plays a role in drug interactions and an individual's ability to metabolically convert drugs using these isoenzymes.[23,75] Poor metabolizers can account for up to 10% of any given population. Some agents that rely on CYP2D6 for metabolism are listed on Table 56–3.

Other Atypical Antidepressants

Venlafaxine

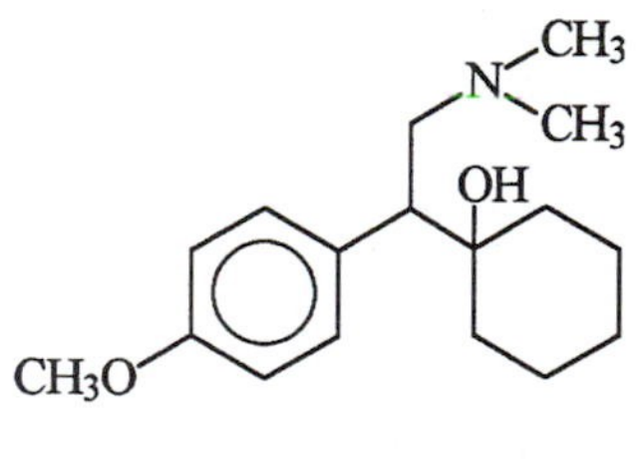

Venlafaxine is an SSRI that, in addition to inhibiting the reuptake of serotonin, inhibits the reuptake of norepinephrine and dopamine.[67] Venlafaxine produces a rapid down-regulation of central beta-adrenergic receptors; which may result in a faster onset of antidepressant effect.[76] Patients acutely exposed to venlafaxine may present with nausea, vomiting, dizziness, central nervous system depression, hyperthermia, and self-limited seizures.[39]

Trazodone

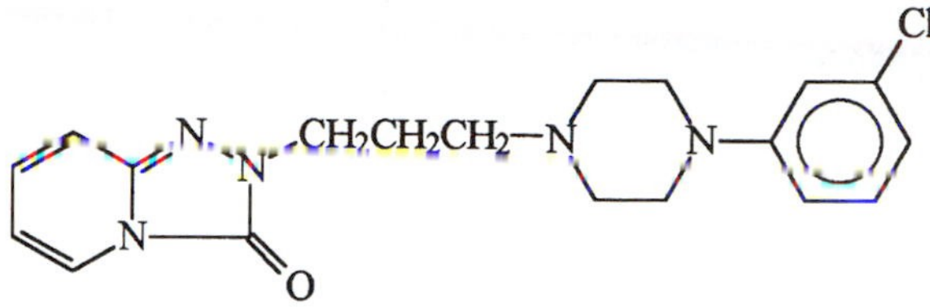

Trazodone is a peripheral serotonin agonist that acts through inhibition of serotonin reuptake. In addition, trazodone may have some peripheral alpha-adrenergic antagonist capability. After acute overdose of trazodone, central nervous system depression is the most common adverse effect, followed by orthostatic hypotension.[26,37] Priapism, reported with the therapeutic use of trazodone, is rarely seen in the overdose setting[11,26] (see Chap. 29). In addition to supportive care, these patients should receive fluids and pressor support, if necessary to maintain blood pressure.

Bupropion

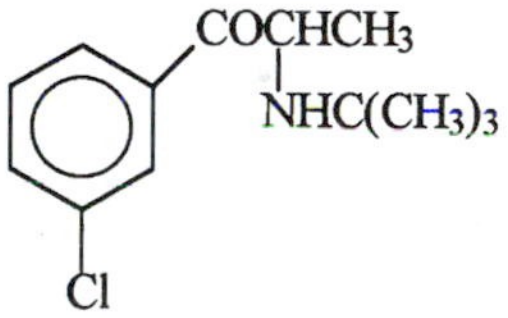

Bupropion is a unicyclic antidepressant. The exact pharmacologic mechanism of bupropion's action is unclear, but either the parent drug or an active metabolite may inhibit the reuptake of biogenic amines or dopamine. At daily doses greater than 450–500 mg/d, patients may be at a substantial increased risk for seizures.[15,43]

Seizure activity after acute overdose 7 hours after an intentional ingestion of 9000 mg was described in one case report.[87] In a case review of 13 patients ingesting doses ranging from 850 to 4500 mg, there was no central nervous system or serious cardiovascular toxicity.[9] However, in a retrospective analysis of 58 patients reported to poison control centers, neurologic toxicity was commonly encountered and included lethargy, tremors, and seizures.[83] There are some data to suggest that the seizures due to bupropion are caused by the metabolite hydroxybupropion.[24,63] In a report of seizure activity when bupropion was used in conjunction with carbamazepine, bupropion levels were nondetectable, whereas hydroxybupropion levels were elevated. In a reported fatality, bupropion levels were found, but were much lower than hydroxybupropion levels.[24,71] Treatment of seizures after bupropion exposure should be supportive and include the judicious use of benzodiazepines, followed by barbiturates as needed.

Nefazodone

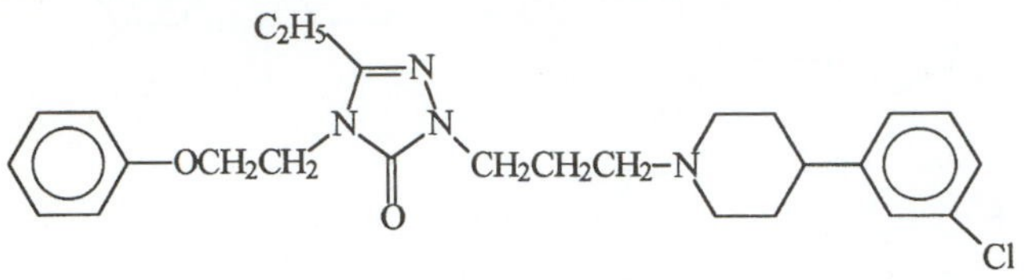

The exact mechanism of action of nefazodone is unclear but may include the inhibition of reuptake of serotonin, antagonism of serotonin $5HT_2$ receptors, down-regulation at these receptor binding sites, inhibition of the reuptake of norepinephrine, and alpha-adrenergic blocking capability.[18,42] Experience with this drug in overdose is limited; however, since it is structurally similar to trazodone, overdoses of nefazodone may be expected to result in similar toxicity.

Mirtazapine

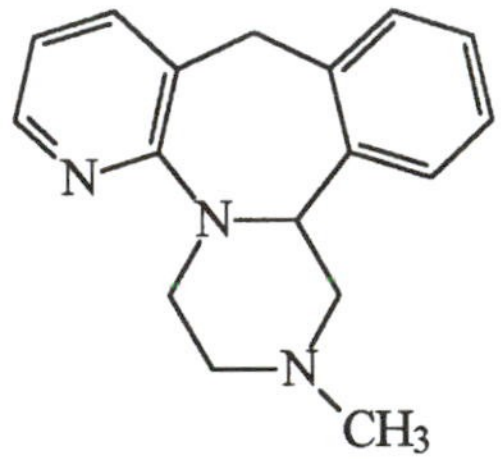

The mechanism of action of mirtazapine is unique in that it increases neuronal serotonin and norepinephrine through $alpha_2$-adrenergic antagonism.[16,38] The main effect seen after acute overdose is mental status depression.[54] In one report of a patient ingesting 975 mg of mirtazapine and 30 mg clonazepam, somnolence and tachycardia developed.[61] Since more overdose data are required before a constellation of symptoms can be attributed to this drug, careful clinical monitoring is advised.

Summary

In summary, the toxicity of acute selective serotonin reuptake inhibitor or atypical antidepressant overdose is usually not life-threatening. Treatment is generally supportive for all of these agents. There are significant drug interactions and adverse drug reactions associated with selective serotonin reuptake inhibitors, however, which may lead to acute life-threatening events.

References

1. Baetz M, Malcolm D: Serotonin syndrome from fluvoxamine and buspirone. Can J Psychiatry 1995;40:428–429.
2. Bakheit AMO, Beehan PO, Prach AT, et al: A syndrome identical to the neuroleptic malignant syndrome induced by LSD and alcohol. Br J Addiction 1990;85:150–151.
3. Baldessarini RJ: Drugs and the treatment of psychiatric disorders. In: Hardman JG, Limbird LE, Molinoff PB, et al, eds: Goodman & Gilman's The Pharmacological Basis of Therapeutics. 9th ed. New York, McGraw-Hill, 1996, pp. 431–459.
4. Bastani JB, Troester MM, Bastani AJ: Serotonin syndrome and fluvoxamine: A case study. Nebr Med J 1996;81:107–109.
5. Bodner RA, Lynch T, Lewis L, Kahn D: Serotonin syndrome. Neurology 1995;45:219–223.
6. Borys DJ, Setzer SC, Ling LJ, et al: Acute fluoxetine overdose: Report of 234 cases. Am J Emerg Med 1992;10; 115–120.
7. Braitberg G, Curry SC: Seizure after isolated fluoxetine overdose. Ann Emerg Med 1995;26:234–237.
8. Brannan SK, Talley BJ, Bowden CL: Sertraline and isocarboxazid cause of serotonin syndrome. J Clin Psychopharmacol 1994;14:144–145. Letter.
9. Bryant SG, Guernsey BG, Ingrim NB: Review of bupropion. Clin Pharm 1983;2:525–537.
10. Cano-Munoz JL, Montejo-Inglesias ML, Yanez-Saez RM, Galvez-Borrero IM: Possible serotonin syndrome following the combined administration of clomipramine and alprazolam. J Clin Psychiatry 1995;56:122. Letter.
11. Carson CC III, Mino RD: Priapism associated with trazodone therapy. J Urol 1988;139:369–370.
12. Cohen RM, Pickar D, Murphy DL: Myoclonus associated hypomania during MAO-inhibitor treatment. Am J Psychiatry 1980;137:105–106.
13. Coplan JD, Gorman JM: Detectable levels of fluoxetine metabolites after discontinuation: An unexpected serotonin syndrome. Am J Psychiatry 1993;150:837. Letter.
14. Crewe HK, Lennard MS, Tucker GT, et al: The effect of selective serotonin re-uptake inhibitors on cytochrome P4502D6 (CYP2D6) activity in human liver microsomes. Br J Clin Pharmacol 1992;34:262–265.
15. Davidson J: Seizures and bupropion: A review. J Clin Psychiatry 1989;50:256–261.
16. deBoer T: The pharmacologic profile of mirtazapine. J Clin Psychiatry 1996;57(suppl 4):19–25.
17. Dursun SM, Mathew VM, Reveley MA: Toxic serotonin syndrome after fluoxetine plus carbamazepine. Lancet 1993; 342:442–443. Letter.
18. Ellingrod VL, Perry PJ: Nefazodone: A new antidepressant. Am J Health Syst Pharm 1995;52:2799–2812.
19. Ferguson JM, Feighrer JP: Fluoxetine-induced weight loss in overweight non-depressed humans. Int J Obesity 1987; 11:163–170.
20. Finley PR: Selective serotonin reuptake inhibitors: Pharmacologic profiles and potential therapeutic distinctions. Ann Pharmacother 1994;28:1359–1369.
21. Fischer P: Serotonin syndrome in the elderly after antidepressive monotherapy. J Clin Psychopharmacol 1995;15: 440–442. Letter.

22. Flint AJ, Crosby J, Genik JL: Recurrent hyponatremia associated with fluoxetine and paroxetine. Am J Psychiatry 1996;114:717–718. Letter.
23. Flockhart DA: Drug interaction and the cytochrome P450 system, the role of cytochrome P1502C19. Clin Pharmacokinet 1995;29:45–52.
24. Friel PN, Logan BK, Fligner CL: Three fatal drug overdoses involving bupropion. J Anal Toxicol 1993;17:436–438.
25. Fuller R: Serotonergic stimulation of pituitary-adrenocortical function in rats. Neuroendocrinology 1985;32:118–120.
26. Gamble DE, Peterson LG: Trazodone overdose: Four years of experience from voluntary reports. J Clin Psychiatry 1986; 47:544–546.
27. George TP, Godleski LS: Possible serotonin syndrome with trazodone addition to fluoxetine. Biol Psychiatry 1996;39: 384–385. Letter.
28. Gerson SC, Baldessarini RJ: Motor effects of serotonin in the central nervous system. Life Sci 1980;27:1435–1451.
29. Gillman PK: Possible serotonin syndrome with moclobemide and pethidine. Med J Aust 1995;162:554. Letter.
30. Goldberg RJ, Huk M: Serotonin syndrome from trazodone and buspirone. Psychosomatics 1992;33:235–236. Letter.
31. Graber MA, Hoens TB, Perry PJ: Sertraline–phenelzine drug interaction: A serotonin syndrome reaction. Ann Pharmacother 1994;28:732–735.
32. Grahame-Smith DC: Studies in vivo on the relationship between brain tryptophan, brain 5-HT synthesis and hyperactivity in rats treated with monoamine oxidase inhibitor and L-tryptophan. J Neurochem 1971;18:1053–1066.
33. Guze BH, Baxter LR Jr: The serotonin syndrome: Case responsive to propranolol. J Clin Psychopharmacol 1986;6: 119–120. Letter.
34. Hansen TE, Dieter K, Keepers GA: Interaction of fluoxetine and pentazocine. Am J Psychiatry 1990;147:949–950.
35. Hansten PD, Horn JR, Koda-Kimble MA, Young LY: Drug Interactions and Updates Quarterly. Drug Interactions Newsletter. A clinical perspective and analysis of current developments. Philadelphia, Lea & Febiger, 1992, pp. 713–716.
36. Heisler MA, Guidry JR, Arnecke B: Serotonin syndrome induced by administration of venlafaxine and phenelzine. Ann Pharmacother 1996;30:84. Letter.
37. Henry JA, Ali CJ, Caldwell R, Flanagan RJ: Acute trazodone poisoning: Clinical signs and plasma concentrations. Psychopathology 1984;17(suppl 2):77–81.
38. Hoes MJ, Zeijpveld JH: Mirtazapine as treatment for serotonin syndrome. Pharmacopsychiatry 1996;29:81. Letter.
39. Holliday SM, Benfield P: Venlafaxine. A review of its pharmacology and therapeutic potential in depression. Drugs 1995;49:280–294.
40. Humphries JE, Wheby MS, Vandenberg SR: Fluoxetine and the bleeding time. Arch Pathol Lab Med 1990;114:727–728.
41. Jackson C, Carson W, Markowitz J, Mintzer J: SIADH associated with fluoxetine and sertraline. Am J Psychiatry 1995; 152:809–810. Letter.
42. John L, Perreault MM, Tao T, Blew PG: Serotonin syndrome associated with nefazodone and paroxetine. Ann Emerg Med 1997;29:287–289.
43. Johnson JA, Lineberry CG, Ascher JA, et al: A 102 center prospective study of seizure in association with bupropion. J Clin Psychiatry 1991;52:450–456.
44. Kaminski CA, Robbins MS, Weibley RE: Sertraline intoxication in a child. Ann Emerg Med 1994;23:1371–1374.
45. Kaskey GB: Possible interaction between MAOI and "ecstasy." Am J Psychiatry 1992;149:411–412.
46. Kline SS, Mauro LS, Scala-Barnett DM, Zick D: Serotonin syndrome versus neuroleptic malignant syndrome as a cause of death. Clin Pharmacol 1989;8:510–514.
47. Kojima H, Terao T, Yoshimura R: Serotonin syndrome during clomipramine and lithium treatment. Am J Psychiatry 1993;150:1897. Letter.
48. Lappin R, Auchincloss E: Treatment of serotonin syndrome with cyproheptadine. N Engl J Med 1994;331:1021–1022.
49. Lejoyeux M, Roullion F, Ades J: Prospective evaluation of the serotonin syndrome in depressed inpatients treated with clomipramine. Acta Psychiatr Scand 1993;88:369–371.
50. Lenzi A, Raffaelli S, Marazziti D: Serotonin syndrome-like symptoms in patients with obsessive-compulsive disorder, following inappropriate increase in fluvoxamine dosage. Pharmacopsychiatry 1993;26:100–101.
51. Martin TG: Serotonin syndrome. Ann Emerg Med 1996; 28:520–526.
52. Miller F, Friedman R, Tanenbaum J, Griffin A: Disseminated intravascular coagulation and acute myoglobinuric renal failure: A consequence of the serotonin syndrome. J Clin Psychopharmacol 1991;11:277–279. Letter.
53. Miyaoka H, Kamijima K: Encephalopathy during amitriptyline therapy: Are neuroleptic malignant syndrome and serotonin syndrome spectrum disorders? Int Clin Psychopharmacol 1995;10:265–267.
54. Montgomery SA: Safety of mirtazapine: A review. Int Clin Psychopharmacol 1995;10(suppl 4):37–45.
55. Montgomery SA: Development of new treatments for depression. J Clin Psychiatr 1985;46:3–6.
56. Muly EC, McDonald W, Steffens D, Book S: Serotonin syndrome produced by a combination of fluoxetine and lithium. Am J Psychiatry 1993;150:1565. Letter.
57. Naranjo CA, Bremner KE: Clinical pharmacology of serotonin-altering medication for decreasing alcohol consumption. Alcohol Alcoholism 1993;2:221–229.
58. Nierenberg DW, Semprebon M: The central nervous system serotonin syndrome. Clin Pharmacol Ther 1993;53:84–88.
59. Nisijima K, Ishiguro T: Cerebrospinal fluid levels of monoamine metabolites and gamma-aminobutyric acid in neuroleptic malignant syndrome. J Psychiatry 1995;29: 233–244.
60. Oates JA, Sjoerdsma A: Neurologic effects of tryptophan in patients receiving monamine oxidase inhibitor. Neurology 1960;10:1076–1078.
61. Organon, Inc. Data on file. West Orange, NJ, 1996.
62. Personne M, Sjoberg G, Persson H: Citalopram overdose—Review of cases treated in Swedish hospitals. J Toxicol Clin Toxicol 1997;35:237–240.
63. Popli AP, Tanquary J, Lamparella V, Masand PS: Bupropion and anticonvulsant drug interactions. Ann Clin Psychiatry 1995;7:90–101.
64. Power BM, Pinder M, Hackett LP, Ilett KF: Fatal serotonin syndrome following a combined overdose of moclobemide, clomipramine and fluoxetine. Anesth Intensive Care 1995; 23:499–502.
65. Preskorn SH, Burke MJ: Somatic therapy for major depres-

sive disorder: Selection of an antidepressant. J Clin Psychiatry 1992;53:5–18.
66. Price LH, Charney DS, Heninger GR: Serotonin syndrome. Am J Psychiatry 1992;149:1116–1117. Letter.
67. Product Information: Effexor(R), venlafaxine. Wyeth-Ayerst Laboratories, Philadelphia, PA 10101, 1995.
68. Reeves RR, Bullen JA: Serotonin syndrome produced by paroxetine and low-dose trazodone. Psychosomatics 1995; 36:159–160. Letter.
69. Rieseman C: Antidepressant drug interactions and the cytochrome p-450 system: A critical appraisal. Pharmacotherapy 1995;15:84S–99S.
70. Rivers N, Horner B: Possible lethal interaction between Nardil and dextromethorphan. Can Med Assoc J 1970;103: 85.
71. Rohrig TP, Ray NG: Tissue distribution of bupropion in a fatal overdose. J Anal Toxicol 1992;16:343–345.
72. Ruiz R: Fluoxetine and the serotonin syndrome. Ann Emerg Med 1994;24:983–985.
73. Safferman AZ, Masiar SJ: Central nervous system toxicity after abrupt monoamine oxidase inhibitor switch: A case report. Ann Pharmacother 1992;26:337–338.
74. Sandyk R: L-dopa induced serotonin syndrome in a parkinsonian patient on bromocriptine. J Clin Psychopharmacol 1986;6:194–195. Letter.
75. Schmid B, Bircher J, Preisig R, Kupfer A: Polymorphic dextromethorphan metabolism: Co-segregation of oxidative *O*-demethylation with debrisoquin hydroxylation. Clin Pharmacol Ther 1985;38:618–624.
76. Schweizer E, Weise C, Clary C, et al: Placebo controlled trial of venlafaxine for the treatment of major depression. J Clin Psychopharmacol 1991;11:233–236.
77. Silbergeld EK, Hurska RE: Lisuride and LSD: Dopaminergic and serotonergic interactions in the serotonin syndrome. Psychopharmacology 1979;65:233–257.
78. Simonsen LLP: Top 200 drugs: Rx prices still moderating as managed care grows. Pharm Times, April 17–23, 1995.
79. Skop BP, Finkelstein JA, Mareth TR, et al: The serotonin syndrome associated with paroxetine, an over-the-counter cold remedy, and vascular disease. Am J Emerg Med 1994; 12:642–644.
80. Smilkstein MJ, Smolinske SC, Rumack BH: A case of MAO inhibitor/MDMA interaction: Agony after ecstacy. J Toxicol Clin Toxicol 1987;25:149–159.
81. Smith B, Prockop DJ: Central nervous system effects of ingestion of L-tryptophan by normal subjects. N Engl J Med 1962;267:1338–1341.
82. Spigset O, Mjorndal T, Lovheim O: Serotonin syndrome caused by a moclobemide-clomipramine interaction. Br Med J 1993;306:248.
83. Spiller HA, Ramoska EA, Krenzelok EP: Bupropion overdose: A 3 year multi-center retrospective analysis. Am J Emerg Med 1994;12:43–45.
84. Sprouse JS, Aghajanian GK: (-)- Propranolol blocks the inhibition of serotonergic dorsal raphe cell firing by 5-HT1A selective agonists. Eur J Pharmacol 1986;128:295–298.
85. Steiner W, Fontaine R: Toxic reaction following the combined administration of fluoxetine and L-tryptophan: Five case reports. Biol Psychiatry 1986;21:1067–1071.
86. Sternbach H: The serotonin syndrome. Am J Psychiatry 1991;148:705–713.
87. Storrow AB: Bupropion overdose and seizure. Am J Emerg Med 1994;12:183–184.
88. Tackley RM, Tregaskis B: Fatality following a monamine oxidase inhibitor/tricyclic interaction. Anaesthesia 1987;42: 760–763.
89. Tordoff SG, Stubbing JF, Linter SPK: Delayed excitatory reaction following interaction of cocaine and monoamine oxidase inhibitor (phenelzine). Br J Anaesth 1991;66: 516–518.
90. Wong DT, Bymaster FP, Horng JS, Molloy BB: A new selective inhibitor for uptake of serotonin into synaptosomes of rat brain: 3-*p*-trifluoromethylphenoxy-*N*-methyl-3 phenylpropylamine. J Pharmacol Exp Ther 1975;193:804–811.
91. Yamada J, Sugimoto Y, Wakita H, Horisaka K: The involvement of serotonergic and dopaminergic systems in hypothermia induced in mice by intracerebroventricular injection of serotonin. Jpn J Pharmacol 1988;48:145–148.

CHAPTER 57

Neuroleptic Agents

Neal A. Lewin

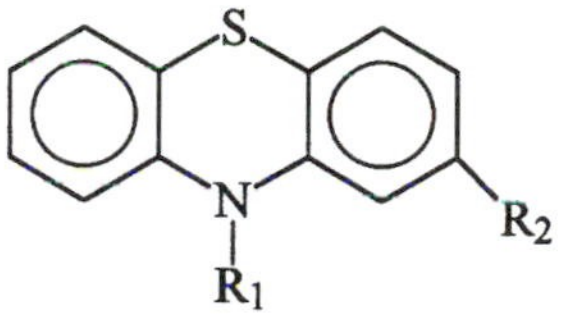

General Structure of Neuroleptics

A comatose 30-year-old man was brought to the emergency department (ED) by the police. He was discovered slumped over the kitchen table in his poorly heated apartment in winter. An empty, unlabeled pill container and a whiskey bottle were at his side. His building superintendent called the police after repeated unsuccessful attempts to arouse the patient. The superintendent reported that the patient had a history of chronic alcoholism, had been hospitalized several times for "hallucinations," and was recently discharged from a "state mental hospital." There was no other medical history available.

His vital signs were: blood pressure, 80/50 mm Hg; pulse, 110 beats/min and regular; respirations, 10 breaths/min and regular; and rectal temperature, 92°F (33°C). The patient's skin was bruised in many places, cool, cyanotic, and anicteric. There was no evidence of head trauma. Numerous carious teeth and gingivitis were noted. An alcoholic fetor was evident. The pupils were slightly miotic but equal and responsive to light. Oculocephalic reflexes were present. The optic discs were sharp with no hyperemia, hemorrhages, or exudates. Coarse rales and rhonchi were heard over the right lower lung area. Heart sounds were normal with no audible murmurs. The abdomen was distended without palpable masses. Bowel sounds were markedly diminished but present. Rectal examination was negative for occult blood. There was trace pitting edema in the extremities. Pulses were palpable and equal bilaterally. The patient was unresponsive to deep pain. Reflexes were normal and equal bilaterally. Plantar flexion was noted bilaterally. There were no localizing neurologic findings.

As his airway and breathing were being assessed, the patient was given 100 mL of 50% dextrose in water (50 g) intravenously, followed by two successive 2-mg IV boluses of naloxone (Narcan), without any response. A 100-mg dose of thiamine was also given intravenously. A cuffed endotracheal tube was inserted and supplemental oxygen was administered. A 1-L infusion of 0.9% sodium chloride solution was administered over 15 minutes and the blood pressure rose to 100/80 mm Hg. The initial room air arterial blood gas was: pH 7.28, PCO_2 53 mm Hg, and PO_2 70 mm Hg. Blood samples drawn prior to the administration of dextrose were sent for electrolytes, glucose, serum calcium, acetaminophen, and complete blood count.

A large-bore (40 French) orogastric tube was placed in the stomach. Aspiration of gastric contents revealed unidentifiable particulate matter. After lavage, 75 g of activated charcoal in a slurry of water was instilled into the stomach, and 1 g/kg sorbitol was given to promote catharsis. An electrocardiogram (ECG) revealed a sinus tachycardia with a prolonged QT interval. An abdominal radiograph showed radiopaque material in the upper small bowel, and a chest radiograph showed an infiltrate with air bronchograms in the right lower lobe. Gram stain of an endotracheal sputum specimen showed mixed organisms and polymorphonuclear white blood cells.

When the patient awakened 24 hours later in the intensive care unit (ICU) he admitted to ingesting a 1-month supply of chlorpromazine pills. When his QT_c interval returned to normal, 60 hours after admission, he was transferred from the ICU to the psychiatric service for a prolonged admission because of his depression and suicidal ideation.

The use of psychotropic agents has increased since their introduction in the 1950s.[9] In the United States today, 10–15% of prescriptions written are for psychiatric disorders. With psychopharmacology becoming a subspecialty and with the emergence of the field of biologic psychiatry, more adverse reactions to psychotropic medications are to be anticipated. The purpose of this chapter is to identify the common neuroleptic agents being used in treating psychiatric illness, the adverse effects as well as the manifestations of intentional and unintentional overdose.

How Are the Neuroleptic Medications Classified?

The term *neuroleptic* has become both synonymous with, and preferred over, "tranquilizing" or "antipsychotic" agents, because all of the medications in these groups are able to suppress extrapyramidal movement disorders that include spontaneous and complex patterns of behavior. However, with the introduction of newer heterocyclic agents, such as clozapine, the use of the term *neuroleptic* may no longer be appropriate for these medications, since clozapine has well-defined antipsychotic effects but only minimal extrapyramidal effects.[31,70,85] In other words, all neuroleptics have antipsychotic effects, but not all antipsychotics have neuroleptic effects. Nevertheless, because of its widespread usage, we will continue to use the term *neuroleptic* in this chapter, despite its limitations.

The phenothiazines, thioxanthenes, butyrophenones, diphenylbutylpiperidines, dibenzodiazepines, dibenzoxazepines, and indoles are the major classes of neuroleptics (Table 57–1). The phenothiazines, commonly used in the treatment of various psychiatric disorders, have a basic three-ring structure (Fig. 57–1). Substitutions at position 2 and the nitrogen atom at position 10 in the middle ring yield compounds that can be divided into three major classes: the aliphatic (eg, chlorpromazine), piperidine (eg, thioridazine), and piperazine (eg, perphenazine) derivatives.[9] All three groups have similar central and peripheral dopaminergic-receptor blockade actions.

The qualitative differences among the three classes of phenothiazines permit a certain amount of flexibility in the management of psychiatric disorders. The extrapyramidal and hypotensive adverse effects are discussed in more detail in the following sections.

TABLE 57–1. SELECTED NEUROLEPTIC DRUGS

Drug Group	Examples
Phenothiazines	
Aliphatic	Chlorpromazine (Thorazine) Triflupromazine (Vesprin)
Piperazine	Trifluoperazine (Stelazine) Prochlorperazine (Compazine) Perphenazine (Trilafon) Fluphenazine (Prolixin)
Piperidine	Thioridazine (Mellaril) Mesoridazine (Serentil)
Thioxanthenes	Chlorprothixene (Taractan) Clopenthixol Flupenthixol Pifluthixol Thiothixene (Narvane)
Butyrophenones (phenyl butylpiperidine)	Droperidol Haloperidol (Haldol)
Indoles	Molindone (Moban)
Dibenzoxazepines	Clothiapine Metiapine Zotapine Loxapine (Loxitane)
Diphenylbutylpiperidines	Pimozide (Orap) Fluspirilene Penfluridol
Dibenzodiazepines	Clozapine (Clozaril) Fluperlapine Olanzapine
Benzisoxazoles	Risperidone (Risperdal)

Adapted, with permission, from Baldessarini RJ: Drugs and the treatment of psychiatric disorders. In: Hardman JG, Limbird LE, Molinoff PB, Ruddon RW, eds: Goodman and Gilman's The Pharmacological Basis of Therapeutics, 9th ed. New York, McGraw Hill, 1996, pp. 404–406.

The thioxanthenes are derivatives of the phenothiazines. A carbon atom replaces the nitrogen at position 10, with a double bond to the side chain. The thioxanthenes and the butyrophenones (such as haloperidol) are similar pharmacologically to the phenothiazines. The butyrophenones, however, are structurally distinct from the other substances. The most studied class of neuroleptics is the phenothiazines, which will be discussed below.

What Are the Mechanisms of Action of the Phenothiazines and Other Neuroleptics?

The phenothiazines have inhibitory effects on a variety of receptors, including dopaminergic, cholinergic, $alpha_1$-, and $alpha_2$-adrenergic, histaminic, and serotonergic receptors ($5HT_2$).[9] The dopamine-receptor blocking activity in the limbic system is thought to account for

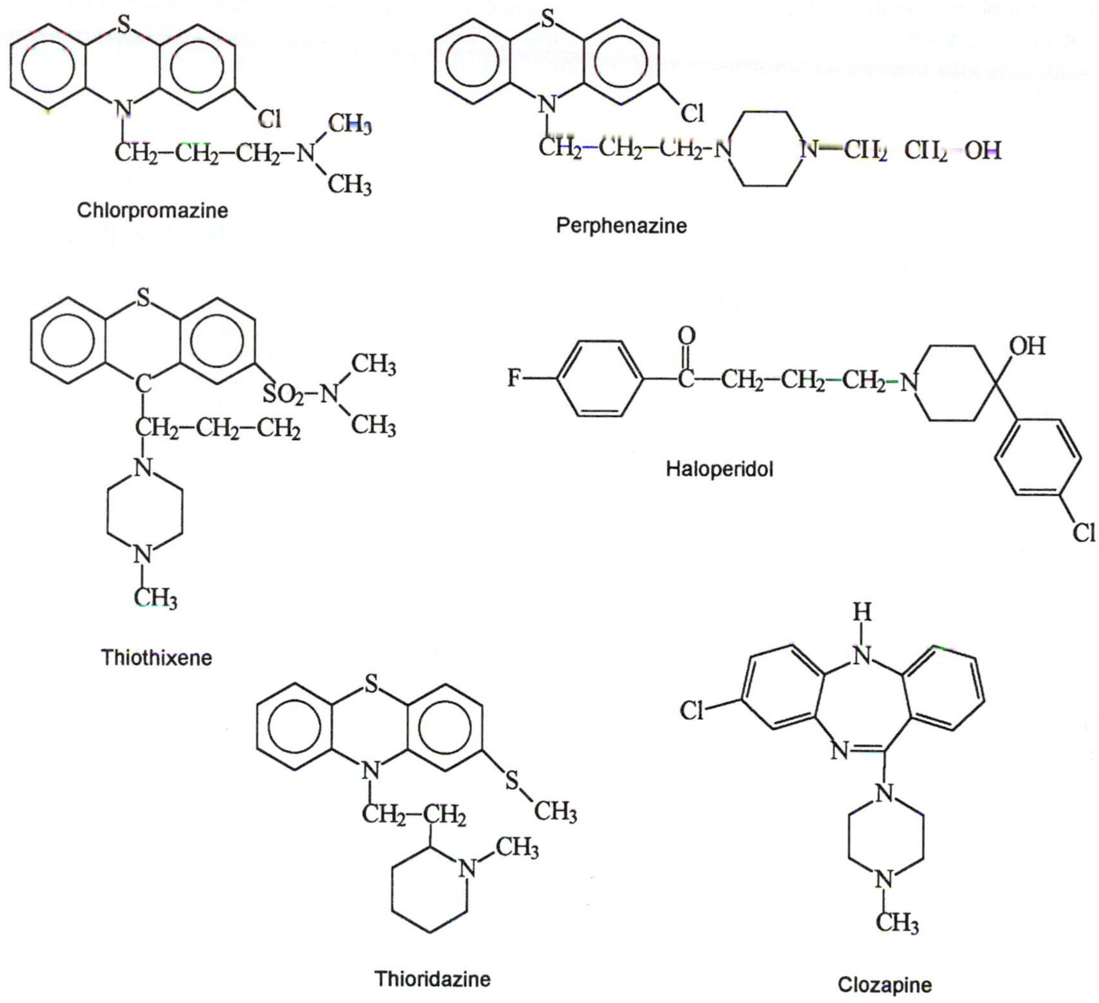

Figure 57–1. The structures of common neuroleptic drugs.

their neuroleptic activity, and the antipsychotic activity is probably mediated by serotonergic receptors. A dopamine-dependent adenylate cyclase enzyme associated with the dopamine receptors has been found in both the limbic system and the basal ganglia. The two basal ganglia sites identified as most important are the substantia nigra and the nucleus accumbens.[9] The former controls movement and the latter controls emotion and cognitive function. There are six distinct dopamine receptor subtypes: D_1, D_{2A}, D_{2B}, D_3, D_4, and D_5 (Table 57–2). Most clinically effective neuroleptic agents have a high affinity for D_2- and D_3-like receptors. There is a strong correlation

TABLE 57–2. SIX TYPES OF POSTSYNAPTIC DOPAMINE RECEPTORS

	D_1 and D_5	D_2	D_{2b}	D_3 and D_4
Effect on cyclic AMP	Increases	Decreases	Increases phosphoinositide turnover	?
Agonists				
Dopamine	Full agonists (weak)	Full agonist (potent)		
Apomorphine	Partial agonists (weak)	Full agonist (potent)		
Antagonists				
Phenothiazines	Potent	Potent		
Thioxanthenes	Potent	Potent		
Butyrophenones	Weak	Potent		
Clozapine	Inactive	Weak	Weak	Potent

Modified with permission from Kandel ER: Disorders of thought: Schizophrenia. In Kandel ER, Schwartz JH, Jessell TM, eds: Principles of Neural Science, 3rd edition. Elsevier, New York, 1991, p 862.

between the clinical potencies of antipsychotic drugs and their ability to block D_2 receptors.[90,91] Some neuroleptics such as the thioxanthenes and phenothiazines bind with high affinity to D_1 and D_2 receptors, and D_3- and D_4-receptor subtypes (see Table 57–2). The heterocyclic substituted agents haloperidol and pimozide have high selectivity as antagonists at D_2 and D_3 dopamine receptors and variable D_4 affinity. The effect of blocking D_1 or D_5 receptors remains unclear.

An atypical neuroleptic agent with low risk of producing extrapyramidal reactions, such as clozapine, has a low affinity for D_2 receptors but is an active alpha-adrenergic antagonist. Clozapine and risperidone also have affinities for 5-HT_2 serotonin receptors. Clozapine has selectivity for D_4 dopamine receptors as well, but the significance of this subtype in the basal ganglia remains unknown. The D_3 receptors are present in limbic areas of the CNS, and agents acting here would have fewer extrapyramidal effects than one acting on dopamine receptors in the basal ganglia.[41]

Normal motor movement patterns depend on a delicate balance between dopamine and acetylcholine in the extrapyramidal system. Excessive stimulation of the cholinergic fibers that project from the basal ganglia to the thalamus results in hyperkinesis. In the physiologic setting, this is prevented by the inhibitory effect of dopamine on cholinergic transmission in the basal ganglia. When neuroleptic agents are used, their antidopaminergic activity can result in excessive cholinergic stimulation and hyperkinesis.

What Are the Pharmacokinetics of the Neuroleptic Drugs?

The phenothiazine can be given orally, intramuscularly, rectally, or intravenously. Gastrointestinal (GI) absorption is diminished due to drug binding in the intestinal wall.[44] Intramuscular absorption is variable, and some phenothiazines, such as chlorpromazine, may cause profound hypotension when administered intravenously or intramuscularly.[94] Chlorpromazine is one of the few neuroleptic agents for which the pharmacokinetics are well studied. This agent is mainly absorbed in the jejunum in a pH-dependent fashion. When patients in one study were placed on H_2 antagonists (ie, cimetidine, famotidine, nizatidine), steady-state plasma chlorpromazine levels decreased.[46] Chlorpromazine has a substantial first-pass metabolism associated with oral dosing, which can be obviated with parenteral dosing. The butyrophenones undergo less first-pass degradation.

Peak chlorpromazine plasma levels are attained within 2–4 hours of oral administration of therapeutic doses.[22] This peak level reaches a plateau for approximately 3–4 hours and then gradually declines. In plasma, 99% of chlorpromazine is bound to albumin.[20]

Biotransformation of this drug occurs in the liver by demethylation and hydroxylation.[44] There are more than 15 postulated metabolites of this drug, half of which are excreted in the urine and stool. Several of these breakdown products, such as 7-hydroxychlorpromazine, have neuroleptic effects.[68,83] Chlorpromazine sulfoxide, another metabolite, is inactive.[55] Drug-responsive patients have high concentrations of the active metabolite but low levels of the sulfoxide. The nonphenothiazine neuroleptics, such as the butyrophenones and the thioxanthenes, have no active metabolites.

Half of the excretion of the phenothiazines occurs by conjugation of oxidized and hydroxylated metabolites with glucuronic acids and sulfates. The conjugated metabolites are excreted by the kidneys.[45] The other half of phenothiazine excretion occurs via the enterohepatic system. Metabolism of the phenothiazines by the liver microsomes may be enhanced by such enzyme inducers as barbiturates and meprobamate, but not by the phenothiazines themselves.[21,34,43,66] A variety of neurotoxic manifestations are reported with concomitant lithium and neuroleptic therapy, including tremors, confusion, ataxia, hypotension, and agitation.[11,24,37,79] Cardiac dysrhythmias have been noted when lithium is discontinued following combined therapy with lithium and phenothiazines.[93,100] The mechanism of toxicity is attributed to an increase in serum phenothiazine levels. Both of these agents affect the absorption of each other, and phenothiazines enhance erythrocyte uptake and renal elimination of lithium.[79,89]

Phenothiazine metabolites are lipophilic and have large volumes of distribution, properties that promote storage in tissues and prolong excretion. As a result, the breakdown products may be found in the urine up to 6 weeks after the last dose of the parent compound.

There is little correlation between dose, serum level, and neuroleptic effect of phenothiazines.[21,68,74] Tolerance to the sedative and hypotensive effects occurs after several weeks of therapy. In general, optimum neuroleptic effects require approximately 1 month of therapy. Chronic therapy with a constant dose results in lowered plasma levels. However, in spite of the lowered plasma levels of phenothiazines, tolerance to their neuroleptic effects does not occur for months.

Sufficient dopaminergic inhibition results in a Parkinson-like syndrome and so-called extrapyramidal effects that may be ameliorated by the anticholinergics trihexyphenidyl (Artane), benztropine mesylate (Cogentin), and diphenhydramine (Benadryl). Chronic dopamine receptor blockade eventually causes an increase in the rate of firing of dopaminergic nigrostriatal neurons, resulting in tardive dyskinesia.

Other important pharmacologic properties of the phenothiazines are central and peripheral cholinergic blockade, adrenergic blockade, and adrenergic action secondary to the inhibition of reuptake of amines.

What Are the Toxic Effects of the Neuroleptics?

Toxicity of the neuroleptic agents can be broadly categorized into central nervous system (CNS) and non-CNS effects (Table 57–3). Toxic manifestations may occur with therapeutic doses but are usually found in patients who have taken a consequential overdose.

The most common non-CNS complication is orthostatic hypotension, usually seen during the initial treatment period. Contributing factors include peripheral alpha-adrenergic blockade, direct vasodilation, central vasomotor reflex depression, and direct myocardial depression.

The depressant action of phenothiazines on the heart is similar to that of the IA antidysrhythmic agents. These drugs prolong PR, QRS, and QT_c intervals, blunt T waves, and depress ST segments. The earliest changes seen with phenothiazine toxicity is prolongation of the QT interval.[49] Supraventricular and ventricular tachydysrhythmias are reported.[61,69] Of all the phenothiazines, thioridazine and mesoridazine are associated with the greatest cardiotoxicity and with marked right-axis deviation of the ECG. A case reported of a suicidal 20-year-old woman who ingested 3.1 g of mesoridazine and then developed marked QT_c prolongation, malignant dysrhythmias, hypocalcemia, and cardiac arrest is representative of the potential cardiotoxicity of mesoridazine.[69]

TABLE 57–3. TOXIC EFFECTS OF NEUROLEPTIC AGENTS

Cardiovascular	Increased QT, QRS, and PR intervals, nonspecific ST and T wave changes, right-axis deviation (terminal 40 msec prolongation)
	Myocardial depression, "quinidine like" effect, orthostatic hypotension
Central nervous system	Akathisia
	Decreased salivation
	Decreased sweating
	Decreased vasomotor reflexes
	Dystonia
	Hypothermia or hyperthermia
	Lowers seizure threshold
	Memory dysfunction
	Parkinsonism
	"Rabbit syndrome" (perioral tremor)
	Somnolence, coma
	Tardive dyskinesia
Endocrine	Amenorrhea
	Decreased ADH secretion
	Decreased gonadotrophins, ACTH, and growth hormone
	Increased prolactin
Gastrointestinal	Dry mouth
	Decreased motility
	Decreased secretions
	Pseudoobstruction
Genitourinary	Inhibited ejaculation
	Priapism
	Urinary retention
Ophthalmologic	Miosis
	Mydriasis

Modified, with permission, from Richelson E: Neuroleptic affinities from human brain receptors and their use in predicting adverse effects. J. Clin Psychiatry 1984; 45:331–335.

TABLE 57–4. NEUROLEPTIC EXTRAPYRAMIDAL ADVERSE EFFECTS

Effect and Time of Maximal Risk	Characteristics	Mechanism	Treatment
Dystonic (acute) 1–5 days	Oculogyric crisis Torticollis Retrocollis Opisthotonos Tortipelvis	Unknown	Anticholinergics (diphenhydramine, benztropine) Benzodiazepines
Akathisia (5–60 days)	Restlessness Inability to sit	Unknown	Reduction in dose of neuroleptic agent Anticholinergics Benzodiazepines
Parkinsonism (5–30 days)	Bradykinesia Shuffling gait Resting tremor Rigidity Masked facies Perioral tremor ("rabbit syndrome")	Antagonism of dopamine	Reduction in dose of neuroleptic agent Anticholinergics
Neuroleptic malignant syndrome (weeks)	Rigidity Autonomic dysfunction (unstable blood pressure) Hyperthermia Altered mental status Catatonia	Antagonism of dopamine	Limit hyperthermia (rapid cooling) Benzodiazepines Central dopamine agonists (bromocriptine, amantadine) Dantrolene
Tardive dyskinesia (months to years)	Involuntary buccolinguomasticatory movements Choreoathetoid movements	Excess dopaminergic activity	Stop offending drug Addition of or increase in neuroleptic dose Cholinergic agents

Modified, with permission, after Baldessarini RJ: Drugs and the treatment of psychiatric disorders. In: Hardman JG, Limbird LE, Molinoff PB, Ruddon RW, eds: Goodman and Gilman's The Pharmacological Basis of Therapeutics, 9th ed. New York, McGraw-Hill, 1996, p. 415.

Haloperidol, both orally and parenterally, is associated with cardiac dysrhythmias including torsades de pointes.[14,32,42,48,62,75,102]

The most common adverse effects of the neuroleptic medications occur in the CNS. These effects are generally reversible and not dose-related. Sedation occurs in all patients with the initiation of neuroleptic therapy. This is a desirable side effect in the psychotic patient when agitation is a prominent symptom. Tolerance to the sedative effects of a constant dose of neuroleptics usually occurs within months.

More serious and disturbing to the patient than the sedation are the movement disorders. Three acute movement disorders occur within 1–60 days of initiating therapy: acute dystonia, parkinsonism (akinesia), and akathisia[5] (Table 57–4). An additional movement disorder, which occurs months to years later, is tardive dyskinesia.[6,101] Acute dystonic reactions occur within 48–72 hours of a single dose and are more common in males and children treated with butyrophenones and piperazines. The reactions may include oculogyric crisis (upward gaze paralysis); jaw, tongue, lip, and throat spasms; torticollis (neck twisting); retrocollis (back of neck spasm); opisthotonos (scoliosis); buccolingual (facial) grimacing; laryngeal dystonia, which has a life-threatening potential;[60,82] and tortipelvis (abdominal wall spasm). The anatomic localization varies according to individual susceptibility and cortical involvement. Rarely, significant hyperthermia may be associated with dystonic reactions. Symptoms rapidly resolve with parenteral antihistamines, anticholinergics, or benzodiazepines. Recommended treatment in adults and children are diphenhydramine (Benadryl) IV 1–2 mg/kg to a maximum of 100 mg, or benztropine mesylate (Cogentin) IV 1–2 mg in adults and older children. Diazepam 0.1 mg/kg IV may be used instead of anticholinergic agents when anticholinergics have failed or in agitated febrile patients who may have impaired thermoregulatory control. After the IV treatment above, therapy with several days of oral benztropine mesylate (Cogentin) 1–2 mg twice daily, trihexyphenidyl (Artane) 2 mg three times daily, or diphenhydramine 1 mg/kg up to 50 mg four times daily is required.[64] If long-term therapy is needed, benztropine mesylate is the agent of choice. Interestingly, agents sold as "street Valium" in a number of cities commonly turn out to be a phenothiazine or haloperidol instead.[25] These agents are easily obtainable and when used, result in the typical dystonic reaction associated with the neuroleptics. When studied, repeated cases of "Valium"-related dystonic reactions, prove to be due to neuroleptic agents.

The elderly are more susceptible to the adverse effects of the neuroleptic agents, other than dystonic reactions, especially tardive dyskinesia (TD).[84] The prevalence of TD in patients over 40 years old is three times the prevalence in those younger than 40 years. The severity and persistence of dyskinesia increases with age.[5,9] Unfortunately, some patients treated with neuroleptics abuse anticholinergic agents often feigning one or more of the movement disorders to receive their anticholinergic agent of choice to achieve euphoria.[78]

Another toxic CNS effect of neuroleptic medications is akathisia, the subjective sensation of restlessness or muscle discomfort.[10] Affected patients are usually elderly and may appear to be agitated, have restless legs, and are unable to sit still. At times the patient may act violently. This symptom usually occurs early in treatment (5–60 days) and is alleviated by reduction of the phenothiazine dose or by the addition of antiparkinsonian drugs, benzodiazepines, or a combination. Parkinsonism (akinesia) is another CNS effect of neuroleptic therapy.[29] In fact, it is the most common extrapyramidal effect, particularly in elderly women. This type of parkinsonism occurs in 90% of susceptible patients within 72 days of initiating neuroleptic therapy and is characterized by a shuffling gait, resting tremor, rigidity, pill rolling, a masklike expression, fine-movement muscle weakness, and bradykinesia. An atypical syndrome of perioral tremor (rabbit syndrome) may merely be a late parkinsonian variant.[54] Reduction of dosage or the addition of antiparkinson agents alleviates the symptoms.

The most serious CNS toxic effect of neuroleptics is tardive dyskinesia,[6,101] which has a reported incidence ranging from 3% to 50%, depending on the type of patient, physician prescribing pattern, and degree of clinical scrutiny. Also called "permanent dyskinesia," this syndrome is characterized by involuntary, repetitive movements of the face, tongue, and lips (buccolinguomasticatory syndrome). The extremities and/or trunk may manifest choreoathetoid movements. Voluntary activity of the involved muscles may reduce the frequency of repetitive cycles. Sleep usually abolishes all abnormal movements. Individuals on long-acting intramuscular depot therapy are most likely to develop the syndrome. It also occurs more frequently in women who have been on butyrophenones or phenothiazine therapy for several years. It may first appear when attempts are made to reduce drug dosage after several years of therapy. Chronic dopamine receptor blockade results in receptor hypersensitivity and increased dopamine secretion.[57] Reduction of phenothiazine dose may thus cause the movement disorder. Similarly, administration of L-dopa, the dopamine precursor, exacerbates the syndrome.[52]

Tardive dyskinesia is a common adverse effect of haloperidol treatment. Although originally thought to be due to striatal damage, neuropathologic examination of the brain does not reveal lesions in patients with tardive dyskinesia. Recent studies in the baboon reveal that haloperidol and its tetrahydropyridine analog are metabolized to potentially neurotoxic pyridinium metabolites haloperidol pyridinium (HPP^+) and reduced pyridinium ($RHPP^+$) respectively.[7] These metabolites are found in the urine of the baboons and have been observed previously in humans; they are believed to cause striatal toxicity by inhibiting mitochondrial respiration in humans and are similar to the structurally related pyridinium neurotoxic metabolite MPP^+ (1-methyl-4-phenylpyridium) of the pro-toxin MPTP (see Chap. 60). HPP^+ in rats is also a potent cytotoxin for dopaminergic and serotonergic neurons. Although the results are as yet unsubstantiated, the study concludes that HPP^+ and $RHPP^+$ neurotoxicity may lead to tardive dyskinesia in haloperidol-treated patients. In another study, the effects of HPP^+ derived from haloperidol on in vivo tyrosine hydroxylation were evaluated in freely moving rats.[50] The study revealed that HPP^+ in vivo caused neurotoxicity, selectively for serotonergic over dopaminergic neurons, and the authors postulated that tardive dyskinesia may be due to this neurotoxicity in chronic haloperidol users. More research in humans is necessary to determine the exact relationship of HPP^+ to tardive dyskinesia, but the linkage is a potentially important breakthrough.

Unfortunately, in many affected patients tardive dyskinesia may be permanent or improve only minimally despite attempts at treatment. Preventive therapy in the form of "drug holidays" (periods of abstinence from drugs) may be effective in avoiding this complication.[59] Avoidance of high-dose, long-term daily therapy may also minimize its incidence.[53] However, if tardive dyskinesia develops, therapy may be difficult. Addition of or increase in dosage of neuroleptic medication may alleviate the symptoms. Haloperidol is frequently used because of its potent blockade of dopamine receptors; however, with this treatment, tardive dyskinesia may be followed by parkinsonism. In some patients, symptoms gradually disappear after complete cessation of the neuroleptic agents, but psychotic symptoms may then again become prominent. If necessary, piperazine phenothiazines or butyrophenones with little anticholinergic effect may be helpful in managing these situations.[59]

Anticholinergic medications do not alleviate tardive dyskinesia and, in fact, may worsen the condition as well as cause a toxic psychosis. This would be the expected result if the postulated mechanism of dopaminergic overactivity with subsequent cholinergic underactivity is valid. Anticholinergics are frequently routinely prescribed with neuroleptics to prevent the appearance of parkinsonism, but this is ill-advised in view of the possibility that anticholinergics facilitate the development of tardive dyskinesia.[47,57,58] Another treatment approach has been to decrease receptor stimulation by decreasing the amount of neurotransmitter available. Reserpine and meclofenoxate deplete catecholamine storage in synaptic vesicles by preventing reuptake of dopamine, thereby decreasing the amount of neurotransmitter available; however, long-term studies have not substantiated this therapy.[35,51]

Cholinergic stimulation using an anticholinesterase (ie, physostigmine) may also be beneficial in the amelioration of tardive dyskinesia.[51,52] The administration of choline, a precursor of acetylcholine, has also improved the symptoms of tardive dyskinesia. Lecithin, a dietary source of choline, has similarly exhibited beneficial effects.[3,39]

What Is the Neuroleptic Malignant Syndrome?

Neuroleptic malignant syndrome (NMS), first described in 1968, is characterized by hyperthermia, muscle rigidity and other extrapyramidal effects, autonomic dysfunction, and altered consciousness.[26] NMS is a rare sequela of neuroleptic-treatment, with an estimated frequency of 0.02–2.4%.[56] Neuroleptics associated with NMS include phenothiazines, butyrophenones, thioxanthenes, and loxapine. Of these, the medications with greater antidopaminergic activity seem to have a greater potential for causing NMS.

Neuroleptic malignant syndrome is believed to be an idiosyncratic reaction, which usually occurs in the course of treatment with neuroleptic drugs. Typically, there is a history of a high initial dose with rapid escalation in usage or a discontinuation of antiparkinson medication.[36,95] A syndrome similar to NMS is described with the withdrawal of dopamine agonists in patients who have Parkinson's disease and in those using lithium.[36,77] The mortality of this disorder was as high as 76% before 1976 but has since declined to 20%, due to early recognition and the institution of appropriate therapy.[87]

The pathophysiology of NMS is thought to be a central dopamine blockade. In essence, it is a severe form of an extrapyramidal reaction, with dystonia at the mild end of the spectrum. This disequilibrium results in a constellation of manifestations, including hyperthermia, muscular hypertonicity, fluctuating mental status, and autonomic irregularities (blood pressure, heart rate, respirations, incontinence, and diaphoresis).[88] The temperature rise can be mild or marked and is believed to result from an altered dopamine response in the hypothalamus and increased heat production due to muscle hyperactivity.[92] Unlike a febrile response to an underlying infection, where there is a hypothalamic-controlled elevation of the temperature set point, NMS-induced hyperthermia is not responsive to antipyretics.[27] The type of muscular activity can vary and includes akinesia, choreoathetosis, tremors, and generalized contractions with "lead pipe" rigidity.[40] There is no specific laboratory test for NMS. Some of the abnormal chemistry findings include metabolic acidosis, liver enzyme abnormalities, leukocytosis, and creatine phosphokinase and creatinine elevations.

The diagnosis of NMS is difficult to establish and is exclusionary. An essential point in the history is a recent change in neuroleptic dose. Medical etiologies for the clinical manifestations must first be excluded. If all of the manifestations of NMS are present and no other obvious causes can be found, then NMS can be considered.

Treatment of NMS includes rapid external cooling with ice and intravenous benzodiazepines to decrease muscle rigidity, and discontinuation of neuroleptic agents.[96] Bromocriptine and amantadine, with central dopamine agonist effects, have been used with anecdotal success in treating NMS.[4,38,73,76,97] However, significant clinical improvement has not occurred for 24–72 hours after initiation of these dopaminergic agents.[81] Dantrolene sodium, which inhibits the release of calcium from the sarcoplasmic reticulum, has also been used with varied success.[19,71,81,98] Because NMS primarily involves the CNS, there is no derangement of calcium transport in the skeletal muscle as in malignant hyperthermia (MH), which responds to dantrolene almost immediately.[98] Although clinically indistinct, pathologically NMS and MH are quite different. Malignant hyperthermia is a hereditary disorder, involving a defect in the skeletal muscle metabolism of calcium.[17,65] Anecdotal evidence has suggested that pancuronium and sodium nitroprusside are effective treatments in NMS.[16,86] Central anticholinergic agents are ineffective in NMS and may contribute to increased morbidity and mortality. The initial management of NMS should consist of good supportive care, aimed primarily at arresting muscle hyperactivity, and evaluation for other potentially life-threatening medical disorders. The benefits of this approach were demonstrated by a prospective controlled clinical trial in which supportive therapy significantly reduced the duration of illness and incidence of complications when compared to dantrolene or bromocriptine (see Chap. 53).[80]

The clinical course of NMS is usually about 10 days, and the patient should not be restarted on neuroleptic agents while symptoms of NMS persist. If neuroleptics are necessary, they should not be reintroduced until 1–2 weeks after symptoms resolve. The neuroleptic chosen should be from a different class than the one that precipitated the NMS and should have minimal extrapyramidal effects. In this setting the atypical antipsychotic clozapine has been recommended.[63]

How Do Laboratory Tests Aid in the Management and Diagnosis of Neuroleptic Overdoses?

Plasma levels of neuroleptics do not correlate well with clinical signs and symptoms.[21,68,72,74] Positive urine phenothiazine colorimetric testing, using the Forrest test, ferric chloride test, or Phenistix reagent strip test can suggest the presence of phenothiazines.[33] An abdominal radiograph may help confirm a deliberate overdose as some solid dosage forms of phenothiazines are radiopaque. However, the frequent lack of this radiographic finding does not exclude the presence of phenothiazines.

What General Management Issues Should Be Considered for the Patient With a Neuroleptic Overdose?

Most neuroleptics are usually safe even when taken in significant overdose. Deaths are rare and are most frequently reported in cases associated with thioridazine and mesoridazine overdose[8,18] or when neuroleptics are taken concomitantly in overdose with sympathomimetics, lithium, antihistamines, or cyclic antidepressants. Routine ECG monitoring before the initiation of neuroleptic therapy, particularly with thioridazine, mesoridazine, and haloperidol is advisable. In the management of an overdose, sympathomimetic agents are relatively contraindicated. It appears that catecholamines modify impulse conduction, permitting reentry of delayed impulse within the conduction system, and promoting dysrhythmias. Catecholamine use should be limited to hypotensive patients who are refractory to fluid resuscitation.

Depression of the CNS occurs with many toxins. The suspicion of mixed drug abuse should guide the clinician in overdose management. The smell of alcohol or evidence of needle tracks should not lull the clinician into a false sense of security that the diagnosis has been established.

Only the use of a precise approach will avoid the potential hazards of a missed diagnosis. Emesis, lavage, multiple-dose activated charcoal (MDAC), and catharsis are the basic tenets of neuroleptic overdose management. Although syrup of ipecac is usually effective (despite the antiemetic properties of phenothiazines), orogastric lavage is preferable if gastric emptying is required to avoid complications should CNS depression develop prior to successful induction of emesis. Forced diuresis or manipulation of urine pH ("ion-trapping") are not helpful in the management of neuroleptic overdoses. Because of the substantial protein binding and large volume of distribution of most neuroleptic agents, hemoperfusion and hemodialysis are of no benefit.[9]

If a vasopressor is needed to manage refractory hypotension, a mixed alpha- and beta-adrenergic receptor agonist such as epinephrine or dopamine should be avoided. Since the phenothiazines are potent alpha-adrenergic antagonists, beta-adrenergic stimulation will cause peripheral vasodilation, further exacerbating the blockade-induced vasodilation and hypotension. The alpha-adrenergic receptor agonists phenylephrine (Neosynephrine), levarterenol (Levophed), and metaraminol (Aramine) are more appropriate drugs in this setting.[13] The use of any vasopressors in this setting requires hemodynamic monitoring.

Dysrhythmias are most common with overdose of the piperidine series and are also seen with the butyrophenone haloperidol. There have been several reports of unexplained sudden deaths attributed to ventricular dysrhythmias in individuals on neuroleptic agents.[1,2,23,28,67] Electrocardiographic abnormalities, including increased QT_c and PR intervals, depressed ST segment, and T and U waves changes, are described.[12,30,49] Electrophysiologic studies with the new phenothiazine analog moricizine, which is an antidysrhythmic (see Chap. 52), have demonstrated its ability to delay intraventricular conduction.[15] These manifestations are similar to those of cyclic antidepressant–induced cardiac toxicity. For this reason, sodium bicarbonate may be an appropriate intervention to treat toxicity from this drug (see Antidotes in Depth: Sodium Bicarbonate). Supraventricular dysrhythmias can usually be managed supportively. Ventricular dysrhythmias should be treated with lidocaine. Conversely, procainamide, quinidine, and disopyramide are contraindicated. If torsades de pointes (polymorphic ventricular tachycardia) is present, magnesium or isoproterenol may be effective.

Neuroleptics should not be given to any patient who may be experiencing hallucinations secondary to drug withdrawal. Phenothiazines will lower the seizure threshold in these patients, who are already particularly susceptible to seizures (see Chap. 70).

Treatment with physostigmine salicylate reverses central as well as peripheral anticholinergic abnormalities caused by phenothiazines, but should not be used in patients with conduction abnormalities[99] (see Antidotes in Depth: Physostigmine).

Which Patients Should Be Admitted for Observation After a Neuroleptic Overdose?

Any patient presenting with ECG abnormalities, such as conduction delays and dysrhythmias or hemodynamic instability, must be admitted to a monitored unit for observation. All other patients should be placed on a cardiac monitor and observed for a minimum of 6 hours. If the patient remains asymptomatic for 6 hours and a repeat ECG is normal, a subsequent dose of activated charcoal may be administered and the appropriate psychiatric or social follow-up begun.

Summary

In summary, the use of neuroleptics has increased since their introduction in the 1950s. Adverse reactions are common, as are intentional and unintentional overdoses; physicians must therefore have knowledge of the pharmacology of these agents and awareness of treatment modalities to be able to manage these potentially lethal reactions.

Acknowledgments

Eddy A. Bresnitz, MD and Richard Y. Wang, MD contributed to this chapter in a previous edition.

References

1. Aherwadkar SJ, Efendigil MC, Coulshed N: Chlorpromazine therapy and associated acute disturbances of cardiac rhythm. Br Heart J 1974;36:1251–1252.
2. Alexander CS, Nino A: Cardiovascular complications in young patients taking psychotropic drugs: A preliminary report. Am Heart J 1969;78:757–769.
3. Alphs LD, Davis JM: Cholinergic treatments for tardive dyskinesia. Mod Probl Pharmacopsychiatry 1983;21:168–186.
4. Amdurski S: A therapeutic trial of amantadine in haloperidol induced malignant neuroleptic syndrome. Curr Ther Res 1983;33:225. Letter.
5. American College of Neuropsychopharmacology—Food and Drug Administration Task Force: Neurologic syndromes associated with antipsychotic drug use. N Engl J Med 1973;289:20–23.
6. American Psychiatric Association Task Force on Late Neurological Effects of Antipsychotic Drugs: Tardive dyskinesia. Am J Psychiatry 1980;137:1163–1172.
7. Avent KM, Etsuko U, Eyles DW, et al: Haloperidol and its tetrahydropyridine derivative (HPTP) are metabolized to potentially neurotoxic pyridinium species in the baboon. Life Sci 1996;59:1473–1482.
8. Baker PB, Merigian KS, Roberts JR, et al: Hyperthermia, hypertension, hypertonia and coma in a massive thioridazine overdose. Am J Emerg Med 1988;6:346–349.
9. Baldessarini RJ: Drugs and the treatment of psychiatric disorders. In: Hardman JG, Limbird LE, Molinoff PB, Ruddon RW, eds: Goodman and Gilman's The Pharmacological Basis of Therapeutics, 9th ed. New York, McGraw-Hill, 1996, pp. 399–420.
10. Ball R: Drug induced akathisia: A review. J R Soc Med 1985;78:748–752.
11. Battaglia J, Thornton L, Young C: Loxapine-lorazepam-induced hypotension and stupor. J Clin Psychopharmacol 1989;9:227–228. Letter.
12. Bausher J, Goldstein HS, Aronson MD, et al: Case report: "Pseudo-giant-p waves" and pericardial friction rub following chlorpromazine therapy. Am J Med Sci 1976;272:357–359.
13. Benowitz NL, Rosenberg J, Becker CE: Cardiopulmonary catastrophes in drug-overdosed patients. Med Clin North Am 1979;63:127–140.
14. Bett JHN, Holt GW: Malignant ventricular tachyarrhythmia and Haldol. Br Med J 1983;287:1264.
15. Bigger JT: Cardiac electrophysiologic effects of moricizine hydrochloride. Am J Cardiol 1990;65:15D–20D.
16. Blue MG, Schneider SM, Noro S, et al: Successful treatment of NMS with sodium nitroprusside. Ann Intern Med 1986;104:56–57.
17. Caroff S, Rosenberg H, Gerber JC: Neuroleptic malignant syndrome and malignant hyperthermia. Drugs 1983;3:120–121.
18. Chouinard G, Ghadirian AM, Jones BD: Death attributed to ventricular arrhythmia induced by thioridazine in combination with a single Contact capsule. Can Med Assoc J 1978;119:729–730.
19. Coons DJ, Hillman FJ, Marshall RW: Treatment of NMS with dantrolene sodium. Ann Intern Med 1982;98:183–184.
20. Curry SH: Relation between binding to plasma protein, apparent volume of distribution, and rate constants of disposition and elimination for chlorpromazine in three species. J Pharm Pharmacol 1972;24:818–819.
21. Curry SH, Davis JM, Janowsky DS, et al: Factors affecting chlorpromazine plasma levels in psychiatric patients. Arch Gen Psychiatry 1970;22:209–215.
22. Dahl SG, Strandjord RE: Pharmacokinetics of chlorpromazine after single and chronic dosage. Clin Pharmacol Ther 1976;21:437–438.
23. Dawling S, Widdop B: Comment: Chlorpromazine sudden death. Drug Intell Clin Pharm 1989;23:510–511. Letter.
24. de la Gandara J, Dominguez RA: Lithium and loxapine: A potential interaction. J Clin Psychiatry 1988;49:126. Letter.
25. Demetropoulos S, Schauben JL: Acute dystonic reactions from "street Valium." J Emerg Med 1987;5:293–297.
26. Diamond JM, Santos AB: Unusual complications of antipsychotic drugs. Am Fam Physician 1982;26:153–157.
27. Dinarello CA, Cannon JG, Wolff SM: New concepts on the pathogenesis of fever. Rev Infect Dis 1988;10:168–190.
28. Dorson PG, Crismon ML: Chlorpromazine accumulation and sudden death in a patient with renal insufficiency. Drug Intell Clin Pharm 1988;22:776–778.
29. Duvoisin R: History of parkinsonism. Pharmacol Ther 1987;32:1–17.
30. Elkayam U, Frishman W: Cardiovascular effects of phenothiazines. Am Heart J 1980;100:397–401.
31. Ereshefsky L, Watanabe MD, Tran-Johnson TK: Clozapine: An atypical antipsychotic agent. Clin Pharm 1989;8:691–709.
32. Fayer SA: Torsades de pointes ventricular tachyarrhythmia associated with haloperidol. J Clin Psychopharmacol 1986;6:375–376.
33. Forrest FM, Forrest IS, Mason AS: Review of rapid urine tests for phenothiazine and related drugs. Am J Psychiatry 1961;118:300–307.
34. Forrest FM, Forrest IS, Serra MT: Modification of chlorpro-

mazine metabolism by some other drugs frequently administered to psychiatric patients. Biol Psychiatry 1970; 2:53–58.
35. Friedman JH: A case of progressive hemichorea responsive to high dose reserpine. J Clin Psychiatry 1986;47: 149–150.
36. Friedman JH, Feinberg SS, Feldman RG: A neuroleptic malignant-like syndrome due to levodopa therapy withdrawal. JAMA 1985;254:2792–2795.
37. Fuller MA, Sajatovic M: Neurotoxicity resulting from a combination of lithium and loxapine. J Clin Psychiatry 1989;50:187–190.
38. Gangadhar BN, Desain G, Channabasarnana SM: Amantadine in the neuroleptic malignant syndrome. J Clin Psychiatry 1984;45:526–529.
39. Gelenberg AJ, Doller-Wojcik JC, Growdon JH: Choline and lecithin in the treatment of tardive dyskinesia: Preliminary results from a pilot study. Am J Psychiatry 1979;136: 772–776.
40. Guze BH, Baxter JR: Neuroleptic malignant syndrome. N Engl J Med 1985;313:163–166.
41. Hacksell U, Jackson DM, Mohell N: Does dopamine receptor subtype selectivity of antipsychotic agents provide useful leads for development of novel therapeutic agents? Pharmacol Toxicol 1995;76:320–324.
42. Henderson RA, Lane S, Henry JA: Life-threatening ventricular arrhythmia (torsades de pointes) after haloperidol overdose. Hum Exp Toxicol 1991;10:59–62.
43. Hicks R, Dysken MW, Davis JM, et al: The pharmacokinetics of psychotropic medication in the elderly: A review. J Clin Psychiatry 1981;42:374–385.
44. Hollister LE: Clinical Use of Psychotherapeutic Drugs. Springfield, IL, Charles C. Thomas, 1973.
45. Hollister LE, Curry SH: Urinary excretion of chlorpromazine metabolites following single doses and in steady state conditions. Res Commun Chem Pathol Pharmacol 1971;2:330–338.
46. Howes CA, Pullar T, Sourindhrin I, et al: Reduced steady state plasma concentrations of chlorpromazine and indomethacin in patients receiving cimetidine. Eur J Clin Pharmacol 1983;24:99–102.
47. Huang CC: Reserpine and alpha methyldopa in the treatment of tardive dyskinesia. Psychopharmacology 1981;33: 359–362.
48. Hunt N, Stern TA: The association between intravenous haloperidol and torsades de pointes. Psychosomatics 1995; 36:541–549.
49. Huston JF, Bell GE: The effect of thioridazine and chlorpromazine on the electrocardiogram. JAMA 1966;198: 134–138.
50. Igarashi K, Matsubata K, Kasuya F, et al: Effect of a pyridinium metabolite derived from haloperidol on the activities of striatal tyrosine hydroxylase in freely moving rats. Neurosci Lett 1996;214:183–186.
51. Izumi K, Tominaga H, Koja T, et al: Meclofenoxate therapy in tardive dyskinesia: A preliminary report. Biol Psychiatry 1986;21:151–160.
52. Jeste DV, Wyatt RJ: Therapeutic strategies against tardive dyskinesia: Two decades of experience. Arch Gen Psychiatry 1982;39:803–816.
53. Jeste DV, Wyatt RJ: In search of treatment for tardive dyskinesia: A review of the literature. Schizophr Bull 1979; 5:251–293.
54. Jus K, Jus A, Gautier J, et al: Studies of the actions of certain pharmacological agents on tardive dyskinesia and on the rabbit syndrome. Int J Clin Pharmacol 1974;9:138–145.
55. Kaul PN, Whitfield LR, Clark ML: Chlorpromazine metabolism. VIII: Blood levels of chlorpromazine and its sulfoxide in schizophrenic patients. J Pharm Sci 1976;65:694–697.
56. Keck PE, Pope HG, Cohen BM, et al: Risk factors for neuroleptic malignant syndrome. Arch Gen Psychiatry 1989; 46:914–918.
57. Klawans HL: Tardive dyskinesia: Review and update. Am J Psychiatry 1980;137:900–905.
58. Klawans HL: Pharmacology of tardive dyskinesias. Am J Psychiatry 1973;130:82–86.
59. Kobayashi RM: Drug therapy of tardive dyskinesia. N Engl J Med 1977;296:257–259.
60. Koek RJ, Pe EH: Acute laryngeal dystonic reactions to neuroleptics. Psychosomatics 1989;30:359–364.
61. Krikler DM, Curry PVL: Torsade de pointes and atypical ventricular tachycardia. Br Heart J 1968;38:117–120.
62. Kriwisky M, Perry GY, Tarchitsky D, et al: Haloperidol-induced torsades de pointes. Chest 1990;98:482–484.
63. Lazarus A, Caroff SN, Mann SC: Beyond NMS: Management after the acute episode. Psychiatry Ann 1991;21: 165–174.
64. Lee A: Drug-induced dystonic reactions. JACEP 1977;6: 351–354.
65. Levenson JL: Neuroleptic malignant syndrome. Am J Psychiatry 1985;142:1137–1145.
66. Loga S, Curry SH, Lader M: Interactions of orphenadrine and phenobarbitone with chlorpromazine: Plasma concentrations and effects in man. Br J Clin Pharmacol 1975;2: 197–208.
67. Lutz EG: Cardiotoxic effects of psychotropic drugs. J Med Soc NJ 1976;73:105–112.
68. Manian AA, Efran DH, Goldberg ME, et al: A comparative pharmacological study of a series of monohydroxylated and methoxylated chlorpromazine derivatives. Life Sci 1965;4:2425–2438.
69. Marrs-Simon P, Zell-Kanter M, Kendzierski DL, et al: Cardiotoxic manifestations of mesoridazine overdose. Ann Emerg Med 1988;17:1074–1078.
70. Matz R, Rich W, Oh D, et al: Clozapine: A potential antipsychotic agent without extrapyramidal manifestations. Curr Ther Res 1974;16:687–695.
71. May DC, Morris SW, Stewart RM, et al: Neuroleptic malignant syndrome: Response to dantrolene sodium. Ann Intern Med 1982;98:183–184.
72. May PRA, Van Putten T, Jenden DJ, et al: Chlorpromazine levels and the outcome of treatment in schizophrenic patients. Arch Gen Psychiatry 1981;38:202–207.
73. McCarron MM, Boettger ML, Peck JJ: A case of neuroleptic malignant syndrome successfully treated with amantadine. J Clin Psychiatry 1982;43:381–382.
74. McIntyre WT, Gershon S: Interpatient variations in antipsychotic therapy. J Clin Psychiatry 1985;46:3–16.
75. Mehta D, Mehta SH, Petit J, et al: Cardiac arrhythmia and Haldol. Am J Psychiatry 1979;136:1468–1469.

76. Mueller PS, Vester JW, Fermaglich J: Neuroleptic malignant syndrome: Successful treatment with bromocriptine. JAMA 1983;249:386–388.
77. Mueller PS, Vester JW, Fermaglich J: Neuroleptic malignant syndrome like state following a withdrawal of anti-parkinsonian drugs. J Nerv Ment Dis 1981;169: 324–327.
78. Pullen GP, Best NR, Maguire J: Anticholinergic drug abuse: A common problem. Br Med J 1984;289:612–613.
79. Rivera-Calimlim L, Kerzner B, Karch FE: Effect of lithium on plasma chlorpromazine levels. Clin Pharmacol Ther 1978;23:451–455.
80. Rosebush PI, Stewart T, Mazurek MF: The treatment of neuroleptic malignant syndrome: Are dantrolene and bromocriptine useful adjuncts to supportive care? Br J Psychiatry 1991;159:709–712.
81. Rosenberg MR, Green M: Neuroleptic malignant syndrome. Arch Intern Med 1989;149:1927–1931.
82. Russell SA, Henner HM, Herson KJ, Stremski ES: Upper airway compromise in acute chlorpromazine ingestion. Am J Emerg Med 1996;14:467–468.
83. Sakalis G, Curry SH, Mould GP, et al: Physiologic and clinical effects of chlorpromazine and their relationship to plasma level. Clin Pharmacol Ther 1972;13:931–946.
84. Saltz BL, Woemer MG, Kane JM, et al: Prospective study of tardive dyskinesia incidence in the elderly. JAMA 1991;266:2402–2406.
85. Sandoz Inc: Clozaril new drug application. Volumes 28–31, 39, 48, 50, 52, 84, 98–100, 103. East Hanover, NJ, August 10, 1987.
86. Sangal R, Dimitrijevic R: Neuroleptic malignant syndrome: Successful treatment with pancuronium. JAMA 1985;254:2795–2796.
87. Shalev A, Hermesh H, Munitz H: Mortality from neuroleptic malignant syndrome. J Clin Psychiatry 1989;50: 18–25.
88. Shalev A, Munitz H: The neuroleptic malignant syndrome: Agent and host interaction. Acta Psychiatr Scand 1986;73:337–347.
89. Sletten I, Pichardo J, Korol B, et al: The effect of chlorpromazine on lithium excretion in psychiatric subjects. Curr Ther Res 1966;8:441–446.
90. Snyder SH: Receptors, neurotransmitters and drug responses. N Engl J Med 1979;300:465–472.
91. Snyder SH: Antischizophrenic drugs and the dopamine receptor. Drug Ther 1978;3:29–34.
92. Srinivassan AV, Murugapappan M, Krishnamurthy SG, et al: Neuroleptic malignant syndrome. J Neurol Neurosurg Psychiatry 1990;53:514–516.
93. Stevenson RN, Blanshard C, Patterson DLH: Ventricular fibrillation due to lithium withdrawal: An interaction with chlorpromazine? Postgrad Med J 1989;65:936–938.
94. Swett C, Cole JO, Hartz SC, et al: Hypotension due to chlorpromazine: Relation to cigarette smoking. Arch Gen Psychiatry 1977;34:661–663.
95. Toru M, Matsuda O, Maleiguchi K, et al: Neuroleptic malignant syndrome-like state following a withdrawal of antiparkinsonian drugs. J Nerv Ment Dis 1981;169:324–327.
96. Vassallo SU, Delaney KA: Pharmacologic effects on thermoregulation: Mechanisms of drug-related heatstroke. J Toxicol Clin Toxicol 1989;27:199–224.
97. Verhoeven WMA, Elderson A, Westernberg HC: Neuroleptic malignant syndrome: Successful treatment with bromocriptine. Biol Psychiatry 1985;20:680–684.
98. Ward A, Chaffman MO, Sorkin EM: Dantrolene: A review of its pharmacodynamic and pharmacokinetic properties and therapeutic use in malignant hyperthermia, the neuroleptic malignant syndrome and an update of its use in muscle spasticity. Drugs 1986;32:130–168.
99. Weisdorf D, Kramer J, Goldberg A, Klawans HL: Physostigmine for cardiac and neurologic manifestations of phenothiazine poisoning. Clin Pharmacol Ther 1978;24: 663–667.
100. Yassa R: A case of lithium chlorpromazine interaction. J Clin Psychiatry 1966;47:90–91.
101. Zaratzian VL: Psychotropic drugs: Neurotoxicity. Clin Toxicol 1980;17:231–270.
102. Zee-Cheng C, Mueller CE, Seifert CF, Gibbs HR: Haloperidol and torsades de pointes. Ann Intern Med 1985;102:418. Letter.

CHAPTER 58

Monoamine Oxidase Inhibitors

Diane Sauter

CASE 1. A 60-year-old female was transported to the emergency department (ED) approximately 4 hours following the ingestion of 50 tablets of phenelzine sulfate (Nardil). The family reported that the patient was depressed recently and talking of suicide.

On arrival, the patient was noted to be somewhat responsive, but rapidly became deeply comatose. Her vital signs were: blood pressure, 130/70 mm Hg; pulse of 87 beats/min; and rapid, shallow respirations at 16 breaths/min. She was afebrile. Her pupils were midsize, round, and reactive to light. She withdrew from painful stimuli but was areflexic. She was rapidly intubated. An intravenous line was inserted and 2 mg of naloxone hydrochloride, 100 mg of thiamine, and 100 mL of $D_{50}W$ were administered IV. No change in neurologic function was noted following the initial interventions. The patient then underwent gastric lavage with a 40 French orogastric tube and 60 g of oral activated charcoal plus a cathartic were administered.

On admission to the intensive care unit the patient had muscular rigidity of both lower extremities with fasciculations of the upper extremities. Her clinical course was remarkable for rapid progression to boardlike rigidity, fever of 40°C (104°F), and an unobtainable blood pressure. She was paralyzed with the use of succinylcholine and then pancuronium. Intravenous fluids and later dopamine were used to treat shock. The patient's laboratory studies were significant for a serum lithium level of > 5.0 mEq/L, for which she underwent hemodialysis. Her clinical course was further complicated by the development of a myocardial infarction. Approximately 24 hours following the ingestion she was noted to have improved. The patient no longer required paralysis and was responsive to voice and touch.

What Is the Therapeutic Approach to the Patient With a Monoamine Oxidase Inhibitor Overdose?

Treatment, as always, begins with the stabilization of abnormal vital signs and the administration of oxygen, dextrose, and thiamine as indicated. Aggressive gastrointestinal decontamination with activated charcoal is appropriate in patients with life-threatening signs or symptoms or in the asymptomatic patient with a history of a recent ingestion. Hyperthermia must be rapidly controlled. Antipyretic agents are too slow in onset of action and inappropriate for use in patients who have pharmacologically induced temperature elevations. Patients with severe hyperthermia must be aggressively cooled with the use of ice baths and/or cold water and fans. Extreme agitation and seizures are best controlled with the use of a benzodiazepine. The use of a nondepolarizing neuromuscular blocking agent may be necessary if seizures persist despite adequate doses of diazepam or phenobarbital. Severe hypertension is most safely and effectively treated with the use of a rapid reversible antihypertensive agent such as nitroprusside. Longer acting agents should not be used in patients with overdoses of monoamine oxidase inhibitors (MAOIs), as hypertension is often rapidly followed by severe hypotension. The persistence of the effects of an antihypertensive agent that cannot be rapidly reversed may worsen the patient's clinical condition. Hypotension should initially be treated with fluid resuscitation. A direct-acting vasopressor, such as norepinephrine, is preferred to agents such as dopamine that require the release of intracellular catecholamines. Cardiac dysrhythmias are generally a premorbid sign and, when present, should be treated with lidocaine or procainamide. Bretylium should be avoided as its use may lead to an increased release of norepinephrine followed by catecholamine depletion and orthostatic hypotension.

Due to the delayed onset of toxicity, all patients with suspected MAOI overdoses, even if asymptomatic, should be admitted for observation to a monitored setting for 24 hours. Symptomatic patients should be monitored until mental status and vital signs have normalized.

What Is the Pharmacology of the Monoamine Oxidase Inhibitors?

The MAOIs (Fig. 58–1) are a chemically heterogeneous group of drugs whose pharmacologic effects result from the inhibition of monoamine oxidase, a flavin-containing enzyme located in the outer mitochondrial membrane of liver and central and peripheral sympathetic nerve terminals.[16] The active form of the enzyme is a dimer consisting of two subunits. Each subunit is covalently bound with one flavin adenine dinucleotide (FAD) and has a molecular weight of approximately 60,000 Daltons. Monoamine oxidase oxidatively deaminates, and thereby inactivates, monoamines that are ingested or synthesized within the body. The reaction consists of two steps. In the first, the amine substrate is oxidized and the FAD is reduced. Hydrolysis of the intermediate imine results in an aldehyde and $FADH_2$. Finally, $FADH_2$ is oxidized by molecular oxygen with H_2O_2 formed as a by-product.[37] Some of these monoamines are essential as neurotransmitters or as modulators of nervous system transmission. These monoamines include the catecholamines norepinephrine (NE), dopamine (DA), and epinephrine (EPI) and the indole alkylamine serotonin (or 5-hydroxytryptamine, 5-HT). Normally, the pool of NE stored in the sympathetic nerve terminals is maintained at steady state through control over synthesis and degradation.[5] MAO is active in the degradation of intraneuronal catecholamines (Fig. 58–2). As a result of MAO inhibition the pool of NE in the presynaptic sympathetic nerve terminal is expanded.[5] The resultant elevation of central nervous system (CNS) NE and DA is thought to result in the antidepressant effects of MAOIs.[16] In addition, considerable attention has been focused on the role of the down-regulation of postsynaptic 5-HT receptors in the treatment of depression. Several weeks after the initiation of MAO therapy, multiple changes occur that affect neurotransmission. The number of beta-adrenergic receptors decreases and the activity of these receptors, as well as those of $alpha_1$- and $alpha_2$-adrenergic receptors, and $5\text{-}HT_1$ and $5\text{-}HT_2$ receptors, is decreased. Dopamine receptors are unaffected.[91,114]

At least two subtypes of MAO exist in tissues: MAO-A is found in liver and GI tract and MAO-B in brain and platelets. Monoaminergic neurons contain predominantly MAO-A. Serotonergic neurons contain both MAO-A and MAO-B.[7] Substrates that are oxidatively deaminated primarily by MAO-A include EPI, NE,

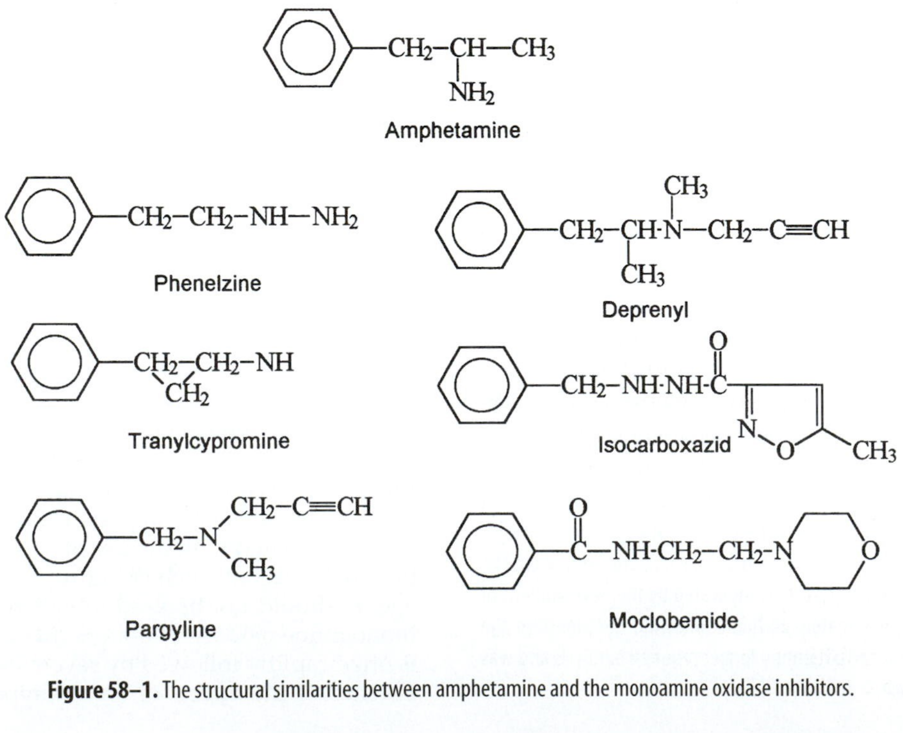

Figure 58–1. The structural similarities between amphetamine and the monoamine oxidase inhibitors.

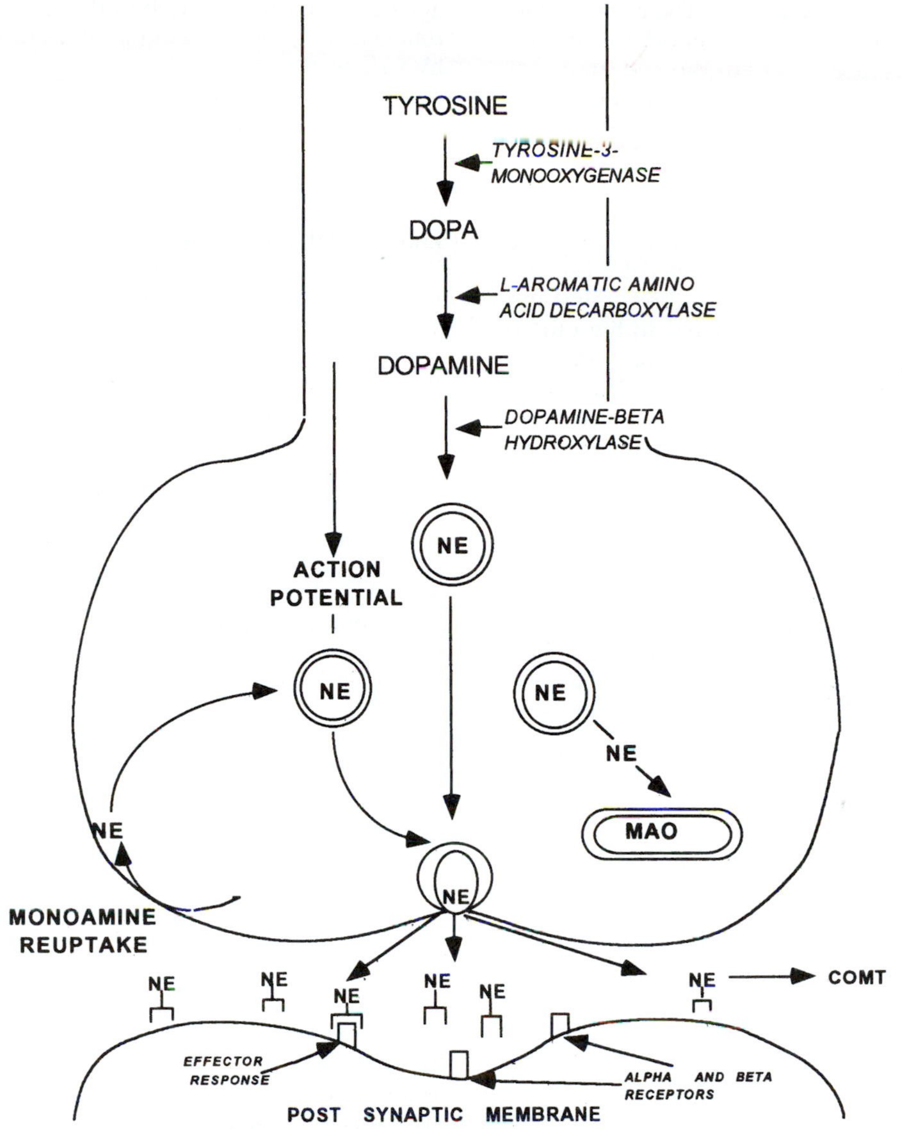

Figure 58–2. The sympathetic nerve terminal. Norepinephrine (NE) is synthesized in the sympathetic nerve cell and stored in vesicles. An action potential causes the vesicles to migrate to and fuse with the presynaptic membrane. NE diffuses across the synaptic cleft and binds with and activates postsynaptic alpha- and beta-adrenergic receptors. NE is then taken back up into the neuron by the monoamine reuptake pump and repackaged into vesicles. NE that is taken up by the neuron but escapes repackaging is inactivated by mitochondrial monoamine oxidase (MAO). NE that diffuses away from the synaptic cleft is inactivated by catechol-*O*-methyl transferase (COMT). *(Reprinted, with permission, from Lefkowitz RJ, Hoffman BB, Taylor P: Drugs acting at synaptic and neuroeffector junctional sites. In: Gilman AG, Rall TW, Nies AS, Taylor P, eds: Goodman and Gilman's The Pharmacologic Basis of Therapeutics, 8th ed. New York, Pergamon Press, 1990, pp. 84–121.)*

metanephrine, and 5-HT. Substrates exclusively degraded by MAO-B include beta-phenylethylamine, phenylethanolamine, tyramine, and benzylamine. Many substrates are metabolized by both including tyramine, dopamine, octopamine, and tryptamine.[114]

Many other enzyme systems are inhibited by MAOIs as well as MAO, including diamine oxidase, pyridoxal phosphokinase, ceruloplasmin, DOPA decarboxylase, L-glutamic acid decarboxylase, and other pyridoxine (B_6)-containing enzyme systems.[40] The clinical implications of the inhibition of these diverse enzyme systems are poorly understood.

History of Monoamine Oxidase Inhibitors

The MAOIs have been in use since the 1950s. Initially marketed for the treatment of tuberculosis and then hypertension, they were noted to have mood-elevating properties and became popular for the treatment of depression.[58] In the 1970s they were largely replaced by the less toxic and apparently more effective tricyclic antidepressants.[7] More recently, it has been found that certain neurotic illnesses with depressive features (anxiety and phobias) as well as treatment-resistant depression respond more favorably to MAOIs.[23,67,91] Their use underwent a resurgence in the 1980s and reports of toxicity reappeared in the literature.[69,100] With the appearance of newer, less toxic, selective serotonin reuptake inhibitors, the use of the MAOIs may once again be on the decline. There have been few fatalities from the use of MAOIs reported to the American Association of Poison Control Centers over the past 5 years.[71–75]

MAOIs are available in oral form only. They are well absorbed from the gut and eliminated by acetylation.[7] Some are structurally related to amphetamine and have amphetamine-like activity unrelated to the inhibition of MAO.[41,61] The oldest MAOIs in use are irreversible inactivators of MAO. Binding of the drug to the enzyme is irreversible and new enzyme must be synthesized before the function of MAO returns to normal. The irreversible inhibitors of MAO-A and MAO-B (nonspecific inhibitors) currently available in the United States include isocarboxazid (Marplan), phenelzine sulfate (Nardil), tranylcypromine sulfate (Parnate), and procarbazine (Matulane), an antitumor agent used in Hodgkin's disease with weak MAO-inhibiting activity.[45] Selegiline (Deprenyl), a relatively selective irreversible MAO-B inhibitor (at doses less than 20 mg/day) is in use for the treatment of Parkinson's disease.[78] Irreversible inhibitors of MAO-A include clorgyline and Lilly 51641 (not currently in clinical use).[114] Reversible inhibitors of MAO-A (brofaromine, cimoxatone, and moclobemide), which retain the antidepressant properties of the older MAOIs without significant tyramine potentiation, have been developed and are in current clinical use.[2,4,14,37,59,78]

What Problems Are Associated With the MAOIs?

The use of MAOIs has been associated with a variety of life-threatening problems. Acute overdoses as well as interactions with various foods and medications have resulted in fatalities.[8,77,92,95]

Monoamine Oxidase Inhibitors Overdose

Overdoses of the irreversible, nonselective MAOIs are infrequently reported and, therefore, data remain scarce. Mortality has occurred with acute ingestions of as little as 170–680 mg of tranylcypromine and 375–1500 mg of phenelzine.[110]

A consistent finding in reports of overdoses is a delay in onset or minimal symptomatology for as long as 12 hours after ingestion.[8,69] The onset of disorientation may occur as late as 32 hours following ingestion.[74] Death resulting from the toxicity of MAOIs may occur as long as 35 hours following ingestion. Death from the complications of toxicity, including disseminated intravascular coagulation, acute respiratory distress syndrome (ARDS), and myoglobinuric renal failure, may occur much later.

Signs and symptoms reported following overdose include headache, hypertension or shock, tachycardia, agitation, delirium and obtundation, nystagmus, hyperreflexia, tremors, myoclonus, muscle rigidity, seizures, hyperthermia and diaphoresis, tachypnea, respiratory depression, and cardiovascular collapse.[70,80]

Whether the inactivation of MAO contributes to the acute toxicity of the MAOIs in overdose is unknown. MAOIs appear to exhibit a combination of sympathomimetic and sympatholytic properties. It is also well known that the MAOIs have amphetamine-like activity,[41,61] which is likely to be an important etiology of the hypertension characteristic of early stages of overdose. The hyperthermia and neuromuscular irritability apparently contribute in important ways to the lethality of these agents. For additional information the reader is referred to Chapter 10.

Initial reports describing the clinical course following overdoses of moclobemide have documented the occurrence of sedation only with no fatalities.[24]

Patients who experience severe hypertension after drug or dietary interactions may be treated with the use of an alpha-adrenergic antagonist (phentolamine) or a rapidly acting oral or parenteral calcium channel blocker (nifedipine).[43,54] These patients usually have early clinical manifestations and may not require hospital admission if the interaction has been mild, resolution of symptoms has been complete, and the patient can be observed in the ED for 4–8 hours. Patients with altered mental status, seizures, or suspected intracranial hemorrhage must be aggressively managed, have appropriate diagnostic studies, and be admitted to the hospital for further studies and observation.

CASE 2. A 28-year-old woman ran into the emergency department (ED) clutching the back of her head, screaming that her head was going to explode. A brief history revealed that she was maintained on tranylcypromine sulfate for depression. Fifteen minutes before the onset of the headache she had been eating dinner in a restaurant and had consumed a salad with a yogurt dressing.

The initial evaluation revealed an alert, oriented but agitated patient who was holding her head with both hands and had her eyes shut tightly. Her skin was markedly flushed and mildly diaphoretic. Initial blood pressure reading was 200/110 mm Hg, with a pulse that was 90 beats /min and irregular, a respiratory rate of 28 breaths/min, and a temperature of 99°F. Cardiac auscultation suggested bigeminy. A neurologic evaluation indicated that the patient had equal round and reactive pupils (although she was photophobic.) She was moving all four extremities equally and had no gross sensory deficits. The remainder of her physical evaluation was unremarkable. At the end of the physical examination, cardiac monitoring demonstrated that the patient was now in a normal sinus rhythm at a rate of 92 beats/min. Simultaneous with the placement of a peripheral intravenous (IV) line, the patient received 10 mg of nifedipine sublingually. She then vomited a large amount of undigested food. Repeat blood pressure was 190/100 mm Hg. The patient continued to complain of a severe throbbing occipital headache. The nifedipine dose was repeated. The blood pressure began to fall within minutes. Over 20 minutes the blood pressure stabilized at 130/80 mm Hg with some resolution of the headache.

On further questioning, the patient denied the ingestion of cheese or wine and denied the use of illicit drugs, specifically amphetamines or cocaine. Due to the persistence of a mild headache and the known risk of cerebral or subarachnoid hemorrhage, a noncontrast computed tomography scan was obtained, and was negative. A lumbar puncture was not performed, as the patient's symptoms resolved completely within 6 hours of observation, and her mental status, vital signs, and neurologic examination remained normal. She was discharged home with instructions for proper diet, medication and drug use.

The patient's clinical presentation was very characteristic of tyramine reaction. As yogurt is one of the foods low in tyramine content, it was thought unlikely that this patient's reaction was secondary to the ingestion of salad dressing. Discussion with her private psychiatrist revealed that the patient was a drug user, particularly of cocaine. Her hypertensive reaction was felt to be secondary to either a pharmacologically active dietary monoamine that she ingested or to cocaine or amphetamine.

Drug and Food Interactions

Multiple food and drug interactions are reported in patients taking MAOIs.[8,35,76,77,92,95,99] These interactions have predominantly occurred after the use of the indirectly acting sympathomimetic agents such as ephedrine and phenylpropanolamine[50,72] (Table 58–1), or the ingestion of foods containing tyramine (Table 58–2) in patients treated with MAOIs.[13,88,108] These drug interactions are particularly problematic in patients taking the older nonspecific, irreversible inhibitors of MAO. The indirect-acting sympathomimetic agents (see Fig. 58–2) act by causing the release of NE stored in the peripheral sympathetic nerve terminal.[54] Tyramine, a pharmacologically active dietary monoamine, has a similar mechanism of action.[54] In the setting of MAO inhibition the pool of NE is expanded. The release of this expanded pool of NE may result in hypertension, tachycardia or bradycardia, severe (typically occipital) headache, hyperthermia, altered mental status, seizures, intracranial hemorrhage, and death. The presence of MAOIs will, therefore, potentiate their toxicity by decreasing their inactivation. Many reports describe hypertensive crises in this setting,[18,31,39,54–56,104,106,111] The agents specifically implicated in case reports or human studies include ephedrine,[39,77] phenylephrine,[18,39] dopamine,[57] mephentermine,[104] methamphetamine,[31] metaraminol,[56] phenylpropanolamine,[53,55,106] amphetamine, and tyramine.[57] Animal studies have confirmed the drug interactions with MAOI and amphetamine,[85,111] phenylethylamine, and tyramine.[52,111] Epinephrine, NE, and isoproterenol are theoretically safe in patients on MAOIs. Rather than release a stored pool of NE, these drugs bind directly with postsynaptic alpha- and beta-adrenergic receptors. Theoretically, no potentiation of their effects should take place in the setting of MAO inhibition. In addition, extraneuronal catecholamines (those that are derived from the adrenal medulla or administered parenterally) are inactivated primarily by catechol-*O*-methyltransferase

TABLE 58–1. SYMPATHOMIMETIC AMINES

Direct acting
Epinephrine
Norepinephrine
Isoetharine
Ethylnorepinephrine
Isoproterenol
Methoxamine
Phenylephrine
Indirect acting
Amphetamine
Hydroxyamphetamine
Benzphetamine
Ritodrine
Methamphetamine
Phenylpropanolamine
Fenfluramine
Propylhexedrine
Phentermine
Tyramine
Both direct and indirect acting
Dopamine
Metaraminol
Ephedrine
Mephentermine

Hypertensive reactions have been reported with the use of MAOIs. Indirect agents or agents having both direct and indirect effects are theoretically dangerous.

Adapted, with permission, from Weiner N: Norepinephrine, epinephrine and the sympathomimetic amines. In: Gilman AG, Goodman LS, Rall TW, Murad F, eds: Goodman and Gilman's The Pharmacological Basis of Therapeutics, 7th ed. New York, Macmillan, 1985.

TABLE 58–2. DIETARY CONSIDERATIONS FOR PATIENTS USING MONOAMINE OXIDASE INHIBITORS

High tyramine content (to be avoided)
Aged, mature cheeses
Smoked, pickled, aged, putrefying meats or fish
Yeast and meat extracts
Red wines
Italian broad beans
Moderate tyramine content (to be eaten only in limited amounts)
Meat extracts
Pasteurized light and pale beers
Ripe avocados
Low tyramine content (permissible)
Distilled spirits
Cottage, cream cheese
Chocolate- and caffeine-containing beverages
Fruits
Soy sauce
Yogurt, sour cream

Adapted, with permission, from Murphy DL: Monoamine oxidase inhibiting antidepressants: A clinical update. Psychiatr Clin North Am 1984;7:549–562.

TABLE 58–3. DIFFERENTIAL DIAGNOSIS IN MAOI REACTIONS

	Drug Interaction		
	Meperidine	*Tyramine*	*Overdose*
Onset of symptoms	Minutes–hours	Minutes–hours	Up to 24 h
Signs and symptoms	Hypertension or hypotension Hyperthermia Muscle rigidity Disorientation Seizures Death	Hypertension Tachycardia or bradycardia Headache Flushing Seizures Intracranial hemorrhage	Hypertension or hypotension Diaphoresis Neuromuscular hyperactivity Obtundation Seizures Cardiovascular collapse Death
Duration of symptoms	Hours	Hours	Days

(COMT), an enzyme not inhibited by MAOIs.[64] The lack of potentiation of the effects of EPI, NE, and isoproterenol is documented in the setting of MAO inhibition.[18,39,52,55,111]

Pharmacologically active dietary monoamines may be found in large quantities in protein foods that contain decarboxylating bacteria.[17,96] Amino acids are converted to monoamines such as tyramine, phenylethylamine, and histamine, which are normally degraded by gut and liver MAO before entering the systemic circulation. In the setting of MAO inhibition, large amounts of these substances may enter the systemic circulation, release stored NE, and result in hypertensive crises.[32] As little as 6 mg of tyramine may result in a significant vasopressor effect in the MAO-inhibited patient.[57] This is 1–10% of the dose normally needed to achieve a vasopressor effect. The amine composition of foods may vary greatly. Analysis found no tyramine in cottage cheese, 1.4 mg/g in cheddar cheese, and 0.025 mg/mL in Chianti wine. A detailed analysis of the tyramine content of various foods and beverages is available.[32] Table 58–3 lists symptoms that may help in differentiating overdoses from drug and food interactions associated with MAOI.

Less danger of a tyramine reaction occurs with the use of the reversible inhibitors of MAO. Tyramine can compete effectively with the reversible MAOIs for MAO.[97] Therefore, less danger exists of hypertensive crisis following the ingestion of tyramine-containing foods. In addition, multiple animal and human studies have demonstrated the lack of pressor effects with combined reversible MAOIs and tyramine.[3,12,15,22,24,25,34,47,65,68,81,82,90]

What Other Drugs Should Be Avoided or Only Used With Caution in Patients on MAOIs?

A potentially fatal interaction between MAOIs and meperidine has been described in human reports[28,113] and confirmed by animal studies.[38,49,86,98] A similar fatal reaction was described in a patient on MAOIs after the ingestion of a dextromethorphan-containing cold preparation.[92] Clinically, the reaction involves the rapid onset of disorientation, muscle rigidity, severe hyperthermia, hypertension or hypotension, coma, seizures, and death. The MAOIs are inhibitors (competitive and noncompetitive) of meperidine-*N*-demethylation, but this is probably not the mechanism that accounts for this drug interaction.[38] Instead, the mechanism is thought to involve an exacerbation by meperidine of an elevated level of CNS serotonin that is known to occur with MAO inhibition.[40,101] The clinical syndrome produced by this drug interaction has been termed the "serotonin syndrome."[63,84,89,105] The ability of various agents to cause hyperthermia in rabbits pretreated with MAOI was in direct proportion to each agent's ability to block the reuptake of serotonin.[98] These agents include fluoxetine, dextromethorphan, and levorphanol. In a similar animal model morphine and pentazocaine were found to lack potentiating effects.[86] Many opioids have not been demonstrated to be safe in this setting and should, therefore, be avoided. The serotonergic effects of the selective, reversible MAO-A inhibitor moclobemide appear to be exacerbated to a considerably lesser degree with the use of meperidine than are the nonselective irreversible inhibitors.[3] However, the simultaneous use of these two agents is not recommended. Morphine sulfate may be used safely.[103] The sedating effects of codeine may be prolonged and potentiated in MAO-inhibited patients.[44] The dose of codeine should therefore be decreased (Table 58–4).

The simultaneous administration of fluoxetine (Prozac) or other selective serotonin reuptake inhibitors (SSRIs) and either selective or nonselective MAOIs is particularly hazardous due to greatly increased serotonergic neurotransmission[21] that results from the combined use.[42,76] Several deaths are reported following their simultaneous administration of these medications.[27] Serotonin syndrome also occurs following the combined use of sertraline and phenelzine.[62] At least 14 days should elapse between the discontinuation of an MAOI and the initiation of SSRI therapy. Fluoxetine and its active metabolite norfluoxetine have relatively long half-lives as well.[27] The manufacturer recommends that the initiation of MAOI therapy should not occur until 5 weeks fol-

TABLE 58–4. MAOI–DRUG INTERACTIONS

Drug	Type of Interaction
Indirect-acting sympathomimetics	Hypertensive crisis, death
Opioids (meperidine, dextromethorphan)	Hyperthermia, death
Antidepressants (imipramine, fluoxetine)	Disorientation, seizures, death
Theophylline, caffeine	Hyperthermia, death (laboratory animals)
Levodopa, tryptophan	Hypertension
Hypoglycemic agents	Potentiation of hypoglycemia
Barbiturates	Potentiation of sedation
Codeine	Potentiation of sedation
Cocaine	Hyperthermia, death (laboratory animals)

lowing the discontinuation of fluoxetine.[27] Although the simultaneous use of an MAOI and a tricyclic antidepressant is common in depressed patients,[115] reports of toxic and fatal reactions appear frequently enough to warrant extreme caution with this combination.[6,19,33,51,79] Most reactions have involved the use of an MAOI and the tricyclic antidepressant imipramine. The clinical presentation includes restlessness, diaphoresis, excitability, opisthotonos, hyperthermia, visual hallucinations, seizures, coma, and death. The etiology of the interaction is unclear but may be mediated by serotonin. Initially the combination of tricyclics and moclobemide was reported to be safe.[3] However, recent information available regarding the combined use of moclobemide and a range of other drugs is conflicting.[35,76] Serotonin syndrome has been reported with the combination of moclobemide and imipramine,[48] clomipramine,[102] or citalopram.[83] It appears that simultaneous or tandem administration either of the older nonselective or a newer selective MAOI and any of the agents that decrease the reuptake of serotonin may precipitate the serotonin syndrome and possibly death. Additional information on the serotonin syndrome may be found in Chapter 56.

Studies of the use of theophylline in MAO treated animals demonstrated significant toxic interactions. Marked toxicity was found in rats pretreated with MAOIs and administered doses of theophylline and caffeine previously shown to be safe.[11] Another study demonstrated a significant reduction in the LD_{50} of both theophylline and caffeine after pretreatment with pargyline.[10,97] The toxic reaction included marked hyperthermia, agitation, and tremors. These effects were blocked by inhibitors of serotonin synthesis. Curiously, reports of these interactions in humans have not appeared in the literature. Nevertheless the animal data are sufficiently alarming so that the use of MAOIs should be avoided in asthmatic patients requiring theophylline as part of their regimen. Toxicity of epinephrine and the inhaled, direct-acting beta-adrenergic agonists isoproterenol and albuterol is not potentiated by the MAOIs.

Many cases of toxic reactions are reported in patients treated with MAOIs and given tryptophan for depression[87,89,109] or levodopa for Parkinson's disease.[94,107] The reaction appears to be similar to the tyramine–MAOI interaction and includes hypertension, facial flushing, and a sensation of warmth. This reaction has been attributed to the administration of precursor amino acids in the setting of decreased degradation[46] (Fig. 58–3). Although there have been no reports of fatalities, these combinations should be avoided or used only with great caution. The use of selegiline, the specific inhibitor of MAO-B, with levodopa is considered safe.

Animal studies and human reports describe a potentiation of the hypoglycemic effects of insulin and sulfonylureas in the presence of MAO inhibition.[1,9,20,29,116] Research demonstrates that tranylcypromine sulfate is a potent insulin secretagogue.[20] Persistent hypoglycemia with the use of selegiline is reported.[93] Doses of hypoglycemic agents should be appropriately adjusted in patients on MAOIs considering the increased risk of hypoglycemic episodes. This hypoglycemic effect is not produced by moclobemide.[3]

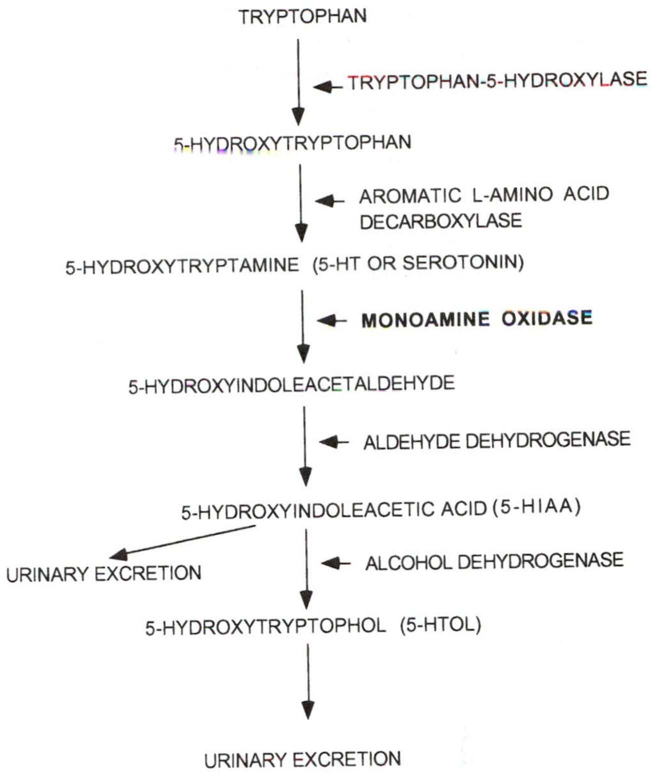

Figure 58–3. The synthesis and metabolism of serotonin from dietary tryptophan. *(Modified, with permission, from Gilman AG, Rall TW: Autocoids: Drug therapy of inflammation. In Garrison JC, Rall TW, Nies AS, Taylor P, eds: Goodman and Gilman's The Pharmacological Basis of Therapeutics, 8th ed. New York, Pergamon Press, 1990, p. 593.)*

The MAOIs inhibit the mixed-function oxidase enzyme systems involved in the metabolism and inactivation of pentobarbital and hexobarbital.[44,66] At least one case of prolonged coma after a standard dose of amobarbital sodium is reported.[36] Doses of the barbiturates should be adjusted in this setting accordingly.

Due to the known toxicity of phenylpropanolamine and dextromethorphan in patients on MAOIs (previously described), these nonprescription cold preparations should be avoided in patients receiving MAO inhibitors.[30,53] In general, a patient on MAOIs should not use nonprescription medications without specific confirmation by a physician and pharmacist that there is no potential risk.

In animals doses of cocaine found nontoxic when administered alone evoked severe signs of toxicity when the animals were pretreated with MAOIs.[26] These toxic signs include tremor, hyperthermia, seizures, and death. Although cocaine is a known toxin in every setting, patients on MAOIs must be specifically warned about the life-threatening dangers of the use of this combination of agents in doses the individual might have used uneventfully before the initiation of the MAOI therapy.

Switching MAOIs

When switching from one MAOI to another, a waiting period of 14 days is recommended. Clearly, in some patients more rapid switching or simultaneous administration may be safe. However, it is impossible to predict who will have a potentially life-threatening adverse reaction and who will not.[112]

When switching from a tricyclic antidepressant to a MAOI, the standard recommendation is to wait 7–10 days between drugs. One survey reported on prescribing practices of psychiatrists at an academic center whose standard practice was to switch from a TCA to an MAOI over the course of 4 days. No adverse events were reported.[60]

Summary

The renewed popularity of MAOIs has highlighted the diversity of drugs that can interact with MAOIs and produce serious or life-threatening events. The frequency of these interactions should make practitioners cautious in the use of any agent that has not specifically been demonstrated to be safe in this setting. In addition, before prescribing or administering any medication to a patient on a MAOI, the practitioner should check for previous reports and any newly described drug interactions by consulting the regional poison center.

References

1. Adnitt PI: Hypoglycemic action of monoamine oxidase inhibitors (MAOIs). Diabetes 1968;17:628–633.
2. Amrein R, Allen SR, Guentert TW, et al: The pharmacology of reversible monoamine oxidase inhibitors. Br J Psych 1989;155(suppl 6):66–71.
3. Amrein R, Guntert J, Dingemanse T, et al: Interactions of moclobemide with concomitantly administered medication: Evidence from pharmacological and clinical studies. Psychopharmacology 1992;106(suppl):S24–31.
4. Antidepressants. In: Sewester CS, Threlkeld DS, Olin B, et al, eds: Drug Facts and Comparisons, 51st ed. St. Louis, Facts and Comparisons, 1997, pp. 1523–1586.
5. Axelrod J, Weinshilboum R: Catecholamines. N Engl J Med 1972;287:237–242.
6. Ayd FJ: Toxic somatic and psychopathologic reactions to antidepressant drugs. J Neuropsychiatry 1961;2:8119–8122.
7. Baldessarini RJ: Drugs and the treatment of psychiatric disorders: Depression and mania. In: Hardman JG, Limbird LE, Molinoff PB, Ruddon RW, Gilman AG, eds: Goodman and Gilman's The Pharmacological Basis of Therapeutics, 9th ed. New York, McGraw-Hill, 1996, pp. 431–460.
8. Baldridge ET, Miller LV, Haverbach JB, et al: Amine metabolism after an overdosage of a monoamine oxidase inhibitor. N Engl J Med 1962;267:421–426.
9. Barrett AM: Modification of the hypoglycemic response to tolbutamide and insulin by mebanazine—An inhibitor of monoamine oxidase. J Pharm Pharmacol 1965;17:19–27.
10. Berkowitz BA, Spector S, Pool W: The interaction of caffeine, theophylline and theobromine with monoamine oxidase inhibitors. Eur J Pharmacol 1971;16:315–321.
11. Berkowitz BA, Tower JH, Spector S: Release of NE in the central nervous system by theophylline and caffeine. Eur J Pharmacol 1970;10:64–71.
12. Berlin I, Zimmer R, Cournot A, et al: Determination and comparison of the pressor effect of tyramine during long-term moclobemide and tranylcypromine treatment in healthy volunteers. Clin Pharmacol Ther 1989;46:344–351.
13. Beswick DT, Rogers ML: Monoamine oxidase inhibitors and low or alcohol free drinks. Br Med J 1990;301:179–180.
14. Bieck PR, Antonin KH: Oral tyramine pressor test and the safety of monoamine oxidase inhibitor drugs: Comparison of brofaromine and tranylcypromine in healthy subjects. J Clin Psychopharmacol 1988;8:237–245.
15. Bieck PR, Antonin KH, Schmidt E: Clinical pharmacology of reversible MAO-A inhibitors. Clin Neuropharmacol 1992;15(suppl 1, pt A):345A–346A.
16. Biel JH, Nuhfer PA, Conway AC: Structure and activity relationships of monoamine oxidase inhibitors. Ann NY Acad Sci 1959;80:568–582.
17. Blackwell B: Adverse effects of antidepressant drugs, Part 1: Monoamine oxidase inhibitors and tricyclics. Drugs 1981;21:201–219.
18. Boaks AJ, Laurence DR, Teich PC, et al: Interactions between sympathomimetic amines and antidepressants in man. Br Med J 1973;1:311–315.
19. Brachfeld J, Wirtshaffer A, Wolfe S: Imipramine-tranylcypromine incompatibility, near fatal toxic reaction. JAMA 1964;183:1172–1173.
20. Bressler R, Vargas-Cordon M, Lebovitz HE: Tranylcypromine: A potent insulin secretagogue and hypoglycaemic agent. Diabetes 1968;17:617–624.
21. Butler J, Leonard BE: Clinical and experimental studies on fluoxetine: Effects on serotonin uptake. Int Clin Psychopharmacol 1990;5:41–48.
22. Callingham BA, Ovens RS: Some in vitro effects of moclobemide and other MAO inhibitors on responses to sympathomimetic amines. J Neural Transm 1988;26(suppl): 17–29.
23. Chaimowitz GA, Links PS, Padgett RW, et al: Treatment resistant depression: A survey of practice habits of Canadian psychiatrists. Can J Psychiatry 1991;36:353–356.
24. Chen DT: Safety of moclobemide in clinical use. Clin Neuropharmacol 1992;15:428A–429A.
25. Chouinard G, Saxena BM, Nair NPV, et al: Efficacy and safety of brofaromine in depression: A Canadian multicenter placebo controlled trial and a review of comparative controlled studies. Clin Neuropharmacol 1992;15 (suppl 1, pt A):426A–427A.
26. Christie JE, Crow TJ: Behavioral studies of the actions of cocaine, monoamine oxidase inhibitors and iminodibenzyl compounds on central dopamine neurons. Br J Pharmacol 1973;47:39–47.
27. Ciraulo DA, Shader RI: Fluoxetine drug-drug interactions: I. Antidepressants and antipsychotics. J Clin Psychopharmacol 1990;10:48–50.

28. Cocks DP, Passmore-Rowe A: Dangers of monoamine oxidase inhibitors. Br Med J 1962;2:1545–1546.
29. Cooper AJ, Ashcroft G: Potentiation of insulin hypoglycaemia by monoamine oxidase in MAOI antidepressant drugs. Lancet 1966;1:407–409.
30. Cuthbert MF, Greenberg MP, Morley SW: Cough and cold remedies: A potential danger to patients on monoamine oxidase inhibitors. Br Med J 1969;1:404–409.
31. Dally PJ: Fatal reaction with tranylcypromine and methylamphetamine. Lancet 1962;1:1235–1236.
32. Da Prada M, Zurchet G, Wuthrich I, et al: On tyramine, food, beverages and the reversible MAO inhibitor moclobemide. J Neural Transm 1988;26(suppl):31–56.
33. Davies G: Side effects of phenelzine. Br Med J 1960;2:1019.
34. Delker A, Gaertner HJ: Tolerability and antidepressive effect of brofaromine, a short-acting reversible MAO inhibitor—An open study. Eur Neuropsychopharmacol 1991;1:177–180.
35. Dingemanse J: An update of recent moclobemide interaction data. Int Clin Psychopharmacol 1993;7:167–180.
36. Domino EF, Sullivan TS, Luby ED: Barbiturate intoxication in a patient treated with a MAO inhibitor. Am J Psychiatry 1962;118:941–943.
37. Dostert P: Can our knowledge of monoamine oxidase (MAO) help in the design of better MAO inhibitors? J Neural Transm 1994;41(suppl):269–279.
38. Eade NR, Renton KW: Effect of monoamine oxidase inhibitors on the *N*-demethylation and hydrolysis of meperidine. Biochem Pharmacol 1970;19:2243–2250.
39. Elis J, Laurence DR, Mattie H, et al: Modification by monoamine oxidase inhibitors of the effect of some sympathomimetics on blood pressure. Br Med J 1967;2:75–78.
40. Erspamer V: Recent research in the field of 5-hydroxytryptamine and related indolealkylamines. Prog Drug Res 1961;3:307–315.
41. Fallon B, Foote B, Walsh BT, et al: "Spontaneous" hypertensive episodes with monoamine oxidase inhibitors. J Clin Psychiatry 1988;49:163–165.
42. Feighner JP, Boyer WF, Tyler DL, et al: Adverse consequences of fluoxetine–MAOI combination therapy. J Clin Psychiatry 1990;51:222–225.
43. Fier M: Safer use of MAOIs. Am J Psychiatry 1991;148: 391–392.
44. Findlay JWA, Butz RF, Williams BB, et al: Effect of monoamine oxidase inhibitors on codeine disposition and pentobarbitone sleep-times in the rat. J Pharm Pharmacol 1981;33:34–47.
45. Foods interacting with MAO inhibitors. Med Lett 1989; 31:11–12.
46. Friend DG, Bell WR, Kline NS: The action of L-dihydroxyphenylalanine in patients receiving nialamide. Clin Pharmacol Ther 1965;6:362–366.
47. Gieschke R, Schmid-Burgk W, Amrein R: Interaction of moclobemide, a new reversible monoamine oxidase inhibitor with oral tyramine. J Neural Transm 1988;26 (suppl):97–104.
48. Gilbar PJ, Brodribb TR, Downey N: Serotonin syndrome due to a moclobemide imipramine interaction. A previously unreported drug interaction? Aust J Hosp Pharm 1995;25;75. Abstract.
49. Gong SNC, Rogers KJ: Role of brain monoamines in the fatal hyperthermia induced by pethidine or imipramine in rabbits pretreated with a monoamine oxidase inhibitor. Br J Pharmacol 1973;48:12–18.
50. Goulet JP, Perusse R, Turcotte JY: Contraindications to vasoconstrictors in dentistry: Part III. Oral Surg Oral Med Oral Pathol 1992;74:692–697.
51. Graham P, Potter JM, Paterson JW: Combination monoamine oxidase inhibitor/tricyclic antidepressant interaction. Lancet 1982;2:440.
52. Griesemer EC, Barsky J, Dragstedt CA, et al: Potentiating effect of iproniazid on the pharmacological action of sympathomimetic amines. Proc Soc Exp Biol Med 1953;84: 669–704.
53. Harrison WM, McGrath PJ, Stewart JW, et al: MAOIs and hypertensive crises: The role of OTC drugs. J Clin Psychiatry 1989;50:64–65.
54. Hesselink JM: Safer use of MAOIs with nifedipine to counteract potential hypertensive crisis. Am J Psychiatry 1991;148:1616. Letter.
55. Hoffman BB, Lefkowitz RJ: Catecholamines, sympathomimetic drugs, and adrenergic receptor antagonists. In: Hardman JG, Limbird LE, Molinoff PB, Ruddon RW, Gilman AG, eds: Goodman and Gilman's The Pharmacological Basis of Therapeutics, 9th ed. New York, McGraw-Hill, 1996, pp. 199–248.
56. Horler AR, Wynne NA: Hypertensive crisis due to pargyline and metaraminol. Br Med J 1965;2:460–461.
57. Horowitz D, Lovenberg W, Engelman K, et al: Monoamine oxidase inhibitors, tyramine and cheese. JAMA 1964;188:1108–1110.
58. Jacobsen E: The early history of psychotherapeutic drugs. Psychopharmacology 1986;89:138–144.
59. Jin YZ, Ramsay RR, Youngster SK, et al: A new class of powerful inhibitors of monoamine oxidase A. Biochem Biophysical Res Commun 1990;172:1338–1341.
60. Kahn D, Silver JM, Opler LA: The safety of switching rapidly from tricyclic antidepressants to monoamine oxidase inhibitors. J Clin Psychopharmacol 1989;9:198–202.
61. Keck PE Jr, Vuckovic A, Pope HG, et al: Acute cardiovascular response to monoamine oxidase inhibitors: A prospective assessment. J Clin Psychopharmacol 1989;9:203–206.
62. Keltner N: Serotonin syndrome: A case of fatal SSRI/ MAOI interaction. Perspect Psychol Care 1994;30:26–31.
63. Kline SS, Slack Mauro L, Scala-Barnett DM, et al: Serotonin syndrome versus neuroleptic malignant syndrome as a cause of death. Clin Pharmacol 1989;8:510–514.
64. Kopin I, Axelrod J: The role of monoamine oxidase in the release and metabolism of norepinephrine. Ann NY Acad Sci 1963;107:848–852.
65. Korn A, Da Prada M, Raffesberg W, et al: Tyramine pressor effect in man: Studies with moclobemide, a novel, reversible monoamine oxidase inhibitor. J Neural Transm 1988;26(suppl):57–71.
66. LaRoche MJ, Brodie B: Lack of relationship between inhibition of monoamine oxidase and potentiation of hexobarbital hypnosis. J Pharmacol Exp Ther 1960;130:134–137.
67. Larsen JK: MAO inhibitors: Pharmacodynamic aspects and clinical implications. Acta Psychiatr Scand 1988;78 (suppl):74–80.

68. Laux G, Beckman H, Classen W, et al: Moclobemide and maprotiline in the treatment of inpatients with major depressive disorder. J Neural Transm 1989;28(suppl):45–52.
69. Linden CH, Rumack BH: Monoamine oxidase inhibitor overdose. Ann Emerg Med 1984;13:1137–1144.
70. Lippman SB, Nash K: Monoamine oxidase inhibitor update: Potential adverse food and drug interactions. Drug Safety 1990;5:195–204.
71. Litovitz TL, Clark LR, Soloway RA: 1993 annual report of the American Association of Poison Control Centers Toxic Exposure Surveillance System. Am J Emerg Med 1994; 12:546–555.
72. Litovitz TL, Felberg L, Soloway RA, et al: 1994 annual report of the American Association of Poison Control Centers Toxic Exposure Surveillance System. Am J Emerg Med 1995;13:551–597.
73. Litovitz TL, Felberg L, White S, et al: 1995 annual report of the American Association of Poison Control Centers Toxic Exposure Surveillance System. Am J Emerg Med 1996; 14:487–537.
74. Litovitz TL, Holm KC, Bailey KM, et al: 1991 annual report of the American Association of Poison Control Centers National Data Collection System. Am J Emerg Med 1992; 10:452–505.
75. Litovitz TL, Holm KC, Clancy C, et al: 1992 annual report of the American Association of Poison Control Centers Toxic Exposure Surveillance System. Am J Emerg Med 1993;2:494–555.
76. Livingston MG, Livingston HM: Monoamine oxidase inhibitors. An update on drug interactions. Drug Safety 1996;14:219–227.
77. Low Beer GA, Tidmarsh D: Collapse after "Parstelin." Br Med J 1963;2:683–684.
78. Mallinger AG, Smith E: Pharmacokinetics of monoamine oxidase inhibitors. Psychopharmacol Bull 1991;27:493–502.
79. McCurdy RL, Kane FJ: Transient brain syndrome as a nonfatal reaction to combined pargyline imipramine treatment. Am J Psychiatry 1964;121:397–398.
80. Meredith TJ, Vale JA: Poisoning due to psychotropic agents. Adverse Drug Reactions Acute Poisoning Rev 1985;4:83–126.
81. Moll E, Hetzl W: Moclobemide (Ro 11–1163) safety in depressed patients. Acta Psychiatr Scand 1990;360 (suppl):69–70.
82. Muller T, Gieschke R, Ziegler WH: Blood pressure response to tyramine-enriched meal before and during MAO-inhibition in man: Influence of dosage regimen. J Neural Transm 1988;26(suppl):105–114.
83. Neuvonen PJ, Pohojla-Sintonen S, Tacke U, et al: Five fatal cases of serotonin syndrome after moclobemide–citalopram or moclobemide–clomipramine overdoses. Lancet 1993;342:1419. Letter.
84. Nierenberg DW, Semprebon M: The central nervous system serotonin syndrome. Clin Pharmacol Ther 1993;53: 84–88.
85. O'Dea K, Rand MJ: Interaction between amphetamine and monoamine oxidase inhibitors. Eur J Pharmacol 1969;6: 115–120.
86. Penn RG, Rogers KJ: Comparison of the effects of morphine, pethidine and pentazocine in rabbits pretreated with a monoamine oxidase inhibitor. Br J Pharmacol 1971;42:485–492.
87. Pope HG, Jonas JM, Hudson JI, et al: Toxic reactions to the combination of monoamine oxidase inhibitors and tryptophan. Am J Psychiatry 1985;142:491–492.
88. Preskorn SH, Goodwin DW: Medical management of the depressed alcoholic patient. Int J Psychiatry Med 1987; 17:117–131.
89. Price WA, Zimmer B, Kucas P: Serotonin syndrome: A case report. J Clin Pharmacol 1986;26:77–78.
90. Provost JC, Funck-Bretano C, Rovei V, et al: Pharmacokinetic and pharmacodynamic interaction between toloxatone, a new reversible monoamine oxidase-A inhibitor, and oral tyramine in healthy subjects. Clin Pharmacol Ther 1992;52:384–393.
91. Rafaelsen OJ: Cheese affects new reversible MAO-A inhibitors: Summary. J Neural Transm 1988;26(suppl): 123–124.
92. Rivers N: Possible lethal reaction between Nardil and dextromethorphan. Can Med Assoc J 1970;103:85.
93. Rowland MJ, Bransome ED Jr, Hendry LB: Hypoglycemia caused by selegiline, an antiparkinsonian drug: Can such side effects be predicted? J Clin Pharmacol 1994;34:80–85.
94. Sandyk R: L-Dopa induced "serotonin syndrome" in a parkinsonian patient on bromocriptine. J Clin Psychopharmacol 1986;6:194–195.
95. Sherman M, Hauser GC, Glover BH: Toxic reactions to tranylcypromine. Am J Psychiatry 1964;120:1019–1021.
96. Shulman KI, Walker SE, MacKenzie S, et al: Dietary restriction, tyramine and the use of monoamine oxidase inhibitors. J Clin Psychopharmacol 1989;9:397–402.
97. Silverstone T: New aspects in the treatment of depression. Int Clin Psychopharmacol 1992;6(suppl 5):41–44.
98. Sinclair JG, Lo GF: The blockade of serotonin uptake and the meperidine monoamine oxidase inhibitor interaction. Proc West Pharmacol Soc 1977;20:373–374.
99. Skoog RE: Monoamine oxidase inhibitors: Pharmacology and implications in the perioperative period. J Post Anesth Nurs 1989;4:264–267.
100. Smilkstein MJ, Smolinske SC, Rumack BH: A case of MAO inhibitor/MDMA interaction. Agony after ecstasy. J Toxicol Clin Toxicol 1987;25:149–159.
101. Spector S: Monoamine oxidase in control of brain serotonin and norepinephrine content. Ann NY Acad Sci 1963; 107:856–864.
102. Spigset O, Mjorndal T: Serotonin syndrome caused by a moclobemide–clomipramine interaction. Br Med J 1993; 306:248.
103. Stack CG, Rogers P, Linter PK: Monoamine oxidase inhibitors and anaesthesia. Br J Anaesth 1988;60:222–227.
104. Stark DCC: Effects of giving vasopressors to patients on MAO inhibitors. Lancet 1962;2:1405–1406.
105. Sternbach H: The serotonin syndrome. Am J Psychiatry 1991;148:705–713.
106. Tanks CM, Lloyd AT: Hazards with monoamine oxidase inhibitors. Br Med J 1965;1:589.
107. Teychenne PF, Calne DB, Lewis PJ, et al: Interactions of levodopa with inhibitors of monoamine oxidase and L-aromatic acid decarboxylase. Clin Pharmacol Ther 1975; 18:273–277.

108. Thakore J, Dinan TG, Kelleher M: Alcohol-free beer and the irreversible monoamine oxidase inhibitors. Int Clin Psychopharmacol 1992;7:59–60.
109. Thomas JM, Rubin EH: Case report of a toxic reaction from a combination of tryptophan and phenelzine. Am J Psychiatry 1984;141:281–283.
110. Tolefson GD: Monoamine oxidase inhibitors: A review. J Clin Psychol 1983;44:280–287.
111. Trinker FR, Flearn HJ, McCullock NW, et al: Experimental observations on the effects of adrenaline after treatment with antidepressant monoamine oxidase inhibitors (MAOI) drugs. Austr Dent J 1967;12:297–303.
112. True L, Alexander B, Carter B: Switching monoamine oxidase inhibitors. Drug Intell Clin Pharm 1985;19:825–827.
113. Vigran IM: Dangerous potentiation of meperidine hydrochloride by pargyline hydrochloride. JAMA 1964;187: 953–995.
114. Wells DG, Bjorksten AR: Monoamine oxidase inhibitors revisited. Can J Anaesth 1989;36:64–74.
115. White K, Pistole T, Boyd JL: Combined monoamine oxidase inhibitor–tricyclic antidepressant treatment: A pilot study. Am J Psychiatry 1980;137:1422–1425.
116. Wickstrom L, Pettersson K: Treatment of diabetics with monoamine oxidase inhibitors. Lancet 1964;2:995–997.

CHAPTER 59

Lithium

Glendon C. Henry

Lithium	
MW	= 6.94 daltons
Lithium levels (serum):	
Therapeutic level for	
Bipolar depression	0.6–1.2 mEq/L (mmol/L)
Action level	
Acute toxicity	> 4.0 mEq/L (mmol/L)
Chronic toxicity	> 1.5 mEq/L (mmol/L)

Values greater than or equal to the action level necessitate clinical intervention. Values less than this level may necessitate intervention based on the clinical condition of the patient.

A 36-year-old stuporous woman was rushed to the emergency department (ED) by her family because of her change in mental status. When aroused, the patient's speech was slurred and she complained of blurred vision, but she was unable to provide any other history. Her family and a clinic psychiatrist who had last seen her several months before admission were, however, helpful. The woman had manifested emotional problems for years and had visited numerous psychiatrists. After looking through the patient's belongings, it was noted that her purse contained bottles of phenothiazines, tricyclic antidepressants, lithium carbonate, and several analgesic mixtures.

On inspection, the patient was unkempt, diaphoretic, and poorly nourished. Her vital signs were blood pressure, 140/85 mm Hg; pulse, 110 beats/min; respirations, 18 breaths/min; temperature, 37.3°C (99.1°F). On HEENT examination she was noted to have poor dentition and her mouth smelled of fresh vomitus. She also had horizontal nystagmus, and possibly thyromegaly.

The chest was clear to auscultation and percussion. The heart rate was regular, with no murmurs, thrills, heaves, or gallop sounds. The abdomen was soft and nontender without organomegaly. Bowel sounds were hyperactive. Rectal examination revealed good tone, and the stool tested negative for occult blood. Her extremities were without clubbing, cyanosis, or edema.

On neurologic examination the patient became agitated after stimulation. She had a faint tremor and fasiculations in both upper extremities. There was no motor weakness, but the deep tendon reflexes were exaggerated. Twice during the examination, clonus of both lower extremities was noted and choreoathetoid movements were observed. All her cranial nerves were normal.

The patient was placed on a nasal canula with low-flow oxygen, and cardiac monitoring was initiated. She had a large-bore intravenous line inserted, and blood specimens were obtained. She was also given 50 mL of 50% dextrose in water, 100 mg of thiamine intravenously, and an ampule of multivitamins was placed in the first liter of D_5W in 0.45% sodium chloride. Her clinical condition did not change.

The initial laboratory data obtained included glucose, BUN, electrolytes, calcium, complete blood count (CBC), an arterial blood gas, and a lithium level.

The electrocardiogram (ECG) showed a regular sinus tachycardia at 110 beats/min with a normal QRS complex, nonspecific ST segment and T wave changes, in addition to U waves. The chest radiograph was normal. A lumbar puncture was performed and all studies on the fluid were normal.

The multiple signs and symptoms in this patient make the differential diagnosis a difficult one. Psychiatric illness should be considered, but placed last on the list, and organicity excluded. Life-threatening disorders such as sedative-hypnotic or alcoholic withdrawal must also be excluded. Metabolic diseases such as thyrotoxicosis and hypoglycemia are some other important considerations.

The patient's differential diagnosis narrowed due to her abnormal movements. Organophosphates, phenytoin, carbamazepine, lithium, and anticholinergic substances commonly produce abnormal movements. Other less likely substances considered included xanthines, strychnine, or nicotine.

The patient continued to receive supportive care. The patient's laboratory values were normal except for the lithium level, which was at 3.6 mEq/L, confirming the diagnosis of lithium intoxication.

The patient continued to improve slowly with supportive therapy only. She did well, and all her neurologic signs and symptoms resolved. This patient may have had more rapid resolution of symptoms with hemodialysis alone or in combination with hemodiafiltration.

History

Lithium, the lightest metal known, has an atomic number of three, and a valence of positive one. Because lithium is in the same column of the periodical table as sodium and potassium, many of its actions are similar to those of these other two cations. Although its consequential medical use began in 1970, lithium had numerous other uses prior to this era.[1]

As early as the mid 19th century, lithium was used in the treatment of arthritis and nephrolithiasis. At one time it was also one of the constituents in the soft drink, Seven-Up.[1] Lithium chloride was popularized as a salt substitute for the treatment of hypertensive patients. In 1949 several patients' deaths were attributed to lithium's toxicity, leading to an FDA withdrawal of its use as a salt substitute. Ironically, this was the same year that lithium was discovered to be beneficial in the treatment of mania. While searching for an agent that could induce mania, several subjects on lithium were overdosed, producing obtundation rather than excitation. It was not until 1970 that lithium was recognized as the treatment of choice for patients with bipolar disorders.

Unfortunately, although it is a rather safe drug when used appropriately, lithium demonstrates a narrow therapeutic–toxic ratio and can induce severe complications if slight changes in dosing or elimination occur. Lithium chloride is also used for several other medical purposes such as prophylaxis for cluster headaches,[30] and as a "cell stimulator" in neutropenic patients.[42]

What Are the Pharmacologic Characteristics of Lithium?

Lithium is rapidly absorbed from the gastrointestinal tract within 1–2 hours; peak levels occur at 2–4 hours, and absorption is complete after 8 hours. Lithium has a volume of distribution of 0.6–0.9 L/kg, which is slightly larger than total body water. Lithium is excreted via the kidney (95%), and its clearance is dependent on the glomerular filtration rate (GFR). The other 5% of this agent is secreted in sweat and saliva, and in the lactating female a small percentage is excreted in breast milk. Eighty percent of the lithium that is handled by the kidney is reabsorbed, while 20% is excreted in the urine unchanged.[22,52] After absorption, lithium undergoes a slow distribution as it transverses cell membranes, at which time it is capable of inducing its biologic effects. This distribution varies throughout the body and therefore accounts for its unexpected apparent volume of distribution.[25] Lithium enters the liver and kidney rapidly, while its passage into muscle, bone, and brain is rather slow.[25] The therapeutic elimination half-life is about one day (20–24 hours), but this may be prolonged in patients who are on lithium therapy for extended periods of time even if they are not poisoned.[21] The time it takes to transverse the cellular membrane seems to correlate with the delay that occurs in eliciting biologic effects in both the therapeutic and overdosed patient.[25] Lithium's precise mechanism of action has not been definitively elucidated. The majority of lithium's actions are neurologic. After entering the cells of the central nervous system, lithium is capable of inducing abnormal movements, a change in mental status, seizures, or coma.

The CNS lithium level ranges from 40 to 80% of that in the serum. Unfortunately, CNS levels do not correlate either with serum levels, therapeutic effect, or toxicity.[45,56]

Lithium may be handled similarly to sodium and potassium because they share the same valence. Lithium's radius is similar to that of magnesium and therefore it may substitute for this ion as well.[36] Although lithium may alter some of magnesium's functions or serve as a false transmitter for either sodium or potassium, it is not felt that lithium's main effect is secondary to the changes induced by its substitution for any of these ions. Recently research has begun to evaluate lithium's effect on phosphatidylinositol metabolism via a second messenger. After inositol is activated by a surface agonist,[7,14,41] it interacts with G proteins that then stimulate phospholipase C to cleave intracellular phosphatidylinositol to intracellular messengers, 1,2-diacylglycerol (DAG), and inositol 1,4,5-triphosphate.[11,29] The latter is a direct stimulator for the release of intracellular calcium, while the former is an activator of protein kinase C. This is important because inositol does not cross the blood–brain barrier; therefore its concentration in the brain is maintained by regeneration and breakdown of phosphorylated components.[3,45] It is postulated that lithium may inhibit the enzyme inositol monophosphatase, which leads to an increase in inositol monophosphate and a decrease in free inositol and the intermediate phosphatidylinositol 4,5-bisphosphate.[10,11,29] The final common pathway is the decrease in the brain's free inositol concentration, which is believed to result in the desired and adverse effects produced. Although this mechanism seems reasonable, it may not be the only pathway altered by lithium, and the effects on protein kinase C and G proteins may be just as important as the depletion of inositol.[36] Norepinephrine's activity may also be attenuated by lithium via a second messenger, cAMP.[5] These numerous chemical interactions may explain the various alterations in biologic functions brought about by lithium as well as its potential in such diverse disease processes. It is now apparent that lithium effects diverse biologic pathways. Although its interactions with cAMP have been extensively evaluated, there is no definitive mechanism of action. The interactions with magnesium metabolism may play a vital role.[37]

Lithium has also been postulated to have its effects on neurotransmitters. It seems to increase the synthesis and turnover of serotonin[35] while producing a down-regulation of the 5-HT_{1A} receptors in the hippocampus[38] by diminishing serotonin binding to its receptors.[29] Although not as well elucidated, the alpha- and beta-adrenergic receptors may also be down-regulated by lithium.[35] Lithium may also have a similar affect on dopaminergic receptors by preventing up-regulation at the D_2 receptors.[2,57] These diverse actions may explain the complex neurologic manifestations.

What Are the Clinical Presentations of Patients With Lithium Intoxication?

Patients who chronically ingest lithium develop signs and symptoms of toxicity that are quite distinct from those with single acute ingestions (see Table 59–1). Patients with an acute ingestion present with gastrointestinal symptoms such as nausea, vomiting, and diarrhea, while initially having no neurologic findings. Cardiovascular complaints such as lightheadedness, dizziness, and orthostatic hypotension are usually secondary to excessive fluid loss rather than from a direct cardiotoxic effect. Electrocardiographic manifestations such as nonspecific T-wave changes may develop, and are usually benign.[17] Although reported in the literature, malignant dysrhythmias and severe cardiac dysfunction are very rare.[53]

Neurologic abnormalities are the major manifestations of both acute or chronic lithium toxicity.[39,46,47] In the acute setting, the initial finding may be merely a fine tremor of the hands. As toxicity progresses, the patient will develop hyperreflexia and agitation. Further toxicity is manifested by fasciculations, muscular irritability, choreathetosis, clonus, and altered mental status. Confusion may be followed by lethargy, coma, and seizures. Dysarthria, nystagmus, and truncal ataxia are also reported.[16,39,55] The electroencephalogram may show diffuse slowing.[46,48] Although the progression of these signs or symptoms may be orderly in that tremor, hyperreflexia, and clonus typically precede the development of an altered mental status, the levels do not necessarily correlate with the toxic manifestations. This may be explained by the slow distribution time for lithium.[19,45,56]

Patients with chronic overdoses of lithium rarely notice or manifest the gastrointestinal symptoms and are usually brought to care due to a change in mental status. Their toxicity develops secondary either to a dosing error or a decrease in lithium excretion. Impaired elimination results from intrinsic renal dysfunction, diuretic therapy, or dehydration and the ensuing relative hyponatremia. With prerenal azotemia, a relative decrease in intravascular sodium leads to a concomitant increased reabsorption of sodium and lithium. The toxicity of the chronically poisoned patient is almost exclusively neurologic and resembles the later stages of acute toxicity. An explanation for the difference is that in the chronic overdose there is a high total body burden of lithium and any additional increase results in immediate toxicity. In the acute setting, there is a substantial delay in tissue distribution prior to the development of therapeutic or toxic effects.

Patients receiving chronic lithium therapy who acutely overdose may be the most difficult to diagnose and manage as they may manifest signs and symptoms of both acute and chronic toxicity. Although these patients may manifest neurologic signs of a chronic overdose, they also have gastrointestinal symptoms, and their toxicity may be more severe and prolonged (see Table 59–1).

TABLE 59–1. TOXICITY OF LITHIUM

	Acute	Chronic
Cardiovascular	Prolonged QT interval ST and T wave abnormalities	Myocarditis
Cutaneous	None	Dermatitis, ulcers, localized edema
Renal	Concentrating defects	Nephrogenic diabetes insipidus Interstitial nephritis Renal failure
Gastrointestinal	Nausea Vomiting	Minimal
Hematologic	Leukocytosis	Aplastic anemia
Neurologic		
Mild	Weakness, lightheadedness Fine tremor	Same
Moderate	Muscle twitching, tinnitus, drowsiness, hyperreflexia, slurred speech, apathy	Same
Severe	Confusion, clonus, coma, seizure, muscular irritability, extrapyramidal symptoms (choreoathetoid movements)	Parkinson's, psychosis, memory deficits, pseudotumor cerebri[47]
Endocrine	None	Hypothyroidism
Congenital	None	Hypothyroidism

Patients who initially appear well may subsequently develop seizures, altered mental status, and cardiac complications.[39] Prolonged exposure of the central nervous system to lithium can cause permanent neurologic sequelae even when enhanced extracorporeal clearance methods such as hemodialysis are used.[24,51] Long-term exposure to sustained levels may lead to diverse CNS manifestations including memory deficits, Parkinson's disease, change in personality, and/or tremors.[51]

What Are the Potential Treatment Modalities?

It is important to define the nature of the patient's ingestion. It must be determined whether the ingestion is suicidal or unintentional and whether one or more agents were ingested. Were the agents sustained- or regular-release products? Was this an acute ingestion, a chronic ingestion, or an acute ingestion following chronic treatment? These characteristics of the history may alter how the patient is treated and the eventual outcome. While the history is being obtained, the patient's airway must be protected. Assessment of the patient's breathing and circulation must be assured, although lithium toxicity does not usually affect the airway or breathing. Cardiovascular collapse and significant dysrhythmias are rare in overdose, but can occur secondary to excessive gastrointestinal and urinary fluid losses. A good history and a thorough physical examination are necessary to elucidate any possible clues or toxidromes that may aid in the diagnosis and treatment of the patient. In most cases of lithium intoxication, neurologic findings predominate, and a detailed neurologic examination is mandatory.

The patient should have an intravenous line placed and bloods drawn for electrolytes, and an initial lithium level. In treating the patient with an acute overdose, it is important to realize that lithium is not adsorbed to activated charcoal.[27,50] In a patient with early presentation of an acute overdose or an acute on chronic overdose of lithium, if vomiting has not already occurred, orogastric lavage may remove pills remaining in the stomach. Therefore activated charcoal plays no role, if the overdose involves solely lithium. If, however, another agent is ingested, or the history is unclear, it is prudent to administer activated charcoal since the benefits far outweigh the risks. If the patient does not have diarrhea, using a cathartic such as sorbitol may also be beneficial in removing lithium from the gastrointestinal tract.[43] Because the initial lithium level may not reflect the actual total body burden, a second level should be drawn about 2 hours after the initial assessment even if the first result is not yet available. The patient should have a saline solution administered at a rate that will promote good urine output. The goal is not to induce forced diuresis, which does not substantially enhance lithium excretion above normal renal function, but rather to correct dehydration or electrolyte depletion that may exist. This will then ensure that lithium is maximally excreted in the urine.

After the patient has been stabilized, enhanced gastrointestinal clearance may be accomplished by initiating whole-bowel irrigation with a balanced polyethylene glycol–electrolyte solution (PEG-ELS). If the patient has ingested a sustained-release lithium preparation, such as Lithobid, then whole-bowel irrigation is of even greater importance.[49] If applicable, PEG-ELS should be administered at 2 L/h in the adult, or 500 mL/h in a child. The endpoint in this therapy is a rectal effluent that has the same appearance as the initial instilled fluid. (See Antidotes in Depth: Whole-Bowel Irrigation.)

What Are the Fluid and Electrolyte Management Concerns ?

In managing the patient with lithium overdose, it is essential that the patient's fluid and electrolyte status be closely monitored and maintained. This approach is obvious in the acutely poisoned patient who presents with nausea, vomiting, and diarrhea. In the chronically overdosed patient, dehydration or an electrolyte disturbance may be the precipitating event for hospitalization.

In those patients with normal renal function, osmotic and saline diuresis have limited roles and have not been shown to increase lithium clearance significantly.[28] In instances of impaired glomerular filtration, volume repletion with 150–300 mL/h of 0.9% sodium chloride solution for several hours should increase renal lithium clearance. Urinary alkalinization may have a limited effect on lithium excretion and clearance, as sodium bicarbonate decreases lithium reabsorption in the proximal tubules. The use of sodium bicarbonate is not recommended, however, because of potential complications such as hypokalemia, alkalemia, and fluid overload and the fact that it offers no better lithium elimination than can be accomplished by giving a balanced salt solution. Diuretics that act on the ascending limb of the loop of Henle or the distal tubule (eg, furosemide, ethacrynic acid, the thiazides, and the mercurials) have limited effects on lithium reabsorption, which maximally occurs in the proximal tubule.[40] They may worsen lithium intoxication, particularly if the patient becomes salt- or water-depleted.

Three classes of agents shown to cause an initial increase in lithium excretion are the osmotic agents (mannitol),[52] carbonic anhydrase inhibitors, and the phosphodiesterase inhibitors (aminophylline). Although these agents initially produce a small increase in lithium excreted, their use is not without risk. Like other diuretics they are capable of inducing mild to moderate dehydration resulting in sodium and lithium retention. Even though these agents will initially lead to a small increase in the amount of lithium excreted by increasing the glomerular filtration rate, this increase will be negated by the dehydration and subsequent retention of sodium and lithium. If the patient's fluid and electrolyte status is not corrected promptly, these diuretics may have a detrimental effect. These medications are not recommended for the patient with lithium toxicity. It is more prudent to achieve good hydration with a saline-containing intravenous solution, promoting sodium and water excretion by increasing the glomerular filtration rate. Hydration will increase lithium filtration as long as renal function is normal. Lithium was believed to be solely reabsorbed in the proximal tubules following filtration,[40] but recent evidence suggests that some lithium is also reabsorbed in the loop of Henle as well as the distal tubules.[5,13,28]

Elderly patients, patients with a history of cardiovascular disease, or anyone who uses a diuretic chronically is at risk for toxicity. Since lithium's resorption may occur almost anywhere in the kidney, almost any diuretic may produce an adverse effect. This occurs because lithium movement parallels that of sodium, and as sodium retention increases so does that of lithium.

Numerous other agents such as the nonsteroidal antiinflammatory agents, ACE inhibitors, and neuroleptics are also capable of producing complications when administered with lithium.

What Other Therapeutic Approaches Are Used for Lithium Toxicity?

Peritoneal dialysis and hemodialysis have been traditionally utilized to enhance lithium elimination. Recently more treatment options have become available, including sodium polystyrene sulfonate (SPS) and continuous venous or arterial hemodiafiltration. Before any of these modalities is considered, it is essential to decide which patients require any of these treatments, because other than SPS all the others are invasive and all including SPS have potentially significant complications.

Peritoneal Dialysis

Although peritoneal dialysis (PD) has previously been advocated in the treatment of lithium overdose, there is no current indication. Peritoneal dialysis is no more efficacious than the kidneys are in removing lithium.[12,59] The clearance of lithium by PD is between 10 and 15 mL/min, which is less than a normally functioning kidney.[58] With this very small clearance and the potential to cause such complications as bowel perforation, peritonitis, or sepsis, PD offers no benefit to the patient who has functioning kidneys. For this reason the only situation where PD may be beneficial is for a patient with renal failure who is already receiving PD and has a working PD catheter in place. In this circumstance PD could be started while more definitive therapy such as hemodialysis was being organized.

Hemodialysis

Lithium is a small ion, has no protein binding, and has a relatively small volume of distribution, making it readily dialyzable.[12] Thus definitive therapy for patients who manifest lithium toxicity and are in need of extracorporeal removal is hemodialysis (HD). Lithium's clearance via hemodialysis is solely dependent on blood flow, and clearances range from 70 to 170 mL/min, far greater than the kidney's potential.[15,18,26] Unfortunately, determining when to institute therapy is not always simple. Patients who are initially poisoned and have high levels but have no signs or symptoms may benefit the most from HD because lithium has not yet fully distributed to tissue compartments that are cleared less well than the plasma. But many of these patients will probably do well without HD, which has potential complications. On the other hand, once lithium has been distributed to the tissues, it is more difficult to remove with HD, and permanent sequelae may occur.[25]

When trying to determine who needs HD, it is best to consider whether or not the patient may become toxic if elimination is not enhanced. Because lithium is not metabolized and only renally excreted, any patient with renal failure or severe neurologic dysfunction should undergo hemodialysis. These patients cannot clear lithium and may suffer long-term complications of toxicity. Patients with altered mental status should undergo hemodialysis.[48] Patients who are stable, but may not be able to tolerate sodium repletion (those with congestive heart failure, pulmonary edema, anasarca), should also be considered candidates for early hemodialysis.

Although a patient with a mild tremor may not warrant HD, that patient must be monitored closely to ensure that further neurologic dysfunction does not occur, which would indicate a need to implement immediate HD. The last group of patients who should undergo hemodialysis is less easily defined. These are the patients with "high" lithium levels. The definition of high is arbitrary and also dependent on the history of the ingestion. In the patient who has an acute ingestion, with no previous body burden of lithium, a level of ≥ 4.0 mEq/L is used as the point when HD should be initiated.[25] At this level, as equilibration begins some lithium will be excreted, and some will cross the cellular membrane, but it is unlikely that the patient will be able to excrete the lithium rapidly enough to prevent a significant amount from entering the central nervous system and causing severe and potentially permanent neurologic toxicity.[4,24] On the other hand, a patient with an acute on chronic overdose or chronic overdose already has a body burden and therefore may suffer toxicity at a lower level.[25] For these patients a lithium level of ≥ 2.5 mEq/L should be used as an indication for HD. In either case the goal is to prevent the delayed neurologic complications.[23]

Patients who are hemodialyzed will frequently develop a "rebound" lithium level after treatment.[25] The reason for this is that dialysis clears only the plasma. A significant amount of lithium is in the intracellular space and redistributes slowly. Following treatment, there will be a rebound level as lithium leaves the intracellular space and reestablishes an equilibration by moving into the plasma.[15] Patients should have a lithium level drawn immediately following hemodialysis, and a repeat level should be performed 6 hours postdialysis. If either level is high, or if the patient continues to show signs of neurologic toxicity, a second dialysis may be needed. With this in mind, most patients should not have their dialysis catheters removed until it can be demonstrated that there will not be a significant rebound effect.

What Is the Role for Continuous Arteriovenous or Continuous Venovenous Hemodiafiltration (CAVH or CVVH)?

Recent studies indicate that CAVH may serve as an alternate therapy to hemodialysis.[6,9] Continuous arteriovenous hemodiafiltration works on the principle that as blood is constantly being filtered, any toxin that is present will be removed gradually from the body (see Chap. 5). The benefits of CAVH are that it is a continuous process; that although filtering takes place in a monitored setting, there is no need for specialized personnel as in HD; and that there may be fewer complications. There are several recent studies promoting this new form of therapy for lithium removal.[6,9,31] In the most recent study,[31] seven patients with severe lithium toxicity were evaluated, four with acute overdoses and three with chronic. The acutely overdosed patients underwent CAVH whereas the chronically overdosed were treated with CVVH. Clearances of 20–62 mL/min were achieved. Although the clearance is far less than that of HD, the total duration of the procedure was much longer, permitting similar total drug elimination. The authors found that CAVH and CVVH were both able to remove a significant amount of total body lithium burden and that all patients improved. In only one of their patients was there a rebound rise in the lithium level, a frequent problem with HD.[25,26] The authors suggested that this particular patient had received CAVH for only 18 hours. The authors concluded that CAVH or CVVH may represent an excellent method for the removal of lithium and in the prevention of a rebound elevation of lithium following the procedure. Because they were able to obtain larger clearances with CVVH, the advantages are the greater clearances over time and limitation of expense and expertise. Some disadvantages are the need to have the patient in a monitored setting for the entirety of the filtration process. HD remains a better modality in terms of speed of toxin removal and therefore may be better at preventing the gravest of complications: permanent neurologic deficits. Although more controlled studies must be performed with hemodiafiltration, it may play an important role in treating patients with lithium toxicity, especially when HD is not available. In addition, it may be useful to attenuate the rebound effect in patients who have completed HD. Currently CAVH and CVVH can not be recommended as the sole therapeutic intervention for lithium removal if HD is available.

Sodium Polystyrene Sulfonate (SPS)

Sodium polystyrene sulfonate, a cation ionic exchange agent commonly known as Kayexalate, is used extensively in patients with hyperkalemia. Its ability to bind potassium in exchange for sodium and then to permit excretion of the excessive potassium in the stool has made it a very valuable agent. Sodium polystyrene sulfonate is an effective treatment for hyperkalemia because the actual amount of potassium to be bound and excreted is small. Because of the similarities between lithium and potassium, SPS has also been considered as a possible agent in the treatment of lithium toxicity. Studies in dogs have shown that orally administered lithium could be cleared more rapidly if SPS was administered.[34] Subsequent animal studies have shown SPS to have beneficial effects in reducing levels when lithium is given intravenously or at a delayed phase of intoxication.[33] There is a single successful human case report.[20]

However, there are substantial concerns with the use of this agent. In the rodent studies, extremely large doses of SPS were needed to obtain significant lithium removal. The animals have received on the order of 10 g/kg of SPS and even the lower doses now under study are much larger than the doses usually given to patients with renal failure. The other major concern is this agent's effect on potassium. In mice the hypokalemia induced can be significant, and if extrapolated to humans this electrolyte shift would contraindicate the use of SPS.[32] Studies in humans present conflicting results of the absence of hypokalemia in patients after a single dose of SPS[8,54] or the need for replacement potassium following multiple doses of SPS.[44] It is reasonable to believe that this agent will induce hypokalemia in any dose comparable to those used in the study of experimental lithium toxicity. The use of this agent for lithium toxicity is theoretically good, but the potential complications of hypokalemia, dysrhythmias, hypernatremia and fluid overload, as well as the substantial amount of this agent that will be needed to achieve success, limit the drug's potential.

Summary

The complications of overexposure of the central nervous system to lithium are great, and therefore patients should be treated aggressively with HD when indicated, since it is difficult to predict which patients will suffer sequelae.

References

1. Aita JF, Aita JA, Aita VA: 7-Up anti-acid lithiated lemon soda or early medicinal use of lithium. Nebr Med J 1990; 75:277–279.
2. Alessi N, Naylor MW, Mohammad G, et al: Update on lithium carbonate therapy in children and adolescents. J Am Acad Child Psychiatry 1994;33:291–303.
3. Allison JH, Stewart MA: Reduced brain inositol in lithium treated rats. Nature N Biol 1971;233:267–268.
4. Apte SN, Langston WJ: Permanent neurological deficits due to lithium toxicity. Ann Neurol 1983;13:452–455.
5. Atherton JC, Doyle A, Gee A, et al: Lithium clearance: Modification by the loop of Henle in man. J Physiol 1990; 437:377–391.
6. Ayuso Gatell A, Leon Regidor MA, Mestre Saura J, et al: Acute lithium poisoning: Treatment with continuous arteriovenous hemofiltration. Rev Clin Exp 1989;185:195–197.

7. Baraban JM, Worley PF, Snyder SH: Second messenger and psychoactive drug action. Focus on the phosphoinositide system and lithium. Am J Psychiatry 1989;146:1251–1260.
8. Belanger DR, Tierne MG, Dickerson G: Effect of sodium polystyrene sulfonate on lithium availability. Ann Emerg Med 1992;21:1312–1315.
9. Bellomo R, Kearly Y, Parkin G: Treatment of life threatening lithium toxicity with continuous arterio-venous hemodiafiltration. Crit Care Med 1991;19:836–837.
10. Berridge MJ, Downes CD, Hanley RR: Neurological and development action of lithium. A unifying hypothesis. Cell 1989;59:411–419.
11. Berridge MJ, Downes CP, Hanley RR: Lithium amplifies agonist-dependent phosphatidylinositol response in brain and salivary gland. Biochem J 1982;206:587–595.
12. Blye E, Lorch J, Cartell S: Extracorporeal therapy in the treatment of intoxication. Am J Kidney Dis 1984;3:321–338.
13. Boer WH, Koomans HA, Dorhout Mees EJ: Lithium clearances in healthy humans suggesting reabsorption beyond the proximal tubules. Kidney Int 1990;37:S39–S44.
14. Chuang DM: Neurotransmitter receptors and phosphoinositide turnover. Annu Rev Pharmacol Toxicol 1989;29:71–110.
15. Clendeninn NJ, Pond SM, Kaysen G, et al: Potential pitfalls in the evaluation of the usefulness of hemodialysis for the removal of lithium. Clin Toxicol 1982;19:341–352.
16. Demers R, Lukesh R, Prichard J: Convulsions during lithium therapy. Lancet 1970;2:315–316.
17. Demers RG, Heninger G: Electrocardiographic changes during lithium therapy. Dis Nerv Syst 1970;31:674–677.
18. Feneves AZ, Emmett M, White MG: Lithium toxicity associated with acute renal failure. South Med J 1984;77:1472–1474.
19. Frazer A, Mendel J, Secunda SK, et al: The prediction of brain lithium concentration from plasma or erythrocyte measure. J Psychiatr Res 1973;10:1–7.
20. Gehrke JC, Watling SM, Gehrke CW, et al: In-vivo binding of lithium using the cation exchange resin sodium polystyrene sulfonate. Am J Med 1996;14:37–38.
21. Goodnick PJ, Fieve RR, Meltzer HC, et al: Lithium elimination half-life and duration of therapy. Clin Pharmacol Ther 1981;29:47–50.
22. Groth U, Prellwitz W, Jahnchen E: Estimation of pharmacokinetic parameter of lithium from saliva and urine. Clin Pharmacol Ther 1974;16:490–498.
23. Hansen HE, Amdisen A: Lithium intoxication. Q J Med 1978;14:123–144.
24. Hartitzch BV, Hoenich NA, Leigh RJ, et al: Permanent neurological sequelae despite hemodialysis. Br Med J 1972;4:757–759.
25. Jaeger A, Sauder P, Kopeferschmitt J, et al: When should dialysis be performed in lithium poisoning? A kinetic study in 14 cases of lithium poisoning. J Toxicol Clin Toxicol 1993;31:429–447.
26. Jaeger A, Sauder P, Kopeferschmitt J, et al: Toxicokinetics of lithium intoxication treated by hemodialysis. J Toxicol Clin Toxicol 1985;23:501–517.
27. Jones J, Mullen MJ, Dougherty J, et al: Repetitive doses of activated charcoal in the treatment of poisoning. Am J Emerg Med 1987;5:305–311.
28. Kirchner K: Lithium as a marker for proximal tubule delivery during low salt intake and diuretic infusion. Am J Physiol 1987;253:F188–F196.
29. Kofman O, Belmaker RH: Biochemical, behavior and clinical studies of the rate of inositol in lithium treatment and depression. Biol Psychiatry 1989;34:839–852.
30. Kudrow L: Lithium prophylaxis for cluster headache. Headache 1977;17:15–18.
31. LeBlanc M, Raymond M, Bonnardeaux A, et al: Lithium poisoning treated by high-performance continuous arterio-venous and venovenous hemodiafiltration. Am J Kidney Dis 1996;27:365–372.
32. Linakis JG, Hull KM, Lacouture PG, et al: Sodium polystyrene sulfonate treatment for lithium toxicity. Effects on serum potassium concentration. Acad Emerg Med 1996;3:333–337.
33. Linakis JG, Hull KM, Lee C, et al: Effects of delayed treatment with sodium polystyrene sulfate on serum lithium concentrations in mice. Acad Emerg Med 1995;2:681–685.
34. Linakis JG, Lacouture PG, Eisenberg MS, et al: Administration of activated charcoal or sodium polystyrene sulfonate (Kayexalate) as gastric decontamination for lithium intoxication: An animal model. Pharmacol Toxicol 1989;65:387–389.
35. Manji HK, Hsaio JK, Risby ED, et al: The mechanism of action of lithium: Effects on serotonergic and noradrenergic systems in normal subjects. Arch Gen Psychiatry 1991;48:505–512.
36. Manji HK, Potter WZ, Lenox RH: Signal transduction pathways. Molecular targets for lithium's action. Arch Gen Psychiatry 1995;52:531–543.
37. Mork A, Geiser A: Mode of action of lithium on the catalytic unit of adenylate cyclase from rat brain. Pharmacol Toxicol 1981;60:241–248.
38. Odagaki Y, Koyama R, Matsubara S, et al: Effects of chronic lithium treatment on serotonin binding sites in rat brain. J Psychiatr Res 1990;24:271–277.
39. Okusa MD, Jovita L, Crystal T: Clinical manifestations and management of acute lithium intoxication. Am J Med 1994;97;383–389.
40. Petersen V, Hvidt S, Thomsen K, et al: Effect of prolonged thiazide treatment on renal lithium clearance. Br Med J 1974;3:143–145.
41. Rana RS, Hokin LE: Role of phosphoinositides in transmembrane signaling. Physiol Rev 1990;70:115–164.
42. Richman CM, Makki MM, Weiser PA, et al: Effect of lithium carbonate on chemotherapy induced neutropenia and thrombocytopenia. Am J Hematol 1984;16:313–323.
43. Riegel JM, Becker CE: Use of cathartics in toxic ingestions. Ann Emerg Med 1981;10:254–258.
44. Roberge RJ, Martin TG, Schneider SM: Use of sodium polystyrene sulfonate in a lithium overdose. Ann Emerg Med 1993;22:1911–1915.
45. Sachs GS, Renshaw PF, Lafer B, et al: Variability of brain lithium levels during maintenance treatment: A magnetic resonance spectroscopy study. Biol Psychiatry 1995;38:422–428.
46. Sansone MEG, Ziegler DK: Lithium toxicity: A review of neurologic complications. Clin Neuropharmacol 1985;8:242–248.

47. Saul RF, Hamburger HA, Selhorst JD: Pseudotumor cerebri secondary to lithium carbonate. JAMA 1985;253:2869–2870.
48. Schou M: Long-lasting neurological sequelae after lithium intoxication. Acta Psychiatr Scand 1984;70:594–602.
49. Smith SW, Ling LJ, Halstenson C: Whole-bowel irrigation as a treatment for acute lithium overdose. Ann Emerg Med 1991;20:536–539.
50. Spyker DA: Activated charcoal reborn: Progress in poison management. Arch Intern Med 1985;145:43–44.
51. Strayhorn JM, Nash JL: Severe neurotoxicity despite "therapeutic" serum lithium levels. Dis Nerv Syst 1977;38: 107–111.
52. Thomsen K, Schou M: Renal lithium excretion in man. Am J Physiol 1968;215:823–827.
53. Tilkian AG, Schroeder JS, Kao JJ: Cardiovascular effects of lithium in man: A review of the literature. Am J Med 1976; 61:665–670.
54. Tomaszewski C, Musso C, Pearson JR, et al: Lithium absorption prevented by sodium polystyrene sulfonate in volunteers. Ann Emerg Med 1992;21:1308–1311.
55. Vacaflor L, Lehmann HE, Ban TA: Side effects and teratogenicity of lithium carbonate treatment. J Clin Pharmacol J New Drugs 1970;10:387–389.
56. White K, Cohen J, Nelson R, et al: Relationship between plasma, RBC and CSF lithium concentrations in human subjects. Int Pharmacopsychiatry 1979;14:185–189.
57. Whitworth P, Kendall DA: Effects of lithium on inositol phospholipid hydrolysis and inhibition of dopamine D_1 receptors mediated cyclic AMP formation by carbacol in rat brain slices. J Neurochem 1989;53:536–541.
58. Wilson JH, Donker AJ, van der Helm GK, et al: Peritoneal dialysis for lithium poisoning. Br Med J 1971;2:749–750.
59. Winchester JF: Evaluation of artificial organs: Extracorporeal removal of drugs. Artif Organs 1986;10:316–323.

CHAPTER 60

Opioids

Lewis S. Nelson

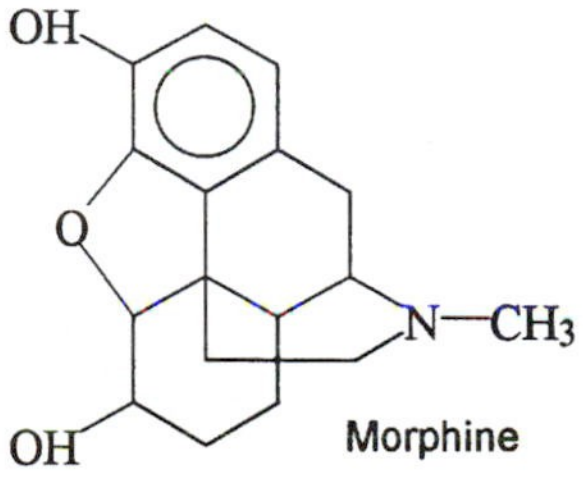

Morphine

The emergency medical service is requested to evaluate a 23-year-old man noted by the caller to be comatose. EMS arrives and finds that the patient is hypoventilating (2 breaths/min), is cyanotic, and has very small pupils. They take the patient to the ED. Earlier the same day the patient was evaluated in another municipal hospital for a similar condition, where he supposedly had a dramatic response to appropriate therapy. He was discharged shortly thereafter.

In the ED the patient is ventilated by bag-valve-mask while preparations are made to perform endotracheal intubation. Naloxone, 2 mg, is administered intravenously. The patient arouses from coma and his respiratory rate rises to 24. He looks uncomfortable, he develops diaphoresis, and his pupils dilate. Physical examination reveals bilateral pulmonary rales, with a normal cardiac examination. An arterial blood gas is performed: pH, 7.38; PCO_2, 28 mm Hg; PO_2 (on 40% Venti-mask), 140 mm Hg. A portable chest radiograph shows diffuse patchy infiltrates.

What Is the History of Opioid Use?

The medicinal value of opium, the dried extract of the poppy plant (*Papaver somniferum*) was recorded as far back as the Ebers papyrus.[95] Although reformulated as laudanum by Paracelsus,[196] as well as paregoric,[85] Dover's powder (pulvis Doveri), and Godfrey's cordial in later centuries, the content remained largely the same: phenanthrene poppy derivatives, such as morphine and codeine (methylmorphine). Over the intervening centuries since the Ebers papyrus, opium and its components have been exploited in two distinct directions. They have been used clinically to produce profound analgesia, and to this day find their widest clinical application in the relief of both acute and chronic suffering. Opioids are available in various formulations that allow administration by virtually any route (oral, parenteral [SQ/IV/IM], transdermal, transmucosal, epidural, intrathecal, transrectal, intranasal, as well as intrapulmonary [smoking]). Patients may also benefit from several of the nonanalgesic effects engendered by certain opioids. For example, codeine finds widespread use as an antitussive agent and diphenoxylate as an antidiarrheal drug.

Unfortunately, the history of the opioids is marred by mankind's quest for the pleasurable effects engendered by drugs. For example, opium smoking was so problematic in China by the early 19th century that the government attempted to prohibit its importation. This act led to the Opium Wars with Britain. China eventually conceded and, in addition to allowing importation and sale of the drug, was forced to turn over Hong Kong to British rule. The euphoric, and addictive, potential of the morphine is immortalized in the works of several famous writers, such as Thomas de Quincey (*Confessions of an English Opium Eater*, 1821), Samuel Coleridge (*Kubla Khan*), and Elizabeth Barrett Browning (*Aroura Leigh*, 1856).[8] Due to mounting concerns about addiction and toxicity, the Harrison Narcotic Act was passed in 1914, which made nonmedicinal use of opioids illegal. During the second half of the 20th century, use of an illicit semisynthetic morphine derivative, heroin (diacetylmorphine), rose to epidemic levels in the United States and today remains a prevalent street drug. Users claim that the modified drug has enhanced euphoric effects. Unfortunately, widespread intravenous use has led to many significant direct and indirect medical complications, particularly endocarditis and AIDS, in addition to fatal and nonfatal overdose. In a recent report it was stated that nearly two thirds of all long-term (>10 years) heroin users in Australia had self-overdosed on heroin.[30] Another group, studying a population of recent-onset heroin users, found that 23% had overdosed on heroin, and 48% had been present when someone else overdosed.[51] Recently, the rising purity and falling price of illicit heroin has fostered a resurgence of use in the United States.[68] However, heroin is now administered intranasally or smoked, routes that are suggested as "safe" alternatives to intravenous use.

What Is the Basis for the Function of Opioid Agents in Humans?

Despite nearly a century of study, the mere existence of opioid receptors was not proposed until 1954.[6] Beckett and Casy, synthetic chemists, noted a pronounced stereospecificity of existing opioids (only the *l*-isomer is active), and postulated the need for the drug to "fit" into a receptor. In 1963, after the study of the clinical interactions of nalorphine and morphine, the theory of receptor dualism was proposed,[98] which postulated the existence of two classes of opioid receptors. However, not until 1973 were such opioid binding sites demonstrated experimentally.[130] Intensive experimental scrutiny with selective agonists and antagonists continues to permit refinement of receptor classification. The current, widely accepted schema postulates the coexistence of three major classes of opioid receptors, each with multiple subtypes, as well as several poorly defined minor classes.

Initially, it was unclear why such an elaborate system of receptors existed, since no endogenous ligand could be identified. Evidence for the existence of such ligands was uncovered in 1975 with the discovery of met- and leu-enkephalin,[66] and the subsequent identification of β-endorphin and dynorphin. As a group, these endogenous ligands for the opioid receptors are called endorphins (*endo*genous mo*rphine*). Each is a five-amino-acid peptide, cleaved from a larger precursor peptide: pro-enkephalin, pro-opiomelanocortin, and pro-dynorphin, respectively. All three major opioid receptors have now been cloned and sequenced.[17] They each consist of seven transmembrane segments, along with an amino and a carboxy terminus. Significant sequence homology exists between their transmembrane regions and that of other members of the G protein–binding receptor superfamily. However, the intracellular and extracellular segments differ from one another. These nonhomologous segments probably represent the ligand binding region, which would be expected to differ between the three classes of receptors.

What Are the Physiologic Functions of the Opioid Receptor Subtypes?

Since there are multiple opioid receptors and each elicits a different effect, determining to which receptor an opioid agent binds preferentially can help predict its clinical effects. However, the binding of a drug is not limited to one receptor type, and it is the relative affinity for differing receptors that accounts for the clinical effects. Even the endogenous opioid peptides exhibit substantial crossover between receptors. A review of the current knowledge regarding opioid receptors is invaluable in understanding the clinical toxicology of these agents (Table 60–1). Although the familiar pharmacologic nomenclature derived from the Greek alphabet is used throughout this textbook, the International Union of Pharmacology (IUPHAR) Committee on Receptor Nomenclature has recommended a nomenclature change to align opioid receptor names with those of other neurotransmitter systems.[36] In this new schema the receptors are denoted by their endogenous ligand (*op*iates) with a subscript identifying their chronologic order of discovery. The δ receptor is therefore renamed as OP_1, κ as OP_2, and μ as OP_3. Interestingly, this group has not incorporated subtype nomenclature into their scheme, but state that addition of a subscripted letter would account for such distinctions (eg, OP_{1A} for μ_1).

TABLE 60–1. CLINICAL EFFECTS RELATED TO OPIOID RECEPTORS

μ_1	Supraspinal analgesia
	Peripheral analgesia
	Euphoria
	Prolactin release
μ_2	Spinal analgesia
	Respiratory depression
	Physical dependence
	Gastrointestinal dysmotility
	Miosis
	Pruritis
	Bradycardia
κ_1	Spinal analgesia
	Miosis
κ_2	Psychotomimesis
	Dysphoria
κ_3	Supraspinal analgesia
δ	Spinal analgesia
	Modulaton of μ receptor function
	Modulation of dopaminergic neurons

Mu Receptor (μ or OP_3)

The early identification of the μ receptor as the *m*orphine binding site has given this receptor its designation.[99] Although many exogenous agents produce supraspinal analgesia via μ receptors, an endogenous ligand has remained elusive. The likely candidate is β-endorphin although the discovery of morphine and other morphinans in mammalian brain[38] raises the possibility of a role for these nonpeptide opioids. Although it is unclear if the mammalian morphinan is a dietary component[55] or is truly endogenous, a tentative biosynthetic pathway in the rat liver has been described.[189] Additionally and equally unexplainable, opioid peptides may be found in cows' milk (morphicetin, casomorphin).[55]

Experimentally, there are two well-defined subtypes (μ_1, μ_2), although there are currently no agents with sufficient selectivity to make this dichotomy clinically relevant. It is the μ_1 subtype that appears to be responsible for supraspinal (brain) analgesia, as well as for the pleasurable euphoria sometimes engendered by these agents. Although stimulation at the μ_2 subtype will produce spinal level analgesia, this also produces respiratory depression. All currently available μ agonists have some activity at the μ_2 receptor and therefore engender some degree of respiratory compromise.[142] It is not unexpected that μ receptors are localized to the regions of the brain involved in analgesia (periaqueductal gray, nucleus raphe magnus, medial thalamus[50]), euphoria (limbic system), and respiratory function (medulla).[109] Also not surprisingly, μ receptors are found in the medullary cough center, peripherally in the gastrointestinal tract, and on sensory nerve endings such as articular surfaces (see Analgesia section).

Kappa Receptor (κ or OP_2)

Although it is now known that dynorphins are the endogenous ligands for κ receptors, these receptors were originally identified by their ability to bind ketocyclazocine (thus κ).[99] Kappa receptors exist predominantly in the spinal cord of higher animals, although they are also found in the antinociceptive regions of the brain[106] as well as the substantia nigra.[190] Stimulation is responsible for spinal analgesia, miosis (less so than μ), and diuresis (via inhibition of ADH release). Unlike μ, however, κ-receptor stimulation is not associated with significant respiratory depression or constipation. The κ receptor has been subclassified based into three subtypes. The κ_1 receptor subtype is responsible for spinal analgesia;[134] this analgesia is not reversed by μ-selective antagonists, supporting the role of κ receptors as independent mediators of analgesia. Although the function of the κ_2 receptor is largely unknown, stimulation of cerebral κ_2 receptors by agents such as pentazocine may produce psychotomimesis (dysphoria) in distinction to the euphoria evoked by μ agonists.[131] The κ_3 receptor is widespread in the brain and appears to participate in supraspinal analgesia. This receptor is primarily responsible for the action of nalorphine, an agonist–antagonist.[128] Nalbuphine, another agonist–antagonist, exerts its analgesic effect via both κ_1 and κ_3 agonism, although it is an antagonist to morphine at the μ receptor.[133]

Delta Receptor (δ or OP_1)

Little is known about δ receptors, although enkephalins appear to be their endogenous ligand. Opioid peptides identified in the skin and brain of *Phyllomedusa* frogs[83] (dermorphin and deltorphin, respectively) are potent agonists at the δ receptor. Delta receptors may be important in spinal and supraspinal analgesia,[136] probably through a noncompetitive interaction with the μ receptor.[147,174] Delta receptors may also mediate dopamine release from the nigrostriatal pathway, where they modulate the motor activity associated with amphetamine.[69] Delta receptors do not modulate dopamine in the mesolimbic tracts and have little behavioral reinforcing role. Subpopulations, δ_1 and δ_2, have been postulated based on in vitro studies, but not confirmed in vivo.[174]

Sigma Receptor (σ)

Although originally conceived as an opioid subtype,[99] the σ receptor is no longer considered to be opioid in nature. Continued investigation into this receptor revealed that it is insensitive to antagonism by naloxone, which is considered to be the sine qua non of opioid character.[181] In addition, the σ receptor prefers ligands with a dextrorotatory stereochemistry, in distinction to all other opioid receptors, which prefer levorotatory isomers. The effects of the σ receptor are none the less relevant to opioid pharmacology since certain opioids, such as dextromethorphan and pentazocine, are σ-receptor agonists. Sigma-receptor stimulation is implicated in psychotomimesis and movement disorders, effects that have been reported with dextromethorphan and pentazocine.[113] Neuroleptic agents, such as haloperidol, bind strongly to the σ receptor.[34,35]

Other Receptors (ϵ, ζ)

The current scheme of opioid receptors while clinically useful has some pharmacologic shortcomings. Two recently discovered opioid receptor subtypes, while largely uncharacterized, may prove valuable following additional research and are worth mentioning. The epsilon receptor (ϵ) is postulated on the basis of in vivo binding assays and has no known clinical role,[120] nor has its presence in humans been identified. The zeta (ζ) receptor has been proposed and may serve as an opioid growth factor receptor.[200] This receptor has not been identified in humans.

What Is the Cellular Mechanism by Which Opioids Produce Their Effects?

Opioid Receptor Signal Transduction Mechanisms

Continuing research into the mechanisms by which an opioid receptor induces an effect on the receptor-bearing cell has produced confusing and often contradictory results (Fig. 60–1). Despite the initial thought that each receptor subtype is linked to a specific transduction mechanism, continued research has found that any receptor subtype may utilize one of several different mechanisms depending on where the receptor is located (eg, presynaptic vs postsynaptic). All opioid receptor subtypes are members of a superfamily of membrane-bound receptors that are coupled to GTP binding proteins or G proteins.[109] The G protein is responsible for signaling the cell that the receptor has been activated and for the initiation of the desired cellular effects. The G proteins are typical of the pertussis-toxin sensitive, inhibitory subtype, known as G_i or G_0. These G proteins consist of three conjoined subunits (α, β, γ), from which the βγ subunit is liberated upon the binding GTP to the α subunit. Upon dissociation from the βγ subunit, the α subunit activates specific effector systems, such as phospholipase C or adenylate cyclase, or it alters a channel or transport protein. The GTP is hydrolyzed by a GTPase intrinsic to the α subunit, which prompts its reassociation with the βγ subunit.[146]

cAMP. Inhibition of adenylate cyclase activity by inhibitory G proteins (G_i or G_0) is the classic mechanism for postsynaptic signal transduction invoked by the μ recep-

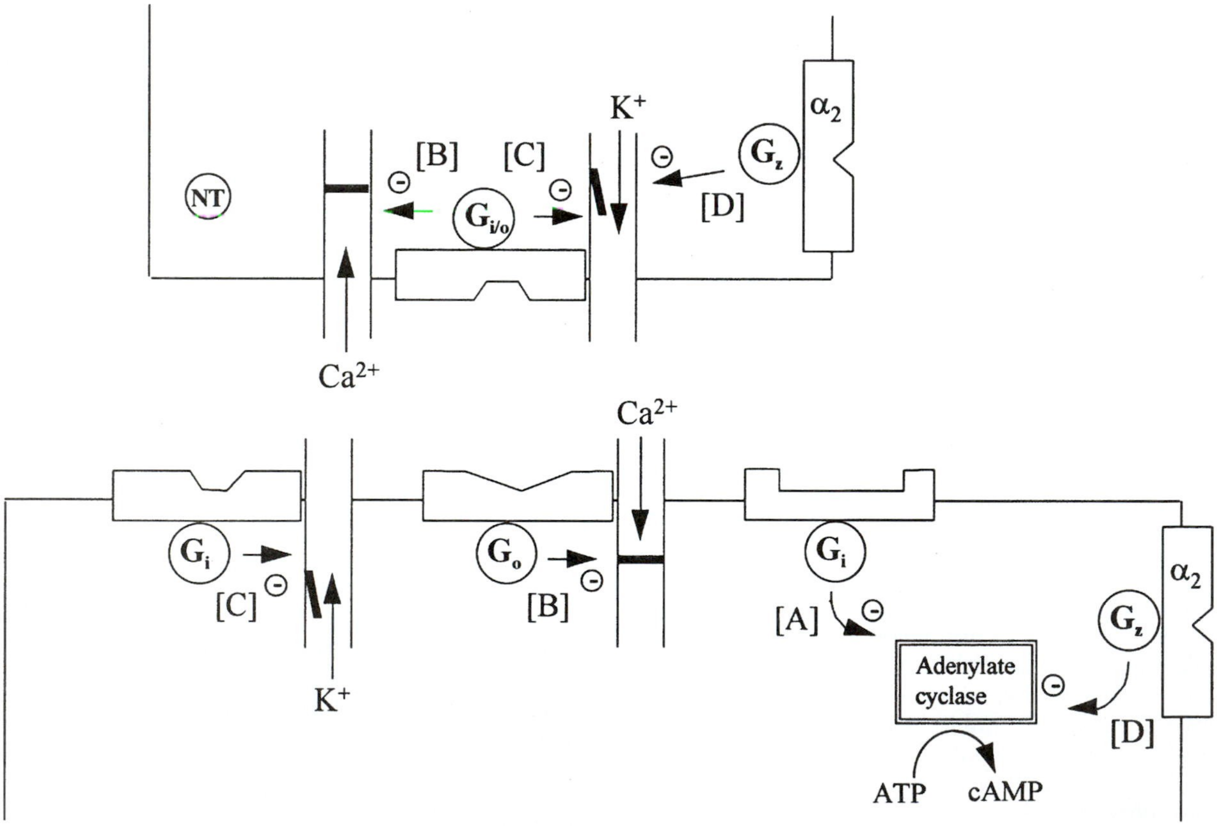

Figure 60–1. Opioid receptor signal transduction mechanisms. Upon binding of an opioid agonist to an opioid receptor, the respective G protein is activated. G_i and G_0 mediate inhibitory effects within the cell. They may [A] reduce the capacity of adenylate cyclase to produce cAMP; [B] close Ca^{2+} ion channels and reduce the signal to release neurotransmitters or perpetuate an action potential; [C] open K^+ channels and hyperpolarize the cell, which indirectly reduces the cell's activity. Each mechanism has been found coupled to each receptor subtype depending on location of the receptor (pre/postsynaptic) as well as of the neuron within the brain (see text). Note that α_2 receptors [D] mediate similar effects, although use a different G protein (G_z).

tor.[176] However, this same mechanism has also been identified in cells bearing either δ or κ receptors.[20,197]

Potassium Channels. Increased conductance through a potassium channel results in membrane hyperpolarization with reduced neuronal excitability. Opening of the potassium channel is mediated by a G protein (G_i or G_0) and has been shown to occur in individual cells bearing one of the three receptor subtypes.[52,121]

Calcium Channels. Presynaptic μ receptors inhibit norepinephrine release from the nerve terminals of cells of the rat cerebral cortex. Adenylate cyclase does not appear to be the modulator for these receptors, since the inhibition of norepinephrine release is not enhanced by raising intracellular cAMP levels by various methods.[153] Opioid-induced blockade is, however, prevented by increased intracellular calcium levels induced either by calcium ionophores, which increase membrane permeability to calcium, or by raising the extracellular calcium concentration.[153] This implies a role for opioid-induced closure of *N*-type calcium channels presumably via a G protein.[59] Reduced intraterminal concentrations of calcium prevent the neurotransmitter-laden vesicles from binding to the terminal membrane and releasing their contents. Nerve terminals containing dopamine appear to have an analogous relationship with inhibitory κ receptors, as do acetylcholine-bearing neurons with δ opioid receptors.[153]

TABLE 60–2. CLINICAL EFFECTS OF OPIOIDS

Cardiovascular	Peripheral vasodilation Orthostatic hypotension
Pulmonary	Respiratory depression Bronchospasm (histamine mediated) Pulmonary edema
Neurologic	Sedation, coma Seizures (meperidine, propoxyphene) Antitussive
Dermatologic	Flushing (histamine) Pruritis
Endocrinologic	Reduced ADH release Reduced gonadotropin release
Gastrointestinal	Reduced motility Reduced gastric acid secretion Increased biliary tract pressure Increased anal sphincter tone
Ophthalmologic	Miosis

What Are the Important Clinical Effects Mediated by the Opioids?

Analgesia

Although classical teaching attributes analgesia to the brain, research into the mechanism of opioid analgesia has uncovered several distinct underlying components (see Table 60–2). Opioids appear to modulate cerebral cortical pain perception at supraspinal, spinal, and peripheral levels. The regional distribution of the opioid receptors confirms that μ receptors are responsible for most of the analgesic effects of morphine within the brain. They are found in highest concentration within areas of the brain classically associated with analgesia, ie, the periaqueductal gray, nucleus raphe magnus, locus ceruleus, and medial thalamus.[127] Microelectrode-induced electrical stimulation of these areas[143] or iontophoretic application of an agonist into these regions results in profound analgesia.[9] Specifically, enhancement of inhibitory outflow from these supraspinal areas to the sensory nuclei of the spinal cord (dorsal roots) dampens nociceptive neurotransmission. Additionally, inactivation of the μ-opioid receptor gene in embryonic mouse cells results in offspring that are insensitive to morphine analgesia.[100] These mice maintain normal concentrations of other opioid receptor subtypes, which are able to bind ligands.

Delta and κ receptors are responsible for mediation of analgesia as well, but they are found in the spinal cord, not in the brain (spinal analgesia). Agents with strong binding affinity for δ receptors in humans produce significantly more analgesia than morphine when both are individually administered intrathecally.[110] Indeed, the utility of spinal and epidural opioid analgesia is predicated on the direct administration of opioid near these receptors. Although agents with specificity toward δ or κ receptors, especially delivered intrathecally, would conceivably produce the most analgesia with the least systemic toxicity, no such agents are clinically available in the United States. Conceptually, these receptors modulate nociceptive impulses in transit to the thalamus via the spinothalamic tract to reduce the brain's perception of the pain.

Recent research has indicated that communication between the immune system and the peripheral sensory nerves occurs in areas of tissue inflammation. In response to inflammatory mediators (eg, interleukin-1[151]), immune cells release opioid peptides locally, which bind and activate peripheral opioid receptors on sensory nerve terminals. Agonism at these receptors reduces afferent pain neurotransmission and may inhibit the release of other pro-inflammatory compounds such as substance P.[164] Of note, intraarticular morphine (1 mg) administered to patients after arthroscopic knee surgery has been shown to produce significant, long-lasting analgesia that can be prevented with intraarticular naloxone.[165] The clinical analgesic effect of 5 mg of intraarticular morphine is equivalent to 5 mg of morphine given intramuscularly.[22] Analgesia appears to be locally mediated by μ receptors.

Euphoria

Many of the drugs abused by humans because they produce pleasurable effects appear to have those effects mediated through the release of dopamine in the mesolimbic system.[37] This final common pathway is shared by the opioids that activate the μ/δ receptor complex in the ventral tegmental area that indirectly induces release of dopamine in the mesolimbic region.[115] Opioids may also have a direct reinforcing effect on heroin self-administration through μ receptors within the mesolimbic system.[58]

The sense of well-being and euphoria associated with strenuous exercise appears to be mediated by endogenous opioid peptides and μ receptors. This so-called runner's high is acutely reversible with naloxone,[32] and naloxone may also produce dysphoria in nonexercising, highly trained persons. Even in normal individuals, high-dose naloxone (up to 4 mg/kg) may produce dysphoric symptoms,[25] but no other adverse effects.

Exogenous opioids do not induce uniform psychologic effects. Some, particularly the highly lipophilic agents such as heroin, result in euphoria and a sense of well-being, while morphine is largely devoid of such pleasurable effects.[160] Morphine is largely analgesic, anxiolytic, and sedating. Fentanyl produces effects that are noted to be subjectively similar to heroin by chronic users.[80] In fact fentanyl rapidly became the most prevalent substance of abuse among anesthesiologists in the 1970s.[183] Interestingly, certain opioids, such as pentazocine, may produce dysphoria. This is presumably related to their affinity for an alternative binding site, likely κ, or the σ receptor.[131]

How Is Opioid Toxicity Diagnosed and Treated?

When used correctly for medical purposes, opioids are remarkably safe and effective agents.[5,88] However, excessive dosing, whether with therapeutic, suicidal, or euphoric intent, may result in significant toxicity. Most of the effects are predictable based on the "opioid" pharmacology of the agents (ie, respiratory depression), although several agents produce unexpected "nonopioid" or agent-specific responses. These drugs are specifically addressed below. In general, patients poisoned by agonist agents are at greater risk of death than are those exposed to agonist–antagonists, partial agonists, or obviously, antagonists.[142] Among the agonist opioids, equianalgesic doses of all agents produce approximately the same degree of respiratory depression.[39,158]

Determining that a patient is suffering from opioid toxicity is generally more important than identifying the specific agent involved. Notwithstanding some minor variations, patients intoxicated by all available opioids predictably develop a constellation of signs known as the opioid toxidrome (see Chap. 17). Mental status depression, hypoventilation, miosis, and reduced bowel motility are classic components. This toxidrome is a logical extension of the known therapeutic and toxic effects of opioids.

The clinically consequential effects of acute opioid poisoning are central nervous system and respiratory depression. Although early support of ventilation and oxygenation is generally sufficient to prevent death, prolonged use of bag-valve-mask ventilation and endotracheal intubation may be avoided by cautious administration of an opioid antagonist. Opioid antagonists, such as naloxone, competitively inhibit the binding of opioid agonists to the opioid receptors, allowing the patient to resume spontaneous respiration. Naloxone competes at all receptor subtypes and is efficacious at reversing almost all adverse effects mediated through opioid receptors. A complete discussion of naloxone and other opioid antagonists can be found in Antidotes in Depth: Opioid Antagonists.

However, since most clinical findings associated with opioid intoxication are nonspecific, the diagnosis requires clinical acumen and a heightened clinical suspicion. Differentiating acute opioid intoxication from other etiologies with similar clinical presentations may be challenging. Patients presenting with a classic opioid toxidrome, found in an appropriate environment, or those with fresh needlemarks require little corroborating evidence. However, subtle presentations of opioid intoxication may be encountered, and other entities superficially resembling opioid poisoning may be seen in patients not exposed to opioids.

Hypoglycemia, hypoxia, and hypothermia are common, readily treatable clinical presentations that share features with opioid intoxication. Each is rapidly diagnosed with routinely available, real-time testing. Other drugs responsible for similar clinical presentations may include clonidine, phencyclidine (PCP), phenothiazines, and sedative-hypnotic agents, primarily benzodiazepines. In such patients, however, clinical evidence usually is available to assist in diagnosis. For example, nystagmus is nearly always noted in PCP-intoxicated patients, hypotension or electrocardiographic abnormalities in phenothiazine-poisoned patients, and coma with virtually normal vital signs in those poisoned by benzodiazepines. Most difficult to differentiate on clinical grounds may be toxicity produced by the centrally acting antihypertensive agents, such as clonidine (see section on clonidine). Of course, myriad traumatic, metabolic, and infectious etiologies must always be considered and evaluated appropriately, and may occur simultaneously.

In the absence of suggestive history or obvious clinical findings, the empiric administration of naloxone may assist in diagnosis. Naloxone, even at extremely high doses, has an excellent safety profile in nonopioid-using patients, such as those with spinal cord injury[11] and acute ischemic stroke.[123] However, adminstration of naloxone to opioid-dependent patients is not without adverse effect. Precipitation of an acute withdrawal syndrome is common. The agitation, hypertension, and tachycardia produced, although rarely life threatening, may produce significant distress to both the patient and the clinical staff. Additionally, emesis commonly occurs in acute withdrawal. This may become problematic in patients who do not regain consciousness immediately after naloxone. Examples of such situations include patients with concomitant intoxication with ethanol or sedative-hypnotic agents or those with head trauma. Particularly challenging are patients on methadone maintenance therapy who present with nonopioid-overdose-related etiologies of altered mental status. All of these groups of patients are at extremely high risk for pulmonary aspiration of gastric contents following acute withdrawal–related emesis.

Small doses of naloxone (0.1–0.4 mg) are generally necessary to reverse intoxication in most patients with an acute opioid overdose. Since precipitation of withdrawal is potentially detrimental and often unpredictable, low initial naloxone doses with rapid escalation is advocated to limit such events yet allow timely treatment of patients needing higher doses. The goal of therapy with naloxone is not necessarily complete arousal, but rather reinstitution of adequate spontaneous ventilation. However, in patients in whom the clinical circumstances are unclear, complete arousal to normal consciousness may be desirable both to diagnose and to prevent misdiagnosis.

Identification of patients likely to respond to naloxone would conceivably reduce the unnecessary and potentially dangerous precipitation of withdrawal in opioid-dependent patients. Routine prehospital administration of naloxone to all patients with subjectively assessed mental status or respiratory depression was not beneficial in 92% of the 813 patients.[198] Another study of unconscious patients presenting to an ED via EMS attempted to determine factors that would predict a response to a therapeutic dose of naloxone (2 mg).[63] Although not perfectly sensitive, the finding of a respiratory rate less than or equal to 12 breaths/min best predicted the response to the naloxone. Interestingly, in hospitalized patients, neither respiratory rate less than 8 breaths/min nor coma was able to predict a response to naloxone.[191] Whether the discrepancy between the latter two studies is due to the definition of respiratory depression (8 vs 12 breaths/min), or if patients with prehospital overdose present differently than those with therapeutic misadventures while in the hospital, is unclear. Regardless, relying on the respiratory rate to assess the need for ventilatory support or naloxone administration is not ideal since hypoventilation secondary to a reduction in tidal volume may precede that due to respiratory rate depression.[145,158]

Since heroin injection is often performed in "shooting galleries," heroin overdose often occurs in the presence of other heroin users. In recent studies of heroin users, 80% of users in Australia and 48% in London had been present when another user overdosed. Based on these factors and the aforementioned excellent safety profile of naloxone, a trial of distribution of naloxone to heroin users has recently been recommended[169] by some. While earlier administration of antidote would certainly be beneficial, certain issues make this approach controversial. The short duration of action of naloxone makes resedation likely and, without appropriate observation, potentially lethal. Even more problematic is the precipitation of acute withdrawal. Also, the inevitable attempt to try to "overcome" the naloxone with high doses of heroin is likely to result in significantly more-profound adverse effects after the naloxone antagonism inevitably ends.

TABLE 60–3. HOW TO USE A NALOXONE INFUSION

1. If naloxone bolus is successful, administer 2/3 of the initial dose per hour by IV infusion; frequently reassess the patient's respiratory status.
2. If respiratory depression is not reversed following the bolus dose:
   Intubate the patient, as clinically indicated. Administer up to 10 mg of naloxone as an intravenous bolus. If the patient does not respond, do not initiate an infusion.
3. If the patient develops withdrawal following the bolus dose:
   Allow the effect of the bolus to abate.
4. If respiratory depression recurs, administer 1/2 the initial bolus dose, and begin an intravenous infusion at 2/3 of the bolus dose per hour. Frequently reassess the patient's respiratory status.
5. If the patient develops withdrawal signs or symptoms during the infusion:
   Stop the infusion until the withdrawal symptoms abate. Restart the infusion at 1/2 the rate; frequently reassess the patient's respiratory status. Exclude withdrawal from other substances.
6. If the patient develops respiratory depression during the infusion:
   Readminister 1/2 of the initial bolus and repeat until reversal occurs. Increase the infusion by 1/2 the initial rate; frequently reassess the patient's respiratory status. Exclude continued absorption, readministration of opioid, or other etiologies for the respiratory depression.

Patients with recurrent or profound poisoning by long-acting opioid agents, such as methadone, or patients with large gastrointestinal burdens ("body packers") may require continuous infusion of naloxone to permit continued adequate spontaneous ventilation (Table 60–3). Pharmacokinetic studies have revealed that an hourly infusion rate of two thirds of the initial reversal dose of naloxone is sufficient to prevent recurrence.[48] Titration of the dose may be necessary, either up or down, as the clinical situation indicates. Although repetitive bolus dosing of naloxone may be effective, it is labor intensive and subject to delay. The availability of long-acting opioid antagonists such as naltrexone and nalmefene[72] may permit single-dose reversal of methadone intoxication. However, the associated risk of precipitation of a persistent withdrawal syndrome argues against the use of these agents for initial reversal.

What Are the Expected Clinical Findings in Opioid-Using Patients?

Respiratory Depression

An experimental rat model utilizing various opioid agonists and antagonists demonstrated that μ_2 receptors were primarily responsible for the respiratory depression associated with morphine.[89] Opioid agonists reduce ventilation by diminishing the sensitivity of the medullary chemoreceptors to hypercapnea.[186] In addition to the loss of hypercarbic stimulation, opioids also depress the ventilatory response to hypoxia.[186] The combined loss of hypercarbic and hypoxic drive leaves virtually no stimulus to breathe, and apnea ensues. Although some opioids, notably the agonist–antagonists, demonstrate a ceiling effect on respiratory depression, this is generally at the expense of analgesic potency.[45] This is likely due to differential effects at the opioid receptor subtypes; ie, agonist–antagonists are predominantly κ receptor agonists, and either partial agonists or antagonists at μ sites. Patients started on methadone maintenance develop chronic hypoventilation, although tolerance to the loss of hypercarbic drive develops over several months.[96] However, such patients never develop complete tolerance to the loss of hypoxic stimulation.[150]

As previously noted, ventilatory depression may be secondary to a reduction either in respiratory rate or in tidal volume. Although more accessible to measure, the respiratory rate is not an ideal index of ventilatory depression. In humans, morphine-induced respiratory depression correlates more closely with changes in tidal volume.[158] Escalating doses of opioids may result in a loss of respiratory rate as well.

Noncardiogenic Pulmonary Edema

Reports linking opioids with the development of noncardiogenic pulmonary edema (NCPE) began to accumulate in the 1960s, although the earliest report can be traced to Osler in 1880[125] and perhaps even earlier.[73] Virtually all opioids have been implicated, and noncardiogenic pulmonary edema is reported in diverse clinical situations. No single pathogenetic mechanism can be consistently invoked, and several prominent theories are each well supported by experimental data. Typically, the patient awakens to an opioid antagonist and over the subsequent several minutes to hours is noted to desaturate and develop pulmonary rales. Occasionally, classic frothy, pink sputum is noted to be present in the mouth or nares, or in the endotracheal tube of an intubated patient. Pulmonary edema was described in 48% of 149 hospitalized heroin overdose patients in New York City in the early 1970s.[31]

Although several authors relate the occurrence of NCPE to the administration of naloxone, the majority of reported patients suffered respiratory arrest and were administered naloxone to reinstitute breathing. It is likely in these patients that naloxone merely "uncovered" NCPE that was masked by the inability to adequately assess breath sounds in hypoventilating patients. The initially reported cases were postoperative patients who were given naloxone because they did not rapidly resume spontaneous breathing.[138,171] In addition to suffering likely apneic events (ie, the reason they needed naloxone) and possibly hypoxia, these patients all received multiple intraoperative medications, further clouding the diagnosis. Pulmonary edema may be the only clinical finding suggesting hypoxic damage, however, and many patients have minimal, if any, indication of hypoxic damage to other organs. However, multisystem organ failure may occur in severely poisoned patients. Whether the lung is selectively more susceptible to hypoxia is unclear.

Although naloxone is overwhelmingly safe when administered to nonopioid-tolerant individuals, the acute induction of withdrawal may be responsible for "naloxone-induced" NCPE. Such acute withdrawal is associated with massive sympathetic discharge from the central nervous system. This same mechanism has been implicated in "neurogenic" NCPE. Indeed, in an interesting series of experiments, induced hypercarbia and precipitated opioid withdrawal in nontolerant dogs was associated with dramatic cardiovascular changes and abrupt elevation of serum catecholamine levels.[107,108] The effect was more dramatic in dogs with elevated PCO_2 than those with normal or low PCO_2 suggesting the need to adequately ventilate patients prior to reversal with naloxone. However, while abrupt precipitation of withdrawal by naloxone may contribute to the development of NCPE, it cannot be the sole effect. Pulmonary edema was noted in nearly 50 to 90% of the postmortem examinations performed on heroin-overdose patients, many of whom were declared dead before arrival to medical care and thus never received naloxone.[57,62] In addition, neither naloxone, nor any other opioid antagonist, was available when Osler and others described their initial cases of pulmonary edema.

A mechanical explanation has also been postulated. Attempted inspiration against a closed glottis (the Müller maneuver) creates a negative pressure within the bronchial tree and alveoli. Creation of this pressure gradient across the alveolar membrane draws fluid into the air sacs and may additionally damage the capillary membranes.[77] This effect may be especially prominent at the time of naloxone administration, in which case breathing may be reinstituted before the return of adequate upper airway function, allowing the vocal cords to block the glottic opening.

Cardiovascular Effects

Arteriolar and venous dilation secondary to opioid use may result in mild reduction in blood pressure.[184] This effect is clinically useful for the treatment of acute pulmonary edema. However, while patients are not expected to develop significant supine hypotension, orthostatic changes in blood pressure and pulse are routinely seen.[201] Bradycardia is uncommon, although slow heart rates are commonly seen and are due to the associated reduction in central nervous system stimulation. Opioid-induced hypotension appears to be mediated by histamine release.[43] Induction of histamine release does not appear to occur through interaction with an opioid receptor. It may be related to the nonspecific ability of certain compounds to activate mast cell G proteins,[4] which directly induce degranulation of histamine-containing vesicles. Many agents share this ability, which seems to be conferred by the presence of a positive charge on a hydrophobic molecule.[4] Accordingly, not all opioids are equivalent in their ability to release histamine.[4] After administration of one of four different opioids to 60 generally healthy patients, meperidine was noted to produce the most, and fentanyl the least, hypotension and elevation of plasma histamine levels.[44] The combination of H_1

and H_2 antagonists is effective in ameliorating the hemodynamic effects of opioids in humans.[132] A beneficial role for naloxone, although claimed to be effective,[142] may occur only with extremely high doses.[49]

Prominent cardiovascular toxicity may be noted with propoxyphene, which induces wide complex dysrhythmias and negative contractility through sodium channel antagonism similar to type IA antidysrhythmic agents (see Propoxyphene). Adulterants or co-ingestants may also produce significant cardiovascular toxicity. For example, quinine adulteration of heroin is associated with dysrhythmias.[92,157] Cocaine, which was surreptitiously added to heroin, contributed to a myocardial infarction suffered by a 24-year-old man.[65] Similarly, concern that naloxone administration may "unmask" cocaine toxicity in patients simultaneously using cocaine and heroin ("speedball") is probably warranted, although never reliably reported.[104]

Miosis

The mechanism by which opioids induce miosis remains controversial, and support for each of several mechanisms may be found. Stimulation of parasympathetic pupilloconstrictor neurons in the Edinger-Westphal nucleus of the oculomotor nerve produces miosis. Additionally, morphine increases firing of pupilloconstrictor neurons to light,[84] which increases the sensitivity of the light reflex (central reinforcement of light reflex).[188] Also, although sectioning of the optic nerve may blunt morphine-induced miosis, the consensual reflex in the denervated eye is enhanced by morphine.[102] Since opioids classically mediate inhibitory neurotransmission, hyperpolarization of sympathetic nerves, or hyperpolarization of inhibitory neurons to the parasympathetic neurons (removal of inhibition), may ultimately be found to mediate the classic "pinpoint pupil" associated with opioid use.

Not all opioid-using patients present with miosis. Meperidine and propoxyphene toxic patients regularly maintain normal pupillary size,[46] and morphine reportedly caused mydriasis in a liver transplant patient.[156] Patients using agents with predominantly κ agonist effects (eg, pentazocine) may not develop miosis. Severely poisoned patients may have hypoxic–anoxic mydriasis. Additionally, concomitant drug use or the presence of adulterants may alter pupillary size. For example, the combination of heroin and cocaine ("speedball") may produce virtually any size pupil depending on the patient's relative intoxication by each drug. Additionally, in the recent epidemic of scopolamine-adulterated heroin, patients routinely were noted to have large, "anticholinergic" pupils.[129]

Seizures

Seizures are a rare complication of the therapeutic use of most opioids. In patients with acute opioid overdose, seizures are likely to be related to hypoxia. However, experimental models in which morphine is microinjected into various brain regions of animals demonstrate a pro-convulsant effect.[175] This effect is not inhibited by naloxone, suggesting that a mechanism other than opioid receptor binding is involved. Interestingly, morphine-induced seizures in humans is only reported in neonates.[78] This may be related to incomplete formation of the neonatal blood–brain barrier.

Naloxone antagonizes the convulsant effects of heroin and propoxyphene in mice, although it is not nearly as effective in preventing seizures from meperidine or its metabolite, normeperidine.[47] Naloxone also potentiates the anticonvulsant effects of benzodiazepines and barbiturates, although it antagonizes that of phenytoin.[67]

Seizures should be anticipated in patients, however, with meperidine, propoxyphene, or tramadol toxicity. These agents are discussed below. The ability of fentanyl to induce seizures remains controversial. After several reported cases of fentanyl-induced seizures,[141] electroencephalograms (EEG) and electromyelograms (EMG) were performed on 127 patients undergoing fentanyl anesthesia.[162] When assessed clinically, about one third were considered to have had a seizure. However, in no case did the corresponding EEG reveal epileptiform activity. It appears likely that the rigidity and myoclonus associated with fentanyl is readily misinterpreted as a seizure.

Rigidity

With rapid intravenous injection of certain high-potency opioids, especially fentanyl, patients may experience acute muscular rigidity. This rigidity primarily involves the trunk and may impair chest wall movement and exacerbate hypoventilation. Although the mechanism is currently unclear, it has been postulated that it is related to blockade of dopamine receptors in the basal ganglia.[40] Indeed dopamine,[182] but not amantadine,[180] has alleviated the rigidity. Recent experimental data suggests that the α_2-adrenergic receptor may also be involved.[187] Regardless of the mechanism, mechanical impairment of ventilation may contribute to lethality during epidemics of fentanyl-adulterated heroin.[79] Chest wall rigidity is common in patients undergoing operative anesthesia and may necessitate administration of neuromuscular blocking agents to allow artificial ventilation. Opioid antagonists may be therapeutic[114] but may produce adverse hemodynamic effects and uncontrollable pain during the intraoperative or postoperative period.

Nausea and Vomiting

Historically, the morphine analog apomorphine was used as an emetic. Emesis induced by apomorphine is mediated through agonism at dopamine-2 receptor subtypes within the chemoreceptor trigger zone of the medulla. It is not clearly established whether these effects are inhibited by naloxone. This is particularly interesting given the aforementioned ability of other opioids to function as antagonists at dopamine receptors and produce rigidity.

Which Opioids Require Special Consideration?

Although the vast majority of opioid-poisoned patients will follow predictable clinical courses, several select opioids may produce atypical toxicity. Some effects can be anticipated, such as fentanyl-induced rigidity, whereas others, such as those induced by contaminants, cannot. Therefore careful clinical assessment and institution of empiric therapy is necessary to ensure proper management (Table 60–4).

Agonist–Antagonist Agents

Most opioids in clinical use tend to have specific binding affinity toward one class of opioid receptor (usually μ). However, this selectivity diminishes as the dose escalates. The mixed agonist–antagonist agents differ in that they interact with multiple receptor types at clinically relevant doses. Also, while most opioids typically produce either agonist or antagonist effects, these agents may have agonist effects at one receptor subtype yet antagonistic effects at another. Pentazocine, for example, may elicit a withdrawal syndrome in a μ opioid–tolerant individual due to antagonist or partial agonist effects at the μ receptor. This effect is the basis for the claim of an "allergy" to pentazocine in methadone-dependent patients. However, this same drug can induce substantial analgesia in nontolerant patients through its agonist effects at κ_1 receptors.

Methadone and Other Long-Acting Opioids

Methadone is a prevalent synthetic opioid that finds its greatest utility as a maintenance agent for patients addicted to heroin. In such circumstances, it replaces the illicit substance with a legal, oral, and long-acting agent and allows patients to abstain from activities associated with procurement and intravenous administration of heroin. Patients are generally given high therapeutic doses to prevent surreptitious illicit drug use.[168] As a μ agonist, methadone is able to prevent (and treat) opioid withdrawal. However, patients taking excessive doses may develop toxicity identical to that of morphine with an important difference: the duration of effect of methadone is very prolonged (about 24 hours). Although patients with uncomplicated heroin overdose may typically be discharged from the ED after an appropriate observation period if they are no longer symptomatic,[159] those with methadone overdose always require hospital admission due to the likelihood of prolonged or recurrent toxicity. In fact, resedation should be expected in patients responding appropriately to naloxone since the duration of effect of naloxone is only about 1 hour. In many cases, continuous infusion of naloxone is needed to maintain adequate ventilation (see Treatment).

Accidental methadone ingestion by children is particularly problematic, as it is often formulated as a palatable liquid and may not have appropriate child-resistant caps. Unfortunate trends toward an increasing number of childhood poisonings with methadone have been noted in England that is likely related to increased prescription of the drug.[7] Death is not infrequent in these children.[7] A newly approved agent, levo-α-acetylmethadol (LAAM, Orlaam), may prove to be even more problematic since its duration of effect is about 3 days.[137,172] Additionally, patients who overdose on sustained-release morphine preparations (eg, MS Contin) should be managed similarly to those with methadone toxicity, with extra emphasis perhaps placed on gastrointestinal decontamination with activated charcoal.

Propoxyphene

Like its structural analog methadone, propoxyphene binds μ opioid receptors producing typical opioid clinical findings, the most life threatening of which is respiratory arrest. However, in overdose, other dangerous pharmacologic properties of propoxyphene may become manifest. Propoxyphene, and its hepatic metabolite, norpropoxyphene, produce fast sodium channel blockade on the myocardium, identical to that seen with class IA antidysrhythmic agents such as quinidine.[91] The result of this blockade is QRS complex widening, as was noted in 19% of 222 propoxyphene-overdose patients.[94] The QRS complex widening may be improved with the parenteral administration of hypertonic sodium bicarbonate[167] or with lidocaine.[192] As in patients with tricyclic antidepressant overdose, the sodium ion component of the sodium bicarbonate enhances sodium influx through a partially occluded sodium channel by augmenting the extracellular to intracellular sodium concentration gradient. The paradoxical effect of lidocaine, another sodium channel blocker, may be explained by the very different dissociation constants of these two agents with the sodium channel.[192] Lidocaine, a minimally toxic agent of the IB class, rapidly associates and dissociates with the sodium channel, effectively competing for binding with the slowly dissociating, and therefore more highly toxic agents, propoxyphene and norpropoxyphene. Naloxone has never been demonstrated to be effective therapy for the cardiotoxic effects of propoxyphene, although in one reported case hemodynamic improvement was related to naloxone-induced propoxyphene (opioid) withdrawal.[54]

Propoxyphene overdose may also produce acute central nervous system toxicity usually manifested as seizures. In one study of propoxyphene-overdose patients, 10% of the subjects developed seizures. Although the exact mechanism is unclear, experimental models demonstrate that only propoxyphene, and not norpropoxyphene, is capable of inducing seizures.[91] Therapy for seizures should follow standard management strategies, including benzodiazepines or barbiturates. Phenytoin has not been studied, but is not expected to be beneficial. Naloxone is reported to prevent propoxyphene-induced seizures in some animal models,[47] although other models have found no effect.

TABLE 60–4. CLASSIFICATION, POTENCY, AND CHARACTERISTICS OF OPIOID AGENTS

Agent (Representative brand name)	Classification[a]	Derivation	Analgesic dose (mg) equivalent to 10 mg morphine SC[b]	Comments[a,c]
Buprenorphine (Buprenex)	P	Semisynthetic	0.4 IM	
Butorphanol (Stadol)	AA	Semisynthetic	2 IM	
Codeine	Ag	Natural	120 PO	Often combined with acetaminophen
Dextromethorphan (Robitussin DM)	NEC	Semisynthetic	Nonanalgesic (10–30 PO)	Antitussive; psychotomimetic via σ receptor
Diphenoxylate (Lomotil)	Ag	Synthetic	Nonanalgesic (2.5 PO)	Antidiarrheal agent, often combined with atropine; difenoxin is potent metabolite
Fentanyl (Sublimaze)	Ag	Synthetic	0.125 IM	Very short acting (< 1 h)
Heroin	Ag	Semisynthetic	5 SC	Diacetylmorphine
Hydrocodone (Hycodan)	Ag	Semisynthetic	10 PO	
Hydromorphone (Dilaudid)	Ag	Semisynthetic	1.3 SC	
Levorphanol (Levodromoran)	Ag	Semisynthetic	2 SC/IM	
Loperamide (Imodium)	Ag	Synthetic	Nonanalgesic (2 PO)	Antidiarrheal agent
Meperidine, pethidine (Demerol)	Ag	Synthetic	75 SC/IM	Seizures due to metabolite accumulation
Methadone (Dolophine)	Ag	Synthetic	10 IM	Very long acting (24 h)
Morphine	Ag	Natural	10 SC/IM	
Nalbuphine (Nubain)	AA	Semisynthetic	10 IM	
Nalmefene (Revex)	Ant	Semisynthetic	Nonanalgesic (0.1 IM)	Long-acting antagonist (4–6 h)
Naloxone (Narcan)	Ant	Semisynthetic	Nonanalgesic (0.1–0.4 IV/IM)	Short-acting antagonist (0.5 h)
Naltrexone (Trexan)	Ant	Semisynthetic	Nonalgesic (50 PO)	Very-long-acting antagonist (24 h)
Oxycodone (Percocet)	Ag	Semisynthetic	10 PO	Often combined with acetaminophen
Oxymorphone (Numorphan)	Ag	Semisynthetic	1 SC	
Paregoric (Parapectolin)	Ag	Natural	25 mL PO	Tincture of opium
Pentazocine (Talwin)	AA	Semisynthetic	50 SC	Psychotomimetic via σ receptor
Propoxyphene (Darvon)	Ag	Synthetic	65 PO	Seizures, cardiac dysrhythmias; often combined with acetaminophen
Tramadol (Ultram)	Ag	Synthetic	50–100 PO	Seizures at therapeutic dose

[a]Agonist antagonists, partial agonists and antagonists may cause withdrawal in tolerant individuals. Ag = full agonist (μ_1, μ_2, κ); AA = agonist–antagonist (κ agonist, μ antagonist); Ant = full antagonist (μ_1, μ_2, κ antagonist); P = partial agonist (μ_1, μ_2, agonist, μ_1, κ antagonist); NEC = not easily classified.
[b]Typical dose (mg) for agents without analgesic effects is given in parenthesis.
[c]Duration of therapeutic clinical effect ~ 3–6 h unless noted; likely to be exaggerated in overdose.

Propoxyphene is often formulated with acetaminophen (Darvocet-N) or salicylates for additive analgesic effects. In the setting of acute overdose, patients may suffer toxicity from either of these two nonopioid analgesics. Since patients may be poisoned by acetaminophen yet be asymptomatic or manifest opioid toxicity, empiric quantitative serum analysis for the drug is indicated. Additionally, delayed peak serum acetaminophen concentrations after ingestion of combination opioid products (such as Darvocet-N®) may occur.[1,173] In such patients, serial assessment of the serum acetaminophen concentration may be necessary to define the need for antidotal therapy.

Meperidine

Meperidine is a widely used agent for the treatment of chronic and acute pain. Although not prevalent as an illicit drug, at least one dramatic epidemic was associated with its attempted synthesis (see MPTP). Patients chronically using meperidine, especially those with renal insufficiency, are at risk for development of normeperidine toxicity.[71] Normeperidine is an active, renally eliminated hepatic metabolite that is associated with excitatory neurotoxicity, typically tremor, myoclonus, or seizures. These seizures are typically not responsive to naloxone. In fact, there is experimental evidence that naloxone may potentiate the seizures due to meperidine, presumably by inhibiting an anticonvulsant effect of meperidine.[28]

Although primarily an opioid, meperidine is capable of exerting effects at other receptor classes. The most consequential are the serotonin effects. Particularly in patients using monoamine oxidase inhibitors (MAOI), meperidine-induced excessive release of presynaptic serotonin may produce the serotonin syndrome,[13] characterized by muscle rigidity, hyperthermia, altered mental status, and death (see Chap. 58). Treatment for this potentially lethal drug interaction involves cooling the patient and administering muscle relaxants (benzodiazepines, nondepolarizing neuromuscular blockers). Occasionally, serotonin antagonists have been administered with questionable benefit. It should be noted that dextromethorphan is also associated with this syndrome. The serotonin syndrome has not been associated with the conjoint use of MAOIs and morphine, fentanyl, or methadone and would not be expected based on the currently appreciated pharmacology of these drugs.

Diphenoxylate and Loperamide

Although structurally similar to meperidine, the extreme insolubility of diphenoxylate limits absorption from the gastrointestinal tract. This factor may enhance its utility as an antidiarrheal agent, which presumably occurs via a local opioid effect at the gastrointestinal μ receptor. The standard adult formulation may result in significant systemic absorption and toxicity in children, and all such ingestions should be deemed consequential. Diphenoxylate is typically formulated with a small dose (0.025 mg) of atropine (as Lomotil), largely to enhance its antidiarrheal effect, but perhaps also to discourage illicit use.

Since both components may be absorbed and since their kinetics differ, a biphasic clinical syndrome is occasionally noted, although such an analysis is unreliable clinically.[101] That is, patients may manifest atropine poisoning (anticholinergic toxidrome) either independently or concomitantly with the opioid effects of diphenoxylate. Delayed onset of toxicity is widely reported and is classically explained as secondary to delayed gastric emptying since both opioids and anticholinergics produce this effect. However, delayed symptomatology following diphenoxylate ingestion is more likely explained by the accumulation of the hepatic metabolite, difenoxine, which is a significantly more potent opioid[148] and possesses a longer serum half-life.[74] A recent review of 36 pediatric reports of Lomotil overdoses found that although naloxone was effective in reversing the opioid toxicity, recurrence of central nervous system and respiratory depression was common.[101] This series included a patient with an asymptomatic presentation 8 hours postingestion, who was observed for several hours and discharged. This patient returned to the ED 18 hours postingestion with marked signs of atropinism.[101] In this same series, children with delayed onset of respiratory depression and other opioid effects were reported,[101] and cardiopulmonary arrest 12 hours postingestion has also been reported.[29] Presumably due to the delayed gastric emptying associated with Lomotil, pills were retrieved by gastric lavage as late as 27 hours postingestion.[149] Naloxone infusion may be appropriate for patients with recurrent signs of opioid toxicity. Due to the delayed and possibly severe consequences, all children, and adult patients with potentially significant ingestions of this substance, should be admitted for monitored observation in the hospital.

Loperamide (Imodium) is another insoluble meperidine analog that is used to treat diarrhea. Since this agent is available without a prescription, the paucity of adverse patient outcomes currently reported in the medical literature suggests that the safety profile of this agent is extremely high.

Pentazocine

Historically, patients abusing pentazocine (Talwin) administered it with tripelennamine (a blue capsule, thus Ts and Blues),[33] but concomitant abuse of pentazocine with methylphenidate is now more frequently reported.[15] Despite its agonist–antagonist effects as mentioned above, pentazocine abuse still occurs.[16] However, at high doses, psychotomimetic effects may be noted, which may be mediated by κ_2 or σ receptors. Since pentazocine is readily dissolved, intravenous injection was a preferred route for its abuse until the commercial formulation was altered in 1983 to include naloxone (Talwin NX®).[135] When ingested, the naloxone is eliminated through first-pass hepatic metabolism. However, if injected, the naloxone is active and prevents the pleasurable effects sought by users. Interestingly, potentiation of pentazocine analgesia by low-dose naloxone has been reported and is presumably due to positive allosteric interactions at the μ or κ receptor.[86]

MPTP

In 1982, several cases of acute, severe parkinsonian symptoms in known intravenous drug users were studied.[82] Due to the severe bradykinesia, these patients were labeled "frozen addicts." Investigation into the source of the disease led to the discovery of MPTP (1-methyl-4-phenyl-1,2,3,6-tetrahydropyridine), an inadvertent product of synthesis of an illicit meperidine analog MPPP

(1-methyl-4-phenyl-4-propionoxy-piperidine). The MPTP was accidentally produced in a clandestine laboratory through incorrect heating of the synthetic mixture. Further experiments revealed that MPTP is metabolized by monoamine oxidase-B in glial cells to MPP^+, a paraquat-like agent capable of selectively destroying dopamine-containing substantia nigra cells[177] through inhibition of mitochondrial oxidative phosphorylation.[117] Pretreatment with deprenyl, a monoamine oxidase-B inhibitor, prevented toxicity.[56] Although the index cases initially responded to standard antiparkinsonian medications, none improved substantially with medical therapy.[2] Although catastrophic for those patients exposed, MPTP is invaluable in experimental models for the study of Parkinson's disease.[53] Interestingly, several of the original "frozen" patients underwent stereotactic implantation of fetal tissue into their basal ganglia and the results are encouraging.[42]

Dextromethorphan

Codeine and dextromethorphan are two opioid agents used as cough suppressants. Dextromethorphan is available over the counter primarily due to its presumed lack of significant addictive potential. However, it is unlikely that cough suppression is mediated via an opioid receptor since the ability of other opioids to suppress the medullary cough centers is not correlated with their analgesia effect. That is, while very low, nonanalgesic, doses of codeine effectively suppress cough,[142] morphine, even at analgesic doses, does not. Dextromethorphan is devoid of analgesic properties altogether, even though it is the optical isomer of levorphanol, a potent opioid analgesic. The receptor pharmacology of dextromethorphan is extremely complex. It appears to bind to opioid receptors and produce miosis and central nervous system depression, but only at high doses. In addition, reversal of toxicity by naloxone is reported in children[155] and adults.[152] Binding to NMDA receptors and inhibition of calcium influx through this receptor channel may account for its role as a neuroprotectant in ischemic injury.[24,166] Movement disorders, described as choreoathetoid or dystonia-like, are reported and may be due to dopaminergic receptor binding. Interaction of dextrorphan, the active metabolite of dextromethorphan, at the σ receptor produces a phencyclidine-like psychosis.[76,170] The formulation of dextromethorphan as the hydrobromide salt accounts for the unusual finding of bromide toxicity in a patient with long-term use[116] (see Chap. 15). Recently, recreational abuse of dextromethorphan was reported, with expectations of euphoria and hallucinations,[112,194] and such abuse has become problematic in some sections of the country.

Clonidine

Although not related to any opioid in structure, clonidine-intoxicated patients may appear identical to those poisoned by morphine or another μ-active opioid. In fact, other imidazoline agents (eg, tetrahydrozaline) as well as other centrally acting α_2 agonists (eg, guanabenz) produce similar toxicity. Patients present with lethargy, miosis, bradycardia, and respiratory depression, although hypotension is generally more pronounced than with opioids. Children, in particular, may develop periodic apnea. Experimentally, there is functional overlap between α_2 and μ receptors. That is, both receptors may be found on the same neuron, and both are coupled via G proteins at a specific K^+ channel.[81] Activation of this K^+ channel produces neuronal hyperpolarization that reduces its rate of firing. This duality of activation of the K^+ channel explains the otherwise odd finding that naloxone, which is opioid specific, improves the level of consciousness and ventilatory status in certain children with clonidine poisoning.[3,193] However, since naloxone does not reduce the duration of symptoms in these children, admission is warranted to observe for recurrent symptoms. The standard dosing regimen used for naloxone in opioid-toxic patients should be used.

Clonidine may be useful in the amelioration of the sympathomimetic symptoms of opioid withdrawal. Since clonidine binds the α_2 receptors in the locus ceruleus, it reduces the enhanced noradrenergic output that remains after the inhibitory effects of opioids resolve. This accounts for the use of clonidine to treat the catecholaminergic symptoms of withdrawal, such as tachycardia, hypertension, agitation, and nausea. Note that the subjective effects such as craving are not ameliorated (see Chap. 70).

Tramadol

Despite nearly 20 years of use worldwide, tramadol has only recently been approved for use in the United States; it is marketed as Ultram. Tramadol is a novel analgesic agent with both opioid and nonopioid mechanisms responsible for its clinical effects. Although it binds only moderately to μ opioid receptors,[140] tramadol exhibits cross-tolerance with morphine in rats,[75] suggesting an opioid-mediated mechanism of analgesia. The demethylated metabolite, M1, exhibits higher affinity binding to μ receptors in vitro and may be important in patients chronically managed with tramadol. However, the role of M1 in the acute analgesic effect is not well defined.[26] Naloxone eliminates only about one third of tramadol-induced analgesia in humans, suggesting that an independent, nonopioid mechanism is important in mediating the clinical effects of tramadol.[26] The nonopioid analgesic effect appears to be mediated by inhibition of reuptake of biogenic amines, specifically serotonin and norepinephrine.[140] Overdose analysis is limited to 115 cases reported to the manufacturer,[119] as well as 71 patients collected in a recent prospective series.[163] Seizures are reported in both therapeutic dosing and overdose.[119,163] Tramadol-related seizures are not responsive to naloxone, but are suppressed with benzodiazepines. In fact, the package insert cautions against the use of naloxone in tramadol overdose, as the risk of seizure is increased and the outcome not improved in animal models treated with naloxone.[178] Additionally, one patient in the prospective series who received naloxone immediately seized.[163] Although patients may develop symptoms typical of an opioid toxidrome, significant respiratory depression is uncommon.[163] Respiratory depression, if noted, should respond to naloxone.[144,163] Drug screening was negative for opioids in all tramadol-intoxicated patients who were tested.[163] Additionally, patients using monoamine oxidase inhibitors are at risk for development of the serotonin syndrome due to the enhanced synaptic concentration of biogenic amines associated with tramadol use.

Heroin Body Packers

In an attempt to transport illicit drugs from one country to another, "mules" or "body packers" ingest large numbers of multiply wrapped packages of concentrated cocaine or heroin. After arrival at their destination, cathartics are self-administered and the packets are passed and delivered. However, after being discovered by authorities, patients may be taken to the hospital for evaluation and observation. Although generally asymptomatic, they are at risk for delayed and prolonged toxicity from packet rupture.[179] An abdominal radiograph is usually sufficient for confirmation of gastrointestinal smuggling[61] but cannot provide information about the contents of the packets. Both ultrasonography[61] and computed tomography[105] are also useful but should be considered only in patients with equivocal radiographs. Regardless of the content, appropriate treatment for asymptomatic patients should include whole-bowel irrigation with polyethylene glycol solution (see Chap. 4 and Antidotes in Depth: Whole Bowel Irrigation). However, unlike patients body packing cocaine in whom surgery is mandatory upon the development of symptoms, those with heroin packets can often be managed nonoperatively with continuous-infusion naloxone,[48] activated charcoal, and whole-bowel irrigation. Although rapid urine testing for drugs of abuse may assist in determining the packet content,[18] the same information is usually obtained more quickly and reliably by asking the patient, determining the country of origin, or identifying toxidromes. Intestinal perforation or obstruction by the packets generally requires surgical intervention. Packets that do not progress beyond the stomach should probably be removed surgically, although endoscopic removal of one or several packets may be carefully performed. However, the need to remove multiple packets requires multiple reinsertions of the endoscope, and packet rupture by the endoscope is possible.

Contaminants

Quinine. The history of heroin contamination alone could fill a textbook chapter. Historically, alkaloids (quinine, strychnine) were used to adulterate heroin in order to mimic the bitter taste of heroin and mislead clients. Quinine may have first been added to quell an epidemic of malaria among intravenous heroin users in New York City in the 1930s[57] and has been implicated as a causative factor in an epidemic of heroin-related deaths in the District of Columbia between 1979 and 1982.[90] Users of quinine-adulterated heroin in New York City[19] and Chicago[87] were noted to suffer from a significantly increased incidence of tetanus during the 1950s and early 1960s, when compared to users of non-quinine-adulterated heroin. Likely due to the extensive tissue destruction caused by extravasated quinine and subcutaneous administration ("skin popping"), this also occurs in patients receiving intramuscular quinine for therapeutic reasons.[199] Interestingly, wound botulism, a rare disease of similar etiology to tetanus, has been reported in several intravenous drug users,[93] although the link with quinine adulteration has not been evaluated. Additional toxicity attributed to quinine in heroin users includes cardiac dysrhythmias (see Cardiovascular Effects), amblyopia,[14] and thrombocytopenia.[23] Whether quinine is still an important adulterant is unclear. Trend analysis of illicit wholesale and retail (street-level) heroin adulteration over a 12-year period in Denmark revealed that while caffeine, acetaminophen, methaqualone, and phenobarbital were all prevalent adulterants, quinine was not found.[70] In Spain from 1985 to 1987, street-level heroin did not contain quinine. A British analysis of wholesale samples from the late 1980s did not report any with quinine adulteration.[124] Data on adulteration in the United States is unavailable.

Fentanyl Analogs. Fentanyl (Sublimaze) is a short-acting, highly potent opioid agonist widely used in clinical medicine. While fentanyl has approximately 50–100 times the potency of morphine, sufentanil, another prevalent anesthetic opioid, is 5–10 times the potency of fentanyl.[142] In some regions of the country, fentanyl and illicit fentanyl analogs (such as 3-methyl fentanyl or para-fluorofentanyl) are prevalent drugs of abuse.[202] Seasoned heroin users could not easily differentiate fentanyl from heroin, although the heroin was noted to provide a more intense "rush."[80] However, regional epidemics of heroin substitution with "superpotent" heroin occasionally produce a dramatic rise in heroin-related fatalities. Typically, the patients present comatose and apneic, with no opioids detected on blood and urine analysis.[12] In most cases, unsuspecting users self-administer their usual dose of heroin, which contains variable amounts of an illicit fentanyl analog. Epidemic death from a fentanyl analog known as "China White" first appeared in Orange County, California, in 1979 and was traced to α-methylfentanyl.[79] Similar epidemics of "China White" poisoning in Pittsburgh (1988) and again in Philadelphia (1992) were experienced, although the adulterant in these cases was 3-methylfentanyl, another potent analog.[60,97] A more recent epidemic in New York City marked the reappearance of 3-methylfentanyl.[118] Due to their profound potency (up to 6000 times more potent than morphine), higher than usual doses of naloxone may be needed to successfully compete for the opioid receptor.

Others. Poisoning by scopolamine-tainted heroin reached epidemic levels in New York City in 1995.[129] Exposed patients presented with acute psychosis and unmistakable anticholinergic signs. Several patients received physostigmine with excellent results. Other reported adulterants have included thallium,[139] lead,[126] cocaine,[65] amphetamines,[21] chloroquine,[122] and strychnine.[64]

In the early 1980s, an epidemic of spongiform leukoencephalopathy appeared in the Netherlands that only affected persons inhaling heroin pyrolysate.[195] These users inhaled the thick white smoke that is generated by vaporizing the heroin with a hand-held flame. Despite extensive investigation, no toxic adulterants were identified, but the epidemiology of the epidemic makes contamination suspect.

Are There Any Special Considerations Regarding the Laboratory Evaluation of Opioid Exposed Patients?

Although it is tempting to seek confirmation of the ingested substance in acutely poisoned patients, current laboratory methodology suffers from several important limitations and confounding variables. In general, the greatest impediment to the use of laboratory testing in the acute care setting is the lack of instantaneous reporting of results. Patients may suffer grave consequences if therapy is withheld pending test results. Opioid-poisoned patients, in particular, are amenable to rapid clinical diagnosis due to the uniqueness of the opioid toxidrome. Additionally, the availability of several distinct classes of agents capable of producing similar opioid effects limits the utility of laboratory tests that rely on structural features to identify drugs, such as immunoassays. There are currently no bioassays, analogous to the botulism assay for example, that are based on the production of observable effects in animals to classify, although not identify, a toxin. Furthermore, since there are remarkable differences in test availability, and the accuracy and sensitivity of each test differs, interpretation of the test results may be difficult. Overall, test results cannot be considered in isolation and must be viewed along with the entire clinical picture. Several well-described problems with laboratory testing for opioids are described in this section, and an overview of laboratory issues is available in Chapter 6.

Cross-reactivity

Many opioids share remarkable structural similarities. Interestingly, structurally similar agents do not necessarily produce consistent clinical characteristics (methadone and propoxyphene for example) (Figure 60–2). Since, as noted, most assays depend on structural features to identify a drug, similar agents may be detected in lieu of the desired drug. Whether a similar drug is noted by the assay depends on the sensitivity and specificity of the assay used, as well as the serum concentration of the agent. Some are predictable such as the cross-reaction of codeine with morphine on a variety of screening tests.[27] Others are less so, as with the cross-reaction of dextromethorphan with the PCP component of the fluorescence polarization immunoassay (Abbott TDx®),[103,185] a widely used drugs-of-abuse screening test (see Chap. 67).

Congeners and Adulterants

Commercial opioid assays are unlikely to detect most of the semisynthetic and synthetic opioids. Oxycodone, hy-

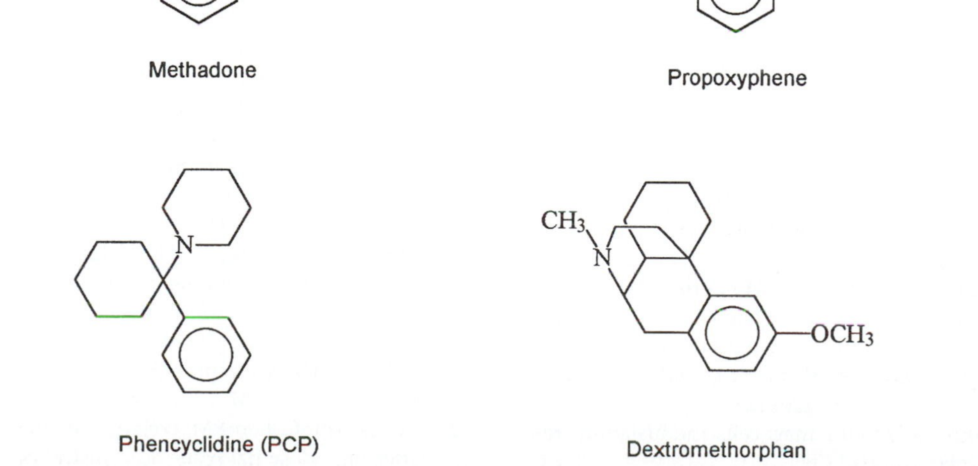

Figure 60–2. The structural similarities between methadone and propoxyphene and between phencyclidine and dextromethorphan.

drocodone, and other prevalent morphine derivatives have variable detectability by different opioid screens.[161] Epidemic fatalities involving fentanyl derivatives remained unexplained despite what appeared to be obvious opioid toxicity, until the ultrapotent fentanyl derivative, α-methylfentanyl, was detected.[79] Adulterants, such as scopolamine, acetaminophen, or salicylates, are obviously not detected as morphine on an opioid screen and may be overlooked.

Drug Metabolism

The metabolism of therapeutic doses of codeine to morphine will produce a positive opioid screen independently of the cross-reactivity just described. However, the metabolism of heroin to morphine forms the basis for the identification of morphine as the screen for heroin use. Since the presence of morphine on a drugs-of-abuse screen may suggest illicit heroin use, determination of the serum codeine is desirable in these patients. Even this is not foolproof, as codeine is often present in the morphine initially used to synthesize heroin.

A similar, and fascinating, problem may arise in patients who ingest moderate to large amounts of poppy seeds.[41] These seeds, which are widely used for culinary purposes, are derived from poppy plants similar to *P. somniferum* and contain both morphine and codeine. Patients may develop dramatically elevated serum morphine and codeine concentrations.[41,154] In patients who test positive for morphine and deny heroin use, assessment of another metabolite of heroin, 6-monoacetylmorphine, should alleviate the confusion.[111] Humans cannot acetylate morphine and therefore cannot make monoacetylmorphine, but can deacetylate heroin (diacetylmorphine) to this detectable product.

Summary

For several important reasons, opioid use is widespread. Overdose and toxicity, both intentional and innocent, remain a major cause of drug-related morbidity and mortality. An appreciation of the pharmacologic differences between the various opioid agents allows rapid diagnosis of poisoned patients and selection of the appropriate therapy.

References

1. Augenstein WL, Kulig KW, Rumack BH: Delayed rise in serum drug levels in overdose patients despite multiple dose charcoal and after charcoal stools. Vet Hum Toxicol 1987;29:491. Abstract.
2. Ballard PA, Tetrud JW, Langston JW: Permanent human parkinsonism due to 1-methyl-4-phenyl-1,2,3,6-tetrahydropyridine (MPTP): Seven cases. Neurology 1985;35:949.
3. Bamshad MJ, Wasserman GS: Pediatric clonidine intoxication. Vet Hum Toxicol 1990;32:220–223.
4. Barke KE, Hough LB: Opiates, mast cells and histamine release. Life Sci 1993;53:1391–1399.
5. Barsan WG, Tomassoni AJ, Seger D, et al: Safety of high-dose narcotic analgesia for emergency department procedures. Ann Emerg Med 1993;22:1444–1449.
6. Beckett AH, Casy AF: Synthetic analgesics: Stereochemical considerations. J Pharm Pharmacol 1954;6:986–1001.
7. Binchy JM, Molyneux EM, Manning J: Accidental ingestion of methadone by children in Merseyside. Br Med J 1994;308:1335–1336.
8. Bishop K: Drugs and art—Thomas DeQuincey and Elizabeth Barrett Browning. J R Soc Med 1994;87:128–131.
9. Bodnar RJ, Williams CL, Lee SJ, Pasternak GW: Role of μ_1-opiate receptors in supraspinal opiate analgesia: A microinjection study. Brain Res 1988;447:25–37.
10. Borsodi A, Toth G: Characterization of opioid receptor types and subtypes with new ligands. Ann NY Acad Sci 1995;757:339–352.
11. Bracken MB, Shepard MJ, Collins WF, et al: A randomized clinical trial of methylprednisolone and naloxone used in the initial treatment of acute spinal cord injury: Results of the Second National Acute Spinal Cord Injury Study. N Engl J Med 1990;322:1405–1411.
12. Brittain JL: China White: The bogus drug. J Toxicol Clin Toxicol 1982;19:1123–1126.
13. Browne B, Linter S: Monoamine oxidase inhibitors and narcotic analgesics: A critical review of the implications for treatment. Br J Psychiatry 1987;151:210–212.
14. Brust JCM, Richter RW: Quinine amblyopia related to heroin addiction. Ann Intern Med 1871;74:84–86.
15. Carter HS, Watson WA: IV pentazocine/methylphenidate abuse—The clinical toxicity of another T's and blues combination. J Toxicol Clin Toxicol 1994;32:541–547.
16. Challoner KR, McCarron MM, Newton EJ: Pentazocine (Talwin) intoxication: Report of 57 cases. J Emerg Med 1990;8;67–74.
17. Chen Y, Mestek A, Liu J, et al: Molecular cloning and functional expression of a μ-opioid receptor from rat brain. Mol Pharmacol 1993;44:8–12.
18. Cherardi RK, Leporc P, Dupeyron JP, et al: Detection of drugs in the urine of body packers. Lancet 1988;i: 1076–1079.
19. Cherubin CE: Epidemiology of tetanus in narcotic addicts. NY State J Med 1970;70:267–271.
20. Chneiweiss H, Glowinski J, Premont J: Mu and delta opiate receptors coupled negatively to adenylate cyclase on embryonic neurons from the mouse striatum in primary cultures. J Neurosci 1988;8:3376–3382.
21. Choudry N, Doe J: Inadvertent abuse of amphetamines in street heroin. Lancet 1986;1:817.
22. Christensen O, Christensen P, Sonnenschein C, et al: Analgesic effect of intraarticular morphine. A controlled, randomized and double-blind study. Acta Anaesthesiol Scand 1996;40:842–846.
23. Christie DJ, Walker RH, Kolins MD, et al: Quinine-induced thrombocytopenia following intravenous use of heroin. Arch Intern Med 1983;143:1174–1175.
24. Church J: Neuromodulatory effects of dextromethorphan: Role of NMDA receptors in responses. Trends Pharmacol Sci 1990;11:146–147.
25. Cohen MR, Cohen RM, Pickar D, et al: Behavioural effects after high dose naloxone administration to normal volunteers. Lancet 1981;2:1110. Letter.

26. Collart L, Luthey C, Dayer P: Multimodal analgesic effect of tramadol. Clin Pharmacol Ther 1993;53:223.
27. Cone E, Dickerson S, Paul B, Mitchell J: Forensic drug testing for opiates. IV. Analytical sensitivity, specificity, and accuracy of commercial urine opiate immunoassays. J Anal Toxicol 1992;16:72–78.
28. Cowan A, Geller EB, Adler MW: Classification of opioids on the basis of change in seizure threshold in rats. Science 1979;206;465–467.
29. Cutler EA, Barrett GA, Craven PW, Cramblett HG: Delayed cardiopulmonary arrest after Lomotil ingestion. Pediatrics 1980;65:157–158.
30. Darke S, Ross J, Hall W: Overdose among heroin users in Sydney, Australia. Addiction 1995;91:405–411.
31. Dauberstein JL, Kaufman DM: A clinical study of an epidemic of heroin intoxication and heroin-induced pulmonary edema. Am J Med 1971;51:704–714.
32. Davis GC: Endorphins and pain. Psychiatr Clin North Am 1983;6:473–487.
33. DeBard ML, Jagger JA: T's and B's—Midwestern heroin substitute. Clin Toxicol 1981;18:1117–1123.
34. Debonnel G: Current hypothesis on sigma receptors and their physiological role: Possible implications in psychiatry. J Psychiatr Neurosci 1993;18:157–172.
35. Debonnel G, de Montigny C: Modulation of NMDA and dopaminergic neurotransmission by sigma ligands: Possible implications for the treatment of psychiatric disorders. Life Sci 1996;58:721–734.
36. Dhawan BN, Cesselin F, Raghubir R, et al: Internation Union of Pharmacology. XII. Classification of opioid receptors. Pharmacol Rev 1996;48:567–592.
37. DiChiara G, Imperato A: Drugs abused by humans preferentially increase synaptic dopamine concentrations in the mesolimbic system of freely moving rats. Proc Natl Acad Sci USA 1988;85:5274–5278.
38. Donnerer J, Oka K, Brossi A, et al: Presence and formation of codeine and morphine in the rat. Proc Natl Acad Sci USA 1986;83:4566–4567.
39. Eckenhoff JE, Oech SR: The effects of narcotics and antagonists upon respiration and circulation in man. Clin Pharmacol Ther 1960;1:483–524.
40. Ellenbroek B, Schwarz M, Sontag KH, et al: Muscular rigidity and delineation of a dopamine-specific neostriatal subregion: Tonic EMG activity in rats. Brain Res 1985;345: 132–140.
41. ElSohly H, ElSohly M, Stanford D: Poppy seed ingestion and opiates urinalysis: A closer look. J Anal Toxicol 1990; 14:308–310.
42. Elsworth JD, Sladek JR Jr, Taylor JR, et al: Early gestational mesencephalon grafts, but not later gestational mesencephalon, cerebellum or sham grafts, increases dopamine in caudate nucleus of MPTP treated monkeys. Neuroscience 1996;72:477–484.
43. Fahmy NR, Sunder N, Soter NA: Role of histamine in the hemodynamic and plasma catecholamine responses to morphine. Clin Pharmacol Ther 1983;33:615–620.
44. Flacke JW, Flacke WE, Bloor BC, et al: Histamine release by four narcotics: A double blind study in humans. Anesth Analg 1987;66:723–730.
45. Gal TJ, DiFazio CA, Moscicki J: Analgesic and respiratory depressant activity of nalbuphine: A comparison with morphine. Anesthesiology 1982;57:367–374.
46. Ghoneim MM, Dhanaraj J, Choi WW: Comparison of four opioid analgesics as supplements to nitrous oxide anesthesia. Anesth Analg 1984;63:405–412.
47. Gilbert PE, Martin WR: Antagonism of the convulsant effects of heroin, *d*-propoxyphene, meperidine, normeperidine and thebaine by naloxone in mice. J Pharmacol Exp Ther 1975;192:538–541.
48. Goldfrank L, Weisman RS, Errick JK, Lo MW: A dosing nomogram for continuous infusion intravenous naloxone. Ann Emerg Med 1986;15:566–570.
49. Gonzalez JP, Brogden RN: Naltrexone. A review of its pharmacodynamic and pharmacokinetic properties and therapeutic efficacy in the management of opioid dependence. Drugs 1988;35:193–213.
50. Goodman RR, Snyder SH, Kuhar MJ, Young WS: Differentiation of δ and μ opiate receptor localization by light microscopic autoradiography. Proc Nat Acad Sci USA 1980; 77:6239–6243.
51. Gossop M, Griffiths P, Powis B, et al: Frequency of nonfatal heroin overdose: Survey of heroin users recruited in non-clinical settings. Br Med J 1996;313:402.
52. Grudt TJ, Williams JT: κ-Opioid receptors also increase potassium conductance. Proc Natl Acad Sci USA 1993;90: 11429–11432.
53. Hantraye P, Brouillet E, Ferrante R, et al: Inhibition of neuronal nitric oxide synthase prevents MPTP-induced parkinsonism in baboons. Nature Med 1996;2:1017–1021.
54. Hantson P, Evenepoel M, Ziade D, et al: Adverse cardiac manifestations following dextropropoxyphene overdose: Can naloxone be helpful? Ann Emerg Med 1995;25: 263–266.
55. Hazum E, Sabatka JJ, Chang KJ, et al: Morphine in cow and human milk: Could dietary morphine constitute a ligand for specific morphine (μ) receptors? Science 1981;213: 1010–1012.
56. Heikkila RE, Manzino L, Cabbat FS, et al: Protection against the dopaminergic neurotoxicity of 1-methyl-4-phenyl-1,2,3,6-tetrahydropyridine by monoamine oxidase inhibitors. Nature 1984;311:467–469.
57. Helpern M, Rho YM: Deaths from narcotism in New York City. Incidence, circumstances, and post mortem findings. NY State J Med 1966;66:2391–2408.
58. Hemby SE, Martin TJ, Co C, Dworkin IS, Smith JE: The effects of intravenous heroin administration on extracellular nucleus accumbens dopamine concentrations as determined by in vivo microdialysis. J Pharmacol Exp Ther 1995;273:591–598.
59. Hescheler J, Rosenthal W, Trautwein W, Schultz G: The GTP-binding protein, G_0, regulates neuronal calcium channels. Nature 1987;325:445–447.
60. Hibbs J, Perper J, Winek CL: An outbreak of designer drug-related deaths in Pennsylvania. JAMA 1991;265: 1011–1013.
61. Hierholzer J, Cordes M, Tantow H, et al: Drug smuggling by ingested cocaine filled packages: Conventional x-ray and ultrasound. Abdom Imaging 1995;20: 333–338.
62. Hine CH, Wright JA, Allison DJ, et al: Analysis of fatalities

from acute narcotism in a major urban area. J Forensic Sci 1982;27:372–384.
63. Hoffman JR, Schriger DL, Luo JS: The empiric use of naloxone in patients with altered mental status: A reappraisal. Ann Emerg Med 1991;20:246–252.
64. Hoffman RS: The toxic emergency: Strychnine. Emerg Med 1994;26:111–112.
65. Hollander JE, Lozano M: Cocaine-associated myocardial infarction secondary to a contaminant. Am J Emerg Med 1993;11:681–682.
66. Hughes J: Isolation of an endogenous compound from the brain with pharmacologic properties similar to morphine. Brain Res 1975;88:295–308.
67. Jackson HC, Nutt DJ: Investigation of the involvement of opioid receptors in the action of anticonvulsants. Psychopharmacology 1993;111:486–490.
68. Jenkins AJ, Keenan RM, Henningfield JE, Cone EJ: Pharmacokinetics and pharmacodynamics of smoked heroin. J Anal Toxicol 1994;18:317–330.
69. Jones DNC, Holtzman SG: Interaction between opioid antagonists and amphetamine: Evidence for mediation by central delta opioid receptors. J Pharmacol Exp Ther 1992; 262:638–645.
70. Kaa E: Impurities, adulterants and diluents of illicit heroin. Changes during a 12 year period. Forensic Sci Int 1994;64:171–179.
71. Kaiko RF, Foley KM, Grabinski PY, et al: Central nervous system excitatory effects of meperidine in cancer patients. Ann Neurol 1983;13:180.
72. Kaplan JL, Marx JA: Effectiveness and safety of intravenous nalmefene for emergency department patients with suspected narcotic overdose: A pilot study. Ann Emerg Med 1993;22:187–190.
73. Karch SB: Narcotics. In: Karch SB: The Pathology of Drug Abuse, 2nd ed. Boca Raton, CRC Press, 1996, pp. 235–353.
74. Karim A, Ranney RE, Evensen KL, Clark ML: Pharmacokinetics and metabolism of diphenoxylate in man. Clin Pharmacol Ther 1972;13:407–419.
75. Kayser V, Besson J-M, Guilbaud G: Effects of the analgesic agent tramadol in normal and arthritic rats: Comparison with the effects of different opioids, including tolerance and cross-tolerance to morphine. Eur J Pharmacol 1991; 195:37–45.
76. Klein M, Musacchio JM: High affinity dextromethorphan binding sites in guinea pig brain. Effect of sigma ligands and other agents. J Pharmacol Exp Ther 1989;251;207–215.
77. Kollef MH, Pluss J: Noncardiogenic pulmonary edema following upper airway obstruction. Medicine 1991;70:91–98.
78. Koren G, Butt W, Pape K, Chinyanga H: Morphine-induced seizures in newborn infants. Vet Hum Toxicol 1985;27:519–520.
79. Kram TC, Cooper DA, Allen AC: Behind the identification of China White. Anal Chem 1981;3:1379A–1386A.
80. LaBarbera M, Wolfe T: Characteristics, attitudes and implication of fentanyl use based on reports from self-identified users. J Psychoactive Drugs 1983;15:293–301.
81. Lai HWL, Minami M, Satoh M, Wong YH: G_z coupling to the rat κ-opioid receptor. FEBS Lett 1995;360:97–99.
82. Langston JW, Ballard P, Tetrud JW, Irwin I: Chronic parkinsonism in humans due to a by-product of meperidine-analog synthesis. Science 1983;219:979–980.
83. Lazarus LH, Bryant SD, Attila M, Salvadori S: Frog skin opioid peptides: A case for environmental mimicry. Environ Health Perspect 1994;102:648–654.
84. Lee HK, Wang SC: Mechanism of morphine-induced miosis in the dog. J Pharmacol Exp Ther 1975;192:415–431.
85. Lerner A, Oerther F: Characteristics and sequelae of paregoric abuse. Ann Intern Med 1966;65:1019–1030.
86. Levine JD, Gordon NC, Taiwo YO, Coderre TJ: Potentiation of pentazocine analgesia by low-dose naloxone. J Clin Invest 1988;82:1574–1577.
87. Levinson AK, Marske RL, Shein MK: Tetanus in heroin addicts. JAMA 1955;157:658–660.
88. Levy MH: Pharmacologic treatment of cancer pain. N Engl J Med 1996;335:1124–1132.
89. Ling GSF, Spiegel K, Lockhart SH, et al: Separation of opioid analgesia from respiratory depression: Evidence for different receptor mechanisms. J Pharmacol Exp Ther 1985;232:149–155.
90. Luke JL, Levy ME: Heroin-related deaths—District of Columbia, 1980–1982. MMWR 1983;32:321–324.
91. Lund-Jacobsen H: Cardio-respiratory toxicity of propoxyphene and norpropoxyphene in conscious rabbits. Acta Pharmacol Toxicol 1978;42:171–178.
92. Lupovich P, Pilewski R, Sapira JD, Juselius R: Cardiotoxicity of quinine as adulterant of drugs. JAMA 1970;212:1216.
93. MacDonald KL, Rutherford GW, Friedman SM, et al: Botulism and botulism-like illness in chronic drug abusers. Ann Intern Med 1985;102:616–618.
94. Madsen PS, Strom J, Reiz S, Sorensen MB: Acute propoxyphene self-poisoning in 222 consecutive patients. Acta Anesthesiol Scand 1984;28:661–665.
95. Mann J: Murder, Magic and Medicine. Oxford, England, Oxford University Press, 1995.
96. Marks CE, Goldring RM: Chronic hypercapnia during methadone maintenance. Am Rev Resp Dis 1973;108: 1088–1093.
97. Martin M, Hecker J, Clark R, et al: China White epidemic: An eastern United States emergency department experience. Ann Emerg Med 1991;20:158–164.
98. Martin WR: Opioid antagonists. Pharmacol Rev 1967; 19:463–521.
99. Martin WR, Eades CG, Thompson JA, et al: The effects of morphine- and nalorphine-like drugs in the nondependent and morphine-dependent chronic spinal dog. J Pharmacol Exp Ther 1976;197:517–532.
100. Matthes HWD, Maldonado R, Simonin F, et al: Loss of morphine-induced analgesia, reward effect and withdrawal symptoms in mice lacking the μ-opioid-receptor gene. Nature 1996;383:819–823.
101. McCarron MM, Challoner KR, Thompson GA: Diphenoxylate-atropine (Lomotil) overdose in children: An update (report of eight cases and review of the literature). Pediatrics 1991;87:694–700.
102. McCrea FD, Eadie GS, Morgan JE: The mechanism of morphine miosis. J Pharmacol Exp Ther 1942;74:239–246.
103. Merigian K: Dextromethorphan crossreacts with the TDx PCP assay. Toxi-Lab News 1991;10:1.
104. Merigian KS: Cocaine-induced ventricular arrhythmias

and rapid atrial fibrillation temporally related to naloxone administration. Am J Emerg Med 1993;11:96–97.

105. Meyers MA: The inside dope: Cocaine, condoms and computed tomography. Abdom Imaging 1995;20:339–340.
106. Millan MJ, Czlonkowski A, Lipkowski A, Herz A: Kappa-opioid receptor-mediated antinociception in the rat. II. Supraspinal in addition to spinal sites of action. J Pharmacol Exp Ther 1989;251:342–350.
107. Mills CA, Flacke JW, Flacke WE, et al: Narcotic reversal in hypercapnic dogs: Comparison of naloxone and nalbuphine. Can J Anaesth 1990;37:238–244.
108. Mills CA, Flacke JW, Miller JD, et al: Cardiovascular effects of fentanyl reversal by naloxone at varying arterial carbon dioxide tensions in dogs. Anesth Analg 1988;67:730–736.
109. Minami M, Satoh M: Molecular biology of the opioid receptors: Structures, functions and distributions. Neurosci Res 1995;23:121–145.
110. Moulin E, Max M, Kaiko RF, et al: The analgesic efficacy of intrathecal [D-Ala^2,D-Leu^5]enkephalin in cancer patients with chronic pain. Pain 1985;23:213–221.
111. Mule SJ, Casella GA: Rendering the "poppy-seed defense" defenseless: Identification of 6-monoacetylmorphine in urine by gas chromatography/mass spectroscopy. Clin Chem 1988;34:1427–1430.
112. Murray S, Brewerton T: Abuse of over-the-counter dextromethorphan by teenagers. South Med J 1993;86:1151–1153.
113. Musacchio JM: The psychotomimetic effects of opiates and the sigma receptor. Neuropsychopharmacology 1990;3:191–200.
114. Negus SS, Pasternak GW, Koob GF, Weinger MB: Antagonist effects of beta-funaltrexamine and naloxonazine on alfentanil-induced antinociception and muscle rigidity in the rat. J Pharmacol Exp Ther 1993;264:739–745.
115. Nestler EJ: Under seige: The brain on opiates. Neuron 1996;16:897–900.
116. Ng YY, Lin WL, Chen TW, et al: Spurious hyperchloremia and decreased anion gap in a patient with dextromethorphan bromide. Am J Nephrol 1992;12:268–270.
117. Nicklas WJ, Youngster SK, Kindt MV, Heikkila RE: MPTP, MPP$^+$ and mitochondrial function. Life Sci 1987;40:721–729.
118. NIDA Capsules. Designer drugs. National Institute on Drug Abuse, Rockville, MD, Number C-86-5, September 1993.
119. Nightingale SL: Important new safety information for tramadol hydrochloride. JAMA 1996;275:1224.
120. Nock B, Biordano AL, Moore BW, Cicero TJ: Properties of the putative epsilon opioid receptor: Identification in rat, guinea pig, cow, pig and chicken brain. J Pharmacol Exp Ther 1993;264:349–359.
121. North RA, Williams JT, Surprenant A, Christie MJ: μ and δ receptors belong to a family of receptors that are coupled to potassium channels. Proc Natl Acad Sci USA 1987;84:5487–5491.
122. O'Gorman P, Patel S, Notcutt S, Wicking J: Adulteration of "street" heroin with chloroquine. Lancet 1987;1:746.
123. Olinger CP, Adams HP, Brott TG, et al: High-dose intravenous naloxone for the treatment of acute ischemic stroke. Stroke 1990;21:721–725.
124. O'Neil PJ, Pitts JE: Illicitly imported heroin products (1984–1989): Some physical and chemical features indicative of their origin. J Pharm Pharmacol 1992;44:1–6.
125. Osler W: Oedema of left lung—Morphia poisoning. Montreal Gen Hosp Rep 1880;1:291–293.
126. Parras F, Patier JL, Ezpeleta C: Lead-contaminated heroin as a source of inorganic-lead intoxication. N Eng J Med 1987;316:755. Letter.
127. Pasternak GW: Multiple morphine and enkephalin receptors and the relief of pain. JAMA 1988;259:1362–1367.
128. Paul D, Pick CG, Tive LA, Pasternak GW: Pharmacological characterization of nalorphine, a kappa$_3$ analgesic. J Pharmacol Exp Ther 1991;257:1–7.
129. Perrone J, Hamilton R, Nelson L, et al: Scopolamine poisoning among heroin users. MMWR 1996;45:457–460.
130. Pert CB, Snyder SH: Opiate receptor: Demonstration in nervous tissue. Science 1973;179:1011–1014.
131. Pfeiffer A, Brantl V, Herz A, Emrich HM: Psychotomimesis mediated by κ opiate receptors. Science 1986;233:774–776.
132. Philbin DM, Moss J, Akins CW, et al: The use of H_1 and H_2 histamine antagonists with morphine anesthesia: A double blind study. Anesthesiology 1981;55:292–296.
133. Pick CG, Paul D, Pasternak GW: Nalbuphine, a mixed kappa$_1$ and kappa$_3$ analgesic in mice. J Pharmacol Exp Ther 1992;262:1044–1050.
134. Piercey MF, Lahti RA, Schroeder LA, et al: U-50,488, a pure κ receptor agonist with spinal analgesic loci in the mouse. Life Sci 1982;31:1197–1200.
135. Poklis A: Decline in the abuse of pentazocine/tripelennamine (T's and Blues) associated with the addition of naloxone to pentazocine tablets. Drug Alcohol Depend 1984;14:135–140.
136. Porreca F, Heyman JS, Mosberg HI, et al: Role of mu and delta receptors in spinal and supraspinal analgesic effects of [D-Pen2, D-Pen5]enkephalin in the mouse. J Pharmacol Exp Ther 1987;241:393–398.
137. Predergast ML, Grella C, Perry SM, Anglin MD: Levo-alpha-acetylmethadol (LAAM): Clinical, research, and policy issues of a new pharmacotherapy for opioid addiction. J Psychoactive Drugs 1995;27:239–247.
138. Prough DS, Roy R, Bumgarner J, Shannon G: Acute pulmonary edema in healthy teenagers following conservative doses of intravenous naloxone. Anesthesiology 1984;60:485–486.
139. Questel F, Dugarin J, Dally S: Thallium-contaminated heroin. Ann Intern Med 1996;124;616. Letter.
140. Raffa RB, Friderichs E, Reimann W, et al: Opioid and nonopioid components independently contribute to the mechanism of action of tramadol, an "atypical" opioid analgesic. J Pharmacol Exp Ther 1992;260:275–285.
141. Rao TLK, Mummaneni N, El-Etr AA: Convulsions: An unusual response to intravenous fentanyl administration. Anesth Analg 1982;61:1020–1021.
142. Reisine T, Pasternak G: Opioid analgesics and antagonists. In: Hardman JG, Limbird LE, Molinoff PB, et al, eds: Goodman and Gilman's The Pharmacologic Basis of Therapeutics, 9th ed. New York, McGraw-Hill, 1996, pp. 521–556.
143. Richardson DE, Akil H: Pain reduction by electrical brain stimulation in man. J Neurosurg 1977;47:178–183.

144. Riedel F, von Stockhausen H: Severe cerebral depression after intoxication with tramadol in a 6-month-old infant. Eur J Clin Pharmacol 1984;26:631–632.
145. Rigg JRA, Rondi P: Changes in rib cage and diaphragm contribution to ventilation after morphine. Anesthesiology 1981;55:507–514.
146. Ross EM: Pharmacodynamics: Mechanisms of drug action and the relationship between drug concentration and effect. In: Hardman JG, Limbird LE, Molinoff PB, et al, eds: Goodman and Gilman's The Pharmacologic Basis of Therapeutics, 9th ed. New York, McGraw-Hill, 1996, pp. 29–42.
147. Rothman RB, Holaday JW, Porreca F: Allosteric coupling among opioid receptors: Evidence for an opioid receptor complex. In: Herz A, Akil H, Simon EJ, eds: Opioids I, Handbook of Experimental Pharmacology, Vol 104/I. Berlin, Springer-Verlag, 1993, pp. 217–237.
148. Rubens R, Verhaegen H, Brugman J, Schuermans V: Difenoxine (R15403), the active metabolite of diphenoxylate (R1132). Arzneim-Forsch Drug Res 1972;22:526–529.
149. Rumack B, Temple A: Lomotil poisoning. Pediatrics 1974;53:495–500.
150. Santiago TV, Pugliese AC, Edelman NH: Control of breathing during methadone addiction. Am J Med 1977; 62:347–354.
151. Schafer M, Carter L, Stein C: Interleukin 1β and corticotropin-releasing factor inhibit pain by releasing opioids from immune cells in inflamed tissue. Proc Natl Acad Sci USA 1994;91:4219–4123.
152. Schneider SM, Michelson EA, Boucek CD, Ilkhanipour K: Dextromethorphan poisoning reversed by naloxone. Am J Emerg Med 1991;9:237–238.
153. Schoffelmeer ANM, Van Vliet BJ, De Vries TJD, et al: Regulation of brain neurotransmitter release and of adenylate cyclase activity by opioid receptors. Biochem Soc Trans 1992;20:449–453.
154. Selavka CM: Poppy seed ingestion as a contributing factor to opiate-positive urinalysis results: The Pacific perspective. J Forensic Sci 1991;36:685–696.
155. Shaul WL, Wandell M, Robertson WO: Dextromethorphan toxicity: Reversal by naloxone. Pediatrics 1977;59:117–118.
156. Shelly MP, Park GR: Morphine toxicity with dilated pupils. Br Med J 1984;289:1071–1072.
157. Shesser R, Jotte R, Olshaker J: The contribution of impurities to the acute morbidity of illegal drugs of abuse. Am J Emerg Med 1991;9:336–342.
158. Shook JE, Watkins WD, Camporesi EM: Differential roles of opioid receptors in respiration, respiratory disease, and opiate-induced respiratory depression. Am Rev Respir Dis 1990;142:895–909.
159. Smith DA, Leake L, Loflin JR, Yealy DM: Is admission after intravenous heroin overdose necessary? Ann Emerg Med 1992;21:1326–1330.
160. Smith GM, Beecher HK: Subjective effects of heroin and morphine in normal subjects. J Pharmacol Exp Ther 1962;136:47–52.
161. Smith M, Hughs R, Levine B, et al: Forensic drug testing for opiates. VI. Urine testing for hydromorphone, hydrocodone, oxymorphone, and oxycodone with commercial opiate immunoassays and gas chromatography-mass spectrometry. J Anal Toxicol 1995;19:18–26.
162. Smith NT, Benthuysen JL, Bickford RG: Seizures during opioid anesthetic induction—Are they opioid-induced rigidity? Anesthesiology 1989;71:852–862.
163. Spiller HA, Gorman SE, Villalobos D, et al: Prospective multi-center evaluation of tramadol exposure. J Toxicol Clin Toxicol 1996;34:578–579.
164. Stein C: The control of pain in peripheral tissues by opioids. N Engl J Med 1995;332:1685–1690.
165. Stein C, Comisel K, Haimerl E, et al: Analgesic effect of intraarticular morphine after arthroscopic knee surgery. N Eng J Med 1991;325:1123–1126.
166. Steinberg GK, Bell TE, Yenari MA: Dose escalation safety and tolerance study of the *N*-methyl-D-aspartate antagonist dextromethorphan in neurosurgery patients. J Neurosurg 1996;84:860–866.
167. Stork CM, Redd JT, Fine K, Hoffman RS: Propoxyphene-induced wide QRS complex dysrhythmia responsive to sodium bicarbonate—A case report. J Toxicol Clin Toxicol 1995;33:179–183.
168. Strain EC, Stitzer ML, Liebson IA, Bigelow GE: Dose-response effects of methadone in the treatment of opioid dependence. Ann Intern Med 1993;119:23–27.
169. Strang J, Darke S, Hall W, et al: Heroin overdose: The case for take-home naloxone. Br Med J 1996;312:1435.
170. Szekely JI, Sharpe LG, Jaffe JH: Induction of phencyclidine-like behavior in rats by dextrorphan but not dextromethorphan. Pharmacol Biochem Behav 1991;40:381–384.
171. Taff RH: Pulmonary edema following naloxone administration in a patient without heart disease. Anesthesiology 1983;59:576–577.
172. Tennant FS, Rawson RA, Pumphrey E, et al: Clinical experiences with 959 opioid-dependent patients treated with levo-alpha-acetylmethadol (LAAM). J Subst Abuse Treat 1986;3:195.
173. Tighe TV, Walter FG: Delayed toxic acetaminophen level after initial four hour nontoxic level. J Toxicol Clin Toxicol 1994;32:431–434.
174. Traynor JR, Elliot J: δ-Opioid receptor subtypes and cross-talk with μ receptors. Trends Pharmacol Sci 1993;14:84–86.
175. Turski WA, Czucawar SJ, Kleinrok Z, et al: Intraamygdaloid morphine produces seizures and brain damage in rats. Life Sci 1983;33:615–618.
176. Ueda H, Harada H, Nozaki M, et al: Reconstitution of rat brain μ opioid receptors with purified guanine nucleotide-binding regulatory proteins. Proc Natl Acad Sci USA 1988;85:7013–7017.
177. Uhl GR, Javitch JA, Snyder SH: Normal MPTP binding in parkinsonian substantia nigra: Evidence for extraneuronal toxin conversion in human brain. Lancet 1985;1:956–957.
178. Ultram package insert. Ortho Pharmaceutical Corporation. Revised 3/12/96.
179. Utecht MJ, Facinelli Stone A, McCarron MM: Heroin body packers. J Emerg Med 1993;11:33–40.
180. Vacanti CA, Silbert BS, Vacanti FX: Fentanyl-induced muscle rigidity as affected by pretreatment with amantadine hydrochloride. J Clin Anesth 1992;4:282–284.
181. Walker JM, Bowen WD, Walker OF, et al: Sigma receptors: Biology and function. Pharmacol Rev 1990;42:355–399.
182. Wand P, Kuschinsk K, Sontag KH: Morphine-induced muscular rigidity in rats. Eur J Pharmacol 1973;24:189–193.

183. Ward CF, Ward GC, Saidman LJ: Drug abuse in anesthesia training programs. JAMA 1983;250:922–925.
184. Ward JM, McGrath RL, Weil JV: Effects of morphine on the peripheral vascular response to sympathetic stimulation. Am J Cardiol 1972;29:659–666.
185. Warner A: Analyte of the month: Dextromethorphan. Am Assoc Clin Chem 1993;14:27–28.
186. Weil JV, McCullough BS, Kline JS, Sodal IE: Diminished ventilatory response to hypoxia and hypercapnia after morphine in normal man. N Engl J Med 1975;21:1103–1106.
187. Weinger MB, Chen DY, Lin T, et al: A role for CNS α-2 adrenergic receptors in opiate-induced muscle rigidity in the rat. Brain Res 1995:669:10–18.
188. Weinhold LL, Bigelow GE: Opioid miosis: Effects of lighting intensity and monocular and binocular exposure. Drug Alcohol Depend 1993;31:177–181.
189. Weitz CJ, Faull KF, Goldstein A: Synthesis of the skeleton of the morphine molecule by the mammalian liver. Nature 1987;330:674–677.
190. Werling LL, Frattali A, Portoghese PS, et al: Kappa receptor regulation of dopamine release from striatum and cortex of rats and guinea pigs. J Pharmacol Exp Ther 1988; 246:282–286.
191. Whipple JK, Quebbeman EJ, Lewis KS, et al: Difficulties in diagnosing narcotic overdoses in hospitalized patients. Ann Pharmacother 1994;28:446–450.
192. Whitcomb DC, Gilliam FR, Starmer CF, Grant AO: Marked QRS complex abnormalities and sodium channel blockade by propoxyphene reversed with lidocaine. J Clin Invest 1989;84:1629–1636.
193. Wiley JF, Wiley CC, Torrey SB, Henretig FM: Clonidine poisoning in young children. J Pediatr 1990;116: 654–658.
194. Wolfe TR, Caravati EM: Massive dextromethorphan ingestion and abuse. Am J Emerg Med 1995;13:174–176.
195. Wolters ECH, van Wijngaarden GK, Stam FC: Leucoencephalopathy after inhaling "heroin" pyrolysate. Lancet 1982;2:1233–1237.
196. Wright-St-Clair RE: Poison or medicine? NZ Med J 1970; 71:224–229.
197. Yasuda K, Raynor K, Kong H, et al: Cloning and functional comparison of kappa and delta opioid receptors from mouse brain. Proc Natl Acad Sci USA 1993;90: 6736–6740.
198. Yealy DM, Paris PM, Kaplan RM, et al: The safety of prehospital naloxone administration by paramedics 1990;19: 902–905.
199. Yen LM, Dao LM, Day NPJ, et al: Role of quinine in the high mortality of intramuscular injection tetanus. Lancet 1994;344:786–787.
200. Zagon IS, Goodman SR, McLaughlin PJ: Demonstration and characterization of zeta (ζ), a growth-related opioid receptor, in a neuroblastoma cell line. Brain Res 1990; 511:181–186.
201. Zelis R, Mansour EJ, Capone RJ, Mason DT: The cardiovascular effects of morphine: The peripheral capacitance and resistance vessels in human subjects. J Clin Invest 1974;54:1247–1258.
202. Ziporyn T: A growing industry and menace: Makeshift laboratory's designer drugs. JAMA 1986;256:3061–3063.

ANTIDOTES IN DEPTH

Opioid Antagonists

Mary Ann Howland

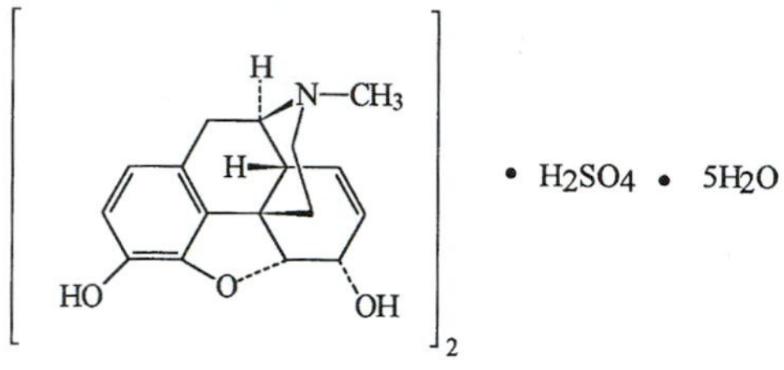

Morphine sulfate

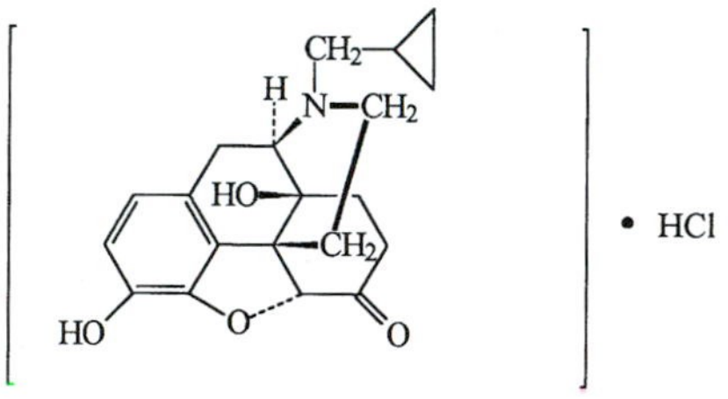

Naltrexone hydrochloride

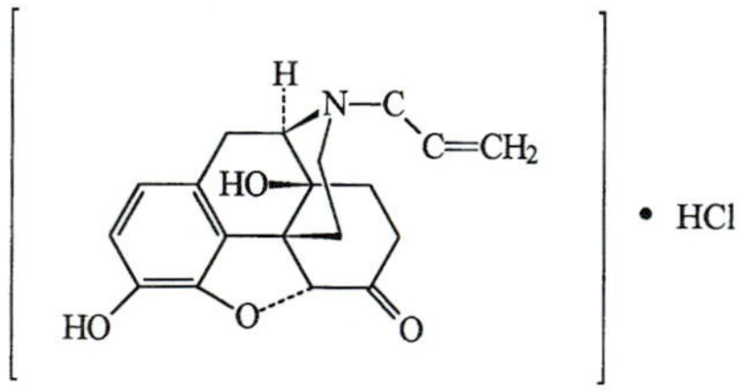

Naloxone hydrochloride

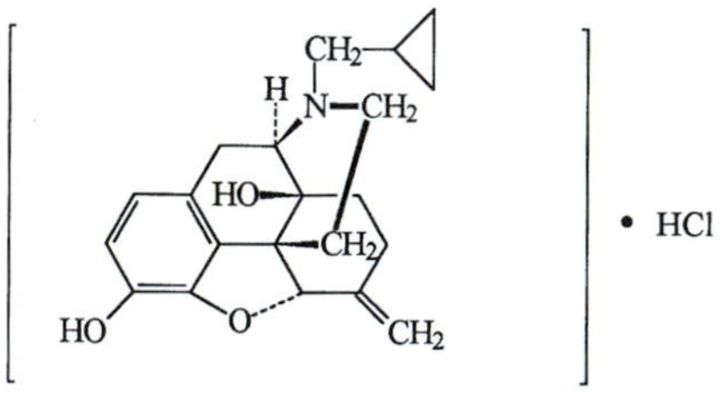

Nalmefene hydrochloride

The effects of opium were recognized as early as the third century B.C.[48] By the 19th century, morphine (named for Morpheus the god of dreams) was isolated from opium. The 20th century revealed the presence of endogenous opioid peptides and families of opioid receptors including mu (μ), delta (δ), and kappa (κ). This century has also witnessed the ever-evolving complication of opioid addiction and abuse. These social problems, and the ability to understand structure activity relationships, have led to the synthesis of many drugs in the hope of producing potent opioid agonists free of abuse potential. Although this has not been achieved, opioid antagonists and partial agonists were developed. *N*-allylnorcodeine was the first opioid antagonist synthesized, in 1915 by J. Pohl, and in the 1940s the pharmacology of *N*-allylnormorphine (nalorphine) was characterized.[30,56] Lasagna and Beecher reported in 1954 that nalorphine, a derivative of morphine, had both agonist and antagonist effects.[48] This led to the development of levallorphan, naloxone, naltrexone, and nalmefene. Naloxone was synthesized by Lewenstein and Fishman in 1960 and naltrexone by Matossian in 1963.[7]

Minor alterations can convert an agonist into an antagonist.[29] The substitution of the *N*-methyl group on morphine with a larger group led to nalorphine and also converted an agonist, levorphanol, to an antagonist, levallorphan.[48] Both nalorphine and levallorphan are weak competitive antagonists at the μ receptor (responsible for analgesia, miosis, euphoria, respiratory depression, and decreased GI motility) and agonists at the κ receptor (responsible for weaker analgesia, miosis, respiratory depression, dysphoria, anxiety, nightmares, and hallucinations).

Patients tolerant to opioid agonists such as morphine exhibit opioid withdrawal reactions (yawning, lacrimation, diaphoresis, rhinorrhea, piloerection, mydriasis, vomiting, diarrhea, myalgias, mild elevations in heart rate and blood pressure, and insomnia) when exposed to opioid antagonists or agonist–antagonists like pentazocine. Nalorphine and levallorphan are no longer marketed because of undesirable κ agonist properties. Naloxone, naltrexone, and nalmefene, derivatives of oxymorphone, are pure competitive opioid antagonists at the μ, κ, and δ receptors. These agents are most potent at the μ receptor, often necessitating higher doses for effects at the κ and δ receptors. These agents bind to the opioid receptor in a competitive fashion, prohibiting the binding of agonists or partial agonists or mixed agonist–antagonists without producing any action of their own. Naloxone, naltrexone, and nalmefene are similar in their potencies but differ primarily in their pharmacokinetics, with both nalmefene and naltrexone having longer durations of action than naloxone. In addition, naltrexone can be administered orally. Antagonists selective for μ, κ, and δ are available and undergoing in vitro and animal testing.[33]

In the proper dose, opioid antagonists reverse all of the effects of endogenous and exogenous opioid agonists at the μ, κ, and δ receptors.[46,48] Effects on other receptors and receptor subtypes are under investigation.[33] Reversal corrects CNS depression, respiratory depression, analgesia, miosis, inhibition of baroreceptor reflexes, some vasodilation, muscular rigidity (commonly seen with fentanyl use), and slowed gastrointestinal motility, all manifestations of opioid receptor effects.[48] Actions of opioid agonists that are not mediated by interaction with opioid receptors, such as direct mast-cell liberation of histamine or the sodium channel blocking effects of propoxyphene, will not be reversed.[4] Opioid-induced seizures in animal models tend to be antagonized by opioid antagonists with the exception of meperidine and tramadol.[8,24,48,55]

Opioid antagonists prevent the actions of opioid agonists if administered as pretreatment, reverse the effects of endogenous and exogenous opioids, and unmask the manifestations of opioid withdrawal in opioid-dependent patients. Pure opioid antagonists produce very few effects in the opioid-nondependent patient, even when administered in high doses.[14,15,36,60] Adverse effects excluding withdrawal and resedation are rare. Opioid withdrawal, although not life threatening, as is the case of sedative-hypnotic withdrawal, can be traumatic for the patient and health care team. In addition, if vomiting occurs due to withdrawal while the patient's airway is unprotected, aspiration pneumonia may complicate the patient's recovery. Resedation is a function of relative duration of action of the opioid antagonist and the opioid agonist. Most opioid agonists have a duration of action longer than naloxone and shorter than naltrexone, whereas the relationship is variable with nalmefene. A long duration of action is advantageous when the antagonist is being used to promote abstinence, but is unwanted when incorrectly administered to an opioid-dependent patient. Rare case reports describe noncardiogenic pulmonary edema, hypertension, and cardiac dysrhythmias in association with naloxone administration.[3,11,21,40,47,50,52] Noncardiogenic pulmonary edema has occurred following heroin overdose in the absence of naloxone. Naloxone is administered to patients who have apparent opioid intoxication, and it may be that naloxone is unmasking the noncardiogenic pulmonary edema previously induced by the opioid, but covert due to the patient's respiratory depression.[12] Hypertension and cardiac dysrhythmias have been most frequently reported following anesthesia and opioid reversal in patients with underlying cardiac or pulmonary disorders. The clinical complexity of the setting and case reports makes it difficult to analyze and attribute these adverse effects solely to naloxone.[10] Unmasking an underlying clinical condition may also be a logical cause of cardiac dysrhythmias developing after naloxone-induced heroin reversal in a patient simultaneously abusing cocaine.[38] In view of the large number of naloxone doses administered, naloxone has a remarkably safe profile.

Opioid dependence is managed by detoxification and prolonged opioid abstinence, or substitution with either methadone or naltrexone.[37] Any pure opioid antagonist could function as a substitute, but naltrexone is chosen based on oral absorption and a very long duration of action as compared to naloxone or nalmefene.[31,36,49] One milligram of naloxone intravenously blocks 25 mg of intravenous heroin for an hour, while 50 mg of oral naltrexone blocks this dose of heroin for 24 hours; 100 mg has a blocking effect of 48 hours, and 150 mg is effective for 72 hours. Nalmefene blocks the actions of 2 μg/kg of intravenous fentanyl with a duration of action that is dose dependent; 0.5 mg IV, 2 mg IV, and 50 mg orally last 4, 8, and 50 hours, respectively.[22,23] Before naltrexone can be administered, the patient must be detoxified from the drug of dependence, and then naloxone is usually administered intravenously to confirm that the patient is no longer physically dependent. Should opioid withdrawal occur, it is short-lived following naloxone, whereas it would be prolonged following naltrexone or nalmefene. Naltrexone does not produce tolerance, although prolonged treatment with naltrexone produces up-regulation of opioid receptors.[65] Naltrexone is also indicated as adjunctive therapy in ethanol dependence. It is theorized that the endogenous opioid system modulates the intake of ethanol.[45] Naltrexone reduces ethanol craving, the number of drinking days, and relapse rates.[45,62]

Endogenous opioids including endorphins, dynorphins, and enkephalins are involved in the regulation of many bodily functions, and opioid receptors are found not only in the CNS but also throughout the body. Often these receptors and endogenous opioids work in concert with other neurotransmitter systems to modulate many effects.[17,19,57,58] For instance, during shock, the release of circulating endorphins produces an inhibition of central sympathetic tone by stimulating κ receptors within the nucleus ceruleus, resulting in vasodilation. By stimulating the nucleus ambiguus, vagal tone is enhanced. The benefit from treatment of patients in septic shock with naloxone has been variable.[13,54] Naloxone may have a temporizing effect through elevation of mean arterial pressure.[28] Although promising in animal models of spinal cord injury, a human investigation of naloxone at doses about 100 times that used in the management of overdoses failed to demonstrate improvement in neurologic recovery.[9] Opioid antagonists have been used in the management of overdoses with nonopioids such as ethanol,[5,16,42,51] clonidine,[64] captopril,[59] and valproic acid.[1] In none of these instances is improvement as dramatic or consistent as in the reversal of the toxic effects of an opioid.

Naloxone is poorly bioavailable orally due to extensive first-pass effect.[20] Naloxone is well absorbed by the intramuscular, subcutaneous, and endotracheal routes of administration. The onset of action after intravenous administration is extremely fast and manifest within 1–2 minutes. The distribution half life of about 5 minutes is rapid due to its high lipid solubility, and the volume of distribution is 0.8–2.64 L/kg.[25,26,44] The elimination half-life is 60–90 minutes in adults and approximately 2–3 times longer in neonates.[10,44] Naloxone is metabolized by the liver to several compounds including a glucuronide.[10] Naloxone's duration of action of approximately 20–90 minutes[6,18] depends on the dose of the agonist, the dose and route of adminstration of the naloxone, and the rate of elimination of the agonist and naloxone.

Naltrexone is rapidly absorbed, with peak plasma concentrations occurring at 1 hour and an oral bioavailability of 5–60%.[27,39,61,63] Distribution is rapid, with a volume of distribution of about 15 L/kg and low plasma-protein binding.[32,35] Naltrexone is metabolized in the liver to β-naltrexol (with 2–8% activity) and 2-hydroxy,3-methoxy-β-naltrexol.[60] Naltrexone has an enterohepatic cycle.[23,63] The plasma elimination half-life is 10 hours for naltrexone and 13 hours for β-naltrexol.[39,61,63] The terminal phase of elimination is 96 hours for naltrexone and 18 hours for β-naltrexol.[2]

Nalmefene is a derivative of naltrexone, with an oral bioavailability of 40%. After oral administration, peak plasma concentrations are ususally reached within 1–2 hours.[14] Protein binding is approximately 45%.[14] Following oral administration, the half-life is 8–9 hours and demonstrates first-order kinetics up to 300-mg doses.[14] Although one study showed the half-life to be 108 ± 38 minutes after intravenous dosing, the study time may have been too short.[25] Another study demonstrated a terminal half life of 10.8 ± 5 hours after a 1-mg intravenous dose.[43] The V_d is 3.9 L/kg for the central compartment and 8.6 L/kg at steady state. Nalmefene is metabolized in the liver to an inactive glucuronide conjugate that then probably undergoes enterohepatic recycling and accounts for about 17% of the drug's reappearance in the feces. Less than 5% is excreted unchanged in the urine.

The initial dose of antagonist is dependent on the dose of the agonist and the relative binding affinity of the agonist to the various opioid receptors in comparison to the antagonist. The presently available antagonists have a greater affinity for the μ receptor than for κ or δ. Therefore the presence of an opioid with a greater affinity for the κ or δ receptor (eg, pentazocine, propoxyphene) will require a larger than ordinary dose of antagonist to cause reversal.[41] The dose of antagonist in a child may equal the adult dose because antagonists are competitive and dependent on the size of the ingested dose of agonist. The duration of action of the antagonist depends on many drug and patient variables such as the dose and clearance of both antagonist and agonist. Evaluation of the return of respiratory depression should be continuous and treated with either a rebolus of the antagonist or a bolus and continuous infusion. The adequacy of the observation period is dependent on many factors. Following the use of naloxone, observation for 4 hours should be adequate to determine if respiratory depression will return. The experience with nalmefene is too limited to allow us to estimate an adequate observation time, although 24 hours seems prudent. An oral dose of 150 mg of naltrexone generally lasts 72 hours and would be adequate for the majority of ingestions with the exception of those opioids, such as levo-alpha-acetylmethadol (LAAM) with extremely long durations of action. Naltrexone should never be administered to a patient who is opioid dependent.[53] A challenge dose of naloxone to verify the lack of opioid dependency is recommended before initiation of naltrexone.

A dose of naloxone of 0.4 mg IV will reverse the respiratory-depressant effects of most opioids and is a good starting dose in the nonopioid-dependent patient. However, this dose in an opioid-dependent patient will usually produce withdrawal. Therefore titration beginning with 0.1 mg is a practical starting dose in most patients, increasing to 0.4 mg then 2 mg and finally 10 mg. If there is no response to 10 mg, then an opioid is unlikely to be responsible for the respiratory depression. Return of respiratory depression requires repeated bolus doses or a continuous infusion.[34] Two thirds of the bolus dose of naloxone that resulted in reversal, when given hourly, will usually maintain the desired effect.[51] This dose can be prepared for an adult by multiplying the effective bolus dose by 6.6, adding that quantity to 1000 mL, and infusing the solution at 100 mL/h. Titration upward or downward is easily accomplished as necessary to maintain adequate ventilation and avoid withdrawal. A continuous infusion of naloxone is not a substitute for continued vigilance. An arbitrary length of time of 12–24 hours is often chosen based on the presumed opioid, the route of administration, and the dosage form. The patient must be observed for about 2 hours after discontinuance of the naloxone to assure that respiratory depression will not recur. Body packers are a unique subset of patients and must have a special management strategy developed for each individual (see Chap. 60).

Naloxone (Narcan) for intravenous, intramuscular, or subcutaneous administration is available at concentrations of 0.02 mg/mL, 0.4 mg/mL, and 1 mg/mL, with and without parabens and in 1-mL and 2-mL ampuls, and in 10-mL multidose vials. Naloxone may be diluted in normal saline or 5% dextrose to facilitate continuous intravenous infusion. Any prepared solution should be used within 24 hours.

Naltrexone is administered orally in a variety of dosage schedules for the treatment of opioid dependence. Fifty milligrams daily Monday through Friday, and 100 mg on Saturdays is a common dosing regimen. Alternatively 100 mg every other day or 150 mg every third day can be administered. Naltrexone is available as 50-mg pale yellow capsule-shaped tablets, scored and imprinted with DuPont on one side and the number 11 on the other side.

The initial intravenous dose of nalmefene is 0.1 mg in a 70 kg person in whom opioid dependency is suspect. If withdrawal does not ensue, 0.5 mg can be given, followed by 1 mg in 2–5 minutes if necessary. If intravenous access is unavailable, the intramuscular or subcutaneous route may be used, but the onset of action is delayed to

5–15 minutes after a 1-mg dose. For the reversal of post-operative opioid depression, a starting dose of 0.25 μg/kg is used, followed by incremental doses of 0.25 μg/kg every 2–5 minutes to the desired effect or to a total of 1 μg/kg. Nalmefene (Revex) is available in a blue-labeled 1-mL ampul containing 100 μg/mL and in a green-labeled 2-mL ampul containing 1 mg/mL.

Acknowledgment

Richard S. Weisman, PharmD contributed to this antidote in a previous edition.

References

1. Alberto G, Erickson T, Popiel R, et al: Central nervous system manifestations of a valproic acid overdose responsive to naloxone. Ann Emerg Med 1989;18:889–891.
2. American Society of Health System Pharmacists Board of Directors, McEvoy G, ed: AMFS 1997 Drug Information Nalmefene, Naloxone, Naltrexone. Bethesda, MD, American Society of Health System Pharmacists, Inc, 1997. pp. 1616–1619.
3. Andree RA: Sudden death following naloxone administration. Anesth Analg 1980;59:782–784.
4. Barke KE, Lindsay BH: Opiates, mast cells and histamine release. Life Sci 1993;18:1391–1399.
5. Barros S, Rodriguez G: Naloxone as an antagonist in alcohol intoxication. Anesthesiology 1981;54:174. Letter.
6. Berkowitz BA: The relationship of pharmacokinetics to pharmacologic activity: Morphine, methadone and naloxone. Clin Pharmacokinet 1976;1:219–230.
7. Blumberg H, Dayton HB: Naloxone, naltrexone, and related noroxymorphones. In: Costa E, Greengard P, Braude MC, et al, eds: Narcotic Antagonists: Advances in Biochemical Psychopharmacology, Vol. 8. New York, Raven Press, 1973, pp. 33–44.
8. Bonfiglio MF: Naloxone in the treatment of meperidine induced seizures. Drug Intell Clin Pharm 1987;21:174–175.
9. Bracken MB, Shepard MJ, Collins WF, et al: A randomized, controlled trial of methylprednisolone or naloxone in the treatment of acute spinal cord injury. N Engl J Med 1990; 322:1405–1411.
10. Chamberlain JM, Klein BL: A comprehensive review of naloxone for the emergency physician. Am J Emerg Med 1994;6:650–656.
11. Cuss FM, Colaco CB, Baron JH: Cardiac arrest after reversal of effects of opiates with naloxone. Br Med J 1984;288: 363–364.
12. Dauberstein JL, Kaufman DM: A clinical study of an epidemic of heroin intoxication and heroin induced pulmonary edema. Am J Med 1971;51:704–714.
13. DeMaria A, Craven DE, Heffernan JJ, et al: Naloxone versus placebo in treatment of septic shock. Lancet 1985;1: 1363–1365.
14. Dixon R, Gentile J, Hsu HB, et al: Nalmefene: Safety and kinetics after single and multiple oral doses of a new opioid antagonist. J Clin Pharmacol 1987;27:233–239.
15. Dixon R, Howes J, Gentile J, et al: Nalmefene: Intravenous safety and kinetics of a new opioid antagonist. Clin Pharmacol Ther 1986;39:49–52.
16. Dole VP, Fishman J, Goldfrank L, et al: Arousal of ethanol-intoxicated comatose patients with naloxone. Alcohol Clin Exp Res 1982;6:275–279.
17. Evans CJ, Hammond DL, Frederickson RCA: The opioid peptides. In: Pasternak GW, ed: The Opiate Receptors. Clifton Park, NJ: Humana Press, 1988, pp. 23–71.
18. Evans JM, Hogg MJ, Lunn JN, Rosen M: Degree and duration of reversal by naloxone of effects of morphine in conscious subjects. Br Med J 1974;2:589–591.
19. Faden AI, Jacobs TP, Monsey E, et al: Endorphins in experimental spinal injury: Therapeutic effect of naloxone. Ann Neurol 1981;10:326–332.
20. Fishman J, Roffwarg H, Hellman L: Disposition of naloxone-7, 8-^{3}H in normal and narcotic dependent men. J Pharmacol Exp Ther 1973;183:575–580.
21. Flacke JW, Flacke WE, Williams GD: Acute pulmonary edema following naloxone reversal of high-dose morphine anesthesia. Anesthesiology 1977;47:376–378.
22. Gal TJ, DiFazio CA: Prolonged antagonism of opioid action with intravenous nalmefene in man. Anethesiology 1986;64: 175–180.
23. Gal TJ, DiFazio CA, Dixon R: Prolonged blockade of opioid effect with oral nalmefene. Clin Pharmacol Ther 1986;40: 537–542.
24. Gilbert PE, Martin WR: Antagonism of the convulsant effects of heroin, *d*-propoxyphene, meperidine, normeperidine and thebaine by naloxone in mice. J Pharmacol Exp Ther 1975;192:538–541.
25. Glass PS, Jhaveri RM, Smith LR: Comparison of potency and duration of action of nalmefene and naloxone. Anesth Analg 1994;78:536–541.
26. Goldfrank LR, Weisman RS, Errick JK, Lo MW: A dosing nomogram for continuous infusion intravenous naloxone. Ann Emerg Med 1986;15:566–570.
27. Gonzalez JP, Brogden RN: Naltrexone: A review of its pharmacodynamic and pharmacokinetic properties and therapeutic efficacy in the management of opioid dependence. Drugs 1988;35:192–213.
28. Hackshaw KV, Parker GA, Roberts JW: Naloxone in septic shock. Crit Care Med 1990;18:47–51.
29. Harris LS: Narcotic antagonists—Structure–activity relationships. In: Costa E, Greengard P, Braude MC, et al, eds: Narcotic Antagonists: Advances in Biochemical Psychopharmacology, Vol. 8. New York, Raven Press, 1973, pp. 13–20.
30. Hart ER, McCawley EL: The pharmacology of *n*-allylnormorphine as compared with morphine. J Pharmacol Exp Ther 1944;82:339–348.
31. Kleber HD, Kosten TR, Gaspari J, Topazian M: Nontolerance to the opioid antagonism of naltrexone. Biol Psychiatry 1985;20:66–72.
32. Kogan MJ, Verebey K, Mule SJ: Estimation of the systemic availability and other pharmacokinetic parameters of naltrexone in man after acute and chronic oral administration. Res Commun Chem Pathol Pharmacol 1977;18:29–34.
33. Kramer TH, Shook JE, Kazmierski W, et al: Novel peptidic *mu* opioid antagonists: Pharmacologic characterization *in vitro* and *in vivo*. J Pharmacol Exp Ther 1989;249:544–551.
34. Lewis JM, Klein-Schwartz W, Benson BE, et al: Continuous naloxone infusion in pediatric narcotic overdose. Am J Dis Child 1984;138:944–946.

35. Ludden TM, Malspeis L, Baggot JD, et al: Tritiated naltrexone binding in plasma from several species and tissue distribution in mice. J Pharm Sci 1976;65:712–716.
36. Martin WR: Naloxone: Diagnosis and treatment; Drugs five years later. Ann Intern Med 1976;85:765–768.
37. Martin WR, Jasinski DR, Mansky PA: Naltrexone, an antagonist for the treatment of heroin dependence: Effects in man. Arch Gen Psychiatry 1973;28:784–790.
38. Merigian KS: Cocaine-induced ventricular arrhythmias and rapid atrial fibrillation temporally related to naloxone administration. Am J Emerg Med 1993;1:96–97.
39. Meyer MC, Straughn AB, Lo MW, et al: Bioequivalence, dose-proportionality and pharmacokinetics of naltrexone after oral administration. J Clin Psychiatry 1984;45:15–19.
40. Michaelis LL, Hickey PR, Clark TA, et al: Ventricular irritability associated with the use of naloxone hydrochloride. Ann Thorac Surg 1984;18:608–624.
41. Moore RA, Rumack BH: Naloxone: Underdosage after narcotic poisoning. Am J Dis Child 1980;134:156–158.
42. Moss LM: Naloxone reversal of nonnarcotic induced apnea. JACEP 1973;2:46–48.
43. Nalmefene. Physician's Desk Reference. Montvale, NJ, Medical Economics Co, 1997, pp. 1863.
44. Ngai SH, Berkowitz BA, Yang JC, et al: Pharmacokinetics of naloxone in rats and man: Basis for its potency and short duration of action. Anesthesiology 1976;44:398–401.
45. O'Malley SS, Jeffe AJ, Chang G, et al: Naltrexone and coping skills therapy for alcohol dependence. Arch Gen Psychiatry 1992;49:881–887.
46. Pasternak GW: Pharmacological mechanisms of opioid analgesics. Clin Neuropharmacol 1993;16:1–18.
47. Prough DS, Roy R, Bumgarner J: Acute pulmonary edema in healthy teenagers following conservative doses of intravenous naloxone. Anesthesiology 1984;60:485–486.
48. Reisine T, Pasternak G: Opioid analgesics and antagonists. In: Hardman JG, Limbird LE, Molinoff PB, et al, eds: Goodman and Gilman's The Pharmacological Basis of Therapeutics, 9th ed. New York, McGraw-Hill, 1996, pp. 521–549.
49. Renault PF: Treatment of heroin dependent persons with antagonists: Current status. In: Willette RE, Barnett G, eds: Naltrexone: Research Monograph. National Institute on Drug Abuse, Rockville, MD, 1980;28:11–22.
50. Schwartz JA, Koenigsberg MD: Naloxone-induced pulmonary edema. Ann Emerg Med 1987;16:1294–1296.
51. Sorenson SC, Mattison K: Naloxone as an antagonist in severe alcohol intoxication. Lancet 1978;2:688–689. Letter.
52. Tanaka GY: Hypertensive reaction to naloxone. JAMA 1974;228:25–26.
53. Tornabene VW: Narcotic withdrawal syndrome caused by naltrexone. Ann Intern Med 1974;81:785–787.
54. Tuggle DW, Horton JW: Effects of naloxone on splanchnic perfusion in hemorrhagic shock. J Trauma 1989;29: 1341–1345.
55. Umans JG, Inturrisi CE: Antinociceptive activity and toxicity of meperidine and normeperidine in mice. J Pharmacol Exp Ther 1982;223:203–223.
56. Unna K: Antagonistic effect of *n*-allyl-normorphine upon morphine. J Pharmacol Exp Ther 1943;79:27–31.
57. Van den Berg MH, Van-Giersbergen PL, Cox-Van-Put J, et al: Endogenous opioid peptides and blood pressure regulation during controlled stepwise hemorrhagic hypotension. Circ Shock 1991;35:102–108.
58. Van Giersbergen PL, Cox-Van-Put J, de-Jong W: Central and peripheral opiate receptors appear to be activated during controlled hemorrhagic hypotension. J Hypertens 1989; 7(suppl):2–27.
59. Varon J, Duncan SR: Naloxone reversal of hypotension due to captopril overdose. Ann Emerg Med 1991;20:1125–1127.
60. Verebey K, DePace A, Jukofsky D, et al: Quantitative determination of 2-hydroxy-3-methoxy-6β-naltrexol (HMN), naltrexone, and 6β-naltrexol in human plasma, red blood cells, saliva and urine by gas liquid chromatography. J Anal Toxicol 1980;4:33–37.
61. Verebey K, Volavka J, Mule SJ, Resnick RB: Naltrexone: Disposition, metabolism, and effects after acute and chronic dosing. Clin Pharmacol Ther 1976;20:315–328.
62. Volpicelli JR, Clay KL, Watson NT, O'Brien CP: Naltrexone in the treatment of alcoholism: Predicting response to naltrexone. J Clin Psychol 1995;56(suppl 7):39–44.
63. Wall ME, Brine DR, Perez-Reyes M: Metabolism and disposition of naltrexone in man after oral and intravenous administration. Drug Metab Disposition 1981;9:369–375.
64. Wedin GP, Edwards LJ: Clonidine poisoning treated with naloxone. Am J Emerg Med 1989;7:343–344.
65. Yoburn BC, Markham CL, Pasternak GW, Inturrisi CE: Upregulation of opioid receptor subtypes correlates with potency changes of morphine and DADLE. Life Sci 1988;43: 1319–1324.

CHAPTER 61

Sedative-Hypnotic Agents

Harold H. Osborn

A comatose and cyanotic 48-year-old woman was brought to the Emergency Department (ED) by ambulance accompanied by the police. The police stated that they had broken into her apartment after her ex-husband had become concerned and called them. The patient was found on the floor of her apartment. Her medicine cabinet was filled with a variety of medications, but no pills or empty bottles were found beside her. The police stated that the couple had recently divorced and that she was currently living alone.

The paramedics noted that the patient was apneic and her ventilations were assisted while on route to the hospital. In the ED she was intubated and placed on a respirator with an FIO_2 of 40%. The initial vital signs were: systolic blood pressure, audible at 70 mm Hg; pulse, 100 beats/min; temperature, 97.4°F (36.2°C). The patient was cyanotic, anicteric, and without pallor. She failed to respond to deep pain. Her pupils were dilated and unresponsive to light. Her fundi were benign. Deep tendon reflexes could not be elicited. Bilateral plantar extension was present. Corneal reflexes were absent and there was no oculocephalic reflex and no response to caloric stimulation. There were no abnormal cutaneous lesions. The rest of the physical examination was unremarkable.

A central venous pressure (CVP) line was inserted and blood was obtained for complete blood cell count (CBC), electrolytes, BUN, glucose, creatinine, and liver function studies. The CVP was 3 cm H_2O. A Foley catheter was inserted. An arterial blood gas analysis was obtained. A fluid challenge of 1 L 0.9% sodium chloride solution was given over 20 minutes. One hundred milliliters of 50% dextrose, 100 mg of thiamine hydrochloride, and a total of 2 mg of naloxone were given intravenously without effect. The blood pressure rose to 110/70 mm Hg. A slow elevation in the CVP to 6 cm H_2O was noted. A 40 French orogastric tube was then passed, the stomach was lavaged, and 60 g of activated charcoal and 30 g of magnesium sulfate were left in the stomach. Orders were written to repeat the activated charcoal in 2 hours. The arterial blood gas results were: pH, 7.15; PCO_2, 50 mm Hg; PO_2, 240 mm Hg. The glucose, BUN, CBC, electrolytes, and prothrombin time were all within normal limits. An ECG showed a sinus tachycardia with nonspecific ST and T-wave changes. Ethanol and acetaminophen were nondetectable. A serum phenobarbital concentration was 95 mg/L, and the diagnosis of barbiturate overdose was made. The patient was admitted to the intensive care unit.

What Are Sedative-Hypnotic Agents?

Sedative-hypnotic agents are commonly prescribed drugs used for a variety of indications including the treatment of insomnia, anxiety, seizures, alcohol withdrawal, and induction of anesthesia. Sedative drugs are those agents that decrease activity, moderate excitement, and exert a calming effect.[82] A hypnotic drug produces drowsiness and facilitates a sleep that resembles natural sleep. Many sedative-hypnotic agents are commonly referred to as tranquilizers because of their calming effects. Recently, the term "anxiolytic" has gained favor for describing sedative-hypnotics that have antianxiety properties. With the exception of the newer drugs buspirone and zolpidem, most of the anxiolytics in use today are benzodiazepines. Many sedative-hypnotics also have anticonvulsant and muscle-relaxing effects. Sedative-hypnotics, as a group, include a wide variety of pharmacologic agents with varying modes of action. The alcohols and opioids are frequently self-administered for their sedative-hypnotic effects, but they are not actually considered sedative-hypnotics. The sedative-hypnotic group can be divided into three main categories: barbiturates nonbarbiturates, and over-the-counter (OTC) compounds (Tables 61–1 and 61–2).

The nonbarbiturate sedative-hypnotic group includes the benzodiazepines, alcohols (chloral hydrate and ethchlorvynol), piperidinediones (glutethimide and methyprylon), meprobamate, bromides, methaqualone, paraldehyde, the anxiolytic buspirone, zolpidem tartrate, and the short-term anesthetic hypnotics propofol and etomidate (see Chap. 53). Paraldehyde, the bromides, and methaqualone have been withdrawn from the U.S. market. The antihistamines (doxylamine, diphenhydramine, pyrilamine, and hydroxyzine) produce sedation as an adverse effect. The OTC compounds and the antihistamines are discussed in Chapter 34.

What Is the History of the Use and Abuse of Sedative-Hypnotic Agents?

Sedative-hypnotic agents are widely used in the United States. Misuse and abuse of these drugs have occurred since their introduction. Chloral hydrate, paraldehyde, bromide, urethane, and sulfonal were among the earliest sedative-hypnotic agents used, and appeared before 1900. Introduced in 1903, the barbiturates quickly supplanted the older agents, and almost as quickly became a major health problem. By the 1950s and 1960s, barbiturates were frequently implicated in self-poisonings and overdoses and were responsible for the majority of all drug-related suicides. As deaths due to barbiturates soared, increasing attention was placed on curbing their abuse and finding safer alternatives[21,26]; the answer was found in the benzodiazepines.

For many years the benzodiazepine diazepam (Valium) was the most widely prescribed drug in the United States. In 1993, the number of barbiturate prescriptions filled nationally in drugstores was one-sixth that of benzodiazepines.[72] There are now many different benzodiazepines on the market in the United States, a reflection of their general acceptance and great financial success.[109] As a safer alternative to the barbiturates, the ingestion of a benzodiazepine alone accounts for relatively few deaths, while morbidity and mortality has occurred from mixed overdoses of benzodiazepines. In addition, an increasing number of nonbenzodiazepine sedative-hypnotics have appeared on the market, adding to the morbidity and mortality of the sedative-hypnotic agents.[42]

The treatment of sedative-hypnotic overdoses has changed dramatically over the past 60 years, with marked improvement in survival. During the late 1940s

TABLE 61–1. PROPERTIES OF FREQUENTLY USED BARBITURATES

Barbiturate	pKa	Plasma Half-life (h)	Duration of Action (h)	Hypnotic Dose	Principle Method of Elimination	Plasma Protein Binding (%)
Ultra-Short Acting						
Methohexital	7.90	3–6	0.3	50–120	Hepatic	73
Thiamylal	NA	NA	0.3	50–100	Hepatic	NA
Thiopental	7.60	6–46	0.3	50–100	Hepatic	80
Short Acting						
Hexobarbital	NA	5–6	3	50–150	Hepatic (3–6% renal)	NA
Pentobarbital	7.96	15–48	3	100	Hepatic (3–6% renal)	45–70
Secobarbital	7.90	15–40	3	50–200	Hepatic (3–6% renal)	52–57
Intermediate Acting						
Amobarbital	7.75	8–42	3–6	65–200	Hepatic (10–12% renal)	NA
Aprobarbital	NA	14–34	3–6	40–160	Hepatic (10–12% renal)	NA
Butabarbital	7.74	34–42	3–6	50–100	Hepatic (10–12% renal)	NA
Long Acting						
Barbital	7.74	5–6	6–12	300–500	Renal (30–35%)	25
Mephobarbital	7.80	11–67	6–12	NA	Renal (35–40%)	40–60
Phenobarbital	7.24	80–120	6–12	100–320	Renal (25–30%)	51
Primidone	13	3.3–22.4	6–12	250–500	Renal (15%)	19

NA = Not available.

TABLE 61–2. NONBARBITURATE SEDATIVE-HYPNOTICS

Generic Name	Trade Name	Plasma Half-life (h)	Protein Binding (%)	V_d (L/kg)
Benzodiazepines				
Alprazolam	Xanax	11.8	80	0.8
Chlordiazepoxide	Librium	5.0–30	96.5	0.3
Chlorazepate	Tranxene	1.1–2.9	97	0.9
Clonazepam	Klonopin	18–50	85.4	
Diazepam	Valium	20–70	98.7	1.1
Estazolam	Prosom	8.0–31	93	
Flurazepam	Dalmane	2.3	97.2	3.4
Halazepam	Paxipam	10.0–20.0		
Lorazepam	Ativan	9.0–19	90	1.0–1.3
Midazolam	Versed	2.0–5.0	95	0.8–1.5
Oxazepam	Serax	23–29	95.5	0.7–1.3
Prazepam	Centrax	0.6–2.0	97	9.3–19.5
Quazepam	Boral	25–41	95	5–19.5
Temazepam	Restoril	10.0–16	97	0.75–1.37
Triazolam	Halcion	1.5–5.5	90	0.7–1.5
Alcohols				
Chloral hydrate	Aquachloral Supprettes	7.0–9.5	35–40	0.6–1.6
Ethchlorvynol	Placidyl	25	30–40	4
Piperidinediones				
Glutethimide	Doriden	12	47–59	2.7
Methyprylon	Noludar	3.0–6.0	60	0.97
Carbamated Propanediol				
Meprobamate	Equanil	11	20	0.75
Quinazoline				
Methaqualone (withdrawn)	Quaalude	19	80–90	5.8–6.0
Cyclic Ethers				
Paraldehyde (withdrawn)	Paral	7		0.9
Azaspirodecanedione				
Buspirone	Buspar	2.0–3.0	95	433
Imidazopyridine				
Zolpidem	Ambien	1.7	92	0.54

and 1950s, CNS stimulants (analeptic agents) were extensively employed.[86] High doses of drugs such as picrotoxin, bemegride (Megimide), ethamivan (Emivan), and nikethamide (Coramine) were used. However, because these agents increase oxygen demand and cause seizures, psychiatric reactions, and hyperthermia, morbidity and mortality actually increased and their use fell out of favor. Another therapy no longer employed is extremely aggressive fluid therapy aimed at producing a "forced diuresis." This approach often resulted in congestive heart failure and fluid overload. Moreover, as most of the sedative-hypnotics are not excreted in the urine to any significant degree, this approach offers little benefit. Since the 1960s, with the identification of shock and hypoxia as the most important pathophysiologic factors, intensive care has become the key to managing patients with sedative-hypnotic overdoses. This "Scandinavian method" relies on antishock measures, maintenance of a patent airway, and adequate respiratory support.[19]

What Is the Mechanism of Action of Sedative-Hypnotics?

The mechanism of action (and presumably of toxicity as well) of the two main classes of sedative hypnotic agents—the barbiturates and the benzodiazepines—is enhancement of the effects of gamma-aminobutyric acid (GABA) mediated in the CNS.[39,79] GABA is the major inhibitory neurotransmitter in the central nervous system. It is synthesized from glutamate in the presynaptic inhibitory neuron, stored in presynaptic vesicles, and released as needed. The GABA receptor is pentamer structurally composed of glycosylated polypeptide subunits (alpha 1-6, beta 1-3, delta 1-2, gamma chains 1-3.)[106] Gamma aminobutyric acid works by producing some of its inhibitory actions via a subclass of $GABA_A$ receptors that gate chloride channels in the subsynaptic membrane.[3] GABA binds to the beta subunit of this receptor complex and causes chloride ions to move from the extracellular to the intracellular space.[3] The increased flow of chloride ions through the chloride ionophore leads to hyperpolarization of the cell and inhibition.

The $GABA_A$ receptor complex and its chloride ionophore are part of a protein complex embedded in the neuronal membrane, which also contains binding sites for benzodiazepines and barbiturates (see Chap. 10).[99] Although both benzodiazepines and barbiturates enhance GABA-mediated chloride currents, they do so by different mechanisms, because they bind to different sites in the GABA receptor–chloride ionophore complex. The benzodiazepine and barbiturate-binding sites exist as separate entities of the $GABA_A$ receptor–chloride ionophore complex.[3,104] Both barbiturates and benzodiazepines act on this complex, but barbiturates appear to hold the ionophore open longer, while benzodiazepines increase the frequency of ionophore opening.[99] GABA and benzodiazepines also increase each other's affinity at their respective binding sites in the receptor complex.

The identification of high-affinity benzodiazepine receptor sites in the central nervous system has led to the classification of three main types of benzodiazepine receptor ligands.[100] The first acts as a classic receptor agonist and includes the benzodiazepines that exert anxiolytic, hypnotic, and anticonvulsant effects. A second group, the anxiogenic compounds or beta-carbolines, are referred to as inverse agonists because they diminish the inhibitory action of GABA, thus producing effects such as anxiety reaction and proconvulsant activity. A representative of the third group of compounds is the benzodiazepine receptor antagonist flumazenil, which blocks the actions of the benzodiazepines.[15]

An important subtype of the benzodiazepine receptor, which represents a distinct molecular entity, is the "peripheral" benzodiazepine receptor located on the postsynaptic neurons.[74,100] Although peripheral receptors are located in diverse tissues, they seem to be concentrated in various glands, including the adrenal, pituitary, testes, and ovaries. Studies show that benzodiazepines differ in their receptor subtype and ligand-binding characteristics, and thus in their neurochemical properties.[74] The functional significance of these differences has not yet been determined.

What Are the Pharmacodynamics of Sedative-Hypnotics?

All the sedative-hypnotics will induce sleep if high enough doses are given. The effect on sleep depends on several factors including the drug used, dose, and frequency of administration. In general, the sedative-hypnotics affect the sleep cycle by decreasing the latency of sleep onset, increasing the duration of stage 2 non-REM sleep, decreasing the duration of REM sleep, and decreasing the duration of slow-wave sleep.[20,52] Use of most sedative-hypnotics for more than a week leads to some tolerance to their effects on sleep patterns. Withdrawal after continued use can result in a "rebound" increase in the frequency of occurrence and duration of REM sleep.

In high doses, sedative-hypnotics will depress the central nervous system to a point known as stage III or general anesthesia. However, the suitability of an agent for use as an anesthetic lies in the properties that determine its rapidity of onset and duration of effect.

Sedative-hypnotic agents, particularly diazepam, are used for muscle relaxation. The benzodiazepines enhance the presynaptic inhibition of afferent neuronal terminals in the primary reflex arc. Selective actions of this type may lead to muscle relaxation.

Many of the sedative-hypnotics can be used to inhibit or decrease epileptiform activity. However, some agents in this category can do so without significant central nervous system depression, so that normal functioning can occur.

Do Sedative-Hypnotic Agents Produce Tolerance?

Tolerance, the progressive diminution of susceptibility to the effects of a drug from its continued administration, is a common feature of the sedative-hypnotics. Pharmacodynamic tolerance to sedative-hypnotics can appear very quickly, even during short-term use. Using an IV infusion of thiopental with a variable rate and a specific EEG pattern, it was demonstrated that the plasma level of thiopental needed to produce a constant state of anesthesia increased hour by hour.[13] The degree of acute tolerance is directly proportional to the degree of CNS depression produced by the drug.[47] Thus, tolerance is dose related and can occur rapidly.

After termination of therapy with any sedative-hypnotic that induces pharmacodynamic tolerance, this tolerance can be lost as the previously desensitized target receptors return to their original level of function. The rate at which this process occurs is governed by the biologic half-life of the particular sedative-hypnotic and any biologically active intermediates produced. In the case of some of the benzodiazepines (eg, diazepam and its metabolite desmethyldiazepam) the process may take 2 to 6 days.[24] This phenomenon explains why withdrawal symptoms appear so late with many of the benzodiazepines. Because cross-tolerance exists among the sedative-hypnotics, one drug may be substituted for another. Thus, benzodiazepines are often used in the treatment of alcohol withdrawal.

What Are the Pharmacokinetics of Sedative-Hypnotics?

Most sedative-hypnotics are taken orally, after which most are absorbed rapidly from the GI tract. Barbiturates and benzodiazepines are primarily absorbed in the intestine. The rate-limiting step is dissolution and dispersion of the drug. The sodium salts of barbiturates are more rapidly absorbed than the nonionized acids. After absorption, the sedative hypnotics act quickly (see Table 61–1). Clinical effects on the CNS are determined by the relative ability of these drugs to penetrate the blood–brain barrier. Agents that are highly lipid soluble penetrate most quickly. The ultra-short-acting barbiturates are taken up maximally within 30 seconds by the most vascular parts of the brain (gray matter first), and sleep is induced within a few circulation times.

After initial distribution, some of the sedative-hypnotics undergo a redistribution phase as they are dispersed to other body tissues, especially fat. Drugs that are redistributed, such as the lipophilic (ultra-short-acting) barbiturates and some of the benzodiazepines (diazepam, midazolam) have a brief clinical effect as the early peak concentrations in the brain rapidly decline. The activity of these drugs is determined by their rapid distribution and redistribution (alpha phase) and not by their elimination (beta phase). However, for some of the benzodiazepines and barbiturates, the half-life (which is based on their metabolism and excretion) may be as long as several days, which explains why there is often no correlation between the duration of action and biologic half-life of these agents in single doses.

Protein Binding

Certain sedative-hypnotics, such as the highly lipid-soluble barbiturates and the benzodiazepines, are highly protein-bound. These agents are poorly filtered in the kidney and elimination is principally by metabolism in the liver. Drugs with a low-lipid-to-water partition coefficient, such as meprobamate and the longer-acting barbiturates, are poorly protein-bound and more subject to renal excretion. This has some implications with regard to treatment in overdose situations, because protein-bound agents and those that are lipid soluble (partitioned in fat) are not easily hemodialyzable.

Metabolism

Metabolism of some of the sedative-hypnotics results in pharmacologically active intermediates. The benzodiazepines are biotransformed by either demethylation and/or hydroxylation or conjugation with glucuronide. The latter proceeds rapidly and leads to inactive products. Thus benzodiazepines like oxazepam, lorazepam, and temazepam, which are biotransformed to inactive products, have shorter half-lives. Other benzodiazepines (eg, diazepam) that undergo demethylation yield active intermediates with a more prolonged biologic half-life than the parent compound. The metabolism of barbiturates in the liver yields few active intermediates.

What Are the Clinical Effects of Individual Sedative-Hypnotic Agents?

Barbiturates

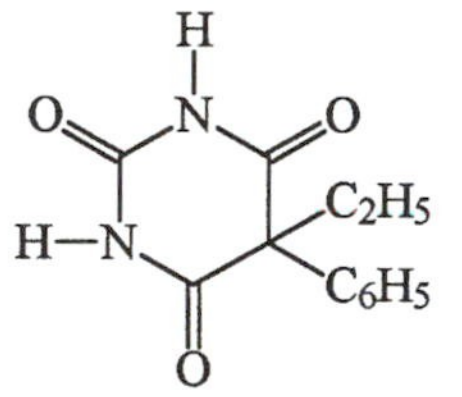

Phenobarbital

The barbiturates are all derivatives of barbituric acid (2,4,6-trioxo-hexa-hydropyrimidine), which by itself has no CNS depressant properties. This family of agents can be divided into four categories based on their elimination half-lives (see Table 61–1). However, the observed clinical effects depend on absorption, redistribution, and the presence or absence of active metabolites. For this reason, the duration of action of barbiturates (like those of benzodiazepines) do not correlate well with biologic half-lives, especially following single doses.

In contrast to the long-acting barbiturates, the ultra-short, short, and intermediate-acting agents tend to be more lipid soluble and more protein bound, have a high pKa, a more rapid onset and shorter duration of action, and are almost completely metabolized in the liver. In the case of the long-acting agent phenobarbital, the liver hydroxylates only 70 to 75% of the drug. Metabolism of barbiturates is more rapid in children and is slower in the elderly. Renal excretion of unchanged drug is significant for the long-acting barbiturates (see Table 61–1); this characteristic, in combination with the relatively low pKa (7.24) for phenobarbital, forms the basis for the use of alkaline diuresis in the treatment of phenobarbital overdoses.

Following a massive overdose of barbiturates, toxicity is manifested initially by slurred speech, ataxia, lethargy, nystagmus, headache, and confusion. As toxicity becomes more severe, the depth of coma increases, and severely poisoned patients may become anesthetized with total loss of neurologic function. Shock may occur due to medullary depression, peripheral vasodilation, or impairment of myocardial contractility. Hypothermia and cutaneous bullae are noted, with a 6.5% incidence of bullae in one series.[10] The EEG may be progressively affected and may mimic brain death in patients with very substantial overdoses.

Early deaths due to barbiturate ingestions are due to respiratory arrest and cardiovascular collapse, while delayed deaths are due to acute renal failure, pneumonia, pulmonary edema, and cerebral edema.[1,37] Mortality rates for barbiturate overdoses vary from 1 to 10%. Higher mortality rates were more common in the past. The potentially fatal dose of phenobarbital is 6 to 10 g and for amobarbital, secobarbital, or pentobarbital, 2 to 3 g.[9] The highest recorded barbiturate blood level from which recovery was reported is 580 mg/L.[53] Adults with barbiturate overdoses almost invariably represent suicide attempts. Earlier notions that a patient could overdose with barbiturates by "automatic" behavior while in a sleepy condition have not withstood close scrutiny.[69]

Tolerance to barbiturates can occur. Pharmacodynamic tolerance occurs when the depressant effect on the CNS decreases after multiple administrations. This affect may be caused by alterations in the $GABA_A$/benzodiazepine–chloride ionophore complex[100] and develops over a period of weeks to months. It usually occurs with long-acting barbiturates and with larger doses of short-acting barbiturates. Metabolic tolerance usually is found with the shorter-acting barbiturates and occurs when a barbiturate accelerates the hepatic inactivation of itself by enzyme induction. Barbiturates cause a marked increase in the enzyme content of the hepatic smooth endoplasmic reticulum and an increased rate of metabolism for a number of drugs and endogenous substances. With chronic administration, tolerance to the effects on mood, sedation, and hypnosis occurs more readily and is greater than that to the anticonvulsant and lethal effects. Thus as tolerance increases, the therapeutic to toxic index decreases.[82] The effective dose of barbiturates with chronic administration may be increased up to six times. This is two or three times greater than would be expected from enhanced hepatic metabolism. The effects of abrupt withdrawal of barbiturates following prolonged exposures vary considerably but may include seizures, delirium, anorexia, tremor, insomnia, cramps, nausea, and orthostatic hypotension.

A variety of drug interactions are reported following the use of barbiturates (Table 61–3). Of note is that barbiturates can interfere with the metabolism of drugs by the hepatic cytochrome P450 system and can cause additive central nervous system depression in combination with other central nervous system depressants. Clinically documented interactions also include increased metabolism of beta-adrenergic antagonists, corticosteroids, doxycycline, estrogens, phenothiazines, quinidine, and theophylline by enzyme reduction. Valproic acid may decrease phenobarbital metabolism.

TABLE 61–3. DRUG INTERACTIONS ASSOCIATED WITH SEDATIVE-HYPNOTIC AGENTS

Barbiturates
Cause hepatic induction and increase the metabolism of anticoagulants, digoxin, quinidine, cyclic antidepressants, phenothiazines, testosterone, corticosteroids, phenytoin, and vitamins D and K
CNS depression with concomitant administration of general anesthetics, aliphatic alcohols, other sedative-hypnotics, and opioids
Displace thyroxine from binding proteins
Increase production of delta-aminolevulinic acid; contraindicated with prophyria
Can be displaced from protein (albumin)-binding sites by salicylates and warfarin
Benzodiazepines
Protentiate the action of other CNS depressants
Cimetidine inhibits hepatic microsomal enzymes and increases half-lives of benzodiazepines with active metabolites
Ethchlorvynol, Methyprylon
Increases production of delta-aminolevulinic acid; contraindicated with porphyria
Glutethimide
Increases hepatic microsomal activity

Benzodiazepines

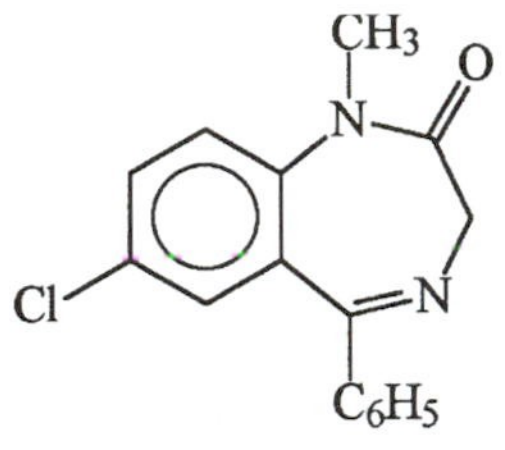

Diazepam

The benzodiazepines became extremely popular after the introduction of diazepam for seizure control in 1965.[32] There are currently millions of prescriptions written annually for the 15 different benzodiazepines available on the U.S. market (see Table 61–2). Benzodiazepines are used principally as anxiolytics to produce sedation. Temazepam (Restoril) and triazolam (Halcion) are exceptions, and are used as hypnotics to produce sleep; and clonazepam (Klonopin) is the only benzodiazepine used as a chronic anticonvulsant agent. Benzodiazepines are also clinically useful in the treatment of neuromuscular diseases, sleep disorders, seizures, alcohol withdrawal, and as preanesthetic agents.[55] This is not surprising given that many of these drugs share a similar metabolic fate and form biologically active intermediates (Fig. 61–1). These active intermediates may have longer half-lives than the parent compounds and may accumulate with chronic use.

Most benzodiazepines are administered orally or by IV injection. When administered by IM injection, drugs such as diazepam and chlordiazepoxide are slowly and erratically absorbed.[73] Midazolam (Versed) and lorazepam (Ativan) are unlike the other benzodiazepines in that their salts are water soluble and they can be given IM. Midazolam is more potent and more lipophilic than diazepam and is eliminated more quickly. The active metabolite is excreted renally and would be expected to accumulate only with long-term administration. Midazolam is ideally suited for use as a preoperative or preinduction agent and as a fast-acting sedative when IV access is not available. Lorazepam was initially used as a sedative-hypnotic agent. It is a 1,4-benzodiazepine (similar to diazepam and oxazepam) and thus is effective as an acute anticonvulsant. It also possesses some advantages that may make it more suited for acute management of seizures. Even though it is less lipophilic than diazepam, it penetrates the blood–brain barrier rather quickly. Because it is less lipophilic it does not redistribute into fat stores as rapidly as diazepam, giving it a longer effective duration of action (up to 12 hours). Initial studies have found that lorazepam is an effective first-line anticonvulsant with no more adverse reactions than diazepam.[58]

Adverse effects of the benzodiazepines consist of weakness, headache, blurred vision, vertigo, nausea, diarrhea, and chest pain. Coingestions, especially with ethanol, can be severe.[41] The incidence and intensity of CNS toxicity increases with age.[73] The benzodiazepines may rarely cause paradoxic psychological and CNS effects. Triazolam (Halcion) has been noted to produce delirium,[105] toxic psychosis,[27] and transient global amnesia,[75] while flurazepam (Dalmane) has been associated with nightmares and hallucinations.[39]

One of the unique properties of the benzodiazepine sedative-hypnotics is their relative safety even following

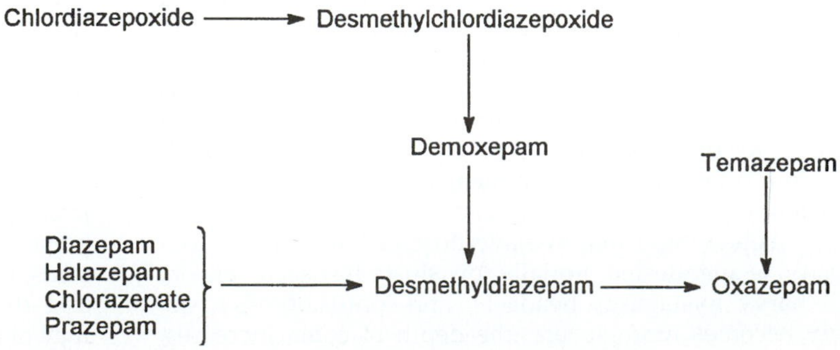

Figure 61–1. Shared metabolic pathway for benzodiazepine metabolism. *(Adapted, with permission, from Rall TW: Hypnotics and Sedatives. In: Gilman AG, Rall TW, Nies AS, Taylor P, eds: Goodman and Gilman's The Pharmacological Basis of Therapeutics, 8th ed. New York, Pergamon, 1990, pp. 345–382.)*

substantial ingestions. Deaths due to benzodiazepines alone are extremely rare; most often deaths are secondary to combined overdoses.[29,62,94] Most obtunded patients become arousable within 12 to 36 hours following a benzodiazepine overdose due to the development of acute tolerance.[88] The duration of coma in elderly patients, however, may be prolonged. Benzodiazepines are not known to cause any specific systemic injury, and their long-term use has not been associated with specific organ toxicity. Of concern is the fact that the newer, shorter-acting benzodiazepines (temazepam, alprazolam, and triazolam) have been associated with several fatalities.[61] It is possible that they have greater potential for significant toxicity, but mixed ingestions particularly with alcohol ingestion often confound analysis.

Tolerance to benzodiazepines exists. Tolerance to the sedative effects of the benzodiazepines occurs more rapidly than does tolerance to the antianxiety effects.[87] Abrupt withdrawal of long-term use of benzodiazepines may precipitate a benzodiazepine withdrawal syndrome, which can be characterized by changes in perception, paraesthesias, headaches, tremors, and weight loss. Treatment of the withdrawal syndrome includes systematic gradual tapering of the dose. Patients who are already in acute withdrawal may require hospitalization.

Flunitrazepam (Rohypnol)—an illegal drug in the United States but sold legally in the Caribbean, Mexico, and Europe—is a common drug of abuse in Florida. It is being used both recreationally and criminally because it causes profound CNS depression without alterations in vital signs if not mixed with alcohol. Much of its popularity seems to surround its long duration of action and its partial amnestic properties. Clinical observation has led to the conclusion that both tolerance and the incidence of withdrawal appears to be high with flunitrazepam.

Chloral Hydrate

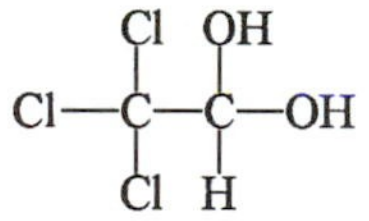

Choral hydrate (2,2,2,-tricholorethane-1,1-diol) belongs to the oldest class of hypnotics, the chloral derivatives. It is well absorbed, although irritating to the GI tract; and once absorbed, it acts quickly. It is rapidly distributed and metabolized. Trichloroethanol, the first active metabolite, is quite lipid soluble and entirely responsible for chloral hydrate's hypnotic effects. Chloral hydrate is metabolized by hepatic alcohol dehydrogenase (Fig. 61–2). Trichloroethanol has a plasma half life of 4 to 12 hours and is metabolized to inactive trichloroacetic acid, conjugated with glucuronide, and then excreted by the kidney as urochloralic acid. Less than 10% is excreted unchanged. The combination of ethanol and chloral hydrate, the infamous "Mickey Finn," has additive CNS depressant effects. Both drugs are CNS depressants; in addition, they influence each other's metabolism. Chloral hydrate competes for alcohol dehydrogenase, thereby prolonging the half-life of ethanol. The activation of ethanol generates NADH, which is needed as a cofactor for the metabolism of choral hydrate to trichloroethanol (the active moiety). Finally, ethanol inhibits the conjugation of trichloroethanol, while trichloroethanol in turn inhibits the oxidation of ethanol.[93] Acute chloral hydrate poisoning resemble acute barbiturate poisoning. Hypotension, miosis, hepatotoxicity, and nephrotoxicity may develop. Cardiac dysrhythmias, also seen with other halogenated hydrocarbons, are the main cause of death and may be atrial or ventricular in nature.[77] AV block and asystole are also reported.[12,111]

Overdose with chloral hydrate can produce nausea, vomiting, hemorrhagic gastritis, and rarely gastric and intestinal necrosis, leading to perforation and esophagitis with stricture formation.[34,107] Hepatic damage and renal failure are also described following overdoses. The compound reduces myocardial contractility, shortens the refractory period, and increases myocardial sensitivity to catecholamines.[36] Persistent cardiac dysrhythmias (ventricular fibrillation, ventricular tachycardia, torsades de pointes) are common terminal events.[54] Standard antidysrhythmic agents are often ineffective.[12,36] A beta-adrenergic antagonist, either noncardioselective or $beta_1$ specific, is currently considered the drug of choice for the treatment of most dysrhythmias secondary to chloral hydrate ingestions.[12,36,98] Chloral hydrate has also recently been shown to be genotoxic,[89] causing chromosome changes and other effects both in vitro and in vivo.[101] In addition, chloral hydrate is a reactive metabolite of trichloroethylene with a chemical similarity to this recognized carcinogen in animals.[89] Death has occurred following ingestion of as little as 4 g of chloral hydrate, and is common with ingestions of 10 g or more. Today, chloral hydrate is used mainly as a sedating agent for children prior to medical procedures in controlled situations.[68,76] Several comprehensive studies of clinical and pharmacologic characteristics of chloral hydrate utilization in neonates and infants suggest that even single-dose administration results in prolonged chloral hydrate, trichloroethanol, and trichloroacetic acid half-lives.[71,86] This latter metabolite was still detectable at 6 days postadministration. These factors are of concern in neonates and those infants exposed to repetitive doses. However, chloral hydrate is still prescribed as a sedating agent for adults in noncontrolled environments. This practice is questionable in light of safer sedating agents, and remains a point of great concern, particularly in the pediatric literature.[101]

Ethchlorvynol

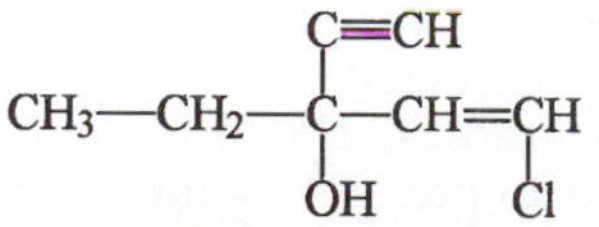

After ingestion, ethchlorvynol (1-chloro-3-ethyl-penten-4-yl-3-ol; Placidyl) is rapidly absorbed and, because of its

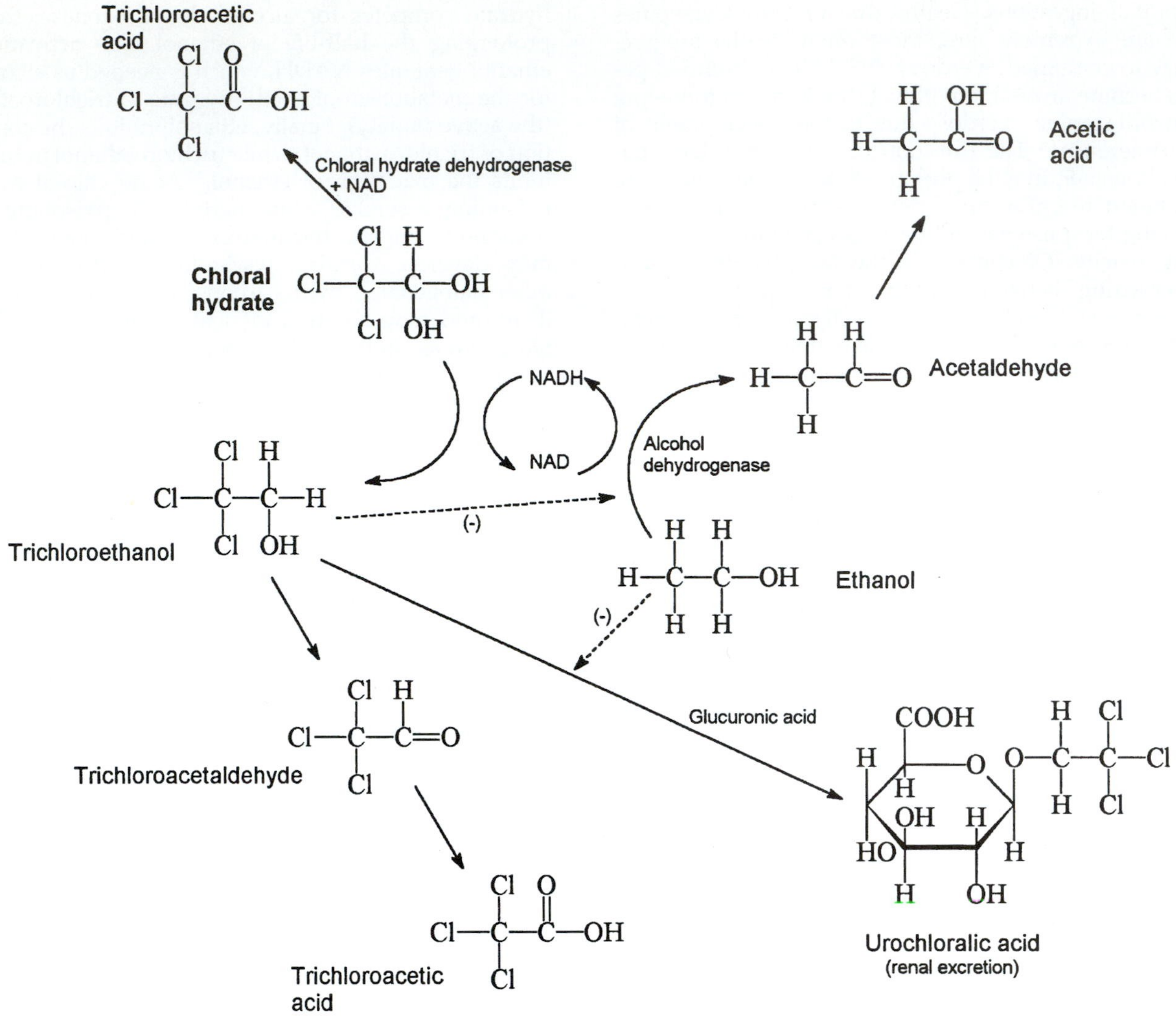

Figure 61–2. Metabolism of chloral hydrate and ethanol, demonstrating the interactions between chloral hydrate and ethanol metabolism. In particular, note the inhibitory (---) effects of ethanol on trichloroethanol metabolism and the converse *(Adapted, with permission, from Sellers EM, Long MA, Koch-Weser J: Clin Pharm Ther 1972;13:4.).*

lipid solubility, stored in adipose tissue. It has a half-life of 25 hours in therapeutic doses and in excess of 100 hours in overdoses. It is metabolized mainly in the liver, and approximately 10% is excreted in the urine unchanged. Ethchlorvynol overdose is characterized by a prolonged deep coma, hypothermia, respiratory depression, hypotension, and bradycardia.[28] In addition, because of its volatility, it produces a characteristic pungent plastic or vinyl-like odor on the breath. Rarely, bullous lesions are noted in comatose patients with ethchlorvynol overdoses. The lesions may be scattered and not confined to pressure points, and ethchlorvynol may be found in blister fluid.[6]

Pulmonary edema may occur secondary to drug-related damage to the pulmonary capillaries and is more common after IV administration.[33,114] Although ethchlorvynol is solubilized in polyethylene glycol, the administration of this vehicle intravenously in a dog model did not result in pulmonary edema, whereas it developed rapidly after IV ethchlorvynol.[33] Ethchlorvynol was also studied in anesthetized, paralyzed, and ventilated swine with rapid elevations of pulmonary vascular resistance, shunting, and dead space almost immediately following intravenous injection, creating another adult respiratory distress model.[48]

Gastric lavage fluids are frequently pink (500-mg capsules) or green (750-mg capsules), depending on the preparation used. Pulmonary aspiration and subsequent pneumonia are common complications. Fatalities have been reported after ingestion of 10 g.[2]

Prolonged coma is a characteristic of ethchlorvynol poisoning.[103] Although hemodialysis increases the rate of removal of the drug from the plasma, because of the significant lipid solubility and volume of distribution (4 L/kg), complete plasma clearance during a 4 to 6 hour dialysis will have little impact on total body clearance, and therefore on management. Hemoperfusion has been suggested as a better choice than hemodialysis.[51] However, even when hemoperfusion is used, a rebound in blood levels occurs due to redistribution from tissues. Prolonged or repeated hemoperfusion may be needed in patients with serious overdoses. Resin hemoperfusion has been reported to be more effective than charcoal hemoperfusion, but is rarely available. Usually, however, hemoperfusion is unnecessary and supportive care is all that is required. Despite safer alternatives, ethchlorvynol remains a drug of abuse and must be considered during the emergency assessment of a comatose patient.

Glutethimide

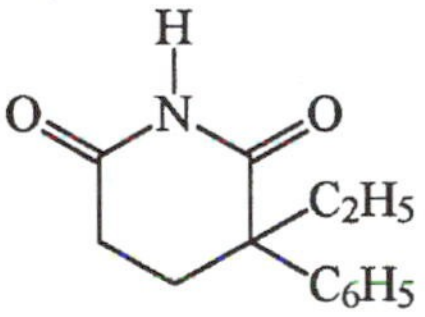

Glutethimide (3-ethyl-3 phenyl-2, 6-piperidinedione; Doriden) is used mainly to treat insomnia and has generally been replaced by safer and more effective medications. Glutethimide is poorly water soluble and hence slowly and erratically absorbed from the GI tract. Absorption may be significantly enhanced by coingestion of ethanol. Due to its lipophilic nature, once the drug is absorbed, it concentrates in fat-containing tissues. It is metabolized in the liver, and over 14 metabolites have been identified, some of which are biologically active and may contribute to its toxicity.[23,40] High lipid solubility and delayed absorption may explain the cyclic variation in CNS depression seen in acute overdosage. In addition, the enterohepatic circulation of metabolites, especially of 4-hydroxy-2-ethyl-2-phenyl-glutarimide (4-HG), which is more potent than the parent compound, may explain the fluctuating clinical course seen in severely intoxicated patients. Symptoms of toxicity in adults appear after ingestion of 3 g or more of glutethimide. Overdose is similar to that seen with the barbiturates. Profound and prolonged coma is encountered with glutethimide as with ethchlorvynol. Sudden apnea (especially during lavage) and focal neurologic findings are described. Convulsions can occur. Glutethimide has anticholinergic properties. It is also reported to produce thick and tenacious bronchial secretions with impairment of ventilation.[18,64,112] Toxic psychosis, seizures, cerebellar ataxia, and peripheral neuropathy are associated with the prolonged use of glutethimide.[18,64]

Methaqualone

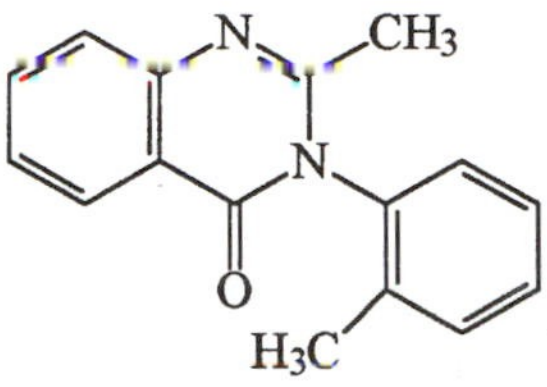

Methaqualone (2-3-disubstituted quinazoline) is a nonbarbiturate sedative hypnotic with anticonvulsant, anesthetic, antihistaminic, and antispasmodic characteristics. The drug's potential for abuse as Mandrax, Quaaludes, or Sopor led to its withdrawal from the market. Its effect as a tranquilizer and mood "elevator" have led to extensive abuse. When large doses are used, a myocardial depressant effect and hypotension are prominent.

The drug is rapidly and completely absorbed from the GI tract within 2 to 3 hours, is highly protein bound (70 to 90%), and almost exclusively metabolized in the liver to 4′ hydroxymethaqualone as well as numerous other hydroxy metabolites.[16]

The CNS depressant effects are similar to other sedative-hypnotic agents. Stupor, fatigue, coma, and respiratory arrest develop. Some patients manifest delirium, myloclonic movements, hypertonia, and hyperflexia. Withdrawal can be associated with agitation, delirium, and seizures.[57,70]

Methyprylon

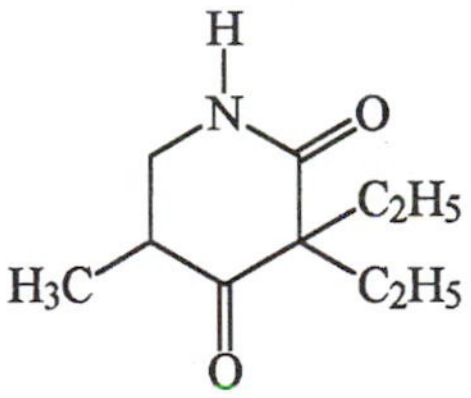

Methyprylon (3,3-diethyl-5-methyl-2,4-piperidinedione; Noludar) is used only as a hypnotic. It is rapidly absorbed in the gastrointestinal tract and its half-life varies between 4 and 16 hours. Approximately 97% of the parent drug is metabolized. Methyprylon is known to stimulate the hepatic microsomal enzyme system as well as delta-ALA synthetase; therefore, it should be avoided in patients with intermittent porphyria. In overdosage, hypotension, pulmonary edema, and shock may occur. Like all sedative-hypnotics, treatment for intoxication is supportive care. However, because methyprylon is water soluble, hemodialysis may be attempted in severe cases.[65,113]

Meprobamate

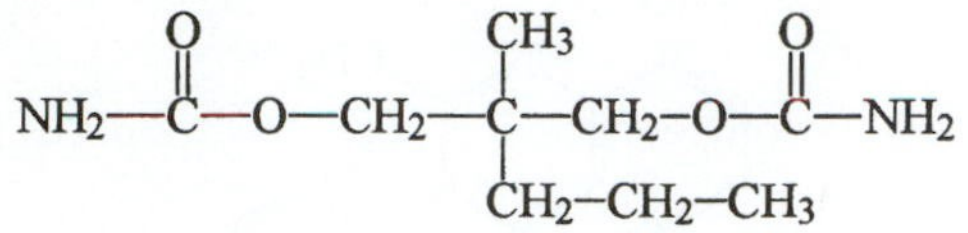

Meprobamate (2-methyl-2-n-propyl-propane-1,3-diol-dicarbamate; Equanil, Meprospan, Miltown, Probate, Trancot) is generally used to relieve nervousness and tension. It is rapidly absorbed from the GI tract. The propanediol carbamates, typified by meprobamate, have pharmacologic effects similar to those of the barbiturates. The drug has a half-life of 11 hours, 20% is bound to protein, and it is metabolized in the liver to inactive hydroxylated and glucuronidated metabolites that are excreted almost exclusively by the kidney. Overdoses in excess of 12 g can be lethal. Fatal intoxications are usually associated with mixed overdoses, whereas death in pure meprobamate poisonings are rare. Of all the nonbarbiturate tranquilizers, meprobamate is the most likely to produce euphoria.[45,46] Massive overdose results in coma, respiratory depression, seizures, hypotension, pulmonary edema, and cardiac dysrhythmias. Profound and protracted hypotension has been noted.[11] This pronounced hypotension seems to be secondary to vasomotor center depression. Large masses or bezoars of pills have been noted at autopsy in the stomach.[49,91] Thus, in a significant meprobamate ingestion, prolonged orogastric lavage with a large-bore tube and multiple-dose activated charcoal may be indicated. In severe cases, and in patients with increasing obtundation, gastroscopy should be performed even if the gastric aspirate contains little apparent drug. Concretions of pills can be removed by lavage after they have been broken up with the aid of an endoscope. Rarely, surgical removal may be necessary. Whole-bowel irrigation may be helpful if multiple pills or small concretions are noted. Because patients can experience recurrent toxic manifestations due to concretion formation and delayed absorption, careful monitoring of the clinical course is essential even following initial improvement. Continuous arteriovenous hemoperfusion with coated activated charcoal has been used in severe meprobamate poisoning.[61] In this report a clearance of 198.8 ± 15.6 mL/min with an extraction ratio of 0.66 ± 0.05 achieved almost complete elimination within 16 hours, but the necessity for this procedure must be questioned.

Bromide

Bromides, once used as a "nerve tonic" and headache remedy, have largely disappeared from the market; acute bromide intoxication is rare today. Bromides are still extensively used in fumigation of soil and warehouses, and fruits and vegetables often contain bromide residues. The drug is irritating to the GI tract and it is difficult to ingest and retain a sufficient amount to achieve a toxic level without vomiting. Bromide intoxication, therefore, usually takes place over a period of time as it tends to accumulate if taken daily. The plasma half-life of bromide is approximately 12 days. Bromide and chloride ions have a similar distribution pattern in the extracellular fluid. It is postulated that the preferential excretion of chloride results from the fact that the bromide ion moves across membranes slightly more rapidly than the chloride ion and is therefore more quickly reabsorbed in the tubules from the glomerular filtrate than the chloride ion. Although osmolar equilibrium persists, CNS function is progressively impaired by a poorly understood mechanism, with resulting inappropriateness of behavior, headache, apathy, irritability, confusion, muscle weakness, anorexia, weight loss, thickened speech, psychotic behavior, tremulousness, ataxia, and eventually coma.[7,17,80,95,96,115] Delusions and hallucinations can occur. A spurious hyperchloridemia may be found due to bromide's interference with the chloride assay (see Chap. 15). Bromide can also lead to hypertension, increased intracranial pressure, and papilledema. Intoxication with bromides during pregnancy may lead to accumulation of bromide in the fetus, resulting in the birth of an infant who may be intoxicated and may exhibit CNS depression.[80] Although bromide intoxication is rare today, it should be considered in the differential diagnosis of obscure or unusual neurologic and psychologic manifestations.[84]

Buspirone

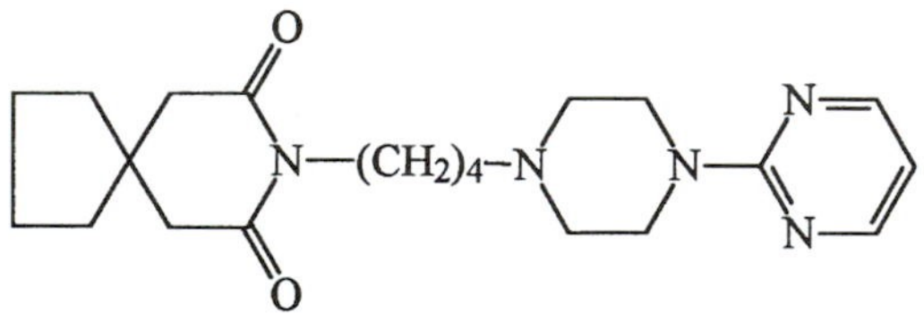

Buspirone (8-[4-[4-(2-pyrimidinyl)-1-piperazinyl]butyl]-8-azaspiro[4.5]decane-7,9-dione monohydrochloride; BuSpar) is an azaspirodecanedione agent not chemically or pharmacologically related to other sedative-hypnotic or anxiolytic agents. It is used mainly in the treatment of generalized anxiety disorder. The mechanism of action is unknown. It does not affect GABA receptors but does interact with serotonergic and central dopamine (D_2) receptors while also increasing norepinephrine metabolism in the locus ceruleus. Buspirone is rapidly absorbed, highly protein bound, and metabolized in the liver, with at least one active metabolite. Fecal elimination accounts for about 20 to 40%. Overdose may produce GI symptoms, dizziness, drowsiness, and miosis. Occasional reports of mild bradycardia and hypotension exist.[102] Buspirone has rarely been associated with dysphoria and extrapyramidal reactions unresponsive to anticholinergic agents. Under controlled circumstances, buspirone has no effect on resting ventilation or on the respiratory center's chemosensitivity.[83] Treatment in the overdose situation is supportive.

Zolpidem

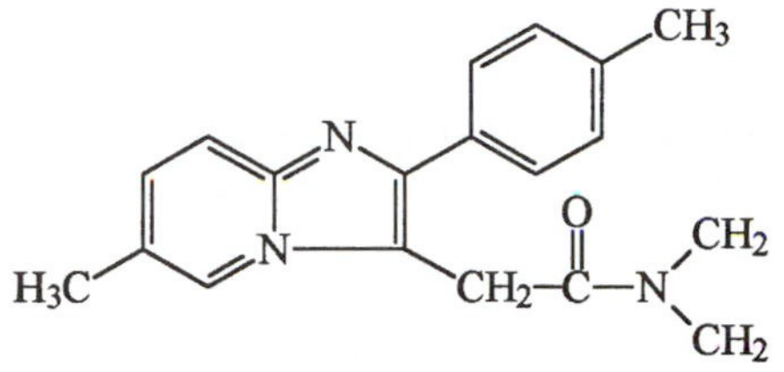

Zolpidem (N,N,6-trimethyl-2-p-toyl-imidazo[1,2-a]pyridine-3-acetamide L-(+)-tartrate (2:1); Ambien, Stilnox, Niotal) is an imidazopyridine hypnotic agent recently approved for short-term treatment of insomnia in the United States. Zolpidem is chemically unrelated to the benzodiazepines, but it binds almost exclusively to one of the benzodiazepine receptor subtypes (BZ, ω_1) in the brain.[90] Unlike the benzodiazepines that prolong the first two stages of sleep and shorten stages 3 and 4 of REM sleep, zolpidem has little effect on the stages of sleep. There appears to be little peripheral effect at the other benzodiazepine receptor sites that mediate anxiolytic, anticonvulsant, or muscle-relaxant effects.[56] Zolpidem is rapidly absorbed from the GI tract with a 70% bioavailability. The drug is highly protein bound (92%) with a volume of distribution of 0.54L/kg. Zolpidem has an elimination half-life of 2.6 hours and is metabolized in the liver and eliminated in the urine. There are now numerous case reports of psychotic reactions,[4,66] hallucinations,[67] and sensory distortion associated with excessive dosing or following therapeutic dosing of this new agent. The safety of zolpidem taken alone in overdosage appears substantial, with drowsiness frequent and coma and respiratory depression exceptionally rare. Even at 40 times the therapeutic dose, no biologic or electrocardiographic abnormalities have been reported.[31] Deaths have occurred when zolpidem was taken in large amounts with other central nervous system depressants.[31] Flumazenil has been used to reverse the effects of the drug,[60] although this approach is of questionable benefit.

Short-Term Anesthetic Sedative-Hypnotics

Propofol

Propofol (2,6-diisopropylphenol; Diprivan) is a rapidly acting intravenous sedative-hypnotic. It is used for either the induction or maintenance of general anesthesia. Propofol is highly lipid soluble and therefore crosses the blood–brain barrier rapidly. Onset of anesthesia usually occurs in less than 1 minute. Its duration of action lasts 3 to 8 minutes due to its rapid redistribution from the central nervous system.[50] Propofol causes dose-related respiratory depression and transient apnea may occur. The drug may also decrease systemic arterial pressure, and cause myocardial depression. It is not known to cause dysrhythmias or myocardial ischemia[92] (see Chap. 53).

Etomidate

Etomidate (Amidate) is a nonbarbiturate hypnotic agent without analgesic properties used principally as an induction agent. The onset of action is less than 1 minute and its duration is less than 5 minutes. Etomidate does not usually cause cardiac or respiratory depression, and hypotension rarely occurs. It may cause involuntary muscle movements. Etomidate may interfere with adrenal steroid production causing plasma cortisol levels to decrease even after a single dose[108] (see Chap. 53).

What Are the Physical Signs of a Sedative-Hypnotic Overdose?

Patients who present with mild to moderate sedative-hypnotic toxicity may manifest slurred speech, ataxia, and incoordination similar to that occurring with ethanol intoxication. Those with moderate to severe toxicity are stuporous or comatose while the most severe cases may lose all neurologic response. Paradoxical excitation is occasionally seen with some of the sedative-hypnotic agents, although it is usually associated with chronic use and is more common in the very young or old patients or those with debilitating diseases. Excitation may also be seen in severe methaqualone poisonings,[57,70] and a toxic psychosis has been described with triazolam, flurazepam, and glutethimide.[27,64] Delirium, extrapyramidal signs (hypertonicity, hyperreflexia, and myoclonus), and convulsions are reported with methaqualone overdoses.[57,70] Seizures are noted in the recovery phase from glutethimide and methyprylon overdoses. Profound and prolonged coma, and sudden apnea, may also follow glutethimide overdoses.[112]

Vital signs may reveal cardiovascular depression manifested by bradycardia or hypotension, or both, leading to shock. This is often due to medullary depression of cardiovascular regulation but also may be a result of dilation of vascular smooth muscle causing ventilation (increased capacitance) and direct depression of cardiac contractility.[97] Tachycardias—both atrial and supraventricular—occur particularly with chloral hydrate and glutethimide overdoses. Hypothermia is often seen following barbiturate and bromide ingestions and may occur due to a direct depression of thermoregulation at the hypothalamic level or the combination of intoxication and exposure. For this reason the temperature must always be measured rectally with a low-reading thermometer. Respiration can be severely affected by several of the sedative-hypnotics. A dose of a barbiturate only three times greater than that used to initiate sleep can essentially eliminate the neurogenic respiratory drive. Such doses can affect the chemoreceptors controlling respiration and all breathing stops.

The odor on a patient's breath may occasionally provide a helpful clue to the etiology of the poisoning. Ethchlorvynol (Placidyl) has a characteristic pungent plastic or vinyl-like odor, whereas chloral hydrate is described as having a pear-like scent. Bullous skin lesions are reported to occur in approximately 6% of barbiturate poisonings[10] (see Color Plate Fig. 10). The lesions are not specific for barbiturates and can also occur in unconscious patients with ethchlorvynol overdoses, carbon monoxide, methaqualone, opioids, meprobamate, glutethimide, cyclic antidepressants, and other compounds.[14] The lesions do not appear to be dependent on depth of coma or associated complications. They may occur in various areas of the body, most typically on the hands, buttocks, and knees. Whereas most drug eruptions are thought to develop on an immune basis, the bullae seen in acute intoxication are believed to be secondary to a direct toxic action of the drugs on the epidermis. In the past, more than 30% of cases of chronic bromide ingestion were associated with a "bromide rash." Typically, the rash begins as an acneiform eruption on the face and may spread to the entire body. Erythema multiforme-like and erythema nodosum-like eruptions have been described as well. Pustular lesions and ulcerations are described. Pemphigus-like bullae may appear and may contain bromide in their transudate.

The ocular examination may not contribute many important findings helpful in establishing a diagnosis of these patients. Depending on the depth of the coma, any of the sedative-hypnotics can cause nystagmus and dysconjugate eye movements. Miosis can be seen early with barbiturate, chloryl hydrate, and methyprylon intoxications. In more severe overdoses of sedative-hypnotics, depressed respiration can lead to hypoxia. Hypoxia together with paralysis of the pupillary sphincter can result in mydriasis.

Sudden cardiac arrest has been described after IV administration of barbiturates, diazepam, and midazolam. Propylene glycol used as a preservative in the parenteral preparation of these drugs may be partially responsible (see Chap. 54).[38] Life-threatening dysrhythmias have been associated with overdoses of meprobamate[63] and chloral hydrate.[114] A hemorrhagic gastritis often follows significant chloral hydrate ingestion.[107]

Is Classification of the Depth of Coma Helpful?

In the 1950s a classification of depth of coma secondary to barbiturate overdose was developed.[85] In the 1970s mortality figures were correlated with barbiturate blood levels and this classification of depth of coma.[37] Other studies[5] have revealed a high mortality in patients with barbiturate poisoning presenting with deep coma. However, because patients differ enormously in their response to barbiturates (and other sedative-hypnotics); and as multiple factors, including treatment modalities, influence outcome; it is impossible to predict survival based on this or any other coma scale alone. In recent years, the Glasgow coma scale (developed for patients with head trauma) has become the most frequently used in the emergency setting. Insofar as it is used to transmit information between providers and to monitor changes in a patient's condition, it is very useful. However, no coma scale should every be used alone to formulate a prognosis with regard to providing or withholding treatment in supposed "hopeless cases." The coma scale is useful for describing more precisely the level of consciousness of a particular patient and for following the change in mental status during the course of treatment.

What Laboratory Studies Are Helpful?

A few laboratory tests should be performed routinely in a patient with a suspected sedative-hypnotic overdose to help distinguish poisoning from the other conditions that cause stupor and coma: metabolic derangements (uremia, liver failure, electrolyte imbalance, hyperglycemia, and hypoglycemia); neurologic conditions (stroke, seizures, CNS infections, and space-occupying lesions); systemic illness; and psychiatric disorders.

These tests include electrolytes, renal profile (BUN and creatinine), glucose, and arterial blood gas analysis (see Chap. 15). Blood should be sent for serum alcohol and phenobarbital levels in cases that remain undiagnosed after a comprehensive history, physical examination, and routine laboratory tests.

Therapy, however, should always be guided by the clinical appearance of the patient. Repeat levels may be of use in the patient who begins to deteriorate. A delayed, rising barbiturate level is suggestive of ongoing absorption from a concretion.

In general, quantitative measurement of sedative-hypnotic levels is not useful or necessary in most overdose situations.[78] The clinical condition of the patient is most important. Phenobarbital serum levels may be useful because management can be enhanced by performing urinary alkalinization.

What Basic Management Is Required for a Patient With a Sedative-Hypnotic Overdose?

Management of a patient with a sedative-hypnotic overdose, as with any overdose of a CNS depressant, must begin with an assessment and stabilization of the airway, manual or mechanical ventilation (if necessary) with supplemental oxygen, and venous access. Once an active gag reflex is elicited or the airway protected by intubation, gastrointestinal (GI) evacuation can proceed. Lavage with a large-bore orogastric tube may be attempted in the most severe cases. The reason is that any of the sedative-hypnotic agents can decrease gut motility, some can cause concretions in the stomach, and others have an enterohepatic circulation. Next, a slurry of 1.0 g/kg of activated charcoal and one dose of a cathartic should be placed in the stomach. For relatively innocuous drugs, such as the benzodiazepines, if the patient's history is reliable, the vital signs are normal, and the patient is stable, the patient can be managed without GI evacuation and with activated charcoal alone as the major approach to decontamination.

Following the initial dose of activated charcoal, repeat doses of 0.5 to 1.0 g/kg should be administered every 2 to 4 hours or by slow continuous nasogastric administration until the patient improves. Repeated doses of activated charcoal significantly decrease the serum half-life of IV phenobarbital by increasing its nonrenal clearance in healthy volunteers.[8,59] In various other studies, activated charcoal adsorbs phenobarbital,[43] meprobamate, and glutethimide[90] effectively. Two series[35,81] of case reports have demonstrated shortening of the half-life of phenobarbital following overdose and subsequent activated charcoal treatment, although clinical benefit remains in doubt probably due to the definition of the therapeutic end-point in these studies. If drug levels rise and the patient continues to deteriorate, endoscopy or a contrast radiographic study should be performed immediately. If a mass (pill concretion) is present, it should be broken up with the endoscope and removed by gastric lavage tube or by gastrotomy, and the patient should be supported with airway protection and multiple-dose activated charcoal. Although it has not been formally studied, there may be potential benefits of whole-bowel irrigation in addition to activated charcoal for those patients who present more than 2 to 3 hours following a sedative-hypnotic overdose and those who ingest slow-release diazepam preparations (diazepam CR).

Is There a Role for Other Therapeutic Modalities?

Acid–Base Manipulation

With phenobarbital (with a pKa of 7.24 and 30% urinary excretion), alkalinization of the urine with sodium bicarbonate to maintain a urinary pH of 7.5 to 8.0 is helpful in promoting excretion. Alkalinization of the urine can increase the amount of phenobarbital excreted 5 to 10-fold. This procedure is not effective for the short-acting barbiturates, as they have higher pKa values, are more protein bound, and are primarily metabolized by the liver with very little excretion by the kidneys.

As these pharmacokinetic concepts were better understood, urinary alkalinization without forced diuresis became more commonplace. Although urinary alkalinization remains in use for phenobarbital intoxication, recent comparisons with multiple-dose activated charcoal (MDAC) in volunteers show that MDAC is far more effective in shortening the elimination half-life (controls 148 hours, alkalinization 47 hours, and MDAC 19 hours).[30] Alkalinization may be accomplished by administering 1 to 2 mEq/kg of sodium bicarbonate by IV bolus, followed by 150 mEq in 1 L of D_5W to maintain an arterial pH of 7.45 to 7.50 and urinary pH of 8.0 (see Antidotes in Depth: Sodium Bicarbonate). Urinary pH, serum electrolytes, and an arterial blood gas should be measured every 2 to 4 hours. Additional potassium should be given if necessary to maintain a serum potassium level greater than 4.0 mEq/L, because urinary alkalinization cannot be achieved in the presence of hypokalemia. Urine output should be maintained above 2 mL/kg per hour.

Hemodialysis and Hemoperfusion

Extracorporeal methods of elimination of sedative-hypnotics are usually not necessary, except in a select few cases. The basic therapeutic principles of evacuation, adsorption, and catharsis with good control of ventilation and circulation usually suffice. Moreover, many of the sedative-hypnotics are unsuitable for hemodialysis or hypoperfusion, having a large volume of distribution and significant protein binding. Hemodialysis and hemoperfusion both have potentially significant complications: infection, thrombosis, hypotension, and bleeding in the former; hypotension, thrombocytopenia, hypocalcemia, hypoglycemia, and bleeding in the latter.

Hemodialysis should be considered only for severe bromide intoxications when a saline diuresis cannot be used or when renal failure is present. Otherwise, in other sedative-hypnotic ingestions when extracorporeal elimination is indicated, hemoperfusion is preferred over hemodialysis because factors such as poor water solubility and plasma protein binding do not limit the efficacy of hemoperfusion to the same degree.

Clinical reports of hemoperfusion treatment in sedative-hypnotic overdoses suggest benefit only in very selected cases.[25,110] Hemoperfusion removes phenobarbital effectively. Meprobamate, with a small volume of distribution (0.65 L/kg) and limited protein binding (20%), has been successfully eliminated with hemoperfusion with isolated reports of clinical improvement.[44] The use of extracorporeal elimination should be considered in the management of overdoses with sedative-hypnotic agents only when the patient's condition is deteriorating despite aggressive therapy. In practice, however, this is rarely necessary.

Are There Any Antidotes to Sedative-Hypnotic Agents?

Flumazenil has been demonstrated to reverse the sedative effects of benzodiazepines and zolpidem (see Antidotes in Depth: Flumazenil).[15] Studies have shown a reversal of coma in the overdose setting, although the effect is short lived and symptoms can return in 0.5 to 1 hour. Flumazenil has the potential to precipitate a withdrawal reaction (including seizures) in benzodiazepine-dependent individuals.[22] Flumazenil should not be used as part of standard therapy ("coma cocktail") in the treatment of unknown or mixed overdoses. Flumazenil may have some role in the reversal of benzodiazepines administered to patients for therapeutic procedures and in the management of patients with selected benzodiazepine overdoses that do not involve other drugs.

Limiting Sedative-Hypnotic Abuse

In some cases, physicians unwittingly provide the means for a patient's suicide. Because barbiturates and nonbarbiturate sedative hypnotics are frequently implicated in suicides (especially when combined with ethanol), it is important for all practitioners to follow stringent guidelines for their use. None of the sedative-hypnotics should be regularly prescribed over a long period of time. Relatively safe hypnotic agents such as the benzodiazepines should be preferentially used whenever possible, especially in emotionally disturbed patients. Combinations of sedative-hypnotics compounds and the single use of these drugs in conjunction with alcohol should be avoided. Chronic hypnotic drug use leads to ineffective control of insomnia, decreased REM sleep, dependency, and drug withdrawal symptomatology.

Acknowledgement

David Malkevich, MD assisted in the preparation of this chapter.

References

1. Afifi AA, Sacks ST, Lui VY, et al: A cumulative prognostic index for patients with barbiturate, glutethimide, and meprobamate intoxication. N Engl J Med 1971;285:1497–1502.
2. Algeri EJ, Katsas GG, Luongo MA: Determination of ethchlorvynol in biologic mediums, and report of two fatal cases. Am J Clin Pathol 1962;38:125–130.
3. American Medical Association: Drugs used for anxiety and sleep disorders. In: Drug Evaluation Annual, Vol. 1. Chicago, AMA Publication, 1990;31:7.
4. Ansseau M, Pichot W, Hansenne M, et al: Psychotic reactions to zolpidem. Lancet 1992;339:809. Letter.
5. Arieff AI, Friedman EA: Coma following non-narcotic drug overdose: Management of 208 adult patients. Am J Med Sci 1973;226:405–426.
6. Armstrong C, Edwards KDG: Multifactorial design for testing oral ion exchange resins, charcoal and other factors in the treatment of aspirin poisoning in the rat. Efficacy of chloestyramine. Med J Aust 1967;2:301–303.
7. Battin D, Varkey T: Neuropsychiatric manifestations of bromide ingestion. Postgrad Med J 1982;58:523–524.
8. Berg MJ, Berlinger WG, Goldberg MJ, et al: Acceleration of the body clearance of phenobarbital by oral activated charcoal. N Engl J Med 1982;307:642–644.
9. Berman LB, Jeghers HJ, Schreiner GE, et al: Hemodialysis: An effective therapy for acute barbiturate poisoning. JAMA 1936;161:820–877.
10. Beveridge AW, Lawson AAH: Occurrence of bullous lesions in acute barbiturate intoxication. Br Med J 1965; 1:835–840.
11. Blumberg AG, Rosett GHL, Dolerow A: Severe hypotensive reactions following meprobamate overdoses. Ann Intern Med 1959;51:609–610.
12. Bowyer K, Glasser SP: Chloral hydrate overdose and cardiac arrhythmias. Chest 1980;77:232–235.
13. Brand L, Mazia V, Roznak AV, et al: Lack of correlation between EEG effects and plasma concentrations of thiopentanol. Br J Anaesth 1961;33:92–96.
14. Brodin M, Redmon W: Bullous eruption due to ethchlorvynol. J Cutan Pathol 1980;7:326–329.
15. Brogden RN, Goa KL: Flumazenil: A reappraisal of its pharmacological properties and therapeutic efficacy as a benzodiazepine antagonist. Drugs 1991;42:1061–1089.
16. Brown SS, Goenechea S: Methaqualone: Metabolism, kinetic and clinical pharmacologic observations. Clin Pharmacol Ther 1973;14:314–324.
17. Carney MW: Five cases of bromism. Lancet 1971;2:525–524.
18. Chazen JA, Garella S: Glutethimide intoxication: A prospective study of 70 patients treated conservatively without hemodialysis. Arch Intern Med 1971;128:215–219.
19. Clemmesen C, Nilsson E: Therapeutic trends in the treatment of barbiturate poisoning: The Scandinavian method. Clin Pharmacol Ther 1960;2:220–229.
20. Consensus Conference: Drugs and Insomnia: The use of medications to promote sleep. JAMA 1984;251:2410–2414.
21. Cooper JR, ed: Sedative-Hypnotic Drugs: Risks and Benefits. Washington, DC, U.S. Dept. of Health, Education, and Welfare, pub. no. (ADM) 1978;78-592.
22. Cumin R, Bonetti EP, Scherschilict R, et al: Use of the specific benzodiazepine antagonist RO 15–788 in studies of physiological dependence on benzodiazepines. Experientia 1982;38:833–834.
23. Curry SC, Hubbard JM, Gerkin R, et al: Lack of correlation between plasma 4-hydroxy glutethimide and severity of coma in acute glutethimide poisoning: A case report and brief review of the literature. Med Toxicol 1987;2:309–316.
24. DeBard M: Diazepam withdrawal syndrome: A case with psychosis, seizure and coma. Am J Psychiatry 1979;136: 104–105.
25. DeGrott G: Hemoperfusion in Clinical Toxicology: A Pharmacokinetic Evaluation. Utrecht, Universitair-Toxicologisch Centrum, 1982.
26. Dorpat TL: Drug automatism, barbiturate poisoning and suicide behavior. Arch Gen Psychiatry 1974;30:216–220.
27. Einarson TR, Yoder ES: Triazolam psychosis. Drug Intell Clin Pharm 1982;16:330.
28. Flemenbaum A, Gunby B: Ethchlorvynol (Placidyl) abuse and withdrawal. Dis Nerv Sys 1971;32:188–192.
29. Finkle BS, McCloskey KL, Goodman LS: Diazepam and drug associated deaths: A survey in the United States and Canada. JAMA 1979;242:429–434.
30. Frenia ML, Schauben JL, Wears RL, et al: Multiple dose activated charcoal compared to urinary alkalinization for the enhancement of phenobarbital elimination. J Toxicol Clin Toxicol 1996;34:169–175.
31. Garnier R, Gueraulte E, Muzard D, et al: Acute zolpidem poisoning-analysis of 344 cases. J Toxicol Clin Toxicol 1994;32:391–404.
32. Gestant H, Naquet R, Roire R, et al: Treatment of status epilepticus with diazepam. Epilepsia 1965;6:167–182.
33. Glauser FL, Smith WR, Caldwell A, et al: Ethchlorvynol (Placidyl)-induced pulmonary edema. Ann Intern Med 1976;84:46–48.

34. Gleich GJ, Moran ES, Vanles DW: Esophageal stricture following chloral hydrate poisoning. JAMA 1967;201:120–121.
35. Goldberg MJ, Berlinger WG: Treatment of phenobarbital overdose with activated charcoal. JAMA 1982;247: 2400–2401.
36. Graham SR, Day RO, Lee R, et al: Overdose with chloral hydrate: A pharmacological and therapeutic review. Med J Aust 1988;149:686–690.
37. Greenblatt DJ, Allen MD, Harnatz JS, et al: Overdosage with pentobarbital and secobarbital: Assessment of factors related to outcome. J Clin Pharm 1979;19:758–768.
38. Greenblatt DJ, Koch-Weser J: Adverse reactions to intravenous diazepam. Am J Med Sci 1973;266:261–266.
39. Greenblatt DJ, Shader RI, Abernathy DR: Current status of benzodiazepines. N Engl J Med 1983;309:354–358.
40. Hansen AR, Kennedy KA, Ambre JA, Fischer LJ: Glutethimide poisoning: A metabolite contributes to morbidity and mortality. N Engl J Med 1975;292:250–252.
41. Hayes SL, Pablo G, Radomski T, Palmer RF: Ethanol and oral diazepam absorption. N Engl J Med 1977;296:186–189.
42. Hoffman RS, Wipfler MG, Maddaloni MA, Weisman RS: Has the New York State triplicate benzodiazepine prescription regulation influenced sedative-hypnotic overdoses? NY State J Med 1991;91:436–439.
43. Holt E, Holz PH: The black bottle. J Pediatr 1963;63:306.
44. Hoy WE, Rivera A, Marin MG, et al: Resin hemoperfusion for treatment of a massive meprobamate overdose. Ann Intern Med 1980;93:455–465.
45. Jacobson D, Frederichsen PS, Knutsen KM, et al: A prospective study of 1212 cases of acute poisoning: General epidemiology. Hum Toxicol 1984;3:93–106.
46. Jacobsen D, Frederichsen PS, Knutsen KM, et al: A prospective study of 1125 consecutively hospitalized adults. Hum Toxicol 1974;3:107–116.
47. Jaffe JH, Martin WR: Opioid analgesics and antagonists. In: Goodman LS, Gilman AG, eds: The Pharmacological Basis of Therapeutics, 6th ed. New York, Macmillan, 1980, pp. 513–514.
48. Jebson PJR, Davies G, Starr J, Tatman D: Swine model of early adult respiratory distress syndrome induced by intravenous ethchlorvynol. Crit Care Med 1989;17:255–260.
49. Jenis EH, Payne AR, Goldbaum LR: Acute meprobamate poisoning. JAMA 1969;207:361–365.
50. Kanto J, Grepts E: Pharmacokinetic implications for the clinical use of propofol. Clin Pharmacokinet 1989;17:308–328.
51. Kathpalia S, Haslitt J, Lim V: Charcoal hemoperfusion for treatment of ethchlorvynol overdose. Artif Organs 1983; 7:246–256.
52. Kay DC, Blackburn AB, Buckingham JA, Karacan I: Human pharmacology of sleep. In: Williams RL, Karacan I, eds: Pharmacology of Sleep. New York, John Wiley and Sons, 1976, pp. 83–210.
53. Kennedy AC, Lindsay RM, Briggs JD, et al: Successful treatment of three cases of very severe barbiturate poisoning. Lancet 1969;1:955–960.
54. King K, England JF: Chloral hydrate (Noctec) overdose. Med J Aust 1983;2:260. Letter.
55. Lader M: Clinical pharmacology of benzodiazepines. Annu Rev Med 1987;38:19–28.
56. Langtry HD, Benfield P: Zolpidem: A review of its pharmacodynamic and pharmacokinetic properties and therapeutic potential. Drugs 1990;40:291–313.
57. Lawson AHH, Brown SS: Acute methaqualone (Mandrax) poisoning. Scott Med J 1967;12:63–68.
58. Leppik IE, Derivan AT, Homan RW, et al: Double blind study of lorazepam and diazepam in status epilepticus. JAMA 1983;249:1452–1454.
59. Levy G: Gastrointestinal clearance of drugs with activated charcoal. N Engl J Med 1982;307:676–678.
60. Lheureux P, Debailleul G, De Witte O, Askenasi R: Zolpidem intoxication mimicking narcotic overdose: Response to flumazenil. Hum Exp Toxicol 1990;9:105–107.
61. Lin JL, Lim PS, Lai BC, Lin WL: Continuous arteriovenous hemoperfusion in meprobamate poisoning. J Toxicol Clin Toxicol 1993;31:645–652.
62. Litovitz T: Fatal benzodiazepine toxicity. Am J Emerg Med 1987;5:472–473. Letter.
63. Longchal J, Tenaillon A, Trunet P, et al: Intoxication par le meprobamate avec incompetence myocardique. Nouv Presse Med 1978;17:1408–1410.
64. Maher JF, Schreiner GE, Westervelt FB Jr: Acute glutethimide intoxication: Clinical experience (22 patients) compared to acute barbiturate intoxication (63 patients). Am J Med 1962;33:70–82.
65. Mandelbaum JM, Simon NM: Severe methyprylon intoxication treated by hemodialysis. JAMA 1971;216:139–140.
66. Markowitz JS, Brewerton TD: Zolpidem-induced psychosis. Ann Clin Psychiatry 1996;8:89–91.
67. Markowitz JS, Rames LJ, Reeves N, Thomas SG: Zolpidem and hallucinations. Ann Emerg Med 1997;29:300–301. Letter.
68. Marti-Bonmati L, Ronchera-Oms CL, Casillas C, et al: Randomized double-blind clinical trial of intermediate- versus high-dose chloral hydrate for neuroimaging of children. Neuroradiology 1995;37:687–691.
69. Matthew H: Drug overdose. Medicine 1972;4:273.
70. Matthew H, Proudfoot AT, Brown SS, et al: Mandrax poisoning: Conservative management of 116 patients. Br Med J 1968;2:101–102.
71. Mayers DJ, Hindmarsh KW, Sankaran K, et al: Chloral hydrate disposition following single dose administration to critically ill neonates and children. Dev Pharmacol Ther 1991;16:71–77.
72. Mendelson WB, Rich CL: Sedatives and suicide: The San Diego study. Acta Psychiatr Scand 1993; 88:337–341.
73. Meyer BR: Benzodiazepines in the elderly. Med Clin North Am 1982;66:1017–1035.
74. Miller LG, Galpren WR, Brynes JJ, Greenblatt DJ: Benzodiazepine receptor binding of benzodiazepine hypnotics: Receptor and ligand specificity. Pharmacol Biochem Behav 1992;43:413–416.
75. Morris HH, Estes ML: Traveler's amnesia: Transient global amnesia secondary to triazolam. JAMA 1987;258: 945–946.
76. Napoli KL, Ingall CG, Martin GR: Safety and efficacy of chloral hydrate sedation in children undergoing echocardiography. J Pediatr 1996;129:287–291.
77. Nordenberg A, Delisle G, Izukawa A: Cardiac arrhythmia in a child due to chloral hydrate intoxication. Br J Surg 1971;59:317–319.

78. Norman TR, Graham BD: Plasma concentrations of benzodiazepines. Prog Neuropsychopharmacol Biol Psychiatry 1984;18:115–126.
79. Paul S, Marangos PJ, Skolnick P: The benzodiazepine GABA–chloride ionophore receptor complex. Biol Psychiatry 1981;16:213–229.
80. Pleasure J, Blackburn M: Neonatal bromide intoxications: Prenatal ingestion of a large quantity of bromides with transplacental accumulation in the fetus. Pediatrics 1975; 55:503–506.
81. Pond SM, Olson KR, Osterloh JD, Tong TG: Randomized study of the treatment of phenobarbital overdose with repeated doses of activated charcoal. JAMA 1984;251: 3104–3108.
82. Rall TW: Hypnotics and sedatives. In: Gilman AG, Rall TW, Nies AS, Taylor P, eds: Goodman and Gilman's The Pharmacological Basis of Therapeutics, 8th ed. New York, Pergamon, 1990, pp. 345–382.
83. Rapoport DM, Greenberg HE, Goldring RM: Differing effects of the anxiolytic agents buspirone and diazepam on control of breathing. Clin Pharmacol Ther 1991;49: 394–401.
84. Raskind MA, Kitchell M, Alcarez C: Bromide intoxication in the elderly. J Am Geriatr Soc 1978;26:222–224.
85. Reed CE, Driggs MF, Foote CG: Acute barbiturate intoxication: A study of 300 cases. Ann Intern Med 1952;37: 301–303.
86. Reimche LD, Sankaran K, Hindmarsh KW, et al: Chloral hydrate sedation in neonates and infants—Clinical and pharmacologic considerations. Dev Pharmacol Ther 1989; 12:57–64.
87. Rickels K, Schweizer E, Csanalosi I, et al: Long term treatment of anxiety and risk of withdrawal: Prospective comparison of clorazepate and buspirone. Arch Gen Psychiatry 1988;45:444–450.
88. Robins AH: The other side of the benzodiazepines. S Afr Cont Med Educ 1984;2:43–48.
89. Salmon AG, Kizer KW, Zeise L, et al: Potential carcinogenicity of chloral hydrate—A review. J Toxicol Clin Toxicol 1995;33:115–121.
90. Salva P, Costa J: Clinical pharmacokinetics and pharmacodynamics of zolpidem. Therapeutic implications. Clin Pharmacokinet 1995;29:142–153.
91. Schwartz HS: Acute meprobamate poisoning with gastrotomy and removal of a drug containing mass. N Engl J Med 1976;295:1177–1178.
92. Sebel PS, Lowden JD: Propofol: New intravenous anesthesia. Anesthesiology 1989;71: 260–277.
93. Sellers EM, Lang BS, Koch-Weser, et al: Interaction of chloral hydrate and ethanol in man. Clin Pharmacol Ther 1971; 13:37–48.
94. Serfaty M, Masterton G: Fatal poisonings attributed to benzodiazepines in Britain during the 1980s. Br J Psychiatry 1993;163:386–393.
95. Serpe S: Bromide intoxication. NY State J Med 1972;72: 2086–2088.
96. Sharpless SK: Hypnotics and sedatives. In: Goodman LS, Gilman A, eds: The Pharmacological Basis of Therapeutics, 4th ed. New York, Macmillan, 1970, pp. 98–120. (Because of the limited therapeutic role of bromides, subsequent editions have not included detailed discussions.)
97. Shubin H, Weil MH: The mechanism of shock following suicidal doses of barbiturate, narcotics and tranquilizer drugs. Am J Med 1965;38:853–857.
98. Sing K, Erickson T, Amitai Y, Hryhorczuk D: Chloral hydrate toxicity from oral and intravenous administration. J Toxicol Clin Toxicol 1996;34:101–106.
99. Sivilotti L, Nistri A: GABA receptor mechanisms in the CNS. Prog Neurobiol 1991;36:35–92.
100. Snyder SH: Drug and neurotransmitter receptors: New perspectives with clinical relevance. JAMA 1989;261: 3126–3129.
101. Steinberg AD: Should chloral hydrate be banned? Pediatrics 1993;92:442–446.
102. Taylor DC: Buspirone: New approach to the treatment of anxiety. FASEB J 1988;2:2445–2452.
103. Teehan BP, Maher JF, Carey JJH, et al: Acute ethchlorvynol (Placidyl) intoxication. Ann Intern Med 1970; 72:875–882.
104. Teicher MH: Biology of Anxiety. Med Clin North Am 1988;72:791–814.
105. Trappler B, Bezeredi T: Triazolam intoxication. Can Med Assoc J 1982;126:893–894. Letter.
106. Twyman RE, Rogers CJ, Macdonald RL: Differential regulation of GABA receptor channels by diazepam and phenobarbital. Ann Neurol 1989;25:213–220.
107. Veller ID, Richardson JP, Doyle JC, et al: Gastric necrosis: A rare complication of chloral hydrate intoxication. Br J Surg 1971;59:317–319.
108. Wagner RL, White PF, Kan PB, et al: Inhibition of adrenal steroidogenesis by the anesthetic etomidate. N Engl J Med 1984;310:1415–1421.
109. Waldron I: Increased prescribing of Valium, Librium and other drugs: An example of the influence of economic and social factors on the practice of medicine. Int J Health 1977;7:37–62.
110. Winchester J, Maher J, Garela S, et al: Artifical organs in acute poisoning: To treat or not to treat with artificial organs. Trans Am Soc Artif Intern Organs 1982;28:666–675.
111. Wiseman HM, Hampel G: Cardiac arrhythmias due to chloral hydrate poisoning. Br Med J 1978;2:970. Letter.
112. Wright N, Roscoe P: Acute glutethimide poisoning. JAMA 1970;214:1704–1706.
113. Xanthaky YG, Freireich AW, Matusiak W, Lukash L: Hemodialysis in methyprylon poisoning. JAMA 1966;198: 1212–1213.
114. Yagi K, Baudendistel LJ, Dahms TE: Ibuprofen reduces ethchlorvynol lung injury: Possible role of blood flow distribution. J Appl Physiol 1992;72:1156–1165.
115. Zatuchni J, Hong K: Methyl bromide poisoning seen initially as psychosis. Arch Neurol 1981;38:529–530.

ANTIDOTES IN DEPTH

Flumazenil

Mary Ann Howland

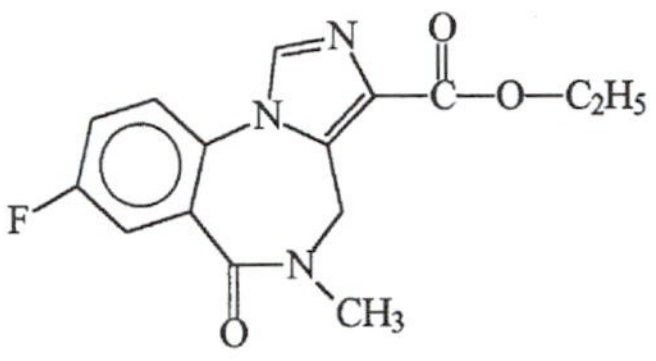

Flumazenil

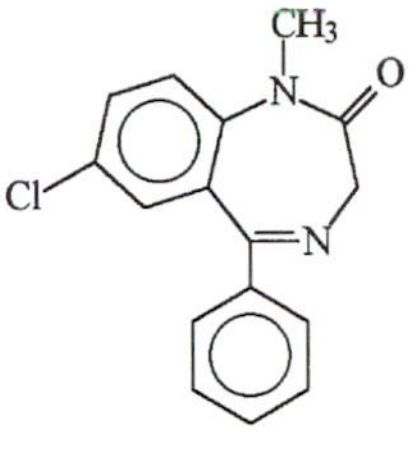

Diazepam

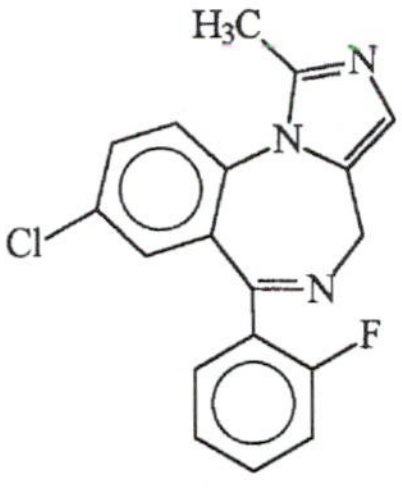

Midazolam

Haefely and Hunkeler's initial work on synthesis of chlordiazepoxide led to an attempt to develop benzodiazepine derivatives that would act as antagonists.[19] This endeavor was unsuccessful at the time, and they investigated the promising gamma-aminobutyric acid (GABA) hypothesis of benzodiazepine mechanism of action. In 1977, the then-new technique of radioligand binding identified specific high-affinity benzodiazepine binding sites. Other investigators had simultaneously isolated a product produced by a *Streptomyces* species that had the basic 1,4-benzodiazepine structure, and subsequently they began to synthesize compounds from this molecule to act as potential tranquilizers. Hunkeler attempted to produce benzodiazepines with potent anxiolytic and anticonvulsant activity and diminished sedative and muscle-relaxing properties. Testing revealed that these derivatives had high in vitro binding affinities but lacked in vivo activity. An inability to enter the central nervous system was considered as an explanation for this discordance. During an experiment that attempted to demonstrate CNS penetration for these derivatives, diazepam was given to incapacitate the animals, and surprisingly had a very weak effect. This lack of potency led to the discovery of a benzodiazepine antagonist. Further modifications led to the synthesis of RO–15–1788, flumazenil.

Flumazenil is a competitive antagonist with very weak agonist properties at the benzodiazepine receptor. Agonists such as diazepam stimulate the benzodiazepine receptor to produce anxiolytic, anticonvulsant, sedative, amnestic, and muscle-relaxant effects at low doses and hypnosis at high doses. Inverse agonists stimulate the benzodiazepine receptor and result in the opposite effects: anxiety, agitation, and seizures. Antagonists, such as flumazenil, competitively occupy the benzodiazepine receptor without causing any functional change and without allowing an agonist or inverse agonist access to the receptor. It has been suggested that the zero set point of intrinsic activity may be influenced by the activity of the GABA system or by chronic treatment with benzodiazepines.[15] Positron emission tomography (PET) investigations reveal that 1.5 mg of flumazenil leads to an initial receptor occupancy of 55%, while 15 mg causes almost total blockade of benzodiazepine receptor sites.[35]

The structures of flumazenil, diazepam, and midazolam are shown in the figure. The physiochemical properties of flumazenil are summarized in Table 61–4.[23]

Flumazenil has been studied in more than 3500 patients worldwide, including healthy volunteers and overdosed or consciously sedated patients. Its safety in healthy volunteers is well established, with no discernible objective or subjective effects. Flumazenil is capable of reversing most benzodiazepine effects. The question to be explored is whether there are subsets of patients for whom the benefits of antagonist use clearly outweigh the risks of withdrawal seizures and, rarely, dysrhythmias.

TABLE 61–4. PHYSIOCHEMICAL AND PHARMACOLOGIC PROPERTIES OF FLUMAZENIL

pKa	Weak base
Partition coefficient at pH 7.4	14 (octanol/aqueous PO_4 buffer)
Volume of distribution	1.06 L/kg
Distribution half-life ($t_{1/2}\ \alpha$)	≤ 5 minutes
Metabolism	Hepatic with three inactive metabolites devoid of benzodiazepine receptor affinity High clearance
Elimination	First order
Protein binding	54–64% (low)
Half-life ($t_{1/2}\ \beta$)	53 minutes
Onset of action	Rapid within 1–2 minutes
Duration of action	Dependent on dose and elimination of benzodiazepine, time interval, dose of flumazenil, and hepatic function

An initial concern was whether flumazenil would be detrimental to patients with epilepsy. It is believed that GABA suppresses abnormal electrical activity, and there was concern that flumazenil might reverse this effect, thereby increasing the risk of seizures. However, studies suggest that flumazenil may actually exhibit anticonvulsant activity in patients with complex partial seizures. Hart and associates found that a dose of 3 mg of flumazenil IV was comparable to 10 mg of diazepam IV, in suppressing interictal electroencephalographic activity.[20] They postulated that flumazenil acted as either a partial agonist or antagonized an endogenous proconvulsant substance. Savec and colleagues found similar results in 6 patients with partial complex seizures but not in 6 patients with generalized seizures.[35] Furthermore, in 3 patients who were tolerant to clonazepam, 1.5 mg of flumazenil IV produced a mild withdrawal syndrome, manifested as 30 minutes of shivering in 2 patients. More important, in the patients who had become tolerant to clonazepam, a clinical response was restored. These studies and others suggest a weak agonist characteristic of flumazenil,[13] or resetting of the benzodiazepine receptors. In animals, there appears to be a curvilinear dose-dependency relationship.

Volunteer studies demonstrate flumazenil's ability to reverse benzodiazepines.[11] Reversal is both immediate and dose dependent. Most individuals achieve complete reversal of benzodiazepine effect with a total IV dose of 1 mg.[1,7] A 3-mg IV dose produces similar effects that last approximately twice as long as the 1-mg dose.

Extensive reviews of the use of flumazenil are published and include patients undergoing conscious sedation for endoscopy or cardioversion.[2,7] Kirkegaard and co-workers conducted a double-blind randomized study involving 40 patients undergoing gastroscopy who received 0.3 to 0.5 mg/kg of diazepam.[25] Flumazenil was initiated at a 0.2-mg dose and titrated in 0.2-mg increments until a total of 1 mg had been given or full reversal of sedation occurred and at least 85% of amnesia was reversed. The median dose was 1 mg. Three patients experienced slight confusion. A similar study performed with midazolam in patients older than 65 years yielded similar results.[24] Another study of 30 patients with midazolam-induced sedation, demonstrated effective reversal with 0.15 mg of flumazenil IV.[6] Five patients reported temporary agitation and restlessness and resedation occurred within 30 to 60 minutes. There are two case reports of patients undergoing endoscopy who developed seizures following benzodiazepine reversal.[38] One patient had a history of seizures and the other had no obvious etiology. Both recovered uneventfully.

When a benzodiazepine is given to achieve conscious sedation during a procedure, flumazenil appears safe and effective in the reversal of sedation and the partial reversal of amnesia. Most patients respond to doses of 0.6 to 1 mg. Administering flumazenil slowly, at a rate of 0.1 mg/min, minimizes the disconcerting symptoms associated with rapid arousal, such as confusion, agitation, and emotional lability. Resedation occurs within 20 to 120 minutes, depending on the dose and pharmacokinetics of the benzodiazepine as well as the dose of flumazenil. For this reason, patients must be carefully monitored, and subsequent doses of flumazenil given as needed. Because the amnestic effect of benzodiazepines is not consistently reversed, posttreatment instructions should be reinforced in writing and given to a responsible caretaker accompanying the patient.[10] Because of the risk of resedation, many endoscopists elect not to use flumazenil.

Flumazenil has not consistently reversed benzodiazepine-induced respiratory depression.[36] If respiratory depression is mediated through the benzodiazepine receptor, then flumazenil should be effective in reversing that effect, as shown by Gross and associates.[17] However, others have not found reversal to occur consistently.[8,28,31,36] Using oxygen saturation measurements and plethysmography to determine minute ventilation volumes, Carter and colleagues examined the effect of IV midazolam on respiratory depression in patients undergoing endoscopy.[8] Flumazenil awakened patients rapidly but failed to affect minute ventilation and had little effect on oxygen saturation. When a benzodiazepine was used concomitantly with an opioid, the effects on ventilation were even more confusing.[41,43] Rebound respiratory depression and prolonged hypoxic episodes were documented. It is suggested that flumazenil may even have a slight respiratory depressant effect when combined with an opioid.[41] Clinical assessment of respiratory rate is inadequate to detect hypoxia. Benzodiazepine-induced apnea should be managed with fundamental procedures such as supplemental oxygen, airway stabilization, bag valve mask ventilation, and endotracheal intubation, if indicated.

The use of flumazenil in the overdose setting has provoked substantial controversy. The first argument against its use is that benzodiazepines rarely cause morbidity and mortality. Höjer and Baehrendtz analyzed 702 patients admitted to a medical intensive care unit over a 14 year time period who had taken benzodiazepines alone or in combination with ethanol or other drugs.[22] Five cases proved fatal (0.7%), and 69 patients (9.8%) experienced complications. By comparison, the fatality rate was 1.6% (55 of 3430) for patients with nonbenzodiazepine-related overdoses. In the pure benzodiazepine group, 2 patients died and 18 of 144 patients (12.5%) had complications, mostly aspiration pneumonitis and decubitus ulcers. Proponents of flumazenil therapy suggest that some of the 29 diagnostic procedures used in these patients would have been unnecessary, and possibly some of the complications that occurred could have been avoided. Opponents of flumazenil suggest that many of the cases of aspiration pneumonitis occurred prior to hospital admission and that these patients also often suffer from trauma and infectious disease, making most diagnostic procedures necessary in any event. In addition, the use of flumazenil may put the patient at risk for seizures by unmasking a toxic effect or by precipitating acute benzodiazepine withdrawal. In addition, flumazenil causes a significant overshoot in cerebral blood flow and may cause a large increase in intracranial pressure in patients previously receiving midazolam for severe head injury.[46]

Because a flumazenil dose of 1 mg or less IV still leaves 50% of benzodiazepine receptors unoccupied, the risk of acute withdrawal should be limited as long as this dose is not exceeded.[33] The ability of flumazenil to precipitate acute benzodiazepine withdrawal seizures in a more controlled setting than the overdose setting was demonstrated by the reversal of long-term benzodiazepine sedation in the ICU. Amrein reported that 14 of 1700 patients studied had adverse drug reactions that could not be excluded as benzodiazepine withdrawal.[2] Following reversal with anesthetic use, 9 patients, 4 of whom had received greater than 1 mg of flumazenil, exhibited anxiety, fear, and confusion. It was suggested that in 7 of these patients the symptoms were probably due to rapid arousal. Of 215 patients treated in the ICU setting, 1 probable (0.5%) and 4 possible (2%) withdrawal reactions occurred.[2] Grand mal seizures occurred in 2 patients with epilepsy, and 1 case of myoclonic seizures and 2 of agitation also occurred. Three of five of these patients had received a large dose of flumazenil. An explanation for this finding may be that small doses of flumazenil allow enough of the benzodiazepine receptor sites to be occupied with benzodiazepine such that abrupt withdrawal seizures are uncommon. The weak intrinsic agonist action of flumazenil may also be protective.

In an attempt to better understand the risks and benefits of flumazenil, Geller and co-workers reviewed 30 published case studies involving a total of 758 patients with drug overdoses; 387 patients were in double-blind study protocols and 371 in open-label studies.[16] Fifty percent of cases involved overdosage with more than one drug. The doses of flumazenil were from 0.2 to 5 mg. In all, there were 5 cases of seizures temporally related to flumazenil administration, all occurring after large bolus doses. Furthermore, in 3 of these 5 patients, tricyclic antidepressants were present in high concentrations in the blood. All of the seizures resolved without treatment or following administration of a small dose of a benzodiazepine. In 2 patients given small doses of flumazenil, cardiac dysrhythmias developed. Again, the presence of an antidepressant has been suggested as a precipitant. Of 497 patients enrolled in two clinical U.S. studies with Hoffman LaRoche Pharmaceuticals,[16] 6 patients developed seizures (5 had coingested tricyclic antidepressants) and one patient who had taken a tricyclic antidepressant and carbamazepine had a junctional tachycardia, which normalized after several minutes. Thus in reviewing 1255 patients, 11 patients seized and 3 developed cardiac dysrhythmias, for an incidence of about 0.9%. The consensus of this group of authors was that (1) flumazenil is not a substitute for primary emergency care; (2) hypoxia and hypotension should be corrected before flumazenil is used; (3) small titrated doses of flumazenil should be used; (4) flumazenil should be avoided in patients with a history of seizures, evidence of seizures or jerking movements, or evidence of a cyclic antidepressant overdose; and (5) flumazenil should not be used by inexperienced clinicians.

Spivey reviewed all published cases of seizures associated with flumazenil or those reported to the manufacturer.[38] The total number of patients studied in the review was approximately 3500. Of the 43 patients who seized, 6 died, but Spivey believed that none of the deaths was attributable to flumazenil. Four patients developed status epilepticus; 2 of these were presumed to be due to concomitant tricyclic antidepressant exposure, and the other 2 patients had received benzodiazepines to treat status epilepticus prior to flumazenil therapy. In 6 of the 43 episodes of seizures, the relationship to flumazenil use was felt to be inadequately defined. The remaining 37 patients were stratified into five categories. In category 1, 7 patients were given flumazenil after they had received a benzodiazepine for treatment of a seizure disorder. Six of these seven patients received more than 1 mg of flumazenil. In category 2, 20 patients received flumazenil for reversal of a benzodiazepine in a mixed-drug overdose. Many of these patients were shown to have coingested tricyclic antidepressants. Thirteen of these patients received more than 1 mg of flumazenil. Two of the patients in this group developed status epilepticus and died, possibly secondary to a severe tricyclic antidepressant overdose. Category 3 included 5 patients receiving benzodiazepines for suppression of nondrug-induced seizures. Two of these five patients received doses of flumazenil greater than 1 mg. Category 4 included 3 patients with acute benzodiazepine overdoses, in the presence of chronic benzodiazepine dependence. Category 5 included 2 patients receiving a benzodiazepine for conscious sedation.

In an effort to develop indications for the safe and effective use of flumazenil, overdosed comatose patients were retrospectively assigned to either a low-risk or non-low-risk group.[18] Low-risk patients had CNS depression with normal vital signs, no other neurologic findings, no evidence of ingestion of a tricyclic antidepressant by history or ECG, no seizure history, and absence of an available history of chronic benzodiazepine ingestion. All other patients fell into the non-low-risk category. Of 35 consecutive comatose patients, 4 patients were assigned to the low-risk group. Flumazenil caused complete awakening in 3 and partial awakening in the fourth patient in the low risk group with no adverse effects. In the non-low-risk group of 31 patients, flumazenil caused complete awakening in 4 and partial awakening in 5. Seizures occurred in 5 patients. Of the 5 patients with seizures, one had a history of seizures, all 5 were long-term benzodiazepine users, 4 had abnormal vital signs, and 3 had evidence of hyperreflexia or myoclonus. Therefore, although the use of flumazenil was safe and effective in the low-risk group, unfortunately very few patients met the criteria. The risk of seizures is substantial in the non-low-risk group.

In conclusion, the benefit of flumazenil appears to outweigh the risks when benzodiazepines are used therapeutically to perform a diagnostic or therapeutic procedure. When benzodiazepines are ingested alone in the overdose setting by nonbenzodiazepine-dependent patients, as very rarely occurs in adults or might be ex-

TABLE 61–5. INDICATIONS FOR FLUMAZENIL IN THE OVERDOSE SETTING

Pure benzodiazepine overdose in a nontolerant individual who has:
- CNS depression
- Normal vital signs
- Normal ECG
- Otherwise normal neurologic examination

pected in children, the risks associated with the use of flumazenil may be limited. Slow IV titration (0.1 mg/min) to a total dose not exceeding 1 mg seems most reasonable. Resedation may occur at 20 to 120 minutes, and it may be necessary to readminister flumazenil. Although not FDA approved, a continuous intravenous infusion in saline or dextrose of 0.25 to 1.0 mg/h has been employed following the loading dose.[45] The risks of flumazenil appear to greatly outweigh the potential benefits of reversal when benzodiazepines are used chronically or acutely to treat a seizure disorder (see Tables 61–5 and Table 61–6).

Flumazenil is best avoided in the overdose setting when there is evidence that a drug capable of causing seizures has been ingested (Table 61–6). Any indication that theophylline, carbamazepine, chloral hydrate, chloroquine, and/or chlorinated hydrocarbons have been ingested is a contraindication to the use of flumazenil.[44] When there is a suggestion, based on history, clinical findings, or ECG findings (increased QRS, increased QT, or increased heart rate), that a cyclic antidepressant is involved, flumazenil should be avoided.[21,27,32,44] In the event of flumazenil-induced seizures, a therapeutic dose of a benzodiazepine such as diazepam should be effective. Flumazenil is a competitive antagonist; higher doses of benzodiazepines will reverse higher doses of flumazenil.

What Is the Role of Flumazenil in Hepatic Encephalopathy?

Hepatic encephalopathy is considered to be a reversible metabolic encephalopathy characterized by a spectrum of CNS effects. Symptoms may progress from confusion and somnolence to coma. The current hypothesis implicates an increase in GABAergic tone as contributory to the encephalopathy.[4,37]

Animal studies of hepatic encephalopathy secondary to galactosamine or thioacetamide (hepatotoxins) demonstrate an increase in GABA effect, which is antagonized by flumazenil, bicuculline (a GABA receptor antagonist), and isopropylbiclophosphate chloride (a calcium channel blocker).[5] Cerebrospinal fluid (CSF) from these animals was shown to contain a benzodiazepine receptor ligand with agonist activity. Rat studies involving hepatic encephalopathy resulting from acute liver ischemia showed only a slight response to flumazenil but significant improvement after administration of a partial inverse agonist.[5,42]

Human studies have also detected benzodiazepine binding activity in the CSF, but not serum, of patients with hepatic encephalopathy. Basile and associates identified 4 to 19 peaks representing benzodiazepine-binding ligands from the frontal cortex of 11 patients who died of hepatic encephalopathy.[3] Two of the peaks were identified as diazepam and *N*-desmethyldiazepam. Six of the patients demonstrated brain concentrations of these substances that were 2 to 10 times higher than normal, and 5 patients had normal concentrations. There have also been several reports of patients with idiopathic recurring stupor who have measurable "endozepines" (endogenous benzodiazepine ligands) in serum and CSF.[34,40]

Flumazenil improves the clinical and electrophysiologic responses of patients with hepatic encephalopathy and idiopathic recurring stupor.[12,14,34,40] Some patients with encephalopathy have improved from stage IV to stage II encephalopathy after IV flumazenil. Maximal improvement after flumazenil lasts about 1 to 2 hours and gradually dissipates within 6 hours. The response rate in case series averages approximately 65%. Not all patients respond, and the proposed explanations for this unresponsiveness include cerebral edema, hypoxia, other systemic diseases or complications, and irreversible CNS damage.

Animal and human data convincingly support the concept that increased GABAergic tone is responsible for hepatic encephalopathy. Evidence for endogenous benzodiazepine ligands that enhance GABA action have also been demonstrated. The source of these benzodiazepine receptor agonists is unclear, but diet and/or production by gut bacteria have been postulated.[4] Most authorities believe endogenous de novo synthesis to be unlikely. Flumazenil can lead to improvement in the clinical condition of a subgroup of patients with hepatic encephalopathy and may prove useful as an addition to conventional therapy. Additional research is necessary to identify prospective responders, dosing considerations, and adverse effects.

TABLE 61–6. CONTRAINDICATIONS TO THE USE OF FLUMAZENIL

- Prior seizure history or current treatment of seizures
- History of ingestion of substance capable of provoking seizures or cardiac dysrhythmias
- Long-term use of benzodiazepines
- ECG evidence (terminal rightward 40 msec axis, QRS or QT prolongation) of tricyclic antidepressants
- Abnormal vital signs

What is the Role of Flumazenil in Ethanol Intoxication?

A number of animal studies indicate that many of the actions of ethanol are mediated through GABA neurotransmission.[39] Acute ethanol administration appears to enhance GABA transmission and inhibit NMDA excitation (excitatory amino acid). Chronic ethanol administration leads to a down-regulation of the GABA system. Ethanol enhances $GABA_A$-induced chloride influx in a dose-dependent fashion without a direct effect on chloride.

Flumazenil does not influence this action of GABA. Chronic ethanol selectively increases the sensitivity to inverse benzodiazepine agonists, invoking a change in coupling or conformation of the receptor. These changes may explain the development of tolerance and the kindling and production of seizures that occur on withdrawal.

Two double-blind studies in patients with benzodiazepine or ethanol overdose evaluated the response to flumazenil. In the study by Martens and colleagues involving 13 patients with suspected ethanol intoxication, 6 had no response to placebo when it was given first, while all 13 patients responded to 5 mg of flumazenil.[30] Improved consciousness occurred after 15 minutes and respiratory rates increased from 14 to 16 breaths/min. There was no effect on heart rate or blood pressure. This 5-mg dose of flumazenil was chosen because when 4 patients were studied with 1 mg of flumazenil, there was no improvement in mental status or vital signs.

Lheureux and Askenasi conducted a comparable study with similar results.[26] One milligram of flumazenil administered to 9 ethanol-intoxicated patients produced the same effects as placebo. Subsequent administration of 2 to 5 mg of flumazenil in the open part of the study produced a clear improvement in the modified Glasgow coma scale in 5 of 11 patients. However, a closer inspection of phase 1 of this study reveals that an arousal reaction occurred in 7 of 9 patients after the flumazenil dose and in 5 of 9 patients following placebo administration. It is conceivable that the improvement in phase 2 was a continuation of this arousal reaction.

A case report by Linowiecki and associates indicates that ethanol-induced respiratory depression was reversed by flumazenil.[29] However, it is unclear whether the actual data supports the author's conclusions.

A randomized double-blind crossover study by Clausen and associates was conducted with eight male volunteers given IV ethanol to achieve a constant blood ethanol concentration of 160 mg/dL.[9] Once stabilized, the volunteers were given either placebo or 5 mg of flumazenil. A number of subjective and objective psychomotor tests were conducted, with no differences noted between volunteers given flumazenil and those given placebo. The probability of ethanol reversal at the suggested doses appears unlikely.

On the basis of this information it is unlikely that flumazenil has a significant effect on ethanol intoxication. Low doses of flumazenil (less than 1 mg) have had no effect, and doses of 5 mg are reported to produce favorable changes in sensorium, but these findings may be the result of confounding factors. Because we would never recommend 5 mg of flumazenil in the overdose setting, because of the increased risk of adverse effects at this dose flumazenil cannot be recommended at this time to treat ethanol intoxication.

References

1. Amrein R, Hetzel W, Hartmann D, Lorscheid T: Clinical pharmacology of flumazenil. Eur J Anaesth 1988;2:65–80.
2. Amrein R, Leishman B, Bentzinger C, Roncari G: Flumazenil in benzodiazepine antagonism: Actions and clinical use in intoxications and anaesthesiology. Med Toxicol 1987;2: 411–429.
3. Basile AS, Hughes RD, Harrison PM, et al: Elevated brain concentrations of 1,4-benzodiazepines in fulminant hepatic failure. N Engl J Med 1991;325:473–478.
4. Benzodiazepine compounds and hepatic encephalopathy. N Engl J Med 1991;325:509–510.
5. Bosman DK, Van Den Buijs CACG, De Haan JC, et al: The effects of benzodiazepine-receptor antagonists and partial inverse agonists on acute hepatic encephalopathy in the rat. Gastroenterology 1991;101:772–781.
6. Breheny FX: Reversal of midazolam sedation with flumazenil. Crit Care Med 1991;20:736–739.
7. Brogden RN, Goa KL: Flumazenil: A reappraisal of its pharmacological properties and therapeutic efficacy as a benzodiazepine antagonist. Drugs 1991;42:1061–1089.
8. Carter AS, Bell GD, Coady T, et al: Speed of reversal of midazolam-induced respiratory depression by flumazenil: A study in patients undergoing upper GI endoscopy. Acta Anaesth Scand 1990;34:59–64.
9. Clausen TG, Wolff J, Carl P, Theilgaard A: The effect of the benzodiazepine antagonist, flumazenil, on psychometric performance in acute ethanol intoxication in man. Eur J Clin Pharmacol 1990;38:233–236.
10. Discussion. Eur J Anaest 1988;2(suppl):233–235.
11. Dunton AW, Schwam E, Pitman V, et al: Flumazenil: US clinical pharmacology studies. Eur J Anaesth 1988;2:81–95.
12. Ferenci P, Grimm G, Meryn S, Gangl A: Successful long-term treatment of portal–systemic encephalopathy by the benzodiazepine antagonist flumazenil. Gastroenterology 1989;96:240–243.
13. File SE, Pellow S: Intrinsic actions of the benzodiazepine receptor antagonist Ro 15–1788. Psychopharmacology 1986; 88:1–11.
14. Flumazenil in the treatment of hepatic encephalopathy. Ann Pharmacother 1993;27:46–47.
15. Gardner CR: Functional in vivo correlates of the benzodiazepine agonist–inverse agonist continuum. Prog Neurobiol 1988;31:425–476.
16. Geller E, Crome P, Schaller MD, et al: Risks and benefits of therapy with flumazenil (Anexate) in mixed drug intoxications. Eur Neurol 1991;31:241–250.
17. Gross JB, Weller RS, Conard P: Flumazenil antagonism of midazolam-induced ventilatory depression. Anesthesiology 1991;75:179–185.
18. Gueye PN, Hoffman JR, Taboulet P. et al: Empiric use of flumazenil in comatose patients: Limited applicability of criteria to define low risk. Ann Emerg Med 1996;27:730–735.
19. Haefely W, Hunkeler W: The story of flumazenil. Eur J Anaesth 1988;2:3–14.
20. Hart YM, Meinardi H, Sander JW, et al: The effect of intravenous flumazenil on interictal electroencephalographic epileptic activity: Results of a placebo-controlled study. J Neurol Neurosurg Pychiatry 1991;54:305–309.
21. Haverkos GP, DiSalvo RP, Imhoff TE: Fatal seizures after flumazenil administration in a patient with mixed overdose. Ann Pharmacother 1994;28:1347–1349.
22. Höjer J, Baehrendtz S: The effect of flumazenil (Ro 15–1788) in the management of self-induced benzodiazepine poison-

ing: A double-blind controlled study. Acta Med Scand 1988; 224:357–365.
23. Hunkeler W: Preclinical research findings with flumazenil (Ro 15–1788, Anexate): Chemistry. Eur J Anaesth 1988;2 (suppl):37–62.
24. Katz JA, Fragen RJ, Dunn KL: Flumazenil reversal of midazolam sedation of the elderly. Regional Anesth 1991;16:247–252.
25. Kirkegaard L, Knudsen L, Jensen S, Kruse A: Benzodiazepine antagonist Ro 15–1788. Anaesthesia 1986;41:1184–1188.
26. Lheureux P, Askenasi R: Efficacy of flumazenil in acute alcohol intoxication: Double blind placebo controlled evaluation. Hum Exp Toxicol 1991;10:235–239.
27. Lheureux P, Vranckx M, Leduc D, Askenasi R: Flumazenil in mixed benzodiazepine/tricyclic antidepressant overdose: A placebo controlled study in the dog. Am J Emerg Med 1992;10:184–188.
28. Lim AG: Death after flumazenil. Br Med J 1989;299:858–859. Letter.
29. Linowiecki K, Paloucek F, Donnelly A, Leikin JB: Reversal of ethanol-induced respiratory depression by flumazenil. Vet Hum Toxicol 1992;34:417–419.
30. Martens F, Köppel C, Ibe K, et al: Clinical experience with the benzodiazepine antagonist flumazenil in suspected benzodiazepine or ethanol poisoning. J Toxicol Clin Toxicol 1990;28:341–356.
31. Mora CT, Torjman M, White PF: Effects of diazepam and flumazenil on sedation and hypoxic ventilatory response. Anesth Analg 1989;68:473–478.
32. Mordel A, Winkler E, Almog S, et al: Seizures after flumazenil administration in a case of combined benzodiazepine and tricyclic antidepressant overdose. Crit Care Med 1992;20:1733–1734.
33. Persson A, Pauli S, Halldin C, et al: Saturation analysis of Specific ^{11}C Ro 15–1788 binding to the human neocortex using positron emission tomography. Hum Psychopharmacol 1989;4:21–31.
34. Rothstein JD, Guidotti A, Tinuper P, et al: Endogenous benzodiazepine receptor ligands in idiopathic recurring stupor. Lancet 1992;340:1002–1004.
35. Savic I, Widen L, Stone-Eldaner S: Feasibility of reversing benzodiazepine tolerance with flumazenil. Lancet 1991;337: 133–137.
36. Shalansky SJ, Naumann TL, Englander FA: Therapy update: Effect of flumazenil on benzodiazepine-induced respiratory depression. Clin Pharm 1993;12:483–487.
37. Skolnick P: The γ-aminobutyric acid A ($GABA_A$) receptor complex. In: Jones EA, moderator. The γ-aminobutyric acid A ($GABA_A$) receptor complex and hepatic encephalopathy: Some recent advances. Ann Intern Med 1989;100: 532–546.
38. Spivey WH: Flumazenil and seizures: Analysis of 43 cases. Clin Ther 1992;14:292–305.
39. Ticku MK, Mhatre M, Mehta AK: Modulation of GABAergic transmission by ethanol. In: Biggio G, Costa E, eds: GABAergic Synaptic Transmission. New York, Raven, 1992, pp. 255–268.
40. Tinuper P, Montagna P, Cortelli P, et al: Idiopathic recurring stupor: A case with possible involvement of the gamma-aminobutyric acid (GABA)ergic system. Ann Neurol 1992;31:503–506.
41. Tolksdorf W, Ney C, Ney R, Amberger M: The influence of flumazenil on respiration after midazolam and/or fentanyl. Anesth Analg 1990;70:S409. Abstract.
42. Van der Rijt CC, de Knegt RJ, Schalm SW, et al: Flumazenil does not improve hepatic encephalopathy associated with acute ischemic liver failure in the rabbit. Metab Brain Dis 1990;3:131–141.
43. Weinbroum A, Geller E: The respiratory effects of reversing midazolam sedation with flumazenil in the presence or absence of narcotics. Acta Anaesth Scand 1990;92:65–69.
44. Weinbroum A, Halpern P, Geller E: The use of flumazenil in the management of acute drug poisoning: A review. Intensive Care Med 1991;17:S32–S38.
45. Winkler E, Shlomo A, Kriger D, et al: Use of flumazenil in the diagnosis and treatment of patients with coma of unknown etiology. Crit Care Med 1993;21:538–542.
46. Whitwan G, Amrein R: Pharmacology of flumazenil. Acta Anaesthesiol Scand 1995;39(suppl 108):3–14.

CHAPTER 62

Ethanol

Harold H. Osborn

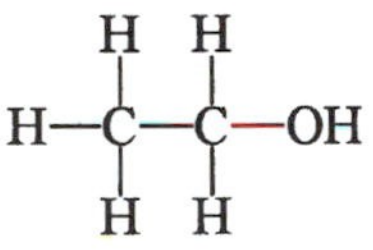

Ethanol

Ethanol	
MW	= 46 D
Level Consistent With Intoxication	= 50–100 mg/dL (10.85–21.7 mmol/L)

A 42-year-old man was brought to the Emergency Department (ED) by his wife with a complaint of nausea and vomiting for 2 days. His wife stated that he was a chronic alcoholic and had been drinking heavily in the preceding days. He had no previous history of hospitalizations or other illnesses. He smoked 1.5 packs of cigarettes a day and was taking no medications.

On physical examination the patient was noted to be a thin man who appeared lethargic with slurred speech. His vital signs were: blood pressure, 90/60 mm Hg; pulse, 110 beats/min supine; respiratory rate, 26 breaths/min; temperature, 100.4°F (38°C). His blood pressure dropped to 70/50 mm Hg, and his pulse rose to 128 beats/min, when sitting.

The patient's tongue and mucous membranes were dry. He was anicteric and without pallor or cyanosis. His head was atraumatic. Eye examination revealed pupils that were 3 mm bilaterally and reacted to light. His extraocular movements were full, and bilateral nystagmus was noted on lateral gaze. Funduscopic examination was normal. His neck was supple and without adenopathy or thyromegaly. Bilateral nontender parotid enlargement was noted. His lungs were clear to percussion and auscultation and his heart sounds were regular, without murmurs, rubs, or gallops. His abdomen was scaphoid and soft. There was hepatomegaly with a palpable liver edge 3 finger breadths below the costal margin (16 cm by percussion overall). There was no splenomegaly or any other abdominal masses noted. Rectal examination revealed brown stool that tested negative for occult blood. Skin evaluation revealed erythema of the palms and face but no evidence of spider angiomata or gynecomastia. There was a normal amount of axillary and pubic hair and no evidence of testicular atrophy. Neurologic examination revealed a lethargic man with intact cranial nerves who responded to voice and touch but was dysarthric and could not answer questions appropriately. His deep-tendon reflexes were 3+ bilaterally, plantar flexion was present bilaterally, and there was no evidence of tremor or asterixis.

An intravenous line was established with 0.9% sodium chloride solution running wide open. A bedside finger stick for blood glucose was less than 120 mg/dL. The patient was given intravenously 50 mL of $D_{50}W$, 100 mg of thiamine, and folate and multivitamins.

A CBC revealed 15,000/mm^3 leukocytes without a left shift; hematocrit, 52%; platelets 150,000/mm^3. Blood chemistries revealed glucose, 100 mg/dL; BUN, 50 mg/dL; creatinine, 1.2 mg/dL, sodium, 148 mEq/L; potassium, 3.6 mEq/L; chloride, 113 mEq/L; carbon dioxide, 15 mEq/L. The ethanol level was 280 mg/dL. The serum amylase level was 200 SU/dL with a serum lipase of 130 U/L. Serum ammonia was normal, at 70 μg/dL. Urinalysis revealed 1 to 2+ ketones, with no glucose, protein, or cells. The prothrombin and partial thromboplastin times were normal. An arterial blood gas analysis revealed a pH of 7.31, PCO_2 of 25 mm Hg, and PO_2 of 93 mm Hg on room air.

During his stay in the ED the patient's mental status improved as did his vital signs, and his metabolic acidosis resolved following several liters of isotonic crystalloid. He was admitted to the hospital for further stablization and rehabilitation.

What Are the Characteristics of Ethanol?

Although ethanol is frequently referred to simply as "alcohol," in reality there are a large number of alcohols. Alcohols are hydroxy derivatives of the aliphatic hydrocarbons. Ethanol, with one hydroxyl (OH) group, is a member of the monohydroxy alcohol series (along with methanol, isopropanol, and others); ethylene glycol possesses two hydroxyl groups and, along with propylene glycol, is a member of the dihydroxy alcohol series. The alcohols in the dihydroxy series are referred to as glycols because of their sweet taste. The propane derivative glycerol or glycerine is the most common example of the trihydroxy series.

Ethanol results from the fermentation of a sugar by yeast. The sugars are derived from cereals, vegetables, or fruits. If a cereal is used as the raw material, it must first be malted to convert the starch to maltose, because yeast will not ferment starch. A malt is produced by moistening barley and allowing it to sprout, leading to a mixture of maltose and the enzyme diastase. The sprouted barley is dried and ground and added to a cereal and water to form a mash. Mash for brewing beer is filtered and the liquid (wort) is then treated with yeast. Whiskey is made by adding the yeast directly to the malted mash. After fermentation, stronger alcoholic beverages are usually distilled. With the most efficient fractioning processes only water and alcohol ("neutral spirits") remain.

The ethanol content of various alcoholic beverages can be expressed by volume percent or by proof, the latter being twice the percentage of alcohol by volume. The ethanol content of beers is usually 2 to 6%, with low-calorie/low-content beers having the weakest concentration. The ethanol content of wines varies from 10 to 20%, averaging approximately 12%. Wines with an ethanol content greater than 16% are usually fortified by adding neutral spirits. Distilled liquors usually contain 40 to 50% ethanol (80 to 100 proof). Other products containing ethanol can occasionally cause intoxication. Mouthwashes may have up to 75% ethanol and colognes may contain 40 to 60% ethanol.[13,91] Ethanol is ubiquitous in the United States and is present in over 700 medicinal preparations as a diluent or solvent in concentrations ranging from 0.3% to 75%.[13,91] Congeners found in alcoholic beverages may contribute to toxicity in heavy drinkers. They include low-molecular-weight alcohols (methanol and butanol), aldehydes, esters, histamines, phenols, tannins, iron, lead, and cobalt. Congeners can be a serious problem in illegally produced alcohol (moonshine) and can result in occasional epidemic poisoning, as occurred when cobalt, used as a defoaming agent in beer, led to "beer drinkers' cardiomyopathy."[76]

Ethanol is a colorless, odorless hydrocarbon composed of weakly charged molecules. It is fully miscible in water and is both water-soluble and lipid-soluble. With a volume of distribution of 0.6 L/kg (roughly equivalent to that of total body water), it diffuses easily across cell membranes and reaches all areas of the body (hence its pervasive effect on most organ systems). Ethanol has a molecular weight of 46 D and yields 7.1 kcal/g when oxidized (Table 62–1). A chronic drinker can obtain sufficient calories from alcohol alone if his or her daily ethanol intake exceeds 5 g/kg body weight (Table 62–2), but can become malnourished in the process due to the absence of all other vital nutrients.

Ethanol is physically addicting. With chronic intake, the degree of tolerance to ethanol is less than that seen with opioids.[95] Withdrawal manifestations seen with the abrupt cessation or relative diminution of ethanol intake are much more severe, however. The consumption of roughly 1 mL/kg of absolute (100% ethanol) alcohol (1 g/kg) raises the blood alcohol level to approximately

TABLE 62–1. CHARACTERISTICS OF ETHANOL

1 g ethanol = 7.1 kcal energy (~7.0)
Volume of distribution = 0.54 L/kg (~0.6)
Specific gravity = 0.7939 g/mL (~0.8)
Milliliters/fluid ounce = 29.9 (~30)
100 mg% = 100 mg/dL = 0.1 g/100 mL = 0.1%
100 mg% = 21.7 mmol/L = 0.217% (vol/vol)
1 mL/kg of 100% ethanol (1 g/kg) produces a blood level of approximately 100 mg/dL
1 oz of whisky, 6-oz glass of wine, or 12-oz bottle of beer raises the blood alcohol approximately 25 mg/dL in an average-sized adult

Metabolism of Ethanol

Maximum rate = 100–125 mg/kg/h (chronic alcoholics, 175 mg/kg/h)
Average adult = 7–10 g/h
Average reduction in level = 15–20 mg/dL/h (chronic alcoholics, 30–40 mg/dL/h)

$$\text{Blood level (mg/dL)} = \frac{\text{dose (mg)}}{\text{Vd (L/kg)} \times \text{body weight (kg)} \times 10}$$

Dose (mg) = amount ingested (mL) × ethanol concentration (mg/dL) × 800
Percent = proof/2
Lethal dose = 5.8 g/kg nontolerant adult
= 3 g/kg child

Adapted with permission from Osborn H: Alcohol toxicodynamics and clinical correlations. In: Schwartz GR, Cayten CG, Mangelsen MA, et al, eds: The Principles and Practice of Emergency Medicine, 3rd ed. Philadelphia, Lea & Febiger, 1992, p. 3021.

TABLE 62–2. CALORIC CONTENT OF ETHANOL

Given

The specific gravity of ethanol is about 0.8 g/mL
Proof is twice the percent of ethanol by volume

Problem

What is the caloric content of 1 quart of 100-proof vodka?

Calculations

1 quart = 32 ounces × 30 mL/ounce = 960 mL
100 proof = 50% by volume
960 mL × 50% = 480 mL of ethanol
480 mL × 0.8 g/mL = 384 g of ethanol
384 g × 7 kcal/g = 2688 kcal

21 to 32 mmol/L (100 to 150 mg/dL). A "standard drink" (roughly 15 g of ethanol), defined as 1 oz (30 mL) of liquor, a 5-oz (150 ml) glass of wine, or a 12-oz bottle of beer, increases blood alcohol level by approximately 5.4 to 7.6 mmol/L (25 to 35 mg/dL). Lethal doses of ethanol are reported to be 5 to 6 g/kg for nontolerant adults and 3 g/kg for children, but the individual response to very high doses is extremely variable.[14] Ethanol freely passes through the placenta, fully exposing the fetus to significant blood alcohol levels if the mother drinks significant amounts. Following complete distribution, ethanol is present in body tissues in a concentration proportional to that of the tissue water content. The concentration in the blood is maintained by back diffusion, which occurs whenever the level in the blood falls below that of the tissues.

What Are the Pharmacokinetics of Ethanol?

The stomach extracts only about 20% of an orally ingested dose and the small intestine extracts the rest.[1] Thus, anything that delays gastric emptying can delay the absorption of ethanol. High concentrations of ethanol itself can do this by causing pylorospasm. Absorption also depends on the volume and character of the alcoholic beverage, the presence or absence of food, GI motility, coexistence of GI disease, coingestion of drugs, concentration of alcohol, the time taken to ingest the drink, and individual variation. Under optimal conditions for absorption, 80 to 90% of an ingested dose is fully absorbed within 30 to 60 minutes. With any one of the conditions mentioned present, absorption may be delayed 2 to 6 hours. Enhanced absorption is seen with rapid gastric emptying, alcohol intake without food, the absence of congeners, dilution of ethanol (maximum absorption occurs at a concentration of 20% volume), and carbonation.

Following an equivalent dose of ethanol, women achieve a higher blood alcohol level than do men as a result of less local metabolism of ethanol in GI tissue.[53] Alcohol dehydrogenase, located in the gastric mucosa, oxidizes a proportion of the ingested ethanol, thus reducing the amount available for absorption. This effect is more pronounced in men than in women and in nonalcoholics than in alcoholics.[27] Moreover, 80% of Japanese are deficient in one of the gastric ADH enzymes.[66] The reduced gastric oxidation of ethanol and its greater bioavailability in women results in enhanced absorption, increased ethanol levels, and presumably an increased susceptibility to alcohol-related disease.

More than 90% of ethanol ingested is eliminated by enzymatic oxidation, with only 5 to 10% excreted unchanged by the kidneys, lungs, and sweat. The excretion of ethanol by the lungs obeys Henry's law: The ratio between the concentration of ethanol in the alveolar air and the blood is constant. Although the alveolar air/blood constant is quite high (1:2100) and very little ethanol is excreted by this route, the fixed relationship forms the basis for the sampling of breath to reliably estimate blood alcohol concentration.

Oxidation of ethanol occurs principally in the liver, and the hepatocytes possess three main ethanol-related metabolic pathways: an alcohol dehydrogenase pathway located in the cell cytosol, a microsomal ethanol-oxidizing system (MEOS: CYP2E1) located on the endoplasmic reticulum, and a relatively unimportant peroxidase-catalase system associated with the hepatic peroxisomes (Fig. 62–1).[16,68]

The alcohol dehydrogenase system is the main pathway for ethanol metabolism in the body and is the rate-limiting step. Ethanol is unique among CNS depressants in that it is metabolized principally by a cytosolic liver enzyme, while the others are cleared by hepatic microsomal enzymes. Alcohol dehydrogenase (ADH), a zinc-containing enzyme, uses nicotinamide adenine dinucleotide (NAD) as a hydrogen acceptor to oxidize ethanol to acetaldehyde. In the alcohol dehydrogenase-mediated pathway, hydrogen is transferred from ethanol to NAD, converting it to its reduced form, NADH. The oxidation of ethanol thus generates an excess of reducing equivalents in the cytosol in the form of NADH, and the ratio of NAD to NADH is dramatically altered. This ratio, also known as the redox potential, determines the ability of the cell to carry on various other oxidative processes. The unfavorable change in redox potential due to ethanol metabolism contributes to the development of numerous metabolic abnormalities associated with alcoholism, such as alcoholic ketoacidosis, impaired gluconeogenesis, and alterations in lipid metabolism. In the final stages of ethanol metabolism, acetaldehyde is converted to acetate by aldehyde dehydrogenase and ac-

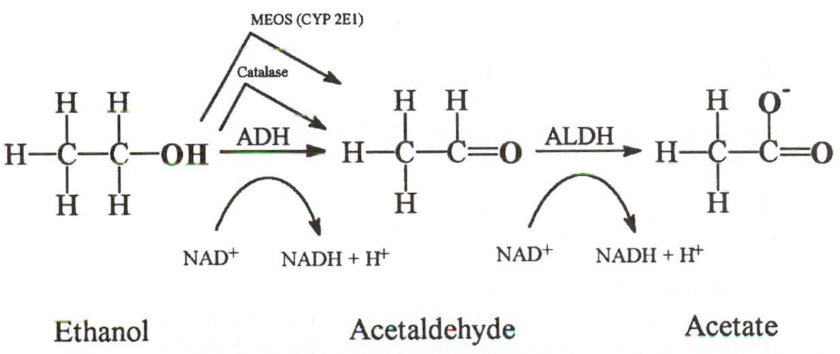

Figure 62–1. Ethanol oxidation. *(Reprinted, with permission, from Hoffman RS, Goldfrank LR: Ethanol-associated metabolic disorders in endocrine metabolic disorders. Emergency Med Clin North Am 1989;7:945.)*

etate is converted to acetylcoenzyme A, which enters the Krebs (citric acid) cycle and is metabolized to carbon dioxide and water. The ability of acetylcoenzyme A to enter the Krebs cycle is indirectly dependent on adequate thiamine stores.

The MEOS system (CYP2E1) is responsible for little ethanol metabolism under normal conditions, but becomes more important as the ethanol concentration rises and ethanol use becomes chronic. The ability of ethanol to stimulate and induce the MEOS system forms the basis for the well-established interactions between ethanol and a host of other drugs metabolized by this system.

The capacity of the ADH enzyme system is saturated at relatively low blood alcohol levels. As the system is saturated, the metabolism moves from first-order (fixed proportion metabolized per unit time) to zero-order (fixed amount metabolized per unit time) kinetics. In adults, the average rate of ethanol metabolism is 100 to 125 mg/kg per hour in occasional drinkers and up to 175 mg/kg per hour in habitual drinkers.[8,32] The average-sized adult metabolizes 7 to 10 g/h and the blood alcohol level falls 15 to 20 mg/dL per hour. Chronic drinkers, by recruiting the CYP2E1 system, may increase their clearance of ethanol to about 30 mg/dL per hour.[8,32] An understanding of these fixed rates of ethanol metabolism is critically important in the correct interpretation of blood alcohol levels in the clinical setting. Most of the studies on ethanol clearance rates have been performed in healthy volunteers or chronic alcoholics. Studies of ethanol clearance in intoxicated patients presenting to the ED indicate that although the average rate is about 20mg/dL per hour, there is considerable individual variation (standard deviation of about 6 mg/dL per hour).[8,32] Thus, to accurately predict the clearance rate in an individual patient a second level should be drawn after several hours.

The mitochondrial form of aldehyde dehydrogenase (ALDH5) is the most important in terms of acetaldehyde metabolism. Approximately 40% of Asians, 80% of Native Americans, and 3 to 29% of Caucasians have an inactive ALDH5 enzyme due to a point mutation in the ALDH5 gene, and hence have a reduced capacity for acetaldehyde metabolism.[33,47] In affected individuals the accumulation of acetaldehyde with even modest ethanol consumption leads to a severe flushing reaction.

What Are the Mechanisms for Ethanol's Intoxicating Effects?

The mechanism of action for ethanol's intoxicating effect is probably multifactorial and has been the subject of much debate.[55,90] Like the volatile anesthetics, ethanol depresses the CNS by dissolving in the cell's lipid membrane and disordering the lipid matrix (referred to as membrane fluidization). However, an effect on membrane organization is only measurable at ethanol concentrations well above the pharmacologic range, and these same changes can be produced by minor changes in temperature that produce no signs of intoxication. Thus, the membrane fluidity mechanism has been challenged and current research has focused on ethanol's interaction with various proteins such as neurotransmittor-gated ion channels.[34,69,90]

Because of the similarity of many of ethanol's behavioral effects with those of sedative-hypnotic agents like barbiturates and benzodiazepines, it was postulated that ethanol acted by enhancing GABA-nergic function. Ethanol does, in fact, augment GABA mediated synaptic transmission by interacting with $GABA_A$ receptors and their associated chloride ion channels.[11,84,102] Recent work has been directed at the suceptibility of particular GABA receptor subtypes to the effects of ethanol.[104] However, pursuit of a GABA-enhancing mechanism has produced controversal results and attempts to demonstrate changes in number or responsiveness of GABA receptors in animals chronically exposed to ethanol have been unsuccessful.[104]

Recently attention has focused on ethanol's effect on excitatory neurotransmittors, in particular the *N*-methyl-*d*-aspartate (NMDA) ligand-gated, glutamate receptor.[105] NMDA receptors mediate neurotoxicity by increasing permeability to calcium currents and regulate neuronal long-term potentiation, which is considered the model for learning and memory.[103] Biochemical and electrophysiologic studies demonstrate that acutely, ethanol inhibits NMDA receptor function, and that chronic ethanol use results in up-regulation of NMDA receptors.[48] This mechanism is attractive because it explains both some of the cognitive changes produced by ethanol as well as the manifestations of ethanol withdrawal. Finally, NMDA receptors play an important role in inhibiting the release of dopamine in the nucleus accumbens and mesolimbic structures, which modulate the reinforcing action of addictive agents like ethanol.[104] By inhibiting NMDA receptor activity, ethanol could increase dopamine release from the nucleus accumbens and ventral tegmental area and could thus create dependence.

What Are the Clinical Effects of Ethanol?

Ethanol is the most commonly used intoxicant. Acutely, ethanol ingestion results in flushed facies, tachycardia, increased sweating, mydriasis, dysarthria, muscular incoordination, ataxia, altered consciousness, emotional lability, increased gregariousness, nystagmus, and occasional antisocial behavior (Table 62–3). Patients may be euphoric, agitated, combative, or comatose. Seizures have been reported, especially in children with ethanol-induced hypoglycemia.[46] A mild hypothermia may occur and may be compounded by exposure, loss of carbohydrate substrate, and ethanol-induced vasodilatation. Acute ethanol intoxication can impair cardiac output in patients with pre-existing cardiac disease,[36] and dysrhythmias (atrial fibrillation and nonsustained ventricular tachycardia) as well as AV block have been docu-

TABLE 62–3. STAGES OF ACUTE ETHANOL INTOXICATION

BLOOD ETHANOL LEVEL	LEVEL OF INTOXICATION
700 mg/dL (0.70%)	POTENTIALLY LETHAL Unconscious Decreased reflexes Respiratory depression
400 mg/dL (0.40%)	SEVERE Hypothermia Hypoglycemia Poor muscle control Poor recall Seizures
300 mg/dL (0.30%)	MODERATE TO SEVERE Slurred speech Sensory loss Visual disturbances
200 mg/dL (0.20%)	MODERATE Staggering gait Nausea, vomiting Mental confusion
150 mg/dL (0.15%)	Altered thought processes Personality/behavior changes
100 mg/dL (0.10%)	PRESUMPTIVE (LEGAL) INTOXICATION MILD TO MODERATE Slow reaction time Altered sensory ability Driving impairment
50 mg/dL (0.05%)	MILD Decreased inhibition Slight incoordination

Reprinted, with permission, from Fourth Special Report to Congress on Alcohol and Health, USDHHS. National Institute on Alcohol Abuse and Alcoholism, 1981.

mented in binge drinkers.[22,38,39] Ethanol-induced angina has been described, but is a rare event.[80]

Ethanol is a selective CNS depressant at low doses and a general depressant at high doses. It depresses first those areas of the brain involved with highly integrated functions. The cortex is released from integrated control, leading to animated behavior and the loss of restraint. As the blood alcohol level increases, there is successive impairment of neural activity and sedation.

At the highest blood alcohol levels, there is loss of protective reflexes, coma, and increasing risk of death from respiratory depression. For most casual drinkers there is a narrow margin between the anesthetic and fatal dose of ethanol. It is essential to remember that a person who is deeply intoxicated with ethanol may be near death and must be managed aggressively.

Intoxication with ethanol has been defined by the National Safety Council as a blood alcohol concentration of 100 mg/dL (0.125% wt/vol or 21.7 mmol/L), and this level has been adopted by many states to define a driver who is legally intoxicated. However, numerous states have now established a lower threshold of 80 mg/dL. Moreover, in certain states drivers can be charged with driving while ability-impaired with a blood alcohol level of 50 to 90 mg/dL. In nonalcoholic individuals, impairment of judgment and of recently learned skills can be documented at a blood alcohol level as low as 25 mg/dL. Gross motor control and orientation may be significantly affected at concentrations of 50 mg/dL,[16,81] while levels as low as 47 mg/dL are associated with an increased risk of motor vehicle accidents. Clinically, ethanol intoxication is usually apparent in nontolerant individuals with levels of 50 to 100 mg/dL. In chronic drinkers, clinical manifestations of intoxication are not noted until levels substantially higher are reached.

The acute effects of ethanol ingestion depend on genetic factors; the rate of consumption, absorption, and elimination; the quantity of alcohol consumed; and the habituation of the drinker. This is mainly due to the development of tolerance, which has a metabolic (pharmacokinetic) and a functional (pharmacodynamic) component.[103] Metabolic tolerance to ethanol is based on enhanced elimination by the ADH enzyme and CYP2E1 system. Functional tolerance (resistance to the effects of ethanol at the cellular level) is a more important determinant of habituation and may be mediated by serotonergic and adrenergic neurons.[54] Thus, although all individuals who drink excessively on an acute basis move through a progressive sequence of events, the association of a particular stage of intoxication with a specific blood alcohol level is not usually possible without knowing the patient's history.

Acutely intoxicated patients may present with nausea and vomiting, abdominal pain, GI bleeding, pulmonary complications secondary to aspiration, or injuries due to falls. Diplopia and visual disturbances may occur as well as nystagmus, which may be due to the toxic effects of ethanol or an acute Wernicke's encephalopathy.

Metabolic derangements in the acutely intoxicated individual include hypoglycemia, metabolic acidosis due to lactate and/or ketoacids, hypokalemia, hypomagnesemia, and hyperamylasemia. An elevated amylase may represent an underlying pancreatitis or salivary gland hyperplasia commonly seen in alcoholics.[6] Contrary to popular thought, ethanol-induced hypoglycemia can occur acutely and does not require chronic drinking or chronic malnutrition. The metabolism of ethanol itself generates NADH and alters the redox (NADH/NAD) ratio, thereby forcing the conversion of pyruvate to lactate and preventing gluconeogenesis (see Figs. 62–1 and 62–2). Even small amounts of ethanol from colognes and other sources have resulted in hypoglycemic seizures and death in young children.[18] A 24% incidence of hypoglycemia was reported in one pediatric series.[64] A small series suggests that although well described, particularly in children and fasting patients, ethanol-induced hypoglycemia may be a relatively uncommon event.[100]

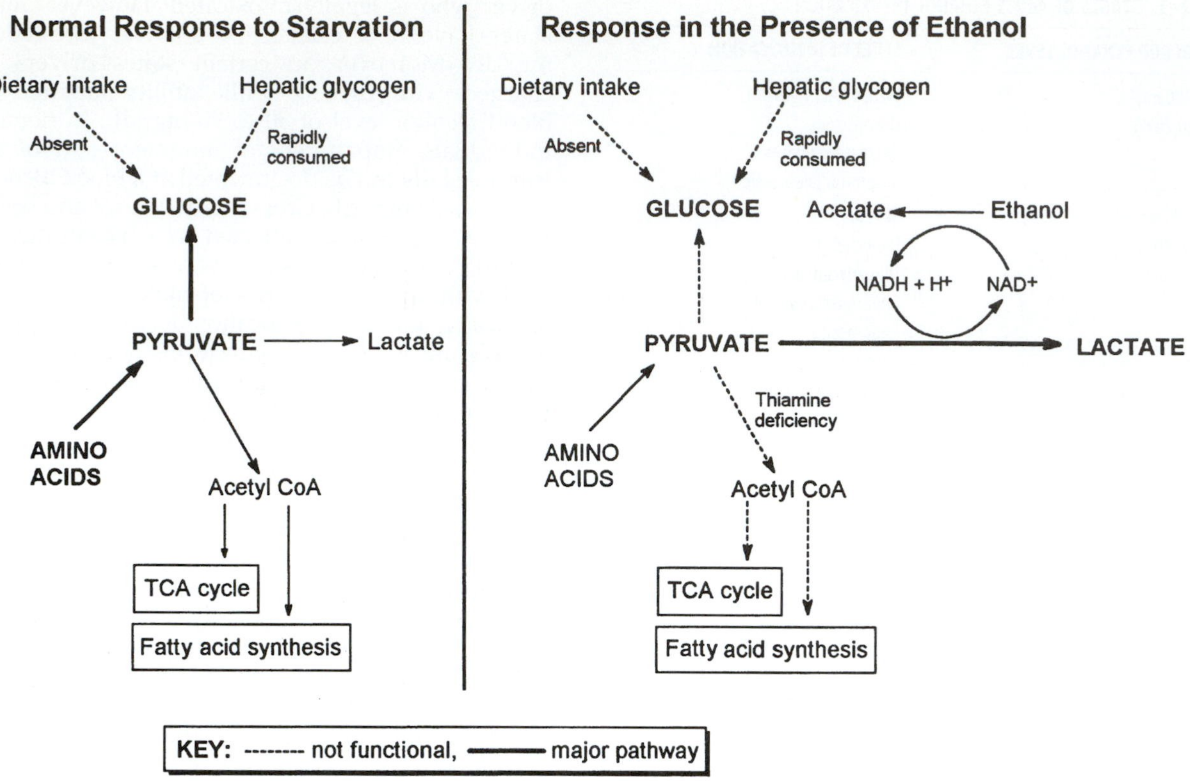

Figure 62–2. Central role of pyruvate in ethanol-induced hypoglycemia. *(Reprinted, with permission, from Hoffman RS, Goldfrank LR: Ethanol-associated metabolic disorders in Endocrine metabolic disorders. Emerg Med Clin North Am 1989;7:949.)*

What Is the Management of the Intoxicated Patient?

The history of drinking, combined with nausea, vomiting, and altered mental status, suggests a range of possibilities, all of which must be considered and systematically excluded. Altered mental status in an alcoholic can be due to a variety of causes including acute ethanol intoxication, head trauma, postictal condition, infection, hypoglycemia, intracranial hematomas (acute or chronic), hepatic encephalopathy, electrolyte derangements, ethanol withdrawal, Wernicke-Korsakoff syndrome, and various drug overdoses (eg, anticonvulsant medication). The challenge of treating a sick alcoholic is the broad range of diagnostic possibilities due to the fact that ethanol can affect virtually every organ system.

As with any other poisoned patient in the ED, the airway must be protected and adequate ventilatory and circulatory support provided. Patients who are combative and violent should be physically restrained prior to chemical sedation. Those who are clinically intoxicated but threaten to sign out AMA or attempt to leave should likewise be restrained. An odor of alcohol on the breath offers no definitive information and may in fact be completely misleading. Some alcoholic beverages create no odor, and some patients with an odor of alcohol will have another reason for their change in mental status.[110] It is imperative to confirm an impression of alcohol intoxication with a blood alcohol level.[45] If it is inconsistent with the patient's condition, it must prompt an exhaustive search for the underlying disorder including toxic-metabolic, trauma-related, neurologic, and infectious etiologies. Coma due to ethanol alone is rare at blood alcohol levels less than 300 mg/dL. Chronic alcoholics are often able to withstand levels substantially higher than this without a significant change in mental status. Thus, blood alcohol levels must be correlated with the individual patient's clinical appearance and drinking history. Comatose patients with levels below 300 mg/dL and those with values in excess of 300 mg/dL who fail to improve during a limited period of close observation, should have a head CT scan, and a lumbar puncture if warranted. Because alcoholics are prone to trauma and coagulopathies, both of which can cause intracerebral bleeding, the threshold for CT scanning in these patients should be low.

Laboratory Testing

A bedside evaluation of the blood glucose level is essential in all alcoholic patients with a change in mental status to identify ethanol-induced hypoglycemia as quickly as possible. A full set of electrolytes, including calcium and magnesium and a CBC, are reasonable for most patients. Patients with an anion gap metabolic acidosis should have a serum osmolality by freezing point depression, serum ketones, and specific levels of other alcohols (methanol, ethylene glycol) performed only as indicated. Ethanol itself will contribute to serum osmolality and the osmolal gap. Ethanol's contribution to osmolality can be estimated by dividing the ethanol level in mg/dL by 4.6 (one-tenth the molecular weight of ethanol). A discrepancy between the ethanol level and measured serum osmolality suggests, but does confirm, the presence of other osmotically active agents (see Chap. 15). Those patients with GI symptoms require a serum amylase and lipase analysis to exclude pancreatitis. Patients who appear encephalopathic, have asterexis, or have other signs of cirrhosis should have an ammonia determination.

Numerous methodologies have been developed over the years to detect the presence of alcohol and quantitate its level. Blood alcohol levels performed by immunoassay or gas chromatography are commonly used in most hospitals. Although accurate, the results of these tests may be delayed several hours, and this delay may hamper decision-making and management in the emergency setting. Breath alcohol analyzers, using microprocessors and infrared spectral analysis, are widely available and are routinely used by law-enforcement agencies as alcohol screening devices. In the emergency department setting they have been shown to accurately predict blood alcohol levels.[111] However, the unconscious or uncooperative patient may not exhale properly. The normal blood/breath ethanol ratio also varies among individuals and within one individual over time.[52] Other potential sources of error include recent use of alcohol products, belching or vomiting of gastric alcohol contents, inadequate expiration, obstructive pulmonary disease, use of metered dose inhalers, and poor technique.[2,63] Attempts have been made to sample the breath of unconscious patients with breath-alcohol devices adapted with mouth cups and nasal tubes.[24,31]

Dipstick tests designed to detect alcohol in saliva are less reliable than breath tests and cannot be recommended.[96] An electrochemical meter using venous blood has also been used for bedside testing of blood alcohol concentrations.[110] Although the specificity of this instrument is poor, its 100% sensitivity and good correlation with blood alcohol levels in the clinically significant range make it a potentially valuable adjunct in the emergency setting. Finally, fatty acid ethyl esters (FAEEs) have recently been shown to be a highly sensitive test for recent ethanol use in a small group of healthy subjects.[20] Because FAEEs remain in the system for at least 24 hours they may have a role as a marker of recent ethanol use even after ethanol is completely metabolized.

What Are the Initial Therapeutic Interventions?

Although ethanol is rapidly absorbed following oral ingestion, the possibility of recent ingestion (within 1 hour of presentation), delayed absorption, and concomitant ingestions makes GI evacuation a reasonable approach to the extremely intoxicated, comatose patient.[79] However, if a coingestion is suspected, the use of activated charcoal is advisable. In addition, a rapid finger stick glucose assessment, provision of 0.5 to 1.0 g of $D_{50}W$ IV when values are normal or low, and administration of 100 mg of thiamine IV are indicated. Failure to administer thiamine is inappropriate care and potentially allows the development of an acute Wernicke's encephalopathy.[109]

Chronic alcohol use is associated with malnutrition and magnesium depletion. Magnesium depletion is due to poor dietary intake, decreased GI absorption secondary to ethanol, and renal wasting due to the ethanol-related diuresis.[101] Alcoholics with documented hypomagnesemia should be given 2 g of magnesium sulfate IV. Multivitamins with folate (1 to 5 mg) should be added to the IV solution of each alcoholic. Hypokalemia and hypophosphatemia are common in alcoholics and should be corrected with the addition of 20 to 40 mEq of potassium phosphate to each liter of infusate once documented and normal renal function is confirmed. Clotting disorders may need to be treated with vitamin K and fresh frozen plasma as needed. Patients with hepatic encephalopathy should be treated with cleansing enemas if GI bleeding is present, followed by 30 mL (20 g) of lactulose in combination with 30 g of 70% sorbitol; alternatively, the patient can be given 20 g of neomycin orally or via enema as needed. Febrile alcoholics should be evaluated aggressively. Fever, especially a high fever, should never be attributed to seizures, alcohol withdrawal, or alcoholic hepatitis without a rigorous search for other causes. If sepsis, meningitis, or peritonitis is suspected, the patient should have blood cultures performed and be started on broad-spectrum antibiotics.

A variety of techniques and agents have been used historically either to hasten the elimination of ethanol or to reverse its intoxicating effects. Neither coffee nor caffeine itself counteract the impaired psychomotor functions seen with acute intoxication.[86] Earlier anecdotal reports suggested a role for naloxone in reversing ethanol intoxication,[40,70] but these reports could not be reliably reproduced.[87] The specific benzodiazepine antagonist flumazenil has no predictable effect on ethanol alone.[26] Because the mechanism of action is complex and not mediated by a single receptor, it is unlikely that a specific ethanol antagonist will ever be discovered. Because of ethanol's relatively small volume of distribution and low molecular weight, its elimination can be enhanced by hemodialysis, but in the absence of a coingestion of other toxic alcohols, this is rarely necessary.

What Are Some of the Indications for Hospitalization?

Most patients with uncomplicated ethanol intoxication can be safely discharged from the ED after an evaluation and observation. No patient should ever be discharged while still clinically intoxicated. The clinical appearance of the patient is far more important in this regard than the blood alcohol level. Patients with altered mental status and a mixed overdose, those with serious trauma, those with significant alcohol withdrawal, and those with another disease (pancreatitis, GI bleeding, etc) should be admitted.

Some chronic drinkers have an organic brain syndrome even when sober. Many others are poor, lack social supports, and cannot follow through with treatment plans. Thus the threshold for admission should be lower for chronic drinkers who are homeless, medically indigent, psychiatrically impaired, or otherwise disadvantaged. Alcoholics who are sober and desire alcohol detoxification can be admitted for "drying out" and rehabilitation. Inpatient alcohol programs have an advantage over outpatient programs in that they enforce abstinence, provide more support and structure, and separate the patient from the social surroundings associated with drinking.[108] For patients who are not admitted, a referral should be offered to Alcoholics Anonymous or another suitable alcohol rehabilitation program.

What Are the Characteristics and Concerns With Regard to Alcoholism?

It is estimated that 5 to 10% of all drinkers of alcohol in the United States are alcohol dependent.[65,112] According to the National Longitudinal Alcohol Epidemiologic Survey (NLAES), the 1-year prevalence of combined alcohol abuse and dependence based on DSM-IV criteria was 7.41%, representing 13,760,000 Americans.[37] The combined rate was almost three times higher among males than females and was also higher in persons under 45 years of age. These data indicate that the rates of alcohol abuse and dependence have been relatively stable since 1984. More than 200,000 Americans die annually of alcoholism, far more than die of all other illicit drugs of abuse combined. Ethanol is the leading killer of persons aged 15 to 45 years. It is associated with 50% of traffic fatalities, 50% of deaths by fire, 67% of drownings, 67% of homicides, and 35% of suicides.[99] Twenty percent of total national expenditure for hospital care is alcohol related, and the annual cost of health expenses and lost productivity is $117 billion. Alcoholism is the leading cause of morbidity and mortality in the United States.[99]

For untreated alcoholics, life expectancy is decreased by 12 to 15 years compared to the normal population.[72] Mortality from the regular use of ethanol begins to increase when 3 to 5 drinks per day are consumed and rises sharply with the consumption of 7 or more drinks per day.[5] Although the daily consumption of 1 or 2 drinks per day may be safe for most people, no amount is currently considered safe for pregnant women. The combination of a national tolerance of drinking and heavy advertising of alcohol makes it especially appealing to young people. In a country increasingly concerned with drug abuse, the excessive use of alcohol constitutes a serious and pervasive problem as well as a major health issue.

Alcoholism has traditionally been defined as a chronic, progressive disease characterized by tolerance and physical dependence to ethanol and pathologic organ changes. Although alcoholism was historically considered to represent a defect in moral character, a more unified and enlightened view now considers it a multifactorial, genetically influenced disorder.[21,35] Alcoholism should be suspected in any patient who presents to the ED with unexplained trauma, seizures, or bizarre behavior. Suggestive physical findings include flushed facies, parotid enlargement, hepatomegaly, stigmata of cirrhosis, fluctuating mild hypertension, peripheral neuropathy, evidence of nutritional deficiencies, and repeated infections.

Concern for early detection and intervention with alcoholism has led to attempts to create reliable diagnostic screening systems. The Brief Michigan Alcoholism Screening Test (MAST)[92] and the Cage questions[74] represent two such devices (Tables 62–4 and 62–5). As can be seen from these screens, the presence of physical tolerance and/or dependence is not essential for a diagnosis of alcoholism. Emphasis instead is placed on the social and behavioral concomitants of heavy drinking.[83] In the ED setting, questions concerning the patient's ability to function physically and psychologically are just as appropriate as quantifying the amount of alcohol consumed per day.

Alcoholism is commonly associated with affective disorders, especially depression[73,97] and there is a higher rate of alcoholism among manic-depressives than in the general population.[115] Ethanol affects mood, judgment, and self-control and creates a situation conducive to self-injury and violence directed at others. Alcoholism is an important risk factor for suicide. Although many people drink in a misguided attempt to ameliorate their depression, all available evidence suggests that alcoholism adversely affects mood and cognitive ability.

Research has pointed to an increased incidence of alcoholism in families,[15] and twin studies suggest that a tendency to drink is partly under genetic control.[4,41] Chromosomal linkage analysis has implicated chromosomes 4, 6, and 11 in the genetic predisposition to alcoholism.[7] An allelic association with alcoholism in the q22-q33 region of the D_2 receptor gene of chromosome 11 suggests that this could mediate susceptibility to ethanol

TABLE 62–4. THE BRIEF MICHIGAN ALCOHOLISM SCREENING TEST

Question	Circle Correct Answer		Points
1. Do you feel you are a normal drinker?	Yes	No	N2
2. Do friends or relatives think you are a normal drinker?	Yes	No	N2
3. Have you ever attended a meeting of Alcoholics Anonymous?	Yes	No	Y5
4. Have you ever lost friends or girlfriends/boyfriends because of drinking?	Yes	No	Y2
5. Have you ever gotten into trouble at work because of drinking?	Yes	No	Y2
6. Have you ever neglected your obligations, your family, or your work for 2 or more days in a row because you were drinking?	Yes	No	Y2
7. Have you ever had delirium tremens (DTs) or severe shaking, or heard voices or seen things that weren't there after heavy drinking?	Yes	No	Y2
8. Have you ever gone to anyone for help about your drinking?	Yes	No	Y5
9. Have you ever been in a hospital because of drinking?	Yes	No	Y5
10. Have you ever been arrested for drunk driving or driving after drinking?	Yes	No	Y2

Score 6 = Probable diagnosis of alcoholism

Reprinted, with permission, from Pokorny AO, Miller BA, Kaplan HB: Am J Psychiatry 1972; 129:342–345. Copyright 1972, American Psychiatric Association.

in some patients.[77] This finding has, however, been questioned by some researchers.[30]

Although a serious disease with important health consequences, alcoholism remains underdiagnosed in the United States. In one study, less than 10% of alcoholics referred for inpatient treatment were referred by physicians.[50] In general, healthcare providers tend to have an overly pessimistic view of the benefits of treating alcoholism. Particularly problematic is the apparent inability of most health care workers to effectively deal with the problem when it affects their colleagues. Success in the efforts to combat alcoholism will require increased public education and greater acceptance of alcoholism as a medical illness amenable to treatment.

Various strategies have been employed to treat alcoholism. A variety of mediations such as serotonin uptake inhibitors, naltrexone, bromocriptine, lithium, and disulfiram have been used to inhibit drinking behavior and/or provide an aversive reaction to drinking.[78,107] Double-blind, placebo controlled trials demonstrate that naltrexone is effective in decreasing the mean number of drinking days per week, the frequency of relapse, and the subjective craving for alcohol without significant side effects.[88,107] Disulfiram is still used to deter drinking, although compliance is often an issue and controlled trials have failed to reveal a consistent effect compared to placebo.[17] The use of supervised disulfiram administration, combined with counseling and support activities, has resulted in greater abstinence and decreased alcohol consumption.[12] Finally, nonpharmacologic treatment for alcoholism has also been shown to be successful. Data derived from several studies and membership surveys indicate that recovery rates of 40 to 80% can be achieved in treatment programs based on the 12-step approach of Alcoholics Anonymous.[42,43,108]

TABLE 62–5. THE CAGE QUESTIONS

1. Have you ever felt you should **C**ut down on your drinking?
2. Have people **A**nnoyed you by criticizing your drinking?
3. Have you ever felt bad or **G**uilty about your drinking?
4. Have you ever had a drink first thing in the morning to steady your nerves or to get rid of a hangover (**E**ye-opener)?

Two or more affirmatives = probable diagnosis of alcoholism

Source: West LJ, Maxwell DS, Noble EP, Solomon DH: Alcoholism. Ann Intern Med 1984;100: 412–420.

What Are the Common Ethanol–Drug Interactions?

Ethanol interacts with a variety of drugs (Table 62–6).[49] Acute intoxication with ethanol can transiently prolong the levels of certain drugs (eg, phenytoin) due to competition for shared metabolic pathways, while alcoholism

TABLE 62–6. ETHANOL DRUG INTERACTIONS

Drugs	Adverse Effects
Acetaminophen	May increase hepatotoxicity[a]
Antihistamines	Enhanced CNS depression
Carbamates	Antabuse-like effect
Cephalosporins	Antabuse-like effect
Chloral hydrate	Enhanced CNS depression
Chloramphenicol	Antabuse-like effect
Chlorpropamide	Antabuse-like effect
Cimetidine	Increased alcohol level
Cocaine	Formation of cocaethylene
Coprinus mushrooms	Antabuse-like effect
Disulfiram (Antabuse)	Nausea, vomiting, abdominal pain, flushing, diaphoresis, chest pain, headache, vertigo, palpitations
Griseofulvin	Antabuse-like effect
Isoniazid	Increased incidence hepatitis, increased metabolism[a]
Methadone	Increased metabolism[a]
Metronidazole	Antabuse-like effect
Nitrofurantoin	Antabuse-like effect
Phenytoin	Increased metabolism
Ranitidine	Increased alcohol level
Sedative-hypnotics	Enhanced CNS depression
Thiuram derivatives	Antabuse-like effect
Tolbutamide	Antabuse-like effect, increased metabolism[a]
Warfarin	Increased metabolism[a]

[a]Effect associated with chronic alcohol consumption.

can increase drug clearance due to enhancement of these same pathways. An increase in the microsomal oxidizing system with chronic drinking leads to accelerated metabolism and shortens the half-lives of drugs such as phenytoin, methadone, tolbutamide, isoniazid, and warfarin.[56]

Ethanol has additive effects when ingested with antihistamines, barbiturates and other sedative-hypnotics, cyclic antidepressants, glutethimide, phenothiazines, opioids, and chloral hydrate ("Mickey Finn"). Ethanol can enhance the aspirin-induced increase in bleeding time. Stimulants, including amphetamines and caffeine, do not reliably counteract the sedative effects of ethanol.

Concomitant use of cocaine and ethanol leads to the formation of an active metabolite, cocaethylene, through transesterification in the liver.[93] Cocaethylene has a longer half-life than cocaine itself (2 hours versus 48 min.), and this may explain some of the delayed cardiovascular effects attributed to cocaine use.[3,114] Both ethanol and cocaethylene inhibit the metabolism of cocaine, thereby prolonging blood levels of cocaine and enhancing its effect.[89]

Histamine-$_2$ receptor antagonists like cimetidine and ranitidine, but not famotidine, increase blood alcohol concentrations.[9,25] This is a result of decreased first-pass metabolism due to inhibition of the activity of alcohol dehydrogenase in the gastric mucosa.[19] In chronic drinkers and those with higher ethanol levels, cimetidine may also delay ethanol clearance by inhibiting the MEOS system (CYP2E1).

Several case reports seem to suggest that chronic ethanol abuse may predispose to acetaminophen hepatotoxicity at doses greater than the recommended limit of 4 g/day.[23,71,75,116] Alcohol use can cause an increase in cytochrome and enzyme content.[106] Because this is also the cytochrome oxidase enzyme involved in the metabolism of acetaminophen to NAPQI, the hepatotoxic intermediate, a theoretical basis for this association exists. Recent fasting, commonly seen in alcoholics, was also associated with a predisposition to acetaminophen hepatotoxicity.[113]

TABLE 62–7. SYSTEMIC EFFECTS OF ALCOHOLISM

Eyes
"Tobacco–alcohol amblyopia"
Ophthalmoplegia (Wernicke's syndrome)

Gastrointestinal
Mouth
- Nutritional stomatitis
- Cheilosis

Esophagus
- Esophagitis
- Diffuse esophageal spasm
- Mallory-Weiss tear
- Rupture with mediastinitis

Stomach and duodenum
- Acute gastritis
- Chronic hypertrophic gastritis
- Peptic ulcer
- Hematemesis
- Malabsorption
- Diarrhea

Liver
- Steatosis
- Alcoholic hepatitis
- Cirrhosis

Pancreas
- Acute pancreatitis
- Chronic pancreatitis
- Pancreatic pseudocyst

Oncologic
Cancer of the mouth, pharynx larynx, and esophagus

Respiratory
Atelectasis
Respiratory depression
Pneumonia
Pneumothorax

Cardiovascular
Alcoholic cardiomyopathy
Wet beriberi
Holiday heart (dysrhythmias)

Genitourinary
Hypogonadism
Impotence
Infertility

Endocrine and Metabolic
Hyperglycemia
Hypoglycemia
Hyperuricemia
Metabolic acidosis
Respiratory acidosis
Hypophosphatemia
Hypokalemia
Hypomagnesemia
Hypertriglyceridemia
Malnutrition
Hypothermia

Neurologic
Acute intoxication
Alcohol withdrawal
Wernicke-Korsakoff syndrome
Cerebellar degeneration
Polyneuropathy
Pellagra
Marchiafava-Bignami disease
Central pontine myelinolysis
Cerebral atrophy (dementia)
Myopathy
CVA (SAH, infarction)

Psychiatric
Suicide and depression
Manic-depressive illness
Alcoholic hallucinosis

Hematologic
Iron, B_{12}, folate deficiency anemias
Hemolysis (Zieve's syndrome, stomatocytosis, spur cell anemia)
Leukopenia
Thrombocytopenia
Coagulopathies

What Are the Common Ethanol-Related Diseases?

Ethanol affects practically every organ system in the body (Table 62–7). In addition to the harmful effects of ethanol itself, there is evidence to suggest that its metabolite, acetaldehyde, is inherently toxic to biologic systems.[10,67] Acetaldehyde is associated with structural and functional alterations of mitochondria and hepatocytes,[57] interferes with phosphorylation, inactivates coenzyme A, and inhibits myocardial protein synthesis.[59] Acetaldehyde can be acutely toxic if its conversion to acetate is blocked due to either congenital dysfunction of acetaldehyde dehydrogenase or inhibition of the enzyme by disulfiram or other agents. Ethanol oxidation also creates an excess of NADH relative to NAD, and this altered redox potential has negative consequences for many cellular functions.

In addition to the direct toxic effects of ethanol, dietary deficiencies, acid–base disorders, and diuretic effects can create low levels of potassium, magnesium, calcium, zinc, and phosphorus. Hypokalemia can lead to muscular paralysis, motor weakness, and areflexia. Hypomagnesemia can lead to changes in mental status, dysrhythmias, and inhibition of parathormone-mediated release of calcium from body stores. Hypocalcemia can result in tetany, motor weakness, and ECG changes (prolonged QT interval). Low levels of zinc have been linked to gonadal dysfunction, delayed wound healing, and depressed immunoresponsiveness. Low phosphate levels can cause myocardial dysfunction, rhabdomyolysis, motor weakness, platelet malfunction, and hemolysis. Finally, hypoglycemia can occur from malnutrition, liver disease, and the inhibition of gluconeogenesis. In the face of a concomitant thiamine deficiency pyruvate cannot enter the tricarboxylic acid cycle and, with an altered redox ratio, there is an impediment to reverse glycolysis and the synthesis of new glucose.

A variety of acid–base disturbances may exist in alcoholic patients. Central hyperventilation due to cirrhosis may result in a chronic respiratory alkalosis. Cirrhosis may also be associated with a non-anion gap renal tubular acidosis (RTA). Finally, alcoholics may manifest a variety of types of high anion gap acidoses that deserve special attention. The differential diagnosis of an anion gap acidosis is the same for an alcoholic as for any other patient (Chap. 15), but special attention in the alcoholic must be paid to the consideration of lactic acidosis (sepsis, hypotension, hypoxia, seizures), ketoacidosis (diabetes and alcoholic ketoacidosis), and ingestions (methanol, ethylene glycol, salicylates, and isoniazid).

Alcoholic Ketoacidosis

Patients with alcoholic ketoacidosis (AKA) are typically chronic drinkers who present several days after a period of heavy drinking followed by a decrease in alcohol and food intake, often due to a GI disturbance such as gastritis or pancreatitis.[28] To compensate for the loss of carbohydrates and depleted glycogen stores, the body mobilizes fat from adipose tissue as an alternative source of energy. This response is mediated by a decrease in insulin and an increased secretion of glucagon, catecholamines, growth hormone, and cortisol. Fatty acids are oxidized and the final product, acetylcoenzyme A, is converted to acetoacetate (Fig. 62–3).[44] In contrast to uncomplicated DKA, in AKA the majority of acetoacetate formed is converted to beta-hydroxybutyrate because of the ethanol-induced low redox state. Because the nitroprusside reaction detects only ketones (acetone and acetoacetate) and not beta-hydroxybutyrate, the assay for ketones in patients with AKA may be only mildly positive and proportionately less than expected from the acid–base data obtained from the ABG. Specific assays for beta-hydroxybutyrate may be performed but are not readily available in most hospital laboratories. Volume depletion in patients with AKA interferes with the renal elimination of acetoacetate and beta-hydroxybutyrate and contributes to the acidosis. Lactic acidosis due to hypoperfusion may coexist with the underlying ketoacidosis. Paradoxically, the arterial pH may be normal due to a compensatory respiratory alkalosis and a primary metabolic alkalosis due to vomiting (see Chap. 15). However, if ketones are absent in an alcoholic with a high anion gap acidosis and lactic acidosis, diabetes, and uremia have been excluded, other causes of acidosis—especially methanol and ethylene glycol ingestion—must be pursued.

Treatment of patients with AKA consists of providing adequate fluid replacement, glucose, and thiamine. Exogenous insulin in a nondiabetic is usually unnecessary. The administration of glucose to these patients stimulates the release of insulin, decreases the concentration of glucagon, and reduces the oxidation of fatty acids. Exogenous glucose also facilitates the synthesis of ATP, which reverses the lactate-to-pyruvate and NADH-to-

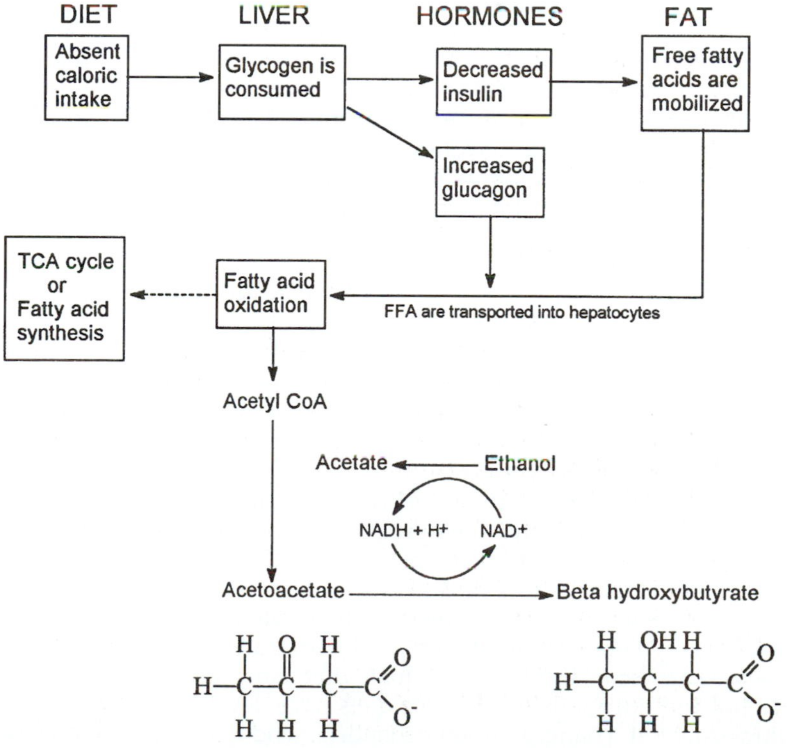

Figure 62–3. Mechanism of alcoholic ketoacidosis. *(Reprinted, with permission, from Hoffman RS, Goldfrank LR: Ethanol-associated metabolic disorders in endocrine metabolic disorders. Emerg Med Clin North Am 1989;7:952.)*

NAD ratios. The provision of thiamine allows pyruvate to enter the Krebs cycle, thus increasing ATP production. Volume replacement restores glomerular flow and improves excretion of organic acids.

Alcoholic Liver Disease

Alcohol-induced liver disease is a frequent cause of death in the alcoholic. Classification of alcoholic liver disease can be made histologically. Fatty liver is present in 90% of chronic drinkers, is usually asymptomatic, and is characterized by hepatocytes distended with cytoplasmic fat.[98] Fatty acids from a variety of sources accumulate as triglycerides in the liver due to enhanced hepatic lipogenesis, decreased hepatic release of lipoproteins, increased mobilization of peripheral fat, and decreased fatty acid oxidation.[66] Steatosis and other alcoholic lesions are most prominent in the perivenular (centrilobular) zone of the hepatic acinus. In animals experimentally fed alcohol, this area of the liver demonstrates defective oxygen utilization. This combined with the low oxygen tension prevailing in this zone, exaggerates the redox shift produced by ethanol.[51] Acetaldehyde produced by ethanol oxidation accumulates in this area and forms adducts with proteins, disrupts electron transport, and generates free radicals that cause lipid peroxidation and membrane injury.[60] In the absence of other complications, fatty liver has a good prognosis and resolves with abstinence from alcohol.

Alcoholic hepatitis is characterized by hepatocyte degeneration and necrosis, often with ballooned cells, and an infiltrate of PMN leukocytes and lymphocytes. Damaged hepatocytes contain Mallory bodies, or alcoholic hyaline, although this finding is not specific for alcoholic hepatitis. Deposition of collagen around the central vein (central hyaline sclerosis) is a precursor of alcoholic cirrhosis. Alcoholic hepatitis is usually accompanied by hyperbilirubinemia, leukocytosis, and abnormal LFTs. In contrast to viral hepatitis, the AST is disproportionally elevated relative to the ALT. Patients may present clinically with nausea and vomiting, abdominal pain, jaundice, fever, and hepatosplenomegaly. Although alcoholic hepatitis may resolve, continued drinking and repeated bouts often lead to hepatic decompensation.

Alcoholic cirrhosis (Laënnec's cirrhosis) is the most common form of cirrhosis in North America, and is usually but not invariably preceded by alcoholic hepatitis. It is characterized by fibroblastic proliferation and the appearance of connective tissue septa in the periportal and pericentral zones. Hepatocyte regeneration is eventually overcome by hepatocyte destruction and the liver becomes shrunken and nodular. Alcoholic cirrhosis is a progressive disease with a poor prognosis, but appropriate therapy and strict abstinence may arrest the process.

Although alcoholic liver disease was historically attributed to poor nutrition, numerous investigators have conclusively demonstrated that the full spectrum of this disease can occur despite an adequate diet. Animals fed alcohol and nutritionally adequate diets have developed ultrastructural changes in mitochondria, endoplasmic reticulum, and plasma membranes, and impairment in respiration, energy production, and fatty acid oxidation.[68] Epidemiologic studies demonstrate a relationship in humans between the development of alcoholic liver injury and the amount of alcohol consumed independent of nutritional factors. Although there is great individual variability in susceptibility to alcoholic liver disease (only 8 to 30% of chronic drinkers develop cirrhosis), its development is closely correlated with the magnitude and duration of alcohol consumption.[61] The typical alcoholic cirrhotic has consumed at least a pint of whisky per day or its equivalent for 10 years or more. Finally, women show a greater susceptibility and more accelerated progression to alcoholic cirrhosis than men. Several studies document a higher incidence of advanced liver injury among women compared to men despite similiar drinking histories.[82]

Alcoholics have a mortality rate that is approximately double that of the normal population[85] due to deaths caused by cirrhosis, infections, accidents, malignancies, and cardiovascular diseases. Alcoholism increases the risk of developing cancer of the tongue, mouth, oropharynx, esophagus, and liver.[112] Many alcoholics also smoke cigarettes, and there appears to be a synergistic effect between ethanol and tobacco that increases the risk of cancer.[47] Light to moderate drinking (< 3 drinks per day) is associated with a decrease in coronary artery disease.[29,58] This may be mediated by increased levels of high-density lipoproteins, decreased platelet adhesiveness, and/or increased release of endogenous tissue plasminogen activator.[29,58,94] Heavier drinking, however, is associated with increased coronary artery disease, hypertension, and heart failure.

Ethanol has a deleterious effect on the reproductive system as well. Male hypogonadism is common among chronic drinkers, and ethanol depresses testosterone production through its effects on the testes and hypothalamus. Finally, fetal alcohol syndrome has been reported to occur in pregnant women who ingest more than 150 g/day of ethanol. The syndrome consists of pre- and postnatal growth retardation, low IQ, microcephaly, short palpebral fissure, maxillary hypoplasia, joint abnormalities, fine tremor, and cardiac malformations.[62] Studies of pregnant women who drink but are not alcoholic have revealed an increased incidence of spontaneous abortion, low birthweight, and altered development. Although the ingestion of less than 3 drinks per day has not been demonstrated to cause fetal damage, the American Medical Association and the Surgeon General have recommended abstension from alcohol during pregnancy (Chap. 104).

Ethanol can cause a potentially serious reaction when combined with disulfiram (Antabuse) due to the inhibition of acetaldehyde dehydrogenase and the buildup of acetaldehyde (Chap. 63). Symptoms include flushing, nausea and vomiting, palpitations, diaphoresis, vertigo, disorientation, headache, and chest pain. The "antabuse reaction" is also described when ethanol is used in combination with cephalosporins (cefoperazone, moxalactam, cefotetan, cefomandole), chloramphenicol, griseofulvin, nitrofurantoin, sulfonamides, chlorpropamide, tolbutamide, chloral hydrate, metronidazole, Coprinus mushrooms, and various industrial chemicals (amides, oximes, carbamates, dithiocarbamates, and thiuram derivatives). Treatment is symptomatic and supportive and involves gut decontamination when appropriate, activated charcoal, IV hydration, antiemetics, and monitoring for seizures and dysrhythmias.

Ethanol remains one of the most common and complex toxicologic and societal problems. The diversity of clinical problems fills our hospitals and represents billions of dollars in excess health care costs.

References

1. Abdulla A, Badawy B: The metabolism of alcohol. Clin Endocrinol Metab 1978;7:247–252.
2. Alobaidi AA, Hill DW, Payne JP: Significance of variations in blood: Breath partition coefficient of alcohol. Br Med J 1976; 2:1479–1481.
3. Bailey DN, Bessler JB, Saucrey BA: Cocaine and cocathylene-creatinine clearance ratios in humans. J Annal Toxicol 1997; 21:41–43.
4. Ball DM, Murray RM: Genetics of alcohol misuse. Br Med J 1994;50:18–35.
5. Becker CE: Alcohol and drug use: Is there a safe amount? West J Med 1984;141:884–890.
6. Block RS, Weaver DW, Bowman DL: Acute alcohol intoxication: Significance of the amylase level. Ann Emerg Med 1983; 12: 294–296.
7. Blum K, Noble EP, Sheridan PJ: Allelic association of human receptor gene in alcoholism. JAMA 1990;263:2055–2060.
8. Brennan DF, Betzelos S, Reed R, Falk JL: Ethanol elimination rates in an ED population. Am J Emerg Med 1995; 13: 276–280.
9. Caballeria J, Barbona E, Podamilens M, Lieber CS: Effects of cimetidine on gastric alcohol dehydrogenase activity and blood ethanol levels. Gastroenterology 1989; 96: 388–392.
10. Cederbaum AI, Lieber CS, Rubin E: Effects of chronic ethanol treatment on mitochondrial functions, I. Arch Biochem Biophys 1974;165:560–570.
11. Charness ME, Simon RP, Greenberg DA: Ethanol and the nervous system. N Engl J Med 1989;321:442–450.
12. Chick J, Gough K, Falkowski W, Kershaw P: Disulfiram treatment of alcoholism. Br J Psychiatry 1992;161: 84–89.
13. Committee on Drugs, 1983–1984, American Academy of Pediatrics: Ethanol in liquid preparations intended for children. Pediatrics 1984;73:405–407.
14. Committee on Medicolegal Problems: Alcohol and the Impaired Driver: A Manual on the Mediocolegal Aspects of Chemical Tests for Intoxication. Chicago, American Medical Association, 1968.
15. Cotton NS: The familial incidence of alcoholism: A review. J Stud Alcohol 1979;40:89–93.
16. Crabb DW, Bosrom WF, Li TK: Ethanol metabolism. Pharmacol Ther 1987;34: 59–73.
17. Critchfield GC, Eddy DM: A confidence profile analysis of the effectiveness of disulfiram in the treatment of chronic alcoholism. Med Care 1987; 25: 566–575.
18. Cummins LH: Hypoglycemia and convulsions in children following alcohol ingestion. J Pediatr 1961; 58: 23–26.
19. Di Padova C, Poine R, Frezza M, et al: Effects of rantidine on blood alcohol levels after ethanol ingestion. JAMA. 1992; 267: 83–86.
20. Doyle KM, Cluette-Brown JE, Dube DM, et al: Fatty acid ethyl esters in the blood as markers of ethanol intake. JAMA 1996; 276: 1152–1156.
21. Eckardt MJ, Harford IC, Kaelber CT: Health hazards associated with alcohol consumption. JAMA 1981;246:648–653.
22. Eilam O, Heyman SN: Wenckebach-type atrioventricular block in severe alcohol intoxication. Am J Emerg Med 1991; 9:1170.
23. Embly DI, Fraser BN: Hepatotoxicity of paracetamol enchanced by ingestion of alcohol. S Afr Med J 1977; 51: 208–209.
24. Falkensson M, Jones W, Sorbo B: Bedside diagnosis of alcohol intoxication with a pocket-size breath alcohol device. Clin Chem 1989; 35: 918–921.
25. Feely J, Wood AJ: Effects of cimetidine on the elimination and actions of ethanol. JAMA 1982; 247: 2819–2821.
26. Fluckiger A, Hartmann D, Leishman B, Zeigler WH: Lack of effect of the benzodiazepine antagonist flumazenil and the performance of healthy subjects during experimentally induced ethanol intoxication. Eur J Clin Pharmacol 1988; 34:273–276.
27. Frezza M, DiRadova C, Pozzato G, et al: High blood alcohol levels in women: The role of decreased gastric alcohol dehydrogenase activity and first pass metabolism. N Engl J Med 1990;322:95–110.
28. Fulop M, Hoberman HD: Alcoholic ketosis. Diabetes 1975; 24:785–790.
29. Gaziano JM, Buring JE, Breslow JL, et al: Moderate alcohol intake, increased levels of high-density lipoprotein and its subfractions, and decreased risk of myocardial infarction. N Engl J Med 1993; 329:1829–1834.
30. Gelernter J, Goldman D, Pisch N: The Ao allele at the D_5 dopamine receptor gene and alcoholism: A reappraisal. JAMA 1993; 269:1673–1677.
31. Gerberich SG, Gerberich BK, Fife D: Analysis of the relationship between blood alcohol and nasal breath alcohol concentrations. J Trauma 1989; 29:338–343.
32. Gershman H, Steper J: Rate of clearance of ethanol from the blood of intoxicated patients in the emergency department. J Emerg Med 1991; 9:307–311.
33. Goedde HW, Harada S, Agarwal DP: Social differences in alcohol sensitivity. Hum Genet 1979;51:331–334.
34. Goldstein DB: The effect of drugs on membrane fluidity. Annu Rev Pharmacol Toxicol 1984; 24:43–64.
35. Goodwin DW: Is Alcoholism Hereditary? New York, Oxford University Press, 1976, pp. 23–26.
36. Gould L: Hemodynamic effects of ethanol in patients with cardiac disease. Q J Stud Alcohol 1972;33:714–722.
37. Grant BF, Harford TC, Dawson DA, Chou P: Prevalence of DSM-IV alcohol abuse and dependence United States 1992. Alcohol Health Res World 1994;18:243–248.
38. Greenspon AJ: Provocation of ventricular tachycardia after consumption of alcohol. N Engl J Med 1979;301: 1049–1156.
39. Greenspon AJ, Schaal SF: The "holiday heart": Electro-

physiological studies of alcohol effects in alcoholics. Ann Intern Med 1983;98:135–140.
40. Guerin J, Friedberg G: Naloxone and ethanol intoxication. Ann Intern Med 1982;97:932–936.
41. Hill SY, Goodwin DW, Cadoret R: Association and linkage between alcohol and eleven serological markers. J Stud Alcohol 1975;36:981–984.
42. Hoffman NG, Harrison PA, Belille CA: Alcoholics anonymous after treatment: Attendance and abstinence. Int J Addict 1983;18:311–313.
43. Hoffman NG, Miller NS: Treatment outcome for abstinence-based programs. Psych Ann 1992;22:402–407.
44. Hoffman RS, Goldfrank LR: Ethanol-associated metabolic disorders. Emerg Med Clin North Am 1989;7:943–961.
45. Holt S, Stewart IC, Dixon JM: Alcohol and the emergency service patient. Br Med J 1980;281:638–640.
46. Hornfeldt CS: A report of acute ethanol poisoning in a child. J Toxicol Clin Toxicol 1992;30:115–121.
47. Hsu LC, Bendel RE, Yoshida A: Genomic structure of the human mitochondrial ALDH gene. Genomics 1988; 2: 57–65.
48. Hu X-J, Ticku MK: Chronic ethanol treatment upregulates the NMDA receptor function and binding in mammalian cortical neurons. Brain Res Mol Brain Res 1995;30:347–356.
49. Interactions of drugs with alcohol. Med Lett Drugs Ther 1981;23:33–34.
50. Isselbacher KJ: Metabolic and hepatic effects of alcohol. N Engl J Med 1977;296:612–616.
51. Jauhonen P, Baraona E, Miyakawa H, Lieber CS: Mechanism for selective perivenular hepatotoxicity of ethanol. Alcohol Clin Exp Res 1982; 6:350–357.
52. Jones AW: Variability of the blood: Breath alcohol ratio in vivo. J Stud Alcohol 1978; 39:1931–1939.
53. Julkunen RJ, DiRadova C, Lieber CB: First pass metabolism of ethanol: A gastrointestinal barrier against the systemic toxicity of ethanol. Life Sci 1985;37:567–573.
54. Kahanna JM, Kalant H, Le AD, et al: Role of serotonergic and adrenergic systems in alcohol tolerance. Prog Neuropsychopharmacol 1981;5:459–465.
55. Kalant H: Ethanol and the nervous system: Experimental neurophysiological aspects. Int J Neurol 1974;9:111–120.
56. Kater RM, Roggin G, Tobon F, et al: Increased rate of clearance of drugs from the circulation of alcoholics. Am J Med Sci 1969;258:35–39.
57. Kissin B, Degleiter H: The Biology of Alcoholism, Vol. 1. New York, Plenum, 1970, pp. 630–637.
58. Klatsky AL: Alcohol, coronary disease, and hypertension. Annu Rev Med 1996; 47:149–160.
59. Klatsky AL, Friedman GD, Sieglaub AB: Alcohol and mortality. Ann Intern Med 1981;95:139–144.
60. Lautenburg BH, Bilzer M: Mechanisms of acetaldehyde hepatotoxicity. J Hepatol 1988; 7:384–390.
61. Lelbach WK: Cirrhosis in the alcoholic and its relation to the volume of alcohol abuse. Ann NY Acad Sci 1975; 252:85–105.
62. Lemoine P, Harousseau H, Borteyou JP: Les enfants de parents alcooliques. Quest Med 1968;21:476–483.
63. Lester D: Breath tests for alcohol. N Engl J Med 1971; 284:1269–1270.
64. Leung AK: Ethyl alcohol ingestion in children. Clin Pediatr 1986; 25:617–619.
65. Lewis DC: Diagnosis and management of the alcoholic patient. RI Med J 1980;63:27–34.
66. Lieber CS: Alcohol and the liver: 1994 update. Gastroenterology 1994;106:1085–1105.
67. Lieber CS: Biochemical and molecular basis of alcohol-induced injury to the liver and other tissues. N Engl J Med 1988;319:1639–1644.
68. Lieber CS, DeCarli LM: Hepatotoxicity of ethanol. J Hepatol 1991;12:394–401.
69. Lovinger DM, White G, Weight FF: Ethanol inhibits NMDA-activated ion current in hippocampal neurons. Science 1989;243:1721–1724.
70. Mackenzie AI: Naloxone in alcohol intoxication. Lancet 1979;1:733–736.
71. Maddrey WC: Hepatic effects of acetaminophen—Enhanced toxicity in alcoholics. J Clin Gastroenterol 1987;9: 180–185.
72. Malin H, Coakley J, Kaelber C: An Epidemiologic Perspective on Alcohol Use and Abuse in the U.S. Alcohol Consumption and Related Problems. Alcohol and Health Monograph no. 1, DHHS pub. no. ADM 82-1190. Washington, DC, U.S. Government Printing Office, 1982.
73. Mayfield D: Alcoholism and affective disorders: Experimental studies. In: Goodwin DW, Erickson CK, eds: Alcoholism and Affective Disorders. New York, SP Medical and Scientific, 1979, pp. 99–107.
74. Mayfield D, McLeod G, Hall P: More detailed interview screening. Am J Psychiatry 1974;131:1121–1126.
75. McClain CJ, Kromhout JP, Peterson FJ, Holtzman JL: Potentiation of acetaminophen hepatotoxicity. JAMA 1980; 244:251–253.
76. McDermott PH, Delaney RL, Egon JD, et al: Myocardosis and cardiac failure in men. JAMA 1966;198: 253–256.
77. Mendleson JH, Miller KD, Mello NK, et al: Hospital treatment of alcoholism: A profile of middle income Americans. Alcohol Clin Exp Res 1982;6:377–383.
78. Miller NS: Pharmacotherapy in alcoholism. J Addict Dis 1995;14:23–46.
79. Minocha A, Herold DA, Barth JT, Gideon DA: Activated charcoal in oral ethanol absorption: Lack of effect in humans. J Toxicol Clin Toxicol 1986; 24:225–234.
80. Miwa K, Igawa A, Miyagi Y: Importance of magnesium deficiency in alcohol-induced variant angina. Am J Cardiol 1994;73:813–816.
81. Modell JG: Behavioral, neurologic, and physiologic effects of acute ethanol ingestion. In Fassler D, ed: The Alcoholic Patient: Emergency Medical Intervention. New York, Gardner Press, 1990, pp. 25–34.
82. Morgan MY, Sherlock S: Sex-related differences among 100 patients with alcoholic liver disease. Br Med J 1977; 1:939–941.
83. Morse RM, Flarin DK: The definition of alcoholism. JAMA 1992; 268: 1012–1014.
84. Nestoros JN: Ethanol specifically potentiates GABA-mediated neurotransmission in feline cerebral cortex. Science 1980;209:708–712.
85. Noble EP: Third Special Report to the U.S. Congress on Alcohol and Health. Rockville, MD, National Institute on Alcohol Abuse and Alcoholism, 1978.
86. Nuotto E: Coffee and caffeine and alcohol effects on psychomotor function. Clin Pharmacol Ther 1982;31:68–72.

87. Nuotto E, Palva ES: Naloxone fails to counteract heavy alcohol intoxication. Lancet 1983;2:167–170.
88. O'Malley S, Jaffe A, Schottenfeld R, Romsaville B: Naltrexone and coping skills therapy in the treatment of alcohol dependence. Alcohol Clin Exp Res 1991;15;382–396.
89. Parker RB, Williams CL, Laizure SC, et al: Effects of ethanol and cocaethylene on cocaine pharmacokinetics in conscious dogs. Drug Metab Dispos 1996; 24:850–853.
90. Peoples RW, Li C, Weight FF: Lipid vs. protein theories of alcohol action in the nervous system. Annu Rev Pharmacol Toxicol 1996;36:185–201.
91. Petroni NC, Cardoni AA: Alcohol content of liquid medicinals. Clin Toxicol 1979;14:407–432.
92. Pokorny AD, Miller BA, Kaplan HB: The brief MAST. Am J Psychiatry 1972;129:342–350.
93. Randall T: Cocaine alcohol mix in body to form even longer lasting, more lethal drug. JAMA 1992;267:1043–1044.
94. Ridker PM, Vaugham DE, Stampfer MJ, et al: Association of moderate alcohol consumption and plasma concentration of endogenous tPA activator. JAMA 1994;272:929–933.
95. Ritchie JM: The aliphatic alcohols. In: Gilman AG, Goodman LS, Rall TW, Murad F, eds: The Pharmacological Basis of Therapeutics, 7th ed. New York, Macmillan, 1985, pp. 372–387.
96. Rodenberg HD, Bennett JR, Watson WA: Clinical utility of a saliva alcohol dipstick estimate of serum ethanol concentrations in the emergency department. DICP Ann Pharmacother 1990;24:358–361.
97. Schuckit MA: Alcoholism and affective disorders: Diagnostic confusion. In: Goodwin DW, Erickson CK, eds: Alcoholism and Affective Disorders. New York, SP Medical and Scientific, 1979, pp. 9–19.
98. Sherman DIN, Williams R: Liver damage: Mechanisms and management. Br Med Bull 1994;50:124–138.
99. Sixth Special Report to Congress on Alcohol and Health. Department of Health and Human Services, National Institute on Alcohol Abuse and Alcoholism. DHHS pub. no. ADM 87-1519, 1987.
100. Sporer KA, Ernst AA, Conte RC, Nick TG: The incidence of ethanol-induced hypoglycemia. Am J Emerg Med 1992; 10:403–405.
101. Sullivan JF, Wolpert PW, Williams R: Serum magnesium in chronic alcoholism. Ann NY Acad Sci 1969;162: 947–955.
102. Suzdak PD, Schwartz RD, Shelwick P, et al: Ethanol stimulates GABA receptor mediated chloride transport in rat brain synaptoneurosomes. Proc Natl Acad Sci USA 1986; 83:4071–4083.
103. Tabakoff B, Cornell N, Hoffman PL: Alcohol tolerance. Ann Emerg Med 1986;15:1005–1010.
104. Tabakoff B, Hoffman PL: Alcohol addiction: An enigma among us. Neuron 1996;16:909–912.
105. Tabakoff B, Hoffman PL: Ethanol and glutamate receptors. In: Deithrich RA, Erwin VG, eds: Pharmacological Effects of Ethanol on the Nervous System. Boca Raton, CRC Press, 1996, pp. 73–93.
106. Takahashi T, Lasker J, Roseman A, Lieber C: Induction of cytochrome P4502E1 in the human liver by ethanol is caused by a corresponding increase in encoding messenger RNA. Hepatology 1993;17:236–245.
107. Volpicelli JR, Alterman AI, Hayashida M, O'Brien CP: Naltrexone in the treatment of alcohol dependence. Arch Gen Psychiatry 1992; 49:876–880.
108. Walsh EC, Himpson RW, Merrigan DM: A randomized trial of treatment options for alcohol abusing workers. N Engl J Med 1991;325:775–782.
109. Watson AJ, Walker JF, Tomkin GN: Acute Wernicke's encephalopathy precipitated by glucose loading. Ir J Med Sci 1981;150:301–305.
110. Wax PM, Hoffman RS, Goldfrank LR: Rapid quantitative determination of blood alcohol concentration in the emergency department using an electrochemical method. Ann Emerg Med 1992;21:254–259.
111. Wenzel J, McDermott FT: Accuracy of blood alcohol estimations obtained with a breath alcohol analyzer in a casualty department. Med J Aust 1985;142:627–628.
112. West LJ, Maxwell DS, Noble EP, Solomon DH: Alcoholism. Ann Intern Med 1984;100:405–406.
113. Whitcomb DC, Block GD: Association of acetaminophen hepatotoxicity with fasting and ethanol use. JAMA 1994; 272:1845–1850.
114. Wilson LD, Hemming RJ, Suttheimer C, et al: Cocaethylene causes dose-dependent reductions in cardiac function in anesthetized dogs. J Cardiovasc Pharmacol 1995;26: 965–973.
115. Winokur G, Clayton P: Family history studies: Sex differences and alcoholism in primary affective illness. Br J Psychiatry 1967;113:973–976.
116. Zimmerman HJ: Effects of alcohol on other hepatotoxins. Alcoholism 1986; 10: 3–15.

ANTIDOTES IN DEPTH

Thiamine Hydrochloride

Robert S. Hoffman

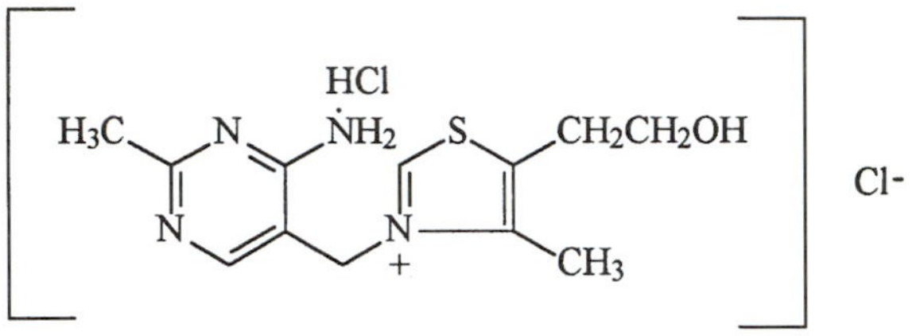

Vitamin B_1
(thiamine hydrochloride)

Thiamine (vitamin B_1) is a water-soluble vitamin essential in the creation and utilization of cellular energy. As a coenzyme in the pyruvate dehydrogenase complex, thiamine diphosphate, the active form of thiamine, accelerates the conversion of pyruvate to acetyl CoA. This reaction is known to occur at thiamine's C2 atom, which is located between the nitrogen and sulfur atoms on the thiazolium ring.[17] In the presence of the protein-rich environment of the enzyme complex, this C2 atom is deprotonated to form a carbanion that rapidly attaches to the carbonyl group of pyruvate, thereby stabilizing it for decarboxylation.[17] In a series of subsequent reactions, the hydroxyethyl group that remains bound to thiamine diphosphate is transferred to lipoamide, where an acetyl group is later broken off and attached to CoA. This process links glycolysis to the Krebs cycle, allowing for aerobic metabolism to produce 36 moles of ATP from each mole of glucose. When the conversion of pyruvate to acetyl CoA is blocked, by thiamine deficiency for example, only 2 moles of ATP can be generated, by anaerobic metabolism, from each mole of glucose. A second enzyme in the Krebs cycle, alpha-ketoglutarate dehydrogenase, also requires thiamine as a cofactor, as does transketolase, an enzyme in the pentose phosphate pathway, in which NADPH is formed for subsequent use in reductive biosynthesis. Thiamine is also important in maintaining normal neuronal conduction.[35,48]

Thiamine is available from natural sources, such as organ meats, yeast, eggs, and green leafy vegetables,[35] in a basic form composed of a substituted pyrimidine ring and a substituted thiazole ring connected by a methylene bridge. This connection between the two rings is weak, and the molecule can be destroyed in alkaline media or with prolonged cooking at high temperatures. In addition, thiamine's high water solubility may allow it to leach out of foods that are washed extensively or cooked in boiling water. When synthesized, however, the hydrochloride salt is usually formed and is quite stable (see figure). Thiamine requirements are determined by total caloric intake, with a minimum daily requirement of 0.5 mg/1000 calories.[35]

Although thiamine is well absorbed from the human gastrointestinal tract, chronic liver disease, steatorrhea, folate deficiency, and other forms of malabsorption all significantly decrease its absorption. This has historic clinical relevance in the alcoholic population.[2,40] In experimental studies, even when healthy volunteers were given small amounts of ethanol, a significant reduction in gastrointestinal thiamine absorption resulted.[40] Thiamine is eliminated from the body largely by renal clearance in a complex process consisting of a combination of glomerular filtration, flow-dependent tubular secretion, and saturable tubular reabsorption.[46]

When thiamine is completely removed from the diet, clinical manifestations of thiamine deficiency typically develop within 2 to 3 weeks, although tachycardia, the first sign of deficiency, has been noted as early as 9 days after cessation of thiamine intake.[48] In the United States, a healthy diet and mandatory supplementation of food products with thiamine protect most people from the manifestations of thiamine deficiency. This is unfortunately not true in other countries. For example, prior to 1991, mandatory thiamine enrichment of the flour used for baking in Australia was not required. A single Australian hospital identified 32 cases of Wernicke's encephalopathy during a 33-month period before the change in legislation.[49] Similarly, a survey of the 17 major public hospitals in the Sydney area identified over 1000 acute cases of either Wernicke's encephalopathy or Korsakoff's psychosis between 1978 and 1993.[22] Mandatory supplementation of flour with thiamine in 1991 resulted in a dramatic reduction in cases during 1992 and 1993.[22]

The alcoholic patient (who consumes ethanol as a major source of calories) is the most easily recognized patient at risk for thiamine deficiency.[31] Consequential thiamine deficiency is also described in inmates,[15] postoperative patients, in those with hyperemesis gravidarum or anorexia nervosa,[31] those receiving parenteral nutrition,[9,16,19,44] patients with acquired immunodeficiency syndrome (AIDS),[5,6] malignancy[4,27,32,42] patients, the institutionalized elderly,[25,26] patients with congestive heart failure on furosemide therapy,[18,34] and patients receiving hemodialysis,[10] among others. Thus, despite dietary supplementation, many people are still at risk because of dietary limitations, alcohol abuse, or underlying medical conditions.

The clinical symptoms of thiamine deficiency are divided into two subsets: "wet" beriberi or cardiovascular disease, and "dry" beriberi, the neurologic disease known as the Wernicke-Korsakoff syndrome. Although many patients display symptoms from both subsets, either cardiovascular or neurologic manifestations can predominate. A genetic abnormality of transketolase activity, combined with low physical activity and low-carbohydrate diet, may predispose to neurologic symptoms, whereas high-carbohydrate diets and increased physical activity lead to cardiovascular symptoms.[3,48]

Wet beriberi results from high-output cardiac failure that is a result of peripheral vasodilatation and the formation of arteriovenous fistulae secondary to thiamine deficiency. Patients complain of fatigue, decreased exercise tolerance, shortness of breath, and peripheral edema. Wernicke's encephalopathy is described by the classic triad of oculomotor abnormalities, ataxia, and global confusion. This syndrome is often seen together with Korsakoff's psychosis, a disorder of learning and processing of new information, characterized by a deficit in short-term memory and confabulation.[43] Traditionally, a 10 to 20% mortality rate is associated with Wernicke's encephalopathy, with survivors having an 80% risk of developing Korsakoff's psychosis.[31] Other manifestations include a peripheral neuropathy with paresthesias and hypesthesias and a myopathy, both related to axonal degeneration.[35] Laboratory studies may reflect a lactic acidosis brought on by excessive anaerobic glycolysis resulting from blocked entry of substrate into the Kreb's cycle.[16,19]

The exact cause for Wernicke's encephalopathy is unclear. In human autopsy studies, brain samples from alcoholic patients with Wernicke-Korsakoff syndrome demonstrated decreased levels of pyruvate dehydrogenase, alpha-ketoglutarate dehydrogenase, and transketolase when compared to controls.[7] Unfortunately, another controlled study comparing enzyme activity of neuronal tissue of alcoholics who died from hepatic coma without ever manifesting signs of Wernicke's encephalopathy to neuronal tissue of controls also revealed that the alcoholic brains had significant reductions in transketolase and pyruvate dehydrogenase activity.[21] Thus while thiamine deficiency is known to produce deficits in critical enzymes in humans, it is unclear whether these deficits are either necessary or sufficient to produce clinical disease. Mice develop signs of encephalopathy 10 days after being rendered thiamine deficient. Immunohistochemistry in these animals demonstrates a breakdown of the blood–brain barrier with resultant extravasation of albumin.[13] Similarly, rats also develop symptoms after 10 days of thiamine deficiency, and reveal failure of the blood–brain barrier with hemorrhage into the mammillary body and other areas of the brain in a pattern similar to findings described in humans with Wernicke's encephalopathy.[8] These findings have been corroborated by other investigators.[29] Finally, thiamine deficiency in rats produces 200 to 640% increases in levels of glutamate, an excitatory amino acid.[20] This excess of glutamate presumably results from blockade of alpha-ketoglutarate dehydrogenase, which shunts alpha ketoglutarate, a natural precursor of glutamate away from the Kreb's cycle. Rats subsequently develop increases in lactate in vulnerable regions of the brain marked by the induction of the proto-oncogene c-fos. Both the histochemical lesions and the gene induction can be blocked by the administration of the calcium channel blocker nicardipine.[23] This suggests a strong role for excitatory amino acid induced alterations in calcium transport in the genesis of thiamine deficient encephalopathy.

Thiamine hydrochloride is included in the initial therapy for any patient with an altered mental status, for both treatment and prevention of Wernicke's encephalopathy. Many of these patients have poor nutritional status or will be hospitalized without oral intake for a number of days because of gastrointestinal disorders or altered consciousness. Although thiamine levels can be measured, either directly or functionally, as determined by erythrocyte transketolase activity at baseline and in response to thiamine diphosphate,[14] these tests are unavailable for clinical use. In the absence of parenteral thiamine supplementation, glucose loading increases thiamine requirements and can thereby exacerbate subtle thiamine deficiencies or even precipitate coma.[31] Although it is commonly believed that acute glucose loading, in the form of hypertonic dextrose administration, can precipitate Wernicke's encephalopathy over several hours in normal individuals, there is only evidence to support this effect in patients who already have grave manifestations of thiamine deficiency.[45] Healthy patients require prolonged dextrose administration in order to develop symptoms. Because the morbidity and mortality associated with Wernicke's encephalopathy are so severe, and treatment is both benign and inexpensive, thiamine hydrochloride must be included as initial therapy in all patients who receive dextrose, all patients with altered consciousness, and every potential alcoholic or nutritionally deprived individual who presents to the emergency department.

Replacement consists of the immediate parenteral administration of 100 mg of thiamine hydrochloride, followed by the same dose on a daily basis. This can be given either intramuscularly or intravenously, but the oral route should be avoided because of its unpredictable absorption. In countries where thiamine propyl disulfide (a lipid-soluble thiamine preparation) is available, the oral route may be equally efficacious for the replacement of serious thiamine deficiencies.[2,40,41] Ophthalmoplegia can respond rapidly to as little as 2 mg of thiamine; however, the other manifestations of thiamine deprivation may necessitate higher doses and respond more slowly, if at all. Some authors suggest that up to 1000 mg of thiamine be used in the first 12 hours if patients have resistant ophthalmoplegia.[24]

The common practice requiring the administration of parenteral thiamine prior to hypertonic dextrose in patients with altered consciousness is not logical. As previously mentioned, the given dose of dextrose is extremely unlikely to produce or exacerbate encephalopathy even if thiamine deficiency is present. In addition, thiamine uptake into cells and activation of enzyme systems is slower than that of glucose uptake, which suggests that even pretreatment with thiamine offers little benefit over posttreatment.[39] Despite these limitations it is prudent to administer 100 mg of parenteral thiamine at the time of hypertonic dextrose administration. The biochemical link between dextrose and thiamine is a useful tool to reinforce that the administration of thiamine is necessary. Although thiamine is unlikely to offer immediate benefits for patients with altered consciousness, it will offer some long-term protection for these individuals and initiate therapy for an uncommon, serious, and easily overlooked disorder.

An additional indication for the administration of thiamine hydrochloride occurs in patients with ethylene glycol poisoning. As shown in Figure 64–2, a minor pathway for the elimination of glyoxylic acid involves its conversion to α-hydoxy-β-ketoadipate by α-ketoglutarate:glyoxylate carboligase, a thiamine and magnesium-requiring enzyme. There are no human data to support an increase in α-hydoxy-β-ketoadipate formation following thiamine administration to either ethylene glycol-poisoned animals or humans. However, animal models of primary hyperoxaluria show increases in urinary oxalate during thiamine deficiency, suggesting at least a potential importance of this pathway.[12,38] Because thiamine therapy is generally considered benign, it is prudent to administer standard doses of thiamine to patients with suspected or confirmed ethylene glycol poisoning. If magnesium supplementation is considered, caution is required because of the risk of renal failure in ethylene glycol poisoned patients.

Very few complications have been associated with the parenteral administration of thiamine. Older literature emphasized intramuscular administration because of numerous reports of anaphylaxis with intravenous thiamine delivery.[11,30,33,37,47] It is generally believed that these reactions resulted from responses to the vehicle (chlorbutanol) or its contaminants rather than thiamine itself. Despite the availability of purer, aqueous preparations of thiamine, rare adverse reports still occur.[1,28,36] Although the intramuscular route is acceptable, many patients requiring thiamine will have low muscle mass or a coagulopathy, making this form of delivery painful and potentially unreliable and therefore impractical. The safety of thiamine use was evaluated in a large case series where nearly 1000 patients received parenteral doses of up to 500 mg of thiamine without significant complications.[50] This suggests that if true anaphylaxis to thiamine exists, it is exceedingly uncommon, and that thiamine can be safely administered to most patients by the intravenous route.

References

1. Assem ESK: Anaphylactic reaction to thiamine. Practitioner 1973;211:565.
2. Baker H, Frank O: Absorption, utilization and clinical effectiveness of allithiamines compared to water-soluble thiamines. J Nutr Sci Vitaminol 1976;22(suppl):63–68.
3. Blass JP, Gibson GE: Abnormality of a thiamine-requiring enzyme in patients with Wernicke-Korsakoff syndrome. N Engl J Med 1977;297:1367–1370.
4. Burbato M, Rodriguez PJ: Thiamine deficiency in patients admitted to a palliative care unit. Palliat Med 1994;8: 320–324.
5. Butterworth RF, Gaudreau C, Vincelette J, et al: Thiamine deficiency in AIDS. Lancet 1991;338:1086. Letter.
6. Butterworth RF, Gaudreau C, Vincelette J, et al: Thiamine deficiency and Wernicke's encephalopathy in AIDS. Metab Brain Dis 1991;6:207–212.
7. Butterworth RF, Kril JJ, Harper CG: Thiamine-dependent enzyme changes in the brains of alcoholics: Relationship to the Wernicke-Korsakoff syndrome. Alcohol Clin Res 1993; 17:1084–1088.
8. Calingasan NY, Baker H, Sheu KF, Gibson GE: Blood–brain barrier abnormalities in vulnerable brain regions during thiamine deficiency. Exp Neurol 1995;134:64–72.
9. Deaths associated with thiamine-deficient total parenteral nutrition. MMWR 1989;38:43–46.
10. Descombes E, Dessibourg CA, Fellay G: Acute encephalopathy due to thiamine deficiency (Wernicke's encephalopathy) in a chronic hemodialyzed patient: A case report. Clin Nephrol 1991;35:171–175.
11. Eisenstadt WS: Hypersensitivity to thiamine hydrochloride. Minnesota Med 1942;85:861–863.
12. Hannet B, Thomas DW, Chalmers AH, et al: Formation of oxalate in pyridoxine or thiamin deficient rats during intravenous xylitol infusions. J Nutr 1977;107:458–465.
13. Harata N, Iwasaki Y: Evidence for early blood–brain barrier breakdown in experimental thiamine deficiency in the mouse. Metab Brain Dis 1995;10:159–174.
14. Herve C, Beyne P, Letteron P, Delacoux E: Comparison of erythrocyte transketolase activity with thiamine and thiamine phosphate ester levels in chronic alcoholic patients. Clin Chim Acta 1995;234:91–100.
15. Jeyakumar D: Thiamine responsive ankle oedema in detention centre inmates. Med J Malaysia 1995;50:17–20.
16. Katamura K, Takahasi T, Tanaka H, et al: Two cases of thiamine deficiency-induced lactic acidosis during total parenteral nutrition. Tohoku J Exp Med 1993;171:129–133.
17. Kern D, Kern G, Neef H, et al: How thiamine diphosphate is activated in enzymes. Science 1997;275:67–70.
18. Kwok T, Falconer-Smith JF, Potter JF, Ives DR: Thiamine status of elderly patients with cardiac failure. Age Ageing 1992;21:67–71.
19. Lange R, Erhard J, Eigler FW, Roll C: Lactic acidosis from thiamine deficiency during parenteral nutrition in a two-year-old boy. Eur J Pediatr Surg 1992;2:241–244.
20. Langlais PJ, Zhang SX: Extracellular glutamate is increased in thalamus during thiamine deficiency-induced lesions and is blocked by MK–801. J Neurochem 1993;61:2175–2182.
21. Lavoie J, Butterworth RF: Reduced activities of thiamine-dependent enzymes in the brains of alcoholics in the absence of Wernicke's encephalopathy. Alcohol Clin Exp Res 1995;19:1073–1077.
22. Ma JJ, Truswell AS: Wernicke-Korsakoff syndrome in Syd-

ney hospitals: Before and after thiamine enrichment of flour. Med J Aust 1995;163:531–534.

23. Munujos P, Vendrell M, Ferrer I: Proto-oncogene c-fos induction in thiamine-deficient encephalopathy. Protective effects of nicardipine on pyrithiamine induced lesions. J Neurol Sci 1993;118:175–180.
24. Nakada T, Knight RT: Alcohol and the central nervous system. Med Clin North Am 1984;68:121–131.
25. O'Keeffe ST, Tormey WP, Glasgow R, Lavan JN: Thiamine deficiency in hospitalized elderly patients. Gerontology 1994;40:18–24.
26. O'Rourke NP, Bunker VW, Thomas AJ, et al: Thiamine status of healthy and institutionalized elderly subjects: Analysis of dietary intake and biochemical study. Age Ageing 1990;19:325–329.
27. Oriot D, Wood C, Gottesman R, Huault G: Severe lactic acidosis related to acute thiamine deficiency. J Parenteral Nutr 1991;12:105–109.
28. Proebstle TM, Gall H, Jugert FK, et al: Specific IgE and IgG serum antibodies to thiamine associated anaphylactic reaction. J Allergy Clin Immunol 1995;95:1059–1060.
29. Rao VL, Butterworth RF: Thiamine phosphatases in human brain: Regional alterations in patients with alcoholic cirrhosis. Alcohol Clin Exp Res 1995;19:523–526.
30. Reingold IM, Webb FR: Sudden death following intravenous injection of thiamine hydrochloride. JAMA 1946; 130:491–492.
31. Reuler JB, Girard DE, Cooney TG: Wernicke's encephalopathy. N Engl J Med 1985;312:1035–1037.
32. Rovelli A, Bonomi M, Murano A, et al: Severe lactic acidosis due to thiamine deficiency after bone marrow transplantation in a child with acute monocytic leukemia. Haematologica 1990;75:579–581. Letter.
33. Schiff L: Collapse following parenteral administration of solution of thiamine hydrochloride. JAMA 1941;117:609.
34. Seligmann H, Halkin H, Rauchfleisch S, et al: Thiamine deficiency in patients with congestive heart failure receiving long-term furosemide therapy: A pilot study. Am J Med 1991;91:151–155.
35. Skelton WP, Skelton N: Thiamine deficiency neuropathy: It's still common today. Postgrad Med 1989;85:301–306.
36. Stephen JM, Grant R, Yeh CS: Anaphylaxis from administration of intravenous thiamine. Am J Emerg Med 1992;10: 61–63.
37. Stiles MH: Hypersensitivity to thiamine chloride with a note on sensitivity to pyridoxine hydrochloride. J Allergy 1941;12:507–509.
38. Takasaki E: The urinary excretion of oxalic acid in vitamin B_1 deficient rats. Invest Urol 1969;7:150–153.
39. Tate JR, Nixon PF. Measurement of Michaelis constant for human erythrocyte transketolase and thiamine diphosphate. Anal Biochem 1987;160:78–87.
40. Thomson AD, Baker H, Leevy CM: Patterns of ^{35}S-thiamine hydrochloride absorption in the malnourished alcoholic patient. J Lab Clin Med 1970;76:34–45.
41. Thomson AD, Frank O, Baker H, Leevy CM: Thiamine propyl disulfide: Absorption and utilization. Ann Intern Med 1971;74:529–534.
42. Van Zaanen HC, van der Lelie J: Thiamine deficiency in hematologic malignant tumors. Cancer 1992;69:1710–1713.
43. Victor M, Adams RD: The effect of alcohol on the nervous system. In: Meritt HH, Hare CC, eds: Metabolic and Toxic Diseases of the Nervous System. Baltimore, Williams & Wilkins, 1953, pp. 526–563.
44. Vortmeyer AO, Hagel C, Laas R: Haemorrhagic thiamine deficient encephalopathy following prolonged parenteral nutrition. J Neurol Neurosurg Psychiatry 1992;55:826–829.
45. Watson AJS, Walker JF, Tomkin GH, et al: Acute Wernicke's encephalopathy precipitated by glucose loading. Ir J Med Sci 1981;150:301–303.
46. Weber W, Nitz M, Looby M: Nonlinear kinetics of the thiamine cation in humans: Saturation of nonrenal clearance and tubular reabsorption. J Pharmacokinet Biopharm 1990; 18:501–523.
47. Weigand CG: Reactions attributed to administration of thiamine chloride. Geriatrics 1950;5:274–279.
48. Wilson JD, Madison LL: Deficiency of thiamine (beriberi), pyridoxine, and riboflavin. In: Isselbacher KJ, Adams RD, Braunwald E, et al, eds: Harrison's Principles of Internal Medicine, 9th ed. New York, McGraw-Hill, 1980, pp. 425–429.
49. Wood B, Currie J: Presentation of acute Wernicke's encephalopathy and treatment with thiamine. Metab Brain Dis 1995;10:52–72.
50. Wrenn KD, Murphy F, Slovis CM: A toxicity study of parenteral thiamine hydrochloride. Ann Emerg Med 1989;18: 867–870.

CHAPTER 63

Disulfiram and Disulfiram-like Reactions

Lewis R. Goldfrank

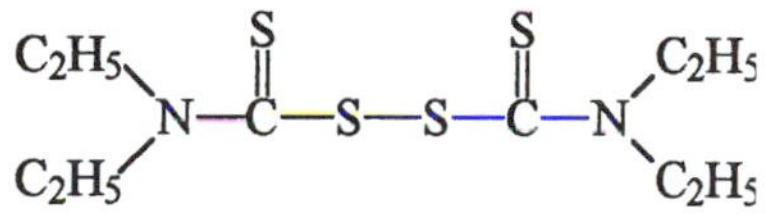

Disulfiram

A 34-year-old known alcoholic man who was being treated with disulfiram (Antabuse) presented to the emergency department (ED) with extreme malaise, weakness, dizziness, and persistent vomiting. Six hours before admission, he had taken "a shot and a half of scotch." Shortly thereafter he began to feel vertiginous and developed a headache. He vomited at least nine times in the 4 hours prior to admission; the last vomitus was described as "blackish."

Physical examination revealed a well-developed, well-nourished man in acute distress. An Antabuse-alert bracelet was on his wrist. Vital signs were: blood pressure, 118/88 mm Hg supine and 112/78 mm Hg seated; pulse, 100 beats/min supine and 120 beats/min seated; respiratory rate, 20 breaths/min; and temperature, 98.2°F (36.8°C). He was alert and oriented. His face was flushed, his trunk erythematous. Pupils and funduscopic examination were normal; the conjunctivae were injected. Head and neck were otherwise unremarkable. The lungs were clear, and the heart was normal. There was no gynecomastia or spider angiomata. Abdominal examination revealed normal bowel sounds and diffuse tenderness without guarding. Bowel sounds were normal. There was no hepatosplenomegaly and no abnormal masses. Rectal examination was negative for occult blood. The vomitus was dark but negative for occult blood; the patient refused nasogastric intubation. Neurologic evaluation and examination of the extremities were unremarkable.

A complete blood count (CBC), prothrombin time, serum electrolytes, BUN, glucose, urinalysis, and ECG were obtained, after which the patient was given 100 mg of thiamine hydrochloride IV and 100 mL of 50% dextrose in water IV; an IV line of normal saline was started with a bolus of 500 mL and maintained at 500 mL/h. The initial laboratory values were only significant for a WBC count of 11,000/mm^3. The ECG showed a sinus tachycardia at 100 beats/min without any acute changes.

After several hours the headache had resolved, there was no further vomiting, and the patient was no longer tachycardic. He was counseled to remain abstinent and return to the care of his therapist.

To appropriately manage the clinical problems associated with disulfiram (Antabuse) and the other thiurams used in industries such as rubber manufacturing and feed grain processing and storage it is important to recognize three clinical patterns: (1) disulfiram (or disulfiram-like)–ethanol reactions; (2) disulfiram overdoses or poisoning; and (3) disulfiram–drug (other than alcohol) interactions. The first consideration is the different basis for evaluating these three clinical syndromes.

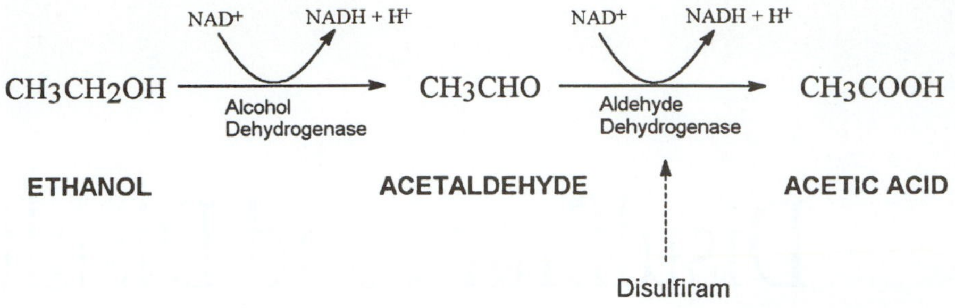

Figure 63–1. Disulfiram's site of action. The irreversible inactivation of aldehyde dehydrogenase results in an increased acetaldehyde level.

What Is Disulfiram?

Disulfiram is a disulfide molecule, tetraethylthiuram, that interferes with the oxidative metabolism of ethanol at the acetaldehyde stage (Chap. 62). Disulfiram competes with nicotinamide adenine dinucleotide (NAD) for aldehyde dehydrogenase moieties, thereby reducing the rate of oxidation of acetaldehyde (Figure 63–1). The resulting increase of acetaldehyde levels produces the characteristic syndrome of adverse effects. The syndrome typically begins 15 to 30 minutes after ingestion or exposure to ethanol.

Diethyldithiocarbamate, the primary metabolite of disulfiram, chelates copper, which is essential for dopamine beta-hydroxylase activity.[3] The inhibition of this metabolic path may be the cause of the hypotension and altered sympathetic tone that are characteristic of disulfiram reactions. Conversely, the experimental injection of acetaldehyde itself usually does not produce these effects but instead actually raises blood pressure.[6] Further support for the effects on other metabolic pathways is offered by the studies of rats given cyanamide, an aldehyde dehydrogenase inhibitor, followed by ethanol. The addition of cyanamide led to an increased mortality and a decreased LD_{50} of ethanol. When these same animals were given the alcohol dehydrogenase inhibitor, 4-methylpyrazole, there was no acetaldehyde accumulation, but there was only a minor effect on mortality.[4] These results also suggest that disulfiram and cyanamide's effects can only be partly explained by the accumulation of acetaldehyde.

Other metals and metalloenzymes including alcohol dehyrogenase may be inhibited by diethyldithiocarbamate. Disulfiram is a relatively nonspecific inhibitor of sulfhydryl-containing enzymes, and decreases the activity of some other hepatic enzymes, such as xanthine oxidase, hexokinase, succinic dehydrogenase, and catalase which has the potential for diverse metabolic manifestations. Diethyldithiocarbamate and one of its metabolites, carbon disulfide, also seem to share these same enzymatic effects with disulfiram. Diethyldithiocarbamate (Imuthiol), a major metabolite of disulfiram, has been reported to inhibit HIV reproduction and to stimulate the immune system.[12] This has led to resurgent use of disulfiram among patients with AIDS or HIV infection. Carbon disulfide, a colorless, fragrant fluid, has been linked to heart disease, peripheral neuropathy, and encephalopathy.[1]

What Is the Metabolic Basis of the Disulfiram Reaction?

A disulfiram–ethanol reaction may result in lethargy, flushing, ataxia, vomiting, and hypotension (Table 63–1). A severe reaction typically occurs in patients on disulfiram who drink enough alcohol to produce a serum ethanol level of 50 to 100 mg/dL (or 0.3 to 0.6 g/kg body weight). However, clinically significant reactions occur at much smaller doses, as seen in patients on disulfiram who take test doses of ethanol or who unknowingly ingest ethanol in one of the 500 to 1000 medicinal preparations that use ethanol as a diluent or solvent. These products range from over-the-counter antitussives to prescribed drugs in almost every therapeutic category, including IV nitroglycerin.[18] In general, the severity and duration of the reaction with disulfiram depend on the amount of ethanol ingested. In diverse medicinal preparations, the ethanol content ranges from less than 1% to 68%.[11] Patients should also be warned about the topical application of ethanol in such products as Sea Breeze (40 to 50% ethanol), Propa pH (30%), and Compound W (77%).

TABLE 63–1. SIGNS AND SYMPTOMS OF DISULFIRAM–ETHANOL REACTIONS

Vital signs	Hypotension Tachycardia Tachypnea
Dermatologic system	Diaphoresis Cutaneous warmth Flushing (face, chest wall) Pruritus
Gastrointestinal system	Abdominal pain Nausea and vomiting
Cardiovascular system	Dysrhythmias Syncope Chest pain and myocardial infarction
Neurologic system	Blurred vision Confusion Dizziness Headache (throbbing, pulsating) Weakness, exhaustion

What Are the Pharmacokinetics of Disulfiram?

About 80% of the oral dose of disulfiram is absorbed from the gastrointestinal tract within 1 hour. Peak effects (manifested by the characteristic adverse reaction with ethanol) occur 8 to 12 hours after taking the drug, when equilibrium is established between tissue-fat and serum. The acetaldehyde dehydrogenase inhibition produced by a disulfiram is irreversible; only the generation of new enzymes allows the metabolism of acetaldehyde to continue. In erythrocytes, disulfiram is metabolized by glutathione reductase to diethyldithiocarbamate and subsequently to diethylamine and carbon disulfide (Fig. 63–2). The diethyldithiocarbamate is conjugated in the liver with glucuronic acid prior to renal excretion as a glucuronide. Small amounts of carbon disulfide are formed, which is metabolized to carbonyl sulfide and sulfur. Urinary excretion is slow, but about 90% of any single dose is removed within 72 hours.[2,13]

As long as the serum activity of acetaldehyde dehydrogenase is diminished, ethanol ingestion will result in an adverse reaction. Depending on hepatic function, this effect may still be present for as long as 2 weeks after the last dose, although 1 week is the more typical duration of action with standard doses. The activity of the microsomal ethanol oxidizing system (MEOS) should rarely be of significance in a patient receiving disulfiram. This system, which increases the metabolism of ethanol by an alternative pathway other than alcohol dehydrogenase, is normally stimulated during chronic exposure to high ethanol concentrations and returns to a low level of activity during abstinence. Of course, it is only during abstinence that disulfiram may be safely given.

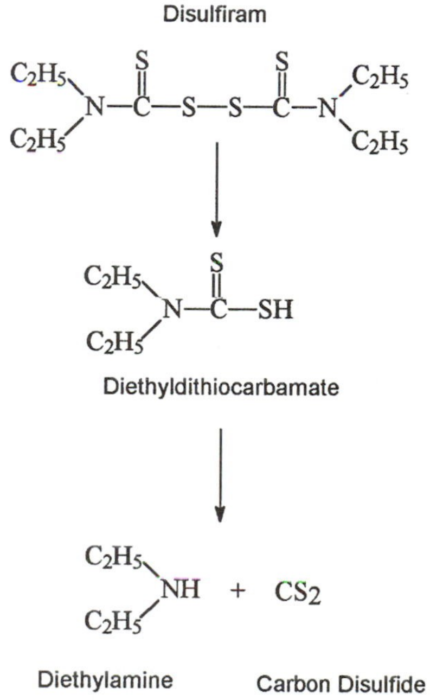

Figure 63–2. Disulfiram metabolism occurs in the liver and erythrocyte. The most consequential metabolites are diethyldithiocarbamate and carbon disulfide.

TABLE 63–2. DISULFIRAM ADVERSE EFFECTS WITH THERAPEUTIC DOSING: SIGNS, SYMPTOMS, AND LABORATORY ABNORMALITIES

System	Signs/Symptoms/Laboratory
Dermatologic	Acneiform eruption
	Urticaria
Gastrointestinal and hepatic	Cholestasis (rare)
	Sulfur or garlic odor on breath
Hematologic	Agranulocytosis
	Eosinophilia
	Thrombocytopenia
	Increased blood nickel
Neuropsychiatric	Ataxia
	Confusion
	Diminished libido and impotence
	Disorientation
	Dysarthria
	Encephalopathy
	Headache
	Irritability
	Lethargy
	Metallic taste
	Optic neuritis
	Paranoia
	Peripheral neuropathy
	Seizures
	Tremor

What Are the Adverse Effects of Disulfiram Use?

Even in the absence of ethanol, disulfiram may produce adverse effects. Many patients report a garlic-like or metallic taste during their first weeks of therapy (Table 63–2). In addition, the breath may have a rotten-egg odor, due to the sulfide metabolites. Some of the other central nervous system manifestations and some of the disagreeable symptoms are attributable to carbon disulfide. Some patients develop pruritus and other dermatologic manifestations. Diverse neuropsychiatric manifestations have been described, such as headache, drowsiness, fatigue, impotence, peripheral neuropathies, catatonia, depression, mania, and acute psychosis.[7,9] Rarely, hepatotoxicity with an increased alkaline phosphatase and bilirubin has occurred.[17] Alcoholics with a history of a psychiatric disorder may experience recurrent symptoms or exacerbations. Both disulfiram and its active metabolite, diethyldithiocarbamate, inhibit brain dopamine beta-hydroxylase, leading to increased brain dopamine and decreased norepinephrine, possibly explaining altered behavior.[5]

What Are the Manifestations of Disulfiram Overdose?

Disulfiram overdose is a consequential risk for either adults and children who have ingested more than 2 to 3 g, although patients of diverse ages have ingested sub-

TABLE 63–3. SIGNS AND SYMPTOMS OF DISULFIRAM OVERDOSE

	Signs/Symptoms
Vital signs	Hypotension
	Tachycardia
	Tachypnea
Gastrointestinal/hepatic systems	Abdominal pain
	Diarrhea
	Sulfur or garlic odor on breath
	Vomiting
Neurologic system	Ataxia
	Agitation
	Choreoathetosis
	Coma
	Dysarthria
	Flaccidity
	Hallucinations
	Headache
	Irritability
	Lethargy
	Parkinsonlike syndrome
	Seizures

stantially greater amounts without symptomatology. In children the manifestations of hypotension can be delayed for 6 to 12 hours. Tachypnea, tachycardia, and hypotension may occur. The neurologic manifestations are quite diverse, including irritability, lethargy, dysarthria, ataxia, seizures, flaccidity, and hallucinations. These various findings are noted in Table 63–3. The slow absorption and potentially delayed onset of symptoms, should they occur, will necessitate observation of 6 to 12 hours following the ingestion prior to discharge, if there are no psychiatric indications for admission.

How Should Patients With Disulfiram-Type Reactions Be Managed?

There are numerous agents other than disulfiram, which when given with ethanol may produce a disulfiram-like reaction (Table 63–4).[14,15] Examples of such drug interactions are cited in Table 63–5. Signs and symptoms similar to those described in this chapter occurring in this population should therefore suggest a disulfiram reaction.

The clinical manifestations of the reaction are usually adequately managed with supportive care. Diphenhydramine has a delayed effect on the flushing response. Diphenhydramine does inhibit alcohol dehydrogenase, delaying metabolism of ethanol; but it also inhibits acetaldehyde dehydrogenase so that acetaldehyde levels remain unchanged. In one clinical study, H_1-receptor antagonists did not modify acetaldehyde accumulation after a disulfiram effect was induced by cyanamide, but did have an effect on the flushing and tachycardia resulting from ethanol.[20] When hypotension develops it is probable that both H_1 and H_2 antagonists will be necessary to achieve a therapeutic benefit for a possible histamine induced vasodilation. This phenomenon was studied in an individual genetically susceptible to ethanol induced flush, but this individual was found to be resistant to H_1 and H_2 antagonists.[21] It remains uncertain whether this vasodilation results from the inhibition of histamine metabolism due to elevated acetaldehyde levels. Inhibitors of prostaglandin synthetase, such as indomethacin, may also limit the flush response.

In patients who experience severe reactions to disulfiram and ethanol, hypotension and refractory vomiting can be life-threatening. For refractory vomiting, a parenteral antiemetic agent, such as ondansetron (4 mg IV), should be preferable to metoclopramide, which due to its alpha-adrenergic antagonist effects could exacerbate hypotension.

General management can be initiated even at a delayed stage when disulfiram is slowly absorbed and symptoms develop 2 to 10 hours after ingestion. Because vomiting typically occurs as part of the reaction, the induction of emesis or orogastric lavage is usually unnecessary. Although disulfiram adsorption to activated charcoal may occur, ethanol is so rapidly absorbed and so poorly adsorbed to activated charcoal that activated

TABLE 63–4. PHARMACEUTICALS AND CHEMICALS PRODUCING DISULFIRAM-LIKE REACTIONS WITH ETHANOL

Pharmaceuticals	Chemicals
Antimicrobial Agents	***Industrial Agents***
Cephalosporins (cefoperazone, cefotetan, cefamandole, and moxalactam)	Butanol oxime
Chloramphenicol	Calcium cyanamide
Diethyldithiocarbamate	Carbon disulfide
Furazolidone	Hydrogen sulfide
Griseofulvin	Tetraethyl lead
Ketoconazole	Tetramethylthiuram disulfide
Metronidazole	Tetrachlorethylene
Nitrofurantoin	Trichlorethylene
Quinacrine	
MAO Inhibitors	
Procarbazine	
Pargyline	
Tranylcypromine	
Sulfonylureas	
Acetohexamide	
Chlorpropamide	
Glipizide	
Glyburide	
Tolazamide	
Tolbutamide	
Miscellaneous	
Animal charcoal	
Calcium carbimide	
Mushrooms (*Coprinus atramentarius, Clitocybe clavipes*)	

TABLE 63–5. REPRESENTATIVE IMPORTANT DISULFIRAM–DRUG INTERACTIONS

Drug	Mechanism/Toxic Manifestations
Alfentanil	May decrease plasma clearance and increase duration of action
Amitriptyline	Organic brain syndrome (unknown causality)
Antipyrine	Inhibits hepatic mixed-function oxidase catalyzed hydroxylation
Benzodiazepines	Decreases clearance of some agents, leading to benzodiazepine accumulation
Coumarin derivatives	Decreases biotransformation of coumarin, leading to prolonged prothrombin time
Ethylene dibromide	Inhibits metabolism, leading to potentially high levels of exposure
Isoniazid	Neurotoxicity for unknown reasons
Metronidazole	Causes visual and auditory hallucinations
Paraldehyde	Metabolism of this acetaldehyde polymer is blocked at acetaldehyde phase, resulting in ethanol–disulfiram type interaction
Phenytoin	Phenytoin metabolism inhibited, leading to phenytoin toxicity
Primidone	Enhanced primidone conversion to phenobarbital
Rifampin	Prolongs half-life of disulfiram
Theophylline	Inhibits metabolism, leading to theophylline accumulation

charcoal is unlikely to be of benefit. Placing the patient in Trendelenberg position and administering IV fluids should be the first form of treatment for orthostatic hypotension. If fluid repletion with normal saline or Ringer's lactate is unsuccessful, a vasopressor may be necessary. Norepinephrine (Levophed) is a more logical choice than dopamine, and is more frequently successful because disulfiram blocks dopamine beta-hydroxylase, which then becomes rate limiting in norepinephrine synthesis.[16] Levophed would be expected to produce a more rapid response to the hypotension or shock.[10] After a massive ingestion of disulfiram and ethanol such as in a suicide attempt, hemodialysis should be considered to remove the ethanol and acetaldehyde if refractory hypotension and protracted vomiting occur. We used hemodialysis on a single occasion to remove ethanol, acetaldehyde, and disulfiram, achieving resolution of the life-threatening reaction in less than 2 hours. The use of 4-methylpyrazole (4-MP) to block alcohol dehydrogenase, has been employed to decrease the production of the toxic metabolite acetaldehyde.[4] 4-MP has no effect on acetaldehyde dehydrogenase and would not inhibit the metabolism of acetaldehyde, the toxic metabolite. Additional studies on 4-MP (see Antidotes in Depth: 4-Methylpyrazole) are necessary before the drug becomes available in the United States. The benefit of 4-MP for a disulfiram–ethanol interaction resulting in hypotension appears limited, as both the persistence of a high ethanol level and the acetaldehyde level contribute to the hemodynamic compromise.

Who Is At Risk of Exposure to Industrial Thiurams?

Disulfiram is a tetraethylthiuram disulfide derivative of thiuram. Many workers in the rubber industry are exposed to thiurams because the derivatives act as accelerators for the vulcanization process. Workers dealing with fungicides, insecticides, larvicides, and seed disinfectants are also exposed to thiurams.[8,19,22] In these settings, enough of the wetted compound may be absorbed to produce a toxic reaction with ethanol similar to the disulfiram–ethanol reaction.

Acknowledgments

Eddy A. Bresnitz, MD, Richard S. Weisman, PharmD, and Menachem Melinek, MD contributed to this chapter in previous editions.

References

1. Davidson M, Feinleib M: Carbon disulfide poisoning: A review. Am Heart J 1972;83:100–114.
2. Eneanya DI, Bianchine JR, Duran DO, et al: The actions and metabolic fate of disulfiram. Annu Rev Pharmacol Toxicol 1981;21:575–579.
3. Goldstein M, Anagnoste B, Lauber E, McKereghan MR: Inhibition of dopamine beta hydroxylase by disulfiram. Life Sci 1964;3:763–767.
4. Hillbom ME, Shrviharju MS, Lindros KO: Potentiation of ethanol by cyanamide in relation to acetaldehyde accumulation. Toxicol Appl Pharmacol 1983;70:133–139.
5. Knee ST, Razani J: Acute organic brain syndrome: A complication of disulfiram therapy. Am J Psychiatry 1974;131:1281–1282.
6. Kupari M, Hillbom M, Lindros K, Nieminen M: Possible cardiovascular hazards of the alcohol-calcium carbimide interaction. J Toxicol Clin Toxicol 1982;19:79–86.
7. Liddon SC, Satran R: Disulfiram (Antabuse) psychosis. Am J Psychiatry 1967;123:1284–1289.
8. Millar JD: Ethylene dibromide and disulfiram toxic interaction. Vet Hum Toxicol 1978;20:434–435.
9. Miller-Fisher C: "Catatonia" due to disulfiram toxicity. Arch Neurol 1989;46:798–804.
10. Motte S, Vincent JL, Gillet JB: Refractory hyperdynamic shock associated with alcohol and disulfiram. Am J Emerg Med 1986;4:323–325.
11. Petroni NC, Cardoni AA: Alcohol content of liquid medicinals. Clin Toxicol 1979;14:407–432.
12. Pompidou A, Delsaux MC, Telvi L, et al: Isoprinosine and Imuthiol, two potentially active compounds in patients with AIDS-related complex symptoms. Cancer Res 1985;45(suppl 9):4671S–4673S.
13. Rall TW: Hypnotics and sedatives: Ethanol. In: Gilman AG, Rall TW, Nies AS, Taylor P, eds: Goodman and Gilman's The Pharmacological Basis of Therapeutics, 8th ed. New York, Pergamon Press, 1990, pp. 378–379.
14. Reynolds WA, Lowe FH: Mushrooms and a toxic reaction

to alcohol: Report of four cases. N Engl J Med 1965;272: 630–631.

15. Roe DA: Interactions between drugs and nutrients. Med Clin North Am 1979;63:985–1007.
16. Rogers WK, Benowitz NL, Wilson KM, Abbot JA: Effect of disulfiram on adrenergic function. Clin Pharmacol Ther 1979;24:469–477.
17. Schade RR, Gray JA, Dekker A, et al: Fulminant hepatitis associated with disulfiram. Arch Intern Med 1983;143: 1271–1273.
18. Seixas FA: Alcohol and its drug interactions. Ann Intern Med 1975;83:86–92.
19. Shelley WB: Golf-course dermatitis due to thiuram fungicide: Cross-hazards of alcohol, disulfiram, and rubber. JAMA 1964;188:415–417.
20. Stowell A, Johnsen J, Ripel A, Moreland J: Diphenhydramine and the calcium carbimide ethanol reaction: A placebo controlled clinical study. Clin Pharmacol Ther 1986;39:521–525.
21. Tan OT, Gaylarde PM, Sarkany K: Blocking of alcohol induced flush with a combination of H_1 and H_2 histamine antagonists. Lancet 1979;2:365. Letter.
22. Webb PK, Gibbs SC, Mathias CT, et al: Disulfiram hypersensitivity and rubber contact dermatitis. JAMA 1979;241: 2061.

CHAPTER 64

Toxic Alcohols

Lewis R. Goldfrank and Neal E. Flomenbaum

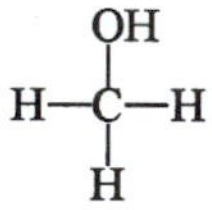

Methanol

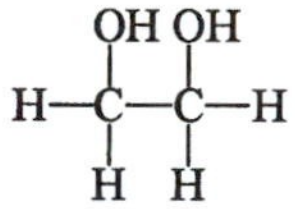

Ethylene glycol

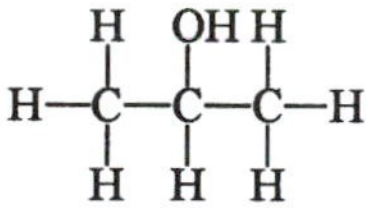

Isopropanol

Ethylene Glycol	
MW	62 D
Action serum level for	
Hemodialysis	>25 mg/dL
	>4.03 mmol/L
Isopropanol	
MW	60 D
Methanol	
MW	32 D
Action serum level for	
Hemodialysis	>25 mg/dL
	>7.8 mmol/L

Values greater than or equal to the action level necessitate clinical intervention.
Values less than this level may necessitate intervention based on the clinical condition of the patient.

A 35-year-old man with an ataxic gait was brought to the Emergency Department (ED). He stated that he had taken something to kill himself. He reported "stomach cramps" and vomiting, but was unable to give any other pertinent history. On physical examination, he appeared well developed and well nourished, mildly agitated, and irritable. His vital signs were: blood pressure, 120/80 mm Hg without orthostatic changes; pulse, 80 beats/min; respiratory rate, 12 breaths/min; temperature, 97.8°F (36.6°C).

His skin was moist, anicteric, and acyanotic. Examination of his head, ears, eyes, nose, and throat revealed only an abrasion on the right cheek. He had nystagmus on extreme lateral gaze and funduscopic examination revealed no hemorrhages, exudates, or papilledema. Examination of the neck, heart, lungs, abdomen and extremities was normal.

An intravenous line was established with a 0.9% sodium chloride solution and blood was drawn and sent for glucose, electrolytes, BUN, creatinine, osmolality, ethanol, and acetaminophen levels, and an extra red-top tube was held pending initial evaluation. Urine was obtained for routine and microscopic examination. An electrocardiogram (ECG) was performed and the patient was placed on a cardiac monitor.

The patient was given 100 mg of thiamine HCl, 10 mL of multivitamins, and 100 mL of 50% dextrose in water ($D_{50}W$) intravenously. Fifty grams of activated charcoal in 35 g of sorbitol were administered orally.

As the examination proceeded, the patient's mental status deteriorated. He became more agitated, requiring physical restraints. Repeat vital signs were blood pressure, 120/80 mm Hg; pulse, 110 beats/min; respiratory rate, 20 breaths/min; temperature, 98.6°F (37°C). The ECG showed a regular sinus tachycardia at a rate of 110 with no abnormalities

Arterial blood gas determination on room air revealed pH, 7.10; PCO_2, 20 mm Hg; PO_2, 95 mm Hg. Electrolytes were Na^+, 145 mEq/L; K^+, 2.7 mEq/L; Cl^-, 105 mEq/L; HCO_3^-, 8 mEq/L; BUN, 20 mg/dL; Ca^{2+}, 9.3 mg/dL; creatinine, 1.0 mg/dL; glucose, 80 mg/dL. These values indicated that the patient had a severe metabolic acidosis with an anion gap of 32 mEq/L (see anion gap discussion in Chap. 15). Urinalysis results were glucose, 4+; ketones, negative; and protein, positive; there were 2 to 5 WBC and 2 to 5 RBC per high-power field. The urine ferric chloride test was negative.

The serum osmolality was measured at 360 mOsm/kg, but the calculated osmolarity was determined to be 303 mOsm/L, from the formula in Figure 64–1.

The ethanol level was only 5 mg/dL and therefore contributed negligibly to the gap calculation. The osmol gap was 57 mOsm/L. This value indicates a substantial gap.

The patient's urine fluoresced brightly under a Wood's lamp in a dark room, a finding highly suggestive of an ethylene glycol (antifreeze) ingestion. This bedside finding together with the high anion gap metabolic acidosis and large osmol gap provided sufficient evidence to establish the diagnosis of ethylene glycol poisoning and to immediately treat the patient with a loading dose of ethanol, followed by a maintenance ethanol infusion and with thiamine and pyridoxine. Ultimately, an initial ethylene glycol level of 350 mg/dL was reported by the reference laboratory.

With the patient receiving IV ethanol, hemodialysis was initiated within 2 hours of admission and two 3-hour hemodialysis treatments were performed. At discharge 1 week after admission, the BUN was 10 mg/dL, creatinine was 0.8 mg/dL, and urine sediment was normal. Follow-up was arranged with the patient's internist and psychiatrist.

This case of ethylene glycol poisoning illustrates many of the features of toxic alcohol poisoning. There are three toxic alcohols commonly associated with toxicologic emergencies: methanol, ethylene glycol, and isopropanol. Several others are uncommonly involved: diethylene glycol, monomethyl ether of ethylene glycol, monobutyl ether of ethylene glycol, and benzyl alcohol. Of the three common toxic alcohols, methanol and ethylene glycol are similar with respect to potential toxicity and lethality; characteristic delayed onset of toxicity, particularly with the presence of ethanol; and treatment, which is ethanol loading and maintenance followed by hemodialysis. The third common toxic alcohol, isopropanol, presents a different and typically less potentially lethal problem that nevertheless requires identification and appropriate medical treatment. The characteristics of ethylene glycol and methanol poisoning will be discussed first, followed by isopropanol and the less common toxic alcohols.

What Are the Pathophysiologic Characteristics of Ethylene Glycol Poisoning?

Ethylene glycol is used extensively as an antifreeze (especially automobile antifreeze), often at concentrations of 95%. It is also used in fire extinguishers, inks, pesticides, adhesives, and air conditioning and solar energy systems. Ethylene glycol is rapidly absorbed from the GI tract and slowly absorbed through the skin or lungs. Usually there are clues to the cause of an exposure, but several reported cases of contamination of the water supply force the clinician to consider ethylene glycol when evaluating an unexplained high anion gap metabolic acidosis. This is essential in preventing an epidemic. In one instance hemodialysis resulted in a fatality because air conditioning cooling fluid containing ethylene glycol contaminated a hospital's water supply.[62]

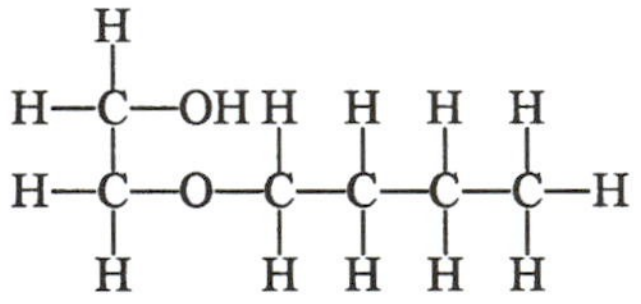

Ethylene glycol butyl ether

There are numerous glycol esters and ethers, some of which may be metabolized to ethylene glycol after exposure.[49] Diethylene glycol is an industrial solvent utilized in

$$2 \times Na^+ \text{ (145 mEq/L)} + \frac{\text{BUN (20 mg/dL)}}{2.8} + \frac{\text{Glucose (80mg/dL)}}{18} + \frac{\text{Ethanol (5mg/dL)}}{4.6} = \text{mOsm/L}$$

OR

$$290 + 7.1 + 4.4 + 1.1 = 303\text{mOsm/L}$$

Figure 64–1. Calculation of osmolarity.

sprinkler antifreeze solutions, lubricants, paints, and cosmetic creams. Diethylene glycol-contaminated glycerin has repetitively been utilized in the preparation of medications, most recently in a Haitian preparation of acetaminophen.[42] Fatalities have commonly resulted from these medication contamination epidemics. (see Chap. 1). Monomethyl ether of ethylene glycol [$CH_3OCH_2CH_2OH$] and monobutyl ether [$CH_3(CH_2)_3OCH_2CH_2OH$] are two commonly used solvents called cellosolves. They are used in resins, paints, and industrial coatings. Following exposure to these ethers, the primary product or its metabolites results in acute tubular necrosis (without oxalaturia); pancreatitis, hepatitis, CNS depression, and metabolic acidosis also occur. Chronic inhalation of these ethers can result in a toxic encephalopathy and bone marrow depression.[16] Awareness of the potential for these agents to cause clinical syndromes of poisoning is important.

As in the case of methanol poisoning, an individual presenting after an ethylene glycol ingestion may rapidly develop somnolence and inebriation. The low vapor pressure of ethylene glycol and its poor cutaneous absorption limit toxicity via the lungs and skin. Ethylene glycol is rapidly absorbed through the gastrointestinal tract and reaches peak levels within 1 to 4 hours. It is rapidly distributed throughout the body due to its high water solubility. In the presence of normal renal function, its apparent half-life is 2.5 to 4.5 hours and less than 20% is excreted unmetabolized by the kidney. The action of alcohol dehydrogenase in the liver is the first rate-limiting step in the breakdown of both methanol and ethylene glycol to toxic metabolites. Ethylene glycol is rapidly metabolized to glycoaldehyde, glycolic acid, and oxalic acid. All of these metabolites are effectively removed with hemodialysis.[21] Once present, the aldehyde and acid metabolites inhibit diverse metabolic pathways in the body, including oxidative phosphorylation (Fig. 64–2). The transformation of

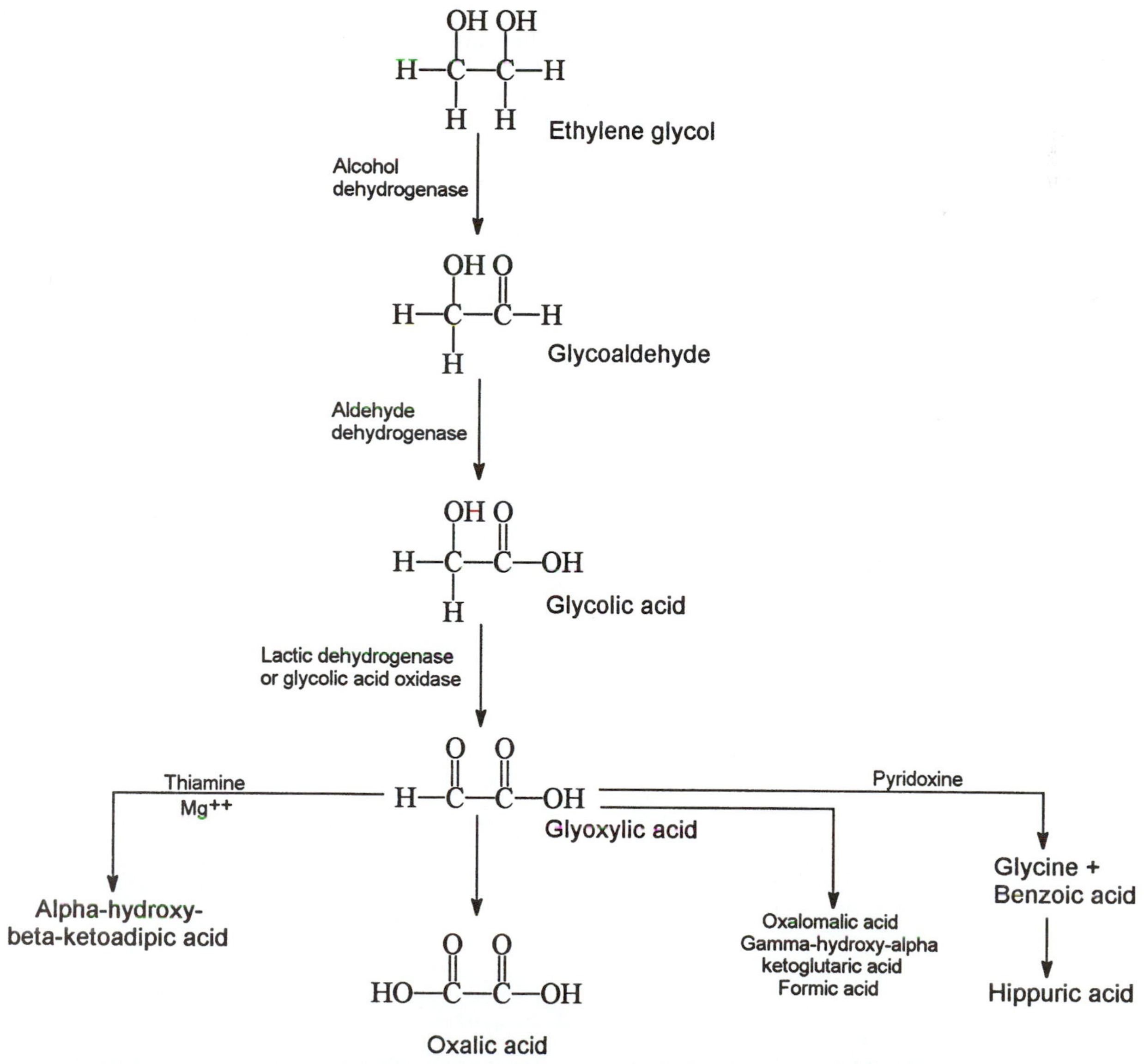

Figure 64–2. Major pathways of ethylene glycol metabolism.

the alcohol, ethylene glycol, to oxalic acid results in a high NADH to NAD ratio, which facilitates the transformation of pyruvate to lactate. This may result in an increased lactic acid level. The metabolites of ethylene glycol are directly toxic to the kidney, lungs, and CNS.

The ingestion of ethylene glycol results in a three-phase intoxication. The first phase is associated with the parent alcohol and its predominant CNS effects. Persistent nausea and vomiting, and the gradual onset of intoxication or inebriation, lethargy, and coma often appear within 4 to 8 hours. Diffuse neurologic abnormalities may be noted, including nystagmus, ataxia, areflexia, myoclonic movements, and seizures. Although reported, pupils with loss of light reflexes, papilledema, and ophthalmoplegia are uncommon with ethylene glycol and more frequently seen with methanol ingestion.

The second phase is mainly metabolic and manifested by cardiopulmonary compromise. A profound anion gap acidosis may also appear within hours after the ingestion.

The third phase is related to the excretion of the toxic metabolites and is renal in nature.

The urine of a patient who has ingested ethylene glycol reveals calcium oxalate (Fig. 64–3) or hippurate crystals in approximately 50% of cases.[13,28] Hippurate crystals are produced by the transamination of glyoxylate to glycine.[55] Calcium oxalate crystals are found either as monohydrates (prism or needle-like) or dihydrates (tent or envelope shaped). The dihydrate form has more commonly been identified in ethylene glycol poisoning and has more diagnostic significance, as the monohydrate form resembles sodium urate crystals too closely to be reliably identified. Red blood cells and protein are also found in the urine after an ethylene glycol ingestion. Acute tubular necrosis secondary to the precipitation of oxalate crystals or the direct toxic effect of ethylene glycol metabolites on the tubules occurs in 12 to 48 hours. Hypocalcemia resulting in a prolonged QTc interval on the ECG, and tetany may develop. Other signs of ethylene glycol poisoning include tachycardia, hyperventilation, leukocytosis, and cerebrospinal fluid pleocytosis. Late findings (after 24 hours) include cardiopulmonary failure and acute renal failure. Cardiac compromise and noncardiogenic pulmonary edema[11] have been reported, as has myositis (Table 64–1).

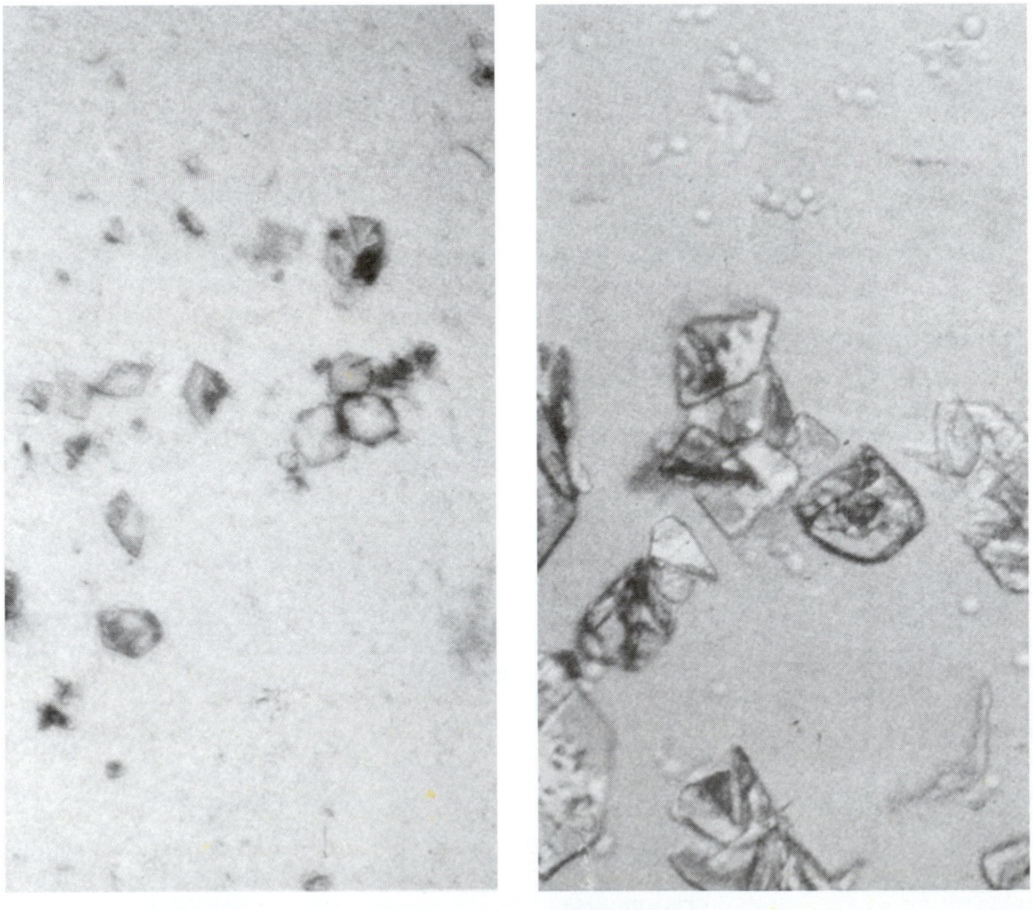

Figure 64–3. Calcium oxalate crystals (dehydrate forms) under low (A) and high (B) power, found in the urine of a patient after ingestion of ethylene glycol.

TABLE 64–1. SIGNS AND SYMPTOMS OF TOXIC ALCOHOL EXPOSURES

Organ System	Ethylene Glycol	Isopropanol	Methanol
Cardiovascular	Tachycardia Hypertension/hypotension Dysrhythmias Myocarditis	Tachycardia Hypotension Myocardial depression	Tachycardia Hypotension
Central nervous	Ataxia Cerebral edema Coma Convulsions CNS depression Inebriation Irritability Myoclonus	Ataxia Areflexia Coma Dizziness Headache Inebriation Muscle weakness Hypothermia	Coma Convulsions Dizziness Headache Hypothermia Inebriation Somnolence
Gastrointestinal	Nausea Vomiting	Abdominal pain, cramping Gastritis Hematemesis Nausea, vomiting	Abdominal pain Anorexia Gastritis Nausea, vomiting Pancreatitis
Ophthalmic	Ophthalmoplegia Nystagmus		"Snow fields" Blurred vision Hyperemic optic discs Mydriasis Papilledema, blindness
Pulmonary	Hyperventilation, tachypnea Pneumonitis Noncardiogenic pulmonary edema	Odor of acetone Respiratory depression Hemorrhagic tracheobronchitis	Noncardiogenic pulmonary edema
Renal	Renal failure Crystalluria	Renal tubular acidosis Rhabdomyolysis	
Uncommon		Hemolytic anemia	

What Are the Pathophysiologic Characteristics of Methanol Poisoning?

Methanol or methyl alcohol is readily available at variable concentrations in numerous products. It is used extensively in windshield washing and deicing solutions (35 to 95%), carburetor cleaners (20%), duplicating fluids (95%), solid canned fuels (4%), shellac, paint removers and thinners, model airplane fuels, denatured alcohol, and embalming fluid. Exposures commonly occur both in the workplace and the household. A colorless liquid, methanol can be absorbed by oral ingestion, inhalation, or transdermally. Toxicity, including death, can result from absorption by all routes.[2,20,32]

When methanol is ingested, peak levels occur within 30 to 60 minutes, but there is often a latent period of about 24 hours (range, 1 to 72 hours) before the development of either toxic symptoms or metabolic acidosis.[7] Methanol has an apparent volume of distribution of 0.6 to 0.7 L/kg About 75 to 85% of methanol is metabolized in the liver by alcohol dehydrogenase and small amounts are excreted unchanged via the lungs (10 to 20%) and the kidneys (3%). In lower amounts, methanol metabolism follows zero-order kinetics at a rate of 8.5 mg/dL per hour,[29] yielding the metabolites formaldehyde and formic acid.[18] Apparent first-order kinetics characterize the metabolism of higher levels, although the variable kinetics may be due to changes in pulmonary clearance.[46] Under typical circumstances the contribution of first-order renal and pulmonary clearance is minimal relative to the substantial zero order hepatic metabolism. [52] At low concentrations and in the absence of ethanol, the apparent half-life of methanol may be 3 hours or less, whereas in 6 patients undergoing ethanol treatment the median half-life was 43.1 hours (range, 30.3 to 52.0 hours).[52] The methanol metabolite formaldehyde is itself rapidly metabolized by aldehyde dehydrogenase, and therefore levels of formaldehyde are only transiently found and have not been measured in any fluids or tissue.[44,46] Rapid oxidation of formaldehyde creates formic acid, which is responsible both for the metabolic acidosis and the retinal toxicity associated with methanol exposures (Fig. 64–4).[63] When formate was administered experimentally at toxic levels to primates, no conversion to formaldehyde was detected.[47] Formate toxicity is noted

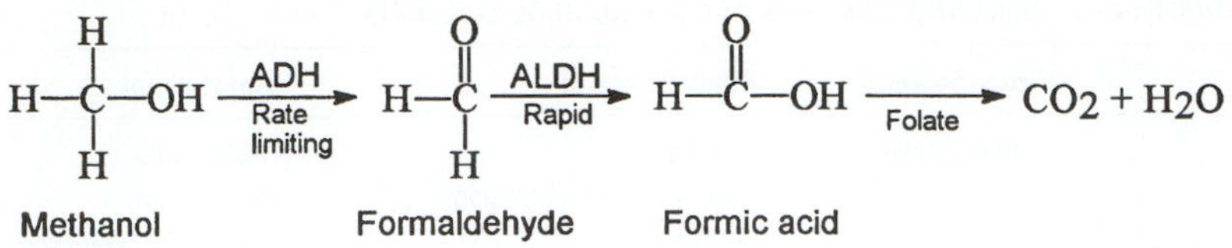

Figure 64–4. Methanol metabolism. Therapy is aimed at interfering with this conversion. Ethanol is a preferential substrate for alcohol dehydrogenase (ADH). 4-Methylpyrazole is a competitive inhibitor of the enzyme ADH. (ALDH = aldehyde dehydrogenase.)

even when experimental conditions allow for buffering at physiologic pH.[47] Formate may inhibit the cytochrome oxidase chain, increasing lactate production and metabolic acidosis. In a folate-dependent step, formic acid is transformed to carbon dioxide and water.

Late recognition of both methanol exposure and symptoms may permit formic acid (formate) to develop to levels that correlate with permanent visual impairment. The two factors of delayed recognition of toxic symptoms for more than 10 hours and elevated formate levels correlate best with poor outcome.[1,40] The most characteristic finding in methanol intoxication is visual disturbances or blindness. Patients often complain of blurred or dimmed vision ("flashes" or a "snowstorm"). Ophthalmologic examination usually reveals dilated pupils with absent or sluggish light reaction and poor accommodation. Hyperemia of the optic disc followed by retinal edema is routinely seen on funduscopic examination in untreated cases. The eye findings correlate better with the acidosis than do any other clinical findings, including hyperventilation; however, in a few fatal cases and in a few cases where the patient actually complained of visual problems, the eye examination was normal. The irreversible sequelae of optic nerve exposure to formic acid are optic atrophy and visual field impairment.[6] Even when the exposure to methanol is recognized early, blindness may result if the poisoning is not aggressively managed (see Chap. 26 for further details).

The CNS symptoms of methanol poisoning include inebriation, headache, dizziness, seizures, and coma. Nausea, vomiting, a stiff neck (meningismus), abdominal pain, obstipation, and malaise are also common complaints. Hypophosphatemia and elevated creatine phosphokinase are commonly noted laboratory findings, as is an elevated amylase accompanying the abdominal pain,[7] although in at least one case of hyperamylasemia the amylase proved to be a salivary type.[17] This same finding has been associated with ethanol intake. Hemorrhagic and nonhemorrhagic necrosis of the putamen have also been described and are often present as characteristic radiologic findings. (Table 64–1).[24,57]

What Special Measures Should Be Taken Early When Methanol or Ethylene Glycol Poisoning Is Suspected?

Like ethanol, methanol and ethylene glycol are odorless (Table 64–2). A crude way to check for the presence of the osmotically active alcohols—methanol, isopropanol, ethylene glycol, and ethanol—is to compare the measured serum osmolality (by freezing point depression) with the (predicted) osmolarity calculated from a routine chemistry profile (Na^+, BUN, and glucose).[60] The difference between the two values is referred to as the osmol gap. An elevated osmol gap suggests the presence of an osmotically active alcohol, but a normal value does not exclude its presence[67] (see Chap. 15). Once metabolism of an ingested alcohol is complete, the osmol gap will be normal even in the presence of life-threatening metabolic acidosis.

In any case of suspected ethylene glycol or methanol ingestion, blood should be sent for a toxicologic analysis of both as well as for ethanol. Methanol and ethanol are quite easy to detect and quantify analytically, where as few laboratories have had the capacity to analyze ethylene glycol. When available all three alcohols—ethanol, methanol, and ethylene glycol—can be analyzed using gas chromatography on a carbowax column (see Chap. 6).

Laboratory reports of low methanol levels are periodically confused with methanol intoxication, because the natural fermentation of wines and distilled fruit spirits may result in methanol levels of 300 mg/L in these beverages. In alcoholics who are binge drinkers, methanol metabolism is inhibited and modest amounts of methanol may accumulate. In a review of 2286 patients with ethanol levels greater than 100 mg/dL, 6% had serum methanol levels of 4.5 mg/dL or more.[41]

The addition of fluorescein to automobile antifreezes by the manufacturers to allow mechanics to identify the souce of any auto radiator leak with an ultraviolet Wood's lamp may also enable the clinician to establish an ethylene glycol ingestion by placing a sample of the patient's urine under a Wood's lamp. A high correlation of positive urine fluorescence was noted when volunteers were given oral fluorescein in doses comparable to that expected with an ethylene glycol ingestion.[70] The incidence of positive findings in ethylene glycol poisoning is unknown and depends on the dose, brand ingested, and time since ingestion. The absence of urine fluorescence should never be used to exclude the diagnosis, particularly if renal shutdown has occurred.

Is Activated Charcoal Useful for Patients With Toxic Alcohol Ingestions?

Activated charcoal has been shown to adsorb 59% of methanol and 68% of ethylene glycol in vitro when used at 5:1 ratios, while even at 1:2 ratios, 48% and 40% were respectively adsorbed.[16a] At a 20:1 ratio of activated charcoal to toxin, 87 to 92% of isopropanol was bound in

TABLE 64–2. TOXIC ALCOHOLS: CHARACTERISTICS, SIGNS, AND SYMPTOMS OF TOXICITY

Substance	Formula	Half-life	Metabolites	High Anion Gap Acidosis	Ketosis	CNS Depression	Characteristic Findings	Commercial Sources
Benzyl alcohol	C_6H_6OH	?	Benzoic acid, hippuric acid	+	−	+	Neonatal "gasping syndrome"	Bacteriostatic preservatives
Ethanol[a]	CH_3CH_2OH	Zero-order kinetics 15–20 mg/dL/h	Acetaldehyde, acetic acid	+	+	+	Intoxication	Solvents, beverages, colognes
Ethylene glycol	CH_2OHCH_2OH	2.5–4.5 h	Oxalic acid, glycolic acid	++	−	+	Renal failure, hypocalcemia, calcium oxalate crystals in urine	Antifreeze (95%), solvents, deicers, air-conditioning units
Glycol ether	$HOCH_2CH_2OR$	?	Ethylene glycol and metabolites	+	−	+	Similar to ethylene glycol	Solvents, industrial coatings
Isopropanol	$CH_3CHOHCH_3$	2.5–3.5 h	Acetone	−	+	++	Hemorrhagic tracheobronchitis, gastritis	Rubbing alcohol, solvents, lacquer
Methanol	CH_3OH	Zero-order kinetics 8.5 mg/dL/h	Formaldehyde, formic acid	++	−	+	Blindness, pink edematous optic disc	Antifreeze, solvents, gasohol denaturant
Propylene glycol	$CH_2OHCHOHCH_3$	2–5 h	Lactic acid, pyruvic acid	+	−	+	Seizures, cardiovascular collapse	Solvents, deicers

+ = Presence and degree of symptoms; — = absence of symptoms.

[a]Only in the case of alcoholic ketoacidosis is there a high anion gap metabolic acidosis with ketonemia.

vitro.[10] Although these data are encouraging, most alcohols are taken in very large quantities and are well absorbed within a half-hour of ingestion, making this approach ineffective in the hospital setting, particularly when patients arrive several hours following ingestion. It is not known how much of the toxic alcohols and their metabolites are secreted or diffused back into the GI tract, and therefore activated charcoal administration is logical but may be without benefit in vivo. Blood ethanol levels in one study were not reduced when activated charcoal was administered 1 and 3 hours after ethanol ingestion, suggesting a very limited clinical benefit for activated charcoal with other alcohols.[31] Multiple-dose activated charcoal is not expected to be useful.

What Treatment Is Indicated for Ethylene Glycol and Methanol Ingestions?

Ethylene glycol and methanol themselves are of limited toxicity, though they are CNS depressants and cause inebriation. More importantly, as noted, the toxic metabolites formed in vivo can cause irreversible damage and death.[27,45,55] Both methanol and ethylene glycol ingestions are managed in nearly the same manner. The first step in management is to avoid the substantial delays that may occur because of false reassurance provided by the seemingly benign initial presentation and concomitant lack of laboratory abnormalities. When methanol or ethylene glycol is concurrently used with ethanol, a "serendipitously therapeutic" level of ethanol may prevent early metabolism of the toxic alcohol and prevent early recognition of what may ultimately become a serious or lethal exposure.[43]

If the history is suggestive, a blood sample should be obtained for stat methanol, ethylene glycol, and ethanol determinations regardless of whether the patient is symptomatic. If the history suggests more than an unintentional sip or the patient has a metabolic acidosis and/or an osmol gap not accounted for by ethanol and the ethanol level is less than 100 mg/dL, ethanol therapy should be started immediately, even before the blood levels are available. As noted previously, the presence of a high anion gap metabolic acidosis is a late finding, dependent on the generation of organic acids by metabolism. Conversely, a low or normal anion gap cannot exclude poisoning, as the presence of ethanol may have inhibited toxin metabolism. If the patient has symptoms and is significantly acidemic, sodium bicarbonate should be administered and titrated to normalize plasma pH in order to enhance formate elimination by ion trapping.[28,29]

Figures 64–2 and 64–4 describe the metabolism of methanol and ethylene glycol. Ethanol is a preferential substrate, with a greater affinity for the enzyme alcohol dehydrogenase than either methanol or ethylene glycol. Administering ethanol to achieve sufficient concentrations (100 to 150 mg/dL) competitively inhibits the formation of the toxic metabolites, eventually allowing the unchanged primary alcohols to be eliminated if adequate urine output can be maintained. An optimal blood ethanol level of 100 to 150 mg/dL or at least an ethanol to methanol or ethylene glycol ratio of 1:4 should be attained quickly by administering a loading dose of ethanol of 0.8 g/kg IV. This rapidly achieves the stoichiometric relationship necessary to achieve competitive inhibition of metabolism of the toxic alcohol (see Antidotes in Depth: Ethanol). This level should then be maintained until blood levels of methanol and ethylene glycol are zero. The maintenance dose of ethanol is 130 mg/kg per hour before hemodialysis begins. When hemodialysis is performed, maintenance doses of 250 to 350 mg/kg per hour are required, as ethanol will be dialyzed out along with the methanol and ethylene glycol.[50] These doses are estimates based on pharmacokinetic principles and past investigations, and for this reason it is essential to check serum ethanol levels frequently to assure that a level of 100 to 150 mg/dL is maintained at all times.[56,57]

In addition to providing and maintaining adequate ethanol levels, the patient's acid–base status must be followed carefully, as large amounts of sodium bicarbonate may be required to keep the pH near normal. There are several advantages to alkalinizing patients with toxic alcohol ingestions. As noted previously, the renal clearance of glycolate can be enhanced by maintaining the molecule in the ionized form.[28] In methanol poisoning the amount of undissociated formic acid may be decreased with higher pH values, thereby limiting access to the CNS. The amount of bicarbonate necessary to achieve alkalinization may be substantial, depending on the amount of the toxic alcohol already metabolized. Management is dictated by frequent arterial blood gas determinations, but at the same time mindful that fluid overload and hyperosmolarity may become significant problems. Good hydration is in and of itself helpful, as ethylene glycol is well excreted by the kidney as long as renal function is maintained.[12]

The metabolic acidosis, if present, should begin to resolve once ethanol is administered, but ethanol inhibits only ethylene glycol and methanol metabolism. The products of the metabolites of ethylene glycol already found will continue to be produced for some time, depending on their rates of metabolism (see Fig. 64–2). The molecules responsible for the acidemia are also responsible for renal and CNS toxicity.

Hemodialysis is effective in removing methanol, ethylene glycol, and their toxic metabolites.[25,33] The apparent half-life of methanol (£3 hours) increases with ethanol therapy to 43 hours and drops to 3.5 hours with ethanol and hemodialysis.[52] The apparent half-life of ethylene glycol (2.5 hours), increases with ethanol therapy to 17 hours but may be reduced to 2.5 to 3.5 hours with hemodialysis and ethanol infusions. Glycolate (with a half-life of 7.0 hours) frequently accounts for the largest component of the anion gap.[28] Hemodialysis should be continued until methanol and ethylene glycol levels approximate 0 mg/dL and the acidosis has cleared. To achieve this, patients may require several 4-hour hemodialysis treatments. In clinical settings where methanol and ethylene glycol levels are not immediately available, hemodialysis must be continued at least until the metabolic acidosis has cleared. Although this is obviously unreliable, the toxic metabolites that correspond to the level of acidosis can be used as markers until the laboratory results are returned.

Hemodialysis should be performed on any patient who is symptomatic, has a significant metabolic acidosis, has a blood level of methanol or ethylene glycol greater than 25 mg/dL, or has any evidence of renal compromise. As noted previously, formate concentrations correlate better with the patient's clinical condition than do methanol levels,[51] and levels in excess of 20 mg/dL can be expected to generate ocular injury and metabolic acidosis. The same concept applies to ethylene glycol; that is, ethylene glycol levels at admission are not predictive of outcome, whereas levels of the toxic acid metabolites—as evidenced by acidemia—are predictive of death.[26] If hemodialysis cannot be accomplished, the patient should be loaded with ethanol, treated with bicarbonate, and transferred expeditiously to a center where hemodialysis can be performed. There is no role for peritoneal dialysis or hemoperfusion in managing methanol or ethylene glycol poisoning.

Some information regarding methanol levels and hemodialysis is available as the result of an epidemic of methanol poisoning in a southern Michigan prison. Of the 150 inmates who stated that they had drunk methanol, only 50 cases of methanol ingestion were confirmed by laboratory analysis. With limited resources and a large potential group of victims, varied therapies were tried. Conservative treatment, including correction of acidosis with bicarbonate and infusion of ethanol, was found to be adequate in some moderately poisoned patients, and the authors suggested that hemodialysis be used only when methanol levels exceed 100 mg/dL.[64] Notwithstanding these positive results reported under adverse conditions, most clinicians believe hemodialysis is indicated when methanol or ethylene glycol levels exceed 25 mg/dL. Moreover, complications such as severe illness, altered mental status, or acidemia accompanying an ingestion have led many to hemodialyze at even lower serum levels. Because heparinization for hemodialysis may be a risk for patients with cerebral hemorrhage complicating methanol intoxication, some authors have suggested the use of albumin-primed biocompatible membranes.[57]

Although limited data are available, continuous arteriovenous hemofiltration dialysis may be effective. It has been utilized in one patient with severe ethylene glycol poisoning and multiple organ dysfunction, deemed too critically ill for transfer to another institution for hemodialysis.[13]

Additional therapeutic measures for ethylene glycol ingestions may include 100 mg of thiamine IV and 50 mg of pyridoxine IV every 6 hours until the ethylene glycol level is zero and no acidosis persists. On theoretical and investigational grounds, pyridoxine in the presence of magnesium shunts the metabolism of ethylene glycol metabolites from glyoxylic acid to the harmless glycine, and thiamine in the presence of magnesium shunts glyoxylic acid to alpha-hydroxy-beta-ketoadipic acid, reducing the production of oxalic acid.[28,59] If the patient becomes hypocalcemic as a result of the precipitation of calcium oxalate crystals, calcium chloride or calcium gluconate should be utilized (see Antidotes in Depth: Calcium).

For methanol poisonings, animal studies suggest that folic acid or 5-formyltetrahydrofolic acid (5-FTHFA; folinic acid, citrovorum factor, a folic acid analog) enhances the elimination of formic acid, decreasing the metabolic acidosis and reducing symptoms.[25] Intravenous folate (folinic or folic acids) should be given at 50 to 75 mg every 4 hours for at least 24 hours.[51]

The use of 4-methylpyrazole (4-MP), a competitive inhibitor of alcohol dehydrogenase, is being investigated in animals[8,9] and humans[5] as an alternative to ethanol therapy for both methanol and ethylene glycol poisonings. It appears that CNS depression, a common problem associated with ethanol therapy, will not occur with 4-MP treatment. However, the potential for adverse effects of 4-MP necessitate futher investigation before 4-MP can be considered standard recommended treatment (see Antidotes in Depth: 4-Methylprazole).

Ethanol infusion therapy or fomepizole followed by hemodialysis has become the standard treatment in all cases in which the serum level of methanol or ethylene glycol exceeds 25 mg/dL. Other therapeutic strategies such as 4 methylpyrazole or ethanol infusion without hemodialysis may actually prolong hospitalization and increase potential risk to the patient.

What Are Other Potential Toxic Alcohols and Glycols?

Two common alcohols, benzyl alcohol and propylene glycol, employed as preservatives or diluents for medications can usually be eliminated rapidly from the differential diagnosis unless a massive ingestion is suspected.

Benzyl Alcohol

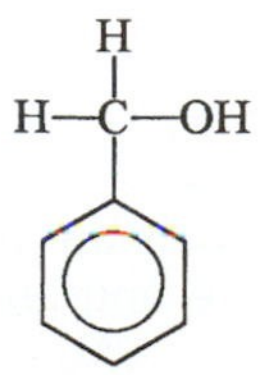

Benzyl alcohol is an aromatic alcohol commonly used in the United States as an antimicrobial preservative in diverse parenteral medications. No adverse results have been noted, when administered to adults, because of the small concentrations (0.9%). In preterm infants, however, lethal consequences have been reported.[23,39] Severe metabolic acidosis has also been reported in a 5-year-old.[37] Metabolic acidosis associated with benzyl alcohol administration results from its hepatic oxidative metabolism to benzoic acid and hippuric acid. Benzoic acid levels 12 times that of controls accounted for the demonstrated anion gap in neonates whose IVs had been flushed with bacteriostatic sodium chloride.[23] A symptom complex in newborns poisoned with benzyl alcohol includes neurologic deterioration, gasping reactions, hypotension, hepatic and renal failure, and death. These small preterm infants have usually received excessive amounts of bacteriostatic 0.9% sodium chloride solution by central venous catheters in intensive care units (ICUs). This misuse of this diluent is reminiscent of problems associated with the use of diethylene glycol as a diluent for some of the early preparations of elixir of sulfanilamide in the 1930s (see Chap. 1).[22] For the reasons described, benzyl alcohol is no longer used in neonatal care. However, the fact that a 5-year-old child who received approximately 180 mg/kg per day of benzyl alcohol for 36 hours as the result of a continous IV diazepam infusion of 2 mg/kg per hour, developed toxicity, suggests that there may be other individuals who cannot effectively metabolize this alcohol without risk.[37]

Propylene Glycol

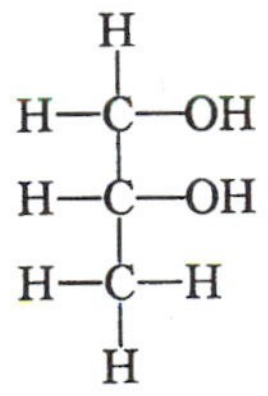

Propylene glycol (1,2 propanediol) is a common diluent for injectable agents such as phenytoin, diazepam, and digoxin. It is considered nontoxic, resulting in toxicity only under unusual circumstances (see Chaps. 1,2,41, and 54).[69] It is used in food and cosmetic preparation and as a deicing agent, although ethylene glycol is cheaper and therefore used more commonly. Most toxicity has resulted from its rapid IV delivery, which may cause profound hypotension, cardiac conduction abnormalities (QRS widening), dysrhythmias, and asystole, particularly when infused in the larger volumes required for phenytoin levels as compared to those employed with diazepam and digoxin.[38]

Transdermal absorption of propylene glycol resulting in hyperosmolarity, hypoglycemia, seizures, and central nervous system (CNS) depression has occurred in children with severe burns exposed to the propylene glycol in silver sulfadiazine cream.[19] Propylene glycol is metabolized to lactic acid, and massive ingestions may be associated with both an osmol gap and a severe high anion gap metabolic acidosis.

Isopropanol

Isopropanol, isopropyl alcohol, or 2-propanol (Fig. 64–5), is readily available as a 70% "rubbing alcohol" solution and in various toiletries, disinfectants, window cleaning solutions, antifreeze, paint removers, and industrial solvents. Because of the frequent ingestion of rubbing alcohol by impaired or suicidal patients, ethanol has replaced isopropanol in the formulation of some "rubbing alcohols" and a blue dye has been added to try to inhibit its use. This isopropanol and dye combination has been referred to as "Blue Heaven" used by some isopropanol abusers.[58] In any possible "rubbing alcohol" ingestion, therefore, the bottle label, if available, and/or serum ethanol and urine ketone (acetone) levels are necessary for proper analysis and to predict the duration of CNS depression and the potential need for hemodialysis.

Isopropanol is a clear, colorless, volatile liquid with a faint odor of acetone and a slightly bitter taste. Oral absorption occurs rapidly, within a half hour,[53] and inhalation,[65] rectal exposure,[4] and cutaneous absorption can be significant, particularly in children.[35,36] The volume of distribution of isopropanol is 0.6 to 0.7 L/kg. Isopropanol alcohol is rapidly metabolized by alcohol dehydrogenase in an apparent concentration-dependent manner (first-order kinetics).[14] The apparent first-order elimination may be the result of significant pulmonary excretion of acetone. Approximately 80% of isopropanol is metabolized to acetone and the remainder is excreted unmetabolized in the urine, with very small amounts of isopropanol excreted via the lungs.[14] The presence of ethanol appears to double the apparent half-life of isopropanol but does not augment the half-life of acetone substantially.[53] Acetone is excreted by the kidneys (majority) and exhaled (minority) if present in high concentrations (Fig. 64–5). Confusion over the CNS depressant effects of isopropanol may relate to the fact that acetone, its metabolite, is also a CNS depressant. Animal studies have suggested that isopropanol is two to three times more potent than ethanol as a CNS depressant and that the potency of acetone is comparable to that of ethanol.[68]

The apparent half-lives of isopropanol and acetone are 2.9 to 16.2 hours and 7.6 to 26.2 hours, respectively, in adults,[53] and half-lives of 5.8 hours and 10.8 hours, respectively, were reported in a 2-month-old infant.[54] In animal models, acetonemia occurred within 15 minutes

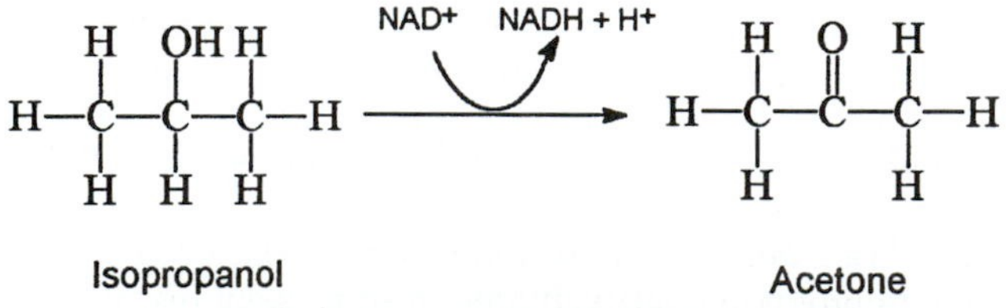

Figure 64–5. Isopropanol metabolism.

of ingestion and continued to rise after isopropanol levels reached a plateau.[30] The levels of acetone and isopropanol showed a linear correlation throughout the study model.

Conversion of isopropanol to acetone may not be a "one-way" phenomenon: The apparent conversion of acetone to isopropanol in the presence of alcohol dehydrogenase and reduced nicotinamide adenine dinucleotide (NADH) has been described in vitro. [15] This same transformation was suggested in vivo in four insulin-dependent diabetics who had diabetic ketoacidosis at the time elevated isopropanol and acetone levels were determined.[3]

Common clinical findings associated with isopropanol ingestion include CNS depression, lethargy, weakness, nausea, headache, ataxia, abdominal pain, odor of acetone, gastritis, hemorrhagic tracheobronchitis, hypotension, and apnea (Table 64–1).

Characteristic laboratory findings of isopropanol ingestion include euglycemia, ketonuria, ketonemia, increased osmolality, and no evidence of metabolic acidosis. The extent of the elevated osmolality is dependent on isopropanol and acetone concentrations, as both exert osmotic forces. In addition, acetone and acetoacetate are known to give a false elevation of the serum creatinine level in those autoanalyzer systems using a colorimetric method.[66] When the acetone level exceeds 40 mg/dL, creatinine values begin to rise at approximately 1 mg/dL creatinine/100 mg/dL acetone.

The treatment for a patient with an isopropanol ingestion is supportive, with attention to any cardiopulmonary complications. If dermal exposure to isopropanol occurs, skin decontamination should be thorough; if exposure is by inhalation, the patient should be rapidly removed from that environment. If the patient is evaluated immediately following ingestion, lavage may be indicated and activated charcoal may be of benefit. A number of reports have suggested that this alcohol, with a small molecular weight, low volume of distribution, and low plasma protein binding, is an ideal molecule for hemodialysis.[34,61] In one case hemodialysis clearance of isopropanol of 137 mL/min and acetone of 165 mL/min was dramatic, respectively removing the agents 32 and 40 times as efficiently as urinary excretion.[61] However, because most patients exposed to isopropanol do well with the conservative treatment described, the question becomes "what is the actual indication for hemodialysis?" Those patients whose isopropanol levels exceed 400 to 500 mg/dL (usually with unmeasured acetone levels) have severe clinical problems, such as hypotension and coma, and typically have the poorest outcomes. When these characteristics are present, hemodialysis should be considered. Although peritoneal dialysis has been attempted by several authors, its marginal benefit over endogenous clearances offers no advantage.[48] Therefore if the patient is ill enough to merit intervention, hemodialysis is the only procedure indicated.

All of these alcohols are readily available from the neonatal intensive care unit and the dialysis unit to the home or the workplace. Many case reports remind us of the potency of these agents, particularly for small children. For children even the proverbial "sip" of several milliliters of a toxic alcohol (such as a solution of 100% methanol in a 10-kg child) can lead to clinical toxicity, the need for hospitalization, and the potential for hemodialysis.

Acknowledgments

Neal A. Lewin, MD and Mary Ann Howland, PharmD contributed to this chapter in a previous edition.

References

1. Anderson TJ, Shnaiba A, Becker WJ: Neurologic sequelae of methanol poisoning. Can Med Assoc J 1987;136: 1177–1179.
2. Aufderheide TP, White SM, Brady WJ, Stueven HA: Inhalational and percutaneous methanol toxicity in two fire fighters Ann Emerg Med 1993;22: 1916–1918.
3. Bailey DN: Detection of isopropanol in acetonemic patients not exposed to isopropanol. J Toxicol Clin Toxicol 1990;28:459–466.
4. Barnett JM, Plotnick M, Fine KC: Intoxication after an isopropyl alcohol enema. Ann Intern Med 1990;113:638–639.
5. Baud FJ, Galliot M, Astier A, et al: Treatment of ethylene glycol poisoning with intravenous 4-methylpyrazole. N Engl J Med 1988;319:97–100.
6. Baumbach GL: Metyl alcohol poisoning. Arch Ophthalmol 1977;95:1859–1865.
7. Bennett IL, Cary FH, Mitchell GL, Cooper MN: Acute methyl alcohol poisoning: A review based on experiences in an outbreak of 323 cases. Medicine 1953;32:431–463.
8. Blomstrand R, Ingemansson SO: Studies on the effect of 4-methylpyrazole on methanol poisoning using the monkey as an animal model: With particular reference to the ocular toxicity. Drug Alcohol Depend 1984;13:343–355.
9. Blomstrand R, Ostling-Witzell H, Lof A, et al: Pyrazoles as inhibitors of alcohol oxidation and as important tools in alcohol research: An approach to therapy against methanol poisoning. Proc Natl Acad Sci 1979;76: 3499–3503.
10. Burkhart KK, Martinez MA: The adsorption of isopropanol and acetone by activated charcoal. J Toxicol Clin Toxicol 1992;30:371–375.
11. Catchings TT, Beamer WC, Lundy L: Adult respiratory distress syndrome secondary to ethylene glycol ingestion. Ann Emerg Med 1985;14:594–596.
12. Cheng JT, Beysolow TD, Kaul B, et al: Clearance of ethylene glycol by kidneys and hemodialysis. J Toxicol Clin Toxicol 1987;25:95–108.
13. Christiansson LK, Kaspersson KE, Kulling PEJ, Ovrebo S: Treatment of severe ethylene glycol intoxication with continuous arteriovenous hemofiltration dialysis. J Toxicol Clin Toxicol 1995;33:267–270.
14. Daniel DR, McAnalley BH, Garriott JC: Isopropyl alcohol metabolism after acute intoxication in humans. J Anal Toxicol 1981;5:110–112.
15. Davis PL, Dal Cortivo LA, Maturo J: Endogenous isopropanol: Forensic and biochemical implications. J Anal Toxicol 1984;8:209–212.
16. Dean BS, Krenzelok EP: Clinical evaluation of pediatric ethylene glycol monobutyl ether poisonings. J Toxicol Clin Toxicol 1992;30:557–563.
16a. Decker WJ, Corby DCT, Hilburn RE, Lynch RE: Adsorption of solvents by activated charcoal, polymers and mineral sorbents. Vet Hum Toxicol 1981;235:44–46.
17. Eckfeldt JH, Kershaw MJ: Hyperamylasemia following methyl alcohol intoxication: Source and significance. Arch Intern Med 1986;146:193–194.
18. Eells TT, Black A, Tedford CE, Tephly TR: Methanol toxicity in the monkey: Effects of nitrous oxide and methionine. J Pharmacol Exp Therap 1983;227:349–353.
19. Fligner CL, Jack R, Twiggs GA, Raisys VA: Hyperosmolality induced by propylene glycol: A complication of silver sulfadiazine therapy. JAMA 1985;253:1606–1609.
20. Frenia ML, Schauben JL: Methanol inhalation toxicity. Ann Emerg Med 1993;22:1919–1923.
21. Gabow PA, Clay K, Sullivan JB, Lepoff R: Organic acids in ethylene glycol intoxication. Ann Intern Med 1986;105: 16–20.
22. Geiling EMK, Cannon PR: Pathologic effects of elixir of sulfanilamide (diethylene glycol) poisoning. JAMA 1938;111:919–926.
23. Gershanik JJ, Boecler G, Ensley H, et al: The gasping syndrome and benzyl alcohol poisoning. N Engl J Med 1982; 307:1384–1388.
24. Glazer M, Dross P: Necrosis of the putamen caused by methanol intoxication: MR findings. Am J Roentgenol 1993;160: 1105–1106.
25. Gonda A, Gault H, Churchill D, et al: Hemodialysis for methanol intoxication. Am J Med 1978;64:749–758.
26. Hylander B, Kjeilstrand CM: Prognostic factors and treatment of severe ethylene glycol intoxication. Intensive Care Med 1996;22: 546–552.
27. Jacobsen D, Bredesen JE, Eide I, Ostborg J: Anion and osmolal gaps in the diagnosis of methanol and ethylene glycol poisoning. Acta Med Scand 1982;212:17–20.
28. Jacobsen D, Hewlett TP, Webb R, et al: Ethylene glycol intoxication: Evaluation of kinetics and crystalluria. Am J Med 1988;84:145–152.
29. Jacobsen D, Webb R, Collins TD, McMartin KE: Methanol and formate kinetics in late diagnosed methanol intoxication. Med Toxicol 1988;3:418–423.
30. Jerrard D, Verdile V, Yealy D, et al: Serum determinations in toxic isopropanol ingestion. Am J Emerg Med 1992;10: 200–202.
31. Katona BG, Siegel EG, Roberts JR, et al: The effect of "superactive" charcoal and magnesium citrate solution on blood ethanol concentrations and area under the curve in humans. J Toxicol Clin Toxicol 1989;27:129–137.
32. Kavet R, Nauss KM: The toxicity of inhaled methanol vapors. Crit Rev Toxicol 1990;21: 21–50.
33. Knepshield JH, Schreiner GE, Lowenthal DT, et al: Dialysis of poisons and drugs: Annual review. Trans Am Soc Artif Intern Organs 1973;19:590–633.
34. Lacouture PG, Wason S, Abrams A, Lovejoy Jr FH: Acute isopropyl alcohol intoxication: Diagnosis and management. Am J Med 1983;75:680–686.

35. Lehman AJ, Chase HF: The acute and chronic toxicity of isopropyl alcohol. J Lab Clin Med 1944;29:561–567.
36. Lewin GA, Oppenheimer PR, Wingert WA: Coma from alcohol sponging. JACEP 1977;6:165–167.
37. Lopez-Herce J, Bonet C, Meana A, et al: Benzyl alcohol poisoning following diazepam intravenous infusion Ann Pharmacother 1995;29:632. Letter.
38. Louis, S, Kutt, H, McDowell F: The cardiocirculatory changes caused by intravenous Dilantin and its solvent. Am Heart J 1967;74:524–529.
39. Lovejoy FH: Fatal benzyl alcohol poisoning in neonatal intensive care units. Am J Dis Child 1982;136:974–975.
40. Mahieu P, Hassoun A, Lauwerys R: Predictions of methanol intoxication with unfavorable outcome. Hum Toxicol 1989;8:135–137.
41. Malandain H, Cano Y: Serum methanol in the absence of methanol ingestion Ann Emerg Med 1996;28:102–103.
42. Malebranche R, Hecdivert C, Lassegue A, et al: Fatalities associated with ingestion of diethylene glycol-contaminated glycerin used to manufacture acetaminophen syrup—Haiti, November 1995 - June 1996. MMWR 1996; 45:649–650.
43. Martensson E, Olofsson U, Heath A: Clinical and metabolic features of ethanol–methanol poisoning in chronic alcoholics. Lancet 1988;1:327–328.
44. Martin-Amat G, McMartin KE, Hayrek SS, et al: Methanol poisoning: Ocular toxicity produced by formate. Toxicol Appl Pharmacol 1978;45:201–208.
45. McCoy HG, Cipolle RJ, Ehlers SM, et al: Severe methanol poisoning. Am J Med 1979;67:804–807.
46. McMartin KE, Makar AB, Martin-Amat G, et al: Methanol poisoning I: The role of formic acid in the development of metabolic acidosis in the monkey and the reversal by 4-methylpyrazole. Biochem Med 1975;13:319–333.
47. McMartin KE, Martin-Amat G, Noker PE, Tephly TR: Lack of a role for formaldehyde in methanol poisoning in the monkey. Biochem Pharmacol 1979;28:645–649.
48. Mecikalski MB, Depner TA: Peritoneal dialysis for isopropanol poisoning. West J Med 1982;137:322–325.
49. Nitter-Hauge S: Poisoning with ethylene glycol monomethyl ether. Acta Med Scand 1970;188:277–280.
50. Noker PE, Eells JT, Tephly TR: Methanol toxicity: Treatment with folic acid and 5-formyltetrahydrofolic acid. Alcohol Clin Exp Res 1980;4:378–383.
51. Osterloh JD, Pond SM, Grady S, Becker CE: Serum formate concentrations in methanol intoxication as a criterion for hemodialysis. Ann Intern Med 1986;104:200–203.
52. Palatnick W, Redman LW, Sitar DS, Tenenbein M: Methanol half life during ethanol administration: Implications for management of methanol poisoning Ann Emerg Med 1995;26:202–207.
53. Pappas AA, Ackerman BH, Olsen KM, Taylor EH: Isopropanol ingestion: A report of six episodes with isopropanol and acetone serum concentration time data. J Toxicol Clin Toxicol 1991;29:11–21.
54. Parker KM, Lera TA: Acute isopropanol ingestion: Pharmacokinetic parameters in the infant. Am J Emerg Med 1992;10:542–544.
55. Parry MF, Wallach R: Ethylene glycol poisoning. Am J Med 1974;57:143–150.
56. Peterson C, Collins A, Mimes J, et al: Ethylene glycol poisoning: Pharmacokinetics during therapy with ethanol and hemodialysis. N Engl J Med 1981;304:21–23.
57. Phang PT, Passerini L, Mielke B, et al: Brain hemorrhage associated with methanol poisoning. Crit Care Med 1988; 16:137–140.
58. Rich J, Scheife RT, Katz N, Caplan LR: Isopropyl alcohol intoxication. Arch Neurol 1990;47:322–324.
59. Roberts JA, Seibold HR: Ethylene glycol toxicity in the monkey. Toxicol Appl Pharmacol 1969;15:624–631.
60. Robinson AG, Loeb JN: Ethanol ingestion: Commonest cause of elevated plasma osmolality? N Engl J Med 1971; 284:1253–1255.
61. Rosansky SJ: Isopropyl alcohol poisoning treated with hemodialysis: Kinetics of isopropyl alcohol and acetone removal. J Toxicol Clin Toxicol 1982;19:265–271.
62. Schultz S, Kinde M, Johnson D, et al: Ethylene glycol intoxication due to contamination of water systems. MMWR 1987;36:611–614.
63. Sejersted OM: Formate concentrations in plasma from patients poisoned with methanol. Acta Med Scand 1983;213: 105–110.
64. Swartz RD, Millman RP, Billi JE, et al: Epidemic methanol poisoning: Clinical and biochemical analysis of a recent episode. Medicine 1981;60:373–382.
65. Vicas IMO, Beck R: Fatal inhalational isopropyl alcohol poisoning in a neonate. J Toxicol Clin Toxicol 1993;31:473–481.
66. Wakins FJ: The effect of ketone bodies on the determination of creatinine. Clin Chim Acta 1967;18:191–196.
67. Walker JA, Schwartzbard A, Krauss EA, et al: The missing gap: A pitfall in the diagnosis of alcohol intoxication by osmometry. Arch Intern Med 1986;146:1843–1844.
68. Wallgren H: Relative intoxicating effects on rats of ethyl, propyl and butyl alcohols. Acta Pharmacol Toxicol 1960; 16:217–222.
69. Wax PM: Elixirs, diluents and the passage of the 1938 Federal Food, Drug and Cosmetic Act. Ann Intern Med 1995; 122:456–461.
70. Winter ML, Ellis MD, Snodgrass WR: Urine fluorescence using a Wood's lamp to detect the antifreeze additive sodium fluorescein: A qualitative adjunctive test in suspected ethylene glycol ingestions. Ann Emerg Med 1990; 19:663–667.

ANTIDOTES IN DEPTH

Folic Acid and Leucovorin (Folinic Acid)

Mary Ann Howland

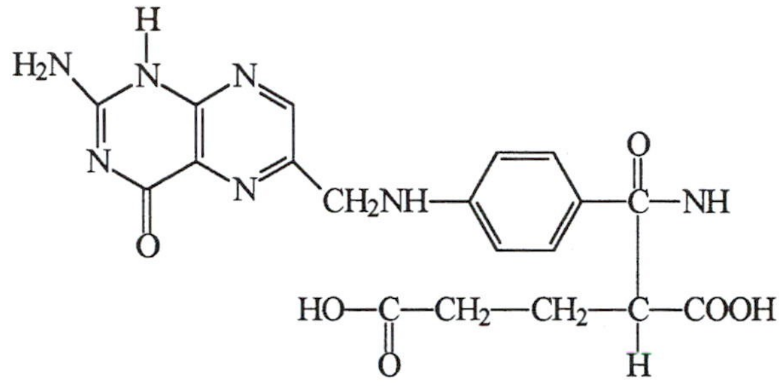

Folic Acid

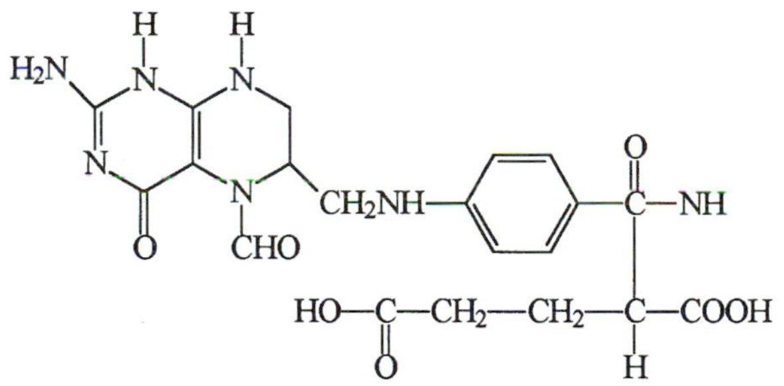

Folinic Acid

Folic acid (pteroylglutamic acid) an essential water-soluble vitamin, is a pteridine ring joined to PABA (p-aminobenzoic acid) and glutamic acid.[1] It is the most common pharmaceutical preparation of folate although other congeners exist in foods. After absorption, folic acid is reduced by dihydrofolic acid reductase (DHFR) to tetrahydrofolic acid, which accepts carbon groups at different positions on the molecule. Tetrahydrofolic acid therefore serves as the precursor for several biologically active forms of folic acid including 5-formyltetrahydrofolic acid (folinic acid, leucovorin, 5-FTHF, and 5-CHO-THF or citrovorum factor). These biologically active forms of folate are enzymatically interconvertable and function as cofactors, providing carbon groups necessary for many intracellular metabolic reactions including the synthesis of thymidylate and purine nucleotides (DNA precursors). The minimum daily requirement of folate is normally 50 μg, but in pregnant women and nutritionally deprived acutely ill patients 100 to 200 μg may be required.[1]

Methanol toxicity in humans is currently believed to develop as a result of reduced formate metabolism secondary to reduced folate concentration. The rat model has not been useful in studying methanol toxicity because that species has a very well-developed folate system, which rapidly oxidizes the toxic formic acid to nontoxic carbon dioxide at a rate two to three times faster than demonstrated in monkeys. Primates and humans are not this fortunate. However, the administration of folic acid to monkeys speeds up formate metabolism.[5] Pretreatment with folic acid for 48 hours or leucovorin administered at 2 mg/kg IV at 0, 4, 8, 12, and 18 hours after methanol administration in monkeys decreased formate levels and the accompanying metabolic acidosis, without affecting the rate of methanol elimination.[6] Leucovorin was still effective in hastening the elimination of formate when given 10 hours following methanol administration. Other studies demonstrate that rats and monkeys made folate-deficient develop methanol toxicity at lower methanol levels.[3]

Total folate, leucovorin, and 10-$HCOH_2$ folate dehydrogenase (which increases leucovorin levels) are all diminished in the livers of methanol-poisoned humans.[3] This finding further supports the hypothesis that methanol toxicity in humans develops as a result of reduced formate metabolism secondary to reduced folate levels.

In an analysis[2] of a single patient who was given folate and ethanol and hemodialyzed, the formate half-life was 1.1 hours.[7] In another methanol-poisoned patient treated without folate, the formate half-life was 2.8 hours.[2] This limited analysis by comparison may be inadequate to draw definitive conclusions, but appears to support the therapeutic role of folate.

Methotrexate, an antimetabolite, is a structural analog of folic acid, differing only in an amino group substituted for a hydroxyl group on the number 4 position of the pteridine ring. Methotrexate binds to the active site of dihydrofolate reductase (DHFR) rendering it incapable of reducing folic acid to its biologically active reduced forms or in regenerating the necessary active forms required for the synthesis of thymidylate, an essential precursor to DNA. Methotrexate's binding to

DHFR is extremely tight at pH 6 with an inhibition constant of about 1 nmol/L. At physiologic pH the binding is more competitive, with an inhibition constant of about 1 micromol/L.[8] Leucovorin is a reduced, active form of folate that does not require DHFR for enzymatic interconversion to the form required for thymidylate formation. Folic acid would not be effective to counteract methotrexate toxicity because DHFR would be unavailable to convert folic acid to the necessary reduced and active forms.

Leucovorin naturally formed in the body exists as the active (l) isomer, while the commercial preparation consists of equal amounts of the inactive (d) and active (l) isomers. The pharmacokinetics of the racemic mixture and its active metabolite were studied after IV infusion of 28 mg/m^2 over 5 minutes and 500 mg/m^2 per day (21mg/m^2 per hour) as a constant infusion over 5.5 days in normal human volunteers. [9] The plasma half-life of the active (l) isomer was 35 minutes, considerably shorter than the 485 minutes of the inactive (d) isomer. During constant infusion the steady-state concentration for the active isomer was 2.33 μmol (1102 μg/L or 1.1 mg/L or 1.1 μg/mL), the half-life 35 minutes, and the volume of distribution 13.6 L. The inactive isomer achieved plasma concentrations 16-fold higher than the active form and was primarily cleared from the plasma by urinary excretion of unchanged drug. In contrast, the active isomer was metabolized to an active metabolite (L-5-CH3-THF) that achieved a plasma concentration of 4.85 μmol, a half-life of 412 minutes, and a volume of distribution of about 40 L; all of these values are greater than that of the parent compound.

The pharmacokinetics of orally administered leucovorin {(d,l)-5-formyltetrahydrofolate)} have been studied in healthy, fasted, male volunteers in single doses ranging from 20 to 100 mg, and 200 mg IV over 5 minutes compared to 200-mg orally.[4] Bioavailability decreased from 100% for the 20-mg dose to 78% for the 40-mg dose and ultimately 31% for the 200-mg dose. A microbiologic assay was used to measure total tetrahydrofolates (reduced and active folates). The peak plasma concentrations for total reduced folates ranges from 318 ng/mL for 20-mg orally to 619 ng/mL for 100-mg orally. The 200-mg oral dose produced a peak plasma concentration of 859 ng/mL (1.82 μmol/L) compared to 12,829 ng/mL (27.1 μmol/L) after the 200-mg IV dose. Normal plasma folate levels are in the range of 6 to 20 ng/mL or 13 to 43 nmol.

When a patient intentionally or unintentionally overdoses on methotrexate or is inadvertently administered methotrexate, a dose of leucovorin estimated to produce the same plasma concentration as the methotrexate dose should be given as soon as possible after the overdose, preferably within 1 hour. One mole of methotrexate weighs 455 D and one mole of leucovorin calcium weighs 511 D; however, only one half of the administered leucovorin is the biologically active isomer. In view of the safety of leucovorin and the toxicity of methotrexate, underdosing of leucovorin should be avoided. Plasma methotrexate concentrations are often closely followed in patients on oncologic regimens including the agent. In the overdose setting it is inappropriate to wait for a methotrexate plasma concentration before treatment with leucovorin is initiated. The toxic threshold for methotrexate is reported to be 2×10^{-8} mol/L (2×10^{-8} mol/L means 0.02×10^{-6} or 0.02 μmol/L or 20 nmol/L). Normal plasma folate levels are in the range of 13 to 43 nmol/L. One mole of methotrexate is 455 g/mol or 455 mg/mmol or 455 μg/μmol or 455 ng/nmol. Therefore 20 nmol equals 9100 ng (455 ng/nmol × 20 nmol) and 20 nmol/L equals 9100 ng/L or 9.1 ng/mL. In a patient not being given methotrexate therapeutically, there is no need for any methotrexate to remain unantagonized by leucovorin. For example, if a child accidentally ingests 100 2.5-mg methotrexate tablets for a total dose of 250-mg, only part of this dose is absorbed because methotrexate absorption is saturable. Methotrexate's bioavailability decreases from 100% with doses below 30 mg/m^2 to about 10 to 20% with doses above 80 mg/m^2. As a safety precaution, assuming a bioavailability of 50% would result in an absorbed dose of methotrexate of 125 mg. For this substantial exposure an intravenous dose of 125 to 250 mg of leucovorin could be given over 10 minutes. The dose should be repeated every 3 to 6 hours until the methotrexate level is less than 1×10^{-8} mol/L and preferably close to zero. The methotrexate half-life may vary from 5 to 45 hours depending on the dose and the patient's renal function. For this reason leucovorin therapy should be continued for 12 to 24 doses (3 days) or even longer. Patients with the potential of third-space storage in ascites or pleural effusion may also require leucovorin dosing for an extended period of time. Patients exhibiting bone marrow toxicity require longer dosing because plasma half-lives of methotrexate do not reflect persistent intracellular concentrations.

A leucovorin dose of 100 mg/m^2 every 6 hours should be effective in all but the most severe overdoses. A constant intravenous infusion of 21 mg/m^2/h has been safely administered for 5 days. A transition to the oral administration of leucovorin will depend on the plasma concentration of the methotrexate and whether adequate plasma concentrations of leucovorin can be achieved by that route. A 200-mg oral dose in an adult produces a peak plasma concentration of 1.82 μmol/L compared to 27.1 μmol/L with a 200-mg IV dose. In addition to leucovorin, other modalities to treat a methotrexate overdose should be performed (activated charcoal, urinary alkalinization), or considered (hemoperfusion, thymidine) under specific circumstances (see Chap. 47).

Folic acid is available parenterally in 10-mL multidose vials with 1.5% benzyl alcohol in concentrations of 5 or 10 mg/mL, from a variety of manufacturers. Once opened this vial must be kept refrigerated.

Leucovorin is available as a powder for injection in 50, 100, and 350-mg vials. Reconstitution with 5 mL to the 50-mg or 10 mL to the 100-mg vial with sterile water for injection results in a final concentration of 10-mg/mL. Adding 17 mL of sterile water for injection to the 350-mg vial will result in a final concentration of 20-mg/mL. Because of the calcium content, the rate of intravenous administration should not be faster than 160 mg/min. Leucovorin is also available orally in a variety of strengths including 5, 10, 15, and 25-mg tablets.

There are rare reports of reactions to parenteral injections of folic acid or leucovorin.[1] The usual dose of leucovorin for methotrexate rescue ranges from 10-mg/m^2 IM or IV every 6 hours for 72 hours to 100-mg/m^2 every 3 hours in patients with renal compromise. Fifty to seventy mg of IV folate has been utilized every 4 hours for the first 24 hours to treat methanol-intoxicated patients without complications.[7] If administration to neonates is necessary, a benzyl alcohol-free preparation must be utilized.

For methotrexate overdoses, a dose of leucovorin twice that of the ingested methotrexate dose should be administered as soon as possible intravenously over 10 minutes (not faster than 160-mg/min). This dose can be repeated every 3 to 6 hours for 3 days or longer depending on renal function, the presence of bone marrow toxicity, and the methotrexate serum concentrations.

Based on the convincing studies in monkeys and the benign nature of the therapy, folic acid or leucovorin should be administered parenterally at the first suspicion of methanol intoxication. It should be continued until the methanol and formate have been eliminated. The precise dose is unknown, but 1 to 2 mg/kg every 4 to 6 hours is probably reasonable. As the first dose is usually administered prior to hemodialysis, a second dose should be administered at the completion of hemodialysis, because hemodialysis probably removes this highly water-soluble vitamin. If leucovorin is not readily available, then folic acid should be given. Folic acid must never be substituted for folinic acid or leucovorin when a patient with methotrexate poisoning is being managed. Folic acid is inadequate treatment for methotrexate intoxication; leucovorin must be used.

References

1. Hillman RS: Vitamin B_{12}, folic acid and the treatment of megaloblastic anemias. In: Gilman AG, Goodman LS, Rall TW, Murad F, eds: Goodman and Gilman's The Pharmacological Basis of Therapeutics, 7th ed. New York, Macmillan, 1985, pp. 1323–1337.
2. Jacobsen D, McMartin KE: Methanol and ethylene glycol poisonings: Mechanism of toxicity, clinical course, diagnosis and treatment. Med Toxicol 1986;1:309–334.
3. Johlin F, Fortman C, Nghiem D, et al: Studies on the role of folic acid and folate dependent enzymes in human methanol poisoning. Mol Pharmacol 1987; 31:557–561.
4. McGuire BW, Sia LL, Haynes JD, et al: Absorption kinetics of orally administered leucovorin calcium. NCI Monogr 1987;5:47–56.
5. McMartin KE, Martin-Amat G, Makar AB, et al: Methanol poisoning. V: Role of formate metabolism in the monkey. J Pharmacol Exp Ther 1977; 201:564–572.
6. Noker PE, Eells MS, Tephly TR: Methanol toxicity: Treatment with folic acid and 5-formyltetrahydrofolic acid. Alcohol Clin Exp Res 1980;4:378–383.
7. Osterloh J, Pond S, Grady S, et al: Serum formate concentrations in methanol intoxication as a criterion for hemodialysis. Ann Intern Med 1986;104:200–203.
8. Salmon SE, Sartorelli AC: Cancer Chemotherapy. In: Katzung BG: Basic and Clinical Pharmacology, 7th ed. Norwalk, CT, Appleton & Lange, 1998, pp. 889–891.
9. Straw JA, Newman EM, Doroshow JH: Pharmacokinetics of leucovorin (dl–5 formyltetrahydrofolate) after intravenous injection and constant intravenous infusion. NCI Monogr 1987; 5:41–45.

ANTIDOTES IN DEPTH

Ethanol

Mary Ann Howland

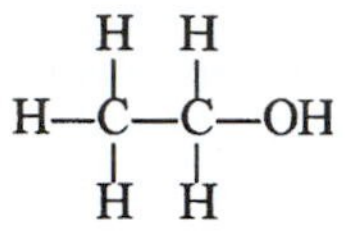

Methanol and ethylene glycol are metabolized to toxic metabolites by the enzyme alcohol dehydrogenase, for which ethanol is a competitive antagonist. The dose of ethanol necessary to achieve competitive inhibition depends on the concentrations of the toxic alcohols and their affinity for the enzyme. Studies in methanol-intoxicated monkeys revealed that when ethanol was administered at a molar ethanol-to-methanol (E/M) ratio of 1:4 and a serum concentration of 204.5 mg/dL of methanol, the metabolism of methanol was reduced by 92%; at a 1:2 E/M ratio, metabolism was reduced by 98%; and at 1:1 E/M ratio, metabolism was reduced by 99%.[11]

Even smaller amounts of ethanol are required to block the metabolism of ethylene glycol, as the affinity of ethylene glycol for alcohol dehydrogenase is less than that of methanol, and much less than that of ethanol.[8,14,15] Most authors[1,8,15] recommend a serum concentration of ethanol of 100 mg/dL or at least a 1:4 molar ratio of ethanol to methanol or ethylene glycol, whichever is greater. One hundred mg/dL (~ 22 mmole/L) protects against 88 mmole/L (286 mg/dL) of methanol and 88 mmole/L (546 mg/dL) of ethylene glycol. Inhibiting the metabolism of methanol and ethylene glycol im-

TABLE 64–3. INTRAVENOUS ADMINISTRATION OF 10% ETHANOL

Loading Dose[c]	Volume (mL)[b] (given over 1 hour as tolerated)					
	10 kg	*15 kg*	*30 kg*	*50 kg*	*70 kg*	*100 kg*
Loading dose of 0.8 g/kg of 10% ethanol (infused over 1 hour as tolerated)	80	120	240	400	560	800
Maintenance Dose[a]	Infusion Rate[b] (mL/h for various weights)[d]					
	10 kg	*15 kg*	*30 kg*	*50 kg*	*70 kg*	*100 kg*
Normal Maintenance Range						
80 mg/kg/h	8	12	24	40	56	80
110 mg/kg/h	11	16	33	55	77	110
130 mg/kg/h	13	19	39	65	91	130
Approximate Maintenance Dose for Chronic Alcoholic						
150 mg/kg/h	15	22	45	75	105	150
Range Required During Hemodialysis						
250 mg/kg/h	25	38	75	125	175	250
300 mg/kg/h	30	45	90	150	210	300
350 mg/kg/h	35	53	105	175	245	350

[a]Infusion to be started immediately following the loading dose. Concentrations above 10% are not recommended for IV administration. The dose schedule is based on the premise that the patient initially has a zero ethanol level. The aim of therapy is to maintain a serum ethanol level of 100–150 mg/dL, but constant monitoring of the ethanol level is required because of wide variations in endogenous metabolic capacity. Ethanol will be removed by hemodialysis, and the infusion rate of ethanol must be increased during hemodialysis. Prolonged ethanol administration may lead to hypoglycemia.

[b]For a 5% concentration, multiply the amount by 2.

[c]A 10% vol/vol concentration yields approximately 100 mg/mL.

[d]Rounded to the nearest mL.

Reprinted, with permission, from Roberts JR, Hedges J, eds: Clinical Procedures in Emergency Medicine. Philadelphia, Saunders, 1985, pp. 1073–1074.

pedes the formation of toxic metabolites and prevents the generation of metabolic acidosis.[6,7,15] Renal, pulmonary, and extracorporeal routes of toxic alcohol removal then become the sole mechanisms for elimination.

Ethanol can be given orally or IV (Tables 64–3 and 64–4). Concentrations of 20 to 30% (orally) and 5 to 10% IV are well tolerated. Intravenous administration has the advantage of complete absorption,[9] avoids gastrointestinal distress, and can be given to an unconscious or uncooperative patient. The disadvantages include the procurement of ethanol, and the preparation of an intravenous solution, the hyperosmolarity of a 5% ethanol solution (about 950 mOsm/L), and the possibility of venous irritation. The drug can also be administered orally, a form which is more readily available. Ethanol is rapidly absorbed orally with peak concentrations achieved in about an hour.[5] The amount of ethanol absorbed after oral administration is dependent on a number of factors but increases with fasting, accelerated gastric emptying, female gender, chronic alcoholism, increasing age, as well as in the presence of certain H_2 antagonists. Sufficient concentrations are generally achieved when 0.8 g/kg of ethanol is given orally over 20 minutes.[2,3,5,10]

The objective, regardless of route, is rapidly to achieve and maintain a level of at least 100 mg/dL of ethanol, which usually proves adequate to achieve enzyme inhibition in most cases. Inhibition is best achieved by administering a loading dose of ethanol followed by a maintenance dose. The volume of distribution for ethanol is approximately 0.6 L/kg.[16] Therefore, the loading dose of ethanol is given by the formula shown in the following figure.

$$\text{Loading dose} = C_p \times V_d$$

$$= 1 \text{ g/L } (100 \text{ mg/dL}) \times 0.6 \text{ L/kg}$$

$$= 0.6 \text{ g/kg}$$

C_p = plasma concentration which for this agent is comparable to the serum concentration

For a 70-kg person, this would be 42 g (70 kg × 0.6 g/kg) of ethanol or 420 mL of 10% V/V ethanol. However, 0.8 g/kg or 8mL/kg loading dose of a 10% ethanol solution is recommended in order to provide a margin of safety due to the metabolism that occurs during administration. The IV loading dose should be administered over 20 to 60 minutes as tolerated by the patient. The 10% ethanol concentration is usually preferred to limit local venous irritation and avoid postinfusion phlebitis. Due

TABLE 64–4. ORAL ADMINISTRATION OF 20% ETHANOL

Loading Dose[b]			**Volume (mL)**			
	10 kg	***15 kg***	***30 kg***	***50 kg***	***70 kg***	***100 kg***
Loading dose of 0.8 g/kg of 20% ethanol, diluted in juice. May be administered orally or via nasogastric over 1 hour.	40	60	120	200	280	400
Maintenance Dose[a]			**mL/h ≤ for various weights**[d]			
	10 kg	***15 kg***	***30 kg***	***50 kg***	***70 kg***	***100 kg***
Normal Maintenance Range						
80 mg/kg/h	4	6	12	20	28	40
110 mg/kg/h	6	8	17	27	39	55
130 mg/kg/h	7	10	20	33	46	66
Approximate Range for Chronic Alcoholic or Patient Receiving Continuous Oral Activated Charcoal						
150 mg/kg/h	8	11	22	38	53	75
Range Required During Hemodialysis						
250 mg/kg/h	13	19	38	63	88	125
300 mg/kg/h	15	23	46	75	105	150
350 mg/kg/h	18	26	53	88	123	175

[a]Concentrations above 30% (60 proof) are not recommended for oral administration. The dose schedule is based on the premise that the patient initially has a zero ethanol level. The aim of therapy is to maintain a serum ethanol level of 100–150 mg/dL, but constant monitoring of the ethanol level is required because of wide variations in endogenous metabolic capacity. Ethanol will be removed by hemodialysis, and the infusion rate of ethanol must be increasing during hemodialysis. Prolonged ethanol administration may lead to hypoglycemia.

[b]A 20% vol/vol concentration yields approximately 200 mg/mL.

[c]Rounded to the nearest mL.

[d]For a 30% concentration, multiply the amount by 0.66.

Reprinted, with permission, from Roberts JR, Hedges J, eds: Clinical Procedures in Emergency Medicine. Philadelphia, Saunders, 1985, pp. 1073–1074.

to the free water content and significant hypertonicity of this solution, the patient should be closely observed for the development of hyponatremia. Due to this concern a second IV line using 0.9% sodium chloride solution may be necessary. Oral administration avoids this potential complication.

To maintain an ethanol concentration of 100 mg/dL, enough ethanol has to be administered to replace that which is being eliminated (66 to 130 mg/kg per hour). The average hourly dose for a 70-kg person is 4.6 g, but higher doses are required in chronic alcoholics (100 to 154 mg/kg per hour) and in those undergoing hemodialysis (250 to 350 mg/kg per hour; see Chap. 5).[4,8,12,13]

Because ethanol elimination varies in each individual, frequent serum ethanol determinations should be made to ensure adequate dosing. Any increase in the anion gap or decrease in bicarbonate concentration implies that the ethanol dose is inadequate to achieve blockade of alcohol dehydrogenase.

Problems encountered with the administration of ethanol include further risk of central nervous system depression, hypoglycemia, dehydration, and fluctuating serum concentrations. Therefore, blood glucose and serum ethanol concentrations should be monitored and attention paid to adequate fluid management. A more practical problem often involves finding or preparing the ethanol to be given. Hospital pharmacies and emergency departments should stock ethanol for such a purpose. Commercial preparations of 5% ethanol in 5% dextrose are available for IV administration. Alternatively, sterile ethanol, USP (absolute ethanol) can be added to 5% dextrose to make a solution of approximately 10% ethanol concentration. A 10% ethanol solution is preferred to limit the volume of fluid administered. Then 55 mL (not 50 mL) of absolute ethanol is added to 500 mL of 5% dextrose, to produce a total end volume of 555 mL (10% = 10 mL in 100 mL, in this case, 55 mL in 555 mL or 55/555). If oral administration is chosen, it is important to remember that 100-proof ethanol is 50% ethanol. Oral ethanol is preferable if this route is acceptable. If there will be any delay in obtaining ethanol for intravenous use, oral therapy with ethanol should be initiated immediately.

When administered appropriately, ethanol is an excellent first step in arresting the further metabolism of methanol and ethylene glycol. However, it does not affect the toxic metabolites that are already present and is not a substitute for hemodialysis.

References

1. Agner K, Hook O, Von Porat B: The treatment of methanol poisoning with ethanol. J Stud Alcohol 1949;9:515–522.
2. Caballeria L: First-pass metabolism of ethanol: Its role as a determinant of blood alcohol levels after drinking. Hepatogastroenterology 1992;39:62–66.
3. Cole-Harding S, Wilson JR: Ethanol metabolism in men and women. J Stud Alcohol 1987;48:380–387.
4. Ekins BR, Rollins DE, Duffy DP, Gregory MC: Standardized treatment of severe methanol poisoning with ethanol and hemodialysis. West J Med 1985;142:337–340.
5. Fraser AG, Hudson M, Sawyer AM, et al: Ranitidine, cimetidine, famotidine have no effect on post-prandial absorption of ethanol (0.8g/kg) taken after an evening meal. Aliment Pharmacol Ther 1992;6:693–700.
6. Grauer G, Thrall MA, Henre B, et al: Comparison of the effects of ethanol on 4-methylpyrazole on the pharmacokinetics and toxicity of ethylene glycol in the dog. Toxicol Lett 1987;35:307–314.
7. Jacobsen D, Jansen H, Wiik-Larsen E, et al: Studies on methanol poisoning. Acta Med Scand 1982;212:5–10.
8. Jacobsen D, McMartin KE: Methanol and ethylene glycol poisonings: Mechanism of toxicity, clinical course, diagnosis and treatment. Med Toxicol 1986;1:309–334.
9. Julkunen RJ, Tannenbaum L, Baradna E, et al: First pass metabolism of ethanol: An important determinant of blood levels after alcohol consumption. Alcohol 1985;2:437–441.
10. Korman MG, Bolin TD: Alcohol and H_2-receptor antagonists. Med J Austral 1992;157:730–731.
11. Makar AB, Tephly TR, Mannering GJ: Methanol metabolism in the monkey. Mol Pharmacol 1963;4:471–483.
12. McCoy HG, Cipolle RJ, Ehlers SM, et al: Severe methanol poisoning: Application of a pharmacokinetic model for ethanol therapy and hemodialysis. Am J Med 1979;67: 804–807.
13. Peterson C: Oral ethanol doses in patients with methanol poisoning. Am J Hosp Pharm 1981;38:1024–1027.
14. Roe O: Methanol poisoning: Its clinical course, pathogenesis and treatment. Acta Med Scand 1946;126(suppl 182): 1–253.
15. Tarr B, Winters L, Moore M, et al: Low dose ethanol in the treatment of ethylene glycol poisoning. J Vet Pharm Ther 1985;8:254–262.
16. Wilkinson P: Pharmacokinetics of ethanol: A review. Alcohol Clin Exp Res 1980;4:6–21.

ANTIDOTES IN DEPTH

4-Methylpyrazole (Fomepizole)

Mary Ann Howland

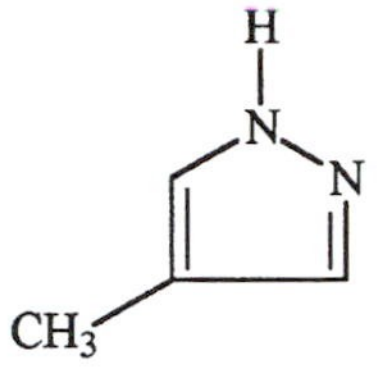

Current management for patients with both ethylene glycol and methanol overdoses includes the use of a loading dose of ethanol followed by a continuous intravenous infusion together with hemodialysis.[3,6,10,16] Ethylene glycol and methanol are metabolized by alcohol dehydrogenase (ADH) to toxic metabolites including glycolic acid and oxalic acid for ethylene glycol and formaldehyde and formic acid for methanol. The formation of these toxic metabolites in vivo is largely responsible for the morbidity and mortality of the parent compounds.

When administered in appropriate doses to patients who have ingested substantial amounts of methanol or ethylene glycol, ethanol will prevent further toxicity by successfully competing for the binding sites of ADH and thereby inhibit the oxidation of methanol or ethylene glycol.[19] Unfortunately, ethanol may contribute to the patient's central nervous system depression, and is technically difficult to administer because of its rapid and often unpredictable rate of metabolism.[21]

In 1963, Theorell and associates described the inhibiting effect of pyrazole on the horse ADH-NAD enzyme–coenzyme system.[17] Pyrazole appeared to block ADH by complexation. Administration to rats and dogs previously poisoned with methanol and ethylene glycol improved survival.[18] However, pyrazole also inhibited other liver enzymes, including catalase and the microsomal ethanol-oxidizing system.[12] The adverse effects of pyrazole administration resulted in bone marrow, liver, and renal toxicity and these effects were increased in the presence of ethanol and methanol.[15] These factors led to further investigations of less toxic compounds.

In 1969, Li and Theorell found that pyrazole and 4-methylpyrazole (4-MP) inhibited ADH found in human liver preparations.[11] Studies in rats and mice using 4-MP found the agent to be relatively nontoxic whether used alone or with ethanol.[5] A single low dose of 4-MP given to humans had a maximal effect on ethanol metabolism at 1.5 to 2 hours.[4]

Subsequent studies in monkeys demonstrated that 4-MP prevents the metabolism of methanol and ethylene glycol, thereby preventing the expected metabolic acidosis and clinical signs and symptoms associated with ethylene glycol and methanol toxicity.[5,15] 4-Methylpyrazole inhibits the metabolism of ethanol, ethylene glycol, and methanol. In a pharmacokinetic study of ethylene glycol in dogs, 4-MP was shown to increase the amount of ethylene glycol excreted in the urine, whereas ethanol did not.[6] 4-Methylpyrazole and ethanol also resulted in increases of the rate constant of ethylene glycol excretion without prolonging ethylene glycol half-life. Investigations with methanol and ethanol showed that 4-MP metabolism is prolonged in monkeys and the duration of action is 12 to 24 hours.[15]

In a rat model, at doses of 10 and 20 mg/kg, 4-MP elimination appeared to obey Michaelis-Menten kinetics, with enzyme saturation and an elimination rate of 10 µmol/L/h at doses in the apparent therapeutic range.[13] The rate of 4-MP elimination decreased by 50% with concomitant administration of ethanol. Urinary excretion was approximately 1% in the absence of ethanol but increased dramatically following its administration. These results demonstrate a mutually inhibitory relationship between 4-MP and ethanol, which may explain why the inhibition of alcohol dehydrogenase is more prolonged than that predicted by the elimination rate of 4-MP alone.[13] The presence of this interaction may prove therapeutically beneficial in the clinical setting.

Because retinol dehydrogenase is an isoenzyme of ADH, and because it is responsible for converting retinol to retinal in the eye, there was concern that 4-MP might inhibit this enzyme and subsequently produce retinal damage.[15] Studies in several species of monkeys and other animals have demonstrated that 4-MP is relatively nontoxic, with no demonstrated signs of ocular toxicity.[3]

4-Methylpyrazole was used to treat 3 patients with ethylene glycol ingestions.[1] It was given at a dose of 15 mg/kg of body weight orally, followed by 5 mg/kg in 12 hours and 10 mg/kg every 12 hours thereafter until ethylene glycol levels were nondetectable. 4-Methylpyrazole appeared to inhibit the metabolism of ethylene glycol; the metabolic acidosis and high anion gap resolved. The half-life of ethylene glycol was about 14 hours during 4-MP therapy. Adverse effects included a skin rash in one individual and eosinophilia in two other patients. Two patients developed a slight increase in serum AST and an increase in serum CPK, but it is uncertain whether this was related to 4-MP administration. Neither visual problems nor ophthalmologic examinations were reported in these patients.

The pharmacokinetics of ethylene glycol after IV 4-MP administration was studied in a patient with an ethylene glycol overdose.[2] This 84.5-kg patient initially received 9.5 mg/kg 9 hours after an ethylene glycol ingestion and then was given progressively smaller doses every 12 hours until the serum ethylene glycol level was only trace positive. The elimination of ethylene glycol after the start of 4-MP demonstrated first-order kinetics, with a half-life of 12 hours. Based on a limited number of determinations, the renal clearance of ethylene glycol averaged 31.5 mL/min during the first 2 days; the corresponding creatinine clearance was 112 mL/min and estimated total body clearance during 4-MP therapy was 57 mL/min. These calculations suggest that the renal clearance of ethylene glycol accounted for only 55% of estimated total body clearance. This patient improved clinically, the metabolic acidosis resolved rapidly, and his serum creatinine remained normal despite a consequential ethylene glycol level of 320 mg/dL. It took about 61 hours for the ethylene glycol level to approximate zero. The kinetics of 4-MP were not studied in this patient, but previous work suggests that a blood concentration of 100 μmol/L is necessary to effect inhibition.[5,15]

An oral placebo-controlled, double-blind, single-dose randomized sequential ascending-dose study was performed in healthy volunteers to determine 4-MP tolerance at 10 to 100 mg/kg.[9] There were no adverse effects in the 10 and 20 mg/kg groups, while at 50 mg/kg 3 of 4 subjects experienced slight to moderate nausea and dizziness within 2.5 hours following medication. All subjects reported comparable symptoms at 100 mg/kg. These symptoms lasted for 30 hours in one individual. There were no concomitant changes in any vital sign or laboratory parameter measured. These authors suggested that a single dose of 10 to 20 mg/kg probably produces 4-MP levels in the therapeutic range without any toxicity. In this human study the elimination of 4-MP followed nonlinear kinetics, renal clearance was low (0.016 mL/min per kg), and only 3% of the administered dose was excreted unchanged in the urine.[7]

Divided daily doses of 4-MP up to 20 mg/kg for 5 days have been administered without any demonstrable toxicity.[14] A transient elevation of aminotransferase levels was reported in 6 of 15 subjects receiving 4-MP.[8] No dose relationship or evidence for hypersensitivity, such as rash, fever, or eosinophilia, was found. These authors suggested that the 4-MP levels that have been utilized[2] are even lower than those employed in their studies to define safe levels. This model used an oral regimen whereas the previous study used an IV dosing regimen. These results are encouraging, but an exact 4-MP dosing regimen remains to be established.

CYP4502E1 isoenzyme oxidizes ethanol and a number of agents to toxic metabolites including acetaminophen, carbon tetrachloride, nitrosamines and benzene. 4-Methylpyrazole like ethanol, isoniazid, and acetone, induces this isoenzyme. In hepatocyte culture 4-MP appears to stabilize and maintain the metabolic activity of the isoenzyme for about a week.[20] Therefore although 4-MP is a potent inhibitor of alcohol dehydrogenase, its action on at least one of the microsomal enzymes of the P450 group is induction.

4-Methylpyrazole has been shown to be a more potent and more specific inhibitor of liver ADH without the toxicity of the parent compound, pyrazole. Adverse reactions include headaches, nausea, dizziness, rash, and eosinophilia. Concurrent administration of both ethanol and fomepizole will reciprocally prolong the elimination of both agents by 40% and 50% respectively. 4-MP is a suitable alternative or adjunct to ethanol dosing in patients with methanol[5a] or ethylene glycol[5b] ingestions. It may also prove useful in patients with severe ethanol-disulfiram reactions. 4-Methylpyrazole has the advantage of being an oral agent with rapid absorption and a rapid onset of action without associated CNS depression. 4-Methylpyrazole has received FDA approval and is now marketed as Fomepizole (Antizol) injection by Orphan Medical. Fomepizole is available in a tray pack containing 4 vials (1.5 mL vials of 1 g/mL) ready to be diluted to 100 mL of D_5W or NS to be administered intravenously over 30 min. The loading dose is 15 mg/kg followed in 12 hours by 10 mg/kg every 12 hours for 4 doses, and then increased to 15 mg/kg every 12 hours as long as necessary. The increase in the maintenance dose from 10 mg/kg to 15 mg/kg is recommended because fomepizole causes autoinduction, stimulating its own metabolism. Patients undergoing hemodialysis require additional doses of fomepizole to replace the amount removed during hemodialysis. It appears likely that 4-MP will effectively replace ethanol as a safe blocker of ADH while patients are being prepared for hemodialysis. The fact that ethanol inhibits 4-MP metabolism may permit synergy in the management of the toxic alcohols.

References

1. Baud F, Bismuth C, Garnier R, et al: 4-Methylpyrazole may be an alternative to ethanol therapy for ethylene glycol intoxication in man. J Toxicol Clin Toxicol 1986;24:463–483.
2. Baud F, Galliot M, Astier A, et al: Treatment of ethylene glycol poisoning with intravenous 4-methylpyrazole. N Engl J Med 1988;319:97–110.
3. Blomstrand R, Ingelmansson S: Studies on the effect of 4-methylpyrazole on methanol poisoning using the monkey as an animal model: With particular reference to the ocular toxicity. Drug Alcohol Depend 1984;13:343–355.
4. Blomstrand R, Theorell H: Inhibitory effect on ethanol oxidation in man after administration of 4-methylpyrazole. Life Sci 1970;9:631–640.
5. Blomstrand R, Wintzell H, Lof A, et al: Pyrazoles as inhibitors of alcohol oxidation and as important tools in alcohol research: An approach to therapy against methanol poisoning. Proc Natl Acad Sci USA 1979;76:3499–3503.
5a. Brent J, McMartin K, Phillips SP, et al: 4-Methylpyrazole

(Fomepizole) therapy of methanol poisoning: Preliminary results of the meta trial. J Toxicol Clin Toxicol 1997;351:567.

5b. Brent J, McMartin K, Phillips SP, et al: 4-Methylpyrazole (Fomepizole) therapy of ethylene glycol poisoning: Preliminary results of the meta trial. J Toxicol Clin Toxicol 1997; 351:567.

6. Grauer GF, Thrall MAH, Henre BA, Hjelle JJ: Comparison of the effects of ethanol and 4-methylpyrazole on the pharmacokinetics and toxicity of ethylene glycol in the dog. Toxicol Lett 1987;35:307–314.

7. Jacobsen D, Barron SK, Sebastian CS, et al: Nonlinear kinetics of 4-methylpyrazole in healthy human subjects. Eur J Clin Pharmacol 1989;37:599–604.

8. Jacobsen D, Sebastian CS, Barron SK, et al: Effects of 4-methylpyrazole, methanol/ethylene glycol antidote, in healthy humans. J Emerg Med 1990;8:455–461.

9. Jacobsen D, Sebastian CS, Blomstrand R, McMartin KE: 4-methylpyrazole: A controlled study of safety in healthy human subjects after single ascending doses. Alcohol Clin Exp Res 1988;12:516–522.

10. Knepshield JH, Shreiner GE, Lowenthal DT, et al: Dialysis of poisons and drugs: Annual review. Trans Am Soc Artif Intern Organs 1973;19:590–633.

11. Li TK, Theorell H: Human liver alcohol dehydrogenase: Inhibition by pyrazole and pyrazole analogs. Acta Chem Scand 1969;23:892–902.

12. Lieber C, Rubin E, DeCarli L, et al: Effects of pyrazole on hepatic function and structure. Lab Invest 1970;22:615–621.

13. McMartin KE, Collins TD: Distribution of oral 4-methylpyrazole in the rat: Inhibition of elimination by ethanol. J Toxicol Clin Toxicol 1988; 26:451–466.

14. McMartin KE, Heath A: The treatment of ethylene glycol poisoning with intravenous 4-methylpyrazole. N Engl J Med 1989;320:125.

15. McMartin K, Hedstrom K, Tolk B, et al: Studies on the metabolic interactions between 4-methylpyrazole and methanol using monkey as an animal model. Arch Biochem Biophys 1980;199:606–614.

16. Parry MF, Wallach R: Ethylene glycol poisoning. Am J Med 1974;57:143–150.

17. Theorell H, Yonetani T, Sjoberg B: On the effects of some heterocyclic compounds on the enzymatic activity of liver alcohol dehydrogenase. Acta Chem Scand 1969;23: 255–260.

18. Van Stee E, Harris A, Horton M, et al: The treatment of ethylene glycol toxicosis with pyrazole. J Pharmacol Exp Ther 1975;192:251–259.

19. Wacker WEC, Haynes H, Druyan R, et al: Treatment of ethylene glycol poisoning with ethyl alcohol. JAMA 1965;194: 1231–1233.

20. Wu DF, Clejan L, Potter B, et al: Rapid decrease of cytochrome P-45011E1 in primary hepatocyte culture and its maintenance by added 4-methylpyrazole. Hepatology 1990; 12:1379–1389.

21. Zahlten RN: Cyclic AMP and corticosteroids. N Engl J Med 1974;290:743–744. Letter.

CHAPTER 65

Cocaine

Judd E. Hollander and Robert S. Hoffman

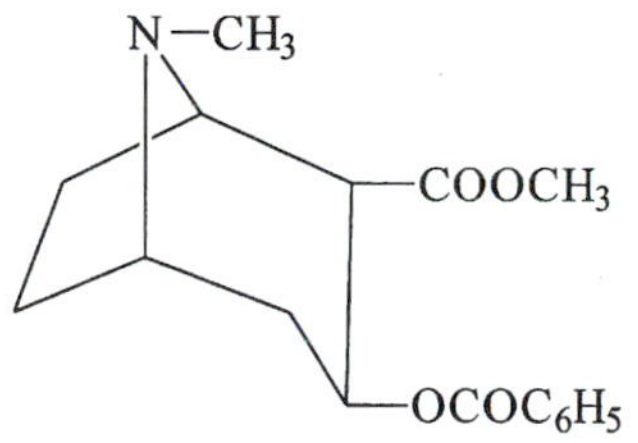

Cocaine

A 22-year-old agitated male was brought to the hospital by ambulance after his family witnessed a "seizure." On arrival at the patient's apartment the paramedics were: told that the patient had shaking movements of all of his extremities, his eyes rolled back, and he began to "foam at the mouth." The family did not know whether the patient had recently used any drugs because he had just returned from a trip to South America.

The patient remained agitated despite reassurance by the medics. Initial vital signs were: blood pressure, 225/130 mm Hg; pulse, 132 beats/min; respiratory rate, 30 breaths/min. An intravenous line was started with 0.9% sodium chloride solution, and 100 mL of 50% dextrose in water ($D_{50}W$) and 100 mg of thiamine were given IV without any clinical response. High-flow oxygen was administered at 8 L/min. The patient was taken immediately to the hospital.

On arrival, the patient appeared to be a well-nourished, well-developed, markedly agitated man. His vital signs were: blood pressure, 215/130 mm Hg; pulse, 130 beats/min and regular with occasional extrasystoles; respiratory rate, 28 breaths/min; and rectal temperature, 103°F (39.4°C). His skin was diaphoretic and flushed. Examination of head, eyes, ears, nose, and throat revealed no head trauma. Blood was noted at the lateral aspect of the tongue. He had dilated (8 mm) pupils that reacted to light bilaterally. Extraocular movements were intact without nystagmus, and funduscopic examination was normal. Examination of the nose revealed an atrophic mucosa with a perforated nasal septum. A dry, white powder was noted on the patient's mustache; it was scraped off and saved for toxicologic examination. The neck was supple without thyromegaly, the trachea was midline. The chest was clear. The heart sounds revealed an S_4 gallop. Examination of his abdomen revealed high-pitched hyperactive bowel sounds, no organomegaly, and mild tenderness throughout without rebound. The patient subsequently vomited bilious material without blood or coffee grounds. On neurologic examination he was noted to be agitated, flailing all extremities with bilateral hyperactive reflexes and plantar flexion. Rectal examination was unremarkable and stool was negative for occult blood.

Initial laboratory studies demonstrated hematocrit, 45%; hemoglobin, 15 g/dL; WBC count, 11,500/ mm^3 with a normal differential; platelets, 200,000/mm^3. Arterial blood gas on room air revealed pH, 7.35; PCO_2, 28 mm

Hg; PO_2, 90 mm Hg. The serum electrolytes were sodium, 140 mEq/L; chloride, 105 mEq/L; bicarbonate, 13 mEq/L; potassium, 4.0 mEq/L; anion gap, 22 mEq/L; calcium, 4.5 mg/dL. The BUN and creatinine were normal and blood glucose was 120 mg/dL.

The ECG revealed a sinus tachycardia with three to four unifocal ventricular premature contractions per minute. The PR, QRS, and QT_c intervals were within normal limits. J-point and 0.5 mm ST-segment elevation was noted. Chest radiograph and urinalysis were normal.

The patient was treated with incremental doses of 5 mg of IV diazepam (total dose of 25 mg) until his vital signs approached normal. Repeat vital signs 20 minutes later were: blood pressure, 140/80 mm Hg; pulse, 95 beats/min; respiratory rate, 20 breaths/min and regular; temperature, 101.0°F (38.3°C). Pupils were 4 mm, equal, and reactive, and the patient was less agitated. The patient stated that he had "snorted snow" and smoked a "joint" that his friends had given him.

What Are the History and Epidemiology of Cocaine Use?

Cocaine is a natural alkaloid contained in the leaves of *Erythroxylon coca*, a shrub that grows abundantly in Mexico, South America, the West Indies, and Indonesia. The 6th-century inhabitants of Peru chewed or sucked on the leaves for social and religious reasons. In the 1100s the Incas used cocaine-filled saliva as local anesthesia for ritual trephinations.[66] Cocaine was noted to be the active alkaloid in the coca leaf in 1857 and was first used as a local anesthetic in 1884.[89] In the early 20th century, cocaine was used briefly as an ingredient in Coca-Cola. Since 1975, the popularity of cocaine has grown due in part to the increased production of the coca crops by international drug trafficking cartels.

The National Institute of Drug Abuse (NIDA) estimated that in 1974, 5.4 million Americans had used cocaine at some time in their lives.[7,66] By 1985, this number had increased drastically, to 25 to 40 million Americans, 3 million of whom were considered regular users. By 1990, over 25 million Americans had tried cocaine at least once and 5 million Americans admitted using cocaine one or more times a month.[148] Cocaine is commonly used along with other illicit drugs or substances of abuse, such as ethanol, opioids, marijuana, and sedative-hypnotics. Current data suggest a marked increase in cocaine use and complications. Cocaine is the most frequent drug-related cause of emergency department visits in the United States.[129]

What Are the Pharmacokinetics and Toxicokinetics of Cocaine?

After extraction from the coca leaf, cocaine (benzoylmethylecgonine) is purified to the hydrochloride salt, a white crystal. Ecgonine is an aminoalcohol base closely related to tropine, the aminoalcohol in atropine. Cocaine is therefore best considered an ester-type local anesthetic of the tropane family.

The onset of action of cocaine depends on the dose and route of administration. When insufflated, the onset of action is within 1 to 3 minutes, and its effects peak in 20 to 30 minutes. When used intravenously or smoked, the onset of action is within seconds and peak action occurs within 3 to 5 minutes. Cocaine can be absorbed through the mucosa of the respiratory, gastrointestinal, and genitourinary tract, including less common routes of absorption such as the urethra, bladder, and vagina.

Cocaine is metabolized by liver esterases and plasma cholinesterase (pseudocholinesterase), and degraded nonenzymatically (Fig. 65–1)[193] Cocaine is rapidly hydrolyzed by cholinesterases to its major metabolite, ecgonine methyl ester (EME), which accounts for 30 to 50% of the parent product. Nonenzymatic hydrolysis results in the formation of the other major metabolite, benzoylecgonine (BE), which accounts for approximately 40% of the parent product. Norcocaine and ecgonine are minor metabolites that constitute the remainder of cocaine's degradation products.

The biologic half-life of cocaine is 0.5 to 1.5 hours. A relatively minor amount is excreted unchanged in the urine.[105] Benzoylecgonine and EME are also excreted in the urine, with half-lives of 5 to 8 and 3.5 to 6 hours, respectively.[105] Due to a long elimination half-life, assays typically detect benzoylecgonine for as long as 48 to 72 hours following cocaine use,[4] although in rare cases benzoylecgonine has been detected in the urine up to 22 days following substantial cocaine use.[210]

The activity of plasma cholinesterase determines the relative concentrations of the various metabolites, and quite possibly affects the degree of toxicity that develops. Serum from patients with plasma cholinesterase deficiency produce decreased concentrations of ecgonine methyl ester.[130] A similar effect is described in animals, and demonstrates a shift of the metabolite profile largely toward an increase in benzoylecgonine, with a smaller, but still substantial increase in norcocaine observed.[107] As a result, patients with pseudocholinesterase deficiency may have a greater potential for adverse reactions than patients with normal metabolism.[41,78,151]

In the setting of decreased cardiac output with decreased hepatic perfusion (hypotension, low-output congestive heart failure), increased cocaine concentrations occur. Consequently, patients with decreased hepatic metabolism of cocaine may also be at increased risk of adverse consequences.

What Are the Pharmacologic Effects of Cocaine?

Cocaine is a unique compound that produces many pharmacologic effects in humans. Through direct blockade of fast sodium channels, cocaine stabilizes the axonal membrane, producing a local anesthetic effect. Similar blockade of fast sodium channels on myocardial tissue imparts type I antidysrhythmic properties to cocaine.[8,213] In addition, cocaine is the only local anesthetic that inter-

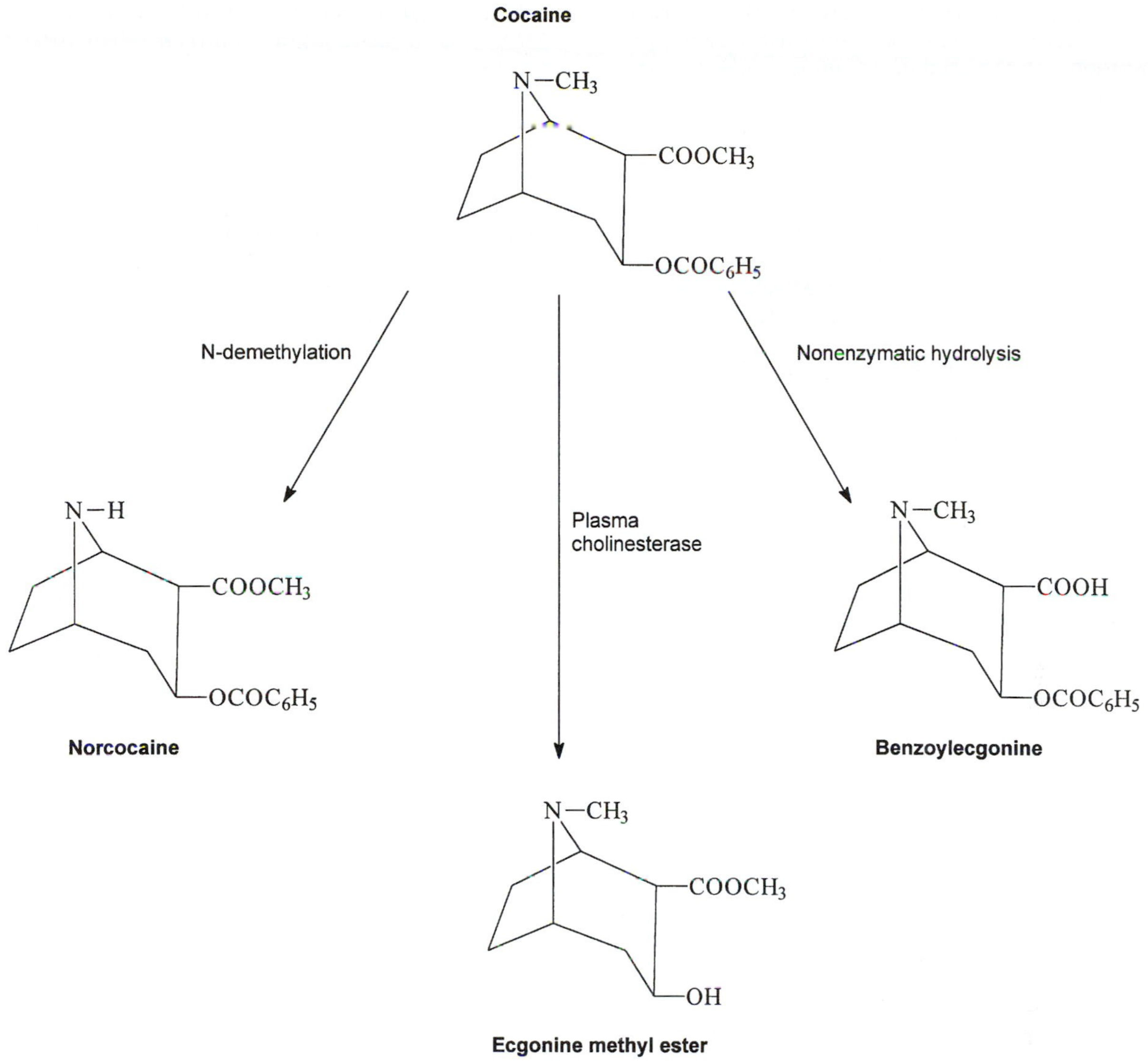

Figure 65–1. Metabolism of cocaine. The three principal metabolic pathways of cocaine are depicted.

feres with the uptake of neurotransmitter by the nerve terminals and simultaneously functions as a vasoconstrictor. These varied mechanisms interact to produce the wide clinical spectrum of cocaine toxicity.

Central nervous system stimulation is probably the most prominent effect of cocaine. The CNS is stimulated in a rostral-to-caudal fashion. The cortex is stimulated first, which may result in restlessness, excitement, and increased motor activity. Later, stimulation of lower motor centers can result in tonic-clonic seizures. Cocaine's effect on the medulla is an initial increase in respiratory rate. Later, depression of medullary respiratory centers occurs, with resultant respiratory failure. The vomiting center may be stimulated early after using cocaine, but emesis is usually self-limited.

The initial effect on the cardiovascular system is bradycardia, secondary to stimulation of the vagal nuclei. The bradycardia is very short-lived and not typically clinically evident. Tachycardia typically ensues, predominantly from increased central sympathetic stimulation. Cocaine's cardiostimulatory mechanism is to produce sensitization to epinephrine and norepinephrine, probably by preventing neuronal reuptake of these catecholamines as well as by increasing the release of norepinephrine from adrenergic nerve terminals. The increased concentrations and persistence of catecholamines near the receptors of the effector organ lead to exaggerated sympathetic effects. Animal investigations reveal that the peak vasopressor effects of cocaine are mediated by norepinephrine of sympathetic neural origin and the peak tachycardic effects of cocaine are mediated by direct release of epinephrine of adrenal medullary origin.[197]

Psychostimulant central nervous system effects secondary to cocaine are at least in part mediated through inhibition of dopamine reuptake in the nucleus accumbens.[71] Genetically engineered absence of the dopamine transporter totally prevents the psychostimulatory effects of cocaine in animals.[58] Cocaine also increases the concentrations of the excitatory amino acids, aspartate and glutamate, in the nucleus accumbens.[190] These excitatory amino acids increase the extracellular concentrations of dopamine. Excitatory amino acid antagonists attenuate the effects of cocaine on extracellular dopamine[152] and block cocaine induced convulsions and death.[169] Dopamine$_1$ (D_1) and dopamine$_2$ (D_2) receptor agonists have opposite effects on cocaine-seeking behavior. The D_2 agonists lead to cocaine-seeking behavior while D_1 agonists diminish craving for cocaine.[182]

What Are the Effects of the Various Metabolites of Cocaine?

The precise degree to which the parent compound and the major metabolites account for the observed clinical effects of cocaine remain unclear. Although studies suggested that cocaine and norcocaine accounted for majority of the vascular effects of cocaine,[12] more recent studies have shown an active role for most of the metabolites. Cocaine, norcocaine, ecgonine, and benzoylecgonine (BE) all cause cerebrovascular vasoconstriction when suffused over the brain surface[117] or when administered directly into the cerebral circulation,[177] although studies have yielded conflicting results regarding the relative potencies of each of the various metabolites. Intravenous administration of cocaine and BE may also lead to cerebral vasoconstriction.[27] In general, most studies suggest that cocaine and norcocaine are the most potent vasoconstrictors followed by BE, and ecgonine. In some studies, however, EME produced mild vasodilation of cerebral blood vessels,[131,177] and in one model was protective against cocaine lethality. With respect to proconvulsant effects, cocaine and norcocaine are most potent, but BE and EME administration may also lead to seizures in some models.[115,137] The sodium channel antagonist effects occur with the parent compound and with norcocaine, but do not result from the administration of BE or EME.[30] The varying potencies of the major metabolites of cocaine explain why augmentation of the metabolism with the use of exogenous plasma cholinesterase may reduce the toxicity of cocaine by shunting degradation away from benzoylecgonine and norcocaine to less toxic metabolites.[80]

The combined use of alcohol and cocaine produces a unique metabolite, cocaethylene.[16] Preclinical studies have found that cocaethylene is equipotent to cocaine in terms of behavioral effects, yet more likely to be lethal. Human studies demonstrate that relative to cocaine, cocaethylene produces milder subjective effects[156] and comparable hemodynamic effects. Cocaethylene has a direct myocardial depressant effect[74] that is not mediated through coronary artery vasoconstriction.[158]

Are There Medical Uses for Cocaine?

Cocaine is still used as a topical anesthetic (4 to 10% solution) for intranasal or bronchoscopic procedures. The older otolaryngologic literature implies that the maximal safe total dose of cocaine is 1 to 3 mg/kg body weight. More concentrated solutions (greater than 10%) are not advantageous clinically and have more adverse effects. The dosage of cocaine used in clinical settings should be decreased in patients with hypermetabolic and febrile conditions, in patients receiving drugs that alter neurotransmitter metabolism, in those with hepatic impairment, and in patients with known pseudocholinesterase deficiency. Cocaine should be used when alternative agents are contraindicated, and only by physicians who understand its pharmacologic and toxicologic properties as well as the appropriate treatments for adverse reactions.

Tetracaine, epinephrine, and cocaine (referred to as TAC) are used as a topical anesthetic in children with scalp and facial lacerations. Pediatric deaths,[32] seizures,[33,34] respiratory distress,[200] and other significant systemic toxicities have been reported.[44,63,175] Until the effective dose of TAC and its potential toxicity are known, it should not be recommended as an anesthetic solution of choice in pediatric facial and scalp lacerations.[63]

In Europe, cocaine is used in the preparation of Brompton's mixture, an analgesic-phenothiazine solution, for the control of pain in oncology patients.

How Is Cocaine Abused?

Cocaine exits as a hydrochloride salt or, in sulfated form, as a powder. It is commonly adulterated with one or more of the following compounds: mannitol, sucrose, lactose, caffeine, talc, amphetamine, heroin ("speedball"), PCP, procaine, lidocaine, ergots, or strychnine.[183] When it is nasally insufflated, various paraphernalia from "head shops" such as little spoons, a rolled-up dollar bill, or straws are used.

"Free-basing" is the home conversion of the hydrochloride form of cocaine to the pure alkaloid cocaine. The "free-base kits" contain such flammable chemicals as ether, benzene, or gasoline. Although cocaine is readily soluble in these solvents, the use of a flame in the conversion process has led to significant burns of some drug users. Unlike cocaine hydrochloride, free-base or crack can be smoked because it vaporizes rather than burns. Because it is fat-soluble, it can readily cross the blood–lung and blood–brain barriers.

On the street, much of what is believed to be cocaine free-base is actually cocaine base. Both products can be smoked and will result in an intense euphoria comparable with IV injection. Cocaine base, cocaine paste, "pasta," or "bazooka" is also manufactured by an extraction process. The raw coca leaves are dried and then digested with sulfuric acid. Cocaine base is then extracted after precipitation with sodium bicarbonate. On assay, cocaine base contains 40 to 85% cocaine sulfate. This similarity has resulted in a great deal of confusion both clinically and in the literature, where the terms cocaine, free-base, crack, and cocaine sulfate are often used synonymously. The distinction between pure cocaine free-base and cocaine (cocaine sulfate) occurs largely in the laboratory as very few clinical differences can be definitively attributed to one particular form of the drug.

The availability of crack, a purified processed smokable form of cocaine, has increased access to cocaine. The agent is available in small chips or rocks that are frequently marketed for as little as $5 to $25. Crack acquired its name because of its rocklike appearance and the crackling sounds made when it is heated.

Cocaine free-base and crack are more stable to pyrolysis than the hydrochloride salt, and therefore can be smoked either using a "coke pipe" or sprinkled on a cigarette or "joint." Crack and free-base cocaine are highly purified (85 to 90%). Crack is of greater risk to the user than ordinary cocaine due to its purity and high rate of absorption. Unlike nasal insufflation of cocaine hydrochloride—which exerts a vasoconstrictor effect on the nasal mucosa, thereby limiting its own absorption—crack smoking offers no such protection.

Crack users do not usually titrate or adjust their dosage, as do intranasal users.[187] Many free-base or crack users employ repetitive doses to achieve the rapid onset of euphoria (seconds) and avoid the rapid dissipation and ensuing depression (5 to 7 minutes). They may continue this use for 12 to 24 hours before becoming exhausted and falling asleep. Intravenous injection and crack use result in high drug concentrations and associated euphoria leading to rapid drug dependence.

What Are the Major Clinical Manifestations of Cocaine Toxicity?

Hyperthermia

By increasing the patient's psychomotor activity, cocaine augments heat production. There is also a decrease in heat dissipation resulting from cocaine-induced vasoconstriction (see Chap. 18). A direct pyrogenic effect is postulated by cocaine's action on thermoregulatory centers in the hypothalamic area, but is not well substantiated. Finally, cocaine's stimulation of the calorigenic activity of the liver is believed to cause hyperthermia.

Animal data underscore the clinical importance of cocaine-induced hyperthermia. One study compared the effects of hypertension and tachycardia, pH, acidosis, seizures, and hyperthermia on cocaine lethality. Only those agents that corrected hyperthermia improved survival.[19]

Neurologic Effects

Most cocaine-intoxicated patients are anxious or agitated. This can be a transient effect of cocaine or reflect underlying organic pathology. Cerebrovascular accidents, including subarachnoid hemorrhage,[125,180] intracerebral hemorrhage,[215] cerebral infarction,[60,123,124,181] transient ischemic attacks,[140] migraine-type headache syndromes,[174] seizures,[26] cerebral vasculitis,[110,116] anterior spinal artery syndrome,[140] and varied psychiatric manifestations have been reported secondary to cocaine use.

Although some patients with neurologic catastrophes have had predisposing cerebrovascular disease[73,174,215] (for example, aneurysms or arteriovenous malformations), most have not. The pathophysiology of cerebrovascular infarction is probably similar to that of coronary arterial insufficiency and includes hypercoagulability, impaired cerebrovascular autoregulation from increased cerebrovascular resistance,[123,124] vasospasm,[60] embolism of particulate matter, and immunologically mediated arteritis or vasculitis.[18,116] In addition, the increased prevalence of anticardiolipin antibodies in cocaine users suggests that immunologic mechanisms may play a role in cocaine toxicity.[54]

Seizures may occur secondary to infarction or hemorrhage or in their absence. The majority of seizures are single, generalized, induced by intravenous or crack cocaine, and are not associated with any lasting neurologic deficits. Multiple or focal seizures are usually associated with concomitant drug use or an underlying seizure disorder. A "washed out" syndrome secondary to cocaine is characterized by a decreased level of consciousness and profound lethargy. These patients are similar to patients with a prolonged postictal period. Patients who remain extremely lethargic and are difficult to arouse for up to 24 hours after cocaine use may have the "cocaine washed out syndrome." These patients assume normal sleep postures and can occasionally be aroused to full orientation, in contrast to lethargic patients with subarachnoid hemorrhage or other intracranial catastrophes.

The visual system can be affected by cocaine through both vascular and direct topical toxicity. Direct instillation of cocaine into the conjunctival sack denudes the corneal epithelium.[165] Particulate matter in smoke produces corneal abrasions and ulcerations ("crack eye").[133] Vascular effects, including central retinal artery occlusion and bilateral blindness from diffuse vasospasm, may also occur.[42,81]

Cardiac Effects

Myocardial ischemia and infarction occur secondary to cocaine insufflation, smoking, intravenous use, and possibly withdrawal.[5,35,57,86,88,90,96,122,138,145,202,218] Myocardial infarctions typically occur in patients 19 to 40 years old without apparent massive exposures to cocaine or without concurrent seizures or agitation. Patients with cocaine-associated myocardial infarctions frequently have atypical chest pain or chest pain delayed for hours to days after their most recent use of cocaine.[86,88,91,92,94] Their ECGs reveal abnormalities consisting of ST-segment elevation and T-wave inversions that often persist during hospitalization;[59,94,97] however, the electrocardiogram is less sensitive and less specific for myocardial infarction in patients who have recently used cocaine.[59,94,97] Cocaine induces vasoconstriction in both the left and right coronary arteries[207] resulting in infarcts within both distributions.[87,89,138] Q-wave and non-Q wave infarctions occur with equal frequency.[5,87,89] Cocaine causes myocardial ischemia through a complex pathophysiology resulting from its acute and chronic effects.[84] Acutely, cocaine results in coronary artery vasoconstriction, tachycardia, systemic arterial hypertension, increased myocardial oxygen demand, platelet aggregation, and in-situ thrombus formation.[86] Chronic cocaine users develop accelerated atherosclerosis and left ventricular hypertrophy, which can further exacerbate the O_2 supply–demand mismatch. There is no evidence suggesting that serum levels or route of administration play a role in the likelihood of developing ischemia.[89] Myocardial ischemia and infarction have occurred in patients without any underlying atherosclerotic disease or other evidence of pre-existing heart disease.[29,100,103,138,154]

In patients with Prinzmetal's angina, ergonovine leads to a rise in systemic pressure, diffuse coronary artery narrowing, and focal vasospasm. In patients with cocaine-induced myocardial infarctions, however, administration of ergonovine uniformly fails to produce focal vasospasm.[100,103,154] One patient with a history of a cocaine-related ischemic event who had a negative ergonovine provocation test developed severe coronary vasospasm when provoked with intranasal cocaine.[102] Therefore, the absence of a response to this testing technique cannot exclude the possibility of cocaine-induced vasospasm.

With the use of ambulatory ECG (Holter) monitoring in patients admitted to an inpatient detoxification center, one group demonstrated spontaneous episodes of ST-segment elevation that occurred for up to 6 weeks after withdrawal of cocaine.[145] The researchers postulated that patients in cocaine withdrawal manifest a dopamine-depleted condition that results in intermittent coronary spasm. Myocardial infarction has been documented in a 42-year-old man with normal coronary arteries, 3 days after his last use of cocaine.[35] Increased adrenergic receptor sensitivity and catecholamine replenishment occurring during the cocaine withdrawal period were offered as an explanation. Further understanding of the pharmacologic characteristics of cocaine withdrawal may better explain these events.

Dysrhythmias. Low-dose cocaine may result in bradycardias, whereas higher doses are associated with virtually all types of tachydysrhythmias. Sinus tachycardia, atrial fibrillation/flutter, other supraventricular tachycardias, ventricular premature contractions, accelerated idioventricular rhythms, ventricular tachycardia, torsades de pointes, and ventricular fibrillation may be the direct result of cocaine use. Laboratory studies demonstrate that high doses of cocaine result in infranodal and intraventricular conduction delays and lethal ventricular dysrhythmias secondary to prolonged QRS and QT intervals.[153,179] Clinical studies also have found a prolonged QT in patients with recent cocaine use.[97] These effects are similar to those observed with type I antidysrhythmic agents[8] and probably are mediated by the local anesthetic properties that result in sodium channel blockade and may help to explain why increasing doses of cocaine appear to have a direct myocardial-depressant effect.[8,69,157,213] In addition to the local anesthetic effects, dysrhythmias also may occur as a result of cocaine-induced myocardial ischemia or infarction.[89,186]

Cardiomyopathy. Chronic cocaine use predisposes patients to the development of a dilated cardiomyopathy either from recurrent or diffuse ischemia with subsequent "stunned" myocardium[209] or from a direct effect on contractility independent of its ischemic effects.[106] In some cases, the left ventricular systolic dysfunction may improve with cessation of cocaine use.[24] Cocaine can cause transplacental myocardial depression as evidenced by the fact that infants born to cocaine-using women had statistically lower cardiac outputs in the first day of life when compared with control infants.[205] The differences resolved by the second day of life. These results are comparable to the catecholamine-induced reversible cardiomyopathies associated with pheochromocytomas[101] and methamphetamine use.[99]

Endocarditis and Endothelial Injury. An increased risk of upper extremity deep vein thrombosis[126,127] and bacterial endocarditis[21] is associated with IV cocaine use. This risk of endocarditis seems to be increased over a similar population of IV heroin users and may result from the increased frequency of injections in cocaine users or direct effects of cocaine on endovascular tissues and the immune system.[20,211]

Aortic Dissection. Several cases of cocaine-induced aortic dissection and rupture have been reported.[2,22,28,50] It is presumed that dissection and rupture result from the increase in shear forces that result from cocaine-induced hypertension and tachycardia.

Pulmonary Effects

Cocaine can result in a broad spectrum of acute pulmonary complications.[67,199] These events range from asthma exacerbations,[171] pneumothorax, pneumomediastinum,[121,185] noncardiogenic pulmonary edema,[31,76,111] diffuse alveolar hemorrhage,[143] recurrent pulmonary infiltrates[150] with eosinophilia, and bronchiolitis obliterans with organizing pneumonia,[155] to pulmonary vascular abnormalities.[36,189,199] Cocaine may increase systemic vascular resistance with resultant left ventricular dysfunction and pulmonary edema.[47] Pulmonary artery hypertrophy, in the absence of foreign particle embolization, may occur with chronic cocaine use.[144]

Chronic effects of cocaine on the lung appear to be related to the route of use, with crack smoking placing patients at highest risk.[3] Studies of pulmonary function in chronic cocaine users have not found significant long-term adverse effects on lung mechanics.[104,194,196] Heavy users of inhaled cocaine do not have abnormal spirometry; however, some studies have revealed a small decrease in the carbon monoxide-diffusing capacity (D_LCO), which is a physiologic marker of the integrity of the alveolar capillary membrane.[196]

Skeletal Muscle Effects

Cocaine use can lead to severe rhabdomyolysis with massive elevations in creatine phosphokinase levels, acute renal failure, profound hypotension, and hyperthermia.[6,14,75,135,136,159,170,172,188,212] Seizures, hyperthermia, hypotension, or prolonged unconsciousness are not necessary for the production of rhabdomyolysis.[217] Cocaine probably causes skeletal muscle ischemia through the same mechanisms by which it affects other vascular beds. Renal failure may result from both myoglobinuria and renal ischemia.[184]

Uteroplacental Effects

Maternal cocaine use decreases the likelihood of term deliveries and has an adverse effect on fetal growth and development.[1,23,25,43,130] An increased incidence of spontaneous abortions, abruptio placentae, fetal prematurity, and intrauterine growth retardation occurs. Experimental evidence in pregnant ewes demonstrated dose-dependent increases in maternal blood pressure with corresponding decreases in uterine blood flow.[142,216] Symptoms of neonatal cocaine withdrawal usually begin within 24 to 48 hours of birth. Withdrawal results in infants with jitteriness, irritability, poor eye contact, and vigorous sucking. In utero cocaine exposure also may result in infants with a small head circumference and low birthweight.

Gastrointestinal, Splenic, and Hepatic Vasculature

The intestinal vasculature is highly sensitive to catecholamines, due to the wide distribution of alpha-adrenergic receptors in the walls of the intestines. Acute mucosal ischemia occurs following all common routes of cocaine use,[46,53,62,139,147] but is especially of concern following direct local toxicity in gastrointestinal drug smugglers.[147] Adverse consequences of cocaine have occurred in all age groups from neonates to adults.[46,62,198] and with various clinical presentations ranging from colitis to intestinal perforation[49,120] (see Color Plate Fig. 23).

In various mouse models, cocaine is hepatotoxic, possibly through the formation of a reactive metabolite, norcocaine nitroxide,[61,108,113,114] or alternatively through the creation of a redox cycle that results in glutathione depletion.[112,113] Isolated hepatotoxicity in humans is uncommon. Elevations of AST and ALT often occur, however, in the setting of hyperthermia or severe cardiovascular instability.

Psychological Effects

Tolerance and physical and psychological addiction to cocaine occur. Animal models, however, suggest that there also may be a "reverse tolerance" to the behavioral reactions of cocaine. It has been theorized that the progressive effects of cocaine with use of smaller amounts may be related to "electrical kindling," a phenomenon in which "repetitive subthreshold electrical stimulation of the limbic system produces increasing effects on electrical activity and behavior, leading to seizures."[161]

The psychological or perceptual effects of cocaine can be disconcerting to the abuser. Some patients experience "cocaine bugs," a crawling sensation under the skin with resultant self-excoriation, leading to irregular scratches and ulcers (Magnan's sign).

The stimulant abstinence syndrome follows a three-phase pattern of crash, withdrawal, and extinction. The crash is associated with intense depression, agitation, and anxiety. Withdrawal is marked by decreased energy, limited interest in the environment, and limited ability to experience pleasure. Extinction is the decrease in craving that occurs over time.[55]

What Is the Treatment for Cocaine Toxicity?

Treatment of cocaine toxicity requires an understanding of the underlying pathophysiology. The clinical approach to treatment requires an understanding of the acute and chronic effects of cocaine, both vascular and nonvascular effects, as well as the fact that cardiovascular and neuropsychiatric complications are inextricably linked (Fig. 65–2).

What Are the Therapeutic Principles and Treatment of Nonvascular Manifestations of Cocaine Intoxication?

Because of the direct pharmacologic and toxicologic relationship between the neuropsychiatric and cardiovascular complications, successful management of the neuropsychiatric manifestations almost invariably has a salutary impact on resolution of the cardiovascular abnormalities, at least from an emergent or initial care perspective. Animal studies uniformly demonstrate that the major causes of death are psychomotor agitation and hyperthermia.[19,65] Sedative-hypnotics are uniformly suc-

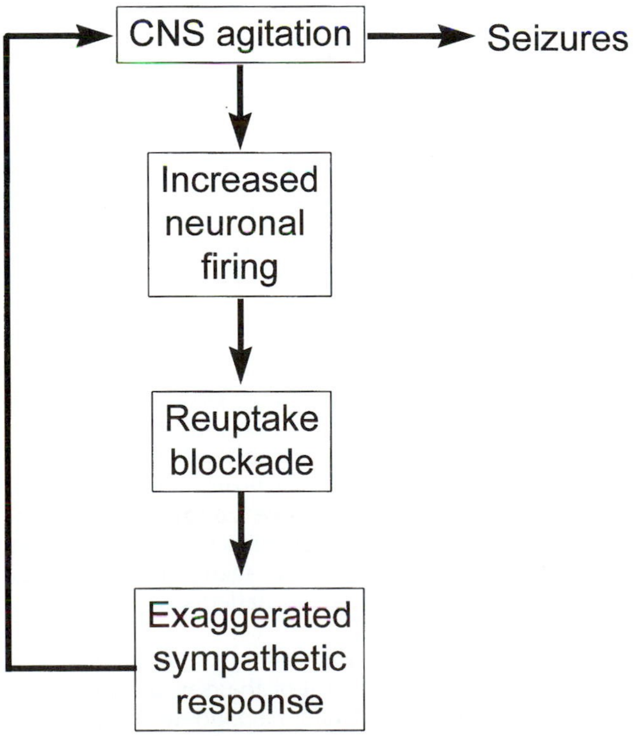

Figure 65–2. Cocaine-induced CNS effects modulate peripheral events.

cessful for the treatment of cocaine toxicity and the prevention of lethality.[19,37,65] Figure 65–2 illustrates the predicted failure of therapeutic interventions directed solely at ameliorating the peripheral manifestations of cocaine toxicity. Thus sedation with a benzodiazepine is chosen, due to demonstrable experimental efficacy[19,37,65] and substantial experience with their use in other clinical conditions associated with severe agitation and catecholamine excess, such as sedative-hypnotic or ethanol withdrawal.

Agitation and seizures are managed in the standard manner, with a focus on rapid control of motor activity while protecting the patient's airway and achieving adequate ventilation and oxygenation. If possible, physical restraints should be avoided, but restraints may need to be applied transiently in order to secure IV access. If a restraining blanket is used, it should be constructed of a strong netting or mesh to avoid increasing the patient's temperature by preventing heat dissipation. Protecting the patient from hypoglycemia and hypoxia are critical; therefore, high-flow oxygen should be routinely administered and 0.5 to 1.0 g/kg of $D_{50}W$ and 100 mg of thiamine should be given as clinically indicated. If the patient manifests severe agitation, IV doses of a benzodiazepine should be used until sedation is achieved (Table 65–1). Neuroleptic agents should be avoided, as they may confuse the clinical picture, impair heat dissipation, exacerbate an anticholinergic crisis, precipitate a dystonic reaction, or in some cases lower the seizure threshold and exacerbate lethality.[19,39,65,214] Diazepam, or another benzodiazepine such as lorazepam, should be used intravenously for initial management of seizures. Although no studies have compared barbiturates to phenytoin for control of cocaine-induced seizures, barbiturates are theoretically preferable because they also produce CNS sedation and are generally more effective for toxin-induced convulsions. If these agents are not rapidly effective, nondepolarizing neuromuscular blockade (eg, with vecuronium) and general anesthesia may be indicated. Succinylcholine, a depolarizing neuromuscular-blocking agent, may increase the risk of hyperkalemia in the setting of severe cocaine-induced rhabdomyolysis. Also the enzyme plasma cholinesterase is responsible for the metabolism of both succinylcholine and cocaine, so that if these two agents are used simultaneously, prolonged clinical effects of either or both agents might result.

Control of the patient's hyperthermia is best achieved by rapid cooling with an ice water bath. Conduction and evaporation are rapidly efficacious. Control of the associated agitation, psychosis, or seizures is essential to maintain cooling while avoiding cerebral, hepatic, and skeletal muscle cell destruction. There is no evidence that other pharmacologic agents (eg, dantrolene) enhance the cooling process in patients with life-threatening hyperthermia.[52]

Atrial tachydysrhythmias that do not respond to sedative-hypnotics or control of the central sympathetic stimulus and cooling should respond to verapamil or diltiazem. The treatment of cocaine-induced ventricular dysrhythmias depends upon the time between cocaine use, dysrhythmia onset, and commencement of treatment. Ventricular dysrhythmias that develop rapidly following cocaine use should be presumed to occur from the local anesthetic effects of cocaine on the myocardium. Animal evidence overwhelmingly demonstrates the importance of the type I antidysrhythmic effects of cocaine.[8,9,64,213] In fact, in some animal models, cocaine-induced wide-complex dysrhythmias respond to the administration of sodium bicarbonate, similar to dysrhythmias produced with other type IA and type IC agents (see Chaps. 52, 55, and 57, and Antidotes in Depth: Sodium Bicarbonate).[9,213] In addition, one animal model suggested that lidocaine exacerbated cocaine-induced seizures and dysrhythmias as a result of similar effects on sodium channels.[40] Although additive cardiac toxicities of lidocaine and cocaine might be anticipated because of lidocaine's IB antidysrhythmic effects, they have not been confirmed in other animal models.[64,72,213] Lidocaine has fast on-off sodium channel binding kinetics, and might be expected to compete with cocaine (which has slow on-off kinetics) for binding to the sodium channel. Because lidocaine rarely affects QRS duration, QRS would be expected to shorten as lidocaine displaces cocaine from sodium channels. In humans with cocaine toxicity, wide-complex dysrhythmias also have been reported.[103,208] Although bicarbonate therapy may be preferable, and has been used effectively,[208] lidocaine may also be beneficial, especially after benzodiazepines have been given to prevent the additive convulsant effects demonstrated in animals.[40,72] In patients who present several hours after the last use of cocaine, the ventricular dysrhythmias may be generated by an ischemic myocardium, and standard management for ventricular dysrhythmias (including lidocaine) is indicated, and appears safe in one clinical case series.[186] Torsades de pointes is a rare complication of cocaine use.[178] Because this probably relates to cocaine's ability to block potassium channels (see Chap. 8), bicarbonate therapy would not be indicated because the resultant hypokalemia would be expected to exacerbate this effect. Torsades de pointes resulting from cocaine toxicity should be managed with magnesium and overdrive pacing.

Patients with significant elevation of creatine kinase or myoglobinuria (rhabdomyolysis) require vigorous hydration to maintain a urine output of at least 3 mL/kg per hour; sodium bicarbonate to alkalinize the urine; and hemodialysis if renal failure occurs.

What Are the Therapeutic Principles and Treatment of the Vascular Manifestations of Cocaine Intoxication?

The vascular effects of cocaine occur through the acute stimulation of coronary artery vasoconstriction, in situ thrombus formation, platelet aggregation, decreased endogenous fibrinolysis, and increased myocardial oxygen demand secondary to hypertension and tachycardia. Chronic cocaine users may have a more exaggerated oxygen supply–demand mismatch because of left ven-

TABLE 65–1. TREATMENT SUMMARY FOR SPECIFIC COCAINE RELATED MEDICAL DISEASES

Medical Problem	Treatments
Dysrhythmias	
Sinus tachycardia	Observation, oxygen, cooling, $D_{50}W$ (as indicated)
	Diazepam 5-10 mg IV or lorazepam 2–4 mg IV titrated to effect (if indicated)
Supraventricular tachycardia	Observation, oxygen, cooling, $D_{50}W$ (as indicated)
	Diazepam 5 mg IV or lorazepam 2–4 mg IV titrated to effect (if indicated)
	Diltiazem 20 mg IV or verapamil 5 mg IV
	Adenosine 6 or 12 mg IV for AV node reentry
	Cardioversion if hemodynamically unstable
Ventricular dysrhythmias	Oxygen, cooling, $D_{50}W$ (as indicated)
	Diazepam 5 mg IV or lorazepam 2–4 mg IV (if indicated)
	Hypertonic sodium bicarbonate
	Lidocaine 1.5 mg/kg IV bolus followed by 2 mg/min infusion
	Defibrillation if hemodynamically unstable
Ischemic chest pain	Oxygen, cooling, $D_{50}W$ (as indicated)
	Diazepam 5 mg IV or lorazepam 2–4 mg IV titrated to effect (if indicated)
	Chewable 325 mg aspirin
	Nitroglycerin 1/150 g sublingual × 3 every 5 min followed by a drip titrated to a mean arterial pressure reduction of 10% or relief of chest pain
	Morphine sulfate 2 mg IV titrated to pain relief
	Phentolamine 1 mg IV; repeat in 5 min
	Verapamil 5–10 mg IV
	Heparin 80 units/kg bolus followed by 18 units/kg/h
	Mechanical reperfusion (angioplasty)
	Thrombolytic therapy
Hypertension	Oxygen, cooling, $D_{50}W$ (as indicated)
	Diazepam 5 mg IV or lorazepam 2–4 mg IV titrated to effect (if indicated)
	Phentolamine 1 mg IV; repeat in 5 min
	Nitroglycerin or nitroprusside drip titrated to effect
Pulmonary edema	Furosemide 20–40 mg IV
	Morphine sulfate 2 mg IV titrated to pain relief
	Nitroglycerin drip titrated to blood pressure or respiratory status
	Consider phentolamine or nitroprusside
Hyperthermia	Oxygen, $D_{50}W$ (as indicated)
	Diazepam 5 mg IV or lorazepam 2–4 mg IV titrated to effect (if indicated)
	Ice baths, Cool water with fans
	Cool environment with minimal activity
Neurologic symptoms	
Anxiety and agitation	Diazepam 5–10 mg IV or lorazepam 2–4 mg IV titrated to effect
Seizures	Diazepam 5–10 mg IV or lorazepam 2–4 mg IV titrated to effect
	Phenobarbital 25–50 mg/min up to 10–20 mg/kg
Intracranial hemorrhage	Neurosurgery consult
Rhabdomyolysis	Cardiac monitoring
	Serial potassium determinations
	IV hydration to maintain urine output at 3 mL/kg/h.
	Sodium bicarbonate titrated to an alkaline urine
	Hemodialysis, as necessary, for renal failure
Cocaine washed-out syndrome	Supportive care
Body packers	Activated charcoal
	Whole-bowel irrigation
	Admission to monitored setting even if asymptomatic
	Laparotomy or endoscopic retrieval for obstruction or symptoms of intoxication

tricular hypertrophy and premature atherosclerosis. Other vascular beds may be involved based on identical mechanisms. Treatment of the vascular manifestations of cocaine intoxication should focus on the reversible causes of oxygen supply–demand mismatch: arterial vasoconstriction, platelet aggregation, thrombus formation, hypertension, and tachycardia.

Coronary Vasoconstriction. Studies in the cardiac catheterization laboratory have helped elucidate the mechanisms of coronary artery vasoconstriction and have evaluated several treatment options. In these studies, adults without prior cocaine use who were undergoing coronary catheterization for evaluation of underlying coronary artery disease were given 2 mg/kg of intranasal cocaine. Patients developed an increase in heart rate, blood pressure, and coronary vascular resistance. Coronary arterial diameter was diffusely narrowed by approximately 13%.[119] The effect of cocaine occurs in both the left and right coronary systems.[207] Following infusion of phentolamine (0.4 mg/min), an alpha-adrenergic antagonist, these parameters returned to baseline.[119] This suggests that cocaine-induced vasoconstriction is caused through an alpha-adrenergic mechanism and that phentolamine may be useful for treatment of cocaine-induced myocardial ischemia. At least one case report supports the use of phentolamine for patients with cocaine-induced myocardial ischemia.[88] Studies in the cardiac catheterization laboratory also demonstrate that nitroglycerin will reverse cocaine-induced vasoconstriction,[15] and clinical case series have found that in patients nitroglycerin relieves cocaine-induced chest pain.[93] Chronic cocaine users, who may be more prone to atherosclerosis, might be at higher risk of ischemia because there is enhanced vasoconstriction at sites of significant coronary artery stenosis.[51] In addition, cigarette smoking enhances cocaine's vasoconstrictive effects.[86]

Data regarding the efficacy of calcium channel blockers for the treatment of cocaine toxicity are contradictory. Some studies of cocaine-intoxicated animals that were pretreated with calcium channel blockers have yielded favorable results in a variety of end-points such as survival, seizures, and cardiac dysrrhythmias.[10,146,204] In contradistinction, other studies have found adverse effects in which these same outcomes were analyzed.[37] In experimental models of cocaine-intoxicated animals that were not pretreated with calcium channel blockers, the subsequent administration of these agents has not been beneficial.[38,68,191] Using the human cardiac catheterization model of cocaine toxicity, verapamil does reverse cocaine-induced coronary artery vasoconstriction.[149] However, large-scale multicenter clinical trials in over 5000 patients with myocardial ischemia unrelated to cocaine did not find beneficial effects of calcium channel blockers on important outcomes such as survival. As a result, the role of calcium channel blockers in patients with cocaine-induced vascular ischemia remains unclear.

Coronary artery vasoconstriction was exacerbated by the administration of propranolol, a beta-adrenergic antagonist, and resulted in anginal symptoms and ST-segment elevation in one of the study patients.[118] Because propranolol inhibits the $beta_2$-adrenergic receptors, an unopposed alpha-adrenergic receptor stimulation may occur, resulting in vasoconstriction and an increased blood pressure. This unopposed alpha-adrenergic effect has been observed in some case series.[162–164,173] The increased afterload along with decreased left ventricular function might adversely effect systemic blood flow and tissue perfusion. These human observations were confirmed in experimental animal models of cocaine toxicity, where the use of beta-adrenergic antagonists led to decreased coronary blood flow, increased seizure frequency, and high fatality rates.[19,65,191,192,204,206] The use of short acting beta-adrenergic antagonists such as esmolol has shown similarly poor results,[160,173] with unopposed alpha effects resulting in significant increases in blood pressure for up to 25% of patients. As a result of the compelling animal and human data, the use of beta-adrenergic antagonists for the treatment of cocaine toxicity must be considered absolutely contraindicated.[70,85,86]

Labetalol does not appear to offer any advantages over pure beta-adrenergic antagonists. Although some case reports have not shown adverse outcomes,[45,56,109] labetalol has substantially more beta-adrenergic antagonism than alpha-adrenergic antagonist effects.[195] Labetalol use results in unopposed alpha effects with severe hypertension in patients with pheochromocytomas,[13] increases the risk of seizure and death in animal models of cocaine toxicity,[191] and does not reverse coronary artery vasoconstriction in humans.[11] The role, if any, for beta and mixed alpha and beta-adrenergic antagonists in the treatment of cocaine intoxication has not been established. The choice of an antihypertensive agent that is rapid-acting and easily and reliably controlled favors the use of vasodilating agents such as nitroprusside, nitroglycerin, or an alpha-adrenergic antagonist such as phentolamine.

Noncoronary Vasoconstriction. Cocaine-induced constriction of the cerebral,[18,124] ophthalmic,[81] pulmonary,[36,189] mesenteric,[53,147] and musculoskeletal[217] vascular beds is well described in human case reports. Additionally, animal models describe cerebral vasoconstriction.[131] Although inadequately studied, all of these effects are presumed to occur by mechanisms similar to those described for cocaine-induced coronary vasoconstriction. As a result, the treatment strategies described should be initiated in patients with clinical signs and symptoms suggestive of vasoconstriction in noncoronary vascular beds. Caution should be exercised, as experimental or clinical support for these therapies is largely absent.

Platelet and Thrombus Formation. Cocaine can directly injure the vascular endothelium, increase platelet aggregation through both direct and indirect pathways, and impair normal fibrinolytic pathways by enhancing the effects of endogenous tissue plasminogen activator inhibitor.[141,166,167,176,201] As a result, the use of aspirin, heparin, and thrombolytic agents makes theoretical sense in the setting of vascular ischemia.[79,83,86,87] When considering the use of thrombolytic agents for acute myocardial infarction, the clinician must recognize that many young patients may have benign early repolarization and that only a small percentage of patients with cocaine-associated chest pain syndromes and J-point/ST-segment elevation will be sustaining an acute infarction.[97] In addition, there are several case reports that document adverse outcomes following thrombolytic administration in patients with recent cocaine use.[17,98,128] The use of thrombolytic agents for vascular ischemia should be reserved for patients who are clearly having myocardial infarction, cannot be taken for invasive reperfusion, fail to respond to vasodilator therapy, and have low risk for cerebrovascular or other serious bleeding catastrophes.[79] The use of thrombolytic therapy for cocaine-induced cerebrovascular or mesenteric ischemia has not been studied.

Hypertension and Tachycardia. The hemodynamic effects of cocaine rarely require specific treatment. Treatments aimed at the resolution of anxiety, agitation, hyperthermia, and ischemia will often lead to resolution of the abnormal hemodynamic parameters. When necessary, treatment aimed at the central effects of cocaine, such as benzodiazepines, will usually lead to reduction in blood pressure and heart rate. When hypertension fails to respond to sedation, it can be managed with sodium nitroprusside (0.5 to 10 μg/kg per min) titrated to achieve and maintain a normal blood pressure. Intravenous phentolamine at doses of 0.4 mg/min or nitroglycerin (starting at a dose of 10 μg/min) are also effective vasodilators and may improve coronary perfusion.[15,119] Cocaine-intoxicated patients should be considered to have an acute elevation in blood pressure. Reduction of the blood pressure to a normal level should therefore occur, without concern of cerebral hypoperfusion, unless there is documentation or clinical evidence of long-standing hypertension.

The other cardiovascular end-organ manifestations of cocaine intoxication may necessitate specific intervention. The general strategies for managing catecholamine excess, myocardial ischemia, and hypertension are summarized in Table 65–1 and allow for very case-specific approaches to complicated examples, such as aortic dissection, mesenteric ischemia, and abruptio placenta. These cases or presentation of the patient in shock necessitate a critical understanding of the risk-to-benefit ratios for pharmacologic, toxicologic, and surgical or obstetric interventions.

What Is the Differential Diagnosis of Cocaine Intoxication?

The differential diagnosis of cocaine toxicity can be subdivided into three areas of consideration: the sympathomimetic toxidrome, specific complaints directly related to cocaine, and disease processes masked or confounded by cocaine.

Sympathomimetic and anticholinergic toxidromes are both characterized by hyperthermia, hypertension, tachycardia, tachypnea, altered mental status, seizures, and mydriasis. Diaphoresis and hyperactive bowel sounds suggest a sympathomimetic toxidrome; while urinary retention, an adynamic ileus, and dry skin characterize an anticholinergic toxidrome. Table 65–2 shows the differential diagnosis for the sympathomimetic toxidrome. Nasal septal ulcerations, perforations, or atrophic mucosa may help identify patients who use intranasal cocaine, but may also result from amphetamine use.

Specific complaints directly related to cocaine may include such signs and symptoms as chest pain, abdominal pain, or shortness of breath. Although cocaine use can result in these symptoms, the differential diagnosis includes disease processes both related to and unrelated to cocaine. For example, chest pain may be caused by chest wall rhabdomyolysis, pneumothorax, or myocardial ischemia resulting from cocaine use or it may be caused by pneumonia or pleurisy unrelated to cocaine. A history of recent cocaine use significantly increases the likelihood of serious etiologies for many otherwise common complaints. Although most cocaine-related adverse events occur within several hours of cocaine use, remote cocaine use (in the past several weeks) is also associated with vascular disasters in patients without other known predisposing factors.

Cocaine-intoxicated patients may have concurrent ethanol ingestions, or mixed overdoses that mask some of the effects of cocaine. On the other hand, serious medical problems should not be falsely attributed to cocaine without excluding underlying medical pathology. For example, patients with an altered mental status may still need to undergo computerized tomography to exclude a subdural hematoma that may not have been caused directly by cocaine. Mental status changes caused by cocaine are short lived. Waiting too long to see if the patient's mental status "clears" after cocaine is metabolized may have adverse consequences.

The evaluation and differential diagnosis of the agitated patient illustrates the difficulty in assessing pa-

TABLE 65–2. DIFFERENTIAL DIAGNOSIS OF THE SYMPATHOMIMETIC TOXIDROME

Toxins
Cocaine, phencyclidine, amphetamines, hallucinogens, caffeine, phenylpropanolamine, theophylline, ephedrine, pseudoephedrine, tyramine, MAO inhibitors
Metabolic Derangements
Pheochromocytoma, hypoglycemia, thyrotoxicosis
Psychiatric Disturbances
Schizophrenia, psychosis, mania
Drug Withdrawal
Ethanol, sedative-hypnotics
Neurologic Abnormalities
Complex status epilepticus

tients with cocaine intoxication. Agitation could be secondary to toxic, metabolic, or structural abnormalities, and various states of withdrawal (sedative-hypnotics and ethanol). Patients intoxicated with hallucinogens, amphetamines, phencyclidine, and cocaine can all present with agitation. Phencyclidine (PCP) generally produces miosis, bidirectional nystagmus, and as in the case of LSD or amphetamines, lasts longer than a cocaine reaction. Hypoglycemia can present with similar derangements. Severe alcohol or sedative hypnotic withdrawal produce almost identical findings. Pheochromocytoma, thyroid storm, and central nervous system structural lesions such as hematoma, tumor, emboli, abscess, or contusion can present with agitation. The thoughtful and thorough evaluation of such patients will lead to the correct diagnosis.

Which Adjunctive Tests Can Be Helpful to Diagnose and Manage Acute Cocaine Intoxication?

Most patients with mild cocaine toxicity do not require laboratory evaluation. When ordered, serum electrolytes may reflect the adrenergic effects of cocaine with hyperglycemia and hypokalemia. Patients with rhabdomyolysis, particularly if they are acidemic, may have hyperkalemia. The serum creatinine may be elevated in cases of rhabdomyolysis, renal failure, or renal infarction. Serial electrolyte determinations are necessary in patients with rhabdomyolysis and/or renal failure. Increases in leukocyte count may also occur. The total creatine kinase (CK) will be elevated in cases of rhabdomyolysis, and in almost half of patients with chest pain, most of whom will have myocardial infarction excluded by isoenzyme analysis.[94] Elevated creatine kinase MB usually indicates a myocardial infarction, but "false positive" elevations may occur.[95,134,202] Use of cardiac troponin I may be needed to confirm a myocardial infarction.[134,202]

Chest radiography should be used to detect pneumonia, pulmonary infarction, pneumothorax, pneumomediastinum, and pneumopericardium.[48] Abdominal radiography may detect cocaine packages. Computerized tomography should be used to detect cerebrovascular events. Magnetic resonance imaging or angiography may be useful for aortic dissection. Additional laboratory or diagnostic testing should be considered depending on the clinical condition. For example, lumbar puncture should be performed in patients with suspected subarachnoid hemorrhage and normal head CTs; ventilation–perfusion scans should be used in patients suspected of pulmonary infarction.

The initial electrocardiogram is less sensitive and less specific for identification of myocardial infarction in patients with cocaine-associated chest pain when compared to traditional patients with chest pain. Myocardial infarction clearly occurs in both patients with normal and abnormal electrocardiograms. ST-segment elevation due to early repolarization is common in young cocaine users without myocardial infarction.[59,94,97] ST-segment elevations that meet standard thrombolysis criteria are present in 11 to 43% of cocaine-associated chest pain patients who are not found to infarct.

TABLE 65-3. LABORATORY ASSAYS FOR COCAINE AND BENZOYLECGONINE (BE)

Laboratory Assay	Specimen	BE[a]	Cocaine (ng/mL)	Sensitivity (ng/mL)
EMIT (enzyme-multiplied immunoassay technique)	Urine	X	—	200–300
RIA (radioimmunoassay)	Urine/blood	X	>50	5–100
TLC (thin-layer chromatography)	Urine	X	—	1000
GC (gas chromatography)	Serum/urine	X	X	200–300
HPLC (high-pressure liquid chromatography)	Serum/urine	X	X	200–300
GC-MS (gas chromatography-mass spectrometry)	Serum/urine	X	X	200–300

X = Detectable.
[a]BE = benzoylecgonine.

Nasal swabs and serum or urine analysis for cocaine can be performed. Laboratory tests available are gas chromatography (GC) and thin-layer chromatography (TLC) (benzoylecgonine in the serum or urine), as well as EMIT (enzyme-multiplied immunoassay techniques) and gas chromatography-mass spectrometry (Table 65–3). Because of the legal and social implications of cocaine use, toxicologic assays have become very important. The relative sensitivity of the screening and definitive assays for cocaine and benzoylecgonine are presented in Table 65–3. Urine immunoassays for cocaine metabolites generally detect the major metabolite of cocaine, benzoylecgonine, at or above concentrations of 300 ng/mL. Usually, the presence of cocaine or its metabolites can be detected for 48 to 72 hours after use.[4] Rarely, using more sensitive methods (GC/MS), cocaine metabolites have been detected for up 3 weeks after the last use.[210]

What Is the Evaluation and Treatment for Body Packers and Body Stuffers?

The act of swallowing containers, condoms, balloons, plastic bags, or packages filled with illegal drugs for the purpose of smuggling is called "body packing" and the individual is called a "mule."[82,132] Patients being arrested who swallow illegal drugs to conceal the evidence are referred to as a "body stuffer."[77,168] Unlike body packers, whose contraband has been very carefully packaged to protect them and the drugs from gastrointestinal absorption, body stuffers do not take such precautions, and drug absorption is common. Body stuffers also tend to

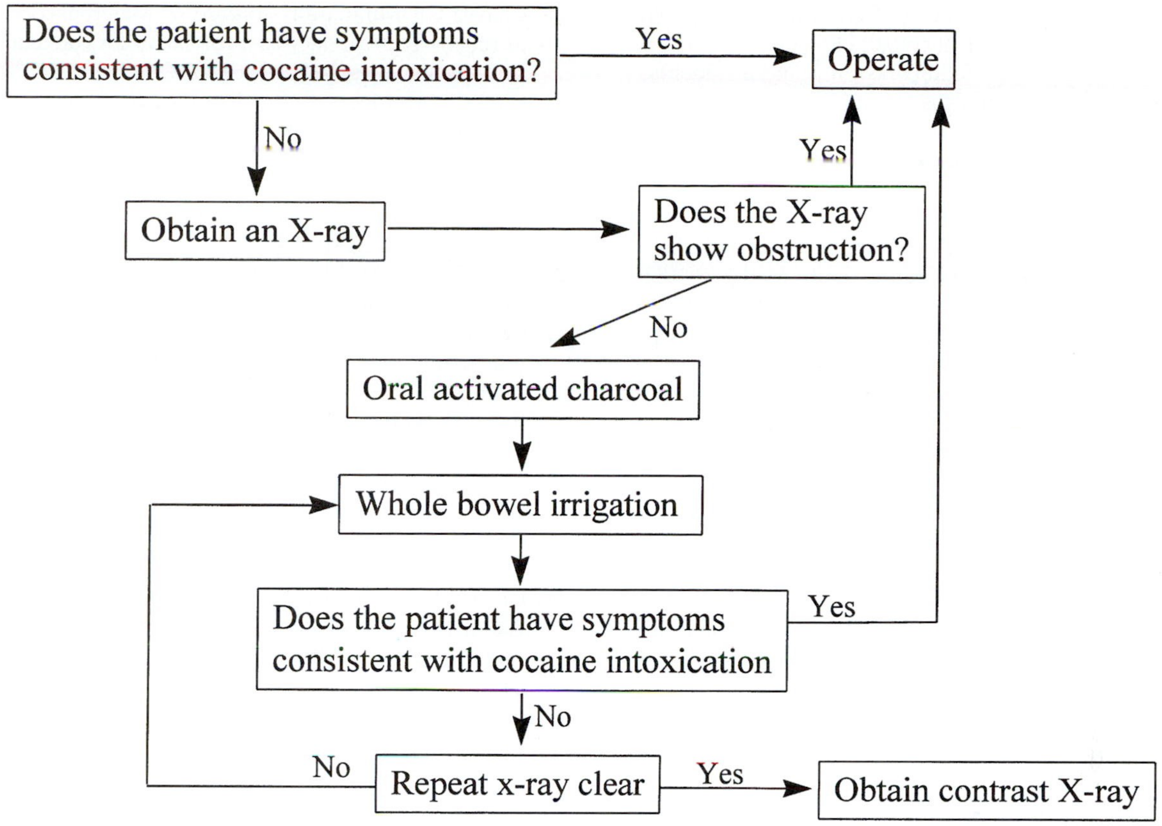

Figure 65–3. Algorithm for the clinical assessment and management of cocaine body packers.

ingest all the drugs they possess, potentially resulting in a polypharmaceutic overdose. Both body packers and body stuffers are unlikely to admit their ingestion. Body packers may be discovered in airports having just arrived from a foreign country known to export illegal drugs. Body stuffers are likely to be found near their homes.

Body stuffers may be seen before symptoms have developed, and recently ingested drugs may be recovered from the stomach by emesis or lavage, preventing absorption. Activated charcoal should be given immediately; multiple-dose activated charcoal and a cathartic or whole-bowel irrigation may be indicated. In body packers, the drugs are usually located in the small and large bowel and are quite difficult to recover. Most body packers may be diagnosed by radiographic means, as the packages used to smuggle drugs are often radiopaque or have a distinct radiographic characteristic.[132] Body stuffers are unlikely to be diagnosed by radiography.[77] Most body packers will be asymptomatic unless leakage occurs. Symptomatic patients should be considered a medical emergency, and be evaluated for surgical removal of the packets. Both body packers and body stuffers should be treated with activated charcoal to limit cocaine absorption and whole-bowel irrigation to decrease gastrointestinal transit time.[82,203] They should be monitored in an intensive care unit setting until the cocaine bags have been eliminated, even if they are asymptomatic. Follow-up plain radiography and a barium swallow with small bowel follow-through offer definitive reassurance that all packages have been evacuated.[82] This treatment plan is summarized in Figure 65–3.

In rare cases, surgical removal may be necessary for bowel obstruction or cocaine toxicity. Obstruction at the ileocecal valve or splenic flexure may necessitate laparotomy with enterotomy. Although some have operated on patients with gastric outlet obstruction, others have successfully retrieved a bag with endoscopic techniques.[82]

Acknowledgment

Neal A. Lewin, MD contributed to this chapter in the previous edition.

References

1. Acker D, Sachs BP, Tracey KJ: Abruptio placentae associated with cocaine use. Am J Obstet Gynecol 1983;146: 220–221.
2. Adkins MS, Gaines WE, Anderson WA, et al: Chronic type A aortic dissection: An unusual complication of cocaine inhalation. Ann Thorac Surg 1993;56:977–979.

3. Albertson TE, Walby WF, Derlet RW: Stimulant induced pulmonary toxicity. Chest 1995;108:1140–1149.
4. Ambre J: The urinary excretion of cocaine and metabolites in humans: A kinetic analysis of published data. J Anal Toxicol 1985;9:241–245.
5. Amin M, Gabelman G, Karpel J, et al: Acute myocardial infarction and chest pain: Syndromes after cocaine use. Am J Cardiol 1990;66:1434–1437.
6. Anand V, Siami G, Stone WJ: Cocaine-associated rhabdomyolysis and acute renal failure. South Med J 1989;82: 67–69.
7. Barash P: Cocaine 1980: An update. Wkly Anesthesiol Update (lesson 9) 1980;3:1–5.
8. Bauman JL, Grawe JJ, Winecoff AP, Hariman RJ: Cocaine-related sudden cardiac death: A hypothesis correlating basic science and clinical observations. J Clin Pharmacol 1994;34:902–911.
9. Beckman KJ, Parker RB, Hariman RJ, et al: Hemodynamic and electrophysiological actions of cocaine: Effects of sodium bicarbonate as an antidote in dogs. Circulation 1991; 83:1799–1807.
10. Billman GE, Hoskins RS: Cocaine-induced ventricular fibrillation: Protection afforded by the calcium antagonist verapamil. FASEB J 1988;2:2990–2995.
11. Boehrer JD, Moliterno DJ, Willard JE, et al: Influence of labetalol of cocaine-induced coronary vasoconstriction in humans. Am J Med 1993;94:608–610.
12. Borne RF, Bedford JA, Buelke JL, et al: Biological effects of cocaine, derivatives I: Improved synthesis and pharmacologic evaluation of norcocaine. J Pharm Sci 1977;66: 119–129.
13. Briggs RSJ, Birtwell AJ, Pohl JEF: Hypertensive response to labetalol in pheochromocytoma. Lancet 1978;1: 1045–1046.
14. Brody SL, Wrenn KD, Wilber MM, Slovis CM: Predicting the severity of cocaine associated rhabdomyolysis. Ann Emerg Med 1990;19:1137–1143.
15. Brogan WC, Lange RA, Kim AS, et al: Alleviation of cocaine-induced coronary vasoconstriction by nitroglycerin. J Am Coll Cardiol 1991;18:581–586.
16. Brookoff D, Rotondo MF, Shaw LM, et al: Cocaethylene levels in patients who test positive for cocaine. Ann Emerg Med. 1996;27:316–320.
17. Bush HS: Cocaine associated myocardial infarction: A word of caution about thrombolytic therapy. Chest 1988; 94:878.
18. Caplan LR, Hier DB, Banks G: Current concepts of cerebrovascular disease: Stroke and drug abuse. Stroke 1982; 13:869–872.
19. Catravas JD, Waters IW: Acute cocaine intoxication in the conscious dog: Studies on the mechanism of lethality. J Pharmacol Exp Ther 1981;217:350–356.
20. Chaisson RE, Bacchetti P, Osmond D, et al: Cocaine use and HIV infection in intravenous drug users in San Francisco. JAMA 1989; 261:561–565.
21. Chambers HF, Morris DL, Tauber MG, Modin G: Cocaine use and the risk for endocarditis in intravenous drug users. Ann Intern Med 1987;106:833–836.
22. Chang RA, Rossi NF: Intermittent cocaine use associated with recurrent dissection of the thoracic and abdominal aorta. Chest 1995;108:1758–1762.
23. Chavez GF, Mulinare J, Cordero JF: Maternal cocaine use during early pregnancy as a risk factor for congenital urogenital anomalies. JAMA 1989;262:795–798.
24. Chokshi SK, Moore R, Pandian NG, et al: Reversible cardiomyopathy associated with cocaine intoxication. Ann Intern Med 1989;111:1039–1040.
25. Chouteau M, Namerow PB, Leppert P: The effect of cocaine abuse on birth weight and gestational age. Obstet Gynecol 1988;72:351–354.
26. Choy-Kwong M, Lipton RB: Seizures in hospitalized cocaine users. Neurology 1989;39:425–427.
27. Covert RF, Schreiber MD, Tebbett IR, Torgerson LJ: Hemodynamic and cerebral blood flow effects of cocaine, cocaethylene and benzoylecgonine in conscious and anesthetized fetal lambs. J Pharmacol Exp Ther 1994;270: 188–126.
28. Cregler LL: Aortic dissection and cocaine use. Am Heart J 1992;124:1665. Letter.
29. Cregler LL, Mark H: Relation to acute myocardial infarction to cocaine abuse. Am J Cardiol 1985;56:794.
30. Crumb WJ, Clarkson CW: Characterization of sodium channel blocking properties of the major metabolites of cocaine in single cardiac myocytes. J Pharmacol Exp Ther 1992;261:910–917.
31. Cucco RA, Yoo OH, Gregler L, et al: Non-fatal pulmonary edema after freebase cocaine smoking. Am Rev Resp Dis 1987;136:179–181.
32. Dailey RH: Fatality secondary to misuse of TAC solution. Ann Emerg Med 1988;17:159–160.
33. Daya MR, Burton BT, Schleiss MR, et al: Recurrent seizures following mucosal application of TAC. Ann Emerg Med 1988;17:646–648.
34. Dehner D, Hamilton GC: Seizures following topical applications of local anesthetics to burn patients. Ann Emerg Med 1984;13:456–458.
35. Del Aguila C, Rosman H: Myocardial infarction during cocaine withdrawal. Ann Intern Med 1990;112:712. Letter.
36. Delaney K, Hoffman RS: Pulmonary infarction associated with crack cocaine use in a previously healthy 23 year old woman. Am J Med 1991;91:92–94.
37. Derlet RW, Albertson TE: Diazepam in the prevention of seizures and death in cocaine-intoxicated rats. Ann Emerg Med 1989;18:542–546.
38. Derlet RW, Albertson TE: Potentiation of cocaine toxicity with calcium channel blockers. Am J Emerg Med 1989;7: 464–468.
39. Derlet RW, Albertson TE, Rice P: The effect of haloperidol in cocaine and amphetamine intoxication. J Emerg Med 1989;7:633–637.
40. Derlet RW, Albertson TE, Tharratt RS: Lidocaine potentiation of cocaine toxicity. Ann Emerg Med 1991;20:135–138.
41. Devenyi P: Cocaine complications and pseudocholinesterase. Ann Intern Med 1989;110:167–168. Letter.
42. Devenyi P, Schneiderman JF, Devenyi RG, Lawby L: Cocaine-induced central retinal artery occlusion. Can Med Assoc J 1988;138:129–130.
43. Doberczak TM, Shanzer S, Senie RT, et al: Neonatal neurologic and electroencephalographic effects of intrauterine cocaine exposure. J Pediatr 1988;113:354–358.
44. Dronen SC: Complications of TAC. Ann Emerg Med 1983;12:333. Letter.

45. Dusenberry SJ, Hicks MJ, Mariani PJ: Labetalol treatment of cocaine toxicity. Ann Emerg Med 1987;16:235. Letter.
46. Endress C, Kling GA: Cocaine-induced small-bowel perforation. Am J Radiol 1990;154:1346–1347.
47. Ettinger NA, Albin RJ: A review of the respiratory effects of smoking cocaine. Am J Med 1989;87:664–668.
48. Eurman DW, Potash HI, Eyler WR, et al: Chest pain and dyspnea related to "crack" cocaine smoking: Value of chest radiography. Radiology 1989;172:459–462.
49. Fishel R, Hamamoto G, Barbul A, et al: Cocaine colitis: Is this a new syndrome? Dis Colon Rectum 1985;28:264–266.
50. Fisher A, Holroyd BR: Cocaine-associated dissection of the thoracic aorta. J Emerg Med 1992;10:723–727.
51. Flores ED, Lange RA, Cigarroa RG, et al: Effect of cocaine on coronary artery dimensions in atherosclerotic coronary artery: Enhanced vasoconstriction at sites of significant stenoses. J Am Coll Cardiol 1990;16:74–79.
52. Fox AW: More on rhabdomyolysis associated with cocaine intoxication. N Engl J Med 1989;321:1271. Letter.
53. Freudenberger RS, Cappell MS, Hutt DA: Intestinal infarction after intravenous cocaine administration. Ann Intern Med 1990;113:715–716.
54. Fritsma GA, Leikin JB, Maturen AJ, et al: Detection of anticardiolipin antibody in patients with cocaine abuse. J Emerg Med 1991;9:37–43.
55. Gawin FH, Kleber HD: Abstinence symptomatology and psychiatric diagnosis in cocaine abusers. Arch Gen Psychiatry 1986;43:107–113.
56. Gay GR, Loper KA: The use of labetalol in the management of cocaine crisis. Ann Emerg Med 1988;17:282–283.
57. Gioia G, Manuel M, Russell J, et al: Myocardial perfusion pattern in patients with cocaine induced chest pain. Am J Cardiol 1995;75:396–398.
58. Giros B, Jaber M, Jones S, et al: Hyperlocomotion and indifference to cocaine and amphetamine in mice lacking the dopamine transporter. Nature 1996;379:606–612.
59. Gitter MJ, Goldsmith ER, Dunbar DN, Sharkey SW: Cocaine and chest pain: Clinical features and outcome of patients hospitalized to rule out myocardial infarction. Ann Intern Med 1991;115:277–282.
60. Golbe LI, Merkin MD: Cerebral infarction in a user of freebase cocaine. Neurology 1986;36:1602–1604.
61. Gottfried MR, Kloss MW, Graham D, et al: Ultrastructure of experimental cocaine hepatotoxicity. Hepatology 1986; 6:299–304.
62. Grafia A, Valverde JL, Borondo JC, et al: Vascular lesions in intestinal ischemia induced by cocaine-alcohol abuse: Report of a fatal case due to overdose. J Forensic Sci 1990; 35:740–745.
63. Grant SA, Hoffman RS: Use of tetracaine, epinephrine and cocaine as a topical anesthetic in the emergency department. Ann Emerg Med 1992;21:987–997.
64. Grawe JJ, Hariman RJ, Winecoff AP, et al: Reversal of the electrocardiographic effects of cocaine by lidocaine, 2. Concentration-effect relationships. Pharmacotherapy 194; 14:704–711.
65. Guinn MM, Bedford JA, Wilson MC: Antagonism of intravenous cocaine lethality in nonhuman primates. Clin Toxicol 1980;16:499–508.
66. Haddad LM: 1978: Cocaine in perspective. JACEP 1979; 8:374–376.
67. Haim DY, Lippman ML, Goldberg SK, Walkenstein MD: The pulmonary complications of crack cocaine. A comprehensive review. Chest 1995;107:233–240.
68. Hale SL, Alker KJ, Rezkalla SH, et al: Nifedipine protects the heart from the acute deleterious effects of cocaine if administered before but not after cocaine. Circulation 1991;83:1437–1443.
69. Hale SL, Alker KJ, Rezkalla S, et al: Adverse effects of cocaine on cardiovascular dynamics, myocardial blood flow, and coronary artery diameter in an experimental model. Am Heart J 1989;118:927–933.
70. Haynes S, Stork CM, Hoffman RS, Goldfrank L: Beta-adrenergic blockade in cocaine toxicity. J Emerg Med 1995;13:537–538. Letter.
71. Heikkila RE, Orlansky H, Cohen G: Studies on the distinction between uptake inhibition and release of dopamine in rat brain tissue slices. Biochem Pharmacol 1975;24: 847–852.
72. Heit J, Hoffman RS, Goldfrank LR: The effects of lidocaine pretreatment on cocaine neurotoxicity and lethality in mice. Acad Emerg Med 1994;1:438–442.
73. Henderson CE, Torbey M: Rupture of intracranial aneurysm associated with cocaine use during pregnancy. Am J Perinatol 1988;5:142–143.
74. Henning RJ, Wilson LD, Glauser JM: Cocaine plus ethanol is more cardiotoxic than cocaine or ethanol alone. Crit Care Med. 1994;22:1896–1906.
75. Herzlich BC, Arsura EL, Pagala M, et al: Rhabdomyolysis related to cocaine abuse. Ann Intern Med 1988;109: 335–336.
76. Hoffman CK, Goodman PC: Pulmonary edema in cocaine smokers. Radiology 1989;172:463–465.
77. Hoffman RS, Chiang WK, Weisman RS, et al: Prospective evaluation of "crack-vial" ingestions. Vet Hum Toxicol 1990;32:164–166.
78. Hoffman RS, Henry GL, Weisman RS, et al: Association between life-threatening cocaine toxicity and plasma cholinesterase activity. Ann Emerg Med 1991;21:247–253.
79. Hoffman RS, Hollander JE: Thrombolytic therapy in cocaine-induced myocardial infarction. Am J Emerg Med. 1996;14:693–695. Editorial.
80. Hoffman RS, Morasco R, Goldfrank LR: Administration of purified human plasma cholinesterase protects against cocaine toxicity in mice. J Toxicol Clin Toxicol 1996;34: 259–266.
81. Hoffman RS, Reimer BI: "Crack" cocaine-induced bilateral amblyopia. Am J Emerg Med 1993;11:35–37.
82. Hoffman RS, Smilkstein MJ, Goldfrank LR: Whole bowel irrigation and the cocaine "bodypacker": A new approach to a common problem. Am J Emerg Med 1990;8:523–527.
83. Hollander JE: Cocaine associated myocardial infarction. J Roy Soc Med 1996;89:443–447. Editorial.
84. Hollander JE: Cocaine associated myocardial ischemia. N Engl J Med 1996;334:536–537. Letter.
85. Hollander JE: Beta-adrenergic blockade in cocaine toxicity. J Emerg Med 1995:13:538–539. Letter.
86. Hollander JE: Management of cocaine associated myocardial ischemia. N Engl J Med 1995;333:1267–1272.
87. Hollander JE, Burstein JL, Shih RD, et al: Cocaine associated myocardial infarction: Clinical safety of thrombolytic therapy. Chest 1995;107:1237–1241.

88. Hollander JE, Carter WC, Hoffman RS: Use of phentolamine for cocaine induced myocardial ischemia. N Engl J Med 1992;327:361. Letter.
89. Hollander JE, Hoffman RS: Cocaine induced myocardial infarction: An analysis and review of the literature. J Emerg Med 1992;10:169–177.
90. Hollander JE, Hoffman RS, Burstein J, et al: Cocaine associated myocardial infarction. Mortality and complications. Arch Intern Med 1995;155:1081–1086.
91. Hollander JE, Hoffman RS, Cocaine Associated Myocardial Infarction Study Group: Cocaine induced "micro-infarcts": A new clinical entity or false positive CK-MB? Vet Hum Toxicol 1994;36:376. Abstract.
92. Hollander JE, Hoffman RS, Gennis P, et al: Cocaine associated chest pain: One year follow-up. Acad Emerg Med 1995;2:179–184.
93. Hollander JE, Hoffman RS, Gennis P, et al: Nitroglycerin in the treatment of cocaine associated chest pain: Clinical safety and efficacy. J Toxicol Clin Toxicol 1994;32:243–256.
94. Hollander JE, Hoffman RS, Gennis P, et al: Prospective multicenter evaluation of cocaine associated chest pain. Acad Emerg Med 1994;1:330–339.
95. Hollander JE, Levitt MA, Young GP, et al: The effect of cocaine on the specificity of cardiac markers. Acad Emerg Med 1997;4:422. Abstract.
96. Hollander JE, Lozano M Jr: Cocaine induced myocardial infarction secondary to a contaminant. Am J Emerg Med. 1993;11:681–682.
97. Hollander JE, Lozano M Jr, Fairweather P, et al: "Abnormal" electrocardiograms in patients with cocaine-associated chest pain are due to "normal" variants. J Emerg Med 1994;12:199–205.
98. Hollander JE, Wilson LD, Leo PJ, Shih RD: Complications from the use of thrombolytic agents in patients with cocaine associated chest pain. J Emerg Med 1996;14: 731–736.
99. Hong R, Matsuyama E, Nur K: Cardiomyopathy associated with the smoking of crystal methamphetamine. JAMA 1991;265:1152–1154.
100. Howard RE, Hueter DC, Davis GJ: Acute myocardial infarction following cocaine abuse in a young woman with normal coronary arteries. JAMA 1985;254:95–96.
101. Imperato-McGinley J, Gautier T, Ehlers HK, et al: Reversibility of catecholamine-induced dilated cardiomyopathy in a child with a pheochromocytoma. N Engl J Med 1987;316:793–796.
102. Isner JM, Chokshi SK: Cocaine and vasospasm. N Engl J Med 1989;321:1604–1607.
103. Isner JM, Estes M, Thompson PD, et al: Acute cardiac events temporally related to cocaine abuse. N Engl J Med 1986;315:1438–1443.
104. Itkonen J, Schnoll S, Glassroth J: Pulmonary dysfunction in "freebase" cocaine users. Arch Intern Med 1984;144: 2195–2197.
105. Jatlow PI: Drug of abuse profile: Cocaine. Clin Chem 1987; 33:66b–71b
106. Johnson MN, Karas SP, Hursey TL, et al: Cocaine "binging" produces left ventricular dysfunction. Circulation 1989;80(4 suppl 2):15. Abstract.
107. Kambam J, Mets B, Hickman RM, et al: The effects of inhibition of plasma cholinesterase and hepatic microsomal enzyme activity on cocaine, benzoylecgonine, ecgonine methyl ester, and norcocaine blood levels in pigs. J Lab Clin Med 1992;120:323–328.
108. Kanel GC, Cassidy W, Shuster L, et al: Cocaine induced liver injury: Comparison of morphologic features in man and experimental models. Hepatology 1990;11:646–651.
109. Karch SB: Managing cocaine crisis. Ann Emerg Med 1988;18:228–229. Letter.
110. Kaye BR, Fainstat M: Cerebral vasculitis associated with cocaine abuse. JAMA 1987;258:2104–2106.
111. Kline JN, Hirasuna JD: Pulmonary edema after freebase cocaine smoking-not due to an adulterant. Chest 1990; 97:1009–1010.
112. Kloss MW, Cavagnaro J, Rosen GM, Rauckman EJ: Involvement of FAD-containing monooxygenase in cocaine-induced hepatotoxicity. Toxicol Appl Pharmacol 1982; 64:88–93.
113. Kloss MW, Rosen GM, Rauckman EJ: Cocaine mediated hepatotoxicity: A critical review. Biochem Pharmacol 1984; 33:169–173.
114. Kloss MW, Rosen GM, Rauckman EJ: Evidence of enhanced in vivo lipid peroxidation after acute cocaine administration. Toxicol Lett 1983;15:65–70.
115. Konkol RJ, Erickson BA, Doerr JK, et al: Seizure induced by the cocaine metabolite benzoylecgonine in rats. Epilepsia 1992;33:420–427.
116. Krendel DA, Ditter SM, Frankel MR, Ross WK: Biopsy-proven cerebral vasculitis associated with cocaine abuse. Neurology 1990;40:1092–1094.
117. Kurth CD, Monitto C, Albuquerque ML, et al: Cocaine and its metabolites constrict cerebral arterioles in newborn pigs. J Pharmacol Exp Ther 1993;265:587–591.
118. Lange RA, Cigarroa RG, Flores ED, et al: Potentiation of cocaine-induced coronary vasoconstriction by beta-adrenergic blockade. Ann Intern Med 1990;112:897–903.
119. Lange RA, Cigarroa RG, Yancy CW, et al: Cocaine-induced coronary-artery vasoconstriction. N Engl J Med 1989;321:1557–1561.
120. Lee HS, LaMaute HR, Pizzi WF, et al: Acute gastrointestinal perforations associated with use of crack. Ann Surg 1990;211:15–17.
121. Leitman BS, Greengart A, Wasser HJ: Pneumomediastinum and pneumopericardium after cocaine abuse. AJR 1988;151:614.
122. Levine MAH, Nishakawa J: Acute myocardial infarction associated with cocaine withdrawal. Can Med Assoc J 1991;144:1139–1140.
123. Levine SR, Brust JCM, Futrell N, et al: Cerebrovascular complications of the use of the "crack" form of alkaloidal cocaine. N Engl J Med 1990;323:699–704.
124. Levine SR, Washington JM, Jefferson MF, et al: "Crack" cocaine-associated stroke. Neurology 1987;37:1849–1850.
125. Lichtenfeld PJ, Rubin DB, Feldman RS: Subarachnoid hemorrhage precipitated by cocaine snorting. Arch Neurol 1984;41:223–224.
126. Lisse JR, Davis CP, Thurmond-Anderle ME: Cocaine abuse and deep venous thrombosis. Ann Intern Med 1989; 110:571–572. Letter.
127. Lisse JR, Davis CP, Thurmond-Anderle ME: Upper ex-

tremity deep venous thrombosis: Increased prevalence due to cocaine abuse. Am J Med 1989;87:457–458.
128. LoVecchio F, Nelson L: Intraventricular bleeding after the use of thrombolytics in a cocaine user. Am J Emerg Med 1996;14:663–664.
129. MacDonald DI: Cocaine leads emergency department drug visits. JAMA 1987;258:2029.
130. MacGregor SN, Keith LG, Chasnoff IJ, et al: Cocaine use during pregnancy: Adverse perinatal outcome. Am J Obstet Gynecol 1987;157:686–690.
131. Madden J, Powers R: Effect of cocaine and cocaine metabolites on cerebral arteries in vitro. Life Sci 1990; 47:1109–1114.
132. McCarron MM, Wood JD: The cocaine body packer syndrome. JAMA 1983;250:1417–1420.
133. McHenry JG, Zeiter JH, Madion MP, Cowden JW: Corneal epithelial defects after smoking crack cocaine. Am J Ophthalmol 1989;108:732.
134. McLaurin MD, Apple FS, Henry TD, Sharkey SW: Cardiac troponin I and T concentrations in patients with cocaine-associated chest pain. Ann Clin Biochem 1996;33:183–186.
135. Menashe PI, Gottlieb JE: Hyperthermia, rhabdomyolysis, and myoglobinuric renal failure after recreational use of cocaine. South Med J 1988;81:379–381.
136. Merigian KS, Roberts JR: Cocaine intoxication: Hyperpyrexia, rhabdomyolysis and acute renal failure. J Toxicol Clin Toxicol 1987;25:135–148.
137. Mets B, Virag L: Lethal toxicity from equimolar infusions of cocaine and cocaine metabolites in conscious and anesthetized rats. Anesth Analg 1995;81:1033–1038.
138. Minor RL, Scott BD, Brown DD, Winniford MD: Cocaine induced myocardial infarction in patients with normal coronary arteries. Ann Intern Med 1991;115:797–806.
139. Mizrahi S, Loar D, Stamler B: Intestinal ischemia induced by cocaine abuse. Arch Surg 1988;123:394.
140. Mody CK, Miller BL, McIntyre HB, et al: Neurologic complications of cocaine abuse. Neurology 1988;38:1189–1193.
141. Moliterno DJ, Lange RA, Gerard RD, et al: Influence of intranasal cocaine on plasma constituents associated with endogenous thrombosis and thrombolysis. Am J Med 1994;96:492–496.
142. Moore TR, Sorg J, Miller L, et al: Hemodynamic effects of intravenous cocaine on the pregnant ewe and fetus. Am J Obstet Gynecol 1986;155:883–888.
143. Murray RJ, Albin RJ, Mergner W, et al: Diffuse alveolar hemorrhage temporally related to cocaine smoking. Chest 1988;93:427–429.
144. Murray RJ, Simialek J, Golle M, Albin RJ: Pulmonary artery medial hypertrophy in cocaine users without foreign particle microembolization. Chest 1989;96:1050–1053.
145. Nademanee K, Gorelick DA, Josephson MA, et al: Myocardial ischemia during cocaine withdrawal. Ann Intern Med 1989;111:876–880.
146. Nahas G, Trouve R, Demus JF, Von Sitron M: A calcium channel blocker as antidote to the cardiac effects of cocaine intoxication. N Engl J Med 1985; 313:519. Letter.
147. Nalbandian H, Sheth N, Dietrich R, Georgiou J: Intestinal ischemia caused by cocaine ingestion: Report of two cases. Surgery 1985;97:374–376.
148. National Institute of Drug Abuse: National household survey on drug abuse. Population estimates, 1991. DHHS number (ADM) 92–1887, Rockville, MD, Department of Health and Human Services, 1992.
149. Negus BH, Willard JE, Hillis LD, et al: Alleviation of cocaine induced coronary vasoconstriction with intravenous verapamil. Am J Cardiol 1994;73:510–513.
150. O'Donnell AE, Mappin G, Sepo TJ, et al: Interstitial pneumonitis associated with "crack" cocaine abuse. Chest 1991; 100:1155–1157.
151. Om A, Ellahham S, Ornato JP, et al: Medical complications of cocaine: Possible relationship to low plasma cholinesterase enzyme. Am Heart J 1993;125:1114–1117.
152. Pap A, Bradberry CW: Excitatory amino acid antagonists attenuate the effects of cocaine on extracellular dopamine in the nucleus accumbens. J Pharmacol Exp Ther 1995; 274:127–133.
153. Parker RB, Beckman KJ, Hariman RJI, et al: The electrophysiologic and arrhythmogenic effects of cocaine. Pharmacotherapy 1989;9:176. Abstract.
154. Pasternack PF, Colvin SB, Baumann FG: Cocaine-induced angina pectoris and acute myocardial infarction in patients younger than 40 years. Am J Cardiol 1985;55:847.
155. Patel RC, Dutta D, Schoenfeld SA: Free base cocaine use associated with bronchiolitis obliterans organizing pneumonia. Ann Intern Med 1987;107:186–187.
156. Perez-Reyes M: Subjective and cardiovascular effects of cocethylene in humans. Psychopharmacol. 1993;113:144–147.
157. Perreault CL, Allen PD, Hague AN, et al: Differential mechanisms of cocaine-induced depression of contractile function in cardiac versus vascular smooth muscle. Circulation 1989;80(4 suppl 2):15. Abstract.
158. Pirwitz MJ, Willard JE, Landau C, et al: Influence of cocaine, ethanol, or their combination on epicardial coronary arterial dimensions in humans. Arch Intern Med 1995; 155:1186–1191.
159. Pogue VA, Nurse HM: Cocaine-associated acute myoglobinuric renal failure. Am J Med 1989;86:183–186.
160. Pollan S, Tadjziechy M: Esmolol in the management of epinephrine and cocaine induced cardiovascular toxicity. Anesth Analg 1989;69:663–664.
161. Post RM, Kopanda RT: Cocaine, kindling, and psychosis. Am J Psychiatry 1976;133:627–634.
162. Ramoska E, Sacchetti AD: Propranolol-induced hypertension in treatment of cocaine intoxication. Ann Emerg Med 1985;14:112–113.
163. Rappolt RT, Gay G, Inaba DS: Use of inderal (propranolo-Ayerst) in 1-a (early stimulative) and 1-b (advanced stimulative) classification of cocaine and other sympathomimetic reactions. Clin Toxicol 1978;13:325–332.
164. Rappolt TR, Gay G, Inaba DS, Rappolt NR: Propranolol in cocaine toxicity. Lancet 1976;2:640–641. Letter.
165. Ravin JG, Ravin LC: Blindness due to illicit use of topical cocaine. Ann Ophthalmol 1979;11:863–864.
166. Rezkalla S, Mazza JJ, Kloner RA, et al: The effect of cocaine on human platelets. Am J Cardiol 1993;72:243–246.
167. Rinder HM, Ault KA, Jatlow PI, et al: Platelet alpha granule release in cocaine users. Circulation 1994;90:1162–1167.
168. Roberts J, Price D, Goldfrank L: The body stuffer syndrome: A clandestine form of drug overdose. Am J Emerg Med 1986;4:21–27.

169. Rockhold RW, Oden G, Ho IK, et al: Glutamate receptor antagonists block cocaine induced convulsions and death. Brain Res Bull 1991;27:721–723.
170. Roth D, Alarcon FJ, Fernandez JA, et al: Acute rhabdomyolysis associated with cocaine intoxication. N Engl J Med 1988;319:673–677.
171. Rubin RB, Neugarten J: Cocaine-associated asthma. Am J Med 1990;88:438–439.
172. Rubin RB, Neugarten J: Cocaine-induced rhabdomyolysis masquerading as myocardial ischemia. Am J Med 1989; 86:551–553.
173. Sand IC, Brody SL, Wrenn KD, Slovis CM: Experience with esmolol for the treatment of cocaine associated cardiovascular complications. Am J Emerg Med 1991;9: 161–163.
174. Satel SL, Gawin FH: Migraine like headache and cocaine use. JAMA 1989;261:2995–2996.
175. Schaffer DJ: Clinical comparison of TAC anesthetic solutions with and without cocaine. Ann Emerg Med 1975; 14:1077–1080.
176. Schnetzer GW: Platelets and thrombogenesis—Current concepts. Am Heart J 1972;83:552–564.
177. Schreiber MD, Madden JA, Covert RF, Torgerson LJ: Effects of cocaine, benzoylecgonine and cocaine metabolites on cannulated pressurized fetal sheep cerebral arteries. J Appl Physiol 1994;77:834–839.
178. Schrem SS, Belsky P, Schwartzman D, Slater W: Cocaine-induced torsades de pointes in a patient with idiopathic long QT syndrome. Am Heart J 1990;120:980–984.
179. Schwartz AB, Janzen D, Jones RT, et al: Electrocardiographic and hemodynamic effects of intravenous cocaine in the awake and anesthetized dogs. J Electrocardiol 1989; 22:159–166.
180. Schwartz KA, Cohen JA: Subarachnoid hemorrhage precipitated by cocaine snorting. Arch Neurol 1984;41:705. Letter.
181. Seaman ME: Acute cocaine abuse associated with cerebral infarction. Ann Emerg Med 1990;19:34–37.
182. Self DW, Barnhart WJ, Lehman DA, Nestler EJ: Opposite modulation of cocaine seeking behavior by D1 and D2 like dopamine receptor antagonists. Science 1996;271: 1586–1589.
183. Shannon M: Clinical toxicity of cocaine adulterants. Ann Emerg Med 1988;17:1243–1247.
184. Sharff JA: Renal infarction associated with intravenous cocaine use. Ann Emerg Med 1984;13:1145–1147.
185. Shesser R, Davis D, Edelstein S: Pneumomediastinum and pneumothorax after inhaling alkaloidal cocaine. Ann Emerg Med 1981;10:213–215.
186. Shih RD, Hollander JE, Hoffman RS, et al: Clinical safety of lidocaine in cocaine associated myocardial infarction. Ann Emerg Med 1995;26:702–706.
187. Siegel RK: Cocaine smoking. J Psychoactive Drugs 1982; 14:286–315.
188. Singhal P, Horowitz B, Quinnones MC, et al: Acute renal failure following cocaine abuse. Nephron 1989;52:76–78.
189. Smith GT, McClaughry PL, Purkey J, Thompson W: Crack cocaine mimicking pulmonary embolism on pulmonary ventilation perfusion scan. A case report. Clin Nuc Med 1995;20:65–68.
190. Smith JA, Mo Q, Guo H, et al: Cocaine increases extraneuronal levels of aspartate and glutamate in the nucleus accumbens. Brain Res Bull 1995;683:264–269.
191. Smith M, Garner D, Niemann JT: Pharmacologic interventions after an LD50 cocaine insult in a chronically instrumented rat model: Are beta blockers contraindicated? Ann Emerg Med 1991;20:768–771.
192. Spivey WH, Schoffstall JM, Kirkpatrick R, et al: Comparison of labetalol, diazepam, and haloperidol for the treatment of cocaine toxicity in a swine model. Ann Emerg Med 1990;19:467–468.
193. Stewart DJ, Inaba T, Lucassen M, Kalow W: Cocaine metabolism: Cocaine and norcocaine hydrolysis by liver and serum esterases. Clin Pharmacol Ther 1979;25:464–468.
194. Suhl J, Gorelick DA: Pulmonary function in male freebase cocaine users. Am Rev Resp Dis 1988;137:A488. Abstract.
195. Sybertz EJ, Sabin CS, Pula KK, et al: Alpha and beta adrenoreceptor blocking properties of labetalol and its R,R-isomer, SCH 19927. J Pharmacol Exp Ther 1981; 218:435–443.
196. Tashkin DP, Khalsa ME, Gorelick D, et al: Pulmonary status of habitual cocaine users. Am Rev Resp Dis 1992;145: 92–100.
197. Tella SR, Schindler CW, Goldberg SR: Cocaine: Cardiovascular effects in relation to inhibition of peripheral neuronal monoamine uptake and central stimulation of the sympathoadrenal system. J Pharmacol Exp Ther 1993;267: 153–162.
198. Telsey AM, Merrit A, Dixon SD: Cocaine exposure in a term neonate. Clin Pediatr 1988;27:547–550.
199. Thadani PV: NIDA conference report on cardiopulmonary complications of crack cocaine use—Clinical manifestations and pathophysiology. Chest 1996;110: 1072–1076.
200. Tipton GA, DeWitt GW, Eisenstein SJ: Topical TAC (tetracaine, adrenaline, cocaine) solution for local anesthesia in children: Prescribing inconsistency and acute toxicity. South Med J 1989;82:1344–1346.
201. Togna G, Tempesta E, Togna AR, et al: Platelet responsiveness and biosynthesis of thromboxane and prostacyclin in response to in vitro cocaine treatment. Haemostasis 1985;15:100–107.
202. Tokarski GF, Paganussi P, Urbanski R, et al: An evaluation of cocaine induced chest pain. Ann Emerg Med 1990;19: 1088–1092.
203. Tomaszewski C, McKinney P, Phillips S, et al. Prevention of toxicity from oral cocaine by activated charcoal in mice. Ann Emerg Med 1993;22:1804–1806.
204. Trouve R, Nahas GG, Maillet M: Nitrendipine as an antagonist to the cardiac toxicity of cocaine. J Cardiovas Pharmacol 1987;9(suppl 4):S49-S53.
205. Van De Bor M, Walther FJ, Ebrahimi M: Decreased cardiac output in infants of mothers who abused cocaine. Pediatrics 1990;85:30–32.
206. Vargas R, Gillis RA, Ramwell PW: Propanolol promotes cocaine induced spasm of porcine coronary artery. J Pharmacol Exp Therap 1991;257:644–646.
207. Vongpatanasin W, Lange RA, Hillis LD: Comparison of cocaine induced vasoconstriction of left and right coronary arterial systems. Am J Cardiol 1997;79:492–493.

208. Wang R: pH dependent cocaine cardiotoxicity. J Toxicol Clin Toxicol 1996;34:561–562. Abstract.
209. Weiner RS, Lockhart JT, Schwartz RG: Dilated cardiomyopathy and cocaine abuse. Am J Med 1986;81:699–701.
210. Weiss RD: Protracted elimination of cocaine metabolites in long term high dose cocaine abuse. Am J Med 1988;85: 879–880.
211. Weiss SH: Links between cocaine and retroviral infection. JAMA 1989;261:607–608.
212. Welch RD, Todd K, Krause GS: Incidence of cocaine associated rhabdomyolysis. Ann Emerg Med 1991;20:154–157.
213. Winecoff AP, Hariman RJ, Grawe JJ, et al: Reversal of the electrocardiographic effects of cocaine by lidocaine. Part 1. Comparison with sodium bicarbonate and quinidine. Pharmacotherapy 1994;14:698–703.
214. Witkin JM, Godberg SR, Katz JL: Lethal effects of cocaine are reduced by the dopamine–1 receptor antagonist SCH 23390 but not by haloperidol. Life Sci 1989;44: 1285–1291.
215. Wojak JC, Flamm ES: Intracranial hemorrhage and cocaine use. Stroke 1987;18:712–715.
216. Woods JR, Plessinger MA, Clark KE: Effect of cocaine on uterine blood flow and fetal oxygenation. JAMA 1987;257: 957–961.
217. Zamora-Quezada JC, Dinerman H, Stadecker MJ, Kelly JJ: Muscle and skin infarction after free-basing cocaine (crack). Ann Intern Med 1988;108:564–566.
218. Zimmerman JL, Dellinger RP, Majid PA: Cocaine associated chest pain. Ann Emerg Med 1991;20: 611–615.

CHAPTER 66

Amphetamines

William K. Chiang

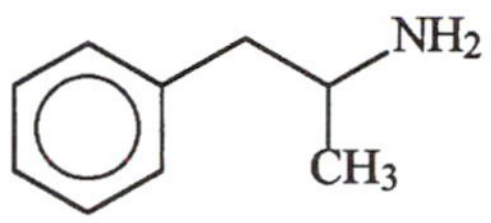

Amphetamine

A-25-year-old woman was brought to the emergency department (ED) by a group of "friends" who left. The woman was delirious, agitated, and paranoid, yet was lucid enough to ask for an injection to "stop the noises." At times she was exceedingly hyperactive, jumping repeatedly on and off the stretcher.

It was impossible to obtain a history. She was suspicious of every question. She refused to identify the people who had brought her to the ED. Frequently, she appeared to be involved with her hallucinations. Her only persistent complaint was severe pain in her left arm.

The physical examination revealed a blood pressure of 170/100 mm Hg, temperature 100.4°F (38°C), pulse of 120 beats/min and regular, and respiratory rate of 16 breaths/min. She appeared wasted, anicteric, acyanotic, and malnourished. Her skin was moist. Her head was normocephalic. Her mouth smelled foul, and her teeth were extensively chipped and carious. Her conjunctivae were not injected, and her extraocular movements were intact. Her pupils were dilated to 7 mm bilaterally, and they reacted slowly to light. Her fundi were normal, with no hemorrhages, exudates, or papilledema. Her neck was supple, exhibiting no thyromegaly. Examination of her heart was unremarkable, except for tachycardia. Her lungs were clear. Her abdomen was soft and nontender; bowel sounds were normal. There was no hepatomegaly.

The radial and ulnar pulses of the patient's left forearm were slightly decreased. There was nonpitting edema to the elbow and a petechial eruption extending from above the elbow to the hand, but there was no impairment of sensory and motor function. Her left arm had no track marks, except for the antecubital fossa, where there appeared to be a fresh puncture. Her right arm showed marked tracking and healing abscesses.

The patient moved all her extremities and had normal symmetric deep-tendon reflexes with plantar flexion. The sensory examination appeared grossly normal, but her delirium and extreme agitation made the findings somewhat unreliable. On admission, her complete blood count and serum electrolytes were normal. The chest radiograph was normal. The ECG revealed a sinus tachycardia. A Rumpel Leede tourniquet test (inflate a sphygmomanometer cuff over the arm to a pressure halfway between the systolic and diastolic pressure for 5 minutes, and observe for petechiae 2 minutes after deflation of the cuff) performed on the right arm was normal, implying no capillary or platelet abnormalities.

This patient was treated with 10 mg of diazepam IV for sedation and was placed in a quiet environment. She became calm and less paranoid.

The lesions in the left arm of the patient resulted from inadvertent intra-arterial injection. Frequent trauma to the artery may cause arterial wall injuries or even thrombosis. The insoluble particles transiently suspended ("cold shaking") before the injection may embolize distally, leading to arteritis.

The physical findings in this case were entirely compatible with inadvertent injection of amphetamines and other material into the brachial artery. The petechiae and edema were compatible with angioedema and vasculitis in the distribution of the brachial artery. Although the pathogenesis is not clear, a proposed mechanism is focal endothelial damage from the active substance, contaminants, or vehicle, with resultant platelet aggregation, vasodilation, and altered vascular permeability.

Therapy for this patient consisted of elevation of her arm, 4 days of anticoagulation with heparin, a full evaluation for sepsis, observation for the development of a compartment syndrome, and prophylaxis for tetanus. An angiogram of the left arm done on admission showed good arterial filling and normal perfusion of the hand and skin of the left arm with vascular occlusions.

The petechiae, edema, erythrema, and pain cleared dramatically, and in these respects the patient had almost returned to normal when she signed out of the hospital against medical advice on the sixth day.

What Are Amphetamines?

Amphetamine (racemic beta-phenylisopropylamine) was first synthesized in 1887 and was marketed as Benzedrine inhaler, a nasal decongestant, in 1932.[14] The stimulant and euphoric effects of amphetamines were widely recognized, resulting in diverse forms of abuse and nonmedicinal use. Amphetamines were used as stimulants by soldiers and prisoners of war in World War II.[14] Widespread amphetamine abuse led to the ban of the Benzedrine inhaler in 1959; the Controlled Substance Act of 1971 began to regulate the diversion of pharmaceutical amphetamines for nonmedicinal uses.[36]

Amphetamine belongs to the phenylethylamine family with a methyl group substitution in the alpha carbon position (Fig. 66–1). Numerous substitutions of the phenylethylamine structure are possible, resulting in different amphetamine-like compounds.[82] Commonly, these compounds are referred to as amphetamines or amphetamine analogs, although *phenylethylamines* would be more precise. Currently, amphetamines can be legally prescribed in the United States for narcolepsy, attention-deficit disorder, and short-term weight reduction[82]; these prescriptive amphetamine analogs include methylphenidate, pemoline, phentermine, dexfenfluramine, fenfluramine, phendimetrazine, amphetamine, dextroamphetamine, and methamphetamine (Table 66–1). Because of structural differences, some amphetamine analogs are marketed as nonamphetamine products in their package inserts.

What Is the Pharmacology of Amphetamines?

The pharmacologic effects of amphetamines are complex and some mechanisms are not completely understood. The primary mechanism of action is the release of catecholamines, particularly dopamine and norepinephrine, from the presynaptic terminals. Although there are conflicting mechanistic models of catecholamine release by amphetamines using dopamine neurons, these variable results may be directly correlated with the different concentrations of amphetamine used in the studies. Two storage pools exist for dopamine in the presynaptic terminals: the vesicular pool and the cytoplasmic pool. The vesicular storage of dopamine and other amines is maintained by an acidic environment inside the vesicles and due to an electrical gradient when compared to the cytoplasm. This is supported by an ATP-dependent active proton transport system.[160] At low doses, amphetamines cause release of dopamine from the cytoplasmic pool by exchange diffusion at the dopamine uptake transporter site in the membrane. At moderate doses, amphetamines can also diffuse through the presynaptic terminal membrane and interact with the vesicular membrane to cause exchange release of dopamine into the cytoplasm. Dopamine is subsequently released into the synapse by reverse transport at the dopamine uptake site.[160,168] At high doses, an additional mechanism is invoked, as amphetamine diffuses through the cellular and vesicular membrane causing an alkalinization of the vesicles, and dopamine is released from the vesicle and carried into synapse by reverse transport.[169,170]

Amphetamines may also block the reuptake of catecholamines similarly to other catecholamine-releasing

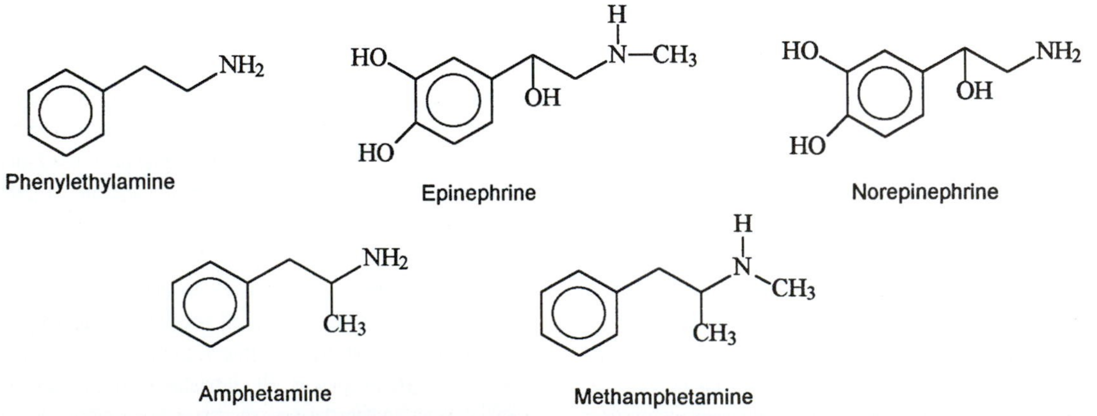

Figure 66–1. Phenylethylamine and related chemicals.

TABLE 66–1. PRESCRIPTION AMPHETAMNES AND AMPHETAMINE ANALOGS AVAILABLE IN THE UNITED STATES

Generic Name	Trade Name	Indications[a]
Amphetamine	Adderall, Biphetamine	A, W
Dextroamphetamine	Dexedrine, DextroStat	A, N
Methamphetamine	Desoxyn	A, W
Methylphenidate	Ritalin, Ritalin SR	A, N
Benzphetamine	Didrex	W
Phendimetrazine	Bontril, Phenzine, Prelu-2	W
Dexfenfluramine	Redux[b]	W
Diethylpropion	Tenuate	W
Fenfluramine	Pondimin[b]	W
Pemoline	Cylert	A
Phentermine	Adipex-P, Fastin, Ionamin, etc	W

[a]A = attention-deficit disorder; N = narcolepsy; W = weight reduction.
[b]Withdrawn from the market, 1997

agents by competitive inhibition.[71,82] However, the effects of this mechanism are considered to be minor. At higher doses, amphetamines can cause the release of serotonin (5-hydroxytryptamine, 5-HT) and affect central serotonin receptors. Certain amphetamines, such as 3,4-methylenedioxymethamphetamine (MDMA) and 4-bromo-2,5-dimethoxyamphetamine (DOB), have more significant serotonergic effects.[66,82] Amphetamines also have weak monoamine oxidase inhibiting activities, but the significance of this inhibition has not been determined.[135]

The most identifiable effects of amphetamines are the catecholamine effects, as the result of stimulation of peripheral alpha and beta-adrenergic receptors. The increased norepinephrine at the locus coeruleus mediates the anorexic and alerting effects, and some of the locomotor-stimulating effects as well.[71] The increase in central dopamine (particular at the neostriatum) mediates stereotypical behavior and some of the other locomotor activities.[35,66,71,95] The activity of dopamine in the neostriatum appears to be linked to glutamate release and inhibition of GABAergic efferent neurons.[66,94,95] Stimulation of the glutamatergic system contributes significantly to the stereotypical behavior, locomotor activities, and neurotoxicity of amphetamines.[15,19,94,95,165,166] The effects of serotonin and dopamine at the mesolimbic system alter perception and cause psychotic behavior.[66,81,122]

Substitution at different positions of the phenylethylamine molecule has some general clinical effects on amphetamines based on animal discrimination studies and human observations. Compounds with methyl substitution at the alpha carbon, such as amphetamine and methamphetamine, possess strong stimulant, cardiovascular, and anorexic properties (see Fig. 66–1).[63] Large group substitution at the alpha carbon reduce the stimulant and cardiovascular effects, but retain the anorexic properties.[9] Substitution at the phenyl ring enhances the hallucinogenic effects of amphetamines.[9,63] Although some of these generalizations enable scientists to understand the effects of amphetamines, there are many exceptions, and such generalization may not apply when large doses are employed.[53] The spectrum of activities of amphetamines varies between the potent cardiovascular effects of amphetamine and methamphetamine, and the potent hallucinogenic effects of 4-bromo-2,5 dimethoxyamphetamine (DOB).[63]

In general, amphetamines are relatively lipophilic (hence they can cross the blood–brain barrier readily) and have large volumes of distribution, varying from 3 to 5 L/kg for amphetamine, to 11 to 33 L/kg for methylphenidate. The half-life of amphetamine ranges from 8 to 30 hours. The major route of elimination is hepatic transformation. A number of active metabolites of ephedrine derivatives are formed.[8] Amphetamines differ from catecholamines in that they lack the catechol structure and therefore cannot be metabolized by catechol-*O*-methyl transferase (COMT), which permits oral efficacy.[82] Repetitive administration, which occurs during binges, may lead to drug accumulation, further prolonging the duration of effect.[88] Renal elimination can be substantial for amphetamine (30%), methamphetamine (40 to 50%), and phentermine (80%).[8]

What Is "Ice" and What Special Problems Are Associated With Its Use?

A pure preparation of methamphetamine hydrochloride marketed in a large crystalline form is termed "ice" by abusers. "Ice" can be smoked, ground and insufflated, or dissolved and administered parenterally.[86] The availability of ice has led to a resurgence in amphetamine abuse in the United States. During the late 1980s, ice became one of the leading drugs of abuse, initially in Hawaii and then subsequently on the West Coast and Midwest regions of the United States.[7,47,121] In fact, ice surpassed cocaine and became the primary substance of abuse in the drug treatment programs of San Diego and San Francisco counties in the 1990s.[70,77] From 1991 to 1994, the number of methamphetamine-related deaths in the United States reported by medical examiners tripled from 151 to 433, with a disproportional distribution from the Los Angeles, San Diego, San Francisco, and Phoenix metropolitan areas. The number of methamphetamine-related emergency department visits also increased from 4900 in 1991 to 17,400 in 1994.[70] Although the initial source of ice was from Pacific rim countries such as Korea and Taiwan, ice currently is primarily produced in the United States, particularly in California and Oregon.[31,57] Because of the ease and low cost of methamphetamine synthesis, the street value of methamphetamine is less than one third that of cocaine.[57] Both the cost and the prolonged duration of effect may contribute to the increasing popularity of methamphetamine.

Methamphetamine abuse in the United States is not new. During the 1950s, 1960s, and 1970s, there were epidemics of methamphetamine abuse.[14] Methamphetamine was and sometimes still is referred to as "crank", "speed", and "go." The pharmacologic profile of methamphetamine is quite similar to amphetamine, although the effects on the central nervous system are more sub-

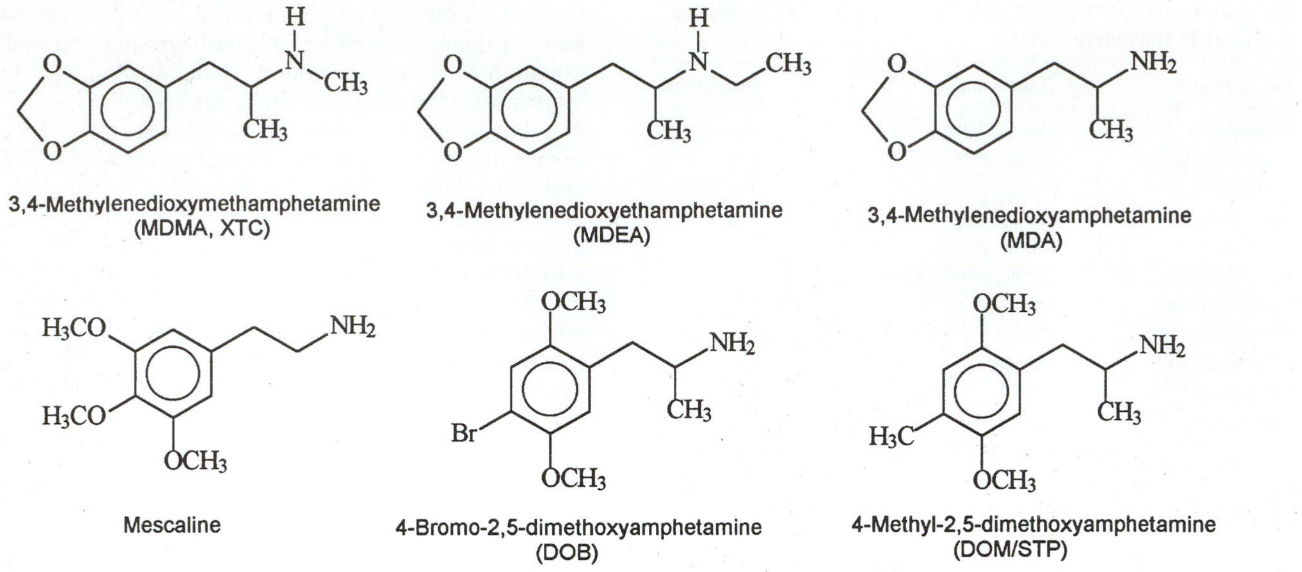

Figure 66–2. Designer amphetamines.

stantial.[31] Ice does not differ pharmacologically from other forms of methamphetamine and thus has similiar medical complications (described later).

The current epidemic and its method of synthesis result in higher activity and purity of the methamphetamine than in previous epidemics.[109] Ice is typically greater than 80 to 90% pure and almost exclusively in the dextroisomer form, which is most active on the CNS. The ephedrine method, using pharmaceutical grade L-ephedrine, produces a product with few contaminants that is stereochemically pure.[30,47] The production of the large crystal is possible by creating a supersaturated solution of methamphetamine hydrochloride.[47] For these reasons, ice is referred to as methamphetamine elsewhere in this chapter, unless a distinction is necessary.

Methamphetamine is currently the most common illicit drug produced by clandestine laboratories in the United States. Methamphetamine can be easily synthesized with the proper chemicals and minimal equipment.[61] The primary ingredient of methamphetamine synthesis is ephedrine, which can be hydrogenated into methamphetamine. Phenyl-2-propanone (P2P), as an alternative ingredient, can be methylated into ephedrine and then into methamphetamine.[22] Because of the strict control of ephedrine and P2P, illicit chemists use phenylacetic acid to synthesize P2P.[22,39] Lead acetate, which is used as a substrate for the reaction, resulted in an epidemic of lead poisoning associated with methamphetamine abuse in Oregon.[2,28] Lead levels reported in drug users were as high as 513 μg/dL, and some samples of illicit manufactured methamphetamine had lead contents as high as 60% by weight.[28] Mercury contamination was also documented, although clinical mercury toxicity has not been reported.[22] The number of potential chemicals involved in the methamphetamine manufacture process is significant, and without any legal monitoring, contamination of the product and the environment is inevitable.[3,22,85,104] In fact, 30% of the illicit methamphetamine manufacturing sites discovered in Oregon were due to laboratory explosion. In California's San Bernadino county alone in 1995, 360 methamphetamine laboratories were identified and closed by drug enforcement agents.[57] Currently, sale of other potential amphetamine synthesis ingredients such as hydriotic acid, hydrochloric gas, red phosphorous, and iodine are also monitored and restricted in the United States.

What Are "Designer Amphetamines?"

The design of therapeutically useful molecules is the hallmark of pharmaceutical research. Congeners of active compounds synthesized for illegitimate use, "Designer drugs," were developed historically to circumvent legal restrictions. The most common designer drugs are analogs of phenylethylamines, fentanyl, meperidine, and phencyclidine.[21,87] Before 1986, the Controlled Substances Act classified drugs as illegal only after they had been synthesized and were formally recognized (by their structure, effects, and illegal usage). During that period any new analogs not formally classified could be sold legally. In 1986, the standard became prospective for any agent that was used as a stimulant, hallucinogen, or depressant and any agent designed as such.[21] In effect, this amendment eliminated the legal "loophole" that was responsible for the designer drug industry. Although the meaning of the term "designer drugs" has changed, many of these analogs are still widely abused, and newer analogs such as methcathinone continue to be developed.[68,177] These agents are responsible for significant morbidity and mortality.[32,44,52,68,78,120,146]

Designer amphetamines are congeners of phenylethylamine, and numerous modifications are possible (Fig. 66–2). Some of the common designer amphetamines are

TABLE 66–2. DESIGNER AMPHETAMINES

2,4,5-Trimethoxyamphetamine (TMA-2)	Similar character as mescaline
4-Methyl-2,5-dimethoxy-amphetamine (DOM/STP) (serenity, tranquility, peace)	Narrow therapeutic index 2–3 mg: Euphoria, perceptual distortion 5 mg: Hallucinations, sympathetic stimulation
Para-methoxyamphetamine (PMA)	Potent hallucinogen Marked stimulant effect
4-Bromo-2,5-dimethoxy-amphetamine (DOB)	Marked psychoactive effect (potency >mescaline) Sold as drug-impregnated paper, like LSD Delayed onset of action Peak 3–4 h Fantasy, mood-altering, for 10 h, resolution 12–24 h Agitation, sympathetic excess
4-Bromo-2,5-methoxyphenyl-ethylamine (2CB, MFT)	Relaxation Sensory distortion Agitation Hallucination Potency (> mescaline)
3,4-Methylenedioxyamphetamine (MDA, love drug)	Low dose: Mild intoxication, empathy, euphoria High-dose: Agitation, delirium, hallucinations, death associated with sympathetic excess
3,4-Methylenedioxymethamphetamine (MDMA, Adam, ecstasy, XTC)	Psychotherapy "facilitator" Euphoria, empathy Nausea, anorexia Anxiety, insomnia Sympathetic excess
3,4-Methylenedioxyethamphetamine (MDEA, Eve)	Comparable to MDMA Sympathetic excess
Methcathinone (cat, Jeff ephedrone)	Comparable to hallucinogen and sympathetic effects of methamphetamine

2,4,5-trimethoxyamphetamine (TMA-2), 4-methyl-2,5-dimethoxyamphetamine (DOM/STP), 3,4-methylenedioxymethamphetamine (MDMA), and 3,4-methylenedioxyethamphetamine (MDEA) (Table 66–2).[87] Although the pharmacologic effects of these congeners vary, taken in large doses the toxicities are similar to amphetamines.[21,108,146,161]

What Is 3,4-Methylenedioxymethamphetamine (MDMA)? What Are Its Clinical Effects?

3,4-Methylenedioxymethamphetamine (MDMA) was first synthesized in 1914, and was rediscovered in the 1970s.[21] It is probably one of the most widely abused designer amphetamines by college students. Over the last few years, MDMA has become extremely popular in large gatherings known as "rave parties" in England, Australia, and the United States.[137,138] It is commonly known as "ecstasy," "E," "Adam," "XTC," "M&M," and "MDM." Other structural relatives of MMDA, 3,4-methylenedioxyethamphetamine (MDEA, "Eve") and 3,4-methylenedioxyamphetamine (MDA, "love drug"), have similar clinical effects and acute and chronic toxicities. People who use MDMA report that it enhances pleasure, heightens sexuality, and expands consciousness without the loss of control.[21] It was also used by psychologists to enhance psychotherapy.[128] 3,4-Methylenedioxymethamphetamine has about one-tenth the CNS stimulant effect of amphetamine. Unlike amphetamine and methamphetamine, MDMA is a potent releaser of serotonin.[24,49,71] In animal models, the stereotypic and the discriminatory effects of MDMA and its congeners can be distinguished from those of other amphetamines.[25,128]

The sympathetic effects of MDMA are mild in low doses. However, when a large amount of MDMA is taken, the clinical presentation is similar to that of other amphetamines and deaths can result from abuse.[52,78] These patients developed dysrhythmias, hyperthermia, rhabdomyolysis, and disseminated intravascular coagulation.[52,78,161] Chronic administration of MDMA causes permanent damage to serotonergic neurons in all animal models tested to date.[123,140,141,143,157] Although these neurotoxic effects are not well studied in humans, indirect evidence of serotonergic effects include lower levels of 5-hydroxyindoleacetic acid (5-HIAA) in the CSF of MDMA users than in controls.[142] Case reports and studies of MDMA users demonstrate alteration in mood, sleep, anxiety, cognition, and impulse control, all functions that are believed to be affected by serotonin.[4,120]

What Is Propylhexedrine?

Propylhexedrine (Fig. 66–3) was introduced in 1949 by Smith, Kline & French as the primary active ingredient in Benzedrex nasal inhaler, to replace the widespread abuse of amphetamine in nasal inhalers.[6,60] Propylhexedrine is an alicyclic aliphatic sympathomimetic amine structurally similar to amphetamine, with a local vasoconstrictive effect and approximately 10% the CNS stimulatory effect of amphetamine.[6] Propylhexedrine abuse became prevalent after the withdrawal of amphetamine in all nasal inhalers. The abusers disassembled the in-

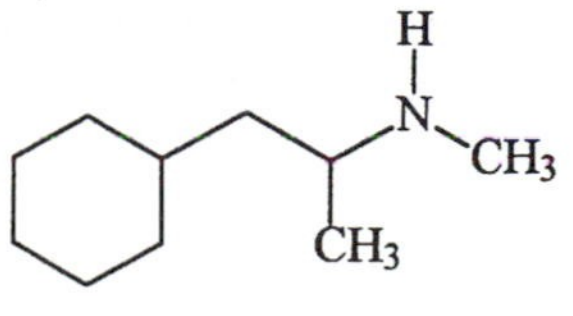

Propylhexedrine

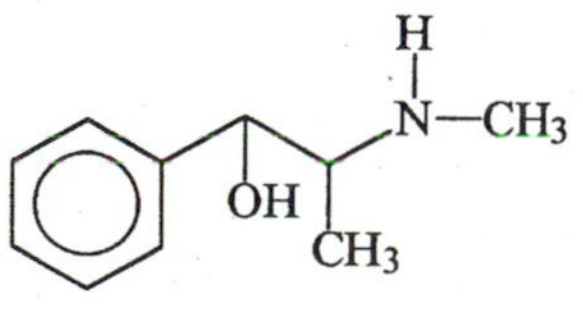

Ephedrine

Figure 66–3. Decongestants.

haler and ingested the cotton pledget vehicle of propylhexedrine itself, diluted it in beverages, or reconstituted the drug for intravenous injection. Numerous toxic effects were reported with propylhexedrine abuse, including sudden death, myocardial infarction, cardiomyopathy, pulmonary hypertension, and acute psychosis.[5,6,37,51,60,110,117,118,174] Although propylhexedrine in nasal inhalers has largely been replaced by safer sympathomimetic agents (see Chap. 34), the drug is still readily available and is abused as an inexpensive, legal "high."

What Are Khat, Cathinone, and Their Derivatives?

Khat (also known as quat and gat), the fresh leaves and stems from the *Catha edulis* shrub, is one of the most commonly used drugs in eastern and central Africa and parts of the Arabian peninsula. The attention to khat was highlighted from the media coverage of Somalia and Ethiopia in the early 1990s. Khat is sold in small bundles of leaves in the local markets of these countries. The leaves and the tender stems are chewed or occasionally concocted into tea. Khat chewing often has a significant role at social gatherings in these countries.[116] When the dried leaves and stems were studied, the primary active ingredient was thought to be cathine (norpseudoephedrine), present as 0.1 to 0.2% of the dried material. Cathine has about one tenth the stimulant effects of D-amphetamine. Numerous other amphetamine-like compounds are also isolated but occur in minute quantities.[92] When the fresh leaves were analyzed, however, cathinone (benzylketoamphetamine), a more potent psychoactive compound, was demonstrated to be the primary active agent.[64,73,92] As the leaves age, cathinone is degraded into cathine, which also explains why dried khat is neither popular nor widely distributed. The primary effects of khat are increased alertness, insomnia, euphoria, anxiety, and hyperactivity. Significant adrenergic complications are much less frequent than associated with amphetamine abuse because of the limited content and dose of khat.

Methcathinone, the methyl-derivative of cathinone, chemically synthesized from ephedrine, has been abused in the Soviet Union since the late 1970s. The potency of methcathinone is comparable to that of methamphetamine.[65,177] Methcathinone—also termed ephedrone, or sold under the street names of "cat," or "Jeff"—is currently widely abused in Russia. Methcathinone abuse, first reported in the United States in Michigan in the early 1990s, is now reported in other states as well.[55] Healthcare providers should monitor the use of methcathinone to define its potential for toxicity.

What Problems Are Associated With Ephedrine or Ma-Huang Herbal Products?

Ephedrine is commonly found in over-the-counter cold preparations (Fig. 66–3). Ephedrine is also the active substance in the Chinese plant ma-huang, which has been used for centuries for the treatment of asthma. Although ephedrine is much less potent than amphetamine, when combined with other catecholamine-stimulating agents or when taken in large quantities, significant toxicity may occur.[20,26,133,155] In the United States, numerous ephedrine products such as "go," "ultimate xphoria," "up your gas," and "ecstasy" are marketed primarily to teenagers. Some of these products are pills containing ephedrine combined with pseudoephedrine, phenylpropanolamine, and caffeine; others contain the plant extract ma-huang.[107,133,134] Many of these products are marketed as legal stimulants or safe herbal stimulants for a natural "high." Unfortunately, these products are linked to more than 15 deaths and numerous adverse reactions.[125,134,176,179] Because these products are sold as food supplements, they are not regulated by the FDA. Only when the FDA can demonstrate a product's hazards, can the federal authority restrict these products. Currently, the FDA is closely monitoring the adverse effects and claims made for these products.

What Substances Are Likely to Be Found in Street Amphetamines?

The Los Angeles County Street Drug Identification Program conducted analysis of street drugs over a 10-year period (1971 to 1980). Street amphetamine and methamphetamine samples actually did not contain any of the alleged drug 50 and 63% of the time, respectively.[99] Substitutions such as caffeine, phenylpropanolamine, ephedrine, pseudoephedrine, lidocaine, and phencyclidine, were common.[99,107,124,139] In addition, materials used to "cut" (adulterate) the active substance included cornstarch, maltose, lactose, talc (magnesium silicate), strychnine, quinine, and a variety of fibrous materials. The vehicle also varied, ranging from bottled water to urine. As a result of the recent epidemic of "ice," the preparation and form of the product increase the chances of getting pure methamphetamine.[46,136]

What Are the Clinical Effects of Amphetamines?

The clinical effects of amphetamines are largely related to the stimulation of central and peripheral adrenergic receptors. These clinical manifestations and complications are similar to those from cocaine use and may be indistinguishable except for the duration of effect of amphetamines, which tends to be longer (up to 24 hours).[47,58] Tachycardia and hypertension are the most common manifestations of cardiovascular toxicity. Most patients present to the emergency department, however, because of the CNS manifestations.[47,86] These patients are anxious, volatile, aggressive, and may have life-threatening agitation. Visual and tactile hallucinations, and psychoses, are common.[17,48,50,76,112,154] Other sympathetic findings include mydriasis, diaphoresis, and hyperthermia (Table 66–3).[48,52]

TABLE 66–3. AMPHETAMINE TOXICITY

Acute Toxicity	*Other Organ Systems*
Cardiovascular System	Rhabdomyolysis
Hypertension	Muscle rigidity
Tachycardia	Pulmonary edema
Dysrhythmias	Ischemic colitis
Myocardial ischemia	
Vasospasm	***Chronic Toxicity***
Central Nervous System	Vasculitis
Hyperthermia	Cardiomyopathy
Agitation	Pulmonary hypertension
Seizures	Permanent damage to dopaminergic and serotonergic neurons?
Intracerebral hemorrhage	
Headache	
Euphoria	***Laboratory Abnormalities***
Anorexia	Leukocytosis
Bruxism	Hyperglycemia
Choreoathetoid movements	Elevated CPK
Hyperreflexia	Elevated liver enzymes
Paranoid psychosis	Myoglobinuria
Other Sympathetic Symptoms	
Diaphoresis	
Tachypnea	
Mydriasis	
Tremor	
Nausea	

Death from amphetamine intoxication most commonly results from dysrhythmias, hyperthermia, and intracerebral hemorrhage.[27,43,91,97,131,147] Direct CNS effects may result in seizures. Tachycardia, hypertension, and vasospasm may lead to cerebral infarction,[69,103,148] intraparenchymal and subarachnoid hemorrhage,[40,75,84,96,167,178] myocardial ischemia or infarction,[59,132] aortic dissection,[40] pulmonary edema,[23,126,127] obstetrical complications, fetal death,[111] and ischemic colitis.[13,79,89] Dysrhythmias vary from premature ventricular complexes to ventricular tachycardia and ventricular fibrillation.[91,113] Agitation, increased muscular activity, and hyperthermia can result in metabolic acidosis, rhabdomyolysis,[38] acute tubular necrosis (acute renal failure), and coagulopathy.[52,62,90,98] Unless these systemic signs and symptoms are rapidly reversed, multiorgan failure and death ensue.

Amphetamine users seeking intense "highs" may go on "speed runs" for days to weeks. Because of the development of acute tolerance, they use increasing amounts of amphetamines during this period, usually without much sustenance or sleep, until they achieve their desired euphoria.[14,36,105,163,171] Acute psychosis resembling paranoid schizophrenia may occur during these binges and has contributed to both amphetamine-related suicides and homicides.[54,101] Return to a normal sensorium occurs within a few days after discontinuation of the drug. Once an amphetamine user experiences psychosis, it is more likely to recur, even after prolonged abstinence, which may be related to a kindling phenomenon.[14,58,129] Amphetamine-induced psychosis has contributed to the understanding of dopamine's function in schizophrenia. Typically after such binges, these subjects may sleep for prolonged periods, feeling hungry and depressed when awake. During this period of depression or withdrawal, the patient has continued craving for amphetamines.[76,102,107]

There are some direct neurologic effects of amphetamines. Compulsive repetitive behavior patterns are reported in humans and animals. Individuals may constantly pick at their skin, grind their teeth, or perform repetitive tasks, such as constantly cleaning their house or car.[14] Choreoathetoid movements, although uncommon, have been reported with acute and chronic amphetamine usage.[100,115,119,140,153,162] The etiology of the choreoathetoid movements may be related to increased dopaminergic activity at the striatal area.

Necrotizing vasculitis is associated with amphetamine abuse.[16,33] Angiography typically demonstrates beading and narrowing of the small and medium-sized arteries (see Fig. 7–22).[149,167] Progressive necrotizing arteritis[40] can involve multiple organ systems, including the central nervous, cardiovascular, gastrointestinal, and renal systems. Complications include cerebral infarction and hemorrhage, coronary disease, pancreatitis, and renal failure.[33,74,114,149,152,167,178] The etiology of the arteritis remains unclear. Although various contaminants associated with parenteral drug abuse were postulated as potential etiologies, oral and IV amphetamine use in animal models is also associated with vasculitis, suggesting that this is a direct amphetamine effect.[150,151,172] Cardiomyopathy is also reported with acute and chronic amphetamine abuse.[23,83,130,164] Excessive catecholamine exposure in pheochromocytomas and chronic cocaine abuse may be responsible for their associated cardiomyopathies; amphetamine-induced cardiomyopathy may be produced by similar mechanisms.[67,93,175]

Primary pulmonary hypertension was reported with chronic methamphetamine and propylhexedrine abuse,[5,51,106,156,176] although it is more commonly associated with fenfluramine and aminorex (2-amino-5-phenyl-2-oxazoline).[18,72] A case-controlled study substantiated the increased risk of primary pulmonary hypertension with amphetamine appetite-suppressant drugs, particularly with fenfluramine.[1] The risk of pulmonary hypertension was increased 23-fold when the cumulative use of anorexic agents totaled more than 3 months.[1] The exact cause of the pulmonary hypertension is unclear, but is postulated to be related to serotonin's pulmonary vasoconstrictive effects.[80,126]

Chronic administration of amphetamines is directly neurotoxic in animals. The depletion of dopamine and serotonin in the neuronal synapses and the subsequent irreversible destruction of those neurons occurs in animals given a variety of amphetamines.[12,143–145,158] A direct correlation between these findings in animals and the effects in humans has not been demonstrated. The potential for permanent neurologic effects associated with chronic amphetamine abuse needs further study.

Finally, multiple medical complications can result from parenteral drug abuse itself. Blood contamination may result in HIV infection, hepatitis, and malaria. Bacterial and foreign body contamination may result in endocarditis, tetanus, wound botulism, osteomyelitis, pulmonary and soft tissues abscesses[29] (see Chaps. 7 and 108).

How Helpful Is the Laboratory in Suspected Amphetamine Toxicity?

Diagnosis by history is rarely reliable, and there is no readily available serum analysis. The prevalence of amphetamine abuse in the local geographic region should heighten the suspicion of amphetamine toxicity. The physical and psychologic assessment is nonspecific, and polydrug abuse is quite common. A qualitative urine testing for amphetamines is available but it is not valuable in the acute setting. Although newer rapid serum qualitative drug screens are available, false-positive and false-negative results are common and may be misleading. In summary, suspicion of amphetamine intoxication cannot be confirmed acutely.

What Is the Management of Patients With Amphetamine Toxicity?

The therapeutic approach to a patient with amphetamine toxicity is discussed here and summarized in Table 66–4. The initial medical assessment of the agitated patient must include the vital signs and a rapid complete physical examination. An often-neglected vital sign is the rectal temperature. Hyperthermia is a frequent and rapidly fatal manifestation in patients with drug-induced delirium, and requires immediate interventions to achieve cooling.[62,90,98] Some patients will require physical restraint to gain clinical control and prevent personal harm to themselves or others. Because agitation and resistance against physical restraint may lead to rhabdomyolysis and continued heat generation, intravenous chemical sedation should be instituted immediately. Blood specimens should be sent for glucose, BUN, and electrolyte assays. Intravenous (IV) glucose ($D_{50}W$, 0.5 to 1 g/kg) and thiamine 100 mg should be given as indicated. An ECG should be obtained to exclude ischemia, hyperkalemia, and drug toxicity (cyclic antidepressant), and cardiac monitoring should be initiated. A CBC, urine analysis, coagulation profile, chest radiograph, computed tomography (CT) of the head, and lumbar puncture may be necessary, depending on the presentation.

TABLE 66–4. MANAGEMENT OF AMPHETAMINE TOXICITY

Agitation
Benzodiazepines (usually adequate for the cardiovascular manifestations)
Diazepam 10 mg IV, repeat until the patient is calm (cumulative dose may be > 100 mg)

Seizures
Benzodiazepines
Barbiturates

Hyperthermia
External cooling
Control agitation rapidly

Gastric Decontamination and Elimination
Activated charcoal for oral ingestions

Hypertension
Control agitation
Alpha-adrenergic antagonist (phentolamine)
Vasodilator (nifedipine, nitroprusside, nitroglycerin)

Delirium or Hallucinations With Abnormal Vital Signs
If agitated: Benzodiazepines

Delirium or Hallucinations With Normal Vital Signs
Consider haloperidol or droperidol

Because the clinician cannot acutely distinguish different etiologies of drug-induced delirium, the choice of chemical sedation should be safe and effective regardless of the etiology. The most appropriate choice of sedation is a benzodiazepine. Benzodiazepines have a high therapeutic index and good anticonvulsant activity. They are effective for the treatment of delirium induced by acute overdose of cocaine, amphetamines, and other agents, and the delirium associated with ethanol and sedative-hypnotic withdrawal.[30,45,48,67] The dose of benzodiazepine should be titrated rapidly intravenously until the patient is calm. In our clinical experience, cumulative benzodiazepine dosages required in the initial 30 minutes to achieve adequate sedation may frequently exceed 100 mg of diazepam or its equivalent. Neuroleptic agents, particularly potent dopamine antagonists such as haloperidol and droperidol, are frequently recommended by others for amphetamine-induced delirium. Neuroleptic agents may actually antagonize some of the effects of amphetamines via dopamine blockade.[45,46,56] In animal models, haloperidol may be superior to diazepam in preventing mortality from amphetamine toxicity.[34,42,45,46] In clinical experience, however, the benzodiazepines appear to be as efficacious as the neuroleptic agents in the management of amphetamine toxicity.[48] Neuroleptic agents lower the seizure threshold, alter temperature regulation, may cause acute dystonia and cardiac dysrhythmias, and do not interact with the benzodiazepine–GABA–chloride channel receptor complex. All of these effects may worsen the clinical outcomes related to amphetamine-induced delirium, which is similar to that of cocaine intoxication and ethanol withdrawal.[30,67,69a]

Rhabdomyolysis from amphetamine toxicity usually results from agitation and hyperthermia.[60,98] Sedation prevents further muscle contraction and heat production. External cooling should be instituted for significant hyperthermia. Adequate IV hydration and cardiovascular support are aimed to maintain urine output of 1 to 2 mL/kg per minute.

Although urinary acidification can significantly increase the elimination and decrease the half-lives of amphetamine, methamphetamine, phentermine, and phendimetrazine,[8,10,11,41] this pH manipulation does not decrease toxicity and in fact may increase the risk of renal compromise and acute tubular necrosis from rhabdomyolysis. Acidification of the urine should not be considered because of the precipitation of ferrihemate in the renal tubules and increased risk of acute renal failure.[38] Patients with acute renal failure, acidemia, and hyperkalemia will likely require urgent hemodialysis.

Amphetamine body packers should be treated similarly to those who transport cocaine (see Chap. 65). Any sympathomimetic symptoms suggesting leakage of the packets will require surgical intervention.[173] Fluids, benzodiazepines, intubation, and external cooling may be necessary to stabilize these patients.

Summary

Amphetamine usage is increasing dramatically throughout various parts of the United States. Similarly, emergency department visits, and morbidity and mortality related to amphetamines, parallel amphetamine usage. Many of these complications are similar to those of cocaine, such as agitation, hyperthermia, rhabdomyolysis, myocardial ischemia, and cerebral infarction. Physicians, more than ever, will need to understand the pathophysiology of amphetamine and be ready to diagnosis and treat its toxicity. The chronic effects of amphetamines as demonstrated in animal models pose serious concerns for the human brain, particularly as amphetamine usage becomes more prevalent; further studies will be required to address this issue.

References

1. Abenhaim L, Moride Y, Brenot F, et al: Appetitite-suppressant drugs and the risk of primary pulmonary hypertension. N Engl J Med 1996;335:609–615.
2. Allcott JV, Barnhart RA, Mooney LA: Acute lead poisoning in two users of illicit methamphetamine. JAMA 1987;258:510–511.
3. Allen A, Cantrell T: Synthetic reductions in clandestine amphetamine and methamphetamine labs. J Forensic Sci 1989;42:183–199.
4. Allen RP, McCann UD, Ricaurte GA: Persistent effects of (±)3,4-methylenedioxymethamphetamine (MDMA, "ecstasy") on human sleep. Sleep 1993;16:560–564.
5. Anderson RJ, Garza HR, Garriott JC, et al: Intravenous propylhexedrine abuse and sudden death. Am J Med 1979;67:15–20.
6. Anderson RJ, Reed WG, Hillis LD: History, epidemiology, and medical complications of nasal inhaler abuse. Clin Toxicol 1982;19:95–107.
7. Bailey DN, Shaw RF: Cocaine and methamphetamine-related deaths in San Diego County (1987): Homicides and accidental overdoses. J Forensic Sci 1989;34:407–422.
8. Baselt RC, Cravey RH: Disposition of Toxic Drugs and Chemicals in Man, 3rd ed. Chicago, Year Book, 1989.
9. Battaglia G, DeSouza EB: Pharmacologic profile of amphetamine derivatives at various brain recognition sites: Selective effects on serotonergic systems. NIDA Res Monogr 1989;94:240–258.
10. Beckett AH, Rowland M: Urinary excretion kinetics of amphetamine in man. J Pharm Pharmacol 1965;17:628–639.
11. Beckett AH, Rowland M, Turner P: Influence of urinary pH on excretion of amphetamine. Lancet 1965;1:303.
12. Berger UV, Grzanna R, Molliver ME: Depletion of serotonin using p-chlorophenylalanine (PCPA) and reserpine protects against the neurotoxic effects of p-chloroamphetamine (PCA) in the brain. Exp Neurol 1989;103:111–115.
13. Beyer KL, Bicker JT, Butt JH: Ischemic colitis associated with dextroamphetamine use. J Clin Gastroenterol 1991;13:198–201.
14. Blum K: Central nervous system stimulants. In: Blum K, ed: Handbook of Arousable Drugs. New York, Gardner, 1984, pp. 305–347.
15. Borowski TB, Kirkby RD, Kokkinidis L: Amphetamine and antidepressant drug effects on GABA- and NMDA-related seizures. Brain Res Bull 1993;30:607–610.
16. Boswick DG: Amphetamine induced cerebral vasculitis. Hum Pathol 1981;12:1031–1033.
17. Bowen JS, Davis GB, Kearney TE, Bardin J: Diffuse vascular spasm associated with 4-bromo-2,5-dimethoxyamphetamine ingestion. JAMA 1983;249:1477–1479.
18. Brenot F, Herve P, Petitpretz P, et al: Primary pulmonary hypertension and fenfluramine use. Br Heart J 1993;70:537–541.
19. Bristow LJ, Thorn L, Tricklebank MD, et al: Competitive NMDA receptor antagonists attenuate the behavioural and neurochemical effects of amphetamine in mice. Eur J Pharmacol 1994;264:353–359.
20. Bruno A, Nolte KB, Chapin J: Stroke associated with ephedrine use. Neurology 1993;43:1313–1316.
21. Buchanan JF, Brown CR: "Designer Drugs": A problem in clinical toxicology. Med Toxicol 1988;3:1–17.
22. Burton BT: Heavy metal and organic contaminants associated with illicit methamphetamine production. NIDA Res Monogr 1991;115:47–59.
23. Call TD, Hartneck J, Dickinson WA, et al: Acute cardiomyopathy secondary to intravenous amphetamine abuse. Ann Intern Med 1982;97:559–560.
24. Callaway CW, Johnson MP, Gold LH, et al: Amphetamine derivatives induce locomotor hyperactivity by acting as indirect serotonin agonists. Psychopharmacology 1991;104:293–301.
25. Callaway CW, Wing LL, Geyer MA: Serotonin release contributes to the locomotor stimulant effects fo 3,4-methylenedioxymethamphetamine in rats. J Pharm Exp Ther 1990;254:456–464.
26. Capwell RR: Ephedrine-induced mania from an herbal diet supplement. Am J Psychiatry 1995;152:647. Letter.
27. Chan P, Chen JH, Lee MH, et al: Fatal and nonfatal methamphetamine intoxication in the intensive care unit 1994;32:147–155.
28. Chandler DB, Norton RL, Kauffman J, et al: Lead poisoning associated with intravenous-methamphetamine use—Oregon, 1988. MMWR 1989;38:830–831.
29. Chiang WK, Goldfrank LG: Medical complications of drug abuse. Med J Aust 1990;152:83–88.

30. Chiang WK, Goldfrank LG: Substance withdrawal. Emerg Med Clin North Am 1990;8:613–631.
31. Cho AK: Ice: A new dosage form of an old drug. Science 1990;249:631–634.
32. Cimbura G: PMA deaths in Ontario. Can Med Assoc J 1974;110:1263–1267.
33. Citron BP, Halpern M, McCarron M, et al: Necrotizing angitis associated with drug abuse. N Engl J Med 1970;283: 1003–1011.
34. Catravas JD, Waters IW, Davis WM, Hickenbottom JP: Haloperidol for acute amphetamine poisoning: A study in dogs. JAMA 1975;231:1340–1341.
35. Costall B, Naylor RJ: Extrapyramidal and mesolimbic involvement with the stereotypic activity of D- and L-amphetamine. Eur J Pharmacol 1974;15:121–129.
36. Council on Scientific Affairs: Clinical aspects of amphetamine abuse. JAMA 1978;240:2317–2319.
37. Croft CH, Firth BG, Hillis LD: Propylhexedrine-induced left ventricular dysfunction. Ann Intern Med 1982;97: 560–561.
38. Curry SC, Chang D, Connor D: Drug- and toxin-induced rhabdomyolysis. Ann Emerg Med 1989;18:1068–1084.
39. Dal Carson TA, Angelos JA, Raney JK: A clandestine approach to the synthesis of phenyl–2-propanone from phenylpropenes. J Forensic Sci 1984;29:1187–1208.
40. Davis GG, Swalwell CI: Acute aortic dissections and ruptured berry aneurysms associated with methamphetamine abuse. J Forsensic Sci 1994;39:1481–1485.
41. Davis JM, Kopin IJ, Lemberger L, et al: Effects of urinary pH on amphetamine metabolism. Ann NY Acad Sci 1971;179:493–501.
42. Davis MW, Logston DG, Hickenbottom JP: Antagonism of acute amphetamine intoxication by haloperidol and propranolol. Toxicol Appl Pharmacol 1974;29:397–403.
43. Delaney P, Estes M: Intracranial hemorrhage with amphetamine abuse. Neurology 1980;30:1125–1128.
44. Delliou D, Bromo DMA: New hallucinogenic drug. Med J Aust 1980;1:83. Letter.
45. Derlet RW, Albertson TE, Rice P: Antagonism of cocaine, amphetamine, and methamphetamine toxicity. Pharmacol Biochem Behavior 1990;36:745–749.
46. Derlet RW, Albertson TE, Rice P: Protection against d-amphetamine toxicity. Am J Emerg Med 1990;8:105–108.
47. Derlet RW, Heischober B: Methamphetamine. Stimulant of the 1990s? West J Med 1990;153:625–628.
48. Derlet RW, Rice P, Horowitz BZ, Lord RV: Amphetamine toxicity: Experience with 127 cases. J Emerg Med 1989;7: 157–161.
49. De Souza EB, Battaglia G: Effects of MDMA and MDA on brain serotonin neurons: Evidence from neurochemical and autoradiographic studies. NIDA Res Monogr 1989; 94:196–222.
50. Devan GS: Phentermine and psychosis. Br J Psychiatry 1990;156:442–443.
51. Di Maio VJM, Garriott JC: Intravenous abuse of propylhexedrine. J Forensic Sci 1977;22:152–158.
52. Dowling GP, McDonough ET, Bost RO: "Eve" and "ecstasy." A report of five deaths associated with the use of MDEA and MDMA. JAMA 1987;257:1615–1617.
53. Edison GR: Amphetamines: A dangerous illusion. Ann Intern Med 1971;74:605–610.
54. Ellinwood EH: Assault and homicide associated with amphetamine abuse. Am J Psychiatry 1971;127:1170–1175.
55. Emerson TS, Cisek JE: Methcathinone ("cat"): A Russian designer amphetamine infiltrates the rural Midwest. Ann Emerg Med 1993;22:1897–1903.
56. Espelin DE, Done AK: Amphetamine poisoning. Effectiveness of chlorpromazine. N Engl J Med 1968;278:1361–1365.
57. Feinstein D: The Methamphetamine Control Act of 1996. HTTP://www.senate.gov/member/ca/feinstein/general/meth.html.
58. Fischman MW: Cocaine and the amphetamines. In: Meltzer HY, ed: Psychopharmacology: The Third Generation of Progress. New York, Raven, 1987, pp. 1543–1553.
59. Furst SR, Fallon SP, Reznik GN, et al: Myocardial infarction after inhalation of methamphetamine. N Engl J Med 1990;323:1147–1148.
60. Gal J: Amphetamines in nasal inhalers. Clin Toxicol 1982; 19:577–578.
61. Gary NE, Saidi M: Methamphetamine intoxication. A speedy new treatment. Am J Med 1978;64:537–540.
62. Ginsberg MD, Hertzman M, Schmidt-Nowara W: Amphetamine intoxication with coagulopathy, hyperthermia, and reversible renal failure. A syndrome resembling heatstroke. Ann Intern Med 1970;73:81–85.
63. Glennon RA: Stimulus properties of hallucinogenic phenalkylamines and related designer drugs: Formulation of structure-activity relationship. NIDA Res Monogr 1989; 94:43–67.
64. Glennon RA, Showwalter D: The effects of cathinone and several related derivatives on locomotor activity. Res Commun Subst Abuse 1981;2:186–191
65. Glennon RA, Yousif M, Naiman N, et al: Methcathinone: A new and potent amphetamine-like agent. Pharmacol Biochem Behavior 1987;26:547–551.
66. Gold LHG, Geyer MA, Koob GF: Neurochemical mechanisms involved in behavioral effects of amphetamines and related designer drugs. NIDA Res Monogr 1989;94: 101–126.
67. Goldfrank LR, Hoffman RS: The cardiovascular effects of cocaine. Ann Emerg Med 1991;20:165–175.
68. Goldstone MS: "Cat": Methcathinone—A new drug of abuse. JAMA 1993;269:2508. Letter.
69. Gospe SM Jr.: Transient cortical blindness in an infant exposed to methamphetamine. Ann Emerg Med 1995;26: 380–382.
69a. Greenblatt DJ, Gross PL, Harris J, et al: Fatal hyperthermia following haloperidol therapy of sedative-hypnotic withdrawal. J Clin Psychiatry 1978;39:673–675.
70. Greenblatt JC, Gfroerer JC, Melnick D: Increasing morbidity and mortality associated with abuse of methamphetamine—United States, 1991–1994. MMWR 1995;44:882–886.
71. Groves PM, Ryan LJ, Diana M, et al: Neuronal actions of amphetamine in the rat brain. NIDA Res Monogr 1989; 94:127–145.
72. Gurtner HP: Aminorex and pulmonary hypertension. Cor Vasa 1985;27:160–171.
73. Halbach H: Medical aspects of the chewing of khat leaves. Bull WHO 1972;27:21–29.

74. Hamer R, Phelphs D: Inadvertent intra-arterial injection of phentermine: A complication of drug abuse. Ann Emerg Med 1981;10:148–150.
75. Harrington H, Heller HA, Dawson D, et al: Intracerebral hemorrhage and oral amphetamine. Arch Neurol 1983; 40:503–507.
76. Hart JB, Wallace J: The adverse effects of amphetamines. Clin Toxicol 1975;8:179–190.
77. Heischober B, Miller MA: Methamphetamine abuse in California. NIDA Res Monogr 1991;115:60–71.
78. Henry JA, Jeffrey KJ, Dawling S: Toxicity and deaths from 3,4-methylenedioxymethamphetamine ("ecstasy"). Lancet 1992;340:384–387.
79. Herr RD, Caravati EM: Acute transient ischemic colitis after oral methamphetamine ingestion. 1991;9:406–409.
80. Herve P, Launay J, Scrobohaci M, et al: Increased plasma serotonin in primary pulmonary hypertension. Am J Med 1995;99:249–254.
81. Hirata H, Ladenheim B, Rothman RB, et al: Methamphetamine-induced serotonin neurotoxicity is mediated by superoxide radicals. Brain Res 1995;677:345–347.
82. Hoffman BB, Lefkowitz RJ: Catecholamines, sympathomimetic drugs, and adrenergic receptor antagonists. In: Hardman JG, Limbird LE, Molinoff PB, et al, eds: Goodman and Gilman's The Pharmacological Basis of Therapeutics, 9th ed. New York, McGraw-Hill, 1996, pp. 199–227.
83. Hong R, Matsuyama E, Nur K: Cardiomyopathy associated with the smoking of crystal methamphetamine. JAMA 1991;265:1152–1154.
84. Imanse J, Vanneste J: Intraventricular hemorrhage following amphetamine abuse. Neurology 1990;40:1318–1319.
85. Irvine GD, Chin L: The environmental impact and adverse health effects of the clandestine manufacture of methamphetamine. NIDA Res Monogr 1991;115:33–46.
86. Jackson JG: Hazards of smokable methamphetamine. N Engl J Med 1989;321:907. Letter.
87. Jerrard DA: "Designer drugs"—A current perspective. J Emerg Med 1990;8:733–741.
88. Johnson LE, Anggaro E, Gunne LM: Blockade of intravenous amphetamine euphoria in man. Clin Pharmacol Ther 1971;12:889–896.
89. Johnson TD, Berenson MM: Methamphetamine-induced ischemic colitis. J Clin Gastroenterol 1991;13:687–689.
90. Jordan SC, Hampson F: Amphetamine poisoning associated with hyperpyrexia. Br J Med 1960;2:844.
91. Kalant H, Kalant OJ: Death in amphetamine users: Causes and rates. Can Med Assoc J 1975;112:299–304.
92. Kalix P: Pharmacological properties of the stimulant khat. Pharmac Ther 1990;48:397–416.
93. Karch SB, Billingham ME: The pathology and etiology of cocaine-induced heart disease. Arch Pathol Lab Med 1988; 112:225–230.
94. Karler R, Calder LD, Thai LH, et al: The dopaminergic, glutamatergic, GABAergic bases for the action of amphetamine and cocaine. Brain Res 1995;671:100–104.
95. Karler R, Calder LD, Thai LH, et al: A dopaminergic-glutamatergic basis for the action of amphetamine and cocaine. Brain Res 1994;658:8–14.
96. Kase CS, Foster TE, Reed JE, et al: Intracerebral hemorrhage and phenylpropanolamine use. Neurology 1987;37: 399–404.
97. Katsumata S, Sato K, Kashiwade H, et al: Sudden death due presumably to internal use of methamphetamine. Forensic Sci Intor 1993;62:209 215.
98. Kendrick WC, Hull AR, Knochel JP: Rhabdomyolysis and shock after intravenous amphetamine administration. Ann Intern Med 1977;86:381–387.
99. Klatt EC, Montgomery S, Nemiki T, et al: Misrepresentation of stimulant street drugs: A decade of experience in analysis program. J Toxicol Clin Toxicol 1986;24:441–450.
100. Klawans HL, Weiner WJ: The effects of D-amphetamine on choreiform movement disorder. Neurology 1974;6: 312–318.
101. Kojima T, Matsushima E, Iwama H, et al: Visual perception process in amphetamine psychosis and schizophrenia. Psychopharmacol Bull 1986;22:768–773.
102. Kokkinidis L, Zacharko RM, Anisman H: Amphetamine withdrawal: A behavioral evaluation. Life Sci 1968;38: 1617–1623.
103. Kokkinos J, Levine SR: Possible association of ischemic stroke with phentermine. Stroke 1993;24:310–313.
104. Kram TC, Kram BS, Kruegel AV: The identification of impurities in illicit methamphetamine exhibits by gas chromatography/mass spectrometry and nuclear magnetic resonance spectroscopy. J Forensic Sci 1976;22:40–52.
105. Kramer JC, Fischman VS, Littlefield DC: Amphetamine abuse. Pattern and effects of high doses taken intravenously. JAMA 1967;201:89–93.
106. Kringsholm B, Christoffersen P: Lung and heart pathology in fatal drug addiction. A consecutive autopsy study. Forensic Sci Int 1987;34:39–51.
107. Lago JA, Kosten TR: Stimulant withdrawal. Addiction 1994;89:1477–1481.
108. Lake C, Quirk R: Stimulants and look-alike drugs. Psychiatr Clin North Am 1984;7:689–701.
109. Lerner MA: The fire of ice. Newsweek, November 27, 1989, pp. 37–40.
110. Liggett SB: Propylhexedrine intoxication: Clinical presentation and pharmacology. South Med J 1982;76:250–251.
111. Little BB, Snell LM, Gilstrap LC: Methamphetamine abuse during pregnancy: Outcome and fetal effects. Obstet Gynecol 1988;72:541–544.
112. Lucas AR, Weiss M: Methylphenidate hallucinosis. JAMA 1971;217:1079–1081.
113. Lucas BB, Gardner DL, Wolkowitz OM, et al: Methylphenidate-induced cardiac arrhythmias. N Engl J Med 1986;315:1485.
114. Lukes SA: Intracerebral hemorrhage from an arteriovenous malformation after amphetamine injection. Arch Neurol 1983;40:60–61.
115. Lundh H, Tunuing K: An extrapyramidal choreiform syndrome caused by amphetamine addiction. J Neurol Neurosurg Psych 1981;44:728–730.
116. Luqman W, Danowski TS: The use of khat (*Catha edulis*) in Yemen social and medical observation. Ann Intern Med 1976;85:246–249.
117. Mancusi-Ungaro HR, Decker WJ: Tissue injuries associated with parenteral propylhexedrine abuse. J Toxicol Clin Toxicol 1983–1984;21:359–372.

118. Marsden P, Sheldon J: Acute poisoning by propylhexedrine. Br Med J 1972;1:730.
119. Mattson RH, Calverley JR: Dextroamphetamine-sulfate-induced dyskinesis. JAMA 1968;204:108–110.
120. McCann UD, Slate SO, Ricaurte GA: Adverse reactions with 3,4-methylenedioxymethamphetamine (MDMA; "ecstasy"). Drug Saf 1996;15:107–115.
121. Miller MA: Trends and patterns of methamphetamine smoking in Hawaii. NIDA Res Monogr 1991;115:72–83.
122. Molliver ME: Serotonergic neuronal systems: What their anatomic organization tells us about function. J Clin Psychopharmacol 1987;7:3S–23S.
123. Molliver ME, Berger UV, Mamounas LA, et al: Neurotoxicity of MDMA and related compounds: Anatomic studies. Ann NY Acad Sci 1990;600:640–661.
124. Morgan JP: Amphetamine and methamphetamine during the 1990s. Pediatr Rev 1992;13:330–333.
125. Nadir A, Agrawal S, King PD, et al: Acute hepatitis associated with the use of a Chinese herbal product, ma-huang. Am J Gastroenterol 1996;91:1436–1438.
126. Naeije R, Wauthy P, Maggiorini M, et al: Effects of dexfenfluramine on hypoxic pulmonary vasoconstriction and emboli pulmonary hypertension in dogs. Am J Respir Crit Care Med 1995;151:692–697.
127. Nestor TA, Tamamoto WI, Kam TH: Acute pulmonary oedema caused by crystalline methamphetamine. Lancet 1989;2:1277–1278.
128. Nichols DE, Oberlender R: Structure-activtity relationships of MDMA-like substances. NIDA Res Monogr 1989; 94:1–29 .
129. Ohmori T, Abekawa T, Muraki A, et al: Competitive and noncompetitive NMDA antagonists block sensitization to methamphetamine. Pharmacol Biochem Behav 1994;48: 587–591.
130. O'Neill ME, Arnolda LF, Coles DM, et al: Acute amphetamine cardiomyopathy in a drug addict. Clin Cardiol 1983;6:189–191.
131. Ong BH: Hazards to health. Dextroamphetamine poisoning. N Engl J Med 1962;266:1321–1322.
132. Packe GE, Garton MJ, Kennings K: Acute myocardial infarction caused by intravenous amphetamine abuse. Br Heart J 1990;64:23–24.
133. Pentel P: Toxicity of over-the counter stimulants. JAMA 1984;252:1898–1903.
134. Perrotta DM, Coody G, Culmo C, et al: Adverse events associated with ephedrine-containing products—Texas, December 1993 to September 1995. MMWR 1996;45: 689–693.
135. Pitts DK, Marwah J: Cocaine and central monoaminergic neurotransmission: A review of electrophysiological studies and comparison to amphetamine and antidepressants. Life Sci 1988;42:949–968.
136. Puder KD, Kagan DV, Morgan JP: Illicit methamphetamine, analysis, synthesis, and availability. Am J Drug Alcohol Abuse 1988;14:463–473.
137. Randall T: Ecstasy-fueled "Rave" parties become dances of death for English youths. JAMA 1992;268:1505–1506.
138. Randall T: "Rave" scene, ecstasy use, leap Atlantic. JAMA 1992;268:1506.
139. Rasmussen S, Cole R, Spiehler V: Methamphetamine prevalence in sheriff's crime lab samples. J Anal Toxicol 1989;12:263–267.
140. Rhee KJ, Albertson TE, Douglas JC: Choreoathetoid disorder associated wtih amphetamine-like drugs. Am J Emerg Med 1988;6:131–133.
141. Ricaurte GA, DeLanney LE, Irwin I, et al: Toxic effects of MDMA on central serotonergic neurons in the primate: Importance of route and frequency of drug administration. Brain Res 1988;446:165–168.
142. Ricaurte GA, Finnegan KF, Irwin I, et al: Aminergic metabolites in cerebrospinal fluid of humans previously exposed to MDMA: Preliminary observations. Ann NY Acad Sci 1990;600:699–710
143. Ricaurte GA, Finnegan KF, Nichols DE, et al: 3,4-Methylenedioxyethylamphetamine (MDE), a novel analogue of MDMA, produces long-lasting depletion of serotonin in the rat brain. Eur J Pharmacol 1987;137:265–268.
144. Ricaurte GA, Guillery RW, Seiden LS, et al: Dopamine nerve terminal degeneration produced by high doses of methylamphetmine in the rat brain. Brain Res 1982;235: 93–103.
145. Ricaurte GA, Seiden LS, Schuster CR: Further evidence that amphetamines produce long-lasting dopamine neurochemical deficits by destroying dopamine nerve fibers. Brain Res 1984;303:359–364.
146. Richards KC, Borgstedt HH: Near fatal reaction to ingestion of the hallucinogenic drug MDA. JAMA 1971;218: 1826–1827.
147. Riley I, Corson J, Haider I, et al: Fenfluramine overdosage. Lancet 1969;2:1162–1163.
148. Rothrock JF, Rubenstein R, Lyden PD: Ischemic stroke associated with methamphetamine inhalation. Neurology 1988;38:589–592.
149. Rumbaugh CL, Bergeron RT, Fang HCH, et al: Cerebral angiographic changes in drug abuse patient. Radiology 1971;101:335–344.
150. Rumbaugh CL, Bergeron RT, Scanlan RL, et al: Cerebral vascular changes secondary to amphetamine abuse in the experimental animal. Radiology 1971;101:345–351.
151. Rumbaugh CL, Fang HCH, Higgins RE, et al: Cerebral microvascular injury in experimental drug abuse. Invest Rad 1976;11:282–294.
152. Salanova V, Taubner R: Intracerebral haemorrhage and vasculitis secondary to amphetamine use. Postgrad Med J 1984;60:429–430.
153. Sallee FR, Stiller RL, Perel JM, et al: Pemoline-induced abnormal involuntary movements. J Clin Psychopharmacol 1989;9:125–129.
154. Sato M: Psychotoxic manifestations in amphetamine abuse. Psychopharmacol Bull 1986;22:751–756.
155. Schaffer CB, Pauli MW: Psychotic reaction caused by proprietary oral diet agents. Am J Psychiatry 1980;137: 1256–1257.
156. Schaiberger PH, Kennedy TC, Miller FC, et al: Pulmonary hypertension associated with long-term inhalation of "crank" methamphetamine. Chest 1993;104:614–616.
157. Schmidt CJ, Wu L, Lovenberg W: Methylenedioxymethamphetamine: A potentially neurotoxic amphetamine analogue. Eur J Pharmacol 1986;124:175–178.
158. Seiden LS: Neurotoxicity of methamphetamine: Mecha-

nisms of action and issues related to aging. NIDA Res Monogr 1991;115:24–32.
159. Seiden LS, Klever MS: Methamphetamine and related drugs: Toxicity and resulting behavorial changes in response to pharmacological probes. NIDA Res Monogr 1989;94:146 160.
160. Seiden LS, Sabol KE, Ricaurte GA: Amphetamine: Effects on catecholamine systems and behavior. Annu Rev Pharmacol Toxicol 1993;32:639–677.
161. Simpson DL, Rumack BH: Methylenedioxyamphetamine. Clinical description of overdose, death, and review of pharmacology. Arch Intern Med 1981;141:1507–1509.
162. Singh BK, Singh A, Chusid E: Chorea in long-term use of pemoline. Ann Neurology 1983;13:218. Letter.
163. Smith DE, Fisher CM: An analysis of 310 cases of acute high dose methamphetamine toxicity in Haight Ashbury. Clin Toxicol 1970;3:117–124.
164. Smith HJ, Roche AHG, Herdson PB: Cardiomyopathy associated with amphetamine administration. Am Heart J 1976;91:792–797.
165. Sonsalla PK: The role of *N*-methyl-d-aspartate receptors in dopaminergic neuropathology produced by the amphetamines. Drug Alcohol Depend 1995;37:101–105.
166. Sonsalla PK, Nicklas WJ, Heikkila RE: Role for excitatory amino acids in methamphetamine-induced nigrostriatal dopaminergic toxicity. Science 1989;243:398–400.
167. Stoessl AJ, Young GB, Feasby TE: Intracerebral haemorrhage and angiographic beading following ingestion of catecholaminergics. Stroke 1985;16:734–736.
168. Sudilovsky A: Disruption of behavior in cats by chronic amphetamine intoxication. Int J Neurol 1975;10:259–275.
169. Sulzer D, Chen TK, Lau YY, et al: Amphetamine redistributes dopamine from synaptic vesicles to the cytosol and promotes reverse transport. J Neurosci 1995;15:4105–4108.
170. Sulzer D, Pothos E, Sung HM, et al: Weak base model of amphetamine action. Ann NY Acad Sci 1992;654:525–528.
171. Tadokoro S, Kuribara H: Reverse tolerance to the ambulation-increasing effect of methamphetamine in mice as an animal model of amphetamine-psychosis. Psychopharmacol Bull 1986;22:757–762.
172. Trugman JM: Cerebral arteritis and oral methylphenidate. Lancet 1988;1:584–585.
173. Watson CJE, Thomson HJ, Johnston PS: Body-packing with amphetamines—An indication for surgery. J Roy Soc Med 1991;84:311–312.
174. White L, DiMaio VJM: Intravenous propylhexedrine and sudden death. N Engl J Med 1977;297:1071. Letter.
175. Wiener RS, Lockhart JT, Schwartz RG: Dilated cardiomyopathy and cocaine abuse. Report of two cases. Am J Med 1986;81:699–701.
176. Wooten MR, Khangure MS, Murphy MJ: Intracerebral hemorrhage and vasculitis related to ephedrine use. Ann Neurol 1983;13:337–340.
177. Young R, Glennon RA: Cocaine-stimulus generalization to two new designer drugs: Methcathinone and 4-methylaminorex. Pharmacol Biochem Behavior 1993;45:229–231.
178. Yu YJ, Cooper DR, Wellenstein DE, et al: Cerebral angiitis and intracerebral hemorrhage associated with methamphetamine abuse. J Neurosurg 1983;58:109–111.
179. Zhinger KY, Dovensky W, Crossman A, et el: Ephedrone: 2-Methylamino-1-phenylpropan-1-one (Jeff). J Forensic Sci 1991;36:915–920.

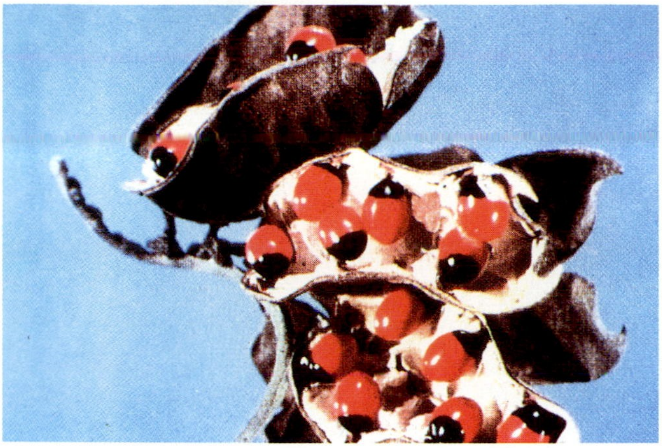

Figure 1. Rosary Pea (*Abrus precatorius*). The fruit is a pea-shaped pod approximately 4 cm in length. When opened and dried, 3 to 5 scarlet pea-sized seeds with a small black spot at the point of attachment are noted. The rosary pea contains the toxalbumin abrin. (See Chap. 77.)

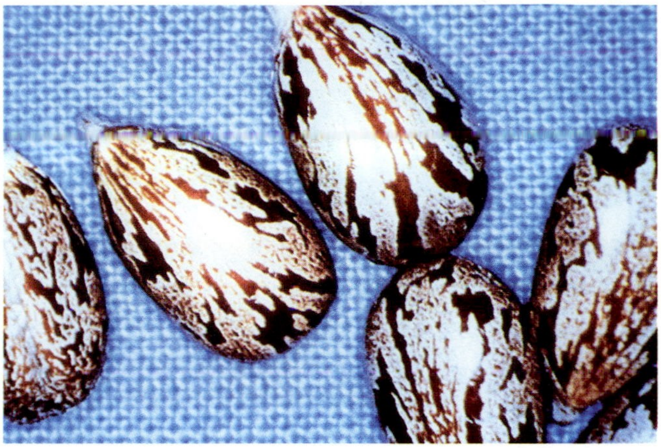

Figure 2. Castor bean (*Ricinus communis*). The bean is white, black, and brown in a variegated pattern somewhat resembling a tick. It contains the toxalbumin ricin. (See Chap. 77.)

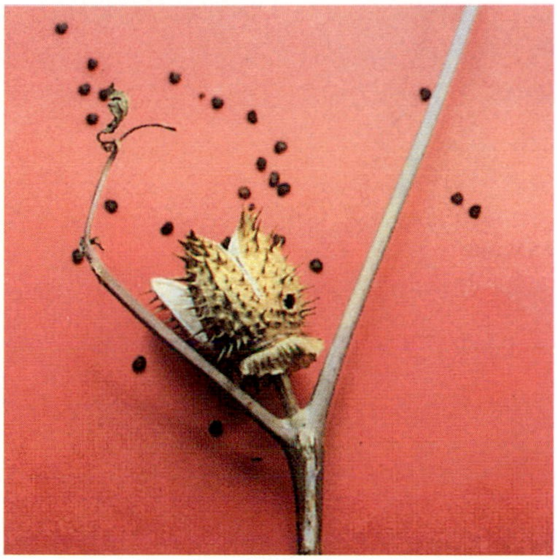

Figure 3. Jimson Weed (*Datura stramonium*). Jimson Weed contains numerous alkaloids (hyoscyamine and hyoscine) in diverse quantities. The plant's flowers, leaves, stem, and seeds are all poisonous. (See Chap. 77.)

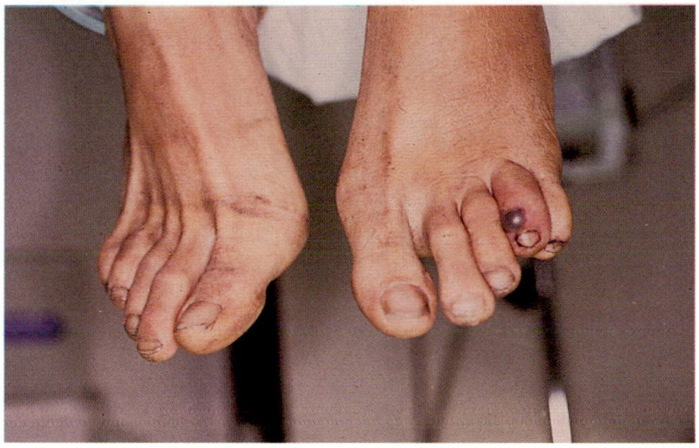

Figure 4. Two hours after the bite of a copperhead (*Agkistrodon contortrix mokason*), a hemorrhagic blister developed at the site of envenomation on the top of the toe, accompanied by swelling of the foot. (*Courtesy of James Roberts, Allegheny University of Health Sciences, MCP Hahnemann School of Medicine.*) (See Chap. 99.)

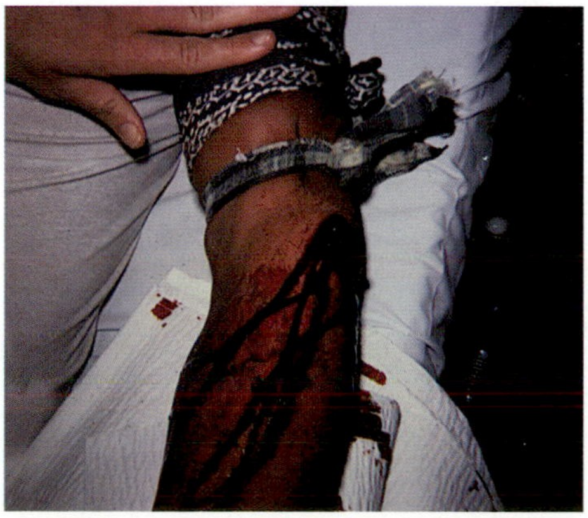

Figure 5. Example of ill-conceived field treatment of a snake bite. An arterial tourniquet was applied and a large vein was severed in attempts to incise the skin and remove venin. The patient developed hemorrhagic shock from blood loss. (*Courtesy of James Roberts, Allegheny University of Health Sciences, MCP Hahnemann School of Medicine.*) (See Chap. 99.)

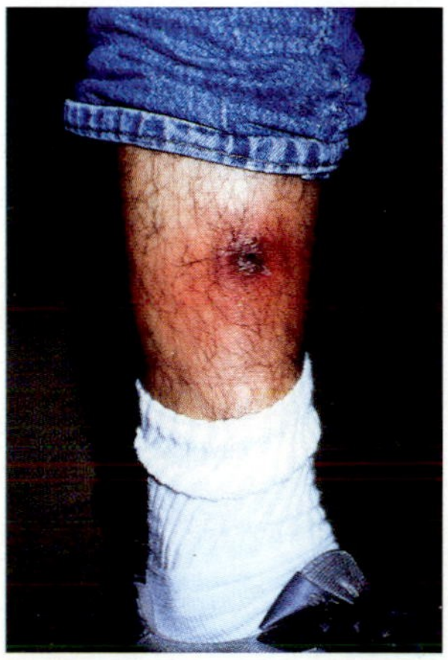

Figure 6. Brown Recluse spider (*Loxosceles reclusa*) bite. This lesion was initially painful. A central bleb developed, which became ecchymotic and necrotic by the fourth day. (See Chap. 100.)

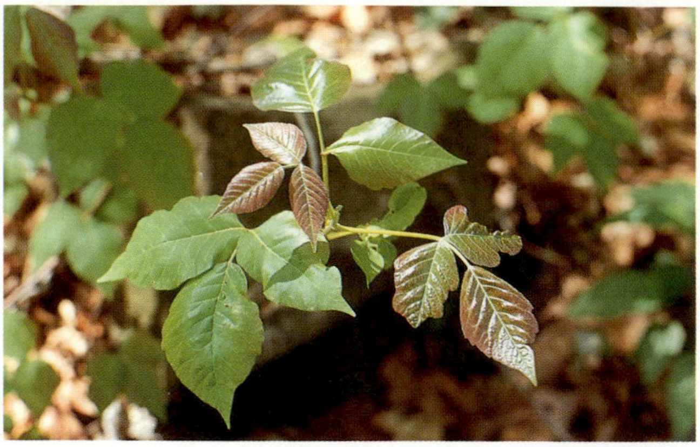

Figure 7. Poison Ivy (*Toxicodendron radicans*). Poison ivy is represented by the characteristic three-leafed patterns, aerial roots, and globular white fruits. This plant's resin, urushiol, is the most common cause of plant dermatitis. (See Chaps. 28 and 77.)

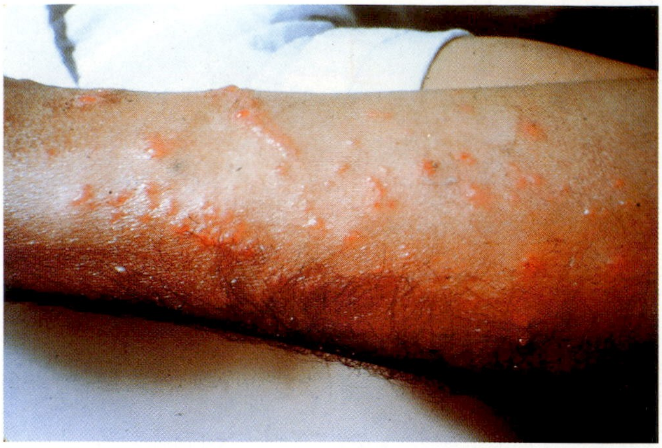

Figure 8. Poison Ivy (*Toxicodendron radicans*). Linear contact dermatitis resulting from exposure to poison ivy. (*Courtesy of New York University, Department of Dermatology*.) (See Chaps. 28 and 77.)

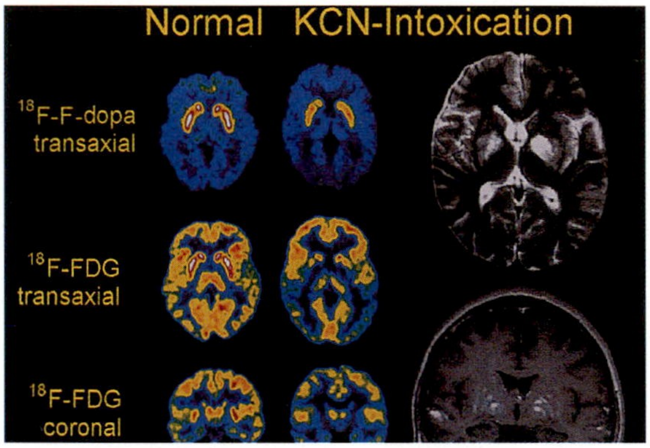

Figure 9. PET (left) and MRI (right) images obtained approximately 2 weeks after an attempted suicide with KCN. There is decreased dopamine uptake and metabolic activity in the basal ganglia on the affected PET scans as indicated by less intense red coloration compared with normal scans. The top axial MRI image (T2-weighted) shows globus pallidus and posterior putamen abnormalities (white). The bottom coronal MRI image (T1-weighted) after gadopentate dimeglumine administration also shows basal ganglia damage (white enhancing areas). (*Reproduced with permission from Rosenow F, Heizholz K, Lanfermann H, et al. Neurological Sequelae of Cyanide Intoxication—The Pattern of Clinical, Magnetic Resonance Imaging and Position Emission Tomography Findings. Ann Neurology 1995;38:828.*) (See Chap. 97.)

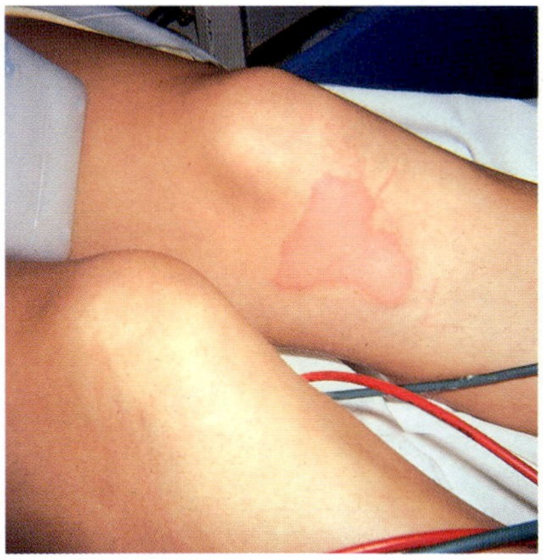

Figure 10. "Barbiturate blisters." Evolving lesions actually were secondary to an ethchlorvynol overdose. (See Chaps. 28 and 61.)

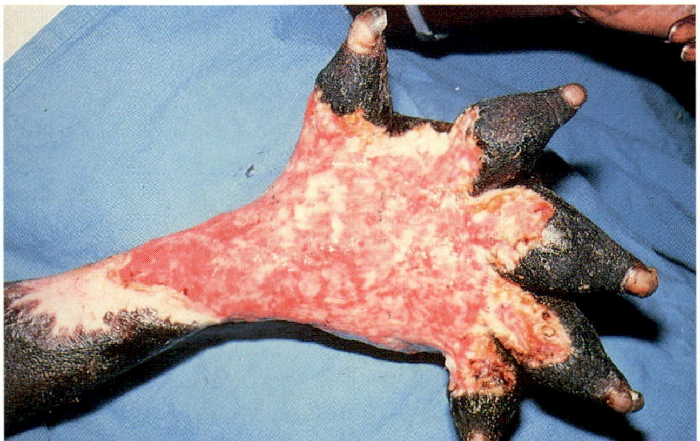

Figure 11. "Hand-claw." Grotesque transformation of a hand from parenteral drug abuse. (See Chaps. 28 and 108.)

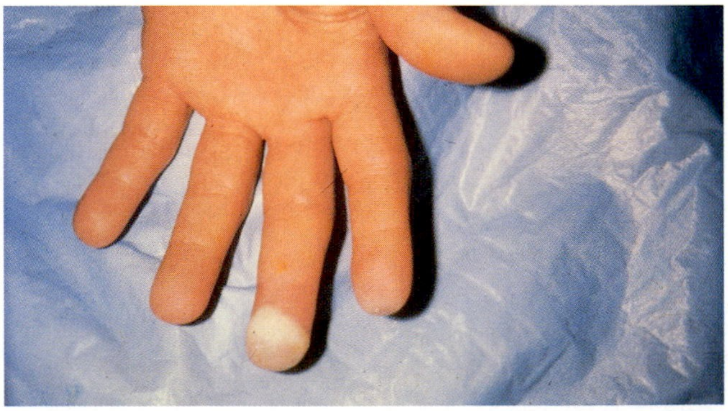

Figure 12. Hydrofluoric acid (HF) burn. As cellular ischemia and tissue necrosis progressed, the exposed tissue of the palmar surface of the third finger throbbed, burned, and blackened. This patient was treated with intra-arterial calcium gluconate. (See Chaps. 28 and 86.)

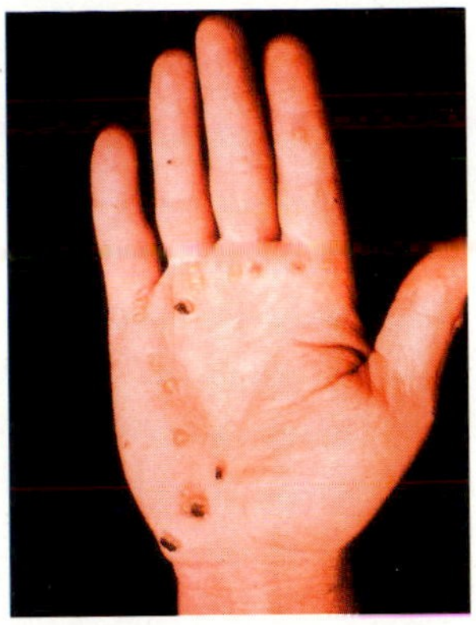

Figure 13. Arsenical keratosis. Long-standing exposure to arsenicals may lead to palmar and plantar discrete, hard, yellow keratotic plaques. These are usually persistent but can be precursors to intraepidermal squamous cell carcinomas. (*Courtesy of New York University, Department of Dermatology.*) (See Chaps. 28 and 78.)

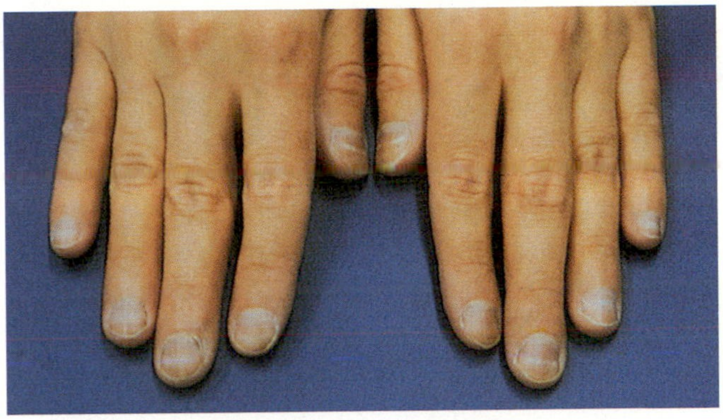

Figure 14. Mee's Lines. On all of this patient's fingernails, horizontal white lines were noted. These lines may appear several weeks after exposure to arsenic and other heavy metals. (See Chaps. 28 and 78.)

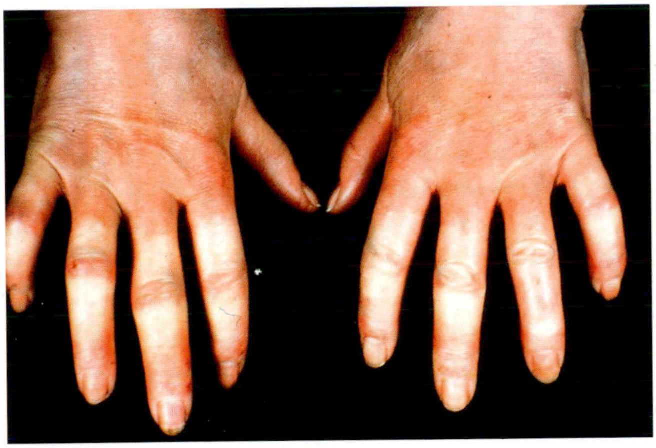

Figure 15. Acrosclerosis. Mottling of the skin of the hands occurred in a worker who was employed in a plant where a high concentration of polyvinyl chloride was found in the air. (*Courtesy of New York University, Department of Dermatology.*) (See Chap. 28.)

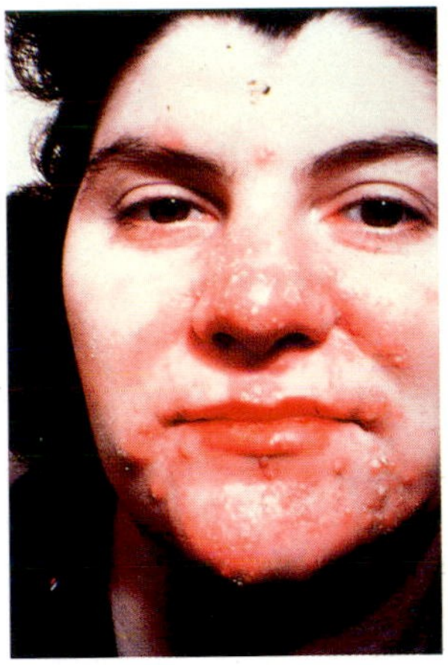

Figure 16. Ioderma. An iodine-related rash that has an acneiform character and may spread extensively on the body. This patient had long-term exposure to iodinated products. (*Courtesy of New York University, Department of Dermatology.*) (See Chaps. 28 and 83.)

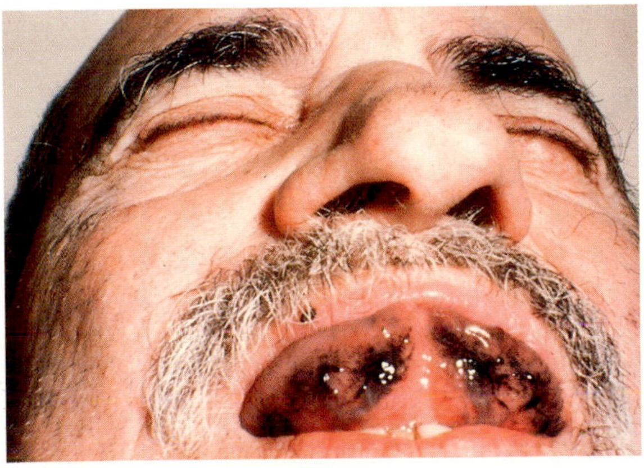

Figure 17. Bismuth lines. Black spots are noted on the mucosa and gums of this patient who chronically ingested bismuth compounds. (*Courtesy of New York University, Department of Dermatology.*) (See Chap. 28.)

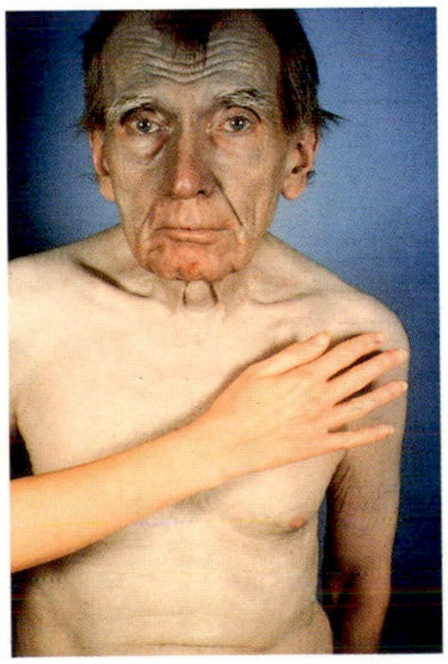

Figure 18. Argyria. This patient not only had deep azure nail pigmentation but also his entire body was dark gray as a manifestation of silver intoxication. Long-term exposure to soluble silver compounds such as $AgNO_3$ in the workplace led to this patient's pigmentation. (*Courtesy of New York University, Department of Dermatology.*) (See Chap. 28.)

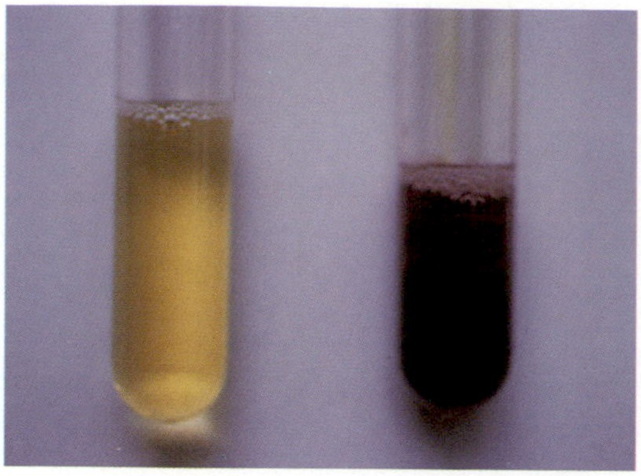

Figure 19. A positive test for salicylates in the urine. The tube on the left shows the urine prior to the addition of $FeCl_3$ (clear yellow), and the tube on the right shows the deep purple color immediately after the addition of 10% ferric chloride. (See Chap. 32 and Fig. 32–3.)

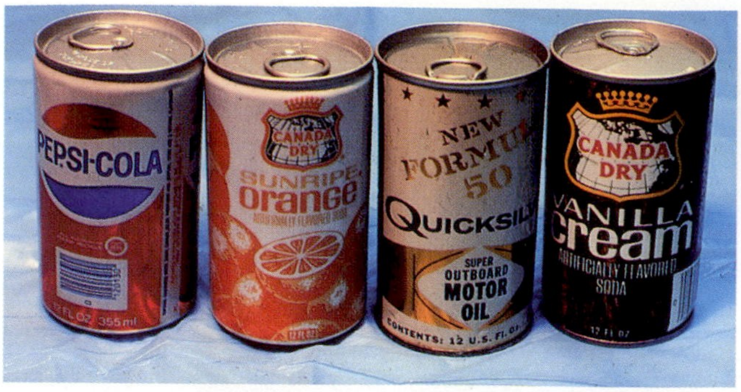

Figure 20. Look-alikes. The can of motor oil in this photograph is a potential source of toxicity for a young child or for a non-reading person. (See Chap. 115.)

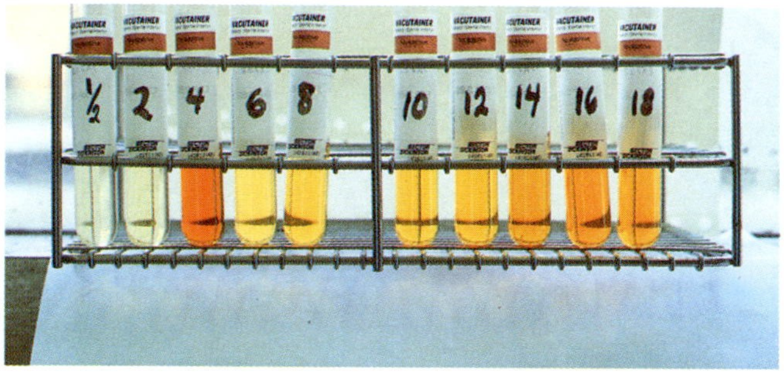

Figure 21. Deferoxamine treatment of a patient with iron poisoning. The initial white-yellow urine prior to therapy evolves with a transition to a deep rose-orange by four hours after therapy and shows the persistence of an orange color for an additional eighteen hours. The high concentration of ferrioxamine maintains the color of the urine as brown-orange or rose. (See Chap. 35.)

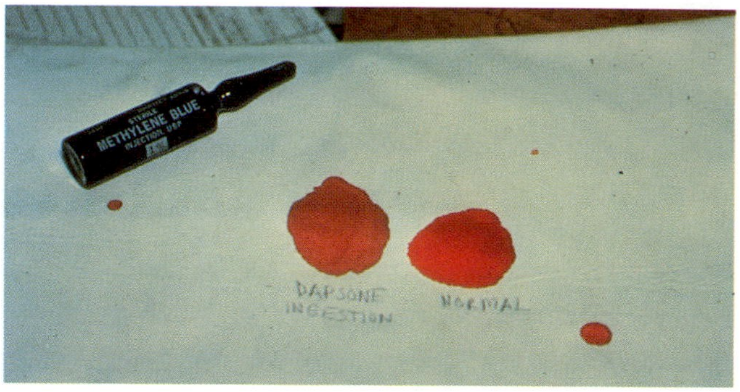

Figure 22. Methemoglobinemia. The drop of blood from the physician (right-red) and from the patient receiving dapsone (left-chocolate brown) demonstrate the visual diagnosis of methemoglobinemia. (See Chap. 93.)

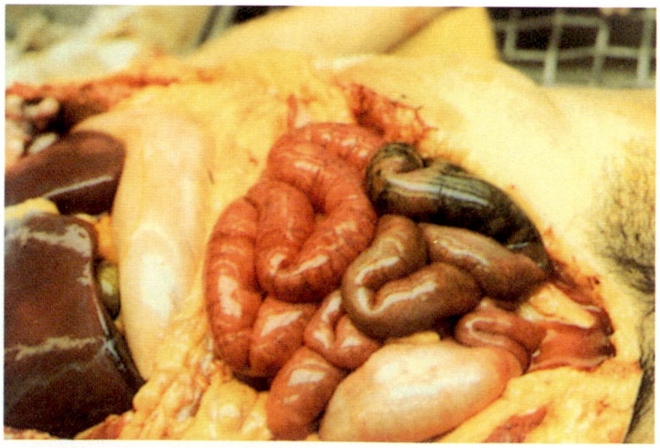

Figure 23. Cocaine-related bowel ischemia. An autopsy was performed on a young woman who died within two hours of smoking cocaine. She developed acute abdominal pain and refactory acidemia in the emergency department. The autopsy demonstrated the necrotic bowel, ischemic bowel, and an area of healthier bowel. (See Chap. 65.)

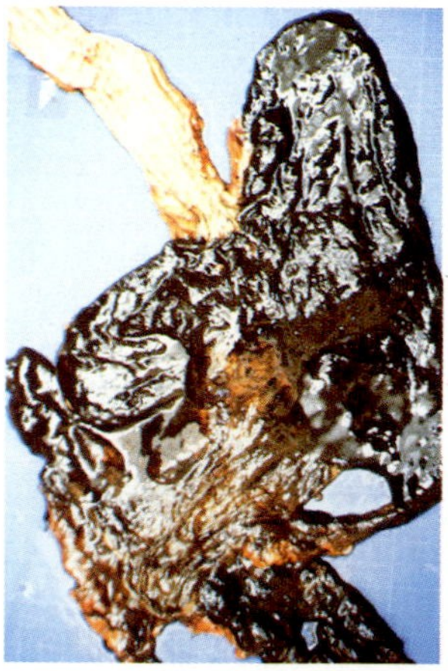

Figure 24. Strong acid ingestion. An autopsy was performed on a patient who ingested hydrochloric (HCl) and phosphoric acids (H_3PO_4). The patient died shortly after the ingestion. The esophagus was normal, but the stomach and duodenum were necrotic at autopsy. (See Chap. 86.)

CHAPTER 67

Phencyclidine

Lewis R. Goldfrank and Neal A. Lewin

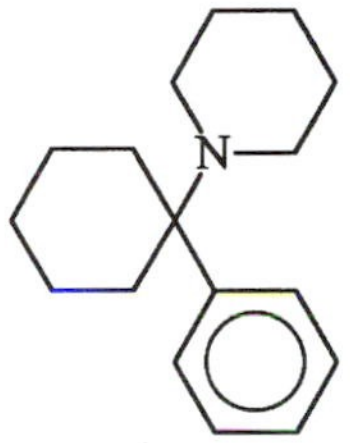

Phencyclidine (PCP)

A 17-year-old male was brought to the Emergency Department (ED) by his school supervisor and two police officers. The boy was extremely agitated. He also had transient periods of blank staring and myoclonic movements of both arms. It took several members of the ED staff to keep him on a stretcher.

Initially, no history was obtainable from the patient, who responded to verbal stimuli with inappropriate physical gestures and a few nonsensical words. The school supervisor reported that the boy had become agitated very suddenly and had created a disturbance in the lunchroom, throwing chairs about the room.

His vital signs were: blood pressure, 130/90 mm Hg; pulse, 110 beats/min; respiratory rate, 18 breaths/min; and temperature, 99.9°F (37.2°C). He was well developed and well nourished, anicteric, and acyanotic. The examination was normal except for a few pertinent findings. The skin was cool and diaphoretic. Conjunctivae were normal; extraocular movements were intact, but there was persistent vertical and horizontal nystagmus; pupils were equal at 4 mm and reactive to light; fundi were normal. The patient moved all extremities, had good strength and normal, symmetric deep tendon reflexes; muscle tone seemed increased and there were periodic myoclonic jerks; plantar flexion was elicited; sensory examination could not be performed due to the patient's unresponsiveness and agitation.

Blood was drawn for initial laboratory tests and an intravenous infusion of 5% dextrose in 0.45% sodium chloride solution was started at 200 mL/h. Fifty milliliters of 50% dextrose and 100 mg of thiamine were given IV. He was placed on 6 L of oxygen via nasal cannula. Fifty grams of activated charcoal were given together with 50 g of sorbitol by mouth.

The initial laboratory data, including CBC, electrolytes, arterial blood gas analysis, and urinalysis, were all normal. An ECG revealed a sinus tachycardia at 110 beats/min and was otherwise normal.

By the time the examination and tests were completed, the patient had become calm and cooperative. He related that while at lunch, one of his friends had put mustard on his sandwich and that it tasted "terrific." He recalled finishing the sandwich and then slowly "freaking out," that is, losing control of his mind and body.

Based on the patient's history and the known prevalence of drug abuse at his school, it was reasonable to assume that his altered mental status was drug-induced. Based on this patient's acute psychotic-like episode, the history he related, and the presence of bidirectional nystagmus, a presumptive diagnosis of phencyclidine (PCP) ingestion was made. The patient's clinical condition had very much improved by the time his mother arrived in the ED. Three hours after arrival he was cooperative and his neuropsychiatric examination was entirely normal. Because he had no prior history of drug abuse, he was discharged home and arrangements were made for follow-up examination with his pediatrician.

What Is the History of Phencyclidine Abuse?

Phencyclidine was developed in the late 1950s as a dissociative anesthetic-analgesic agent and was marketed under the name Sernylan. It was the prototype of a drug combining analgesic and anesthetic actions without respiratory or cardiovascular depression. The dissociation from any perception of the environment while remaining conscious and achieving anesthesia defines this group of anesthetic agents. After surgery, however, many patients experienced psychotomimetic effects, and the drug was taken off the market.

In the mid–1960s, PCP arrived in San Francisco as a street drug called the "PeaCe Pill." Initially it was not popular, as users noted its devastating dysphoric effects and oral absorption was erratic and unpredictable.[27] Phencyclidine was often misrepresented by drug dealers as other substances, such as tetrahydrocannabinol, cocaine, LSD, mescaline, and amphetamines, as it had consciousness-altering and hallucinogenic properties. Sprinkled on tobacco or marijuana cigarettes and smoked, the effects of PCP were immediate. A nationwide resurgence of use occurred in the 1970s,[7] and has continued to the present. PCP is easily and cheaply synthesized from readily obtainable ingredients. Its popularity may also be due to a bravado or macho image, associated with its usage as teenagers try to prove themselves by using the most dangerous drug they can get—"killer weed." Studies demonstrate that the average PCP user is a polydrug abuser who begins with illicit drugs other than PCP, first uses PCP at the age of 14, and rarely takes PCP alone.[31]

Several congeners of PCP, such as ketamine and arylhexylamine derivatives, are still used clinically or are under investigation for use in anesthesiology (see Chap. 53). Many PCP analogs and metabolites are also used on the streets.[25] Some of these—such as TCP (a thiophene analog, 1-(1-cyclohexyl) piperidine); PHP (phenylcyclohexylpyrrolidine); PCE (1-phenyl-cyclohexylethylamine), which causes a barbituratelike sedation; and PCC (1-piperidonocyclohexanecarbinol)—are considered acceptable substitutes by street users, and some of them are more toxic than PCP itself. These drugs are aliphatic or aromatic substituted amines, ketones, or halides appearing quite similar to the parent compound. To thwart the manufacture of these "designer" agents the federal government has restricted the sale of piperidine, which is used as a precursor in the synthesis of PCP. Designer chemists responded by using 4-methylpiperidine to make phenylcyclohexyl-4-methylpiperidine,[26] and pyrrolidine to make PHP.[8] These chemical variations led to a diversity of similar products that were sold on the street as PCP. It is for this reason that toxicologic assessment for PCP may yield negative results, although the agent was sold as PCP and the clinical manifestations are similar.[17] Until 1986, those caught selling drugs similar but not identical to illicit substances could escape criminal prosecution. This loophole in the law was responsible for the so-called "designer drug phenomenon," Designer drugs are drugs synthesized to duplicate the effects of illicit substances, but with modified structural formulas. After 1986, creation of such illicit substances became illegal.

What Is the Clinical Pharmacology of Phencyclidine?

Phencyclidine is 1-(1-phenylcyclohexyl)piperidine, hence the acronym PCP. It is a highly lipid-soluble drug that is also soluble in water and alcohol. Blood-to-plasma ratio is approximately 1.0, and plasma protein binding is 65%.[12] It has a large volume of distribution of 6.2 L/kg.[12,33] Phencyclidine is a weak base with a pKa between 8.6 and 9.4. It is metabolized by the liver and excreted by the kidneys, mainly as the inactive monohydroxypiperidine complex.[9] Under experimental circumstances the drug is removed almost exclusively by metabolism. More than half of an administered dose of PCP is metabolized to the hydroxyl and glucuronide metabolites and then excreted in the urine within 12 hours. Only 9% of the active drug can be found in the urine.[12] Phencyclidine antagonizes the action of glutamate at the NMDA (*N*-methyl-*d*-aspartate) receptor. Both phencyclidine and the related ketamine appear to bind within the ion channel (PCP binding site) to block Ca^{2+} influx, which results from glutamate binding (see Chap. 10).[32]

Phencyclidine can be abused by smoking, insufflating, or ingestion. When ingested orally, subjective responses are noted in 15 to 30 minutes; when inhaled by smoking, responses may be noted in 2 to 5 minutes and are maximal at 15 minutes. Sedation is produced by doses of 1 to 5 mg ingested orally, whereas only 0.25 mg is required to produce sedation with IV injection. The relationship between dose or serum levels and clinical effects is not reliable or predictable with PCP. Phencyclidine is commonly sold on the street as capsules, tablets (about 5 mg), powder, a solution in water or alcohol, or as "rock salt" crystal. PCP may be insufflated, smoked, or injected IV or SC. It has been mixed with mint, oregano, and parsley, or with marijuana. A typical PCP joint contains about 1 mg per 150 mg of plant product, totaling anywhere from 1 to 10 mg of the drug per joint. Finally, as in the case that begins this chapter, PCP may be placed on food and ingested deliberately or unintentionally.[7,11]

Toxic effects often persist, and detectable serum levels may be noted up to a week later. The drug's high lipid solubility accounts for its entry into and storage in adipose and brain tissue; also, as a weak base it is concentrated in the slightly more acidic environment of the cerebrospinal fluid (CSF). Because of ion trapping, CSF levels are approximately four times as high as simultaneous serum concentrations. This "reservoir" explains in part the long-lasting CNS effects of the drug. The apparent terminal phase half-lives averaged 21 ± 3 hours (range, 7 to 46 hours) under both control and overdose settings.[12,18] The data indicates first-order elimination over both toxic and nontoxic levels. The duration of action of PCP may range from 7 to 16 hours and may be longer in chronic users. Continued absorption from a concretion or "body pack" should be considered if signs of toxicity persist beyond 24 hours.[35]

Placental transfer of PCP has been documented both in animal models and clinically.[20] Various physical and neuropsychiatric findings in the newborn suggest prenatal exposure to PCP.[16,28]

What Are the Typical Signs and Symptoms of Phencyclidine Toxicity?

PCP abuse typically produces relatively small pupils, nystagmus (horizontal and/or vertical and/or rotary), hypertension, tachycardia, salivation, flushing, sweating, ataxia, and central nervous system stimulation or depression. In the largest case series reported to date, nystagmus and hypertension were noted in 57% of patients who had taken PCP (Table 67–1).[21] The symptoms are, in fact, quite variable, showing a remarkable mixture of CNS stimulant and depressant effects. Miosis, choreoathetosis, and seizures appear more frequently in children than in adults.[19] Cholinergic, anticholinergic, muscarinic, and sympathomimetic effects, and cerebellar manifestations, can all be seen in those patients who have overdosed on PCP.[5,8,29]

Some authors have attributed particular symptoms to the dose of PCP taken, but because the clinical manifestations are so variable, and because so many patients simultaneously abuse other drugs, this attribution is neither exact nor reliable.[2,9]

TABLE 67–1. PCP CLINICAL AND LABORATORY FINDINGS

Central Nervous System
Calm, unresponsive, incompletely responsive, or comatose; excited, disordered thought processes, amnesia, disorientation, paranoia, dysphoria, dysarthria, jargonaphasia, hallucinations (auditory and visual), seizures, violent or bizarre behavior, agitation, hyperthermia

Ophthalmic
Blank stare, dysconjugate gaze, nystagmus (horizontal and/or vertical and/or rotatory), blurred vision, miosis, rarely mydriasis

Sensory-motor
Hyperactivity, tremor, myoclonic movements, dystonic movements (opisthotonos, facial grimacing, tortipelvis, torticollis), abnormal stereognosis and proprioception, variable deep tendon reflexes

Cardiovascular
Systolic and diastolic hypertension, sinus tachycardia

Gastrointestinal
Vomiting

Muscle
Rhabdomyolysis

Pulmonary
Tachypnea, increased minute and tidal volumes, irregular respiratory pattern, and apnea (rare)

Laboratory
Leukocytosis, hyperkalemia, metabolic acidosis, muscle enzyme abnormalities (CPK, LDH, AST), ketonuria, myoglobinuria, diffuse slowing with theta and delta waves on EEG

After exposure to PCP, a user's mental state may vary widely. The person may appear calm or agitated, intoxicated, violent, stuporous, or comatose. Some authors report that the true extent and incidence of violent behavior is less than previously suggested.[6] Patients may also have amnesia or disordered thought processes (including disorientation to time, place, and person), paranoia, dysphoria, dysarthria, jargonaphasia, and auditory and visual hallucinations.[14] In contrast, vomiting, hyperthermia,[1] and seizures are uncommon.

Patients may complain of blurred vision. Hyperactivity, tremor, myoclonic and dystonic movements, opisthotonos, torticollis, tortipelvis, and facial grimacing have been reported. Abnormal stereognosis and proprioception are seen. The effect on deep tendon reflexes is highly variable. Profound agitation and self-induced trauma may lead to rhabdomyolysis, myoglobinuria, and acute tubular necrosis.[19]

Cardiovascular examination reveals sinus tachycardia with systolic and diastolic hypertension.[13,22] The finding of abnormal behavior, miosis, and hypertension in children strongly suggests PCP poisoning.[19] Irregular respiratory patterns are seen, and both tachypnea and apnea are frequently noted. Tachypnea when present typically results in increases in both minute ventilation and tidal volumes.

The most common abnormalities on physical examination are behavioral changes and nystagmus.[4] It is useful to distinguish between PCP-induced psychosis and PCP-dependent psychologic effects. In the former, the patient exhibits evidence of psychosis that persists even after the drug is eliminated from the body. A possible explanation for this occurrence is that the patient had an underlying psychiatric condition that was unmasked by the effects of the drug. On the other hand, direct chemical action of the drug is thought to be responsible for PCP-dependent clinical effects.

Ironically, the very characteristics that were thought to make phencyclidine ideal for anesthesia—the preservation of muscle tone and cardiopulmonary function—magnify the difficulties in managing an individual who manifests dysphoria after an overdose. Respiratory depression or pulmonary edema have only rarely been reported. Central nervous system stimulation is maintained and seizures are rarely seen, except with high doses.

The course of delirium, stupor, and coma associated with PCP is extremely variable and depends on the route of administration, dose taken, number and type of other drugs ingested, and the patients' predrug state.

What Therapeutic Measures Should Be Used for Patients With Phencyclidine Poisoning?

Conservative management is indicated and includes maintaining adequate respiration, circulation, and thermoregulation. To prevent self-injury, a common form of PCP-induced morbidity and mortality, the patient must be safely restrained, initially physically and then chemically.

Although it is always important to ask the patient the names, quantities, times, and route of all drugs taken, this information is notoriously unreliable. Many street psychoactive agents are mixtures; therefore pharmacologic management is complex and often sign- or symptom-dependent. Although some authors have attempted to define the appropriate therapy for specific PCP congeners,[15] we have not found such an approach to be beneficial.

During the initial management phase an IV line must be established and blood drawn for electrolytes, glucose, BUN, and creatinine determinations. The use of 100 mL of $D_{50}W$ and thiamine should be considered following an immediate bedside determination of glucose.

Patients with a history of recent oral consumption of PCP are candidates for gastrointestinal decontamination, but they should be considered too unstable for the use of the syrup of ipecac, as uncontrolled agitation, seizures, or respiratory compromise may rapidly develop. Gastric lavage may be initiated with a nasogastric tube, although agitation may preclude this approach as well until the patient is adequately sedated. As soon as possible activated charcoal, 1 g/kg, should be administered, and repeated every 4 hours for several doses. Activated charcoal will effectively adsorb PCP and increase its nonrenal clearance, and even without prior gastric evacuation is usually adequate.[24] Unless there are specific contraindications, a single dose of a cathartic, such as sorbitol, should be given.

Theoretically, toxic substances that are weak bases, such as PCP, are eliminated more rapidly if the urine is acidified. Athough we do not recommend this approach, urinary acidification with ammonium chloride has been recommended for this reason by some authors.[2] As the urine pH is reduced from 7.00 to 5.00 and diuresis is forced using a diuretic such as furosemide, PCP urinary clearance is increased 100-fold as the molecule becomes ionized in the acidic urine and cannot be reabsorbed. The fallacy of this theory is that although this ion trapping technique does increase the urinary load of PCP, only 10% of the active drug is excreted by the kidneys, making this route clinically insignificant; 90% of the drug is metabolized by the liver. The risks associated with acidifying the urine—simultaneously inducing a systemic acidosis, thereby potentially increasing urinary myoglobin precipitation—outweigh any perceived benefits. Because of the large volume of distribution (6.2 ± 0.3 L/kg) of PCP along with its substantial protein binding, high lipid solubility, and limited renal excretion, hemoperfusion and hemodialysis have not proved to be beneficial.[3]

The same principle described may be utilized to remove PCP via the GI tract: ion trapping results in the active mobilization of PCP into gastric secretions. Phencyclidine is in a substantially ionized (and therefore non-lipid-soluble) form in the acid of the stomach and can be absorbed only when it reaches the more alkaline intestine. Gastric suction, therefore, can remove a significant amount of the drug and also interrupt the gastroenteric circulation (by which the drug is secreted into the acid environment of the stomach only to be reabsorbed again in the small intestine).[2] Continuous gastric suction, however, may be dangerous. Moreover, it is not necessary routinely and is usually reserved for stuporous or comatose patients. Continuous suction may result in trauma to the patient and fluid and electrolyte loss, which can further complicate management and possibly interfere with drug clearance by inhibiting the efficacy of activated charcoal. For these reasons the administration of multiple-dose activated charcoal rather than continuous nasogastric suction seems to be the safest and most effective way to remove ion-trapped drug from the stomach.

A detailed psychiatric assessment is usually impossible prior to initial therapeutic intervention. When the etiology of the agitation (functional versus drug-induced) cannot be determined and pharmacologic management is necessary, once hypoglycemia is excluded it is probably best to start with an intravenous dose of a benzodiazepine. A benzodiazepine such as diazepam, administered in titrated doses of up to 10 mg IV every 5 to 10 minutes until agitation is controlled, is usually safe and effective for control of agitation regardless of the etiology. In contrast, phenothiazines may lower the seizure threshold, and both phenothiazines and butyrophenones may cause acute dystonic reactions. Phenothiazines may also cause significant hypotension, worsen hyperthermia, and add even more anticholinergic effects to those resulting from the drugs the patients initially ingested. The differential diagnosis of drug-induced agitation is broad and includes PCP, cocaine, amphetamines, and withdrawal from alcohol or sedative hypnotics.

Most patients rapidly regain normal CNS function 45 minutes to several hours after using the drug. However, those who have taken exceedingly high doses or have an underlying psychiatric disorder may remain comatose or exhibit bizarre behavior for days or even weeks before returning to normalcy. Those who regain normal function rapidly should be monitored for several hours and then, after a psychiatric consultation, receive drug counseling and whatever additional social support is available. Patients whose recovery is delayed should be treated supportively and monitored carefully in an intensive care unit.

Many patients become depressed and anxious during the "post-high" period, and chronic users may manifest a variety of psychiatric disturbances.[34] These individuals have a very grim prognosis, with repeated drug use, hospitalizations, and poor psychosocial functioning in the long term.

The major toxicity of PCP appears to be behaviorally related: self-inflicted injuries, injuries resulting from exceptional physical exertion, and injuries sustained as a result of resisting the application of physical restraints are frequent, as patients appear to be unaware of their surroundings and sometimes even oblivious to pain due to the agent's dissociative anesthetic effects. In addition to major trauma, rhabdomyolysis and resultant myoglobinuric renal failure account in large measure for the high morbidity and mortality associated with PCP intoxication. (See Chapter 114 for detailed indications and techniques of restraint application.)

If significant rhabdomyolysis[10,23] has occurred, myoglobinuria may be present. Early fluid therapy should be used to avoid deposition of pigment into the kidneys, leading to renal failure. Urinary alkalinization as part of the treatment regimen for rhabdomyolysis would potentially increase PCP reabsorption and deposition in fat stores, but this is of limited clinical concern when weighed against the potential for renal protection.

How Is the Laboratory Diagnosis of Phencyclidine Poisoning Made?

Although most laboratories do not perform quantitative analysis of PCP, most can do a qualitative test for the presence of the drug. PCP may not be part of a routine toxicologic screen and it may therefore be necessary to request it specifically. Routine toxicologic screen reported back as negative may lead to the erroneous conclusion that PCP exposure has been excluded. The qualitative test for PCP is almost always more important than a quantitative determination, as the precise serum concentration does not correlate closely with the clinical effects. If it is necessary to confirm the suspicion that PCP is the offending agent, we use urine, although serum and possibly gastric contents can be employed. However, rarely is it essential to make this determination. One of the most common false-positive reactions involves the use of dextromethorphan (Fig. 67–1). It has been verified that dextromethorphan cross-reacts with Syva EMIT and TDx PCP assays (see Chap. 6).[30]

Laboratory findings resulting from PCP abuse may include leukocytosis, hypoglycemia, and elevated muscle enzymes.[21] As a result of seizures, myoclonus, or trauma, rhabdomyolysis can lead to myoglobinuria and, potentially, acute renal failure.[10,19] The EEG reveals diffuse slowing with theta and delta waves, but this test may return to normal before the patient improves clinically.

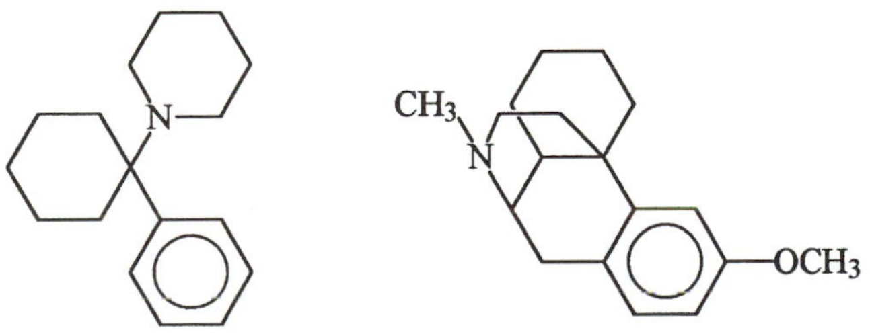

Phencyclidine (PCP) Dextromethorphan

Figure 67–1. Chemical structures of dextromethorphan and phencyclidine demonstrate the similarity between the two. This close chemical relationship is responsible for false-positive drug testing.

In spite of the common complications associated with the drug's use, it remains a frequently abused drug in the late 1990s.

Acknowledgement

Harold Osborn, MD contributed to this chapter in a previous edition.

References

1. Armen R, Kanel G, Reynolds T: Phencyclidine-induced malignant hyperthermia causing submassive liver necrosis. Am J Med 1984;77:167–172.
2. Aronow R, Done AK: Phencyclidine overdose: An emerging concept of management. JACEP 1978;7:56–59.
3. Bailey DN: Clinical findings and concentrations in biological fluids after non-fatal intoxication. Am J Clin Pathol 1979; 72:795–799.
4. Barton CH, Sterling ML, Naziri ND: Phencyclidine intoxication: Clinical experience with 27 cases confirmed by urine assay. Ann Emerg Med 1981;10:243–246.
5. Barton CH, Sterling ML, Naziri ND: Rhabdomyolysis and acute renal failure associated with phencyclidine intoxication. Arch Intern Med 1980;140:568–569.
6. Brecher M, Wang BW, Wong H, Morgan JP: Phencyclidine and violence: Clinical and legal issues. J Clin Psychopharmacol 1988;8:397–401.
7. Brown JK, Malone HH: Street drug analysis: Four years later. Clin Toxicol Bull 1974;4:139–160.
8. Budd RD: PHP, a new drug of abuse. N Engl J Med 1980; 303:588. Letter.
9. Burns RS, Lerner SE, eds: Phencyclidine: A symposium. Clin Toxicol 1976;9:473–600.
10. Cogen FC, Rigg G, Simmons JL, Domino EF: Phencyclidine associated acute rhabdomyolysis. Ann Intern Med 1978; 88:210–212.
11. Cohen S: Angel dust. JAMA 1977;238:515–516.
12. Cook CE, Brine DR, Jeffcoat AR, et al: Phencyclidine disposition after intravenous and oral doses. Clin Pharmacol Ther 1982;31:625–634.
13. Eastman JW, Cohen SN: Hypertensive crisis and death associated with phencyclidine poisoning. JAMA 1975;231: 1270–1271.
14. Fauman B, Baker F, Coppleson LW: Psychosis induced by phencyclidine. JACEP 1975;4:223–225.
15. Giannini AJ, Price WA, Loiselle RW, Malone DW: Treatment of phenylcyclohexylpyrrolidine (PHP) psychosis with haloperidol. J Toxicol Clin Toxicol 1985;23:185–189.
16. Golden NL, Sokol RJ, Rubin IL: Angel dust: Possible effects on the fetus. Pediatrics 1980;65:18–20.
17. Heveran JE: Radioimmunoassay for phencyclidine. J Forensic Sci 1980;25:79–87.
18. Jackson EJ: Phencyclidine pharmacokinetics after a massive overdose. Ann Intern Med 1989;111:613–615.
19. Karp HN, Kaufman ND, Anand SK: Phencyclidine poisoning in young children. J Pediatr 1980;97:1006–1009.

20. Kaufman KR, Petrucha RA, Pitts FN Jr, et al: Phencyclidine in umbilical cord blood: Preliminary data. Am J Psychiatry 1983;140:450–452.
21. McCarron M, Schulze BW, Thompson GA, et al: Acute phencyclidine intoxication: Incidence of clinical findings in 1000 cases. Ann Emerg Med 1981;10:237–242.
22. McMahon B, Ambre J, Ellis J: Hypertension during recovery from phencyclidine intoxication. Clin Toxicol 1978;12: 37–40.
23. Patel R, Connor G: A review of thirty cases of rhabdomyolysis associated acute renal failure among phencyclidine users. J Toxicol Clin Toxicol 1985–1986;23:547–556.
24. Picchioni AC, Consroe PF: Activated charcoal: A phencyclidine antidote, or hog in dogs. N Engl J Med 1979;300:202.
25. Shulgin AT, Maclean DE: Illicit synthesis of phencyclidine (PCP) and several of its analogs. Clin Toxicol 1979;9:553–560.
26. Soine WH, Balster RL, Berglund KE, et al: Identification of a new phencyclidine analog, 1-(1-phenylcyclohexyl)-4-methylpiperidine, as a drug of abuse. J Anal Toxicol 1982;6: 41–43.
27. Stillman R, Petersen RC: The paradox of phencyclidine (PCP) abuse. Ann Intern Med 1979;90:428–429.
28. Strauss AA, Modanlou HD, Bosu SK: Neonatal manifestations of maternal phencyclidine (PCP) abuse. Pediatrics 1981;68:550–552.
29. Tong TG, Benowitz NL, Becker CE, et al: Phencyclidine poisoning. JAMA 1975;234:512–516.
30. Warner A: Dextromethorphan: Analyte of the month. In: American Association of Clinical Chemistry: In Service Training and Continuing Education. 1993;14(2):27–28.
31. Welch MJ, Correa GA: PCP intoxication in young children and infants. Clin Pediatr 1980;19:510–514.
32. Wong EHF, Kemp JA: Sites for antagonism of *N*-methyl-*d*-aspartate receptor channel complex. Annu Rev Pharmacol Toxicol 1991;31:401–425.
33. Woodworth JR, Owens SM, Mayersohn M: Phencyclidine (PCP) disposition kinetics in dogs as a function of dose and route of administration. J Pharmacol Exp Ther 1985;234: 654–661.
34. Wright HH, Cole EA, Batey SR, Hanna K: Phencyclidine-induced psychosis: Eight-year follow-up of ten cases. South Med J 1988;81:565–567.
35. Young JD, Crapo LM: Protracted phencyclidine coma from an intestinal deposit. Arch Intern Med 1992;152:859–860.

Lysergic Acid Diethylamide and Other Hallucinogens

Jeffrey R. Tucker and Robert P. Ferm

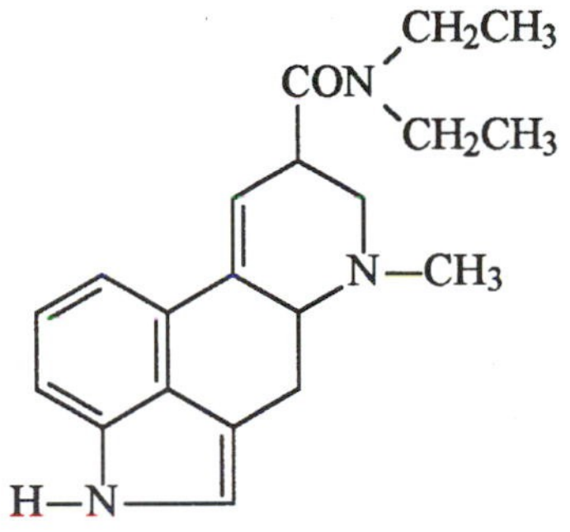

LSD

A 17-year-old male was brought to the Emergency Department (ED) by his friends because he was acting bizarrely on the way home from school. He told a friend that he had done "acid" after school and now could not stop staring at the bright lights. He kept telling his friends to join with him to enjoy the "peace of the lights."

Physical examination in the ED revealed an agitated male staring at the overhead lights. Vital signs were: blood pressure, 150/100 mm Hg; pulse, 112 beats/min; respiratory rate, 28 breaths/min; and temperature, 100.4°F (38°C). His skin was moist and pale. HEENT examination revealed 6 mm slowly reactive pupils and no nystagmus. He had occasional faint, scattered end-expiratory wheezes. Cardiac auscultation was normal. The abdomen was soft and nontender, with hyperactive bowel sounds. There was no clubbing, peripheral cyanosis, or edema. The neurologic examination initally revealed an agitated, frightened, but oriented young male who appeared distracted. He described vivid colors around lights that he could hear. The remainder of the neurologic examination was intact with the exception of a fine tremor. The patient admitted that he had taken lysergic acid diethylamide (LSD). He previously used LSD at concerts with others, but this was the first time that he used it alone. Although he knew where he was and that he was experiencing drug effects, he was frightened and extremely anxious of losing his mind. He was placed in a quiet location with minimal stimuli and an intravenous line was established. He received 10 mg diazepam by slow IV push. A rapid bedside blood glucose was 120 mg/dL. Electrolytes were normal.

After approximately 8 hours observation, the patient was fully alert and oriented and was at his baseline functional status. His primary care provider was notified about the ingestion and a referral was made for drug-abuse counseling. He was discharged with family members.

Historical Perspectives

Hallucinogenic substances have been used by different cultures for religious or mystical experiences. In the Hindu holy book, the Rig Veda, a sacramental substance called soma is described both as a god and an intoxicating substance. Soma was derived from the juice of a plant proposed to be the hallucinogenic mushroom *Amanita muscaria*.[71,76] In Eastern Europe during the 16th century, morning glory seeds were recognized as a cause of hallucinations. Natural ergot (*Claviceps purpurea*) was associated with hallucinations, altered mental status, seizures, gangrene, limb loss, and death. Hallucinogens have been implicated in the behavior of the alleged witches of Salem, Massachusetts.[14]

Synthetic hallucinogen use is often said to have begun with the discovery and ingestion of of LSD-25. The synthesis of LSD was the result of extensive research with the ergot alkaloids at Sandoz laboratories. In 1938, while searching for a new analeptic agent, the Swiss chemist Albert Hofmann synthesized LSD-25. (The number 25 denotes that it was the 25th substance synthesized within the series.) LSD-25 was inadvertently tested 5 years later when Hofmann accidentally became exposed to the agent by the percutaneous route and subsequently developed hallucinations.[3,17,37] Sandoz began marketing LSD under the trademark Delysid starting in 1947. In the 1950s, LSD was also used by psychiatrists as an adjunct for analytic psychotherapy.[85] It was thought that the administration of LSD could aid the patient in releasing repressed material. The CIA experimented with the use of LSD as tool for interrogating suspected communists and as a mind control agent.[7,83]

In the 1950s, LSD became popular as a recreational drug with the concept of "fifth freedom": the right of all individuals to alter the consiousness as they saw fit. Timothy Leary popularized LSD as a way to "Tune in, Turn on, Drop out."[85] In 1966, due to concerns about a public health problem, LSD was banned by federal law.[64] Reports of LSD-induced chromosomal breakage appeared in the 1960s.[6,16,39,46] These studies were poorly controlled and did not consider causes known to induce chromosomal damage such as significant cigarette smoking, malnutrition, infection, and the use of other drugs and agents with teratogenic potential.[41] Better-controlled studies in animals and reviews of the original data have suggested that there is no more evidence for a teratogenic effect with the use of hallucinogens than with the use of other drugs of abuse.[23,86]

Hallucinogen use diminished in the 1970s and early 1980s, but recent statistics show an increasing popularity. Presently, LSD is classified as a schedule I agent with high abuse potential, lack of established safety even under medical supervision, and no known use in medical treatment. LSD use is more widespread than cocaine among some high school students.[29] Use is more prevalent in suburbs than in the inner city. Several studies have shown a prevalence of use in high school students approaching 10%.[65] Approximately 14% of adolescents

TABLE 68–1. PHARMACOLOGIC AGENTS CLASSIFIED AS HALLUCINOGENS

Lysergamides
D-lysergic acid diethylamide
Convolvulaceae (morning glory family)
Ipomoea violacea
Ololiuqui (South American morning glory)
Argyreia (wood rose)
Isoergine, chanoclavine, lysergol, ergonovine
Indolealkylamines
Psilocybin
Psilocin
Bufotenine
N,N-Dimethyltryptamine
Phenylethylamines
Mescaline
Methamphetamine
TMA-2 (2,4,5-trimethoxyamphetamine)
DOM/STP (4-methyl-2,5-dimethoxyamphetamine)
PMA (para-methoxyamphetamine)
DOB (4-bromo-2,5-dimethoxyamphetamine)
2-CB/MFT (4-bromo-2,5-methoxyphenylethylamine)
MDA (3,4-methylenedioxyamphetamine)
MDMA (3,4-methylenedioxymethamphetamine)
MDEA (3,4-methylenedioxyethamphetamine)
MMDA (3-methoxy-4,5-methylenedioxyamphetamine)
Arylhexylamines
Phencyclidine (PCP) and congeners
Ketamine
Tetrahydrocannabinols (THC)
Marijuana
Hashish
Opioids
Pentazocine
Meperidine analogs
MPTP (1-methyl-4 phenyl-1,2,3,6-tetrahydropyridine)
Cocaine
Anticholinergics
Antihistamines
Tricyclic antidepressants
Phenothiazines
Belladonna alkaloids
Jimsonweed (*Datura stramonium*)
Mandrake (*Mandragora officinarum*)
Henbane (*Hyoscyamus niger*)
Deadly nightshade (*Atropa belladonna*)
Matrimony vine (*Lycium halimifolium*)
Miscellaneous Plants
Yohimbine (*Corynanthe yohimbe*)
Catnip (*Nepeta cataria*)
Juniper (*Juniper macropoda*)
Kavakava (*Piper methysticum*)
Nutmeg and Mace (*Myristica fragans*)
Periwinkle (*Catharanthus roseus*)
Mate (*Ilex paraguayensis*)

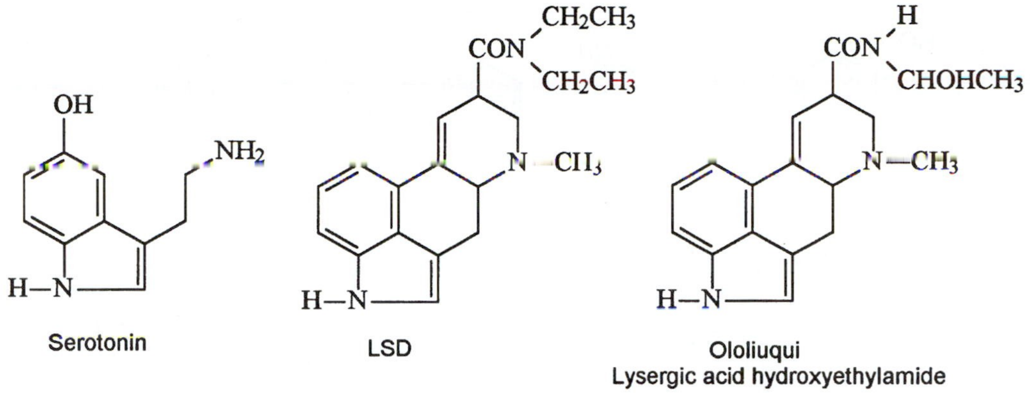

Figure 68–1. Hallucinogens of the lysergamide chemical class and their chemical similarity to serotonin.

have used hallucinogens, and this class is the third most frequently abused drug, following alcohol and marijuana.[77] Hallucinogenic drugs were a regular experience at Greatful Dead Concerts for almost 30 years, are used at rave parties, and are an important part of the Acid House Movement.[20,50,63]

What Are Illusions and Hallucinations?

Hallucinogens are a diverse group of drugs that alter and distort perception, thought, and mood. To understand the effects of these drugs, an understanding of the concepts of altered perception is important. An illusion is a mental impression that is derived from misinterpretation of an actual experience. Synesthesias are sensory misperceptions such as hearing color or seeing sounds. Both illusions and synesthesias usually require an outside stimulus for their initiation. An hallucination is a false perception that has no basis in external stimulation. The term is derived from the Latin "to wander in mind." Alterations in mood and thought are more consistent findings with hallucinogens, because true hallucination does not occur with each exposure.[89] Other terms have been used to describe the effects of the drugs, including psychedelic (mind manifesting), entheogen (generating religious experience), oneirogen (producing dream), and phanerothyme (making feeling visible).[81]

What Are the Common Hallucinogens?

The major structural classes of hallucinogens are the lysergamides, indolealkyamines, phenylethylamines, and cannabinols (Table 68–1). Lysergamides include LSD and ololihqui (Fig. 68–1). Psilocybin and bufotenine are the major indolealkylamines (Fig. 68–2). The most significant phenylethylamines include mescaline and amphetamine derivatives such as MDMA (3,4-methylenedioxymethamphetamine) (see Chap. 66). Cannabinols are discussed in Chapter 69.

Lysergic acid diethylamide is the synthetic diethylamide derivative of ergot alkaloids. It was originally synthesized from the ergot alkaloids produced by the fungus *Claviceps purpurea,* which is a contaminant of rye and wheat flour (see Chap. 45). Although four LSD isomers exist, only the D (–) is active. Lysergic acid diethylamide is an extremely potent hallucinogen and is a water-soluble, colorless, tasteless, and odorless powder. Currently, most LSD is synthesized and typically sold as liquid-impregnated blotter paper, microdots (tiny tablets), window panes (gelatin squares), liquid, powder, or tablets.[77] Ingestion is the most common route of exposure. Other routes of administration include intranasal, parenteral, sublingual, smoking, and conjunctival instillation. It is rapidly absorbed by the gastrointestinal tract. Typical street doses range from 50 to 300 μg, with a minimum effective dose of 25 μg.[36,44] Plasma protein binding is over 80% and volume of distribution is 0.28 L/kg. It is concentrated within the visual cortex and the limbic and reticular activating systems and has an elimination half-life is about 2.5 hours. Onset of psychological effects occurs 30 to 60 minutes after ingestion with peak effect at 3 to 5 hours. It is metabolized via the liver and excreted predominately as a pharmacologically inactive compound. Only small amounts are eliminated unchanged in the urine.

Lysergamides are found naturally in several species of morning glory (*Rivea corymbosa*) or Hawaiian baby woodrose (*Ipomoea violacea*). Morning glory seeds contain lysergic acid hydroxyethylamide, which has one-tenth the potency of LSD. Hallucinogenic effects require about 200 to 300 seeds. The seed must be pulverized, because the intact seed coat prevents drug absorption.

Peyote (*Lophophora williamsii*) is a small blue-green spineless cactus that grows in dry and rocky slopes throughout the southwestern United States and northern Mexico. Peyote buttons are the round fleshy tops of the cactus which have been sliced off and dried.[76] The Native American Church uses peyote buttons in their religious ceremonies.[9] Mescaline is the active hallucinogenic alkaloid found in the peyote cactus. Mescaline

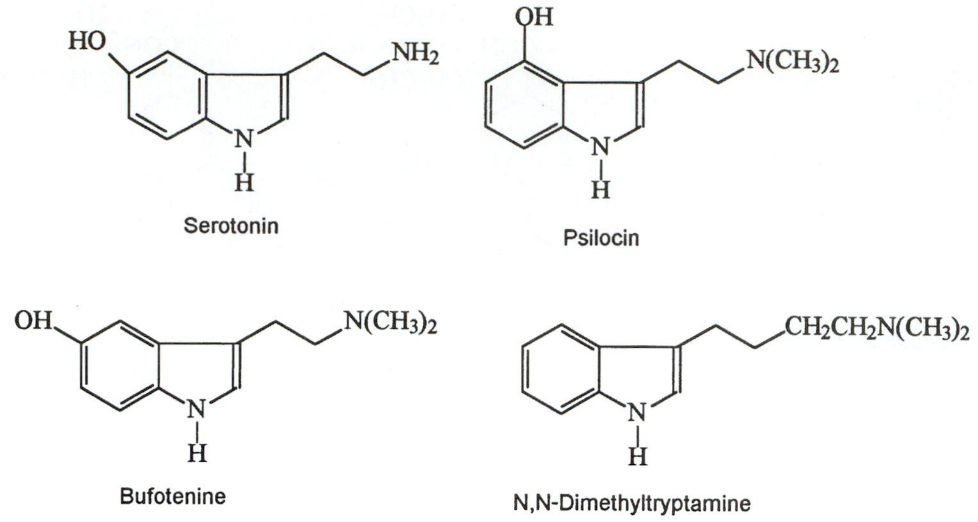

Figure 68–2. Hallucinogens of the indolealkylamine chemical class and their chemical similarity to serotonin.

pills contain synthetic mescaline or ground peyote compressed into a tablet. Mescaline is absorbed rapidly from the gastrointestinal tract. Six to twelve buttons (270 to 540 mg) are the common dose to produce hallucinogenic effects. The buttons are bitter tasting and nausea, vomiting, and diaphoresis often precede the psychological effects.

Psilocybin can be found in three major genera of mushrooms: *Psilocyba, Panaelous,* and *Conocybe* (see Chap. 75).[78] Psilocybin mushrooms are found in the southern United States, usually in cow pastures. The mushroom may be recognized by a greenish blue color it assumes after bruising, but misidentification is common.[2,32] Psilocybin was first isolated in 1958 by Albert Hofmann. The effects are similar to LSD, but with a shorter duration of action of about four hours.

DMT (N,N-dimethyltryptamine) is a potent short-acting hallucinogen. It is found naturally in the bark of the Yakee plant (*Virola calophylla*), which grows in the Amazon basin and has been used by shamans as an hallucinogenic snuff.[76] DMT is not absorbed from the gastrointestinal tract and is typically smoked, snorted, or injected. Since DMT is smoked or injected, peak effects often occur in 5 to 20 minutes, with a duration of 30 to 60 minutes. This has earned it the name "businessman's trip."

The toad of the genus *Bufo* has secretions that contain a complex mixture of cardiotoxins and neurotransmitters such as bufotenine (5-hydroxydimethyltryptamine), 5-Me0-DMT (5-methoxy,-N,N dimethyltryptamine), bufotenidine, and dehydrobufotenine. Severe reactions and death have occurred from oral ingestion of toad venom.[35,59,68,79] There is uncertainty about the hallucinogenic potential of bufotenine.[15,49] Recent evidence suggests that 5-Me0-DMT may be the component with hallucinogenic potential, is only present in the *Bufo alvarius,* and is only active when smoked.[88]

What Are the Mechanisms of Action of Hallucinogens?

The mechanisms of action for most of these drugs are poorly characterized, but are presumed to involve various neurotransmitters in the central nervous system.[12] The effect of LSD on thought and perception is due primarily to actions on serotonergic neurons.[10,11,18,48,56,57,67,84,90] Serotonin (5-hydroxytryptamine) is involved in the regulation of smooth muscle function in the gastrointestinal tract and cardiovascular system, and in the regulation of platelet function, and it occurs as a neurotransmitter in the brain.[33,34] Although the exact site of action has not been defined, serotonin modulates many psychological and physiological processes including mood, personality, affect, appetite, motor function, sexual activity, temperature regulation, pain perception, and sleep induction. An appreciation of serotonin receptor subtypes is important to understand the mechanism of hallucinogens.

LSD is structurally related to serotonin and is an agonist at the 5-HT_1 receptor.[67] 5-HT_1 neuronal cell bodies are clustered in median raphe nuclei of the brainstem. LSD inhibits central raphe neurons through stimulation of the 5-HT_1 receptors, which are coupled to adenyl cyclase. Psilocybin and DMT also inhibit 5-HT_1 neurons in the raphe nucleus, while phenethylamine hallucinogens do not inhibit 5-HT neurons. Stimulation of 5-HT_{1A} receptors results in inhibitory effect on raphe neurons of the brainstem by a voltage-gated calcium channel. LSD action at the 5-HT_{1A} receptors is shared by a number of selective 5-HT_{1A} agonists such as buspirone, which has an anxiolytic rather than a hallucinogenic effect. LSD is also an agonist at 5-$HT_{2A,2C}$.[27,55] 5-HT_2 receptors are not located presynaptically on serotonergic cell bodies, but on certain subpopulations of neurons in postsynpatic regions. The majority of 5-HT_2 receptors in the brain are located in the cerebral cortex. There is very good correlation between the affinity of both indolealkylamine and phenylethylamine hallucinogens for 5-HT_2 receptors and hallucinogenic potency in humans.[21,28] Atypical neuroleptics such as clozapine and risperidone are antagonist at the 5-HT_2 receptors.[22] 5-HT_2 antagonists such as ketanserin and ritanserin are effective in blocking the electrophysiologic and behavioral effects of hallucinogenic drugs in animal model systems and may be a potential treatment for adverse reactions to hallucinogens.[60,61,72] Recent work suggests that activation of D_1 dopamine receptors may contribute to the neurochemical effect of LSD.[87]

What Is the Clinical Presentation of Patients With Hallucinogen Poisoning?

Most drug-induced conditions associated with perceptual changes are accompanied by physiologic abnormalities. The physical effects may be due to direct drug effect or a response to the disturbing or enjoyable experience. Sympathomimetic effects are common, occur shortly after ingestion, and often precede the hallucinogenic effects. Findings may include dilated pupils, tachycardia, hypertension, tachypnea, hyperthermia, diaphoresis, piloerection, dizziness, hyperactivity, ataxia, altered mental status, and coma.[17,45] Other clinical findings that have been reported include muscle weakness, ataxia, and hippus (spasmodic rhythmical pupillary dilation and constriction).[45] Oral ingestion of peyote buttons produces nausea and vomiting preceding the psychedelic effects. Patients who are on therapeutic doses of lithium or a selective serotonin reuptake inhibitor and ingest LSD are at greater risk for seizures or flashbacks.[40,53]

The psychological effects of LSD are dose related and affect changes in arousal, emotion, perception, thought process, and self-image. The response to the drug is related to the person's mindset, emotions, or expectations at the time and can be altered by the group or setting.[4] The person experiencing the effects of a hallucinogen is usually fully awake, alert, and oriented but confronted with diverse perceptual anomalies and varied sensations. The person may experience euphoria or dysphoria, can be emotionally labile, but generally realizes that he or she is under the influence of a drug. Perceptual distortions are common with loss of body image (people's faces and body parts appear distorted) and alteration in visual perceptions (objects undulate, their boundaries are lost and merge). There is an acute attention to details with excessive attachment of meaning to ordinary objects and events. Usual thoughts seem novel and profound. Many people report an intensification of their sensory perceptions such as sound magnification and distortion; colors seem brighter with halo-like lights around objects. Frequently the person relates a sense of depersonalization and separation from the environment. The hallucinating person may perceive that he or she is observing an event as opposed to being involved in one. The person's body image may become distorted as well as the boundaries of objects in the environment. Synesthesias are frequent.[47,51] True hallucinations are spontaneous and without an external stimulus and appear real to the hallucinating person. Hallucinations may be visual, auditory, tactile, or olfactory, although those of a visual nature are the most common.[89] The altered perceptual conditions typically last for 6 to 12 hours.

What Is the Appropriate Management for Patients With Hallucinogen Poisoning?

Most patients with hallucinogenic experiences are never brought to medical attention because these are the desired effect of the drug. For any patient who presents to the emergency department with hallucinations or psychosis, even if an ingestion of a hallucinogen is suspected, the basic approach for altered mental status should include consideration of the administration of dextrose, thiamine, and naloxone as indicated, and the vigorous search for other etiologies. Acute adverse psychiatric effects of hallucinogens include panic reactions, true hallucinations, psychosis, and major depressive dysphoric reactions. Acute panic reactions, the most common adverse effect, present with frightening illusions, tremendous anxiety, apprehension, and a terrifying sense of loss of self-control. The patient can be placed in a quiet location with minimal stimuli and a nonjudgmental advocate should attempt to reduce the patient's anxiety, provide reality testing, and remind the individual that a drug has been ingested and the effect will wear off in a couple of hours.[26,30]

Significant agitation, dysphoria, or a "bad trip," combined with some of the signs of autonomic instability, can usually be treated by the parenteral administration of a benzodiazepine.[1,77] Benzodiazepines remain the cornerstone of therapy as the sedating effect will diminish both endogenous and exogenous sympathetic effects.[62] Phenothiazines and butyrophenes should be avoided due to adverse effects such as hypotension and reduction of seizure threshold. Gastrointestinal decontamination with activated charcoal may be considered for asymptomatic patients with recent ingestions, but is probably not helpful once clinical symptoms appear and attempts may lead to further agitation. Excessive physical restraint should be avoided due to concerns for hyperthermia and rhabdomyolysis.

The psychedelic agents rarely produce life-threatening problems. Sedation with benzodiazepines is usually sufficient to treat hypertension and tachycardia. In rare cases, hypertension, tachycardia, and hyperthermia may require more aggressive therapy. Phentolamine, nifedipine, or nitroprusside are all useful in treating the hypertension depending upon its severity and end-organ effects.[3] A beta-adrenergic antagonist is contraindicated, as many of these drugs have both alpha and beta-adrenergic effects. Unopposed alpha-adrenergic induced hypertension may develop from the use of a pure beta antagonist or the mixed alpha- and beta-adrenergic antagonist labetalol.[5,69,70] Hyperthermia must be aggressively treated with hydration, active external cooling, and muscle relaxants ranging from benzodiazepines to paralytic agents depending upon the severity of the individual's condition. Morbidity and mortality typically result from the complications of hyperthermia including rhabdomyolysis and myoglobinuric renal failure, hepatic necrosis, and disseminated intravascular coagulopathy. For the most part, however, hydration, a supportive environment, and meticulous supportive care will prove adequate.[13,17,47]

What Is the Differential Diagnosis of Hallucinosis?

Hallucinosis is the abnormal organic mental condition of persistent hallucinations. The major causes of hallucinosis can be divided into structural, infectious, functional, and toxic–metabolic origins (Table 68–2). The differential diagnosis of toxic hallucinosis is large as almost every drug class can cause hallucinations in a small part of the population. The diagnosis of hallucinogen ingestion often must be made on the basis of history and physical examination alone. Sympathomimetic effects such as mydriasis, tachycardia, hypertension, diaphoresis, and hyperactivity are generally less prominent in LSD ingestion than in phenylethylamine intoxication. The person who has ingested hallucinogens is oriented and will often give a history of ingestion, while under the effect of the drug. This is in contrast to a drug-induced delirium where orientation is by definition altered.

TABLE 68–2. DIFFERENTIAL DIAGNOSES FOR HALLUCINATIONS

Structural	***Metabolic***
Cerebral neoplasm	Sedative-hypnotic withdrawal
Seizures	Heat-related illness
CNS trauma	Organic brain syndromes
Cerebral edema	Porphyria
Functional	Altitude sickness
Schizophrenia	Electrolyte disturbances
Psychosis	Hypoxia
Toxins	Endocrine abnormalities
Analgesics	Myxedema, thyrotoxicosis
Anesthetics	Cushing's syndrome
Antidysrhythmics	Pheochromocytoma
Antibiotics	Hypoglycemia
Antispasmodics	Hyperglycemia
Antihypertensives	
Corticosteroids	
Drugs of abuse	
Ethanol	
Plant and fungal-derived agents	
Infectious	
Meningitis	
Encephalitis	
AIDS related illness	
Toxoplasmosis	
Cryptococcosis	
Viral encephalitis (herpes, HIV)	
Endocarditis	
Cerebral abscess	

Drugs such as amphetamine, cocaine, phencyclidine (PCP), and anticholinergics produce delirium or psychosis at doses capable of producing hallucinations. Amphetamine intoxication typically presents with an elaborate and paranoid delusion as well as visual hallucinations. Functional causes of perceptual changes such as psychosis or schizophrenia typically present with auditory hallucinations. Disorientation, panic reactions, and combative behavior are more common with anticholinergic toxicity than LSD. Patients with central anticholinergic toxicity usually present with incoherent mumbling and may be unaware that the hallucinations are drug induced.[31] The presence of marked hyperthermia, uncontrollable behavior, or extreme agitation should suggest an alternative exposure such as cocaine or PCP.

Laboratory tests are available to confirm an LSD exposure, but are not widely used.[19] Two radioimmunoassays test for the presence of LSD and its urinary metabolite, 2-oxy-LSD.[54] It is important to recognize that most standard drug of abuse screens do not detect hallucinogens.[29]

Can Hallucinogens Induce Tolerance?

Tolerance can be physiological or psychological, depending on the response of the person and also on the substance. LSD, mescaline, and amphetamines all induce tolerance in animals. Tolerance to LSD occurs within 2 to 3 days with daily dosing but rapidly dissipates if the drug is withheld for 2 or more days. Cross-tolerance among mescaline, psilocybin, and LSD occurs in animals and is reported in humans. Cross-tolerance has not been documented among any members of that group with the amphetamines.[74] Tolerance has been demonstrated to a limited extent between psilocybin and cannabinoids such as marijuana.[8,38,66]

What Are the Long-Term Effects of Hallucinogen Use?

When LSD was initially popularized, some patients were noted to behave in a manner similar to schizophrenia and were admitted to psychiatric facilities. In volunteer studies, panic reactions, flashbacks, and extended psychoses were noted. When the drug was used for alleviation of anxiety and personality abnormalities, flashbacks and extended psychosis were reported.[24] It has been suggested that these individuals had pre-existing compensated psychological disturbances. The acute depersonalization and perceptual alterations associated with psychedelic use may have been the stimulus for the noted decompensation. The commonly noted panic reactions are often responsive to supportive measures including placing the patient in a stable environment with supportive reassurance that the abnormal feelings are drug induced and will subside.[25,42,43,58,73,82]

Long-term consequence of LSD use may include prolonged psychotic reactions, severe depression, exacerbation of pre-existing psychiatric illness, and hallucinogen persisting perception disorder (HPPD).[1,52,75,77,80] HPPD (flashbacks) is an infrequent but significant chronic problem of LSD abuse and is listed in the *Diagnostic and Statistical Manual of Mental Disorders,* fourth edition revised. Patients have described this perceptual disorder as living in "purple haze." HPPD is a chronic disorder, following cessation of hallucinogen use, of one or more of the perceptual symptoms that were experienced while intoxicated and results in clinically significant distress. Flashbacks (HPPD) can be triggered during times of stress, illness, and exercise and are often virtual recurrence of the initial hallucinations. The etiology of flashbacks is unknown. HPPD (flashbacks) may occur up to 18 months after ingestion.

Acknowledgment

Cynthia K. Aaron, MD contributed to this chapter in a previous edition.

References

1. Abraham HD, Aldridge AM: Adverse consequences of lysergic acid diethylamide. Addiction 1993;88:1327–1334.
2. Badham ER: Ethnobotany of psilocybin mushrooms, especially Psilocybe cubensis. J Ethnopharmacol 1984;10:249–254.
3. Benowitz NL, Goldschlager N: Cardiac disturbances. In: Haddad LM, Winchester JM, eds: Clinical Management of Poisoning and Drug Overdose, 2nd ed. Philadelphia, Saunders, 1990, pp. 63–101.
4. Bowers MB, Freedman DX: Psychedelic experiences in acute psychoses. Arch Gen Psychiatry 1966;15:240–248.
5. Briggs RSJ, Birtwell AJ, Pohl JEF: Hypertensive response to labetalol in phaeochromocytoma. Lancet 1978;11:1045–1046.
6. Buchanan J, Brown CR: "Designer drugs": A problem in clinical toxicology. Med Toxicol 1988;3:1–17.
7. Buchman J: Brainwashing, LSD, and CIA. Historical and ethical perspective. Int J Soc Psychiatry 1977; 23:8–19.
8. Buckholtz NS, Zhou D, Freedman DX: Serotonin$_2$ agonist administration downregulates rat brain serotonin$_2$ receptors. Life Sci 1988;42:2439–2445.
9. Bullis RK: Swallowing the scroll: Legal implications of the recent supreme court peyote cases. J Psychoactive Drugs 1990;22:325–332.
10. Burris KD, Breeding M, Sanders-Bush E: (+)Lysergic acid diethylamide, but not its nonhallucinogenic congeners, is a potent serotonin 5HT1C receptor agonist. J Pharmacol Exp Ther 1991;258:891–896.
11. Burris KD, Sanders-Bush E: Unsurmountable antagonism of brain 5-hydroxytryptamine-2 receptors by (+)-lysergic acid diethylamide and bromo lysergic acid diethylamide. Mol Pharmacol 1992;42:826–830.
12. Caldwell J, Sever PS: The biochemical pharmacology of abused drugs. Clin Pharmacol Ther 1974;16:625–638.
13. Callaway CW, Clark RF: Hyperthermia in psychostimulant overdose. Ann Emerg Med 1994;24:68–76.
14. Caporeal LR: Ergotism: The satan loosed in Salem? Science 1976;192:21–26.
15. Chilton WS, Bigwood J, Jensen RE: Psilocin, bufotenine and serotonin: Historical and biosynthetic observations. J Psychoactive Drugs 1979;11:61–69.
16. Cohen MM, Hirshhorn K, Frosch W: In vivo and in vitro chromosomal damage induced by LSD–25. N Engl J Med 1967;277:1043–1049.
17. Cohen S: The hallucinogens and the inhalants. Psychiatr Clin North Am 1984;7:681–688.
18. Darmani NA, Martin BR, Pandey U, Glennon RA: Pharmacological characterization of ear-scratch response in mice as a behavioral model for selective 5-HT2-receptor agonists and evidence for 5-HT1B- and 5-HT2-receptor interactions. Pharmacol Biochem Behav 1990;37:95–99.
19. Dupont RL, Verebey K: The role of the laboratory in the diagnosis of LSD and ecstasy pyschosis. Psychiatr Ann 1994; 24:142–144.
20. Erickson TB, Aks SE, Koenigsberg M, Bunney EB: Drug use patterns at major rock concerts events. Ann Emerg Med 1996;28:22–26.
21. Fink H, Morgenstern R, Oelssner W: Studies of the relationship between molecular structure and hallucinogenic. Pharmacol Biochem Behav 1986;24:335–340.
22. Fink H, Morgenstern R, Oelssner W: Clozapine—A serotonin antagonist? Pharmacol Biochem Behav 1984;20: 513–517.
23. Fody RP, Walker EM: Effects of drugs on the male and female reproductive systems. Ann Clin Lab Sci 1985;15: 451–458.
24. Frankel FH: The concepts of flashbacks in historical perspective. Int J Clin Exp Hypn 1994;152:321–326.
25. Frosch WA, Robbins ES, Stern M: Untoward reactions to lysergic acid diethylamide (LSD) resulting in hospitalization. N Engl J Med 1965; 273:1235–1239.
26. Gay GR, Smith DE: A free clinic approach to drug abuse. Prev Med 1973;2:543–553.
27. Glennon RA: Do classical hallucinogens act as 5-HT2 agonists or antagonists? Neuropsychopharmacology 1990; 3:509–517.
28. Glennon RA, Titeler M, McKenney JD: Evidence for 5-HT2 involvement in the mechanism of action of hallucinogenic agents. Life Sci 1984;35:2505–2511.
29. Gold MS, Dackis CA: Role of the laboratory in the evaluation of suspected drug abuse. J Clin Psychiatry 1986;47 (suppl):17–23.
30. Haddad LM: Management of hallucinogen abuse. Am Fam Physician 1977;14:312–314.
31. Hall RC, Popkin MK, McHenry LE: Angels' trumpet psy-

chosis: A central nervous system anticholinergic syndrome. Am J Psychiatry 1977;134:312–314.
32. Hanrahan JP, Gordon MA: Mushroom poisoning: Case reports and a review of the treatment. JAMA 1984;251: 1057–1061.
33. Harrington MA, Zhong P, Garlow SJ, Ciarnello RD: Molecular biology of serotonin receptors. J Clin Psychiatry 1992: 53(suppl):8–27.
34. Heym J, Jacobs BL: Serotonergic mechanisms of hallucinogenic drug effects. Monogr. Neural Sci 1987;13:55–81.
35. Hitt M, Ettinter DD: Toad toxicity. N Engl J Med 1986; 314:517.
36. Hoffer A: D-Lysergic acid diethylamide (LSD): A review of its present status. Clin Pharmacol Ther 1965;6:183–255.
37. Hofmann A: How LSD originated. J Psychedelic Drugs 1979;11:53–60.
38. Jacobs BL, Trulson ME, Stern WC: An animal behavior model for studying the actions of LSD and related hallucinogens. Science 1977;194:741–743.
39. Jacobson CB, Berlin CM: Possible reproductive detriment in LSD users. JAMA 1972;222:1367–1373.
40. Jackson TW, Hornfeldt CS: Seizures activity followed recreational LSD use in patients treated with lithium and fluoxetine. Vet Hum Toxicol 1991;33:387. Abstract.
41. Kato T, Jarvik LF: LSD–25 and genetic damage. Dis Nerv Syst 1969;20:42–46.
42. Klepfisz A, Racy J: Homicide and LSD. JAMA 1973;223: 429–430.
43. Kulick AR, Ahmed I: Substance-induced organic mental disorders: A clinical and conceptual approach. Gen Hosp Psychiatry 1986;8:168–172.
44. Kulig K: LSD. Emerg Med Clin North Am 1990;8:551–558.
45. Leikin JB, Krantz AJ, Zell-Kanter M, et al: Clinical features and management of intoxication due to hallucinogenic drugs. Med Toxicol Adverse Drug Exp 1989;4:324–350.
46. Louria DB: Current concepts: Lysergic acid diethylamide. N Engl J Med 1968;278:435–438.
47. Lyles A: LSD: A review. Pharmalert 1979;11:1–4.
48. Lyon RA, Titeler M, Seggel MR, Glennon RA: Indolealkylamine analogs share 5-HT_2 characteristics with phenylalkylamine hallucinogens. Eur J Pharmacol 1988;145: 291–297.
49. Lyttle T, Goldstein D, Gartz J: Bufo toads and bufotenine: Fact and fiction surrounding an alleged psychedelic. J Psychoactive Drugs 1996;28:267–290.
50. Lyttle T, Monagne, M: Drugs, music and ideology: A social pharmacological interpretation of the acid house movement. Int J Addicit 1992;27:1159–1177.
51. Mace S: LSD. Clin Toxicol 1979;15:219–224.
52. Madden JS: LSD and post-hallucinogen perceptual disorder. Addiction 1994;89:762–763.
53. Markek H, Lee A, Holmes RD, et al: Flashback syndrome exacerbated by selective serotonin reuptake inhibitor antidepressant in adolescents. J Pediatr 1994;125:817–819.
54. McCarron MM: Phenycyclidine. In: Rippe JM, Irwin RS, Fink MP, Cerra FB, eds: Intensive Care Medicine, 3rd ed. Boston, Little, Brown, 1996, pp. 1657–1663.
55. McClue SJ, Brazell C, Stahl SM: Hallucinogenic drugs are partial agonists of the human platelet shape change response: A physiological model of the 5-HT_2 receptors. Biol Psychiatry 1989;26:297–302.
56. McKenna DJ, Nazarali AJ, Hoffman AJ, et al: Common receptors for hallucinogens in rat brain: A comparative autoradiographic study using [^{125}I]LSD and [^{125}I]DOI, a new psychotomimetic radioligand. Brain Res 1989;476:45–56.
57. McKenna DJ, Repke DB, Lo L, Peroutka SJ: Differential interactions of indolealkylamines with 5-hydroxytryptamine receptor subtypes. Neuropharmacology 1990;29:193–198.
58. McLellan AT, Woody GE, O'Brien CP: Development of psychiatric illness in drug abusers, possible role of drug preference. N Engl J Med 1979;301:1310–1314.
59. McLeod WR, Sitaram BR: Bufotenine reconsidered. Acta Psychiatr Scand 1985;72:447–450.
60. Meert T, Clincke G: Evidence for a possible role of the 5-HT_2 antagonist ritanserin in drug abuse. Ann NY Acad Sci 1992;654:483–486.
61. Meert TF, de Haes P, Janssen PAJ: Risperidone (R 64 766), a potent and complete LSD antagonist in drug discrimination by rats. Psychopharmacology 1989;97:206–212.
62. Miller PL, Gay GR, Ferris KC, Anderson S: Treatment of acute adverse psychedelic reactions: "I've tripped and I can't get down." J Psychoactive Drugs 1992;24:277–279.
63. Millman RB, Beeder AB: The new psychedelic culture: LSD, ectasy, "rave parties" and the Grateful Dead. Psychiatr Ann 1994;24:145–147.
64. Neill JR: "More than medical significance": LSD and American Psychiatry 1953–1966. J Psychoactive Drugs 1979;19: 39–45.
65. O'Malley PM, Johnston LD, Bachman JG: Adolescent substance use: Epidemiology and implications for public policy. Pediatr Clin North Am 1995;42:241–260.
66. Owens MJ, Knight DL, Ritchie JC, Nemeroff CB: The 5-hydroxytryptamine$_2$ agonist, (+–)-1-(2,5-dimethoxy-4-bromophenyl)-2-aminopropane stimulates the hypothalamic–pituitary–adrenal (HPA) axis: II. Biochemical and psychological evidence for the development of tolerance after chronic administration. J Pharmacol Exp Ther 1991;256: 795–800.
67. Pierce PA, Peroutka SJ: Hallucinogenic drug interactions with neurotransmitter receptor binding sites in human cortex. Psychopharmacology 1989;97:118–122.
68. Radford DJ, Gilles AD, Hinds JA, Duffy P: Naturally occuring cardiac glycosides. Med J Aust 1986;144:540–544.
69. Ramoska E, Sacchetti AD: Propranolol-induced hypertension in treatment of cocaine intoxication. Ann Emerg Med 1985;14:1112–1113.
70. Reach G: Effect of labetalol on blood pressure and plasma catecholamine concentrations in patients with pheochromocytoma. Br Med J 1980;280:1300–1301.
71. Riedlinger TJ: Wasson's alternative candidates for soma. J Psychoactive Drugs 1993;25:149–156.
72. Sadzot B, Baraban JM, Glennon RA, et al: Hallucinogenic drug interactions at human brain 5-HT_2 receptors: Implications for treating LSD-induced hallucinogenesis. Psychopharmacology 1989;98:495–499.
73. Saidel DR, Babireau R: Prolonged LSD flashbacks as conversion reactions. J Nerv Ment Dis 1976;163:352–355.
74. Schechter M, Rosecrans J: Lysergic acid diethylamide (LSD)

as a discriminative cue: Drugs with similar stimulus properties. Psychopharmacologia 1972;26:313–316.

75. Schneier FR, Siris SG: A review of psychoactive substance use and abuse in schizophrenia: Patterns of drug choice. J Nerv Ment Dis 1987;175:641–652.
76. Schultes RE: Hallucinogens of plant origin. Science 1969; 163:245–254.
77. Schwartz RH: LSD. Its rise, fall and renewed popularity among high school students. Ped Clin North Am 1995;42: 403–413.
78. Schwartz RH, Smith DE: Hallucinogenic mushrooms. Clin Pediatr 1988;27:70–73.
79. Siegel DM, McDaniel SH: The frog prince: Tale and toxicology. Am J Orthopsychiatry 1991;61:558–562.
80. Smith DE, Seymour RB: LSD: History and toxicity. Psychiatr Ann 1994;24:145–147.
81. Strassman RJ: Hallucinogenic drugs in psychiatric research and treatment. J Nerv Ment Dis 1995;183:127–138.
82. Strassman RJ: Adverse reactions to psychedelic drugs: A review of the literature. J Nerv Ment Dis 1984;172: 577–595.
83. Szulc J: The CIA's electric Kool Aid acid test. Psychol Today 1977;11:92–153.
84. Titeler M, Lyon RA, Glennon RA: Radioligand binding evidence implicates the brain 5-HT_2 receptor as a site of action for LSD and phenylisopropylamine hallucinogens. Psychopharmacology 1988;94:213–216.
85. Ulrich RF, Patten BM: The rise, decline and fall of LSD. Perspect Biol Med 1991;34:561–578.
86. Van Went GF: Mutagenicity testing of three hallucinogens: LSD, psilocybin, and delta 9-THC, using the micronucleus test. Experientia 1978;34:324–325.
87. Watts VJ, Lawler CP, Fox DR, et al: LSD and structural analogs: Pharmacological evaluation at D1 receptors. Psychopharmacology 1995;118:401–409.
88. Weil AT, Davis W: Bufo alvarius: A potent hallucinogen of animal origin. J Ethnopharmacol 1995;41:1–8.
89. Weller M, Wiedmann P: Visual hallucinations. Int Ophthalmol 1989;13:193–199.
90. Wing LL, Tapson GS, Geyer MA: 5HT_2 mediation of acute behavioral effects of hallucinogens in rats. Psychopharmacology 1990;100:417–425.

CHAPTER 69

Marijuana

Edward J. Otten

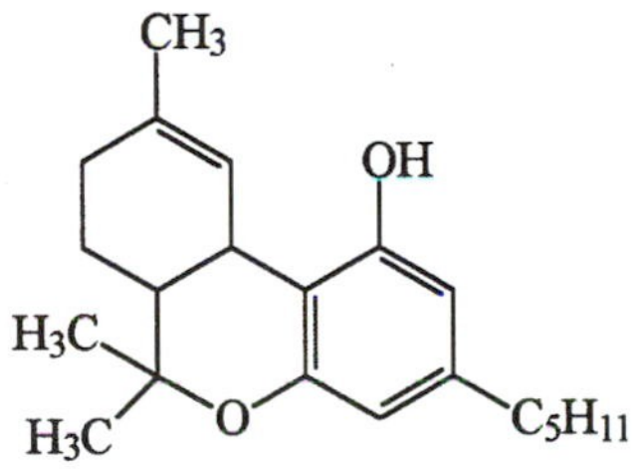

Δ^9-tetrahydrocannabinol (THC)

A 20-year-old male was brought to the emergency department by the police, after they had stopped his automobile for reckless driving. The patient's vehicle was weaving along the highway and had crossed the center line several times. The police initially thought that the patient was intoxicated, but his breath analysis was neglible for ethanol. They felt that he might have some medical problem and he was brought to the emergency department.

The patient was drowsy but easily arousable to verbal stimuli. He stated that he had been to a party earlier that evening and thinks that someone may have put something in his drink. He stated that he had not been drinking alcohol and does not use drugs in any form. He complained of a slight headache and inability to focus. He had no other complaints. His past medical history was negative. He had no known allergies and took no medications regularly. Vital signs were: temperature, 99.0°F (37.2°C); pulse, 112 beats/min; respiratory rate, 18 breaths/min; blood pressure, 138/84 mmHg. He was drowsy but arousable, oriented to person, place, time, and situation. His pupils were 5 mm equal and reacted to light, his conjunctiva were injected, and his extraocular movements were normal without nystagmus. His lungs were clear to auscultation and his heart examination revealed a rapid, regular rhythm without murmur or rub. His neurologic examination was normal except for difficulty maintaining a normal stance. His gait was not ataxic and his finger to nose examination was normal. His oxygen saturation was 95% on room air and his fingerstick blood glucose was 120 to 140 mg/dL.

The patient rapidly improved while in the emergency department and no further diagnostic studies were done. The patient's brother reported that the patient had been arrested on several previous occasions for driving under the influence of drugs and had a significant past history of drug abuse, especially marijuana. When confronted with the brother's information, the patient admitted to smoking several "joints" of marijuana prior to attempting to drive home. The patient was referred to outpatient drug counselling and discharged to the custody of his brother.

What Is Marijuana?

Marijuana is a common name for material obtained from the leaves and flowers of the Indian hemp plant, *Cannabis sativa*. It is one of many names for cannabis, which contains the psychoactive substance delta-9-

tetrahydrocannabinol (THC). Other names include ace, birck, bush, Colombian ganga, hashish, Indiana hay, Jamaican, joint, kif, maryjane, Panama red, pot, reefer, rope, smoke tea, weed, and yerba. THC is found in both the male and female plants. *Cannabis sativa* is the only species belonging to the genus *Cannabis*. There are a number of cultivated varieties used in the manufacture of fiber for rope and clothing, and these have erroneously been thought to be separate species. This plant has been cultivated for thousands of years for numerous uses including medical and religious as well as for fiber and recreation. *Cannabis sativa* contains a number of other resins known as cannabinoids, including cannabidiol, cannabinol, cannabidolic acid, cannabicyclol, and cannabigerol. In all, approximately 60 other cannabinoids and 200 other chemical compounds have been identified in *Cannabis* plant material. These compounds usually are found in small concentrations and have less or no psychoactivity compared to THC, although they do have some chemical activity and may contribute to the acute and chronic medical problems seen with marijuana use. Thus THC is the primary constituent of marijuana, but not the only one; and THC is not pharmacologically equivalent to marijuana. The percentage of THC found in plants depends on ecotypic variables including amount of light, moisture, soil type, trace elements, and nutrients. The common myths associated with potency of various types of marijuana based on origin, sex of the plant, and color are probably related to this fact. The amount of active THC found in a sample will also deteriorate with time. Hashish and hashish oil are derivatives of the Cannabis plant that contain higher concentrations of THC and are smoked either in pipes (hashish) or mixed with tobacco and smoked (hashish oil). Marijuana is also commonly used in conjunction with other drugs such as opium, alcohols, cocaine, heroin, phencyclidine, ketamine, and formaldehyde.[2,12,15,20]

What Is the Extent of Marijuana Usage in the United States?

After nicotine, alcohol, and caffeine, marijuana is probably the most commonly abused substance in the world. Marijuana is the most commonly used illegal substance in the United States, where an estimated 20 million people use it.[33] It is thought by many to be a "gateway" drug, leading to use of other more dangerous substances such as heroin, cocaine, or amphetamines. Marijuana was shown to be a gateway drug, although alcohol was not included in this study of serious drug abusers in New York City.[14] The Drug Enforcement Agency has classified marijuana as a Schedule I substance.The latest Center for Disease Control and Prevention statistics and National Institute on Drug Abuse (NIDA) data show a rise in the use of marijuana in the general population and in particular among teenagers. The NIDA survey on drug use showed an increase in the prevalance of marijuana usage in all groups of teenagers in 1994. Eighth graders' use increased by 13%, 10th grader use by 25%, and 12th grader use by 31% over 1993. From a historical peak of marijuana use in 1978, there was a decrease in use from 1979 to 1991. This trend reversed in 1992, and the prevalance rate has increased annually since then. The Substance Abuse and Mental Health Services Administration (SAMHSA) National Household Survey on Drug Abuse, SAMHSA's Drug Abuse Warning Network (DAWN), and the National Institute of Justice Drug Use Forecasting (DUF) system data all showed increases in marijuana use in 1995.[14,19,21,33]

What Pharmacologic and Pathophysiologic Changes Occur With Marijuana Usage?

Acute Effects

The onset of the effects of marijuana depend on the route of administration and the concentration of THC in the product. Smoking marijuana usually leads to immediate effects, while oral ingestion has a slow and unpredictable effect due to the instability in the acidic environment of the stomach.[29] The smoking dynamics or manner in which the marijuana is smoked is the most important factor in determining the bioavailability of THC.[3,7] Depending on the initial concentration of THC, pyrolysis of THC, loss in sidestream smoke, and mucosal concentration, on average about half of the THC in the marijuana is delivered to the lungs. It takes about 15 seconds for the lungs to absorb the THC and transport it to the brain.[30] A specific cannabinoid receptor is located in the cerebral cortex and may explain the pharmacologic effects of marijuana. Certain neuronal membranes contain receptors that bind to THC and are responsible for the pharmacologic effects. The naturally occuring substance anandamide behaves similiarly to THC, and binds these same receptors.[28] After smoking, the effects peak in 10 to 30 minutes and may last for 1 to 4 hours, depending on the dose inhaled.[6]

The effects of marijuana may be both physiologic and psychologic based on previous experience and expectations of the user.[6,16] The usual psychological effects are fairly predictable and include alterations in sensation, peception, cognition, and psychomotor functions. Although users report enhanced perception and sensation, this has not been observed experimentally. A sense of euphoria, relaxation, and various sensory alterations are generally the effects that are sought with marijuana use.[6,16] An acute psychosis is described with marijuana use; it is not clear whether pre-existing psychopathology is responsible or whether this behavioral alteration is related to the dose of THC or the inexperience of the user. Studies of patients without prior psychopathology who developed acute psychotic reactions following the use of marijuana have shown that the reaction is usually transient.[25,27] Marijuana does have an acute effect on performance of neuropsychiatric tests, especially digit recall and arithmetic, that covaries with THC levels.[10,31]

Although the psychological effects may or may not be dose dependent, the physiologic effects are generally dose related. Increase in heart rate is common but blood pressure response is variable. Acutely, muscle tremors and weakness can be noted as well as bronchodilatation. Conjunctival injection, increased appetite, decreased intraocular pressure, decreased testosterone levels, and urinary retention are all commonly noted with acute marijuana usage.[3,16,17,29]

Chronic Effects

Tolerance is clearly associated with repeated use, just as with many other psychoactive drugs. Similar to these other drugs, tolerance can lead to dependence, both physiologic and psychologic, and a withdrawal syndrome. This syndrome can be reproduced experimentally and includes sleep disturbances, irritability, decreased appetite, nausea and restlessness, all of which can be reversed by small doses of THC. Heavy marijuana use (more than 27 days out of 30) has been shown to have a residual neuropsychological effect not seen with light users (less than 3 days out of 30).[31]

Smoking marijuana can lead to chronic lung disease and carcinogenesis similar to tobacco smoking.[38] Marijuana smoking showed a fivefold increase in blood carboxyhemoglobin level and threefold increase in the amount of tar inhaled when compared with tobacco.[39] Some studies indicate that because of the smoking dynamics, a fourfold greater respiratory burden of particulates occurs with marijuana smoking, making this form of inhalation potentially more dangerous than tobacco.[30] Marijuana seems to have a greater impact on central airway function, while tobacco's predominant effect is on peripheral airways. Significantly worse values for specific airway conductance and airway resistance were found with marijuana smoking when compared with nonsmokers or tobacco smokers.[38] Bronchoaveolar lavage fluid from the lungs of marijuana smokers demonstrated an increase in macrophages and other inflammatory cells that was independent of, and additive to, that of tobacco.[38,39] Base fractions of marijuana are more mutagenic than tobacco, and high-dose base fractions were sevenfold more mutagenic than either tobacco or low-dose marijuana base fractions.[37] Studies in female smokers demonstrate that there are a number of neonatal neurobehavioral disturbances that correlate with marijuana usage during pregnancy; they seem to disappear during infancy and reappear later in early childhood.[1,9,13,32] THC interferes with testicular function by a number of mechanisms causing decreased sperm motility and number and increased abnormal morphology.[18] THC has a dose-dependent effect in diminishing the cytolytic activity of large granular lymphocytes against K562 tumor cells and decreasing the synthesis of tumor necrosis factor by macrophages. Both B and T-cell activity are depressed by THC; however, cell-mediated immunity is more sensitive.[22,40]

Which Laboratory Tests Detect Marijuana?

THC is hydrophobic and therefore accumulates in lipid tissue; it is highly protein bound (97 to 99%), has a V_d of 10 L/kg, and it is enterohepatically recirculated. All of these characteristics result in slow elimination from the body. Any of the 20 metabolites of THC may cross-react with the immunoassay used for the screening of urine for marijuana. The screening test is designed to detect THC at levels of 20, 50, or100 ng/mL, depending on for what purpose the test is ordered. THC is oxidatively metabolized to the active compound 11-hydroxy-delta9-tetra hydrocannabinol, which is further oxidized to the inactive 11 nor-9-carboxy-delta9-THC. This last compound is the basis for the confirmation test using GC/MS with a cutoff level of 15 ng/mL.[17,35] The pattern of excretion is similar for most users of marijuana. What differs is the length of each phase of excretion, and this varies with the pattern of usage of the individual. Therefore, screening and confirmation tests may be positive for up to 70 or more days, depending on the cutoff levels used and the individual's lipid stores of THC. The general detection times for THC is 1 to 3 days for single acute use and 10 days to 4 weeks for daily use.[11]

Passive exposure to marijuana smoke, depending on room air concentration, may give positive screening results for several days even after a single exposure.[8] False-positive results may occur with therapeutic use of naproxen, ibuprofen, and fenoprofen. False negatives may result from dilution, diuretic use, table salt, or other contaminants. Concomitant testing of urine specific gravity, pH, temperature, and creatinine have eliminated most of these confounders.[17,35]

What Are the Documented Medical Uses of Marijuana?

Although marijuana has been shown to be useful in treating the nausea and vomiting associated with cancer chemotherapy, these studies were done prior to the approval of ondansetron and other newer antiemetics. Marijuana may also be useful in stimulating the appetite of AIDS patients and others. The use of THC in the treatment of glaucoma, multiple sclerosis, and asthma has been recommended, but currently there are no scientific studies showing marijuana to be useful for these conditions. The dose of THC in marijuana that is smoked cannot be controlled, and therefore scientific studies are difficult to interpret as to efficacy and therapeutic drug levels. There are no studies showing THC to be better than standard antiemetic therapy. Currently there is one prescription product, dronabinol (Marinol), that contains synthetic THC. This drug has a standard concentration of THC and therefore the amount that the patient receives can be controlled. Dronabinol is a Schedule II drug and can be prescribed for nausea and vomiting or anorexia. In November 1996, two states, California and Arizona, passed propositions legalizing marijuana for medical purposes. The US Senate Judiciary Committee and the Drug Enforcement Agency have not supported these laws at the time of this writing.[2,23,34]

What Is the Management of Patients With Marijuana Intoxication?

The true danger related to acute marijuana intoxication is more related to the loss of motor skills and judgment than to the toxicity of THC. Operating a motor vehicle or other machinery while under the influence of marijuana could lead to potential loss of life or limb. The magnitude of the problem of motor vehicle injuries or work-related injuries that are due to marijuana usage is unknown. Studies have implicated marijuana in motor vehicle fatalities, especially in the 15 to 30-year-old age group. After alcohol, marijuana was the most common drug found, being detected in 11 to 33% of the cases.[5,26,36] Airline pilots had impairment when using a simulator for as long as 24 hours after a single dose of marijuana; this was compounded with age and the difficulty of the flying task.[24] The various regulatory agencies of the federal government require drug testing for the crew of commercial carriers involved in major accidents. An acute psychotic reaction commonly involving paranoid delusions and hallucinations may occur with marijuana usage and can be managed with benzodiazepines.[27] Pneumomediastinum has been described secondary to deep inhalation, leading to alveolar overdistention and rupture during marijuana smoking.[4] This may be responsible for dyspnea and chest pain, but is rarely life threatening. There are no known cases of lethal marijuana intoxication.

References

1. Astley SJ, Little RE: Maternal marijuana use during lactation and infant development at one year. Neurotoxicol Teratol 1990;12:161–168.
2. Beal JE, Olson R, Laubenstein L, et al: Dronabinol as a treatment for anorexia associated with weight loss in patients with AIDS. J Pain Symptom Manage 1995;10:89–97.
3. Benowitz NL, Jones RT: Cardiovascular and metabolic considerations in prolonged cannabinoid adminstration in man. J Clin Pharmacol 1981;21:214–223.
4. Brody SL, Anderson GV, Gutman JB: Pneumomediastinum as a complication of "crack" smoking. Am J Emer Med 1988; 6:241–243.
5. Brookoff D, Cook CS, Williams C, Mann CS: Testing reckless drivers for cocaine and marijuana. N Engl J Med 1994; 331:518–522.
6. Chait LD, Burke KA: Preference for high- versus low-potency marijuana. Pharmacol Biochem Behav 1994;49: 643–647.
7. Chiang CN, Barnett G: Marijuana pharmacokinetics and pharmacodynamics. In: Redda KK, Walker CA, Barnett G, eds: Cocaine, Marijuana, Designer Drugs: Chemistry, Pharmacology, and Behavior. Boca Raton, CRC Press, 1989, pp. 113–126.
8. Cone EJ, Johnson RE, Darwin WD, et al: Passive inhalation of marijuana smoke: Urinalysis and room air levels of delta-9-tetrahydrocannabinol. J Anal Toxicol 1987;11:89–96.
9. Day NL, Richardson GA, Goldschmidt L, et al: Effect of prenatal marijuana exposure on the cognitive development of offspring at age three. Neurotoxicol Teratol 1994;16: 169–175.
10. Deadwyler SA, Heyse CJ, Michaelis RC, Hampson RE: The effects of delta-9-THC on mechanisms of learning and memory. In: Erinoff L, ed: Neurobiology of Drug Abuse: Learning and Memory. NIDA research monograph 97. Washington, DC, USDHHS, 1990, pp. 79–93.
11. Ellis GM, Mann MA, Judson BA, et al: Excretion patterns of cannabinoid metabolites after last use in a group of chronic users. Clin Pharmacol Ther 1985;38:572–578.
12. Evans RP, Clement W: Compendium of drug abuse jargon. J Fam Pract 1977;4:67–71.
13. Fried PA: Behavioral outcome in preschool and school-age children exposed prenatally to marijuana: A review and speculative interpretation. In: Wetherington CL, Smeriglio VL, Finnegan LP, eds: Behavioral Studies of Drug-Exposed Offspring: Methodological Issues in Human and Animal Research. NIDA research monograph 164. Washington, DC, USDHHS, 1996, pp. 242–260.
14. Golub A, Johnson BD: The shifting importance of alcohol and marijuana as gateway substances among serious drug abusers. J Stud Alcohol 1994;55:607–614.
15. Hawks, RL: The constituents of Cannabis and the disposition and metabolism of cannabinoids. In: Hawks RL: The Analysis of Cannabinoids in Biological Fluids, NIDA research monograph 42. Washington, DC, USDHHS, 1982, pp. 125–317.
16. Heishman SJ, Huestis MA, Henningfield JE, Cone EJ: Acute and residual effects of marijuana: Profiles of plasma THC levels, physiological, subjective, and performance measures. Pharmacol Biochem Behav 1990;37:561–565.
17. Huestis M: Pharmacology and toxicology of marijuana. Ther Drug Monit 1993;14:131–138.
18. Husain S: Marijuana abuse: Its pharmacology and effects on testicular function. In Redda KK, Walker CA, Barnett G, eds: Cocaine, Marijuana, Designer Drugs: Chemistry, Pharmacology and Behavior. Boca Raton, CRC Press, 1989.
19. Johnston LD, O'Malley PM, Bachman JG: National Survey Results on Drug Use from Monitoring the Future Study, 1975–1994. Washington, DC, USDHHS, 1996.
20. Joyce CRB, Curry SH: The Botany and Chemistry of Cannabis. London, J&A Churchill, 1970, pp. 1–60.
21. Kann L, Warren CW, Harris WA, et al: Youth risk behavior surveillance—United States, 1995. MMWR 1996;45(SS4): 1–83.
22. Kusher DI, Dawson LO, Taylor AC, Djeu, JY: Effect of the psychoactive metabolite of marijuana, delta-9-tetrahydrocannabinol (THC), on the synthesis of tumor necrosis factor by human large granular lymphocytes. Cell Immunol 1994;154:99–108.
23. Lane M, Vogel CL, Ferguson J, et al: Dronabinol and prochlorperazine in combination for the treatment of cancer

chemotherapy-induced nausea and vomiting. J Pain Symptom Manage 1991; 6:352–359.
24. Leirer VO, Yesavage JA, Morrow DG: Marijuana, aging and task difficulty effects on pilot performance. Aviat Space Environ Med 1989;60:1145–1152.
25. Linszen DH, Dingemans PM, Lenior ME: Cannabis abuse and the course of recent-onset schizophrenic disorders. Arch Gen Psychiatry 1994; 51:273–279.
26. Logan BK, Schwilke EW: Drug and alcohol use in fatally injured drivers in Washington State. J Forensic Sci 1996; 41:505–510.
27. Mathers DC, Ghodse AH: Cannabis and psychotic illness. Br J Psychiatry 1992;161:648–653.
28. Matsuda LA, Lolait SJ, Brownstein MJ, Bonner TI: The THC receptor and its implications. In: Korenman SG, Barchas JD, eds: Biological Basis of Substance Abuse. Oxford, Oxford University Press, 1993, pp. 95–106.
29. Ohlsson A, Lingren JE, Wahlen A, et al: Plasma delta-9-tetrahydrocannabinol concentrations and clinical effects after oral and intravenous administration and smoking. Clin Pharmacol Ther 1980;28:409–416.
30. Perez-Reyes M: Marijuana smoking: Factors that influence the bioavailability of tetrahydrocannabinol. In: Chiang CN, Hawks RL, eds: Research Findings on Smoking of Abused Substances. NIDA research monograph 99. Washington, DC, USDHHS, 1990, pp. 42–62.
31. Pope HG, Yurgelun-Todd D: The residual cognitive effects of heavy marijuana use in college students. JAMA 1996; 275:521–527.
32. Richardson GA, Day NL, McGauhey PJ: The impact of prenatal marijuana and cocaine use on the infant and child. Clin Obstet Gynecol 1993;36:302–318.
33. Rouse BA: Epidemiology of illicit and abused drugs in the general population, emergency department drug-related episodes, and arrestees. Clinic Chem 1996;42:1330–1336.
34. Schwartz RH, Beveridge RA: Marijuana as an antiemetic drug: How useful is it today? Opinions from clinical oncologists. J Addict Dis 1994;13:53–65.
35. Schwartz RH, Hawks RL: Laboratory detection of marijuana use. JAMA 1985; 254:788–792.
36. Soderstrom EA, Trifillis AL, Shankar BS, et al: Marijuana and alcohol use among 1023 trauma patients. Arch Surg 1988;123:733–737.
37. Sparacino CM, Hyldburg PA, Hughes TJ: Chemical and biological analysis of marijuana smoke condensate. In: Chiang CN, Hawks RL, eds: Research Findings on Smoking of Abused Substances. NIDA research monograph 99. Washington, DC, USDHHS, 1990, pp. 121–140.
38. Tashkin DP, Coulson AH, Clark VA, et al: Respiratory symptoms and lung function in habitual heavy smokers of marijuana alone, smokers of marijuana and tobacco, smokers of tobacco alone and nonsmokers. Am Rev Resp Dis 1987;135:209–216.
39. Wu TC, Tashkin DP, Djahed B, Rose JE: Pulmonary hazards of smoking marijuana as compared with tobacco. N Engl J Med 1988;318:347–351.
40. Zheng ZM, Specter S, Friedman H: Inhibition by delta-9-tetrahydrocannabinol of tumor necrosis factor alpha production by mouse and human macrophages. Int J Immunopharmacol 1992;14:1145–1152.

CHAPTER 70

Substance Withdrawal

Richard J. Hamilton

CASE 1. A 46-year-old male arrived in the Emergency Department. He had been in police custody for 18 hours and requested evaluation by a physician because he had a seizure disorder and needed his daily dose of phenytoin. He stated that he was a frequent drinker but denied drug use. His seizures began 10 years ago, and he had been taking phenytoin ever since. He had been noncompliant with his phenytoin, possibly for 2 months. He denied any physical complaints and wanted to be seen and discharged.

His vital signs were: blood pressure, 130/80 mm Hg; respiratory rate, 12 breaths/min; pulse, 105 beats/min without orthostatic changes; and rectal temperature, 99.9°F (37.2°C). The man was well developed, poorly nourished, and appeared older than his stated age. He was garrulous and somewhat anxious. He was alert and oriented to time, place, and person. The pertinent positives on physical examination included a fine hand and tongue tremor, scattered spider nevi, and hepatomegaly of 14 cm. Auscultation of the heart and lungs revealed no abnormalities.

The history and initial physical examination appeared consistent with the diagnosis of alcoholism and suspected alcohol withdrawal. The patient was to be observed while serum laboratory test results returned. Blood was drawn for complete blood count, serum chemistries, liver function tests, and serum alcohol and phenytoin levels. A rapid reagent blood sugar was 70 mg/dL. One liter 0.9% sodium chloride was administered at 500 mL/h with multivitamins and 100 mg of thiamine. In addition, 25 mL of 50% dextrose solution was administered over 2 minutes.

One hour later, the patient began to shout at nursing staff that he was being held against his will and that he must leave. Repeat vital signs were: blood pressure, 130/80 mm Hg; respiratory rate, 12 breaths/min; pulse, 130 beats/min; room air pulse oximetry, 98% saturation; and rectal temperature, 100.3 °F (37.9°C). The patient was diaphoretic. The pupils were 5 mm, equal and briskly reactive. The tremor was now coarse. The patient demanded to be released and could not remember why he asked to be evaluated or who brought him to the hospital.

The patient's clinical condition was unchanged after 20 mg of diazepam was given as two 10-mg IV boluses 15 minutes apart. A portable chest radiograph was within normal limits. The electrocardiogram demonstrated a sinus tachycardia. A room air arterial blood gas analysis was reported as pH, 7.41; PCO_2, 37.4 mm Hg; PO_2, 73 mm Hg; HCO_3, 24 mEq; oxygen saturation, 95%. Diazepam was repeated as 10-mg IV boluses to a total of 100 mg, and the patient was placed in four-point soft restraints after he began to remove his intravenous line and climb off the stretcher. His diaphoresis and tachycardia continued. He picked at the restraints, scratched his skin, and shouted nonsensical words occasionally.

Diazepam administered to a total dose of 220 mg did not improve the patient's agitation; the pulse was 110 beats/min; respiratory rate, 12 breaths/min; and temperature, 101.0°F (38.3°C). Toxicology consultation recommended phenobarbital intravenously. This was administered as 130-mg boluses over 3 minutes and repeated four times (520 mg total); the patient was sleeping and the heart rate was 100 beats/min. The patient was electively intubated using thiopental and placed on a mechanical ventilator for airway protection. The patient remained sedate and required only an additional 40 mg of diazepam over the next 24 hours. He developed a right lower lobe infiltrate on day 2 of his hospitalization and was treated with ampicillin/sulbactam. He recovered uneventfully and was extubated 48 hours later.

Why Do Patients Experience Withdrawal?

The central nervous system must balance excitation and inhibition to control physiologic function. The most intuitive way to balance this might be to increase excitatory nerve impulses for a physiologic action, and to increase inhibitory impulses whenever a physiologic action must be stopped. The CNS uses a more efficient method: Excitatory neurons fire regularly, and inhibitory neurons inhibit the transmission of these impulses. Whenever action is required, the inhibitory neurons decrease their firing and permit the excitatory nerve impulses to travel to their end organs. Thus, all action in human neurophysiology is dysinhibition. [71,133,146]

When administered chronically, many drugs and toxins affect the transmission of all classes of inhibitory neurons. Some act to increase the inhibitory effect with subsequent adaptive modulation (such as benzodiazepines and the $GABA_A$ receptor, opioids on the opioid receptor, or clonidine on the central $alpha_2$ receptor). Others act to block the inhibitory effect with subsequent adaptive modulation (caffeine on the adenosine receptor). Still others appear to increase the inhibitory effect with subsequent adaptive modulation of both inhibitory and excitatory neurons (ethanol and the $GABA_A$ and NMDA receptors).[48,123] A withdrawal syndrome occurs when the drug or toxin is removed or reduced and the adaptive changes persist, producing dysfunction instead.

Thus, every withdrawal syndrome has two characteristics: (1) a pre-existing physiologic adaptation to a drug or toxin, the continuous presence of which prevents physiologic derangement; and (2) decreasing concentrations of that substance. In contrast, simple tolerance to a drug is characterized as a physiologic adaptation that shifts the dose–response curve to the right. Patients with withdrawal syndromes have often developed tolerance, but tolerance does not require the continued presence of the drug to prevent physiologic derangement.

Finally, drugs and toxins that stimulate the excitatory neuronal pathways, such as cocaine, can produce a postintoxication syndrome that often results in lethargy, hypersomnolence, movement disorders, and irritability. Despite the fact that this syndrome meets DSM-IV criteria for a withdrawal syndrome, it does not meet a toxicologic definition because the continuous use of this drug does not prevent this physiologic derangement. This postintoxication syndrome, so called "crack crash" or "washed out syndrome," is caused by prolonged use of the drug, and patients return to their premorbid function without intervention.[106,124,131,132,145]

Withdrawal syndromes are best described and treated based on the class of receptors that are mostly affected. This concept will organize the approach to patient care as well.

What Is GABAminergic Withdrawal?

Ethanol, benzodiazepines, and barbiturates enhance GABAminergic tone. This is the mechanism by which they produce sedation. $GABA_A$ receptors are postsynaptic receptors that, when activated, hyperpolarize the postsynaptic neuron by an inward chloride current without a G protein messenger.[71] These receptors have separate binding sites for GABA, barbiturates, benzodiazepines, and picrotoxin. Barbiturates and benzodiazepines bind to their receptor sites and enhance the affinity for GABA at its receptor site.[5] Chronic exposure to benzodiazepines appears to decrease $GABA_A$ receptor sensitivity.[78,139] Only high-dose barbiturates can open the GABA chloride channel without concomitant binding of a GABA molecule, and this has been especially demonstrated with phenobarbital and pentobarbital.[44,57]

Many drugs, (eg, ethanol, etomidate) have GABA receptor activity without a clearly identified binding site. Ethanol, benzodiazepines, etomidate, and propofol are examples of drugs that merely enhance $GABA_A$ chloride channel activity and are classified as indirect GABA agonists. Acute exposure to ethanol appears to affect membrane fluidity and cross-couple the five proteins that construct the GABA receptor, interact with a portion of the receptor, and enhance GABA release.[23,69,103,119,120] Although the mechanism is unclear, the result is an enhancement in GABA chloride channel activity, apparently without enhancing GABA binding to its recognition site on the receptor.[72] The adaptation to chronic exposure to ethanol is a modified $GABA_A$ receptor expression without a change in receptor sensitivity to GABA or benzodiazepines.[22,72,73,107,108,113,139] Recent evidence demonstrates that chronic ethanol exposure first increases and then ultimately decreases mRNA expression of certain $GABA_A$ subunit proteins.[22,67,72] These subunit proteins ($alpha_1$, $alpha_3$, $alpha_6$, $gamma_{2s}$, $gamma_{2l}$, and $gamma_3$) are assembled in multiple combinations to form GABA receptor complexes with slightly different characteristics in different areas of the brain. Ultimately, withdrawal symptoms may represent the clinical manifestation of a change in GABA receptor complex characteristics, and thus cause diminished effectiveness, rather than a simple change in receptor numbers.[34]

Although the exact mechanism is not completely known, what is clear is that during withdrawal, GABA synaptic activity is so diminished that inhibitory control of excitatory neurotransmitters and pathways such as glutamate, NMDA, norepinephrine, and dopamine is lost.[41,117] This results in the clinical syndrome of withdrawal–CNS excitation (seizures, tremor, hallucinations), and autonomic stimulation (tachycardia, hypertension hyperthermia, diaphoresis).[49,70]

What Is the Mechanistic Treatment for GABAminergic Withdrawal?

Restoration of inhibitory control by administration of $GABA_A$ agonists is essential for resolution of this life-threatening syndrome. Long-acting $GABA_A$ agonists that can be administered in a loading dose are the ideal agents for the treatment of withdrawal. Diazepam is the benzodiazepine with the best profile. Phenobarbital has been used successfully because of its long half-life. Because benzodiazepines only enhance GABA binding, and GABAminergic transmission is lowered in withdrawal because of either decreased GABA receptor complex production and/or decreased receptor efficacy, the indirect-acting agents may be ineffective even at higher doses than normal. For this reason, high-dose intravenous barbiturates are advantageous in refractory cases because they can open GABA chloride channels without GABA binding.[44]

Up-regulation in the excitatory neuronal pathways is also important in GABAminergic withdrawal and the NMDA subtype of glutamate receptor (especially the MK801 binding site) appears to be the major contributor.[59,148] Enhanced excitatory neurotransmission is a characteristic of ethanol withdrawal that appears to explain the "kindling" hypothesis, in which withdrawal events become progressively more severe.[9,12,17,20,151] The activity of an excitatory neuronal pathway increases the more it fires, a phenomenon known as long-term potentiation.[48] This may be a result of increased activity of mRNA and receptor protein expression.[32] Thus, as NMDA receptors increase in number and function, and $GABA_A$ receptor activity diminishes, withdrawal becomes more severe.[33,78,88,112] Knowledge of this phenomenon should prompt the clinician toward aggressive treatment of even minor withdrawal symptoms, in the hopes of attenuating the progression to subsequently more severe withdrawal episodes.[162]

How Does Delirium Tremens Serve As a Model for Diagnosis and Treatment of This Patient?

Delirium tremens is the best studied of all the withdrawal phenomena, and its proper management serves as a guide to managing any agitated patient with an elevated temperature. Because of the confusion generated by use of the terms "pure DTs," "impending DTs," and "florid DTs," the findings of morbidity studies are of limited value. Careful examination of the literature on DTs reveals that many published reports included patients who were calm, cooperative, and readily taking fluids and medication by mouth.

In the early 1950s, Victor and Adams,[152] Mendelson and LaDou,[91] and Isbell and co-workers[63] identified the etiology of DTs as alcohol withdrawal in a chronically (usually at least 2 to 3 weeks) dependent individual. Delirium tremens was not found to be caused by alcohol intoxication, electrolyte or fluid disturbances, shock, infection, or trauma, as previously postulated, but only by withdrawal. All of these investigators demonstrated the similarity of alcoholic DTs and barbiturate and paraldehyde withdrawal. As Victor and Adams[152] noted:

> Delirium tremens in its full-blown form is the most dramatic and gravest of all the alcoholic complications. It develops in a variety of settings. The patient, an excessive and steady drinker . . . may have been admitted for an unrelated illness, accident, operation, or infection. . . . He may have suffered through several days of tremulousness, hallucinosis or seizures.
>
> The patient is restless and agitated, requiring restraints, . . . constantly pulling at his bed clothes, . . . swept over by a wave of apprehension and tremulousness, . . . conversation being garbled and unintelligible. Autonomic overactivity is manifested by dilated pupils, tachycardia, and an elevated temperature, attributable occasionally to no cause other than delirium. Drenching sweats may result in severe dehydration.

Bowman and co-workers noted that abnormal mental states may cause physical reactions that in turn lead to hyperthermia.[18] They stated that physical manifestations and complications of agitation were common to all markedly disturbed patients, regardless of the type of mental illness (alcohol or organic delirium, manic–depressive psychosis, schizophrenia, or dementia paralytica). Because of the severity of the agitation, febrile patients often received inadequate fluid replacement, resulting in dehydration.

What Are the Characteristics of Ethanol Withdrawal?

The classic works of Victor and Adams in 1953 as well as Isbell and co-workers in 1955 provide excellent descriptive studies of ethanol withdrawal.[63,152] The keen observations and classifications of the symptoms associated with withdrawal make worthwhile reading and can still contribute to the clinician's understanding of the natural history of this disorder. Much of the terminology used in these reports continues to this day and unfortunately adds to a confusing assortment of terms. The term "rum fit" appears to have originated as a description of the convulsions and/or behavior of sailors who were denied their daily rum rations. The term is used to describe a typical alcohol withdrawal seizure—brief, generalized, and occasionally recurrent. "Delirium tremens" was originally described as the "distinct clinical condition characterized by psychomotor, speech, and autonomic overactivity, disorientation, confusion, disordered sense perception, and frequently fatal outcome."[152]

Nearly half a century later, our understanding of neurotransmitters and neurologic function makes a more precise understanding of this disorder possible. Alcohol withdrawal is a neurologic disorder with a continuum of progressively worsening symptoms caused by the effects of chronic ethanol on the central nervous system, and is often exacerbated by the clinical manifestations of alcoholism (nutritional depletion, impaired immunity, anemia, cirrhosis, head trauma).[76] The morbidity and mortality from this condition largely arise from inappropriate resuscitative efforts (failure to correct hypovolemia and lower temperature), inappropriate treatments (neuroleptics), and failure to identify concurrent illness (infection, CNS trauma; Fig. 70–1). The 15% mortality observed by Victor and Adams largely occurred in the patients with concurrent illness. Half of all patients with delirium tremens and two thirds of the patients with fatal delirium tremens had concurrent illness. This

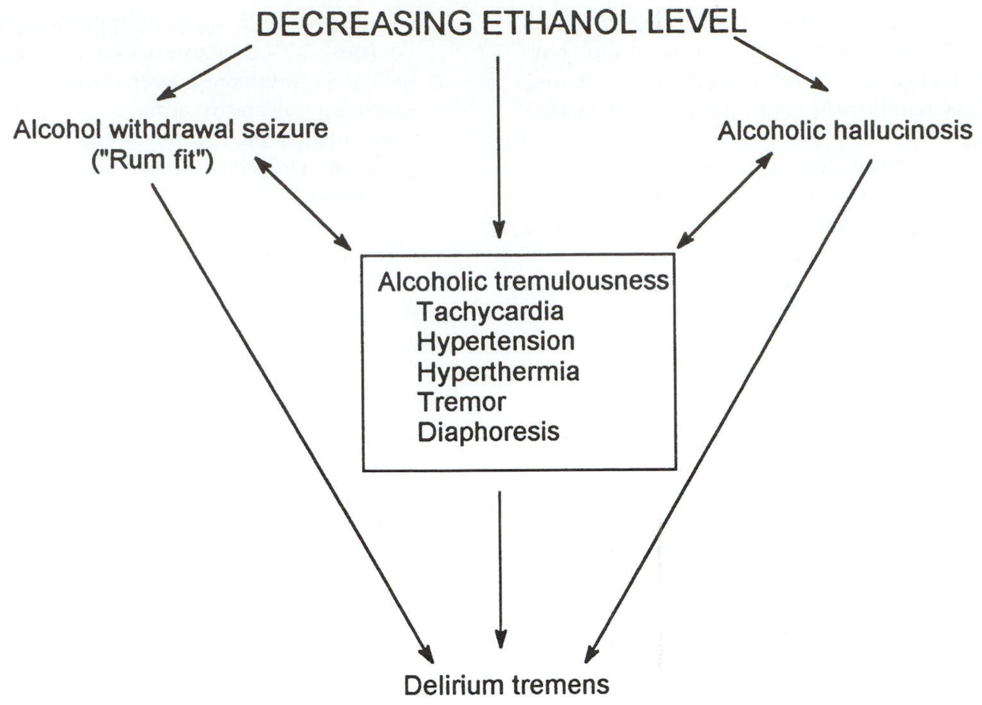

Figure 70–1. Schematic representation of alcohol withdrawal. As ethanol levels fall, patients may develop alcohol withdrawal seizures ("rum fits"), alcoholic hallucinosis, or alcoholic tremulousness. Following this stage, the patient can recover, develop another early manifestation of withdrawal, or progress to delirium tremens.

mortality was reduced to below 5% within a decade of their work when aggressive fluid resuscitation, cooling, and supportive care became the goal of therapy.[140,141] Now, we expect the mortality from this condition to be zero unless the patient is inadequately treated.[127]

Patients who drink continuously, as opposed to "binge drinkers," are theoretically at highest risk for withdrawal.[104] The majority of patients arrive at the hospital seeking care for the illness or circumstance that prevented them from drinking, such as an upper respiratory infection that confined them to bedrest or imprisonment. If the patient has an elevated ethanol level on admission, the severity of withdrawal is predictably worse.[153] A sizable portion of patients will present to the ED after a seizure. They may even have a history of a seizure disorder and be taking anticonvulsant medications largely because alcohol withdrawal seizures (AWS) cannot be differentiated from a generalized seizure disorder at the bedside.

Rum fits may occur without other signs of withdrawal and are characteristically brief tonic–clonic events with a short postictal period. They may recur, but status epilepticus is distinctly unusual in withdrawal (40% single seizures and 3% status epilepticus).[152] All patients with first-time AWS should receive a thorough evaluation, including CBC, serum electrolytes, calcium and magnesium, chest radiograph, urinalysis, CT scan of the brain, and lumbar puncture. The yield on these clinical investigations is extraordinarily high, and often reveals complications or phenomena associated with alcoholism that require treatment (occult infection, remote and/or recent head trauma, anemia, electrolyte abnormalities, and so forth).[40] Cortical atrophy is a common finding on a CT scan of the head in alcoholic patients, but temporal lobe volume deficits may correlate with AWS either as a cause or sequela.[138] It is unclear whether these AWS invariably progress to a permanent seizure disorder with chronic neurologic dysfunction or are merely a marker for the problems associated with severe alcoholism such as recurrent head trauma, infections, and hypoxia, which cause CNS injury.[10]

A rapid recovery and normal mental status belie the seriousness of this event. For one third of all patients with alcohol withdrawal characterized by delirium (delirium tremens), the sentinel event is an isolated AWS. This seizure may occur despite the presence of an elevated serum ethanol level. In fact, an AWS that occurs despite an elevated ethanol level is a poor prognostic indicator because the relative protection of an elevated ethanol level will continue to be lost as the level drops.[153] An asymptomatic period after an alcoholic abstinence seizure may last for several hours or the CNS excitation will progress without recovery.

Progressive CNS excitation characterizes the next phase of withdrawal. We suggest that patients with alcohol withdrawal be clinically classified into those with an intact and those with an altered consciousness. The advantage to this simple classification is that it avoids clinical descriptors that are only confusing, such as delirium, DTs, or florid DTs. Tachycardia, fever, and hypertension are identifiable markers for worsening withdrawal.

The central nervous system excitation begins as a fine intention tremor that can be detected in the outstretched hands or protruding tongue.[92] This appears to be a variation of physiologic tremor except that patients with alcohol have a tremor with a significantly higher amplitude compared to the tremor normally associated with anxiety or emotional stress.

Formication, or the sensation of ants crawling on the skin, often promotes repeated itching and leads to excoriations. Disorders of thought, anxiety, agitation, and lability of mood also manifest to varying degrees. Hallucinations are largely visual and appear to occur especially in patients with inadequate thiamine stores.[60] When these CNS manifestations are present with normal vital signs, the patient may be anxious, display a fine tremor, and appear otherwise normal. Because these symptoms will invariably progress, all patients should be treated with sedation. Indeed, there is evidence to support the notion that withdrawal that is allowed to become severe invariably leads to progressively more severe episodes of withdrawal during subsequent periods of abstinence.[147,151]

Patients with a history of alcoholism who develop CNS excitation and then manifest abnormal vital signs are experiencing clinical deterioration. Tachycardia, elevated temperature, hypertension, and diaphoresis mark the autonomic manifestations of this worsening withdrawal syndrome. If untreated or undertreated, the central nervous system excitation of these patients progresses to uncontrollable agitation, seizures, involuntary tremor, hyperthermia, rhabdomyolysis, and death.

How Was Delirium Tremens Managed and What Was Its Mortality?

In 1916, Osler recommended confinement to bed, no restraints, withdrawal of alcohol, and judicious use of potassium bromide, chloral hydrate, trional, hyoscine, and, possibly, opium.[101] He suggested that cold douches or baths be used to reduce fever and thereby produce sedation. He also emphasized the importance of feeding milk or broth. Using these methods, mortality was 14% according to several studies at the time.

In 1927, Cecil wrote that there were "no specific treatments," but that it was essential to produce sleep, stimulate the neurologic and circulatory systems, and feed the patient.[25] Paraldehyde, chloral hydrate, and hyoscyamine were considered acceptable hypnotics, but barbiturates were not recommended and morphine use was avoided. Strychnine and ergot were recommended for the treatment of tremor. Sheet restraints were suggested as replacements for old-fashioned canvas jackets. Sodium bicarbonate and cathartics were given hourly to patients with gastritis. Despite these innovations proposed by Cecil, mortality for uncomplicated cases approached that found in studies following Osler's recommendations. When DTs were associated with infections such as pneumonia, mortality was even higher; if associated with trauma, mortality reached 50%.

By the early 1940s, studies demonstrated that previously promoted theories on the benefits of dehydration were totally inappropriate and that carbohydrates, sodium chloride, and fluids were essential. However, mortality remained the same. On the other hand, by the mid–1930s at Boston City Hospital the fatality rate for all cases declined, which Moore and Gray attributed to improved nursing care.[93]

In the late 1950s and early 1960s, paraldehyde and chloral hydrate were compared with phenothiazines in the treatment of DTs.[45] The phenothiazines were associated with slower control of fever and greater morbidity and mortality. A controlled study in 1964 demonstrated a 35% mortality rate with promazine and a 4.5% mortality rate with paraldehyde.[142] Causes of death were similar: fever, tachycardia, stupor, cyanosis, and cardiovascular collapse without defined pathology. Phenothiazines and butyrophenones are now generally considered inappropriate for any form of withdrawal, because they increase the incidence of hypotension, hyperthermia, seizures, and mortality.[15,49,51,52,100]

A comprehensive review of 39 fatal cases of DTs found dehydration in all cases in which volume status was noted.[141] The review included psychotic patients displaying mania or hyperactivity, and patients with DTs who also exhibited increased somatic activity (tremor, seizures) associated with dehydration. Approximately 50% of patients had temperatures greater than 40°C (104°F), including 9 of 12 patients with seizures; in 11 cases, hyperthermia was attributed solely to the delirium. Thus, regardless of etiology, hyperthermia, increased motor activity, and fluid depletion in the setting of DTs carried a grave prognosis. However, recognition and treatment of complications along with better fluid replacement and supportive care seemed to be the most important determinants of survival. Mortality at Philadelphia General Hospital decreased to 5.4% in the late 1950s (as compared to 18.5% in the early 1950s) using this approach.[140]

In a 1975 controlled trial of diazepam and paraldehyde for severe DTs, Thompson and colleagues found that parenteral diazepam calmed patients more rapidly than did rectal paraldehyde.[144] There was no mortality in diazepam-treated patients. Adverse reactions and mortality, however, were significant in patients treated with paraldehyde. The suggested diazepam regimen was 10 mg IV followed by 5 mg IV every 5 minutes until calm. If no response was noted, the diazepam dose was increased. When the loading dose is administered, most patients, if adequately sedated, will not require additional sedation, as diazepam and desmethyldiazepam have long half-lives, thus permitting the primary agent and the metabolite to be endogenously tapered and avoiding drug-induced cyclic variations.[2,3,126] Some patients who manifest withdrawal while their ethanol levels are persistently elevated necessitate additional doses of benzodiazepine, as the ethanol is rapidly metabolized. Physicians who choose short half-life benzodiazepines (oxazepam and lorazepam) must readminister the agents every 6 hours and begin tapering regimens by the second day.

Sedation (to produce calm, restful sleep), substrate repletion (dextrose, thiamine, folic acid, pyridoxine), fluid and electrolyte balance, oxygen, and control of hyperthermia and agitation improve survival. Although some patients still die from complications such as trauma, CNS hemorrhage, pancreatitis, infection, liver disease, and electrolyte- or alcoholic cardiomyopathy-related dysrhythmias,[76,82] DTs themselves should not be fatal if properly managed. The effects of rapid cooling and hydration in combination with sedation have virtually eliminated mortality from uncomplicated DTs.[143]

A similar approach to all agitated patients significantly reduces mortality and morbidity related to hyperthermia, rhabdomyolysis, and dehydration. Hyperthermia in the agitated patient carries a particularly high risk. Unlike fevers of infectious etiologies, temperatures may exceed 106°F (41.1°C), with resultant tissue damage. Rapid cooling, titration of sedation with a benzodiazepine, and adequate hydration are essential early steps in the management of the agitated patient, regardless of the etiology.

How Is Alcohol Withdrawal Treated?

There are four important principles in the management of the patient in withdrawal.

1. Restore inhibitory tone to the central nervous system using long acting benzodiazepines or barbiturates.
2. Identify and correct fluid, electrolyte, and nutritional deficiencies.
3. Evaluate the patient for concurrent infection.
4. Allow the patient to rest peacefully without pulling out intravenous lines, decrease the need for restraints, and decrease the risk of rhabdomyolysis while participating in all necessary diagnostic studies.

The application of these principles is derived from our understanding of the protean effects of alcoholism and the nature of withdrawal as a neurologic disorder.

Patients with alcohol withdrawal are disinhibited. They have amplified excitatory neuronal pathways and impaired inhibitory neuronal pathways that require the continuous presence of ethanol to approximate normal physiology. The goal of therapy is to rapidly restore the inhibitory tone—to reinhibit them. The patient should be rapidly brought to the point of a continuously controlled peaceful state and the vital signs normalized. Once this is achieved, metabolites of the initial drug continue the treatment of the patient. Many patients are effectively treated with an initial agent although some require periodic additional dosing of the primary agent. Instead of the patient accumulating small, ineffective doses and becoming progressively more sedated, the patient is brought to a calm peaceful point of sedation. As the initial maximum CNS depression gradually improves over days, the metabolism of the drug proceeds. Numerous studies support this "loading" or "symptom-triggered therapy" principle, in which a benzodiazepine with active metabolites is administered in an escalating bolus fashion.[85,121,155] Although the initial doses may be quite high, withdrawal is ultimately better managed with less total benzodiazepine and fewer symptoms.[121,154] In addition, studies indicate that the hospital can realize a cost savings (50%) by using a tapered diazepam regimen.[156] Properly sedated patients also improve staff perceptions of the safety of the environment, because of a decrease in patient violence and agitation using the loading technique.[58]

Even with substantial benzodiazepine doses, respiratory compromise and the need for airway support are unlikely. Concerns about dosing benzodiazepines in patients with liver failure and the elderly are justified, but these patients also benefit from this approach, as the modest prolongation in half-life is not deleterious and patients do not have greater CNS depression but only a potentially more prolonged phase.[19,55,102,162]

The selection of a benzodiazepine is important to the success of this loading principle. Chlordiazepoxide has been used, but offers no unique benefits over diazepam. Lorazepam is considered inferior to diazepam because it is short acting, must be dosed at frequent intervals, and may even be less effective at providing steady control of the CNS manifestations.[65,98,113] In fact, it is precisely because large boluses of diazepam are metabolized to active metabolites (desmethyldiazepam) over the typical period of withdrawal (48 to 72 hours) that diazepam is the only benzodiazepine needed to treat this disorder.[3,163] A retrospective review reported that the use of a single benzodiazepine rather than multiple benzodiazepines was a marker for treatment success in surgical patients experiencing alcohol withdrawal during surgical admission.[95] Ultimately, this approach has the added benefit of greatly simplifying management.

The typical starting dose for a patient in alcohol withdrawal is 10 mg of diazepam given intravenously repeated every 15 minutes until the patient is sedated and the vital signs have normalized. Twenty milligrams may be all that is needed for slightly more than one third of the patients; one quarter of all patients in ethanol withdrawal will require 200 mg.[122] Patients who begin to experience withdrawal with an elevated ethanol level will require immediate treatment plus additional therapy as the ethanol level continues to decrease. An alcoholic can take as long as 10 hours to eliminate a serum ethanol level of 150 mg/dL (see Chap. 62). In addition, the previously coupled chloride channel and the benzodiazepine receptor becomes uncoupled, and this may render benzodiazepines ineffective. These patients can remain symptomatic despite doses of diazepam that approach 1 g.[77,97] In fact, doses can be so high (eg, gram quantities of diazepam) that the excipients such as propylene glycol may approach toxicity, although this has never been reported for a diazepam loading regimen.[13,75,150] One report describes the use of 2335 mg of diazepam intravenously and 21,225 mg of oxazepam orally without control of agitation from alcohol withdrawal.

There was no evidence of an abnormal pharmacokinetic profile.[161] When this level of benzodiazepine "resistance" is noted, it is more efficacious to add a barbiturate to attain a synergistic effect on the $GABA_A$ receptor chloride channel and bypass the ineffectual benzodiazepine receptor.[44,64]

Intravenous phenobarbital should be given as a bolus of 260 mg (phenobarbital is supplied in 130-mg ampules) over 5 minutes. Repeat dosing should be considered in 30 minutes. This is accomplished by giving a bolus of 130 mg of phenobarbital over 3 minutes. Studies and clinical experience with this drug show that most patients will require 8.5 mg/kg to achieve the endpoint of light sedation. Side effects of this drug regimen include hypotension (6%) that is easily reversed with fluid administration.[164] In addition, airway protection should always be considered when phenobarbital is given after benzodiazepines. The dose of phenobarbital can be as high as 20 mg/kg, as in status epilepticus, but most patients with alcohol withdrawal will respond to a dose of 15 mg/kg.[96] Phenobarbital levels are unnecessary, as the patient is loaded to a clinical effect and only treated as symptoms occur.[86,164]

Ultimately, very high dose anesthetic type doses of barbiturates never fail to treat withdrawal because they directly open the $GABA_A$ chloride channel.[37,49] If anesthetic doses are utilized, the patient should be intubated and placed on mechanical ventilation. Intravenous pentobarbital given as a 3 to 5-mg/kg bolus and 100-mg/h drip should be an effective starting point. The initial pentobarbital bolus should be used as the induction agent for the rapid sequence intubation.

Phenytoin does not protect against AWS seizures and is in fact no better than placebo.[6,27,109] Alcoholics may be on phenytoin for primary epilepsy or a seizure disorder acquired from the manifestations of their disease (CNS infections, trauma, cortical atrophy). The original work by Victor and Adams is still helpful in making the clinical determination. Alcohol withdrawal seizures are brief, and recurrent, but rarely progress to status epilepticus. If seizure focality is evident other CNS pathology is invariably present.[125] AWS are often first recognized in patients in their third and fourth decades. All other seizures should be considered to have a cause, other than alcoholism itself.[152]

The liberal use of radiologic and laboratory testing is encouraged to evaluate the patient needs for the second and third goals of therapy. In general, the more severe the alcohol withdrawal, the more likely a concurrent illness.[39]

Hypoglycemia is an important problem in alcohol withdrawal because of increased CNS glucose requirements.[36] Thus, all patients with withdrawal require supplemental glucose and thiamine to assist in its transport and metabolism (see Chap. 62).[158]

Magnesium continues to be a source of controversy in alcohol withdrawal. Though many reports suggest a beneficial effect and animal models point to a role in NMDA antagonism, prospective trials fail to find a benefit. Because deficiencies of this electrolyte can mimic ethanol withdrawal and alcoholics are often magnesium depleted, measuring magnesium levels and repleting a patient with a magnesium deficiency is important. There appears to be no role for its empiric use in this setting.[16,42,47,159]

All first-time seizures in an alcoholic require an emergency CT scan of the head. This study has a high yield for identifying useful diagnostic information such as evidence of CNS trauma and cortical atrophy, although intervention is uncommon.[35,68,74] A lumbar puncture should be routinely performed to determine if there are any manifestations of a CNS infection. Chest radiography often reveals evidence of chronic pulmonary infections, aspiration pneumonia, and cardiomyopathy.

The use of antihypertensive agents, phenothiazines, neuroleptics, and sedative hypnotics (other than benzodiazepines and barbiturates) is without foundation. A number of studies that use vital signs as surrogate markers for severity of withdrawal support the use of clonidine and beta-adrenergic antagonists.[11,61] However, these patients often experience more of the CNS manifestations of withdrawal, such as anxiety, agitation, and delirium.[3,155] The use of these drugs has largely arisen because of a lack of understanding of the pathophysiology of withdrawal. Although these drugs obviously will block the peripheral manifestations of alcohol withdrawal, they fail to treat the primary neurologic derangement responsible for these symptoms. For example, although the use of antipyretic agents are an important adjunct in treating patients with bacterial infection and fever, one would never consider reducing the dose of antibiotics if the fever resolved with acetaminophen. Vital sign abnormalities are the peripheral manifestations or markers for the severity of the neurologic derangement, and should be aggressively treated with drugs (benzodiazepines and barbiturates) that primarily affect the CNS. In addition, other therapies may actually exacerbate toxicity. Alcohol withdrawal treated with neuroleptics has a mortality of 6%.[8] These drugs lower the seizure threshold, impair heat regulation, and fail to correct the neurologic origin of this disorder. [7,10,15,51,52,149] Their use is only justified to treat underlying medical problems other than withdrawal. Patients with CNS excitation with normal vital signs are candidates for oral therapy and can often be managed by an alcohol detoxification service.[14,54]

What Are the Clinical Characteristics and Treatment of Benzodiazepine and Barbiturate Withdrawal?

The similarity between the two forms of withdrawal was identified by Victor and Adams who noted the work of Isbell on chronic barbiturate intoxication and withdrawal.[62] Patients who are addicted to benzodiazepines, barbiturates, and other sedative-hypnotic drugs display withdrawal symptoms that are similar to alcohol withdrawal symptoms except that they may develop as late as 14 days after cessation of drug administration depending on the pharmacokinetic profile of the abused drug. Diazepam, chlorazepate, and chlordiazepoxide are converted to active metabolites with half-lives of up to 200 hours. Phenobarbital's half life is as long as 2 to 6 days. These patients may have symptoms such as anxiety or insomnia for many days before objective manifestations of withdrawal develop. Alprazolam is a short-acting benzodiazepine without active metabolites and can cause withdrawal symptoms within 24 hours of cessation of use.

Benzodiazepine withdrawal has most of the same charactersitics as severe ethanol withdrawal, except the expected time course for resolution of withdrawal symptoms can last for 10 days. Patients develop the dysinhibitory syndrome characterized by progressively worsening agitation, tachycardia, hypertension, fever, hyperthermia, and seizures.

No controlled studies have been done addressing the comparative efficacy of various treatment regimens. However, considering this entity as another form of $GABA_A$minergic withdrawal, diazepam and barbiturates become the logical choices.

For patients with benzodiazepine withdrawal who still have normal vital signs, some believe that phenobarbital is a useful first choice, because patients perceive that the addicting drug has been eliminated. In addition, its long half-life will allow an appropriate taper of drug levels without complicating management.[116] One approach is to start the patient on a phenobarbital dose that is considered a sedative-hypnotic equivalent (each 10 mg of diazepam is equated with 30 mg phenobarbital), and then each day the patient is administered 10% less of the total dose.

For benzodiazepine withdrawal with abnormal vital signs or seizures, diazepam loading in a fashion similar to ethanol withdrawal is an appropriate first choice. Phenobarbital loading can be used in this situation as well. One interesting and apparently successful strategy is the use of a phenobarbital drip until the point of a continuously controlled, peaceful sleep is achieved. The dose was 0.03 to 0.04 mg/kg per minute and the infusion time to reach the clinical end point was 7.8 ± 1.1 hours, the total dose was 992 ± 144 mg, and the peak serum phenobarbital concentration was 26.1 ± 5.1 μg/mL. The mean serum half-life ($t_{½}$) was 57.5 ± 4.9 hours for 7 sedative-hypnotic abusers and 86 ± 3 hr for 8 normal volunteers (*P* > 0.001). Only the patient with the shortest $t_{½}$ (36.4 hours) required oral phenobarbital supplements to prevent withdrawal symptoms. The use of infusions may be perilous in anything but a closely monitored situation, and even then overshoot remains a concern. Periodic boluses after which the patient can be closely observed prevent the possibility of infusion errors. However, the total dose and half-life described in this study correspond to our clinical experience with phenobarbital boluses.[86]

Benzodiazepine Treatment Regimen for the Patient With Sedative-Hypnotic or Ethanol Withdrawal

An appropriate treatment regimen follows.

1. Assume the patient has a significant ethanol or sedative-hypnotic dependency.
2. Plan to admit the patient to a well-staffed hospital setting. Exclude serious intoxications, trauma, and infectious processes, and then initiate therapy.
3. Titrate the benzodiazepine intravenously to a dose that will produce mild intoxication, manifested by slurred speech, nystagmus, and ataxia without making the patient somnolent. A reasonable starting dose is 10 mg of diazepam. If this dose produces intoxication, sedative-hypnotic dependency is questionable, and another etiology for the symptom complex should be sought. The peak respiratory depressant effect from IV diazepam occurs within 5 minutes, allowing for rapid repetitive dosing as clinically needed. If the patient shows no intoxication at 5 minutes, a second dose may be given and repeated every 5 minutes until mild intoxication is achieved. Despite using an agent such as diazepam with long-acting metabolites, the CNS depression will never be greater than that noted in the initial acute phase of management. This "5-minute rule" is well established by clinical experience with diazepam and short-acting barbiturates such as pentobarbital. It may not be applicable to other IV benzodiazepines such as lorazepam, for which further experience is necessary to determine a safe dosing schedule.
4. The dose required is variable and should not be of concern. However, recently we have noted patients who were refractory to doses of diazepam in the thousands of milligrams who responded to IV amobarbital or phenobarbital. These patients may be manifesting clinically the imperfect cross-tolerance between sedative-hypnotic agents that has been demonstrated in animal studies of sedative-hypnotic dependence. The failure of benzodiazepine therapy to reverse completely the mental status changes associated with delirium tremens may be another example of incomplete cross-tolerance at a neurochemical level.[1] Nevertheless, in most cases the cross-tolerant benzodiazepines or barbiturates relieve the most life-threatening effects of delirium tremens and facilitate safe passage through the crisis. Adding a second agent should be considered as an unusual and exceedingly high-risk gesture, particularly with regard to CNS and respiratory depression.
5. The patient should not manifest such signs or symptoms of withdrawal as anxiety, insomnia, hyperactivity, or hallucinations. If withdrawal symptoms occur, the agent that initially controlled the symptoms should be further titrated until control is once again achieved. Recurrent withdrawal symptoms are uncommon because of the very long half-life of these benzodiazepines and, in the case of diazepam, its metabolites.[105,128] If withdrawal occurs it is usually because of continued metabolism of the primary agent of intoxication (eg, ethanol, a short-acting barbiturate, or benzodiazepine), leading to renewed manifestations of withdrawal and indicating a need for further therapy.
6. Careful neurologic assessment must be performed at the time each dose is given. Each dose should be ordered separately and administered intravenously so

that incomplete or slowed absorption does not cause confusion in dosing. No oral sedation is necessary and no standing orders should ever be written. The patient should be easily arousable but sleeping peacefully. This allows the patient to relax psychologically and physiologically. It should not be difficult to feed the patient orally. This therapy eliminates the most dangerous complications of withdrawal-related agitation, resulting in trauma, rhabdomyolysis, and hyperthermia.

7. In most cases, once the patient is controlled no further sedative therapy is required.[128] The agents with long half-lives self-taper, which accomplishes delayed as well as acute withdrawal management simultaneously. This regimen also limits reinforcement of drug-seeking behavior associated with detoxification with drugs with shorter half-lives. It is for this reason that diazepam and its long-acting metabolites may represent an advantage over lorazepam, which has a shorter half-life. This concept necessitates clinical investigation.
8. Long-term social and psychologic supportive care is essential in addition to this acute management, if the withdrawal effort is to be successful.

How Should Flumazenil-Induced Withdrawal Be Treated?

Flumazenil is a short-acting benzodiazepine receptor antagonist that is capable of rapidly inducing a withdrawal syndrome in patients who are habituated to benzodiazepines (see Antidotes in Depth: Flumazenil in Chap. 61). It is for this reason that its use is discouraged in the overdose setting.[53,157,160] Flumazenil may have a role in reversing intoxications in pediatric patients, because the likelihood of chronic use is low. Flumazenil can produce seizures without the onset of consciousness, a particularly dangerous combination. The clinician should expect these seizures to require higher than normal doses of benzodiazepines because of the benzodiazepine receptor antagonism. This need for increased benzodiazepines can last from 1 to 2 hours depending on the dose of flumazenil used. In refractory cases, intravenous pentobarbital intubation and mechanical ventilation may become necessary. Flumazenil is unable to reverse alcohol intoxication.[26]

$GABA_B$ Withdrawal

Baclofen

$GABA_B$ receptors mediate presynaptic inhibition (by preventing Ca^{2+} influx) and postsynaptic inhibition (by increasing K+ efflux). The postsynaptic receptors appear to have a similar inhibitory effect as the $GABA_A$ receptors. The presynaptic receptors provide feedback inhibition of GABA release. Unlike $GABA_A$ receptors, these are mediated through G protein messengers. Baclofen is the only clinically important $GABA_B$ agonist. The pre- and postsynaptic inhibitory properties of baclofen allow it to paradoxically cause seizures in both acute overdose and withdrawal. When the drug is withdrawn, a disinhibition similar to $GABA_A$ withdrawal occurs. This effect is probably a result of the reduction of the chronic inhibitory effect of baclofen on postsynaptic $GABA_B$ receptors. Although it is more typically sedating in overdose, baclofen also stimulates presynaptic $GABA_B$ autoreceptors to decrease release of $GABA_A$. The subsequent dysinhibition leads to seizures, hypertension, and coma.

Interestingly, many case reports of baclofen withdrawal describe hallucinations and psychosis as prominent symptoms. However, these may be no different than the withdrawal symptoms of $GABA_A$ agonists. The fact that many patients experience double vision is difficult to explain.[114,129]

The development of this withdrawal syndrome typically occurs 24 to 48 hours after discontinuation of baclofen during an admission to the hospital for an unrelated medical problem. Case reports highlight the development of seizures, hallucinations, psychosis, dyskinesia, and visual disturbances. Intrathecal baclofen pumps have become an effective replacement for oral dosing, but withdrawal can occur following the use of this modality as well. Reinstatement of the prior baclofen dosing schedule appears to resolve these symptoms within 24 to 48 hours. Benzodiazepines and $GABA_A$ agonists, not phenytoin, are the appropriate treatment for seizures induced by baclofen withdrawal.

Gamma-Hydroxybutyrate

Gamma-hydroxybutyrate (GHB) is a compound found in mammalian brain, which has been investigated as an anesthetic and for treatment of narcolepsy, alcohol dependence, and opioid dependence. It is abused for its euphoric, sedative, and purported anabolic effects. Its mechanism of action is not fully known, but appears to have its effect on the GABA receptors. A withdrawal syndrome which resolves in 3 to 12 days has been reported that appears consistent with this mechanism—insomnia, anxiety, and tremor.[46]

CASE 2. A 45-year-old male was brought to the Emergency Department by police officers. The patient was agitated, vomiting, diaphoretic, and complained that he was withdrawing from his methadone. He was incarcerated 24 hours earlier and had not received his methadone for 72 hours. His vital signs were: blood pressure, 165/90 mm Hg; respiratory rate, 22 breath/min; pulse, 110 beats/min without orthostatic changes; and rectal temperature, 99.9°F (37.2°C). The man was well developed, well nourished, and appeared older than his stated age. He had mydriasis, profuse diaphoresis, hyperactive bowel sounds, piloerection, and diarrhea. He was given 10 mg of diazepam intravenously. Thirty minutes later he was noted to be sleeping, but when awakened continued to appear agitated. The remainder of his symptoms persisted.

Methadone 10 mg was administered IM, and his vomiting, diarrhea, piloerection, and hyperactive bowel sound resolved.

What Is the Pathophysiology of Opioid Withdrawal?

Opioids inhibit neurons and alleviate pain by activating a G_s protein, which then stimulates a rectifying K^+ efflux current. The opioid receptors are also linked to the $G_{i/o}$ proteins. These act through adenyl cyclase and activate inward Na^+ current, thus enhancing the intrinsic excitability of a neuron.[30] Chronic exposure to opiates (only drugs directly derived from opium) and opioids (all drugs with opioid receptor efficacy) results in a decreased efficacy of this receptor to open potassium channels by altering postreceptor, intracellular pathways. The expression of adenyl cyclase increases through activation of the transcription factor cAMP response element-binding protein (CREB). This results in an upregulation of cAMP pathway proteins such as the inward Na+ channels responsible for excitability. The enhanced excitability and an increased firing rate can only be blocked by higher levels of opioids. Without them, the patient experiences withdrawal symptoms, largely because of uninhibited activity at the locus coeruleus.[28,83,87,94] Opioid receptors and central alpha$_2$ receptors share a similar effect on the potassium channel in the locus coeruleus. This may explain the partial efficacy of clonidine as a therapy for opioid withdrawal and naloxone for clonidine overdose (Fig. 70–2).[50]

What Are the Clinical Characteristics of Opioid Withdrawal?

Symptoms progress from drug craving, yawning, rhinorrhea, and piloerection to nausea, vomiting, diarrhea, diaphoresis, myalgias, arthralgias, anxiety, fear, and mild tachycardia. Chronicity relates to pharmacology of the opioid of abuse. Methadone withdrawal starts 24 hours after the last dose and persists for 3 to 7 days. Heroin withdrawal will begin 6 hours after the last dose and is usually fully manifest at 24 hours. Withdrawal is physically and emotionally painful, but not life threatening as long as adequate hydration and nutritional support are maintained and morbidity from emesis and dehydration can be minimized. See Table 70–1 for a comparison between opioid withdrawal and sedative-hypnotic or ethanol withdrawal.

What Is the Treatment of Opioid Withdrawal?

Treatment with methadone (10 mg IM or 20 mg PO) is enough to blunt withdrawal symptoms without providing euphoria, although it may not eliminate drug craving. Maintenance programs often use higher daily doses

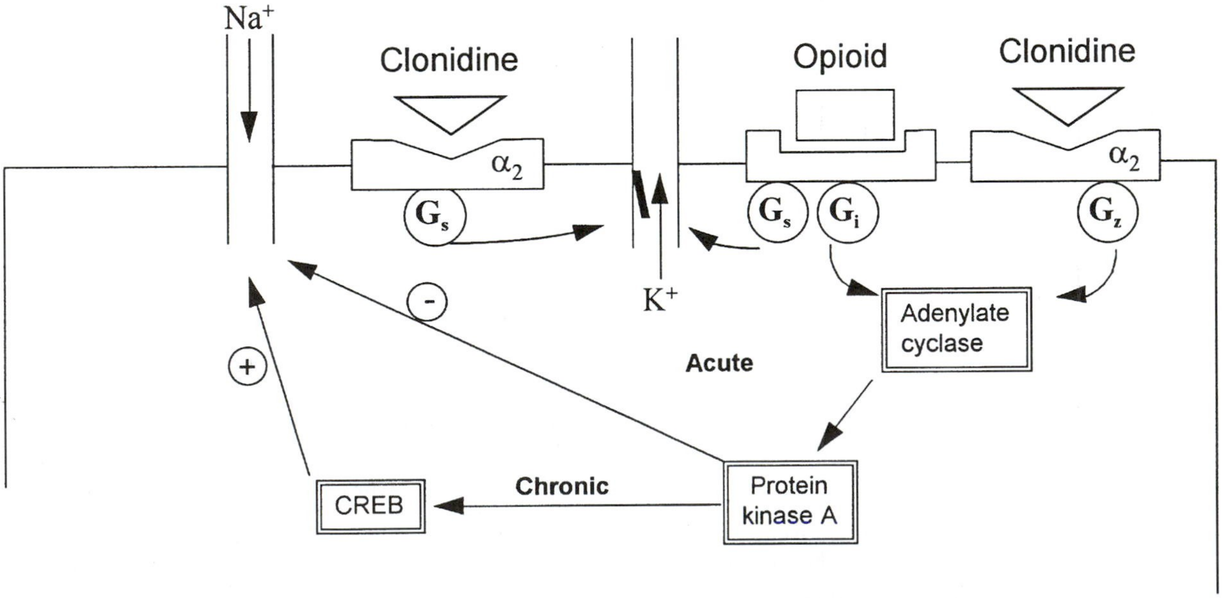

Figure 70–2. Immediate and long-term effects of opioids. The acute effects of both opioids and alpha$_2$-adrenergic agonists are to increase inhibition through enhanced potassium efflux and inhibited sodium influx. Chronic effects alter gene expression to enhance sodium influx and restore homeostasis.

TABLE 70–1. CLINICAL DIFFERENTIATION OF DRUG WITHDRAWAL

	Opioids	Sedative-Hypnotics/Ethanol
Vital Signs		
Blood pressure	Hypertension, normal or orthostatic hypotension when volume depleted	Normal, hypertension, then orthostatic hypotension when volume depleted
Pulse	Tachycardia	Tachycardia
Respiratory rate	Tachypnea	Tachypnea
Temperature	Normal	Hyperthermia
Mental Status		
	Normal	Abnormal
	Anxiety	Restlessness
		Irritability
		Psychosis, visual hallucinations more common than auditory
		Disorientation
Physical Signs and Symptoms		
	Yawning	Tremulousness
	Lacrimation	Muscle fasciculations
	Rhinorrhea	Diaphoresis
	Mydriasis	Seizures
	Tremor	
	Piloerection	
	Restlessness	
	Emesis, nausea	
	Diarrhea with increased bowel sounds	
	Seizures in neonates (only)	
	Muscle pain and spasm	

to achieve this latter effect. Very high doses (greater than 100 mg of methadone per day) are used to flood opioid receptors so that intercurrent heroin abuse will not result in euphoria, thereby deterring drug-seeking behavior.[24,136,137]

Clonidine is an effective adjuvant in opioid withdrawal. It acts on the locus coeruleus to open the same potassium channels that opioids open, and corrects many aspects of the withdrawal syndrome.[4,43,50] Doses start at 5 to 6 μg/ kg per day and can get as high as 25 μg/kg per day. Clonidine is most useful in conjunction with methadone maintenance and a structured detoxification program. Clonidine can be considered as a therapeutic alternative in situations where hospital policy does not permit methadone administration.

Opioid withdrawal can be induced by the use of opioid receptor antagonists or mixed agonist-antagonists in opioid habituated patients. Often, this is the result of administering large doses of naloxone to opioid addicted patients who present with an opioid overdose. The frequency of this problem can be decreased by using a low initial starting dose, supporting oxygenation, gauging the therapeutic effect, and redosing based on clinical grounds. If acute withdrawal makes the patient a behavioral problem, diazepam can be administered for sedation. Withdrawal symptoms should resolve within 1 hour as the naloxone is eliminated and there is a reemergence of the primary opioid's effects.

Rapid Heroin Withdrawal

Protocols for the rapid antagonism and withdrawal of patients addicted to opioids are based on the belief that naloxone and naltrexone-induced withdrawal only produces severe symptoms for the first few hours after administration. For this period, patients are placed under general anesthesia and then treated with a combination of antiemetics, sedatives, and clonidine, and a rapid institution of naltrexone therapy.[79–81,111] Some poorly designed studies support this approach; however, its safety and efficacy are not proven and the possibility of protracted withdrawal remains consequential. The potential complications have not been thoroughly investigated.

Clonidine Withdrawal (Alpha$_2$ Receptors)

Alpha$_2$ receptors are located in the central and peripheral nervous system. Clonidine is a central and peripheral alpha$_2$ agonist. Stimulation of peripheral postsynaptic alpha$_2$ receptors results in vasoconstriction, bradycardia, and hypertension and prevents acetylcholine release. This results in some anticholinergic symptoms, especially dry mouth. The peripheral effects manifest only in the initial period after a toxic dose. Stimulation of central presynaptic alpha$_2$ receptors inhibits sympathomimetic output and results in bradycardia, and hypotension.[38]

Within 24 hours after the discontinuation of clonidine, norepinephrine levels rise as a result of enhanced efferent sympathetic activity.[118] Patients who use the clonidine patch may experience withdrawal later than 24 hours, if at all, because a reservoir of the drug in the skin generally allows levels to persist for days. Clonidine elimination half-life is 14 hours, and most patients who manifest withdrawal still have a low level of clonidine in the initial phase. Simultaneous use of beta-adrenergic antagonists will exacerbate withdrawal, as alpha-adrenergic receptor stimulation is unopposed by beta-adrenergic antagonism.

The first symptoms occur 24 hours after discontinuation of clonidine and include headache, flushing, sweating, hallucinations, and anxiety.[19] Hypertensive encephalopathy and death have been reported in rare cases. Within 48 hours the patient's blood pressure rises to near or above pretreatment levels. There appears to be an association with high-dose therapy (greater than 1.2 mg/day) or concomitant beta-adrenergic antagonism therapy and an increased likelihood and severity of withdrawal.[21,110]

Treatment requires reinstatement of the drug by the oral route. Patients unable to swallow may be treated with sublingual clonidine. Beta-adrenergic antagonists are absolutely contraindicated.

Caffeine (Adenosine$_1$ Receptors)

The release of neurotransmitters is accompanied by passive release of adenosine as a byproduct of ATP breakdown. This adenosine acts on the presynaptic adenosine$_1$ autoreceptors to decrease further release of neurotransmitters, and on the postsynaptic adenosine$_1$ receptors to terminate neuronal transmission. Adenosine$_2$ receptors are found on the cerebral vasculature and peripheral vasculature and promote vasodilation.

Caffeine antagonizes the inhibitory effect of adenosine (see Chap. 38). As a result, acute exposure results in increases in heart rate, ventilation, gastrointestinal motility, gastric acid secretion, and motor activity. Chronic exposure results in tolerance to the effects of large acute administration of the drug. This effect appears to be associated with caffeine's occupancy of adenosine$_1$ receptors. Chronic caffeine exposure regulates adenosine$_1$ receptors by a variety of theoretical mechanisms, such as increases in receptor number, increases in receptor affinity, or enhancing receptor coupling to the G protein. An animal study demonstrates that the adenosine receptor has a three-fold increase in affinity for adenosine at the height of withdrawal symptoms. This model suggests that chronic caffeine administration results in increase in receptor affinity for adenosine, thus restoring a state of physiologic balance (normal motor inhibitory tone). When caffeine is withdrawn, the enhanced receptor affinity results in a strong adenosine effect and clinical symptoms of withdrawal: headache (cerebral vasodilation), fatigue, and hypersomnia (motor inhibition).[130,135]

Symptoms of anxiety, depression, headaches, sleepiness, and decreased alertness and activity peak at 24 to 48 hours and decrease over 1 week. Most patients will correctly identify the source of their symptoms and medicate with the appropriate dose and preferred form of caffeine. Caffeine dependence and withdrawal have been demonstrated in patients who take as little as 129 mg/day of caffeine—the equivalent of an average 5 oz cup of coffee. Clinicians should consider this entity in the patient who is being evaluated for headache symptoms.[66]

Nicotine Withdrawal

Nicotinic receptors are a type of acetylcholine receptors located in the autonomic ganglia, adrenal medulla, CNS, spinal cord, neuromuscular junction, and carotid and aortic bodies. Nicotinic receptors are fast-response cation channels that are not coupled to G proteins. This distinguishes them from muscarinic receptors, which are coupled to G proteins. They have both excitatory and inhibitory effects. Much remains unknown about these receptors and how they affect addiction and withdrawal (see Chap. 71).[99,134]

Smoking cessation is the primary cause for nicotine withdrawal, although discontinuation of any tobacco product can lead to this syndrome. Cigarette craving is an important problem for hospitalized patients who are not permitted to smoke.

Nicotine withdrawal manifests largely as cigarette craving and subjective dysphoric symptoms. There are some symptoms of irritability, restlessness, and a decrease in heart rate and blood pressure. Cardiac symptoms resolve over 3 to 4 weeks, but cigarette craving may persist for months to years.

The nicotine transdermal system (patch) and nicotine polacrilex (gum) can be used to provide nicotine without the carcinogens in tobacco and are now available over the counter. The patches utilize a stepwise reduction in subcutaneous delivery to gradually decrease the nicotine dose and appear to have greater compliance than the gum. Acute relief from withdrawal symptoms is most easily achieved with use of the gum, as rapid chewing releases an immediate dose of nicotine. However, the dose is approximately half of that which the average smoker receives in one cigarette, and the onset of action is 30 minutes instead of 10 or less. These pharmacologic changes in delivery minimize the reinforcement and self-reward effects that are so prominent with the rapid nicotine delivery of cigarette smoking.

Neonatal Withdrawal Syndromes

Alcohol and GABA$_A$ Agonists

Maternal addiction to alcohol can result in a neonatal withdrawal syndrome that begins within 3 days after birth. It is characterized by varying degrees of tremor, nystagmus, clonus, opisthotonos, hypertonia, seizures, sleeplessness, crying, asymmetric or hyperactive reflexes, abnormal Moro reflex, excessive mouthing or rooting, diarrhea, vomiting, inability to feed, startle, sweating, and inability to thermoregulate. This syndrome is not directly correlated with the fetal alcohol syndrome. The syndromes are related to the use of alcohol at different times during pregnancy. Children of mothers addicted to benzodiazepine and barbiturate will display the same symptoms.[29]

Neonatal alcohol withdrawal should be treated as with adult alcohol withdrawal. The drug with the most clinical use for this condition in pediatrics is phenobarbital. The loading dose is 16 mg/kg over 24 hours to produce a 24-hour serum level of 20 to 30 μg/mL. This can be maintained with a dose of 2 to 8 mg/kg per 24 hours. Once withdrawal symptoms are controlled for 72 hours, the phenobarbital dose should be tapered at 10% per day. Elixirs of phenobarbital contain 14 to 25% ethyl alcohol; parenteral forms contain 67.8% propylene glycol, 10% ethyl alcohol, and 1.5% benzyl alcohol. Both of these preparations have potential risk to the neonate and should be considered possible explanations for metabolic abnormalities (see Chaps. 54 and 104).[31,115]

Opioids

The neonatal opioid withdrawal syndrome shares characteristics of the adult opioid withdrawal syndrome: gastrointestinal distress (vomiting and diarrhea), irritability, yawning, sneezing, hypertonicity, hyperacusis, diaphoresis, lacrimation, and tremulousness. It typically occurs within 2 weeks of birth. In neonates, the usual adult opioid withdrawal symptoms are accompanied by mottling, fever, myoclonic jerks, and seizures. This latter symptom is only characteristic of opioid withdrawal in neonates and occurs in roughly 8% of children born to mothers on methadone maintenance and only 1% of those born to mothers who use heroin.[56,84] Paregoric appears to be more effective than diazepam in controlling and preventing these seizures while preserving the suck reflex. Paregoric is a combination of anhydrous morphine (0.4 mg/mL), camphor, alcohol 46%, and benzoic acid (4 mg/mL). Some clinicians prefer a 1:25 dilution of opium tincture because it contains only 0.7% alcohol and no camphor or benzoic acid. Dosage for either drug is 0.2 mL every 3 hours, increased by 0.05 mL at each dose until withdrawal symptoms are controlled up to a maximum of 0.7 mL per dose. Once the patient is stable, therapy is continued for 3 to 5 days and decreased gradually over a 2 to 4-week period. Parenteral morphine should be reserved for short-term therapy of only severe withdrawal symptoms because it contains sodium bisulfite and phenol, which may cause anaphylactic reactions and hyperbilirubinemia, respectively, when administered chronically. Methadone has been used for neonatal withdrawal, but its use is discouraged because the long half-life (26 hours) makes dosing adjustments difficult.[7]

Caffeine

An infant with irritability, jitteriness, and vomiting may be suffering from caffeine withdrawal. One study detected caffeine in the serum of 6 of 8 infants with these symptoms. All mothers gave a history of heavy caffeine use and none were dependent on other drugs or alcohol. The children's symptoms persisted for several days and then resolved spontaneously.[89,90]

Acknowledgements

Kathleen A. Delaney, MD and Neal E. Flomenbaum, MD contributed to this chapter in a previous edition.

References

1. Aaronson LM, Hinman DJ, Okamoto M: Effects of diazepam on ethanol withdrawal. J Pharmacol Exp Ther 1982;221:319–325.
2. Adinoff B: Double-blind study of alprazolam, diazepam, clonidine, and placebo in the alcohol withdrawal syndrome: Preliminary findings. Alcohol Clin Exp Res 1994; 18:873–878.
3. Adinoff B, Bone HGA, Linnoila M: Acute ethanol poisoning and the ethanol withdrawal syndrome. Med Toxicol 1988; 3:172–196.
4. Aghajanian GK: Tolerance of locus coeruleus neurons to morphine and suppression of withdrawal response to clonidine. Nature 1978;276:186–188.
5. Allan AM, Baier LD, Zhang X: Effects of lorazepam tolerance and withdrawal on $GABA_A$ receptor operated chloride channels in mice selected for differences in ethanol withdrawal severity. Life Sci 1992;51:931–943.
6. Alldredge BK, Lowenstein DH, Simon RP: Placebo-controlled trial of intravenous diphenylhydantoin for short-term treatment of alcohol withdrawal seizures. Am J Med 1989;87:645–648.
7. American Academy of Pediatrics Committee on Drugs: Neonatal drug withdrawal. Pediatrics 1983:72;895–902.
8. Athen D: Comparative investigation of chlormethiazole and neuroleptic agents in the treatment of alcoholic delirium. Acta Psychiatr Scand Suppl 1986;329:167–170.
9. Ballenger JC, Post RM: Kindling as a model for alcohol withdrawal syndromes. Br J Psychiatry 1978;133:1–14.
10. Bartolomei F, Suchet L, Barrie M, Gastaut JL: Alcoholic epilepsy: A unified and dynamic classification. Eur Neurol 1997;37:13–17.
11. Baumgartner GR, Rowen RC: Clonidine vs chlordiazepoxide in the management of acute alcohol withdrawal syndrome. Arch Intern Med 1987;147:1223–1226.
12. Becker HC, Hale RL: Repeated episodes of ethanol withdrawal potentiate the severity of subsequent withdrawal seizures: An animal model of alcohol withdrawal "kindling." Alcohol Clin Exp Res 1993;17:94–98.
13. Bedichek E, Kirschbaum B: A case of propylene glycol toxic reaction associated with etomidate infusion. Arch Intern Med 1991;151:2297–2298.

14. Beshai NN: Providing cost efficient detoxification services to alcoholic patients. Public Health Rep 1990;105:475–481.
15. Blum K, Eubanks JD, Wallace JE, Hamilton H: Enhancement of alcohol withdrawal convulsions in mice by haloperidol. Clin Toxicol 1976;9:427–434.
16. Bluntzer ME, Blachley JD: Acid–base and electrolyte disturbances induced by alcohol. J Crit Illness 1986;1:19–26.
17. Booth BM, Blow FC: The kindling hypothesis: Further evidence from a U.S. national study of alcoholic men. Alcohol Alcoholism 1993;28:593–598.
18. Bowman KM, Wortis H, Joliff E: Treatment of disturbed patients with sodium chloride orally and intravenously in hypertonic solutions. Arch Neurol Psychiatry 1939;41: 702–710.
19. Brower KJ, Mudd S, Blow FC, et al: Severity and treatment of alcohol withdrawal in elderly versus younger patients. Alcohol Clin Exp Res 1994;18:196–201.
20. Brown ME, Anton RF, Malcom R, Ballenger JC: Alcohol detoxification and withdrawal seizures: Clinical support for a kindling hypothesis. Biol Psychiatry 1988;23:507–514.
21. Brown M, Salmon D, Rendell M: Clonidine hallucinations. Ann Intern Med 1980;93:456–457.
22. Buck KJ, Hahner L, Sikela J, Harris RA: Chronic ethanol treatment alters brain levels of gamma-aminobutyric acid A receptor subunit mRNAs: Relationship to genetic differences in ethanol withdrawal seizure severity. J Neurochem 1991;57:1452–1455.
23. Buck KJ, Harris RA: Benzodiazepine agonist and inverse agonist actions on $GABA_A$ receptor-operated chloride channels. II. Chronic effects of ethanol. J Pharmacol Exp Ther 1990;253:713–719.
24. Caplehorn JR, Bell J, Kleinbaum DG, Gebski VJ: Methadone dose and heroin use during maintenance treatment. Addiction 1993;88:119–124 .
25. Cecil RL: A Textbook of Medicine. Philadelphia, Saunders, 1927, pp 516–518.
26. Chan AW, Leong FW, Schanley DL, et al: Flumazenil (Ro15–788) does not affect ethanol tolerance and dependence. Pharmacol Biochem Behav 1991;39:659–663.
27. Chance JF: Emergency department treatment of alcohol withdrawal seizures with phenytoin. Ann Emerg Med 1991;20:520–522.
28. Christie MJ, Williams JT, North RA: Cellular mechanism of opioid tolerance: Studies in single brain neurons. Mol Pharmacol 1987;32:633–638.
29. Coles CD, Smith IE, Fernhoff PM, et al: Neonatal ethanol withdrawal: Characteristics in clinically normal, nondysmorphic neonates. J Pediatr 1984:105;445–451.
30. Crain SM, Shen KF: Modulatory effects of G_s-coupled excitatory opioid receptor functions on opioid analgesia, tolerance, and dependence. Neurochem Res 1996;21: 1347–1351.
31. D'Apolito KC, McRorie TI: Pharmacologic management of neonatal abstinence syndrome. J Perinat Neonat Nurs 1996;9:70–80.
32. Dave JR, Tabakoff B: Ethanol withdrawal seizures produce increased c-fos mRNA in mouse brain. Mol Pharmacol 1990;37:367–371.
33. Davidson M, Shanley B, Wilce P: Increased NMDA-induced excitability during ethanol withdrawal: A behavioural and histological study. Brain Res 1995; 674:91–96.
34. Diamond I, Gordon AS: Cellular and molecular neuroscience of alcoholism. Physiol Rev 1977;77:1–20.
35. Earnest MP, Yarnell PR: Seizure admissions to a city hospital: The role of alcohol. Epilepsia 1976;17:387–393.
36. Eckardt MJ, Campbell GA, Marietta CA, et al: Ethanol dependence and withdrawal selectively alter localized cerebral glucose utilization. Brain Res 1992;584:244–250.
37. Essig CF, Jones E, Lam RC: The effect of pentobarbital on alcohol withdrawal in dogs. Arch Neurol 1969;20: 554–558.
38. Farsang C, Kaposci J, Vajda L, et al: Reversal by naloxone of the antihypertensive action of clonidine: Involvement of the sympathetic nervous system. Circulation 1984;69: 461–467.
39. Ferguson JA, Suelzer CJ, Eckert GJ, et al: Risk factors for delirium tremens development. J Gen Intern Med 1996; 11:410–414.
40. Feussner KR: Computed tomography brain scanning in alcohol withdrawal seizures. Ann Intern Med 1981;94: 519–524.
41. Fifkova E, Eason H, Bueltmann K, Lanman J: Changes in GABAergic and non-GABAergic synapses during chronic ethanol exposure and withdrawal in the dentate fascia of LS and SS mice. Alcohol Clin Exp Res 1994;18:989–997.
42. Frankushen D: Significance of hypomagnesemia in alcoholic patients. Am J Med 1964;37:802–807.
43. Franz DN, Hare BD, McCloskey KL: Spinal sympathetic neurons: Possible site of opiate-withdrawal suppression by clonidine. Science 1982;215:1643–1645.
44. French-Mullen JMH, Barker JL, Rogawski MA: Calcium current block by (–)pentobarbital, phenobarbital, and CHEB but not (+)pentobarbital in acutely isolated hippocampal CA1 neurons: Comparison with effects on GABA-activated Cl-current. J Neurosci 1993;13:3211–3221.
45. Friedhoff AJ, Zitrin A: A comparison of the effects of paraldehyde and chlorpromazine in delirium tremens. NY State J Med 1959;59:1060–1063.
46. Galloway GP, Frederick SL, Staggers FE Jr, et al: Gamma-hydroxybutyrate: An emerging drug of abuse that causes physical dependence. Addiction 1997;92:89–96.
47. Geiderman JM, Goodman SL, Cohen DB: Magnesium: The forgotten electrolyte. JACEP 1979;8:204–209.
48. Glue P, Nutt D: Overexcitement and disinhibition. Dynamic neurotransmitter interactions in alcohol withdrawal. Br J Psychiatry 1990;157:491–499.
49. Golbert TM, Sanz CJ, Rose HD, et al: Comparative evaluation of treatments of alcohol withdrawal syndromes. JAMA 1967;201:99–102.
50. Gold MS, Redmond DE, Kleber HD: Clonidine blocks acute opiate withdrawal symptoms. Lancet 1978;2:599–602.
51. Greenblatt DJ, Gross PL, Harris J, et al: Fatal hyperthermia following haloperidol therapy of sedative hypnotic withdrawal. J Clin Psychiatry 1978;39:673–675.
52. Greenland P, Southwick WH: Hyperthermia associated with chlorpromazine and full sheet restraint. Am J Psychiatry 1978;135:1234–1235.
53. Haverkos GP, DiSalvo RP, Imhoff TE: Fatal seizures after

flumazenil administration in a patient with mixed overdose. Ann Pharmacother 1994;28:1347–1349.
54. Hayashida M, Alterman A, McLellan T, et al: Is inpatient medical alcohol detoxification justified?: Results of a randomized, controlled study. NIDA Res Monogr 1988;81: 19–25
55. Heinala P, Piepponen T, Heikkinen H: Diazepam loading in alcohol withdrawal: Clinical pharmacokinetics. Int J Clin Pharmacol Ther Toxicol 1990;28:211–217.
56. Herzlinger RA, Kandall SR, Vaughan HG Jr: Neonatal seizures associated with narcotic withdrawal. J Pediatr 1977:91;638–641.
57. Hobbs RW, Rall TW, Verdoorn TA: Hypnotics and sedatives: Ethanol. In: Hardman JG, Limbird LE, Molinoff PB, Ruddon RW, eds: Goodman and Gilman's The Pharmacological Basis of Therapeutics, 9th ed. New York, Macmillan, 1996, pp. 374–377 .
58. Hoey LL, Nahum A, Vance-Bryan K: A retrospective review and assessment of benzodiazepines in the treatment of alcohol withdrawal in hospitalized patients. Pharmacotherapy 1994;14:572–578.
59. Hoffman PL: Glutamate receptors in alcohol withdrawal-induced neurotoxicity. Metab Brain Dis 1995;10:73–79.
60. Holzbach E: Thiamine absorption in alcoholic delirium patients. J Stud Alcohol 1996;57:581–584.
61. Horwitz RI, Gottlieb LD, Kraus ML: The efficacy of atenolol in the outpatient management of the alcohol withdrawal syndrome. Results of a randomized clinical trial. Arch Intern Med 1989;149:1089–1093.
62. Isbell H, Altschul S, Kornetsky AB, et al: Chronic barbiturate intoxication: An experimental study. Arch Neurol Psychiatry 1950;64:1–28.
63. Isbell H, Fraser HF, Wikler A, et al: An experimental study of the etiology of "rum fits" and delirium tremens. Q J Stud Alcohol 1955;16:1–33.
64. Ives TJ, Mooney AJ 3rd, Gwyther RE: Pharmacokinetic dosing of phenobarbital in the treatment of alcohol withdrawal syndrome. South Med J 1991;84:18–21.
65. Kaim SC, Klett CJ: Treatment of delirium tremens: A comparative evaluation of four drugs. Q J Stud Alcohol 1972; 33:1065–1072.
66. Kaplan GB, Greenblatt DJ, Kent MA, Cotreau-Bibbo MM: Caffeine treatment and withdrawal in mice: Relationships between dosage, concentrations, locomotor activity and A1 adenosine receptor binding. J Pharm Exp Ther 1993;266: 1563–1571.
67. Keir WJ, Morrow AL: Differential expression of $GABA_A$ receptor subunit mRNAs in ethanol-naive withdrawal seizure resistant (WSR) vs. withdrawal seizure prone (WSP) mouse brain. Brain Res Mol Brain Res 1994;25: 2000–2008.
68. Koranyi EK, Ravindran A, Seguin J: Alcohol withdrawal concealing symptoms of subdural hematoma—A caveat. Psychiatr J Univ Ott 1990;15:15–17.
69. Korpi ER: Role of $GABA_A$ receptors in the actions of alcohol and in alcoholism: Recent advances. Alcohol Alcoholism 1994;29:115–129.
70. Kosobud AE, Crabbe JC: Sensitivity to *N*-methyl-*d*-aspartic acid-induced convulsions is genetically associated with resistance to ethanol withdrawal seizures. Brain Res 1993; 610:176–179.
71. Krogsgaard-Larsen P, Scheel-Kruger J, Kofod H, eds: GABA-neurotransmitters: Pharmacological, Biochemical, and Pharmacological Aspects. New York, Academic Press, 1979, pp. 102–103.
72. Kuriyama K, Ueha T: Functional alterations in cerebral $GABA_A$ receptor complex associated with formation of alcohol dependence: Analysis using GABA-dependent $^{36}Cl^-$ influx into neuronal membrane vesicles. Alcohol Alcoholism 1992;27:335–343.
73. Kuriyama K, Ueha T, Hirouchi M, et al: Functional alterations in $GABA_A$ receptor complex induced by ethanol. Alcohol Alcoholism 2 (suppl) 1993:321–325
74. Lacy JR: Brain infarction and hemorrhage in young and middle-aged adults. West J Med 1984;141:329–335.
75. Levy ML, Aranda M, Zelman V, Giannotta SL: Propylene glycol toxicity following continuous etomidate infusion for the control of refractory cerebral edema. Neurosurgery 1995;37:363–371.
76. Lieber CS: Medical disorders of alcoholism. N Engl J Med 1995;333:1058–1065.
77. Lineaweaver WC, Anderson K, Hing DN: Massive doses of midazolam infusion for delirium tremens without respiratory depression. Crit Care Med 1988;16:294–297.
78. Little HJ: The benzodiazepines: Anxiolytic and withdrawal effects. Neuropeptides 1991;19 (suppl):11–14.
79. Loimer N, Lenz K, Schmid R, et al: Techniques for greatly shortening the transition from methadone to naltrexone maintenance of patients addicted to opiates. Am J Psychiatry 1991;148:933–935.
80. Loimer N, Schmid R, Lenz K, et al: Acute blocking of naloxone-precipated opiate withdrawal. Brit J Psychiatry 1990;157:748–752.
81. Loimer N, Schmid W, Presslich O, Lenz K: Continous naloxone administration suppresses opiate withdrawal symptoms in human opiate addicts during detoxification treatment. J Psychiatr Res 1989;23:81–86.
82. Lowenstein SR, Gabow PA, Cramer J, et al: The role of alcohol in new-onset atrial fibrillation. Arch Intern Med 1983;143:1882–1885.
83. Maldonado R, Blendy JA, Tzavara E, et al: Reduction of morphine abstinence in mice with mutation in the gene encoding CREB. Science 1996;273:657–659.
84. Malpas TJ, Darlow BA, Lennox R, Horwood LJ: Maternal methadone dosage and neonatal withdrawal. Aust NZ J Obstet Gynaecol 1995;35:175–177.
85. Manikant S, Tripathi BM, Chavan BS: Loading dose diazepam therapy for alcohol withdrawal state. Indian J Med Res 1993;98:170–173.
86. Martin PR, Bhushan CM, Kapur BM, et al: Intravenous phenobarbital therapy in barbiturate and other hypnosedative withdrawal reactions. Clin Pharmacol Ther 1979; 26:256–264.
87. Matthes HWD, Maldonado R, Simonin F, et al: Loss of morphine-induced analgesia: Reward effect and withdrawal symptoms in mice lacking the m-opioid-receptor gene. Nature 1996;383:819–823.
88. McCown TJ, Breese GR: A potential contribution to

ethanol withdrawal kindling: Reduced GABA function in the inferior collicular cortex. Alcohol Clin Exp Res 1993; 17:1290–1294.
89. McGowan JD, Altman RE, Kanto WP Jr: Neonatal withdrawal symptoms after chronic maternal ingestion of caffeine. South Med J 1988:81;1092–1094.
90. McKim EM: Caffeine and its effects on pregnancy and the neonate. J Nurse Midwifery 1991;36:226–231.
91. Mendelson JH, LaDou J: Experimentally induced chronic intoxication and withdrawal in alcoholics: 2. Psychophysiological findings. Q J Stud Alcohol 1964; 2(suppl): 14–39.
92. Milanov I, Toteva S, Georgiev D: Alcohol withdrawal tremor. Electromyogr Clin Neurophysiol 1996;36:15–20.
93. Moore M, Gray MG: Delirium tremens: A study of cases at the Boston City Hospital, 1915–1936. N Engl J Med 1939; 220:953–956.
94. Nestler EJ: Under siege: The brain on opiates. Neuron 1996;16:897–900.
95. Newman JP, Terris DJ, Moore M: Trends in the management of alcohol withdrawal syndrome. Laryngoscope 1995;105:1–7.
96. Nicol CF: Status Epilepticus. JAMA 1975;234:419–420.
97. Nolop KB, Natow A: Unprecedented sedative requirements during delirium tremens. Crit Care Med 1985;13: 246–249.
98. O'Brien JE, Meyer RE, Thoms DC: Double blind comparison of lorazepam and diazepam in the treatment of the acute alcohol abstinence syndrome. Curr Ther Res 1983;34: 825–830.
99. Ochoa EL, Li L, McNamee MG: Desensitization of central cholinergic mechanisms and neuroadaptation to nicotine. Mol Neurobiol 1990;4:251–287.
100. Oldham AJ, Bott M: The management of excitement in a general psychiatric ward by high dosage of haloperidol. Acta Psychiatr Scand 1971;47:369–376.
101. Osler W: The Principles and Practice of Medicine, 8th ed. New York, Appleton, 1916, pp. 398–400.
102. Peppers MP: Benzodiazepines for alcohol withdrawal in the elderly and in patients with liver disease. Pharmacotherapy 1996;16:49–57.
103. Peris J, Coleman-Hardee N, Burry J, Pecins-Thompson M: Selective changes in GABAergic transmission in substantia nigra and superior colliculus caused by ethanol and ethanol withdrawal. Alcohol Clin Exp Res 1992;16: 311–319.
104. Pohorecky LA, Roberts P: Development of tolerance to and physical dependence on ethanol: Daily versus repeated cycles treatment with ethanol. Alcohol Clin Exp Res 1991;15:824–833.
105. Pond SM, Phillips M, Benowitz N, et al: Diazepam kinetics in acute alcohol withdrawal. Clin Pharmacol Ther 1979; 25:832–836.
106. Prakash A, Das G: Cocaine and the nervous system. Int J Clin Pharmacol Ther Toxicol 1993;31:575–581.
107. Rassnick S, Krechman J, Koob GF: Chronic ethanol produces a decreased sensitivity to the response-disruptive effects of GABA receptor complex antagonists. Pharmacol Biochem Behav 1993;44:943–950.
108. Rastogi SK, Thyagarajan R, Clothier J, Ticku MK: Effect of chronic treatment of ethanol on benzodiazepine and picrotoxin sites on the GABA receptor complex in regions of the brain of the rat. Neuropharmacology 1986;25: 1179–1184.
109. Rathlev N, D'Onofrio G, Fish S, et al: The lack of efficacy of phenytoin in the prevention of recurrent alcohol-related seizures. Ann Emerg Med 1994;23:513–518.
110. Reid JL, Dargie HJ, Davies DS, et al: Clonidine withdrawal in hypertension. Lancet 1977;1:1171–1174.
111. Resnick RB, Kestenbaum RS, Washton A, Poole D: Naloxone-precipitated withdrawal: A method for rapid induction onto naltrexone. Clin Pharmacol Therap 1977;21: 409–413.
112. Ripley TL, Little HJ: Ethanol withdrawal hyperexcitability in vitro is selectively decreased by a competitive NMDA receptor antagonist. Brain Res 1995;699:1–11.
113. Ritson B, Chick J: Comparison of two benzodiazepines in the treatment of alcohol withdrawal: Effects on symptoms and cognitive recovery. Drug Alcohol Depend 1986;18: 329–334.
114. Rivas DA, Chancellor MB, Hill K, Freedman MK: Neurological manifestations of baclofen withdrawal. J Urol 1993;150:1903–1905.
115. Robe LB, Gromisch DS, Iosub S: Symptoms of neonatal ethanol withdrawal. Curr Alcohol 1981;8:485–493.
116. Robinson GM, Sellers EM, Janacek E: Barbiturate and hypnosedative withdrawal by a multiple oral phenobarbital loading dose technique. Clin Pharmacol Ther 1981;30: 71–76.
117. Rossetti ZL, Carboni S, Brodie BB: Ethanol withdrawal is associated with increased extracellular glutamate in the rat striatum. Eur J Pharmacol 1995;283:177–183.
118. Rupp H, Maisch B, Brilla CG: Drug withdrawal and rebound hypertension: Differential action of the central antihypertensive drugs moxonidine and clonidine. Cardiovasc Drugs Ther 1996;10(suppl 1):251–262.
119. Saito T, Hashimoto E: Membrane effects of ethanol in the brain. J Clin Exp Med 1990;154:869–873.
120. Saito T, Lee JM, Tabakoff B: Effects of chronic ethanol treatment on the beta adrenergic receptor coupled adenylate cyclase system of mouse cerebral cortex. J Neurochem 1987;48:1817–1822.
121. Saitz R, Mayo-Smith MF, Roberts MS, et al: Individualized treatment for alcohol withdrawal. A randomized double-blind controlled trial. JAMA 1994;272:519–523.
122. Salloum IM, Cornelius JR, Daley DC, Thase ME: The utility of diazepam loading in the treatment of alcohol withdrawal among psychiatric inpatients. Psychopharmacol Bull 1995;31:305–310.
123. Sanna E, Serra M, Cossu A, et al: Chronic ethanol intoxication induces differential effects on $GABA_A$ and NMDA receptor function in the rat brain. Alcohol Clin Exp Res 1993;17:115–123.
124. Satel SL, Price LH, Palumbo JM, et al: Clinical phenomenology and neurobiology of cocaine abstinence: A prospective inpatient study. Am J Psychiatry 1991;148: 495–498.
125. Schwartz HS, Yarnell PR, VanderArk G: Focal motor seizures in patients with alcoholism. JACEP 1974;3:394.
126. Sellers EM: Clinical pharmacology and therapeutics of benzodiazepines. Can Med Assoc J 1978;118:1533–1538.

127. Sellers EM, Kalant H: Alcohol intoxication and withdrawal. N Engl J Med 1976;294:757–769.
128. Sellers EM, Naranjo CA, Harrison M, et al: Diazepam loading: Simplified treatment of alcohol withdrawal. Clin Pharmacol Ther 1983;34:822–826.
129. Siegfried RN, Jacobson L, Chobal C: Development of an acute withdrawal syndrome following the cessation of intrathecal baclofen therapy in a patient with spasticity. Anesthesiology 1992;77:1048–1050.
130. Silverman K, Evans SM, Strain EC, et al: Withdrawal syndrome after the double-blind cessation of caffeine consumption. N Engl J Med 1992;327:1109–1114.
131. Spies CD, Nordmann A, Brummer G, et al: Intensive care unit stay is prolonged in chronic alcoholic men following tumor resection of the upper digestive tract. Acta Anaesthesiol Scand 1996;40:649–656.
132. Sporer KA, Lesser SH: Cocaine washed-out syndrome. Ann Emerg Med 1992;21:112. Letter.
133. Squires RF, ed: GABA and Benzodiazepine Receptors, Vol 1. Boca Raton, CRC Press, 1991, pp. 2–10.
134. Stolerman IP, Shoaib M: The neurobiology of tobacco addiction. Trends Pharmacol Sci 1991;12:467–473.
135. Strain EC, Mumford GK, Silverman K, et al: Caffeine dependence syndrome. JAMA 1994;272:1043–1048.
136. Strain EC , Stitzer ML , Liebson IA , Bigelow GE: Dose–response effects of methadone in the treatment of opioid dependence. Ann Intern Med 1993;119:23–27 .
137. Strain EC, Stitzer ML, Liebson IA, Bigelow GE: Methadone dose and treatment outcome. Drug Alcohol Depend 1993;33:105–117.
138. Sullivan EV, Marsh L, Mathalon DH, et al: Relationship between alcohol withdrawal seizures and temporal lobe white matter volume deficits. Alcohol Clin Exp Res 1996;20:348–354.
139. Tamborska E, Marangos PJ: Brain benzodiazepine binding sites in ethanol dependent and withdrawal states. Life Sci 1986;38:465–472.
140. Tavel ME: A new look at an old syndrome: Delirium tremens. Arch Intern Med 1962;109:129–134.
141. Tavel ME, Davidson W, Batterton TD: A critical analysis of mortality associated with delirium tremens: Review of 39 fatalities in a 9-year period. Am J Med Sci 1961; 242:58–69.
142. Thomas DW, Freedman DX: Treatment of alcohol withdrawal syndrome: Comparison of promazine and paraldehyde. JAMA 1964;188:316–318.
143. Thompson WL: Management of alcohol withdrawal syndromes. Arch Intern Med 1978;138:278–283.
144. Thompson WL, Johnson AD, Maddrey WL, et al: Diazepam and paraldehyde for treatment of severe delirium tremens: A controlled trial. Ann Intern Med 1975;82: 175–180.
145. Trabulsy ME: Cocaine washed out syndrome in a patient with acute myocardial infarction. Am J Emerg Med 1995;13:538–539.
146. Tunniclif G, Raess BU: GABA Mechanism in Epilepsy. New York, Wiley, 1992, pp. 54–55.
147. Ulrichsen J, Bech B, Allerup P, et al: Diazepam prevents progression of kindled alcohol withdrawal behaviour. Psychopharmacology (Berl) 1995;121:451–460.
148. Ulrichsen J, Bech B, Ebert B, et al: Glutamate and benzodiazepine receptor autoradiography in rat brain after repetition of alcohol dependence. Psychopharmacology (Berl) 1996;126:31–41.
149. Uzbay IT, Akarsu ES, Kayaalp SO: Effects of bromocriptine and haloperidol on ethanol withdrawal syndrome in rats. Pharmacol Biochem Behav 1994;49: 969–974.
150. Van de Wiele B, Rubinstein E, Peacock W, Martin N: Propylene glycol toxicity caused by prolonged infusion of etomidate. J Neurosurg Anesthesiol 1995; 7:259–262.
151. Veatch LM, Gonzalez LP: Repeated ethanol withdrawal produces site-dependent increases in EEG spiking. Alcohol Clin Exp Res 1996;20:262–267.
152. Victor M, Adams RD: The effect of alcohol on the nervous system. Res Publ Assoc Res Nerv Ment Dis 1953;32: 526–573.
153. Vinson DC, Menezes M: Admission alcohol level: A predictor of the course of alcohol withdrawal. J Fam Pract 1991;33:161–167.
154. Wartenberg AA, Nirenberg TD, Liepman MR, et al: Detoxification of alcoholics: Improving care by symptom-triggered sedation. Alcohol Clin Exp Res 1990;14: 71–75.
155. Wasilewski D, Matsumoto H, Kur E, et al: Assessment of diazepam loading dose therapy of delirium tremens. Alcohol 1996;31:273–278.
156. Watling SM, Fleming C, Casey P, Yanos J: Nursing-based protocol for treatment of alcohol withdrawal in the intensive care unit. Am J Crit Care 1995;4:66–70.
157. Weinbroum A, Rudick V, Sorkine P, et al: Use of flumazenil in the treatment of drug overdose: A double-blind and open clinical study in 110 patients. Crit Care Med 1996;24:199–206.
158. Williams HE: Alcoholic hypoglycemia and ketoacidosis. Med Clin North Am 1984;68:33–45.
159. Wilson A, Vulcano B: A double blind, placebo controlled trial of magnesium sulfate in the ethanol withdrawal syndrome. Alcohol Clin Exp Res 1984;8:542–545.
160. Winkler E, Almog S, Kriger D, et al: Use of flumazenil in the diagnosis and treatment of patients with coma of unknown etiology. Crit Care Med 1993;21:538–542.
161. Woo E, Greenblatt DJ: Massive benzodiazepine requirements during acute alcohol withdrawal. Am J Psychiatry 1979;36:821–823.
162. Worner TM: Relative kindling effect of readmissions in alcoholics. Alcohol Alcohol 1996;31:375–380.
163. Wretlind M, Pilbrant A, Sundwall A, Vessman J: Disposition of three benzodiazepines after single oral administration in man. Acta Pharmacol Toxicol (Copenh) 1977; 40:28–39.
164. Young GP, Rores C, Murohy C, Dailey RH: Intravenous phenobarbital for alcohol withdrawal and convulsions. Ann Emerg Med 1987;16:847–850.

CHAPTER 71

Nicotine and Tobacco Preparations

Morton E. Salomon

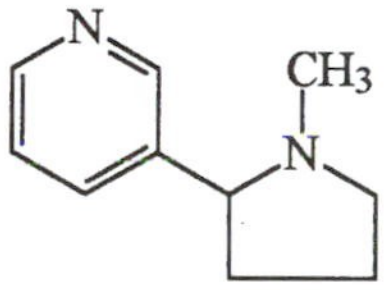

Nicotine
MW = 162 daltons
Toxic blood level = 50 ng/mL
Toxic dose = 1–2 mg (children)
4–8 mg (adults)

At 8:15 A.M. an 11-month-old boy was found eating cigarette butts out of an ashtray. The parents cleaned his lips and mouth with cold water. Twenty minutes later the child vomited three times. The parents contacted their regional poison center, which advised them to bring the child immediately to an emergency department (ED). En route, via ambulance, the child vomited again. On presentation to the ED at 9:00 A.M., the child was noted to be tremulous and diaphoretic with excessive salivation. He had a glassy-eyed look and did not interact with his parents. His vital signs were: blood pressure, 128/78 mm Hg; pulse, 150 beats/min; respiratory rate, 28 beats/min; and temperature, 99.7°F (37.6°C). Pupils were 3 mm and reactive to light. The skin was pale without rashes or bruises. The anterior fontanel was open (1 cm) and flat. The mouth was clear of particulate matter. Examination of the chest, heart, and abdomen was unremarkable. Pulses were strong. The neurologic examination was nonfocal. Pulse oximetry measured 96% saturation on room air.

At 9:10 A. M., the child had a generalized seizure lasting less than 15 seconds. There was no incontinence, eye rolling, or focal features. The ED staff placed a 28 French orogastric tube into the stomach and lavaged with 100 mL aliquots of 0.9% sodium chloride. Lavaging produced a scant amount of brown particulate material along with other stomach contents. Once the stomach contents were cleared, 10 g of activated charcoal were delivered through the orogastric tube, which was then replaced by a nasogastric tube.

Over the next half hour, the child became increasingly lethargic. Neurologic examination demonstrated progressively more hypotonia, and his deep tendon reflexes became undetectable. His respiratory rate decreased to 18 breaths/min and he was breathing diaphragmatically with little intercostal muscle movement. The pulse had decreased to 84 beats/min and blood pressure to 76/50 mm Hg. His skin was mottled and cool. The pulse oximeter registered 88–89%. An arterial blood gas analysis done prior to placing the child on oxygen showed: pH, 7.44; PCO_2, 46 mm Hg; PO_2 57 mm Hg. At 9:45 A.M. the child was intubated and placed on a ventilator. Copious secretions were noted from the mouth and endotracheal tube and the child was given 0.2 mg of atropine IV. The CBC, electrolytes, glucose, calcium, magnesium, and renal function tests done at the time of admission were within normal limits.

Four hours after presentation, the child was more alert and breathing more effectively and began fighting the ventilator. He was sedated with a continuous midazolam infusion, but was gradually weaned from the respirator and extubated 11 hours after the ingestion. He was discharged home 48 hours after ingestion in stable condition. Follow-up examination 15 days later revealed no apparent sequelae.

What Are the Physiologic Effects of Nicotine?

Nicotine binds stereospecifically to select acetylcholine receptors, generally referred to as nicotine receptors.[6,33] There are nicotine receptors throughout the body, particularly in the autonomic ganglia, adrenal medulla, central nervous system, spinal cord, neuromuscular junctions, and chemoreceptors of the carotid and aortic bodies.[6,33] In the CNS, the highest density of nicotine receptors can be found in the limbic system, midbrain, and brainstem.[6]

The physiologic effects on the CNS are similarly multiple, complex, and dose-dependent. At the usual doses experienced with tobacco use there is stimulation of the reticular activating system and an alerting pattern on electroencephalogram (EEG).[33,69] There is a facilitation of memory and attention, with a decrease in aggression and irritability.[33] Although nicotine might reduce skeletal muscular tone and decrease deep tendon reflexes, its central and neuromuscular stimulatory effects can also produce tremor.[33,65] At very high doses, nicotine induces seizures. Studies in mice suggest that nicotine-induced seizures can be controlled by the neuroinhibitory agent, 3-alpha-OH-DHP. It is therefore postulated that nicotine produces seizures at high doses by a CNS disinhibition mechanism.[43]

Gastrointestinal effects are probably created by nicotine stimulation of vagal centers in the medulla oblongata. Even at low doses, nicotine exposure produces nausea and vomiting, and these symptoms can be seen in inexperienced, nontolerant tobacco users. Nicotine also increases gastroesophageal reflux, probably by either lowering sphincter pressure or increasing acid secretion.[60] Diarrhea can be stimulated by larger doses of nicotine, which is probably mediated by both central and parasympathetic excitation.[22,33]

Nicotine exerts a number of endocrinologic effects either by acting directly on nicotine receptors in the endocrine gland or by stimulating neurohumoral pathways in the CNS. It enhances release of catecholamines. It also stimulates the production of vasopressin (ADH), growth hormone, ACTH, cortisol, prolactin, serotonin, and beta-endorphins. Nicotine also affects pancreatic exocrine functions. Rats pretreated with nicotine doses comparable to the exposure of moderate smokers exhibit increased amylase, trypsin, and chymotrypsin activity.[17] With repeated exposure, tolerance develops to many of these effects.[6]

Nicotine suppresses the appetite for food, especially sweet foods, while increasing basal energy expenditures. These effects explain why nicotine promotes weight loss. Smokers weigh, on average, 6–10 lb less than nonsmokers. With repeated exposure, tolerance develops to many of these effects.[6,33] Habitual use of nicotine also decreases estrogen levels in female smokers, probably by promoting hydroxylation of estradiol. As a result, women who smoke are at increased risk for osteoporosis.

What Are the Pharmacologic Characteristics of Nicotine?

The pharmacologic characteristics of nicotine are summarized in Table 71–1.

Nicotine is a tertiary amine. It is a colorless, bitter-tasting, highly water-soluble, volatile liquid that is weakly alkaline (pK_a = 8.0–8.5).[6] The principal source of nicotine today is the tobacco plant, *Nicotiana tabacum*, from which nicotine was first isolated in 1826.[13] Nicotine also can be isolated from multiple plant species in the Solanaceae family. *Nicotiana tabacum* is not the only tobacco plant in this family: The first tobacco to be brought back from the New World to Europe was *Nicotiana rustica*, which contains a much higher concentration of nicotine (approximately 18%) and is still used in "Turkish tobacco."[39] Nicotine is also found in small concentrations in plants outside the *Nicotiana* genus and even in plants outside the Solanaceae family. In addition, there are a number of alkaloids with chemical structures and physiologic activity similar to that of nicotine in tobacco plants and botanical species related to tobacco.[39] Nornicotine, anabasine, and anabatine are structurally similar alkaloids also found in tobacco. Anabasine is the principal alkaloid found in *Nicotiana glauca*.[65] Lobeline, derived from *Lobelia inflata*, or "Indian tobacco," is frequently used as a nicotine substitute.[33] Cystisine, found in mescal beans, is used for its mind-altering properties. Coniine, the lethal alkaloid in "poison hemlock," is also chemically related to nicotine.

Absorption

Nicotine is readily absorbed from the buccal mucosa, respiratory tract, intestinal tract, and skin. The usual site of absorption is the lungs. Inhaled nicotine from cigarette smoke reaches the brain in approximately 8 seconds, with CNS levels of nicotine rising rapidly and then declining rapidly as the drug is redistributed to other tissues.[6,33] The cigarette smoker achieves a blood nicotine concentration of 5–30 ng/mL after a single cigarette. The typical smoker will adjust his or her use of cigarettes and pattern of smoking to maintain an average nicotine concentration of 30 ng/mL.[6]

TABLE 71–1. PHARMACOLOGIC CHARACTERISTICS OF NICOTINE

Absorption	Lungs, oral mucosa, skin, intestinal tract; gastric acidity inhibits absorption
Volume of distribution	Approximately 1 L/kg
Protein binding	5–20%
Metabolism	80–90% metabolized in the liver, remainder in lung and kidney; principle metabolites are cotinine, nicotine-1'-*N*-oxide
Half-life	1–4 h, shorter in smokers (average, 2 h); half-life of cotinine is 19 h
Elimination	2–35% excreted unchanged in urine

Cigar and pipe tobacco as well as chewing tobacco, snuff, and nicotine resin chewing gum are generally absorbed through the buccal mucosa. Pipe and cigar tobacco are air-cured to achieve an alkaline pH of 8.50. Smokeless tobaccos and nicotine gum are buffered. The alkaline pH of all of these products enhances buccal absorption.[6] Smokeless tobacco users generally achieve nicotine concentrations comparable to those of cigarette smokers. Pipe and cigar smokers usually average lower nicotine concentrations, unless they inhale the smoke from these products.[6]

Ingested tobacco is poorly absorbed across the gastric mucosa because the acidic pH of the stomach keeps the nicotine ionized.[33,39] Nicotine absorption increases again in the alkaline milieu of the intestines.

Nicotine generally achieves a volume of distribution of 1 L/kg. It crosses the placenta readily and is also transmitted in small concentrations in breast milk.[6]

Metabolism/Elimination

Habitual tobacco users generally metabolize 80–90% of their nicotine intake, excreting 10–20% in urine unchanged. Metabolism takes place primarily in the liver, but also, to a lesser extent, in the kidney and lung.[9,33] The two major oxidative metabolites of nicotine are cotinine and nicotine–1-*N*-oxide. Both of these compounds are pharmacologically inactive and are also excreted primarily by the kidney.[6,33]

The half-life of nicotine is 1–4 hours but generally averages 2 hours in chronic users.[6,33] Since nicotine metabolism in the liver is an inducible transformation, smokers metabolize the drug more rapidly than nonsmokers. The elimination half-life of cotinine is approximately 19 hours, making cotinine levels in the urine a better marker of recent tobacco use and total tobacco exposure.[6,33]

Renal excretion of unchanged nicotine can vary from 2 to 35% of the total dose,[6] depending on urine flow and urine pH. Experimentally, acidification of the urine traps nicotine ions and enhances direct elimination.[6,22] Nonsmokers eliminate a larger proportion of nicotine unchanged in the urine because of their slower liver metabolism.[36]

Drug Interactions

A number of studies have demonstrated that smokers have altered metabolism of many commonly used medications. Smokers metabolize the compounds listed in Table 71–2 more quickly than nonsmokers.[33,36] As discussed above, nicotine itself is metabolized more rapidly in smokers. The therapeutic effectiveness of opioids, benzodiazepines, nifedipine, and beta-adrenergic antagonists is diminished in smokers.[33] Smokers with peptic ulcer disease are also more likely to fail treatment with H_2 antagonists and antacids.[6] The presumed mechanism for this change in drug metabolism is induction of microsomal enzyme systems. However, because there are 3000 components to tobacco smoke, it is difficult to know exactly which components affect metabolism. In all likelihood, nicotine is not responsible for the induction. For example, IV nicotine does not effect theophylline metabolism in humans.[6] It is more likely that polynuclear aromatic hydrocarbons (PAH), released by the combustion of tobacco, are responsible for the induction of P448 microsomal enzymes in the liver.[36] Drugs whose metabolism is affected by smoking are in part metabolized by this system. In contrast, drugs using the P450 system exclusively are not affected by chronic smoking.[36]

TABLE 71–2. DRUGS WITH ENHANCED METABOLISM IN SMOKERS

Benzodiazepines	Opioids
Caffeine	Phenacetin
H_2 antagonists	Propranolol
Imipramine	Theophylline
Nicotine	

Nicotine and ethanol are frequently used concomitantly. Animal studies demonstrate that pretreatment with ethanol exaggerates cardiovascular responses to IV nicotine. Heart rate and blood pressure increase in an additive way. Since ethanol does not influence the rate of nicotine metabolism, this additive response is thought to be catecholamine mediated. Smokers are more apt to suffer from dysrhythmias and sudden death during alcohol use. It is likely that this is the result of increased oxygen demand triggered by this additive cardiovascular stimulation.[7]

What Are the Symptoms of Acute Nicotine Poisoning?

Over 60% of nicotine exposures produce no toxicity and only 1% produced moderate to major toxicity. This low proportion of serious poisoning is not surprising, because 98% of exposures are unintentional and over 90% occur in children younger than 6 years of age. Nonetheless, serious exposures do occur, even in young children, and seem to be dose related. In one report, approximately 45% of 51 childhood exposures to nicotine resulted in some degree of symptomatology. Only eight of these (16%) required evaluation by a physician and only four patients (8%) developed significant symptomatology (lethargy, unresponsiveness, limb jerking).[71] Similarly, another study reported that only 1 of 20 children who ingested nicotine became moderately ill and required 24 hours of hospitalization.[8] Most unintentional exposures in small children result from the ingestion of tobacco products. The tobacco itself usually induces spontaneous vomiting, which limits absorption of the toxin.

A child who ingests one or more cigarettes or three or more cigarette butts has a 90% chance of becoming symptomatic. Conversely, ingestion of smaller amounts will produce symptomatology only half the time.[71] In a retrospective review of 10 childhood cigarette ingestions, the 4 children who became severely poisoned each ingested at least two whole cigarettes.[45] One-half piece or more of 2-mg nicotine chewing gum usually produces symptomatology in a child.[71]

Symptoms associated with acute nicotine exposure are outlined in Table 71–3. Clinical signs of low concentrations of nicotine, such as those seen routinely in smokers, include tremor and increased heart rate, respiratory rate, blood pressure, and alertness.

In marked contrast to these relatively mild effects seen in cigarette smoking, when nicotine is taken in "toxic" quantities, as in an ingestion or insecticide exposure, the effects are more severe. The symptoms may follow a biphasic pattern in which there is initial stimulation followed quickly by inhibition.[65] Early symptoms of toxicity often include nausea, vomiting, diaphoresis, and increased salivation. Cardiovascular signs include tachycardia, hypertension, and pallor (secondary to vasoconstriction). Early neurologic manifestations include headache, dizziness, ataxia, and, in more severe cases, confusion as well as visual and auditory distortions.[8,65]

In more severe exposures, these generally mild symptoms can be quickly overshadowed by signs of more extreme stimulation, such as seizures, muscle fasciculations, and atrial fibrillation.[8,65,69] Although seizures do occur, there have been no reports of nicotine-induced status epilepticus in nonexperimental conditions. These symptoms are often succeeded by signs of multisystem depression, such as bradycardia and hypotension, and a curare like neuromuscular blockade that leads to muscle paralysis, particularly respiratory paralysis.[55,65,69] Death is generally attributable to respiratory depression or paralysis (particularly of the intercostal muscles) complicated by increased bronchial secretions or to cardiovascular collapse.[9,55,65] Timely and adequate respiratory and cardiovascular support generally leads to full recovery without sequelae.[9,55]

Vomiting is the most common symptom of nicotine poisoning, occurring in more than 50% of symptomatic patients. However, it is not a reliable sign of toxicity.[71] Patients can present with lethargy and respiratory depression without prior vomiting or any other signs of central nervous system (CNS) stimulation.[9] Moreover, nicotine chewing gum ingestions in children produce vomiting less frequently (20% incidence) than do cigarette ingestions.[71]

Following the ingestion of tobacco products, children usually manifest symptoms within 30–90 minutes. When children chew nicotine gum (Nicorette), symptoms are usually apparent within 15–30 minutes, due to more rapid absorption through the buccal mucosa.[69,71] When death occurs, it usually occurs within 1 hour of exposure. In mild exposures, symptoms generally last only 1–2 hours after exposure. With severe intoxication, however, full recovery might take 48–72 hours.[69]

As little as 1 mg of nicotine can produce symptoms in a small child. Four to 8 mg of nicotine might produce symptoms in an adult, especially a nonhabituated victim.[22] Forty to 60 mg of nicotine is generally accepted as the lethal dose in adults.[22,25,45] Table 71–4 lists the nicotine content of tobacco products and substitutes. In a prospective study of nicotine ingestions in children, the three most severely poisoned infants ingested a minimum of 1.4 mg/kg. The 25 asymptomatic children ingested a mean of 0.5 mg/kg, and all asymptomatic children ingested less than 1 mg/kg.[71] These numbers indicate a very narrow range between nontoxic and significantly toxic doses.

What Is the Treatment for Patients With Acute Nicotine Poisoning?

Unintentional ingestions of nicotine in small children almost invariably involve small amounts, with spontaneous vomiting providing adequate decontamination. Thus, many patients do not need medical evaluation. Individuals who have ingested one or more cigarettes or three or more cigarette butts, who acquired their exposures from a more toxic source (a nicotine insecticide or a tobacco enema), who have developed symptoms other than vomiting, or who are potentially suicidal should be referred to an ED without delay. Patients with mild symptoms and no complicating circumstances can gener-

TABLE 71–3. SIGNS AND SYMPTOMS OF ACUTE NICOTINE POISONING

	Gastrointestinal	Respiratory	Cardiovascular	Neurologic	
Early (15–60 min)	Abdominal pain Nausea Salivation Vomiting	Bronchorrhea Hyperpnea	Hypertension Tachycardia Pallor	Agitation/anxiety Ataxia/dizziness Blurred vision Confusion Distorted hearing	Headache Hyperactivity Muscle fasciculation Seizures Tremor
Delayed (0.5–4 h)	Diarrhea	Apnea Hypoventilation	Bradycardia Dysrhythmias Hypotension Shock	Coma Hyporeflexia Hypotonia	Lethargy Weakness Muscle paralysis

TABLE 71–4. SOURCES OF NICOTINE

Source	Nicotine Content (mg)	Nicotine Delivered (mg)[a]
1 whole cigarette	13–30	0.5–2.0
1 low-yield cigarette	3–8	0.1–1.0
1 cigarette butt	5–7	—
1 cigar	15–40	0.2–1.0
1 g of snuff (wet)	12–16	2.0–3.5
1 g of chewing tobacco	6–8	2.0–4.0
1 piece of nicotine gum	2 or 4	1.0–2.0
1 nicotine patch	8.3–114	5.0–22/24 h
1 nicotine nasal spray	0.5	0.2–0.4

[a]Delivered through intended use of standard dose.

ally be observed for 4 hours in the ED and then released if symptoms have resolved.[65]

Initial Management

The patient with a significant recent oral exposure, who has not vomited prior to presentation, should be decontaminated by orogastric lavage. Emesis induced by syrup of ipecac should be avoided because nicotine poisoning may cause seizures or respiratory depression.[9,71] Activated charcoal effectively binds nicotine and should be used in gastrointestinal (GI) exposures to reduce absorption. Pharmacokinetic studies have indicated that nicotine appears in the GI tract even when administered IV.[71] Since this would suggest that nicotine undergoes enteroenteric or enterohepatic circulation, multiple-dose activated charcoal would theoretically be of value in patients with serious exposures.

In cases of skin exposure to wet tobacco leaves, concentrated nicotine liquid, or nicotine pesticide powder, the patient's clothing should be promptly removed and the skin thoroughly washed. The medical staff must be gloved and gowned during these procedures to avoid secondary exposure.

Use of the Laboratory

Toxicologic assay for nicotine or its metabolites is of limited value in the management of a patient with an acute overdose. The presence of nicotine or cotinine in the urine might reflect coincidental passive smoke exposure and therefore does not confirm nicotine as the cause of poisoning.[69] Serum nicotine levels must be determined shortly after exposure and are difficult to interpret. A serum nicotine level greater than 50 ng/mL generally predicts serious toxicity, but lower levels can also be significant in the nontolerant patient.[65]

Symptom-Directed Treatment

Because of the variety of stimulatory and depressant effects in the neuromuscular, sympathetic, parasympathetic, and central nervous systems, treatment of nicotine toxicity is a complex therapeutic problem. Treatment is based on a symptom analysis. Seizures are usually treated with a benzodiazepine. Loading the patient with longer-acting anticonvulsants is generally unnecessary.[9,45,65] Cardiovascular compromise is treated with atropine for bradycardia and fluids for hypotension.[65] If hypotension does not respond to fluids, a vasopressor such as dopamine or norepinephrine is recommended.[69] Atropine is used to overcome excessive muscarinic stimulation. By reversing muscarinic effects, there is some risk of creating unopposed catecholamine effects. For this reason, some authors also suggest using phentolamine, an alpha-adrenergic antagonist agent, in the treatment of nicotine overdose.[22,65] Such an approach is unnecessary, however, as adrenergic stimulation is rarely life-threatening in nicotine poisoning and adrenergic antagonism can exacerbate hypotension in the delayed phase. Respiratory compromise, caused by respiratory depression and bronchial secretions, is generally treated with oxygen, intubation, positive pressure ventilation, and atropine, if indicated.

Enhancing Elimination

As nicotine is a weak base (pK_a = 8.0–8.5), excretion can theoretically be enhanced by acidification of the urine, but this approach is not advisable.[9,65] The risks of acidification in a patient with seizures and possible rhabdomyolysis outweigh the benefits.[65] Furthermore, since the symptoms in nicotine poisoning are generally short-lived, acidification is unnecessary. Fluid diuresis may also enhance elimination and is safer but also is unnecessary due to the limited urinary elimination.[9]

Antidotes

There is no specific antidote for nicotine poisoning. Pempidine and mecamylamine demonstrate both competitive and noncompetitive antagonism to the central effects of nicotine,[47] and hexamethonium, a ganglionic blocking agent, prevents nicotine-induced seizures in animals.[65] None of these agents has been used, either experimentally or clinically, to treat overdoses in humans. Although their application is theoretically of interest, new approaches with these agents are not likely to be developed because severe nicotine poisoning is rare and nonspecific supportive measures are almost always adequate when initiated in a timely manner.

What Are the Sources of Nicotine?

The principal sources of nicotine exposure and poisoning are tobacco products: cigarettes, cigars, pipe tobacco, chewing tobacco, and snuff. Nicotine is also the essential component of smoking-cessation products such as nicotine gum, nicotine patches, and nicotine nasal spray. Nicotine had a brief application as an animal tranquilizer and was used extensively as an agricultural insecticide in the 1920s and '30s; formulations of this product are still available.

Cigarettes

Cigarettes are the most widely used tobacco products in Western culture and the most likely culprit in nicotine poisoning. When a cigarette is burned, the smoker inhales both gaseous and particulate matter. Nicotine is found in the particulate phase of cigarette smoke, along with tar. The total nicotine content of a "regular" American cigarette varies between 13 and 20 mg. "Low-nicotine" cigarettes contain half this amount, and many European cigarettes contain up to 30 mg of nicotine.[8,22,71] When a cigarette is smoked, more than half the nicotine escapes in the sidestream smoke and a large fraction remains in the butt and filter.[2] As a result, a typical cigarette delivers 0.5–2.0 mg of nicotine (average = 1.0 mg) to the smoker.[33] This amount depends on not only the total nicotine content of the cigarette but also the individual's smoking technique. The nicotine content written on a cigarette package is determined by burning cigarettes on mechanical smoking machines in a standardized manner.[46] A smoker, on the other hand, extracts variable amounts of nicotine from a cigarette to maintain a steady blood nicotine level. Smokers vary the degree of nicotine extraction by altering the rate of puffing, the puff volume, the depth of inhalation, and the size of the residual butt.[6,46] When smokers switch from "regular" to "low-yield" cigarettes, they often maintain a similar nicotine intake by increasing the number of cigarettes they smoke and by puffing in a more vigorous manner.[46]

Not all cigarettes are made from pure tobacco. It is common, especially in Asia, to create cigarettes out of a mixture of tobacco and other products. "Kreteks" are cigarettes composed of 60% tobacco and 40% ground clove. In 1984, 66 billion of these cigarettes were sold worldwide. In the United States they are especially popular with adolescents. Unfortunately, kreteks are more addicting than tobacco alone. Moreover, eugenol, the major active ingredient in cloves, is believed to be the probable cause of the severe lower respiratory complications—acute pulmonary edema and hemorrhage—seen in some users.[39]

Smokeless Tobacco

Smokeless tobacco, especially snuff, has regained popularity in the United States, particularly among adolescent boys.[12] There are an estimated 10–22 million smokeless tobacco users in the United States. About 3 million of these are younger than 21 years. Twenty percent of high school students report having tried smokeless tobacco products. Sales of smokeless tobacco products increased approximately 11% per year throughout the 1980s and early '90s.[11–13,27,70] Their use is particularly prevalent among professional baseball players.[11,20]

The rising use of smokeless tobacco has paralleled the decline in cigarette smoking in the United States. Many users have switched to smokeless tobacco as a way to quit cigarettes. Conversely, many adolescents who start using smokeless tobacco will eventually progress to smoking cigarettes. Because smoking is not involved, the public generally believes that smokeless tobacco is more socially acceptable and less of a health risk.[27,39] In fact, there is as much as 48 times the risk of oropharyngeal cancers among long-time users of smokeless tobacco, as well as other oral and nonoral health hazards.[12,13,39]

Smokeless tobacco comes in two varieties: chewing tobacco and snuff. Snuff is a finely cut tobacco powder packaged dry or moist. In Europe, especially England, small pinches of dry snuff are inhaled through the nostrils. In the United States dry and wet snuff are usually "dipped." This involves placing a bite-size amount of tobacco (a "quid") between the mucous membranes and the gums. Chewing tobacco is generally packaged as "twists"—leaf tobacco twisted into ropelike portions—or "plugs"—shredded tobacco pressed into cakes. These are chewed or simply placed between the mucous membranes and the gums. Generally, the nicotine from smokeless tobacco dissolves in the saliva and is absorbed through the mucous membranes of the mouth. However, approximately one-third of smokeless tobacco users swallow their saliva, absorbing additional nicotine in the intestinal tract.[12,13,70]

Snuff contains approximately 14 mg of nicotine per gram of tobacco. A typical quid contains 1.5–2.5 g of tobacco, which the user "dips" for 20–30 minutes. Ten percent of the available nicotine crosses the oral mucosa, producing a total nicotine dose of 2.0–3.5 mg/dip. Tobacco chewers use approximately 7 g of tobacco at a time. The nicotine content of a typical "chaw" is 7.8 mg/g of tobacco. Only 8% of this nicotine is absorbed through the oral mucosa, because the pH of chewing tobacco is only 6.5. Ultimately, the tobacco chewer gets approximately the same dose of nicotine or slightly more than the tobacco snuffer.[11] The smokeless tobacco user who takes 8–10 dips or chaws per day gets a nicotine dose equivalent to 30–40 cigarettes per day, and cotinine concentrations found in their urine are similar to those found in the urine of smokers.[5,11]

Less Common Sources

Although poisoning from smokeless tobacco usually occurs by unintentional ingestion in children, one case report of nicotine poisoning occurred when a child licked the contents of a spittoon.[25] Another unusual source of nicotine poisoning is tobacco enemas. On occasion, tobacco has been soaked in water and the juice of this extract added to enemas for the treatment of pinworm. This practice has produced at least one reported case of severe nicotine poisoning.[22]

Green-leaf tobacco sickness (GTS) occurs when a tobacco harvester handles dew-laden tobacco leaves. The nicotine dissolves in the water and is absorbed through the worker's skin, if cutaneous precautions are not taken. This generally produces a mild to moderate illness consisting of nausea, vomiting, headaches, dizziness, pallor, and diaphoresis.[6,23,39] However, in two recent outbreaks in Kentucky nearly 25% of the affected tobacco workers required hospitalization. A significant portion of these poisoned workers were under 18 years.[3,49] Nicotine poisoning has also been reported in smugglers who have hidden tobacco leaves under their clothing.[39] Nicotine salts such as nicotine sulfate were popular pesticides in the 1920s and '30s. These compounds generally contain 40% nicotine; when they come in contact with moist skin, significant doses of nicotine are absorbed. Several cases of severe nicotine poisoning from insecticide skin exposure or ingestion, including deaths, have occurred.[9,39,55] Although the manufacture of nicotine insecticides was discontinued by 1950, these products may still be available in old barns and homes.

Gum

Nicotine is prepared in the form of gum to assist smokers with withdrawal symptoms. Nicotine resin gum (Nicorette) is packaged in two strengths, 2 mg and 4 mg. It is designed to be chewed slowly and intermittently. When used correctly, blood concentrations of nicotine are less than those achieved through cigarette smoking, even when 4-mg gum is chewed. Approximately 53–72% of the nicotine in the gum is absorbed through the buccal mucosa. Additional amounts can be absorbed through swallowed saliva.[6] However, when the gum is chewed rapidly and vigorously, nicotine concentrations in the blood can rise rapidly, producing adverse effects, especially in children.[71] Severe nicotine poisoning in a 20-month-old child occurred from the use of nicotine gum.[69] Moreover, adverse effects have been reported in adults who have used the gum while continuing to smoke.[51,71] If the gum is swallowed, it is less likely to be toxic because the nicotine is released and absorbed slowly, during GI transit, producing low blood concentrations.[6]

Patches

There are currently four nicotine-releasing adhesive patches available to aid in the treatment of smoking cessation. These patches, designed for 16–24 hours of use, vary in size and nicotine release rates and contain 8.3–114 mg of nicotine per patch.

One study exposed dogs transdermally and orally to three different commercially available nicotine patch systems. The topical adminstration provided 1–2 mg/kg over 24 hours, producing plasma concentration as high as 43 ng/mL. Two of 12 applications elicited mild symptomatology (salivation and vomiting). Oral exposure up to 13 mg/kg produced maximal plasma concentrations of 73 ng/mL, with only mild symptoms (vomiting) in two of 12 trials.[48]

Recently published reports from a 2-year postmarketing surveillance study by 34 poison centers discuss toxicity from misuse and unintentional exposure to transdermal nicotine patches (TNPs). Transdermal exposure of 2–20 TNPs in nine adults resulted in very serious toxicity. Eight patients were admitted to intensive care, four had refractory seizures, and four required assisted ventilation. However, seven of the nine patients ingested co-intoxicants in suicide attempts, and the maximum nicotine level recorded was only 27 ng/mL.[84] Thirty-six exposures in children were less severe. Half the children had topical exposures, while half had bitten, chewed, or swallowed the patches. Nearly 40% developed symptoms but only 27% required medical evaluation and only 5% were hospitalized for 24 hours.[83] It seems, therefore, that unintentional exposure to nicotine patches has not yet produced serious toxicity.

Nasal Spray and Inhaler

In 1996, a nicotine nasal spray (Nicotrol) was released in the United States as another treatment modality for withdrawal symptoms during smoking cessation. The metered dose inhaler contains 100 mg of nicotine in a concentration of 10 mg/mL and is designed to deliver 200 equivalent puffs. Each puff contains 0.5 mg of nicotine of which slightly more than half will pass into the circulation through the nasal mucosa.[50] Absorption is diminished slightly by rhinitis and delayed by the use of alpha-adrenergic decongestants.[41] The recommended dose is 2 sprays (1 mg)—one in each nostril—every 30–60 minutes. The user titrates the dosing frequency to withdrawal symptoms, using a maximum of 40 doses (80 puffs) per day and creating a steady-state serum nicotine level of 6–18 ng/mL. No overdoses with this product have been reported yet in the literature, but prospective postmarketing surveillance is underway.

A nicotine metered-dose oral inhaler has also been developed for smoking cessation, but not yet released. The device is designed to mimic smoking by providing airway stimulation as well as nicotine replacement. Absorption of nicotine occurs primarily through the buccal and pharyngeal mucosa, but slow deep inhalation can redirect some absorption to the pulmonary tree. An average steady-state serum nicotine level of 7 ng/mL was achieved in a 2-day trial of 15 subjects.[42]

Tobacco Dependancy and Nicotine

Fifty million Americans—30% of the adult population—smoke cigarettes despite antismoking public education campaigns, widespread knowledge of its health consequences, and decreasing social acceptance.[6,79] In the United States, 350,000 deaths annually are attributable to cigarette smoking, making it the single most important cause of preventable premature mortality.[57] It is now widely accepted that tobacco use is addicting and that nicotine is the component primarily responsible for dependency.[73]

Tobacco use meets all of the World Health Organization (WHO) definitions of addiction. There is an overpowering compulsion to continue taking the drug. There is a tendency to develop tolerance to its effects and therefore keep increasing the dosage. Psychologic and physical dependency develops, and the absence of tobacco produces discomfort in the smoker. Finally, tobacco has detrimental effects on both the individual user and society at large.[52]

Tobacco addiction seems to occur with forms of tobacco besides cigarettes, especially with smokeless tobacco. Of course, many smokeless tobacco users switch to this product to wean themselves from cigarettes.[52,59] About one-third of baseball players using smokeless tobacco report trying to stop but being unable to do so despite the development of oral health problems from continued use.[11]

Individuals dependent on tobacco, like any other substance-dependent individuals, go through multiple cycles of quitting and relapsing. While spontaneous quitting without any special treatment program is the most common route to abstinence, the achievement rate by this method is only 1% of users per year.[6,37] Women cigarette smokers have a lower success rate than men. It has been shown that women who quit during the second half of their menstrual cycles undergo a stronger withdrawal syndrome than men or than women quitting in the first half of their menstrual cycle.[56]

Smokers are much more likely than nonsmokers to have other substance dependencies.[37] Conversely, 80–95% of alcohol and drug abusers also smoke cigarettes. In a survey of 1000 drug users seeking treatment for their addictions, 57% thought it would be harder to achieve abstinence from cigarettes than from the substance for which they were seeking treatment. They generally felt the urge to smoke a cigarette was greater than the urge to use their problem drug, despite the fact that cigarettes were less pleasurable.[37] It has been suggested that nicotine use promotes the release of endogenous endorphins. Therefore, withdrawal from nicotine might have a strong biochemical resemblance to withdrawal from opioids.[18] In fact one study was able to precipitate withdrawal symptoms in nicotine-dependent rats with subcutaneous naloxone and then reverse the abstinence symptoms with morphine sulfate.[44]

With so many substances involved in cigarette smoking, it is quite likely that tobacco dependency is a complex addiction, involving both psychological components, such as oral gratification, and physical dependency. It is now widely accepted that the primary addictive component of tobacco is nicotine,[53,59,79] but this has been the subject of some controversy and is supported primarily by indirect evidence. As previously discussed, smokers will adjust their smoking behavior to compensate for reductions in nicotine content and maintain nicotine concentrations in their blood by changing their inhalation behavior when smoking low-nicotine-content cigarettes. This supports the concept that they smoke to dose themselves with nicotine.[2,53] Furthermore, when mecamylamine, a nicotine central antagonist, is administered to smokers, their smoking increases.[38] Moreover, it has been demonstrated that animals will self-administer nicotine without any other reward for this behavior.[53] Finally, tobacco withdrawal symptoms are significantly mitigated by treatment with nicotine substitutes (see below).

However, nicotine is undoubtedly not the entire cause of tobacco dependency. When IV nicotine is administered to abstinent smokers, it reduces, but does not completely eliminate, their ad libitum smoking. There seems to be a compulsion to smoke even when usual blood nicotine levels are obtained by IV administration.[38]

What Are the Symptoms and Signs of Nicotine Withdrawal?

Manifestations of nicotine withdrawal can occur within 2–8 hours of the last cigarette. In fact, most moderate to heavy smokers experience some withdrawal symptoms as they wake up each morning. Withdrawal reaches maximum intensity at 24–48 hours, then diminishes over a 2-week period of abstinence. After 1 month, symptoms are gone, except for the cravings for cigarettes and an increase in appetite.[6,67] Approximately 80% of smokers experience withdrawal symptoms when quitting, and withdrawal is nearly universal among smokers using 20 or more cigarettes per day.[6] Nicotine withdrawal is not confined to cigarette smokers alone. The same syndrome is reported in smokeless tobacco users and chronic users of nicotine chewing gum.[6,52]

Most of the symptoms associated with tobacco withdrawal are subjective, leading to an overall feeling of dysphoria. These manifestations, widely described in the literature, are summarized in Table 71–5.[16,32,33,38,52,81] The most dramatic and intense symptom of tobacco abstinence is a craving for cigarettes, which can continue for months to years.[6] Cravings for cigarettes are less intense and diminish more quickly in people who are totally abstinent, as compared to those who are only partially abstinent.[67]

One study evaluated seven smokers in a battery of computerized performance tasks over a 24-hour period of abstinence. With increasing abstinence, the smoker's

TABLE 71–5. CLINICAL MANIFESTATIONS OF NICOTINE WITHDRAWAL

Subjective	Objective
Anger/aggression/hostility	Decreased arousal pattern on EEG
Anxiety	Decreased blood pressure
Blurred vision	Decreased heart rate
Confusion	Diminished psychomotor performance
Constipation	Impaired short-term memory
Craving for cigarettes	Reduced plasma catecholamines
Drowsiness	Weight gain
Gastrointestinal upset	
Headache	
Hunger	
Impaired concentration	
Irritability/impatience	
Moodiness	
Restlessness	
Sleep disturbance	

responses showed increased latencies and decreased accuracy.[72] Moreover, EEG studies evaluating smokers in withdrawal show a decrease in high-frequency activity and an increase in low-frequency activity, consistent with diminished arousal.[33]

The most common objective physical manifestation of nicotine abstinence is a decrease in heart rate by a mean of 9 beats/min within the first day of abstinence; it is a unique feature of nicotine withdrawal syndrome.[32] This decrease remains constant when measured over the next 5 weeks of abstinence, suggesting that heart rate reduction in tobacco abstinence reflects the absence of stimulation from nicotine, rather than withdrawal symptomatology.[82] Plasma levels of epinephrine and norepinephrine also decrease in abstinent smokers. This is probably another manifestation of the absence of nicotine effect and undoubtedly contributes to the reduction in mean heart rate.[19]

How Are Patients With Acute Nicotine Withdrawal Treated?

In clinical practice, nicotine withdrawal syndrome is encountered when tobacco users attempt to quit in the interest of their long-term health or when acute illness forces abstinence. The discomfort is a primary obstacle to smoking cessation and contributes significantly, but not solely, to the low success rate of attempts to quit smoking. Therefore, any treatment approach that lessens nicotine withdrawal symptoms, without reinitiating the use of tobacco products, is more likely to aid the effort to quit, which in turn will have many long-term health benefits.

Nicotine Replacement Therapy

One approach to the treatment of nicotine abstinence syndrome is to provide nicotine without tobacco. This therapy offers nicotine in a safer, more clinically controllable form that minimizes nicotine withdrawal symptoms. Once the patient breaks the smoking habit, the nicotine replacement is gradually tapered.[30,62]

Nicotine gum, the oldest of the nicotine substitution therapies, ameliorates many, but not all, symptoms of nicotine withdrawal. It is especially effective in relieving feelings of irritability, aggression, and dysphoria. However, it seems less effective in eliminating cigarette craving and increased hunger.[10]

The effectiveness of nicotine chewing gum in promoting long-term smoking abstinence has been extensively studied.[35,75,76] A meta-analysis of all these studies, with special emphasis on double-blind, randomized, placebo-controlled trials with 1 or more years of follow-up study, indicates that nicotine chewing gum in conjunction with a formal program of behavioral therapy can produce 1-year abstinence rates of 29–49%.[1,6,34,78] It is likely that nicotine gum treatment is most useful with the most nicotine-dependent smokers.[4] Some studies also support the conclusion that 4-mg gum is more effective than 2-mg gum in treating highly dependent smokers, but no more effective than 2-mg gum in treating moderate- to low-dependency smokers.[6,64,75] On the other hand, when nicotine gum is used in general medical practice, without structured behavioral interventions, improvement in smoking abstinence is short-lived and smoking cessation rates at 6–12 months are similar to those of placebo-treated patients.[4,6,35]

Unfortunately, many smokers who use nicotine gum to quit develop dependency on the gum itself. As an adjunct to smoking cessation, nicotine gum should be used for a maximum of 3 months. However, several studies have reported continued use of the gum at 1-year follow-up (6–38% of users.).[6,29,31] Extended use of the gum is particularly prevalent among lapse-free smoking abstainers.[29]

There are other problems that make nicotine gum less than perfect as a smoking-cessation therapy. The gum has to be chewed correctly, and many patients are unable to master the technique. If the gum is not chewed slowly, for limited periods of time, and then placed between the cheek and gums, patients can develop adverse effects such as nausea, heartburn, oral irritation, and hiccups. Some users find the peppery taste unpleasant. Moreover, gum chewing is not socially permissible in all situations.[63,67,79] Finally, self-administration of the gum may reinforce some of the behavioral patterns that sustain smoking. It can be argued that the behavioral components of the addictive process must be decisively interrupted for successful treatment of the addiction.[59]

Transdermal nicotine systems (TNSs) have supplanted chewing gum as the preferred nicotine replacement therapy. Because nicotine patches are easier to use (they require once-a-day application) compliance is better. The dose of nicotine delivered to the patient is more predictable, nicotine steady-state levels in the blood are higher, and the different-size patches make tapering easier to control. Finally, because no specific behavioral action is required of the patient, other than putting the patch on in the morning, a TNS does not require self-administration of nicotine by the user and therefore does not mimic smoking behavior.[59,62]

There are four patch systems currently available, each of which has several different doses of nicotine. Three of the patch systems are designed for 24-hour use, and the newest is made for 16-hour use to approximate more closely nicotine concentrations of the smoker.[54] The patches generally deliver steady-state nicotine plasma concentrations of 10–15 ng/mL, which are maintained throughout the application of the patch.[28] Whenever studied, the patches have effectively diminished some but not all subjective nicotine withdrawal symptoms. As with nicotine gum, negative affect and dysphoria are more effectively diminished by the patch than are cigarette craving and increased appetite.[62]

Several double-blind, placebo controlled studies have demonstrated that, at 6–12-month follow-up, TNS users achieve abstinence two to four times more frequently than placebo users.[16,21,26,78,79] And many studies have now demonstrated that this long-term efficacy is present even with little or no formal behavioral intervention accompanying the program.[1,14,16,78]

Nicotine patches are generally better tolerated and produce fewer adverse effects than nicotine gum. The most consistent adverse effect of the patches is skin irritation at the side of the patch. Generally this consists of transient erythema, which resolves within 24 hours of patch removal.[16] Some patients develop a persistent contact dermatitis, which may require topical corticosteroids and antihistamine treatment.[62] In one trial, approximately 5% of patients withdrew from the study because they could not tolerate the cutaneous irritation.[1]

Other adverse effects of TNSs include nausea, vertigo, and headache,[78] which are more likely to occur if the patient continues to smoke while using the patch. Because patch systems generally are available in only two or three sizes, it is difficult to achieve the appropriate dosage in some instances. For example, it is not possible to increase the dose slightly to treat persistent cigarette cravings or lower the dose slightly to prevent unwanted adverse effects.[78]

As TNS treatment has become widespread, a number of cases of myocardial ischemia associated with patch use have been reported. Acute MIs were reported in users, with and without a previous history of heart disease, who continued to smoke or remained abstinent.[15,58,80] However, it is important to remember that smoking places the patient at greater risk for ischemic events than nicotine replacement therapy alone, by producing higher maximal serum nicotine levels and reducing blood oxygen. Moreover, lower dose TNSs have not been associated with a higher frequency of cardiac events in patients with stable coronary artery disease[85] and offer a higher probability of achieving abstinence than untreated quitting.

For a short period of time, "smoke-free cigarettes" were marketed in the United States as a healthier alternative to smoking. These are aerosol rods designed to deliver puffs of nicotine vapor without lighting up. They offered the possibility of delivering nicotine to the lungs in the same bolus fashion as cigarettes without any of the other harmful effects of smoking. However, it was discovered that normal puffing on these rods delivered no detectable nicotine in the blood or urine.[66] Only intensive puffing over time generates a very slow increase in blood nicotine, and most of this nicotine is probably absorbed in the mouth, not through the alveoli.[63] These products have been removed from the market.

Both nicotine nasal spray and nicotine oral inhalers reduce withdrawal symptoms and promote abstinence more effectively than placebo.[42,74,77] Both treatment modalities are based on the belief that airway stimulation will mimic smoking more closely and therefore be more effective in reducing cigarette cravings. Although this is probably correct, the reproduction of smoking's airway sensations might actually make long-term abstinence more difficult to achieve.

To date there have been no head-to-head comparisons of any of the nicotine replacement therapies (NRTs). TNSs seems to be more effective than nicotine gum in reducing cigarette craving and increased appetite.[62] In one study, TNSs effectively controlled weight gain: Placebo patients gained an average of 4.4 kg more than TNS-treated patients.[1] A meta-analysis of 53 NRT trials, with data from over 17,000 patients, concluded that all modalities were better than placebo in promting abstinence at 6 or more months. The nicotine oral inhaler had the best abstinence odds ratio, but this is based on data from only one study, while nicotine gum had the lowest odds ratio.[68]

Other Treatment Modalities

Clearly, nicotine replacement therapies are moderately effective in promoting smoking cessation, especially in the short run. To be successful, the patient must eventually face the inevitable—withdrawal from nicotine itself. Ideally, if other treatment modalities effectively promote tobacco abstinence without the use of nicotine replacement they would have a substantial advantage. Other drugs studied in smoking cessation experiments include clonidine, doxepin, sertraline, and mecamylamine.

Clonidine is an $alpha_2$-adrenergic agonist that is somewhat successful in the treatment of opioid and alcohol withdrawal. Although the exact mechanism is not fully understood, it is theorized that clonidine is effacacious in all withdrawal syndromes because it inhibits noradrenergic neurons in the locus ceruleus. Adrenergic hyperactivity in the locus ceruleus might be the common thread of many withdrawal syndromes. In a placebo-controlled trial of 71 smokers, oral clonidine in doses of 150–200 μg/day for 4 weeks was successful in promoting abstinence. At 6-month follow-up, 27% of the clonidine-treated patients were still abstinent, compared to only 5% of the placebo-treated patients. Clonidine proved particularly successful with women smokers. However, abstinence was measured only by self-report.[24] A later study tested the effect of transdermal clonidine patches on withdrawal symptoms. Clonidine patches deliver steady-state dosing for 7 days and produce fewer adverse effects than tablets. This trial demonstrated that clonidine significantly decreased feelings of irritability, anxiety, and restlessness associated with tobacco abstinence and that it was particularly effective in treating the craving for cigarettes. However, there was no effective reduction in hunger or impairment of concentration. Moreover, 6 of the 19 patients who received clonidine patches were unable to complete the study due to adverse effects of hypotension, tachycardia, headache, sedation, visual disturbances, and dizziness.[57] This high incidence of intolerable effects would seem to limit the applicability of clonidine in smoking-cessation treatment. It is possible, however, that a lower-dose patch might be as effective, with fewer adverse effects.

Doxepin, a cyclic antidepressant, has been applied to smoking withdrawal treatment regimens based on the theory that it might relieve the dysphoric symptoms of withdrawal, particularly irritability, anxiety, diminished concentration, and depression. In one small pilot study,

8 women receiving doxepin for 5 weeks were compared to 21 women receiving no pharmacologic intervention. At the end of 5 weeks twice as many women in the doxepin group were abstinent. These patients also experienced significantly less withdrawal symptom severity.[18] Sertraline (Zoloft), a serotonin reuptake inhibitor, reduced hyperphagia and weight gain during nicotine withdrawal in nicotine-dependent rats.[40] The efficacy of doxepin and other cyclic antidepressants in the treatment of nicotine withdrawal and smoking cessation as a primary or adjuvant therapy deserves further consideration.

One fascinating study compared the combination of mecamylamine—a competitive nicotine antagonist—and nicotine patch to patch alone in a placebo-controlled, double-blind trail of smoking cessation in 48 smokers. The mecamylamine plus patch group reported fewer withdrawal symptoms, and abstinence rates for this agonist–antagonist group were significantly better at 7 weeks and 12 months.[61]

Finally, it should be noted that although several agents will reduce the severity of nicotine withdrawal, long-term smoking cessation is more difficult to achieve. In many approaches to smoking treatment, the overall mean 6–12-month success rate seems to be approximately 25%.[59] This is, of course, much better than the spontaneous abstinence rate of 1%, but 70–80% of patients who achieve initial abstinence will be smoking again after 1 year.[18] Whatever approach one takes in treating tobacco abstinence, it seems the patient must start with a strong desire to quit, avoid unusually stressful situations, and have a social support network that encourages the effort to stop smoking. The most successful programs are multimodality treatments that combine counseling or other behavioral therapies with a pharmacologic intervention.

References

1. Abelin T, Muller P, Buehler A, et al: Controlled trial of transdermal nicotine patch in tobacco withdrawal. Lancet 1989;1:7–10.
2. Armitage AK, Dollery CT, George CF, et al: Absorption and metabolism of nicotine from cigarettes. Br Med J 1975;4: 313–316.
3. Ballard T, Ehler J, Freund E, et al: Green tobacco sickness: Occupational poisoning in tobacco workers. Arch Environ Health 1995;50:384–389.
4. Benowitz NL: Nicotine replacement therapy during pregnancy. JAMA 1991;266:3174–3177.
5. Benowitz NL: Nicotine and smokeless tobacco. CA: Cancer J Clin 1988;38:244–247.
6. Benowitz NL: Pharmacologic aspects of cigarette smoking and nicotine addiction. N Engl J Med 1988;319:1318–1330.
7. Benowitz NL, Jones RT, Jacob P: Additive cardiovascular effects of nicotine and ethanol. Clin Pharmacol Ther 1986; 40:420–424.
8. Bonadio WA, Anderson Y: Tobacco ingestions in children. Clin Pediatr 1989;28:592–593.
9. Borys DJ, Seltzer SC, Ling LJ: CNS depression in an infant after the ingestion of tobacco: A case report. Vet Hum Toxicol 1988;30:20–22.
10. Cherek DR, Bennett RH, Grabowski J: Human aggressive responding during acute tobacco abstinence: Effects of nicotine and placebo gum. Psychopharmacology 1991;104: 317–322.
11. Connolly GN, Orleans CT, Kogan M: Use of smokeless tobacco in major-league baseball. N Engl J Med 1988;318: 1281–1284.
12. Consensus Conference: Health applications of smokeless tobacco use. JAMA 1986;255:1045–1048.
13. Council on Scientific Affairs: Health effects of smokeless tobacco. JAMA 1986;255:1038–1044.
14. Cummings KM, Biernbaum RM, Zevon MA, et al: Use and effectiveness of transdermal nicotine in primary care settings. Arch Fam Med 1994;3:682–689.
15. DaCosta A, Guy JM, Tardy B, et al: Myocardial infarction and nicotine patch: A contributing or causative factor? Eur Heart J 1993;14:1709–1711.
16. Daughton DM, Heatley SA, Prendergast JJ, et al: Effect of transdermal nicotine delivery as an adjunct to low-intervention smoking cessation therapy. Arch Intern Med 1991; 151:749–752.
17. Dubick MA, Palmer R, Lau PP, et al: Altered exocrine pancreatic function in rats treated with nicotine. Toxicol Appl Pharmacol 1988;96:132–139.
18. Edwards NB, Simmons RC, Rosenthal TL, et al: Doxepin in the treatment of nicotine withdrawal. Psychosomatics 1988;29:203–206.
19. Elgerot A: Psychological and physiological changes during tobacco-abstinence in habitual smokers. J Clin Psychol 1978; 34:759–764.
20. Ernster VL, Grady DG, Greene JC, et al: Smokeless tobacco use and health effects among baseball players. JAMA 1990; 264:218–224.
21. Fiore MC, Smith SS, Jorenby DE, Baker TB: Effectiveness of nicotine patch for smoking cessation. A meta-analysis. JAMA 1994;271:1940–1947.
22. Garcia-Estrada H, Fischman C: An unusual case of nicotine poisoning. Clin Toxicol 1977;10:391–393.
23. Gelbach SH: Green tobacco sickness. JAMA 1974;229: 1880–1883.
24. Glassman AH, Stetner F, Walsh T, et al: Heavy smokers, smoking cessation and clonidine. JAMA 1988;259: 2863–2866.
25. Goepferd SJ: Smokeless tobacco: A potential hazard to infants and children. J Am Dent Assoc 1986;113:49–50.
26. Gourlay S: The pros and cons of transdermal nicotine therapy. Med J Aust 1994; 160:152–159.
27. Gross JY, D'Alessandri R, Powell VL, Rodeheaver A: Smokeless tobacco: Health hazard on the rise. South Med J 1988;81:1089–1091.
28. Gupta SK, Okerholm RA, Coen P, et al: Single and multiple dose pharmacokinetics of Nicoderm. J Clin Pharmacol 1993;33:169–174.
29. Hajek P, Jackson P, Belcher M: Long-term use of nicotine chewing gum: Occurrence, determinants and effect on weight gain. JAMA 1988;260:1593–1596.
30. Henningfield JE: Improving the diagnosis and treatment of nicotine dependence. JAMA 1988; 260:1613–1614.

31. Hughes JR, Gust SW, Keenan R, et al: Long-term use of nicotine versus placebo gum. Arch Intern Med 1991;151: 1993–1998.
32. Hughes JR, Higgins ST, Bickel WK: Nicotine withdrawal versus other drug withdrawal syndromes: Similarities and dissimilarities. Addiction 1994;89:1461–1470.
33. Jaffe JH: Drug addiction and drug abuse. In: Gilman AG, Rall TW, Nies AS, Taylor P, eds: Goodman and Gilman's The Pharmacological Basis of Therapeutics, 8th ed. New York, Pergamon Press, 1990, pp. 545–549.
34. Jarvik ME: Beneficial effects of nicotine. Br J Addict 1991; 86:571–575.
35. Jensen EJ, Schmidt E, Pedersen B, Dahl R: Effect of nicotine, silver acetate and ordinary gum in combination with group counseling on smoking cessation. Thorax 1990;45:831–834.
36. Jusko WJ: Influence of cigarette smoking on drug metabolism in man. Drug Metab Rev 1979; 9:221–236.
37. Kazlowski LT, Wilkinson DA, Skinner W, et al: Comparing tobacco cigarette dependence with other drug dependencies. JAMA 1989;261:898–901.
38. Kumar R, Cooke EC, Lader MH, Russell MAH: Is nicotine important in tobacco smoking? Clin Pharmacol Ther 1976; 21:520–529.
39. Kunkel DB: The toxic emergency: Tobacco and friends. Emerg Med 1985;17:142–158.
40. Levin ED, Briggs SJ, Christopher NC, Rose JE: Sertraline attenuates hyperphagia in rats following nicotine withdrawal. Pharmacol Biochem Behav 1993;44:51–61.
41. Lunell E, Molander L, Andersson M: Relative bioavailability of nicotine from a nasal spray in infectious rhinitis and after use of a topical decongestant. Eur J Clin Pharmacol 1995;48:71–75.
42. Lunell E, Molander L, Leischow SJ, Fagerstrom KO: The effect of nicotine vapour inhalation on the relief of tobacco withdrawal symptoms. Eur J Clin Pharmacol 1995;48: 235–240.
43. Luntz-Leybman V, Freund RK, Collins AC: 5-alpha-Pregnane-3 alpha-ol-20-one blocks nicotine-induced seizures and enhanced paired-pulse inhibition. Eur J Pharmacol 1990;185:239–242.
44. Malin DH, Lake JR, Carter VA, et al: Naloxone precipitates nicotine abstinence syndrome in the rat. Psychopharmacology 1993;112:339–342.
45. Malizia E, Andreucci E, Alfani F, et al: Acute intoxication with nicotine alkaloids and cannabinoids in children from ingestion of cigarettes. Hum Toxicol 1983;2:315–316.
46. Marion DJ, Fortmann SP: Nicotine yield and measures of cigarette smoke exposure in a large population. Am J Public Health 1987;77:546–549.
47. Martin TJ, Suchocki J, May EL, Martin BR: Pharmacological evaluation of the antagonism of nicotine's central effects by mecamylamine and pempidine. J Pharmacol Exp Ther 1990; 251:45–51.
48. Matsushima D, Prevo ME, Gorsline J: Absorption and adverse effects following topical and oral administration of three transdermal nicotine products to dogs. J Pharm Sci 1995;84:365–369.
49. McKnight RH, Levine EJ, Rodgers GC: Detection of green tobacco sickness by a regional poison center. Vet Hum Toxicol 1994;36:505–510.
50. McNeil Consumer Products Co: Manufacturer's Product Information. March 1996.
51. Mensch AR, Holden M: Nicotine overdose after a single piece of nicotine gum. Chest 1984; 86:801–802.
52. Morse RM, Norvich RC, Graf JA: Tobacco chewing: An unusual case of drug dependence. Mayo Clin Proc 1977;52: 358–360.
53. Mulligan SC, Masterson JG, Devane JG, Kelly JG: Clinical and pharmacokinetic properties of a transdermal nicotine patch. Clin Pharmacol Ther 1990;47:331–337.
54. Nicotine patches. Med Lett 1992;34:37–38.
55. Obsert BB, McIntyre RA: Acute nicotine poisoning. Pediatrics 1953;11:338–340.
56. O'Hara P, Portser SA, Anderson BP: The influence of menstrual cycle changes on the tobacco withdrawal syndrome in women. Addict Behav 1989;14:595–600.
57. Ornish KA, Zisook S, McAdams LA: Effects of transdermal clonidine treatment on withdrawal systems associated with smoking cessation. Arch Intern Med 1988;148:2027–2031.
58. Otterranger JP, Festen JM, deVries AG, Stricker BH: Acute myocardial infarction while using the nicotine patch. Chest 1995;107:1765–1766.
59. Peters JA: Nicotine-replacement therapy in cessation of smoking. Mayo Clin Proc 1990;65:1619–1623.
60. Rahal PS, Wright RA: Transdermal nicotine and gastroesophageal reflux. Am J Gastroenterol 1995;90:919–921.
61. Rose JE, Behm FM, Westman EC, et al: Mecamylamine combined with nicotine skin patch facilitates smoking cessation beyond nicotine patch alone. Clin Pharmacol Ther 1994;56: 86–99.
62. Rose JE, Levin ED, Behm FM, et al: Transdermal nicotine facilitates smoking cessation. Clin Pharmacol Ther 1990;47: 323–330.
63. Russell MAH, Jarvis MJ, Sutherland G, Feyerabend C: Nicotine replacement in smoking cessation: Absorption of nicotine vapor from smoke-free cigarettes. JAMA 1987;257: 3262–3265.
64. Sach DP: Effectiveness of the 4-mg dose of nicotine polacrilex for the initial treatment of high-dependent smokers. Arch Intern Med 1995;155:1973–1980.
65. Saxena K: Suicide plan by nicotine poisoning: A review of nicotine toxicity. Vet Hum Toxicol 1985;27:495–497.
66. Sepkovic DW, Colosimo SG, Axelrad CM, et al: The delivery and uptake of nicotine from an aerosol rod. Am J Public Health 1986;76:1343–1344.
67. Shiffman SM, Jarvik ME: Smoking withdrawal symptoms in two weeks of abstinence. Psychopharmacology 1976;50: 35–39.
68. Silagy C, Mant D, Fowler G, Lodge M: The effectiveness of nicotine replacement therapies in smoking cessation. Online J. Curr Clin Trials 1994; Doc# 113.
69. Singer J, Janz T: Apnea and seizures caused by nicotine ingestion. Pediatr Emerg Care 1990;6:135–137.
70. Smokeless Tobacco. Facts and Comparisons. Lawrence Review of Natural Products, June 1990.
71. Smolinske SC, Spoerke DG, Spiller SK, et al: Cigarette and nicotine chewing gum toxicity in children. Hum Toxicol 1988;7:27–31.
72. Sunder FR, Davis FC, Henninfield JE: The tobacco withdrawal syndrome: Performance decrements assessed on a

computerized test battery. Drug Alcohol Depend 1989;23: 259–266.

73. Surgeon General's Report: The health consequences of smoking. Nicotine addition: A report of the Surgeon General. U. S. Dept. of Health and Human Services, 1988.
74. Sutherland G, Stapleton JA, Russell MAH, et al: Randomized controlled trial of nasal nicotine spray in smoking cessation. Lancet 1992;340:324–329.
75. Tonnesen P, Fryd V, Hansen M, et al: Effect of nicotine chewing gum in combination with group counseling on the cessation of smoking. N Engl J Med 1988;318: 15–18.
76. Tonnesen P, Fryd V, Hansen M, et al: Two and four milligram nicotine chewing gum and group counseling in smoking cessation. Addict Behav 1988;13:17–27
77. Tonnesen P, Norregaard J, Mikkelsen K, et al: A double-blind trial of a nicotine inhaler for smoking cessation. JAMA 1993;269:1268–1271.
78. Tonnesen P, Norregaard J, Simonsen K, Sawe U: A double-blind trial of a 16-hour transdermal nicotine patch in smoking cessation. N Engl J Med 1991;325:311–315.
79. Transdermal Nicotine Study Group: Transdermal nicotine for smoking cessation. JAMA 1991;266:3133–3138.
80. Warner JG, Little WC: Myocardial infarction in a patient who smoked while wearing a nicotine patch. Ann Intern Med 1994;120:695. Letter.
81. West R, Russell MA. Loss of acute nicotine tolerance and severity of cigarette withdrawal. Psychopharmacology 1988;94:563–565.
82. West R, Schneider N: Drop in heart rate following smoking cessation may be permanent. Psychopharmacology 1988; 94:566–568.
83. Woolf A, Burkhart K, Caraccio T, Litovitz T: Childhood poisoning involving transdermal nicotine patches. Pediatrics (electronic pages) 1997;99:724(e4).
84. Woolf A, Burkhart K, Caraccio T, Litovitz T: Self-poisoning among adults using multiple transdermal nicotine patches. J Toxicol Clin Toxicol 1996;34:691–698.
85. Working Group for the Study of Transdermal Nicotine in Patients with Coronary Artery Disease: Nicotine replacement therapy for patients with coronary artery disease. Arch Intern Med 1994;154:989–995.

CHAPTER 72

Food Poisoning

Michael G. Tunik and Lewis R. Goldfrank

CASE 1. A 29-year-old man was admitted to the emergency department (ED) complaining of persistent vomiting, abdominal cramps, and diarrhea. The patient related that every year his family gathers to perform the "rites of spring." Each participant brings his or her own culinary specialty for the feast. The patient was well before the meal; he took no medication, did not smoke, and drank only wine socially. At the feast he ate numerous hors d'oeuvres, freshly prepared: home-grown eggplant; deviled eggs; gefilte fish with fresh, homemade horseradish; liver paté; and assorted cheeses. He ate large portions of several main courses, which included exotic Chinese, Italian, and Middle Eastern preparations. Dessert included several slices of Boston cream pie and rhubarb pie, and the feast was concluded with coffee and chocolate dessert truffles. Participants concluded the "rites of spring" by consuming ice-cold water drawn from a local spring.

The patient became nauseated and dizzy about 15 minutes after dessert. Shortly thereafter he began retching and vomiting. The vomitus was initially particulate; then it became bilious, and finally it contained persistently bloody material. He also had several bouts of bloody diarrhea mixed with mucus.

The patient's history was unremarkable, and review of systems was entirely negative. Physical examination showed him to be well-nourished and ill-appearing. His vital signs were: blood pressure, 130/75 mm Hg, with no orthostatic changes; pulse, 120 beats/min and regular; respirations, 20 breaths/min; and temperature, 101.3°F (38.5°C).

His skin, eyes, ears, nose, throat, heart, and lung and neurologic examinations were normal. Abdominal examination showed voluntary guarding, active bowel sounds, and no hepatosplenomegaly or masses. A nasogastric tube was inserted, and the aspirate was positive for occult blood. Rectal examination revealed blood and mucus.

The 12-lead ECG demonstrated sinus tachycardia at 120 beats/min with a normal QT_c interval. Chest and abdominal radiographs were normal. A complete blood count revealed a hematocrit of 53% with a normal platelet estimate and a WBC count of 7700/mm^3. The differential count showed 80% polymorphonuclear forms, 10% bands, and 10% lymphocytes. Electrolytes, BUN, creatinine, amylase, and urinalysis were normal.

A Gram stain and methylene blue stain of the stool showed many polymorphonuclear cells, mononuclear cells, and diverse enteric flora. A saline preparation showed no parasites. Sigmoidoscopy showed hyperemic nonfriable mucosa. The patient's vomitus, stool, and blood were cultured. While these diagnostic and therapeutic procedures were being performed, an attempt was made to contact other family members who attended the party.

Which Agents Cause a Combination of Bloody Diarrhea, Hematemesis, and an Elevated Temperature?

The initial differential diagnosis for acute diarrhea involves several etiologies: infectious (bacterial, viral, parasitic, and fungal), structural (including surgical), metabolic, functional, toxin-induced, and food-induced. The differential diagnosis is described in greater detail in Chapter 22.

The most common causes of foodborne disease include bacterial: *Salmonella* spp, *Shigella* spp, *Clostridium perfringens*, *Staphylococcus aureus*, *Campylobacter* spp, *Bacillus cereus*, *Escherichia coli*, group A *Streptococcus*, *Clostridium botulinum*, *Vibrio cholera*, viral: hepatitis A, E, F, and G, Norwalk virus; parasitic: *Giardia lamblia*, *Trichinella spiralis;* fishborne: scombrotoxin, ciguatoxin, paralytic shellfish; and chemical: heavy metals, mushrooms, monosodium glutamate[13] (Table 72–1).

An elevated temperature may be caused by invasive organisms, including *Salmonella* spp, *Shigella* spp, *Campylobacter* spp, invasive *E. coli*, *Vibrio parahaemolyticus*, and *Yersinia* spp, as well as some viruses. Episodes of acute gastroenteritis not associated with fever are usually caused by organisms producing toxins, including *S. aureus*, *B. cereus*, *C. perfringens*, enterotoxigenic *E. coli*, and viruses.[94]

Fecal leukocytes are typically found in patients with shigellosis, salmonellosis, campylobacter enteritis, typhoid fever, invasive *E. coli* colitis, *V. parahaemolyticus*, *Y. enterocolitica*, and ulcerative colitis. In all of these except typhoid fever, the leukocytes are primarily polymorphonuclear, whereas in typhoid they are mononuclear. No stool leukocytes are noted in cholera, viral diarrhea, noninvasive *E. coli* diarrhea, or nonspecific diarrhea.[57]

The onset of diarrhea after exposure or incubation period can be useful. Extremely short incubation periods of less than 6 hours are typical for *Staphylococcus*, *B. cereus* (type I) and enterotoxigenic *E. coli*,[88,122,146] preformed enterotoxins, as well as roundworm larvae ingestions. Intermediate incubation periods of 8–24 hours are found with *C. perfringens*, *B. cereus* (type II enterotoxin), enteroinvasive *E. coli*, [30,93] and salmonella. Longer incubation periods are seen in other bacterial causes of acute gastroenteritis (Table 72–2).

In Case 1, the three etiologies most likely involved are infectious, drug or chemical toxin–induced, and food-induced. The differential diagnosis must be made among these groups. The time from exposure to onset of symptoms was 2–4 hours, which serves to eliminate all of the nonbacterial etiologies (viral, parasitic, fungal, and algal) except for upper GI invasion by roundworm larvae. Anisakiasis is unlikely, as no raw fish that carry anisakiasis were consumed. The possibility of a bacterial etiology with enterotoxin production should be considered. All bacterial causes except *S. aureus*, *B. cereus* (type I), and enterotoxigenic *E. coli* were eliminated by the time from exposure to onset of symptoms (Table 72–1).[38,48]

TABLE 72–1. EPIDEMIOLOGY OF FOODBORNE POISONINGS REPORTED TO THE CDC 1988–1992

Etiology	Cases	Outbreaks	Deaths
Salmonella spp	21,177	549	38
Shigella spp	4,788	25	0
Clostridium perfringens	3,801	40	1
Hepatitis A	2,109	43	6
Staphylococcus aureus	1,678	50	0
Campylobacter spp	732	27	2
Scombroid	514	76	1
B. cereus	433	21	0
Norwalk virus	292	2	0
E. coli[a]	244	11	0
Trichinosis	195	36	0
Giardia spp	184	7	0
Ciguatera	176	42	0
Group A *Streptococcus*	135	2	0
C. botulinum	133	60	11
Shellfish	65	5	2
V. cholera	34	4	1
Heavy metals	26	3	0
V. parahaemolyticus	21	4	0
Mushrooms	18	5	0

[a]The fatality rate of *E. coli* 0157:H7 increased dramatically in the late 1990s.

What Epidemiologic Techniques Can Be Used to Assist in the Diagnosis?

Epidemiologic analysis is of immediate importance, particularly when gastrointestinal (GI) diseases strike more than one person in a group. The questions raised in Table 72–3 must be answered.[125] If available, the infectious disease consultant or the infection control staff should be called for assistance. Alternatively, state and local health departments should become involved. Often only the Centers for Disease Control or state health department have the resources to confirm a presumptive diagnosis in an outbreak. Sophisticated techniques such as detection of a toxin, matching the organism in the food by phage type with a food handler, matching an organism by phage type with numerous persons, the isolation of 10 or more organisms per gram of implicated food,[30,38] or polymerase chain reaction identification of bacterial or plasmid DNA are potentially useful although generally not possible using the laboratory and personnel available in most hospitals. [47,59,139]

In Case 1, several other family members were located who were also ill. The duration of the illness in the other family members was 2–4 hours. However, none of the other afflicted members reported vomiting and diarrhea to the extent experienced by our patient, and none reported a bloody component in the diarrhea. The patient's history and epidemiologic survey of the family enabled structural, metabolic, and functional causes to be eliminated. In these diseases neither a significant grouping of cases nor a limited clinical history is generally present. Foodborne parasites such as *Trichinella spiralis* (trichinosis), *Toxoplasma gondii* (toxoplasmosis), and *G. lamblia* (giardiasis) must be considered, but none was likely in this episode as the symptom complexes are distinctly different.

In cases of suspected food poisoning with a short incubation period, the physician should first assess the risk for staphylococcal causes. The usual foods to consider as the milieu of staphylococcal toxin production include milk products and other proteinaceous foods, cream-filled baked goods (Boston cream pie), potato and

TABLE 72–2. COMMON FOODBORNE DISEASE: GASTROINTESTINAL (PRIMARY PRESENTING SYMPTOM)

		Symptoms							
Etiology	**Onset**	***A***	***V***	***Di***	***Dy***	***F***	**Source**	**Pathogenesis**	**Therapy**
Staphylococcus spp	2–6 h	+	+	+	−	−	Prepared foods: meats, pastries, salads	Heat-stable enterotoxin	Volume expansion
Bacillus cereus									
Type I	1–6 h	+	+	+	−	−	Fried rice	Heat-labile toxins	Volume expansion
Type II	12 h	+	−	+	−	−	Meats, vegetables	Heat-labile toxins	
Anasikiasis	1–12 h	+	+	−	−	−	Raw fish, sushi, Eustrongyloides, minnows, salmon, cod, herring, squid, tuna	Intestinal larvae	Endoscopy Laparotomy Removal
Clostridium perfringens	8–24 h	+	±	+	+	−	Poultry, heat-processed meats	Heat-labile enterotoxin	Volume expansion
Salmonella spp	8–24 h	±	±	+	±	+	Poultry, egg Pets (turtles, lizards, chicks)	Bacteria, endotoxin (Bacteremia)	Antibiotics
E. coli	24–72 h						Water, food,	Enterotoxin,	Volume expansion
Enterotoxigenic		±	−	±	±	+	Enteric contact	heat stable	Electrolytes
Invasive							Bacteria (invasive)		Antibiotics
Hemorrhagic							Shiga like toxin		Renal, hematologic support
Vibrio cholera	24–72 h	±	±	+	−	±	Water, food Enteric contact	Enterotoxin Heat labile	Electrolyte replacement
Shigella spp	24–72 h	+	±	+	+	±	Institutional food handler Household, preschool, enteric contact	Bacteria, Endotoxin	Antibiotics
Campylobacter jejuni	1–7 d	+	+	+	±	+	Milk, poultry Unchlorinated water Mimic appendicitis	Bacteria Heat-labile enterotoxin	Antibiotics
Yersinia spp	1–7 d	+	+	+	±	+	Pork, milk, pets: (arthritis pharyngitis); rash	Bacteria Enterotoxin	Antibiotics

A = abdominal pain; V = vomiting; Di = diarrhea; Dy = dysentery; F = fever.

chicken salads, sausages, ham, tongue, and gravy. The crust of the pie acts as an insulator, maintaining the temperature of the cream filling and occasionally permitting toxin production even during refrigeration.[4] An assessment must routinely be made for the presence of lesions on the hand or nose of the food handlers. Unfortunately, "carriers" of enterotoxigenic staphylococci are difficult to recognize as they usually lack lesions and appear healthy.[59]

A fixed association between a particular food and an illness would be most helpful epidemiologically, but clinically this rarely occurs. Factors such as environment, host resistance, nature of the agent, and dose make the results surprisingly variable.

Staphylococcus Species

Patients with staphylococcal food poisoning rarely have a significant temperature elevation, although in a review of 2992 documented cases 16% had a subjective sense of fever.[59] Abdominal pain, nausea followed by vomiting, and diarrhea dominate the clinical findings. Diarrhea does not occur in the absence of nausea and vomiting. The mean incubation period is 4.4 hours with a mean duration of illness of 20 hours.

Salmonella Species

Salmonella enteritidis infections have become a great concern in the United States. Two particular outbreaks define very special problems. In the 1980s there were recurrent outbreaks associated with grade A eggs or food containing such eggs. In the past, such outbreaks of salmonella enteritis have been attributed to infection of the egg with salmonella (from the chicken's gastrointestinal tract) through cracks in the shell. More recently, outbreaks have involved noncracked, nonsoiled eggs.[95] In these cases, presumably the salmonella has infected the eggs before the shell was formed. In either case, people who consume raw or undercooked eggs are most at risk for salmonella enteritis. Raw eggs may be found as ingredients of chocolate mousse, hollandaise sauce, eggnog, raw egg–based milkshakes, caesar salads, and homemade ice cream. Whole, partially cooked eggs may be eaten as sunny-side-up or poached eggs.[138]

The second group of outbreaks was associated with

TABLE 72–3. EPIDEMIOLOGIC ANALYSIS OF GASTROINTESTINAL DISEASE

1. Is the occurrence of the disease in a large group significant enough to be consistent with foodborne disease (two or more cases)?
2. Is the symptomatology in affected individuals well defined and similar?
3. Is the onset time similar among affected group members (incubation)? Duration of illness?
4. What are the possible modes of transmission (ie, contact, food, water)?
5. Is there a relationship between the time of exposure of the group and the mode of transmission?
6. Do attack rates differ for age, gender, or occupation?
7. Can it be determined which foods were served and to whom? Can the items which were not eaten by those who did not become ill be identified?
8. What is the food-specific attack rate?
9. How was the food procured? How was it stored?
10. Was cooking technique adequate?
11. Was personnel hygiene acceptable?
12. Was there animal contamination?

raw milk,[113] which has become very popular in certain communities for unclear reasons. Inadequate microwave cooking also may cause small outbreaks.[34] Chronic diarrheal syndromes [104] of an ill-defined nature result. These outbreaks are of great concern because they frequently involve multiple drug-resistant salmonella infections.[143] Campylobacteriosis, brucellosis, listeriosis, and tuberculosis also result from consuming raw milk. Drinking pasteurized milk may not be protective. An outbreak of salmonellosis resulting in more than 16,000 culture-proven cases was traced to one Illinois dairy. The probable cause of the outbreak was a transfer line connecting raw and pasteurized milk containment tanks.[121]

Additional concern has developed over the widespread use of antibiotics in animal feed. Meats, poultry, and manure-fertilized vegetables now frequently contain resistant bacterial strains that place virtually the entire population at risk.[121,143]

The ownership of pet animals known to harbor salmonella also places families at risk. Chicks, turtles, and iguanas carry salmonella and frequently transmit the organism to household contacts, including infants, who are at particular risk for invasive disease.[2]

Campylobacter jejuni

Campylobacter jejuni, a curved gram-negative rod, is a major cause of bacterial enteritis. The organism is most commonly isolated in children younger than 5 years of age and in adults 20–40 years of age. *Campylobacter* enteritis outbreaks are more common in the summer months in temperate climates. Although most cases of *Campylobacter* enteritis are sporadic, outbreaks are associated with contaminated food and water.[145] The most frequent sources of *Campylobacter* in food are unpasteurized milk[160] and raw or undercooked poultry products.[35] Birds are a common reservoir, and small outbreaks are associated with contamination of milk by birds pecking milk-container tops.[134] Contaminated water supplies are also a frequent source of *Campylobacter* enteritis involving large numbers of individuals.[20] *C. jejuni* is heat-labile; cooking of food, pasteurization of milk, and chlorination of water prevent human transmission.

The incubation period for *Campylobacter* enteritis varies from 1 to 7 days (mean, 3 days). Typical symptoms include diarrhea, abdominal cramps, and fever. Other symptoms may include headache, vomiting, excessive gas, and malaise. The diarrhea may contain gross blood, and frequently leukocytes are present on microscopic examination.[35] Illness usually lasts 5–6 days (range, 1–8 days). Rarely, symptoms may last for several weeks. Severe presentations include lower GI hemorrhage, abdominal pain mimicking appendicitis, a typhoid like syndrome, reactive arthritis, and meningitis. The organism may be detected using polymerase chain reaction identification techniques.[44] Treatment is supportive emphasizing volume resuscitation. Oral erythromycin decreases fecal shedding of the organism but may not decrease the duration or severity of symptoms.

Group A *Streptococcus*

Bacterial infections not usually associated with food or food handling may occasionally be transmitted by food or food handling. Streptococcal pharyngitis has been associated with food prepared by an employee recuperating from pharyngitis. The food implicated was a rice dressing, which was not primarily composed of milk, eggs, or meat.[28]

Clostridium botulinum

Home-canned fruits and vegetables as well as commercial fish products are among the common foods causing botulism. The incubation period is usually 12–36 hours; typical symptoms include some initial GI symptoms, followed by malaise, fatigue, diplopia, dysphagia, and rapid development of small muscle incoordination.[81] In botulism, the toxin is irreversibly bound to the neuromuscular junction, where it impairs the presynaptic release of acetylcholine.[74] The diagnosis of botulism must be made immediately, and aggressive respiratory therapy must be initiated if the patient is to survive. Additional therapeutic measures include administering antitoxin (Chap. 73 and Antidotes in Depth: Botulinum Antitoxin). The differential diagnosis of botulism includes myasthenia gravis, atypical Guillain-Barré syndrome, tick-induced paralysis, and certain chemical ingestions (see Tables 73–1, 73–5).

Yersinia enterocolitica

Yersinia enterocolitica is a gram-negative coccobacillus that causes enteritis most frequently in children and young adults. Typical clinical features include fever, abdominal pain, and diarrhea, which usually contains mucus and blood.[8,142,156] Other associated symptoms include nausea, vomiting, anorexia, and weight loss. The incubation period may be 1 day to 1 week or more. Less common features include prolonged enteritis, arthritis, pharyngeal and hepatic involvement, and rash. *Yersinia* is a common pathogen in many animals, including dogs and pigs. Sources of human infection include milk products, raw pork products, infected household pets, and person-to-person transmission.[18,52,82] Infections may be diagnosed based on cultures of food, stool, blood, and, less frequently, skin abscesses, pharyngeal cultures, or cultures from other organ tissues (mesenteric lymph nodes, liver). *Yersinia* may also be identified with polymerase chain reaction.[66] Therapy is usually supportive; however, patients with invasive disease (eg, bacteremia, bacterial arthritis) should be treated with intravenous antibiotics. Ciprofloxacin and third-generation cephalosporins are highly bacteriocidal against *Yersinia* spp.

Listeria monocytogenes

Listeriosis transmitted by food usually occurs in pregnant women, their fetuses, the elderly, and immunocompromised individuals (corticosteroid use, malignancy, diabetes, renal disease, HIV infection).[15,129,152] Typical food sources include unpasteurized milk, soft cheeses such as feta, and undercooked chicken. Individuals at risk should avoid the usual sources and should be evaluated for listeriosis if typical symptoms of fever, severe headache, muscle ache, and pharyngitis develop. Treatment with intravenous ampicillin or trimethoprim–sulfamethoxazole is indicated for systemic listerial infections.

Drug- and Toxin-Induced Diseases

Careful assessment of the possibility of a foodborne pesticide poisoning is essential. Aldicarb contamination has occurred in hydroponically grown vegetables, and eating watermelons contaminated with pesticides has resulted in extensive anticholinesterase poisoning[50] (see Chap. 87).

The possibility of accidental acute heavy metal ingestion must also be considered. This type of poisoning most typically occurs when very acidic fruit punch is served in metal-lined containers. Antimony, zinc, copper, tin, or cadmium in a container may be dissolved by an acid food or juice medium. Insecticides, rodenticides, arsenic, lead, or fluoride preparations can be mistaken for a food ingredient. These poisonings usually have a rapid onset of signs and symptoms after the exposure.

Mushroom-Induced Disease

Some species produce major GI effects. *Amanita phalloides*, the most poisonous mushroom, usually causes GI symptoms as well as hepatotoxic effects, but its incubation period (6–10 hours) is slightly longer than was seen in this case (see Chap. 75).

Spicy Food

Certain religious or cultural customs, such as eating bitter herbs at a Passover seder[119] or wasabi [135] at a sushi bar, are associated with syncope. The precipitant in both instances is horseradish. No hematemesis, hematochezia, or fever is typically noted with horseradish. Gastric mucosal contact with pepperoni and jalapeno peppers (capsaicin) does not typically cause severe gastritis or gastric hemorrhage in normal individuals.[49]

Intestinal Parasitic Infections or "Japanese Restaurant Syndrome"

The popularity of eating raw fish, usually from Japanese restaurants, has led to an increase in reported intestinal parasitic infections. The etiologic agents are typically roundworms (*Eustrongylidis anisakis*) or fish tapeworms (*Diphyllobothrium* spp). Symptoms of anisakiasis or eustrongylidiasis that are localized to the stomach typically occur 1–12 hours after eating raw fish, while symptoms of lower intestinal involvement may be delayed for days or weeks. Typical gastric symptoms include nausea, vomiting, and severe crampy abdominal pain that may mimic a gastric ulcer; typical lower intestinal symptoms include abdominal cramping and, with perforation of the intestinal wall by the larvae, severe localized abdominal pain, rebound, and guarding, which may mimic an acute abdomen (appendicitis). Without an adequate dietary history (of eating raw fish), the diagnosis may be almost impossible to establish. Therapy would be directed toward the most likely diagnostic entity (gastric ulcer or appendicitis). Diagnosis is usually established on visual inspection of the larvae (on endoscopy, laparotomy, or pathologic examination), which are typically pink or red. Raw fish that may contain eustrongylides include minnows (*Fundulus* spp) and other bait fish. *Anisakis simplex* and *Pseudotterranova decipiens* are anisakidae that may be found in several frequently consumed raw fish, including mackerel, cod, herring, rockfish, and salmon as well as yellowfin tuna and squid. Reliable methods of preventing ingestion of live anisakid larvae are freezing (–4°F for 60 hours) or cooking (140°F for 5 minutes).[63,72,120,127,159]

Diphyllobothriasis (fish tapeworm disease) is caused by eating uncooked fish that harbor the parasite. Hosts include but are not limited to herring, salmon, pike, and whitefish. The symptoms are less acute than with intestinal roundworm ingestions, and usually begin 1–2 weeks after ingestion. Signs and symptoms include nausea, vomiting, abdominal cramping, flatulence, abdominal distension, diarrhea, and anemia (megaloblastic). Diagnosis is established based on history of the ingestion of raw fish and on identification of the tapeworm proglottids in stool. Treatment with niclosamide, praziquantel, or paromomycin is usually effective.[1,151]

Monosodium Glutamate or "Chinese Restaurant Syndrome"

The so-called Chinese restaurant syndrome is induced by ingestion of monosodium glutamate (*l*-sodium glutamate; MSG). Individuals present with burning, facial pressure, headache, flushing, chest pain, GI symptoms usually limited to nausea and vomiting, and, infrequently, life-threatening bronchospasm[3] and angioedema.[137] Intensity and duration of the symptoms are dose-related, with significant variation in individual responses.[128] Monosodium glutamate causes "shudder attacks" or a seizure-like syndrome in young children. Absorption is more rapid following fasting, and the typical burning symptoms rapidly spread over the back, neck, shoulders, abdomen, and occasionally the thighs. Gastrointestinal symptoms are rarely prominent. Symptoms can usually be prevented by prior ingestion of food. When symptoms do occur, they usually last approximately 1 hour.

The syndrome is not limited to patrons of Chinese restaurants; it occurs in areas where Chinese restaurants are rare. Monosodium glutamate is also marketed as a flavor enhancer. Many sausages and canned soups contain heavy doses of MSG.

MSG (regarded as "safe" by the Food and Drug Administration) can also be the cause of acute and bizarre neurologic symptoms. The actual pathophysiology has not been clarified, although studies implicate arterial receptors such as aortic chemoreceptors.

Another Chinese restaurant syndrome is associated with the reheating of fried rice and *B. cereus* type I overgrowth, which causes consequential early-onset nausea and vomiting, and *B. cereus* type II, which has a delayed onset of similar symptoms and diarrhea.[43]

Anaphylaxis and Anaphylactic Like Presentations

Some foods and foodborne toxins may cause allergic or anaphylactic like manifestations, that are also referred to as "restaurant syndromes"[131] (Table 72–4). The similarity of these syndromes complicates a patient's future approach to safe eating. Isolating the precipitant is essential so that the risk can be effectively assessed. Manufacturers of processed foods should provide an unambiguous listing of ingredients on package labels, and sensitive individuals (or their parents) must be rigorously attentive.[124,162] Confirmation may necessitate controlled double-blind oral challenge tests, and those with severe reactions should be protected by the immediate availability of epinephrine and antihistamine. Attempts to avoid allergic reactions to dairy products by avoiding dairy-containing foods may fail. Nondairy foods may still contain flavor enhancers of a dairy origin (partially hydrolyzed sodium caseinate, etc) and cause morbidity and death in allergic individuals.[42] Individuals with known food allergies frequently fail to carry prescribed epinephrine, believing that the allergen is easily identifiable and avoidable.[68] Food additives to consider include antibiotics, aspartame, butylated hydroxyanisole (BHA), butylated hydroxytoluene (BHT), nitrates or nitrites, and parabens esters.[84] Regulation of these preservatives is limited, and agents such as sulfites are so ubiquitously used that it may be hard to predict which guacamole, cider, vinegar, fresh or dried fruits, wines or beers do or do not contain these sensitizing agents.

Vegetables and Plants

The rhubarb plant (*Rheum rhaponticum*) is a hardy perennial herb easily grown in parts of the United States with abundant moisture. The typical thick, leafy stalks are harvested from early spring into the summer on the Eastern seaboard. The critical issue is that only the stalk is edible; the leafy part of the plant is not edible either raw or cooked. The leaves contain anthraquinones and water-soluble oxalates (Chap. 77). The stalk contains citric and malic acids, which would not result in toxic manifestations.

The case was finally resolved when it became apparent that another amateur gourmet botanist had dug and harvested in error. In search of horseradish for the feast, he had unearthed another quite similar-appearing root: pokeweed (*Phytolacca americana*), commonly found throughout the eastern United States. The plant, which has many names (pokeberry, Virginia poke, scoke, pigeon berry, garget, inkberry, and American cancer,

TABLE 72–4. COMMON FOODBORNE DISEASE SYMPTOMS: FLUSHING, BRONCHOSPASM, HEADACHE (PRIMARY PRESENTING SYMPTOMS)

	Onset	Symptoms	Cause	Therapy
Anaphlaxis (anaphylactoid)	Minutes to hours	Urticaria, angioedema, bronchospasm, hypotension	Allergens—nuts, eggs, milk, fish, shellfish, peanuts	Oxygen, epinephrine, Beta-$_2$ agonists Corticosteroids, volume expansion, H-$_1$ & H-$_2$ blockers
MSG (monosodium glutamate)	10–20 min	Flushing, ↓ BP, palpitations, facial pressure, headaches, bronchospasm Shivering (children)	Monosodium glutamate flavor enhancer, Chinese food, fast food	Oxygen, beta-$_2$ agonists, volume expansion, avoidance
Metabisulfites	Minutes	Flushing, low BP, bronchospasm	Preservative: wines, salad (bars), fruit, juice, shrimp	See Anaphylaxis, Avoidance
Scrombroid	Minutes to hours	Flushing, low BP, urticaria, headache, pruritis, GI symptoms	Large fish—poorly refrigerated: tuna, bonito, albacore, mackerel, mahi mahi (histidine)	See Anaphylaxis, Avoidance
Tyramine	Minutes to hours	Headache, hypertension (INH use increases risk)	Wines, aged cheeses	Avoidance As for hypertension, migraines
Tartrazine	1–2 h	Urticaria, angioedema, bronchospasm	Yellow coloring Food additive	See Anaphylaxis, Avoidance

among others), grows 6–12 feet tall and dies down to the ground each fall.[56,76] As it is strong-smelling with interesting stalk colors and berries, young children are frequently attracted to its reddish-purple poisonous berries. Unfortunately, its roots are often mistaken for horseradish and parsnips. The toxic ingredients, *Phytolacca* toxin and related triterpenes, are most concentrated in the root, although the leaves, stems, and fruits are also toxic in decreasing order.[65] The common use of the youngest parts of the plant suggest that toxicity increases with plant maturity, although some suggest that the mature berries are nontoxic.[76] The fatal dose has not been determined. The classic GI manifestations are attributable to the triterpenes. More severe manifestations may include blurred vision, hypoventilation, diaphoresis, weakness, convulsions, dysrhythmias, and death.

Plants[136] and even products such as honey[75] can be perilous to the uninitiated. Before seeking attractive plants or leaving any plants within the reach of young children, a review of botanical and chemical information is necessary[70,71] (Table 77–1). Pokeweed is available canned and is eaten fresh by many Americans, who consider it a staple in their diet. It is used in numerous herbal and folk remedies as well. Children covered with the purple pokeberry juice have reportedly developed toxicity from ingestion, yet poke wine is used commonly in the south of the United States. The common method for preparation of the fresh materials is parboiling.

Pokeweed has a nonspecific mitogenic character. In addition, pokeweed mitogen stimulates human lymphocytes in the production of an antiviral substance that is biologically, chemically, and physically identical to human interferon. Studies demonstrate that all parts of the plant, from the berries to the roots, have leukoagglutinating and hemagglutinating activity and that these are distinctly different from phytohemagglutinin.[12] In experimental studies, as well as in several case reports, these substances have been shown to produce significant mitotic and morphologic alterations in lymphocytes and plasma cells.

These toxicologic manifestations may be associated with only minimal contact.[12] Previously it was shown that with doses of pokeweed inadequate to produce other systemic effects, large immature basophilic lymphocytes, atypical plasma cells, and "plasmablasts" have persisted in the serum for at least 8 weeks in some cases. In vitro cytoplasmic vacuolization, cytoplasmic basophilia, and azurophilic granules are also observed.

Therapy includes emesis and catharsis, which are frequently accomplished by the agent itself. Emesis, activated charcoal adsorption, and catharsis may be indicated as the initial therapy if vomiting and diarrhea are not prominent. Thereafter, supportive care is indicated, with the ultimate prognosis being excellent. Recovery usually occurs in 18–36 hours.

CASE 2. A 4-year-old child presented to the emergency department with a history of diarrhea, vomiting, and intermittent abdominal pain for 1 week. The family became concerned when blood and mucus became evident in the stool after 4 days. At that time blood tests and stool cultures were obtained at another hospital. Antipyretics were prescribed for fever and instructions regarding hydration were given. No antibiotics or other therapy were offered and the child's diarrhea and other symptoms began to resolve. The parents became concerned when they noticed the child appeared pale, more irritable than usual, had a decreased urine output, and was uninterested in eating at a favorite fast food restaurant. The child was brought to the ED for evaluation after a brief generalized seizure. The child was otherwise healthy with no significant medical history, other medication use, or intoxications. The child was attending preschool.

Physical examination revealed an afebrile child with normal respirations, blood pressure 125/80 mm Hg, and heart rate 150 beats/min. The child appeared pale and irritable. The remainder of the physical examination was significant for a systolic flow murmur, mild abdominal pain without rebound or guarding, and a liver edge palpated 3 cm below the right costal margin. No meningeal signs were evident, and the neurologic examination was nonfocal. Laboratory studies were significant for a white blood count of 22,000/mm^3; hematocrit of 25%; platelet count of 80,000/mm^3; blood smear revealed many schistocytes and helmet cells. Serum sodium was 128 mEq/L; potassium, 5.9 mEq/L; BUN, 40 mg/dL; creatinine, 2.2 mg/dL; ALT, 180 U/L. Coagulation studies and CSF analysis were normal.

What Is the Differential Diagnosis of a Child Presenting With Gastroenteritis, Anemia, Thrombocytopenia, and Azotemia?

This constellation of findings are typical for the hemolytic uremic syndrome (HUS), which is frequently due to a bacterial gastroenteritis. The most common organism responsible is E. coli O157:H7. Other bacteria producing a shiga-like toxin can also cause the same findings. Agents and toxins also implicated as causes of HUS include estrogen-containing oral contraceptives, mitomycin-C, cyclosporin-A, and radiation therapy.[111] Other nontoxicologic causes of this clinical picture include autoimmune disease, Kawasaki syndrome, eclampsia of pregnancy, and bacterial enteritis/sepsis leading to disseminated intravascular coagulopathy (DIC) and shock.

Laboratory analysis typically includes a microangiopathic hemolytic anemia, thrombocytopenia, and acute intrinsic renal failure. Other laboratory findings include hyperkalemia, metabolic acidosis, hyponatremia and hypocalcemia. Liver aminotransferases may be elevated, and pancreatic involvement may produce hyperamylasemia, elevated pancreatic lipase, and hyperglycemia.

Most children with hemolytic uremic syndrome are under 6 years of age; many are less than 2. HUS begins with a prodrome of diarrhea 90% of the time. The diarrhea lasts for 3–4 days and frequently becomes bloody. Abdominal pain due to colitis is also common. Other frequent findings include vomiting, altered mental status (irritability or lethargy), pallor, and low-grade fever. At the time of presentation, many children have oliguria or anuria. About 10% of children will present with a generalized seizure at the onset of HUS.[132]

Postdiarrheal HUS is endemic in Argentina.[87] Frequent epidemics occur in North America, and many of these reports describe the association of enterohemorrhagic *E. coli* (EHEC) or *E. coli* O157:H7 with postdiarrheal HUS.[23,89,103,105,118,157] Postdiarrheal HUS is seen most frequently during the summer months, matching the peak incidence of positive stool cultures in cattle (the most common source of the organism).[55] Food products from cattle (ground beef, milk, yogurt, cheese) and water contaminated with fecal material are the common sources.[29,51,140] Contaminated water used in gardens and unpasteurized apple cider have also caused bloody diarrhea and HUS due to EHEC.[16,27]

Enterohemorrhagic *E. coli* (EHEC), including *E. coli* O157:H7, produces a toxin similar to the toxin produced by *Shigella dysenteriae* type I, referred to as shiga-like toxin (SLT) or verotoxin.[39,117] The proposed mechanism for SLT damage is intestinal absorption, bloodstream access to renal glomerular endothelium, intracellular adsorption via glycolipid receptors, ribosomal inactivation, and cell death.[111] In animal models organ damage is more severe if endothelial cells have high concentrations of globotriaosylceramide receptors. This may explain the propensity for renal, gastrointestinal, and central nervous system involvement in children. Endothelial cell damage and other pathologic processes, including platelet and leukocyte activation, triggering of the coagulation cascade, as well as the production of cytokines, also occur.[67,154] More than one type of SLT exists; SLT–1, SLT–2 as well as variants on SLT–2 structure have been identified.[17]

Detection of *E. coli* O157:H7 through stool culture early in the course of disease is useful. The recovery decreases after the first week of illness.[111,144] *E. coli* O157:H7 almost always produces SLT; therefore if stool cultures are negative, EIA and polymerase chain reaction test should be used to detect SLT in the stool.[24]

Treatment of HUS should focus on meticulous supportive care, with fluid and electrolyte balance being a priority. Peritoneal dialysis or hemodialysis should be instituted early for azotemia, and for hyperkalemia, acidosis, or fluid overload. Red blood cells are transfused to maintain a hemoglobin above 6 g/dL, and platelets to maintain hemostasis, especially before invasive procedures. Hypertension may be treated with short-acting calcium channel blockers (nifedipine 0.25–0.5 mg/kg/dose po), and seizures with benzodiazepines. Many therapies have been used for HUS, including heparin, fibrinolytics, IV immunoglobulin, fresh frozen plasma, vitamin E, and antiplatelet agents. None has been obviously beneficial and some deleterious.[130] Plasmapheresis has been used in nondiarrheal HUS and in recurrent HUS after renal transplants. In a controlled trial, antibiotics did not change the course or outcome of children with postdiarrheal HUS.[114] Anti-SLT–2 antibodies have protected mice from SLT–2 toxicity, but intravenous immunoglobulin with SLT–2 activity has not improved outcome in children with HUS. A phase 1 study of the feasibility of using synthetic SLT receptors attached to a chromosorb to prevent HUS is in progress.[5]

The mortality from HUS with good supportive care is approximately 5%; another 5% of victims suffer end-stage renal disease or severe cerebral ischemic events and chronic neurologic impairment. Prolonged anuria (more than 1 week) or oliguria (more than 2 weeks) or severe extrarenal disease may be as severe as markers for higher mortality and morbidity.[111]

Strategies to prevent the spread of *E. coli* O157:H7 and subsequent HUS include public education regarding thorough cooking of beef (no pink hamburgers), pasteurization of milk and apple cider, and thorough cleaning of vegetables. Public health measures include education of clinicians to consider *E. coli* O157:H7 in patients with bloody diarrhea, and routine capability of microbiology laboratories to culture *E. coli* O157:H7 and provide for EIA or PCR determination of SLT. Public health departments should provide active surveillance systems to identify early outbreaks of *E. coli* O157:H7 infection.

CASES 3 AND 4. A 30-year-old woman and her 32-year-old husband, on a scuba diving vacation in Puerto Rico, had a local dinner of rice, beans, a large red snapper, home-canned fruit preserves, and wine. That night, approximately 5 hours after dinner, they were both awakened by abdominal discomfort and nausea, followed by vomiting and diarrhea. Although they were unsure of the order of events, a throbbing headache, rapid breathing, numbness of the arms, legs, and mouth ensued. Each patient described a feeling of bone and tooth pain with "deep aches in the joints." The most bizarre symptom, noted by the woman, was temperature misinterpretation. When she reached for a warm washcloth to rub on her "freezing skin," it seemed to her that the warm washcloth felt cold. This distressing symptom lasted for 2 days. The vomiting abated during the early morning hours, but the nausea and diarrhea continued for several days. Mild, crampy abdominal pain persisted for approximately 4 days. The following morning, the couple spoke with some of the local inhabitants. Many of them described similar symptoms that appeared after they would eat a large fish, such as sea bass, red snapper, grouper, or barracuda. As so many people had the same symptoms, the couple did not seek medical help. On their return to the mainland 10 days later, there were no clinical or physical complaints. They did not seek medical care.

What Is the Differential Diagnosis of Foodborne Poisoning Presenting With Neurologic Symptoms?

The differential diagnosis of foodborne poisoning presenting with neurologic symptoms is vast (Tables 72–5, 72–6). Many of theses cases are ichthyosarcotoxic (involving toxins from muscles, viscera, skin, gonads, and

TABLE 72–5. DIFFERENTIAL DIAGNOSIS OF POSSIBLE FOODBORNE POISONING PRESENTING WITH NEUROLOGIC SYMPTOMS

Myasthenia gravis
Botulism
MSG (monosodium glutamate)
Poliomyelitis
Encephalitis
Tick paralysis
Carbon monoxide
Organophosphates
Anticholinergic poisoning
Postanesthesia paralysis
Heavy metals
Diphtheria
Eaton-Lambert syndrome
Bacterial food poisoning
Plant ingestions (poison hemlock, buckthorn)
Migraine
Bends type I, II, III (caisson disease)

mucous surfaces of the fish); rarely, toxicity follows consumption of the fish blood or skeleton. Shellfish poisoning must also be considered. Most episodes of poisoning are not species specific, although particular forms of toxicity from Tetraodontiformes (puffer fish) and *Gymnothoraces* (moray eels) have been recognized.

Deep-sea fish, eels, mussels, clams, and crabs are all implicated in diarrheal syndromes. In cases of ciguatera poisoning, the major symptoms are usually neurotoxic and the GI symptoms are minor. In cases of scombroid poisoning, facial flushing, headache, and dysphagia may overshadow nausea and vomiting.

Knowing where the fish was caught is often helpful, but refrigerated transport of foods and rapid worldwide travel can complicate the assessment. Scombroid fish poisoning has been traced to frozen mahi mahi shipped to the Midwest.[100] Travelers to Caribbean and Pacific islands, as well as individuals traveling within the United States, have suffered from ciguatera poisoning.[78] In geographically disparate regions of Canada, 107 individuals suffered from domoic acid intoxication caused by the ingestion of cultivated mussels from Prince Edward Island.

In the differential diagnosis, activities other than eating must always be considered. In particular, sport divers often perform their activities in high-risk areas (Florida, California, and Hawaii) and often during the high-risk periods (May through August). They often spearfish many of the toxic fish in question and might have an unrecognized bite, a sting from a stingray tail, or a laceration from a deltoid or pectoral fin spine of a lion fish or stonefish that can cause consequential marine toxicity (Chap. 101). Divers who surface too quickly might also have caisson disease. It is important to assess all of these possibilities when a diver with sudden cutaneous and neurologic symptoms is evaluated. The presence of one or more of these possibilities makes assessment particularly difficult.

TABLE 72–6. COMMON FOODBORNE NEUROLOGIC DISEASES (PRIMARY PRESENTING SYMPTOMS)

	Onset/Duration*	Symptoms	Toxin Source/Toxin*/Mechanism+	Diagnosis/Therapy*
Ciguatera	2–30 h *Months to years	t, p n, v, d	Large reef fish: barracuda, snapper, parrot, sea bass, moray (dinoflagellate, source) *Ciguatoxin +Increased sodium channel permeability	Clinical, mouse bioassay, immunoassay *Supportive, mannitol
Tetrodon	Minutes to hours *Days	p, r, ↓bp n, v, d	Puffer fish, *fugu*, blue-ringed octopus, newts, horseshoe crab *Tetrodotoxin +Blocks sodium channel	*Respiratory support
Neurotoxic shellfish poisoning	15 minutes to 18 hours *Days	b, t, n, v, d, p	Mussels, clams, scallops, oysters, *P. brevis:* "red tide" *Brevitoxin +↑ Sodium channel permeability	Clinical, mouse bioassay of food, HPLC
Paralytic shellfish poisoning	30 minutes *Days	r, p, n, v, d	Mussels, clams, scallops, oysters, *P. catanella, P. tamarensis* *Saxitoxin +Decreases sodium channel permeability	Clinical, mouse bioassay of food, HPLC * Respiratory support
Amnestic shellfish poisoning	15 minutes to 38 hours *Years	a n, v, d, p, r	Mussels, possibly other shellfish; *N. pungens;* *Domoic acid +Glutamate analog	Clinical, mouse bioassay of food, HPLC * Respiratory support
Botulism	12–73 h	r	Home canned foods, ? honey, corn syrups, *C. botulinum* *Botulinum toxin; +Binds to presynapse, blocks acetylcholine release	Immunoassay *Antitoxin, respiratory support

n = nausea; v = vomiting; d = diarrhea; p = paresthesias; r = respiratory depression; b = bronchospasm; t = temperature reversal sensation; a = amnesia, ↓bp = hypotension.

Ciguatera Poisoning

Ciguatera poisoning is the most commonly reported vertebrate fishborne poisoning, accounting for more than 50% of reported cases. It is endemic to warm-water, bottom-dwelling shore reef fish living around the globe between 35 degrees north and 35 degrees south latitude, including tropical areas such as the Indian Ocean, the South Pacific, and the Caribbean. Hawaii and Florida report 90% of all cases in the United States, most commonly during the spring and summer months.[53]

The fish species involved probably exceed 500 in number, with the barracuda, sea bass, parrot fish, red snapper, grouper, amber jack, kingfish, and sturgeon the most common sources. The common factor is the comparably large size of the fish involved.

Large fish (4–6 lbs or more) become vectors of ciguatera poisoning according to the complex feeding patterns inherent in aquatic life. Ciguatoxin can be found in blue-green algae, protozoa, and the free algae dinoflagellates. Photosynthetic dinoflagellates *Gambierdiscus toxicus* and bacteria within the dinoflagellate are the origins of ciguatoxin.[32,60,86] These dinoflagellates are the main nutritional source for small herbivorous fish; as these small fish are the major food source for larger carnivorous fish, the ciguatoxin becomes increasingly concentrated in the flesh, adipose tissue, and viscera of larger and larger fish.[11]

Ciguatoxin is heat-stable, lipid-soluble, acid-stable, odorless, and tasteless. When purified, the toxin is a large (MW, 1100 D), complex ester that does not harm the fish but is stored in tissues.[85,115] The structure is a polyether ladder, which binds to the sodium channel in diverse tissues and increases the sodium permeability of the channel.[10,116,141] Multiple ciguatoxins have been identified in the same fish, perhaps explaining the variability of symptoms and differing severity.[86] People have been afflicted after eating fresh or properly frozen fish prepared by all common methods: boiling, baking, frying, stewing, or broiling.

By history, the meal is usually unremarkable. The majority of episodes occur 2–6 hours after ingestion, 75% within 12 hours, and all but 4% within 24 hours.[11] Symptoms include acute onset of diaphoresis; abdominal pain with cramps, nausea, vomiting, a profuse watery diarrhea; and a constellation of dramatic neurologic symptoms.[158] Headaches are common. The feeling of loose, painful teeth may occur. Typically, dysesthesias and paresthesias predominate. Watery eyes, tingling, and numbness of the tongue, lips, throat, and perioral area rapidly ensue. A strange metallic taste has frequently been reported. A striking manifestation is the reversal of temperature discrimination: hot substances feel cold or cold substances feel hot. In addition, patients often describe their extremities as burning or feeling extremely warm superficially but cold under the skin. This temperature perception disturbance is most likely the result of an exaggerated nerve depolarization in peripheral small A-delta myelinated (C-polymodal nociceptor) fibers.[25] Myalgias, most often in the lower extremities, arthralgias, ataxia, and weakness are commonly experienced.[11] Dysuria[46] and symptoms of dyspareunia and vaginal and pelvic discomfort may occur in women after sexual intercourse with men who are ciguatoxic.[77] Ciguatoxin may also be transmitted in breast milk[21] and can cross the placenta.[108] Vertigo, seizures, and visual disturbances (eg, blurred vision, manifestations of scotomata, and transient blindness) are also described.

Although deaths are reported, none has been documented in the United States.[13] Mortality is due to respiratory paralysis and seizures apparently managed without adequate life support. Bradycardia and orthostatic hypotension are also described.[41] The orthostatic hypotension may respond to atropine and sympathomimetic agents.

The GI symptoms usually subside within 24–48 hours; however, cardiovascular and neurologic symptoms may persist for several days to weeks, depending on the amount of ingested toxin. Delayed symptoms may include protracted itching and hiccoughs.

Laboratory analysis using an ELISA (enzyme-linked immunosorbent assay) test for ciguatera toxin can be performed; alternatively, HPLC (high-pressure liquid chromatograph) is accurate. The original mouse bioassay was the standard, but was slow, involved the destruction of animals, and did not differentiate the variants in ciguatoxin structure. A rapid test is under development for field use (dipstick immunobead assay) that will allow testing of fish without laboratory processing of the toxin-containing tissues.[10,58,107] Other useful laboratory tests are those that may exclude other diagnostic possibilities and determine the need for, or extent of, specific therapeutic interventions.

Initial treatment should include standard supportive care for a toxic ingestion.[79,158] In most patients elimination of toxin is accelerated by vomiting (40%) and also diarrhea (70%). Unless the patient develops symptoms and seeks medical care within 2 hours of the meal, syrup of ipecac is probably of little benefit. There may be some benefit from the administration of activated charcoal and a cathartic. A cathartic (sorbitol, magnesium sulfate, or magnesium citrate) should be given only to patients who do not have diarrhea. In patients with significant GI fluid loss through vomiting and/or diarrhea, intravenous fluid and electrolyte repletion is essential.

The use of IV mannitol may produce a marked decrease in neurologic and muscular dysfunctional symptoms associated with ciguatera. Gastrointestinal symptoms are less responsive to mannitol.[106,109] Mannitol should be used with caution, as it may cause hypotension. Vascular re-expansion and cardiovascular stability should be initial treatment priorities. A dose of 1 g/kg of mannitol over 30–45 minutes seems efficacious. Additional controlled clinical studies with mannitol are needed to define its mechanism(s) of action and therapeutic indications.

Admission to the hospital for cautious supportive care is essential for anyone with an uncertain diagnosis, volume depletion, or any consequential manifestations. The differential diagnosis of botulism, organophosphate poisoning, and other potentially life-threatening processes (Tables 72–5, 72–6) must be rapidly resolved. Diaphoresis is a common clinical finding and an important factor in the differential diagnosis (Chap. 28). Pralidoxime, nifedipine, amitriptyline, atropine sulfate, tocainide, corticosteroids, multivitamins, and calcium gluconate have been used to treat ciguatera poisoning; however, none of these measures has yielded significant or consistent success.

Ciguatera Like Poisoning

Moray, conger, and anguillid eels carry a ciguatoxin like neurotoxin in their viscera, muscles, and gonads that does not affect the eel itself. The toxin has a complex ester structure that may be structurally very similar to ciguatoxin and is thermostable.[102] These same eels also possess an ichthyohemotoxin that can be destroyed by heating to greater than 65°C but is resistant to drying.

Individuals may manifest neurotoxic symptomatology similar to that which occurs with ciguatoxin, or they may show signs of cholinergic toxicity, such as hypersalivation, nausea, vomiting, and diarrhea. Shortness of breath, mucosal erythema, and cutaneous eruptions may ensue. These findings may be present along with the neurotoxic symptoms.[54] Management is solely supportive. Mortality is related to the complications of neurotoxicity, such as seizures and respiratory paralysis.

Scombroid

Scombroid poisoning was originally described with the Scombroidae fish (including the large dark meat marine tuna, albacore, bonito, mackerel, and skipjack). However, the most commonly ingested vectors identified by the Centers for Disease Control and Prevention are nonscombroid fish, such as mahi mahi and amber jack.[13] All of the implicated fish species live in temperate or tropical waters, particularly around California or Hawaii. The ingestion of bluefish in New Hampshire was the probable cause of scombroid poisoning in five people,[33] and mackerel the likely offender in 28 cases in a prison.[13] The incidence of this disease is probably far greater than was originally perceived. This poisoning differs from other fishborne causes of illness in that it is entirely preventable if the fish is properly stored after it is removed from the water.

Scombroid poisoning may occur with cooked, smoked, canned, or raw fish. These fish all have a high concentration of histidine in their dark meat. *Morganella morganii*, *E. coli*, and *Klebsiella pneumoniae*, commonly found on the surface of the fish, contain a histidine decarboxylase enzyme that acts on a warm (unrefrigerated), freshly killed fish to convert histidine to histamine, saurine, and other heat-stable substances. Saurine has been suggested as the causative toxin of scombroid poisoning. Chromatographic analysis has demonstrated that the only difference between histamine and saurine is that histamine is found as histamine phosphate and saurine is merely histamine hydrochloride.[37] The term *saurine* originated from saury, a Japanese dried fish delicacy often associated with scombroid intoxication. Recently histamine was identified as the likely causative toxin in scombroid fish poisoning.[98] The extent of spoilage usually correlates with histamine levels. Histamine levels in healthy fish are less than 0.1 mg/100 g of fish; left at room temperature this level rapidly increases, reaching toxic levels of 100 mg/100 g fish within 12 hours.

The appearance, taste, and smell of the fish is usually unremarkable.[6] Rarely, the skin has an abnormal "honeycombing" character, or a pungent, peppery taste may be a clue to its toxicity (Chap. 27). Usually, within minutes to several hours after eating the fish, the individual experiences numbness, tingling, or a burning sensation of the mouth, dysphagia, headache, and, of particular significance for scombroid poisoning, a peculiar flush characterized by an intense diffuse erythema of the face, neck, and upper torso.[69] Rarely, pruritus, urticaria, angioedema, or bronchospasm ensues. Nausea, vomiting, dizziness, palpitations, abdominal pain, diarrhea, and prostration may develop.[45,69,73,92]

The prognosis is good with appropriate supportive care and parenteral antihistamines such as diphenhydramine or any of the H_2-receptor antagonists such as cimetidine or ranitidine.[19] The toxic substance should be removed or absorbed from the gut. Inhaled beta$_2$-adrenergic agonists and epinephrine may be necessary if bronchospasm is prominent. Patients usually show significant improvement within a few hours.

The diagnosis can be confirmed by elevated serum or urine histamine levels. If any uncooked fish remains, the isolation of causative bacteria from the flesh is suggestive but not diagnostic. A new capillary electrophoretic assay makes histamine detection rapid.[96] Levels of histamine greater than 50 mg/100 g of fish are considered hazardous by the FDA. Isoniazid may increase the severity of the reaction to scombroid fish by inhibiting enzymes that break down histamine.[62,153]

The patient may be reassured that he or she is not allergic to fish if other individuals experience a similar reaction to eating the same fish at the same time, or if any remaining fish can be preserved and tested for elevated levels of histamine. If this information is not available, an anaphylactic reaction to the fish must be considered. The differential diagnosis of flushing, bronchospasm, and headache is found in Table 72–4. Because many people often consume alcohol with fish, alcohol must be considered as an independent variable. The differential diagnosis of flushing associated with alcohol ingestion includes ethanol plus chloral hydrate, tyramine-containing drinks and monoamine oxidase inhibitors, alcohol–disulfiram-type reactions, and simply ethanol in certain Asians and Native Americans with a genetic predisposition to an ethanol "flush" (Chap. 28).

The differential diagnosis of the scombrotoxic flush not associated with concomitant ethanol ingestion includes excessive levels of niacin or nicotinic acid, carcinoid syndrome, Zollinger-Ellison syndrome, pheochromocytoma, and migraine or cluster headaches. The history and clinical evolution usually establish the diagnosis quickly.

Shellfish Poisoning

Healthy mollusks living between 30 degrees north and 30 degrees south latitude ingest and filter large quantities of dinoflagellates. These plankton members of the phylum Protozoa are single-celled, motile, flagellated, pigmented organisms. Thriving through photosynthesis, these dinoflagellates form the major source of available ocean food during the "non-R" months (May through August), when they are responsible for the "red tides" that may be seen from California to Alaska, from New England to St. Lawrence, and across the west coast of Europe.[90] The number of toxic dinoflagellates may be so overwhelming that birds and fish die, and humans who walk along the beach may suffer respiratory symptoms due to aerosolized toxin.[91]

Ingestion of shellfish, including oysters, clams, mussels, scallops, contaminated by dinoflagellates or algae may cause neurotoxic, paralytic, and amnestic symptoms. The dinoflagellates most frequently implicated are *Ptychodiscus brevis* (formerly *Gymnodinium breve*), the diatom causing neurotoxic shellfish poisoning; *Protogonyaulax catanella* and *P. tamarensis*, which cause paralytic shellfish poisoning; and *Nitzschia pungens*, the diatom implicated in amnestic shellfish poisoning. *Ptychodiscus brevis* causes neurotoxic shellfish poisoning due to the production of brevitoxin, while *P. catanella* and *P. tamarensis* are responsible for paralytic shellfish poisoning due to the production of saxitoxin. Proliferation of *P. brevis* may cause a red tide, but shellfish poisoning may occur even in the absence of this extreme proliferation.

Paralytic shellfish poisoning (PSP) typically occurs during the months of May through November, when water temperature is highest. The shellfish implicated are usually clams, oysters, mussels, and scallops. An increased number of shellfish consumed is associated with more severe symptoms. The onset of symptoms is usually within 30 minutes of ingestion. Neurologic symptoms predominate and include paresthesias and numbness of the mouth and extremities, a sensation of floating, headache, ataxia, vertigo, muscle weakness, paralysis, and cranial nerve dysfunction manifested by dysphagia, dysarthria, dysphonia, and transient blindness. Gastrointestinal symptoms are less common and include nausea, vomiting, abdominal pain, and diarrhea. Fatalities may occur due to respiratory failure, usually within the first 12 hours after symptom onset. Muscle weakness may persist for weeks. Saxitoxin blocks the voltage-sensitive sodium channel. Treatment is supportive, with early intervention for respiratory failure. Orogastric lavage and cathartics have been used to remove unabsorbed toxin from the GI tract.[31,61,83,97,123] Antibodies against saxitoxin have reversed cardiorespiratory failure in animals,[14] but this therapy has yet to be used in humans. Assays for saxitoxin include a mouse bioassay, ELISA, and HPLC.[155] HPLC has good interlaboratory accuracy,[155] but the differences in saxitoxin derivatives makes standardization of an analytic test difficult.[10,80]

Neurotoxic shellfish poisoning (NSP) is characterized by gastroenteritis with associated neurologic symptoms. Gastrointestinal symptoms include abdominal pain, nausea, vomiting, diarrhea, and rectal burning. Neurologic features include paresthesias, reversal of hot and cold temperature sensation, myalgias, vertigo, and ataxia. Other symptoms may include headache, malaise, tremor, dysphagia, bradycardia, decreased reflexes, and dilated pupils. Paralysis is not seen. The combination of bradycardia and mydriasis is unusual, but is also seen with phenylpropanolamine toxicity. The incubation period is 3 hours (range, 15 minutes to 18 hours). The GI and neurologic symptoms appear simultaneously. Duration of symptoms is 17 hours (range, 1–72 hours).[97] Treatment is supportive and severe respiratory depression is very uncommon. Brevitoxin, produced by *P. brevis*, is a lipid-soluble, heat-stable polyether ladder toxin. It acts by stimulating sodium flux through the sodium channels of both nerve and muscle.[7,26] Brevitoxin can be assayed using mouse bioasssay or ELISA, and more recently by antibody RIA and reconstituted sodium channels.[112,150] Other manifestations of brevitoxin toxicity include respiratory irritation, cough, and bronchospasm, which occur when *P. brevis* is aerosolized by wave action during red tides. Therapy includes removal of the patient from the environment, and bronchodilators. NSP is not fatal.

Amnestic shellfish poisoning (ASP) is characterized by GI symptoms of nausea, vomiting, abdominal cramps, and diarrhea and neurologic symptoms of memory loss and, less frequently, coma, seizures, hemiparesis, ophthalmoplegia, purposeless chewing, and grimacing. Other symptoms include unstable blood pressure and cardiac dysrhythmias. The onset of symptoms after ingestion of mussels is 5 hours (range, 15 minutes to 38 hours). The mortality rate is 2%, with death most frequently occurring in older patients, who suffer more severe neurologic symptoms. Ten percent of victims may suffer long-term antegrade memory deficits as well as motor and sensory neuropathy. Postmortem examination has revealed neuronal damage in the hippocampus and amygdala.[147] The etiologic agent is domoic acid, a structural analog of glutamic and kainic acids produced by the diatom *Nitzschia pungens*. The only documented outbreak occurred in Canada in 1987 and affected 107 individuals who had consumed mussels harvested from cultivated river estuaries on Prince Edward Island.[110] The possibility for other outbreaks exists, since the diatom *N. pungens* f. *multiseries* has been isolated in shellfish from other areas.[40] Pelican deaths due to domoic acid–laden anchovies were reported in 1991. Canada instituted monitoring for domoic acid after this outbreak.[148]

Tetrodon Poisoning

This type of fish poisoning involves only the order Tetraodontiformes, not restricted geographically but eaten most frequently in Japan, California, Africa, South

America, and Australia.[54] Approximately 100 fresh- and saltwater species of fish exist, including the puffer-like fish: globe fish, balloon fish, blowfish, and toad fish.[99] Tetrodotoxin has been isolated from the blue-ringed octopus[36] and the gastropod mullusc[161] and has caused fatalities from ingestion of horseshoe crab eggs.[61] In Japan, a local variety of puffer fish—*fugu*—is considered a delicacy, but special licensing is required to prepare this exceedingly toxic fish. In 1989 the Food and Drug Administration legalized the importation of puffer fish, but prior to exportation from Japan the fish must be laboratory tested and certified by two Japanese organizations to be tetrodotoxin-free. In addition, certain tetrodotoxin-containing newts (taricha, notophthalmus, triturus, and cynops), in particular the *Taricha granulosa*, found in Oregon, California, and southern Alaska, can be fatal when ingested. Most newts and salamanders with bright colors and rough skins contain toxins.[22]

Tetrodotoxin is a heat-stable (except in alkaline milieu), water-soluble, nonprotein, aminoperhydroquanizole found mainly in the fish skin, liver, ovary, intestine, and, possibly muscle.[54,126] Because of the ovary's high concentration of the toxin, the female is most poisonous if eaten during the spawning season. Tetrodotoxin is detected by mouse bioassay. It is unstable heated to 100°C in acid, distinguishing it from saxitoxin. It may also be detected using flourescent spectrometry.[9] Neurotoxicity is produced by inhibition of sodium–potassium pump activity and blockade of neuromuscular transmission.[101]

Symptoms of tetrodon poisoning typically occur within minutes of ingestion. Headache, diaphoresis, dysesthesias, and paresthesias of the lips, tongue, mouth, face, fingers, and toes evolve rapidly. Buccal bullae and salivation may develop. Dysphagia, dysarthria, nausea, vomiting, and abdominal pain may ensue. Generalized malaise, loss of coordination, weakness, fasciculations, and an ascending paralysis (with risk of respiratory paralysis) occur in 4–24 hours. Other cranial nerves may be involved. In more severe toxicity hypotension is present. In some studies, mortality has approached 50%.[133]

Therapy is supportive. Removal of the toxin and prevention of absorption are the essential measures. Supportive respiratory care emphasizing airway protection, including intubation, if necessary, is extremely important. To date, there is no clinical experience with the use of extracorporeal techniques for this condition.[149]

Less Common Poisonings: Echinoderms

The sea urchin usually causes toxicity by contact with its spinous processes, but this Caribbean delicacy is also toxic on ingestion. In preparing it as food, the venom-containing gonads should be removed, as they contain an acetylcholine-like substance that causes profuse salivation, abdominal pain, nausea, vomiting, and diarrhea. The starfish is also considered by some to be edible, although there are reports of an asterotoxin with saponin-like activity that produces nausea and vomiting.

Other Types of Shellfish Poisoning

Oyster poisoning can be caused by a highly toxic venerupin extracted from dinoflagellates. Oyster poisoning has a high fatality rate and is localized to Japan. Callistin poisoning is caused by choline- or histamine-like substances, which generate an acute allergic reaction, and is localized to Japan. Adalone poisoning is caused by a photosensitizer that is extracted from Japanese seaweed. Red whelk poisoning is precipitated by a tetramine that produces curare-like symptoms and is frequently reported in Japan.

Prevention of Marine Foodborne Disease

Careful evaluation of the symptoms and meticulous reports to local and state health departments as well as the Centers for Disease Control and Prevention (CDC) will allow for more precise analysis of epidemics of poisoning from contaminated or poisonous food or fish. Many states and countries have developed rigorous health codes with regard to harvesting certain species of fish in certain areas at certain times. A review of foodborne intoxications reported to the CDC over a 5-year period may be representative of the number and severity of food poisoning in the United States (Table 72–1).

Some examples of actions taken by state and foreign health agencies in controlling epidemics of fishborne food poisoning are:

1. In 1972 the 3230-km Massachusetts coastline was declared unsafe for shellfish harvesting. A health emergency was declared due to a blooming of red tide. The state confiscated shellfish and prohibited the marketing, export, and serving of shellfish.[90]
2. The Miami, Florida, health code prohibits the sale of barracuda and warns against eating fillets from the large and potentially ciguatera toxic fish.
3. The Japanese closely regulate preparation and selling of the puffer fish ("*fugu*"), requiring special training and licensing of preparers.
4. The Canadian government marks the location and time of harvesting of mussels, and mussels are tested for the presence of domoic acid.[40,110]

Other Forms of Fishborne Poisoning

Filefish forms the toxin aluterin, which produces vomiting and diarrhea. Herring, sprat, sardines, and tarpon may contain clupeotoxin, which causes GI and neurologic symptoms. Ratfish, elephantfish, or chimeras may cause rapid central nervous system depression. Lampreys and hagfish may cause cyclostome poisoning with GI complications. Snek, mackerel, and caster-oil fish may cause gemblid poisoning, characterized by dramatic purgation. Mullet, goatfish, and rudderfish may cause hallucinogenic responses. Sawara (mackerel) and ishingh (sea bass), two Japanese fish, and sandfish can cause a hypervitaminosis A syndrome.

Acknowledgment

Robert H. Kirstein, MD contributed to this chapter in a previous edition.

References

1. Abramowicz M, ed: Drugs for parasitic infections. Med Lett 1990;32:29.
2. Ackman DM, Drabkin P, Birkhead G, Cieslak P: Reptile-associated salmonellosis in New York State. Pediatr Infect Dis J 1995;14:955–959.
3. Allen DH, Baker GJ: Chinese restaurant asthma. N Engl J Med 1981;305:1154–1155.
4. Anunciacao LL, Linardi WR, do Carmo LS, Bergdoll MS: Production of staphylococcal enterotoxin A in cream-filled cake. Int J Food Microbiol 1995;26:259–263.
5. Armstrong GD, Rowe PC, Goodyer P, et al: A phase I study of chemically synthesized verotoxin (Shiga-like toxin) Pk-trisaccharide receptors attached to chromosorb for preventing hemolytic-uremic syndrome. J Infect Dis 1995;171:1042–1045.
6. Arnold SH, Brown WD: Histamine toxicity from fish products. Adv Food Res 1978;24:113–154.
7. Asai S, Krzanowski JJ, Lockey R, et al: The site of action of *Ptychodiscus brevis* toxin within the parasympathetic axonal sodium channel h gate in airway smooth muscle. J Allerg Clin Immunol 1984;73:824–828.
8. Attwood SE, Healy K, Caffarkey MT, et al: Yersinia infection and abdominal pain. Lancet 1987;1:529–533.
9. Baden DG, Flemeing LE, Bean JA: Marine toxins. In: de Wolf FA, ed: Handbook of Clinical Neurology: Intoxication of the Nervous System. II. Clinical Toxins and Drugs. Elsevier, Amsterdam, 1994.
10. Baden DG, Melinek R, Sechet V, et al: Modified immunoassays for polyether toxins: Implications of biological matrixes, metabolic states, and epitope recognition. J Assoc Off Anal Chem 1995;78:499–508.
11. Bagnis R, Kubergki T, Laugier S: Clinical observations on 3,009 cases of ciguatera (fish poisoning) in the South Pacific. Am J Trop Med Hyg 1979;28:1067–1073.
12. Barker BE, Farnes P, LaMarche PH: Peripheral blood plasmacytosis following systemic exposure to *Phytolacca americana* (pokeweed). Pediatrics 1966;38:490–493.
13. Bean NH, Goulding JS, Lao G, Angulo FJ: Surveillance for foodborne-disease outbreaks—United States, 1988–1992. MMWR 1996;45:SS–5; 1–55.
14. Benton BJ, Rivera VR, Hewetson JF, et al: Reversal of saxitoxin-induced cardiorespiratory failure by a burro-raised-STX antibody and oxygen therapy. Toxicol Appl Pharmacol 1994;124:39–51.
15. Berenguer J, Solera J, Diaz MD, et al: Listeriosis in patients infected with human immunodeficiency virus. Rev Infect Dis 1991; 13:115–119.
16. Besser RE, Lett SM, Weber JT, et al: An outbreak of diarrhea and hemolytic uremic syndrome from *Escherichia coli* O157:H7 in fresh pressed apple cider. JAMA 1993;269: 2217–2220.
17. Bitzan M, Ludwig K, Klemt M, et al: The role of *Escherichia coli* O 157 infections in the classical (enteropathic) haemolytic uraemic syndrome: Results of a Central European, multicentre study. Epidemiol Infect 1993;110:183–196.
18. Black RE, Jackson RJ, Tsai T, et al: Epidemic *Yersinia enterocolitica* infection due to contaminated chocolate milk. N Engl J Med 1978;298:76–79.
19. Blalesly ML: Scombroid poisoning: Prompt resolution of symptoms with cimetidine. Ann Emerg Med 1983;12: 104–106.
20. Blaser MJ, Keller LB: *Campylobacter* enteritis. N Engl J Med 1981;305:1444–1452.
21. Blythe DG, Desilva DP: Mother's milk turns toxic following a fish feast. JAMA 1990;264:2074.
22. Bradley SG, Klika LJ: A fatal poisoning from the Oregon rough-skinned newt (*Taricha granulosa*). JAMA 1981; 246:247.
23. Brandt HR, Fouser LS, Watkins SL, et al: Escherichia coli O157:H7-associated hemolytic uremic syndrome after ingestion of contaminated hamburgers. J Pediatr 1994;125: 519–526.
24. Brian MJ, Frosolono M, Murray BE, et al: Polymerase chain reaction for diagnosis of enterohemorrhagic *Escherichia coli* infection and hemolytic-uremic syndrome. J Clin Microb 1992;30:1801–1806
25. Cameron J, Capra MF: The basis of the paradoxical disturbance of temperature perception in ciguatera poisoning. J Toxicol Clin Toxicol 1993;31:571–579.
26. Catterall WA, Trainer V, Baden DG: Molecular properties of the sodium channel: A receptor for multiple neurotoxins. Bull Soc Pathol Exot 1992;85:481–485.
27. Cieslak PR, Barrett TJ, Griffen PM, et al: *Escherichia coli* O157:H7 infection from a manured garden. Lancet 1993; 342:367. Letter.
28. Decker MD, Lavely GB, Hutcheson RH, Schaffner W: Food-borne streptococcal pharyngitis in a hospital pediatrics clinic. JAMA 1985;253:679–681.
29. Deschenes G, Casenave C, Grimont F, et al: Clusters of haemolytic uremic syndrome due to unpasteurized cheese. Pediatr Nephrol 1996;10:203–205.
30. Dupont HL, Formal HB, Hornick RB, et al: Pathogenesis of *Escherichia coli* diarrhea. N Engl J Med 1971;285:1–9.
31. Eastaugh JE, Shepherd S: Infections and toxic syndromes from fish and shellfish consumption: A review. Arch Intern Med 1989;149:1735–1740.
32. Endean R, Monks SA, Griffith JK, Llewellyn LE: Apparent relationships between toxins elaborated by the cyanobacterium *Trichodesmium erythraeum* and those present in the flesh of the narrow-barred Spanish mackerel *Scomberomorus commersoni*. Toxicon 1993;31:1155–1165.
33. Etkind P, Wilson ME, Gallagher K, et al: Bluefish associated scombroid poisoning. JAMA 1987;258:3409–3410.
34. Evans MR, Parry SM, Ribeiro CD: Salmonella outbreak from microwave cooked food. Epidemiol Infect 1995;115: 227–230.
35. Finch MJ, Blake PA: Foodborne outbreaks of campylobacteriosis: The United States experience. Am J Epidemiol 1985;122:262–267.
36. Flachsenberger WA: Respiratory failure and lethal hy-

potension due to blue-ringed octopus and tetrodotoxin envenomations observed and counteracted in animal models. J Toxicol Clin Toxicol 1987;24:485–502.
37. Foo LY: Scombroid poisoning: Isolation and identification of saurine. J Sci Food Agric 1976;27:807–810.
38. Foster EM: Foodborne hazards of microbial origin. Fed Proc 1978;37:2577–2581.
39. Fritsche TR, Tarr P: Shiga-like toxin-producing *Escherichia coli* in Seattle children: A prospective study. Gastroenterology 1993;105:1724–1731.
40. Fritz L, Quillam MA, Walter JA, et al: An outbreak of domoic acid poisoning attributed to the pennate diatom *Pseudonitzschia australis*. J Phycol 1992;28:439–442.
41. Geller RJ, Benowitz NL: Orthostatic hypotension in ciguatera fish poisoning. Arch Intern Med 1992;152: 2131–2133.
42. Gern JE, Yang E, Evrard HM, et al: Allergic reactions to milk-contaminated "nondairy" products. N Engl J Med 1991;324:976–979.
43. Giannella RA, Brasile A: Hospital food-borne outbreak of diarrhea caused by *Bacillus cereus*: Clinical, epidemiologic, and microbiologic studies. J Infect Dis 1979;139:366–370.
44. Giesendorf BA, Quint WG: Detection and identification of *Campylobacter* spp. using the polymerase chain reaction. Cell Mol Biol 1995;41:625–638.
45. Gilbert RJ, Hobbs G, Murray CK, et al: Scombrotoxic fish poisoning: Features of the first fifty incidents to be reported in Britain (1976–1979). Br Med J 1980;2:71–72.
46. Gillespie RJ, Lewis JH, Pearn ATC, et al: Ciguatera in Australia: Occurrence, clinical features, pathophysiology, and management. Med J Aust 1986;145:584–590.
47. Goossens H, Giesendorf BA, Vandamme P, et al: Investigation of an outbreak of *Campylobacter upsaliensis* in day care centers in Brussels: Analysis of relationships among isolates by phenotypic and genotypic typing methods. J Infect Dis 1995;172:1298–1305.
48. Grady GF, Keush GT: Pathogenesis of bacterial diarrheas. N Engl J Med 1971;285:831–841,891–900.
49. Graham DY, Smith JL, Opekun AR: Spicy food and the stomach: Evaluation by endoscopy. JAMA 1988;260: 3473–3475.
50. Green MA, Henmann MA, Wehr HM, et al: An outbreak of watermelon-borne pesticide toxicity. Am J Public Health 1987;77:1431–1434.
51. Griffin PM, Tauxe RV: The epidemiology of infections caused by *Escherichia coli* O157:H7, other enterohemmorhagic *E. coli*, and the associated hemolytic uremic syndrome. Epidemiol Reviews 1991;13:60–98.
52. Gutman LT, Ottesen EA, Quan TJ, et al: An inter-familial outbreak of *Yersinia enterocolitica* enteritis. N Engl J Med 1973;288:1372–1377.
53. Habekost RC, Fraser IM, Halstead BW: Observations on toxic marine algae. J Wash Acad Sci 1955;45:101–103.
54. Halstead BW: Poisonous and Venomous Animals of the World. Princeton, NJ, Darwin Press, 1978.
55. Hancock DD, Besser TE, Kinsel ML, et al: The prevalence of *Escherichia coli* O157.H7 in dairy and beef cattle in Washington State. Epidemiol Infect 1994;113:199–207.
56. Hardin JW, Arena JM: Human Poisoning from Native and Cultivated Plants. Chapel Hill, NC, Duke University Press, 1969, pp. 69–73.
57. Harris JC, Dupont HL, Hornic RB: Fecal leukocytes in diarrheal illness. Ann Intern Med 1972;76:697–703.
58. Hokama Y, Asahina AY, Shang ES, et al: Evaluation of the Hawaiian reef fishes with the solid phase immunobead assay. J Clin Lab Anal 1993;7:26–30.
59. Holmberg SD, Blake PA: Staphylococcal food poisoning in the United States: New facts and old misconceptions. JAMA 1984;251:487–489.
60. Holmes MJ, Lewis RJ, Poli MA, et al: Strain dependent production of ciguatera precursors (gambiertoxins) by *Gambierdiscus toxicus* (Dinophyceae) in culture. Toxicon 1991;29:761–765.
61. Hughs JM, Merson MH: Fish and shellfish poisoning. N Engl J Med 1976;295:1117–1120.
62. Hui JY, Taylor SL: Inhibition of in vivo histamine metabolism in rats by foodborne and pharmacologic inhibitors of diamine oxidase, histamine-*N*-methyl transferase, and monoamine oxidase. Toxicol Appl Pharmacol 1985;81: 241–249.
63. Intestinal perforation caused by larval Eustrongylides—Maryland. MMWR 1982;31:383–389.
64. Kanchanapongkul J, Krittayapoositpot P: An epidemic of tetrodotoxin poisoning following ingestion of the horseshoe crab *Carcinoscorpius rotundicauda*. Southeast Asian J Trop Med Public Health 1995;26:364–367.
65. Kang SS, Woo WS: Triterpenes from the berries of *Phytolacca americana*. J Nat Prod 1980;43:510–513.
66. Kapperud G, Vardund T, Skjerve E, et al: Detection of pathogenic *Yersinia enterocolitica* in foods and water by immunomagnetic separation, nested polymerase chain reactions, and colorimetric detection of amplified DNA. Appl Environ Microbiol 1993;59:2938–2944.
67. Karpman D, Andreasson A, Thysell H, et al: Cytokines in childhood hemolytic uremic syndrome and thrombotic thrombocytopenic purpura. Pediatr Nephrol 1995;9: 694–699.
68. Kemp SF, Lockey RF, Wolf BL, Lieberman P: Anaphylaxis. A review of 266 cases. Arch Intern Med 1995;155: 1749–1754.
69. Kim R: Flushing syndrome due to mahimahi (scombroid fish) poisoning. Arch Dermatol 1979;115:963–964.
70. Kingsbury JM: Phytotoxicology: Major problems associated with poisonous plants. Clin Pharmacol Ther 1969;10: 163–169.
71. Kingsbury JM: Poisonous Plants of the United States and Canada. Englewood Cliffs, NJ, Prentice-Hall, 1964.
72. Kliks MM: Human anisakiasis: An update. JAMA 1986; 255:2605. Letter.
73. Kow-Tong C, Malison MD: Outbreak of scombroid fish poisoning, Taiwan. Am J Public Health 1987;77: 1335–1336.
74. Lamanna C, Carr CJ: The botulinal, tetanal and enterostaphylococcal toxins: A review. Clin Pharmacol Ther 1967;8:286–332.
75. Lampe KF: Rhododendrons, mountain laurel and mad honey. JAMA 1988;259:2009.
76. Lampe KF, McCann MA: AMA Handbook of Poisonous

and Injurious Plants. Chicago, American Medical Association, 1985.
77. Lange WR, Lipkin KM, Yang GC: Can ciguatera be a sexually transmitted disease? J Toxicol Clin Toxicol 1989;27: 193–197.
78. Lange WR, Snyder FR, Fudala PJ: Travel and ciguatera fish poisoning. Arch Intern Med 1992;152:2049–2053.
79. Lawrence DN, Enriquez MB, Lumish RM, Maceo A: Ciguatera fish poisoning in Miami. JAMA 1980;244: 254–258.
80. Laycock MV, Thibault P, Ayer SW, Walter JA: Isolation and purification procedures for the preparation of paralytic shellfish poisoning toxin standards. Nat Toxins 1994; 2:175–183.
81. Le Cour H, Ramos H, Almeida B, et al: Foodborne botulism: A review of 13 outbreaks. Arch Int Med 1988;148: 578–580.
82. Lee LA, Gerber AR, Lonsway DR, et al: *Yersinia enterocolitica* 0:3 infections in infants and children associated with the household preparation of chitterlings. N Engl J Med 1990;322:984–987.
83. Levin R: Paralytic shellfish toxins: Their origin, characteristics and methods of detection: A review. J Food Biochem 1991;15:405–407.
84. Levine AS, Labuza TP, Morley JE: Food technology: A primer for physicians. N Engl J Med 1985;312:628–634.
85. Lewis RJ, Holmes MJ: Origin and transfer of toxins involved in ciguatera. Comp Biochem Physiol 1993;106: 615–628.
86. Lewis RJ, Sellin M: Multiple ciguatoxins in the flesh of fish. Toxicon 1992;30:915–919.
87. Lopez EL, Contrini MM, Devoto S, et al: Incomplete hemolytic uremic syndrome in Argentinean children with bloody diarrhea. J Pediatr 1995;127:364–367.
88. Lumish RM, Ryder RW, Anderson DC, et al: Heat-labile enterotoxigenic *Escherichia coli* induced diarrhea aboard a Miami-based cruise ship. Am J Public Health 1980;111: 432–436.
89. Martin DL, MacDonald KL, White KE, et al: The epidemiology and clinical aspects of the hemolytic uremic syndrome in Minnesota. N Engl J Med 1990;323:1161–1167.
90. Massachusetts Department of Health: The red tide: A public health emergency. N Engl J Med 1973;288:1126–1127.
91. McCollum JPK, Pearson RCM, Ingham HR, et al: An epidemic of mussel poisoning in north-east England. Lancet 1968;2:767–770.
92. Merson MH, Baine WB, Gangarosa EJ, et al: Scombroid fish poisoning: Outbreak traced to commercially canned tuna fish. JAMA 1974;228:1268–1269.
93. Merson MH, Morris GK, Sack DA, et al: Travelers diarrhea in Mexico: A prospective study of physicians and family members attending a congress. N Engl J Med 1976;294: 1299–1305.
94. Metcalf TG: Indication of viruses in shellfish-growing waters. Am J Public Health 1979;69:1093–1094.
95. Mishu B, Griffen PM, Tauxe RV, et al: *Salmonella enteritidis* gastroenteritis transmitted by intact chicken eggs. Ann Intern Med 1991;115:190–194.
96. Mopper B, Sciacchitano CJ: Capillary zone electrophoretic determination of histamine in fish. J Assoc Off Anal Chem 1994;77:881–884.
97. Morris PD, Campbell DS, Taylor TJ, et al: Clinical and epidemiological features of neurotoxic shellfish poisoning in North Carolina. Am J Public Health 1991;8:471–474.
98. Morrow JD, Margolis GR, Rowland J, et al: Evidence that histamine is the causative toxin of scombroid-fish poisoning. N Engl J Med 1991;324:716–720.
99. Mosher HS, Fuhrman FA, Buckwald HD, et al: Taricha-toxin-tetrodotoxin, a potent neurotoxin. Science 1964;144: 1100–1110.
100. Murray LR, Edwards LC, Martin RJ, et al: Scombroid fish poisoning—Illinois, South Carolina. MMWR 1989;38: 140–141.
101. Narahashi T: Mechanism of action of tetrodotoxin and saxitoxin on excitable membranes. Fed Proc 1972;31: 1117–1123.
102. Nukina M, Koyangi LM, Scheur PJ: Two interchangeable forms of ciguatoxin. Toxicon 1984;22:169–176.
103. Orr P, Lorencz B, Brown R, et al: An outbreak of diarrhea due to verotoxin-producing *Escherichia coli* in the Canadian Northwest Territories. Scand J Infect Dis 1994;26: 675–684.
104. Osterholm MT, MacDonald KL, White KE, et al: An outbreak of a newly recognized chronic diarrhea syndrome associated with raw milk consumption. JAMA 1986;256: 484–490.
105. Ostroff SM, Kobayashi JM, Lewis JH: Infections with *Escherichia coli* O157:H7 in Washington state: The first year of statewide disease surveillance. JAMA 1989;262: 355–359.
106. Palafox NA, Jain LG, Pinano AZ, et al: Successful treatment of ciguatera fish poisoning with mannitol. JAMA 1988;259:2740–2742.
107. Park DL: Evolution of methods for assessing ciguatera toxins in fish. Rev Environ Contam Toxicol 1994;136:1–20. Review.
108. Pearn J, Harvey P, De Ambrosis W, et al: Ciguatera and pregnancy. Med J Aust 1982;1:57–58.
109. Pearn JH, Lewis RJ, Ruff T, et al: Ciguatera and mannitol: Experience with a new treatment regimen. Med J Aust 1989;151:77–80.
110. Perl TM, Bedard L, Kosatsky T, et al: An outbreak of toxic encephalopathy caused by eating mussels contaminated with domoic acid. N Engl J Med 1990;322:1775–1780.
111. Pickering LK, Obrig TG, Stapleton FB: Hemolytic-uremic syndrome and enterohemorrhagic *Escherichia coli.* Pediatr Infect Dis J 1994;13:459–475.
112. Poli MA, Rein KS, Baden DG: Radioimmunoassay for PbTx–2-type brevetoxins: Epitope specificity of two anti-PbTx sera. J Assoc Off Anal Chem 1995;78:538–542.
113. Potter ME, Kaufman AF, Blake PA, Feldman RA: Unpasteurized milk: The hazards of a health fetish. JAMA 1984;252:2050–2054.
114. Proulx F, Turgeon JP, Delage G, et al: Randomized, controlled trial of antibiotic therapy for *Escherichia coli* O157:H7 enteritis. J Pediatr 1992;121:299–303.
115. Ragelis EP: Ciguatera seafood poisoning—Overview. In: Ragelis EP, ed: Seafood Toxins. ACS Symposium Series, 262. Washington, D.C., American Chemical Society, 1984, pp. 25–36.

116. Rayner MD, Kosaki T, Felmeth EL: Ciguatoxin: More than an anticholinesterase. Science 1968;160:70–71.
117. Rowe PC, Orrbine E, Ogborn M, et al: Epidemic *Escherichia coli* O157:H7 gastroenteritis and hemolytic-uremic syndrome in a Canadian Inuit community: Intestinal illness in family members as a risk factor. J Pediatr 1994;124:21–26.
118. Rowe PC, Orrbine E, Wells GA, et al: Epidemiology of hemolytic uremic syndrome in Canadian children from 1987 to 1988. J Pediatr 1991;119:218–224
119. Rubin HR, Wu AW: The bitter herbs of seder: More on horseradish horrors. JAMA 1988;259:1943. Letter.
120. Ruttenberg M: Safe sushi. N Engl J Med 1989;320:900–901.
121. Ryan CA, Nickels MK, Hargrett-Bean NT, et al: Massive outbreak of antimicrobial-resistant salmonellosis traced to pasteurized milk. JAMA 1987;258:3269–3274.
122. Sack DA, Kaminsky DC, Sack RB, et al: Enterotoxigenic *Escherichia coli* diarrhea of travelers: A prospective study of Peace Corps volunteers. Johns Hopkins Med J 1977;141: 63–70.
123. Sakamoto Y, Lockey RF, Krzanowski JJ: Shellfish and fish poisoning related to the toxic dinoflagellates. South Med J 1987;80:868–872.
124. Sampson HA, Mendelson L, Rosen J: Fatal and near fatal anaphylactic reactions to food in children and adolescents. N Engl J Med 1992;27:380–384.
125. Sartwell PE, ed: Maxcy-Rosenau Public Health and Preventive Medicine, 13th ed. Norwalk, CT, Appleton & Lange, 1992.
126. Schantz EJ, Johnson EA: Properties and use of botulinum and other microbial neurotoxins in medicine. Microbiol Rev 1989;56:80–99.
127. Schantz PM: The dangers of eating raw fish. N Engl J Med 1989;320:1143–1145.
128. Schaumburg HH, Byck R, Gerstl R, Mashman JH: Monosodium glutamate: Its pharmacology and role in the Chinese restaurant syndrome. Science 1969;163:826–828.
129. Schuchat A, Deaver KA, Wenger JD, et al: Role of foods in sporadic listeriosis. I. Case control study of dietary risk factors. JAMA 1992;267:2041–2045.
130. Seigler RL: Management of hemolytic-uremic syndrome. J Pediatr 1988;112:1014–1020.
131. Settipane GA: The restaurant syndromes. Arch Intern Med 1986;146:2129–2130.
132. Siegler RL, Pravia AT, Christofferson RD, et al: A 20 year population based study of post diarrheal hemolytic uremic syndrome in Utah. Pediatrics 1994;94:35–40.
133. Sims JK, Ostman DC: Pufferfish poisoning: Emergency diagnosis and management of mild human tetrodotoxication. Ann Emerg Med 1986;15:1094–1098.
134. Southern JP, Smith RM, Palmer S: Bird attack on milk bottles: Possible mode of transmission of *Campylobacter jejuni* to man. Lancet 1990;336:1425–1427.
135. Spitzer DR: Horseradish horrors—Sushi syncope. JAMA 1988;259:218–219.
136. Spoerke DG, Hall AH, Dodson CD, et al: Mystery root ingestion. J Emerg Med 1987;5:385–388.
137. Squire EN: Angioedema and monosodium glutamate. Lancet 1987;1:988.
138. St. Louis ME, Morse D, Potter ME, et al: The emergence of grade A eggs as a major source of salmonella enteritis infections: New implications for the control of salmonellosis. JAMA 1988;259:2103–2107.
139. Surveillance for epidemics. MMWR 1990;38:694–696.
140. Swerdlow DL, Woodruff BA, Brady RC, et al: A waterborne outbreak in Missouri of *Escherichia coli* 0157:H7 associated with bloody diarrhea and death. Ann Intern Med 1992;117:812–819.
141. Swift AE, Swift TR: Ciguatera. J Toxicol Clin Toxicol 1993; 31:1–29.
142. Tacket CO, Ballard J, Harris N, et al: An outbreak of *Yersinia enterocolitica* infections caused by contaminated tofu (soybean curd). Am J Epidemiol 1985;121:705–710.
143. Tacket CO, Dominguez LB, Fisher HJ, Cohen ML: An outbreak of multiple-drug-resistant salmonella enteritis from raw milk. JAMA 1985;253:2058–2060.
144. Tarr PI, Neill MA, Clausen CR, et al: *Escherichia coli* O157:H7 and the hemolytic uremic syndrome: Importance of early cultures in establishing the etiology. J Infect Dis 1990;162:553–556.
145. Tauxe RV, Hargrett-Bean N, Patton CM: *Campylobacter* isolates in the United States, 1982–1986. MMWR 1988;37: SS:1–13.
146. Taylor WR, Schell WL, Wells JG, et al: A foodborne outbreak of enterotoxigenic *Escherichia coli* diarrhea. N Engl J Med 1982;306:1093–1095.
147. Teitelbaum JS, Zatorre RJ, Carpenter S, et al: Neurologic sequelae of domoic acid intoxication due to ingestion of contaminated mussels. N Engl J Med 1990;322:1781–1787.
148. Todd ECD: Domoic acid and amnesic shellfish poisoning—A review. J Food Prot 1993;56:69–83.
149. Torda TA, Sinclair E, Ulyatt DB: Puffer fish (tetrodotoxin) poisoning: Clinical record and suggested management. Med J Aust 1973;1:599–602.
150. Trainer VL, Baden DG, Catterall WA: Detection of marine toxins using reconstituted sodium channels. J Assoc Off Anal Chem 1995;78:570–573.
151. Turner JA, Sorvillo FJ, Murray RA, et al: Diphyllobothriasis associated with salmon. MMWR 1981;30:331–338.
152. Update: Foodborne listeriosis United States, 1988–1990. MMWR 1992;41:251–252.
153. Uragoda CG, Kottegoda SR: Adverse reaction to isoniazid and ingestion of fish with a high histamine content. Tubercle 1977;58:83–89.
154. van de Kar NC, van Hinsbergh VW, Brommer EJ, et al: The fibrinolytic system in the hemolytic uremic syndrome: In vivo and in vitro studies. Pediatr Res 1994;36:257–264.
155. van Egmond HP, van den Top HJ, Paulsch WE, et al: Paralytic shellfish poison reference materials: An intercomparison of methods for the determination of saxitoxin. Food Addit Contam 1994;11:39–56.
156. Vantrappen G, Geboes K, Ponette E: *Yersinia* enteritis. Med Clin North Am 1982;66:639–653.
157. Waters JR, Sharp JC, Dev VJ: Infection caused by *Escherichia coli* O157:H7 in Alberta, Canada and in Scotland: A five year review, 1987–1991. Clin Infect Dis 1994;19: 834–843.
158. Withers NW: Ciguatera fish poisoning. Annu Rev Med 1982; 33:97–111.
159. Wittner M, Turner JW, Jacquette G, et al: Eustrongylidia-

sis—A parasitic infection acquired by eating sushi. N Engl J Med 1989;320:1124–1126.

160. Wood RC, MacDonald KL, Osterholm MT: *Campylobacter* enteritis outbreaks associated with drinking raw milk during youth activities. A 10-year review of outbreaks in the United States. JAMA 1992;268:3228–3230.

161. Yang CC, Han KC, Lin TJ, et al: An outbreak of tetrodotoxin poisoning following gastropod mollusc consumption. Hum Exp Toxicol 1995;14:446–450

162. Yunginger JW, Sweeney KG, Sturner WQ, et al: Fatal food-induced anaphylaxis. JAMA 1988;260: 1450–1452.

CHAPTER 73

Botulism

Lewis R. Goldfrank and Neal E. Flomenbaum

A 27-year-old woman had been in excellent health until 3 days before admission, when the family gathered for dinner following the funeral of the patient's mother-in-law. Shortly thereafter, the patient began experiencing dysphagia and dysarthria and seemed generally anxious. She saw her family physician, who prescribed diazepam. The day prior to her admission, the patient became dyspneic. She began to communicate by writing when talking became impossible. Writing soon became difficult as well, and the patient complained of having trouble walking and lifting her head. She would not eat and vomited food when she was force-fed. She then began to look straight ahead without moving her eyes.

The next day she was taken to the closest hospital, where the physicians in attendance noted the peculiarity of the symptoms, the fact that she was taking diazepam, and the temporal relationship to her mother-in-law's funeral. The family physician was called and told of the new symptoms that had developed in the previous 2 days. The private physician was struck by the resemblance to the mother-in-law's symptoms prior to her death of a presumed myocardial infarction. He recommended an IM injection of saline as a placebo and discharge of the patient.

Shortly after the patient arrived home, she became increasingly dyspneic and cyanotic, and then had a cardiopulmonary arrest. The husband initiated CPR until the paramedics arrived and took over.

Physical examination on admission revealed an apneic, intubated, comatose young woman with a blood pressure of 90/40 mm Hg, pulse of 80 beats/min, and rectal temperature of 97.0°F (36.1°C). The left pupil was 4 mm, the right 3 mm; both were sluggishly responsive to light.

The heart and lungs were unremarkable. The abdomen was soft, and bowel sounds were diminished. The stools were negative for occult blood. There was no response to painful stimuli or cold-water caloric testing. Her upper extremities were flaccid, with absent reflexes. She had increased extensor tone in her legs, 2+ patellar reflexes, ankle clonus, and generalized myoclonic jerks. Cerebrospinal fluid (CSF) examination was normal. Edrophonium (Tensilon) testing was normal. An electromyogram (EMG) demonstrated increased muscle action potentials with rapid repetitive stimulation and posttetanic potentiation.

Botulism was diagnosed and the patient was given 2 vials of trivalent botulinal antitoxin and two 375-mg doses of guanidine over 6 hours.* Her condition steadily deteriorated and she died 3 days after admission. Postmortem examination revealed cerebral edema and herniation. Her stomach contents revealed undigested mushrooms, from which *Clostridium botulinum* type B was isolated.

The mother-in-law's hospitalization was reviewed. Twelve days before the daughter-in-law first had symptoms, the mother-in-law had had nausea, vomiting, abdominal cramps, and distention and was treated with an antiemetic. Three days later, she complained of a dry throat, dysphagia, and chest pains. Two days after that, she had dyspnea as well; an electrocardiogram (ECG) revealed inverted T waves in the precordial leads and occasional premature ventricular contractions, and she was admitted to "rule out myocardial infarction." The day after admission she was even more dyspneic and stuporous and had dilated, sluggishly reactive pupils. She was intubated and became more alert. When extubated the next day, she developed respiratory distress and required reintubation. The next day a tracheostomy was performed. The patient became febrile and died 2 days later.

Following the daughter-in-law's hospitalization and death, the body of the mother-in-law was exhumed, and an autopsy revealed bronchopneumo-

*The patient described presented in 1974. Guanidine is rarely if ever used currently in the management of botulism. See discussion p. 1183.

nia, an enlarged heart, and mushroom fragments in the small intestines. The mushroom fragments yielded *C. botulinum* type B.

When the diagnosis of botulism was first entertained, and before the mushrooms were implicated, all family members who had been at the funeral meal were admitted to the hospital for observation. At that time, a third member of the family reported having had difficulty swallowing. She was the only other family member who had eaten mushrooms at the funeral meal. She was given one vial of trivalent botulinal antitoxin, and her symptoms resolved in 3 days. Her stool specimens later revealed *C. botulinum* type B. Twenty days after being given the antitoxin, she developed severe arthralgias and fever suggestive of serum sickness secondary to the antitoxin.

The mother-in-law had canned peppers, eggplant, artichokes, and mushrooms without pressure cooking. When examined, only the home-canned mushrooms contained *C. botulinum* type B. Many of the other family members were understandably anxious and some complained of dry throat, headache, or tingling in their extremities, although none had eaten any of the mushrooms, and none had stools positive for *C. botulinum* type B. Most were discharged from the hospital within 24–48 hours.[25]

What Are the Characteristics of *C. Botulinum*?

Clostridium botulinum is a spore-forming, anaerobic, gram-positive bacillus. Eight distinct strains (designated types A through G, with C_{alpha} and C_{beta}) have been identified. All produce similar neurotoxins with identical mechanisms of action. Spores are dormant and highly resistant to damage. They can withstand boiling at 100°C for hours, although 30 minutes of moist heat at 120°C usually destroys them. Germination of spores in food is promoted if the pH is greater than 4.5, the sodium chloride content is less than 3.5%, or a low nitrite level is present. Most viable organisms produce toxin under anaerobic conditions and temperatures above 27°C, although some strains produce toxins even when conditions are not optimal. Some strains (especially type E) can produce toxin at temperatures as low as 5°C. Thus, at the temperatures used in freezing, toxin can be produced. To prevent germination, acidifying agents such as phosphoric or citric acid are employed in canning or bottling foods that are low in acid content, such as green beans, corn, beets, asparagus, chili peppers, mushrooms, spinach, figs, olives, and certain nonacidic tomatoes. As opposed to the spores, the toxin is heat-labile and can be destroyed by heating to 80°C for 30 minutes or 100°C for 10 minutes. In certain high altitude areas the boiling point is as low as 94.7°C, which may not be adequate to destroy the toxin unless boiling continues for 30 minutes. Under high-altitude conditions pressure cooking at 13–14 lb of pressure is often necessary to achieve appropriate temperatures.

Clostridium botulinum spores are ubiquitous and are present in soil, sea water, and air. Botulism outbreaks can occur anywhere around the world and in recent years have been reported from such diverse areas as Iran, the former Soviet Union, Japan, France, Belgium, Portugal,[32] Scandinavia, and Canada. Type B is the only strain thus far reported from Portugal[65] and is the most commonly found in all European countries except the Baltic states, where type E is the predominant form.[30] These distributions are general and not absolute. In the United States, type A strain is found west of the Mississippi,[9,37] B east of the Mississippi,[6] and E in the Pacific northwest.[53] Types A and B are typically produced in poorly processed meats and vegetables. Type G has not been associated with naturally occurring disease.

Food contaminated by *C. botulinum* types A and B often do not look or smell normal and appear putrified because of the action of proteolytic enzymes. In contrast, type E organisms are saccharolytic and not proteolytic, and food contaminated with type E toxin may look and taste normal. Rare instances of both adult and infant botulism have now been attributed to *C. barati* and *C. butyricum*.[43]

What Is the Pathophysiology of Botulism?

Botulinum toxin is the most poisonous substance known. The LD_{50} for mice is 3 million molecules injected intraperitoneally. The oral human lethal dose is 1 pg (10^{-12} g) per kilogram. Since the toxin is often demonstrated in the stool and is presumably biodegraded or inactivated in great part in the gastrointestinal tract, it is difficult to determine what percentage of the toxin is actually absorbed.[15] The toxin is a protein consisting of a single polypeptide chain, with a MW of 900,000 D, which includes the nontoxic protein hemaglutinin and the 150,000 MW neurotoxic component. To become fully active, the single-chain molecule must be cleaved by proteolysis to generate a heavy chain (MW 100,000) that is linked by a disulfide bond to a light chain (MW 50,000). It is the dichain form of the molecule that is responsible for both the toxicity and the therapeutic benefits.[52] The protein enters the preganglionic nerve terminal by endocytosis and binds rapidly and irreversibly to the cell membrane. Once inside the cell it inhibits calcium-dependent exocytosis, thereby preventing release of acetylcholine and resulting in presynaptic blockade.[29,48] The toxin acts as a zinc-dependent endoprotease to cleave polypeptides that are essential for exocytosis. This reduction in presynaptic function impairs cholinergic transmission at all acetylcholine-dependent synapses in the peripheral nervous system (Fig. 73–1). There is no effect on the central nervous system or on axonal conduction. Anticholinesterase (cholinergic) drugs, such as edrophonium (Tensilon), have no effect on the action of the toxin. The prolonged and variable period of recovery is directly related to the extent of the neuromuscular blockade and the nerve ending and presynaptic membrane regeneration rates.[22]

The recent use of 1 ng or more of botulinum toxin type A (Oculinum) injected under electromyographic control into extraocular muscles as a treatment for blepharospasm or as a supplement to corrective strabismus surgery is of related clinical interest.[27,52] This injec-

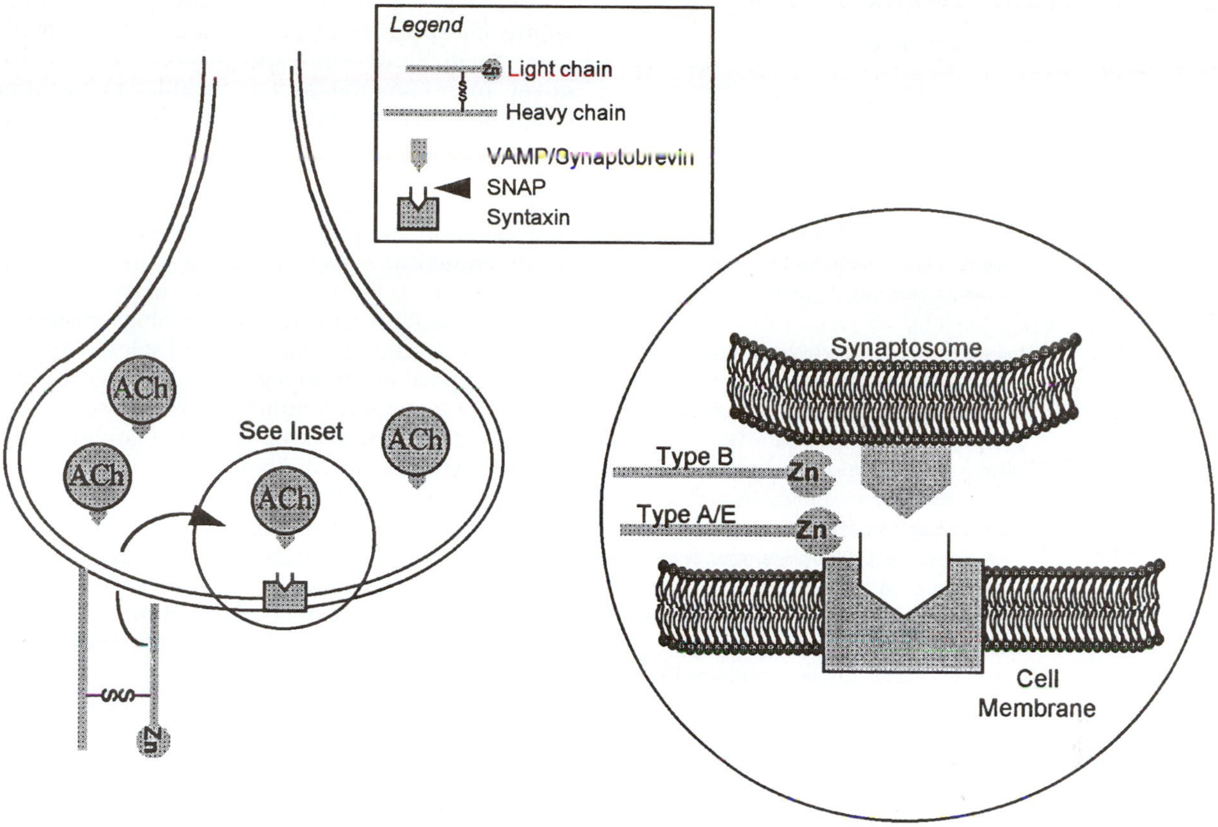

Figure 73–1. Botulinum toxin consists of two peptides linked by disulfide bonds. The heavy chain is responsible for specific binding to acetylcholine-containing neurons (the heavy chain of tetanus toxin is specific for glycine-containing neurons). The light chain, which is shared by tetanus toxin, contains a zinc-requiring endopeptidase. After translocation into the nerve cell cytoplasm, the zinc-endopeptidase cleaves proteins required by the docking–fusing complex that are critical to neuroexocytosis. Type B botulinum toxin (and tetanus toxin) targets VAMP/synaptobrevin, a docking protein located on the acetylcholine-containing synaptic vesicles (synaptosome). Types A and E botulism toxins proteolyse SNAP, a component of the presynaptic cell–membrane docking complex (associated with syntaxin). After destruction of these important components of the docking complex, neurotransmitter release cannot proceed, resulting in clinical findings consistent with acetylcholine (botulism) or glycine (tetanus) deficiency. VAMP: vesicle-associated membrane protein; SNAP: synaptosomal-associated protein.

tion selectively weakens and irreversibly blocks the release of acetylcholine at the local neuromuscular junction. These muscles then weaken by atrophy over a 3-week period but recover within 2–4 months as nerve transmission is restored.[1] This agent is also used to create the temporary weakness necessary to treat facial nerve disorders, achalasia, dystonia, torticollis, and voice and speech disorders (spasmodic dysphonia), although repetitive doses may be indicated.[27,34] Such therapeutic advances are now recognized in the fields of ophthalmology, otolaryngology, neurology, and gastroenterology.

Although there are no known adverse effects of the botulinal toxin injection, there is concern that an inadvertent excessive or misdirected dose of toxin may potentially cause weakness and respiratory compromise. Futhermore, following repeated injections, patients develop neutralizing antibodies which may subsequently limit the toxin's efficacy.[10] On the other hand, recurrent episodes of foodborne botulism have been documented in the same individual, suggesting that minute quantities of toxin exposure do not result in long-term immunity.[8,48]

What Are the Signs and Symptoms of Botulism?

Foodborne Botulism (Adult Type) [in vitro]

Although botulism is the most dreaded of all food poisonings, the initial phase of the disease, which occurs during the first day after ingestion, is often so subtle as to go unnoticed. Unfortunately, botulism is often misdiagnosed on the first visit to a physician or emergency department.[11,67] When gastrointestinal symptoms are striking, and food poisoning is suspected, the differential diagnosis should also include more acute poisonings, such as heavy metals, plants, mushrooms, and the common bacterial, viral, and parasitic agents found in Chapter 72.

Because the initial presentation of botulism is often subtle, and because physicians are so infrequently confronted with the disease (especially compared with the relatively more common diseases included in the differential diagnosis), there are often serious delays in initiating appropriate management (Table 73–1). This is particularly true of type E botulism, where initial gastrointestinal signs may be much more prominent than neurologic signs.[5] The first victim in an epidemic or an isolated victim is often misdiagnosed at a stage when the person could still be saved.[12,13] The definitive diagnosis of botulism is made when a patient presents with a neurologic disorder manifested by a descending paralysis and at least one of the following: typical electromyographic findings; *C. botulinum* in stool or a wound; botulinum toxin in serum, stool, or implicated food samples; or a compatible clinical illness in a person who is epidemiologically linked to a laboratory-confirmed case[35] (Chap. 117).

The early GI symptoms of botulism include nausea, vomiting, abdominal distention, and pain. There may or may not be a time lag (from 12 hours to several days) before one or more of the following symptoms appears: constipation; dry or sore mouth and throat; difficulty with visual accommodation; dysphonia; diplopia; descending, bilaterally symmetric motor paralysis beginning with abducens (VI) or oculomotor (III) nerve palsy; dysphagia (at times predominant and severe); mydriasis (often fixed); respiratory insufficiency; and urinary retention (Table 73–2). Many of these initial signs and symptoms are anti-

TABLE 73–1. BOTULISM: CLUES IN THE DIFFERENTIAL DIAGNOSIS

Condition	Diagnostic Findings
Aminoglycoside poisoning	Postanesthetic paralysis, intraoperative exposure
Anticholinergic poisoning	Mydriasis, vasodilation, fever, tachycardia, ileus, dry mucosa, altered mental status
Buckthorn (*Karwinskia humboldtiana*)	Progressive ascending paralytic neuropathy
Carbon monoxide	Headache, nausea, altered sensorium, tachypnea, elevated carboxyhemoglobin
Cerebrovascular accident (midbrain)	Asymmetric focal findings, abnormal CT
Diphtheria (polyneuritis)	Exudative pharyngitis, cranial polyneuropathy, cardiac manifestations, hypotension
Eaton-Lambert syndrome	Neoplasm, ophthalmoplegia (rare), no respiratory paralysis, posttetanic facilitation on EMG
Elapidae (coral snake) envenomation	Following envenomation euphoria, lightheadedness, fasciculations, tremor, weakness, salivation, nausea, vomiting followed by bulbar palsy, paralysis including slurred speech, diplopia, ptosis, dysphagia, dyspnea, and respiratory compromise
Encephalitis	Fever; mental status abnormalities, seizures, elevated CSF protein, and pleocytosis
Food poisoning (bacterial)	Rapid onset of disease, absence of cranial nerve findings
Guillain-Barré syndrome (Miller-Fisher variant)	Elevated CSF protein without cells, denervation and prolonged nerve conduction velocity on EMG
Inflammatory myelopathies (acute myelitis, transverse myelitis, necrotic myelopathy)	Complete (transverse) or incomplete spinal syndrome: posterior column myelopathy with ascending paresthesias or ascending spinothalamic findings or Brown-Sequard syndrome. Typically follows viral illness, back pain, progressive paraparesis, asymmetric ascending paresthesias in legs CSF: 5–50 lymphocytes/mm^3
Magnesium intoxication	Oral or intravenous exposure to magnesium, respiratory compromise, diffuse flushing, weakness, hypermagnesemia
Multiple sclerosis	Weakness, visual blurring (optic neuritis), sensory disturbances, diplopia, ataxia. Lesions separated in space and time. Mononuclear cell pleocytosis in CSF. Evoked response testing: slow or abnormal conduction in visual, auditory, somatosensory, or motor pathways; abnormal MRI or occasionally CT
Myasthenia gravis	Aggravation of fatigue with exercise, positive edrophonium (Tensilon) test
Organophosphates	Salivation, lacrimation, urination, defecation, fasciculations, bronchorrhea
Paralytic shellfish poisoning	Incubation < 1 h, dysesthesias, paresthesias, impaired mentation, respiratory paralysis
Poliomyelitis	Fever, GI symptoms, asymmetric neurologic findings, CSF pleocytosis
Tetanus	Cranial nerve defects (rare), spasticity, rigidity
Tick (*Dermacentor* spp)-related paralysis	Focal findings, progressive large muscle weakness, ascending paralysis, presence of an embedded tick

TABLE 73–2. COMMON SYMPTOMS AND SIGNS OF FOODBORNE BOTULISM

General	Normal mental status	
	Fatigue	
	Sore throat	
	Dizziness	
	Orthostatic hypotension	
Gastrointestinal	Nausea	
	Vomiting	
	Abdominal distress	
	Constipation	
	Diarrhea	
	Ileus	
Neurologic	***Symptoms***	***Signs***
	Blurred vision	Ophthalmoplegia
	Diplopia	Mydriasis
	Dysphagia	Nystagmus
	Dysarthria	Cranial nerve deficits
	Dry mouth	Ptosis
	Extremity weakness	Facial paresis
	Dyspnea	Lingual weakness
	Difficulty urinating	Decreased gag reflex
		Extremity weakness
		Paralysis, descending
		Hyporeflexia
		Ataxia
		Urinary retention

TABLE 73–3. FOCUSED DIFFERENTIAL DIAGNOSIS: BOTULISM VERSUS GUILLAIN-BARRÉ SYNDROME

	Botulism	Guillain-Barré Syndrome	Miller Fisher Variant of Guillain-Barré
Fever	Absent	May be present	May be present
Motor			
Pupillary reactivity	Dilated or unreactive (50%)	Normal	Normal
Ophthalmoplegia	Present early	Present late	Present
Paralysis	Descending	Ascending	Descending
Deep tendon reflexes	Present	Absent	Absent
Ataxia	Absent	Present	Present
Sensory			
Paresthesias	Absent	Present	Present
Laboratory			
CSF Protein	Normal	Elevated	Elevated

cholinergic, while mental status, sensory examination, and reflexes all usually remain normal. When medial rectus palsy, ptosis, and sluggish pupillary reactivity occur, there is a high correlation with subsequent respiratory insufficiency. As weakness progresses, deep tendon reflexes may diminish. The pulse is frequently normal or slow, and temperature in adults is normal. The normal mental status, absence of fever, and presence of ophthalmoplegia seen with botulism but not anticholinergic poisoning allow the clinician to move rapidly toward appropriate management.[61] The most difficult and frequently encountered problem is differentiating between botulism and the Guillain Barré syndrome. The Miller Fisher variant of Guillain Barré is the descending paralytic form of this acute inflammatory polyneuropathy (Table 73–3).

The index or first cases noted are usually the most seriously affected: They have been exposed to the greatest amount of toxin and therefore have the shortest incubation period. A lack of symptoms in others is not necessarily reassuring.

How Is Botulism Diagnosed? Which Laboratory Studies Are Useful?

Specific tests that are helpful in the differential diagnosis of botulism include the following:

Tensilon Test

Edrophonium (Tensilon) is a rapid-acting anticholinesterase used to diagnose myasthenia gravis and occasionally used to differentiate myasthenia gravis from suspected botulism. An intravenous (IV) injection of 10 mg is prepared and then 1–2 mg are administered slowly, to avoid the commonly associated nausea and vomiting. The remainder of the Tensilon is given over the next 5 minutes. The strength of patients who have myasthenia gravis will dramatically improve within 30–60 seconds, and this improvement will last 3–5 minutes. This drug prevents the available acetylcholine from being metabolized, permitting continued reaction with the reduced number of postsynaptic acetylcholine receptors. In rare cases of botulism there is a small improvement in strength, which is far less dramatic than that seen in patients with myasthenia gravis.[16,46] In botulism, the release of acetylcholine is impaired and the prevention of its metabolism is of limited importance.

Electromyography

The EMG pattern in all forms of botulism is characterized by brief, small, abundant motor unit action potentials (BSAPs; or low-amplitude, short-duration potentials). Motor nerve conduction velocity is normal. Primary muscle diseases also show normal conduction velocity and a BSAP pattern, but in botulism, serum levels of muscle enzymes and muscle biopsy are normal. Another typical EMG finding in botulism is an increment of small compound muscle action potential (CMAP) amplitude directly related to the release of acetylcholine following repetitive stimulation at 20–50 Hz[44] (Fig. 73–2). Posttetanic facilitation may be noted in cases of botulism as well as other entities, including the Eaton-Lambert paraneoplastic syndrome, aminoglycoside-associated paralysis, and hypermagnesemia. Therefore, although not pathognomonic, EMG findings interpreted in the light of the total clinical presentation can help to establish the diagnosis of botulism.[2,64]

Specimens

Samples of serum, stool, vomitus, gastric contents, and suspect foods should be tested for *C. botulinum* and botu-

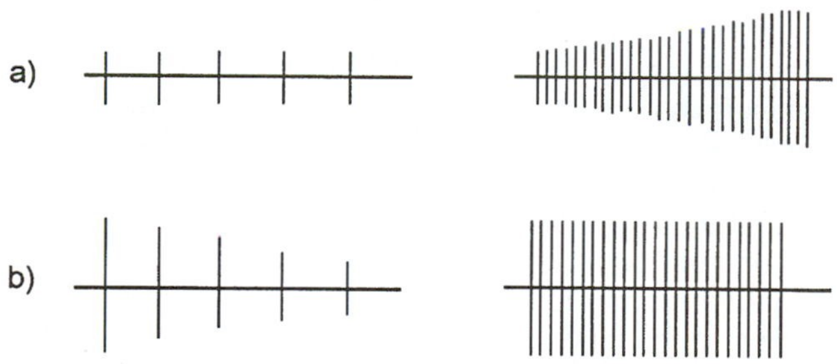

Figure 73–2. Electromyographic findings. Schematic representations of repetitive nerve stimulation at low (5/sec) and high (50/sec) frequencies. In botulism (a) repetitive stimulation produces a small muscle action potential that facilitates (increases in amplitude) at higher frequencies. This effect results from increased acetylcholine release at high-frequency stimulation because of increased intracellular calcium concentration. In contrast, myasthenia gravis (b) is associated with a normal muscle action potential amplitude and a decremental response at low-frequency stimulation with a normal response at high-frequency stimulation. Myasthenia gravis, a disorder of the muscle endplate, produces this decremental response at low freqencies because the natural reduction in acetylcholine response with subsequent stimulation falls below threshold. *(See references 4, 44, 62.)*

TABLE 73–4. LABORATORY ASSESSMENT IN THE DIAGNOSIS OF BOTULISM

Classification	Food	Infant	Wound Infection	Infant Type Adult Botulism
Toxin type	A,B,E,F,G in humans, C,D in animals	A,B,C,F	A,B	A?
Route	Ingestion	Ingestion	Wound, abscess (sinusitis)	Ingestion of bacteria and spores
Specimens	Stool: positive for bacteria/spores and toxin	Stool: positive for bacteria/ spores and toxin for up to 8 wk after recovery	Wound site: Gram stain, aerobic and anaerobic cultures	Stool: positive for bacteria/ spores and toxin
Toxin in serum	Yes	Yes	Yes	Yes
Toxin, bacteria/spores in food	Yes (all)	Bacteria/spores: yes Toxin: no	No	Bacteria/spores: yes Toxin: no
Family and friends	At risk if same foods were eaten	Unaffected	Unaffected (unless shared needle)	Unaffected

linum toxins (Table 73–4). If wound botulism is suspected, serum, stool, exudate, debrided tissue, and swab samples should be collected. In infants, feces and serum samples should be obtained. The specimens should be handled cautiously, refrigerated, and examined as soon as possible after collection. Serum samples should be taken prior to administration of antitoxin. Stool and serum samples are used for a mouse bioassay. Stool specimens are incubated anaerobically and subcultured on an egg yolk agar.[36] Routine laboratory studies, including CSF analysis, are normal in botulism.

How Is Botulism Treated?

Supportive Care

Respiratory compromise is the usual cause of death from botulism. Therefore, hospital admission of both the patient and all individuals suspected of exposure to the possible source is mandatory. Careful continuous monitoring of respiratory status using precise parameters such as vital capacity, peak expiratory flow rate (PEFR), negative inspiratory force (NIF), pulse oximetry, and gag reflex is essential to determine the need for intubation or tracheostomy as the patient begins to manifest signs of bulbar paralysis.[50] In a single study, approximately 80% of children with botulism required intubation for a reduced vital capacity; 25% of these children had frank respiratory compromise.[50] When suspicion of disease is high and the vital capacity is less than 30% of predicted, intubation should be strongly considered.[59]

Gastric Decontamination

An attempt should be made to remove the spores and toxin from the gut. Although most patients present after a delay in time, the etiologic agent may still be present hours or even days later. Activated charcoal should be part of routine supportive care as it has been shown to adsorb *C. botulinum* type A toxin in vitro.[21] Gastric lavage or emesis should be initiated only for a cohort who has recently ingested a known contaminated food. If a cathartic is chosen, sorbitol is probably the cathartic of choice. Magnesium salts may potentially depress neuromuscular transmission and should theoretically be avoided in this situation. Whole-bowel irrigation theoretically may have a role in decontamination, but has not been thoroughly evaluated in this situation.

Botulinum Antitoxin

The efficacy of antitoxin to type B strain is unknown; antitoxins to A and E are probably beneficial.[59] Antitoxin can prevent paralysis but does not affect already paralyzed muscles. Therefore, to be most effective, antitoxin must be employed immediately upon consideration of the disease in both the afflicted and those who have been exposed but have not yet developed symptomatology. However, the possible benefits of antitoxin must be weighed against the incidence of anaphylaxis and serum sickness. Antitoxin is not employed in children with infant botulism because circulating toxin is believed to be at very low levels, and the antitoxin has no effect on toxin-producing organisms in the gut.[49]

In a review of 132 cases of type A foodborne botulism, a lower fatality rate and a shorter course were demonstrated for those who received trivalent antitoxin, even after controlling for age and incubation period.[59] The earlier a patient received antitoxin, the shorter was the clinical course. In addition, no respiratory arrests occurred more than 5 hours after antitoxin was administered. In view of the high mortality rate with foodborne botulism and limited statistical data, the antitoxin should be given IV to all exposed patients. Botulinum antitoxins types A, B, AB (bivalent), E, ABE (trivalent), and F are available. The type-specific antitoxins are ineffective against any other antigen. Although specific foods tend to correlate relatively well with botulinum type, this should not restrict the use of the trivalent antitoxin (7500 U type A, 5500 U type B, and 8500 U type E) until more specific type information is available. Each vial of trivalent antitoxin contains 10 mL (monovalent type E has 5000 IU/2 mL vial), which should be given as a 1:10 vol/vol dilution in 0.9% sodium chloride. If epidemiologic work identifies the organism, subsequent type-specific antitoxin therapy may be instituted. Hypersensitivity testing for horse serum is officially recommended, but its utility is questionable. Epinephrine should be readily available, owing to the risk of hypersensitivity and anaphylaxis. The overall rate of adverse reactions is 9–17%, with an incidence of anaphylaxis as low as 1.9%.[5,40]

Guanidine

At one time guanidine was used to enhance acetylcholine release, although its merits have never been substantiated.[17] In poorly controlled studies, 15–40 mg/kg/day of guanidine orally resulted in possible EMG improvement. The most striking improvement was in the ocular muscles and the least consequential was in the respiratory muscles. Significant nausea and epigastric pain are associated with guanidine. These adverse effects, the fact that many patients present with intestinal ileus, and the absence of a parenteral form of the drug make interpretation of drug efficacy difficult. For all of these reasons the drug is now rarely used clinically.[45]

Penicillin

Penicillin has no role in the management of botulism caused by preformed toxin and it has not been shown to prevent gut spores from germinating. For these reasons, penicillin is not considered useful in infantile and infant variant adult botulism. Penicillin G is one of many drugs with excellent in vitro efficacy against *C. botulinum* and is used for wound botulism.[58]

Epidemiologic and Therapeutic Assistance

Whenever botulism is suspected or proven, the state health department or the Enteric Disease Branch, Bacterial Diseases Division, Bureau of Epidemiology, Centers for Disease Control (404–639–2206 days or 404–639–2888 nights, weekends, or holidays) should be contacted for diagnostic, consultative, and laboratory testing services, for the use of trivalent botulinum antitoxin, and for assistance in epidemiologic investigations. This can be done by the local physician, hospital, or poison control center. Any possibly contaminated foods should be preserved for epidemiologic investigation.

What Are the Other Forms of Botulism?

Infant Botulism [in vivo]

Infant botulism was first described in 1976 in California.[3,26,28,63] As of 1994, 1270 hospitalized cases have been documented,[43] making this the most common form of botulism. Of these cases 95% occurred in the United States and 99% were from botulinum neurotoxin type A or B.[43] Affected children are always less than 1 year of age (usually 1–3 months) and characteristically have had normal gestations and births. The first signs of infant botulism are constipation, feeding difficulty, feeble crying, and a "floppy" baby with diffuse decreased muscle tone, particularly apparent in the limbs and neck. Ophthalmoplegia, loss of facial grimacing, dysphagia, diminished gag reflex, poor anal sphincter tone, and respiratory failure have been noted, but fever and enteric symptoms have not. The differential diagnosis of infant botulism initially includes dehydration, a failure to thrive, hypotonia of unknown etiology, sepsis, or a viral syndrome. Many of the syndromes cited in Table 72–1 are also relevant to the evaluation of children as are many rarer neurologic, myopathic, and congenital syndromes that occur in the first year of life.[28]

Only certain infants are susceptible to this condition. Some young children may be immunologically unprepared for spore control, a deficiency that allows subsequent germination and toxin development. As opposed to the better understood foodborne botulism variants, infant botulism may be the result of the ingestion of *C. botulinum* organisms with subsequent in vivo production of toxin followed by gut absorption. An infant's gastrointestinal tract lacks bile acids and gastric acid, which may inhibit clostridial growth in the older child and adult. Some authors have suggested that bacterial growth associated with breast feeding (70% of cases) favors *Bifibobacterium* development as opposed to *Coliforme* spp, *Enterococcus* spp, and *Bacteroides* spp, all three of which may inhibit *C. botulinum*.[23,62] Thus, the absence of these typical organisms may facilitate *C. botulinum* multiplication. Since the toxin in infant botulism is absorbed gradually as it is produced, the clinical manifestations of botulism may be less dramatic than in severe cases of foodborne botulism, where large amounts of preformed toxin are absorbed at one time.

Certain studies have shown a correlation between the presence of *C. botulinum* organisms and toxin and sudden infant death syndrome (SIDS).[54] These disorders have a common age distribution as well. However, the survival rate in infant botulism to date is approximately 97%, which is quite different from SIDS.[4]

Although infant botulism has been detected in approximately half of the states in the United States and in England and Australia, 50% of reported cases emanate from California, Utah, and New Mexico. In California, aggressive surveillance and educational efforts with regard to infant botulism have been practiced since 1976.

Cases of infant botulism must be managed in the hospital, preferably in an ICU for at least the first week, when the risk of respiratory arrest is greatest. In a group of 57 patients aged 18 days to 7 months, 77% of patients were intubated and 68% required mechanical ventilation. The loss of airway protection was the best indicator for aggressive management, whereas neither hypoxia nor hypercarbia was a reliable indicator.[51]

Several children with infant botulism have had multiple respiratory arrests.[4] Often the respiratory difficulties were associated with such procedures as lumbar punctures or radiographs. Although nothing should ever take precedence over basic cardiopulmonary support, these functions often are unintentionally compromised during procedures.[28,33]

Whether there is any role for antitoxin or antibiotics in infant botulism is at present unclear. There are documented cases of children surviving without either antitoxin or parenteral antibiotics. In any case, antitoxin is not recommended, as it has no effect on toxin-producing organisms in the gut,[28,33] nor is it expected to halt the syndrome's progression. Moreover, in fully recovered children, toxin as well as spores have been found for months in the stools, despite either oral or parenteral antibiotics and antitoxin administration.

Prevention in infants includes limiting exposure to spores by thoroughly washing foods and objects that might be placed in a child's mouth. In addition, honey should not be given to infants. Epidemiologic studies indicate that ingestion of honey was associated with 34.7% of hospitalized cases of infant botulism worldwide. Moreover, of all nutritional items tested in one study, only honey was found to contain *C. botulinum* spores.[3] When *C. botulinum* spores have been isolated from honey, the identical toxin serotype has been isolated from the infant. As noted previously, no preformed toxin has been isolated. Testing on a human-derived botulism immune globulin (BIG) is under investigation for the treatment of infant botulism.[18,39]

Wound Botulism [in vivo]

Wound contamination is the least common cause of botulism. The first case was not reported until 1943, and the Centers for Disease Control (CDC) had identified only approximately 75 cases by 1995. The "classic" presentation is that of a patient injured in an automobile accident sustaining a deep muscle laceration, crush injury, or compound fracture treated with open reduction. The wound is frequently quite dirty, usually associated with inadequate debridement, subsequent purulent drainage, and local tenderness. Although the wound may subsequently appear unremarkable, 4–18 days later cranial nerve palsies and the other neurologic findings typical of botulism (eg, dysphagia, dysphonia, dyspnea, and dysarthria) appear.[38] Other classic signs of food-related botulism may be absent and there are no GI manifestations.

In this form of botulism, fever may be prominent and associated with the sinusitis, abscess, or other tissue infection presumed to harbor the clostridial organisms. The patient may need to be managed for wound-related problems or the wound may appear healthy and uninfected. No particular vehicle, vector, or pathophysiology has been identified. Recognition of the entity in the differential diagnosis of wound infections is essential for appropriate therapy.

In 1982 and 1983 three parenteral drug abusers presented to emergency departments in New York City with dysphagia, dysarthria, dry mouth, and progressive neurologic impairment. The symptoms were typical for botulism except that one patient did not have ocular symptoms and two did not have cutaneous infections prior to the onset of cranial nerve dysfunction. In one case a subcutaneous cystic lesion (site of a previous attempted injection) yielded anaerobic gram-positive bacilli, and material that was positive for type B botulinum toxin by mouse bioassay. Remarkably, in all three cases, dysphagia was the most prominent symptom; in fact, two patients were initially admitted to otolaryngology services. The CDC evaluated three additional patients with botulism-like illnesses in whom no organism or toxin was found in serum, stool, or skin lesions.[36] The clinical course and electromyographic patterns of these cases were compatible with botulism.

The three New York City cases were the first recognized cases among drug abusers, but botulism would appear to be a logical complication of septic parenteral drug abuse. Thorough wound debridement is the most critical aspect of the management and should be performed even if the wound appears unremarkable.[24,35] Antibiotic therapy alone is inadequate as there are several case reports of disease despite antibiotic therapy. One of the three patients chronically used cocaine and had a purulent sinusitis, which may have been the source of the type A *C. botulinum* toxin found in the serum, although nothing was cultured from sinus drainage or stool. More recently cocaine[46,57] and heroin,[11] particularly a "black tar heroin" that is often used subcutaneously, have been associated with increasing numbers of cases of wound botulism.[20]

Classification Undetermined (Infant Type Adult Botulism) [in vivo]

This fourth class of botulism established by the CDC includes any patient older than 1 year for whom it has been impossible to implicate a particular food source. It is postulated that some of the cases in this group represent a variant form of botulism similar to infant botulism.[40] A case of adult botulism resulting from the ingestion of a food source contaminated with *C. botulinum* type A with no preformed toxin has been well documented.[14] In this case a long incubation period with toxin present in the serum and stool for 3 weeks after exposure and the absence of disease in the patient's spouse suggested in vivo intraluminal elaboration of toxin. This patient may have been a very unusual host in that she had peptic ulcer disease treated with truncal vagotomy, antrectomy, and a Billroth I anastomosis. She also had received perioperative antibiotics 5 weeks prior to the development of botulism. All of these factors may have compromised the gastric and bile acid barrier, gut flora, and motility, thus allowing spore germination, altered bacterial growth, and toxin development. Other cases have occurred in a patient with ileal bypass surgery and Crohn's disease[7] and a necrotic volvulus.[35] The general risk factors favoring organism persistence and *C. botulinum* colonization include recent antibiotic therapy, gastric achlorhydria (either surgically or pharmacologically induced) and previous intestinal surgery.

What Are the Epidemiologic Characteristics of Botulism?

Contrary to popular opinion, multiple cases per occurrence are not necessarily expected in outbreaks of the disease. Between 1976 and 1984, 124 outbreaks occurred, involving 308 persons. Sixty-eight percent involved only one person, 20% two persons, and only 12% more than two persons (mean number of 2.7 cases per outbreak). There are approximately 1.25 cases of foodborne botulism per 10 million people annually.[35]

Only 4% of foodborne outbreaks are associated with food purchased in restaurants, but these usually affect large numbers of individuals and account for more than 40% of the total number of reported cases.[35] Commercial food processing accounts for 2% of reported cases. Vegetables (peppers, beans, mushrooms, tomatoes, and beets), with or without meat, are thought to be the causative agents in about 70%, meat in 17%, and fish in 13% of cases. Common home-canning errors include failure to pressure cook and allowing food to putrefy at room temperature. In recent years outbreaks of botulism have been associated with specialty foods consumed by different ethnic groups: chopped garlic in soy oil by Chinese in Vancouver, British Columbia;[41,56] fried lotus rhizome solid mustard in Japan;[42] uneviscerated salted fish—called *kapchunka* by Russian immigrants in New York City[31,60] and called *maloha* by Egyptians in Egypt; and fermented salmon eggs, seal, and whale skin by Inuits and Native Americans in Alaska.[65] It is important to be aware of new trends and unusual presentations of botulism. Preventive education is also necessary. Ninety percent of type E outbreaks have occurred in Alaska, and all type E outbreaks have implicated home-processed fish or meat from marine animals.[19,35]

The case fatality ratio for type A is about 12% and for types B and E approximately 10%.[32,40,59] When the type of toxin is unknown, the case fatality rate may be as high as 50%, as have been mortality rates in the past.[32,40,59] The improvement in case fatality rates for all types of botulism probably represents increasing awareness of the problem, the use of antitoxin, and better and more easily accessible life-support techniques.

What Is the Prognosis in Botulism?

If the patient has had excellent respiratory support during the acute phase prior to hypoxia or aspiration pneumonitis and receives parenteral nutrition, residual neurologic disability may not occur. Although the initial course may be protracted, almost total functional recovery can follow within several months to a year. Common long-term sequelae are dysgeusia (Chap. 27), dry mouth, constipation, dyspepsia, arthralgia, exertional dyspnea, tachycardia, and easy fatigability.

The long-term status of 13 patients who survived a type B botulinum outbreak 2 years earlier was characterized by persistent dyspnea and fatigue, although, surprisingly, pulmonary function tests had returned to normal in all patients.[66] Inspiratory muscle weakness persisted in 4 of 13 patients. Maximal oxygen consumption and maximal workload during exercise were diminished. These patients had more rapid shallow breathing and a higher dyspnea score than controls. The reason for premature exercise termination may be multifactorial: Although persistent respiratory muscle weakness may be an explanation, most dyspnea and fatigue appeared to be related to reduced cardiovascular fitness, leg fatigue, and diminished nutrition. Nevertheless, because long-term prognosis can be so good, early recognition of the disease and supportive care are essential.

There are now at least three reports of botulism occuring during pregnancy. One occurred during the second trimester[47] and two during the third trimester.[20,55] Although botulinal toxin or *C. botulinum* were isolated in the mother in two of the cases prior to antitoxin therapy, no detectable toxin was isolated from the neonate in either of the third-trimester cases. The large molecular weight of the neurotoxic component (150,000 D) of the toxin makes passive diffusion unlikely and, although a possiblity, no active transport system has been identified.[55] In these cases, neurologic findings in the neonate noted at birth were most likely the result of complications of delivery, not botulinal disease in the infant. It appears that appropriate care of the mother and preparation for maternal complications of delivery should assure the best potential for a normal infant.

Acknowledgment

Richard S. Weisman, PharmD contributed to this chapter in a previous edition.

References

1. Alderson K, Holds JB, Anderson RL: Botulinum induced alteration of nerve-muscle interactions in human orbicularis oculi following treatment for blepharospasm. Neurology 1991;41:1800–1805.
2. Argov MD, Mastaglia FL: Disorders of neuromuscular transmission caused by drugs. N Engl J Med 1979;301: 409–413.
3. Arnon SS, Midura TF, Damus K, et al: Honey and other environmental risk factors for infant botulism. J Pediatr 1979; 94:331–336.
4. Arnon SS, Midura TF, Damus K: Intestinal infection and toxin production by *Clostridium botulinum* as one cause of sudden infant death syndrome. Lancet 1978;1:1273–1277.
5. Badhey H, Cleri DJ, D'Amato RF, et al: Two fatal cases of type E adult foodborne botulism with early symptoms and terminal neurologic signs. J Clin Microbiol 1986;23:616–618.
6. Barker WH, Weissman MD, Dowell VR, et al: Type B botulism outbreak caused by a commercial food product. JAMA 1977;237:456–459.
7. Bartlett JC: Infant botulism in adults. N Engl J Med 1986; 315:254–255.
8. Beller M, Middaugh JP: Repeated type E botulism in an Alaskan Eskimo. N Engl J Med 1990;322:855. Letter.
9. Blake PA, Horwitz MD, Hopkins L, et al: Type A botulism from commercially canned beef stew. South Med J 1977;70: 5–7.
10. Borodic GE, Pearce LB. New concepts in botulinum toxin therapy. Drug Safety 1994;11:145–152.
11. Burningham MD, Walter FG, Mechem C, et al: Wound botulism. Ann Emerg Med 1994;24:1184–1187.

12. Case records of the Massachusetts General Hospital, Case 48—1980. N Engl J Med 1980;303:1347–1355.
13. Cherington M: Botulism: Ten-year experience. Arch Neurol 1974;30:432–437.
14. Chia JK, Clark JB, Ryan CA, Pollack M: Botulism in an adult associated with foodborne intestinal infection with *Clostridium botulinum*. N Engl J Med 1986;315:239–241.
15. Dowell UR Jr, McCroskey LM, Hatheway CL, et al: Coproexamination for botulinal toxin and *Clostridium botulism*. JAMA 1977;238:1829–1832.
16. Edell TA, Sullivan CP Jr, Osborn KM, et al: Wound botulism associated with a positive Tensilon test. West J Med 1983;139:218–219.
17. Faich GA, Graebner RW, Sato S: Failure of guanidine therapy in botulism A. N Engl J Med 1971;285:773–776.
18. Frankovich TL, Arnon SS: Clinical trial of botulism immune globulin for infant botulism. West J Med 1991;154:103.
19. French G, Pavlick A, Felsen A, et al: Outbreak of type E botulism associated with an uneviscerated, salt cured fish product: New Jersey, 1992. MMWR 1992;41:521–522.
20. Gollober M, Beyer RA, Kwan S, et al: Wound botulism: California, 1995. MMWR 1995;44:889–892.
21. Gomez HF, Johnson R, Guven H, et al: Adsorption of botulinum toxin to activated charcoal with a mouse bioassay. Ann Emerg Med 1995;25:818–822.
22. Gutmann L, Pratt L: Pathophysiologic aspects of human botulism. Arch Neurol 1976;33:175–179.
23. Hentges D: The intestinal flora and infant botulism. Rev Infect Dis 1979;1:668–673.
24. Hikes DC, Manoli A II: Wound botulism. J Trauma 1981;21:68–71.
25. Horwitz MA, Marr JS, Merson MH, et al: A continuing common-source outbreak of botulism in a family. Lancet 1975;2:861–863.
26. Infant botulism: A newly recognized syndrome. Calif Morbid 1976;34 (suppl):1–2.
27. Jankovic J, Brin MF: Therapeutic use of botulinum toxin. N Engl J Med 1991;324:1186–1193.
28. Johnson RO, Clay SA, Arnon SS: Diagnosis and management of infant botulism. Am J Dis Child 1979;133:586–593.
29. Kao I, Drachman DB, Price DL: Botulinum toxin: Mechanism of presynaptic blockade. Science 1976;193:1256–1258.
30. Koenig M, Spickard A, Cardella M, et al: Clinical and laboratory observations on type E botulism in man. Medicine 1964;43:517–545.
31. Kotev S, Leventhal A, Bashary A, et al: International outbreak of type E botulism associated with ungutted, salted white fish. MMWR 1987;36:812–813.
32. LeCour H, Ramos H, Almeida B, Barbosa R: Food borne botulism: A review of 13 outbreaks. Arch Intern Med 1988;148:578–580.
33. Long SS: Botulism in infancy. Pediatr Infect Dis J 1984;3:266–271.
34. Ludlow CL: Treatment of speech and voice disorders with botulinum toxin. JAMA 1990;264:2671–2675.
35. MacDonald KL, Cohen ML, Blake PA: The changing epidemiology of adult botulism in the United States. Am J Epidemiol 1986;124:794–799.
36. MacDonald KL, Rutherford GW, Friedman SM, et al: Botulism and botulism-like illness in chronic drug users. Ann Intern Med 1985;102:616–618.
37. MacDonald KL, Spengler RF, Hatheway CL, et al: Type A botulism from sauteed onions: Clinical and epidemiologic observations. JAMA 1985;253:1275–1278.
38. Merson MH, Dowel VR: Epidemiologic, clinical and laboratory aspects of wound botulism. N Engl J Med 1973;289:1005–1010.
39. Metzger JF, Lewis GE Jr: Human derived immune globulin for the treatment of botulism. Rev Infect Dis 1979;1:689–692.
40. Morris JG Jr, Hatheway CL: Botulism in the United States, 1979. J Infect Dis 1980;142:302–305.
41. Morse DL, Pichard LK, Guzewich JT, et al: Garlic in oil associated botulism: Episode leads to product modification. Am J Public Health 1990;80:1372–1373.
42. Otofugi T, Tokiwa H, Takahashi K: A food poisoning incident caused by *Clostridium botulinum* toxin A in Japan. Epidemiol Infect 1987;99:167–172.
43. Paisley JW, Lauer BA, Arnon RS: A second case of infant botulism type F caused by *Clostridium baratii*. Pediatr Infect Dis J 1995;14:912–914.
44. Pickett JB III: AAEE case report #16: Botulism. Muscle Nerve 1988;11:1201–1205.
45. Puggiari M, Cherington M: Botulism and guanidine. JAMA 1978;240:2276–2277.
46. Rapoport S, Watkins PB: Descending paralysis resulting from occult wound botulism. Ann Neurol 1984;16:359–361.
47. Robin L, Herman D, Redett R: Botulism in a pregnant woman. N Engl J Med 1996;335:823–824.
48. Schantz EJ, Johnson EA: Properties and use of botulinum toxin and other microbial neurotoxins in medicine. Microbiol Rev 1992;56:80–99.
49. Schmidt RD, Schmidt TW: Infant botulism: A case series and a review of the literature. J Emerg Med 1992;10:713–718.
50. Schmidt-Nowara WW, Samet JM, Rasario PA: Early and late pulmonary complications of botulism. Arch Intern Med 1983;143:451–456.
51. Schreiner MS, Field E, Ruddy R: Infant botulism: A review of 12 years experience at the Children's Hospital of Philadelphia. Pediatrics 1991;87:159–165.
52. Simpson LL: Botulinum toxin: A deadly poison sheds its negative image. Ann Intern Med 1996;125:616–617.
53. Smith LDS: The occurrence of *Clostridium botulinum* and *Clostridium tetani* in the soil of the United States. Health Lab Sci 1978;15:74–80.
54. Sonnabend OAR, Sonnabend WFF, Krech V, et al: Continuous microbiological and pathological study of 70 sudden and unexpected infant deaths: Toxigenic intestinal *Clostridium botulinum* infection in 9 cases of sudden infant death. Lancet 1985;1:237–241.
55. St. Clair EH, DiLiberti JH, O'Brien ML: Observations of an infant born to a mother with botulism. J Pediatr 1975;87:658.
56. St. Louis ME, Peck SHS, Bowering D, et al: Botulism from chopped garlic, delayed recognition of a major outbreak. Ann Intern Med 1988;108:363–368.
57. Swedberg J, Wendel TH, Deiss F: Wound botulism. West J Med 1987;147:335–338.
58. Swenson JM, Thornsberry C, McCroskey LM, et al: Susceptibility of *Clostridium botulinum* to thirteen antimicrobial agents. Antimicrob Agents Chemother 1980;18:13–19.
59. Tacket CO, Shandera WX, Mann JM, et al: Equine antitoxin use and other factors that predict outcome in type A foodborne botulism. Am J Med 1984;76:794–798.

60. Telzak EE, Bell EP, Kauter DA, et al: An international outbreak of type E botulism due to uneviscerated fish. J Infect Dis 1990;161:340–342.
61. Terranova W, Palumbo JN, Breman JG: Ocular findings in botulism type B. JAMA 1979;241:475–477.
62. Thompson JA, Glascow LA, Warpinski JR, et al: Infant botulism. Clinical spectrum and epidemiology. Pediatrics 1980;6:936–942.
63. Turner HD, Brett EM, Gilbert RJ, et al: Infant botulism in England. Lancet 1978;1:1277–1278.
64. Valli G, Barbieri S, Scarlato G: Neurophysiological tests in human botulism. Electromyogr Clin Neurophysiol 1983;23: 3–11.
65. Wainwright RB, Heyward WL, Middaugh JP, et al: Foodborne botulism in Alaska, 1947–1985: Epidemiology and clinical findings. J Infect Dis 1988;157:1158–1162.
66. Wilcox P, Andofatto C, Fairbain MS, Pardy RL: Long-term follow-up of symptoms, pulmonary function, respiratory muscle strength and exercise performance after botulism. Am Rev Respir Dis 1989;139:157–163.
67. Wolfe L: Death by botulism: A medical mystery story. New York Magazine 1980;13:56–60.

ANTIDOTES IN DEPTH

Botulinum Antitoxin

Lewis R. Goldfrank

Trivalent botulinum antitoxin (types A, B, and E) is an equine globulin preparation that has been available in the United States since the late 1960s.[1] All of the individuals treated during the initial decade of the antitoxin's availability (1967–1977) were studied to define hypersensitivity reaction rates and efficacy of the antitoxin in preventing botulism.

The antitoxin is produced by healthy horses immunized against botulinum toxin and is then defibrinated, digested, dialyzed, and prepared as a 20% protein antitoxin.[2] Like many other heterologous proteins, this horse serum–derived preparation produces substantial adverse effects.[8] Botulinum antitoxin is distributed from the nine regional centers of the Centers for Disease Control (CDC) on a named patient basis once a probable diagnosis of botulism has been established. Because of the lethality of botulinum toxin, the risk of adverse drug reaction is considered acceptable for anyone with presumed illness as well as individuals potentially exposed to the toxin. Pregnancy is not a contraindication to antitoxin administration and has been used successfully in this setting.[5]

The currently available trivalent botulinum antitoxin contains 7500 IU (2381 US units) of type A botulinum antitoxin, 5500 IU (1839 US units) of type B antitoxin, and 8500 IU (8500 US units) of type E antitoxin in each 10-mL vial.[6] Although evidence for the efficacy of types B and E antitoxin have not been established, the proportion and quantity of types A and B antitoxin are assumed to be adequate to neutralize corresponding circulating toxins, and the level of type E antitoxin exceeds the level shown to be efficacious.[2,6]

Limited data exist with regard to the relationship of dose and route of administration, the amount of circulating antitoxin found in treated patients, the toxin-neutralizing capacity of this material, and the half-life of the antitoxin. Peak serum levels of antitoxin have been measured at 10–1000 times higher than necessary to achieve toxin neutralization. There appears to be little depletion of antitoxin when patients who had circulating type A toxin prior to treatment have been studied.[7] In one patient, the half-life for antitoxin persistence was calculated at 6.5, 7.6, and 5.3 days for antitoxin types A, B, and E, respectively.[7] In another patient 90% of the activity of the equine antitoxin administered was detected when all the circulating toxin had been neutralized.[9] The prolonged half-life of the antitoxin and the exceedingly small quantities of toxin measured explain the limited depletion of antitoxin even after toxin–antitoxin binding has occurred.

Type E botulinum antitoxin was used succesfully to treat 100 Egyptians who presumably had ingested botulinum toxin–contaminated fish.[4] The type E antitoxin was available as 5000 IU per 2-mL vials in Egypt as a consequence of the military preparedness for the Persian Gulf War. Prophylactic doses were considered 1000–5000 IU of the monovalent antitoxin administered IM, based on the estimated quantity of toxin ingested. The safety of this human-derived preparation allowed for repetitive dosing if clinical findings developed.[4]

Small repetitive dosing was based on the belief that effective treatment could be achieved with antitoxin doses exceeding the level of toxin dose when administered before circulating toxin became tissue-bound. There is no evidence that antitoxin will reverse symptoms, but it may inhibit progression of symptoms. In the presence of disease one vial of the antitoxin is administered slowly IV as a 1:10 vol/vol dilution in 0.9% sodium chloride. This dose may be complemented by an IM dose of a single vial given simultaneously. Subsequently doses may be given IV every 2–4 hours, depending on clinical findings.[2,6]

The issue of sensitivity to equine proteins and conjunctival or intradermal testing is discussed in detail in this text in Antidotes in Depth: Antivenin (Crotalid and Elapid). However, once the need for botulinum antitoxin has been established, hypersensitivity to equine proteins is not a contraindication to antitoxin administration, as botulism is fatal. Anaphylaxis should be anticipated, and the clinician should be prepared to treat it immediately with epinephrine. The smaller quantities of botulinum antitoxin used for botulism present a far smaller risk for serum sickness[1] than do the larger amounts of antitoxin used to treat snake envenomation. The risk of serum sickness with the refined serum proteins may be approximately 5–10%.[1,6] Patients who have received antitoxin in the first 24 hours have been shown to have a shorter course but a comparable mortality rate to those who received antitoxin later.[13] Only in animal models have botulinum antitoxins been shown definitively to reduce mortality.[10] Morbidity and mortality studies are difficult to perform for a disorder that is so rare and often recognized at a delayed stage, after the toxin is already tightly bound to the neuromuscular junction. Most of the reported case series involve patients who have received varying degrees of supportive care, further making evaluation or comparison unreliable.

Future possible treatments for botulism may involve two additional types of immunotherapy.

1. *Pentavalent (A, B, C, D, E) toxoid.* Although a pentavalent toxoid (A, B, C, D, E) has been studied for almost 40 years,[9] it remains investigational. Its use had been suggested only for laboratory personnel who work intimately with *Clostridium botulinum* and was developed at the U.S. Army Medical Research Institute of Infectious Diseases at Fort Detrich, Maryland. Clinical trials with a human-derived pentavalent botulism immune globulin (BIG) are currently underway through an orphan drug infant botulism prevention program.[3]

2. *Human botulism immune globulin (BIG) for infant botulism.* Results of the clinical trial of the human BIG for infant botulism suggests many advantages over the current equine antitoxin therapy. This pentavalent (types A, B, C, D, and E) immune globulin is harvested by plasmapheresis from human donors who received multiple immunizations with pentavalent botulinal toxoid.[11,14] A longer biologic half-life with a prolonged effective level should be possible with BIG,[9] and this form of human immune globulin obviously avoids the use of foreign equine proteins and its inherent risk of hypersensitivity. Both of these are substantial clinical advantages, particularly in the infant form, where toxin is slowly and continuously absorbed as ongoing intestinal production occurs.

Human-derived botulism immune globulin (BIG) became available in California in 1991 for clinical trials.[3] Human BIG has been used successfully for a 3-year-old child who, following bone marrow transplant, developed altered gut microbial flora and botulism. This may be termed an infant form of adult botulism in a child.[12]

Summary

Consultation with the regional poison center and health department will improve access to rapid diagnostic tests and therapeutic modalities that appear to be decreasing morbidity and enhancing survival after typical food-borne botulism. Current research on infant botulism will demonstrate whether there is enough circulating toxin present in that variant to be amenable to antitoxin treatment. Presumably antitoxin may be useful if, as suggested, a low level of absorbed toxin is present in these disorders.9 The BIG study should clarify this issue and allow adequate treatment for the infant form of botulism, which has become the most prevalent form of botulism encountered today.

References

1. Black RE, Gunn RA: Hypersensitivity reactions associated with botulinal antitoxin. Am J Med 1980;69:567–570.
2. Food and Drug Administration, Biological Products, Bacterial Vaccines and Toxoids: Implementation of efficacy review: Proposed rule. Fed Reg 1985;50:51002–51117.
3. Frankovich TL, Arnon SS: Clinical trial of botulism immune globulin for infant botulism. West J Med 1991;154:103.
4. Goldsmith MF: Defensive biological warfare researchers prepare to counteract "natural enemies" in battle, at home. JAMA 1991;266:2522–2523.
5. Gollober M, Beyer RA, Kwan S, et al: Wound botulism—California, 1995. MMWR 1995;44:889–892.
6. Grabenstein JD: Immunoantidotes: II. One hundred years of antitoxins. Hosp Pharm 1992;27:637–646.
7. Hatheway CH, Snyder JD, Seals JE, et al: Antitoxin levels in botulism patients treated with trivalent equine botulism antitoxin to toxin types A, B, and E. J Infect Dis 1984;150: 407–412.
8. Merson MH, Hughes JM, Dowell VR: Current trends in botulism in the United States. JAMA 1974;229:1305–1308.
9. Metzger JF, Lewis LE: Human-derived immune globulins for the treatment of botulism. Rev Infect Dis 1979;1: 689–692.
10. Oberst FW, Crook JW, Cresthull P, House MJ: Evaluation of botulinum antitoxin, supportive therapy, and artificial respiration in monkeys with experimental botulism. Clin Pharmacol Ther 1968;9:209–214.
11. Pickett J, Berg B, Chaplin E, Brunstetter-Shafer MA: Syndrome of botulism in infancy: Clinical and electrophysiologic study. N Engl J Med 1976;295:770–772.
12. Shen WP, Felsing N, Lang D, et al: Development of infant botulism in a 3 year old female with neuroblastoma following autologous bone narrow transplantation: Potential use of human botulism immune globulin. Bone Marrow Transplant 1994;13:345–347.
13. Tacket CO, Shandera WX, Mann JM, et al: Equine antitoxin use and other factors that predict outcome in type A food-borne botulism. Am J Med 1984;76:794–798.
14. Thilo EH, Townsend SF, Deacon J: Infant botulism at 1 week of age: Report of two cases. Pediatrics 1993;92:151–153.

CHAPTER 74

Air and Water Pollution

Jeffrey R. Brubacher

Air Pollution

CASE 1. For centuries coal was the primary source of heating fuel used in London, England, and it was not unusual for "great stinking fogs" to form over the city. The association of these fogs with increased death rates and respiratory illness was noted as early as 1661.[34] In the winter of 1952, a severe temperature inversion settled over London, England, and caused vast quantities of smoke from coal fires and other sources of pollution to form a thick fog over the city. At the same time clinicians attended to an increased number of persons complaining of respiratory symptoms and noted a marked increase in the number of deaths occurring among the elderly and persons with respiratory diseases. During the 1952 London Fog Incident it was estimated that the daily mortality rate almost tripled, resulting in 4000 excess deaths.[69]

CASE 2. On December 3, 1984, the densely populated area surrounding the Union Carbide pesticide plant in Bhopal, India, suffered the "world's worst industrial accident." Just after midnight, an explosion at the plant resulted in the release of over 24 metric tons of methyl isocyanate (MIC) into the air. Although MIC was used by the ton as an intermediary in the synthesis of the carbamate pesticide carbaryl, little was known at the time about its toxicity. MIC is now recognized as a potent respiratory irritant and the disaster that unfolded was consistent with this. By the morning, over 1000 persons had died of pulmonary edema and the death toll soon exceeded 3000. Over 200,000 people developed symptoms of toxicity, and medical practitioners were overwhelmed as 90,000 persons sought health care in the first day after the tragedy. Between 20,000 and 50,000 of the survivors suffered chronic ocular and pulmonary effects from MIC exposure.[29,75,129]

What Agents Are in Polluted Air and What Are Their Associated Adverse Health Effects?

Air pollution is a complex mixture of suspended particles, aerosols, and gases that are released from motor vehicle exhaust, industrial activity, and residential sources such as barbeques and furnaces. Natural sources of air pollution include pollinating plants, forest fires, and volcanoes. Sources of air pollution are categorized as "mobile sources" (eg, trucks and automobiles), "point sources" (eg, factories and power plants), and "area sources" (numerous small sources that together constitute a significant source, eg, gas stations or fireplaces). The most important air pollutants are carbon monoxide, lead, ozone, nitrogen dioxide, sulfur dioxide, and fine particulate matter. EPA regulation of these "criteria pollutants" is discussed below. In addition, there are hundreds of chemicals that may be released into the air in quantity by industrial sources.

Carbon Monoxide. Carbon monoxide results from the incomplete combustion of carbon-based fuels. The most important source of ambient carbon monoxide is motor vehicle exhaust. Other important sources include fires, industry, natural-gas stoves, and coal furnaces. High levels of carbon monoxide are known to cause headache, confusion, coma, permanent brain damage, myocardial ischemia, dysrhythmias, and death (Chap. 96). Low levels of carbon monoxide such as those found in polluted city air may also have adverse health effects. Healthy persons exposed to low levels of carbon monoxide resulting in carboxyhemoglobin levels of approximately 5% have decreased exercise performance. Patients with ischemic heart disease have decreased time to onset of angina with COHb levels as low as 2%.[11,55] Some, but not all, studies have suggested that low levels of carbon monoxide may also be associated with an increased risk of cardiac dysrhythmias.[11] Low levels of carbon monoxide may also cause higher mortality rates in persons with coronary artery disease,[23] and chronic occupational exposure to carbon monoxide may cause an increased incidence of cardiovascular disease.[60,117]

Lead. Lead toxicity is well recognized and involves multiple organ systems (Chap. 79). Even slightly elevated blood lead levels in the fetus and young children may result in neurologic impairment.[8,86] Chronic exposure to low levels of lead is associated with hypertension and has been implicated in other cardiovascular diseases including myocardial infarction and cerebrovascular accidents.[11] Airborne lead may be inhaled and absorbed through the lungs or settle onto roadside dust and garden soil and be ingested.[2] Ambient levels of airborne lead in the United States and many other countries have declined greatly since the 1970s, when the use of alkyl lead as an octane booster in gasoline was greatly reduced. Between 1976 and 1980, there was a 50% reduction in the amount of lead used in gasoline, paralleled by a 37% decrease in the average blood lead level in the U.S. population.[2] In the United States, lead released from industrial sources results in local ambient levels that exceed EPA regulations in several states, and use of leaded gasoline in agricultural implements may pose a health threat to certain individuals.[10,11] Airborne lead remains a problem in countries that still use leaded gasoline.[89]

Nitrogen Dioxide. Nitrogen dioxide and other oxides of nitrogen are pulmonary irritants of low solubility, and prolonged exposure to high concentrations of these compounds can result in pulmonary edema and death (Chap. 94). Nitric oxide and to a lessor extent nitrogen dioxide and other oxides of nitrogen are formed from nitrogen and oxygen during high-temperature combustion. Nitric oxide, in turn, is oxidized to nitrogen dioxide, which is an important precursor in the formation of ozone. The primary source of nitric oxide and nitrogen dioxide in outdoor air is motor vehicle exhaust. Other important sources include power plants and industries that burn fossil fuels. Nitric oxide is unique among the criteria pollutants in that it is often found at higher levels indoors than outdoors. Important indoor sources of nitric oxide include gas stoves and kerosene heaters. Zamboni machines used for ice resurfacing in indoor skating rinks may produce significant amounts of nitric oxide as well as carbon monoxide[65] and hockey players have developed respiratory symptoms and pulmonary edema from this source of nitrogen dioxide.[82] Important industrial sources of nitrogen dioxide include silo gas and welding fumes (Chaps. 94, 110). In polluted air the most important toxicity from nitrogen dioxide is probably due to its conversion to ozone. There are no consistently documented ill effects in healthy persons following acute exposure to nitrogen dioxide at levels up to 4.0 ppm,[11,67] although some studies have demonstrated increased airway reactivity following low-level nitrogen dioxide exposure.[78] Asthmatics in particular may develop increased airway reactivity after nitrogen dioxide exposure[79,90] but this has not been consistently found in all studies.[67,83] Some authors have concluded that chronic nitrogen dioxide exposure predisposes to respiratory infections,[101,113] but others have been unable to confirm these results.[93,103]

Ozone. In contrast to its beneficial effects in the stratosphere, ozone in the air that we breath is harmful. Trophospheric ozone is formed through photochemical reactions from oxides of nitrogen and volatile organic compounds. Motor vehicle exhaust and power plant and other industrial emissions are the most important sources of ozone precursors. Because these reactions require sunlight, ozone pollution is more common in the summer months and in warmer climates. In the United States, southern California has the highest ozone levels, but excessive summertime levels are found in many other areas throughout the country. Indoor levels of ozone are much lower than outdoor levels because ozone is removed during reactions with water found on numerous surfaces within buildings.[10,64]

Ozone is a highly reactive, low-solubility irritant that is directly toxic to pulmonary epithelium. Inhaled ozone is completely removed in the lungs, presumably because it is depleted in reactions with lung constituents. Animal studies demonstrate epithelial cell injury along the entire respiratory tract following ozone exposure.[33] Bronchoalveolar lavage in human volunteers experimentally exposed to low levels of ozone confirms lower airway inflammation and damage with neutrophilia, increased LDH, and significant increases in mediators of inflammation such as interleukins, prostaglandins, coagulation factors, and plasminogen activator.[22,27,59] Similar findings have been found in joggers following exposure to ambient levels of ozone in polluted city air.[52] Acute exposure to ozone results in decreases in functional vital capacity (FVC) and forced expiratory volume in one second (FEV_1) in children,[54] healthy volunteers,[15,44] asthmatics,[45] and persons with chronic obstructive pulmonary disease (COPD).[39] These effects are apparent at ozone levels less than the EPA-regulated limit of 0.12 ppm[15] and become more prominent with physical exertion, at higher levels, and with prolonged duration of exposure.[10] The changes in airway function following ozone exposure are independent of inflammation.[9] There is marked variability in the response to ozone, with some individuals consistently demonstrating marked decrements in airway function and others less severely affected.[73] Healthy persons exposed to ozone may also complain of decreased exercise capacity and respiratory symptoms such as cough and chest pain.[10,92]

The airway response of asthmatics to ozone is the same as[62,106] or greater than[45] that of the normal population. Since asthmatics start with lower FVC and FEV_1, they are more likely to develop symptoms such as shortness of breathe, cough, and wheezing after ozone exposure.[45,62] Some studies have also found that following ozone exposure, asthmatics develop more severe airway inflammation than nonasthmatics.[106] These findings may explain the increased incidence of emergency department visits[48,130] and hospital admissions for respiratory diseases[16] that occur with higher ozone levels even when they remain within the EPA guidelines.[16,130]

In experimental animals, chronic exposure to ozone damages the nasal epithelium and causes a chronic lung disease characterized by bronchiolitis, collagen deposition, and chronic inflammation. [10] The effects of chronic ozone exposure on humans has been difficult to study, but a recent preliminary study found that persons who lived in areas with higher ozone levels had lower mid- and end-expiratory flow rates.[63] Chronic ozone exposure may also cause respiratory cancers, and persons exposed to high ozone levels in Mexico City were found to have increased number of DNA single strand breaks compared to controls.[17]

Sulfur Dioxide. Sulfur dioxide is a highly water-soluble pulmonary irritant that is formed during the combustion of sulfur-containing fossil fuels. Point sources such as coal- and oil-fueled power plants and metal smelters are the main sources of airborne sulfur dioxide. Fossil-fuel combustion also results in the release of particulate matter and acidic aerosols (see below). Occupational exposure to sulfur dioxide may occur in the petroleum-refining industry, paper-production plants, refrigeration plants, and fruit processing plants. [10,126]

Like other highly soluble irritants (Chap. 94), sulfur dioxide's primary effects are on the upper airway. Inhaled sulfur dioxide reacts with water in the lungs to form hydrogen (H^+), bisulfite (HSO_3^-), and sulfite (SO_3^{2-}) ions. These irritants are responsible for sulfur dioxide's toxic effect. High concentrations of sulfur dioxide may cause eye, nose, and throat irritation, cough, and, with prolonged exposure, upper airway obstruction or pulmonary edema. These effects often occur at sulfur dioxide concentrations much higher than those found in polluted air. Healthy individuals are relatively resistant to the effects of sulfur dioxide and tolerate acute exposure to levels as high as 1.0 ppm without adverse effects. Asthmatics, in contrast, may develop bronchospasm, decreased FEV_1, shortness of breath, and cough with exposure to levels of sulfur dioxide as low as 0.25 ppm.[112] These effects often occur within 2 minutes of exposure and generally resolve within an hour after removal from exposure.[10] Bronchodilators shorten the duration of symptoms.[112] Not all asthmatics are sensitive to sulfur dioxide and some may tolerate exposure to levels as high as 2.0 ppm without developing bronchospasm or increased reactivity.[10]

Particulate Matter. Particulate air pollution is a complex mix of suspended solids and aerosols made up of dusts, smoke, fumes, and fog (see Chap. 94). Particulate air pollution, like sulfur dioxide, is largely from fossil-fuel combustion. The EPA regulates the total amount of suspended particulate matter that is less than 10 μm in diameter (PM_{10}). Particles larger than this are less toxic because they are filtered out in the nose, pharynx, and upper airways, and removed by sneezing, coughing, or mucociliary clearance. Smaller particles may gain access to the terminal bronchiolar tree and alveoli, where they are cleared by lung macrophages. In animal models, inhaled particles decrease vital capacity and diffusing capacity,[19] are cytotoxic to macrophages,[41] and may cause pulmonary inflammation and edema.[10] Ozone and inhaled particulate matter have synergistic toxicity in animal models.[20] Acidic aerosols are an important component of particulate air pollution and cause greater reductions in vital capacity and diffusing capacity than other particles.[19] Sulfate (SO_4^{2-}) and bisulfate (HSO_4^-) ions are the most important component of acid aerosols. Acid aerosols induce bronchospasm, cause pulmonary irritation, and reduce mucociliary clearance.[10]

Increased ambient levels of sulfur dioxide and particulate pollution are associated with an increased incidence of hospital visits and admissions for asthma and other pulmonary diseases. In addition, these pollutants appear to be responsible for increased short-term total, pulmonary, and cardiac mortality and increased long-term mortality from cardiopulmonary disease and from lung cancer. These relations are discussed in more detail below.

How Is Air Quality Assured?

The "London Fog Incident" and other episodes of severe air pollution in the United States and around the world prompted legislative measures to assure adequate air quality. In the United States this resulted in the Clean Air Act of 1955 and subsequent amendments. The Environmental Protection Agency (EPA) has defined National Ambient Air Quality Standards (NAAQS) for six "criteria pollutants." Individual states are responsible for implementing adequate plans to achieve and maintain the NAAQS for these pollutants and are subject to EPA sanctions if they fail to do so. The criteria pollutants are carbon monoxide, lead, ozone, nitrogen dioxide, particles less than 10 μm in diameter (PM_{10}), and sulfur dioxide. The NAAQS values for these pollutants are given in Table 74–1. The EPA has also identified a list of 189 "toxic" pollutants, which are considered to be potentially dangerous to human health[94] (Table 74–2). Under the "air toxics" provisions of the 1990 Clean Air Act amendments, the EPA sets standards regulating industrial emissions of these "toxic" pollutants. These standards, known as Maximum Achievable Control Technology (MACT) require that all industries reduce emissions to a technically feasible low level. These levels are generally

TABLE 74–1. NATIONAL AMBIENT AIR QUALITY STANDARDS OF THE SIX "CRITERIA POLLUTANTS" REGULATED BY THE EPA

Pollutant	Health Effects	NAAQS Level
Carbon monoxide (see Chap. 96)	Acute: Headache, altered level of consciousness, encephalopathy, lowered angina threshold, decreased exercise tolerance	10 $\mu g/m^3$ (9 ppm) 8-h average
	Chronic: Cardiac disease (?)	40 $\mu g/m^3$ (35 ppm) 1-h average
Lead (see Chap. 79)	Acute: Vomiting, abdominal pain, altered level of consciousness, encephalopathy	1.5 $\mu g/m^3$
	Chronic: Decreased IQ, hypertension, renal impairment, anemia	
Nitrogen dioxide	Acute: Increased bronchial reactivity (?)	100 $\mu g/m^3$ (0.053 ppm) annual mean
	High levels: Pulmonary inflammation and edema	
	Chronic: Increased incidence of respiratory infections (?)	
Ozone	Acute: Cough, chest pain, bronchospasm, pulmonary inflammation, decreased FVC and FEV_1	235 $\mu g/m^3$ (0.12 ppm)
	Chronic: Lung cancer (?)	Maximum annual daily 1-h average
Fine particles (PM_{10})	Acute: Bronchospasm, pulmonary irritation	50 $\mu g/m^3$ annual average
	Chronic: Increased cardiopulmonary mortality, increased incidence of lung cancer	150 $\mu g/m^3$ 24-h average
Sulfur dioxide	Acute: Bronchospasm in asthmatics	80 μg (0.03 ppm) annual mean
	High levels: Mucosal membrane irritation, cough	365 $\mu g/m^3$ (0.14 ppm) max 24-h mean
	Chronic: Increased cardiopulmonary mortality, increased incidence of lung cancer	

as low as those from the best controlled similar industrial source. If a significant public health threat remains after industries comply with MACT, the EPA is required to enact further measures, including the establishment of more stringent "residual risk standards" for industry and regulation of area sources of the pollutant.[21]

What Are the Beneficial Effects of Ozone?

Ozone may be beneficial or harmful depending on where in the atmosphere it is located. Wavelengths of ultraviolet (UV) radiation between 290 and 320 nanometers are referred to as UVB radiation and are responsible for sunburns, photoaging of the skin, and numerous cases of skin cancer. Many kilometers above ground, stratospheric ozone, which is formed from the action of UV light on oxygen, absorbs UVB radiation. Under stratospheric conditions, chlorofluorocarbons (CFCs) used in refrigerators and air conditioners and as aerosol propellants undergo chemical reactions that deplete ozone and allow greater penetration of UVB radiation. These reactions are favored by the very low temperatures found in winter in the polar regions. In 1985, an area of marked ozone depletion was detected over Antarctica. Ozone depletion by CFCs is not restricted to the arctic regions. In fact, stratospheric ozone has been decreasing at a rate of aproximately 1% per year since 1979. Although CFCs have little direct toxicity, the control of their release is of vital health importance. It is hoped that regulations controlling the amount of CFCs released into the atmosphere will prevent further decline in stratospheric ozone levels.[98]

Ozone generators are marketed as air fresheners and purported to be capable of removing odors from rooms, destroying air contaminants, neutralizing carbon monoxide, and preventing the "sick building syndrome." These generators can produce ozone in quantities that exceed the EPA limit of 0.12 ppm. In fact, one device marketed for home use can generate ozone concentrations "well over" 4.0 ppm. The manufacturer states that at this level ozone can cause uncomfortable stinging of the eyes and mouth and states that humans should avoid this environment "even though it is harmless."[88] There is little evidence that these products actually prevent symptoms of the sick building syndrome and the harmful effects of ozone at these levels are well described.

Ozone has also been popularized as "oxygen therapy" with the potential for miraculous cures for the acquired immune deficiency syndrome (AIDS), cancer, heart disease, arthritis, and many other diseases. These therapies, which include drinking ozonated water, intravenous or intraarterial injections of ozone, and rectal insufflation of ozone, are supported by dramatic claims and personal testimonies. Unfortunately, few of these claims are tested in rigorous clinical trials. One "ozone therapy" known as ozone autohemotherapy was tested in Europe for patients with peripheral vascular disease. In this procedure blood is removed, exposed to ozone, and reinjected into the patient. Blood treated in this way is less viscous, and this treatment may be beneficial for patients with peripheral vascular disease.[127] Other benefits of ozone therapy are less well established. A Canadian pilot study showed no measurable benefit of ozone therapy in patients with AIDS.[37] As may be expected, persons with incurable diseases who have become disillusioned with standard medical treatment are willing to pay substantial sums of money for these largely unproved therapies. Medical practitioners should discourage the use of such unproven therapies except as part of a clinical trial.

Who Is Affected by Air Pollution?

No source of air is completely free of contamination so everyone is exposed to some degree of air pollution. It was estimated that over 80 million U.S. citizens live in counties that exceeded the NAAQS limits for at least one

TABLE 74–2. "TOXIC" POLLUTANTS REGULATED BY THE 1990 AMENDMENT TO THE CLEAN AIR ACT

Acetaldehyde
Acetamide
Acetonitrile
Acetophenone
2-Acetylaminofluorene
Acrolein
Acrylamide
Acrylic acid
Acrylonitrile
Allyl chloride
4-Aminobiphenyl
Aniline
o-Anisidine
Asbestos
Benzene (including benzene from gasoline)
Benzidine
Benzotrichloride
Benzyl chloride
Biphenyl
Bis(2-ethylhexyl)phthalate (DEHP)
Bis(chloromethyl)ether
Bromoform
1,3-Butadiene
Calcium cyanamide
Caprolactam
Captan
Carbaryl
Carbon disulfide
Carbon tetrachloride
Carbonyl sulfide
Catechol
Chloramben
Chlordane
Chlorine
Chloroacetic acid
2-Chloroacetophenone
Chlorobenzene
Chlorobenzilate
Chloroform
Chloromethyl methyl ether
Chloroprene
Cresols/cresylic acid (isomers and mixture)
o-Cresol
m-Cresol
p-Cresol
Cumene
2,4-D, salts and esters
DDE
Diazomethane
Dibenzofurans
1,2-Dibromo-3-chloropropane
Dibutylphthalate
1,4-Dichlorobenzene(p)
3,3-Dichlorobenzidene
Dichloroethyl ether (bis(2-chloroethyl)ether)
1,3-Dichloropropene
Dichlorvos
Diethanolamine
N,N-Diethyl aniline (*N,N*-dimethylaniline)
Diethyl sulfate
3,3-Dimethoxybenzidine
Dimethyl aminoazobenzene
3,3′-Dimethyl benzidine
Dimethylcarbamoyl chloride
Dimethyl formamide
1,1-Dimethylhydrazine
Dimethyl phthalate
Dimethyl sulfate
4,6-Dinitro-*o*-cresol, and salts
2,4-Dinitrophenol
2,4-Dinitrotoluene
1,4-Dioxane (1,4-diethylenedioxide)
1,2-Diphenylhydrazine
Epichlorohydrin (l-chloro-2,3-epoxypropane)
1,2-Epoxybutane
Ethyl acrylate
Ethyl benzene
Ethyl carbamate (urethane)
Ethyl chloride (chloroethane)
Ethylene dibromide (dibromoethane)
Ethylene dichloride (1,2-dichloroethane)
Ethylene glycol
Ethyleneimine (aziridine)
Ethylene oxide
Ethylene thiourea
Ethylidene dichloride (1,1-dichloroethane)
Formaldehyde
Heptachlor
Hexachlorobenzene
Hexachlorobutadiene
Hexachlorocyclopentadiene
Hexachloroethane
Hexamethylene-1,6-diisocyanate
Hexamethylphosphoramide
Hexane
Hydrazine
Hydrochloric acid
Hydrogen fluoride (hydrofluoric acid)
Hydrogen sulfide
Hydroquinone
Isophorone
Lindane (all isomers)
Maleic anhydride
Methanol
Methoxychlor
Methyl bromide (bromomethane)
Methyl chloride (chloromethane)
Methyl chloroform (1,1,1-trichloroethane)
Methyl ethyl ketone (2-butanone)
Methyl hydrazine
Methyl iodide (iodomethane)
Methyl isobutyl ketone (hexone)
Methyl isocyanate
Methyl methacrylate
Methyl *tert* butyl ether
4,4-Methylene bis(2-chloroaniline)
Methylene chloride (dichloromethane)
Methylene diphenyl diisocyanate (MDI)
4,4′-Methylenedianiline
Naphthalene
Nitrobenzene
4-Nitrobiphenyl
4-Nitrophenol
2-Nitropropane
N-Nitroso-*N*-methylurea
N-Nitrosodimethylamine
N-Nitrosomorpholine
Parathion
Pentachloronitrobenzene (quintobenzene)
Pentachlorophenol
Phenol
p-Phenylenediamine
Phosgene
Phosphine
Phosphorus
Phthalic anhydride
Polychlorinated biphenyls (aroclors)
1,3-Propane sultone
beta-Propiolactone
Propionaldehyde
Propoxur (Baygon)
Propylene dichloride (1,2-dichloropropane)
Propylene oxide
1,2-Propylenimine (2-methyl aziridine)
Quinoline
Quinone
Styrene
Styrene oxide
2,3,7,8-Tetrachlorodibenzo-*p*-dioxin
1,1,2,2-Tetrachloroethane
Tetrachloroethylene (perchloroethylene)
Titanium tetrachloride
Toluene
2,4-Toluene diamine
2,4-Toluene diisocyanate
o-Toluidine
Toxaphene (chlorinated camphene)
1,2,4-Trichlorobenzene
1,1,2-Trichloroethane
Trichloroethylene
2,4,5-Trichlorophenol
2,4,6-Trichlorophenol
Triethylamine
Trifluralin
2,2,4-Trimethylpentane
Vinyl acetate
Vinyl bromide
Vinyl chloride
Vinylidene chloride (1,1-dichloroethylene)
Xylenes (isomers and mixture)
o-Xylenes
m-Xylenes
p-Xylenes
Antimony compounds
Arsenic compounds (inorganic including arsine)
Beryllium compounds
Cadmium compounds
Chromium compounds
Cobalt compounds
Coke oven emissions
Cyanide compounds
Glycol ethers
Lead compounds
Manganese compounds
Mercury compounds
Fine mineral fibers
Nickel compounds
Polycylic organic matter
Radionuclides (including radon)
Selenium compounds

From Pollutants and sources. Unified air toxics website. Office of Air Quality Planning and Standards. US Environmental Protection Agency. http://www.epa.gov/oar/oaqps/airtox/pollsour.htm.

criteria pollutant.[10] For a variety of reasons, ethnic minorities and the poor are exposed to higher levels of air pollution. This disparity may contribute to the health problems of these populations.[110] In heavily polluted areas, outdoor air is generally more polluted than indoor air so persons who spend more time outdoors have greater exposure.

Asthmatics and other persons with respiratory disease appear to be most affected by air pollution, with more symptoms, an increased admission rate, and increased mortality during periods with higher levels of air pollution (see below). Young children may suffer higher rates of sudden infant death syndrome (SIDS) during these periods.[56] Increased mortality during times of higher pollution also affects the elderly (see below).

What Are the Respiratory Effects of Air Pollution?

Ozone, nitrogen dioxide, sulfur dioxide, and suspended particles (especially acidic aerosols) cause acute pulmonary toxicity, including bronchospasm and pulmonary inflammation. These effects are more marked in asthmatics and others with pulmonary disease and are demonstrated in controlled exposure studies and in persons exposed to ambient air (see above). Given these facts, it is not surprising that numerous studies document an association between air pollution and exacerbations of respiratory diseases.

Increased ambient levels of sulfur dioxide and particulates were associated with an increased number of hospital admissions for respiratory causes in Milan, Italy,[128] and in Paris, France.[25] Respiratory admissions were positively associated with ozone, suspended sulfates, and total suspended acid aerosols in Toronto, Ontario,[123] with ozone in London, England,[95] and with both ozone and particulates in Spokane, Washington.[109] Daily admissions for chronic obstructive pulmonary disease (COPD) were correlated with daily levels of sulfur dioxide and black smoke (a measure of particulate pollution) in Barcelona, Spain.[120] In the Japanese city of Kushiro, a dense acidic fog occurs every summer and results in an increased number of admissions for asthma.[122] Increased levels of suspended particulates and ozone caused cough, wheezing, sputum production, and a decreased peak expiratory flow rate in a group of asthmatics in Mexico City.[99] Naturally occurring pollutants such as the dust from the Mount St. Helens eruption also cause an increased number of hospital visits for respiratory complaints in asthmatics.[12]

In addition to the acute conditions described above, exposure to air pollution may cause chronic pulmonary toxicity. Polluted air has been implicated as a cause of asthma.[74,100] Chronic exposure to air pollution may impair pulmonary function[63] and predispose to respiratory infections.[101,113] Polluted air contains numerous carcinogens, including benzo(a)pyrene and other polyaromatic hydrocarbons,[87] so it is not surprising that persons chronically exposed to polluted air have an increased incidence of lung cancer. The link between lung cancer and air pollution is statistically significant but weaker than that with smoking or occupational exposure.[31,96] On occasion, severe pollution may make the association more apparent, as was dramatically demonstrated by an "epidemic" of lung cancer deaths occurring in persons living downwind of a foundry in Armsdale, Scotland.[68]

What Is the Relationship Between Air Pollution and Mortality?

Prior to the 1950s, air quality in most industrial countries was unregulated and severe urban air pollution was not uncommon. In addition to the famous London Fog Incident, other episodes of severe air pollution with marked excess mortality were documented in the Meuse Valley, Belgium, in 1930 and in Donora, Pennsylvania, in 1948. Since the introduction of clean air acts in the United States and other industrialized countries, episodes of severe air pollution such as these are unlikely to recur, and the association between air quality and mortality is less striking. Recent studies, nevertheless, suggest that there remains an association between air pollution and mortality.

Studies correlating short-term mortality rates with measured levels of pollutants were performed in several European and American cities. Following uniform methodology, several groups of investigators compared daily air-quality data with short-term mortality rates and other health outcomes in 15 European cities with a combined population of over 25 million persons. The air-quality parameters included sulphur dioxide, particulate matter, nitrogen dioxide, and ozone. The measured health outcomes included hospital admissions, total nontraumatic mortality, and cause specific mortality.[49] In most of these cities, increased ambient levels of sulfur dioxide and particulate air pollution were positively associated with increased short-term total, respiratory, or cardiovascular mortality.[25,115,119,124,128,133,137] Similar results were recorded recently in Philadelphia, Pennsylvania,[108] London, England,[5] Steubenville, Ohio,[109] Southern Ontario, Canada, and in Santa Clara and Los Angeles counties, California.[91] One review found that, on average, a 10 $\mu g/m^3$ increase in small suspended particles resulted in a 0.96% increase in total mortality.[91] Ozone was associated with increased mortality in Barcelona, Spain,[119] and in Los Angeles,[53] but other studies have failed to confirm this association.

In addition to short-term mortality, several authors have found a relationship between chronic exposure to air pollution and long-term mortality. In a prospective cohort study, 14–16 year mortality data was collected on 8111 adults from 6 American cities. After adjusting for smoking and other risk factors, there remained a significant association between fine particulate air pollution and total mortality, lung cancer mortality, and cardiopulmonary mortality. The adjusted mortality rate in the most polluted city was 1.26 times that of the least polluted city.[30] Another prospective study correlated average ambient sulfate and fine particulate pollution with 7-year mortality data on 552,138 adults from 151 cities across the United States. After controlling for smoking, total mortality, lung cancer mortality, and cardiopulmonary mortality were highest in the areas with the most sulfate pollution, and total mortality and cardiopulmonary mortality were greatest in the areas with the highest levels of fine particulate pollution. These correlations were true for smokers and nonsmokers, and for both sexes.[96] In both of these studies, mortality rates were more strongly associated with cigarette smoking than with air pollution.

What Are the Difficulties Encountered in Air Pollution Research?

Air pollution research asks several important questions. What are the acute and chronic health effects of exposure to polluted air? Do these effects exist at present-day levels of pollution? What specific agents are responsible? Epidemiologic studies can determine associations between adverse health outcomes and potential exposure to various pollutants but do not prove cause and effect. These studies are complicated by the fact that the chronic health effects of air pollution are overshadowed by occupational exposures and by "lifestyle" exposures such as smoking or diet. Furthermore, the mix of contaminants in polluted air fluctuates from hour to hour and varies between regions within a city so that it is impossible to determine what toxins a given individual or population was exposed to. Measuring pulmonary function or other endpoints in human volunteers during days with different levels of ambient pollution may give valuable information concerning the effects of acute exposure on certain populations. Personal-exposure monitors may increase the validity of these studies. Controlled human-volunteer exposure studies may shed light on the acute effects of exposure to low levels of certain pollutants but cannot be used for studying the effects of high levels of pollutants nor for chronic toxicity studies. Animal studies of acute and chronic toxicity are useful but are limited by species differences, the difficulty associated in mimicking the constantly changing mix of pollutants in the air we breathe, and the long follow-up required to detect certain outcomes such as malignancies. Studies examining the effects of exposure to a single pollutant cannot account for synergy with other pollutants. Despite these difficulties, the public health implications justify ongoing research.

What Is the "Sick Building Syndrome"?

Since the 1970s there have been numerous reports of subjective complaints occurring in a large percentage of persons who work in certain buildings. This phenomenon, which occurs most often in energy-efficient, airtight buildings with limited ventilation with outside air, has become known as the sick building syndrome (SBS) or tight building syndrome. Affected persons report headache, fatigue, dizziness, decreased concentration, nausea, perception of objectionable odors, cough, irritation of the eyes, mouth, and nose, and other subjective complaints. These complaints are so nonspecific and common that in any large building some occupants will report having these symptoms in the previous 2 weeks. The SBS is often said to occur when over 15% of persons in a building report these complaints.[18,118] Secondhand tobacco smoke, overgrowth of micororganisms in the air conditioning system, and release of volatile organic compounds (VOCs) from building materials, carpets, insulation, cleaning products, paints, hydraulic systems, and other sources have all been implicated in the SBS.[118,131] The rate of air exchange in a building appears to play an important role in the development of the SBS. Workers in buildings with lower ventilation rates are more likely to report symptoms of the SBS than those in well-ventilated buildings,[46] and moving from a poorly ventilated to a well-ventilated building was associated with a decrease in these symptoms.[14] Surprisingly, a blinded study, in which the ventilation rate of a building was randomly varied, failed to show an association between ventilation rate and the incidence of symptoms of the SBS.[77] The etiology of the SBS is likely multifactorial and may vary from building to building. Further work is required to better define the cause and best preventive method of this bothersome syndrome.

As well as the VOCs implicated in SBS, indoor air may become polluted by toxic gases, dusts, and microbial agents. Carbon monoxide is the most important of these and is responsible for numerous deaths (Chap. 96). Other toxic compounds that may contaminate indoor air include asbestos, nitrogen dioxide, and radon. Prior to widespread recognition of its adverse health effects, asbestos was used in many building products for insulating and as a fire retardant. Chronic exposure to asbestos causes severe pulmonary fibrosis and mesothelioma. Nitrogen dioxide is a common combustion by-product. Gas stoves are probably the most important source of nitrogen dioxide, and homes with gas stoves have higher nitrogen dioxide levels than those with electric stoves. Health effects of nitrogen dioxide are discussed above. Radon is a gas found in soil, rocks, and water and in some granite building materials. Radon gains access to houses by diffusing through cracks in the foundation. The most important toxicity associated with radon is its ability to act in synergy with tobacco smoke to cause lung cancer.[104]

What Is Acid Rain?

When large amounts of sulfur dioxide are released close to the ground, it is quickly removed through reactions with vegetation, buildings, and other surfaces, including human lungs. Under certain weather conditions, this sulfur dioxide will rapidly react with foggy air masses to form high concentrations of sulfuric-acid mist. This is believed to have been the cause of the London fog of 1952. In an attempt to minimize local concentrations, large power plants have built tall smoke stacks that release sulfur dioxide high above the ground-based mixing layer. At these heights, sulfur dioxide remains airborne for a considerably longer period of time and is slowly oxidized to form sulfuric acid aerosols. This phenomenon is most marked in summer months. In North America, the highest concentrations of acidic atmosphere occurs downwind of several large power plants in the Ohio River valley. Precipitation formed in these conditions will also be acidic.[126]

Acidic precipitation is usually buffered by naturally occurring alkaline chemicals found in bedrock. Acid rain has numerous environmental sequelae, which are most severe in regions with limited buffering capacity. When acid rain is not neutralized, there is damage to forests, commercial crops, and aquatic ecosystems. The pH in lakes will drop with loss of beneficial species of plankton, overgrowth of mosses, and death of fish. Waterfowl that depend on aquatic life for food will also be affected. Acid rain can leach minerals from soil and increase the concentration of harmful metals such as aluminum, copper, and lead. Plants exposed to acid rain are less likely to germinate and become more susceptible to disease. Ironically, much of the damage from acid rain occurs far from the original source of sulfur dioxide. Prevailing winds in the eastern parts of North America are generally from southwest to northeast so that acidic pollutants from the midwestern states are deposited in the northeastern United States and southeastern Canada. It is estimated that half of the sulfate deposited in Canada is derived from sources in the United States.[1]

Water Pollution

CASE 3. On April 5, 1993, the Wisconsin Division of Health was alerted to an outbreak of diarrheal illness affecting hospital employees, schoolchildren, and teachers in Milwaukee. Standard stool cultures failed to demonstrate an increased incidence of bacterial pathogens, but special cultures grew cryptosporidium in stool samples from 285 persons. Telephone surveys confirmed an increase in the incidence of diarrheal illnesses among persons living in the southern part of the city. In fact, over 50% of the interviewed residents from this part of the city had a diarrheal illness during March or April of 1993. The peak incidence of this illness was on April 6. The widespread distribution of cases suggested a common source such as food or water.

Milwaukee drinking water is drawn from Lake Michigan and treated in one of two water-treatment plants. These plants treat the water with chlorine and polyaluminum chloride before it is filtered and stored in a large well. The turbidity of the treated water is monitored as a marker of microbial purity. For the 10-year period ending in January 1993, the turbidity of water from the southern treatment plant was consistently less than 0.4 nephelometric turbidity units (NTU). From March 18, 1993, until April 9, 1993, when the plant was temporarily closed, the turbidity was consistently above 0.45 NTU with a peak of 1.7 NTU. Despite the elevated turbidity, the treated water consistently failed to grow excess numbers of coliform bacteria. Analysis of aliquots of ice frozen from water treated on March 25 and on April 16 demonstrated the presence of cryptosporidium. Review of plant operations showed several problems. These facts strongly suggested that the outbreak of diarrheal illness was caused by cryptosporidium due to a problem in the malfunctioning water-treatment plant. A telephone survey of 1663 Milwaukee residents suggested that 403,000 persons were affected by this outbreak. This was the largest documented outbreak of waterborne disease in the United States.[70]

What Measures Assure the Safety of Our Drinking Water?

Under the Safe Drinking Water Act of 1986, the EPA is authorized to set standards for drinking-water contaminants that may pose a health risk.[102] There are two categories of drinking water regulations: the National Primary Drinking Water Regulations, which regulate levels of microbial and toxic chemical contaminants, and the National Secondary Maximum Contaminant Levels, which are concerned with aesthetic qualities of the water such as color, odor, and taste. The National Primary Drinking Water Regulations consist of nonenforceable Maximum Contaminant Level Goals (MCLGs), which represent a "safe" contaminant level below which no adverse health effects are anticipated, and enforceable Maximum Contaminant Levels (MCLs) that take into consideration technical and economic limitations. For example, the MCL for benzene is 0.005 mg/L, but since benzene is a carcinogen with no known threshold level, the MCLG is set at zero. MCLs are established for metals, pesticides, radioactive contaminants, and organic compounds (Table 74–3).[102,114]

Microbial purity of drinking water is as important as chemical purity, and the EPA has established standards for microbial contaminants. The total coliform count is used as a marker of water quality. Not all coliforms are pathogenic, but absence of coliforms correlates well with absence of pathogenic bacteria and presence of coliforms indicates inadequate water decontamination. The 1989 MCL for coliforms requires that fewer than 5% of the water samples collected each month be positive for coliforms. Any positive sample must be tested for fecal coliforms and for *E. coli,* and repeated within 24 hours. Fecal coliforms or *E. coli* must be reported to the state agency and mandate further testing. Recognizing that any pathogenic organisms are potentially harmful to our health, the EPA has established MCLGs of zero for *Giardi lamblia*, viruses, Legionella, and total coliforms.

Water purification serves to remove or destroy microbial contamination, improve taste and clarity, and remove chemical contamination. Removal of suspended particles and colloidal material is achieved by the processes of coagulation, flocculation, and sedimentation. After addition of coagulants such as aluminum sulfate or ferric sulfate, the water is gently stirred in flocculation tanks. This process causes particles to clump together, forming flocs, which settle to the bottom in the quiet water of sedimentation tanks. The next step is filtration of the water to remove persistent small flocs and some microorganisms. Typically a bed of sand or other fine particles about 1 meter deep is used for this purpose. Specialized treatment may require the use of ion-exchange resins or activated charcoal filters. Following filtration, most water sources require disinfection to remove remaining bacterial and parasitic contamination. Methods of disinfection include use of ozone, hydrogen peroxide, ultraviolet light, and silver ions. Chlorination is the most widely used disinfection method. Recently concern has been raised about potential harmful effects of these disinfectants, and the EPA has proposed MCLs for disinfectants and disinfectant by-products and is now collecting information on the levels of these compounds in public water systems. Aeration of the water adds oxy-

TABLE 74–3. WATER CONTAMINANTS REGULATED BY THE SAFE DRINKING ACT

Contaminant	MCL (mg/L)	MCLG (mg/L)	Contaminant	MCL (mg/L)	MCLG (mg/L)
1,1,1-Trichloroethane	0.2	0.2	Endrin	0.002	0.002
1,1,2-Trichloroethane	0.005	0.003	Epichlorohydrin	TT	0
1,1-Dichloroethylene	0.007	0.007	Ethylbenzene	0.7	0.7
1,2,4-Trichlorobenzene	0.07	0.07	Ethylenedibromide	0.00005	0
1,2-Dichloroethane	0.005	0	Fluoride	4	4.0
1,2-Dichloropropane	0.005	0	Glyphosate	0.7	0.7
2,3,7,8-TCDD (dioxin)	3×10^{-8}	0	Heptachlor	0.0004	0
2,4,5-TP (Silvex)	0.05	0.05	Heptachlorepoxide	0.0002	0
2,4-D	0.07	0.07	Hexachlorobenzene	0.001	0
Acrylamide	TT	0	Hexachlorocyclopentadiene	0.05	0.05
Alachlor	0.002	0	Lead	0.015	
Aldicarb	0.003	0.001	Lindane	0.0002	0.0002
Aldicarb sulfone	0.002	0.001	Mercury	0.002	0.002
Aldicarb sulfoxide	0.004	0.001	Methoxychlor	0.04	0.04
Antimony	0.006	0.0006	Monochlorobenzene	0.1	0.1
Arsenic	0.05		Nickel	0.1	0.1
Asbestos fibers/liter	7×10^6	7×10^6	Nitrate	10	10
Atrazine	0.003	0.003	Nitrite	1	1
Barium	2	2	*o*-Dichlorobenzene	0.6	0.6
Benzene	0.005	0	Oxamyl (Vydate)	0.2	0.2
Benzo[*a*]pyrene (PAHs)	0.0002	0	*para*-Dichlorobenzene	0.075	0.075
Beryllium	0.004	0.004	Pentachlorophenol	0.001	0
Cadmium	0.005	0.005	Picloram	0.5	0.5
Carbofuran	0.04	0.04	Polychlorinated biphenyls	0.0005	0
Carbon tetrachloride	0.005	0	Selenium	0.05	0.05
Chlordane	0.002	0	Simazine	0.004	0.004
Chromium	0.1	0.1	Styrene	0.1	0.1
cis-1,2-Dichloroethylene	0.07	0.07	Sulfate	500	500
Copper	1.3		Tetrachloroethylene	0.005	0
Cyanide (as free cyanide)	0.2	0.2	Thallium	0.002	0.0005
Dalapon	0.2	0.2	Toluene	1	1
Di(2-ethylhexyl) adipate	0.4	0.4	Total nitrate and nitrite	10	10
Di(2-ethylhexyl) phthalate	0.006	0	Total trihalomethanes	0.1	0
Dibromochloropropane	0.0002	0	Toxaphene	0.003	0
Dichloromethane	0.005	0	*trans*-1,2-Dichloroethylene	0.1	0.1
Dinoseb	0.007	0.007	Trichloroethylene	0.005	0
Diquat	0.02	0.02	Vinyl chloride	0.002	0
Endothall	0.1	0.1	Xylenes (total)	10	10

Federal maximum contaminant levels (MCLs) and maximum contaminant level goals (MCLGs) as of July 1996. This list may be modified as new health data come to light. The maximum permissible level of a contaminant that may be delivered in drinking water is the MCL; MCLGs represent the maximum level for which there is no known or anticipated adverse health effect. In the case of suspected or known carcinogens, the MCLG is set at zero. Lead and copper are monitored separately based on levels measured at the consumer's tap.
Data from references 102, 114.

gen and removes dissolved carbon dioxide and hydrogen sulfide, resulting in improved taste and color.

How Safe Is the Water in Our Hospitals?

Even when the municipal water supply to a hospital is adequately treated, chemical or microbial contamination can occur in the hospital. Water used in hospitals has become contaminated when hardware within the hospital water-distribution system becomes colonized with microorganisms. This was the cause of an outbreak of pseudomonal sepsis in a burn unit.[57] Outbreaks of Legionnaires' disease have also occurred for this reason.[76] Chemical contamination with ethylene glycol of water used in hemodialysis units has occurred due to a connection between the hospital's potable water system and air conditioning system.[32] In another hemodialysis unit, malfunctioning of a water deionization device caused fluoride contamination of dialysis fluid, resulting in an outbreak of fluoride intoxication with three deaths.[6]

Minimizing the adverse impact of such potentially devasting outbreaks requires early recognition and correction of the problem. Interim solutions may range from using an alternate water source, to closing certain units within the hospital, to evacuating the entire hospital. Permanent solutions involve cooperation between clinicians and laboratory and maintenance personnel to facilitate early detection and correction of the source of the contamination. Hospital disaster plans should incorporate strategies for such eventualities.

What Acute Health Effects Are Caused by Drinking Polluted Water?

The most important adverse health effects from drinking polluted drinking water are caused by infectious agents. For the 9-year period from 1986 through 1994, over 150 disease outbreaks affecting more than 450,000 people caused by water intended for drinking were reported to the CDC (Table 74–4). *Giardia lamblia* and *Cryptosporidium parvum* are resistant to chlorination so that any breach in the water filtration system can result in contamination of drinking water with these organisms and, in fact, these parasites were responsible for the majority of reported outbreaks. The largest outbreak of waterborne disease ever reported in the United States occurred in Milwaukee in 1993, with an estimated 403,000 persons developing diarhea following *C. parvum* contamination of the city water supply (see Case 3). Acute illness caused by these protozoa is characterized by watery diarrhea. Nausea, bloating, and abdominal discomfort may also be present. Immunocompromised patients with cryptosporidial infections typically develop severe unremitting diarrhea, whereas the disease is self-limiting and requires only supportive care in the immunocompetent. Giardiasis can cause chronic symptoms characterized by loose soft greasy stools, flatulence, belching, and weight loss. Antibiotic treatment with either quinacrine or metronidazole is required for persons infected with *Giardia*. Bacterial pathogens such as *Shigella*, *Campylobacter*, and *E. coli* 0157:H7 as well as viruses are also occasionally implicated in the United States and may pose major health threats in areas where drinking water is inadequately treated or becomes contaminated with sewage. Sewage contamination of a rural Missouri town's drinking water resulted in an outbreak of *E. coli* O157:H7, which affected 243 persons, with 32 hospitalizations and 4 deaths out of a population of 2090.[121] Another example of the catastrophic outcome associated with transmission of bacterial diseases in drinking water occurred in 1976 in Sangli Town, India. In previous years, this city of 135,000 had had 60–75 cases of typhoid per year. During the 12-week period between December 1975 and February 1976, fecal contamination of the city's drinking water combined with inadequate chlorination resulted in an epidemic of typhoid fever that affected over 9000 persons.[105] In many cases of waterborne-disease outbreak no pathogen is discovered; these outbreaks are classified as acute gastrointestinal illness of unknown etiology.

TABLE 74–4. WATERBORNE DISEASE OUTBREAKS IN THE USA, 1985–1992[a]

	Outbreaks		Cases	
Responsible Agent	***No.***	***%***	***No.***	***%***
Parasitic				
Giardia lamblia	28	17.8	3,115	0.6
Cryptosporidium[b]	9	5.7	419,822	92.4
Total Parasitic	37	23.6	422,937	93.1
AGI[c]	74	47.1	19,637	4.3
Bacterial	21	13.4	4,853	1.1
Chemical				
Nitrates	5	3.2	8	<0.1
Chlorine	1	0.6	31	<0.1
Fluorine	4	2.5	357	0.1
Other	6	3.8	52	<0.1
Total Chemical	16	10.2	448	0.1
Viral	7	4.5	6,409	1.4
Other	2	1.3	93	<0.1
Total	157	100	454,377	100

[a]Outbreaks of disease caused by drinking water reported to the CDC from 1985 to 1994. The actual number of waterborne disease outbreaks is probably much greater.
[b]The majority of the cases of cryptosporidium (403,000) occured in a single huge outbreak in Milwaukee in 1993. (See reference 70.)
[c]AGI-acute gastrointestinal illness of unknown etiology; outbreaks for which the etiology was not determined.
Data from references 43,61,66,70,80,116.

Compared with infectious organisms, disease caused by chemical contamination of drinking water is relatively rare. Nitrate is the most important cause of chemical water contamination. Nitrate poisoning commonly occurs when wells become contaminated with surface water that contains fertilizers or sewage. The symptoms of nitrate ingestion are due to methemoglobin production (Chap. 93). Bottle-fed infants are particularly at risk. Acute illness from other types of chemical contamination occur sporadically. An epidemic of fluoride toxicity occured in Hooper Bay, Alaska, when overflouridation of the town's drinking water caused nausea, vomiting, diarrhea, and tingling of the face and extremities in an estimated 296 patients; there was one death.[38] The River Dee in southern Wales provides drinking water to almost 2 million persons in England and Wales. In 1984, contamination of the river with phenol imparted a foul taste to the water and an outbreak of gastrointestinal illness among those persons who drank it.[47] In 1987, 29 persons at a picnic in North Dakota developed symptoms attributed to ethylene glycol poisoning when the water used for preparing a soft drink was cross-contaminated with fluid from an air conditioning system that contained ethylene glycol.[32]

What Chronic Health Effects Are Associated With Drinking Polluted Water?

In addition to acute illness from microbial and chemical contamination, long-term ingestion of polluted water has been implicated as a cause of cancer. Throughout the United States, many tons of hazardous industrial waste have been disposed of in metal drums buried in the ground at thousands of hazardous waste sites (HWS). These wastes may leach into groundwater and pose a health threat to nearby communities. Groundwater near a HWS may be contaminated with numerous chemicals, including carbon tetrachloride, trichloroethylene, and other organic solvents. The EPA has identified 538 HWS that pose a significant health risk because of their location close to a population that uses groundwater as a drinking source. Comparison of cancer mortality data from counties with these HWS with that from non-HWS counties suggests that females living close to these sites are at increased risk for breast and rectal carcinoma and that males are at increased risk of bladder, esophageal, colonic, and rectal cancer.[40] A high incidence of esophageal carcinoma among persons living in the Gassim region of Saudi Arabia was linked to groundwater contamination with petroleum oils and numerous minerals, including chromium. Drinking water collected from some wells in this region was found to be mutagenic by the Ames test.[4]

In the 1970s tetrachloroethylene (TCE) was used as a solvent to add a vinyl lining to water pipes in Massachusetts and other New England states. The purpose of the liner was to decrease palatability problems associated with the action of water on the currently used asbestos cement pipes. It was assumed that the TCE would vaporize and not be present in drinking water. Unfortunately this was not the case, and TCE concentrations ranged from 1.5 to 80 μg/L in regularly used pipes and up to 7750 μg/L in low-use sites. Before this problem was detected and addressed by regularly flushing and bleeding the water pipes, thousands of Massachusetts residents had been exposed to TCE for periods of up to 10 years. A case control study found an increased incidence of leukemia and bladder cancer among persons with high TCE exposure by this route.[7] Another study found an association between contamination of drinking water with volatile organic solvents such as TCE and a higher incidence of leukemia in exposed females.[35] In some areas of England, rivers are used both as sources of drinking water and, unfortunately, as drainage routes for sewage effluent. An epidemiologic study found that persons living in regions where more sewage effluent drained into the river that supplied drinking water had a higher incidence of gastric and urinary tract cancer.[13]

Polluted drinking water has been cited as a cause of spontaneous abortions. An intriguing Californian study found that women who drank bottled water had a lower risk of spontaneous abortions than those who used tap water and that the risk was highest when the tap water came from a groundwater source. No specific contaminants in the water could be found to explain these observations.[42] An association between drinking tap water and spontaneous abortions was confirmed in another Californian study.[26] Occupational-solvent exposure is associated with spontaneous abortions,[132] and it was originally suspected that the results of these studies could be explained by solvent contamination of the drinking water. Closer analysis of these data showed that the association between tap water consumption and spontaneous abortions held not only in areas were the drinking was contaminated with solvents but also in areas without solvent contamination.[134,135] Water pollution may also cause birth defects. A recent case control study conducted in Massuchusetts examined the relation between contaminants in the community drinking water and pregnancy outcome for 1039 congenital anomalies, 77 stillbirths, 55 neonatal deaths, and 1177 healthy neonates as controls. The results of this study suggested that exposure to chlorinated surface water was associated with an increased frequency of stillbirths, that exposure to water with detectable lead levels was associated with both stillbirths and cardiovascular system defects, that exposure to water with elevated potassium levels was associated with central nervous system defects, and that exposure to water with higher silver levels was associated with head and neck anomalies. Most of these relations did not reach statistical significance and the study was unable to prove causality. Nevertheless the results are intriguing and warrant further study.[7] Perhaps the most dramatic example of congenital anomalies caused by water pollution is the Minamata methyl mercury disaster in Japan (Chap. 80). In North America, fish in the Great Lakes contain potentially toxic levels of both methylmercury and polychlorinated biphenyls.[97]

Heavy-metal contamination of water is a problem in many areas of the world. This may occur directly, as metals from industrial waste or mining operations leach into drinking water sources, or indirectly from changes in water pH, which increase the solubility of various metals. Persons may be affected by drinking contaminated water or by eating contaminated seafood, as occurred in Minimata. Chronic lead poisoning in children is associated with delayed development and lower intelligence and remains an important health problem (see Chap. 79). Contaminated drinking water is an important source of lead exposure in the United States and around the world. It is estimated that 3.8 million children in the United States drink water with elevated lead levels and that this source is the cause of elevated lead levels in 240,000 of them.[85] This is particularly important in infants fed formula reconstituted with tap water.[111] Persons with chronic renal failure are also at risk of lead poisoning from drinking water.[51] When leaded pipes are the source of drinking water lead, altering the water pH effectively lowers the lead content of the water and the blood lead levels in consumers.[81] Flushing tap water for 10 minutes before morning use also significantly reduces lead concentrations.[84] Arsenic contamination of well water is an important problem in some countries. A unique peripheral vascular disease associated with chronic arsenic poisoning and known as blackfoot disease is endemic to the southwestern coast of Taiwan, where the primary drinking water source is from artesian wells contaminated with arsenic. A study of 42 villages in this area also demonstrated a dose–response relationship between artesian well arsenic levels and the incidence of bladder, kidney, skin, and lung cancers.[136] A well supplying drinking water to a Japanese village was heavily contaminated with arsenic during the 5-year period from 1955 to

1959. Death reports over the next 33 years demonstrated that heavily exposed persons had increased odds of developing lung cancer and urinary tract cancer.[125] Arsenic contamination of well water also causes health problems in regions of Thailand[36] and Calcutta, India.[72] Numerous metals in addition to those discussed above can also contaminate drinking water.

What Adverse Health Effects Are Associated With Swimming in Polluted Water?

Several investigators have studied the acute effects of swimming in polluted water, and it appears that persons who swim in polluted water are at risk of developing a mild illness with fever, respiratory complaints, vomiting, diarrhea, or pruritis. An Australian survey of 2839 ocean-beachgoers found that almost a quarter developed respiratory, gastrointestinal, ocular, or ear complaints during 10 day follow-up, and that those who entered the water were twice as likely to report symptoms as those who did not. The authors also found that these symptoms were more likely to occur following days when the water was more polluted.[24] A British study investigated symptoms in 857 children at a beach with water that exceeded European Community Standards for total coliforms, fecal coliforms, salmonellae, and enteroviruses. These investigators found that children who entered the water were more likely to develop vomiting, diarrhea, pruritis, fever, lack of energy, and loss of appetite than those who remained on the beach.[3] A Hong Kong study gathered data from 18,741 beachgoers at 9 beaches over a 2-year period. They found that those who swam at more polluted beaches were more likely to report gastrointestinal, respiratory, dermatologic, and "total illness" complaints than those who swam at less polluted beaches. The best predictor of symptoms in this study was the *E. coli* count. Similar results were obtained in an American study comparing symptoms of gastroenteritis, otitis, conjunctivitis, and skin infection in persons who windsurfed on polluted water with nonwater-going controls. The windsurfers were 2.9 times as likely to develop at least one of these symptoms and 5.5 times as likely to develop gastrointestinal symptoms. In this study, relative risk increased with the number of falls into the water.[28] Skin contact with polluted water may be sufficient to cause symptoms. A group of workers involved in a cleanup operation had prolonged contact with water polluted with low levels of methyl isocyanate from a pesticide spill. Of the 42 persons involved, 27 developed dermatitis of the feet and ankles.[58]

In addition to the relatively benign illnesses described above, more serious infectious diseases have been contracted by swimmers who enter polluted water. An outbreak of hemorrhagic colitis caused by *E. coli* O157:H7 and *Shigella sonni* occurred in 59 persons who swam in a lake near Portland, Oregon, that was contaminated with these bacteria. Three of these persons required hospitalization. Bathers who reported swallowing water were more likely to develop symptoms.[50] A public pool was the probable source of an outbreak of hepatitis A that affected 20 of 822 campers at a commercial campground. Investigators found that the design of the pool's filtering system may have allowed contamination of the intake water with sewage and they believed this to be the source of the infection outbreak.[71]

Summary

Air and water pollution have the potential of harming large numbers of persons. Most developed countries have set standards for air and water quality that are designed to protect the public from pollution disasters similar to those that occurred earlier this century. In spite of these measures, adverse health effects may still occur. Concentrations of airborne pollutants can exceed regulated levels following unpredictable industrial or natural accidents or when local weather conditions prevent their dissipation. Chronic exposure to low levels of these pollutants may cause cancer, respiratory illness, and premature mortality in susceptible persons. Drinking water quality is maintained by treatment plants that remove harmful organisms, debris, and some chemicals. Failure of some part of this process may expose numerous persons to disease-causing organisms or harmful chemicals. Furthermore, many harmful chemicals are not removed during the water-treatment process and are not routinely tested for. Accidental or intentional disposal of these chemicals into a community's water source may result in acute or chronic toxicity. Toxic chemicals may also be leached from municipal or building water pipes. Some persons may drink untreated water out of ignorance or unconcern of the health risks involved. Swimming in polluted water or eating seafood grown in polluted water may also expose people to significant health risks. Continued study is required to further define the health risks associated with chronic exposure to low levels of pollutants, and vigilance and education are needed to prevent breaches of the current environmental regulations.

References

1. Acid Rain. In: A Primer on Environmental Citizenship. Environment Canada. 1997 http://www.ns.doe.ca/aeb/ssd/acid/acidfaq.htm.
2. Air quality criteria for lead. Research Triangle Park, North Carolina: Environmental criteria and assessment office, US Environmental Protection Agency; 1986. EPA publication EPA-600/8-83-028.
3. Alexander LM, Heaven A, Tennant A, Morris R: Symptomatology of children in contact with sea water contaminated with sewage. J Epidemiol Community Health 1992; 46:340–344.
4. Amer MH, El-Yazigi A, Hannan MA, Mohamed ME: Water contamination and esophageal cancer at Gassim Region, Saudi Arabia. Gastroenterology 1990;98:1141–1147.
5. Anderson HR, Ponce de Leon A, Bland JM, Bower JS, Strachan DP: Air pollution and daily mortality in London: 1987–92. Br Med J 1996;312:665–669.

6. Arnow PM, Bland LA, Garcia-Houchins S, et al: An outbreak of fatal fluoride intoxication in a long term hemodialysis unit. Ann Intern Med 1994;121:339–344.
7. Aschengrau A, Zierler S, Cohen A: Quality of community drinking water and the occurrence of late adverse pregnancy outcomes. Arch Environ Health 1993;48:105–113.
8. Baghurst PA, McMichael AJ, Wigg NR, et al: Environmental exposure to lead and children's intelligence at the age of seven years: The Port Pirie cohort study. N Engl J Med 1992;327:1279–1284.
9. Balmes JR, Chen LL, Scannell C, et al: Ozone-induced decrements in FEV_1 and FVC do not correlate with measures of inflammation. Am J Respir Crit Care Med 1996; 153:904–909.
10. Bascom R, Bromberg PA, Costa DL, et al: Health effects of outdoor air pollution. Part I. Am J Respir Crit Care Med 1996;153:3–50.
11. Bascom R, Bromberg PA, Costa DL, et al: Health effects of outdoor air pollution. Part II. Am J Respir Crit Care Med 1996;153:477–498.
12. Baxter PJ, Ing R, Falk H, Plikaytis B: Mount St. Helens eruptions: The acute respiratory effects of volcanic ash in a North American community. Arch Environ Health 1983; 38:138–143.
13. Beresford SA: Cancer incidence and reuse of drinking water. Am J Epidemiol 1983;117:258–268.
14. Bourbeau J, Brisson C, Allaire S: Prevalence of the sick building syndrome symptoms in office workers before and after being exposed to a building with an improved ventilation system. Occup Environ Med 1996;53:204–210.
15. Brauer M, Blair J, Vedal S: Effect of ambient ozone exposure on lung function in farm workers. Am J Respir Crit Care Med 1996;154:981–998.
16. Burnett RT, Brook JR, Yung WT, et al: Association between ozone and hospitalization for respiratory diseases in 16 Canadian cities. Environ Res 1997;72:24–31.
17. Calderon-Garciduenas L, Osnaya-Brizuela N, Ramirez-Martinez L, Villarreal-Calderon A: DNA strand breaks in human nasal respiratory epithelium are induced upon exposure to urban pollution. Environ Health Perspect 1996; 104:160–168.
18. Chang CC, Ruhl RA, Halpern GM, Gershwin ME: The sick building syndrome. I. Definition and epidemiological considerations. J Asthma 1993;30:285–295.
19. Chen LC, Lam HF, Kim EJ, et al: Pulmonary effects of ultrafine coal ash inhaled by guinea pigs. J Toxicol Environ Health 1990;29:169–184.
20. Chen LC, Miller PD, Lam HF, et al: Sulfuric acid-layered ultrafine particles potentiate ozone-induced airway injury. J Toxicol Environ Health 1991;34:337–352.
21. Clean air act. Pro-act fact sheet. July 1996. http://www.afcee.brooks.af.mil/pro_act/main/fact/caa7_96/0796fact.ht.
22. Coffey MJ, Wheeler CS, Gross KB, et al: Increased 5-lipoxygenase metabolism in the lungs of human subjects exposed to ozone. Toxicology 1996;114:187–197.
23. Cohen SI, Deane M, Goldsmith JR: Carbon monoxide and survival from myocardial infarction. Arch Environ Health 1969;19:510–517.
24. Corbett SJ, Rubin GL, Curry GK, Kleinbaum DG: The health effects of swimming at Sydney beaches. The Sydney Beach Users Study Advisory Group. Am J Public Health 1993;83:1701–1706.
25. Dab W, Medina S, Quenel P, et al: Short term respiratory health effects of ambient air pollution: Results of the APHEA project in Paris. J Epidemiol Community Health 1996;50(suppl)1:42–46.
26. Deane M, Swan SH, Harris JA, Epstein DM, Neutra RR: Adverse pregnancy outcomes in relation to water consumption: A re-analysis of data from the original Santa Clara County Study, California, 1980–1981. Epidemiology 1992;3:94–97.
27. Devlin RB, McDonnell WF, Mann R, et al: Exposure of humans to ambient levels of ozone for 6.6 hours causes cellular and biochemical changes in the lung. Am J Respir Cell Mol Biol 1991;4:72–81.
28. Dewailly E, Poirier C, Meyer FM: Health hazards associated with windsurfing on polluted water. Am J Public Health 1986;76:690–691.
29. Dhara VH, Kriebel D: The Bhopal gas disaster, it's not too late for sound epidemiology. Arch Environ Health 1993; 48:436–437.
30. Dockery DW, Pope AC 3d, Xu X, et al: An association between air pollution and mortality in six U.S. cities. N Engl J Med 1993;329:1753–1759.
31. Engholm G, Palmgren F, Lynge E: Lung cancer, smoking, and environment: A cohort study of the Danish population. Br Med J 1996;312:1259–1263.
32. Ethylene glycol intoxication due to contamination of water systems. MMWR 1987;36:611–614.
33. Evans MJ, Johnson LV, Stephens RJ, Freeman G: Cell renewal in the lungs of rats exposed to low levels of ozone. Exp Mol Pathol 1976;24:70–83.
34. Evelyn J: Fumifugium, or the inconvenience of the aer and smoake of London dissipated. In: Lodge JP Jr, ed: The Smoke of London; Two Prophecies. Elmstead, NY: Maxwell Reprint Co., 1969, p. 55
35. Fagliano J, Berry M, Bove F, Burke T: Drinking water contamination and the incidence of leukemia: An ecologic study. Am J Public Health 1990;80:1209–1212.
36. Foy HM, Tarmapai S, Eamchan P, Metdilogkul O: Chronic arsenic poisoning from well water in a mining area in Thailand. Asia-Pacific J Public Health 1992–93;6:150–152.
37. Garber GE, Cameron DW, Hawley-Foss N, et al: The use of ozone-treated blood in the therapy of HIV infection and immune disease: A pilot study of safety and efficacy. AIDS 1991;5:981–984.
38. Gessner BD, Beller M, Middaugh JP, et al: Acute fluoride poisoning from a public water system. N Engl J Med 1994;330:95–99.
39. Gong H Jr, Shamoo DA, Anderson KR, Linn WS: Responses of older men with and without chronic obstructive pulmonary disease to prolonged ozone exposure. Arch Environ Health 1997;52:18–25.
40. Griffith J, Duncan RC, Riggan WB, Pellom AC: Cancer mortality in U.S. counties with hazardous waste sites and ground water pollution. Arch Environ Health 1989;44: 69–74.
41. Hatch GE, Boykin E, Graham JA, et al: Inhalable particles and pulmonary host defense: in vivo and in vitro effects of ambient air and combustion products. Environ Res 1985; 36:67–80.

42. Hertz-Picciotto I, Swan SH, Neutra RR, Samuels SJ: Spontaneous abortions in relation to consumption of tap water: An application of methods from survival analysis to a pregnancy followup study. Am J Epidemiology 1989;130: 79–93.
43. Herwaldt BL, Craun GF, Stokes SL, et al: Waterborne disease outbreaks, 1989–1990. MMWR Surveillance Summaries 1991;40:1–21.
44. Hiltermann TJ, Stolk J, Hiemstra PS, et al: Effect of ozone exposure on maximal airway narrowing in non-asthmatic and asthmatic subjects. Clin Sci 1995;89:619–624.
45. Horstman DH, Ball BA, Brown J, et al: Comparison of pulmonary responses of asthmatic and nonasthmatic subjects performing light exercise while exposed to a low level of ozone. Toxicol Ind Health 1995;11:369–385.
46. Jaakkola JJ, Miettinen P: Ventilation rate in office buildings and sick building syndrome. Occup Environ Med 1995;52:709–714.
47. Jarvis SN, Straube RC, Williams ALJ, Bartlett CLR: Illness associated with contamination of drinking water supplies with phenol. Br Med J 1985;290:1800–1802.
48. Jones GN, Sletten C, Mandry C, Brantley PJ: Ozone level effect on respiratory illness: An investigation of emergency department visits. South Med J 1995;88:1049–1056.
49. Katsouyanni K, Schwartz J, Spix C, et al: Short term effects of air pollution on health: A European approach using epidemiologic time series data: The APHEA protocol. J Epidemiol Community Health 1996;50(suppl 1):12–18.
50. Keene WE, McAnulty JM, Hoesly FC, et al: A swimming associated outbreak of hemorrhagic colitis caused by *Escherichia coli* O157:H7 and *Shigella sonnei*. N Engl J Med 1994;331:579–584.
51. Kessler M, Durand PY, Hestin D, et al: Elevated blood lead burden from drinking water in end stage renal failure. Nephro Dialy Transplant 1995;10:1648–1653.
52. Kinney PL, Nilsen DM, Lippmann M, et al: Biomarkers of lung inflammation in recreational joggers exposed to ozone. Am J Respir Crit Care Med 1996;154:1430–1435.
53. Kinney PL, Ozkaynak H: Associations of daily mortality and air pollution in Los Angeles county. Environ Res 1991;54:99–120.
54. Kinney PL, Ware JH, Spengler JD, et al: Short-term pulmonary function change in association with ozone levels. Am Rev Respir Dis 1989;139:56–61.
55. Kleinman MT, Davidson DM, Vandagriff RB, et al: Effects of short term exposure to carbon monoxide in subjects with coronary artery disease. Arch Environ Health 1989; 44:361–369.
56. Knobel HH, Chen CJ, Liang KY: Sudden infant death syndrome in relation to weather and optimetrically measured air pollution in Taiwan. Pediatrics 1995;96:1106–1110.
57. Kolmos HJ, Thuesen B, Nielson SV, et al: Outbreak of infection in a burn unit due to *Pseudomonas aeruginosa* originating from contaminated tubing used for irrigation of patients. J Hosp Inf 1993;24:11–21.
58. Koo D, Goldman L, Baron R: Irritant dermatitis among workers cleaning up a pesticide spill: California 1991. Am J Ind Med 1995;27:545–553.
59. Koren HS, Devlin RB, Graham DE, et al: Ozone-induced inflammation in the lower airways of human subjects. Am Rev Respir Dis 1989;139:407–415.
60. Koskela RS: Cardiovascular diseases among foundry workers exposed to carbon monoxide. Scand J Work, Environ Health 1994;20:286–293.
61. Kramer MH, Herwaldt BL, Craun GF, et al: Surveillance for waterborne-disease outbreaks—United States, 1993–1994. Centers for Disease Control and Prevention. CDC Surveillance Summaries, April 12, 1996. MMWR 1996; 45(no. SS–1):1–34.
62. Kreit JW, Gross KB, Moore TB, et al: Ozone-induced changes in pulmonary function and bronchial hyperresponsiveness in asthmatics. J Appl Physiol 1989;66: 217–222.
63. Kunzli N, Lurmann F, Segal M, et al: Association between lifetime ambient ozone exposure and pulmonary function in college freshmen—Results of a pilot study. Environ Res 1997;72:8–23.
64. Lambert WE, Samet JM, Dockery DW: Community air pollution. In: Rom WN, ed: Environmental and Occupational Medicine, 2nd ed. Boston, Little, Brown, 1992, pp. 1223–1242.
65. Lee K, Yanagisawa Y, Spengler JD, Nakai S: Carbon monoxide and nitrogen dioxide exposures in indoor ice skating rinks. J Sports Sci 1994;12:279–283.
66. Levine WC, Stephenson WT: Waterborne disease outbreaks, 1986–1988. MMWR Surveillance Summaries 1990; 39:87–98.
67. Linn WS, Solomon JC, Trim SC, et al: Effects of exposure to 4 ppm nitrogen dioxide in healthy and asthmatic volunteers. Arch Environ Health 1985;40:234–238.
68. Lloyd OL, Williams FL, Gailey FA: Is the Armadale epidemic over? Air pollution and mortality from lung cancer and other diseases, 1961–82. Br J Ind Med 1985;42:815–823.
69. Logan WPD: Mortality in the London fog incident, 1952. Lancet 1953;264:336–338.
70. MacKenzie WR, Hoxie NJ, Proctor ME, et al: A massive outbreak of cryptosporidium infection transmitted through the public water supply. N Engl J Med 1994; 331:161–167.
71. Mahoney FJ, Farley TA, Kelso KY, et al: An outbreak of hepatitis A associated with swimming in a public pool. J Infect Dis 1992;165:613–618.
72. Mazumder DN, Das Gupta J, Chakraborty AK, et al: Environmental pollution and chronic arsenicosis in south Calcutta. Bull WHO 1992;70:481–485.
73. McDonnell WF, Horstman DH, Abdul-Salaam S, House DE: Reproducibility of individual responses to ozone exposure. Am Rev Respir Dis 1985;131:36–40.
74. Meggs WJ: RADS and RUDS—The toxic induction of asthma and rhinitis. J Toxicology Clin Toxicology 1994;32: 487–501.
75. Mehta PS, Mehta AS, Mehta SJ, Makhijani AB: Bhopal tragedy's health effects. JAMA 1990;264:2781–2787.
76. Memish ZA, Oxley C, Contant J, et al: Plumbing system shock absorbers as a source of *Legionella pneumophila*. Am J Inf Con 1992;20:305–309.
77. Menzies R, Tamblyn R, Farant JP, et al: The effect of varying levels of outdoor-air supply on the symptoms of sick building syndrome. N Engl J Med 1993;328:821–827.
78. Mohsenin V: Airway responses to 2.0 ppm nitrogen dioxide in normal subjects. Arch Environ Health 1988;43: 242–246.

79. Mohsenin V: Airway responses to nitrogen dioxide in asthmatic subjects. J Toxicology Environ Health 1987;22:371–380.
80. Moore AC, Herwaldt BL, Craun GF, et al: Surveillance for waterborne disease outbreaks—United States, 1991–1992 MMWR CDC Surveillance Summaries 1993;42:1–22.
81. Moore MR, Richards WN, Sherlock JG: Successful abatement of lead exposure from water supplies in the west of Scotland. Environ Res 1985;38:67–76.
82. Morgan WK: "Zamboni disease." Pulmonary edema in an ice hockey player. Arch Intern Med 1995;155:2479–2480.
83. Morrow PE, Utel MJ: Responses of susceptible populations to nitrogen dioxide. Res Rep Health Effects Inst 1989;23:1–44.
84. Murphy EA: Effectiveness of flushing on reducing lead and copper in school drinking water. Environ Health Perspect 1993;101:240–241.
85. Mushak P, Crocetti AF: Determination of numbers of lead-exposed American children as a function of lead source: Integrated summary of a report to the U.S. Congress on childhood lead poisoning. Environ Res 1989;50:210–229.
86. Needleman HL, Schell A, Bellinger D, et al: The long term effects of exposure to low doses of lead in childhood: An 11-year followup report. N Engl J Med 1990;322:83–88.
87. Nielsen T, Jorgensen HE, Larsen JC, Poulsen M: City air pollution of polycyclic aromatic hydrocarbons (PAH) and other mutagens: Occurrences, sources, and health effects. Sci Total Environ 1996;189–190:41–49.
88. Odatus product advertisement. http://www.odatus.com/ May 1997.
89. Ogunsola OJ, Oluwole AF, Asubiojo OI, et al: Environmental impact of vehicular traffic in Nigeria: Health aspects. Sci Total Environ 1994;146–147:111–116.
90. Orehek J, Massari JP, Gayrard C, et al: Effect of short term, low level nitrogen dioxide exposure on bronchial sensitivity of asthmatic patients. J Clin Invest 1976;57:301–307.
91. Ostro B: The association of air pollution and mortality: Examining the case for inference. Arch Environ Health 1993;48:336–342.
92. Ostro BD, Lipsett MJ, Mann JK, et al: Air pollution and respiratory morbidity among adults in southern California. Am J Epidemiology 1993;137:691–700.
93. Pilotto LS, Douglas RM: Indoor nitrogen dioxide and childhood respiratory illness. Aust J Public Health 1992;16:245–250.
94. Pollutants and sources. Unified air toxics website. Office of Air Quality Planning and Standards. US Environmental Protection Agency. http://www.epa.gov/oar/oaqps/airtox/pollsour.htm.
95. Ponce de Leon A, Anderson HR, Bland JM, et al: Effects of air pollution on daily hospital admissions for respiratory disease in London between 1987–88 and 1991–92. Epidemiol Community Health 1996;50(suppl 1):63–70.
96. Pope CA 3rd, Thun MJ, Namboodiri MM, et al: Particulate air pollution as a predictor of mortality in a prospective study of U.S. adults. Am J Respir Crit Care Med 1995;151:669–674.
97. Rice DC: Neurotoxicity of lead, methylmercury, and PCBs in relation to the Great Lakes. Environ Health Perspect 1995;103(suppl):71–87.
98. Rom WN: Chlorofluorocarbons and destruction of the ozone layer. In: Rom WN, ed: Environmental and Occupational Medicine, 2nd ed. Boston, Little, Brown, 1992, pp. 1299–1304.
99. Romieu I, Meneses F, Ruiz S, et al: Effects of air pollution on the respiratory health of asthmatic children living in Mexico City. Am J Respir Care Med 1996;154:300–307.
100. Rusznak C, Devalia JL, Davies RJ: The impact of pollution on allergic disease. Allergy 1994;49(18 suppl):21–27.
101. Rutishauser M, Ackermann U, Braun C, et al: Significant association between outdoor NO_2 and respiratory symptoms in preschool children. Lung 1990;168(suppl):347–352.
102. Safe Drinking Water Act. Pro-act fact sheet. July 1996. http://www.afcee.brooks.af.mil/pro_act/main/fact/sdw9_96/0996fact.ht.
103. Samet JM, Lambert WE, Skipper BJ, et al: Nitrogen dioxide and respiratory illnesses in infants. Am Rev Respir Dis 1993;148:1258–1265.
104. Samet JM, Spengler JD: Indoor air pollution. In: Rom WN, ed: Environmental and Occupational Medicine, 2nd ed. Boston, Little, Brown, 1992, pp. 1243–1254.
105. Sathe PV, Karandikar VN, Gupte MD, et al: Investigation report of an epidemic of typhoid fever. Int J Epidemiology 1983;12:215–219.
106. Scannell C, Chen L, Aris RM, et al: Greater ozone-induced inflammatory responses in subjects with asthma. Am J Respir Crit Care Med 1996;154:24–29.
107. Schwartz J: Air pollution and hospital admissions for respiratory disease. Epidemiology 1996;7:20–28.
108. Schwartz J, Dockery DW: Increased mortality in Philadelphia associated with daily air pollution concentrations. Am Rev Respir Dis 1992;145:600–604.
109. Schwartz J, Dockery DW: Particulate air pollution and daily mortality in Steubenville, Ohio. Am J Epidemiol 1992;135:12–19.
110. Sexton K, Gong H Jr, Bailar JC 3rd, et al: Air pollution health risks: Do class and race matter? Toxicology Ind Health 1993;9:843–878.
111. Shannon MW, Graef JW: Lead intoxication in infancy. Pediatrics 1992;89:87–90.
112. Sheppard D, Wong WS, Uehara CD, et al: Lower threshold and greater bronchomotor responsiveness of asthmatic subjects to sulfur dioxide. Am Rev Respir Dis 1980;122:873–891.
113. Shy CM, Creason JP, Pearlman ME, et al: The Chattanooga school children study. Part II. Effect of community exposure to nitrogen dioxide. J Air Pollut Control Assoc 1970;50:582–588.
114. Sidhu KS: Standard setting process and regulations for environmental contaminants in drinking water: State versus federal needs and viewpoints. Reg Toxicol Pharm 1991;13:293–308.
115. Spix C, Wichmann HE: Daily mortality and air pollutants: Findings from Koln, Germany. J Epidemiol Community Health 1996;50(suppl 1):52–58.
116. St. Louis ME: Water-related disease outbreaks, 1985. MMWR Surveillance Summaries 1988;37:13–20.
117. Stern FB, Halperin WE, Hornung RW, et al: Heart disease mortality among bridge and tunnel officers exposed to carbon monoxide. Am J Epidemiol 1988;128:1276–1288.
118. Stolwijk JA: Sick-building syndrome. Environ Health Perspect 1991;95:99–100.

119. Sunyer J, Castellsague J, Saez M, et al: Air pollution and mortality in Barcelona. J Epidemiol Community Health 1996;50(suppl 1):76–80.
120. Sunyer J, Saez M, Murillo C, et al: Air pollution and emergency room admissions for chronic obstructive pulmonary disease: A 5-year study. Am J Epidemiology 1993;137: 701–705.
121. Swerdlow DL, Woodruff BA, Brady RC, et al: A waterborne outbreak in Missouri of *Escherichia coli* O157:H7 associated with bloody diarrhea and death. Ann Intern Med 1992;117:812–819.
122. Tanaka H, Honma S, Nishi M, et al: Two-year follow-up study of the effect of acid fog on adult asthma patients. Int Med 1995;35:100–104.
123. Thurston GD, Ito K, Hayes CG, et al: Respiratory hospital admissions and summertime haze air pollution in Toronto, Ontario: Consideration of the role of acid aerosols. Environ Res 1994;65:271–290.
124. Touloumi G, Samoli E, Katsouyanni K: Daily mortality and "winter type" air pollution in Athens, Greece—A time series analysis within the APHEA project. J Epidemiol Community Health 1996;50(suppl 1):47–51.
125. Tsuda T, Babazono A, Yamamoto E, et al: Ingested arsenic and internal cancer: A historical cohort study followed for 33 years. Am J Epidemiology 1995;141:198–209.
126. Utell MJ, Framptom MW: Sulfur dioxide and sulfuric acid aerosols. In: Rom WN, ed: Environmental and Occupational Medicine, 2nd ed. Boston, Little, Brown, 1992, pp. 519–527.
127. Verrazzo G, Coppola L, Luongo C, et al: Hyperbaric oxygen, oxygen-ozone therapy, and rheologic parameters of blood in patients with peripheral occlusive arterial disease. Undersea Hyperbar Med 1995;22:17–22.
128. Vigotti MA, Rossi G, Bisanti L, et al: Short term effects of urban air pollution on respiratory health in Milan, Italy, 1980–89. J Epidemiol Community Health 1996;50(suppl 1):71–75.
129. Wax PM: The ultimate poison center call—Bhopal. J Toxicol Clin Toxicol 1995;33:18.
130. Weisel CP, Cody RP, Lioy PJ: Relationship between summertime ambient ozone levels and emergency department visits for asthma in central New Jersey. Environ Health Perspect 1995;103(suppl 2):97–102.
131. Weschler CJ, Shields HC, Rainer D: Concentrations of volatile organic compounds at a building with health and comfort complaints. Am Ind Hyg Assoc J 1990;51: 261–268.
132. Windham GC, Shusterman D, Swan SH, et al: Exposure to organic solvents and adverse pregnancy outcomes. Am J Ind Med 1991;20:241–259.
133. Wojtyniak B, Piekarski T: Short term effect of air pollution on mortality in Polish urban populations—What is different? J Epidemiol Community Health 1996;50(suppl 1):36–41.
134. Wrensch M, Swan S, Lipcomb J, et al: Pregnancy outcomes in women potentially exposed to solvent-contaminated drinking water in San Jose, California. Am J Epidemiol 1990;131:283–300.
135. Wrensch M, Swan S, Murphy PJ, et al: Hydrogeologic assessment of exposure to solvent-contaminated drinking water: Pregnancy outcomes in relationship to exposure. Arch Environ Health 1990;45:210–216.
136. Wu MM, Kuo TL, Chen CJ: Dose-response relation between arsenic concentration in well water and mortality from cancers and vascular disease. Am J Epidemiology 1989;130:1123–1132.
137. Zmirou D, Barumandzadeh T, Balducci F, et al: Short term effects of air pollution on mortality in the city of Lyon, France, 1985–90. J Epidemiol Community Health 1996; 50(suppl 1):30–35.

CHAPTER 75

Mushrooms: Toxic and Hallucinogenic

Lewis R. Goldfrank

A 58-year-old woman presented to the emergency department (ED) with severe crampy abdominal pain and profuse diarrhea. She had spent the summer morning picking wild mushrooms in a local park, as she had done for many years. She found numerous edible species and ate quite a few while picking them. Her symptoms began within 1 hour after returning from the park.

The woman was pale and diaphoretic, with persistent gagging. She explained that she was an expert in selecting edible mushrooms, picked at the same place every year, and never had had trouble before. She had foraged in the woods of Poland for years without difficulty. She insisted that the mushrooms could not be at fault as they were found growing on dead wood, and that several were mutilated by slugs.

The patient had type 2 diabetes mellitus, well controlled with chlorpropamide 500 mg daily, took no other medications, had no known allergies, and did not drink alcohol or smoke cigarettes. No other family members had been ill recently.

Physical examination revealed a diaphoretic, dyspneic, and anxious woman. Her blood pressure was 110/60 mm Hg and pulse was 120 beats/min supine with orthostatic changes. When she stood up, her blood pressure was 90/40 mm Hg and pulse was 145 beats/min. Her respiratory rate was 24 breaths/min and temperature was 98.6°F (37°C).

The head was atraumatic, pupils were 4 mm, equal, and reactive, sclerae were anicteric, and the conjunctivae were not pale. The mucosa were moist with no excessive lacrimation or salivation, and the throat was unremarkable. There were no cutaneous abnormalities. The lungs were clear. Heart sounds were normal. Abdominal examination showed diffuse tenderness with hyperactive bowel sounds, but the liver and spleen were unremarkable. The extremities were normal.

When it was suggested that she stay in the hospital, the patient resisted vehemently. Her dizziness in the erect position, however, convinced her to remain. Blood samples were drawn, an IV was started with 0.9% sodium chloride at 300 mL/h, a fingerstick blood glucose was >180 mg/dL, and the patient was admitted for observation and volume repletion.

As the patient prepared for admission, she gave her belongings and clothes to her daughter. At that point the staff noticed a large bag filled with mushrooms. The patient was so convinced of the benignity of these mushrooms that she wanted to give them to her daughter to take home, but she was eventually persuaded to leave the mushrooms in the ED for further examination.

The CBC showed a hematocrit of 42% with 8300 WBC/mm^3 (72% polys, 20% lymphocytes, 4% monocytes, and 4% eosinophils). The prothrombin time was 13 seconds, control 12 seconds. The glucose was 220 mg/dL; BUN, 21 mg/dL; sodium, 140 mEq/L; potassium, 3.7 mEq/L; chloride, 101 mEq/L; and bicarbonate, 30 mEq/L. The chest radiograph was normal. Abdominal radiographs showed a nonspecific ileus pattern.

Despite the patient's confidence concerning the edibility of the mushrooms, her presentation encouraged the staff to have them investigated. Microscopic spore assessment methods of identifying toxic mushrooms by a mycologist confirmed that this patient had made a classic mistake: She had picked the jack-o'-lantern (*Omphalotus olearius*), an orange, bioluminescent mushroom[4] often mistaken for the edible species of chanterelle (*Cantharellus cibarius*), an error often reported by others.[21,69]

Which Mushroom Ingestions Lead to Poison Center Calls?

Unintentional exposures to mushrooms represent a relatively constant percentage of exposures reported from American Association of Poison Control Centers.[35–45,71] Using these data and those of the Mushroom Poisoning Registry of the North American Mycological Association, it has been estimated that approximately 5 mushroom exposures per 100,000 population occur per year, with geographic and climatic conditions as well as mycologic habitats leading to variations.[68] Although the analysis of mushroom ingestions has changed over the 12 years of the AAPCC National Data Collection Systems analyses, the relative benignity of these ingestions, the inadequacy of the identification of the ingested mushroom, and the rarity of lethal ingestions are most evident. Summation analysis of the data available shows that mushrooms represented approximately 0.5% of the more than 16,000,000 exposures. It is estimated that more than 95% of the exact species were unidentified,[68] approximately 90% of the toxin groups ingested were unknown, more than 50% of the individuals had no symptoms, 25% of the patients were treated in healthcare facilities, annually 10–15% of these had minor manifestations of toxicity, less than 5% had moderate toxicity, and approximately 0.2% had major toxicity. During this 12-year period approximately 15 patients died of their ingestion. Of those mushrooms identified 11 of 12 were probably *Amanita* species and one was a *Boletus* spp. All patients involved were adults. Of the mushroom groups identified (approximately 10% of the ingested mushrooms) the following approximate the group's incidence: hallucinogenic (4%), gastrointestinal (2%), miscellaneous nontoxic (1.5%), monomethylhydrazine (0.8%), cyclopeptide (0.5%), ibotenic (0.2%), coprine (0.1%), muscarine (0.1%), and orellanine (0.1%). The fact that about 90% of the reported mushroom exposures generally remain unidentified forces the clinician to make significant decisions with incomplete data.

How Should the Victim of a Suspected Mushroom Poisoning Be Managed?

Because the ingestion of certain mushrooms may lead to toxicity, with substantial mortality from 10 to 50% for *Amanita* spp.,[17] suspected mushroom ingestions may require vigorous management. A consequential effort at precise identification of the genus and species involved will make assessment, management, and follow-up easier and more logical. Initially, the basic regimen of emesis, adsorption, and catharsis should be followed. Often, the unknown mushroom toxins produce sufficient emesis, obviating the need for the routine use of syrup of ipecac or lavage. Once vomiting stops, the patient should be given activated charcoal, 1 g/kg.

Appropriate life-support measures should be instituted as necessary. Fluid, electrolyte, and glucose repletion are essential. There is wide variability in quantity and type of toxin present in mushrooms according to geography and local conditions and in individual susceptibility. The routine use of specific antidotes should be avoided, as they may provoke an unanticipated adverse reaction.

How Are Mushroom Poisonings Classified Clinically? What Is the Specific Management Strategy for Each Group?

Because mushroom species vary widely in the toxins they contain and because identifying them with certainty is difficult, a clinical rather than a taxonomic system of classification is useful (Table 75–1). Eight groups of toxins are identifiable: cyclopeptides, monomethylhydrazine, muscarine, coprine, ibotenic acid, and muscimol, psilocybin, general gastrointestinal (GI) toxins, and orellanine.[23,31] The management and prognosis can be determined with a high degree of confidence from the history and initial symptoms.[23,31,32]

I. Cyclopeptide-containing Mushrooms

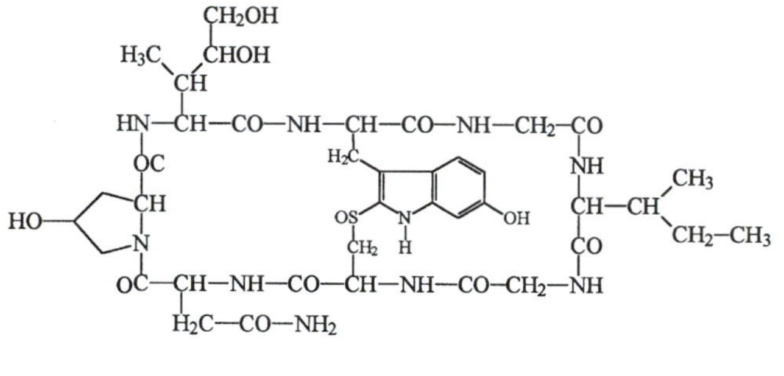

α-Amanitin

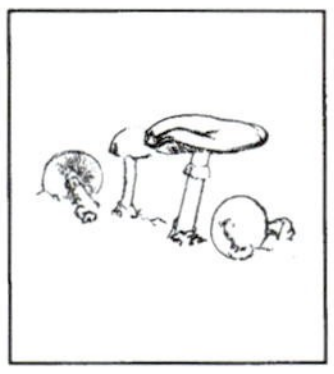

Ninety-five percent of all mushroom fatalities in North America are associated with the cyclopeptide-containing species.[5] These mushrooms include a number of *Amanita* species, including *A. verna*, *A. virosa*, and *A. phalloides*, as well as *Galerina autumnalis*, *G. marginata*, *G. venenata*, *Lepiota helveola*, *L. chlorophyllum*, and *L. brunneoincarnata*. In general, the mortality rate is higher in children than in adults.[49]

Unfortunately, early differentiation of cyclopeptide poisonings from other types of mushroom poisoning is very difficult. Patients poisoned with cyclopeptides may present to an ED with a seemingly innocuous picture of nausea, vomiting, abdominal pain, and diarrhea, which is often attributed to other causes. Such patients are frequently sent home, only to return moribund on a subsequent day. The delayed onset of symptoms is typical of cyclopeptide poisoning and should be a critical consideration in assessing any potential poisoning.

The first phase of cyclopeptide poisoning resembles

TABLE 75–1. MUSHROOM TOXICITY

Genus/Species	Toxin	Onset of Action	Site of Toxicity	Symptoms	Mortality	Therapy
I. *Amanita* *phalloides* *tennifolia* *virosa* *Galerina* *autumnalis* *marginata* *venenata* *Lepiota* *josserandii* *helveola*	Cyclopeptides Amatoxins Phallotoxins Virotoxins	6–10 h	Hepatic (primarily)	Phase 1: GI toxicity—nausea, vomiting, diarrhea Phase 2: Quiescent, ↑ enzymes Phase 3: hematuria, proteinuria, gastroenteritis, jaundice, ↑AST, ↑ALT	10-50 % (lethal at < 0.1 mg/kg)	Activated charcoal Fluids Electrolytes Intensive care
II. *Gyromitra* *ambigua* *esculenta* *infula*	Gyromitrin (monomethylhydrazine)	6–10 h	CNS	Seizures, abdominal pain, nausea, vomiting, hepatorenal failure, weakness	Rare	Pyridoxine, 25 mg/kg IV if indicated
III. *Clitocybe* *dealbata* *dilatata* *illudens* Most *Inocybe* spp.	Muscarine	0.5–2 h	Autonomic nervous system	Muscarinic effects—salivation, lacrimation, urination, defecation	Rare	Atropine, 1–2 mg IV (adults), 0.02 mg/kg (children)
IV. *Coprinus atramentarius*	Coprine ? Metabolite 1-aminocyclopropanol	0.5-2 h	Acetaldehyde dehydrogenase	Disulfiram-like effect with ethanol flush, tachycardia, nausea, vomiting	Rare	IV fluids, electrolytes
V. *Amanita* *gemmata* *muscaria* *pantherina*	Ibotenic acid, muscimol	0.5–2 h	CNS	GABAergic effects, rare delirium, hallucinations, dizziness, ataxia, seizures, mixed muscarinic and atropinic effects	Rare	Benzodiazepines during excitatory phase
VI. *Psilocybe* *caerulipes* *cubensis* *Gymnopilus* *spectabilis* *Psathyrella* *foenisecii*	Psilocybin, psilocin	0.5–1 h	CNS	Ataxia, hyperkinesis, hallucinations	Rare	Benzodiazepines
VII. *Clitocybe* *nebularis* *Chlorophyllum* *molybdites* *esculentum* *Lactarius* sp. *Paxillus* *involutus*	Gastrointestinal	0.5–3 h	GI	Malaise, nausea, vomiting, diarrhea	Rare	Fluids, electrolytes
VIII. *Cortinarius* *orellanus* *speciosissimus* *rainierensis*	Orelline, orellanine	>24 h Days–weeks	Renal (primarily)	Nausea, vomiting, oliguria, renal failure	Rare	Fluids, electrolytes, hemodialysis for renal failure

Adapted, with permission, from Lincoff G, Mitchel DH: Toxic and Hallucinogenic Mushroom Poisoning: A Handbook for Physicians and Mushroom Hunters. New York, Van Nostrand Reinhold, 1977, pp. 246–247.

severe gastroenteritis, with profuse, watery diarrhea, occurring not before 6–12 hours after ingestion. Supportive fluid and electrolyte replacement leads to transient improvement during phase 2, at 12–24 hours. However, a third devastating phase, manifested by hepatic,[5] renal,[5] and, rarely, pancreatic[18] toxicity and death, ensues 1–6 days after ingestion. The initial hepatotoxicity begins within the second phase, and hepatic necrosis is evident with bilirubin, AST, and ALT elevations, hypoglycemia, jaundice, and hepatic coma within 2–3 days. Hypoglycemia is a marker of grave hepatic damage and a grim prognosis. Pathologic manifestations are steatosis, central zonal necrosis, and centrilobular hemorrhage.[5] Viable hepatocytes are at the rims of the larger triads, although lobular architecture remains intact.

Endocrine abnormalities have been found involving the hormones that regulate glucose, calcium, and thyroid homeostasis.[27] Insulin and C-peptide concentrations may be elevated, suggesting that hypoglycemia was not solely associated with hepatic failure. Serum calcitonin concentrations may be elevated in conjunction with hypocalcemia. Thyroxine concentrations may be depressed and triiodothyronine concentrations undectable, while thyroid-stimulating hormone concentrations may not be elevated. These findings have been reported in a single study and merit further investigation.[27]

In a series of 10 patients poisoned by diverse *Lepiota* spp. 50% of the patients developed a mixed polyneuropathy. In most of these cases, a spontaneous recovery was noted within 1 year, although a single additional patient had progressive deterioration.[54]

Amanita phalloides contains a number of cyclopeptides of approximately 900 daltons, of which amatoxins (cyclic octapeptides), phallotoxins (cyclic heptapeptides), and virotoxins (cyclic heptapeptides) are responsible for human poisoning following ingestion.[15,29,74] Approximately 1.5–2.5 mg of amanitin can be obtained from 1 g of dry *Amanita phalloides* or as much as 3.5 mg/g for some *Lepiota* spp.[50,53] Therefore these mushrooms (a 20-g specimen might contain as much as 50 mg for an *Amanita* or 70 mg for a *Lepiota*) can contain well in excess of the 0.1 mg/kg hypothesized lethal doses.[14] Of these chemically similar molecules, phalloidin appears to be a rapid-acting toxin while amanitin leads to more delayed manifestations.[59] Phalloidin interrupts actin polymerization and impairs cell membrane function, but has a limited absorption and therefore toxicity, and may be restricted to the GI manifestations. The amatoxins appear to be more toxic in humans, leading to hepatic, renal, and central nervous system (CNS) damage. These polypeptides are heat stable and are insoluble in water, and they lose activity very slowly over years after drying.[15] In vitro studies have shown that alpha-amanitin is cytotoxic on the basis of its interference with RNA polymerase II, preventing the transcription of DNA.[62] The LD_{50} in mice of alpha-amanitin has been shown to be 0.1–0.75 mg/kg and 0.2–0.4 mg/kg for the gamma-amanitin.[14] These molecules are poorly but rapidly absorbed from the GI tract.[26] The target organs are those with the highest rate of cell turnover, including the gastrointestinal tract epithelium, liver hepatocytes, and kidneys. These amatoxins show limited protein binding and are present in the plasma at low concentrations for 24–48 hours.[26] Amatoxins are eliminated in the urine, gastroduodenal fluids, and feces for days following ingestion. The toxins can be detected in poisoned patients from gastroduodenal fluid, serum, urine, stool, and liver and kidney biopsies using high-performance liquid chromatography,[26] thin-layer chromatography, and radioimmunoassay for several days.

The search for therapies has been vigorously pursued in Europe because of the large number of victims each year and high mortality rates: currently 20–30% and previously up to 50–60%.[17] Thioctic acid (alpha-lipoic acid) was initially reported to be beneficial in the treatment of liver disease in laboratory animals.[25] A number of uncontrolled clinical trials in humans followed. In 1963 thioctic acid was credited with the survival of 39 of 40 patients poisoned by *Amanita phalloides*,[30] in contrast to the previously high fatality rates. Thioctic acid was subsequently utilized in *Amanita* poisoning in the United States involving 11 patients, of whom all 10 patients who received thioctic acid early in the course survived.[5]

Investigators have not substantiated the protective effect of thioctic acid in the mouse[20] or dog,[1,2] even with adequate glucose replacement.[19] Hypoglycemia is a common feature of thioctic acid therapy for *Amanita* poisoning, although it is not clear whether it results from direct toxicity of the drug or is secondary to hepatic damage.

Additional investigators have cared for *Amanita phalloides*–poisoned patients using supportive care, fluid and electrolyte repletion, high-dose penicillin G, dexamethasone, and thioctic acid, with resultant survival in excess of 90%.[12,48] Other substances, including massive doses of penicillin at 1 million U/kg/day and silibinin (an extract of silymarin from the milk thistle *Silybum marianum*),[72] both suggested to inhibit alpha-amanitin hepatocellular penetration, have also been used in humans but have shown no clear advantage over management in a good intensive care unit.

More recently, activated charcoal has been shown to adsorb amanitin and improve survival in laboratory animals.[14] Cimetidine, a potent cytochrome P450 system inhibitor, may have a hepatoprotective effect in animals against alpha-amanitin[57] but shows no protective affect against phalloidin toxicity.[59] Cimetidine at 4–6 g/day has been suggested as a therapeutic intervention.[58] Emesis, lavage, and catharsis are not usually necessary, as emesis and catharsis are usually induced by the toxin. Activated charcoal is safe, logical, and the most valuable part of any therapeutic intervention. Alpha-amanitin may be enterohepatically recirculated.[9] Although the clinical presentation is often delayed, 1 g/kg body weight of activated charcoal orally every 2–4 hours if the patient is not vomiting or by continuous nasogastric infusion appears appropriate. Fluid and electrolyte resuscitation and treatment of hepatic compromise are essential. Intravenous fluid repletion with 0.9% sodium chloride solution, electrolytes, and $D_{50}W$ or $D_{10}W$ may be necessary due to substantial diarrheal volume loss and glycogen depletion.

Forced diuresis, hemodialysis, plasmapheresis, hemofiltration, and hemoperfusion[13,16,21] have all been suggested, but there is no clinical evidence of benefit nor supportive pharmacokinetic data for any of these therapies.[52,53,70,73] Plasmapheresis has not been shown to remove more than 10 µg of amatoxin. Some of the toxicokinetic analyses demonstrate 12–23 µg of amatoxin excretion in the urine, of which 60–80% occurred during the first 2 hours of collection. The extreme variability of the type and quantity of ingestant, the host, and the management has made interpretations exceedingly difficult. It should be noted that maximal urinary retrieval of 20 µg of amanitin was achieved in one series.[70] In another series total maximal urinary alpha- and beta-amanitin excreted were 3.19 mg and 5.21 mg, respectively. Two thirds of the patients had a total excretion of ≥ 1.5 mg amanitin toxins.[26] Because of the absence of prospective controlled studies for these agents, in addition to the extreme variability of success with many regimens, multiple-dose activated charcoal and supportive care remain the standard therapy.

The criteria and timing for transplantation are far less well-developed than those available for decision analysis for fulminant viral hepatitis where grade III or IV hepatic encephalopathy, marked hyperbilirubinemia, and azotemia are indications for transplantation.[51] Early identification is essential due to the rapid progression of hepatic failure and the temporal delay necessary to find an appropriate organ. Individuals have been transplanted whose resected livers showed 0–30% hepatocyte viability. In these cases the authors did not wait for progression past grade II encephalopathy, nor did they allow for the development of azotemia or marked hyperbilirubinemia.[51] The development of criteria for patient selection is essential to avoid risking unnecessary hepatic transplantation while offering the potential for survival for those individuals who have no functional liver. The grim prognosis[49,66] in hepatic coma secondary to *Amanita* poisoning has led several transplant groups to consider the role of hepatic transplantation in encephalopathic patients with prolonged prothrombin times despite factor replacement with fresh frozen plasma, persistent hypoglycemia, metabolic acidosis, increased serum ammonia, increased AST, and hypofibrinogenemia.[22,28,51] There are now numerous case reports of successful liver transplantation for fulminant hepatic failure from presumed *Amanita ocreata*,[28,75] *A. phalloides*[26,51] *Lepiota helveola*,[47] and *L. brunneoincarnata* poisoning.[54]

Most studies suggest that no circulating amatoxin will be present by the time transplantation is considered indicated.[13] Several authors suggest those individuals who manifest symptoms suggestive of hepatotoxic *Amantia, Galerina*, or *Lepiota* species should be counseled with regard to the potential need for transplantation and rapidly transferred to a regional liver transplantation center should it be indicated.

II. Monomethylhydrazine-containing Mushrooms

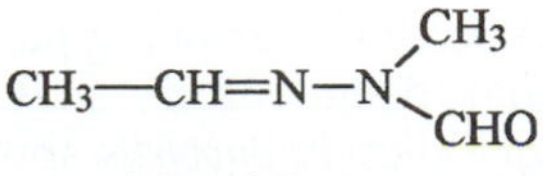

Gyromitrin

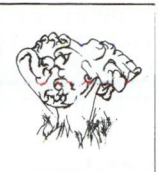

These mushrooms are found commonly in the Spring under conifers and are easily recognized by their brain-like appearance. *Gyromitra* mushrooms contain gyromitrin (*N*-methyl-*N*-formyl hydrazone), which on hydrolysis splits into acetaldehyde and *N*-methyl-*N*-formyl hydrazine. This molecule, on later hydrolysis, yields monomethylhydrazine. Due to its instability it is unlikely that gyromitrin exists in its free form. The hydrazine moiety reacts with pyridoxine, resulting in inhibition of pyridoxal phosphate–related enzymatic reactions. This interference with pyridoxal phosphate disrupts the function of gamma-amino butyric acid as an inhibitory neurotransmitter (GABA). The implications of this decrease in GABA, which is thought to contribute to intractable seizures with INH or gyromitrin toxicity, is discussed in Antidotes in Depth: Pyridoxine. The clinical effects of eating these mushrooms include headache, nausea, vomiting, and, occasionally seizures and hepatorenal failure. The onset of toxicity is approximately 6–10 hours after ingestion, and previously high mortality rates are no longer reported.[35–45,68,71] Pyridoxine, in doses of 25 mg/kg, may be useful in limiting toxicity, particularly seizures (see Antidotes in Depth: Pyridoxine).

Members of the monomethyl hydrazine (MMH) group include *G. esculenta, G. californica, G. brunnea*, and *G. infula*. *Gyromitra esculenta* is a good example of a mushroom with a "Jekyll and Hyde" personality, enjoying a reputation of being edible in the western United States but of being poisonous in other areas. Certain cooking methods may eliminate the toxin, but inhalation of the fumes while cooking may cause poisoning. Because of the potential for toxicity, members of this mushroom family should not be eaten.

III. Muscarine-containing Mushrooms

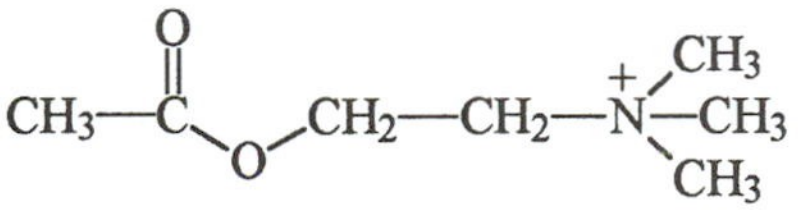

Acetylcholine

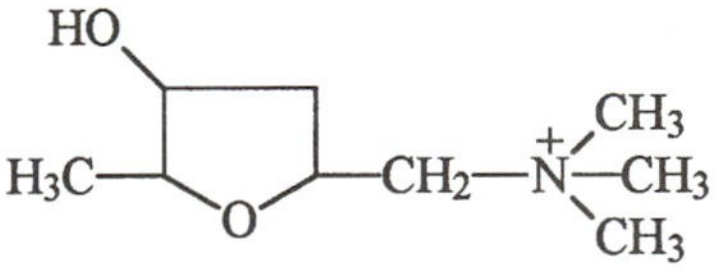

Muscarine

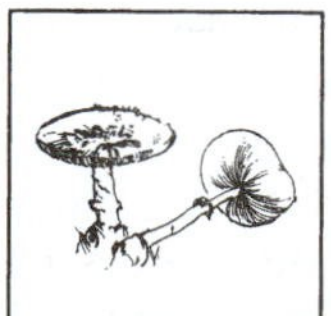

Muscarinic effects on the autonomic nervous system by this class of mushrooms include salivation, lacrimation, bronchorrhea, urination, and defecation. Symptoms usually develop within 0.5–2 hours of ingestion.

Lethality is extremely rare. Muscarine produces a peripheral cholinergic effect but does not cross the blood–brain barrier, since it is a quarternary ammonium compound. Atropine, 1–2 mg given IV slowly (for adults or 0.5–1.0 mg for children), can be titrated and can be repeated as frequently as indicated to reverse symptomatology. Mushrooms that contain muscarine include *Clitocybe dealbata* ("the sweater"), *C. illudens* (*Omphalotus olearius*), and *Inocybe lacera*; usually only traces are present in *A. muscaria.*

IV. Coprine-containing Mushrooms

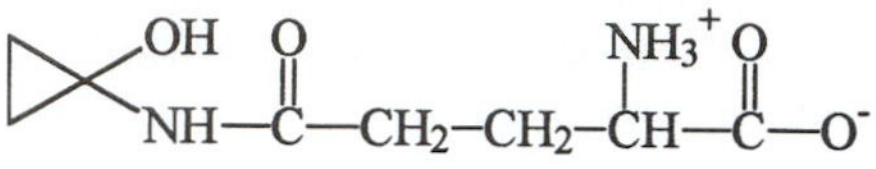

Coprine

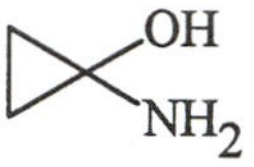

1-aminocyclopropanol

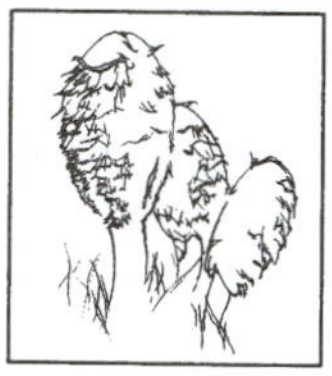

Coprinus mushrooms, particularly *C. atramentarius,* contain the toxin coprine. They are known as "inky caps" because the gills autodigest into an inky liquid shortly after picking. Coprine, an amino acid, or, more likely, its metabolite 1-aminocyclopropanol,[11,46,67] has a disulfiram-like effect, blocking acetaldehyde dehydrogenase and thereby allowing for the buildup of acetaldehyde with its accompanying effects. These effects occur if the patient ingests alcohol concomitantly or up to 48–72 hours after mushroom ingestion. Within 0.5–2 hours after ingestion, an acute disulfiram effect is noted, with tachycardia, flushing, nausea, and vomiting. This group of mushrooms rarely causes fatalities (see Chap. 63 for further discussion of disulfiram).

V. Ibotenic Acid- and Muscimol-containing Mushrooms

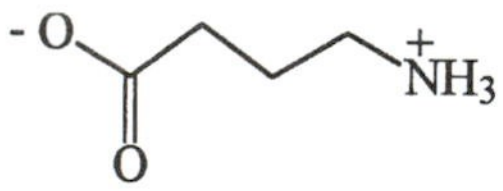

GABA

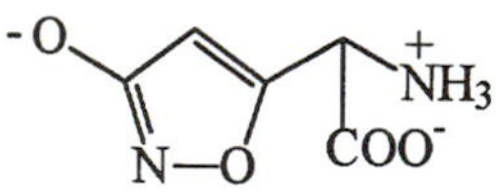

Ibotenic acid

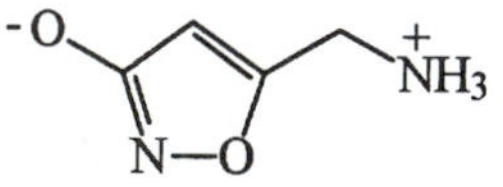

Muscimol

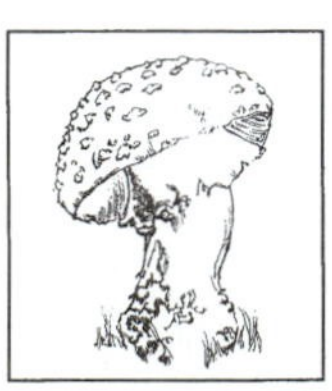

The fifth class of mushrooms contains the isoxazole derivative ibotenic acid and muscimol, its decarboxylated metabolite. Within 0.5–2 hours after ingestion, these compounds produce somnolence, hallucinations, and delirium in adults as well as myoclonic movements, seizures, and other neurologic findings in children.[6] Ibotenic acid, which is structurally similar to the stimulatory neurotransmitter glutamic acid, is decarboxylated in vivo to muscimol. The stereochemistry of muscimol is very similar to that of the depressant neurotransmitter gamma-amino butyric acid (GABA) and may stimulate GABA receptors, with typical GABA manifestations. Mushrooms in this group include *Amanita gemmata, A. muscaria,* and *A. pantherina.* Stimulatory effects of this group of mushrooms can be treated with benzodiazepines.

VI. Psilocybin-containing Mushrooms

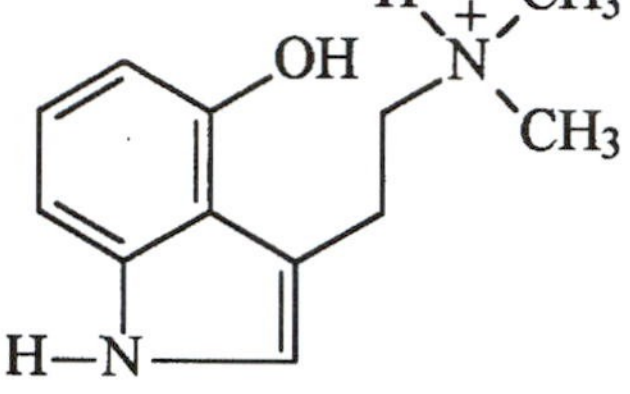

Psilocybin

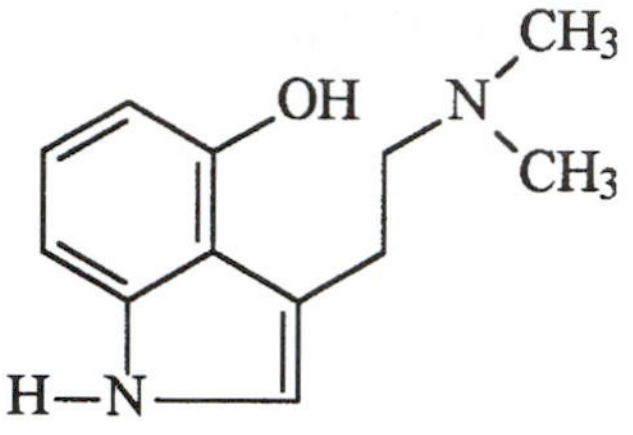

Psilocin

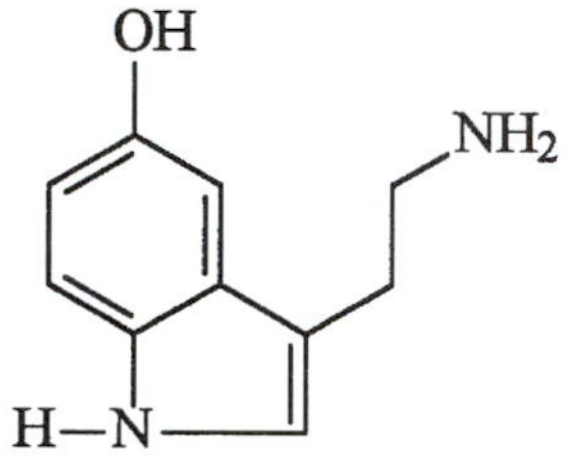

Serotonin

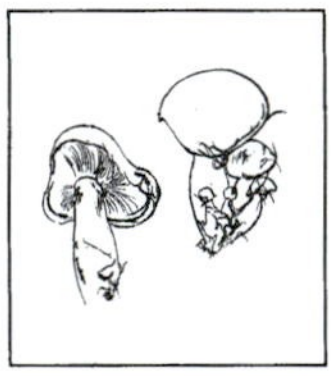

Psilocybin-containing mushrooms constitute the sixth diagnostic group. Toxicity in this group is substantial because of the popularity of hallucinogens. The psilocybin and psilocin indoles are similar to those of lysergic acid diethylamide (LSD) in rapidly (within 0.5–1 hour after ingestion) producing CNS effects, including ataxia, hyperkinesis, and hallucinations.[24] Serotonin, psilocin, and psilocybin are all structurally very similar molecules. Psilocybin's effects as an agonist and antagonist of serotonin is discussed in Chapter 10. Mortality is rare.

The IV use of an extract of *Psilocybe* mushrooms has been reported in which the patient's course was characterized initially by chills, rigors, dyspnea, headache, severe myalgias, vomiting, and extreme weakness. Hyperthermia, hypoxemia, and mild methemoglobinemia were also noted.[12]

Domestic cultivation of these so-called "magic mushrooms" has become a growing part of the drug culture. One popular drug culture magazine advertised mail-order kits of *Psilocybe cubensis* spores that could be grown at home. Psilocybin-containing mushrooms include *Psilocybe caerulescens, Conocybe cyanopus, Panaeolus foenisecii, Gymnopilus spectabilis,* and *Psathyrella foenisecii.*

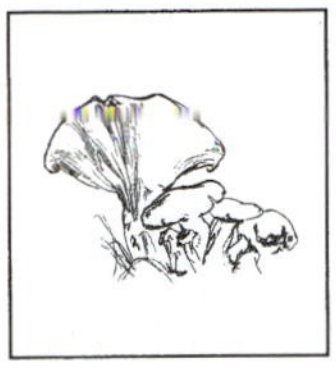

VII. Gastrointestinal Toxins

The seventh diagnostic classification, and by far the largest, is a diverse group of mushrooms containing a variety of ill-defined GI toxins. This group contains hundreds of mushrooms, many of which fall into the "little brown mushroom" group. Some *Boletes, Lactarius, Rhodophyllus, Tricholoma, Chlorophyllum molybdites,* and *C. esculentum* are mistaken for edible or hallucinogenic species. Gastrointestinal toxicity is seen 0.5–3 hours after ingestion. Severe epigastric distress, malaise, nausea, vomiting, and diarrhea are evident. Rare clinical presentations can be life-threatening, with hypovolemic shock necessitating fluids and vasopressors.[63] Resolution of symptoms usually occurs within 6–24 hours. The irritant chemicals have not been defined, and the clinical courses of the specific mushrooms are variable.[6] Death is rare.

VIII. Orelline- and Orellanine-containing Mushrooms

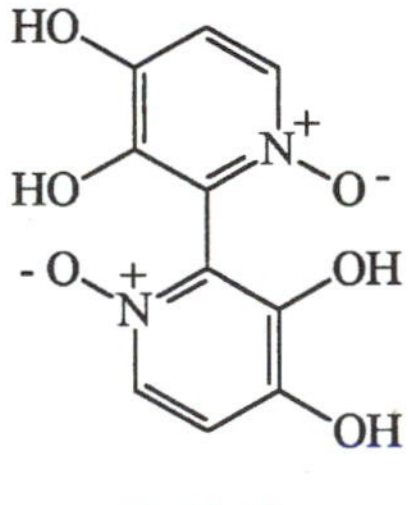

Orellanine

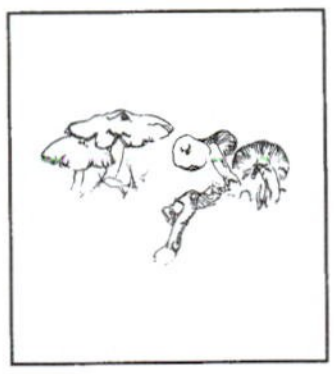

The eighth diagnostic group is associated with *Cortinarius* mushrooms. *Cortinarius speciosissimus* and *C. orellanus* result in interstitial nephritis and tubular damage with relative glomerular sparing.[10,60] The *C. orellanus* toxins orelline and orellanine are bipyridyl agents and are present also in the North American species *C. rainierensis.*[10,60]

The initial symptoms occur 24–36 hours after ingestion and include headache, chills, anorexia, nausea, and gastritis. Hepatotoxicity has been reported.[7] Several days to weeks after the initial symptoms, oliguric renal failure may develop. Hemoperfusion, hemodialysis, and renal transplantation have been employed.[7] The data are inadequate to define management or prognosis precisely, as most patients improve rapidly while some (4 of 26 in one series) demonstrate months of chronic renal failure.[7] There were no laboratory or clinical parameters to assist in predicting the individual reactions to the toxins.

The toxic compound orellanine was shown to be a hydroxylated and amine oxidized bipyridine compound. Orellanine can be detected long after clinical exposure only by performing thin-layer chromatography on renal biopsy material. Orellanine is rapidly concentrated in the urine in a soluble form, but has not been detected in urine, blood, or dialysate at the time of clinical symptoms.[55]

How Is the Appropriate Disposition Made?

It is important to remember that many mushroom ingestions present as mixed poisonings. Whereas some produce "purer" symptom complexes than others, many mushrooms (eg, *A. muscaria*) have muscarinic, atropinic, GI, and CNS effects. Treatment or partial treatment may further complicate the assessment.

Because the clinical course in mushroom poisoning can be deceptive, all patients who remain symptomatic despite supportive care with suspected poisoning from groups I–VIII (Tables 75–1, 75–2) should be admitted, as should patients who cannot be followed safely or reliably as outpatients. Figure 75–1 shows the characteristic times of appearance and evolution of symptoms. Confusion may result from atypical clinical manifestations or, commonly, the ingestion of several kinds of mushrooms, some of which may produce early symptoms and some late symptoms. Patients with certain types of ingestions may appear to improve initially with only supportive care. This latency, which is characteristic of *Amanita* spp., may not be appreciated when several species are eaten simultaneously. However, because hepatotoxicity leading to death may not appear until 3–6 days after ingestion (group I) and nephrotoxicity may not appear for 3–21 days (group VIII), all patients with symptoms require subsequent follow-up.

What Is Lycoperdonosis?

Lycoperdonosis is neither related to a toxic nor an hallucinogenic characteristic of a mushroom. This syndrome is manifested by the acute inhalation of spores as a folk medical therapy for epistaxis[64] or for adolescent pleasure.[65] In both reports patients have inhaled, insufflated, or chewed puff ball mushrooms (*Lycoperdon perlatum, L. pyriforme,* or *L. gemmatum*). These mushrooms, edible in the Fall, upon decay or drying can release large numbers of spores by compression or agitation. Massive inhalation of spores leads to rapid development of nasopharyngitis, nausea, vomiting, and pneumonitis within hours. Over a period of several days cough, shortness of breath, myalgias, fatigue, and fever develop.

Several patients have been intubated because of diffuse reticulonodular infiltrates. Lung biopsy demonstrated an inflammatory process with the presence of *Lycoperdon* spores.[64] Patients treated with prednisone and antifungal agents such as amphotericin B recovered within several weeks without sequelae.

TABLE 75–2. PHYSICAL CHARACTERISTICS OF COMMON TOXIC MUSHROOMS

Name	Color of Pileus	Spore Print Color	Spore Shape/Melzer Reaction	Gill Attachment	Veils	Habitat	Season
Amanita virosa	White	White	R/amyloid	F	U;P±	G	A
Amanita phalloides	Yellow-green to green-blue	White	R/amyloid	F	U;P±	G	A
Amanita muscaria	Red to red-orange to yellow-orange	White	E/—	F	U;P±	G	A/W
Galerina	Brown	Brown	Er/—	A	P±	G/W	
Gyromitra	Brown-rust		E/—			G under conifers	Sp
Coprinus	Gray-brown	Black	E/—	F/A	U±;P±	G/W/D	P
Clitocybe	White	White	E/—	A/D	—	G	P
Inocybe	Variable: white to gray-brown	Brown	E/—	A	P±	G	A
Psilocybe	Brown	Purple-brown	E/—	A/D	P±	G/W/D	A
Cortinarius orellanus	Orange-brown	Rust	Oval-r/—	A	U±;P	G under conifers	S/A
Paxillus involutus	Brown	Clay brown	E/—	D/S	—	G/W	S/A

E = ellipsoid, R = round, r = roughened, F = free, A = attached, D = decurrent, S = stipeless and shelflike, P = partial veil or veil remnants present, P± = partial veil or veil remnants present in some species, U = universal veil or veil remnants present, U± = universal veil or veil remnants present in some species, — = no veils, G = ground, W = wood, D = dung, A = autumn, Sp = spring, W = winter, S = summer, P = perennial.

Source: Lincoff GH: The Audubon Society Field Guide to North American Mushrooms. New York, Chanticleer Press, 1981.

Mushroom Poisoning Principles

1. Persons unfamiliar with wild mushrooms should never eat them unless absolute identification can be confirmed by an experienced mycologist. Even experts have trouble identifying some mushrooms, yet some foragers boldly imply that distinguishing edible from toxic mushrooms is "as easy as telling brussel sprouts from broccoli." Remember the saying, "There are old mushroom hunters, and bold mushroom hunters; but there are no old, bold mushroom hunters."
2. The toxicology of any species may vary, depending on the area of growth.
3. If poisoning is suspected, attempt to find the mushrooms eaten and identify them. Each ED should have a readily available resource such as one of the major guides in field mycology.[3,8,33,34,55,61] However, identification is best made with the aid of a consultant mycologist, if available.
4. Mushrooms are often blamed for an illness when infections or other diseases are responsible. The mode of preparation and the cooking utensils (the sauce, pot, or wine) may also be responsible for the illness.
5. There are no absolute generic approaches for evaluating a mushroom's potential toxicity. Myths regarding the safety or lack of it by the staining of silver, the presence of insects or slugs, peeling off the mushroom cap, or the area of growth are valueless. Neither odor nor taste is a good predictor of toxicity. A good general rule is that pure white mushrooms, little brown mushrooms (LBMs), large brown mushrooms, and red- or pink-pored boletes should be considered potentially toxic.
6. Cooking may inactivate some toxins but not others. In general, no wild mushroom should be eaten raw or in large quantities. Examples include *Armillariella mellea* (honey mushroom), which is usually well tolerated cooked but not raw, and *Verpa bohemica* (a morel-like mushroom), which is considered edible but causes illness if eaten in excess.
7. Associated phenomena may be responsible for or contribute to toxicity. Could insecticides have been sprayed on the mushrooms? Is it an alcohol-related response? Besides the well-known disulfiram reaction involving *C. atramentarius*, other good edibles, including the black morel (*Morchella angusticeps*) and the sulfur polypore (*Laetiporus sulfureus*), can cause adverse reactions if consumed with alcohol. The etiology of these adverse reactions is not understood.
8. Even "edible" mushrooms, if allowed to deteriorate, become toxic. Therefore, only young, recently matured specimens should be eaten.
9. The finding that only some people who ate a species of mushroom manifested characteristic toxicity should not exclude the diagnosis of mushroom poisoning. Toxicity may be dose-related or genetically determined, or a patient may have a pathologic condition predisposing him or her to toxicity.
10. Mushroom allergy can manifest as anaphylaxis.
11. Most poisonous mushrooms resemble edible mushrooms at some phase of their growth. Even careful examination of the ring, cap, consistency, form, and

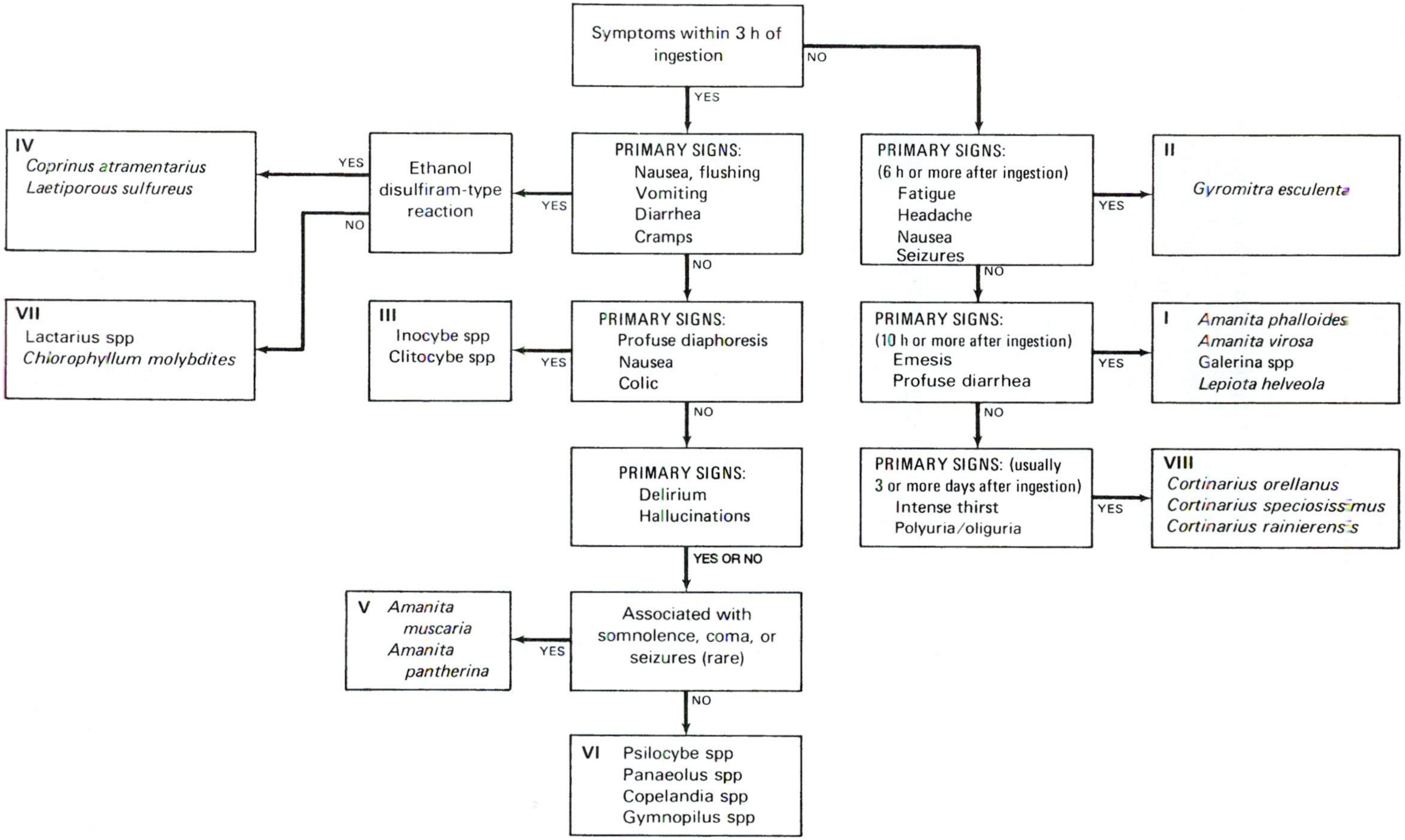

Figure 75–1. Clinical differentiation of mushroom poisoning. *(Modified from Lampe KF: Mushroom poisoning in children, updated. Pediatrician 1977;6:289–299.)*

color may not identify the edible species. Also, mushrooms with supposedly characteristic features may not have them under certain conditions. The deadly *A. phalloides* and *A. virosa* usually have remnant patches of tissue from the universal veil that envelops the mushroom in its "button" stage, but rain may wash them off. Similarly, the subterranean basal cup may not be noticed if the mushroom is cut at the ground level by a novice forager (Fig. 75–2).

Mycology for the Clinician: How to Identify a Toxic Mushroom

Although mushroom identification is a difficult science, this section may be helpful to the clinician faced with a suspected case of mushroom toxicity. However, it is generally best to rely on symptomatology, not mushroom appearances, to confirm a diagnosis. As a general rule, positive identification of the mushroom should be left to the mycologist or toxicologist.

The most important of the edible and poisonous mushrooms are grossly described by their pileus, stipe, lamellae or gills, and volva. The typical basic forms include:

- Pileus—the broad, caplike structure from which hang the gills (lamellae), tubes, or teeth.
- Stipe—the long stalk or stem supporting the cap; not present in some species.
- Lamellae—the platelike or gill-like structures on the undersurface of the pileus that radiate out like spokes of a wheel. The spores are found on the lamellae. Some mushrooms have pores or toothlike structures on their pilei, which contain the spores. The mode of attachment of the lamellae to the stipe is noteworthy in making an identification (Fig. 75–3).
- Volva—the partial remnant of the veil found around the base of the stipe in some species.
- Veil—a membrane that may completely or partially cover the lamellae, depending on the stage of development. The "universal" veil covers the underside, the spore-bearing surface of the pileus.
- Annulus—the ringlike structure that may surround the stipe at some point below the junction with the cap is a remnant of the partial veil.
- Spores—microscopic reproductive structures, resistant to extremes in temperature and dryness, that are produced in the millions on the spore-bearing surface (see lamellae, above). Spores represent the least variable characteristic, although many mushrooms have similar-appearing spores. A spore print is helpful in making an identification (Fig. 75–4). Colors of spores range from white to black, with shades of pink, salmon, buff, brown, and purple in between. The spore color is, in general, constant for a species.

Steps in Identifying the Unknown Mushroom

1. The most important distinction to make is whether the ingested mushroom could have been one of the deadly varieties, especially *Amanita*. Onset of GI symptoms within 3 hours of ingestion (when no other mushrooms were eaten within the previous 12 hours) is not the result of *Amanita* poisoning (see Fig. 75–1).
2. Attempt to obtain the mushrooms collected or a detailed description of their features. Transport the mushroom in a dry paper bag; do not moisten or refrigerate as this will alter its structure. Gastric contents may contain spores that can be crucial for analysis.
3. If the mushroom cap is available, make a spore print by placing the pileus spore-bearing surface side down on a piece of paper for at least 4–6 hours in a windless area. The spores that collect on the paper can then be

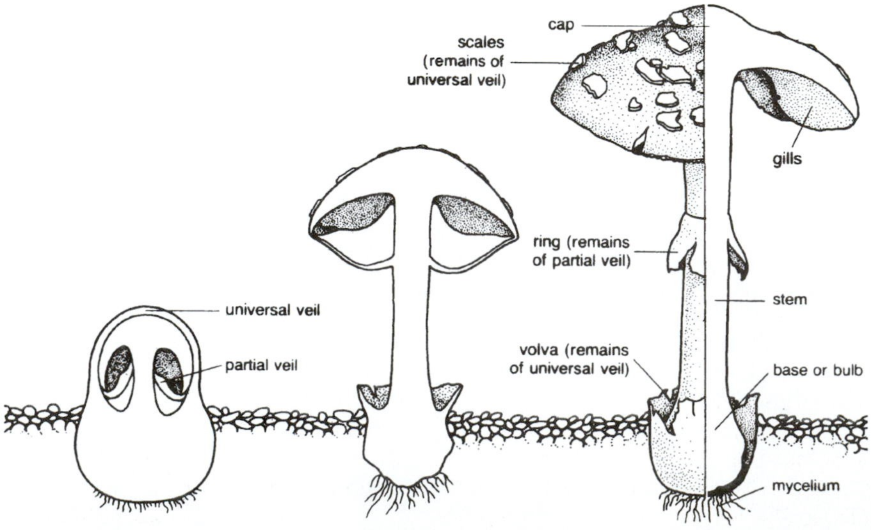

Figure 75–2. In the more highly specialized and evolved mushrooms, various protective tissues cover the fruit body and its constituent parts during its development. In the toadstool shown, an *Amanita* species, two veils of tissue are involved, one an outer enclosing bag, the universal veil, which ruptures as the fruit body expands to leave a volva at the base and fragments on the cap, the other an inner partial veil covering the developing gills, which is pulled away as the cap opens to leave a ring on the stem. *(Reprinted, with permission, from Kibby G: Mushrooms and Toadstools, A Field Guide. Oxford, Oxford University Press, 1979, p. 14.)*

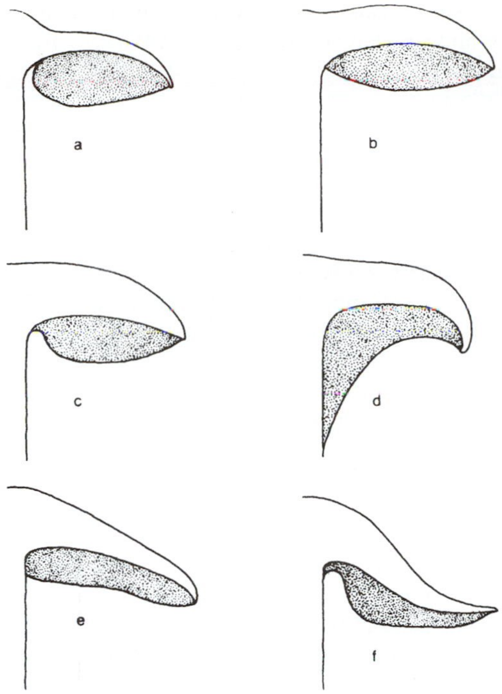

Figure 75–3. Gill attachment. The way the gill approaches and joins the stem is often specific for certain genera and most species. Any gills will be of one of the following types (or a combination of two types, such as sinuate-decurrent): **(a)** free; **(b)** adnexed (just reaching the stem); **(c)** sinuate (with sudden notch or upward curve by the stem; emarginate); **(d)** decurrent (running down the stem to a greater or lesser extent); **(e)** adnate (joined to the stem by the full depth of the gill, but not running down the stem); **(f)** sinuate, with a decurrent "tooth" running down the stem. *(Reprinted, with permission, from Kibby G: Mushrooms and Toadstools: A Field Guide. Oxford, Oxford University Press, 1979, p. 16.)*

analyzed for color. White spore prints can be more easily visualized on white paper by tilting the paper and looking at it from an angle. (For details of a slightly refined technique, see Fig. 75–4.)

4. Concomitant with step 3, contact and use the best resources available for identification. A botanical garden usually has staff members with expertise in mycology, or the local mycology club (there is at least one in every state) can locate a mycologist. The North American Mycological Association can be contacted for this information. A regional poison control center can usually provide all of the above information.
5. In the event that none of the resources in step 4 is accessible, a vial of Melzer's reagent (a solution of 20 mL of water, 1.5 g of potassium iodide, 0.5 g of iodine, and 20 g of chloral hydrate) may be useful. Staining a sample of the spores with 1 drop of reagent and then viewing it under a microscope will at least help to determine whether the mushroom is a deadly *Amanita*, with bluish black "amyloid" reacting round spores (Table 75–2).

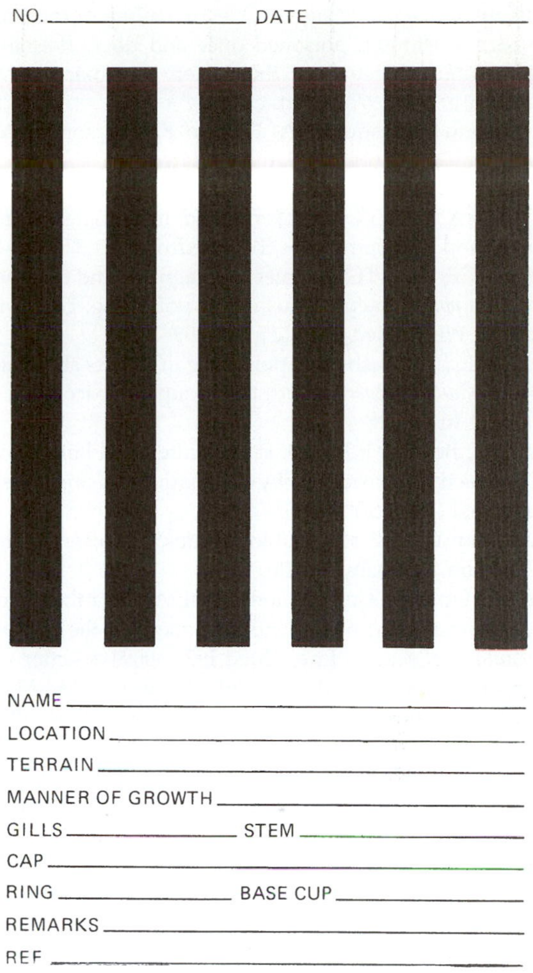

Figure 75–4. Spore print format. To make the print, cut off the stem (stipe) from the cap (pileus), as close to the cap underside as possible. Lay the cap, underside down, on the pattern. Cover with a bowl or can overnight. In the absence of air currents, the spores will drift down onto the paper rather than blowing away. After several hours usually a sufficient pileup of loose spores will be quite visible. The print may be "fixed" onto the paper with artist's fixative or hair spray. It is wise to enter any data on the print sheet before cutting off the stipe. *(The spore print format was invented by D.A. Wolfthal; it was first reported briefly in* The Mycophile, *published by The North American Mycological Association, and then completely presented in* The Journal of Wild Mushrooming. *Published with inventor's permission.)*

Acknowledgments

Alan G. Kulberg, MD, Kenneth E. Lampe, PhD (deceased), and Eddy A. Bresnitz, MD contributed to this chapter in a previous edition. Pamela Ryder, Nurse Practitioner, contributed the mushroom illustrations.

References

1. Alleva FR: Thioctic acid and mushroom poisoning. Science 1975;187:216. Letter.

2. Alleva FR, Balazs T, Sager AO, et al: Failure of thioctic acid to cure mushroom poisoned mice and dogs. Presented at 14th Annual Meeting of the Society of Toxicology, Williamsburg, VA, 1975. Abstract 155.
3. Ammirati JF, Traquair JA, Horgen PA: Poisonous Mushrooms of the Northern United States and Canada. Minneapolis, University of Minnesota Press, 1985.
4. Ayer WA, Browne LM: Terpenoid metabolites of mushrooms and basidiomycetes. Tetrahedron 1981;37:2199–2248.
5. Becker CE, Tong TG, Boerner U: Diagnosis and treatment of *Amanita phalloides*-type mushroom poisoning: Use of thioctic acid. West J Med 1976;125:100–109.
6. Benjamin DR: Mushroom poisoning in infants and children: The *Amanita pantherina/muscaria* group. J Toxicol Clin Toxicol 1992;30:13–22.
7. Boujet J, Bousser J, Pats B, et al: Acute renal failure following collective intoxication by *Cortinarius orellanus*. Intensive Care Med 1990;16:506–510.
8. Bresinsky A, Besl H: A Colour Atlas of Poisonous Fungi. Wurzburg, Germany, Wolfe, 1990.
9. Busi C, Fiume L, Costantino D, et al: *Amanita* toxins in gastroduodenal fluid of patients poisoned by the mushroom *Amanita phalloides*. N Engl J Med 1979;300:800. Letter.
10. Carder CA, Wojciechlowski NJ, Skoutakis VA: Management of mushroom poisoning. Clin Toxicol Consult 1983; 5:103–118.
11. Carlson A, Henning P, Lindberg P, et al: On the disulfiram-like effect of coprine, the pharmacologically active principle of *Coprinus atramentarius*. Acta Pharmacol Toxicol 1978;42: 292–297.
12. Curry SC, Rose MC: Intravenous mushroom poisoning. Ann Emerg Med 1985;14:900–902.
13. Fantozzi R, Ledda F, Caramelli L, et al: Clinical findings and follow-up evaluation of an outbreak of mushroom poisoning: Survey of *Amanita phalloides* poisoning. Klin Wochenschr 1986;64:38–43.
14. Faulstich H: New aspects of *Amanita* poisoning. Klin Wochenschr 1979;57:1143–1152.
15. Faulstich H: Structure of poisonous components of *Amanita phalloides*. Curr Probl Clin Biochem 1977;7:2–10.
16. Feinfeld DA, Mofenson HC, Caraccio T, Kee M: Poisoning by amatoxin containing mushrooms in suburban New York—Report of Four Cases. J Toxicol Clin Toxicol 1994; 32:715–721.
17. Floersheim GL: Treatment of human amatoxin mushroom poisoning: Myths and advances in therapy. Med Toxicol 1987;2:1–9.
18. Floersheim GL: Treatment of mushroom poisoning. JAMA 1984;252:3130–3132.
19. Floersheim GL: Antagonistic effects against single lethal doses of *Amanita phalloides*. Naunyn-Schmiedebergs Arch Pharmacol 1976;293:171–174.
20. Floersheim GL: Rifampicin and cysteamine protect against the mushroom toxin phalloidin. Experientia 1974;30: 1310–1311.
21. French AL, Garrettson LK: Poisoning with the North American jack o'lantern mushroom: *Omphalotus illudens*. J Toxicol Clin Toxicol 1988;26:81–88.
22. Galler GW, Weisenberg E, Brasitus TA: Mushroom poisoning: The role of orthotopic liver tranplantation. J Clin Gastroenterol 1992;15:229–232.
23. Hanrahan JP, Gordon MA: Mushroom poisoning: Case reports and a review of therapy. JAMA 1984;251:1057–1061.
24. Hatfield GM, Brady LR: Toxins of higher fungi. Lloydia 1975;38:36–55.
25. International Symposium on Thioctic Acid, Naples, 1955: Thioctic acid, physics, chemistry, and biology. Chem Abstr 1957;51:8153–8155.
26. Jaeger A, Jehl F, Flesch F, et al: Kinetics of amatoxins in human poisoning: Therapeutic implications. J Toxicol Clin Toxicol 1993;31:63–80.
27. Kelner MJ, Alexander NM: Endocrine hormone abnormalities in amanita poisoning. J Toxicol Clin Toxicol 1987;25: 21–37.
28. Klein AS, Hart J, Brems JJ, et al: *Amanita* poisoning: Treatment and the role of liver transplantation. Am J Med 1989;86:187–193.
29. Kostansek EC, Lipscomb WN, Yocum RR, et al: The crystal structure of the mushroom toxin β-amanitin. J Am Chem Soc 1977;99:1273–1274.
30. Kubicka J: Neue Moglichkeiten in der Behandlung von Vergiftung mit dem grunen Knollenblatterpilz—*Amanita phalloides*. Mykol Mitteil 1963;7:92–94.
31. Lampe KF: Toxic fungi. Annu Rev Pharmacol Toxicol 1979;19:85–104.
32. Lampe KF, McCann MA: Differential diagnosis of poisoning by North American mushrooms with particular emphasis on *Amanita phalloides*-like intoxication. Ann Emerg Med 1987;16:956–962.
33. Lincoff GH: The Audubon Society Field Guide to North American Mushrooms. New York, Knopf, 1981.
34. Lincoff G, Mitchel DH: Toxic and Hallucinogenic Mushroom Poisoning: A Handbook for Physicians and Mushroom Hunters. New York, Van Nostrand Reinhold, 1977.
35. Litovitz, TL, Bailey KM, Schmitz BF, et al: 1990 Annual Report of the American Association of Poison Control Centers National Data Collection System. Am J Emerg Med 1991; 9:461–508.
36. Litovitz TL, Clark LR, Soloway RA: 1993 Annual Report of the American Association of Poison Control Centers National Data Collection System. Am J Emerg Med 1994;12: 546–515.
37. Litovitz TL, Felberg MA, Soloway RA, et al: 1994 Annual Report of the American Association of Poison Control Centers National Data Collection System. Am J Emerg Med 1995;13:551–597.
38. Litovitz TL, Holm KC, Bailey KM, Schmitz RF: 1991 Annual Report of the American Association of Poison Control Centers National Data Collection System. Am J Emerg Med 1992;10:452–505.
39. Litovitz TL, Holm KC, Clancy C, et al: 1992 Annual Report of the American Association of Poison Control Centers National Data Collection System. Am J Emerg Med 1993;11: 494–555.
40. Litovitz TL, Martin TG, Schmitz B: 1986 Annual Report of the American Association of Poison Control Centers National Data Collection System. Am J Emerg Med 1987;5: 405–445.
41. Litovitz TL, Normann SA, Veltri JC: 1985 Annual Report of the American Association of Poison Control Centers National Data Collection System. Am J Emerg Med 1986;4: 427–458.

42. Litovitz TL, Schmitz BF, Bailey KM: 1989 Annual Report of the American Association of Poison Control Centers National Data Collection System. Am J Emerg Med 1990; 8:394–442.
43. Litovitz TL, Schmitz BF, Holm KC: 1988 Annual Report of the American Association of Poison Control Centers National Data Collection System. Am J Emerg Med 1989;7: 495–545.
44. Litovitz TL, Schmitz BF, Matyunas N, Martin TG: 1987 Annual Report of the American Association of Poison Control Centers National Data Collection System. Am J Emerg Med 1988;6:479–515.
45. Litovitz TL, Veltri JC: 1984 Annual Report of the American Association of Poison Control Centers National Data Collection System. Am J Emerg Med 1985;3:423–450.
46. Marchner H, Tottmar O: A comparative study on the effects of disulfiram, cyanamide, and 1-aminocyclopropanol on the acetaldehyde metabolism in rats. Acta Pharmacol Toxicol 1978;43:219–232.
47. Meunier BC, Camus CM, Houssin DP, et al: Liver transplantation after severe poisoning due to amatoxin containing *Lepiota*—report of three cases. J Toxicol Clin Toxicol 1995;33:165–171.
48. Moroni F, Fantozzi R, Masini E, Mannaioni PF: A trend in the therapy of *Amanita phalloides* poisoning. Arch Toxicol 1976;36:111–115.
49. Paaso B, Harrison DC: A new look at an old problem: Mushroom poisoning—Clinical presentations and new therapeutic approaches. Am J Med 1975;58:505–508.
50. Paydas S, Kocak R, Erturk F, et al: Poisoning due to amatoxin containing *Lepiota* species. Br J Clin Pract 1990;44: 450–453.
51. Pinson CW, Daya MR, Benner KG, et al: Liver transplantation for severe *Amanita phalloides* mushroom poisoning. Am J Surg 1990;159:493–499.
52. Piqueras J, Duran-Suarez JR, Massuet L, Hernandez-Sanchez JM: Mushroom poisoning: Therapeutic apheresis or forced diuresis. Transfusion 1987;27:116–117.
53. Pond SM, Olson KR, Woo OF, et al: Amatoxin poisoning in Northern California, 1982–1983. West J Med 1986;145: 204–209.
54. Ramirez P, Parrilla P, Sanchez-Bueno F, et al: Fulminant hepatic failure after *Lepiota* mushroom poisoning. J Hepatology 1993;19:51–54.
55. Rohrmoser M, Kirchmair M, Feifet E, et al: Orellanine poisonings: Rapid detection of the fungal toxin in renal biopsy material. J Toxicol Clin Toxicol 1997;35:63–66.
56. Rumack BH, Salzman E, eds: Mushroom Poisoning: Diagnosis and Treatment. Boca Raton, FL, CRC Press, 1978.
57. Schneider SM, Borochovitz D, Krenzelok EP: Cimetidine protection against alpha amanitin hepatotoxicity in mice: A potential model for the treatment of *Amanita phalloides* poisoning. Ann Emerg Med 1987;16: 1136–1140.
58. Schneider SM, Cochran KW, Knenzelok EP: Mushroom poisoning: Recognition and emergency management. Emerg Med Rep 1991;12:81–88.
59. Schneider SM, Vanscoy G, Michelson EA: Failure of cimetidine to affect phalloidin toxicity. Vet Hum Toxicol 1991;33: 17–18.
60. Schumacher T, Hoiland K: Mushroom poisoning caused by species of the genus *Cortinarius* fries. Arch Toxicol 1983; 53:87–106.
61. Smith AH: The Mushroom Hunter's Field Guide. Ann Arbor, University of Michigan Press, 1969. (Essential for anyone who wants to be sure out in the field; good descriptions and color photographs of common poisonous and edible species.)
62. Sperti S, Montanaro L, Fiume L, Mattioli A: Dissociation constants of the complexes between RNA polymerase II and amanitins. Experientia 1973;29:33–34.
63. Stenklyft PH, Augenstein WL: Chlorophyllum molybdites: Severe mushroom poisoning in a child. J Toxicol Clin Toxicol 1990;28:159–168.
64. Strand RD, Neuhauser EBD, Sornberger CF: Lycoperdonosis. N Engl J Med 1967;277:89–90.
65. Taft TA, Cardillo RC, Letzer D, et al: Respiratory illness associated with inhalation of mushroom spores. Wisconsin, 1994. MMWR 1994;43:525–526.
66. Teutsch C, Brennan RW: *Amanita* poisoning with recovery from coma: A case report. Ann Neurol 1978;3:177–179.
67. Tottmar O, Lindberg P: Effect on rat liver acetaldehyde dehydrogenases *in vitro* and *in vivo* by coprine, the disulfiram-like constituent of *Coprinus atramentarius*. Acta Pharmacol Toxicol 1977;40:476–481.
68. Trestrail JH III: Mushroom poisoning in the United States: An analysis of 1989 United States Poison Center Data. J Toxicol Clin Toxicol 1991;29:459–465.
69. Vander Hoek TL, Erickson T, Hryhorczuk D, et al: Jack o'lantern mushroom poisoning. Ann Emerg Med 1991;20: 559–561.
70. Vesconi S, Langer M, Iapichino G, et al: Therapy of cytotoxic mushroom intoxication. Crit Care Med 1985;13:402–406.
71. Veltri JC, Litovitz TL: 1983 Annual Report of the American Association of Poison Control Centers National Data Collection System. Am J Emerg Med 1984;2:420–443.
72. Vogel G: The anti-*Amanita* effect of silymarin. In: Faulstich H, Kommerell B, Wieland T, eds: Amanita Toxins and Poisoning: International Amanita Symposium, Heidelberg. Gerhard Witzstrock, Baden-Baden, 1980, pp. 180–189.
73. Wauters JP, Rossel C, Farquet JJ: *Amanita phalloides* poisoning treated by early charcoal hemoperfusion. Br Med J 1970;2:1465.
74. Wieland TH, Faulstich H: Amatoxins, phallotoxins, phallolysin, and antamanide: The biologically active components of poisonous *Amanita* mushrooms. CRC Crit Rev Biochem 1978;5:185–260.
75. Woodle ES, Moody RR, Cox KL, et al: Orthotopic liver transplantation in a patient with *Amanita* poisoning. JAMA 1985;253:69–70.

CHAPTER 76

Herbal Preparations

Oliver L. Hung, Neal A. Lewin, and Mary Ann Howland

A 21-year-old female, 5–6 weeks pregnant, presented to the emergency department (ED) complaining of 2 days of abdominal pain and bilious vomiting. She reported that she purchased several abortifacients from an herbalist including "slippery elm" powder to be brewed as a tea, "blue cohosh" tincture for ingestion, and "parsley" and "slippery elm" douches. For 4 days, she ingested approximately 15 cups/day of slippery elm tea and 10–20 doses/day of blue cohosh. She had also used the parsley and slippery elm douches the day before presentation. The patient denied any history of medical illness, allergies, or medications. She denied cigarette smoking.

On examination, the patient was flushed and diaphoretic. Vital signs were: blood pressure 149/62 mmHg; pulse 148 beats/min; respiratory rate 24 breaths/min; temperature 102.2°F (39°C) (rectal). Her heart sounds were normal and her lungs were clear to auscultation. She was noted to have fasciculations of her abdominal muscles. The pelvic examination was unremarkable. Neurologic examination revealed diffuse muscular weakness. Her pupils were equal, reactive, and normal size. Laboratory tests including serum electrolytes and complete blood count were normal. The EKG revealed a sinus tachycardia without conduction abnormalities. An urinalysis revealed large ketones. The patient was admitted to the hospital for intravenous hydration. An ultrasound revealed a viable intrauterine gestation. With appropriate social services follow-up, she was discharged home without complications the following day.

In this case, the patient's history and physical findings are consistent with acute nicotinic poisoning. The recent use of herbal preparations in a previously healthy woman suggest that the poisoning may be related to a toxic constituent of one or several of these preparations. Although the popularity of herbal preparations may in part be related to the belief that they are safe, one of the herbal products used by this patient is known to have toxic side effects. Blue cohosh (*Caulophyllum thalictroides*) is also known as squaw root and papoose root. The word "cohosh" is an Algonquin name. It is a traditional Native American herb found in the woods of eastern North America. Historically, blue cohosh was used by the American Indians to facilitate childbirth. It continues to be used today as a uterine stimulant, antispasmodic, antirheumatic, emmenagogue, and abortifacient.[11] The oxytocic activity of the plant is believed to be due to the glycosides caulosaponin and caulophyllosaponin, derivatives of the saponin hederagenin. The plant also contains the alkaloid methylcytisine, which has nicotinic effects. Methylcytisine has approximately one-fortieth the potency of nicotine. Nicotine-like poisoning was previously reported following use of this herbal preparation. Many other herbal preparations are popularly used as abortifacients, including aloe, bitter melon, black cohosh, canthardin, compound Q, ergots, feverfew, juniper, mugwort, nutmeg, pennyroyal oil, quinine, rue, sage, and white cohosh.

How Are Herbal Preparations Regulated?

There is very little federal regulation of the herbal industry. In 1994, Congress passed the Dietary Supplement and Health Education Act which reduced the Food and

Drug Administration's (FDA) oversight of products categorized as dietary supplements.[57] This includes vitamins, minerals, herbals, amino acids, and any product that had been sold as a "supplement" before October 15, 1994. As a result of this act, the FDA now has very little authority regulating herbal products.[45]

Herbal products can be marketed without any testing for efficacy or safety. The FDA must prove an herbal product is unsafe before it can be challenged. These products are manufactured without any federal standards of quality control. Although packaging claims to cure or prevent a specific disease are not permitted, claims detailing how a product affects the "body's structure or function" are acceptable. Substantiation of these claims is required, but this has not been defined. In reality, no proof is necessary unless the manufacturer is challenged by regulators. No FDA approval is required with regard to packaging or marketing.

Historical Background

Since ancient times and perhaps prehistoric times, peoples of all cultures have utilized herbal preparations to treat disease and to promote health.[40] A 60,000-year-old Iraqi burial site was found to contain eight different medicinal plants suggesting very early historical usage.[121] The earliest surviving written account of medicinal plants is the Egyptian Ebers papyrus c. 1500 B.C., which lists dozens of medicinal plants and uses. In India, the *Vedas,* epic poems written in about 1500 B.C., contain references to herbal preparations of the time. In China, the *Divine Husbandman's Classic* written in the 1st century A.D., lists 252 herbal preparations. In ancient Europe, herbal medicines were also the mainstay of healing. In the 1st century, the Greek physician Dioscorides wrote one of the first European herbal books, *De Materia Medica,* which listed 600 herbals and was translated into many languages. Shamans and folk healers from America, Africa, and Asia continue to include herbals for spiritual and medicinal purposes based on oral traditions passed from generation to generation.

During the Scientific Revolution, European scientists began to isolate purified extracts of plant products for medicinal agents. In 1806 and 1832, morphine and codeine were isolated from the sap of the poppy plant, *Papaver somniferum.*[106] In the current century, research in an attempt to develop nonaddictive opioid analgesics resulted in the development of synthetic agents such as fentanyl and methadone. In the mid-18th century, Edward Stone described the success of the bark of the willow tree in the cure of "agues" (fever) in a letter to the president of the Royal Society of Medicine.[71] In 1829, the active ingredient of the willow bark, salicin, was identified and in 1875 its derivative sodium salicylate was marketed as a treatment for rheumatic fever and as an antipyretic. The enormous success of this drug led to the synthesis of acetylsalicylic acid in 1899. The original brandname, aspirin (*a*cetyl *spiric* acid), is said to have been derived from *Spirea,* the plant genus from which salicylic acid was once prepared. Further chemical modifications to the salicylic acid molecule in the present century to improve its action and reduce side effects resulted in a diverse class of nonsteroidal antiinflammatory drugs (NSAIDs). In 1992, over 100 million prescriptions costing over $1 billion were written for NSAIDs in the United States alone.[12] Prescriptions from plant-derived medicines accounted for 25% of prescriptions dispensed in the United States between 1959 and 1980.[2]

Today, herbal preparations continue to be the dominant form of healing in the developing world because of the high cost of "Western" medical treatment and the scarcity of "Western" trained medical personnel.[47,78,81,90] The World Health Organization estimates that 4 billion people, 80% of the world population, use herbal preparations for some aspect of primary health care.[2] In the developed world, there appears to be a resurgence of herbal preparation usage.[54] Sales of herbal preparations in the United States in 1994 were estimated to be approximately $1.6 billion and are growing at an annual rate of 15% a year.[15,88]

Herbal preparation usage is widespread in our society (Tables 76–1 and 76–2). For most people, herbal preparations are easily obtained through health food stores, neighborhood pharmacies, complementary practitioners, and mail order companies. Although these preparations are not classified as medications by the FDA, they are often used to prevent or treat medical illness. Despite reports of toxicity associated with their usage, no systematic evaluation of herbal efficacy or safety is required. Since patients often do not consider herbal preparations as medications, they may not provide a history of usage unless directly questioned. In one recent study, 21.7% of respondents in an urban emergency department survey reported the use of herbal

TABLE 76–1. HERB PRODUCT USAGE BY TYPE—HEALTH FOOD MARKET

Delivery Forms	Herb Supplement Types
Capsules 53%	Single herbs 52.5%
Tablets 15%	Herb combinations 34.8%
Teas 11.4%	Herbs combined with nonherbal ingredients 11.5%
Tinctures 7.3%	Other 1.2%
Extracts 7.4%	
Bulk herbs 5.3%	
Other 0.6%	

Reprinted, with permission, from HerbalGram 1996;36:52.

TABLE 76–2. TOP TEN HERB SALES IN SELECTED HEALTH FOOD STORES

Echinacea	9.9%	Aloe	4.3%
Garlic	9.8%	Ma huang and other ephedra products	3.5%
Goldenseal	7.0%	Siberian ginseng	3.1%
Ginseng	5.9%	Cranberry	3.0%
Ginkgo biloba	4.5%		
Saw palmetto	4.4%		

Reprinted, with permission, from HerbalGram 1996;36:54.

preparations.[68] For 15.6% of these users, the herbal preparation was being used to treat aspects of the patient's presenting chief complaint. Thirty-seven percent of herbal users reported that their physicians were unaware of their herbal preparation usage.[68] Although a national survey determined that only 3% of respondents indicated that they had used herbal preparations in the past year, herbal preparation use appears to vary greatly depending on the community surveyed.[53] Surveys of rural areas of Mississippi and southwestern West Virginia reported that 71% and 73% of respondents used herbal remedies in the past week and past year, respectively.[31,44] Among Chinese-Americans in New York City and Hispanic-Americans in west Texas, herbal preparation use was also reported to be very high, 43% and 50%, respectively.[87,100] Herbal preparations use also appears to be higher among populations with chronic illness such as AIDS, rheumatoid arthritis, and cancer.[74,75,89,130] In the United States, increased herbal preparation usage is associated with multiple factors, including concurrent illness and diverse socioeconomic and cultural influences.

Definition of Herbal Preparation

The botanical definition of the term *herb* is specific for certain leafy plants without woody stems. However, herbal preparations often include nonherb plant materials, even animal and mineral products. The definition of herbal preparation is unclear. Broadly, it includes any "natural" or "traditional" remedy, but these terms are poorly defined. Often, these products are called medications. However, the use of the term *medication* may be inaccurate. Many herbal preparations are used for their nonspecific adaptogenic properties and lack any disease-specific effects. Herbal preparations such as herbal stimulants and sedatives may contain active ingredients, but their intended use is without specific medicinal value. Since many herbal users and herbalists do not consider herbal preparations as medications, the use of the term "herbal medicine" by the clinician may convey a different and perhaps unintended meaning. For these reasons, it may be inappropriate and unhelpful to refer to these products as medications.

The study of herbal preparations is complicated by a lack of standardized nomenclature. As discussed earlier, these preparations are often derived from many ingredients, including plants, animals, and minerals. For some herbal products, these ingredients are still unknown. Although most herbal preparations are derived from a single plant source, the diversity of common and botanical names may increase confusion. A single plant preparation may have many common names in addition to a botanical name. For example, *Datura stramonium* is also known as Jimson Weed, datura, stramonium, apple of Peru, Jamestown weed, thornapple, and tolguacha. Likewise, a common name for a plant such as gordolobo may refer to several botanical plants such as *Verbascum thapsus* and *Gnaphalium macounii*.[69] An accurate classification of herbal preparations is very difficult, thus limiting effective study.

Background of Herbal Toxicology

There is a growing awareness of the widespread use of herbal preparations in the United States. Frequently, it is only after the patient demonstrates toxicity that the physician seeks information about the use of these products. Some well-publicized examples of toxicity from herbal preparation usage include six cases of anticholinergic poisoning in New York City in 1994, from contaminated Paraguay tea;[21,67] three cases of life-threatening bradycardia in Colorado in 1993, following consumption of *Jin Bu Huan* tablets;[26] and four cases of agranulocytosis with 1 death following consumption of *Chui Fong Tou Ku Wan* in San Francisco in 1975.[109] Although few studies have examined this issue, most herbal preparations used in developed countries appear to be safe. In Hong Kong in 1990, Chinese herbal medicines and proprietary medicines accounted for only 0.2% of all acute medical admissions despite their widespread use in the colony (40–60% of population). Meanwhile, Western medications were responsible for 4.4% of acute medical admissions.[35,36] From 1983 to 1989, the National Poisons Unit, London, received 1070 inquiries following exposures to herbal extracts, of which 270 (25.2%) cases were symptomatic. They were able to demonstrate probable association between exposure and effect in only 32 of the 270 cases.[101] However, in developing countries, the toxicity from herbal preparation usage may be much higher. In South Africa, traditional medicines and herbal preparations account for 15.8% of acute poisonings and were responsible for 51.7% of all deaths from acute poisonings.[72] In the United States, there is little information concerning herbal toxicity, with no major U.S. toxicologic databases recording epidemiologic data on herbal preparation use and toxicity.

Herbal Pharmacologic Principles

The pharmacologic activity of herbal (plant-containing) preparations can be classified by five active constituent classes: volatile oils, resins, alkaloids, glycosides, and fixed oils.[122]

Volatile oils are odorous plant ingredients. They are also called ethereal or essential oils, because they evaporate at room temperatures. Most are mucous membrane irritants with some central nervous system activity. Examples of herbs containing volatile oils include catnip *(Nepata cataria)*, chamomile *(Chamamilla recutita)*, and garlic *(Allium sativum)*.

Resins are complex chemical mixtures of acrid resins, resin alcohols, resinol, tannols, esters, and resenes. These substances are often strong gastrointestinal irritants. Examples of resin-containing herbs include dandelion *(Taraxacum officinale)*, elder *(Sambucus* spp.), and black cohosh root *(Cimicifuga racemosa)*.

Alkaloids are a heterogeneous group of alkaline, organic, and nitrogenous compounds (see Fig. 76–1). The alkaloid compound is usually found throughout the plant. Alkaloids are often the most pharmacologically active and

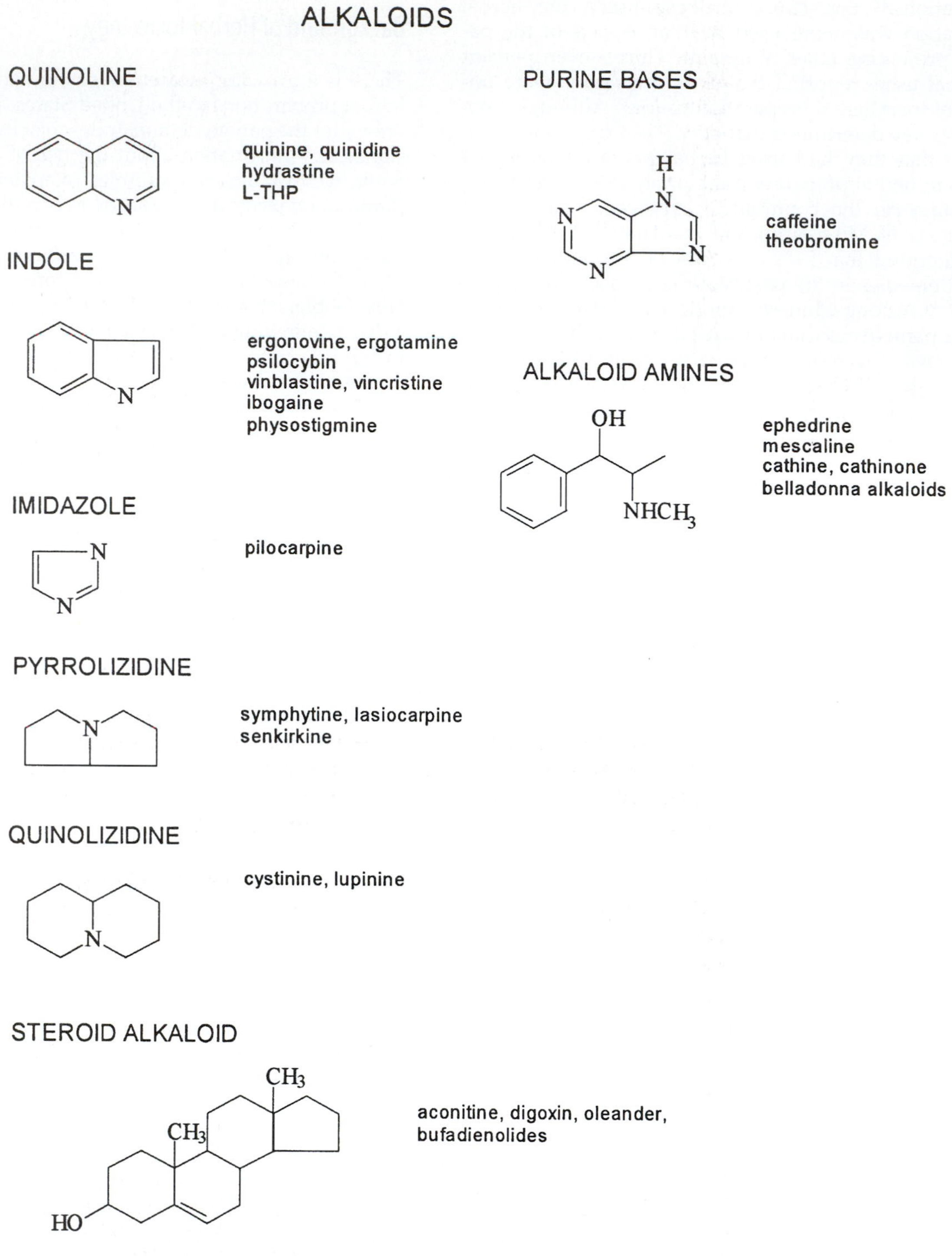

Figure 76–1. The heterogenous structures of plant alkaloids.

most toxic compounds. Their pharmacologic actions may be CNS depression or stimulation. The pyrrolizidine alkaloids, present in thread-leafed groundsel *(Senecio longilobus)* and comfrey *(Symphytum officinale)*, have been found to cause hepatic veno-occlusive disease.[125] Other examples of alkaloid-containing herbs include Goldenseal *(Hydrastis canadensis)* and Jimson weed *(Datura stramonium)*.

Glycosides are sugar esters containing a sugar component (glycol) and a nonsugar (aglycone), which yields one or more sugars during hydrolysis. These include the anthroquinones, saponins, cyanophores, and lactone glycosides. The anthroquinones [senna *(Cassia acultifolia)* and aloe *(Aloe vera)*] are irritating cathartics. Saponins [licorice *(Glycyrrhiza lepidata)* and ginseng *(Panax ginseng* and *quinquefolium)*] are mucous membrane irritants, may destroy red blood cells, and have steroid activity. Cyanophores found in apricot, cherry, and peach pits release cyanide. Lactone glycosides [tonka beans *(Dipteryx odorata)*] have anticoagulant activities.

Fixed oils are esters of long-chain fatty acids and alcohols. Herbs containing fixed oils are generally used as emollients, demulcents, and bases for other agents. Generally, these are the least active and least dangerous of all herbal preparations. Examples include olive *(Olea europaea)*, and peanut *(Arachis hypogaea)* oil.

Factors Contributing to Herbal Toxicity

The toxicity of a plant may vary widely depending on certain conditions.[69] The time of year or developmental stage at which the plant is collected may affect its toxicity. For example, the pyrrolizidine alkaloid content of *Senecio* leaves vary widely from month to month and year to year. In some cases, only selective parts of a plant used to prepare an herbal preparation may be responsible for its toxicity. For example, the pyrrolizidine content of comfrey-pepsin capsules has been found to vary from 270 mg/kg to 2900 mg/kg depending on whether the leaves or roots were used in the preparation.[68] The area in which the plant is collected may affect its toxicity. *Senecio longilobus* from Gardner Canyon, Arizona, may contain up to 18% pyrrolizidine alkaloids by dry weight, the highest level recorded for any *Senecio* plant species (normal concentration = 0.5%). Finally, conditions of storage and length of storage may affect its toxicity. The toxicity of *Crotalaria* decreases with storage because of the breakdown of pyrrolizidines.

Probably, few alleged poisonings are the result of the inherent toxicity of the herbal. Most are the result of misuse, misidentification, misrepresentation, or contamination of the product. Heavy metal poisonings from lead, cadmium, mercury, copper, zinc, and arsenic are associated with herbal preparation usage.[28,32,36,46,49,52,99,101,106] High levels of these elements may be the result of contamination during the manufacturing process of some herbal or patent medications. In some cases such as cinnabar (mercuric sulfide) and calomel (mercurous chloride), these ingredients are intentionally included for purported medicinal benefit.[73] Patent medications may also contain Western drugs such as acetaminophen, aspirin, antihistamines, or corticosteroids.[37,49] Many of these Western medicines are unlisted on the packaging and may not even be approved for use in the United States. An example of toxicity of an herbal preparation containing Western medication is the four cases of agranulocytosis that were reported following consumption of *Chui Fong Tou Ku Wan*.[109] This preparation contained aminopyrine (which is not approved for OTC sales in the United States) and phenylbutazone, but did not list these ingredients on the packaging. Both aminopyrine and phenylbutazone are known to cause agranulocytosis.

Classification of Toxicity

Herbal preparations are associated with a wide variety of toxicologic manifestations. In addition, many individual herbal preparations are associated with multiple types of toxicologic effects. To better understand these effects, it may be useful to organize herbal toxicity into several general categories.[48]

Indirect Health Risks

Herbal usage may result in toxicity by altering previous conventional medication therapy. A patient may discontinue or become less compliant with previous therapy with untoward consequences. Alternatively, the addition of an herbal preparation may affect the pharmacologic effect (eg, bioavailability or clearance) of concurrent conventional therapy with resulting increase risk of toxicity.

Direct Health Risks

Direct health risks include pharmacologically predictable and dose-dependent toxic reactions, idiosyncratic toxic reactions, long-term toxic effects, and delayed toxic effects. An example of a pharmacologically predictable toxic reaction is that due to aconite. Ingestion of aconite tea in the appropriate dosage predictably results in tachydysrhythmias and hypotension in all patients. Idiosyncratic toxic reactions cannot be predicted on the basis of principal pharmacologic properties. For example, ingestion of chamomile tea results in anaphylactic reactions in a subset of patients. Long-term toxic effects result only after chronic usage. For example, long-term use of herbal anthranoid laxatives results in muscular weakness from hypokalemia. Delayed toxic effects include carcinogenicity and teratogenicity. For example, sassafras root contains safrole, which is a hepatocarcinogen in laboratory animals.

Toxicity of Specific Herbal Preparations

Cardiovascular Toxins

Aconite. Aconites (caowu and chuanwu) are the dried rootstocks of the *Aconitum* plant.[124] In China, aconite is usually derived from *A. carmichaeli* (chuanwu) or *A. kuznezoffii* (caowu). In Europe and the United States, aconite is derived from *A. napellus*, commonly known as monkshood or wolfsbane. The tubers are the most toxic part of the plant, and when ingested both cardiac and neurologic symptoms occur. Aconite poisoning is far more common in Asia, especially China and Hong Kong.[39] In Hong Kong, it is responsible for the majority of serious poisonings from Chinese herbal preparations.[37,39]

Aconite toxicity is due to C19 diterpinoid-ester alkaloids, including aconitine, mesaconitine, and hypaconitine.[18] The mechanism involves increased sodium influx through the sodium channel, delaying the final repolarization phase of the action potential and initiating premature excitation.[66] Symptoms can occur from 5 minutes to 4 hours after ingestion. Paresthesias of the oral mucosa and entire body may be followed by nausea, vomiting, diarrhea, and hypersalivation and then progressive skeletal muscle weakness. Sinus bradycardia and ventricular tachycardia and fibrillation can occur.[38] Fatalities may occur with doses as low as 5 mL of aconite tincture, 2 mg of pure aconite, or 1 g of plant. There is no antidote available. Atropine may be of value in treating bradycardia or hypersalivation.[124] Anecdotal reports have suggested the use of amiodarone, flecainide, bretylium, and procainamide for tachydysrhythmias.[124] Pharmacologic principles would suggest the use of a sodium channel blocker such as procainamide or flecainide. One case of aconite-induced refractory tachydysrhythmia was successfully managed with a ventricular assist device.[56]

Ch'an Su. Ch'an Su is a traditional herbal remedy derived from the secretions of the parotid and sebaceous glands of a toad, *Bufo bufo gargarizans* or *Bufo melanosticus*. It is used as a topical anesthetic and cardiac medication.[76] In New York City, it is also marketed as an aphrodisiac and is sold under names such as "Stone," "Love Stone," "Black Stone," and "Rock Hard." Ch'an Su contains two groups of toxic compounds: cardioactive steroids consisting of bufadienolides, and bufotenine, a hallucinogenic compound. Symptoms of toxicity are similar to digoxin toxicity including nausea, vomiting, abdominal pain, cramping, and dysrhythmias. Between 1993 and 1996 in New York City, several fatalities were associated with the ingestion of Ch'an Su marketed as a topical aphrodisiac.[23] Severe toxic reactions or death are also reported after mouthing toads, "toad licking," and following ingestion of an entire toad, toad soup, or toad eggs.[16] Assays for serum digoxin may cross-react with bufadienolides and aid in establishing the diagnosis. Digoxin-specific Fab (10 vials Digibind®) has been used to successfully treat Ch'an Su toxicity and should be empirically administered for any suspected case of Ch'an Su cardiotoxicity.[16] Other indications for antidotes are listed in Table 76–3.

Oleander. Oleander (*Nerium oleander*) is also known as adelfa, laurier rose, rosa laurel, rose bay, and rosa francesca. Oleander, commonly used as an ornamental plant, has also been traditionally used in the treatment of cardiac illnesses, asthma, cancer, corns, and epilepsy. All parts of the plant contain the cardiac glycosides, oleandrin, and neriin, as well as the cardenolides gentiobiosyloeandrin and olorside A. Deaths are reported in children who have ingested a handful of flowers and in an adult who mistakenly drank herbal tea prepared from oleander.[5,64] Symptoms of toxicity are similar to digoxin toxicity including nausea, vomiting, abdominal pain, cramping, and dysrhythmias. Assays for serum digoxin may cross-react with oleander cardiac glycosides and help with the diagnosis. Since digoxin-specific Fab has been used to successfully treat human oleander toxicity,

TABLE 76–3. LABORATORY ANALYSIS AND TREATMENT GUIDELINES FOR SPECIFIC HERBAL PREPARATIONS

Herbal Preparation	Laboratory Analysis	Antidote
Cardiac Toxins		
Ch'an Su	Serum digoxin level	Digoxin Fab
Foxglove	Serum digoxin level	Digoxin Fab
Oleander	Serum digoxin level	Digoxin Fab
Squill	Serum digoxin level	Digoxin Fab
Central Nervous System Toxins		
Henbane	None required	Physostigmine
Jimson weed	None required	Physostigmine
Mandrake	None required	Physostigmine
Gastrointestinal Toxins		
Aloe	Serum potassium	KCl
Buckthorn	Serum potassium	KCl
Cascara	Serum potassium	KCl
Fo-Ti	Serum potassium	KCl
Senna	Serum potassium	KCl
Heavy Metals	Ag, As, Au, Cd, Cr, Cu, Hg, Pb, Th, or Zn as indicated; radiography	Heavy metal chelator
Hematologic Toxins		
Dong Quai	Serum prothrombin time	Vitamin K_1
Tonka bean	Serum prothrombin time	Vitamin K_1
Woodruff	Serum prothrombin time	Vitamin K_1
Hepatotoxins		
Pennyroyal oil	AST/ALT	*N*-acetylcysteine
Pyrrolizidine alkaloids	AST/ALT	N/A
Salicylates		
Medicated oils, etc	Serum salicylate level	Sodium bicarbonate, multiple-dose activated charcoal, hemodialysis
Cellular Toxins		
Apricot pits (cyanide)	Lactate	Cyanide antidote kit
Autumn crocus (colchicine)	None required	Consider glutamic acid
Elder (cyanide)	Lactate	Cyanide antidote kit
Periwinkle (vinca alkaloids)	None required	Consider glutamic acid
Podophyllum (podophyllin)	None required	Consider glutamic acid
Miscellaneous		
Licorice	Serum potassium	KCl
Quinine	None required	Consider diazepam/epinephrine / sodium bicarbonate

it should be empirically administered for known or suspected oleander cardiotoxicity.[111,116] Other herbal sources of cardiac glycosides include squill (*Urginea maritima*), lily-of-the-valley (*Convallaria majalis*), and yellow oleander (*Thevetia peruviana*).

Central Nervous System Toxins

Absinthe. Wormwood (*Artemisia absinthium*) extract was the main ingredient in absinthe, a toxic liquor, now outlawed in the United States, that caused absinthism: pyschosis, hallucinations, and intellectual deterioration. The volatile oil is a mixture of alpha- and beta-thujone.[133] A thujone-free wormwood extract is now used in flavoring vermouth. One of the most famous cases of absinthism may have involved Van Gogh, who is thought to have suffered from it in the later part of his life. He is suggested to have had pica, eating paint and drinking turpentine and camphor for its terpene content when he craved absinthe.[6] The CNS effects of thujone are comparable to those of camphor. Both tetrahydrocannabinol and thujone have an affinity for a common CNS receptor binding site and for similar oxidative metabolic pathways.[133] Treatment remains supportive. Other psychoactive herbal preparations are listed in Table 76–4.

Anticholinergic Agents: Henbane, Jimson Weed, Mandrake. Many plants contain the belladonna alkaloids: atropine (*d,l*-hyoscyamine), and scopolamine (*l*-hyoscine). They are often used as asthma remedies or as hallucinogens. Occasionally, these plants are misidentified and are ingested

TABLE 76–4. PSYCHOACTIVE SUBSTANCES USED IN HERBAL PREPARATIONS

Labeled Ingredient	Scientific Name	Suggested Use	Active Ingredients	Reported Effects
Broom	*Cytisus* spp.	Smoked for relaxation	Cytisine	Sedative-hypnotic
California poppy	*Eschscholtzia californica*	Smoked as marijuana substitute	Alkaloids and glycosides	Euphoriant
Catnip	*Nepeta cataria*	Smoke or tea as marijuana substitute	Nepetalactone	Reputed euphoriant
Ch'an su	*Bufo bufo gargarizans* *Bufo bufo melanosticus*	Smoked or licked for hallucinations	Bufotenin	Hallucinogen
Cinnamon	*Cinnamomum camphora*	Smoked with marijuana	?	Stimulant
Cloves	*Syzgium aromaticum*	Smoked in cigarette/ "kreteks"	Eugenol	Stimulant
Damiana	*Tumera diffusa*	Smoke as marijuana substitute	?	Reputed stimulant/hallucinogen
Goldenseal	*Hydrastis canadensis*	Ingested to mask detection of opioid, marijuana, or cocaine in urine drug screen	—	No evidence supporting purported use
Hops	*Humulus lupulus*	Smoke or tea as sedative and marijuana substitute	Humulone, lupulone → methylbutenol	Purported sedative, but concentrations probably too low to produce effect
Hydrangea	*Hydrangea paniculata*	Smoke as marijuana substitute	Hydrangin, saponin, cyanogens	Stimulant
Ibogaine	*Tabernanthe iboga*	Stimulant, hallucinogen	Ibogaine	Hallucinogen
Juniper	*Juniper macropoda*	Smoke as hallucinogen	?	Hallucinogen
Kavakava	*Piper methysticum*	Smoke or tea as marijuana substitute	Kava lactones	Hallucinogen
Kola nut	*Cola* spp.	Smoke, tea, or capsules as stimulant	Caffeine, theobromine, kolanin	Stimulant
Lobelia	*Lobelia inflata*	Smoke or tea as marijuana substitute	Lobeline	Euphoriant
Mandrake	*Mandragora officinarum*	Tea as hallucinogen	Scopolamine, hyoscamine	Hallucinogen
Mate	*Ilex parguayensis*	Tea as stimulant	Caffeine	Stimulant
Mormon tea	*Ephedra nevadensis*	Tea as stimulant	Ephedrine	Stimulant
Morning glory	*Ipomoea violacea*	Seeds has hallucinogens	*d*-Lysergic acid diethylamide (ergine)	Hallucinogen
Nutmeg	*Myristica fragrans*	Tea as hallucinogen	Myristicin	Hallucinogen
Passion flower	*Passiflora incarnata*	Smoke, tea, or capsules as marijuana substitute	Harmala alkaloids	Mild stimulant
Periwinkle	*Catharanthus roseus*	Smoke or tea as euphoriant	Indole alkaloids	Hallucinogen
Prickly poppy	*Argemone mexicana*	Smoke as euphoriant	Protopine, bergerine, isoquinoline	Analgesic
Snakeroot	*Rauwolfia serpentina*	Smoke or tea as tobacco substitute	Reserpine	Tranquilizer
Thorn apple	*Datura stramonium*	Atropine, scopolamine	Smoke or tea as tobacco substitute or hallucinogen	Strong hallucinogen
Tobacco	*Nicotiana* spp.	Nicotine	Smoke as tobacco	Strong stimulant
Valerian	*Valeriana officinalis*	Chatinine, velerine alkaloids	Tea or capsules as tranquilizer	Tranquilizer
Wild lettuce	*Lactuca sativa*	Smoke as opium substitute	Unknown	Reputed mild analgesic
Wormwood	*Artemisia absinthium*	Smoke or tea as relaxant	Thujone	Analgesic
Yohimbe	*Pausinystalia yohimbe*	Smoke or tea as stimulant	Yohimbine	Mild hallucinogen

Adapted, with permission, from Siegel RK: Herbal intoxication. JAMA 1976;236:473–476.

in the form of herbal teas.[33] Examples of plants with anticholinergic properties include henbane (hyoscyamine, hyoscine), Jimson weed (atropine, hyoscyamine, stramonium), and mandrake (scopolamine, hyoscyamine). Signs and symptoms of anticholinergic poisoning include mydriasis, diminished bowel sounds, urinary retention, dry mouth, flushed skin, tachycardia, and agitation. Mild cases usually respond to supportive care and central nervous system sedation with intravenous benzodiazepines. Although intravenous physostigmine reverses anticholinergic poisoning, its use should be limited for selected severely affected patients because of the risk of seizures and dysrhythmias (see Chap. 34).

Ephedra. Members of the genus *Ephedra* are generally erect evergreen plants resembling small shrubs. Common names include sea grape, ma-huang, yellow horse, desert tea, squaw tea, and Mormon tea. These plants have a long history of use as stimulants and for the management of bronchial disorders. They contain the alkaloids, ephedrine, and in some species, pseudoephedrine.[127] In large doses, ephedrine causes nervousness, headache, insomnia, dizziness, palpitations, skin flushing, tingling, vomiting, anxiety, restlessness, mania, and psychosis. Case reports of seizure, cerebrovascular accident, myocardial infarct, and death are described following the ingestion of pills known as "herbal ecstacy," which contain ephedra and were used as stimulants.[20] Supportive care is usually sufficient treatment for ephedra toxicity.

Khat. One of the most common forms of drug abuse in East Africa involves chewing the leaves and stems of the khat plant (*Catha edulis*) and swallowing the juice.[53,85] Khat is used by herbalists to treat depression, fatigue, obesity, and gastric ulcers. The two active compounds in khat are cathine (norpseudoephedrine) and cathinone (alpha-aminopropiophenone), the more active stimulant. More than 30 other minor compounds are also found in khat. Red khat contains more cathinone than white khat and is a more potent stimulant. This herb produces euphoria, dysphoria, stimulation, and sedation. The two major components have a direct action on neuromuscular junctions and also interact with dopaminergic pathways. It is suggested that these amphetamine-like compounds have a stimulatory effect between that of caffeine and amphetamine. True psychotic reactions are rare and physical dependence has not been reported, but psychologic dependency is common in chronic abusers. Chronic abuse is implicated in causing hypertension in young adults, which is reversible with cessation of khat. Stomatitis, constipation, esophagitis, and gastritis result from ingestion of khat tannins. Norpseudoephedrine is found in the urine and breast milk of women who use khat. Severe reactions to khat use include myocardial infarction, cerebral hemorrhage, and pulmonary edema. Cirrhosis, decreased libido, anorexia, and impotence are also reported. Oral carcinomas are described in khat chewers in Saudi Arabia. Because of increased availability in the United States, the use of this herb has become more prevalent.

Nicotinic Agents: Betel Nut, Blue Cohosh, Broom, Chestnut, Lobelia, Tobacco. Betel (*Areca catechu*) is chewed by an estimated 200 million people worldwide for its euphoric effect. The active ingredient is arecholine, a nicotinic agent and volatile alkaloid, which produces increased central acetylcholine. The betel leaf contains a phenolic volatile oil and an alkaloid capable of producing cocaine-like reactions. Arecholine is a bronchoconstrictor, although it is weaker than methacholine, and may cause exacerbation of bronchospasm in asthmatic patients chewing betel nut.[126] Treatment for betel nut toxicity is supportive. Long-term use of betel nut is associated with leukoplakia and squamous cell carcinoma of the oral mucosa.

Many other herbal preparations have nicotinic effects. Examples of plants and their nicotinic ingredient include: blue cohosh, methylcytisine; broom, *l*-sparteine; chestnut, esculin; lobelia, lobeline; and tobacco, nicotine.

Nutmeg and Mace. Nutmeg and mace are products of the evergreen tree *Myristica fragrans*, indigenous to the Spice Islands and cultivated in the Caribbean. The fruits of *M. fragrans* resemble apricots or peaches. When ripe, the husk splits open and a single glossy brown nut (nutmeg) is revealed, enclosed by a scarlet net like aril, which when dried is called mace.

Nutmeg has been used by herbalists to treat dyspepsia, musculoskeletal and arthritic disorders, psychiatric conditions, and narcosis and as an emmenagogue and abortifacient. Many recent nutmeg ingestions are among prisoners, college students, and adolescents attempting to achieve euphoria, although intoxications have occurred with the accidental misuse of the herbal preparation. The essential oil is thought to be the active component, containing allylbenzene derivatives and terpenes. The nutmeg contains 5–15% of this volatile oil, depending on the geographic region. Myristicin, one of the components of the oil, was initially considered the active compound; it has weak monoamine oxidase inhibitor properties that are responsible for some of the cardiovascular symptoms.[1,96,118] However, myristicin alone does not account for the total effects of nutmeg. It may be metabolized in vivo to the psychotomimetic amphetamine-like compound 3-methoxy-4,5-methylenedioxyamphetamine (MMDA), and elemicin, another ingredient in the oil, is converted to 3,4,5-trimethoxyamphetamine (TMA).[96,120] Eugenol, isoeugenol, borneol, safrole, and linalol are also active components.

Symptoms of nutmeg poisoning (including nausea, vomiting, and CNS effects) occur within several hours of ingesting 5–15 g of nutmeg. Within 24 hours, after an acute delirium and subsequent deep sleep, the patient usually recovers uneventfully. With exceedingly large doses, symptoms may persist for days. Hypothermia may be a consequence of ingesting large amounts of nutmeg.

Gastrointestinal Toxins

Goldenseal. Goldenseal (*Hydrastis canadensis*) was originally used by the Cherokee and other Native Americans as a dye and an internal remedy.[62] Today, it is used as an astringent, a remedy for the mucous membranes or gastrointestinal tract, and as a treatment of menorrhagia. Goldenseal is reputed to be able to mask the presence of illicit drugs on urine drug screens. The basis for this myth originated from the murder-mystery *Stringtown on the Pike* (1900), which was written by an internationally known plant pharmacist, Uri Lloyd. In this novel, one of the major characters is accused of murder by poisoning with strychnine, but is posthumously exonerated with evidence that hydrastine (the active alkaloid in goldenseal) and morphine cross-react to produce a false-positive color assay for strychnine.[58] Multiple studies indicate that goldenseal does not affect the results of urinary drug screens.[42,93,98] Appropriate usage of this herbal is thought to be safe, but large ingestions can cause vomiting, diarrhea, convulsions, paralysis, and respiratory failure. In such cases, the patient should receive supportive care.

Pokeweed. Pokeweed (*Phytolacca americana* or *Phytolacca decandra*) is also known as inkberry, Viginia poke, scoke, pigeon berry, garget, and American cancer. It is often mistaken for horseradish, parsnips, or Jerusalem artichoke. Gastrointestinal effects are very common after ingestion; in severe cases, there may also be neurologic symptoms, such as decreased vision, respiratory depression, seizures, weakness, and cardiac dysrhythmias. The root is the most toxic part of the plant, although the leaves, stems, and berries also possess the enterotoxin.[83] Toxins include triterpene, saponins, and glycoproteins. Pokeweed can cause mitotic and morphologic changes in lymphocytes and plasma cells by a nonspecific mitogenic effect. Symptoms typically begin within several minutes of exposure and last 24–48 hours. Treatment remains supportive.

Hepatotoxins

Pennyroyal. Pennyroyal oil is a volatile oil extract from the leaves of *Mentha pulegium* and *Hedeoma pulegioides* plants. It is cited as the causative agent in several well-documented cases of hepatic failure following ingestion of as little as 15 mL of the oil.[4] The postulated mechanism is direct hepatotoxicity from the cyclohexanone pulegone and its cytochrome P450 toxic metabolites, which include menthofuran. Pulegone and menthofuran also cause neurotoxicity, renal toxicity, and bronchiolar epithelial cell destruction. Since pulegone depletes glutathione stores in the liver, *N*-acetylcysteine treatment may be beneficial. In two case reports, hepatotoxicity may have been prevented by early administration of *N*-acetylcysteine.[4,17] Other effects of pennyroyal oil ingestion include a minty odor on the breath, GI bleeding, seizures, hematuria, and vaginal bleeding. On autopsy, vacuolization of the white matter of the midbrain is reported in both a human case of pennyroyal fatality and in animal models.[8,97] Herbalists use pennyroyal oil as an abortifacient and to regulate menstruation. The abortive effect is thought to be due to irritation and contraction of the uterus.[123] It is usually ingested as a strong tea prepared from the leaves or as the oil itself. *N*-acetylcysteine treatment similar to the dosing regimen used in acetaminophen overdose should be considered as first-line therapy for patients with pennyroyal associated hepatoxicity.

Pyrrolizidine Alkaloids. Pyrrolizidine alkaloids are hepatotoxins found in many plant families. *Heliotropium, Senecio, Crotolaria,* and *Symphytum* are the most common sources of pyrrolizidine alkaloids.[103,108] Conversion to the toxic, active principles probably occurs in vivo and probably involves metabolism in the liver to pyrroles, which serve as biologic alkylating agents.[70] They cause hepatic veno-occlusive disease, hepatomegaly, cirrhosis, and possibly hepatic carcinoma. Chronic low doses may cause pulmonary toxicity, resulting in pulmonary artery hypertension and right ventricular hypertrophy. Many cases of hepatic veno-occlusive disease follow the consumption of pyrrolizidine alkaloid containing herbal teas. Consumption of "bush" tea, prepared from the leaves of the surrounding scrubland, is considered an endemic problem in Jamaica. Epidemics have also occurred in Afghanistan and India, where ingestion of contaminated cereals containing *Heliotropium* and *Crotolaria* seeds resulted in 1632 and 60 cases of veno-occlusive disease, respectively.[92,127] In Western countries, ingestion of herbal products containing *Senecio* and comfrey have led to several cases of hepatic veno-occlusive disease.[103] Treatment of hepatic veno-occlusive disease is supportive. Examples of plants and products containing pyrrolizidine alkaloids include borage (*Borago officinalis*), coltsfoot (*Tussilago farfara*), comfrey (*Symphatum officinale*), gordolobo (*Senecio longilobo*), heliotrope (*Crotolaria spectabulis, Heliotropium europeaum*), T'u-san-chi'i (*Gynura segetum*), and Jamaican "bush tea" (probably *Crotolaria* species).[70,77,107]

Other Hepatotoxins

Several herbal preparations are also associated with hepatotoxicity. These include chapparel (*Larrea tridentata*),[22,63] germander (*Teucrium chamaedrys*),[80] impilia (*Callilepsis laureola*),[79] atractylis (*Atractylis gummifera*), and sassafras (*Sassafras albidum*).[115]

Heavy Metals

Heavy metal poisoning from arsenic, cadmium, lead, and mercury is associated with various types of herbal preparations.[27,46,107] Treatment consists of stopping consumption of the herbal product and use of an appropriate chelating agent when indicated.

Hai Ge Fen (clamshell powder) was contaminated with copper, chromium, arsenic, or lead in several case reports.[65,86] Pay-Loo-Ah, a red and orange powder used by the Hmong people as a fever and rash remedy, was contaminated with lead in one case report.[24] Ghasard,

Bola Goli, Kandu, Moha Yogran Guggulu, traditional Indian remedies for abdominal pain, are associated with lead poisoning.[27,113] One fatality from lead poisoning from Ghasard, Bola Goli, and Kandu was reported in the United States. Ayurvedic remedies often contain metals such as gold, silver, copper, zinc, iron, lead, tin, and mercury.[105]

Azarcon (lead tetroxide) and Greta (lead oxide) are used by an estimated 7.2–12.1% Mexican-Hispanic families for treatment of *empacho*. In Spanish, *empacho* means "blocked intestine" but it refers to any type of chronic digestive problem, including diverse symptoms such as constipation, diarrhea, nausea, vomiting, anorexia, apathy, and lethargy.[29,34] Azarcon and Greta are fine powders with total lead contents varying from 70% to greater than 90%.[13,30]

Surma and kohl, eye makeup used in India, Middle East, and Africa, contains over 50% lead.[3,7,104,119] Lead poisoning and fatalities have been reported. Herbal balls, hand-rolled mixtures of herbs and honey produced in China, are often associated with arsenic and mercury contamination.[55] Examples include An Gong Niu Huang Wan, Da Huo Luo Wan, and Niu Huang Chiang Ya Wan.

Colloidal silver proteins are promoted by health food stores as antimicrobials, immune system stimulants, and antiinflammatory agents. Silver toxicity is associated with argyria or bluish skin discoloration.[59] Chronic usage is associated with neurologic deficits, silver deposition in visceral organs, and renal damage.

Renal Toxins

Aristolochia. Aristolochia (*Aristolochia clematis*), also known as birthwort, heartwort, and fangji, was associated with progressive interstitial renal fibrosis in Belgium when substituted for another Chinese herbal, *Stephania tetranda*, in the formulation of a weight loss regimen.[128,129] Out of 70 identified cases of renal fibrosis, 30 patients developed terminal renal failure. Aristolochia contains aristolochic acid, which is a known nephrotoxin. The fibrosing process typically becomes clinically apparent 12–24 months after the initial injury.

Miscellaneous

Garlic. Garlic (*Allium sativum*) has been used as a food and a medicine since ancient times.[60] The intact cells of garlic contain the odorless, sulfur-containing amino acid derivative (+)-S-allyl-L-cysteine sulfoxide, also known as alliin. When crushed, alliin is converted to allicin (diallyl thiosulfinate), which has antibacterial activity and gives the herb its characteristic odor and flavor. Garlic is used as a traditional remedy for a host of infections and a treatment for hypertension, colic, and cancer. Side effects of using garlic extracts include contact dermatitis, gastroenteritis, nausea, and vomiting. Patients who are already taking anticoagulant medications should only consume garlic with caution because of its antiplatelet metabolite, ajoene. Treatment remains supportive.

Ginseng. Ginseng is the common name for deciduous, perennial plants of the genus *Panax*. *Panax ginseng* is native to Korea, China, Japan, and Russia. In North America, *Panax quinquefolium* is the common species. Ginseng preparations have been used in China for the treatment of respiratory illnesses, gastrointestinal disorders, impotence, fatigue, and stress ("adaptogenic effect"). It is regarded as a tonic and panacea (hence the name Panax: "all healing"). Its only recognized use in America is as an external demulcent.[61,82,91] However, an estimated 6 million people regularly ingest ginseng in herbal teas or apply it as a cosmetic. Ginseng provides a good example of the complexity of the biochemical and pharmacologic effects of herbs. The active components of ginseng include panaxin, panax acid, panaquilin, panacen, sapogenin, and ginsenin. Its general metabolic effects include decreased serum glucose levels and serum cholesterol levels; increased erythropoiesis, hemoglobin production, and iron absorption from the gut; increased blood pressure and heart rate; and GI motility and CNS stimulation. Ironically because of the lack of oversight in the health food industry, many ginseng products may not actually contain significant quantities of ginseng. In one study, 54 ginseng products were analyzed for ginseng. Sixty percent of those analyzed contained pharmacologically insignificant amounts of ginseng and 25% contained no ginseng at all.[84] Long-term use of ginseng is associated with Ginseng Abuse Syndrome (GAS), consisting of hypertension, nervousness, sleeplessness, and morning diarrhea.[117]

Chamomile Tea. Chamomile tea is a popular herbal drink made from chamomile flower heads. Anaphylactic reactions can occur in patients allergic to ragweed, asters, chrysanthemums, or other members of the Compositae family.[9,19] Such reactions are rare but can be life-threatening. The patient need not have severe allergies or be highly atopic to experience a cross-reaction.

Rattlesnake Capsules. Rattlesnake capsules are a common Mexican folk remedy used to treat cancer, arthritis, and skin disorders. They contain dried, pulverized rattlesnake powder and are sold under various names: *vibora de cascabel, polvo de vibora,* and *carne de vibora,* without prescriptions. Infection with *Salmonella arizonae* has been described following ingestion.[10,43,95,110,131]

Chinese Patent Medications

These medications are mass produced and are available as tablets, capsules, syrups, powders, ointment, and plasters.

Jin Bu Huan is a traditional Chinese preparation used as a sedative and analgesic.[132] The active ingredient, an isoquinoline alkaloid levo-tetrahydropalmatine (L-THP), is responsible for the morphine-like properties of Jin Bu Huan. In two case reports, three pediatric patients developed life-threatening bradycardia and seven adult patients developed hepatitis while using Jin Bu Huan.[25,26] Hepatotoxicity may be related to L-THP, which is structurally similar to the hepatotoxic pyrrolizidine alkaloids.[132] Although the package insert for Jin Bu Huan in these cases indicates that *Polygala chinensis* was the plant source for L-THP, *Polygala chinensis* does not contain L-THP. Plants from the genera *Stephania* and *Corydalis* are also known as Jin Bu Huan and contain appreciable amounts of L-THP, and it is probable that this product was simply mislabeled by the manufacturer.

Nan Lien Chiu Fong Toukuwan (now withdrawn from the market) was found to contain aminopyrine, phenacetin, phenylbutazone, indomethacin, mefenamic acid, diazepam, hydrochlorothiazide, dexamethasone, mercuric sulfide, lead, and cadmium, depending on the manufacturer.[37] Several cases of agranulocytosis were reported after ingestion of this preparation.[109]

Dr. Tong Shap Yee's asthma pills were found to contain theophylline.[37]

Leng Pui Kee cough pills were found to contain bromhexine.[37]

Tung Shueh, also known as black ball, contains diazepam and mefenamic acid and is associated with acute interstitial nephritis.[50]

Gan Mao Tong Pian, an herbal cold remedy, contains phenylbutazone and has caused aplastic anemia in one case report.[94]

Chui Feng Su Ho Wan, which contains *Glycyrrhiza glabra*, was associated with hypokalemia-induced torsades de pointes in an elderly woman.[37]

Several Chinese patent medicines contain the mercurials cinnabar (mercuric sulfide) and calomel (mercurous chloride). Tse Koo Choy and Qing Fen, which contain calomel, have been associated with several cases of mercury poisoning.[73]

Many Chinese medicated oils contain oil of wintergreen, methylsalicylate. Although these oils are intended for external use, it is a common practice to ingest a few drops undiluted or in a hot drink as a general tonic or specific remedy. Examples of medicated oils include White Flower Medicine Oil (40% wintergreen, 30% menthol, 6% camphor), Red Flower Oil (67% wintergreen, 22% turpentine oil), and Kwan Loong Medicated Oil (menthol 25%, methyl salicylate 15%, camphor 10%).[37] Additional examples are shown in Table 76–5.

Herbal Preparations and AIDS Therapies

Many patients infected with human immunodeficiency virus (HIV) have turned to alternative treatments in the hope of finding more effective and/or less toxic therapy than the conventional modalities currently available. In a study of 114 HIV-positive patients in a university-based AIDS clinic, 22% used one or more herbal products in a 3-month period.[74] Twenty-four percent of these patients were unable to state which herbs they were taking. Adverse effects included dermatitis, nausea, vomiting, diarrhea, thrombocytopenia, coagulopathies, altered mental status, hepatotoxicity, and electrolyte imbalances. Twenty percent of patients stated their physicians were unaware of their use of herbs.

Two herbals currently used for AIDS therapy are Saint John's Wort (*Hypericum perforatum*) and Chinese cucumber (*Trichosanthes kirilowii*).[41,112] Saint John's Wort is a

TABLE 76–5. THE 20 MOST POPULAR ASIAN PATENT MEDICINES THAT CONTAIN TOXIC INGREDIENTS

Product Name	Manufacturer	Toxic Ingredients
Ansenpenaw Tablets	Chung Lien Drug Works (Hankow, China)	Mercury chloride
Bezoar Sedative Pills	Lanzhou Fo Ci Pharmaceutical Factory (Lanzhou, China)	Mercury chloride 2% or 10%
Compound Kangweiling	Wo Zhou Pharmaceutical Factory (Zhe Jiang, China)	Centipede (scolopendra) 10%
Dahuo Luodan	Beijing Tun Jen Tang (Beijing, China)	Centipede (scolopendra)
Danshen Tabletco	Shanghai Chinese Medicine Works (Shanghai, China)	Borneol
Fructus Persica Compound Pills	Lanzhou Fo Ci Pharmaceutical Factory (Lanzhou, China)	Cannabis indica seed
Fuchingsung-N Cream	Tianjin Pharmaceutical Corp. (Tianjin, China)	Fluocinolone acetanide
Kwei Ling Chi	Changchun Chinese Medicines and Drugs Manufactory (Chang Chun, China)	Mercury chloride
Kyushin Heart Tonic	Kyushin Seikyaku Co., Ltd. (Tokyo, Japan)	Toad venom, borneol
Laryngitis Pills	China Dzechuan Provincial Pharmaceutical Factory (Chengtu Branch, China)	Borax 30%, toad-cake 10%
Leung Pui Kee Cough Pills	Leung Pui Kee Medical Factory (Hong Kong)	Dover's powder (opium powder)
Lu-Shen-Wan	Shanghai Chinese Medicine Works (Shanghai, China)	Toad secretion
Nasalin	Kwangchow Pharmaceutical Industry Co. (Kwangchow, China)	Centipede 5%
Nui Huang Chieh Tu Pien	Tung Jen Tang (Beijing, China)	Borneo camphor
Niu Huang Xiao Yan Wan Bezoar Antiphlogistic Pills	Soochow Chinese Medicine Works (Kiangsu, China)	Realgar 19.23%
Pak Yuen Tong Hou Tsao Powder	Kwan Tung Pak Yuen Tong Main Factory (Hong Kong)	Scorpion 10%
Po Ying Tan Baby Protector	Po Che Tong Poon Mo Um (Hong Kong)	Camphor 20%
Superior Tabellae Berberini HCl	Min-Kang Drug Manufactory (I-Chang, China)	Berberini HCl
Watson's Flower Pagodo Cakes	A.S. Watson & Co., Ltd. (Hong Kong)	Piperazine phosphate
Xiao Huo Luo Dan	Lanzhou Fo Ci Pharmaceutical Factory (Lanzhou, China)	Aconite 42%

Reprinted from Appendix E. Alternative Medicine: Expanding Medical Horizons. A report to the National Institutes of Health on alternative medical systems and practices in the United States. Presented under the auspices of the workshop on alternative medicine. Chantilly, VA, Sept 14–16, 1992.

perennial, native to Europe but now found in the United States and Canada. The plant has been used by herbalists since the Middle Ages. Recently, it has been used to treat anxiety and depression, as a diuretic, and for gastritis. It contains tannin, hypericin, a red dianthrone pigment, rutin, flavinoids, and hyperoside. Studies are currently being conducted with hypericin as an immunomodulator in patients with AIDS. Toxicity appears to be limited to photosensitization reactions.

Chinese cucumber, or Compound Q, is employed in Chinese medicine to reduce fevers, swelling, and coughing, to control diabetes, and as an abortifacient.[41] Trichosanthin appears to be synonymous with Compound Q. It has also been called Gualougen and GLQ–223. According to some herbalists this compound is supposed to be able to block HIV replication in infected T4 cells and destroy HIV-infected macrophages. Extracts of Chinese cucumber are extremely toxic, especially if administered parenterally. There are reports of pulmonary and cerebral edema, cerebral hemorrhage, and myocardial damage. Seizures and fevers occurred in patients with AIDS who had used Chinese cucumber parenterally.

Other herbal preparations, including astragalus, blue-green algae, allicin, artemisia, astragalus, bee pollen, bitter melon capsules, cat's claw, chlorella, chromium picolinate, coenzyme Q10, curcumin, dandelion root, echinacea, evening primrose oil, flaxseed oil, germanium-132, *Ginkgo biloba*, glycyrrhizin, grapeseed, iscador, prunellin, saw palmetto, shark cartilage, shiitake mushrooms, Sho-Saiko-To (SSKT), Siberian ginseng, and silymarin, have been used for the treatment of HIV infection.[14,51,89,114]

What Is the Treatment Approach to Patients With Herbal Preparation Toxicity?

A specific treatment strategy should emphasize identification of the specific herbal preparation(s) used by the patient, concurrent medication(s), and medical illness(es). Since herbal preparation toxicity varies greatly depending on the preparation used, careful examination may be aided by knowledge of the herbal preparation. In most cases, supportive care and discontinuation of the herbal preparation(s) is sufficient. Some herbal toxicities may require specific laboratory analysis and therapy. Additional information concerning specific herbals including use, potential toxicity, and popularity are summarized in Table 76–6. All adverse events associated with herbal preparations should be reported to the FDA Medwatch at 1-800-FDA-1088.

TABLE 76–6. SELECTED HERBAL PREPARATIONS, POPULAR USE, AND POTENTIAL TOXICITIES

Herbal Preparation	Scientific Name	Other Common Names	Traditional and Popular Usage	Toxic Ingredient(s)	Adverse Effects
Aconite	*Acontium napellus, kusnezoffi, carmichael*	Monkshood, wolfbane caowu, chuanwu, bushi	Topical analgesic Neuralgia, asthma, and heart disease	Aconite alkaloids (C19 diterpinoid esters)	Gastrointestinal upset, cardiac dysrhythmias
Agrimony	*Agrimonia eupatoria*	Cocklebur, stickwort, liverwort	Catarrh, gall bladder disease, astringent		Photodermatitis
Aloe	*Aloe vera* and other spp.	Cape, Zanzibar, Socotrine, Curacao, Carrisyn	Heals wounds, emollient, laxative, abortifacient	Anthraquinones, barbaloin, isobarbaloin	Gastrointestinal upset, dermatitis
Apricot pits	*Prunus armeniaca*	—	(Laetrile) cancer remedy	Amygdalin	Cyanide poisoning
Aristolochia	*Aristolochia clematis*	Birthwort, heartwort, fangchi	Uterine stimulant	Aristolochic acid	Nephrotoxin
Artemisa	*Artemisa vulgaris, dracunculus, lactiflora*	Mugwort, felon herb, moxa, guizhou	Depression, dyspepsia, menstrual disorder, abortifacient		Gastrointestinal upset
Atractylis	*Atractylis gummifera*		Chewing gum, antipyretic, diuretic, gastrointestinal remedy	Potassium atractylate and gummiferin: mitochondrial toxin	Hepatitis, altered mental status, seizures, vomiting, hypoglycemia
Autumn crocus	*Colchicum autumnale*	Crocus, fall crocus, meadow saffron, mysteria, vellorita	Gout, rheumatism, prostate >hepatic disease, cancer, gonorrhea	Colchicine	Gastrointestinal upset, renal disease, agranulocytosis
Bee pollen, royal jelly	Derived from *Apis mellifera*	—	Increase stamina, athletic ability, longevity		Allergic reactions, anaphylaxis
Bee venom	Derived from *Apis mellifera*	—	Immunomodulator		Allergic reactions, anaphylaxis
Betel nut	*Areca catechu*	Areca nut, pinlang, pinang	Stimulant	Arecholine	Possible bronchospasm, chronic use associated with leukoplakia and squamous cell carcinoma
Bitter melon	*Momordica charantia*	MAP-30 (protein extract)	Abortifacient, diabetes, gastrointestinal disorder, diabetes, cancer, HIV therapy	—	None

(*continued*)

TABLE 76–6. SELECTED HERBAL PREPARATIONS, POPULAR USE, AND POTENTIAL TOXICITIES (continued)

Herbal Preparation	Scientific Name	Other Common Names	Traditional and Popular Usage	Toxic Ingredient(s)	Adverse Effects
Black cohosh	*Cimicifuga racemosa*	Black snakeroot, squawroot, bugbane, baneberry	Abortifacient, menstrual irregularity, astringent, dyspepsia		Dizziness, nausea, vomiting, headache
Blue cohosh	*Caulophyllum thalictroides*	Squaw root, papoose root	Abortifacient, menstrual disorders, antispasmodic	Methylcytisine (1/40 potency of nicotine)	Nicotinic toxicity
Borage	*Borago officinalis*	—	Diuretic, antidepressant, antiinflammatory	Pyrrolizidine alkaloids, amabiline	Possible hepatotoxicity
Boron		Boron	Topical astringent, wound remedy	Boron	Dermatitis, gastrointestinal upset, renal and hepatic toxicity, seizures, coma, death
Boneset	*Eupatorium perfoliatum*	Thoroughwort, vegetable antimony, feverwort	Antipyretic	Pyrrolizidine alkaloids	Possible hepatotoxicity, dermatitis, milk sickness
Broom	*Cytisus scoparius*	Bannal, broom, broom top	Cathartic, diuretic, induce labor, drug of abuse	*l*-sparteine	Nictotine-like poisoning
Buchu	*Barosma betulina*	Bookoo, buku, diosma, bucku, bucco	Diuretic, stimulant, carminative, urine infections, insect repellant	—	None
Buckthorn	*Rhamnus frangula*		Laxative	Anthraquinones	Diarrhea, weakness
Burdock root	*Arctium lappa, Arctium minus*	Great burdock, gobo, lappa, beggar's button, hareburr, niu bang zi	Diuretic, cholerectic, induce sweating, skin disorders, burn remedy	Atropine (possible contaminant)	Potential anticholinergic toxicity
Calendula	*Calendula officinalis*	Marigold, garden marigold, pot marigold, gold bloom, holligold	Wounds, dysmenorrhea, fever; pesticide	—	None
Cantharidin	*Cantharidin* beetle	Spanish fly, blister beetles	Aphrodisiac, abortifacient, blood purifier	Terpenoid: cantharidin	Gastrointestinal upset, urinary tract and skin irritant, renal toxicity
Caraway	*Umbellifarae carvi*		Antispasmodic, carminative		
Cascara	*Cascara sagrada*		Laxative	Anthraquinones	Diarrhea, weakness
Cat's claw	*Uncaria tomentosa Uncaria guianensis*	*Uña de gato*	AIDS, cancer arthritis, ulcers, menstrual cramp, wounds, contraceptives	—	None
Catnip	*Nepata cataria*	Cataria, catnip, catmint	Indigestion, colic, sedative, headaches, emmenagogue	Nepetalactone	Sedative
Chamomile	*Chamomilla recutita Chamomilla nobile*	In Mexico, manzanilla	Digestive disorders, skin disorders, cramps	Allergens	Contact dermatitis, allergic reaction, anaphylaxis very rare
Carp bile (raw)	*Ctenopharyngodon idellus,*	Grass carp	Improve visual acuity and health	? Cyprinol, C27 bile alcohol	Hepatitis, renal failure
	Cyprinus carpio	Common carp			
Ch'an Su	*Bufo bufo gargarizans Bufo bufo melanosticus*	Stone, lovestone, black stone, rock hard, chu an wu, kyushin	Topical anesthetic, aphrodisiac, cardiac medication	Bufadienolides Bufotenin	Cardiac dysrhythmias Hallucinations
Chaparral	*Larrea tridentata*	Creosote bush, greasewood, hediondilla	Bronchitis, analgesic, retard aging, possible cancer treatment	Nondihydroguaiaretic acid (NDGA)	Hepatotoxicity (chronic)
Chestnut	*Aesulus* spp.	Horse chestnut, California buckeye, Ohio buckeye, buckeye	Arthritis, rhematism, varicose veins, hemorrhoids	Esulin, nicotine, quercitin, quercitrin, rutin, saponin, shikimic acid	Fasciculations, weakness, incoordination, gastrointestinal upset, paralysis, stupor
Clove	*Syzgium aromaticum*	Caryophyllum	Expectorant, antiemetic, counterirritant, antiseptic, carminative	Eugenol (4-allyl-2-methoxyphenol)	Pulmonary toxicity (cigarettes)
Coltsfoot	*Tussilago farfara*	Coughwort, horse-hoof, kuandong hua	Dry cough, throat irritation, asthma, bronchitis	Pyrrolizidine alkaloid, senkirkine	Occasional allergy, potential hepatotoxicity, hepatic tumors (rats)
Comfrey	*Symphytum officinale* and other species *S. uplandicum*	Knitbone, bruisewort, blackwort, slippery root, Russian comfrey	Ulcers, hemorrhoids, bronchitis, heal burns, sprains, swelling, bruises	Pyrrolizidine alkaloids: symphytine, echimidine, lasiocarpine	Hepatic veno-occlusive disease, hepatocellular adenomas (rats)

(*continued*)

TABLE 76–6. SELECTED HERBAL PREPARATIONS, POPULAR USE, AND POTENTIAL TOXICITIES (continued)

Herbal Preparation	Scientific Name	Other Common Names	Traditional and Popular Usage	Toxic Ingredient(s)	Adverse Effects
Compound Q	*Trichosanthes kirilowii*	Gualougen, GLQ-223, chinese cucumber root	Fevers, swelling, expectorant, abortifacient, diabetes, AIDS	Trichosanthin	Pulmonary and cerebral edema, cerebral bleed, seizures, fevers
Chuenlin	*Coptis chinensus, japonicum*	Huanglien, mahuang	Infant tonic	Berberine: displace bilirubin from protein	Neonatal hyperbilirubinemia
Damiana	*Tumera diffusa* var. *aphrodisiaca*		Stimulant, purgative, aphrodisiac, antidepressant		Genitourinary irritation
Dandelion	*Taraxacum officinale*		Diuretic, detoxifying remedy; bitter	—	None
Dong Quai	*Angelica polymorpha*	Tang kuei, dang gui	Blood purifier, menstrual disorders, improve circulation	Coumarin, psoralens, safrole in essential oil	Anticoagulant effects, photodermatitis, possible carcinogen in oil
Echinacea	*Echinacea angustifolia* *Echinacea purpurea*	American cone flower, purple cone flower, snakeroot	Infections, immunostimulant	—	None
Elder	*Sambucus* spp.	Elderberry, sweet elder, sambucus	Diuretic, laxative, astringent, cancer	Cyanogenic glycoside sambunigrin in leaves	Vomiting, abdominal cramps, weakness if ingesting uncooked leaves
Ephedra	*Ephedra* spp.	Ma-huang, Mormon tea, yellow horse, desert tea, squaw tea	Stimulant, bronchial disorder therapy	Ephedrine, pseudoephedrine	Headache, insomnia, dizziness, palpitations, occasional seizures, cerebrovascular accidents, myocardial infarction, and death
Evening primrose	*Oenothera biennis*	Oil of evening primrose	Coronary disease, multiple sclerosis, cancer, rheumatoid arthritis, menstruation	—	None
Fennel	*Foeniculum vulgare*	Common, sweet, or bitter fennel	Gastroenteritis, expectorant, emmenagogue, stimulate lactation	Volatile oils: transanethole, fenchone; estrogens: dianethole and photoanethole	Ingestion of volatile oils: vomiting, seizures, pulmonary edema; dermatitis, estrogen effects
Feverfew	*Tanacetum parthenium*	Featherfew, altamisa, bachelor's button, featherfoil, febrifuge plant, midsummer daisy, nosebleed, wild quinine	Migraine headache, menstrual pain, asthma, dermatitis, arthritis, antipyretic, abortifacient		Oral ulcerations, "postfeverfew syndrome," rebound of migraine symptoms, anxiety, and insomnia following cessation of use
Fo-Ti	*Polygonum multiflorum*	Climbing knotwood, ho shou-wu	Scrofula, cancer, and constipation therapy; promote longevity	Anthraquinones: chrysophaol and emodin	Cathartic effects
Foxglove	*Digitalis purpurea* *Digitalis lanata* *Digitalis lutea* *Digitalis* spp.	Purple foxglove, throatwort, fairy finger, fairy cap, lady's thimble, scotch mercury, witch's bells, dead man's bells	Asthma therapy; sedative and diuretic/cardiotonic; in India, used to treat wounds and burns	Digitalis glycosides (eg, digitoxin, gitoxin, digoxin, digitalin, gitaloxin)	Miosis, blurred vision, gastrointestinal upset, dizziness, muscle weakness, tremors, cardiac dysrhythmias
Garlic	*Allium sativum*	Allium, stinking rose, rustic treacle, nectar of the gods, da suan	Therapy for infections and coronary artery disease; antihypertensive agent	Ajoene	Contact dermatitis, gastroenteritis, antiplatelet effects
Gentian	*Gentiana lutea* *Gentiana* spp.	Bitter root, gall weed Longdancao	Bitter, digestive stimulant, emmenagogue	—	None
Germander	*Teucrium chamaedrys*	Wall germander	Relief of fever, abdominal disorders, wounds, diuretic, choleretic		Hepatitis, cirrhosis
Ginkgo	*Ginkgo biloba*	Maidenhair tree, kew tree, tebonin, tanakan, rokan, kaveri	Asthma, chillblains, digestive aid, cerebral dysfunction therapy, improve memory		Extracts: gastrointestinal upset, headache, skin reaction; whole plants: allergic reactions

(*continued*)

TABLE 76–6. SELECTED HERBAL PREPARATIONS, POPULAR USE, AND POTENTIAL TOXICITIES (continued)

Herbal Preparation	Scientific Name	Other Common Names	Traditional and Popular Usage	Toxic Ingredient(s)	Adverse Effects
Ginseng	*Panax ginseng, quinquefolium, pseudoginseng*	Ren shen	Respiratory illnesses, gastrointestinal disorders, impotence, fatigue, stress, adaptogenic; external demulcent		Ginseng abuse syndrome
Glucomannan	*Amorphophallus konjac*	Konjac, konjac mannan	Weight reducing agent: "grapefruit diet"	Polysaccharides to increase viscosity and decrease gastric emptying	Esophageal and lower gastrointestinal obstruction
Glucosamine	2-amino-2-deoxyglucose	Chitosamine	Wound-healing polymer, antiarthritic	—	None
Goat's rue	*Galega officinalis*	French lilac, French honeysuckle	Antidiabetic	Galegine, paragalegine	Hypoglycemia
Goldenseal	*Hydrastis candensis*	Orange root, yellow root, turmeric root	Astringent; gastrointestinal disorder and menstrual bleeding therapy		Gastrointestinal upset, paralysis, and respiratory failure in large ingestions
Gordolobo yerba	*Senecio longiloba, aureus, vulgaris, spartoides*	Groundsel Liferoot	Gargle and cough medicine Emmenagogue	Pyrrolizidine alkaloids	Hepatic veno-occlusive disease
Gotu kola	*Centella asiatica*	Hydrocotyle, Indian pennywort, talepetrako	Wound healing, tonic		Contact dermatitis
Hawthorn	*Crataegus oxyacantha*	English hawthorn, haw, maybush, whitethorn	Blood pressure and dysrhythmia therapy; antispasmodic, sedative	Dehydrocatechins	Low doses: safe; High dose: potential for hypotension and sedation
Heliotrope	*Crotalaria specatabulis, Heliotropium europeaum*	Rattlebox, groundsel, viper's bugloss, bush tea		Pyrrolizidine alkaloids	Hepatic veno-occlusive disease
Henbane	*Hyoscyamus niger*	Fetid nightshade, poison tobacco, insane root, stinky nightshade	Sedative, painkiller, antispasmodic, asthma remedy	Hyoscyamine, hyoscine	Anticholinergic toxicity
Holly	*Ilex aquifolium* *Ilex opaca* *Ilex vomitoria*	Holly, English holly, Oregon holly, American holly	Tea: emetic, CNS stimulant, coronary artery disease therapy	Saponins	Gastrointestinal upset
Hydrangea	*Hydrangea paniculata*	Seven bark, wild hydrangea	Diuretic, stimulant, carminative; cystitis, renal calculi, and asthma therapy	—	Dizziness, chest pain, gastrointestinal upset
Iboga	*Tabernanthe iboga*	Ibogaine	Aphrodisiac, stimulant, hallucinogen; addiction treatment	Indole alkaloid: ibogaine	Hallucinations, cholinergic hyperactivity
Impila	*Callipesis laureola*		Zulu traditional remedy	Potassium atractylate-like compound	Vomiting, hypoglycemia, centrilobular hepatic necrosis
Jalap	*Ipomoea purga*	—	Cathartic	Convolvulin	Profuse watery diarrhea
Jimson weed	*Datura stramonium*	Datura, stramonium, apple of Peru, Jamestown weed, thornapple, tolguacha	Asthma remedy	Atropine, scopolamine, hyoscyamine, stramonium	Anticholinergic toxicity
Juniper	*Juniperus communis*	Oil of sabinol	Tonic, diuretic, urinary antiseptic, emmenogogue, abortifacient	Oil: terpinen-4-ol	Renal irritation
Kava kava	*Piper methysticum*	Awa, kava-kava, kew, tonga	Relaxation beverage Uterine relaxation, headaches, colds, wounds, aphrodisiac	Kava lactones Flavokwain A and B	Mild euphoria, muscle weakness Skin discoloration
KH-3	Procaine HCl	Gerovital-H3, GH-3, Gero-vita	Cerebral atherosclerosis, dementia, arthritis, hair loss, hypertension	Procaine	Procaine toxicity

(*continued*)

TABLE 76–6. SELECTED HERBAL PREPARATIONS, POPULAR USE, AND POTENTIAL TOXICITIES (continued)

Herbal Preparation	Scientific Name	Other Common Names	Traditional and Popular Usage	Toxic Ingredient(s)	Adverse Effects
Khat	*Catha edulis*	Qut, kat, chaat, Kus es Salahin, Tchaad, Gat	CNS stimulant Depression, fatigue, obesity, and ulcers remedy	Cathine and cathinine	Euphoria, dysphoria, stimulation, sedation, psychological dependence
Kola nut	*Cola acuminata*	Botu cola, cola nut	Digestive aid, tonic, aphrodisiac, headache remedy, diuretic	—	None
Kombucha	Mixture of bacteria and yeast	Kombucha tea, kombucha mushroom, Manchurian tea	Memory loss, premenstrual syndrome, cancer therapy	—	None
Levant berry	*Anamirta cocculus*	Fish killer, fishberry, hockle elderberry, Indian berry, louseberry, poisonberry	Vermifuge, symptomatic relief for malaria	Picrotoxin	Stimulant, gastrointestinal upset
Licorice	*Glycyrrhiza glabra*	Spanish licorice, Russian licorice, gancao	Gastric irritation	Glycoside: glycyrrhizin	Flaccid weakness, hypokalemia, lethargy
Lobelia	*Lobelia inflata*	Indian tobacco	Antispasmodic, respiratory stimulant, relaxant	Pyridine-derived alkaloids (lobeline)	Nicotine toxicity
Mace	*Myristica fragrans*	Mace, muscade, seed cover of nutmeg	Diarrhea, mouth sores, insomnia, rheumatism	Myristicin (methoxysafrole)	Hallucinations
Mandrake	*Mandragora officinarum*		Hallucinogen	Scopolamine, hyoscyamine	Anticholinergic toxicity
Mate	*Ilex paraguayensis*	Paraguay tea	Stimulant (caffeine)	—	None
Milk thistle	*Carduus marianus* *Silybum marinaum*	Mary thistle	Liver disease, antidepressant, HIV therapy	—	None
Mistletoe	*Viscum album, Phoradendron leucarpum*	Iscador	Antispasmodic, calmative, cancer and HIV therapy	Viscotoxins, pharotoxins	Gastrointestinal upset, bradycardia, delirium
Morning glory	*Ipomoea purpurea, Ipomoea violacea*	Heavenly blue, blue star, flying saucers	Drug of abuse	LSD	LSD toxicity
Myrrh	*Commiphora molmol*	Mulmul, ogo, heerabol	Astringent, antiseptic, emmenagogue, antispasmodic, cancer	—	None
Nutmeg	*Myristica fragrans*	Mace, rou dou kou	Hallucinogen, abortifacient, aphrodisiac, gastrointestinal disorders, emmenogogue	Myristicin	Hallucinogen, gastrointestinal upset
Oleander	*Nerium oleander*	Adelfa, laurier rose, rosa laurel, rose bay, rose francesca	Cardiac illness, asthma, corns, cancer, and epilepsy	Oleanrin, neriin, gentiobiosyloeandrin, odoroside A	Gastrointestinal upset, diarrhea, dysrhythmias
Ostrich fern	*Matteuccia struthipteris*	—	Laxative	—	Gastrointestinal upset if eaten undercooked
Parsley	*Petroselinum crispum*	Rock parsley, garden parsley	Diuretic, uterine stimulant, abortifacient	Myristicin, apiol, furocoumarin, psoralen	Uterine stimulant, photosensitization
Passion flower	*Passiflora incarnata*	Passiflora, maypop	Insomnia, analgesic	—	None
Pau d'Arco	*Tabebuia* spp.	Ipe roxo, lapacho, taheebo tea	Tonic, blood builder, cancer remedy, AIDS therapy	Naphthoquinone derivative: lapachol	Gastrointestinal upset, anemia, bleeding
Pennyroyal oil	*Hedeoma pulegioides, Mentha pulegium*	American pennyroyal, squawmint, mosquito plant	Abortifacient, regulate menstruation, digestive tonic	Pulegone, menthofuran	Hepatotoxicity
Periwinkle	*Catharanthus roseus*	Red periwinkle, Madagascar or Cape periwinkle, old maid, church-flower, ram-goat rose, "myrtle," magdalena	Ornamental; used to treat ocular inflammation, diabetes and hemorrhage, insect stings, cancers	Vincristine, vinblastine	Vincristine/vinblastine toxicity
Podophyllum	*Podophyllum peltatum, Podophyllum hexandrum, Podophyllum emodi*	Mandrake, mayapple, American podophyllum, Indian podophyllum, guijiu	Cathartic, purgative	Podophyllin	Podophyllin toxicity
Pokeweed	*Phytolacca americana* *Phytolacca decandra*	American nightshade, cancer jalap, inkberry poke, scoke	Chronic rheumatisms, arthritis, emetic, purgative	Saponins: phytolaccigenin, jaligonic acid, phytolaccagenic acid, pokeweed mitogen	Gastroenteritis, blurry vision, weakness, respiratory distress, seizures, leukocytosis

(*continued*)

TABLE 76–6. SELECTED HERBAL PREPARATIONS, POPULAR USE, AND POTENTIAL TOXICITIES (continued)

Herbal Preparation	Scientific Name	Other Common Names	Traditional and Popular Usage	Toxic Ingredient(s)	Adverse Effects
Quinine	*Cinchona succirubra, Cinchona calisya, Cinchona ledgeriana*	Red bark, Peruvian bark, Jesuit's bark, China bark, cinchona bark, quinaquina, fever tree	Malaria, fever, indigestion, cancer, hemorrhoids, varicose veins, abortifacient	Quinine	Cinchonism
Red bush tea	*Aspalathus linearis*	Rooibos tea	Common tea substitute	—	None
Rehmennia	*Rehmannia glutinosa*	Sheng di huang, Chinese foxglove root	Longevity herb, lowers blood pressure, kidney and liver tonic	—	None
Rue	*Ruta graveolens*	Herb of grace, herb grass	Emmenagogue, antispasmodic, abortifacient	Fucocoumarins, bergapten and xanthoxanthin	Photosensitization
Sage	*Salvia officinalis*	Garden sage, true sage, scarlet sage, meadow sage	Antiseptic, astringent, hormonal stimulant, carminative, abortifacient	Thujone	None
Saint John's wort	*Hypericum perforatum*	Klamath weed, john's wort, goatweed, sho-ren-gyo	Anxiety, depression, gastritis, insomnia, promote healing, AIDS	—	Photosensitization
Sassafras	*Sassafras albidum*	—	Stimulant, antispasmodic, purifier	Safrole	Hepatotoxicity, carcinogen (?)
Saw palmetto	*Serenoa repens*	Sabal, American dwarf palm tree, cabbage palm	Genitourinary disorders, increase sperm production, sexual vigor, decrease prostate size	—	Diarrhea
Schisandra	*Schisandra chinensis*	Wu zei zi	Tonic, aphrodisiac, liver treatment, sedative	—	None
Scullcap	*Scutellaria laterifolia*	Skullcap, helmetflower, hood wort	Reputed tranquilizer, tonic, antispasmodic	—	None
Senna	*Cassia acutifolia Cassia angustifolia*	Alexandrian senna	Stimulant, laxative, Diet tea	Anthraquinone Glycosides (sennosides)	Diarrhea, CNS effects
Shark cartilage	*Squalus acanthias, Sphyrna lewini*	—	Cancer cure—inhibit tumor Angiogenesis, arthritis	—	None
Siberian ginseng	*Acanthopanax senticos*	Devil's shrub, eleuthra, eleutherococ	Adaptogens; blood pressure therapy; immune system stimulant	—	None
Slippery Elm	*Ulmus rubra Ulmus fulva*	Elm, elm bark, red elm	Acne, boils, indigestion, abortifacient	Oleoresin	Contact dermatitis
Soapwort	*Saponaria officinalis*	Bruisewort, bouncing bet, dog cloves, fuller's herb, latherwort	Acne psoriasis, eczema, boils; used to make natural soaps	Saponins	(IV) highly toxic; (po) none
SOD	Superoxide dismutase	Orgotein, ormetein, palosein	Improve health, lengthen life span; chronic bladder disease, paraquat poisoning	—	None
Squill	*Urginea maritima, Urginea indica*	Sea onion	Diuretic, emetic, cardiotonic, expectorant	Cardiac glycoside: scillaren A	Emesis
Tonka bean	*Dipteryx odorata Dipteryx oppositifolia*	Tonquin bean, cumaru	Food and cosmetics	Coumarin	Anticoagulant effect
T'u-san-chi	*Gynura segetum*	—	Herbal tea	Pyrrolizidine alkaloids	Hepatic veno-occlusive disease
Tung seed	*Aleurities moluccana*	Tung, candlenut, candleberry, barnish tree, balucanat, otaheite	Wood preservative (oil), purgative (oil), asthma treatment (seed)		Gastrointestinal upset, Hyporeflexia, death; latex: dermatitis
Valerian	*Valeriana officinalis*	Radix valerianae, Indian valerian, red valerian	Anxiety, insomnia, antispasmodic	—	None
White cohosh	*Actaea alba Actaea rubra*	Baneberry, snakeberry, doll's eyes, coralberry	Emmenagogue	Toxic glycosides	Headache, gastrointestinal upset, delirium, circulatory failure
Wild lettuce	*Lactuca virosa*	Lettuce opium, prickley lettuce	Sedative, cough suppressant, opioid substitute	—	None
Woodruff	*Galium odoratum*	Sweet woodruff	Wound healing, tonic, varicose vein treatment, antispasmodic	Coumarin	None

(continued)

TABLE 76–2. SELECTED HERBAL PREPARATIONS, POPULAR USE, AND POTENTIAL TOXICITIES (continued)

Herbal Preparation	Scientific Name	Other Common Names	Traditional and Popular Usage	Toxic Ingredient(s)	Adverse Effects
Wormwood	*Artemisa absinthium*	Absinthem	Sedative, analgesic, antihelminthic	Thujone	Psychosis, hallucinations, seizures
Yarrow	*Archillea millefolium*	Bloodwort, carpenter's grass, dog daisy, nosebleed	Heal wounds, cold and flu remedy, digestive disorder treatment, diuretic		Contact dermatitis
Yew	*Taxus baccata* and other spp.	Yew	Antispasmodic, cancer remedy	Taxin (Na^+-K^+ channel blocker)	Dizziness, dry mouth, bradycardia, cardiac arrest
Yohimbe	*Pausinystalia yohimbe*	Yohimbi, yohimbehe	Body building, aphrodisiac, hallucinogen	*Alkaloid:* yohimbine (bark)	Hypotension, abdominal pain, weakness, paralysis

What Recommendations Can Be Offered for the Use of Herbal Preparations?

The popularity of herbal preparations is expected to increase in this country for the foreseeable future. Although most herbal users will suffer no ill effect, both herbal users and clinicians should be aware that these preparations are pharmacologically active with the potential for toxicity. They may interact with prescription medications to increase the toxicity of the medication or decrease its therapeutic effect. Patients with specific medical conditions may have increased risk of toxicity when using herbal preparations.

Herbal users should be aware that these preparations are poorly studied. Scientific proof of efficacy is lacking for many preparations. In the United States, no standards exist for their manufacture. Many herbal products do not contain the purported amount of the active ingredient. Some herbal products do not contain the correct active ingredient. Many herbal products are adulterated with prescription medications or contain contaminants such as heavy metals.

Many herbal stores are staffed by untrained personnel who may dispense incorrect medical advice and unfounded claims concerning their products.[102] Trained herbalists (eg, Chinese herbalists) may dispense potent traditional remedies with potential for serious toxicity as the result of improper identification of the correct herbal or improper preparation of the herbal product by the herbalist or herbal user.[37] Most herbal users, including many herbalists, may be unaware of their products' potential for toxicity.

Clinicians should be familiar with herbal preparations and their potential for drug interactions and adverse effects. Every patient history should include questions assessing the concurrent use of herbal preparations.

References

1. Abernethy MK, Becker L: Acute nutmeg intoxications. Am J Emerg Med 1992;10:429–430.
2. Akerele O: Summary of WHO guidelines for the assessment of herbal medicines. HerbalGram 1993;28:13–20.
3. Ali A, Smales O, Aslam M: Surma and lead poisoning. Br Med J 1978;2:915–916.
4. Anderson IB, Mullen WH, Meeker JE, et al: Pennyroyal toxicity: Measurement of toxic metabolite levels in two cases and review of the literature. Ann Intern Med 1996;124:726–734.
5. Ansford A, Morris N: Fatal oleander poisoning. Med J Aust 1981;1:360–361.
6. Arnold WN: Vincent van Gogh and the thujone connection. JAMA 1988;260:3042–3044.
7. Aslam M, Healy MA, Daris SS, et al: Surma and blood lead in children. Lancet 1980;1:568–569.
8. Bakerink JA, Gospe SM, Dimand RJ, et al: Multiple organ failure after ingestion of pennyroyal oil from herbal tea in two patients. Pediatrics 1996;98:944–947.
9. Benner M, Lee H: Anaphylactic reaction of chamomile tea. J Allergy Clin Immunol 1973;52:307–308.
10. Bhatt BD, Zuckerman MJ, Foland JA, et al: Rattlesnake meat ingestion—A common Hispanic folk remedy. West J Med 1988;149:605. Letter.
11. Blue cohosh. Lawrence Review of Natural Products. May 1985.
12. Bond WS: Non-steroidal anti-inflammatory drugs: Are there significant differences? Facts Comp Drug Newsletter 1992;11:81–83.
13. Bose A, Vashishta K, O'Loughlin BJ: Azarcon por emphacho—Another cause of lead toxicity. Pediatrics 1983;72:106–110.
14. Braun JF, Powderly WG, Steinberg CL, et al: A guide to underground AIDS therapies. Patient Care 1993;27:53–70.
15. Brevoort P: The US botanical market—An overview. HerbalGram 1996;36:49–57.
16. Brubacher JR, Ravikumar PR, Bania T, et al: Treatment of toad venom poisoning with digoxin-specific Fab fragments. Chest 1996;110:1282–1288.
17. Buechel DW, Haverlah VC, Gardner ME: Pennyroyal oil ingestion: Report of a case. J Am Osteopath Assoc 1983;82:793–794.
18. But PP, Tai YT, Young K: Three fatal cases of herbal aconite poisoning. Vet Hum Toxicol 1994;34:212–215.
19. Casterline C: Allergy to chamomile teas. JAMA 1980;244:330–331.
20. CDC: Adverse events associated with ephedrine-containing products—Texas. MMWR 1996;45:689–693.

21. CDC: Anticholinergic poisoning associated with an herbal tea—New York City. MMWR 1995;44:193–195.
22. CDC: Chaparrel-induced toxic hepatitis—California and Texas. MMWR 1992;41:812–814.
23. CDC: Deaths associated with a purported aphrodisiac—New York City. MMWR 1995;44:853–861.
24. CDC: Folk remedy-associated lead poisoning in Hmong children. MMWR 1983;32:555–556. Also JAMA 1983;250; 3149–3150.
25. CDC: Jin Bu Huan toxicity in adults—Los Angeles. MMWR 1993;42:920–922.
26. CDC: Jin Bu Huan toxicity in children—Colorado. MMWR 1993;42:633–636.
27. CDC: Lead poisoning associated death from Asian Indian folk remedies—Florida. MMWR 1984;33:638–645.
28. CDC: Lead poisoning associated with traditional ethnic remedies—California, 1991–1992. MMWR 1993;42:521–524
29. CDC: Lead poisoning from lead tetroxide used as a folk remedy—Colorado. MMWR 1982;30:647–648.
30. CDC: Lead poisoning from Mexican folk remedies—California. MMWR 1983;32:554. Also JAMA 1983;250:3149.
31. CDC: Self-treatment with herbal and other plant-derived remedies—rural Mississippi, 1993. MMWR 1995;44:204–207.
32. CDC: Use of lead tetroxide as a folk remedy for gastrointestinal illness. MMWR 1981;30:546–547.
33. Chan JCN, Chan TYK, Chan KL, et al: Anticholinergic poisoning from Chinese herbal medicines. Aust NZ J Med 1994;24:317. Letter.
34. Chan TYK: Aconitine poisoning: A global perspective. Vet Human Toxicol 1994;36:326–328.
35. Chan TYK, Chan AYW, Critchley JAJH: Hospital admissions due to adverse reactions to Chinese herbal medicines. J Trop Med Hyg 1992;95:296–298.
36. Chan TYK, Chan JCN, Tomlinson B, et al: Chinese herbal medicines revisited: A Hong Kong perspective. Lancet 1993;342:1532–1534.
37. Chan TYK, Critchley JAJH: Usage and adverse effects of Chinese herbal medicines. Hum Exp Toxicol 1996;15:5–12.
38. Chan TYK, Tomlinson B, Chan WWM, et al: A case of acute aconitine poisoning caused by chuanwu and caowu. J Trop Med Hyg 1993;96:62–63.
39. Chan TYK, Tse LKK, Chan JCN, et al: Aconitine poisoning due to Chinese herbal medcines: A review. Vet Hum Toxicol 1994;36:452–455.
40. Chevalier A: The Encyclopedia of Medicinal Plants. New York, DK Publishing, 1996.
41. Chinese cucumber. Lawrence Review of Natural Products, Apr 1990.
42. Combie J, Nugent TE, Tobin T: Inability of goldenseal to interfere with the detection of morphine in urine. Equine Vet Sci, Jan/Feb 1982, pp. 16–21.
43. Cone LA, Boughton WH, Cone LA, et al: Rattlesnake capsule-induced *Salmonella arizonae* bacteremia. West J Med 1990;153;315–316.
44. Cook C, Baisden D: Ancillary use of folk medicine by patients in primary care clinics in southwestern West Virginia. South Med J 1986;79:1098–1101.
45. Cowley G: "Herbal warning." Newsweek, May 6, 1996, pp. 60–65.
46. D'Arcy PF: Adverse reactions and interactions with herbal medicines. Adverse Drug React Toxicol Rev 1991;10: 189–208.
47. Danesi MA, Adetunji JB: Use of alternative medicine by patients with epilepsy: A survey of 265 epileptic patients in a developing country. Epilepsia 1994;35:344–351.
48. DeSmet PA: Health risks of herbal remedies. Drug Safety 1995;13:81–93.
49. DeSmet PA: Toxicological outlook on the quality assurance of herbal remedies. Adverse Effects Herbal Drugs 1992;1:1–72.
50. Diamond JR, Pallone PL: Acute interstitial nephritis following use of Tung Shueh pills. Am J Kidney Dis 1994; 24:219–221.
51. Direct AIDS Alternative Information Resources: Buyer's Club Product Catalog, Dec 15, 1996.
52. Dolan G, Blumsohn A: Lead poisoning due to Asian ethnic treatment for impotence. J R Soc Med 1991;84:630–631.
53. Duke JA: CRC Handbook of Medicinal Herbs. Boca Raton, FL, CRC Press, 1985.
54. Eisenberg DM, Kessler RC, Foster C, et al: Unconventional medicine in the United States. N Engl J Med 1993;328: 246–252.
55. Espinoza EO, Mann MJ, Bleasdell B: Arsenic and mercury in traditional Chinese herbal balls. N Engl J Med 1995; 333:803–804. Letter.
56. Fitzpatrick AJ, Crawford M, Allan RM, et al: Aconite poisoning managed with a ventricular assist device. Anaesth Intensive Care 1994;22:714–717.
57. Food and Drug Administration: Federal register. Part II 21 CFR Part 101. Food labeling; Final Rule and Proposed Rules. Dec 28, 1995.
58. Foster S: Goldenseal: Masking of drug tests. HerbalGram 1989;21:7–8.
59. Fung MC, Weinbraub M, Bowen DL: Colloidal silver proteins marketed as health supplements. JAMA 1995;274: 1196–1197. Letter.
60. Garlic. Lawrence Review of Natural Products, Apr 1994.
61. Ginseng. Lawrence Review of Natural Products, Sept 1990.
62. Goldenseal. Lawrence Review of Natural Products, May 1994.
63. Gordon DW, Rosenthal G, Hart J, et al: Chaparral ingestion. JAMA 1995;273:489–490.
64. Haynes BE, Bessen HA, Wightman WD: Oleander tea: Herbal draught of death. Ann Emerg Med 1985;14:350–353.
65. Hill GJ: Lead poisoning due to Hai Ge Fen. JAMA 1995; 273:24–25.
66. Honerjager P, Meissner A: The positive inotropic effect of aconitine. Arch Pharmacol 1983;322:49–58.
67. Hsu CK, Leo P, Shastry D, et al: Anticholinergic poisoning associated with herbal tea. Arch Intern Med 1995;155: 2245–2248.
68. Hung OL, Shih RD, Chiang WK, et al: Herbal preparation usage among urban emergency department patients. Acad Emerg Med 1997;4:209–213.
69. Huxtable RJ: The harmful potential of herbal and other plant products. Drug Safety 1990;5(suppl 1):126–136.
70. Huxtable RJ: Herbal teas and toxins: Novel aspects of pyrrolizidine poisoning in the United States. Perspect Biol Med 1980;24:1–14.

71. Insel PA: Analgesic-antipyretic and antiinflammatory agents and drugs employed in the treatment of gout. In: Hardman JG, Limbird LE, eds: Goodman and Gilman's The Pharmacological Basis of Therapeutics, 9th ed. New York, McGraw-Hill, 1996.
72. Joubert PH: Poisoning admissions in black South Africans. J Toxicol Clin Toxicol 1990;28:85–94.
73. Kang-Yum E, Oransky SH: Chinese patent medicine as a potential source of mercury poisoning. Vet Hum Toxicol 1992; 34:235–238.
74. Kassler WJ, Blanc P, Greenblatt R: The use of medicinal herbs by human immunodeficiency virus-infected patients. Arch Intern Med 1991;151:2281–2288.
75. Kestin M, Miller L, Littlejohn G, et al: The use of medicinal herbs by human immunodeficiency virus-infected patients. Arch Intern Med 1991;151:2281–2288.
76. Ko RJ, Greenwald MS, Loscutoff SM, et al: Lethal ingestion of Chinese herbal tea containing Ch'an Su. West J Med 1996:164:71–75.
77. Kumana CR, Ng M, Lin HJ, et al: Herbal tea induced hepatic veno-occlusive disease: Quantification of toxic alkaloid exposure in adults. Gut 1985;26:101–104.
78. Lam CL, Catarivas MG, Munro C, et al: Self-medication among Hong Kong Chinese. Soc Sci Med 1994;39:1641–1647.
79. Larrey D, Pageaux GP: Hepatoxicity of herbal remedies and mushrooms. Semin Liver Dis 1995;15:183–188.
80. Larrey D, Vial T, Pauwels A, et al: Hepatitis after germander (*Teucrium chamaedrys*) administration: Another instance of herbal medicine hepatotoxicity. Ann Intern Med 1992;117:129–132.
81. LeGrand A, Sri-Ngernyuang L, Streefland PH: Enhancing appropriate drug use: The contribution of herbal medicine promotion. Soc Sci Med 1993;36:1023–1035.
82. Lewis W: Ginseng revisited. N Engl J Med 1980;243:31.
83. Lewis WH, Smith P: Poke root herbal tea poisoning. JAMA 1979;242:2759–2760.
84. Liberti LE, DerMarderosian A: Evaluation of commercial ginseng products. J Pharm Sci 1978;67:1487–1489.
85. Louman W, Danouske MD: The use of khat (*Catha edulis*) in Yemen social and medical observations. Ann Intern Med 1976;85:246–249.
86. Markowitz SB, Nunez CM, Klitzman S, et al: Lead poisoning due to Hai Ge Fen. The porphyric content of individual erythrocytes. JAMA 1994;271:932–934.
87. Marsh WW, Hentges K: Mexican folk remedies and conventional medical care. Am Fam Physician 1988;37:257–262.
88. Marwick C: Growing use of medicinal botanicals force assessment by drug regulators. JAMA 1995;273:607–609.
89. McKnight I, Scott M: HIV and complementary medicine. Med J Aust 1996;165:143–145.
90. Michie CA: The use of herbal remedies in Jamaica. Ann Trop Paediatr 1992;12:31–36.
91. Minor JR: Ginseng: Fact or fiction. Hosp Formul 1979; 186–192.
92. Mohabbat O, Younos MS, Merzad AA, et al: An outbreak of hepatic veno-occlusive disease in north-western Afghanistan. Lancet 1976;2:269–271.
93. Nebelkopf E: Herbal therapy in the treatment of drug use. Int J Addictions 1987;22:695–717.
94. Nelson L, Shih R, Hoffman R: Aplastic anemia induced by an adulterated herbal preparation. J Toxicol Clin Toxicol 1995;33:467–470.
95. Noskin GA, Clarke JT: *Salmonella arizonae* bacteremia as the presenting manifestation of human immunodeficiency virus infection following rattlesnake meat ingestion. Rev Infect Dis 1990;12:514–517.
96. Nutmeg. The Lawrence Review of Natural Products. Levittown, PA, Pharmaceutical Information Associates, Sept 1987.
97. Olsen P, Thorup I: Neurotoxicity in rats dosed with peppermint oil and pulegone. Arch Toxicol 1984;7(suppl): 408–409.
98. Ostrenga UJ, Perry D: Goldenseal. Pharmchem Newsl 1975;4.
99. Parsons JS: Contaminated herbal tea as a potential source of chronic arsenic poisoning. NC Med J 1981;42:38–39.
100. Pearl WS, Leo P, Tseng WO: Use of Chinese therapies among Chinese patients seeking emergency department care. Ann Emerg Med 1995;26:735–738.
101. Perharic L, Shaw D, Colbridge M, et al: Toxicological problems resulting from exposure to traditional remedies and food supplements. Drug Safety 1994;11:285–294.
102. Phillips LG, Nichols MH, King WD: Herbs and HIV: The health food industry's answer. South Med J 1995;88: 911–913.
103. Pillans PI: Toxicity of herbal products. NZ Med J 1995; 108:469–471.
104. Pontifex AH, Gary AK: Lead poisoning from an Asian Indian folk remedy. Can Med Assoc J 1985;133:1227–1228.
105. Prpic-Majic D, Pizent A, Jurasovic J, et al: Lead poisoning associated with the use of Ayurvedic meta-mineral tonics. J Toxicol Clin Toxicol 1996;34:417–423.
106. Reisine T, Pasternak G: Opioid analgesics and antagonists. In: Hardman JG, Limbird E, Molinoff PB, et al, eds: Goodman and Gilmans' The Pharmacological Basis of Therapeutics, 9th ed. New York, McGraw-Hill, 1996.
107. Ridker PM: Toxic effects of herbal teas. Arch Environ Health 1987;42:133–136.
108. Ridker PM, Okhuma S, McDermott WV, et al: Hepatic venocclusive disease associated with the consumption of pyrrolizidine containing dietary supplements. Gastroenterology 1985;88:1050–1054.
109. Ries CA, Sahud MA: Agranulocytosis caused by Chinese herbal medicines. JAMA 1975;231:352–355.
110. Riley KB, Antoniskis D, Maris R, et al: Rattlesnake capsule-associated *Salmonella arizonae* infections. Arch Intern Med 1988;148:1207–1210.
111. Safadi R, Levy I, Amitai Y, et al: Beneficial effect of digoxin-specific Fab antibody fragments in oleander intoxication. Arch Intern Med 1995;155:2121–2125.
112. Saint John's Wort. Lawrence Review of Natural Products, Jan 1995.
113. Saryan LA: Surreptitious lead exposure from an Asian Indian medication. J Anal Toxicol 1991;15:336–338.
114. Scott-Harland B: Common alternative therapies for AIDS. http://www.critpath.org/aric/altern
115. Segelman AB, Segelman FP, Karliner J, et al: Sassafras and herb tea: Potential health hazards. JAMA 1976;236:477.
116. Shumaik GM, Wu AW, Ping AC, et al: Oleander poison-

ing: Treatment with digoxin-specific Fab antibody fragments. Ann Emerg Med 1988;17:732–735.
117. Siegel RK: Ginseng abuse syndrome. JAMA 1979;241: 1614–1615.
118. Siegel RK: Herbal intoxication: Psychoactive effects from herbal cigarettes, tea, and capsules. JAMA 1976;236: 473–476.
119. Snodgrass G, Ziderman D, Gulati V, et al: Cosmetic plumbism. Br Med J 1973;27:230.
120. Snow LG: Folk medical beliefs and their implications for care of patients: A review based on studies among black patients. Ann Intern Med 1974;81:82–96.
121. Solecki RS: Shanidar IV, a neanderthal flower burial of northern Iraq. Science 1975;190:880.
122. Spoerke DG: Herbal medication: Use and misuse. Hosp Formul 1980;15:941–951.
123. Sullivan JB, Rumack BH, Thomas H, et al: Pennyroyal oil poisoning and hepatoxicity. JAMA 1979;242:2873–2874.
124. Tai YT, But PP-H, Young K, et al: Cardiotoxicity after accidental herb-induced aconite poisoning. Lancet 1992;340: 1254–1256.
125. Tandon BN, Handon HD, Tandon RK, et al: An epidemic of veno-occlusive disease of liver in central India. Lancet 1976;2:271–272.
126. Taylor RFH, Al-Jarad N, John LME, et al: Betel-nut chewing and asthma. Lancet 1992;330:1134–1136.
127. The Ephedras. Lawrence Review of Natural Products, Nov 1995.
128. Vanhaelen M, Vanhaelen-Fastre R, But P, et al: Identification of aristolochic acid in Chinese herbs. Lancet 1994;343: 174. Letter.
129. Vanherweghem JL, Depierreux M, Tielemans C, et al: Rapidly progressive interstitial renal fibrosis in young woman: Association with slimming regimen including Chinese herbs. Lancet 1993;341:387–391.
130. Verhoef MJ, Sutherland LR, Brkich L: Use of alternative medicine by patients attending a gastroenterology clinic. Can Med Assoc J 1990;142:121–125.
131. Waterman SH, Juarez G, Carr SJ, et al: *Salmonella arizonae* infections in Latinos associated with rattlesnake folk medicine. Am J Public Health 1990;80:286–289.
132. Woolf GM, Petrovic JM, Rojter SE: Acute hepatitis associated with the Chinese herbal product Jin Bu Huan. Ann Intern Med 1994;121:729–735.
133. Wormwood. Lawrence Review of Natural Products, Apr 1991.

Bibliography

Chevalier A: The Encyclopedia of Medicinal Plants. New York, DK Publishing, 1996.

The Lawrence Review of Natural Products Monograph System (ISSN 0734-4961). Levittown, PA, Pharmaceutical Information Associated.

Lewis WH, Elvin-Lewis MP: Medical Botany: Plants Affecting Man's Health. New York, Wiley, 1977.

Robbers JE, Speedie MK, Tyler VE: Pharmacognosy and Pharmacobiotechnology. Philadelphia, Williams & Wilkins, 1996.

Tyler VE: Herbs of Choice: The Therepeutic Use of Phytomedicinals. New York, Pharmaceutical Products Press, 1994.

Tyler VE: The Honest Herbal: A Sensible Guide to the Use of Herbs and Related Remedies, 3 ed. New York, Pharmaceutical Products Press, 1993.

CHAPTER 77

Plants

Richard D. Shih and Lewis R. Goldfrank

CASE 1. An 18-month-old child was brought to the emergency department (ED) by his mother. The woman held four large leaves in her hand and reported that she had discovered the child playing with several of the plants in her living room. She feared he had ingested some of the leaves.

The child was screaming and salivating profusely. Vital signs were: blood pressure, 90/60 mm Hg; pulse, 120 beats/min; respiratory rate, 20 breaths/min; temperature, 99°F (37.2°C).

The child's mouth showed diffuse erythema and swelling of the lips, buccal mucosa, and tongue. There was a 1-cm bullous lesion on the anterior aspect of the tongue. The uvula was normal in size and color, and there was no stridor. Indirect laryngoscopy revealed a normal pharynx and vocal cords. Heart and lung examinations were unremarkable. Bowel sounds were normal with no abdominal tenderness. The extremities were normal. Milk was offered, but the child was unable to swallow.

The four different leaves the mother brought were easily identified as African violet, coleus, wandering Jew, and dumbcane (*Dieffenbachia*). Swelling of the lips and buccal mucosa is characteristic of dumbcane and implicated this plant as the toxic agent. The child was admitted for observation and intravenous hydration. Admission is rarely indicated unless there is severe edema and concern for protection of the upper airway. The swelling decreased overnight and the child was discharged the subsequent day. The mother was advised to "poison-proof" her home and was given several suggestions for safety in and around her home.

CASE 2. Four adolescents, aged 12–17 years, presented to the ED one evening in late August. One of the boys was actively hallucinating; another complained of diminished vision and an intensely dry mouth. The other two youths were anxious but quite cooperative.

They said they had been at a beach party drinking wine and a tea made of weeds growing wild on the beach. They had been using this "locoweed" to stay high during their summer vacation.

The 15-year-old was agitated and actively communicating with an invisible girlfriend. He believed he was still at the beach and refused to change from his bathing trunks. His vital signs were: blood pressure, 100/60 mm Hg; pulse, 120 beats/min; respiratory rate, 20 breaths/min; temperature, 100.4°F (38°C). His skin was slightly moist and acyanotic, but the oral mucosa was dry. His pupils were equal, dilated (8 mm), unresponsive to light. Extraocular movements were intact. The lungs, heart, and abdomen examinations were unremarkable except for diminished bowel sounds, and the bladder was distended to the level of the umbilicus.

The patient was not oriented to person, place, or time. Short-term memory was impaired, and he continued to hallucinate, claiming that the beach was full of "little people." He said his girlfriend was so small she could be "put into my pocket." Neurologic examination revealed mild ataxia. Deep tendon reflexes and cranial nerves were grossly intact.

The patient's initial presentation was that of anticholinergic toxicity. Given the known local distribution and frequent association with the street name "locoweed," the initial diagnosis was that of Jimson weed (*Datura stramonium*) poisoning. Because of the strong anticholinergic effects of the plant, the patient was given 2 mg of physostigmine IV over 5 minutes (see Antidotes in Depth: Physostigmine). Within 10 minutes he became cooperative. Within 30 minutes his pupils became reactive and decreased to 3 mm. Mucosal secretions returned to normal, his heart rate decreased to 70 beats/min, and he voided 1100 mL of urine.

Subsequently he was given activated charcoal (50 g) and magnesium sulfate (30 g). The patient's CBC, BUN, glucose, electrolytes, and ECG were normal except for a WBC count of 14,600 mm^3.

During the initial night in the hospital, the patient had several recurrent episodes of hallucinations. He was given 0.5–1.0 mg of physostigmine IV on two additional occasions, which controlled the symptoms.

By the end of the first hospital day, the patient's hallucinations had ceased and the WBC count had returned to normal. The following morning he was discharged. The other adolescents were managed in the ED with supportive therapy, activated charcoal, and cathartic. They were discharged after 4 hours of observation to the care of their parents.

How Common Are Plant Ingestions? Who Is Most Likely to Ingest Plants?

Five to ten percent of all human exposures reported to poison control centers involve plants. Probably because plants are so accessible and attractive to youngsters, in approximately 80% of these cases the individuals are younger than 6 years of age.[97–101] As indoor plants have become more popular, the incidence of plant ingestion has increased. Data compiled by the American Association of Poison Control Centers (AAPCC) gives some indication of which plants are most commonly involved in exposures.[96–105]

Table 77–1 lists the plants most frequently reported to poison control centers.[96–105] Although household plants are most commonly reported, these plants typically have relatively limited toxicity (Table 77–2). More than 80% of those patients exposed to plants reported to the AAPCC were asymptomatic. Fewer than 20% had minor to moderate symptomatology. Fewer than 7% required a visit to a health care facility. Fatalities occurred in fewer than 0.001% of reported outcomes.[97–99,101,102]

What Should Be Done if the Plant Involved in an Exposure Is Unknown?

The majority of plant exposures to young children involve an unknown plant. The approach to a patient exposed to an unknown plant depends on the presenting symptomatology and the availability of the plant for inspection. With the myriad of possible plant species, toxins, and clinical presentations, plant identification is an essential step in patient evaluation and management.[170] Specific antidotal therapy depends on the knowledge of the plant toxin involved. If samples of the plant are not available, it is very useful to return to the site of exposure to obtain the plant or a part of it for identification. Simultaneously, decontamination measures need to be considered, and if any symptoms are present, supportive care should be rendered and a differential diagnosis developed.

TABLE 77–1. MOST FREQUENTLY REPORTED PLANT EXPOSURES (IN ORDER OF FREQUENCY)

Botanical Name	Common Name
Brassaia and *Schefflera* spp.	Umbrella tree
Capsicum annum	Pepper
Crassula spp.	Jade plant
Dieffenbachia spp.	Dumbcane
Euphorbia pulcherrima	Poinsettia
Ilex spp.	Holly
Philodendron spp.	Philodendron
Phytolacca americana	Pokeweed
Spathiphyllum spp.	Peace lily
Toxicodendron radicans	Poison ivy

Data compiled from American Association of Poison Control Centers data collection system annual reports, references 96–105.

If the plant or part of it is available, then plant identification should occur. Involvement of a local botanist or poison center is recommended. Several computer database systems have been developed that may be useful to help in plant identification.[28] These systems were originally developed for veterinary use but are also applicable to human exposures. Another potential aid in the identification of an unknown plant is to fax a photocopy of the plant in question to someone with greater botanical skills.[112] The limits of this technique are not adequately studied and should be employed only when an onsite botanist is unavailable. In addition to standard texts and references, the World Wide Web is another source of botanical information. An increasing number of rapidly changing websites are easily found for this purpose. It is unclear how accurate the information from these internet sources are; however, one particular website administered by the Food and Drug Administration offers over 18,000 bibliographic references on poisonous plants (Poisonous Plant Database, "PLANTOX").[170]

What Are the Characteristics of the Most Commonly Reported Plant Exposures?

The plants that are most commonly involved in human exposures tend to be relatively nontoxic and typically of the household type (Table 77–2). These plants will be dis-

TABLE 77–2. NONTOXIC HOUSEPLANTS

Common Name	Botanical Name
African violet	*Saintpaulia ionantha or Episcia reptans*
Aluminum plant	*Pilea cadierei*
Aralia, false	*Dizygotheca elegantissima or Fatsia japonica*
Baby's tears	*Helxine soleirolii*
Begonia	*Begonia semperflorens*
Bird's nest fern	*Asplenium nidus*
Boston fern	*Nephrolepis exaltata*
Bridal veil	*Tradescantia*
Christmas cactus	*Schlumberga bridgesii*
Coleus	*Coleus blumei*
Corn plant	*Dracena fragrans*
Creeping Charlie	*Pilea nummularifolia, Plectranthus australis*
Creeping Jenny	*Lysimachia nummularia*
Donkey tail	*Sedum morganianun*
Emerald ripple	*Peperomia caperata*
Fiddleleaf fig	*Ficus lyrata*
Gardenia	*Gardenia radicans*
Grape ivy	*Cissus rhombifolia*
Hawaiian ti	*Cordyline terminalis*
Hen and chicks	*Echeveria* spp., *Sempervivum tectorus*
Jade tree	*Crassula argentea*
Lipstick plant	*Aeschynanthus lobbianus*
Monkey plant	*Ruellia makoyana*
Monther-in-law's tongue	*Sansevieria trifasciata*
Parlor palm	*Chamaedorea elegans*
Peacock plant	*Calathea makoyana*
Piggy-back plant	*Tolmiea menziesii*
Pink polka dot plant	*Hypoestes phyllostachya*
Prayer plant	*Maranta leuconeura*
Rosary vine[a]	*Ceropegia woodii*
Rosary pearls[a]	*Senico rowleyanus or Senico herreianus*
Rubber plant	*Ficus elastica*
Sensitive plant	*Mimosa pudica*
Snake plant	*Sansevieria trifasciata*
Spider plant	*Chlorophytum comosum*
String of hearts	*Creopegia woodii*
Swedish ivy	*Plectranthus australis*
Umbrella plant (Schefflera)	*Brassaia actinophylla*
Wandering Jew	*Tradescantia albiflora, Zebrina pendula*
Wax plant	*Hoya camosa* or *Hoya exotica*
Weeping fig	*Ficus benjamina*
Zebra plant	*Aphelandra squarrosa*

It should be noted that several different species have identical common names. Some may cause diarrhea in infants.

[a]Should not be confused with the fatally toxic rosary pea (*Abrus precatorius*).

Modified after Mary Bridge Children's Health Center Poison Information Service, San Francisco Bay Area Poison Center, and the New York Botanical Gardens.

cussed in this section and will be listed in alphabetical order.

Brassaia and *Schefflera* spp. (Umbrella Tree)

Brassaia and *Schefflera* species are popular indoor trees commonly known as the umbrella tree, Australian umbrella tree, rubber tree, and starleaf. Ingestion of this plant is thought to be nontoxic. Although these trees contain calcium oxalate crystals, the severity of toxicity is not as great as that following ingestion of other plants containing similar concentrations of calcium oxalate, such as *Dieffenbachia* (dumbcane).[149,151] The reason for this is unclear but may be due to the organization or packaging of the calcium oxalate in this plant (see the section on *Dieffenbachia* below).[47,49,52]

Skin exposures to this species during gardening are commonly reported. Contact dermatitis has been reproduced by patch testing with falcarinol,[63] which is found throughout these plants.

Capsicum annum (Chili Pepper)

This genus includes most of the cultivated peppers of North America. They are used as spices, ornamental plants, or as an active ingredient in protective repellents such as dog repellents and mace-like agents.[173] Common names include chili pepper, cherry pepper, cone pepper, cluster pepper, cayenne pepper, Christmas pepper, and red pepper.

The toxicity is related to the irritant effects of the alkaloid capsaicin and four naturally occurring associated derivatives: dihydrocapsaicin, nordihydrocapsaicin, homocapsaicin, and homodihydrocapsaicin. These alkaloids are irritants theorized to cause their effects by depleting nerve terminals of substance P.[18,167] Blocking substance P–induced dilation of local blood vessels and stimulation of sensory nerve endings results in local swelling and pain.[18,159] This initial intense excitation of sensory nerve endings is thought to be followed by a period of relative insensitivity to various stimuli and is the physiologic basis for its use as an active ingredient in some analgesic creams.[11] These alkaloids have no specific effects on the motor system.[159]

Even transient exposure to mucous membranes or nonintact skin elicits intense and immediate symptoms. Prolonged exposure to intact skin, however, can also produce symptomatology.[168,174] This effect depends on length of exposure, individual sensitivity, and the area of skin involved (related to the thickness of the stratum corneum).[168] Symptoms following cutaneous exposure include burning, stinging, and/or pain.[168,174] Nausea, vomiting, abdominal cramping, and burning diarrhea may occur with large oral exposures.[35] Eye exposure causes intense tearing, pain, conjunctivitis, and blepharospasm.[159]

Although exposed individuals experience severe pain and discomfort, they do not suffer long-term sequelae. Treatment involves copious local irrigation and/or systemic analgesics.[73] Eye exposures, despite their initial dramatic presentations, are treated similarly, with irrigation and local analgesics, and usually resolve without sequelae in 24 hours.[57]

Crassula spp. (Jade Plant)

The jade plant is a popular houseplant. No toxin has been isolated from this plant and it is considered nontoxic.[149] There is a single reported case of a 1-year-old

TABLE 77–3. PLANT TOXICITY, WITH AN EMPHASIS ON PLANTS APPROPRIATELY OR MISTAKENLY INGESTED AS FOODS

I. Plants that are gastroenteric irritants
- A. Plants producing irritation primarily of the mouth and throat: edema, bullae, salivation, dysphagia, dysarthria
  Precipitant: water-insoluble calcium oxalate crystals and a proteolytic enzyme
  1. Philodendron (*Philodendron* spp.)
  2. Dumbcane (*Dieffenbachia* spp.)
  3. Caladium (*Caladium* spp.)
  4. Jack-in-the-pulpit (*Arisaema triphyllum*)
  5. Elephant ear (*Colocasia* spp.)
  6. Skunk cabbage (*Symplocarpus foetidus*)
  7. Pothos (*Scindapsus aureus*)
- B. Irritation chiefly of gastric mucosa
  Symptoms: local and centrally initiated emesis
  1. Daffodil (*Narcissus pseudonarcissus*)
  2. Spider lily (*Liliaceae* spp.)
  3. Narcissus (*Narcissus* spp.)
  4. Balsam pear (*Mornordica charantia*) ψ
  5. Amaryllis (*Hippeastrum equestre*)
  6. Hyacinth (*Hyacinthus orientalis*)
- C. Irritation chiefly of intestinal mucosa
  Symptoms: emesis, abdominal pain, colic, diarrhea, and melena
  1. **Horse chestnut (*Aesculus hippocastanum*)**
  2. English ivy (*Hedera helix*)
  3. **Pokeweed (*Phytolacca americana*)** ψ
  4. Yew (*Taxus* spp.)
  5. Baneberry (*Actaea* spp.)
- D. Plants producing delayed gastroenteritis
  1. Lectin (toxalbumin) group
     Symptoms: burning in mouth, nausea, vomiting, diarrhea, dehydration, headache, CNS depression, seizures, shock
     - a. Castor bean (*Ricinus communis*) (color plate Fig. 2)
     - b. Rosary pea (*Abrus precatorius*) (color plate Fig. 1)
     - c. Black locust (*Robinia pseudoacacia*)
     - d. Sandbox tree (*Hura crepitans*)
  2. Solanine group, glycoalkaloids
     Symptoms: nausea, vomiting, diarrhea, headache, muscle weakness
     - **a. Potato (*Solanum tuberosum*)**
     - b. Black nightshade (*Solanum nigrum*)
     - c. Tomato (*Lycopersicon esculentum*)
     - d. Jerusalem cherry (*Solanum pseudocapsicum*)
     - e. Ground cherry (*Physalis heterophylla*)
  3. Colchicine group
     Symptoms: nausea, crampy abdominal pain, diarrhea, hematochezia
     - a. Autumn crocus (*Colchicum autumnale*)
     - b. Glory lily (*Gloriosa superba*)
- E. Diverse symptoms, including gastrointestinal
  1. Bleeding heart (*Dicentra* spp.)
  2. Bloodroot (*Sanguinaria canadensis*)
  3. Buttercup (*Ranunculus* spp.)
  4. Mayapple (*Podophyllum peltatum*)
  5. **Rhubarb (*Rheum rhaponticum*)** ψ

II. Plants producing cardiovascular disturbances
- A. Cardiac glycoside group
  Symptoms: nausea, vomiting, cardiac dysrhythmias
  1. Lily of the valley (*Convallaria majalis*)
  2. Foxglove (*Digitalis purpurea*)
  3. Yellow oleander (*Thevetia peruviana*)
  4. Oleander (*Nerium oleander*)
- B. Aconitine group
  Symptoms: nausea, vomiting, dysesthesias, hypotension, bradycardia, respiratory failure, ventricular dysrhythmias
  1. Monkshood (*Aconitum napellus*)
- C. Veratrum group
  Symptoms: nausea, vomiting, diarrhea, dysesthesias hypotension, bradycardia
  1. False or green hellebore (*Veratrum viride*)
- D. Grayanotoxins (Veratrine and Andromedotoxin) group
  Symptoms: salivation, lacrimation, rhinorrhea, emesis, weakness, bradycardia, hypotension
  1. Death camas (*Zigadenus*)
  2. Azalea (*Rhododendron* spp.)
  3. Rhododendron (*Rhododendron* spp.)
  4. Mountain laurel (*Kalmia latifolia*)

III. Plants having a nicotinelike action
Symptoms: salivation, headache, nausea, vomiting, ataxia, coma, seizures, hypotension, respiratory compromise
1. Poison hemlock (*Conium maculatum*)
2. Wild tobacco (*Nicotiana glauca*)
3. Golden chain (*Laburnum anagyroides*)

IV. Belladonna alkaloid–containing plants
Anticholinergic symptoms: mydriasis, dry skin, vasodilation, ileus, dysrhythmias, altered mental status
1. Belladonna, deadly nightshade (*Atropa belladonna*)
2. Angel's trumpet (*Solandra* spp.)
3. **Jimson weed (*Datura stramonium*) (color plate 3)**

V. Plants acting primarily on the central nervous system
- A. Convulsants
  1. Water hemlock (*Cicuta maculata*)
- B. Hallucinogens
  1. Peyote (*Lophophora williamsii*)
  2. **Nutmeg and mace (*Myristica fragrans*)**
  3. Morning glory (*Ipomoea* spp.)

VI. Cyanogenic plants: amygdalin, cyanogenic glycosides
Symptoms: Delayed onset, vomiting, rapid deterioration with symptoms of tissue hypoxia
1. Elderberry (*Sambucus canadensis*)
2. Hydrangea (*Hydrangea macrophylla*)
3. Tapioca plant (*Manihot esculenta*)
4. **Almond, apricot, cherry (*Prunus* spp.)**

VII. Hepatotoxic plants
1. **Akeé (*Bilghia sapida*)**
2. Comfrey (*Symphytum officinale*) } carcinogenic
3. Sassafras (*Sassafras albidum*) } carcinogenic

VIII. Miscellaneous Christmas poisonous plants
1. Mistletoe (*Phoradendron flavescens*)
2. Holly (*Ilex* spp.)
3. Poinsettia (*Euphorbia pulcherrima*)

IX. Plant dermatitis
- A. Mechanical injury
  1. Dumbcane (*Dieffenbachia maculata*)
  2. Philodendron (*Philodendron* spp.)
  3. Cow's horn (*Euphorbia grandicornis*)
- B. Chemical injury
  1. Creeping spurge (*Euphorbia myrsinites*)
  2. Pencil cactus (*Euphorbia tirucalli*)
  3. Candelabra cactus (*Euphorbia lactea*)
  4. Manchineel, beach apple (*Hippomane mancinella*)

(*continued*)

TABLE 77–3. PLANT TOXICITY, WITH AN EMPHASIS ON PLANTS APPROPRIATELY OR MISTAKENLY INGESTED AS FOODS (continued)

C. Allergic contact dermatitis
  1. Poison ivy (*Toxicodendron radicans*) (color plate Fig. 7)
  2. Poison oak—eastern (*Toxicodendron toxicarium*), western (*Toxicodendron diversilobum*)
  3. Poison sumac (*Toxicodendron vernix*)
  4. Gingko (*Gingko biloba*)
  5. Cashew (*Anacardium occidentale*)
  6. Mango (*Mangifera indica*)

D. Contact urticaria
  1. Stinging nettle (*Urtica dioica*) and wood nettle (*Laporatea canadensis*)
  2. Cowitch (*Mucuna pruriens*)
  3. Bull nettle (*Cridoscolus stimulosus*)
  4. Agave, century plant (*Agave americana*)
  5. Primrose (*Primula* spp.)

E. Phytophotodermatitis
  1. Cow parsnip (*Heracleum lanatum*)
  2. Wild parsnip (*Pastinaca sativa var pratensis*)
  3. Lime (*Citrus anrantiifolia*)

Those substances taken as food are in **bold type.** Ψ = edible with special preparation.

TABLE 77–4. POISONOUS AND INJURIOUS PLANTS OUTSIDE THE HOME

Common Name	Botanical Name
Poisonous plants and flowers of the flower garden	
Amaryllis	*Amaryllis belladonna*
Autumn crocus	*Colchicum autumnale*
Bleeding heart	*Dicentra spectabilis*
Daffodil	*Narcissus pseudonarcissus*
Foxglove	*Digitalis purpurea*
Glory lily	*Gloriosa superba*
Hyacinth	*Hyacinthus* spp.
Hydrangea	*Hydrangea* spp.
Iris	*Iris* spp.
Larkspur	*Delphinium ajacis*
Lily of the valley	*Convallaria majalis*
Monkshood	*Aconitum napellus, Aconitum columbianum*
Narcissus	*Narcissus* spp.
Nicotiana	*Nicotiana* spp.
Primrose	*Primula* spp.
Spider lily	*Crinum asiaticum*
Poisonous ornamental plants and flowers	
American holly	*Ilex opaca*
Azalea	*Rhododendron* spp.
Common privet	*Ligustrum vulgare*
Daphne	*Daphne mezereum*
English ivy	*Hedera* spp.
Golden chain	*Laburnum anagyroides*
Jessamine (yellow, Carolina)	*Gelsemium sempervirens*
Lantana	*Lantana camara*
Mountain laurel	*Kalmia* spp.
Nightshade	*Atropa belladonna*
Oleander	*Nerium oleander*
Rhododendron	*Rhododendron* spp.
Wisteria	*Wisteria* spp.
Yew	*Taxus* spp.

Common Name	Botanical Name
Poisonous trees and shrubs with toxic seeds, fruits, or other parts	
Apple	*Malus* spp.
Black locust (seeds and bark)	*Robinia pseudoacacia*
Buckeye, horse chestnut	*Aesculus* spp.
Chinaberry tree	*Melia azedarach*
Cherry (choke)	*Prunus* spp.
Elderberry	*Sambucus* spp.
Gingko	*Gingko biloba*
Oleander (all parts)	*Nerium oleander*
Sand box tree	*Hura crepitans*
Yew	*Taxus* spp.
Poisonous wild flowers of the woods	
Bloodroot	*Sanguinaria canadensis*
Hellebore (false)	*Veratrum viride*
Jack-in-the-pulpit	*Arisaema* spp.
Mayapple (except the fruit)	*Podophyllum peltatum*
Skunk cabbage	*Symplocarpus foetidus*
Water hemlock	*Cicuta* spp.
Poisonous wild flowers of the fields	
Buttercup	*Ranunculus* spp.
Death camas	*Zigadenus* spp.
Jimson weed	*Datura stramonium*
Nettles (stinging, bull)	*Urtica dioica, Cridoscolus stimulosus*
Nightshades	*Solanum* spp.
Poison hemlock	*Conium maculatum*
Pokeweed	*Phytolacca americana*
Tobacco	*Nicotiana glauca*

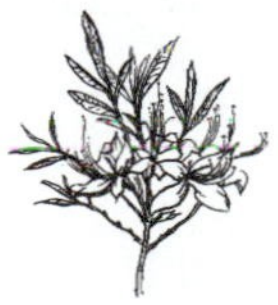
Azalea

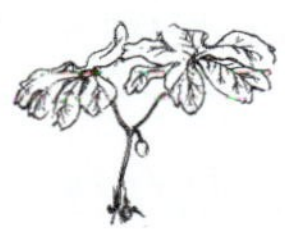
Mayapple

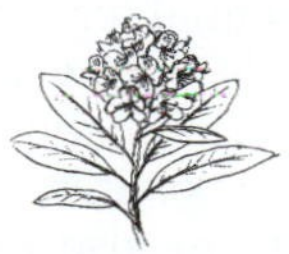
Rhododendron

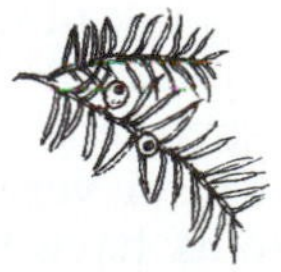
Yew

child who ingested a large number of leaves and had symptoms of persistent diarrhea and perianal dermatitis.[142]

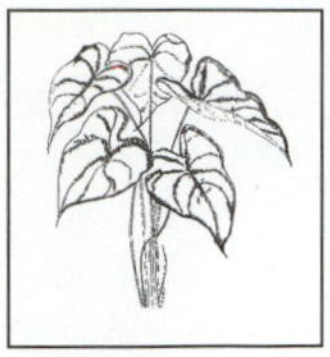

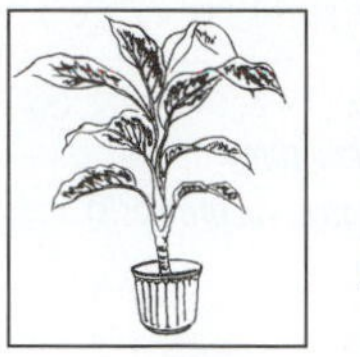

Dieffenbachia spp. (Dumbcane)

The leaves of the *Dieffenbachia* are large, smooth, and green on the periphery and mottled white in the center. Common names for this plant include dumbcane, dumbplant, mother-in-law's tongue, and tuftroot. Ingestion of any part of this plant causes severe local symptoms, especially when the leaves are chewed.[118] Immediate pain and swelling result, limiting further exposure.[42,49,118] The mechanism for the production of these local effects is controversial. The calcium oxalate crystals are spearlike and packaged in raphides.[130] One to two hundred raphides are bundled together and located in idioblasts.[130,140] These idioblasts are cigar-shaped structures with specialized nozzles at each end, capable of firing the needlelike raphides in a projectile fashion.[130] The idioblasts also contain proteolytic enzymes, which are released when the raphides are fired.[130] When a mechanical force is applied to a *Dieffenbachia* leaf, such as biting into the leaf, thousands of idioblasts fire the needlelike calcium oxalate crystals, which penetrate mucous membranes and deposit proteolytic enzymes.[130] These proteolytic enzymes, reported to have trypsin-like activity, may stimulate a cascade of events leading to bradykinin and histamine release and, ultimately, local swelling and pain. Bradykinin release has been demonstrated in vitro.[87,88] In one human study histamine levels were shown to be increased after local application of *Dieffenbachia* to the tongue.[47] Since other plants, such as *Philodendron* spp., *Brassaia* spp., and *Schefflera* spp., contain similar concentrations of calcium oxalate crystals but do not produce similar local irritant effects, calcium oxalate crystals alone do not account for the toxic effects.[47,151]

Patients may describe oral exposure to *Dieffenbachia* leaf as biting down on a hornet's nest or chewing ground glass. Although most cases involve unintentional ingestion by children, some cases have resulted from pranks in which the patient was fed a salad or sandwich made from these leaves.

Most cases of dumbcane toxicity involve oral exposure causing immediate and severe symptoms of pain and local swelling.[8] Local treatment with cold milk or ice cream as a demulcent is sufficient in most cases. Severe exposures may progress to profuse salivation, dysphagia, pain, loss of speech, and the potential for respiratory compromise.[36,44,107] Parenteral opioids, intravenous fluids, corticosteroids, and endotracheal intubation may be indicated in very rare and large exposures. Systemic symptoms have been reported but are also extremely rare because local symptoms typically limit the amount of plant ingested.[149] Ocular exposure to sap may result in severe pain, chemical conjunctivitis, corneal abrasions, and, rarely, permanent corneal opacifications.[95] Calcium oxalate crystals have been identified on the corneal epithelium, but in animal experiments other toxic irritants play a more important role in the pathologic process.[40,117] Copious irrigation, systemic analgesics, and ophthalmologic consultation are necessary for this type of exposure.

Euphorbia pulcherrima (Poinsettia)

This popular ornamental Christmas plant has large, 4–6-inch leaves with serrated margins. Leaves become bright red, yellow, or pink in the fall. The poinsettia is a member of the Euphorbiaceae, more commonly known as the spurges. There are more than 7000 species in this family; many of them produce a milky latex.

This plant has inappropriately gained a reputation of significant toxicity capable of causing mortality. A single inadequately documented case report from Hawaii in 1919 involving the death of a 2-year-old child is most likely responsible for frequent citations expressing this concern.[136] The vast majority of thousands of reported poinsettia ingestions have not been associated with consequential toxic manifestations.[81,177]

Oral ingestion usually causes no symptoms or minimal GI complaints of nausea, vomiting, and abdominal cramping.[108] Oral mucosal burns were reported in one case of an 8-month-old child who chewed one of the leaves, but this is uncommon.[37] Severe contact dermatitis has been infrequently reported.[31] The diterpene esters found throughout the plant are thought to be responsible for the dermatologic manifestations.[31]

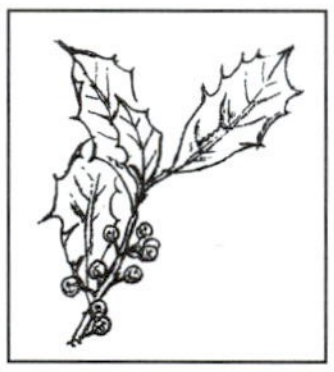

Ilex spp. (Holly)

The *Ilex* genus, with more than 300 species, are trees or shrubs characterized by green leaves with sharp spines on the margins and attractive red or black berries (Tables 77–3 and 77–4). Exposures frequently involve young children during the winter holidays, when the plant is commonly used as an ornament.

Ingestions usually involve the berries, as the leaves have numerous sharp spines that inhibit ingestion. Gastrointestinal symptoms, when present, include nausea, vomiting, abdominal cramping, and diarrhea.[137] Although alkaloids, polyphenols, saponins, steroids, and triterpenes have been extracted from *Ilex* spp., it is unclear which toxin is responsible for these symptoms.[175]

Treatment is often unnecessary but in severe cases may involve activated charcoal, fluid resuscitation, and supportive care.

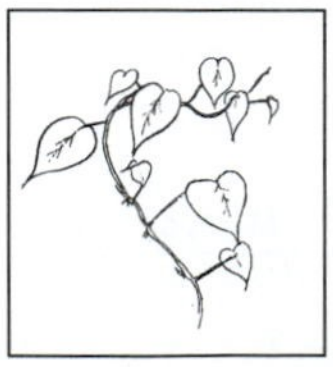

Philodendron spp.

Philodendron spp., with variously shaped, glossy, dark green leaves, are very popular houseplants. Common names for these plants include panda plant and parlor ivy. Ingestion is generally associated with minimal symptoms, although there are anecdotal reports of mucosal irritation, local swelling, and GI irritation.[90,111] These plants contain calcium oxalate crystals, but exposure usually does not lead to the same severity of toxicity experienced with other plants containing similar concentrations (eg, dumbcane and caladium).[47,49,133,145] The reason for this is unclear but may be due to the packaging of the calcium oxalate in *Philodendron* (see section on *Dieffenbachia*).[130]

In sensitized individuals, cutaneous exposure to the leaves produces a delayed contact dermatitis that is reproducible by patch testing. The responsible substance is thought to be the alkyl agent, resorcinol, found throughout the plant.[132]

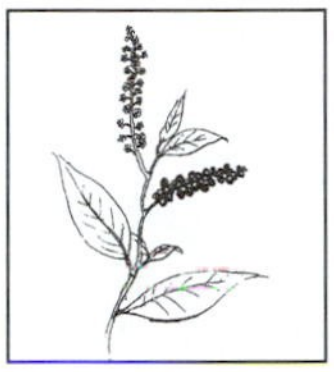

Phytolacca americana (Pokeweed)

A native shrublike plant of the eastern United States, this is a popular plant used in salads (after detoxification), especially in the southeast. *Phytolacca* grows to a height of 5–10 ft and produces attractive berries that mature from green to deep purple. Common names include pokeweed, pokeberry, poke, inkberry, scoke, pigeonberry, American cancer, and garget. All parts of the plant contain the toxins phytolaccine and pokeweed mitogen.[135] The root has the highest concentration and the more mature purple berries are less toxic.[38] Phytolaccine is a potent GI irritant, and pokeweed mitogen causes mitosis of lymphoid cells.[6,7,135] In preparation for eating, the plant is typically detoxified by a double-boiling technique known as parboiling. The leaves are boiled twice and the water is changed between boiling. Despite the use of this technique, there are reported cases of toxicity from ingestion.[17]

Toxic exposures typically involve ingestion of poorly detoxified pokeweed salad or pokeroot tea. Symptoms begin 0.5–6 hours after ingestion and include severe recurrent nausea, vomiting, abdominal cramping, and diarrhea. Severe cases have been reported to cause hemorrhagic gastritis.[20,135] A lymphocytosis is usually seen 2–4 days after exposure secondary to the pokeweed mitogen. This effect resolves spontaneously within 10 days and is without consequence.[6,7]

Treatment is supportive, often necessitating antiemetics and intravenous rehydration. Activated charcoal can be given in hopes of adsorbing the GI toxin. Symptoms usually resolve within 24 hours without other sequelae.

Spathiphyllum spp. (Peace Lily)

Spathiphyllum species are common houseplants with large, glossy, green leaves that contain calcium oxalate crystals.[115] Common names include peace lily, white anthurium, spathe flower, snowflower, and Mauna Loa.

There are no published case reports of serious ingestions, but because of the calcium oxalate crystals, symptoms similar to those of *Dieffenbachia* (dumbcane) ingestion can be anticipated.[149] The majority of ingestions reported to poison control centers result in no toxicity or minimal GI symptoms.

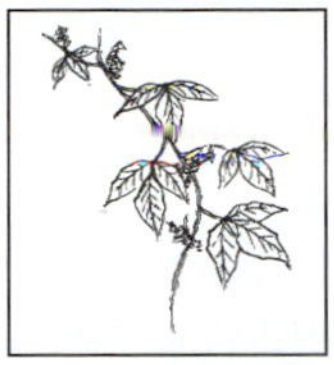

Toxicodendron radicans (Poison Ivy) and Other Plant-Induced Dermatitis

The major types of dermatitis are mechanical injury, chemical injury, allergic contact dermatitis (see Color Plate Fig. 8), contact urticaria, and phytophotodermatitis (see Chap. 28).[90] The most important type of plant dermatitis is *Toxicodendron* dermatitis, because of its frequency. This results from exposure to poison ivy (*Toxicodendron radicans*; see above), poison oak (*Toxicodendron diversilobum* and *Toxicodendron quercifolium*), or poison sumac (*Toxicodendron vernix*), all members of the Anacardiaceae family.

Toxicodendron diversilobum thrives on the west coast of the United States, while *T. radicans* is abundant everywhere except the west coast. These plants may be climbing vines or crawling species. The clustered three leaflets are green and waxy in spring and yellow or red in the fall, with white berries.

Toxicodendrol, the oily resin present in these plants, contains the active principle urushiol, which is a mixture of antigenic catechols. The toxicodendron antigens act as haptens that, on contact, penetrate the skin and bind to form complete antigens.[128]

The Anacardiaceae are responsible for more cases of contact dermatitis than any other plant or product and commonly bring patients to the ED. Most individuals are sensitized to this antigen and very few are immune to these ubiquitous plants.[45]

What Plants Are Most Likely to Cause Serious Toxicity?

In cases of plant toxicity, the history is usually poor. The plant in question may not have been brought with the patient or identification may be difficult. Fortunately, the symptomatology of various plants can be grouped into general categories, such as gastrointestinal (GI), central nervous system (CNS), and cardiovascular (see Table 77–3). Uncommon plant exposures are beyond the scope of this chapter. The plants most likely to cause serious toxicity are discussed in this section. Groups of plants with common toxins or individual plants will be presented in alphabetical order.

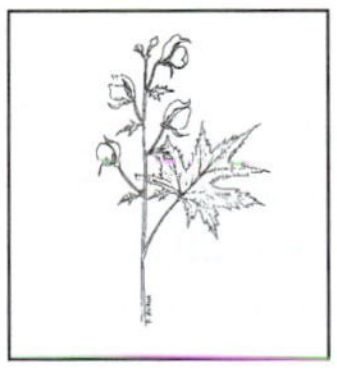

Aconitine. Representative Plant: *Aconitum napellus* (Monkshood)

The aconitum family consists of hundreds of different species that contain varying amounts of aconitine alkaloids. Several dozen of these alkaloids are found in these plants. They are all diterpene or norditerpine alkaloids with cardiovascular effects. A common plant of this family frequently reported in exposures is the monkshood. Other common names for this plant include aconite, wolfsbane, helmet flower, soldiers' cap, old wife's hood, aconitine, and friar's cap. This perennial herb is distinguished by its flowers, which are situated at the end of its stalk, resemble a helmet, and come in several colors (blue, whitish-pink, and purple).

The toxin's mechanism is not well understood but seems to be related to augmentation of the parasympathetic system mediated by the vagal nerve.[1,79] Bradycardic effects may be reversed with atropine. Further, increased ventricular automaticity via a direct cardiac effect has been proposed.[171]

Aconitine alkaloids are rapidly absorbed in the GI tract. Symptom onset is rapid and is initially manifested by paresthesias and numbness throughout the body. Later-developing symptoms include severe nausea, vomiting, abdominal cramping, and diarrhea. Severe cases manifest CNS and respiratory effects. Atrioventricular blocks, multifocal premature ventricular contractions, torsades de pointes, ventricular tachycardia, ventricular fibrillation, and respiratory muscle paralysis have been reported.[46,114,155,160,171]

No specific antidote exists for this toxin. In the past, tannic acid or potassium permanganate were recommended as lavage solutions to inactivate the toxins.[155] These modalities, however, are not supported experimentally, have additional side effects, and are not recommended.

Aggressive supportive care including decontamination may be necessary. A 32-year-old male ingested an aconite herbal preparation and developed refractory hypotension and ventricular dysrhythmias. He was treated with multiple antidysryhthmic agents without success and finally responded to cardiac pacing and the use of a left ventricular assist device.[114]

Belladona Alkaloids. Representative Plant: *Datura stramonium* (Jimson Weed)

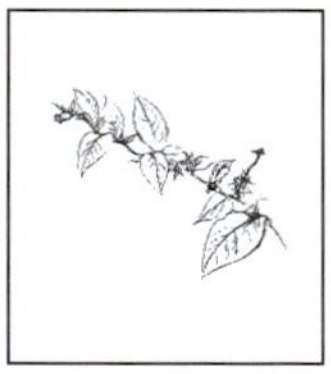
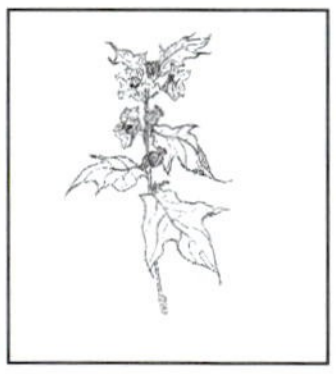 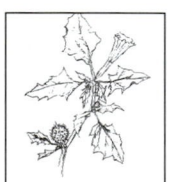

Native to Asia, *Datura stramonium* is a hearty weed with a characteristic rank malodor that now can be found throughout the United States. The plant is able to thrive along roadsides, in cornfields, in pastures, and in waste areas.[17] It has dark green, pointed leaves and grows to a height of 3–5 feet. Its flowers are tubular-shaped and white, blooming in late summer and fall. The fruit has an unappealing round spiny capsular shape that contains 50–100 black seeds[17] (see Color Plate Fig. 3).

This plant has been recognized throughout history as a toxin. In the *Odyssey,* Homer talked of this plant as a poison. Cleopatra is said to have used *Datura stramonium* to woo Caesar; Marc Antony's retreating troops were reported to have eaten the plants as they left Parthia in A.D. 38, with stupor, confusion, and fatalities resulting.[165]

In 1676, the term *Jamestown weed* came into use when British troops sent to halt Bacon's Rebellion invaded Jamestown, Virginia. The soldier's mistakenly prepared a meal of *Datura stramonium* and suffered acute poisoning. The following passage from Beverly's *History and Present State of Virginia*[12] describes the event:

> The plant was gathered very young for a boiled salad by some of the soldiers sent thither to Virginia to quell the rebellion of Bacon. Some of them ate plentifully of it, the effect of which was a very pleasant comedy, for they turned natural fools upon it for several days: One would blow up a feather in the air; another would dart straws at it with very much fury; and another stark naked, was sitting in the corner like a monkey. A thousand such simple tricks they played, after eleven days returned to themselves again, not remembering anything that had passed.

Over the years *Jamestown weed* was abbreviated to *jimson weed.* Other common names for this plant include locoseed, locoweed, apple of Peru, green dragon, devil's apple, devil's trumpet, stinkweed, and datura.[56]

In the 1970s and '80s, the cause of jimson weed overdoses changed from predominantly unintentional childhood poisonings to inadvertent overdoses in persons experimenting with the plant for its hallucinogenic properties.[4,23,27,58,60,61,64]

Datura stramonium and other plants that cause anticholinergic poisoning contain Belladonna alkaloids (Table 77–5).[69] These alkaloid toxins, including atropine, hyoscyamine, scopolamine, and mandragorine, have potent anticholinergic effects. The various plants contain differing concentrations of the alkaloids are listed in Table 77–5.[62,64,69,70,164,165,166] Individual plants also differ in toxin concentrations depending on factors such as soil and climate conditions.[116]

All parts of the plants are toxic, but the seeds have the highest concentration of toxins, with 100 seeds containing the equivalent of approximately 6 mg of atropine.[83] Exposure causes the classic anticholinergic toxidrome characterized by tachycardia, mydriasis, dry flushed skin, decreased bowel sounds, urinary retention, sedation, and hallucinations.[56,60,83] Although symptoms typically begin within 1–4 hours of ingestion, drinking tea or smoking the plant may result in a more rapid onset.[4,23,165] Symptoms usually resolve within 1–2 days but have been reported to last as long as 1–2 weeks.[56]

Treatment consists of supportive care and the consideration of gastric decontamination. Symptoms are usually mild and resolve in a calm environment. If central nervous system effects occur such as stupor, coma, hallucinations, or seizures, the use of physostigimine, should be considered.[61,147] Other signs of severe anticholinergic poisoning and potential indications for physostigmine include high fever and severe agitation (see Antidotes in Depth: Physostigmine).[165]

TABLE 77–5. HYOSCYAMINE AND HYOSCINE CONTAINING PLANTS

Latin Name	Common Name	Description	Distribution	Toxin
Atropa belladonna	Belladonna, deadly nightshade	Fleshy, erect stem; hairy leaves; purple flowers; purple-black many-seeded berry when ripe	Cultivated in Eastern states; rarely survives in wild form	Hyoscyamine, hyoscine
Cestrum nocturnum, Cestrum diurnum	Night-blooming jessamine; day-blooming jessamine	Large, attractive shrubs; fragrant small trumpet flowers; small berry	Coastal plains in South and Southwest	Saponins, gastroenterotoxins
Datura stramonium (color plate Fig. 3)	Tolguacha, apple of Peru, jimson weed, Jamestown weed, devil's apple, thorn apple, devil's trumpet, stinkweed, loco seeds, locoweed	Large erect plant; funnel-shaped white or purple flowers; spreading branches; hard, prickly, ovate, many-seeded fruit	Cultivated or uncultivated fields; widespread in U.S.	Hyoscyamine (leaves, roots, seeds); hyoscine (roots)
Hyoscyamus niger	Henbane, black henbane	Tall, erect stem; multibranched stem with fetid odor, yellowish flowers, encapsulated seeds	Weed in U.S.	Hyoscyamine, hyoscine
Lycium halimifolium	Matrimony vine	Vine or shrub; bell-shaped flowers; ovoid orange-red berry	Northern U.S.	Hyoscyamine

Blighia sapida (Ackee)

This large fruit-bearing tree is native to Africa and tropical areas. It is well distributed in the Caribbean, south Florida, and southern California. The fruit is edible when ripe and serves as a staple in many Caribbean diets. Because of the prevalence of this plant in Jamaica, poisonings are often referred to as *Jamaican vomiting sickness*.

Ackee contains several toxins, of which the two principal substances are hypoglycin A (beta-methylene cyclopropyl-L-alpha-aminopropionic acid) and hypoglycin B (a dipeptide of hypoglycin A and glutamic acid). The exact mechanism of toxicity of these toxins is unclear but may be due to inhibition of fatty acid beta-oxidation or inhibition of glucose–6-phosphatase activity.[16,41,71,156,169] These biochemical effects lead to the major clinical effects of hypoglycemia and hepatic cell destruction.

These hypoglycins are metabolized to methylene cyclopropylacetic acid, which is excreted in the urine and can be used to verify exposure.[156–158]

Fruit ingestion is dangerous when toxin concentrations are high. This occurs when the ackee has not opened itself (unripe) or is damaged or decayed.[143] Symptoms are typically delayed for several hours after ingestion, but once they begin, progression is rapid.

Initial symptoms consist of severe nausea and vomiting. This is followed shortly by manifestations of hypoglycemia (mental status change, seizures, and hypothermia). Fatalities were reported commonly in the 1950s but are less common with improved attention to glucose and supportive measures.[67,68,72,163] In these fatalities seizures were reported in 85% of the cases. Liver function abnormalities that are seen include potentially reversible elevations in bilirubin, aminotransferases, and alkaline phosphatase. Biopsy in one well-documented case revealed centrilobular necrosis.[92] Nonketotic metabolic acidosis is also often seen and is due to the metabolic production of dicarboxylic acids.[156,158] Treatment consists of administration of glucose for hypoglycemia, gastric decontamination, and supportive care. L-Carnitine has been suggested as a possible antidote, with mixed results, in animal studies.[15,41]

Cardiac Glycosides. Representative Plant: *Nerium oleander* (Oleander)

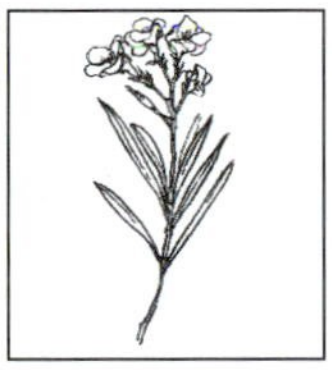

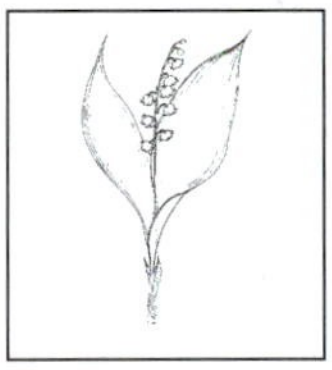

A shrub or tree native to the Mediterranean, the oleander is cultivated throughout the Southern United States as a flowering shrub in gardens and along roadsides. It has been known since the ancient times to be toxic to humans. [176] Africans used it as an arrow poison and the ancient Greeks believed it to be poisonous to "all four-footed beasts.[79,80,129] The shrub grows to a height of 25 feet and has green leaves that produce a clear, thick sap. Attractive white, red, or yellow flowers appear in the summer.

All parts of the plant contain cardiac glycosides. The highest concentrations are found in seeds, stems, and roots with highest toxin concentration occurring during the peak flowering stages.[65] Numerous different types of cardiac glycosides have been isolated from oleander: oleandrin, digitoxigenin, nerium folinerium, and rosagenin.[126,129] All have digoxin-like effects; they inhibit sodium–potassium ATPase. The relative toxicity of these glycosides is not well understood. Relative concentrations of these toxins differ throughout the plant: The leaves contain the highest oleandrin concentration and red flowers possess the highest total glycoside concentration.

Cardiac glycosides in nature abound in the plant kingdom and are even found naturally occurring in

TABLE 77–6. PLANTS CONTAINING CARDIAC GLYCOSIDES

Apocyanaceae	Liliaceae
Nerium oleander (oleander)	*Convallaria majalis* (lily of the valley)
Strophanthus (dogbane)	*Urginea maritima* } (squill)
Thevetia peruviana spp. (yellow oleander)	*Urginea indica* } (squill)
Asclepiadaceae	
Asclepias (milkweed)	
Calotropis (crown flower)	
Celastraceae	Ranunculaceae
Euonymus europaeus (spindle tree)	*Helleborus niger* (henbane)
Cruciferae	Scrophulariaceae
Cheiranthus } wall flower	*Digitalis purpurea* } foxglove
Erysimum } wall flower	*Digitalis lanata* } foxglove

animal species, such as the cane toad (*Bufo marinus*).[26] More than 400 different cardiac glycosides have been isolated (see, eg, Table 77–6).[129] Digitalis is derived from the plants *Digitalis purpurea* and *Digitalis lantana*. It is the most well-known of the cardiac glycosides and has a long and significant medical history. As a plant ingestion, digitalis rarely causes significant toxicity, because of its relatively low toxin concentration. However, oleander, lily of the valley (*Convallaria majalis*), and yellow oleander (*Thevetia peruviana*) are highly toxic because of their potency, with well-documented cases of severe poisoning.[3,78,79,129]

Toxicity from oleander as well as from cardiac glycosides derived from other plants is quite similar to digoxin poisoning.[26,74,146,154] Gastrointestinal and cardiac symptoms predominate. Nausea and vomiting occur within several hours, followed by dysrhythmias. Any rhythm induced by digoxin can be expected with oleander and other naturally occurring cardiac glycosides (Chap. 48).

Because many of the plant-derived cardiac-glycosides are cross-reactive with the frequently used radioimmunoassays for digoxin, an elevated level may help confirm the clinical impression of toxicity.[126,129] The absolute digoxin level, however, is difficult to interpret, and does not correlate clinically. Thus, any elevation in the digoxin level in this setting may represent a serious, potentially fatal cardiac glycoside poisoning.

Treatment for oleander and other plant-derived cardiac glycoside poisoning is similar to that for digoxin toxicity (see Chap. 48; Antidotes in Depth: Digoxin-specific Antibody Fragments [Fab]). Because of the cross-reactivity of digoxin radioimmunoassay, digoxin-specific fragments have been suggested as an antidote for poisoning. There are several anecdotal case reports of digoxin-specific Fab's efficacy in oleander poisoning.[26,148] Digoxin-specific Fab effectively bound proscillaridin and scilliroside, cardiac glycosides derived from the red squill plant, in an in vitro model.[139] Digoxin-specific fragments are recommended in severely poisoned patients, using the same indications as for digoxin toxicity. However, as discussed, absolute digoxin levels should not be used to evaluate the severity of toxicity. Furthermore, because of the possibility of incomplete cross-reactivity, higher than expected doses of digoxin-specific fragments may be needed. Dosing depends on the initial response to therapy and clinical signs of continued or recurrent toxicity (see Antidotes in Depth: Digoxin-specific Antibody Fragments [Fab]).

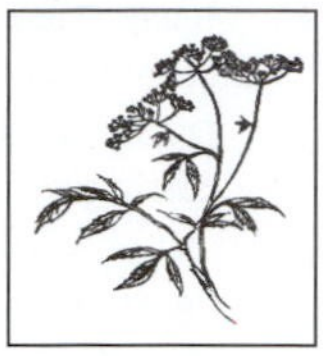

Cicuta maculata (Water Hemlock)

The water hemlock is a weed that grows most commonly along lakes, streams, and marshes. It is characterized by its thick, hollow, tuberous roots but is easily mistaken for several wild edible plant species such as *Daucus carota* (Queen Anne's lace).

All parts of the plant contain the toxin cicutoxin, but the highest concentrations are found in the root.[54] Cicutoxin is among the most potent toxins and has accounted for numerous deaths, with a reported mortality rate of 30% in one series of 83 patients.[69]

Ingestion of this plant leads to rapid onset (within 60 minutes) of GI symptoms of nausea, vomiting, and abdominal pain.[91] This is followed by status epilepticus refractory to standard anticonvulsants in severe cases.[91] Mortality most commonly is secondary to status epilepticus.[91,103,105,150] The mechanism for these seizures is unclear but may be related to cicutoxin-induced overstimulation of central cholinergic pathways.[21,122]

No antidote is available for toxicity. Therefore, aggressive supportive care is the main mode of treatment. Gastric decontamination with gastric lavage and activated charcoal should be performed. If seizures occur, diazepam and a rapid-acting barbiturate should be initiated. If seizures continue, general anesthesia may be necessary. Hemodialysis was used successfully in one anecdotal case of refractory status epilepticus,[85] but limited data on the efficacy of hemodialysis or hemoperfusion for water hemlock exposure are available.

Conium maculatum (Poison Hemlock)

Used in ancient times as a means of execution (Socrates is reported to have been killed by this plant,[34,43] poison hemlock is a weed that has fernlike leaves. It grows along roads, ditches, and in wooded areas throughout the United States. Because it resembles edible wild plants, poisonings most often occur because of misidentification.

Conium contains several toxins in the piperdine alkaloid class of compounds, conine being the most well-known and well-studied. These toxins are structurally similar to nicotine and posses similar clinical features in toxicity.[43] All parts of the plant contain the toxins but the concentration varies depending on the age of the plant (more mature plants have higher concentrations), time of year, and geographic area where the plant is grown.[29]

Clinically, patients initially manifest symptoms of stimulation that include tachycardia, tremors, diaphoresis, mydriasis, and seizures.[34,122,123] Gastrointestinal symptoms of nausea, vomiting, and abdominal pain are common as well.[134] This initial phase is followed in severe cases by a depressant period characterized by bradycardia, ascending motor paralysis, and coma.[29,43] If death occurs, it is typically due to motor weakness and subsequent respiratory failure.[134]

No specific antidote exists for this poisoning. Because of the risk of severe toxicity, aggressive GI decontamination, including gastric lavage and activated charcoal, should be instituted.

Cyanogenic Plants

Cyanogenic glycosides are predominantly found in the trees of the *Prunus* species (Table 77–7).[93,141] These trees contain the toxin amygdalin. Although the toxin is found in all parts of the plant, the highest concentrations are in young leaves. Amygdalin is not harmful until it is metabolized by the enzyme emulsin, which is found in the seeds of these plants.[19] Certain bacteria that have been isolated in human intestinal flora also possess this enzyme and can catalyze this reaction in the absence of seeds (see Fig. 97–1B).[19,93,141]

Warming or crushing the seeds of these plants leads to the typical bitter almond or peach pit odor associated with cyanide poisoning. Some investigators attribute this odor to benzaldehyde formation,[78,79] while most believe hydrocyanic acid causes the odor. This aroma, which can be detected by approximately 60% of the population, is also produced when leaves or branches are burned. The ability to detect this odor is thought to be a sex-linked recessive characteristic, with a male to female ratio of 3:1 in the incidence of the inability to detect this odor.[78]

Toxicity from amygdalin is related to the amount of plant or seed ingested and thus the amount of hydrocyanic acid that is released. The symptoms of headache, dizziness, vertigo, stupor, coma, seizures, and hyperthermia are identical to those of cyanide poisoning from other sources (Chap. 97).[59,138,162]

Treatment for exposures to cyanogenic plants is also similar to that for cyanide poisoning and involves use of the cyanide antidote kit (Antidotes in Depth: Cyanide Antidotes).[59] Gastric emptying should be considered. Gastric lavage and/or activated charcoal may be useful to prevent further metabolism of amygdalin to hydrocyanic acid.

TABLE 77–7. PLANTS CONTAINING A CYANOGENIC GLYCOSIDE

Christmas berry	
Prunus spp. (leaves, bark, and seeds may contain amygdalin)	
Apple (seeds)	Jetberry bush (jet bead)
Apricot	Lima beans
Bamboo (sprouts of some species)	Mountain mahogany
Bitter almond	Peach
Cassava (beans and roots)	Pear (seeds)
Cherry laurel	Pin cherry
Crab apple (seeds)	Plum
Choke cherry (stone fruit)	Western choke cherry
Elderberry (leaves and shoots)	Wild black cherry
Hydrangea (leaves and buds)	

Grayanotoxin. Representative Plant: *Rhododendron* spp. (Rhododendron)

Grayanotoxins are diterpenes found in all parts of plants of the *Ericaceae*. The different species of this family are distributed throughout the United States and Europe. Rhododendron, the most common of these plants, is green and shrublike and has flowers of varying color. Exposures occur from ingestion of the plant or contaminated honey. Contaminated honey results from honey bees harvesting nectar in areas densely populated with plants from this family.[14,144,178]

Grayanotoxin binds to myocardial sodium channels and increases permeability by opening sodium channels. Variable cardiovascular effects have been reported. Most commonly a mild increased inotropy and bradydysrhythmias are seen.[21,152] Reports of hypotension and tachydysrhythmias are less common.[13,174]

Other effects include early gastrointestinal complaints and nonspecific findings of paresthesias, lethargy, and weakness.[94] Rarely, in severe cases, mental status change, liver function abnormalities, ataxia, and seizures have been documented.[55,89]

Most cases of plant exposure manifest minimal or no toxicity.[82] In severe exposures aggressive decontamination and supportive care are sufficient treatment.

Nicotine. Representative Plant: *Nicotiana tabacum* (Tobacco)

The *Nicotiana* contain a number of species that contain the toxin nicotine. *Nicotiana tabacum* is native to the United States and is cultivated extensively for commercial purposes. Acute poisoning most commonly occurs in two scenarios: ingestion of cigarettes or cigars by young children or skin exposure to workers harvesting the plant.[22] Symptoms usually begin shortly after exposure and begin with nausea and vomiting. Most cases resolve without sequelae. Cigarette ingestions unassociated with nausea and vomiting do not manifest any other toxicity.[110]

Tobacco workers harvesting this plant are frequently reported to manifest toxicity, termed *green tobacco sickness*.[50–53] Nicotine is absorbed through the intact skin; absorption is enhanced when handling wet leaves.[52,53,76] Poisoning can be prevented in the majority of cases with the use of rubber or cotton gloves.[50,52,53]

Patients with larger exposures manifest symptoms of diaphoresis, hypertension, and tachycardia. Seizures, respiratory muscle failure (nicotinic receptor overstimulation), and hyperthermia are very rare but can be responsible for fatalities.[20,109]

No specific antidote is available. Treatment is aimed at prevention of absorption and supportive measures.

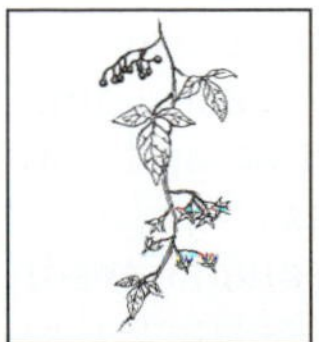

Solanaceous Alkaloids

Solanaceous alkaloids are found predominantly in the *Solanum* plants (Table 77–8).[75] The predominant toxin, solanine,

TABLE 77–8. SOLANINE- AND SOLANIDINE-CONTAINING PLANTS

Latin	Common Name	Description	Distribution
Lycopersicon esculentum	Tomato	Vines and suckers of tomato plant	Worldwide
Physalis heterophylla	Ground cherry	Perennial; solitary flowers; many-seeded	Eastern North America
Physalis longifolia	Husk tomato	Yellow berry	Weed meadows; pastures
Solandra spp.	Trumpet flower, chalice vine	Large, showy yellow or white flowers	Greenhouse or warmest parts of U.S.
Solanum aculeatissimum	Devil's apple, bull nettle		
Solanum carolinense	Horse nettle, ball nettle	Varied but similar	
Solanum dulcamara	European bittersweet, blue nightshade, woody nightshade, climbing nightshade	Shrub or slender vine; purple flowers; bright red berry; various seeds	Along fences, streams, ditches; most common in the east and north central U.S.
Solanum eleagnifolium	White horse nettle, silver leaf nightshade, tropillo	Varied	Throughout U.S.
Solanum gracile	Bull nettle, wild tomato	Varied	Throughout U.S.
Solanum nigrum americanum	Black nightshade, poison berry, common nightshade	Multibranched vines or bushes; white flowers; purple-black berries	In fields, woods, waste places; widespread in U.S.
Solanum pseudocapsicum	Jerusalem cherry, natal cherry	Ornamental plant; orange, cherry-like berries	Various species throughout U.S.
Solanum rostratum	Buffalo burr, sandburr, Colorado burr, Texas thistle	Varied	Throughout U.S.
Solanum sodomeum	Apple of sodom, popalo	Varied	Throughout U.S.
Solanum trifolium	Three-flowered nightshade, cut-leafed nightshade	Varied	Throughout U.S.
Solanum tuberosum	Irish potato, common potato	Vines, "eyes" and sprouts; peelings or tubers exposed to light, turning green	Mainly in northeast, northwest U.S.
Solanum villosum	Hairy nightshade	Varied	Throughout U.S.

has been isolated in many of the 1700 different *Solanum* species. *Solanum tuberosum*, the common potato plant, is most often involved in poisoning because of its relatively high toxin concentration and its popularity as a food staple.[62]

Solanine is a glycoalkaloid that contains three sugar molecules attached to a steroid-like moiety, the aglycone portion. Other solanaceous alkaloids that are also found in these plants (ie, chaconine) contain the basic aglycone portion but differ in the number and type of glucose molecules.[119,120] These toxins are found throughout the plant, but the concentration varies widely in different parts of the plant and also depends on environmental factors.[119,120] Solanine occurs in highest concentration in unripe fruit; "green" potatoes are most commonly responsible for human poisonings.[62] Other factors that increase toxin concentration include increased exposure to light, shallow planting, prolonged periods of storage, and physiologic stresses to the plant during its growth, such as cold temperatures.[25,62]

Toxicity from solanaceous alkaloids predominantly affects the GI and central nervous systems. Although the mechanism of human toxicity is unclear, in animal models solanine inhibits cholinesterase activity[30,119,127,129] and has cardiac glycoside effects.[120] Despite these in vitro findings, cholinergic poisoning and cardiac glycoside effects are not observed in human or animal poisoning. Symptoms of nausea, vomiting, diarrhea, and abdominal pain typically begin 2–24 hours after ingestion and may last several days in cases of severe exposures.[127]

Neurologic findings generally involve alterations in mental status. Delirium, hallucinations, and coma have been reported and typically resolve over several days.[113] Deaths have been reported in the older literature, typically involving malnourished individuals,[2,62,113] but no deaths have been reported since the 1960s.

Initial treatment involves consideration for gastric decontamination. No specific antidote exists, and supportive care with attention to fluid and electrolyte management is sufficient for the majority of exposures.

Toxalbumins. Representative Plant: *Abrus precatorius* (Jequirty Pea)

The toxalbumin-containing plants of toxicologic significance are *Abrus precatorius* (jequirty pea) and *Ricinus communis* (castor bean). These plants have attractive seeds and are used for ornamental purposes. They contain potent cellular toxins (toxalbumins)—abrin in the jequirty pea and ricin in the castor bean—which are proteins with similar structures. They are composed of two subunits, the A and B chains, that are covalently linked by a single disulfide chain (Fig. 77–1).[10] The B chain binds to cell surface glycoproteins and by an unknown mechanism affects entry of the toxin into the cell.[66] The A chain, once in the cell, acts on the 60S ribosomal subunit, preventing binding of elongation factor 2, thus inhibiting protein synthesis and leading to cell demise.[9,66] This basic structure of two peptide chains linked by a single disulfide chain is similar to that of botulinal toxin, tetanus toxin, cholera toxin, diptheria toxin, and insulin.[5]

Abrus precatorius, the jequirty pea (also known as

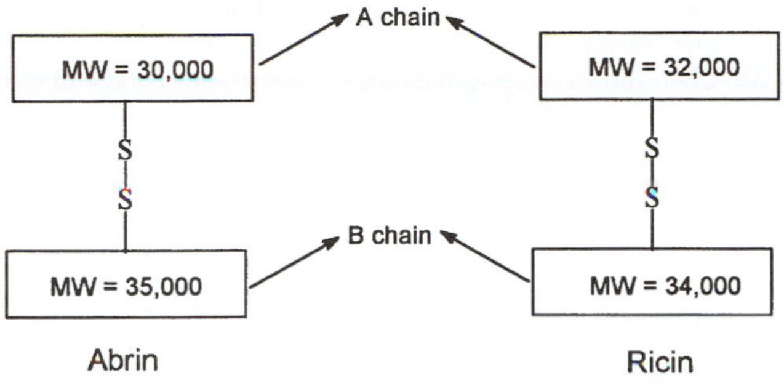

Figure 77–1. Toxalbumin structure. *(Adapted from Olsnes S, Refnes K, Pihl A: Mechanism of action of the toxic lectins arbin and ricin. Nature 1974;249:627–631.)*

rosary pea, Indian bean, crab's eye, Buddhist's rosary bead, and prayer bead) is a green vine native to India, but it is also found in the Caribbean and Florida. The distinctive part of the plant is the seeds, which are oval and approximately 5 mm in diameter. They have an attractive hard glossy outer shell that is red with a black center, black with a white center, or white with a black center (see Color Plate Fig. 1).

Because this seed is commonly used in jewelry, most reports of exposure involve children who ingest seeds from broken necklaces or other ornaments. All parts of the plant are toxic, but the seeds contain the highest concentration of toxins. Abrin has been implicated as responsible for the severe toxicity, but this plant also contains small amounts of glycyrrhizin, abric acid, and *N*-methyltryptophan, the significance of which is unclear.[32,33]

Ingestion of seeds rarely result in symptoms. The potent toxins are encased within the hard shell of the seed; if this is not broken or digested there is minimal toxicity. However, if the toxins are released, by chewing or digestion, and absorbed, symptoms of severe gastroenteritis ensue; fatalities have occurred over a course of 3–4 days. Seizures, CNS depression, cerebral edema, and cardiac dysrhythmias have been reported, the mechanisms of which are unclear.[32] Autopsy studies have shown GI hemorrhage, edematous bowl, cerebral edema, and congested liver and kidneys.[9,33]

Treatment for jequirty pea ingestion is supportive, as no specific antidote is available. Because of the potential for serious toxicity, gastric decontamination should be administered. Older references have recommended urinary alkalinization for potential hemolysis and prevention of renal tubular damage.[33] This phenomenon is reported to occur in vitro, but has not been substantiated in animal models or reported in humans.[9,77,121] Urinary alkalinization is not recommended. Whole-bowel irrigation has been suggested to decrease transit time of the seeds, but in the only case report of its use for this purpose seeds were still noted in the stool 3 days later.[153]

Ricinus communis is a large, leafy plant reaching a height of 10–12 feet. It produces brown capsules, each containing three shiny, hard-coated, grayish-brown seeds. The toxalbumin ricin is found throughout the plant but is most concentrated in the seeds (see Color Plate Fig. 2). When the seeds are ingested, if the hard exterior coat is not damaged by mastication or digestion, no toxin is released and toxicity does not occur. If the ricin is released and absorbed, symptoms similar to abrin poisoning (described above) ensue.[39]

The plant is cultivated commercially as a source of castor oil, which is used medicinally as a purgative and as a lubricant for engines. Human exposures typically involve adults who ingest the seeds while playing with jewelry or ornaments or after finding seeds strewn from the plant.[66,77,108]

Historically, castor bean ingestions have been reported to be lethal,[84] with one chewed bean sufficient to cause death in a child. Review of the available case reports shows this not to be true.[24,26,78,86,131,172] Although ricin is lethal when parenterally injected in animals or humans, its lethality is greatly diminished when ingested orally because of its poor GI absorption.[24,48,66,86,131] Many documented cases exist of mastication of multiple seeds without fatal outcome.[86,131] This exaggerated concern over ricin's lethality may stem in part from the highly celebrated case of Georgi Markov, an exiled Bulgarian broadcaster. Markov was waiting for a bus in London one day in 1978, when an unidentified man jabbed the back of his thigh with an umbrella. Over the next 3 days he developed severe gastroenteritis marked by high fevers, which culminated in his death. At autopsy, a metallic sphere 1.5 mm in diameter was found at the wound site on his thigh. The sphere had two tiny holes bored through it, with a volume of 0.28 mm^3 available for a toxic agent. Although no toxin was isolated from the sphere, due to the symptomatology and small dose, ricin was virtually the only toxin capable of causing this. The coroner recreated the scenario by injecting a pig with a similar dose of ricin, which resulted in death in a similar manner within 26 hours.[66,86]

Allergic reactions from exposure, reproducible with patch testing, are well recognized.[108] Anaphylaxis has been reported from handling necklaces made with the seeds, but most cases involve occupational exposures in factories producing oil from this plant.[33,106,108,161]

Treatment of suspected cases of ricin poisoning is similar to that for abrin. No specific antidote exists and the majority of patients have an excellent outcome.

Summary

Plant exposures are a common medical problem. There are thousands of potentially dangerous species, and this chapter focuses on those most likely to cause serious toxicity and those most commonly reported to poison control centers. For information on plants not covered in this chapter, the reader is referred to more inclusive texts.[79,90,115,117]

Acknowledgment

Pamela Ryder, Nurse Practitioner, contributed the plant illustrations.

References

1. Agarwal B, Agarwal R, Misra D: Malignant arrhythmias induced by accidental aconite poisoning. Ind Heart J 1977; 29:246–248.
2. Alexander RF, Forbes GB, Hawkins ES: A fatal case of solanine poisoning. Br Med J 1948;2:518.
3. Ansford AJ, Morris HP: Fatal oleander poisoning. Med J Aust 1981;1:360–362.
4. Anticholinergic poisoning associated with an herbal tea—New York City, 1994. MMWR 1995;44:193–195.
5. Balint GA: Ricin: The toxic protein of castor oil seeds. Toxicology 1974;2:77–102.
6. Barker BE, Farnes P: Histochemistry of blood cells treated with pokeweed mitogen. Nature 1967;214, 787–789.
7. Barker BE, Farnes P, LaMarche PH: Peripheral blood plasmacytosis following systemic exposure to *Phytolacca americana* (pokeweed). Pediatrics 1966;38:490–493.
8. Barnes B, Fox L: Poisoning by Dieffenbachia. J History Med 1953;10:173–181.
9. Barri ME, el Dirdiri NI, Abu Damir H, et al: Toxicity of *Abrus precatorius* in Nubian goats. Vet Hum Tox 1990;32: 541–545.
10. Benson S, Olsnes S, Pihl A: On the mechanism of protein-synthesis inhibition by abrin and ricin. Eur J Biochem 1975;58:573–580.
11. Bernstein JE, Swift RM , Soltani K, et al: Inhibition of axon reflex vasodilation by topically applied capsaicin. J Invest Dermatol 1981;76:394–395.
12. Beverly R: History and Present State of Virginia. Ann Arbor, MI, Books on Demand, 1968.
13. Bhattacharya SK, Somani PN, Srivastava PK: Cardiac changes in *Thevetia nerifolia* poisoning. Acta Cardiol 1976; 31:169–174.
14. Biberoglu S, Biberoglu K , Biberoglu B: Mad honey. JAMA 1988;269:1943. Letter.
15. Borum PR: Carnitine. Annu Rev Nutr 1983;3:233–259.
16. Bressler R, Corredor C, Brendel K: Hypoglycin and hypoglycin-like compounds. Pharmacol Rev 1969;21:105–130.
17. Callhan R, Piccola F, Gensheimer K, et al: Plant poisonings: New Jersey. MMWR 1981;30:65–66.
18. Carpenter SE, Lynn B: Vascular and sensory responses of human skin to mild injury after topical treatment with capsaicin. Br J Pharmacol 1981;73:755–758.
19. Carter JH, Goldman P: Bacteria-mediated cyanide poisoning by apricot kernels in children from Gaza. Pediatrics 1981;68:5–7.
20. Castorena JL, Garriott JC, Barnhardt FE, et al: A fatal poisoning from *Nicotiana glauca*. J Toxicol Clin Toxicol 1987; 25:429–435.
21. Catterall WA: Neurotoxins that act on voltage-sensitive sodium channels in excitable membranes. Annu Rev Pharmacol Toxicol 1980;20:15–43.
22. Centers for Disease Control and Prevention: Ingestion of cigarettes and cigarette butts by children. JAMA 1997; 277:785–786
23. CDC: Jimson weed poisoning—Texas, New York, and California, 1994. MMWR 1995;44:41–44.
24. Challoner KR, McCarron MM: Castor bean intoxication. Ann Emerg Med 1990;19:1177–1183
25. Chaube S, Swinyard CA: Teratological and toxicological studies of alkaloidal and phenolic compounds from *Solanum tuberosum*. Toxicol Appl Pharmacol 1976;36: 227–237.
26. Cheung K, Urech R, Taylor L, et al: Plant cardiac glycosides and digoxin Fab antibody. J Pediatr Child Health 1991;27:312–313.
27. Coremans P, Lambrecht G, Shepens P, et al: Anticholinergic intoxication with commercially available thorn apple tea. J Toxicol Clin Toxicol 1994;32:589–592.
28. Cornell J, Weathers P, Pokras M: Poisonous plant identification: A comparison of databases designed for veterinary use. Vet Hum Toxicol 1995;37:482–485.
29. Cromwell BT: The separation, micro-estimating and distribution of the alkaloids of hemlock (*Coinium maculatum L*). Biochem J 1956;64:259–266.
30. Dalvi RR, Bowie WC: Toxicology of solanine: An overview. Vet Hum Toxicol 1983;25:13–15.
31. D'Archy WG: Severe contact dermatitis from poinsettia. Arch Dermatol 1974;109:909–910.
32. Davies JH: *Abrus precatorius* (rosary pea): The most common lethal plant poison. J Fla Med Assoc 1978;65:188–191.
33. Davison AG, Britton MG, Forrester JA, et al: Asthma in merchant seamen and laboratory workers caused by allergy to castor beans: Analysis of allergens. Clin Allergy 1983;13:553–561.
34. De Boer J: The death of Socrates: A historical and experimental study on the action of coniine and conium maculata. Arch Int Pharmacodyn 1950; 83:473–490.
35. Diehl AK, Bauer RL: Jalaproctitis. N Engl J Med 1978; 299:1137–1138.
36. Drach G, Maloney WH: Toxicity of the common houseplant *Dieffenbachia*. JAMA 1963;184:1047.
37. Edwards N: Local toxicity from a poinsettia plant: A case report. J Pediatr 1983;102:404–405.
38. Edwards N: Pokeberry pancake breakfast—or—it's gonna be a great day! Vet Hum Toxicol 1982;24(suppl):135–137.
39. El Badwi SMA, Adam SEI, Hapke HJ: Experimental *Ricinus communis* poisoning in chicks. Phytother Res 1992;6: 205–208.
40. Ellis W, Barfort P, Mastman GJ: Keratoconjunctivitis with corneal crystals caused by the *Dieffenbachia* plant. Am J Ophthalmol 1973;76:143–147.
41. Entman M, Bressler R: The mechanism of action of hypoglycin on long-chain fatty acid oxidation. Mol Pharmacol 1967;3:333–340.
42. Evans CRH: Oral ulceration after contact with the houseplant *Dieffenbachia*. Br Dent J 1987;162:467–468.
43. Fairbairin JW, Challen SB: The alkaloids of hemlock (*Conium maculatum L*). Biochem J 1958;72:556–561.
44. Faivre M, Barral C: La toxicité d'une plante ornamentale: un cas d'intoxication par *Dieffenbachia picta*. Nouv Presse Med 1974;3:1313–1314.

45. Fisher AA: The poison "rhus" plants. Cutis 1965;1:230–236.
46. Fitzpatrick AJ, Crawford M, Allan RM, Wolfenden H: Aconite poisoning managed with a ventricular assist device. Anaesth Intensive Care 1994;22:714–717.
47. Fochtman FW, Manno JE, Eisek CL, et al: Toxicity of the genus *Dieffenbachia.* Toxicol Appl Pharmacol 1969;15: 38–45.
48. Fodstad O, Johannessen JV, Schjerven L, et al: Toxicity of abrin and ricin in mice and dogs. J Toxicol Environ Health 1979;5:1073–1084.
49. Gardner DG: Injury to the oral mucous membranes caused by the common houseplant, dieffenbachia. Oral Surg Oral Med Oral Pathol 1994; 78:631–633.
50. Gehlbach SH, Willilam WA, Perry LD, et al: Nicotine absorption by workers harvesting green tobacco. Lancet 1975;1:478–480.
51. Gehlbach SH, William WA, Perry LD, et al: Green tobacco sickness: An illness of tobacco harvesters. JAMA 1974; 229:1880–1883.
52. Ghosh SK, Gokani VN, Doctor PB, et al: Intervention studies against "green symptoms" among Indian tobacco harvesters. Arch Environ Health 1991;46:316–317.
53. Ghosh SK, Gokani VN, Parikh JR, et al: Protection against "green symptoms" from tobacco in Indian harvesters: A preliminary intervention study. Arch Environ Health 1987;42:121–124.
54. Gompertz LM: Poisoning with water hemlock (*Cicuta maculata*). A report of 17 cases. JAMA 1926;87:1277–1278.
55. Gossinger H, Hruby K, Haubenstock A: Cardiac arrhythmias in a patient with grayanotoxin-honey poisoning. Vet Hum Toxicol 1983;25:328–329.
56. Gowdy JM: Stramonium intoxication: A review of symptomatology in 212 cases. JAMA 1972;221:585–587.
57. Grant WM: Toxicology of the Eye, 3rd ed. Springfield, IL, Charles C. Thomas, 1986.
58. Guharoy SR, Barajas M: Atropine intoxication from the ingestion and smoking of jimson weed (*Datura stromonium*). Vet Hum Toxicol 1991;33:588–589.
59. Hall AH, Linder CH, Kulig KW, et al: Cyanide poisoning from laetrile ingestion: Role of nitrite therapy. Pediatrics 1986;78:269–272.
60. Hall RW, Popkin MK, McHenry LE: Angel trumpet psychosis: A central nervous system anticholinergic syndrome. Am J Psychiatry 1977;134:312–314,
61. Hanna JP, Schmidley JW, Braselton WE: Datura delirium. Clin Neuropharmacol 1992;15:109–113.
62. Hansen AA: Two fatal cases of potato poisoning. Science 1925;61:348–349.
63. Hansen L, Hammershoy O, Boll PM: Allergic contact dermatitis from falcarinol isolated from *Shefflera arboricola.* Contact Derm 1986;14:91–93.
64. Haymen HJ: Datura poisoning: The angel's trumpet. Pathology 1985;17:465–466.
65. Haynes BE, Bessen HA, Wrightman WD: Oleander tea: Herbal draught of death. Ann Emerg Med 1985;14:350–353.
66. Henry GW, Schwenk GR, Bohnert GA: Umbrellas and mole beans: A warning about acute ricin poisoning. J Indiana State Med Assoc 1981;74:572–573.
67. Hill KR: The vomiting sickness of Jamaica. A review. West Indian Med J 1952;1:243–264.
68. Hill KR, Bras G, Clearkin KP: Acute toxic hypoglycemia occurring in the vomiting sickness of Jamaica. Morbid anatomical aspects. West Indian Med J 1955;4:91–104.
69. Hopkins J. The glycoalkaloids: Naturally of interest (but a hot potato?). Food Chem Toxicol 1995;33:323–328.
70. Hudson MJ: Acute atropine poisoning from ingestion of *Datura rosei.* NZ Med J 1973;77:245–248.
71. Hue L, Sherratt HSA: Inhibition of gluconeogenesis by hypoglycin in the rat. Biochem J 1986;240:765–769.
72. Jelliffe DB, Stuart KL: Acute toxic hypoglycemia in the vomiting sickness of Jamaica. Br Med J 1954;1:75.
73. Jones LA, Tandberg D, Troutmann WG: Household treatment for "chile burns" of the hands. J Toxicol Clin Toxicol 1987;25:483–491.
74. Kakrani AL, Rajput CS, Khandare SK, et al: Yellow oleander seed poisoning with cardiotoxicity: A case report. Indian Heart J 1981;33:31–33.
75. Karawya MS, Balboa SI, Khayyal SE: Estimation of cardenolides in Nerium oleander. Planta Med 1973;23: 70–73.
76. Keeler RF, Baker DC, Gaffield W: Spirosolane-containing *Solanum* species and induction of congenital craniofacial malformations. Toxicon 1990;28:873–884.
77. Kinamore PA: Abrus and ricinus ingestion: Management of three cases. Clin Toxicol 1980;17:401–405.
78. Kingsbury JM: Phytotoxicology. I: Major problems associated with poisonous plants. Clin Pharmacol Ther 1969; 10:163–169.
79. Kingsbury JM: Poisonous Plants of the United States and Canada. Englewood Cliffs, NJ, Prentice-Hall, 1964.
80. Kirtikar KR: The poisonous plants of Bombay. J Bombay Nat Hist Soc 1897;11:251–261.
81. Kkug S, Saleena C, Honcharuk L, et al: Toxicity potential of poinsettia: Is the plant really toxic? Vet Hum Toxicol 1990;32:368. Abstract.
82. Klein-Schwartz W, Litovitz T: Azalea toxicity: An overrated problem? J Toxicol Clin Toxicol 1985;23:91–101.
83. Klein-Schwartz W, Oderda GM: Jimson weed intoxication in adolescents and young adults. Am J Dis Child 1984; 138:737–739.
84. Knight B: Ricin: A potent homicidal poison. Br Med J 1979; 1:350–351.
85. Knutsen OH, Paszkowshi P: New aspects in the treatment of water hemlock poisoning. J Toxicol Clin Toxicol 1984; 22:157–166.
86. Kopferschmitt J, Flesch F, Lugnier A, et al: Acute voluntary intoxication by ricin. Hum Toxicol 1983;2:239–242.
87. Kuballa B, Lugnier AJ, Anton R: Study of *Dieffenbachia*-induced edema in mouse and rat hindpaw: Respective role of oxalate needles and trypsin-like protease. Toxicol App Pharmacol 1981;58:444–451.
88. Ladiera AM, Andrade SO, Sawaya P: Studies on *Dieffenbachia picta* Schott: Toxic effects in guinea pigs. Toxicol Appl Pharmacol 1975;34:363–373.
89. Lampe KF: Rhododendrons, mountain laurel, and mad honey. JAMA 1988;259:2009.
90. Lampe KF, McCann MA: AMA Handbook of Poisonous

and Injurious Plants. Chicago, American Medical Association, 1985.
91. Landers D, Seppi K, Blauer W: Seizures and death on a white river float trip: Report of water hemlock poisoning. West J Med 1985;142:637–640.
92. Larson J, Vender R, Camuto P: Cholestatic jaundice due to ackee fruit poisoning. Am J Gastroenterol 1994;89: 1577–1578
93. Lasch EE, El Shawa R: Multiple cases of cyanide poisoning by apricot kernels in children from Gaza. Pediatrics 1981; 68:5–7.
94. Leach DG: That's why the lady is a tramp. J Am Rhododendron Soc 1982:151–152.
95. Lim KH: External eye allergy from sap of *Dieffenbachia picta*. Singapore Med J 1977;18:176–177.
96. Litovitz TL, Bailey KM, Schmitz BF, et al: 1990 annual report of the American Association of Poison Control Centers national data collection system. Am J Emerg Med 1991;9:461–509.
97. Litovitz TL, Clark LR, Soloway RA: 1993 annual report of the American Association of Poison Control Centers Toxic Exposure Survellance System. Am J Emerg Med 1994; 12:546–584.
98. Litovitz TL, Felberg L, Soloway RA, et al: 1994 annual report of the American Association of Poison Control Centers Toxic Exposure Surveillance System. Am J Emerg Med 1995;13:551–597.
99. Litovitz TL, Felberg L, White S, Klein-Schwartz W: 1995 annual report of the American Association of Poison Control Centers Toxic Exposure Surveillance System. Am J Emerg Med 1996;14:487–537.
100. Litovitz TL, Holm KC, Bailey KM, et al: 1991 annual report of the American Association of Poison Control Centers national data collection system. Am J Emerg Med 1992;10: 452–505.
101. Litovitz TL, Holm KC, Clancy C, et al: 1992 annual report of the American Association of Poison Control Centers Toxic Exposure Surveillance System. Am J Emerg Med 1993;11:494–555.
102. Litovitz TL, Normann SA, Vetri JC: 1985 annual report of the American Association of Poison Control Centers national data collection system. Am J Emerg Med 4:427–458, 1986.
103. Litovitz TL, Schmitz BF, Bailey KM: 1989 annual report of the American Association of Poison Control Centers national data collection system. Am J Emerg Med 1990;8: 394–442.
104. Litovitz TL, Schmitz BF, Holm KL: 1988 annual report of the American Association of Poison Control Centers national data collection system. Am J Emerg Med 1989;7: 495–545.
105. Litovitz TL, Schmitz BF, Matyunas N, et al: 1987 annual report of the American Association of Poison Control Centers national data collection system. Am J Emerg Med 1988 6:479–515.
106. Lockey AD Jr, Dunkelberger L: Anaphylaxis from an Indian necklace. JAMA 1968;206:2900–2901.
107. Mack RB: The Arum family. NC Med J 1982;43:36.
108. Malizia E, Sarcinelli L, Andreucci G: Ricinus poisoning: A familiar epidemy. Acta Pharmacol Toxicol 1977;41:351–361.
109. Manoguerra AS, Freeman D: Acute poisoning from the ingestion of *Nicotiana glauca*. J Toxicol Clin Toxicol 1982–83; 19:861–864.
110. McGee D, Brabson T, McCarthy J, Picciotti M: Four year review of cigarette ingestions in children. Pediatr Emerg Care 1995;11:13–16.
111. McIntire MS, Guyest JR, Porterfield JF: Philodendron: An infant death. J Toxicol Clin Toxicol 1990;28:177–183.
112. McKinney PE, Gomez HF, Phillips S, Brent J: The fax machine: A new method of plant identification. J Toxicol Clin Toxicol 1993;31:663–665. Letter.
113. McMillan M, Thompson JC: An outbreak of suspected solanine poisoning in schoolboys: Examination of solanine poisoning. Q J Med 1979;48:227–243.
114. Merchant HD, Choksi ND, Ramamoorthy K, et al: Aconite poisoning and cardiac arrhythmias. Report of 3 cases. Indian J Med Sci 1963;17:857.
115. Mitchell JC, Rook A: Botanical Dermatology. Plants Injurious to the Skin. Vancouver, Greengrass, 1979.
116. Moore DW: The autumnal high: Jimson weed in North Carolina. NC Med J 1976;37:492–494.
117. Morton JF: Plants Poisonous to People in Florida and Other Warm Areas. Miami, Hurricane House, 1971.
118. Mrvos R, Dean BS, Krenzelok EP: Philodendron/dieffenbachia ingestions: Are they a problem? J Toxicol Clin Toxicol 1991;29:485–491.
119. Nishie K, Fitzpatrick TJ, Swain AP, et al: Positive inotropic action of Solanaceae glycoalkaloids. Res Commun Chem Pathol Pharmacol 1976;15:601–607.
120. Nishie K, Gumbann MR, Keyl AC: Pharmacology of solanine. Toxicol Appl Pharmacol 1971;19:81–92.
121. Niyogi SK: The toxicology of *Abrus precatorius linnaeus*. J Forensic Sci 1970;15:529–536.
122. North DJ, Nelson RB: Anticholinergic agents in cicutoxin poisoning. West J Med 1985;143:250.
123. Ober WB: Did Socrates die of hemlock poisoning? NY State J Med 1977;254–258.
124. Olsnes S, Refnes K, Pihl A: Mechanism of action of the toxic lectins abrin and ricin. Nature 1974;249:627–631.
125. Orgell WH: Inhibition of human plasma cholinesterase in vitro by alkaloids, glycosides and other natural substances. Lloydia 1963;26:36–43.
126. Osterloh J, Harold S, Pond S: Oleander interference in the digoxin radioimmunoassay in a fatal ingestion. JAMA 1982;247:1596–1597.
127. Patil BC, Sharma RP: Evaluation of solanine toxicity. Food Cosmet Toxicol 1972;10:395–398.
128. Poison Ivy. The Lawrence Review of National Products. Levitown, PA, Pharmaceutical Information Associates, Sept. 1988.
129. Radford DJ, Gillies AD, Hinds JA, Duff P: Naturally occurring cardiac glycosides. Med J Aust 1986;144:540–544.
130. Rauber A: Observations on the idioblasts of *Dieffenbachia*. J Toxicol Clin Toxicol 1985;23:79–90.
131. Rauber A, Heard J: Castor bean toxicity re-examined. Vet Hum Toxicol 1985;27:498–502.
132. Reffstrup T, Hammershoy O, Boll PM, et al: *Philodendron scandens Koch et sello* subsp: Oxycardium (Schott) bunting, a new source of allergenic alkyl resorcinols. Acta Chem Scand 1982;36:291–294.

133. Rekhis J: The poisonous plant *Oxalis cernua*. Vet Hum Toxicol 1994; 36:23.
134. Rizzi D, Basile L, DiMaggio A, et al: Rhabdomyolysis and acute tubular necrosis in coniine (hemlock) poisoning. Lancet 1989;2:1461–1462.
135. Roberge R, Brader E, Martin ML, et al: The root of evil pokeweed intoxication. Ann Emerg Med 1986;15:470–473.
136. Rock JF: The poisonous plants of Hawaii. Hawaiian Forest Agric 1920;17:61.
137. Rodrigues TD, Johnson PN, Jeffrey LP: Holly berry ingestion: Case report. Vet Hum Toxicol 1984;26:157–158.
138. Rubino MJ, Davidoff F: Cyanide poisoning from apricot seeds. JAMA 1979;241:359. Letter.
139. Sabouraud AE, Urtizberea M, Garnier R, et al: Specific antidigoxin Fab fragments: An available antidote for proscillaridin and scilliroside poisoning? Hum Exp Toxicol 1990; 9:191–193.
140. Sakai WS, Nagao MA: Raphide structure in *Dieffenbachia maculata*. J Am Soc Hort Sci 1980;105:124–126.
141. Sayre JW, Kaymalealan S: Cyanide poisoning from apricot seeds among children in central Turkey. N Engl J Med 1964;270:1113–1115.
142. Schilling R, Marderosian AD, Speaker J: Incidence of plant poisonings in Philadelphia noted as poison information calls. Vet Hum Toxicol 1980;22:148–150.
143. Scott HH: On the vomiting sickness in Jamaica. Ann Trop Med 1916;10:1.
144. Scott PM, Caldwell BB, Wiberg GS: Grayanotoxins. Occurrence and analysis in honey and a comparison of toxicities in mice. FD Cosmet Toxicol 1971;9:179–184.
145. Sellers SJ, King M, Aronson CE, et al: Toxicologic assessment of *Philodendron oxycardium* Schoot (*Araceae*) in domestic cats. Vet Hum Toxicol 1978;20:92–95.
146. Shaw D, Pearn J: Oleander poisoning. Med J Aust 1979; 2:267–269.
147. Shenoy RS: Pitfalls in the treatment of jimson weed intoxication. Am J Psychiatry 1994;151:1396–1397.
148. Shumaik GM, Wu AW, Ping AC: Oleander poisoning: Treatment with Digoxin-specific Fab antibody fragments. Ann Emerg Med 1988;17:732–735.
149. Spoerke DG, Smolinske SC: Toxicity of Houseplants. Boca Raton, FL, CRC Press, 1990.
150. Starreveld E, Hope CE: Cicutoxin poisoning (water hemlock). Neurology 1975;25:730–734.
151. Stowe CM, Fangman G, Trumpel D: *Schefflera* toxicosis in a dog. J Am Vet Med Assoc 1975;167:79.
152. Sutlupinar N, Mat A, Satganoglu Y: Poisoning by toxic honey in Turkey. Arch Toxicol 1993;67:148–150.
153. Swanson-Bierman B, Dean BS, Krenzelok EP: Failure of whole bowel irrigation to decontaminate the GI tract following massive jequirity bean ingestion. Vet Hum Toxicol 1992;34:352. Abstract.
154. Szabuniewicz M, McCrady JD, Camp BJ: Treatment of experimentally induced oleander poisoning. Arch Int Pharmacodyn Ther 1971;189:12–21.
155. Tai YT, But PP, Young K et al: Cardiotoxicity after accidental herb-induced aconite poisoning. Lancet 1992;340: 1254–1256.
156. Tanaka K: Inhibition of gluconeogenesis by hypoglycin: Alternate interpretations. Hepatology 1987; 7:1377–1378.
157. Tanaka K, Isselbacker KJ, Shih V: Isovaleric and alpha methylbutyric acidemias induced by hypoglycin A: Mechanism of Jamaican vomiting sickness. Science 1972;175: 69–71.
158. Tanaka K, Kean EA, Johnson B: Jamaican vomiting sickness, biochemical investigation of two cases. N Engl J Med 1976;295:461–467.
159. Tominack RL, Spyker DA: Capsicum and capsaicin—A review: Case report of the use of hot peppers in child abuse. J Toxicol Clin Toxicol 1987;25:591–601.
160. Tomlinson B, Chan TYK, Chan JCN, et al: Herb-induced aconitine poisoning. Lancet 1993;341:370–371.
161. Topping MND, Henderson RTS, Luczynska CM, et al: Castor bean allergy among workers in the felt industry. Allergy 1982;37:603–608.
162. Townsend WA, Boni B: Cyanide poisoning from ingestion of apricot kernals. MMWR 1975;24:428.
163. Toxic hypoglycemic syndrome—Jamaica, 1989–1991. MMWR 1992;41:53–55.
164. Trabattoni G, Visintini D, Terzano GM, et al: Accidental poisoning with deadly nightshade berries: A case report. Hum Toxicol 1984;3:513–516.
165. Vanderhoff BT, Mosser KH: Jimsonweed toxicity: Management of anticholinergic plant ingestion. Am Fam Physician 1992;46:526–530.
166. Viachos P, Poulos L: A case of mandrake poisoning. J Toxicol Clin Toxicol 1982;19:521–522.
167. Virus RM, Bebhart T: Pharmacologic actions of capsaicin: Apparent involvement of substance P and serotonin. Life Sci 1979;25:1273–1283.
168. Vogl TP: Treatment of Hunan hand. N Engl J Med 1982; 306:178. Letter.
169. Von Holt C, Von Holt CM, Bohn H: Metabolic effects of hypoglycin and methylenecyclopaneacetic acid. Biochem Biophys Acta 1960;25:11–21.
170. Wagstaff DJ, Raisbeck M, Wagstaff AT: Poisonous Plant Information System (PPIS). Vet Hum Toxicol 1989;31: 237–238.
171. Wedd AM, Tenney SM: Effects of aconite on cold blooded heart. Proc Soc Exp Biol Med 1953; 4:199–203.
172. Wedin GP, Neal JS, Everson GW, et al: Castor bean poisoning. Am J Emerg Med 1986;4:259–261.
173. Weidner J: Possible harmful effects from a capsaicin base aerosol dog repellent. Vet Hum Toxicol 1980;22:18–19.
174. Weinberg RB: Hunan hand. N Engl J Med 1981;305:1020. Letter.
175. West LG, McLaughlin JL, Eisenbeiss GK: Saponins and triterpenes from *Ilex opaca*. Phytochemistry 1977;16: 1846–1847.
176. Westbrooks RG, Preacher JW: Poisonous plants of eastern North America. Columbia, SC, University of South Carolina Press, 1986.
177. Winek CL, Butala J, Shanor SP, et al: Toxicology of poinsettia. Clin Toxicol 1978;13:27–45.
178. Yavuz H, Ozel A, Akkus I, et al: Honey poisoning in Turkey. Lancet 1991;1:789–790.

CHAPTER 78

Arsenic

Marsha D. Ford

Arsenic	
MW	= 74.9 daltons
Normal range (whole blood)	< 5 μg/L
	< 0.665 μmol/day
Normal range (24-h urine)	< 50 μg/day
	< 6.65 μmol/day
Action level (24-h urine)	> 100 μg/day
	> 13.3 μmol/day

Values greater than or equal to the action level necessitate clinical intervention.
Values less than this level may necessitate intervention based on the clinical condition of the patient.

A 55-year-old Asian female was hospitalized for diarrhea, nausea, vomiting, and weakness of unknown etiology. The patient had diabetes and had been in her usual state of health until 5 weeks earlier when, after eating noodle paste, she and her husband developed persistent nausea, vomiting, and diarrhea. Both were admitted with dehydration and hypokalemia and treated for 1 week. On discharge the patient's weakness necessitated the use of a cane for walking. Approximately 3 weeks later, the patient's husband complained of weakness, then vomited and had a syncopal episode. He was resuscitated with intravenous (IV) fluids and admitted to the hospital. The following day he suddenly became hypotensive, had a cardiopulmonary arrest, and died. Four days later, the patient again developed nausea, vomiting, diarrhea, and weakness. She also noted numbness in her hands and feet, described as "pins and needles." She distinguished this from the numbness in her toes previously ascribed to diabetic neuropathy. The patient had also been bedridden for the past 10 days due to weakness and inability to walk. There were no further neurologic complaints.

Her past medical history revealed adult onset diabetes for 3 years, hypertension, and an episode of an unknown heart dysrhythmia. Her medications included NPH insulin, digoxin, ranitidine, multivitamins, and thiamine. There was no history of alcohol abuse. Review of systems was pertinent for a 20-lb weight loss over the past month and diffuse tissue swelling,

Physical examination revealed a weak Asian female lying in bed. Vital signs were: blood pressure, 120/75 mm Hg; pulse, 90 beats/min; respirations, 20 beats/min; and temperature, 100.4°F (38°C). HEENT examination demonstrated periorbital edema and bilateral carotid bruits. Lungs were clear to auscultation, and the cardiac examination revealed normal rate with a 2/6 systolic ejection murmur radiating to the aortic region. Abdominal examination revealed mild distention with bowel sounds present, with no tenderness or organomegaly. Pulses were 1+ in all the extremities. Neurologic exam revealed orientation to person, place, and time; cranial nerves II–XII intact; motor examination with muscle strength 4 to 5/5 except for quadriceps and iliopsoas strength of 3/5 bilaterally; deep tendon reflexes 1+ biceps with absent brachioradialis, knee, and ankle reflexes. Plantar reflexes were normal. Sensory examination revealed absent position sense and decreased vibration and pin prick in the lower extremities, and decreased vibration, position sense, and pin prick in the upper extremities.

During the next 3 days the patient's muscle strength diminished in a caudal-to-rostral pattern, and she was transferred to the ICU with a diagnosis of Guillain-Barré syndrome. Review of the records from the first hospitalization revealed a prolonged QT_c interval on routine ECG and a finding of mild hypotension requiring 6 days of intravenous crystalloid infusions, an unusual requirement for the presumed diagnosis of gastroenteritis. In the ICU, laboratory examination revealed a hemoglobin (Hb) of 8.1 g/dL with a mean corpuscular volume (MCV) of 93.3 μ^3, and a white blood count (WBC) of 2400 cells/mm^3. Other laboratory tests were within normal limits, including serum iron, cortisol, vitamin B_{12}, folate, and thyroid function tests. Westergren sedimentation rate was normal at 19 mm/h. Her ECG demonstrated a normal sinus rhythm, QRS axis of +60 degrees, and a QT_c of 0.61 seconds. Lumbar puncture measured a normal opening pressure of 135 mm H_2O and the CSF contained 5 WBC/mm^3, 0 RBC/mm^3, protein 0.042 g/L, and glucose 98 mg/dL. Radiopaque material was noted on a plain abdominal radiograph. The toxicologic consultant ordered a stat spot urine for arsenic, which measured 16,422 μg/L. The patient underwent chelation therapy until the urinary arsenic was less than 50 μg/L. During recovery the patient experienced extreme pain with even light touch to the extremities. Ten months later the patient had gradually recovered from her peripheral neuropathy to the point that she could feed herself.

TABLE 78–1. SOURCES OF ARSENIC

Inorganic (Arsenite [As^{3+}], Arsenate [As^{5+}], elemental)
Insecticides/Pesticides
Arsenic trioxide
Sodium arsenite
Calcium arsenite
Arsenic acid
Ant poisons (now banned by EPA)
Herbicides
Cacodylic acid
Occupational sources
Ethylene oxide manufacture
Electronic device manufacture
Radioactive tracers
Dyes
Semiconductors (gallium arsenide)
Fossil-fuel combustion
Forestry
Agriculture
Decorative glass making
Mining
Smelting/refining
Metallurgy
Medicines/contaminated drugs
Asian folk remedies
Homeopathic remedies
Depilatory
Herbals
Opium
"Moonshine" ethanol
Kelp
Other
Wood preservatives (chromium–copper–arsenate)
Contaminated well water
Organic
Seafood
Melarsoprol (trypanocidal)
Parasitic chemotherapy (veterinary)

What Are the Pharmacologic Properties and Toxicologic Effects of Arsenic?

Arsenic, an element situated between phosphorous and antimony in group Vb of the Periodic Table, assumes characteristics of the elements near it and thus is characterized as a metalloid. Multiple forms exist: elemental, gaseous (arsine), organic, and inorganic (arsenite [trivalent] and arsenate [pentavalent]). The diversity of sources of arsenic is described in Table 78–1. The gaseous form is highly toxic; its effects are covered in Chapter 24. Of the remaining forms, inorganic arsenite, as arsenic trioxide (As_2O_3), is the most prevalent natural form, and the trivalent compounds are also the most toxic.[118] Arsenic metal is thought to be nonpoisonous due to its insolubility in water or bodily fluids,[5,118] and the toxicity of exogenous organic forms is low.[34] Therefore this chapter will discuss the properties and toxicity of inorganic arsenic only.

Tasteless and odorless, arsenic is well-absorbed via the gastrointestinal, respiratory, and parenteral routes. Gastrointestinal absorption of inorganic arsenic depends on the solubility of the arsenical compound. For most trivalent and pentavalent arsenical compounds dissolved in water, the gastrointestinal absorptive rate exceeds 90% in human and animal studies,[97,135,138] with greatest absorption occurring predominantly in the small intestine, followed by the colon.[94] Poorly soluble compounds such as arsenic trioxide are less well absorbed.[135] Smaller particle size may facilitate absorption whereas dietary factors such as casein are inhibitory.[93,121,135] Inhaled arsenic is absorbed either through the lungs or via the gastrointestinal tract after being swallowed. Large arsenic particles will deposit in the upper respiratory tract, where ciliary action results in removal and transfer to the gastrointestinal tract, while respirable particles will deposit in the air exchange region of the respiratory tract. Either scenario can result in approximately 80% systemic absorption.[97,102,126] Minimal dermal absorption occurs through intact skin,[1] but prolonged topical administration can cause skin irritation, which may promote systemic absorption.[114] Mucous membrane absorption can be consequential. Administration via enema has also resulted in fatality.[30]

Blood clearance of arsenic occurs in three phases, with significant extraplasma distribution resulting within 15 minutes after intravenous injection.[86] In phase 1, a rapid decline occurs within 2–3 hours; some estimate greater than 90% of arsenic clears from the blood with a half life ($t_{1/2}$) of 1–2 hours.[85,135] For the remaining arsenic, a more gradual decline occurs in phase 2, from 3 hours to 7 days (estimated $t_{1/2}$ = 30 hours). This is followed by phase 3, a slower elimination phase with an estimated $t_{1/2}$ = 200 hours.[86,135] Acutely, tissue levels are highest in liver and kidney with distribution also occurring in virtually all other body tissues.[30,65,92,135] Brain partitioning ensues rapidly; in a human study of the fate of injected radiolabeled trivalent arsenic in normal brain, the greatest percentage of the injected dose was found in the first hour after injection.[86] Chronic ingestion of small amounts of arsenic result in highest concentrations in hair, nails, and skin, tissues rich in cysteine-containing proteins.[6,85] Chronic accumulation also occurs in lungs.[6] Arsenic crosses the placenta and can accumulate in the fetus.[17,53,135]

Metabolism of inorganic arsenic occurs via methylation. If the arsenic is in pentavalent form, it must first be reduced to the trivalent form.[134] The methylation process forms methylarsonic acid (MMA) followed by dimethylarsinic acid (DMA).[23,25,84] Methylation also renders the arsenic less reactive to tissues and increases elimination from the body.[23,135] Each added methyl group decreases the acute toxicity of the arsenic by an order of magnitude, although this effect may not be true for chronic toxicity and carcinogenecity.[85] For man, the estimated LD_{50} of arsenic trioxide is 1.43 mg/kg, while that of MMA is 50 mg/kg and that of DMA is 500 mg/kg. Both unchanged arsenic and its methylated metabolites are excreted predominantly by the kidneys in an elaborate process involving glomerular filtration, tubular secretion, and active reabsorption.[132,138] Human volunteer studies demonstrate renal arsenic elimination of 46–63% of a dose within 4–5 days postingestion.[23,103,135] Another 30% is cleared with a $t_{1/2}$ greater than 1 week, while the remainder demonstrates a $t_{1/2}$ of greater than 1 month.[85,103] Fecal excretion may eliminate 5% of an oral dose,[135] less for parenterally administered arsenic.[86] Some biliary excretion occurs independent of fecal elimination.[29,105] Knowledge of this excretion assumes importance when ongoing gastrointestinal decontamination is considered; if unremoved, this secreted arsenic may be reabsorbed by the small intestine. Very small amounts of arsenic are eliminated via sweating and skin desquamation.[88,135]

Inorganic arsenic elimination also depends on the chemical form, the route of administration, and the dose. The pentavalent form, oral administration, and smaller doses favor a faster elimination rate.[31,136] Glutathione depletion decreases arsenic elimination by inhibiting methylation since reduced glutathione is necessary for this process.[22,56] Thus, individuals with glutathione deficiency, such as alcoholic or malnourished patients, may be more susceptible to arsenic toxicity.

The toxicologic mechanisms of inorganic arsenic differ for the trivalent and pentavalent forms. For trivalent arsenic (As^{3+}), inhibition of the pyruvate dehydrogenase (PDH) complex is the primary biochemical lesion.[106,110] Dysfunction of this complex, which is comprised of three enzymes, occurs when As^{3+} binds to the sulfhydryl groups of dihydrolipoamide, preventing regeneration of lipoamide, which is a necessary cofactor in the conversion of pyruvate to acetyl coenzyme A (acetyl CoA)[99] (Fig. 78–1). Diminished acetyl CoA levels, in turn, reduce

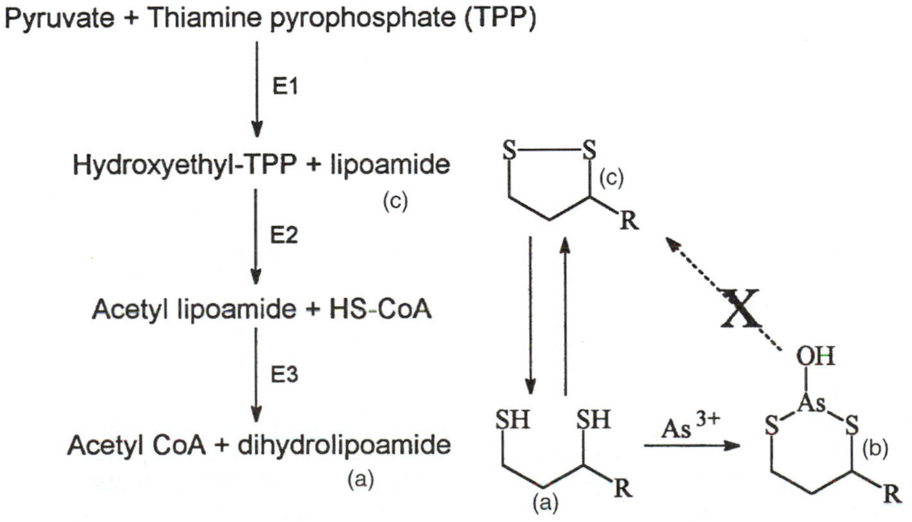

Figure 78–1. Effect of trivalent arsenicals (As^{3+}) on pyruvate dehydrogenase complex. (a) = dihydrolipoamide, (b) = arsenic binding preventing the regeneration of lipoamide, (c) = lipoamide, E1 = pyruvate dehydrogenase, E2 = dihydrolipoamide acetyltransferase, E3 = dihydrolipoamide dehydrogenase.

citric acid cycle activity with resulting decreased production of adenosine triphosphate (ATP). Direct effects of As^{3+} on the alpha-ketoglutarate dehydrogenase complex, which contains a dihydrolipoyl dehydrogenase identical to that in the PDH complex, further reduce citric acid cycle activity.

Arsenic^{3+} also interferes with glucose production and uptake. The drop in acetyl CoA levels, discussed above, also inhibits the activity of pyruvate carboxylase, which catalyzes the conversion of pyruvate to oxaloacetate, the initial step in gluconeogenesis.[127] Animal studies demonstrate that As^{3+} has the greatest effect on gluconeogenesis from pyruvate with lesser effects on gluconeogenesis from other substances such as lactate, amino acids, and glycerol.[128] Impaired gluconeogenesis combined with carbohydrate depletion due to the stress of poisoning can result in hypoglycemia.[108,110,128] Arsenic^{3+} also affects other sulfhydryl-containing enzymes, including membrane transport enzymes involved with insulin-independent cellular glucose uptake.[74–76] Thus cellular lack of glucose may be a consequential problem in As^{3+} poisoning,[107,128] although it remains unproven in humans.

The importance of the inhibition of thiolase, which catalyzes the final step in fatty acid oxidation, is less clear.[111] Diminished fatty acid oxidation results in decreased acetyl CoA production. This results in decreased ATP production due to the loss of acetyl CoA units and to the loss of NADH and $FADH_2$, electron carriers reduced during fatty acid breakdown whose subsequent oxidation yields ATP.[127] However, this cause of diminished ATP production may be insignificant compared to the effect of PDH inhibition.[128] Trivalent arsenic also inhibits glutathione synthetase, glucose-6-phosphate dehydrogenase, and glutathione reductase.[24] This results in decreased levels of reduced glutathione, which facilitates arsenic metabolism, protects red blood cells (RBCs) from oxidative damage, and maintains hemoglobin in the ferrous form [Fe^{2+}].[128] Dermal toxicity may result from As^{3+}-induced production of growth-promoting cytokines and growth factors in keratinocytes.[45]

The toxicity of arsenate (As^{5+}) may be partially due to its transformation to arsenite (As^{3+}).[58,137] However, arsenate resembles phosphate chemically and structurally,[6,127] may share a common transport system for cellular uptake with phosphate,[58] and can uncouple oxidative phosphorylation by substituting for inorganic phosphate (P_i) in the glycolysis reaction catalyzed by glyceraldehyde 3-phosphate dehydrogenase (Fig. 78–2).[12] The resulting unstable product, 1-arseno-3-phosphoglycerate, spontaneously hydrolyzes to 3-phosphoglycerate, so glycolysis continues. However, the ATP normally produced during conversion of 1,3-bisphosphoglycerate to 3-phosphoglycerate is lost. Uncoupling may also occur if adenosine diphosphate (ADP) forms ADP-arsenate instead of ATP in the presence of As^{5+}. The ADP-arsenate rapidly hydrolyzes, thus uncoupling oxidative phosphorylation.[50]

What Are the Signs and Symptoms of Arsenic Toxicity?

Signs and symptoms of arsenic toxicity vary depending on the amount and form ingested; the rate of absorption, metabolism, and excretion; and the time course of ingestion (acute, subacute, or chronic ingestion). Both arsenite and arsenate compounds can produce toxicity. In a review of 149 cases suspected of ingesting arsenate ant killer (typically 2.28% sodium arsenate) reported to a regional poison center, based on mild, limited symptoms of vomiting and diarrhea developing in only 3 patients, the authors concluded that "toxicity from single, acute, accidental ingestions of sodium arsenate . . . appears minimal."[62] This conclusion is problematic for the following reasons: 137 cases were children 3 years of age or less, who presumably ingested very small amounts; arsenic levels were performed in only 1 patient, thus leaving in doubt whether the other 148 cases, all unintentional ingestions, consumed a significant amount of sodium arsenate; and the one case of suicidal ingestion was chelated immediately with dimercaprol (BAL), which contributed to his relative lack of symptoms. Other reported cases of suicidal or homicidal arsenate ingestions have exhibited clinical manifestations similar to those seen with arsenite toxicity.[83,123] Thus, patients with arsenate exposures should be treated no differently from those with arsenite exposures.

Acute toxicity typically begins with gastrointestinal symptoms of nausea, vomiting, abdominal pain, and diarrhea which may be rice water or cholera like, occurring 10 minutes to several hours postingestion.[15,46,54,61,69,117,125,142] Cardiovascular instability often accompanies or quickly follows these symptoms. Manifestations of this instability range from sinus tachycardia and orthostatic hypotension to a frank shock, which can mimic sepsis or acute myocardial infarction.[10,15,17,39,47,69] Intravascular volume depletion, capillary leak myocardial dysfunction, and diminished systemic vascular resistance contribute to the hypotension.[17,21,89,120] Patients with severe poisoning may also quickly develop acute encephalopathy with delirium, seizures, coma, dysrhythmias, fever, pulmonary edema, ARDS and respiratory failure, hepatitis, rhabdomyolysis, hemolytic anemia, acute renal failure, and death.[1,15,17,37,46,47,49,125,129] The encephalopathy may develop over several days following an acute ingestion and is attributed to underlying cerebral edema and focal microhemorrhages.[32,39,46,47,120] Seizures may be secondary to direct CNS toxicity, cerebral edema, or an underlying cardiac dysrhythmia.[120] In three reported cases, seizures secondary to torsades de pointes associated with a prolonged QT_c developed 4 days to 5 weeks after acute arsenic ingestion.[15,46,125] Thus, an underlying dysrhythmia should be investigated in any seizing patient with arsenic toxicity. Fever may occur[1,35,125] and further reinforce a misdiagnosis of sepsis. Hepatitis can develop[37,129] and may be due to altered intrahepatic heme metabolism resulting in increased synthesis of bilirubin, and/or altered protein transport be-

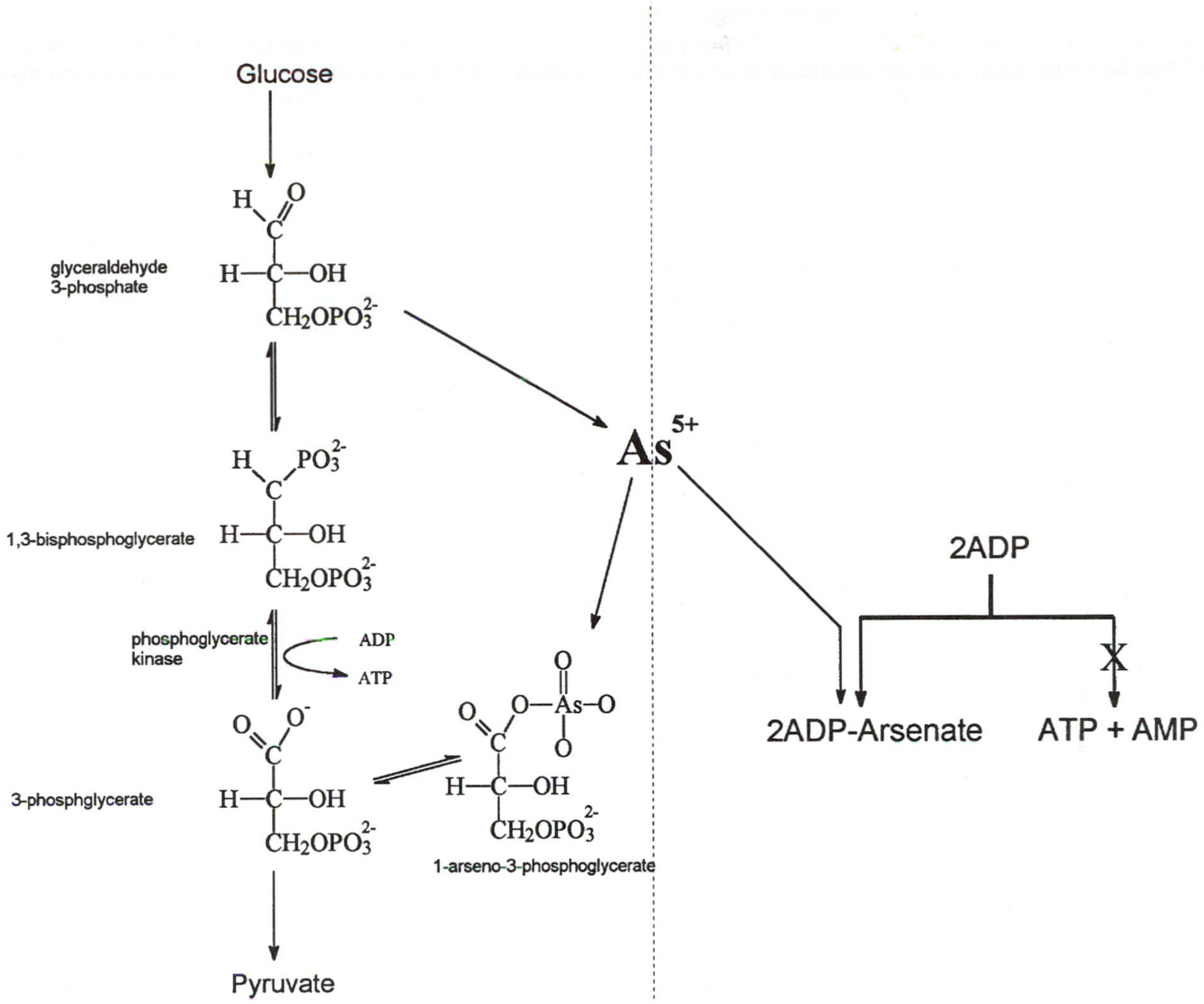

Figure 78–2. Proposed toxic effects of pentavalent arsenic (As^{5+}) on glycolysis.

tween hepatocytes.[3] Rhabdomyolysis with biopsy-proven acute myopathy has been reported,[37] as well as acute hemolytic anemia.[10] Acute renal failure has occurred in many cases. The etiology may be multifactorial, including renal ischemia secondary to hypotension, myoglobinuric- and hemoglobinuric-induced failure, renal cortical necrosis, and a direct toxic effect on renal tubules.[19,44,133] Glutathione depletion, which can exist in malnourished patients and alcoholics, may enhance the nephrotoxicity of arsenic.[56] Unilateral facial nerve palsy, acute pancreatitis, pericarditis, and pleuritis were reported in one case.[147] Fetal demise in pregnant women has occurred with toxic levels of arsenic reported in the fetal organs.[17,78]

Acutely poisoned patients with less severe illness may experience persistent gastroenteritis and mild hypotension, necessitating hospitalization and intravenous fluids for days.[69] This prolonged course is atypical for most viral and bacterial enteric illnesses and should alert the physician to consider arsenic toxicity, especially if the gastroenteritis recurs. Patients may complain of a metallic taste. The garlicky breath odor attributed to arsenic has also developed after exposure to arsine gas. Arsenic irritates mucous membranes. Patients unwittingly ingesting arsenic-laden chocolate complained of a burning oral sensation.[17] The irritated mucous membranes can mimic pharyngitis,[53] leading to a misdiagnosis of upper respiratory tract infection. Gastrointestinal ulcerative lesions and hemorrhage can occur.[39,47] Toxic erythroderma and exfoliative dermatitis result from a hypersensitivity reaction to arsenic.[129]

Further signs and symptoms may develop subacutely in the days to weeks following the acute toxic episode. Peripheral neuropathy due to axonal degeneration typically develops 1–3 weeks after arsenic ingestion, although one case series reported nine patients who developed maximal neuropathy within 24 hours.[28,54,69] Sensory symptoms predominate early, with patients complaining of "pins and needles" or electrical shock like pains in the lower extremities.[28,54,82] Early physical examination may demonstrate isolated diminished or absent vibratory sense.[54] As the neuropathy progresses, symptoms include numbness, tingling, and formication with physical findings of diminished to absent pain, touch, temperature, and deep tendon reflexes in a stocking–glove distribution.[28,54,69] Motor weakness may then develop. The worst cases manifest an ascending flaccid paralysis mimicking Guillain-Barré syndrome.[17,28,54,69] Encephalopathic symptoms of headache, confusion, decreased memory, personality change, irritability, hallucinations, delirium, and seizures may develop or persist.[10,32,35,43,54,82,98] Sixth cranial nerve palsy and bilateral sensorineural hearing loss have been reported during this subacute period.[1,28,46] Superficial touch of the extremities may elicit severe or deep aching pains.[54,82] Dermatologic lesions can include patchy alopecia, oral herpetic-appearing lesions, a diffuse pruritic macular rash, and a brawny, nonpruritic desquamation.[10,35,54,82,96,129,142] Mee's lines of the nails, horizontal 1–2 mm white lines, which represent arsenic deposition, uncommonly occur after acute episodes of poisoning[4,87] (see Color Plate Fig. 14). A series of 74 chronic and acute arsenical cases found Mee's lines in only 5% of patients.[1] In thoses cases where Mee's lines are found, a delay of 30–40 days after ingestion is required for the lines to extend visibly beyond the nail lunalae.[54,125] Facial and peripheral edema may develop,[1,10,54,96] as well as diaphoresis.[28,39,54] Respiratory manifestations including dry hacking cough, rales, hemoptysis, chest pain, and patchy interstitial infiltrates have been reported.[54,98] Again, the possibility for a misdiagnosis of bronchitis, viral pneumonia, or persistent upper respiratory infection exists. Other potential toxic manifestations include pancytopenia, nephropathy, fatigue, anorexia with weight loss, and torsades de pointes dysrhythmia as well as persistence of acute gastrointestinal symptoms.[10,82]

With chronic, low-level arsenic exposure, many subacute symptoms may develop or persist, including headache, chronic encephalopathy, peripheral sensorimotor neuropathy, malaise, chronic cough, and peripheral edema. Gastrointestinal symptoms may be absent, although cases with colicky abdominal pain, nausea, and persistent diarrhea have been reported.[18,24,54,98] Numerous dermatologic lesions can develop. In a survey of a Mexican population chronically exposed to arsenate and arsenite in well water, hypopigmentation (thought to be the first skin change), hyperpigmentation, palmoplantar keratoses, papular keratoses and ulcerative lesions (epidermoid/basal cell carcinomas at autopsy) were observed[24] (see Color Plate Fig. 13). These skin lesions have been detected in other chronically exposed cases[1,18,82,129,131] and in a population cohort.[33] Squamous cell carcinomas and Bowen's disease of the skin have also been observed.[129]

Other cancers are noted in patients exposed to arsenic via medicinal preparations, industrial or mining processes, or contaminated well water.[14,16,26,60,131] Increased rates of lung cancer are documented in chemical and smelter workers,[95,101,143] with reported latency periods of 34–51 years between arsenic exposure and disease.[11,70,130] Animal studies indicate that free radicals generated during metabolism of dimethylarsinic acid may cause pulmonary DNA damage.[112,144,145] Increased rates of renal and bladder cancer are also reported.[14] Hepatic angiosarcomas, as well as cirrhosis and noncirrhotic portal hypertension, are linked to chronic arsenic exposure.[51,60,68,90,104,113]

An obliterative arterial disease of the lower extremities, Blackfoot's disease, occurs on the southwest coast of Taiwan, where elevated arsenic levels exist in well water.[27,131] The incidence of disease increases with age and with arsenic content of well water.[131] Finally, three cases of aplastic anemia and eleven cases of agranulocytosis have been documented following arsenic exposure.[35]

What Are the Neurologic Sequelae of Arsenic Toxicity?

Slow, partial recovery from peripheral neuropathy most commonly occurs, with mild cases having a better prognosis.[17,54] In a case series of 40 patients followed for variable time periods, 60% experienced partial recovery over 5 months to 5 years, 15% had full recovery from 40 days to 6 years, while 5% had no recovery over 5 years. The remainder either died or were lost to follow-up.[28] Administration of BAL after the development of peripheral neuropathy is generally felt to be ineffective. In this same case series, 50% of patients treated with variable BAL regimens had minimal to no improvement, while 60% not treated with BAL had a similar outcome.[28] Improvement in the peripheral neuropathy is often accompanied by transient severe pains in the extremities.[54] Patients who develop encephalopathy may recover poorly.[39]

What Laboratory Studies Can Assist in This Patient's Diagnosis?

The utility of laboratory diagnostic studies depends on whether the exposure is acute, acute-on-chronic, chronic, or remote with residual clinical effects. Failure to understand the time course of arsenic metabolism, clearance, and effect on laboratory parameters can mislead the clinician in assessing a case of possible arsenic toxicity. In acute and acute-on-chronic poisoning, an abdominal radiograph will likely demonstrate radiopaque material in the gastrointestinal tract,[2,47,55] which may be misinterpreted as the residua of a barium radiographic study. How long this material can be seen after ingestion remains unknown but will depend on the dose and form of arsenic, gastrointestinal motility, the presence of co-ingestants, the underlying condition of the gastrointestinal mucosa, and the effects of any gastric decontamination procedures. Diagnosis ultimately depends on finding an elevated urinary arsenic level. In an emergency, a spot urine may be sent prior to beginning chelation therapy. An elevated arsenic level verifies the diagnosis whereas a low level does not exclude arsenic toxicity.[140] In nine acute, symptomatic patients, initial spot urine arsenic levels ranged from 192 to 198,450 μg/L.[61] Because urinary excretion of arsenic is intermittent,[30] definitive diagnosis hinges upon finding a level of ≥ 50 μg/L or a total of ≥ 100 μg arsenic in a 24-hour urine collection. When interpreting slightly elevated urinary arsenic levels, laboratory findings must be correlated with the clinical findings, since seafood ingestion has been reported to transiently elevate urinary arsenic excretion up to 1700 μg/L.[9] Where seafood arsenic is a consideration, speciation of arsenic can be accomplished either using liquid chromatography separation followed by graphite furnace atomic absorption analysis[91] or by ion chromatography coupled with inductively coupled plasma mass spectrometry.[72,115] These techniques separate arsenobetaine (the predominant arsenic form in seafood), As^{3+}, As^{5+}, MMA, and DMA. All urines should be collected in metal-free containers. If testing is performed by an outside reference laboratory, specimens from acutely ill patients should be sent via express transportation with a request for a rapid result.

Laboratory evaluation of chronic toxicity, including laboratory parameters that become abnormal within days to weeks following an acute exposure, should focus on complete blood count (CBC), renal and liver function tests, and urinalysis (UA) as well as 24-hour urinary arsenic determinations. Complete blood count findings can include a normocytic, normochromic, or megaloblastic anemia; an initial leukocytosis followed by leukopenia, with neutrophils depressed more than lymphocytes, and a relative eosinophilia; thrombocytopenia; and a rapidly declining hemoglobin indicative of hemolytic anemia or a gastrointestinal hemorrhage.[10,67,142] Basophilic stippling of RBCs may be seen;[36,67,125,147] this can occur in other toxic and clinical disorders (see Chaps. 24, 79). Karyorrhexis, a rupture of the RBC cell nucleus with chromatin disintegration into granules that are extruded from the cell, and dyserythropoeisis are reported in both lead- and arsenic-toxic patients. Both findings are due to arsenic-induced inhibition of DNA synthesis and damage to the nuclear envelope.[38] The karyorrhexis can occur within 4 days and resolve by 2 weeks after poisoning[67,73,77] and may be an early indication of arsenic toxicity.[36] Elevated serum creatinine, aminotransferases, and bilirubin and depressed haptoglobin levels may develop.[10] Urinalysis may reveal proteinuria, hematuria, and pyuria.[10,142] Cerebral spinal fluid examination in patients with CNS findings can be normal[28,54,82] or exhibit mild protein elevation to 0.265 g/L,[54] in contradistinction to patients with Guillain-Barré syndrome, who usually exhibit a protein concentration > 0.55 g/L after the first week of illness with a cell count < 10 cells/mm³ (see Table 78–2).[116] Urinary arsenic excretion varies inversely with the postexposure time period, but low-level excretion may continue for months after exposure.[30,54] In a study of 41 cases of arsenic-induced peripheral neuropathy, most patients with a neuropathy of 4–8 weeks' duration had total 24-hour urinary arsenic measurements of 100–400 μg.[54] In cases of suspected arsenic toxicity in which the urinary arsenic measurements fall below accepted toxic levels, analysis of hair and nails may permit a diagnosis. Arsenic can be detected in the proximal portions of hair within 30 hours of ingestion.[146] Hair grows at a rate of 0.4 mm/day while nail grows at 0.1 mm/day. Total replacement of a fingernail requires 3–4 months while toenails require 6–9 months of growth.[52,79] These facts, plus the frequency of hair cutting, should be considered when estimating the utility of measuring arsenic levels in these tissues. Reference laboratory normal values should be used to determine the presence of elevated arsenic levels. The utility of a chelation mobilization test to unmask occult arsenic toxicity is doubtful, since arsenic is not appreciably stored in body tissues. Penicillamine chelation for 1 week failed to elevate urinary arsenic levels in two symptomatic patients who had elevated nail and hair levels.[98] In cases of remote toxicity, hair and nail arsenic measurements may or may not be elevated, depending on the time elapsed since exposure.

TABLE 78–2. DIFFERENTIAL DIAGNOSIS OF INORGANIC ARSENIC TOXICITY

Neurologic	Mercury
Encephalopathy	Paralytic shellfish poisoning
Korsakoff's syndrome	Buckthorn
Viral	Organophosphates
AIDS	***Dermatologic***
Peripheral neuropathy	Dermatitis
Guillain-Barré syndrome	Stasis
Diabetic	Atrophic
Alcohol induced	Contact
Nutritional	Exfoliative
Endocrinopathy	Lichen planus
Hypothyroidism	Lichen planus simplex
Hyperthyroidism	Malignancy
Addison's disease	***Infectious***
Hematologic	Sepsis
Porphyria	Pharyngitis
Hemolytic anemia	Upper respiratory infection
Iron deficiency anemia	***Cardiovascular***
Gastrointestinal	Myocardial ischemia/infarction
Gastroenteritis	Myocarditis
Hepatitis	Peripheral vascular disease
Toxins	***Other***
Thallium	Depression

What Are the Key Management Issues?

Initial

Any patient suspected of having a progressive ascending neuropathy should be hospitalized in intensive care and undergo frequent negative inspiratory force (NIF) testing to detect deteriorating respiratory function. A detailed history, including recent illnesses or immunizations, licit or illicit drug use, ingestions, unusual dietary or health habits such as use of herbal or homeopathic medications, hobbies and occupational or other exogenous chemical exposures should be obtained (see Table 78–1). Routine laboratory tests, including electrolytes, BUN, glucose, complete blood count with differential, metabolic chemistry profile, and urinalysis are indicated, as is thyroid function testing. An electrocardiogram, chest radiograph, and lumbar puncture (LP) should be performed.

General Management for Arsenic

Acute arsenical toxicity is life-threatening and mandates aggressive treatment. Advanced life-support monitoring and therapies should be initiated when necessary. Hypotension can be treated with crystalloid fluids, pressor agents such as dopamine and levarterenol, and blood products if gastrointestinal hemorrhage occurs. Careful attention to fluid balance is important, since cerebral and pulmonary edema may be present. Ventricular tachycardia and fibrillation can be treated with lidocaine, bretylium, and electrical defibrillation. Agents that prolong the QT_c, such as the class IA, IC, and III antidysrhythmic agents, should be avoided. Potassium, magnesium, and calcium levels should be maintained within normal range to avoid exacerbating a prolonged QT_c. Torsades de pointes dysrhythmia may respond to magnesium, isoproterenol, and overdrive pacing therapies. Seizures should be treated with benzodiazepines, phenobarbital, phenytoin, and general anesthesia, as required. If radiopaque material is seen in the gastrointestinal tract, lavage with a large-bore orogastric tube followed by instillation of activated charcoal for possible co-ingestants is indicated. This should be followed by whole-bowel irrigation (see Antidotes in Depth: Whole-bowel Irrigation) until the radiopaque material is no longer seen on repeat abdominal radiograph. Continuing nasogastric suction may be important in removing arsenic resecreted in the gastric or biliary secretions.[105] In three patients arsenite was still detectable in the gastric aspirate 5–7 days following an ingestion.[80] Early parenteral nutrition with careful attention to glucose metabolism is essential to avoid the deleterious effect of hypoglycemia on the brain.

In cases of chronic toxicity the patient should be removed from the arsenic source and gastric decontamination performed if there is evidence of arsenic in the gastrointestinal tract. For all cases, if homicidal intent is suspected, patients should be advised against accepting food or drink from anyone. Hospital visitors should be closely monitored and outside nutritional products should be forbidden.

Specific Management for Arsenic

Chelation therapy should begin as soon as acute arsenic toxicity is suspected and should not be withheld pending laboratory confirmation of the diagnosis. In cases of subacute and chronic toxicity, chelation therapy can await rapid laboratory verification unless the patient's clinical condition is deteriorating. Three agents are available in the United States for accelerated removal of arsenic: 2,3-dimercaptopropanol (British Anti-Lewisite, or BAL), 2,3-dimercaptosuccinic acid (DMSA), and D-penicillamine (see Antidotes in Depth: Dimercaprol for discussion). BAL and DMSA form dimercaptan–arsenic complexes that concomitantly remove arsenic from tissues and render it more water soluble and thus more readily excreted.[81] BAL has been the standard therapy for inorganic arsenic toxicity. It is administered IM in doses of 3–5 mg/kg every 4–6 hours until the 24-hour urinary arsenic excretion is less than 50 μg/L or until another agent is substituted. In case series BAL has been reportedly efficacious in acute toxicity, especially if given early. Of 33 severely ill patients, 24 were treated with BAL within 6 hours (mean = 1 hour) and 75% survived, while the remaining 9 patients were treated later with BAL (range 9 to 72 hours, mean = 30 hours) and only 45% survived.[35] Of 4 patients with a massive unintentional arsenic exposure, 3 treated early with BAL recovered while the fourth, inadequately chelated, died.[35] Of 15 patients with encephalopathy, 14 improved clinically within 24 hours of initiating BAL therapy.[35] British Anti-Lewisite may also be efficacious in treating skin eruption, dermatitis, and agranulocytosis.[35] When initiated for peripheral neuropathy in subacute cases, BAL therapy accelerated recovery but did not affect the overall recovery rate.[28]

Adverse effects may occur with BAL (Table 78–3), especially at doses of 4 mg/kg or greater. In vitro and animal experiments have raised concerns that BAL may actually worsen arsenic toxicity, perhaps by facilitating cellular entry of arsenic to its active sites, especially the brain.[7,8,41,57,66,106,119] However, many of these studies focus on tissue levels of arsenic rather than survival rates. Other studies demonstrate the effectiveness of BAL in removing tissue arsenic.[40,124] Additionally, in a cellular model BAL reversed inhibition of cellular glucose uptake more readily than either DMSA or DMPS.[75] At this writing BAL remains the only chelation agent that can be administered parenterally to critically ill patients who may have decreased gastrointestinal motility or residual arsenic in the gastrointestinal tract.

2,3-Dimercaptosuccinic acid, an oral analog of BAL, has been approved by the Food and Drug Administration only for lead chelation in children. Nonetheless DMSA has been used successfully to chelate arsenic in humans.[42,63,72] In mice given an LD_{99} dose of arsenite, the therapeutic index of DMSA exceeded that of BAL.[8] Studies in rabbits, mice, and guinea pigs indicate DMSA to be equal or superior to BAL in eliminating arsenic.[59,66,81,119] 2,3-Dimercaptosuccinic acid increased biliary elimination of arsenic, whereas BAL had no effect in a guinea pig model.[109] Thus use of DMSA may be advantageous in patients with renal insufficiency. Oral DMSA can be substituted for BAL as soon as gastrointestinal motility returns in acutely ill patients and may be the therapy of choice in subacute and chronically toxic patients with functioning gastrointestinal tracts. In acutely toxic patients, gastrointestinal decontamination should precede

TABLE 78–3. ADVERSE EFFECTS OF CHELATING AGENTS USED FOR ARSENIC INTOXICATION

Chelating Agent	Adverse Effects
BAL	Hypertension
	Febrile reaction, diaphoresis
	Painful injection, injection site sterile abscess
	Nausea/vomiting, salivation
	Headache
	Lacrimation, salivation, rhinorrhea
	Hemolysis in G-6-PD deficient patients
	BAL–iron complex very toxic
D-Penicillamine	Nausea/vomiting
	Fever
	Rash
	Leukopenia, thrombocytopenia
	Eosinophilia
	Hemolytic anemia
	Stevens-Johnson syndrome
DMSA	Nausea, vomiting, diarrhea
	Abdominal gas, pain
	Transient elevated AST, alkaline phosphatase
	Rash, pruritus
	Sore throat, rhinorrhea
	Drowsiness, paresthesia
	Thrombocytosis, eosinophilia

DMSA administration. Whether DMSA will enhance gastrointestinal absorption of arsenic remains unknown, although this has not been a problem in treating lead toxicity. 2,3-Dimercaptosuccinic acid dosage follows the guidelines approved for lead: 10 mg/kg/dose every 8 hours for 5 days, followed by 10 mg/kg/dose every 12 hours until the urinary arsenic is less than 50 μg/L/24 hours or for an additional 14 days. If urinary arsenic remains elevated, this regimen may be extended. Liver function tests should be monitored, as well as essential metal levels if prolonged therapy is required. A significant decrease in zinc was reported in one human case,[42] and increased copper excretion was found in one rodent study.[48]

D-Penicillamine has been used as an oral chelating agent in cases of arsenic toxicity[100,141] without experimental evidence validating this treatment. A comparison of the effectiveness of D-penicillamine, BAL, DMSA, and 2,3-dimercapto-1-propanesulfonic acid (DMPS) in murine, guinea pig, and in vitro rat renal tubule models found D-penicillamine ineffective in treating arsenic toxicity in all three models.[64] D-Penicillamine should be used only if BAL and DMSA are unavailable. The recommended dose is 25 mg/kg/dose (maximum 1 g/24 hours) every 6 hours until the urinary arsenic is less than 50 μg/L/24 hours.

Hemodialysis may be an effective adjunct therapy in patients with decreased renal function. Reported clearance values have ranged from 76 to 87.5 mL/min, with or without concomitant BAL therapy.[83,139] Two acutely toxic patients with renal failure received BAL therapy and then underwent multiple hemodialysis treatments.[139] Total arsenic removed in a single 4-hour dialysis exceeded 24-hour urinary excretion in each patient. When renal function returned, however, urinary arsenic excretion far exceeded the amount removed by hemodialysis. Thus hemodialysis may be most useful in patients with diminished renal function.

Other therapies either experimental or not approved for use in the United States include:

1. 2,3-Dimercapto-1-propanesulfonic acid (DMPS). Used as the primary chelating agent in the former Soviet Union. Animal studies show DMPS equal to or better than DMSA and BAL in ameliorating arsenic toxicity.[7,59,109]
2. Monoesters of DMSA. Engineered to increase lipophilicity compared to the parent DMSA. A rodent study indicates that these monoesters may be comparable to or more effective than DMSA in chelating arsenic, with no elevation in brain arsenic measured.[65]
3. *N*-Acetylcysteine (NAC). Supplies monothiol groups whose adducts with arsenic are not as stable as those formed by dithiols, such as DMSA and BAL.[20,41] In animal models cysteine and NAC have ameliorated arsenic toxicity.[13,122]
4. Antibodies to arsenic. In one murine study antibodies formed to arsenic conferred protection from low-dose but not high-dose arsenic.[71]
5. 2,3-Dithioerythritol (DTE). A BAL derivative with polarity intermediate between BAL and DMSA. DTE demonstrated improved survival in cells exposed to phenyldichloroarsine when compared to BAL and DMSA.[20]
6. Sulfo-adenosyl-L-methionine. Donates methyl groups that may facilitate methylation and elimination of arsenic.

References

1. Abernathy CO, Ohanian EV: Non-carcinogenic effects of inorganic arsenic. Environ Geochem Health 1992;14:35–41.
2. Adelson L, George RA, Mandel A: Acute arsenic intoxication shown by roentgenograms. Arch Intern Med 1961; 107:401–404.
3. Albores A, Cebrian ME, Bach PH, et al: Sodium arsenite induced alterations in bilirubin excretion and heme metabolism. J Biochem Toxicol 1989;4:73–78.
4. Aldrich CJ: Leuconychia striata arsenicalis transversus: With report of three cases. Am J Med 1904;127:702–709.
5. Ambient Water Quality Criteria Doc: Arsenic. 1980; (EPA 440/5-80-021:A-1). Abstract.
6. Aposhian HV: Biochemical toxicology of arsenic. Rev Biochem Toxicol 1989;10:265–299.
7. Aposhian HV, Aposhian MM: Newer developments in arsenic toxicity. J Am Coll Toxicol 1989;8:1297–1305.
8. Aposhian HV, Carter DE, Hoover TD, et al: DMSA, DMPS, and DMPA as arsenic antidotes. Fund Appl Toxicol 1984;4:S58–S70.
9. Arbouine MW, Wilson HK: The effect of seafood consumption on the assessment of occupational exposure to

arsenic by urinary arsenic speciation measurements. J Trace Elem 1992;6:153–160.
10. Armstrong CW, Stroube RB, Rubio T, et al: Outbreak of fatal arsenic poisoning caused by contaminated drinking water. Arch Environ Health 1984;39:276–279.
11. Axelson O, Dahlgren E, Jansson CD, Rehnlund SO: Arsenic exposure and mortality: A case-referent study from a Swedish copper smelter. Br J Indian Med 1978;35:8–15.
12. Azzone GF, Ernster L: Compartmentation of mitochondrial phosphorylations as disclosed by studies with arsenate. J Biol Chem 1961;236:1510–1517.
13. Baker DH, Czarnecki-Maulden GL: Pharmacologic role of cysteine in ameliorating or exacerbating mineral toxicities. J Nutr 1987;117:1003–1010.
14. Bates MN, Smith SH, Hopenhayn-Rich C: Arsenic ingestion and internal cancers: A review. Am J Epidemiol 1992; 135:462–476.
15. Beckman KJ, Bauman JL, Pimental PA, et al: Arsenic-induced torsades de pointes. Crit Care Med 1991;19:290–291.
16. Bencko V, Symon K, Stalnik L, et al: Rate of malignant tumor mortality among coal burning power plant workers occupationally exposed to arsenic. J Hyg Epidemiol Microbiol Immunol 1980;24:278–284.
17. Bolliger CT, van Zijl P, Louw JA: Multiple organ failure with the adult respiratory distress syndrome in homicidal arsenic poisoning. Respiration 1992;59:57–61.
18. Borgono JM, Vincent P, Venturino H, Infante A: Arsenic in the drinking water of the city of Antofagasta: Epidemiological and clinical study before and after the installation of a treatment plant. Environ Health Perspect 1977;19: 103–105.
19. Bouletreau P, Ducluzeau R, Bui-Xuan B, et al: Acute renal complications of acute intoxications. Acta Pharmacol Toxicol 1977;41(suppl):49–63.
20. Boyd VL, Harbell JW, O'Connor RJ, McGown EL: 2,3-Dithioerythritol, a possible new arsenic antidote. Chem Res Toxicol 1989;2:301–306.
21. Brown CE, McNamara DH: Acute interstitial myocarditis following administration of arsphenamines. Arch Derm Syph 1940;42:312–321.
22. Buchet JP, Lauwerys R: Role of thiols in the in-vitro methylation of inorganic arsenic by rat liver cytosol. Biochem Pharmacol 1988;37:3149–3153.
23. Buchet JP, Lauwerys R, Roels H: Comparison of the urinary excretion of arsenic metabolites after a single oral dose of sodium arsenite, monomethylarsonate or dimethylarsinate in man. Int Arch Occup Environ Health 1981;48:71–79.
24. Cebrian ME, Albores A, Aguilar M, Blakely E: Chronic arsenic poisoning in the north of Mexico. Hum Toxicol 1983; 2:121–133.
25. Challenger F: Biological methylation. Chem Rev 1945;36: 315–361.
26. Chen C, Chuang Y, Lin T, Wu HY: Malignant neoplasms among residents of a Blackfoot disease-endemic area in Taiwan: High-arsenic artesian well water and cancers. Cancer Res 1985;45:5895–5899.
27. Chen GS, Asai T, Suzuki Y, et al: A possible pathogenesis for Blackfoot disease: Effects of trivalent arsenic (As_2O_3) on cultured human umbilical vein endothelial cells. J Dermatol 1990;17:599–608.
28. Chuttani PN, Chawla LS, Sharma TD: Arsenical neuropathy. Neurology 1967;17:269–274.
29. Cikrt M, Bencko V, Tichy M, Benes B: Biliary excretion of ^{74}As and its distribution in the golden hamster after administration of ^{74}As (III) and ^{74}As (V). J Hyg Epidemiol Microbiol Immunol 1980;24:384–388.
30. Copeman PR, Bodenstein JC: An investigation of cases of arsenical poisoning. J Forensic Med 1955;2:196–216.
31. Crecelius EA: Changes in the chemical speciation of arsenic following ingestion by man. Environ Health Perspect 1977;19:147–150.
32. Danan M, Dally S, Conso F: Arsenic-induced encephalopathy. Neurol 1984;34:1524. Letter.
33. Das D, Chatterjee A, Badal K, et al: Arsenic in ground water in six districts of West Bengal, India: The biggest arsenic calamity in the world. Part 2. Arsenic concentration in drinking water, hair, nails, urine, skin-scale and liver tissue (biopsy) of the affected people. Analyst 1995;120: 917–924.
34. Done AK, Peart AJ: Acute toxicities of arsenical herbicides. Clin Toxicol 1971;4:343–355.
35. Eagle H, Magnuson HJ: The systemic treatment of 227 cases of arsenic poisoning (encephalitis, dermatitis, blood dyscrasias, jaundice, fever) with 2,3-dimercaptopropanol (BAL). Am J Syph Gonor Ven Dis 1946;30:420–441.
36. Eichner ER: Erythroid karyorrhexis in the peripheral blood smear in severe arsenic poisoning: A comparison with lead poisoning. Am J Clin Pathol 1984;81:533–537.
37. Fernandez-Sola J, Nogue S, Grau JM, et al: Acute arsenical myopathy: Morphological description. J Toxicol Clin Toxicol 1991;29:131–136.
38. Feussner JR, Shelburne JD, Bredehoeft S, Cohen HJ: Arsenic-induced bone marrow toxicity: Ultrastructural and electron-probe analysis. Blood 1979;53:820–827.
39. Fincher RE, Koerker RM: Long-term survival in acute arsenic encephalopathy: Follow-up using newer measures of electrophysiologic parameters. Am J Med 1987;82:549–552.
40. Fleay RF, Thomas BW: Test of chelation process to remove arsenic from a biological system using neutron activation. Aust Radiol 1975;19:384–386.
41. Fluharty A, Sanadi DR: Evidence for a vicinal dithiol in oxidative phosphorylation. Proc Natl Acad Sci 1960;46: 608–616.
42. Fournier L, Thomas G, Garnier R, et al: 2,3-Dimercapto-succinic-acid treatment of heavy metal poisoning in humans. Med Toxicol 1988;3:499–504.
43. Freeman JW, Crouch JR: Prolonged encephalopathy with arsenic poisoning. Neurology 1978;28:853–855.
44. Gerhardt RE, Hudson JB, Rao RN, Sobel RE: Chronic renal insufficiency from cortical necrosis induced by arsenic poisoning. Arch Intern Med 1978;138:1267–1269.
45. Germolec DR, Yoshida T, Gaido K, et al: Arsenic induces overexpression of growth factors in human keratinocytes. Toxicol Appl Pharmacol 1996;141:308–318.
46. Goldsmith S, From AHL: Arsenic-induced atypical ventricular tachycardia. N Engl J Med 1980;303:1096–1098.
47. Gousios AG, Adelson L: Electrocardiographic and ra-

diographic findings in acute arsenic poisoning. Am J Med 1959;27:659–663.
48. Graziano JH, Cuccia D, Friedheim E: The pharmacology of 2,3-dimercaptosuccinic acid and its potential use in arsenic poisoning. J Pharmacol Exp Ther 1978;207:1051–1055.
49. Greenberg C, Davies S, McGowan T, et al: Acute respiratory failure following severe arsenic poisoning. Chest 1979;76:596–598.
50. Gresser MJ: ADP-arsenate: Formation by submitochondrial particles under phosphorylating conditions. J Biol Chem 1981;256:5981–5983.
51. Guha Mazumder DN, Chakraborty AK, Ghose A, et al: Chronic arsenic toxicity from drinking tubewell water in rural West Bengal. Bull WHO 1988;66:499–506.
52. Habif TP: Nail Disease in Clinical Dermatology: A Color Guide to Diagnosis and Therapy, 3rd ed. St. Louis, Mosby, 1996, p. 758.
53. Hanlon DO, Ferm VH: Placental permeability of arsenate ion during early embryogenesis in the hamster. Experientia 1977;33:1221–1222.
54. Heyman A, Pfeiffer JB, Willett RW: Peripheral neuropathy caused by arsenical intoxication: A study of 41 cases with observations on the effects of BAL (2,3-dimercaptopropanol). N Engl J Med 1956;254:401–409.
55. Hilfer RJ, Mandel A: Acute arsenic intoxication diagnosed by roentgenograms. N Engl J Med 1962;266:663–664.
56. Hirata M, Tanaka A, Hisanaga A, Ishinishi N: Effects of glutathione depletion on the acute nephrotoxic potential of arsenite and on arsenic metabolism in hamsters. Toxicol Appl Pharmacol 1990;106:469–481.
57. Hoover TD, Aposhian HV: BAL increases the arsenic-74 content of rabbit brain. Toxicol Appl Pharmacol 1983;70: 160–162.
58. Huang R, Lee T: Cellular uptake of trivalent arsenite and pentavalent arsenate in KB cells cultured in phosphate-free medium. Toxicol Appl Pharmacol 1996;136:243–249.
59. Inns RH, Rice P, Bright JE, Marrs TC: Evaluation of the efficacy of dimercapto chelating agents for the treatment of systemic organic arsenic poisoning in rabbits. Hum Exp Toxicol 1990;9:215–220.
60. Kasper ML, Schoenfield L, Strom RL, Theologides A: Hepatic angiosarcoma and bronchioloalveolar carcinoma induced by Fowler's solution. JAMA 1984;252:3407–3408.
61. Kersjes MP, Maurer JR, Trestrail JH: An analysis of arsenic exposures referred to the Blodgett regional poison center. Vet Hum Toxicol 1987;29:75–78.
62. Kingston RL, Hall S, Sioris L: Clinical observations and medical outcome in 149 cases of arsenate ant killer ingestion. J Toxicol Clin Toxicol 1993;31:581–591.
63. Kosnett MJ, Becker CE: Dimercaptosuccinic acid as a treatment for arsenic poisoning. Vet Hum Toxicol 1987;29:462. Abstract.
64. Kreppel H, Reichl FX, Forth W, Fichtl B: Lack of effectiveness of D-penicillamine in experimental arsenic poisoning. Vet Hum Toxicol 1989;31:1–5.
65. Kreppel H, Reichl FX, Kleine A, et al: Antidotal efficacy of newly synthesized dimercaptosuccinic acid (DMSA) monoesters in experimental arsenic poisoning in mice. Fund Appl Toxicol 1995;26:239–245.
66. Kreppel H, Reichl FX, Szinicz L, et al: Efficacy of various dithiol compounds in acute As_2O_3 poisoning in mice. Arch Toxicol 1990;64:387–392.
67. Kyle RA, Pease GL: Hematologic aspects of arsenic intoxication. N Engl J Med 1965;273:18–23.
68. Lander JJ, Stanley RJ, Sumner HW, et al: Angiosarcoma of the liver associated with Fowler's solution (potassium arsenite). Gastroenterology 1975;68:1582–1586.
69. Le Quesne PM, McLeod J: Peripheral neuropathy following a single exposure to arsenic: Clinical course in four patients with electrophysiological and histological studies. J Neurol Sci 1977;32:437–451.
70. Lee AM, Fraumeni JF: Arsenic and respiratory cancer in man: An occupational study. J Natl Cancer Inst 1969;42: 1045–1052.
71. Leikin JB, Goldman-Leikin RE, Evans MA, et al: Immunotherapy in acute arsenic poisoning. J Toxicol Clin Toxicol 1991;29:59–70.
72. Lenz K, Hruby K, Druml W, et al: 2,3-Dimercaptosuccinic acid in human arsenic poisoning. Arch Toxicol 1981;47: 241–243.
73. Lerman BB, Ali N, Green D: Megaloblastic, dyserythropoietic anemia following arsenic ingestion. Ann Clin Lab Sci 1980;10:515–517.
74. Liebl B, Muckter H, Doklea E, et al: Influence of 2,3-dimercaptopropanol and other sulfur compounds on oxophenylarsine-mediated inhibition of glucose uptake in MDCK cells. Analyst 1995;120:771–774.
75. Liebl B, Muckter H, Doklea E, et al: Reversal of oxophenylarsine-induced inhibition of glucose uptake in MDCK cells. Fund Appl Toxicol 1995;27:1–8.
76. Liebl B, Muckter H, Doklea E, et al: Influence of organic and inorganic arsenicals on glucose-uptake in MDCK-cells. Analyst 1992;117:681–684.
77. Limarzi LR: The effect of arsenic (Fowler's solution) on erythropoiesis. Am J Med Sci 1943;206:339–347.
78. Lugo G, Cassady G, Palmisano P: Acute maternal arsenic intoxication with neonatal death. Am J Dis Child 1969; 117:328–330.
79. Lynch PJ: Dermatology for the House Officer. Baltimore, Williams & Wilkins, 1982, pp. 7–9.
80. Mahieu P, Buchet JP, Roels HA, Lauwerys R: The metabolism of arsenic in humans acutely intoxicated by As_2O_3: Its significance for the duration of BAL therapy. Clin Toxicol 1981;18:1067–1075.
81. Maiorino RM, Aposhian HV: Dimercaptan metal-binding agents influence the biotransformation of arsenite in the rabbit. Toxicol Appl Pharmacol 1985;77:240–250.
82. Massey EW, Wold D, Heyman A: Arsenic: Homicidal intoxication. South Med J 1984;77:848–851.
83. Mathieu D, Mathieu-Nolf M, Germain-Alonso M, et al: Massive arsenic poisoning—Effect of hemodialysis and dimercaprol on arsenic kinetics. Intensive Care Med 1992; 18:47–50.
84. McBride BC, Merilees H, Cullen WR: Anaerobic and aerobic alkylation of arsenic. In: Brinckman FE, Bellama JM, eds: Organometals and Organometalloids (ACS Symp Ser No 82). Washington, DC, American Chemical Society, 1978, pp. 94–115.

85. McKinney JD: Metabolism and disposition of inorganic arsenic in laboratory animals and humans. Environ Geochem Health 1992;14:43–48.
86. Mealey J, Brownell GL, Sweet WH: Radioarsenic in plasma, urine, normal tissues, and intracranial neoplasms. Arch Neurol Psychiatry 1959;8:310–320.
87. Mees RA: Nails with arsenical polyneuritis. Ned Tijdschr Geneeskd 1919;1:391.
88. Molin L, Wester PO: The estimated daily loss of trace elements from normal skin by desquamation. Scand J Clin Lab Invest 1976;36:679–682.
89. Nelson RL: Acute diffuse myocarditis following exfoliative dermatitis. Am Heart J 1934;9:813–816.
90. Nevens F, Fevery J, Van Steenbergen W, et al: Arsenic and non-cirrhotic portal hypertension: A report of eight cases. J Hepatol 1990;11:80–85.
91. Nixon DE, Moyer TP: Arsenic analysis II. Rapid separation and quantification of inorganic arsenic plus metabolites and arsenobetaine from urine. Clin Chem 1992;38:2479–2483.
92. North DW: Risk assessment for ingested inorganic arsenic: A review and status report. Environ Geochem Health 1992;14:59–62.
93. Nozaki S, Tsutsumi S, Tamura S: Effect of casein on enteral absorption of arsenic trioxide. Jpn J Pharmacol 1975; 25:122P–123P.
94. Otani K: Studies on the absorption and distribution of arsenic. Sappori Igaku Zasshi 1957;11:285–294. English summary.
95. Ott MG, Holder BB, Gordon HL: Respiratory cancer and occupational exposure to arsenicals. Arch Environ Health 1974;29:250–255.
96. Park MJ, Currier M: Arsenic exposures in Mississippi: A review of cases. South Med J 1991;84:461–464.
97. Pershagen G, Vahter M: Arsenic: A Toxicological and Epidemiological Appraisal. Stockholm, Department of Environmental Hygiene of the Karolinska Institute and the National (Swedish) Environment Protection, 1979.
98. Peters HA, Croft WA, Woolson EA, et al: Seasonal arsenic exposure from burning chromium-copper-arsenate treated wood. JAMA 1984;251:2393–2396.
99. Peters RA: I. Present state of knowledge of biochemical lesions induced by trivalent arsenical poisoning. Bull Johns Hopkins Hosp 1955;87:1–20.
100. Peterson RG, Rumack BH: D-Penicillamine therapy of acute arsenic poisoning. J Pediatr 1977;91:661–666.
101. Pinto SS, Bennett BM: Effect of arsenic trioxide exposure on mortality. Arch Environ Health 1963;7:583–591.
102. Pinto SS, Varner MO, Nelson KW, et al: Arsenic trioxide absorption and excretion in industry. J Occup Med 1976; 18:677–680.
103. Pomroy C, Charbonneau SM, McCullough RS, Tam GK: Human retention studies with ^{74}As. Toxicol Appl Pharmacol 1980;53:550–556.
104. Regelson W, Kim U, Ospina J, Holland JF: Hemangioendothelial sarcoma of liver from chronic arsenic intoxication by Fowler's solution. Cancer 1968;21:514–522.
105. Reichl F, Hunder G, Liebl B, et al: Effect of DMPS and various adsorbents on the arsenic excretion in guinea-pigs after injection with As_2O_3. Arch Toxicol 1995;69:712–717.
106. Reichl F, Kreppel H, Forth W: Pyruvate and lactate metabolism in livers of guinea pigs perfused with chelation agents after repeated treatment with As_2O_3. Arch Toxicol 1991;65:235–238.
107. Reichl F, Kreppel H, Szinicz L, et al: Reduction of arsenic trioxide toxicity in mice by repeated treatment with glucose. Arch Toxicol 1991;14(suppl):225–228.
108. Reichl F, Kreppel H, Szinicz L, et al: Effect of glucose treatment on carbohydrate content in various organs in mice after acute As_2O_3 poisoning. Vet Hum Toxicol 1991;33: 230–235.
109. Reichl F, Muckter H, Kreppel H, Forth W: Effect of various antidotes on biliary excretion of arsenic in isolated perfused livers of guinea pigs after acute experimental poisoning with As_2O_3. Pharmacol Toxicol 1992;70: 352–356.
110. Reichl F, Szinicz L, Kreppel H, Forth W: Effects of arsenic on carbohydrate metabolism after single or repeated injection in guinea pigs. Arch Toxicol 1988;62:473–475.
111. Rein K, Borrebaek B, Bremer J: Arsenite inhibits B-oxidation in isolated rat liver mitochondria. Biochim Biophys Acta 1979;574:487–494.
112. Rin K, Kawaguchi K, Yamanaka K, et al: DNA-strand breaks induced by dimethylarsinic acid, a metabolite of inorganic arsenics, are strongly enhanced by superoxide anion radicals. Biol Pharm Bull 1995;18:45–48.
113. Roat JW, Wald A, Mendelow H, Pataki KI: Hepatic angiosarcoma associated with short-term arsenic ingestion. Am J Med 1982;73:933–936.
114. Robinson TJ: Arsenical polyneuropathy due to caustic arsenical paste. Br Med J 1975;3:139.
115. Roehl R: New LC-ICP-MS techniques. Proceedings of the Fifth Annual Hazardous Materials Management Conference West. Anonymous Glen Ellyn, IL: Tower Conference Management Company, 1989, pp. 555–562.
116. Ropper AH: The Guillain-Barré syndrome. N Engl J Med 1992;326:1130–1136.
117. Roses OE, Garcia Fernandez JC, Villaamil EC, et al: Mass poisoning by sodium arsenite. J Toxicol Clin Toxicol 1991; 29:209–213.
118. Savory J, Sedor FA: Arsenic poisoning. In: Brown SS, ed: Clinical Chemistry and Chemical Toxicology of Metals. New York, Elsevier/North Holland, 1977, pp. 271–286.
119. Schafer B, Kreppel H, Reichl FX, et al: Effect of oral treatment with BAL, DMPS or DMSA arsenic in organs of mice injected with arsenic trioxide. Arch Toxicol 1991;14 (suppl):228–230.
120. Schoolmeester WL, White DR: Arsenic poisoning. South Med J 1980;73:198–208.
121. Schwartze EW: The so-called habituation to "arsenic": Variation in the toxicity of arsenious oxide. J Pharmacol Exp Ther 1922;20:181–203.
122. Shum S, Skarbovig J, Habersang R: Acute lethal arsenite poisoning in mice: Effect of treatment with *N*-acetylcysteine, D-penicillamine and dimercaprol on survival time. Vet Hum Toxicol 1981;23(suppl):39–42.
123. Shum S, Whitehead J, Vaughn L, Hale T: Chelation of organoarsenate with dimercaptosuccinic acid. Vet Hum Toxicol 1995;37:239–242.
124. Snider TH, Wientjes MG, Joiner RL, Fisher GC: Arsenic distribution in rabbits after Lewisite administration and

treatment with British anti-Lewisite (BAL). Fund Appl Toxicol 1990;14:262–272.

125. St. Petery J, Gross C, Victorica BE: Ventricular fibrillation caused by arsenic poisoning. Am J Dis Child 1970;120: 367–371.
126. Stevens JT, Hall LL, Farmer JD, et al: Disposition of ^{14}C and/or ^{74}As-cacodylic acid in rats after intravenous, intratracheal, or peroral administration. Environ Health Perspect 1977;19:151–157.
127. Stryer L: Biochemistry, 4th ed. New York, Freeman, 1995, pp. 503, 514–517.
128. Szinicz L, Forth W: Effect of As_2O_3 on gluconeogenesis. Arch Toxicol 1988;61:444–449.
129. Tay CH, Seah CS: Arsenic poisoning from anti-asthmatic herbal preparations. Med J Aust 1975;2:424–428.
130. Tokudome S, Kuratsune M: A cohort study on mortality from cancer and other causes among workers at a metal refinery. Int J Cancer 1976;17:310–315.
131. Tseng W: Effects and dose-response relationships of skin cancer and Blackfoot disease with arsenic. Environ Health Perspect 1977;19:109–119.
132. Tsukamoto H, Parker HR, Gribble DH: Metabolism and renal handling of sodium arsenate in dogs. Am J Vet Res 1983;44:2331–2335.
133. Tsukamoto H, Parker HR, Gribble DH, et al: Nephrotoxicity of sodium arsenate in dogs. Am J Vet Res 1983;44: 2324–2330.
134. Uthe JF, Reinke J: Arsenate ion reduction in non-living biological materials. Environ Lett 1975;10:83–88.
135. Vahter M: Metabolism of arsenic. In: Fowler BA, ed: Biological and Environmental Effects of Arsenic. New York, Elsevier, 1983, pp. 171–198.
136. Vahter M: Biotransformation of trivalent and pentavalent inorganic arsenic in mice and rats. Environ Res 1981;25: 286–293.
137. Vahter M, Marafante E: Intracellular interaction and metabolic fate of arsenite and arsenate in mice and rabbits. Chem Biol Interac 1983;47:29–44.
138. Vahter M, Norin H: Metabolism of ^{74}As-labeled trivalent and pentavalent inorganic arsenic in mice. Environ Res 1980;21:446–457.
139. Vaziri ND, Upham T, Barton CH: Hemodialysis clearance of arsenic. Clin Toxicol 1980;17:451–456.
140. Wagner SL, Weswig P: Arsenic in blood and urine of forest workers. Arch Environ Health 1974;28:77–79.
141. Watson WA, Veltri JC, Metcalf TJ: Acute arsenic exposure treated with oral D-penicillamine. Vet Hum Toxicol 1981; 23:164–166.
142. Weinberg SL: The electrocardiogram in acute arsenic poisoning. Am Heart J 1960;60:971–975.
143. Welch K, Higgins I, Oh M, Burchfiel C: Arsenic exposure, smoking, and respiratory cancer in copper smelter workers. Arch Environ Health 1982;37:325–335.
144. Yamanaka K, Hasegawa A, Sawamura R, Okada S: Cellular response to oxidative damage in lung induced by the administration of dimethylarsinic acid, a major metabolite of inorganic arsenics, in mice. Toxicol Appl Pharmacol 1991;108:205–213.
145. Yamanaka K, Hasegawa A, Sawamura R, Okada S: Dimethylated arsenics induce DNA strand breaks in lung via the production of active oxygen in mice. Biochem Biophys Res Commun 1989;165:43–50.
146. Young EG, Smith RP: Arsenic content of hair and bone in acute and chronic arsenical poisoning: Review of 2 cases examined posthumously from medico-legal aspect. Br Med J 1942;1:251–253.
147. Zaloga GP, Deal J, Spurling T, et al: Case report: Unusual manifestations of arsenic intoxication. Am J Med Sci 1985;289:210–214.

ANTIDOTES IN DEPTH

Dimercaprol (BAL)

Mary Ann Howland

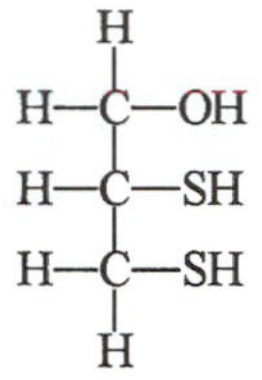

2,3-Dimercaptopropanol (BAL)

Dimercaprol (British Anti-Lewisite; BAL) is an effective metal chelator used clinically in the treatment of inorganic mercury toxicity and arsenic toxicity (not arsine) and in conjunction with calcium disodium EDTA ($CaNa_2EDTA$) for lead toxicity. The dose and duration of BAL therapy depends on the metal being chelated and the severity of toxicity.[15,20]

Chelation theory of metals states that soft metals (Hg^{2+}, Au^+, Cu^+, Ag^+) form the most stable complexes with sulfur donors.[1,2,22] Soft metals are therefore referred to as sulfur seekers and have large atomic radii with a large number of electrons in the outer shell. The chelator or ligand, in this case a sulfur-containing compound such as BAL, forms a coordinate bond with the metal by donating a pair of free electrons. Hard metals (Na^+, K^+, Mg^{2+}, Ca^{2+}, and Al^{3+}) or oxygen seekers form the best complexes with hard ligands containing a COO^- group such as EDTA. Borderline metals (Pb^{2+}, Cd^{2+}, Cu^{2+}, As^{3+}, Zn^{2+}) prefer nitrogen-donating species but will also react with hard or soft ligands. Metal antidotes often contain more than one donating group, making them effective for more than one type of metal. BAL has two adjacent sulfur groups, making it a dithiol; being a dithiol permits the formation of a ring structure with the metal, thereby enhancing chelator stability. The most useful chelators have a relatively low order of toxicity, form stable complexes with their respective metals, and have tissue distribution characteristics similar to the metal to be chelated. Desirable aspects of the metal-chelator complex are elimination from the body without breakdown, no redistribution to the brain or other critical organs and a low order of toxicity. Unfortunately, no chelator available at present has all of these attributes. Currently, redistribution characteristics of metal chelator complexes are being rigorously investigated.

During World War II the threat of chemical warfare with lewisite (dichloro-(2-chlorovinyl)-arsine) and mustard gas (dichloro-diethyl-sulfide) led Peters and his group to develop an antidote to these vesicant gases.[25] They determined that when arsenicals combined with protein sulfhydryl (SH) groups, tissue damage resulted. Investigation into the use of sulfur donors as antidotes led to the discovery of the dithiol 2,3-dimercaptopropanol, called British anti-lewisite (see Figure). As a chelator, BAL combines with lewisite to form a very stable five-membered ring.

The assumption that lewisite would be sprayed over the land and its population, and the knowledge that it caused skin lesions, led researchers to believe that BAL's limited water solubility and high lipid solubility would be valuable for potential cutaneous application.[27] Studies in rodents demonstrated that topical BAL was very effective at low concentrations both in preventing lewisite-induced toxicity and in reversing toxicity if administered up to 1 hour after skin contamination.[23,25] In rabbits topical BAL proved effective in preventing ocular destruction if applied within 20 minutes of exposure.[15] Urinary arsenic concentrations were significantly increased after the application of topical BAL.[25]

The effectiveness and toxicity of parenteral single-dose and multiple-dose BAL were studied in rabbits against lewisite and other arsenicals. If given within 2 hours of exposure, four injections of 4 mg/kg BAL at 4-hour intervals saved 50% of rabbits exposed to lewisite. This was demonstrated to be one-seventh of the maximum tolerated dose of BAL.[10] Experiments in human volunteers with minute amounts of arsenic confirmed the ability of BAL to increase urinary arsenic concentration by about 40%, with maximum excretion occurring within 2–4 hours after BAL administration.[29]

Dimercaprol was subsequently used in the treatment of arsenical dermatitis that resulted from therapy with organic arsenicals. When applied on affected skin, topical BAL produced erythema, pruritus, and dysesthesias, but on unaffected skin BAL had no adverse effects. When given intramuscularly through both affected and unaffected skin, abscesses occasionally resulted. Intramuscular BAL produced subjective and objective improvement, limited the duration of the dermatitis, and was accompanied by elevated arsenic levels in the urine.[6,17,18] In a study of 227 patients with arsenic poisoning who were given BAL intramuscularly at multiple dose ranges, 3 mg/kg every 4 hours for 48 hours and then twice a day for 7–10 days achieved maximum effectiveness with minimum toxicity.[9] Six of 7 patients with severe arsenic-induced encephalitis recovered completely with this regimen. This study demonstrated the importance of administering BAL as soon as possible after the exposure. Of 33 patients with severe arsenic-induced encephalitis, 18 of 24 treated within 6 hours survived, versus only 4 of 9 treated 72 hours or later.[9] The effectiveness of BAL was also demonstrated in three patients mistakenly given 10–20 times the therapeutic dose of Mapharsen (oxophenarsine hydrochloride) who were treated with appropriate doses of BAL. A fourth patient, who was treated with inadequate doses of BAL, died.[9] This study supported the effectiveness of BAL for arsenic-induced agranulocytosis, encephalitis, dermatitis, massive overdose of Mapharsen, and probably arsenical fever.[9] The recent controversy with regard to in vitro and animal studies on the facilitation of arsenical entry into the cells is discussed in Chapter 78.

Ocular damage caused by lewisite is due in part to the liberation of hydrochloric acid, which results in an acid injury causing localized superficial opacity of the cornea and deep penetration of lewisite into the cornea and aqueous humor with resultant rapid necrosis. A 5% BAL ointment or solution applied within 2 minutes prevents development of a significant reaction; application at 30 minutes lessens the reaction but does not prevent permanent damage.[13]

Because mercury also reacts with sulfhydryl groups, animal studies were performed to assess the affinity of thiols and their ability to competitively chelate mercury, preventing toxicity. As with arsenic toxicity, the dithiols BAL and BAL glucoside were more effective than the monothiol 1-thiosorbitol in preventing mercury-induced death and uremia.[12] The clinical efficacy of BAL in inorganic mercury poisoning was substantiated in patients who ingested mercury bichloride.[16] It is particularly useful in patients who have ingested the mercuric salt, as their associated gastrointestinal toxicity limits the potential of an orally administered antidote. Dimercaprol also antagonizes the actions of gold.

Dimercaprol is used in combination with calcium disodium EDTA to treat severe lead poisoning. In lead encephalopathy it is very important to administer the dimercaprol first and then the EDTA 4 hours later with the second dose of dimercaprol. This technique is used to prevent the possibility of EDTA facilitating the redistribution of lead into the brain.[7,8] Cerebral edema is often a critical factor in lead encephalopathy and, therefore, meticulous attention must be made to lowering elevated intracranial pressure and achieving fluid restriction.

In rats, the LD_{50} of BAL by SC administration is 110 mg/kg.[15] The toxicity of BAL in humans is dose-dependent and affected by urinary pH. In patients receiving 2.5 mg/kg every 4–6 hours for four doses less than 1% of 700 IM injections resulted in minor reactions, mostly pain at the site of injection.[9] When doses of 4 mg/kg and 5 mg/kg were given, the incidence of adverse effects rose to 14% and 65%, respectively.[9] At these doses the following symptoms were reported in decreasing order of frequency: nausea, vomiting, headache, burning sensation of lips, mouth, throat, and eyes, lacrimation, rhinorrhea, salivation, muscle aches, burning and tingling of extremities, teeth pain, diaphoresis, chest pain, anxiety, and agitation.[17] These effects were maximal within 10–30 minutes and usually subsided within 30–50 minutes.[9]

Elevations in systolic and diastolic blood pressure and tachycardia commonly occur and are correlated with increasing doses.[15,20] Thirty percent of children given BAL may develop a fever, which may persist during therapy.[15] A transient reduction in the percentage of polymorphonuclear leukocytes may also occur.[15] In the presence of arsenic-induced liver damage, BAL is not very effective.[18] Moreover, rats whose livers were previously damaged showed toxicity with BAL and arsenic; therefore, unless the patient has postarsenical jaundice, BAL is contraindicated when liver dysfunction is noted.[25]

Dissociation of the BAL–metal chelate takes place in an acid urine; therefore, maintenance of an alkaline urine may protect the kidney during therapy.[15] Dimercaprol should be used with caution in patients with glucose-6-phosphate dehydrogenase (G6PD) deficiency, as it may cause hemolysis.[14] A risk to benefit analysis must be made as most G6PD-deficiency syndromes are partial in nature. Another consideration is that chelators are relatively nonspecific and may bind metals other than those desired, thus causing a deficiency of an essential metal. For example, when BAL was given to mice, their elimination of copper increased to three times normal.[4]

Animal models demonstrate that if BAL is administered to chelate short-chain organic mercury compounds, increased brain levels may result.[3,5] Based on this, most authors recommend against BAL when these toxins are present.[2,15] However, in a rat model, if BAL therapy was initiated within 1 day of exposure to short-chain organic mercury compounds, neurologic toxicity could be prevented.[30] No effect on established neurotoxicity was evident when treatment was delayed for 12 days.

Plasma concentrations of BAL peak about 30 minutes after IM administration and persist for at least 12 hours.[26] BAL is concentrated in the kidney, liver, and small intestine, with 20% of a dose appearing in the urine within 8 hours.[24] BAL can also be found in the feces.

The toxicity of BAL appears to be dose-related. Hemodialysis may be needed to remove the BAL–metal chelate in cases of renal failure.[15,19,28] Dimercaprol should not be used in patients with hepatic damage or in those poisoned by methylmercury. The urine of patients receiving dimercaprol should be alkalinized to prevent renal liberation of the metal. Dimercaprol is formulated in peanut oil; therefore, the patient should be evaluated for peanut allergy. Medicinal iron should not be given to patients receiving BAL because the BAL–iron complex is reported to cause severe vomiting and decreased the efficacy of chelation, although this recommendation may have a limited scientific basis.[7,8,11]

A pharmaceutical formulation that stabilized BAL against oxidation was developed and contained 5% wt/vol peanut oil and a benzyl benzoate-to-BAL ratio of 2:1.[10] Dimercaprol is a relatively colorless liquid with a sulfur odor. It is available in 3-mL ampules containing 100 mg/mL of BAL, 200 mg/mL of benzyl benzoate, and

700 mg/mL of peanut oil. It is available only for deep intramuscular (IM) injection.

References

1. Aaseth J: Recent advances in the therapy of metal poisonings with chelating agents. Hum Toxicol 1983;2:257–272.
2. Aposhian HV, Maiorino RM, Gonzalez-Ramirez D, et al: Mobilization of heavy metals by newer, therapeutically useful chelating agents. Toxicology 1995;97:23–38.
3. Berlin M, Ullberg S: Increased uptake of mercury in mouse brain caused by 2,3 dimercaptopropanol. Nature 1963;197: 84–85.
4. Cantilena LR, Klaassen CD: The effect of chelating agents on the excretion of endogenous metals. Toxicol Appl Pharmacol 1982;63:344–350.
5. Canty AJ, Kishimoto R: British anti-lewisite and organ-mercury poisoning. Nature 1972;253:123–125.
6. Carleton AB, Peters RA, Stocken LA, et al: Clinical uses of 2,3-dimercaptopropanol (BAL): VI. The treatment of complications of arseno-therapy with BAL. J Clin Invest 1946; 25:497–527.
7. Chisolm JJ Jr: The use of chelating agents in the treatment of acute and chronic lead intoxication childhood. J Pediatr 1968; 73:1–38.
8. Committee on Drugs: Treatment guidelines for lead exposure in children. Pediatrics 1995;96:155–160.
9. Eagle H, Magnuson HJ: The systemic treatment of 227 cases of arsenic poisoning (encephalitis, dermatitis, blood dyscrasias, jaundice, fever) with 2,3-dimercaptopropanol (BAL). Am J Syph Gonor Ven Dis 1946;30:420–441.
10. Eagle H, Magnuson HJ, Fleischman R: Clinical uses of 2,3-dimercaptopropanol (BAL): I. The systemic treatment of experimental arsenic poisoning (Mapharsen, lewisite, phenyl arsenoxide) with BAL. J Clin Invest 1946;25:451–466.
11. Edge WD, Somers GF: The effect of dimercaprol (BAL) in acute iron poisoning. Q J Pharm Pharmacol 1948;21: 364–369.
12. Gilman A, Allen RP, Philips FS, et al: Clinical uses of 2,3-dimercaptopropanol (BAL): X. The treatment of acute systemic mercury poisoning in experimental animals with BAL, thiosorbitol and BAL glucoside. J Clin Invest 1946; 25:549–556.
13. Hughes WF: Clinical uses of 2,3-dimercaptopropanol (BAL): IX. The treatment of lewisite burns of the eye with BAL. J Clin Invest 1946;25:541–548.
14. Janakiraman N, Seeler RA, Royal JE, et al: Hemodialysis during BAL chelation therapy for high blood lead levels in two G6PD deficient children. Clin Pediatr 1978;17:485–487.
15. Klaassen CD: Heavy metals and heavy metal antagonists. In: Gilman AG, Goodman LS, Rall TW, Murad F, eds: The Pharmacological Basis of Therapeutics, 7th ed. New York, Macmillan, 1985, pp. 1605–1627.
16. Longcope WT, Luetscher JA, Calkins F, et al: Clinical uses of 2,3-dimercaptopropanol (BAL): XI. The treatment of acute mercury poisoning by BAL. J Clin Invest 1946;25:557–567.
17. Longcope WT, Luetscher JA, Wintrobe MM, et al: Clinical uses of 2,3-dimercaptopropanol (BAL): VII. The treatment of arsenical dermatitis with preparations of BAL. J Clin Invest 1946;25:528–533.
18. Luetscher JA, Eagle H, Longcope WT: Clinical uses of 2,3-dimercaptopropanol (BAL): VIII. The effect of BAL on the excretion of arsenic in arsenical intoxication. J Clin Invest 1946;25:534–540.
19. Maher JF, Schreiner GE: The dialysis of mercury and mercury-BAL complex. Clin Res 1959;7:298.
20. Mahieu P, Buchet JP, Roels HA, et al: The metabolism of arsenic in humans acutely intoxicated by As_2O_3: Its significance for the duration of BAL therapy. J Toxicol Clin Toxicol 1981;18:1067–1075.
21. Oehme FW: British anti-lewisite (BAL): The classic heavy metal antidote. Clin Toxicol 1972;5:215–222.
22. Pearson RG: Hard and soft acids and bases; NSAB. Part II. Underlying theories. J Chem Educ 1968;45:643–648.
23. Peters RA: Biochemistry of some toxic agents. J Clin Invest 1955;34:1–20.
24. Peters RA, Spray GH, Stocken LA, et al: The use of British anti-lewisite containing radioactive sulfur for metabolism investigations. Biochem J 1947;41:370–373.
25. Peters RA, Stocken LA, Thompson RM: British anti-lewisite (BAL). Nature 1945;156:616–618.
26. Spray GM, Stocken LA, Thompson RMS: Further investigations on the metabolism of 2,3-dimercaptopropanol. Biochem J 1947;41:363–366.
27. Stocken LA, Thompson RM: Reactions of British-lewisite with arsenic and other metals in living systems. Physiol Rev 1949;29:168–194.
28. Vaziri ND, Upham T, Barton CM: Hemodialysis clearance of arsenic. Clin Toxicol 1980;17:451–456.
29. Wexler J, Eagle M, Tatum MJ, et al: Clinical uses of 2,3-dimercaptopropanol (BAL): II. The effect of BAL on the excretion of arsenic in normal subjects after minimal exposure to arsenical smoke. J Clin Invest 1946;25:467–473.
30. Zimmer LJ, Carter DE: The effect of 2,3-dimercaptopropanol and D-penicillamine on methyl mercury induced neurological signs and weight loss. Life Sci 1978;23: 1025–1034.

CHAPTER 79

Lead

Fred M. Henretig

Lead	
MW	= 207 daltons
Normal range (whole blood)	< 10 μg/dL
	< 0.48 μmol/L
Action level (children)	10–14 μg/dL
	> 0.48–0.62 μmol/L

Values greater than or equal to the action level necessitate clinical intervention.

Values less than this level may necessitate intervention based on the clinical condition of the patient.

A three-year-old boy was rushed to the emergency department (ED) by rescue squad after having had a 20-minute seizure at home. He initially appeared postictal, with flaccid muscle tone and minimal response to painful stimulation. His blood pressure was 130/80 mm Hg with heart rate 110 beats/min, his respirations were shallow, at a rate of 10 breaths/min, and his temperature was 98.6°F (37°C). Pulse oximetry was 85% on room air. The child improved with suctioning, placement of a nasopharyngeal airway, and oxygen by face mask. Intravenous lines were placed, blood for laboratory studies drawn, and intravenous fluid administered. The ECG monitor revealed a normal sinus rhythm. An effort was made to elicit more history of the child's illness and to perform a more systematic examination, but within a few minutes the child began to convulse. Diazepam, 0.2 mg/kg IV was infused, with prompt cessation of seizure activity. However, respiratory effort also diminished, and the child underwent endotracheal intubation. A rapid bedside test for glucose estimated the blood glucose at 194 mg/dL. Arterial blood gas determination after intubation revealed normal ventilation and oxygenation, with a minimal metabolic acidosis. Five minutes later, another generalized seizure occurred, but resolved immediately with a second dose of 0.2 mg/kg of diazepam.

Further history revealed that this child had been in his usual state of health until 3 days prior to admission, when he developed symptoms of an upper respiratory infection. Two days later he developed tactile fever, vomited once, and appeared less active. On the day of admission he seemed drowsy, vomited several times, and in the evening developed twitching and abnormal eye movements, prompting a call to the rescue squad.

His past medical history was notable for developmental delay, primarily in the speech and personal/social spheres. He spoke only single words, was not toilet trained, and was unable to dress himself. The mother denied any history of head trauma or recent ingestion, but did comment that 3 weeks previously she had had to remove paint chips from the child's mouth.

Physical examination revealed an intubated child with blood pressure of 84/50 mm Hg, heart rate of 120 beats/min, a manually ventilated respiratory rate of 25 breaths/min, and temperature of 100.9°F (38.3°C). There were no signs of external trauma. Cardiac, pulmonary, and abdominal examinations were normal. The neurologic examination revealed an obtunded child with intermittent withdrawal to pain. At times tonic extensor posturing was noted. Pupils were 3 mm and sluggishly reactive, with normal fundi. Deep tendon reflexes were 3+ to 4+ on the left leg and 2+ to 3+ on the right leg. There was bilateral sustained ankle clonus. Plantar extension was present on the left and the response was equivocal on the right.

This patient's persistently abnormal mental status, lateralizing findings, and extensor posturing were all suggestive of increased intracranial pressure and raised the concern of serious intracranial pathology . The development of fever also suggested possible intracranial infection. The child's age, history of developmental delay, and observation of paint chip ingestion were all highly suspicious for childhood lead poisoning . A comprehensive evaluation with urgent institution of specific therapy was indicated. Thus, the patient went immediately to computed tomography scan, which revealed diffuse cerebral edema and loss of gray–white matter differentiation (Fig. 79–1). Recurrent seizure activity necessitated first phenobarbital loading and then midazolam

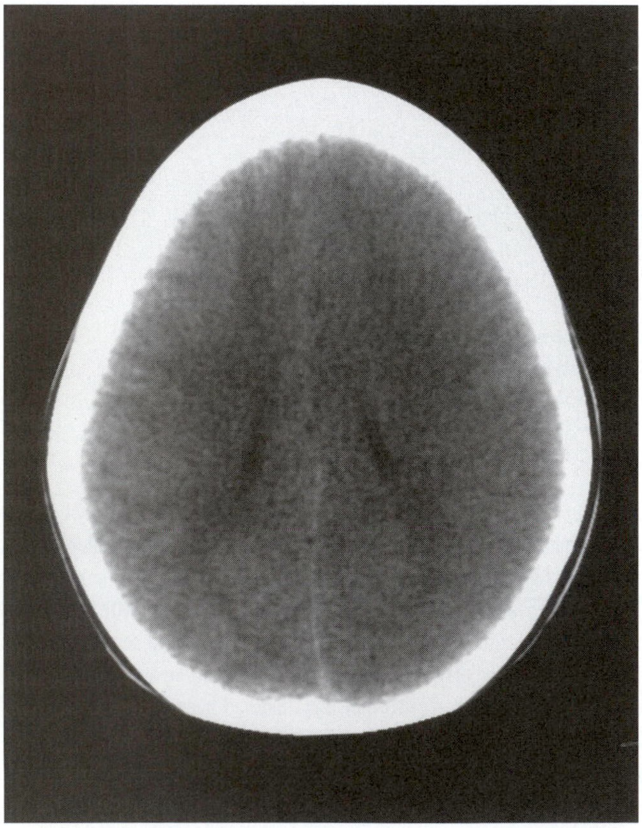

Figure 79–1. Computerized tomography scan of the head reveals diffuse cerebral edema and loss of gray–white matter differentiation. *(Courtesy of Department of Radiology, St. Christopher's Hospital for Children, Philadelphia, PA.)*

infusion. The child was also treated with modest hyperventilation and dexamethasone for presumed increased intracranial pressure, and empirically with ceftriaxone and acyclovir for possible central nervous system (CNS) infection. A lumbar puncture was performed, revealing opening pressure of 46 cm H_2O, clear, colorless fluid, and closing pressure of 15 cm H_2O. The cell count was 3 WBC/mm^3 and 0 RBC/mm^3, with CSF protein of 96 mg/dL and glucose of 108 mg/dL. One dose of mannitol was given after the lumbar puncture and confirmed elevated intracranial pressure. The results of other admission laboratory tests included white blood count 11,300/mm^3, hemoglobin 6.6 g/dL, MCV 50 μm^3, platelet count 473,000/mm^3, peripheral blood smear positive for RBC basophilic stippling; sodium 139 mEq/L, potassium 4.3 mEq/L, chloride 105 mEq/L, bicarbonate 22 mEq/L, blood urea nitrogen 15 mg/dL, creatinine 0.3 mg/dL, glucose 170 mg/dL, calcium 9.4 mg/dL, magnesium 1.8 mg/dL, phosphorus 3.5 mg/dL, ammonia 44 mol/L, ALT 83 U/L, and AST 118 U/L. Urinalysis revealed 4+ glucose, 5–10 WBC, 0–5 RBC, and 1+ protein. Radiographic studies were negative for radiopaque foreign bodies of the abdomen, but positive for dense metaphyseal bands at the wrist (Fig. 79–2). Blood lead level was 220 μg/dL and erythrocyte protoporphyrin was 649 μg/dL.

Despite anticonvulsant therapy with phenytoin, phenobarbital, and midazolam infusion, a continuous reading electroencephalogram demonstrated periodic epileptiform activity. Pentobarbital was added to the therapeutic regimen, resulting in intermittent burst suppression of up to 40-second duration. The child underwent chelation therapy with dimercaprol (British anti-lewisite, BAL) and calcium disodium edetate ($CaNa_2EDTA$). The BAL was dosed at 75 mg/m^2/dose IM every 4 hours for 5 days. The $CaNa_2EDTA$ was begun with the second dose of BAL, as a continuous infusion of 1500 mg/m^2/day diluted in normal saline to a concentration of 0.5%, and continued also for 5 days. After a 2-day interval, the child received a second 5-day course of chelation, resulting in a blood lead level of 33 μg/dL.

Despite chelation, the patient required high-dose pentobarbital for 6 days and continuous midazolam infusion for 14 days in order to suppress seizure activity. He was hospitalized for 23 days prior to transfer to a chronic care rehabilitative facility. His neurologic examination prior to transfer was notable for choreoathetoid movements and generalized hypotonia, inability to localize visual or auditory stimuli, and nonpurposeful movements of the extremities. A magnetic resonance image on day 22 revealed cerebral and cerebellar cortical atrophy with multiple areas of infarct involving the frontal and parietal lobes (Fig. 79–3).

What Are the Physical Properties of Lead?

Lead is a silvery-gray, soft, metal with atomic weight 207.21 D and atomic number 82. It has a low melting point, 327.4°C, and boils at 1620°C at atmospheric pressure. It is widely distributed geologically, and occurs prinicipally as two isotopes, ^{206}Pb and ^{208}Pb. Natural lead ore deposits are found in the Western hemisphere in Canada, the United States, Mexico, and Peru, and in Europe, Asia, and Australia. The most abundant lead ore is galena (PbS).[246] Lead is relatively insoluble in water and dilute acids, but will dissolve in nitric, acetic, and hot, concentrated sulfuric acids. In compounds, lead assumes valence states of +2 and +4. Inorganic lead compounds

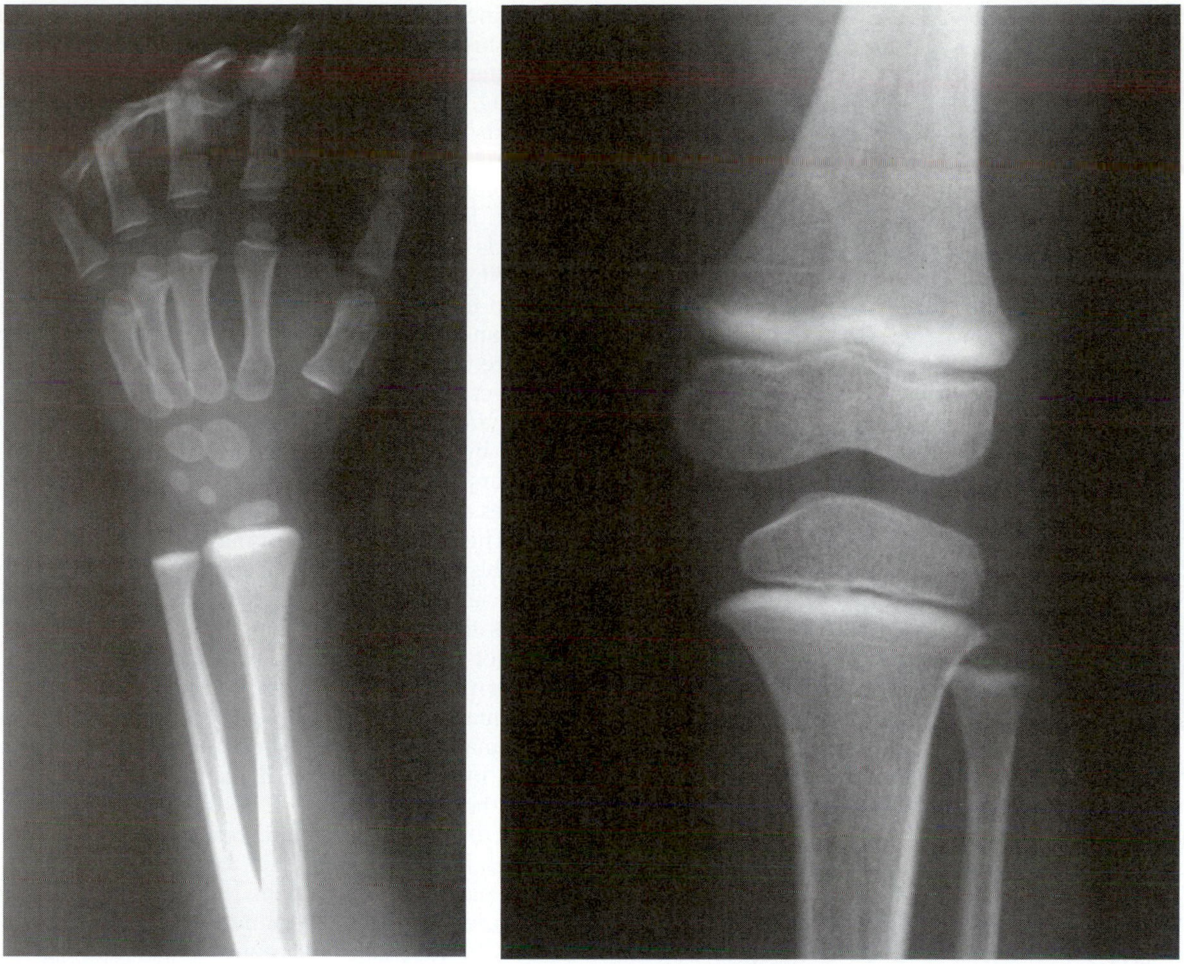

A B

Figure 79–2. A. Radiograph of the wrist reveals increased bands of calcification: "lead lines." *(Courtesy of Department of Radiology, St. Christopher's Hospital for Children, Philadelphia, PA.)* **B.** Similar radiographic findings in another patient at the knee. *(Courtesy of Richard Markowitz, MD, Department of Radiology, Children's Hospital of Philadelphia, Philadelphia, PA.)*

may be brightly colored and vary widely in water solubility; several are used extensively as pigments. Lead also forms organic compounds, of which two, tetramethyl and tetraethyl lead, have found commercial use as gasoline additives.[126] These are essentially insoluble in water, but readily soluble in organic solvents.[214] Lead complexes with ligands containing sulfur, oxygen, or nitrogen as electron donors and forms stable complexes with several ligands common to biologic molecules, including –OH, $-H_2PO_3$, –SH, and $-NH_2$. Complexes with sulfhydryl (–SH) groups are thought to be of most toxicologic importance. There is no known physiologic role for lead, and any lead found in human body fluids represents environmental contamination.[182] Major lead compounds are summarized in Table 79–1.

What Is the History of Lead Poisoning?

Lead's low melting point and malleability made it one of the first metals smelted and used by early human societies.[14,254] Lead-based ocher paints have been recovered from the Neanderthal-era Mousterian burial mounds dating to approximately 40,000 BC. Lead artifacts were

TABLE 79–1. REPRESENTATIVE LEAD COMPOUNDS

Compound	Molecular Formula	Major Use / Comment
Lead arsenate	$Pb_3(AsO_4)_2$	Insecticide
Lead azide	$Pb(N_3)_2$	Cartridge primers, primer cord
Lead carbonate	$2PbCO_3Pb(OH)_2$	Paint pigment (basic white lead)
Lead chromate	$PbCrO_4$	Paint pigment (chrome yellow)
Lead oxide	Pb_3O_4	Paint pigment (red lead) commonly used as primer, for rust protection on metal. Other oxides used as pigments and in glazes.
Lead silicate	$PbSiO_3$	Glazes for china, porcelain, tiles
Lead sulfide	PbS	Most abundant lead ore (galena); responsible for gingival lead line
Tetraethyl lead	$Pb(C_2H_5)_4$	Anti-knock additive to gasoline

Adapted and compiled, with permission, from references 126, 214.

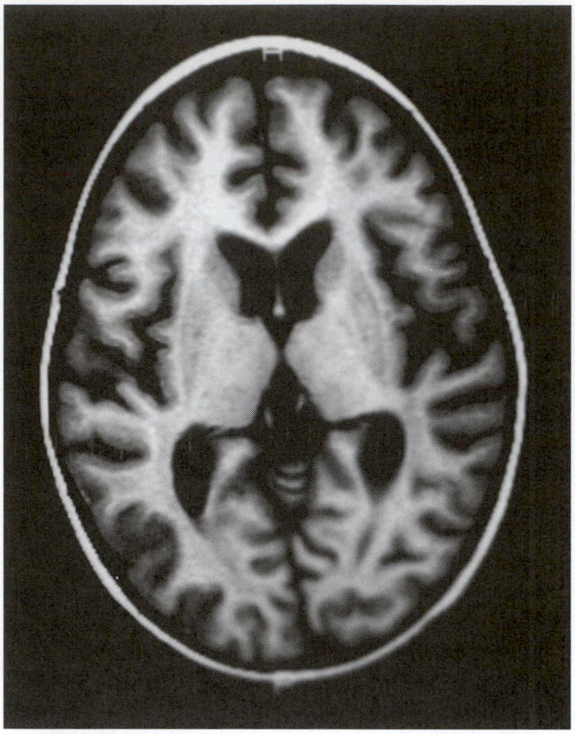

Figure 79–3. Magnetic resonance image of the head reveals cortical atrophy and multiple infarcts. *(Courtesy of Eric Faerber, MD, Department of Radiology, St Christopher's Hospital for Children, Philadelphia, PA.)*

unearthed in a Neolithic site in Turkey dating to 6200 BC. Ancient Egyptians and Hebrews used lead, and the Phoenicians established lead mines in Spain circa 2000 BC. The Greeks and Romans produced lead during the process of extracting silver intended for coinage. Roman society found many uses for lead, including pipes, cooking utensils, and ceramic glazes, and a common practice was to use sapa, a grape syrup simmered down in lead vessels, as a sweetener and preservative.[176,253] Postindustrial lead use increased dramatically, and today, lead is the most widely used nonferrous metal, with global production on the order of 9 million tons annually. The U.S. annual production of lead averages 1.1 million tons, of which about 0.5 million tons are newly mined and 0.6 million tons are recycled from scrap metal.[126,263] Lead is used widely in industry for its waterproofing and electrical- and radiation-shielding properties. Both metallic lead (as grids) and lead oxide (in paste) are used in electric storage batteries, and this use accounts for almost two-thirds of annual U.S. use. Since batteries last only 27 months on average, and about 80% of battery lead is resmelted as scrap, this single product accounts for the largest source of raw lead to the secondary smelting and refining industry.[214] Lead alloys are used to shield power and telephone cables, in the printing industry to produce type, and in solders. Solder is used in many industries, including tin can production, plumbing and repair operations, and the automobile industry, particularly radiator production and repair. Sheet lead lines chemical reaction containers and is used in medical and industrial radiation shields. Metallic lead is also used for ammunition manufacturing, bronze and brass production, and for annealing, galvanizing, and plating. Inorganic lead compounds have historically been considered among the highest quality paint pigments for their bright colors, durability, and weather resistance and are still used today for nonresidential outdoor paints. Lead compounds are used as stabilizers in the production of polyvinylchloride plastics, in glazes for ceramicware, and in the manufacture of glass intended for crystal, optical, and electronic applications such as color television picture tubes. Lead azide and stephanate are used in explosives.[126,214] Use of both lead-based paint for house paint and leaded gasoline have been essentially eliminated by regulation in the United States since the 1980s, but persistence of lead paint in our older houses still constitutes an enormous environmental challenge.[5,165]

The problem of human poisoning from lead, plumbism, dates back to antiquity. Dioscorides, a Greek physician in the second century BC, observed that lead makes the mind "give way."[142] Pliny cautioned the Romans of the danger of inhaled fumes from lead smelting.[167] Modern authors have suggested that extensive use of sapa in Roman aristocratic society contributed to the downfall of Roman dominance.[176] Lead poisoning was also recognized in Colonial times. Benjamin Franklin observed in 1763 the "dry gripes" (abdominal colic) and "dangles" (wrist drop) that afflicted tinkers, painters, and typesetters, as well as the "gripes" due to rum distillation in leaden condensing coils.[155] With the 19th-century Industrial Revolution, lead poisoning became a common occupational disease. Charles Dickens's account of lead mill workers in his 1863 *The Uncommercial Traveler* is haunting. Dickens visits a home near the mill, sees a woman bent over in a corner, and inquires of his guide as to her condition:

> And tis the lead, sur.
> The what?
> The lead, sur. Sure, tis the lead-mills, where the woman gets took on at eighteen-pence a day, sur . . . and her constitooshun is lead-poisoned, bad as can be, sur; and her brain is coming out her ear and it hurts her dreadful. . . .[69,167]

The reproductive effects of lead poisoning were also noted by the turn of the century. A 1911 article described the high rate of stillbirths, infertility, and abortions among women in the pottery industry, or who were married to pottery workers.[177] The modern history of childhood plumbism can be traced to the recognition of lead-paint poisoning in Brisbane, Australia, in 1897.[242] By 1914, a law banning the use of lead house paint was passed in Australia. It took another 57 years for a similar law to be effected in the United States.[167] Lead poisoning was reported in U.S. children in 1917,[24] and a classic article by Byers and Lord in 1943 established that children recovered from clinical plumbism were frequently left with neurologic sequelae and intellectual impairment.[33]

Symptomatic childhood lead poisoning was a frequent occurence in U.S. pediatric medical centers throughout the 1950s and 1960s, a period during which much research established effective chelation therapy protocols with BAL and CaEDTA.[49,52,53] In the 1970s and '80s, the research thrust in childhood lead poisoning centered on the recognition and quantification of more subtle neurocognitive impairment due to subclinical lead poisoning.[138,167,168] Over this time period, the U.S. Centers for Disease Control and Prevention (CDC) has steadily revised downward the definitions of blood lead levels in children representing undue absorption and lead poisoning. The CDC definition of lead poisoning was 60 μg/dL in the early 1960s, while currently 10 μg/dL represents undue absorption, and 15–20 μg/dL suggests the need for medical case management.[41] Current research directions involve seeking the most effective preventive and screening strategies, as well as addressing the question of whether chelation therapy can have impact on the neurocognitive effects of low-level lead poisoning.[4,5,88,202]

How Extensive Is the Lead Problem in the United States Today ? Who Is Getting Poisoned?

Although substantial progress has been made in prevention due to hazard reduction and early screening, specific diagnostic tests, and treatment, lead poisoning remains a pervasive environmental and toxicologic problem today. Lead poisoning affects persons of all ages, but tends to cluster into several distinct populations at risk. The scope and clinical significance of the problem is most severe in young children, aged 1–6 years, whose primary source of exposure is deteriorated lead paint in their home. The U.S. Department of Health and Human Services has recently declared such childhood lead poisoning "the most important environmental health problem for young children."[5] The second large affected group is adults exposed at their worksite, whose occupation involves lead smelting or reclamation, construction or demolition, or the manufacture or repair of lead-containing materials.[32,68,214] General environmental exposures from contaminated air, water, and food are uncommon in advanced societies today, but may still effect an entire community under special circumstances. Exotic sources are also reported sporadically, including exposures to contaminated folk medications, cosmetics, ingested lead foreign bodies, retained bullets, artists' or other hobby materials, firing ranges, illicit distilled alcoholic beverages, and substances of abuse.[206]

Population Surveys

Several recent national and regional surveys have evaluated current U.S. population-based trends in blood lead levels and sociodemographic correlates. The Third National Health and Nutrition Examination Survey (NHANES III) examined over 13,000 U.S. citizens of ages 1 to beyond 70 years, in a nationally representative cross-sectional survey.[32] The survey, done between 1988 and 1991, determined mean blood lead levels and their sociodemographic correlates. The mean blood lead for this sample of the U.S. population was 2.8 μg/dL, with the highest mean lead levels observed in 1–2 year olds (4.1 μg/dL). Among adults, elderly persons had higher mean levels than younger adults, with a mean of 4.0 μg/dL in the 50–69-year-old and > 70-year-old categories. In general, lead levels were higher for males, blacks, central city residents, persons of low income and educational attainment, and residents of the Northeast region of the United States. The estimated prevalence of lead levels > 10 μg/dL for children aged 1–5 years was 8.9%, or approximately 1.7 million children; however, this prevalence rose to 36.7% for non-Hispanic black children residing in central cities of > 1 million population. When these findings are compared to the previous NHANES II survey carried out in 1976–1980,[141] a 78% decline in blood lead levels overall is observed.[192]

Such a dramatic improvement might be interpreted as evidence that the general problem of environmental lead pollution has been largely conquered in the United States. The current overall mean blood lead level in the United States is comparable to that measured in children living in the relatively pristine environment of the Himalayas.[188,190] Further, several studies of urban and suburban private fee-for-service or health manintenance organization pediatric practices have confirmed the relative infrequency (<5%) of finding middle- to upper-income children with elevated lead levels.[23,173,240] Nevertheless, for young minority children and the poor who reside in our nation's deteriorating central cities, the battle is far from won.[38,92] In some of these inner-city neighborhoods, such as West Philadelphia, the majority of children age 1–5 years have lead levels > 10 μg/dL, and as many as 15% have levels > 20 μg/dL,[186] a level at which the CDC recommends medical intervention.[41] A recent study of Philadelphia children visiting two pediatric emergency departments for acute illnesses, and who used Medicaid predominantly as their health insurance, found that more than 50% had lead levels > 10 μg/dL and that 7% had levels > 25 μg/dL.[259]

The CDC has estimated that 95% of adults with lead levels above 25 μg/dL are exposed primarily through occupational exposure.[39] Nevertheless, NHANES III demonstrated that similar demographic correlates as noted for children apply to adult populations, and thus urbanization and poverty are likely important factors for adult lead poisoning as well as for children.[32]

What Are the Sources of Human Lead Exposure?

Numerous sources of lead exposure exist. Environmental exposures affect the entire population, particularly young children, and include leaded paint, soil and dust contaminated by lead paint, leaded gasoline automobile exhaust, and industrial waste, airborne lead from automobile exhaust and industrial emissions, water con-

TABLE 79–2. ENVIRONMENTAL LEAD SOURCES

Source	Comment
Leaded paint	Especially pre-1978 homes
Dust	House dust from deteriorated lead paint
Soil	From yards contaminated by deteriorated lead paint, lead industry emissions, roadways with high leaded gasoline usage
Water	Leached from leaded plumbing (pipes, solder), cooking utensils, water coolers
Air	Leaded gasoline (pre-1976 US, still prevalent worldwide), industrial emissions
Food	Lead solder in cans (pre-1991 US, still prevalent in imported canned foods); "natural" calcium supplements; "moonshine" whiskey; lead-foil covered wines; contaminated flour, paprika
Exotic	Folk remedies, cosmetics; ingested lead foreign bodies, retained lead bullets; illicit substance abuse (heroin, methamphetamine, leaded gasoline "huffing"); burning batteries, leaded paper, or wood for fuel; use of lead-glazed ceramics; hand–mouth contact with pool cue chalk, glazes, leaded ink

taminated via lead pipes and lead solder, and food contaminated via lead-soldered cans (Table 79–2). Adults with occcupational or recreational exposure to lead constitute another large group of persons at risk. For convenience, these categories of lead exposure are discussed separately, though there is considerable overlap. For example, workers who fail to change lead dust–covered work clothes or shoes may bring this lead hazard home to affect their children.[13,206]

What Are the Environmental Sources of Lead?

Paint

In the 20th century, the toxicologic hazard associated with lead paint has been recognized and resulted in widespread regulation. Lead content in many white house paints (typically lead carbonate) was 50% by weight in the pre–World War II era. A thumbnail-sized chip of 50% leaded paint might contain up to 200 mg of lead (vs a typical dietary intake of 50–100 μg/day for a young child).[56] Since 1978, paint intended for interior or exterior residential surfaces, toys, or furniture may contain no more than 0.06% lead.[5] However, an estimated 3 million tons of lead remain in 57 million exisiting U.S. homes built prior to 1980 and painted with lead-based paint.[245] Most dangerous are the 3.8 million homes with deteriorated paint in which 2 million young children reside.[5,165] This aging housing stock has created an enormous environmental hazard of lead exposure to these children, and to adult homeowners, house painters, and construction workers who become involved in sanding, scraping, and restoration of painted surfaces in these homes. Further, lead-based paint is still allowed for industrial, military, marine, and some outdoor uses such as structural components of bridges and highways; occasionally some of this paint is inadvertently used in homes.[41] Attempts to abate lead-painted outdoor structures can pollute entire communities.[132]

Paint-derived lead exposure to children has historically been blamed on pica, the common pediatric behavior of eating nonfood items, and attributed to ingestion of macroscopic paint chips. Unproven inferences were made suggesting such children were victims of inadequate parenting.[167] A more recent understanding is that, while pica may play a role for some children, most lead paint exposure in childhood relates to the crumbling, peeling, flaking, or chalking of aging paint.[41,51] These fine paint particles are incorporated into household dust and yard soil, where ordinary childhood hand–mouth activity results in ingestion.[45,215] Lead paint is typically found in these older homes on kitchen and bathroom walls, and particularly on any wood surfaces such as the doors, windows, stairway bannisters, decorative trim or moldings, and exterior wood surfaces, especially on porches. Surfaces subject to friction, especially sash windows, are particularly dangerous, as every opening and closing adds to the lead dust burden of the home.[81] Window sills have also been noted to be likely sites of mouthing for toddlers playing near or looking out the window.[52]

Dilapidated homes in the inner city are not the only source of lead-paint hazard. Pre–1960 dwellings in any area, particularly if paint is visibly deteriorated or the home is undergoing renovation, are likely to be hazardous.[36,51,216] Adults as well as children may develop lead poisoning when homeowners renovate Victorian-era homes in rural[148] or regentrifying urban neighborhoods (the latter has been dubbed "yuppie plumbism").[6,216]

Soil

Closely related to the exposure due to lead-based paint is that of soil contaminated by residue of deteriorated exterior house paint and leaded gasoline emissions. In addition, some communities are further contaminated by proximity to lead smelters or lead-using industries.[1] Although lead emissions from gasoline contributing to soil lead has largely been eliminated, it is estimated that more than 4 million tons of gasoline-derived lead remain in our dust and soil.[1] The same normal hand–mouth and play activities of children that have impact on lead paint–contaminated house dust exposure are operative in terms of outdoor soil to which children have access. Children's blood lead levels rise 3–7 μg/dL for every 1000 ppm rise in their environmental soil or dust concentrations.[1,29]

Water

Ground and surface water generally have low lead levels. Lead contaminates drinking water via lead-based plumbing, connectors, lead-soldered joints, and/or lead-containing brass faucets. Water that is low in mineral content (soft), acidic, and hot is more likely to leach lead; the time of standing in contact with lead piping or solder is also correlated with higher lead content.[1] Many homes in the United States built prior to 1920 have lead pipes, and many newer homes have lead-containing solder or brass fixtures. An estimated 16% of household water supplies have lead in excess of 20 μg/L (the current standard is 15 μg/L).[75] Older water-coolers in schools and public buildings also may contain lead-solder, with resulting high water lead levels. Their intermittent use, with water standing for some time (eg, over a weekend), may exacerbate this phenomenon.[41] Elevated lead levels in infancy are associated with the use of hot tap water that has been further boiled down to prepare infant formula,[229] as has water boiled in an imported Iranian kettle.[86]

Air

Studies of glacial icecaps have shed fascinating insight into the history of worldwide lead consumption and resultant atmospheric pollution.[214] The lead contained in Greenland ice layers increased 400% from 1735 to 1935, representing primarily the effect of industrial emissions. Between 1935 and 1965, icecap lead tripled, presumably the effect of leaded gasoline use. The regulated removal of lead from gasoline in the United States between 1976 and 1990, and EPA standards for industrial emissions, have resulted in dramatic decreases in overall air lead content, with concomitant decreases in mean U.S. blood lead levels, as noted above. In 1976, more than 200,000 tons of lead were used in gasoline in the United States. By 1990, lead use in gasoline had dropped to just over 500 tons, representing a 99.8% decrease.[192] Remaining sources of airborne lead in the United States include point sources such as mines and smelters and the allowed use of leaded gasoline in agricultural vehicles.[206] Unfortunately, many third-world and former Eastern-bloc countries have not yet been able to institute leaded-gasoline and industrial-emission controls, with the result that airborne lead remains for them a significant source of exposure.[41] A recent report from China, for example, found average blood lead levels in young children ranging from 21 to 67 μg/dL in industrial and heavily trafficked areas.[231]

Food

Lead in food is the result of several factors, including atmospheric lead falling onto leafy vegetables, soil lead being taken up by plants, and lead-solder in food cans leaching into contents. Declines in leaded gasoline use have indirectly decreased food lead exposure via improved atmospheric quality resulting in decreased food lead content.[41,165] A further dramatic reduction in food exposure can be attributed to the regulation of lead-soldered cans. Studies of canned tuna have found a 200-fold increase in lead content due to lead-soldered canning.[227] In 1980, 47% of food and beverage cans were lead soldered, versus less than 1% in 1990.[192] The Food and Drug Administration has estimated that typical daily food lead intake for a 2-year-old child averaged 30 μg/day in 1982, and has decreased to 1.9 μg/day in 1991.[28] Lead-soldered food or soft-drink cans have not been manufactured in the United States since November 1991, but some foreign cans still have lead-soldered seams.[165]

Food supplements and beverages may be contaminated with lead. Exposures are described secondary to the use of "natural" calcium supplements derived from animal bones;[159] alcoholic beverages stored in lead crystal decanters;[8] foods and beverages, especially if acidic, stored in improperly lead-glazed, often imported, ceramics;[133] bootleg whiskey made in automobile radiators or distilled in lead-containing or soldered piping;[43,237] lead-pigmented lettering on plastic bread bags;[165] wine from older European wineries capped with lead-foil covered corks;[167] flour contaminated from being ground in a mill repaired with lead;[128] and Hungarian ground paprika contaminated with lead tetroxide (red lead).[123]

Other Environmental Sources

A number of additional, somewhat "exotic," sources of lead exposure resulting in occasional cases of lead poisoning have been described.[41,165] One such source is ethnic folk remedies or cosmetics common to immigrant populations in the United States.[37] Hispanic-Americans have used metal-containing remedies for an illness often referred to as "empacho" (colic or gastroenteritis symptoms). Two such remedies are azarcon, which is an orange, 86–95% lead tetroxide powder, and greta which may also contain mercury. Patients ingesting these preparations may demonstrate intestinal radiopaque matter on abdominal radiographs.[30] Other names for azarcon and greta include alarcon, coral, rueda, liga, and Maria Luisa.[206] Lead-containing ethnic folk remedies used by Asian communities include paylooah which can contain arsenic, used for rash and fever, and chuifong tokuwan, ghasard, bali goli, and kandu.[37,206] A lead-contaminated Chinese herbal tea is hau ge fen.[153] Similarly, Middle Eastern and Indo-Pakistani remedies and eye cosmetics are maha yogran guggulu, surma, kohl, alkohl, saoott, satrinj, bint dahab, and cebagin.[213,264] Of note, many families are initially hesitant to report these remedies when their child's history is taken, or fail to consider them as "medicine" at all. It may enhance reporting to specifically ask about them in their common name.[37]

Another significant group of unusual exposures relates to ingestion of metallic lead objects or gunshot wounds with lead ammunition. Several cases have been reported of pediatric lead intoxication due to lead curtain weight, bullet, or fishing weight ingestions (Fig. 79–4).[109,112,139] Ingested foreign bodies do not generally cause toxicity unless they are retained in the intestinal tract for 2 weeks or more.[73] Lead poisoning from retained lead bullets, shrapnel, or shot after gunshot wounds is an uncommon complication of gunshot wounds, but was recognized during the Roman wars and was reported (without the benefit of lead levels) more than 100 years ago.[108,239] Most cases result from lead ammunition particles being bathed by synovial, serosal, or, possibly, spinal fluids.[71,157,222,239] The surface area of lead fragments exposed to body fluids also appears to influence the rapidity of developing elevated blood levels, with buckshot injuries resulting in lead poisoning much faster (eg, average interval of 8 months) than shrapnel (average 10 years) or single bullets (average 17 years).[71,222]

Several additional exposures are reported as lead hazards. Illicit substance abuse has caused lead poisoning via methamphetamine containing lead acetate in Oregon,[2] heroin contaminated with lead in Spain,[181] and

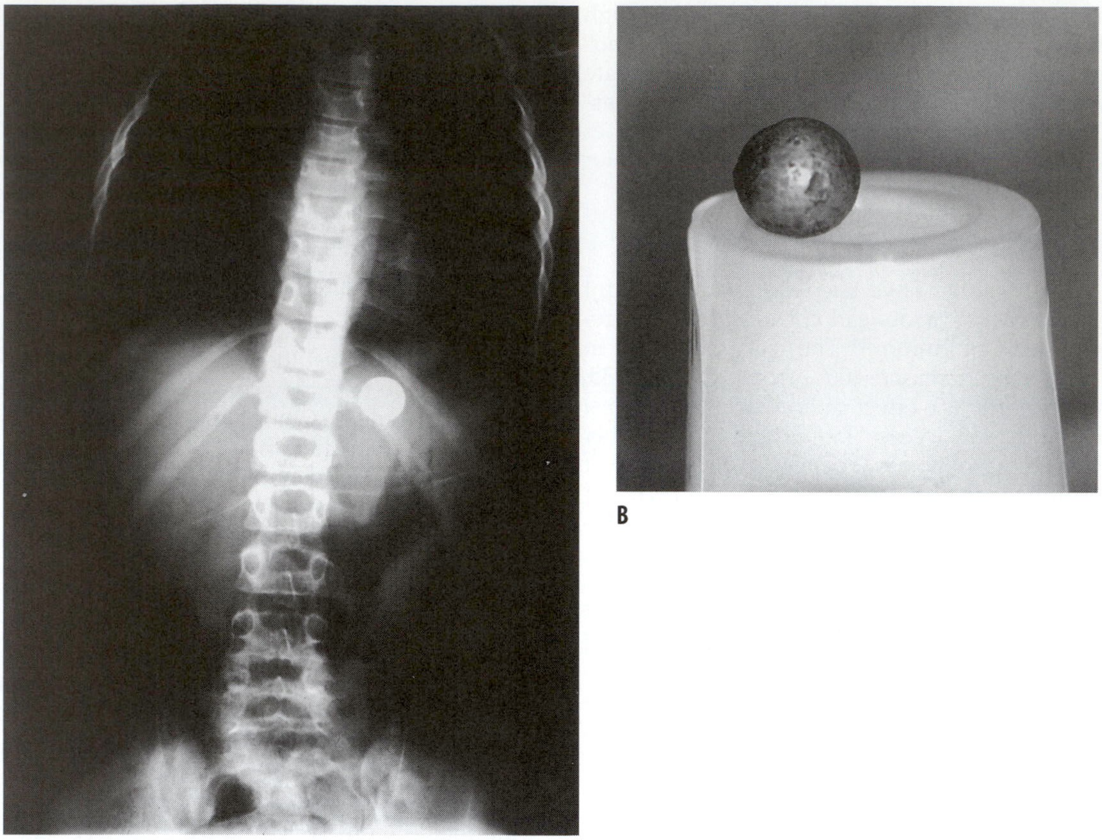

A

B

Figure 79–4. A. Radiograph of the abdomen reveals ingested metallic foreign body. **B.** The ingested foreign body was a Civil War era musketball from the collection of the father of the patient. *(Courtesy of Evaline Allessandrini, MD, Division of Emergency Medicine, Children's Hospital of Philadelphia, Philadelphia, PA.)*

chronic gasoline sniffing (with leaded gasoline).[125] Lead poisoning has resulted from burning of lead-painted wood,[41] rolled newspaper logs,[178] or recycled storage battery casings for heating fuel.[72] Lead poisoning has also resulted from the ingestion or hand-to-mouth contact of several unusual lead-containing nonfood items: ceramic glazes (nursing home residents in art class)[250] (see Chap. 111); ink (a scriptural scribe who frequently licked his pen);[55] hair spray (intentional adult overdose);[196] pool cue chalk (pediatric exposure);[158] and plastic wire insulation (an electrician who chewed wires).[85]

What Are the Typical Occupational and Recreational Sources of Lead?

It is estimated that more than one million workers in the United States, employed in over 100 occupations are exposed to lead.[206] The most important route of absorption in occupational settings is inhalation of lead dust and fumes. In addition, workers may eat, drink, or smoke in lead-dust-contaminated areas, resulting in some ingestion as well. However, presence of lead in the workplace, per se, does not imply a significant risk of poisoning. The risk is correlated with several factors that contribute to the occurrence of respirable lead fumes or dust particles (< 5 μm in diameter) in the worksite atmosphere.[214] There are three general categories of such factors. The first relates to the degree of hazard inherent in the work process itself, including high temperatures (eg > 1000°C), significant aerosol, dust, or fume production, and less mechanized technology. Second, the adequacy of dust elimination, such as local and general ventilation, is critical. The third category is that of worksite and personal hygiene, including proper use of protective clothes and equipment, and thorough housekeeping. In general, small shops employing few workers are more hazardous than large factories with hundreds or thousands of employees. The small, sometimes "backyard" plants are less likely to adhere to industry safety regulations, are less automated, and have less environmental control, and the relatively few workers are less educated about potential risks and protective equipment usage. A good example of this distinction is that between primary and secondary lead smelting.[68,137] The primary smelter produces pig lead from raw ore. Such facilities tend to be very large, but few in number. Secondary smelters reclaim lead from scrap metal, particularly discarded automobile storage batteries. These shops tend to be small in size and workforce, but many in number (a 1984 government analysis found 82 foundries with > 500 workers, and 2633 with < 50).[166] Despite the above-noted risk factors that may be specific to each worksite, there are some types of lead-related work that are more hazardous than others, based on actual surveys of blood lead levels and reported incidence of clinical poisoning (see Table 79–3).[146,206,214]

The highest risk group of occupational exposures include any that involve welding, cutting, or burning of metallic lead or lead-coated materials.[111,147,214] Such occupations include shipbreaking,[154] and welding or cutting of lead-painted or galvanized steels as in the structural metal of highways and bridges.[147] These jobs often involve the use of very-high-temperature (3500°C) oxyacetylene torches, resulting in effective vaporization of lead. Another high-temperature operation is that of primary and secondary lead smelting.[68] Storage battery manufacture involves considerable exposure to lead oxide dust, in addition to fumes from welding of battery connectors. Additional high-risk occupations are noted in Table 79–3.[63,72,82,93,214]

In moderate-risk occupations exposure potential is significant, but typical job circumstances result in relatively low incidence of clinical poisoning and/or prevalence of elevated biologic markers of excessive body lead burden.[83,214] These include lead miners, solderers, plumbers, wire and cable workers, type founders, ship repair workers, automobile factory workers and repair mechanics, lead glass blowers, pottery glazers, shot makers, welders, enamelers, and varnish makers.

Several occupations occasion lead exposure beyond normal background levels, but with minimal health risk.[214] These include persons exposed to heavy fumes or automobile exhaust (where leaded gasoline has been in use) such as traffic police, taxi drivers, garage workers, turnpike tollbooth operators, and gas station attendants. Additional workers at slightly elevated risk include manufacturers of rubber products or electronics, jewelers, pipefitters, and printers.

Exposure to alkyl leads, particularly tetraethyl lead (TEL), is currently much less common with the near elimination of leaded gasoline production and institution of industry safety standards in production and distribution.[214] The most important remaining exposure occurs during the cleaning or repair of leaded gasoline storage tanks, which tend to accumulate a sludge with high TEL content on the bottom.

Hobbies and recreational pursuits using lead-containing materials under circumstances similar to occupational exposures are obviously a source of potential risk.[41,214] Lessened time spent in these activities in comparison to full-time occupational exposures may be offset by less vigilant adherence to safety principals. An important example includes amateur crafting of pottery and ceramics using leaded frits and glazes.[133] In addition to the potter's exposure, improperly glazed ceramicware may pose a hazard to persons using the product. Inadequate firing temperature (<1150°C) results in the glaze not fusing properly, allowing acidic foods and beverages, such as fruit juices, cider, wine, or vinegar, particularly, to leach lead. This phenomenon is common in pottery imported from Latin America and Mediterranean countries. Other hobbies and recreational activities at risk include car, boat, furniture, and home repair, remodeling, or refinishing; stained glass making using lead solder; painting with artists' leaded pigments; target shooting; or recasting molten lead for bullets, toy soldiers, or fishing weights.

TABLE 79–3. OCCUPATIONAL AND RECREATION LEAD SOURCES

High-risk Occupations
Shipbreaking
Metal welders, cutters (includes bridge and highway reconstruction workers)
Lead smelters, refiners
Storage battery manufacturers, repairers, recyclers
Painters, construction workers (sanding, scraping, spraying of lead paint; demolition of lead-painted sites)
Polyvinyl chloride plastic manufacturers
Crystal glass makers
Automobile radiator repairers
Firing range instructors
Moderate-risk Occupations
Lead miners
Welders
Solderers
Plumbers
Wire and cable workers
Type founders
Ship repairers
Automobile factory workers and mechanics
Glass blowers
Pottery glazers
Enamelers
Varnish makers
Shot makers
Low-risk Occupations
Traffic police officers, taxi drivers, garage workers, turnpike tollbooth operators, gas station attendants (exposed to leaded gasoline exhaust fumes)
Rubber product manufacturers
Electronics manufacturers
Jewelers
Pipefitters
Printers
Recreational and Hobby Sources
Crafters of ceramics
Repair of automobiles, boats
Home remodeling, refinishing
Furniture refinishing, restoring
Stained glass making
Painting (fine artists' pigments)
Target shooting, recasting lead for bullets

What Is the Toxicology of Lead?

Pharmacodynamics

Absorption. Lead is absorbed primarily through inhalation and via the gastrointestinal tract. In adults with occupational exposures, inhalation is the predominant form of absorption, while for children gastrointestinal absorption is primary. Cutaneous absorption is essentially nonexistent for inorganic lead, but does occur with alkyl leads.

Inhalation of particles < 0.5–1 μm in size are most likely to reach the alveoli, where they are almost completely absorbed.[97,98] Larger particles deposit in airways, are cleared by mucociliary activity, and are eventually swallowed, acting as ingested lead. The overall absorption of inhaled lead averages 30–40%. Of note, both minute ventilation and the concentration of lead in air determine airborne lead exposure, and thus a worker engaged in vigorous physical activity will absorb considerably more lead than a person in the same atmosphere at rest. Likewise, children, with relatively greater volume of inhaled air per unit of body size due to higher metabolic rates, are proportionally at greater risk in a given degree of atmospheric lead pollution. It has been estimated that children have a 2.7-fold higher lung deposition rate of lead than do adults.[1]

Gastrointestinal (GI) absorption is less efficient than pulmonary. Adults absorb an estimated 10–15% of ingested lead in food, and children have a higher GI absorption rate, averaging 40–50%.[1,98] However, it should be noted that fasting and diets deficient in iron, calcium, and zinc enhance GI absorption of lead, factors that are frequent among groups of young children.[98,140] A study of adults under fasting conditions found a lead absorption rate from beverage consumption of almost 60%.[115] The role of essential trace elements in decreasing lead absorption is assumed due to competitive absorption processes; recently an iron-binding protein, mobilferrin, initially identified in rat duodenum, has been found in human duodenal mucosa and competitively binds lead.[57]

Cutaneous absorption of inorganic lead is low; one study found an average absorption of 0.06% through intact skin.[162] Alkyl leads may have appreciable cutaneous absorption that is capable of causing toxicity.[214]

Transplacental lead transfer is critical in fetal and neonatal lead exposure, which has come under increasing scrutiny in recent years.[18] Lead readily crosses the placental barrier throughout gestation, and lead uptake is cumulative until birth.[197]

Distribution. Absorbed lead enters the bloodstream, where at least 99% is bound to erythrocytes.[97] From blood, lead is distributed into both a relatively labile soft tissue pool and a more stable bone compartment. The classic three-compartment model may be somewhat of an oversimplification. Currently, at least two bone compartments are recognized, a more labile pool in trabecular bone, and a more stable pool in cortical bone. In adults, about 95% of body lead burden is stored in bone, versus only 70% for children. The remainder is distributed to the major soft tissue lead storage sites, including liver, kidney, bone marrow, and brain. Most of the toxicity associated with lead is due to soft tissue uptake, so that the relative decrease in bone storage is another comparative disadvantage to lead-poisoned children.

Lead uptake into soft tissues occurs in a complex fashion that depends on numerous factors, including blood lead levels, external exposure factors, and specific tissue kinetics.[1] In general, lead levels in populations without very excessive exposure average 200–500 parts per billion (ppb); rises above this with excessive exposure rapidly produce overt toxicity. For example, brain lead content in humans with overt encephalopathy is on the order of 1–2 parts per million (ppm) or less (eg, only twice the above noted range). Blood lead levels of only 100–150 ppb (10–15 μg/dL) are now recognized as being associated with subtle toxic effects in critical target organs.

Lead in the central nervous system (CNS) is of particular toxicologic importance, and studies have addressed specific storage sites. Lead preferentially concentrates in gray matter and certain nuclei.[97] Fetal brain uptake is relatively higher than with postnatal exposure in animal models.[205] The highest brain concentrations are found in hippocampus, cerebellum, cerebral cortex, and medulla.

Unlike soft tissue storage, bone lead accumulates throughout life. Bone storage begins in utero, and occurs across all ranges of exposure, so that there is no threshold for bone lead uptake.[1] Total body accumulation of lead may range from 200 mg to over 500 mg in workers with heavy occupational exposure.[97] Bone lead is thought to be relatively metabolically inert, but recent evidence suggests that it can be mobilized from the more labile compartment and contributes as much as 50% of blood lead concentration. This may be of particular importance during pregnancy and lactation, in elder persons with osteoporosis,[233] and in children with immobilization due to fracture or neurologic disease.[152] Lead also accumulates in teeth, particularly the dentine of children's teeth, a phenomenon that has been used to quantify cumulative lead exposure in young children by researchers.[168,170]

Excretion. Absorbed lead that is not retained is excreted primarily in urine (about 65%) and bile (about 35%).[1] A miniscule amount is lost via sweat, hair, and nails. Children excrete less of their daily uptake than adults, with an average retention of 33% versus 1–4%, respectively.[265] Biologic half-lives for lead are estimated as follows[1,144,198]: blood (adults, short-term experiments), 25 days; blood (children, natural exposure), 10 months; soft tissues (adults, short-term exposure), 40 days; bone (labile, trabecular pool), 90 days; bone (cortical, stable pool), 10–20 years.

Alkyl lead compounds have unique pharmacokinetics that are less well characterized.[27] Tetraethyl lead is lipid soluble, easily absorbed through intact skin, and distributed widely to lipophilic tissues including the brain. Tetraethyl lead is metabolized to triethyl lead, which is believed to be the major toxic compound.[27] Alkyl leads may slowly release lead as the inorganic form, with subsequent kinetics as noted above.

What Are the Pathophysiologic Effects of Lead?

General Effects

Lead, similar to many heavy metals, is a complex toxin exerting numerous pathophysiologic effects in many organ systems.[97] At the biomolecular level, lead functions in three general ways. First, its affinity for biologic electron-donor ligands, especially sulfhydyl groups, allows it to bind and have impact on numerous structural and enzymatic proteins. Second, lead is chemically similar to calcium and interferes with numerous metabolic pathways, particularly in mitochondria and in second messenger systems regulating cellular energy metabolism. Lead may function as an inhibitor or agonist of calcium-dependent processes. For example, lead inhibits neuronal voltage-sensitive calcium channels[11] and membrane-bound Na,K-ATPase,[235] but activates calcium-dependent protein kinase C.[149] Third, lead exhibits mutagenic and mitogenic effects in mammalian cells in vitro and is carcinogenic in rats and mice.[161] Evidence for human carcinogenicity is lacking, however.[77]

CNS Neurotoxicity

Overt neurotoxicity classically manifests as an acute encephalopathy. The pathogenesis of this syndrome involves failure of the blood–brain barrier.[96] When lead accumulates in brain microvasculature above a critical level, capillary function is disrupted by alteration of cellular calcium metabolism, resulting in separation of the tight intercellular junctions that normally seal endothelial cells. Proteinaceous fluid extravasates, and since brain tissue is without lymphatic drainage, brain edema occurs rapidly. The cerebellum and cerebral occipital lobes are effected predominantly, but the process is widespread, resulting in increased intracranial pressure, coma, seizures, and permanent neuronal loss.

More subtle neurotoxic effects, such as those that underly cognitive impairment without overt symptomatology, are less well understood but probably include altered neurotransmitter function in both children and adults, and subtle morphologic changes, particularly in the developing brain in utero and early childhood.[94,98] Neuronal cell bodies of the cerebral cortex and basal ganglia begin to form during the first trimester of gestation and have migrated to their adult location by the end of the second trimester.[94,232] At birth, synaptic connections are sparse, however. Over the first 2 years of life, the multiple connections and neural networks characteristic of the mature brain are rapidly developing and are actually twice as dense at age 2 years as in adulthood. The next several years of life, through late childhood, allow considerable postnatal reorganization and progressive "pruning" of synapses.[120] Synapse persistence is likely determined by individual synpase activity, which in turn is determined by environmental factors involving motor and sensory stimulation, as well as nutritive and potentially toxic influences.[17]

These events are taking place at precisely the time that brain lead is peaking in lead-exposed young children. Animal models have demonstrated also that the immature endothelium lining capillaries of the developing brain allow greater egress of lead into astrocytes and neurons.[95,241]

Lead is known to have impact on cell differentiation and several biochemical pathways that may interfere with this postnatal reorganization of brain microanatomy. In rodent models, lead decreases oligodendrite density, myelin deposition, and cortical synaptogenesis.[185] Lead induces glial cells to undergo precocious differentiation, potentially altering the migration path of neurons.[58] Lead blocks voltage-sensitive calcium channels, and thus may reduce stimulated synaptic conduction.[11] At the same time, lead either facilitates calcium entry or functions as a calcium agonist within nerve terminals, resulting in enhanced background release of neurotransmitters.[160] Thus, stimulated neurotransmitter release is decreased while spontaneous neurotransmitter release is facilitated, resulting in a decreased "signal-to-noise" ratio in the developing brain.[94] Synaptic pruning may become disorganized, leaving a cortex with approximately normal synaptic density but suboptimal architecture. Such changes are likely to be long-lasting if not permanent.

An additional consideration is the impact of lead on protein kinases. These enzymes are believed to influence neurotransmitter function in several ways, including regulation of release, ion flux, and gene activation involved in memory function.[116] Low levels of lead directly stimulate brain protein kinases.[149] This effect could also alter synapse development and pruning. Lead-induced changes in brain capillary endothelial cells that are less severe than occur in encephalopathy may also allow altered fluid dynamics and cellular milieu in astrocytes and neurons. Thus lead may exert both direct effects on neurons and indirect effects via the brain's support system that result in abnormal synaptic anatomy and function.[94]

Lead exerts neuropharmacologic effects that may be relevant to cortical function in both developing and mature nervous systems. Lead impairs several neurotransmitter systems, including the classic acetylcholine-, dopamine-, norepinephrine-, and gamma-aminobutyrate (GABA)-dependent systems.[97] This effect of lead is also found in the more recently recognized systems dependent on glutamate and particularly, the *N*-methyl-D-aspartate receptor complex, which is believed to be important in memory function.[59] Lead also interferes with normal neural cell adhesion molecule sialylation, and thus impairs cell–cell adhesion and learning in adult animal models.[199]

Low-level lead exposure is also toxic to the auditory and visual neural systems, as well as neuromotor performance and fine motor coordination. Elevated blood lead levels are associated with hearing deficits in children.[220]

Recent studies have found higher threshold for auditory nerve action potentials and segmental demyelination and axonal degeneration of the cochlear nerve in lead-exposed animals. Similar deficits of retinal function have been observed in rats with lead levels < 20 μg/dL.[179] Studies of 6-year-old children with modest lead burdens (mean blood lead at age 2 years of 17 μg/dL range 6–49 μg/dL) found an association of higher lead levels with poorer performance in bilateral coordination, visual-motor control, upper-limb speed and dexterity, and overall fine motor coordination.[70]

Peripheral Neuropathy

Peripheral neuropathy is a classic effect of occupational lead poisoning. It is accompanied by Schwann cell destruction, followed by segmental demyelination and axonal degeneration.[97] Sensory nerves are less effected than motor nerves. Using a sensitive test such as nerve conduction velocity, peripheral nerve dysfunction can be demonstrated at blood lead levels as low as 40 μg/dL.[226] Peripheral neuropathy is rarely reported in children, but has been described occasionally in children with hemoglobinopathy.[79]

Hematologic

Lead is a potent inhibitor of several enzymes in the heme synthesis pathway, as well as other enzymes of hematologic importance. Lead poisoning results in anemia, which is believed due to both decreased erthrocyte survival and decreased hemoglobin synthesis. Some authors have further postulated a defect in erythropoietin function secondary to associated renal damage.[107,204]

Shortened erythrocyte life span is believed due to increased membrane fragility. Inhibition of Na,K-ATPase and pyrimidine–5′-nucleotidase may impair erythrocyte membrane stability by altering energy metabolism. The inhibition of pyrimidine–5′-nucleotidase is also thought to underlie the appearance of stippling in erythrocytes, representing clumping of degraded RNA, which is normally eliminated by this enzyme.[180] Several steps in the heme synthesis pathway are impaired (Fig. 79–5).

The most sensitive effect of lead is inhibition of mitochondrial delta-aminolevulinc acid dehydratase (ALA-D). Genetic polymorphism of the ALA-D gene (alleles D^1 and D^2) may contribute to individual sensitivity to lead-induced heme toxicity, with the D^2 allele providing a basis for increased lead sensitivity.[10] Accumulation of ALA-D in blood and urine is the earliest easily measurable marker of lead toxicity and occurs at blood levels > 10 μg/dL. Lead also depresses function of coproporphyrinogen oxidase and ferrochelatase. The former effect results in elevated urinary coproporphyrin III, a phenomenon that in the past has been used in a bedside test for acute plumbism. The ferrochelatase inhibition results in decreased heme formation and increased erythrocyte protoporphyrin concentration. The latter is complexed with zinc in vivo, at the site normally occupied by iron. Erthrocytes with increased zinc-protoporphyrin fluoresce intensely, and the quantification of this effect

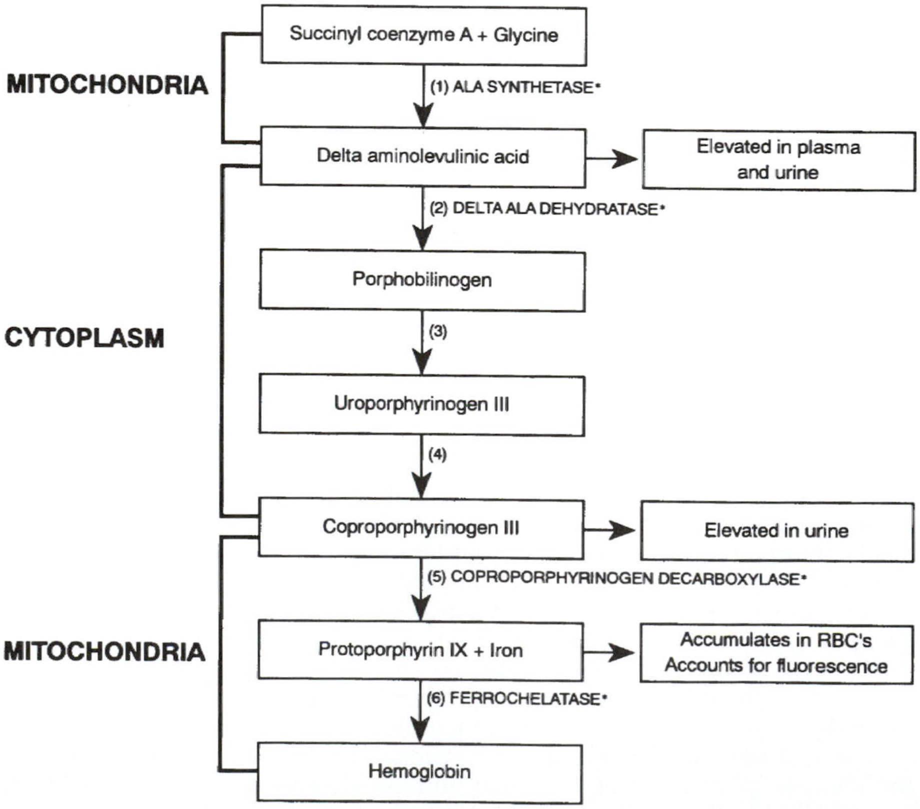

Figure 79–5. The heme synthesis pathway. The enzymatic steps inhibited by lead are marked with an asterisk (*).

serves as the basis of a commonly used screening test and marker of lead's hematologic toxicity.[189] Erythrocyte protoporphyrin is also increased in iron-deficiency anemia, due to lack of available iron for incorporation into heme, and the rare condition erythropoietic protoporphyria. Iron deficiency is a common concomitant of lead exposure, as noted above, and probably contributes significantly to much of the hypochromic, microcytic anemia actually observed in childhood.[54]

The reduced heme body pool may also have impact on other organ systems, but for convenience in the context of understanding lead's impairment of heme synthesis, is commented on here. It has been suggested that impaired heme synthesis might impair several heme-dependent metabolic systems, including decreased cytochrome function with resultant impaired energy metabolism in the CNS, reduced 1,25-$(OH)_2$-vitamin D synthesis with consequent alterations in calcium metabolism, and reduced activity of liver enzymes resulting in altered xenobiotic detoxification and endogenous agonist metabolism.[1,99] Elevations of ALA per se may be neurotoxic at higher levels, impacting GABA receptors.[31]

Renal

Nephropathy is one of the oldest described toxic effects of lead. It is typically a hazard for the heavily exposed adult worker,[97] and is inconsistently reported in adult survivors of severe childhood plumbism.[74] Lead is a renal carcinogen in rodent models, but its status in humans is uncertain.[77,97]

Functional changes associated with acute lead nephropathy include decreased energy-dependent transport, resulting in a Fanconi like syndrome of aminoaciduria, glycosuria, and phosphaturia. These changes are believed related to disturbed mitochondrial respiration and phosphorylation and are reversible with discontinuation of exposure and/or treatment. Ultrastructural studies have revealed swollen mitochondria with distorted cristae.[103] An additional microscopic finding is characteristic nuclear inclusion bodies in renal tubular cells, composed of lead–protein complex. These may be present in shed cells in the urinary sediment of heavily exposed workers. When affected persons are chelated, these inclusion bodies disappear coincident with increased urinary lead excretion. It is thought that these inclusion bodies account for the major fraction of renal intracellular lead and provide a significant pathway for lead excretion.[101] As lead nephropathy becomes more chronic, inclusion bodies become less common, and renal tubules begin to atrophy with the progressive appearance of interstitial fibrosis. These morphologic changes are typically associated with mild renal azotemia and decreased creatinine clearance. This progression from acute, reversible nephropathy to chronic, irreversible fibrosis has not been clearly demonstrated in humans, but has in rodent models.[100]

There does not appear to be a specific biologic marker for lead nephropathy. Chronic pathologic changes as noted are usually observed in workers with levels > 60 μg/dL. Some studies have found correlation between markers of renal dysfunction such as urinary *N*-acetyl-beta-D-glucosaminadase, and blood and urinary beta$_2$-microglobulin with elevated blood lead levels, but these findings are not consistent.[89] One study found markers of altered renal eicosanoid synthesis (decreased urinary 6-keto-prostaglandin F1 and increased thromboxane) in exposed workers with normal renal function,[34] while another recent study found urinary alpha$_1$-microglobulin to correlate with chronic lead exposure,[46] suggesting potential future value for such tests.

The asssociation of plumbism with gout ("saturnine gout") was noted more than 100 years ago by a pioneer in occupational medicine, the English physician Garrod.[88] Lead decreases uric acid renal excretion, with resulting elevated blood urate levels and urate crystal deposition in joints. Renal function is virtually always impaired. Patients with gout and renal disease have higher lead excretions after chelation than do patients with gout who are free of renal dysfunction (Table 79–4).[14,16]

Increased blood pressure is probably the most sensitive adverse health effect observed from lead exposure in adults. Several epidemiologic studies have found significant associations between increased blood pressure and body lead burdens.[78,193] The association is particularly strong for adult men aged 40–59, with an approximate 1.5–3.0 mm Hg rise in systolic pressure for every doubling of blood lead beginning at 7 μg/dL.[243] Hypertension does not appear to be consistently associated with elevated lead levels in children.[224] As noted above for gout, lead excretion after chelation challenge was found to be higher in patients with decreased renal function and hypertension than in patients with hypertension alone, or renal failure of known, but not lead-related etiology (Table 79–4).[14] The primary mechanism of lead-related hypertension is believed to be altered calcium-activated changes in contractility of vascular smooth muscle cells, secondary to decreased Na,K-ATPase activity and stimulation of the Na–Ca exchange pump. Lead may also

TABLE 79–4. RELATION OF LEAD BURDEN, RENAL INSUFFICIENCY, GOUT, AND HYPERTENSION

	N	Age (y)	SCr (mg/dL)	BPb (μg/dL)	EDTA Provocation (μg lead/3 day)
Gout, no RI	22	53	1.3	24	470
Gout and RI	22	57	3.0[a]	26	806[b]
HTN, no RI	21	55	1.2	18	340
HTN and RI	27	57	3.2[a]	19	860[a]
RI of known etiology (controls)	22	54	3.4	15	440

[a]$p < 0.001$ compared to HTN, no RI and controls
[b]$p < 0.005$ compared to gout, no RI and controls
SCr = serum creatinine; BPb = blood lead; RI = renal insufficiency; HTN = hypertension. Values given are group means.
Adapted, with permission, from Batuman V: Lead nephropathy, gout and hypertension: Am J Med Sci 1993;305:241-247

affect vessels by altering neuroendocrine input or sensitivity to such stimuli. Elevated plasma renin activity is found in persons after periods of modest exposure, though levels may drop to normal or lower in chronic severe exposure.[251] Lead has been found to increase Na–lithium countertransport in vitro (a phenomenon believed linked to renal Na–hydrogen exchange) in erythrocytes from healthy normotensive persons.[15] Similar findings are also observed in patients with essential hypertension, suggesting that there may be some common pathophysiologic mechanisms, as well as that some proportion of "essential" hypertension may actually represent occult lead nephropathy.[14]

Reproductive System

Impairment of both male and female reproductive function has been long associated with overt plumbism. Historically, infertility and stillbirths were common among heavily exposed women lead workers. Gametotoxic effects in animals of both sexes and chromosomal abnormalites in workers with blood lead levels above 60 μg/dL are reported.[97,238] More recent studies found reduced sperm counts, impaired sperm motility, and abnormal morphology in battery workers with lead levels > 40 μg/dL,[9] and increased incidence of menstrual irregularity and spontaneous abortion in lead-exposed female workers in China.[121] Prematurity is more common in pregnancies associated with elevated maternal lead levels.[165] Testicular endocrine hypofunction occurs in smelter workers with lead levels in the 60 μg/dL range.[203]

Congenital anomalies are reported after maternal lead exposure. An infant with the VACTERL association (vertebral anomalies, anal atresia, cardiac defect, tracheoesophageal fistula, renal and limb anomalies) was born to a mother with first-trimester high lead levels.[134] At least two young infants are reported, who presented at ages 2 days[90] and 2 months[225] repectively, with convulsions and very high blood lead levels believed due to intrauterine exposure. In addition, the 2-month-old infant manifested an unusual finding of "metallic brownish" fingernail discoloration, and was found to have an extremely elevated nail lead content of 4157 μg/g.

Endocrine

Reduced thyroid and adrenopituitary function are reported in adult lead workers.[210,211] Children with elevated lead levels have depressed secretion of human growth hormone and insulin-like growth factor.[119]

Skeletal System

In addition to the skeletal system's importance as the largest repository of lead body burden, recent studies have suggested that bone metabolism is adversely affected by lead as well. Hormonal response is altered by reduced 1,25-dihydroxyvitamin D_3 levels and by inhibition of osteocalcin. Both new bone formation and coupling of normal osteoblast and osteoclast function may thus be impaired.[97] Bands of increased metaphyseal density on radiographs of long bones in young children with heavy lead exposure demonstrate increased calcium deposition in the zones of provisional calcification (see Fig. 79–2). Impaired bone growth and shortened stature are associated with childhood lead poisoning.[219] It has been suggested that impaired calcium or cyclic AMP messenger systems underly these cellular effects.[97]

Gastrointestinal

Gastrointestinal symptoms typically appear with higher levels of blood lead and include abdominal pain, anorexia, vomiting, and constipation. It is suggested that these symptoms may be partly explained by spasmodic contraction of intestinal wall smooth muscle, analogous to that believed to occur in vascular walls.[214] Hepatitis and pancreatitis are reported in association with an acute intravenous exposure to lead,[175] and in cases of acute ingestion of lead compounds.[174] A metallic taste has been described in patients with lead poisoning.[110] A purple-blue gingival "lead line" (or Burton's line) representing precipitation of lead sulfide is also observed occasionally in adults with lead exposure and poor gingival hygiene.[3]

Cardiac

Rarely, myocarditis and cardiac dysfunction are reported in both adult[130] and pediatric[167,234] patients with clinical plumbism. Animal models demonstrate increased sensitivity to norepinephrine-induced dysrhythmias and decreased myocardial contractility, protein phosphorylation and high energy phosphate generation.[129] Electrocardiographic abnormalities include atrial dysrhythmias, tachycardia, and inverted T waves.[234] Recent descriptions of cardiac toxcity are scarce, although one adult worker with blood lead 213 μg/dL developed frequent multifocal premature ventricular contractions in addition to colic and anemia.[201] It seems plausible that lead-induced impairment of intracellular calcium metabolism is likely to have impact on cardiac effects.

What Is the Clinical Presentation of Lead Poisoning?

Inorganic Lead

The numerous observed lead-induced pathophysiologic effects accurately predict that the clinical manifestations of lead poisoning are diverse. These manifestations of lead toxicity are often characterized as falling into distinct syndromes of acute and chronic symptomatology. In most cases, these distinctions really describe a continuum of severity, with more severely exposed persons manifesting the classic "acute" lead intoxication syndrome. Rarely, patients with massive acute inhalational exposure, intentional overdose of soluble lead compounds, or intravenous administration of lead-contaminated substances of abuse present with a clinical picture that is somewhat unique, but overlaps considerably with the more severe cases of chronic lead exposure. By far, the most important contexts of lead toxicity in the United

TABLE 79–5. CLINICAL MANIFESTATIONS OF LEAD POISONING IN CHILDREN

Clinical Severity	Typical Blood Lead Levels (μg/dl)
Severe	>70–100
CNS: Encephalopathy (coma, altered sensorium, seizures, bizarre behavior, ataxia, apathy, incoordination, loss of developmental skills; papilledema, cranial nerve palsy, signs of increased ICP)	
GI: Persistent vomiting	
Heme: Pallor (anemia)	
Mild/moderate (preencephalopathic)	
CNS: Hyperirritable behavior, intermittent lethargy, decreased interest in play, "difficult" child	>50–70
GI: Intermittent vomiting, abdominal pain, anorexia	
Asymptomatic	
CNS: Impaired cognition, behavior	>10
PNS: Impaired fine motor coordination	
Misc: Impaired hearing, growth	

CNS = central nervous system; ICP = intracranial pressure; PNS = peripheral nervous system; GI = gastrointestinal; Heme = hematologic; Misc = miscellaneous

States today are related to chronic environmental exposure in children and chronic occupational exposure in adult workers. These are sufficiently distinct in epidemiology, clinical manifestations, and current recommended management approaches that they will here be described separately (Tables 79–5 and 79–6). Severe symptomatic poisoning is rare today among persons of all ages, though it is still reported. There were 139 deaths attributed to lead poisoning in the United States between 1979 and 1988, with the majority occurring among adults, in whom the primary reported exposure was illegal moonshine whiskey.[237] However, the largest public health concern currently is the detection and management of persons with asymptomatic but potentially toxic elevated lead levels.

TABLE 79–6. CLINICAL MANIFESTATIONS OF LEAD POISONING IN ADULTS

Clinical Severity	Typical Blood Lead Levels (μg/dL)
Severe	>100–150
CNS: Encephalopathy (coma, seizures, obtundation, delirium, focal motor disturbances, headaches, papilledema, optic neuritis, signs of increased ICP)	
PNS: Foot drop, wrist drop	
GI: Abdominal colic	
Heme: Pallor (anemia)	
Renal: Nephropathy	
Moderate	> 80
CNS: Headache, memory loss, decreased libido, insomnia	
GI: Metallic taste, abdominal pain, anorexia, constipation	
Renal: Nephropathy with chronic exposure	
Misc: Mild anemia, myalgias, muscle weakness, arthralgias	
Mild	>40
CNS: Tiredness, falling asleep easily, moodiness, lessened interest in leisure activities	
Misc: Impaired psychometrics, reproduction; elevated blood pressure	

CNS = central nervous system; ICP = intracranial pressure; PNS = peripheral nervous system; GI = gastrointestinal; Heme = hematologic; Misc = miscellaneous

It should be first reemphasized that the occurrence of overt clinical symptoms in lead-exposed persons is in most cases the culmination of a long history of lead exposure. As total dose increases, these symptoms are almost always preceded first by measureable biochemical and physiologic impairment, and followed in turn by subtle prodromal clinical effects that may only become apparent in hindsight (Fig. 79–6). In general, it has been considered that children are more susceptible than adults to toxicity for a given dose (eg, measured blood lead level); however, the data for this regard primarily concerns effects on the CNS, reflecting the aforementioned issues of blood–brain barrier immaturity and early childhood neurodevelopment.

Symptomatic Children. Acute lead encephalopathy is the most severe presentation of pediatric plumbism. Encephalopathy is characterized by pernicious vomiting and apathy, bizarre behavior, loss of recently acquired developmental skills, ataxia, incoordination, seizures, altered sensorium, or coma. Physical examination may reveal papilledema, oculomotor or facial nerve palsy, diminished deep tendon reflexes, or other evidence of increased intracranial pressure.[40,260] There may be pallor if there is coexisting anemia. Encephalopathy is usually associated with lead levels > 100 μg/dL, though it has been reported with levels as low as 70 μg/dL,[191] and tends to occur more commonly in summer months,[52] for reasons that are poorly understood. Milder but ominous symptoms that may portend incipient encephalopathy include sporadic vomiting, hyperirritable or aggressive behavior, periods of lethargy interspersed with lucid intervals, and decreased interest in play activities. Many patients seek medical advice for vomiting and lethargy during the 2–7 days prior to onset of frank encephalopathy.[52] Additional symptoms include anorexia, constipation, and intermittant abdominal pain.[49,191] Physical examination of such children is usually without specific abnormalities. Subencephalopathic symptomatic plumbism is usually associated with blood lead levels > 70 μg/dL, but may be seen with levels as low as 50 μg/dL. These presentations are most likely in children 1–5 years old, with encephalopathy particularly in the 15–30 month range. Unfortunately, common complaints in well children of this age ("terrible two's," with functional constipation and who don't eat as much as parents expect) often overlap with the milder range of reported symptoms of lead poisoning. It is not infrequent that parents whose child was diagnosed by routine blood screening recognize milder symptoms only in hindsight, after chelation treatment ("it seemed as if the child was going through a phase").[87] This is especially true currently, when sympatomatic plumbism is rarely reported.[40,41]

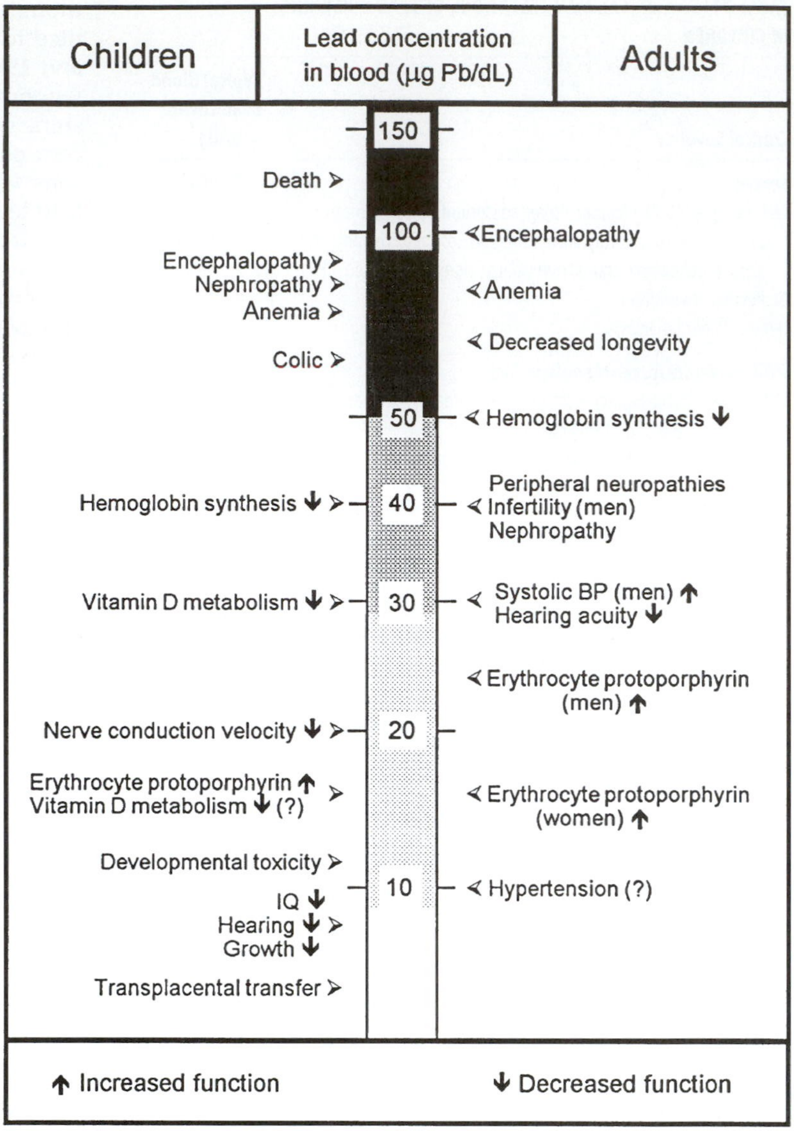

Figure 79–6. The biochemical and clinical effects of lead in children and adults. *(From Royce SE, Needleman HL: Case Studies in Environmental Medicine. Lead Toxicity. Atlanta, Agency for Toxic Substances and Disease Registry, 1992.)*

Other uncommon clinical presentations are described,[49] including isolated seizures without encephalopathy (indistinguishable from idiopathic epilepsy), chronic hyperactive behavior disorder, isolated developmental delay, progressive loss of cortical function simulating degenerative cerebral disease, peripheral neuropathy (reported particularly in children with hemoglobinopathy),[79] and a syndrome of colicky abdominal pain, vomiting, constipation, and myalgias of trunk and proximal girdle muscles.

Death and serious neurologic sequelae occurred frequently when encephalopathy was common.[50] Mortality was 65% in the pre-chelation era, dropping to < 5% with the advent of effective chelation. The incidence of permanent neurologic sequelae, including mental retardation, seizure disorder, blindness, and hemiparesis, is 25–30% in patients who develop encephalopathic symptoms prior to onset of chelation.[49]

Asymptomatic Children. Children with elevated body lead burdens but without overt symptoms represent the largest group of persons believed to be at risk of chronic lead toxicity. Almost 2 million children aged 1–5 years have lead levels > 10 μg/dL, the currently accepted level of concern. As noted previously in the discussion of pathophysiologic effects, the subclinical toxicity of lead in this population centers around subtle effects on growth, hearing, and neurocognitive development. The latter, in particular, has been the subject of intense research interest and scrutiny.[67]

Numerous studies have attempted to elucidate and quantify cognitive and behavioral deficits in children with blood lead levels below those typically associated with symptomatic plumbism (<50–70 μg/dL). Early cross-sectional or retrospective studies, carried out in the early 1970s, demonstrated subtle but statistically significant deficits in cognitive performance, in the range of 1–5 point decrement on standardized intelligence quotient (IQ) tests, in children with elevated lead levels.[66,184] Many of these studies, however, lacked sufficient numbers of patients, adequate markers of lead burden, or careful controls to be fully convincing. The first large, well-controlled study that addressed the majority of methodologic criticisms was reported 1979.[168] These authors compared the neurocognitive performance of 58 children in whom the dentine of shed primary teeth showed a high lead content (top 10th percentile) versus that of 100 control children with the lowest 10th percentile lead content. The subjects were Boston first- and second-grade schoolchildren, and none had been identified as having had lead poisoning. The high- and low-lead-content groups were carefully controlled for confounding variables, including medical history; parental education, social class, and IQ; and parental attitudes toward education and school. There was a 4-point deficit in IQ in the high-lead group (102.1 vs 106.6). In addition, more than 2000 children with known dentine levels were blindly evaluated by teachers in ratings of several classroom behaviors. The occurrence of nonadaptive behaviors such as distractibility and impulsiveness was asssociated in dose-related fashion to dentine lead content. Of note, prior lead levels were determined from medical record review for some of the study participants and averaged 23.8 μg/dL for 23 of 50 in the low-lead cohort and 35.5 μg/dL for 58 of 100 in the high-lead cohort. Both the strength and dose–response effect of these associations was impressive, particularly since the study population was a large random sample of ostensibly normal school children. Despite these strengths, criticisms of the Boston study have been noted.[80] These include lack of concordance on multiple dentine lead analyses, high subject exclusion rate, focus on one measure of cognitive performance, the IQ test, rather than including tests of academic achievement, and failure to correct for confounders in the analysis of classroom behavior by teachers. However, a number of similar cross-sectional studies using a variety of controls for potential confounders and either blood lead or tooth lead as markers of body burden have found similar associations.[41,98,208,262]

The Boston researchers provided an 11-year follow-up on these schoolchildren.[171] Persistent high lead effects included failure to graduate high school, frequency of learning disability, and lower class rank. Recently, socially maladaptive behaviors, in addition to IQ per se, were also studied in schoolchildren. Body lead burden, measured by K x-ray fluorescence spectroscopy of tibia, correlated with antisocial or delinquent behaviors.[69]

Additional studies have attempted to extend the potential lower threshold for both lead body burden and critical age by using a longitudinal design and enrolling children at birth, or even prenatally. Bellinger et al[18] reported on 249 Boston children from birth to 2 years of age, and found a 4.8 point IQ deficit between high- and low-lead-exposure groups. However, they subsequently reported that by age 5 years, the association between prenatal lead exposure and cognitive index diminished greatly, except in children with higher concurrent lead exposure.[19] The persistence of cognitive deficit was related primarily to higher postnatal lead exposure and less favorable markers of socioeconomic status. Similar studies and results were found in Cincinnati and Cleveland in the United States, and Sydney and Port Pirie in Australia (the latter is a smelter town with rural surroundings).[12,98,194] An effort to rigorously evaluate all three types of recent (since 1979), carefully done studies of the low-lead and intelligence association (cross-sectional studies with blood or tooth lead, and prospective studies) and combine their results with a statistical meta-analysis technique has been recently reported.[194] The overall finding was that, while the majority of individual studies failed to acheive statistical significance, taken together, there was a significant inverse association between lead exposure and IQ, on the order of 1–2 IQ points for a doubling of body lead burden (blood lead increase from 10 to 20 μg/dL or tooth lead from 5 to 10 μg/g). A schematic overview of several representative lead–intelligence relationship studies is presented in Fig. 79–7.

It should be noted that several issues relating to the ability of observational epidemiologic studies to infer causality need to be considered in interpreting these findings. On the one hand, they share several features of classic epidemiologic criteria for such inference: temporal relationship, strong statistical association, dose–response gradient, control for confounding variables, relatively consistent findings across studies, and biologic plausibility (including support from animal studies). On the other hand, it is difficult to control for all confounders, especially those that relate to individual parent–child and other mini-environmental factors. In this regard, the possibility of reverse causality should also be considered. It is possible that children with lower IQ manifest behaviors that would enhance lead absorption. This has been evaluated statistically, using data derived from many of the aforementioned studies, and reveals that every 10-point decrement in IQ is associated with a 1.5–3.0% increase in blood lead, a relatively small but obviously important effect, were it to occur.[194] While many questions remain for future research, the cumulative weight of these studies certainly adds to the conviction that occult lead poisoning is a potential cause of cognitive deficit. These results are those of populations, not individuals, and the magnitude of change may seem small for the majority of exposed children. However, it has been observed that mean population changes on the order of 4 IQ points result in a 5% decrease in the number of children who score in the superior range (IQ > 125), and a fourfold increase in those with a severe deficit (IQ < 80)[98,167] This would obviously represent an enormous societal loss.

Additional subtle clinical findings in asymptomatic children with elevated lead burdens have been alluded to in the discussion of pathophysiologic effects. These findings do not usually present as recognized concerns in individual patients, but to review, have included measurable deficits in growth,[219] hearing,[220] and fine motor coordination.[70]

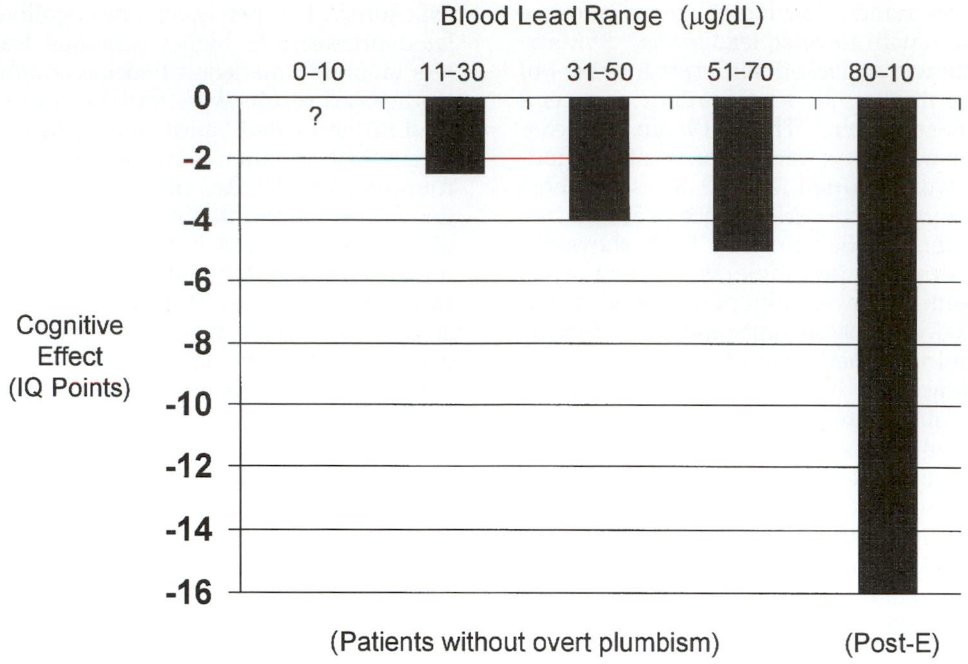

Figure 79–7. The relationship between blood lead and neurocognitive impairment. IQ = full-scale intelligence quotient scores; Post-E = postencephalopathic children. *(Adapted from reference 98. Composite data from references 66, 67, 168, 194, 208, 262.)*

Adults. Adults with occupational lead exposure may manifest numerous signs and symptoms representing disorders of several organ systems. True acute poisoning is seen rarely after very high respiratory exposures,[126] large ingestions,[174] or intravenous exposures.[1,175] Such patients may present with colic, hepatitis, pancreatitis, hemolytic anemia, and encephalopathy in days or weeks. Most adult plumbism is related to chronic respiratory exposure, though some authors have used the term *acute poisoning* to include patients with such exposure whose symptoms are severe and of relatively recent onset (within 6 weeks of presentation) and whose exposure is relatively brief (average 1 year or less).[62]

Acute encephalopathy has rarely been reported in adults since the 1920s.[62] The majority of modern cases are not associated with occupational exposures, but rather with ingestion of illicit "moonshine" whiskey. Of fatal adult cases in the United States between 1979 and 1988, moonshine was the lead source in 22 of 25 patients for which the lead source was identified.[237] Encephalopathy in adults is manifested by seizures (75% of cases), obtundation, confusion, focal motor disturbances, papilledema, headaches, and optic neuritis.[258] Encephalopathy is characterized by diffuse pathologic changes and cerebral edema and is usually associated with very high blood levels (typically > 150 μg/dL).

Other manifestations of symptomatic lead poisoning in adults involve CNS, peripheral nerve, hematologic, renal, gastrointestinal, rheumatologic, and endocrine/reproductive findings.[126,206,214] Subencephalopathic CNS findings include changes in mood and cognition. Subtle neurocognitive abnormalities demonstrable by neuropsychiatric testing are being found in adults as well as children with modest elevations in blood lead. Such studies have documented abnormal psychometrics and nerve conduction in workers recently exposed to lead as blood levels rose to above 30 μg/dL.[143] Early symptoms, at blood levels 40–80 μg/dL, include increased tiredness at the end of the day, disinterest in leisure-time pursuits, falling asleep easily, moodiness, and irritability. As for children, these early symptoms may be so subtle as to be recognized only in hindsight after the patient has been away from the exposure. Subclinical effects on reproductive function and blood pressure may be apparent in this range of exposure, as detailed in the section on pathophysiologic effects. As exposure increases (blood lead >80 μg/dL, or air levels of 0.3 to 0.5 mg/m^3), new symptoms develop, including headache, memory loss, decreased libido, and insomnia. Gastrointestinal effects may appear, including metallic taste in the mouth, abdominal pain, decreased appetite, weight loss, and constipation. Musculoskeletal and rheumatologic complaints at this stage include muscle pain, muscle weakness (especially upper extremity, dominant side), joint tenderness, numbness of the legs, occasional paresthesias, tremor, and hyperreflexia. Many patients at this stage will have mild anemia. Patients with prolonged exposure at this level are at risk for chronic nephropathy. As exposure increases further (blood levels > 100 μg/dL), attacks of colic may appear, anemia is virtually always present, and the patient is at significant risk for peripheral nerve palsy or encephalopathy.

Physical examination findings will vary with degree

of severity. Mild and moderate symptoms ususally occur in patients with normal examination findings.[68] In encephalopathic patients, typical changes of stupor, coma, posturing, and papilledema are noted. Milder abnormal neurologic findings include dominant wrist or hand weakness, paresthesia, or tremor. Grayish stippling of the retina circumferential to the optic disk has been described by one author,[236] but disputed by others.[183] A bluish-purple gingival lead line (Burton's line) is described rarely in adult patients with poor oral hygiene, representing lead sulfide precipitation. Abdominal guarding and tenderness are occasionally observed. Patients with gout may have typical joint findings of acute arthritis. Severely anemic patients may exhibit pallor. Careful neuropsychologic testing may reveal abnormalities of memory span, rapid motor tapping, visual motor coordination, and grip strength.[62] Table 79–6 summarizes the spectrum of symptoms and signs associated with adult lead poisoning.[206]

Organic Lead

Clinical symptoms of TEL toxicity are usually nonspecific initially, including insomnia and emotional instability.[27,214] Nausea, vomiting, and anorexia may occur. The patient may exhibit tremor and increased deep tendon reflexes. In more severe cases, these symptoms progress to an encephalopathy with delusions, hallucinations, and hyperactivity, which may resolve or deteriorate to coma and, occasionally, death. Severe cases may also develop hepatic and renal injury. Of note, patients with TEL toxicity do not become anemic or develop biomarkers of heme pathway dysfunction, and blood lead levels are not markedly elevated in many affected patients.

How Are Patients at Risk for Lead Poisoning Assessed?

Clinical Diagnosis in Symptomatic Patients

The physician must consider the diagnosis of lead poisoning in order to recognize the uncommon symptomatic patient. For all patients in whom plumbism is considered, based on clinical manifestations, the medical evaluation should first include a comprehensive history into occupational and recreational history of all home occupants; family use of ethnic folk medicines; use of imported, glazed ceramics; age and condition of residence and/or any recent renovation activity; source and use of drinking water; and proximity of residence to lead-using industry. Children may be at further risk if they are 1–5 years in age and have persistent vomiting, lethargy, irritability, clumsiness or loss of recently acquired developmental skills; afebrile seizures; a strong history of pica, including acute accidental ingestions,[113] or aural, nasal, or esophageal foreign body;[261] residence in a pre–1960s home, especially with deteriorated paint, or that has undergone recent remodeling; a family history of lead poisoning; iron deficiency anemia; and evidence of child abuse or neglect.[84,223]

The differential diagnosis of plumbism is broad. Adult patients may be misdiagnosed as having carpal tunnel syndrome, Guillain-Barré syndrome, sickle cell crisis, acute appendicitis, renal colic, and infectious encephalitis. Children are often initially considered to have viral gastroenteritis, or even to have insidious symptoms passed off as a difficult developmental phase.

The patient who presents to the ED with acute encephalopathy that may represent lead poisoning presents the physician with a dilemma: severe lead intoxication requires urgent diagnosis, but confirmatory blood lead assays are usually not available on an immediate basis.[117] For adults, a history of occupational exposure is often available from past medical records or family members, and lead encephalopathy can be strongly considered with positive supportive laboratory findings (usually available on urgent basis) such as anemia, basophilic stippling, elevated erythrocyte protoporphyrin (especially > 250 μg/dL), and abnormal urinalysis. In this context, it would probably be appropriate to institute presumptive chelation therapy while awaiting lead levels. In children, a similar indication for presumptive treatment would be suggested by a constellation of clinical features and ancillary studies: age 1–5 years; a prodromal illness of several days' to weeks' duration (suggestive of milder lead-related symptoms); occurrence in summer; history of pica and source of lead exposure; the laboratory features noted above, which are equally helpful in young children; and radiologic findings of dense metaphyseal "lead lines" at wrists or knees (Fig. 79–2), and/or evidence of recent pica for lead paint particles on abdominal radiographs (Fig. 79–8). In both adults and children, the decision to institute empiric chelation treatment should not deter additional emergent diagnostic efforts to exclude or confirm other important entities while blood lead levels are pending. An important consideration in this context may be the suspicion of an acute, potentially treatable CNS infection (eg, bacterial meningitis or herpetic encephalitis). Lumbar puncture may be dangerous in patients with lead encephalopathy due to the risk of cerebral herniation. If immediate lumbar puncture is felt to be highly desirable, a computed tomography scan would allow determination of severe cerebral edema, midline shift, or other evidence of especially high risk for herniation. If performed, the minimal amount of fluid necessary for diagnosis (< 1 mL) should be removed through a small gauge needle. Alternatively, empiric treatment for infectious processes can be initiated while the lead level is pending, and delayed lumbar puncture can be performed if blood lead level is normal.

Laboratory Considerations

Laboratory testing is used to augment the evaluation of both lead exposure and lead toxicity. Traditionally, the direct measurement of lead in blood was costly and posed technical obstacles, and a reliance developed on utilization of biomarkers derived from lead-induced abnormalities of the heme synthesis pathway and of enhanced urine lead excretion after chelating agent admin-

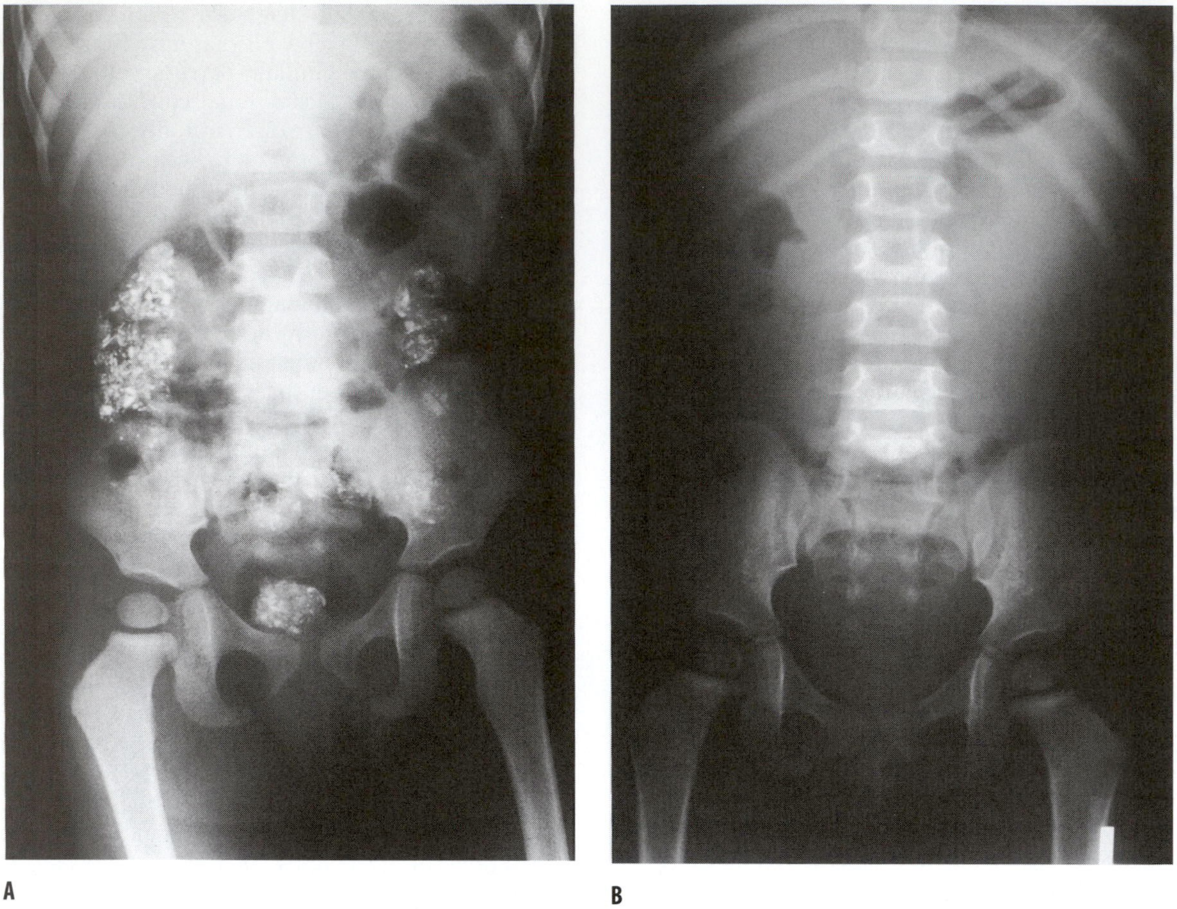

Figure 79–8. A. Abdominal radiograph of a child who had massive paint chip ingestion. **B.** Follow-up radiograph after whole-bowel irrigation. *(Courtesy of Department of Radiology, St. Christopher's Hospital for Children, Philadelphia, PA.)*

istration. These indirect assays have waned in utility as levels of concern for lead exposure have decreased concomitantly with technical advances in direct blood lead measurement.[104] Several of the indirect biomarkers are here reviewed briefly; for a more in-depth discussion the interested reader is referred to several comprehensive reviews.[104,187]

Routine Laboratory Tests. As detailed in the sections on hematologic and renal pathophysiolgic effects, lead may cause several changes in routine complete blood count, urinalysis, or renal function tests. These are usually observed only in moderate to severe degrees of exposure. The patient may manifest normochromic or hypochromic microcytic anemia and red blood cell stippling. The urinalysis may be positive for protein and glucose. Renal function tests may reveal elevated blood urea nitrogen and creatinine in patients with chronic lead nephropathy.

Radiographic evaluation may be helpful occasionally. The growing long bones, particularly at wrists and knees, in children about 9 months to 5 years of age may reveal characteristic "lead lines" of increased calcification in the zone of provisional calcification (see Fig 79–2). These dense metaphyseal bands take 4–8 weeks of heavy exposure to develop. They are more likely to be significant if the smaller ulna and fibula are involved as well as the larger radius and tibia.[25] Lead lines may also be present in flat bones such as ribs, clavicles, and the iliac crest.[264] Abdominal radiographs may reveal radiopacities representing lead paint chips or particles and rarely lead-containing folk medicines or foreign bodies (see Figs. 79–4 and 79–8).[30] These findings are usually present for 24–36 hours postingestion.[187] A recent survey found that 26% of children with lead levels > 55 μg/dL had abdominal radiopacities.[156]

Biomarkers of Lead Exposure and Toxicity. The effect of lead on the heme synthesis pathway (see Fig. 79–5) and the ease of sampling blood and urine has led to several tests based on enzyme inhibition or accumulation of substrates. The erythrocyte delta-aminolevulinic acid dehydratase activity is a sensitive marker of lead exposure and shows 50% inhibition at lead levels of only 15 μg/dL. However, the enzyme must be assayed within 24 hours of blood sampling and is so sensitive it cannot distinguish between moderate and severe exposure.[104,172] The measurement of accumulated delta-aminolevulinic acid (ALA) in urine may serve as a useful tool for tracking lead exposure in occupational settings, but today is considered relatively insensitive since it does not rise appreciably until blood lead is > 40 μg/dL. The relatively low-cost test of urine ALA continues its value in areas of the world with extensive lead contamination but limited financial resources.[104,221]

Erythrocytes accumulate protoporphyrin in the presence of iron deficiency or inhibition of heme synthetase by lead. The red cell has an average life span of 120 days, so that erythrocyte protoporphyrin (EP) levels reach a steady state over 3 months and reflect relatively long-term lead exposure.[187] Piomelli et al developed a simple fluorometric technique for assaying red cell EP in the early 1970s,[189] and for two decades this test became the method of choice for lead surveillance. It could utilize a finger-stick drop of blood, was not influenced by surface lead-dust contamination, and also screened for iron deficiency, another prevalent conditon of young children. Of note, the terms EP, free erthrocyte protoporphyrin (FEP), and zinc protoporphyrin (ZPP) have often been used interchangeably in the past. This reflects a confusion based on older extraction techniques of measuring red cell protoporhyrins.[187] In lead-poisoned or iron-deficient red cells, most of the increased EP is bound to zinc. Most current tests measure total red cell EP and obviate the need for extraction and for distinguishing FEP from ZPP. The EP first increases at lead levels of about 17 μg/dL, and thus is also insensitive to lead levels in the 10–25 μg/dL range.[104] As such, it is no longer recommended as a surveillance test for childhood lead poisoning. The EP may still be useful for tracking response to therapy and distinguishing acute from chronic lead exposure and as an adjunct to the emergency diagnosis of symptomatic plumbism.

Chelatable Lead. The baseline excretion of lead in urine is not generally considered a sensitive biomarker of lead exposure. However, lead excretion after a single dose of the chelator $CaNa_2EDTA$ is correlated with blood lead and several heme pathway markers.[48,104] A lead "challenge," "mobilization," or "provocative" test was developed to evaluate the size of the mobilizable pool of body lead burden, with the hope of pinpointing which asymptomatic patients with modestly elevated blood lead levels would most benefit from a full course of chelation therapy.[209] Standardized doses of $CaNa_2EDTA$ were administered and 24-hour[209] or 8-hour[151] urine collections tested for lead excretion, with various formulas proposed for a "positive" test. Several assumptions about the validity of this test are not obvious.[104] It is not clear if positive responders will continue to excrete more lead than poor responders. Conversely, it is not clear that negative tests would imply lack of any value for subsequent chelation. One large series of lead mobilization tests found that the test was positive in only 28% of children with blood lead levels of 40–49 μg/dL, and 66% of children with lead levels of 50–69 μg/dL.[256] Most authorities would currently recommend chelation for all patients in the latter group, and many of those in the former.[41] It is also possible that single doses of $CaNa_2EDTA$ may translocate lead from less vulnerable sites, such as bone, to more vulnerable, such as the brain; this has in fact been demonstrated in rats.[48,61] Finally, the test is cumbersome, difficult technically in children who are not toilet trained, and requires parenteral drug administration, and thus is not risk free. This test is no longer recommended by the American Academy of Pediatrics[4] and seems to be falling out of favor in occupational medicine practice as well.[68,104,214]

Blood Lead. For many years the use of blood lead as a biomarker for lead exposure was avoided by researchers and clinicians.[104] As noted earlier, blood lead has complex kinetics, reflecting the redistribution of lead from other compartments, primarily bone, to blood. Blood sampling required relatively large volumes (5–7 mL) and was costly and technically difficult. However, recently several factors have favored the use of whole blood as the primary biomarker for both research and clinical practice. The evolution of atomic absorption spectrophotometry (AAS) has allowed reliable, sensitive determinations of blood lead as low as 1 μg/dL. The equipment is widely available and some techniques (eg, graphite furnace AAS) require only 0.25 mL blood; newer modifications also allow application to capillary blood samples.[214] All the alternative biomarkers discussed above have some inherent limitations, particularly lack of sensitivity at the lower body lead burdens curently of concern. Lastly, virtually all of the recent research associating low-level lead exposure with adverse clinical outcomes, especially neurocognitive deficits in children or renal function in adults, have utilized blood lead as the primary biomarker.[104]

Whole venous blood for lead testing may be collected, after careful skin preparation, through standard stainless steel needles into special lead-free (tan top) or trace element-free (dark blue top) evacuated tubes (eg, Vacutainers from Becton Dickinson Co). If these are not readily available, standard heparinized tubes (green top) may be used, but elevated values should probably be verified.[214] The blood should be mixed thoroughly as soon as possible to ensure anticoagulation.

Pediatric blood lead testing has often been hampered by the requirement for venipuncture and relatively large blood volumes. An alternative is the use of capillary sampling by fingerstick puncture. This technique is safe and quick and can be applied to mass screening settings. Its principal drawback is the potential for contamination by lead-soiled fingertips, and thus an excessive rate of false positive testing. A recent study found that, at least in a controlled research protocol, capillary test results were highly correlated with matched venous samples, with mean capillary-venous differences of less than 1 μg/dL.[217] It is imperative that fingers be swabbed thoroughly with alcohol prior to puncture. Venous confirmation of elevated capillary lead levels is still considered mandatory prior to chelation or other significant interventions. The capillary test is considered too inaccurate in the context of adult occupational exposure to be of any value.[214]

Other Lead Assays

Lead can also be quantified in urine, teeth, and hair.[187] Urine assays are considered insensitive, and hair is unreliable due to surface contamination.[187] Shed primary teeth have been used in research studies as biomarkers of cumulative childhood lead exposure,[168] but obviously would be impractical in clinical patient management.

Research Methodologies. X-ray fluorescence (XRF) technology estimates tooth[26] and bone[118] lead, and thus indirectly is a cumulative measure of body lead exposure in epidemiologic studies. Protocols have not yet acheived the standardization that would be required for a clinically useful test. The tests are relatively costly and require the patient to remain still for up to 30 minutes, involve low-dose radiation exposure, and are not widely available.[104] The XRF technique may have promise in research studies of issues concerning past chronic heavy lead exposure and a variety of current health outcomes.[255]

How Should Persons Be Screened for Lead Exposure?

Children

As evidence accumulated in the 1970s and 1980s that low-level lead exposure was a significant pediatric public health issue, it simultaneously became apparent that the only way to detect elevated lead burdens early in childhood would be to screen widely.[42] In October of 1991, the CDC recommended that every child in the United States be screened at age 1 year , and preferably, at age 2 years as well, by whole blood lead determination. A blood lead of > 10 μg/dL was defined as the intervention level.[41] However, over the next few years, numerous studies appeared that found a very low prevalence of elevated lead levels in selected communities.[23,173,240] Several of these found that a few simple questions regarding housing age and condition were predictive for the few children who did have elevated lead levels.[23,114,173] Concern grew that overemphasis and misappropriation of resources on universal screening would further compromise higher priority efforts for targeted screening of the most at-risk populations.[114,218] A national survey in 1994 found that only 29% of children living in homes built prior to 1960, and only 30% of children in families earning less than $20,000 per year, had been screened.[22] At the same time, remarkable cases of extremely elevated blood lead levels (> 100 μg/dL) detected on routine screening continue to be reported, especially in minority, inner-city children.[65] In response to these developments, the CDC proposed new recommendations in 1997,[35] outlined in Table 79–7. This approach emphasizes targeted screening and follow-up.

TABLE 79–7. PEDIATRIC SCREENING AND FOLLOW-UP GUIDELINES

Screening

Screen

1. All high-risk children at 1 and 2 y (3–6 y if not previously screened)
2. Selected low-risk children (any affirmative answer to risk questions)
   (high risk community = 12% of young children with elevated BPb, 27% of homes built before 1950)

Personal Risk Questionaire

1. Does your child live in or regularly visit a home built before 1950?
2. Does your child live in or regularly visit a home built before 1978 undergoing remodeling or renovation (or has been within 6 mo) ?
3. Specific exposure questions:
   Personal, family history of lead poisoning
   Occupational, industrial, hobby exposures
   Proximity to major roadway
   Hot tap water for consumption
   Cultural exposures (folk remedies, cosmetics, ceramic food containers, trips, residence outside US)
   Migrant farm workers, receipt of poverty assistance
   History of pica for paint chips, dirt
   History of iron deficiency

Follow-Up

BPb (μg/dL)	*Recommended Action*
< 9	Retest in 1 y
10–14	Retest in 3 mo; education
15–19	Retest in 2 mo; education; if 15–19 twice, refer for case management
20–44	Clinical evaluation; education; environmental investigation
45–69	Clinical evaluation and case management within 48 h; education; environmental investigation; chelation therapy
≥ 70	Hospitalize child; immediate chelation therapy; education; environmental investigation

BPb = venous blood lead
Educational interventions as per Table 79–9.
Chelation therapy as per Tables 79–10, 79–11
Reprinted, with permission, from Centers for Disease Control and Prevention: Screening young children for lead poisoning: Guidance for state and local public health officials. US Dept of Health and Human Services, Public Health Service, Federal Register, Feb 21, 1997.

Adults

The Occupational Safety and Health Administration (OSHA) developed a lead standard for U.S. workers in 1978, formulated to reduce workplace exposure to lead, decrease symptomatic lead poisoning, and provide quality medical care to workers with elevated blood lead levels.[249] This regulation requires employers to ensure workplace standards for environmental control and employee education, to regularly monitor environmental contamination and employee lead status, and to provide free medical surveillance and necessary treatment, while continuing the salary of any worker removed from the worksite because of lead exposure. The OSHA permissible exposure level for lead in worksite air is 50 μg/m^3 averaged over an 8-hour day. Employees at risk for the action level of 30 μg/m^3 for > 30 days per year must be screened periodically, as outlined in Table 79–8.[248] It is illegal to provide medicinal dietary interventions or prophylactic chelation prior to routine screening. It should be noted that the law's intent is not simply to remove lead-poisoned workers from the worksite, only to replace them with newer employees whose lead burdens are less extensive, but rather to recognize an opportunity to improve workplace hygiene.[214] Where the lead standard has been invoked, such as the lead smelting and battery manufacturing industries, clinical lead poisoning and av-

TABLE 79–8. OSHA ADULT LEAD STANDARD SCREENING AND FOLLOW-UP SUMMARY

BPb (μg/dL)	Recommended Action
> 60 on a single test; or average > 50 of last 3 samples, or all samples over prior 6 mo (requires confirmation within 2 wk)	Immediate removal from worksite; BPb every month
> 40–60	Repeat BPb in 2 mo
< 40	Repeat BPb in 6 mo; BPb at which a worker who has been medically removed from the worksite may return (requires confirmation BPb within 2 wk)

BPb = blood lead (μg/dL)

Compiled, with permission, from references 68 and 249.

erage blood lead levels have decreased impressively.[248] In 1993, the lead standard was extended to the construction industry,[247] but is not yet applied to agricultural workers.

How Is Lead Poisoning Treated?

There are several caveats about the treatment of lead poisoning. First, the most important aspect of treatment, for all degrees of toxicity, in patients of all ages, is removal from exposure to lead. Unfortunately, effective implementation of this therapy is often beyond the control of the clinician, but rather depends on a complex interplay of public health, social, and political actions. Currently, the ability to control exposure is generally more applicable to adults with occupational exposures than to children exposed to residential hazards. Second, in children for whom some residual lead exposure continues, optimization of nutritional status is vital in order to minimize absorption. Finally, pharmacologic therapy with chelation agents, while a mainstay of therapy for symptomatic patients, is an inexact science, with numerous unanswered questions despite almost 50 years of clinical use.[4,7,131] The rationale for chelation therapy of lead-poisoned patients is that chelation drugs are known to complex with lead, forming a chelate that is excreted in urine, feces, or both. Chelation therapy does increase lead excretion, reduce blood levels, and reverse hematologic markers of toxcity during therapy. Reports from the 1950s found symptomatic improvement of adults chelated for lead colic.[252] The institution of effective combination chelation treatment of childhood lead encephalopathy in the 1960s certainly contributed to the dramatic decline in mortality and morbidity of that devastating degree of plumbism.[49] However, the same era saw major advances in pediatric critical care in general, and medical management of increased intracranial pressure in particular.[131] The situation of chelation therapy for asymptomatic patients with mildly to moderately increased body burdens of lead is even less clear. Questions asked today include: (1) Do chelating drugs materially decrease body burdens of lead in the context of chronic exposure, or merely enhance excretion briefly, only to be offset by slowed "natural" excretion subsequently?[150] (2) To what degree does increased excretion of a toxic metal reverse established toxicity?[102,131] (3) Does the process of chelation result in dangerous redistribution of metal from less vulnerable (eg, bone) to more vulnerable target organs (eg, brain)?[48,131] Long-term reduction of target tissue lead content or reversal of toxicity has not been demonstrated in human trials.[150,164] For example, two recent studies examined the impact of $CaNa_2EDTA$ therapy on neurotoxic effects of low to moderate lead exposure. A study in rats failed to find improvement in a lever-pressing-for-food model,[60] and a study in children found modest improvement in cognitive index after treatment, but failed to demonstrate any additional benefit of $CaNa_2EDTA$ per se over dietary supplementation and home abatement.[207]

Decreasing Exposure

All patients with significantly elevated lead levels warrant specific environmental interventions. In adults, this usually involves changes in their worksite, as noted in the discussion above on screening.[68,214] Remedial actions might include improvements in ventilation, modification of personal hygiene habits, and optimal use of respiratory apparatus. It is vital to prohibit smoking, eating, and drinking in a lead-exposed work area. Workclothes should be changed after each shift and should not be lockered together with street clothes.

Several specific educational guidelines may be offered to parents of lead-exposed children and are summarized in Table 79–9.[5,41,51] While home lead-paint abatement, or relocation, is mandatory, renovations must be done by trained and experienced workers, with the family out of the home, and with appropriate clean-up instituted prior to the family's return. In many communities, assistance with home inspection and abatement is available through public health agencies.[76,244] In addition, simple, inexpensive home dust-reduction techniques correlate with decreased blood lead levels.[44,127] Simple efforts to decrease soil lead exposure may also help, such as planting grass or large shrubs in affected areas (usually close to the house).[41] Formal soil removal and replacement has been studied and found to be very costly (average $9600 per home) and minimally effective (average decline in blood lead of 1 μg/dL).[257] Nutritional evaluation and counseling to optimize diet will minimize lead absorption. All lead-exposed children should be tested for concommitant iron deficiency and treated with pharmacologic iron preparations as necessary. Even in the absence of overt iron deficiency, or after successful treatment, a diet rich in iron, calcium, and frequent nutritious snacks is optimal[212](Table 79–9).

Chelation Therapy

The indications for and specifics of chelation therapy are determined by patient age, blood lead level, and clinical

TABLE 79–9. REDUCING LEAD EXPOSURE

Adults
Implement OSHA lead standard
Improve ventilation
Utilize respiratory apparatus
Wear protective clothing, change from workclothes before leaving worksite
Modify personal hygiene habits
Prohibit eating, drinking, smoking in worksite

Children
Notify local health department
Home lead paint abatement (professional contractors if possible, utilize plastic sheeting, low dust-generating paint removal, replacement of lead-painted windows, floor treatment, final clean-up with high-efficiency particle air vacuum, wet-mopping)
Avoid most hazardous areas of home, yard
Dust control: wet-mopping, sponging with high-phosphate detergent; frequent hand, toy, pacifier washing
Soil lead exposure reduction by planting grass, shrubs around house
Use only cold, flushed tap water for consumption
Optimize nutrition: avoid fasting; iron, calcium sufficient diet; iron and/or calcium supplementation as necessary
Avoid food storage in open cans
Avoid imported ceramic containers for food, beverage use
Evaluate parental occupations, hobbies

symptomatology (Table 79–10). Three chelation agents are currently recommended as drugs of choice for the treatment of lead poisoning: BAL and $CaNa_2EDTA$ are used parenterally for more severe cases, and succimer (dimercaptosuccinic acid) is available for oral therapy.[64] Pharmacologic profiles of these three agents are detailed in Antidotes in Depth: Succimer and Antidotes in Depth: Calcium Disodium Edetate. Capsule summaries in relation to therapeutic adverse effects and monitoring issues are presented in Table 78–3.

A fourth drug, D-penicillamine, has been used orally for patients with mild to moderate excess lead burdens, and its use will be described here briefly. Since 1991, the role of D-penicillamine in lead poisoning treatment has been largely replaced by succimer. Chelation using D-penicillamine shares the advantage of oral administration with succimer. Typical dosing regimens begin with one dose of 10 mg/kg/day, increased as tolerated in a week to 20 mg/kg/day (in 2 doses), and then a week or more later to 30 mg/kg/day (in 2 or 3 doses).[135] Unfortunately, D-penicillamine has a toxicity profile that includes serious, life-threatening hematologic disorders and reversible but serious dermatologic and renal effects, though these are reported primarily in adults on high-dose treatment. In children, adverse effects may occur in up to 33% of patients, but are milder, with gastrointestinal upset, reversible leukopenia or thrombocytopenia, rash, and proteinuria/hematuria dominating.[135,230] Nevertheless, courses of therapy have averaged 10 weeks in duration, and it seems unlikely that patients unable to successfully complete succimer therapy will do better with D-penicillamine. It has been our practice to utilize inpatient $CaNa_2EDTA$ chelation with the rare child who fails succimer treatment; the American Academy of Pediatrics recommends D-penicillamine use only when unacceptable adverse reactions to both succimer and $CaNa_2EDT$ occur, and yet it remains important to continue chelation.[4]

As noted above, chelation is not a panacea for lead poisoning. It is a relatively inefficient process, with a typical course of therapy decreasing body content of heavy metal by 1–2%.[131,164] Further, there is little evidence that chelating agents have significant access to critical sites in target organs, particularly in the brain. Assumptions that reducing blood lead level will improve subtle neurocognitive dysfunction or other subclinical organ toxicity are appealing theoretically, but unproven.

Pediatric Therapy. Lead encephalopathy is an acute life-threatening emergency and should be treated under the guidance of a multidisciplinary team in the intensive care unit of a hospital experienced in the management of critically ill children. Encephalopathy requires treatment by combination parenteral chelation therapy with maximum dose BAL and $CaNa_2EDTA$ and meticulous supportive care.[4,41,49]

Chelation is instituted with intramuscular (IM) BAL 75 mg/m^2/day (or 25 mg/kg/day) in six divided doses.[4,41] The second dose of BAL is given 4 hours later, followed immediately by intravenous (IV) $CaNa_2EDTA$, in maximun concentration of 0.5% solution, at 1500 mg/m^2/day (or 50 mg/kg/day)[4] as a continuous infusion over several hours or in divided-dose infusions.[4,41,191] The delay in initiating $CaNa_2EDTA$ infusion is based on past observations of clinical deterioration in encephalopathic patients treated with this agent alone.[4,49] Therapy is typically continued with both agents for 5 days, although in milder cases with prompt resolution of encephalopathy and decrease of blood lead to < 50 μg/dL, BAL may be discontinued after 3 days, with continuation of $CaNa_2EDTA$ alone for 2 more days. The presence of radiopaque material in the gastrointestinal tract on radiography has raised concern that parenteral chelation might enhance absorption of residual gut lead. This issue has not been settled fully,[48,122] but most authors advocate initiation of chelation without delay in seriously symptomatic patients. It would seem reasonable to simultaneously attempt bowel decontamination,[4] as with a whole-bowel irrigation solution (see Fig. 79–8).

Oral fluids, feedings, and medications are witheld for at least the first several days. Careful provision of adequate intravenous fluids will optimize renal function while avoiding overhydration and the risk of exacerbating cerebral edema. Appropriate fluid therapy is approximated by maintenance fluid requirements (1 cc/kcal/day; kcal = 100/kg for first 10 kg, plus 50/kg for next 10 kg, plus 20/kg thereafter) and replacement of ongoing losses. Such a regimen should result in the desired urine output of 0.5 mL/kcal/day (or 350–500 mL/m^2/day).[49,117] The occurrence of inappropriate secretion

TABLE 79–10. CHELATION THERAPY GUIDELINES[a]

Condition, BPb(μg/dL)	Dose	Regimen/Comments
Adults		
Encephalopathy	BAL 450 mg/m²/d +	75 mg/m² IM every 4 h for 5 d
	$CaNa_2EDTA$ 1500 mg/m²/d[a]	Continuous infusion, or 2–4 divided IV doses, for 5 d (start 4 h after BAL)
Symptomatic, BPb > 100	BAL 300–450 mg/m²/d+	50–75 mg/m² every 4 h for 3–5 d
	$CaNa_2EDTA$ 1000–1500 mg/m²/d[a]	Continuous infusion, or 2–4 divided IV doses, for 5 d (start 4 h after BAL)
		Base dose, duration on BPb, severity of symptoms (see text)
Mild symptoms, or BPb 70-100	Succimer 700-1050 mg/m²/d	350 mg/m² tid for 5 d, then bid for 14 d
Asymptomatic, BPb < 70	Usually not indicated	Remove from exposure
Children		
Encephalopathy	BAL 450 mg/m²/d +	75 mg/m² IM every 4 h for 5 d
	$CaNa_2EDTA$ 1500 mg/m²/d[a]	Continuous infusion, or 2–4 divided IV doses, for 5 d (start 4 h after BAL)
Symptomatic, BPb > 70	BAL 300–450 mg/m²/d +	50–75 mg/m² every 4 h for 3–5 d
	$CaNa_2EDTA$ 1000–1500 mg/m²/d[a]	Continuous infusion, or 2–4 divided IV doses, for 5 d (start 4 h after BAL)
		Base dose, duration on BPb, severity of symptoms (see text)
Asymptomatic, BPb 45–69	Succimer 700–1050 mg/m²/d or $CaNa_2EDTA$, 1000 mg/m²/d[a] (or, rarely, D-penicillamine)	350 mg/m² tid for 5 d, then bid for 14 d Continuous infusion, or 2–4 divided IV, for 5 d (see text)
BPb 20–44	Routine chelation not indicated. Consider succimer for: BPb 35–44, younger child (< 2 years), elevated EP and rising BPb despite exposure reduction measures, hint of mild symptoms	Await current studies (eg, NIEHS TLC) If succimer used, same regimen as per above group
BPb < 20	Chelation not indicated. Attempt exposure reduction	See Table 79–9

[a]Doses expressed in mg/ kg: BAL 450 mg/m² (24 mg /kg); 300 mg/m² (18 mg/kg). $CaNa_2EDTA$ 1000 mg/m² (25–50 mg/kg); 1500 mg/m² (50–75 mg/kg) (adult maximum 2–3 g/day). Succimer 350 mg/m² (10 mg/kg).

Subsequent treatment regimens based on postchelation BPb and clinical symptoms (see text). BPb = blood lead (μg/dL); EP = erythrocyte protoporphyrin; IM = intramuscular; IV = intravenous; NIEHS TLC = National Institute of Environmental Health Sciences supported multicenter study: Treatment of lead-exposed children

Compiled, with permission, from references 4, 41, 126, 164, 191, 195.

of antidiuretic hormone has been suspected in lead encephalopathy,[49] so that urine volume, specific gravity, and serum electrolytes should be closely monitored, especially as fluids are gradually liberalized with clinical improvement.

Seizure control is usually accomplished with benzodiazepines (pediatric dosing: diazepam 0.1–0.3 mg/kg, or lorazepam 0.05–0.1 mg/kg); ongoing anticonvulsant therapy is typically continued with phenytoin, loading dose 15–20 mg/kg, then 5–10 mg/kg/day; or phenobarbital, loading dose 10–15 mg/kg, then 3–6 mg/kg/day). Rarely, continuous infusions of midazolam or high-dose pentobarbital therapy may be necessary.[260]

Recent advances in management of cerebral edema and increased intracranial pressure have not been critically evaluated in the currently rare context of lead encephalopathy. Lumbar puncture should be avoided if lead encephalopathy is highly suspected, and acute infectious processes are not. It seems reasonable that noninvasive measures such as modest hyperventilation, low-dose mannitol or glycerol hyperosmotic therapy, and steroids might have a salutory effect at minimal risk of increased iatrogenic morbidity.[4,49,53,260] Whether more aggressive measures such as intracranial pressure monitoring, induced hypothermia, or pentobarbital coma would decrease mortality or morbidity further is unknown.

Patients with milder symptoms, and/or lead levels > 70 μg/dL, should be chelated with a regimen similar to that recommeded for encephalopathy. It is likely that this group of patients will require only 3 days of BAL, in addition to 5 days $CaNa_2EDTA$. Intensive care monitoring may be prudent for this group of patients as well, at least during the initiation of chelation therapy.[164,191]

Chelation therapy is widely recommendeded for asymptomatic patients with lead levels between 45 and 70 μg/dL.[4,7,41,164] Children without overt symptoms may be treated with succimer, which has had considerable efficacious and safe use since its FDA approval in 1991.[21,106,136,164] Succimer is initiated at 30 mg/kg/day (or 1050 mg/m²/day) orally in three divided doses; this is continued for 5 days, then decreased to 20 mg/kg/day (or 700 mg/m²/day) in two divided doses for 14 additional days.[4,105] It has been noted that the original data establishing this empiric dosing regimen was based on surface area rather than body weight,[105] and that for younger children the alternative dosing by body weight would result in suboptimal dosing.[202] Though the ability to chelate children orally with succimer makes it tempting to prescribe this medication routinely for outpatient therapy, and some animal evidence suggests succimer does not enhance lead absorption,[124] clinical reports suggest that children must be protected from continued lead exposure during succimer chelation.[47] Home abatement and reinspection should be accomplished before initiation of ambulatory succimer therapy; if this is not feasible, then hospitalization is still warranted. Alternative regimens (for rare patients with succimer intolerance or allergy, or parental noncompliance) would include parenteral inpatient chelation with $CaNa_2EDTA$ at 25 mg/kg/day for 5 days[4] or an oral course of D-penicillamine.

After initial chelation therapy, decisions to retreat are based on clinical symptoms and follow-up blood lead levels. Patients with encephalopathy or any severe symptoms, or initial blood lead > 100 μg/dL, will often require repeated courses of treatment. It is suggested that at least 2 days elapse before restarting chelation. The precise regimen and dosing of chelating agents will be determined by ongoing symptomatology and the repeat blood lead levels (see Table 79–10). A third course of chelation should rarely be necessary sooner than 5–7 days after the second.[191] For patients will milder degrees of plumbism (eg, asymptomatic, initial blood lead < 70 μg/dL), it is reasonable to allow 10–14 days of reequilibration before restarting treatment.[4]

The management of children with lead levels of 20–44 μg/dL is currently controversial.[4,20,91,135,145,163,164,202] Current CDC[35] and American Academy of Pediatrics[4] recommendations include aggressive environmental and nutritional interventions with close monitoring of blood lead levels, but not routine chelation therapy, for children with this degree of elevated body lead burden. To assess potential additional benefit of chelation therapy for these children, the National Institute of Environmental Health Sciences is currently sponsoring a multicenter, randomized, placebo-controlled study of succimer therapy in children aged 12–32 months with blood lead levels of 20–44 μg/dL, the Treatment of Lead-exposed Children (TLC) trial.[202] Outcome measures will include scores on development, behavior, and growth 3 years after randomization. Until the results of this, and similar, studies are available, the optimal approach to chelation for these children is unknown. Reasonable current guidelines for chelation treatment in this group have been proposed and include blood lead levels at the higher end of the range (eg, 35–44 μg/dL), levels that remain the same or rise over several months after rigorous environmental controls are instituted, younger children (eg, < 2 years old), or evidence of biochemical toxicity (elevated EP, after iron supplementation if necessary).[164] Any hint of subtle symptoms might also persuade the clinician to institute chelation as a therapeutic trial.

Blood lead levels of 10–19 μg/dL are defined by CDC as representing excessive exposure to lead, but do not require chelation therapy. Close monitoring (for the 10–14 μg/dL range) and careful environmental investigation and interventions as necessary (particularly for the 15–19 μg/dL range) are appropriate and sufficient (see Table 79–7).[4,41] The educational approaches outlined earlier (see Table 79–9) should be included in the case management of all children with even modestly elevated lead levels.

Adult Therapy. The first principle in the treatment of adults with lead poisoning is that chelation therapy may not substitute for adherence to OSHA lead standards at the worksite and should never be given prophylactically.[68,126,195,200,214,228] In addition to the guidelines for decreasing lead exposure noted earlier, chelation therapy is indicated in adults with significant symptoms (encephalopathy, abdominal colic, severe arthralgias or myalgias), evidence of target organ damage (neuropathy or nephropathy), and possibly in asymptomatic workers with markedly elevated blood lead levels and/or evidence of biochemical toxicity or increased chelatable lead. Chelation therapy regimens for adults are outlined in Table 79–10. Treatment of patients with TEL toxicity is largely supportive, with sedation as necessary. If blood lead levels are significantly elevated, chelation as described above may be considered, but has not been found clinically efficacious.[214]

References

1. Agency for Toxic Substances and Disease Registry: The nature and extent of lead poisoning in children in the United States: A report to Congress. Atlanta: ATSDR, 1988.
2. Allcott JV III, Barnhart RA, Mooney LA: Acute lead poisoning in two users of illicit methamphetamine. JAMA 1987;258:510–511.
3. Aly MH, Kim HC, Renner SW, et al: Hemolytic anemia associated with lead poisoning from shotgun pellets and the response to succimer treatment. Am J Hematol 1993;44: 280–283.
4. American Academy of Pediatrics, Committee on Drugs: Treatment guidelines for lead exposure in children. Pediatrics 1995;96:155–160.
5. American Academy of Pediatrics, Committee on Environmental Health: Lead poisoning: From screening to primary prevention. Pediatrics 1993;92:176–183.
6. Amitai Y, Graef JW, Brown MJ, et al: Hazards of "deleading" homes of children with lead poisoning. Am J Dis Child 1987;141:758–760.
7. Angle CR: Childhood lead poisoning and its treatment. Annu Rev Pharmacol Toxicol 1993;32:409–434.
8. Appel BR, Kahlon JK, Ferguson J, et al: Potential lead exposures from crystal decanters. Am J Public Health 1992; 82:1671–1673.
9. Assenato G, Paci C, Molinnini R, et al: Sperm count suppression without endocrine dysfuction in lead-exposed men. Annu Rev Pharmacol Toxicol 1986;30:41:387–390.
10. Astrin KH, Bishop DF, Wetmur JG, et al: Delta-aminolevulinic acid dehydratase isoenzymes and lead toxicity. Ann NY Acad Sci 1987;514:23–29.
11. Audesirk G: Electrophysiology of lead intoxciation: Effects on voltage-sensitive ion channels. Neurotoxicology 1993; 14:137–147.

12. Baghurst P, McMichaelm A, Wigg N, et al: Environmental exposure to lead and children's intelligence at the age of 7 years. N Engl J Med 1992;327:1279–1284.
13. Baker EL Jr, Folland DS, Taylor TA, et al: Lead poisoning in children of lead workers: Home contamination with industrial dust. N Engl J Med 1977,296:260 261.
14. Batuman V: Lead nephropathy, gout and hypertension Am J Med Sci 1993;305:241–247.
15. Batuman V, Dreisbach A, Chun E, Naumoff M: Lead increases red cell sodium–lithium countertransport. Am J Kidney Dis 1989;14:200–203.
16. Batuman V, Maesaka JK, Haddad B, et al: The role of lead in gout nephropathy. N Engl J Med 1981;304:520–523.
17. Bear MF, Cooper LN, Ebner E: A physiologic basis for a theory of synapse modification. Science 1987;237:42–48.
18. Bellinger D, Leviton A, Waternaux C, et al: Longitudinal analyses of prenatal and postnatal lead exposure and early cognitive development. N Engl J Med 1987;316:1037–1043.
19. Bellinger D, Sloman J, Leviton A, et al: Low-level lead exposure and children's cognitive function in the pre-school years. Pediatrics 1991;87:219–227.
20. Berlin CM, Banner W: Treatment of lead-exposed children. Pediatrics 1996;98:163. Letter.
21. Besunder JB, Anderson RL, Supeer DM: Short-term efficacy of oral dimercaptosuccinic acid in children with low to moderate lead intoxication. Pediatrics 1995;96:683–687.
22. Binder S, Matte TD, Kresnow M, et al: Lead testing of children and homes: Results of a national telephone survey. Public Health Rep 1996;111:342–346.
23. Binns HJ, LeBailly SA, Poncher J, et al: Is there lead in the suburbs? Risk assessment in Chicago suburban pediatric practices. Pediatrics 1994;93:164–171.
24. Blackfan KD: Lead poisoning in children with special reference to lead as a cause of convulsions. Am J Med Sci 1917;153:877–887.
25. Blickman JG, Wilkinson RF, Graef JW: The radiologic "lead band" revisited. Am J Radiol 1986;146:245–247.
26. Bloch P, Garavaglia G, Mitchell G, et al: Measurement of lead content of children's teeth in situ by x-ray fluorescence. Phys Med Biol 1976;20: 56–63.
27. Bolanowska W, Piotrowski J, Garczynski H: Triethyl lead in the biologic material in cases of acute tetraethyl lead poisoning. Arch Toxicol 1967;22:278–282.
28. Bolger PM, Carrington CD, Capar SG, Adams MA: Reductions in dietary lead exposure in the United States. Chem Speciation Bioavailability 1991;3:3–36.
29. Bornschein RL, Succop PA, Krafft KM, et al : Exterior surface dust lead, interior house dust lead and childhood exposure in an urban environment. In: Hemphill D, ed: Trace Substances in Environmental Health. Columbia, MO, Universiy of Missouri, 1986, pp. 322–332.
30. Bose A, Vashistha K, O'Loughlin BJ: Azarcon por empacho—Another cause of lead toxicity. Pediatrics 1983;72:106–108.
31. Brennan MJW, Cantrill RC: Delta-aminolevulinic acid is a potent agonist for GABA receptors. Nature 1979;280: 514–515.
32. Brody DJ, Pirkle JL, Kramer RA, et al: Blood lead levels in the US population. Phase 1 of the Third National Health and Nutrition Examination Survey (NHANES III, 1988 to 1991). JAMA 1994;272:277–283.
33. Byers RK, Lord EE: Late effects of lead poisoning on mental development. Am J Dis Child 1943;66:471–483.
34. Cardenas A, Roels H, Bernard AM, et al: Markers of early renal changes induced by industrial pollutants. II. Application to workers exposed to lead. Br J Indian Med 1993;50;28–36.
35. Centers for Disease Control and Prevention: Screening young children for lead poisoning: Guidance for state and local public health officials. US Dept of Health and Human Services, Public Health Service, Federal Register, Feb 21, 1997.
36. Centers for Disease Control and Prevention: Children with elevated blood lead levels attributed to home renovation and remodeling activities—New York, 1993–1994. MMWR 1996;45:1120–1123.
37. Centers for Disease Control and Prevention: Lead poisoning associated with use of traditional ethnic remedies—California, 1991–1992. MMWR 1993;42:521–524.
38. Centers for Disease Control and Prevention: Blood lead levels among children in high-risk areas—California, 1987–1990.MMWR 1992;41:291–294.
39. Centers for Disease Control and Prevention: Elevated blood lead levels in adults—United States, second quarter, 1992. MMWR 1992;41:715–716.
40. Centers for Disease Control and Prevention: Fatal pediatric poisoning from leaded paint—Wisconsin, 1990. MMWR 1991;40:193–195.
41. Centers for Disease Control and Prevention: Prevention of lead poisoning in young children: A statement by the Centers for Disease Control. Atlanta, US Dept of Health and Human Services, Public Health Service, 1991.
42. Centers for Disease Control and Prevention: Strategic plan for elimination of childhood lead poisoning. US Dept of Health and Human Services, Public Health Service, 1991.
43. Centers for Disease Control and Prevention: Elevated blood lead levels associated with ilicitly distilled alcohol—Alabama, 1990–1991. MMWR 1992;41:294.
44. Charney E, Kessler B, Farfel M, Jackson D: Childhood lead poisoning: A controlled trial of the effect of dust-control measures on blood lead levels. N Engl J Med 1983;309: 1089–1093.
45. Charney E, Sayre J, Coulter M: Increased lead absorption in inner city children: Where does it come from. Pediatrics 1980;65:226–231.
46. Chia KS, Jeyaratnam J, Lee J, et al: Lead-induced nephropathy: Relationship between various biologic exposure indices and early markers of nephrotoxicity. Am J Indian Med 1995;27:883–895.
47. Chisolm JJ Jr: BAL, EDTA, DMSA, and DMPS in the treatment of lead poisoning in children. J Toxicol Clin Toxicol 1992;30:493–504.
48. Chisolm JJ Jr: Mobilization of lead by calcium disodium edetate: A reappraisal. Am J Dis Child 1987;141:1256–1257.
49. Chisolm JJ Jr: The use of chelating agents in the treatment of acute and chronic lead intoxication in childhood. J Pediatr 1968;73:1–38.
50. Chisolm JJ Jr, Barltrop D: Recognition and management of children with increased lead absorption. Arch Dis Child 1979;54:249–362.

51. Chisolm JJ Jr, Farfel MR: Environmental control and deleading. Pediatr Ann 1994;23:627–633.
52. Chisolm JJ Jr, Harrison HE: The treatment of acute lead encephalopathy in children. Pediatrics 1957;19:2–20.
53. Coffin R, Phillips JL, Staples WI, Spector S: Treatment of lead encephalopathy in children. J Pediatr 1966;69: 198–206.
54. Cohen AR, Trotzky MS, Pincus D: Reassessment of the microcytic anemia of lead poisoning. Pediatrics 1981;67:904–906.
55. Cohen N, Modai D, Golik A, et al: An esoteric occupational hazard for lead poisoning. J Toxicol Clin Toxicol 1986;24:59–67.
56. Colorado Department of Health: Colorado Disease Bulletin,Vol XV, Issue 9, May 1, 1987.
57. Conrad ME, Umbrier JN, Moore EG, Rodning CR: Newly identified iron-binding protein in human duodenal mucosa. Blood 1992;79: 244–247.
58. Cookman GR, Hemmens SE, Keane GJ, et al: Chronic low-level lead exposure precociously induces rat glial development in vitro and in vivo. Neurosci Lett 1988;86:33–37.
59. Corey-Slechta DA: Relationships between lead-induced learning impairments and changes in dopaminergic, cholinergic, and glutamatergic neurotransmitter system functions. Annu Rev Pharmacol Toxicol 1995;35:391–415.
60. Corey-Slechta DA, Weiss B: Efficacy of the chelating agent CaEDTA in reversing lead-induced changes in behavior. Neurotoxicology 1989;10:685–698.
61. Corey-Slechta DA, Weiss B, Cox C: Mobilization and redistribution of lead over the course of CaEDTA chelation therapy. J Pharmacol Exp Ther 1987;243:804–813.
62. Cullen MR, Robins JM, Eskenazi B: Adult inorganic lead intoxication: Presentation of 31 new cases and a review of the literature. Medicine 1983;62:221–247.
63. Curran JP, Nunez JR: Lead poisoning during home renovation. NY State J Med 1989;89:679–680.
64. Dart RC, Hurlbut KM, Maiorino RM, et al: Pharmacokinetics of meso–2,3-dimercaptosuccinic acid in patients with lead poisoning and in healthy adults. J Pediatr 1994; 125:309–316.
65. Davoli CT, Serwint JR, Chisolm JJ Jr: Asymptomatic children with venous lead levels > 100 μg/dL. Pediatrics 1996;98:965–968.
66. De la Burde B, Choate MS: Early asymptomatic lead exposure and development at school age. J Pediatr 1975;87: 637–642.
67. De la Burde B, Choate MS: Does asymptomatic lead exposure in children have latent sequelae? J Pediatr 1972;81: 1088–1096.
68. DeRoos FJ: Smelters and metal reclaimers. In: Greenberg MI, Hamilton R, Phillips S, eds: Occupational, Industrial and Environmental Toxicolgy. St. Louis, Mosby–Year Book, 1997, pp. 291–301.
69. Dickens C: The Uncommercial Traveller: A Collection of Short Stories. London, T. Nelson & Sons, 1861.
70. Dietrich KN, Berger OG, Succop PA: Lead exposure and the motor developmental status of urban six-year old children in the Cincinnati prospective study. Pediatrics 1993;91:301–307.
71. Dillman RO, Crumb CK, Lidsky MJ: Lead poisoning from a gunshot wound. Am J Med 1979;66:509.
72. Dolcourt JL, Finch C, Coleman GD, et al: Hazard of lead exposure in the home from recycled automobile storage batteries. Pediatrics 1981;68:225–229.
73. Durback LF, Wedin GP, Seidler DE: Management of lead foreign body ingestion. J Toxicol Clin Toxicol 1989;27: 173–182.
74. Emmerson BT: Chronic lead nephropathy. Kidney Int 1973;4:1–5.
75. Environmental Protection Agency: Maximum contaminant level goals and national primary drinking water regulations for lead and copper. Federal Register 1991;56: 26469–26470.
76. Environmental Protection Agency: Strategy for reducing lead exposures: Report to Congress. Washington, DC, EPA, 1991.
77. Environmental Protection Agency: Evaluation of Potential Carcinogenicity of Lead and Lead Compounds. EPA/ 600/8–89/0454A, US Environmental Protection Agency, Office of Health and Environmental Assessment, Washington, DC, 1989.
78. Environmental Protection Agency: Supplement to the 1986 Air Quality Criteria for Lead. Addendum EPA/ 600/8–89/049A. Office of Health and Environmental Assessment. Washington, DC: US Environmental Protection Agency, 1989;1:A1-A67.
79. Erenberg G, Rinsler SS, Fish BG: Lead neuropathy and sickle cell disease. Pediatrics 1974;54:438–441.
80. Ernhardt CB, Landa B, Schell NB: Lead levels and intelligence. Pediatrics 1981;68:903–905. Letter.
81. Farfel MR, Chisolm JJ Jr: Health and environmental outcomes of traditional and modified practices for abatement of residential lead-based paint. Am J Public Health 1990; 80:1240–1245.
82. Fishbein A: Lead poisoning: I. Some clinical and toxicological observations on the effects of occupational lead exposure among firearms instructors. Isr J Med Sci 1992; 28:560–572.
83. Fishbein A, Thornton J, Blumberg WE, et al: Health status of cable splicers with low-level exposure to lead: Results of a clinical survey. Am J Public Health 1980;70:697–700.
84. Flaherty EG: Risk of lead poisoning in abused and neglected children. Clin Pediatr 1995;34:128–132.
85. Franco G, Cottica D, Minoia C: Chewing electric wire coatings: An unusual source of lead poisoning. Am J Ind Med 1994;25:291–296.
86. Frankel M, Rogers P, Pursell R, et al: Severe lead intoxication in an infant from an imported kettle. Vet Hum Toxicol 1992;34:355. Abstract.
87. Friedman JA, Weinberger HL: Six children with lead poisoning. Am J Dis Child 1990;144:1039–1044.
88. Garrod AB: A Treatise on Gout and Rheumatic Gout (Rheumatoid Arthritis), 3rd ed. London: Longmans, Green & Co., 1876.
89. Gennart JP, Bernard A, Lauwerys R: Assessment of thyroid, testis, kidney, and autonomic nervous system function in lead-exposed workers. Int Arch Occup Health 1992;64:49–58.
90. Ghafour SY, Khuffash FA, Ibrahim HS, Reavey PC: Congenital lead intoxication with seizures due to prenatal exposure. Clin Pediatr 1984;23:282–283.

91. Glotzer DE: Management of childhood lead poisoning: Strategies for chelation. Pediatr Ann 1994;23:606–615.
92. Goldman LR, Carra J: Childhood lead poisoning in 1994. JAMA 1994;272:315–316.
93. Goldman RH, Baker El, Hannan M, et al: Lead poisoning in automobile radiator mechanics. N Engl J Med 1987; 317:214–218.
94. Goldstein GW: Neurologic concepts of lead poisoning in children. Pediatr Ann 1992;21:384–388.
95. Goldstein GW: Lead poisoning and brain cell function. Environ Health Perspect 1990;89:91–94.
96. Goldstein GW: Brain capillaries: A target for inorganic lead poisoning. Neurotoxicology 1984;5:167–175.
97. Goyer RA: Toxic effects of metals. In: Klaassen CD, ed: Casarett and Doull's Toxicolgy: The Basic Science of Poisons, 5th ed. New York, McGraw-Hill, 1996, pp. 691–709.
98. Goyer RA: Lead toxicity: Current concerns. Environ Health Perspect 1993;100:177–187.
99. Goyer RA: Lead toxicity: From overt to subclinical to subtle health effects. Environ Health Perspect 1990;86: 177–181.
100. Goyer RA: Lead and the kidney. Curr Topics Pathol 1971; 55:147–176.
101. Goyer RA: Lead toxicity: A problem in environmental pathology. Am J Pathol 1971;64:167–182.
102. Goyer RA, Cherian MG, Jones MM, Reigart JR: Role of chelating agents for prevention, intervention and treatment of exposures to toxic metals. Environ Health Perspect 1995;103:1048–1052.
103. Goyer RA, Rhyne B: Pathologic effects of lead. Int Rev Exp Pathol 1973;12:1–77.
104. Graziano JH: Validity of lead-exposure markers in diagnosis and surveillance. Clin Chem 1994;40:1387–1390.
105. Graziano JH, LoIacono NJ, Meyer P: Dose–response study of oral 2,3-dimercaptosuccinic acid in children with elevated blood lead concentrations. J Pediatr 1988;113: 751–757.
106. Graziano JH, LoIacono LJ, Moulton T, et al: Controlled study of meso–2,3-dimercaptosuccinic acid for the management of childhood lead intoxication. J Pediatr 1992; 120:133–139.
107. Graziano JH, Slavkovic V, Factor-Litvak P, et al: Depressed serum erythropoietin in pregnant women with elevated blood lead. Arch Environ Health 1991;46:347–350.
108. Greenough FB: A case of probable lead poisoning, resulting fatally from a bullet lodged in the knee joint twelve years previously. Boston Med Surg J 1874;91:472.
109. Greensher J, Mofenson HC, Balakrishnan C, et al: Lead poisoning from ingestion of lead shot. Pediatrics 1974;54: 641–643.
110. Grimsley EW, Adams-Mount L: Occupational lead intoxication: Report of four cases. South Med J 1994;87:689–691.
111. Grondona C: Lead revisited: A case study on lead exposed painters. AAOHN J 1993;41:33–38.
112. Hagelmeyer CD, Moorehead JC, Horenblas L, Bayer MJ: Fatal lead encephalopathy following foreign body ingestion: Case report. J Emerg Med 1988;6:397–400.
113. Hammer LD, Ludwig S, Henretig F: Increased lead absorption in children with accidental ingestions. Am J Emerg Med 1985;3:301–304.
114. Harvey B: Should blood lead screening recommendations be revised? Pediatrics 1994;93:201–204.
115. Heard MJ, Chamberlain AC: Effect of minerals and food on uptake of lead from the gastrointestinal tract in humans. Hum Toxicol 1982;1:411–415.
116. Hemings HC, Nairn AC, McGuinness TL, et al: Role of protein phosphorylation in neuronal signal transduction. FASEB J 1989;3:1581–1592.
117. Henretig FM, Shannon M: Toxicologic emergencies. In: Fleisher GR, Ludwig S, eds: Textbook of Pediatric Emergency Medicine, 3rd ed. Baltimore, Williams & Wilkins, 1993, pp. 779–781.
118. Hu H, Milder FL, Burger DE: The use of k xray fluorescence for measuring lead burden in epidemiological studies: High and low lead burdens and measurement uncertainty. Environ Health Perspect 1991;94:107–110.
119. Huseman CA, Varma MM, Angle CR: Neuroendocrine effects of toxic and low blood lead levels in children. Pediatrics 1992;90:186–189.
120. Huttenlocher PR, de Courten C: The devlopment of synapses in striate cortex of man. Hum Neurobiol 1987;6:1–9.
121. Jiang X, Liang Y, Wang Y: Studies of lead exposure on reproductive system: A review of work in China. Biomed Environ Sci 1992;5:266–275
122. Jugo S, Malikovic T, Kostial K: Influence of chelating agents on the gastrointestinal absorption of lead. Toxicol Appl Pharmacol 1975;34:259–263.
123. Kakosy T, Hudak A, Naray M: Lead intoxication epidemic caused by ingestion of contaminated ground paprika. J Toxicol Clin Toxcicol 1996;34:507–511.
124. Kapoor SC, Wielopolski L, Graziano JH, LoIacono NJ: Influence of 2,3-dimercaptosuccinic acid on gastrointestinal lead absorption and whole body lead retention. Toxicol Appl Pharmacol 1989;97:525–529.
125. Kaufman A, Wiese W: Gasoline sniffing leading to increased lead absorption in children. Clin Pediatr 1978; 17:475–477.
126. Keogh JP: Lead. In Sullivan JB Jr, Krieger GR, eds: Hazardous Materials Toxicology: Clinical Principals of Environmental Health. Baltimore, Williams & Wilkins, 1992, pp. 834–844.
127. Kimbrough RD, LeVois M, Webb DR: Management of children with slightly elevated lead levels. Pediatrics 1994;93:188–191.
128. Kocak R, Anarat A, Altinas G, et al: Lead poisoning from contaminated flour in a family of 11 members. Hum Toxicol 1989;8:385–386.
129. Kopp SJ, Glonek T, Erlander M, et al: The influence of chronic low-level cadmium and/or lead feeding on myocardial contractility related to phosphorylation of cardiac myofibrillar proteins. Toxciol Appl Pharmacol 1980;54: 48–56.
130. Kosmider S, Petelenz T: Electrocardiographic changes in elderly patients with chronic lead poisoning. Pol Arch Med Wewn 1962;32:437–442.
131. Kosnett MJ: Unanswered questions in metal chelation. J Toxicol Clin Toxicol 1992;30:529–547.
132. Landrigan PJ, Baker EL Jr, Himmelstein JS, et al: Exposure to lead from the Mystic River bridge: The dilemma of deleading. N Engl J Med 1982;306:673–676.

133. Lecos CW: Pretty poison: Lead and ceramic ware. FDA Consumer July/August 1987:6–9.
134. Levine F, Muenke M: VACTERL association with high prenatal lead exposure: Similarities to animal models of lead teratogenicity. Pediatrics 1991;87:390–392.
135. Liebelt EL, Shannon MW: Oral chelators for childhood lead poisoning. Pediatr Ann 1994;23:616–626.
136. Liebelt EL, Shannon M, Graef JW: Efficacy of oral meso-2,3 dimercaptosuccinic acid therapy for low-level childhood plumbism. J Pediatr 1994;1214:313–317.
137. Lilis R, Fischbein A, Eisinger J, et al: Prevalence of lead disease among secondary lead smelter workers and biologic indicators of lead exposure. Environ Res 1977;14: 255–285.
138. Lin-Fu JS: Undue absorption of lead among children—A new look at an old problem. N Engl J Med 1972;286: 702–710.
139. Lyons JD, Filston HC: Lead intoxication from a pellet entrapped in the appendix of a child: Treatment considerations. J Pediatr Surg 1994;29:1618–1620.
140. Mahaffey KR: Nutrition and lead: Strategies for public health. Environ Health Perspect 1995;103:191–196.
141. Mahaffey KR, Annest JL, Roberts J, Murphy RS: National estimates of blood lead levels: United States 1976–1980. N Engl J Med 1982;307:573–579.
142. Major RH: A History of Medicine. Springfield, IL: Charles C Thomas, 1954.
143. Mantere P, Hanninen H, Hernberg S, Luukkonen R: A prospective follow-up study on psychological effects in workers exposed to low levels of lead. Scand J Work Environ Health 1984;10:43–50.
144. Marcus AH: Multicompartment kinetic modules for lead: Linear kinetics and variable absorption in humans without excessive lead exposures. Environ Res 1985;36:459–472.
145. Marcus SM: Treatment of lead-exposed children. Pediatrics 1996;98:161–162. Letter.
146. Marcus SM: Lead poisoning from industrial exposure. Occup Med 1978;1:1–4.
147. Marino PE, Franzblau A, Lilis R, et al: Acute lead poisoning in construction workers: The failure of current protective standards. Arch Environ Health 1989;44:140–145.
148. Marino PE, Landrigan PJ, Graef J, et al: A case report of lead paint poisoning during renovation of a Victorian farmhouse. Am J Public Health 1990;80:1183–1185.
149. Markovac J, Goldstein GW: Picomolar concentrations of lead stimulate brain protein kinase C. Nature 1988;334: 71–73.
150. Markowitz ME, Bijur PE, Ruff H, Rosen JF: Effects of calcium disodium versenate ($CaNa_2EDTA$) chelation in moderate childhood lead poisoning. Pediatrics 1993;92: 265–271.
151. Markowitz ME, Rosen JF: Assessment of lead stores in children: Validation of an 8 hour $CaNa_2EDTA$ provocation test. J Pediatr 1984;104:337–341.
152. Markowitz ME, Weinberger HL: Immobilization-related lead toxicity in previously lead-poisoned children. Pediatrics 1990;86:455–457.
153. Markowitz SB, Nunez CM, Klitzman S, et al: Lead poisoning due to hai ge fen: The porphyrin content of individual erythrocytes. JAMA 1994;271:932–934.
154. McCallum RI, Sanderson JT, Richards AE: The lead hazard in shipbreaking: The prevalence of anemia in burners. Ann Occup Hyg 1968;11:101–113.
155. McCord CP: Lead and lead poisoning in early America. Benjamin Franklin and lead poisoning. Industr Med Surg 1953;22:394–399.
156. McElvaine MD, DeUngria EG, Matte TD, et al: Prevalence of radiographic evidence of paint chip ingestion among children with moderate to severe lead poisoning, St. Louis, Misssouri, 1989 through 1990. Pediatrics 1992; 89:740–742.
157. Meggs WJ, Gerr F, Aly M et al: The treatment of lead poisoning from gunshot wounds with succimer (DMSA). J Toxicol Clin Toxicol 1994;32:377–385.
158. Miller MB, Curry S, Kunkel D, et al: Pool cue chalk: A source of environmental lead. Pediatrics 1996;97:916–917.
159. Miller SA: Lead in calcium supplements. JAMA 1987; 257:1810.
160. Minnema DJ, Michelson IA, Cooper GP: Calcium efflux and neurotransmitter release from rat hippocampal synaptosomes exposed to lead. Toxicol Appl Pharmacol 1988;92:351–357.
161. Moore MR, Meredith P: The carcinogenicity of lead. Arch Toxicol 1979;42:87–94.
162. Moore MR, Meredith PA, Watson WS, et al: The percutaneous absorption of lead-203 in humans from cosmetic preparations containing lead acetate, as assessed by whole-body counting and other techniques. Food Cosmet Toxicol 1980;18:399–405.
163. Mortensen ME: Succimer chelation: What is known? J Pediatr 1994;125:233–234.
164. Mortensen ME, Walson PD: Chelation therapy for childhood lead poisoning—The changing scene in the 1990s. Clin Pediatr 1993; 32: 284–291.
165. Mushak P, Davis JM, Crocewtti AF, Grant LD: Pre-natal and post-natal effects of low-level lead exposure: Integrated summary of a report to the US Congress on childhood lead poisoning. Environ Res 1989;50:11–36.
166. National Institute for Occupational Safety and Health: Recommendations for control of occupational safety and health hazards—Foundries. Washington, DC, Sept 1985, US Government Printing Office.
167. Needleman HL: The persistant threat of lead: Medical and sociological issues. Curr Probl Pediatr 1988;18:702–744.
168. Needleman HL, Gunnoe C, Leviton A, et al: Deficits in psychological and classroom performance of children with elevated dentine lead levels. N Engl J Med 1979; 300:689–695.
169. Needleman HL, Riess JA, Tobin MJ, et al: Bone lead levels and delinquent behavior. JAMA 1996;275:363–369.
170. Needleman HL, Shapiro IM: Dentine lead levels in asymptomatic Philadelphia school children: Subclinical exposure in high and low risk groups. Environ Health Perspect 1974;7:27–31.
171. Needleman HL, Schell A, Bellinger D, et al: The long-term effects of exposure to low doses of lead in childhood: An 11-year follow-up report. N Engl J Med 1990;322:83–88.
172. Nieburg PI, Weiner LS, Oski BF, Oski FA: Red blood cell-aminolevulinic acid dehydratase activity. Am J Dis Child 1974;127:348–350.

173. Nordin JD, Rolnick SJ, Griffen JM: Prevalence of excess lead absorption and associated risk factors in children enrolled in a midwestern health maintenance organization. Pediatrics 1994;93:172–177.
174. Nortier JWR, Sangster B, Van Kestern RG: Acute lead poisoning with hemolysis and liver toxicity after ingestion of red lead. Vet Hum Toxicol 1980;22:145–147.
175. Norton RL, Weinstein L, Rafalski T, et al: Acute intravenous lead poisoning in a drug abuser: Associated complications of hepatitis, pancreatitis, hemolysis and renal failure. Vet Hum Toxicol 1989;31:340. Abstract.
176. Nriagu JO: Saturnine gout among Roman aristocrats. N Engl J Med 1983;308:660–663.
177. Oliver P: A lecture on lead poisoning and the race. Br Med J 1911;1:1096–1098.
178. Oski FA, Perkins KC: Elevated blood lead in a six-month old breast fed infant: The role of newsprint logs. Pediatrics 1976;57:426–427.
179. Otto DA, Fox DA: Auditory and visual dysfunction following lead exposure. Neurotoxicology 1993;14:191–207.
180. Paglia DE, Valentine WN, Dahlgner JG: Effects of low level lead exposure on pyrimidine–5′-nucleotidase and other erythrocyte enzymes. J Clin Invest 1976;56: 1164–1169.
181. Parras F, Patier JL, Ezpeleta C: Lead-contaminated heroin as a source of inorganic lead intoxication. N Engl J Med 1987;316:755. Letter.
182. Patterson CC: Contaminated and natural lead environments of man. Arch Environ Health 1965;11:344–348.
183. Pearce WG: More on retinal stippling. N Engl J Med 1964;270:533–534. Letter.
184. Perino J, Ernhardt CB: The relation of subclinical lead levels to cognitive and sensorimotor impairment in black preschoolers. J Learning Disabilities 1974;7:616–620.
185. Petit TL, LeBoutillier JC: Effects of lead exposure during development on neocortical dendritic and synaptic structure. Exp Neurol 1979;64:482–492.
186. Philadelphia Department of Public Health, Childhood Lead Poisoning Prevention Program: Venous lead levels, Quarterly report, Jan 1, 1993–March 31, 1993.
187. Philip AT, Gerson B: Lead poisoning—Part II: Effects and assay. Clin Lab Med 1994;14:651–670.
188. Piomelli S: Childhood lead poisoning in the 90s. Pediatrics 1994;93:508–510.
189. Piomelli S: A micromethod for free erythrocyte protoporphyrins: FEP test. J Lab Clin Med 1973;81:932–940.
190. Piomelli S, Corash L, Corash MB, et al: Blood lead concentrations in a remote Himalayan population. Science 1980;210:1135–1137.
191. Piomelli S, Rosen JF, Chisolm JJ Jr, Graef JW: Management of childhood lead poisoning. J Pediatr 1984;105:523–532.
192. Pirkle JL, Brody DJ, Gunter EW, et al: The decline in blood lead levels in the United States. The National Health and Nutrition Examination Surveys (NHANES). JAMA 1994; 272:284–291.
193. Pirkle JL, Schwartz J, Landis JR, Harlan WR: The relationship between blood lead levels and blood pressure and its cardiovascular risk implications. Am J Epidemiol 1985; 121:246–258.
194. Pocock SJ, Smith M, Baghurst P: Environmental lead and children's intelligence: A systematic review of the epidemiological evidence. Br Med J 1994;309:1189–1197.
195. Porru S, Alessio L: The use of chelating agents in occupational lead poisoning. Occup Med 1996;46:41–48.
196. Raasch FO, Rosenberg JH, Abraham JL: Lead poisoning from hair spray ingestion. Am J Forensic Med Pathol 1983;4:159–164.
197. Rabinowitz MB, Needleman HL: Temporal trends in the lead concentrations of umbilical cord blood. Science 1982; 216:1429–1431.
198. Rabinowitz MB, Wetherill GW, Kopple JD: Kinetic analysis of lead metabolism in healthy humans. J Clin Invest 1976;58:260–270.
199. Regan CM: Neural cell adhesion molecules, neuronal development and lead toxicity. Neurotoxicology 1993;14: 69–74.
200. Rempel D: The lead-exposed worker. JAMA 1989; 262:532–534.
201. Restek-Samarzija N, Samarzija M, Momcilovic B: Ventricular arrhythmia in acute lead poisoning: A case report. Presented at the EAPCCT XVI International Congress, Vienna, Austria, April, 1994. Abstract.
202. Rhodes GG, Rogan WJ: Treatment of lead-exposed children. Pediatrics 1996;98:162–163. Letter.
203. Rodamilans M, Martinez-Osaba MJ, To-Figueras J, et al: Lead toxicity on endocrine testicular function in an occupationally exposed population. Hum Toxicol 1988;7:125–128.
204. Romeo R, Aprea C, Boccalon P, et al: Serum erythropoietin and blood lead concentrations. Int Arch Occup Environ Health 1996;69:73–75.
205. Rossouw J, Offermeier J, von Rooyen JM: Apparent central neurotransmitter receptor changes induced by low-level lead exposure during different developmental phases in the rat. Toxicol Appl Pharmacol 1987;91:132–139.
206. Royce SE, Needleman HL: Case Studies in Environmental Medicine. Lead Toxicity. Atlanta, Agency for Toxic Substances and Disease Registry, 1992.
207. Ruff H, Bijur PE, Markowitz M, et al: Declining blood lead levels and cognitive changes in moderately lead-poisoned children. JAMA 1993;269:1641–1646.
208. Rummo JH, Routh DK, Rummo NJ, Brown JF: Behavioral and neurological effects of symptomatic and asymptomatic lead exposure in children. Arch Environ Health 1979;34:120–124.
209. Saenger P, Rosen JF, Markowitz M: Diagnostic significance of edetate disodium calcium testing in children with increased lead absorption. Am J Dis Child 1983;136: 312–315.
210. Sandstead HH, Orth DN, Abe K, et al: Lead intoxication: Effect on pituitary and adrenal function in man. Clin Res 1970;18:76.
211. Sandstead HH, Stant EG, Brill AB, et al: Lead intoxication and the thyroid. Arch Intern Med 1969;123:632–635.
212. Sargent JD: The role of nutrition in the prevention of lead poisoning in children. Pediatr Ann 1994;23:636–642.
213. Saryan LA: Surreptitious lead exposure from an Asian Indian medication. J Anal Toxicol 1991;15:336–338.
214. Saryan LA, Zenz C: Lead and its compounds. In: Zenz C, Dickerson OB, Horvath EP Jr, eds: Occupational Medicine, 3rd ed. St. Louis, Mosby, 1994, pp. 506–541.

215. Sayre JW, Charney E, Vostal J, Pless IB: House and hand dust as a potential source of childhood lead exposure. Am J Dis Child 1974;127:167–170.
216. Schaeffer SJ, Campbell JR: The new CDC and AAP lead poisoning recommendations: Consensus versus controversy. Pediatr Ann 1994;23:592–599.
217. Schlenker TL, Fritz CJ, Mark D, et al: Screening for pediatric lead poisoning: Comparability of simultaneously drawn capillary and venous blood samples. JAMA 1994; 271:1346–1348.
218. Schoen EJ: Childhood lead poisoning: Definitions and priorities. Pediatrics 1993;91:504–505.
219. Schwartz J, Angle C, Pitcher H: Relationship between childhood blood lead levels and stature. Pediatrics 1986; 77:281–288.
220. Schwartz J, Otto D: Blood lead, hearing thresholds, and neurobehavioral development in children and youth. Arch Environ Health 1987;42:153–164.
221. Selander S, Cramer K: Interrelationships between lead in blood, lead in urine and ALA in urine during lead work. Br J Ind Med 1970;27:28–39.
222. Selbst SM, Henretig F, Fee MA, et al: Lead poisoning in a child with a gunshot wound. Pediatrics 1986;77:413–416.
223. Selbst SM, Henretig FM, Pierce J: Lead encephalopathy in a child with sickle cell disease. Clin Pediatr 1985;24:280–285.
224. Selbst SM, Sokas RK, Henretig FM, et al: The effect of blood lead on blood pressure in children. J Environ Pathol Toxicol Oncol 1993;12:213–218.
225. Sensirivatana R, Supachadhiwong O, Phancharoen S, Mitrakul C: Neonatal lead poisoning: An unusual clinical manifestation. Clin Pediatr 1983;22:582–584.
226. Seppalainen AM, Hernberg S: Subclinical lead neuropathy. Am J Ind Med 1989;1:413–420.
227. Settle DM, Patterson CC: Lead in albacore: Guide to lead pollution in Americans. Science 1980;207:1167–1176.
228. Seward JP: Occupational lead exposure and management. West J Med 1996;165:222–224.
229. Shannon MW, Graef JW: Lead intoxication in infancy. Pediatrics 1992;89:87–90.
230. Shannon MW, Graef J, Lovejoy FH Jr: Efficacy and toxicity of D-penicillamine in low-level lead poisoning. J Pediatr 1988;112:799–804.
231. Shen X, Rosen JF, Guo D, Wu S: Childhood lead poisoning in China. Sci Total Environ 1996;181:101–109.
232. Sidman RL, Rakie P: Neuronal migration, with special reference to developing human brain. Brain Res 1973;62: 1–35.
233. Silbergeld EK, Scwartz J, Mahaffey K: Lead and osteoporosis: Mobilization of lead from bone in post-menopausal women. Environ Res 1988;47:79–94.
234. Silver W, Rodriguez-Torres R: Electrocardiographic studies in children with lead poisoning. Pediatrics 1968;41: 1124–1127.
235. Simons TJB: Cellular interactions between lead and calcium. Br Med Bull 1986;42:431–434.
236. Sonkin N: Stippling of the retina—A new physical sign in the early diagnosis of lead poisoning. N Engl J Med 1963;269:779–780.
237. Staes C, Matte T, Staeling N, et al: Lead poisoning deaths in the United States, 1979–1988. JAMA 1995;273:847–848. Letter.
238. Stowe HD, Goyer RA: The reproductive ability and progeny of F_1 lead-toxic rats. Fertil Steril 1971;22:755–760.
239. Stromberg BV: Symptomatic lead toxicity secondary to retained shotgun pellets: Case report. J Trauma 1990;30: 356–357.
240. Taubman B, Wiley C, Henretig F: Prevalence of elevated blood lead levels in a suburban middle class private practice. Arch Pediatr Adol Med 1994;148:757–760.
241. Toews AD, Kolber A, Hayward J, et al: Experimental lead encephalopathy in the suckling rat: Concentration of lead in cellular fractions enriched in brain capillaries. Brain Res 1978;147:131–138.
242. Turner AJ: Lead poisoning among Queensland children. Aust Med Gazette 1897;16:475–479.
243. Tyroler HA: Epidemiology of hypertension as a public health problem: An overview as background for evaluation of blood lead-blood pressure relationship. Environ Health Perspect 1988;78:3–8. Symposium.
244. US Department of Housing and Urban Development: A comprehensive and workable plan for the abatement of lead-based paint in privately owned housing. Report to Congress. Washington, DC, Housing and Urban Development, 1990.
245. US Department of Housing and Urban Development: Lead-based paint: Interim guidelines for hazard identification and abatement in public and Indian housing. Fed Reg 1990;55:14556–14614.
246. US Department of the Interior: Minerals yearbook for 1990, vol 1. Washington, DC, Government Printing Office, 1991.
247. US Department of Labor, Occupational Safety and Health Administration: Lead exposure in construction—Interim final rule. 29CFR part 1926.62. Federal Register, 5/4/93.
248. US Department of Labor, Occupational Safety and Health Administration: Lead standard, 20CFR1910.1025 (revised July 1, 1990). Washington, DC, 1990, US Government Printing Office.
249. US Department of Labor, Occupational Safety and Health Administration: Occupational health and safety standard: Occupational exposure to lead. (29 CR 1910.1025) Fed Reg Nov 14, 1978; 42:52952–53014.
250. Vance MV, Curry SC, Bradley JM, et al: Acute lead poisoning in nursing home and psychiatric patients from the ingestion of lead-based ceramic glazes. Arch Intern Med 1990;150:2085–2092.
251. Vander AJ: Chronic effects of lead on renin-angiotensin system. Environ Health Perspect 1988;78:77–83.
252. Wade JF, Burnum JF: Treatment of acute and chronic lead poisoning with disodium calcium versenate. Ann Intern Med 1955;42:251–259.
253. Waldron HA: Lead poisoning in the ancient world. Med Hist 1973;17:391–399.
254. Wedeen RP: Poison in the Pot: The Legacy of Lead. Carbondale: Southern Illinois University Press, 1984.
255. Wedeen RP, Ty A, Udasin I, et al: Clinical application of in vivo tibial K-XRF for monitoring lead stores. Arch Environ Health 1995;50:355–361.
256. Weinberger HL, Post EM, Schneider T, et al: An analysis

of 248 initial mobilization tests performed on an ambulatory basis. Am J Dis Child 1987;141:1266–1270.
257. Weitzman M, Aschengrau A, Bellinger D, et al: Lead-contaminated soil abatement and urban children's blood lead levels. JAMA 1993;269:1647–1654.
258. Whitfield CL, Ch'ien LT, Whitehead JD: Lead encephalopathy in adults. Am J Med 1972;52:289–297.
259. Wiley JF II, Bell LM, Rosenblum LS, et al: Lead poisoning: Low rates of screening and high prevalence among children seen in inner-city emergency departments. J Pediatr 1995;126:392–395.
260. Wiley J, Henretig F, Foster R: Status epilepticus and severe neurologic impairment from lead encephalopathy, November, 1994. J Toxicol Clin Toxicol 1995;33:529–530. Abstract.
261. Wiley JF II, Henretig FM, Selbst SM: Blood lead levels in children with foreign bodies. Pediatrics 1992;89: 593–596.
262. Winneke G, Brockhaus A, Ewers U, et al: Results from the European multicenter study on lead neurotoxicity in children: Implications for risk assessment. Neurotoxicol Teratol 1990;12:553–559.
263. Woodbury WD: Lead. In: Minerals Yearbook, 1987. Washington, DC, Bureau of Mines. US Department of Commerce, 1987, pp. 541–567.
264. Woolf DA, Riach ICF, Deerwesh A, et al: Lead lines in young infants with acute lead encephalopathy: A reliable diagnostic test. J Trop Pediatr 1990;36:90–93.
265. Ziegler EE, Edwards BB, Jensen RL, et al: Absorption and retention of lead by infants. Pediatr Res 1978;12:29–34.

ANTIDOTES IN DEPTH

Succimer (2,3-Dimercaptosuccinic Acid, DMSA)

Joseph H. Graziano and Mary Ann Howland

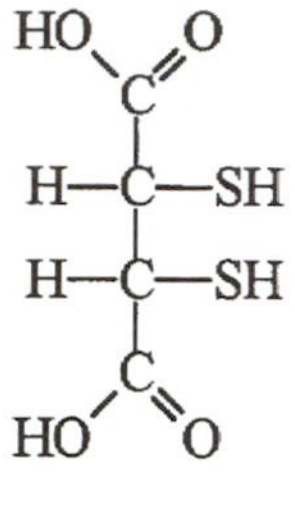

DMSA
(2,3-dimercapto succinic acid)

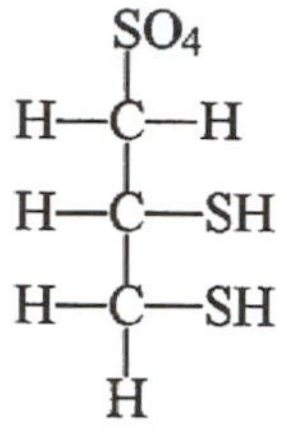

DMPS
(2,3-dimercapto-1-propane sulfonic acid)

Succimer (2,3-meso-dimercaptosuccinic acid, DMSA) is a relatively selective, orally active, water-soluble chelating agent for the treatment of lead, arsenic, and organic and inorganic mercury poisoning.[3,4,6,7,26] The drug can be considered a hydrophilic, less toxic analog of British antilewisite (BAL). It was first synthesized in 1940 by Ernst Friedheim, who incorporated the molecule into the structure of Mel W, a drug for the treatment of schistosomiasis.[22] Succimer was first used as an antidote for heavy-metal poisoning in 1965 in China, by Wang et al.[53] Its use by the Chinese can probably be traced to a visit by Friedheim to China in the early 1960s. The drug has been subsequently used rather widely in Asia[42,43,50,53,54,56] and Europe.[11,19,21,23,34,51] Succimer is the mesoform of 2,3-dimercaptosuccinic acid. The potential efficacy of the racemic mixture is being investigated.[20]

Until recently, conventional chelation therapy for heavy-metal poisoning has largely relied on the parenteral use of BAL and/or calcium disodium edetate ($CaNa_2EDTA$) and D-penicillamine, drugs that are not specific for heavy metals and that have been associated with unpleasant and potentially dangerous adverse effects.[32,46] In the United States, succimer was approved by the Food and Drug Administration (FDA) in 1991 for the treatment of asymptomatic children with lead levels greater than 45 µg/dL. Although not FDA approved, succimer has also been used for the treatment of organic and inorganic mercury and arsenic (see Fig. 79–9).

Several controlled clinical trials of succimer have been conducted. A study evaluating oral succimer dose ranges in 18 men with occupational lead intoxication found a 5-day course with 30 mg/kg/day of succimer (in three divided doses daily) to be more effective than 10 or 20 mg/kg/day of succimer.[29] The response to 30 mg/kg/day was considered to be excellent, since the mean blood lead concentrations fell from 79 to 23 µg/dL, while mean urinary lead excretion totaled 18,901 µg over 5 days. Computations indicate that the lead content of the blood, soft tissue, and skeletal compartments was depleted by succimer; more lead was eliminated on the first day alone than was contained in the blood and soft tissue lead compartments combined prior to treatment. In addition, succimer was more effective than IV $CaNa_2EDTA$ in lowering blood lead concentration.[26] Unlike IV $CaNa_2EDTA$, however, oral succimer did not have a clinically significant effect on the excretion of essential minerals, including calcium, magnesium, iron, copper, and zinc. Two of the 18 men who received succimer had a mild, transient rise in serum alanine aminotransferase (ALT), but no other adverse effects were noted.

Similar dose-defining study of oral succimer was conducted in 21 children with blood lead concentration of 30–49 µg/dL.[27] 2,3-Dimercaptosuccinic acid is available as microspheres in hard gelatin capsules. For children, the capsules, which contain 1000 mg of succimer, can be opened immediately prior to use and their contents mixed with juice, apple sauce, or ice cream. A 5-day course of 1050 mg/m²/day of succimer in three divided doses daily, was significantly more effective than IV $CaNa_2EDTA$ (1000 mg/m²/day) or lower doses of succimer (350 and 700 mg/m²/day) in lowering blood lead concentration and restoring red cell gamma-aminolevulinic acid dehydratase (ALA-D) activity. The succimer

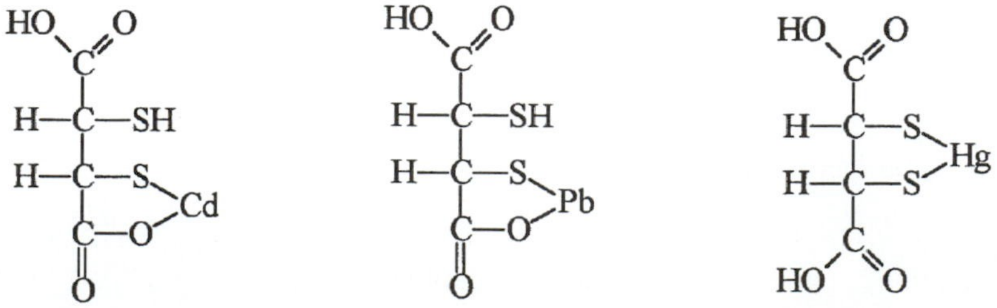

Figure 79–9. The chelation of cadmium, lead, and mercury with succimer (DMSA).

was well tolerated, and no elevations of ALT or other adverse effects were found. The succimer was highly specific for lead and had no effect on the elimination of essential minerals; $CaNa_2EDTA$ caused a clinically significant rise in zinc excretion and lesser rises in copper, iron, and calcium excretion.

A more recent study of oral succimer (1050 mg/m^2/day) in children with moderately severe lead intoxication (50–69 µg/dL) also found an excellent response to succimer, without adverse effects.[20] Results from 19 children treated with oral succimer and 4 children treated with IV $CaNa_2EDTA$ (1000 mg/m^2/day) indicated that succimer is more effective than $CaNa_2EDTA$ in decreasing blood lead concentration, restoring red cell ALA-D activity, and increasing urinary lead excretion. Furthermore, the rebound typically seen early after $CaNa_2EDTA$ treatment was delayed with succimer. A retrospective study of 28 children with low to moderate levels of lead intoxication also supports the short-term efficacy of succimer.[12]

Thus, controlled clinical studies of succimer indicate that a 5-day course of 30 mg/kg/day in adults or 1050 mg/m^2/day in children is safe and effective in treating lead intoxication. As with other chelating agents,[32,46] however, a rebound in blood lead concentration occurs following the completion of the 5-day course.[26,27,29] The lead burden associated with chronic lead ingestion cannot be eliminated in 5 days, nor would it seem wise to attempt to do so. The above-described, ongoing study has established that following a 5-day course of 30 mg/kg/day of succimer, a 14-day course with 20 mg/kg/day in adults or 700 mg/m^2/day in children (but not less) is capable of delaying and blunting the eventual rebound in blood lead concentration.[28] However, the duration of treatment required to prevent the rebound entirely has not yet been established. Because there is relatively little experience with long-term succimer administration, caution should be exercised regarding long-term (>19 days) continuous use.

In addition to controlled trials, several case reports document the safety and efficacy of succimer in adults with chronic lead poisoning.[25,52]

Chelating agents, particularly D-penicillamine, have been known to increase the absorption of lead from the gastrointestinal tract. Pediatricians have therefore been wary of administering D-penicillamine on an outpatient basis. Animal studies indicate that, unlike D-penicillamine, succimer does not increase and may actually decrease the gastrointestinal absorption of lead.[31] A recent human trial also suggests that the use of succimer in children with ongoing lead exposures not only enhanced lead elimination but also reduced total blood lead concentration and ALA-D levels.[45] Obviously, removal of lead from the child's environment should remain the first strategy in the management of lead intoxication. However, in the event of unintentional exposure to a new lead source, concomitant oral succimer should not pose a particular risk.

The published foreign experience with oral succimer for heavy-metal poisoning includes nearly 100 adult cases. At least 74 additional cases have been successfully treated parenterally (IM or IV) with the sodium salt of succimer. These foreign studies add an important dimension to our estimation of efficacy, in that they describe the effectiveness of succimer in extremely severe, life-threatening cases of lead poisoning not evaluated in the controlled studies conducted in the United States. Clinical improvement has been described in many reports.[9,11,21,23] In a series of eight severely lead-poisoned subjects, encephalopathy (2 individuals) and abdominal pain (4 individuals) resolved in all with these symptoms. A 3-day course of oral succimer administered to lead-intoxicated workers showed more than 80% success in disappearance or reduction of a variety of symptoms.[9]

Human and animal studies indicate that succimer is effective for the treatment of arsenic and mercury poisoning as well. Of 53 construction workers who were exposed to mercury vapor, 11 received succimer and *N*-acetyl-*d,l*-penicillamine in a cross-over study.[13] Mercury elimination was increased during the period of succimer administration when compared to the period of *N*-acetyl-*d,l*-penicillamine administration. Since the chelators were administered for only 2 weeks late in the clinical course, therapeutic benefit could not be evaluated. A variety of animal studies have demonstrated succimer's ability to enhance urinary mercury elimination, decrease tissue concentrations, and/or decrease brain mercury levels following exposure to methyl mercury.[1,2,6,38] Embryo lethality was also decreased in pregnant mice given methyl mercury chloride. When succimer was given to victims of an Iraq methyl mercury disaster, blood methyl mercury half-life decreased from 63 days to 10 days.[3] Succimer has been shown to improve survival, decrease kidney damage, and enhance elimination of mercury following inorganic mercury exposure in animals.[3,14,37,47,55] Succimer has been used in China and the Soviet Union since 1965 for arsenic toxicity. Rodent studies also support the beneficial effects of succimer following arsenic exposures, as do a few human case reports.[8,9,17,33,48,49]

Aside from the occasional elevation of serum aspartate aminotranferase (AST) (which may in fact be lead-related), reported adverse effects of oral succimer have been rare and mild, largely confined to abdominal complaints, such as flatus, diarrhea, or pain.[24,39,44] A single patient with severe hyperthermia and hypotension reportedly related to succimer administration has been described.[44] Rarely chills, fever, urticaria, rash, and reversible neutropenia are reported.[16] The Chinese, however, have reported a high incidence of more serious adverse effects (including dizziness and weakness) in response to IV or IM succimer.[54,56] This discrepancy is undoubtedly related to the fact that the oral bioavailability of succimer due to the first-pass hepatic metabolism is relatively low (approximately 20%),[40] and parenteral administration delivers a substantially greater dose. An obvious limitation of our conclusions concerning the safety of succimer is that there is still relatively limited clinical experience with the drug, particularly with regard to long-term administration.

Subhuman primate studies of IV and oral ^{14}C-succimer indicate that following an IV dose, radiolabel is eliminated almost exclusively via the kidney, with only trace amounts (less than 1%) excreted via feces or expired air.[40] Following the administration of a single oral dose of 10 mg/kg, succimer is rapidly and extensively metabolized.[36] Approximately 20% of the administered dose was recovered in the urine, presumably reflecting the quantity of drug absorbed from the gut. Of the total drug eliminated in the urine, 89% was metabolized (as disulfides of *l*-cysteine) and 11% was excreted as free succimer.[36] One mixed disulfide contained one *l*-cysteine residue per succimer molecule, and a second contained two *l*-cysteine residues per succimer molecule. Maximal excretion of succimer occurred in urine specimens collected between 2 and 4 hours after administration.

The pharmacokinetics of a single oral dose of succimer were determined in three children and three adults with lead poisoning and in five healthy adult volunteers.[18] Children received 350 mg/m^2 of succimer and adults received 10 mg/kg of succimer. The peak blood concentration and the time to peak blood concentration of total succimer (parent and oxidized metabolites) was similar for all three groups. The half-life of total succimer was $1\frac{1}{2}$ times longer in the children than in either adult group. The renal clearance of total succimer was greater in healthy adults than in lead-poisoned patients. Distribution of succimer (parent and/or oxidized metabolites) into erythrocytes appeared greater in poisoned patients than in the healthy adults.[18]

The metabolism of succimer was studied in lead-poisoned children and then in normal adults.[10] The results indicate that succimer undergoes an enterohepatic circulation facilitated by GI microflora. This study suggests that a metabolite of succimer is the active chelator. Similar to the previous pharmacokinetic study, moderate lead exposure impaired the renal elimination of succimer.

DMPS (racemic-2,3-dimercapto-1-propanesulfonic acid, Na salt) is an investigational heavy-metal chelator which, like succimer, is a water soluble analog of BAL.[3,6,15] DMPS has been used in the Soviet Union since the late 1950s and is marketed in both oral and parenteral form in Germany as Dimaval. DMPS seems promising in mercury and arsenic poisoning.[3,6,15] More research needs to be done to determine whether DMPS is more advantageous than succimer given its lower LD_{50} in rodents (5.22 mmol/kg vs 16.5 mmol/kg for succimer).

Succimer appears to offer five major advantages over conventional therapy with BAL and $CaNa_2EDTA$: (1) succimer is less toxic, with an LD_{50} of approximately 5000 mg/kg, as compared to 100 and 1000 mg/kg for BAL and $CaNa_2EDTA$, respectively; (2) succimer is orally active and highly effective; (3) succimer is a relatively specific chelator that, unlike $CaNa_2EDTA$, does not induce a substantial elimination of essential minerals such as zinc, copper, and iron; (4) while BAL reportedly can cause hemolysis in patients with G6PD deficiency,[32,46] succimer has been given to two patients with confirmed G6PD deficiency with no resultant hemolysis; and (5) while iron supplementation cannot be given concomitantly with BAL because the BAL–iron complex may be a potent emetic, iron has been given concomitantly to patients receiving succimer without any adverse effects.[30]

The observation that succimer is effective and safe in children receiving concomitant iron supplementation is important. The prevalence of both iron deficiency and elevated blood lead levels is highest among poor, inner-city children.[35] In this group pediatricians are often faced with the need to treat combined lead poisoning and iron deficiency, both of which result in deficits in heme synthesis. As heme is a constituent of all cells, including those of the brain, it appears clinically prudent to provide iron supplementation during chelation therapy, when the heme pathway is freed of the inhibitory effects of lead.

Succimer (Chemet) is available as 100 mg bead-filled capsules. In patients who cannot swallow the capsule whole, the capsule can be separated and sprinked onto a small amount of soft food or put in a spoon and should be followed by a fruit drink. The dosage is 350 mg/m^2 in children three times a day for 5 days followed by 350 mg/m^2 twice a day for 14 days. In adults the dosage is 10 mg/kg in the same regimen as above. Using 10 mg/kg in children rather than dosing based upon body surface area as done during the premarketing trials may result in patient underdosing.[41]

References

1. Aaseth J: Treatment of mercury and lead poisonings with dimercaptosuccinic acid and sodium dimercaptopropanesulfonate. Analyst 1996;120:853–854.
2. Aaseth J, Friedheim EA: Treatment of methyl mercury poisoning in mice with 2,3-dimercaptosuccinic acid and other complexing thiols. Acta Pharmacol Toxicol 1978;42:248–252.
3. Aposhian HV: DMSA and DMPS—Water soluble antidotes for heavy metal poisoning. Annu Rev Pharmacol Toxicol 1983;23:193–215.
4. Aposhian HV, Aposhian MM: Meso–2,3-dimercaptosuccinic acid: Chemical, pharmacological and toxicological properties of an orally effective metal chelating agent. Annu Rev Pharmacol Toxicol 1990;30:279–306.
5. Aposhian HV, Maiorino RM, Dart RC, et al: Urinary excretion of meso–2,3 dimercaptosuccinic acid in human subjects. Clin Pharmacol Ther 1989;45:520–526.
6. Aposhian HV, Maiorino RM, Gonzalez-Ramirez D, et al: Mobilization of heavy metals by newer, therapeutically useful chelating agents. Toxicology 1995;97:23–38.
7. Aposhian HV, Maiorino RM, Rivera M, et al: Human studies with the chelating agents, DMPS and DMSA. J Toxicol Clin Toxicol 1992;30:505–528.
8. Aposhian HV, Mershon MM, Brinkley, Hsu CA: Anti-lewisite activity and stability of meso-dimercaptosuccinic acid and 2,3-dimercapto-1-propanesulfonic acid. Life Sci 1982;31:2149–2156.
9. Aposhian HV, Taklock CH, Moon TE: Protection of mice against the lethal effects of sodium arsenite: A quantitative

comparison of a number of chelating agents. Toxicol Appl Pharmacol 1981;61:385–392.

10. Asiedu P, Moulton T, Blum, et al: Metabolism of meso-2,3-dimercaptosuccinic acid in lead-poisoned children and normal adults. Environ Health Perspect 1995;103:735–739.
11. Bentur Y, Brook JG, Behar R, Taitelman U: Meso-2,3-dimercaptosuccinic acid in the diagnosis and treatment of lead poisoning. J Toxicol Clin Toxicol 1987;25:39–51.
12. Besunder JB, Anderson RL, Super DM: Short-term efficacy of oral dimercaptosuccinic acid in children with low to moderate lead intoxication. Pediatrics 1995;96:683–687.
13. Bluhm RE, Bobbitt RG, Welch LW, et al: Elemental mercury vapour toxicity, treatment, and prognosis after acute, intensive exposure in chloralkali plant workers. I: History, neuropsychological findings and chelator effects. Hum Exp Toxicol 1992;11:201–210.
14. Buchet JP, Lauwerys RR: Influence of 2,3 dimercaptopropane-1-sulfonate and dimercaptosuccinic acid on the mobilization of mercury from tissues of rats pretreated with mercuric chloride, phenylmercury acetate or mercury vapors. Toxicology 1989;54:323–333.
15. Campbell JR, Clarkson TW, Omar MD: The therapeutic use of 2,3-dimercaptopropane-1-sulfonate in two cases of inorganic mercury poisoning. JAMA 1986;256:3127–3130.
16. Committee on Drugs: Treatment guidelines for lead exposure in children. Pediatrics 1995;96:155–160.
17. Cullen NA, Wolf LR, St. Clair D: Pediatric arsenic ingestion. Am J Emerg Med 1995;13:432–435.
18. Dart RC, Hurlbut KM, Maiorino RM, et al: Pharmacokinetics of meso-2,3-dimercaptosuccinic acid in patients with lead poisoning and in healthy adults. J Pediatr 1994;125: 309–316.
19. Devars DuMayne JF, Prevost C, Gaudin B, et al: Lead poisoning treated with 2,3-dimercaptosuccinic acid. Presse Med 1984;13:2209.
20. Fang X, Fernando Q: Synthesis, structure, and properties of *rac*–2,3-dimercaptosuccinic acid, a potentially useful chelating agent for toxic metals. Chem Res Toxicol 1994;7:148–156.
21. Fournier L, Thomas G, Garnier R, et al: 2,3-Dimercaptosuccinic acid treatment of heavy metal poisoning in humans. Med Toxicol Adverse Drug Exp 1988;3:499–504.
22. Friedheim E, DaSilva JR: Treatment of schistosomiasis mansonii with antimony a, a/-dimercapto-potassium succinnate (TWSb). Am J Trop Med Hyg 1954;3:714–727.
23. Friedheim E, Graziano JH, Popovac D, et al: Treatment of lead poisoning by 2,3 dimercaptosuccinic acid. Lancet 1978; 2:1234–1235.
24. Glotzer DE: The current role of 2,3-dimercaptosuccinic acid (DMSA) in the management of childhood lead poisoning. Drug Safety 1993;9:85–92.
25. Grandjean P, Jacobsen IA, Jorgensen PJ: Chronic lead poisoning treated with dimercaptosuccinic acid. Pharmacol Toxicol 1991;68:266–269.
26. Graziano JH: Role of 2,3-dimercaptosuccinic acid in the treatment of heavy metal poisoning. Med Toxicol 1986;1: 155–162.
27. Graziano JH, LoIacono N, Meyer P: A dose-response study of oral 2,3-dimercaptosuccinic acid (DMSA) in children with elevated blood lead concentrations. J Pediatr 1988;113: 751–757.
28. Graziano JH, LoIacono NJ, Moulton T, et al: Controlled study of meso-2,3-dimercaptosuccinic acid for the management of childhood lead intoxication. J Pediatr 1992;120: 133–139.
29. Graziano JH, Siris E, LoIacono N, et al: 2,3-Dimercaptosuccinic acid as an antidote for lead intoxication. Clin Pharmacol Ther 1985;37:431–438.
30. Haust HL, Inwood M, Spence JD, et al: Intramuscular administration of iron during long-term chelation therapy with 3,2-dimercaptosuccinic acid in a man with severe lead poisoning. Clin Biochem 1989;22:189–196.
31. Kapoor SC, Wielopolski L, Graziano JH, LoIacono NJ: Influence of 2,3-dimercaptosuccinic acid on gastrointestinal lead absorption and whole body lead retention. Toxicol Appl Pharmacol 1989;97:525–529.
32. Klaassen CD: Heavy metals and heavy-metal antagonists. In: Gilman AG, Goodman LS, Rall TW, Murad F, eds: Goodman and Gilman's The Pharmacological Basis of Therapeutics, 7th ed. New York, Macmillan, 1985, pp. 1605–1627.
33. Kreppel H, Paepcke U, Thiermann H, et al: Therapeutic efficacy of new dimercaptosuccinic acid (DMSA) analogues in actue arsenic trioxide poisoning in mice. Arch Toxicol 1993; 67:580–585.
34. Lenz K, Hruby K, Druml W, et al: 2,3-Dimercaptosuccinic acid in human arsenic poisoning. Arch Toxicol 1981;47: 241–243.
35. Mahaffey KR: Factors modifying susceptibility to lead. In: Mahaffey KR, ed: Dietary and Environmental Lead: Human Health Effects. New York, Elsevier, 1985, pp. 373–419.
36. Maiorino RM, Bruce DC, Aposhian HV: Determination and metabolism of dithiol chelating agents: VI. Isolation and identification of the mixed disulfides of meso-2,3-dimercaptosuccinic acid with l-cysteine in human urine. Toxicol Appl Pharmacol 1989;97:338–349.
37. Magos L: The effects of dimercaptosuccinic acid on the excretion and distribution of mercury in rats and mice treated with mercuric chloride and methylmercury chloride. Br J Pharmacol 1976;56:479–484.
38. Magos L, Peristianis GC, Snowden RT: Postexposure preventive treatment of methylmercury intoxication in rats with dimercaptosuccinic acid. Toxicol Appl Pharmacol 1978;45:463–475.
39. Mann KV, Travers JD: Succimer, an oral lead chelator. Clin Pharm 1991;10:914–922.
40. McGown EL, Tillotson JA, Knudsen JJ, Dumlao CR: Biological behavior and metabolic fate of the BAL analogues DMSA and DMPS. Proc West Pharmacol Soc 1984;27: 169–176.
41. Mortensen ME: Succimer chelation: What is known? J Pediatr 1994;125:233–234.
42. Ni W, Feng Y, Yu J, et al: A study of oral DMSA in the treatment of lead poisoning. Personal communication, 1989.
43. Okonishnokova IE, Rosenberg EE: Succimer as a means of chemoprophylaxis against occupational poisonings of workers handling mercury. Gig Tr Prof Zabol 1971;15: 29–32.
44. Okose P, Jennis T, Honcharuk L: Untoward effects of oral dimercaptosuccinic acid in the treatment of lead poisoning. Vet Hum Toxicol 1991;33:376. Abstract.

45. Pappas JB, Ahlquist T, Winn P, et al: The effect of oral succimer on ongoing exposure to lead. Vet Hum Toxicol 1992;34:361. Abstract.
46. Piomelli S, Rosen JF, Chisolm JJ Jr, Graef JW: Management of childhood lead poisoning. J Pediatr 1984;105:523–532.
47. Planas-Bohne F: The influence of chelating agents on the distribution and biotransformation of methylmercuric chloride in rats. J Pharmacol Exp Ther 1981;217:500–504.
48. Schafer B, Kreppel H, Reichl FX, et al: Effect of oral treatment with BAL, DMPS or DMSA in organs of mice injected with arsenic trioxide. Arch Toxicol 1991;14(suppl): 228–230.
49. Shum S, Whitehead J, Vaughn L: Chelation of organoarsenate with dimercaptosuccinic acid. Vet Human Toxicol 1995; 37:239–242.
50. Singh PK, Jones MM, Xu Z, et al: Mobilization of lead by esters of meso-2,3-dimercaptosuccinic acid. J Toxicol Environ Health 1989;27:423–434.
51. Thomas G, Fournier L, Garnier R, Dally S: Nail dystrophy and dimercaptosuccinic acid. J Toxicol Clin Exp 1987;7: 285–287.
52. Thomas PS, Ashton C: An oral treatment for lead toxicity. Postgrad Med J 1991;67:63–65.
53. Wang SC, Ting KS, Wu CC: Chelating therapy with NaDMS in occupational lead and mercury intoxication. Chin Med J 1965;84:437–439.
54. Xue H, Ni W, Xie Y, Cao T: Comparison of lead excretion of patients after injection of five chelating agents. Chung Kuo Yao Li Hsuch Pao 1982;3:41–44.
55. Zalups RK: Influence of 2,3-dimercaptopropoane-1-sulfonate (DMPS) and *meso*-2,3-dimercaptosuccinic acid (DMSA) on the renal disposition of mercury in normal and uninephrectomized rats exposed to inorganic mercury. J Pharmacol Exp Ther 1993;267:791–799.
56. Zhang J: Clinical observations in ethyl mercury chloride poisoning. Am J Ind Med 1984;5:251–258.

ANTIDOTES IN DEPTH

Calcium Disodium Edetate

Mary Ann Howland

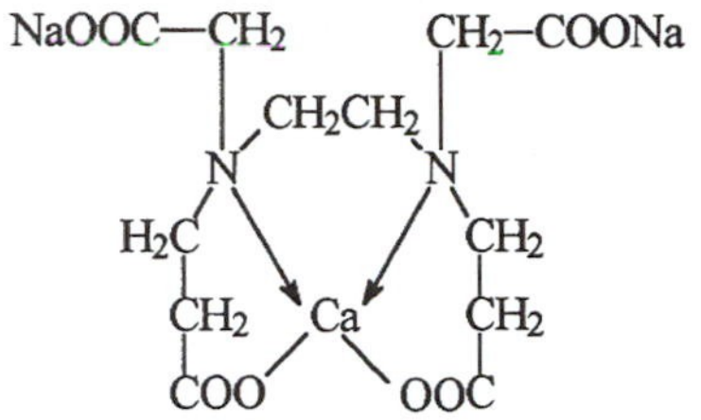

Calcium Disodium EDTA

Calcium disodium edetate (ethylenediamine tetraacetic acid, EDTA; $CaNa_2EDTA$) belongs to the family of polyaminocarboxylic acids. It is capable of chelating many heavy metals, but is used primarily in the management of lead intoxication. The term *chelate* has its origin in the Greek word *chele*, which means "claw," implying an ability to tightly grasp the metal.[25] Implicit in chelation is the formation of a ring-structured complex. When EDTA chelates lead, the calcium is displaced and the lead takes its place, to form a stable-ring compound.[13]

Calcium disodium EDTA is an ionic, freely water-soluble compound. The volume of distribution is small because of its polar nature, approximates that of the extracellular fluid compartment in normal individuals,[13] and is smaller in patients with renal dysfunction (0.05–0.23 L/kg).[18] It therefore appears to penetrate cells such as erythrocytes poorly.[1] Less than 5% of $CaNa_2EDTA$ gains access to the spinal fluid.[13] Oral administration is of limited value due to an oral bioavailability of less than 5%. Renal elimination approximates the glomerular filtration rate,[17] which can be correlated with creatinine clearance[18] and results in 50% of EDTA excreted in the urine in 1 hour and more than 95% in 24 hours.[13] Dosage adjustments are therefore necessary if $CaNa_2EDTA$ is used in patients with renal dysfunction.[17,18] The half-life is about 20–60 minutes.[2,13]

When EDTA combines with lead extracted from soft tissues and body fluids, it forms a stable, soluble, nonionized compound that is subsequently excreted in the urine. Following EDTA administration, urinary lead excretion is increased 20- to 50-fold.

Early treatment with EDTA with or without BAL is capable of preventing the effects of lead on hemoglobin synthesis and in limiting progression of toxicity.[6] Although EDTA has been used for more than two decades, rigorous clinical studies evaluating whether EDTA is capable of reversing the neurobehavioral effects produced by lead are only currently being conducted.[20] A recent study in children with blood lead levels of 25–50 μg/dL given 5 days of EDTA found very little difference in blood lead, bone lead, or erythrocyte protoporphyrin levels, once initial blood lead levels were considered.[15]

The principal toxicity of EDTA is related to the metal chelate. In mice the LD_{50} of various EDTA metal chelates when administered IP are calcium EDTA, 14.3 mmol/kg; lead EDTA, 3.1 mmol/kg; and mercury EDTA, 0.01 mmol/kg.

The site of major toxicity when EDTA is given to patients with lead poisoning is the proximal tubule, although more limited effects are noted in the distal tubule and glomeruli.[13] This toxicity may be caused by the release of lead in the kidneys during excretion.[13] Of 130 children receiving dimercaprol and calcium disodium edetate, 3% developed acute oliguric renal failure, which resolved over time without hemodialysis, and 13% had biochemical evidence of nephrotoxicity.[14] Other studies failed to demonstrate renal failure in over 1000 courses of therapy when EDTA was given at a divided daily dose of 1000 mg/m^2 IV over 1 hour, every 6 hours.[16] Lead intoxication also causes renal damage independent of chelation. It is therefore important to monitor renal function closely during EDTA administration and to adjust the dose and schedule appropriately.[17,18] Nephrotoxicity is limited by keeping total daily doses to 1 g in children or 2 g in adults, although doses may need to be higher in the presence of encephalopathy. Small doses, widely spaced, while maintaining good hydration seem to increase efficacy and decrease toxicity.[17] Other adverse effects include malaise, fatigue, thirst, chills, fever, myalgias, dermatitis, headache, anorexia, urinary frequency and urgency, sneezing, nasal congestion, lacrimation, glycosuria, anemia, transient hypotension, increased prothrombin times, and inverted T waves.[13] Usually reversible mild elevations in ALT and AST and decreases in alkaline phosphatase are frequently reported. Extravasation may result in the development of painful calcinosis at the injection site.[21] Depletion of endogenous metals, particularly zinc, iron, and manganese, may result from chronic therapy.[4,24] A decrease in serum dopamine beta-hydroxylase, a copper-dependent enzyme, occurred after a single injection of calcium disodium edetate in three adult lead welders without any demonstrable decrease in serum copper.[9] The clinical relevance of this is unknown.[9] Since $CaNa_2EDTA$ replaced sodium EDTA as the EDTA preparation of choice, hypocalcemia no longer develops as a clinical problem.

The safety of EDTA is not established in pregnancy, and a risk to benefit analysis must be made if its use is considered. In a model of lead poisoning in pregnant rats, a decrease in fetal resorption and an increase in the number of live fetuses resulted when EDTA was used, although the placental levels of lead were increased.[11] Zinc levels were not affected. Another study, however, found that when calcium EDTA was given to pregnant rats without lead intoxication, increases in submucous clefts, cleft palate, adactyly/syndactyly, curly tail, and abnormal ribs and vertebrae occurred.[3] These teratogenic effects occurred with doses of EDTA comparable to human doses and without causing noticeable changes in the mother except for weight gain. Use of zinc calcium EDTA and zinc EDTA preparations caused no teratogenic effects at low dose but resulted in the development of submucous cleft palates in 30% of the offspring receiving the higher dose of zinc calcium EDTA.[3] This suggests that the incorporation of zinc may be protective in pregnant rats.

Calcium disodium EDTA should be administered IM or IV with careful attention to total fluid requirements in children and patients who have or are at risk for lead encephalopathy[13,19] (see Chap. 79). Procaine sufficient to produce a final concentration of 0.5% is added to the $CaNa_2EDTA$ for IM injection to minimize pain at the injection site (1 mL of a 1% procaine solution for each mL of chelator).[13] The total daily dose of chelator is divided into two or three equal doses spaced 12 or 8 hours apart, respectively. Rapid intravenous infusions may worsen lead encephalopathy associated with cerebral edema and increased intracranial pressure. Calcium disodium EDTA diluted in 250–500 mL of 0.9% sodium chloride or 5% dextrose solution for adults or diluted to < 0.5% solution for children, may be given, by slow infusion of at least 1 hour. EDTA is not compatible with other solutions. Infusion times should be at least 2 hours in symptomatic adults and preferably over 8–24 hours. Concentrations greater than 0.5% may lead to thrombophlebitis and should be avoided. The dose of $CaNa_2EDTA$ is determined by the patient's body surface area or weight (up to a maximum dose) and severity of the poisoning (Chap. 79 and Table 79–10).[6,15,19] Usually the total daily dose of $CaNa_2EDTA$ is administered intravenously as a single prolonged daily infusion over 8–24 hours for up to 5 days, followed by a rest period of at least 2–4 days. The rest period allows time for redistribution of the lead. Before a blood lead concentration is measured, the calcium EDTA infusion should be interrupted for 1 hour to avoid a falsely elevated value. Lead encephalopathy should be treated with a combination of British anti-lewisite (BAL) and $CaNa_2EDTA$.[5] This combination therapy begins with intramuscular BAL. The second dose of intramuscular BAL is given 4 hours later, followed immediately by the $CaNa_2EDTA$ dose. This regimen appears to be more effective than starting $CaNa_2EDTA$ before or with BAL when treating children with acute lead encephalopathy.[15] Calcium disodium edetate alone, without BAL, may promote redistribution of lead from soft tissue to brain.[6,7,8]

There is limited evidence to suggest that folic acid, pyridoxine, and thiamine may increase the antidotal properties of $CaNa_2EDTA$.[22]

The use of EDTA for diagnostic purposes as part of the lead mobilization test has recently come under scrutiny. The authorities cited difficulties with administration, its unreliability as a predictor of total body lead burden, expense, and the potential risks of worsening toxicity through redistribution of lead to either the kidney or brain as reasons to render the EDTA mobilization test obsolete.[6,7] Advocates reason that the EDTA lead mobilization test can be cost saving as it attempts to identify the one third of moderately lead-poisoned children (25–45 μg/dL) who are most able to excrete lead at an enhanced rate.[16] They cite institution of outpatient 6–8-hour protocols as minimizing administration difficulties.[16] Finally, they suggest that the potential risk of redistribution of lead to the brain has only been demonstrated in rats,[7] and is purely theoretical in humans.[16] There are no data to support a detrimental CNS effect of the EDTA challenge test in moderately poisoned children.

Animal studies continue to be performed to investigate the benefits of combining EDTA with succimer (DMSA) and 2,3-dimercapto-1-propane-sulfonic acid (DMPS).[10,12,23] The combination of EDTA with DMSA appears more potent than any individual agent in promoting urine and fecal lead excretion, and decreasing blood and liver lead levels, but this approach may increase nephrotoxicity and zinc depletion.

The treatment of atherosclerosis with disodium EDTA cannot be recommended. Although proponents cite the theoretical benefit of chelating calcium from atherosclerotic plaques, there is no scientific evidence to support this approach. In addition the administration of disodium EDTA can lead to life-threatening hypocalcemia.[1]

Calcium disodium EDTA is available as calcium disodium Versenate in 5-mL ampules containing 200 mg of $CaNa_2EDTA$ per milliliter.[13] Disodium edetate (sodium EDTA) should not be confused with or used instead of calcium disodium edetate because of the risk of life-threatening hypocalcemia.

In summary, EDTA is very effective in the treatment of acute lead poisoning. It is used in conjunction with BAL in patients with lead levels greater than 70 μg/dL and in lead encephalopathy with the first dose of BAL preceding calcium disodium edetate by 4 hours. It is used in chronic lead poisoning and as a diagnostic aid in determining which patients are appropriate for chelation. Both of these uses have recently been questioned, however.[6,8] Recommended doses and dosage schedules should not be exceeded. Patients should be well-hydrated and an adequate urine flow established prior to and maintained during EDTA therapy. Dosage adjustment is necessary when creatinine clearance is reduced.

References

1. Aposhian HV, Maiorinao RM, Gonzalez-Ramirez D, et al: Mobilization of heavy metals by newer, therapeutically useful chelating agents. Toxicology 1995;97:23–38.
2. Bowazzi P, Lanzoni J, Marcussi F: Pharmacokinetic studies of EDTA in rats. Eur J Drug Metab Pharmacokinet 1981;6: 21–26.
3. Brownie CF, Brownie C, Noden D, et al: Teratogenic effect of Ca EDTA in rats and the protective effect of zinc. Toxicol Appl Pharmacol 1986;82:426–443.
4. Cantilena LR, Klaassen CD: The effect of chelating agents on the excretion of endogenous metals. Toxicol Appl Pharmacol 1982;63:344–350.
5. Coffin R, Phillips LJ, Staples WL, et al: Treatment of lead encephalopathy in children. J Pediatr 1966;69:198–206.
6. Committee on Drugs: Treatment guidelines for lead exposure in children. Pediatrics 1995;96:155–160.
7. Cory-Slechta D, Weiss B, Cox C: Mobilization and redistribution of lead over the course of calcium disodium ethylenediamine tetraacetate chelation. J Pharmacol Exp Ther 1994; 13:253–256.
8. Cory-Slechta DA, Weiss B, Cox C: Mobilization and redistribution of lead over the course of calcium disodium ethylenediamine tetraacetate chelation therapy. J Pharmacol Exp Ther 1987;243:804–813.
9. Deparis P, Caroldi S: In vivo inhibition of serum dopamine B hydroxylase by Ca Na_2EDTA injection. Hum Exp Ther 1994;13:253–256.
10. Flora GJS, Seth PK, Prakas A, et al: Therapeutic efficiency of combined meso-2,3-dimercaptosuccinic acid and calcium disodium edetate treatment during acute lead intoxication in rats. Hum Exp Toxicol 1995;14:410–413.
11. Flora SJ, Tandon SK: Influence of calcium disodium edetate on the toxic effects of lead administration in pregnant rats. Indian J Physiol Pharmacol 1987;31:267–272.
12. Flora SJS, Bhattacharga R, Vijayaraghauan R: Combined therapeutic potential of meso-2,3-dimercaptosuccinic acid and calcium disodium edetate on the mobilization and distribution of lead in experimental lead intoxication in rats. Fund Appl Toxicol 1995;25:233–240.
13. Klaassen CD: Heavy metals and heavy metal antagonists. In: Gilman AG, Goodman LS, Rall TW, Murad F, eds: Goodman and Gilman's The Pharmacological Basis of Therapeutics, 9th ed. New York, McGraw-Hill, 1996, pp. 1664–1665.
14. Kumark, N: Reversible nephrotoxic reactions to a combine 2,3 dimercapto–1-propanol and calcium disodium ethylene diaminetetraacetic acid regimen in asymptomatic children with elevated blood lead levels. Pediatrics 1982;70:259–262.
15. Markowitz M, Bijur P, Ruff M, et al: Effects of calcium disodium versenate ($CaNa_2$-EDTA) chelation in moderate childhood lead poisoning. Pediatrics 1993;92:265–271.
16. Markowitz M, Rosen J, Piomelli S, Weinberger H: Personal communication, 1995.
17. Morgan JW: Chelation therapy in lead nephropathy. South Med J 1975;68:1001–1006.
18. Osterloh J, Becker CE: Pharmacokinetics of $CaNa_2$-EDTA and chelation of lead in renal failure. Clin Pharmacol Ther 1986;40:686–693.
19. Piomelli S, Rosen JF, Chisolm JJ Jr, Graef JW: Management of childhood lead poisoning. J Pediatr 1984;105:523–532.
20. Rosen JF, Markowitz ME: Trends in the management of childhood lead poisonings. Neurotoxicology 1993;14: 211–217.
21. Schumacher HR, Osterman AL, Choi SJ, et al: Calcinosis at the site of leakage from extravasation of calcium disodium edetate intravenous chelator therapy in a child with lead poisoning. Clin Orthop 1987;219:221–225.
22. Tandon SK, Flora ST, Singh S: Chelation in metal intoxication: influence of various components of vitamin B complex on the therapeutic efficacy of Ca EDTA in lead intoxication. Pharmacol Toxicol 1987;60:62–65.
23. Tandon SK, Singh S, Jain VK: Efficiency at combined chelation in lead intoxication. Chem Resin Toxicol 1994;7: 585–589.
24. Thomas DJ, Chisolm J: Lead, zinc, copper decorporation during Ca EDTA treatment of lead poisoned children. J Pharmacol Exp Ther 1986;229:829–835.
25. Williams DR, Halstead BW: Chelating agents in medicine. J Toxicol Clin Toxicol 1982–1983;19:1081–1115.

CHAPTER 80

Mercury

Young-Jin Sue

Mercury		
MW		200.59 daltons
Normal levels	blood	<10 μg/L
		< 50 nmol/L
	urine	< 20 μg/L
		<100 nmol/L
Action levels	blood	>35 μg/L
		>175 nmol/L
	urine	>150 μg/L
		>750 nmol/L

Values greater than or equal to the action level necessitate clinical intervention. Values less than this level may necessitate intervention based on the clinical condition of the patient.

A 16-year-old male presented to the emergency department approximately 40 minutes after having intentionally ingested "several teaspoons" of mercuric oxide (HgO) from his chemistry set. On arrival, he was alert and oriented but diaphoretic and vomiting. He complained of midepigastric pain and a metallic taste in his mouth. Initial vital signs were a blood pressure of 130/80 mm Hg, pulse of 110 beats/min, respiratory rate of 18 breaths/min, and temperature of 99.7°F (37.6°C). Physical examination revealed an anxious, somewhat pale young man who was repeatedly vomiting blood-tinged, nonbilious material. He had no respiratory distress or drooling. Other than a grayish discoloration of the buccal mucosa, examination of the oropharynx was unremarkable. The lungs were clear. The cardiac examination was without abnormalities except for a sinus tachycardia. The abdominal examination revealed a nondistended, soft abdomen, moderately tender to deep palpation in the epigastric region; no masses or organomegaly were appreciated. Examination of the rectum revealed no trace of blood. Examination of the skin was unremarkable. The neurologic examination was normal except for mild tremulousness.

The patient was placed on a cardiac monitor and given 1 L of 0.9% sodium chloride solution (IV). Complete blood count (CBC), electrolytes, BUN, creatinine, glucose, prothrombin time (PT), partial thromboplastin time (PTT), and liver function tests were determined to be within normal limits. Blood was obtained for whole blood mercury levels, and the bladder was catheterized to collect urine for 24-hour urine mercury quantitation. Initial urinalysis revealed 2+ proteinuria.

Due to the possible caustic effects of mercuric oxide, endoscopic examination of the upper gastrointestinal (GI) tract was recommended. However, based on this patient's clinical presentation, the treating physician determined that he was at low risk for penetrating mucosal injury. Gastric lavage via nasogastric tube with milk followed by 0.9% sodium chloride solution was performed. After lavage, 1 g/kg of activated charcoal was instilled.

The electrocardiogram (ECG) was normal except for sinus tachycardia. Upright chest and abdominal radiographs revealed no extraluminal air and confirmed the presence of a radiopaque substance scattered throughout the GI tract Figs. 80–1A, B are radiographs of a patient with a similar course. Whole-bowel irrigation with polyethylene glycol electrolyte lavage solution was begun and continued until the rectal effluent which had contained flecks of gross blood returned clear and serial abdominal radiographs confirmed the disappearance of radiopaque densities.

When Should Mercury Poisoning Be Suspected?

Mercury is a complex toxin whose toxicologic manifestations have become known through thousands of years of medicinal applications, industrial use, and environmental tragedies.[44,58] These manifestations vary by route of exposure, the chemical form of mercury involved, and acuity of intoxication. Acute mercury intoxication usually follows either inhalation or ingestion, although rare cases follow parenteral exposure. Acute inhalation of elemental mercury vapor produces respiratory distress and pneumonitis. Ingestion of inorganic mercuric salts results in symptoms of a corrosive gastroenteritis with third-spacing of fluids and gastrointestinal hemorrhage, which may be followed by acute renal failure. Following subacute or chronic exposure to mercury compounds, the predominant findings are neuropsychiatric abnormalities, renal dysfunction, and characteristic dermal manifestations. Acrodynia, thought to be a hypersensitivity reaction to mercury, may occur alone or in combination with the other manifestations of mercury poisoning. The co-existence of neuropsychiatric and renal abnormalities that are otherwise unexplained in an individual should alert the examiner to strongly consider the diagnosis of mercurialism. The presence of an at-risk occupation or access to a mercurial product (Tables 80–1 and 80–2) may alert the examiner to the otherwise unsuspected possibility of mercury as the etiologic agent.

TABLE 80–1. POTENTIAL OCCUPATIONAL EXPOSURES TO MERCURY

Elemental	Salts	Organic
Amalgam makers	Disinfectant makers	Bactericide makers
Barometer makers	Dye makers	Drug makers
Bronzers	Explosives makers	Embalmers
Ceramic workers	Fireworks makers	Farmers
Chlorine workers	Fur processors	Fungicide makers
Dentists	Laboratory workers	Histology technicians
Electroplaters	Tannery workers	Insecticide makers
Jewelers	Taxidermists	Pesticide workers
Mercury refiners	Vinyl chloride makers	Seed handlers
Paint makers		Wood preservative workers
Paper pulp workers		
Photographers		
Thermometer makers		

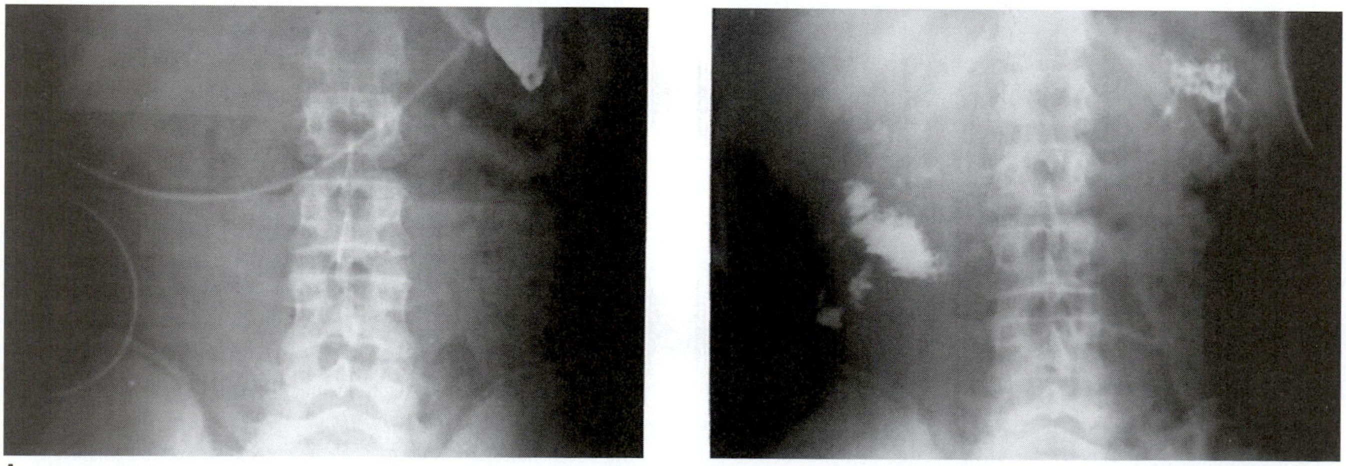

A B

Figure 80–1. A chemist ingested mercuric oxide in a suicide attempt. **A.** Initial plain abdominal radiograph reveals the radiopaque liquid in the stomach. **B.** A second radiograph shows progression of the toxin through the bowel. The patient was followed radiographically as the substance was eventually expelled into the feces.

TABLE 80–2. NONOCCUPATIONAL EXPOSURES TO MERCURY

Medical	Food	Other
Antiseptics	Fish	Button batteries
Calomel teething powders	Grains and seed, treated	Chemistry sets
Dental amalgam	Livestock, fed treated grain	Home amalgam extraction
Diuretics		Lightbulbs
Laxatives		Self-injection
Sphygmomanometers		Preservatives
Stool fixatives		"Magico-religious" use
Thermometers		
Weighted nasogastric tubes		

TABLE 80–3. CLASSES OF MERCURY COMPOUNDS

	Formula	Example
Elemental mercury	Hg^0	Quicksilver
Inorganic mercury salts	Hg^+	Mercurous ion
	HgCl	Calomel
	Hg^{2+}	Mercuric ion
	$HgCl_2$	Mercuric chloride
Organic mercury compounds	Short-chain,	Methyl mercury
	alkyl-mercury compounds	Ethyl mercury
	Long-chain,	Phenylmercury
	aryl-mercury compounds	Methoxyethylmercury

What Is the Pathophysiology of Mercury Poisoning?

Mercury's pervasive disruption of normal cell physiology is believed to arise from its avid covalent binding to sulfur, replacing the hydrogen ion in the body's ubiquitous sulfhydryl groups. Mercury also reacts with phosphoryl, carboxyl, and amide groups, resulting in widespread dysfunction of enzymes, transport mechanisms, membranes, and structural proteins.[34] Mercury deposition has been found in all tissues. Not surprisingly, the clinical manifestations of mercury intoxication involve multiple organ systems with variable features and intensity.

Necrosis of proximal renal tubules, which occurs shortly after mercuric salt intoxication, is thought to result from direct toxic effects of mercuric ions upon the kidney, whereas an immune mechanism is attributed to the membranous glomerulonephritis and acrodynia associated with the use of mercurial ointments.[10,25] Magnetic resonance images of patients with organic mercury poisoning revealed atrophy of the cerebellar hemispheres, postcentral gyri, and calcarine area of the brain. This correlates with the clinical findings of ataxia, sensory neuropathy, and visual field constriction.[36] Neuronal atrophy is especially severe and widespread in victims exposed prenatally.[35,43]

What Are the Forms of Mercury and Their Distinct Kinetic Properties?

With respect to toxicodynamics and toxicokinetics, mercury exists as three important classes of compounds (Table 80–3). These three classes of mercurials produce distinct clinical patterns of intoxication, which stem in part from their individual and combined kinetic features (Table 80–4). Within each class, the specific manifestations are determined by route of intoxication (eg, inhalational, oral, dermal, or parenteral), rate of exposure, distribu-tion and biotransformation within the body, and relative accumulation or elimination from the target organ systems.

Absorption

Elemental mercury gains access to the circulation primarily via inhalation of vapor, although slow absorption following subcutaneous deposition and direct intra-

TABLE 80–4. DIFFERENTIAL CHARACTERISTICS OF MERCURY EXPOSURE

	Elemental	Inorganic (Salt)	Organic (alkyl)
Primary route of exposure	Inhalation	Oral, cutaneous	Oral
Primary tissue distribution	CNS, kidney	Kidney	CNS, kidney, liver
Clearance	Renal, GI	Renal, GI	Methyl: fecal Aryl: renal, fecal
Clinical effects			
CNS	Tremor	Tremor, erethism	Paresthesias, ataxia, tremor, tunnel vision, dysarthria
Pulmonary	+++	–	–
Gastrointestinal	+	+++ (caustic)	+
Renal	+	+++ (ATN)	+
Acrodynia	+	++	–
Therapy	BAL, DMSA	BAL, DMSA	DMSA

venous embolization are reported.[37,47,70] Although metallic mercury is moderately volatile at room temperature, volatilization increases significantly when heated. Vaporization may also be hastened by aerosolization, which occurs when metallic mercury is vacuumed.[22,54] When inhaled by human volunteers, 75–80% of a stable and radioactive mercury vapor mixture was retained.[27,41] Elemental mercury is usually considered nontoxic when ingested because of negligible absorption from normally functioning gut. Abnormal GI motility prolongs mucosal exposure to mercury and increases the degree of biotransformation to a more readily absorbed form. Abnormal GI morphology, eg, fistulae or perforation, may be associated with extravasation of mercury into the peritoneal space.

In contrast, the principle route of absorption for the inorganic salts and organic compounds is the GI tract. Absorption of inorganic mercurial salts occurs following dissociation of ingested soluble divalent mercuric salts such as mercuric chloride ($HgCl_2$). Approximately 10% of such compounds are absorbed from the gut. The absorption of the relatively insoluble monovalent mercurous compounds, such as calomel (HgCl), is thought to depend on oxidation to the divalent form.[34,48] Inorganic mercurials are also absorbed across skin and mucous membranes, as evidenced by urinary excretion of mercury following the dermal application of mercurial ointments and powders.[66] The degree of dermal absorption varies by concentration of mercury, skin integrity, and the lipid solubility of the vehicle. Dermal absorption may be difficult to distinguish from concomitant absorption via other routes.

Organic mercury compounds are well absorbed from the GI tract. Methyl mercury, considered the prototype of the short-chain alkyl compounds, is about 90% absorbed from the gut.[34] Similarly aryl and long-chain alkyl compounds are better absorbed than the inorganic salts, with greater than 50% gastrointestinal absorption reported.[48] Dermal and inhalational absorption is known to occur, though precise quantitation and exclusion of concomitant absorption by ingestion may be difficult to determine.[15,18,68,69]

Distribution and Biotransformation

Once absorbed, mercury distributes widely to all tissues, predominantly the kidneys, liver, spleen, and central nervous system (CNS).[60] The initial distributive pattern of elemental mercury differs from that of the inorganic salts by its relatively high penetration of nervous tissue, enabled by its greater lipid solubility. Although delayed peak levels of elemental mercury are reached in the CNS with respect to other organs (2–3 days vs 1 day),[9] significant accumulation in the CNS may occur following an acute, intense exposure to elemental mercury vapor. Conversion to the charged mercuric cation within the CNS exacerbates retention and local accumulation of the metal.

As Hg^0 (elemental mercury) does not covalently bind to other compounds, its toxicity depends on its oxidation initially to the mercurous ion (Hg^+) then to the mercuric ion (Hg^{2+}). This reaction requires the enzyme catalase (Table 80–5).[41] Since at steady state this oxidation–reduction reaction favors the mercuric cation, the distribution and clinical manifestations of metallic mercury intoxication resemble those of inorganic mercuric salt poisoning during the later stages, following endogenous transformation.[41] Conversely, and to a lesser extent, inorganic mercuric ions are reduced to the elemental state, although the site and mechanism of this reaction are not well understood.[9,48]

Inorganic mercurials are known to undergo organification in marine life (eg, Minamata Bay), but the importance of this conversion in humans is unknown.[15] The greatest concentration of mercuric ions is found in the kidneys, particularly within renal tubules. Very little mercury exists as free mercuric ions. In blood it exists within the red blood cells and bound to plasma proteins in approximately equal proportions. Blood concentration is greatest immediately following inorganic mercury exposure, with rapid waning as distribution to other tissues occurs. Although penetration of blood–brain barrier is poor due to low lipid solubility, slow elimination and prolonged exposure contribute to consequential CNS accumulation of mercuric ions. Within the CNS, mercuric ions are concentrated in the cerebral and cerebellar cortices. Animal studies demonstrate that the placenta functions as an effective barrier to mercuric ions.[48]

Once absorbed, aryl and long-chain alkyl mercury compounds differ from the short-chain alkyl mercurials (ie, methyl mercury) in an important way. The former possess a labile carbon–mercury bond, which is cleaved shortly following absorption, releasing the inorganic mercuric ion. Thus, the distribution pattern and toxicologic manifestations produced by the aryl and long-chain alkyl compounds beyond the immediate postabsorptive phase are comparable to that of inorganic mercurials, but the organification has facilitated absorption. In contrast, methyl mercury possesses a relatively stable carbon–mercury bond, and it is the intact compound believed to be responsible for the profound neurotoxicity associated with methyl mercury exposure. Only a very small proportion is converted to the mercuric cation.[68] Being lipophilic, methyl mercury readily undergoes blood–brain barrier penetration and placento–fetal transfer. An important consequence of these properties is the devastating neurologic degeneration seen in prenatally exposed infants (Minamata disease).

Once in brain tissue, the fate of methyl mercury is uncertain. Animal evidence exists that supports the conversion of methyl mercury to inorganic mercury in brain tissue.[39] In primates fed oral methyl mercury daily for periods exceeding 1 year, those killed within a few days

TABLE 80–5. OXIDATION STATES OF MERCURY

$2Hg^0$ [elemental]	<—catalase—>	$(Hg^+)_2$ (unstable) [mercurous]	<—>	$2Hg^{2+}$ [mercuric]

of termination of exposure had an average brain inorganic mercury fraction of 19%. When the postexposure period was extended to 150–650 days, the inorganic mercury fraction was 88%. Similarly, greater quantities of inorganic mercury relative to total mercury were found in brains of long-term survivors of methyl mercury poisoning.[16] In one patient who survived 22 years following methyl mercury ingestion, autopsy results revealed brain mercury that was nearly completely the inorganic form.

Methyl mercury concentrates in red blood cells to a much greater degree than do mercuric ions, with an RBC to plasma ratio of about 10:1.[48] Despite its relative affinity for nervous tissue and red blood cells, the kidneys and liver are the sites of greatest methyl mercury concentration. The deposition of methyl mercury in hair at concentrations approximately 250 times that found in whole blood has encouraged attempts to quantify degree of exposure to methyl mercury by hair analysis.[23,33,59]

Elimination

Elimination of mercury occurs primarily by urinary and fecal excretion. Mercuric ions are excreted in the kidney by both glomerular filtration and tubular secretion and in the GI tract by transfer across gut mesenteric vessels into feces. Small amounts are reduced to mercury vapor and volatilized from skin and lungs. The total-body half-life of inorganic mercury is estimated at approximately 30–60 days.[41]

In contrast to the mercury salts, the elimination pattern of methyl mercury is predominantly fecal. Enterohepatic recirculation contributes to its somewhat longer half-life of about 70 days. Less than 10% of methyl mercury is excreted in urine and feces as the inorganic divalent or mercuric cation.[68]

What Are the Clinical Syndromes of Mercury Poisoning?

The clinical presentation of mercury poisoning may be characterized by five syndromes:

1. Acute toxicity by inhalation of elemental mercury
2. Acute toxicity by ingestion of mercuric salts
3. Subacute or chronic toxicity by
   a. Delayed or chronic exposure to elemental mercury
   b. Delayed or chronic exposure to inorganic mercury salts
   c. Exposure to aryl and long-chain alkyl mercurials
4. Acrodynia
5. Methyl mercury intoxication

An individual case of mercury poisoning may become manifest as one or more of these syndromes, serially or in combination.

Acute Inhalation of Elemental Mercury Vapor

Symptoms of acute elemental mercury inhalation occur within hours of exposure and consist of cough, chills, fever, and shortness of breath. Gastrointestinal complaints include nausea, vomiting, and diarrhea. These may be accompanied by a metallic taste, dysphagia, salivation, weakness, headaches, and visual disturbances. A chest radiograph during the acute phase may reveal interstitial pneumonitis and both patchy atelectasis and emphysema. Thrombocytopenia is also described during the acute phase.[22,54]

Symptoms may resolve or progress to pulmonary edema, respiratory failure, and death. Survivors of severe pulmonary manifestations may develop interstitial fibrosis and residual restrictive pulmonary disease. The acute respiratory symptoms may coexist with or subsequently lead to the development of subacute inorganic mercury poisoning manifested by tremor, renal dysfunction, and gingivostomatitis. Though elemental mercury toxicity usually results from inhalation of vapor, massive endobronchial hemorrhage followed by death has been reported following direct aspiration of metallic mercury into the tracheobronchial tree.[72]

The workplace threshold limit value (TLV) for mercury vapor is 50 $\mu g/m^3$ for an 8-hour workday, 40-hour work week; the ceiling value (TLV-C) is 100 $\mu g\ Hg/m^3$.[41] A self-limited syndrome of cough, chills, fever, and headache known as "metal fume fever" may follow occupational inhalation of mercury vapor. The lethal dose of inhaled elemental mercury has not been determined due to variability of individual tidal volumes and duration of exposure.

While acute exposure to elemental mercury vapor occurs most commonly in the occupational setting, poisonings due to mishandling of the metal in the home continue to be reported.[30,46,57,61] A number of attempts at home alchemy with metallic mercury have resulted in fatalities. In one case, ambient air concentrations of mercury in the home were found to be as high as 900 $\mu g/m^3$, requiring demolition of the home following futile attempts at decontamination.

Younger individuals may possess greater sensitivity to the pulmonary toxicity of mercury vapor. A case report describes this potential increased risk, although exposure times were not available. A 7-month-old infant and the family's 6-month-old kitten were the first to succumb to fumes generated during attempts to heat metallic mercury on the kitchen stove.[46]

Acute Ingestion of Mercuric Salts

Acute ingestion of mercuric salts produces a characteristic spectrum from severe irritant to caustic gastroenteritis. Immediately, a grayish discoloration of mucous membranes and metallic taste may accompany local oropharyngeal pain, violent nausea, vomiting, and diarrhea. In addition to abdominal pain, hematemesis and hematochezia may develop. The lethal dose has been estimated at 30–50 mg/kg of mercuric chloride.[9] The hallmarks of severe acute mercuric salt ingestion are hemorrhagic gastroenteritis, massive fluid loss resulting in shock, and acute tubular necrosis. In a typical case, a 27-year-old man presented with hematemesis 24 hours after ingesting 6 g of mercuric chloride. Shortly after admission, he developed hypotension and oliguric renal failure. He underwent gastrectomy for total gastric necrosis and was maintained on hemodialysis until the time of his death due to sepsis 3 months later.[53]

Oropharyngeal burns, nausea, hematemesis, hematochezia, and abdominal pain were prominent symptoms in a series of 54 patients who presented after ingesting up to 4 g of mercuric chloride.[62] In this group, a fatal outcome was associated with the early development of oliguria (within 3 days). The development of anuria in these patients appeared to be related to the dose of mercuric chloride ingested. The histopathologic finding of proximal tubular necrosis following mercuric salt intoxication is thought to result both from direct toxicity of mercuric ion upon renal tubules and from renal hypoperfusion due to shock.[25]

Acute ingestion of mercuric salts is usually intentional, but unintentional ingestion occurs sporadically in children as well as adults.[31] Disc batteries and mercury-containing stool preservatives are potential sources of unintentionally ingested inorganic mercury. A 2-year-old girl passed a melanotic stool 2 days after swallowing a mercury-containing disc battery.[42] Abdominal radiograph revealed two battery halves surrounded by radiopaque material in the stomach and proximal gut. Upon surgical removal of the battery fragments, areas of ulceration and bleeding were found in the gastric mucosa. Although ingestion of button batteries containing mercuric oxide is associated with a greater incidence of fragmentation than with other batteries, clinical mercury toxicity by this route has not been reported.[40] Two young children presented with bloody gastroenteritis and proteinuria after ingesting 10–20 mL of a polyvinyl alcohol preservative which contained 4.5% mercuric chloride.[55] One child had a relatively benign course and was discharged following 5 days of oral chelation. The other went on to require dialysis for renal failure but recovered without apparent sequelae. Two adults also developed gastrointestinal toxicity and elevated urine and blood mercury levels following the ingestion of stool fixatives.[65] The need for clear labeling, careful instructions (particularly to non-English-speaking patients) regarding proper use and limitation of availability of these potentially toxic substances must be emphasized.

Chinese patent medicines are yet another source of unintentional inorganic mercury intoxication.[32] Not subjected to FDA regulation and available over the counter, these substances are often inadequately labeled and of variable composition.

Subacute or Chronic Inorganic Mercury Intoxication

Subacute or chronic inorganic mercury intoxication occurs via several routes. In addition to prolonged subacute inhalation of vapor (minimal risk level or MRL for chronic inhalation is 0.06 μg/m^3)[9] or ingestion of inorganic mercuric salts, mercuric ions are formed in vivo by oxidation of elemental mercury and by the dissociation of the carbon–sulfur bonds of organic mercurial compounds, primarily the aryl and long-chain alkyl mercurials. Historically, experience with inorganic mercury toxicity was

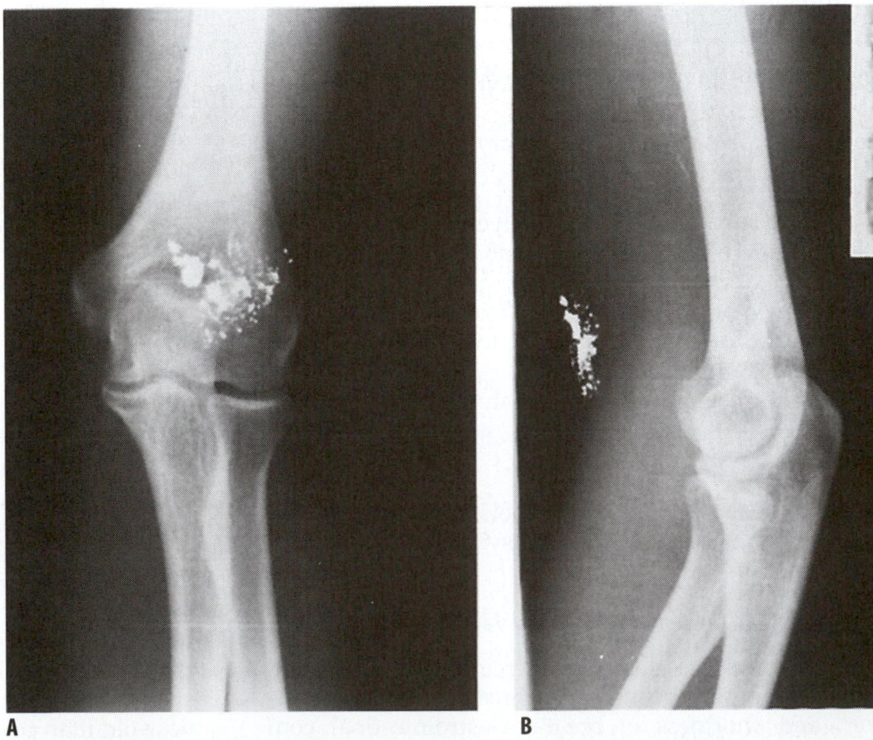

A B

Figure 80–2. A-P **(A)** and lateral **(B)** view of the elbow after an unsuccessful suicidal attempt involving an intravenous injection of mercury in the antecubital fossa. Note extensive mercury deposition, which was partially removed by surgical intervention. *(Courtesy of Diane Sauter, MD.)*

supplied by the medicinal practice of administering mercury-containing powders, ointments, and diuretics.[66] Currently, although inorganic mercury toxicity is primarily a hazard of industrial occupations, slow volatilization of elemental mercury has resulted in toxicity from improper handling of the metal in the home.[45,54,61]

The clinical significance of mercury exposure from dental amalgams for both the dentist and patient has been a point of contention for years. Current thinking debunks the idea that mercury poisoning from dental amalgams occurs. Several comprehensive reviews of the subject agree that (1) dental occupational exposure to amalgam is acceptably low provided that recommended preventive measures are enforced, (2) the quantity of mercury vaporized from dental amalgam by mechanical forces such as chewing is clinically insignificant, and (3) hypersensitivity to mercury amalgam may necessitate removal of the amalgam in rare cases.[17,19,20,21,38,56]

Unusual cases of toxicity have resulted from intentional subcutaneous or intravenous injection of elemental mercury (see Figs. 7–5C and 80–2A,B).[29,47] Aside from management specific to mercury toxicity, local wound care and excision of localized deposits of mercury were additional therapeutic challenges presented by these cases. Unintentional rupture of Cantor tubes used for small-bowel decompression has resulted in substantial exposure (see Fig. 80–3A,B).

The predominant manifestations of subacute or chronic inorganic mercury toxicity include gastrointestinal symptoms, neurologic abnormalities, and renal dysfunction. Gastrointestinal symptoms consist of a metallic taste and burning sensation in the mouth, loose teeth and gingivostomatitis, hypersalivation, and nausea.[66] The neurologic manifestations of chronic inorganic mercurialism are described by the overlapping syndromes of neurasthenia and erethism. Neurasthenia is a symptom complex that includes fatigue, depression, headaches, hypersensitivity to stimuli, psychosomatic complaints, weakness, and loss of concentrating ability. Erethism describes the symptoms of anxiety, emotional lability, irritability, forgetfulness, insomnia, anorexia, weight loss, timidity, and delirium associated with chronic inorganic mercurialism. The mercurial tremor is well described in numerous case reports as a central, intention tremor that

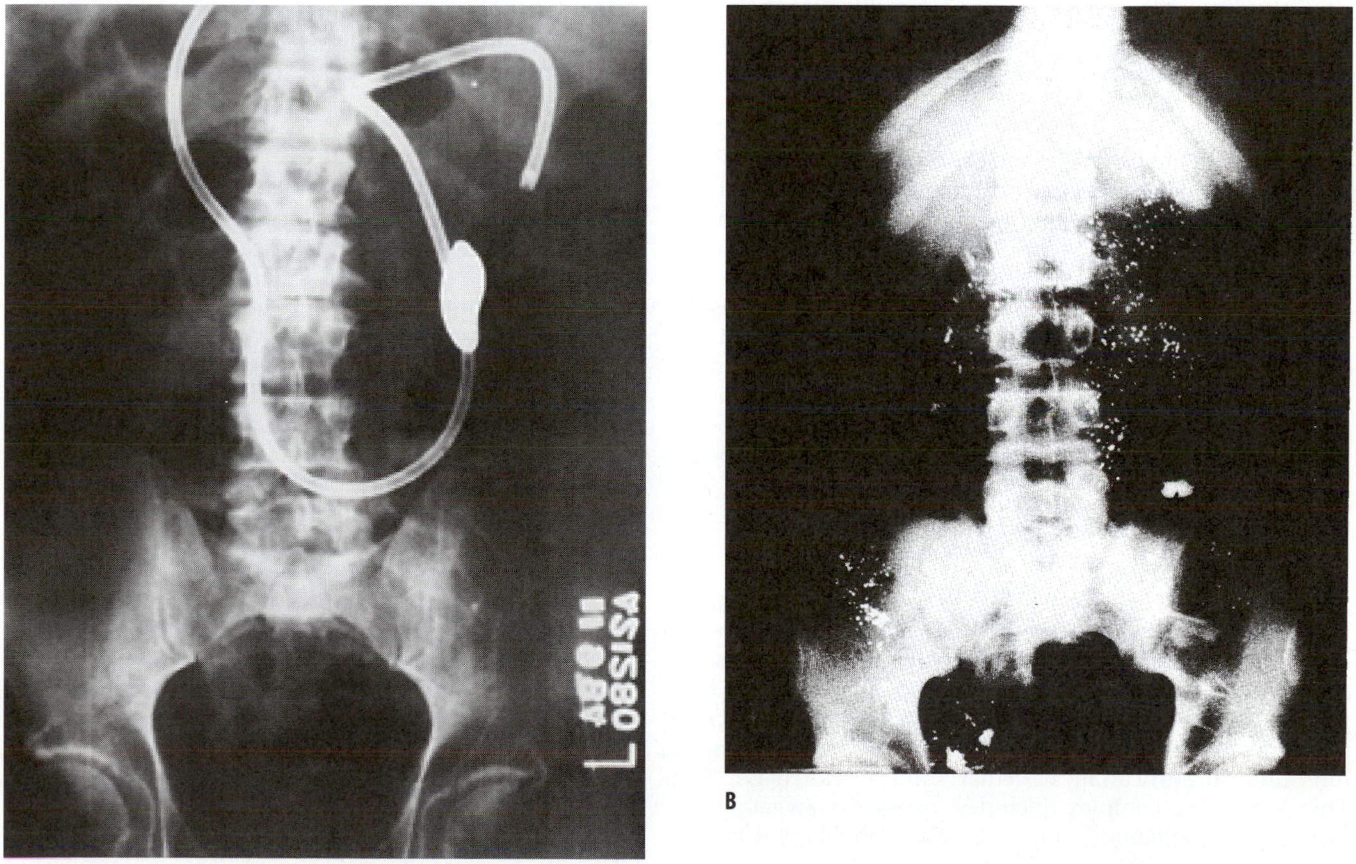

A

B

Figure 80–3. A. An abdominal radiograph with a Cantor tube and mercury contents intact. **B.** An abdominal radiograph demonstrating an accidental rupture of a Cantor tube, which was uneventful as the patient was treated conservatively for a small bowel obstruction (day 3); elemental mercury is found throughout the large bowel with some remaining in the small bowel. *(Courtesy of Richard Lefleur, MD, Associate Professor of Radiology, New York University.)*

is abolished during sleep. These symptoms, which occurred in workers exposed to mercury in the felt hat industry, gave rise to such expressions as the "mad hatter" and the "Danbury shakes" (Danbury, CT, was a U.S. center of felt hat manufacturing).[58] In its most severe form, choreoathetosis and spasmodic ballismus may be present. Other neurologic manifestations of inorganic mercurialism include a mixed sensorimotor neuropathy, ataxia, concentric constriction of visual fields ("tunnel vision"), and anosmia.

In a typical case of domestic exposure to inorganic mercury, two siblings presented with ataxia several weeks after approximately 20 mL of elemental mercury was spilled in their home. Evaluation revealed distal paresthesias, mild weakness, and absent deep tendon reflexes.[61] One child had residual weakness, visual field defects, and emotional lability despite chelation.

Therapeutic application of mercury-containing solutions has also resulted in toxicity. An 18-month-old child with chronic otitis media and bilateral tympanostomy tubes developed neurologic symptoms after receiving a total of 1.2 L of merthiolate (600 mg mercury) over 4 weeks. Although the merthiolate was administered as an ear irrigant, a substantial amount was believed to have been swallowed after draining through the tympanostomy tubes.[51] Merthiolate contains 0.1% thimerosal, an aryl organic mercurial compound (see Chap. 54). Examination of the child revealed irritability, ataxia, tremors, and opisthotonic posturing. Despite chelation with *N*-acetyl penicillamine (NAP), the child died 3 months following hospital admission.

Chronic intoxication with mercuric ions is associated with renal dysfunction, which ranges from asymptomatic, reversible proteinuria to nephrotic syndrome with edema and hypoproteinemia. Renal histology of patients with mercury-associated nephrotic syndrome is suggestive of an immune glomerulonephritis.[10] Postmortem examination of the kidneys of two women who died following chronic abuse of mercurous chloride–containing laxatives revealed severe proximal tubular atrophy and mercury deposition within the cortical interstitium and renal macrophages.[64]

Acrodynia

An idiosyncratic hypersensitivity to mercury is thought to be the underlying pathophysiologic etiology for acrodynia or "pink disease," an erythematous, edematous, and hyperkeratotic induration of the palms, soles, and face and a pink papular rash seen in some children exposed to mercurial powders. The rash is described as morbilliform, urticarial, vesicular, and hemorrhagic.[66] This symptom complex includes excessive sweating, tachycardia, irritability, anorexia, photophobia, insomnia, tremors, paresthesias, decreased deep tendon reflexes, and weakness. The acral rash may progress to desquamation and ulceration. The prognosis is favorable with withdrawal from mercury exposure. Acrodynia was vividly described in 41 children, many of whom had been treated with calomel-containing powders or ointments.[66] The authors observed that the development of acrodynia following exposure to mercury was more common in younger children, did not seem to correlate with dose, and was not necessarily related to urine concentrations of mercury.

The incidence of childhood acrodynia has become uncommon since the use of mercurial teething powders and diaper rinses has been abandoned. Occasional case reports are noted. An 8-year-old child developed acrodynia after playing with elemental mercury for several days.[3] Her symptoms included a scarlatiniform rash, irritability, and myalgias. Particularly striking were the presence of an unremittingly pruritic, vesicular eruption of the hands and feet, profuse diaphoresis which necessitated four or five changes of clothes a day, and the maintenance of a rigid fetal position. Another 23-month-old child developed acrodynia following exposure to mercury from shattered fluorescent light bulbs.[63] A 4-year-old boy developed acrodynia and increased urinary mercury excretion 10 days after the interior of his home was painted with phenyl mercury–containing paint. The paint used was subsequently found to contain approximately three times the concentration of mercury recommended by the Environmental Protection Agency (EPA). In 1990, the EPA banned mercury-containing compounds from interior paints.[2] However, mercury-containing paints manufactured prior to that ruling can still be sold.

Methyl Mercury Intoxication

Methyl mercury is the prototype of the short-chain alkyl mercury compounds and historically the most important, having been implicated in large outbreaks of food-related poisoning in Japan and Iraq. In contrast to the inorganic mercurials, it produces an almost purely neurologic disease that is usually permanent except in the mildest of cases. Methyl mercury accumulates in marine life following the release of both methyl mercury and inorganic mercuric compounds in industrial waste effluent. The latter are biotransformed in marine life to the organic compounds.[15,67] Methyl mercury also finds its way into the environment through its agricultural use as a fungicide.

Although the predominant syndrome associated with methyl mercury is a delayed neurotoxicity, acutely, gastrointestinal symptoms, tremor, respiratory distress, and dermatitis may occur.[15,68] Characteristically, clinical manifestations follow the initial intoxication by a latent period of weeks to months. Consequently, the lethal dose is difficult to determine for methyl mercury. The Agency for Toxic Substances and Disease Registry minimal risk level with respect to developmental effects has been set at 0.04 μg/kg for acute oral exposure.[9] Several properties of methyl mercury may contribute to its profound neurologic effects.[18]

During a decade of contamination of Minamata Bay by a nearby vinyl chloride plant during the 1940s, methyl mercury accumulated in the Japanese bay's marine life and resulted in the poisoning of the local fishing community. Although the initial epidemic listed only 121 victims, over thousands more are believed to have been affected by what has subsequently been described as Minamata disease.[49,60] The most severely affected victims of this outbreak were those infants exposed in utero. Often born to mothers with little or no manifestation of methyl mercury intoxication themselves, these infants exhibited decreased birth weight and muscle tone, profound developmental delay, seizure disorders, deafness, blindness, and severe spasticity. The development of neurologic symptoms in infants exclusively breast-fed by women exposed to methyl mercury after delivery and the detection of mercury in the milk of lactating women is evidence for the risk of mercury intoxication via breast milk.[18,35]

The neurologic manifestations of methyl mercury poisoning correlate with pathologic findings in the brains of both adults and children believed to have been prenatally exposed.[43,60] Grossly, atrophy of the brain was more severe in children, prenatally or postnatally acquired, when compared with the brains of most adult cases. Neuronal necrosis and glial proliferation were most prominent in the calcarine cortex of the cerebrum and in the cerebellar cortex of adult brains. In fetal Minamata disease, similar lesions were present but in a more diffuse and severe form.

The largest outbreak of methyl mercury poisoning occurred in Iraq in late 1971. Approximately 95,000 tons of seed grain treated with methyl mercury intended for planting was baked into bread for direct consumption.[4,13,52] After a latent period of several weeks, cases of paresthesias involving the lips, nose, and distal extremities began to appear. These patients also noted headaches, fatigue, and tremor. More serious cases progressed to ataxia, dysarthria, visual field constriction, and blindness. Other neurologic deficits included hyperreflexia, hearing disturbances, movement disorders, salivation, and dementia. The most severely affected patients lay in a mute rigid posture altered only by spontaneous crying, primitive reflexive movements, or feeding efforts.[52] By the spring of 1972, the mass poisoning had resulted in 6530 hospital admissions and 459 hospital deaths. While the outlook for methyl mercury neurotoxicity is generally considered dismal, observations over the subsequent two years of 49 Iraqi children poisoned during the 1971 outbreak showed complete resolution or at least partial improvement in all but the most severely affected.[4] Of 40 symptomatic children, 33 mildly to severely affected children showed some to complete resolution of symptoms. The 7 children classified as "very severely poisoned" remained physically and mentally incapacitated.

While neurologic disease is by far the dominant manifestation of methyl mercury poisoning, dermatitis, electrocardiographic abnormalities (ST segment changes), and renal tubular dysfunction have been associated with this form of toxic exposure.[18,28]

Initial Management of the Mercury-Poisoned Patient

After initial assessment and stabilization, the early toxicologic management of mercury poisoning includes termination of exposure (removal from vapors, washing exposed skin, gastrointestinal decontamination), supportive measures (hydration, humidified oxygen), baseline diagnostic studies (serum laboratories, radiographs, electrocardiogram), consideration of co-intoxicants, and meticulous monitoring.

Mercury spilled onto solid surfaces should be adsorbed to sand or, ideally, the contents of a mercury decontamination kit. The resulting mixture should then be swept into tightly covered containers. The decontamination kits contain a compound such as calcium polysulfide which, containing excess sulfur, converts mercury to the water-insoluble mercuric sulfide. Absorbable surfaces such as carpets should be removed. Vacuuming spilled mercury compounds could volatilize the substances and should be avoided.[12] Decontamination of major spills and disposal of materials should be guided by the local Hazardous Materials Agency.

Inhalation of mercury vapors or aspiration of metallic mercury may result in life-threatening respiratory failure, and stabilization of cardiorespiratory function is the initial priority. Postural drainage and endotracheal suction may be effective in removing aspirated metallic mercury. Ingestion of inorganic mercuric salts may likewise lead to cardiovascular collapse due to severe gastroenteritis and third-space fluid loss. Parenteral deposition of subcutaneous or intramuscular mercury may be amenable to surgical excision if well localized (see Fig. 80–2A,B)

Gastrointestinal decontamination of ingested inorganic salts of mercury is particularly problematic because of the salts' caustic nature and risk for perforating injury. Endoscopic examination of the upper gastrointestinal tract may be considered prior to attempts at gastric emptying and lavage. Several series of mercuric chloride poisoning, however, report recovery without long-term gastrointestinal sequelae in patients who do not succumb to renal failure.[62] Therefore, unless there is high suspicion for penetrating gastrointestinal mucosal injury, removal of mercury from absorptive surfaces should take priority.

Lavage with protein-containing solutions such as milk or egg whites has been advocated with the belief that mercury may be bound to the administered proteins and thereby be more readily removed by subsequent lavage.[7] While this has not been rigorously studied, it is probably not harmful and may be of benefit. Heavy metals are among the substances that are not well adsorbed to activated charcoal. Nevertheless, the serious nature of late sequelae following mercury absorption, the typically small quantities of mercury ingested, and evidence that mercuric compounds have substantial adsorption to activated charcoal (800 mg mercuric chloride to 1 g activated charcoal in one in vitro study) justify administration of the adsorbent.[5] Whole-bowel irrigation with polyethylene glycol solution may be useful in removing residual mercury as revealed by serial radiographs.

How Can a Diagnosis of Mercury Poisoning Be Confirmed?

Occupational or environmental exposure and a consistent clinical picture may be suggestive of mercury poisoning, but demonstration of mercury in blood, urine, or tissues is necessary for confirmation of exposure. Of the many methods available to measure mercury, cold atomic absorption spectrometry is rapid, sensitive, and accurate. Thin-layer and gas chromatographic techniques can be used to distinguish organic from inorganic mercury.[15] Blood should be collected into a trace-element collection tube obtained from the laboratory performing the assay. Urine should be collected for 24 hours into an acid-washed container obtained from the laboratory. Attempts to measure or otherwise handle the specimen should be avoided to prevent contamination.

There is considerable overlap among concentrations of mercury found in the normal population, asymptomatic exposed individuals, and patients with clinical evidence of poisoning. There is no definitive correlation between blood and urine mercury levels with mercury toxicity.[9,23] However, mercury is virtually undetectable in the nonpoisoned individual, and levels less than 10 μg/L and 20 μg/L for whole blood and urine, respectively, are generally considered normal. Following long-term exposure to mercury vapor, levels as low as 35 μg/L for blood and 150 μg/L for urine may be associated with nonspecific symptoms.[24]

Urine mercury levels may correlate roughly with exposure severity and neuropsychiatric symptoms associated with inorganic mercury poisoning,[9,50] but the relationship to total body burden is probably poor. Urine mercury values have their greatest utility in confirming exposure and monitoring the efficacy of chelation therapy. Because of the very minimal urinary excretion of methyl mercury, urine mercury levels are not useful in evaluating methyl mercury intoxication. Blood levels may acutely reflect inorganic mercury load but become less reliable as redistribution to tissues takes place. Due to the relative concentration of methyl mercury in red blood cells, total body methyl mercury burden may be best reflected by blood levels.[15] Correlation of increasing blood mercury levels with prevalence of paresthesias was suggested in a population of Iraqis studied early in the course of methyl mercury poisoning.[14] Unfortunately, in another group of patients, blood levels were not found to correlate with severity of methyl mercury poisoning.[52] This apparent discrepancy is not difficult to accept considering that paresthesias are among the earliest reported symptoms of methyl mercury poisoning. Blood levels may well reflect the acute body burden of methyl mercury. As methyl mercury distributes to and accumulates in brain, the severity of clinical manifestations probably reflects the degree of the irreversible neuronal destruction that has taken place rather than the current body burden of mercury.

Since mercury accumulates in hair, efforts to develop hair analysis as a useful tool for measuring mercury burden have been attempted. Its utility has been criticized as being limited by the fact that metal incorporation reflects past exposure and that hair avidly binds mercury from the environment. Nevertheless, a number of authors support its utility.[33] One analysis comparing organic mercury concentrations in distal scalp hair and organs of cadavers demonstrated significant correlation, with correlation coefficients ranging from 0.59 to 0.82 for the cerebrum and 0.65 to 0.76 for the kidney.[59] The hair was prepared by washing in a nonionic detergent and acid digestion.

In addition to mercury assays, neuropsychiatric testing, nerve conduction studies and urine assays for *N*-acetyl β-D-glucosaminidase and beta-2-microglobulin are advocated for early detection of subclinical inorganic and organic mercury intoxication.[20,28,50]

What Is the Specific Treatment of Mercury Poisoning?

After initial stabilization and decontamination (see Initial Management), the early institution of chelating agents may minimize or prevent the widespread toxicity of mercury, which results from its affinity for essential cellular sulfhydryl groups. A high degree of protein binding and distribution to the brain are responsible for the lack of efficacy of other measures such as peritoneal dialysis and hemodialysis to increase mercury clearance.[53] However, hemodialysis may be necessitated by the acute renal failure that often follows mercuric chloride poisoning.

Chelating agents themselves have thiol groups that are believed to compete with endogenous sulfhydryl groups for the binding of mercury and thereby prevent inactivation of sulfhydryl-containing enzymes and other essential proteins (see Antidotes in Depth: BAL and Antidotes in Depth: Succimer for further discussion). A history of significant exposure and the presence of typical symptoms are indications for the institution of chelation therapy. Elevated blood and urine mercury concentrations are contributory and can help in the decision to begin chelation therapy in unclear cases and may be used to guide duration of therapy.

For clinically significant acute inorganic mercury intoxication, dimercaprol (BAL) may be administered for 10 days in decreasing dosages, eg, 5 mg/kg IM once, 2.5 mg/kg IM every 8–12 hours for 1 day, then 2.5 mg/kg IM every 12–24 hours thereafter until clinically improved.[34] This dosing regimen, which was derived from its application in lead poisoning, may be adjusted according to clinical response and occurrence of adverse reactions. Animal evidence suggests that BAL may increase mercury concentrations in brain. However, phenylmercury and BAL were administered simultaneously. It is unclear whether the increased brain mercury represents altered distribution due to a phenylmercury–BAL complex or BAL-driven redistribution of inorganic mercury.[11] When the patient is able to take oral medications, therapy may be augmented with 2,3-dimercaptosuccinic acid (DMSA) at 10 mg/kg po three times a day for 5 days. Adverse effects such as headache, nausea, vomiting, abdominal pain, and diaphoresis may result from both the primary ingestion as well as the chelation therapy itself, especially with BAL. Psychiatric intervention should be initiated during the recovery period. In a patient who is not acutely ill or has been chronically poisoned, initiation of therapy with oral DMSA is recommended.

D-Penicillamine (DPCN) is an orally administered monothiol whose adverse effects include gastrointestinal distress, rashes, leukopenia, thrombocytopenia, and proteinuria. Though seen uncommonly in therapeutic doses, these adverse effects are felt by many to seriously limit the utility of the drug. The use of DPCN has been supplanted by the availability of DMSA. The DPCN–mercury chelation compound is excreted exclusively into urine; thus other agents should be utilized in the event of renal failure. DPCN is available as 125-mg and 250-mg capsules and is administered in 4 daily divided doses totaling 20–30 mg/kg (250 mg qid for adults). The duration of therapy should be guided by serial 24-hour urine mercury levels and clinical evaluation.[34] Should prolonged therapy be required, it has been recommended that treatment courses of 1–2 weeks should alternate with brief interruptions to minimize the risk for adverse reactions. *N*-Acetyl-*d,l*-penicillamine (NAP), an investigational analog of DPCN, has been used with variable success for mercury poisoning.[8,26] It is thought to be a superior chelator of mercury than DPCN perhaps due to its greater stability.[6,34] The penicillamines should be administered only after complete gastrointestinal decontamination, as the absorption of mercury may theoretically be enhanced following chelation by penicillamine.

The neurotoxicity of methyl mercury is relatively resistant to treatment, and the optimum mode of therapy is not clear. In rats treated with BAL or DPCN following injection with methyl mercury, both agents were effective at reducing tissue mercury and preventing neurologic toxicity when administered within the first day following methyl mercury injection.[71] However, neither agent produced reversal of neurologic toxicity when administered 12 days after injection of methyl mercury despite a decrease of tissue mercury in rats treated with DPCN. 2,3-Dimercapto-1-propanesulphonate (DMPS), an investigational water-soluble analog of BAL, led to a striking reduction of blood half-life of mercury, ie, 60 days vs 10 days, when compared with DPCN, NAP, and a thiolated resin (half-lives of 24 days, 23 days, and 19 days, respectively) during the outbreak of methyl mercury poisoning in Iraq in 1971.[14] Clinical improvement was not observed in any treatment group, but it is reasonable to postulate that reducing the total body burden of methyl mercury may prevent or limit progression of disease. When studied in mice poisoned with methyl mercury,[1] DMSA was found to be superior to NAP, DMPS, and a thiolated resin in decreasing brain mercury and increasing urinary excretion. Brain mercury was decreased to 35% of control, and total body burden fell to 19%. A nonabsorbed polythiol resin may reduce the elimination half-life of methyl mercury, presumably by interrupting its enterohepatic reabsorption.[14,18]

As the neurologic impairment associated with methyl mercury is both profound and essentially irreversible, early recognition of poisoning and prevention of neurotoxicity are critical. Although further investigation is necessary, DMSA may prove to be the treatment of choice for methyl mercury poisoning because of its apparently low toxicity and reported efficacy in animal trials. Mercury is a complex toxicologic problem with immensely varying clinical presentations. An ever-present awareness coupled with the knowledge of its differing physical forms may serve to guide recognition of is occurrence. Although some chelating agents show promise in the treatment of mercury poisoning, neurologic sequelae, particularly of organic mercury, remain a largely irreversible problem. Prevention of mercury intoxication and public education regarding the dangers of mercury deserve equal consideration in the allocation of resources dedicated to mercury research.

References

1. Aaseth J, Friedheim EAH: Treatment of methyl mercury poisoning in mice with 2,3-dimercaptosuccinic acid and other complexing thiols. Acta Pharmacol Toxicol 1978;42: 248–252.
2. Agocs MM, Etzel RA, Parrish G, et al: Mercury exposure from interior latex paint. N Engl J Med 1990;323: 1096–1100.
3. Alexander JF, Rosario R: A case of mercury poisoning: Acrodynia in a child of 8. Can Med Assoc J 1971;104:929–930.
4. Amin-Zaki L, Majeed MA, Clarkson TW, Greenwood MR: Methylmercury poisoning in Iraqi children: Clinical observations over two years. Br Med J 1978;1:613–616.
5. Andersen AH: Experimental studies on the pharmacology of activated charcoal; III. Adsorption from gastrointestinal contents. Acta Pharmacol 1948;4:275–284.
6. Aposhian HV, Aposhian MM: *N*-acetyl-*d,l*-penicillamine, a new oral protective agent against the lethal effects of mercuric chloride. J Pharmacol 1959;126:131–135.
7. Arena JM: Treatment of mercury poisoning. Mod Treat 1971;8:619–625.
8. Aronow R, Fleischmann LE: Mercury poisoning in children. Clin Pediatr 1976;15;936–945.
9. ATSDR: Toxicologic profile for mercury. Atlanta, GA, USDHHS, 1992. Draft.
10. Becker CG, Becker EL, Maher JF, Schreiner GE: Nephrotic syndrome after contact with mercury. Arch Intern Med 1962;110:178–186.
11. Berlin M, Rylander R: Increased brain uptake of mercury induced by 2,3-dimercaptopropanol (BAL) in mice exposed to phenylmercuric acetate. J Pharmacol Exp Ther 1964;146: 236–240.
12. Campbell D, Gonzales M, Sullivan JB: Mercury. In: Sullivan JB, Krieger GR, eds: Hazardous Material Toxicology. Baltimore, Williams & Wilkins, 1992, pp. 824–833.
13. Clarkson TW, Amin-Zaki L, Al-Tikriti SK: An outbreak of methylmercury poisoning due to consumption of contaminated grain. Fed Proc 1976;35:2395–2399.
14. Clarkson TW, Magos L, Greenwood MR, et al: Tests of efficacy of antidotes for removal of methylmercury in human

poisoning during the Iraq outbreak. J Pharmacol Exp Ther 1981;218:74–83.
15. Dales LG: The neurotoxicity of alkyl mercury compounds. Am J Med 1972;53:219–232.
16. Davis LE, Kornfeld M, Mooney HS, et al: Methylmercury poisoning: Long-term clinical, radiological, toxicological, and pathological studies of an affected family. Ann Neurol 1994;35:680–688.
17. Eley BM, Cox SW: Mercury from dental amalgam fillings in patients. Br Dent J 1987;163:221–225.
18. Elhassani SB: The many faces of methylmercury poisoning. J Toxicol Clin Toxicol 1982–1983;19:875–906.
19. Englund GS, Dahlquist R, Lindelof B, et al: DMSA administration to patients with alleged mercury poisoning from dental amalgams—A placebo controlled study. J Dent Res 1994;73:620–628.
20. Eti S, Weisman RS, Hoffman RS, Reidenberg MM: Slight renal effect of mercury amalgam fillings. Pharmacol Toxicol 1995;76:47–49.
21. Fung YK, Molvar MP: Toxicity of mercury from dental environment and from amalgam restorations. J Toxicol Clin Toxicol 1992;30:49–61.
22. Fuortes LJ, Weismann DN, Graeff ML, et al: Immune thrombocytopenia and elemental mercury poisoning. J Toxicol Clin Toxicol 1995;33:449–455.
23. Gosselin RE, Smith RP, Hodge HC: Mercury. In: Gosselin RE, Smith RP, Hodge HC, eds: Clinical Toxicology of Commercial Products, 5th ed. Baltimore, Williams & Wilkins, 1984, pp. 262–275.
24. Goyer RA: Toxic effects of metals. In: Amdur MO, Doull J, Klaassen CD, eds: Casarett and Doull's Toxicology: The Basic Science of Poisons, 4th ed. New York, Pergamon Press, 1991, pp. 623–680.
25. Hewitt WR, Goldstein RS, Hook JB: Toxic responses of the kidney. In: Amdur MO, Doull J, Klaassen CD, eds: Casarett and Doull's Toxicology: The Basic Science of Poisons, 4th ed. New York, Pergamon Press, 1991, pp. 354–382.
26. Hryhorczuk DO, Meyers L, Chen G: Treatment of mercury intoxication in a dentist with *N*-acetyl-*d,l*-penicillamine. Clin Toxicol 1982;19:401–408.
27. Hursh JB, Clarkson TW, Cherian MG, et al: Clearance of mercury (Hg-197, Hg-203) vapor inhaled by human subjects. Arch Environ Health 1976;31:302–309.
28. Iesato K, Wakashin M, Wakashin Y, Tojo S: Renal tubular dysfunction in Minamata disease: Detection of renal tubular antigen and beta-2-microglobulin in the urine. Ann Intern Med 1977;86:731–737.
29. Johnson HRM, Koumides O: Unusual case of mercury poisoning. Br Med J 1967;1:340–341.
30. Jung RC, Aaronson J: Death following inhalation of mercury vapor at home. West J Med 1980;132:539–543.
31. Kahn A, Denis R, Blum D: Accidental ingestion of mercuric sulphate in a 4-year-old child. Clin Pediatr 1977;16:956–958.
32. Kang-Yum E, Oransky SH: Chinese patent medicine as a potential source of mercury poisoning. Vet Hum Toxicol 1992;34:235–238.
33. Katz SA, Katz RB: Use of hair analysis for evaluating mercury intoxication of the human body: A review. J Appl Toxicol 1992;12:79–84.
34. Klaassen C: Heavy metals and heavy-metal antagonists. In: Gilman AG, Rall TW, Nies AS, Taylor P, eds: Goodman and Gilman's The Pharmacological Basis of Therapeutics, 8th ed. New York, Pergamon Press, 1990, pp. 1592–1614.
35. Koos BJ, Longo LD: Mercury toxicity in the pregnant woman, fetus, and newborn infant: A review. Am J Obstet Gynecol 1976;126:390–409.
36. Korogi Y, Takahashi M, Shinzato J, Okajima T: MR findings in seven patients with organic mercury poisoning (Minamata disease). Am J Neuroradiol 1994;15:1575–1578.
37. Krohn IT, Solof A, Mobini J, Wagner DK: Subcutaneous injection of metallic mercury. JAMA 1980;243:548–549.
38. Langan DC, Fan PL, Hoos AA: The use of mercury in dentistry: Critical review of the recent literature. J Am Dent Assoc 1987;115:867–879.
39. Lind B, Friberg L, Nylander M: Preliminary studies on methylmercury biotransformation and clearance in the brain of primates: II. Demethylation of mercury in brain. J Trace Elements Exp Med 1988;1:49–56.
40. Litovitz T, Schmitz BF: Ingestion of cylindrical and button batteries: An analysis of 2382 cases. Pediatrics 1992;89: 747–757.
41. Magos L. Mercury. In: Seiler HG, Sigel H, eds: Handbook on Toxicity of Inorganic Compounds. New York, Marcel Dekker, 1988, pp. 419–436.
42. Mant TGK, Lewis JL, Mattoo TK, et al: Mercury poisoning after disc-battery ingestion. Hum Toxicol 1987;6:179–181.
43. Matsumoto H, Koya G, Takeuchi T: Fetal Minamata disease: A neuropathological study of two cases of intrauterine intoxication by a methyl mercury compound. J Neuropathol Exp 1964;24:563–574.
44. Maurissen JPJ: History of mercury and mercurialism. NY State J Med 1981;81:1902–1909.
45. Mortensen ME, Powell S, Sferra TJ: Elemental mercury poisoning in a household. MMWR 1990;39:424–425.
46. Moutinho ME, Tompkins AL, Rowland TW, et al: Acute mercury vapor poisoning. Am J Dis Child 1981;135:42–44.
47. Murray KM, Hedgepeth JC: Intravenous self-administration of elemental mercury: Efficacy of dimercaprol therapy. Drug Intel Clin Pharm 1988;22:972–975.
48. Nordberg GF, Skerfving S: Metabolism. In: Friberg L, Vostal J, eds: Mercury in the Environment: An Epidemiological and Toxicological Appraisal. Cleveland, OH, CRC Press, 1972, pp. 29–90.
49. Powell PP: Minamata disease: A story of mercury's malevolence. South Med J 1991;84:1352–1358.
50. Rosenman KD, Valciukas JA, Glickman L, et al: Sensitive indicators of inorganic mercury toxicity. Arch Environ Health 1986;41:208–215.
51. Royhans J, Walson PD, Wood GA, MacDonald WA: Mercury toxicity following merthiolate ear irrigations. J Pediatr 1984;104:311–313.
52. Rustam H, Hamdi T: Methyl mercury poisoning in Iraq. Brain 1974;97:499–510.
53. Sauder PH, Livardjani F, Jaeger A, et al: Acute mercury chloride intoxication: Effects of hemodialysis and plasma exchange on mercury kinetic. J Toxicol Clin Toxicol 1988;26: 189–197.
54. Schwartz JG, Snider TE, Montiel MM: Toxicity of a family from vacuumed mercury. Am J Emerg Med 1992;10: 258–261.
55. Seidel J: Acute mercury poisoning after polyvinyl alcohol preservative ingestion. Pediatrics 1980;66:132–134.

56. Snapp KR, Boyer DB, Peterson LC, Svare CW: The contribution of dental amalgam to mercury in blood. J Dent Res 1989;68:780–785.
57. Snodgrass W, Sullivan JB, Rumack BH, Hashimoto C: Mercury poisoning from home gold ore processing. JAMA 1981;246:1929–1931.
58. Sunderman FW: Perils of mercury. Ann Clin Lab Sci 1988; 18:89–101.
59. Suzuki T, Hongo T, Yoshinaga J, et al: The hair-organ relationship in mercury concentration in contemporary Japanese. Arch Environ Health 1993;48:221–229.
60. Takeuchi T: Pathology of Minamata disease. Acta Pathol Jpn 1982;32:73–99.
61. Taueg C, Sanfilippo DJ, Rowens B, et al: Acute and chronic poisoning from residential exposures to elemental mercury—Michigan, 1989–1990. J Toxicol Clin Toxicol 1992;30:63–67.
62. Troen P, Kaufman SA, Katz KH: Mercuric bichloride poisoning. N Engl J Med 1951;244:459–463.
63. Tunnessen WW, McMahon KJ, Baser M: Acrodynia: Exposure to mercury from fluorescent light bulbs. Pediatrics 1987;79:786–789.
64. Wands JR, Weiss SH, Yardley JH, Maddrey WC: Chronic inorganic mercury poisoning due to laxative abuse. Am J Med 1974;57:92–101.
65. Wang RY, Henry GC, Fine J, et al: Mercuric chloride poisonings from stool fixative ingestion. Vet Hum Toxicol 1992;34:341. Abstract.
66. Warkany J, Hubbard DM: Adverse mercurial reactions in the form of acrodynia and related conditions. Am J Dis Child 1951;81:335–373.
67. Wheatley B, Barbeau A, Clarkson TW, Lapham LW: Methylmercury poisoning in Canadian Indians—The elusive diagnosis. Can J Neurol Sci 1979;6:417–422.
68. Winship KA: Organic mercury compounds and their toxicity. Adv Drug React Ac Pois Rev 1986;3:141–180.
69. Yeh TF, Pildes RS, Firor HV: Mercury poisoning from mercurochrome treatment of an infected omphalocele. Clin Toxicol 1978;13:463–467.
70. Yotsuyanagi T, Yokoi K, Sawada Y: Facial injury by mercury from a broken thermometer. J Trauma Injury Infect Crit Care 1996;40:847–849.
71. Zimmer LJ, Carter DE: The effect of 2,3-dimercaptopropanol and D-penicillamine on methyl mercury induced neurological signs and weight loss. Life Sci 1978;23: 1025–1034.
72. Zimmerman JE: Fatality following metallic mercury aspiration during removal of a long intestinal tube. JAMA 1969; 208:2158–2160.

CHAPTER 81

Cadmium and Other Metals and Metalloids

Robert J. Nadig

A 35-year-old male welder felt weak and dizzy but finished his shift and went home after brazing for an estimated maximum of 2.5 hours of the 6.5 hours he worked that day. He did not return to work because he developed severe cough and chest pain, in addition to shortness of breath, increased malaise, and fever. He attributed his symptoms to welder's fever (metal fume fever). When he saw a physician 1 day later, a diagnosis of "chemical bronchitis" was made and antibiotics and a cough suppressant were given. The next day, the fourth day of his illness, he was found dead sitting up in his bedroom.[25,26] The cause of death was determined to be noncardiogenic pulmonary edema secondary to cadmium chemical pneumonitis.

How Is a Differential Diagnosis Regarding Exposure to Various Heavy Metals Formulated?

The term "heavy metal" is historically used to describe elements such as lead, mercury, arsenic, cadmium, and chromium. In fact, many metals and metalloids are often loosely considered together with the traditional heavy metals and are often grouped together as a single category during the initial refinement of a differential diagnosis for a poisoned patient. Generalizations concerning the heavy metal group and metalloids have limited utility. However, heavy metals, particularly heavy metal compounds with other inorganic and organic elements, manifest diverse toxicities (Table 81–1). A number of the heavy metals, such as lead, mercury, arsenic, and thallium, are discussed in separate chapters due to the relatively high prevalence of intoxication and the associated toxicity.

In general, all of the inorganic forms of metals cause GI irritation, resulting in nausea, vomiting, abdominal pain, and diarrhea. The next most consistent toxicity for the metals as a group, but not for every metal, is renal toxicity, in particular renal tubular toxicity with acute and subacute exposure and interstitial nephritis with chronic exposure. A further generalization is that each member of the metal group tends to cause multi-organ toxicity. Many metals cause cutaneous abnormalities, such as irritant and allergic contact dermatitis, urticaria, keratoses, and premalignant and malignant lesions. Several of the metals, such as lead and mercury, produce central nervous system toxicity. Depending on the compound, the toxicity attributed to a particular metal varies. For example, zinc oxide produces a relatively benign metal fume fever syndrome after inhalation, while inhalation of zinc chloride can cause a severe chemical pneumonitis.

The toxicities of many of the metals can be misdiag-

TABLE 81–1. COMPARISON OF THE TOXICITY OF SOME COMMONLY ENCOUNTERED METALS AND METAL SALTS

	Acute	Chronic
Cadmium	GI irritation Pneumonitis Pulmonary edema Nephrotoxicity: Proximal tubular dysfunction with small molecular weight proteinuria, glycosuria, and aminoaciduria	Nephrotoxicity: Interstitial nephritis Nephrolithiasis Osteomalacia Prostate cancer Lung cancer (possible)
Chromium	Dermatitis Skin and mucus membrane ulcers Caustic burns Acute renal failure Nephrotoxicity : Proximal tubular dysfunction with small molecular weight proteinuria, glycosuria, and aminoaciduria Hemolysis Liver damage	Nephrotoxicity: Interstitial nephritis Inflammatory airway disorders Respiratory tract cancer Nasal ulcers (chrome holes) Acute tubular necrosis Skin ulcers
Cobalt	Dermatitis Asthma-like syndrome	Cardiomyopathy Hypothyroidism Polycythemia Interstitial lung fibrosis
Copper	Dermatitis Respiratory tract GI irritation and ulceration Hemolysis Hepatotoxicity	Pulmonary fibrosis, liver disease, lung cancer (inhalation of copper sulfate) Blindness, cirrhosis, encephalopathy in individuals with a genetic deficiency of ceruloplasmin (Wilson's disease)
Manganese	Dermatitis, conjunctivitis GI caustic (potassium permanganate) Pneumonitis (MnO_2)	Psychosis Parkinson like syndrome Pulmonary fibrosis
Nickel	Dermatitis, conjunctivitis GI irritation, hemorrhagic gastritis Pneumonitis, sinusitis	Respiratory tract cancer Anosmia, nasal polyps, and perforation
Selenium	Dermatitis, conjunctivitis GI irritation and ulceration	Fatigue Alopecia Nail loss
Tin	Encephalopathy Cerebral edema, death (organotin compounds)	Benign pneumoconiosis (inorganic tin compounds) Chronic encephalpoathy (organotins)
Zinc	Pneumonitis ($ZnCl_2$) GI irritation Metal fume fever	Sideroblastic anemia

nosed as a viral or other illness, particularly when the presentation involves multiple organs. Conversely, simple viral syndromes can be inappropriately attributed to metal toxicity when no toxicity has in fact occurred, because many of the early symptoms of intoxications due to metals are nonspecific.

Metalworking: Vapors, Fumes, Soldering, Brazing, and Welding

Knowledge of metalworking is often crucial in the differential diagnosis of metal poisoning. Welding describes the joining of metals by melting and fusing together. Welders also cut and grind metal objects and add filler metals by soldering or brazing. Soft soldering is the joining of metal using filler metal (solder) with a melting point less than 316°C (600°F); hard solder is used in the range of 316 to 427°C (600 to 800°F). Soldering does not have to be performed as a welding operation, because the high temperatures of welding techniques are not necessary. Soldering differs from brazing, in which a filler metal with a melting point greater than 427°C (800°F) is used. The temperature of the operation is important: at higher temperatures the vapor pressure of the metals is higher and the operator is exposed to higher concentrations of metal fumes. In gas or torch welding, lead, zinc, and cadmium release are of particular concern. These types of welding utilize the burning of oxygen with another fuel (eg, acetylene, propane, butane, or hydrogen). Lead, zinc, and cadmium have significant vapor pressures at the temperatures present in gas or torch welding. Although brazing is commonly identified as a soldering operation in industry, it is more properly identified as a welding process because of the high temperatures involved. Brazing is used widely in the manufacture of refrigerators, electronics, jewelry, and aerospace components.[31]

In metalworking operations the entire process and the materials used must be analyzed to determine the potential hazards involved. Insulation on wire must be stripped to allow soldering or brazing. Stripping can be accomplished by mechanical, chemical, or thermal methods. Caustic agents are used in chemical stripping. Thermal stripping of insulation derived from polytetrafluoroethene polymer (Teflon) may result in polymer fume fever. In addition, asbestos release may result from the disruption of insulation on wires. The metal must also be cleaned to remove oils, grease, wax, and other surface debris, so that subsequent flux agents can work. Chlorinated solvents are often used in these degreasing operations. Finally, all metals have a film or tarnish that must be removed to achieve a good bonding. A flux agent, which may be a gas, solid, or liquid, is designed to remove any adsorbed contaminants from the metal surface and keep it clean until the solder or brazing metal is applied. Diverse organic and inorganic materials, often in complex combinations, are used as soldering and welding fluxes. Examples of inorganic fluxes are hydrochloric acid, hydrofluoric acid, orthophosphoric acid, zinc chloride, and ammonium chloride salts. Examples of organic fluxes are rosin, phthalic acid, and aniline hydrochloride. These flux agents can be dissolved in organic solvents.[31]

Diverse metals and other agents may be responsible for pulmonary illness in metalworking operations. A study of brazing in a ship pipe shop surveyed for cadmium fumes (from the filler metal), fluorides (from the flux), and nitrogen dioxide (from the torch) revealed that cadmium comprised 10 to 24% of the filler metal used in most of the brazing operations. In one episode of pulmonary illness initially attributed to cadmium fumes, it was discovered that the filler metal did not contain cadmium. In that instance, the nitrogen dioxide concentrations reached dangerous levels and accounted for pulmonary disease with characteristics similar to those from exposure to cadmium fumes.[3]

Cadmium

Sources of Exposure to Cadmium

Cadmium is a bluish, silver-white metal that is very ductile, malleable, and lustrous and can be polished to a high gloss. It is also highly resistant to corrosion and is consequently widely used in industry and in arts and crafts. In air, cadmium burns readily when heated and produces orange-brown, odorless, initially nonirritating cadmium oxide fumes. The melting point of cadmium is 321°C (610°F), and its boiling point is 767°C (1413°F).[55]

About 50% of cadmium is used for electroplating coatings. Electroplated cadmium items are used in automobile engine parts, aircraft parts, radio and television parts, and nuts and bolts. Cadmium alloys, such as cadmium-nickel, cadmium-silver-copper, and cadmium-silver, are the next most commonly used cadmium products. Cadmium-silver alloy and solder are used in jewelry manufacture. The third largest use of cadmium is in solders in combination with copper, lead, tin, zinc, or silver.[145]

Cadmium is also found in nickel cadmium batteries. Cadmium bromide ($CdBr_2$) and cadmium iodide (CdI_2) are used rarely in photography. In the manufacture of polyvinylchloride film, cadmium stearate is used as a stabilizer.[144] Cadmium salts are also used as pigments in paints.[88]

Exposure to cadmium can occur during the smelting of impure zinc ore to separate cadmium. Lead is also present. Other exposures occur when cadmium alloys or solders are melted, remelted (scrap metal recycling), or subjected to cutting or grinding without recognition of the presence of the hazardous metal. Fatal cases of cadmium poisoning have occurred among workers who flanged cadmium-plated steel pipe with a blowtorch.[91,144] Exposures may also occur during the production of phosphate fertilizers, because of the presence of significant amounts of cadmium in crude phosphate.[60]

The use of cadmium-silver solders in arts and crafts or in small jewelry manufacturing shops is of particular concern. These solders are available in coils, rods, and sheets or plaques, initially packed together in a large box. In some instances, only the box cover or front is labeled to indicate that cadmium is present. Often an individual purchases only a small amount and therefore does not receive the box with the warning label. Sometimes a single warning tag is attached to a coil. If that tag is detached, subsequent users of the coil in a classroom or shop are unaware of the presence of cadmium.[26]

Food represents the second major source of exposure to cadmium.[36] Sources of food contamination may be pots and pans with cadmium-containing glazing and cadmium soldering used in vending machines for hot and cold drinks.[55] Children have been sickened by 13 to

15 ppm of cadmium in frozen ices, 67 ppm in punch, and 530 ppm in gelatin.[145] Persons in areas near cadmium-emitting plants can have significant exposures from air contamination.[48]

Routes of Exposure to Cadmium

Inhalation and ingestion are the two major routes of exposure to cadmium compounds. Cadmium vapor and fumes account for most inhalation exposures, but dusts of respirable size (less than 10 μm) can also be inhaled.[55] It is estimated from animal experiments that 10 to 40% of inhaled cadmium[88] and 2 to 6% of ingested cadmium is absorbed, although cadmium absorption from the GI tract may reach 20% of a given dose in iron-deficient individuals.[55]

After absorption, cadmium is transported to the liver, where it is bound to metallothionein, a low-molecular-weight protein synthesized in the liver. The metallothionein–cadmium complex is transported via blood to the kidney, where it is filtered by the glomeruli, but then is reabsorbed by proximal tubular cells and subsequently degraded. The renal tubular cells are able to synthesize metallothionein capable of binding cadmium. Cadmium toxicity occurs when the metallothionein-producing ability of the proximal tubular cells is exceeded and the cells are left unprotected from cadmium.[55,130]

The highest concentrations of cadmium are found in the kidney and liver. In the absence of significant renal damage and loss of proximal tubular cells, the concentration of cadmium in the kidney can be 15 times that of the liver.[55] Cadmium is also distributed to the bone, testes, pancreas, spleen, various endocrine organs, brain, and muscle tissue.[88] Cadmium is excreted in breast milk.

The elimination of cadmium from the body is slow, with a half-life of 7 to 30 years. Thus, cadmium accumulates in the body with increasing duration of exposure.[55]

Pathophysiology of Cadmium Exposure

The ingestion of cadmium-contaminated solutions causes nausea, vomiting, and diarrhea. Large concentrations of cadmium or cadmium compounds, which are caustic, may cause gastritis. The acute effects of inhalation exposure to cadmium oxide fumes include delayed chemical pneumonitis with accompanying noncardiac pulmonary edema.[11,19,25,26,133]

The chronic toxicity of cadmium compounds includes kidney damage with proteinuria of low-molecular-weight molecules. A Japanese epidemic of cadmium poisoning, called itai-itai ("ouch, ouch") disease, was believed to be the result of chronic ingestion of cadmium from environmental pollution. Findings included altered renal tubular function with impaired regulation of calcium and phosphorus, manifesting bone demineralization, osteomalacia, and pathologic fractures.[46,53,55]

In workers with occupational cadmium exposure, renal dysfunction manifested as proteinuria is often detected, as have amino aciduria, glucosuria, impaired concentration ability, and abnormalities in calcium, phosphorus, and uric acid excretion. There are some reports of decreased glomerular filtration rates, and an increase in nephrolithiasis with calcium phosphate stones was found.[71,72,86,131,144]

Chronic inhalation exposure to cadmium is associated with emphysema.[87] Inhibition of alpha$_1$-antitrypsin is suggested as a possible mechanism,[36] although others[23] have reported conflicting in vitro findings and no evidence for decreased alpha$_1$-antitrypsin levels in workers with significant long-term exposure to cadmium. Anemia, liver function abnormalities, and anosmia[54,88,122] are also noted to follow exposure to cadmium.

Cadmium is an animal carcinogen and mutagen.[46] Epidemiologic studies of cadmium workers demonstrate an increased risk of prostate and respiratory tract cancer.[55] The National Institute for Occupational Safety and Health (NIOSH) recommends that cadmium be regarded as a potential occupational carcinogen.[105] The Environmental Protection Agency (EPA) considers cadmium to be a probable carcinogenic in humans (category 2A).[46]

In male and female animal studies, cadmium adversely affects the reproductive system and reproductive function. Cadmium is also teratogenic in animals, but teratogenicity in humans has not been demonstrated.[46]

Serum concentrations of cadmium are not usually a useful indicator of acute poisoning. This is because cadmium manifests its acute toxicity at the site of absorption in the lungs and GI tract, and most cadmium thereafter is protein-bound in the liver and kidneys.[88] However, on at least one occasion, serum cadmium determinations were used to help in the differential diagnosis of pneumonitis.[15]

Urinary concentrations of cadmium do not reflect acute exposure unless it is overwhelming, but can be used as a marker of body burden in chronic exposure unless significant destruction of renal tissue is present.[88,93,156] Smokers often have concentrations twice those of nonsmokers.[85] Urinary concentrations greater than 10 μg/L are believed by OSHA to be abnormal and to require medical investigation.[104,108]

Low-molecular-weight urinary proteins, such as beta$_2$-microglobulin and metallothionein, can be used as indirect markers of cadmium exposure. Urinary retinol-binding protein is a nonspecific finding when tubular reabsorption is decreased due to any cause, including cadmium.[61,86]

Because of the potential to cause cancer and kidney disease, there is an 8-hour time-weighted average (TWA) permissible exposure limit (PEL) of 5 $\mu g/m^3$ in air. If the ambient exposure is above an action level of 2.5 $\mu g/m^3$ (TWA), then the employer must comply with all sections of the standard, including establishing a medical surveillance program for employees.[102,108]

Emergency examinations following acute exposure are mandated, especially looking for chemical pneumonitis and noncardiac pulmonary edema following inhalation exposures.[108] Removal of the employee from exposure is required when the urine cadmium exceeds 15 μg/g of creatinine, or beta$_2$-microglobulin exceeds 1500 μg/g of creatinine and urine cadmium exceeds 3 μg/g of creatinine or blood cadmium exceeds 5 μg/L whole blood.[108]

Treatment

When there is a question of acute cadmium salt ingestion, gastric evacuation should be performed, unless the patient has vomited spontaneously. Catharsis may assist in elimination of the ingested cadmium before absorption. Persons with acute inhalation should be removed from exposure, hospitalized, and given supportive therapy for pulmonary sequelae. No specific treatment for acute or chronic cadmium poisoning is available. Chelation agents such as British antilewisite (BAL) and calcium disodium EDTA are contraindicated for cadmium because there is evidence that the large concentration of cadmium brought to the kidneys will only exacerbate renal toxicity. There is histopathologic evidence for increased toxicity in animals when calcium disodium EDTA is used.[53,55,56]

Chromium

Sources and Routes of Exposure to Chromium

Chromium is used extensively in electroplating as well as in combination with other metals in alloys. Lead chromate (chrome yellow) is a common chromium pigment. Calcium chromate and zinc chromate are primers and corrosion inhibitors. Chromium compounds are also used as catalysts and wood preservatives and in videotape and ceramics manufacture, leather tanning, textile printing, and lithography.[145] It may also be present in cement, particularly in that used outside the United States.[1]

The primary routes of chromium intoxication are via the lungs, GI tract, and skin. Chromium 3^+ is poorly absorbed by all routes. Chromium 6^+ is more readily absorbed, particularly via the lungs. It is estimated that only 1% of dietary chromium 3^+ is absorbed. Chromium is distributed throughout the body, but the liver, kidney, and (in occupational exposures) lungs have the highest concentrations.[63] When Cr^{6+} enters the body, it is an oxidizing agent and is reduced to Cr^{3+}. When Cr^{6+} enters the red blood cells, it is reduced to insoluble Cr^{3+} and is trapped for the life (100 to 120 days) of the red blood cell.[50] Three hours after an oral ingestion of potassium dichromate, 80 to 90% of the chromium in blood was found in the red blood cell fraction, and the chromium was in the trivalent state.[70] Chromium is excreted primarily via the kidneys but also via the bile and feces. Minor routes of excretion include breast milk, sweat, hair, and nails. The proportion of excretion via the feces is increased after inhalation uptake.[63]

Dermal and respiratory exposure to chromium may occur in mining and refining operations. Numerous sites of residual chromium contamination exist in residential areas of New Jersey as a result of using waste from refining operations as landfill. The risk of skin or respiratory exposure and inadvertent ingestion has been termed low, but full characterization of the risk is still underway. The sites have been isolated from contact with residents. Hexavalent chromium (Cr^{6+}) is released in the machining and welding of stainless steels.[24] Chromium mist can be produced in electroplating, spray painting operations, or with other uses of chromium solutions.[145]

Drinking water can become contaminated with low levels of chromate anticorrosive compounds when improper procedures have been employed during refrigeration plumbing work. Chromate crystals and solutions have been ingested both intentionally and accidentally. Unintentional pediatric ingestions have resulted from the attractive colorful characteristics of some chromate solutions.[119]

Recently, Cr^{3+} picolinate supplements have become popular without apparent scientific basis. Chromium accumulation is predicted to occur.[143] There is a single case report of chronic interstitial nephritis with renal failure attributed to such supplements.[161]

Pathophysiology of Chromium Exposure

Hexavalent chromium compounds (chromate, chromic acid) are irritating and corrosive to the skin, mucous membranes, and GI tract. Toxicity is manifested as an irritant contact dermatitis, although sensitization may occur and some individuals may develop an allergic dermatitis.[138] Chromium causes approximately 8% of all cases of contact dermatitis. The proportion of sensitized persons in a workplace is directly related to the amount of chromium in the work environment.[132] The dermatitis can persist despite removal from exposure. Ulcerations of the skin (chrome holes) and perforation of the nasal septum may occur. This ulceration typically begins as a painless papule. There may also be irritation of the sinuses and the entire respiratory tract, with resultant pneumonitis. Pulmonary sensitization may also occur.[110,138] Systemic sensitization was documented in a welder exposed to chromium by inhalation who developed a delayed anaphylactoid reaction.[98] Chrome in cement has resulted in dermatitis and skin ulcers.[1] Timber preserved with chromium salts has produced dermatitis, as have solutions and mists containing chromium in electroplating shops, woolen mills, air conditioning services, and shops where the cooling systems for diesel locomotives are repaired.[144]

Systemic effects of severe chromate poisoning include acute renal tubular necrosis, hemolysis, and liver damage. Systemic poisoning typically occurs via ingestion or skin contact if the skin barrier has been compromised secondary to a caustic (often from the chromate compound itself) or thermal burn.[138,145] Trivalent chromium (Cr^{3+}) compounds have a low order of acute toxicity and infrequently cause allergic sensitization, probably due to their low solubility.

Cancer of the respiratory tract is the overriding concern with chronic exposure to chromium. Excess rates of lung cancer occur in persons exposed to the production of chromates from ore as well as after exposure to zinc and lead-chromate pigments.[24,123] Nasal and other upper respiratory tract cancers are also suspected.[129] Trivalent chromium compounds and some of the highly soluble hexavalent chromium compounds are often considered noncarcinogenic. These highly soluble hexavalent chromium compounds include chromium oxide (chromic acid anhydride), the monochromates and bichromates (dichromates) of hydrogen, lithium, sodium, potassium, rubidium, cesium, and ammonia.[74,84,107] Some suggest that these highly soluble compounds are also carcinogenic.[66]

Chronic bronchitis, sinusitis, and rhinitis, as well as asthma and a type of pneumoconiosis, are associated with long-term exposure to chromium.[138] Nephrotoxicity occurs in welders exposed to fumes containing hexavalent chromium.[101,111]

Clinical Chemistry of Chromium

Chromium can be measured in the blood and urine. Measurement of blood or red blood cell chromium is fraught with difficulties due to contamination during collection and analysis. Thus, these values are unreliable.[50] In an occupational setting, biologic monitoring of chromium is not believed to be a useful component of a medical surveillance program, although elevated urine concentrations can indicate exposure.[50,138] Respiratory or dermal manifestations of allergy to chromium can be difficult to assess via laboratory testing, because provocative respiratory or dermal testing may itself induce sensitization.

Treatment of Chromium Poisoning

Because of the carcinogenic potential of hexavalent chromium compounds, prevention of exposure, particularly respiratory exposure, is required. When skin becomes contaminated with chromium solutions, contaminated clothing should be removed. If the contaminated area is extensive, skin cuts or abrasions contaminated with chromium 6^{+} must be immediately lavaged by deluge shower. A 10% topical solution of ascorbic acid is recommended as a reducing agent to convert chromium from the toxic hexavalent to the relatively nontoxic trivalent form.[79,126] If the hexavalent chromium is reduced to trivalent chromium, then a 10% topical solution of calcium disodium EDTA can theoretically be used to chelate the metal.[24]

Supportive treatment and hemodialysis are not effective for the treatment of severe chromium poisoning. In vitro experimentation has shown that ascorbic acid is an effective reducing agent of hexavalent chromium to trivalent chromium in serum and blood. The dose of ascorbic acid necessary to eliminate peak levels of hexavalent chromium in severe poisoning cases can be achieved clinically, and this regimen has a limited role and will not have any appreciable intrinsic toxicity. Severe hexavalent chromium poisoning secondary to extensive chromate burns was successfully treated with ascorbic acid.[64] Ascorbic acid and calcium disodium EDTA therapy[115] prevented acute nephrotoxicity in animals poisoned with hexavalent chromium.

Based on the above evidence, IV ascorbic acid, 3 g divided into 1-g doses every 10 to 20 minutes, should be used initially to treat severe chromium poisoning in adults. Because of the rapid excretion of ascorbic acid in the urine, IV ascorbic acid dosing should be repeated frequently, although no specific schedule is suggested.[79]

For burns, in addition to 10% topical ascorbic acid, 10 g of ascorbic acid should be given orally while awaiting further intravenous therapy. As with ingestion of strong acids and alkalis, inducing vomiting after the ingestion of chromic acid is not recommended. Chromate salts are not strong acids, but they are very corrosive because of their oxidizing properties. If vomiting is not spontaneous, then careful orogastric lavage with 1% ascorbic acid solution is recommended, as well as leaving 10 g of ascorbic acid in the stomach (10 g/100 mL).[64] In rats, *N*-acetylcysteine (NAC) appears to be more effective than calcium disodium EDTA or 2,3-dimercaptosuccinic acid (DMSA) for increasing the excretion of chromium.[17] *N*-acetylcysteine is also believed to have significant clinical antioxidant efficacy.[97] A 25-year-old man survived a severe ingestion of 16 g hexavalent chromium when NAC treatment and hemodialysis were employed.[157] With chromium ingestion, in addition to intravenous ascorbic acid therapy, NAC orally or via nasogastric tube, in doses comparable to that employed for acetaminophen toxicity, appears to be a logical adjunctive therapy.

Cobalt

Dermal exposure to cobalt compounds typically produces an irritant contact dermatitis, but allergic contact dermatitis is also possible (see Chap. 28).[2] Inhalation exposure to cobalt dust in the manufacture of cemented tungsten carbides and in the grinding and cutting of these tools is of concern.[142] Both asthma-like syndromes and chronic interstitial fibrosis with impairment of lung function can result.[16,37,47,76,82,125,164] Low-dose cyclophosphamide therapy has been used with some success.

Ingestion of cobalt compounds is rare. Cobalt chloride was once used therapeutically (with some success) to stimulate erythropoiesis in anephric individuals on hemodialysis. Clinical hypothyroidism was noted in one patient and high-tone deafness developed in another.[45] Cobalt therapy for anemia has also been reported to produce thyroid hyperplasia and hypothyroidism.[60,80] Epidemiologic studies of exposed workers revealed mild hypothyroidism.[154]

After a cobalt compound was added to beer as a foam stabilizer, epidemics of cardiomyopathy were attributed to the ingestion of cobalt in combination with excessive alcohol intake and nutritional deficiencies, most notably thiamine.[7,27,92,99] There are also reports of cardiomyopathies,[12,28,73,75] increases and decreases in red cell count, and increases in erythropoietin levels from occupational exposures to cobalt.[12] Two young men developed noninflammatory cardiomyopathy manifested as congestive heart failure while employed in a dusty facility where mineral assays were performed on metal ores.[73] Workers in industries with potential cobalt exposure, such as grinders, filers, fitters, polishers, buffers, and tool sharpeners, have an increased risk of ischemic heart disease and acute myocardial infarction.[135]

Ingestion of a large number of magnets by a child produced polycythemia, thyromegaly with hypothyroidism, metabolic acidosis, and cardiomyopathy.[67]

Clinical Chemistry of Cobalt

Blood and urine analysis can be used to monitor exposure to cobalt. [9,12]

Treatment of Cobalt Poisoning

Under most circumstances of dermal and inhalation exposure, therapy consists of removing the patient from further exposure, treating symptoms, and medical surveillance. Surgical removal of the magnets followed by chelation with $CaNa_2$ EDTA resulted in clinical improvement in a case of magnet ingestion.[67]

Sources and Routes of Exposure to Cobalt

Cobalt is essential for humans and it is found in vitamin B_{12}. Normally a total of only 1 mg of cobalt is stored in the adult human body. Cobalt is present naturally in food, and is poorly absorbed in the GI tract and excreted in the urine. Inhalation exposure to cobalt compounds results in immediate increases in blood and urine concentrations.[63] There appears to be an initial fast elimination phase in the urine of a few days, and then a slower elimination phase of undetermined length. The half-life of cobalt after pulmonary uptake is 5 to 10 years, allowing for accumulations in target tissues such as the myocardium.[12,107]

Copper

Sources and Routes of Exposure to Copper

A major use of copper is in the manufacture of electrical equipment. Copper is also useful in alloys with metals such as zinc (brass), tin (bronze), nickel (money), aluminum, beryllium, cadmium, chromium, gold, lead, silicon, and phosphorus. Copper compounds are found in insecticides, fungicides, and algicides intended for environmental application and used as preservatives for wood, fabric, and paints. Copper chromates and other copper compounds (eg, red copper oxide; CuO) are used as pigments and catalysts.[38]

Persons may be exposed to copper fumes via welding, grinding, or polishing of copper metal or alloys. Significant amounts of copper dust may be generated from large copper bushings used in heavy industrial machinery.[77] Inhalation or dermal exposure to copper compounds as dusts may occur in the manufacture of ceramics, paints, and pesticides.[146] Furniture polishers have developed allergic dermatitis to the copper sulfate added to commercial alcohol as a coloring agent.[43] Ingestion of copper compounds may occur intentionally as a suicidal or criminal act or from inadvertent contamination of food, particularly liquids. Acidic water conditions may result in leaching of copper from pipes into drinking water. Carbonated water, citrus fruit juices, and other acidic beverages will also dissolve copper metal containers. Copper salts are reported to impart a taste to water at concentrations of 1 to 5 mg/L.[10]

Copper Absorption and Metabolism

After ingestion, copper can be absorbed via the GI tract under the acidic conditions of the stomach. Copper has also been absorbed systemically via dialysis solutions, where it dissolved from the tubing under acidic conditions.[78] Copper from intrauterine contraceptive devices can be absorbed systemically as well.[20] Absorption secondary to dermal exposure would be expected only when the integrity of the skin barrier has been breached.[66,67] Inhalation of copper dusts and mists is not believed to result in significant systemic absorption unless substantial amounts of copper reach the GI tract, where systemic copper absorption occurs more easily.

Copper is considered an essential mineral for the functioning of enzymes such as catalase and peroxidase, and a minimum daily dietary intake of 2 to 3 mg is recommended for adults.[58] Wilson's disease is an autosomal recessive genetic disorder due to a deficiency in the plasma copper protein, ceruloplasmin.[57] For those who do not suffer from Wilson's disease, 93% of serum copper is in ceruloplasmin and the rest is combined with albumin and other proteins. Two to five milligrams of copper are ingested each day in typical diets. Practically all of it is excreted via bile into the feces, and the total body content of copper remains constant at 100 to 150 mg.[10] In patients with Wilson's disease, rather than being bound in ceruloplasmin or excreted in the bile, copper is deposited to many organs (particularly the liver, kidney, brain, and cornea), resulting in accumulation of copper in the body.[146]

Elevated levels of serum copper and ceruloplasmin occur in women taking oral contraceptives. Whether or not there is increased deposition in tissues has not been determined.[125]

Pathophysiology of Copper Exposure

Gastrointestinal symptoms are reported with ingestion of as little as 15 mg of copper sulfate.[128] Gastrointestinal irritation, manifested by nausea, vomiting, and diarrhea, can result from drinking well water with high levels of copper or carbonated water or citrus juices left in contact with copper vessels.[131] Symptoms after suicidal ingestion of 1 to 12 g of copper sulfate included metallic taste, epigastric burning, vomiting, and diarrhea. Gastric ulceration and hemorrhage, hemolysis, hemoglobinuria, and jaundice develop subsequently. Liver toxicity in fatal cases includes centrilobular necrosis and biliary stasis. Early deaths were due to shock, whereas death occurring later was attributed to hepatic or renal failure or both.[5,38] It was not clear whether the renal injury was secondary to hypovolemia and hemoglobinuria or whether the copper compound also had a clinically significant primary toxic effect on the kidney.[5,38] A religious ritual involving copper-contaminated water induced hemolysis and subsequent acute renal failure.[139]

Acute inhalation of copper dusts or fumes can cause upper respiratory irritation, resulting in sore throat and cough. Conjunctivitis, palpebral edema, and sinus irritation may also occur. Atrophic changes in the nasal mucous membranes may occur with perforation. Pneumonitis and pulmonary edema result in animals exposed to copper acetate dust.[146] Inhalation of copper oxide fumes in humans more typically results in systemic toxicity manifested as metal fume fever. Inhalation exposure to dusts and fumes may also result in ingestion by swallowing particles causing local GI irritation with nausea, abdominal pain, and diarrhea.[131]

Dermal exposure to copper compounds may cause an irritant contact dermatitis or an allergic contact dermatitis.[3] Excessive dermal exposure may cause a greenish-blue discoloration of the skin (which does not correlate with the severity of systemic toxicity). Copper salts used in the treatment of extensive burns can cause systemic toxic manifestations identical to those of severe ingestion.[22,68]

Chalcosis is the lodging of metallic copper or copper alloy foreign bodies in the eye. Uveitis, abscess, and loss of the eye can result following industrial injuries.

Pulmonary fibrosis,[112] lung cancer,[159] and liver granulomas occur with chronic exposure to copper sulfate neutralized with hydrated lime (Bordeaux mixture) in vineyard sprayers in Portugal. The spectrum of liver disease in a series of 30 vineyard sprayers using Bordeaux mixture also included liver fibrosis, cirrhosis, angiosarcoma, and idiopathic portal hypertension.[113,114] Copper miners have an increased incidence of lung cancer.[35]

Copper dissolved in dialysis solutions has been shown to produce a syndrome of pancreatitis and myoglobinemia, as well as GI symptoms, leukocytosis, metabolic acidosis, and hemolysis. Significant increases in hepatic copper have also been found.[78] Systemic absorption of copper from the wire in certain intrauterine contraceptive devices is believed not to cause significant toxicity but has been rarely associated with a generalized eczematous dermatitis.[20,52] A syndrome of liver, CNS, kidney, bone, and eye dysfunction and structural damage are the classic manifestations of chronic copper toxicity in Wilson's disease. Increased daily ingestion can occur in persons who eat large amounts of shellfish, liver, mushrooms, nuts, and chocolate and those who are occupationally exposed to copper dusts.[131,146] Clinical disease has not, however, been observed in individuals with daily intakes of copper 10 times the average daily ingestion of 2 to 5 mg.[131]

Laboratory Findings and Copper Exposure

In India, where copper sulfate poisoning is one of the leading causes of suicidal death, whole blood copper concentrations in a series of suicidal ingestions ranged from 383 to 684 μg/dL. An association of whole blood copper, but not serum copper, concentrations with the clinical severity of the poisoning was demonstrated.[38] Beyond acute massive poisoning, laboratory testing has limited utility in the evaluation of an individual patient suspected to be suffering from copper intoxication from environmental sources, for example. Whole blood copper values are reported to range from 16 to 348 μg/dL (mean, 89 μg/dL) in patients studied in 19 American cities.[81] Several of the higher values were thought to result from environmental exposure in areas adjacent to smelters, but the levels did not correlate with clinical illness.[57] In Wilson's disease, the mean urinary copper concentration is 602 μg/L, compared with a mean of 33 μg/L in normal individuals,[57] while fecal and serum copper concentrations are generally found to be below normal values.[128]

Treatment of Copper Poisoning

Treatment of intentional ingestions of significant quantities of copper compound should include gastric emptying and catharsis. Corticosteroid therapy has been suggested in the past, but only general supportive therapy, including hydration, can be recommended at this time.[146] Chelation therapy with D-penicillamine is used in Wilson's disease, but this agent would not be clinically useful in the case of suicidal ingestion, particularly if significant renal insufficiency were present. Triethylenetetraamine dihydrochloride has also been shown to be effective in removal of copper in Wilson's disease.[128]

Dimercaprol was initially used in Wilson's disease for removal of copper[128] and might be useful parenteral therapy after accidental or intentional ingestion of copper compounds. Renal excretion is necessary for maximum efficacy, although the bile is a major route of elimination for the BAL-metal complex. Other than for treatment of Wilson's disease, use of chelation therapy, including DMSA, has not been adequately studied. In the case of exposures that are not life threatening, termination of exposure and medical surveillance of copper excretion are probably sufficient.

Manganese

Sources and Routes of Exposure to Manganese

Manganese is present in many alloys, and its compounds are used as animal food additives and in the manufacture of electrical coils, ceramics, matches, glass, dyes, pharmaceuticals, fertilizer, and welding rods.

Exposure to manganese most commonly occurs via two manganese compounds, inorganic manganese dioxide and organic methylcyclopentadienyl manganese tricarbonyl (MMT),[155] as well as via manganese supplements to total parental nutrition regimens.[51] Manganese dioxide is present during mining operations and during welding. There is usually no risk of exposure to manganese in electroplating operations. Manganese radiography contrast agents have also been considered as a possible exposure risk.[96]

Methylcyclopentadienyl manganese tricarbonyl (MMT) is used as an antiknock agent in gasoline and is found in about 2% of leaded gasoline in the United States and in both leaded and unleaded gasoline in Canada. Long-term epidemiologic studies of MMT workers have not been reported. Besides concern about workplace exposures, the potential health effects of the release of manganese into the environment from gasoline must also be evaluated. The use of MMT has been curtailed because it interferes with the efficacy of the catalytic converters currently used to control automobile exhaust emissions.

Chronic exposure to naturally occurring elevated levels of manganese in drinking water was not shown to result in increased manganism.[158]

Pathophysiology of Manganese Exposure

Manganese is an essential element for humans, but neurotoxicity develops at higher body burdens. Increased body burdens of manganese have been reported in the presence of chronic liver disease, and it has been postulated that much of the extrapyramidal syndrome associated with chronic liver disease may be due to manganese.[32,65]

Many manganese compounds are mild irritants to the skin and mucous membranes; potassium permanganate, however, is a strongly corrosive oxidant.[140] Acute inhalation of high levels of manganese dioxide causes pneumonitis.[140]

Chronic exposure to manganese dioxide produces a neurologic syndrome with morbidity and disability similar to that of Parkinson's disease.[121] The classic cases were described in mining operations, but a railroad worker repairing and recycling railroad track containing manganese alloy was also reported to develop manganism.[104] In addition, there have been two reported manganism cases associated with maneb (manganese dithiocarbamate), although the dithiocarbamates may have contributed to the neurotoxic presentations.[95]

The onset of manganese neurotoxicity may occur as long as 10 years after cessation of exposure. In true parkinsonism, the substantia nigra is the area of the brain most affected; in manganism, the striatum and pallidum are the key areas affected. Magnetic resonance imaging (MRI) and positron emission tomography (PET) scanning may be useful in the diagnosis.[33,104] Three stages are described in chronic manganese poisoning. Initially, the chronically exposed worker may be asymptomatic or experience irritability, anorexia, fatigue, headaches, leg weakness, and muscular cramps. Neurobehavioral testing may detect early neurotoxicity and may also differentiate from parkinsonism.[90,136] Dysarthria, disturbances of gait, and excessive salivation along with emotional instability or even organic psychosis occur in the next stage. In the final stage, a neurologic syndrome similar to that of Parkinson's disease occurs. A patient with manganese poisoning exhibits more dystonia and an intention tremor, as opposed to the resting tremor noted in parkinsonism.[41,155]

Treatment of Manganese Poisoning

Manganese neurologic syndrome may be reversible in the early stages, if exposure ceases.[41,155] Chelation therapy with calcium disodium EDTA may be helpful in accelerating elimination and may produce at least temporary improvement in the clinical syndrome.[41,155] A Chinese report claimed improvement in chronic manganese poisoning treating with sodium para-aminosalicylic acid[83]; however, there are no other confirming reports. Dimercaptosuccinic acid has not had a substantial clinical effect.[13]

Nickel

Sources and Routes of Exposure to Nickel

Dermal contact with nickel compounds does not result in significant systemic absorption. When nickel dusts or aerosols of nickel solutions are inhaled most of the nickel is retained in the lung, although some systemic absorption also occurs. There is systemic absorption of 1 to 5% of nickel from the GI tract. The highest concentrations of nickel are found in bone, with lesser concentrations in the lung, kidney, liver, and heart in individuals without any known exposure other than that normally present in food. Nickel is bound to albumin in the serum and extracted from the serum by the kidney and then excreted. A half-life of 53 hours for an initial rapid elimination phase is estimated for nickel inhaled by welders, but a slower elimination phase of weeks to months is also believed to exist.[151]

The nickel compounds in common use are solid powders. Nickel is used in steel, other alloys, and electroplating. In electroplating, nickel provides a hard surface that does not tarnish and can be polished.[150] Exposure to nickel occurs in the mining, milling, and manufacture of nickel products. Finely ground nickel is used as a catalyst, and nickel compounds are used in ceramic glazes, and nickel-cadmium storage batteries, and to color glass green.[147]

Nickel carbonyl is a colorless gas that may be associated with a "sooty" odor. Nickel carbonyl ($NiCO_4$), formed as an intermediate in the refining of nickel, is also manufactured for use as a chemical reagent and is used in the metallurgic and electronic industries for vapor plating of nickel and in the plastics industry as a catalyst.[148] An episode of nickel carbonyl poisoning took place involving maintenance and repair workers in a facility manufacturing acrylics where nickel carbonyl was used as a catalyst. The workers were poisoned while repairing an exhaust scrubber that was not in operation but harbored the toxic gas.[150]

Pathophysiology of Nickel Exposure

Oral ingestion of nickel compounds is generally unintentional. Sequelae of nickel ingestion can be severe. A 25-year-old woman became stuporous and developed nuchal rigidity, erythema, dilated pupils, tachycardia, and pulmonary congestion after ingestion of 10 to 15 g of nickel sulfate hexahydrate crystals (2.2 to 3.3 g nickel) from a chemistry hobby set. Autopsy revealed a hemorrhagic gastritis.[42]

Contamination of the drinking water supply in an electroplating plant resulted in ingestion of nickel sulfate and chloride by 32 workers. The amount of nickel ingested per individual was estimated to be 0.5 to 2.5 g. Symptoms of nausea, vomiting, abdominal discomfort, diarrhea, giddiness, lassitude, headache, cough, and shortness of breath generally lasted several hours but persisted for 1 to 2 days in some cases. Transient proteinuria developed in several cases. The reticulocyte counts were transiently elevated. Hydration with intravenous fluids improved the elimination of nickel.[152] A biochemical marker study of renal changes in workers exposed to nickel compounds revealed increased urinary small molecular weight proteins such as lysozyme and *N*-acetyl-beta-D-glucosaminidase (NAG).[160]

Twenty-three dialysis patients suffered nausea, vomiting, weakness, and headache when their dialysate was contaminated with nickel from a water heater tank that was improperly plated when manufactured. These symptoms reportedly resolved spontaneously after removal from the source of exposure.[162] In 1997, a major retailer recalled all of its home water filters due to possible nickel chloride contamination and the threat of abdominal cramping, nausea, vomiting, and diarrhea.[14]

In a survey of patients attending a general dermatology practice, allergic contact dermatitis due to nickel was second only to the *Anacardiacae* family of plants (poison ivy, poison oak, etc).[109] Sensitized individuals require only minute amounts of nickel to incite or exacerbate their dermatitis. After removal from exposure, the dermatitis may be very recalcitrant, possibly due to the retention of nickel in the epidermis. Nickel also causes an irritant contact dermatitis. Exposure of the conjunctivae to nickel can cause conjunctivitis, and sensitization may occur with subsequent episodes of allergic conjunctivitis (see Chap. 28).[4,149]

Inhalation exposure to nickel causes rhinitis and sinusitis. Anosmia, nasal polyposis, and perforation may occur. Chronic pulmonary irritation and bronchitis are also reported.[148]

Studies of workers at nickel smelters and refineries indicate that nickel is a potent carcinogen in those industries, producing nasal and pulmonary cancers. There is also some evidence for an excessive cancer risk in nickel-using industries, but concurrent exposure to other carcinogens may confound these studies.[59]

Immediate symptoms of inhalation of nickel carbonyl are nausea, vertigo, headache, GI symptoms, dyspnea, and chest pain. Initial symptoms are not necessarily dramatic and usually abate. Twelve to 36 hours later, a diffuse interstitial pneumonitis may develop, resulting in cough, dyspnea, cyanosis, and hypoxia. Deaths result from interstitial pneumonitis, cerebral edema, and hemorrhage. Sequelae in survivors include pulmonary fibrosis.[149]

Laboratory Evaluation of Nickel Exposure

Urinary nickel measurements can be useful in acute nickel toxicity, both to confirm the diagnosis and to monitor therapy (described in the next section). Unfortunately, the assays may not be readily available to guide the initial diagnosis or management. Urinary nickel measurements are useful in predicting the severity of acute pneumonitis secondary to nickel carbonyl poisoning. Blood and urine measurements of nickel are useful for surveillance of exposure to nickel, although specific risks to health cannot be predicted based on these findings.[148,151]

Treatment of Nickel Poisoning

Intravenous hydration is helpful in enhancing the elimination of nickel from the body, but no alleviation of symptoms has been documented with this treatment.[154] Sodium diethyldithiocarbamate (Dithiocarb) is recommended as a chelating agent in the treatment of nickel carbonyl poisoning (Fig. 81–1).[151] Sodium diethyldithiocarbamate has been used as the nickel-binding reagent in the routine method for measuring nickel in urine since the 1950s. Subsequent animal and clinical studies demonstrated that IV Dithiocarb is the chelating agent of choice, while D-penicillamine and calcium disodium EDTA are not effective and BAL is only partially effective.[81] The utility of DMSA remains to be investigated.

Disulfiram has been used to treat allergic nickel dermatitis[4] and has increased urinary excretion of nickel.[153] Patients with nickel allergic contact dermatitis must avoid nickel-containing objects, but this is extremely difficult because nickel is used in coins, jewelry, cooking utensils, and other common products. The amount of nickel leaching from a product may be determined by the Fisher's test (dimethylglyoxime and ammonium hydroxide), allowing the individual to avoid objects with high amounts of leaching.[4]

Selenium

Selenium is an essential nonmetallic element found commercially in steel and copper alloys, metal bluing solution, glass and paint pigments, and antifungal shampoos. Many selenium compounds are very irritating or even caustic to the skin, mucous membranes, and respiratory

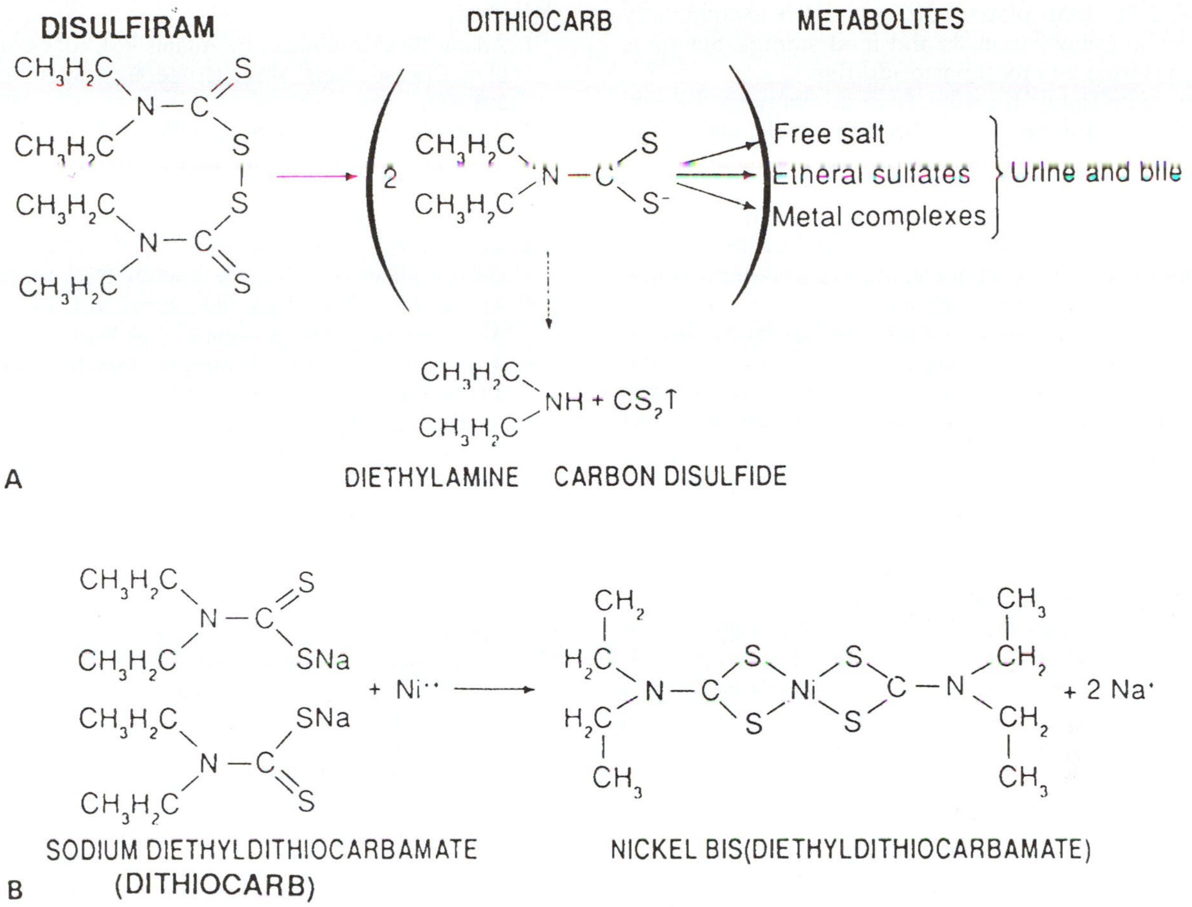

Figure 81–1. A. Metabolism of disulfiram and sodium diethyldithiocarbamate. **B.** Chelation of nickel by Dithiocarb. *(Reprinted, with permission, from Sunderman FW: Efficacy of sodium diethyldithiocarbamate [Dithiocarb] in acute nickel carbonyl poisoning. Ann Clin Lab Sci 1979;9:1–10. Copyright 1979 by the Institute for Clinical Science, Inc.)*

tract. Selenium oxychloride destroys skin on contact. Selenious acid (hydrogen selenide), used by gun owners as a "gun bluing" agent, is very caustic when ingested. Fatalities from unintentional ingestion of gun bluing agents by children are reported.[34]

There is some evidence that selenium is a naturally occurring antioxidant in the body and may be anticarcinogenic.[8,21,89] It is beyond the scope of this chapter to review this discussion, but because of these suggestive findings, selenium in various forms is being consumed in megadoses as a dietary supplement. The Centers for Disease Control and Prevention reported 12 persons with nausea, vomiting, nail changes, fatigue, and irritability from excessive selenium intake. About half of the patients experienced hair loss, and about one-third lost nails. Other symptoms included watery diarrhea, abdominal cramps, dryness of hair, paresthesias, and garlic breath odor.[39,44,134,142] Chronic selenosis is manifested by garlic breath odor, GI distress, upper airway irritation, metallic taste in the mouth, and anosmia.[6,21,40] Endemic selenium consumption and intoxication has been associated with all of these symptoms, and polyneuritis is described.[163]

The differential diagnosis of a garlic odor includes garlic consumption, phosphorous, arsenic, tellurium, dimethyl sulfoxide, and selenium. Urine concentrations are used to monitor excessive exposure to selenium, but are not helpful in the management of acute selenium toxicity, because toxicity may be localized to the respiratory tract or GI tract.[120] Only supportive treatment can be offered for patients with selenium toxicity. Nephrotoxic selenium complexes are formed with BAL, calcium disodium EDTA, and D-penicillamine.[6] Activated charcoal and a cathartic have been recommended.[137]

Tin

Tin is used in many alloys, such as copper-tin alloys, called bronzes. The main use of tin today is in solders. Tin and stannous sulfate, chloride, fluoride, and fluoroborate salts, and potassium and sodium stannates are also used in electroplating processes. Tin is commonly used for household utensils and food storage. Stannous fluoride is used as a toothpaste additive.

Some inorganic tin salts, such as stannous chloride and stannous sulfate, can be strongly acidic, and potassium and sodium stannate can form strong alkaline solutions. Inhalations of tin oxide can result in a "benign" pneumoconiosis in which there is radiographic evidence of dust or fiber deposition in the lungs but no evidence of pulmonary function abnormalities or long-term sequelae, such as pulmonary malignancies.

Some organic tin compounds used as fungicides, algicides, and bacteriocides in paints and wood, and catalysts and stabilizers in the production of rubber and other polymers, are highly toxic and readily absorbed through the skin. The trialkyl compounds, particularly triethyltin, can cause encephalopathy and cerebral edema. Diethyltin diiodide was used to treat staphylococcal skin disorders in the 1950s, and resulted in an epidemic of neurologic illness with 102 deaths and hundreds of cases of permanent sequelae.[116]

British anti-Lewisite (BAL) has been suggested for the treatment of poisoning by dialkyl tin compounds. DMSA might therefore also be useful. Because trialkyl tin compounds do not readily react with sulfhydral groups, BAL would not be helpful in these cases.[18]

Zinc

Zinc is a silvery white metal that is present in common alloys such as brass and bronze. It is used as an anticorrosion agent to produce galvanized iron or steel. Zinc most commonly causes GI distress and diarrhea after ingestion, but as much as 12 g of elemental zinc has been consumed over a 2-day period without evidence of hematologic, hepatic, or renal toxicity. Beverages have been contaminated with elemental zinc after storage in galvanized containers or use of galvanized utensils, with resulting gastrointestinal upset.[62] Unintentional ingestion of liquid zinc chloride flux caused severe local burns and metabolic acidosis (see Chap. 86). A severe chemical pneumonitis can result from inhalation of zinc chloride.[69] Zinc chloride also causes contact dermatitis.[117]

Welding with alloys or galvanized items containing zinc produces zinc oxide, a cause of metal fume fever. Zinc chloride is used as a flux agent and wood preservative, in paper manufacturing, in dyes and deodorants, and to produce smokescreens.[117]

Zinc has become a common dietary supplement. Zinc gluconate lozenges are reported to reduce the duration of symptoms of the common cold.[100] Excessive oral ingestion of zinc supplements in one case[118] and zinc coins in another resulted in reversible sideroblastic anemia and bone marrow depression. The mechanism for the anemia was thought to be a zinc-induced copper deficiency.[127] Both patients recovered after cessation of excess zinc intake.[30] Excessive intake of zinc is also associated with pure white cell aplasia.[49] A fatal case of intravenous zinc intoxication has also been reported.[29]

References

1. Adams RM: Chromium. In: Adams RM, ed: Occupational Skin Disease. New York, Grune & Stratton, 1983, pp. 208–217.
2. Adams RM: Cobalt. In: Adams RM, ed: Occupational Skin Diseases. New York, Grune & Stratton, 1983, pp. 217–220.
3. Adams RM: Copper. In: Adams RM, ed: Occupational Skin Disease. New York, Grune & Stratton, 1983, p. 220.
4. Adams RM: Nickel. In: Adams RM, ed: Occupational Skin Disease. New York, Grune & Stratton, 1983, pp. 225–230.
5. Ahasan HA, Chowdhury MA, Azhar MA, Rafiqueuddin AK: Copper sulphate poisoning. Trop Doct 1994;24:52–53.
6. Alderman LC, Bergin JJ: Hydrogen selenide poisoning: An illustrative case with review of the literature. Arch Environ Health 1986;41:354–358.
7. Alexander CS: Cobalt-beer cardiomyopathy. Am J Med 1972;53:395–417.
8. Alexander J: Risk assesment of selenium. Scand J Work Environ Health 1993;19 (suppl 1):122–123.
9. Alexandersson T: Blood and urinary concentrations as estimators of cobalt exposure. Arch Environ Health 1988;43:299–303.
10. American Conference of Govermental Industrial Hygienists (ACGIH): Copper as Cu: Documentation of Threshold Limit Values for Substances in Workroom Air. Cincinnati, ACGIH, 1983.
11. Ando Y, Shibata E, Tsuchiyama F, Sakai S: Elevated urinary cadmium concentrations in a patient with acute cadmium pneumonitis. Scand J Work Environ Health 1996; 22:150–153.
12. Angerer J, Heinrich R: Cobalt. In Seiler HG, Sigel H, eds: Handbook on Toxicity of Inorganic Compounds. New York, Marcel Dekker, 1988, pp. 251–261.
13. Angle CR. Dimercaptosuccinic acid (DMSA): Negligible effect on manganese in urine and blood. Occup Environ Med 1995;52:846. Letter.
14. Anonymous. Product alert: Home water filter nickel chloride contamination. Infect Dis Child Newsletter. American Academy of Pediatrics, 1997;10:58.
15. Baker EL, Peterson WA, Holtz JL, et al: Subacute cadmium intoxication in jewelry workers: An evaluation of diagnostic procedures. Arch Environ Health 1979;39:173–177.
16. Balmes JR: Respiratory effects of hard-metal dust exposure. State Art Rev Occup Med 1987;2:327–344.
17. Banner W Jr, Koch M, Capin DM, et al: Experimental chelation therapy in chromium, lead, and boron intoxication with *N*-acetylcysteine and other compounds. Toxicol Appl Pharmacol 1986;83:142–147.
18. Barnes JM, Magos L: The toxicity of organometallic compounds. Organometal Chem Rev 1968;3:137–141.
19. Barnhart S, Rosenstock L: Cadmium chemical pneumonitis. Chest 1984;86:789–791.
20. Barranco VP: Eczematous dermatitis caused by internal exposure to copper. Arch Dermatol 1972;106:386–387.
21. Bedwal RS, Nair N, Sharma MP, Mathur RS: Selenium—Its biological perspectives. Med Hypotheses 1993;41: 150–159. Review.
22. Bentur Y, Koren G, McGuigan M, Spielberg SP: An unusual skin exposure to copper: Clinical and pharmacokinetic evaluation. J Toxicol Clin Toxicol 1988;26:371–380.
23. Bernard A, Roels H, Buchet SP, et al: Alpha 1-antitrypsin

in cadmium toxicity: An evaluation of its suggested role. Toxicology 1978;9:249–253.
24. Bidstrup PL, Wagg R: Chromium, alloys and compounds. In: Parmeggiani L, ed: Encyclopedia of Occupational Health and Safety, 3rd ed. Geneva, International Labor Organization, 1985, pp. 468–473.
25. Blejer HP: Death due to cadmium oxide fumes. Ind Med Surg 1996;35:362–364.
26. Blejer HP: Cadmium-silver solders: An example of regulatory, medical and other failures. In: McCann M, Barazoni S, eds: Health Hazards in the Arts and Crafts. Washington, DC, Society for Occupational and Environmental Medicine, 1980, pp. 166–175.
27. Bonenfant JL, Miller G, Roy PE: Quebec beer-drinkers cardiomyopathy: Pathological studies. Can Med Assoc J 1967;97:910–916.
28. Borborik M Dusek J: Cardiomyopathy accompanying industrial cobalt exposure. Br Heart J 1972;34:113–166.
29. Brocks JA, Reid H, Glazer G: Acute intravenous zinc poisoning. Br Med J 1977;28:1390–1391.
30. Broun ER, Greist A, Tricot G, Hoffman R: Excessive zinc ingestion. JAMA 1990;264:1441–1443.
31. Burgess WA: Recognition of Health Hazardous in Industry: A Review of Materials and Processes. New York, Wiley, 1995.
32. Butterworth RF, Spahr L: Manganese toxicity, dopaminergic dysfunction and hepatic encephalopathy. Metab Brain Dis 1995;10:259–267.
33. Calne DB, Chu NS, Huang CC, et al: Manganism and idiopathic parkinsonism: Similarities and differences. Neurology 1994;44:1583–1586.
34. Carter RF: Acute selenium poisoning. Med J Aust 1966; 1:525–528.
35. Chen R, Wei L, Huang H: Mortality from lung cancer among copper miners. Br J Ind Med 1993;50:505–509.
36. Chowdhury P, Louria DB: Influence of cadmium and other trace metals on human alpha 1-antitrypsin: An in vitro study. Science 1976;191:480–481.
37. Christensen JM, Poulsen OM: A 1982–1992 surveillance programme on Danish pottery painters. Biological levels and health effects following exposure to soluble or insoluble cobalt compounds in cobalt blue dyes. Sci Total Environ 1994;150:95–104.
38. Chuttani HK, Gupta PS, Gulati S, et al: Acute copper sulfate poisoning. Am J Med 1965;39:849–854.
39. Clark RF, Strukle E, Williams SR, Manoguerra AS: Selenium poisoning from a nutritional supplement. JAMA 1996;275:1087–1088. Letter.
40. Combs GF Jr: Essentiality and toxicity of selenium with respect to recommended dietary allowance and reference doses. Scand J Work Environ Health 1993;19(suppl 1): 119–121.
41. Cook DG, Fahn S, Brait KA: Chronic manganese intoxication. Arch Neurol 1974;30:59–64.
42. Dalrup T, Haarhoff K, Szathmary SC: Toedliche nickelsulfate-intoxication. Beitr Berichtl Med 1983;41:141–144.
43. Dhir GG, Rao DS, Mehrotra MP: Contact dermatitis caused by copper sulfate used as coloring material in commercial alcohol. Ann Allergy 1977;39:204.
44. Diskin CJ, Tomasso CL, Alper JC, et al: Long term selenium exposure. Arch Intern Med 1979;139:824–826.
45. Duckham JM, Lee HA: The treatment of refractory anaemia of chronic renal failure with cobalt chloride. Q J Med 1976;178:277–294.
46. Dunnick JK, Fowler BA: Cadmium. In: Seiler HG, Sigel H, eds: Handbook on Toxicity of Inorganic Compounds. New York, Marcel Dekker, 1988, pp. 155–174.
47. Figueroa S, Gerstenhaber B, Welch L, et al: Hard metal interstitial pulmonary disease associated with a form of welding in a metal parts coating plant. Am J Ind Med 1992;21:363–373.
48. Fishbein L: Environmental metallic carcinogens: An overview of exposure levels. J Toxicol Environ Health 1976;2:77–109.
49. Forsyth PD, Davies JM: Pure white cell aplasia and health food products. Postgrad Med J 1995;71:557–558.
50. Franchin R Mutti A, Cavatorta E, et al: Nephrotoxicity of chromium. Contrib Nephrol 1978;10:98–110.
51. Fredstrom S, Rogosheske J, Gupta P, Burns LJ: Extrapyramidal symptons in a BMT recipient with hyperintense basal ganglia and elevated manganese. Bone Marrow Transplant 1995;15:989–992.
52. Frentz G, Teilum D: Cutaneous eruptions and intrauterine contraceptive copper device. Acta Derm Venereol 1979;60: 69–71.
53. Friberg L: Cadmium. In: Friberg L, Nordberg GF, Vouk VB, eds: Handbook on the Toxicology of Metals. New York, Elsevier North-Holland, 1979, pp. 355–377.
54. Friberg L: Proteinuria and kidney injury among workmen exposed to cadmium and nickel dust. J Ind Hyg Toxicol 1948;30:32–36.
55. Friberg L, Elinder CG: Cadmium and compounds. In: Parmeggiani L, ed: Encyclopedia of Occupational Health and Safety, 3rd ed. Geneva, International Labor Organization, 1985, pp. 356–357.
56. Friberg L, Piscator M, Nordberg GF, Kjellstrom T: Cadmium in the Environment, 2nd ed. Cleveland, CRC Press, 1974.
57. Goldstein NP, Owen CA: Sympsium on copper metabolism and Wilson's disease. Mayo Clin Proc 1974;49: 361–367.
58. Grandjean P: Diseases associated with metals. In: Last JM, ed: Public Health and Preventive Medicine, 23rd ed. Norwalk, CT, Appleton-Century-Crofts, 1986, pp. 587–616.
59. Grandjean P, Andersen O, Nielsen G: Carcinogenicity of occupational nickel exposures: An evaluation of the epidemiological evidence. Am J Ind Med 1988;13:193–209.
60. Gross RT, Kriss JP, Spaet TH: The hematopoietic and goitrogenic effects of cobaltous chloride in patients with sickle cell anemia. Pediatrics 1955;15:284–290.
61. Grum EE: Cadmium toxicity. In: Bresnitz EA, ed: Case Studies in Environmental Medicine. Agency for Toxic Substances and Disease Registry, Public Health Service, U.S. Department of Health and Human Services, 1990.
62. Guyer RA: The Toxic Effects of Metals. In: Amdur MD, Doull J, Klasseen CD, eds: Cassaret and Doull's Toxicology. New York, Pergamon Press, 1991, pp. 623–680.
63. Hamilton JW, Wetterhahn KE: Chromium. In: Seiler HG, Sigel H, eds: Handbook on Toxicity of Inorganic Compounds. New York, Marcel Dekker, 1988, pp. 240–248.
64. Hathaway JA: Treatment of acute chromate poisoning. In:

Serrone DM, ed: Chromium Symposium, 1986: An Update. Pittsburg, Industrial Health Foundation, 1986, pp. 87–99.
65. Hauser RA, Zesiewicz TA, Rosemurgy AS, et al: Manganese intoxication and chronic liver failure. Ann Neurol 1994;36:871–875.
66. Hayes RB, Lilienfeld AM, Snell LM: Mortality in chromium chemical production workers: A prospective study. Int J Epidemiol 1979;8:365–374.
67. Henretig F, Joffe M, Baffa G, et al: Elemental cobalt toxicity and effects of chelation therapy. Vet Human Toxicol 1988;30:372. Abstract.
68. Holtzman NA, Elliot DA, Heller, RH: Copper intoxication. N Engl J Med 1966;275:347–352.
69. Homma S, Jones R, Quist J, et al: Pulmonary vascular lesions in the adult respiratory distress syndrome caused by inhalation of zinc chloride smoke: A morphometric study. Hum Pathol 1992;23:45–50.
70. Iverson KV, Banner W, Froede RC, Derrick MR: Failure of dialysis therapy in potassium dichromate poisoning. J Emerg Med 1983;1:143–149.
71. Jarup L, Persson B, Edling C, Elinder CG: Renal function impairment in workers previously exposed to cadmium. Nephron 1993;64:75–81.
72. Jarup L, Persson B, Elinder CG: Decreased glomerular filtration rate in solderers exposed to cadmium. Occup Environ Med 1995;52:818–822.
73. Jarvis JQ, Hammond E, Meier R, Robinson C: Cobalt cardiomyopathy: A report of two cases from mineral assay laboratories and a review of the literature. J Occp Med 1992;34:620–626.
74. Katz SA, Salem H: The toxicology of chromium with respect to its chemical speciation: A review. J Appl Toxicol 1993;13:217–224.
75. Kennedy A, Dornan JD, King R: Fatal myocardial disease associated with industrial exposure to cobalt. Lancet 1981; 1:412–414.
76. Kennedy SM, Chan-Yeung M, Marion S, et al: Maintenance of stellite and tungsten carbide saw tips: Respiratory health and exposure–response evaluations. Occup Environ Med 1995;52:185–191.
77. Keogh J: Personal communication. Baltimore, March 1986.
78. Klein WJ, Metz EN, Price AN: Acute copper intoxication. Arch Intern Med 1972;129:578–582.
79. Korallus U. Hartdort C, Lewalter J: Experimental cases for ascorbic acid therapy of poisoning by hexavalent chromium compounds. Int Arch Occup Environ Health 1984; 53:247–256.
80. Kriss JP, Carnes WH, Gross RT: Hypothyroidism and thyroid hyperplasia in patients treated with cobalt. JAMA 1955;157:117–121.
81. Kubota J, Lazar VA, Losee F: Copper, zinc, cadmium, and lead in human blood from 19 locations in the United States. Arch Environ Health 1968;16:788–793.
82. Kusaka Y, Iki M, Kumagai S, Goto S: Decreased ventilatory function in hard metal workers. Occup Environ Med 1996;53:194–199.
83. Ky SQ, Deng HS, Xie PY, HU W: A report of two cases of chronic serious manganese poisoning treated with sodium para-aminosalicylic acid. Br J Ind Med. 1992;49:66–69.
84. Langard S: Role of chemical species and exposure characteristics in cancer among persons occupationally exposed to chromium compounds. Scand J Work Environ Health 1993;19(suppl 1):81–89.
85. Lauwerys R: The Toxicology of Cadium. Environment and Quality of Life Series, EUR 7649. Luxembourg, Commission of the European Communities, 1982.
86. Lauwerys RR, Bernard AM, Roels HA, Buchet JP: Cadmium: Exposure markers as predictors of nephrotoxic effects. Clin Chem 1994;40:1391–1394.
87. Leduc D, de Francquen P, Jacobovitz D, et al: Association of cadmium exposure with rapidly progressive emphysema in a smoker. Thorax 1993;48:570–571.
88. Lee JS, White KL: Cadmium. In: Rom WN, ed: Environmental and Occupational Medicine. Boston, Little, Brown, 1983, pp. 465–472.
89. Longnecker MP: Selenium: The public health connection. Health Environ Dig 1989;3:1–3.
90. Lucchini R, Selis L, Folli D, et al. Neurobehavioral effects of manganese in workers from a ferroalloy plant after temporary cessation of exposure. Scand J Work Environ Health 1995;21:143–149.
91. Mangold, CA, Beckett RR: Combined occupational exposure of silver brazers to cadmium oxide, nitrogen dioxide and fluorides at a naval shipyard. Am Ind Hyg Assoc J 1971;32:115–118.
92. McDermott PH, Delancy RL, Egan JD, Sullivan JF: Myocardosis and cardiac failure in men. JAMA 1966;198: 253–256.
93. McDiarmid MA, Freeman CS, Grossman EA: Biological monitoring results for cadmium exposed workers. Am Ind Hyg Assoc J 1996;57:1019–1023.
94. McKinney PE, Brent J, Kulig K: Acute zinc chloride ingestion in a child: Local and systemic effects. Ann Emerg Med 1994;23:1383–1387.
95. Meco G, Bonifati V, Vanacore N, Fabrizio E: Parkinsonism after chronic exposure to the fungicide maneb (manganese ethylene-bis-dithiocarbamate). Scand J Work Environ Health 1994;20:301–305.
96. Misselwitz B, Muhler A, Weinmann HJ: A toxicolgic risk for using manganese complexes? A literature survey of existing data through several medical specialties. Invest Radiol 1995;30:611–620.
97. Mitchell JR: Acetaminophen toxicity. N Engl J Med 1988; 319:1601–1602. Editorial.
98. Moller DR, Brooks JM, Bernstein DI, et al: Delayed anaphylactoid reaction in a worker exposed to chromium. J Allergy Clin Immunol 1986;77:451–456.
99. Morin YL, Foley AR, Martineau G, Roussel J: Quebec beer-drinkers' cardiomyopathy: Forty-eight cases. Can Med Assoc J 1967;97:881–883.
100. Mossad SB, Macknin ML, Medendorp SV, Mason P: Zinc gluconate Lozenges for treating the common cold. A randomized, double-blind, placebo-controlled study. Ann Intern Med 1996;125:81–88.
101. Mutti A, Cavatorta A, Pedroni C, et al: The role of chromium accumulation in the relationship between airborne and urinary chromium in welders. Int Arch Occup Environ Health 1979;43:123–133.
102. National Institute for Occupational Safety and Health: Cadmium. Curr Intell Bull 1984;42.
103. National Institute for Occupational Safety and Health: Cri-

teria for a Recommended Standard: Occupational Exposure to Cadmium (DHEW pub. no. 76–192). Cincinnati, NIOSH, 1976.
104. Nelson K, Golnick J, Korn T, Angle C: Manganese encephalopathy: Utility of early magnetic resonance imaging. Br J Ind Med 1993;50:510–513.
105. New York State Reporting Standards for Heavy Metal Levels in Blood and Urine. Albany, New York State Department of Health, 1988.
106. Newton D, Rundo J: The long-term retention of inhaled cobalt-60. Health Phys 1970;21:377–384.
107. NIOSH: Pocket Guide to Chemical Hazards. Washington, DC, U.S. Department of Health and Human Services (pub. no 85–114), 1987.
108. Occupational Exposure to Cadmium: Final rule, 29 CFR Parts 1910, 1915 and 1920 Fed Reg, 1992;57(178).
109. Occupational Exposure to Formaldehyde: Final rule, 29 CFR Parts 1910 and 1926: Fed Reg, 1987;52(233):46175.
110. Park HS, Yu HJ, Jung KS: Occupational asthma caused by chromium. Clin Exp Allergy 1994;24:676–681.
111. Petersen R, Mikkelsen S, Thomsen OF: Chronic interstitial nephropathy after plasma cutting in stainless steel. Occup Environ Med 1994;51:259–261.
112. Pimental JC, Marques F: Vineyard sprayer's lung. Thorax 1969;24:678–688.
113. Pimental JC, Menezes AP: Liver disease and vineyard sprayer's lungs. Gastroenterology 1977;72:275–283.
114. Pimental JC, Menezes AP: Liver granulomas containing copper in vineyard sprayer's lung. Am Rev Respir Dis 1975;111:189–195.
115. Powers WJ, Gad SC, Siino KM, et al: Effects of therapeutic agents on chromium-induced acute nephrotoxicity. In: Serrone DM, ed: Chromium Symposium, 1986: An Update. Pittsburgh, Industrial Health Foundation, 1986, pp. 87–99.
116. Raffle PAB, Lee WR, McCallum RI, Murray R, eds: Diseases of Occupations. Boston, Little, Brown, 1987, pp. 310–311.
117. Raffle PAB, Lee WR, McCallum RI, Murray R, eds: Diseases of Occupations. Boston, Little, Brown, 1987, pp. 288–289.
118. Ramadurai J, Shapiro C, Kozloff M, Telfer M: Zinc abuse and sideroblastic anemia. Am J Hematol 1993;42: 227–228.
119. Reichelderfer TE: Accidental death of an infant caused by ingestion of ammonium dichromate. South Med J 1968; 61:96–97.
120. Robberecht JH, Deelstra HA: Selenium in human urine: Concentration levels and medical implications. Clin Chem Acta 1984;136:107–120.
121. Roels H, Lauwerys R, Buchet JP, et al. Epidemiological survey among workers exposed to manganese: Effects on lung, central nervous system, and some biological indices. Am J Ind Med 1987;11:307–327.
122. Rose CS, Heywood PG, Costanzo RM: Olfactory impairment after chronic occupational cadmium exposure. J Occup Med 1992;34:600–605.
123. Rosenman KD, Standbury M: Risk of lung cancer among former chromium smelter workers. Am J Ind Med 1996; 29:491–500.
124. Rubinfeld Y, Maor Y, Simon D, et al: A progressive rise in serum copper levels in women taking oral contraceptives: A potential hazard? Fertil Steril 1979;32:599–601.
125. Ruokonen EL, Linnainmaa M, Seuri M, et al: A fatal case of hard-metal disease. Scand J Work Environ Health 1996;22:62–65.
126. Samitz MH: Prevention of occupational skin diseases from exposure chromic acid and chromates: Use of ascorbic acid. Cutis 1974;13:569–574.
127. Sandstead HH: Requirements and toxicity of essential trace elements, illustrated by zinc and copper. Am J Clin Nutr 1995;62(suppl 3):6215–6245.
128. Sarkar B: Copper. In: Seiler HG, Sigel H, eds: Handbook on Toxicity of Inorganic Compounds. New York, Marcel Dekker, 1988, pp. 266–272.
129. Satah N, Fukuda S, Takizawa M, et al, Chromium-induced carcinoma in the nasal region: A report of four cases. Rhinology 1994;32:47–50.
130. Savolainen H: Cadmium-associated renal disease. Ren Fail 1995;17:483–487.
131. Scheinberg HI: Copper. In: Parmeggiani L, ed: Encyclopedia of Occupational Health Safety, 3rd ed. Geneva, International Labor Organization, 1985, pp. 546–548.
132. Schwartz L, Dunn JE: Dermatitis occurring in a woolen mill. Ind Med Surg 1942;11:432–435.
133. Seidal K, Jorgensen N, Elinder CG, et al: Fatal cadmium-induced pneumonitis. Scand J Work Environ Health 1993; 19:429–431.
134. Selenium intoxication—New York. MMWR 1984;33: 157–158.
135. Sieber WK, Sundin DS, Frazier TM, Robinson CF: Development, use and availability of a job exposure matrix based on national occupational hazard survey data. Am J Ind Med 1991;20:163–174.
136. Sjogren B, Iregren A, Frech W, et al. Effects on the nervous system among welders exposed to aluminum and manganese. Occup Environ Med 1996;53:32–40.
137. Smith THF: Selenium, tellurium, and osmium. In: Zenz C, ed: Occupational Medicine, 2nd ed. Chicago, Year Book, 1988, pp. 614–618.
138. Smith TJ, Blough S: Chromium, manganese, nickel and other elements. In: Rom W, ed: Environmental and Occupational Medicine. Boston, Little, Brown, 1983, pp. 491–510.
139. Sontz E, Schwieger J: The green water syndrome: Copper-induced hemolysis and subsequent acute renal failure as a consequence of a religious ritual. Am J Med 1995;98: 311–315.
140. Southwood T, Lamb CM, Freeman J: Ingestion of potassium permanganate crystals by a 3-yr-old boy. Med J Aust 1987;146:639–640.
141. Sprince NL, Oliver C, Eisen EA, et al: Cobalt exposure and lung disease in tungsten carbide production. Am Rev Respir Dis 1988;138:1220–1226.
142. Srivastava AK, Gupta BN, Bihari V, Gaur JS: Generalized hair loss and selenium exposure. Vet Hum Toxicol 1995; 37:468–469.
143. Sterns DM, Belbruno JJ, Wetterhahn KC: A prediction of chromium (III) accumulation in humans from chromium dietary supplements. FASEB J 1995;9:1650–1657.
144. Stokinger HE: Cadmium. In: Clayton GD, Clayton FE, eds: Patty's Industrial Hygiene and Toxicology. New York, Wiley, 1981, pp. 1563–1582.

145. Stokinger HE: Chromium. In: Clayton GC, Clayton FE, eds: Patty's Industrial Hygiene and Toxicology. New York, Wiley, 1981, pp. 1589–1604.
146. Stokinger HE: Copper. In: Clayton GC, Clayton FE, eds: Patty's Industrial Hygiene and Toxicology. New York, Wiley, 1981, pp. 1620–1630.
147. Stokinger HE: Nickel. In: Clayton GC, Clayton FE, eds: Patty's Industrial Hygiene and Toxicology. New York, Wiley, 1981, pp. 1820–1841.
148. Sunderman FW: Nickel. In: Seiler HG, Sigel H, eds: Handbook on Toxicity of Inorganic Compounds. New York, Marcel Dekker, 1988, pp. 451–464.
149. Sunderman FW: Nickel and compounds. In: Parmeggiani L, ed: Encyclopedia of Occupational Health and Safety, 3rd ed. Geneva, International Labor Organization, 1985, pp. 1438–1440.
150. Sunderman FW: Efficacy of sodium diethyldithiocarbamate (Dithiocarb) in acute nickel carbonyl poisoning. Ann Clin Lab Sci 1979;9:1–10.
151. Sunderman FW, Aitio A, Morgan LG, Norseth T: Biological monitoring of nickel. Toxicol Ind Health 1986;2:17–78.
152. Sunderman FW, Dingle B, Hopfer SM, Swift T: Acute nickel toxicity in electroplating workers who accidentally ingested a solution of nickel sulfate and nickel chloride. Am J Ind Med 1988;14:257–266.
153. Suvorov IM, Cekunova MP: Cobalt, alloys and compounds. In: Parmeggiani L, ed: Encyclopedia of Occupational Health and Safety, 3rd ed. Geneva, International Labor Organization, 1985, pp. 493–495.
154. Swennen B, Buchet JP, Stanescu D, et al: Epidemiological survey of workers exposed to cobalt oxides, cobalt salts, and cobalt metal. Br J Ind Med 1993;50:835–842.
155. Tanaka S: Manganese and its compounds. In: Zenz C, ed: Occupational Medicine, 2nd ed. Chicago, Year Book, 1988, pp. 583–589.
156. Trevisan A, Nicoletto G, Maso S, et al: Biological monitoring of cadmium exposure: Reliability of spot urine samples. Int Arch Occup Environ Health 1994;65:373–375.
157. Vasallo S, Howland MA: Severe dichromate poisoning: Survival after therapy with intravenous *N*-acetylcysteine and hemodialysis. Vet Human Toxicol 1988;30:347.
158. Vieregge P, Heinzow B, Korf G, et al. Long term exposure to manganese in rural well water has no neurological effects. Can J Neurol Sci. 1995;22:286–289.
159. Villar TG: Vineyard sprayer's lung. Am Rev Respir Dis 1969;110:545–555.
160. Vyskocil A, Senft V, Viau C, et al: Biochemical renal changes in workers exposed to soluble nickel compounds. Hum Exp Toxicol 1994;13:257–261.
161. Wasser WG, Feldman NS, D'Agati VD: Chronic renal failure after ingestion of over-the-counter chromium picolinate. Ann Intern Med 1997;126:410. Letter.
162. Webster JD Parker TF, Alfrey AC, et al: Acute nickel intoxication by dialysis. Ann Intern Med 1980;92:631–633.
163. Yang G, Wang S, Zhou R, et al: Endermic selenium intoxication of humans in China. Am J Clin Nutr 1983;37: 872–881.
164. Zanelli R, Barbic F, Migliori M, Michetti G: Uncommon evolution of fibrosing alveolitis in a hard metal grinder exposed to cobalt dusts. Sci Total Environ 1994;150:225–229.

CHAPTER 82

Thallium

Maria Mercurio and Robert S. Hoffman

Thallium
MW = 204.39 daltons

Normal Levels	
Blood: <2μg/L	<9.78 nmol/L
Urine: <5μg/L	<24.5 nmol/L

Action Levels	
Blood: >100μg/L	>0.490 μmol/L
Urine: >200μg/L	>0.980 μmol/L

Values greater than or equal to the action level necessitate clinical intervention. Values below this level may necessitate intervention based on the clinical condition of the patient.

A 21-year-old female college student developed mild, but persistent abdominal pain that was interspersed with periods of severe colicky pain. Three days after the initial pain, her hair began to fall out. She became constipated, and noted a delay in the onset of her menses. Within 5 days of her initial symptoms, she was completely bald. On day 18, she was hospitalized, where routine physical examination only revealed lines on her fingernails. Her routine chemistry tests and several special studies for autoimmune disease were all normal. Her overall condition responded to nutritional support, her symptoms gradually resolved, her hair regrew, and she was discharged almost 2 months after the onset of symptoms without a diagnosis.

The patient returned to school. One month later, she felt pain in both her hands and feet, and developed difficulty speaking, dizziness, blurred vision, and vertigo. She was taken to the hospital once again. On admission, her blood pressure was 140/110 mm Hg; other vital signs were normal. Examination of her extremities showed good muscular strength in her legs but poor muscle coordination, and hyperesthetic pain in a stocking-and-glove distribution. Her deep-tendon reflexes were hypoactive in both legs, but normal in her upper extremities. Cranial nerve examination revealed horizontal and vertical nystagmus, and palsies of the abducens (CN VI) and facial (CN VII) nerves. Routine chemistries and a lumbar puncture were again essentially normal.

Four days later, still without a diagnosis, her symptoms of vertigo and tremulousness worsened. Her doctors noted that she was showing signs of oculogyric crisis, and her mental status deteriorated. Her alopecia returned. An MRI of her brain was interpreted as normal, and an EEG was felt to be nondiagnostic. Her condition progressed very rapidly with the development of bulbar palsy, involuntary chewing movements of her mouth, and spastic clonus of both upper limbs. Her level of consciousness changed from mild agitation to lethargy. Tonic movements of both upper extremities and episodic oculogyric crisis were noted.

Five days after her hospitalization, she became comatose. Negative studies included arsenic, antinuclear antibody, anti-double-stranded DNA antibody, rheumatoid factor, HIV, and lyme disease titers. Routine urinalysis was normal. She was treated with several broad-spectrum antibiotics, antiviral agents, hormones, and intravenous injections of gammaglobulin, none of which had any appreciable effect on her signs and symptoms.

Because her spontaneous respiratory efforts became progressively weaker and irregular, a tracheostomy was performed and she was placed on a ventilator. At that point, the diagnosis of acute disseminated encephalomyelitis was considered. Plasmapheresis of 1400 to 2000 mL at a time was initiated and seven exchanges, for a total of 10 L, were completed over the following 3 weeks. No change in her condition was noted.

Finally, the diagnosis of thallium intoxication was considered. Blood, urine, and CSF thallium levels were reported as 275, 532, and 31 μg/L, respectively. Nail and hair levels were 22,824 and 532 μg/kg, respectively. The patient was started on a regimen of intravenous potassium (100 mEq/day), oral Prussian blue (250 mg/kg per day divided q4h in 50 mL of 15% mannitol), and daily hemodialysis. Her symptoms slowly improved, and she intermittently regained consciousness about 2 months after hospitalization.

One year after the initial event, her orientation and memory improved and her IQ was estimated at 128, with good mathematical and verbal abilities. The patient was able to sit in a wheelchair for a prolonged period of time and could move herself 20 to 30 meters. She still could not move her legs. Her vision remained poor, but periodically she was able to see clearly.

What Are the Physical Properties of Thallium and How Has It Been Used?

Thallium, a toxic metal with atomic number 81, is located between mercury and lead on the periodic table. Thallium is a commonly found constituent of granite, shale, volcanic rock, and pyrites (which are used to make sulfuric acid), and is also recovered as flue dust from iron, lead, cadmium, and copper smelters. Thallium metal, which is soft and pliable like lead, melts at 300°C, boils at 1482°C, and forms univalent thallous and trivalent thallic salts. It has been used in alloys as an anticorrosive, in optical lenses to increase the refractive index, in artist's paints, in lamps to improve tungsten filaments, in imitation jewelry, as a catalyst, and in fireworks. In the early 1900s, thallium was used medicinally to treat syphilis, gonorrhea, tuberculosis, and ringworm of the scalp, and as a depilatory.[3,50] Although the usual oral dose given for epilation in the treatment of ringworm of the scalp was 7 to 8 mg/kg, fatal doses ranged from 6 to 40 mg/kg.[9,42] Many cases of severe thallium poisoning resulted from this practice, with one author summarizing nearly 700 cases and 46 deaths.[52]

Because thallium sulfate is odorless and tasteless, it was also successfully used as a rodenticide. Commercially available as Thalgrain, Echol's Roach Powder, Mo-Go, Martin's Rat Stop liquid, and Senco Corn Mix, thallium sulfate was very efficient at killing rats, prairie dogs, and other unwanted pests. In response to numerous case reports of unintentional poisonings,[53,61] its use as a household rodenticide was restricted in the United States in 1965. Ultimately even commercial use of thallium as a rodenticide was banned in the United States in 1975 because of continued human toxicity. Unfortunately, severe unintentional poisonings still occur in other countries where thallium is commonly used as a rodenticide.[59,75] Cases of severe thallium poisoning are still reported in this and other countries as a result of its use as a homicidal agent[14,45,49,55] and through contamination of herbal products[65] and cocaine.[29] Presently, trace amounts of thallium are used as a radioactive contrast agent to image tumors and to visualize cardiac function.[50]

What Are the Toxicokinetics of Thallium?

Exposures usually occur via one of three routes: *inhalation* of dust, *ingestion*, and *absorption* through intact skin. Thallium is rapidly absorbed, distributed throughout most of the body following three-compartment toxicokinetics,[60] and eliminated slowly via the kidneys and gastrointestinal tract. The volume of distribution for thallium is very large, and is estimated to be about 3.6 L/kg.[13] Thallium is found in all organs, with the highest concentrations in the large and small intestine, followed by the kidney, heart, brain, and muscles.[3]

The toxicokinetics of thallium can be described in a three-phase model. In the first phase, which occurs rapidly in the 4 hours following exposure, thallium is distributed to a central compartment (blood) and to well-perfused peripheral organs such as the kidney, liver, and muscle. In the second phase, which can last between 4 and 48 hours, thallium is distributed into the central nervous system.[60] This distribution phase is generally completed within 24 hours of ingestion. The third, or elimination, phase starts about 24 hours after ingestion. The primary mechanism of thallium elimination is secretion into the intestine, but enteral reabsorption results in the excretion of only a small portion of the thallium initially present in the bile.[12,49] The duration of the elimination phase depends on the route of exposure, dose, and treatment that is given. Unlike many other metals (such as lead), thallium does not have a major reservoir where it persists in the body. As such, reported elimination half-lives are as short as 1.7 days in humans with thallium poisoning.[27]

Thallium is excreted primarily via the feces (51.4%) and the urine (26.4%).[41] It is glomerularly filtered, and approximately 50% is reabsorbed in the tubules. Thallium is secreted into the tubular lumen in a manner similar to potassium.[2] Renal function remains normal in mild cases of thallium poisoning even though the kidney accumulates a higher concentration of thallium than any other organ. Changes in renal function in patients with severe thallotoxicosis include oliguria, diminished creatinine clearance, elevated blood urea nitrogen, and albuminuria.[2,45,48,50] Morphologic studies of rats with thallium poisoning show abnormalities in the renal medulla, mainly in the thick ascending limb of the loop of Henle, that occur by the second day after exposure and resolve by the tenth day.[2]

What Is the Pathophysiology of Thallium Poisoning?

The mechanism of action of thallium toxicity is not well established. In the body, thallium behaves biologically like potassium because of their similar ionic radii (0.147 nm for thallium and 0.133 nm for potassium). Because cell membranes cannot differentiate between thallium and potassium ions, thallous ions accumulate in areas with high potassium concentrations such as central and peripheral nervous, hepatic, and muscular tissues.[47,75] This principle underlies the use of radioactive thallium in cardiac imaging studies. Thallium replaces potassium in the activation of potassium-dependent enzymes.[47] In low concentrations, thallium stimulates these enzyme systems, but in high concentrations, it inhibits them.[48] Thallium is known to inhibit several potassium-dependent systems. Pyruvate kinase, a magnesium-dependent glycolytic enzyme that requires potassium to achieve maximum activity, has a 50 times greater affinity for thallous ions than potassium ions.[34] Succinic dehydrogenase, an essential enzyme in the Krebs cycle, is inhibited by small doses of thallium in rats.[25] Sodium-potassium ATPase, which is responsible for active transport of monovalent ions across cell membranes, can utilize thallous ions at low concentrations with a 10-fold greater affinity than potassium ions,[5,20] but is inhibited by thallium at higher concentrations.[30] Thallium also impairs depolarization of muscle fibers.[50] Mitochondrial energy is decreased due to the inhibition of pyruvate dehydrogenase complex and succinate dehydrogenase, resulting in a decrease of ATP generation via oxidative phosphorylation. Enzymatic destruction results in swelling and vacuolization of the mitochondria after exposure to thallium.[67] At low levels, thallium can activate other potassium-dependent enzymes such as phosphatase, homoserin dehydrogenase, vitamin B_{12}-dependent diol dehydrogenase, L-threonine dehydrogenase, and AMP deaminase.[50]

Thallous ions have been used to isolate riboflavin from milk in the form of a reversible precipitate. It is possible to conclude that thallous ions also form insoluble complexes and cause intracellular sequestration of riboflavin in vivo.[7] Riboflavin is the vitamin precursor of the flavin coenzyme FAD (flavin adenine dinucleotide). Due to a decrease in riboflavin, metabolic reactions dependent upon flavoproteins will decrease, causing disruption of the electron transport chain and a subsequent further decrease or impairment in the generation of cellular energy.[7] A decrease in cellular energy may lead to decreased mitotic activity and cessation of hair follicle formation resulting in the clinical sign of alopecia. Subsequent hair loss is the result of combined arrested formation and local destruction of hairshaft cells in the hair bulb.[7,61] Studies demonstrate that the dermatologic, neurologic, and cardiac effects of thallium toxicity mirror the side effects of thiamine deficiency (beriberi), highlighting the inhibitory effect of thallium on pyruvate dehydrogenase complex.[7,50] It is unclear whether thiamine administration has any beneficial effect in patients with thallium poisoning.

Thallium, like many other metals, has a high affinity for sulfhydryl groups. Sulfhydryl groups, present in enzymes and other proteins, form complexes with thallium. Keratin, a structural protein, consists of many cysteine residues that cross-link and form disulfide bonds. These disulfide bonds, add strength to keratin. Thallium interferes with the formation of disulfide bonds, which may contribute to findings such as alopecia and defects in nail growth resulting in Mees lines.[22,50,55,64] Additionally, the complexation of sulfhydryl groups with thallium results in a decrease in glutathione production (secondarily to a decrease in cysteine). This results in the accumulation of lipid peroxides in the brain, specifically the cerebellum, which appears as dark, pigmented, lipofuscin-like areas.[24]

Thallium also adversely affects protein synthesis in animals by damaging ribosomes, particularly the 60S subunit.[28] Although ribosomes are primarily dependent on potassium and magnesium, they will utilize thallium if present. At low concentrations, thallium has a protective effect, such as when the ribosome is confronted with irreversible inactivation from potassium deficiency. But as the concentration of thallium increases, its protective effect diminishes, resulting in progressive destabilization and destruction of the ribosomes. Ribosomal destruction can also be produced with potassium but at concentrations of 4.5 to 20 times higher than is required with thallium.[28]

Pathologic studies of the central nervous system in patients with thallium poisoning reveal localized areas of edema found in the cerebral hemispheres and brainstem. Chromatolytic changes are prominent in neurons of the motor cortex, third-nerve nuclei, substantia nigra, and pyramidal cells of the globus pallidus. In chronic exposures, there are signs of edema of the pial and arachnoidal membranes, and changes in the ganglion cells of the ventral and dorsal horns of the spinal cord consisting of chromatolysis, swelling, and fatty degeneration.[3,61]

The peripheral nervous system, which is usually clinically affected before the central nervous system, exhibits axonopathy in a classic dying back or Wallerian degeneration pattern.[3,16] That thallium affects the longer peripheral fibers—first sensory, then motor, and finally the shorter fibers—explains the primary toxic effects occurring in the lower extremities. Fragmentation and degeneration of associated myelin sheaths is accompanied by activation of Schwann cells.[3,7,8]

What Is the Clinical Presentation of Thallium Toxicity?

Many of the effects of thallium poisoning are somewhat nonspecific and occur over a variable time course.[39] When combined, however, a clear toxidrome can be defined (Table 82–1). Alopecia and the painful ascending peripheral neuropathy are the most characteristic find-

TABLE 82–1. CLINICAL STAGES OF THALLIUM POISONING[a]

Immediate (3–4 h)
Constipation
Diarrhea
Nausea
Vomiting
Intermediate (hours to days)
Alopecia
Altered mental status
Autonomic instability
Dysrhythmias
Ophthalmoplegia and cranial neuropathies
Painful ascending peripheral neuropathy
Pleuritic chest pain
Proteinuria
Seizures
Late (2–4 wk)
Alopecia
Mees lines
Persistent neurologic toxicity
Residual Neurologic Toxicity (months)
Impaired memory and cognition
Motor neuropathy
Ophthalmoplegia
Optic neuritis

[a]Substantial overlap of these findings and variability of the time course have been noted in many patients.

Adapted, with permission, from Lovejoy FH: Thallium. Clin Toxicol Rev 1982;4:1–2.

ings.[18,49] Because of the delayed development of alopecia, the diagnosis of thallotoxicosis is often overlooked. In fact, depending on the dose, a latent period of hours to days may follow an acute exposure.[39,50] When death occurs, it is usually the result of coma, respiratory paralysis, and cardiac arrest.

Unlike most other metal salt poisonings, in cases of thallium toxicity, gastrointestinal symptoms are usually modest or may even be absent.[9] Symptoms range from vague abdominal pains or anorexia to such severe symptoms as hematemesis, bloody diarrhea, or ulceration of the mucosal lining. The most common symptom is abdominal pain, which is sometimes accompanied with vomiting and either diarrhea or constipation.[14,39,45,48,64,76] Constipation may be due to decreased intestinal motility and peristalsis due to direct involvement of the vagus nerve.[9,50]

Pleuritic chest pain was described in one small series of poisoned patients.[45] Another patient was reported to have developed "chest tightness" shortly after drinking thallium-poisoned tea.[49] No etiology for this finding has been proposed.

Tachycardia and hypertension frequently occur in patients with thallotoxicosis and usually develops by the second week following an acute ingestion. The more persistent and pronounced the tachycardia, the worse the prognosis. No exact mechanism has been determined for the cardiovascular effects of thallium intoxication. Some authors theorize that these effects result from autonomic neuropathic dysfunction directly related to vagus nerve involvement, but others have noted electrocardiographic changes, such as T-wave flattening or inversion and nonspecific ST-segment abnormalities, that might suggest direct myocardial damage.[4,8,48,50] Another theory suggests a stimulating effect of thallium on ATPase in the chromaffin cells can lead to increased output of catecholamines resulting in sinus tachycardia.[2,49]

Neurologic effects usually appear 2 to 5 days postexposure. Patients may present with severely painful, rapidly progressive ascending peripheral neuropathies.[3,4,16,45] Pain and paresthesias are present in lower extremities (especially the soles of the feet), and although numbness is present in fingers and toes, there is also decreased sensation to pinprick, touch, temperature, vibration, and proprioception.[4,65] The weight of the bedsheets on the lower extremeties may be sufficient to cause excrutiating pain.[45] Motor weakness is always distal in distribution, with the lower limbs more affected than the upper limbs.[8,50]

Symptoms of confusion, delirium, psychosis, hallucination, seizures, headache, insomnia, anxiety, tremor, ataxia, and choreoathetosis are common. Ataxia can develop within 48 hours after ingestion. Insomnia occurs in almost every patient and may progress to total reversal of sleep rhythym. Coma may occur, especially in patients with larger exposures.[8,39,50,64] All cranial nerves—with the possible exception of I, V, and VIII—can be affected by thallium. Third cranial nerve involvement, as evidenced by ptosis, is common, and may be present asymmetrically.[8] Nystagmus, another common finding, demonstrates fourth and sixth cranial nerve involvement.[8] Optic neuropathies can lead to optic atrophy and a permanent decrease in visual acuity. In early stages, the optic disk shows signs of neuritis with a poorly defined and red papilla, followed by the development of a pale or white papilla resulting from atrophy of the optic nerve. In cases of a large single ingestion of thallium, approximately 25% of patients may develop severe lesions of the optic nerve.[50,64] In patients exposed to small multiple doses, close to 100% can be affected.[48] Other ocular effects that have been described are noninflammatory keratitis, cataracts, and the color vision defect of tritanomaly (blue color defect).[70,71]

Alopecia is the most common and classic effect of thallium intoxication.[49] Typically seen as a presenting symptom in patients with chronic ingestions, epilation begins approximately 10 days after an acute ingestion, and total hair loss usually occurs within a month.[18,49] Facial and axillary hair, especially the inner one third of the eyebrows, may be spared, but in some cases full beards as well as scalp hair are lost.[61] Microscopic studies show thallium deposition as dark brown or black pigmentation located in the roots of hair samples. These deposits can be seen within 3 to 5 days of initial exposure.[6,48] In patients with chronic exposures, several bands may be noted on the hair shaft, demonstrating multiple exposures. Initial hair regrowth is very fine and unpigmented, but in patients who completely recover, hair regrowth becomes normal.[48] In patients with severe exposures, alopecia may be permanent. Dermatologic effects that have been observed in thallotoxicosis include acne, palmar erythema, and dry scaly skin that can be due to damage of the sebaceous glands. White lines or bands known as Mees lines appear within 2 to 4 weeks after exposure (see Color Plate Fig. 14).[49,55,64]

Other less common findings in thallium toxicity include hepatic injury[29] and hypochloremic metabolic acidosis.[64] Although anemia and thrombocytopenia are occasionally reported,[40,64] these findings are much less commonly noted than in patients with lead toxicity.

What Are the Effects of Thallium Toxicity on the Developing Fetus?

In animal models, thallium is teratogenic.[21,23] One study evaluated 297 children born in an area where thallium levels were higher than normal due to industrial contamination.[15] Urine thallium levels in the exposed children were as high as 76.5 μg/L. Although these children had a slightly higher than expected incidence of congenital abnormalities, no causal relationship could be established between this finding and the thallium exposure.[15]

There are few human reports of acute thallium poisoning during pregnancy. Thallium appears to cross the placenta slowly and is able to cause characteristic fetal toxicity,[17,54] which manifests as decreased fetal movement, possibly due to fetal paralysis. The classic adult signs and symptoms of thallium poisoning have been described in the neonate following delivery and the fetus following abortion.[17,48,54,59] However, outcome of the pregnancy may be normal despite significant maternal toxicity.[17,31] At least one author recommends continuing the pregnancy as long as the mother is clinically improving.[17] It is reasonable to conclude that a fetus exposed during organogenesis has the potential for permanent injury. Those exposed later in the pregnancy may recover without deficit if their exposures are limited and the mother recovers. If the exposure occurs closer to term, the child may be born with overt toxicity such as alopecia, dermatitis, nail growth disturbances, and permanent central nervous system lesions.[48]

These few case reports and animal studies provide confusing and sometimes contradictory results. It seems that fetal outcome is determined both by the stage of pregnancy and the extent of maternal toxicity. However, because there are insufficient data to predict the outcome of pregnancy complicated by maternal thallium poisoning, all patients should receive individualized care.

What Is the Assessment of Patients With Thallium Overdose?

Most patients with acute and consequential thallium toxicity will present to the emergency department soon after exposure with the severe alterations in gastrointestinal, cardiovascular, and neurologic function described previously. Establishing the correct diagnosis at this early stage is essential to assure a satisfactory outcome. Unfortunately, many patients with either smaller acute exposures or chronic thallium poisoning first present for health care days to weeks after their initial exposure, and diagnosis is often delayed. In these instances, obtaining a history may be difficult. Gastrointestinal symptoms may not have occurred, or may have been dismissed because of their mild and transient nature. These patients usually present for health care because of alopecia or the acute onset of neuropathy.

The differential diagnosis of the neuropathy includes disorders such as poisoning by arsenic, colchicine, and vinca alkaloids; botulism; and Guillain-Barré syndrome. Both the painful character of the neuropathy and the preservation of reflexes help differentiate thallium-induced neuropathy from Guillain-Barré syndrome and most other causes of acute neuropathy.[8] When gastrointestinal symptoms are present along with neuropathy and other end-organ effects, poisoning with metal salts such as arsenic and mercury should be considered (see Chaps. 78 and 80). The differential diagnosis of abrupt and complete alopecia is smaller, but includes arsenic, selenium, colchicine, and vinca alkaloid poisoning (see Table 28–4). When Mees lines are present, they indicate past exposure to metals, mitotic inhibitors, or antimetabolites, and as such are nonspecific for thallium (see Chaps. 28, 78, and 80)

Thallium is radiopaque and its presence can be documented in tampered food products[45] and on abdominal radiograph.[22] Although abdominal radiography may be indicated shortly following suspected exposure, the sensitivity and specificity of this test is unknown. Similarly, the yield from other routine studies such as the complete blood count, electrolytes, urine analysis, and ECG are limited in that they are often normal, or demonstrate nonspecific findings at most.

Microscopic inspection of the hair is felt to yield a diagnostic pattern of black pigmentation of the hair roots of the scalp in approximately of 95% of poisoned patients.[6,49,64] However, to the untrained observer this test is unlikely to be conclusive. The definitive clinical diagnosis of thallium poisoning can only be established by demonstrating elevated thallium levels. Thallium can be recovered in the hair, nails, feces, saliva, blood, and urine, and standard assays and normal values for most of these sources can be found.[50] Urine spot tests notoriously give false-negative results, require the use of dangerous materials that are not routinely available (20% nitric acid), and should therefore be avoided.[64] The standard toxicologic method is to obtain a 24-hour urine sample for thallium to be assayed by atomic absorption spectroscopy.[10,77] Normal urine values are below 5 μg/L. Some authors suggest a potassium mobilization test (similar to the EDTA mobilization test previously used for lead poisoning) to assist in the diagnosis of thallium exposure by enhancing urinary elimination.[6,29,64] We advise against this practice because of its lack of proven utility and its potential to exacerbate neurologic toxicity (see the discussion of potassium in the next section of this chapter).

What Is the Treatment of Patients With Thallium Poisoning?

The goals of treating a patient with thallium poisoning are identical to those of all poisoned patients: initial stabilization, prevention of absorption, and enhanced elimination. Following the initial assessment and stabilization of the patient's airway, breathing, and circulatory status, aggressive gastrointestinal decontamination should be instituted in patients with known thallium ingestions because of the severe outcome of a significant exposure.

Patients who present for health care shortly after ingestion should be considered candidates for ipecac-induced emesis or orogastric lavage (see Chap. 4). If the patient presents more than a few hours after ingestion or has had substantial spontaneous emesis, these techniques should be avoided. Unlike many heavy metal salts, thallium salts are substantially adsorbed to activated charcoal in vitro.[37] Because thallium undergoes enterohepatic recirculation, activated charcoal may be useful both to prevent absorption following a recent ingestion and to enhance elimination of thallium in patients who present in the postabsorptive phase.[72] In fact, a rat model of thallium poisoning demonstrated that multiple-dose activated charcoal (given as 0.5 g/kg twice daily for 5 days) increased the fecal elimination of thallium by 82% and produced a substantial improvement in survival.[41] Other data demonstrate that activated charcoal alone is superior to either forced diuresis or potassium chloride therapy.[38] In patients with severe thallium intoxication constipation is common, such that the addition of mannitol[43] or another cathartic to activated charcoal seems logical. While no studies address the utility of whole-bowel irrigation with polyethylene glycol electrolyte lavage solution, this technique may prove useful, especially when radiopaque material is present in the intestine as demonstrated by an abdominal radiograph.

The similarities between the cellular handling of potassium and thallium ions led to the natural investigation of a role for potassium in the treatment of thallium poisoning. In humans, potassium administration is associated with an increase in urinary thallium elimination.[9,19,56] The magnitude of this increase is reported to be on the order of two to threefold.[56] This is supported by animal models that demonstrate some benefit in terms of either enhanced thallium elimination or survival.[20,38,41] It is believed that potassium administration blocks tubular reabsorption of thallium and mobilizes thallium from tissue stores, thereby raising thallium levels available for glomerular filtration.[51,64] However, it is this second mechanism that is of concern. Many authors report either the development of acute toxicity or the severe exacerbation of neurologic symptoms during potassium administration.[4,19,45,56,63,73] Others cite data demonstrating that potassium's augmentation of thallium elimination in humans is quite limited.[35] Some animal models demonstrate that potassium loading enhances lethality[44] and permits thallium redistribution into the CNS.[25] For these reasons, the routine use of potassium in thallium-poisoned patients should be considered speculative and potentially dangerous. Some authors recommend forced diuresis, especially in conjunction with potassium chloride.[12,72] However, no convincing experimental evidence can support the use of forced diuresis with or without potassium at this time.

Thallium does not respond to traditional chelation therapy. Studies have shown that the use of ethylenediamine tetra-acetic acid (EDTA) and diethylenetriamine penta-acetic acid are without benefit.[50,64] Dimercaprol (British anti-Lewisite, BAL) and D-penicillamine also fail to enhance thallium excretion in experimental models.[50,64] In one model where D-penicillamine was able to enhance thallium elimination, it did so at the cost of substantial thallium redistribution into vital organs.[62] Similarly, a protective effect of sulfur-containing compounds such as cysteine or *N*-acetyl cysteine (NAC) has not been demonstrated.[41,46] Another chelator, diphenylthiocarbazone (dithizone), forms a minimally toxic complex with thallium, resulting in a 33% increase in fecal elimination of thallium in rats.[66] Unfortunately, dithizone was found to be goitrogenic and diabetogenic in animal studies.[41,50,72] Dithiocarb (sodium diethyldithiocarbamate), an intermediate metabolite of tetraethylthiuram disulfide (disulfiram, or Antabuse) (see Chap. 81), also increases the urinary excretion of thallium.[66,69] Prior to thallium elimination, however, the formation of a lipophilic thallium–diethyldithiocarbamate complex can result in the redistribution of thallium into the central nervous system.[32,69] After decomposition of the chelate complex, thallium may remain in the central nervous system, thereby exacerbating neurologic symptoms.[32,69] Because of the potential for harmful side effects from dithizone, and the redistribution of thallium following dithiocarb use, neither are recommended in the treatment of patients with thallium intoxication.

Prussian blue is a crystal lattice of potassium ferric hexacyanoferrate ($KFe(Fe(CN)_6)$) and can be used as a chelator for thallium toxicity.[36] In vitro adsorption of thallium to Prussian blue is superior to that of activated charcoal.[33,36] When given orally, Prussian blue acts as an ion exchanger for univalent cations, with its affinity increasing with the increasing ionic radius of the cation. As such, Prussian blue interferes with the enterohepatic circulation by exchanging potassium ions, from its lattice, for thallium ions in the gastrointestinal system. This results in the formation of a concentration gradient causing an increased flow of thallium into the gut.

Oral Prussian blue reduces the half-life of elimination of thallium in rats by 50%.[60] Other animal studies overwhelmingly support both the safety and the superiority of Prussian blue as an antidote over all other agents in thallium poisoning.[26,32,36,44,46,62] Humans with thallium poisoning are routinely given Prussian blue with suggestive clinical and numerical benefit.[10,11,13,45,58,68,73,74,76] One series of 11 thallium-poisoned patients demonstrated both the safety of Prussian blue and its ability to substantially increase fecal thallium elimination.[68] Because there are no controlled trials in humans that compare Prussian blue to other agents, and many of the patients reported above received multiple therapies, the true utility of Prussian blue is unknown.

Reports suggest that Prussian blue is not absorbed from the gastrointestinal system,[28,68] but clinical experience has shown us that prolonged therapy results in blue discoloration of the sweat and tears. Presently, Prussian blue is not commercially available, nor has it been approved for use in the United States by the Food and Drug Administration. It is available from chemical supply companies, in variable preparations with variable efficacy.[36,68] The colloidal or soluble form seems to be more efficacious than the insoluble form.[68] The dose of Prussian blue is 250 mg/kg per day orally via a nasogastric tube in two to four divided doses per day.[68] If patients are constipated, the Prussian blue may be dissolved in 50 mL of 15% mannitol.[72] Although any cathartic may be appropriate, most reports use mannitol, possibly due to concerns regarding magnesium use in patients with neurologic findings and sorbitol in patients with poor gastrointestinal mobility.

Extracorporeal drug removal may have a limited role in patients with thallium toxicity, especially if begun shortly after the initial exposure while serum concentrations are high and distribution is incomplete. As is the case with other toxins, the use of peritoneal dialysis is probably ineffective in removing thallium.[35] A frequently quoted review attests to the benefits of hemodialysis.[48] The actual data, however, show that hemodialysis at various stages of poisoning is no better than forced diuresis.[11,57] Reported thallium removal rates by hemodialysis are trivial: 143 mg of thallium were removed by 120 hours,[58] 222.8 mg were removed by 121 hours,[11] and 128 mg were removed by 54 hours of hemodialysis.[11] These values can be placed in perspective knowing that the minimum lethal adult dose of thallium is estimated to be on the order of 1 gram,[50] and that many reported cases involve ingestions ten times greater. Charcoal hemoperfusion may be two to three times more efficient than hemodialysis, providing clearance rates as high as 139 mL/min.[11] Furthermore, combined hemoperfusion and hemodialysis has been used in several cases[1,11,13] and has been reported to remove as much as 93 mg of thallium in 3 hours of therapy.[1] While extracorporeal therapy alone is probably insufficient for patients with significant poisoning and unnecessary in those with small exposures, it may have some role in combination with other therapies, especially in patients with renal insufficiency. Table 82–2 summarizes suggested therapy for thallium-poisoned patients.

TABLE 82–2. TREATMENT FOR THALLIUM POISONING

Early (patients who present in the first hours postexposure)

- Stabilize airway, breathing, and circulation if necessary
- Consider ipecac-induced emesis or orogastric lavage if the patient has not vomited
- Consider whole-bowel irrigation with polyethylene glycol electrolyte lavage solution for patients with large ingestions or the presence of radiopaque material on abdominal radiograph
- Begin multiple-dose activated charcoal therapy; add a cathartic to the first dose if the patient does not have diarrhea
- Give Prussian blue 250 mg/kg/day in 2 or 4 divided doses, dissolved in water, or 50 mL of 15% mannitol if the patient does not have diarrhea
- Consider simultaneous charcoal hemoperfusion and hemodialysis, especially if the patient has renal insufficiency

Late (patients who present more than 24 hours postexposure or with chronic toxicity)

- Stabilize airway, breathing, and circulation if necessary
- Begin multiple-dose activated charcoal therapy; add a cathartic to the first dose if the patient does not have diarrhea
- Give Prussian blue 250 mg/kg/day in 2 or 4 divided doses, dissolved in water, or 50 mL of 15% mannitol if the patient does not have diarrhea

Summary

The elimination of thallium salts from common use as depilatories and rodenticides substantially reduced the incidence of both intentional and unintentional thallium toxicity in the United States. Despite this fact, cases of significant poisoning still occur in countries where thallium-containing rodenticides are used today, and in this country as well as a result of attempted homicide by intentional tampering of foods and illicit drugs. Early recognition of the thallium toxidrome and prompt initiation of safe and appropriate therapy will substantially improve the patient's prognosis. When treatment is delayed, morbidity and mortality can be consequential.[61]

References

1. Aoyama H, Yoshida M, Yamamura Y: Acute poisoning by intentional ingestion of thallous malonate. Hum Toxicol 1986;5:389–392.
2. Appenroth D, Gambaryan S, Winnefeld K, et al: Functional and morphological aspects of thallium induced nephrotoxicity in rats. Toxicology 1995;96:203–215.
3. Bank WJ: Thallium. In: Spencer PS, Schaumburg HH, eds: Experimental and Clinical Neurotoxicology. Baltimore, Williams & Wilkins, 1980, pp. 570–577.
4. Bank WJ, Pleasure DE, Suzuki K, et al: Thallium poisoning. Arch Neurol 1972;26:456–464.
5. Britten JS, Blank M: Thallium activation of the (Na^+-K^+)-activated ATPase of rabbit kidney. Biochim Biophys Acta 1968; 159:160–166.
6. Burnett JW: Thallium poisoning. Cutis 1990;46:112–113.
7. Cavanagh JB: What have we learned from Graham Frederick Young? Reflections on the mechanism of thallium neurotoxicity. Neuropath Appl Neurobiol 1991;17:3–9.
8. Cavanagh JB, Fuller NH, Johnson HRM, Rudge P: The effects of thallium salts with particular reference to the nervous system changes. Q J Med 1974;43:293–319.
9. Chamberlain PH, Stavinoha WB, Davis H, et al: Thallium poisoning. Pediatrics 1958;12:1170–1182.
10. Chandler HA, Archbold GPR, Gibson JM, et al: Excretion of a toxic dose of thallium. Clin Chem 1990;36:1506–1509.

11. De Backer W, Zachee P, Verpooten GA, et al: Thallium intoxication treated with combined hemoperfusion–hemodialysis. Clin Toxicol 1982;19:259–264.
12. De Groot G, van Heijst ANP: Toxicokinetic aspects of thallium poisoning: Methods of treatment by toxin elimination. Sci Total Environ 1988;71:411–418.
13. De Groot G, van Heijst ANP, van Kesteren RG, Maes RAA: An evaluation of the efficacy of charcoal hemoperfusion in the treatment of three cases of acute thallium poisoning. Arch Toxicol 1985;57:61–66.
14. Desenclos JC, Wilder MH, Coppenger GW, et al: Thallium poisoning: An outbreak in Florida, 1988. South Med J 1992; 85:1203–1206.
15. Dolgner R, Brockhaus A, Ewers U, et al: Repeated surveillance of exposure to thallium in a population living in the vicinity of a cement plant emitting dust containing thallium. Int Arch Occup Environ Health 1983;52:79–94.
16. Dumitru D, Kalantri A: Electrophysiologic investigation of thallium poisoning. Musc Nerv 1990;13:433–437.
17. English JC: A case of thallium poisoning complicating pregnancy. Med J Aust 1954;1:780–782.
18. Feldman J, Levisohn DR: Acute alopecia: Clue to thallium toxicity. Pediatr Dermatol 1993;10:29–31.
19. Gastel B: Clinical conferences at Johns Hopkins Hospital. Thallium poisoning. Johns Hopkins Med J 1978;142:27–31.
20. Gehring PJ, Hammond T: Prussian blue: The interrelationship between thallium and potassium in animals. Pharmacol Exp Ther 1967;155:187–201.
21. Gibson JE, Becker BA: Placental transfer, embryotoxicity, and teratogenicity of thallium sulfate in normal and potassium-deficient rats. Toxicol Appl Pharmacol 1970;16: 120–132.
22. Grunfeld O, Hinostroza G: Thallium poisoning. Arch Intern Med 1964;114:132–138.
23. Hall BK: Critical periods during development as assessed by thallium-induced inhibition of growth of embryonic chick tibiae in vitro. Teratology 1985;31:353–361.
24. Hasan M, Ali SF: Effects of thallium, nickel, and cobalt administration on the lipid peroxidation in different regions of the rat brain. Toxicol Appl Pharmacol 1981;57:8–13.
25. Hasan M, Chandra S, Dua PR, et al: Biochemical and electrophysiological effects of thallium poisoning on the rat corpus striatum. Toxicol Appl Pharmacol 1977;41:353–359.
26. Heydlauf H: Ferric-cyanoferrate (II): An effective antidote in thallium poisoning. Eur J Pharmacol 1969;6:340–344.
27. Hologgitas J, Ullucci P, Driscoll J: Thallium elimination kinetics in acute thallotoxicosis. J Anal Toxicol 1980;4:68–73.
28. Hultin T, Naslund PH: Effects of thallium (I) on the structure and functions of mammalian ribosomes. Chem Biol Interact 1974:8:315–328.
29. Insley BM, Grufferman S, Ayliffe HE: Thallium poisoning in cocaine users. Am J Emerg Med 1986;4:545–548.
30. Inturrisi CE: Thallium-induced dephosphorylation of a phosphorylated intermediate of the (sodium+thallium-activated) ATPase. Biochim Biophys Acta 1969;78:630–633.
31. Johnson W: A case of thallium poisoning during pregnancy. Med J Aust 1960;47:540–542.
32. Kamerbeek HH, Rauws AG, ten Ham M, van Heijst ANP: Dangerous redistribution of thallium by treatment with sodium diethyldithiocarbamate. Acta Med Scand 1971;189: 149–154.
33. Kamerbeek HH, Rauws AG, ten Ham M, van Heijst ANP: Prussian blue therapy in thallotoxicosis. Acta Med Scand 1971;189:321–324.
34. Kaye JF: Thallium activation of pyruvate kinase. Arch Biochem Biophys 1971;143:232–239.
35. Koshy PM, Lovejoy FK: Thallium injection with survival: Ineffectiveness of peritoneal dialysis and potassium chloride diuresis. Clin Toxicol 1981;18:521–525.
36. Krazov J, Rios C, Altagracia M, et al: Relationship between physicochemical properties of Prussian blue and its efficacy as antidote against thallium poisoning. J Appl Toxicol 1993; 13:213–216.
37. Lehmann PA, Favare L: Parameters for the absorption of thallium ions by activated charcoal and Prussian blue. J Toxicol Clin Toxicol 1984;22:331–339.
38. Leloux MS, Lich NP, Claude JR: Experimental studies on thallium toxicity in rats. J Toxicol Clin Exp 1990;10:147–156.
39. Lovejoy FH: Thallium. Clin Toxicol Rev 1982;4:1–2.
40. Luckit J, Mir N, Hargreaves M, et al: Thrombocytopenia associated with thallium poisoning. Hum Exp Toxicol 1990;9:47–48.
41. Lund A: The effect of various substances on the excretion and the toxicity of thallium in the rat. Acta Pharmacol Toxicol 1956;12:260–268.
42. Lynche GR, Lond MB, Scovell JMS: The toxicology of thallium. Lancet 1930;12:1340–1344.
43. Malbrain MLNG, Lambrecht GLY, Zandijk E, et al: Treatment of severe thallium intoxication. J Toxicol Clin Toxicol 1997;35:97–100.
44. Meggs WJ, Goldfrank LR, Hoffman RS: Effects of potassium in a murine model of thallium poisoning. J Toxicol Clin Toxicol 1995;33:559–559. Abstract.
45. Meggs WJ, Hoffman RS, Shih RD, et al: Thallium poisoning from maliciously contaminated food. J Toxicol Clin Toxicol 1994;32:723–730.
46. Meggs WJ, Morasco RC, Shih RD, et al: Effects of Prussian blue and *N*-acetylcysteine on thallium toxicity in mice. J Toxicol Clin Toxicol 1997;35:163–166.
47. Melnick RL, Monti LG, Motzkin SM: Uncoupling of mitochondrial oxidative phosphorylation by thallium. Biochem Biophys Res Comm 1976;69:68–73.
48. Moeschlin S: Thallium Poisoning. Clin Toxicol 1980;17: 133–146.
49. Moore D, House I: Thallium poisoning: Diagnosis may be elusive but alopecia is the clue. Br Med J 1993;306: 1527–1529.
50. Mulkey JP, Oehme FW: A review of thallium toxicity. Vet Hum Toxicol 1993;35:445–453.
51. Mullins LJ, Moore RD: The movement of thallium ions in muscle. J Gen Physiol 1960;43:759–773.
52. Munch JC: Human thallotoxicosis. JAMA 1934;102: 1929–1933.
53. Munch JC, Ginsburg HM, Nixon CE: The 1932 thallotoxicosis outbreak in California. JAMA 1933;100:1315–1319.
54. Neal JB, Appelbaum E, Gaul LE, Masselink RJ: An unusual occurrence of thallium poisoning. NYS J Med 1935;35: 657–659.

55. Pai V: Acute thallium poisoning: Prussian blue therapy in 9 cases. West Ind Med J 1987;36:256–258.
56. Papp JP, Gay PC, Dodson VN, Pollard HM: Potassium chloride treatment in thallotoxicosis. Ann Intern Med 1969;71:119–123.
57. Paulson G, Vergara G, Young J, Bird M: Thallium intoxication treated with dithizone and hemodialysis. Arch Intern Med 1972;129:100–103.
58. Pedersen RS, Olesen AS, Freund LG, et al: Thallium intoxication treated with long-term hemodialysis, forced diuresis and Prussian blue. Acta Med Scand 1978;204:429–432.
59. Rangel-Guerra R, Martinez HR: Thallium poisoning: Experience with 50 patients. Gac Med Mex 1990;126:487–494.
60. Rauws AG: Thallium pharmacokinetics and its modification by Prussian blue. Arch Pharmacol 1974;284:295–306.
61. Reed D, Crawley J, Faro SN, et al: Thallotoxicosis: Acute manifestations and sequelae. JAMA 1963;183:516–522.
62. Rios C, Monroy-Noyola A: D-Penicillamine and Prussian blue as antidotes against thallium intoxication in rats. Toxicology 1992;74:69–76.
63. Roby DS, Fein AM, Bennett RH, et al: Cardiopulmonary effects of acute thallium poisoning. Chest 1984;84:236–240.
64. Saddique A, Perterson CD: Thallium poisoning: A review. Vet Hum Toxicol 1983;25:16–22.
65. Schaumberg HH, Berger A: Alopecia and sensory polyneuropathy from thallium in a Chinese herbal medication. JAMA 1992;268:2430–2431. Letter.
66. Schwetz BA, O'Neil PV, Voelker FA, Jacobs DW: Effects of diphenylthiocarbazone and diethyldithiocarbamate on the excretion of thallium by rats. Toxicol Appl Pharmacol 1967;10:79–88.
67. Spencer PS, Peterson ER, Madrid RA, et al: Effects of thallium salts on neuronal mitochondria in organotypic cord ganglia-muscle combination cultures. J Cell Biol 1973;58:79–85.
68. Stevens W, van Peteghem C, Heyndrickx A, Barbier F: Eleven cases of thallium intoxication treated with Prussian blue. Int J Clin Pharmacol 1974;10:1–22.
69. Sunderman FW: Diethyldithiocarbamate therapy of thallotoxicosis. Am J Med Sci 1967;2:107–118.
70. Tabandeh H, Crowston JG, Thompson GM: Ophthalmologic features of thallium poisoning. Am J Ophthalmol 1994;117:243–245.
71. Tabandeh H, Thompson GM: Visual function in thallium toxicity. Br Med J 1993;307:324. Letter.
72. Thompson DF: Management of thallium poisoning. Clin Toxicol 1981;18:979–990.
73. Van Der Merwe CF: The treatment of thallium poisoning: A report of 2 cases. S Afr Med J 1972;46:960–961.
74. Vergauwe PL, Knockaert DC, Van Tittelboom TJ: Near fatal subacute thallium poisoning necessitating prolonged mechanical ventilation. Am J Emerg Med 1990;8:548–550.
75. Villanueva E, Hernandez-Cueto C, Lachica E, et al: Poisoning by thallium: A study of five cases. Drug Saf 1990;5:384–389.
76. Wainwright AP, Kox WJ, House IM, et al: Clinical features and therapy of acute thallium poisoning. Q J Med 1988;69:939–944.
77. Wakid NW, Cortas NK: Chemical and atomic absorption methods for thallium in urine compared. Clin Chem 1984;30:587–588. Letter.

CHAPTER 83

Antiseptics, Disinfectants, and Sterilants

Paul M. Wax

A 40-year-old man was brought to the Emergency Department (ED) from a psychiatric hospital 1 hour after he was found to be drinking povidone-iodine solution (Betadine). Apparently the patient had walked into a utility room where he found the antiseptic solution. An attendant stated that at least 6 oz (180 mL) of povidone-iodine were missing from the bottle. The patient had a past medical history that was significant for chronic paranoid schizophrenia. His medications included haloperidol and benztropine mesylate.

In the ED the patient was cooperative. He stated that he had ingested about one-half of the bottle of povidone-iodine. He admitted to mild epigastric distress and nausea but denied vomiting or diarrhea. His vital signs were: blood pressure, 120/80 mm Hg; pulse, 82 beats/min and regular; respiratory rate, 20 breaths/min; and temperature, 98.6°F (37°C). The patient was disheveled but otherwise well appearing. He was in no distress. Examination of the head, eyes, ears, nose, and throat (HEENT) was significant for faint brownish discoloration of the tongue and buccal mucosa. The neck was supple. The chest was clear to auscultation bilaterally with a normal cardiac auscultation. Abdominal examination was soft and nontender with normoactive bowel sounds. Rectal examination was negative for occult blood. Extremity and neurologic examinations were normal.

The patient was observed in the ED for 6 hours, during which time he never developed significant toxicity and his epigastric distress and nausea resolved. He was able to take oral fluids well and was discharged back to the psychiatric hospital.

What Are the Differences Between Iodine, Iodophor, and Iodide?

Iodine usually refers to molecular iodine also known as I_2, free iodine, or elemental iodine. This chemical is the active ingredient of iodine-based antiseptics. Iodophors are substances in which molecular iodine is compounded to a high-molecular-weight carrier or solubilizing agent. Povidone-iodine (Betadine), a commonly used iodophor, consists of iodine linked to polyvinylpyrrolidone (povidone). Problems associated with the use of iodine include unpleasant odor, skin irritation, allergic reactions, clothes staining, and poor stability. Iodophors, which limit the release of molecular iodine and are generally less toxic, have become the standard iodine-based antiseptic preparations. Iodophor preparations are formulated as solutions, ointments, foams, surgical scrubs, and vaginal preparations. The most common preparation is a 10% povidone-iodine solution that contains 1% "available" iodine (referring to all oxidizing iodine species) but only 0.001% free iodine (referring only to molecular iodine).[17,59]

Iodide refers to the reduced form of iodine, I^-. This can be found in the iodine salts, potassium iodide and sodium iodide. Potassium iodide is used as an expectorant and in the treatment of hyperthyroidism and radiation exposure. Saturated solution of potassium iodide (SSKI), containing 1 g/mL, is an example of a potassium iodide preparation. Sodium iodide is found as a dietary supplement in table salt. Although iodides by themselves are not used as antiseptics, iodine-containing antiseptic compounds may consist of a mixture of molecular iodine and an iodide salt. Lugol's solution, for instance, consists of 5% iodine and 10% potassium iodide. Tincture of iodine consists of 2% iodine, 2.4% sodium iodide, 47% alcohol, and water.

The organic iodides are another group of iodine-containing compounds. Radiologic contrast agents such as diatrizoate sodium (Hypaque) and sodium methylglucamine diacetylamino-triiodobenzoates (Renografin) are examples of commonly used organic iodides. Other iodine-containing compounds include the antidysrhythmic amiodarone and the antifungal vioform. Isotopes of iodine are another group of agents that contain iodine. The most commonly used isotope, I^{131}, is used in the diagnosis of thyroid disorders and treatment of hyperthyroidism.

What Are the Typical Toxic Effects of Iodine Poisoning?

Iodine and iodide exposures can be divided into five major subtypes: oral ingestion of iodine, oral ingestion of iodophor, topical absorption of iodine/iodophor, acute ingestion of iodide, and chronic ingestion of iodide. Iodine is much more toxic than iodide because of its propensity to cause significant local tissue injury. Because iodide is not caustic, treatment of iodine ingestions includes conversion of iodine to the less toxic iodide.

Iodine is one of the oldest topical antiseptics. It is also used to disinfect medical equipment and drinking water. It is effective against bacteria, viruses, protozoa, and fungi.[39] It has been used both prophylactically and therapeutically. Iodine is cytotoxic; it is also an oxidant. It is thought to work by binding amino and heterocyclic nitrogen groups, oxidizing sulfhydryl groups, and saturating double bonds. Iodine also iodinates tyrosine groups.[59]

Although occasional cases of iodine ingestions are still reported, iodine ingestions are much less common than in the past as a result of the change in antiseptic use from iodine to iodophor antiseptics.[41] During the early part of the 20th century, however, iodine ingestions were quite routine. A study at Boston City Hospital from 1915 to 1936 revealed that iodine ingestions (usually tincture of iodine) were the most common cause of poisoning, accounting for 27% of all patients admitted for suicide attempts.[103] Molecular iodine may cause severe caustic injury of the gastrointestinal (GI) tract similar to what occurs after exposure to a strong alkali or acid (see Chap. 86). A 1937 study reported 18 cases of oral iodine ingestions, usually involving tincture of iodine, that resulted in death.[44] The amount ingested was recorded in 9 of these cases, and ranged from 30 to 250 mL (0.6 to 5.0 g of iodine). Symptoms consisted of vomiting, diarrhea, abdominal pain, GI bleeding, delirium, anuria, and vasomotor collapse. Death usually occurred within the first 48 hours after ingestion and resulted from hypovolemia and circulatory collapse. Postmortem examination revealed that most of the patients had significant GI injury. Gastrointestinal strictures can also occur after the ingestion of tincture of iodine.[166]

Until recently, cases of adverse consequences from iodophor ingestions could not be found in the literature. In a recent single case report, however, a 9-week-old infant died within 3 hours of receiving povidone-iodine by mouth.[82] In this unusual case, the child was administered 15 mL of povidone-iodine mixed with 135 mL polyethylene glycol by nasogastric tube over a 3-hour period for the treatment of infantile colic. Postmortem examination showed an ulcerated and necrotic intestinal tract. A blood iodine level of 14,600 μg/dL (normal 5 to 8 μg/dL) was recorded. Significant toxicity from intentional ingestions of iodophors in adults has not been documented.

Attention has been directed to the problem of systemic absorption of topical iodine and iodophor preparations.[115] Markedly elevated iodine levels do occur in patients who have received topical iodophor treatments to areas of dermal breakdown, such as burn injuries.[85] Significant absorption has also occurred when iodophors were applied to the vagina, perianal fistulas, umbilical cords, and the skin of low-birthweight neonates.[161] A fatality following intraoperative irrigation of a hip wound with povidone-iodine was also reported.[36] The serum iodine level, reported at necropsy, in this case was 1000 times normal.

Acid–base disturbances are among the most significant abnormalities associated with topical absorption of iodophors. Metabolic acidosis was reported in several burn patients after receiving multiple applications of povidone-iodine ointment.[85,117] These patients had elevated serum iodide concentrations and normal lactate levels. The exact etiology of the acidosis remains unclear. Postulated mechanisms for the acidosis have included the povidone-iodine itself (pH 2.43), bicarbonate consumption from the conversions of I_2 to NaI, or decreased renal elimination of H^+ due to iodine toxicity.[117] Metabolic acidosis associated with a high lactate level after iodine absorption was also reported.[39]

Electrolyte abnormalities are also associated with the topical absorption of iodophors. A patient with decubitus ulcers who received prolonged wound care with povidone-iodine-soaked gauze developed metabolic acidosis, renal failure, hypernatremia, and hyperchloremia.[39] The hyperchloremia was thought to be due to a spurious elevation of measured chloride ions due to iodine's interference with the chloride assay. This interference occurs on the Technicon STAT/ION autoanalyzer but does not occur when the silver halide precipitation assay is used.[39] Spurious hyperchloremia from iodine (or iodide) may result in the calculation of a low or negative anion gap (see Chap. 15).[23]

Other problems associated with topical absorption

of iodine containing preparations include hypothyroidism (particularly in neonates),[23,141] hyperthyroidism, elevated liver function tests, neutropenia, and hypoxemia.[39] Due to the lack of consistency between iodine levels and symptomatology, and because many of these patients had significant secondary medical problems that may have accounted for their symptoms, the exact relationship between iodine absorption and the development of a specific clinical syndrome remains speculative. Contact dermatitis can result from repetitive applications of iodophors.[96] A fatal case of exfoliative dermatitis from repeated local applications of tincture of iodine has also been described.[134]

What Is Iodism?

Iodism, first described in 1902, refers to a variety of reactions to iodides. The term has been used to describe both dose-dependent reactions and hypersensitivity reactions ("iodine idiosyncrasy").[21,70] Duration of exposure may be chronic (most often) or acute.

The most noticeable manifestations of chronic dose-dependent iodide toxicity include skin eruptions (ioderma), salivary gland swelling, and goiter. Acute parotitis may be the most recognizable finding; hence this syndrome may be referred to as "iodide mumps."[21,57] Salivary swelling is thought to be due to ductal inflammation and blockage. Significant salivary gland enlargement may result in dysphagia and possible airway obstruction.[15] Other manifestations of iodism include metallic taste, gingivitis, sialorrhea, bronchorrhea, coryza, nausea, and vomiting.[15,70] Drug-induced fever has also been attributed to iodide administration.[155] Unlike iodine ingestions, however, iodide ingestions do not produce GI burn injuries.

Hypersensitivity reactions associated with iodides include the development of eosinophilia, lymphadenopathy, arthralgias, submucosal hemorrhages, arthritis, skin reactions, hematuria, proteinuria, and fever.[70] A periarteritis nodosa type of reaction from iodide exposure has also been described.[124] Rapid onset of acute painful salivary gland swelling (sialoadenitis) at times may occur within hours of ingesting small therapeutic doses of iodides.[21,57,164] Whether this reaction represents a true hypersensitivity reaction is not clear.

Ioderma refers to the protean group of dermal lesions usually associated with chronic exposure to iodides (see Color Plate Fig. 16). These skin eruptions are quite varied, ranging from pustular/bullous eruptions to generalized erythema and urticaria.[134] Although ioderma is usually related to iodide exposure, it is also reported to occur as a systemic manifestation of povidone-iodine exposure from wound irrigation.[16]

Iodides are also implicated in a variety of thyroid disorders, including goiter,[168] thyrotoxicosis,[46] and myxedema.[104]

Acute overdose of iodide medications is rare. In one case, a patient inadvertently ingested 15 g of potassium iodide and developed myocardial irritability and face, neck, and mouth swelling within 12 hours of ingestion.[156] Subsequent recovery was uneventful.

Reactions to iodinated radiologic contrast agents are well known.[33] Anaphylactoid reactions are idiosyncratic in nature and not dose dependent. Salivary gland swelling is also described as a sequela to intravenous urography using these agents.[152] The use of iodides such as radiologic contrast media in early pregnancy is potentially teratogenic and may lead to cretinism.

What Is the Management of Patients With Iodine and Iodide Ingestions?

The patient who has ingested an iodine preparation requires expeditious evaluation, stabilization, and decontamination. Due to the potential for reexposure to the iodine if emesis is induced, syrup of ipecac is contraindicated. Careful nasogastric aspiration followed by gastric lavage may be performed to limit the caustic effect of the iodine if signs of perforation are absent. Irrigation with a starch solution will convert iodine to the much less toxic iodide, and in the process turn the gastric effluent dark blue-purple. This change in color may serve as a useful guide in determining when lavage can be terminated. If starch is not available, milk may be a useful alternative. Instillation of a solution of 1 to 5% sodium thiosulfate may also convert any remaining iodine to the much less toxic iodide. Activated charcoal binds iodine and may be useful, particularly in the presence of a mixed ingestion.[38] Whether any one of the agents named offers a distinct advantage over the others has not been studied. Minimal GI absorption of iodine occurs because of its conversion to iodide in the GI tract.[30] Early endoscopy may help assess the extent of the burn injury. Judicious use of corticosteroids for circumferential second-degree burn injuries may be helpful in preventing stricture formation (see Chap. 86).

Most cases of iodophor ingestions require only supportive management. The use of starch or sodium thiosulfate may be considered in symptomatic patients. Endoscopy is recommended in patients with persistent symptoms.

Management of acute iodide ingestions is basically supportive. Activated charcoal may be considered in large ingestions. Because absorbed iodide competes with chloride in the proximal tubule, sodium chloride diuresis may enhance the elimination of iodide. Due to the conversion of iodine to iodide, patients treated for iodine ingestions may be at risk for subsequent iodide toxicity. Systemic corticosteroids have been used with success in the management of iodide-induced sialoadenitis[164] and ioderma.[5]

What Are the Differences Between Antiseptics, Disinfectants, and Sterilants?

Antiseptics, disinfectants, and sterilants are a diverse group of antimicrobial agents used to prevent infection (Table 83–1). Although these terms are sometimes used interchangeably (and some of these agents are used for

TABLE 83–1. ANTISEPTICS, DISINFECTANTS, STERILANTS, AND RELATED COMPOUNDS

Chemical	Commercial Product	Use	Toxic Effects	Therapeutics and Evaluation
Acids				
Boric acid	Borax Sodium perborate Dobell's solution	Antiseptic, mouthwash, eyewash, roach killer	Blue-green emesis and diarrhea Boiled-lobster appearance CNS; renal	GI decontamination Hemodialysis (rare)
Alcohols (see Chaps. 62, 64)				
Ethanol	Rubbing alcohol (70% ethanol)	Antiseptic, disinfectant	CNS depression Respiratory depression Dermal irritant	Supportive
Isopropanol	Isopropyl rubbing alcohol (70% isopropanol)	Antiseptic, disinfectant	CNS depression Respiratory depression Ketonemia, ketonuria GI irritation/bleeding Hemorrhagic tracheobronchitis Hypotension Dermal irritant	Hemodialysis (rare)
Aldehydes				
Formaldehyde	Formalin (37% formaldehyde, 12% to 15% methanol)	Disinfectant, fixative, urea insulation	Caustic gastroenteritis Acidosis CNS depression Dermatitis	Gastric lavage Hemodialysis Sodium bicarbonate Folic acid
Glutaraldehyde	Cidex (2% glutaraldehyde)	Sterilant	Mucosal and dermal irritant	
Chlorhexidine	Hibiclens	Antiseptic	GI irritation	
Chlorinated Compounds				
Chlorine		Disinfectant	Irritant	
Chlorophors (sodium hypochlorite)	Chlorine bleach (5% NaOCl) Dakin's solution (1 part 5% NaOCl, 10 parts H_2O)	Disinfectant	Mild GI irritation	Endoscopy (rare)
Ethylene Oxide		Sterilant, plasticizer	Irritant CNS depression Peripheral neuropathy Carcinogen?	
Heavy Metals				
Organic mercurials (see Chap. 80)	Merbromin 2% (Mercurochrome) Thimerosal (Merthiolate)	Antiseptic (obsolete)	CNS Renal	DMSA?
Iodinated Compounds				
Iodine	Tincture of iodine: 2% free iodine, 2% sodium iodide, 50% ethanol	Antiseptic	Caustic gastroenteritis	Milk, starch, sodium thiosulfate Endoscopy
Iodophors	Povidone-iodine (Betadine)	Antiseptic	Limited	Same as iodine if symptomatic
Iodide	SSKI	Expectorant	Iodism	Steroids for significant salivary gland enlargement
Oxidants				
Chlorates	Sodium chlorate Potassium chlorate	Antiseptic, mouthwash, matches, herbicide	Hemolytic anemia Methemoglobinemia Renal failure	Methylene blue? Exchange transfusion Hemodialysis
Hydrogen peroxide	H_2O_2 3%—household use H_2O_2 30%—industrial use	Disinfectant	Oxygen emboli GI caustic	Lavage Radiographic evaluation Endoscopy
Potassium permanganate		Antiseptic	Oxidizing agent, caustic Manganese elevation Methemoglobinemia	Decontamination Endoscopy as needed Methylene blue

(*continued*)

TABLE 83–1. ANTISEPTICS, DISINFECTANTS, STERILANTS, AND RELATED COMPOUNDS (continued)

Chemical	Commercial Product	Use	Toxic Effects	Therapeutics and Evaluation
Phenols				
Nonsubstituted	Phenol (carbolic acid)	Disinfectant	Caustic gastroenteritis Dermal burns Cutaneous absorption CNS effects	Decontamination: Polyethylene glycol or water Endoscopy as needed
Substituted	Hexachlorophene	Disinfectant	CNS disturbances	
Quaternary Ammonium Compound				
Benzalkonium chloride	Zephiran	Disinfectant	GI caustic at high concentrations	Endoscopy if significant GI symptoms

both antisepsis and disinfection), the distinguishing characteristics between the groups are important to emphasize. An antiseptic is a chemical agent that is applied to living tissue to kill or inhibit microorganisms. Iodophors, chlorhexidine, and the alcohols (ethanol and isopropanol) are commonly used antiseptics. A disinfectant is a chemical or physical agent that is applied to inanimate objects to kill microorganisms. Chlorine bleach (sodium hypochlorite), phenolic compounds, and formaldehyde are examples of currently used disinfectants. A sterilant is a chemical or physical agent that is applied to inanimate objects to kill all living organisms, including spores. Ethylene oxide and glutaraldehyde are examples of sterilants. Neither antiseptics nor disinfectants have complete sporicidal activity. Not surprisingly, many of these chemicals used to kill microbiologic organisms also demonstrate considerable human toxicity.[17,59]

Although sulfur, vinegar (acetic acid), and mercurial compounds were used as antiseptics as long as 2000 years ago, it was not until the 19th century that the use of antiseptics became commonplace. Some of the epochal figures in medicine were the first to extol the importance of antiseptics. Semmelweis implemented the practice of hand washing with chloride of lime as a means of preventing the dreaded puerperal fever. Lister experimented extensively with phenol as an antiseptic. Koch used mercury bichloride. Other agents introduced as antiseptics during the 19th century include tincture of iodine (used extensively during the Civil War), hydrogen peroxide, isopropanol, and ethanol.[59]

The use of these agents evolved during the 20th century as their toxicity and the principles of microbiology became better understood. Two of the more toxic antiseptics—iodine and phenol—were gradually replaced by the less toxic iodophors and substituted phenols. Mercury bichloride was superseded by the organic mercurials (eg, merbromin, thimerosal), which also proved toxic. More recently, newer compounds, such as quaternary ammonium compounds, ethylene oxide, and glutaraldehyde, have been introduced.

Chlorhexidine

Chlorhexidine (Fig. 83–1) is another commonly used antiseptic agent that is especially useful as a dental antiseptic. This cationic biguanide compound has been in use since the early 1950s. It is found in a variety of skin cleansers, usually as a 4% emulsion (eg, Hibiclens), and may also be found in mouthwash. Chlorhexidine is reported to have low toxicity.

Few cases of deliberate oral ingestion of chlorhexidine can be found in the literature. Symptoms are usually mild and gastrointestinal irritation is the most likely effect after oral ingestion.[24] Chlorhexidine has poor enteral absorption. In one case, ingestion of 150 mL of a 20% chlorhexidine gluconate solution resulted in oral cavity edema and significant caustic injury of the esophagus.[98] In the same case, liver function tests rose to 30 times normal on the fifth day after ingestion. Liver biopsy showed lobular necrosis and fatty degeneration. Subsequently, the liver function tests normalized. In another case, the ingestion of 30 mL of a 4% solution by an 89-year-old woman did not result in any GI injury.[43]

Intravenous administration of chlorhexidine is associated with hemolysis, although this may have been due to the hypotonicity of the solution.[26] Inhalation of va-

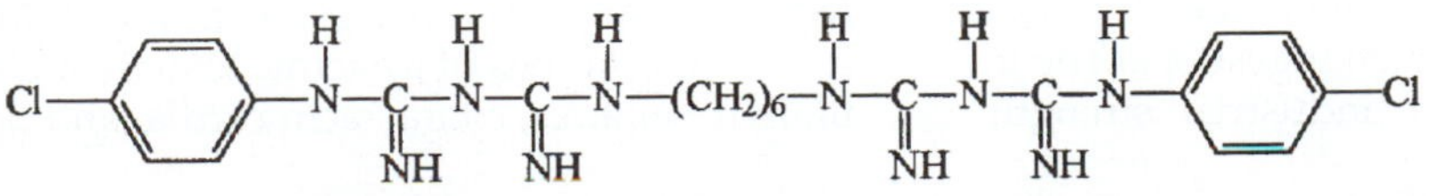

Figure 83–1. Structure of chlorhexidine.

porized chlorhexidine is reported to cause methemoglobinemia due to the conversion of chlorhexidine to p-chloraniline.[159] The rectal administration of 4% chlorhexidine resulted in acute ulcerative colitis.[58]

Topical absorption of chlorhexidine is negligible. Contact dermatitis is reported in up to 8% of patients who received repetitive topical applications of chlorhexidine.[59] More ominously, anaphylactic reactions are associated with dermal application.[109] Eye exposure may result in corneal damage.[153]

Treatment guidelines for chlorhexidine exposure are similar to those for other potentially caustic agents. Patients with significant symptoms may require endoscopy, but the need for this sort of aggressive intervention is quite uncommon.

The Alcohols

Isopropanol and ethanol are commonly used as skin antiseptics. Sold as rubbing alcohol, the standard concentration for these solutions is usually 70%. Their antiseptic action is thought to be due to their ability to coagulate proteins. Isopropanol is slightly more germicidal than ethanol.[59] These agents have limited efficacy against viruses or spores. Isopropanol tends to be more irritating than ethanol and may cause more pronounced central nervous system depression.[162] The greater toxicity of isopropanol has caused some emergency departments to switch rubbing alcohol formulations from isopropanol to ethanol (see Chaps. 62 and 64).

Chlorine and Chlorophors

Chlorine, one of the first antiseptics, is still used in the treatment of the community water supply and in swimming pools. Chlorine is a potent pulmonary irritant and may cause severe bronchospasm and pulmonary edema. Further discussion of chlorine can be found in Chapter 94.

Sodium hypochlorite, found in chlorine bleach (eg, Clorox) and Dakin's solution, remains a commonly used disinfectant. First used in the late 1700s to bleach clothes, its utility arises from its oxidizing capability, measured as "available chlorine," and its ability to release hypochlorous acid slowly. It is used to clean blood spills and sterilize certain medical instruments. Toxicity from hypochlorite is mainly due to its irritant effects. The ingestion of large amounts of household liquid bleach (5% sodium hypochlorite) on rare occasions can result in esophageal burns with subsequent stricture formation.[47] In a cat model, bleach caused a high incidence of mucosal injury and stricture formation.[165] However, the vast majority of ingestions in humans do not cause significant GI injuries.[83,118] Accordingly, aggressive evaluation with endoscopy is usually not warranted when assessing most patients with household liquid bleach ingestions. The ingestion of a more concentrated "industrial strength" bleach preparation increases the likelihood of local tissue injury and should be managed accordingly (see Chap. 86).

Although direct inhalation of sodium hypochlorite vapors by itself is usually not problematic, the erroneous mixing of sodium hypochlorite bleach with ammonia or acids can lead to the production of toxic vapors resulting in significant pulmonary symptomatology. Mixing sodium hypochlorite ($NaOCl$) with ammonium hydroxide (NH_3OH) produces chloramine; mixing sodium hypochlorite with acid-containing toilet bowl cleaners (eg, hydrochloric acid, phosphoric acid) produces chlorine. When chloramine comes in contact with the moist mucous membranes of the pulmonary tree, hypochlorous acid ($HOCl$) and oxygen free radicals are produced. Hypochlorous acid subsequently decomposes to hydrochloric acid and oxygen. Chlorine contact with moist airway tissues also produces hypochlorous acid, hydrochloric acid, and oxygen.

Phenol

Phenol (carbolic acid) is one of the oldest antiseptic agents. Although at one time it was the standard antiseptic to which other antiseptics were compared and was used as a preoperative antiseptic and in wound dressings, phenol's toxicity limited its usefulness. It is rarely used as an antiseptic today and has been replaced by one of the many phenolic derivatives. Currently phenol is used as a disinfectant, chemical intermediary, and nail cauterizer. The last application uses a highly potent 89% solution. Phenol is also a component (0.1 to 4.5%) of various lotions, ointments, gels, gargles, lozenges, and throat sprays.[59] Campho-phenique and Chloraseptic contain 4.7% and 1.4% phenol, respectively. Cresol, a mixture of three isomers of methyl phenol, has better germicidal activity than phenol and is a commonly used disinfectant. Although not quite as toxic as phenol, it remains quite irritating and toxicity can occur.[59]

Phenol acts as a general protoplasmic poison. Toxicity is due to its ability to cause cell wall disruption, protein denaturation, and coagulation necrosis. Phenol demonstrates excellent skin penetrance. The lethal dose may be as little as 1 g.[69]

Although many cases of phenol poisoning were reported in the past, acute oral overdoses of phenol-containing solutions are relatively uncommon today.[54] Clinical manifestations can be divided into local and systemic symptoms. Local toxicity to the GI tract may result in nausea, vomiting, bloody diarrhea, and severe abdominal pain. White patches in the oral cavity may be detected. Serious GI burns are uncommon and strictures are rare.[65,133]

Systemic symptoms from GI or dermal absorption of phenol are usually more dangerous than the local effects and can result in significant morbidity and mortality. Manifestations of systemic toxicity include CNS stimulation, seizures, coma, tachycardia, and dysrhythmias.[56]

Bradycardia, hypotension, hypothermia, metabolic acidosis, methemoglobinemia, and pulmonary disturbances may also develop.[12,69] A sweet aromatic odor may be detected on the breath, due to pulmonary elimination of phenol metabolites. In a recent study of patients who had ingested Creolin (26% phenol), CNS symptoms predominated.[144] Nine of 52 patients evaluated at the hospital developed lethargy and 2 patients developed coma. Seizures were not reported. Only one of the 17 patients who underwent endoscopy in this study had a significant esophageal burn.[144]

Environmental phenol exposure resulting from the ingestion of phenol-contaminated water caused an outbreak of an illness that featured many of these same symptoms: nausea, vomiting, diarrhea, burning sensation in the mouth, mouth sores, and dark urine.[6,75]

"Phenol marasmus" was a term used in the 19th century to describe patients (usually physicians) who developed a typical characteristic syndrome after chronic exposure to aerosolized phenol. These symptoms included anorexia, weight loss, vertigo, headache, and salivation. A brown or even black discoloration of the urine was usually noted.[99] In a more recent case of occupational exposure to vaporized phenol dark urine (bilirubin-negative) was also a prominent feature.[99]

Although many dermal exposures to phenol are limited to a light brown staining of the skin, severe dermal burns with subsequent phenol absorption and systemic toxicity may occur in some cases. Excessive dermal absorption of phenol during chemical peeling procedures is associated with dysrhythmias.[163] Extensive topical exposure to a brush that had been soaking in phenol resulted in rapid onset of seizures, apnea, and death.[88] Nausea, vomiting, bradycardia, hypoxemia, and elevated serum and urinary phenol levels were associated with a 20% partial-thickness skin burn from phenol.[69] Parenteral administration of phenol has also resulted in death.[90]

A variety of solutions have been suggested for dermal and gastric decontamination of phenol. Olive oil was recommended in the past as an irrigant fluid because it was thought to dissolve phenol and prevent absorption.[51] Animal studies, however, show that systemic phenol absorption is actually increased when olive oil is used as a decontaminant.[32] More recently, cutaneous decontamination with a low-molecular-weight polyethylene glycol solution was shown to decrease mortality, systemic effects, and dermal burns in a rat model.[19] Although this study suggested that polyethylene glycol was superior to water as a decontamination agent, a subsequent study using a swine model could not demonstrate a difference between these two agents.[121] Given the lack of definitive efficacy data, either low-molecular-weight polyethylene glycol (eg, PEG 300 or 400) if it is readily available in the ED, or water, is currently recommended for dermal irrigation and careful gastric decontamination. Appropriate endoscopic evaluation as needed to determine the extent of GI injury and good supportive care are also recommended.

Substituted Phenols

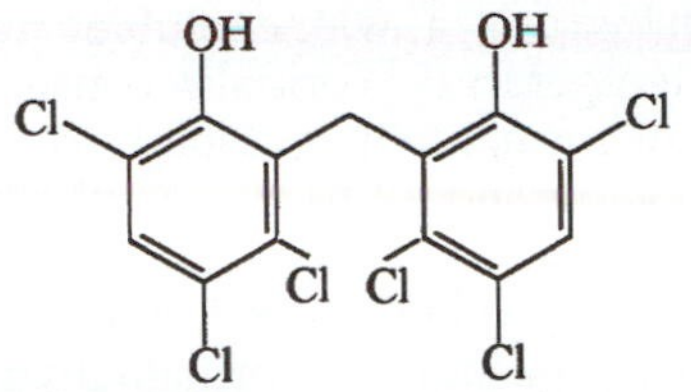

Hexachlorophene

Substituted phenols (phenol molecules with additional groups, usually halogens) have also been used as antiseptic and disinfectant agents. Hexachlorophene (pHisoHex), a trichlorinated bis-phenol, is one of the best known substituted phenols. Hexachlorophene is considered generally less tissue-toxic than phenol. This agent was formerly used extensively as a detergent in hospitals. During the 1970s an association was observed between repetitive whole-body washing of premature infants with 3% hexachlorophene and the development of vacuolar encephalopathy and cerebral edema.[97] There were multiple reports of significant neurologic toxicity and death in children who became toxic after ingesting hexachlorophene.[64] Fatalities also occurred after patients absorbed substantial amounts of hexachlorophene during the treatment of burn injuries.[27] Since these reports, the use of hexachlorophene has declined significantly.

Phisoderm, another antiseptic agent with a similar sounding name to pHisoHex, contains sodium octylphenoxyethoxyethyl ether sulfonate and lanolin. These chemicals act as soaps and detergents. No reports of significant toxicity from Phisoderm can be found in the literature. Irritative effects (nausea, vomiting, diarrhea) would be the main problems to anticipate with oral exposure.

A recent study showed that "Dettol" liquid, a household disinfectant that contains 4.8% chloroxylenol, pine oil, and isopropanol, accounted for 10% of poisoning admissions to Hong Kong hospitals.[25] Aspiration (perhaps in part due to the pine oil) occurred in 8% of these patients, resulting in upper airway obstruction, pneumonia, and adult respiratory distress syndrome. More common symptoms included nausea, vomiting, sore mouth, sore throat, drowsiness, abdominal pain, and fever.

Formaldehyde

Although formaldehyde was once widely used as a disinfectant and fumigant, its role as a disinfectant is now largely confined to the disinfection of hemodialysis machines. Nonetheless, formaldehyde has many other applications. Healthcare workers are probably most familiar with the use of formaldehyde as a tissue fixative. Formaldehyde is also used in the textile industry and in the production of resins and plastics. Formaldehyde is a major component of urea formaldehyde foam, used extensively for insulation.[22]

Formaldehyde is a water-soluble, highly reactive gas at room temperature. Formalin consists of an aqueous solution of formaldehyde usually containing about 37% formaldehyde and 12 to 15% methanol. Formaldehyde is quite irritating to the upper airways, and its odor is readily detectable at low concentrations.

The acute ingestion of formaldehyde (as formalin) may result in both local and systemic symptoms. Formaldehyde is a protoplasmic poison and potent caustic. It causes coagulation necrosis, protein precipitation, and tissue fixation. Ingestions of formalin may result in significant gastric injury, including hemorrhage, diffuse necrosis, perforation, and stricture.[4,9,129] Emergent gastrectomy has sometimes been required.[4,9,81] Chemical fixation of the stomach has been described at laparotomy.[150] The most extensive damage appears in the stomach, with only occasional involvement of the small intestine and colon.[79] Esophageal involvement is not very prominent, and if present is usually limited to its distal segment.[79]

The most striking systemic manifestation of formaldehyde poisoning is acidosis resulting from the conversion of formaldehyde to formic acid. This reaction occurs rapidly. On initial presentation, the patient may already have a profound acidemia accompanied by a large anion gap. Although the methanol component of the formalin solution is readily absorbed and has resulted in methanol levels of 40 mg/dL,[20,42] the rapid metabolism of formaldehyde to formic acid appears to be responsible for much of the acidosis (see Chap. 64). The development of extensive tissue necrosis leading to lactate production may also be a factor.

Patients presenting after acute formaldehyde ingestions complain of the rapid onset of severe abdominal pain, which may be accompanied by vomiting and diarrhea. Altered mental status and coma usually follow rapidly. Examination may demonstrate epigastric tenderness, hematemesis, cyanosis, hypotension, and tachypnea. It is not clear how much of the hypotension can be attributed to fluid losses from local tissue injury and how much is secondary to the systemic effects of the formaldehyde. Early endoscopic findings include ulceration, necrosis, perforation, and hemorrhage of the stomach, with little esophageal involvement. Acute intravascular hemolysis is described in hemodialysis patients whose dialysis equipment contained residual formaldehyde after undergoing routine cleaning.[112,122]

Occupational and environmental exposure to formaldehyde has received considerable attention. In particular, concern has arisen over the potential off-gassing of formaldehyde from the widely used urea formaldehyde building insulation such as particle boards.[110] Headache, nausea, skin rash, sore throat, nasal congestion, and eye irritation have been associated with the use of these urea formaldehyde polymers.[35] Formaldehyde, at concentrations as low as 1 ppm, may cause significant irritation to mucous membranes of the upper respiratory tract and conjunctivae.[67,92] Formaldehyde is also considered a potential sensitizer in immune-mediated reversible bronchospasm,[62] where it may act as a hapten. The exact immunologic mechanism, however, has not been elicited.[92] Acute chemical pneumonitis is associated with significant inhalational exposure.[120] Hepatotoxicity is also related to formaldehyde exposure.[11] Recently, four cases of membranous nephropathy were associated with occupational or environmental formaldehyde exposure.[18] Significant neurobehavioral impairment and seizures are associated with long-term occupational exposure to formaldehyde (although phenol exposure may have contributed to the problems).[77] In addition, formaldehyde is thought to be a dermal sensitizer.[142] Although both animal and human data suggest that formaldehyde exposure is associated with an increased incidence of nasopharyngeal carcinoma,[3,128] its role in the pathogenesis of cancer in humans has not been proven.[1,114]

The initial management of a patient with a significant formaldehyde exposure should include immediate dilution with water. Although such an approach may be useful in reducing the caustic effect, strong evidence for a beneficial result is lacking. Careful gastric aspiration with a small-bore nasogastric tube may limit systemic absorption. The role of activated charcoal has not been studied. Significant acidosis should be treated with sodium bicarbonate and folic acid. Immediate hemodialysis may remove the accumulating formic acid as well as parent formaldehyde and methanol.[42] An ethanol infusion or 4-methylpyrazole may block the metabolism of methanol, but neither of these agents will block the conversion of formaldehyde to formic acid (see Chap. 64). Early endoscopy is recommended for all patients with significant GI symptoms to assess the degree of burn injury. Surgical intervention may be required for those with severe burns.

Quaternary Ammonium Compounds

Quaternary ammonium compounds are a type of cationic surfactant (surface-active agent) used as disinfectants, detergents, and sanitizers. Chemically, the quaternary ammonium compounds are synthetic derivatives of ammonium chloride. They are structurally similar to other quaternary ammonium derivatives, such as the cholinesterase inhibitors (eg, neostigmine) and the neuromuscular blockers (eg, succinylcholine). Other cationic surfactants include the pyridinium compounds and the quinolinium compounds. Benzalkonium chloride (Zephiran) was one of the most commonly employed quaternary ammonium compounds in the past, but with the development of many newer quaternary ammonium compounds over the years, its use has substantially decreased. However, nebulized solutions used for the treatment of asthma including albuterol and ipratropium bromide may contain small amounts of benzalkonium chloride. Newer quaternary ammonium compounds are currently used as hospital disinfectants, including Coverage 256, which contains 6% alkyl dimethyl ammonium chloride and 5% octyldecyldimethyl ammonium chloride, and Render, which contains 5% alkyl dimethyl benzyl ammonium chloride.

Quaternary ammonium compounds generally have a low order of toxicity compared to phenol or formaldehyde. Of the infrequent complications that have been described, most result from ingestions of benzalkonium chloride. Complications of these ingestions include burns to the mouth and esophagus, CNS depression, elevated liver function tests, metabolic acidosis, and hypotension.[158,167] The unintentional ingestion, in a 45-year-old woman, of less than 1 oz (30 mL) of methyldodecylbenzyltrimethyl ammonium chloride was associated with rapid onset of altered mental status, respiratory distress, and generalized twitching, resulting in death within 30 minutes.[2] The lethal course of events was postulated to have occurred in part as a result of cholinesterase inhibition, although no enzymatic determinations were performed. Muscle paralysis is also occasionally described as a complication of these ingestions.[54] Chronic inhalational exposure is associated with occupational asthma.[14] Topical use of the quaternary ammonium compounds can cause contact dermatitis.[137] Few data are available on the toxicity of the newer quaternary ammonium compound ingestions.

Ingestions of other cationic surface active agents, such as the pyridinium agent cetrimonium bromide (Cetrimide), are associated with caustic burns to the mouth, lips, and tongue.[105] Peritoneal irrigation with cetrimonium bromide can produce metabolic abnormalities, hypotension, and methemoglobinemia.[7,102]

Treatment recommendations following the ingestion of the quaternary ammonium compounds and other cationic surface active agents are similar to those for other potentially caustic ingestions. Emergency department evaluation should be considered for all ingestions other than an unintentional taste of a dilute (less than 1%) solution. Therapy is mainly supportive. Endoscopy may be warranted if symptoms suggest the possibility of a burn injury.

Potassium Permanganate

Potassium permanganate ($KMnO_4$) is a violet water-soluble compound that is usually sold as crystals or tablets. Historically, it was used as an abortifacient, urethral irrigant, lavage fluid for alkaloid poisoning, and snake bite remedy. Currently, potassium permanganate is most often used as an antiseptic, particularly for patients with eczema.

Potassium permanganate poisoning may result in local and systemic toxicity.[143] Fatalities from oral ingestions are reported.[101,111] Potassium permanganate is a strong oxidizing agent. Upon contact with mucus membranes, potassium permanganate reacts with water to form manganese dioxide, potassium hydroxide, and molecular oxygen. Local tissue injury is the result of contact with the nascent oxygen as well as the caustic effect of potassium hydroxide. A brown-black staining of the tissues occurs from the manganese dioxide.

Initial symptoms include nausea and vomiting. Laryngeal edema and ulceration of the mouth, esophagus, and to a lesser extent the stomach may result from these caustic effects. Gastrointestinal perforation and hemorrhage may occur. Esophageal strictures and pyloric stenosis may be late complications.

Although potassium permanganate is not well absorbed from the GI tract, systemic absorption may occur, resulting in life-threatening toxicity. Systemic effects include hepatotoxicity, renal damage, methemoglobinemia, hemolysis, hemorrhagic pancreatitis, acute respiratory distress syndrome, disseminated intravascular coagulation, and cardiovascular collapse.[95,101,111] Elevation in blood or serum manganese concentration may also occur, confirming systemic absorption (normal levels: blood manganese 3.9 to 15.0 μg/L, serum manganese 0.9 to 2.9 μg/L).

Chronic ingestion of potassium permanganate may result in manganese poisoning. A 66-year-old man who mistakenly ingested 10 g of potassium permanganate over a 4-week period (due to medication mislabeling) developed neurosensory, autonomic, visual, and concentration symptoms. He also developed abdominal pain, gastric ulceration, and alopecia. Serum manganese was elevated. Nine months later the patient's neurologic examination displayed extrapyramidal signs consistent with parkinsonism.[68]

Initial treatment of a patient with potassium permanganate ingestion should include assessment for evidence of airway compromise. Endotracheal intubation may be required in cases with airway edema. Syrup of ipecac induced emesis is not recommended. Dilution with milk or water may be useful. The use of neutralizing agents such as egg whites or sodium hypochlorite has been reported.[143] Efficacy of activated charcoal is not known.

Patients with symptoms consistent with caustic injury should undergo early endoscopy. Corticosteroid agents along with antibiotics may be warranted in some cases, especially if laryngeal edema is present. Liver and renal function tests, amylase, serum manganese, and methemoglobin levels should be performed when systemic toxicity is suspected. Methemoglobinemia should be treated with methylene blue. Dermal irrigation with dilute oxalic acid has been recommended to remove cutaneous staining.[143]

Hydrogen Peroxide

Hydrogen peroxide, an oxidizing agent with weak antiseptic properties, has been used for many years as an antiseptic and a disinfectant. This agent is generally available in two strengths: dilute hydrogen peroxide, with a concentration of 3 to 9% (usually 3%), sold for home use; and concentrated hydrogen peroxide, with a concentration greater than 10%, used primarily for industrial purposes. Commercial-strength hydrogen peroxide is most commonly found as a 27.5 to 70% solution. Home uses for dilute hydrogen peroxide include ear cerumen removal, mouth gargle, vaginal douche, enema, and hair bleaching. Dilute hydrogen peroxide is also sometimes used as a veterinary emetic. Commercial uses of the more concentrated solutions include bleaching and cleansing textiles and wool, and producing foam rubber and rocket fuel. In the last few years, 35% hydrogen peroxide became available to the general public in health food stores and is sold as "hyper-oxygenation therapy" for a variety of conditions including AIDS and cancer.[71]

Hydrogen peroxide has two main mechanisms of toxicity: local tissue injury and gas formation. The extent of local tissue injury is determined by the strength of the hydrogen peroxide. Dilute hydrogen peroxide is an irritant and concentrated hydrogen peroxide is a caustic. Gas formation results when hydrogen peroxide interacts with tissue catalase, liberating molecular oxygen and water. One milliliter of 3% hydrogen peroxide can liberate 10 mL of oxygen at standard temperature and pressure. Gas formation can result in life-threatening embolization. The use of hydrogen peroxide in closed spaces such as operative wounds, or its use under pressure during wound irrigation, increases the likelihood of embolization.

An increasing number of hydrogen peroxide ingestions have been reported and involve the formation of life-threatening oxygen emboli after the ingestion of 35% hydrogen peroxide. Symptoms consistent with sudden oxygen embolization include rapid deterioration in mental status, cyanosis, acute respiratory failure, seizures, and ischemic ECG changes.[48] A 2-year-old boy died after ingesting 4 to 6 oz (120 to 180 mL) of 35% hydrogen peroxide.[28] Antemortem chest radiograph showed gas in the right ventricle, mediastinum, and portal venous system. Portal vein gas has also been a prominent feature in other cases.[94] Arterialization of gas oxygen embolization may result in cerebral infarction.[136]

Other findings from ingestion of concentrated hydrogen peroxide include GI disturbances, such as vomiting, hematemesis, abdominal pain, and abdominal bloating.[71,94] Endoscopy may show significant gastric mucosal erosions; esophageal injury is usually minimal. Rupture of a hollow viscus such as the stomach is a major concern considering the caustic and gas-producing properties of concentrated hydrogen peroxide. Cases of perforation, however, have not been reported. Airway compromise manifested by stridor, drooling, apneic episodes, and radiographic evidence of subepiglottic narrowing may also occur.[40] Death from intravenous injection of 35% hydrogen peroxide is also reported.[87]

Clinical sequelae from the ingestion of dilute hydrogen peroxide are usually much more benign.[40,63] Nausea and vomiting are the most common symptoms.[40] A whitish discoloration may be noted in the oral cavity. Gastrointestinal injury is usually limited to superficial mucosal irritation, but multiple gastric and duodenal ulcers accompanied by hematemesis have been reported.[63] Portal venous gas embolization may also occur as a result of the ingestion of 3% hydrogen peroxide.[29,123]

The use of 3% hydrogen peroxide for wound irrigation may result in significant complications. Extensive subcutaneous emphysema occurred after a dog bite to a human's face was irrigated under pressure with 60 mL of 3% hydrogen peroxide.[140] Systemic oxygen embolism causing hypotension, ischemic ECG changes, and coma resulted from the intraoperative irrigation of an infected herniorrhaphy wound.[10] Gas embolism resulting in intestinal gangrene was reported to occur following colonic lavage with 1% hydrogen peroxide during surgical treatment of meconium ileus.[135] Multiple cases of acute colitis are reported as a complication of administering 3% hydrogen peroxide enemas.[100] The use of 3% hydrogen peroxide as a mouth rinse is associated with the development of oral ulcerations.[125] Ocular exposures may result in conjunctival injection, burning pain, and blurry vision.[40]

The treatment of patients with hydrogen peroxide ingestions depends to a large degree on whether the patient has ingested a dilute or concentrated solution. Those with ingestions of concentrated solutions require expeditious evaluation. Careful nasogastric aspiration of hydrogen peroxide may be helpful if the patient presents immediately after ingestion. Dilution with milk or water may be useful but has not been studied. Syrup of ipecac induced emesis is contraindicated. Activated charcoal should be used only in cases of suspected mixed ingestions. A careful examination should be performed to detect any evidence of gas formation. A chest radiograph may reveal gas in the cardiac chambers, mediastinum, or pleural space. An abdominal radiograph may show gas in the GI tract or portal system and define the extent of bowel distension. Patients with abdominal distension from gas formation should be treated with nasogastric suctioning. Those with clinical or radiographic evidence of gas in the heart should be placed in the Trendelenburg position to prevent gas from blocking the right ventricular outflow tract. Careful aspiration of air through a central venous line may be attempted in patients in extremis.[28] Immediate hyperbaric oxygen therapy is indicated in cases of life-threatening gas embolization after hydrogen peroxide ingestion.[94] Endoscopic evaluation may be necessary in patients who ingest concentrated hydrogen peroxide to determine the extent of burn injury. Asymptomatic patients who have unintentionally ingested small amounts of 3% hydrogen peroxide can be safely watched at home.

Boric Acid

Boric acid (H_3BO_3), prepared from borax (sodium borate), was first used as an antiseptic agent by Lister in the late 19th century. Although used extensively over the years for antisepsis and irrigation, boric acid has proven to be only weakly bacteriostatic. As a result of its germicidal limitations and its inherent toxicity, boric acid has become obsolete in modern antiseptic therapy. Nonetheless, it continues to be used as an antimicrobial to treat such conditions as vulvovaginal candidiasis.[160] Boric acid is also employed in the treatment of cockroach infestation and as a soap, contact lens solution, toothpaste, and food preservative.

Boric acid is readily absorbed through the GI tract, wounds, abraded skin, and serous cavities. Absorption does not occur through intact skin. Boric acid is predominantly eliminated unchanged by the kidney. Small amounts are also excreted into sweat, saliva, and feces.[49] Boric acid is concentrated in the brain and liver.

The exact mechanism of action of boric acid's toxicity remains unclear. Although it is an inorganic acid, it does not behave as a caustic agent. Local effects are limited to tissue irritation.

Over the years boric acid has developed a reputation as an exceptionally potent toxin. This reputation was derived in great part from a series of reports involving neonatal exposures to boric acid resulting in high morbidity and mortality. Life-threatening toxicity resulted from the repetitive topical application of boric acid for the treatment of diaper rash or the use of infant formulas accidently contaminated with boric acid.[49,169] Fatality rates greater than 50% were reported in some series.[169] Although infants appear to be the most sensitive to the toxic effects of boric acid, many cases of significant adult toxicity were also reported. These cases date predominantly from the time when boric acid was widely used as an irrigant. Routes of exposure to boric acid resulting in fatalities included wound irrigation, pleural irrigation, rectal washing, bladder irrigation, and vaginal packing.[116,157]

Classic boric acid poisoning as described in these reports usually involved multiple exposures over a period of days. Gastrointestinal, dermal, CNS, and renal manifestations predominate. The initial symptoms—nausea, vomiting, diarrhea, and occasionally crampy abdominal pain—may be confused with an acute gastroenteritis. At times, the emesis and diarrhea are greenish blue.[169] Following the onset of GI symptoms, the majority of patients develop a characteristic intense generalized erythroderma.[169] This rash, described as having a "boiled lobster" appearance, may appear indistinguishable from toxic epidermal necrolysis or staphylococcal scalded skin syndrome in the neonate.[130] The rash may be especially noticeable on the palms, soles, and buttocks.[49] Typically, extensive desquamation takes place within 1 to 2 days. At times prominent mucous membrane involvement of the oral cavity and conjunctivae are also apparent.[169] At about the time of the development of the erythroderma, patients, particularly young infants, may develop prominent signs of CNS irritability resembling meningeal irritation. Seizures, delirium, and coma can occur.[49] Renal injury is common, and due to the renal elimination of this compound.[49] Other complications of boric acid poisoning include hepatic injury, hyperthermia, and cardiovascular collapse.

The abandonment of boric acid as an irrigant and its removal from the nursery have led to a marked decrease in the incidence of significant boric acid poisoning. Two retrospective studies on boric acid ingestions suggest that a single acute ingestion of boric acid is generally quite benign.[89,91] In these studies, 79 to 88% of patients remained asymptomatic. Symptoms, when present, primarily consist of GI irritative symptoms, such as nausea and vomiting. None of the 1184 patients in these two studies manifested generalized erythroderma so commonly described in previous reports. Central nervous system manifestations of acute overdose were limited to occasional lethargy and headache. Renal toxicity did not generally occur following single acute ingestions.

Several recent reports have suggested, however, that significant toxicity from acute ingestion of boric acid can still occur. Fatality resulted from a single ingestion of two cups of boric acid crystals in a 45-year-old man.[126] Symptoms on presentation (two days after ingestion) included nausea, vomiting, green diarrhea, lethargy, hypotension, renal failure, and a prominent "boiled lobster" rash on his trunk and extremities. In another case, the ingestion of 30 g of boric acid by a 77-year-old man resulted in similar symptoms and death 63 hours postingestion despite hemodialysis.[72]

Long-term chronic exposure to boric acid has resulted in alopecia in adults and seizures in children.[52,112,151] A 32-year-old woman who had been chronically ingesting mouthwash containing boric acid over a 7-month period developed progressive hair loss.[151] The chronic application of a borax and honey mixture to pacifiers resulted in the development of recurrent seizures in 9 infants, which resolved after the mixture was withheld.[52,113]

Treatment of boric acid toxicity is mainly supportive. Activated charcoal is not recommended because of its relatively poor adsorptive capacity for boric acid.[38] In cases of massive oral overdose or renal failure, hemodialysis may be helpful in shortening the half-life of boric acid.[91,154]

Mercurials

Both inorganic mercurials, such as mercury bichloride, and organic mercurials, such as merbromin (Mercurochrome) or thimerosal (Merthiolate), have been used in the past as topical antiseptic agents. Thimerosal contains 49% mercury. Their relatively weak bacteriostatic properties along with the many problems associated with mercury toxicity significantly limits their usefulness (see Chaps. 54 and 80). Repeated application of topical mercurials has resulted in significant absorption and systemic toxicity.[127] The use of high-dose hepatitis-B immunoglobulin (HBIG) in liver transplantation may cause mercury toxicity due to the use of thimerosal as a preservative in the HBIG preparation.[93] In one case, a 44-year-old male patient received 250 mL of HBIG (containing about 30 mg thimerosal) over 9 days following liver transplantation. He developed speech difficulties, tremor, and chorea. His blood mercury level was 104 μg/L.

Chlorates

The chlorate salts, sodium chlorate and potassium chlorate, were at one time used as medicinal agents to treat inflammatory and ulcerative lesions of the oral cavity and could be found in various mouthwash, toothpaste, and gargle preparations.[145] Although their use as local antiseptics has become obsolete, chlorates are used as herbicides and in the manufacture of matches, explosives, and dyestuffs.[73] Most recent cases of chlorate poisoning have resulted from the ingestion of the sodium chlorate-containing weed killers, or dispensing errors confusing sodium chlorate for sodium sulfate or sodium chloride.[73,78] Sodium chlorate in the form of white crystals has also been mistaken for table sugar.[60] A case of significant toxicity from the inhalation of atomized chlorates is also reported.[73]

Sodium chlorate ($NaClO_3$) is a strong oxidizing agent. It is rapidly absorbed from the GI tract and eliminated predominantly unchanged from the kidneys.[74] Its systemic effects are chiefly hematologic and renal. Chlorate's major mechanism of toxicity is its ability to oxidize hemoglobin and increase red blood cell membrane rigidity.[138] Consequently, significant methemoglobinemia and hemolytic anemia may result. Chlorates may also be directly toxic to the proximal renal tubule.[86] The hemolytic anemia and the resultant hemoglobinuria may secondarily cause disseminated intravascular coagulation and potentiate renal toxicity. The worsening renal function is especially problematic because of its adverse effect on chlorate elimination. The methemoglobinemia may be severe and cause significant hypoxic stress. Earlier reports suggested that methemoglobinemia was predominantly extracellular, occurring only after the development of significant hemolysis,[53] but more recent reports suggest that methemoglobinemia may occur prior to hemolytic anemia.[107,148] Chlorates may also act locally as a GI irritant, and cause mild CNS depression after absorption.[54]

Clinical signs and symptoms of chlorate poisoning usually begin 1 to 4 hours after ingestion.[80] The earliest symptoms are GI, including nausea, vomiting, diarrhea, and crampy abdominal pain. Subsequently, the patient may exhibit cyanosis from the methemoglobinemia and black-brown urine from the hemoglobinuria. Anuria may ensue. Laboratory studies may show methemoglobinemia, anemia, Heinz bodies, ghost cells, fragmented spherocytes, decreased platelet count, and abnormal coagulation studies. Hyperkalemia may be particularly problematic if the patient ingests potassium chlorate preparations.[37]

Treatment of a patient with a significant chlorate ingestion should include gastric lavage and activated charcoal.[60] It has been suggested that administration of sodium thiosulfate may inactivate the chlorate ion by reducing it to the chloride ion,[60] but an in vitro study did not confirm this hypothesis.[149] Although methylene blue may be used in the treatment of symptomatic methemoglobinemia in an attempt to reduce methemoglobin to hemoglobin, its efficacy in the treatment of chlorate-induced methemoglobinemia may be limited compared to its efficacy in the treatment of other oxidant-induced methemoglobinemias.[107,148] This may be due to the inactivation by chlorates of glucose-6-phosphate dehydrogenase, an enzyme that is required for methylene blue's reduction of methemoglobin.[139] Exchange transfusion, peritoneal dialysis, and hemodialysis have all been advocated in the treatment of patients with severe chlorate poisoning.[107,148] Because the chlorate ion is easily dialyzable, hemodialysis (or peritoneal dialysis if hemodialysis is unavailable) is capable of removing this toxin as well as treating any concomitant renal failure that may have developed.[60,73,80,86]

Ethylene Oxide

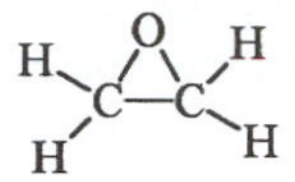

Ethylene oxide (C_2H_4O) is a gas that is commonly used to sterilize heat-sensitive material in healthcare facilities. Unlike antiseptics and disinfectants, which generally do not exhibit full sporicidal activity, sterilants such as ethylene oxide inactivate all organisms. Ethylene oxide is also used in the synthesis of many chemicals, including ethylene glycol, surfactants, rocket propellants, and petroleum demulsifiers, and has been used as a pesticide fumigant. Chemically, ethylene oxide has a cyclic ester structure known as an epoxide. It acts as an alkylating agent, reacting with most cellular components including DNA and RNA.

Medical attention regarding ethylene oxide toxicity has centered on its mutagenic and possible carcinogenic effects.[84] Approximately 270,000 workers (including 96,000 hospital workers) in the United States are at risk for occupational exposure to ethylene oxide.[147] Retrospective studies have suggested a possible excess incidence of leukemia and gastric cancer in ethylene oxide-exposed workers.[66,147] These studies have not been conclusive, and the carcinogenicity of ethylene oxide remains subject to debate. It has also been suggested that an increased incidence of spontaneous abortions may be associated with occupational exposure to ethylene oxide (see Chap. 109).[61]

The acute toxicity of ethylene oxide is mainly due to its irritant effects. Conjunctival, upper respiratory tract, GI, and dermal irritation may occur. Dermal burns from acute exposure to ethylene oxide have also been described.

Ethylene oxide also has central and peripheral nervous system effects. Acute exposure to a broken ethylene oxide ampule by a 43-year-old recovery room nurse resulted in nausea, light-headedness, malaise, syncope, and recurrent seizures.[132] There were no long-term complications. In another case of acute exposure, coma was followed by an irreversible parkinsonism.[8] Chronic exposure to ethylene oxide has resulted in motor and sensory neuropathies.[55,108]

Treatment for patients with ethylene oxide exposure is supportive.

Glutaraldehyde

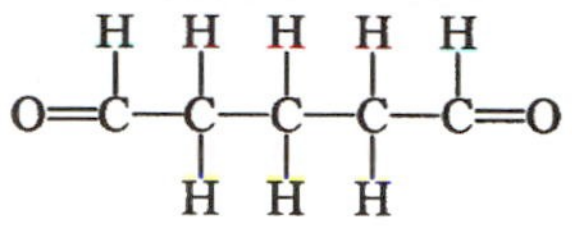

Glutaraldehyde [$HCO(CH_2)_3CHO$] is a liquid solution used in the cold sterilization of nonautoclavable endoscopic, surgical, and dental equipment. It is also employed as a tissue fixative, embalming fluid, preservative, and tanning agent, in radiographic solutions, and in the treatment of warts.[50] Glutaraldehyde is a dialdehyde with two active carbonyl groups. It kills all microorganisms, including viruses and spores. It is prepared as a 2% alkaline solution in 70% isopropanol (Cidex). Approximately 35,000 workers are occupationally exposed to glutaraldehyde (see Chap. 109).[119]

Data on human toxicity from glutaraldehyde are limited. Clinical signs and symptoms are thought to be comparable to those of formaldehyde exposure. However, animal studies have shown that glutaraldehyde administered enterally or topically is less toxic than an equal concentration of formaldehyde.[131]

No cases of deliberate or unintentional ingestion of glutaraldehyde have been reported. Glutaraldehyde is a mucosal irritant. Coryza, epistaxis, headache, asthma, chest tightness, palpitations, tachycardia, and nausea are all associated with glutaraldehyde vapor exposure.[13,31,106] Contact dermatitis and ocular inflammation may also occur.[34,50,76,106] To date, no significant GI, renal, neurologic, or acid–base disturbances have been associated with glutaraldehyde.

Preliminary animal evidence suggests that glutaraldehyde, like formaldehyde, may be a potent nasal carcinogen.[146] Additional research is needed in this controversial area. Treatment recommendations are similar to those for patients with formaldehyde exposure.

Summary

A chemically diverse group of antiseptic, disinfectant, and sterilant agents have been reviewed. Many of the more toxic agents—such as iodine, phenol, and chlorates—are no longer commonly used as cleansing agents but have not disappeared and may still be available in some settings. Formaldehyde exposures, while also uncommon, can also cause significant problems. Frequently employed antiseptics such as chlorhexidine, Phisoderm, and many of the currently used quaternary ammonium compounds have a relatively low degree of toxicity. Ingestions of the iodophors do not usually cause significant toxicity, but absorption through other routes may still produce significant adverse effects. Ingestions of hydrogen peroxide, particularly the more concentrated formulations, may be more problematic.

References

1. Acheson ED, Gardner MJ, Pannett B, et al: Formaldehyde in the British chemical industry: An occupational cohort study. Lancet 1984;1:611–616.
2. Adelson L, Sunshine I: Fatal poisoning due to a cationic detergent of the quaternary ammonium compound type. Am J Clin Pathol 1952;22:656–661.
3. Albert RE, Sellakumar AR, Laskin S, et al: Gaseous formaldehyde and hydrogen chloride induction of nasal cancer in the rat. J Natl Cancer Inst 1982;68:597–603.
4. Allen RE, Thoshinsky MJ, Stallone RJ, Hunt TK: Corrosive injuries of the stomach. Arch Surg 1970; 100:409–413.
5. Aquilina JT: Fungating ioderma treated with hydrocortisone. JAMA 1955;158:727–728.
6. Baker EL, Landrigan PJ, Bertozzi PE, et al: Phenol poisoning due to contaminated drinking water. Arch Environ Health 1978;33:89–94.
7. Baraka A, Yamut F, Wakid N: Cetrimide-induced methaemoglobinemia after surgical excision of hydatid cyst. Lancet 1980;2:88–89.
8. Barbosa ER, Comerlatti LR, Haddad MS, Scaff M: Parkinsonism secondary to ethylene oxide exposure. Arq Neuropsiquiatr 1992;50:531–533.
9. Bartone NF, Grieco V, Herr BS: Corrosive gastritis due to ingestion of formaldehyde. JAMA 1968;203:50–51.
10. Bassan MM, Dudai M, Shalev O: Near-fatal systemic oxygen embolism due to wound irrigation with hydrogen peroxide. Postgrad Med J 1982;58:448–450.
11. Beall JR, Ulsamer AG: Formaldehyde and hepatotoxicity: A review. J Toxicol Environ Health 1984;13:1–21.
12. Bennett IL, James DF, Golden A: Severe acidosis due to phenol poisoning: Report of two cases. Ann Intern Med 1950;32:324–327.
13. Benson WG: Exposure to glutaraldehyde. J Soc Occup Med 1984;34:63–64.
14. Bernstein JA, Stauder T, Bernstein DI, Bernstein IL: A combined respiratory and cutaneous hypersensitivity syndrome induced by work exposure to quaternary amines. J Allergy Clin Immunol 1994;94:257–259.
15. Bianco RP, Smith PJ, Keen RR, Jordan JE: Iodide intoxication: Report of a case. Oral Surg 1974;32:876–880.
16. Bishop ME, Garcia RL: Ioderma from wound irrigation with povidone-iodine. JAMA 1978;240:249–250.
17. Block SS: Definition of terms. In: Block SS, ed: Disinfection, Sterilization, and Preservation, 4th ed. Philadelphia, Lea & Febiger, 1991, pp. 18–25.
18. Breysse P, Couser WG, Alpers CE, et al: Membranous nephropathy and formaldehyde exposure. Ann Intern Med 1994;120:396–397.
19. Brown VK, Box VL, Simpson BJ: Decontamination procedures for skin exposed to phenolic substances. Arch Environ Health 1975;30:1–6.
20. Burkhart KK, Kulig KW: Formate levels following a formalin ingestion. Vet Hum Toxicol 1990;32:135–137.
21. Carter JE: Iodide "mumps." N Engl J Med 1961;264: 987–988.
22. Casteel SW, Vernon RJ, Bailey EM: Formaldehyde: Toxicology and hazards. Vet Hum Toxicol 1987;29:31–33.
23. Chabrolle JP, Rossier A: Goiter and hypothyroidism in the

newborn after cutaneous absorption of iodine. Arch Dis Child 1978;53:495–498.
24. Chan TY. Poisoning due to Savlon (cetrimide) liquid. Hum Exp Toxicol 1994;13:681–682.
25. Chan TYK, Lau MSW, Critchley JA: Serious complications associated with Dettol poisoning. Q J Med 1993;86: 735–738.
26. Cheung J, O'Leary JJ: Allergic reaction to chlorhexidine in an anaesthetized patient. Anaesth Intens Care 1985;13: 429–439.
27. Chilcote R, Curley A, Loughlin HH, et al: Hexachlorophene storage in burn patients associated with encephalopathy. Pediatrics 1977;59:457–459.
28. Christensen DW, Faught WE, Black RE, et al: Fatal oxygen embolization after hydrogen peroxide ingestion. Crit Care Med 1992;20:543–544.
29. Cina SJ, Downs JC, Conradi SE: Hydrogen peroxide: A source of lethal oxygen embolism. Am J Forensic Med Pathol 1994;15:44–50.
30. Cohn BN: Absorption of compound solution of iodine from the gastro-intestinal tract. Arch Intern Med 1932; 49:950–956.
31. Connaughton P: Occupational exposure to glutaraldehyde associated with tachycardia and palpitations. Med J Aust 1993;159:567. Letter.
32. Conning DM, Hayes MJ: The dermal toxicity of phenol: An investigation of the most effective first-aid measures. Br J Ind Med 1970;27:155–159.
33. Crocker D, Vandam LD: Untoward reactions to radiodiagnostic contrast media. Clin Pharmacol Ther 1963;4:654–662.
34. Dailey JR, Parnes RE, Aminlari A: Glutaraldehyde keratopthy. Am J Opthmol 1993;115:256–258.
35. Dally KA, Hanrahan LP, Woodbury MA, Kanarek MS: Formaldehyde exposure in nonoccupational environments. Arch Environ Health 1981;36:277–284.
36. D'Auria J, Lipson S, Garfield JM: Fatal iodine toxicity following surgical debridement of a hip wound: Case report. J Trauma 1990;30:353–355.
37. Davies P: Potassium-chlorate poisoning with oliguria. Lancet 1956;1:612–613.
38. Decker WJ, Combs HF, Corby DG: Adsorption of drugs and poison by activated charcoal. Toxicol Appl Pharmacol 1968;13:454–460.
39. Dela Cruz F, Brown DH, Leikin JB, et al: Iodine absorption after topical administration. West J Med 1987; 146:43–45.
40. Dickson KF, Caravati EM: Hydrogen peroxide exposure—325 exposures reported to a regional poison control center. J Toxicol Clin Toxicol 1994;32:705–714.
41. Dyck RF, Bear RA, Goldstein MB, Halperin ML: Iodine/iodide toxic reaction: Case report with emphasis on the nature of the metabolic acidosis. Can Med Assoc J 1979;120:704–706.
42. Eells JT, McMartin KE, Black K, et al: Formaldehyde poisoning: Rapid metabolism to formic acid. JAMA 1981;246: 1237–1238.
43. Emerson D, Pierce C: A case of a single ingestion of 4% Hibiclens. Vet Hum Toxicol 1988;30:583.
44. Finkelstein R, Jacobi M: Fatal iodine poisoning: A clinicopathologic and experimental study. Ann Intern Med 1937;10:1283–1296.
45. Fischman RA, Fairclough GF, Cheigh JS: Iodide and negative anion gap. N Engl J Med 1978;298:1035–1036.
46. Fradkin JE, Wolff J: Iodide-induced thyrotoxicosis. Medicine 1983;62:1–20.
47. French RJ, Tabb HG, Rutledge LJ: Esophageal stenosis produced by ingestion of bleach: Report of two cases. South Med J 1970;63:1140–1144.
48. Giberson TP, Kern JD, Pettigrew DW, et al: Near-fatal hydrogen peroxide ingestion. Ann Emerg Med 1989;18: 778–779.
49. Goldbloom RB, Goldbloom A: Boric acid poisoning: A report of four cases and a review of 109 cases from the world literature. J Pediatr 1953;43:631–643.
50. Goncalo S, Brandao M, Pecegueiro M, et al: Occupational contact dermatitis to glutaraldehyde. Contact Derm 1984; 10:183–184.
51. Goodman L, Geiger AJ: Therapy in carbolic acid poisoning: With special reference to the use of oil antidotes. Am J Med Sci 1935;190:206–219.
52. Gordon AS, Prichard JS, Freedman MH: Seizure disorders and anemia associated with chronic borax intoxication. Can Med Assoc J 1973;108:719–724.
53. Gordon S, Brown JA: Potassium chlorate poisoning: Report of a case. Lancet 1947;2:503–504.
54. Gosselin RE, Smith RP, Hodge HC: Clinical Toxicology of Commercial Products, 5th ed. Baltimore, Williams & Wilkins, 1984.
55. Gross JA, Haas ML, Swift TR: Ethylene oxide neurotoxicity: Report of four cases and review of the literature. Neurology 1979;29:978–983.
56. Haddad LM, Dimond KA, Schweistris JE: Phenol poisoning. JACEP 1979;8:267–269.
57. Harden RM: Submandibular adenitis due to iodide administration. Br Med J 1968;1:160–161.
58. Hardin RD, Tedesco FJ: Colitis after Hibiclens enema. J Clin Gastroenterol 1986; 8:572–575.
59. Harvey SC: Antiseptics and disinfectants; fungicides; ectoparasiticides. In: Gilman AG, Rall TW, Nies AS, Taylor P, eds: Goodman and Gilman's The Pharmacological Basis of Therapeutics, 7th ed. New York, Pergamon Press, 1985, pp. 959–979.
60. Helliwell M, Nunn J: Mortality in sodium chlorate poisoning. Br Med J 1979;1:1119.
61. Hemminki K, Mutanen P, Saloniemi I, et al: Spontaneous abortions in hospital staff engaged in sterilising instruments with chemical agents. Br Med J 1982;285:1461–1463.
62. Hendrick DJ, Land DJ: Occupational formalin asthma. Br J Ind Med 1977;34:11–18.
63. Henry MC, Wheeler J, Mofenson HC, et al: Hydrogen peroxide 3% exposures. J Toxicol Clin Toxicol 1996;34: 323–327.
64. Herskowitz J, Rosman NP: Acute hexachlorophene poisoning by mouth in a neonate. J Pediatr 1979;94:495–496.
65. Hodge GE, Scharfe EE: Stricture of the esophagus. Can Med Assoc J 1937;37:541–547.
66. Hogstedt C, Aringer L, Gustavsson A: Epidemiologic support for ethylene oxide as a cancer-causing agent. JAMA 1986;255:1575–1578.
67. Holness DL, Nethercott JR: Health status of funeral service

workers exposed to formaldehyde. Arch Environ Health 1989;44:222–228.
68. Holzgraefe M, Poser W, Kijewski H, Beuche W: Chronic enteral poisoning cause by potassium permanganate. J Toxicol Clin Toxicol 1986;24:235–244.
69. Horch R, Spilker G, Stork GB: Phenol burns and intoxications. Burns 1994;20:45–50.
70. Horn B, Kabins SA: Iodide fever. Am J Med Sci 1972; 64:467–471.
71. Humberston CL, Dean BS, Krenzelok EP: Ingestions of 35% hydrogen peroxide. J Toxicol Clin Toxicol 1990;28:95–100.
72. Ishii Y, Fujizuka N, Takahashi T, et al: A fatal case of acute boric acid poisoning. J Toxicol Clin Toxicol 1993;31: 345–352.
73. Jackson RC, Elder WJ, McDonnell H: Sodium-chlorate poisoning complicated by acute renal failure. Lancet 1961;2: 1381–1383.
74. Jansen H, Zeldenrust J: Homicidal chronic sodium chlorate poisoning. Forensic Sci 1972;1:103–105.
75. Jarvis SN, Straube RC, Williams AL, Bartlett CL: Illness associated with contamination of drinking water supplies with phenol. Br Med J 1985;290:1800–1802.
76. Jordan WP, Dahl MV, Albert HL: Contact dermatitis from glutaraldehyde. Arch Dermatol 1972;105:94–95.
77. Kilburn KH: Neurobehavioral impairment and seizures from formaldehyde. Arch Environ Health 1994;49:37–44.
78. Klendshoj NC, Burke WJ, Anthone R, Anthone S: Chlorate poisoning. JAMA 1962;180:1133–1134.
79. Kline BS: Formaldehyde poisoning. Arch Intern Med 1925;36:220–228.
80. Knight RK, Trounce JR, Cameron JS: Suicidal chlorate poisoning treated with peritoneal dialysis. Br Med J 1967;3: 601–602.
81. Koppel C, Baudisch H, Schneider V, Ibe K: Suicidal ingestion of formalin with fatal complications. Intensive Care Med 1990;16:212–214.
82. Kurt TL, Morgan ML, Hnilica V, et al: Fatal iatrogenic iodine toxicity in a 9-week old infant. J Toxicol Clin Toxicol 1996;34:231–234.
83. Landau G, Saunders WH: The effect of chlorine bleach on the esophagus. Arch Otolaryngol 1964;80:174–176.
84. Landrigan PJ, Meinhardt TJ, Gordon J, et al: Ethylene oxide: An overview of toxicologic and epidemiologic research. Am J Ind Med 1984;6:103–115.
85. Lavelle KJ, Doedens DJ, Kleit SA, Forney RB: Iodine absorption in burn patients treated topically with povidone-iodine. Clin Pharmacol Ther 1975;17:355–362.
86. Lee DB, Brown DL, Baker LR, et al: Haematological complications of chlorate poisoning. Br Med J 1970; 2:31–32.
87. Leiken J, Sing K, Woods K: Fatality from intravenous use of hydrogen peroxide for home "superoxygenation therapy." Vet Hum Toxicol 1993;35;342. Abstract.
88. Lewin JF, Cleary WT: An accidental death caused by the absorption of phenol through skin: A case report. Forensic Sci Int 1982;19:177–179.
89. Linden CH, Hall AH, Kulig KW, Rumack BH: Acute ingestions of boric acid. J Toxicol Clin Toxicol 1986;24: 269–279.
90. Litovitz TL, Holm KC, Bailey KM, et al: 1991 annual report of the American Association of Poison Control Centers national data collection system. Am J Emerg Med 1992;10: 452–505.
91. Litovitz TL, Klein-Schwartz W, Oderda GM, Schmitz BF: Clinical manifestations of toxicity in a series of 784 boric acid ingestions. Am J Emerg Med 1988;6:209–213.
92. Loomis TA: Formaldehyde toxicity. Arch Pathol Lab Med 1979;103:321–324.
93. Lowell JA, Burgess S, Shenoy S, et al: Mercury poisoning associated with hepatitis-B immunoglobulin. Lancet 1996; 347:480. Letter.
94. Luu TA, Kelley MT, Strauch JA, Avradopoulos K: Portal vein gas embolism from hydrogen peroxide ingestion. Ann Emerg Med 1992;21:1391–1393.
95. Mahomedy MC, Mahomedy YH, Canham PA, et al: Methemoglobinemia following treatment dispensed by witch doctors: Two cases of potassium permanganate poisoning. Anesthesia 1975;30:190–193.
96. Marks JG: Allergic contact dermatitis to povidone-iodine. J Am Acad Dermatol 1982;6:473–475.
97. Martinez AJ, Boehm V, Hadfield MG: Acute hexachlorophene encephalopathy: Cliniconeuropathological correlation. Acta Neuropathol 1974;28:93–103.
98. Massano G, Ciocatto E, Rosabianca C, et al: Striking aminotransferase rise after chlorhexidine self-poisoning. Lancet 1982;1:289. Letter.
99. Merliss RR: Phenol marasmus. J Occup Med 1972;14: 55–56.
100. Meyer CT, Brand M, DeLuca VA, Spiro HM: Hydrogen peroxide colitis: A report of three patients. J Clin Gastroenterol 1981;3:31–35.
101. Middleton SJ, Jacyna M, McClaren D, et al: Hemorrhagic pancreatitis—A cause of death in severe potassium permanganate poisoning. Postgrad Med J 1990;66:657–658.
102. Momblano P, Pradere B, Jarrige N, et al: Metabolic acidosis induced by cetrimonium bromide. Lancet 1984; 2:1045.
103. Moore M: The ingestion of iodine as a method of attempted suicide. N Engl J Med 1938; 219:383–388.
104. Morgans ME, Trotter WR: Two cases of myxedema attributed to iodide administration. Lancet 1953;2:1335–1337.
105. Mucklow ES: Accidental feeding of a dilute antiseptic solution (chlorhexidine 0.05% with cetrimide 1%) to five babies. Hum Toxicol 1988;7:567–569.
106. Norback D: Skin and respiratory symptoms from exposure to alkaline glutaraldehyde in medical services. Scand J Work Environ Health 1988; 14:366–371.
107. O'Grady J, Jarecsni E: Sodium chlorate poisoning. Br J Clin Pract 1971;25:38–39.
108. Ohnishi A, Murai Y: Polyneuropathy due to ethylene oxide, propylene oxide, and butylene oxide. Environ Res 1993;60:242–247.
109. Okano M, Nomura M, Hata S, et al: Anaphylactic symptoms due to chlorhexidine gluconate. Arch Dermatol 1989;125:50–52.
110. Olsen JH, Dossing M: Formaldehyde induced symptoms in day care centers. Am Ind Hyg Assoc J 1982;43: 366–370.
111. Ong KL, Tan TH, Cheung WL: Potassium permanganate poisoning—A rare cause of fatal self-poisoning. J Accid Emerg Med 1997;14:43–45.
112. Orringer EP, Mattern WD: Formaldehyde-induced hemol-

ysis during chronic hemodialysis. N Engl J Med 1976;294: 1416–1420.
113. O'Sullivan K, Taylor M: Chronic boric acid poisoning in infants. Arch Dis Child 1983;58:737–749.
114. Partanen T, Kauppinen T, Nurminen M, et al: Formaldehyde exposure and respiratory and related cancer. Scand J Work Environ Health 1985;11:409–415.
115. Pennington JA: A review of iodine toxicity reports. J Am Diet Assoc 1990;90:1571–1581.
116. Pfeiffer CC, Hallman LF, Gersh I: Boric acid ointment: A study of possible intoxication in the treatment of burns. JAMA 1945;128:266–273.
117. Pietsch J, Meakins JL: Complications of povidone-iodine absorption in topically treated burn patients. Lancet 1976; 1:280–282.
118. Pike DG, Peabody JW, Davis EW, Lyons WS: A re-evaluation of the dangers of Clorox ingestion. J Pediatr 1963;63: 303–305.
119. Pinnas JL, Meinke GC: Other aldehydes. In: Sullivan JB, Krieger GR, eds: Hazardous Materials Toxicology. Baltimore, Williams & Wilkins, 1992, pp. 981–986.
120. Porter JA: Acute respiratory distress following formalin inhalation. Lancet 1975;2:603–604.
121. Pullin TG, Pinkerton MN, Johnston RV, Kilian DJ: Decontamination of the skin of swine following phenol exposure: A comparison of the relative efficacy of water versus polyethylene glycol/industrial methylated spirits. Toxicol Appl Pharmacol 1978;43:199–206.
122. Pun KK, Yeung CK, Chan TK: Acute intravascular hemolysis due to accidental formalin intoxication during hemodialysis. Clin Nephrol 1984;21:188–190.
123. Rackoff WR, Merton DF: Gas embolization after ingestion of hydrogen peroxide. Pediatrics 1990;85:593–594.
124. Rasmussen H: Iodide hypersensitivity in the etiology of periarteritis nodosa. J Allergy 1955;26:394–407.
125. Rees TD, Orth CF: Oral ulcerations with use of hydrogen peroxide. J Peridontal 1986;57:689–692.
126. Restuccio A, Mortensen ME, Kelley MT: Fatal ingestion of boric acid in an adult. Am J Emerg Med 1992; 10:545–547.
127. Rohyans J, Walson PD, Wood GA, MacDonald WA: Mercury toxicity following merthiolate ear irrigations. J Pediatr 1984;104:311–313.
128. Roush GC, Walrath J, Stayner LT, et al: Nasopharyngeal cancer, sinonasal cancer and occupations related to formaldehyde: A case-control study. J Natl Cancer Inst 1987;79:1221–1224.
129. Roy M, Calonje MA, Mouton R: Corrosive gastritis after formaldehyde ingestion. N Engl J Med 1962;266: 1248–1250.
130. Rubenstein AD, Musher DM: Epidemic boric acid poisoning simulating staphylococcal toxic epidermal necrolysis of the newborn infant: Ritter's disease. J Pediatr 1970;77: 884–887.
131. Rumack B: Glutaraldehyde: POISINDEX, 1997.
132. Salinas E, Sasich L, Hall DH, et al: Acute ethylene oxide intoxication. DICP 1981;15:384–386.
133. Schulenburg CA: Corrosive stricture of the stomach without involvement of esophagus. Lancet 1941;2:367–368.
134. Seymour WB: Poisoning from cutaneous application of iodine. Arch Intern Med 1937;59:952–966.
135. Shaw A, Cooperman A, Fusco J: Gas embolism produced by hydrogen peroxide. N Engl J Med 1967; 277:238–241.
136. Sherman SI, Boyer LV, Sibley WA: Cerebral infarction immediately after ingestion of hydrogen peroxide solution. Stroke 1094;25:1065–1067.
137. Shmunes E, Levy EJ: Quaternary ammonium compound contact dermatitis from a deodorant. Arch Dermatol 1972; 105:91–93.
138. Singelmann E, Steffen C: Increased erythrocyte rigidity in chlorate poisoning. J Clin Pathol 1983;36:719.
139. Singelmann E, Wetzel E, Adler G, Steffen C: Erythrocyte membrane alterations as the basis of chlorate toxicity. Toxicology 1984;30:135–147.
140. Sleigh JW, Linter SP: Hazards of hydrogen peroxide. Br Med J 1985;291:1706.
141. Smerdely P, Boyages SC, Wu D, et al: Topical iodine-containing antiseptics and neonatal hypothyroidism in very-low-birthweight infants. Lancet 1989;2:661–664.
142. Sneddon IB: Dermatitis in an intermittent haemodialysis unit. Br Med J 1968; 1:183–184.
143. Southwood T, Lamb CM, Freeman J: Ingestion of potassium permanganate crystal by a three-year old boy. Med J Aust 1987;146:639–640.
144. Spiller HA, Quadrani-Kushner DA, Cleveland P: A five year evaluation of acute exposure to phenol disinfectant. J Toxicol Clin Toxicol 1993;31:307–313.
145. Stavrou A, Butcher R, Sakula A: Accidental self-poisoning by sodium chlorate weed-killer. Practitioner 1978;221:397–399.
146. St. Clair MD, Goross EA, Morgan KT: Interactions of glutaraldehyde with nasal epithelium. Toxicologist 1989; 9:37.
147. Steenland K, Stayner L, Greife A, et al: Mortality among workers exposed to ethylene oxide. N Engl J Med 1991; 324:1402–1407.
148. Steffen C, Seitz R: Severe chlorate poisoning: Report of a case. Arch Toxicol 1981;48:281–288.
149. Steffen C, Wetzel E: Pathophysiological aspects of chlorate poisoning. Hum Toxicol 1985;4:541–542.
150. Steigmann F, Dolehide RA: Corrosive (acid) gastritis. N Engl J Med 1956;254:981–986.
151. Stein KM, Odom RB, Justice GR, Martin GC: Toxic alopecia from ingestion of boric acid. Arch Dermatol 1973;108: 95–97.
152. Sussman RM, Miller J: Iodide "mumps" after intravenous urography. N Engl J Med 1956;255:433–434.
153. Tabor E, Bostwich DC, Evans CC: Corneal damage due to eye contact with chlorhexidine gluconate. JAMA 1989; 261:557–558.
154. Teshima D, Morishita K, Ueda Y, et al: Clinical management of boric acid ingestion: Pharmacokinetic assessment of efficacy of hemodialysis for treatment of acute boric acid poisoning. J Pharmacobiodyn 1992; 15:287–294.
155. Thurm RH, Finkel HE: Drug fever due to potassium iodide. NY State J Med 1965;65:2263–2265.
156. Tresch DD, Sweet DL, Keelan MH, Lange RL: Acute iodide intoxication with cardiac irritability. Arch Intern Med 1974;134:760–762.
157. Valdes-Dapena MA, Arey J: Boric acid poisoning: Three fatal cases with pancreatic inclusions and a review of the literature. J Pediatr 1962;61:531–546.

158. Van Berkel M, de Wolff FA: Survival after acute benzalkonium chloride poisoning. Hum Toxicol 1988;7:191–193.
159. Van der Vorst MM, Tamminga P, Wijburg FA, Schutgens RB: Severe methaemoglobinaemia due to para-chloraniline intoxication in premature neonates. Eur J Pediatr 1990;150:73. Letter.
160. Van Slyke KK, Michel VP, Rein MF: Treatment of vulvovaginal candidiasis with boric acid powder. Am J Obstet Gynecol 1981;141:145–148.
161. Vorherr H, Vorherr UF, Mehta P, et al: Vaginal absorption of povidone-iodine. JAMA 1988;244:2628–2629.
162. Wallgren H: Relative intoxicating effects of ethyl, propyl and butyl alcohol. Acta Pharmacol et Toxicol 1960;16: 217–220.
163. Warner MA, Harper JV: Cardiac dysrhythmias associated with chemical peeling with phenol. Anesthesiology 1985; 62:366–367.
164. Waugh WH: Use of cortisone by mouth in prevention and therapy of severe iodism. Arch Intern Med 1954;93: 299–303.
165. Weeks RS, Ravitch MM: Esophageal injury by liquid chlorine bleach: Experimental study. J Pediatr 1969;74: 911–916.
166. Wilensky AO, Kaufman PA: Pyloric stenosis following the ingestion of tincture of iodine. Am J Surg 1939; 43:779–782.
167. Wilson JT, Burr IM: Benzalkonium chloride poisoning in infant twins. Am J Dis Child 1975;129:1208–1209.
168. Wolff J: Iodide goiter and the pharmacologic effects of excess iodide. Am J Med 1969;47:101–124.
169. Wong LC, Heimbach MD, Truscott DR, Duncan BD: Boric acid poisoning: Report of 11 cases. Can Med Assoc J 1964; 90:1018–1023.

CHAPTER 84

Camphor and Moth Repellents

Lewis R. Goldfrank

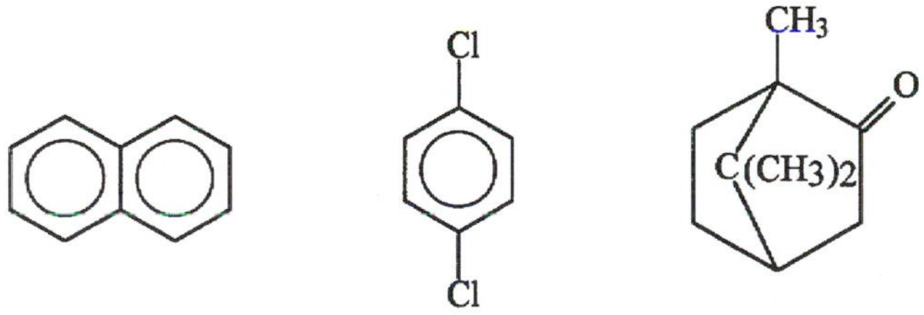

Naphthalene   Paradichlorobenzene   Camphor

A 64-year-old woman with Alzheimer's disease was brought to the Emergency Department (ED) after a day of ingesting a large number of mothballs that had been spread about her room to deodorize the smell of urine. Initial evaluation revealed a patient with no complaints, a blood pressure of 150/100 mm Hg, pulse of 90 beats/min, a respiratory rate of 16 breaths/min, and a temperature of 98.6°F (37°C). The remainder of the examination was unremarkable except for her profound dementia and a relative lack of personal hygiene.

The patient was given 60 g of activated charcoal and 50 g of sorbitol orally. Blood was drawn for initial laboratory tests, an intravenous (IV) line was established with D_5W and 0.45% sodium chloride solution at 100 mL/h, and the patient was admitted to the hospital. She subsequently passed numerous whole mothballs in her stool. The patient remained well and asymptomatic with normal laboratory data. On the third day of her hospitalization a lactate dehydrogenase level (LDH) was markedly elevated to 800 IU. On the fourth day she became weak and dizzy and was noted to have brisk hemolysis and a hemoglobin level of 6 g/dL requiring three transfusions over several days.

What Are Moth Repellents?

Today naphthalene and paradichlorobenzene are the sole ingredients in balls, flakes, and crystals used to repel moths (Table 84–1). "Moth repellents" are also placed on lawns and shrubs as deer, rodent (moles, voles), and rabbit repellents. Until the 1980s camphor was also commonly used as a moth repellent. Rapid identification of the type of mothball can sometimes be made based on the product's odor. Unfortunately, however, a confounding odor may be added by the manufacturer to mask the primary ingredients. It is extremely important to identify the type of moth repellent ingested, because unintentional acute ingestions of paradichlorobenzene are of little consequence, whereas ingestions of naphthalene may necessitate expeditious therapy. Fortunately, many man-

TABLE 84–1. MOTH REPELLENTS: DIFFERENTIAL CHARACTERISTICS

	Naphthalene	Paradichlorobenzene	Camphor
Toxicity	Substantial (≤ 1 mothball)	Minimal > 1 mothball	Substantial (≤ 1 mothball)
Special risk groups	Newborns (dermal) G-6-PD deficiency	None	None
Absorption	Oral, dermal, inhalation	Oral, inhalation	Oral, dermal, inhalation
Toxic metabolites	Alpha-naphthol	None	None
Clinical manifestations			
Acute	Hemolytic anemia (pallor) Hemoglobinuria (dark urine) Methemoglobinemia Fever Nausea, vomiting, diarrhea Abdominal pain Lethargy Seizures	Mucosal irritation Jaundice Methemoglobinemia(?) Hemolysis (?)	Burning of mouth Confusion, restlessness, Tremor, seizures Nausea, vomiting, ↑AST, ↑ALT Mydriasis, conjunctival injection
Chronic	Aplastic anemia Centrilobular hepatic necrosis Nausea, vomiting, ascites Jaundice	Hepatitis Pulmonary granulomatosis	Hepatotoxicity (transient) Encephalopathy
Diagnostic Evaluation	CBC Peripheral smear G-6-PD level Renal function studies Methemoglobin level	None	Observe for agitation, seizures
Treatment	Emesis, activated charcoal ? Catharsis; if hemolysis: transfusion, IV fluids, exchange transfusion	Usually none	Activated charcoal Cathartic Sedation

ufacturers have now recognized the limited toxicity of paradichlorobenzene and have substituted this chemical for the much more toxic naphthalene in mothballs and also toilet bowl, urinal, and diaper pail deodorizers.

What Laboratory Techniques Can Be Used to Differentiate Mothballs?

A rapid laboratory determination of the type of repellent ingested can be accomplished using any of the tests listed in Table 84–2. The two most practical and valuable laboratory and radiographic studies are cited below. The other tests have been cited in the table but are of limited practical value and are rarely if ever used. Rapid confirmation that paradichlorobenzene was the ingestant by an asymptomatic patient may obviate the need for therapeutic intervention, additional laboratory studies, or prolonged observation.

Test 1. Camphor mothballs float in water and in a saturated solution of table salt. Paradichlorobenzene mothballs sink in water and a saturated solution of table salt. Naphthalene mothballs sink in water but float in a saturated solution of table salt.[15] A saturated solution of table salt may be made by adding 3 tablespoons (45 g) of salt to 100 mL water and then stirring vigorously for 45 seconds to reach a concentration of about 20% by weight and a specific gravity of 1.15. Place the mothball in water. If it floats it is probably camphor. If it sinks in water add salt as described, and if the mothball still sinks it is paradichlorobenzene, whereas if it floats it is naphthalene.

Test 2. Paradichlorobenzene and naphthalene can be x-rayed in air and in water. Due to the presence of chlorine atoms in paradichlorobenzene these mothballs are densely radiopaque,[26] whereas naphthalene mothballs are only faintly radiopaque (Fig. 84–1).

What Are the Characteristic Clinical Manifestations of a Patient With a Paradichlorobenzene Ingestion?

Paradichlorobenzene is much less toxic acutely than camphor or naphthalene. Ingestion may cause nausea and vomiting. Hemolytic anemia has been rarely reported.[11] Hepatotoxicity manifested by hepatic necrosis following serious overdose or extended chronic exposure has also been rarely described.[5] Due to the limited toxicity, gastric emptying is considered only when large quantities are ingested. If there is any question as to

TABLE 84–2. MOTHBALLS: LABORATORY DIFFERENTIATION

	Naphthalene	Paradichlorobenzene	Camphor
Weight	3.6 g/mothball	5.0 g/mothball	No longer available
Appearance	Clear, white, dry crystalline balls	Clear white, wet, oily crystalline balls	Wet, oily crystalline
Specific gravity[8]	1.094–1.100	1.429–1.437	0.999
Radiography[28]	Faintly opaque	Densely opaque	—
Flotation in water[16]	Sinks	Sinks	Floats
Flotation in saturated solution table salt[16]	Floats	Sinks	Floats
Chloroform + aluminum chloride test[1]	Immediate blue color	No reaction	Not tested
Bunsen burner test: touch crystals to copper wire[1]	Initial flame yellow-orange	Initial yellow-orange, then bright green	Not tested
Differentiation by melting point by placing in 60°C water bath[20]	Solid until 80°C	Early liquefaction in 3 min at 53°C	Solid until 178°C
Solubility in turpentine	Poor (64–75%) Incomplete at 60 min	Excellent (98%) Complete at 60 min	Not tested
Solubility in water	None	None	None
Differential solubility in alcohols[31] (methanol, ethanol, isopropanol)	None	None	None
Odor (have reference mothballs available)	Pungent aromatic	Pungent aromatic	Pungent aromatic

whether the product may contain naphthalene, emesis or lavage should be performed immediately. Activated charcoal should be used in either case and may be an adequate therapeutic intervention. Fatty meals should be avoided, as they enhance absorption and the potential for toxicity.

What Are the Characteristic Clinical Manifestations of a Naphthalene Ingestion?

Naphthalene is readily absorbed and is toxic from oral,[4,8,17] inhalation,[27] and dermal exposure.[23] Organic solvents enhance absorption from any surface. Water does not adequately remove naphthalene from skin or fabrics. Therefore, soap and water should be used for decontamination. Naphthalene, a polycyclic aromatic hydrocarbon, is metabolized by the liver to numerous hydroxylated byproducts, including alpha-naphthol, beta-naphthol, a naphthoquinone, and beta-naphthoquinone.[8] Naphthalene itself does not induce hemolysis; only alpha-naphthol, its metabolite,[2,20] is capable of acting as a potent hemolytic agent in vivo. When hemolysis does occur as a result of exposure to naphthalene, the onset is usually delayed for several days as naphthalene must be converted to alpha-naphthol for hemolysis to occur.

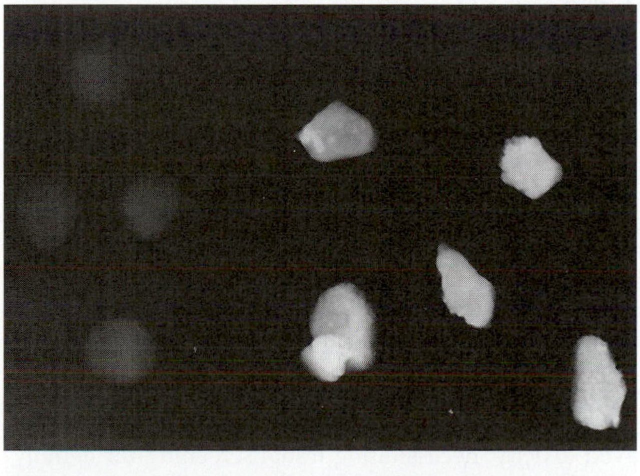

Figure 84–1. Radiograph of mothballs. Paradichlorobenzene (on the right) is densely radiopaque, whereas naphthalene (on the left) is faintly radiopaque.

The ingestion of less than one naphthalene mothball by a patient with G-6-PD deficiency can cause significant toxicity. In patients who are not G-6-PD deficient, small quantities of naphthalene are well tolerated.

The nonhemolytic clinical manifestations of naphthalene toxicity are fever, nausea, vomiting, abdominal pain, and diarrhea developing 24 to 48 hours after ingestion, although in some cases the delay before toxic effects occur may be more substantial. Lethargy and seizures may also result from exposure.

Signs of hemolysis include pallor from a rapid decrease in hemoglobin and hematocrit, weakness, dark urine, jaundice, and cyanosis. Other hematologic findings are an elevation in white blood count, fragmented RBCs, anisocytosis, Heinz bodies, and poikilocytosis; after several days, a brisk reticulocytosis and methemoglobinemia may also develop. The acute hemolytic reaction is much more severe in a patient with a G-6-PD deficiency. Hemolysis increases in proportion to the severity of G-6-PD deficiency, because G-6-PD assists in maintaining reduced glutathione levels, which limits oxidative stress (Chaps. 24 and 93). The metabolism of naphthalene to alpha-naphthol results in the depletion of glutathione. When oxidative stress increases, alpha-naphthol complexes with and precipitates hemoglobin, resulting in Heinz body formation.

This complexation of hemoglobin sulfhydryl groups results in hemolytic anemia. The inability of newborns to conjugate alpha-naphthol with reduced glutathione leads to hemolysis in the presence of normal G-6-PD levels.[27,29] Africans, African Americans (15 to 20%), and Mediterranean Jews (10%) have a high incidence of G-6-PD deficiency, with the former possessing 5 to 15% and the latter less than 1% of normal erythrocyte G-6-PD activity, which therefore places them at increased risk of toxicity. The youngest RBCs in circulation have normal G-6-PD levels, but levels decline as the RBCs age, increasing the risk of hemolysis. It is for this reason that a G-6-PD level determined after the onset of hemolysis may be misleadingly low.

What Is Camphor?

Camphor is an aromatic volatile terpene ketone ($C_{10}H_{16}O$) that is readily soluble in volatile oils and organic solvents. It is a colorless or white compound occurring as crystals, granules, or a translucent mass, with a pungent odor and taste. Camphor is derived from the wood of *Cinnamomum camphora* or synthesized from turpentine oil.

Camphor is available in numerous over-the-counter (OTC) forms of spirits or liniments and as a topical rubefacient and antipruritic agent.[6] Previously camphor was the major chemical constituent of mothballs, moth repellents, and moth flakes, but naphthalene and paradichlorobenzene have largely replaced camphor today. Even ingestions of less than 1 g of camphor represent a limited clinical risk.[24] Fatalities in children and adults have resulted from ingestion of 1 to 2 g of camphor-containing products.[10,12,25] When used as an illicit abortifacient, intrauterine instillation of camphor has produced significant maternal toxicity and fetal demise.[22]

Camphor is rapidly absorbed cutaneously, by inhalation, by insufflation, and orally. Toxic effects can occur within 10 to 20 minutes of ingestion and usually peak within 90 minutes. Hepatic metabolism of camphor rapidly ensues, with the glucuronidation of a metabolite campherol followed by urinary excretion of inactive compound. The rapid onset of toxicity suggests that camphor itself, as opposed to its alcohol metabolites (campherol, borneol or hydroxy-camphor), is responsible for toxicity.[16]

What Are the Effects of Camphor Poisoning?

Symptoms of camphor poisoning include nausea, vomiting, epigastric distress, and a sensation of warmth. The odor of camphor is recognizable easily and an important clue to the identity of an unknown ingestion. There may be evidence of CNS hyperactivity such as excitement, restlessness, vertigo, confusion, delirium, tremors, and seizures followed by CNS depression, characterized by apnea and coma (see Table 84–1). Chronic ingestions in children may mimic Reye's syndrome, with catastrophic hepatic and neurotoxic manifestations.[13] Most patients survive acute camphor ingestion with limited toxic effects if treatment with effective supportive and possibly sedative measures begins early enough.

What Is the Treatment for Camphor Poisoning?

As in most cases of poisoning, the general principle is to remove as much of the substance as soon as possible before it is absorbed, to adsorb and hasten the elimination of what remains in the GI tract, and to provide close monitoring and support of the patient. In addition, if a patient poisoned by camphor has overt manifestations of central nervous system hyperactivity—such as tremors, extreme agitation, or seizures—only an anticonvulsant with sedative-hypnotic characteristics such as a benzodiazepine should be considered. Both the seizures and the toxicity are limited, and therefore maintenance anticonvulsant therapy is not indicated.

Most patients who ingest camphor vomit shortly after ingestion; however, in the event that emesis has not occurred, syrup of ipecac should not be used because the danger of aspiration exists when the level of consciousness becomes impaired. Even in the home setting, the delay in the onset of action of syrup of ipecac outweighs its potential benefits.[3]

Gastric lavage and emesis have no role in the management as the symptoms usually begin to resolve prior to ED arrival. Although the adsorption of camphor is poorly defined, activated charcoal may decrease gastrointestinal absorption and has no inherent toxicity.[19,21] If a cathartic is given, sorbitol or a magnesium cathartic should be used and not an oil-based cathartic, which may enhance camphor absorption.[10] In the past, lipid hemodialysis with soybean or safflower oil had been used to adsorb camphor from the blood,[2,9,14] but this technique remains experimental and probably unnecessary.

What Is the Treatment for an Unknown Moth Repellent Ingestion?

The size of most mothballs exceeds that of any orogastric tube. Assuming that current mothballs are unlikely to contain camphor, syrup of ipecac can be used for the ingestion of small numbers of mothballs in the first 1 to 2 hours following ingestion. Activated charcoal and a cathartic or whole-bowel irrigation may be used to prevent further absorption. Fatty meals should be avoided, as they enhance absorption. Cutaneous exposure should be managed by removing contaminated clothing, washing exposed skin with soap and water, and ultimately discarding the contaminated clothing, which may act as a toxin reservior for reexposure.

Naphthalene ingestions may cause acute and delayed toxicity, necessitating initial screening for hemolysis with a hematocrit and blood smear. The very young and those with known or potential G-6-PD deficiency may require more prolonged observation. Patients who can be followed closely can be discharged, for if hemolysis occurs it may be delayed for days. On discharge, the patient or parent should be instructed with regard to the delayed manifestations of toxicity, particularly those associated with hemolysis (anemia, hemoglobinemia, jaundice, and weakness). Any question of cyanosis necessitates a methemoglobin level and potential treatment with methylene blue. The clinician should be prepared to treat massive hemolysis with IV fluids, RBC transfusions, and possibly exchange transfusion.

Acknowledgment

Eddy A. Bresnitz, MD, Richard S. Weisman, PharmD, and Theodore C. Bania, MD contributed to this chapter in previous editions.

References

1. Ambre J, Ruo TI, Smith-Coggins R: Mothball composition: Three simple tests for distinguishing paradichlorobenzene from naphthalene. Ann Emerg Med 1986;15:724–726.
2. Antman E, Jacob G, Volpe B, Finkel S: Camphor overdosage. NY State J Med 1978;78:895–896.
3. Aronow R, Spiegel RW: Implications of camphor poisoning. Drug Intel Clin Pharm 1976;10:631–634.
4. Chusid E, Fried CT: Acute hemolytic anemia due to naphthalene ingestion. Am J Dis Child 1955;87:612–614.
5. Cotter LH: Paradichlorobenzene poisoning from insecticides. NY State J Med 1953;53:1690–1692.
6. Dickinson WL: External analgesics. In: Griffenhagen GB, Hawkins CC, eds: Handbook of Nonprescription Drugs. Washington, DC, American Pharmaceutical Association, 1973, pp. 138–142.
7. Fukuda T, Koyama K, Yamashita M, et al: Differentiation of naphthalene and paradichlorobenzene mothballs based on their difference in specific gravity. Vet Hum Toxicol 1991; 33:313–314.
8. Gidron E, Leuren J: Naphthalene poisoning. Lancet 1956;1: 228–230.
9. Ginn HE, Anderson KE, Mercier RK, et al: Camphor intoxication treated by lipid dialysis. JAMA 1968;203:230–231.
10. Gosselin RE, Hodge HC, Smith RP: Clinical Toxicology of Commercial Products, 4th ed. Baltimore, Williams & Wilkins, 1976.
11. Hallowell M: Acute hemolytic anemia following the ingestion of paradichlorobenzene. Arch Dis Child 1959;34: 74–75.
12. Jacobziner H, Raybin HW: Camphorated oil, talcum powder, and lead poisonings. NY State J Med 1963;63: 3575–3577.
13. Jimenez JF, Brown AL, Arnold WC, Byrne WJ: Chronic camphor ingestion mimicking Reye's syndrome. Gastroenterology 1983;84:374–398.
14. Kopelman R, Miller S, Kelly R, Sunshine I: Camphor intoxication treated by resin hemoperfusion. JAMA 1979;241: 727–728.
15. Koyama K, Yamashita M: A simple test for mothball component differentiation using water and a saturated solution of table salt: Its utilization for poison information service. Vet Hum Toxicol 1991;33:425–427.
16. Kressel JJ: Camphor. Clin Toxicol Rev 1982;4:1.
17. Mackell JV, Rieders F, Brieger H, Bauer EL: Acute hemolytic anemia due to ingestion of naphthalene mothballs. I: Clinical aspects. Pediatrics 1951;7:722–725.
18. Phelan W: Camphor poisoning: Over-the-counter dangers. Pediatrics 1976;57:428–431.
19. Reeves RR, Pendarvis RO: Mothball melting points. Ann Emerg Med 1986;15:1377. Letter.
20. Reid F: Accidental camphor ingestion. JACEP 1979;8: 339–340. Letter.
21. Rieders F, Brieger H: Hemolytic action of naphthalene and its oxidation products. Pediatrics 1951;7:725–728 .
22. Riggs J, Hamilton R, Hormel S, et al: Camphorated oil intoxication in pregnancy. Obstet Gynecol 1965;25:255–258.
23. Schafer WB: Acute hemolytic anemia related to naphthalene: Report of a case in a newborn infant. Pediatrics 1951; 7:172–174.
24. Siegel E, Wason S: Camphor toxicity. Pediatr Clin North Am 1986;33:375–379.
25. Smith A, Margolis G: Camphor poisoning. Am J Pathol 1954;30:857–868.
26. Sue YJ, Saperstein A, Zawin J, et al: Radiopacity of paradichlorobenzene-containing products. Vet Hum Toxicol 1992;34:350. Abstract.
27. Valaes T, Psyros AD, Phaedron F: Acute hemolysis due to naphthalene inhalation. J Pediatr 1963;63:904–915.
28. Winkler JV, Kulig K, Rumack BH: Mothball differentiation: Naphthalene from paradichlorobenzene. Ann Emerg Med 1985;14:30–32.
29. Zinkham WH, Child B: A defect of glutathione metabolism in erythrocytes from patients with naphthalene induced hemolytic anemia. Pediatrics 1958;22:461–471.

CHAPTER 85

Hydrocarbons

Richard D. Shih

PATIENT 1. A 15-month-old male presented to the Emergency Department after being found with an empty bottle of furniture polish (99% mineral seal oil). The child had spilled much of the contents of the bottle on his clothing. His mother did not recall him coughing or having any difficulty breathing but stated that he vomited once.

On examination, the child had a "hydrocarbon" odor. The child interacted appropriately for his age. He did not appear ill and appeared normal to his mother. His vital signs were: heart rate, 110 beats/min; respiratory rate, 20 breaths/min; temperature, 99.5°F (37.5°C); and pulse oximetry, 99% saturation on room air. The skin, pulmonary, cardiac, and abdominal examination were unremarkable.

After 4 hours of observation in the Emergency Department, he remained asymptomatic. His CXR revealed a right lower lobe infiltrate.

PATIENT 2. A $2\frac{1}{2}$-year-old boy was exploring in the kitchen and found a familiar soda bottle with a clear liquid in it (a similar type of confusion is demonstrated in Color Plate 20). The bottle was sealed with aluminum foil. As he began to drink the liquid, he suddenly started to cough violently. His mother heard the sounds of distress and found him lying on the kitchen floor near the sink, appearing blue with respiratory difficulty. He was only mildly responsive to vocal stimuli.

The child vomited once on the way to the hospital. On arrival in the ED, he was cyanotic and in severe respiratory distress. Vital signs were: blood pressure, 110/60 mm Hg; pulse, 160 beats/min; respiratory rate, 40 breaths/min; and temperature, 99.6°F (37.9°C). Physical examination revealed the child to be responsive only to deep pain. Pulmonary examination revealed diffuse rhonchi and wheezes bilaterally, predominantly in the lower lung fields.

A 5.0-mm endotracheal tube was inserted and bag mask ventilatory assistance with 100% oxygen was given. Initial suctioning of the tube produced a frothy serosanginous fluid. Blood was drawn for a complete blood count, BUN, electrolytes, and an ABG. An intravenous line with 5% dextrose and 0.3% sodium chloride solution was begun at a maintenance rate.

The initial ABG (after 2 minutes on oxygen) revealed: pH, 7.34; PCO_2, 27 mm Hg; and PO_2, 70 mm Hg. The endotracheal tube was attached to a volume-cycled ventilator (intermittent mandatory ventilation) with 4 cm positive end-expiratory pressure (PEEP). Within 45 minutes the child's vital signs had normalized and the PO_2 was 86 mm Hg on an FIO_2 of 50%. A chest radiograph showed bilateral hazy densities in the left perihilar region and at both bases.

The product was later identified as Pine Sol, a pine-scented household cleaner with 20 to 35% pine oil.

PATIENT 3. A 15-year-old boy was inhaling from a rag that had been soaked in typewriter correction fluid while he was at school. When one of his teachers witnessed him performing this act, the boy turned and ran the opposite direction. Within several seconds, while running, he collapsed. The teacher found him unconscious and not breathing.

Upon paramedic arrival, he was awake and responding normally to questions. He recalled feeling his heart beating very rapidly and then waking up on the floor. On emergency department arrival his physical examination was entirely normal. His ECG revealed normal sinus rhythm at 90 beats/min with no abnormalities. Chest radiograph, electrolytes, and liver function tests were unremarkable.

What Are Hydrocarbons?

Hydrocarbon-containing products are essential and ubiquitous in our industrial society (Table 85–1). In 1859, the petroleum industry initiated drilling of the first commercial oil well and opening of the first refineries that processed crude oil into kerosene. Modern distillation techniques now refine millions of barrels of oil daily into a multitude of different products.

The nomenclature of hydrocarbons has caused confusion for several reasons. The term "hydrocarbons" has been used incorrectly to represent only compounds derived from petroleum distillation. A more appropriate and broader definition is one that includes all organic compounds made of predominantly carbon and hydrogen molecules. This expands the number of compounds to include products derived from other sources such as plants (pine oil, vegetable oil), animal fats (cod liver oil), and coal (coal-based kerosene). Although the majority of cases of hydrocarbon poisoning result from products of petroleum distillation, products derived from these other sources produce similar toxicity and will be discussed together in this chapter.

Hydrocarbons are organic compounds that contain from 1 to 60 carbon molecules. The physical properties of a given compound depend on the number and arrangement of these molecules. Compounds that contain from 1 to 4 carbon molecules are gaseous; 5 to 19, liquids; and 20 to 60, solids. Hydrocarbons are classified into four types, based on the arrangement of the carbon atoms: aliphatic (paraffins), aromatic, cycloparaffins (naphthenes), and alkenes (olefins).

Aliphatic compounds are saturated (contain no carbon–carbon double or triple bonds) molecules that have either straight or branched-chain arrangements. Examples include propane, isobutane, and hexane (Fig. 85–1).

Aromatic compounds contain at least one benzene ring. They are unsaturated compounds and may contain double-fused (naphthalenes) or multifused aromatic rings (polynuclear compounds). Examples include benzene, toluene, and naphthalene, as shown in Figure 85–1.

Cycloparaffins are saturated hydrogen compounds that are arranged in closed rings. The most common compounds have five and six carbon rings.

Alkene compounds contain one carbon–carbon double bond in the molecule. Molecules containing two and three double bonds are known as dienes (diolefins) and trienes (triolefins) respectively. These compounds are not typically found in natural crude oil but are formed by catalytic and thermal processing techniques. They are more reactive than their saturated counterparts, and are useful for manufacturing other hydrocarbon products such as the halogenated hydrocarbons.

Another issue that further complicates nomenclature is the imprecise nature of the specific hydrocarbon compounds found in different products. Some hydrocarbon-containing products are specific compounds that are highly separated and contain almost 100% of one specific compound (eg, toluene, benzene, n-hexane). Most household products, however, are complex mixtures of different compounds (> 100) that are grouped together by processing techniques because of similar physical properties (boiling point, number of carbon molecules). These properties are typically the basis for their separation and processing by methods of distillation.

The general process of petroleum distillation begins with crude oil that is heated in large columns. As the oil is heated, the hydrocarbons are volatilized and separated on the basis of their boiling point, in different condensors (Table 85–2). The subsequent product contains complex mixtures of different hydrocarbons with varying percentages of aliphatic hydrocarbons, aromatic hydrocarbons, and cycloparaffins. Gasoline contains over 100 different individual hydrocarbon compounds, each with 4 to 10 carbon molecules. Aliphatic hydrocarbons, aromatic hydrocarbons, cycloparaffins, and unsaturated hydrocarbons can be found in proportions of 53, 36, 5, and 6%, respectively, with less than 1% unknown substances.[112,138] The relative amounts of the different hydrocarbons found in these mixtures (eg, kerosene, gasoline, mineral seal oil, naphtha) varies from one region to another. This is due, to a lesser degree, to differences in distillation techniques, and more importantly to the region of origin of the crude oil.

TABLE 85–1. HOUSEHOLD PRODUCTS CONTAINING HYDROCARBONS

Adhesives (glues)	Mothballs
Baby oil	Motor oils
Car waxes	Naphtha
Cod liver oil	Paint removers
Contact cement	Paint thinners
Furniture polishes	Paraffin
Furniture refinishers	Paste waxes
Gasoline	Petroleum jelly
Home heating fuel	Pine oils
Kerosene	Plastic cement
Kitchen waxes	Solvents
Lacquers	Stain removers
Laxatives	Sterno fuel
Lighter fluids	Stoddard solvent
Liquid solder	Turpentine
Liquid steel	Typewriter correction fluids
Mineral oil	Varnish removers
Mineral seal oil	Wax
Mineral spirits	

Which Patients Are At Risk for Hydrocarbon Poisoning?

The American Association of Poison Control Centers (AAPCC) reports an annual incidence of about 60,000 hydrocarbon exposures. Ninety-five percent of the cases

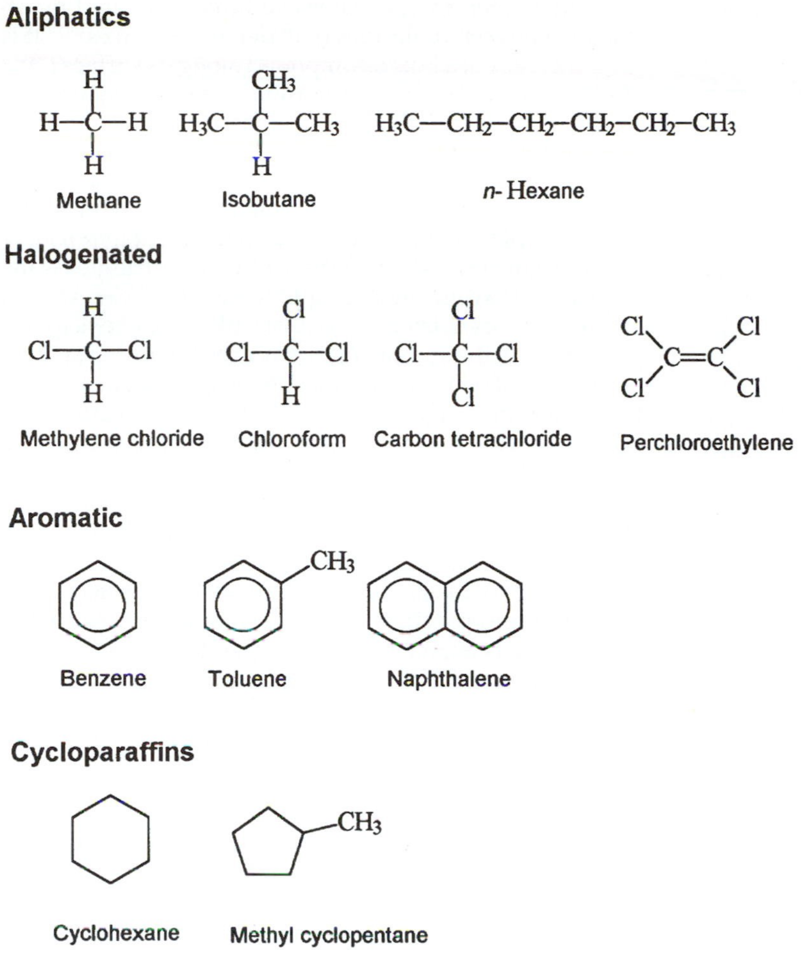

Figure 85–1. Chemical structures of hydrocarbons of each representative class.

are unintentional. Approximately 20% are treated at a healthcare facility, with about 50% of these demonstrating minimal toxic effects. Approximately 20 deaths are attributed to hydrocarbon poisoning annually. One third of these cases involved gasoline; Freon/propellants, mineral spirits/varsol, lubricating/motor oils, lighter fluid/naphtha, and kerosene accounted for 11, 9, 7, 7, and 5%, respectively.[103–107]

About 60% of these exposures involve children.[103–107] In one study, hydrocarbons accounted for 18% of all pediatric admissions for poisoning.[44] Ninety percent of hydrocarbon-related deaths involved children less than 5 years old.[134]

What Organ Systems Are Affected by the Acute Ingestion of a Hydrocarbon?

The pulmonary system is predominantly affected by acute hydrocarbon ingestion. The central nervous, gastrointestinal, cardiac, and dermatologic systems are also

TABLE 85–2. COMMON PETROLEUM DISTILLATION FRACTIONS AND PHYSICAL PROPERTIES

Distillate Fraction	Boiling Point (°C)	Carbon Atoms per Molecule	Volatility	Viscosity
Gases	< 30	1–4	H	L
Gasoline	30–210	4–10	H	L
Naphtha	100–200	8–12	H	L
Kerosene	200–300	5–15	L	L
Mineral seal	300–500	13–17	L	L
Heavy fuel oil	315–540	20–45	L	H

H = high; L =low; high viscosity is greater than 100 Saybolt seconds universal (SSU); low viscosity is less than 60 SSU.

commonly affected, with rare reports of hematologic, hepatic, and renal effects.

How Do Hydrocarbons Cause Pulmonary Toxicity?

Since the first reported cases of hydrocarbon toxicity in the late 1800s, a long and heated debate occurred regarding the pathogenesis of pulmonary injury.[75,85] Early clinical and laboratory investigators debated whether the pulmonary toxicity was due to gastrointestinal absorption of hydrocarbons and subsequent pulmonary secretion, or due to direct aspiration into pulmonary parenchyma.[22,45,51,63,81,82,99,137,141,177]

In studies of rats and baboons utilizing radiolabeled toluene and hexadecane, it is clear that hydrocarbons are absorbed by the gastrointestinal tract and can be recovered from many tissues including the lungs.[9,109] Based on the amounts absorbed in these animal studies, however, the amount of hydrocarbon that would be needed to cause pulmonary toxicity would be huge.

In addition, a number of different animal models (dogs, monkeys, and baboons) utilizing transected and ligated esophagi with gastric instillation of hydrocarbon, demonstrated the lack of pulmonary toxicity when aspiration did not occur.[48,82,183,189] It is currently believed that aspiration is the main route of injury from these toxins.

The mechanism of pulmonary injury caused by these agents, however, is not completely understood. Intratracheal instillation of small amounts (0.2 mL/kg) of kerosene causes physiologic abnormalities in lung mechanics (decreased compliance and total lung capacity) and pathologic changes such as interstitial inflammation, polymorphonuclear exudation, intra-alveolar hemorrhage and edema, hyperemic blood vessels, bronchial and bronchiolar necrosis, and vascular thrombosis.[63,65,71,76,144,145] The cause for these changes is most likely a combination of direct toxicity to pulmonary tissue and the disruption of the lipid surfactant layer.[67,149,182]

What Factors Influence the Risk for Aspiration After Hydrocarbon Ingestion?

Several factors are associated with pulmonary toxicity after hydrocarbon ingestion. These factors include specific physical properties of the hydrocarbon ingested and historical information involving the amount of toxin ingested and the occurrence of vomiting.

The properties of viscosity, surface tension, and volatility of a particular hydrocarbon are the main determinants of its aspiration potential (see Table 85–2).[64,82] Viscosity is the tendency of a substance to resist flow ("the ability to resist stirring"). One form of measuring viscosity is by the rate of flow through a calibrated orifice measured in Saybolt seconds universal (SSU). Substances with lower viscosities (SSU < 60; turpentine, gasoline, naphtha) are associated with a higher tendency for aspiration in animal models.

Surface tension is a cohesive force generated by attraction between molecules (van der Waals forces).[129] It is the adherence of a liquid compound along its surface ("the ability to creep"). Surface tension is measured using a modified Wilhelmy balance.[82] In theory, the lower the surface tension, the higher the aspiration risk.[64,82]

Volatility is the tendency for a liquid to become a gas. Hydrocarbons with high volatility will tend to vaporize, displace oxygen, and lead to transient hypoxia.

It is not clear which of these physical attributes is the most important in predicting toxicity. However, several studies have evaluated the risk of pulmonary toxicity associated with the amount of hydrocarbon ingested and the occurrence of one or more episodes of spontaneous vomiting. Some investigators have found an association between the volume ingested and the risk for pulmonary toxicity, while others have not.[17,20,42] Similar findings have been reported with vomiting.[17,20,30,124,126] Further, these studies have been questioned because of their retrospective methodology and exceedingly poor response rates with regard to the amount of hydrocarbon ingested.

Only one prospectively collected study addressing these issues is available, the Co-Operative Kerosene Poisoning Study (COKP). Forty-six hospitals participated in this study with 760 cases. Of these, 54% had the amount ingested estimated. Twenty-nine percent of patients were reported to have ingested more than 30 mL; 35%, 10 to 30 mL; and 35%, less than 10 mL. No association was found between amount ingested and the age of the patient. In patients who ingested more than 30 mL, there was a 52% chance of developing pulmonary complications.[134] Those patients who ingested this amount were found to have a higher chance of developing central nervous system complications than those who ingested less than 30 mL.

With regard to spontaneous vomiting and pulmonary complications, the cooperative study was only able to provide data on 273 of the 760 patients. They found a 54% incidence of pulmonary toxicity with vomiting and 39% when no history of vomiting was elicited.[134]

Although these factors may be useful for predicting the possibility of hydrocarbon-induced pulmonary toxicity, none of these parameters are 100% predictive. Serious poisoning is less likely with agents that have higher viscosity and higher surface tension, such as mineral oil. However, severe hydrocarbon pneumonitis has been associated with "low-risk" hydrocarbons as well.[143] Furthermore, patients have been severely injured with low-volume (< 5 mL) ingestions as well as ingestions without a history of coughing, gagging, and vomiting.[5]

What Are the Clinical Signs and Symptoms of Acute Hydrocarbon Poisoning?

Pulmonary

Many patients who develop pulmonary toxicity will have an episode of coughing, gagging, and choking. This occurs shortly after ingestion, usually within 30 minutes, and is presumptive evidence of pulmonary aspiration.[110]

More severely affected patients may rapidly develop progressive pulmonary toxicity over the next hours to days. This is manifested as rales, rhonchi, bronchospasm, tachypnea, hypoxia, hemoptysis, pulmonary edema (hemorrhagic or nonhemorrhagic), and signs of respiratory distress.[166] Cyanosis develops in approximately 2 to 3% of patients.[115] This may be due to simple asphyxiant effects from volatilized hydrocarbon, ventilation–perfusion mismatch, or rarely due to methemoglobinemia (aniline, nitrobenzene, nitrite-containing hydrocarbons). Clinical findings often worsen over several days but typically resolve in 5 to 7 days. Deaths are rare (< 2%) and are typically due to severe progressive respiratory insult marked by hypoxia, ventilation–perfusion mismatch, and barotrauma.[15,55,78,114,151,176,193]

Radiographic evidence of pneumonitis develops in 40 to 88% of admitted patients.[13,17,20,51,99,126,137] Findings can develop as early as 15 minutes or as late as 24 hours after exposure (Fig. 85–2).[42,59,76,89,134,173] Ninety percent of patients who develop radiographic abnormalities will develop evidence by 4 hours postingestion.[42] The majority of patients who have respiratory signs and symptoms beyond the initial history of gagging, choking, and coughing will develop radiographic pneumonitis.[5] Clinical signs of pneumonia (rales, rhonchi, etc) are evident in 40 to 50% of patients.[51] A small percentage (< 5%) will be completely asymptomatic after a period of observation but have radiographic findings.[5]

The radiologic findings include perihilar densities, bronchovascular markings, bibasilar infiltrates, and pneumonic consolidation.[13,66] Right-sided involvement occurs in 75% of the cases and bilateral involvement in approximately 50%; upper lobe involvement is uncommon.[13,26,77] Pleural effusions develop in 3% of cases,[112] with one third appearing within 24 hours. Pneumothorax, pneumomediastinum, and pneumatoceles are not commonly reported.[12,18,31,50,97,147,184] Early upright radiographs may reveal two liquid densities in the stomach, known as the "double-bubble" sign.[41] This represents an air–hydrocarbon and a hydrocarbon–fluid interface as the hydrocarbon is not miscible with water and may have a specific gravity less than water.

Radiographic changes often progress over several days, typically reaching a maximum at 5 to 7 days with resolution over several weeks. Radiographic resolution does not correlate with clinical improvement, usually lagging behind by several days to weeks.[63]

Long-term follow-up in patients with hydrocarbon pneumonitis is limited.[26,59,72,137,164,169] Frequent respiratory tract infections are described in individuals after hydrocarbon pneumonitis, but these studies are poorly controlled.[59,139,166] Bronchiectasis and pulmonary fibrosis are reported, but appear to be uncommon.[69,113,137] In one study, 82% of patients seen 8 to 14 years after hydrocarbon-induced pneumonitis had asymptomatic minor pulmonary function abnormalities.[72] The abnormalities were consistent with small-airway obstruction and loss of elastic recoil. The authors hypothesized that this group may be predisposed to chronic obstructive pulmonary disease.

Central Nervous System

Ingestions of hydrocarbons are commonly associated with CNS manifestations. Coma and seizures are reported in 1 to 3% of cases.[99,126,128,137,192] The etiology of the CNS effects are unclear. Based on animal studies, it is doubtful that gastrointestinal absorption of hydrocarbons plays a role, as substantial amounts would need to be absorbed to cause CNS manifestations.[9,11] Most likely, a combination of pulmonary absorption of volatilized hydrocarbon and hypoxia from severe pulmonary effects accounts for these findings.[109,186]

Gastrointestinal

Hydrocarbons are irritants to the gastrointestinal mucous membranes. Nausea and vomiting are common. As discussed earlier, vomiting is variably associated with an increased risk of pulmonary toxicity.[20,124,126,143] Hematemesis can occur, and was reported in 5% of cases in one study.[124] Gastrointestinal ulcerations may occur and have been found in animal studies.[9,90]

Cardiac

Dysrhythmias, pneumopericardium, cardiomegaly, and myocardial infarction can occur after hydrocarbon ingestion, but are uncommon.[87,97,156] The most worrisome of these manifestations is the possibility of myocardial sensitization and dysrhythmias.[14,140] This phenomenon is well described with halogenated hydrocarbons and less so for aromatic compounds. Reports of sudden death due to this mechanism are quite common when patients are exposed to high concentrations secondary to substance abuse of volatile hydrocarbons or inhalational anesthetics. Although dysrhythmias are uncommon after hydrocarbon ingestions, this is a potential concern.

Dermatologic

Hydrocarbons are irritating to the skin. Acute prolonged exposure can cause dermatitis and severe full-thickness burns.[74] Hydrocarbons are toxic to the lipid components of the stratum corneum layer of the epithelium ("defatting effect"). Chronic exposure to kerosene can cause severe acne.[169] A disulfiram-like reaction, "degreaser's flush," is associated with concomitant ethanol and trichloroethylene exposure.

Other Organ Systems

Hemolysis has been sporadically reported to occur with hydrocarbon ingestion.[2,4,159] One retrospective study of 12 patients showed hemolysis in three individuals and disseminated intravascular coagulation in another.[4] Although one of these patients required transfusion, the hemolysis is usually mild and does not require RBC administration.

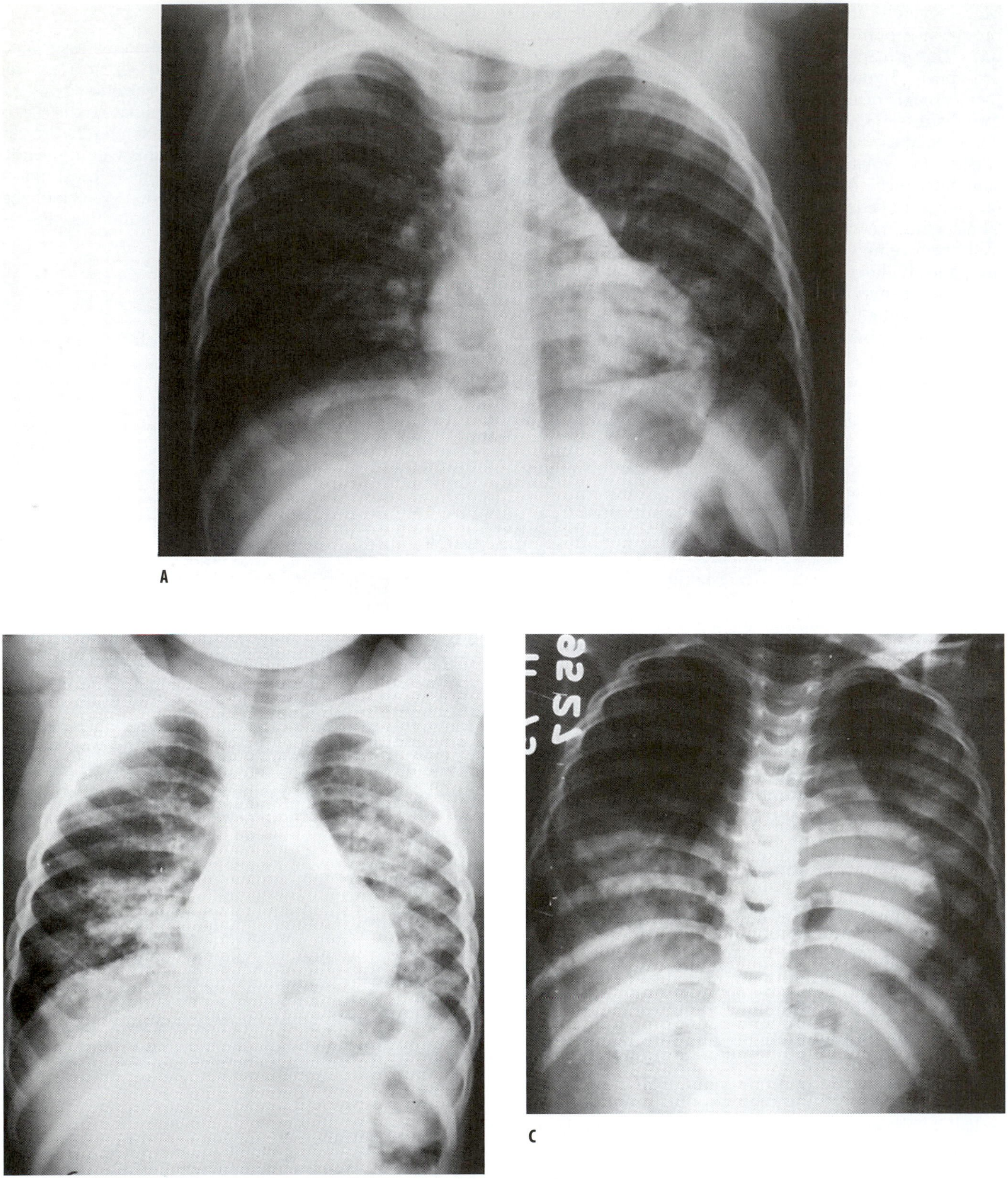

Figure 85–2. Three sequential radiographs of a young girl with severe hydrocarbon aspiration pneumonitis. **A.** Initial: Patchy densities appear in basilar areas of both lung fields with increased interstitial markings and peribronchial thickening. **B.** Day 2: More extensive diffuse alveolar infiltrates are apparent. **C.** Day 6: Dense consolidation and atelectasis are evident in the right lower lobe. *(Courtesy of Nancy Genieser, MD, Professor of Radiology, New York University.)*

Should Gastric Emptying Be Employed?

Gastric emptying in the management of hydrocarbon ingestions remains controversial and has been rigorously debated for decades.[14,45,118,119,125,187,189] Initial arguments centered around whether gastrointestinal absorption and subsequent lung secretion were the major route by which hydrocarbon induced pulmonary toxicity occurred. Many clinical studies have addressed the issue of gastric lavage or ipecac-induced vomiting to prevent pulmonary toxicity.[5,17,30,42,122–124,126,134] Equivocal results are reported. The majority of studies were retrospective and nonrandomized. Because it is more likely that sicker patients had gastric emptying performed, this methodology is inherently biased against the ability to show a benefit from gastric emptying. Furthermore, spontaneous vomiting was frequently included in the gastric emptying group.[42] Unfortunately, these studies are further biased as vomiting is an independent variable associated with an increased risk of pneumonitis.[42,134]

Two studies utilized prospective randomized protocols employing gastric lavage. However, one of these studies, the COKP trial, was only able to randomize patients at 7 of 46 hospitals. Neither of the studies had uniform criteria for the performance of gastric lavage. In the subset of randomized patients from COKP, 44% of the lavaged versus 47% of the nonlavaged patients had pulmonary complications. The other study reported pulmonary complications in 47 versus 61% in the lavaged versus nonlavaged patients.

The presently available studies do not offer a definitive answer as to the utility of gastric emptying in this setting, although many authors have opinions favoring a specific method.[6,7,63,102,118,119,178,180] Gastric emptying is only indicated in rare situations, and a rational approach for utilization is offered.

Patients who have no symptoms at home and at initial medical evaluation do not need gastric emptying. Two studies suggest that these patients do not develop subsequent toxicity.[5,108] For patients requiring gastric emptying, it is not clear whether gastric lavage or syrup of ipecac-induced emesis is the superior method.[122,123,134] If induced emesis is chosen, the patient must be awake, alert, and able to protect his or her own airway. Other toxic co-ingestions that may suddenly affect mental status or airway protection represent contraindications for use of this procedure. If gastric lavage is utilized, a small nasogastic tube (18 F, not a large-bore tube) should be employed. If there is no gag reflex, an endotracheal tube (preferably cuffed) should be placed prior to lavage. There are no studies evaluating the safety and efficacy of paralysis and intubation to facilitate the performance of this procedure in a patient who is awake and has normal airway protective mechanisms.[19]

When there are no contraindications, gastric emptying may be potentially useful in several circumstances. The first is when the hydrocarbon has inherent toxicity, has been used to solubilize a toxin, or has been ingested with a toxin. The second is when a large volume of hydrocarbon is ingested (> 30 mL). Intentional ingestions frequently are characterized by large ingestions (Table 85–3).

TABLE 85–3. GASTRIC EMPTYING FOR HYDROCARBON INGESTION

Contraindications

- Occurrence of spontaneous vomiting
- Asymptomatic initially and at initial medical evaluation

Potential Benefits from Gastric Emptying

- Large volume of hydrocarbon ingested: (> 30 mL)
- Intentional ingestions
- A hydrocarbon with inherent systemic toxicity (CHAMP)
    - C: camphor
    - H: halogenated hydrocarbons
    - A: aromatic hydrocarbons
    - M: hydrocarbons associated with metals
    - P: hydrocarbons associated with pesticides

Which Patients Need to Be Admitted?

In the older literature, routine admission was frequently recommended for patients who had ingested hydrocarbons, due to concern for possible delayed symptom onset and progression of toxicity.[30,42,70] Several reports documented patients with relatively asymptomatic presentations who rapidly decompensated with respiratory compromise.[5,70,108] However, progressive symptoms after hydrocarbon ingestion are very rare.[5,108] In a study of 950 patients, only 14 (1.5%) had progression of pulmonary toxicity.[5] Seven of these patients had persistence of their symptoms for only 24 hours.

In this study, a large retrospective cohort of 950 patients was evaluated to determine which patients could be treated safely as outpatients. Eight hundred patients were asymptomatic on initial evaluation with normal chest radiographs, remained asymptomatic after 6 to 8 hours of observation, and had a normal repeat radiograph. No patients in this group had progressive symptoms and all were discharged without clinical manifestations. Seventy-one of the 950 patients had initial respiratory symptoms but were asymptomatic at initial medical evaluation. Of the 71 patients, 36 had radiographic evidence of pneumonitis. Among these 36 patients, 2 (6%) developed progression of pulmonary symptoms during their 6-hour observation period. Of the 35 who had a normal radiograph, 2 (6%) developed pulmonary symptoms and radiographic pneumonitis during their 6-hour observation period. The 4 patients with progression of symptoms who were hospitalized, became asymptomatic over the next 24 hours, and had no complications.

A poison center-based study that also evaluated 120 asymptomatic patients for an 18-hour telephone follow-up period, found that no individual developed progressive symptoms.[108] Sixty-two patients had initial pulmonary symptoms that quickly resolved. One of these patients (1.6%) developed progressive pulmonary toxicity. This patient was hospitalized and had resolution of symptoms within 24 hours without complications.

It is clear that the vast majority of patients exposed to a hydrocarbon will not need to be hospitalized.[5,103–108] A number of investigators have suggested protocols for determining which patients can be safely discharged.[5,7,90,102,108] None of these protocols have been prospectively validated. However, rational guidelines for hospitalization can be recommended.

Those patients who have clinical evidence of toxicity, and most individuals with intentional ingestions, should be hospitalized. Patients who do not have any initial symptoms, have normal chest radiographs at 6 hours after ingestion, and do not develop symptoms during a 6-hour observation period can be safely discharged. Care should be individualized for patients who are asymptomatic with radiographic evidence of hydrocarbon pneumonitis, and for patients who have initial respiratory symptoms but quickly become asymptomatic during medical evaluation. Reliable patients may be considered for possible discharge with next day follow-up.

Should Prophylactic Antibiotics Be Administered?

Antibiotics are frequently administered in the setting of hydrocarbon pneumonitis to treat possible bacterial superinfection.[42,82,84,124,134,150,173] In experimental models this occurs as rapidly as 7 hours after aspiration.[82] Using radiolabelled *Staphylococcus aureus*, hydrocarbon-injured lungs were shown by 4 hours after insult to have a decreased ability to clear bacteria.[28]

Several investigators utilizing guinea pigs, dogs, and baboons demonstrated that antibiotics are not useful in the laboratory setting.[25,155,185] One of these studies also showed that bacterial flora were altered by antibiotic administration as the lung cultures in these treated animals demonstrated predominantly gram-negative organisms as compared to gram-positive infections in the control animals.[25]

These studies led to a decreased utilization of prophylactic antibiotics, and clinical assessment of infection became the indication for antibiotic use for most clinicians.[51] This approach, however, is not without its limitations. Abnormal lung auscultation, fever, leukocytosis, and abnormal radiographic findings are the initial manifestaions of bacterial pneumonia and hydrocarbon pneumonitis. Abnormal temperatures are reported to occur in 50 to 90% of patients with hydrocarbon toxicity.[17,30,42,63,99,124,126] An elevated temperature is often initially noted, and the temperature reaches a maximum at 8 to 12 hours and then subsides over several days.[42,126] A leukocytosis is also frequently reported. Fifty to 60% of patients will have an elevated white blood cell count (WBC).[99,124,126,137]

Ideally, pulmonary cultures should be used to guide antibiotic administration. This, however, is often delayed and not useful in critically ill patients. Antibiotic usage may be justified in severly poisoned patients. Some practitioners continue to utilize prophylactic antibiotics in all cases. Others recommend close observation of temperature and WBC curves; delayed elevation (24 hours after presentation) of temperature and/or WBC may signal bacterial superinfection. No human studies are available to support either approach and this issue remains controversial.

Should Prophylactic Corticosteroids Be Offered?

Corticosteroids, like antibiotics, have been prophylactically administered in the setting of hydrocarbon pulmonary toxicity.[32,69,85,88,113,117,134,172] The rationale for their use is the prevention and limitation of the inflammatory response in the lungs after hydrocarbon injury.

Animal experiments do not show benefits with corticosteroid administration.[3,25,155,188] In fact, one study showed that corticosteroid administration increased the risk for bacterial superinfection with or without coadministration of antibiotics.[98] Furthermore, two controlled human trials failed to show a benefit from corticosteroid administration.[75,111]

It is clear that corticosteroid use does not improve the acute course of hydrocarbon pulmonary toxicity. None of the experimental or human studies, however, addressed long-term effects such as pulmonary fibrosis, chronic obstructive pulmonary disease, or bronchiectasis. The incidence of long-term effects is poorly studied, but they appear to be relatively uncommon. Coupled with the possible increased risk of bacterial superinfection, corticosteroid administration in this setting cannot be advocated.

What Are Important Management Concerns in Severely Poisoned Patients?

Patients who have severe manifestations of hydrocarbon toxicity pose some unique problems that may need to be considered. Respiratory distress requiring mechanical ventilation in this setting may be associated with large ventilation–perfusion mismatch. The use of positive end-expiratory pressure (PEEP) is often beneficial.[143,193] However, very high levels of PEEP may be required with subsequent increased risk of barotrauma.[29,143] High-frequency jet ventilation (HFJV), utilizing very high respiratory rates (220 to 260) with small tidal volumes, has been useful to decrease the need for PEEP.[29,143] One patient who continued to have severe ventilation–perfusion mismatch despite PEEP and then HFJV was successfully treated with extracorporeal membrane oxygenation (ECMO).[143] ECMO appears to be a useful option in severe pulmonary toxicity after other treatments have failed.

Patients who are hypotensive have several additional considerations. The etiology for hypotension in this setting is often compromise of cardiac output due to high levels of PEEP. Hydrocarbons do not have significant direct cardiovascular effects, and decreasing the PEEP may correct this problem. The use of catecholamines (dopamine, epinephrine, isoproterenol, norepinephrine, etc) should be avoided if possible, as hydrocarbons sensitize the myocardium and predispose to dysrhythmias.[15,58,139,140]

Cyanosis is uncommon after hydrocarbon toxicity. Although this manifestation is most often due to severe hypoxia, methemoglobinemia associated with hydrocarbon exposure is reported.[40,94] The potential for methemoglobinemia should be investigated in patients who remain cyanotic following oxygen administration.

Methylene chloride is metabolized to carbon monoxide; a finding that is otherwise infrequently associated with hydrocarbon ingestion (Table 85–4).[49,136,157,158]

Significant cutaneous toxicity and hydrocarbon absorption can occur.[164] All exposed clothing should be removed, and exposed skin areas should be irrigated with copious amounts of water and then washed with soap. Medical personnel need to be protected from exposure with adequate gloves and aprons (see Chap. 92).

What Are Other Therapies for Severe Hydrocarbon Poisoning?

Activated Charcoal

Activated charcoal has limited ability to decrease gastrointestinal absorption of hydrocarbons.[93,120] As discussed earlier, absorption of hydrocarbons plays only a small role in hydrocarbon toxicity. Furthermore, activated charcoal administration may distend the stomach and predispose patients to vomiting and aspiration.[179] Its usage may be justified in patients with mixed overdoses, but its role in isolated hydrocarbon ingestions is limited.

Additives (Olive Oil and Mineral Oil)

Giving olive oil or mineral oil with hydrocarbon ingestion was suggested in the past.[6,9,17,21,59,120,192] These hydrocarbon oils have very high viscosities and low aspiration potential. Theoretically, adding these oils to ingested hydrocarbon will raise the viscosity of the resultant combi-

TABLE 85–4. CHLORINATED HYDROCARBONS

	Methylene Chloride (CH_2Cl_2)	Carbon Tetrachloride (CCl_4)	Trichloroethylene ($Cl_2C=CHCl$)	Tetrachloroethylene ($Cl_2C=CCl_2$)
Uses	Solvent, paint stripper, degreaser, fumigant, refrigerant	Solvent, propellant, refrigerant	Degreasant, typewriter correction fluid, paint/spot remover	Dry cleaning, engine cleaning, plastics, chemical industry
Exposure				
Inhalation	++	++	++	++
Cutaneous	+	+	+	+
Ingestion	++	++	++	++
OSHA permissible exposure limit (ppm)[a]	500	10	50	25
Toxicity				
Acute				
CNS	++	++	++	+
Respiratory	+	+	+	+
CVS	++	−	+	−
Dermal	+	+	+	+
Ocular	+	−	+	+
GI/hepatic	+	++	+	−
Renal	−	+	+	−
Metabolic	−	−	−	−
Hematologic	+	±	−	−
Chronic	Neoplasms (animal), cardiovascular, hepatic	Neoplasms (animal), hepatic (human liver?), leukemia	Neoplasms (animal), CNS	Neoplasm (animal), liver/kidney
Elimination				
Exhalation	+	50–80%	+ (small)	80%
Metabolism	CO, CO_2, HCOH	CO_2	Trichloroacetic acid (10–30%), chloral hydrate, trichloroethanol (30–50%)	< 2% trichloroacetic acid, trichloroethanol

++ = significant; + = present; ± = equivocal; − = absent.
[a]Highest level averaged over 8-hour work shift.

nation and thus decrease aspiration risk. Animal studies failed to prove any benefit,[21,120] and these additives can rarely cause hydrocarbon pneumonitis and lipoid pneumonia themselves.[16,23,46,61,68,82,96,132,133,143,148,165] The addition of these agents may distend the stomach and increase the risk of vomiting and aspiration. No role for olive oil or mineral oil administration in hydrocarbon ingestions can be recommended.

Cathartics

The use of cathartics for hydrocarbon ingestions has not been studied well in the laboratory or in clincal trials. Because hydrocarbon absorption plays little role in toxicity, their theoretical use cannot be justified.

A single study showed that baboons administered metoclopramide had less hydrocarbon in their stomach 2 hours after gastric instillation compared to controls. The authors suggest that the promotility effect coupled with the antiemetic effect may decrease aspiration risk when administered in this setting.[185] Further study is needed to delineate the role of this agent in acute hydrocarbon ingestions.

Surfactant

As discussed, the toxic mechanism for hydrocarbon-induced pulmonary damage may in part be due to detrimental effects on surfactant.[67] Several commercial surfactant preparations are available and are useful for other disease conditions associated with inadequate surfactant function. One animal model did not show benefit, while another showed increased survival and improved pulmonary function with administration.[149,182] No studies are currently available to assess the clinical effectiveness in human toxicity, and further study is warranted.

Hyperbaric Oxygen

The use of hyperbaric oxygen (HBO) was studied in a rat model of severe kerosene-induced pneumonitis.[146] The use of high-pressure HBO (4 ATA) showed some benefit in 24-hour survival rates. No follow-up studies have been performed. The use of HBO can reverse hypoxia for short periods of time in severely toxic patients serving as a temporizing agent to allow tissue recovery. The use of HBO for prolonged periods is associated with oxygen toxicity. HBO is unlikely to be useful for severe hydrocarbon toxicity because pulmonary recovery occurs slowly over several days to weeks. Hydrocarbon poisonings associated with carbon tetrachloride and methylene chloride, however, may include a role for hyperbaric oxygen (see Chap. 96). [27,157,158,167]

What Are the Volatile Substances of Abuse? How Are Inhaled Hydrocarbons Abused?

Aromatic and short-chained hydrocarbons are volatile at room temperature and, upon inhalation, have a rapid onset of intoxicating effects. These products are inexpensive, accessible, and legal. The reported incidence of abuse was 13% in a group of teenagers in Great Britain, and 24% in adolescents from a socioeconomically deprived area of Brazil.[33,62] The epidemiology of these agents is not well studied in the United States, with the full extent of abuse most likely underreported.[56,154,190]

Users are typically adolescents with poor family structure and poor socioeconomic backgrounds. Abuse is often a group activity, often to enhance sexual pleasure. Other groups with high incidence of abuse include native Americans and chemical workers with easy access to industrial solvents.[101,130]

The hydrocarbon is typically poured into a container for "sniffing"; a rag or sock for "huffing"; or a plastic/paper bag for "bagging." The concentration of the inhaled hydrocarbon increases from "sniffing," to "huffing," to "bagging." Consequently, abusers often begin with "sniffing" lower concentrations and progress to "huffing" and "bagging" with higher levels of exposure.[101]

The volatilized hydrocarbon used is well absorbed through the lungs and rapidly distributed to the CNS. One or two huffs will begin to intoxicate the user in several seconds and lasts several hours. Chronic users can maintain a prolonged high with periodic inhalations every few hours. Some chronic abusers have maintained intoxication thoughout their waking hours during years of use.

A vast array of hydrocarbons have been utilized (Table 85–5). However, the most commonly abused substances include toluene from paints and adhesives; gasoline; butane from cigarette lighter fluids; butyl and isobutyl nitrite; and halogenated hydrocarbons from typewriter correction fluids, propellants, and dry cleaning fluids.[36,37,57,101,127,154]

What Is the Acute Toxicity from Volatile Substance Use?

The major toxic effects from volatile substance use are cardiac and neurologic.[34,35] Central nervous system effects include stupor, lethargy, excitation, agitation, hallucinations (auditory and visual), seizures, ataxia, headache, dizziness, nystagmus, and respiratory depression.[154]

Cardiac effects are the most dangerous acute effects. High concentrations of hydrocarbons sensitize the myocardium to catecholamines.[15,58,139,140] Dysrhythmias and sudden death are frequently reported. Termed "sudden sniffing death," in the typical scenario an intoxicated user suddenly exerts himself or herself.[15,58,139] The halogenated hydrocarbons and benzene are the most frequent etiologies, although toluene and gasoline have been reported to cause cardiotoxicity.[14]

Other less common acute effects include methemoglobinemia from butyl and isobutyl nitrites[35,36,40]; carbon monoxide toxicity from methylene chloride[49,136,157,158]; hepatitis from the chlorinated hydrocarbons (carbon tetrachloride especially; see Table 85–4); and muscle weakness, metabolic acidosis, rhabdomyolosis, renal tu-

TABLE 85–5. COMPOSITION OF ABUSED HYDROCARBON SOLVENTS

Inhalant	Chemical Constituents
Acrylic paint	Toluene
Aerosol propellant	Fluorocarbons (chlorodifluoromethane, dichlorodifluoromethane), trichlorofluoromethane, nitrous oxide
Anesthetics	Enflurane, halothane, isoflurane, nitrous oxide
Dyes	Acetone, methylene chloride
Fire extinguishing agent	Bromochlorodifluoromethane (BCF)
Gas (bottled), torches	Propane, butane
Gasoline	Hydrocarbons, tetraethyl lead
Glues/adhesives	Toluene, benzene, xylene, acetone, naphtha, *n*-hexane, trichlorethylene, ethyl acetate, tetrachloroethylene, trichloroethane, carbon tetrachloride, methylethyl ketone (MEK)
Lighter fluid	Butane
Nail polish remover	Acetone, amyl acetate, isopropanol
Paint stripper	Methylene chloride
Paints/varnishes/lacquers	Trichloroethylene, toluene, mineral spirits
Polystyrene cements	Acetone, toluene, trichloroethylene, *n*-hexane
Refrigerants	Fluorochloromethanes
Rubber cement	Benzene, *n*-hexane, trichloroethylene
Shoe polish	Chlorinated hydrocarbons, toluene
Solvent (laboratory)	Carbon tetrachloride, chloroform, diethyl ether, *n*-hexane, methyl isobutyl ketone (MIBK)
Spot remover	Trichloroethane, trichloroethylene, carbon tetrachloride
Typewriter correction fluid	Trichloroethane, trichloroethylene, perchloroethylene

Modified, with permission, from Meredith TJ, Ruprah M, Liddle A, Flanagan RJ: Diagnosis and treatment of acute poisoning with volatile substances. Human Toxicol 1989: 8:277–286; and Wyse DG: Deliberate inhalation of volatile hydrocarbons: A review. Can Med Assoc J 1973;108:71–74.

bular acidosis, and hypokalemia from toluene toxicity.[38,52,56,98,116,161,163]

What Are the Chronic Effects Associated With Hydrocarbon Exposure?

Chronic occupational exposure and volatile substance abusers are susceptible to a number of long-term risks.[10,131,135,142] The central nervous, peripheral nervous, and hematologic systems are most affected. Occupations with high solvent exposure, and chronic volatile substance users, can develop a neurobehavioral syndrome characterized by memory loss, cognitive impairment, sleep disorder, depression, anxiety, neurasthenia, and personality changes.[80] This entity, termed chronic painter syndrome, is an organic brain syndrome or organic solvent-induced encephalopathy. The CT scans of these patients show areas of atrophy, EEGs may show abnormalities, and neuropsychiatric testing often reveals distinctive deficit patterns.[95]

Cerebellar dysfunction with chorea has been reported following chronic gasoline sniffing. Lead poisoning associated with gasoline abuse has been associated with the prior use of tetraethyl lead.[60] The incidence of lead toxicity from gasoline has decreased substantially with the reduction of lead content in gasoline (see Chap. 79).

Peripheral neuropathy is well described following the occupational exposure to *n*-hexane (see Chap. 19). Similar effects have been reported with volatile substance abuse and may be due to exposure to *n*-hexane, *n*-heptane, methylethyl ketone, methyl *n*-butyl ketone, and methyl isobutyl ketone.[1,100] This neuropathy typically begins with sensory involvement in the distal extremities and progresses proximally to include the motor system. With discontinuation of exposure many of the effects reverse over weeks to months.[77,135,191]

Chronic occupational exposure to benzene is associated with a number of hematologic effects. An increased number of cases of leukemia, aplastic anemia, and multiple myeloma are found in long-time workers exposed to benzene. Other aromatic hydrocarbons have been reported to cause similar hematologic effects in animals. These effects are most likely due to benzene contamination of the hydrocarbons, and an excess risk has not been demonstrated in groups with long-term exposure to toluene, xylene, or other aromatic hydrocarbons.[8,43,142,174,181]

What Is Pine Oil? What Are Terpenes?

Pine oil is an active ingredient in many household cleaning and disinfectant products. It is a mixture of unsaturated, nonaromatic, cyclic hydrocarbons from the classes of compounds known as terpenes, camphenes, and pinenes. The major components are terpenes, which are found in plants and flowers. These products are derived by oleoresin distillation of the particular plant. Wood distillates are products from pine trees and include pine oil and turpentine.

As opposed to patients who ingest petroleum distillates, those who ingest pine oil often have a strong pine odor. In addition, wood distillates are more readily absorbed and may cause CNS and pulmonary toxicity from this route. Despite the absorption risk, little information is available on the efficacy of gastric emptying. Toxicity from gastrointestinal absorption appears to be limited.[24,39,53,86,92,152,153]

Aspiration pneumonitis remains the main clinical concern. Acute toxicity is similar to petroleum distillate ingestions and management principles are similar. Other rare reported problems associated with wood distillates include turpentine-associated thrombocytopenic purpura, acute renal failure, and hemorrhagic cystitis.[93,175]

Other Routes of Hydrocarbon Exposure

Intravenous and subcutaneous injection of hydrocarbons are rarely reported.[169,170] Severe hydrocarbon pneumonitis has occurred following intravenous exposure.[169,170] Animal experiments have shown that intravascular injections of hydrocarbons cause injury to the first capillary bed or sinusoid system that is encountered.[22] Intravenous injection leads to pulmonary toxicity and portal vein injection to hepatic injury.[22,45,82,141,185,189] The clinical course of the individuals exposed to IV hydrocarbons was not dissimilar to aspiration-induced injury.

Soft-tissue injection of hydrocarbon is locally toxic, leading to tissue necrosis. Secondary infection with cellulitis, abscess formation, and fasciitis can occur. Infectious complications are treated with meticulous wound care and surgical debridement as necessary. A particularly destructive injury involves high-pressure injection gun injury. These injuries typically involve the extremities with high-pressure injection of grease or paint into the fascial planes and tendon sheaths. Emergent surgical debridement is necessary in many of these cases.[54,121]

Tar and Asphalt Injury

Tar and asphalt injury is a common occupational hazard among construction workers. These hot hydrocarbon mixtures can cause severe burns on exposure to skin. The material quickly hardens and is very difficult to remove. Immediate cooling with cold water is important to limit further thermal injury. Complete removal is then essential to ensure proper burn management and limit infectious complications.

Mechanical attempts to remove the hardened tar or asphalt often cause further tissue damage. Dissolving the material with mineral oil, petroleum jelly, and antibacterial ointments (Neosporin, Polysporin) has been attempted with variable success. Surface-acting agents in combination with a hydrocarbon ointment (De-Solv-it, Tween–80, Polysorbate 80) are more effective.[47,160,168]

Another problem related to asphalt is the potential for toxic gas exposure. Unused roofing asphalt is typically cooled in well-ventilated tanks with release of a number of toxic gases. Without proper dispersion of these gases, high concentrations of hydrogen sulfide, carbon monoxide, propane, methane, and volatilized hydrocarbons can accumulate with subsequent severe poisoning.[79]

References

1. Abel Rahman MS, Hetland LB, Couri D: Toxicity and metabolism of methyl *n*-butyl ketone. Am Ind Hyg Assoc J 1976;37:95–102.
2. Adler R, Robinson RG, Binkin NJ: Intravascular hemolysis: An unusual complication of hydrocarbon ingestion. J Pediatr 1976;89:679.
3. Albert WC: The efficacy of steroid therapy in the treatment of experimental kerosene pneumonitis. Am Rev Respir Dis 1968;98:888–889.
4. Algren JT, Rodgers GC: Intravascular hemolysis associated with hydrocarbon poisoning. Pediatr Emerg Care 1992;8:34–35.
5. Anas N, Namasonthi V, Ginsburg CM: Criteria for hospitalizing children who have ingested products containing hydrocarbon. JAMA 1981;246:840–843.
6. Arena J: Hydrocarbon poisoning—Current management. Pediatr Ann 1987;16:879–883.
7. Arena J: Petroleum distillate ingestion. Pediatr Ann 1978; 7:513. Letter.
8. Ashford NA: New scientific evidence and public health imperatives. N Engl J Med 1987;316:1084–1085.
9. Ashkenazi AE, Berman SE: Experimental kerosene poisoning in rats: Use of C^{14} labeled hendecane as indicator of absorption. Pediatrics 1961;26:642–649.
10. Askergren A, Allgen LG, Karlsson C, et al: Studies on kidney function in subjects exposed to organic solvents. I. Excretion of albumin and beta-2-microglobulin in the urine. Acta Med Scand 1981;209:479–483.
11. Baghdassarian OM, Weiner S: Pneumatocele formation complicating hydrocarbon pneumonitis. Am J Roentgenol 1965;95:104–111.
12. Baldachin BJ, Melmed RN: Clinical and therapeutic aspects of kerosene poisoning. A series of 200 cases. Br Med J 1964;2:28–30.
13. Barbour O: Kerosene poisoning. JAMA 1926;87:488.
14. Bass M: Death from sniffing gasoline. N Engl J Med 1978;299:203. Letter.
15. Bass M: Sudden sniffing death. JAMA 1970;212:2075–2079.
16. Baumgartner L, Angevine DM: Lipoid pneumonia and conditions that may favor its occurrence. Am J Med Sci 1936;192:252–257.
17. Beamon RF, Siegel CJ, Landers G, et al: Hydrocarbon ingestion in children: A six-year retrospective study. JACEP 1976;5:771–775.
18. Bergeson PS: Pneumatoceles following hydrocarbon ingestion. Am J Dis Child 1975;129:49–54.
19. Blattner RJ: Kerosene poisoning. J Pediatr 1951;39:391–392.
20. Bonte FJ, Reynolds J: Hydrocarbon pneumonitis. Radiology 1958;71:391–397.
21. Bothe J, Braun W, Conhardt A: Untersuchungen zur Antidotwirkung von Paraffinol bei Vergiftungen mit Kohlenwasserstoffen an der Maus. Arch Toxikol 1973;30:243–250.

22. Bratton L, Haddon JE. Ingestion of charcoal lighter fluid. J Pediatr 1975;87:633–636.
23. Bromer RS, Wolman IJ: Lipoid pneumonia in infants and children. Radiology 1939;32:1–7.
24. Brook MP, McCarron MM, Mueller JA: Pine oil cleaner ingestion. Ann Emerg Med 1989;18:391–395.
25. Brown J III, Burke B, Dajani AS, et al: Experimental kerosene pneumonia: Evaluation of some therapeutic regimens. J Pediatr 1974;84:396–401.
26. Brunner S, Rovsing H, Wulf H: Roentgenographic change in the lungs of children with kerosene poisoning. Am Rev Respir Dis 1964;89:250–254.
27. Burkhart KK, Hall AH, Gerace R, et al: Hyperbaic oxygen treatment for carbon tetrachloride poisoning. Drug Saf 1991;6:332–338.
28. Burley S, Huber G: The effect of toxic agents commonly ingested by children on antibacterial defenses in the lung. Proc Soc Pediatr Res 1971;16:83.
29. Bysani GK,Rucoba RJ, Noah ZL: Treatment of hydrocarbon pneumonitis; High-frequency jet ventilation as an alternative to extracorporeal membrane oxygenation. Chest 1994;106:300–303.
30. Cachia EA, Fenech FF: Kerosene poisoning in children. Arch Dis Child 1964;39:502.
31. Campbell JB: Pneumatocele formation following hydrocarbon ingestion. Am Rev Respir Dis 1970;101:414–418.
32. Carithers HA: Accident prevention in childhood—The kerosene hazard. JAMA 1955;159:109–111.
33. Carlini-Cotrim B, Carlini EA: The use of solvents and other drugs among children and adolescents from a low socioeconomic background: A study in Sao Paulo, Brazil. Int J Addict 1988;23;1145–1156.
34. Carpenter C: Animal and human response to vapors of Stoddard solvent. Tox Appl Pharmacol 1975;32: 282–297.
35. Carpenter CP, Geary DL, Myers RC, et al: Petroleum hydrocarbon toxicity studies, XIII. Animal and human response to vapors of toluene concentrate. Toxicol Appl Pharmacol 1976;36:473–490.
36. Cohen S: The volatile nitrites. JAMA 1979;241:2077–2078.
37. Cohen S: Glue sniffing. JAMA 1975;231:653–654.
38. Cohr KH, Stolkholm J: Toluene, A toxicologic review. Scand J Work Environ Health 1979;5:71–90.
39. Cubells JM, Martinez RA, Youssef W: Poisoning by spirits of turpentine or turpentine oil. Review of its treatment. Ann Esp Pediatr 1952;83:446–453.
40. Curry S: Methemoglobinemia. Ann Emerg Med 1982;11: 214–221.
41. Daffner RH, Jimenez JP: The double gastric fluid level in kerosene poisoning. Pediatr Radiol 1973;106:383–384.
42. Daeschner CW, Blattner RJ, Collins VP: Hydrocarbon pneumonitis. Pediatr Clin North Am 1957;4:243–253.
43. Decoufle P, Blattner WA, Blair A: Mortality among chemical workers exposed to benzene and other agents. Environ Res 1983;30:16–25.
44. Deeths TM, Breeden JT: Poisoning in children—A statistical study of 1,057 cases. J Pediatr 1971;78:299–305.
45. Deichmann WB, Kitzmiller KV, Witherup S, et al: Kerosene intoxication. Ann Intern Med 1944;21:803–823.
46. De la Rocha SR, Cunningham JC, Fox E: Lipoid pneumonia secondary to baby oil aspiration: A case report and review of the literature. Pediatr Emerg Care 1985;1:74–80.
47. Demling RH, Buerstatte WR, Perea A: Management of hot tar burns. J Trauma 1980;20:242.
48. Dice WH, Ward G, Kelley J, et al: Pulmonary toxicity following gastrointestinal ingestion of kerosene. Ann Emerg Med 1982;11:138–142.
49. Di Vincenzo GD, Kaplan CJ: Uptake, metabolism and elimination of methylene chloride vapors by humans. Toxicol Appl Pharmacol 1981;59:130–140.
50. Dragsted PJ: Pseudocysts of the lungs in kerosene poisoning. Dis Chest 1965;48:87–90.
51. Eade NR, Taussig LM, Marks MI: Hydrocarbon pneumonitis. Pediatrics 1974;54:351–357.
52. Echeverria D, Fine L, Langolf G, et al: Acute neurobehavioral effects of toluene. Br J Indust Med 1989;46: 483–495.
53. Erickson T, Popiel R, Hryhorczuk DO, et al: Pine oil cleaners in prison. Ann Emerg Med 1990;19:445–448.
54. Failkov, Freiberg A: High pressure injection injuries: An overview. J Emerg Med 1991;9:367–371.
55. Farabaugh JC: Kerosene poisoning. Minnesota Med 1936; 19:780–781.
56. Fischman C, Oster VR: Toxic effects of toluene. JAMA 1979;241:1713–1715.
57. Flanagan RJ, Ruprah M, Meredith TJ, Ramset JR: An introduction to the clinical toxicology of volatile substances. Drug Saf 1990;5:359–383.
58. Flowers NC, Horan LG: Nonanoxic aerosol arrhythmias. JAMA 1972;219:23–27.
59. Foley JC, Dreyer NB, Soule AB, et al: Kerosene poisoning in young children. Radiology 1954;62:817–829.
60. Fortenberry JD: Gasoline sniffing. Am J Med 1985;79: 740–744.
61. Freiman DG, Engelberg H, Merrit WH: Oil aspiration (lipoid) pneumonia in adults. Arch Intern Med 1940;66: 11–38.
62. Gayu M, Meller R, Stanley S: Drug abuse monitoring: A survey of solvent abuse in the county of Avon. Hum Toxicol 1982;1:257–263.
63. Geehr E: Management of hydrocarbon ingestions. Topics Emerg Med 1979;1:97–110.
64. Gerarde HW: Toxicological studies on hydrocarbons: IX. The aspiration hazard and toxicity of hydrocarbons and hydrocarbon mixtures. Arch Environ Health 1963;6:329–341.
65. Gerarde HW: Toxicological studies on hydrocarbons: V. Kerosene. Toxic Appl Pharmacol 1959; 1:462–469.
66. Gershon-Cohen J, Bringhurst LS, Byrne RN: Roentgenography of kerosene poisoning. Am J Roentgenol 1953;69: 557.
67. Giammona ST: Effects of furniture polish on pulmonary surfactant. Am J Dis Child 1967;113:658–663.
68. Goodwin TC: Lipoid cell pneumonia. Am J Dis Child 1934;48:309–326.
69. Graham JR: Pneumonitis following aspiration of crude oil and its treatment by steroid hormones. Trans Am Clin Climatol Assoc 1955–56;67:104–112.
70. Griffin JW, Daeschner CV, Collins VP, et al: Hydrocarbon pneumonitis following furniture polish ingestion. J Pediatr 1954;13:13–26.

71. Gross P: Kerosene pneumonitis: An experimental study with small doses. Am Rev Resp Dis 1963;88:656–663.
72. Gurwitz D, Katten M, Levison H, et al: Pulmonary function abnormalities in symptomatic children after hydrocarbon pneumonitis. Pediatrics 1978;62:789–794.
73. Hamilton WC: Death from drinking coal oil. Med News 1897;71:214.
74. Hansbrough JF, Saputa-Sirvent R, Dominic W, et al: Hydrocarbon contact injuries. 1985;25:250–252
75. Hardman G, Tolson R, Hadhdassarian O: Prednisone in the management of kerosene pneumonia. Indian Practitioner 1960;13:615–620.
76. Heacock CH: Pneumonia in children following the ingestion of petroleum products. Radiology 1949;53:793.
77. Herskowitz A, Ishh N, Schaumburg H: *N*-hexane neuropathy: A syndrome occurring as a result of industrial exposure. N Engl J Med 1971;285:82–85
78. Higgins JM: Rapidly fatal result in a child from ingestion of kerosene. Penn Med J 1932;36:526–527.
79. Hoidal CR, Hall AH, Robinson ND, et al: Hydrogen sulfide poisoning from toxic inhalations of roofing asphalt fumes. Ann Emerg Med 1986;15:826–830.
80. Hormes JT, Filley CM, Rosenberg NL: Neurologic sequelae of chronic solvent vapor abuse. Neurology 1986;36: 698–702.
81. Huxtable KA, Bolande RP, Klaus M: Experimental furniture polish pneumonia in rats. Pediatrics 1964;34:228–235.
82. Ikeda K: Oil aspiration pneumonia (lipoid pneumonia): Clinical, pathologic and experimental consideration. Am J Dis Child 1935;49:985–1006.
83. Jackson WH: A case of poisoning by kerosene. Aust Med J 1871;16:200–201.
84. Jacobziner H: Accidental chemical poisonings, kerosene, and other petroleum distillate poisonings. NY J Med 1963;63:3428.
85. Jacobziner H, Raybin HW: Mixture of tranquilizers, lighter fluid, paint thinner, and iodine poisonings. NY State J Med 1962;62:862.
86. Jacobziner H, Raybin HW: Turpentine poisoning. Arch Pediatr 1961;78:357–364.
87. James FW, Kaplan S, Bensing G: Cardiac complications following hydrocarbon ingestion. Am J Dis Child 1971; 121:431–433.
88. Jamison KE, Wallace ER: Kerosene pneumonitis treated with adrenal steroids. Calif Med 1964;100:43.
89. Karlson KH: Hydrocarbon poisoning in children. South Med J 1982;75:839–840.
90. Klein BL, Simon JE: Hydrocarbon poisonings. Pediatr Clin North Am 1986;33:411–419.
91. Klein FA, Hackler RH: Hemorrhagic cystitis associated with turpentine ingestion. Urology 1980;16:187. Letter.
92. Koppel C, Tenczer J, Tonnesmann U, et al: Acute poisoning with pine oil—Metabolism of monoterpenes. Arch Toxicol 1981;49:73–78.
93. Laass W: Therapy of acute oral poisonings by organic solvents: Treatment by activated charcoal in combination with laxatives. Arch Toxicol 1980;4(suppl):406–409.
94. Lareng L: Acute toxic methemoglobinemia from accidental ingestion of nitrobenzene. Eur J Toxicol 1974;7:12–16.
95. Larsen F, Leira HL: Organic brain syndrome and long term exposure to toluene: A clinical psychiatric study of vocationally active printing workers. J Occup Med 1988; 30:875–878.
96. Laughlen GF: Studies on pneumonia following nasopharyngeal injections of oil. Am J Pathol 1925;1: 407–414.
97. Lavenstein AF: Ingestion of kerosene complicated by pneumonia, pneumothorax, pneumopericardium, and subcutaneous emphysema. J Pediatr 1945;26:395–400.
98. Lazar RB, Ho SU, Melen O, et al: Multifocal central nervous system damage caused by toluene abuse. Neurology 1983;33:1337–1340.
99. Lesser LI, Weens HS, McKey JD: Pulmonary manifestations following ingestion of kerosene. J Pediatr 1943;23: 352–364.
100. Liira J, Riihimaki V, Pfaffli P: Kinetics of methyl ethyl ketone in man. Int Arch Occup Environ Health 1988;60: 195–200.
101. Linden CH: Volatile substances of abuse. Emerg Med Clin North Am 1990;8:559–578.
102. Litovitz TL: Hydrocarbon ingestions. Ear Nose Throat J 1983;62:142–147.
103. Litovitz TL, Clark LR, Soloway RA: 1993 annual report of the American Association of Poison Control Centers Toxic Exposure Surveillance System. Am J Emerg Med 1994; 12:546–584.
104. Litovitz TL, Felberg L, Soloway RA, et al: 1994 annual report of the American Association of Poison Control Centers Toxic Exposure Surveillance System. Am J Emerg Med 1995; 13:551–597.
105. Litovitz TL, Felberg L, White S, et al: 1995 annual report of the American Association of Poison Control Centers Toxic Exposure Surveillance System. Am J Emerg Med 1996, 14:487–537.
106. Litovitz TL, Holm KC, Bailey KM, et al: 1991 annual report of the American Association of Poison Control Centers national data collection system. Am J Emerg Med 1992;10: 452–505.
107. Litovitz TL, Holm KC, Clancy C, et al: 1992 annual report of the American Association of Poison Control Centers Toxic Exposure Surveillance System. Am J Emerg Med 1993;11:494–555.
108. Machado B, Cross K, Snodgrass WR: Accidental hydrocarbon ingestion cases telephoned to a regional poison center. Ann Emerg Med 1988;17:804–807.
109. Mann MD, Pirie DJ, Wolfsdorf J: Kerosene absorption in primates. J Pediatr 1977;91:495–498.
110. Marandian MH, Youssefian H, Saboury M, et al: Intoxication accidentelle par ingestion de petrole chex l'enfant: Etude clinique, radiologique, biologique et anatomopathologique, a propos de 3462 cas. Ann Pediatr 1981;28: 601–609.
111. Marks MI, Chicoine L, Legere G, et al: Adrenocorticosteroid treatment of hydrocarbon pneumonia in children—A cooperative study. J Pediatr 1972;81:366–369.
112. Matsumoto T, Koga M, Sata T, et al: The changes of gasoline compounds in blood in a case of gasoline intoxication. J Toxicol Clin Toxicol 1992;30:653–662.
113. Mayock RL, Zinsser HF: Kerosene pneumonitis treated with adrenal steroids. Ann Intern Med 1961;54:559.

114. McLean CC: Kerosene poisoning. JAMA 1933;101:1987. Letter.
115. McNally WD: Kerosene poisoning in children. J Pediatr 1956;48:296–299.
116. Meulenbelt J, De Groot G, Savelkoul TJF: Two cases of toluene intoxication. Br J Ind Med 1990;47:417–420
117. Mintz AA: Furniture polish intoxication. South Med J 1966;59:1010–1014.
118. Mofenson HC: The new correct answer to an old question on kerosene ingestion. Pediatrics 1977;59:788. Letter.
119. Mofenson HC, Greensher J: Controversies in the prevention and treatment of poisonings. Pediatr Ann 1977; 6:717–725.
120. Morgan DP: Effectiveness of activated charcoal, mineral oil, and castor oil in limiting gastrointestinal absorption of a chlorinated hydrocarbon pesticide. Clin Toxicol 1977;11: 61–70.
121. Mrvos R, Dean BS, Krenzelok EP: High pressure injection injuries: A serious occupational hazard. J Toxicol Clin Toxicol 1987;25:297–304.
122. Ng RC: Using syrup of ipecac for ingestion of petroleum distillates. Pediatr Ann 1977;6:708–710.
123. Ng RC, Darwish H, Stewart DA: Emergency treatment of petroleum distillate and turpentine ingestion. Can Med Assoc J 1974;3:537–538.
124. Nouri L, Al-Rahim K: Kerosene poisoning in children. Postgrad Med J 1970;46:71.
125. Nunn JA, Martin FM: Gasoline and kerosene poisoning in children. JAMA 1934;103:472–475.
126. Olstad RB, Lord RM, Jr: Kerosene intoxication. Am J Dis Child 1952;83:446–453.
127. Osterloh J: Butyl nitrite abuse and overdose. Vet Hum Toxicol. 1984;26:416. Abstract.
128. Ottelio C, Giagheddu M, Marrosu F: Altered EEG pattern in aromatic hydrocarbon intoxication: A case report. Acta Neurologica 1993;15:357–362.
129. Padday JF: Theory of surface tension. In: Matijevic E, ed: Surface and Colloid Science, Vol. 1. New York, Wiley-Interscience, 1969.
130. Parker SE: Use and abuse of volatile substances in industry. Human Toxicol 1989;8:271–275.
131. Pedersen LM, Rasmussen JM: The hematological and biochemical pattern in occupational organic solvent poisoning and exposure. Int Arch Occup Environ Health 1982; 51:113–126.
132. Pierson JW: Some unusual pneumonias associated with the aspiration of fats and oils in the lungs. Am J Radiol 1932;27:572–579.
133. Pinkerton H: Oils and fats: Their entrance into and fate in the lungs of infants and children: A clinical and pathologic report. Am J Dis Child 1927;33:259–285.
134. Press E: Cooperative kerosene poisoning study: Evaluation of gastric lavage and other factors in the treatment of accidental ingestion of petroleum distillate products. Pediatrics 1962;29:648–674.
135. Prockop L: Neurotoxic volatile substances. Neurology 1979;29:862–865.
136. Ratney RS, Wegman DH, Elkins HB: In vivo conversion of methylene chloride to carbon monoxide. Arch Environ Health 1974;28:223–236.
137. Reed ES, Leikin S, Kerman HD: Kerosene intoxication. Am J Dis Child 1950;79:623–632.
138. Reese E, Kimbrough RD: Acute toxicity of gasoline and some additives. Environ Health Perspec 1993;101(suppl): 115–131.
139. Reinhardt CF, Aza A, Maxfield ME, et al: Cardiac arrhythmias and aerosol sniffing. Arch Environ Health 1971;22: 265–279.
140. Reinhardt CF, Mullin LS, Maxfield ME: Epinephrine-induced cardiac arrhythmia potential of some common industrial solvents. J Occup Med 1973;15:953–955.
141. Richardson JA, Pratt-Thomas HR: Toxic effects of varying doses of kerosene administered by different routes. Am J Med Sci 1951;221:531–536.
142. Rinsky RA, Smith AB, Hornung R, et al: Benzene and leukemia: An epidemiologic risk assessment. N Engl J Med 1987;316:1044–1050.
143. Scalzo AJ, Weber TR, Jaeger RW, et al: Extracorporeal membrane oxygenation for hydrocarbon aspiration. Am J Dis Child 1990;144:867–871.
144. Scharf SM, Heimer D, Goldstein J: Pathologic and physiologic effects of aspiration of hydrocarbons in the rat. Am Rev Respir Dis 1981;124:625–629.
145. Scharf SM, Prinsloo I: Pulmonary mechanics in dogs given different doses of kerosene intratracheally. Am Rev Respir Dis 1982;126:695–700.
146. Schwartz SI, Breslau RC, Kutner F, et al: Effects of drugs and hyperbaric oxygen environment on experimental kerosene pneumonitis. Dis Chest 1965;47:353–359.
147. Scott EP: Pneumonia, pneumothorax and emphysema following ingestion of kerosene. J Pediatr 1944;25:31–34.
148. Sexena S, Gupta U: Lipoid pneumonia: Review of the literature with a case report. J Indian Med Assoc 1966;47: 169–172.
149. Shih RD, Mercurio M, Morasco R, et al: Artificial surfactant administration in an animal model of severe hydrocarbon induced pulmonary toxicity. J Toxicol Clin Toxicol 1996;34:139. Abstract.
150. Shirkey HC: Treatment of petroleum distillate ingestion. Mod Treatment 1967;4:580–592.
151. Soule AB, Foley JC: Poisoning from petroleum distillates. The hazards of kerosene and furniture polish. J Maine Med Assoc 1957;48:103–110.
152. Sperling F: In vivo and in vitro toxicology of turpentine. Clin Toxicol 1969;2:21–35.
153. Sperling F, Marcus W, Collins C, et al: Acute effects of turpentine vapor on rats and mice. Toxicol Appl Pharmacol 1967;10:8–20.
154. Spiller HA, Krenzolak EP: Epidemiology of inhalant abuse reported to two regional poison centers. J Toxicol Clin Toxicol 1997;35:167–173.
155. Steele RW, Conklin RH, Mark HM: Corticosteroids and antibiotics for the treatment of fulminate hydrocarbon aspiration. JAMA 1972;219:1434–1437.
156. Steiner MM: Syndromes of kerosene poisoning in children. Am J Dis Child 1947;74:32–44.
157. Stevens JL, Ratnayake JH, Anders MW: Metabolism of dihalomethanes to carbon monoxide: Studies in isolated rat hepatocytes. Toxicol Appl Pharmacol 1980;55:484–489.
158. Stewart RD, Fisher TN, Hosko MJ, et al: Experimental

human exposure to methylene chloride. Arch Environ Health 1972;25:342–348.
159. Stockman JA: More on hydrocarbon-induced hemolysis. J Pediatr 1977;90:848. Letter.
160. Strata RJ, Saffle JR, Kravitz M, et al: Management of tar and asphalt injuries. Am J Surg 1983;146:766–769.
161. Streicher HZ, Gabow PA, Moss AN, et al: Syndromes of toluene sniffing in adults. Ann Intern Med 1981;94: 758–762.
162. Susten AS, Niemeier RW, Simon SD: In vivo percutaneous absorption studies of volatile organic solvents in hairless mice II. Toluene, ethylbenzene, and aniline. J Appl Toxicol 1990;10:217–225.
163. Taher SM. Anderson RJ, McCartney R, et al: Renal tubular acidosis associated with toluene "sniffing." N Engl J Med 1974;290:765–768.
164. Taussig LM, Castro E, Landau LI, et al: Pulmonary function 8–10 years after hydrocarbon pneumonitis. Clin Pediatr 1977;16:57–59.
165. Tchertkoff IG, Ornstein GG: Bronchopulmonary disease attributed to the use of intranasal instillation of oily substances: A report of 10 cases. Q Bull Sea View Hosp 1936;1:139–159.
166. Truemper E, Reyes de la Rocha SR, et al: Clinical characteristics, pathophysiology, and management of hydrocarbon ingestion: Case report and review of the literature. Pediatr Emerg Care 1987;3:187–193.
167. Truss CD, Killenberg PG: Treatment of carbon tetrachloride poisoning with hyperbaric oxygen. Gastroenterology 1982;82;767–769.
168. Tsou TJ, Hutson HR, Bear M, et al: De-solv-it for hot paving asphalt burn: Case report. Acad Emerg Med 1996;3:88–89.
169. Upreti RK, Das M, Shanker R: Dermal exposure to kerosene. Vet Hum Toxicol 1989;31:16–20
170. Vaziri ND, Smith PJ, Wilson A: Toxicity with intravenous injection of naphtha in man. Clin Toxicol 1980;16: 335–343.
171. Vaziri ND, Smith PJ, Wilson AF: Hemorrhagic pneumonitis after intravenous injection of charcoal lighter fluid. Ann Intern Med 1979;90:795–796.
172. Verhulst HL, Page LA: Adrenocortical steroids in the treatment of kerosene pneumonia. New Drugs 1961;1: 147–153.
173. Victoria MS, Nangia BS: Hydrocarbon poisoning: A review. Pediatr Emerg Care 1987;3:184–186.
174. Vigliano EC, Saita G: Benzene and leukemia. N Eng J Med 1964;271:872–876.
175. Wahlberg P, Nyman D: Turpentine and thrombocytopenic purpura. Lancet 1969;2:215–216.
176. Waldowski D, Meyer RJ: Hydrocarbon poisoning: A continuing childhood hazard. Virg Med Monthly 1967;94: 409–411.
177. Waring JI: Pneumonia in kerosene poisoning. Am J Med Sci 1933;185:325–330.
178. Wasserman GS: Hydrocarbon poisoning. Crit Care Q 1982;4:33–41.
179. Watson WA, Weinman SA, ACE Study Group: Activated charcoal (AC) dosing and the prevalence and predictors of emesis. J Toxicol Clin Toxicol 1995;33:489–490. Abstract.
180. White LE, Driggers DA, Wardinsky TD: Poisoning in childhood and adolescence: A study of 111 cases admitted to a military hospital. J Fam Pract 1980;11:27–31.
181. White MC, Infante PF, Chu KC: A quantitative estimate of leukemia mortality associated with occupational exposure to benzene. Risk Anal 1982;2:195–204.
182. Widmer LR, Goodwin SR, Berman LS, et al: Artificial surfactant for therapy in hydrocarbon-induced lung injury in sheep. Crit Care Med 1996;24:1524–1529.
183. Wolfe BM, Brodeur AE, Shields JB: The role of gastrointestinal absorption of kerosene in producing pneumonitis in dogs. J Pediatr 1970;76:867–873.
184. Wolfe RR: Pneumatoceles complicating hydrocarbon pneumonitis. J Pediatr 1967;71:711–714.
185. Wolfsdorf J: Experimental kerosene pneumonitis in primates: Relevance to the therapeutic management of childhood poisoning. Clin Exp Pharmacol Physiol 1976;3:539–544.
186. Wolfsdorf J: Kerosene intoxication: An experimental approach to the etiology of the CNS manifestations in primates. J Pediatr 1976;88:1037–1040.
187. Wolfsdorf J: Massive ingestion of kerosene: A study of gastric clearance in primates. Clin Exp Pharm Physiol 1975;2:405–409.
188. Wolfsdorf J, Kundig H: Dexamethasone in the management of kerosene pneumonia. Pediatrics 1974;53:86–90.
189. Wolfsdorf J, Kundig H: Kerosene poisoning in primates. S Afr Med J 1972;46:619–621.
190. Wyse DG: Deliberate inhalation of volatile hydrocarbons: A review. Can Med J 1973;108:71–74.
191. Yamamura Y: n-Hexane polyneuropathy. Folia Psychiatr Neurol Jap 1969;23:45–57.
192. Zieserl E: Hydrocarbon ingestion and poisoning. Compr Ther 1979;5:35–42.
193. Zucker AR, Berger S, Wood LDH: Management of kerosene-induced pulmonary injury. Crit Care Med 1986; 14:303–304.

CHAPTER 86

Caustics and Batteries

Rama B. Rao and Robert S. Hoffman

A 34-year-old male ingested a cup of liquid drain opener (sodium hydroxide) in an attempted suicide. He vomited once and presented to the Emergency Department 30 minutes later complaining of chest and abdominal pain. His physical examination revealed a heart rate of 100 beats/min, a respiratory rate of 22 breaths/min, blood pressure of 130/80 mm Hg, and a temperature of 99°F (37.2°C). His oropharynx was only mildly erythematous. There was no stridor, and his lungs were clear. His heart was regular in rhythm without murmurs or gallops. Bowel sounds were present, and the abdomen was soft with mild left upper quadrant tenderness. His stool was negative for occult blood. The patient's extremities were warm and well perfused, and his neurologic examination was unremarkable.

Two large-bore intravenous lines were started with 0.9% sodium chloride at 250 mL/h. Blood was sent for serum electrolyte, hemoglobin, platelet, coagulation profile, type and cross-match, and arterial blood gas analyses. A fiber-optic inspection of the nasopharynx revealed a patent airway with no edema of the larynx. Chest and abdominal radiographs were unremarkable. Over the next few hours his vital signs remained unchanged, as did the rest of his physical examination. The arterial blood gas analyses returned with pH 7.30; PCO_2 30 mm Hg; and PO_2 88 mm Hg. Endoscopy performed 4 hours after the ingestion revealed a second-degree noncircumferential burn of the midesophagus and third-degree circumferential burn of the distal esophagus with significant necrosis precluding safe passage of the endoscope into the stomach. Repeat vital signs at that time were heart rate, 120 beats/min; respiratory rate, 26 breaths/min; blood pressure, 90/60 mm Hg; and temperature, 100°F (37.8°C). His examination became significant for inspiratory rales in the left lower lung field, and a repeat chest radiograph revealed a small effusion at the left lung base. His abdomen remained soft with the same degree of tenderness as he had on presentation.

The patient was taken to the operating room for exploratory surgery. A bronchoscopy, done simultaneously, was unremarkable. Laparotomy revealed dark discoloration and necrosis of the serosal surface of the gastric antrum necessitating resection. Further evaluation of the esophagus via thoracotomy revealed a perforation of the distal esophagus above the lower esophageal sphincter. The patient underwent esophagogastrectomy with placement of bilateral chest tubes for drainage, and placement of a jejunostomy tube for subsequent feeding. Postoperatively the patient developed a pneumonia and responded well to antibiotic therapy. He had intensive medical and psychiatric care in the hospital. After several weeks in the hospital, he was discharged with postoperative and psychiatric follow-up.

What Are Caustics?

A caustic agent is a substance that causes both functional and histologic damage on contact with body surfaces. The injury is incurred as neutralization of the substance takes place at the expense of the tissues, releasing thermal energy and inducing burns. The extent of injury is determined by duration of contact; ability of the substance to penetrate tissues; volume, pH, and concentration of the agent; and a property known as titratable acid or alkaline reserve (TAR). TAR defines the volume of neutralizing substance needed to bring the pH of a caustic to that of physiologic tissues. The larger the titratable alkaline reserve, the more caustic, or damaging the agent.[7,26,53,66,72] Some agents with a pH between 3 and 11 can cause severe burns due to the molecular properties of the substance and its TAR. Both zinc chloride and phenol are examples of caustics with a near physiologic pH. These factors, along with the presence or absence of food in the stomach, may play a role in the severity of injury sustained by caustic exposure.[149]

Though there are many ways to categorize caustic agents, they are most typically classified as acids or alkalis. An acid is a proton donator and causes significant injury, generally at a pH below 3. Common sources of acid exposure include toilet bowl cleaners, soldering flux, swimming pool products, and battery fluid (Table 86–1). An alkaline agent is a proton acceptor with significant caustic injury generally occurring at a pH above 11. Household sources of alkaline agents include drain openers, lye, hair permanent products,[52] and oven cleaners (Table 86–1). These come in solid and liquid forms with different viscosities and concentrations of solution.

Skin, eyes, gastrointestinal tract, and the respiratory tract can all be sites of caustic injury. By far the most life-threatening and long-term morbidity of caustic exposure results from ingestion.

TABLE 86–1. SOURCES OF COMMON CAUSTIC CHEMICALS

Chemical Agent	Commercial Applications
Acetic acid	Permanent wave neutralizers, photographic stop bath
Acids (tungstic, picric, tannic)	Industrial use
Ammonia (ammonium hydroxide)	Toilet bowl cleaners, metal cleaners and polishes, hair dyes and tints, antirust products, jewelry cleaners, floor strippers, glass cleaners, wax removers
Benzalkonium chloride	Detergents
Boric acid	Roach powders, water softeners, germicide
Cantharides (Spanish fly)	Aphrodisiac (in animals), hair tonic, illicit abortifacient
Formaldehyde (formic acid)	Deodorizing tablets, plastic menders, fumigant, embalming agent
Hydrochloric acid (muriatic acid)	Metal and toilet bowl cleaners
Hydrofluoric acid	Antirust products, glass etching, microchip etching
Iodine	Antiseptics
Mercuric chloride ($HgCl_2$)	Preservative
Methylethyl ketone peroxide	Industrial synthetic agent
Oxalic acid	Disinfectants, household bleach, metal cleaning liquids, antirust products, furniture polish
Phenol (creosol, creosote)	Antiseptics, preservatives
Phosphoric acid	Toilet bowl cleaners
Phosphorous	Matches, rodenticides, fireworks, insecticides
Potassium permanganate	Illicit abortifacient, antiseptic solution
Selenious acid	Gun bluing
Sodium hydroxide	Detergents, Clinitest tablets, washing powders, paint removers, drain cleaners and openers, oven cleaners
Sodium borates, carbonates, phosphates, and silicates	Detergents, electric dishwasher preparations, water softeners
Sodium hypochlorite	Bleaches, cleansers
Sulfuric acid	Automobile batteries, drain cleaners
Zinc chloride	Soldering flux

What Is the Pathophysiology and Natural History of Alkali Ingestions?

Alkaline agents cause tissue injury within seconds of contact, resulting in almost immediate pain. The histologic injury is classically described as liquefactive, in which the agent saponifies the tissues, causing deep and progressive damage as it penetrates mucosal surfaces.[7,66] Animal studies demonstrate that within seconds of contact there is the erythema and edema of the mucosa and a subsequent inflammatory reaction extending to the submucosa and muscular layers of the esophagus. Ulcers may form. On microscopic inspection there is evidence of transmural thrombosis, and cell death occurs early in this necrotic phase.[7,88,101,184]

As wound healing progresses, neovascularization and fibroblast proliferation take place, laying down new collagen and replacing the damaged esophageal layers with granulation tissue. Ulcers may persist for up to 8 weeks as remodeling occurs. The esophagus subsequently undergoes shortening.[197] If the initial injury penetrates deeply enough, there is progressive narrowing of the esophageal lumen. The dense scar formation presents clinically as a stricture.[41,66] Strictures can evolve over a period of weeks to months, leading to dysphagia and significant nutritional deficits.[153,161,197] Both the histologic and clinical patterns of injury in experimental animals are repeatedly described in human case reports, histologic inspection of surgical specimens, and postmortem studies.[1,54,61,117,133,158] Strictures may require repeated dilation or surgical repair, becoming a chronic problem over the course of months to years.

The risk of stricture formation can be determined clinically by the initial depth of injury noted on endoscopic visualization of the esophagus. A grading system has evolved describing esophageal burns in a classification similar to that applied to dermal burns. Grade I burns are generally accepted as hyperemia or edema of the mucosa without evidence of ulcer formation. These burns carry no risk of stricture formation.[38,86,207] Grade II burns include submucosal lesions, ulcerations, and exudates. Grade II lesions have a variable progression to stricture formation. This may depend on the distribution of the lesions across the esophagus. As such, some studies have further divided grade II lesions into IIa, noncircumferential lesions, which rarely form strictures; and grade IIb, near-circumferential injuries,[33] which lead to stricture formation in about 75% of cases. Grade III burns are defined as deep ulcers and necrosis into the periesophageal tissues.[56,60,68,86] These lesions invariably progress to stricture formation and are also at a high risk of perforation.[4,69,133,195]

The evolution of injury and repair can be attended by significant complications at various stages of wound recovery. Most importantly, these include airway compromise, spontaneous perforations of the gastrointestinal tract with the development of mediastinitis or peritonitis, and other overwhelming infections from bacteria residing in the oropharynx. Other complications reported include motility abnormalities of the pharynx and esophagus,[42] formation of aorto- and tracheo-esophageal fistulas, delayed massive hemorrhage from erosion into a great vessel, and pulmonary thrombosis.[18,69,86,140,147,166,168] Long-term survivors of moderate and severe injury of the esophagus have a risk of esophageal carcinoma that is one-thousand times higher than the general population and appear to present with a 40-year latency.[6]

What Signs and Symptoms Predict Significant Caustic Injury?

The clinical evolution of patients with alkaline ingestions is attended by severe pain on contact. Depending upon the amount of agent swallowed and its formulation (solid versus liquid), the patient may complain of chest and abdominal pain. Spontaneous vomiting may occur, followed by rapid airway compromise if significant burns of the oropharynx or aspiration have occurred.

Several studies have attempted to identify patients who are not at risk for serious esophageal injury in order to limit unnecessary endoscopy. The presence or absence of oropharyngeal burns identified on examination has repeatedly been found to be a poor predictor of distal esophagogastric injury.[2,27,38,56,60,151,192] In one study there was a 37.5% incidence of esophageal lesions in the absence of oropharyngeal lesions and 22.2% of these were second and third-degree burns.[151]

Abdominal pain and the abdominal examination are also unreliable indicators of the severity of injury. The presence of abdominal pain suggests tissue injury of variable grades, but the absence of pain or findings on abdominal examination does not preclude significant gastrointestinal damage.[51,78,153,166,204] Peritoneal signs and mental status changes are more ominous findings, usually indicating severe injury.

The presence of pleural fluid is suggestive of perforation and can be used as an indication for surgical management.[204] A gastric pH greater than 7.30 also correlated retrospectively with severe alkaline injury. The prospective utility of this information is limited, as obtaining gastric secretions without direct visualization may be dangerous.

Some authors report using serum pH below 7.20 as an indication for surgery.[204] A prospective study of serum pH as a predictor of significant injury in patients with alkaline ingestions has yet to be undertaken, but it may be a useful indicator of the extent of injury, as significant tissue necrosis would be expected to generate a lactic acidosis.[166, 204]

Other clinical signs and symptoms have been examined in an attempt to better identify patients at risk for esophagogastric injury. A retrospective study of 378 children admitted for a caustic injury found that signs or symptoms could not be used to predict significant esophageal injury defined as greater than grade I lesions identified on endoscopy.[56] In a prospective study of 79 children evaluated for vomiting, drooling, or stridor, a combination of two or more of these signs was found to be a predictor of significant esophageal injury on endoscopy. It was concluded that asymptomatic children may not require endoscopy. Another retrospective study also found that children with unintentional caustic ingestions who are asymptomatic did not have significant lesions on endoscopy.[33]

A prospective study of alkaline ingestions by both adults and children found that stridor was 100% specific for significant esophageal injury based on 3 patients with this sign. No other single sign or symptom was predictive of the presence of an esophageal injury.[60]

It can be concluded that the presence of stridor, apart from the obvious necessity to protect the airway, should always prompt an investigation of distal esophagogastric injury even as an isolated finding. Children with unintentional caustic ingestions who remain completely asymptomatic and tolerate liquids after a few hours of observation can probably be discharged from the hospital. Further evaluation by endoscopy should be entertained in pediatric patients with a single symptom and definitively provided if more than one symptom is present.

Until disproved by endoscopy, serious injuries should be presumed in all suicidal patients, those with an altered mental status, and those who co-ingest analgesics as reliable indicators of injury are not established.

What Is the Initial Care of Patients With Alkaline Ingestions?

The primary goal of initial management is airway assessment and stabilization followed by obtaining a thorough history of the exposure. Although children who unintentionally ingest caustic agents can have serious injuries, there are data to support management based on specific clinical indicators and predictors of injury. Adults, however, are often exposed to caustics as a result of suicidal intent, and larger volumes of alkaline agents are swallowed. Clinical parameters may not be as reliable in these patients as co-ingestants may mask signs and symptoms, or patients may not wish to describe the severity of symptoms. One study noted that although children comprised 39% of admissions for caustic ingestions, adults comprised 81% of patients requiring treatment.[69]

For both adults and children, simple inspection of the oropharynx, vital signs, mental status, and assessment for stridor or respiratory distress is critical to preparing for the treatment of airway compromise. Large-bore intravenous access in adults is crucial, and blood work should be sent for type and cross-match, hematocrit, coagulation parameters, and electrolytes, as these patients may require emergent surgical intervention. Direct visual inspection of the vocal cords with a fiberoptic nasopharyngoscope will provide additional information regarding the need for intubation. Any signs of airway edema or depressed mentation should prompt consideration of airway protection, as edema may rapidly evolve over a period of minutes to hours making subsequent attempts at intubation or bag-valve mask ventilation difficult. Patients who clearly have a need for intubation are best served by direct visualization of the airway, as perforation of edematous tissues of the pharynx and larynx is a grave complication. Fiber-optic intubation or orotracheal intubation with a laryngoscope may be attempted. Paralytic agents for induction are best avoided, if possible, as airway edema and bleeding may distort the ability to successfully intubate or ventilate via bag-valve mask. Patients with significant ingestions may require emergent surgical airway intervention. These decisions are dependent upon the status of the patient, the ability to endotracheally or nasotracheally intubate via fiberoptic scope, and the comfort of the physician in performing the technique of a surgical airway. If airway involvement is significant enough to warrant intubation, electively or otherwise, it is best to mobilize a team of the most skilled physicians early in the event of unforeseen complications in attempting to gain control of the airway. Nonsurgical airway placement is recommended whenever possible, as it is less likely to interfere with the surgical field if esophageal repair is required.[204]

Subsequent assessment of heart rate and blood pressure will provide some information regarding the severity of the ingestion, and should be followed serially. Hypotension is a grave finding and often indicates perforation and significant blood loss. Intravenous fluids and assessment for operative intervention should be considered. The majority of adult patients, however, will fall into the category of significant injury without immediate life-threatening manifestations. Their assessment will subsequently require direct inspection of the esophagus via endoscopy, which is discussed later.

Should Gastric Decontamination Be Performed in Alkaline Ingestions?

The ability to decontaminate patients with alkaline ingestions is limited. Gastric emptying via blind passage of an orogastric or nasogastric tube carries the risk of perforation of damaged tissues and thus should be avoided. Activated charcoal is contraindicated, as it will interfere with tissue evaluation by endoscopy and preclude a subsequent management plan. Additionally, most caustics are not adsorbed to activated charcoal. Syrup of ipecac is also contraindicated, as it may cause reintroduction of the caustic agent to the upper gastrointestinal tract and airway.

What Is the Role of Dilutional Therapy?

The use of dilutional therapy has been examined in both in vitro and in vivo models. The theory behind dilution is to limit tissue contact with the caustic agent and potentially attenuate the damage incurred. The generation of heat and intraluminal pressure from the addition of a dilutional agent was also investigated in different models. Early in vitro models demonstrated a dramatic increase in temperature when either water or milk was added to crystal Drano or Clinitest tablets.[164] Another in vitro model of dilution found smaller changes in temperature and pH despite large volumes of diluent. It was suggested that dilution would have limited utility.[118] An in vivo canine model of alkaline injury demonstrated that water dilution did not cause an increase in either temperature or intraluminal pressures.[77] Alternatively, an ex vivo study of harvested rat esophagi examined the histopathologic effects of saline dilution after an alkali injury and found that damage occurred to tissue within seconds to minutes and was attended by an increase in temperature. The utility of dilution appeared to decrease as time from exposure lengthened, with minimal efficacy noted in as little as 30 minutes.[74,75] The extrapolation of these variable results to humans with caustic exposures may be limited, but many of these studies demonstrate that injuries of the gastrointestinal tract are almost instantaneous[7,101,184] and that histologic damage can only be attenuated by milk or water when administered within the first seconds to minutes of the ingestion.[74–77] For solid substances, such as crystal lye or Clinitest tablets, there may be some value for dilution later than for liquid caustics, because tissue contact time is increased with solid agents and their concentration is usually 100% over a small surface area. Milk may be the best agent with regard to its ability to attenuate the heat generated.[118] Caution should be used in advising patients or family members about the use of dilutional agents. A child who refuses to swallow or take oral liquids should not be forced to do so. There is concern about the airway, extent of damage, potential for nausea, abdominal distention, and vomiting that may worsen the injury. Though never explicitly studied, vomiting in these patients can lead to re-exposure to the caustic agent and should be avoided whenever possible.[164]

The use of milk or water should therefore be limited to patients within the first few minutes after exposure who readily accept liquids, have no airway compromise or vomiting, are alert, and not complaining of significant abdominal pain or nausea and who are old enough to speak.

What Is the Role of Neutralization Therapy for Alkaline Ingestions?

The basic theory behind neutralization is to alter the properties of the caustic agent before tissues incur injury. Even more than dilution, this technique has the potential to worsen tissue damage by forming gas and generating an exothermic reaction. In vitro and ex vivo models demonstrate that neutralization of caustics generates heat, requires large volume to attain a physiologic pH, and may have limited utility in preventing histologic damage after the first few minutes postexposure.[73,118,163] In an in vivo canine model, however, orange juice was used to neutralize sodium hydroxide-induced gastric injury and demonstrated no change in temperature or intraluminal pressure.[77] There is no in vivo evidence of an improvement in outcome with this technique. Extrapolation of these different findings to human exposures is limited, and more definitive evidence of the safety of neutralization therapy is needed before its use can be advocated.

What Is the Role of Endoscopy?

Endoscopy is a standard diagnostic tool in the management of caustic ingestions. The candidates for endoscopy include all patients with stridor once their airways have been stabilized, children with both vomiting and drooling (and potentially just one of these symptoms), adults with intentional ingestions, and any adult with an unintentional ingestion who manifests any symptomatology potentially related to the exposure, as this group has not been adequately studied. Patients who do not need endoscopy are asymptomatic children with unintentional ingestions, and those who meet criteria for immediate operative repair (discussed later). Patients should have the procedure performed within 12 hours, and preferably no later than 24 hours postingestion. Numerous case series demonstrate that the procedure is safe during this period; it offers a rapid means of obtaining diagnostic and treatment information, and shortens the period of time that patients forego nutritional support.[33,41,44,51,65,68,94,109,132,166,167,195,198,207] There is a period of wound softening beginning on the second or third day postinjury and lasting for roughly 2 weeks during which there is an increased risk of perforation if endoscopy is performed.

The choice of rigid versus flexible endoscopy is dependent on the comfort and experience of the endoscopist. The flexible endoscope has a smaller diameter but may require gentle insufflation of air for visualization. A prospective evaluation of fiberoptic endoscopy recommends the following guidelines for a safe approach: direct visualization of the esophagus prior to advancing the instrument, minimal insufflation of air, passage into the stomach unless there was a severe esophageal burn (particularly circumferential burns), and no retroversion or retroflexion of the instrument within the esophagus.[207] Adherence to this regimen should minimize the risk of iatrogenic perforation of the upper gastrointestinal tract. Most cases of perforation clearly linked to endoscopy have occurred when the endoscope was advanced through a severely eroded esophagus.[195] The advantage of visualization of the gastric mucosa has been demonstrated by several case reports of patients with minimal esophageal damage, yet severe necrosis and ulceration of the stomach, sometimes necessitating surgical resection.[132,181,192,207] Some authors advocate the presence of a surgeon during endoscopy to assist in the assessment for potential surgical intervention.[166]

How Are the Results of Endoscopy Used?

The extent of tissue injury will dictate the subsequent management and disposition of patients. Patients with isolated grade I injuries of the esophagus do not develop strictures and are not at increased risk of carcinoma. Their diet can be resumed as tolerated and they can potentially be discharged from the hospital once this diagnosis is established with endoscopy, they are able to eat and drink,[14,192] and their psychiatric status is defined as stable. If the endoscopy reveals grade IIa lesions of the esophagus and sparing of the stomach, a soft diet can be resumed as tolerated, or a nasogastric tube can be passed to provide interim enteral support. Patients with higher grades of injury must be followed for the complications of perforation, infection, and stricture. The metabolic demands of these burn patients increase significantly,[176] and oral intake may be poorly tolerated or contraindicated if there is a risk of perforation. For these patients feeding via gastrostomy or jejunostomy, or total parenteral nutrition, can be instituted as indicated. Patients with grade IIb lesions often develop strictures, and interventions such as corticosteroids and stents for lesional bypass can be entertained (see the later section on corticosteroids). One author recommends further division of grade III injuries into IIIa reflecting small areas of necrosis; and IIIb, as extensive necrosis.[207] In general, patients with grade III injuries progress to stricture formation that is not altered by corticosteroids. Severely injured tissue (grade IIIb) is at a high risk of complications including perforations and infections, which may be masked or worsened by corticosteroid therapy. This group needs close attention to several clinical parameters to aid in deciding on the need for surgery. Endoscopy can be used to follow the progress of patients provided they remain stable and other imaging procedures such as contrast radiography or computed tomography are used during the period of wound softening.

Patients with stricture formation require long-term endoscopic follow-up for the presence of neoplastic changes of the esophagus that may occur with a delay of several decades.[6]

There are several limitations to endoscopy. Significant circumferential burns to the esophagus may preclude the visualization of distal portions of the upper GI tract, which may contain more severe lesions. The evolution of caustic injury is a dynamic process, and although most endoscopies performed early give an adequate idea of the grading, continued tissue damage may occur. Perforations, in fact, often occur during the remodeling phase between days 7 and 14.[184] Additionally, it is an operator-dependent procedure in which distinguishing between a grade II and grade III injury can be difficult. The

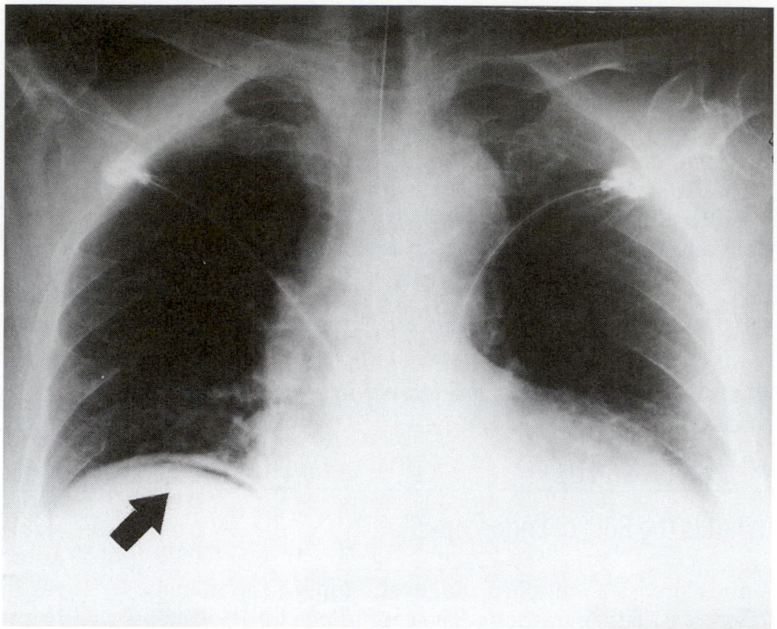

Figure 86–1. Chest radiograph demonstrating free air under the right hemidiaphragm. This patient ingested concentrated hydrochloric acid and had a perforated viscus. The patient required emergent laparotomy for repair. *(Courtesy of the New York City Poison Center Toxicology Fellowship.)*

endoscopist is only able to appreciate the mucosal surface, and not the serosal side, limiting the utility of the results. This is especially evident in stomach ulcerations, which may appear black and necrotic from a true burn through the layers of the stomach, or from the effect of stomach acid on the blood exposed from a shallower lesion. Only direct serosal inspection allows for the distinction, and in questionable circumstances surgical inspection will provide the definitive evaluation.

What Is the Role of Radiographic Investigations?

Both chest and abdominal radiographs can provide additional information in the initial stages of management only if radiographic findings are present (Fig. 86–1). Pneumomediastinum, pleural effusion, and pneumoperitoneum are indicators of viscus perforation. An upright lateral chest radiograph may be more sensitive than a postero-anterior film in detecting free peritoneal air.[203] In general, however, these studies have a low sensitivity, and an absence of radiographic findings does not preclude presence of perforations of the upper gastrointestinal tract.[204] Even contrast studies can fail to detect perforations,[78] but dye extravasation outside of the gastrointestinal tract is diagnostic when present.[208]

Contrast radiography does not give adequate information regarding the nature of lesions if used alone immediately postinjury. There may be some role for water-soluble contrast studies in patients with grade III injuries in which the presence of perforation is uncertain or where circumferential burns of the esophagus preclude visualization of the remainder of the upper GI tract.[54] Esophageal dilation, displacement of the pleural reflection, and widening of the pleuroesophageal line are suggestive of significant necrosis and impending perforation.[117] In general, the results should be interpreted within the context of the patient's clinical status, as the information can be unreliable.[18,35,65,78,117] There may be a role for computed tomography (CT), although the use of CT has yet to be investigated in acute caustic ingestions (Fig. 86–2).

The most valuable use of radiographic procedures is to noninvasively follow the patient once initial evaluation and stabilization have occurred. In a group of patients followed with serial contrast studies, radiographic findings included blurred esophageal margins or "scalloped and straightened margins," linear collections of contrast materials corresponding to intramural dissection and ulcers, retained contrast secondary to esophageal dysmotility, dilation of the esophagus, and displacement of the pleural reflection.[117] Esophageal narrowing develops later (Fig. 86–3).[117] This information can be utilized in management of patients, and one author recommends routine use of contrast radiography to follow patients postoperatively.[185]

Other radiographic studies recently reported in the management of patients with caustic ingestion include esophageal ultrasound to determine the depth of injury,[138] and chest contrast tomography of strictures to determine width as a potential indicator for response to dilation.[99]

What Is the Role of Corticosteroids?

Corticosteroid therapy for treatment of caustic injury was first investigated in animals in the 1950s. The theory was to arrest the process of inflammatory repair and potentially prevent stricture formation. Unfortunately, most animals died of overwhelming sepsis. When com-

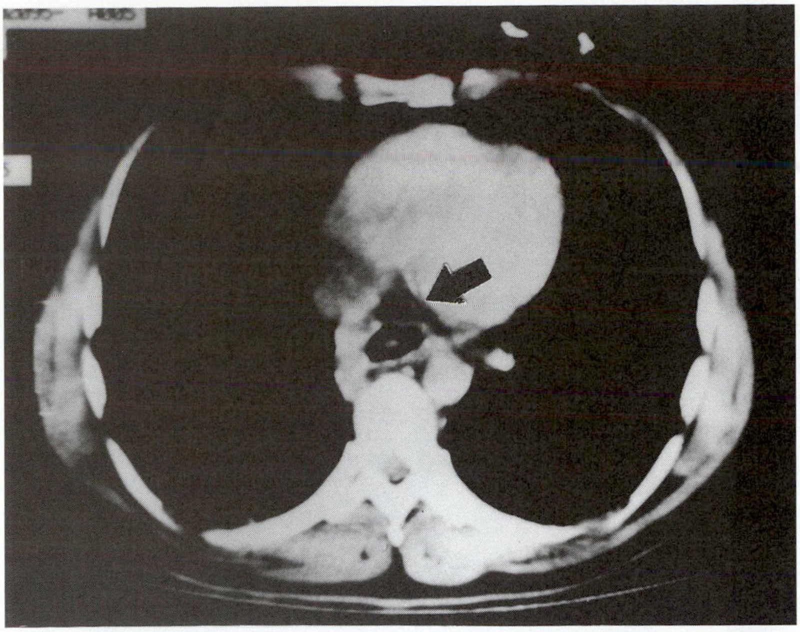

Figure 86–2. Computed tomograph of a patient who ingested an acid. This transverse view through the chest demonstrates mediastinal air (arrow) from a perforated esophagus that was not evident on plain radiographs. *(Courtesy of the New York City Poison Center Toxicology Fellowship.)*

bined with antibiotic therapy, the death rate diminished.[161]

Adequate human data demonstrating the efficacy of corticosteroids with or without antibiotics has yet to be generated. There are a multitude of case series that use different criteria for the institution of corticosteroid and antibiotic therapy. Most of these are retrospective and do not differentiate the outcome of second and third-degree lesions. First-degree burns of the esophagus do not progress to stricture formation, and as such would not be expected to benefit from corticosteroid therapy.[4,35,79,133,135,166,195] Third-degree burns as described in different studies have variable definitions, and there is some evidence that they may progress to stricture regardless of therapy.[4,69,133,195] Third-degree burns also have a high degree of complications including fistula formation, infection, and perforation. Corticosteroids may mask infection and make the friable, necrotic tissue more prone to perforation. A meta-analysis of the efficacy of corticosteroid therapy in 361 patients with caustic injury found that there is no role for corticosteroids in first-degree burns.[79] For patients with second and third-degree burns, strictures formed in 24% of the corticosteroid-treated group and 52% of the untreated group. The authors concluded that prospective trials are necessary to better define the role of corticosteroids in caustic injury.[79] The only prospective, randomized study of corticosteroid efficacy for caustic injury of the esophagus spanned an 18-year period during which a total of only 60 children could be randomized to corticosteroid therapy plus antibiotics or no corticosteroid therapy. In this study, third-degree burns were distinguished from second degree by their circumferential pattern. The incidence of stricture was not different between the treated and untreated groups, and it appeared that the circumferential burns were more likely to develop strictures than the ulcerative noncircumferential lesions.[4] Although the study failed to have the power to detect a meaningful difference in the treatment and nontreatment groups, no other study has prospectively enrolled sufficient patients to answer the question of corticosteroid efficacy. If corticosteroids are employed, the appropriate dose is 2 mg/kg per day of prednisolone or its equivalent in children, and methylprednisolone 40 mg every 8 hours in adults. The course of therapy is 14 to 21 days followed by a corticosteroid taper. Concomitant antibiotic therapy is indicated once corticosteroids are begun. The antibiotic chosen should treat oral flora, including anaerobic bacteria. Intravenous penicillin, ampicillin, or clindamycin are appropriate for infectious prophylaxis.

What Is the Role of Antibiotics?

There is some evidence that the tissue disruption caused by caustic agents can provide a pathway for infection deep to the mucosa, even in the absence of a clinical perforation.[66,161] The use of antibiotics is routinely advocated for patients receiving corticosteroids, as it lowers the risk of infection that attends corticosteroid use. No major outcome studies have investigated the use of antibiotics alone as prophylactic treatment for stricture or burns, although some case series include antibiotics in the therapeutic regimen. The tissue turnover caused by caustic burns is high and the risk of perforation or softening of the mucosa rises between 7 and 14 days postingestion. Fever and infection may indicate a potential or impending perforation and may be masked by the prophylactic use of antibiotics alone. It is probably best to reserve antibiotics for an identified source of infection unless corticosteroids are being employed as therapy.

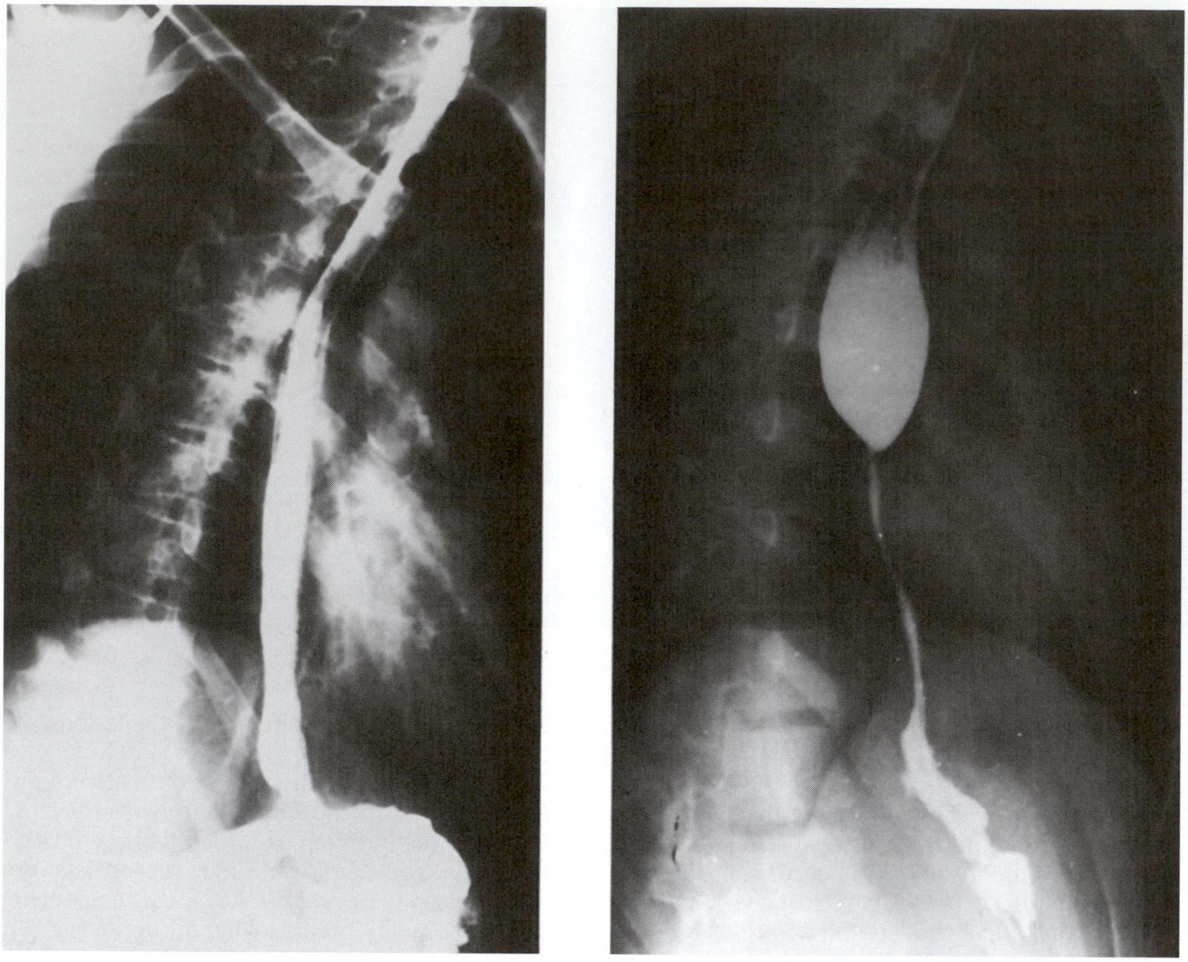

Figure 86–3. **(A)** Barium swallow several days after ingestion of liquid lye shows the esophagus to be atonic. There is poor coating of the esophagus, suggesting edema and intramural penetration. Note that the initial evaluation immediately following a caustic ingestion to assess the extent of injury is esophagoscopy, rather than a contrast esophagram. **(B)** Four months later, a repeat barium esophagram shows a severe stricture below the middle third of the esophagus. The barium barely passes the stricture and the remainder of the esophagus is pencil thin. *(Courtesy of Emil J. Balthazar, MD, Professor of Radiology, New York University.)*

How Do Acid Ingestions Differ from Alkaline Ingestions?

Acid ingestions differ histologically from alkaline ingestions. A cat model of the effects of sulfuric acid on the esophagus revealed a coagulative necrosis of the mucosa with whitish discoloration of the tissues and underlying smooth muscle spasm.[7] On gross inspection an inflammatory response ensues,[119] and edema, mucosal sloughing, motility dysfunction, and esophageal shortening are demonstrated in animal models.[172,175] The subsequent burns incurred are not unlike those seen with alkaline ingestion. Acid ingestions frequently give rise to gastric damage with pooling of the agent in the antrum probably secondary to pylorospasm.[32,39,44,45,63,78,89,99,119,139,179,180,200,207] In most series, both the gastric and esophageal mucosa are equally affected.[45,78,208] On occasion, the esophagus may be spared damage while severe injury is noted in the stomach (see Color Plate Fig. 24).[39,63,69,181] This tends to be a rarer finding than concomitant injury to both stomach and esophagus, and is probably related to the rapid transit time of liquid acids through the upper gastrointestinal tract. Skip lesions from acid ingestions may be a function of viscosity and contact time.[69]

Following ingestion, acids can rapidly traverse the stomach mucosa and cause systemic acidemia. Hydrochloric acid ingestions may result in a non-anion gap metabolic acidosis, as both the hydrogen and chloride ions dissociate in the serum and are both accounted for in the measurement of the anion gap. Other acids, such as sulfuric acid, may also be absorbed and precipitate a rapid anion gap metabolic acidosis as the anion, sulfate (SO_4^{-2}), in this case is not directly measured in the calculation of the anion gap.

In addition, acids tend to disproportionally damage extraintestinal organs such as the spleen, biliary tract, and pancreas due to the penetrating characteristics of these agents.[29,74,193,197]

In general, patients who have ingested acid have similar initial presentation as those who have ingested alkalis, consisting largely of chest and abdominal pain, vomiting, and respiratory distress. Management is also similar. The airway should be evaluated immediately. There may be a role for water or milk dilution early after the ingestion with the same caveats as those described for alkaline agents.[75] Syrup of ipecac and activated charcoal should be avoided. In patients with large intentional ingestions of acid who present within 30 minutes, some consideration can be given to gentle placement of narrow nasogastric tube suction to remove remaining acid in the gut.[149] This technique has never been studied, and although there is a risk of perforation, the outcome for these patients is often grave and options for treatment limited. Therefore early, cautious removal of some portion of the ingested material may have potential benefit.

Patients with severe acid injuries may lack abdominal pain, abdominal tenderness on examination, and radiographic findings.[45,78,208] Due to the systemic effects of acids, a depressed mental status, a serum pH below 7.20, and a shock index (pulse to systolic blood pressure ratio) greater than 1 seem to be predictors of poor outcome due to extensive injury.[78] Large-volume ingestions ranging between 40 and 200 mL and a delay in surgical repair are also associated with increased mortality.[45,78,204]

Endoscopy must visualize the entire gastric mucosa except in those patients who have clinical evidence for immediate surgical intervention. The tissue damage can be graded using the same scale applied to alkaline burns.[45,119,208] A depressed mental status, unstable vital signs, or acidemia are grave findings, and these patients should be considered for emergent surgical intervention. The role of corticosteroids is unproved, but they should be used in conjunction with antibiotics as these patients are at risk for overwhelming sepsis.[157] Patients may benefit from nutritional support via jejunostomy tube or TPN.[44,45,208]

Clinically, patients who ingest acids experience a wide variety of complications comparable to those who ingest alkalis, including airway compromise and stricture formation. Acid injuries also predispose to gastric atony, decreased acid secretion, pseudodiverticuli, and gastric outlet obstruction that presents several weeks postingestion.[28,59,89,144,179,208] The subsequent risk of carcinoma is not adequately studied in this population, but three cases of squamous cell cancer of the stomach (a rare form of stomach cancer) are described in patients with prior history of acid ingestion.[48] It is suggested that this may arise from a downgrowth of esophageal tissue into the gastric mucosa during repair. Long-term studies are required to determine the risk of neoplasm after acid ingestion.

What Is the Role of Surgery in Patients Who Ingest Caustic Agents?

The decision to perform emergent surgery for patients with caustic ingestions is most obvious in those who have evidence of perforation either on endoscopic examination or radiographic studies, severe abdominal rigidity, or hypotension. Many patients, however, will not have such evidence, and yet may be in grave danger of perforation, necrosis, sepsis, or delayed hemorrhage during recovery, all of which may be avoided if surgery is performed early in the management.[143] Identifying these patients in a timely fashion is challenging. Some studies demonstrate increased morbidity and mortality for patients who have delayed surgical repair.[51,78,81,157,166] In some cases these patients may not have manifested evidence of significant tissue damage earlier in their clinical course and the parameters utilized for surgical intervention were variable.[78,166,204] Surgical intervention can include laparotomy for inspection and resection or repair of perforations; or possibly laparoscopy for tissue visualization, although this may not allow inspection of posterior portions of the stomach. Gastrostomy or enterostomy can be performed to provide a nutritional conduit. Delayed surgery is also used for stricture repair and repair of gastric outlet obstruction.

Endoscopy may provide some useful information in otherwise hemodynamically stable patients. Some surgeons advocate laparotomy for all patients with second- and third-degree burns of the esophagus.[51,132] This aggressive approach allows for direct inspection of serosal surfaces and an opportunity for repair.[51,132]

Several retrospective and prospective series of surgical patients with caustic ingestions have found that patients with large ingestions of caustics (greater than 150 mL), shock, agitation, acidemia, or coagulation disorders tend to have severe findings on surgical exploration. The abdominal examination was frequently unreliable.[166,204,208]

Dilation of the esophageal margins on chest radiograph may herald an impending perforation[117] that can be addressed surgically, but the absence of this finding does not preclude severe esophageal injury. Contrast radiographs may be employed in these cases, and water-soluble contrast is recommended as it is less irritating to tissues in cases of perforation.[54] Computed tomography may become a more valuable tool early in the management of patients in whom the need for surgery is unclear.

One author utilized a stepwise approach of bronchoscopy, endoscopy, and abdominal sonography to provide additional information regarding extent of injury prior to surgery. Hemoglobinuria, respiratory distress, ascites, pleural fluid, and a serum pH below 7.2 were used as indications for surgery.[204]

It is clear that no single criterion can determine which patients without obvious perforation require surgery. Serial clinical evaluation of mental status, vital signs, acid–base status, radiographs, coagulation studies, history of massive or intentional ingestions, and type of caustic agent may collectively aid in the decision to operate. A timely decision for those patients who need surgery appears to improve outcome following acid ingestions[31] and it is likely that the same holds true for alkaline ingestions.

Are Lathryogens Indicated?

The natural repair of tissue causes collagen production, which increases scar formation and can ultimately result in stricture formation. Lathyrogens such as beta-amino proprionitrile (BAPN), penicillamine, and other agents such as *N*-acetylcysteine (NAC) and colchicine interfere with collagen synthesis and/or breakdown. These agents have been examined as treatment for the prevention of strictures in various animal models. Colchicine, which increases collagen synthesis but also increases collagenase activity, did not prevent stricture formation in rabbits with sodium hydroxide-induced esophageal burns.[186] Both penicillamine and NAC were of some benefit in preventing strictures in rats and rabbits.[57,108,186] BAPN was examined in a dog model in conjunction with dilation, and there was some suggestion that it was useful.[113] More recently, rats treated with epidermal growth factor and interferon gamma had decreased collagen production and stenosis following sodium hydroxide burns.[13]

All of these modalities are still experimental for the treatment of caustic burns, and their routine use is not advocated in human exposures at this time.

How Are Strictures Managed?

Stricture formation is a debilitating complication of both acid and alkaline ingestions that can evolve over a period of weeks or months (Fig. 86–3). A variety of management strategies have been used in an attempt to prevent strictures or to minimize the sequelae of esophageal obstruction. The placement of intraluminal stents and nasogastric tubes may have some potential benefit.[134,198] Both animal models[155] and human case series[71,134,154] report the use of silicone rubber tubing to maintain the patency of the esophageal lumen. The stent is placed via direct visualization and attached to a feeding tube secured in the nasopharynx. The internal diameter is $\frac{3}{8}$ of an inch in adults and $\frac{1}{4}$ inch in children, allowing the patient to receive feedings through the stent without interference in esophageal repair. The device is left in place for 3 weeks,[154,155] and these patients are given corticosteroids as well as antibiotics. Outcomes are variable in the prevention of strictures. In animal models, the use of a stent for 3 weeks appears to be superior in maintaining patency to corticosteroids with antibiotics alone.[155] The potential disadvantage is the concomitant mechanical trauma of the stent or tube at the site, and the potential for increased reflux, which may inhibit repair.[175] A cat model of stented sodium hydroxide burns also reported deaths from aspiration and mediastinitis.[155] Large series of human exposures managed with stents and corticosteroids are lacking.

The more common approach is endoscopic dilation, which is usually done over a wire with a device designed for esophageal dilation. There are a variety of types of dilators, and generally, multiple dilations are required. The safest time for dilation is after confirmation of stricture formation and after acute repair of the esophagus has taken place so that the risk of perforation is decreased. This is usually no earlier than 4 weeks postingestion. Contrast CT can be utilized to determine maximal esophageal wall thickness as a predictor of response to dilation.[99] In one study, patients with a maximal esophageal wall thickness of 9 mm or greater required more than seven sessions to achieve adequate dilation. This was significantly higher than in patients with a smaller maximal wall thickness.[99] Measurement of maximal wall thickness may be useful in determining the long-term follow-up, type of nutritional support, and potential need for surgical repair as an alternative to dilations. It may also provide an indication for those who should undergo dilations under fluoroscopy to limit the risk of perforation.

The risks of perforation from dilation has been well reported in several series.[69,86,99,152,195] Following perforation, patients may complain of dyspnea or chest pain and may have subcutaneous emphysema or pneumomediastinum. A CT scan or contrast radiograph may identify the perforation and provide information for emergent surgical repair if the diagnosis is unclear.[99,152]

What Other Household Agents Are Caustic?

Clinitest Tablets

Clinitest tablets are used to test for glucosuria by directly adding the tablet to the urine. The reagent contains copper sulfate, sodium carbonate, sodium hydroxide, and citric acid. In the presence of glucose and moisture, cupric sulfate is converted to cupric oxide, inducing a detectable color change in the urine and releasing carbon dioxide and heat.[24,98,145] Unfortunately, this tablet formulation can be easily misinterpreted as an oral medication and can be ingested unintentionally or in an attempted suicide with the potential for severe alkaline caustic injury. As the tablet takes minutes to dissolve, the tissue destruction incurred is generally well localized, especially if minimal fluid is ingested and the tablet is lodged in the upper gastrointestinal tract. The range of reported toxicity is highly variable. One patient who swallowed at least 47 tablets over several days secondary to misunderstanding the use of the pills had relatively benign findings and outcome,[114] yet unintentional ingestion of just one pill has also resulted in death from an aortoesophageal fistula induced by the burn.[143] Single tablet ingestions in children frequently result in stricture formation perhaps because they are often consumed without fluids.[24,58,147] Gastroduodenal ulcers are also reported.[36,194]

Patients can present with vomiting, chest and abdominal pain, and, rarely oral lesions, which are unreliable indicators of the severity of exposure.[114,145] A case of fatal laryngeal edema was reported.[114] Management of these injuries is similar to those caused by other caustic alkaline agents. The airway should be quickly assessed. Dilutional therapy should be considered in an attempt to decrease the local concentration of the caustic components. An in vitro study noted that the heat released on contact with water is increased when less water is present, or when the number of tablets in solution is increased. Orange juice appeared to minimize the pH elevation of the resulting solution most efficaciously.[98] An extrapolation of these results would warrant at least cold tap water dilution, and, if possible cold orange juice only if the patient is alert and can tolerate fluids. Subsequent management includes endoscopic evaluation of the upper gastrointestinal tract. Fortunately Clinitest use has decreased dramatically since safer glucose testing of capillary blood has become more widely available.

Is Ammonia Ingestion Dangerous?

Ammonia products are weak bases that can cause significant esophageal burns depending on the concentration and volume ingested.[14,69,166,181,184] Household ammonium hydroxide ranges in concentration from 3 to 10%. Management of these patients should proceed similarly to other alkaline ingestions. Strictures have evolved in patients who ingested 28% ammonia solutions.[142]

How Safe Is Exposure to Bleach?

Sodium hypochlorite is the major component in most industrial and household bleach preparations. Large case series and reports have found that grade II and grade III injuries occur only in patients with large-volume ingestions of concentrated bleach products.[44] A series of 393 household bleach ingestions reported no stricture formation,[100] and a canine model found that although regurgitation was a common effect of bleach, no esophageal lesions were noted, and perforation only occurred with prolonged contact.[100] Most patients do well with supportive care.[14,33,69,180] Patients who complain of pain or who have either high-concentration or high-volume ingestions should have endoscopic evaluation of the esophagus, as there is little data regarding these severe exposures.

What Are the Consequences of Phenol Exposure?

Phenols have historically been used as antiseptic agents and are currently present in household cleaning agents and disinfectants in 2 to 5% solutions.[80] Phenolic compounds are strongly acidic agents that can induce severe dermal and mucosal injury. The acidity attributed to phenols is not from the ability to donate protons, but rather the ability to accept an electron pair to form a covalent bond. The aromatic ring in phenol confers a property known as resonance stabilization, which allows the electron pair to reside at different sites on the molecule. As such the potential energy in the compound can cause caustic injury including liquefactive necrosis. Phenols are insoluble in water, and irrigation with water can potentially increase tissue penetration. If water is the only irrigant immediately available for dermal burns, it can be employed, preferably with soap, and then followed by low molecular weight polyethylene glycol (PEG) solution or isopropyl alcohol when available.[80,137,177] Oral ingestion of phenol has caused significant esophageal burns.[10,14,177] Concentrated phenol ingestion has resulted in coma and severe acidosis, most likely from tissue destruction.[10] One retrospective study found that patients presented with cough, vomiting, a change in urine color to dark green, stridor, and in 3 cases, coma of rapid onset.[177] Endoscopy and supportive care are recommended.

Are Detergents Caustic?

Household detergents contain silicates, carbonates, and phosphates and can potentially induce caustic burns and strictures even when ingested unintentionally.[34,181] Airway compromise can occur,[34,49,115] but the majority of unintentional exposures result in minor toxicity.[93] These agents are frequently present in laundry powders and automatic dishwashing detergents.

Cationic detergents include quinilinium compounds, pyridinium compounds, and quarternary ammonium agents. These are frequently found in products for industrial use as well as household fabric softeners. A concentration of greater than 7.5% of the agent can cause severe burns.[110] These agents bind well to activated charcoal[110]; however, because no large series has been evaluated with this therapy, all patients with symptoms or signs of caustic injury, intentional ingestions, or exposures to concentrations greater than 7.5% should be evaluated endoscopically and activated charcoal should be avoided.[110]

Are Exposures to Zinc Chloride and Mercuric Chloride Managed Differently?

Zinc chloride ($ZnCl_2$) and mercuric chloride ($HgCl_2$) are corrosive agents with severe systemic toxicity.[30,128,129,150] Ingestion of these substances causes life-threatening illness from heavy metal exposure. The local corrosive effects, though of great concern, are less consequential than the manifestations of systemic absorption. For this reason, aggressive decontamination with gentle nasogastric tube aspiration, and placement of activated charcoal, serve as primary gestures in the initial management of patients with these ingestions, as there is some in vitro data to suggest adequate charcoal binding.[3] Some of these patients will also require chelation therapy (see Chaps. 80 and 81). The local effects of these agents can be managed supportively and directly assessed once systemic absorption has been prevented or treated.

How Are Ophthalmic Exposures to Caustic Agents Managed?

Ophthalmic exposures to caustic agents frequently occur from splash injuries, and more recently, the alkaline byproducts of sodium azide release in automobile airbag deployment.[196] The mainstay of therapy for these patients is immediate irrigation of the eye for a minimum of 15 minutes with normal saline, lactated Ringer's solution, or tap water, if it is the only agent available. Acid exposures can be severe, but the tissue damage is usually self-limited once irrigation has been completed, as the coagulative necrosis tends to prevent further penetration into deeper layers of the eye. Alkaline injuries are of considerable concern as the liquefactive necrosis and saponification of the tissue allows for deep penetration of the substance. Several liters of irrigation fluid are recommended for these patients. The normal pH of ophthalmic secretions is close to 7.4. This can be tested colorimetrically using a urine dipstick, which can test a range of pH from 5 to 9 using a color chart.[130] Litmus paper can be utilized in the same fashion. Another option is nitrazine paper, which changes color from yellow to dark blue at a pH above 6.5,[55] and may be especially useful in acid exposures. These different test strips can be applied to the ocular secretions to test the baseline pH, and followed with intermittent evaluations after 15 minutes to determine the adequacy of irrigation. If these agents are not readily available, irrigation should not be delayed, as the depth of penetration of the caustic agent can determine outcome. Anterior chamber irrigation may be required and is performed emergently by an ophthalmologist. A thorough eye examination should be completed and follow-up should be arranged (see Chap. 26).

How Is Hydrofluoric Acid Different from Other Caustics?

Hydrofluoric acid (HF) has unique properties that can cause life-threatening complications following seemingly trivial exposure. The less common anhydrous form is greater than 99% hydrofluoric acid and used almost exclusively for industrial purposes. More common, in both industry and household products, is the aqueous form of HF, which generally ranges in concentrations from 3 to 70%. Hydrofluoric acid is used for glass etching, brick cleaning, etching chips in the semiconductor industry, electroplating, leather tanning, rust removal, and the cleaning of porcelain.[43,85]

Hydrofluoric acid is formed as the product of gaseous sulfuric acid and calcium fluoride, which is subsequently cooled to a liquid.[111] The pKa of aqueous HF is 3.5×10^{-4}, behaving in part as a weak acid. As such, it is roughly one thousand times less dissociated than equimolar hydrochloric acid. A permeability coefficient of $1.4 \times {}^{10-4}$ cm/sec allows it to penetrate deeply into tissues prior to dissociating into hydrogen ions and highly electronegative fluoride ions.[64] These fluoride ions avidly bind to intracellular stores of calcium and magnesium, ultimately leading to cellular dysfunction and cell death.[16,104,123]

There are several theories regarding the fate of the calcium and fluoride ions in the tissues. Formation of insoluble calcium fluoride is proposed as the etiology for the precipitous fall in serum calcium and the severe pain associated with tissue toxicity. There is also some in vitro evidence that fluorapatite [$3(Ca_3(PO_4)_2Ca(F_2)$] is formed in the presence of phosphate and hydroxyapatite and may be a more likely pathway for deposition of the fluoride ion.[16]

Exposures to hydrofluoric acid occur via dermal, ocular, inhalation, and oral routes with one reported case of toxicity from an HF enema.[25] The extent of tissue injury in dermal exposures is determined by the volume, concentration, and contact time with the tissues. Fatal dermal exposures are reported from burns of 2.5% body surface area with exposure to 100% (anhydrous) HF.[183] Because of the ability of HF to penetrate tissues, systemic toxicity can occur via any route, and this poses a greater threat to the patient than local injury if not rapidly decontaminated and treated.[17,22,62,165,171,187,188] The natural history of these fatal exposures shares the similar features of hypocalcemia, hypomagnesemia, and in most cases, hyperkalemia as preterminal events.[8,19,62,97,111,116,125,126,183] In some circumstances the hypocalcemia is so severe that the coagulation cascade is disrupted and patients are noted to be coagulopathic on postmortem examination.[116,127,131] Patients who die invariably do so from sudden-onset myocardial conduction failure and ventricular fibrillation. The evidence regarding the mechanism of myocardial irritability is variable. Some postmortem cases reveal significant myocardial injury.[127] These findings are inconsistently encountered in humans, but dog studies in which animals die of cardiac arrest have not demonstrated any histologic abnormalities of the myocardium.[40,122] Most theories regarding myocardial irritability relate to the hypocalcemia causing an efflux of potassium ions into the extracellular space.[40,104,127] The subsequent hyperkalemia may alter the automaticity and resting potential of the heart, making it more prone to fatal dysrhythmias.[126] Dogs treated with quinidine, a potassium efflux blocker, seem to be protected from fatal doses of intravenous sodium fluoride.[40] However, the mechanism of toxicity may be much more complicated.[205] A child with systemic fluoride toxicity, who was appropriately repleted with calcium, and who had reportedly "normal electrolytes" still experienced ventricular fibrillation and was successfully resuscitated. Perhaps this is because serum potassium levels only partly represent levels near the tissues.[16,17,40,125,126]

How Is the Severity of the Hydrofluoric Acid Exposure Assessed?

Not all exposures to HF are fatal; in fact, the vast majority of exposures are to the surfaces of fingertips with low concentrations of the agent. Most household rust removal products have concentrations ranging between 6 and 12%, and the time to evolution of pain at the site of contact may be delayed as long as 24 hours.[191] These presentations are much less likely to result in life-threatening systemic toxicity. Determining which exposures are life threatening can be achieved by following certain historical and clinical features of an exposure. All oral ingestions and inhalational exposures should be considered potentially fatal, as well as burns of the face and neck regardless of HF concentration. Concentrations of greater than 20% HF are worrisome irrespective of the surface area exposed. As a general rule, patients who experience severe pain within minutes of contact are most likely exposed to a very high concentration of HF and can deteriorate rapidly. An otherwise well-appearing patient may have a precipitous demise without any clinical manifestations of hypocalcemia. In some reported cases, this may be because these findings were not sought, and in others, the signs did not exist, despite a very low serum calcium. Other cases report carpal spasm and Chvostek's sign.[62,165] Electrocardiographic findings of both hypocalcemia (prolonged QT) and hyperkalemia (peaked T wave) found both in human case reports and dog studies may be more reliable.[8,22,62,131,144,183]

What Is the Presentation and Management of Patients With Hydrofluoric Acid Exposure?

For all types of exposures, the mainstay of management is to prevent systemic absorption, assess for systemic toxicity, and aggressively correcting any electrolyte imbalances. To prevent absorption from dermal, oral, or inhalational routes, a solution of calcium or magnesium salt is delivered to the affected area to prevent HF penetration and provide an alternative source of cations for the damaging electronegative fluoride ions. Intravenous access should be obtained. An ECG should be examined for signs of hypocalcemia and hyperkalemia, and serum levels of these electrolytes should be obtained.

If there is a clinical suspicion of severe toxicity by the parameters described, the immediate administration of calcium and magnesium is recommended. Intravenous preparations of calcium are available in two forms. Ten percent calcium gluconate contains 0.45 mEq/mL and comes in 10-mL vials of 1 g/vial. It can safely be administered in a peripheral line at 1 g over 5 minutes, or by rapid intravenous push if the patient suddenly deteriorates. Calcium chloride contains 1.36 mEq/mL of solution. It is also available in 10-mL vials of 1 g each. It is considerably more irritating to the tissues and may be more appropriately administered through a central venous access site (see Antidotes in Depth: Calcium). Patients can require several grams of calcium to treat HF toxicity.[62,178] Intravenous magnesium can be administered to adults as 20 mL of a 20% solution (4 g) over 20 minutes. An approach of using both intravenous calcium, magnesium, and calcium or magnesium gels locally to prevent absorption may protect against life-threatening hypocalcemia. Ionized calcium should be monitored serially along with magnesium and potassium.[62] Serial screening with both the electrocardiogram and physical examination can help to guide the aggressiveness of therapy. Additional information may be obtained from an arterial blood gas analysis. As systemic toxicity progresses, there is potential for development of metabolic acidosis.[16] An animal model of hydrogen fluoride toxicity found that maintaining a normal acid–base balance was protective against HF toxicity,[156] hence it may be beneficial to correct any significant acidemia with hydration and intravenous sodium bicarbonate. This may simultaneously protect against life-threatening hyperkalemia.

A Foley catheter should be placed to follow urine output as most of the fluoride ions are eliminated renally.[12,82,92,165] If renal function is compromised, then hemodialysis should be considered in the patient with severe HF poisoning. There is one reported case of successful clearance of fluoride ions via hemodialysis.[12] The clearance rate, however, was not significantly different than that of normally functioning kidneys and therefore is not recommended in cases in which renal function is preserved. The use of quinidine, though protective in dogs,[127] has not been studied or utilized in humans and would not be considered appropriate treatment for severe HF poisoning at this time.

For patients dying from overwhelming dermal exposure, both the intravenous calcium and magnesium treatment described, and local decontamination should occur simultaneously. This can be achieved by the topical application of a calcium containing gel, or by intradermal injections of calcium, which is described later. There is a case report of a woman dying from severe HF toxicity with multiple manifestations of systemic toxicity, who was treated surgically with amputation of the affected limb and subsequently survived. Though not routinely recommended, this may be an alternative measure for patients not responding adequately to all other therapeutic modalities.[21,91]

Are There Special Airway Concerns for Patients Exposed to Hydrofluoric Acid?

Rapid airway assessment and protection should occur early in patients with potential inhalation, respiratory distress, or burns significant enough to cause a change of mental status. Inhalational exposure should be assumed for all skin burns with a body surface area greater than 5%, soaked clothing, HF concentration greater than 50%, and head and neck burns.[84] Inhaled hydrogen fluoride is a particular risk with concentrations greater than 60 or 70%. The inhalational effects of HF studied in rats demonstrate that most of the HF is absorbed from the proximal upper airways.[136] It is unclear if these data can be extrapolated to humans. Thirteen oil refinery workers exposed to low-concentration hydrofluoric acid mist experienced, at most, minor upper respiratory tract irritation.[102] Alternatively, in a mass exposure to HF in a community in Texas, throat burning and shortness of breath were among the common chief complaints. Some patients showed evidence of altered pulmonary function tests and hypoxemia on arterial blood gas analysis. Sixteen percent of patients had hypocalcemia from the gaseous exposure. Stridor, wheezing, and rhonchi were described on the physical examinations of these patients as well as erythema and ulcers of the upper respiratory tract. Eye pain was another complaint noted with these patients and it can occur simultaneously with gaseous HF exposure.[102,121,136,160,202] Patients with inhalational injuries can be treated with nebulized calcium gluconate. A report of patients exposed to a low concentration of HF and treated with 4 mL of a 2.5% nebulized solution demonstrated no adverse effects to treatment.[102] All patients who inhaled HF should have intravenous access, serial ECG monitoring, physical examination, and serum calcium, magnesium, and potassium levels to assess for systemic toxicity.

How Should Hydrofluroic Acid Ingestions Be Managed?

Intentional ingestion of concentrated hydrofluoric acid (or NaF, which results in the formation of HF when mixed with stomach acid) causes significant gastritis while sparing the remainder of the GI tract. Systemic absorption is rapid and usually fatal. There is even one case report of a patient with an ingestion of a low concentration of HF resulting in survival to discharge despite multiple episodes of ventricular fibrillation.[178] Patients who survive to reach the hospital may present with vomiting or depressed mental status and are at risk for airway compromise.[19,105,116,178] Gastrointestinal decontamination of patients with intentional ingestion of hydrofluoric acid should proceed with gastric emptying via nasogastric tube as these exposures are almost universally fatal.[8,19,116,131] Because aqueous hydrofluoric acid is a weak acid, the risk of perforation by passage of a nasogastric tube is significantly lower than the risk of death from systemic absorption.[8,116] It may be that in the acidic environment of the stomach, more of the weak acid solution remains less ionized, penetrating the gastric mucosa and causing rapid systemic poisoning. Oral calcium or magnesium-containing solution should be delivered to the stomach as soon as gastric emptying has been completed. Magnesium citrate (standard cathartic dose), magnesium sulfate, or any of the calcium solutions can be administered orally to prevent absorption. There have been no controlled trials of this therapy in animals or humans, but there may be a potential benefit in limiting absorption of HF. These patients should be assessed for systemic HF poisoning.

How Should Ophthalmic Exposure to Hydrofluoric Acid Be Managed?

Ocular exposures from liquid splashes or HF gas result in pain, corneal opacification, sloughing of the cornea, revascularization, and sometimes keratoconjunctivitis sicca (dry eye) as a long-term complication.[11,124,162] Patients with ocular exposures should receive vigorous irrigation of 1 L of normal saline, lactated Ringer's or water to the affected eye.[124] Although there are limited data, repetitive irrigation is described as causing a worsened outcome.[120] A complete ophthalmic examination should be performed once the patient is deemed stable, and an ophthalmic consultation should be obtained. One case report demonstrated a good outcome of ocular HF exposure with the use of 1% calcium gluconate eye drops.[11] This has yet to be adequately studied and is not indicated at this time. There is no role for gel therapy or intraocular injection in these patients as most calcium and magnesium preparations are potentially toxic to ocular tissues and may actually worsen outcome.[124]

What Is the Presentation and Management of Dermal Hydrofluoric Acid Exposure?

The skin is most readily contaminated, and most frequently affected, especially the digits. Often in dermal exposure, the higher the concentration, the sooner the onset of excruciating pain at the site of contact.[50,111,183] For household products there is often a delay of several hours before patients develop pain.[50,173,190,191] The initial site may appear benign despite the complaints of the patient. Over time the tissue may become hyperemic, with subsequent blanching with whitish discoloration and coagulative necrosis of the tissue as calcium is precipitated.[141] Ulcerations may form at a rate dependent on the concentration and duration of contact (see Color Plate Fig. 12).[43,87,112]

Most important for skin exposures is rapid removal of clothing and irrigation of the affected area with copious amounts of water or saline, whichever is more readily available.[5,92,103,112] For high-concentration HF or a more than 5% body surface area burn, electrocardiographic monitoring and large-bore intravenous access should be established, and laboratory studies sent for calcium, magnesium, serum electrolytes, type, crossmatch, and coagulation profiles. This should be followed by the application of a topical calcium gel to the affected area, which can be prepared by mixing 3.5 g of calcium gluconate powder in 5 ounces of sterile water soluble lubricant, or 25 mL of 10% calcium gluconate in 75 mL of sterile water-soluble lubricant.[5,23,84] If calcium gluconate is unavailable, calcium chloride or calcium carbonate can be utilized in a similar formulation.[29] If none of these are available, a sterile magnesium solution (3.48 g of magnesium gluconate in 5 ounces lubricating jelly) has also demonstrated some efficacy in the treatment of HF burns.[23] Topical therapy for both severe and non-life-threatening exposures may scavenge the fluoride ions prior to dermal penetration. An animal study examining the efficacy and mechanism of topical calcium gel therapy found the fluoride ion concentration of the gel significantly higher than in the non-calcium-containing gel controls. Though a limited study, these animals also had a decrease in urinary fluoride ion concentration compared to controls, suggesting less overall absorption of the HF into the tissues.[92] Quarternary ammonium compounds, such as topical benzalkonium chloride, have also been advocated in the treatment of HF burns and can be utilized when available[112]; however, calcium-containing gels appear to be more efficacious.

Intradermal injection of calcium and magnesium salts and intravenous infusions of magnesium may also be therapeutic. Their use is discussed in the next section.

How Should Hydrofluoric Acid Hand Injuries Be Treated?

Hand exposures are by far the most common presentation of hydrofluoric acid exposure. There are several options for therapy that have been studied and described in animal models for treatment of topical HF burns. Unfortunately, many study designs use histologic or subjective wound inspection as outcome parameters,[23,146] some with unblinded inspection.[20,47,91,92] These animal models do not address the parameters of pain reduction, cosmesis, and functionality that are important clinically. There are four types of therapies that have had variable success in human exposures. These include the application of calcium via topical, intradermal, intravenous, and intra-arterial routes.

The first step in management of digital hydrofluoric acid burns is irrigation. Thereafter, a gel solution of calcium carbonate or gluconate can be mixed directly into a sterile surgical glove and then placed onto the patients hand for 30 minutes. Two case series report limited success with this therapy.[5,29] Some patients describe prompt and dramatic relief of pain within minutes. Magnesium hydroxide and magnesium gluconate gel used in rabbit models show some histologic evidence of efficacy,[23] but their use has not been reported in humans.

Alternatively or simultaneously, pain control can be administered orally or intravenously as needed, but preferably not to the point of sedation, because local pain control response will guide therapy. For this reason, digital blocks with subcutaneous lidocaine are also best avoided in management.[46]

These patients should be observed over 4 to 6 hours as the pain is likely to recur and reapplication of the gel or alternative therapy may be necessary. In addition, wound margins may become apparent and require debridement, and even if successful pain control is achieved the patient will require special follow-up or wound care.

If topical gel therapy fails within the first few minutes of application, consideration should be given to intradermal therapy with calcium gluconate, since the benefit in pain control is often seen almost immediately. This treatment may have limited utility in small spaces such as fingertips. Histologic studies in animal models demonstrate that 10% calcium chloride solution can be damaging to the tissues and ought to be avoided.[46,67] The preferable method is to approach the wound from a distal point of injury and inject intradermally no more than 0.5 mL/cm^2 of 5% calcium gluconate. One author recommends a palmar fasciotomy whenever this method of treatment is utilized.[5] This seems extreme, and is not currently recommended unless a compartment syndrome is present, as the potential for iatrogenic injury is increased. The limits of intradermal injection include potential to increase soft-tissue damage without adequate relief, infection, and inadequate space to safely inject without causing a compartment syndrome. This is especially problematic under the nail. Some authors have recommended removal of the nail. This has some advantages in accessing the affected area; however, it is a painful procedure that is often cosmetically undesirable and the outcome is not always significantly improved.

If the wound is large or in a section of the fingerpad or an area that is not amenable to intradermal injections, then consideration should be given to the use of intra-arterial calcium gluconate. This procedure delivers calcium directly to the affected tissue from a proximal artery. Usually radial or brachial arteries are used. The method of obtaining access is somewhat debated. Because of the potential to sclerose and damage the endothelial lining of the artery, and because extravasation can have potentially devastating consequences, the placement of an intra-arterial infusion line was originally recommended with confirmation of an arteriogram or placement under direct visualization of the vessel. This is recommended in cases where cannulation of the artery is expected to be difficult owing to prior surgery or deformity. If the arterial line is carefully placed in a single attempt and a good confirmatory arterial tracing is obtained, the infusate can be started. The recommended drip consists of 10 mL of 10% calcium gluconate in either 40 mL of D_5W or normal saline to run over 4 hours.[5,90,148,173,190,191] This gives a 2% calcium gluconate solution for arterial infusion. An animal model examined the effect of undiluted 10% calcium gluconate intra-aortically in rats. Though the model did not include HF, there was significant tissue injury in the vessel wall compared to 2% calcium gluconate.[46] Calcium chloride has also been used successfully, although the potential for vessel injury may increase and complications of calcium chloride extravasation can lead to significant tissue necrosis itself.[189,206] The overall complications of intra-arterial calcium infusion in several case series were relatively benign including radial artery spasm, hematoma, and inflammation at the puncture site, and in some cases a fall in serum magnesium.[173,190]

Once the drip begins, patients typically experience significant pain relief. Patients requiring an arterial line for treatment should be admitted to the hospital, as the majority will require more than one treatment, and some may require as many as five separate infusions of calcium gluconate. In addition, wounds may require debridement,[5] and one author suggests that after the drip, tissue can be salvaged that initially would not have been considered viable.[191] There have been no reported cases of clinically significant hypercalcemia with this therapy, though serum calcium levels were not recorded in every series.

Other reported therapies have included an intravenous Bier block technique using 25 mL of 2.5% calcium gluconate. The effects lasted 5 hours and there were no adverse events.[70] It has not been utilized with any reported frequency and has yet to be studied as an alternative therapy.

A rabbit model of empiric intravenous magnesium therapy for the management of dermal HF burns suggested an efficacy for wound healing when compared to untreated controls.[37] Another animal model suggested a potential benefit to wound healing with empiric therapy as well.[199] Both of these models are limited, and this therapy has never been well examined in humans. If used carefully, however, intravenous magnesium may have a potential role in the management of dermal injuries.

An approach of both local and systemic therapy with calcium and magnesium may be required to provide adequate relief for patients with HF hand injuries.

How Are Button Battery Ingestions Managed?

Button batteries present a unique problem of both foreign body ingestion and potential caustic injury. Button or disk batteries are found in small devices such as hearing aids, watches, and hand-held calculators and computer games. These batteries range in size from 6.8 to 23 mm and they are easily ingested by children.[107] Each contains a metal salt and a variety of caustic alkaline substances such as sodium and potassium hydroxide, which can induce significant burns and subsequent strictures if the contents leak.[96,174]

In vitro models of button batteries placed in a liquid with a pH of 5.5 led to an increase in pH to 11.5 with a

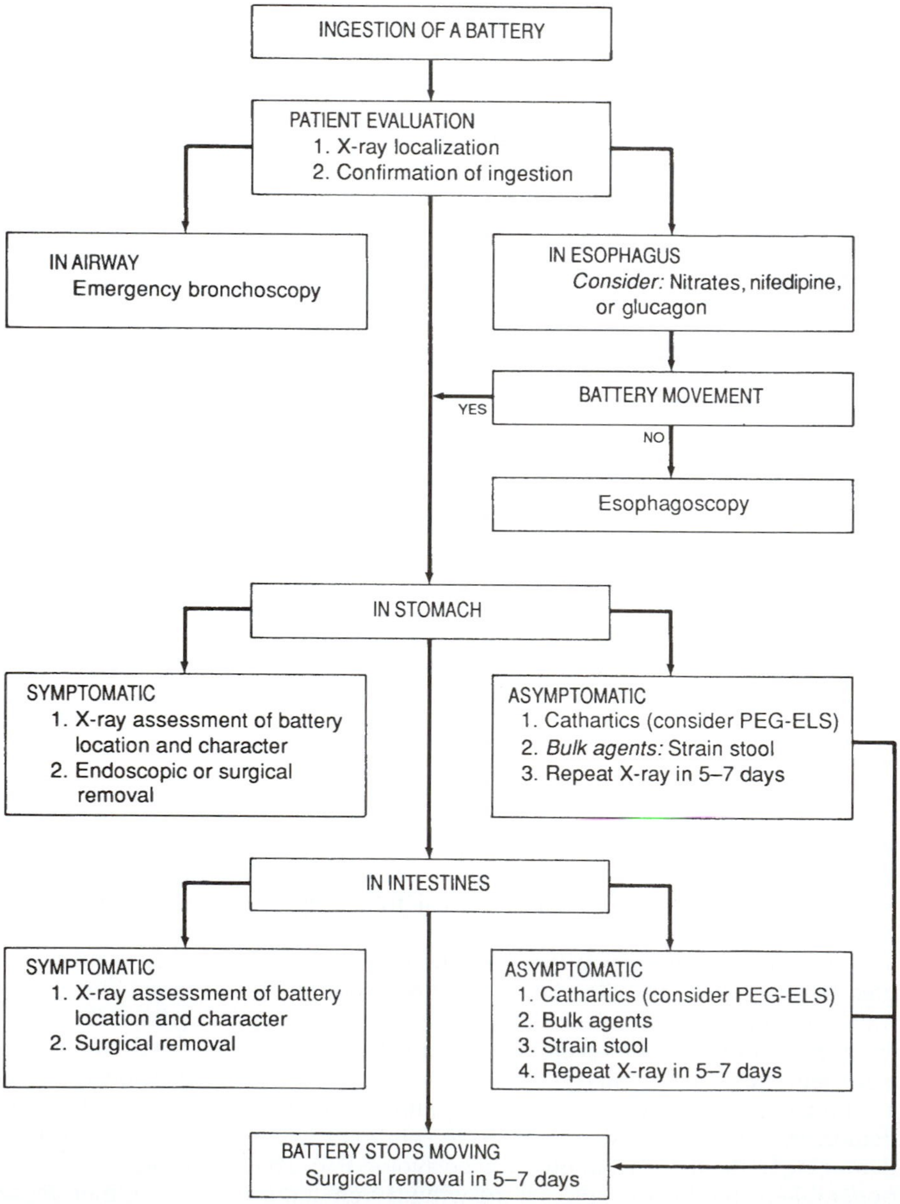

Figure 86–4. Algorithm for the management and assessment of patients with button battery ingestions.

brownish discoloration when leakage occurred from the seal or crimp of the two sides of the battery.[159,193] Animal models of button batteries placed on esophageal surfaces result in serosal edema, and tissue discoloration, and degree of burns that correlates with duration of contact.[120,159,193]

A review of 2382 cases of button battery ingestions revealed that the majority of batteries pass uneventfully in the stool, with 86% completing the transit through the gastrointestinal tract within 4 days.[107] Two patients in the series developed strictures and 10% of the batteries had dissolution of the crimp or seal. Unfortunately, fatal cases of transesophageal fistula and perforation of the aortic arch were reported in 2 patients with a significant delay in diagnosis.[15,169] For this reason a thorough evaluation and follow-up of patients with button battery ingestion are mandatory.

Initial management includes airway assessment and stabilization followed by antero-posterior and lateral chest radiographs that visualize the neck, chest, and abdomen in that order, particularly in children.[170] Patients with batteries in the airway or lower respiratory tract are usually symptomatic and require emergent removal via bronchoscopy. Intact batteries located past the pylorus in patients who are asymptomatic can be followed at home with serial stool examinations checking for battery passage, as 99% will be eliminated within 7 days.[106] Patients should return for abdominal pain, vomiting, fever, or failure of the battery to pass within 7 days.

For children younger than 6 years old in whom the battery is located in the stomach, battery size should be assessed on the radiograph, as batteries greater than 15 mm are less likely to pass the pylorus spontaneously.[170] These patients should be reassessed in 48 hours by physical examination and repeat radiograph to check for movement of the battery past the pylorus. Endoscopic retrieval of the battery should be considered when the battery has failed to pass the pylorus.[163,170] The role of polyethylene glycol solution in whole-bowel irrigation has not been adequately investigated, although its use can be considered in patients with batteries in the stomach or with poor mobility in the intestines.[182]

If the battery is visualized in the esophagus, it requires immediate endoscopic removal by forceps or magnet.[201] There are no studies of the use of glucagon or other agents to lower the esophageal sphincter pressure and allow movement of the battery into the stomach. Glucagon should be used with caution, as it can induce vomiting and nausea, and patients are at risk of battery aspiration. Other means of battery removal have been attempted, such as syrup of ipecac or Foley balloon passage to retrieve the battery, but these procedures have met with little success and incur the risk of foreign body aspiration. Endoscopy allows for both battery removal and tissue inspection (Fig. 86–4).[163, 201]

Heavy metal leakage of mercury was reported in patients with a concomitant elevation in urine mercury excretion.[9,95] Though heavy metal poisoning is a potential concern, especially when the battery is split on the radiograph, there have been no reported cases of symptomatic heavy metal poisoning from these exposures.

In addition to leakage of battery contents, pressure necrosis and an electrical gradient across the moist tissue from the battery surfaces may contribute to damage, but this appears to be less significant than the alkaline exposure of battery contents.

Tissue damage can occur at other sites of battery placement including the nares and ear canal. These exposures have resulted in severe otorhinologic burns and perforations.[83] These too, should be removed when identified.

References

1. Aceto T, Terplan K, Fiore RR, Munschauer RW: Chemical burns of the esophagus in children and glucocorticoid therapy. J Med 1970;1:101–109.
2. Alford BR, Harris HH: Chemical burns of the mouth pharynx and esophagus. Ann Otol 1959;68:122–128.
3. Andersen AH: Experimental studies on the pharmacology of activated charcoal. III. Adsorption from gastro-intestinal contents. Acta Pharmacol 1948;4:275–284.
4. Anderson KD, Rouse TM, Randolph JG: A controlled trial of corticosteroids in children with corrosive injury of the esophagus. N Engl J Med 1990;323:637–640.
5. Anderson WJ, Anderson JR: Hydrofluoric acid burns of the hand: Mechanism of injury and treatment. J Hand Surg 1988;13:52–57.
6. Appelqvist P, Salmo M: Lye corrosion carcinoma of the esophagus: A review of 63 cases. Cancer 1980;45: 2655–2658.
7. Ashcraft KW, Padula RT: The effect of dilute corrosives on the esophagus. Pediatrics 1974;53:226–232.
8. Baltazar RF, Mower MM, Reider R, et al: Acute fluoride poisoning leading to fatal hyperkalemia. Chest 1980;78: 660–663.
9. Bass DH, Millar AJW: Mercury absorption following button battery ingestion. J Pediatr Surg 1992;27:1541–1542.
10. Bennet IL, James DF, Golden A: Severe acidosis due to phenol poisoning: Report of two cases. Ann Intern Med 1950;32:324–327.
11. Bentur Y, Tannenbaum S, Yaffe Y, Halpert M: The role of calcium gluconate in the treatment of hydrofluoric acid eye burn. Ann Emerg Med 1993;22:1488–1490.
12. Berman L, Taves D, Mitra S, Newmark K: Inorganic fluoride poisoning: Treatment by hemodialysis. N Engl J Med 1973;289:922.
13. Berthet B, Di Costanzo J, Arnaud C, et al: Influence of epidermal growth factor and interferon gamma on healing of oesophageal corrosive burns in the rat. Br J Surg 1994;81: 395–398.
14. Bikhazi HB, Thompson ER, Shumrick DA: Caustic ingestions—Current status: A report of 105 cases. Arch Otolaryngol 1969;89:112–115.
15. Blatnik BS, Toohill RJ, Leman RH: Fatal complications from alkaline foreign body in the esophagus. Ann Otol Rhinol Laryngol 1977;86:611–615.
16. Boink ABTJ, Wemer J, Meulenbelt J, et al: The mechanism

of fluoride-induced hypocalcemia. Hum Exp Toxicol 1994; 13:149–155.
17. Bordelon BM, Saffle JR, Morris SE: Systemic fluoride toxicity in a child with hydrofluoric acid burns: Case report. J Trauma 1993;34:437–439.
18. Borja AR, Ransdell HT, Thomas TV, Johnson W: Lye injuries of the esophagus: Analysis of ninety cases of lye ingestion. J Thorac Cardiovasc Surg 1969;57:533–538.
19. Bost RO, Springfield A: Fatal hydrofluoric acid ingestion: A suicide case report. J Anal Toxicol 1995;19:535–536.
20. Bracken WM, Cuppage F, McLaury RL, et al: Comparative effectiveness of topical treatments for hydrofluoric acid burns. J Occup Med 1985;27:733–739.
21. Buckingham FM: Surgery: A radical approach to severe hydrofluoric acid burns—A case report. J Occup Med 1988;30:873–874.
22. Burke WJ, Hoegg UR, Philips RE: Systemic fluoride poisoning resulting from a fluoride skin burn. J Occup Med 1973;15:39–41.
23. Burkhart KK, Brent J, Kirk MA, et al: Comparison of topical magnesium and calcium treatment for dermal hydrofluoric acid burns. Ann Emerg Med 1994;24:9–13.
24. Burrington JD: Clinitest burns of the esophagus. Ann Thorac Surg 1975;20:400–404.
25. Cappell MS, Simon, T: Fulminant acute colitis following a self-administered enema. Am J Gastroenterol 1993;88: 122–126.
26. Cardona JC, Daly JF: Current management of corrosive esophagitis: An evaluation of results in 239 cases. Ann Otol Rhinol Laryngol 1971;80:521–526.
27. Cello JP, Fogel RP, Boland CR: Liquid caustic ingestion—Spectrum of injury. Arch Intern Med 1980;140:501–504.
28. Chaudhary A, Puri AS, Dhar P, et al: Elective surgery for corrosive-induced gastric injury. World J Surg 1996;20: 703–706.
29. Chick LR, Borah G: Calcium carbonate gel therapy for hydrofluoric acid burns of the hand. Plastic Reconstr Surg 1990;86:935–939.
30. Chobanian SJ: Accidental ingestion of liquid zinc chloride: Local and systemic effects. Ann Emerg Med 1981;10:91–93.
31. Chodak GW, Passaro E: Acid ingestion—Need for gastric resection. JAMA 1978;238:225–226.
32. Chong SC, Beahrs OH, Payne WS: Management of corrosive gastritis due to ingested acid. Mayo Clin Proc 1974; 49:861–865.
33. Christensen BT: Prediction of complications following unintentional caustic ingestion in children. Is endoscopy always necessary? Acta Paediatr 1995;84:1177–1182.
34. Clausen JO, Nielsen TLF, Fogh A: Admission to Danish hospitals after suspected ingestion of corrosives. Dan Med Bull 1994;41:234–237.
35. Cleveland WW, Thorton N, Chesney JG, Lawson RB: The effect of prednisone in the prevention of esophageal stricture following the ingestion of lye. South Med J 1958;51: 861–864.
36. Colbert PM, Sanders PD, Frankl H: Isolated antral ulceration from ingestion of a single Clinitest tablet. Gastrointest Endosc 1977;24:82–83.
37. Cox RD, Osgood KA: Evaluation of intravenous magnesium sulfate for the treatment of hydrofluoric acid burns. J Toxicol Clin Toxicol 1994;32:123–136.
38. Crain EF, Gershel JC, Mezey, AP: Caustic ingestions—Symptoms as predictors of esophageal injury. Am J Dis Child 1984;138:863–865.
39. Cullen ML, Klein MD: Spontaneous resolution of acid gastric injury. J Pediatr Surg 1987;22:550–551.
40. Cummings CC, McIvor ME: Flouride-induced hyperkalemia—The role of calcium dependent potassium channels. Am J Emerg Med 1986;6:1–3.
41. Daly JF, Cardona JC: Acute corrosive esophagitis. Arch Otolaryngol 1961;74:41–46.
42. Dantas RO, Mamede RCM: Esophageal motility in patients with esophageal caustic injury. Am J Gastroenterol 1996;91:1157–1161.
43. Dibbell DG, Iverson RE, Jones W, et al: Hydrofluoric acid burns of the hand. J Bone Joint Surg 1970;52:931–936.
44. Di Costanzo J, Noirclerc M, Jouglard J, et al: New therapeutic approach to corrosive burns of the upper gastrointestinal tract. Gut 1980;21:370–375.
45. Dilawari JB, Singh S, Rao PN, Anand BS: Corrosive acid ingestion in man—A clinical and endoscopic study. Gut 1984;25:183–187.
46. Dowbak G, Rose K, Rohrich RJ: A biochemical and histological rationale for the treatment of hydrofluoric acid burns with calcium gluconate. J Burn Care Rehabil 1994; 15:323–327.
47. Dunn BJ, MacKinnon MA, Knowlden NF, et al: Hydrofluoric acid dermal burns—An assessment of treatment efficacy using an experimental pig model. J Occup Med 1992;34:902–909.
48. Eaton H, Tennekoon GE: Squamous carcinoma of the stomach following corrosive acid burns. Br J Surg 1972; 59:382–387.
49. Einhorn A, Horton L, Altieri M, et al: Serious respiratory consequences of detergent ingestions in children. Pediatrics 1989;84:472–474.
50. El Saadi MS, Hall AH, Hall PK, et al: Hydrofluoric acid dermal exposure. Vet Hum Toxicol 1989;31:243–247.
51. Estrera A, Taylor W, Mills LJ: Corrosive burns of the esophagus and stomach: A recommendation for an aggressive surgical approach. Ann Thorac Surg 1986;41: 276–283.
52. Forsen JW, Muntz HR: Hair relaxer ingestion: A new trend. Ann Otol Rhinol Laryngol 1993;102:781–784.
53. Friedman EM, Lovejoy Jr FH: The emergency management of caustic ingestions. Emerg Med Clin North Am 1984;2:77–86.
54. Gago O, Ritter FN, Martel W, et al: Aggressive surgical treatment for caustic injury of the esophagus and stomach. Ann Thorac Surg 1972;13:243–250.
55. Garite TJ, Spellacy WN: Premature rupture of membranes. In: Scott JR, DiSaia PJ, Hammond CB, Spellacy WN, eds: Danforth's Obstetrics and Gynecology, 7th ed. Philadelphia, Lippincott, 1994, p. 30.
56. Gaudreault P, Parent M, McGuigan MA, et al: Predictability of esophageal injury from signs and symptoms: A study of caustic ingestion in 378 children. Pediatrics 1983;71:767–770.

57. Gehanno P, Geudon C: Inhibition of experimental esophageal lye strictures by penicillamine. Arch Otolaryngol 1981;107:145–147.
58. Genieser NB, Becker MH: "Clinitest strictures" of the esophagus. Clin Pediatr 1969;8:17A–19A.
59. Gillis DA, Higgins G, Kennedy R: Gastric damage from ingested acid in children. J Pediatr Surg 1985;20:494–496.
60. Gorman RL, Khin-Maung-Gyi MT, Klein-Schwartz W, et al: Initial symptoms as predictors of esophageal injury in alkaline corrosive ingestions. Am J Emerg Med 1992;10: 189–194.
61. Gossot D, Safarti E, Celerier M: Early blunt esophagectomy in severe caustic burns of the upper digestive tract: Report of 29 cases. J Thorac Cardiovasc Surg 1987;94: 188–191.
62. Greco RJ, Hartford CE, Haith LR, Patton ML: Hydrofluoric acid induced hypocalcemia. J Trauma 1988;28: 1593–1596.
63. Gupta S: A technique of repairing acid burns of the stomach. Ann Roy Coll Surg Engl 1988;70:74–75.
64. Gutknecht J, Walter A: Hydrofluoric and nitric acid transport through lipid bilayer membranes. Biochim Biophys Acta 1981;644:153–156.
65. Haller JA, Andrews HG, White JJ, et al: Pathophysiology and management of acute corrosive burns of the esophagus: Results of treatment in 285 children. J Pediatr Surg 1971;6:578–583.
66. Haller JA, Bachman K: The comparative effect of current therapy on experimental caustic burns of the esophagus. Pediatrics 1964;34:236–245.
67. Harris JC, Rumack BH, Bregman DJ: Comparative efficacy of injectable calcium and magnesium salts in the therapy of hydrofluoric acid burns. Clin Toxicol 1981;18: 1027–1032.
68. Hawkins DB: Dilatation of esophageal strictures: Comparative morbidity of anterograde and retrograde methods. Ann Otol Rhinol Laryngol 1988;97:460–465.
69. Hawkins DB, Demeter MJ, Barnett TE: Caustic ingestion: Controversies in management: A review of 214 cases. Laryngoscope 1980;90:98–109.
70. Henry JA, Hla KK: Intravenous regional calcium gluconate perfusion for hydrofluoric acid burns. J Toxicol Clin Toxicol 1992;30:203–207.
71. Hill JL, Norberg HP, Smith MD, et al: Clinical technique and success of the esophageal stent to prevent corrosive strictures. J Pediatr Surg 1976;11:443–450.
72. Hoffman RS, Howland MA, Kamerow HN, Goldfrank LR: Comparison of titratable acid/alkaline reserves an pH in potentially caustic household products. J Toxicol Clin Toxicol 1989;27:241–261.
73. Homan CS, Maitra SR, Lane BP, et al: Effective treatment for acute alkali injury to the esophagus using weak-acid neutralization therapy: An ex-vivo study. Acad Emerg Med 1995;2:952–958.
74. Homan CS, Maitra SR, Lane BP, et al: Histopathologic evaluation of the therapeutic efficacy of water and milk dilution for esophageal acid injury. Acad Emerg Med 1995; 2:587–591.
75. Homan CS, Maitra SR, Lane BP, et al: Therapeutic effects of water and milk for acute alkali injury of the esophagus. Ann Emerg Med 1994;24:14–19.
76. Homan CS, Maitra SR, Lane BP, Geller ER: Effective treatment of acute alkali injury of the rat esophagus with early saline dilution therapy. Ann Emerg Med 1993;22:178–182.
77. Homan CS, Singer AJ, Henry MC, Thode HC: Thermal effects of neutralization therapy and water dilution for acute alkali exposure in canines. Acad Emerg Med 1997;4:27–32.
78. Horvath OP, Olah T, Zentai G: Emergency esophagogastrectomy for the treatment of hydrochloric acid injury. Ann Thorac Surg 1991;52:98–101.
79. Howell JM, Dalsey WC, Hartsell FW, Butzin CA: Steroids for the treatment of corrosive esophageal injury: A statistical analysis of past studies. Am J Emerg Med 1992;10: 421–425.
80. Hunter DM, Timerding BL, Leonard RB, et al: Effects of isopropyl alcohol, ethanol, and polyethylene glycol/industrial methylated spirits in the treatment of acute phenol burns. Ann Emerg Med 1992;21:1303–1307.
81. Hwang TL, Shen-Chen SM, Chen MF: Nonthoracotomy esophagectomy for corrosive esophagitis with gastric perforation. Surg Gynecol Obstet 1987;164:537–540.
82. Juncos LI, Donadio JV: Renal failure and fluorosis. JAMA 1972;222:783–785.
83. Kavanaugh K, Litovitz T: Miniature battery foreign bodies in auditory and nasal cavities. JAMA 1986;255:1470–1472.
84. Kirkpatrick JR, Burd DAR: An algorithmic approach to the treatment of hydrofluoric acid burns. Burns 1995;21: 495–499.
85. Kirkpatrick JR, Enion DS, Burd DAR: Hydrofluoric acid burns: A review. Burns 1995;21:483–493.
86. Kirsch MM, Peterson A, Brown JW, et al: Treatment of caustic injuries of the esophagus: A ten year experience. Ann Surg 1978;188:675–678.
87. Klauder JV, Shelanski L, Gabriel K: Industrial uses of compounds of fluorine and oxalic acid. Arch Environ Health 1955;12:412–419.
88. Knox WG, Scott JR, Zintel HA, et al: Bougeniage and steroids used singly or in combination in experimental corrosive esophagitis. Ann Surg 1967;166:930–940.
89. Kocchar R, Mehta S, Nagi B, Goenka MK: Corrosive acid-induced esophageal intramural pseudodiverticulosis—A study of 14 patients. J Clin Gastroenterol 1991;13:371–375.
90. Kohnlein HE, Achinger R: A new method of treatment of the hydrofluoric acid burns of the extremities. Chir Plast 1982;6:297–305.
91. Kohnlein HE, Merkle P, Springorum HW: Hydrogen fluoride burns: Experiments and treatment. Surg Forum 1973; 24:50.
92. Kono K, Yoshida Y, Watanabe M, et al: An experimental study on the treatment of hydrofluoric acid burns. Arch Environ Contam Toxicol 1992;22:414–418.
93. Kost KM, Shapiro RS: Button battery ingestion—A case report and review of the literature. J Otolaryngol 1987;16: 252–254.
94. Krenzelok EP: Liquid automatic dishwashing detergents: A profile of toxicity. Ann Emerg Med 1989;18:60–63.
95. Kuhn JR, Tunell WP: The role of cineesophagoscopy in caustic esophageal injury. Am J Surg 1983;146:804–806.

96. Kulig K, Rumack C, Rumack B, Duffy J: Disk battery ingestion—Elevated urine mercury levels and enema removal of battery fragments. JAMA 1983;249:2502–2504.
97. Kwok MC, Svancarek WP, Creer M: Fatality due to hydrofluoric acid exposure. J Toxicol Clin Toxicol 1987;25: 333–339.
98. Lacouture PG, Gaudreault P, Lovejoy FH: Clinitest tablet ingestion: An in vitro investigation concerned with initial emergency management. Ann Emerg Med 1986;15: 143–146.
99. Lahoti D, Broor SL, Basu P, et al: Corrosive esophageal strictures: Predictors of response to endoscopic dilatation. Gastrointest Endosc 1995;41:196–200.
100. Landau GD, Saunders WH: The effect of chlorine bleach on the esophagus. Arch Otolaryngol 1964;80:174–176.
101. Leape LL, Ashcraft KW, Scarpelli DG, Holder TM: Hazard to health—Liquid lye. N Engl J Med 1971;284:578–581.
102. Lee DC, Wiley JF, Snyder JW: Treatment of inhalational exposure to hydrofluoric acid with nebulized calcium gluconate. J Occup Med 1993;35:470. Letter.
103. Leonard LG, Scheulen JJ, Munster AM: Chemical burns: Effect of prompt first aid. J Trauma 1982;22:420–423.
104. Lepke S, Paasow H: Effects of fluoride on potassium and sodium permeability of the erythrocyte membrane. J Gen Physiol 1968;51:365S–372S.
105. Lidbeck WL, Hill IB, Beeman JA: Acute sodium fluoride poisoning. JAMA 1943;121:826–827.
106. Litovitz T, Butterfield AB, Holloway RR, Marion LI: Battery ingestion: Assessment of therapeutic modalities and battery discharge state. J Pediatr 1984;105:868–873.
107. Litovitz T, Schmitz BF: Ingestion of cylindrical and button batteries: An analysis of 2382 cases. Pediatrics 1992;89: 747–757.
108. Liu A, Richardson M, Robertson WO: Effects of *N*-acetylcysteine on caustic burns. Vet Hum Toxicol 1985;28:316.
109. Lowe JE, Graham DY, Boisaubin EV, Lanza FL: Corrosive injury to the stomach: The natural history and role of fiberoptic endoscopy. Am J Surg 1979;137:803–806.
110. Mack RB: Decant the wine, prune back your long-term hopes. North Carol Med J 1987;48:593–595.
111. MacKinnon MA: Hydrofluoric acid burns. Dermatol Clin 1988;6:67–74
112. MacKinnon MA: Treatment of hydrofluoric acid burns. J Occup Med 1986;28:804. Letter.
113. Madden JW, Davis WM, Butler C, Peacock EE: Experimental esophageal lye burns II: Correcting established strictures with beta-aminoproprionitrile and bougeniage. Ann Surg 1973;178:277–284.
114. Mallory A, Schaefer JW: Clinitest ingestion. Br Med J 1977;2:105–107.
115. Mandarikan BA: Ingestion of dishwasher detergent by children. Br J Clin Pract 1990;44:35–36.
116. Manoguerra AS, Neuman TS: Fatal poisoning from acute hydrofluoric acid ingestion. Am J Emerg Med 1986;4: 362–363.
117. Martel W: Radiologic features of esophagogastritis secondary to extremely caustic agents. Diagnos Radiol 1972; 103:31–36.
118. Maull KI, Osmand AP, Maull CD: Liquid caustic ingestions: An in vitro study of the effects of buffer, neutralization, and dilution. Ann Emerg Med 1985;14:1160–1162.
119. Maull KI, Scher LA, Greenfield LJ: Surgical implications of acid ingestion. Surg Gynecol Obstet 1979;148:895–898.
120. Maves MD, Carrithers JS, Brick HG: Esophageal burns secondary to disc battery ingestion. Ann Otol Rhinol Laryngol 1984;93:364–369.
121. Mayer L, Guelich, J: Hydrogen fluoride (HF) inhalation and burns. Arch Environ Health 1963;7:445–447.
122. Mayer TG, Gross PL: Fatal systemic fluorosis due to hydrofluoric acid burns. Ann Emerg Med 1985;14:149–153.
123. McClure FJ: A review of fluorine and its physiologic effects. Physiol Rev 1933;13:277–300.
124. McCulley JP, Whiting DW, Petitt MG, Lauber SE: Hydrofluoric acid burns of the eye. J Occup Med 1983;25: 447–450.
125. McIvor ME: Delayed fatal hyperkalemia in a patient with acute fluoride intoxication. Ann Emerg Med 1987;16: 1165–1167.
126. McIvor M, Baltazar RF, Beltran J, et al: Hyperkalemia and cardiac arrest from fluoride exposure during hemodialysis. Am J Cardiol 1983;51:901–902.
127. McIvor ME, Cummings CE, Mower MM, et al: Sudden cardiac death from acute fluoride intoxication: The role of potassium. Ann Emerg Med 1987;16:777–781.
128. McKinney PE: Zinc chloride ingestion in a child—Exocrine pancreatic insufficiency. Ann Emerg Med 1995;25:562.
129. McKinney PE, Brent J, Kulig K: Acute zinc chloride ingestion in a child—Local and systemic effects. Ann Emerg Med 1994;23:1383–1387.
130. McNeely MDD: Urinalysis. In: Sonnenwirth AC, Jarrett L, eds: Gradwohl's Clinical Laboratory Methods and Diagnosis. St. Louis, Mosby, 1980, p. 483.
131. Menchel SM, Dunn WA: Hydrofluoric acid poisoning. Am J Forens Med Pathol 1984;5:245–248.
132. Meredith W, Kon ND, Thompson JN: Management of injuries from liquid lye ingestion. J Trauma 1988;28: 1173–1180.
133. Middelkamp JN, Ferguson TB, Roper CL, Hoffman FD: The management and problems of caustic burns in children. J Thorac Cardiovasc Surg 1969;57:341–347.
134. Mills LJ, Estrera AS, Platt MR: Avoidance of esophageal stricture following severe caustic burns by the use of an intraluminal stent. Ann Thorac Surg 1979;28:63–65.
135. Mitani M, Hirata K, Fukuda M, Kaneko M: Endoscopic ultrasonography in corrosive injury of the upper gastrointestinal tract by hydrochloric acid. J Clin Ultrasound 1996;24:40–42.
136. Moazam F, Talbert JL, Miller D, Mollitt DL: Caustic ingestion and its sequelae in children. South Med J 1987;80: 187–190.
137. Morris JB, Smith FA: Regional deposition and absorption of inhaled hydrogen fluoride in the rat. Toxicol Appl Pharmacol 1982;62:81–89.
138. Mozingo DW, Smith AA, McManus WF, et al: Chemical burns. J Trauma 1988;28:642–647.
139. Muhletaler CA, Gerlock AJ, de Soto L, Halter SA: Acid corrosive esophagitis: Radiographic findings. Am J Radiol 1980;134:1137–1140.

140. Mutaf O, Avanoglu A, Ozok G: Management of tracheoesophageal fistula as a complication of esophageal dilatations in caustic esophageal burns. J Pediatr Surg 1995; 30:823–826.
141. Noonan T, Carter EJ, Edelman PA, Zawacki BE: Epidermal lipids and the natural history of hydrofluoric acid (HF) injury. Burns 1994;20:202–206.
142. Norton RA: Esophageal and antral strictures due to ingestion of household ammonia—Report of two cases. N Engl J Med 1960;262:10–12.
143. Ochi K, Ohashi T, Sato S, et al: Surgical treatment for caustic ingestion injury of the pharynx, larynx, and esophagus. Acta Otolarygol 1996;522(suppl):116–119.
144. O'Connor HJ, Dixon MF, Grant AC, et al: Fatal accidental ingestion of Clinitest in an adult. J Roy Soc Med 1984;77:963–965.
145. O'Neil K: A fatal hydrogen fluoride exposure. J Emerg Nurs 1994;20:451–453.
146. Paley A, Seifter J: Treatment of experimental hydrofluoric acid corrosion. Proc Soc Exp Biol Med 1941;46:190–192.
147. Payten RJ: Clinitest tablet stricture of the esophagus. Br Med J 1972;4:728–729.
148. Pegg SP, Siu S, Gillett G: Intra-arterial infusions in the treatment of hydrofluoric acid burns. Burns 1985;11: 440–443.
149. Penner GE: Acid ingestion—Toxicology and treatment. Ann Emerg Med 1980;9:374–379.
150. Potter JL: Acute zinc chloride ingestion in a young child. Ann Emerg Med 1981;10:267–269.
151. Previtera C, Guisti F, Guglielmi M: Predictive value of visible lesions (cheeks, lips, oropharynx) in suspected caustic ingestion: May endoscopy reasonably be omitted in completely negative pediatric patients? Pediatr Emerg Care 1990;6:176–178.
152. Ragheb MI, Ramadan AA, Khalia MA: Management of corrosive esophagitis. Surgery 1976;79:494–498.
153. Ray III JF, Myers WO, Lawton BR, et al: The natural history of liquid lye ingestion—Rationale for an aggressive surgical approach. Arch Surg 1974;109:436–439.
154. Reyes HM, Hill JL: Modification of the experimental stent technique for esophageal burns. J Surg Res 1976;20: 65–70.
155. Reyes HM, Lin CY, Schlunk FF, Repogle RL: Experimental treatment of corrosive esophageal burns. J Pediatr Surg 1974;9:317–327.
156. Reynolds KE, Whitford GM, Pashley DH: Acute fluoride toxicity: The influence of acid–base status. Toxicol Appl Pharmacol 1978;45:41–427.
157. Ribet ME: Esophagogastrectomy for acid injury. Ann Thorac Surg 1992;53:738–742.
158. Ritter FN, Newman MH, Newman DE: A clinical and experimental study of corrosive burns of the stomach. Ann Otol Rhinol Laryngol 1968;77:830–842.
159. Rivera EA, Maves MD: Effects of neutralizing agents on esophageal burns caused by disk batteries. Ann Otol Rhinol Laryngol 1987;96:362–366.
160. Rose L: Further evaluation of hydrofluoric acid burns to the eye. J Occup Med 1984;26:483. Letter.
161. Rosenberg N, Kunderman PJ, Vroman L, Moolten SE: Prevention of experimental esophageal stricture by cortisone II. Arch Surg 1953;66:593–598.
162. Rubinfeld RS, Silbert DI, Arentsen JJ, Laibson PR: Ocular hydrofluoric acid burns. Am J Ophthalmol 1992;114: 420–423.
163. Rumack BH, Burrington JD: Caustic ingestions: A rational look at diluents. Clin Toxicol 1977;11:27–34.
164. Rumack CM, Rumack BH: Battery ingestions. Pediatrics 1992;89:771–772.
165. Sadove R, Hainsworth D, Van Meter W: Total body immersion in hydrofluoric acid. South Med J 1990;83: 698–700.
166. Safarti E, Gossot D, Assens P, Celerier M: Management of caustic ingestion in adults. Br J Surg 1987;74:146–148.
167. Schild JA: Caustic ingestion in adult patients. Laryngoscope 1985;95:1199–1201.
168. Scott JC, Jones B, Eisele DW, Ravich WJ: Caustic ingestion injuries of the upper aerodigestive tract. Laryngoscope 1992;102:1–8.
169. Shabino CL, Feinberg AN: Esophageal perforation secondary to alkaline battery ingestion. JACEP 1979;8:360–362.
170. Sheikh A: Button battery ingestions in children. Pediatr Emerg Care 1993:224–229.
171. Sheridan RL, Ryan CM, Quinby WC Jr, et al: Emergency management of major hydrofluoric acid exposures. Burns 1995;21:62–64.
172. Shirazi S, Schulze-Delrieu K, Custer-Hagen T, et al: Motility changes in opossum esophagus from experimental esophagitis. Dig Dis Sci 1989;34:1668–1676.
173. Siegel DC, Heard J: Intra-arterial calcium infusion for hydrofluoric acid burns. Aviat Space Environ Med 1992;63: 206–211.
174. Sigalet D, Lees G: Tracheoesophageal injury secondary to disc battery ingestion. J Pediatr Surg 1988;23:996–998.
175. Sinar DR, Fletcher JR, Cordova CC, et al: Acute acid-induced esophagitis impairs esophageal peristalsis in baboons. Gastroenterol 1981;80:1286.
176. Souba WW: Nutritional support. N Engl J Med 1997; 336:41–48.
177. Spiller HA, Quadrani-Kushner DA, Cleveland P: A five-year evaluation of acute exposures to phenol disinfectant (26%). J Toxicol Clin Toxicol 1993;31:307–313.
178. Stremski ES, Grande GA, Ling LJ: Survival following hydrofluoric acid ingestion. Ann Emerg Med 1992;21: 1396–1399.
179. Subbarao KSVK, Kakar AK, Chandrasekhar V, et al: Cicatrical gastric stenosis caused by corrosive ingestion. Aust NZ J Surg 1988;58:143–146.
180. Sugawa C, Lucas CE: Caustic injury of the upper gastrointestinal tract in adults: A clinical and endoscopic study. Surgery 1989;106:802–807.
181. Sugawa C, Mullins RJ, Lucas CE, Leibold WC: The value of early endoscopy following caustic ingestion. Surg Gynecol Obstet 1981;153:553–556.
182. Tenenbein M: Whole bowel irrigation for toxic ingestions. J Toxicol Clin Toxicol 1985;23:177–184.
183. Tepperman PB: Fatality due to acute systemic fluoride poisoning following a hydrofluoric acid skin burn. J Occup Med 1980;22:691–692.

184. Tewfik TL, Schloss MD: Ingestion of lye and other corrosive agents—A study of 86 infant and child cases. J Otolaryngol 1980;9:72–77.
185. Thompson JN: Corrosive esophageal injuries I: A study of nine cases of concurrent accidental caustic ingestions. Laryngoscope 1987;97:1060–1066.
186. Thompson JN: Corrosive esophageal injuries II: An investigation of treatment methods and histochemical analysis of esophageal strictures in a new animal model. Laryngoscope 1987;97:1191–1202.
187. Trevino MA, Hermann GH, Sprout WL: Treatment of severe hydrofluoric acid exposures. J Occup Med 1983;25: 861–863.
188. Upfal M, Doyle C: Medical management of hydrofluoric acid exposure. J Occup Med 1990;32:727–731.
189. Upton J, Mulliken JB, Murray JE: Major intravenous extravasation injuries. Am J Surg 1979;137:497–506.
190. Vance MV, Curry SC, Kunkel DB, et al: Digital hydrofluoric acid burns: Treatment with intraarterial calcium infusion. Ann Emerg Med 1986;15:890–896.
191. Velvart J: Arterial perfusion for hydrofluoric acid burns. Hum Toxicol 1983;2:233–238.
192. Viscomi GJ, Beekhuis GJ, Whitten CF: An evaluation of early esophagoscopy and corticosteroid therapy in the management of corrosive injury of the esophagus. J Pediatr 1961;59:356–360.
193. Votteler TP, Nash JC, Rutledge JC: The hazard of ingested alkaline disc batteries in children. JAMA 1983;249: 2504–2506.
194. Warren JB, Grifin DJ, Olson RC: Urine sugar reagent tablet ingestion causing gastric and duodenal ulceration. Arch Intern Med 1984;144:161–162.
195. Webb WR, Koutras P, Ecker RR, Sugg WL: An evaluation of steroids and antibiotics in caustic burns of the esophagus. Ann Thorac Surg 1970;9:95–101.
196. White JE, McClafferty K, Orfon RB, et al: Ocular alkali burn associated with automobile air-bag activation. Can Med Assoc J 1995;153:933–934.
197. Wiesskopf A: Effects of cortisone on experimental lye burn of the esophagus. Ann Otol Rhinol Laryngol 1952;61: 681–691.
198. Wijburg FA, Beukers MM, Heymans HS, et al: Nasogastric intubation as sole treatment of caustic esophageal lesions. Ann Otol Rhinol Laryngol 1985;94:337–341.
199. Williams JM, Hammad A, Cottington EC, Harchelroad FC: Intravenous magnesium in the treatment of hydrofluoric acid burns in rats. Ann Emerg Med 1994;23:464–469.
200. Wilson DAB, Wormald PJ: Battery acid—An agent of attempted suicide in black South Africans. S Afr Med J 1994;84:529–531.
201. Wilson JA, Phillips EM: Endoscopic retrieval of a miniature battery. Gut 1985;26:215. Letter.
202. Wing JS, Sanderson LM, Brender JD, et al: Acute health effects in a community after a release of hydrofluoric acid. Arch Environ Health 1991;46:155–159.
203. Woodring JH, Heiser MJ: Detection of pneumoperitoneum on chest radiographs: Comparison of upright lateral and posteroanterior projections. Am J Radiol 1995;165:45–47.
204. Wu MH, Lai WW: Surgical management of extensive corrosive injuries of the alimentary tract. Surg Gynecol Obstet 1993;177:12–16.
205. Yolken R, Konecny P, McCarthy P: Acute fluoride poisoning. Pediatrics 1976;58:90–93.
206. Yosowitz P, Ekland DA, Shah RC, Parsons RW: Peripheral intravenous infiltration necrosis. Ann Surg 1975;182:553–556.
207. Zargar SA, Kochhar R, Mehta S, Mehta SK: The role of fiberoptic endoscopy in the management of corrosive ingestion and modified endoscopic classification of burns. Gastrointest Endosc 1991;37:165–169.
208. Zargar SA, Kochhar R, Nagi B, et al: Ingestion of corrosive acids: Spectrum of injury to upper gastrointestinal tract and natural history. Gastroenterology 1989;97:702–707.

ANTIDOTES IN DEPTH

Dilution and Neutralization

Richard S. Weisman and Christine M. Stork

Dilution and neutralization have been advocated for treatment of all forms of poisoning for nearly 300 years. It has been suggested that dilution will make a poison less potent, while neutralization will render a poison inactive and harmless.

Dilution (Noncaustics)

With the exception of ingestions that cause local tissue irritation or destruction, dilution as a technique for gastrointestinal decontamination is probably detrimental. In the animal model, dilution of orally ingested salicylate, pentobarbital, and quinine increases the rate of absorption and toxicity.[2,4,5]

In the rat, salicylate levels were significantly higher when equal amounts of sodium salicylate were administered as a dilute solution as compared to a concentrated solution.[2] It was also shown that the time to onset of sleep is inversely correlated with the concentration of pentobarbital solution administered to rats. This suggests that absorption was augmented by fluid due to hastened gastric emptying and exposure of a larger percentage of the absorptive surface to drug.

The effects of dilution volume on absorption were also studied in a rat model.[5] Following the administration of a standardized mg/kg oral dose of pentobarbital, quinine, and salicylate, control animals received 1 mL/kg and test animals 20 mL/kg of oral water. Serum drug assays were performed at times ranging from 5 to 320 minutes after drug administration. Statistically significantly higher levels of pentobarbital and quinine were measured in the animals that received the larger volume of water. A statistical difference was not shown for salicylate absorption. The authors concluded that dilution will always increase absorption by increasing the absorptive surface area for the ingested drug or chemical. They recommended that dilution not be employed as a first-aid treatment for ingested systemic toxins.

The absorption characteristics of 12 different toxins were evaluated in groups of 20 fasted, Sprague-Dawley rats. The animals received the toxins in quantities of water equal to 5, 2.5, and 1.25% of their body weight. "In all cases, with both organic and inorganic compounds, the results showed the same trend. The greater the dilution of the toxic dose, the greater was the death rate."[4]

In 1982, the American Association of Poison Control Centers' policy statement advised that dilution with fluids should not be considered a first-aid procedure for noncaustic ingestions.[3]

Dilution (Caustics)

The oral dilution of an ingested alkaline or weak acid caustic with fluids may be beneficial if it is performed immediately after the exposure. The immediate administration of fluids may help to decrease the caustic's contact time with the oropharyngeal, esophageal, or gastric mucosa. Dilution may also dissipate heat produced from the chemical reactions of hydration and neutralization. Milk may have a limited capacity to achieve neutralization.

Dilution/neutralization should not be performed for patients who have ingested a concentrated acid until an attempt has been made to remove as much of the acid as possible through a nasogastric tube. The addition of water to concentrated acid is likely to produce a substantial increase in heat.

In an in vitro rat model, it was observed that early dilution of either acid or alkalies with water, milk, normal saline, orange juice, or a cola beverage reduced esophageal damage. Histologic analysis demonstrated a statistically significant decrease in tissue damage with early dilution.[6–9]

When water was used for in vitro dilution of concentrated sulfuric acid, there was an instantaneous increase in temperature.[13] However, if the amount of water was increased 20-fold, the temperature increase was less. The authors cautioned that the addition of any water to concentrated acid would be likely to cause boiling and explosive steam formation.[13] They advocated extracting as much of the acid as possible from the stomach through a nasogastric tube prior to lavage with large volumes of cold milk or cold water.

Several in vitro studies demonstrated that injury to the esophagus will occur within seconds of exposure to both strong acid and strong alkaline caustics.[1,11]

Dilutional Therapy for the Patient With a Caustic Ingestion

If dilution is to reduce the extent of tissue damage from a caustic ingestion, fluids must be administered as soon as possible after the exposure to have a beneficial effect.

Upon discovery that a patient has ingested an alkaline or weak acid caustic, the first available nontoxic, cool liquid should be given to the victim to voluntarily swallow. The most immediately available liquid will often be either water or milk. If the patient is an adult, 250 mL (8 ounces) should be given or 15 mL/kg if the victim is a child (not to exceed 250 mL). Larger quantities of fluid are avoided to reduce the likelihood of distending the stomach and causing vomiting.

If the patient has impaired consciousness, is unable to swallow, is unable to protect the airway from aspiration, or has respiratory difficulty or severe abdominal pain, fluids should *not* be offered and the patient should be transported to the nearest healthcare facility for emergency care.

The immediate administration of fluids following an alkali (any strength) or weak acid caustic ingestion may be able to reduce the extent of tissue damage prior to the patient being brought to emergency care. The *immediate* availability of water or milk may make them more beneficial than other, less available fluids that may have a *potential* for increased efficacy in neutralization.

Following the ingestion of a strong acid, the patient should immediately be referred to the nearest healthcare facility for emergency care and nothing should be given by mouth. If treatment can be initiated within the first 90 minutes and there are no signs of perforation, a nasogastric tube should be placed and as much of the acid removed from the stomach as possible. Dilution with cold milk or water can then be performed if there are no signs of perforation.

Neutralization (Caustics)

Neutralization, the process of returning pH toward neutrality (pH = 7), has only been considered for caustic ingestions. The controversy surrounding the use of neutralizing agents for caustic ingestions results from an absence of controlled human or animal studies. In vitro studies[1,11,13,14] demonstrated that the use of small volumes of a neutralizing solution could result in a substantial temperature increase. In a subsequent study, larger volumes of a neutralizing solution were shown to minimize the temperature changes.[10]

The administration of an antacid for acid ingestions, or a weak acid for alkaline ingestions, may be more effective than water or milk in neutralizing a caustic. However, if the former agents are not immediately available, the time necessary to obtain them may limit their benefit.[12]

In an in vitro study designed to examine the diluent effect of 1.5 mL of lemon juice, vinegar, water, and milk on 1.5 g of Drano crystals (54.2% sodium hydroxide, 4.1% aluminum shavings) and Clinitest tablets (232 mg sodium hydroxide, 80 mg sodium carbonate, 20 mg copper sulfate, 300 mg citric acid), peak temperature was measured in addition to the time to return to baseline temperature.[14] Milk blunted the rise in temperature more effectively than water, lemon juice, or vinegar. Water and milk produced a more rapid return to baseline temperature than did lemon juice or vinegar.

The major criticism of this study is that the increase in temperature would have been insignificant if a larger quantity of diluent (250 mL) had been used for neutralization.

In another in vitro dilution study, 55.4 mL of 91.6% sulfuric acid was diluted with 55 mL of water. It was found that there was an instantaneous increase in temperature of 79°C.[13] If the amount of water was increased to 1000 mL, the temperature increase was only 14°C.

Magnesium hydroxide antacid was also studied for the in vitro neutralization of one mole (98 g) of concentrated sulfuric acid.[13] To achieve neutralization to a bisulfite salt, a total of 365 mL of antacid was required and a temperature increase of 73°C occurred. The pH of this partially neutralized sulfuric acid was still less than 1.0. To completely neutralize the acid to the bisulfate salt, an additional 365 mL of antacid was required and an increase in temperature of 62°C occurred.

The major criticism of this study is that the conclusion is based upon the neutralization of a relatively large amount of acid. The amount of heat produced in this in vitro study may not accurately reflect that which would be seen in a small unintentional ingestion.

In an in vitro neutralization study of 1.8% sodium hydroxide and 9.5% hydrochloric acid, 5% acetic acid was used as a neutralizing agent for the sodium hydroxide and an antacid (aluminum hydroxide and magnesium hydroxide) as a buffering agent for hydrochloric acid.[12] Fifty milliliters of the caustic were placed in a beaker and the neutralizing or buffer agent was added in 10 mL increments up to 200 mL. Acetic acid was found to decrease pH and cause a minimal increase in temperature when added to sodium hydroxide. The addition of antacid to hydrochloric acid increased the pH without significantly increasing temperature. When water was added to hydrochloric acid or sodium hydroxide, neither pH nor temperature were significantly affected.

The major criticism of this particular study is that neutralization of an acid in a beaker is an oversimplification of a complex reaction at the interface of the acid and tissue. The study also did not evaluate the effect of solid caustics and the changes in temperature and pH at the interface of a solid caustic and tissue.

In examining the changes in temperature, pH, and dissolution rates of Clinitest tablets as the quantity of diluent and the number of tablets were varied, it was found that increasing the volume of water had no effect on Clinitest tablet dissolution time, minimized the increase in temperature, and had a minimal effect on solution pH.[10] Increasing the number of tablets prolonged tablet dissolution time, had a variable effect on temperature, and had no effect on pH.

In an in vitro rat model, early dilution of a weak acid with normal saline was capable of reducing esophageal damage. At time zero, harvested esophagi maintained in an oxygen-perfused saline bath at 37°C were canulated and perfused with 1 mL of 50% sodium hydroxide. Study groups were then irrigated with 3 mL of normal saline at either time 0, 5 minutes, or 30 minutes. Histologic analysis demonstrated a statistically significant decrease in tissue damage with early dilution.[6]

The effects of dilute (less than 10% strength) drain cleaner (sulfuric acid, potassium hydroxide, or sodium hydroxide) were studied on the esophagus with relationship to time and the effect of copious irrigation with water. The authors reported that 9% sulfuric acid, 8% potassium hydroxide, and 8.3% sodium hydroxide all produced both gross and microscopic burns to the esophagus within 30 seconds. This damage could not be prevented with copious water irrigation of the esophagus at 30 seconds.[1]

The neutralization effects of dilute acetic acid were studied in the feline esophagus following the administration of 1 to 5 mL aliquots of 30% sodium hydroxide by nasogastric tube.[11] At 3, 5, and 10 seconds after the alkaline exposure, the esophagus was irrigated with 0.2 N acetic acid (in a quantity previously determined in vitro to neutralize the sodium hydroxide) to pH 7. At a dose of 5 mL, 30% sodium hydroxide was uniformly fatal to the cat following an exposure of 3 seconds or more. One of 3 cats survived 1 mL of 30% sodium hydroxide with a 5-second contact time before dilution and neutralization, and 2 of 3 cats survived 1 mL of 30% sodium hydroxide exposure for 3 seconds prior to dilution and neutralization.[11]

In a continuation of this study, cotton pledgets soaked with 30% sodium hydroxide were placed in the esophagus of anesthetized cats and then the esophagus was flushed with either 50 mL of physiologic saline or with 25 mL of 0.2 N acetic acid. At postmortem, 24 hours after exposure, the cats were examined for esophageal burns. At 24 hours after a 1-second exposure to 30% sodium hydroxide all animals had lesions that had progressed to ulceration with an intense inflammatory reaction. It was concluded that "therapeutic approaches to these exposures are of little benefit."[11]

In conclusion, it appears logical to immediately give an adult patient who has swallowed a strong alkali or a weak acid several glasses of water to drink to dilute and reduce tissue injury. If the patient has ingested more than a taste of a strong acid, it should be removed with a nasogastric tube before water is administered.

References

1. Ashcraft KW, Padula RT: The effect of dilute corrosives on the esophagus. Pediatrics 1974; 53:226–232.
2. Borowitz JL, Moore PF, Yim GKW, et al: Mechanism of enhanced drug effects produced by dilution of the oral dose. Toxicol Appl Pharmacol 1971; 19:164–168.
3. Dean BL, Peterson R, Garrettson LK, et al: American Association of Poison Control Centers policy statement: Gastrointestinal dilution with water as a first aid procedure for poisoning. J Toxicol Clin Toxicol 1982; 19:531–532.
4. Ferguson HC: Dilution of dose and acute oral toxicity. Toxicol Appl Pharmacol 1962; 4:759–762.
5. Henderson ML, Picchioni AL, Chin L: Evaluation of oral dilution as a first aid measure in poisoning. J Pharm Sci 1966; 55:1311–1313.
6. Homan CS, Maitra SR, Lane BP, et al: Effective treatment for acute alkali injury to the esophagus using weak-acid neutralization therapy: An ex-vivo study. Acad Emerg Med 1995; 2:952–958.
7. Homan CS, Maitra SR, Lane BP, et al: Histopathologic evaluation of the therapeutic efficacy of water and milk dilution for esophageal acid injury. Acad Emerg Med 1995; 2:587–591.
8. Homan CS, Maitra SR, Lane BP, et al: Therapeutic effects of water and milk for acute alkali injury of the esophagus. Ann Emerg Med 1994; 24:14–20.
9. Homan CS, Maitra SR, Lane BP, Geller ER: Effective treatment of the rat esophagus with early saline dilution therapy. Ann Emerg Med 1993; 22:178–182.
10. Lacouture PG, Gaudreault P, Lovejoy FH: Clinitest tablet ingestion: An in vitro investigation concerned with initial emergency management. Ann Emerg Med 1986;15:143–146.
11. Leape LL, Ashcraft KW, Scarpelli DG, et al: Hazard to health—Liquid lye. N Engl J Med 1971; 284:578–581.
12. Maull KI, Osmand AP, Maull CD: Liquid caustic ingestions: An in vitro study of the effects of buffer, neutralization, and dilution. Ann Emerg Med 1985; 14:1160–1162.
13. Penner GE: Acid ingestion: Toxicology and treatment. Ann Emerg Med 1980; 9:374–379.
14. Rumack BH, Burrington JD: Caustic ingestions: A rational look at diluents. Clin Toxicol 1977; 11:27–34.

ANTIDOTES IN DEPTH

Calcium

Mary Ann Howland

Calcium
1 mg/dL = 0.25 mmol/L = 0.50 mEq/L

Normal Range
- Total
  - 8.4–10.2 mg/dL
  - 2.10–2.55 mmol/L
  - 4.20–5.10 mEq/L
- Ionized
  - 4.48–4.92 mg/dL
  - 1.12–1.23 mmol/L
  - 2.24–2.46 mEq/L

Calcium is essential in maintaining the normal function of the heart, vascular smooth muscle, skeletal system, and nervous system. It is vital to many enzymatic reactions, intimately involved in neurohormonal transmission, and critical for the maintenance of cellular integrity.[22,34] Excess calcium raises the threshold for nerve and muscle excitation, resulting in muscle weakness, lethargy, and coma.[22] Insufficient calcium facilitates stimulation of nerves and muscles, resulting in tetany and seizures.[22] The endocrine system keeps the serum calcium concentration within the physiologic range. Approximately half of the total serum calcium is ionized and active, and the rest is bound primarily to albumin.

In the clinical practice of medical toxicology, calcium is administered to overcome the effects of calcium channel blockers (CCBs), to correct the hypocalcemia induced by ethylene glycol and fluoride, to complex with fluoride to limit tissue destruction, to treat iatrogenic magnesium poisoning, and to counteract the cardiac effects of hyperkalemia (except when associated with cardiac glycosides). The use of calcium in the management of beta-adrenergic antagonist overdoses is being investigated, and the role of calcium to counteract muscle spasms resulting from black widow spider envenomations is being questioned.

Calcium channel blocker overdoses result in hypotension, myocardial depression, bradycardia, AV block, asystole, altered mental status, nausea, vomiting, constipation, hyperglycemia, and, rarely, seizures.[39] Of the numerous ways for calcium to enter the cell, the calcium channel blockers may selectively block either the voltage-dependent L channels in cardiac and smooth muscles.[2,53] CCBs do not alter receptor-operated channels, the release of calcium from intracellular stores, or serum calcium concentrations.[53] In patients who overdose with calcium channel blockers, the serum calcium concentration therefore remains normal.

Intravenous administration of small doses of calcium to dogs poisoned with verapamil or diltiazem improves cardiac output secondary to an increase in inotropy.[2,21] Heart rate and cardiac conduction are affected minimally, if at all, unless greater amounts of calcium are given.[19,21,45] Case reports and reviews of the literature suggest similar findings in humans.[1,9,18,23,31,41,42,51] Calcium should be administered to symptomatic patients and often produces a beneficial response. Unfortunately in the sickest patients, this response is often inadequate, and other measures are required. Calcium administration to a patient with digoxin toxicity could prove quite harmful. In the event of concurrent overdose with both digoxin and a calcium channel blocker, early use of digoxin-specific antibody fragments should make the subsequent use of calcium less dangerous.

The amount of calcium needed to treat calcium channel blockers is not known. In animal experiments there appears to be a dose-related improvement.[9,21] The customary approach has been to administer an initial intravenous dose of 1 g of calcium chloride or 3 g of calcium gluconate to adults and to repeat this dose every 10 to 20 minutes for 3 to 4 additional doses, as needed.[39]

Dosing in children must rely on the current recommended pediatric dose of calcium for hypocalcemia, which is 5 to 7 mg/kg of elemental calcium (calcium chloride 10% contains 27.2 mg/mL of elemental calcium and calcium gluconate 10% contains 9 mg/mL of elemental calcium) infused slowly at a rate ≤ 100 mg/min and repeated once in 10 minutes. Therefore, a starting dose in children should be about 0.2 mL/kg of calcium chloride 10%. Serum calcium concentration should be monitored when more than two doses are administered, to avoid hypercalcemia. One author successfully used 6 g of calcium gluconate intravenously over 20 minutes, followed by 6 g over the second hour and then 2 g/h for a total of 30 g of calcium gluconate.[9] The patient's peak serum calcium reached 4.8 mmol/L, but decreased to 3.07 mmol/L the following day and was normal within 4 days.[9] Although hyperphosphatemia followed by hypophosphatemia accompanied this therapy, the authors were not able to attribute any adverse clinical effects to the hypercalcemia.[13] Another author administered 18 g of calcium gluconate over 3 hours to a patient who overdosed on sustained-release verapamil. The serum calcium rose to 3.04 mmol/L without obvious toxicity and the patient survived.[30]

Ethylene glycol intoxication results in the generation of directly toxic metabolites that frequently produce central nervous system, cardiovascular, renal, and metabolic abnormalities. The generation of oxalic acid and its complexation with calcium and subsequent precipitation in the kidneys, brain, and elsewhere is believed to account for the hypocalcemia seen in a number of cases.[1,24,38,49,52] Serum calcium and albumin levels should be monitored. Other signs of hypocalcemia are widening of the QT interval, the presence of Chvostek and Trousseau signs, and tetanic seizures. Intravenous calcium should be given in the customary doses to patients with these findings, with frequent monitoring of serum calcium.

Body contact with hydrofluoric acid via any route of exposure can result in extensive burns and death, depending on the concentration of hydrofluoric acid and duration of exposure. The pathophysiologic mechanism is thought to be threefold: (1) release of free hydrogen ions; (2) complexation of fluoride with calcium and magnesium to form insoluble salts, which cause cellular necrosis and the liberation of potassium ions; and (3) cellular dehydration.[5,6,10,17,32,33,35,54] Following hydroflouric acid exposure, calcium is used topically and subcutaneously to manage minor to moderate cutaneous burns, intravenously to treat systemic hypocalcemia, and intraarterially to manage significant burns.[1,5,7,10–12,15,17,20,32,33,35,40,44,46,48,54–56,58] Experimental studies demonstrate that concentrated hydrofluoric acid burns that are immediately flushed with water and then covered with 2.5% calcium gluconate gel or topical DMSO/10% calcium gluconate plus subcutaneous 10% calcium gluconate showed a significant reduction in burn size.[7,58] Unfortunately, neither DMSO nor a commercial calcium gluconate gel is readily available. A topical calcium gel can be prepared from calcium carbonate tablets and a water-soluble jelly such as K-Y Jelly. Calcium chloride should not be injected subcutaneously as it may lead to tissue necrosis. Deaths from hypocalcemia secondary to skin, gastrointestinal, and inhalational hydrofluoric acid toxicity have occurred.[11,20] Aggressive intravenous calcium may be required, along with frequent serum calcium determinations. To facilitate maximum amounts of calcium, simultaneous administration of oral and nebulized calcium (2.5% calcium gluconate = 0.11 mEq/mL) should also be given if there are no contraindications. One patient required a total of 267 mEq of calcium over 24 hours.[20] An ingestion of 30 mL of 70% hydroflouric acid is equivalent to 660 mEq of fluoride. For moderate to severe burns (generally hydrofluoric acid concentrations greater than 10%) of the fingers and hands, an intraarterial calcium infusion may be more effective than local therapy, although it is more invasive[40,48,55,56] and therefore more hazardous.[48] One group used 10 mL of 10% calcium gluconate solution mixed in 40 to 50 mL of 5% dextrose over 4 hours with repeated infusions after 4 hours if pain persisted.[55] Serum calcium and serum magnesium concentrations should be carefully monitored in all severely poisoned patients.[48,55]

Hypermagnesemia causes both direct and indirect depression of skeletal muscle, resulting in neuromuscular blockade, loss of reflexes, and profound muscular paralysis.[22] Excess magnesium also causes widening of the PR interval and QRS complex and slows the SA node, ultimately resulting in cardiac arrest. Intravenous calcium serves as a physiologic antagonist to the effects of magnesium.

Hyperkalemia causes significant myocardial depression. The height of the T wave increases, the PR interval and QRS complex widen, impulse generation and conduction are depressed, and cardiac arrest occurs.[22] Intravenous calcium serves as a physiologic antagonist to the cardiac effects of hyperkalemia. However, if hyperkalemia is secondary to the toxic effects of digoxin on the Na^+/K^+-ATPase pump, then intravenous calcium would potentially exacerbate an already excessive intracellular calcium concentration and is therefore contraindicated.

In vitro studies suggest that the negative inotropic action of propranolol and analogs is related to interference of both the forward and reverse transport of calcium in the sarcoplasmic reticulum and to inhibition of microsomal and mitochondrial calcium uptake[16,36] In a canine model of propranolol poisoning, the administration of a bolus of calcium chloride followed by a continuous infusion improved mean arterial pressure, maximal left ventricular pressure change over time, and peripheral vascular resistance, but had no effect on bradycardia or QRS prolongation.[29] Several case reports attest to the beneficial effects of calcium in beta-adrenergic antagonist overdose.[8,25,47] As long as no contraindications exist, a trial of intravenous calcium seems reasonable.

Envenomation by a black widow spider (*Lactrodectus spp*) leads to local and systemic symptoms. Excruciating abdominal or back pain that begins within several hours of envenomation is the most common finding in severe cases.[13] It is unclear exactly how the venom works, but the release of synaptic transmitters, including norepinephrine and acetylcholine, is believed to be involved.[43] Intravenous calcium along with analgesics, benzodiazepines, and muscle relaxants are used to relieve the pain and muscle spasms.[13,26] Rarely, antivenin may be indicated. Animal studies suggest that the venom induces changes in the permeability of calcium that may be antagonized by increasing the extracellular concentration of calcium.[27,37] One prospective collection of cases noted improvement in 6 of 13 patients treated with calcium gluconate.[26] Recently, however, a large retrospective study of 163 patients cast doubt on calcium's effectiveness.[13] The authors reported that very few patients received adequate pain relief from calcium, and all but one patient also required opioids.[13] More research is necessary to clarify calcium's utility, if any, in the management of black widow spider envenomation.

The adverse effects of hypercalcemia (independent of the rate of administration) include nausea, vomiting, constipation, hypertension if intravascular volume is maintained, shortened QT interval, polyuria, polydypsia, cognitive difficulties, hyporeflexia, coma, and enhanced sensitivity to digitalis.[3] Significant hypercalcemia may lead to myocardial depression. The symptoms exhibited depend on the patient's age, rate of increase in the serum calcium, and duration of the hypercalcemia.[3] Severe hypercalcemia is defined by a serum calcium concentration greater than 3.5 mmol/L in a patient with a normal albumin concentration.

A variety of calcium salts are available for parenteral administration. The two most commonly used are calcium chloride and calcium gluconate. A 1-g vial (10 mL) of 10% calcium chloride contains 1.36 mEq/mL of Ca^{2+}, while a 1-g vial (10 mL) of 10% calcium gluconate delivers only 0.45 mEq/mL of Ca^{2+}. Calcium chloride is an acidifying salt and is extremely irritating to tissue. It should never be given intramuscularly, subcutaneously, or perivascularly.[22,34] Calcium gluconate is less irritating, but care should be taken to avoid extravasation. There is some evidence to suggest that during intravenous infusion calcium chloride produces slightly larger increases in ionic calcium than calcium gluconate.[57] Intravenous calcium must be administered slowly, at a rate not exceeding 0.7 to 1.8 mEq/min or one 10-mL vial of calcium chloride over 10 minutes. In cases of extreme life-threatening hypocalcemia or for a patient in extremis, faster rates may be required. More rapid administration may lead to vasodilation, hypotension, bradycardia, dysrhythmias, syncope, and cardiac arrest.[4,14,28,34,50]

In summary, intravenous calcium is an effective remedy for the hypocalcemia induced by ethylene glycol and hydrofluoric acid. It serves as a physiologic antagonist to the cardiac and/or neurologic effects of hypermagnesemia and hyperkalemia (except when associated with cardiac glycosides) and counteracts the effects of calcium channel blocker overdoses. The efficacy of calcium in the management of patients with black widow spider envenomation has yet to be clarified. Great care must be taken to avoid extravasation. Calcium chloride, in particular, can be quite toxic to tissue. There is some debate as to whether the calcium chloride preparation delivers more ionic or active calcium. It must be recognized that 30 mL of a 10% solution of calcium gluconate is necessary to equal 10 mL of a 10% calcium chloride solution (13.6 mEq of calcium). Electrocardiographic monitoring and frequent serum calcium determinations are required to prevent iatrogenic toxicity.

References

1. Anderson WJ, Anderson JR: Hydrofluoric acid burns of the hand: Mechanism of injury and treatment. Am J Hand Surg 1988;13:52–57.
2. Bean BP: Classes of calcium channels in vertebrate cells. Annu Rev Physiol 1989;51:367–384.
3. Belezekian JP: Management of acute hypercalcemia. N Engl J Med 1992;326:1196–1215.
4. Berliner K: The effect of calcium injections on the human heart. Am J Med Sci 1936;191:117.
5. Bertolini JC: Hydrofluoric acid: A review of toxicity. J Emerg Med 1992;10:163–168.
6. Boink ABTJ, Wemer J, Meulenbelt J, et al: The mechanism of fluoride-induced hypocalcemia. Hum Exp Toxicol 1994;13:149–155.
7. Bracken WM, Cuppage F, McLaury RL, et al: Comparative effectiveness of topical treatments for hydrofluoric acid burns. J Occup Med 1985;27:733–739.
8. Briacombe JR, Scully M, Swainston R: Propranolol overdose. A dramatic response to calcium chloride. Med J Aust 1991;155:267–268.
9. Buckley N, Dawson AH, Howarth D, Whyte IM: Slow-release verapamil poisoning. Med J Aust 1993;158:202–204.
10. Caravati EM: Acute hydrofluoric acid exposure. Am J Emerg Med 1988;6:143–150.
11. Chan KM, Svancarek WP, Creer M: Fatality due to acute hydrofluoric acid exposure. J Toxicol Clin Toxicol 1987; 25:333–339.
12. Chick LR, Borah G: Calcium carbonate gel therapy of hydrofluoric acid burns of the hand. Plast Reconstruct Surg 1990;86:935–940.
13. Clark RF, Wathern-Kestner S, Vance M, Gerkin R: Clinical presentation and treatment of black widow spider envenomation: A review of 163 cases. Ann Emerg Med 1992;21: 782–787.
14. Clarke NE: The action of calcium on the human electrocardiogram. Am Heart J 1941;22:367.
15. Conway EE, Sockolow R: Hydrofluoric acid burn in a child. Pediatr Emerg Care 1991;7:345–347.
16. Dhalla NS, Lee SL: Comparison of the actions of acebutolol, practolol, and propranolol on calcium transport by heart microsomes and mitochondria. Br J Pharmacol 1976;57: 215–221.
17. Edinburg M, Swift R: Hydrofluoric acid burns of the hands: A case report and suggested management. Aust NZ J Surg 1989;59:88–91.
18. Erickson F, Ling L, Grande G, et al: Diltiazem overdose? Case report and review. J Emerg Med 1991;9:357–366.
19. Gay R, Algeo S, Lee R, et al: Treatment of verapamil toxicity in intact dogs. J Clin Invest 1986;77:1805–1811.

20. Greco RJ, Hartford CE, Haith LR, Patton ML: Hydrofluoric acid-induced hypocalcemia. J Trauma 1988;28:1593–1596.
21. Hariman RJ, Mangiardi LM, McAllister RG, et al: Reversal of the cardiovascular effects of verpamil by calcium and sodium: Differences between electrophysiologic and hemodynamic responses. Circulation 1979;59: 797–804.
22. Hayes RC: Agents affecting calcification: Calcium, parathyroid hormone, calcitonin, vitamin D, and other compounds. In: Gilman AG, Rall T, Nies A, Taylor P, eds: Goodman and Gilman's The Pharmacologic Basis of Therapeutics, 8th ed. New York, Pergamon, 1990, pp. 1496–1501.
23. Hofer CA, Smith JK, Tenholder MF: Verapamil intoxication: A literature review of overdoses and discussion of therapeutic options. Am J Med 1993;95:431–438.
24. Introna F Jr, Smialek JE: Antifreeze (ethylene glycol) intoxications in Baltimore: Report of six cases. Acta Morphol Hung 1989;37:245–263.
25. Jones JL: Metoprolol overdose. Ann Emerg Med 1982; 11:114–115.
26. Key GF: A comparison of calcium gluconate and methocarbamol (Robaxin) in the treatment of lactrodectism (black widow spider envenomations). Am J Trop Med Hyg 1981; 30:273–277.
27. Kobernick M: Black widow spider bites. Am Fam Physician 1984;29:241–245.
28. Kuhn M: Severe bradyarrhythmias following calcium pretreatment. Am Heart J 1991;121:1812–1813.
29. Love J, Hanfling D, Howell J: Hemodynamic effects of calcium chloride in a canine model of acute propranolol intoxication. Ann Emerg Med 1996; 28:1–6.
30. Luscher TF, Noll G, Sturmer T, Muser B et al: Calcium gluconate in severe verapamil intoxication. N Engl J Med 1994;330:718–719. Letter.
31. MacDonald D, Alguire P: Case reports: Fatal overdose with sustained release verapamil. Am J Med Sci 1992;303: 115–117.
32. MacKinnon MA: Hydrofluoric acid burns. Dermatol Clin 1988;6:67–74.
33. McCulley JP: Ocular hydrofluoric acid burns: Animal model, mechanism of injury and therapy. Am Ophthalmol Soc 1990;88:649–683.
34. McEvoy G, ed: AHFS Drug Information, 1993. Baltimore, American Society of Hospital Pharmacists, 1997.
35. Mistry DG, Wainwright DJ: Hydrofluoric acid burns. Am Fam Physician 1992;45:1748–1754.
36. Noack E, Kurzmack M, Verjovski-Almeida Sand Inesi G: The effect of propranolol and its analogs on Ca^{++} transport by sarcoplasmic reticulum vesicles. J Pharmacol Exp Ther 1978;206:281–288.
37. Pardel JF: Influence of calcium on 3H-noradrenaline release by *Lactrodectus* venom gland extract on arterial tissue of the rat. Toxicon 1979;17:455–465.
38. Parry MF, Wallach R: Ethylene glycol poisoning. Am J Med 1974;57:143–150.
39. Pearigen PD, Benowitz NS: Poisoning due to calcium antagonists: Experience with verapamil, diltiazem and nifedipine. Drug Saf 1991;6:408–430.
40. Pegg SP, Siu S, Gillet G: Intra-arterial infusions in the treatment of hydrofluoric acid burns. Burns 1985;11: 440–443.
41. Proano L, Chiang WK, Wang RY: Calcium channel blocker overdose. Am J Emerg Med 1995;13:444–450.
42. Ramoska EA, Spiller HA, Winter M, Borys D: A one year evaluation of calcium channel blocker overdoses: Toxicity and treatment. Ann Emerg Med 1993;22:196–200.
43. Rauber A: Black widow spider bites. J Toxicol Clin Toxicol 1983–1984;21:473–485.
44. Roberts JR, Merigian KS: Acute hydrofluoric acid exposure. Am J Emerg Med 1989;7:125–126.
45. Sabatier J, Pouyet T, Shelvey G, Cavero I: Antagonistic effects of epinephrine, glucagon and methylatropine but not calcium chloride against atrio-ventricular conduction disturbances produced by high doses of diltiazem in conscious dogs. Fundam Clin Pharmacol 1991;5:93–106.
46. Sadove R, Hainsworth D, Van Meter W: Total body immersion in hydrofluoric acid. South Med J 1990;83:698–700.
47. Sangster B, de Wildt D, van Dijk A: A case of acebutolol intoxication. J Toxicol Clin Toxicol 1983;20:69–77.
48. Siegel DC, Heard JM: Intra-arterial calcium infusion for hydrofluoric acid burns. Aviat Space Environ Med 1992;63: 206–211.
49. Simpson E: Some aspects of calcium metabolism in a fatal case of ethylene glycol poisoning. Ann Clin Biochem 1985;22:90–93.
50. Smallwood RA: Some effects of the intravenous administration of calcium in man. Aust Acad Med 1967;16:126–131.
51. Spiller HA, Meyers A, Ziemba T, Riley M: Delayed onset of cardiac arrhythmias from sustained release verpamil. Ann Emerg Med 1991;20:201–203.
52. Tarr BD, Winters LJ, Moore MP, et al: Low dose ethanol in the treatment of ethylene glycol poisoning. J Vet Pharmacol Ther 1985;8:254–262.
53. Triggle DJ: Calcium-channel antagonists: Mechanisms of action, vascular selectivities, and clinical relevance. Cleve Clin J Med 1992;59:617–626.
54. Upfal M, Doyle C: Medical management of hydrofluoric acid exposure. J Occup Med 1990;32:726–731.
55. Vance MV, Curry SC, Kunkel DB, et al: Digital hydrofluoric acid burns: Treatment with intraarterial calcium infusion. Ann Emerg Med 1986;15:890–896.
56. Velvart J: Arterial perfusion for hydrofluoric acid burns. Hum Toxicol 1983;2:233–238.
57. White RD, Goldsmith RS, Rodriquez R, et al: Plasma ionic calcium levels following injection of chloride, gluconate, and gluceptate salts of calcium. J Thorac Cardiovasc Surg 1976;71:609–613.
58. Zachary LS, Reus W, Gottlieb J, et al: Treatment of experimental hydrofluoric acid burns. J Burn Care 1986;7:35–39.

CHAPTER 87

Insecticides: Organophosphates and Carbamates

Cynthia K. Aaron and Mary Ann Howland

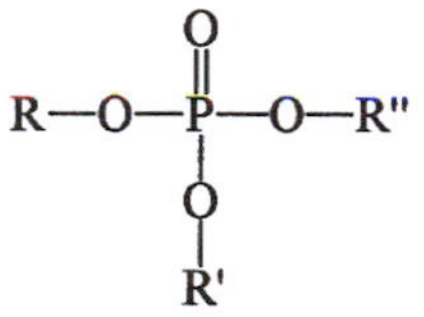

Organophosphate

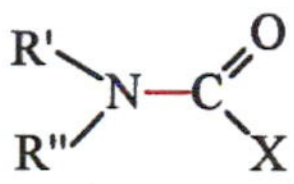

Carbamate

A 34-year-old male was found by co-workers at his place of employment, lying on the ground vomiting, holding his abdomen, and acting as if he were in pain. Although the patient was awake, he was markedly confused and unable to give any history. EMS was called and found him to be awake, oriented to name only, and groaning. Initial vital signs were an irregularly irregular heart rate of 130 beats/min, respiratory rate of 32 breaths/min, and blood pressure of 90 mm Hg palpable. The ambulance run sheet noted marked salivation and drooling. Lungs were filled with rhonchi and the patient continued to vomit en route to the hospital. The paramedics started an IV line of normal saline, placed him on a 100% nonrebreather oxygen mask, and attempted to monitor his cardiac rhythm, however, electrodes would not stick to his diaphoretic skin. En route to the hospital, he was increasingly agitated.

This patient presented a confusing constellation of signs and symptoms. He was unable to communicate but clearly quite ill. His vital signs were abnormal. The paramedics followed the ABCs and placed him on oxygen, started an IV, attempted to monitor his cardiac rhythm, and transported. Because of the difficulty in keeping electrodes on his skin and the need for two people to restrain him, the paramedics elected to transport immediately to the nearest hospital, which was only 5 minutes away, rather than intubate him in the field. The paramedics noted his marked secretions and they suggested an ingestion when they called medical control.

Upon arrival in the hospital, the patient was confused, drooling, vomiting, and incontinent. He smelled strongly of solvents. He had diffuse myoclonus and tremors. The vital signs were unchanged and his temperature 34°C (93.4°F). His clothing was soaked with sweat. As he was being transferred to the stretcher, the worksite called to notify the hospital that they had found an empty can of Roach Control Spray and an empty wet glass. All unprotected healthcare workers immediately were sent away from the bedside to wash, fully gown and glove, and mask. The paramedic transport team was sent to disrobe and decontaminate in the shower. The patient was moved into an isolation room and stripped.

Within 2 minutes of arrival, the patient was restrained, being bagged with 100% oxygen. A pulse oximeter was placed and read 88%. Spontaneous respiratory movements were clearly uncoordinated and ineffectual. The monitoring strip showed atrial fibrillation at a rate of 130 beats/min. Two milligrams of IV atropine were administered without effect while intubation equipment was prepared. Additional atropine was administered as 4 mg and then 8 mg IV. Bagging increased his pulse oximetry to 94% and oral secretions decreased, although he was now coughing up frothy sputum. The patient was sedated with 5 mg midazolam and 120 mg succinylcholine intravenously and was rapidly intubated. The endotracheal tube immediately filled with frothy sputum and needed to be continually suctioned. A nasogastric tube was placed and drained copious amounts of fluids. Additional atropine was given while 2 g of pralidoxime were obtained. A Foley catheter was placed. By 10 minutes after arrival, 24 mg of atropine had been administered and the patient's bronchorrhea had diminished. He was sedated with 10 mg of diazepam intravenously. Two additional intravenous lines were started and a fingerstick glucose was 210 mg/dL. Blood work was drawn and sent. He remained in atrial fibrillation at 120 beats/min. The 2 g of pralidoxime were administered intravenously over 15 minutes.

Thirty minutes after arrival, the peak ventilation pressures had dropped to under 50 mm Hg and bronchial secretions had markedly decreased. Although still diaphoretic, the patient converted to a sinus tachycardia at 120 beats/min. His blood pressure was now 112/60 and pulse oximetry was 98% on 100% oxygen. One hundred grams of activated charcoal without cathartic were administered via the nasogastric tube. The patient was then washed off with a weak bleach solution. His hair was also washed, and all bedding was changed. His clothing had been collected in double plastic bags and were segregated for toxic waste disposal.

Forty-five minutes after arrival, the patient remained paralyzed. An ECG showed sinus rhythm with a mildly prolonged QT_c of 490 msec and nonspecific ST-T changes. The chest radiograph was consistent with pulmonary edema or ARDS. His wife arrived and was able to give the history that he had been depressed lately and had made an appointment to see his family doctor. She had noted that the previous weekend, he had bought a large amount of lawn and garden products.

One hour after presentation, he had a metabolic acidosis, glucose of 240 mg/dL, and potassium of 3.4 mEq/L. His complete blood count showed a leukocytosis of 18,600 and a normal differential. His hepatic enzymes were mildly elevated. The patient was kept sedated. An additional 4 mg of atropine was administered when he began to vomit around the NG tube.

Two hours after admission, pralidoxime was started as an infusion at a rate of 500 mg/h. His pulmonary status had improved and he was weaned down to 50% FIO_2. Salicylate and acetaminophen levels were negative, and ethanol was 135 mg/dL. The patient was transferred to the ICU as he began to make spontaneous movements. Several of the ambulance personnel reported feeling "ill" but none showed any evidence of muscarinic and nicotinic symptoms. All were admitted to the ED and observed for 6 hours. A level was determined for plasma cholinesterase on the paramedic who had had the closest contact with the patient. Both the isolation room and the ambulance were cleaned with a dilute bleach solution. All leather items worn by the medics were discarded.

During his ICU stay, pralidoxime was continued for 48 hours. He did not require additional atropine. His pulmonary status deteriorated and he developed a fever. Chest radiograph was consistent with an aspiration pneumonia. After 4 days of mechanical ventilation and antibiotics, he was weaned from the ventilator and extubated. At that time he admitted to spraying several cans of the roach killer into a glass and drinking this mixed with beer. Once his medical problems resolved, he was transferred for psychiatric care.

One week after discharge, the patient's plasma cholinesterase level returned markedly decreased. The RBC cholinesterase level had been drawn in the wrong tube and could not be ascertained. The paramedic's plasma cholinesterase was "low normal," and he was advised to avoid general anesthetics and all organophosphates and carbamates for 4 to 6 weeks.

Pathophysiology

Pest control sprays are an example of cholinesterase inhibitors and include organophosphorus compounds and carbamates. Cholinesterase inhibitors exert their toxicity by interfering with the normal function of acetylcholine, an essential neurotransmitter throughout the autonomic and central nervous system. Acetylcholine is the neurotransmitter at pre- and postganglionic parasympathetic synapses, sympathetic preganglionic synapses, and at the neuromuscular junction. When an action potential stimulates the nerve terminal, specific quanta of acetylcholine are released via exocytosis into the synapse. The acetylcholine binds the postsynaptic receptors (G proteins for muscarinic receptors and ligand linked ionchannels for the nicotinic receptors). Activation of the receptor alters the flow of K^+, Na^+, and Ca^{2+} ionic currents and alters membrane potential of the postsynaptic membrane, leading to propagation of the action potential.[16] At the autonomic and neuromuscular synapses, acetylcholine is immediately hydrolyzed by acetylcholinesterase to choline and acetic acid, preventing continued stimulation of the local receptors and eventual paralysis of the nerve or muscle (see Fig. 10–4).

Organophosphates and carbamates are powerful inhibitors of carboxylic ester hydrolases including chymotrypsin, acetylcholinesterase, plasma or butyrlcholinesterase (pseudocholinesterase), plasma and hepatic carboxylesterases (aliesterases), paraoxonases (A-esterases), and other nonspecific proteases. Functioning acetylcholinesterase is found in human nervous tissue and skeletal muscles and is also genetically expressed on the membrane of erythrocytes; hence its activity can be assessed by red blood cell acetylcholinesterase measurements. The RBC cholinesterase activity level parallels functioning nervous system acetylcholinesterase. Butyryl-cholinesterase is a hepatic derived protein that is found in human plasma, liver, heart, pancreas, and brain. Its activity can be measured by plasma or butyrylcholinesterase (pseudocholinesterase) measurements, although its endogenous function is not fully understood.

The active acyl pocket in the center of acetylcholinesterase is a narrow cleft 2 nm deep and surrounded by tetramers. Two additional domains on the enzyme include a peripheral anionic site and a choline subsite of the active center. These three sites confer the steriospecificity for other ligands to bind. At the base of the cleft, the enzymatic active site contains a serine 203 residue. Coiled nearby are a histidine 447 residue and a glutamate 334. When acetylcholine enters the binding area, it is attracted by local atomic forces into a tetrahedral structure with the serine, histadine, and glutamate, and forms a nucleophilic serine hydroxyl intermediate. The acetylcholine is hydrolyzed to acetic acid and choline, which then leave the site and the enzyme reforms its allosteric structure. Turnover time for this reaction is 150 microseconds. (Fig. 87–1A).[88,90,100,110,122]

Although carbamates and organophosphorus compounds differ structurally from acetylcholine, they can bind to the acetylcholinesterase molecule at the active site and either carbamoylate or phosphorylate/phosphonate the serine moiety. When this occurs, the resultant conjugate is infinitely more stable than the acetylcholine–acetylcholinesterase conjugate, although endogenous hydrolysis does occur. Depending upon the amount of stability and charge distribution, the time to hydrolysis is increased. Carbamoylated enzyme spontaneously degrades in minutes to hours so that the enzyme site is eventually regenerated. Most carbamate poisonings spontaneously revert within 24–48 hours. Phosphorylated or phosphonylated enzymes, however, degrade over days to weeks, making the acetylcholinesterase essentially inactive. In order for the physiologic enzyme activity to return, new enzyme must be generated or antidote given (Fig 87–1B).[56,105,122,128]

Once the acetylcholinesterase is phosphorylated, over the next 24 to 48 hours, an alkyl group is eventually lost from the conjugate, further exacerbating the clinical situation. As this "aging" occurs the enzyme can no longer spontaneously hydrolyze and is permanently inactivated.[100,110,122]

Carbamates and organophosphates are used in industry as insecticides, miticides, and aphicides. Fortunately, both morbidity and mortality associated with carbamates are limited as a result of the transient nature of cholinesterase inhibition and the rapid enzyme reactivation. Another important distinction between organophosphates and carbamates is that carbamates do not penetrate the CNS to the same extent, resulting in limited CNS toxicity. With respect to all other clinical manifestations, there is little difference between organophosphates and carbamates.[56,105]

Pharmacology and Pharmacokinetics

The organophosphorous insecticides are a closely related family of chemicals varying in structure (Fig. 87–2). The various attached groups to the different sites of the phosphorus or sulfur moiety influences the relative tightness of the bond to acetylcholinesterase, the time for hydrolysis, potency, and latency of onset of symptoms. This latent period may vary with route of administration, degree of exposure, fat solubility, ability of the substance to be endogenously hydrolyzed, affinity to the cholinesterase active site, inherent toxicity of the particular organophosphate, and whether the toxin is a direct-acting agent or must first undergo conversion to an active metabolite. Organophosphorous compounds may be absorbed by virtually any route including transdermal, transconjunctival, inhalational, across the GI or GU mucosa, and through direct injection.[12–14,46,55,58,59,61,82,88]

Onset of systemic symptoms is most rapid following inhalation and least rapid following percutaneous absorption. Symptom onset may occur in less than 5 minutes with massive ingestions or inhalational exposures or may be delayed. Except for the fat-soluble organophosphates such as fenthion or clorfenthion, or if significant metabolic activation must occur for activity (parathion), most patients become symptomatic within 12 hours of exposure. A single exposure to fenthion may not immediately depress acetylcholinesterase because its effect may be cumulative. Over time, however, enough inhibitor is leached out of fat stores, and the additive effects of cholinesterase depression becomes clinically significant, leading to symptom onset. This delay has implications not only in determining who becomes sick from a fenthion exposure, but also in treating with antidotes and in determining the meaning of blood cholinesterase depression.[14,126]

The pharmacologic and toxicologic effects of organophosphates and carbamates are due predominately to inhibition of acetylcholinesterase and accumulation of acetylcholine at the synapse (Fig. 87–3). The excess acetylcholine paralyzes the cholinergic synaptic transmission within the CNS, somatic nerves, autonomic ganglia, parasympathetic nerve endings, and some sympathetic nerve endings such as the sweat glands.

In the presence of cholinesterase inhibition, excess acetylcholine accumulates at the parasympathetic, sympathetic, and somatic sites of neurotransmission. Each organophosphate has a different affinity for the histidine-serine esteratic subsite on the acetylcholinesterase molecule. This affinity will determine how strongly the organophosphate is bound at each site. The degree of affinity as well as the route of absorption, amount of metabolism, local blood flow, and active site of concentration will determine which signs and symptoms predominate.[1,56,105,122,128]

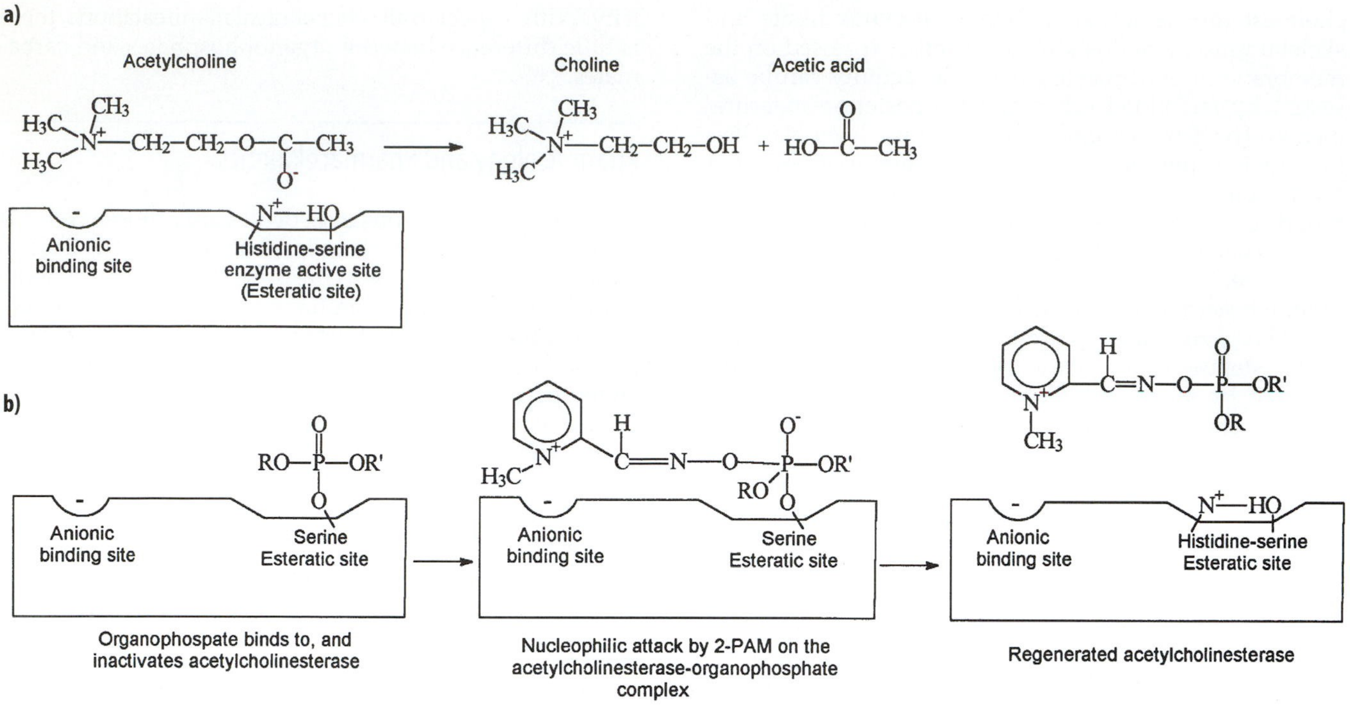

Figure 87–1. (a) Hydrolysis of acetylcholine by acetylcholinesterase. **(b)** Reactivation of alkylphosphorylated acetylcholinesterase. *(Modified, with permission, from Taylor P: Anticholinesterase agents. In: Gilman AG, Goodman LS, Rall TW, Murad F, eds: Goodman and Gilman's The Pharmacological Basis of Therapeutics, 7th ed. New York, Macmillan, 1985, p. 112.)*

Signs and Symptoms

The signs and symptoms of cholinesterase poisoning can be classified into three categories: (1) muscarinic or hollow-organ parasympathetic manifestations, (2) nicotinic or autonomic ganglionic and somatic motor (NMJ) effects, and (3) CNS effects. The muscarinic signs and symptoms involve the bronchial tree, sweat and lacrimal glands, heart, gastrointestinal and genitourinary systems, pupils, and ciliary bodies. Muscarinic effects can be remembered by the acronym "SLUDGE": salivation, lacrimation, urination, diarrhea, gastrointestinal distress, and emesis. Bronchorrhea and bronchoconstriction with compromised pulmonary function may occur secondary to the muscarinic effects. Cardiac effects are mostly re-

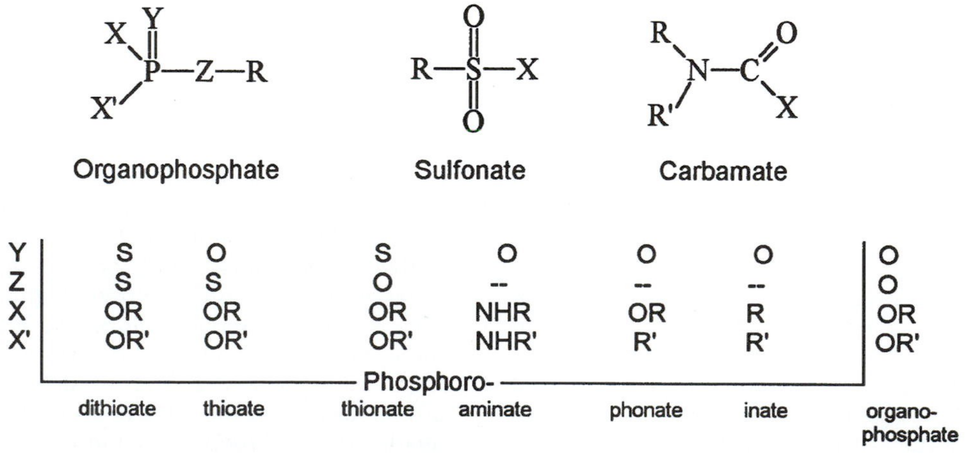

Figure 87–2. Structure of organophosphates, sulfonates, and carbamates.

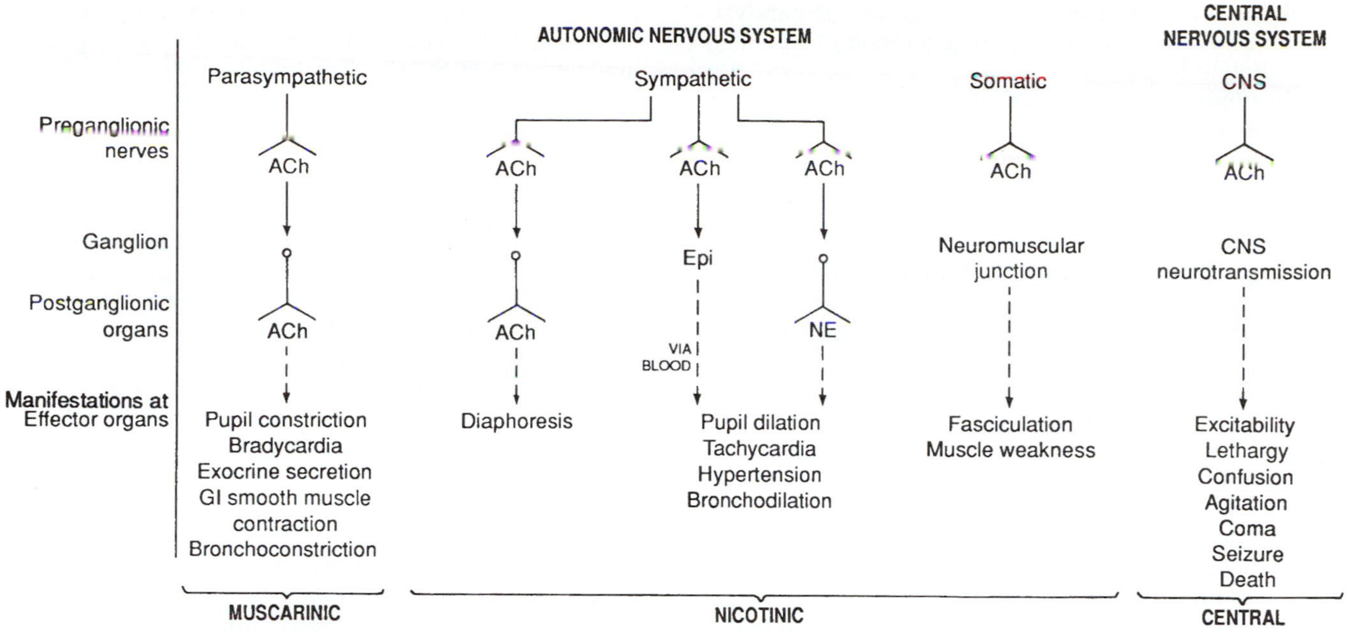

Figure 87–3. Schematic representation of the autonomic nervous system and effector organ manifestations of toxicity. *(Adapted, with permission, from Tafuri J, Roberts J: Organophosphate poisoning. Ann Emerg Med 1987;16:196. As modified from Rymer WZ: Organization of the Autonomic Nervous System, Northwestern University Medical School, 1981.)*

lated to the augmented vagal tone with increase in the refractory period and conduction time in the sinoatrial and atrioventricular nodes, decrease the effective refractory period of atrial muscle fibers, and possibly coronary blood flow restriction.[14,15,46,84,106]

Nicotinic manifestations include muscle fasciculations, cramping and weakness, and diaphragmatic failure, and can progress to paralysis, areflexia, and respiratory failure. Autonomic effects include hypertension, tachycardia, pupillary dilation, and pallor. Electrophysiologically, nicotinic effects may lead to persistent depolarization of the cell membrane.[38,56,91,97,114,115]

Central nervous system effects include restlessness, emotional lability, headache, tremor, drowsiness, confusion, slurred speech, ataxia, generalized weakness, delirium, seizures, psychosis, and death.[38,91,97,120]

Miosis is a characteristic sign found in many patients with severe and moderately severe poisoning. However, miosis can appear late and mydriasis can be present in up to 100% of patients. Thus if miosis is absent, treatment should not be delayed following exposure to these compounds.[120] Ocular exposures from vapor or aerosols may result in a covert form of exposure that necessitates specific decontamination with large quantities of irrigating fluid. Ocular exposure may be a reason for persistent miosis and may require topical atropine or scopolamine instillation.[97]

The usual cause of death from an organophosphate exposure is respiratory failure, resulting from weakness of the respiratory muscles and central depression of the respiratory drive.[121] This may be aggravated by the inability to oxygenate because of bronchospasm and severe bronchorrhea. Patients suffering pulmonary effects of poisoning are also susceptible to multiple complications of prolonged mechanical ventilation, including aspiration pneumonia and barotrauma. Agents with significant CNS penetration may contribute to mortality by causing prolonged seizures with hypoxia, hyperthermia, and seizure-induced rhabdomyolysis with acute tubular necrosis. Those organophosphates requiring hepatic metabolism for activation are also directly hepatotoxic.[91,97]

Treatment

Treatment of cholinesterase inhibition is directed toward reversing the synaptic biochemical abnormalities and reversing the cholinesterase blockade. This is done pharmacologically via the administration of two complementary medications. Atropine, a competitive antagonist of acetylcholine at the muscarinic postsynaptic membrane and in the CNS, will block the muscarinic manifestations of poisoning. Pralidoxime, or 2-PAM, a nucleophilic oxime, will regenerate acetylcholinesterase at muscarinic, nicotinic, and CNS sites (Fig. 87–1B). The two medications are synergistic in their effects. Because atropine will only affect postsynaptic muscarinic receptors, it will have no effect on muscle weakness or paralysis and will not affect the rate of regeneration of inhibited acetylcholinesterase.

In symptomatic poisoned adult patients, atropine is administered with an initial test dose of 1 to 2 mg (0.05 mg/kg in children) intravenously although it may be given intramuscularly if there is no IV access. If there is no effect, then the dose is doubled every 5 to 10 minutes until muscarinic symptoms are relieved. Glycopyrrolate (0.05 mg/ kg) may be substituted if there is no evidence of central toxicity. Glycopyrrolate will not penetrate the CNS, and substituting it for atropine will eliminate the potential for a central anticholinergic syndrome in a patient with an initially clear sensorium. The endpoint to anticholinergic treatment is clearing of the secretions from the tracheobronchial tree and drying of most secretions. Pupillary dilation is an early response to atropine but it is not a therapeutic endpoint. Tachycardia is not a contraindication to atropine treatment, as it may represent hypoxia and autonomic stimulation. The patient's heart rate may slow as oxygenation is improved, although an increase of 10 to 20 beats/min is not unusual. Once signs of adequate atropinization occur, the dose should be adjusted to maintain this effect for at least 24 hours.[34,69,70,90,114,115]

In massive exposures, hundreds of milligrams of atropine may be needed. An atropine drip may be compounded using the powdered form of the drug or the 20-mL multidose vial. Once the patient is adequately stabilized, atropine may be carefully withdrawn while maintaining close observation. Anticholinergic therapy should be reinstituted at the first signs of cholinergic symptoms.

Some authors have commented on the need to maximize oxygenation prior to atropine administration to prevent ventricular dysrhythmias associated with hypoxia. Unfortunately, atropine may be needed to maximize oxygenation if copious secretions and bronchospasm are present. Once atropine has been administered, the patient should be admitted for observation for at least 24 hours.[34,91,96,97,120]

Isolated pulmonary manifestations may respond to local administration of nebulized atropine or ipratropium. Only a small amount of nebulized atropine is systemically absorbed, so if the patient develops widespread systemic symptoms, IV atropine is still indicated.

Pralidoxime and other oximes restore acetylcholinesterase activity by regenerating the phosphorylated acetylcholinesterase (see Fig 87–1B). They may also prevent continued toxicity by scavenging the remaining organophosphate molecules. Oximes function by nucleophilic attack on the phosphorylated enzyme, removing the bulky sterically hindering phosphate moiety. This completely restores normal acetylcholinesterase activity. Once the phosphorylated enzyme has "aged," then the phosphate group becomes irreversibly bound to the enzyme and oxime therapy is no longer as effective. This time sequence is extremely variable, however; review of the literature shows that the restriction of 2-PAM use to 48 hours is unjustified and may actually have deleterious effects (see Antidotes in Depth: Pralidoxime).[4,11–14,55,58,59,61,88,96,102] Treatment with 2-PAM is most effective when started early and if used with acute rather than chronic organophosphate poisonings.[6,25,34,38,48,91,94,96,97,102,110]

In acute poisonings, 2-PAM should be administered as soon as the diagnosis is made and toxicity is present. Although it is most effective when administered early, it continues to have a salutary effect for a prolonged period of time after exposure. This is particularly true for highly fat-soluble compounds such as fenthion but may also be appropriate for most other organophosphates. There are many reports of the effectiveness of 2-PAM given days after intoxication with organophosphates.[1,4,14,27–29,88,96,102]

Pralidoxime may be administered via bolus injections or as a continuous infusion (see Antidotes in Depth: Pralidoxime). As a bolus, 1 to 2 grams (20 to 40 mg/kg) of 2-PAM are dissolved into 0.9% normal saline solution and infused over 30 minutes. The dose may be repeated in one hour if necessary. Rapid IV bolus administration should be avoided because respiratory and cardiac arrest have occurred. Other side effects of bolus dosing include diastolic hypertension, dizziness, and blurred vision.[88] Although 2-PAM is also effective when given IM or orally, IV infusion is the preferred route as it has the most rapid onset of action and the most reliable kinetics. Amelioration of muscle weakness and fasciculations, plus the additive antimuscarinic effects with atropine, will occur within 10 to 40 minutes. Some patients may require multiple doses of 2-PAM before a significant clinical effect is noted, as regeneration is dependent upon plasma concentration of the organophosphate. If the organophosphate concentration is high enough, it will inhibit the newly synthesized enzyme or inhibit the reactivated acetylcholinesterase.[126] Several studies have looked at the minimal serum level necessary to achieve therapeutic efficacy of pralidoxime. Based on animal data, a serum level of 4 μg/L is suggested as the minimum therapeutic threshold. When pralidoxime is given as a bolus infusion in nonpoisoned volunteers, concentrations will fall below this level by 2 hours postinfusion.[87] Although the manufacturer suggests rebolusing every 3 to 8 hours, this will lead to subtherapeutic levels for a large part of the dosing interval.

Subsequent dosing regimens based on a computerized pharmacokinetic simulation have suggested an infusion of 500 mg/h as an alternative way to maintain serum levels greater than 4 μg/L. Most recently, several authors have tested a treatment protocol using a loading dose followed by a continuous weight-based infusion. One author, using poisoned patients, infused a 4.42 mg/kg load administered over 30 minutes followed by 2.14 mg/kg per hour,[127] and a different group, in normal volunteers, infused 4 mg/kg over 15 minutes followed by 3.2 mg/kg per hour for 3.75 hours.[87] Both groups achieved consistent serum pralidoxime levels greater than 4 μg/mL with minimal side effects. However, the presence of organophosphate residues may bind the circulating free 2-PAM and lower the serum concentration of the oxime; thus empiric adjustments to this formula based on clinical symptoms may be necessary. Dosing should be continued for 24 to 48 hours after presentation as the effect of pralidoxime is dependent upon the body load of organophosphate. Some organophosphates have been shown to persist for several days to weeks after exposure, including several not normally associated with increased fat solubility.[126] Patients exposed to fat-soluble organophosphates or those showing severe symptoms may require prolonged therapy. In these situations, the endpoint of treatment should be determined by the absence of signs and symptoms when 2-PAM therapy is withheld. Patients in whom the causative agent is an organophosphate implicated in the intermediate syndrome, should be observed in a controlled environment for a more prolonged time period or have continued pralidoxime therapy after resolution of cholinergic toxicity (Table 87–1). These patients may develop respiratory arrest after apparent complete resolution of their cholinergic crises (see below). There is a possibility that electromyographic and nerve conduction studies may show decremental conduction prior to development of IMS symptoms.[8,9,27] If this is the case, then continuous 2-PAM dosing after symptom resolution may be justified.

Some evidence suggests that 2-PAM is also capable of reversing the CNS effects of organophosphates.[14,79,80,91] Human toxicity studies have shown 2-PAM to have a high therapeutic index. Large doses given over prolonged periods have failed to document toxicity.[25,79,80,98,108]

TABLE 87–1. TREATMENT OF ORGANOPHOSPHATE POISONING[a]

Severity	Signs/Symptoms	Treatment
Mild	Nausea, malaise, fatigue, minimal muscle weakness, cramping without diarrhea	Remove from exposure until cholinesterase returns to 75% of baseline
Moderate	SLUDGE and/or tremors, weakness, fasciculations, confusion, lethargy, anxiety, bronchorrhea	Administer atropine until bronchial secretions clear **plus** 2-PAM 1 g q4–6h or infusion for minimum of 24–48 h or longer until signs/symptoms resolve
Severe	SLUDGE, respiratory insufficiency, weakness, fasciculations, coma, paralysis, seizures, autonomic dysfunction	Administer atropine until bronchial secretions clear (may require repetitive dosing) **plus** 2-PAM as infusion **plus** diazepam for seizures. Continue 2-PAM until all signs/symptoms resolve, minimum 24–48 h. Consider longer therapy for fat-soluble agents or others as defined by EMG

[a]This treatment is in addition to normal decontamination procedures and basic management.
SLUDGE = Salivation, lacrimation, urination, diarrhea, gastrointestinal distress, and emesis.

Atropine and 2-PAM given together are synergistic against the signs and symptoms of cholinesterase inhibition, thus decreasing atropine requirements. Atropine can provide the immediate blockade of muscarinic effects and 2-PAM will regenerate all cholinesterase enzymes regardless of location. There is now suggestion that although immediate symptoms may be resolved with prompt treatment, organophosphate residues remain detectable for days to weeks after exposure.[82,126] Pralidoxime and other oximes may also function as a scavenger for free organophosphate.[68,103] These findings support the administration of 2-PAM if the patient requires atropine for symptomatic relief of muscarinic signs and symptoms, even in the absence of nicotinic or CNS effects. The immediate regeneration of acetylcholinesterase and other cholinesterases may also assist in preventing later subacute and chronic sequelae.[8,24,26,28,29,97]

Carbamate insecticides are also cholinesterase inhibitors but their action is more transient than that of organophosphates. Toxicity should be treated with atropine to relieve signs and symptoms of carbamoylated acetylcholinesterase. Most acetylcholinesterase will spontaneously hydrolyze within 24 hours, but the patient may be acutely ill prior to regeneration. Controversy exists over the use of 2-PAM in treating symptomatic carbamate exposures. Some researchers believe that in the presence of carbaryl, acetylcholinesterase inhibition may increase and atropine efficacy may decrease if 2-PAM is given. This adverse effect was documented in a study using LD_{50} doses of obidoxime (Toxigonin) on rats. Pralidoxime mesylate (p2S) caused no significant difference in lethality in the same model.[98,108,117] Pralidoxime-enhanced carbaryl toxicity has been supported in a subsequent study using in vitro eel cholinesterase and an in vivo murine model.[78] Although initially the enhanced toxicity was believed to result from a more toxic carbamylated oxime, this has not been shown. The current mechanism is still under investigation, but some authors suspect that certain oximes may function as allosteric effectors on the acetylcholinesterase.[78] Many clinicians will use 2-PAM in the presence of carbamates unless carbaryl is known to be involved.

The addition of diazepam to atropine and 2-PAM improves survival. In multiple animal studies, the addition of diazepam to other oximes in the treatment of organophosphates and nerve gases (sarin, soman, tabun, VX) has increased survival and decreased seizures and neuropathy.[68–70,72,79,93,107] Diazepam decreases cardiac and brain morphologic damage resulting from organophosphate seizures.[85,86,114,115]

The use of other medications, including opioids for sedation or pulmonary edema, may worsen CNS manifestations and the degree of respiratory depression. However, if patient care is compromised by agitation, then judicious use of sedation is indicated after oxygenation has been maximized and maintained. Many opioids are partially metabolized through the pseudocholinesterase pathway and may have a prolonged duration of action. If seizure activity develops, oxygenation and large doses of benzodiazepines along with antidotal therapy should precede the use of barbiturates. Because of the membrane-stabilizing and autonomic effects of phenytoin, its use is not recommended. Increased pulmonary secretions and bronchospasm should be treated with oxygen, atropine, pralidoxime, positive pressure ventilation, and/or intubation. It is critical not to confuse or misdiagnose organophosphate poisoning as congestive heart failure or noncardiogenic pulmonary edema. Patients with cardiogenic pulmonary edema will have an excess of bronchial secretions, bronchospasm, will be tachycardic, may be hypertensive and diaphoretic, may be confused, and will show severe air hunger. If endogenous sympathetic tone is high, pupils may be dilated. Additional muscarinic signs and symptoms, however, should be absent, including sialorrhea, excessive tearing, diarrhea, urinary incontinence, and gastrointestinal cramping. Nicotinic myojunctional findings such as tremor, myoclonus, and fasciculations will also be absent. Unless the patient is moribund, respiratory movement is coordinated and active in pulmonary edema whereas the cholinesterase-inhibited patient will develop uncoordinated gasping and diaphragmatic paralysis. Organophosphate-poisoned patients inadvertently treated for cardiogenic pulmonary edema will not respond and may worsen with conventional therapy such as diuretics (further depleting intravascular volume), nitrates (preload is diminished), and cardiotonic agents (dysrhythmogenic). Other medications metabolized via plasma cholinesterases such as succinylcholine, mivacurium, ester anesthetics (cocaine and tetracaine), and esmolol have an increased duration of effect in organophosphate poisoned patients, and should be avoided when possible.[99] Alternatively, the nondepolarizing paralytics (vecuronium, pancuronium) rely on acetylcholine effect at the neuromuscular junction and patients may be resistant to their effects.

Deaths from acute organophosphate poisonings usually occur within 24 hours in untreated cases and within 10 days in unsuccessfully treated cases. In the absence of posthypoxic brain damage, complete symptomatic recovery occurs within 10 days in patients treated early and not exposed to those substances that can cause delayed neurotoxicity. Patients with fat-soluble organophosphate exposures or those treated later, may remain partially symptomatic and pralidoxime dependent for prolonged time periods.[14,83,88] Following symptomatic occupational exposure, patients should not work with these pesticides until acetylcholinesterase levels have returned to at least 75% of normal or plateau level.[22]

Decontaminaton Issues

Many organophosphates and carbamates are formulated in a hydrocarbon or solvent base to enhance environmental dispersion. Others can be found as granular or powder forms. Regardless, they are persistent on the body and in clothing. Because most organophosphates will penetrate skin, they will also penetrate tanned skin products such as leather. The majority of products can be removed with copious washing with simple soap and water. Although tincture of green soap is frequently recommended, the advantage of using an alcohol-based soap substance to solubilize hydrocarbons is lost in the time required to find this now rarely used cleaning agent.[90] Gentle cleansing is recommended, as abrading the skin with rigorous rubbing will enhance absorption. Clothing should be discarded, preferably before the patient is transported from the scene to prevent contamination of the treating personnel and ambulance. Clothing is considered toxic waste and should be double bagged or washed down with large amounts of water. Depending upon the toxicity and concentration of the organophosphate, the wash water may also be a potential toxic product. Organophosphate agents can be deactivated with a mild hypochlorite (bleach) solution; the chlorine radical reacts with the active portion of the organophosphate molecule. This can be used on the skin if immediately available, but should never be used in the eyes.[37,114]

Because hydrocarbons can freely penetrate many nonpolar substances, the treating personnel should be protected with water-impermeable gowns, masks with eyeshields, and shoe covers. Latex and vinyl gloves provide inadequate protection; neoprene or nitrile gloves should be substituted until the person is fully decontaminated. If these are not immediately available, caregivers should at a minimum double glove and watch for loss of glove integrity. Persons who have ingested organophosphates or had large surface exposures will have toxic secretions. Caregivers can be poisoned from unprotected handling of the patient.

In symptomatic patients with organophosphate/carbamate ingestions, the need for gastric decontamination maneuvers is simplified. The majority of these patients will have already vomited repeatedly. Activated charcoal should be administered in the normal dosing of 1 g/kg. Cathartics are unnecessary as intestinal motility is markedly enhanced; any oral treatment will move rapidly throughout the GI tract. Patients with ocular exposures should have copious eye irrigation with normal saline or lactated Ringer's solution. If these are not available, tap water can be used. Inhalational exposures should be treated with removal from the offending vapor and administration of oxygen. Workers who knowingly use organophosphate or carbamate dusts or vapors should wear an approved respirator for that agent.

Diagnostic Testing

The essential finding in laboratory diagnosis is depression of cholinesterase activity. However, the diagnosis of organophosphate poisoning is usually confirmed retrospectively, as the majority of facilities cannot perform these tests on an immediate basis. Additionally, a single isolated cholinesterase level may neither confirm nor exclude exposure, because a normal cholinesterase level is based on population estimates. This has been established for men, women, and children. Neonates and infants have baseline cholinesterase activity that is lower than adults.[22,24,66,89] There is a wide distribution in the definition of normal; someone with a baseline "high normal" level, may be symptomatic with a "low normal" activity.[129] Although these absolute values still fall within the population normal distribution, this still may represent a drop of 50% in activity.[119] Ideally, diagnosis is based on a drop of 50% from baseline cholinesterase determinations (see Table 87–2). Most people, however, do not have a known baseline level. In this case, unless the value is markedly abnormal, the diagnosis can be confirmed by a progressive increase in cholinesterase value until the values plateau over time. In acute poisonings, signs and symptoms generally occur after more than 50% of cholinesterase is inhibited, and the severity of symptoms parallels the degree of cholinesterase depression. Mild poisoning is defined as a depression in cholinesterase activity to 20 to 50% of normal; moderate poisoning occurs when activity is 10 to 20% of normal; and severe poisoning occurs at less than 10% enzyme activity. Almost as important as the degree of enzyme depression is the rate at which it occurs. Small repeated exposures may gradually depress the cholinesterase activity to very low levels, often resulting in minimal symptoms. Thus a very low cholinesterase level does not always correlate with clinical illness. In every case, the exposure history, symptoms, and clinical findings must be considered carefully no matter what the cholinesterase activity.[24,39,40,47,89,104]

TABLE 87–2. INTERPRETATION OF CHOLINESTERASE LEVELS

	Red Blood Cell Cholinesterase	Plasma Cholinesterase
Advantage	Better reflection of synaptic inhibition	Easier to assay, declines faster
Site	CNS gray matter, RBC, motor end-plate	CNS white matter, plasma, liver, pancreas heart
Regeneration (untreated)	1%/day	25–30% in first 7–10 days
Normalization (untreated)	35–49 days	28–42 days
Use	Unsuspected prior exposure with elevated plasma cholinesterase	Acute exposure
False depression	Pernicious anemia, hemoglobinopathies, antimalarial treatment, oxalate blood tubes	Liver dysfunction (cirrhosis), malnutrition, hypersensitivity reactions, drugs (succinylcholine, codeine, morphine), pregnancy, genetic deficiency

Both erythrocyte and plasma cholinesterase levels can be obtained and used for testing. Although there are some major differences between them, for the most part they both can be affected by organophosphates and carbamates. There are a number of exceptions (eg, OMPA which preferentially depresses plasma cholinesterase) but as a group, the cholinesterases react in a parallel manner.[128] Because the enzyme is expressed on the RBC surface, erythrocyte acetylcholinesterase represents the acetylcholinesterase found in peripheral nerve tissue, muscle, and brain. Plasma cholinesterase is chiefly a liver acute phase protein and circulates in the blood plasma. RBC cholinesterase is considered the more accurate of the two; however, plasma cholinesterase activity is easier to assay and generally more available.[22–24,38,41,55,97]

In an untreated patient, plasma cholinesterase activity takes approximately 4 to 6 weeks to return to normal pre-exposure levels whereas RBC acetylcholinesterase requires 5 to 7 weeks. Plasma cholinesterase activity increases by 25 to 30% within the first 7 to 10 days after exposure and then is followed by a gradual increase over time. RBC acetylcholinesterase activity increases following first-order kinetics; it changes by approximately 1% per day. The establishment of a plateau in changes determines when the individual is back at baseline, and if this is an occupational exposure, when the person can safely return to work.[23,39,89,122]

Plasma cholinesterase levels can be depressed by factors other than organophosphates and carbamates. Because it is a liver protein, plasma cholinesterase activity drops in low protein conditions such as malnutrition, cirrhosis, neoplasia, and infection. Certain drugs such as succinylcholine, lidocaine, codeine, and morphine can depress, cholinesterase activity.[99] During pregnancy, the activity of plasma cholinesterase is also depressed, more substantially during the first two trimesters than the third. There is also a genetic variant in which plasma cholinesterase activity is depressed. Erythrocyte acetylcholinesterase is affected by factors that influence the circulating life of the erythrocyte such as hemoglobinopathies (sickle cell and thalassemia) and other anemias.[23,39,66,89,119]

Administration of oxime nucleophiles such as pralidoxime, will reactivate a majority but not all membrane-bound acetylcholinesterase. Consequently, RBC acetylcholinesterase, being membrane-bound, will reflect this dichotomy. Plasma cholinesterase is not as predictable. There are multiple references in which plasma cholinesterase is unaffected by the administration of oximes, and yet there are others in which plasma cholinesterase activity was restored to normal. Although organophosphates and carbamates are usually considered together as one homogenous group, there are significant differences between the families, and the presumed group response of cholinesterases to oxime therapy should no longer be considered dogma.[34,35,48,54,64,72,102,109,113,114,126,130]

When the decision is made to obtain cholinesterase activity levels, it is important to obtain the sample in the appropriate blood tubes. Gray-top tubes containing fluoride will permanently inactivate the enzyme, yielding falsely low activity levels, and should not be used. Erythrocyte acetylcholinesterase level usually is drawn into a tube containing a chelating anticoagulant such as EDTA (lavender tube) to prevent clot formation. Plasma cholinesterase can be drawn into a lavender or red-top tube. This is not universal, however, and each laboratory may use a different reference system, so the laboratory should be contacted to ascertain which is the appropriate venipuncture container. If either test will not be immediately performed, the tubes should be spun and frozen. Freezing reversibly halts cholinesterase activity.

Ancillary Laboratory Testing

Patients with exposure to cholinesterase inhibitors will show laboratory abnormalities consistent with stress reactions. A complete blood count may show a stress leukocytosis with a relatively normal differential. The hematocrit may be high secondary to hemoconcentration from large fluid losses. The patient may develop an anion gap acidosis from poor tissue perfusion; this can be used to help guide fluid replacement and inotropic support. The patient's serum glucose will be elevated and potassium and magnesium will be lowered secondary to catecholamine excess. Blood urea nitrogen, creatinine, and urine specific gravity can be used in determining the patients hydration status.

Continuous pulse oximetry or arterial blood gases will help with monitoring oxygenation status. Because patients will have bronchorrhea and bronchospasm, continuous end-tidal carbon dioxide waveform monitoring can give an early indication of return of bronchospasm and need for additional atropine administration.

Delayed and Long-Term Neurologic Sequelae

In addition to acute toxicity, patients poisoned with organophosphates may develop more persistent effects that last from several weeks to months. These findings are primarily referable to the central and peripheral nervous system and include peripheral neuropathies, memory impairment, personality changes, depression, confusion, and thought disorders. One case report also documents morphologic changes in the basal ganglia as detected by SPECT scanning.[14] The early use of pralidoxime may prevent some of these findings, although this has yet to be definitively proven.[39,65,75]

Organophosphates have become increasingly popular as insecticides because of their greater environmental safety when compared to DDT and other chlorinated hydrocarbons.[91,101] Ironically, while chlorinated hydrocarbons are deemed hazardous chemicals because of their persistence in nature, the immediate human toxicity of organophosphates is far more severe. In addition to the known direct effects on cholinesterases, many organophosphates with mild cholinergic toxicity have been implicated in epidemics of delayed peripheral neurotoxicity. In the 1930s, "Jamaican ginger paralysis" affected thousands of people in the Caribbean because a popular remedy was adulterated with the organophosphate tri-orthocresyl phosphate (TOCP).[92] This epidemic and subsequent studies have demonstrated that acetylcholinesterase activity inhibition and delayed sensorimotor polyneuropathy are largely independent.[36,92,132,133]

Typically, organophosphate-induced delayed neurotoxicity (OPIDN) or polyneuropathy (OPIDP) occurs 1 to 3 weeks after exposure. The patient initially complains of symmetric lower extremity weakness and glove and stocking paresthesias, leg cramping, and calf pain. Atrophy and paralysis of the peroneal muscles lead to foot drop and eventually to ataxia. Steppage gate develops and a positive Romberg sign. The Achilles and ankle jerk reflexes are eventually lost. This ultimately progresses to the upper extremities. In some cases, a bilateral symmetric flaccid paralysis occurs. Sensory symptoms resolve over the ensuing 1 to 2 months but paralysis remains. Mild cases may recover over 15 months to several years but the more severe cases have persistent symptoms including spasticity resulting from spinal cord or upper motor neuron damage. Abnormal electromyograms and nerve conduction studies may help to differentiate this from other similar neurologic disorders such as Guillain-Barré syndrome.[2,7,18,19,44,57,63,111,112,118,124]

The neuropathologic findings of OPIDN demonstrate that the large distal neurons tend to be affected first and axonal degeneration precedes myelin degeneration. The nerves are reported to "die back." Onset of degeneration coincides with development of ataxia and paralysis.[95] Recovery may occur gradually or not at all. The phenomenon of OPIDN was first demonstrated in the hen model; this model has served to recreate the human pathologic changes. A membrane-bound target esterase named neuropathy target esterase (NTE, previously named neurotoxic esterase) is the primary target in OPIDN. Specific organophosphorous compounds bind to this axonal membrane-bound enzyme at its active site. The target protein is first structurally modified, and then undergoes one of two processes. If the binding compound is a phosphate, phosphonate, or phosphoraminate, the enzyme rapidly "ages" or loses one of the carbon groups from the P–O-carbon linkage. The leaving group probably permanently binds to an adjacent macromolecular site as yet undetermined. If the cholinesterase-binding compound is a phosphinate, sulfonate, or carbamate, then the enzyme cannot "age" and NTE is protected.[62] Some theories suggest that the enzyme involved in NTE is associated with calmodulin kinase II. Once calmodulin kinase II is phosphorylated, calmodulin becomes active, increasing axoplasmic calcium concentration, disruption of the cytoskeletal proteins, and ultimately causing axonal degeneration.[62] The most commonly used organophosphorus compounds have been tested in the hen model and have been found to have some level of neurotoxicity. Unfortunately, some of these compounds were active only in the hen brain and not in the peripheral nervous system; there appears to be a dose-related response in the peripheral system. Although onset of symptoms may be delayed by days to weeks, the damage probably occurs immediately after exposure. A critical mass approximating 70% of NTE must be inhibited to cause clinical symptoms. The delay in symptom onset may be explained in that not all axons will degenerate at the same time and the nerve may continue to function until significant numbers of axons are involved.[62]

In an attempt to develop an in vitro test for neuropathic potential, a lymphocyte and platelet assay was developed. Initially, this was hoped to be a simple way to test for NTE inhibition without using the in vivo hen assay. Unfortunately there is a large interindividual variability in human lymphocyte NTE activity, making preexposure measurements necessary for the interpretation of postexposure response. Parallel activity, between lymphocyte NTE activity and neuronal response has not yet been documented in humans. Other problems have shown that the lymphocyte NTE is unstable and has a very short usable period. There are also multiple subpopulations of lymphocytes in the circulation, and cells sustaining any damage are immediately removed from circulation, thereby altering the assay. Finally, lymphocytes will proliferate in response to infection, again altering the total activity. Both platelet and RBC NTE are currently under study as an in vitro assay.[95] Another block in the study of in vitro NTE testing lies in the fact that many organophosphorus compounds have a chiral center. Subsequently, the test substance is a mixture of sterioisomers. Unfortunately, studies have shown that there is strong stereochemistry involved in the binding of the toxic compound to NTE; one enantiomer may be toxic and the other protective.[62]

The third neurologic finding associated with organophosphorus compounds is the "intermediate syndrome" (IMS). IMS was first described in 1987 and occurs approximately 24 to 96 hours after resolution of an acute severe cholinergic crisis.[111] Clinically, patients develop acute respiratory paralysis, weakness in the bulbar musculature, nuchal weakness, proximal limb weakness, and depressed reflexes. Electromyographic studies show decremental conduction with repetitive nerve stimulation and suggest both pre- and postsynaptic impairment. Animal studies have suggested that activity of acetylcholinesterase must be at 20% or lower before muscle activity is affected. As the patient improves, there is incremental conduction improvement and normalization preceding resolution of neurologic symptoms. Recovery can take 2 to 4 times longer than development,[9] and the majority of patients with IMS will recover providing the patient does not suffer hypoxic brain damage. Muscle biopsies of the involved muscles have shown scattered necrotic fibrils but not enough to explain the severe muscle weaknesses seen with the syndrome.

Staining for acetylcholinesterase at the motor endplates ranges from normal to decreased and absent activity. Initially there was thought to be a component of OPIDN associated with IMS, but that has since been disproved.[42,84]

IMS is associated with certain organophosphorus compounds: dimethoate, monocrotophos, methamidofos, parathion and methylparathion, diazinon, Bidrin, malathion, and fenthion. Subsequent investigations have found the symptoms occur simultaneously with depression of acetylcholinesterase and butyrlcholinesterase. Organophosphorus compounds are still detectable in the patient's urine and gastric fluid during onset and duration of IMS. As the serum levels of the organophosphorus compound begin to fall, the endplate shows its greatest decremental response. This may reflect a period where there is final distribution of the organophosphorus compound from the serum to the tissue compartments such as the motor endplate.[9–11,26,27,29–32,45,74,82,112]

Although many of the patients with IMS received large doses of atropine and moderate oxime therapy, the consensus appears that IMS may result from inadequate therapy with oximes. The symptom complex begins at a time when the cholinesterase function is extremely low and organophosphorus compound is still detectable in the body. Prior therapy with atropine and oximes may have been successful in treating the acute cholinergic crises. However, as the organophosphate blood levels fall and organophosphate tissue redistribution occurs, it may be that the motor end-plate is rechallenged with the cholinesterase inhibitor in the presence of inadequate circulating oxime.[73] Because IMS seems to occur preferentially with certain organophosophorus compounds and fenthion (fat soluble with prolonged toxicity), there may be significant stereochemistry involved with the effect of the oximes on the neuromuscular junction. Finally, not all oximes have identical effects on all organophosphorus compounds; obidoxime and pralidoxime may be less effective than HI-6 and HLÖ-7 on regeneration of the end-plate acetylcholinesterase. There may be a preferential dose (as yet undetermined) for treatment of the delayed end-plate cholinesterase inhibition versus the dose required for immediate reversal of the acute cholinergic crises. This question remains unresolved.[8,27–29,50,73]

Finally, there is one case report of a 38-year-old female exposed to a combination of phosphorothionate, pyrethrin, piperonyl butoxide, and petroleum distillates who developed a sensory peripheral neuropathy and abnormal SPECT scanning with basal ganglia involvement. She was incompletely treated at outset and did not receive pralidoxime or atropine.[17] This study is again suggestive that the combination of agents may have more toxicity than originally believed.

Chemical Warfare Agents

In the search for better insecticides, in 1936 the German chemist Schrader synthesized tabun (GA), the first of three German or "G" military agents. Sarin (GB) and soman (GD) followed quickly. A fourth agent, VX was synthesized in England a decade later.[37,49,67,104,115] Recently another agent, cyclohexylmethylphosphonofluoridate (CMPF, or GF), was declassified.[68] The G agents are very potent, with an inhaled lethal dose in the milligram range. This makes them about 30 times more potent than phosgene. VX is an oily liquid, less volatile but more rapidly absorbed through the skin and more persistent in the environment. In comparison to the insecticides, these five agents are extremely potent and rapid acting, with death occurring within minutes of exposure.[104]

Inactivation of cholinesterase is believed to be of major importance in the toxicity of these agents. However, these agents may have other effects possibly mediated through other neurotransmitters such as GABA and NMDA, direct interaction with the nicotinic acetylcholine ligand receptor–ionic channel complex, and direct binding to cardiac muscarinic receptors.[37,49,104,115] Aging and destruction of the acetylcholinesterase nerve agent complex occurs extremely rapidly with GB and GD (minutes to hours), but requires 4 to 38 hours with GF and over 40 hours with GA.[68] Consequently, the former two agents are more sensitive to the classical oximes than the latter.

In the Persian Gulf War, a large number of key military personnel were pretreated with the carbamate pyridostigmine. Animal studies have demonstrated pretreatment with carbamates such as pyridostigmine enhanced successful postexposure treatment of soman in combination with atropine and pralidoxime. This is based on the rationale that the carbamate acts to protect the acetylcholinesterase by screening it from the nerve agent and then, when the carbamate spontaneously disengages, regenerates the acetylcholinesterase. Pyridostigmine was chosen over physostigmine because the former does not cross the blood–brain barrier and has a better therapeutic index. This contributes to fewer adverse effects in treated individuals, but would be of lesser therapeutic benefit should a nerve gas be employed.[37,43,67,115]

As in the management of organophosphate insecticides, decontamination, intensive respiratory support, atropine, and pralidoxime are essential. In addition, animal studies confirm that the use of benzodiazepines is additive to the antidotal therapy in preventing seizures and preventing morphologic brain damage. For these reasons, military physicians recommended prophylactic use of diazepam in all severely poisoned personnel.[69–71,85,86,93,107]

The Persian Gulf War stimulated research into development of new nucleophiles for cholinesterase regeneration. Pralidoxime is a moderate regenerator of cholinesterase inhibited by the "G" agents. Other oximes used internationally (obidoxime and pyrimidoxime) have variable effects on these agents. A new group of nucleophiles, the Hagedorne group, has been tailored for effect against the nerve agents. The agents showing the best activity with least side effects are HI-6 and HLÖ-7. In multiple animal studies, HI-6 and HLÖ-7 have varying success against poisoning with soman, tabun, sarin, VX, and GF. In each case, both of the H series were overall more effective than pralidoxime and obidoxime.[20,21,33,35,69,71,81,106,113,131] The antidotal efficacy of these agents and the oximes is enhanced with high-dose atropine. Two studies show marked improvement in animal survival with cumulative atropine doses of 13 to 16 mg/kg. Additionally, diazepam 2 mg/kg enhanced soman protection in a rodent model.[69,70]

Other nonnucleophilic agents showing promise as prophylactic treatments against poisoning with nerve agents and organophosphates include human butyrlcholinesterase and acetylcholinesterase, paraoxonase, and phosphotriesterase. The underlying philosophy for use is that exogenously administered cholinesterase (acetylcholinesterase or butyrlcholinesterase) acts as a scavenger for the nerve agent, binding and inactivating it before it can affect the active site on native acetylcholinesterase.[103] In a rodent model, 1 active site on the exogenously administered human butyrlcholinesterase will bind 0.5 moles of soman in less than 5 seconds and has a prolonged circulating half-life without engaging an immunologic response.[5,103] Paraoxonase is believed to work by hydrolyzing paraoxon and other organophosphate-oxon molecules prior to the organophosphate engaging native acetylcholinesterase. Again, it functions as a scavenger and affords CNS protection.[76,77] Phosphotriesterase is another scavenger being studied and is believed to work by breaking the cholinesterase–organophosphate bond, or if it is already spontaneously broken, by hydrolyzing the organophosphate before it can reinhibit a new molecule of acetylcholinesterase.[116,123,125]

Subsequent to the Persian Gulf War, veterans have complained about an entity that has been entitled the Gulf War syndrome. At this point in time, there is no good explanation for the constellation of signs and symptoms associated with this illness. The service personnel were exposed to multiple biologic, chemical, and psychological stressors, which makes it difficult to locate a discreet causal agent.[60] A recent article evaluated neurotoxicity in hens resulting from exposure to the combination of pyridostigmine bromide, DEET, and permethrin. This combination was used by the military: DEET as a skin insect repellent, permethrin on clothing as an insecticide, and pyridostigmine as a nerve gas protectant. Animals treated with a combination of all three agents developed signs of neurotoxicity. Neuropathologic changes were varied and ranged from mild axonal changes to axonal degeneration. Although there are flaws in the paper including marked cholinesterase inhibition from pyridostigmine, the ideas suggested may lead to an increased understanding of the syndrome.[3] Recently, studies have identified six syndrome groups associated with complaints of illness in Gulf War veterans.

Three of the syndromes (I, "impaired-cognition"; II, "confusion-ataxia"; and III, "arthro-myo-neuropathy") were strongly associated with risk factors for exposure to six cholinesterase-inhibiting chemicals, although a direct cause and effect relationship has not been established. There is some suggestion that these three syndromes may be associated with OPIDN, but more study is required.[51–53,60]

New Avenues of Research

Several authors have suggested that inhibition of acetylcholinesterase is not the sole cause of the severe toxicity of organophosphate insecticides and chemical warfare agents, and research should be redirected.[40,104] These questions have been raised because: (1) some compounds that show protective activity do not reactivate acetylcholinesterase; (2) research suggests there are direct effects on the nicotinic acetylcholine receptor-ionic channel complex; (3) it is not possible to predict in vivo efficacy of oxime reactivators based on in vitro potencies; (4) carbamates may work as prophylactic agents because of direct effects on the affinity or sensitivity of the nicotinic acetylcholine receptor; (5) evidence suggests that respiratory depression is a central phenomenon perhaps independent of cholinesterase inhibition; and (6) morphologic brain damage can be decreased in animals with the use of diazepam. Some of the newer nucleophiles may function not only as a cholinesterase reactivator but prevent secondary inhibition of phosphorylated enzyme, or increase the endogenous catabolism of the organophosphate.[40,104,115]

References

1. Aaron CK, Smilkstein MJ: Organophosphate poisoning: Intermediate syndrome or inadequate therapy. Vet Hum Toxicol 1988;30:370. Abstract.
2. Abou-Donia MB, Lapadula DM: Mechanisms of organophosphorus ester-induced delayed neurotoxiciuy: Type I and type II. Annu Rev Pharmacol Toxicol 1990;30:405–440.
3. Abou-Donia MB, Wilmarth KR, Jensen KP, et al: Neurotoxicity resulting from coexposure to pyrodistigmine bromide, DEET, and permethrin. J Toxicol Environ Health 1996;48:101–122.
4. Amos WC Jr, Hall A: Malathion poisoning treated with protopam. Ann Intern Med 1965;62:1013–1016.
5. Ashani Y, Shapira S, Levy D, et al: Butyrylcholinesterase and acetylcholinesterase prophylaxis against soman poisoning in mice. Biochem Pharmacol 1991;41:37–41.
6. Ayerst Laboratories Professional Bulletin: Protopam Chloride (pralidoxime chloride).
7. Baron RL ed: Pesticide-Induced Delayed Neurotoxicity: Proceedings of a Conference. Co-sponsored by the Environmental Protection Agency and the National Institute for Environmental Health Sciences, February, 1976. EPA-600/1–76–025.
8. Benson BJ, Tolo D, McIntire M: Is the intermediate syndrome in organophosphate poisoning the result of insufficient oxime therapy? J Toxicol Clin Toxicol 1992;30: 347–349.
9. Besser R, Gutmann L, Weilemann LS: Inactivation of the end-plate acetylochlinesterase during the course of organophosphate intoxications. Arch Toxicol 1989;63: 412–415.
10. Besser R, Weilmann LS, Gutmann L: Efficacy of obidoxime in human organophospate determination by neuromuscular transmission studies. Muscle Nerve 1995;18:15–22.
11. Betrosian AP, Balla M: Multiple system organ failure, intermediate syndrome, congenital myasthenic syndrome, and anticholinesterase treatment: The linkage is puzzling—Author's reply. J Toxicol Clin Toxicol 1996;34:247.
12. Blaber LC, Creasey NH: The mode of recovery of cholinesterase activity in vivo after organophosphorus poisoning: I. Erythrocyte cholinesterase. Biochem J 1960; 77:591–596.
13. Blaber LC, Creasey NH: The mode of recovery of cholinesterase activity in vivo after organophosphorus poisoning: II. Brain cholinesterase. Biochem J 1960;77: 597–604.
14. Borowitz SM: Prolonged organophosphate toxicity in a twenty-six-month-old child. J Pediatr 1988;112:302–304.
15. Brill D, Maisel A, Prabhu R: Polymorphic ventricular arrhythmias in organophosphate insecticide poisoning. J Electrocardiol 1984;17:97–102.
16. Brown JH, Taylor J: Muscarinic receptor agonists and antagonists. In: Hardman JG, Limbird LE, Molinoff PB, et al, eds: Goodman & Gilman's The Pharmacological Basis of Therapeutics, 9th ed. NY, McGraw-Hill, 1996, pp. 141–160.
17. Callender TJ, Morrow L, Subramanian K: Evaluation of chronic neurological sequelae after pesticide exposure suing SPECT brain scans. J Toxicol Environ Health 1994;41:275–284.
18. Centers for Disease Control: Neurological findings among workers exposed to fenthion in a veterinary hospital–Georgia. MMWR 1985;26:402–403.
19. Cherniack MG: Organophosphorus esters and polyneuropathy. Ann Intern Med 1986;104:264–266.
20. Clement JG: Toxicity of the combined nerve agents GB/GF in mice: Efficacy of atropine and various oximes as antidotes. Arch Toxicol 1994;68:64–66.
21. Clement JG, Hansen AS, Boulet CA: Efficacy of HI6–7 and pyrimidoxime as antidotes of nerve managent poisoning in mice. Arch Toxicol 1992;66:216–219.
22. Coye MJ, Barnett PG, Midtling JE, et al: Clinical confirmation of organophosphate poisoning by serial cholinesterase analysis. Arch Intern Med 1987;147:438–442.
23. Coye MJ, Barnett PG, Midtling JE, et al: Clinical confirmation of organophosphate poisoning in agricultural workers. Am J Med 1986;10:399–409.
24. Coye MJ, Lowe JA, Maddy KT: Biological monitoring of agricultural workers exposed to pesticides: I. Cholinesterase activity determinations. J Occup Med 1986; 28:619–627.
25. Davies DR, Green AL: The kinetics of reactivation by

oximes, of cholinesterase inhibition by organophosphorus compounds. Biochemistry 1956;63:529–535.
26. DeBleeker JL: Multiple system organ failure: Link to intermediate syndrome indirect. J Toxicol Clin Toxicol 1996;34: 249–250.
27. DeBleecker JL: The intermediate syndrome in organophosphate poisoning: An overview of experimental and clinical observation. J Toxicol Clin Toxicol 1995;33: 683–686.
28. DeBleecker JL. Intermediate syndrome: Prolonged cholinesterase inhibition. J Toxicol Clin Toxicol 1993;31:197–199.
29. DeBleecker J, Van Den Neucker K, Colardyn F: Intermediate syndrome in organophosphorus poisoning: A prospective study. Crit Care Med 1993;21:1706–1711.
30. DeBleecker J, Van Den Neucker K, Willems J: The intermediate syndrome in organophosphate poisoning: Presentation of a case and review of the literature. J Toxicol Clin Toxicol 1992;30:321–329.
31. DeBleecker J, Vogelaers D, Ceuterick C, et al: Intermediate syndrome due to prolonged parathion poisoning. Acta Neurol Scand 1992;86:421–424.
32. DeBleecker J, Willems J, Van Den Neucker K, et al: Prolonged toxicity with intermediate syndrome after combined parathion and methyl parathion poisoning. J Toxicol Clin Toxicol 1992;30:333–345.
33. DeJong LPA, Verhagen MAA, Langenberg JP, et al: The bispyridinium-dioxime HLÖ-7. A potent reactivator for acetylcholinesterase inhibited by the stereoisomers of tabun and soman. Biochem Pharmacol 1989;38: 633–640.
34. DiKart WL, Kiestra SH, Sangster B: The use of atropine and oximes in organophosphate intoxication: A modified approach. J Toxicol Clin Toxicol 1988;26:199–208.
35. De la Manche IS, Verge DE, Bouchard C, et al: Penetration of oximes across the blood–brain barrier. A histochemical study of the cerebral cholinesterases reactivation. Experientia 1979;35:531–532.
36. Drug CD: The central nervous systems affinity of triorthocresyl phosphate. Brain 1972;65:34–47.
37. Dunn MA, Sidell FR: Progress in medical defense against nerve agents. JAMA 1989;262:649–652.
38. Durham WF, Hayes WJ Jr: Organic phosphorus poisoning and its therapy. Arch Environ Health 1962;5:21–47.
39. Edmiston S, Maddy KT: Summary of illnesses and injuries reported in California by physicians in 1986 as potentially related to pesticides. Vet Hum Toxicol 1987;29:391–397.
40. Ellin RI: Anomalies in theories and therapy of intoxication by potent organophosphorus anticholinesterase compounds. Gen Pharmacol 1982;13:457–466.
41. Ellman GL, Courtney KD, Andres Jr V, Featherstone RM: A new and rapid calorimetric determination of acetylcholinesterase activity. Biochem Pharmacol 1961;7:88–95.
42. Eyer P: Neuropsychopathological changes by organophosphorus compounds—A review. Human Exp Toxicol 1995; 14:857–864.
43. Francesconi R, Hubbard R, Matthew C, et al: Oral pyridostigmine administration in rats: Effects on thermoregulation, clinical chemistry and performance in the heat. Pharmacol Biochem Behav 1986;25:1071–1075.
44. Gadoth N, Fisher A: Late onset of neuromuscular block in organophosphorus poisoning. Ann Intern Med 1978;88: 654–655.
45. Ganendran A, Balabaskaran S: Cholinesterase reactivation: In vitro studies. Anaesth Intensive Care 1975;3:60–61.
46. Goldberg L, Shupp D, Weitz H: Injection of household spray insecticide. Ann Emerg Med 1982;11:626–629.
47. Green MA, Henmann MA, Wehr HM, et al: An outbreak of watermelon-borne pesticide toxicity. Am J Public Health 1987;77:1431–1434.
48. Grob D, Johns RJ: Use of oximes in the treatment of intoxication by anticholinesterase compounds in normal subjects. Am J Med 1968;24:497–511.
49. Gunderson CH, Lehmann CR, Sidell FR, Jabbari B: Nerve agents: A review. Neurology 1992;42:946–950.
50. Haddad LM: Organophosphate poisoning: Intermediate syndrome? J Toxicol Clin Toxicol 1992;30:331–332.
51. Haley RW, Hom J, Roland PS, et al. Evaluation of neurologic function in Gulf War veterans: A blinded case control study. JAMA 1997;277:223–230.
52. Haley RW, Kurt TL: Self-reported exposure to neurotoxic chemical combinations in the Gulf War: A cross-section epidemiological study. JAMA 1997;277:231–237.
53. Haley RW, Kurt TL, Hom J: Is there a Gulf War syndrome? Search for syndromes by factor analysis of symptoms. JAMA 1997;277:215–222.
54. Hassan RM, Pesce AJ, Sheng P, Hanenson IR: Correlation of serum pseudocholinesterase and clinical course in two patients poisoned with organophosphate insecticides. J Toxicol Clin Toxicol 1981;18:401–406.
55. Hawkins RD, Gunter JM: Studies on cholinesterase: 5. The selective inhibition of pseudocholinesterase in vivo. Biochem J 1946;40:192–197.
56. Hayes WJ Jr: Epidemiology and general management of poisoning by pesticides. Pediatr Clin North Am 1970; 17:629–644.
57. Hierons R, Johnson MK: Clinical and toxicological investigations of a case of delayed neuropathy in man after acute poisoning by an organophosphorus pesticide. Arch Toxicol 1978;40:279–284.
58. Hobbinger F: Chemical reactivation of phosphorylated human and bovine true cholinesterase. Br J Pharmacol 1956;11:295–303.
59. Holmstedt B: Pharmacology of organophosphorus cholinesterase inhibitors. Pharmacol Rev 1956;11:567–688.
60. Hyams KC, Wignal S, Roswell R: War syndromes and their evaluation: From the U.S. Civil War to the Persian Gulf War. Ann Intern Med 1997;125:398–405.
61. Jandorf BJ, Michel HO, Schaffer NK, et al: The mechanism of reaction between esterases and phosphorus-containing antiesterases. Disc Farady Soc 1955;20:134–147.
62. Johnson MK: Organophosphages and delayed neuropathy—Is NTE alive and well? Toxicol Appl Pharmacol 1990;102:385–399.
63. Johnson MK: The delayed neuropathy caused by some organophosphorus esters: Mechanism and challenge. CRC Crit Rev Toxicol 1975;3:289–316.
64. Kaliste-Korhonen E, Ryhanen R, Ylitalo P, Hanninen O: Cold exposure decreases the effectiveness of atropine-oxime treatment in organophosphate intoxication in rats and mice. Gen Phamac 1989:20:805–809.

65. Kaplan JG, Kessler J, Rosenberg N, et al: Sensory neuropathy associated with Dursban (chlorpyrifos) exposure. Neurology 1993;43:2193–2196.
66. Karlsen RL, Sterri S, Lyngaas S, Fonnum F: Reference values for erythrocyte acetylcholinesterase and plasma activities in children: Implications for organophosphate intoxications. Scand J Clin Lab Invest 1981;4:301–302.
67. Keeler JR, Hurst CG, Dunn MA: Pyridostigmine used as a nerve agent pretreatment under wartime conditions. JAMA 1991;266:693–695.
68. Koplovitz I, Gresham VC, Dochterman LW, et al: Evaluation of the toxicity, pathology, and treatment of cyclohexylmethylphosphonofluoridate (CMPF) poisoning in rhesus monkeys (GF). Arch Toxicol 1992;66:622–628.
69. Koplovitz I, Mento R, Matthews C, et al: Dose-response effects of atropine and HI-6 treatment of organophosphorus poisoning in guinea pigs. Drug Chem Toxicol 1995;18: 119–136.
70. Koplovitz I, Stewart JR: A comparison of the efficacy of Hl-6 and 2-PAM against soman, tabun, sarin, and VX in the rabbit. Toxicol Lett 1994;70:269–279.
71. Kusic R, Boskovic B, Vojvodic V, Jovanovic D: HI-6 in man: Blood levels, urinary excretion, and tolerance after intramuscular administration of the oxime to healthy volunteers. Fund Appl Toxicol 1985;55:89–97.
72. Kusic R, Jovanovic D, Randjelovic S, et al: HI-6 in man: Efficacy of the oxime in poisoning by organophosphorus insecticides. Human Exp Toxicol 1991;10:113–118.
73. Laiwani K: Acute organophosphorous insecticide poisoning. Anaesthesia 1993;48:141–142.
74. Leon SFE, Pradilla AG, Gamboa N, et al: Multiple system organ failure, intermediate syndrome, congenital myasthenic syndrome, and anticholinesterase treatment: The linkage is puzzling. J Toxicol Clin Toxicol 1996;34: 245–246.
75. Levin HS, Rodnitzky RL: Behavioral effects of organophosphate pesticides in man. J Toxicol Clin Toxicol 1976; 9:391–405.
76. Li WF, Costa LG, Furlong CE: Serum paraoxonase status: A major factor in determining resistance to organophosphates. J Toxicol Environ Health 1993;40:337–346.
77. Li WF, Furlong CE, Costa LG: Paraoxonase protects against chlorpyrifos toxicity in mice. Toxicol Lett 1995;76: 219–226.
78. Lieske CN, Clark JH, Maxwell DM, et al: Studies of the amplification of carbaryl toxicity by various oyimes. Toxicol Lett 1992;62:127–137.
79. Lotti M: Treatment of acute organophosphate poisoning. Med J Aust 1991;154:51–55.
80. Lotti M, Becker CE: Treatment of acute organophosphate poisoning: Evidence of a direct effect on central nervous system by 2-PAM (pyridine–2-aldoxime methyl chloride). J Toxicol Clin Toxicol 1982;19:121–127.
81. Lundy PM, Hansen AS, Hand BT, Boulet CA: Comparison of several oximes against poisoning by soman, tabun, and GF. Toxicology 1992;72:99–105.
82. Lyon J, Taylor H, Ackerman B: A case report of intravenous malathion injection with determination of serum half-life. J Toxicol Clin Toxicol 1987;25:243–249.
83. Mahieu P, Hassoun A, VanBinst R, et al: Severe and prolonged poisoning by fenthion: Significance of the determination of the anticholinesterase capacity of plasma. J Toxicol Clin Toxicol 1982;19:425–432.
84. Marks TC: Oganophosphate poisoning. Pharmac Ther 1993;58:51–66.
85. McDonough JH, Jaax NK, Crowley RA, et al: Atropine and/or diazepam therapy protects against Soman-induced neural and cardiac pathology. Fund Appl Toxicol 1989;13:256–276.
86. McLoed CG: Pathology of nerve agents: Perspectives on medical management. Fund Appl Toxicol 1985;5: 510–516.
87. Medicis JJ, Stork CM, Howland MA, et al: Pharmacokinetics following a loading plus a continuous infusion of pralidoxime compared with the traditional short infusion regimen in human volunteers. J Toxicol Clin Toxicol 1996;34: 289–295.
88. Merril DG, Mihn FG: Prolonged toxicity of organophosphate poisoning. Crit Care Med 1982;10:550–551.
89. Midtling JE, Barnett PG, Coye MJ, et al: Clinical management of field worker organophosphate poisoning. West J Med 1985;142:514–518.
90. Milby T: Prevention and management of organophosphate poisoning. JAMA 1971;216:2131–2133.
91. Minton NA, Murray SG: A review of organophosphate poisoning. Med Toxicol 1988;3:350–375.
92. Morgan JP: The Jamaica ginger paralysis. JAMA 1982;248: 1864–1867.
93. Murphy MR, Blick DW, Dunn MA, et al: Diazepam as a treatment for nerve agent poisoning in primates. Aviat Space Environ Med 1993; 64:110–115.
94. Murphy SD: Toxic effects of pesticides. In: Klaasen CD, Amdur MO, Doull J, eds: Cassarett and Doull's Toxicology: The Basic Science of Poisons, 3rd ed. New York, Macmillan, 1986, pp. 535–539.
95. Mutch E, Blain PG, Williams FM. Interindividual variations in enzymes controlling organophosphate toxicity in man. Human Exp Toxicol 1992;11:109–116.
96. Namba T, Hiraki K: PAM (pyridine–2-aldoxime methiodide) therapy for alkylphosphate poisoning. JAMA 1958; 166:1834–1839.
97. Namba T, Nolte C, Jackrel J, Grob D: Poisoning due to organophosphate insecticides. Am J Med 1971; 50:475–492.
98. Natoff IL, Reiff B: Effect of oximes on the acute toxicity of acetylcholinesterase carbamates. Toxicol Appl Pharmacol 1973;25:569–575.
99. Nelson TC, Burritt MF: Pesticide poisoning, succinylcholine induced apnea and pseudocholinesterase. Mayo Clin Proc 1986;61:750–755.
100. O'Brien RD: Phosphorylation and carbamylation of cholinesterase. Ann NY Acad Sci 1969;169:204–214.
101. Peoples SA, Maddy KT: Organophosphate pesticide poisoning. West J Med 1978;129:273–277.
102. Quimby GE: Further therapeutic experience with pralidoxime in organic phosphorus pesticide poisoning. JAMA 1964;187:114–118.
103. Raveh L, Grunwald J, Marcus D, et al: Human butyrylcholinesterase as a general prophylactic antidode for nerve agent toxicity. In vitro and in vivo quantitative characterization. Biochem Pharmacol 1993;45:2465–2474.

104. Rickett DJ, Glenn JF, Houston WE: Medical defense against nerve agents: New directions. Mil Med 1987;152: 35–41.
105. Rotenberg M, Shefi M, Dany S, et al: Differentiation between organophosphate and carbamate poisoning. Clin Chim Acta 1995;234:11–21.
106. Rousseaux CG, Dua AK: Pharmacology of HI-6, an H-series oxime. Can J Physiol Pharmacol 1989;67:1183–1189.
107. Rump S, Raszewski W, Gidynska T, Galecka E: Effects of CGS 9896 in acute experimental intoxication with fluostigmine (DFP). Arch Toxicol 1990;64:412–413.
108. Sanderson DM: Treatment of poisoning by anticholinesterase insecticides in the rat. J Pharm Pharmacol 1961;13:435–442.
109. Saravanapavananthan T: Serum pseudocholinesterase estimation in the management of organophosphate poisoning cases and the effects of PAM on regenerating it. Singapore Med J 1987;28:166–171.
110. Segall Y, Waysbort D, Barak D, et al: Direct observation and elucidation of the structures of aged and nonaged phosphorylated cholinesterases by ^{31}P NMR spectroscopy. Biochemistry 1993;32:13441–13450.
111. Senanayake N, Karalliede L: Neurotoxic effects of organophosphorus insecticides: An intermediate syndrome. N Engl J Med 1987;316:761–763.
112. Senanayake N, Sanmuganathan PS: Extrapyramidal manifestations complicating an organophosphorus poisoning. Human Exp Toxicol 1995;14:600–604.
113. Shih TM: Comparison of several oximes on reactivation of soman-inhibited blood, brain, and tissue cholinesterase activity in rats. Arch Toxicol 1993;67:637–646.
114. Sidell FR: Soman and Sarin: Clinical manifestations and treatment of accidental poisoning by organophosphates. J Toxicol Clin Toxicol 1974;7:1–17.
115. Sidell FR, Borak J: Chemical warfare agents: II. Nerve agents. Ann Emerg Med 1992;21:865–871.
116. Spoljar MS, Simeon V: Reactions of usual and atypical human serum cholinesterase phenotypes with progressive and reversible inhibitors. J Enzyme Inhib 1993;7:169–174.
117. Sterri SH, Rognerud B, Fishum SE, Lyngaas S: Effect of toxigonin and P2S on the toxicity of carbamates and organophosphorus compounds. Acta Pharmacol Toxicol 45:16–19.
118. Stuart LD, Oehme FW: Organophosphorus delayed neurotoxicity: A neuromyelopathy of animals and man. Vet Hum Toxicol 1982;24:107–118.
119. Sumerford WT, Hayes WJ Jr, Johnston JM, et al: Cholinesterase response and symptomatology from exposure to organic phosphorus insecticides. Arch Indust Hygiene Occup Med 1953;7:383–398.
120. Tafuri J, Roberts J: Organophosphate poisoning. Ann Emerg Med 1987;16:193–202.
121. Takahashi H, Kojima T, Ikeda T et al: Differences in the mode of lethality produced through intravenous and oral administration of organophosphorus insecticides in rats. Fundam Appl Toxicol 1991;16:459–468.
122. Taylor P: Anticholinesterase agents. In: Hardman JG, Limbird LE, Molinoff PB, et al, eds: Goodman & Gilman's The Pharmacological Basis of Therapeutics, 9th ed. New York, Macmillan, 1996, pp. 161–176.
123. Tuovinen K, Kaliste-Korhonen E, Rausehl FM, Hanninen O: Phosphotriesterase—A promising candidate for use in detoxification of organophosphates. Fund Appl Toxicol 1994;23:578–584.
124. Wadia RS, Sadagopan C, Amin RD, Sardesai HV: Neurological manifestations of organophosphorus insecticide poisoning. J Neurol Neurosurg Psychiatry 1974;37: 841–847.
125. Wang EIC, Braid PR: Oxime reactivation of diethylphosphoryl human serum cholinesterase. J Biol Chem 1967; 242:2683–2687.
126. Willems JL, De Bisschop HC, Verstraete AG, et al: Cholinesterase reactivation in organophosphorus poisoned patients depends on the plasma concentrations of the oxime pralidoxime methylsulphate and of the organophosphate. Arch Toxicol 1993;67:79–84.
127. Willems JL, Langenberg JP, Verstaete AG, et al: Plasma concentrations of pralidoxime methylsulphate in organophosphorus poisoned patients. Arch Toxicol 1992; 66:260–266.
128. Wilson IB, Hatch MA, Ginsburg S: Carbamylation of acetylcholinesterase. J Biol Chem 1960;235:2312–2315.
129. Wofsie JH, Winter GD: Statistical analysis of normal human red blood cell and plasma cholinesterase activity values. Arch Indust Hygiene Occup Med 1952;6:43–49.
130. Woodard CL, Calamaio CA, Kaminskis A, et al: Erythrocyte and plasma cholinesterase activity in male and female rhesus monkeys before and after exposure to Sarin. Fund Appl Toxicol 1994;23:342–347.
131. Xue SZ, Ding XJ, Ding Y: Clinical observation and comparison of the effectiveness of several oxime cholinesterase reactivations. Scand J Work Environ Health 1985;11: 46–48.
132. Zavon M: Poisoning from pesticides: Diagnosis and treatment. Pediatrics 1974;54:332–336.
133. Zavon M: Treatment of organophosphorus and chlorinated hydrocarbon insecticide intoxications. Mod Treatment 1971;8:503–510.

ANTIDOTES IN DEPTH

Pralidoxime

Mary Ann Howland and Cynthia K. Aaron

Pralidoxime

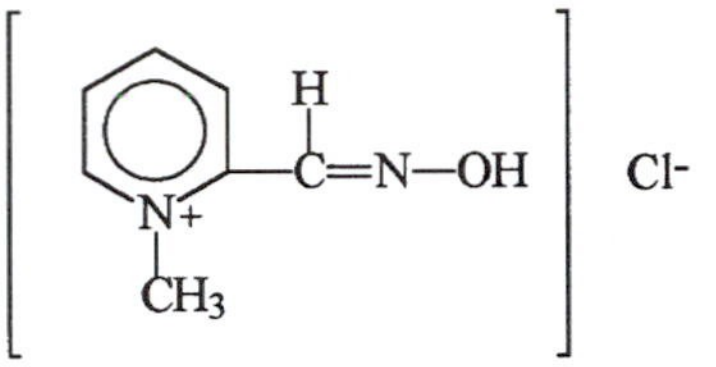

Obidoxime
(Toxigonin)

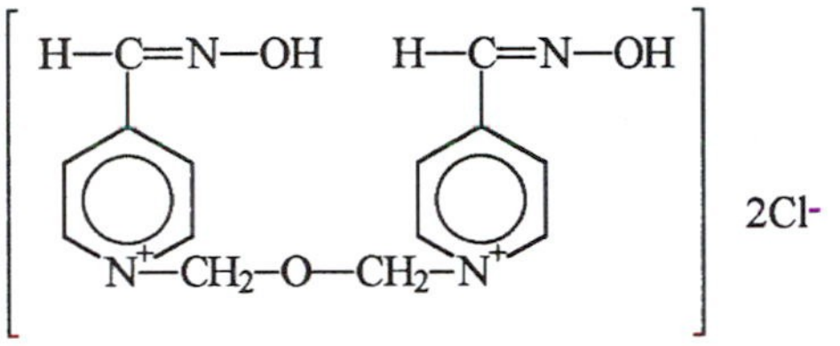

HI-6
HJ-6

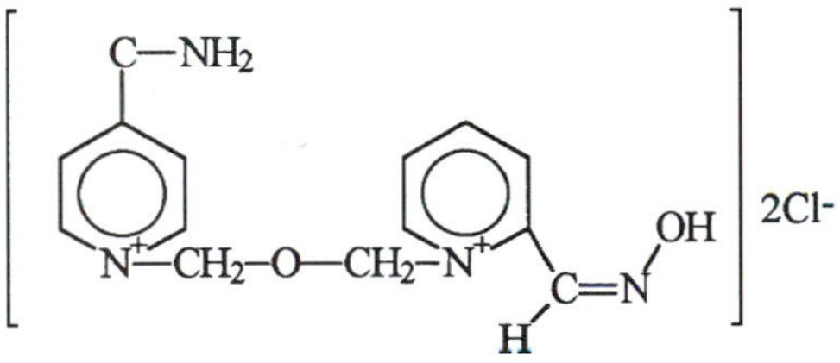

Pralidoxime (2-hydroxyiminomethyl-1-methyl pyridinium chloride; 2-PAM) is the only currently available cholinesterase-reactivating agent in the United States.[22] It is employed with atropine in the management of organophosphate pesticide poisonings. These agents are powerful inhibitors of carboxylic esterase enzymes, including acetylcholinesterase (true cholinesterase, found in red blood cells, nervous tissue, and skeletal muscle) and pseudocholinesterase or butyrlcholinesterase (found in plasma, liver, heart, pancreas, and brain).[34] The organophosphate compound binds firmly to the esterase enzyme, inactivating it by phosphorylation.[34,46] This results in the accumulation of acetylcholine at muscarinic, nicotinic, and CNS synapses, leading to the manifestations of organophosphate intoxication. Once the organophosphate pesticide binds to cholinesterase, the enzyme is inactivated and can undergo three processes: endogenous hydrolysis of the phosphorylated enzyme; reactivation by a strong nucleophile, such as 2-PAM; and biochemical changes that render the phosphorylated molecule inactive ("aged").

Endogenous hydrolysis of organophosphates can be extremely slow and, for the most part, is considered insignificant. Pralidoxime works by competing for the phosphate moiety of the organophosphorus compound and releasing it from the acetylcholinesterase enzyme.[33] This action liberates the enzyme and allows it to work again. Early in vitro evidence suggested that to be successful, cholinesterase reactivators must be administered within 24 to 48 hours of exposure to the organophosphorus compounds; otherwise the acetylcholinesterases would be irreversibly inactivated. The 48-hour limit was derived from in vitro experiments using a small number of tightly bound compounds and reactivators such as nicotinehydroxamic acid methiodide (NHA), monoisonitrosoacetone (MINA), and oximes (obidoxime and pralidoxime methiodide). These studies used data from plasma pseudocholinesterase enzyme activity, which is now recognized to be relatively unaffected by oxime nucleophilic attack. These data were generally accepted without consideration of such factors as their relevance to human systems, the use of newer and less tightly bound compounds, temperature and pH variation, blood flow, fat solubility, and species specificity. An in vitro experiment assessed the effect of aging on the ability of pralidoxime to regenerate rat erythrocyte and brain cholinesterases using three different organophosphates.[49] The rate of reactivation of erythrocyte and brain cholinesterases by pralidoxime was significantly decreased with time for fenitrothion and methylparathion, with no reactivation occurring at 48 hours. In contrast, a very high reactivation rate for ethylparathion was still apparent at 48 hours. This demonstrates that the structure of the organophosphate plays a significant role in the rate of aging and reactivation with pralidoxime. Fenitrothion and methylparathion are both O′O dimethylorganophosphates while ethylparathion is an O′O diethylorganophosphate.[49] Other studies have also suggested that 2-PAM and obidoxime are effective long after the previously suggested 48-hour window of therapy.[2–4,7,10,11,13,18,19,31,33]

Acetylcholinesterase inactivated by carbamates spontaneously reactivates with plasma elimination half-lives of 1 to 2 hours and clinical recovery in several hours and rarely more than 24 hours.[25] Although pralidoxime is rarely indicated, it was previously suggested that pralidoxime was contraindicated following exposure to a carbamate. This approach was based solely on data derived from the study of a single carbamate—carbaryl (Sevin)—and inappropriately generalized to all carbamates. In vitro experiments have demonstrated that pralidoxime had no effect on the reactivation of erythrocyte acetylcholinesterase carbamylated by aldicarb, methoxyl, and carbaryl.[25] Pralidoxime decreased the rate of carbamylation by 16 insecticidal carbamates and only modestly increased the rates for 3, one of which was carbaryl.[12] Animal studies have demonstrated the beneficial effects of pralidoxime and obidoxime in doubling the lethal dose for a number of carbamate insecticides.[35,44] However, with carbaryl (Sevin), obidoxime and pralidoxime mesylate worsened intoxication, possibly because the carbamate–oxime complex may be a more potent cholinesterase inhibitor than carbaryl alone.[17,35,41,44] Even in the presence of carbaryl, atropine and the oxime resulted in survival data comparable to that of atropine alone.[17] This evidence suggests that although pralidoxime is not usually a necessary adjunct to atropine in a pure carbamate overdose, it may occasionally improve morbidity and mortality.[8] Pralidoxime should always be used in conjunction with atropine and should not be the sole therapy. Pralidoxime should not be withheld in a seriously poisoned patient due to the possibility that the agent may be a carbamate.

Pralidoxime's action is most striking at nicotinic sites, often improving muscle strength within 10 to 40 minutes after administration.[34,46] Pralidoxime is effective at muscarinic sites and also appears to be synergistic with atropine at these sites.[14] The primary effect of atropine is to block the muscarinic and CNS symptoms of organophosphate poisoning. Pralidoxime and atropine work synergistically, and 2-PAM should rarely be used alone.[14] Some organophosphates respond much better to 2-PAM than others.

The CNS effects of 2-PAM, a quaternary nitrogen compound,[34] are controversial as the molecule is not expected to cross the blood–brain barrier.[28,34] Animal studies offer conflicting results possibly due to the use of brain hemogenate models rather than cortical slices.[30] Rat studies using radiolabeled pralidoxime demonstrated a lack of any radioactivity in the CNS after IV administration.[48] Intravenous administration of pralidoxime in rats failed to improve survival after IV fenitrothion or to reactivate brain cholinesterase, whereas intramedullary pralidoxime afforded complete survival and partially restored brain cholinesterase.[48] Clinical observations have certainly suggested a CNS action, with a return of consciousness in some cases.[33,34,37,51] A $3\frac{1}{2}$-year-old child who was comatose from parathion intoxication was given 500 mg of 2-PAM IV over 15 minutes with continuous electroencephalographic (EEG) monitoring. Within 2 minutes there was a dramatic response on the EEG, followed by normalization of consciousness.[26]

To improve the central effect of pralidoxime, the dihydropyridine derivative of pralidoxime (2-PAM) was synthesized.[5] This derivative, known as pro-2-PAM, acts as a "pro drug," or drug carrier, which allows passage through membranes such as the blood–brain barrier. Once across the membranes, in vivo oxidation converts pro-2-PAM to the active species, demonstrating a 13-fold higher level of 2-PAM in the brain than PAM administered under similar conditions. Further experiments supported the significantly increased central effects of pro-2-PAM.[40] The use of sugar oximes (the molecular combination of glucose with 2-PAM derivatives) to promote CNS penetration appears promising.[38] Obidoxime (Toxogonin) is an oxime used outside the United States that contains two active sites per molecule and is considered by some to be more effective than 2-PAM.[14] The H series of oximes (named after Hagedorn) have been developed to act against the chemical warfare nerve agents. They may have superior effectiveness in organophosphate insecticide poisoning, although their toxicity profile awaits further study.[9,24,27,39] In addition to reactivating acetylcholinesterase, they have direct central and peripheral anticholinergic effects.[39]

The signs and symptoms of organophosphate poisoning are usually manifested within 12 to 24 hours of exposure.[34] Delayed manifestations occur with the fat-soluble organophosphorus compounds, such as fenthion or chlorfenthion, and other compounds requiring metabolic conversion to active agents, such as parathion, which undergoes hepatic conversion to paraoxon. The route of exposure may also influence onset of systemic symptoms; for example, there may be a delay following dermal contact as opposed to ingestion or inhalation. When symptoms are delayed or prolonged, or when treatment is delayed, prolonged therapy with 2-PAM may be indicated.[1,7,31] In one case of poisoning with the fat-soluble organophosphate fenthion there was a 5-day delay before cholinergic symptoms appeared and some symptoms persisted for 30 days.[31] Pralidoxime and atropine were administered continuously in varying doses for most of that period.

Pralidoxime is characterized by a two-compartment model, with a steady-state volume of distribution of about 0.8 L/kg in volunteers.[20] Pralidoxime is renally excreted, and within 12 hours 80% of the dose has been recovered unchanged in the urine.[43] Thiamine administered intravenously at 100 mg/h for 2.5 hours prolonged the half-life, increased the volume of distribution and peak plasma concentrations, and decreased the plasma, intercompartmental, and renal clearances when pralidoxime (5 mg/kg) was given intravenously.[21] Thiamine and pralidoxime are both strong bases, and thiamine might decrease renal clearance through competition for renal secretion.[21] The benefit of using thiamine in poisoned patients to prolong the plasma half-life of pralidoxime has never been tested. In poisoned patients, the pharmacokinetics of 2-PAM appear to be altered. A volume of distribution of 2.77 L/kg and an elimination half-life of 3.44 hours has been reported.[51]

A dose of 10 mg/kg of 2-PAM IM or IV results in peak plasma concentrations of 6 μg/mL (reached 5 to 15 minutes after IM injection) and a plasma half-life of approximately 75 minutes.[43] Animal data suggest that a plasma level greater than 4 μg/mL is effective against nicotinic symptoms.[6,45] However, 1.5 hours after a standard IV 30-minute infusion dose of 1 g of 2-PAM in a 70-kg man, the plasma level was less than 4 μg/mL. In a simulated model, a continuous infusion of 500 mg/h of 2-PAM leads to a level greater than 4 μg/mL after 15 minutes, which can be maintained throughout the infusion.[47] In a human volunteer study an intravenous loading dose of 4 mg/kg over 15 minutes followed by 3.2 mg/kg per hour for a total of 4 hours maintained pralidoxime serum concentrations greater than 4 μg/mL for 257 minutes. The same total dose, 16 mg/kg, administered over 30 minutes only maintained those concentrations for 118 minutes.[29] Oral administration of salts of 2-PAM (not used clinically due to anticholinesterase poisoning induced vomiting) demonstrated peak concentrations at 2 to 3 hours, a biologic half-life of 1.7 hours, and an average urine recovery of 27% of unchanged 2-PAM.[23]

Adverse effects of therapeutic doses of 2-PAM in humans have been absent or minimal and may not be evident unless plasma levels are greater than 400 μg/mL.[15,16,32–34,37,47] Transient dizziness, blurred vision, and elevations in diastolic blood pressure may be related to the rate of administration.[20,21,29] Rapid IV administration has produced sudden cardiac and respiratory arrest.[36,42,52]

Pralidoxime is an effective reactivator of acetylcholinesterase in many organophosphate poisonings. It primarily reverses neuromuscular manifestations but has some CNS effects. New oximes should improve CNS penetration and efficacy in general. Pralidoxime and atropine are synergistic and should be used together in the management of organophosphate intoxications. If a patient requires atropine for muscarinic symptoms, then the use of 2-PAM is indicated. In symptomatic patients, acetylcholinesterase is partially inactivated and will remain so until new enzyme is endogenously created, which can be a prolonged process. The resolution of all signs or symptoms with atropine alone indicates only that the percentage of inactivation is less than 50% and that endogenous hydrolysis of phosphorylated enzyme is sufficient to eliminate symptoms. This does not mean, however, that the enzyme systems are fully active; patients may still benefit from enzyme regeneration with the relatively nontoxic antidote pralidoxime.

Finally, because newer fat-soluble organophosphates are being employed as pesticides, it may be necessary to administer atropine and 2-PAM for much longer periods of time than has been previously suggested.[50]

Pralidoxime chloride (Protopam) is supplied in 20-mL vials containing 1 g of powder, ready for reconstitution with sterile water for injection.[22] The adult dose is 1 to 2 g in 100 to 150 mL of 0.9% sodium chloride solution given intravenously over 30 minutes. The pediatric dose is 20 to 40 mg/kg to a maximum of 1 g/dose. This dose can be repeated in 1 hour if muscle weakness and fasciculations are not relieved. This dose should be repeated at 6 to 12-hour intervals for 24 to 48 hours to ensure distribution to all affected sites. This may result in reappearance of toxicity before the next dose, because serum concentrations would be expected to fall to less than therapeutic within several hours. Alternatively, a 2.5% concentration of 2-PAM can be given as a loading dose followed by a maintenance infusion. Serious intoxication may require continuous infusion of 500 mg/h in adults and 9 to 19 mg/kg per hour in children. Continuous infusion may be more effective than multiple single injections.[32,34] In the case of pulmonary edema, it can be given as a 5% solution (concentrations above 35% wt/vol produce muscle necrosis in animals).[43] Rapid administration (bolus or >200 mg/min) can lead to respiratory and cardiac arrest. Occasionally, long-term dosing may be necessary, depending on the patient's clinical condition.

References

1. Aaron CK, Smilkstein M: Intermediate syndrome or inadequate therapy. Vet Human Toxicol 1988;30:370. Abstract.
2. Amos WC Jr, Hall A: Malathion poisoning treated with protopam. Ann Intern Med 1965;62:1013–1016.
3. Blaber LC, Creasey NH: The mode of recovery of cholinesterase activity in vivo after organophosphorus poisoning: I. Erythrocyte cholinesterase. Biochem J 1960; 77:591–596.
4. Blaber LC, Creasey NH: The mode of recovery of cholinesterase activity in vivo after organophosphorus poisoning: II. Brain cholinesterase. Biochem J 1960;77: 597–604.
5. Bodor N, Shek E, Higuchi T: Delivery of a quaternary pyridinium salt across the blood–brain barrier by its dihydropyridine derivative. Science 1975;190:155–156.
6. Bokowjic D, Jovanovic D, Jokanovic M, et al: Protective effects of oximes HI-6 and PAM 2 applied by osmotic minipumps in quinalphos poisoned rats. Arch Int Pharmacodyn Ther 1987;288:309–318.
7. Borowitz SM: Prolonged organophosphate toxicity in a twenty-six-month-old child. J Pediatr 1988;112:303–304.
8. Burgess JL, Bernstein JN, Hurlbut K: Aldicarb poisoning a case report with prolonged cholinesterase inhibition and improvement after pralidoxime therapy. Arch Intern Med 1994;154:221–224.
9. Clement JG, Bailey DG, Madill HD, et al: The acetylcholinesterase oxime reactivator HI-6 in man: Pharmacokinetics and tolerability in combination with atropine. Biopharm Drug Dispos 1995;16:415–425.
10. Davies DR, Green AL: The kinetics of reactivation, by oximes, of cholinesterase inhibited by organophosphorus compounds. Biochemistry 1956;63:529–535.
11. Davison AN: Return of cholinesterase activity in the rat after inhibition by organophosphorus compounds: I. Diethyl *p*-nitrophenyl phosphate (E600, Paraoxon). Biochem J 1953;54:583–590.
12. Dawson RM: Oximes in treatment of carbamate poisoning. Vet Rec 1994;134:687. Letter.
13. Durham WF, Hayes WJ Jr: Organic phosphorus poisoning and its therapy. Arch Environ Health 1962;5:21–47.
14. Finkelstein Y, Taitelman U, Biegon A: CNS involvement in acute organophosphate poisoning: Specific pattern of toxi-

city, clinical correlates and antidotal treatment. Ital J Neurol Sci 1988;9:437–446.
15. Grob D, Jones RJ: Use of oximes in the treatment of intoxication by anticholinesterase compounds in normal subjects. Am J Med 1958;24:497–511.
16. Hagerstrom-Portnoy G, Jones R, Adams AJ, Jampolsky A: Effects of atropine and 2-PAM chloride on vision and performance in humans. Aviat Space Environ Med 1987;10: 47–53.
17. Harris LW, Talbot BG, Lennox WJ, et al: The relationship between oxime induced reactivation of carbamylated acetylcholinesterase and antidotal efficacy against carbamate intoxication. Toxicol Appl Pharmacol 1989;98: 128–133.
18. Hobbinger F: Chemical reactivation of phosphorylated human and bovine true cholinesterase. Br J Pharmacol 1956;11:295–303.
19. Hobbinger F: Effect of nicotinehydroxamic acid methiodide on human plasma cholinesterase inhibited by organophosphates containing dialkylphosphate groups. Br J Pharmacol 1955;10:356–362.
20. Jager BV, Staff GN: Toxicity of diacetyl monoxime and of pyridine-2-aldoxime methiodide in man. Bull Johns Hopkins Hosp 1958;102:203–211.
21. Josselson J, Sidell FR: Effect of intravenous thiamine on pralidoxime kinetics. Clin Pharmacol Ther 1978;24:95–100.
22. Kastrup E, ed: Facts and Comparisons. Philadelphia, Lippincott, 1983.
23. Kondritzer A, Zvirblis P, Goodman A, Paplanus S: Blood plasma levels and elimination of salts of 2-PAM in man after oral administration. J Pharm Sci 1968;57: 1142–1145.
24. Kusic R, Jovanovic D, Randjelovic A, et al: HI-6 in man: Efficacy of the oxime in poisoning by organophosphorus insecticides. Hum Exp Toxicol 1991;10:113–118.
25. Lifshitz M, Rotenberg M, Sofer S, et al: Carbamate poisoning and oxime treatment in children: A clinical and laboratory study. Pediatrics 1994;93:652–655.
26. Lotti M, Becker C: Treatment of acute organophosphate-poisoning: Evidence of a direct effect on central nervous system by 2-PAM (pyridine-2-aldoxime methyl chloride). J Toxicol Clin Toxicol 1982;19:121–127.
27. Lundy PM, Hansen AS, Hand BT, Boulet CA: Comparison of several oximes against poisoning by soman, tabun and GF. Toxicology 1992;72:99–105.
28. Matin M, Siddiqui R: Modification of the level of acetylcholinesterase activity by two oximes in certain brain regions and peripheral tissues of paraoxon treated rats. Pharmacol Res Commun 1982;4:241–246.
29. Medicis JJ, Stork CM, Howland MA, et al: Pharmacokinetics following a loading plus a continuous infusion of pralidoxime compared with the traditional short infusion regimen in human volunteers. J Toxicol Clin Toxicol 1996;34: 289–295.
30. Milosevic MP, Andjelkovic D: Reactivation of paraoxon-inactivated cholinesterase in the rat cerebral cortex by pralidoxime chloride. Nature 1966;210:206.
31. Merrill D, Mihm F; Prolonged toxicity of organophosphate poisoning. Crit Care Med 1982;10:550–551.
32. Namba T: Diagnosis and treatment of organophosphate insecticide poisoning. Med Times 1972;100:100–126.
33. Namba T, Hiraki K: PAM (pyridine-2-aldoxime methiodide) therapy for alkyl-phosphate poisoning. JAMA 1958;166:1834–1839.
34. Namba T, Nolte C, Jackrel J, Grob D: Poisoning due to organophosphate insecticides: Acute and chronic manifestations. Am J Med 1971;50:475–492.
35. Natoff IL, Reiff B: Effect of oximes on the acute toxicology of acetylcholinesterase carbamates. Toxicol Appl Pharmacol 1973;25:569–575.
36. Pickering EN: Organic phosphate insecticide poisoning. Can J Med Technol 1966;28:174–179.
37. Quimby G: Further therapeutic experience with pralidoximes in organic phosphorus poisoning. JAMA 1963; 187:202–206.
38. Rachaman E, Ashani Y, Leader H, et al: Sugaroximes, new potential antidotes against organophosphorus poisoning. Arzneimittelforschung 1979;29:875–876.
39. Rousseaux CG, Du AK: Pharmacology of HI-6, an H-series oxime. Can J Physiol Pharmacol 1989;67:1183–1189.
40. Rump S, Faff J, Borkowska G, et al: Central therapeutic effects of dihydro-derivative of pralidoxime (pro-2-PAM) in organophosphate intoxication. Arch Int Pharmacodyn Ther 1978;232:321–331.
41. Sanderson DM: Treatment of poisoning by anticholinesterase insecticides in the rat. J Pharm Pharmacol 1961;13:435–442.
42. Scott RJ: Repeated asystole following PAM in organophosphate self-poisoning. Anesth Intensive Care 1986;4: 458–460.
43. Sedell FR, Groff WA: Intramuscular and intravenous administration of small doses of 2-pyridinium aldoxime methylchloride to man. J Pharm Sci 1971;60:1224–1228.
44. Sterri S, Rognerud B, Fiskum S, Lyngaas S: Effect of toxigonin and P2S on the toxicity of carbamates and organophosphorus compounds. Acta Pharmacol Toxicol 1979;45:9–15.
45. Sundwall A: Minimum concentrations of n-methyl pyridinium-2-aldoxime methane sulphonate (PS2) which reverse neuromuscular block. Biochem Pharmacol 1961;8: 413–417.
46. Taylor P: Anticholinesterase agents. In: Hardman JG, Limbind LE, Molinoff PB, Ruddoev RW, eds: Goodman and Gilman's The Pharmacological Basis of Therapeutics, 9th ed. New York, Macmillan, 1996, pp. 100–119.
47. Thompson DF, Thompson GD, Greenwood RB, Trammel HL: Therapeutic dosing of pralidoxime chloride. Drug Intell Clin Pharm 1987;21:1590–1593.
48. Uehara S, Hiromori T, Isobe N, et al: Studies on the therapeutic effect of 2-pyridine aldoxime methiodide (2-PAM) in mammals following organophosphorous compound (op)-poisoning (report III): Distribution and antidotal effect of 2-PAM in rats. J Toxicol 1993;18:265–275.
49. Uehara S, Hiromori T, Suzuki T, et al: Studies on the therapeutic effect of 2-pyridine aldoxime methiodide (2-PAM) in mammals following organophosphorous compound (op)-poisoning (report II): Aging of op-inhibited mammalian cholinesterase. J Toxicol 1993;18:179–183.

50. Willems JL, BeBisschop HC, Verstraete AG, et al: Cholinesterase reactivation in organophosphorus poisoned patients depends on the plasma concentrations of the oxime pralidoxime methylsulfate and of the organophosphate. Arch Toxicol 1993;97:79–84.
51. Willems JL, Langenberg JP, Verstraete AC, et al. Plasma concentrations of pralidoxime methyl sulfate in organophosphorus poisoned patients. Arch Toxicol 1992;66: 260–266.
52. Wislicki L: Differences in the effect of oximes on striated muscle and respiratory centre. Arch Int Pharmacodyn Ther 1960; 120:1–19

CHAPTER 88

Insecticides: Chlorinated Hydrocarbons, Pyrethrins, and DEET

Mary Ann Howland

A 2-year-old boy was brought to the Emergency Department (ED) after having vomited and having a 1-minute seizure. On admission, the child was alert and oriented with normal vital signs. The only history available was that the child had a cold and a "skin condition." By pursuing the connection between seizures and a skin condition, the poison information specialist obtained further history that implicated lindane. The child's grandmother (who was unable to read the instructions on the bottle) had given him 1 teaspoon (5 mL) of lindane orally three times a day. She assumed the medication was to be given orally to treat the skin condition. The child probably received a total of six doses, the last dose being approximately 3 hours prior to admission.

Because the child was no longer seizing and was now alert and oriented with normal vital signs, 1 g/kg of activated charcoal in a water slurry was given to adsorb any lindane remaining in the gastrointestinal tract. The child was observed in an intensive care setting for 6 to 12 hours.

The ingestion of 1% lindane usually results in one or two generalized seizures of short duration followed by a postictal period of variable duration. The length of observation is dictated by the individual case.

What Are the Characteristics of the Organochlorine Pesticides?

Chlorinated hydrocarbon pesticides and chlorinated hydrocarbon solvents and fumigants are organochlorines with varying molecular size, volatility, and CNS effects. Chlorinated pesticides are cyclic in structure, have molecular weights generally in the range of 300 to 550 D, have limited volatility, and are CNS stimulants.[18] Chlorinated hydrocarbon solvents and fumigants, on the other hand, are more volatile, smaller, and generally CNS depressants (see Chap. 85).[18]

The organochlorine pesticides can be divided into four categories based on their chemical structures: (1) dichlorodiphenyltrichloroethane (DDT) and related analogs; (2) hexachlorocyclohexane (benzene hexachloride, a chemical misnomer in common usage, or lindane); (3) cyclodienes and related compounds; and (4) toxaphene and related compounds (Table 88–1; Fig. 88–1).[18] These compounds differ substantially between and within groups with respect to toxic doses, skin absorption, fat storage, metabolism, and elimination.[18] The signs and symptoms of toxicity in humans, however, are remarkably similar. In animals there may be significant interspecies variation.

What Is the Mechanism of Toxicity?

Electrophysiologic studies demonstrate that DDT affects the neuronal membrane, especially that of the axon, perhaps through effects on Ca^{2+}-ATPase.[18] In particular, DDT affects the sodium channel and sodium conductance by

TABLE 88–1. CATEGORIES OF ORGANOCHLORINE PESTICIDES AND THEIR TOXIC POTENTIAL

	Acute Oral Toxicity
DDT and Analogs	
DDT	Low to moderate
Methoxychlor	Low
Benzene Hexachloride	
Gamma-hexachlorocyclohexane (Lindane)	Moderate
Cyclodienes and Related Compounds	
Aldrin	High
Dieldrin	High
Endosulfan (Thiodan)	High
Endrin	High
Isobenzan	High
Chlordane	Moderate
Chlordecone (Kepone)	Moderate
Heptachlor	Moderate
Mirex (Dechlorane)	Low
Toxaphene and Related Compounds	
Toxaphene	Moderate

lengthening the time the sodium channel is open.[51] Other effects include alterations in the metabolism of serotonin, norepinephrine, and acetylcholine. Dogs given large IV doses of DDT were sensitized to endogenous and exogenous epinephrine and died of ventricular fibrillation,[18] an effect similar to that seen with trichloroethylene and the chlorinated hydrocarbons (see Chap. 85). Death in small animals is attributed to respiratory arrest.[18] The cyclodienes and lindane appear to inhibit the GABA-mediated chloride channels in the CNS.[5,17,30] Although intracerebral injection into mice potentiated the toxicity of the cyclodienes as compared to intraperitoneal administration, that was not the case for lindane. This suggests that lindane also has significant peripheral nervous system toxicity, affecting $GABA_A$ receptors in the dorsal root ganglia, myenteric plexus in the gut, and voltage-dependent chloride channels in nerve and skeletal muscle.[5,57] Cholecystokinin, a peptide neurotransmitter, is often found jointly with GABA and also acts as an anticonvulsant.[57] Administration of a cholecystokinin antagonist facilitated the incidence of lindane-induced seizures.[57] The release of endogenous cholecystokinin may therefore play a role in the brief nature of lindane-induced seizures.[57] Acute and chronic doses of lindane given to rats also decreases the concentrations of dopamine in the diencephalon. Research in rats with repetitive dosing of endosulfan (thiodan) implicates indirect effects on serotonin.[2] Methysergide (Sansert, an ergot), a 5-hydroxytryptamine blocker, reversed the aggressive behavior pattern induced in these rats.[2]

What Are the Pharmacokinetics and Associated Drug Interactions of These Agents?

All of these pesticides can be absorbed transdermally, orally, and via inhalation. Absorption by any route may

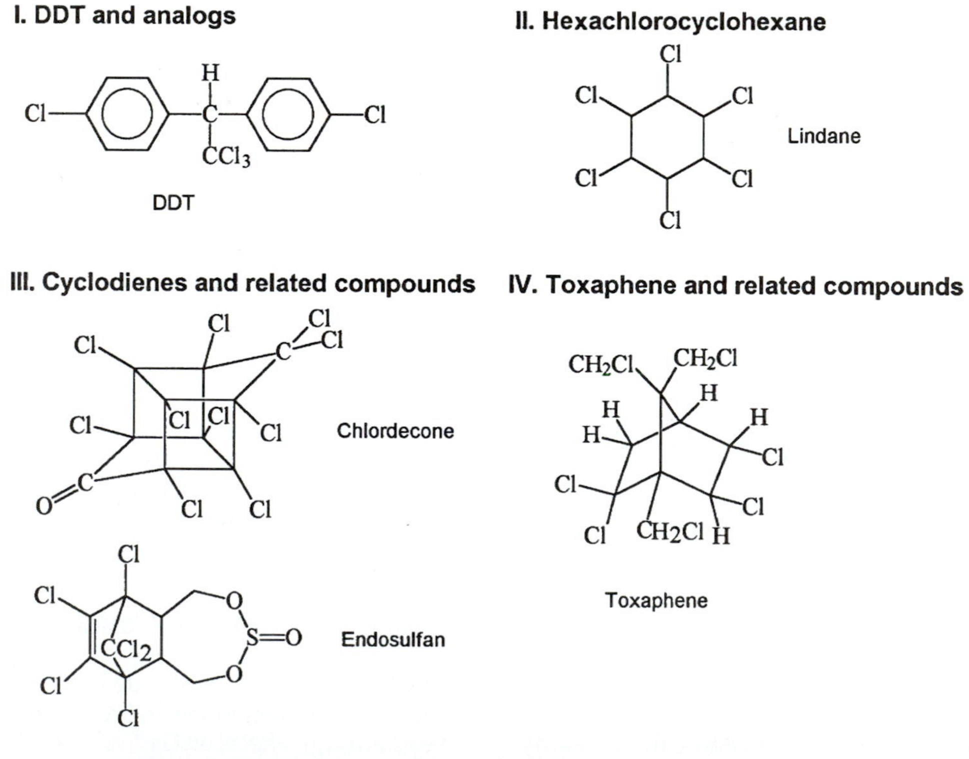

Figure 88–1. The varied chemical structures of organochlorine pesticides by category.

be affected by the vehicle as well as the physical state (solid or liquid) of the pesticide. Dichlorodiphenyltrichloroethane (DDT) is the least well absorbed transdermally, whereas dieldrin is so well absorbed by this route that toxicity by the dermal route is approximately 50% that of the oral route.[18] These compounds have limited volatility, so that air concentrations are usually low but solid particles of the right size and shape can be inhaled and absorbed.[41]

These agents are highly lipid soluble. When liver metabolism is impaired or fecal excretion delayed with agents such as dieldrin, adipose tissue storage is increased.[18] Agents that are rapidly metabolized and eliminated, such as endrin, an isomer of dieldrin, do not persist in body tissues.[18] Mirex and chlordecone, as compared to the cyclodienes, are very slowly metabolized.

Most chlorinated hydrocarbon pesticides are capable of inducing the hepatic microsomal enzyme systems.[10,18,56] This can lead to self-induction, with more rapid metabolism of the offending compound, and interaction with other chemicals and drugs using these enzyme systems. In certain animal models the acute toxicity of organophosphates and carbamates may be reduced by the administration of several chlorinated hydrocarbons (eg, aldrin, chlordane). This protective effect can be blocked by piperonyl butoxide, an inhibitor of the rat liver microsomal enzyme system.[18,56]

However, metabolism may result in the production of a more toxic metabolite. Hydrocarbon pesticide induction of the microsomal enzymes has also led to changes in ascorbic acid and glucuronic acid pathways. This induction has produced an ascorbic acid deficiency, which in turn decreases the biodegradation of the pesticide.[47]

Other consequences of liver enzyme induction include enhanced metabolism of therapeutic drugs and reduced efficacy. Enhanced oral contraceptive metabolism induced by chlordane has reportedly led to dysfunctional uterine bleeding.[16] This hepatic induction might be clinically important when an anticonvulsant such as phenobarbital is administered for seizure control in poisoned patients.

Some of these agents undergo an enterohepatic and enteroenteric recirculation.[6,9] Central nervous system redistribution of chlorinated hydrocarbons to the blood and then to fat may account for the apparent rapid CNS recovery in spite of the persistent substantial total body burden. In the rat model there appears to be a relationship between the concentration of DDT or dieldrin in the brain and the clinical signs produced after a single dose of the agents.[13,18] Blood levels document exposure, but they may have no other clinical value. Most humans studied have measurable DDT levels. In a study of a community with a very large exposure to DDT, serum DDT levels continued to increase with age. These increasing levels were not associated with any apparent health effects, but there was an association with increasing gamma glutamyltranspeptidase levels.[24] In a group of factory workers with a prolonged exposure to chlordecone (Kepone), clinical signs and symptoms of toxicity seemed to correlate with blood levels.[9]

What Are the Signs and Symptoms of Organochlorine Poisoning?

Acute Exposure

In sufficient doses, this class of agents will lower the seizure threshold and produce CNS stimulation, to result in seizures, respiratory failure, and death.[4,7,8,17,18,21,22,29,38,40] In the case of DDT, tremor may be the only initial manifestation. Nausea; vomiting; hyperesthesia of the mouth and face; paresthesias of face, tongue, and extremities; headache; dizziness; myoclonus; opsoclonus, rapid, irregular, dysrhythmic ocular movements; leg weakness; agitation; and confusion may occur prior to or independent of seizures.[18,22,29] Agents other than DDT may have no prodomal signs or symptoms, and the first manifestation of toxicity may be a seizure.[4,7,18,22,29,38,46] If seizures develop, they often do so within 1 to 2 hours postingestion if the stomach is empty, but the delay may be as long as 5 to 6 hours if the ingestion follows a substantial meal.[18] The seizures are often self-limited but may recur and result in status epilepticus. If the seizures are brief and hypoxia has not occurred, recovery is usually complete. Electroencephalographic (EEG) abnormalities have been recorded before, during, and sometimes following seizures.[22] Fever secondary to central mechanisms, increased muscle activity, and/or aspiration pneumonitis is common.[18]

The ingestion of combinations of agents may result in significantly increased toxicity due to synergy. This has been demonstrated for DDT and lindane.

Chronic Exposure

Chlordecone, unlike the other agents, produces an insidious picture of chronic toxicity related to its extremely long persistence in the body. Pseudotumor cerebri, oligospermia, and decreased sperm motility are reported in factory workers with a prolonged exposure to chlordecone.[9] Other symptoms include weight loss, tremor, weakness, opsoclonus, ataxia, mental status changes, rash, and abnormal liver function tests.[18] Chlordane and heptachlor exposures are associated with leukemias and thrombocytopenic purpura, although firm proof is lacking.[18] Several reports also suggest an association between long-term exposure to organochlorine pesticides and aplastic anemia.[37,39]

Are These Agents Carcinogenic?

The organochlorines can induce liver tumors in mice but have not been shown to do so in rats or hamsters. There is no convincing evidence that any of these agents are carcinogenic in humans.[18] Workers heavily exposed to DDT and dieldrin have not had an increased incidence of neoplasms. Epidemiologic evidence suggests that the incidence of deaths from liver cancer has steadily decreased since 1930, which includes the 50 years since the introduction of these agents.[18] There is some evidence that DDT can be a facilitator of carcinogenesis induced by another agent such as aflatoxin and chlordane may have the same facilitative character with regard to diethylnitrosamine.[18]

What Clues Can Assist in the Diagnosis of Organochlorine Poisoning?

The history is probably the most important piece of information. By law, the package label of these products must contain certain information, and this can be very helpful in determining which agents, what quantity, and what vehicle are involved. The potential use of the insecticide may be helpful in determining possible ingredients (Table 88–2). The presence of an unusual odor in the mouth, in the vomitus, or on the skin may be helpful. An abdominal radiograph may reveal the presence of a radiopaque chlorinated pesticide.[14] Radiopacity may be correlated with the number of chlorine atoms per molecule (Chap. 7).[14] A limited number of other toxins lead to seizures as the first manifestation of toxicity; these include strychnine, camphor, fluoroacetate, isoniazid, water hemlock, and picrotoxin (see Chaps. 10 and 19).

Who Is at Risk for Toxicity?

Patients are at risk for developing central nervous system toxicity from 1% lindane from improper topical therapeutic use, unintentional oral ingestion, and, rarely, proper therapeutic use.[3,12,15,23,25,32,35,36,45,48] An evaluation of published English-language case reports and those submitted to the Food and Drug Administration divided toxicity into those associated with concentrations of lindane greater than or less than 1%.[23] An algorithm to determine the likelihood that the adverse drug reaction was lindane related was applied. Only 6 of 26 cases could be considered probably related to 1% lindane; 4 of these 6 were secondary to ingestion or inappropriate skin application. Young animals of various species and young children appear at greatest risk, possibly because of greater skin permeability, increased body surface area/mass, immature liver enzymes, and oral absorption from licking the skin. The elderly may also be at risk. Three of 19 elderly patients treated topically with 1% lindane developed a single seizure of 5 to 10 minutes duration 4 to 5 days after application.[49] Although it was not recommended, all of the patients had had a hot bath prior to lindane application. This combined with atrophic skin, a generalized dermatitis in one patient, and perhaps an age-related increased sensitivity may have predisposed these patients to seizures.

Review of data when lindane was ingested therapeutically as an anthelmintic demonstrates that 40 mg/day for 3 to 14 days often produced no symptoms.[18] A number of serious cases related to lindane occurred in the 1960s and 1970s, when lindane pellets were used in vaporizers and unintentionally ingested by children.[18] An epidemic of lindane poisoning related to the unintentional substitution of lindane for sugar in the preparation of Nescafe demonstrated a delay of 20 minutes to 3 hours to the onset of nausea, vomiting, dizziness, facial pallor, severe cyanosis of the face and extremities, collapse, convulsions, and hyperthermia.[18]

Animal studies and case reports suggest that the young, malnourished, and those receiving repeated doses may have increased fat storage and increased risk for seizures.[35] Cutaneous penetration is enhanced by hot baths, the vehicle for the lindane, and a disturbed cutaneous integrity.[45] Impaired hepatic metabolism may also be contributory.[18] Lindane is heat stable and easily vaporized, and toxicity has also occurred following inhalation.[18]

Single acute oral doses of 10 mg/kg or more of DDT are usually necessary to produce symptoms.[18]

TABLE 88–2. COMMON HOUSEHOLD PESTICIDES

Pest	Usual Recommendation
Ants	Baygon, bendiocarb, chlorpyrifos, diazinon, permethrin, resmethrin, silica gel-pyrethrum, baits containing boric acid
Bedbugs	Permethrin
Cockroaches	Baygon, bendiocarb, chlorpyrifos, diazinon, permethrin, resmethrin, silica gel pyrethrum, tetramethrin, boric acid
Fleas	Baygon, bendiocarb, chlorpyrifos, d-limonene, permethrin, pyrethrins, silica gel pyrethrum, resmethrin, tetramethrin
Flies (house)	Allethrin, pyrethrum, resmethrin, tetramethrin
Mosquitoes	Allethrin, pyrethrum, pyrethrins, resmethrin, tetramethrin
Silverfish	Baygon, bendiocarb, boric acid, chlorpyrifos, diazinon, silica gel pyrethrum
Spiders	Baygon, bendiocarb, chlorpyrifos, diazinon, permethrin, pyrethrins, resmethrin, tetramethrin
Termites	Effective pesticides restricted in use for application by certified applicators
Ticks	Baygon, chlorpyrifos, diazinon, malathion, tetramethrin

Reproduced, with permission, from Pest Management Around the Home. Cornell Cooperative Extension Bulletin 74. Ithaca, NY: Cornell University Media and Technology Services.

How Should Patients Exposed to Chlorinated Hydrocarbon Pesticides Be Managed?

The airway, breathing, and adequate circulation should be assured and maintained. These agents may result in hypoxia secondary to seizures, aspiration of vomitus, or respiratory failure. Hyperthermia as a consequence of seizures or from a central mechanism may occur. Patients who present with an altered mental status should receive dextrose and thiamine as indicated. Skin decontamination is essential and must always be considered. Clothing should be removed and placed in a plastic bag and the skin washed with soap and water. Healthcare providers should be protected with rubber gloves and aprons. Because these pesticides are almost invariably liquids, a nasogastric tube can be used to suction and lavage gastric contents. This is most appropriate if the ingestion occurred within several hours. Activated charcoal can be used after gastric lavage or in place of gastric lavage, when lavage is not indicated.[18,28] The ability of activated charcoal to bind various organochlorines has never been adequately studied. A murine model of lindane toxicity following intragastric administration showed a trend but not a statistically significant benefit of activated charcoal use.[20] The use of cholestyramine in the same murine model did show statistical significance by raising both the convulsive dose and the lethal dose.[20] The doses of activated charcoal or choleystyramine were 2.25 g/kg, or about 12 to 28 times the lethal and convulsive doses of lindane, respectively. Oil-based cathartics should never be used, as they may facilitate absorption.

Seizures should be controlled promptly with a benzodiazepine followed by phenobarbital if further intervention is indicated. Phenytoin is probably less effective than phenobarbital in these cases.[51,52] If these measures are inadequate, more aggressive measures should be instituted rapidly, such as a pentobarbital infusion and, if necessary, neuromuscular blockade to control the peripheral manifestations of seizures, thereby preventing metabolic acidosis and rhabdomyolysis. Hyperthermia should be managed aggressively with cooling.

Cholestyramine, a nonabsorbable bile acid-binding anion exchange resin, should be administered to all patients symptomatic from chlordecone. Chlordecone undergoes both enterohepatic and enteroenteric recirculation, which can be interrupted by cholestyramine at a dosage of 16 g/day.[9] Cholestyramine increases the fecal elimination of chlordecone 3- to 18-fold in industrial workers exposed to this chemical for many months.[9] The extent of toxicity appears to be related to the tissue levels of chlordecone and improves following cholestyramine therapy.

Adverse effects associated with cholestyramine include a gritty texture in the mouth, nausea, abdominal discomfort, and constipation.[22] Hypoprothrombinemia, hyperchloremic metabolic acidosis, and transient increases in alkaline phosphatase and hepatic aminotransferases have been reported.[2] Steatorrhea and malabsorption of fat-soluble vitamins may also occur.[22] Because therapeutic drugs may be affected by cholestyramine, they should be ingested 1 hour before or 4 hours after a dose of cholestyramine.

What Laboratory Tests Are Available to Measure the Organochlorines?

Gas chromatography can detect organochlorine pesticides in serum, adipose tissue, and urine.[11,44] If confirmation is necessary for legal purposes, it may be necessary to measure concentrations of organochlorines. If the patient's history and toxidrome are obvious, then laboratory evaluation is unnecessary, as this determination will not alter the course of management. At present there are no data correlating health effects and tissue concentrations. Routine surveillance of serum levels in the occupationally exposed is not currently performed.[11]

What Toxicity Is Associated With the Pyrethrins?

Pyrethrum is the first identified of the pyrethrins, which are the active extracts from the *Chrysanthemum cinerariaefolium.* There are over 1000 pyrethroids, which are the synthetic analogs of these natural products.[18,34] Pyrethrins and pyrethroids are found in more than 2000 commercially available products. These insecticides quickly incapacitate ("knock down") insects. Most mammalian species are relatively resistant, because they can rapidly metabolize and detoxify the agents.[18] Toxicity of the pyrethrins and pyrethroids is enhanced in insects by combination with synergists like piperonyl butoxide or *N*-octyl bicycloheptene dicarboximide, which further impairs the insect's capacity to detoxify the pyrethrins. There appear to be no effects of pyrethrins in mammals because of the small amounts necessary to achieve this effect, species specificity, and affinity characteristics of the agents.[18]

Pyrethrum has an LD_{50} of over 1 g/kg. Most cases of toxicity associated with the pyrethrins are the result of allergic reactions.[34,35] At highest risk are those patients who are sensitive to ragweed pollen, which may cross-react with chrysanthemums.[34] It appears that the synthetic pyrethroids are less likely to induce allergic reactions than the pyrethrins.[18] Contact dermatitis and acute systemic allergic reactions should be treated in the usual manner.

The pyrethroids can be divided into two types based on their structures and their clinical manifestations in overdose. Type 1 pyrethroids (permethrin) do not contain a cyano group while the type 2 agents (cypermethrin, deltamethrin, fenpropathrin, fenvalerate) do.[30] Like DDT, the pyrethroids prolong the inactivation of the sodium channel by binding to it in the open state.[18,30] Type 2 agents are more potent in this regard and lead to significant after-potentials, which can produce repetitive depolarizations and eventual nerve conduction block. Type 2 agents may also inhibit GABA-mediated inhibitory chloride channels.[18] In animals, type 1 poisoning most closely resembles DDT with extensive tremors, twitching, increased metabolic rate, and hyperthermia. Excluding the rare possibility of skin irritation or allergy, the type 1 agents are unlikely to cause systemic toxicity in humans. The type 2 agents cause profuse salivation, ataxia, coarse tremor, choreoathetosis, and seizures in animals. In humans, type 2 agents cause paresthesias (secondary to sodium channel effects in sensory nerves), nausea, vomiting, dizziness, fasciculations, altered mental status, coma, seizures, and pulmonary edema.[18,26] A review of over 500 cases of acute pyrethroid poisoning from China highlights some similar manifestations between a massive acute type 2 pyrethroid overdose and an organophosphate overdose. Treatment is entirely supportive and symptomatic with atropine for secretions and benzodiazepines for tremor and seizures. Cutaneous paresthesias may respond to topical vitamin E.[19]

What Toxicity Has Been Associated With DEET?

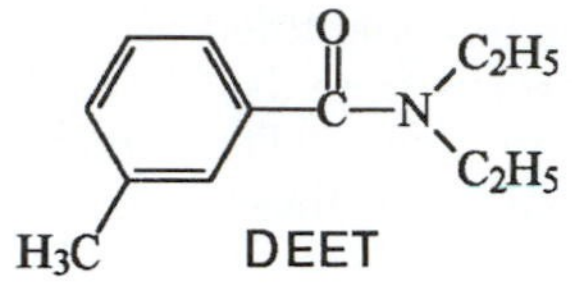

DEET

N,N-diethyltoluamide (DEET) was patented by the U.S. Army in 1946 and marketed in the United States since 1956, with widespread use by over 50 to 100 million persons since that time.[27] It can be purchased over the counter in concentrations ranging from 5 to 100%, and is often combined with isopropyl or ethyl alcohol. Fewer than 20 cases have reported major morbidity (encephalopathy, ataxia, convulsions, respiratory failure, hypotension, anaphylaxis) or death, particularly after ingestion or dermal exposure to large amounts.[31,33,50,53] Single large acute oral doses (1 to 3 g/kg) in rats produced ataxia, prostration, EEG evidence of seizures, and spongiform myelinopathy in the cerebellar roof nuclei.[54] Toxicity was statistically increased with younger age, female gender, and in the presence of piperonyl butoxide. Smaller acute doses (500 mg/kg and less) and chronic multigenerational dosing in another rat study produced no obvious toxicity.[42] Teratogenicity studies in rats and rabbits have failed to demonstrate toxicity, with the exception of reduced fetal weight in one study at the highest dose of 750 mg/kg, although incidently, ataxia was noted.[43,58] In view of the number of applications, the number of reports of toxicity appears relatively small, suggesting a substantial margin of safety.[33,49,53]

It seems prudent to avoid the overuse of DEET. One application lasts 4 to 8 hours. Soaking the skin is not more effective and may contribute to toxicity. Pediatric patients, pregnant women, patients whose skin is damaged or rendered permeable, and those who ingest the DEET may be presumed at high risk for toxicity. Other options of protection include mechanical means, such as mosquito netting. If DEET is to be used, it can be used safely if applied to clothing and as directed to skin. Solutions of lower concentrations seem preferable as they offer nearly as much protection as those that are 100% DEET.[1] Care should be taken to avoid exposure to eyes and sensitive skin areas.

What Are the Legal Standards for an Insecticide Label?

The label on the original container of these products is usually instructive. For this reason the container should always be brought to the medical facility. The label provides the following information:

- Brand name
- Intended product use
- Active and inert ingredients and their percent composition
- Directions for use
- Pests to be controlled—crops, animals, or sites to be treated
- Dosage, time interval, and method of application
- Warnings to protect users, consumers of treated foods, beneficial plants, animals, and endangered species
- "Keep out of reach of children"
- Antidotes and first-aid instruction
- Net content
- Name and address of manufacturer
- EPA registration number and signal word based on the LD_{50}

What Does the Signal Word on the Package Label Mean?

The signal word implies the degree of toxicity based on an oral LD_{50}. The criteria were established by the Federal Insecticide, Fungicide and Rodenticide Act of 1962 (Table 88–3).

Consumers asking for help in choosing the most effective and safest pesticides should be told to contact their county agricultural or cooperative extension agents. It is important to choose an effective pesticide as well as a product formulated for use in the requisite area (indoors versus outdoors), because concentrations and residues vary. Instructions must always be read carefully and followed, as failure to do so may lead to toxicity (Table 88–2).

TABLE 88–3. CRITERIA ESTABLISHED BY THE FEDERAL INSECTICIDE, FUNGICIDE, AND RODENTICIDE ACT OF 1962

Signal Word	Toxicity	Acute Oral LD_{50}
Danger Poison Skull and crossbones Call physician immediately Keep out of reach of children	High	0–50 mg/kg
Warning No antidote Keep out of reach of children	Moderate	50–500 mg/kg
Caution No antidote Keep out of reach of children	Low	500–5000 mg/kg
No Signal Word Keep out of reach of children	Relatively safe	>5000 mg/kg

References

1. Abramowicz M, ed: Insect repellents. Med Lett 1989;792: 45–47.
2. Agrawal AK, Anand M, Zaidi NF, et al: Involvement of serotonergic receptors in endosulfan neurotoxicity. Biochem Pharmacol 1983;32:3591–3593.
3. Aks SE, Krantz A, Hryhorczuk DO, et al: Acute accidental lindane ingestion in toddlers. Ann Emerg Med 1995;26: 647–651.
4. Anonymous: Acute convulsions with endrin poisoning: Pakistan. MMWR 1986;33:687–688, 693.
5. Bloomquist JR: Intrinsic lethality of chloride-channel-directed insecticides and convulsants in mammals. Toxic Lett 1992;60:289–298.
6. Boylan JJ, Cohn WJ, Egle JL, et al: Excretion of chlordecone by the gastrointestinal tract: Evidence for a nonbiliary mechanism. Clin Pharmacol Ther 1979;25:579–585.
7. Carvalho WA, Matos GB, Cruz SLB, Rodrigues DS: Human aldrin poisoning. Brazilian J Med Biol Res 1991;24:883–887.
8. Coble Y, Hildebrandt P, Davis J, et al: Acute endrin poisoning. JAMA 1967;202:153–157.
9. Cohn WJ, Boylan JJ, Blanke RV, et al: Treatment of chlordecone (kepone) toxicity with cholestyramine. N Engl J Med 1978;298:243–248.
10. Conney AH, Welch RM, Kuntzman R, et al: Effects of pesticides on drug and steroid metabolism. Clin Pharmacol Ther 1966;8:1–10.
11. Coye MJ, Lowe JA, Maddy KJ: Biological monitoring of agricultural workers exposed to pesticides: II. Monitoring of intact pesticides and their metabolites. J Occup Med 1986;28:628–636.
12. Crosby AD, D'Andrea GH, Geller RJ: Human effects of veterinary biological products. Vet Hum Toxicol 1986;28:569–571.
13. Dale WE, Gaines TB, Hayes WJ: Poisoning by DDT: Relationship between clinical signs and concentrations in rat brain. Science 1963;142:1474–1476.
14. Dally S, Garnier R, Bismuth C: Diagnosis of chlorinated hydrocarbon poisoning by x-ray examination. Br J Ind Med 1987;44:424–425.
15. Fischer TF: Lindane toxicity in a 24-year-old woman. Ann Emerg Med 1994;24:972–974.
16. Garrettson LK, Guzelian PS, Blanke RV: Subacute chlordane poisoning. J Toxicol Clin Toxicol 1984–85;22:565–571.
17. Grutsch JF, Khasuwinah A: Signs and mechanisms of chlordane intoxication. Biomed Environ Sci 1991;4:317–326.
18. Hayes WJ: Chlorinated hydrocarbon insecticides. In: Hayes WJ, Lawes ER, eds: Pesticides Studied in Man. San Diego, Academic Press, 1991, pp. 731–868.
19. Hayes WJ, Lawes ER, ed: Handbook of Pesticide Toxicology. San Diego, Academic Press, 1991.
20. Kassner JT, Maher TJ, Hull KM, Woolf, AD: Cholestyramine as an adsorbent in acute lindane poisoning: A murine model. Ann Emerg Med 1993;22:1392–1397.
21. Kintz P, Baron L, Tracqui A, et al: A high endrin concentrate in a fatal case. Forensic Sci Int 1992;54:177–180.
22. Klaassen CD: Nonmetallic environmental toxicants. In: Gilman AG, Rall TW, Nies AS, Taylor P, eds: Goodman and Gilman's The Pharmacologic Basis of Therapeutics, 8th ed. New York, Pergamon Press, 1985, pp. 1615–1639.
23. Kramer MS: Operational criteria for adverse drug reactions in evaluating suspected toxicity of a popular scabicide. Clin Pharmacol Ther 1980;27:149–155.
24. Kriess K, Zack MM, Kimbrough RD, et al: Cross-sectional study of a community with exceptional exposure to DDT. JAMA 1981;245:1926–1930.
25. Lee B, Groth P: Scabies transcutaneous poisoning during treatment. Pediatrics 1977;59:643.
26. Le Quesne PM, Maxwell IC, Butterworth STG: Transient facial sensory symptoms following exposure to synthetic pyrethroids: A clinical and electrophysiological assessment. Neurotoxicology 1980;2:1–11.
27. Miller E: Dangers of DEET: An insect repellent. Hosp Pharm Hotline 1987;1:6–7.
28. Morgan DP, Dotson TB, Lin LI: Effectiveness of activated charcoal, mineral oil, and castor oil in limiting gastrointestinal absorption of a chlorinated hydrocarbon pesticide. Clin Toxicol 1977;11:61–70.
29. Murphy SD: Toxic effects of pesticides. In: Klaassen CD, Amdur MO, Doull J, eds: Casarett and Doull's Toxicology: The Basic Science of Poisons. New York, Macmillan, 1986, pp. 543–553.
30. Narahashi T, Frey JM, Ginsburg, Roy ML: Sodium and GABA-activated channels as the targets of pyrethroids and cyclodienes. Toxicol Lett 1992;64/65:429–436.
31. Oransky S, Roseman B, Fish D, et al: Seizures temporally associated with use of DEET insect repellent—New York and Connecticut. MMWR 1989;38:678–680.
32. Ortiz Martinez A, Martinez-Conde E: The neurotoxic effects of lindane at acute and subchronic dosages. Ecotoxicol Environ Saf 1995;30:101–105.
33. Osimitz TG, Grothaus RH: The present safety assessment of DEET. J Am Mosquito Control Assoc 1995;11:274–278.
34. Paton DL, Walker JS: Pyrethrin poisoning from commercial strength flea and tick spray. Am J Emerg Med 1988;6: 232–235.
35. Pramanik A, Hansen R: Transcutaneous gamma benzene hexachloride absorption and toxicity in infants and children. Arch Dermatol 1979;115:1224–1225.
36. Rasmussen J: The problem of lindane. J Am Acad Dermatol 1981;3:507–516.
37. Rauch A, Kowalsky S, Lesar T, et al: Lindane (Kwell)-induced aplastic anemia. Arch Intern Med 1990;150: 2393–2395.
38. Rowley DL, Rab MA, Hardjutunojo W, et al: Convulsions caused by endrin poisoning in Pakistan. Pediatrics 1987;79: 928–934.
39. Rugman FP, Cosstick R: Aplastic anemia associated with organochlorine pesticide: Case reports and review of evidence. J Clin Pathol 1990;43:98–101.
40. Runhaar EA, Sangster B, Greve PA, Voortman M: A case of fatal endrin poisoning. Hum Toxicol 1985;4:241–247.
41. Schenker MB, Albertson TE, Saiki CL: Pesticides. In: Rom WN, ed: Environmental and Occupational Medicine, 2nd ed. Boston, Little, Brown, 1992, pp. 887–902.
42. Schoenig GP, Hartnagel RE, Schardein JL, Vorhees CV: Neurotoxicity evaluation of *N,N*-diethyl-*m*-toluamide in rats. Fundam Appl Toxicol 1993;22:355–365.
43. Schoenig GP, Neeper-Bradley TL, Fisher LC, Hartnagel RE: Teratologic evaluations of *N,N*-diethyl-*m*-toluamide

(DEET) in rats and rabbits. Fundam Appl Toxicol 1994;23: 63–69.
44. Smith RA, Lewis D: A potpourri of pesticide poisonings in Alberta in 1987. Vet Hum Toxicol 1988;30:118–120.
45. Solomon L, Fahrner L, West D: Gamma benzene hexachloride toxicity. Arch Dermatol 1977;113:353–357.
46. Starr M, Clifford N: Acute lindane intoxication. Arch Environ Health 1972;25:374–375.
47. Street JC, Chadwick RW: Ascorbic acid requirements and metabolism in relation to organochlorine pesticides. Ann NY Acad Sci 1975;258:132–143.
48. Telch J, Jarvis DA: Acute intoxication with lindane (gamma benzene hexachloride). Can Med Assoc J 1982;126: 662–663.
49. Tennebein M: Seizures after lindane therapy. J Am Geriatr Soc 1991;39:394–395.
50. Tenenbein M: Severe toxic reactions and death following the ingestion of diethyltoluamide-containing insect repellents. JAMA 1987;258:1509–1511.
51. Tilson HA, Hong JS, Mactutus CF: Effects of 5,5 diphenylhydantoin (phenytoin) on neurobehavioral toxicity of organochlorine pesticides and permethrin. J Pharmacol Exp Ther 1985;233:285–289.
52. Tilson MA, Shaw S, McLamb RL: The effects of lindane, DDT and chlordecone on avoidance responsing and seizure activity. Toxicol Appl Pharmacol 1987;88:57–65.
53. Veltri JC, Osimitz TG, Bradford DC, Page BC: Retrospective analysis of calls to poison control centers resulting from exposure to the insect repellent *N,N*-diethyl-*m*-toluamide (DEET) from 1985–1989. J Toxicol Clin Toxicol 1994;32:1–16.
54. Verschoyle RD, Brown AW, Nolan C, et al: A comparison of the acute toxicity, neuropathology, and electrophysiology of *N,N*-diethyl-*m*-toluamide and *N,N*-dimethyl-1,2-diphenylacetamide in rats. Fundam Appl Toxicol 1992;18:79–88.
55. Wax PM, Hoffman RS, Goldfrank LR: Fatality associated with inhalation of a pyrethrin insecticide. J Toxicol Clin Toxicol 1994;32:457–460.
56. Williams CH, Casterline JL: Effects on toxicity and on enzyme activity of the interactions between aldrin, chlordane, piperonyl butoxide and banol in rats. Proc Soc Exp Biol Med 1970;135:46–49.
57. Woolley DE: Differential effects of benzodiazepines, including diazepam, clonazepam, Ro 5-4864 and devazepide, on lindane-induced toxicity. Proc West Pharmacol Soc 1994; 37:131–134.
58. Wright DM, Hardin BD, Goad PW, Chrislip DW: Reproductive and developmental toxicity of *N,N*-diethyl-*m*-toluamide in rats. Fundam Appl Toxicol 1992;19:33–42.

CHAPTER 89

Rodenticides

Neal E. Flomenbaum

PATIENT 1. A 4-year-old boy who frequently played with other children in a remote part of an industrial park site was brought to the Emergency Department (ED) after his mother learned that he had been ingesting unknown "cereal" from a dish on the grounds that day and possibly on other occasions. The boy previously had been healthy.

On presentation to the ED, the boy was awake, alert, fearful, but otherwise acting "normally," according to his mother. Vital signs were: blood pressure, 90/60 mm Hg; pulse, 112 beats/min; respiratory rate, 20 breaths/min; rectal temperature, 97.6°F (36.5°C). Physical examination was entirely normal.

The emergency physician made arrangements to contact the security firm responsible for the site in an attempt to identify the rodenticide. Not expecting an early positive identification, the physician inserted an intravenous line and obtained samples for a complete blood count and electrolyte analysis. An ECG was interpreted as normal for age, and an abdominal radiograph failed to detect any radiopaque matter. The child was given a single 1-g/kg dose of activated charcoal. A security officer from the site arrived 2 hours later with the licensed pest control operator employed by the company and the dish the boy had eaten from. The dish contained a corn and sugar mixture identified as Quintox brand of cholecalciferol bait by the pest control operator.

The boy was hydrated with 5% dextrose in 1/3 N sodium chloride solution at twice the maintenance rate. All initial laboratory studies were normal including a serum calcium of 9.2 mg/dL. The child was admitted to the hospital and observed overnight. The next day when the physical examination and repeat calcium determination were normal, he was discharged home. A repeat serum calcium by the boy's pediatrician obtained 48 hours after ingestion also was normal and afterwards no further interventions were considered necessary.

PATIENT 2. An 18-month-old boy was brought to the ED by his parents 1 hour after he had ingested an unknown quantity of "rat poison." He had been playing on the kitchen floor when his mother noticed that the plastic dish containing yellow cornmeal and rodenticide was overturned and empty. The child had some cornmeal clutched in his hand and also around his mouth. On physical examination the child was well developed, well nourished, and appeared to be apprehensive and somewhat irritable. His conjunctivae were slightly injected and there was dried mucus in and around his nares. The parents did not know the name or type of rodenticide used. The father was asked to return home and bring back the remainder of the rodenticide in its original container.

The father returned with a package labeled Black Jack Mouse and Rat Poison that contained 0.025% warfarin and 99.97% inert ingredients. A decision was made not to induce emesis or perform lavage. There was no overt evidence of child abuse. The parents were given poison prevention advice and told to purchase syrup of ipecac and activated charcoal from their pharmacy to keep at home. They were instructed to administer the syrup of ipecac or activated charcoal only on the advice of a poison center or their physician. The child was discharged home to be observed by his parents.

These two cases are presented together here because although each involves the single acute ingestion of a small quantity of a relatively harmless rodenticide (when ingested in this manner), the approach in the ED differed based on the ability to rapidly identify the rodenticide and on the setting in which the exposure took place. Although the vast majority of rodenticide exposures are uneventful, rarely a very toxic or lethal agent may be ingested. The goal is to rapidly identify and manage the toxic agents and not overtreat the single acute nontoxic ingestions. The management of long-acting anticoagulant exposures is described in detail in Chapter 42.

What Is Rodenticide or "Rat Poison?"

A rodenticide is any product commercially marketed to kill rodents, including mice, squirrels, gophers, and other small animals. The "perfect rodenticide," one that effectively kills rodents but is not toxic to humans or nonrodent pets, has yet to be discovered. For this reason, a wide variety of rodenticides are available, which differ with respect to chemical composition, mechanism for killing rodents, and toxicity to humans.[22,35,36,50,55] In addition to the most commonly available warfarin-type or cholecalciferol rodenticides and the more toxic but rarely used varieties, occasionally a new, supposedly "effective and harmless" product is introduced only to be subsequently withdrawn as its true human toxicities become known. Unfortunately, some of these products remain in basements or on hardware store shelves or continue to be available to professional pest control operators long after they are officially withdrawn from sale. Hence, the single most important piece of information necessary to deal effectively with a "rat poison" ingestion is the full name or type of rodenticide actually ingested.

Rodenticides are a disparate group of organic and inorganic compounds and substances bearing no relationship to one another other than their usage currently or historically as rodenticides. They have been classified in several ways: Arena and Drew divided them into inorganic compounds, including arsenic, thallium, phosphorus, barium carbonate, and zinc phosphide; and organic compounds, including sodium fluoroacetate, ANTU, warfarin, red squill, strychnine, norbormide, and PNU.[3]

Another means of classifying rodenticides is by animal selectivity. For example, the cardiac glycoside and potent emetic, red squill, takes advantage of the fact that rats cannot vomit whereas humans and other animals (hopefully) would regurgitate the poison before experiencing the cardiotoxic effects. Norbormide, an irreversible smooth muscle constrictor, causes widespread ischemic necrosis and death in rats but does not appear to affect other animals or humans, presumably because it acts on a specific smooth muscle norbormide receptor found only in rats.

Alpha naphthyl thiourea (ANTU) is also relatively selective. A derivative of phenyl thiourea, without the bitter taste characteristic of the thiourea, it causes pulmonary edema in rats that have not developed tolerance to it. It is, however, only *relatively* selective: although the rat is most sensitive (LD_{50}, 3 mg/kg), in large doses (> 4 g/kg) ANTU can also be lethal to primates.

All of the rodenticides classified as inorganic, as well as organic ones such as strychnine and sodium fluoroacetate, are nonselective and of concern after human and domestic-animal ingestions. For the most part, use of this entire group of rodenticides is restricted to commercial pest control operators and government agencies.

A rodenticide classification system based purely on the nature and onset of symptoms may be unreliable and may possibly create a false sense of security leading to inappropriate management and inadequate follow-up. Many rodenticides cause neurologic and/or gastrointestinal signs and symptoms, and characteristic or pathognomonic signs such as "risus sardonicus" from strychnine, or alopecia from thallium, may not be recognized, may not occur consistently with very small amounts ingested, or, in the case of thallium, would not be expected to occur for days after an acute ingestion. Classifying rodenticides by the *onset* of symptoms may isolate some of the least toxic (regular warfarin type, cholecalciferol) and most toxic (thallium, long-acting warfarin types) rodenticides in the late-onset group, possibly leading to inappropriate discharge and inadequate follow-up.

Probably the most clinically useful way of classifying rodenticides at present is by toxicity based on LD_{50} data in rats. The relative degree of toxicity and characteristic adverse effects generally hold among different mammals, allowing the physician dealing with a possible rodenticide exposure to utilize a combination of historical and characteristic physical evidence to diagnose or, in some cases, exclude various rodenticides in deciding on an optimal management plan. In utilizing such a classification system, however, the physician should understand its limitations: (1) in rare cases the LD_{50} may vary widely among species (eg, Vacor); and (2) repeated ingestions of less toxic rodenticides (eg, regular anticoagulants, cholecalciferol) may in fact make them highly toxic (Table 89–1).

Highly Toxic Rodenticides (Signal Word: "Danger")

According to the Federal Insecticide, Fungicide and Rodenticide Act, highly toxic rodenticides are those substances with a single-dose LD_{50} of less than 50 mg/kg body weight. The label "Danger" is the Consumer Product Safety Commission's highest level of warning for potential hazard of toxicity. The other lower levels of hazard are described by "Warning" and "Caution" (Table 88–3; see also Chap. 9). The highly toxic group includes thallium, sodium monofluoroacetate (SMFA, compound 1080), fluoroacetamide (compound 1081), strychnine, zinc phosphide, elemental phosphorus, arsenic, barium carbonate, and PNU (Vacor).

Thallium

Thallium sulfate is an odorless, tasteless compound absorbed easily by inhalation, through unbroken skin, and through the GI tract. It may also cause death secondarily, that is, when a thallium-poisoned animal is eaten. The use of thallium as a commercial rodenticide ended in 1965, but it is still used by industry and in homeopathic remedies; thallium is occasionally implicated in attempted suicides or homicides.[12,13,23,28,42,49,51,54]

Thallium appears to have a large volume of distribution (estimates range from 3.6 L/kg in humans to 20

TABLE 89–1. MANAGEMENT OF SPECIFIC RODENTICIDE INGESTIONS

Toxin Name	Physical Characteristics	Toxic Mechanism	Estimated Fatal Dose	Diagnostic Presenting Signs and Symptoms	Onset	Antidote and/or Treatment
Highly Toxic Signal word: DANGER[a] (LD_{50}<50 mg/kg)						
Thallium	White, crystalline, odorless, tasteless	Combines with mitochondrial sulfhydryl groups, interfering with oxidative phosphorylation	14 mg/kg	Anorexia, abdominal pain, diarrhea, paresthesias, myalgias, painful neuropathy, delirium, coma, seizures, alopecia (late), Mees line	GI symptoms acutely, other symptoms 12–24 h delay	Activated charcoal, ferric ferrocyanide, (Berlin or Prussian blue)
Sodium monofluoroacetate (SMFA compound 1080);	White, crystalline, odorless, tasteless, water soluble	Converts fluoroacetate to fluorocitrate; interferes with TCA (Krebs) cycle, especially in cardiac and CNS cells	3–7 mg/kg	Seizures, coma, tachycardia, PVCs, VT, VF, ST-T wave changes	2–20 h	Experimental regimens: glycerol monoacetate, ethanol loading Lavage, activated charcoal
Sodium fluoroacetamide (compound 1081)	Same as SMFA	Same as SMFA	13–14 mg/kg	Same as SMFA	Same as SMFA	Same as SMFA
Strychnine	Bitter taste	Competitive antagonism of the neurotransmitter glycine at the postsynaptic spinal cord motor neuron	Children: 15 mg Adults: 5–10 mg/kg	Restlessness, anxiety, twitching, hyperextension alternating with relaxation, intense pain, trismus or facial grimacing ("risus sardonicus"), inability to swallow, opisthotonos, skeletal fractures secondary to muscle contractions	10–20 min	Quiet room, IV, benzodiazepines, neuromuscular blockade Lavage (after airway protection), activated charcoal
Zinc phosphide	Heavy, gray crystalline powder, water insoluble, "rotten fish" or "phosphorus" odor; normally used as 1% concentration	Releases phosphine on contact with water or acid or in GI tract	40 mg/kg in rats	Phosphorus or "rotten fish" breath odor, black vomitus, GI and cardiovascular toxicity, pulmonary edema, agitation, coma, seizures, hepatic/renal toxicity	Within hours; inhalation may have delayed onset	Dilution with water, milk, or $NaHCO_3$; followed by orogastric lavage, activated charcoal, and a cathartic; supportive care
Elemental phosphorus (yellow phosphorus)	Yellow, waxy paste, fat soluble, water insoluble	Local irritation and burns on contact followed by GI, liver, and renal damage, and interferes with clotting	1 mg/kg (more toxic if dissolved in alcohol, fats, oils)	Skin and GI burns, "smoking" luminescent vomitus and stools with garlic odor, jaundice, dysrhythmias, coma, delirium, seizures, cardiac arrest	1–2 h	Orogastric lavage with 0.1% $KMnO_4$ or 2% H_2O_2 activated charcoal, catharsis, hypertonic dextrose, benzodiazepines as indicated
Arsenic	White, crystalline powder	Combines with sulfhydryl groups and interferes with a variety of enzymatic reactions	120 mg	Dysphagia, nausea and vomiting, bloody diarrhea with mucus shreds, seizures, cardiovascular collapse, garlic odor, altered mental status, late sensory/motor neuropathy	Symptoms: 1 h Death: 1–24 h	Orogastric lavage, activated charcoal, succimer, dimercaprol or penicillamine until urine arsenic level: < 50 μg/24 h. Hemodialysis to remove chelation compound if renal failure

(continued)

TABLE 89–1. MANAGEMENT OF SPECIFIC RODENTICIDE INGESTIONS (continued)

Toxin Name	Physical Characteristics	Toxic Mechanism	Estimated Fatal Dose	Diagnostic Presenting Signs and Symptoms	Onset	Antidote and/or Treatment
Barium (soluble forms: carbonate, chloride, hydroxide)	Yellow, white, slightly lustrous lump	Neuromuscular blockade, hypokalemia	20–30 mg/kg	Headache, paresthesias, peripheral weakness, paralysis, nausea, vomiting, diarrhea, abdominal pain, ECG abnormalities (secondary to hypokalemia?), dysrhythmias, cardiac and pulmonary failure	1–8 h	Emesis (early) or orogastric lavage with Na_2SO_4, potassium replacement
PNU (*N*-3-pyridylmethyl-*N*′-p-nitrophenyl urea, Vacor)	Yellow, resembling cornmeal or yellow-green powder in bait; odor: peanuts	Interferes with nicotinamide metabolism in pancreas (destroying pancreatic beta cells), central and peripheral nervous system, and heart	5 mg/kg	Nausea and vomiting abdominal pain, severe orthostatic hypotension, hyperglycemia with or without ketoacidosis, GI perforations, pneumonia, neuropathy	4–48 h	Emesis or orogastric lavage followed by activated charcoal Nicotinamide (Niacinamide) 500 mg IV or IM followed by 200 mg IV or IM every 2 h to a total of 3 g/24 h. 100 mg PO 3 times/d for 2 weeks Manage diabetic ketoacidosis with insulin
Moderately Toxic Signal Word: WARNING[a] ***(LD_{50}, 50–500 mg/kg)***						
Alpha-naphthylthiourea (ANTU)	Odorless, slightly bitter, fine, blue-gray powder, water-insoluble	Increases permeability and damage of lung capillaries, causing pulmonary edema	>4 g/kg	Dyspnea, rales, clear pulmonary froth, cyanosis, hypothermia	?	Emesis or orogastric lavage followed by activated charcoal and catharsis
Cholecalciferol (vitamin D_3)	0.075% pellets, 364 pellets/oz; (1 pellet = 2308 U vitamin D)	Metabolized to alpha-dihydroxycalciferol, which mobilizes calcium and causes hypercalcemia	?	Headache, lethargy, weakness, fatigue, renal injury and failure, "metastatic" calcifications, due to hypercalcemia	Hours to days	Gastric decontamination, fluids; if severe: furosemide, prednisone, calcitonin, biphosphates
Low Toxicity Signal Word: CAUTION[a] ***(LD_{50}, 500–5000 mg/kg)***						
Red squill	Bitter taste	A cardiac glycoside; massive doses cause ventricular irritability (PVCs, VT, VF), death	?	Mycocardial irritability, nausea, protracted vomiting, diarrhea, abdominal pain, blurred vision	30 min–6 h	Orogastric lavage, activated charcoal, treat dysrhythmias with lidocaine, digoxin-specific Fab, atropine
Norbormide (dicarboximide)	Yellow cornmeal bait, peanut butter, 1% concentration	Vasoconstriction and ischemia in rats only via specific norbormide receptor in rat smooth muscle	?	Transient hypothermia and hypotension with doses up to 300 mg	?	Emesis or orogastric lavage, activated charcoal and cathartic
Bromethalin	7.5% concentrate, green pellets, cornmeal with Bitrex (denatonium benzoate)	Uncouples oxidative phosphorylation in mitochondria decreasing ATP, increasing fluid and pressure on axons, interrupting nerve impulse conduction	?	Muscle tremors Myoclonic jerks, flexion of major muscles, coma ?, ataxia, focal motor seizures	Immediate	Symptomatic, supportive care, airway, seizure control and, ventilatory assistance

(*continued*)

TABLE 89–1. MANAGEMENT OF SPECIFIC RODENTICIDE INGESTIONS (continued)

Toxin Name	Physical Characteristics	Toxic Mechanism	Estimated Fatal Dose	Diagnostic Presenting Signs and Symptoms	Onset	Antidote and/or Treatment
Anticoagulants: Short Acting						
Warfarin	Yellow cornmeal, rolled oats (0.025%)	Capillary injury and anticoagulation via interference with clotting factors II, VII, IX, X; death from hemorrhage	$>$ 5–20 mg/d for $>$ 3 5 d	Continual ingestion produces bleeding with elevated INR	12–48 h	Acute ingestions: None Chronic ingestions: Vitamin K_1, fresh frozen plasma (FFP), whole blood if available
Prolin	Warfarin (0.025%) plus sulfaquin-oxalin (0.025%)	Anticoagulant antibiotic combination eliminates intestinal vitamin K producing organisms				
Anticoagulants: Long Acting						
HYDROXYCOUMARINS						
4-Hydroxycoumarin (Brodifacoum, Difenacoum)	0.005% grain-based bait	Anticoagulant	?	Bleeding with elevated INR	Delayed several days	GI decontamination, vitamin K_1, fresh frozen plasma
Warfacide (Coumafuryl)	0.5% for dilution to 0.025% white powder, tasteless, odorless, to be diluted for use to 0.025%					
INDANDIONES						
Pindone (Pival)	Moldy, acrid odor, fluffy yellow powder, concen-trations 0.005–2.5%	Anticoagulant	?	Chronic ingestion possibly produces cardiac and neurologic symptoms as well as bleeding with elevated INR	Delayed several days	GI decontamination, vitamin K_1, fresh frozen plasma, whole blood if available
Pivalyn	0.5%					
Diphacinone	0.005–2.0%					
Chlorophacinone	0.005–2.5%					
Valone	0.005–2.5%					

[a]The LD_{50} values used in this table are derived from data on acute oral ingestions of the commercial product by rats. In some cases the commercial product contains a very small percentage of active ingredient. The signal words that appear on labels of registered products may differ from the signal word assigned to the acute oral LD_{50} test because the label may also reflect another study (acute dermal or inhalational LD_{50}) requiring a more severe signal word. See Chapters 9 and 88 for the Consumer Product Safety Commission definitions and use of signal words as indicators of potential hazard of toxicity.
Peacock D, Biologist, Registrations Division Office of Pesticide Programs, EPA, Washington, DC.

L/kg in rats) and is excreted by both the kidneys and liver. The human elimination half-life is 2 to 15 days.[42,50] Gastrointestinal signs appear 0.5 to 2 days following ingestion or exposure and include nausea, vomiting, hematemesis, bloody diarrhea, abdominal pain, and, later, ileus. Neurologic sequelae typically occur 2 to 5 days after exposure and include headache, lethargy, muscle weakness, painful paresthesias in the extremities, tremors, ptosis, ataxia, myoclonus, seizures, delirium, and coma. Nonfatal exposures have resulted in long-term neurologic impairment such as painful neuropathies, paresis, optic nerve atrophy, ataxia, choreiform movements, and dementia (see Chap. 82).

Sodium Monofluoroacetate

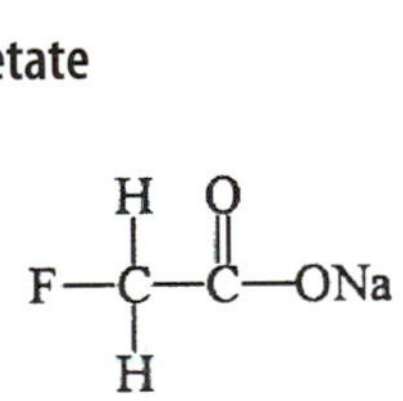

Sodium monofluoroacetate (SMFA, compound 1080) is another highly toxic rodenticide whose toxicity is not related to its fluoride content[62] but rather to its interference with the Krebs cycle.[56] Its use in the United States is limited to commercial exterminators. Derived from *Palicourea spp* (South America), *Acacia spp* (Australia), and a few other plants, SMFA is a white, odorless, tasteless, water-soluble salt that looks like flour or baking soda; it is tasteless as a powder but has a weak vinegar taste in dilute solution.[22] Unlike thallium, SMFA cannot be absorbed through unbroken skin. However, it is toxic when ingested, inhaled in dusts, or absorbed through open wounds.

Toxic effects primarily involve the CNS and the heart and include nausea and apprehension followed by cardiac dysrhythmias, seizures, and coma. Death may result from ventricular tachycardia and fibrillation or respiratory failure secondary to pulmonary edema or bronchopneumonia.[9,20,62]

Recently, investigators from Taiwan retrospectively analyzed 38 consecutive cases of SMFA poisoning presenting over a 5-year period (1988–1993). Seven of the 38 patients died; 74% had nausea or vomiting, which was the most common finding; 65% had hypokalemia; 42% had hypocalcemia; and the most common ECG pattern was nonspecific, ST-T and T-wave abnormalities. Hypotension, elevated serum creatinine, and decreased blood pH proved to be the most accurate prognostic indicators of mortality.[11] Animals that die of SMFA poisoning develop a characteristic extensor rigor mortis rapidly and are found with their extremities in hyperextension. The toxic effects of SMFA are delayed 1 to several hours and result from the conversion of the nontoxic fluoroacetate ions to fluorocitric acid, which in turn blocks the tricarboxylic acid cycle that is essential to energy production in mammalian cells (see Chap. 12).[56]

There is no known antidote for SMFA. Lavage followed by the use of activated charcoal and a sorbitol cathartic are recommended, although adsorption by activated charcoal is probably not significant. Glycerol monoacetate has been used experimentally in monkeys (0.1 to 0.5 mL/kg body weight IV or 0.55 g/kg IM of glycerol monoacetate every half hour for several hours) as an antidote to serve as substrate in the blocked Krebs cycle.[10] To inhibit the conversion of fluoroacetate to fluorocitrate, 500 mL of 10% acetamide in 5% dextrose over 30 minutes every 4 hours, or a 10% solution of ethyl alcohol, has been used experimentally with limited success.[9] An ethanol loading regimen is described in Antidotes in Depth: Ethanol. A combination of calcium gluconate (to correct hypocalcemia) and sodium succinate (to supplement the blocked trichloroacetic acid cycle) reduced mortality from sodium fluoroacetate in mice, but only when the calcium gluconate and sodium succinate were administered simultaneously.[53]

Fluoroacetamide

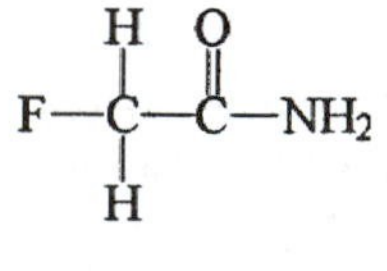

Fluoroacetamide (compound 1081) is a related fluoroacetate derivative with a slightly higher LD_{50} (13 to 14 mg/kg)[22] and a somewhat slower onset of symptoms. Both fluoroacetamide and sodium monofluoroacetate are generally shunned even by licensed pest control operators.

Strychnine

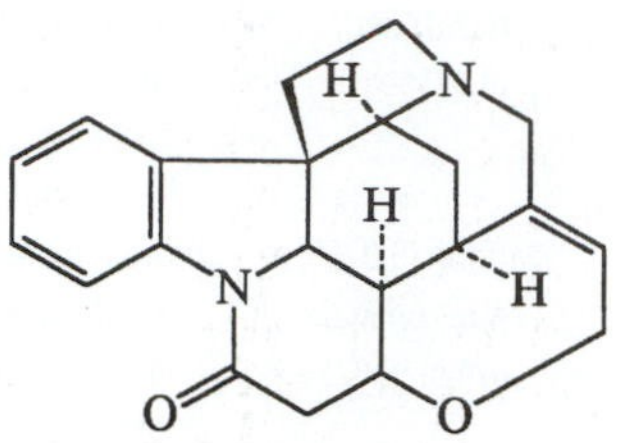

Strychnine, a naturally occurring alkaloid from the seeds of the tree *Strychnos nux vomica*, is a highly toxic rodenticide used for this purpose since the 16 century. Strychnine is an odorless, colorless crystal or a bitter white powder that is absorbed through the GI tract or nasal mucosa. It is a CNS stimulant that causes muscle twitching, extensor spasm, opisthotonos, trismus or facial grimacing (risus sardonicus), characteristic painful strychnine "seizures" during which the patient is conscious, and medullary paralysis resulting in death.[52,71,73] Signs and symptoms often begin within 15 to 20 minutes of ingestion. Strychnine results in the competitive antagonism of the inhibitory neurotransmitter glycine at the postsynaptic spinal cord motor neuron.[25,32] The patient may remain awake with relaxed muscles between episodes of opisthotonos and muscle contractions.

Early useful intervention includes the use of activated charcoal[1,2] and orogastric lavage. However, once symptoms appear, any manipulation or excitement may precipitate the opisthotonos or convulsions, and for this reason the patient should be kept in a quiet environment and treated with benzodiazepines and possibly pain medication. Hepatic metabolism appears to be the major route of strychnine elimination after massive ingestion.[67] Although acidification of the urine may significantly enhance urinary excretion of strychnine after an ingestion of minimal amounts and theoretically shorten the duration of action in symptomatic ingestions, acidification is not without risk: Renal excretion of strychnine after significant poisonings may be minimal, and the benefit is probably outweighed by the risk of acidifying the urine in the presence of (probable) myoglobinuria secondary to rhabdomyolysis[7] as well as profound lactic acidosis. This same problem (and the management of rhabdomyolysis) is discussed at length with regard to phencyclidine ingestion in Chapter 67.

The extensor spasm, opisthotonos, and convulsions may be controlled initially with a benzodiazepine such as diazepam (0.1 to 0.5 mg/kg, IV slowly) followed by a barbiturate such as pentobarbital IV or a neuromuscular blocking agent. If these prove ineffective, the immediate use of general anesthesia and/or neuromuscular blockade with a nondepolarizing neuromuscular blocker should be considered.[25,71] Intubation and mechanical ventilation are obviously required and will permit further gastric evacuation by orogastric lavage.

As suggested, emesis or lavage in the unintubated patient is theoretically extremely dangerous because of the potential for generalized muscle contractions; in this scenario, activated charcoal alone given by nasogastric tube may be effective. Apart from its danger to humans, strychnine is not even an adequate rodenticide, because rats quickly learn to avoid the bitter taste it imparts to the bait. For both of these reasons, strychnine is rarely used today as a rodenticide. Unbelievably, however, it is still a component of some tonics and cathartic pills available in health food stores. Crimidene is a synthetic chlorinated pyrimidine compound related to strychnine that produces similar CNS signs and symptoms.[50]

Zinc Phosphide

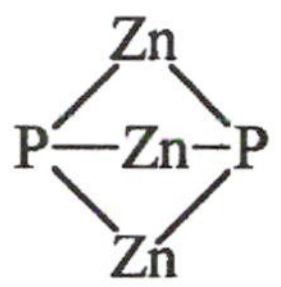

The dark gray color, odor of rotten fish, and taste of zinc phosphide make it unattractive to animals other than rats. Usually mixed with a tartar emetic, it nevertheless is highly toxic because it releases phosphine and zinc on contact with water and acid. Poisoned patients manifest nausea and vomiting, excitement, chills, chest tightness, cough, hypotension, dyspnea, pulmonary edema, circulatory collapse, cardiac dysrhythmias, convulsions and coma, renal damage, anuria, tetany (hypocalcemia), leukopenia, and death in 4 days to 2 weeks. Inhalation of dust may induce pulmonary edema. Treatment includes dilution with sodium bicarbonate, milk, or water; gastric lavage; and administration of activated charcoal, a cathartic, and possibly a proton pump inhibitor.

Yellow Phosphorus

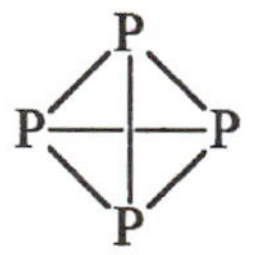

Elemental phosphorous

Yellow (or "white") phosphorus, the form of elemental phosphorus used as a rodenticide, is highly poisonous: A human ingestion of 50 mg or 1 mg/kg may be fatal.[14,65,70] The other form of elemental phosphorus, red phosphorus, is the only form of phosphorus still used in matches, and in contrast to yellow phosphorus, is relatively harmless. When used as a rodenticide (which is now rare), yellow phosphorus is usually mixed with molasses or peanut butter and spread on bread as bait for rodents or roaches. For obvious reasons, when used in this manner it is occasionally ingested unintentionally by children. Contact with yellow phosphorus causes second and third-degree skin burns within a few minutes to hours. It is most toxic to the GI tract and liver and on ingestion is usually followed by vomiting, which is said to be "smoking," luminescent, and with a garlicky odor. Resultant stools may also be luminescent and "smoking."[70]

Delirium, coma, and death from cardiovascular collapse may ensue.[58,72] Yellow phosphorus appears to have a direct toxic effect on the myocardium and peripheral vessels. Experimentally, acute phosphorus poisoning depresses rat myocardial protein synthesis.[72] If a patient survives the acute effects, a relatively symptom-free period of a few weeks may ensue, only to be followed by a third stage of systemic toxicity involving the GI tract, liver, heart, kidney, and CNS.

Treatment includes orogastric lavage with potassium permanganate 0.1% solution or 3% hydrogen peroxide diluted to a 2% solution to oxidize the phosphorus to harmless phosphates, followed by the use of activated charcoal and a cathartic (magnesium and mineral oil cathartics should not be used). Neither corticosteroids, previously recommended nor exchange transfusion appear to be useful: In one group of 49 suicidal patients from Colombia, corticosteroids did not prevent either coma or death from hepatic injury.[43] In another group of 15 patients with hepatic encephalopathy, 3 of 5 treated with exchange transfusions survived, compared to 3 of the 10 not treated with exchange transfusions.[43]

Red phosphorus is nonvolatile, insoluble, and not absorbed through the GI tract; it is, therefore, harmless when ingested.[70]

Arsenic

Another highly toxic rodenticide still in use is arsenic, a white, crystalline powder that causes dysphagia, muscle cramps, convulsions, vomiting, and bloody diarrhea. Death is due to cardiovascular collapse. Immediate treatment is lavage followed by activated charcoal and a cathartic. Dimercaptosuccinic acid (DMSA, succimer),[31,68] dimercaprol or penicillamine is used to chelate this heavy metal after it is absorbed. Between 1956 and 1974, arsenicals were identified as the single most common cause of accidental rodenticide-related deaths. Because of arsenic's toxicity, pest control operators have avoided its use (see Chap. 78).

Barium Carbonate

Barium carbonate is a highly toxic substance used in the past as a rodenticide and currently, in some parts of the world, as a male depilatory. Insoluble forms of barium, such as the barium sulfate commonly used in radiographic procedures, are harmless. However, *soluble* forms—such as the acetate, carbonate, chloride, hydroxide, nitrate, and sulfide—cause profound weakness and gastrointestinal, neurologic, cardiovascular, pulmonary, and possibly renal dysfunction.[57,77]

Most of the toxic effects of barium result from its direct stimulation of all types of muscle, including cardiac muscle, and from its ability to cause a profound reduction in serum potassium together with an increase in intracellular potassium.[64,77] Death results from hypokalemia, cardiac dysrhythmias, congestive heart failure, and pulmonary toxicity.

A similar mechanism has been proposed for the hypokalemic paralysis that results from barium poisoning, chronic potassium deficiency, and thyrotoxicosis[33]: The large active and passive influx of extracellular potassium into the muscle turns off the Na-K pump causing depolarization and paralysis. However, in one case report involving barium carbonate, the degree of weakness correlated with the plasma *barium* concentrations and not the potassium concentrations.[57] The author suggests that barium itself is responsible for membrane depolarization by causing release of acetylcholine[69] and by competitively reducing the permeability of all membranes to potassium[33] with the resultant intensity of neuromuscular blockade correlating directly with the plasma barium concentrations.

Renal toxicity and acute renal failure following ingestion of a teaspoonful of barium chloride may have resulted from treatment with *intravenous* $MgSO_4$, saline, and furosemide (in addition to the previously recommended oral $MgSO_4$).[77] The intravenous combination of medication may have caused barium sulfate to precipitate in the renal tubules.

Treatment for the ingestion of soluble forms of barium includes emesis, if it can be accomplished rapidly outside the hospital, or orogastric lavage with sodium sulfate in the hope of converting the barium carbonate to barium sulfate.[3,55] Rapid, aggressive potassium replacement intravenously as indicated by frequent serum potassium monitoring is the most important aspect of management.[22,55,77]

Vacor (*N*-3-pyridylmethyl-*N'*-p-nitrophenyl urea) (PNU)

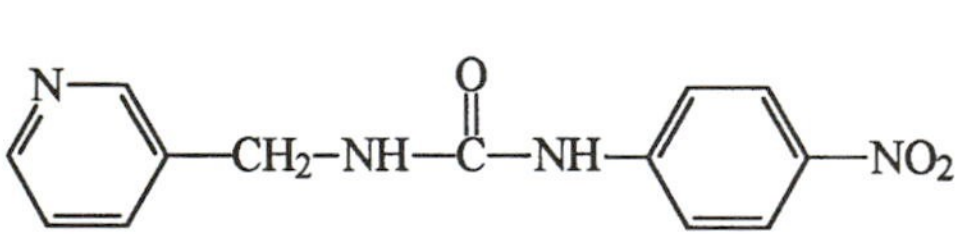

The quest for a safe, highly effective single-dose rodenticide occasionally leads to the introduction of extremely toxic substances with tragic consequences to humans who consume them. One of the most unfortunate examples is *N*–3-pyridylmethyl-*N'*-p-nitrophenyl urea (PNU; Vacor). Marketed in the United States under trade names such as House Mouse Tracking Powder, Vacor was introduced in 1975 as safe for humans. Shortly after its introduction, 7 South Koreans who ate rice contaminated with Vacor died. In the United States there were more than 100 poisonings and more than 12 deaths between 1975 and 1980. Death has occurred after ingestion of a single (30-g) package. Although the manufacturer withdrew Vacor from sale in June 1979 and requested the return of unsold Vacor, they did not issue a public recall. In 1986 a patient ingested the contents of a package of Vacor that had been sold and placed many years earlier: At that time the local hospital ED no longer kept the antidote niacinamide.[26] Vacor exposures are still being reported yearly.[37–41]

Vacor is a structural analog of alloxan and streptozotocin and, like them, destroys pancreatic beta cells.[30] Pentamidine also produces a picture of islet cell necrosis without an accompanying lymphocytic infiltrate.[21] Although the lethal mechanism in rodents had never been fully described, PNU, like alloxan and streptozotocin, was known to interfere with niacinamide metabolism in pancreatic beta cells, liver, and brain cells.[24,29,34] In vitro studies demonstrated that this toxin is incorporated into various intracellular nucleotides, which are then unable to act as hydrogen carriers in oxidoreductase systems, thereby inhibiting the activities of certain enzyme systems. When substituted for niacinamide in the synthesis of nicotinamide-adenine dinucleotide (NAD) or nicotinamide-adenine dinucleotide phosphate (NADP), major abnormalities of the pentose phosphate pathway result, causing defects in intermediary metabolism and RNA production.[24]

Patients who ingest PNU present within hours with an insulin-deficient hyperglycemia or diabetic ketoacidosis, together with severe postural hypotension and peripheral and autonomic neuropathies.[29,34,47,59,61] Reported deaths were due to ketoacidosis, GI perforation, cardiac dysrhythmias, and pneumonia.

Based on both the in vitro studies already noted above and in vivo studies involving rats, a treatment plan for PNU (or alloxan or streptozotocin) ingestion was formulated calling for 500 mg of niacinamide (nicotinamide) IM or IV, immediately followed by 100 to 200 mg IM or IV every 4 hours for up to 48 hours. If signs of PNU toxicity developed, the dosing frequency of niacinamide was increased to every 2 hours, without exceeding 3 g/day in an adult. For small children, approximately one-half the adult dose was to be administered. When the patient was able to take oral medications, 100 mg of niacinamide was administered 3 to 5 times daily for 2 weeks. Fludrocortisone was often necessary for persistent postural hypotension.

In addition to niacinamide (nicotinamide) therapy for patients who ingest PNU, emesis or orogastric lavage, activated charcoal and a cathartic are indicated. Ketoacidosis should be managed with insulin, and silent, nonpainful GI perforation should be rigorously sought.

Initially, authors cautioned against the substitution of niacin (nicotinic acid) for niacinamide (nicotinamide) because the vasodilatory effects of nicotinic acid might exacerbate the problems of blood pressure control.[34] Moreover, nicotinic acid was thought to be less effective and also known to cause glucose intolerance.[48] However, when intravenous niacinamide became unavailable in this country, the possibility of substituting niacin as the only available alternative became more logical.

Patients who survived PNU ingestions after manifesting symptoms, almost invariably required insulin therapy to manage their newly acquired diabetes. The major long-term management problem, however, was the neuropathy, especially the resultant postural hypotension, which is both severe and extremely resistant to therapy.

The Vacor tragedy continues to be of more than historical interest for a number of reasons. First, every year through 1995 (the latest information currently available) 1 to 5 Vacor exposures (including 5 in 1995), have been reported in the United States.[37–41] Second, the Vacor story serves as a model of how even with presumably methodical testing, a potent toxin can be introduced commercially with lethal consequences: Because of widely varying LD_{50}s, rats and humans appear to be among the most affected by the toxic effects of Vacor.[22] Third, as was true of the MPTP/parkinsonism syndrome (see Chap. 60), new insights into possible environmental etiologies for diseases may be provided. Fourth, the toxin itself may prove to be an extremely important research tool: Recently, investigators incubated mitochondria and submitochondrial particles from beef and rat heart and rat liver with various concentrations of Vacor and demonstrated that Vacor specifically inhibits the NADH–ubiquinone reductase activity of respiratory complex I in mammalian mitochondria; this in turn correlates quantitatively with the inhibition of insulin release in insulinoma cells and pancreatic islets. Moreover, the inhibition is entirely consistent with the effect of the doses of Vacor that have been reported in human poisoning. How these new findings relate to the previously published studies suggesting that Vacor interferes with nicotinamide metabolism is not yet clear. Remarkably, the site of Vacor inhibition is at the level of ubiquinone reduction by complex I, near the site of action of the same neurotoxin metabolite of MPTP that induces parkinsonism.[18] Thus, Vacor poisoning may be a biochemical paradigm for the metabolic induction of insulin-dependent diabetes mellitus, as well as some of its associated vascular and neurologic problems.

Vacor-induced diabetes mellitus closely mimics the "naturally occurring" disease. Of 18 patients who developed diabetes mellitus after Vacor ingestions, 44% had retinopathy, 28% had proteinuria, and all had (muscle) capillary membrane thickening similar to that in insulin-dependent diabetes after a mean duration of 6.2 years postingestion.[19]

Moderately Toxic Rodenticides (Signal Word: "Warning")

The moderately toxic rodenticides, those with an LD_{50} of 50 to 500 mg/kg body weight, include the "selective" rodenticide ANTU and cholecalciferol (vitamin D_3), one of the newest and increasingly popular rodenticides.

Alpha-Naphthyl-Thiourea

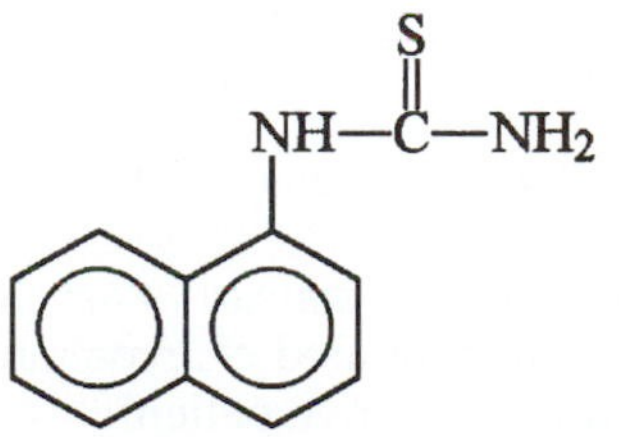

Alpha-naphthyl-thiourea (ANTU) kills rats by causing pulmonary edema and pleural effusion probably because of damage to the lung capillaries resulting in increased permeability.[5,63] The heart appears to be unaffected by ANTU.[5,63] Patients who ingest large quantities of ANTU may present with hypothermia and dyspnea, rales, and cyanosis secondary to pulmonary edema or pleural effusions. Recommended treatment for ANTU ingestions is orogastric lavage followed by administration of activated charcoal and a cathartic.[50]

Cholecalciferol

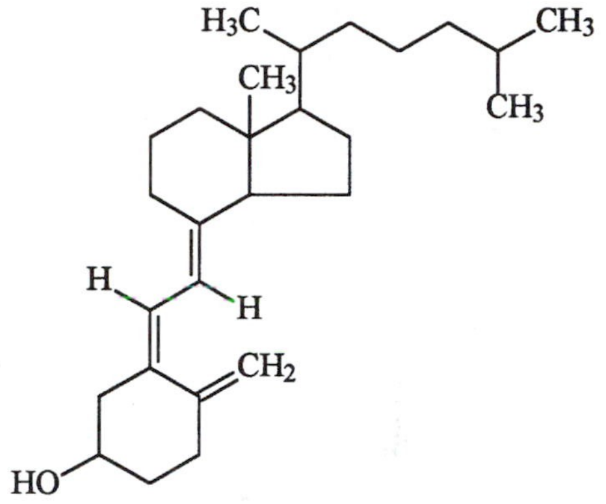

Cholecalciferol (vitamin D_3) was first registered and marketed in the United States in late 1984. It is now widely used by professional pest control operators as Quintox and by the general public as Rampage. In rodents and rabbits, cholecalciferol mobilizes calcium from bones and in toxic doses produces hypercalcemia, osteomalacia, and metastatic calcification of the cardiovascular system, kidneys, stomach, and lungs; death typically occurs in 2 to 5 days.[44–46] All animals are susceptible to the effects of cholecalciferol, but because of their size, rats and mice succumb to much lower doses than other animals.[44–46]

Cholecalciferol appears to be an effective rodenticide when a large amount is consumed in one meal or when smaller amounts are consumed over a 2 to 3-day period.[46,60] Because death is not immediate and the cholecalciferol does not impart unusual characteristics to the bait, the type of bait shyness seen with zinc phosphide, ANTU, strychnine, and other rodenticides does not occur.[44–46] Rabbits and presumably other small animals are also very susceptible to the toxic effects of cholecalciferol, as are, to a lesser degree, dogs and cats. The closely related calciferol (vitamin D_2 or ergocalciferol) has been used as a rodenticide in Europe and Canada since 1978, with no genetic resistance reported to date.[44–46]

Although rats manifest the signs of severe acute hypercalcemia, including lethargy and ultimately death from myocardial infarction in 2 to 5 days,[60] no serious human toxicity or death from the rodenticide form of cholecalciferol has been reported to date. All of the advice for managing human ingestions is based on experience with treating therapeutic forms of vitamin D intoxication and hypercalcemia. One case of cholecalciferol poisoning in an industrial setting may be particularly relevant because, as in the case of a child who might repeatedly ingest small amounts of rodenticide, the exposure described was to small doses over a 32-day period and resulted in prolonged hypercalcemia.[27]

Immediate intervention after a large acute ingestion should include gastric emptying by emesis or orogastric lavage followed by gastric decontamination with activated charcoal and sorbitol. Repetitive dosing of activated charcoal has been recommended, but data are insufficient to confirm its usefulness.

Treatment for moderate to severe degrees of hypercalcemia (greater than 11.5 mg/dL) include IV fluid therapy with 0.9% sodium chloride solution if the patient is hypovolemic and can tolerate a fluid load. Potassium and magnesium levels should be monitored and maintained. Furosemide should be administered (adult doses range from 20 to 80 mg IV, or 40 to 120 mg orally in divided doses). Prednisone (0.5 to 1.0 mg/kg daily) appears to be particularly effective for hypercalcemia secondary to vitamin D intoxication. Calcitonin (salmon calcitonin, Calcimar) 4–8 IU/kg SC or IM every 6 to 12 hours may reduce serum calcium levels by 1 to 3 mg/dL over a few hours by inhibiting osteoclastic bone resorption while promoting calciuria.

A normal serum calcium level obtained 48 hours after an acute ingestion almost certainly excludes any significant toxicity.

Low-Toxicity Rodenticides (Signal Word: "Caution")

The remaining rodenticides, with one exception, are of low toxicity (LD_{50}, 500 to 5000 mg/kg). This category includes red squill (*Urginea maritima*) and norbormide, along with the "warfarin-type" anticoagulant rodenticides, which are still the most commonly used rodenticides today.

Red Squill

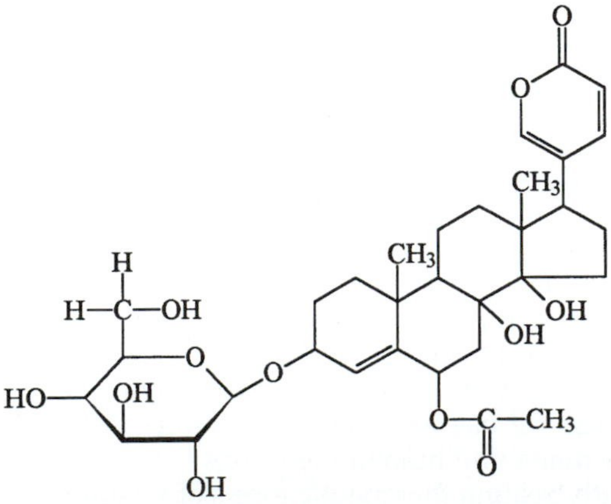

Red squill is a naturally occurring rodenticide found in the sea onion plant *Urginea maritima* of the *Liliaceace* family. It contains scillaren A and B, which are cardiac glycosides. The effects of red squill on humans are chiefly GI: abdominal pain, nausea, and vomiting. Red squill is considered to be so potent an emetic in humans, that the expected cardiotoxicity (ie, ventricular irritability, premature ventricular contractions, ventricular fibrillation, etc) is rarely, if ever, seen as a result of ingesting the commercial rodenticide. However, a recent case report of a human who ingested two bulbs of the plant documents the subsequent nausea, vomiting, seizures, hyperkalemia, atrioventricular block, ventricular dysrhythmias, and death, that would be expected after a massive cardiac glycoside poisoning.[74] Evaluation should include cardiac monitoring, electrolyte (particularly potassium) analysis, and a digoxin assay with which these cardiac glycosides may show cross-reactivity. There is no current data with regard to cross-reactivity, but this concept is discussed for many other plant and animal cardiac glycosides. When pres-ent, the cardiotoxicity of red squill would best be treated with lidocaine for the ventricular dysrhythmias and digitalis-specific antibody fragments (see Antidotes in Depth: Digoxin Specific Antibody Fragments (Fab)).[66]

Norbormide

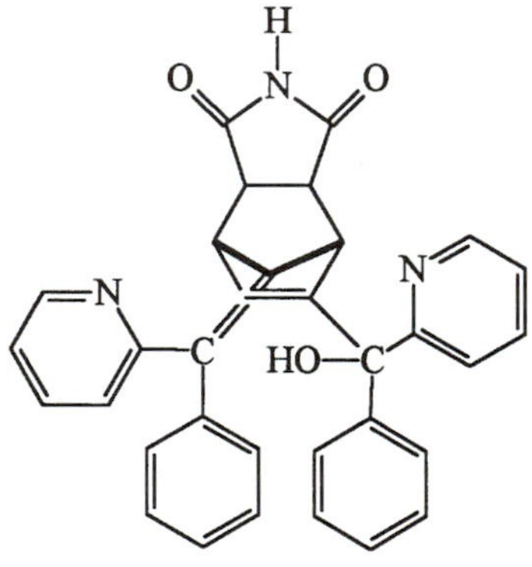

Norbormide, the irreversible smooth muscle constrictor, appears to be specific for rats and has no known human toxicity. Rats die as a result of intense generalized vasoconstriction, resulting in tissue anoxia.[50] In vitro norbormide promotes calcium entry into smooth muscle cells, inducing a myogenic contraction selective for the small vessels in rats, whereas in the arteries of other mammals (and in the rat aorta), norbormide behaves like a calcium channel entry blocker.[6] Although emesis and catharsis may be considered if they can be easily performed, it is probably safer instead to accomplish gastric decontamination with activated charcoal and a cathartic, especially for an uncooperative patient.

Anticoagulants

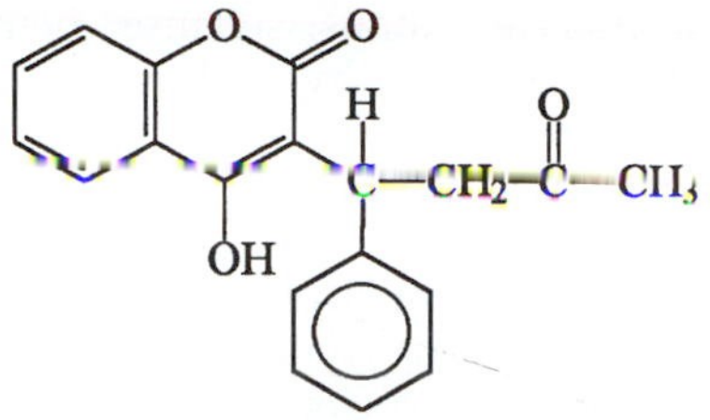

Warfarin

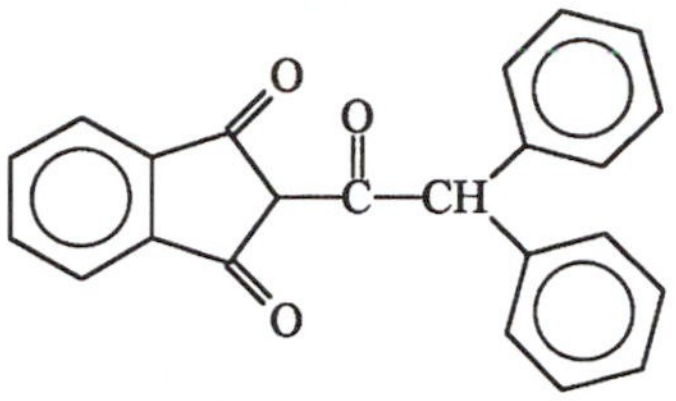

Diphacinone

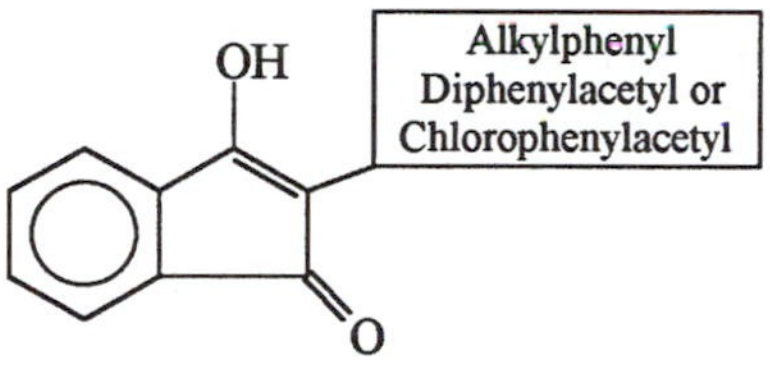

4-Hydroxycoumarins

The anticoagulant, or warfarin-type, rodenticides are far and away the most commonly implicated rodenticides in calls to poison centers as a result of a rodenticide ingestion.[37–41]

Prior to the last decade, both human and rodent toxicity of the anticoagulant rodenticides depended on repeated exposure to relatively small doses. Although this property resulted in virtually no toxicity to humans after a single exposure, the inability to ensure that rats would repeatedly eat the bait made them less effective as rodenticides. In addition, a selection process led to the prevalence of resistant rats ("super rats") in some areas. For both reasons, more toxic rodenticides continue to be used and new ones introduced.

Newer types of anticoagulant rodenticides have been introduced that are acutely toxic. A single ingestion of one of the new "superwarfarin" rodenticides, such as difenacoum and brodifacoum, may result in marked anticoagulation effects for up to 7 weeks. (For a detailed discussion on the classification, mechanism of action, diagnosis, and treatment of warfarin and long-acting anticoagulants, see Chap. 42.)

Because an acute single-dose ingestion of most of the currently available anticoagulant rodenticides does not usually result in immediate toxic effects, initially there are no clinical findings. The history then becomes essential in attempting to exclude exposure to the long-acting compounds; if the details of the history are in doubt, baseline CBC and prothrombin time are especially important. An abnormal prothrombin time will serve to identify either the chronic ingester or a patient who presents several hours or days after exposure to a long-acting coumarin.[4] In either case, if the prothrombin time is abnormal, a careful search for bleeding complications should be performed.

Bromethalin

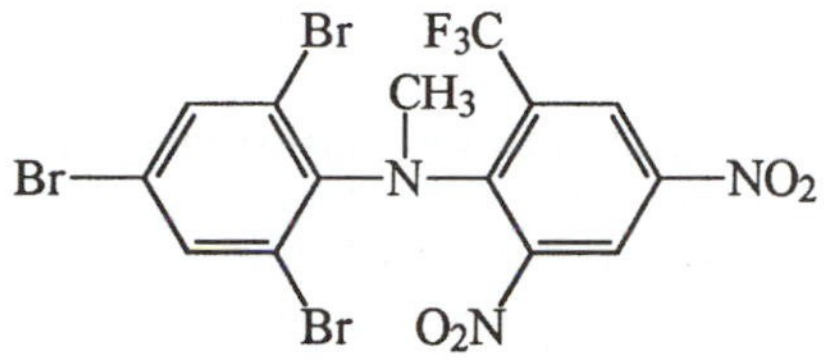

The newest rodenticide considered of low toxicity by its *commercial product* LD_{50} *of >500 mg/kg* in rats is bromethalin, which was registered with the EPA in 1982 and which became available in 1986. Bromethalin is available commercially in the United States as green pellets mixed with cornmeal (which gives it a fresh corn odor) and Bitrex. Of all the currently used rodenticides, less is known about bromethalin, marketed as Assault or Vengeance, than about any of the other rodenticides. From the time bromethalin became available, concern was expressed about its potential toxicity.[44] However, the first possible bromethalin-induced case of human toxicity was not reported until 1996,[8] perhaps because as late as 1997, bromethalin had been registered in only 6 states (including California and New York, in both of which states it became available in 1996).

Bromethalin is considered a highly effective single-feeding rodenticide with a mode of action reportedly involving the uncoupling of oxidative phosphorylation in the mitochondria, resulting in decreased ATP production, increased fluid accumulation, and consequent increased pressure on nerve axons interrupting nerve impulse conduction.[45]

The pathologic changes resulting from a 1.5 mg/kg oral dose administered to cats included spongy changes, hypertrophied fibrous astrocytes, and hypertrophied oligodendrocytes in the white matter of the cerebrum, cerebellum, brainstem, spinal cord, and optic nerve.[15,17] Prior to sacrifice, the clinical manifestations of bromethalin poisonings included ataxia, focal motor seizures, decerebrate posture, decreased proprioception, and depressed level of consciousness. Dogs given oral doses of 6.25 mg/kg of bromethalin developed hyperexcitability, tremors, seizures, depression, and death within 15 to 63 hours after exposure.[16] Death in animals is also usually preceded by paralysis and loss of tactile sensation.[75,76]

In 1996, the first case of possible bromethalin-induced human toxicity was reported: A 28-year-old male was found unconscious with two different open packages of rat poison, carisoprodol, and empty beer bottles. Tactile stimulation produced muscle tremors and severe myoclonic jerks with flexion of major muscle groups. He was placed on a respirator, lavaged, and given phenytoin, mannitol, dexamethasone, and diazepam. Blood and urine analyses were positive for therapeutic levels of his prescribed fluoxetine with negative carisoprodol and ethanol levels. EEG demonstrated only bihemispheric slowing with a normal head CT scan. After 24 hours the patient responded to noxius stimuli and was free of tremors and myoclonus. He was discharged 2 days later.[8]

Because there is no known antidote for bromethalin, it is hoped that the symptomatic and supportive care provided to the patient described will be sufficient to achieve a good outcome after significant human exposures. In rats, administration of a commercially available extract of *Gingko biloba* immediately after 1.0 mg/kg of bromethalin resulted in a statistically significant decrease in the severity of adverse neurologic effects.[15]

Managing the Patient Exposed to an Unknown Rodenticide

For the patient exposed to an unknown rodenticide, the approach is more complicated than for a patient who ingests a single dose of a known common commercial rodenticide, such as warfarin or cholecalciferol. First, as always, adequate breathing and circulation must be assured and the patient briefly examined. If the patient is initially stable, the next priority is to make every effort to fully identify the type and quantity of rodenticide ingested.

If the rodenticide and its package material are not brought with the patient, someone should be sent to bring them back to the ED. Identifying a harmless rodenticide ingestion early on is more cost effective and less traumatic to the patient than treating for an unknown ingestion. If the rodenticide container is labeled, and the information is telephoned back to the ED, care should be taken to obtain the full name, not just the brand name. For example, until 1986 there was a line of rodenticides all carrying the "Pied Piper" name on a variety of very different products: Pied Piper for Rats and Mice, for example, was alpha-naphthyl-thiourea (ANTU) and warfarin; while Pied Piper Kwik-Kill Mouse Seed was strychnine; and Pied Piper Rodenticide was red squill. Many manufacturers still use similar names for very dissimilar poisons.

While awaiting full identification of the rodenticide, a careful physical examination should be performed, searching for toxic signs that indicate specific rodenticides. Gastrointestinal symptomatology, paresthesias, and the late onset of hair loss, for example, are characteristic of thallium. Sodium monofluoroacetate (SMFA) and fluoroacetamide produce irritability or "apprehension" followed by seizures, coma, and death from respiratory failure or ventricular tachycardia and fibrillation. Central nervous system stimulation, opisthotonos, prolonged recurrent motor seizures or convulsions, and medullary paralysis followed by death suggest strychnine poisoning. Hypotension, vomitus with a rotten or "fishy" odor, cardiopulmonary collapse, coma, renal damage, and leukopenia suggest zinc phosphide poisoning. Oral and skin burns, luminescent "smoking" vomitus and stools with a garlic odor, and GI and biliary damage characterize yellow phosphorus poisoning.

Dysphagia, muscle cramps, seizures, hematemesis, and bloody diarrhea followed by cardiovascular collapse suggest arsenic. The combination of striking hyperglycemia with or without ketoacidosis, and severe postural hypotension, autonomic and peripheral neuropathies, ileus, and esophageal or GI perforation characterize *N*-3-pyridylmethyl-N′-p-nitrophenyl urea (PNU or Vacor) poisoning. Muscle tremors, myoclonic jerks with flexion of major muscle groups, and unresponsiveness may be the human manifestations of bromethalin poisoning.

Dyspnea, rales, pulmonary edema, pleural effusions, and hypothermia are seen with massive ingestions of ANTU. Nausea, vomiting, diarrhea, and abdominal pain will probably be the only effects of ingesting red squill, but when combined with signs of ventricular irritability (premature ventricular contractions and ventricular fibrillation) certainly identify this potent emetic and cardiac glycoside. Signs or symptoms of a bleeding disorder point to either acute ingestion of a superwarfarin rodenticide, such as brodifacoum, or repeated (chronic) ingestion of a regular warfarin-type rodenticide. Finally, evidence of hypercalcemia following (massive or chronic) rodenticide ingestion suggests a new and popular product, cholecalciferol (vitamin D_3).

If a toxic syndrome is identified, aggressive management, including the use of specific antidotes, may be necessary (see Table 89–1). Prior to the development of signs and symptoms of toxicity, there is no rodenticide currently in use for which lavage or, in most cases, emesis followed by activated charcoal and a cathartic is *contraindicated*, although they may be unnecessary for the older warfarin-type rodenticides. Once the patient becomes symptomatic, however, emesis or orogastric lavage, activated charcoal, and catharsis must be individualized according to the specific toxin and the patient's clinical condition.

If every effort to identify the rodenticide fails, the following diagnostic evaluation may be indicated. A complete blood count and prothrombin time will help diagnose and manage acute or chronic ingestions of the newer "superwarfarin" anticoagulant rodenticides and repetitive ingestions of the older warfarin-type rodenticides. (The latter consideration is important for children with pica as well as institutionalized emotionally disturbed adults who may nibble grainlike rodenticides repeatedly.) Serum glucose, potassium, and bicarbonate determinations will identify hyperglycemia and ketoacidosis caused by PNU (Vacor), and an elevated serum calcium concentration suggests cholecalciferol (vitamin D_3) ingestion. Liver enzymes, blood urea nitrogen (BUN), and creatinine are useful baseline determinations for rodenticides that cause renal or hepatic damage (eg, zinc phosphide, yellow phosphorus, cholecalciferol).

A serum sample and 50 mL of urine should be obtained and sent to the toxicology laboratory with the request to hold it for possible heavy metals screening, especially if the patient is vomiting. Finally, if indicated by history or symptomatology, additional specimens may be collected for specific rodenticide determinations (eg, thallium, strychnine); chest and abdominal radiographs may be useful because of the radiopaque nature of some of the uncommonly used rodenticides (see Chap. 7).

Following the diagnostic evaluation, if there is any doubt about either the nature of the rodenticide or the reliability of the patient (or parents), the patient may be admitted or held in the ED for observation. No matter what type of rodenticide was ingested, a determination should be made as to whether the ingestion was unintentional, a suicide gesture or attempt, or a manifestation of abuse or neglect.[4] A psychiatric assessment is, of course, indicated for any possible suicide attempt.

In summary, the key to managing the patient who ingested a rodenticide is to identify the rodenticide, the quantity ingested, its potential toxicity, and any available specific antidote. Toxic ingestions should be excluded or treated immediately; conversely, the most common acute anticoagulant or cholecalciferol exposures should not be overtreated.

Who Ingests Rodenticides?

As in the cases at the start of the chapter, young children are most commonly associated with rodenticide ingestions. Between 1991 and 1995, there were approximately 15,000 to 17,000 reported exposures to rodenticides annually in the United States, of which almost 90% involved children younger than 6 years of age. Remarkably, there have been fewer than 6 deaths per year from 1991 through 1995 reportedly related to rodenticides.[37–41]

In addition to children, suicidal persons, victims of attempted homicide, exterminators, and intoxicated, psychiatric, or impaired elderly persons are at risk. Finally, the occasional person who unintentionally ingests a rodenticide because it was placed in a container commonly used for an edible product illustrates the danger of transferring toxic substances to other containers (Chap. 115).

If the patient is a child or infant, the emergency physician should review the principles of poison prevention with his or her parents (Chap. 115) and should consider the possibility that the incident represents child abuse or neglect. The emotional state of the parents must be noted if the physician is contemplating sending the child home for continued observation in the absence of history, physical, or laboratory evidence suggesting a serious exposure.

Acknowledgments

Mary Ann Howland, PharmD and Richard S. Weisman, PharmD contributed to this chapter in a previous edition.

References

1. Anderson AH: Experimental studies on the pharmacology of activated charcoal: III. Absorption from gastrointestinal contents. Acta Pharmacol 1948;4:275–284.
2. Anderson AH: Experimental studies on the pharmacology of activated charcoal: I. Absorption power of charcoal in aqueous solutions. Acta Pharmacol 1946;2:69–78.
3. Arena JM, Drew RH: Rodenticides, fungicides, herbicides, fumigants and repellents. In: Arena JM, Drew RH, eds: Poisoning: Toxicology, Symptoms, Treatment, 5th ed. Springfield, IL, Thomas, 1986, pp. 222–251.
4. Babcock J, Hartman K, Pedersen A, et al: Rodenticide-induced coagulopathy in a young child. A case of Münchausen syndrome by proxy. Am J Pediatr Hematol Oncol 1993;15:126–130.
5. Bohm G.M. Changes in lung arterioles in pulmonary oedema induced in rats by alpha-naphthyl-thiourea. J Pathol 1973; 110:343–345.
6. Bova S, Travis L, Debetto P et al: Vasorelaxant properties of norbormide, a selective vasoconstrictor agent for the rat microvasculature. Brit J Pharmacol 1996;117:1041–1046.
7. Boyd RE, Brennan PT, Deng JF, et al: Strychnine poisoning: Recovery from profound lactic acidosis, hyperthermia, and rhabdomyolysis. Am J Med 1983;74:507–512.
8. Buller G, Heard J, Gorman S: Possible bromethalin-induced toxicity in a human. A case report. J Toxicol Clin Toxicol 1996; 34:572. Abstract.
9. Chenoweth MB: Monofluoroacetic acid and related compounds. Pharm Rev 1949;1:383–424.
10. Chenoweth MB, Kandel A, Johnson LB, Bennett DR: Factors influencing fluoroacetate poisoning: Practice treatment with glycerol monoacetate. J Pharmacol Exp Ther 1951; 102:31–49.
11. Chi CH, Chen KW, Chan SH, et al: Clinical presentation and prognostic factors in sodium monofluoroacetate intoxication. J Toxicol Clin Toxicol 1996;34:707–712.
12. DeBacker W, Zachee P, Verpooten GA, Majelyne W: Thallium intoxication treated with combined hemoperfusion–hemodialysis. J Toxicol Clin Toxicol 1982;19:259–264.
13. Desenclos JC, Wilder MH, Coppenger GW, et al: Thallium poisoning: An outbreak in Florida, 1988. South Med J 1992; 85:1203–1206.
14. Diaz-Rivera RS, Collazo PJ, Pons ER, et al: Acute phosphorus poisoning in man: A study of 56 cases. Medicine 1950; 29:269–298.
15. Dorman DC, Cote LM, Buck WB: Effects of an extract of Gingko biloba on bromethalin-induced cerebral lipid peroxidation and edema in rats. Am J Vet Res 1992;53:138–142.
16. Dorman DC, Simon J, Harlin KA, Buck WB: Diagnosis of bromethalin toxicosis in the dog. J Vet Diagn Invest 1990; 2:123–128.
17. Dorman DC, Zachary JF, Buck WB: Neuropathologic findings of bromethalin toxicosis in the cat. Vet Pathol 1992; 29:138–144.
18. Esposti MD, Myers MA: Inhibition of mitochondrial complex I may account for IDDM induced by intoxication with the rodenticide Vacor. Diabetes 1996;45:1531–1534.
19. Feingold KR, Lee TH, Chung MY, Sipehstein MD: Muscle capillary basement membrane width in patients with Vacor-induced diabetes mellitus. J Clin Invest 1986;78: 102–107.
20. Gajdusek DC, Luther G: Fluoroacetate Poisoning: A review and report of a case. Am J Dis Child 1950;79:310–320.
21. Hauser L, Sheehan P, Simpkins H: Pancreatic pathology in

pentamidine-induced diabetes in acquired immunodeficiency syndrome patients. Hum Pathol 1991; 22:926–929.
22. Hayes WJ: Pesticides Studied in Man. Baltimore, Williams & Wilkins, 1982.
23. Heath A, Ahlmen J, Branegard B, et al: Thallium poisoning: Toxin elimination and therapy in three cases. J Toxicol Clin Toxicol 1983;20:451–463.
24. Herken H: Antimetabolic action of 6-amino-nicotinamide on the pentose phosphate pathway in the brain. In: Aldridge N, ed: Mechanism of Toxicity. London, St. Martin's, 1970, p. 189.
25. Heiser JM, Daya MR, Magnussen AR, Norton RL: Massive strychnine intoxication: Serial blood levels in a fatal case. J Toxicol Clin Toxicol 1992; 30:269–283.
26. Howland MA, Weisman R, Sauter D, Goldfrank L: Nonavailability of poison antidotes. N Engl J Med 1986;314: 927–928.
27. Jibani M, Hodges NH: Prolonged hypercalcemia after industrial exposure to vitamin D_3. Br Med J 1985; 290:748–749.
28. Kamerbeek HH, Rauws AG, Ham MT, et al: Dangerous redistribution of thallium by treatment with sodium diethyldithiocarbamate. Acta Med Scand 1971;189:149–154.
29. Karam JH, LeWitt PA, Young CH, et al: Insulinopenic diabetes after rodenticide (Vacor) ingestion: A unique model of acquired diabetes in man. Diabetes 1980;29:971–978.
30. Kenney RM, Michaels IAL, Flomenbaum NE, Yu GSM: Poisoning with *N*-3-pyridylmethyl-*N'*-p-nitrophenyl urea (Vacor). Arch Pathol Lab Med 1981;105:367–370.
31. Kosnett MJ, Becker CE: Dimercaptosuccinic acid: Utility in acute and chronic arsenic poisoning. Vet Hum Toxicol 1988; 30:369. Abstract.
32. Kuno M, Weakly JN: Quantal components of the inhibitory synaptic potential in spinal mononeurones of the cat. J Physiol (Lond) 1972;224:287–303.
33. Layzer RB: Periodic paralysis and the sodium–potassium pump. Ann Neurol 1982;11:547–552.
34. LeWitt PA: The neurotoxicity of the rat poison Vacor: A clinical study of 12 cases. N Engl J Med 1980;302:73–77.
35. Lisella FS, Long KR, Scott HG: Toxicology of rodenticides and their relation to human health. J Environ Health 1970; 33:231–237.
36. Lisella FS, Long KR, Scott HG: Toxicology of rodenticides and their relation to human health. J Environ Health 1970; 33:361–365.
37. Litovitz TL, Clark LR, Soloway RA, et al: 1993 Annual Report of the American Association of Poison Control toxic exposure surveillance system. Am J Emerg Med 1994;12: 546–599.
38. Litovitz TL, Felberg L, Soloway RA, et al: 1994 Annual report of the American Association of Poison Control Centers toxic exposure surveillance system. Am J Emerg Med 1995; 13:551–597.
39. Litovitz TL, Felberg L, White S, Klein-Schwartz W: 1995 Annual report of the American Association of Poison Control Centers toxic exposure surveillance system. Am J Emerg Med 1996;14:487–537.
40. Litovitz TL, Holm KC, Bailey KM, et al: 1991 Annual report of the American Association of Poison Control Centers National Data Collection System. Am J Emerg Med 1992;10: 452–505.
41. Litovitz TL, Holm KC, Clancy C, et al: 1992 Annual Report of the American Association of Poison Control Centers toxic exposure surveillance system. Am J Emerg Med 1993; 11:494–555.
42. Lovejoy FH: Thallium. Clin Toxicol Rev 1982;5:1–2.
43. Marin GA, Mantoya CA, Sierra JL, Senior JR: Evaluation of corticosteroid and exchange transfusion treatment of acute yellow phosphorous intoxication. N Engl J Med 1961;284: 125–128.
44. Marsh R: Personal communication, June 29, 1993.
45. Marsh RE: Currrent (1987) and future rodenticides for commensal rodent control. Bull Soc Vector Ecol 1988;13: 102–107.
46. Marsh R, Tunberg A: Characteristics of cholecalciferol: Rodent control—Other options. Pest Control Technol 1986;14: 43–45.
47. Miller LV, Stokes JD, Silpipat C: Diabetes mellitus and autonomic dysfunction after Vacor rodenticide ingestion. Diabetes Care 1978;1:73–76.
48. Molner GD, Berge KG, Rosenveas JW, et al: The effect of nicotinic acid in diabetes mellitus. Metabolism 1974;13: 181–189.
49. Moore D, House I, Dixon A, et al: Grand rounds, Guy's Hospital—Thallium poisoning. Br Med J 1993;306:1527–1529.
50. Morgan DP: Recognition and Management of Pesticide Poisonings, 4th ed. Washington, DC, United States Environmental Protection Agency, 1989.
51. Nogué S, Mas A, Parés A, et al: Acute thallium poisoning: An evaluation of different forms of treatment. J Toxicol 1982;19:1015–1021.
52. O'Callaghan WA, Joyce N, Counihan HE, et al: Unusual strychnine poisoning and its treatment: Report of 8 cases. Br Med J 1982;285:478.
53. Omara F, Sisodia CS: Evaluation of potential antidotes for sodium fluoroacetate in mice. Vet Hum Toxicol 1990;32: 427–431.
54. Pedersen RS, Olesen AS, Freund LG, et al: Thallium intoxication treated with long-term hemodialysis, forced diuresis and Prussian blue. Acta Med Scand 1978;204:429–432.
55. Pelfrene AF: Synthetic rodenticides. In: Hayes WJ, Laws ER, eds: Handbook of Pesticide Toxicology. San Diego, Academic Press, 1991, pp. 1271–1316.
56. Peters RA: Lethal synthesis. Proc Roy Soc Lond 1952;13: 139–143.
57. Phelan DM, Hagley SR, Guerin MD: Is hypokalaemia the cause of paralysis in barium poisoning? Br Med J 1984; 289:662.
58. Pietras RJ, Stavrakos C, Gunnar RM, Tobin JR: Phosphorus poisoning stimulating acute myocardial infarction. Arch Intern Med 1968;122:430–434.
59. Pont A, Rubino JM, Bishop D, Peal R: Diabetes mellitus and neuropathy following Vacor ingestion in man. Arch Intern Med 1979;139:185–187.
60. Product Information Sheet. Quintox. Madison, WI, Bell Laboratories, 1985.
61. Prosser PR, Karm JH: Diabetes mellitus following rodenticide ingestion in man. JAMA 1978;239:1148–1150.
62. Reigart JR, Brueggeman JL, Keil JE: Sodium fluoroacetate poisoning. Am J Dis Child 1975;129:1224–1226.

63. Richter CP: The development and use of alpha-naphthylthiourea (ANTU) as a rat poison. JAMA 1945;129:927–931.
64. Roza O, Berman LB: The pathophysiology of barium, hypokalemia and cardiovascular effects. J Pharmacol Exp Ther 1971;177:433–439.
65. Rubitsky HJ, Myerson RM: Acute phosphorus poisoning. Arch Intern Med 1949;83:164–178.
66. Sabouraud AE, Ortizberea M, Cano N, et al: Specific antidigoxin Fab fragments: An available antidote for proscillandin and scilliroside poisoning. Hum Exp Toxicol 1990;9:191–193.
67. Sgaragli GP, Mannaioni PF: Pharmacokinetic observations on a case of massive strychnine poisoning. Clin Toxicol 1973;6:533–540.
68. Shum S, Whitshead J, Vaughan L, et al: Chelation of organoarsonate with dimercapton succinic acid. Vet Hum Toxicol 1995;37:239–242.
69. Silinsky EM: On the role of barium in supporting the asynchronous release of acetylcholine quanta by motor nerve impulses. J Physiol 1978;274:157–171.
70. Simon FA, Pickering LK: Acute yellow phosphorus poisoning. JAMA 1976;235:1343–1366.
71. Smith BA: Strychnine poisoning. J Emerg Med 1990;8: 321–325.
72. Talley RC, Linhart JW, Trevino AJ, Moore L: Acute elemental phosphorous poisoning in man: Cardiovascular toxicity. Am Heart J 1972;84:139–140.
73. Teitelbaum DT, Ott JE: Acute strychnine intoxication. Clin Toxicol 1970;2:267–273.
74. Tuncok Y, Kozan O, Caudar C, et al: Urginea maritima (squill) toxicity. J Toxicol Clin Toxicol 1995;33:83–86.
75. Van Lier RBL, Ottosen D: Studies on the mechanism of toxicity of bromethalin, a new rodenticide. Theoret Toxicol 1981;1:114.
76. Velsicol Chemical Corp: Vengeance Rodenticide Technical Manual 1986, p. 19.
77. Wetherill SF, Guarino MJ, Cox RW: Acute renal failure associated with barium chloride poisoning. Ann Intern Med 1981;95:187–188.

CHAPTER 90

Herbicides: Paraquat and Diquat

Susan M. Pond

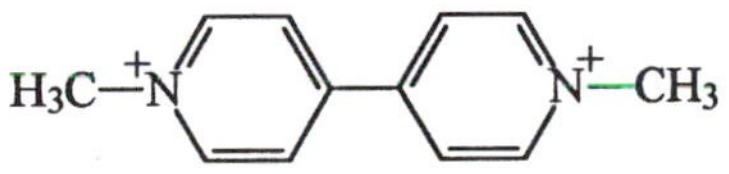

Paraquat

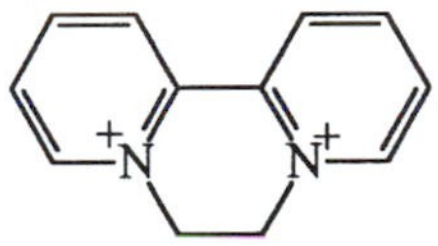

Diquat

A 22-year-old, 60-kg male was brought by the police to the Emergency Department of a large urban hospital at 2 AM, about 1 hour after deliberately swallowing about 100 mL of 20% paraquat. He had decanted the paraquat into a soft drink bottle at his sugar cane farm the day before and drank it in a hotel room in the center of the city. He had been drinking heavily and had not eaten for about 12 hours. He vomited several times soon after the ingestion and then ran down into the downtown shopping mall where he told the police what he had done. In the Emergency Department, he was cooperative but restless and agitated. His clothing and hands were stained blue. He complained of burning in the mouth, throat, and stomach and shortness of breath. He kept on repeating "I want to die." The pulse was 105 beats/min, blood pressure 170/70 mm Hg, respiratory rate 40 breaths/min, and temperature, 97.3°F (36.3°C). Physical examination was normal except for superficial buccal ulceration and pharyngeal erythema.

An intravenous line was inserted and fluid therapy with normal saline and potassium chloride were administered. Gastrointestinal decontamination was initiated immediately with 100 g of activated charcoal mixed into a slurry with 100 mL of 70% sorbitol by mouth. The patient vomited most of the dose and became increasingly agitated and uncooperative. To proceed further with therapy, the patient was paralyzed, intubated, and ventilated with room air. A nasogastric tube was inserted and another dose of charcoal/sorbitol run in over 20 min. He was transferred to the ICU.

By 4 AM, the patient's parents had been contacted. They conveyed the history that he had been admitted to a psychiatric hospital three times over the past year for treatment of depression. The day before he checked in to the hotel, he had lost his job. He had left home that day having read an article in the local newspaper about the toxicity of paraquat.

On admission, the chest radiograph was normal and the ECG showed sinus tachycardia. The complete blood count was normal except for a mild neutrophilia; serum electrolytes were normal except for a potassium level of 2.6 mEq/L and creatinine of 2.0 mg/dL; serum enzymes were normal except for a slight increase in alanine aminotransferase and lactate dehydrogenase. An arterial blood gas on room air showed pH, 7.43; PO_2, 68.5 mm Hg; PCO_2, 23.3 mm Hg; bicarbonate, 15.5 mEq/L.

The spot test for paraquat performed on admission in the urine was strongly positive. Three hours after the ingestion a catheter was inserted into the right femoral vein and charcoal hemoperfusion commenced, and continued for 6 hours. The blood flow across the cartridge was 150 mL/min.

At 10 AM an upper GI endoscopy was performed. The pharynx was edematous and inflamed. There was mild erythema in the upper esophagus. The stomach had generalized diffuse erythema and confluent areas of superficial ulceration with adherent membrane, especially in the antrum. There was minor oozing of blood from some of these surfaces.

By 3 PM, the serum paraquat had been measured quantitatively by high-performance liquid chromatography. At 2:30 AM it was 106 μg/mL, and at the beginning of hemoperfusion at 4 AM it was 36 μg/mL. The concentration in urine at 2:30 AM was 1.6 mg/mL.

By 5 PM, the urine output had fallen to less than 5 mL/h and the blood pressure to 50/30, despite a normal intravascular volume. On room air, the O_2 saturation was 75%. The patient died at 9 PM from cardiogenic shock.

What Is the Epidemiology of Paraquat Poisoning?

When stored, diluted, and applied correctly, paraquat is a relatively safe herbicide. Education and training programs about safe use, handling, and disposal are essential. Most occupational injuries reported involve the contact-related irritative effects of paraquat on the skin, nasal mucosa, and eyes.[19,38]

Most cases of paraquat poisoning are due to the deliberate ingestion of one of the liquid formulations containing 20 to 40% paraquat.[38] By 1977, 600 deaths from paraquat had been documented, most of them following intentional ingestion and most of them in adults. Unintentional ingestions do occur, however, particularly when the product has been handled or stored incorrectly.[19,38] The occasional use of paraquat as a homicide weapon has been reported, as has death after massive dermal exposure or intravenous administration.[19,38,52]

Suicidal ingestion of paraquat has been a disproportionate problem in some countries including the United Kingdom, Western Samoa, Fiji, Sri Lanka, Malaysia, and Japan.[38] Up until 1985, there had been more than 1900 deaths due to paraquat reported in Japan. Thickened or gel formulations with reduced concentrations of paraquat were introduced in an attempt to curb the incidence of unintentional ingestions and reduce the mortality rate.[56] In many countries, regulatory action has restricted open sale of paraquat and implemented improved labeling on the products and education programs about correct use.

Exposures to paraquat and/or diquat reported to U.S. poison centers between 1983 and 1992 were summarized recently.[18] They represented 1973 (0.02%) of the total of 12.5 million exposures; only 89 were reported as being intentional. Of the 1173 for which the outcome was known, 18 died from paraquat poisoning, 17 after ingestion and 1 after inhalation and dermal exposure. Diquat accounted for 2 deaths, both after ingestion. In the 1970s, concern was expressed in the United States about the inhalation of paraquat from contaminated marijuana. This was proven to have been insignificant. Rapid pyrolysis of paraquat during smoking precludes inhalation of the herbicide from the cigarette.

What Is Paraquat?

Paraquat (1,1′dimethyl-4-4′-bipyridylium dichloride) was synthesized first in 1882 and used as a redox indicator known as methyl viologen after the rediscovery in 1932 of its reduction to a blue radical by alkaline sodium dithionite.[10] It was serendipitously recognized when a field observation in the 1950s recorded that a quaternary salt used as a surfactant for a test herbicide was itself herbicidal.[9] Synthesis of more active compounds led to the rediscovery of both paraquat and diquat and their introduction onto the market in the early 1960s as nonselective contact herbicides.[9]

Paraquat is highly soluble in water and is marketed most commonly as a concentrate containing 200 g paraquat dichloride/L (20% wt/vol), sometimes in combination with diquat or other herbicides. Working solutions of paraquat for spraying are prepared by dilution of the concentrate with water to yield 1 to 5 g/L (0.1 to 0.5% wt/vol). The concentrate also usually contains agents to wet, spread, promote retention of moisture, adhere to the plants, and reduce foaming. Many liquid concentrate formulations contain an emetic, a distinctive blue dye and a stenching agent (a pyridine derivative). If no dye is added, the concentrate is dark brown like cola, for which it can be mistaken if decanted into a soft drink bottle. These additives may prevent unintentional ingestion, or reduce the amount swallowed and absorbed. They do not seem to influence those truly intent on suicide.

What Are the Kinetics of Paraquat?

Inhalation of the correctly diluted and generated spray leads to minimal if any systemic exposure. The large droplets that are generated by the spraying apparatus only reach the nose and upper airways. Likewise, absorption of paraquat from the eye and intact skin is minimal. Repeated or continuous dermal contact may lead to some absorption into the bloodstream if the integrity of the stratum corneum is impaired.[52]

When a liquid formulation of paraquat is ingested, it will enter the intestine quickly, particularly if the stomach is empty. Absorption takes place predominantly from the small intestine and is incomplete (<30% of the dose) but rapid because of active transport of the herbicide across the mucosal cells.[23] When the integrity of the GI mucosa is destroyed, the percentage absorbed is likely to be higher because of an additional large diffusive flux. Plasma concentrations of paraquat peak from within minutes to about 2 hours after the ingestion.[47]

Paraquat distributes to most organs in the body, but the highest concentrations are found in the kidneys and the lungs.[47] The high renal concentrations reflect the role of the kidney in the elimination of paraquat. The high concentrations in the lung are due to the time and energy-dependent uptake of paraquat by type I and II alveolar epithelial cells via the polyamine uptake pathway. The uptake results from the structural similarity between paraquat and the endogenous diamines and polyamines, such as putrescine and spermidine.[47] These are taken up actively into the lung by a membrane transport system that has specificity for molecules with two positively charged quaternary nitrogen atoms separated by a distance of approximately 0.6 to 0.7 nm (Fig. 90–1).[17] The volume of distribution of paraquat is about 1 to 2 L/kg.[24]

More than 90% of the absorbed dose of paraquat is eliminated by the kidneys as the parent compound within the first 12 to 24 hours after the ingestion.[6] Even in patients who have ingested a toxic dose, renal function and paraquat clearance remain unaffected for several hours. When renal function is normal, the renal clearance of paraquat is higher than that of creatinine because of net tubular secretion of the molecule. As renal function deteriorates, clearance of paraquat falls concurrently and the half-life becomes prolonged, from about 12 hours to more than 24.[24] The efflux from lung and muscle into the bloodstream is slow, with a half-life of about 24 hours.[47] This ac-

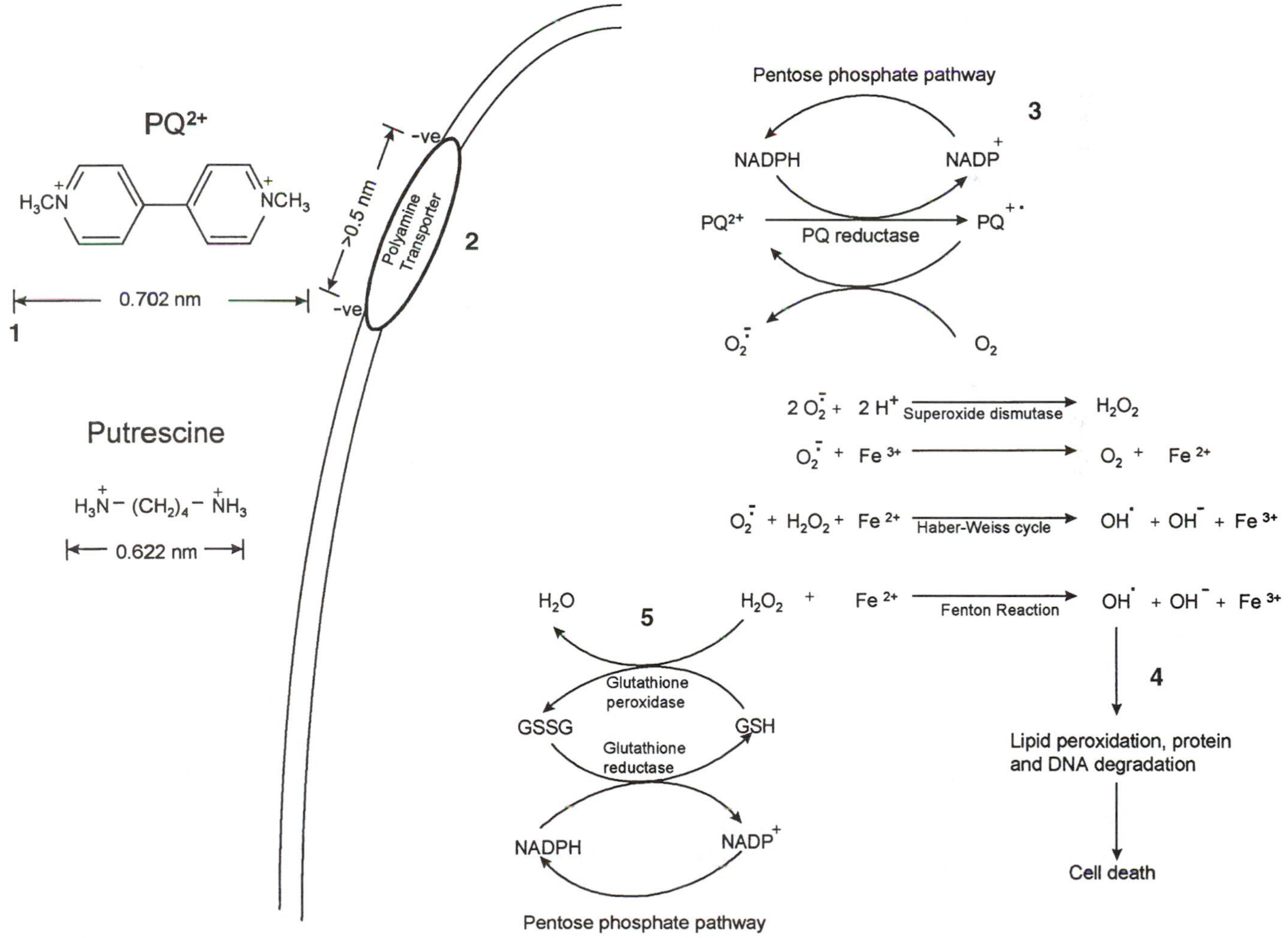

Figure 90–1. Mechanisms of toxicity of paraquat in the type II alveolar epithelial cell. **1.** Structure of paraquat and putrescine, showing the distance between the two nitrogen atoms. **2.** Putative receptor responsible for the active uptake of paraquat by the alveolar epithelial cells. **3.** Redox cycling of paraquat and oxygen. **4.** Formation of the OH radical. **5.** Detoxification of hydrogen peroxide (H_2O_2). *(Reprinted, with permission, from Smith LL: Mechanism of paraquat toxicity in lung and its relevance to treatment. Hum Toxicol 1987;6:31–36.)*

counts for the detection of low concentrations of paraquat in the urine for several days after the ingestion.[6]

What Are the Mechanisms of Paraquat Toxicity?

The caustic effects of paraquat produce mechanical damage in the upper GI tract and mediastinum. The mechanisms of damage by very high concentrations of paraquat to organs such as kidney, heart, liver, pancreas, and muscle are assumed to be related to redox cycling and oxygen toxicity, but this has not been proven. The mechanisms of toxicity have been determined most clearly in the lung when it is exposed to lower concentrations consistent with an ingested dose of 20 to 40 mg ion/kg. In the pneumocyte, cellular injury is initiated by the NADPH-dependent reduction of paraquat to the monocation radical (PQ^+; Fig. 90–1).[47] Spontaneous, rapid reaction with molecular oxygen yields the superoxide radical (O_2^-) and reforms the paraquat dication, ready to be reduced again. This process, known as redox cycling, is sustained by the extensive supply of electrons and oxygen in the lung. This and the subsequent reactions explain why oxygen enhances the toxicity of paraquat and paraquat enhances the toxicity of oxygen.[28,47] Two superoxide species form hydrogen peroxide in a reaction catalyzed by superoxide dismutase. Hydrogen peroxide can be inactivated by metabolism to water by catalases or peroxidases. However, superoxide and hydrogen peroxide also undergo a series of iron-catalyzed reactions to yield the hydroxyl radical ($OH^•$), which is thought to be the ultimate toxic species derived from paraquat. The $OH^•$ generates further reactive oxygen species by interacting with biomolecules such as proteins or membrane fatty acids. For example, the abstraction of hydrogen from polyunsaturated fatty acids by $OH^•$ forms a lipid radical and subsequently lipid peroxides or hydroperoxide. This process, known as lipid peroxidation, leads to degradation of cell membranes. The reactive oxygen species, in interacting with DNA, proteins, and cell membranes, disrupt cellular function and lead to cell death. The amplified generation of oxygen radicals explains why the cellular injury from paraquat far exceeds that produced by the initial reaction products.

Cell injury and death are due in part also to the depletion of NADPH, which is consumed during the reduction of paraquat and by the glutathione peroxidase and reductase enzyme systems as they detoxify the superoxide radicals and their products.[47] In response, the pentose phosphate and fatty acid synthesis pathways are activated to regenerate NADPH. This promotes the redox reaction involving paraquat and oxygen and thus the generation of more toxic oxygen species.

The toxicity of paraquat in plants is also due to the production of reactive oxygen species, which damage the envelope of photosynthesizing chloroplasts. As in the alveolar epithelial cells, there may be a specific uptake mechanism for paraquat in plant cells.[10]

In contrast to the rapid production of reactive oxygen species, the capacity of the antioxidant systems, such as the enzymes superoxide dismutase, catalase, and glutathione peroxidase, and vitamins C and E, is limited, and there is a lag time in their adaptation.[47] This imbalance explains why the dose–response curve for paraquat toxicity is very steep.

What Is the Pathology in the Lung?

The biochemical effects of the redox reaction are reflected pathologically in two phases, the destructive and proliferative.[47] The destructive phase is characterized by loss of type I and II alveolar cells, loss of surfactant, infiltration by inflammatory cells, and hemorrhage. Patients can develop hemorrhagic pulmonary edema. The subsequent proliferative phase is characterized by loss of alveolar integrity, proliferation of fibroblasts, and deposition of collagen in the interstitium and alveolar spaces. The fibrosis, which is in part cytokine mediated,[1] is not specific for paraquat-induced injury but is seen in response to acute alveolitis induced by many pulmonary toxins.

What Are the Clinical Features of Paraquat Toxicity?

The clinical features of paraquat poisoning are summarized in Table 90–1.[4,5,43,48,49,52] Eye irritation due to stripping of the superficial epithelium of the cornea and conjunctiva develops gradually, reaching a maximum about 12 to 24 hours after exposure. The severity of the injury is directly proportional to the concentration of the formulation. Dermatitis and nail damage can follow contact with paraquat, particularly if it is not washed off quickly.[43] The nails can become deformed by white bands, ridging, disruption of the nail bed, and impaired growth. When the spray droplets impact on the upper respiratory tract mucosa, the patient can develop epistaxis, inflammation, cough, and chest pain.

In patients who ingest paraquat, the toxicity can be divided into three categories.[52] Patients classified as having mild poisoning—less than 20 mg paraquat ion/kg (less than 10 mL of the 20% paraquat dichloride concentrate in a 70-kg person)—may be asymptomatic or develop only those symptoms and signs referable to the GI tract, such as oral mucosal ulceration and diarrhea. They recover without any sequelae.

Patients who ingest between 20 to 40 mg paraquat ion/kg (10 to 20 mL of the 20% concentrate in a 70-kg person) usually die 5 days to several weeks after the ingestion. The most characteristic features of toxicity in these patients are the early development of upper GI tract corrosion and acute renal tubular necrosis, and the later development of pulmonary fibrosis. The renal failure usually resolves in accordance with the natural history of acute tubular necrosis. Death is due to the extensive pulmonary injury.

Patients who ingest more than 40 mg paraquat ion/kg usually die 1 to 5 days after ingestion from multiorgan failure or the corrosive effects of paraquat in the

TABLE 90–1. CLINICAL FEATURES OF PARAQUAT POISONING

Skin and Mucus Membranes Corrosion of skin, nails, cornea, conjunctivae, and nasal mucosa	***Cardiovascular System*** Hypovolemia, shock, dysrhythmias
Gastrointestinal Tract Oropharyngeal ulceration and corrosion; nausea, vomiting, hematemesis, diarrhea; dysphagia, perforation of esophagus; pancreatitis; centrilobular hepatic necrosis; cholestasis	***Central Nervous System*** Coma, convulsions, cerebral edema
Genitourinary System Oliguria or nonoliguric renal failure due to acute tubular necrosis. Proximal tubular dysfunction	***Endocrine System*** Adrenal insufficiency due to adrenal necrosis as part of multiple organ failure
Respiratory System Cough, aphonia; prominent pharyngeal membranes (pseudodiphtheria); mediastinitis; pneumothorax; hemoptysis, pulmonary edema, and hemorrhage; pulmonary fibrosis	***Hematopoietic System*** Polymorphonuclear leukocytosis early; anemia late

GI tract. Death from esophageal perforation and mediastinitis can occur within 2 to 3 days of the ingestion.

On occasion, the history of paraquat exposure or ingestion is not forthcoming, because the patient does not know the chemical nature of the material or because of homicidal intent. In these cases, the diagnosis can be missed. Such patients have been treated for spurious illness such as diphtheria, as was the case in 3 patients who presented with prominent membranes on the tongue and pharynx.[48]

What Immediate Therapeutic Interventions Are Indicated?

Early treatment is a very important determinant of survival in paraquat-poisoned patients. Therefore, any patient who has been exposed to paraquat should be treated as a medical emergency, even if there are no symptoms or signs of toxicity at the time of presentation. This is particularly true when the patient has been exposed to one of the concentrated liquid formulations.

An accurate history should be taken to determine the formulation involved, the route or routes of exposure, and the dose. The questions listed in Table 90–2 form the basis of this history. Because ingestion exposes the patient to the highest dose, this route should be asked about specifically, even in those patients who appear only to have inhalational, dermal, or ocular contact.

If paraquat has only just been ingested, measures to prevent its absorption from the gastrointestinal tract should be instituted immediately. If there is to be any delay in reaching a medical facility and it is not precluded by vomiting, the patient can be asked to eat one or two handfuls of dirt, preferably clay, or be given something to eat.

The clothing should be removed immediately and the skin decontaminated by washing the patient thoroughly with soap and water. Scrubbing brushes should not be used because they abrade the skin and this could increase transdermal absorption of paraquat. If the eyes have been splashed, ocular irrigation with copious amounts of water should continue for 15 minutes. These patients should be seen by an ophthalmologist for further management.

Supplemental oxygen should never be given as an initial measure, because oxygen potentiates paraquat toxicity.

What Procedures Should Be Used to Decontaminate the Gastrointestinal Tract?

Patients who have ingested paraquat concentrate almost invariably will vomit because of its irritant effects or the emetogenic properties of the theophylline-like compound that is added to many liquid formulations. Even if the patient has vomited, further gastrointestinal decontamination should be undertaken. Syrup of ipecac should not be employed due to the time delay involved between its administration and subsequent emesis.

An adsorbent should be given orally as quickly as possible.[32] This could be 1 to 2 g/kg of activated charcoal, 1 to 2 g/kg of Fuller's earth in a 15% (wt/vol) aqueous suspension, or 1 to 2 g/kg bentonite in a 7% (wt/vol)

TABLE 90–2. QUESTIONS THAT SHOULD BE ASKED ABOUT EXPOSURE TO PARAQUAT OR DIQUAT

- Name of product
- Concentration of paraquat/diquat in the formulation
- Name and concentration of any other pesticides in the product
- Type of formulation—liquid, granular, gel
- Route(s) of administration or exposure
- Delay between ingestion or exposure and admission
- Age of patient
- Circumstances of poisoning (unintentional/suicidal)
- Amount ingested
- Time and extent of vomiting after ingestion
- Delay between last meal and the ingestion

aqueous slurry. All three adsorbents bind and retain paraquat effectively, but activated charcoal is used most frequently because of its ready availability. The adsorbent should be given with a cathartic such as a magnesium salt or 70% sorbitol (2 mL/kg). In some countries, the manufacturer provides hospitals or local company representatives with kits containing Fuller's earth and a cathartic. If the patient vomits the first dose of the adsorbent, another should be given through a nasogastric tube if necessary.

Conventional gastric lavage is unsatisfactory for reducing absorption because it takes 20 to 30 minutes to perform and empties only the stomach. During this time, any paraquat that has reached the intestine would be absorbed. In cats, absorption of paraquat was reduced more by an oral adsorbent than by lavage.[12] In addition, given the possible mucosal damage in the esophagus and stomach, perforation by the large bore lavage tube is a risk.

What Other Aspects of Initial Management Are Important?

Fluids and electrolytes should be administered IV in sufficient volume to replace losses from the GI tract due to the mucosal corrosion, emesis, and the cathartic. To prevent prerenal failure, urine output should be measured and maintained at least at normal flow rates.

Supportive and palliative care are most important components of the management of paraquat-poisoned patients. Attention should be paid to analgesia for the pain associated with the mucosal ulceration. Patients should be monitored frequently for the development and progression of renal and respiratory failure. Supplemental oxygen is administered only when the arterial oxygen tension falls below 50 mm Hg and/or the patient has symptoms of respiratory distress.

Should Hemodialysis or Hemoperfusion Be Performed?

Methods to maintain or increase the rate of elimination of paraquat from the body should be considered. Some advocate the use of forced diuresis,[51] although it does not increase the renal clearance of paraquat significantly.[6] The additional clearance of paraquat by conventional peritoneal dialysis is not sufficient to increase the total body clearance of paraquat significantly.[6]

Although the clearance of paraquat by hemodialysis can equal or exceed renal clearance, particularly when renal function is impaired, hemodialysis has not been shown clinically to reduce mortality.[21] Therefore, hemodialysis should be performed only for the usual indications in patients with acute renal failure.

Hemoperfusion, across a cartridge containing activated charcoal, enhances elimination of paraquat from the blood. When hemoperfusion was performed once in dogs 2 to 12 hours after an LD_{50} or LD_{100} dose of paraquat, mortality was reduced significantly.[20,54] On the other hand, there is no clinical evidence that hemoperfusion is efficacious.[21] This is because of the many times greater than LD_{100} dose ingested in most cases; the long delay after the ingestion before patients present; the high renal compared to hemoperfusion clearance of paraquat when renal function is normal; the elimination of most of the absorbed dose of paraquat by the kidneys during the first 12 hours after the ingestion; and the later limitation of the removal rate of paraquat from the body by its slow efflux from the muscles and lung to the plasma.[36] Taking all of these factors into account, we recommend that charcoal hemoperfusion be begun and continued for 6 to 8 hours only if it can be initiated *within 4 hours* of ingestion. Based on current clinical and experimental evidence, there is no indication for repeated hemoperfusion.

Although continuous arteriovenous hemofiltration can reduce the marked rebound in plasma paraquat concentrations seen after hemoperfusion due to the redistribution of paraquat from the tissues,[35] no clinical benefit of this procedure has been demonstrated.

Are There Antidotes to Paraquat?

None of the proposed "antidotes" for paraquat toxicity have been shown to be effective clinically.[2,4] Treatments examined experimentally, and in some cases clinically, include those that could prevent the accumulation of paraquat by the lung (various polyamines, D-propranolol); increase efflux of paraquat from the lung (cyclophosphamide, D-propranolol); reduce or prevent the consequences of the redox cycling (reduction of FIO_2, vitamin E, superoxide dismutase, ascorbic acid, deferoxamine, selenium, niacin, or *N*-acetylcysteine); or reduce the extent of pulmonary fibrosis (corticosteroids, immunosuppressive agents, fibrinolytic agents, colchicine, and radiotherapy). Some groups administer vitamin C (4000 mg/day) and vitamin E (250 mg/day) routinely[51]; these have very few contraindications or side effects, even if efficacy is unproven. Few controlled trials of these approaches have been performed. In one study, when 33 patients given high doses of cyclophosphamide and dexamethasone ($n = 33$) were compared prospectively with 14 given standard therapy (gastrointestinal decontamination and fluids; $n = 14$), there was no significant difference in the mortality in the two groups (63 and 61%, respectively).[34]

Despite having theoretical benefit or demonstrated effectiveness in animal models,[15,42] reduction of inspired oxygen concentration in paraquat-poisoned patients has not been demonstrated to be effective clinically. Although low-dose inhaled nitric oxide has been reported to reduce the intrapulmonary shunt in a paraquat-poisoned patient, it is not indicated, because it could add to the toxicity by reacting with the superoxide anion forming the peroxynitrite anion and the hydroxyl radical.[3,30]

Paraquat-specific IgG antibodies and their Fab fragments have been shown in vitro to reduce the uptake and toxicity of paraquat in type II cells.[11] However, in vivo use of intact antibodies or Fab fragments is complicated by their reduction of the renal clearance of paraquat because of the protein–paraquat complex formation and the protein load of antibody required to reduce or prevent toxicity. Assuming that a 70-kg patient ingested 30 mg paraquat ion/kg, the absorbed dose to be "neutralized" (5% absorption) would be 105 mg. Thus, a stoichiometric dose of Fab fragments would be 28 g. If less than a stoichiometric dose can shift the patient's position on the dose toxicity curve to the left sufficiently far to prevent death, the dose would be less. It would be even less for a recombinant, single-chain antibody (sFv), which is half the molecular weight of Fab fragments. The volume of a 14-g (0.2 g/kg) dose of a sFv corresponds to 200 mL of plasma. In addition, compared to intact IgG and Fab fragments, the volume of distribution (V_d) and renal clearance of sFvs are larger.[13] These kinetic properties would be advantageous for treatment of PQ poisoning because of its large V_d and high renal clearance. It may be possible to deliver lower doses of anti-PQ sFv by inhalation, more or less topically to the target cells. Unfortunately, such therapy with sFvs has not been developed clinically to date because of the prohibitive costs of manufacturing sufficient amounts of such recombinant products even to test in animals. Any efficacy of such antibody therapy, however, will be limited by the practical issues such as the length of time before the patient presents to a medical facility. The "window of opportunity" for any effective treatment of paraquat poisoning is very short, only a few hours at most.

What About Lung Transplantation?

Lung transplantation has been performed in a few patients, but none have survived.[27,31,44] Nevertheless, if a patient survives for 3 weeks and is well, apart from life-threatening respiratory failure, bilateral lung transplantation can be considered. In this context, it is possible that other serious, long-term effects of paraquat will be revealed. For example, one group reported that a patient who had two lung transplants and survived for about 6 months after being exposed to paraquat developed a progressive toxic myopathy.[44]

What Laboratory Tests Should Be Requested in Patients With Paraquat Toxicity?

Urine and plasma should be sent to the laboratory promptly for qualitative and, if the service is available, quantitative determination of paraquat concentrations. If possible, specimens should be shipped in plastic containers, because paraquat binds to glass. Treatment of the patient should continue until the results are available.

Rapid, qualitative analysis in urine is performed by reducing paraquat to its blue monocation radical with sodium dithionite under alkaline conditions and comparison with the appropriate positive and negative controls.[7,10] In our laboratory, we make up a fresh alkaline sodium dithionite solution by adding 100 mg of sodium dithionite (nonoxidized) to 5 mL of 5M NaOH. An aliquot sample (250 μL) of this solution is added to 1 mL urine. If paraquat is present in a concentration of 2 μg/mL or greater, a blue-black color, depending on the concentration, is evident. Diquat is reduced similarly to form a yellow-green color.

Plasma or urine paraquat concentrations can be measured quantitatively by a variety of techniques, the most common being radioimmunoassay, gas chromatography, spectroscopy, and high-performance liquid chromatography.[7,16,45] It is usually relatively easy to identify a laboratory that can perform the spot test but more difficult to find one to do the quantitative measurements. Many manufacturers support a 24-hour emergency service that should provide this information for each country. The telephone number for the service can be found either on the product label or via a poison center or other emergency facility. In many countries and areas, quantitative assays are not available in a timely manner to assist with management of the patient. In this case, the management must be guided by the clinical and other laboratory findings.

Clinical chemistry abnormalities reflect the development of acute renal tubular necrosis and necrosis of the liver, lung, pancreas, and muscle.[47] If paraquat concentrations in blood exceed about 10 mg/L, measured values of creatinine and LDH may be elevated artificially because of interference with the colorimetric methods used to measure them.[14]

Hematologic abnormalities, if any, are usually nonspecific and related to bleeding or infection. Methemoglobinemia with hemolysis has been reported[33] but was thought to be due to the monolinuron in the formulation, not the paraquat.[40]

Caustic injury to the esophagus and mediastinum can be associated with pneumomediastinum and pneumothorax. The changes in the lung parenchyma are obvious on the chest radiograph, first as cystic and linear opacities and later as consolidation, particularly in the perihilar regions.[26] The chest radiograph, taken on the 9th day after the ingestion of paraquat in a patient who died 3 days later, is shown in Figure 90–2. It shows diffuse consolidation most marked in the perihilar regions.

What Determines the Prognosis of Paraquat Poisoning?

Not all patients who ingest paraquat die, but the mortality in some series of patients has been as high as 75%.[4,46,52] There have been a few survivors reported with residual pulmonary fibrosis,[25] but typically a patient who survives does not develop pulmonary injury and has no residual effects.

The outcome is determined by the dose ingested. Patients who ingest paraquat intentionally usually take a higher dose than those who ingest it unintentionally and therefore have a worse prognosis. Similarly, the inci-

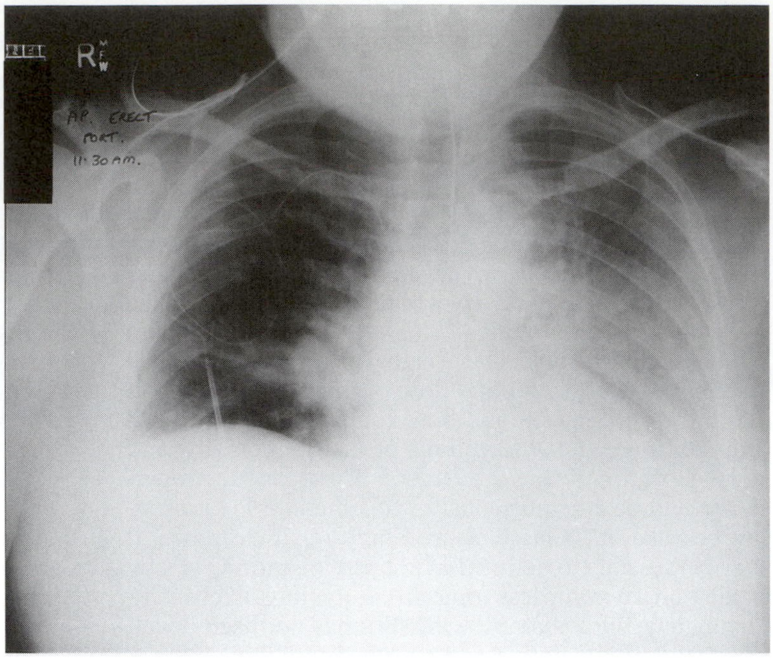

Figure 90–2. Chest radiograph taken 9 days after the ingestion of 70 mL of 20% paraquat, demonstrating diffuse alveolar consolidation most marked in the perihilar regions.

dence of death is higher the more concentrated the formulation ingested.

Plasma concentrations of paraquat measured within 28 hours after the ingestion are useful in estimating the prognosis according to the nomogram presented in Figure 90–3.[22,39] This nomogram was derived empirically from clinical data and not by statistical means. Thus, it is not infallible. Patients with higher concentrations than those expected from the nomogram to be associated with survival have survived; conversely, those with lower concentrations have died.[39] When experience with the nomogram in 166 cases was reviewed, it correctly predicted the outcome in 93% of cases who died and in 64% who survived.[39] Therefore, reports in the literature of unexpected survival in individual patients, unexpected according to the nomogram, should only be attributed with caution to one or another innovative treatment because of the imperfections of the predictive line. The extension of this nomogram beyond 28 hours[45,46] has similar predictive efficacy as do compilations of indices using physiologic and clinical data.[41,45,50] It appears that whenever the initial plasma concentration of paraquat exceeds 3 μg/mL, mortality is 100%.[21] The mode of death is cardiogenic shock within 24 hours of the ingestion in those whose paraquat levels exceed 10 μg/mL.[39]

Concentrations of paraquat in urine obtained within the first 24 hours of ingestion can be used to estimate prognosis.[45,46] Of 53 patients studied, 15 who had urinary concentrations of paraquat below 1 μg/mL within the first 24 hours survived. Urinary concentrations in those who died within 24 hours ranged from approximately 10 to 10,000 μg/mL; concentrations in those who died later from pulmonary fibrosis were between 1 and 1000 μg/mL.

Several factors can moderate the amount of paraquat absorbed and thus the plasma and urinary concentrations. When paraquat is swallowed on a full stomach, its absorption is reduced because of delayed gastric emptying and the adsorption of the herbicide by the food.[5] The presence of ulceration in the upper gastrointestinal tract is a poor prognostic sign because it may reflect the concentration and the dose of paraquat in the formula-

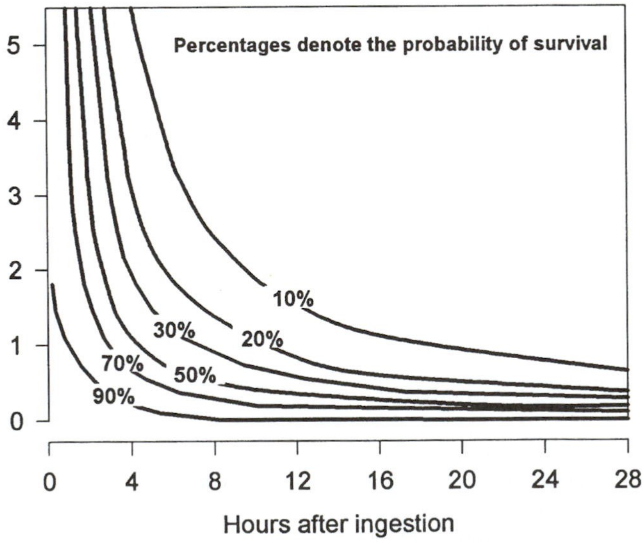

Figure 90–3. Nomogram showing the relationship between the plasma concentrations of paraquat on the ordinate (μg/mL), time after ingestion on the abscissa, and the probability of survival. *(Reprinted, with permission, from Hart RB, Nevitt A, Whitehead A: A new statistical approach to the prognostic significance of plasma paraquat concentrations. Lancet 1984;2:1222–1223. Letter.)*

tion. In one series of patients who had upper GI endoscopy between 3 hours and 3 days after the ingestion, 9 of 14 patients with gastric and esophageal ulcerations died.[5] Conversely, all 6 who had no gastric ulcerations survived.

The development of renal failure heralds a poor prognosis. Of 20 patients in one series who developed renal failure, 19 died.[5]

Diquat

Diquat (1,1′-ethylene-2,2′-dipyridylium dibromide)[8] is used agriculturally for the same indications as paraquat as well as for the control of aquatic weeds and is included in several formulations of paraquat. In terms of caustic effects, kinetics, and mechanisms of toxicity, diquat is similar to paraquat[49] with one important exception. Diquat lacks the structural features necessary for active transport by the polyamine uptake pathway. Therefore, the extent of pulmonary injury and fibrosis in patients who take toxic doses of diquat is much less than that after paraquat. Overall, however, the LD_{50} of the two compounds in animals is of the same order of magnitude.[49] In a review of 11 cases, Vanholder and colleagues concluded that the lethal adult human dose of diquat was 6 to 12 g.[53]

In comparison to paraquat, there have been relatively few cases of diquat poisoning. Most of the cases reported in the literature involved patients who died, despite treatment such as forced diuresis, hemoperfusion, and the administration of antioxidants.[29,37,53,55]

Treatment of diquat-exposed patients proceeds along the same lines as for those exposed to paraquat.

References

1. Barabás K, Serényi P, Selypes A: Inhibition of lung damage caused by paraquat with lymphokines or cytokines. Exp Pathol 1990;38:189–195.
2. Bateman DN: Pharmacological treatments of paraquat poisoning. Hum Toxicol 1987;6:57–62.
3. Berisha HI, Pakbaz H, Absood A, Said SI: Nitric oxide as a mediator of oxidant lung injury due to paraquat. Proc Natl Acad Sci USA 1994;91:7445–7449.
4. Bismuth C, Garnier R, Baud FJ, et al: Paraquat poisoning. An overview of the current status. Drug Saf 1990;5:243–251.
5. Bismuth C, Garnier R, Dally S, et al: Prognosis and treatment of paraquat poisoning: A review of 28 cases. J Toxicol Clin Toxicol 1982;19:461–474.
6. Bismuth C, Scherrmann JM, Garnier R, et al: Elimination of paraquat. Hum Toxicol 1987;6:63–67.
7. Braithwaite RA: Emergency analysis of paraquat in biological fluids. Hum Toxicol 1987;6:83–86.
8. Brian RC, Homer RF, Stubbs J, Jones RL: A new herbicide: 1,1′-ethylene-2,2′-dipyridylium dibromide. Nature 1958;191: 446–447.
9. Calderbank A, Brian RC, Allen HP, et al: Bipyridylium herbicides. In: Peacock FC, ed: Jealott's Hill. Fifty Years of Agricultural Research 1928–1978. Birmingham, Kynock Press, 1978, pp. 67–86.
10. Calderbank A, Farrington JA: The chemistry of paraquat and its radical. In: Bismuth C, Hall AH, eds: Paraquat Poisoning. Mechanisms, Prevention, Treatment. New York, Marcel Dekker, 1995, pp. 89–106.
11. Chen N, Bowles MR, Pond SM: Prevention of paraquat toxicity in suspensions of alveolar type II cells by paraquat-specific antibodies. Hum Exp Toxicol 1994;13:551–557.
12. Clark DG: Inhibition of the absorption of paraquat from the gastrointestinal tract by adsorbents. Br J Indust Med 1971; 28:186–188.
13. Devlin CM, Bowles MR, Gordon RB, Pond SM: Production of a paraquat-specific murine single chain Fv fragment. J Biochem 1995;118:480–487.
14. Fairshter RD, Miyada DS, Ulich TR, Tipper P: The effects of paraquat dichloride on clinical chemistry measurements. J Anal Toxicol 1986;10:162–164.
15. Fogt F, Zilker T: Total exclusion from external respiration protects lungs from development of fibrosis after paraquat intoxication. Hum Toxicol 1989;8:465–474.
16. Fuke C, Ameno K, Ameno S, et al: A rapid, simultaneous determination of paraquat and diquat in serum and urine using second-derivative spectroscopy. J Anal Toxicol 1992; 16:214–216.
17. Gordonsmith RH, Brooke-Taylor S, Smith LL, Cohen GM: Structural requirements of compounds to inhibit pulmonary diamine accumulation. Biochem Pharmacol 1983; 32:3701–3709.
18. Hall AW: Paraquat and diquat exposures reported to U.S. poison centers, 1983–1992. In: Bismuth C, Hall AH, eds: Paraquat Poisoning. Mechanisms, Prevention, Treatment. New York, Marcel Dekker, 1995, pp. 33–64.
19. Hall AH, Becker CE: Occupational health and safety considerations in paraquat handling. In: Bismuth C, Hall AH, eds: Paraquat Poisoning. Mechanisms, Prevention, Treatment. New York, Marcel Dekker, 1995, pp. 249–266.
20. Hampson ECGM, Effeney DJ, Pond SM: Efficacy of single or repeated hemoperfusion in a canine model of paraquat poisoning. J Pharmacol Exp Ther 1990;254:732–740.
21. Hampson ECGM, Pond SM: Failure of hemoperfusion and hemodialysis to prevent paraquat poisoning. A retrospective review of 42 patients. Med Toxicol 1988;3: 64–71.
22. Hart TB, Nevitt A, Whitehead A: A new statistical approach to the prognostic significance of plasma paraquat concentrations. Lancet 1984;2:1222–1223.
23. Heylings JR: Gastrointestinal absorption of paraquat in the isolated mucosa of the rat. Toxicol Appl Pharmacol 1991; 107:482–493.
24. Houzé P, Baud FJ, Mouy R, et al: Toxicokinetics of paraquat in humans. Hum Exp Toxicol 1990;9:5–12.
25. Hudson M, Patel SB, Ewen SWB, et al: Paraquat induced pulmonary fibrosis is three survivors. Thorax 1991;46: 201–204.
26. Im J-G, Lee KS, Han MC, et al: Paraquat poisoning: Findings of chest radiography and CT in 42 patients. Am J Radiol 1991;157:697–701.
27. Kalmholz S, Veith FJ, Mollenkopf F, et al: Single lung transplantation in paraquat intoxication. NY State J Med 1984; 84:81–85.
28. Keeling PL, Pratt IS, Aldridge WN, Smith LL: The enhance-

ment of paraquat toxicity in rats by 85% oxygen: Lethality and cell-specific lung damage. Br J Exp Pathol 1981;62: 643–654.

29. Mahieu P, Bonduelle Y, Bernard A, et al: Acute diquat intoxication. Interest of its repeated determination in urine and the evaluation of renal proximal tubule integrity. J Toxicol Clin Toxicol 1984;22:363–369.
30. Maruyama K, Takeuchi M, Chikusa H, Muneyuki M: Reduction of intrapulmonary shunt by low-dose inhaled nitric oxide in a patient with late-stage respiratory distress associated with paraquat poisoning. Intensive Care Med 1995; 21:778–779.
31. Matthew H, Logan A, Woodruff MFA, Heard B: Paraquat poisoning. Lung transplantation. Br Med J 1968;3:759–763.
32. Meredith TJ, Vale JA: Treatment of paraquat poisoning in man: Methods to prevent absorption. Hum Toxicol 1987;6: 49–55.
33. Ng LL, Naik RB, Polak A: Paraquat ingestion with methemoglobinemia treated with methylene blue. Br Med J 1982; 284:1445–1446.
34. Perriëns JH, Benimadho S, Kiauw IL, Wisse J, et al: High-dose cyclophosphamide and dexamethasone in paraquat poisoning: A prospective study. Hum Exp Toxicol 1992;11: 129–134.
35. Pond SM, Johnston SC, Schoof DD, et al: Repeated hemoperfusion and continuous arteriovenous hemofiltration in a paraquat poisoned patient. J Toxicol Clin Toxicol 1987;25: 305–316.
36. Pond SM, Rivory LP, Hampson ECGM, Roberts MS: Kinetics of toxic doses of paraquat and the effects of hemoperfusion in the dog. J Toxicol Clin Toxicol 1993;31:229–246.
37. Powell D, Pond SM, Allen TB, Portale AA: Hemoperfusion in a child who ingested diquat and died from pontine infarction and hemorrhage. J Toxicol Clin Toxicol 1983;20: 405–420.
38. Pronczuk de Garbino J: Epidemiology of paraquat poisoning. In: Bismuth C, Hall AH, eds: Paraquat Poisoning. Mechanisms, Prevention, Treatment. New York, Marcel Dekker, 1995, pp. 37–52.
39. Proudfoot A: Predictive value of early plasma paraquat concentrations. In: Bismuth C, Hall AH, eds: Paraquat Poisoning. Mechanisms, Prevention, Treatment. New York, Marcel Dekker, 1995, pp. 275–284.
40. Proudfoot AT: Methemoglobinemia due to monolinuron—not paraquat. Br Med J 1982;285:812.
41. Ragoucy-Sengler C, Pileire B. A biological index to predict patient outcome in paraquat poisoning. Hum Exp Toxicol 1996;15: 265–268.
42. Rhodes ML, Zavala DC, Brown D: Hypoxic protection in paraquat poisoning. Lab Invest 1976;5:496–500.
43. Samman PD, Johnston ENM: Nail damage associated with handling of paraquat and diquat. Br Med J 1969;1:818–819.
44. Saunders NR, Alpert HM, Cooper JD: Sequential bilateral lung transplantation for paraquat poisoning. A case report. J Thorac Cardiovasc Surg 1985;89:734–742.
45. Scherrmann JM: Analytical procedures and predictive value of late plasma and urine concentrations. In: Bismuth C, Hall AH, eds: Paraquat Poisoning. Mechanisms, Prevention, Treatment. New York, Marcel Dekker, 1995, pp. 285–298.
46. Scherrmann JM, House P, Bismuth C, Bourdon R: Prognostic value of plasma and urine paraquat concentration. Hum Toxicol 1987;6:91–93.
47. Smith LL: The toxicity of paraquat. Adv Drug React Pois Rev 1988;1:1–17.
48. Stephens DS, Walker DH, Schaffner W, et al: Pseudodiphtheria: Prominent pharyngeal membrane associated with fatal paraquat ingestion. Ann Interrn Med 1981;94: 202–204.
49. Stevens JT, Sumner DD: Herbicides. In: Hayes WJ, Laws ER, eds: Handbook of Pesticide Toxicology, Vol. 3. Classes of Pesticides. Boston, Academic Press, 1991, pp. 1356–1408.
50. Suzuki K, Takasu N, Arita S, et al: A new method for predicting the outcome and survival period in paraquat poisoning. Hum Toxicol 1989;8:33–38.
51. Talbot AR, Barnes MR, Ting RS: Early radiotherapy in the treatment of paraquat poisoning. Br J Radiol 1988;61: 405–408.
52. Vale JA, Meredith TJ, Buckley BM: Paraquat poisoning: Clinical features and immediate general management. Hum Toxicol 1987;6:41–47.
53. Vanholder R, Colardyn F, DeRueck J, et al: Diquat intoxication. Report of two cases and review of the literature. Am J Med 1981;76:1267–1271.
54. Widdop BM, Medd RK, Braithwaite RA: Charcoal hemoperfusion in the treatment of paraquat poisoning. Proc Eur Soc Toxicol 1976;18:156–159.
55. Williams PF, Jarvie DR, Whitehead AP: Diquat intoxication: Treatment by charcoal hemoperfusion and description of a new method of diquat measurement in plasma. J Toxicol Clin Toxicol 1986;24:11–20.
56. Yoshioka T, Sugimoto T, Kinoshita N, et al: Effects of concentration reduction and partial replacement of paraquat by diquat on human toxicity: A clinical survey. Hum Exp Toxicol 1992;11:241–245.

CHAPTER 91

Industrial Poisoning: Information and Control

Eddy A. Bresnitz, Harriet Rubenstein, and Kathleen M. Rest

A 38-year-old woman presented to the emergency department (ED) with a 6-month history of progressive cough and shortness of breath. She had been relatively well until 3 years earlier, when she had similar complaints. Her physician at that time ordered several tests that confirmed a diagnosis of sarcoidosis. She was treated for 9 months with prednisone, resulting in improvement of her symptoms. She continued to have minimal complaints of shortness of breath on exertion, and 6 months earlier her dyspnea progressed and she developed a cough. She was concerned that she had had a relapse and required more prednisone.

The patient's symptoms had increasingly limited her activities over the previous 6 months. On some weekdays, for example, these symptoms were associated with a dry, nonproductive cough that was worse at night. The shortness of breath and cough appeared together and did not seem to be associated with exercise or relieved with rest. Her symptoms were unassociated with chest pain, hemoptysis, sore throat, tingling in the arms or shoulders, nausea, vomiting, wheezing, sputum production, or weight loss.

In addition to her respiratory complaints, the patient complained of intermittent headache and burning eyes. At times these headaches occurred while she was at work, but she was not sure they were related to her job. She thought the eye irritation was definitely work-related because she experienced this symptom only while at work (but not every day). Moreover, on the days she had this problem, it seemed to disappear within a couple of hours of leaving the factory.

The patient had a history of pulmonary embolism 10 years earlier, documented by angiography and requiring a 3-month course of coumadin. Her physician at that time thought birth control pills were the cause of the embolus. At the time of her pulmonary embolism, she was also noted to have cervical and mediastinal lymphadenopathy that eventually led to the diagnosis of sarcoidosis.

The patient denied any past medical history of pneumonia, asthma, bronchitis, heart disease, or heart murmurs. She stated that she had hay fever as a child but had not developed any new allergies as an adult. She had no other medical problems.

On physical examination, she appeared to be well-developed and well-nourished and in no acute respiratory distress. Her vital signs were: blood pressure, 140/90 mm Hg; pulse, 84 beats/min and regular; respiratory rate, 20 breaths/min and regular; and temperature, 99°F (37.2°C). Examination of the head, ears, eyes, nose, and throat was within normal limits. Chest examination revealed good air entry bilaterally, with diffuse wheezes on forced expiration.

There were no rales or rhonchi. The cardiovascular examination showed normal S_1 and S_2 without murmurs. The abdomen was soft and nontender and the bowel sounds were normal. The liver was 11 cm in span and nontender. The extremities showed no evidence of clubbing, cyanosis, or edema. The neurologic examination was also within normal limits.

The resident diagnosed acute asthma based on clinical evaluation and a reduced peak flow measurement that improved with inhaled bronchodilators. The patient began to feel better soon after inhalation treatment. Because of the temporal relationship of the patient's symptoms to her work, the examining physician suspected her complaints might be work-related. He sent a medical student to take a detailed occupational history from the patient.

What Are the Important Issues in Taking an Occupational History From a Patient With a Suspected Workplace-Related Illness?

One risk factor that may provide a wealth of information in assessing a patient but that is frequently overlooked is the patient's occupation. The occupational and environmental history is composed of three important elements: present job, past work, and nonoccupational exposures.

Current Work History

The reasons for collecting data on a person's present job are obvious: They reveal what his or her present exposures may be, which can influence both acute and

TABLE 91–1. COMPONENTS OF AN OCCUPATIONAL HISTORY

Current Work History
Specifics of the job
Employer's name
Duration of employment
Process description
Job description
Adjacent processes
Hazardous exposures
Health effects
Suspicious health problems
Temporality of symptoms
Affected co-workers
Medical surveillance records
Biologic monitoring
Control measures
Environmental sampling and monitoring
Engineering controls
Work practice protocols
Administrative controls
Personal protective equipment
Worker education and training
Medical monitoring
Past Work History
Nonoccupational Exposures
Secondary employment
Hobbies
Outdoor activities
Residential exposures
Community contamination

chronic health problems. These data can be systematically collected by focusing on four areas: specifics of the job, hazardous exposures, health effects, and control measures (Table 91–1).

Specifics of the Job. It is not sufficient simply to inquire what the patient does for a living. Like healthcare professionals, workers in other industries have their own jargon. When asked for a job title, a patient may respond with one that has meaning only in his or her trade. Even if the job title is recognizable, it may not provide any useful information and, in fact, may be misleading. A secretary working in a small plastics manufacturing plant may have occupational exposures quite different from the secretary who works for a law firm.

The important specific information requested should include: name of employer, duration of employment, process description, job description, and adjacent processes. The employer may be able to provide information about materials used at the plant. The patient's permission should always be obtained before calling the employer. A patient may be fired or otherwise discriminated against (despite legal interdictions) if he or she suggests that the health problems are work-related.

The patient said she was employed by Zipco, a zipper tape manufacturer located in an industrial park. The building had been in use since the late 1800s and was last renovated several years earlier when it was bought by the current owner. The company operated two shifts per day.

The duration of employment information gives an indication of the duration of possible exposure to hazardous substances or conditions in the workplace. The patient had worked for the company for the past 10 years, in several different positions. She had held her current position for 5 years, 2 of those years before the diagnosis of sarcoidosis. She stated that her job had not changed at all during this 5-year period. She always worked in the finishing department, but in different locations. She began working in her current location about 7 months earlier, when the plant upgraded its equipment and all activities were relocated to accommodate the new machinery.

It is important to learn what actually happens in the patient's immediate work environment, because the work process itself may make chemicals more toxic. If possible, the patient should be asked for a diagram of the work area. The patient should also be questioned about job process changes. A previously safe job may have been changed to a potentially dangerous one without a change in the patient's job title.

The company's major products were zipper tapes and bindings. Cloth tape purchased from outside manufacturers was sewn to metal or plastic zippers. Before the zipper was sewn to the tape, the tape was treated with various substances that act as flame retardants or shrink resistors, according to the customer's specifications, and were often dyed. Finished tapes were cut and packaged on the finishing floor. The patient stated that she had never handled any of the chemicals or dyes used in the tape-finishing process.

The patient should describe exactly what he or she does on any given day and for how long. Unusual and nonroutine tasks, such as those performed during overtime, maintenance, or in an emergency, should also be described. The primary job may not involve chemicals, but the patient may nevertheless perform tasks that entail unprotected exposure to a toxic chemical. The patient had a very simple job: She stood or sat at a workbench and processed customers' orders. Since starting this job 5 years ago, she had not done any other kind of work in the plant.

It is important to know what processes occur in the patient's immediate work area. Although the patient may not work directly with chemicals, adjacent co-workers may use them in their jobs. The patient worked about 15 feet from the "dipping" tanks, where the zipper tapes were dipped in solutions, including flame retardants, shrink resistors, adhesive emulsions, lubricants, dyes, and bleaches. The tapes were automatically unwound from a large spool, continuously run through an open dip tank 15 feet from the patient's work station, and then rewound on a hot roller to hasten drying. At times, she noticed steam emanating from the hot rewinding rollers.

Hazardous Exposures. The names and/or types of all chemicals or substances to which the patient may be exposed are important in determining potential adverse effects and any relationship to the patient's complaints. It is important to elicit any recent changes in suppliers of these products, as even a slight change in the formulation of a chemical may cause adverse effects in an individual who had no problems working with that compound previously. This information may be obtained from the material safety data sheet (MSDS), an important but not always reliable source of information about the chemical. In addition to adverse health effects, it contains information on chemical reactivity, safety precautions, and other data. As an initial step, it should be requested and reviewed; however, information provided on health effects should be cross-checked with other resources.

Most patients know what they are, or have been, exposed to, even if they do not know the exact name of the substance or its medical effects. The patient had a list of the substances used at the company. She thought that she may have been exposed to the vapors and gases of the chemicals used to treat zipper tapes. The substances included Pyrocrest 007, Daratak 17.200, and Triton X-100.

Health Effects. Significant occupational exposures usually cause medical effects, although some do so only after a substantial latency period. Key areas of interest include suspicious health problems, temporality of symptoms, affected co-workers, medical surveillance records, and biologic monitoring data. All of these data can help in determining whether the patient is suffering a work-related illness. Patients may suspect that their illness or complaint is work-related, especially when symptoms occur at the workplace and improve or disappear over the weekend or during a vacation. Co-workers with similar complaints (not necessarily of the same severity) should raise suspicion that a workplace exposure is responsible for a particular symptom complex.

Patients may also know if their workplace has an active medical surveillance program. A surveillance program that includes periodic spirometry and respiratory questionnaires usually indicates that the patient works with a potential respiratory toxin. A medical surveillance program that includes biologic monitoring for a specific substance may also provide an immediate clue to what may be causing the patient's complaints. Finally, if the patient knows exactly what he or she is working with, the physician can usually determine quickly whether any of the substances are compatible with the patient's complaints.

The patient suspected that she had a work-related problem because of the temporal relationship between her symptoms and her work. She indicated that her symptoms were exacerbated particularly when the finishing department used Pyrocrest 007 and Triton X-100, substances used in a batch process run only every other week. The patient stated that although co-workers had complained of burning eyes during this operation, none of them experienced the shortness of breath and chest tightness she felt. She indicated that there was no ongoing medical surveillance program at work.

Control Measures. It is important to determine whether the workplace employs any control measures, including environmental sampling and monitoring, engineering controls, work practice protocols, administrative controls, personal protective equipment, worker education and training, and medical surveillance. The existence of control measures usually indicates that the employer recognizes and has attempted to deal with a hazardous exposure.

To the patient's knowledge there had been no environmental sampling or monitoring in her workplace. She stated that the factory had large fans stationed throughout the plant, which cooled the factory, especially in summer, when all the windows were open. The windows were kept closed in the winter, and the lack of adequate ventilation seemed to exacerbate her problems. She was not aware of any specific local exhaust ventilation in the vicinity of the "dipping" tanks.

The patient had not been instructed to follow any specific procedure at work. Some of her co-workers wore paper surgical masks when they poured chemicals from large open pails into the "dipping" tanks to replenish the supply of liquids, which was sometimes done several times per day, depending on the volume of orders. None of the workers left their posts when the tanks were being filled or when the machines were being cleaned. The patient did not think her symptoms were worse during these operations.

Her supervisor was somewhat accommodating in attempting to deal with her symptoms. Since her symptoms were exacerbated when tapes were processed through the flame-retardant (Pyrocrest 007) or shrink-resistor (Triton X-100) chemicals, her supervisor let her know when these batch runs would be done, and the patient did not work on those days. As a result, her job had become part-time. However, her symptoms reappeared even on days when these chemicals were not used. She said she could smell the chemicals in the air when she returned to work even after several days' absence.

The patient tried to use paper dust masks to prevent inhalation of the dust and vapors, but they did not help. She was unaware of other available types of masks. None of the plant employees received any education or training about the chemicals used in the plant. The patient had never heard of right-to-know legislation and did not know there were information sheets (MSDSs) available for every chemical used in the plant. She said she would determine the manufacturers' names from the labels on the chemical drums.

Normally, such a patient would not present to an ED; she would likely present at an earlier stage to an in-plant medical provider or to a private physician. However, this non-unionized plant had no in-house medical department and did not provide healthcare benefits for its workers. Zipco did not require preplacement or periodic physical examinations of its workers, so there were no available records to determine baseline health status. The company did not perform routine spirometry or chest radiographs. Individuals who became sick or ill at work were sent to the local hospital's ED. In situations such as this, EDs must be prepared to develop the type of occupational history outlined above.

Past Work History

It is important not to limit the occupational history to the patient's current workplace and job. Many occupational diseases have long latency periods between exposure to a toxic agent(s) and initial development of clinical symptoms. In addition, patients may have been exposed to substances at work that make them more sensitive to other environmental agents. Thus, for example, someone who developed asthma secondary to a previous workplace exposure may suffer asthma attacks on exposure to simple irritants in their current workplace. When taking an in-depth occupational history, issues relevant to the current work history should be ascertained for each previous job.

The patient indicated that before taking a job at her present company, she worked as a quality control inspector for 5 years at a furniture manufacturing plant in North Carolina. She worked in several areas of the plant, each of them adjacent to areas heavily contaminated with wood dust. She did not recall having any specific respiratory problems related to her work. Other employees had complained of respiratory irritation when they had to trim foam cushions with hot knives, but she never did that type of work. She had no other jobs before her employment at the furniture manufacturing plant.

Nonoccupational Exposures

Workers may be exposed to toxic substances in the course of pursuing secondary employment, hobbies, or outdoor activities in contaminated or industrial areas. Residential exposures, such as those from gas and wood stoves, chemically treated furniture and fabrics, and pest control, may also be relevant. It is important to ask patients about these potential exposures before focusing entirely on exposures in their primary place of employment. The patient stated that she had no hobbies aside from reading and swimming, did not have a second job, and lived in a residential, nonindustrial neighborhood. She knew of no sources of indoor air pollution in her home.

This patient was experiencing both upper and lower respiratory system symptoms that appeared to be work-related. She indicated possible chemical exposures at work but did not know the generic identity of the chemicals involved. She gave a list of chemical trade names to the ED staff. The problem was to discover the specific nature of these chemicals to determine their potential for respiratory toxicity, which would explain her symptoms. She was referred to the medical clinic for diagnosis and follow-up.

What Information Resources Are Available to Help Determine Whether a Patient's Occupational or Environmental Exposure(s) Are Related to His or Her Complaints?

Health care professionals require information on industrial toxins in a number of situations, ranging from caring for an acutely ill patient in an ED, when information must be obtained quickly, to caring for a patient with chronic symptoms that may reflect an occupational disease. The Suggested Reading section at the end of this chapter lists resources that provide concise information on toxicology, acute and chronic health effects, diagnosis, and treatment; assists in screening and surveillance; and provides information on groups at risk, product uses, and sources of further information. The use of these resources depends on the proper identification of the substance in question; if the substance, its generic name, and ingredients are not known, the research process becomes more difficult.

The practitioner should take a logical approach to seeking information about industrial toxins. First, the substance must be identified by its generic name. This can be done by reviewing the MSDS or contacting poison control centers, the employer, manufacturer, unions, and government agencies. Again, the patient's consent must be obtained before the employer or union is contacted.

Poison Control Centers

Regional poison control centers (PCCs) can provide assistance even when the exact chemical name is unknown, because information on toxic substances and their management may be cross-referenced by trade name and manufacturer. Moreover, PCC personnel can usually suggest additional resources. Most PCCs (and some hospital pharmacies) have computerized listings of poisons that are updated regularly. The best known system is Poisindex (Micromedex, Englewood, CO). Subscribers to this system receive quarterly updates of an alphabetically organized listing of approximately 500,000 industrial and nonindustrial chemicals and compounds. The system includes trade names. The components and their concentrations, when available, of each compound are listed; these are cross-referenced to management protocols. The name of the manufacturer is also listed.

The patient presented to the medical clinic 2 weeks after her ED visit. She had asked her supervisor to provide copies of the MSDSs of the chemicals used in the plant, but he was able to provide only their trade names and manufacturers: Pyrocrest 007, manufacturer A; Triton X-100, manufacturer B; and Daratak 17.200, manufacturer C. The medical resident had no idea what chemicals were contained in these products. He called the regional PCC, where information specialists consulted Poisindex. They discovered that Triton X-100 contains octylphenoxypolyethoxy-ethanol, a nonionic surfactant listed as an irritant. They could not locate the other chemicals in the Poisindex database. At this point, the resident advised the patient that he would call the product manufacturers for further information before her next visit.

Employers and Manufacturers

Many state and federal laws require employers and manufacturers to generate, retain, and disclose information that may help physicians care for persons with work-related health problems. Scientific information, exposure data, information on health effects, and collected medical data are included in the types of information that must be retained.

The Chemical Transportation Emergency Center (CHEMTREC; 1-800-424-9300; WWW.CMAHQ.COM) sponsored by the Chemical Manufacturers Association, has as its primary responsibility to provide information to healthcare practitioners responding to hazardous spills. However, it will also provide information on commercial products found in a patient's workplace.

The Occupational Safety and Health Act requires chemical manufacturers to create a MSDS for each chemical they produce, and employers who use chemicals must retain the MSDS in the workplace. Required information includes chemical and common names; physical, safety, and health-hazard data; exposure limits; precautions for safe handling and use; generally applicable control measures; and emergency and first aid procedures. Individual employers are required to provide employees with information on the chemical and physical agents used in their workplaces. With the patient's permission, a call to the plant manager, foreperson, or safety officer may be all that is necessary to determine the name of the substance in question. Employers may also be able to provide information on exposure levels in the patient's work environment. In addition, company medical departments (where they exist) may have results of medical testing done on the patient.

The next day the resident called the manufacturers for information on their products. The product manager of Daratak 17.200 referred the resident to the plant's safety person, who told him Daratak 17.200 is a polyvinyl acetate, homo polymer emulsion adhesive similar to Elmer's glue. It also contains a polyvinyl alcohol that acts as a stabilizer. When shipped, it has 0.5% free monomer that dwindles to 0% after 3–4 weeks. This substance may have some irritant effects.

The operations manager of the Triton X-100 manufacturer sent the MSDS, which confirmed the irritant effects of Triton X-100 outlined in Poisindex. The plant manager of the Pyrocrest 007 manufacturer sent an MSDS upon receipt of a written request. The MSDS indicated that Pyrocrest 007 contains ammonium salts and that thermal decomposition results in sulfur and nitrogen oxides. The health hazard section indicated that "long-term exposure may cause skin blemishes." The emergency and first aid procedures stated: "If swallowed, call physician." There was no mention of respiratory effects, although the special protection section of the MSDS recommended use of a respirator.

To ascertain the effects of these oxides, the resident consulted a reference that indicated that ammonium salts and oxides of both nitrogen and sulfur are respiratory irritants that cause or exacerbate bronchoconstriction. His investigation indicated that several chemicals in the patient's workplace were respiratory irritants that would explain her symptoms. He supported his diagnosis by noting that the patient's history met many of the criteria needed to diagnose workplace-related illness (Table 91–2).

TABLE 91–2. CRITERIA FOR ESTABLISHING WORK-RELATEDNESS OF OCCUPATIONAL DISEASE

Known and documented occupational exposure to a suspected causative agent
Symptoms compatible with the suspected workplace exposure
Suggestive or diagnostic physical signs
Similar problems in co workers or workers in related occupations
Periodicity of complaints related to work
Confirmatory industrial hygiene or other environmental monitoring data
Scientific biologic plausibility
Biologic (tissue or fluid) confirmation
Lack of an obvious nonoccupational cause

This case illustrates an important point about MSDSs: Some are excellent; others are incomplete and inadequate. Health care providers should not rely on these sheets as the sole source of information. Although this information may be easily obtained from large companies, smaller employers may have little written information available. In this patient's case, direct communication with the chemical manufacturer was necessary. Chemical manufacturers generate scientific and health data in the course of seeking approval from the Environmental Protection Agency (EPA) to manufacture chemical substances and mixtures. In addition, Section 8(c) of the Toxic Substances Control Act (TSCA) requires chemical manufacturers to report records of significant adverse reactions to human health or the environment. When contacting chemical manufacturers, physicians should ask to speak with a toxicologist, chemist, or someone in the products information department.

Unions

Labor unions should not be overlooked as sources of information on toxic exposures. At the local level, union officers, health and safety committee members, and shop stewards may be able to provide material safety data sheets, exposure data, medical and epidemiologic information, and reports of incidents or cases of interest in a particular plant. The health and safety department of the American Federation of Labor and Congress of Industrial Organizations (AFL-CIO) in Washington, D.C., can provide information on occupational health and safety activities as well as advice on which member unions may be of specific help. At the international level, unions often have well-trained health and safety professionals who may provide or suggest sources of helpful information. In addition, some cities have a coalition of occupational safety and health groups that may provide information about other known exposed/affected workers.

Government Agencies

Appendix A describes the most relevant government agencies, and Table 91–3 lists their telephone numbers.

Telecommunications and On-line Databases

Printed material is often adequate to determine the adverse health effects of chemical exposures, but some re-

TABLE 91–3. NATIONAL CHEMICAL INFORMATION TELEPHONE NUMBERS

Agency	Telephone Number and On-Line Services
Agency for Toxic Substances and Disease Registry, Division of Toxicology	404–639–6300 (.ATSDRI.ATSDR.CDC.GOV:8080\)
National Institute for Occupational Safety and Health	800–356–4674 FAX 513–533–8573 (PUBSTAFT@NIOSHBT1.CDC.GOV)
National Toxicology Program, Public Information Office	919–541–3991 (WWW.NIEHS.NIH.GOV)
Toxic Substance Control Act Assistance Office	202–554–1404 (WWW.EPA. GOV)

sources may be unavailable to physicians, and textbook publication usually lags 2 years or more behind new information. As a result, up-to-date findings and reports may be missed if the practitioner relies solely on printed material. Table 91–4 lists available databases likely to provide useful, up-to-date information on all aspects of toxic exposures. Unfortunately, not all of these databases are available to practitioners, but database vendors can provide access to them (Table 91–5).

What Are the Obligations of the Health Care Provider to the Individual Patient, Co-workers, Government, and Community?

Occupational diseases and injuries are in principle preventable. Physicians who diagnose a work-related disease or injury have an opportunity, and even an ethical obligation, to participate in the identification and control of workplace hazards and the prevention of further occupational illness and injury. Physicians can choose from a range of possible follow-up measures, the goals of which are to prevent recurrence or worsening of the disease or injury in the patient and to prevent the development of disease or injury in other potentially exposed workers. Some of these activities may necessitate contact with occupational medicine physicians, toxicologists, industrial hygienists, lawyers, journalists, government officials, management personnel, and union officials.

Obligations to the Patient

Inform the Patient That the Illness May Be Work-Related. When it is determined that the workplace is a factor in the etiology or aggravation of the patient's illness, this fact and its implications should be discussed with the patient. It should never be assumed that the patient is fully aware of the health risks associated with any workplace exposure. He or she should be provided information regarding the nature of workplace hazards, their health risks, and preventive measures as well as recommendations regarding continued exposure.

Suggest How the Patient Can Reduce the Exposure. In some cases the patient can take steps to reduce exposure. Adjustments in work habits that may be helpful may include using a respirator or other personal protective equipment provided by the employer, using workplace shower and change rooms to avoid carrying toxic chemicals from the workplace to the home, and avoiding ingestion of workplace toxins by careful handwashing before eating or smoking and by taking lunch, coffee, and smoking breaks away from the work station. Obviously, these recommendations assume that the employer provides the appropriate equipment and facilities, which is often not the case. The most effective hazard-control measures require significant commitment by and cooperation from the employer (Appendix B).

The resident advised the patient that her respiratory symptoms appeared to be exacerbated by her workplace exposures. He suggested that he call her supervisor to discuss the problem; she agreed. The supervisor indicated that he was aware of the patient's symptoms and had tried to accommodate her by warning her not to come in when the suspect chemicals were used. The resident expressed concern that, although it seemed to help, this solution did not prevent exposure entirely and, in fact, resulted in continued risk to other workers.

The resident made several suggestions to reduce the potential for exposure and perhaps prevent this patient's symptoms and the development of symptoms in other workers, which included enclosing the dipping process or installing better local exhaust ventilation over the dip tanks, improving general ventilation, and instituting an educational program to teach the employees how best to handle the chemicals, for example, when they refilled the dip tanks. The resident suggested that the employer contact the factory's insurance carrier, which may have a staff industrial hygienist who could coordinate all of these activities, as well as provide environmental sampling and monitoring.

Suggest the Patient Remove Himself or Herself from the Exposure. The employer may be willing to transfer the patient to a location away from the offending hazard. This may result in a reduction in pay, seniority, or other benefits, which may be compensable under Workers Compensation. The employment provisions of the Americans with Disabilities Act require employers to make "reasonable accommodations" for both work- and non-work-related disabilities. Nevertheless, the employer may decide to terminate rather than accommodate the patient. The patient should be counseled carefully, and other options should be explored.

The patient's situation was made easier by an accommodating employer. Because her job involved mostly paperwork, she was moved out of the production area, into the offices located on a separate floor of the plant. Her supervisor agreed that this was a relatively

TABLE 91–4. DATABASES WITH INFORMATION ON INDUSTRIAL TOXIC EXPOSURES

Database	Producer	Description	On-Line Services[a]
CA Search	CA Service	Chemical reference	1, 2, 11
Chemical Carcinogenesis Research Information System	NIH, National Cancer Institute	Records of bibliographic references/data on test conditions and results of co-carcino-genicity, mutagenicity	3, 5, 8, 9
Chemical Exposure	Science Applications Internat. Corp	Citations to chemicals identified in human biologic media	3
Chemtox Online	Health/Environmental Information Resource Consultants, Inc.	Integrates toxicologic and regulatory information on more than 6400 chemicals	3
Chemical Regulations and Guidelines System (CRGS)	CRC Systems, Inc.	U.S. regulations on chemical substances	3
Chemical Safety Newsbase	Royal Society of Chemistry	Information on hazardous effects of chemicals and processes in industry and laboratories	3
Clinical Toxicology of Commercial Products (CTCP)	Dartmouth Medical School, University of Rochester	Corresponds to Gosselin: *Clinical Toxicology of Commercial Products*	9
Dermal Absorpt Data Base	Office of Pesticides and Toxic Substances (EPA)	Information on health effects related to approximately 655 chemical substances entering via a dermal route	9
EMBASE	Elsevier Science Publisher	Biomedical literature related to human medicine	3, 8, 12
Environmental Bibliography	Environmental Studies Institute	Environmental hazards (including health hazards)	3
Hazardline	Occupational Health Services, Inc.	Data on over 78,000 hazardous chemicals	2, 8
Hazardous Substances Data Bank	NLM-Toxicology Info Program	Data on over 4100 known toxic substances	5, 7, 12
HEALTHSAFE	Cambridge Scientific Abstracts	Worldwide literature relating to public health, safety, and industrial hygiene	12
Laboratory Hazards Bulletin	Royal Society of Chemistry	Over 5000 citation on hazards encountered in chemistry laboratories	11, 12
Medical Science Research	Elsevier Applied Science Publishers Ltd.	Full text research papers in field of medicine	2, 8
MEDLINE	NLM	Worldwide biomedical literature	3, 8, 12
MSDS-CCOHS	Canadian Centre for Occupational Health and Safety	Material Safety Data Sheets in the workplace	12
NIOSHTIC	NIOSH	Over 138,000 citations since 1973 on all aspects of OS&H	3
NTIS	National Technical Info Service	Technical reports in biologic and other sciences	1, 2, 3, 11
Occupational Safety & Health Reporter	Bureau of National Affairs, Inc.	Full text of OS&H Reporter—recent developments in OS&H	
Registry of Toxic Effects of Chemical Substances (RTECS)	NIOSH	Toxicologic evaluation of chemical substances	3, 5, 9, 12
SCI Search	Institute for Scientific Information	Wide range of scientific technologic disciplines (corresponds to coverage in Science Citation Index and Current Contents)	3
TOXLINE	NLM Toxicology Info Programs	15 discrete files relating to all areas of toxicology	3, 5
TSCA Chemical Substances Inventory	DIALOG and EPA	Dictionary listing of all chemical substances in commercial use in the U.S. since 1979	3

EPA = Environmental Protection Agency; NIOSH = National Institute for Occupational Safety and Health; NIH = National Institutes of Health; NLM = National Library of Medicine.
[a]Numbers refer to services listed in Table 91–5.

easy accommodation that could allow the patient to work more regularly.

Advise the Patient to Notify the Employer and to Consider Obtaining Legal Advice. Patients who are suffering from a work-related illness may be entitled to Workers Compensation benefits, Social Security disability, or other government-sponsored benefit programs. In addition, they may have a valid claim against the manufacturer of a chemical, a defective product, or another third party. The degree and extent of disability necessary to bring a successful claim varies.

TABLE 91–5. KEY TO ON-LINE SERVICES

1. **CISTI**
National Research Council Canada
Ottawa, Ontario K1A0S2
Canada
800–668–1222
WWW.CISTI.NRC.CA/CISTI/CISTI.HTML

2. **Information Handling Services**
15 Inverness Way East
PO Box 1154
Englewood, CO 80150
303–790–0600
800–241–7824
TWX 910–935–0715
WWW.IHS.COM

3. **KNIGHT RIDDER Information Services, Inc.**
2440 El Camino Real
Mountain View, CA 94040–1400
800–334–2564
415–528–7709
TWX 910–339–9221
WWW.KRINFO.COM

4. **Lexus-Nexus**
PO Box 933
Dayton, OH 45401
937–865–6800
WWW.LEXUS-NEXUS.COM

5. **National Library of Medicine**
Toxicology Information Program
8600 Rockville Pike
Bethesda, MD 20894
800–638–8480
WWW.NLM.NIH.GOV

6. **National Technical Information Service**
Office of Product Management
5285 Port Royal Road
Springfield, VA 22161
703–487–4929
TELEX 899405
WWW.NTIS.GOV

7. **Oak Ridge National Laboratory** (TIRC)
Toxicology Information Response Center
1060 Commerce Park MS-6480
Oak Ridge, TN 37831–6050
423–576–1746

8. **OVID Technologies**
333 7th Avenue
4th Floor
New York, NY 10001
212–563–3006
800–289–4277 = Utah
WWW.OVID.COM

9. **OXFORD Molecular**
810 Gleneagles Court
Suite 300
Baltimore, MD 21286
410–821–5980
800–247–8737
WWW.OXMOL.COM

10. **PaperChase**
350 Longwood Avenue
Boston, MA 02115
800–722–2075
WWW.PAPERCHASE.COM

11. **QUESTAL • ORBIT Inc.**
8000 Westpark Drive
Suite 301
McLean, VA 22102
703–442–0900
WWW.QUESTAL.ORBIT.COM\PATIENTS

12. **STN International**
c/o Chemical Abstracts Service
2540 Olentangy River Road
PO Box 3012
Columbus, OH 43210
800–848–6533
800–848–6538
TELEX 6842086 CHMAB
TWX 810–482–1606
WWW.CAS.ORG

13. **U.S. Dept. of Health and Human Services**
Public Health Service
National Institute for Occupational Safety and Health
Registry of Toxic Effects of Chemical Substances
4676 Columbia Parkway
Cincinnati, OH 45220–1998
800–356–4674
PUBSTAFT@NIOSH DT1.CDC.GOV

14. **U.S. Environmental Protection Agency**
Office of Prevention, Pesticides, and Toxic Substances
401 M Street, SW, MS-7407
Washington, DC 20460
202–260–3944
WWW.EPA.GOV

Once a patient is informed that he or she has a work-related illness, strict time limits are set in motion, and failure to use them can preclude the patient from successfully filing a claim or receiving needed benefits. The patient should be advised to provide written notice immediately to his or her employer of a work-related illness (supported by a physician's letter) and to seek legal advice about statutes of limitations and other requirements. If there is a union at the workplace, it may be able to advise and assist the patient.

The patient planned to file for Workers Compensation benefits for payment of her medical bills and lost salary.

Initiate Periodic Health Surveillance. Depending on the exposure or the diagnosis, periodic monitoring for changes in health status may be recommended (Appendix B).

Obligations to Co-workers

A patient with a work-related illness should be advised to inform co-workers about his or her condition. If the patient belongs to a union, he or she should inform the union representative. If there is no union, the patient may contact OSHA or discuss the situation with the employer.

If the patient is a union member and agrees, the physician should contact the union, which may assist in hazard investigation, identify and warn other workers potentially affected by the hazard, and pressure the employer to take corrective action if it is unwilling to do so. The union can also help the patient to obtain any available benefits. The patient can sometimes identify appropriate contacts, such as shop stewards, members of the union's health and safety or workers compensation committees, an occupational health specialist employed by the union at the local or national level, or an official of the union local.

Committees on Occupational Safety and Health (COSH), coalitions of labor, health, and legal professionals and community and environmental activists working to prevent job related illness and injury may be able to help with both diagnosis and follow-up of an occupational disease. These groups provide education and technical assistance nationwide on a range of topics, including the health effects of specific hazards, control measures, how to use government agencies, and the legal rights of disabled workers.

Obligations to Notify the Government

States may have laws that require reporting of occupational disease. If management and the company medical department are uncooperative despite notification that a hazardous situation exists, OSHA should be contacted, with the patient's consent. In addition to the federal agencies specifically empowered to protect worker health and safety, physicians may contact the state or local health department, which may initiate action or may refer the problem to one of the federal agencies.

Obligation to Inform Colleagues and the Public

It is not implausible that an individual primary care physician or specialist would be the first to suspect a link between a workplace exposure and a serious health problem, especially if he or she practices in a small town or industrial area or provides health care to worker groups through a company or union. Armed with an increased index of suspicion and the occupational history, the physician may be able to alert workers and companies and prevent the occurrence of a major health problem. Even if the physician chooses not to be involved in subsequent investigation or research, it is important that information about suspected problems and hazards be made available to workers and employers in similar industrial settings, government agencies, healthcare professionals, and, perhaps, the public at large. Case reports in the medical literature, at medical meetings, or through the media can be very helpful in this regard.

Appendix A

The Occupational Safety and Health Administration (OSHA) of the U.S. Department of Labor is responsible for setting and enforcing workplace health and safety standards. It is empowered to investigate occupational health and safety complaints and can inspect worksites and levy fines for violations of its standards. In approximately half of the 50 states, the OSHA program is implemented by a state agency. Individual workers, their representatives (unions), or their physicians can file a complaint with the state or federal OSHA program and request an inspection. Although OSHA regulations protect workers from discrimination and punishment by their employer, who may be angered by their filing a complaint, this protection is usually difficult to enforce and discrimination is difficult to prove.

Some state OSHA agencies have separate enforcement and consultation arms. This means that companies can request assistance from the occupational health specialists in the consultation branch without fear of reprisal from the enforcement branch. Healthcare workers should be familiar with the functions of their state agency and workers' rights under the law.

The National Institute for Occupational Safety and Health (NIOSH) of the U.S. Department of Health and Human Services is part of the Centers for Disease Control. It is not a regulatory agency. Briefly, NIOSH is responsible for researching the causes of occupational disease and injury and methods for their prevention and control; evaluating workplace conditions; recommending exposure limits to OSHA for standard setting; and training occupational health and safety professionals. It is empowered to conduct on-site evaluations of health hazards in response to requests from employee representatives or employers. After conducting these evaluations, NIOSH investigators immediately contact OSHA, the employees, and the employer if they find that the workers are in imminent danger.

As part of the process of recommending exposure standards to OSHA, NIOSH develops comprehensive documents that critically evaluate all available scientific data on particular chemicals. These "criteria documents" review the chemical's properties, production methods, uses, and workers at risk as well as studies of exposure effects in humans and animals. Methods of screening, surveillance, and control are presented. The agency periodically issues technical reports and special occupational hazard reviews of specific occupations. In conjunction with OSHA, NIOSH develops and disseminates health hazard alerts to inform employers, employees, and healthcare professionals of serious health effects of particular chemicals.

Physicians and other healthcare professionals can be placed on the NIOSH mailing list by writing to Publications Dissemination, DTS, NIOSH, 4676 Columbia Parkway, Cincinnati OH 45226-1998. Through its computerized database of trade name ingredients gathered from the National Occupational Hazard Survey, NIOSH also provides information by telephone (free of charge) when only a trade name is known (Table 91–4).

The Environmental Protection Agency (EPA) is charged with protecting the nation's land, air, and water. The agency administers a number of laws designed to preserve the public health and environment, one of which is the Toxic Substances Control Act (TSCA). This act authorizes the EPA to collect information on chemical risks from manufacturers and processors. The act requires the agency to review information on new chemicals and new uses of chemicals before they are manufactured. Unless designated a trade secret, this information is subject to disclosure and is, therefore, available. The TSCA assistance office may be most useful when resource materials and government documents contain no information about the chemicals or processes in question.

The National Toxicology Program (NTP) is a federal program established in 1978 to develop scientific information on exposure to toxic chemicals. The Public Information Office responds to requests for information on specific chemicals.

The Agency for Toxic Substances and Disease Registry (ATSDR) is part of the Public Health Service created by Congress to implement the health-related sections of laws that protect the public from hazardous wastes and environmental spills of hazardous substances. In 1986, the Superfund Amendments and Reauthorization Act (SARA) made amendments to the initial enabling legislation of 1980 and broadened ATSDR's responsibilities in the areas of health assessment, toxicologic databases, information dissemination, and medical education. One of its offices, the Office of Health Assessment, provides emergency response for toxic and environmental disasters, consults in public health emergencies, assesses hazardous waste sites, provides technical assistance to agencies and organizations, and estimates health risks to humans from exposure to hazardous substances. The program areas in which ATSDR operates include health assessments, toxicologic profiles, emergency response, and exposure and disease registries.

Appendix B—Industrial Hygiene Control Measures

Initial Workplace Evaluation

The Occupational Safety and Health Act (OSHA) places legal responsibility for providing a safe and healthy workplace squarely on the employer, who is in the best position to make any modifications necessary to prevent additional work-related illness and injury. The physician may wish to initiate a dialogue with a patient's employer to promote preventive action but should do so only with the patient's consent, as the law may not always protect a worker who has suffered a job-related illness or injury from harassment, discrimination, or termination. Consent is necessary even if the patient is not referred to by name.

Because the initial contact may influence subsequent events, it is important to identify the appropriate person, perhaps someone in the company medical department, the patient's supervisor, the plant's safety officer, or the shop manager. If management is willing to examine the hazardous conditions, a plant walk-through inspection can provide unique insight and information usually unavailable in an office setting. A walk-through helps persons involved understand the work environment, identify safety and health hazards, assess control measures, and recognize opportunities for prevention, and also facilitates a good working relationship with key personnel in management and labor. The physician with a number of patients who work in the plant or who provides health services to the workers through the company or labor union may wish to be involved in the walk-through. Assistance with plant inspections can be obtained from occupational health specialists, such as occupational physicians or industrial hygienists.

Methods of Prevention Available to Management

Industrial Hygiene Sampling and Monitoring. Equipment exists to measure airborne concentrations of toxic chemicals, noise levels, radiation levels, temperature, and humidity. Employees can be fitted with pumps and other devices to measure individual exposure levels at the breathing zone, where, depending on what controls are used, concentrations may vary from those in the general work area. These results can then be compared with OSHA and other available standards to help determine the extent of the hazard and to formulate a control plan. OSHA requires that employers monitor the levels of only a few specific hazards, including asbestos, formaldehyde, lead, vinyl chloride, noise, and ethylene oxide; ongoing sampling of the remaining 60,000 chemicals used in the workplace is not required. Where industrial hygiene sampling has been performed, OSHA's medical access standard gives any exposed worker or his or her representative the right to review and copy all sampling data.

Engineering Controls. Health and safety professionals prefer, and OSHA regulations require, where feasible, the use of engineering controls to reduce worker exposure to hazardous substances or agents. Engineering controls are preferred because they intercept hazards at their source or in the workplace atmosphere before they reach the worker. Control methods directed at the worker, such as personal protective equipment, are the least favored measures.

Engineering controls include substitution of less toxic agents or substances, redesign or modification of process or equipment to reduce hazardous emissions, isolation of a process through enclosure, automation of an operation, and installation of exhaust systems that remove hazardous dusts, fumes, and vapors. Local exhaust systems, such as hoods, are preferable to general dilution ventilation because the former removes contaminants closer to their source and at relatively high rates.

Engineering controls have several advantages over control measures focused on the worker. Properly installed and maintained engineering controls are reliable and consistent, and their effectiveness does not depend on human supervision or interaction. They can limit exposure through several routes, such as inhalation and skin absorption, simultaneously. In addition, engineering controls do not place a burden on the worker or interfere with worker comfort or safety.

Work Practices. Work practices are procedures that the worker can follow to limit exposure to hazardous agents. Examples are the use of high-powered vacuum cleaners instead of compressed air cleaning and pouring techniques that direct hazardous material away from the worker. Although not as effective as engineering controls, work practice can be a useful component of an overall hazard control program.

Administrative Controls. Administrative controls reduce the duration of exposure for any individual worker or reduce the total number of workers exposed to a hazard. Examples are rotation of workers into and out of hazardous areas so that no one worker is exposed full time and scheduling procedures likely to generate high levels of exposure, such as cleaning or maintenance activities, during nights or weekends. The latter sometimes exposes more workers to a hazard that causes effects at low doses.

Personal Protective Equipment. Personal protective equipment, such as respirators, earplugs, gloves, and hard hats, is the least effective but most commonly used control method. Employers favor personal protective equipment over the institution of more costly engineering controls, safe work practices, and administrative controls.

Respirators and other forms of personal protective equipment are generally hot, uncomfortable, and awkward to wear and may make it difficult for workers to breathe, speak, or hear, depending on the equipment involved. Consequently, workers often remove or refuse to wear the protection. Respirators put extra stress on the heart and the lungs. Both respirators and earplugs limit conversation and therefore present a safety hazard in themselves.

Because personal protective equipment does not stop a hazard from getting into the environment, if it fails the worker is entirely vulnerable to exposure. In addition, generally only one route of exposure is protected. For example, the commonly used half-mask respirator still leaves the skin and eyes exposed.

Choosing the right piece of personal protective equipment can be difficult and may depend on the nature and extent of the hazard. For example, each type of respirator is rated for the amount of protection it provides; as would be expected, the cost of a respirator increases with its protection factor. Use of the wrong type of respirator can leave the worker insufficiently protected.

Half-mask respirator cartridges are available in various colors, coded to the contaminant filtered out of the breathing environment. If the wrong cartridge is used, the worker is effectively unprotected from the hazardous contaminant. To be effective, a respirator must be meticulously fit to the individual worker. Failure to achieve a proper seal negates the respirator's usefulness. High cheek bones, dentures, scars, perspiration, talking, head movements, and facial hair can prevent a proper seal. This is often ignored or overlooked by employers who adopt a "one-size-fits-all" policy.

Even assuming that each employee is provided the proper respirator, the respiratory protection program may not be effective. OSHA requires that employers institute a program of proper fit testing, cleaning, maintenance, and storage of respirators, which can be at least as costly as the institution of engineering controls.

In some instances, the use of personal protective equipment may be unavoidable. An employer may need to control a hazardous exposure through a combination of measures, such as engineering controls and personal protective equipment. Ideally, the employer is using personal protective equipment as a control of last resort and in strict compliance with OSHA standards.

Worker Education and Training. Regardless of the control measures employed, workers and supervisors need to be educated in the recognition and control of workplace hazards and the prevention of work-related illness and injury. The OSHA Hazard Communication Standard requires that employers train workers in how to detect the presence or release of hazardous chemicals, their physical and health hazards, methods of protection against the hazards, and proper emergency procedures, as well as how to read the labeling system and how to read and use a Material Safety Data Sheet.

With the passage of federal, state, and local right-to-know laws, many consulting companies now offer hazard communication training. These programs are of uneven quality. Those that focus on acute hazards, ignore chronic effects, and emphasize personal protective equipment over other control measures may not be effective in training workers to recognize and control chemical hazards.

Medical Monitoring. Together with worker education and industrial hygiene, a medical program can form the foundation of an effective occupational disease prevention program. Medical monitoring, however, is fraught with technical and ethical pitfalls. Medical monitoring encompasses both medical screening and medical surveillance. Medical screening refers to the cross-sectional testing of a population of workers for evidence of excessive exposure or early stages of disease that may or may not be related to work and that may or may not influence the ability to tolerate or perform work. Medical surveillance refers to the ongoing evaluation, by means of periodic examinations, of high-risk individuals or potentially exposed workers to detect early pathophysiologic changes indicative of significant exposure. OSHA requires little in the way of medical surveillance, although several OSHA standards require employers to institute medical surveillance programs, for example, for workers exposed to asbestos, arsenic, vinyl chloride, lead, and ethylene oxide. Depending on the potential exposure, medical surveillance can include a history and physical examination, chest radiograph, pulmonary function test, blood and urine tests, and other laboratory evaluations.

A medical surveillance program can also include biologic monitoring, the purpose of which is not to identify the occurrence of disease but to measure the uptake or presence of a particular substance or its metabolites in body fluids or organs. Ideally, this occurs before any pathophysiologic damage has been done. Consequently, biologic monitoring is potentially a primary preventive measure. For example, several volatile organic compounds, such as benzene and toluene, if inhaled or absorbed through the skin, produce metabolites that can be measured in urine.

Biologic monitoring can have some advantages over

air monitoring because it measures the absorption of a substance by the body as opposed to ambient levels in the workplace. The amount of a chemical absorbed may not be closely correlated to ambient levels for several reasons, including differences in individual work habits, use and effectiveness of personal protective equipment, dermal absorption of chemicals unrelated to their concentration in the air, and nonoccupational exposures.

Biologic monitoring, however, has several very significant limitations. For most chemicals, there are no standards of "normal" or "safe" levels against which results can be compared. Obtaining specimens may be difficult, expensive, and invasive (eg, fat biopsies to detect dioxin). The timing of specimen collection is critical, as different chemicals have different biologic half-lives. The storage and handling of specimens and interpretation of results are also vulnerable to error. Nevertheless, if carefully designed and implemented, biologic monitoring can be a useful complement to a comprehensive industrial hygiene program.

With the exception of biologic monitoring, medical monitoring programs identify disease processes already underway and are therefore, at best, a form of secondary prevention. Medical and biologic monitoring programs are abused by employers who use results to remove workers instead of remediating the hazard. To be an effective preventive measure, these programs must be coordinated with environmental monitoring programs that identify the nature, source, and extent of workplace hazards; implementation of engineering controls and other measures that control hazards as close as possible to the source; and worker education programs that, at a minimum, inform workers of exposures, their effects, and proper control measures.

Preemployment and preplacement physical examinations are another type of medical screening, often favored by employers. The new Americans with Disabilities Act (ADA) regulates the timing, scope, content, and use of these examinations and the information gathered. The ADA prohibits medical examinations and inquiries before a firm job offer has been made. After a job offer has been made, examinations and inquiries can be conducted to determine whether an applicant can perform a job safely and effectively. The physician evaluates past medical history, current symptoms, and physical laboratory findings to determine whether an individual currently has the physical or mental abilities necessary to perform the essential functions of the job and whether the individual can do so without posing a "direct threat" to the health or safety of self or others. (This threat must be more than theoretical and cannot be based on some future time; the threat must be concrete and relatively immediate.)

There are few tests and few conditions that are good predictors of either ability to perform a task or increased susceptibility to a particular exposure. Many workers and their advocates see preplacement examinations as a way for employers to choose the "fittest" worker and to avoid their legally mandated obligation to provide a safe and healthy workplace for all workers. Physicians asked by an employer to perform preplacement examinations should be sure that each component of the examination relates to the actual job the individual is being hired to perform and the actual risks he or she will encounter on the job. Both the law and sound occupational medicine practice dictate that the employer's attention and efforts be directed toward redesign of the job and its hazards, so that it is safe and healthy for all workers to perform.

Both medical monitoring programs and preplacement examinations raise issues of doctor–patient confidentiality. Employee medical records should be available only to the corporate medical or first aid department, and not to the personnel office and general management. Unless required by statute, employers should never be told the results of history, physical, or diagnostic examinations unless the patient gives his or her written consent. The examining physician need only inform the employer that an individual is or is not capable of performing a particular job with or without specified restrictions; the physician should not disclose diagnostic information about medical conditions.

Suggested Reading

Americans with Disabilities Act. PL No. 101-336; 42 USC 12101 et seq (1990).

Bresnitz E, Rest K, Miller N: Clinical industrial toxicology: An approach to information retrieval. Ann Intern Med 1985; 103:967–972.

Burgess WA: Recognition of Health Hazards in Industry: A Review of Materials amd Processes, 2nd ed. New York, Wiley, 1995. Excellent descriptions of industrial processes and general types of exposures. Not to be used when you already know the chemical name(s).

Clayton GD, Clayton FE, eds: Patty's Industrial Hygiene and Toxicology, 4th ed. New York, Wiley, 1995. Excellent reference on occupational health and general toxicologic data.

Comprehensive, Environmental Response, Compensation and Liability Act (CERCLA or Superfund) of 1980.

Equal Employment Opportunity Commission, Department of Labor. Equal Employment Opportunity for Individuals with Disabilities, Final rule. Fed Reg 1991;56:35725–35755.

Gosselin RE, Smith RP, Hodge HC: Clinical Toxicology of Commercial Products, 5th ed. Baltimore, Williams & Wilkins, 1984. Useful as a first step for identifying trade name products and their ingredients, addresses and telephone numbers of companies, and estimates of relative toxicities of various chemicals.

Hamilton A, Hardy HL, Finkel AJ: Hamilton and Hardy's Industrial Toxicology, 4th ed. Boston, John Wright PSG, 1983. Describes occupational diseases secondary to known exposures.

Himmelstein JS, Frumkin H: The right to know about toxic exposures: Implications for physicians. N Engl J Med 1985; 312:687–690.

Key MM: Occupational Diseases: A Guide to Their Recognition. Washington, DC, US Department of Health, Education, and Welfare, 1977. DHEW publ. no. (NIOSH) 79-116. Helpful in identifying chemicals associated with various occupations and routes of entry; not comprehensive.

Levy B, Wegman D, eds: Occupational Health, 2nd ed. Boston,

Little Brown, 1988. Excellent general reference on occupational health. Not a compendium of chemical substances, but presents a good overall approach and good for more common hazardous substances.

Lewis RJ: Hazardous Chemicals Desk Reference, 4th ed. New York, Van Nostrand Reinhold, 1996. A compendium of over 20,000 chemicals, including specific health hazards, chemical and physical properties, relevant regulations, and more. A good first book to use if you know the specific chemical(s).

Mackison FW, Stricoff RS, Partridge LJ Jr, eds: Occupational Safety and Health Guidelines for Chemical Hazards. Washington, DC, Department of Health and Human Services and Department of Labor, 1995, DHHS publ. no. (NIOSH) 81-123, Gordon Press. A looseleaf compendium describing chemical properties, health hazard information, recommended medical practices, monitoring and measurement procedures, personal protective equipment, and waste removal and disposal. Exposure limits may be out of date for some substances, but this is a good resource for identifying the health effects of several hundred chemicals.

Mackison FW, Stricoff RS, Partridge LJ Jr, eds: NIOSH Pocket Guide to Chemical Hazards. Cincinnati, US Department of Health and Human Services, Public Health Service, Centers for Disease Control, National Institute for Occupational Safety and Health, 1993, DHHS (NIOSH) publ. no. 90-117, Diane Publishing. General industrial hygiene and medical monitoring practices, chemical structures or formulas, identification codes, synonyms, exposure limits, chemical and physical properties, incompatibilities and reactivities, measurement methods, respirator selections, signs and symptoms of exposure, and procedures for emergency treatment.

Occupational Safety and Health Act of 1970. PL 91-596, [bu10]2(b), 1970.

Plunket ER: Handbook of Industrial Toxicology. New York, Chemical Publishing, 1987. Suggests potential chemical exposures for one or more signs or symptoms.

Plunket ER: Occupational Diseases: A Syllabus of Signs and Symptoms. Stamford, CT, Bartlett, 1977. Suggests potential chemical exposures for one or more sign or symptom.

Poisindex: Rocky Mountain Poison and Drug Center, Emergency Information Center, and University of Colorado Health Sciences Center. Microfiche or CD-ROM database listing chemicals and trade names as well as detailed treatment and management protocols.

Proctor NH: Chemical Hazards of the Workplace, 3rd ed. New York: Van Nostrand Reinhold, 1991. Mainly monographs on chemical substances with entries on nomenclature, physical form of substance uses, means of exposure, toxicology, treatment, and medical control. A reasonable book to consult initially.

Rest KM, Hake JC, Cordes DH: The Occupational and Environmental History. Tucson, Arizona Center of Occupational Safety and Health, 1983.

Rom W, ed: Environmental and Occupational Medicine, 2nd ed. Boston, Little Brown, 1992. Excellent general textbook on occupational medicine. Not comprehensive for many specific chemicals, but excellent discussions of pathophysiologic mechanisms.

Rosenstock L, Cullen MR: Clinical Occupational Medicine. Philadelphia, Saunders, 1986. A new housestaff-type manual. Brief and not comprehensive.

Sullivan JB, Krieger GR: Hazardous Materials Toxicology: Clinical Principles in Environmental Health. Baltimore, Williams & Wilkins, 1992. Excellent reference with sections on basic science and clinical principles of hazardous materials toxicology, organ system toxicity with principles of immediate treatment and evaluation, specific hazardous substances and general industries, and regulatory, health, and safety aspects of hazardous materials.

Superfund Amendments and Reauthorization Act (SARA) of 1986.

Sweet D, ed: Registry of Toxic Effects of Chemical Substances: A Comprehensive Guide. Cincinnati, US Department of Health and Human Services, National Institute for Occupational Safety and Health, 1993, Diane Publishing. Brief descriptions of substances for which acute or other toxic effects have been reported in the literature, as well as references to government regulations and standards. Also online at National Library of Medicine.

Toxic Substances Control Act. PL 94-469, [bu10]90, stat 2003, Oct 11, 1976.

Wexler P: Information Resources in Toxicology, 2nd ed. New York, Elsevier, 1988. No specific information on exposures but the best compendium of all the available information resources in toxicology, including print, audiovisual, government documents, journals, books, databases, newsletters, organizations, and international resources.

Zenz C, ed: Occupational Medicine Principles and Practice, 3rd ed. Chicago, Mosby–Year Book, 1993. Broad, detailed overview of occupational health issues. Not the first book to consult for the hazardous effects of a specific substance.

CHAPTER 92

Hazardous Materials Release and Decontamination

Robert J. Nadig

What Is Meant by "Hazardous Materials"?

Hazardous materials are substances that can potentially cause adverse health effects in individuals via skin or mucous membrane contact and/or skin, respiratory, or gastrointestinal (GI) absorption. Hazardous materials include chemicals, biologic agents, and radioactive substances, which may be in the solid, liquid, or gaseous state.

Before discussing the hospital management of a patient, it is important to review the prehospital management of patients in a hazardous material (HAZMAT) incident. These principles are important, particularly when the patient enters the ED without the benefit of prehospital management.

What Is the Likelihood That a Patient Involved in a Hazardous Materials Release Will Come to a Particular ED?

In the United States in 1991 there were 25,800 reported hazardous materials incidents. Injuries were reported in 893 incidents, evacuations were determined to be necessary at 352 sites, and 97 reports involved deaths. A significant number of incidents—7335—were transportation-related. A train derailment resulted in the release of the pesticide methyldithiocarbamate into the Sacramento River. The pesticide reacted with water to form methylisothiocyanate, a severe respiratory and dermal irritant. Evacuations at times involved a substantial number of people. For example, 50,000 residents of Duluth, Minnesota, and Superior, Wisconsin, were evacuated as a result of the release of aromatic hydrocarbon vapor.

Hazardous waste sites remain a consequential concern with respect to hazardous materials release. At least 10,000 sites have been identified for the federal Superfund program. The EPA estimated that approximately 255 million metric tons of hazardous waste is generated annually in the United States. Furthermore, in the past, only about 10% of hazardous waste was disposed of properly. Experience has shown that there are probably more hazardous waste sites yet to be identified. The sites already identified are in rural, suburban, and urban location, so no geographic area is without risk of a hazardous materials incident.

What Is of Primary Concern at Any Hazardous Materials Release?

The primary concern at any hazardous materials release is the protection of the responders. Prevention of secondary contamination of responders or areas outside the "hot zone" (see below) is of utmost importance. The goal of an emergency response is to prevent or limit overall casualty numbers and severity, but it is recognized that the situation is never improved when the rescuer also becomes a victim. Injury to the responder is very likely at a hazardous materials incident unless the appropriate precautions are taken.

What Is the Key to a Successful Response to a Hazardous Materials Release? What Is Secondary Contamination?

Organization is the key to a successful response to a hazardous materials release. This requires planning, preparation, and training before the incident and coordination throughout the incident. With protection of responders, the next priority is to restrict access (and thus potential exposure) only to personnel essential for extrication of the victims. Similarly, egress must be controlled so that all potentially contaminated individuals, whether rescuers or victims, are decontaminated and contamination is not extended to medical personnel, equipment, and facilities (secondary contamination).

Thus, the ideal hazardous materials release scenario would be organized so that medical providers, including emergency medical service (EMS) providers, would ordinarily be excluded from any risk of secondary contamination or exposure. Figure 92–1 demonstrates the typical organization of a hazardous materials response. There are three basic zones at a hazardous materials incident: the hot zone, the decontamination zone, and the support zone. The hot zone is the area immediately around the incident, where there is a danger of exposure. Only firefighters or specialized hazardous materials responders should operate in this zone. The decontamination zone includes the firefighters, specialized responders, and decontamination personnel. All other personnel should remain in the support zone.

An access control point is used to limit access to any particular zone by the essential personnel. Protection from contamination cannot be compromised by medical activities. Rescue and decontamination must occur first. When an EMS provider is part of the response team in the hot zone, he or she should have appropriate training and perform with level A protection (see below), just like any other response team member.

Table 92–1 summarizes the goals of an EMS hazardous materials responder.

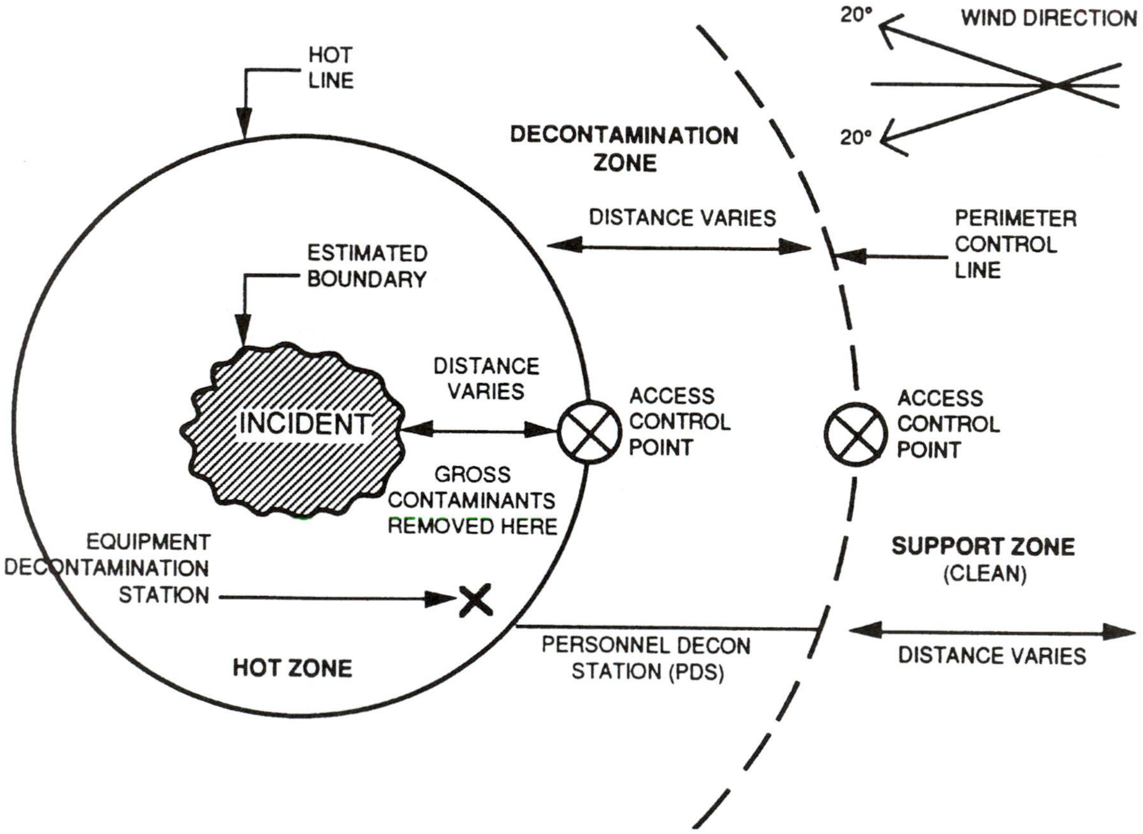

Figure 92–1. Organization of a hazardous materials incident. *(From ATSDR: Medical Management Guidelines for Acute Chemical Exposures U.S. Department of Health and Human Services. 1992.)*

TABLE 92–1. GOALS OF AN EMERGENCY RESPONDER AT A HAZARDOUS MATERIALS INCIDENT

1. Protect yourself. Approach the scene cautiously, arriving upwind. Maintain a safe distance and inspect the scene from a nearby elevated area, such as a hill. Respect established exclusion zone and resist the temptation to rush in to attempt a rescue. Report to the incident commander. Maintain a buddy system, if feasible.
2. Attempt to identify the chemical product. [Become familiar with the Department of Transportation (DOT) placard system, Material Safety Data Sheets (MSDSs) or shipping papers, and the National Fire Protection Association (NFPA) hazardous labeling system.] After identifying the chemical, contact the regional poison center for information about health effects, medical treatment, and decontamination guidelines.
3. Determine the potential for secondary contamination. Know whether the substance is likely to create a risk to you or others in the support zone, ambulance, or hospital if decontamination is not completed at the scene.
4. Be certain that adequate decontamination measures have been performed.
5. Provide basic and advanced life support as required and transport victims to an appropriate medical facility as soon as possible.

Reprinted, with permission, from ATSDR: Managing Hazardous Materials Incidents, vol 3: Medical Management Guidelines for Acute Chemical Exposures. U.S. Department of Health and Human Services, 1992.

What Can Be Done to Prevent Emergency Personnel From Becoming Victims Themselves?

In 1989, the Occupational Safety and Health Administration (OSHA) mandated training for emergency responders via the Hazardous Waste Operations and Emergency Response Standard (29 CFR 1910.120). Training is required for all employees "who participate, or are expected to participate, in an emergency response to hazardous substance accidents."

The OSHA standard mandates that all emergency responders be familiar with U.S. Department of Transportation regulations concerning the meaning of placards placed on vehicles warning about and identifying hazardous materials. The placards incorporate universal symbols to identify types of substances. In addition, the United Nations Classification numbering system may be present on vehicles that transport hazardous materials (Table 92–2 and Fig. 92–2).

Although not specifically mandated by the OSHA standard for all categories of emergency responders in all settings, training usually includes a thorough review of the OSHA Hazard Communication Standard (HazCom), which includes labeling at manufacturing sites. This system is the familiar placard divided into quadrants, each of which supplies certain information about the chemical (Fig. 92–2). In addition, HazCom training teaches the use of a Material Safety Data Sheet (MSDS), which provides detailed information about the chemical (see Chap. 91).

What Are the Levels of Personal Protective Equipment?

Both respiratory protective equipment and dermal protective clothing are needed to protect against potential chemical exposures. Respiratory protective equipment can be divided into devices that purify the air before it reaches the worker and those that supply fresh air to the worker from a pure source. Air-purification devices are lighter-weight and less expensive than air-supply devices, but they rely on filters. Filters have a limited capacity, usually are effective for only a limited range of chemical types, and were developed for use at room temperature. Air-supply devices seriously limit the mobility of the worker as a result of bulky hoses or heavy tanks, and the self-contained breathing apparatus (SCBA) offers only a limited air supply.

Chemical protective clothing is either fully encapsulating or nonencapsulating. Fully encapsulating clothing achieves airtight protection of the skin and respiratory tract. Nonencapsulating clothing protects against skin contamination from splashes and sprays but does not provide skin protection against gases, vapors, or dusts.

TABLE 92–2. UNITED NATIONS CLASSIFICATION SYSTEM

United Nations Class or Division numbers may be displayed at the bottom of placards or in the hazardous materials description on shipping papers. In certain cases, this Class or Division number may replace the written name of the hazard class in the shipping paper description. The Class and Division numbers have the following meanings:

Class 1	*Explosives*
Division 1.1	With a mass explosion hazard
Division 1.2	With a projection hazard
Division 1.3	With predominantly a fire hazard
Division 1.4	With no significant blast hazard
Division 1.5	Very insensitive explosives
Class 2	*Gases*
Division 2.1	Flammable
Division 2.2	Nonflammable
Division 2.3	Poisonous
Division 2.4	Corrosive (Canadian)
Class 3	*Flammable liquids—flashpoint*
Division 3.1	$<-18°C$ (0°F)
Division 3.2	$>-18°C$ (0°F) but $<23°C$ (73°F)
Division 3.3	$>23°C$ up to 61°C (141°F)
Class 4	*Flammable solids, spontaneously combustible materials, and materials that are dangerous when wet*
Division 4.1	Flammable solid
Division 4.2	Spontaneously combustible materials
Division 4.3	Materials that are dangerous when wet
Class 5	*Oxidizers and organic peroxides*
Division 5.1	Oxidizers
Division 5.2	Organic peroxides
Class 6	*Poisonous and etiologic (infectious) materials*
Division 6.1	Poisonous materials
Division 6.2	Etiologic (infectious) materials
Class 7	*Radioactive materials*
Class 8	*Corrosives*
Class 9	*Miscellaneous hazardous materials*

Reprinted, with permission, from 1987 Emergency Response Book: Guideline for Initial Response to Hazardous Materials Incidents. U.S. Department of Transportation, publ. No P5800.4.

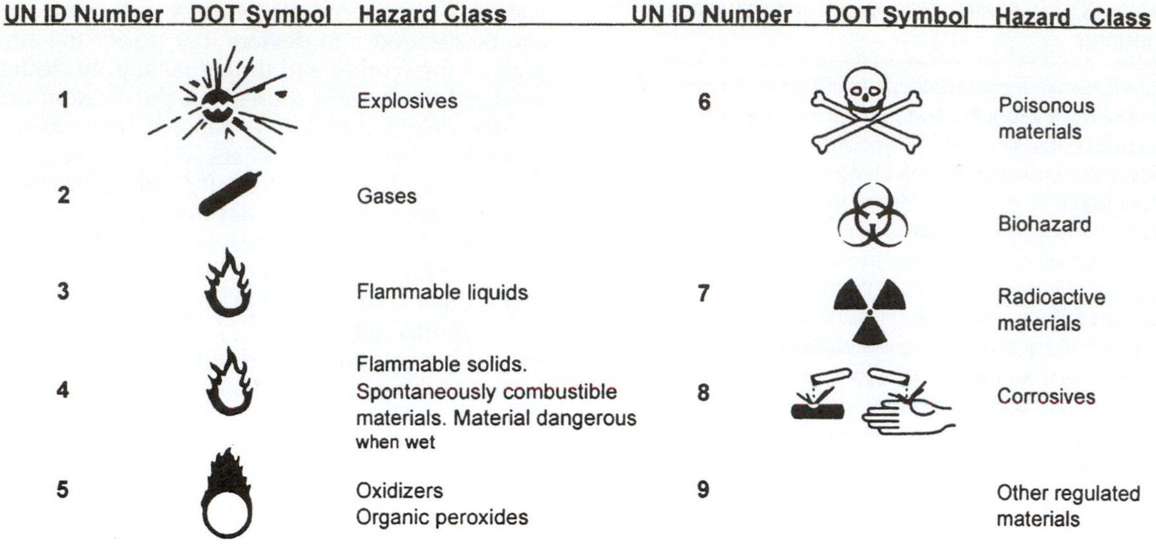

UN ID Number
DOT Symbol
Hazard Class
1
Explosives
2
Gases
3
Flammable liquids
4
Flammable solids. Spontaneously combustible materials. Material dangerous when wet
5
Oxidizers Organic peroxides
UN ID Number
DOT Symbol
Hazard Class
6
Poisonous materials
Biohazard
7
Radioactive materials
8
Corrosives
9
Other regulated materials

Health (Typically in blue on placard)

0 None	Not generally considered hazardous.
1 Slight	Can cause irritation.
2 Moderate	Can cause injury. Requires prompt treatment.
3 High	Can cause serious injury despite medical treatment.
4 Extreme	Can cause death or major injury.

Flammability (Typically in red on placard)

0 None	Will not burn.
1 Slight	Can ignite after considerable preheating.
2 Moderate	Can ignite after moderate preheating. Combustible liquid.
3 High	Can ignite at normal temperatures. Flammable liquid.
4 Extreme	Very flammable gas or very volatile flammable liquid.

Reactivity (Typically in yellow on placard)

0 None	Normally stable. Not reactive to water.
1 Slight	Normally stable. Unstable at high temperature and pressure, or if water added.
2 Moderate	Normally unstable, may be explosive if water added.
3 High	Explosive with strong initiating force, heat or water.
4 Extreme	Readily explosive under normal conditions.

Figure 92–2. Chemical Hazard Rating Signs; 4 = extreme, 3 = high, 2 = moderate, 1 = slight, 0 = insignificant. *(From Borak J, Callan M, Abbott W: Hazardous Materials Exposure: Emergency Response and Patient Care. Englewood Cliffs, NJ, Prentice Hall, 1991.)*

The Environmental Protection Agency (EPA) has designated four levels of personal chemical protective equipment, with level A providing the greatest and level D the lowest level of protection (Table 92–3). Level A protection is required when the potential for high-level contamination of the atmosphere exists. Use of level A protection is standard at all unknown hazardous materials incidents. When the risk from dermal contact with gases, vapors, or dusts is very remote, level B protection is sometimes considered because of the increased ease of dressing and movement and overall greater comfort compared to level A equipment. It is often possible to only wear level B protection in the decontamination zone when the risk of inhaling off-gassing vapor is low and the decontamination zone is far enough removed from the hot zone that there is no risk of exposure. Firefighters typically enter structural (not chemical) fires wearing the level B protection. Level C is used when the hazardous materials have been identified and likely air contamination levels characterized, allowing determination of what air-purification device (respirator) is needed. Use of level C protection also assumes that there is no risk of dermal or mucous membrane absorption from air contamination, as it provides only skin and mucous membrane protection against splashes and sprays. Level D protection actually provides no specific respiratory or skin protection. The category was created to describe what *not* to wear. Table 92–4 describes various types of protective gloves.

How Should the Emergency Department Manage a Hazardous Materials Incident?

Table 92–5 outlines the goals of the ED provider in hazardous material incidents. The Joint Commission for the Accreditation of Health Care Organizations (JCAHO) requires that hospitals have standing disaster committees and perform at least one internal and one external disaster drill per year. The reader is referred to any standard emergency medicine text for review. In addition, hospitals should be an integral part of the local emergency response plan. In 1986, the EPA, through legislation that

TABLE 92–3. LEVELS OF PERSONAL CHEMICAL PROTECTIVE EQUIPMENT

A	Positive-pressure self-contained breathing apparatus Fully encapsulating chemical-resistant suit Double layer of chemical resistant gloves Chemical resistant boots Airtight seals between the suit, gloves, and boots
B	Positive-pressure self-contained breathing apparatus Chemical-resistant, long-sleeved suit Double layer of chemical resistant gloves Chemical resistant boots
C	Full-face air purification device Chemical-resistant suit Chemical-resistant outer gloves Chemical-resistant boots
D	No respiratory protection device Common work clothes

Adapted, with permission, from ATSDR: Managing Hazardous Materials Incidents, vol 3: Medical Management Guidelines for Acute Chemical Exposures. U.S. Department of Health and Human Services, 1992.

reauthorized the SuperFund (Title III of Superfund Amendments and Reauthorization Act of 1986; SARA), required the development of emergency response plans at local, state, and regional levels nationwide. SARA Title III specifically mandates the establishment of regional emergency planning committees to include representatives of all parties necessary to respond to a hazardous materials incident. Reporting of the presence and use of hazardous materials to the local committees is also mandated. In addition, access by emergency responders and the community to the database of locations and identities of hazardous material is authorized.

The emergency planning is designed to call upon greater local, state, and regional resources, as required. When the level of resources required or the threat posed is significant, the Federal Emergency Management Agency (FEMA) becomes directly involved in coordinating the overall response.

TABLE 92–5. GOALS OF THE HOSPITAL PROVIDER IN HAZARDOUS MATERIALS INCIDENTS

1. Assess the potential for secondary contamination. If there is a risk assure that decontamination takes place at the scene or outside the main ED prior to medical treatment.
2. Quickly move victims without prior decontamination to a predesignated decontamination area.
3. Obtain toxicity information from a regional poison center.
4. Provide basic and advanced life support.
5. Perform adequate and appropriate laboratory testing.
6. Determine the need for prolonged observation, hospital admission, and follow-up.

Adapted, with permission, from ATSDR: Managing Hazardous Materials Incidents, vol 3: Medical Management Guidelines for Acute Chemical Exposures. U.S. Department of Health and Human Services, 1992.

How Should a Contaminated Person Be Treated in the Emergency Department?

Unfortunately, not all hazardous materials releases are responded to ideally. It is always possible that the ED will be confronted with the issue of contamination from a patient who walks in. Planning and organization are key to preventing untoward medical outcomes for both the patient, other patients at the health care facility, and health care providers. An additional important consideration is that if decontamination is not handled appropriately in the ED, it may compromise the entire hazardous materials response. Furthermore, the expense of remediating otherwise preventable widespread contamination of the ED, for example with asbestos, is expensive and time consuming.

Table 92–6 outlines a strategy for confronting a potentially contaminated patient. The overriding goal is to

TABLE 92–4. CHEMICAL PROTECTIVE GLOVES

Type	General Comments	Useful For	Poor Utility
Natural rubber	Limited protection	Alcohols and dilute bases	Most organic chemicals and solvents
Nitrile rubber	Good overall protection	Alcohols, oils and fuels, alkalis, amines, and phenols	Aromatic and halogenated hydrocarbons, ketones, and esters
Neoprene rubber	More expensive protection than nitrile rubber gloves	Strong alkalis, dilute acids, alcohols, phenols, oils and fuels, aliphatic hydrocarbons	Aromatic and halogenated hydrocarbons, ketones, and concentrated acids
Butyl rubber	Twice the cost of neoprene gloves	Alkalis and many organic compounds	Aliphatic, aromatic, halogenated hydrocarbons, gasoline
Viton	Ten times more costly than the most expensive glove listed above	Organic solvents (aliphatic, aromatic, and halogenated hydrocarbons) acids	Ketones, esters, aldehydes amines

Note: The latex or vinyl gloves typically found in medical facilities offer protection only from aqueous biologic fluids are of no protection in a hazardous chemical release.

Adapted, with permission, from Borak J, Callan M, Abbott W: Protection of the health care system. In: Hazardous Materials Exposure: Emergency Response and Patient Care. Englewood Cliffs, NJ, Prentice-Hall, 1991, p. 184.

TABLE 92–6. GUIDELINES FOR PROTECTION OF PERSONS IN THE EMERGENCY DEPARTMENT

1. Perform triage outdoors, if possible.
2. Use separate entrance, if possible.
3. Use designated treatment room.
4. Restrict access.
5. Use protective clothing if necessary.
6. Attempt to limit ED from contaminants.
7. Maintain log of persons involved in treatment.
8. Isolate drainage and ventilation and monitor clean-up.

Adapted, with permission, from ATSDR: Managing Hazardous Materials Incidents: Emergency Medical Services—A Planning Guide for the Management of Contaminated Patients. U.S. Department of Health & Human Services; and Borak J, Callan M, Abbott W: Hazardous Materials Exposure: Emergency Response and Patient Care. Englewood Cliffs, NJ, Prentice Hall, 1991.

restrict access and adequately protect responders to avoid secondary contamination. The first step is to decontaminate the patient. If a dedicated decontamination space is not available, as is usually the case, it may be necessary to cover the floors and walls with plastic and possibly shut off the ventilation to prevent spread of contamination. Table 92–7 lists materials and supplies necessary for decontamination.

Two examples of gurneys outfitted for self-contained decontamination are shown in Figure 92–3. Figure 92–4 is a flowchart of the protocol in the decontamination zone at the incident site. The same principles and protocol must be followed in the ED if there is a risk that the patient is significantly contaminated.

When there is no risk of significant secondary contamination, or after decontamination, health care providers should proceed with medical management as for any other patient. If the patient has ingested a chemical, then provisions should be made for the immediate isolation of any vomitus.

TABLE 92–7. EMERGENCY DECONTAMINATION SUPPLIES

Item	Use
Geiger-Müller counter	Surveying for radioactive contamination
Spare batteries	For Geiger-Müller survey meter
Plastic bags of all sizes	Disposing of contaminated materials
Plastic sheeting	Covering ventilation ducts, if necessary, and contaminated areas
Remote handling tongs	Handling contaminated objects
Radiation warning rope or ordinary rope or cord	Roping off and securing contaminated areas
Radiation caution signs and labels	Labeling contaminated areas and objects
Containers of various volumes or plastic bags	Collecting contaminated materials (ie, liquids)
Masking tape	Sealing plastic bags and other containers
Soap and water	Decontamination
Cotton swabs	Decontamination
Absorbent materials	Decontamination
Waste containers (lined with removable plastic bags)	Radioactive waste disposal
Rubber gloves	Handling contaminated materials
Shoe covers or boots	Avoiding contamination of shoes
Gowns and masks	Avoiding contamination
Shower with self-contained water drainage, or plastic hose and child's plastic pool	Avoiding contamination

How Can It Be Determined Whether a Patient Is Significantly Contaminated and Whether There Is a Risk of Secondary Contamination?

The significance of contamination and the risk of secondary contamination depends on the nature of the agent, the route of exposure, and the extent of contamination. As a practical matter, when there is insufficient information, proceed conservatively and institute the decontamination protocol. Victims exposed to only gases or vapor are not significantly contaminated if their clothes are not soaked or there is no gross residue on their skin or clothing. Vomitus may still present a risk, however.

A Geiger-Müller counter or similar instrument should be available to check for radioactive contamination. Usually, the hospital radiology department can provide this equipment.

How Should a Patient Be Decontaminated?

The first step in decontamination is to remove all clothes and any other reservoirs of contamination. Wiping or brushing off visible liquids and dusts is the second step, if the dust does not become airborne. Dilution with water and a mild soap is the most readily available means of decontamination. Special attention should be given to decontamination of the body hair, skin folds, orifices, toes, fingernails, and eyes, especially in a critically ill patient. Burns and wounds should be debrided and irrigated. For some substances there may be specific agents that are preferred for decontamination. For example, low-molecular-weight polyethylene glycol is recommended for the removal of phenols from skin.

Radioactive materials require special consideration. There are three types of exposures that might occur in a radioactive hazardous materials incident: irradiation, contamination, and incorporation. When irradiation, such as exposure to gamma or x-rays, occurs, the victim is not radioactive and no decontamination precautions are necessary. If the victim is contaminated with a radioactive dust, solid, or liquid, decontamination would be the same as for any other hazardous dust, solid, or liquid, but the Geiger-Müller counter may be used to monitor the success of decontamination. Incorporation occurs when radioactive material is inhaled or ingested or contaminates a wound. Decontamination (decorporation) involves trying to neutralize or remove the radioactive isotope from the body. Diethylenetriaminepentaacetic acid (DTPA) has been

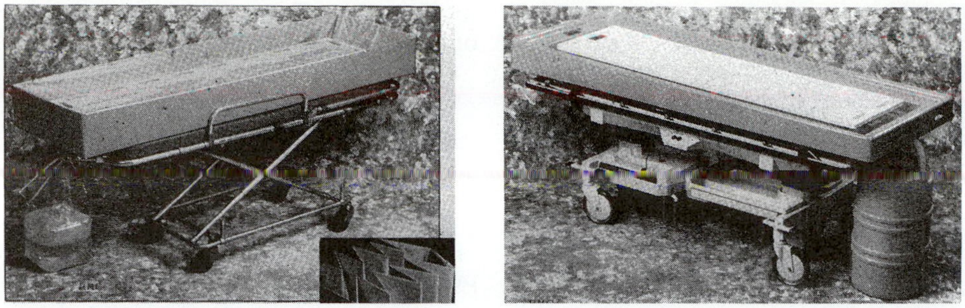

Figure 92–3. Examples of commercial decontamination stretchers with self-contained collection systems. *(Courtesy of Radiation Management Consultants, Philadelphia, PA. From Borak J, Callan M, Abbott W: Hazardous Materials Exposure Emergency Response and Patient Care. Englewood Cliffs, NJ, Prentice Hall, 1991.)*

used to chelate actinide isotopes and enhance elimination by excretion. Another example of decorporation includes iodide supplements to block uptake of radioactive iodide into the thyroid. Antacids have been used to precipitate many metals in the stomach as insoluble hydroxides. Aluminum phosphate gel can effectively reduce intestinal absorption of radioactive strontium.

Is the Reactivity of Some Substances With Water a Concern?

One of the first questions regarding chemical contamination concerns the danger of reactivity with water. Water reactivity is a worksite safety concern due to explosions

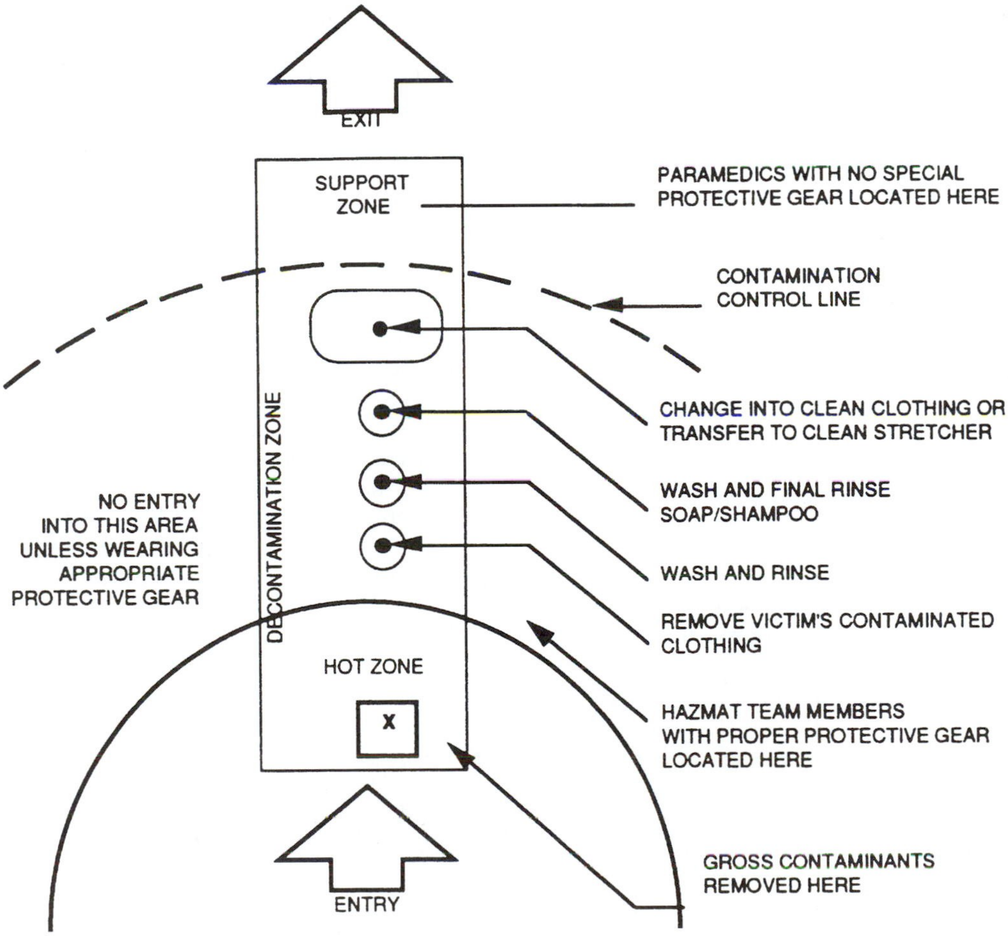

Figure 92–4. Detail of decontamination zone. *(From ATSDR: Medical Management Guidelines for Acute Chemical Exposures. U.S. Department of Health and Human Services, 1992.)*

with bulk amounts of chemicals. Decontamination of victims should not be delayed due to this concern. The flushing actions of the water is very important in separating the hazardous materials from the skin or mucous membranes. Although there may be some reaction when water is applied externally, a hazardous substance that is highly water-reactive will presumably already be reacting with the skin or mucous membranes, since these tissues contain large amounts of water.

What Should Be the Emergency Department Management Strategy for an Unknown or Uncertain Exposure?

In patients with an unknown or uncertain exposure, management is guided by the patient's presentation and history of symptoms and the findings on physical examination. Laboratory testing is directed by symptoms and the physical examination, unless specific information about the identity of the hazardous substance prompts certain testing. For example, a known or suspected carbon monoxide leak would prompt a carboxyhemoglobin level determination. Three important principles influence medical management in a hazardous materials emergency:

1. The onset of severe toxicity may be precipitous.
2. The onset of severe toxicity may be delayed.
3. Although it is usually uncommon, there may be a risk of exposure to more than one agent.

Often the hardest clinical task is not to miss the truly exposed, the truly at risk, and the truly sick. Hazardous materials releases often generate large numbers of "worried well." This is to be expected, but health care personnel must be careful to evaluate fully all persons, so as not to miss the ill patient who may be lost among a crowd of anxious patients.

What Resources Are Immediately Available for Help Clinically?

The regional poison center is the best resource for immediate, up-to-date information on toxicity and clinical management. Chapter 91 details an approach to retrieval of information on chemicals.

Acknowledgment

Lorraine Hartnett, MD contributed to this chapter in a previous edition.

Suggested Readings

ATSDR: Managing Hazardous Materials Incidents, vol 1: Emergency Medical Services—A Planning Guide for the Management of Contaminated Patients. U.S. Department of Health and Human Services, 1992.

ATSDR: Managing Hazardous Materials Incidents, vol 2: Hospital Emergency Departments—A Planning Guide for the Management of Contaminated Patients. U.S. Departments of Health and Human Services, 1992.

ATSDR: Managing Hazardous Materials Incidents, vol 3: Medical Management Guidelines for Acute Chemical Exposures. U.S. Department of Health and Human Services, 1992.

Borak J, Callan M, Abbott W: Hazardous Materials Exposure: Emergency Response and Patient Care. Englewood Cliffs, NJ, Prentice Hall, 1991.

Gough AR, Markus K: Hazardous materials protections in ED practice: Laws and logistics. J Emerg Nurs 1989;15:476–480.

Hazardous Materials Medical Management Protocols. The State of California, Emergency Medical Services Authority, 1992.

Hazardous Substance and Public Health, vol 2(3). U.S. Department of Health and Human Services, The Public Health Service, Agency for Toxic Substance and Disease Registry, July/Aug 1992.

Leonard RB, Ricks RC: Emergency department radiation, accident protocol. Ann Emerg Med 1980;9:462–470.

Merritt NL, Anderson MJ: Malathion overdose: When one patient creates a departmental hazard. J Emerg Nurs 1989; 15:463–465. Case review.

1987 Emergency Response Book: Guidebook for Initial Response to Hazardous Materials Incidents. U.S. Department of Transportation, pub. no. P5800.4.

Rom WN: Environmental and Occupational Medicine, 2nd ed. Boston, Little Brown, 1992.

CHAPTER 93

Methemoglobinemia

Dennis Price

Normal serum level:	1%, slightly higher in infants
Action serum level:	20%: Asymptomatic patient
	10–20%: Symptomatic patient

Values greater than or equal to the action level usually necessitate clinical intervention. Values less than this level may necessitate intervention based on the clinical condition of the patient.

A 27-year-old man was brought to the emergency department (ED) by ambulance because of shortness of breath. The patient had a history of acquired immunodeficiency syndrome (AIDS), complicated by *Candida* esophagitis and two episodes of *Pneumocystis carinii* pneumonia. His medical regimen included zidovudine for a CD4 count of 200/mm^3, fluconazole for his esophagitis, and dapsone for *Pneumocystis carinii* prophylaxis. He previously had an allergic reaction while on trimethoprim and sulfamethoxazole . The patient stated that he recently become depressed over the death of a close friend and took "all of his medications" in a suicide attempt. He vomited once at home and began getting short of breath about 2–3 hours later.

On physical examination, the patient appeared cachectic and acutely short of breath. His vital signs were: blood pressure, 90/40 mm Hg; pulse, 140 beats/min; respiratory rate, 40 breaths/min; rectal temperature, 100.2°F (37.9°C). A pulse oximeter read 88% saturation. The skin was diaphoretic with old track marks. Examination of the head, eyes, ears, nose, and throat was remarkable for perioral cyanosis. His neck was supple and without jugular venous distention. The chest was clear to auscultation with good air flow. Cardiac examination revealed a tachycardia but normal S_1 and S_2 heart sounds with 1/6 systolic ejection murmur heard best at the left lower sternal border. The abdomen was nontender with good bowel sounds and no hepatomegaly. The extremities were without clubbing or edema, but marked cyanosis of the nail beds was noted. Neurologic assessment demonstrated intact orientation, concentration, and memory. No cranial nerve abnormalities were noted; deep tendon reflexes were intact and symmetric; and plantar extension was noted. Motor and sensory testing were grossly normal.

The patient was placed on a 100% nonrebreathing oxygen mask and connected to a cardiac monitor. An intravenous (IV) line was started and blood samples were obtained for a complete blood count, electrolytes, BUN, glucose, and acetaminophen level. After a few minutes of oxygen therapy, the patient's heart rate decreased to 128 beats/min, but he was still cyanotic and tachypneic and the pulse oximeter continued to read 86–88% oxygen saturation. Arterial blood gas analysis (on oxygen) was obtained, but the house officer was concerned that it was a venous specimen because it was darkly colored. The results were: pH, 7.34; PCO_2, 30 mm Hg; PO_2, 400 mm Hg; calculated oxygen saturation, 99%. The patient was given 60 g of activated charcoal in a slurry of water and 50 mL of 70% sorbitol orally.

The electrocardiogram (ECG) showed a sinus tachycardia with normal axis, intervals, ST segments, and T waves. The chest radiograph was normal. Acetaminophen was not detected. The rest of the laboratory evaluation was not remarkable. Co-oximetry testing revealed: total hemoglobin, 8.4 g/dL; oxyhemoglobin, 64%; methemoglobin, 33%; deoxyhemoglobin, 1%; carboxyhemoglobin, 2%.

The patient received 60 mg of methylene blue (0.1 mL/kg of 1% solution) IV over 20 minutes. His pulse oximeter transiently dropped to 73–75% for several minutes. About 40 minutes later, he was noted to be less cyanotic, and a repeat methemoglobin level was 6%. Three hours later he was again short of breath and cyanotic, and his methemoglobin had risen to 24%. Another 60 mg of methylene blue was given with a good response. Another dose of activated charcoal was administered 4 hours after the first dose.

Over the first 24 hours, the patient required a total of 3 doses of methylene blue therapy. His hemoglobin subsequently fell to 6.2 g/dL, and he was transfused with 2 units of packed red blood cells. While in the hospital, he was seen by a psychiatrist and enrolled in an AIDS support group. The patient was discharged 6 days after admission with a hemoglobin of 9.7 g/dL and normal co-oximetry values.

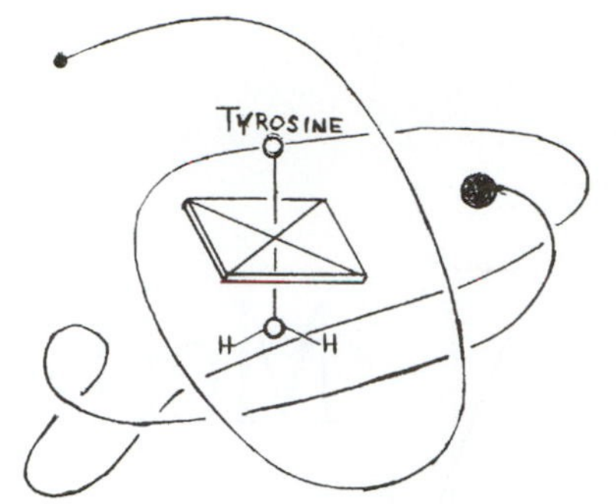

Figure 93–2. Hemoglobin M occurs when histidine is replaced by tyrosine in the amino acid sequence of the polypeptide chain. Hemoglobin M is more easily autooxidized (as shown) to methemoglobin.

What Is the Molecular Biology of Hemoglobin and Methemoglobin?

Hemoglobin consists of four polypeptide chains noncovalently attracted to one another, each of these subunits carries one heme molecule deep within its structure. This protects the iron moiety from ready oxidation (Fig. 93–1). Changes in the amino acid sequence of the polypeptide chain, as occurs in Hemogoblin M, influence this protective "pocket," allowing for easier iron oxidation (Fig. 93–2). This is referred to as hemogoblin autooxidation.[44]

Each heme molecule has an iron atom in the center. This iron is held in position by six coordination bonds.

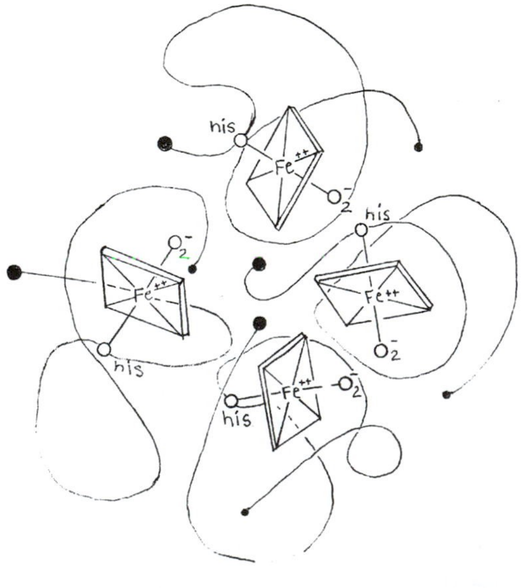

Figure 93–1. The hemoglobin molecule is symbolically represented with its heme center being surrounded by the globin portion of the molecule.

Four of these bonds are with the nitrogen atoms of the protoporphyrin ring, and the fifth and sixth sites are above and below the protoporphyrin plane. The fifth site is occupied by histidine of the polypeptide chain. The sixth coordination site is where most of the activity within hemoglobin occurs. Oxygen transport occurs here and additionally this site is altered with methemoglobinemia and carbon monoxide poisoning (Fig. 93–3).

Hemoglobin will transport the oxygen molecule only when its iron atom is in the reduced ferrous state (Fe^{2+}). During oxygen transport, the iron atom actually transfers an electron to oxygen; thus oxygen is transported as a superoxide charged particle $Fe^{3+}O_2^{-1}$. When oxygen leaves, the ferrous ion is restored and hemoglobin is ready to accept another oxygen molecule. Interestingly, a small percent of oxygen leaves hemoglobin with this shared electron, leaving iron in an oxidized state. This oxidized state of hemoglobin is methemoglobin. (This site then becomes occupied by a water molecule.) This abnormal unloading of oxygen contributes to the baseline level of methemoglobin found in normal individuals. In summary, the differences between hemoglobin and methemoglobin are subtle and involve only a small part of the hemoglobin molecule, but make methemoglobin incapable of oxygen transport.

Oxidant stresses from exogenous sources, such as drugs and toxins, may bring about the loss of an electron from iron and raise the methemoglobin level above baseline. Therapy for methemoglobinemia aims to restore the lost electron.

What Are the Major Diagnostic Considerations When a Patient Presents With Cyanosis?

The majority of patients presenting to the emergency department with cyanosis will do so because of an elevated level of deoxyhemoglobin. Five grams of deoxyhemoglobin will give a patient a bluish discoloration. Tachypnea, tachycardia, and cyanosis may suggest a pulmonary eti-

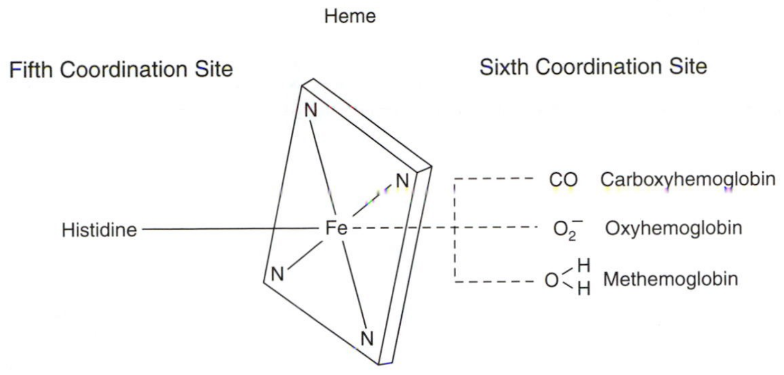

Figure 93–3. The heme molecule is depicted with its bonding sites. Oxyhemoglobin, carboxyhemoglobin, and methemoglobin all involve the sixth coordination bonding site of iron.

ology; however, a failure to respond to oxygen as expected and an arterial blood gas analysis with an elevated PO_2 exclude this diagnosis.

Cyanosis occurs when just 1.5 g/dL (ie, 10% methemoglobin if baseline hemoglobin is 15 g/dL) of hemoglobin has been converted to methemoglobin. Additionally, sulfhemoglobin, another darkly pigmented hemoglobin, will produce a detectable bluish color when the level is 0.5 g/dL.

These abnormal hemoglobin species, which are incapable of oxygen transport and dark in color, must be considered in the evaluation and differential diagnosis of the cyanotic patient. Additionally, some patients may present a mixed etiology for their cyanosis, having both hypoxia for cardiopulmonary reasons and methemoglobinemia from other causes. The blood oxygen-carrying capacity in such situations may be drastically reduced (Fig. 93–4).

How Can the Correct Diagnosis Be Confirmed?

What Is the Role of the Arterial Blood Gases, the Co-oximeter and the Pulse Oximeter?

The key findings in methemoglobinemia are cyanosis unresponsive to oxygen therapy and a normal cardiopulmonary examination. These findings in conjunction with the history of ingestion of a known oxidizing compound suggest the presence of an abnormal hemoglobin, methemoglobinemia. The diagnosis is further suspected by arterial blood gas sampling which reveals a characteristic chocolate brown color (see color plate Fig. 22) and a normal PO_2. The PO_2 reflects the partial pressure of the oxygen dissolved in the blood and thus the adequacy of pulmonary function to deliver oxygen to the blood effectively. It does not measure the more important physiologic parameter, that is, the hemoglobin oxygen saturation or oxygen content of the blood. When the partial pressure of oxygen is known and oxyhemoglobin and deoxyhemoglobin are the only species of hemoglobin, oxygen saturation can be accurately calculated from the arterial blood gas: If, however, other hemoglobins are present, such as methemoglobin or carboxyhemoglobin, then the oxygen-carrying capacity of the hemoglobin must be determined on the co-oximeter (see Chap. 20).

The co-oximeter is a laboratory instrument that evaluates the absorptive characteristics of hemoglobin species at different wavelengths. Most instruments today are capable of measuring blood content of oxyhemoglobin, deoxyhemoglobin, carboxyhemoglobin, and methemoglobin. Some newer instruments can also measure fetal hemoglobin and sulfhemoglobin.[22,70]

The oximeter used at the bedside is a pulse oximeter. These instruments are calibrated to measure only oxyhemoglobin and deoxyhemoglobin in pulsatile blood. The instrument reports only oxyhemoglobin. Because the pulse oximeter measures at only two wavelengths (those wavelengths that optimize the evaluation of oxyhemoglobin and deoxyhemoglobin), pulse oximeters are not accurate when blood contains methemoglobin[50] or other substances that have absorptive characteristics similar to oxyhemoglobin or deoxyhemoglobin, ie, methylene blue.[37,39,67]

Methemoglobin interferes with these readings in a complicated fashion. Initially, the pulse oximeter saturation determination will drop with increasing methemoglobin levels. This fall in saturation is not exactly proportional to the fraction of methemoglobin, however, as the pulse oximeter overestimates the level of oxygen saturation. At methemoglobin concentrations approaching 30%, the pulse oximeter saturation approaches 85% and will show no additional change in saturation, regardless of further increases in methemoglobin concentration.[2,66]

Although the pulse oximeter reading in methemoglobinemia may not be accurate, it may be helpful when we compare it with that of the arterial blood gas. If there is a difference between the measured oxyhemoglobin of the pulse oximeter and the calculated oxyhemoglobin of the arterial blood gas, then a "saturation gap" exists and methemoglobin may be the cause. Methemoglobin can be measured directly on the co-oximeter (Table 93–1).

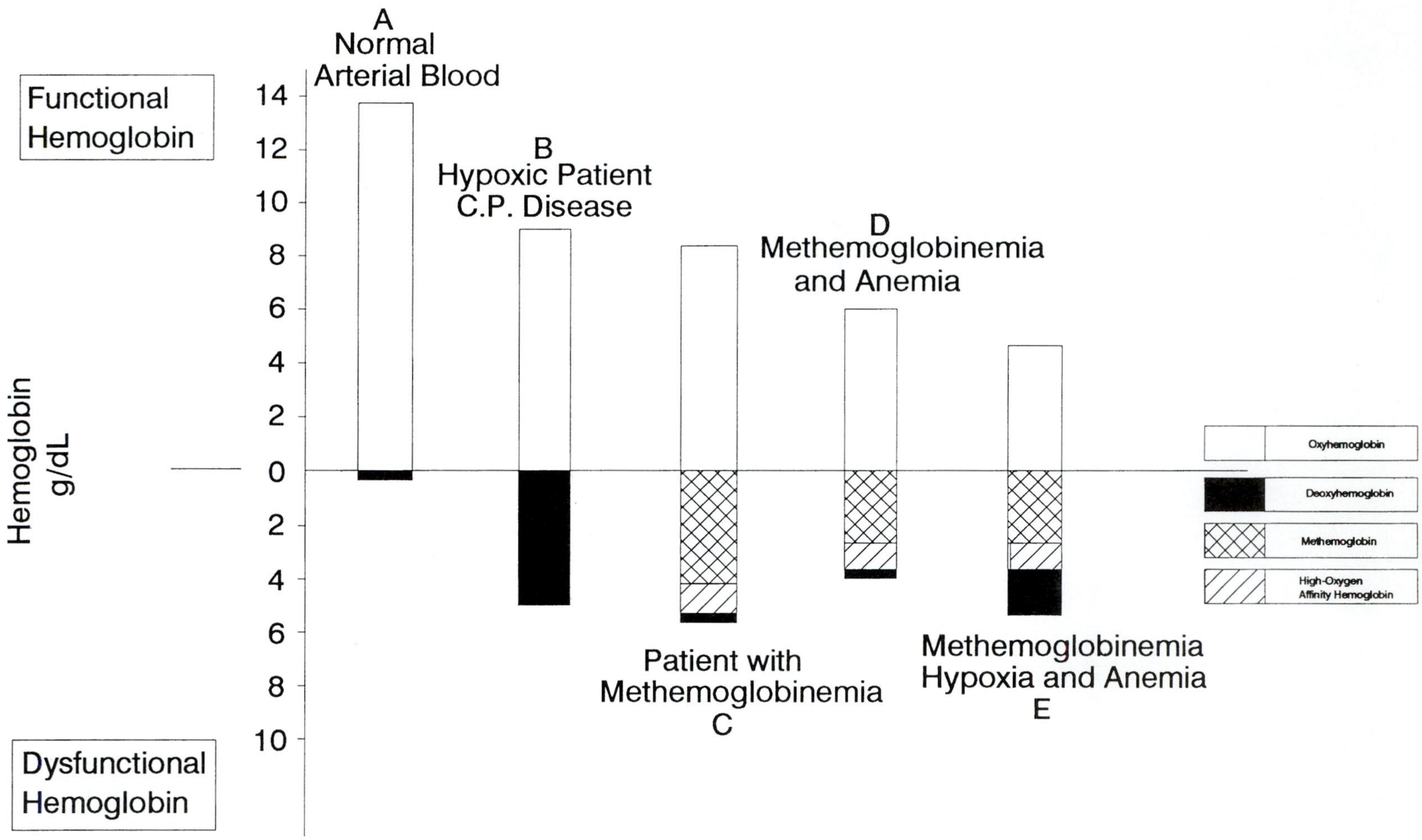

Figure 93–4. Clinical manifestations of methemoglobinemia depend on the level of methemoglobin as well as host factors, such as preexisting disease, anemia, and hypoxemia. **(A)** Blood gas from a normal individual with 14 g/dL of hemoglobin. Almost all hemoglobin is saturated with oxygen. **(B)** Blood gas from a patient with cardiopulmonary (C.P.) disease producing cyanosis in which only 9 g/dL of hemoglobin is capable of oxygen transport. **(C)** Methemoglobin concentration of 28% in an otherwise normal individual will reduce hemoglobin available for oxygen transport at less than 9 g/dL (approximately 4 g/dL of methemoglobin and 1.3 g/dL of high-oxygen-affinity hemoglobin due to the left shift of the oxyhemoglobin dissociation curve). **(D)** The same degree of methemoglobin as in **(C)** but in a patient with a hemoglobin of 10 g/dL. Only 6 g/dL of hemoglobin would be capable of oxygen transport. **(E)** Methemoglobinemia and anemia to the same degree as **(D)** but in a hypoxic patient.

TABLE 93–1. HEMOGLOBIN OXYGENATION ANALYSIS

Measuring Device	Source	What Is Measured	How Are Data Expressed?	Benefits	Pitfalls	Insight
Blood gas analyzer	Blood	Partial pressure of dissolved oxygen in serum	PO_2	Also gives information about pH and PCO_2	Calculates SaO_2 from the partial pressure of oxygen in serum; inaccurate if forms of Hb other than oxyHb and deoxyHb are present	If gap exists between ABG and pulse oximeter an abnormal Hb form may exist
Co-oximeter	Blood	Directly measures absorptive characteristics of oxyhemoglobin, deoxyhemoglobin, methemoglobin, carboxyhemoglobin at different wavelength bands in vitro	SaO_2 % Methb % CoHb % OxyHb %DeoxyHb	Measures hemoglobin species directly	Provides data on hemoglobin only; most instruments will not measure sulfhemoglobin, Hb M, and some other forms of Hb	Most accurate method to determine oxygen content of blood
Pulse oximeter	Monitor	Absorptive characteristics of oxyhemoglobin in pulsatile blood assuming the presence of only oxy- and deoxy-hemoglobin in vivo	Percent oxyhemoglobin	Moment-to-moment bedside data	Inaccurate data if interfering substances are present: methemoglobin, sulfhemoglobin, carboxyhemoglobin, methylene blue	Maximum depression 85% regardless of how much methemoglobin present

Hyperlipidemia interferes with accurate co-oximeter evaluation of blood. Triglyceride levels above 500 mg/dL also produce falsely elevated methemoglobin levels. Lipemic serum should be washed free of this interfering substance in order to evaluate for methemoglobinemia.[46,65]

What Causes Methemoglobin to Rise Above Baseline Levels?

An increase in the concentration of methemoglobin above the normal level can result from (1) the presence of an inherited abnormal hemoglobin structure resulting from various amino acid substitutions, making the hemoglobin more susceptible to oxidation or unsuitable for reduction, such as with Hemoglobin M; (2) hereditary deficiencies of the various methemoglobin reductases (responsible for enzymatically reducing oxidized hemoglobin); or (3) exposure to oxidant stress from various drugs or chemicals that increase the rate of hemoglobin oxidation beyond the reductive capacity of the erythrocyte.

What Are Some Commonly Encountered Oxidant Compounds?

Nitrites, which are powerful oxidizing agents, represent one of the most common groups of methemoglobin-forming compounds.[1] The reaction, which occurs in vivo and in vitro, is complex and poorly understood. When ingested, nitrates are reduced to nitrites by bacteria in the intestinal tract (especially in infants) and can then be absorbed, ultimately leading to methemoglobin production. This conversion is not essential, however, because nitrates themselves can oxidize hemoglobin.[23,27,63] Nitrates have been an all too common cause for well water contamination and infant fatalities associated with methemoglobinemia.[14,43] A number of reports from the midwestern United States demonstrate the problems of poorly constructed shallow wells that permit contamination by surface waters containing varied chemicals, pesticides, fertilizers, and microorganisms.[45] In several South Dakota studies, 20–50% of wells contained coliform bacteria, and the water exceeded the Environmental Protection Agency (EPA) permissible 10 ppm (10 mg/L) of nitrogen as nitrate.[33] These analyses demonstrate the high potential for nitrate contamination of well water.

Nitroglycerin (glyceryl trinitrate) and organic nitrates are more effectively absorbed through mucous membranes and intact skin than from the gastrointestinal (GI) tract. The onset of action is also more rapid and the total effect is much greater through the former.[15,19,53]

Aromatic amino and nitro compounds may indirectly produce methemoglobin. These agents do not form methemoglobin in vitro and are therefore assumed to do so by chemical conversion to some extremely active in vivo intermediate compounds.[9,64]

Elevated methemoglobin and carboxyhemoglobin levels are noted in victims of gas poisoning, fires, and exhaust fume poisoning.[6,32,34,38,61] Heat-induced hemoglobin denaturation and the inhalation of nitrogen oxides are suggested as causative factors for methemoglobin formation. The most common causes of methemoglobinemia are listed in Table 93–2.

How Does the Red Cell Handle Methemoglobin?

Multiple intracellular erythrocyte mechanisms function to maintain the normal level of methemoglobin at less than 1%.[7] All of these systems act as electron donors to the oxidized iron atom. The quantitatively most important reductive system requires nicotinamide-adenine dinucleotide (NADH), which is generated in the Embden-Meyerhof glycolytic pathway (Fig. 93–5). This electron donor, along with the enzyme NADH methemoglobin reductase, reduces the ferric (Fe^{3+}) iron of the heme moiety to the more favorable ferrous (Fe^{2+}) iron state. There are numerous cases of hereditary deficiencies of the enzyme NADH methemoglobin reductase.[30,41,56] Homozygotes for the deficiency usually have methemoglobin levels of 10–50% under normal conditions, without provocation. Heterozygotes do not ordinarily demonstrate methemoglobinemia, except when subjected to the effects of oxidant stresses. This enzyme system lacks full activity until about the age of 4 months; consequently, all infants are more susceptible than adults to oxidizing stresses.[48,68]

TABLE 93–2. COMMON ETIOLOGIES OF METHEMOGLOBINEMIA

Hereditary

Hemoglobin M

NADH methemoglobin reductase deficiency (homozygote and heterozygote)

Acquired

A. Medications

- Amyl nitrite
- Benzocaine
- Dapsone
- Lidocaine
- Nitroglycerin
- Nitroprusside
- Phenacetin
- Phenazopyridine
- Prilocaine (local anesthetic)
- Quinones (chloroquine, primaquine)
- Sulfonamides (sulfanilamide, sulfathiazide, sulfapyridine, sulfamethoxazole)

B. Chemicals agents

- Aniline dye derivatives (shoe dyes, marking inks)
- Butyl nitrite
- Chlorobenzene
- Fires (heat-induced denaturation)
- Food adulterated with nitrites
- Food high in nitrates
- Isobutyl nitrite
- Naphthalene
- Nitrophenol
- Nitrous gases (seen in arc welders)
- Silver nitrate
- Trinitrotoluene
- Well water (nitrates)

Pediatric

Reduced NADH methemoglobin reductase activity in infants (up to 4 months).

Seen in association with low birth weight, prematurity, dehydration, acidosis, diarrhea, and hyperchloremia.

Oxidized iron can be reduced nonenzymatically using ascorbic acid and reduced glutathione as electron donors, but this method is much slower and quantitatively less important under normal circumstances. Within the red cell there is another enzyme system for reducing oxidized heme, dependent on nicotinamide-adenine dinucleotide phosphate (NADPH) generated in the hexose monophosphate shunt pathway (Fig. 93–6). This NADPH, acting as an electron donor, is responsible for only a small percentage of methemoglobin reduction under normal circumstances, while the NADH-dependent methemoglobin reductase plays the major role. Patients with a deficiency of this enzyme therefore do not exhibit methemoglobinemia under normal clinical circumstances.[60] When supplied with an exogenous electron carrier (such as methylene blue), however, this system is accelerated.[24] Methylene blue is reduced to leukomethylene blue using NADPH-dependent methemoglobin reductase and NADPH as the electron donor. Leukomethylene blue directly reduces the heme iron (see Chap. 24). This provides the rationale for the use of methylene blue in situations of severe methemoglobinemia.

The hereditary types of methemoglobinemia are exceedingly rare, with only several hundred cases reported in the literature.[30,40,41,56] Even acquired methemoglobinemia, although more common, remains infrequent, due in part to increased federal regulation of industrial manufacturing methods and food processing,[51] and in part to the limited clinical manifestations at the lower methemoglobin concentrations.

What Is the Symptomatology of Methemoglobinemia?

Symptomatology is determined not only by the absolute concentration of methemoglobin but also by its rate of formation and elimination. Levels of methemoglobin that may be clinically benign when caused by hereditary defects are likely to produce more severe signs if they are acutely acquired. Healthy subjects do not have the compensatory mechanisms that develop over a lifetime with such hereditary compromise (eg, erythrocytosis, increased 2,3-diphosphoglyceric acid).

Certain compounds have characteristics that result in prolonged methemoglobinemia. For instance, dapsone has a very long half-life in overdose situations and is metabolized to a methemoglobin-forming metabolite. Aniline has numerous toxic metabolites capable of oxidizing

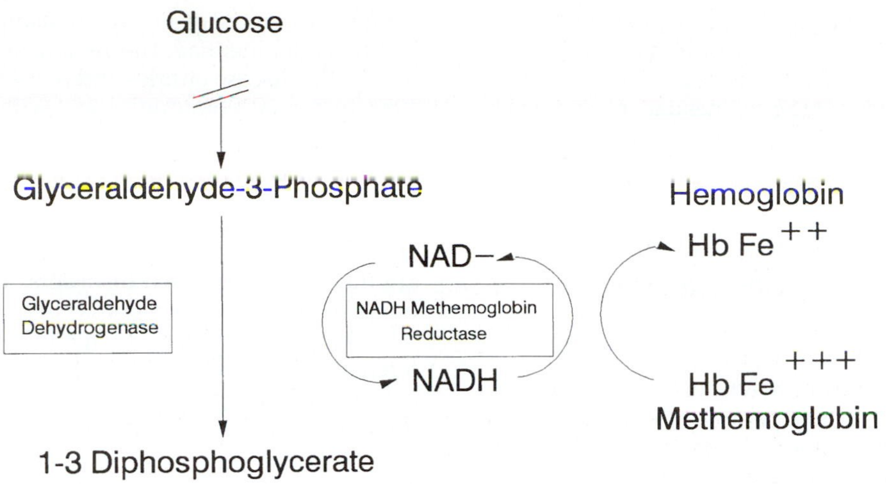

Figure 93–5. The role of glycolysis in the Embden–Meyerhof pathway in the reduction of methemoglobin.

hemoglobin. In the presence of renal failure, drugs such as phenazopyridine (Pyridium) are slowly eliminated, causing prolonged methemoglobinemia. In addition, the compounds producing the oxidant stress may have toxicities unrelated to methemoglobinemia, such as seizures with benzocaine and lidocaine or hypotension with the nitrates.[52]

Since the symptomatology associated with methemoglobinemia is related to impaired oxygen delivery to tissues, prior disease such as congestive heart failure, chronic obstructive pulmonary disease, or pneumonia may greatly increase the toxicity of methemoglobinemia. Anemia has profound effects as well (see Fig. 93–4). Therapy must address diverse issues in any patient with methemoglobinemia. Predictions of symptoms and recommendations for therapy are based on methemoglobin concentrations in previously healthy individuals with normal hemoglobin levels.

The manifestations of toxicity in acquired methemoglobinemias are usually more severe than those produced by a corresponding degree of anemia. This discordance occurs because methemoglobin, as in the case of carboxyhemoglobin, not only decreases the available oxygen-carrying pigment, but also increases the affinity of the unaltered hemoglobin for oxygen, shifting the oxygen hemoglobin dissociation curve to the left, thus further impairing oxygen delivery. (see Chap. 20).[16] This effect has been attributed to the formation of heme compounds intermediate between normal reduced hemoglobin (all four iron atoms are ferrous) and methemoglobin, in which one or more of the iron moieties are in the ferric state.[4,16] The degree to which this high-oxygen-affinity hemoglobin reduces oxygen delivery to the tissues from arterial blood is unclear, because the work was done at partial pressures of oxygen found in venous blood.[16]

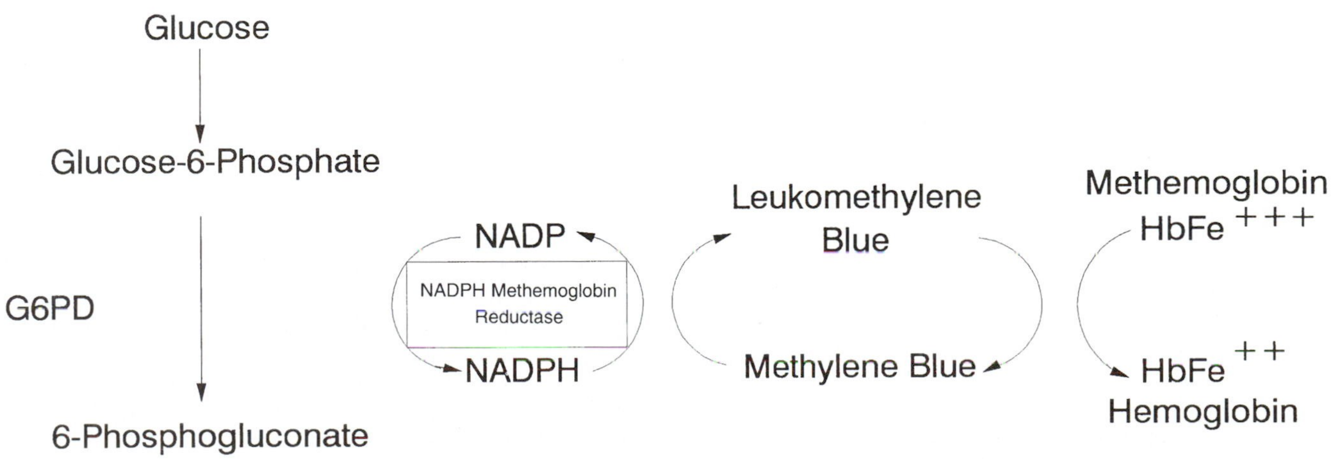

Figure 93–6. The role of hexose monophosphate shunt in the reduction of methemoglobin.

In previously healthy individuals, methemoglobin concentrations of 10–20% usually result in cyanosis without apparent adverse clinical manifestations. At 20–50% concentration, dizziness, fatigue, headache, and exertional dyspnea may develop. Lethargy and stupor usually appear at about 50%, and the lethal concentration is probably greater than 70% (Table 93–3).

What Is the Relationship of Methemoglobinemia to Infancy?

Methemoglobinemia of unknown origin is often reported in infants.[55,59,69] These patients are usually ill for other reasons with an associated methemoglobinemia. Most of these patients are very young (under 6 months) and many are small for their age.[31] Dehydration, acidosis, diarrhea, and hyperchloremia are frequently reported findings in small infants with methemoglobinemia. This may be due to these infants' immature enzyme system with its inability to reduce oxidized hemoglobin.

What Is the Relationship of Methemoglobinemia to Hemolysis?

A review of hemolysis shortly after the discovery of the enzyme defect responsible for oxidant-induced hemolysis (glucose-6-phosphate dehydrogenase) addressed the confusion regarding the relationship of hemolysis and methemoglobinemia.[5] The review stressed the separateness of the disease entities and reaffirmed this position in 1991 (personal communication with E. Beutler). However, confusion persists for a number of reasons. Both hemolysis and methemoglobinemia are caused by the oxidant stress induced by oxidizing compounds. Hemolysis is seen following episodes of methemoglobinemia. Certain erythrocytic protective mechanisms against oxidants are the same in the two disorders. Treatment of methemoglobinemia itself is reported to produce hemolysis.[25,29]

Oxidants produce damage to the erythrocyte at different locations in the two disease entities. Hemolysis occurs when oxidants damage the erythrocyte by acting directly as electron acceptors or through the formation of hydrogen peroxide or other oxidizing free radicals. These compounds are highly reactive and form irreversible bonds with sulfhydryl groups of hemoglobin and the cell membrane.[11] This causes denaturation and precipitation of the protein. These precipitates are sufficient quantitatively to form Heinz bodies within the cell. Cells with large numbers of Heinz bodies are removed by the reticuloendothelial system, producing hemolysis. Methemoglobin formation occurs when the oxidant affects only the iron atom of the hemoglobin in a reversible fashion. Methemoglobinemia does not necessarily progress to hemolysis if unchecked, although the mechanism for the combined occurrence is unclear.

Numerous cases are reported in which methemoglobinemia has been followed by hemolysis. This sequence of events is associated with dapsone,[17,18,49] phenazopyridine (Pyridium),[13,21,26,47,62] amyl nitrite,[10] and aniline.[28,35,42] Most poisonings with these compounds do not manifest both types of toxicity. These combined instances may represent the incidental toxicity of an oxidizing agent or be the result of eventual depletion of all cellular defenses against oxidants. Currently it is not possible to predict when hemolysis will follow methemoglobinemia with any level of certainty; however, there is an association.

Another source of confusion is that reduced glutathione (GSH) is required to protect against both hemolysis and methemoglobinemia. Erythrocytes are able to withstand hemolytic oxidant damage as long as they can maintain adequate levels of reduced glutathione, the principle cellular antioxidant. Glutathione is maintained in its reduced form using NADPH as its reducing agent. Cells with reduced capacity to produce NADPH (ie, cells of patients with G-6-PD deficiency or cells with depleted reduced glutathione/NADPH) are susceptible to hemolysis. In the presence of methemoglobinemia, reduced glutathione plays a minor role as a reducing agent, but NADPH is necessary for successful antidotal therapy. This co-dependence on the reducing power of NADPH generated by the hexose monophosphate shunt links the two disorders. Competition for NADPH by oxidized glutathione and exogenously administered methylene blue has been postulated to be the cause of methylene blue–induced hemolysis (ie, competitive inhibition of glu-

TABLE 93–3. SIGNS AND SYMPTOMS ASSOCIATED WITH METHEMOGLOBIN CONCENTRATIONS IN HEALTHY PATIENTS WITH NORMAL HEMOGLOBIN CONCENTRATIONS

Methemoglobin Concentration (%)	Signs and Symptoms
1–<3	Normal level
3–15	Possibly none
	Slate gray cutaneous coloration
	Pulse oximeter will read low SaO_2
15–20	Cyanosis
	Chocolate brown blood
20–50	Dyspnea
	Exercise intolerance
	Headache
	Fatigue
	Dizziness, syncope
	Weakness
50–70	Tachypnea
	Metabolic acidosis
	Dysrhythmias
	Seizures
	CNS depression
	Coma
>70	Grave hypoxic symptoms
	Death

tathione reduction). The clinical importance of the phenomenon is uncertain.

It may be easier to consider hemolysis and methemoglobin formation as subclasses of disorders of oxidant stress. They should be considered separate clinical entities sharing limited characteristics.

What Therapeutic Interventions Are Indicated and Why Might They Fail?

For most patients with mild methemoglobinemia, no therapy is necessary other than withdrawal of the offending agent and oxygen administration, as reduction of the methemoglobin will occur by means of intact normal reconversion mechanisms (NADH methemoglobin reductase). The reconversion rate in normal individuals is about 15%/h.[20] This assumes no ongoing methemoglobin production. In the clinical setting, continued absorption, prolonged half-life, and toxic intermediate metabolites may prolong methemoglobinemia. Patients should be examined carefully for signs of stress related to decreased oxygen delivery to the tissue (Fig. 93–7). Obviously, changes in mental status, such as stupor or lethargy, or ischemic chest pain necessitate immediate treatment, but subtle changes in behavior or inattentiveness also may be signs of global hypoxia and should be treated as well. Abnormal vital signs, such as tachycardia and tachypnea, thought to be due to tissue hypoxia or the functional anemia of methemoglobinemia, should be treated. Patients who develop acidosis or ischemic ECG changes should be treated as well. A methemoglobin level alone is generally not adequate to indicate the need for therapy. The most widely accepted treatment is to administer methylene blue, 1–2 mg/kg body weight as a 1% solution, given IV over 5 minutes. The slow infusion helps prevent a painful local response, which can also be minimized by flushing the IV rapidly with at least 15–30 mL of fluid following the infusion. Improvement should be noted within 1 hour of the methylene blue administration. If cyanosis has not disappeared within 1 hour, a second dose should be given and other factors considered (Fig. 93–8).

The use of methylene blue in patients with G-6-PD deficiency is controversial. Deficiency of this enzyme has been estimated to occur in 200 million people worldwide. Its incidence in the United States is highest among African Americans (11%).[3] These patients have been excluded from most treatment protocols because methylene blue has been classified as a mild oxidant and case reports have suggested methylene blue's toxicity. However, most patients with no known history of G-6-PD deficiency who need treatment receive methylene blue therapy before their G-6-PD status is known, because of the lack of immediate availability of the test. Many patients with G-6-PD deficiency have undoubtedly been treated unknowingly, yet few case reports of toxicity exist. While assessing the hemolytic potency of varied drugs, methylene blue in doses of 390–780 mg proved to be only a moderate hemolytic agent, producing a mild anemia.[36] Even the authors of the article most frequently cited as a rationale for withholding methylene blue treatment were unsure that the methylene blue given to their G-6-PD-deficient patient produced hemolysis.[58] The dose of methylene blue was small in the patient under study, and the patient had taken other agents capable of producing hemolysis. Patients with G-6-PD deficiency have variable activity of the enzyme and manifest different levels of disease in response to oxidant stress. The judicious use of methylene blue is warranted in most of these patients.

If methylene blue treatment fails to relieve significant methemoglobinemia, a number of possibilities should be considered. The etiology of the oxidant stress may not have been adequately removed, allowing for continuing oxidation. In such situations, decontamination of the gut (emesis, lavage, activated charcoal, or possibly whole-bowel irrigation) and skin must be resumed. Additional doses of methylene blue are also indicated.

The treatment of dapsone toxicity deserves special consideration. The *N*-hydroxylation of dapsone to its hydroxylamine metabolite is in part responsible for methemoglobin formation in both therapeutic use and overdose. This *N*-hydroxylation is a cytochrome P450-mediated reaction. Cimetidine is an inhibitor of this metabolic pathway and has been shown to reduce methemoglobin levels during therapeutic dosing.[57] In overdose there may be some protective effects as well and its use should be considered.

Some drugs that produce methemoglobinemia have also been reported to produce sulfhemoglobinemia. Sulfhemoglobin is a dark-colored hemoglobin with a sulfur atom incorporated into the heme molecule, but not attached to iron. The sulfur atom's exact location in the porphyrin ring is unclear. Sulfhemoglobin is a darker pigment than methemoglobin, producing cyanosis when only 0.5 g/dL of blood has been affected. The cyanosis produced is similar to that produced by methemoglobinemia. It is characterized in the laboratory by its spectrophotometric appearance and its lack of reaction with cyanide. Its absorption peak is at 620 mm on the spectrophotometer, the same as that of methemoglobin, but does not disappear upon addition of cyanide to the mixture. Isoelectric focusing further defines the substance. It is an extremely stable compound that is eliminated when the red blood cell is removed naturally by the circulation.[12] Although the oxygen-carrying capacity of the hemoglobin is reduced by sulfhemoglobinemia, unlike methemoglobinemia there is a decreased affinity for oxygen in the remaining "unaltered" hemoglobin, thereby making oxygen more available to the tissues (the oxyhemoglobin dissociation curve is shifted to the right) (see Fig. 20–1). This, fortunately, reduces the effect of sulfhemoglobin at the tissue level. Sulfhemoglobin can be produced in vitro by the action of hydrogen sulfide on hemoglobin and was produced in dogs fed elemental sulfur.[40] A number of drugs have induced sulfhemoglobinemia in humans, including acetanilid, phenacetin, ni-

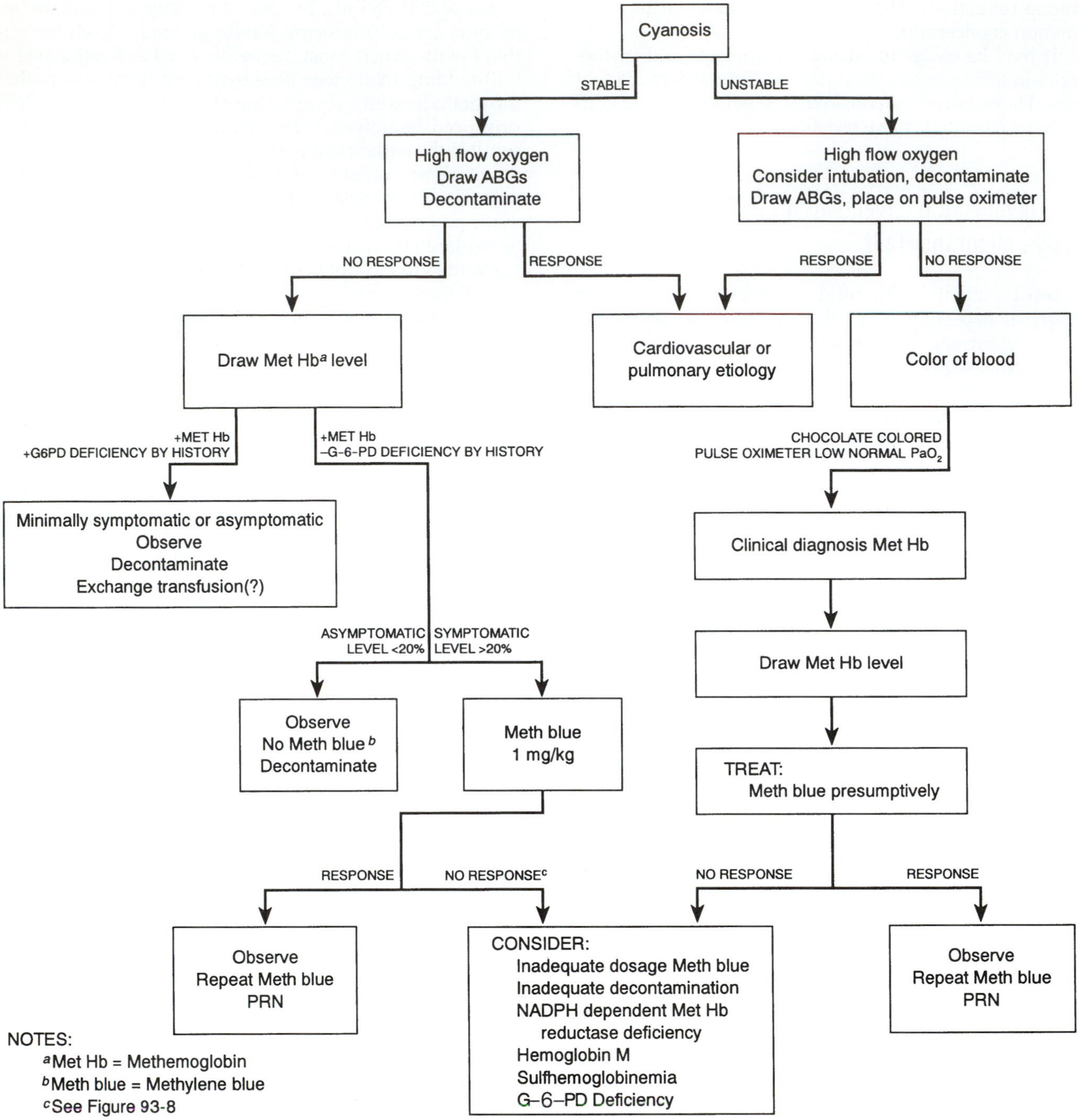

Figure 93–7. Toxicologic assessment of the cyanotic patient.

trates, trinitrotoluene, and sulfur compounds. It has also been seen in individuals with chronic constipation and those who purge.[40]

There is theoretical evidence to suggest that either exchange transfusion or hyperbaric oxygen may be beneficial when methylene blue is ineffective. Both interventions take time, but hyperbaric oxygen may allow the dissolved oxygen time to protect the patient while the body reduces the methemoglobin. Ascorbic acid has no place in the management of acquired methemoglobinemia because the rate at which it reduces methemoglobin is considerably slower than that of the normal intrinsic mechanism.[8] Methylene blue has no therapeutic effect on sulfhemoglobinemia.[54]

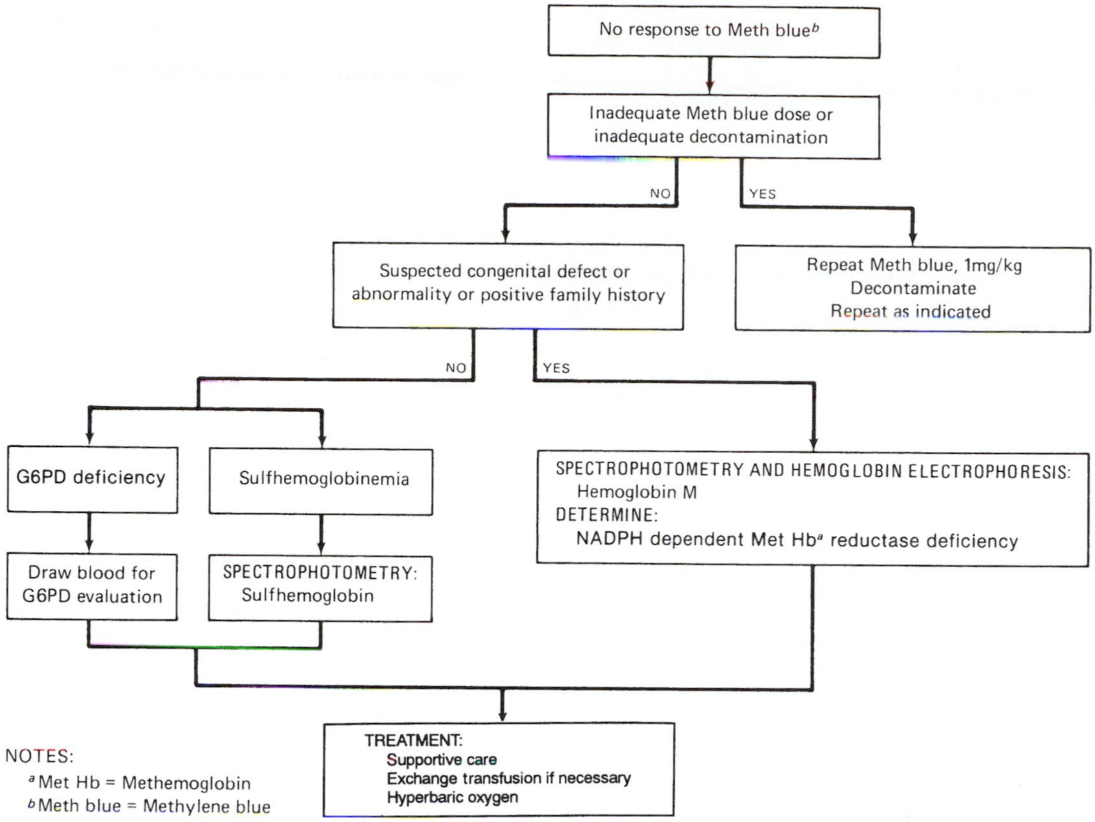

Figure 93–8. Management algorithm for patients with suspected methemoglobinemia unresponsive to initial therapy.

Acknowledgment

Robert H. Kirstein, MD contributed to this chapter in a previous edition.

References

1. Bakshi SP, Fahey JL, Pierce LE: Sausage cyanosis-acquired methemoglobinemic nitrite poisoning. N Engl J Med 1967; 277:1072.
2. Barker SJ, Tremper KK, Hyatt J: Effects of methemoglobinemia on pulse oximetry and mixed venous oximetry. Anesthesiology 1989;70:112–117.
3. Beutler E: Glucose-6-phosphate dehydrogenase deficiency. N Engl J Med 1991;324:169–174.
4. Beutler E: Methemoglobinemia and sulfhemoglobinemia. In: Williams JW, Beutler E, Ersleu AJ, Licthman MA, eds: Hematology, 4th ed. New York, McGraw-Hill, 1990, pp. 379–388.
5. Beutler E: The hemolytic effect of primaquine and related compounds: A review. J Hematol 1959;14:103–139.
6. Birky M, Malek D, Paabo M: Study of biological samples obtained from victims of MGM Grand Hotel fire. J Anal Toxicol 1983;7:265–271.
7. Bodansky O: Methemoglobinemia and methemoglobin producing compounds. Pharmacol Rev 1951;3:144–196.
8. Bolyai JZ, Smith RP, Gray CT: Ascorbic acid and chemically induced methemoglobinemias. Toxicol Appl Pharmacol 1972; 21:176–185.
9. Bower PJ, Peterson JN: Methemoglobinemia after sodium nitroprusside therapy. N Engl J Med 1975;293:865.
10. Brandes JC, Bufill JA, Pisciotta AV: Amyl nitrite-induced hemolytic anemia. Am J Med 1989;86:252–254.
11. Caprari P, Bozzi A, Ferroni L, et al: Membrane alterations in G6PD- and PK-deficient erythrocytes exposed to oxidizing agents. Biol Med Metabol Biol 1991;45:16–27.
12. Cartwright GI: Methemoglobinemia and sulfhemoglobinemia. In: Wintrobe M, Thorn GW, Adams RD, Braunwald RW, eds: Harrison's Principles of Internal Medicine, 7th ed. New York, McGraw-Hill, 1974, pp. 1644–1646.
13. Cohen BL, Bovasso GJ: Acquired methemoglobinemia and hemolytic anemia following excessive Pyridium (phenazopyridine hydrochloride) ingestion. Clin Pediatr 1971;10:537–540.
14. Comly HH: Cyanosis in infants caused by nitrates in well water. JAMA 1945;129:112–116.
15. Craun GF, Greathouse DG, Gunderson DH: Methemoglobin levels in young children consuming high nitrate well water in the United States. Int J Epidemiol 1981;10:309–317.
16. Darling RC, Roughton FJW: The effect of methemoglobin on the equilibrium between oxygen and hemoglobin. Am J Physiol 1942;137:56–66.
17. Dawson AH, Whyte IM: Management of dapsone poisoning complicated by methemoglobinemia. Med Toxicol Adverse Drug Exp 1989;4:387–392.

18. Elonen E, Neuvonen PJ, Halmekoski J, Mattila MJ: Acute dapsone intoxication: A case with prolonged symptoms. Clin Toxicol 1979;14:79–85.
19. Fibuch EE, Cecil WT, Reed WA: Methemoglobinemia associated with organic nitrate therapy. Anesth Analg 1979; 58:521–523.
20. Finch CA: Treatment of intracellular methemoglobinemia. Bull N Engl Med Center 1947;6:241–245.
21. Fincher ME, Campbell HT: Methemoglobinemia and hemolytic anemia after phenazopyridine hydrochloride (Pyridium) administration in end-stage renal disease. South Med J 1989;82:372–374.
22. Fogh-Andersen N, Siggarrad-Andersen O, Lundsgaard FC, Wimberly PD: Diode-array spectrophotometry for simultaneous measurement of hemoglobin pigments. Clin Chim Acta 1987;166:283–289.
23. Fung H: Pharmacokinetic determinants of nitrate action. Am J Med 1984;76:22–27.
24. Gaetani GD, Parker JC, Kirkman HN: Intracellular restraint: A new basis for the limitation in response to oxidative stress in human erythrocytes containing low-activity variants of glucose-6-phosphate dehydrogenase. Proc Natl Acad Sci USA 1974;9:3584–3587.
25. Goldstein BD: Exacerbation of dapsone-induced Heinz body hemolytic anemia following treatment with methylene blue. Am J Med Sci 1974;267:291–297.
26. Greenberg MS, Wong H: Methemoglobinemia and Heinz body hemolytic anemia due to phenazopyridine hydrochloride. N Engl J Med 1964;271:431–435.
27. Harris JC, Rumack BH, Peterson RG, McGuire BM: Methemoglobinemia resulting from absorption of nitrates. JAMA 1979;242:2869–2871.
28. Harrison MR: Toxic methemoglobinemia: A case of acute nitrobenzene and aniline poisoning tested with exchange transfusion. Anaesthesia 1977;32:270–272.
29. Harvey JW, Keitt AS: Studies of the efficacy and potential hazards of methylene blue therapy in aniline-induced methemoglobinemia. Br J Haematol 1983;54:29–41.
30. Hegesh E, Hegesh J, Kaftory A: Congenital methemoglobinemia with a deficiency of cytochrome b5. N Engl J Med: 1985;314:757–761.
31. Hjelt K, Lund JT, Scherling B, et al. Methemoglobinemia among neonates in a neonatal intensive care unit. Acta Paediatr 1995;84:365–370.
32. Hoffman RS, Sauter D: Methemoglobinemia resulting from smoke inhalation. Vet Hum Toxicol 1989;31:40–42.
33. Johnson CJ, Bonrud PA, Dosch TL, et al: Fatal outcome of methemoglobinemia in an infant. JAMA 1987;257: 2796–2797.
34. Katsumata Y, Aoki M, Oya M, et al: Simultaneous determination of carboxyhemoglobin and methemoglobin in victims of carbon monoxide poisoning. J Forensic Sci 1980;25: 546–549.
35. Kearney TE, Manoguerra AS, Dunford JV: Chemically induced methemoglobinemia from aniline poisoning. West J Med 1984;140:282–286.
36. Kellermeyer RW, Tarlov AR, Brewer GJ, et al: Hemolytic effect of therapeutic drugs: Clinical considerations of the primaquine-type hemolysis. JAMA 1962;180:128–134.
37. Kirlangitis JJ, Middaugh RE, Zablocki A, Rodriquez F: False indication of arterial oxygen desaturation and methemoglobinemia following injection of methylene blue in urological surgery. Milit Med 1990;155:260–262.
38. Laney RF, Hoffman RS: Methemoglobinemia secondary to automobile exhaust fumes. Am J Emerg Med 1992;10: 426–428.
39. Larsen VH, Freudendal-Pedersen A, Fogh-Andersen NF: The influence of patent blue V on pulse oximetry and haemoximetry. Acta Anesthesiol Scand 1995;39:53–55.
40. Lehman H, Huntsman RG, Cosey R, et al: Hemoglobinopathies associated with unstable hemoglobin. In: Williams JW, Beutler E, Ersleu AJ, Lichtman MA, eds: Hematology, 4th ed. New York, McGraw-Hill, 1990, pp. 746–751.
41. Leroux A, Junien C, Kaplan JC, Bamberger J: Generalized deficiency of cytochrome b5 reductase in congenital methemoglobinemia with mental retardation. Nature 1975;258: 619–620.
42. Lubash GD, Phillips RE, Shields JD, Bonsnes RW: Acute aniline poisoning treated by hemodialysis. Arch Intern Med 1964;114:530–532.
43. Lukens JN: The legacy of well water methemoglobinemia. JAMA 1987;257:2793–2795.
44. Mansouri A, Lurie AA: Concise review: Methemoglobinemia. Am J Hematol 1993;42:7–12.
45. Methemoglobinemia in an infant—Wisconsin. MMWR 1993;42:217–219.
46. Murray KM, Meth B: Methemoglobin, MEDLINE, and hyperlipemia. Crit Care Med 1987;15:797–798.
47. Nathan DM, Siegel AJ, Bunn F: Acute methemoglobinemia and hemolytic anemia with phenazopyridine. Arch Intern Med 1977;137:1636–1638.
48. Nathan GD, Oski FA: Hematology of Infancy and Childhood, 2nd ed. Philadelphia, Saunders, 1981, pp. 675–686.
49. Neuvonen PJ, Elonen E, Haapanen EJ: Acute dapsone intoxication: Clinical findings and effect of oral charcoal and hemodialysis on dapsone elimination. Acta Med Scand 1983;214:215–220.
50. Nijland R, Jongsma HW, Nijhuis JG, et al: Notes on the apparent discordance of pulse oximetry and multiwavelength hemoglobin photometry. Acta Anaesthesiol Scand 1995;107: 49–52.
51. Nitzan M, Volovitz B, Topper E: Infantile methemoglobinemia caused by food additives. Clin Toxicol 1979;15:273–280.
52. Odonohue WJ, Moss LM, Angelillo VA: Acute methemoglobinemia induced by topical benzocaine and lidocaine. Arch Intern Med 1980;140:1508–1509.
53. Paris PM, Kaplan RM, Steward RD, Weiss LD: Methemoglobin levels following sublingual nitoglycerin in human volunteers. Ann Emerg Med 1986;15:171–173.
54. Park CM, Nagel RL: Sulfhemoglobinemia: Clinical and molecular aspects. N Engl J Med 1984;310:1579–1584.
55. Pollack ES, Pollack CV: Incidence of subclinical methemoglobinemia in infants with diarrhea. Ann Emerg Med 1994; 24:652–656.
56. Prchal JT, Borgese N, Moore MR, et al: Congenital methemoglobinemia due to methemoglobin reductase deficiency in two unrelated American black families. Am J Med 1990; 89:516–522.
57. Rhodes LE, Tingle MD, Park BK, et al: Cimetidine improves

the therapeutic/toxic ratio of dapsone in patients on chronic dapsone therapy. Br J Dermatol 1995;132:257–262.

58. Rosen PJ, Johnson C, Mcgehee WG, Beutler E: Failure of methylene blue treatment in toxic methemoglobinemia. Ann Intern Med 1971;76;83–86.
59. Sager S, Garyson GH, Feig SA: Methemoglobinemia associated with acidosis of probable renal origin. J Pediatr 1995; 126:59–61.
60. Sass MD, Caruso CJ, Farhangi M: TPNH-methemoglobin reductase deficiency: A new red-cell enzyme defect. J Lab Clin Med 1967;5:760–767.
61. Schwerd W, Schulz E: Carboxyhemoglobin and methemoglobin findings in burnt bodies. Forensic Sci Int 1978;12: 233–235.
62. Sharon M, Puente G, Cohen LB: Phenazopyridine (Pyridium) poisoning: Possible toxicity of methylene blue administration in renal failure. Mt Sinai J Med 1986;3: 280–282.
63. Smith ER, Smiseth IK, Maryari D, et al: Mechanism of action of nitrates. Am J Med 1984;76:14–22.
64. Smith R, Olson M: Drug-induced methemoglobinemia. Semin Hematol 1973;10:253–268.
65. Spurzem JR, Bonchat HW, Shigeoka JW: Factitious methoglobinemia caused by hyperlipemia. Chest 1984;88:84–86.
66. Tremper KK, Barker SJ: Using pulse oximetry when dyshemoglobin levels are high. J Crit Illness 1988;11:103–107.
67. White CD, Weiss LD: Varying presentations of methemoglobinemia: Two cases. J Emerg Med 1991;9:45–49.
68. Wintrobe M: Clinical Hematology, 7th ed. Philadelphia, Lea & Febiger, 1974, pp. 1009–1016.
69. Yano SS, Danish EH, Hsia YE: Transient methemoglobinemia with acidosis in infants. J Pediatr 1982;100:415–418.
70. Zijlstra WG, Buursma A, Zwart A: Performance of an automated six-wavelength photometer (Radiometer OSM3) for routine measurement of hemoglobin derivatives. Clin Chem 1988;34:149–152.

ANTIDOTES IN DEPTH

Methylene Blue

Mary Ann Howland

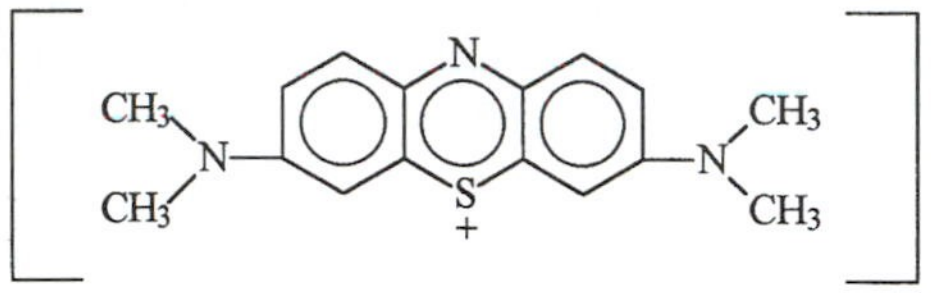

Methylene blue was initially recommended for use as an intestinal and urinary antiseptic and subsequently recognized as a weak antimalarial agent.[13] In 1933, Williams and Challis successfully used methylene blue to treat aniline-induced methemoglobinemia.[32]

Methylene blue is tetramethyl thionine chloride,[13] which is reduced (is an electron acceptor) in the presence of NADPH and methemoglobin reductase to leukomethylene blue (see Fig. 93–6). Leukomethylene blue then becomes available to reduce methemoglobin to hemoglobin.[7,13] In the absence of methylene blue, this reaction is quantitatively limited, whereas in its presence methemoglobin reduction via this pathway is dramatically increased (four to five times in dogs), making methylene blue the treatment of choice for methemoglobinemia.

Spectrophotometric assays to study the pharmacokinetics of methylene blue and leukomethylene blue have been developed.[7] Methylene blue has a pK_a close to –1, making it completely ionized in the gastrointestinal (GI) tract.[8] Administration of 10 mg of methylene blue in capsule form to seven volunteers demonstrated good oral absorption, with an average urinary recovery of 74%.[8] The majority of the volunteers (78%) excreted leukomethylene blue stabilized as a salt complex with the remainder as methylene blue. A similar canine experiment revealed distinctly different results, with oral absorption of only 2–4%.[8] These data may be responsible for reports that suggest that methylene blue is poorly absorbed orally.

In a canine model, intravenous administration of increasing doses of methylene blue led to two divergent interpretations: a nonlinear single-compartment model and a classic linear, two-compartment, open model (volume of distribution, 0.22–0.87 L/kg; plasma clearance, 1.98–2.65 L/kg/h).[9] Subsequent studies in rats have shown rapid tissue uptake and reduction of methylene blue and support the nonlinear canine model.[9]

In the initial studies 100 mL of a 1% concentration of methylene blue was used intravenously to treat aniline-induced methemoglobinemia.[32] Subsequently 50 mL of 1% methylene blue IV was studied in 18 volunteers.[21] The dose used, about 7 mg/kg, was recommended as the average therapeutic dose when methylene blue was used to treat carbon monoxide and cyanide toxicity.[11] Methemoglobin levels measured when symptoms were most pronounced were found to be approximately 1.0 g/dL (0.4–8.3% of total hemoglobin). Electrocardiographic manifestations included ST-T wave changes and a decrease in R wave amplitude, which resolved within 2 hours of therapy. Other consequential adverse effects included shortness of breath, tachypnea, chest discomfort, burning sensation of the mouth and stomach, initial bluish tinged skin and mucous membranes, paresthesias, restlessness, apprehension, tremors, nausea and vomiting, dysuria, and excitation. One patient complained of a feeling of impending death. Urine and vomitus had a blue color. Intraamniotic injection of methylene blue may result in infants born with skin dyed blue leading to inaccurate pulse oximetry readings, methemoglobin, hemolysis, or intestinal obstruction.[6,20,22,25,28] One infant exposed in utero at 5½ weeks was born normal.[16] Infiltration of IV methylene blue was painful and resulted in tissue necrosis. Methylene blue doses of 1–2 mg/kg IV or 65–130 mg orally every 4 hours were suggested to reverse sulfanilamide-induced methemoglobinemia.[14,30] With these regimens a very rapid fall in methemoglobin occurred concurrently with a disappearance of cyanosis.

Later investigations confirmed the effectiveness and safety of IV doses of 1–2 mg/kg of methylene blue in reversing the methemoglobinemia produced by sulfanilamide,[29] aniline dye,[10] and silver nitrate, among other agents.[27]

The apparent paradoxical effects of methylene blue suggest an equilibrium between the ability of methylene blue to oxidize hemoglobin directly to methemoglobin and the ability of methylene blue (through the NADPH–methemoglobin reductase pathway and leukomethylene blue production) to reduce methemoglobin to hemoglobin.[2,3] Methylene blue at doses of 1–2 mg/kg does not produce methemoglobin. An equilibrium seems to be established in favor of the reducing properties of methylene blue unless excessively large doses of methylene blue are given[1,12,31] or the NADPH–methemoglobin reductase system is abnormal. This equilibrium constant may vary substantially, as 20 mg/kg IV in dogs and 65 mg/kg intraperitoneally in rats failed to produce methemoglobinemia.[26] In high doses, methylene blue can also induce an acute hemolytic anemia in the absence or presence of methemoglobinemia.[12,19] In dose–response studies in G-6-PD deficient homozygous black males, daily doses with hemolytic potential were 390–780 mg (5.5–11 mg/kg) of methylene blue.[18] This was comparable to 15 mg of primaquine base.[18] Due to the sensitivity of neonates (Hb F and diminished NADH reductase) to these risks, the smallest effective dose should be employed.[15,19] Since oxidizing agents can independently result in chemical-induced Heinz body hemolytic anemia, the contribution of methylene blue is often difficult to elucidate.[17]

Methylene blue may be ineffective in reversing a toxic methemoglobinemia in patients with G-6-PD deficiency,[24] because the G-6-PD in the hexose monophosphate shunt is essential for the generation of NADPH. Without NADPH methylene blue cannot act as a reducing agent in the transformation of methemoglobin to oxyhemoglobin. However, G-6-PD deficiency is an X-linked hereditary deficiency with more than 400 variants. The red cells containing the more common G-6-PD A^- variant found in 11% of black Americans retains 10% residual activity, mostly in younger erythrocytes and reticulocytes. The enzyme is barely detectable in those of Mediterranean descent who have inherited the defect. Therefore, it is impossible to predict prior to the use of methylene blue who will or will not respond and to what extent. A risk-to-benefit ratio must be determined when administering methylene blue to achieve methemoglobin reversal. However, when therapeutic doses of methylene blue fail to have an impact on the methemoglobin level, the possibility of G-6-PD deficiency should be considered. Further doses of methylene blue should not be administered in these cases because the risk of methylene blue-induced hemolysis exists in the absence of any potential benefit. In these cases exchange transfusion and hyperbaric oxygen are potential alternatives (see Chap. 93). It must always be excluded that there is continued toxin absorption and/or continued methemoglobin production.

Methylene blue is a dye. It will alter pulse oximeter readings.[4] Large doses may interfere with a clinician's ability to detect a decrease in cyanosis, and therefore repeat co-oximeter readings and arterial blood gas analysis should be used in conjunction with clinical findings.

When there is continued absorption or slow elimination of the chemical producing the methemoglobinemia, repetitive dosing of methylene blue may be required in conjunction with efforts to decontaminate the GI tract and perhaps stop the formation of the methemoglobin-inducing metabolite with the use of inhibitors of drug metabolism such as cimetidine.[5,23] Methylene blue is indicated when patients are symptomatic from methemoglobinemia. This usually occurs at methemoglobin levels greater than 20% but may occur at lower levels in anemic patients or those with cardiovascular, pulmonary, or central nervous system compromise. Methylene blue is ineffective in patients with an absolute G-6-PD deficiency. Fortunately most individuals have a variable expression of this deficiency and differ in their responses to oxidant stress. Judicious use of methylene blue is warranted in patients with questionable levels of G-6-PD deficiency. Very large doses of methylene blue may produce methemoglobinemia or a hemolytic anemia in the absence of a G-6-PD deficiency, but this is extremely rare at doses of 1–2 mg/kg IV. Methylene blue is ineffective in treating other entities, such as sulfhemoglobinemia (see Chap. 93).

In summary, methylene blue is a very effective reducer of toxin-induced methemoglobinemia. In most cases, doses of 1–2 mg/kg IV given over 5 minutes followed immediately by a 15–30-mL fluid flush to minimize local pain is both effective and relatively safe. In neonates doses of 0.3–1 mg/kg are often effective.[15] The onset of action is quite rapid, with maximum effects usually seen within 30 minutes. Methylene blue is available in 10-mL 1% ampules containing 10 mg/mL.

References

1. Blass N, Fung D: Dyed but not dead—methylene blue overdose. Anesthesiology 1976;45:458–459.
2. Bodansky O: Methemoglobinemia and methemoglobin-producing compounds. Pharmacol Rev 1951;3:144–196.
3. Bodansky O: Mechanism of action of methylene blue in treatment of methemoglobinemia. JAMA 1950;142:923.
4. Coleman MD, Coleman NA: Drug-induced methaemoglobinemia. Drug Safety 1996;14:394–405.
5. Coleman MD, Rhodes LA, Scott AK, et al: The use of cimetidine to reduce dapsone-dependent methemoglobinemia in dermatitis herpetiformis patients. Br J Clin Pharmacol 1992; 34:244–249.
6. Crooks J: Haemolytic jaundice in a neonate after intra-amniotic injection of methylene blue. Arch Dis Child 1982; 57:872–886.
7. DiSanto AR, Wagner JG: Pharmacokinetics of highly ionized drugs. I: Methylene blue—whole blood, urine and tissue assays. J Pharm Sci 1972;61:598–602.
8. DiSanto AR, Wagner JG: Pharmacokinetics of highly ionized drugs. II: Methylene blue—absorption, metabolism and excretion in man and dog after oral absorption. J Pharm Sci 1972;61:1086–1090.
9. DiSanto AR, Wagner JG: Pharmacokinetics of highly ionized drugs. III: Methylene blue—blood levels in the dog and tissue levels in the rat following intravenous administration. J Pharm Sci 1972;61:1090–1094.
10. Etteldorf JN: Methylene blue in the treatment of methemoglobinemia in premature infants caused by marking ink. J Pediatr 1951;38:24–27.
11. Geiger JC: Cyanide poisoning in San Francisco. JAMA 1932;99:1944–1945.
12. Goluboff N, Wheaton R: Methylene blue-induced cyanosis and acute hemolytic anemia complicating the treatment of methemoglobinemia. J Pediatr 1961;58:86–89.
13. Goodman LS, Gilman A: The Pharmacological Basis of Therapeutics. New York, Macmillan, 1941, p. 869.
14. Harman A, Perley A, Barnett H: A study of some of the physiological effects of sulfanilamide. II: Methemoglobin formation and its control. J Clin Invest 1938;17:699–710.
15. Hjelt K, Lund JT, Scherling B, et al: Methemoglobinemia

among neonates in a neonatal intensive care unit. Acta Pediatr 1995;84:365–370.

16. Katz Z, Lancet M: Inadvertent intrauterine injection of methylene blue in early pregnancy. N Engl J Med 1981;304: 1427. Letter.
17. Kearney T, Manoguerra A, Dunford JV: Chemically induced methemoglobinemia from aniline poisoning. West J Med 1984;140:282–286.
18. Kellermeyer RW, Tarlov A, Brewer G, et al: Hemolytic effect of therapeutic drugs. JAMA 1962;180:128–134.
19. Kirsch I, Cohen M: Heinz body hemolytic anemia from the use of methylene blue in neonates. J Pediatr 1980;96: 276–278.
20. McEnerney JK, McEnerney LN: Unfavorable neonatal outcome after intra-amniotic injection of methylene blue. Obstet Gynecol 1983;61:35S–37S.
21. Nadler JE, Green M, Rosenbaum A: Intravenous injection of methylene blue in man with reference to its toxic symptoms and effect on the electrocardiogram. Am J Med Sci 1934; 188:15–21.
22. Nicolini U, Monni G: Intestinal obstruction in babies exposed in utero to methylene blue. Lancet 1990;336: 1258–1259.
23. Rhodes LE, Tingle MD, Park BK, et al: Cimetidine improves the therapeutic/toxic ratio of dapsone in patients on chronic dapsone therapy. Br J Derm 1995;132:257–262.
24. Rosen PJ, Johnson C, McGehee WG, Beutler E: Failure of methylene blue treatment in toxic methemoglobinemia. Ann Intern Med 1971;76:83–86.
25. Serota FT, Bernbaum JC, Schwartz E: The methylene blue baby. Lancet 1979;2:1142–1143.
26. Stossel TP, Jennings RB: Failure of methylene blue to produce methemoglobinemia in vivo. Am J Clin Pathol 1966; 45:600–604.
27. Strauch B, Buch W, Grey W, et al: Successful treatment of methemoglobinemia secondary to silver nitrate therapy. N Engl J Med 1969;281:257–258.
28. Troche BI: The methylene blue baby. N Engl J Med 1989; 320:1756–1757.
29. Wendel WB: The control of methemoglobinemia with methylene blue. J Clin Invest 1939;18:179–185.
30. Wendel WB: Use of methylene blue in methemoglobinemia from sulfanilamide poisoning. JAMA 1937;109: 1216.
31. Whitwam JG, Taylor AR, White JM: Potential hazard of methylene blue. Anesthesiology 1979;34:181–182.
32. Williams JR, Challis FE: Methylene blue as an antidote for aniline dye poisoning. J Lab Clin Med 1933;19:166–171.

CHAPTER 94

Simple Asphyxiants and Pulmonary Irritants

Lewis S. Nelson

In an attempt to clean a grimy bathtub in a newly purchased house, a 37-year-old woman mixed together several over-the-counter cleaning products. Seconds after creating the mixture, an acrid cloud of green-tinted gas filled the room. The woman was able to escape the fumes rapidly, but quickly began feeling pain in her eyes and throat. She remained at home for a half an hour but her symptoms progressed. She arrived in the emergency department with significant dyspnea, cough, and mild, nonlocalized chest discomfort.

Her vital signs were: blood pressure, 120/85 mm Hg, pulse, 120 beats/min; respiratory rate, 32 breaths/min; temperature 99°F (37.2°C). A pulse oximeter revealed a saturation of 83% and she was placed on 2 L nasal oxygen. Pertinent findings on her physical examination included teary, red eyes with normal vision. Her oropharyngeal mucosa was unremarkable, although she was salivating. She had no stridor, hoarseness, or dysphagia. Her lung examination demonstrated bilateral rales, and her heart sounds were normal, albeit tachycardic. An arterial blood gas was: pH, 7.50; PCO_2, 25 mm Hg; and PO_2, 50 mm Hg on 2 L of oxygen by nasal cannula. She was placed on a nonrebreather with FIO_2 100% oxygen facemask, and her oxygen saturation climbed to 94%. Her electrocardiogram revealed a sinus tachycardia. The chest radiograph, done at the bedside, showed a significant bilateral alveolar filling pattern with a normal-size heart.

She received one dose of nebulized bicarbonate and several doses of albuterol and was admitted to the ICU for observation. Over the next 24 hours her symptoms and abnormal pulmonary findings resolved and she was able to be discharged. On follow-up, she was asymptomatic and had a normal physical examination.

On a daily basis our bodies are exposed to a variety of potentially damaging external influences. While most organs remain relatively protected from such influence, the skin and respiratory tract, by their nature, maintain constant contact with the external environment. Several critical systems exist within the respiratory system to prevent or ameliorate toxicity from without and allow life to persist in what actually is a hostile environment. Although these efficient systems provide substantial protection under normal circumstances, they may be overburdened occasionally.

The respiratory tract, as discussed in Chapter 20, performs several important functions. Transfer of oxygen to hemoglobin across the pulmonary endothelium and its subsequent distribution throughout the body allows cellular respiration to continue. Different toxins act at unique points in this distribution pathway to ultimately produce tissue hypoxia. For example, toxins may induce hypoventilation (eg, opioids, paralytic agents) or prevent binding of oxygen to hemoglobin (eg, carbon monoxide or methemoglobin inducers). Certain toxins prevent adequate oxygenation of hemoglobin at the level of pulmonary gas exchange. Two mechanistically distinct groups of agents are capable of interfering with gas exchange: simple asphyxiants and pulmonary irritants. Impairment of transpulmonary oxygen diffusion, regardless of the etiology, reduces the oxygen content of the blood and can result in tissue hypoxia.

What Are Simple Asphyxiants?

Simple asphyxiants displace oxygen from ambient air and reduce the partial pressure of available oxygen. The partial pressure is a measure of the oxygen contribution to the total inspired air and is based on both percentages of oxygen and barometric pressure. For example, since the ambient pressure at sea level (less water vapor) is 713 mm Hg and the percentage of oxygen is 21%, the partial pressure of oxygen is 150 mm Hg. Displacement of oxygen from air by a simple asphyxiant gas effectively lowers the contribution of oxygen to air to below 21%. Thus, the partial pressure of oxygen falls. Under most circumstances, however, carbon dioxide exchange is not impaired and hypercapnia does not occur. Since dyspnea, or the sensation that breathing is difficult, develops more rapidly from hypercapnia than hypoxemia, the breathlessness associated with physical asphyxiation does not develop until severe hypoxemia intervenes.[72,96]

In general simple asphyxiants have no pharmacologic activity, and it is their presence in significant quantity that induces hypoxemia. Due to the need for exceedingly high ambient concentrations of the gas, most asphyxiant-poisoned patients are exposed in either confined spaces or to extremely concentrated forms of the gas. Asphyxiation by gas at the work site is unfortunately common.[143] The widespread use of liquefied gas, which expands several hundredfold on depressurization or warming, may account for a substantial number of these cases.[104] A patient exposed to any simple asphyxiant gas will develop characteristic symptoms of hypoxia (Table 94–1), which are directly related to the partial pressure of the gas in the air, or more correctly, to the reduction in ambient oxygen partial pressure.[103] At sea level, the oxygen concentration, or fraction of inspired oxygen (FIO_2), is a convenient substitute for partial pressure of oxygen. However, this relationship is not applicable at other barometric pressures. For example, the reduced ambient partial pressure of oxygen at the summit of a mountain (despite a normal FIO_2 of 21%) is often incapable of producing an adequate oxygen saturation, and supplemental oxygen may be needed. Additional exposure to simple asphyxiant gases at elevation may further reduce the oxygen partial pressure to life-threatening levels. Alternatively, underwater divers could, in theory, reduce their FIO_2 to less than 21% by adding helium and still maintain adequate oxygenation. This is because the elevated barometric pressure raises the partial pressure of oxygen to normal levels despite the addition of an asphyxiant gas such as helium.

TABLE 94–1. CLINICAL FINDINGS ASSOCIATED WITH A REDUCTION OF INSPIRED OXYGEN

FIO_2[a,b]	Symptoms/Signs
16–12	Tachypnea, hyperpnea (resultant hypocapnia), tachycardia, reduced attention and alertness, euphoria, headache, mild incoordination
14–10	Altered judgment, incoordination, muscular fatigue, cyanosis
10–6	Nausea, vomiting, lethargy, air hunger, severe incoordination, coma
<6	Gasping respirations, seizures, coma, death

[a]At sea level barometric pressure (1 ATM); appropriate adjustments must be made for altitude and depth exposures.
[b]Normal FIO_2 is 21%.
Adapted, with permission, from Miller TM, Mazur PO: Oxygen deficiency hazards associated with liquefied gas systems: derivation of a program of controls. Am Ind Hyg Assoc J 1984;45:293–298.

Treatment for all patients poisoned by simple asphyxiants begins with removal from exposure and ventilatory assistance. Provision of supplemental oxygen is preferable, but normal air should suffice. Restoration of oxygenation, through spontaneous or mechanical ventilation, occurs after only several breaths. Support of vital functions is the mainstay of therapy, but is generally not needed after brief exposures. There is no role for hyperbaric oxygen therapy, nor is it contraindicated if the patient is concomitantly exposed to a toxin such as carbon monoxide. Since poisoning in effect results from hypoxemia, the complications of simple asphyxiants are predictable.[29] Myocardial and central nervous system damage predominate as these tissues have with the greatest oxygen requirements. With severe hypoxemia, multisystem organ failure and death may occur.

Noble Gases: Helium, Neon, Argon, Xenon

Noble gases are used in welding operations, lasers, and other illumination. In their radioactive gaseous form they have diagnostic medical applications. Helium is the smallest member of the noble gas family of elements. Due to its lower lipid solubility, helium is used as a replacement gas for nitrogen by underwater divers to prevent nitrogen narcosis at depth (see Nitrogen). Even at diving gas mixtures of 50% helium, divers suffer no adverse effects as long as the partial pressure of oxygen is maintained in the mixture. In addition, due to the lower density of helium compared with nitrogen, its resistance to flow is markedly less (ie, lower viscosity). This property is the basis for the use of helium in patients with increased airway resistance (eg, asthma), and also makes breathing easier at depth, where the volumes inspired per breath are severalfold larger than at sealevel. Additionally, low viscosity accounts for the use of helium as an inflation gas for an intraaortic balloon. Rupture of the balloon may result in helium bubble embolism, an effect unrelated to the simple asphyxiant property of the gas.[48] All noble gases, when compressed, form cryogenic liquids, which expand rapidly to their gas phase upon decompression. Transport or use of these agents in closed spaces may result in asphyxiation or freezing injuries.

Argon and neon, both used in lighting manufacture, are simple asphyxiants and may produce asphyxiation.[72,143] Xenon, in addition, is anesthetic at sea level pressures due to its high lipid solubility.[39,82] The other noble gases have no other known direct toxicity, although several, such as radon, emit ionizing radiation.

Short-chain Aliphatic Hydrocarbon Gases: Methane, Ethane, Propane, Butane

Methane is also known as "swamp gas" and may be present in high ambient concentrations in bogs of decaying organic matter. Compressed natural gas has recently been introduced as an alternative fuel for automotive use. Although unreported, leakage into the passenger compartment with resultant poisoning may occur. Methane exposure is also an occupational hazard for miners, who have historically carried canaries into their workplace to assess for toxic gases and oxygen depletion. Conceptually, the higher metabolic and respiratory rate of small animals (and children) make them more rapidly susceptible to both. Interestingly, animals can breath air which is 80% methane and 20% oxygen without manifesting hypoxic symptoms since the FIO_2 is essentially normal.

Perhaps because of its ubiquity as a home cooking fuel, methane is considered by the public to be a very dangerous gas. However, as with all simple asphyxiants, ambient levels must be significantly elevated to produce symptoms.[19] Methane itself is odorless, and therefore undetectable without sophisticated equipment. Accumulation to life-threatening levels could potentially occur without notice, producing both toxicologic and explosive consequences. For this reason, natural gas is intentionally adulterated with a small concentration of alkyl mercaptan, a stenching agent responsible for the well recognized sulfur odor of natural gas. Cooking with natural gas may lead to increased respiratory symptoms and pulmonary dysfunction in young female homemakers.[74] However, methane itself is unlikely to be the etiology, since its combustion is generally complete and ambient levels are negligible. It is likely that exposure to the combustion product, nitrogen dioxide, is the explanation for these symptoms (see Oxides of Nitrogen).

Ethane is a similar, odorless gas that is occasionally implicated as a simple asphyxiant. It is found in natural gas and used as a refrigerant. Propane is widely used in compressed form as an industrial and domestic fuel and as an industrial solvent. Butane is also a prevalent fuel and solvent. Deliberate butane inhalation from cigarette lighters by adolescents may cause myocardial infarction[5] and cerebral damage.[5,55]

What Are the Effects of Carbon Dioxide (CO_2) and Nitrogen (N_2) Gas?

Although not strictly simple asphyxiant gases since they produce physiologic effects, carbon dioxide and nitrogen most closely resemble simple asphyxiants from a toxicologic viewpoint. Both are nonirritating and odorless, and neither acutely interferes with critical biochemical processes in the body. Carbon dioxide gas has many practical uses. For example, it is responsible for the carbonation of soft drinks and is used as a shielding gas during welding. Carbon dioxide is widely used as a fire extinguisher, the basis of which is its ability to displace oxygen from the fire environment.

Buildup of carbon dioxide to dangerous concentrations in enclosed spaces has resulted in poisoning in several situations. For example, a 37-year-old man developed coma, seizures, hypoxemia and acidosis when solid carbon dioxide ("dry ice") evaporated in his car.[146] Additionally, a child undergoing general anesthesia was accidentally ventilated with 99.97% carbon dioxide instead of oxygen.[75] Cardiac asystole occurred, but rapid recognition of the mistake and institution of resuscitative efforts allowed a full recovery. The large-scale emission of carbon dioxide from Lake Nyos, a volcanic crater lake in Cameroon, West Africa, resulted in nearly 2000 human and many more livestock deaths.[82] Simple asphyxiation was likely since medical evaluation of both survivors and casualties found no signs of skin or pulmonary irritation[156] and toxicologic evaluation was unrevealing. Investigators noted that death was so rapid that casualties appeared to "die in their tracks."[83]

Carbon dioxide dissolves in the serum to form carbonic acid. Thus respiratory acidosis occurs; the physiologic response to acidosis is to increase ventilation. Unfortunately, this increases the uptake of carbon dioxide unless the patient is removed from the exposure. Closed anesthesia systems use scrubber systems, which contain sodium hydroxide, to chemically eliminate carbon dioxide. Failure of the scrubber system results in increasing depth of anesthesia due to hypercapnia-induced hyperventilation.

Nitrogen gas finds many uses in manufacturing. It is used as a carrier gas for chromatography, as a fertilizer, and as a cryogenic agent for surgery. Liquid nitrogen toxicity is relatively common and is usually related to its extremely cold temperature.[90] Rarely, bubbles introduced through the skin may embolize through the vascular system and impair organ blood flow.[36] Nitrogen gas poisoning is uncommon. Inadvertent connection of air-line respirator hoses to nitrogen and other inert gas sources results in acute asphyxiation, with unconsciousness in about 12 seconds[72,104,143] and death shortly thereafter. More indolent inhalational poisoning by nitrogen is characterized by impairment of intellectual function and judgment, giddiness, and euphoria with more severely poisoned patients manifesting lethargy or coma.[45] Systemic absorption is not rapid, however, and prolonged, high-level exposure is required for poisoning. Nitrogen poisoning, also known as nitrogen narcosis, is most commonly seen in underwater divers breathing air (70% nitrogen) at depth. It has been called "rapture of the deep" (*l'ivresse des grandes profondeurs*)[26] and has unfortunately led to many foolish maneuvers and deaths in the dangerous subaquatic environment. Although the underlying mechanism of nitrogen narcosis is unknown, the simple structure and relatively high lipophilicity of nitrogen suggests a membrane-related mechanism similar to that of other anesthetic gases.[6,45,47] To avoid nitrogen narcosis, less lipid-soluble inert gases such as hydrogen or helium are generally substituted for nitrogen.[82] Oxygen substitution, while logical, is not acceptable due to the risk of oxygen toxicity (see Oxygen).

How Are the Irritant Gases Classified?

Irritant gases share the ability to damage the respiratory tract. However, the irritant gases are a heterogeneous group of chemicals that produce toxic effects via a final common pathway, by destruction of the integrity of the mucosal barrier (Table 94–2). Regardless of the mechanism by which the mucosa is damaged, the clinical presentations of patients exposed to irritant gases are similar. Those exposed to agents that are rapidly irritating (ie, within seconds) generally develop mucosal irritation limited to the upper respiratory tract. The rapid onset of symptoms is usually a sufficient signal to escape the exposure. Patients may present with oral, nasal, and pharyngeal pain along with associated drooling, mucosal edema, cough, or stridor. Conjunctival irritation or chemosis, as well as dermatologic irritation, is often noted since concomitant ocular and skin exposure to the gaseous agent is usually unavoidable. Agents that are less rapidly irritating may not provide an adequate signal of their presence and do not prompt escape. Prolonged breathing thus allows entry of the toxic gas further into the bronchopulmonary system, where delayed toxic effects may subsequently be noted. Tracheobronchitis, bronchiolitis, bronchospasm, and noncardiogenic pulmonary edema are typical inflammatory responses of this anatomic region and represent the spectrum of acute lower respiratory tract injury.

Exceptions to this relationship of an agent and its expected toxicity are, however, not uncommon. For example, in situations where escape from ongoing exposure is prevented, patients may develop lower respiratory tract injury following the prolonged exposure to acutely irritating gases. Alternatively, rapid onset of upper respiratory irritation may be noted in patients following substantial exposures to agents that are generally associated with delayed symptomatology. Exposure to exceedingly high concentrations of any gas may produce hypoxemia analogous to that seen with exposure to the simple asphyxiants.

The most characteristic and worrisome clinical man-

TABLE 94–2. CHARACTERISTICS OF SEVERAL IRRITANT GASES

Gas	Solubility (g%)[a]	Odor threshold (ppm)[b]	STEL[c]	IDLH[d]
Ammonia	90	5	35 ppm (24 mg/m^3)	500 ppm
Cadmium fumes	—	—	None	9 mg/m^3
Carbon dioxide	—	—	30,000 ppm (54,000 mg/m^3)	50,000
Chloramine	—	—	—	—
Chlorine	0.5	0.3	1 ppm (2.9 mg/m^3)	10 ppm
Copper fumes	—	—	None	100 mg/m^3
Formaldehyde	—	0.8	0.1 ppm ceiling (NIOSH)	20 ppm
Hydrogen chloride	82	1–5	5 ppm ceiling (NIOSH)	50 ppm
Hydrogen sulfide	0.3	25 ppb	15 ppm (21 mg/m^3)	300 ppm
Mercury vapor	—	—	0.3 mg/m^3	10 mg/m^3
Methane	—	200	None	—
Methyl bromide	—	—	None	2000 ppm
Nitrogen	—	—	None	—
Nitrogen dioxide	sl[e]	5	5 ppm (9.4 mg/m^3)	20 ppm
Osmium tetroxide	7.24	0.02 mg/L	0.0006 ppm (0.0047 mg/m^3)	1 mg/m^3
Ozone	$<$0.1	0.05	0.1 ppm (0.2 mg/m^3)	5 ppm
Phosgene	sl	0.5	0.2 ppm (0.8 mg/m^3) ceiling	2 ppm
Propane	—	5000	None	2100 ppm
Sulfur dioxide	23	1	5 ppm (13 mg/m^3)	100 ppm
Vanadium pentoxide	0.8	n/a	0.5 mg/m^3 ceiling	35 mg/m^3
Zinc chloride fumes	—	—	2 mg/m^3	50 mg/m^3
Zinc oxide (fume fever)	—	odorless	10 mg/m^3	500 mg/m^3

[a]g% = grams of gas per 100 mL water

[b]If applicable.

[c]STEL = short-term exposure limit; a 15-minute time-weighted average exposure level that should not be exceeded at any time during the workday. Ceiling: an exposure level that should not be exceeded at any time during the workday. The STEL permits brief excursions above the limit value if compensatory time during the 15-minute exposure interval is spent below the limit value (ie, it is an average exposure over time).

[d]IDLH = Immediately dangerous to life or health.

[e]sl = slightly

Source: Zenz C, ed: Occupational Medicine Principles and Practice, 3rd ed. Chicago, Mosby–Yearbook, 1993.

ifestation of irritant gas exposure is "acute lung injury" (ALI).[7] Acute lung injury is a syndrome consisting of clinical, radiographic, and physiologic abnormalities caused by pulmonary inflammation and alveolar filling that must be both acute in onset and not explained solely by pulmonary capillary hypertension (eg, congestive heart failure). The most severe manifestation of ALI is the acute respiratory distress syndrome (ARDS).[7] The criteria for the diagnosis of ARDS (versus ALI) hinges on the ratio of the partial pressure of dissolved oxygen (PaO_2) to the inspired oxygen fraction (FIO_2). Patients with an appropriate history and clinical presentation, with a PaO_2/FIO_2 less than 200 would be classified as having ARDS. Importantly, positive end-expiratory pressure (PEEP) is not part of the oxygenation criteria. Both ALI and ARDS, however, are nonspecific and are noted in patients suffering severe physiologic insults from countless etiologies, such as sepsis or trauma. Patients with ALI may present with dyspnea, chest tightness, chest pain, cough, frothy sputum, arterial hypoxemia, wheezing, or rales.[85] Typical radiographic abnormalities include bilateral pulmonary infiltrates suggestive of alveolar filling with a normal cardiac silhouette suggesting the absence of congestive heart failure.[84]

Pathologically, irritant chemicals damage both the more prevalent type I pneumocytes and the surfactant-producing type II pneumocytes, and also disrupt the integrity of the capillary endothelial cells. This damage results in accumulation of cellular debris and plasma exudate in the alveolar sacs, producing the characteristic clinical findings of ALI. Interestingly, the specific mechanisms by which the irritant gases damage the pulmonary endothelial and epithelial cells vary. Many irritant gases require dissolution in the lung water to liberate the ultimate toxicant, which is often an acid (eg, chlorine produces hydrochloric acid). Other gases induce pulmonary damage through free radical–mediated oxidative stress (eg, oxygen) on the cellular membranes. Several gases produce both acid and free radical oxidants (eg, nitrogen dioxide) and others induce pulmonary irritation through different mechanism (eg, metals).

What Is RADS?

Substantial exposure to irritant gas results in the development of a persistent asthma like syndrome which has been variously termed "reactive airways dysfunction syndrome" (RADS)[16] or "irritant-induced asthma."[147] It has often been compared to occupational asthma, since both are chemically induced disorders, most frequently occurring following chemical exposure in the workplace. However, in comparison with those who develop occupational asthma, patients who develop RADS have a lower incidence of atopy and are exposed to agents not typically considered to be immunologically sensitizing.[147] In addition, the airflow improvement with β_2-adrenergic agonist therapy is significantly better in patients with occupational asthma.[52] Bronchial biopsy performed in patients with RADS generally reveals a chronic inflammatory response.[16,52] The inflammation in RADS may have a neurogenic etiology,[12] as opposed to an immunologic origin as in patients with occupational asthma,[102] which may differentiate these clinically similar diseases on a mechanistic basis. Neurogenic inflammation results from increased vascular permeability, presumably due to release of substance P from unmyelinated sensory neurons (C-fibers).[93] Neurogenic inflammation is inhibited by substance P depletors such as capsaicin[93] and enhanced by substances that inhibit neutral endopeptidase, the enzyme responsible for the degradation of substance P.[102] Recovery may take months, with the delay related to either ongoing low-level exposures to endopeptidase inhibitors[35] or to persistent irritation of impaired tissue by environmental irritants (ie, pollution).

Which Agents Produce Toxicity Through Acid–Base Effects?

As already mentioned, irritant gases require dissolution in the mucosal water to reach the pneumocytes and endothelial cells. Agents that are highly water soluble rapidly produce clinical effects, prompting the patients to remove themselves from the exposure if possible. Thus, unless the gas is very concentrated or the escape prevented, the gas does not proceed past the upper respiratory tract. Since poorly soluble agents are not generally acutely irritating at low or moderate concentration, prolonged exposure often occurs. Therefore, pulmonary toxicity is common and is often delayed due to the need for the gas to dissolve in the mucosal water. Experimental models assessing the water solubility of a gas to predict the location of its associated lesions have largely agreed with the clinical data.[81] The exact mechanism by which acids produce toxicity is unclear, but oxidation of intracellular proteins causing rapid cytoskeletal shortening may be involved.[148]

Highly Water-soluble Agents

Ammonia (NH_3). Ammonia is a common industrial and household chemical that is used in the synthesis of plastics and explosives, and as a fertilizer, a refrigerant, and a cleaning agent. The characteristic odor is an unmistakable warning of exposure. The high water solubility (forming ammonium hydroxide, NH_4OH and heat) produces such rapid and severe upper airway irritation that patients seldom remain exposed for more than an instant. However, patients with exposures to highly concentrated gas or exposure for prolonged duration may develop tracheobronchial or pulmonary inflammation. For example, in a World War II London bomb shelter, which was actually a converted brewery cellar, a bomb fragment pierced an ammonia-carrying condenser pipe.[20] Exposed patients, especially those closest to the source, suffered acute lung injury and the overall mortality rate was 63%. Similarly, in more conventional situations, sloughing of the bronchial mucosa with subsequent airway obstruction may develop in patients inhaling concentrated ammonia refrigerant fumes.[44] Upon recovery from the acute event, patients may develop the reactive airways dysfunction syndrome.[44,107]

Chloramines. Chloramines are a series of chlorinated nitrogen compounds, the most important of which are monochloramine (NH_2Cl) and, less so, dichloramine ($NHCl_2$)(Fig. 94–1).[62] Chloramine is most commonly generated de novo through the admixture of ammonia with hypochlorite (bleach), often in a misguided attempt to potentiate the cleaning ability of one agent with a second.[63] Upon dissolution in the mucosal water, hypochlorous acid and ammonia gas are released, both of which are irritants. Although less water soluble than ammonia, chloramine generally produces rapid onset of symptoms.[49] However, the symptoms may not be so severe as to prompt immediate escape, with resultant prolonged or recurrent exposure.[125] Interestingly, chloramine toxicity may occur after the addition of hypochlorite to septic systems due to mixture of the bleach with urine.[105]

Hydrogen Chloride (HCl). Hydrochloric acid production is the most important use of hydrogen chloride gas, and hydrochloric acid use is widespread. Dissolution of hydrogen chloride gas in lung water after inhalation also produces hydrochloric acid. Respiratory dysfunction and pathologic lung changes are seen in experimental models of hydrogen chloride exposure.[17] Pyrolysis of polyvinylchloride, a plastic commonly used in pipe, generates hydrogen chloride[112] and is an occupational hazard of firefighters.[37] Because of adsorption to respirable carbonaceous particles generated in the fire, deposition of hydrogen chloride at the alveolar level may produce pulmonary toxicity. In addition, generation of hydrogen chloride gas from inadvertent mixing of chemicals may result in acute poisoning.[119] As with most irritants, reactive airways dysfunction syndrome has been reported after exposure to highly concentrated hydrogen chloride gas.[42,119]

Hydrogen Fluoride (HF). Unlike the former acid-forming gases, hydrogen fluoride gas dissolves in mucosal water to form a weak acid, hydrofluoric acid. That is, few free hydronium ions are liberated due to the high electronegativity of the fluoride ion. Following low-dose inhalational exposure, patients may develop typical irritant symptoms,[161] and large exposure may cause bronchial and pulmonary parenchymal destruction.[15] Death following inhalation may be due to acute lung injury,[98] but is usually due to systemic causes.[158] The undissociated, and therefore uncharged, hydrogen fluoride complex penetrates the mucosal cell. Once inside, the highly electronegative fluoride ion preferentially binds calcium ions and intracellular calcium stores become rapidly depleted. This interferes with cellular metabolic processes and results in mucosal cell death. Calcium follows the gradient into the cell, causing systemic hypocalcemia, and cellular destruction liberates potassium. Dermal exposure is significantly more common than is inhalational, but since the majority of severe toxicity is systemic rather than local in nature, this distinction is blurred (see Caustics in Chap. 86)

Management of hydrogen fluoride inhalation is similar to that with other irritants. The use of nebulized 2.5% calcium gluconate should be considered, which limits systemic fluoride absorption (made as 1.5 mL 10% calcium gluconate + 4.5 mL normal saline or water).[88] The exogenous calcium binds the fluoride locally and prevents fluoride-induced cellular and systemic toxicity. Systemic calcium salts should be administered as needed to correct hypocalcemia (see Hydrofluoric Acid in Chap. 86 and Antidotes in Depth: Calcium). Monitoring of the electrocardiogram and aggressive correction of serum electrolytes is critical to prevent death.

Hydrogen Sulfide (H_2S). Hydrogen sulfide, along with hydrogen fluoride, is unique among the irritant gases due to its ability to produce significant systemic toxicity. Hydrogen sulfide is both a mucosal irritant and an inhibitor of mitochondrial respiration. Hydrogen sulfide exposures occur most frequently in the petroleum-refining industry.[18] However, poisoning is described in asphalt production workers,[68] in hospital workers using acid to clean drains clogged with plaster of paris sludge,[116] and in workers in the synthetic rubber and nylon industries. It is present in natural sources such as from volcanic emission, in caves, and in sulfur springs. Interestingly, life forms, such as the vent tube worm, which lives around deep-sea hydrothermal vents, have evolved blood-borne factors that scavenge sulfides and allow existence in these otherwise lethal environments.[118] Hydrogen sulfide is also a decay product of organic material found in sewers or manure pits.[113] Due to the extreme potency and rapidity of action of hydrogen sulfide, would-be rescuers frequently become victims themselves.[113,140] The distinctive odor of "rotten eggs," while helpful in diagnosis, is not specific for this agent. Despite an odor threshold of several parts per billion,[124] rapid olfactory fatigue occurs, which provides a false sense that the exposure is abating (see Chap. 27). At low and moderate levels (up to 500 ppm), upper respiratory tract mucosal irritation is the principle toxicity. This irritant potential of hydrogen sulfide is highlighted by a large series of acutely exposed patients in whom acute lung injury was evident in 20%.[18]

The rapidity of death in patients exposed to high-level hydrogen sulfide makes it likely that cytochrome oxidase inhibition is the mechanism of lethality. In the largest study of sulfide poisonings to date, 10 of the 14 deaths occurred before arrival at the hospital.[18] Although

$$\text{a. } NH_4^+ + HOCl \rightarrow H^+ + H_2O + NH_2Cl$$

$$\text{b. } NH_2Cl + HOCl \rightarrow H_2O + NHCl_2$$

Figure 94–1. Formation of monochloramine (a) and dichloramine (b) from hypochlorous acid and ammonia.

the mechanism of toxicity is analogous to cyanide, the binding of hydrogen sulfide to cytochrome, unlike that of cyanide or carbon monoxide, is rapidly reversible.[139] Therefore, cautious removal of victims from exposure, only by rescuers wearing protective breathing apparatus, and rapid institution of on-scene supportive care may permit time for sulfide dissociation from the cytochrome complex. Oxygen is essential to encourage release of hydrogen sulfide from the cytochrome complex. In patients with pulmonary edema, positive end-expiratory pressure may be needed to provide adequate oxygenation. The utility of hyperbaric oxygen (HBO) therapy in hydrogen sulfide poisoned patients, while controversial, has theoretical benefits and is indicated in patients who do not demonstrate rapid clinical improvement.[138] While attractive as a method to improve oxygenation, patients with pulmonary edema have never been shown to benefit from hyperbaric oxygen therapy. Since the affinity of methemoglobin for hydrogen sulfide exceeds that of cytochrome oxidase,[138] methemoglobin generation may be beneficial, although this remains unproved in humans. The use of sodium nitrite should be reserved for patients who are not rapidly improving clinically. However, the thiosulfate portion of the cyanide antidote kit should not be used since thiosulfate is generated during sulfide metabolism. In addition, rhodanese, the enzyme for which thiosulfate is a co-substrate, is not involved in detoxification of hydrogen sulfide. As with CO and CN, persistent[140] or delayed[153] neurologic symptoms may be seen. It is currently unclear whether HBO can prevent these sequelae.

Sulfur Dioxide/Sulfuric Acid (SO_2/H_2SO_4). Sulfur dioxide has multiple industrial applications and is a by-product found in smelting and oil refining. It is a principle component of atmospheric smog. In addition, it may be generated de novo through inadvertent mixing of chemicals, such as acid with sodium bisulfite ($NaHSO_3$).[1] Sulfur dioxide is highly water soluble and fortunately has a characteristic pungent odor to provide warning of its presence at concentrations well below those that are irritating. Upon dissolution in water, sulfur dioxide converts to sulfurous acid (H_2SO_3),[95] which is responsible for mucosal cell edema and epithelial sloughing as well as altered mucous production.[126] The most important effect of exposure to sulfur dioxide is dose-related bronchospasm,[111] which is most pronounced, and difficult to treat, in asthmatic patients.[84] Large acute exposure produces the expected acute irritant response of both the upper and lower respiratory tract,[21] and RADS may persist for several years.[2,121] In the presence of catalytic metals (Fe, Mn), environmental sulfur dioxide is readily converted to sulfuric acid within water droplets. Sulfuric acid is a major environmental concern and the cause of "acid rain." In addition, periods of peak atmospheric levels are associated with significant health risk. The London fog incident in 1952, which produced 4000 deaths primarily from respiratory causes, as well as the Donora, Pennsylvania, fog in 1946 with 20 deaths, were attributed to sulfur dioxide and sulfuric acid.[92]

Intermediate Water Solubility

Chlorine (Cl_2). Chlorine gas (Fig. 94–2) is a valuable oxidizing agent with many industrial uses, making occupational exposure common. Chlorine gas was the first successful (albeit limited) large-scale chemical warfare gas, used by both the French and the Germans in World War I.[38] Although chlorine gas is not generally available for use in the home, domestic exposure to chlorine gas is common. The acidification of household bleach (ie, sodium hypochlorite) liberates chlorine gas.[63] As such, inappropriate mixing of cleaning agents is the cause of most nonoccupational exposures.[109] Since the anionic component of the acid is not involved in the reaction, combining hypochlorite with virtually any acid may release chlorine gas (eg, phosphoric,[63,145] hydrochloric,[50] sulfuric). Although almost always unintentional, some patients have intentionally generated chlorine gas in this manner for "pleasurable" purposes.[122] Chlorine gas is generated by stored swimming pool chlorination tablets, which are usually calcium hypochlorite [$Ca(OCl)_2$] or trichloro-s-triazinetroine (TST).[97] The vapors may be so concentrated that even brief inhalational exposures may produce pulmonary toxicity.[162] Mixing of the two different types of chlorinating tablets for additive effect generates chlorine gas and, in addition, is explosive.[97] Acute chlorine toxicity may occur when compressed chlorine gas is used for the direct chlorination of swimming pools[30,155] or drinking-water systems.[43] Although most episodes involve one or two patients, mass poisoning may occur. For example, several deaths occurred after puncture of a railroad tank car carrying 90 tons of liquid chlorine.[77]

Mucosal irritation, cough, and bronchospasm are the most common initial findings in patients exposed to chlorine gas. The odor threshold for chlorine is low, but it is difficult to distinguish toxic from permissible air levels until irritating, and potentially hazardous, ambient concentrations are attained. The intermediate solubility characteristics of chlorine make it only mildly irritating in moderate concentrations and allow substantial time to elapse, typically several hours, before patients develop symptoms. Acute lung injury may occur quickly, however, in patients with large acute exposures.[162] Pneumo-

a. $HCl + HOCl \leftrightarrow Cl_2 + H_2O$

b. $Cl_2 + H_2O \leftrightarrow 2\ HCl + \{O\}$ $\{O\}$ is nascent oxygen

Figure 94–2. Chlorine gas. (a) Formation of chlorine gas from hypochlorous acid; (b) hydration of chlorine gas to form hydrochloric acid and nascent oxygen.

mediastinum may occur, presumably due to the acute increase in intrathoracic pressure induced by the bronchospasm and pulmonary edema.[50]

Chlorine dissolves in the lung water and generates hydrochloric (HCl) and hypochlorous (HClO) acids. The hypochlorous acid rapidly degenerates into HCl and nascent oxygen (O^-). The unpaired oxygen molecule produces additional pulmonary damage by initiating a free-radical cascade. Symptomatic relief for patients with acute chlorine toxicity has been reported with nebulized sodium bicarbonate (see below).[155] Whether the chloride ion is absorbed systemically is unclear, although one patient developed a mild hyperchloremic metabolic acidosis after accidentally inhaling the chlorine gas generated through the mixture of household cleaning agents.[145] Reactive airways dysfunction syndrome appears to be relatively frequent following significant chlorine gas inhalation.[32]

Poorly Water Soluble Agents

Phosgene (Carbonyl Chloride) ($COCl_2$). During World War I,[38] phosgene was an important weapon of mass destruction that produced countless deaths. Intentional poisoning is, fortunately, now uncommon, but occupational exposure to phosgene occasionally produces, unintentional poisoning.[33] Phosgene finds industrial applications in the synthesis of various organic compounds, especially isocyanates. It is also a by-product of heating or combustion of various chlorinated organic compounds.[141] Intense exposure to phosgene may produce acute mucosal irritation,[40] but with more moderate exposure irritation is typically absent. In fact, the pleasant odor of fresh hay, rather than prompting escape, may ironically promote deep and prolonged breathing of the toxic gas.

By virtue of its use as a war agent, phosgene poisoning has received more investigation than most other irritant gases. The most consequential clinical effect related to phosgene exposure is delayed onset of acute lung injury. Due to the accumulation of a significant alveolar burden of phosgene, symptoms are generally severe once they occur. Since the delay in onset may be nearly a day, prolonged observation of patients thought to be phosgene poisoned is warranted.

The most important therapeutic maneuver remains support of pulmonary function and oxygenation, including positive end-expiratory pressure and high inspired-oxygen concentrations. Although its use has not been reported, nebulized sodium bicarbonate has theoretical value in phosgene-poisoned patients.

The mechanism of phosgene toxicity is complex. To some extent, dissolution of the gas into the mucosal water to liberate hydrochloric acid is important. The acid reacts with functional groups on epithelial and endothelial cell membranes and, via cellular messengers, engenders a systemic inflammatory response. Phosgene stimulates the synthesis of lipoxygenase-derived leukotrienes, and pulmonary edema may be prevented in rabbits by tomelukast, a leukotriene-receptor antagonist.[60] Methylprednisolone, which blocks leukotriene synthesis, also prevents pulmonary edema in experimental models but does not appear to offer postexposure benefit.[60] In addition, ibuprofen, a nonsteroidal antiinflammatory agent, reduces phosgene-induced pulmonary edema.[133] Leukotrienes are important chemotactic factors for neutrophils, accumulation of which is related to the development of oxidant-induced pulmonary edema.[46] Other agents capable of reducing neutrophil influx, such as colchicine and cyclophosphamide, reduce lung injury and mortality in mice when given 30 minutes postexposure.[53] Intratracheal DBcAMP, a cAMP analog, inhibits the release of leukotrienes.[135] This may be the same mechanism by which other cAMP enhancers, such as terbutaline or aminophylline, limit the development of pulmonary capillary leakage in phosgene-exposed rabbits.[80] Intratracheal *N*-acetylcysteine, administered 45 minutes postexposure to phosgene-poisoned rabbits, resulted in decreased formation of leukotrienes and limited the development of pulmonary edema.[134] Presumably administration via nebulization would prove similarly effective. Intravenous administration of *N*-acetylcysteine to nonpoisoned patients with mild to moderate acute lung injury improved systemic oxygenation and reduced the need for ventilatory support.[144] However, the progression to frank ALI/ARDS was not altered. Since damage to the lung had already occurred, the observed benefit may be related to improved hemodynamic function rather than an antioxidant effect.[62]

Which Agents Are Toxic due to Free-radical Mechanisms?

Rather than acidic or alkaline metabolites, free radicals mediate the pulmonary toxicity of certain irritant gases. Examples of oxygen free radicals include superoxide ($O_2^{-\bullet}$), hydroxyl radical (OH^-), hydrogen peroxide (HOOH), and singlet oxygen ($O^\bullet$).[130] These highly reactive oxygen derivatives bind to and destroy tissue near their site of generation. Ironically, free radicals generated by inflammatory cells contribute to the pulmonary damage. Fortunately, the lung has antioxidant systems, both enzymatic (eg, superoxide dismutase, glutathione peroxidase, catalase) and nonenzymatic (glutathione, ascorbate) in nature, that detoxify virtually all free radicals present in the lung.[120] However, the oxidant burden imposed by oxidant gases can overwhelm the detoxifying systems and produce cellular damage.

Oxygen (O_2). Oxygen toxicity is uncommon in the workplace, but ironically is common in hospitalized patients. Although oxygen may produce central nervous system and retinal toxicity, pulmonary damage is most common. Based on several clinical studies, it appears that humans can tolerate 100% oxygen at sea level for up to 48 hours without significant acute pulmonary damage.[31] Under hyperbaric conditions (2.0 atmospheres absolute), such as during compressed air diving or while inside a pressurized hyperbaric chamber, oxygen toxicity may develop within 3–6 hours.[24] Delayed pulmonary fibrosis, presumably due to healing of subclinical injury, may be found, however, in patients breathing lower concentrations at sea level for shorter periods.[25] Techniques to prevent pulmonary oxygen toxicity currently emphasize reduction of the inspired oxygen concentration with the use of positive end-expiratory pressure ventilation, although this approach failed to prove beneficial in at least one clinical trial.[115]

Although it seems paradoxical that oxygen, a molecule without which we could not live, may be deleterious at elevated concentrations, it is not. In mitochondria, oxygen plays a critical role as the ultimate acceptor for electrons, completing the electron transport chain. It is this same potent oxidizing activity that allows oxygen to remove electrons from other compounds, generating toxic oxygen radicals.

Although several other oxidant chemicals, notably paraquat, produce their toxicity through the induction of apoptosis, or programmed cell death, oxygen toxicity produces cellular necrosis.[79] Oxygen increases pulmonary capillary permeability,[160] which may be prevented by the administration of either parenteral *N*-acetylcysteine,[132] a chemical antioxidant, or superoxide dismutase, an enzymatic antioxidant.[152] Although several other agents have shown promise in preventing oxygen-mediated toxicity, none has yet proven to be therapeutic for patients already manifesting pulmonary toxicity. In the future, magnetic resonance imaging enhanced by a gadolinium derivative may allow early diagnosis and quantitation of endothelium damage in patients at risk for iatrogenic pulmonary oxygen toxicity.[14] This technique should be useful for patients exposed to other pulmonary irritants as well and may help guide the evaluation of potential therapeutic modalities.

Oxides of Nitrogen. The oxides of nitrogen are a series of variably oxidized compounds containing both oxygen and nitrogen.[51] Included in this series are stable compounds such as nitrogen dioxide (NO_2), nitrogen tetraoxide (ie, dinitrogen tetraoxide: N_2O_4), nitrogen trioxide (N_2O_3), nitrous oxide (N_2O), and nitric oxide (NO). These compounds either react directly with pulmonary tissues or generate free radicals such as peroxynitrites ($ONOO^-$) that damage the lung. In addition to generating free radicals, dissolution in the respiratory tract water generates nitric (HNO_3) and nitrous acid (HNO_2), which produce injury consistent with other inhaled acids.[59] In fact, inhalation of nitric acid produces the same clinical syndrome.[61] Antioxidants afford significant protection to human endothelial cells exposed to nitrogen dioxide, implying an important role for free radicals in the toxicology of these agents.[150]

The oxides of nitrogen have limited value in industrial operations, although they may be generated during welding and brazing. Nitrogen dioxide, in addition to hydrogen cyanide, is also produced in the pyrolysis of nitrocellulose, which is a substantial component of radiographic film. For example, the fire in the radiology department of the Cleveland Clinic in 1929 resulted in 125 casualties, virtually all of whom died of cyanide or nitrogen oxide gas poisoning.[57] Nitrogen dioxide toxicity is seen in indoor ice skating rinks when the gas is generated by the propane-driven ice-cleaning machines (ie, Zamboni).[64] Military exposure to high levels of nitrogen dioxide may occur during closed-space fires (eg, submarines) or during combat.[99] Nitrogen dioxide is also the cause of "silo filler's disease," in which the toxic gas generated from decomposing (oxidized) fertilizer accumulates within the silo shortly after grain storage[34] (see Chap. 110). Prior to ventilation, such high concentrations may accumulate in the silo that entrance may result in asphyxiation due to the depletion of oxygen. Additionally, substantial quantities of nitrogen dioxide remaining after incomplete ventilation may produce the delayed pulmonary toxicity characteristic of the silo filler's disease. Chronic indoor exposure to nitrogen dioxide[74] or outdoor exposure to smog[131] may predispose to the development or exacerbation of chronic lung diseases, including infection, asthma,[151] and cancer.

Ozone (O_3). Ozone is formed in the stratosphere (region between 5 and 31 miles above the planet) by the action of ultraviolet light on oxygen molecules and thus reduces the amount of solar ultraviolet irradiation reaching Earth.[89] The high ozone concentration at this altitude may occasionally cause symptoms in occupants of high flying planes.[123] Ozone is an important component in photochemical smog and may contribute to chronic lung disease.[91] It is produced in significant quantities by welding and high-voltage electrical equipment and in more moderate doses by photocopying machines and laser printers. Due to its high electronegative oxidation potential (only fluorine is higher), ozone is one of the most potent oxidizing agents available. For this reason it is used as a bleaching agent, particularly as an alternative to chlorine in water purification and sewage treatment.

The pulmonary toxicity associated with ozone is primarily due to its high reactivity toward unsaturated fatty acids and amino acids with a sulfhydryl functional group.[154] Ozonation and free radical damage to the lipid component of the membrane initiates an inflammatory cascade, with resultant influx of inflammatory cells.[86] Increased permeability of the pulmonary epithelium results in alveolar filling from the transudation of proteins and fluids[86] (ie, ALI). Antioxidant agents, such as vitamin E, which react preferentially with free radicals before membrane damage occurs, prevent or limit the pulmonary toxicity of ozone.[54,127]

Other Irritant Gases

Acrolein

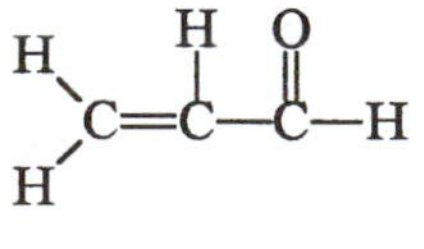

Acrolein is a highly water-soluble, three-carbon aldehyde, which exerts a potent irritant effect on the upper respiratory tract.[94] It is an important pyrolysis product of hydrocarbon polymers such as polypropylene when burned in an oxygen-containing atmosphere.[112] It is also used in industrial applications as an oxidizing agent. Despite the high water solubility of acrolein, patients exposed to polypropylene fires commonly develop pulmonary edema, even in the absence of prolonged exposure. As with hydrogen chloride, it is likely that acrolein is carried by carbon containing particles to the lower respiratory tract[73] (see Chap. 95).

Methylisocyanate

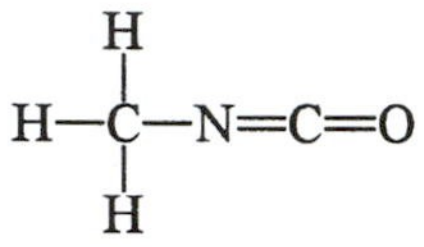

Methylisocyanate (MIC) is one of a series of compounds sharing a similar isocyanate (N=C=O) moiety. Isocyanates important in the polymer industry include toluene diisocyanate (TDI) and diphenylmethane diisocyanate (MDI). Despite the mass devastation seen after the inadvertent release of MIC in Bhopal, India, in 1984, MIC toxicity is relatively uncommon. The Union Carbide plant in Bhopal used MIC for the manufacture of carbaryl, a carbamate pesticide, which is the primary industrial role for MIC. The MIC gas, which escaped after water had leaked into its holding tank, produced immediate eye and respiratory symptoms in approximately 200,000 local inhabitants.[103] Many had pulmonary edema, demonstrated both clinically[106] and radiographically.[136] Approximately 2500 deaths, most due to respiratory dysfunction, were reported. Many survivors suffered persistent respiratory symptoms consistent with RADS and had abnormal tests of pulmonary function.[78] Methylisocyanate is a significantly more potent respiratory irritant than the other regularly used isocyanate derivatives.[41] Although not irritating, TDI frequently produces pulmonary effects through immunologic sensitization. There is no specific therapy for patients exposed to MIC, although decontamination and supportive care should be provided. Despite the nomenclature, cyanide poisoning does not occur and empiric antidotal therapy is not indicated.

Riot Control Agents: Capsaicin, CS, and CN. Historically, riot control agents consisted primarily of chloroacetophenone (CN) or chlorobenzylidenemalononitrile (CS) (Fig. 94–3). Both are white solids that are dispersed as an aerosol. This is generally accomplished through mixture with a pyrotechnic agent such as a grenade or with a volatile organic solvent in a personal-protection canister.[9] After low-level exposure, ocular discomfort and lacrimation alone are expected (thus the name "tear gas") and are probably due to enhanced release of substance P from sensory nerve terminals. These effects are transient, and recovery is usually complete within 30 minutes. Closed space[149] or close range[56] exposure may produce significant ocular toxicity[56] or dermal burns[149] in addition to pulmonary toxicity. Exposed patients may develop chest pain, cough, and bronchospasm rapidly in these situations, and may subsequently develop RADS.[70,129]

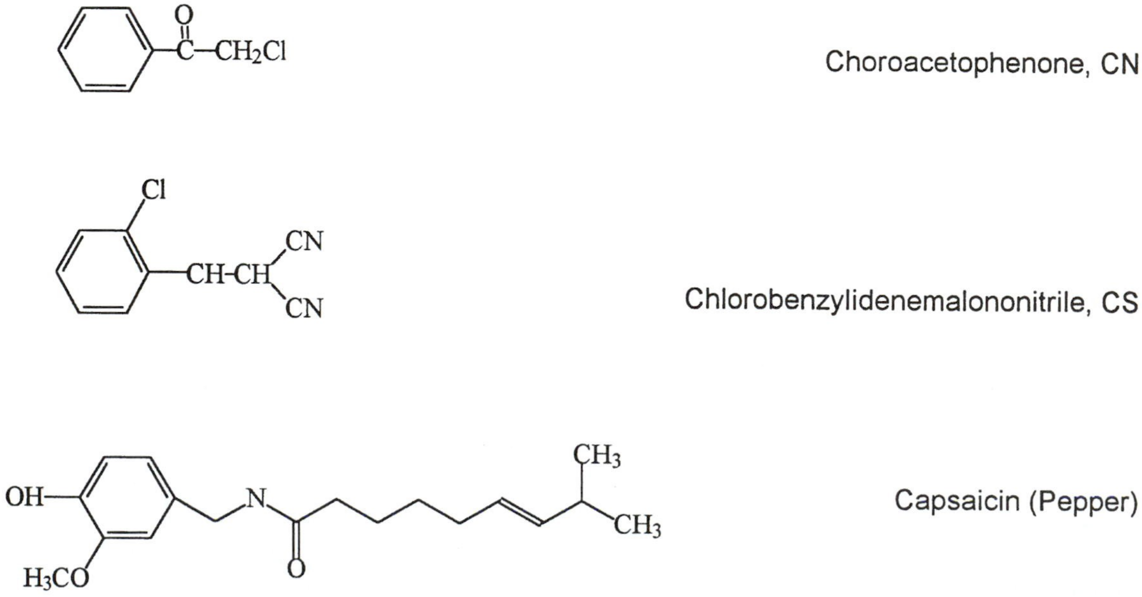

Figure 94–3. Chemical structures of commonly used lacrimating agents (tear gases).

Delayed noncardiogenic pulmonary edema, consistent with acute lung injury, is also seen in these situations[149] and is likely related to the ability of these agents to alkylate tissues in a manner similar to mustard agents.[27] Since the delivery systems remain relatively primitive and subject to prevailing environmental conditions, dosing is unpredictable and toxicity common.

Due to their high potential for severe toxicity, CN and CS were replaced for civilian use by oleoresin capsicum, or pepper spray. Although capsaicin, the active component of pepper spray, is considerably less toxic, pneumonitis[10] and death[142] unfortunately still occur. Capsaicin invokes the release of substance P, a neuropeptide involved with the transmission of pain impulses.[69] Substance P also induces neurogenic inflammation which, in the lung, results in pulmonary edema and bronchoconstriction[142] (see section on RADS). Current therapy for inhalation of capsaicin, or of any tear gas, is primarily supportive. Extracorporeal membrane oxygenation has been used in children to maintain oxygenation in the presence of severe pulmonary toxicity.[10] Substance P antagonists, which are currently not available for clinical use, show promise in experimental models.[110]

Metal Fume Fever/Polymer Fume Fever. Metal fume fever is a recurrent flu-like syndrome that develops shortly after exposure to metal oxide fumes generated during welding, galvanizing, or smelting (see Table 94–3). Although most symptoms of metal fume fever are similar to those expected with irritant gas exposures (dyspnea, cough, chest pain), the presence of fever, typically between 38° and 39°C, distinguishes the syndromes.[12] In addition, patients may experience headache, metallic taste, myalgias, and chills.[12] Direct pulmonary toxicity probably does not occur, and patients with metal fume fever generally have normal chest radiographs. Interestingly, acute tolerance develops so that repeat daily exposure produces more mild symptoms, but after a short work hiatus, such as a weekend, the tolerance is lost.[128] Many metals are capable of eliciting this syndrome, but most frequently it is noted in patients who have welded galvanized steel, which contains zinc.[128] Serum and urine zinc levels are not elevated[128] after the acute event, although they may be chronically elevated due to daily occupational exposure.

The etiology of metal fume fever is still debated, but the syndrome has features suggestive of both an immunologic and a toxic etiology.[11] Antigen release with immunologic response appears to be responsible for the induction of symptoms.[100] On subsequent exposure, proinflammatory cytokines, such as tumor necrosis factor-alpha, and various interleukins can be detected in bronchoalveolar lavage fluid.[87] However, since symptoms can occur with the patient's first exposure to fumes, a direct toxic effect on the respiratory mucosa presumably exists. Significant exposure to certain metals fumes, such as cadmium, may produce direct toxic effects on the pulmonary parenchyma. Patients with metal-induced pneumonitis present with pulmonary edema. Metal pneumonitis is distinguishable from other causes of ARDS only by history[67] or, retrospectively, by finding elevated serum or urine metal levels.[3]

The management of patients with metal fume fever is supportive and includes analgesics and antipyretics. There is no specific antidote. Patients with ALI are probably suffering from metal toxicity (eg, cadmium pneumonitis). The natural course of metal fume fever involves spontaneous resolution within 48 hours. Persistent symptoms are rare and should prompt investigation for metal toxicity. Patients with acute cadmium or zinc pneumonitis should be hospitalized and receive corticosteroids.

A remarkably similar syndrome occurs subsequent to inhaling pyrolysis products of fluorinated polymers (eg, Teflon), which is aptly termed "polymer fume fever."[137] Patients develop self-limited viral-illness-like symptoms several hours after exposure to the fumes. As with metal fumes, very large exposures to polymer fumes may result in direct pulmonary toxicity. Supportive care remains the therapy of choice.

TABLE 94–3. EXPOSURE FORMS OF INHALATIONAL TOXINS

Gas	A substance in a gaseous physical state at room temperature (70°F) and standard pressure (760 mm Hg).
Aerosol	A suspension of fine particles (solid or liquid) in a gas (eg, air); fog, mist, and smoke are aerosols.
Fog	A liquid aerosol formed from the condensation from a gaseous to a liquid state.
Mist	A liquid aerosol formed by dispersion of a liquid (eg, atomization) or by gas entrainment of a liquid.
Smoke	A solid aerosol resulting from the incomplete combustion of organic materials.
Fume	A suspension of fine solid particles in a gas resulting from condensation; generally applied to metals and their oxides.
Dust	A suspension of solid organic or inorganic material in a gas formed through a disintegration process (eg, grinding).
Vapor	A gaseous form of a substance that generally exists as a solid or liquid under standard conditions.

What Is the General Approach to Managing Patients With Irritant Gas Exposure?

Management of patients with acute respiratory tract injury begins with meticulous support of airway patency, bronchial and pulmonary secretions, and oxygenation. Although various theoretical and experimental treatment modalities have been proposed, supportive care remains the mainstay of therapy.[85] Supplemental oxygen, bronchodilators, and airway suctioning should be used if clinically indicated. The similarity of the pulmonary pathology among patients with irritant gas exposure and other etiologies of ARDS permit the broad application of certain general management principles. For example, positive end-expiratory pressure (PEEP) and inverse ratio ventilation are successful in enhancing the oxygenation of patients with ARDS of various etiologies.[108] Although not specifically evaluated, there are sound theoretical reasons to believe these modalities should improve oxygenation in poisoned patients as well. While it is always important to reduce the inspired concentration of oxygen to below 50% as rapidly as possible, patients poisoned by irritant gases may be even more susceptible to oxygen toxicity due to depletion of endogenous antioxidant barriers.[114] Similarly, hyperbaric oxygen therapy may be deleterious.[114] Nitrovasodilators, diuretics, and morphine have little role in the management of ARDS, although low-dose morphine may prove beneficial as an anxiolytic.[117] Recent experience with partial liquid ventilation using perfluorocarbon in patients with nonchemically induced ARDS suggests that exfoliated tissue, and presumably toxin if still present, may be effectively lavaged from the bronchopulmonary tree.[65] This approach may ultimately prove important since bronchopulmonary decontamination is otherwise severely limited by virtue of its anatomy. In addition, partial liquid ventilation improves oxygenation in experimental models[27,66] as well as in humans with ARDS.[65]

Several other recent developments may prove useful in the general management of patients with ARDS. Surfactant replacement therapy initially received attention as a treatment for patients with ARDS due to its beneficial effects in infant respiratory distress syndrome.[76] Conceptually, surfactant therapy is beneficial in patients with ARDS since surfactant levels are diminished in this population. This decrease is due both to destruction of surfactant-producing cells and alteration of the structure and function of existing surfactant by protein exudates.[58] Although several experimental and clinical studies[157,159] suggested the safety and efficacy of surfactant therapy in patients with ARDS, large, randomized, controlled clinical trials failed to show a benefit.[4] However, these studies generally included patients with sepsis-related ARDS and most of these patients died of septic complications, not of pulmonary failure. Thus the inability to show a beneficial effect may not adequately reflect the potential of surfactant in irritant gas–induced ARDS. In fact, a promising model of oxygen-induced lung injury in primates noted a beneficial effect of aerosolized surfactant.[71] Conversely, early corticosteroid therapy designed to reduce the host inflammatory response appears to provide little benefit to patients with ARDS,[8] although it may reduce the late fibroproliferative phase.[101] Although there is an intriguing report of better outcome with steroid treatment in one of two sisters with simultaneous, equivalent chlorine exposure, there is little reason to suspect any specific benefit in most poisoned patients.[22]

A therapy unique to several of the acid–base-forming irritant gases is chemical neutralization. Although contraindicated in acid or alkali injury of the gastrointestinal tract, the large surface area of the lung allows dissipation of the heat generated during neutralization. Case studies suggest that nebulized 2% sodium bicarbonate may be beneficial in patients poisoned by acid-forming irritant gases.[155] However, formal evaluation in poisoned patients for either safety or efficacy has not been attempted. Caution should be observed that the sodium bicarbonate is sufficiently dilute, since sodium bicarbonate itself may prove irritating. Typically, a 1:3 dilution of 8.4% sodium bicarbonate solution with sterile water is sufficient (resulting in a 2.1% solution for nebulization). Although apparently safe if properly diluted, it is uncertain whether such therapy alters the natural course of the pulmonary damage. Nebulized 4% sodium bicarbonate administered to chlorine-poisoned sheep improved oxygenation but failed to improve mortality.[23] Therefore, patients receiving nebulized bicarbonate therapy require observation beyond the period of symptom resolution. Why previously evaluated neutralizing agents, such as Tris buffer (trishydroxymethylaminomethane, THAM) and methenamine (hexamethylenetetramine, HMT), are no longer utilized despite potential efficacy is unclear.[32] No neutralizing agent for alkaline irritants has been evaluated.

Summary

Although the spectrum of agents capable of causing pulmonary toxicity is large, the pathologic changes are rather limited. Gases that have little or no irritant potential or systemic toxicity cause simple asphyxiation, in which the ambient air is devoid of oxygen. Parenchymal irritation, with severely toxic patients progressing to ARDS, is common to both acid-forming as well as free radical generating toxic gases. Treatment of all such exposures centers on supportive and respiratory care. In addition, RADS has been described in patients following exposure to virtually all of the irritant gases.

References

1. MMWR. Acute occupational exposure to sulfur dioxide—Missouri. MMWR 1983:32:541–542.
2. Alford PT, McLees BD, Case LD, Faust JR: Reactive airways dysfunction syndrome (RADS) in workers post exposure to sulfur dioxide (SO_2). Chest 1988;94 (suppl):87S. Abstract.
3. Ando Y, Shibata E, Tsuchiyama F, Sakai S: Elevated urine cadmium concentrations in a patient with acute cadmium pneumonitis. Scand J Work Environ Health 1996;22: 150–153.
4. Anzueto A, Baughman RP, Guntupalli KK, et al: Aerosolized surfactant in adults with sepsis-induced adult respiratory distress syndrome. N Engl J Med 1996;334: 1417–1421.
5. Bauman JE, Dean BS, Krenzelok EP: Myocardial infarction and neurodevastation following butane inhalation. Vet Hum Toxicol 1991;33:389. Abstract.
6. Bennett PB, Papahadjopoulos D, Bangham AD: The effect of raised pressure of inert gas on phospholipid membranes. Life Sci 1967;6:2527–2533.

7. Bernard GR, Artigas A, Brigham KL, et al: The American-European Consensus Conference on ARDS: Definitions, mechanisms, relevant outcomes, and clinical trial coordination. Am J Respir Crit Care Med 1994;149:818–824.
8. Bernard GR, Luce JM, Sprung CL, et al: High-dose corticosteroids in patients with the adult respiratory distress syndrome. N Engl J Med 1987;317:1565–1570.
9. Beswick FW: Chemical agents used in riot control and warfare. Hum Toxicol 1983;2:247–256.
10. Billmire DF, Vinocur C, Ginda M, et al: Pepper-spray-induced respiratory failure treated with extracorporeal membrane oxygenation. Pediatrics 1996;98:961–963.
11. Blanc P, Wong H, Bernstein MS, Boushey HA: An experimental human model of metal fume fever. Ann Intern Med 1991;114:930–936.
12. Blount BW: Two types of metal fume fever: Mild vs. serious. Milit Med 1990;155:372–377.
13. Bozic CR, Lu B, Hopken UE, et al: Neurogenic amplification of immune complex inflammation. Science 1996;273: 1722–1725.
14. Brasch RC, Berthezene Y, Vexler V, et al: Pulmonary oxygen toxicity: Demonstration of abnormal capillary permeability using contrast-enhanced MRI. Pediatr Radiol 1993; 23:495–500.
15. Braun J, Stoss H, Zober A: Intoxication following the inhalation of hydrogen fluoride. Arch Toxicol 1984;56: 50–54.
16. Brooks SM, Weiss MA, Bernstein IL: Reactive airways dysfunction syndrome. Case reports of persistent asthma syndrome after high level irritant exposure. Chest 1985;88: 376–384.
17. Burleigh-Flayer HK, Wong KL, Alarie Y: Evaluation of the pulmonary effects of HCl using CO_2 challenges in guinea pigs. Fund Appl Toxicol 1985;5:978–985.
18. Burnett WW, King EG, Grace M, Hall WF: Hydrogen sulfide poisoning: Review of 5 years' experience. Can Med Assoc J 1977;117:1277–1280.
19. Byard RW: Methane. Death scene gas analysis in suspected methane asphyxia. Am J Forensic Med Pathol 1992;13:69–71.
20. Caplin M: Ammonia-gas poisoning. Forty-seven cases in a London shelter. Lancet 1941;2:95–96.
21. Charan NB, Myers CG, Lakshminarayan S, Spencer TM: Pulmonary injuries associated with acute sulfur dioxide inhalation. Am Rev Respir Dis 1979;119:555–560.
22. Chester EH, Kaimal J, Payne CB, Kohn PM: Pulmonary injury following exposure to chlorine gas: possible beneficial effects of steroid treatment. Chest 1977;72:247–250.
23. Chisholm CD, Singletary EM, Okerberg CV, Langlinais PC: Inhaled sodium bicarbonate for chlorine inhalation injuries. Ann Emerg Med 1989;18:466. Abstract.
24. Clark JM, Lambertsen CJ: Rate of development of pulmonary O_2 toxicity in man during O_2 breathing at 2.0 Atm abs. J Appl Physiol 1971;30:739–752.
25. Collins JF, Smith JD, Coalson JJ, et al: Variability of lung collagen amounts after prolonged support for respiratory failure. Chest 1984;85:641–646.
26. Cousteau JY: The Silent World. London, The Reprint Society, 1954.
27. Cucinell SA, Swentzel KC, Biskup R, et al: Biochemical interactions and metabolic fate of riot control agents. Fed Proc 1971;30:86–91
28. Curtis SE, Peek JT, Kelly DR: Partial liquid ventilation with perflubron improves arterial oxygenation in acute canine lung injury. J Appl Physiol 1993;75:2696–2702.
29. DeBehnke DJ, Hilander SJ, Dobler DW, et al: The hemodynamic and arterial blood gas response to asphyxiation: A canine model of pulseless electrical activity. Resuscitation 1995;30:169–175.
30. Decker WJ: Chlorine poisoning at the swimming pool revisited: Anatomy of two minidisasters. Vet Hum Toxicol 1988;30:584–585.
31. Deneke SM, Fanburg BL: Normobaric oxygen toxicity of the lung. N Engl J Med 1980;303:76–86.
32. Deschamps D, Soler P, Rosenberg N, et al: Persistent asthma after inhalation of a mixture of sodium hypochlorite and hydrochloric acid. Chest 1994;105:1895–1896.
33. Diller WF: Medical phosgene problems and their possible solution. J Occup Med 1978;20:189–193.
34. Douglas WW, Hepper NGG, Colby TV: Silo-filler's disease. Mayo Clin Proc 1989;64:291–304.
35. Dusser DJ, Djokic TD, Borson DB, Nadel JA: Cigarette smoke induces bronchoconstrictor hyperresponsiveness to substance P and inactivates airway neutral endopeptidases in the guinea pig. Possible role of free radicals. J Clin Invest 1989;84:900–906.
36. Dwyer DM, Thorne AC, Healey JH, et al: Liquid nitrogen instillation can cause venous gas embolism. Anesthesiology 1990;73:179–181.
37. Dyer RF, Esch VH: Polyvinyl chloride toxicity in fires. JAMA 1976;235:393–397.
38. Eckert WG: Mass deaths by gas or chemical poisoning: A historical perspective. Am J Forensic Med Pathol 1991;12: 119–125.
39. Edmonds C, Lowry C, Pennefather J: Diving and Subaquatic Medicine. Oxford, England, Butterworth-Heinemann Ltd, 1992, pp. 215–225.
40. Everett ED, Overholt EL: Phosgene poisoning. JAMA 1968;205;103–105.
41. Ferguson JS, Schaper M, Stock MF, et al: Sensory and pulmonary irritation with exposure to methyl isocyanate. Toxicol Appl Pharmacol 1986;82:329–335.
42. Finnegan MJ, Hodson ME: Prolonged hypoxaemia following inhalation of hydrogen chloride vapor. Thorax 1989; 44:238–239.
43. Fleta J, Calvo C, Zuñiga M, et al: Intoxication of 76 children by chlorine gas. Hum Toxicol 1986;5:99–100.
44. Flury KE, Dines DE, Rodarte JR, Rodgers R: Airway obstruction due to inhalation of ammonia. Mayo Clin Proc 1983;58:389–393.
45. Fowler B, Ackles KN, Porlier G: Effects of inert gas narcosis on behaviour—A critical review. Undersea Biomed Res 1985;12:369–402.
46. Fox RB, Hoidal JR, Brown DM, Repine JE: Pulmonary inflammation due to oxygen toxicity: Involvement of chemotactic factors and polymorphic leukocytes. Am Rev Respir Dis 1981;123:521–523.
47. Franks NP, Lieb WR: Do general anesthetics act by com-

petitive binding to specific receptors? Nature 1984;310: 599–601.
48. Frederiksen JW, Smith J, Brown P, et al: Arterial helium embolism from a ruptured intraaortic balloon. Ann Thorac Surg 1988;46:690–692
49. Gapany-Gapanavicius M, Molho M, Tirosh M: Chloramine-induced pneumonitis from mixing household cleaning agents. Br Med J 1982;285:1086.
50. Gapany-Gapanavicius M, Yellin A, Almog S, Tirosh M: Pneumomediastinum: A complication of chlorine exposure from mixing household cleaning agents. JAMA 1982;248: 349–350.
51. Gaston B, Drazen JM, Loscalzo J, Stamler JS: The biology of nitrogen oxides in the airway. Am J Respir Crit Care Med 1994;149:538–551.
52. Gautrin D, Boulet LP, Boutet M, et al: Is reactive airways dysfunction syndrome a variant of occupational asthma? J Allergy Clin Immunol 1994;93:12–22.
53. Ghio AJ, Kennedy TP, Hatch GE, Tepper JS: Reduction of neutrophil influx diminishes lung injury and mortality following phosgene inhalation. J Appl Physiol 1991;71: 657–665.
54. Goldstein BD, Levine MR, Cuzzi-Spada R, et al: *p*-Aminobenzoic acid as a protective agent in ozone toxicity. Arch Environ Health 1972;24:243–247.
55. Gray MY, Lazarus JH: Butane inhalation and hemiparesis. J Toxicol Clin Toxicol 1993;31:483–485.
56. Gray PJ: Treating CS gas injuries to the eye: Exposure at close range is particularly dangerous. Br Med J 1995; 311:871. Letter.
57. Gregory KL, Malinoski VF, Sharp CR: Cleveland Clinic fire survivorship study, 1929–1965. Arch Environ Health 1969;18:508–515.
58. Gregory TJ, Longmore WJ, Moxley MA, et al: Surfactant chemical composition and biophysical activity in adult respiratory distress syndrome. J Clin Invest 1991;88: 1976–1981.
59. Guidotti TL: Toxic inhalation of nitrogen dioxide: Morphologic and functional changes. Exp Mol Pathol 1980; 33:90–103
60. Guo YL, Kennedy TP, Michael JR, et al: Mechanism of phosgene-induced lung toxicity: Role of arachidonate mediators. J Appl Physiol 1990;69:1615–1622.
61. Hajela R, Janigan DT, Landrigan PL, et al: Fatal pulmonary edema due to nitric acid inhalation in three pulp-mill workers. Chest 1990;97:487–489.
62. Harrison PHM, Wendon JA, Grimson AES, et al: Improvement by acetylcysteine of haemodynamics and oxygen transport in fulminant hepatic failure. N Engl J Med 1991;324:1852–1857.
63. Hattis RP, Greer JR, Dietrich S, et al: Chlorine gas toxicity from mixture of bleach with other cleaning products—California. MMWR 1991;40;619–629.
64. Hedberg K, Hedberg CW, Iber C, et al: An outbreak of nitrogen dioxide-induced respiratory illness among ice hockey players. JAMA 1989;262:3014–3017.
65. Hirschl RB, Pranikoff T, Wise C, et al: Initial experience with partial liquid ventilation in adult patients with adult respiratory distress syndrome. JAMA 1996;275:383–389.
66. Hirschl RB, Tooley R, Parent A, et al: Improvement of gas exchange, pulmonary function, and acute lung injury with partial liquid ventilation: A study model in a setting of severe respiratory failure. Chest 1995;108:500–508.
67. Hjortso E, Qvist J, Bud MI, et al: ARDS after accidental inhalation of zinc chloride smoke. Intensive Care Med 1988; 14:17–24.
68. Hoidal CR, Hall AH, Robinson MD, et al: Hydrogen sulfide poisoning from toxic inhalations of roofing asphalt fumes. Ann Emerg Med 1986;15:826–830.
69. Holzer P: Capsaicin: Cellular targets, mechanisms of action, and selectivity for thin sensory neurons. Physiol Rev 1991;43:143–201.
70. Hu H, Fine J, Epstein P, et al: Tear gas—Harassing agent or toxic chemical weapon? JAMA 1989;262:660–663.
71. Huang YC, Caminiti SP, Fawcett TA, et al: Natural surfactant and hyperoxic lung injury in primates. I. Physiology and biochemistry. J Appl Physiol 1994;76:991–1001.
72. Hudnall JB, Suruda A, Campbell DL: Deaths involving air-line respirators connected to inert gas sources. Am Ind Hyg Assoc J 1993;54:32–35.
73. Jakab GJ: The toxicologic interactions resulting from inhalation of carbon black and acrolein on pulmonary antibacterial and antiviral defenses. Toxicol Appl Pharmacol 1993;121:167–175.
74. Jarvis D, Chinn S, Luczynska C, Burney P: Association of respiratory symptoms and lung function in young adults with use of domestic gas appliances. Lancet 1996;347: 426–431.
75. Jawan B, Lee JH: Cardiac arrest caused by an incorrectly filled oxygen cylinder: A case report. Br J Anaesth 1990; 64:749–751.
76. Jobe AH: Pulmonary surfactant therapy. N Engl J Med 1993;328:861–868.
77. Jones RN, Hughs JM, Glindmeyer H, Weill H: Lung function after acute chlorine exposure. Am Rev Respir Dis 1986;134:1190–1195.
78. Kamat SR, Patel MH, Kolhatkar VP, et al: Sequential respiratory changes in those exposed to the gas leak at Bhopal. Indian J Med Res 1987;86(suppl):20–38.
79. Kazzaz JA, Xu J, Palaia TA, et al: Cellular oxygen toxicity. Oxidant injury without apoptosis. J Biol Chem 1996;271: 15182–15186.
80. Kennedy TP, Michael JR, Hoidal JR, et al: Dibutyryl cAMP, aminophylline, and β-adrenergic agonists protect against pulmonary edema caused by phosgene. J Appl Physiol 1989;67:2542–2552.
81. Kimbell JS, Gross EA, Joyner DR, et al: Application of computational fluid dynamics to regional dosimetry of inhaled chemicals in the upper respiratory tract of the rat. Toxicol Appl Pharmacol 1993;121:253–263.
82. Kindwall EP: Medical aspects of commercial diving and compressed-air work. In: Zenz C, Dickerson OB, Horvath EP, eds: Occupational Medicine, 3rd ed. St. Louis, Mosby–Year Book, 1996, pp. 343–383.
83. Kling GW, Clark MA, Compton HR, et al: The 1986 Lake Nyos gas disaster in Cameroon, West Africa. Science 1987;236:169–175.
84. Koenig JQ, Pierson WE, Horike M, Frank R: Effects of SO_2

plus NaCl aerosol combined with moderate exercise on pulmonary function in asthmatic adolescents. Environ Res 1981;25:340–348.
85. Kollef MH, Schuster DP: The acute respiratory distress syndrome. N Engl J Med 1995;332:27–37.
86. Koren HS, Devlin RB, Graham DE: Ozone-induced inflammation in the lower airways of human subjects. Am Rev Respir Dis 1989;139:407–415.
87. Kuschner WG, D'Alessandro A, Wentermeyer SF, et al: Pulmonary responses to purified zinc oxide fume. J Invest Med 1995;43:371–378
88. Lee DC, Wiley JF, Snyder JW: Treatment of inhalational exposure to hydrofluoric acid with nebulized calcium gluconate. J Occup Med 1993;35:470.
89. Lehmann P: The ozone hole. Med J Aust 1995;163:576–578.
90. Leu HJ, Clodius L: An unusual cause of gangrene: Cold injury caused by liquid nitrogen. Schweiz Med Wochenschr 1989;119:192–195.
91. Lippmann M: Health effects of ozone: A critical review. J Air Pollut Control Assoc 1989;39:672–695.
92. Logan WPD: Mortality in the London fog incident, 1952. Lancet 1953;1:336–339.
93. Lundberg JM, Saria A: Capsaicin-induced desensitization of airway mucosa to cigarette smoke, mechanical and chemical irritants. Nature 1983;302:251–253.
94. Lyons JP, Jenkins LJ, Jones RA, et al: Repeated and continuous exposure of laboratory animals to acrolein. Toxicol Appl Pharmacol 1970;17:726–732.
95. Manahan SE: Toxic inorganic compounds. In: Manahan SE, ed: Toxicologic Chemistry, 2nd ed. Boca Raton, FL, Lewis Publishers, 1992, pp. 303.
96. Manning HL, Schwartzstein RM: Pathophysiology of dyspnea. N Engl J Med 1995;333:1547–1553.
97. Martinez TT, Long C: Explosion risk from swimming pool chlorinators and review of chlorine toxicity. J Toxicol Clin Toxicol 1995;33:349–354.
98. Mayer L, Guelich J: Hydrogen fluoride (HF) inhalation and burns. Arch Environ Health 1963;7:445–447.
99. Mayorga MA: Overview of nitrogen dioxide effects on the lung with emphasis on military relevance. Toxicology 1994;89:175–192.
100. McCord CP: Metal fume fever as an immunological disease. Ind Med Surg 1960;29:101–107.
101. Meduri GU, Belenchia JM, Estes RJ, et al: Fibroproliferative phase of ARDS: Clinical findings and effects of corticosteroids. Chest 1991;100:943–952.
102. Meggs WJ: RADS and RUDS—The toxic induction of asthma and rhinitis. J Toxicol Clin Toxicol 1994;32: 487–501.
103. Mehta PS, Mehta AS, Mehta SJ, Makhijani AB: Bhopal tragedy's health effects: A review of methylisocyanate toxicity. JAMA 1990;264;2781–2787.
104. Miller TM, Mazur PO: Oxygen deficiency hazards associated with liquefied gas systems: Derivation of a program of controls. Am Ind Hyg Assoc J 1984;45:293–298.
105. Minami M, Katsumata M, Miyake K, et al: Dangerous mixture of household detergents in an old-style toilet: A case report with simulation experiments of the working environment and warning of potential hazard relevant to the general environment. Hum Exp Toxicol 1992;11: 27–34.
106. Misra NP, Pathak R, Gaur KJBS, et al: Clinical profile of gas leak victims in acute phase after Bhopal episode. Indian J Med Res 1987;86(suppl):11–19.
107. Montaguo TJ, Macneil AR: Mass ammonia inhalation. Chest 1980;77:496–498.
108. Morris AH, Wallace CJ, Menlowe RL, et al: Randomized clinical trial of pressure-controlled inverse ratio ventilation and extracorporeal CO_2 removal for adult respiratory distress syndrome. Am J Respir Crit Care Med 1994;149: 295–305.
109. Mrvos R, Dean BS, Krenzelok EP: Home exposures to chlorine/chloramine gas: Review of 216 cases. South Med J 1993;86:654–657.
110. Murai M, Morimoto H, Maeda Y, Fujii T: Effects of the tripeptide substance P antagonist, FR 113680, on airway constriction and airway edema induced by neurokinins in guinea-pigs. Eur J Pharmacol 1992;217:23–29.
111. Nadel JA, Salem H, Tamplin B, Tokiwa Y: Mechanism of bronchoconstriction during inhalation of sulfur dioxide. J Appl Physiol 1965;20:164–167.
112. Orzel RA: Toxicologic aspects of firesmoke: Polymer pyrolysis and combustion. Occup Med 1993;8:415–429.
113. Osbern LN, Crapo RO: Dung lung: A report of toxic exposure to liquid manure. Ann Intern Med 1981;95:312–314.
114. Pelled B, Schechter Y, Alroy G, et al: Deleterious effects of oxygen at ambient and hyperbaric pressure in the treatment of nitrogen dioxide-poisoned mice. Am Rev Respir Dis 1973;108:1152–1157.
115. Pepe PE, Hudson LD, Carrico CJ: Early application of positive end-expiratory pressure in patients at risk of the adult respiratory distress syndrome. N Engl J Med 1984; 311:281–286.
116. Peters JW: Hydrogen sulfide poisoning in a hospital setting. JAMA 1981;246:1588–1589.
117. Pino F, Puerta H, D'Apollo MD, et al: Effectiveness of morphine in non-cardiogenic pulmonary edema due to chlorine gas inhalation. Vet Hum Toxicol 1993;35:36.
118. Powell MA, Somero GN: Blood components prevent sulfide poisoning of respiration of the hydrothermal vent tube worm *Riftia pachyptila*. Science 1983;219:297–299.
119. Promisloff RA, Lenchner GS, Cichelli AW: Reactive airway dysfunction syndrome in three police officers following a roadside chemical spill. Chest 1990;98:928–929.
120. Quinlan T, Spivak S, Mossman BT: Regulation of antioxidant enzymes in lung after oxidant injury. Environ Health Perspect 1994;102:79–87.
121. Rabinovitch S, Greyson ND, Weiser W, et al: Clinical and laboratory features of acute sulfur dioxide inhalation poisoning: Two year follow up. Am Rev Respir Dis 1989;139: 556–558.
122. Rafferty P: Voluntary chlorine inhalation: A new form of self-abuse? Br Med J 1980;281:1178–1179.
123. Reed D, Glasser S, Kaldor J: Ozone toxicity symptoms among flight attendants. Am J Ind Med 1980;1:43–54.
124. Reiffenstein RJ, Hulbert WC, Roth SH: Toxicology of hydrogen sulfide. Annu Rev Pharmacol Toxicol 1992;32: 109–134.

125. Reisz GR, Gammon RS: Toxic pneumonitis from mixing household cleaners. Chest 1986;89:49–52.
126. Riechelmann H, Maurer J, Kienast K, et al: Respiratory epithelium exposed to sulfur dioxide—Functional and ultrastructural alterations. Laryngoscope 1995;105:295–299.
127. Roehm JN, Hadley JG, Menzel DB: The influence of vitamin E on the lung fatty acids of rats exposed to ozone. Arch Environ Health 1972;24:237–242.
128. Ross DS: Welder's metal fume fever. J Soc Occup Med 1974;24:125–129.
129. Roth VS, Franzblau A: RADS after exposure to riot-control agent: A case report. J Occup Environ Med 1996;38: 863–865.
130. Ryrfeldt A, Bannenberg G, Moldeus P: Free radicals and lung disease. Br Med Bull 1993;49:588–603.
131. Samet JM, Utell MJ: The environment and the lung: Changing perspectives. JAMA 1991;266:670–675.
132. Sarnstrand B, Tunek A, Sjodin K, Hallberg A: Effects of *N*-acetylcysteine stereoisomers on oxygen-induced lung injury in rats. Chem Biol Interact 1995;94:157–164.
133. Sciuto AM, Stotts RR, Hurt HH: Efficacy of ibuprofen and pentoxifylline in the treatment of phosgene-induced acute lung injury. J Appl Toxicol 1996;16:381–384.
134. Sciuto AM, Strickland PT, Kennedy TP, Gurtner GH: Protective effects of *N*-acetylcysteine treatment after phosgene exposure in rabbits. Am J Respir Crit Care Med 1995;151:768–772.
135. Sciuto AM, Strickland PT, Kennedy TP, et al: Intratracheal administration of DBcAMP attenuates edema formation in phosgene-induced acute lung injury. J Appl Physiol 1996; 80:149–157.
136. Sharma PN, Gaur KJBS: Radiological spectrum of lung changes in gas exposed victims. Indian J Med Res 1987; 86(suppl):39–44.
137. Shusterman DJ: Polymer fume fever and other fluorocarbon pyrolysis-related syndromes. Occup Med 1993;8:519–531.
138. Smilkstein MJ, Bronstein AC, Pickett HM, Rumack BH: Hyperbaric therapy for severe hydrogen sulfide poisoning. J Emerg Med 1985;3:27–30.
139. Smith L, Kruszyna H, Smith RP: The effect of methemoglobin on the inhibition of cytochrome c oxidase by cyanide, sulfide or azide. Biochem Pharmacol 1977;26: 2247–2250.
140. Snyder JW, Safir EF, Summerville GP, Middleberg RA: Occupational fatality and persistent neurological sequelae after mass exposure to hydrogen sulfide. Am J Emerg Med 1995;13:199–203.
141. Snyder RW, Mishel HS, Christensen GC: Pulmonary toxicity following exposure to methylene chloride and its combustion product, phosgene. Chest 1992;101:860–861.
142. Steffee CH, Lantz PE, Flannagan LM, et al: Oleoresin capsicum (pepper) spray and "in custody deaths." Am J Forensic Med Pathol 1995;16:185–192.
143. Suruda A, Agnew J: Deaths from asphyxiation and poisoning at work in the United States, 1984–1986. Br J Ind Med 1989;46:541–546.
144. Suter PM, Domenighetti G, Schaller MD, et al: *N*-Acetylcysteine enhances recovery from acute lung injury in man: A randomized, double-blind, placebo-controlled clinical study. Chest 1994;105:190–194
145. Szerlip HM, Singer I: Hyperchloremic metabolic acidosis after chlorine inhalation. Am J Med 1984;77:581–582.
146. Takaoka M, Morinaga K, Karakowa K, et al: A case report of acute carbon dioxide intoxication by dry ice. Jpn J Toxicol 1988;1:87–90.
147. Tarlo SM, Broder I: Irritant-induced occupational asthma. Chest 1989;96;297–300.
148. Tatsumi T, Fliss H: Hypochlorous acid and chloramines increase endothelial permeability: Possible involvement of cellular zinc. Am J Physiol 1994;267:H1597–H1607.
149. Thorburn KM: Injuries after use of the lacrimatory agent chloroacetophenone in a confined space. Arch Environ Health 1982:182–186.
150. Tu B, Wallin A, Moldeus P, Cotgreave I: The cytoprotective roles of ascorbate and glutathione against nitrogen dioxide toxicity in human endothelial cells. Toxicology 1995;98:125–136.
151. Tunnicliffe W, Burge P, Ayres J: Effect of domestic concentration of nitrogen dioxide on airway responsiveness to inhaled allergen in asthmatic patients. Lancet 1994;344: 1733–1736.
152. Turrens JF, Crapo JD, Freeman BA: Protection against oxygen toxicity by intravenous injection of liposome-entrapped catalase and superoxide dismutase. J Clin Invest 1984;73:87–95.
153. Tvedt B, Edland A, Skyberg K, Forberg O. Delayed neuropsychiatric sequlae after acute hydrogen sulfide poisoning: Affection of motor function, memory, vision and hearing. Acta Neurol Scand 1991;84:348–351.
154. Uppu RM, Cueto R, Squadrito GL, Pryor WA: What does ozone react with at the air/lung interface? Model studies using human red blood cell membranes. Arch Biochem Biophys 1995;319:257–266.
155. Vinsel PJ: Treatment of acute chlorine gas inhalation with nebulized sodium bicarbonate. J Emerg Med 1990;8: 327–329.
156. Wagner GN, Clark MA, Koenigsberg EJ, Decata SJ: Medical evaluation of the victims of the 1986 Lake Nyos disaster. J Forensic Sci 1988;33:899–909.
157. Walmrath D, Günther A, Ghofrani HA, et al: Bronchoscopic surfactant administration in patients with severe adult respiratory distress syndrome and sepsis. Am J Respir Crit Care Med 1996;154:57–62.
158. Watson AA, Oliver JS, Thorpe JW: Accidental death due to inhalation of hydrofluoric acid. Med Sci Law 1973;13: 277–279
159. Weg JG, Balk RA, Tharratt RS, et al: Safety and efficacy of an aerosolized surfactant in human sepsis-induced adult respiratory distress syndrome. JAMA 1994;272:1433–1438.
160. Weir KL, O'Gorman EN, Ross JA, et al: Lung capillary albumin leak in oxygen toxicity. A quantitative immunochemical study. Am J Respir Crit Care Med 1994;150: 784–789.
161. Wing JS, Sanderson LM, Brender JD, Perrota DM, Beauchanp RA: Acute health effects in a community after release of hydrofluoric acid. Arch Environ Health 1991;46:155–160.
162. Wood BR, Colombo JL, Benson BE: Chlorine inhalation toxicity from vapors generated by swimming pool chlorinator tablets. Pediatrics 1987;79:428–430.

CHAPTER 95

Smoke Inhalation

Mark A. Kirk and Christopher P. Holstege

Firefighters discovered an unresponsive 39-year-old man in an apartment building fire. His vital signs were: systolic blood pressure, 70 mm Hg; pulse, 160 beats/min, and apneic. A large amount of soot was noted in the patient's upper airway during endotracheal intubation. He was placed on 100% oxygen during transport. On arrival at the emergency department (ED), he was still unresponsive to painful stimuli and had a palpable systolic blood pressure of 100 mm Hg. Physical examination showed pupils that were equal and reactive to light. Intense conjunctival irritation and corneal burns were noted. He had singed nasal hairs and soot in his oropharynx. Carbonaceous material was suctioned from his endotracheal tube. He had no evidence of head trauma or skin burns. Breath sounds were equal, with diffuse wheezes in all lung fields. In the ED he was placed on a ventilator with 100% oxygen and administered aerosolized albuterol. His blood pressure continued to improve with intravenous (IV) fluid therapy. He had no response when given 2 mg of naloxone, 100 mg of thiamine, and 25 g of 50% dextrose ($D_{50}W$) IV.

Admission laboratory data were: WBC, 14,000 cells/mm^3; hemoglobin, 11.3 g/dL; sodium, 141 mEq/L; potassium, 3.5 mEq/L; chloride, 111 mEq/L; bicarbonate, 12 mEq/L; BUN, 27 mg/dL; creatinine, 0.7 mg/dL; and blood glucose, 80 mg/dL. Arterial blood gas analysis on 100% oxygen showed: pH, 7.17; PCO_2, 30 mm Hg; PO_2, 150 mm Hg. Co-oximeter measured a carboxyhemoglobin concentration of 38% and a methemoglobin concentration of 0.8%. A blood ethanol concentration was 179 mg/dL. A blood lactate concentration was 14 mEq/L. Chest radiograph was unremarkable. Electrocardiogram (ECG) showed a sinus tachycardia without evidence of ischemia.

Because of his critical condition and the presence of metabolic acidosis, 12.5 g of sodium thiosulfate was given IV. The patient was taken to the intensive care unit, where mechanical ventilation and fluid resuscitation continued. He had no further significant hemodynamic instability. Within 4 hours of admission he received hyperbaric oxygen therapy. He had a progressive improvement in mental status and was awake 6 hours after admission. The patient had complete recovery with no neurologic deficits. Admission blood cyanide concentration of 1.80 μg/mL was reported 12 hours later.

What Is the Toxicologic Significance of Fire Injuries?

Fire injuries can result from an array of inhaled toxic chemicals and/or thermal burns. In 1942, toxic inhalation was considered unusual from dwelling fires. That year a fire at the Cocoanut Grove Night Club in Boston proved that toxic gases may be generated in typical dwelling fires: "The complications encountered were similar to those resulting from inhalation of certain war gases. . . . From the experience of the Cocoanut Grove fire, we know that such pulmonary complications are to be found not solely in warfare, but may be encountered at any moment in civilian life."[93]

Disastrous fires are frequent reminders of the role of inhalation injuries in fire deaths.[29,63] From 1955 to 1972, a threefold increase in death from inhalational injury was reported and was attributed to abundant use of newer synthetic materials for building and furnishings.[11] The National Fire Protection Agency reported 17,900 fire-related deaths over the past 5 years (3600/year) and averaged over 29,000 injuries per year over the same time.[58] An estimated 50–80% of these fire deaths were due to inhalation injuries rather than burns or trauma.[11,49,84,133] Compared with other countries, the United States has one of the highest fire death rates in the world.[74]

How Are Toxins Generated in Fires?

Combustion, or pyrolysis, is the rapid decomposition or cleavage of a substance (fuel) by heat. This process is the oxidation of a fuel with atmospheric oxygen and generates flame (light), heat, and smoke as combustion products. Smoke is a complex mixture of heated air, suspended solid and liquid particles, gases, fumes, aerosols, and vapors. Chemical composition of the fuel, oxygen availability, and temperature determine the combustion products.[48,112] Table 95–1 lists toxic combustion products of common fuels.[8,23,34,38,94,98,99,112] Combustion products are difficult to predict in a fire; in fact, the composition of smoke often is quite variable within the same fire environment.[8,29,94] Polyvinyl chloride produces at least 75 potentially toxic agents and wood as many as 200.[34,84] The variety of materials now used in our environment contributes to a broad spectrum of combustion products present in typical smoke.[23]

Combustion of organic material produces finely divided carbonaceous particulate matter (soot) suspended in hot air and gases. These particles are not just composed of carbon; but organic acids, aldehydes, and reactive chemical radicals are adsorbed to their surfaces.[34,52,109,131]

TABLE 95–1. COMMON MATERIALS AND THEIR COMBUSTION PRODUCTS

Products	Combustion Products
Wool	Carbon monoxide, hydrogen chloride, phosgene, chlorine, cyanide
Silk	Sulfur dioxide, hydrogen sulfide, ammonia, cyanide
Nylon	Ammonia, cyanide
Wood, cotton, paper	Carbon monoxide, acrolein, acetaldehyde, formaldehyde, acetic acid, formic acid, methane
Petroleum products	Carbon monoxide, acrolein, acetic acid, formic acid
Polystyrene	Styrene
Acrylic	Acrolein, hydrogen chloride, carbon monoxide
Plastics	Cyanide, hydrogen chloride, aldehydes, ammonia, nitrogen oxides (methemoglobinemia), phosgene, chlorine
Polyvinyl chloride	Carbon monoxide, hydrogen chloride, phosgene, chlorine
Polyurethane	Cyanide, isocyanates
Melamine resins	Ammonia, cyanide
Rubber	Hydrogen sulfide, sulfur dioxide
Sulfur-containing material	Sulfur dioxide
Nitrogen-containing material	Cyanide, isocyanates, oxides of nitrogen (methemoglobinemia)
Nitrocellulose	Oxides of nitrogen (methemoglobinemia), acetic acid, formic acid
Fluorinated resins	Hydrogen fluoride
Fire retardant materials	Hydrogen chloride, hydrogen bromide

What Toxins Are Generated by Fires?

Toxic substances generated by combustion are in the form of gases, vapors, aerosols, fumes, and coated particulates. Toxic combustion products are classified as simple asphyxiants, irritants, or chemical asphyxiants (Table 95–2). Particulate and gaseous fractions (eg, carbon dioxide) can act as simple asphyxiants by exerting a space-occupying effect, filling an enclosed space at the expense of oxygen.[29,34,109,131] In addition to displacing oxygen, combustion (oxidation) uses oxygen, producing an oxygen-deprived environment.[29]

Irritant toxins are chemically reactive compounds that exert a local effect on the respiratory tract. Many irritant chemicals react with the moisture of respiratory mucosa, generating caustics that cause chemical burns and inflammatory reactions (see Chap. 94). Acrolein is one of the most common irritant gases generated by fires.[69] High concentrations have been measured in air samples from fire environments and in the blood of fire victims.[1,124] Acrolein penetrates cell membranes easily because it is lipid soluble and injures cells by denaturing proteins and nucleic acids.[39,133] Ammonia is generated when wool, silk, nylon, or synthetic resins are burned. It reacts with the mucosa to produce the alkaline agent ammonium hydroxide.[24,65] Sulfur dioxide, a combustion product of sulfur-containing material, is found in more than 50% of air samples from fires.[16] Sulfuric acid is a strong caustic that forms when sulfur dioxide reacts with the moisture of the respiratory mucosa. Polyvinyl chloride (PVC) is widely used in home and office furnishings, floor coverings, and electrical insulation; therefore, high concentrations of its combustion products, hydrogen chloride, chlorine, and phosgene, are present in many fires.[12,29,34,71] In the presence of mucosal water, chlorine generates hydrogen chloride and oxygen free radicals that cause an oxidative injury.[30] Phosgene produces delayed alveolar injury. Isocyanates, combustion

TABLE 95–2. TOXIC COMBUSTION PRODUCTS

Simple asphyxiants	***Irritants***
Carbon dioxide	Highly water soluble
Methane	(upper airway injury)
Oxygen-deprived environment	Acrolein
	Sulfur dioxide
Chemical asphyxiants	Ammonia
Carbon monoxide	Hydrogen chloride
Hydrogen cyanide	Intermediately water soluble
Hydrogen sulfide	(upper & lower respiratory injury)
Oxides of nitrogen	Chlorine
(Methemoglobinemia)	Isocyanates
	Low water solubility
	(pulmonary parenchymal injury)
	Oxides of nitrogen
	Phosgene

products generated from upholstery, cause intense irritation of the upper and lower respiratory tract.

Inhalation of soot particles and aerosols enhances the exposure to toxins in a fire environment. Soot adheres to the mucosa of the airways, allowing adsorbed irritant chemicals to react with the mucosal surface moisture. The deposition of these particles in the respiratory tract depends on their size, with those 1–3 μm reaching the alveoli.[79] Experimental animals have markedly decreased lung injury when exposed to smoke filtered to remove particulates.[61] Also, irritant gases can "piggyback" on aerosol droplets and alter the site of deposition of the gas.[50] For example, sulfur dioxide is often found adsorbed onto the surface of carbonaceous particles and the combustion of PVC generates a large amount of particulate-filled smoke coated with hydrogen chloride, chlorine, and phosgene.[16,34,71]

Chemical asphyxiants exert toxic effects at tissues distant from the lung. Incomplete combustion of organic materials generates carbon monoxide, considered the most common serious acute hazard to victims of inhalation injury (see Chap. 96).[10,29,124,133] Significant concentrations of carbon monoxide are measured in most fires. Cyanide is produced from combustion of nitrogen-containing products such as plastics, melamine resins, polyurethanes, wool, silk, nylon, nitrocellulose, polyacrylonitriles, synthetic rubber, and paper[94] (see Chap. 97). High concentrations of cyanide have been measured in air samples from fires, and elevated blood cyanide concentrations have been reported in both fire survivors and fire fatalities.[2,7,8,20,29,47,57,105,107,110,128] Nitrogen-containing materials also generate oxides of nitrogen, which are irritants and methemoglobin inducers (see Chap. 93). Burning sulfur-containing materials generates hydrogen sulfide, which acts as an irritant gas and chemical asphyxiant.

Depending on the fuel, other combustion products are generated that act by local irritation or systemic toxicity. Such compounds as metal oxides, hydrocarbons, hydrogen fluoride, and hydrogen bromide may contribute to toxicity. A variety of cyclic and straight-chained hydrocarbons have been measured in fire environments.[29] Benzene has been detected from combustion of petroleum products and plastics.[124] Antimony, bromine, cadmium, chromium, cobalt, gold, iron, lead, and zinc have been recovered in air samples taken during fires and from soot removed from the surface of the trachea and bronchi of fire victims.[10,29] In addition, combustion produces highly reactive free radicals that interact with tissues to cause lipid peroxidation.[131] Dwelling fires generate many combustion products already discussed. Unusual fires from industries, clandestine drug laboratories, transportation accidents, or natural disasters (eg, volcanoes) produce additional toxic inhalants.

For the most part, studies evaluate isolated effects of harmful combustion products. However, as seen in patients with smoke inhalation, exposure to a combination of toxins may have additive or synergistic adverse effects.

What Are the Effects of Smoke Inhalation on the Respiratory System?

Smoke inhalation is a respiratory and systemic disease. The final common pathway to morbidity is hypoxia (Fig. 95–1). Smoke inhalation's pathophysiologic effects impair the body's ability to acquire oxygen from the environment and the ability to deliver and use oxygen at every step of respiration, including its final step in oxidative phosphorylation. The natural course of inhalation injury is rapid compromise from cyanide or carbon monoxide poisoning or upper airway obstruction, then progression over several hours to days to acute respiratory failure due to atelectasis, airway obstruction, pulmonary edema, pneumonia, acute lung injury (ALI), or adult resiratory distress syndrome (ARDS).[126]

The many irritant chemicals generated during combustion may injure the upper airway, tracheobronchial tree, or pulmonary parenchyma. Water solubility is the most important chemical characteristic in determining the level of the respiratory tract injury. Highly water-soluble gases react with the upper airway mucosa to produce intense upper mucosal injury and inflammatory reaction. Unless toxic gas concentrations are extremely high or duration of exposure prolonged, injury is limited to the mucosa of the upper respiratory tract. Conversely, chemicals with low water solubility do not react with the upper airway mucosa and reach the lung parenchyma, where they react slowly to create a delayed toxic effect. In addition to water solubility, concentration of the substance inhaled, duration of exposure, particle size, respiratory rate, absence of protective reflexes, and preexisting disease influence the level of the respiratory tract injury.

The upper airway functions to thermoregulate and humidify inspired air, filter particulates from the air, and protect lower airways from aspiration. Caustic injury from water-soluble chemicals and thermal injury occurs in the upper airway.[15,80,98] Both thermal and chemical insults damage mucosal cells, stimulating release of mediators of inflammation and oxygen free radicals. This intense inflammatory response increases microvascular permeability and movement of fluid from the intravascular space into the tissues of the upper airway. The loosely attached underlying tissue of the supraglottic larynx, the usual site of edema, may become massively swollen.[54] An edematous upper airway may develop in minutes to hours and progress to occlude the upper airway completely.[101] Furthermore, irritant chemicals may produce a reflex laryngospasm.

Tracheobronchial injuries are due to inhaled particulates and toxic gases that cause increased airway resistance from intraluminal debris, airway mucosal edema, inspissated secretions, and bronchospasm. Thermal injury is rare at this level unless steam is inhaled.[15,98] Toxic chemicals induce an intense inflammatory reaction in response to caustic injury to mucosal cells.[22,70,119] Damaged

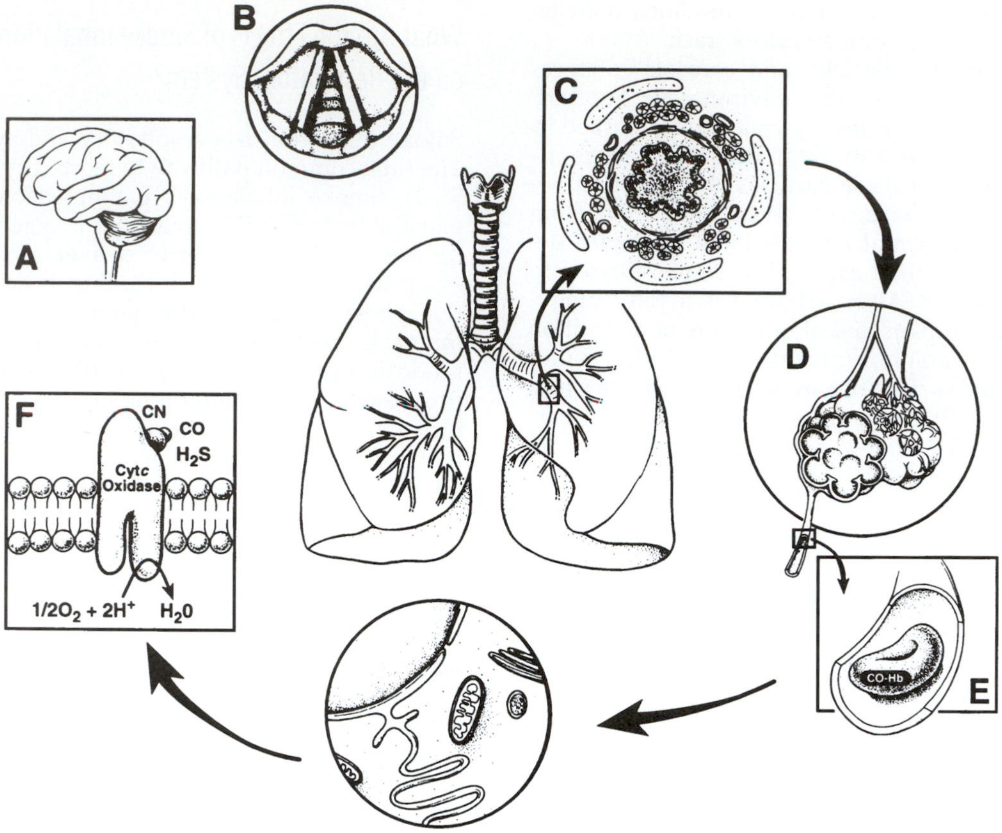

Pathophysiology	Signs and Symptoms	Management
A) Direct CNS toxic effects	Coma Hypoventilation	Oxygen; Secure unprotected airway Naloxone; Dextrose and thiamine
B) Upper airway edema	Hypoxemia; Respiratory distress Stridor Hoarse voice	Oxygen Direct visualization of vocal cords Endotracheal intubation
C) Bronchiolar airway obstruction Mucosal edema Intraluminal debris and casts Inspissated secretions Bronchospasm	Respiratory distress Hypoxemia Wheezes Cough Increased peak airway pressures	Oxygen Removal of debris and secretions Chest physiotherapy Frequent airway suctioning Therapeutic bronchoscopy Inhaled beta-adrenergic agonists
D) Atelectasis Surfactant destruction Pulmonary edema	Respiratory distress Hypoxemia Rales Chest radiographic changes	Oxygen Continuous positive airways pressure Mechanical ventilation Positive end expiratory pressure
E) Impaired oxygen carrying capacity (carbon monoxide or methemoglobinemia)	CNS depression or seizures Myocardial ischemia Dysrhythmias Metabolic acidosis	Oxygen Consider hyperbaric oxygen Consider methylene blue
F) Impaired oxygen use at tissues (cyanide, hydrogen sulfide or carbon monoxide)	CNS depression or seizures Myocardial ischemia Dysrhythmias Metabolic acidosis	Oxygen Assure adequate tissue perfusion Consider treating suspected cyanide toxicity with sodium thiosulfate Consider hyperbaric oxygen

Figure 95–1. The final common pathway for all pathophysiologic changes that occur in smoke inhalation is hypoxia. All treatments should be focused on improving oxygen delivery and oxygen utilization.

cells release chemotactic factors that stimulate production of an exudate rich in protein and inflammatory cells.[126] This reaction eventually results in sloughing of the mucosa. Exudate, mucosal sloughing, and reactive bronchorrhea combine to create casts of the airways. In animal models and victims of smoke inhalation, casts are found to block major airways, increase airway resistance, and prevent passage of oxygen to the alveoli.[22,119,126] Increased tracheobronchial vascular permeability causes interstitial edema of the airways and increased airway resistance. Bronchoconstriction is caused by a response to mediators of inflammation—a reflex response to toxic mucosal injury.[46,122]

Toxic chemicals reaching the alveoli injure the lung parenchyma.[88] At autopsy, carbon particles have been found in alveoli.[26] Caustics, proteolytic enzymes, free radicals, and mediators of inflammation all contribute to parenchymal lung injury.[122,131] Pathophysiologic changes of the parenchyma decrease lung compliance and bacterial defense, cause ventilation–perfusion mismatch and intrapulmonary shunt, and increase extravascular lung water and microvascular permeability.[22,40,122,126] Decreased lung compliance from atelectasis is produced when toxic chemicals deactivate pulmonary surfactant.[22,88,95,126] In animals, patchy atelectasis occurs rapidly after smoke is inspired.[22,88,126] In addition, ventilation–perfusion mismatch occurs when pulmonary blood flow is diverted by hypoxia and vasoactive mediators of inflammation.[66,67,87,122] Toxins further damage the normal pulmonary defense systems by impairing mucociliary clearance, altering alveolar macrophage function, and impairing phagocytosis of bacteria, which contribute to the subsequent development of pulmonary infections and sepsis.[9,37,51,100]

Caustic effects of toxins and an intense inflammatory response injure the alveolar epithelium and capillary endothelium, thus increasing the permeability of the alveolar–capillary barrier.[40,129] Damage to the integrity of the alveolar–capillary barrier causes pulmonary edema without an increased pulmonary-capillary wedge pressure. In animals, the irritant chemical acrolein and the combustion products of PVC produce pulmonary edema in addition to mucosal injury to the larger airways.[34,39,40,133] The combination of inflammatory response and slowed toxic effects of some inhaled chemicals may delay the initial manifestations of parenchymal injury for up to 24 hours after smoke exposure. The clinical presentation includes progressive respiratory failure, decreased compliance (stiff lungs), and diffuse alveolar infiltrates on chest radiograph.

Even if oxygen can enter the blood through the alveoli, systemic toxins may impair tissue oxygenation. Carbon monoxide prevents oxygen from binding to hemoglobin, creating a "relative anemia." It also hinders the release of oxygen at the tissues by shifting the oxyhemoglobin dissociation curve to the left. Other mechanisms, such as lipid peroxidation, may contribute to the toxicity of carbon monoxide[114] (see Chap. 96). Oxides of nitrogen produce methemoglobin, which impairs the oxygen-carrying ability of hemoglobin (see Chap. 93). Once oxygen reaches the tissues, cyanide prevents its use in oxidative phosphorylation. Cyanide has at least an additive, if not synergistic, effect in smoke inhalation toxicity[7,78,91,97,99] (see Chap. 97).

The complex interactions of lung injury, together with the inflammatory effects of skin burns, produce a more serious systemic illness.[33,116,131] Burn victims with inhalation injury have a higher morbidity and mortality than those with burns only; the incidence of acute respiratory failure is 61% versus 12%, respectively.[6,22,118,129,132] In addition, burn edema is accentuated and nonburned tissue has increased vascular permeability when associated with inhalation injuries.[32]

What Diagnostic Studies Are Useful in Evaluating the Patient With Smoke Inhalation?

Smoke inhalation injury causes hypoxia; therefore diagnostic studies should focus on assessing oxygenation and ventilation. Arterial blood gas (ABG) analysis, measured oxygen saturation, carboxyhemoglobin concentration, methemoglobin concentration, and chest radiography are the most important laboratory tests to obtain.

Arterial blood gas analysis assesses both arterial oxygenation and alveolar ventilation. Serial measurements are helpful in identifying hypoxemia or ventilatory failure. The presence of acidemia may be an early clue to tissue hypoxia.

The accuracy of oxygen saturation measurement depends on the method used. Oxygen saturation calculated from an ABG may be unreliable, but measured oxygen saturation determined by co-oximeter accurately reflects the percent saturation of oxygenated hemoglobin. Transcutaneous monitoring is unreliable in the patient with smoke inhalation because it has been shown to overestimate oxygen saturation in the presence of carboxyhemoglobin[5] (see Chap. 20). Pulse oximetry is also unreliable in the presence of methemoglobin (see Chap. 93).[35,90,125]

An elevated carboxyhemoglobin concentration in a fire victim indicates substantial exposure to combustion products and a greater possibility of developing smoke inhalation toxicity.[21,132] In fact, clinical series have suggested that carboxyhemoglobin elevation may be considered an index of cyanide poisoning because of a significant correlation between measured concentrations of both toxins.[3,7,20,72,107] To the contrary, postmortem studies do not support this correlation.[4,68] Carboxyhemoglobin concentration alone is a poor predictor of the severity of toxicity, because a low or nondetectable concentration does not exclude the possibility of inhalation injury.[76,108] Admission carboxyhemoglobin measurements are inaccurate predictors of peak concentrations.[77] Admission nomograms for peak concentrations have not been prospectively evaluated and may be very inaccurate (see Chap. 96). Elevated methemoglobin concentrations have been reported in fire victims and should be assessed in the initial laboratory evaluation.[53,104] A co-oximeter will provide an accurate methemoglobin measurement. Blood cyanide analysis is of little clinical use because it takes hours to obtain results. Therapy should not await laboratory confirmation of elevated blood cyanide. Accurate measurement depends on acquiring the sample soon after exposure, because cyanide is rapidly eliminated from the blood following smoke inhalation.[7,60]

Lactic acidosis, common in patients with smoke inhalation, is the result of oxygen deprivation, carbon monoxide poisoning, cyanide poisoning, and/or tissue hypoperfusion. Hypoxia, from any cause, impairs aerobic metabolism and generates lactic acid. High lactate concentrations are correlated with elevated concentrations of cyanide and carbon monoxide.[7,108] Elevated lactate concentrations may signal cyanide or carbon monoxide toxicity, but in the clinical setting of smoke inhalation these concentrations are nonspecific indicators of tissue hypoxia.

A chest radiograph is most commonly normal in the early course of smoke inhalation and is therefore an insensitive indicator of pulmonary injury.[21,96,130] Subtle findings within 24 hours of exposure include perivascular haziness, peribronchial cuffing, bronchial wall thickening, and subglottic edema.[64,111] Serial chest radiographs following a baseline study are extremely helpful in detecting pulmonary disease following smoke inhalation.[46] Widespread airways disease is usually seen more than 24 hours after inhalation injury and may represent ALI, ARDS, aspiration, volume overload, infection, or even cardiogenic pulmonary edema.[111]

Nuclear imaging and pulmonary function testing, although not readily available for initial evaluation, can detect pulmonary injury after smoke inhalation. Xenon ventilation studies can detect small airway and alveolar injury before radiographic changes occur.[46,81] Abnormal flow volume curves can indicate early upper airway obstruction.[45] Abnormal spirometry, especially forced expiratory volume (FEV_1), detects early obstructive pulmonary defects of smoke inhalation, which may precede abnormalities of arterial blood gases or radiography.[46,82]

How Should the Patient With Smoke Inhalation Initially Be Managed?

Critical airway compromise may be present on arrival at the hospital or may develop suddenly or insidiously.[27,45,101] A major pitfall in managing a patient with smoke inhalation is failure to appreciate the potential for rapid deterioration. History and physical findings help to determine significant smoke exposure and the potential for clinical deterioration (Table 95–3). The clinical effects of smoke exposure and their appropriate treatment are described in Figure 95–1. Upper airway patency must be rapidly established. When obvious oropharyngeal burns are observed, upper airway injury is almost certain. If such obvious injuries are not present, the degree of injury may be underestimated because of nonspecific history and physical findings.[45] Direct evaluation of the upper airway is essential in assessing patients at high risk for inhalation injury.[27,45,46,54] Fiberoptic endoscopy is the preferred method, but when not possible, empiric, prophylactic intubation is justified. When evidence of upper airway injury exists, early endotracheal intubation should be performed under controlled circumstances instead of emergently when a patient abruptly decompensates. Relative indications for early intubation include CNS depression, visible burns or edema of the oropharynx, stridor, or full-thickness circumferential neck burns.[6,45,46,101] Massive fluid resuscitation of the burned patient contributes to upper airway edema formation.[45,46,83,101] Therefore, early intubation may be necessary in the patient with dermal burns undergoing aggressive fluid management.[45]

TABLE 95–3. FACTORS THAT INCREASE RISK OF SMOKE INHALATION INJURY

History	***Signs***
Closed space exposure	CNS depression
Loss of consciousness	Carbonaceous sputum
Entrapment	Edema of posterior pharynx
Symptoms	Face or neck burns
Respiratory distress	Hoarseness
	Singed nasal hairs
	Stridor

Although inhaled beta$_2$-adrenergic agonists are effective and considered the first line of therapy for acute reversible bronchoconstriction due to asthma or chronic obstructive pulmonary disease (COPD), their efficacy has not been evaluated in patients with smoke inhalation.[13,73] Pathophysiologic changes induced by irritant toxins in smoke are partially reversible, suggesting beta$_2$-adrenergic agonists will improve airflow obstruction.[55,75] Aminophylline is no longer considered part of the initial management of acute bronchospasm because of significant adverse effects and questionable efficacy.[55] Clinical studies fail to show any benefit from the use of aminophylline when used in early management of bronchospasm secondary to acute asthma.[36,106] Benefits of corticosteroids for smoke inhalation injury have not been demonstrated in either clinical or animal studies.[86,102] Corticosteroids are effective in the management of refractory acute asthma but should be avoided in patients with burns and inhalation injury because mortality and infection rates are increased in these patients.[81] Corticosteroids may be considered in selected patients with isolated inhalation injury and refractory bronchospasm.

Pathophysiologic changes in the lung may cause progressive hypoxia over hours to days. Treatment of progressive respiratory failure includes mechanical ventilation, continuous positive airways pressure, positive end-expiratory pressure, and vigorous clearing of pulmonary secretions.[85] Frequent airway suctioning, chest physiotherapy, and therapeutic bronchoscopy can clear inspissated secretions, plugs, and casts. Inhalation injury can progress to ARDS. Researchers are investigating the use of high-frequency ventilation, inhaled nitric oxide, instillation of natural surfactant, continuous infusion of heparin, and deferoxamine–hetastarch complex for improving inhalation injury.[19,25,31,62,89,92]

Respiratory compromise and other conditions may not be due to smoke inhalation but rather to trauma or underlying medical problems. Trauma from falls or explosions must be suspected and treatment begun simultaneously with treatment of burns and inhalation injury. Comatose patients should be considered to have other etiologies and should receive naloxone, thiamine, and hypertonic dextrose as indicated. Inhaled toxins, such as carbon monoxide, can directly cause altered mental status, but drug and ethanol intoxication contribute significantly to adult fire fatalities and injuries. Blood ethanol concentrations correlate with elevated concentrations of carbon monoxide and cyanide, implying that intoxication impairs escape and prolongs toxic smoke exposure.[4,10,84]

Toxins may injure the skin or mucous membranes in addition to the respiratory mucosa.[24] A chemical's duration of contact with tissue is one important factor in determining the extent of injury to the skin and eyes. Rapid removal of soot from skin or eyes may prevent continued injury. The eyes should be evaluated for corneal burns caused by thermal or irritant chemical injury. Patients with signs of ocular irritation should have their eyes irrigated (see Chap. 26). Dermal decontamination should be considered to prevent dermal burns from toxin-laden soot adherent to the skin.

How Is Carbon Monoxide Poisoning Treated in Patients With Smoke Inhalation?

The treatment for carbon monoxide poisoning is supplemental oxygen therapy, administered by high flow, tight-fitting mask, endotracheal tube, or hyperbaric oxygen therapy. Studies suggest that hyperbaric oxygen is superior to normobaric 100% oxygen in correcting toxicity and preventing delayed sequelae.[113,117,120] In addition, hyperbaric oxygen used to treat carbon monoxide toxicity has been shown to decrease burn edema of the skin and airways, preserve marginally viable burn tissue, promote wound closure, enhance host defenses, reduce extravascular lung water in pulmonary injury, and possibly treat methemoglobin or cyanide poisoning.[47,76]

Unfortunately, there are no prospective, randomized, controlled studies that fully evaluate hyperbaric oxygen's role in the clinical outcome of patients with smoke inhalation. Based on current literature, patients with low carboxyhemoglobin (COHb) concentrations and without a history of loss of consciousness, coma, neurologic findings, cardiovascular instability, or pregnancy are at low risk for significant sequelae and can be treated with 100% oxygen therapy.[115,127] If readily available, hyperbaric oxygen should be used in patients with a history of loss of consciousness, coma, focal neurologic findings, pregnancy, or elevated COHb concentration (consider if greater than 25%).[115] Any seriously ill patient with isolated smoke inhalation injury should be considered for transport to a facility with hyperbaric oxygen capabilities. Hyperbaric oxygen should be administered to patients with significant associated trauma, burns covering more than 40% of the body, or hemodynamic instability only after life-threatening conditions have been treated and the patient's condition has stabilized. Controversy surrounds the lengthy transportation of critically ill patients to a facility solely for hyperbaric oxygen therapy. If a major burn is involved with inhalation injury, consultation with the burn center before transporting to a hyperbaric oxygen facility is necessary. It is recommended that these patients receive hyperbaric oxygen, but not at the expense of expedient, experienced resuscitation and burn care. Many burn units in the United States do not use hyperbaric oxygen.[127] Further scientific evidence (ie, controlled studies) is necessary to define the risks and benefits of hyperbaric oxygen in burn and inhalation injury care.

How Should Cyanide Poisoning Be Treated in the Presence of Smoke Inhalation?

The amount of cyanide exposure and its contribution to the overall toxicity of a patient with smoke inhalation is not predictable. Cyanide toxicity causes agitation, coma, seizures, cardiovascular compromise, and metabolic acidosis. Other toxins and hypoxia may create similar signs and symptoms in the patient with smoke inhalation. Furthermore, no rapid laboratory test exists to confirm cyanide toxicity. Cyanide poisoning should be suspected in seriously ill patients with smoke inhalation. Only after life-support measures, including 100% oxygen therapy, are instituted should specific treatment for cyanide toxicity be considered.[7,78,91,97,98,107] Treatment options include supportive care alone, administration of all or part of the Lilly Cyanide Antidote Kit, and hyperbaric oxygen therapy (see Antidotes in Depth: Cyanide Antidotes; Hyperbaric Oxygen). Patients with a potentially lethal cyanide concentration treated with oxygen therapy and supportive care survived.[14,103] Hyperbaric oxygen has been suggested to improve the outcome of cyanide toxicity, although the data supporting its use alone are not convincing.[47,123] Currently, hyperbaric oxygen therapy is considered only an adjunct treatment for cyanide poisoning in the presence of concomitant carbon monoxide poisoning.[121]

The Cyanide Antidote Kit (amyl nitrite, sodium nitrite, and sodium thiosulfate) is the only antidote for cyanide poisoning available in the United States. Amyl nitrite and sodium nitrite produce methemoglobinemia. Detoxification occurs when methemoglobin binds cyanide to form cyanomethemoglobin, but alternate mechanisms to methemoglobin formation have been proposed.

Sodium thiosulfate donates sulfur to the enzyme rhodanese, which converts cyanide to thiocyanate. Nitrite-induced methemoglobin and sodium thiosulfate work synergistically to detoxify cyanide.[17,18] Sodium thiosulfate has few adverse side effects and can be safely administered to all patients seriously ill from smoke inhalation. When coma, seizures, cardiac dysrhythmias, hypotension, or metabolic acidosis is present, sodium thiosulfate alone should be given empirically. Unfortunately, methemoglobin is a dysfunctional hemoglobin that is unable to carry oxygen; in addition, its presence increases the affinity of the remaining hemoglobin for oxygen, which prevents its release at the tissues.[28] Impairing oxygen-carrying capacity and oxygen delivery to tissues with nitrite-induced methemoglobinemia is a valid concern in the presence of tissue hypoxia from carboxyhemoglobinemia and other factors.

Because cyanomethemoglobin is not measured as cyanide or methemoglobin by current clinical laboratory methods, there is a theoretical concern that formation of the cyanomethemoglobin complex may underestimate the total amount of impaired hemoglobin. Thus, the measured methemoglobin does not reflect true impairment in oxygen-carrying capacity. However, measured peak methemoglobin concentrations after a single dose of sodium nitrite are not well studied. Volunteers (obviously without cyanide poisoning) administered approximately one ampule (300 mg) of sodium nitrite generated methemoglobin concentrations of only 7% methemoglobin.[59] These concentrations are similar to the peak concentrations of only 9% measured in successfully treated cyanide-poisoned patients.[56]

In a small series of fire victims treated with sodium nitrite, methemoglobin concentrations peaked at 7.8–13.4% between 35 and 70 minutes after slow intravenous infusion.[60] Corresponding carboxyhemoglobin concentrations decreased prior to attaining peak methemoglobin concentrations. To the contrary, a case of hypotension and prolonged impairment of oxygen-carrying capacity in a smoke-inhalation victim following the rapid infusion of sodium nitrite was reported.[41] Because the safety of nitrites has not been studied in a large population of concomitant cyanide and carbon monoxide poisoning and the effect of cyanomethemoglobin on oxygen-carrying capacity is not understood, it is reasonable to treat with thiosulfate alone initially and reserve nitrite for refractory cases. If it is given, it should be in a clinical setting where carboxyhemoglobin and methemoglobin can be measured rapidly.[98] In the presence of elevated concentrations of carboxyhemoglobin, nitrite should be withheld. When hyperbaric oxygen therapy is available, sodium nitrite may be administered just prior to entering the hyperbaric chamber, if still clinically indicated, without concern of impairing oxygen-carrying capacity.[42] Hydroxocobalamin binds cyanide and is a safe and effective antidote.[7,44] It is not yet approved in the United States but because of its apparent safety and efficacy, it can be given empirically to patients seriously ill with smoke inhalation, thus eliminating the need for nitrites.[7,44]

How Should Methemoglobinemia From Smoke Inhalation Be Treated?

Although rarely reported in fire victims, methemoglobinemia can result from inhalation of certain toxic combustion products.[53,104] Elevated concentrations of methemoglobin in the presence of elevated carboxyhemoglobin concentrations increase tissue hypoxia. In cases of smoke inhalation, initial treatment with oxygen and, if readily available, hyperbaric oxygen is best. Oxygen therapy alone should be effective for most cases. Methylene blue should be administered only in the presence of elevated methemoglobin concentrations (more than 20–30%) and/or serious symptoms.

Methemoglobinemia from smoke inhalation may be more common than is generally believed, going unrecognized because it is bound as cyanomethemoglobin and not measured. Combustion products producing methemoglobinemia may be protective of cyanide poisoning from smoke inhalation. Theoretically, methylene blue administered in the presence of cyanomethemoglobin could release free cyanide and potentially worsen toxicity.[43] The primary goal of therapy is to improve tissue oxygenation. With this in mind, methylene blue should not be withheld in situations where it is clinically indicated.

References

1. Anderson RA, Cheng KN, Harland WA: The toxicology of fire deaths. Acta Med Leg Soc 1984;34:110–121.
2. Ansell M, Lewis FA: A review of cyanide concentrations found in human organs. J Forensic Med 1970;17:148–155.
3. Barillo DJ, Goode R, Esch V: Cyanide poisoning in victims of fire: Analysis of 364 cases and review of the literature. J Burn Care Rehabil 1994;15:46–57.
4. Barillo DJ, Goode R, Rush BF, et al: Lack of correlation between carboxyhemoglobin and cyanide in smoke inhalation. Curr Surg 1986;43:421–423.
5. Barker SJ, Tremper KK: The effect of carbon monoxide inhalation on pulse oximetry and transcutaneous PO_2. Anesthesiology 1987;66:677–679.
6. Bartlett RH, Niccole M, Tavis MJ, et al: Acute management of the upper airway in facial burns and smoke inhalation. Arch Surg 1976;111:744–749.
7. Baud FJ, Barriot P, Toffis V, et al: Elevated blood cyanide concentrations in victims of smoke inhalation. N Engl J Med 1991;325:1761–1766.
8. Becker CE: The role of cyanide in fires. Vet Hum Toxicol 1985;27:487–490.
9. Bidani A, Wang CZ, Heming TA: Early effects of smoke inhalation on alveolar macrophage functions. Burns 1996; 22:101–106.
10. Birky MM, Clarke FB: Inhalation of toxic products from fires. Bull NY Acad Med 1981;57:997–1013.
11. Bowes PC: Casualties attributed to toxic gas and smoke at fires: A survey of statistics. Med Sci Law 1976;16:104–110.
12. Brandt-Rauf PW, Fallon LF, Tarantini T: Health hazards of

fire fighters: Exposure assessment. Br J Ind Med 1988;45: 606–609.
13. Brenner BE: Bronchial asthma in adults: Presentation to the emergency department. Am J Emerg Med 1983;3: 306–333.
14. Brivet F, Delfraissy JF, Duche M, et al: Acute cyanide poisoning: Recovery with non-specific supportive therapy. Intensive Care Med 1983;9:33–35.
15. Cahalane M, Demling RH: Early respiratory abnormalities from smoke inhalation. JAMA 1984;251:771–773.
16. Charan NB, Meyers CG, Lakshminarayan S, et al: Pulmonary injuries associated with acute sulfur dioxide inhalation. Am Rev Respir Dis 1979;119:555–560.
17. Chen KK, Rose CL: Nitrite and thiosulfate in cyanide poisoning. JAMA 1952;149:113–119.
18. Chen KK, Rose CL, Clowes GH: Comparative values of several antidotes in cyanide poisoning. Am J Med Sci 1934;188:767–781.
19. Cioffi WG, deLemos RA, Coalson JJ, et al: Decreased pulmonary damage in primates with inhalation injury treated with high-frequency ventilation. Ann Surg 1993;218: 328–337.
20. Clark CJ, Campbell D, Reid WH: Blood carboxyhaemoglobin and cyanide levels in fire survivors. Lancet 1981;1: 1332–1335.
21. Clark WR, Bonaventura M, Meyers W: Smoke inhalation and airway management at a regional burn unit: 1974–1983. J Burn Care Rehabil 1989;10:52–62.
22. Clark WR, Nieman GF: Smoke inhalation. Burns 1988;14: 473–494.
23. Clarke FB: Toxicity of combustion products: Current knowledge. Fire J 1983;77:84–101.
24. Close LG, Catlin FI, Cohn AM: Acute and chronic effects of ammonia burns of the respiratory tract. Arch Otolaryngol 1980;106:151–158.
25. Cox CS, Zwischenberger JB, Traber DL, et al: Heparin improves oxygenation and minimizes barotrauma after severe smoke inhalation in an ovine model. Surg Gynecol Obstet 1993;176:339–349.
26. Cox ME, Heslop BF, Kempton JJ, et al: The Dellwood fire. Br Med J 1955:942–946.
27. Crapo RO: Smoke-inhalation injuries. JAMA 1981;246: 1694–1696.
28. Curry S: Methemoglobinemia. Ann Emerg Med 1982;11: 214–221.
29. Davies JW: Toxic chemicals versus lung tissue—An aspect of inhalation injury revisited. J Burn Care Rehabil 1986; 7:213–222.
30. Decker WJ, Koch HF: Chlorine poisoning at the swimming pool: An overlooked hazard. Clin Toxicol 1978;13:377–381.
31. Demling R, LaLonde C, Ikegami K: Fluid resuscitation with deferoxamine hetastarch complex attenuates the lung and systemic response to smoke inhalation. Surgery 1996;119:340–348.
32. Demling R, Lalonde C, Youn YK, et al: Effect of graded increases in smoke inhalation injury on the early systemic response to a body burn. Crit Care Med 1995;23:171–178.
33. Demling RH, Knox J, Youn Y, et al: Oxygen consumption early postburn becomes oxygen delivery dependent with the addition of smoke inhalation injury. J Trauma 1992; 32:593–599.
34. Dyer RF, Esch VH: Polyvinyl chloride toxicity in fires: Hydrogen chloride toxicity in fire fighters. JAMA 1976;235: 393–397.
35. Eisenkraft JB: Pulse oximeter desaturation due to methemoglobinemia. Anesthesiology 1988;68:279–282.
36. Fanta CH, Rossing TH, McFadden ER: Emergency room treatment of asthma: Relationships among therapeutic combinations, severity of obstruction, and time course of response. Am J Med 1982;72:416–422.
37. Fein A, Leff A, Hopewell PC: Pathophysiology and management of the complications resulting from fire and the inhaled products of combustion: Review of the literature. Crit Care Med 1980;8:94–98.
38. Guzzardi L: Toxic products of combustion. Top Emerg Med 1985;7:45–51.
39. Hales CA, Barkin PW, Jung BW, et al: Synthetic smoke with acrolein but not HCl produces pulmonary edema. J Appl Physiol 1988;64:1121–1133.
40. Hales CA, Musto SW, Janssens S, et al: Smoke aldehyde component influences pulmonary edema. J Appl Physiol 1992;72:555–561.
41. Hall AH, Kulig KW, Rumack BH: Suspected cyanide poisoning in smoke inhalation: Complications of sodium nitrite therapy. J Toxicol Clin Exp 1989;9:3–9.
42. Hall AH, Kulig KW, Rumack BH: Toxic smoke inhalation. Am J Emerg Med 1989;7:121–122. Editorial.
43. Hall AH, Rumack BH: Increasing survival in acute cyanide poisoning. Emerg Med Rep 1988;9:129–136.
44. Hall AH, Rumack BH: Hydroxocobalamin/sodium thiosulfate as a cyanide antidote. J Emerg Med 1987;5: 115–121.
45. Haponik EF, Meyers DA, Munster AM, et al: Acute upper airway injury in burn patients. Am Rev Respir Dis 1987;135:360–366.
46. Haponik EF, Summer WR: Respiratory complications in burned patients: Diagnosis and management of inhalation injury. J Critical Care 1987;2:121–143.
47. Hart GB, Strauss MB, Lennon PA, et al: Treatment of smoke inhalation by hyperbaric oxygen. J Emerg Med 1985;3:211–215.
48. Hartzell GE: Overview of combustion toxicology. Toxicology 1996;115:7–23.
49. Harwood B, Hall JR: What kills in fires: Smoke inhalation or burns? Fire J 1989;84:29–34.
50. Henderson RF, Schlesinger RB: Symposium on the importance of combined exposures in inhalation toxicology. Fund Appl Toxicol 1989;12:1–11.
51. Herlihy JP, Vermeulen MW, Joseph PM, et al: Impaired alveolar macrophage function in smoke inhalation injury. J Cell Physiol 1995;163:1–8.
52. Hill IR: Particulate matter of smoke inhalation. Ann Acad Med Singapore 1993;22:119–123.
53. Hoffman RS, Sauter D: Methemoglobinemia resulting from smoke inhalation. Vet Hum Toxicol 1989;31:168–170.
54. Hunt JL, Agee RN, Pruitt BA: Fiberoptic bronchoscopy in acute inhalation injury. J Trauma 1975;15:641–649.
55. Jagoda A, Shepherd SM, Spevitz A, et al: Refractory

asthma, Part 1: Epidemiology, pathophysiology, pharmacologic interventions. Ann Emerg Med 1997;29:262–274.
56. Johnson WS, Hall AH, Rumack BH: Cyanide poisoning successfully treated without "therapeutic methemoglobin levels." Am J Emerg Med 1989;7:437–440.
57. Jones J, Mcmullen MJ, Dougherty J: Toxic smoke inhalation: Cyanide poisoning in fire victims. Am J Emerg Med 1987;5:318–321.
58. Karter MJ: NFPA's latest fire loss figures. National Fire Protection Admin (NFPA) J 1996;90:52–59.
59. Kiese M, Weger N: Formation of ferrihaemoglobin with aminophenols in the human for the treatment of cyanide poisoning. Eur J Pharmacol 1969;7:97–105.
60. Kirk MA, Gerace R, Kulig KW: Cyanide and methemoglobin kinetics in smoke inhalation victims treated with the cyanide antidote kit. Ann Emerg Med 1993;22:1413–1418.
61. Lalonde C, Demling R, Brain J, et al: Smoke inhalation injury in sheep is caused by the particle phase, not the gas phase. J Appl Physiol 1994;77:15–22.
62. LaLonde C, Ikegami K, Demling R: Aerosolized deferoxamine prevents lung and systemic injury caused by smoke inhalation. J Appl Physiol 1994;77:2057–2064.
63. Layton TR, Elhauge ER: U.S. fire catastrophes of the 20th century. J Burn Care Rehabil 1982;3:21–28.
64. Lee MJ, O'Connell DJ: The plain chest radiograph after acute smoke inhalation. Clin Radiol 1988;39:33–37.
65. Levy DM, Divertie MB, Litzow TJ, et al: Ammonia burns of the face and respiratory tract. JAMA 1964;190:873–876.
66. Loick HM, Traber LD, Stothert JC, et al: Smoke inhalation causes a delayed increase in airway blood flow to primarily uninjured lung areas. Intensive Care Med 1995;21: 326–333.
67. Loick HM, Traber LD, Tokyay R, et al: The effects of dopamine on pulmonary hemodynamics and tissue damage after inhalation injury in an ovine model. J Burn Care Rehabil 1992;13:305–315.
68. Lundquist P, Rammer L, Sorbo B: The role of hydrogen cyanide and carbon monoxide in fire casualties: A prospective study. Forensic Sci Int 1989;43:9–14.
69. Mahut B, Delacourt C, de Blic J, et al: Bronchiectasis in a child after acrolein inhalation. Chest 1993;104:1286–1287.
70. Mallory TB, Brickley WJ: Management of the Cocoanut Grove burns at Massachusetts General Hospital. Pathology: With special reference to the pulmonary lesions. Ann Surg 1943;117:865–884.
71. Markowitz JS, Gutterman EM, Schwartz S, et al: Acute health effects among firefighters exposed to a polyvinyl chloride (PVC) fire. Am J Epidemiol 1989;129:1023–1031.
72. Matsubara K, Akane A, Maseda C, et al: "First pass phenomenon" of inhaled gas in the fire victims. Forensic Sci Int 1990;46:203–208.
73. McFadden ER: Therapy for acute asthma. J Allergy Clin Immunol 1989;84:151–158.
74. McNeil DG: Why so many more Americans die in fires? New York Times 1991:3, Dec 22,1991, Section E, p. 3.
75. Mellins RB, Park S: Respiratory complications of smoke inhalation in victims of fires. J Pediatr 1975;87:1–7.
76. Meyer GW, Hart GB, Strauss MB: Hyperbaric oxygen therapy for acute smoke inhalation injuries. Postgrad Med 1991;89:221–223.
77. Meyers RA, Britten JS: Are arterial blood gases of value in treatment decisions for carbon monoxide poisoning? Crit Care Med 1989;17:139–142.
78. Moore SJ, Ho IK, Hume AS: Severe hypoxia produced by concomitant intoxication with sublethal doses of carbon monoxide and cyanide. Toxicol Appl Pharmacol 1991;109: 412–420.
79. Morgan WK: The respiratory effects of particles, vapours, and fumes. Am Ind Hyg Assoc J 1986;47:670–673.
80. Moritz AR, Henriques FC, McLean R: The effects of inhaled heat on the air passages and lungs: An experimental investigation. Am J Pathol 1945;21:311–331.
81. Moylan JA, Chan C: Inhalation injury—An increasing problem. Ann Surg 1977;188:34–37.
82. Musk AW, Smith TJ, Peters JM, et al: Pulmonary function in firefighters: Acute changes in ventilatory capacity and their correlates. Br J Ind Med 1979;36:29–34.
83. Navar PD, Saffle JR, Warden GD: Effect of inhalation injury on fluid requirements after thermal injury. Am J Surg 1985;150:716–720.
84. Nelson GL: Regulatory aspects of fire toxicology. Toxicology 1987;47:181–199.
85. Nieman GF, Clark WR, Goyette DA: Positive end expiratory pressure (PEEP) efficacy following wood smoke inhalation. Am Rev Respir Dis 1986;133:A347. Abstract.
86. Nieman GF, Clark WR, Hakim T: Methylprednisolone does not protect the lung from inhalation injury. Burns 1991;17:384–390.
87. Nieman GF, Clark WR, Paskanik AM, et al: Unilateral smoke inhalation increases pulmonary blood flow to the injured lung. J Trauma 1994;36:617–623.
88. Nieman GF, Clark WR, Wax SD, et al: The effects of smoke inhalation on pulmonary surfactant. Ann Surg 1980;191: 171–181.
89. Nieman GF, Paskanik AM, Fluck RR, et al: Comparison of exogenous surfactants in the treatment of wood smoke inhalation. Am J Respir Crit Care Med 1995;152:597–602.
90. Nijland R, Jongsma HW, Nijhuis JG, et al: Notes on the apparent discordance of pulse oximetry and multi-wavelength haemoglobin photometry. Acta Anaesthesiol Scand 1995;107:(suppl)49–52.
91. Norris JC, Moore SJ, Hume AS: Synergistic lethality induced by the combination of carbon monoxide and cyanide. Toxicology 1986;40:121–129.
92. Ogura H, Saitoh D, Johnson AA, et al: The effects of inhaled nitric oxide on pulmonary ventilation–perfusion matching following smoke inhalation injury. J Trauma 1994;37:893–898.
93. Oliver O: Management of the Cocoanut Grove burns at the Massachusetts General Hospital. Ann Surg 1943;117: 801–802.
94. Orzel RA: Toxicologic aspects of firesmoke: Polymer pyrolysis and combustion. Occup Med 1993;8:414–429.
95. Oulton MR, Janigan DT, MacDonald JM, et al: Effects of smoke inhalation on alveolar surfactant subtypes in mice. Am J Pathol 1994;145:941–950.
96. Peitzman AB, Shires GT, Teixidor HS, et al: Smoke inhalation injury: Evaluation of radiographic manifestations and pulmonary dysfunction. J Trauma 1989;29:1232–1239.
97. Pitt BR, Radford EP, Gurtner GH, et al: Interaction of car-

bon monoxide and cyanide on cerebral circulation and metabolism. Arch Environ Health 1979;34:354–355.

98. Prien T: Toxic smoke compounds and inhalation injury—A review. Burns 1988;14:451–460.
99. Purser DA, Woolley WD: Biological studies of combustion atmospheres. J Fire Sci 1983;1:118–144.
100. Riyami BM, Kinsella J, Pollok AJ, et al: Alveolar macrophage chemotaxis in fire victims with smoke inhalation and burns injury. Eur J Clin Invest 1991;21:485–489.
101. Robinson L, Miller RH: Smoke inhalation injuries. Am J Otolaryngol 1986;7:375–380.
102. Robinson NB, Hudson LD, Riem M, et al: Steroid therapy following isolated smoke inhalation injury. J Trauma 1982;22:876–879.
103. Saincher A, Swirsky N, Tenenbein M: Cyanide overdose: Survival with fatal blood concentration without antidotal therapy. J Emerg Med 1994;12:555–557.
104. Schwerd W, Schulz E: Carboxyhaemoglobin and methaemoglobin findings in burnt bodies. Forensic Sci Int 1978; 12:233–235.
105. Shusterman D, Alexeeff G, Hargis C, et al: Predictors of carbon monoxide and hydrogen cyanide exposure in smoke inhalation patients. J Toxicol Clin Toxicol 1996;34: 61–71.
106. Siegel D, Sheppard D, Gelb A, et al: Aminophylline increases the toxicity but not the efficacy of an inhaled beta-adrenergic agonist in the treatment of acute exacerbations of asthma. Am Rev Respir Dis 1985;132:283–286.
107. Silverman SH, Purdue GF, Hunt JL, et al: Cyanide toxicity in burned patients. J Trauma 1988;28:171–176.
108. Sokal JA, Kralkowska E: The relationship between exposure duration, carboxyhemoglobin, blood glucose, pyruvate and lactate and the severity of intoxication in 39 cases of acute carbon monoxide poisoning in man. Arch Toxicol 1985:196–199.
109. Stone JP, Hazlett RN, Johnson JE, et al: The transport of hydrogen chloride by soot from burning polyvinyl chloride. J Fire Flammability 1973;4:42–51.
110. Symington IS, Anderson RA, Oliver JS, et al: Cyanide exposures in fires. Lancet 1978;2:90–92.
111. Teixidor HS, Rubin E, Novick GS, et al: Smoke inhalation: Radiologic manifestations. Radiology 1983;149:383–387.
112. Terrill JB, Montgomery RR, Reinhardt CF: Toxic gases from fires. Science 1978;200:1343–1347.
113. Thom SR: Antagonism of carbon monoxide-mediated brain lipid peroxidation by hyperbaric oxygen. Toxicol Appl Pharmacol 1990;105:340–344.
114. Thom SR: Carbon monoxide mediated brain lipid peroxidation in the rat. J Appl Physiol 1990;63:997–1003.
115. Thom SR, Keim LW: Carbon monoxide poisoning: A review of epidemiology, pathophysiology, clinical findings, and treatment options including hyperbaric oxygen. J Toxicol Clin Toxicol 1989;27:141–156.
116. Thom SR, Mendiguren I, Van Winkle T, et al: Smoke inhalation with a concurrent systemic stress results in lung alveolar injury. Am J Respir Crit Care Med 1994;149: 220–226.
117. Thom SR, Taber RL, Mendiguren II, et al: Delayed neuropsychologic sequelae after carbon monoxide poisoning: Prevention by treatment with hyperbaric oxygen. Ann Emerg Med 1995;25:474–480.
118. Thompson PB, Herdon DN, Traber DL, et al: Effects on mortality of inhalation injury. J Trauma 1986;26:163–165.
119. Thorning DR, Howard ML, Hudson LD, et al: Pulmonary responses to smoke inhalation: Morphologic changes in rabbits exposed to pine wood smoke. Hum Pathol 1982;13:355–364.
120. Tomaszewski CA, Rudy J, Rosenberg N, et al: Prevention of neurologic sequelae from carbon monoxide by hyperbaric oxygen in rats. Neurology 1992;42:196. Abstract.
121. Tomaszewski CA, Thom SR: Use of hyperbaric oxygen in toxicology. Emerg Med Clin North Am 1994;12:437–459.
122. Traber DL, Linares HA, Herndon DN: The pathophysiology of inhalation injury—A review. Burns 1988;14: 357–364.
123. Trapp WG: Massive cyanide poisoning with recovery: A boxing-day story. Can Med Assoc J 1970;102:517.
124. Treitman RD, Burgess WA, Gold A: Air contaminants encountered by firefighters. Am Ind Hyg Assoc J 1980;41: 796–802.
125. Tremper KK, Barker SJ: Using pulse oximetry when dyshemoglobin levels are high. J Crit Illness 1988;3: 103–107.
126. Wang CZ, Li A, Yang ZC: The pathophysiology of carbon monoxide poisoning and acute respiratory failure in a sheep model with smoke inhalation injury. Chest 1990;97: 736–742.
127. Weiss LD, Van Meter KW: The applications of hyperbaric oxygen therapy in emergency medicine. Am J Emerg Med 1992;10:558–568.
128. Wetherell HR: The occurrence of cyanide in the blood of fire victims. J Forensic Sci 1966;11:167–173.
129. Witten ML, Quan SF, Sobonya RE, et al: New developments in the pathogenesis of smoke inhalation-induced pulmonary edema. West J Med 1988;148:33–36.
130. Wittram C, Kenny JB: The admission chest radiograph after acute inhalation injury and burns. Br J Radiol 1994; 67:751–754.
131. Youn Y, Lalonde C, Demling R: Oxidants and the pathophysiology of burn and smoke inhalation injury. Free Radic Biol Med 1992;12:409–415.
132. Zawacki BE, Jung RC, Joyce J, et al: Smoke, burns, and the natural history of inhalation injury in fire victims: A correlation of experimental and clinical data. Ann Surg 1977; 185:100–110.
133. Zikria BA, Ferrer JM, Floch HF: The chemical factors contributing to pulmonary damage in "smoke poisoning." Surgery 1972;71:704–709.

CHAPTER 96

Carbon Monoxide

Christian Tomaszewski

Carbon Monoxide	
MW	= 28.01 D
Gas density	= 0.968 (air = 1.0)
Carboxyhemoglobin levels	
Nonsmokers	1 – 2 %
Smokers	5–10 %
Action level	> 10%
TLV – TWA	= 50 ppm

A 35-year-old female was found sitting outside of a warehouse. Her boss stated she had been operating a forklift in an enclosed building all morning. She came stumbling out complaining of dizziness and headaches. Co-workers in an adjoining building also complained of mild headache. After collapsing outside, she regained consciousness immediately but still appeared confused to co-workers. Prehospital personnel started an IV of 0.9% sodium chloride and placed her on 100% oxygen at the scene prior to transport.

On arrival to the ED, the patient was still somewhat drowsy, oriented only to person and place and complaining of a severe headache. Initial vital signs were: blood pressure, 92/58 mm Hg; pulse, 112 beats/min; respirations, 26 breaths/min; and rectal temperature 100°F (38°C). Examination of the head revealed mid-size reactive pupils with a supple neck. Chest examination revealed clear lungs with a regular tachycardia. Neurologic examination revealed good strength and sensation bilaterally with normal reflexes. The patient refused to stand because of weakness and dizziness.

The boss arrived and stated that the patient was probably suffering from the flu or food poisoning. Several other employees had been complaining of similar symptoms all week. This was not surprising because the local health department had reported record cases of influenza A this season.

The patient was placed on a cardiac monitor and 100% oxygen by nonrebreather face mask. A fingerstick bedside blood glucose was 60–80 mg/dL. As the health care worker obtained an arterial blood gas for carboxyhemoglobin determination, she was reassured by the pulse oximeter reading of 98% saturation. The patient then related that she had been having palpitations and mild chest pain. An ECG was ordered.

Laboratory results finally returned. The ECG revealed normal sinus rhythm without ischemic changes. Arterial blood gas results were: pH, 7.32; PCO_2, 32 mm Hg; PO_2, 124 mm Hg. The carboxyhemoglobin was 18%. Further questioning of EMS personnel revealed that patient transport was delayed and the patient was on 100% oxygen for at least 30 minutes prior to the blood drawing in the emergency department.

After 2 hours on 100% the patient remained somewhat drowsy and still complained of a severe headache. On brief mental status examination the patient was still amnestic for the events that occurred and was only oriented to person and place. She could apparently remember only two out of three objects at five minutes. She had difficulty with serial threes and saying the days of the week backward. In addition, when standing she still had problems walking a straight line heel to toe. The health care worker decided to consult a local poison center to see if further neurologic evaluation was warranted. After discussing the case with the poison center, the health care worker felt that she should transfer the patient to the nearest hyperbaric facility for further treatment.

The patient was transferred by helicopter, requiring less than an hour to reach the hyperbaric center. On arrival she mentioned her concern for HBO treatment when in fact she might be pregnant. A pregnancy test was promptly done on urine, testing positive. After being explained the risks and benefits of the procedure, she decided to go ahead with HBO treatment. After one dive her symptoms improved, but 4 hours later she still complained of a mild headache. The health care provider decided to treat the patient again with HBO, 6 hours after her initial treatment. She refused, stating that she is severely claustrophobic and refuses to reenter the confines of the monoplace unit.

On the subsequent day the patient felt much better. She returned to work in 3 days. At 3-week follow-up, she reported no untoward symptoms. A bedside mini-mental status examination revealed good attention and memory. A more formal neuropsychological battery revealed no deficiencies. Seven months later she gave birth to an apparently normal infant boy.

How Prevalent Is Carbon Monoxide Poisoning?

Carbon monoxide (CO) is the leading cause of poisoning morbidity and mortality in the United States.[108] A comprehensive review of death certificate data compiled by the National Center for Health Statistics shows an average of 5613 deaths each year (1979–1988) from CO poisoning.[28] A more significant problem may be the morbidity associated with this poisoning. One source has estimated that approximately 10,000 people seek medical attention or lose at least 1 day of normal activity due to CO intoxication each year.[148] The most serious complication of this poisoning is persistent or delayed neurologic dysfunction in 14–40% of discharged patients.[121,159] These numbers may underestimate the real problem, because many more patients may be treated and released for a myriad of complaints when in reality they have unrecognized CO poisoning.

What Are the Sources of Carbon Monoxide Poisoning?

Although CO is found naturally in the body as a byproduct of heme degradation, it does not reach toxic concentrations unless inhaled from exogenous sources.[30] External sources of CO include incomplete combustion of any carbonaceous fossil fuel. In a 10-year review of CO-related deaths, over half of unintentional deaths were caused by motor vehicle exhaust.[28] Occupants of motor vehicles are not the only victims of exhaust gases. Carbon monoxide poisoning is also reported in children riding in the back of pickup trucks.[68] Workers also become symptomatic from use of propane-powered equipment indoors such as fork lifts[46,50] and ice skating rink resurfacers.[83] Even occupants of boats are not immune to this insidious toxin.[156]

In the past 10 years, unintentional CO exposures from nonvehicular sources have resulted in an average of 500 deaths per year in the United States.[28] Predominantly, these have involved the burning of charcoal, wood, or natural gas for heating and cooking.[34,51,53,67] Furnaces for heating are often the culprit, especially when the flue is blocked.[13,64,72] Gas kitchen stoves are an important source of CO in indigent populations with marginal heating systems.[162] In fact, the use of gas stoves for supplemental heat is predictive of high COHb levels in patients with headache and dizziness.[73]

Fires are another important source of CO exposure. In the past 10 years, CO was listed as the cause of or major contributor to 15,523 fire deaths.[28] Carbon monoxide is considered to be the most common hazard to smoke inhalation victims.[13,38,153,179] Exposure to smoke that may include cyanide, another by-product of fire combustion, can result in morbidity and mortality greater than that predicted by the amount of CO exposure alone[11] (see Chap. 95).

Methylene chloride, a paint stripping agent, is another source of CO. It is readily absorbed through the skin or by inhalation and is metabolized in the liver to CO.[164] After a delay of 8 hours or longer, peak levels of COHb can range from 10–50%.[48,93,101,143] Because of ongoing production of CO, the apparent COHb half-life is prolonged to 13 hours.[141] Carboxyhemoglobin (COHb) levels after methylene chloride exposure appear to be proportional to the concentration and duration of exposure.[154]

How Does Carbon Monoxide Poison?

Carbon monoxide's most obvious effect is binding to hemoglobin, rendering it incapable of delivering oxygen to the cells. Carbon monoxide has an affinity for hemoglobin 200–250 times greater than does oxygen.[42] Therefore, in spite of adequate partial pressures of oxygen in blood (PO_2), there is decreased arterial oxygen content. Further insult occurs because CO causes a leftward shift of the oxyhemoglobin dissociation curve, thus decreasing the offloading of oxygen from hemoglobin to tissue.[146] This may be partially due to a decrease in erythrocyte 2,3-diphosphoglycerate concentration.[6,174] The net effect of all these processes is the decreased ability of oxygen to be carried by the bloodstream and released to cells.

Carbon monoxide toxicity cannot be attributed solely to COHb-mediated hypoxia.[142] Neither clinical effects nor the phenomena of delayed neurologic deficits can be completely predicted by the extent of binding between hemoglobin and CO.[171] Furthermore, it does not explain why negligible levels of COHb (4–5%) can result in cognitive impairment.[98] An early study showed that dogs breathing 13% CO died within an hour with COHb levels 54–90%; however, exchange transfusion of this same blood into healthy dogs caused no untoward effects.[60] Comparable levels of anemia also lacked adverse effects. The conclusion was that inherent to CO toxicity is its delivery to target organs such as the brain and heart.[59,60]

The delivery of CO intracellularly and its binding to hemoproteins other than hemoglobin may also account for its toxicity. Ten to 15% of the total body store of CO is extravascular.[29] Some of this CO may be interfering with cellular respiration by binding to mitochondrial cytochrome oxidase, as has been shown in vitro.[7,22] Initial studies showed that this binding was especially exaggerated under conditions of hypoxia and hypotension.[18] Further damage comes from displacement of nitric oxide by CO from platelets that in turn form peroxynitrites, strong inactivators of cytochrome oxidase.[172]

The inactivation of cytochrome oxidase may be only a temporary event in the initiation of a cascade of events resulting in an ischemic reperfusion injury to the brain after CO poisoning. During recovery from the initial poisoning, white blood cells are attracted and adhere to the brain microvasculature.[172] This attraction may be partly attributable to endothelial changes from initial cytochrome oxidase dysfunction.[167] After attaching, the leukocytes release proteases that convert xanthine dehydrogenase to xanthine oxidase, an enzyme that promotes formation of oxygen free radicals.[168] The end result of this process is delayed lipid peroxidation of the brain, as demonstrated in a rat model.[169]

Myoglobin is another hemoprotein that binds CO. A dog model demonstrates that this binding is enhanced under hypoxic conditions.[31] This binding may partially explain the myocardial impairment seen in both animal studies[35] and low-level exposures in patients with ischemic heart disease.[5] Isolated rat heart studies demonstrate that this toxic effect on the heart exists regardless of COHb formation.[23] The combination of COHb formation, which decreases oxygen-carrying capacity, in addition to the production of reduced myoglobin in the heart, which decreases oxygen extraction, may explain the preterminal dysrhythmias seen in animal studies.[55] Volunteers, especially in those with preexisting heart disease, develop an increase in life-threatening dysrhythmias and ischemic changes with low-level exposures (resulting in COHb levels up to 6%) during stress testing.[1,151]

Several recent studies suggest that CO effects on the cardiovascular system may be essential for the ischemic reperfusion injury of the brain. Carbon monoxide is a presumed neural messenger that activates guanyl cyclase, which in turn relaxes smooth muscle.[181,183] Also, CO can act on platelets to displace nitric oxide, which in turn is a potent vasodilator.[90] These factors may partially account for the hypotension that accompanies high doses of CO toxicity.[58,66] Such an episode of hypotension may represent the syncope or loss of consciousness that accompanies serious CO poisoning and portends a worse outcome.[26,52,112] In the rhesus monkey, cerebral white matter lesions correlate better with decreases in blood pressure than with COHb percentages.[58,127] Lipid peroxidation of the brain in rats develops an hour after a CO exposure that has terminated in syncope and hypotension.[169] This delay is comparable to that necessary to produce mitochondrial destruction from oxidative stress in rats exposed to CO.[191] In a feline model, central nervous system damage comparable to that associated with CO can be reproduced only when hypoxia is accompanied by an interval of ischemia, confirming the ischemic-reperfusion model for central nervous system insult after CO poisoning.[126]

CO neuronal damage may not be a simple matter of cytochrome oxidase inactivation accompanying ischemic-reperfusion injury. In addition, glutamate increases in rat brains after CO poisoning.[147] Glutamate is an excitatory amino acid that can bind at *N*-methyl-D-aspartate receptors and cause intracellular calcium release, resulting in delayed neuronal cell death.[14] Blockade of receptors can prevent the neuronal death and learning deficits that accompany a model of serious CO poisoning in a mouse.[170]

What Are the Unique Signs and Symptoms of Acute Carbon Monoxide Poisoning?

The earliest symptoms associated with CO poisoning are often nonspecific and readily confused with other illnesses, typically viral syndromes[20] (Table 96–1). The initial symptom reported by volunteers within 4 hours of exposure to 200 ppm (COHb levels 15–20%) is headache; shorter exposures at 500 ppm lead to nausea as well.[165] The incidence of CO poisoning (COHb levels ≥ 10%) in symptomatic patients presenting with flu-like symptoms to emergency departments in the winter ranges from 3–24% in some series.[25,41,70,73] Because the typical presenting complaints are headache, dizziness, and nausea, and the most frequent exposures are winter time, influenza becomes the most common misdiagnosis.[41,64] Carbon

TABLE 96–1. CLINICAL MANIFESTATIONS OF CARBON MONOXIDE POISONING

Severity[a]	Symptoms	Signs
Mild	Headache	Vomiting
	Nausea	
	Dizziness	
Moderate	Chest pain	Tachycardia
	Difficulty thinking	Tachypnea
	Blurred vision	Cognitive deficits
	Dyspnea on exertion	Myonecrosis
	Weakness	Ataxia
Severe	Chest pain	Seizures
	Palpitations	Coma
	Disorientation	Ventricular dysrhythmias
		Hypotension
		Myocardial ischemia
		Skin bullae (associated)

[a]Increasing severity is associated with addition of signs and symptoms listed.

monoxide poisoning is also frequently misdiagnosed as food poisoning,[9] gastroenteritis,[53,77] and even colic in an infant.[136] Children also show nonspecific symptoms, eg, nausea, headache, and vomiting, with CO poisoning, making the diagnosis equally as difficult.[36]

Continued exposure to CO can lead to symptoms attributable to another extremely oxygen-dependent organ, the heart. Low-level exposures (COHb 2–4%) in volunteers with stable angina results in decreased exercise tolerance, as well as signs and symptoms of myocardial ischemia.[1,2,4] At higher levels (COHb 6%) there is a greater frequency of premature ventricular contractions during exercise.[151] Myocardial infarction, life-threatening dysrhythmias, and cardiac arrest are commonly described in victims of CO poisoning.[3,105,149,157] In fact, acute mortality from CO is usually due to ventricular dysrhythmias, probably predominantly caused by the accompanying hypoxia.[1,3,35,149]

The central nervous system is the most sensitive area to CO poisoning. Acutely, otherwise healthy patients may manifest headache, dizziness, and ataxia at COHb levels as low as 15–20%; with longer exposures, syncope, seizures, or coma can result.[20,44,95,175,187] Patients may present with symptoms of an acute stroke.[9,86] The EEG can show diffuse frontal slow-wave activity.[52,124] Within a day of exposures that result in coma, the CT scan can show decreased density in the central white matter and globus pallidus (Fig. 96–1).[155,176] Autopsies show involvement of other areas including the cerebral cortex, hippocampus, cerebellum, and substantia nigra.[94]

Although the brain and heart are the most sensitive organs, other areas are also subject to the effects of CO poisoning. Retinal hemorrhages can develop with exposures greater than 12 hours.[39,86] One fifth to one third of severe cases, eg, requiring intubation, go on to develop cardiogenic pulmonary edema.[63,161] This does not appear to be a direct effect of CO. Studies of sheep with prolonged exposure to CO, resulting in COHb levels greater than 50%, showed no anatomic or physiologic change in lung function.[152] Mild cases may be accompanied by respiratory alkalosis to compensate for the reduction in oxygen-carrying capacity and delivery.[107] Longer exposures with decreased levels of consciousness result in metabolic acidosis, from the lactate production that accompanies tissue hypoxia.[160] Although myonecrosis and even compartment syndromes occur, patients rarely develop renal failure.[12,150] Cherry-red color is seen only after excessive exposure (2–3% of cases referred to one hyperbaric center) and may represent a combination of CO-induced vasodilation with concomitant tissue ischemia.[122,144] Another uncommon phenomenon is the development of cutaneous bullae following severe exposures.[120] These bullae are thought to be due to a combination of pressure necrosis and possibly direct CO effects in the epidermis.[79,99]

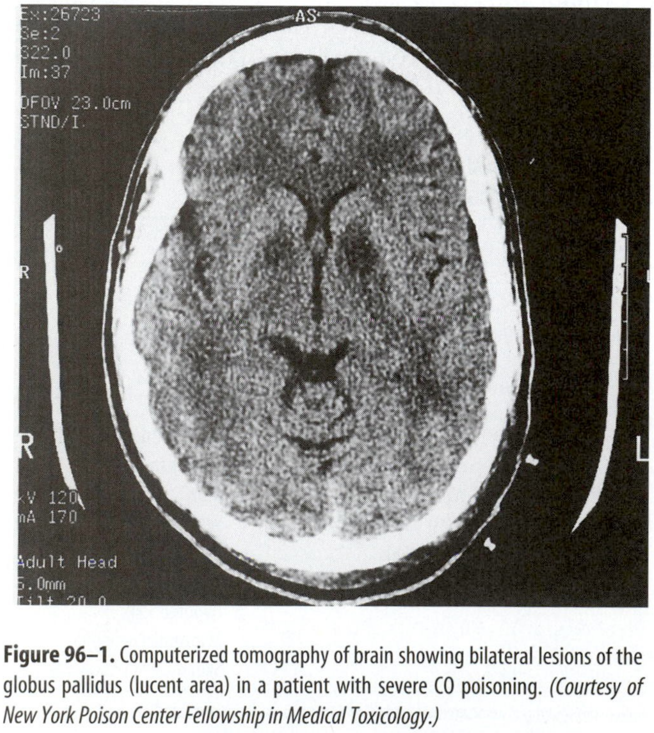

Figure 96–1. Computerized tomography of brain showing bilateral lesions of the globus pallidus (lucent area) in a patient with severe CO poisoning. *(Courtesy of New York Poison Center Fellowship in Medical Toxicology.)*

What Are the Delayed Effects of Carbon Monoxide Poisoning?

The persistent or delayed effects of acute CO poisoning are varied and include dementia, amnestic syndromes, psychosis, parkinsonism, paralysis, chorea, cortical blindness, apraxia and agnosias, peripheral neuropathy, and incontinence.[54,100] The neurologic deterioration can be preceded by a lucid period of 2–40 days after the initial CO poisoning.[26] In patients admitted to an intensive care unit for severe CO intoxication and treated with 100% oxygen, 14% of survivors had permanent neurologic impairment.[90] In a Korean series of 2360 CO-poisoned patients, almost 3% continued to show memory failure or parkinsonian features 1 year postexposure.[26] In contrast, another series of 63 seriously poisoned patients showed memory impairment in 43% and deterioration of personality in 33% at 3-year follow-up.[159] Children have shown behavioral and school difficulties after severe poisoning.[92] However, older patients (greater than 30 years old) appear to be much more susceptible to developing delayed sequelae.[26] Most cases of delayed neurologic sequelae are associated with loss of consciousness in the acute phase of intoxication.[26,52,159]

Delayed neurologic sequelae probably involve lesions of the cerebral white matter.[54] Weeks postexposure, autopsies show necrosis of the white matter, globus pallidus, cerebellum, and hippocampus.[52] Computerized tomography and MRI confirm the damage to the white matter and hippocampus.[78,127,155,176] Animal studies show that marked COHb alone cannot cause similar white-matter lesions; there must be an episode of hypotension.[58,126] The fact that the areas permanently damaged in serious CO poisoning cases are the areas with the poorest vascular supply in the brain is consistent with these animal findings.

What Initial Treatment Is Indicated in Patients With Carbon Monoxide Poisoning?

The mainstay of treatment is initial attention to the airway. One hundred percent oxygen should be provided as soon as possible by either nonrebreather face mask or endotracheal tube. The immediate effect of oxygen will be to enhance the dissociation of COHb.[146] In volunteers this reduces the half-life of COHb from a mean of 5 hours (range 2–7 hours) in room air to approximately 1 hour in 100% oxygen at normal atmospheric pressure.[130,135] Actual poisonings show a range in half-lives of 30–150 minutes when breathing 100% oxygen; the longer elimination half-lives appear to be most often associated with long, low-level exposures.[118] With oxygenation and intensive care treatment, hospital mortality rates for serious exposures range from 1 to 30%.[52,90]

Cardiac monitoring and intravenous access are necessary in any CO-poisoned patient with altered mental status. Hypotension can initially be treated with intravenous fluids; inotropic agents may also be necessary to treat any myocardial depression.[104] Standard ACLS protocols can be followed for the treatment of life-threatening dysrhythmias.

Patients with depressed mental status should have a rapid blood glucose check. This should precede the administration of intravenous glucose because of the theoretical potential for exacerbation of cerebral damage in the presence of hyperglycemia (see Antidotes in Depth: Dextrose).[133,138,139] However, animal studies of CO poisoning suggest that hypoglycemia can be deleterious as well.[131,132,134] Correction of any acidemia with bicarbonate is controversial and could result in further cell hypoxia secondary to a left shift of the oxyhemoglobin dissociation curve.

What Initial Diagnostic Tests Are Indicated in Patients With Carbon Monoxide Poisoning?

The most useful diagnostic test obtainable in a suspected CO poisoning is a COHb level. Normal levels of COHb range from 0–5%, with levels at the high range in neonates and patients with hemolytic anemia[188] as carbon monoxide is a natural by-product of the breakdown of protoporphyrin to bilirubin.[29,109] Carboxyhemoglobin levels average 6% in one-pack-per-day smokers but can range as high as 10%.[163,188] Although high COHb levels confirm exposure to CO, particular levels are not necessarily predictive of symptoms or outcome. In fact, COHb can return to normal or be zero if the patient has been treated with oxygen before obtaining the blood test.[116,125,160]

The usual method for measuring COHb is with a co-oximeter, which spectrophotometrically reads the percentage of total hemoglobin saturated with CO.[10,32] Traditionally arterial blood is used for this determination; however, venous blood levels from a heparinized (lithium heparin tube) specimen are just as accurate.[178] Bedside tests with ammonia or sodium hydroxide are unable to differentiate reliably various levels of COHb versus controls.[129] Breath sampling methods may be used for screening patients; however, ethanol, a common co-intoxicant, can falsely elevate breath levels unless an activated charcoal filter is used.[91,135,180] Because of the similarities in extinction coefficients, COHb is misinterpreted as oxyhemoglobin on pulse oximetry (see Chap. 20).[8] The pulse oximetry reading overestimates oxyhemoglobin by the approximate amount of carboxyhemoglobin present.[19]

Additional laboratory tests may be useful in severe poisoning cases. An arterial blood gas will confirm the presence of metabolic acidosis, a complication of CO poisoning associated with neurologic sequelae and death.[96] This acidosis is presumably a reflection of high lactate, an index more reliable than COHb in determining severity of toxicity.[160] Unfortunately, arterial pH does not correlate with either COHb level or initial neurologic examination, making it a poor criterion for deciding the need for hyperbaric oxygen (HBO) treatment.[116] Mild elevations of CPK are common (ranging 20–1315 IU/L in one series of 65 cases), but severe rhabdomyolysis and its complications are also reported.[150] Cardiac monitoring as well as a 12-lead ECG is essential to document ischemia or dysrhythmias in patients with preexisting coronary artery disease or severe exposure.

Does a Particular Carboxyhemoglobin Level Dictate Treatment or Predict Outcome?

The problem with using COHb levels to base treatment is that there is a wide variation in clinical manifestations with identical COHb levels.[115,121] Furthermore, particular COHb levels are not predictive of symptoms or final outcome.[107,116,125,160] In the largest prospective study of CO poisoning, COHb levels did not correlate with loss of consciousness and were not predictive of delayed neurologic sequelae.[140] Part of the problem is that admission COHb levels are inaccurate predictors of peak levels.[116] The use of nomograms to extrapolate to earlier levels have not been validated. Their credibility is also suspect because of the great variability in COHb half-lives and differences in treatment with oxygen.

Is Neuroimaging or Neurologic Evaluation Useful in Patients With Carbon Monoxide Poisoning?

The extent of neurologic insult from CO can be assessed with a variety of tests. The most basic is documentation of a normal neurologic examination with a quick mini-mental status examination. A more sensitive indicator of the acute effects of CO on cortical function is a detailed neuropsychiatric test battery developed specifically for CO patients.[119] The advantages of such testing, which usually takes about 30 minutes, is that: (1) it can reliably distinguish 79% of the time between CO-poisoned patients and controls, and (2) it shows improvement with appropriate HBO treatment.[110] Unfortunately, such testing shows only a sensitivity of 77% and specificity of 80% for CO poisoning.[145] There may be practice effects as well, if repeated testing is performed. The biggest problem with such neuropsychiatric testing is that it is unclear if deficits in the test during the acute CO intoxication are at all predictive of which patients will develop neurologic sequelae and therefore require HBO treatment.

Acute changes on CT scan of the brain have been seen within 12 hours of CO exposure that resulted in loss of consciousness.[84,113,123] Symmetrical low-density areas in the region of the globus pallidus, putamen, and caudate nuclei are frequently seen.[80,87,123] Although a normal initial CT usually predicts a favorable outcome, changes in the globus pallidus and subcortical white matter early within the first day after poisoning are associated with poor outcomes[113,137] (Fig. 96–1). The use of contrast may enhance early isodense changes that may not be visible on initial CT scan.[190] MRI appears to be superior in detecting basal ganglia lesions.[78,85] Neuroimaging usually does not influence patient management and can be reserved for patients who show poor response or have an equivocal diagnosis.

More recently, EEG and cerebral blood flow studies have been performed on CO-poisoned patients. Although initial studies show that many patients have regional EEG abnormalities after poisoning, it is undetermined if these are predictive of persistent or delayed neurologic problems.[40,43] More promising is single-photon emission computed tomography (SPECT), which can gauge regional blood flow noninvasively using an iodine or technetium tracer.[40] In one series of 13 patients with delayed neurologic sequelae, all cases showed patchy hypoperfusion throughout the cerebral cortex initially.[27] The utility of SPECT scans for predicting patients at risk for neurologic sequelae appears promising, but as yet is untested. In addition, there is the real risk that definitive treatment with hyperbaric oxygen will be delayed for any neurologic assessment beyond a routine bedside mental status examination.

What Are the Benefits of Hyperbaric Oxygen in Patients With Carbon Monoxide Poisoning?

Hyperbaric oxygen therapy appears to be the treatment of choice for significant CO exposures.[125] One hundred percent oxygen at ambient pressure reduces the half-life of COHb to 40 minutes; at 2.5 atmospheres absolute it is reduced to 20 minutes.[130,135,147] Actual CO-poisoned victims treated with HBO show half-lives ranging 4–86 minutes.[118] Hyperbaric oxygen also increases the amount of dissolved oxygen by about 10 times, which is sufficient alone to supply cerebral needs.[14] But this is not the most important clinical issue, because most patients have already been stabilized and have appreciably decreased carboxyhemoglobin levels just with ambient oxygen, prior to mobilization of chamber.

More important clinically is the fact that hyperbaric, but not normobaric, oxygen therapy prevents lipid peroxidation in rat brains after loss of consciousness from CO exposure.[170] This is because HBO appears to prevent ischemic reperfusion injury by a variety of mechanisms. First, in animal models HBO accelerates regeneration of inactivated cytochrome oxidase, which may be the initiating site for CO neuronal damage.[17] Second, HBO also prevents the subsequent leukocyte adherence to brain microvascular endothelium, a process essential for amplification of central nervous system damage from CO.[24,166] This may explain why HBO, but not 100% oxygen at atmospheric pressure, prevented delayed deficits in a learning and memory maze model.[177]

Clinical studies of the effectiveness of HBO in preventing neurologic damage from CO are not as convincing as basic science studies would suggest. In uncontrolled human clinical series, persistent neuropsychiatric symptoms, including memory impairment, range 12–43% in patients treated with 100% oxygen, and have been as low as 0–4% in patients treated with HBO.[63,107,120,125,159] The most comprehensive randomized study to date failed to show a benefit from HBO in patients who had no initial loss of consciousness.[140] Unfortunately, flaws in this study included significant delays to treatment and use of suboptimal pressure. A smaller, more recent, controlled study avoided these flaws and showed that HBO was able to decrease delayed neurologic sequelae to 0 from 23% in the control group.[173] Both of these studies failed to randomize seriously ill CO-poisoned cases, which is currently being undertaken. Although HBO may not be completely proven therapy for CO poisoning, life-threatening complications, which can usually be anticipated, are usually less than 5% with HBO use in such patients.[157]

What Are the Indications for Hyperbaric Oxygen Therapy in Carbon Monoxide Poisoning?

Specific indications for HBO after acute CO poisoning are listed (Table 96–2), but these have not been prospectively evaluated. The patients most likely to benefit are those most at risk for persistent or delayed neurologic sequelae, such as patients presenting in coma.[63,88,122,158,189,192] Other potential markers for delayed neurologic sequelae include a history of syncope.[26,52,112,159] This may represent the episode of hypotension, which is necessary for causing neuronal damage from CO-induced ischemic-reperfusion injury in animal models.[58,127] Patients with long exposures, or "soaking" periods, are also at greater risk for neurologic sequelae.[15,184] The presence of a significant metabolic acidosis may be a reliable marker for this.[96,160] Some authors advocate ongoing myocardial ischemia as

TABLE 96–2. INDICATIONS FOR HBO

On initial presentation
Syncope
Coma
Seizures
Glasgow coma scale < 15
Any focal neurologic deficits or
COHb ≥ 25%
COHb ≥ 15% in pregnancy
Myocardial ischemia or
Venticular dysrhythmias
After initial treatment and stabilization with 2–4 h of oxygen
Persistent neurologic symptoms (headache, ataxia, confusion)

an indication for HBO; however, in our experience these patients already meet neurologic criteria for treatment (eg, loss of consciousness, ongoing mental status changes). Isolated cardiac ischemia, more importantly, deserves immediate proven myocardial salvaging therapy rather than delayed treatment with an unproven therapy such as HBO.

Some authors advocate treating all patients with COHb levels of 40% or greater with HBO.[81,117] Many HBO centers arbitrarily use a more conservative level of 25% as an indication for HBO. More important than actual level are patient history and examination. If the patient had loss of consciousness or significant neurologic symptoms (eg, coma, seizures, focal neurologic deficits, GCS < 15), he or she should be treated with HBO regardless of COHb levels. It is still unclear if mild neurologic symptoms (eg, confusion, headache, dizziness, visual blurring) or abnormal mental status testing on initial presentation is prognostic of delayed sequelae. These symptoms simply represent CO intoxication, which at COHb levels approaching 20% in volunteers can cause some temporary mental impairment.[97,165] Patients with these mild signs and symptoms deserve several hours of oxygen by nonrebreather face mask; then if symptoms do not resolve, HBO can be considered. However, any delay in HBO may decrease its efficacy.[63]

Beyond good supportive care, these patients require 100% oxygen as soon as possible. Hyperbaric oxygen may provide additional benefits as outlined above. This might be especially useful in smoke-inhalation victims, to treat concomitant cyanide poisoning, chemical pneumonitis, and thermal burns.[69] Some authors recommend selective use of HBO, because of cost and difficulties in transport if the primary facility lacks a chamber.[128] However, complications that may make such transfers and treatment unsafe are rare.[157] Although HBO cannot be recommended for every patient with CO poisoning, it is a relatively safe treatment that should be considered in all serious exposures. Fortunately, three quarters of cases with delayed neurologic sequelae will resolve, albeit after several months.[26] Hopefully, completion of well-designed and scientifically controlled clinical studies will allow clarification of the indications for HBO.

Is Hyperbaric Oxygen Therapy Still Useful in Carbon Monoxide Poisoning if Given Late or After Chronic Poisoning?

The optimal timing and number of HBO treatments for CO poisoning is unclear at this time. Patients treated later than 6 hours tend to fare worse in terms of delayed sequelae (30% vs 19%) and mortality (30% vs 14%).[63] However, others suggest that late treatment may still be useful. Patients who have experienced unconsciousness from CO have been shown to benefit from an initial treatment of HBO as late as 6 hours postexposure with no evidence of delayed neurologic sequelae.[121,192] In addition, patients who did not receive HBO initially and have already developed neuropsychologic sequelae have shown benefit from HBO as late as 21 days postexposure.[120]

The problem with studies showing HBO benefits days after an acute poisoning, or after chronic poisoning, is that these cases are all anecdotal and lack controls. In fact, most cases of delayed neurologic sequelae resolve 100% within 2 months in mild poisoning[173] and 75% within 1 year in severe poisoning.[26] In fact, positive benefits in these delayed or chronic cases may simply represent the salutary effects of HBO. A preliminary study shows that HBO improves memory scores by over 50% in normal volunteers.[82]

Does Pregnancy Change the Treatment of Carbon Monoxide–Poisoned Patients?

The management of CO exposure in the pregnant patient is difficult because of the potential adverse effects of both the toxin and its treatment. A literature review of all CO exposures during pregnancy revealed a high incidence of fetal central nervous system damage and stillbirth after severe maternal poisonings.[182] A series of three severely symptomatic patients who did not receive HBO had adverse fetal outcomes: two stillbirths and one case of cerebral palsy.[89] There have even been cases of limb malformations, cranial deformities, and a variety of mental disabilities in children poisoned in utero.[21,102]

Maternal COHb levels do not accurately reflect fetal hemoglobin or tissue levels.[33,37,61,106] In primate studies, a single CO exposure insufficient to cause clinical disease in a rhesus mother led to intrauterine hypoxia, fetal brain injury, and increased rates of fetal death.[56,57] One problem is that CO absorption and elimination are slower in the fetal circulation than maternal circulation.[56,103] A mathematical model predicted that elimination of CO from the fetus would take 3.5 times longer than maternal CO elimination.[75]

Treatment of pregnant patients with HBO is not without theoretical risk. Animal studies show conflicting results on the effects of HBO on fetal development.[182]

Some studies have shown that HBO causes developmental abnormalities in the central nervous, cardiovascular, and pulmonary systems of the fetus.[111] This is in marked contrast to the extensive Russian experience, where hundreds of pregnant women have been treated with HBO, apparently without significant perinatal complications and with improvement in fetal/maternal status for their underlying conditions (eg, toxemia, anemia, diabetes).[114] Cases in this country where HBO has been used for CO poisoning have resulted in normal infants at birth.[45,76,89,182] In contrast, relatively minor exposures with no loss of consciousness in pregnant mothers, especially with prolonged exposure, have resulted in poor fetal outcomes.[21,89]

There currently is no scientific validation for an absolute level at which to dive a pregnant patient for CO exposure. Arbitrarily, COHb levels greater than 20% are touted as an indication to dive a pregnant patient regardless of symptoms.[182] Pregnant patients should not be treated any differently if they meet criteria for HBO that have already been mentioned (see Table 96–2). Additional criteria would include any signs of fetal distress, such as abnormal fetal heart rate, if developmentally available. Elevated levels of COHb (> 15%), especially with a symptomatic mother, warrant HBO if locally available. This will facilitate more efficient treatment of the mother because of the necessity for prolonged oxygen therapy in pregnant patients with the uncertainty of what actual fetal COHb levels are.

Is There Any Proven Benefit to Repeat Treatment With Hyperbaric Oxygen Therapy?

The number of HBO treatments necessary remains unclear. In one series, repeated HBO treatment reduced the incidence of delayed sequelae from 50% to 18%.[62] However, a recent controlled study showed no difference in outcome between one and two HBO treatments for those individuals who had loss of consciousness.[140] Based on the known physiology of the poisoning, there is nothing to support repeat treatment at this time. Any late effects from HBO treatment may represent spontaneous symptom resolution.

How Are Carbon Monoxide Exposures Prevented?

Early diagnosis will prevent much of the associated morbidity and mortality associated with CO poisoning, especially in unintentional exposures. The increased quality of home carbon monoxide–detecting devices will allow personal intervention in the prevention of exposure. Routine screening of emergency department patients during the winter is not very efficacious in diagnosing unsuspected CO poisoning; the yield is less than 1% when patients are tested in whom the diagnosis of CO exposure was already excluded by history.[71,180] Instead, selecting patients with CO-related complaints, such as headache, dizziness, or nausea, increases the yield to 5–11%.[65,180] During winter, risk factors, such as gas heating or symptomatic cohabitants in patients with flu-like symptoms (eg, headache, dizziness, nausea) will be the most useful method for deciding when to obtain COHb levels on potential cases.[13,70,72,73]

The issue of symptomatic cohabitants is especially important from a preventive standpoint. A common oversight is neglecting the history of multiple involvement in a single household.[86] Alerting other cohabitants to this danger and effecting evacuation may prevent needless deaths.[185] Most communities have multiple resources for on-site evaluation. Usually the local fire department or utility company can either check home appliances or measure ambient CO levels with portable monitoring equipment. Current workplace standards for ambient CO exposures are 35 ppm for a 1-hour limit and 9 ppm for an 8-hour limit.[47] Until they arrive, natural-gas-fueled appliances should be turned off and the area evacuated, leaving all windows and doors open.

Unintentional exposures to CO can be easily misdiagnosed. Carbon monoxide should be suspected in any patient with coma, acidosis, or signs of cardiac ischemia that may be attributable to suicide. Fire victims, in addition to airway problems and potential cyanide toxicity, may succumb to CO toxicity.[11] The mainstay of treatment in all these cases is good supportive care with early oxygenation to increase the elimination of CO. Because of the overwhelming clinical successes with HBO and its limited risks, early use of this treatment modality in severe exposures is encouraged. Discussion with a poison control center or hyperbaric facility will help in identifying those patients most likely to benefit from such treatment.

How Do Patients Get Carbon Monoxide Poisoned?

The onset of headache and dizziness, especially with involvement of co-workers, strongly suggested an airborne toxin in our case sample. With poor air circulation, there could be a buildup of various air pollutants, microbial agents, and allergens that could result in sick building syndrome. Although patients suffering from sick building syndrome often have a headache, this is usually accompanied by irritation of the airways and mucous membranes, which would not be seen with CO poisoning.[16] The forklift was a likely culprit for an exposure in this case. Propane, the typical fuel of indoor forklifts, is an asphyxiant and at low doses can cause euphoria[186] (see Chap. 94). However, the accompanying mercaptans would have alerted workers to a dangerous leak. Nitrogen dioxide, an occasional combustion product of propane, can cause delayed respiratory symptoms, but does not typically cause headache.[74] The most likely gas exposure responsible for these symptoms is CO. For optimal performance propane-powered forklifts are typically adjusted to produce no less than 10,000 ppm CO in exhaust, and in fact average more than 30,000 ppm.[49] In an enclosed warehouse, with poor ventilation, CO levels could exceed toxic levels within an hour at this rate of production. Workers, as in the case example, would succumb to its toxic effects without warning because CO is a clear, odorless, nonirritating gas.

References

1. Allred EN, Bleecker ER, Chaitman BR, et al: Short-term effects of carbon monoxide exposure on the exercise performance of subjects with coronary artery disease. N Engl J Med 1989;321:1426–1432.
2. Anderson EW, Andelman RJ, Strauch JM, et al: Effect of low-level carbon monoxide exposure on onset and duration of angina pectoris. A study in ten patients with ischemic heart disease. Ann Intern Med 1973;79:46–50.
3. Anderson RF, Allensworth DC, DeGroot WJ: Myocardial toxicity from carbon monoxide poisoning. Ann Intern Med 1967;67:1172–1182.
4. Aronow W, Isbell MW: Carbon monoxide effect on exercise-induced angina pectoris. Ann Intern Med 1973;79: 392–395.
5. Aronow WS, Cassidy J, Vangrow JS, et al: Effect of cigarette smoking and breathing carbon monoxide on cardiovascular hemodynamics in anginal patients. Circulation 1974;50:340–347.
6. Astrup P: Intraerythrocyte 2,3-diphosphoglycerate and carbon monoxide exposure. Ann NY Acad Sci 1970;174: 252–254.
7. Ball EG, Strittmatter CF, Cooper O: The reaction of cytochrome oxidase with carbon monoxide. J Biol Chem 1951;193:635–647.
8. Barker SJ, Tremper KK: The effect of carbon monoxide inhalation on pulse oximetry and transcutaneous pO_2. Anesthesiology 1987;66:677–679.
9. Barret L, Canel V, Faure J: Carbon monoxide poisoning, a diagnosis frequently overlooked. J Toxicol Clin Toxical 1985;23:309–313.
10. Barrows GH, Thomas BB, Short CS, et al: A simple carbon monoxide screening method on hemoglobin absorbance ratios. Am J Clin Pathol 1986;85:387. Abstract.
11. Baud FJ, Barriot P, Toffis V, et al: Elevated blood cyanide concentrations in victims of smoke inhalation. N Engl J Med 1991;325:1761–1766.
12. Bessoudo R, Gray J: Carbon monoxide poisoning and nonoliguric renal failure. Can Med Assoc J 1978;119:41–44.
13. Birky MM, Clarke FB: Inhalation of toxic products from fires. Bull NY Acad Med 1981;57:997–1013.
14. Boerema I, Meyne, I, Brummelkamp WH, et al: Life without blood. Arch Chir Neder 1959;11:70–83.
15. Bogusz M, Cholewa L, Pach J, et al: A comparison of two types of acute carbon monoxide poisoning. Arch Toxicol 1975;33:141–149.
16. Bourbeau J, Brisson C, Allaire S: Prevalence of the sick building syndrome symptoms in office workers before and after being exposed to a building with an improved ventilation system. Occup Environ Med 1996;53:204–210.
17. Brown SD, Piantadosi CA: Recovery of energy metabolism in rat brain after carbon monoxide hypoxia. J Clin Invest 1992;89:666–672.
18. Brown SD, Piantadosi CA: In vivo binding of carbon monoxide to cytochrome oxidase in rat brain. J Appl Physiol 1990;68:604–610.
19. Buckley RG, Aks SE, Eshom JL, et al: The pulse oximety gap in carbon monoxide intoxication. Ann Emerg Med 1994;24:252–255.
20. Burney RE, Wu S: Mass carbon monoxide poisoning: Clinical effects and results of treatment in 184 victims. Ann Emerg Med 1982;11:394–399.
21. Caravati EM, Adams CJ, Joyce SM, et al: Fetal toxicity associated with maternal carbon monoxide poisoning. Ann Emerg Med 1988;17:714–717.
22. Chance BC, Erecinska M, Wagner M: Mitochondrial responses to carbon monoxide. Ann NY Acad Sci 1970; 174:193–203.
23. Chen KC, McGrath JJ: Response of the isolated heart to carbon monoxide and nitrogen anoxia. Toxicol Appl Pharmacol 1985;81:363–370.
24. Chen Q, Banick PD, Thom SR: Functional inhibition of rat polymorphonuclear leukocyte B2 integrins by hyperbaric oxygen is associated with impaired cGMP synthesis. J Pharmacol Exp Ther 1996;276:929–933.
25. Chisolm CD, Reilly J, Berejan B: Carboxyhemoglobin levels in patients with headache. Ann Emerg Med 1986; 16:497. Abstract.
26. Choi HS: Delayed neurological sequelae in carbon monoxide intoxication. Arch Neurol 1983;40:433–435.
27. Choi IS, Kim SK, Lee SS, Choi YC: Evaluation of outcome of delayed neurologic sequelae after carbon monoxide poisoning by technetium-99m hexamethylpropylene amine oxime brain single photon emission computed tomography. Eur Neurol 1995;35:137–142.
28. Cobb N, Etzel RA: Unintentional carbon monoxide-related deaths in the United States, 1979 through 1988. JAMA 1991;266:659–663.
29. Coburn RF: The carbon monoxide body stores. Ann NY Acad Sci 1970;174:11–22.
30. Coburn RF: Endogenous carbon monoxide production. N Engl J Med 1970;282:207–209.
31. Coburn RF, Mayers LB: Myoglobin oxygen tension determined from measurements of carboxyhemoglobin in skeletal muscle. Am J Physiol 1971;220:66–74.
32. Commins BT, Lawther PJ: A sensitive method for the determination of carboxyhemoglobin in a finger prick sample of blood. Br J Ind Med 1965;22:139–143.
33. Copel JA, Bowen F, Bolognese RJ: Carbon monoxide intoxication in early pregnancy. Obstet Gynecol 1982;59: 26S–28S.
34. Cox BD, Wichelow MJ: Carbon monoxide levels in the breath of smokers and nonsmokers: Effect of home heating systems. J Epidemiol Community Health 1985;39: 75–78.
35. Cramlet SH, Erickson HH, Gorman HA: Ventricular function following carbon monoxide exposure. J Appl Physiol 1975;39:482–486.
36. Croker PJ, Walker JS: Pediatric carbon monoxide toxicity. J Emerg Med 1985;3:443–448.
37. Curtis GW, Alger EJ, McDay AJ, et al: The transplacental diffusion of carbon monoxide. Arch Pathol Lab Med 1955;59:677–690.
38. Davies JWL: Toxic chemicals versus lung tissue—An as-

pect of inhalation injury revisited. J Burn Care Rehabil 1986;7:213–222.
39. Dempsey LC, O'Donnell JJ, Hoff JT: Carbon monoxide retinopathy. Am J Ophthalmol 1976;82:692–693.
40. Denays R, Makhoul E, Dachy B, et al: Electroencephalographic mapping and 99mTc HMPAO single-photon emission computed tomography in carbon monoxide poisoning. Ann Emerg Med 1994;24:947–952.
41. Dolan MC, Haltom TL, Barrows GH, et al: Carboxyhemoglobin levels in patients with flu-like symptoms. Ann Emerg Med 1987;16:782–786.
42. Douglas CG, Haldane JS, Haldane JBS: The laws of combustion of hemoglobin with carbon monoxide and oxygen. J Physiol (London) 1912;44:275–304.
43. Ducasse JL, Celsis P, Marc-Vergnes JP: Non-comatose patients with acute carbon monoxide poisoning: Hyperbaric or normobaric oxygenation. Undersea Hyperb Med 1995; 22:9–15.
44. Durnin C: Carbon monoxide poisoning presenting with focal epileptiform seizures. Lancet 1987;1:1319. Letter.
45. Elkharrat D, Faphael JC, Korach JM, et al: Acute carbon monoxide intoxication and hyperbaric oxygen in pregnancy. Intensive Care Med 1991;17:289–292.
46. Ely EW, Moorehead B, Haponik EF: Warehouse workers' headache: Emergency evaluation and management of 30 patients with carbon monoxide poisoning. Am J Med 1995;98:145–155.
47. Environmental Protection Agency: Air Quality Criteria for Carbon Monoxide. Research Triangle Park, NC. Environmental Criteria and Assessment Office, Office of Health and Environmental Assessment, 1997, EPA 600–8/90/045.
48. Fagin J, Bradley J, Williams D: Carbon monoxide poisoning secondary to inhaling methylene chloride. Br Med J 1980;281:1461.
49. Fawcett TA, Moon RE, Fracica PJ, et al: Warehouse workers' headache: Carbon monoxide poisoning from propane-fueled forklifts. J Occup Med 1992;34:12–15.
50. Fort L, Griggs P: Carbon monoxide poisoning in North Carolina. NC Med J 1987;48:317–321.
51. Foutch RG, Henrichs W: Carbon monoxide poisoning at high altitudes. Am J Emerg Med 1988;6:596–598.
52. Garland H, Pearce J: Neurological complications of carbon monoxide poisoning. Q J Med 1967;36:445–455.
53. Gasman JD, Varon J, Gardner JP: Carbon monoxide poisoning. West J Med 1990;153:656–657.
54. Ginsberg MD: Carbon monoxide intoxication: Clinical features, neuropathology, and mechanisms of injury. J Toxicol Clin Toxicol 1985;23:281–288.
55. Ginsberg MD, Myers RAM: Experimental carbon monoxide encephalopathy in the primate. I. Physiologic and metabolic aspects. Arch Neurol 1974;30:202–208.
56. Ginsberg MD, Myers RE: Fetal brain injury after maternal carbon monoxide intoxication: Clinical and neuropathologic aspects. Neurology 1976;26:15–23.
57. Ginsberg MD, Myers RE: Fetal brain damage following maternal carbon monoxide intoxication: An experimental study. Acta Obstet Gynecol Scand 1974;53:309–317.
58. Ginsberg MD, Myers RE, McDonaugh BF: Experimental carbon monoxide encephalopathy in the primate. II. Clinical aspects, neuropathology and physiologic correlation. Arch Neurol 1974;30:209–216.
59. Goldbaum LR, Orellano T, Dergal E: Mechanism of the toxic action of carbon monoxide. Ann Clin Lab Sci 1976;6:372–376.
60. Goldbaum LR, Ramirez RG, Absalon KB: XIII. What is the mechanism of carbon monoxide toxicity? Aviat Space Environ Med 1975;46:1289–1291.
61. Goldstein DP: Carbon monoxide poisoning in pregnancy. Am J Obstet Gynecol 1965;92:526–528.
62. Gorman DF, Clayton D, Gilligan JE, et al: A longitudinal study of 100 consecutive admissions for carbon monoxide poisoning to the Royal Adelaide Hospital. Anaesth Intensive Care 1992;20:311–316.
63. Goulon M, Barios A, Raphin M, et al: Carbon monoxide poisoning and acute anoxia due to breathing coal gas and hydrocarbons. Ann Med Interne 1969;120:335–349.
64. Grace TW, Platt FW: Subacute carbon monoxide poisoning: Another great imitator. JAMA 1981;246:1698–1700.
65. Greene C, Lumpkin JR, Baker FJI: Association between unsuspected carbon monoxide exposure and headache. Ann Emerg Med 1983;12:244–245. Abstract.
66. Halebian B, Robinson N, Barie P, et al: Whole body oxygen utilization during acute carbon monoxide poisoning and isocapneic nitrogen hypoxia. J Trauma 1986;26: 110–117.
67. Hampson NB, Kramer CC, Dunford RG, et al: Carbon monoxide poisoning from indoor burning of charcoal briquets. JAMA 1994;271:52–53.
68. Hampson NB, Norkool DM: Carbon monoxide poisoning in children riding in the back of pickup trucks. JAMA 1992;267:538–540.
69. Hart GB, Strauss MB, Lennon PA, et al: Treatment of smoke inhalation by hyperbaric oxygen. J Emerg Med 1985;3:211–215.
70. Heckerling PS: Occult carbon monoxide poisoning: A cause of winter headache. Am J Emerg Med 1987;5: 201–204.
71. Heckerling PS, Leiken JB, Maturen A, et al: Screening hospital admissions from the emergency department for occult carbon monoxide poisoning. Am J Emerg Med 1990;8:301–304.
72. Heckerling PS, Leikin JB, Maturen A: Occult carbon monoxide poisoning: Validation of a prediction model. Am J Med 1988;84:251–256.
73. Heckerling PS, Leiken JB, Maturen A, et al: Predictors of occult carbon monoxide poisoning in patients with headache and dizziness. Ann Intern Med 1987;107: 174–176.
74. Hedberg K, Hedberg CW, Iber C, et al: An outbreak of nitrogen dioxide-induced respiratory illness among ice hockey players. JAMA 1990;263:3024–3025.
75. Hill EP, Hill JR, Power GG, et al: Carbon monoxide exchanges between the human fetus and mother: A mathematical model. Am J Physiol 1977;232:H311–H323.
76. Hollander DI, Nagey DA, Welch R, et al: Hyperbaric oxygen therapy for the treatment of acute carbon monoxide poisoning in pregnancy: A case report. J Reprod Med 1987;32:615–617.

77. Hopkinson JM, Pearce PJ, Oliver JS: Carbon monoxide poisoning mimicking gastroenteritis. Br Med J 1980;281: 214–215.
78. Horowitz AL, Kaplan R, Sarpel G: Carbon monoxide toxicity: MR imaging in the brain. Radiology 1987;162: 787–788.
79. Howse AJ, Seddon H: Ischaemic contracture of muscle associated with carbon monoxide and barbiturate poisoning. Br Med J 1966;1:192–195.
80. Ikeda T, Kondo T, Mogami H, et al: Computerized tomography in cases of acute carbon monoxide poisoning. Med J Osaka Univ 1978;29:253–262.
81. Ilano AL, Raffine TA: Management of carbon monoxide poisoning. Chest 1990;97:165–169.
82. Jackson WR: Hyperbaric oxygenation effects on the cognitive function of memory. Undersea Biomed Res 1992; 19(suppl):62. Abstract.
83. Johnson EJ, Moran JC, Paine SC, et al: Abatement of toxic levels of CO in Seattle skating rinks. Am J Public Health 1975;65:1087–1090.
84. Jones JS, Lagasse J, Zimmerman G: Computed tomographic findings after acute carbon monoxide poisoning. Am J Emerg Med 1994;12:448–451.
85. Kanaya N, Imaizumi H, Nakayama M, et al: The utility of MRI in acute stage of carbon monoxide poisoning. Intensive Care Med 1992;18:371–372.
86. Kelley JS, Sophocleus GJ: Retinal hemorrhages in subacute carbon monoxide poisoning: Exposure in homes with blocked furnace flues. JAMA 1978;239:1515–1517.
87. Kim KS, Weinberg PE, Suh JH, et al: Acute carbon monoxide poisoning: Computed tomography of the brain. Am J Neuroradiol 1980;1:399–402.
88. Kindwall EP: Carbon monoxide poisoning treated with hyperbaric oxygen. Respir Ther 1975;5:29–33.
89. Koren G, Sharav T, Pastuszak A, et al: A multicenter, prospective study of fetal outcome following accidental carbon monoxide poisoning in pregnancy. Reprod Toxicol 1991;5:397–403.
90. Krantz T, Thisted B, Strom J, et al: Acute carbon monoxide poisoning. Acta Anaesthesiol Scand 1988;32:278–282.
91. Kurt TL, Anderson RJ, Weed WG: Rapid estimation of carboxyhemoglobin by breath sampling in an emergency setting. Vet Hum Toxicol 1990;32:227–229.
92. Lacey DJ: Neurologic sequelae of acute carbon monoxide poisoning. Am J Dis Child 1981;135:145–147.
93. Langehennig PL, Seeler RA, Berman E: Paint removers and carboxyhemoglobin. N Engl J Med 1976;295:1137.
94. Lapresle J, Fardeau M: The central nervous system and carbon monoxide: II. Anatomical study of brain lesions following intoxication with carbon monoxide (22 cases). Prog Brain Res 1976;24:31–74.
95. Larcan A, Lambert H: Current epidemiological, clinicobiological and therapeutic aspects of acute carbon monoxide poisoning. Bull Acad Natl Med 1981;165:471–478.
96. Larkin JM, Brahos GJ, Moylan JA: Treatment of carbon monoxide poisoning: Prognostic factors. J Trauma 1976;16: 111–114.
97. Laties V: Carbon monoxide and behavior. Arch Neurol 1980;167:68–72.
98. Laties V, Merigan WH: Behavioral effects of carbon monoxide on animals and man. Ann Rev Pharmacol Toxicol 1979;19:357–392.
99. Leavell UW, Farley CH, McIntyre JS: Cutaneous changes in a patient with CO poisoning. Arch Dermatol 1969;99: 429–433.
100. Lee MS, Marsden CD: Neurological sequelae following carbon monoxide poisoning: Clinical course and outcome according to the clinical types and brain computed tomography scan findings. Mov Disord 1996;9:550–558.
101. Leiken JB, Kaufman D, Lipscomb JW, et al: Methylene chloride report of 5 exposures and 2 deaths. Am J Emerg Med 1990;8:534–537.
102. Longo LD: The biologic effects of carbon monoxide on the pregnant woman, fetus and newborn infant. Am J Obstet Gynecol 1977;129:69–103.
103. Longo LD, Hill EP: Carbon monoxide uptake and elimination in fetal and maternal sheep. Am J Physiol 1977; 232:H324–H330.
104. Lowe-Ponsford FL, Henry JA: Clinical aspects of carbon monoxide poisoning. Adv Drug React Acute Poisoning Rev 1989;8:217–240.
105. Marius-Nunex AL: Myocardial infarction with normal coronary arteries after acute exposure to carbon monoxide. Chest 1990;97:491–494.
106. Martland HS, Martland HSJ: Placental barrier in carbon monoxide, barbiturate, and radium poisoning. Am J Surg 1950;80:270–279.
107. Mathieu D, Nolf M, Durocher A, et al: Acute carbon monoxide poisoning: Risk of late sequelae and treatment by hyperbaric oxygen. J Toxicol Clin Toxicol 1985;23: 315–324.
108. McBay AJ: Carbon monoxide poisoning. N Engl J Med 1965;272:252–253.
109. McFaul SJ, McGrath J: Studies on the mechanism of carbon monoxide-induced vasodilation in the isolated perfused rat heart. Toxicol Appl Pharmacol 1987;87:464–473.
110. Messier LD, Myers RAM: A neuropsychological screening battery for emergency assessment of carbon monoxide poisoned patients. J Clin Psychol 1991;47:675–684.
111. Miller PD, Telford ID, Haas GR: Effect of hyperbaric oxygen on cardiogenesis in the rat. Biol Neonate 1971;17: 44–52.
112. Min SK: A brain syndrome associated with delayed neuropsychiatric sequelae following acute carbon monoxide intoxication. Acta Psychiatr Scand 1986;73:80–86.
113. Miura T, Mitomo M, Kawai R, et al: CT of the brain in acute carbon monoxide intoxication: Characteristic features and prognosis. Am J Neuroradiol 1985;6:739–742.
114. Molzhaninov EV, Chaika VK, Domanova AI, et al: In: 1. Experience and prospects of using hyperbaric oxygenation in obstetrics. Anonymous Proceedings of the Seventh International Congress on Hyperbaric Medicine, Moscow, 1981. Moscow, Nauka, 1983, pp. 139–141.
115. Myers RAM: Carbon monoxide poisoning. J Emerg Med 1984;1:245–248.
116. Myers RAM, Britten JS: Are arterial blood gases of value in treatment decisions for carbon monoxide poisoning? Crit Care Med 1989;17:139–142.

117. Myers RAM, Goldman B: Planning an effective strategy for carbon monoxide poisoning. Emerg Med Rep 1987; 8:193–200.
118. Myers RAM, Jones DW, Britten JS: Carbon monoxide half life. Proceedings of the VIII International Congress on Hyperbaric Medicine, Long Beach, CA, 1987, p. 263. Abstract.
119. Myers RAM, Mitchell JT, Cowley RA: Psychometric testing and carbon monoxide poisoning. Disaster Med 1983;1: 279–281.
120. Myers RAM, Snyder SK, Emhoff TA: Subacute sequelae of carbon monoxide poisoning. Ann Emerg Med 1985;14: 1163–1167.
121. Myers RAM, Snyder SK, Linberg S, et al: Value of hyperbaric oxygen in suspected carbon monoxide poisoning. JAMA 1981;246:2478–2480.
122. Myers RAM, Snyder SK, Majerus TC: Cutaneous blisters and CO poisoning. Ann Emerg Med 1985;14:603–606.
123. Nardizzi LR: Computerized tomographic correlate of carbon monoxide poisoning. Arch Neurol 1979;36:38–39.
124. Neufeld MY, Swanson JW, Klass DW: Localized EEG abnormalities in acute carbon monoxide poisoning. Arch Neurol 1981;38:524–527.
125. Norkool DM, Kirkpatrick JN: Treatment of acute carbon monoxide poisoning with hyperbaric oxygen: A review of 115 cases. Ann Emerg Med 1985;14:1168–1171.
126. Okeda R, Funata N, Takano T, et al: Comparative study on pathogenesis of selective cerebral lesions in carbon monoxide poisoning and nitrogen hypoxia in cats. Acta Neuropathol 1982;56:265–272.
127. Okeda R, Funata N, Takano T, et al: The pathogenesis of carbon monoxide encephalopathy in the acute phase—Physiological and morphological conditions. Acta Neuropathol 1981;54:1–10.
128. Olson KR: Carbon monoxide poisoning: Mechanisms, presentation, and controversies in management. J Emerg Med 1984;1:233–243.
129. Otten EJ, Rosenberg J, Tasset JT: An evaluation of carboxyhemoglobin spot tests. Ann Emerg Med 1985;14:850–852.
130. Pace N, Stajman E, Walker EL: Acceleration of carbon monoxide elimination in man by high pressure oxygen. Science 1950;111:652–654.
131. Penney DG: Acute carbon monoxide poisoning in an animal model: The effects of altered glucose on morbidity and mortality. Toxicology 1993;80:85–101.
132. Penney DG, Helfman CC, Dunbar JC, et al: Acute severe carbon monoxide exposure in the rat: Effects of hyperglycemia and hypoglycemia on mortality, recovery, and neurological deficit. Can J Physiol 1991;69:1168–1177.
133. Penney DG, Helfman CC, Hull JA, et al: Elevated blood glucose is associated with poor outcome in the carbon-monoxide-poisoned rat. Toxicol Lett 1990;54:287–298.
134. Penney DG, Sharma P, Sutariya BB, et al: Development of hypoglycemia is associated with death during carbon monoxide poisoning. J Crit Care 1990;5:169–179.
135. Peterson JE, Stewart RD: Absorption and elimination of carbon monoxide by inactive young men. Arch Environ Health 1970;21:165–171.
136. Piatt JP, Kaplan AM, Bond GR, et al: Occult carbon monoxide poisoning in an infant. Pediatr Emerg Care 1990;6:21–23.
137. Pracyk JB, Stolp BW, Fife CE, et al: Brain computerized tomography after hyperbaric oxygen therapy for carbon monoxide poisoning. Undersea Hyperb Med 1995;22:1–7.
138. Pulsinelli WA, Levy DE, Sigsbee B, et al: Increased damage after ischemic stroke in patients with hyperglycemia with or without established diabetes mellitus. Am J Med 1983;74:540–544.
139. Pulsinelli WA, Waldman S, Rawlinson D, et al: Moderate hyperglycemia augments ischemic brain damage: A neuropathologic study in the rat. Neurology 1982;32: 1239–1246.
140. Raphael JC, Elkharrat D, Jars-Guincestre MC, et al: Trial of normobaric and hyperbaric oxygen for acute carbon monoxide intoxication. Lancet 1989;2:414–419.
141. Ratney RS, Wegman DH, Elkins HB: In vivo conversion of methylene chloride to carbon monoxide. Arch Environ Health 1974;28:223–236.
142. Raybourn MS, Cork C, Schimmerling W, et al: An in vitro electrophysiological assessment of the direct cellular toxicity of carbon monoxide. Toxicol Appl Pharmacol 1978; 46:769–779.
143. Rioux JP, Myers RAM: Hyperbaric oxygen for methylene chloride poisoning: Report on two cases. Ann Emerg Med 1989;18:691–695.
144. Riser D, Bonsch A, Schneider B: Should coroners be able to recognize unintentional carbon-monoxide related deaths immediately at the death scene? J Forensic Sci 1995;40: 596–598.
145. Rottman SJ: Carbon monoxide screening in the ED. Am J Emerg Med 1991;9:204–205.
146. Roughton FJW, Darling RC: The effect of carbon monoxide on the hemoglobin dissociation curve. Am J Physiol 1944;141:17–31.
147. Sasaki T: One-half clearance time of carbon monoxide hemoglobin in blood during hyperbaric oxygen therapy. Bull Tokyo Med Dent Univ 1975;22:63–77.
148. Schaplowsky AF, Oglesbay FB, Morrison JH, et al: Carbon monoxide contamination of the living environment: A national survey of home air and children's blood. J Environ Health 1974;36:569–573.
149. Scharf SM, Thames MD, Sasrgent RK: Transmural myocardial infarction after exposure to carbon monoxide in coronary-artery disease. N Engl J Med 1974;291:85–86.
150. Shapiro AB, Maturen A, Herman G, et al: Carbon monoxide and myonecreosis: A prospective study. Vet Hum Toxicol 1989;31:136–137.
151. Sheps DS, Herbst MC, Hinderliter AL, et al: Production of arrhythmias by elevated carboxyhemoglobin in patients with coronary artery disease. Ann Intern Med 1990;113: 343–351.
152. Shimazeu T, Ikeuchi H, Hubbard GB, et al: Smoke inhalation injury and the effect of carbon monoxide in the sheep model. J Trauma 1990;30:170–175.
153. Shusterman D, Alexeeff G, Hargis C, et al: Predictors of carbon monoxide and hydrogen cyanide exposure in smoke inhalation patients. J Toxicol Clin Toxicol 1996;34: 61–71.
154. Shusterman D, Quinlan P, Lowengart R, et al: Methylene chloride intoxication in a furniture refinisher. J Occup Med 1990;32:451–454.

155. Silver DA, Cross M, Fox B, Paxton RM: Computed tomography of the brain in acute carbon monoxide poisoning. Clin Radiol 1996;51:480–483.
156. Silvers SM, Hampson NB: Carbon monoxide poisoning among recreational boaters. JAMA 1995;274:1614–1616.
157. Sloan EP, Murphy DG, Hart R, et al: Complications and protocol considerations in carbon monoxide-poisoned patients who require hyperbaric oxygen therapy: Report from a ten-year experience. Ann Emerg Med 1989;18: 629–634.
158. Smith GI, Sharp GR: Treatment of carbon monoxide poisoning with oxygen under pressure. Lancet 1960;2:905–906.
159. Smith JS, Brandon S: Morbidity from acute carbon monoxide poisoning at 3 years follow-up. Br Med J 1973;1: 318–321.
160. Sokal JA, Kralkowska E: The relationship between exposure duration, carboxyhemoglobin, blood glucose, pyruvate and lactate and the severity of intoxication in 39 cases of acute carbon monoxide poisoning in man. Arch Toxicol 1985;57:196–199.
161. Sone S, Higashihara T, Kotake T, et al: Pulmonary manifestations in acute carbon monoxide poisoning. Am J Roentgenol Radium Ther Nucl Med 1974;120:865–871.
162. Sterling TD, Sterling E: Carbon monoxide levels in kitchens and homes with gas cookers. J Air Poll Control Assoc 1979;29:238–241.
163. Stewart R, Baretta ED, Platte LR, et al: Carboxyhemoglobin levels in American blood donors. JAMA 1974;229: 1187–1195.
164. Stewart RD: Paint remover hazard. JAMA 1976;235: 398–401.
165. Stewart RD, Peterson JE, Baretta ED, et al: Experimental human exposure to carbon monoxide. Arch Environ Health 1970;21:154–164.
166. Thom SR: Functional inhibition of leukocyte B2 integrins by hyperbaric oxygen in carbon monoxide-mediated brain injury in rats. Toxicol Appl Pharmacol 1993;123:248–256.
167. Thom SR: Leukocytes in carbon monoxide-mediated brain oxidative injury. Toxicol Appl Pharmacol 1993;123: 234–247.
168. Thom SR: Dehydrogenase conversion to oxidase and lipid peroxidation in brain after carbon monoxide poisoning. J Appl Physiol 1992;73:1584–1589.
169. Thom SR: Carbon monoxide-mediated brain lipid peroxidation in the rat. J Appl Physiol 1990;68:997–1003.
170. Thom SR: Antagonism of carbon monoxide-mediated brain lipid peroxidation by hyperbaric oxygen. Toxicol Appl Pharmacol 1990;105:340–344.
171. Thom SR, Keim LW: Carbon monoxide poisoning: A review of epidemiology, pathophysiology, clinical findings, and treatment options including hyperbaric oxygen therapy. J Toxicol Clin Toxicol 1989;27:141–156.
172. Thom SR, Ohnishi ST, Ischiropoulos H: Nitric oxide release by platelets inhibits neutrophil B2 integrin function following acute carbon monoxide poisoning. Toxicol Appl Pharmacol 1994;128:105–110.
173. Thom SR, Taber RL, Mendiguren I, et al: Delayed neuropsychological sequelae after carbon monoxide (CO) poisoning: Prevention by treatment with hyperbaric oxygen. Ann Emerg Med 1995;25:474–480.
174. Thomas MF, Penney DG: Hematologic responses to carbon monoxide and altitude: a comparative study. J Appl Physiol 1977;43:365.
175. Thompson N, Henry JA: Carbon monoxide poisoning: Poisons unit experience over five years. Hum Toxicol 1983;2:335–338.
176. Tom T, Abedon S, Clark RI, Wong W: Neuroimaging characteristics in carbon monoxide toxicity. J Neuroimaging 1996;6:161–166.
177. Tomaszewski C, Rosenberg N, Wathen J, et al: Prevention of neurological sequelae from carbon monoxide by hyperbaric oxygen in rats. Neurology 1992;42(suppl 3):196. Abstract.
178. Touger M, Gallagher EJ, Tyrell J: Relationship between venous and arterial carboxyhemoglobin levels in patients with suspected carbon monoxide poisoning. Ann Emerg Med 1995;25:481–483.
179. Treitman RD, Burgess WA, Gold A: Air contaminants encountered by firefighters. Am Ind Hyg Assoc J 1980; 41:796–802.
180. Turnbull TL, Hart RG, Strange GR, et al: Emergency department screening for unsuspected carbon monoxide exposure. Ann Emerg Med 1988;17:478–483.
181. Utz J, Ullrich V: Carbon monoxide relaxes ileal smooth muscle through activation of guanylate cyclase. Biochem Pharmacol 1991;41:1195–1201.
182. Van Hoesen KB, Camporesi EM, Moon RE, et al: Should hyperbaric oxygen be used to treat the pregnant patient for acute carbon monoxide poisoning? A case report and literature review. JAMA 1989;261:1039–1043.
183. Verma A, Hirsch DJ, Glatt CE, et al: Carbon monoxide: A putative neural messenger. Science 1993;259:381–384.
184. Wasowaski J, Myslack Z, Graczyk M, et al: An attempt at comparing the results of carboxyhemoglobin level in blood and gasometric determination in capillary blood in cases of carbon monoxide poisoning when treatment began at the place of accident. Anaesth Resusc Intensive Ther 1976;4:245–249.
185. Wharton M, Bistowish JM, Hutcheson RH, et al: Fatal carbon monoxide poisoning at a motel. JAMA 1989;261: 1177–1178.
186. Wheeler MG, Rozycki AA, Smith RP: Recreational propane inhalation in an adolescent male. J Toxicol Clin Toxicol 1992;30:135–139.
187. Winter PM, Miller JN: Carbon monoxide poisoning. JAMA 1976;236:1502.
188. Wright GR, Shephard RJ: Physiological effects of carbon monoxide. Int Rev Physiol 1979;20:311–368.
189. Yee LM, Brandon GK: Successful reversal of presumed carbon monoxide-induced semicoma. Aviat Space Environ Med 1983;54:641–643.
190. Zeiss J, Brinker R: Role of contrast enhancement in cerebral CT of carbon monoxide poisoning. J Comput Assist Tomogr 1988;12:341–343.
191. Zhang J, Piantadosi CA: Mitochondrial oxidative stress after carbon monoxide hypoxia in the rat brain. J Clin Invest 1992;90:1193–1199.
192. Ziser A, Shupak A, Halpern P, et al: Delayed hyperbaric oxygen treatment for acute carbon monoxide poisoning. Br Med J 1984;289:960.

ANTIDOTES IN DEPTH

Hyperbaric Oxygen

Stephen R. Thom

Hyperbaric oxygen therapy (HBO) is a treatment modality involving inhalation of oxygen at a pressure greater than 1 atmosphere absolute (ATA). The clinical entities that can be effectively treated with HBO are defined by the Undersea and Hyperbaric Medical Society[39] and updated approximately every 3 years. Hyperbaric oxygen has a number of mechanisms of action that are based on elevation of both hydrostatic pressure and oxygen partial pressure. Elevation of hydrostatic pressure causes a reduction in volume of gas according to Boyle's law. This action has direct relevance to pathologic conditions where gas bubbles are present in the body, such as arterial gas embolism and decompression sickness. Hyperoxygenation precipitates a number of biochemical and physiologic effects.[45] Elevations of oxygen partial pressure in tissues is directly dependent on the delivery of blood. Because hemoglobin is virtually saturated with oxygen on passage through the pulmonary microvasculature under normal environmental conditions, the primary effect of HBO is to increase oxygen content of plasma. Application of each atmosphere of oxygen partial pressure increases dissolved oxygen concentration in the plasma by 2.2 mL O_2/dL (vol%) (see Chap. 20).

In toxicology, hyperbaric oxygen is most commonly used for treatment of carbon monoxide (CO) poisoning. There is also scientific evidence to consider its use when managing life-threatening poisonings with cyanide (CN), hydrogen sulfide (H_2S), or carbon tetrachloride (CCl_4). Hyperbaric oxygen has been used experimentally for diverse additional poisonings, and this literature has been reviewed elsewhere.[84] Hyperbaric oxygen treatment can be delivered in either a mono- or multiplace hyperbaric chamber. Monoplace chambers, which accommodate only a single patient, are pressurized with pure oxygen. Larger walk-in, or multiplace, chambers accommodate two or more patients as well as support staff for hands-on patient care. These chambers are pressurized with air while patients breathe pure oxygen via mask, head tent, or endotracheal tube. Recent technological advances have allowed fabrication of portable "chambers" made of synthetic textile materials that can be inflated to a pressure of 2 ATA. Their principal use to date has been for emergency treatment of high-altitude sickness, although they have been investigated for use as an emergency monoplace chamber in wilderness situations.[43,46,79]

Injuries from CO occur primarily in the cardiovascular and central nervous systems. Traditionally, these injuries have been viewed as occurring due to the hypoxic stress mediated by an elevated carboxyhemoglobin (COHb) level. Data derived from human and animal studies indicate that major cardiac injury may indeed be due primarily to CO-induced hypoxic stress.[2,27,34] However, the predominant morbidity associated with CO poisoning occurs in the CNS, and the mechanism of CO-mediated brain injury is incompletely understood. Hypoxia per se does not adequately explain the development of neurologic injuries, which have not been found to be correlated with elevated COHb levels.[19,32,61,83,93]

Use of supplemental oxygen is a cornerstone to the treatment of CO poisoning. The hypoxic stress mediated by COHb and use of supplemental oxygen have been recognized for more than 100 years.[6,52] The rate of COHb dissociation is proportional to the arterial oxygen partial pressure, and HBO can provide a physiologic benefit by hastening dissociation of CO from hemoglobin.[29,64] Approximately 10–15% of the total amount of CO taken up by the body is bound to extravascular heme-containing proteins.[22] Included among these proteins are myoglobin, reduced cytochromes, soluble guanylate cyclase, and nitric oxide synthase.[12,18,23,92] The pathophysiologic impact of binding to these proteins has not been clearly defined. There is evidence in animals that despite a relatively low affinity for cytochrome aa_3, CO can bind in vivo during severe poisoning and compromise oxidative metabolism.[11] Hyperbaric oxygen has been shown to markedly accelerate CO dissociation from cytochrome oxidase in this model.[11] Improved survival with HBO treatment versus ambient pressure O_2 in another animal model has been ascribed to both COHb dissociation and cellular effects, possibly related to mitochondrial function.[65]

Morphologic features of CO-mediated brain injuries are most often localized to cerebral white matter, globus pallidus, and hippocampus.[33] Carbon monoxide appears to disturb the blood–brain barrier, and demyelination occurs in a perivascular distribution.[26,58,67] Clinical pathologic examiners have stressed the extent of the perivascular injury in brain, and more recent imaging studies have detected blood flow abnormalities in symptomatic patients.[28,49,55,71] Acute vascular and perivascular changes are also found in several animal models of CO poisoning.[31,40] Vascular changes triggered by CO precipitate leukocyte sequestration and a cascade of biochemical events that result in global oxidative injury.[40] In this model, HBO prevented brain injury by inhibiting leukocyte sequestration.[81] Hyperbaric oxygen has been found to mediate the same effect in human neutrophils, with the maximum benefit occurring after exposure to 2.8 ATA O_2.[82]

Based on the foregoing discussion, there are at least three possible mechanisms of therapeutic action for HBO in CO poisoning: enhanced dissociation of CO from hemoglobin, enhanced dissociation of CO from cytochrome oxidase, and temporary inhibition of leukocyte β_2 integrin adhesion molecules to blunt the cascade of vascular injury. To date, at least nine clinical studies have been published in the peer-reviewed literature that have examined the effect of HBO in CO poisoning.[28,35,36,47,57,58,61,62,68,83] They all conclude with a recommendation for using HBO in at least some clinical settings. Among these reports, three are prospective, randomized trials.[28,68,83] The first suggested that HBO should be used in patients who have suffered an interval of unconsciousness, an aspect of the clinical history that is considered to be evidence of serious poisoning.[68] However, much of the data in this study do not demonstrate clinical efficacy of HBO. Difficulties with the methodology used prevent substantiation of many of the conclusions.[10] The second reported that HBO reduced the time to initial recovery and the incidence of delayed neurologic sequelae among 13 patients who were compared with 13 patients treated with ambient pressure O_2.[28] The patients in this study had a mean COHb level of 23% and the majority had suffered an interval of unconsciousness. Another recent study examined the incidence of delayed neurologic sequelae between patients treated with ambient pressure O_2 and HBO.[83] Twenty-three percent (7 of 30 patients) treated with ambient pressure O_2 developed neurologic sequelae, whereas none of 30 (0%, $p < 0.05$) treated with HBO developed sequelae. It is important to note that this study was performed on patients who were considered to have suffered only mild or moderately severe poisoning, as none had lost consciousness. This raises what is probably the most pressing problem associated with the clinical management of CO poisoned patients: an absence of reliable methods for prospectively estimating the severity of CO poisoning. This problem and what methods to use to evaluate patient outcome are important issues to be considered in both day-to-day practice and future clinical investigations.

Clinical indications for HBO in CO poisoning are reviewed in Chapter 96. Important caveats regarding HBO include the observation that treatment efficacy may diminish severely if treatment is delayed for more than 6 hours after poisoning.[36] There also is discussion in the literature that patient outcome may be improved if more than a single treatment is administered.[35]

Carbon monoxide (CO) and cyanide (CN) poisonings can occur together in victims of smoke inhalation,[3,4,20] and experimental evidence suggests that these agents can produce synergistic toxicity.[60,63,66] Toxicity from CN stems from binding to cytochrome aa_3 and inhibiting oxidative phosphorylation.[88] Animal studies demonstrate that ambient pressure 100% O_2 can enhance protection from CN toxicity[72] and also enhance CN metabolism to thiocyanate when thiosulfate is used concomitantly.[8] Hyperbaric oxygen may have direct effects in reducing CN toxicity[25,41,42,73,80] or augmenting antidote treatments.[17,72,90] However, not all animal studies have found HBO to improve outcome,[89] and clinical experience regarding CN treatment with HBO is sparce. In a series of smoke-inhalation victims with both toxic CO and CN levels who received both HBO and treatment for CN involving sodium nitrite and thiosulfate, 4 of 5 patients survived without apparent neurologic damage.[37] The results with HBO in clinical cases of isolated CN poisonings refractory to standard antidote treatment (nitrite plus thiosulfate) have been equivocal. One case showed dramatic improvement,[85] whereas another was without any response.[53] Further research in this area is necessary. Because cyanide is among the most lethal poisons, and intoxication is rapid, standard antidotal therapy for isolated CN poisoning is of primary importance. Hyperbaric oxygen may be an adjunct to be considered in refractory cases.

Methylene chloride (CH_2Cl_2) is an organic solvent used commercially as a paint stripper. It is readily absorbed through the skin or by inhalation and metabolized by the mixed function oxidase system to yield CO.[77] This process is slow and although peak COHb levels may not be reached for 8 hours or more, they can be substantial (10–50%).[30,44,48,77] Methylene chloride toxicity can have many of the same acute manifestations as CO poisoning.[75] Acute signs and symptoms are attributable to the direct effects of this solvent on the central nervous system and to concomitant hypoxia. Effects that are present after 1 hour or more, especially if the COHb level is elevated, may be partially due to CO toxicity. Treatment with HBO in this setting has been reported.[38,70]

Hydrogen sulfide (H_2S) binds to cytochrome aa_3 and impairs oxidative phosphorylation. Hence, its mechanism of toxicity is similar to that of CN, although it is more readily dissociated from cytochrome oxidase by O_2.[78] Clinical manifestations of toxicity are similar to those with CO and CN.[78] Management of patients with serious H_2S poisoning principally involves oxygenation and cardiovascular support, as well as consideration of sodium nitrite. In animals, HBO may be more effective than nitrite in preventing mortality.[7] There are several instances where HBO has appeared to be beneficial.[16,75,91] Relatively late treatment with HBO, 10 or more hours after poisoning, has also been reported beneficial in some,[87] but not all cases.[1] There are no definitive data regarding use of HBO in H_2S poisoning, but it should be considered in refractory cases.

Carbon tetrachloride (CCl_4) hepatotoxicity may be diminished by HBO. Mortality has been decreased in a number of animal studies,[5,15,54,59,69] and there are several case reports of patients surviving potentially lethal ingestions with HBO therapy.[50,76,86,94] Hyperbaric oxygen inhibits the mixed-function oxidase system that is responsible for conversion of CCl_4 to hepatotoxic free radicals.[14,56] Trichloromethyl radicals ($\cdot CCl_3$) pose a greater risk for centrilobular necrosis than the oxidized peroxytrichloromethyl radical ($\cdot CCl_3OO$).[15] Conversion to $\cdot CCl_3OO$ is hastened by HBO, and $\cdot CCl_3OO$ is quickly detoxified by thiols such as glutathione.[13] Because there are no proven antidotes for CCl_4 poisoning, use of HBO should be considered with potentially severe CCl_4 exposures. However, there may be a delicate balance between oxidative processes that are therapeutic compared with those that mediate hepatotoxicity.[9] If HBO is considered, it is prudent to initiate treatments prior to onset of liver-function abnormalities.

When arranging for treatment with HBO, probably the first consideration must be the logistic requirements to transport a patient to a hyperbaric facility. One group examined this question in their review of 297 consecutive CO-poisoned patients and concluded that transfer need not be deferred because of a concern over cardiac or respiratory arrest, myocardial infarction, or deterioration in mental status if these events had not occurred prior to transfer.[74] The potential adverse effects of HBO per se are relatively rare, and they are usually mild and self-limited. However, relative risks must always be considered in any therapeutic setting. The most common complaint of patients undergoing HBO is otic barotrauma due to difficulty equalizing pressure in the middle ear space. This problem is usually minor, but effusion, hemorrhage, and/or rupture of the tympanic membrane can occur. Preexisting conditions that require some forethought and possible management prior to initiating HBO include claustrophobia, sinus congestion, and patients with scarred or noncompliant structures in the middle ear such as those with otosclerosis.[45] Central nervous system oxygen toxicity, manifested as a grand mal seizure, occurs with an incidence of less than 1 in 10,000 patients.[45] Although this can present an acute management challenge, there is no evidence that an oxygen-induced convulsion causes permanent parenchymal damage.[21] Oxygen exposures associated with HBO do not typically produce evidence of pulmonary O_2 toxicity, as the tolerance limits of the lung are not exceeded.[21] However, previous exposure to the chemotherapeutic agent bleomycin is considered a relatively strong contraindication to HBO. Bleomycin exacerbates pulmonary oxygen toxicity through an unknown mechanism, and although there are no reports of bleomycin patients having received HBO, there are reports of fulminant pulmonary injury following exposure to inspiratory oxygen concentration of more than 30%.[24,51] Therefore, on a case-by-case basis, careful consideration of this risk must be weighed against the potential benefits of HBO. The only well-recognized absolute contraindication for HBO therapy is an unvented pneumothorax, based on the obvious risk of exacerbating this condition while in the hyperbaric chamber and especially on decompression.

References

1. Al-Mahasneh QM, Cohle SD, Haas E: Lack of response to hyperbaric oxygen in a fatal case of hydrogen sulfide poisoning. Vet Hum Toxicol 1989;31:353. Abstract.
2. Anderson EW, Andelman RJ, Strauch JM: Effects of low-level carbon monoxide exposure on onset and duration of angina pectoris. Ann Intern Med 1973;79:46–50.
3. Barillo DJ, Goode R, Rush BF, et. al: Lack of correlation between carboxyhemoglobin and cyanide in smoke inhalation injury. Curr Surg 1986;46:421–423.
4. Baud FJ, Barriot P, Toffis V, et al: Elevated blood cyanide concentrations in victims of smoke inhalation. N Engl J Med 1991;325:1761–1766.
5. Bernacchi A, Myers R, Trump BF, Margello L: Protection of hepatocytes with hyperoxia against carbon tetrachloride induced injury. Toxicol Pathol 1984;12:315–323.
6. Bernard C: Le Cons Sur les Effects des Substances Toxiques et Medicamenteuses. Paris, J.B. Bailliere, 1857.
7. Bitterman N, Talmi Y, Lerman A: The effect of hyperbaric oxygen on acute experimental sulfide poisoning in the rat. Toxicol Appl Pharmacol 1986;84:325–328.
8. Breen PH, Isserles SA, Westley J, et. al: Effect of oxygen and sodium thiosulfate during combined carbon monoxide and cyanide poisoning. Toxicol Appl Pharmacol 1995;134: 229–234.
9. Brent JA, Rumack BH: Role of free radicals in toxic hepatic injury: I. Free radical biochemistry. J Toxicol Clin Toxicol 1993;31:173–196.
10. Brown SD, Piantadosi CA: Hyperbaric oxygen for carbon monoxide poisoning. Lancet 1989;1:1032–1033. Letter.
11. Brown SD, Piantadosi CA: Reversal of carbon monoxide-cytochrome C oxidase binding by hyperbaric oxygen in vivo. Adv Exp Biol Med 1989;248:747–754.
12. Brune B, Schmidt KU, Ullrich V: Activation of soluble guanylate cyclase by carbon monoxide and inhibition by superoxide anion. Eur J Biochem 1990;192:683–688.
13. Burk RF, Lane JM, Patel K: Relationship of oxygen and glutathione in protection against carbon tetrachloride-induced hepatic microsomal lipid peroxidation and covalent binding in the rat. J Clin Invest 1984;74:1996–2001.
14. Burk RF, Patel K, Lane JM: Reduced glutathione protection against rat liver microsomal injury by carbon tetrachloride. Biochem J 1983;215:441–445.
15. Burk RF, Reiter R, Land JM: Hyperbaric oxygen protection against carbon tetrachloride hepatotoxicity in the rat: Association with altered metabolism. Gastroenterology 1986;90: 812–818.
16. Burnett WW, King EG, Grace M: Hydrogen sulfide poisoning: Review of 5 years' experience. Can Med Assoc J 1977; 117:1277–1280.
17. Burrows GE, Way JL: Cyanide intoxication in sheep: Therapeutic value of oxygen or cobalt. Am J Vet Res 1977;38: 223–227.
18. Chance B, Erecinska M, Wagner M: Mitochondrial responses to carbon monoxide toxicity. Ann NY Acad Sci 1970;174:193–204.
19. Choi S: Delayed neurologic sequelae in carbon monoxide intoxication. Arch Neurol 1983;40:433–435.
20. Clark CJ, Campbell D, Reid WH: Blood carboxyhaemoglobin and cyanide levels in fire survivors. Lancet 1981;1: 1332–1335.
21. Clark JM,Thom SR: The toxicity of oxygen, carbon dioxide and carbon monoxide. In: Bove AA, Davis JC, eds: Bove and Davis' Diving Medicine. 3rd edition. Philadelphia, Saunders, 1997.
22. Coburn RF: The carbon monoxide body stores. Ann NY Acad Sci 1970;174:11–22.

23. Coburn RF, Mayers LB: Myoglobin O_2 tension determined from measurements of carboxymyoglobin in skeletal muscle. Am J Physiol 1971;220:66–74.
24. Comis RL: Bleomycin pulmonary toxicity: Current status and future directions. Semin Oncol 1992;19:64–70.
25. Cope C: The importance of oxygen in the treatment of cyanide poisoning. JAMA 1961;175:1061–1064.
26. Courville CB: The process of demyelination in the central nervous system. Demyelination as a delayed residual of carbon monoxide asphyxia. J Nerv Ment Dis 1957;125:504–546.
27. Cramlet SH, Erickson HH, Gorman HA: Ventricular function following acute carbon monoxide exposure. J Appl Physiol 1975;39:482–486.
28. Ducasse JL, Celsis P, Marc-Vergnes JP: Non-comatose patients with acute carbon monoxide poisoning: Hyperbaric or normobaric oxygenation? Undersea Hyperb Med 1995;22:9–15.
29. End E, Long CW: Oxygen under pressure in carbon monoxide poisoning. J Ind Hyg Toxicol 1942;24:302–306.
30. Fagin J, Bradley J, Williams D: Carbon monoxide poisoning secondary to inhaling methylene chloride. Br Med J 1980;281:1461.
31. Funata N, Okeda R, Takano T, et al: Electron microscopic observations of experimental carbon monoxide encephalopathy in the acute phase. Acta Pathol Jpn 1982;32:219–229.
32. Garland H, Pearce J: Neurological complications of carbon monoxide poisoning. Q J Med 1967;144:445–455.
33. Ginsberg MD: Carbon monoxide intoxication: Clinical features, neuropathology and mechanisms of injury. J Toxicol Clin Toxicol 1985;23:281–288.
34. Ginsberg MD, Myers RE: Experimental carbon monoxide encephalopathy in the primate. I. Physiologic and metabolic aspects. Arch Neurol 1974;30:202–208.
35. Gorman DF, Clayton D, Gilligan JE, Webb RK: A longitudinal study of 100 consecutive admissions for carbon monoxide poisoning to the Royal Adelaide Hospital. Anaesth Intensive Care 1992;20:311–316.
36. Goulon M, Barois A, Rapin M, et al: Carbon monoxide poisoning and acute anoxia due to breathing coal gas and hydrocarbons. Ann Med Interne 1969;120:335–349. (English translation in J Hyperb Med 1986;1:23–41.)
37. Hart GB, Strauss MB, Lennon PA, Whitcraft DD: Treatment of smoke inhalation by hyperbaric oxygen. J Emerg Med 1985;3:211–215.
38. Horowitz BZ: Carboxyhemoglobinemia caused by inhalation of methylene chloride. Am J Emerg Med 1986;4:48–51.
39. Hyperbaric Oxygen Therapy: A Committee Report. Undersea and Hyperbaric Medical Society, Bethesda, MD, 1996, pp. 1–73.
40. Ischiropoulos H, Beers MF, Ohnishi ST, et al: Nitric oxide production and perivascular tyrosine nitration in brain after carbon monoxide poisoning in the rat. J Clin Invest 1996;97:2260–2267.
41. Isom GE, Way JL: Effect of oxygen on cyanide intoxication. VI. Reactivation of cyanide inhibited glucose metabolism. J Pharmacol Exp Ther 1974;189:235–243.
42. Ivanov KP: The effect of elevated oxygen pressure on animals poisoned with potassium cyanide. Pharmacol Toxicol 1959;22:476–479.
43. Jay GD, Tetz DJ, Hartigan LF, et al: Portable hyperbaric oxygen therapy in the emergency department with a modified Gamow bag. Ann Emerg Med 1995;26:707–711.
44. Kaufman D, Lipscomb JW, Leikin JB: Methylene chloride report of 5 exposures and 2 deaths. Vet Hum Toxicol 1989;31:352
45. Kindwall EP, ed: Hyperbaric Medicine Practice. Flagstaff, Arizona, Best Publishing Co, 1994.
46. King SJ, Greenbee RR: Successful use of the Gamow hyperbaric bag in the treatment of altitude illness at Mt. Everest. J Wilderness Med 1990;1:193–202.
47. Lamy M, Hauguet M: Fifty patients with carbon monoxide intoxication treated with hyperbaric oxygen therapy. Acta Anaesthesiol Belg 1969;1:49–53.
48. Langehennig PL, Seeler RA, Berman E: Paint removers and carboxyhemoglobin. N Engl J Med 1976;295:1137. Letter.
49. Lapresle J, Fardeau M: The central nervous system and carbon monoxide poisoning. Prog Brain Res 1967;24:31–74.
50. Larcan A, Lambert H: Current epidemiological, clinical, biological, and therapeutic aspects of acute carbon monoxide intoxication. Bull Acad Natl Med (Paris) 1981;165:471.
51. Lazo JS, Sebati SM, Schellens JH: Bleomycin. Canc Chemother Biol Respir Modifiers 1996;16:39–47.
52. Linas AJ, Limousin S: Asphyxie lente et graduelle par le charbon, traitment et guerison par les inspirations d'oxygène. Bull Mem Soc Ther 1868;2:32.
53. Litovitz TL, Larkin RF, Myers RAM: Cyanide poisoning treated with hyperbaric oxygen. Am J Emerg Med 1983;1:94–101.
54. Lowe-Ponsford FL, Henry JA: Clinical aspects of carbon monoxide poisoning. Adv Drug React Acute Poisoning Rev 1989;8:217–240.
55. Maeda Y, Kawasaki Y, Jibiki I, et al: Effect of therapy with oxygen under high pressure on regional cerebral blood flow in the interval form of carbon monoxide poisoning: Observation from subtraction of technetium–99m HMPAOSPECT brain imaging. Eur Neurol 1991;31:380–383.
56. Marzella L, Muhvich K, Myers RAM: Effect of hyperoxia on liver necrosis induced by hepatotoxins. Virchows Arch 1986;51:497–507.
57. Mathieu D, Nolf M, Durocher A, et al: Acute carbon monoxide poisoning risk of late sequelae and treatment by hyperbaric oxygen. J Toxicol Clin Toxicol 1985;23:315–324.
58. Meyer A: Experimentelle erfahrungen uber die kohlenoxydverguftung des zentralnervens systems. Z Gesamte Neurol Psychiatr 1928;112:187–212.
59. Montani S, Perret C: Oxygenation hyperbare dans l'intoxication experimentale au tetrachlorure de carbon. Rev Fr Etudes Clin Biol 1967;12:274–278.
60. Moore SJ, Norris JC, Walsh DA, Hume AS: Antidotal use of methemoglobin forming cyanide antagonists in concurrent carbon monoxide/cyanide intoxication. J Pharmacol Exp Ther 1987;242:70–73.
61. Myers RAM, Snyder SK, Emhoff TA: Subacute sequelae of carbon monoxide poisoning. Ann Emerg Med 1985;14:1163–1167.
62. Norkool DM, Kirkpatrick JN: Treatment of acute carbon monoxide poisoning with hyperbaric oxygen: A review of 115 cases. Ann Emerg Med 1985;14:1168–1171.
63. Norris JC, Moore SJ, Hume AS: Synergistic lethality in-

duced by the combination of carbon monoxide and cyanide. Toxicology 1986;40:121–129.

64. Pace N, Strajman E, Walker EL: Acceleration of carbon monoxide elimination in man by high pressure oxygen. Science 1950;111:652–654.
65. Pearce EC, Zacharias A, Alday JM Jr, et al: Carbon monoxide poisoning: Experimental hypothermic and hyperbaric studies. Surgery 1972;72:229–237.
66. Pitt, BR, Radford EP, Gurtner GH, Traystman RJ: Interaction of carbon monoxide and cyanide on cerebral circulation and metabolism. Arch Environ Health 1979;34:354–359.
67. Putnam TJ, McKenna JB, Morrison LR: Studies in multiple sclerosis. JAMA 1991;97:1591–1596.
68. Raphael JC, Elkharrat D, Guincestre MCJ, et al: Trial of normobaric and hyperbaric oxygen for acute carbon monoxide intoxication. Lancet 1989;2:414–419.
69. Rapin M, Got C, Le Gall JR: Effect de l'oxygene hyperbare sur la toxicite tetrachlorure de carbone chez le rat. Rev Fr Etudes Clin Biol 1967;12:594–599.
70. Rudge FW: Treatment of methylene chloride induced carbon monoxide poisoning with hyperbaric oxygen. Milit Med 1990;155:570–572.
71. Sesay M, Bidabe AM, Guyot M, et al: Regional cerebral blood flow measurements with xenon-CT in the prediction of delayed encephalopathy after carbon monoxide intoxication. Acta Neurol Scand 1996;166:22–27.
72. Sheehy M, Way JL: Effect of oxygen on cyanide intoxication: III. Mithridate. J Pharmacol Exp Ther 1968;161: 163–168.
73. Skene WG, Norman JN, Smith G: Effect of hyperbaric oxygen in cyanide poisoning. In: Brown IW, Cox B, eds: Proceedings of the Third International Congress on Hyperbaric Medicine. Washington, DC, National Academy of Sciences, National Research Council, 1966, pp. 705–710.
74. Sloan EP, Murphy DG, Hart R, et al: Complications and protocol considerations in carbon monoxide-poisoned patients who require hyperbaric oxygen therapy: Report from a ten-year experience. Ann Emerg Med 1989;18:629–634.
75. Smilkstein MJ, Bronstein AC, Pickett HM: Hyperbaric oxygen therapy for severe hydrogen sulfide poisoning. J Emerg Med 1985;3:27–30.
76. Stewart RD, Boettner EA, Southworth RR: Acute carbon tetrachloride intoxication. JAMA 1963;183:994–997.
77. Stewart RD, Hake CL: Paint remover hazard. JAMA 1976;235:398–401.
78. Stine RJ, Slosberg B, Beacham BE: Hydrogen sulfide intoxication. Ann Intern Med 1976;85:756–758.
79. Taber RL: Protocols for the use of a portable hyperbaric chamber for the treatment of high altitude disorders. J Wilderness Med 1990;1:181–192.
80. Takano T, Miyazaki Y, Nashimoto I, Kobayashi K: Effect of hyperbaric oxygen on cyanide intoxication: In situ changes in intracellular oxidation reduction. Undersea Biomed Res 1980;7:191–197.
81. Thom SR: Functional inhibition of leukocyte β_2 integrins by hyperbaric oxygen in carbon monoxide-mediated brain injury in rats. Toxicol Appl Pharmacol 1993;123:248–256.
82. Thom SR, Mendiguren I, Hardy KR, et al: Inhibition of human neutrophil β_2 integrin-dependent adherence by hyperbaric oxygen. Am J Physiol 1997;272:770–771.
83. Thom SR, Taber RL, Mendiguren II, et al: Delayed neuropsychologic sequelae after carbon monoxide poisoning: prevention by treatment with hyperbaric oxygen. Ann Emerg Med 1995;25:474–480.
84. Tomaszewski CA, Thom SR: Use of hyperbaric oxygen in toxicology. Emer Med Clin North Am 1994;12:437–459.
85. Trapp WG, Lepawsky M: 100% survival in five life-threatening acute cyanide poisoning victims treated by a therapeutic spectrum including hyperbaric oxygen. In: First European Conference on Hyperbaric Medicine, Amsterdam, 1983.
86. Truss CD, Killenberg PG: Treatment of carbon tetrachloride poisoning with hyperbaric oxygen. Gastroenterology 1982; 82:767–769.
87. Vicas I, Fortin S, Uptigrove OF: Hydrogen sulfide exposure treated with hyperbaric oxygen. Vet Hum Toxicol 1989;31: 353. Abstract.
88. Way JL: Cyanide intoxication and its mechanism of antagonism. Annu Rev Pharmacol Toxicol 1984;24:451–481.
89. Way JL, End E, Sheehy MH, et al: Effect of oxygen on cyanide intoxication. Toxicol Appl Pharmacol 1972;22: 415–421.
90. Way JL, Gibbon SL, Sheehy M: Effect of oxygen on cyanide intoxication. I. Prophylactic protection. J Pharmacol Exp Ther 1966;13:381–382.
91. Whitcraft DD, Bailey TD, Hart GB: Hydrogen sulfide poisoning treated with hyperbaric oxygen. J Emerg Med 1985;3:23–25.
92. White KA, Marletta MA: Nitric oxide synthase is a cytochrome P-450 type hemoprotein. Biochemistry 1992;31: 6627–6631.
93. Winter PM, Miller JN: Carbon monoxide poisoning. JAMA 1976;236:1502–1504.
94. Zearbaugh C, Gorman DF, Gilligan JE: Carbon tetrachloride/chloroform poisoning: case studies of hyperbaric oxygen in the treatment of lethal dose ingestion. Undersea Biomed Res 1988;15:44.

CHAPTER 97

Cyanide and Hydrogen Sulfide

William P. Kerns II and Mark A. Kirk

Cyanide	
MW:	26.02 D
Whole blood reference:	< 1 μg/mL
	38.5 μmol/L
Airborn	
Immediately fatal	270 ppm
Life threatening	110 ppm > 30 min
Hydrogen Sulfide	
MW:	34.08 D
Airborne concentrations:	
Odor threshold	0.02–0.13 ppm
Olfactory fatigue	100–150 ppm
Immediately fatal	700 ppm

Cyanide Toxicity

CASE 1. Co-workers discovered a 28-year-old graduate student unconscious in his biochemistry laboratory. They summoned paramedics who found a comatose, cyanotic male with no palpable blood pressure, faint pulse of 60 beats/min, and agonal respirations. Paramedics intubated him orotracheally and ventilated him with a bag-valve-mask using 100% oxygen. Following the establishment of intravenous access, the patient received 2 mg naloxone, 25 g dextrose, 100 mg thiamine, and 1 mg atropine IV without a change in his condition. A 500-mL bolus of 0.9% saline produced no change in blood pressure. Soon after, the patient's pulse was lost and CPR was begun. The paramedics noted a bottle of potassium cyanide nearby.

Cardiac pulmonary resuscitation was continued upon arrival in the emergency department. A focused physical examination revealed a well-developed, but comatose male without pulse or blood pressure. Cardiac monitoring revealed a wide complex with a rate of 20 beats/min. Skin examination showed no evidence of trauma, track marks, or burns. No unusual odors were detected. Pupils were 4 mm and nonreactive to light. He had clear breath sounds. Because of the history supplied by the paramedics, physicians administered the Lilly Cyanide Kit. They also gave 2 ampules of sodium bicarbonate (100 mEq) IV. Soon after, the patient developed a blood pressure of 70 mm Hg and a heart rate of 120 beats/min. Crystalloids and a dopamine infusion raised the systolic blood pressure to 96 mm Hg. Orogastric lavage was performed via a 40 Fr tube with return of clear fluid.

Arterial and venous blood was obtained upon arrival. The initial arterial pH was 7.12; PCO_2, 29 mm Hg; PO_2, 258 mm Hg. The measured oxygen saturation was 98%. Electrolyte values included: sodium 140 mEq/L; chloride 107 mEq/L; bicarbonate 9 mEq/L. Serum lactate was 15 mEq/L. The anion gap was 24 mEq/L. Following the cyanide antidote kit and bicarbonate therapy, the pH was 7.33; PCO_2, 29 mm Hg; PO_2, 280 mm Hg. A methemoglobin level was 7.5%. The patient's hemodynamic status stabilized and he regained consciousness over the next several hours. In the next 24 hours, he was extubated. He appeared neurologically normal. However, he was despondent and acknowledged ingesting potassium cyanide due to a social situation. A whole blood cyanide level was 5.5 μg/mL. He was transferred to an inpatient psychiatric facility for further care of his depression.

One month after discharge, he visited the campus physician complaining of tremors and stiffness. Physical examination revealed signs of parkinsonism including: masked facies, intention tremor, and cogwheel rigidity. He had no family history of parkinsonism and was taking no medications except fluoxetine, prescribed for his depression. He was referred to a neurologist, who confirmed the extrapyramidal findings. An MRI scan was performed, demonstrating abnormal signals in the basal ganglia, especially the globus pallidus. The parkinsonian symptoms were felt to be secondary to cyanide. The neurologist prescribed a dopamine agonist, which provided mild symptomatic relief.

How Are Persons Exposed to Cyanide?

The case example represents a common scenario of cyanide exposure: a dramatic and potentially successful suicide. According to American Association of Poison Control Center data for 1991 to 1996,[83–87] suicide accounted for 26 of 31 cyanide deaths. Suicides frequently involve chemists or technicians working in laboratories where cyanide salts are common reagents.[24,31,48,49,71,88,142,152] A dramatic mass suicide occurred at Jonestown, Guyana, in 1978, involving 900 followers of a religious fanatic.[52]

Fire is also a cyanide source. Aside from thermal injury and smoke inhalation, carbon monoxide was previously felt to be the primary toxin responsible for mortality from fires. However, the contribution of cyanide to mortality was recently recognized.[14,91,109,121] This is not surprising as the combustion of many materials including wool, silk, synthetic rubber, polyurethane, and nitrocellulose form cyanide. Elevated blood cyanide and thiocyanate levels were found in autopsy cases and prospective studies of fire victims. Cyanide is synergistic with carbon monoxide.[98,101] Hence, patients may be severely ill and have unimpressive blood levels of either toxin.

Many industrial processes utilize cyanide reagents, including electroplating, metal refining, photography, and fumigation. Despite potential hazard, deaths due to occupational exposures are rare. In 1988 workers mistakenly used hydrogen chloride to clean a vat containing zinc cyanide sludge. The resulting release of cyanide gas killed five workers.[89] A review of 5 years of occupational data from the Netherlands found only one death attributed to cyanide.[81]

Other rare exposures to cyanide may occur. Tampering of consumer products, especially over-the-counter medications, resulted in cyanide poisoning. Cyanide-laced acetaminophen caused seven deaths in Chicago in 1982. The tampering was engineered by an individual attempting to coverup a homicide of one of the victims.[28] In February 1991, three persons in Washington State were poisoned with an over-the-counter decongestant intentionally contaminated with cyanide. Physicians suspected cyanide in one case and successfully treated with the antidote kit.[67] Food tampering has also occurred. In 1988, contaminated yogurt resulted in severe toxicity.[94] The Department of Agriculture found traces of cyanide in fruit imported from Chile in 1989. A terrorist threat led to the inspection of the food and subsequent discovery of the cyanide.[58]

Ingestion of cyanogenic chemicals represents another source of exposure. Cyanogenic chemicals liberate cyanide during metabolism. Acetonitrile is a clinically relevant cyanogen. Acetonitrile is relatively nontoxic, but metabolism via cytochrome P450 forms a cyanohydrin that readily breaks down to an aldehyde and cyanide. Unintentional poisoning with acetonitrile-based artificial-nail remover by children was first reported in 1988.[37,53,80,90] As expected, the clinical manifestations of acetonitrile poisoning are similar to those of inorganic cyanide poisoning. However, symptoms appeared in a delayed fashion, range 3–24 hours, due to metabolism from parent compound to toxic metabolite (Fig. 97–1). Delayed manifestations provide the opportunity for early diagnosis, observation, and administration of antidote. In contrast, lack of initial symptoms, coupled with the lack of knowledge of nitriles, may lead to misdiagnosis and result in an unfavorable outcome.[37] Adults ingesting acetonitrile also develop signs and symptoms several hours after exposure.[73,96,138] Other nitriles, such as proprionitrile, caused cyanide symptoms from occupational exposure.[23]

Many plants contain cyanogenic compounds including the *Prunus* species, the pitted fruits—apricots, bitter almond, cherry, and peaches. Pits contain amygdalin, D-mandelonitrile-ß-*d*-glucoside, that by itself has little toxicity. Intravenous laetrile, the amygdalin-containing, purported antineoplastic agent, does not cause cyanide toxicity. However, when laetrile is ingested, intestinal β-*d*-glucosidase biotransforms amygdalin to glucose, aldehyde, and cyanide, with resultant cyanide toxicity (see Fig. 97–1).[60,62] Cassava (*Manihot*) is another cyanogenic glycoside-containing plant. Two cyanogens, linamarin and lotaustralin, are found in the tuber. After harvesting, enzymes catalyze the breakdown into glucose, acetone, and cyanide. While of little consequence in the United States, cassava is a staple, inexpensive food source in developing countries. Proper fermentation techniques are described that remove the cyanide. Unfortunately, economic pressures to export higher quality plants result in a relative shortage of cassava and less meticulous attention to proper detoxification that results in cyanide poisoning.[3,7,30]

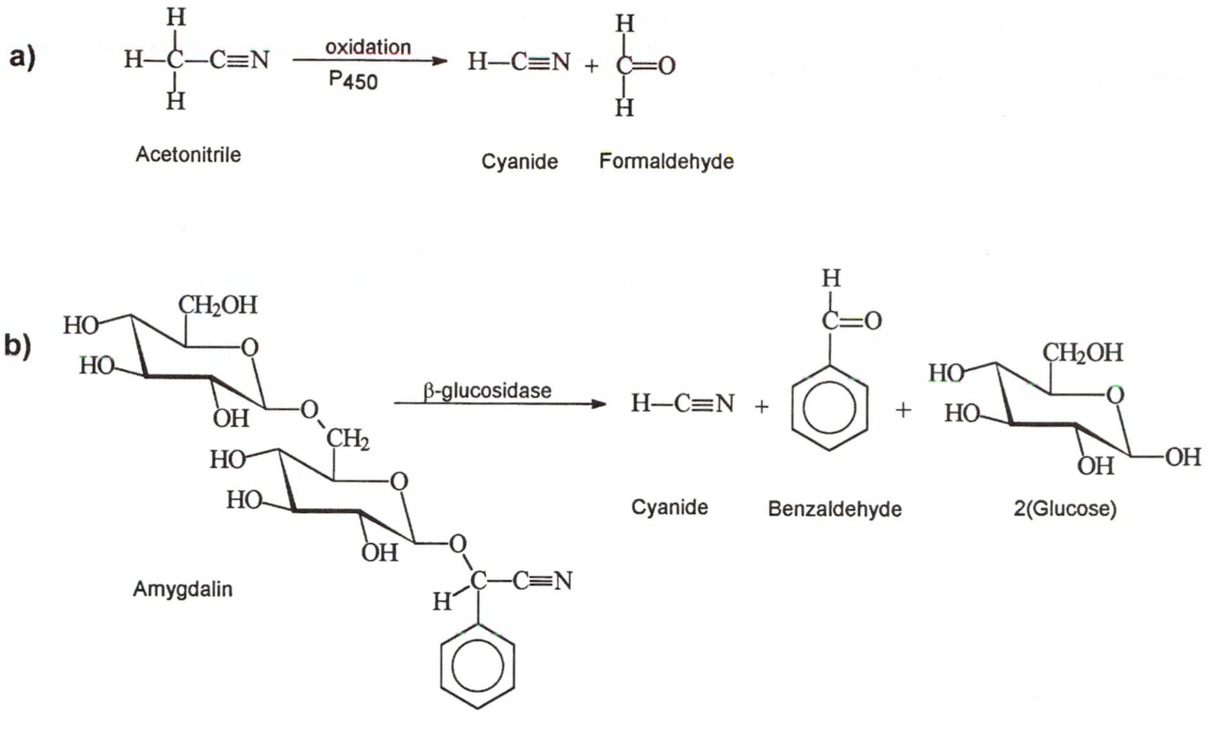

Figure 97–1. Biotransformation of the cyanogens (a) acetonitrile and (b) amygdalin to cyanide.

Last, cyanide intoxication may occur iatrogenically during nitroprusside administration. Sodium nitroprusside is a potent vasodilator with several favorable pharmacologic properties that make it a popular antihypertensive agent and afterload reducer. The disadvantage of nitroprusside is the in vivo release of cyanide. Each nitroprusside molecule contains five cyanide molecules. If thiosulfate stores are depleted, as in the malnourished or postoperative patient, cyanide may accumulate even with therapeutic nitroprusside infusion rates (2–10 μg/kg/min). Manifestations appear within hours to days and include alterations in mental status, acidosis, or tachyphylaxis to nitroprusside. Concurrent administration of thiosulfate[41,114] or hydroxocobalamin[40] with nitroprusside may prevent toxicity.

What Is the Mechanism of Cyanide Toxicity?

Cyanide is a nonspecific inhibitor of enzymes, including succinic dehydrogenase, superoxide dismutase, carbonic anhydrase, cytochrome oxidase, and many others.[9,148] Of these, the interaction of cyanide and cytochrome oxidase is best understood. Cytochrome oxidase is an iron-containing metalloenzyme essential for oxidative phosphorylation and, hence, aerobic energy production. It functions in the electron transport chain within mitochondria, converting catabolic products of glucose into high-energy molecules, adenosine triphosphate (ATP). Cyanide induces cellular hypoxia by inhibiting cytochrome oxidase[148] at the cytochrome aa_3 portion of the enzyme (Fig. 97–2). Thus, cyanide blocks efficient ATP production (see Chap. 12). In addition to decreased ATP production, two other metabolic abnormalities occur: lactic acidosis and decreased oxygen utilization.

Lactate production is the result of anaerobic energy production, a less efficient, alternate pathway for formation of ATP. Pyruvate no longer enters into the Krebs cycle, but is instead converted to lactate, which accumulates and results in metabolic acidosis.[14,22,53,55,67,77,80,120,122]

Central nervous system manifestations and histopathology[141,145] are consistent with inhibited oxygen utilization. Cranial imaging from survivors of cyanide poisoning reveals injury to the most oxygen-sensitive area of the brain, the basal ganglia.[20,27,48,117,118] However, experimental evidence demonstrates additional mechanisms that likely contribute to central nervous system toxicity.

Cyanide causes direct neurotoxicity through lipid peroxidation.[70] The exact mechanism is undefined but may be due to inhibition of antioxidant enzymes such as catalase, glutathione dehydrogenase, glutathione reductase, or superoxide dismutase.[5] Cyanide-induced lipid peroxidation displays tissue specificity. Lipid peroxidation occurs to the greatest extent in the brain, whereas the liver and heart have no reactive oxygen species following experimental cyanide exposure.[6] This tissue specificity explains the predominance of neurologic findings in cyanide toxicity.

There is also compelling evidence that excitatory amino acids, such as glutamate, mediate cyanide neuro-

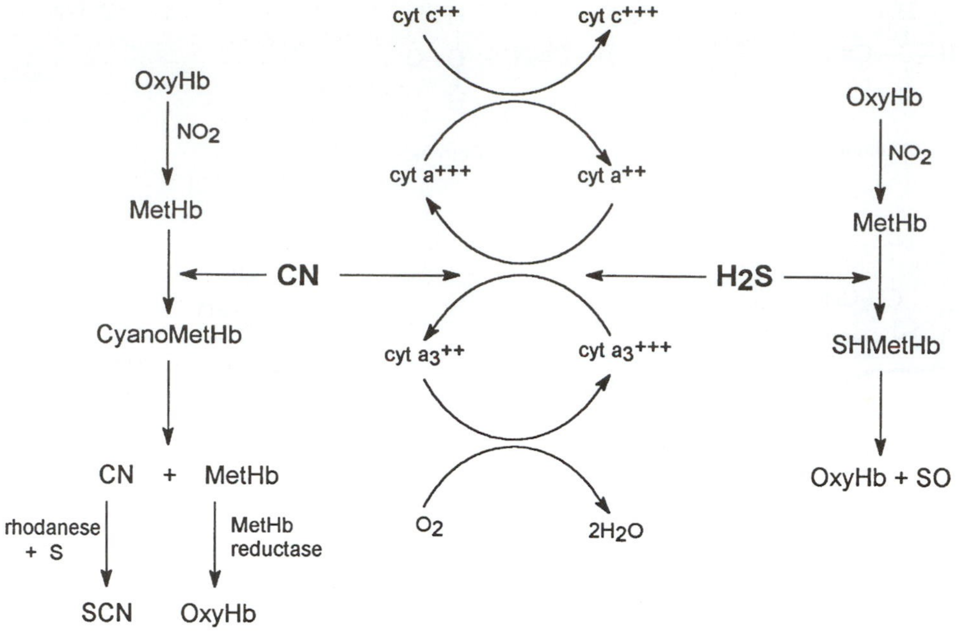

Figure 97–2. Pathway of cyanide and hydrogen sulfide toxicity and detoxification.

toxicity. Glutamate stimulation of *N*-methyl-*d*-aspartate (NMDA) receptors results in calcium and sodium entry into the cytosol of neurons (see Chap. 10). Cyanide releases glutamate,[104] directly stimulates NMDA receptors,[105,106] and augments cytosolic calcium release due to excitatory amino acids.[35] Ultimately, excess calcium results in cell death. Experimental studies demonstrate that NMDA inhibitors, such as dextrophan and MK-801 (dizocilpine), attenuate cyanide histopathology and lethality.[64,145]

The interaction of cyanide and cytochrome oxidase is reversible through endogenous detoxification pathways, including sulfur transfer enzymes, oxidation, and binding to cystine or hydroxocobalamin.[9] These pathways are the basis for research into effective antidotes.

Sulfurtransferase metabolism is crucial for detoxification. Three enzymes have been characterized: thiosulfate-cyanide sulfurtransferase (rhodanese), β-mercaptopyruvate-cyanide sulfurtransferase,[69] and cystathionase γ-lyase.[110] Sulfurtransferases catalyze the attachment of sulfur to cyanide, forming thiocyanate. This is a favorable reaction in that the sulfation of cyanide is essentially irreversible and the sulfation product, thiocyanate, has little inherent toxicity. Many compounds, including thiosulfate found in the Lilly antidote kit, can contribute the sulfur moiety.

Cyanide-induced metabolic derangements may decrease enzyme detoxification. Lowered ATP, reactive oxygen species, and increased cytosolic calcium stimulate protein kinase C activity that inactivates rhodanese.[92] NMDA and protein-kinase inhibitors increase detoxification.[92,93,111]

In addition to the above-mentioned pathways, the red blood cell may provide some protective effect against cyanide toxicity by sequestering cyanide.[143] While no cyanide degradation occurs within the RBC, there are no mitochondria present to be poisoned either. Hence, the RBC may help limit the amount of cyanide available to poison cells that participate in oxidative phosphorylation.

What Are the Clinical Manifestations of Cyanide Intoxication?

Cyanide is an extremely potent toxin, ranking closely with tabun, sarin, amanitin, and mustard gas for consideration as chemical warfare agents.[19] An oral lethal dose of KCN is approximately 200 mg.[10] An airborne concentration of 270 ppm may be immediately fatal, and exposures over 110 ppm for greater than 30 minutes are generally considered life-threatening.[136]

The amount of cyanide, duration of exposure, route of exposure, and premorbid condition of the individual influence onset and severity of illness. A critical combination of these factors overwhelms endogenous detoxification pathways, leading to illness.

The duration of exposure will also affect toxicity. Rapid, concentrated exposure to cyanide causes serious toxicity, while exposure to low levels over a lengthy period may not cause illness.

Toxicity may occur through a variety of routes, including inhalation, ingestion, dermal, conjunctival, and parenteral. Cyanide readily crosses membranes because it has a low molecular weight and is non-ionized. Rapid diffusion across alveolar membranes followed by direct distribution to target organs accounts for the lethality of inhalation. Parenteral exposure also provides a direct path to target organs. Oral exposures demonstrate a slightly longer time to death (20 minutes) as compared to parenteral exposure (5 minutes).[9] Cutaneous exposure, especially in abraded skin, will also induce toxicity.

However, correlation of clinical toxicity in human cases with dermal exposure is difficult because accidental exposures commonly involve both dermal and inhalation routes and it is accepted that vapor inhalation is more toxic.[26,122]

There is no reliable pathognomonic symptom or toxidrome associated with acute cyanide poisoning. The bitter almond odor is not uniformly present and when present, is not detectable by 40% of the population[79] (see Chap. 27). Clinical manifestations reflect dysfunction of oxygen-sensitive organs, with central nervous and cardiovascular findings predominating. The time to onset of symptoms is rapid with inorganic and gaseous forms—usually in minutes. Symptoms occur hours later following poisoning with cyanogens, due to metabolic requirements.

Central nervous system signs and symptoms are typical of progressive hypoxia and include headache, anxiety, agitation, confusion, convulsions, lethargy, coma, and death. A central tachypnea occurs initially, followed by bradypnea.

The cardiovascular responses to cyanide are complex. Studies of isolated heart preparation and intact animal models show that the principle cardiac insult is progressive failure, with slowing of rate and loss of contractile force due to ATP depletion.[11,144] Several reflex mechanisms, including catecholamine release and central vasomotor activity, may modulate myocardial performance and vascular response in cyanide poisoning. In laboratory investigations, there is a brief period of increased inotropy due to reflex compensatory mechanisms just prior to myocardial depression. Clinically, there may be an initial bradycardia and hypertension, then hypotension with reflex tachycardia, but the terminal event is consistently bradycardia and hypotension. Ventricular dysrhythmias do not appear to be an important factor.

Both cardiogenic and noncardiogenic pulmonary edema occur regularly and are found at necropsy.[37,49,55,77,120] Postulated causes of noncardiogenic pulmonary edema in cyanide poisoning include neurogenic or membrane leak from direct cellular toxicity.

Gastrointestinal symptoms occur infrequently. Abdominal pain, nausea, and vomiting occur following ingestion of inorganic cyanide and cyanogens.[3,37,53,55,73,80,90,94,120] These symptoms are due to hemorrhagic gastritis identified on necropsy and are thought to be secondary to the alkaline nature of cyanide salts.[49]

Cutaneous manifestations may vary. Traditionally, a cherry-red skin color is described.[31,122] The proposed etiology is increased hemoglobin oxygen saturation in venous blood due to decreased utilization of oxygen at the tissue level. This phenomenon may be more evident on funduscopic examination, where veins and arteries may appear similar in color.[71] Cyanosis has also been described, and is likely due to shock.[88,142,152]

TABLE 97–1. CYANIDE POISONING: EMERGENCY MANAGEMENT GUIDELINES

Supportive Care

Control airway, ventilate, and give 100% oxygen

Establish intravenous access

Crystalloids and vasopressors for hypotension

Administer $NaHCO_3$ according to ABG and serum HCO_3

Antidote

Amyl nitrite pearls are crushed into gauze and inhaled by the patient or placed over the intake valve of the ambu bag during assisted ventilation. Amyl nitrite should be inhaled alternatively with 100% oxygen every 30 sec while sodium nitrite is prepared. If sodium nitrite is readily available, it should be given in lieu of the pearls.

Give sodium nitrite ($NaNO_2$) as a 3% solution over 15–20 min IV:

- Adult dose: 10 mL (300 mg)
- Pediatric dose: See Table 97–2

Caution: Monitor blood pressure frequently and treat hypotension by slowing infusion rate and giving crystalloids and vasopressors. Obtain methemoglobin level 30 min after dose and consider possible excessive methemoglobin formation if patient deteriorates during therapy.

Give sodium thiosulfate (NaS_2O_3) as a 25% solution IV:

- Adult dose: 50 mL (12.5 g)
- Pediatric dose: See Table 97–2

Decontamination

Cutaneous: carefully remove all clothing and flush the skin

Ingestion: lavage with a large-bore orogastric tube and instill 1 g/kg activated charcoal

Laboratory

Arterial blood gas

Central venous blood gas

Electrolytes and glucose

Serum lactate

Serum cyanide concentration (for later confirmation only)

How Are Patients With Suspected Cyanide Poisoning Managed?

The initial care for the cyanide-poisoned patient begins in a fashion similar to the severely ill-appearing, comatose patient (see Table 97–1): direct attention to airway patency and support of ventilation and oxygenation. After establishing intravenous access, dextrose, naloxone, and thiamine should be given as indicated. Venous blood for renal function, glucose, and electrolyte determinations should be sent. A cyanide level may be requested, but will take hours to days to obtain results in most hospitals and, therefore, will be of little value during the acute care of the patient. An arterial blood gas specimen and serum lactate level will help assess the acid–base status.

The Lilly Antidote Kit should be administered as soon as cyanide poisoning is suspected. The kit contains amyl nitrite, sodium nitrite, and sodium thiosulfate. Nitrites oxidize hemoglobin to methemoglobin, which has a higher affinity for cyanide than does cytochrome oxidase. Methemoglobin draws cyanide away from cytochrome oxidase, regenerating enzyme function (Fig. 97–2). The resulting cyanomethemoglobin eventually breaks down to cyanide and methemoglobin, but at a rate within the capability of rhodanese to detoxify the cyanide. Methemoglobin is then available to bind to another molecule of cyanide or is reduced to hemoglobin.

Intravenous sodium nitrite induces approximately 7–14% methemoglobin.[76] Amyl nitrite is contained within pearls that are crushed and intermittently inhaled or intermittently introduced into the ventilator system to initiate methemoglobin formation. The pearls should only be used when intravenous access is delayed or not possible, as the pearls induce less methemoglobin, approximately 3%.

Experimental work demonstrating the efficacy of nitrite without methemoglobinemia suggests an alternate or additional mechanism to methemoglobin formation.[148] This may be due in part to conversion of nitrites to nitric oxide (NO), a potent vasodilator. In isolated, perfused liver, nitrite-induced vasodilation increases blood flow and detoxification.[133] In other experiments, NO-releasing compounds antagonized cyanide toxicity.[12,13,131]

Adverse effects of nitrites include excessive methemoglobin formation and, because of potent vasodilation, hypotension and tachycardia. Avoiding rapid infusion, monitoring blood pressure, and adhering to dosing guidelines will prevent adverse effects. The case of a toddler who died from excessive methemoglobinemia during nitrite treatment prompted the development of pediatric dosing guidelines.[18] Based on the premise that nitrite oxidizes hemoglobin on a mole-for-mole ratio, doses were calculated for various hemoglobin concentrations (Table 97–2). These values may also be useful if the patient is anemic. However, if giving nitrites empirically, care should be based on the 12-g hemoglobin concentration. Do not delay treatment while awaiting a hemoglobin measurement.

The goal of nitrite therapy has been to achieve a methemoglobin level of 20–30%. This level is not based on clinical data, but represents the maximum tolerated concentration without adverse symptoms from methemoglobin in a healthy individual. Clinical response occurs with lower methemoglobin levels, 3.6–9.2%.[45,71,72] These case reports are not conclusive, as levels were not drawn serially and peak levels may have been missed. Also, low levels do not reflect methemoglobin bound with cyanide in the form of cyanomethemoglobin, which is not typically detected. Therefore, lower than expected methemoglobin concentrations may represent indirect evidence of cyanide poisoning.

The issue of the safety of nitrites and degree of methemoglobin formation is especially important in cases of combined cyanide and carbon monoxide toxicity. Caution, to the point of withholding nitrite, has been advocated in this circumstance due to fear of critically reducing blood oxygen-carrying capacity by methemoglobin in the presence of carboxyhemoglobin. Recent data might allay this concern: In a small series of fire victims treated with nitrite,[76] methemoglobin concentrations peaked at 7.9–13.4% between 35 and 70 minutes after infusion. Corresponding carboxyhemoglobin levels decreased prior to peak methemoglobin levels. Because the safety of nitrites has not been studied in a large population of concomitant cyanide and carbon monoxide poisoning and the effect of cyanomethemoglobin on oxygen-carrying capacity is not understood, it is still reasonable to treat with thiosulfate alone initially and reserve nitrite for refractory cases.

Thiosulfate is the second component of the cyanide antidote kit. It is supplied as 50 mL of a 25% solution. Thiosulfate provides sulfur for conversion of cyanide to thiocyanate by rhodanese. It has several favorable properties as an antidote. Thiosulfate increases cyanide biotransformation 13-fold.[150] It is a substrate for a reaction that is essentially irreversible, converting a highly toxic entity to a relatively harmless compound. (Thiocyanate does, however, have its own toxicity in the presence of renal failure, including abdominal pain, vomiting, rash, and central nervous system dysfunction.[41]) There are no adverse reactions to thiosulfate itself. The pediatric dose of thiosulfate is adjusted for weight.

Combined nitrite and thiosulfate are more efficacious than either agent alone.[39] Additionally, co-administered oxygen increases the efficacy of these combined agents.[149]

Decontamination of cyanide-poisoned patients should occur concurrently with initial resuscitation. Exposure occurs by multiple routes including ingestion, inhalation, dermal, or parenteral. The route of exposure affects decontamination technique and poses potential hazards to health care personnel. For patients with cutaneous exposure, the clothing should be removed and the skin flushed with water. Particular attention should be given to open wounds since cyanide is readily absorbed through abraded skin. Skin decontamination should begin at the scene, with emergency personnel taking appropriate precautions to avoid self-contamination. For inhalation exposure, removal from the exposure area is critical. In general, first responders should exercise extreme caution when entering potentially hazardous areas such as chemical plants and laboratories where a previously healthy person is "found down."

For oral exposure, orogastric lavage may prevent further cyanide absorption (although absorption is rapid). Instillation of activated charcoal has previously been considered ineffective due to low binding of cyanide (1 g charcoal : 35 mg cyanide).[4] However, the lethal oral dose of cyanide is 100–200 mg and case reports cite ingested amounts in the hundreds of milligrams range. This amount of cyanide is within the adsorptive capacity of a standard dose of activated char-

TABLE 97–2. CYANIDE MANAGEMENT: PEDIATRIC NITRITE INFUSION

Hemoglobin (g)	$NaNO_2$ (mg/kg)	3% $NaNO_2$ solution (mL/kg)
7.0	5.8	0.19
8.0	6.6	0.22
9.0	7.5	0.25
10.0	8.3	0.27
11.0	9.1	0.30
12.0	10.0	0.33
13.0	10.8	0.36
14.0	11.6	0.39
Pediatric thiosulfate dose: 1.65 mL/kg of 25% solution		

Adapted, with permission, from Berlin CM: The treatment of cyanide poisoning in children. Pediatrics 1976;46:793–796.

coal. Additionally, prophylactic superactivated-charcoal administration improved survival in animals given LD_{100} doses of potassium cyanide.[82] Based on the potential benefits compared to minimal risks, activated charcoal administration is advocated.

Acidemia should be treated with adequate ventilation and sodium bicarbonate administration based on arterial pH and serum bicarbonate determination.

Patients who do not survive cyanide poisoning may be suitable organ donors. Heart, liver, kidney, pancreas, cornea, skin, and bone were successfully transplanted following cyanide poisoning.[33,63,85,132]

What Laboratory Tests Facilitate Assessment?

As mentioned, serum cyanide determination can confirm toxicity but is not available in a timely manner. Plasma thiocyanate levels are of little value in assessing patients with acute poisoning as there is little correlation with symptoms. Because of nonspecific symptoms and delay in laboratory testing, historical circumstances must be relied upon to raise suspicion of cyanide poisoning and institute therapy (see Table 97–3). There are however, some laboratory findings that support cyanide intoxication.

Metabolic acidosis secondary to lactate production is the metabolic manifestation of cyanide poisoning. An elevated venous oxygen saturation occurred in two cases.[60,71] Tissue extraction partly determines venous oxygen content. If tissue utilization decreases, venous oxygen saturation approaches arterial saturation. A venous oxygen saturation greater than 90% from superior vena cava or pulmonary artery blood indicates decreased oxygen utilization.[71] This is not specific for cyanide and could represent cellular poisoning from other agents such as carbon monoxide or hydrogen sulfide.

A saturation gap, the difference between measured and calculated arterial oxygen saturation, has been suggested to indicate cyanide poisoning. The saturation gap is based on the premise that cyanide combines with hemoglobin, forming cyanohemoglobin, which does not bind oxygen, thereby diminishing the oxygen-carrying capacity of the blood. However, an in vitro study shows no evidence for such a gap.[42]

Cyanide results in nonspecific electrocardiographic findings.[11] There is initial bradycardia, followed by transient tachycardia, and then recurrent bradycardia. Myocardial injury pattern may develop. AV conduction blocks also occur.

TABLE 97–3. CYANIDE POISONING: SUGGESTIVE CLINICAL SETTINGS

When to Suspect Cyanide
Sudden collapse of laboratory or industrial worker
Fire victim with coma or acidosis
Suicide or unexplained coma and acidosis
Ingestion of artificial-nail remover
ICU patient with decreased mental status, acidosis, and tachyphylaxis to nitroprusside

Are There Other Potential Therapies?

Although the Lilly Cyanide Kit is the mainstay of antidotal therapy in the United States, other treatments are currently in use abroad and others are investigational. In Europe, 4-dimethylaminophenol (4-DMAP) is the oxidizing agent of choice to induce methemoglobin. It is has a more rapid onset of methemoglobin production than does sodium nitrite. Methemoglobin peaks at 5 minutes after 4-DMAP as opposed to 30 minutes following sodium nitrite.[78,99,150] The dose of 4-DMAP is 3 mg/kg and is co-administered with thiosulfate. As with sodium nitrite, its major adverse effect is excessive methemoglobin.

Several agents that directly bind cyanide have been investigated and are in use. Stroma-free methemoglobin, oxidized hemoglobin in which the cell membrane has been removed, attenuates lethality and prevents hemodynamic changes in animal models.[29,134,135] The advantage to this treatment lies in providing exogenous methemoglobin without compromising oxygen-carrying capacity of native hemoglobin. Removal of the cell membrane eliminates the problem of antigenicity.

Dicobalt edetate is a cyanide chelator, but has serious adverse effects. These include hypotension, cardiac dysrhythmias, decreased cerebral blood flow, and angioedema.[30,100,150] Because these adverse reactions are magnified when in fact a patient does not have cyanide intoxication, its use has been reserved for confirmed cyanide poisonings. The inherent problems in delaying treatment while waiting for confirmation is obvious and relegates this antidote to very limited usefulness.

Hydroxocobalamin, a vitamin B_{12} precursor, is another cobalt-containing chelator. It displaces cyanide from the cytochrome enzyme, forming cyanocobalamin. Then either cyanocobalamin (vitamin B_{12}) is excreted in the urine or the cyanide moiety is released at a rate sufficient to allow detoxification by rhodanese. For this reason, thiosulfate is co-administered with hydroxocobalamin. One molecule of hydroxocobalamin binds one molecule of cyanide, yielding a molecular weight binding ratio of 50 : 1. Four grams of hydroxocobalamin is the standard, initial dose and is expected to bind 200 mg of cyanide. The dose may be repeated in cases of massive poisoning. Typically, 8 g of thiosulfate is co-administered. Hydroxocobalamin has few adverse effects. It does not form abnormal hemoglobin. In a canine model given human therapeutic doses, no hemodynamic changes occurred.[115] Exposure of isolated cardiac muscle to hydroxocobalamin does not alter contractility.[17] However, allergic reaction and a reddening of the skin are reported.[32,61] Currently, hydroxocobalamin is used in Europe for acute and chronic poisoning.[24]

Alpha-ketoglutaric acid is a promising antidote. It has a molecular configuration that renders it amenable to nucleophilic binding of cyanide. Prophylactic treatment studies demonstrate reduced lethality and synergy with sodium thiosulfate.[21,46,68,102] The advantage to alpha-ketoglutarate is direct binding of cyanide without generation of methemoglobin.

Delivery of exogenous rhodanese and sulfur donors by encapsulation into RBCs increases the LD_{50} of cyanide in a murine model.[36,108]

Hyperbaric oxygen (HBO) has been used in cyanide treatment, often with dramatic clinical improvement.[43,48,54,88,117,119,137] However, patients received multiple therapies during resuscitation and improvement cannot be attributed to HBO alone. Experimental data supporting HBO efficacy are contradictory. In a murine model, survival increased with 100% oxygen at 2 atmospheres absolute (ATA) compared to normobaric oxygen.[123] However, HBO in combination with nitrite and thiosulfate did not confer additional protection compared to normobaric oxygen with nitrite and thiosulfate.[149] Currently, the Undersea and Hyperbaric Medical Society supports hyperbaric therapy for cyanide poisoning when complicated by coincident carbon monoxide intoxication.[151] Until further studies clearly demonstrate the efficacy of hyperbaric therapy for isolated cyanide, it should not supplant the combination of normobaric oxygen, nitrite, and thiosulfate.

Are There Any Chronic Illnesses Related to Cyanide Exposure?

Survivors of serious, acute poisoning may develop delayed neurologic sequelae.[20,27,38,48,56,95,117,118,141] Parkinsonian symptoms, including dystonia, dysarthria, rigidity, and bradykinesia, are most common. Symptoms typically develop over weeks to months, but subtle findings can be present within a few days. Cranial computerized tomography and magnetic resonance imaging consistently reveal basal ganglia (globus pallidus, putamen, and hippocampus) damage, with radiologic changes appearing several weeks after onset of symptoms (see Color Plate Fig. 9). The extrapyramidal manifestations may progress or resolve. Response to pharmacotherapy with antiparkinsonian agents is disappointing. It is unclear if delayed manifestations result from direct cellular injury or secondary hypoxia. Chronic, low-grade exposure to cyanide may result in insidious syndromes, including tobacco amblyopia, tropical ataxic neuropathy, and Leber's hereditary neuropathy.

Tobacco amblyopia is a progressive loss of visual function occurring almost exclusively in males who smoke. Affected smokers have lower plasma cyanocobalamin and thiocyanate levels than unaffected smoking counterparts, suggesting a reduced ability to detoxify cyanide. Cessation of smoking and administration of hydroxocobalamin often reverses symptoms.[50]

Tropical ataxic neuropathy is a demyelinating disease associated with cassava consumption. Neurologic manifestations include paresthesias, sensory ataxia, optic atrophy, and sensorineural hearing loss. Concomitant dermatitis and glossitis led investigators to the association of high dietary intake of cassava. Elevated thiocyanate levels in affected individuals suggested cyanide as an etiology. Removal of dietary cassava and institution of vitamin B_{12} therapy alleviates symptoms.[3,154]

Leber's hereditary optic atrophy, a condition of subacute visual failure affecting men, is thought due to rhodanese deficiency.[50,154]

Hydrogen Sulfide Toxicity

CASE 2. A 23-year-old male entered an empty petroleum storage tank for repairs. He rapidly collapsed and fell unconscious. Two co-workers attempted a rescue, but both collapsed immediately after entering the tank. Firefighters wearing self-contained breathing apparatus entered the tank and removed all three victims. Both of the would-be-rescuers regained consciousness after removal from the tank. The first worker to collapse was removed and noted to be cyanotic, with minimal respiratory effort. When paramedics arrived on the scene, he was immediately intubated.

He arrived in the emergency department intubated, receiving 100% oxygen by assisted ventilation. He had shallow, spontaneous respirations and responded only to deep painful stimuli. Vital signs included: blood pressure, 110/72 mm Hg; pulse, 140 beats/min; respiratory rate, 34 breaths/min; rectal temperature, 102°F (38.4°C). Pertinent findings on physical examination included dilated pupils, marked conjunctival injection, and diffuse rales in all lung fields.

Laboratory data showed an ABG: pH 7.21; PCO_2 30 mm Hg; PO_2 48 mm Hg; and calculated bicarbonate 11 mEq/L. The carboxyhemoglobin level was 1.5%. A serum lactate was 10.5 mEq/L. Electrocardiogram showed sinus tachycardia with normal intervals and axis. Chest radiograph showed diffuse alveolar infiltrates and a normal sized heart.

The patient was placed on a ventilator with 100% oxygen and positive end-expiratory pressure of 10 cm H_2O. Over the next hour, his oxygenation improved and his PO_2 was 335 mm Hg. He rapidly required less ventilatory support. The lactic acidosis resolved over the next 8 hours. His neurologic status slowly improved over the next 20 hours, at which point he appeared alert and would follow commands. Following extubation, a repeat neurologic examination was normal. Follow-up 1 week later did not show any adverse effects. Air samples of the tank were taken the day after the accident. Analysis showed hydrogen sulfide 880 ppm; methane 420 ppm; carbon dioxide 400 ppm; carbon monoxide 50 ppm; oxygen 18%.

What Are the Sources of Hydrogen Sulfide Exposure?

Hydrogen sulfide (H_2S) is produced naturally by bacterial decomposition of proteins and is used or produced in many industrial activities. Industrial sources of hydrogen sulfide include pulp paper mills, heavy-water production, the leather industry, petroleum distillation and refining, roofing asphalt tanks, vulcanizing of rubber, viscose rayon production, and coke manufacturing from coal.[34,65,103,116,126] It is a major industrial hazard in oil and gas production, particularly in sour gas fields (natural gas containing sulfur).[59] Decay of sulfur-containing products, such as fish, sewage, and manure, also produces hydrogen sulfide. Several farm workers and rescuers have died from exposure to hydrogen sulfide generated in liquid manure pits.[47,103] Natural sources are volcanoes, caves, sulfur springs, vent tube worms, and underground deposits of natural gas.[2,44,65,113,116]

How Does Hydrogen Sulfide Produce Toxicity?

Hydrogen sulfide is a colorless gas, more dense than air, with an odor of "rotten eggs" and high lipid solubility, which allows easy penetration of biologic membranes. Systemic absorption usually occurs through inhalation.[113] The tissues most sensitive to hydrogen sulfide are those with exposed mucous membranes and those with high oxygen demands. Hydrogen sulfide not only has systemic effects but produces intense local irritation to mucous membranes and the skin. It reacts with the moisture on the surface of mucous membranes to form sodium sulfide, which produces the irritant chemical effect. Despite skin irritation, it has little dermal absorption.

Hydrogen sulfide, like cyanide, is a potent inhibitor of cytochrome oxidase, interrupting oxidative phosphorylation.[125,128] Hydrogen sulfide binds to the ferric (Fe^{3+}) moiety of cytochrome aa_3 oxidase complex (Fig. 97–2). The resulting inhibition of oxidative phosphorylation produces cellular hypoxia and anaerobic metabolism.[125] In addition to producing cellular hypoxia, hydrogen sulfide causes potassium channel–mediated hyperpolarization of neurons and potentiates other neuronal inhibitory mechanisms. It also alters brain neurotransmitter content and release.[1,113] A proposed mechanism of death is poisoning of the brainstem respiratory center due to selective uptake by lipophilic white matter in this region.[146]

The major pathways of hydrogen sulfide detoxification are enzymatic and nonenzymatic oxidation of sulfides and sulfur to thiosulfate and polysulfides.[25] Oxyhemoglobin catalyzes this reaction.[16] Other pathways play a lesser role in detoxification and elimination. Hydrogen sulfide binds to heme compounds such as endogenously produced methemoglobin to form sulfmethemoglobin. Only small amounts are excreted in urine or exhaled into the air. Sulfhemoglobin is not found in significant concentrations in the blood of animals or fatally poisoned humans.[126]

What Are the Clinical Manifestations of Hydrogen Sulfide Toxicity?

The primary target organs of hydrogen sulfide poisoning are those of the central nervous system and respiratory system. The clinical findings reported in two large series[8,34] are shown in Table 97–4. The intensity of exposure likely accounts for the diverse clinical findings in reported cases. A distinct dose–response to hydrogen sulfide has been identified. The odor threshold is between 0.02 and 0.13 ppm. It has a strong, intense odor at 20–30 ppm. Mild mucous membrane irritation occurs at 50–100 ppm and olfactory fatigue or paralysis occurs at 100–150 ppm (see Chap. 27). Ability to perceive the odor is rapidly extinguished because of olfactory nerve paralysis at higher levels. Prolonged exposure can occur when the disappearance of the odor is misinterpreted as dissipation of the gas. Strong irritation of the upper respiratory tract and eyes, as well as pulmonary edema, occurs at 200–300 ppm. At greater than 500 ppm H_2S become a systemic toxin. Rapid unconsciousness and cardiopulmonary arrest occur at concentrations greater than 700 ppm.[15,113]

TABLE 97–4. HYDROGEN SULFIDE POISONING: CLINICAL MANIFESTATIONS

When to Suspect Hydrogen Sulfide Poisoning	
Person rapidly loses consciousness ("knocked down")	
Smell of rotten eggs	
Signs and Symptoms	
CNS	Headache, weakness, dysequilibrium, convulsions, coma
CV	Chest pain, bradycardia
Pulmonary	Dyspnea, cyanosis, hemoptysis, pulmonary edema
GI	Nausea and vomiting
HEENT	Conjunctivitis and pharyngitis

Symptoms of mucous membrane irritation occur early and at low levels of exposure. Mucous membrane irritation of the eye produces keratoconjunctivitis. If exposure persists, damage of the epithelial cells will produce reversible corneal ulcerations ("gas eye") and, rarely, irreversible corneal scarring.[97] The irritant effects of the respiratory tract include rhinitis, bronchitis, and pulmonary edema. A significant number of victims develop pulmonary edema.[34]

In one series, 75% of 221 patients with acute hydrogen sulfide exposure lost consciousness at the site of exposure.[34] In acute, massive exposures, rapid loss of consciousness is due to paralysis of the respiratory center of the brain.[126] If the patient is removed from the exposure rapidly, recovery may be rapid and complete. Secondary neurologic effects can result from hypoxia due to respiratory compromise.[113] Neurologic outcome can be quite variable, ranging from no neurologic impairment to permanent sequelae. Delayed neuropsychiatric sequelae have occurred after acute exposures.[34,65,74,129,130,139,140,147] The role of cerebral hypoxia versus the direct neurotoxic effect of hydrogen sulfide is unclear. Neuropsychiatric changes reported include memory failure (amnestic syndrome), lack of insight, disorientation, delirium, and dementia.[147] Neurosensory abnormalities include transient hearing impairment, vision loss, and anosmia. Motor symptoms are likely due to injury of the basal ganglia and result in ataxia, position/intention tremor, and muscle rigidity.[140] Common neuropathologic findings observed on CT scan and at autopsy are subcortical white matter demyelination and globus pallidus degeneration.[51,139]

Acute exposures affect other organ systems. Myocardial hypoxia or direct toxic effects of hydrogen sulfide on cardiac tissue may cause cardiac dysrhythmias, myocardial ischemia, or myocardial infarction.[57] Since unresponsiveness is rapid, trauma due to falls may be significant.[8]

What Bedside Observations and Diagnostic Studies Are Helpful in the Diagnosis of Hydrogen Sulfide Poisoning?

Management decisions must be made based on history and clinical presentation. No rapid method of detection exists that is of clinical diagnostic use. At the bedside, the smell of rotten eggs on clothing or emanating from the blood, exhaled air, or gastric secretions suggests hydrogen sulfide exposure.[66] In addition, blackening of copper and silver coins in a patient's pocket or darkening of jewelry are clues to exposure. Rapid diagnostic tests are nonspecific. Metabolic acidosis reflected by elevated serum lactate concentrations is expected but not specific for hydrogen sulfide poisoning. Since sulfhemoglobin is not generated in hydrogen sulfide poisoning, an oxygen saturation gap is not expected.[126] Specific tests for laboratory confirmation of hydrogen sulfide exposure are not readily available in clinical laboratories. The presence of hydrogen sulfide is best confirmed by directly measuring the gas in the environment. It can be detected in atmospheric air samples by monitoring devices such as colorimetric tubes or toxin-specific air sampling devices. In biologic specimens, sulfide ions can be measured by microdiffusion isolation with colorimetry determination or with an ion-selective electrode.[113] Whole blood sulfide levels greater than 0.05 mg/L are considered abnormal. Reliable measurements are ensured only if the level is obtained within 2 hours after the exposure and analyzed immediately, because sulfide concentrations rise with tissue decomposition.[113]

How Are Patients With Hydrogen Sulfide Poisoning Managed?

Hydrogen sulfide poisoning should be suspected whenever a person is found unconscious in an enclosed space, especially if the odor of rotten eggs is noted. No rescuer should enter until proper self-contained breathing apparatus (SCBA) is available. Hydrogen sulfide is also known as "knock down" gas, because of its ability to produce rapid unconsciousness. Unintentional exposure can lead to injuries and even death to well-meaning rescuers without proper protective equipment. There are cases of multiple rescuers injured in an attempt to remove one victim from an environment with high concentrations of hydrogen sulfide.[44,47,75,103,129]

The initial treatment (Table 97–5) is immediate removal of the victim from the contaminated area into a fresh-air environment. High-flow oxygen should be administered as soon as possible. Optimal supportive care and advanced cardiac life support have the greatest influence on the patient's outcome. Because death is rapid from inhalation of hydrogen sulfide, limited human cases are reported in the literature. Most patients have significant delays before receiving treatment. Therefore, specific treatments and antidotal therapies have not shown definitive improvement in patient outcome.

Animal studies and human case reports suggest that oxygen therapy is beneficial for hydrogen sulfide poisoning.[16,25,112] However, one animal study concluded contradictory findings.[127] Studies showing benefit of hyperbaric oxygen (HBO) for cyanide toxicity have led to the use of HBO in hydrogen sulfide poisoning. In rats, HBO was more effective in preventing mortality from sulfide poisoning.[25] Case reports suggest that HBO is beneficial.[124,153] Proposed mechanisms for oxygen's beneficial effects are competitive reactivation of oxidative phosphorylation by inhibiting hydrogen sulfide–cytochrome binding, enhanced detoxification by catalyzing oxidation of sulfides and sulfur, and improved oxygenation in the presence of pulmonary edema.[16,124] All patients suspected of hydrogen sulfide poisoning should receive supplemental oxygen and HBO when readily available.[151] Since data on the efficacy of HBO are limited, it is not necessary to transfer the patient solely for HBO therapy.

TABLE 97–5. HYDROGEN SULFIDE POISONING: EMERGENCY MANAGEMENT GUIDELINES

Supportive Care

Prehospital
- Attempt rescue only if using SCBA.
- Move victim to fresh air.
- During extrication, consider traumatic injuries from falls.
- Administer 100% oxygen.
- Administer advanced cardiac life support as indicated.

Emergency Department
- Maximize ventilation and oxygenation.
- Consider PEEP.
- Treat acidosis based on ABG and serum HCO_3 analysis.
- Administer crystalloids and vasopressors for hypotension.

Antidote

Give sodium nitrite (3% $NaNO_2$) IV over 15–20 min:
- Adult dose: 10 mL (300 mg)
- Pediatric dose: See Table 97–2

Caution
- Monitor blood pressure frequently.
- Obtain methemoglobin level 30 min after dose.
- Consider hyperbaric oxygen if immediately available.

The similarities in the toxic mechanism between hydrogen sulfide and cyanide created an interest in the use of nitrite-induced methemoglobin as an antidote. Methemoglobin protects animals from toxicity of hydrogen sulfide poisoning in both pretreatment and postexposure experiments.[25,126,127] Nitrite-generated methemoglobin acts as a scavenger of sulfide. Hydrogen sulfide's affinity for methemoglobin is greater than that of cytochrome oxidase.[125] When hydrogen sulfide binds to methemoglobin, it forms sulfmethemoglobin.[16] Since hydrogen sulfide poisoning is rare, no studies exist to evaluate the clinical outcome of patients treated with sodium nitrite. Animal studies suggest that nitrite must be given within minutes of exposure to ensure effectiveness.[16] However, several human case reports showed rapid return of normal sensorium when nitrites were administered soon after exposure.[65,107,130] Patients with suspected hydrogen sulfide poisoning with altered mental status, coma, hypotension, or dysrhythmias should probably receive sodium nitrite by slow infusion.

Treatment of patients with hydrogen sulfide poisoning requires optimum supportive care. Treatments and antidotes beyond supportive care are not of proven clinical benefit. Since hydrogen sulfide toxicity is severe and reports suggest the occurrence of delayed sequelae, the potential benefits of nitrite therapy and hyperbaric oxygen should be considered for seriously ill patients exposed to hydrogen sulfide. Use of these therapies occurs after ensuring optimum supportive care.

References

1. Abe K, Kimura H: The possible role of hydrogen sulfide as an endogenous neuromodulator. J Neurosci 1996;16: 1066–1071.
2. Afane ZE, Roche N, Atchou G: Respiratory symptoms and peak expiratory flow in survivors of the Nyos disaster. Chest 1996;110:1278–1281.
3. Akintonwa A, Tunwashe OL: Fatal cyanide poisoning from cassava-based meal. Hum Exp Toxicol 1992;11:47–49.
4. Andersen AH: Experimental studies on the pharmacology of activated charcoal. I. Adsorption power of charcoal in aqueous solutions. Acta Pharmacol 1946;2:69–78.
5. Ardelt BK, Borowitz JL, Isom GE: Brain lipid peroxidation and antioxidant protectant mechanisms following acute cyanide intoxication. Toxicology 1989;56:147–154.
6. Ardelt BK, Borowitz JL, Maduh EU, et al: Cyanide-induced lipid peroxidation in different organs: Subcellular distribution and hydroperoxide generation in neuronal cells. Toxicology 1994;89:127–137.
7. Aregheore EM, Agunbiade BS: The toxic effects of cassava (Manihout esculenta grantz) diets on humans: A review. Vet Hum Toxicol 1991;33:274–275.
8. Arnold IM, Dufresne RM, Alleyne BC: Health implication of occupational exposures to hydrogen sulfide. J Occup Med 1985;27:373–376.
9. Ballantyne B: Toxicology of cyanides. In: Ballantyne B, Marrs TC, eds: Clinical and Experimental Toxicology of Cyanides. Bristol, England, IOP Publishers, 1987, p. 42.
10. Baselt RC, Craven RH: Disposition of Toxic Drugs and Chemicals in Man, 3rd ed. Chicago, Year Book, 1989, pp. 224–227.
11. Baskin SI: The cardiac effects of cyanide. In: Baskin SI, ed: Principles of Cardiac Toxicology. Boca Raton, FL, CRC Press, 1991, pp. 419–430.
12. Baskin SI, Neally EW, Lempka JC: Cyanide toxicity in mice pretreated with diethylamine nitric oxide complex. Hum Exp Toxicol 1996;15:13–18.
13. Baskin SI, Neally EW, Lempka JC: The effects of EDRF/NO releasers or calcium ionophore A23187 on cyanide toxicity in mice. Toxicol Appl Pharmacol 1996; 139:349–355.
14. Baud FJ, Barriot P, Toffis V, et al: Elevated blood cyanide concentrations in victims of smoke inhalation. N Engl J Med 1991;325:1761–1766.
15. Beauchamp RO, Bus JS, Popp JA: A critical review of the literature on hydrogen sulfide toxicity. Crit Rev Toxicol 1984;13:25–97.
16. Beck JF, Bradbury CM, Connors AJ: Nitrite as an antidote for acute hydrogen sulfide intoxication? Am Ind Hyg J 1981;42:805–809.
17. Beregi JP, Riou B, Lecarpentier Y: Effects of hydroxocobalamin on rat cardiac papillary muscle. Intensive Care Med 1991;17:175–177.
18. Berlin CM: The treatment of cyanide poisoning in children. Pediatrics 1976;46:793–796.
19. Beswick FW: Chemical agents used in riot control and warfare. Hum Toxicol 1983;2:247–256.
20. Bhatt MH, Obeso JA, Marsden CD: Time course of postanoxic akinetic-rigid and dystonic syndromes. Neurology 1993;43:314–317.
21. Bhattacharya R, Vijayaraghavan R: Cyanide intoxication in mice through different routes and its prophylaxis by α-ketoglutarate. Biomed Environ Sci 1991;4:452–459.
22. Binder L, Frederickson L: Poisoning in laboratory personnel and health care professionals. Am J Emerg Med 1991; 9:11–15.
23. Bismuth C, Baud FJ, Djeghout H, et al: Cyanide poisoning from proprionitrile exposure. J Emerg Med 1987;5: 191–195.
24. Bismuth C, Baud FJ, Pontal PG: Hydroxocobalamin in chronic cyanide poisoning. J Toxicol Clin Exp 1988;8: 35–38.
25. Bitterman N, Talmi Y, Lerman A: The effect of hyperbaric oxygen on acute experimental sulfide poisoning in the rat. Toxicol Appl Pharmacol 1986;84:325–328.
26. Blanc P, Hogan M, Mallin K, et al: Cyanide intoxication among silver-reclaiming workers. JAMA 1997;253: 367–371.
27. Borgohain R, Singh AK, Radhakrishna H, et al: Delayed onset generalised dystonia after cyanide poisoning. Clin Neurol Neurosurg 1995;97:213–215.
28. Brahams D: Medicine and the law: "Sudafed" capsules poisoned with cyanide. Lancet 1991;337:968.
29. Breen PH, Isserles SA, Tabac E, et al: Protective effect of stroma-free methemoglobin during cyanide poisoning in dogs. Anesthesiology 1996;85:558–564.
30. Brian MJ: Case reports: Cyanide poisoning in children in Goroka. Papua New Guinea Med J 1990;33:151–153.
31. Brivet F, Delfraissy JF, Duche M, et al: Case reports: Acute cyanide poisoning—Recovery with nonspecific supportive care. Intensive Care Med 1983;9:33–35.
32. Brouard A, Blaisot B, Bismuth C: Hydroxocobalamine in cyanide poisoning. J Toxicol Clin Exp 1987;7:155–168.
33. Brown PWG, Buckels JAC, Jain AB, McMaster P: Successful cadaveric renal transplantation from a donor who died of cyanide poisoning. Br Med J 1987;294:1325.
34. Burnett WW, King EG, Grace M: Hydrogen sulfide poisoning: Review of 5 years' experience. Can Med Assoc J 1977;117:1277–1280.
35. Cai Z, McCaslin PP: Selective effects of cyanide (100 mM) on the excitatory amino acid-induced elevation of intracellular calcium levels in neuronal culture. Neurochem Res 1992;17:803–808.
36. Cannon EP, Leung P, Hawkins A, et al: Antagonism of cyanide intoxication with murine carrier erythrocytes containing rhodanese and sodium thiosulfate. J Toxicol Environ Health 1994;41:267–274.
37. Caravati EM, Litovitz TL: Pediatric cyanide intoxication and from an acetonitrile-containing cosmetic. JAMA 1988; 260:3470–3473.
38. Carella F, Grassi MP, Savoiardo M, et al: Dystonic-parkin-

sonian syndrome after cyanide poisoning: Clinical and MRI findings. J Neurol Neurosurg Psychiatry 1988;51: 1345–1348.
39. Chen KK, Rose CL: Nitrite and thiosulfate therapy in cyanide poisoning. JAMA 1952;149:113–119.
40. Cottrell JE, Casthely P, Brodie JD, et al: Prevention of nitroprusside-induced cyanide toxicity with hydroxocobalamin. N Engl J Med 1978;298:809–811.
41. Curry SC, Arnold-Capell P: Toxic effects of drugs used in the ICU: Nitroprusside, nitroglycerine, and angiotensin-converting enzyme. Crit Care Clin North Am 1991;7: 555–581.
42. Curry SC, Patrick HC: Lack of evidence for a percent saturation gap in cyanide poisoning. Ann Emerg Med 1991; 20:523–528.
43. Davis FM, Ewer T: Acute cyanide poisoning: Case report of the use of hyperbaric oxygen. J Hyperb Med 1988;3: 103–106.
44. Deng JF, Chang SC: Hydrogen sulfide poisoning in hot springs reservoir cleaning: Two case reports. Am J Ind Med 1987;11:447–451.
45. DiNapoli J, Hall AH, Drake R, Rumack BH: Cyanide and arsenic poisoning by intravenous injection. Ann Emerg Med 1989;18:308–311.
46. Dulaney MD, Brumley M, Willis JT, Hume AS: Protection against cyanide toxicity by oral alpha-ketoglutaric acid. Vet Hum Toxicol 1991;33:571–575.
47. Fatalities attributed to entering manure waste pits—Minnesota, 1992. MMWR 1993;42:325–329.
48. Feldman JM, Feldman MD: Sequelae of attempted suicide by cyanide ingestion: A case report. Int J Psychiatry Med 1990;20:173–179.
49. Fernando GCA, Busuttil A: Cyanide ingestion: Case studies of four suicides. Am J Forensic Med Pathol 1991;12: 241–246.
50. Freeman AG: Optic neuropathy and chronic cyanide intoxication: A review. J R Soc Med 1988;81:103–106.
51. Gaitonde UB, Sellar RJ: Long term exposure to hydrogen sulphide producing subacute encephalopathy in a child. Br Med J 1987;294:614.
52. Gee DJ: Cyanides in murder, suicides, and accident. In: Ballantyne B, Marrs TC, eds: Clinical and Experimental Toxicology of Cyanides Bristol, England, IOP Publishers, 1987, p. 212.
53. Geller RJ, Ekins BR, Iknoian RC: Cyanide toxicity from acetonitrile-containing false nail remover. Am J Emerg Med 1991;9:268–270.
54. Goodhart GL: Patient treated with antidote kit and hyperbaric oxygen survives cyanide poisoning. South Med J 1994;87:814–816.
55. Graham DL, Laman D, Theodore J, Robin ED: Acute cyanide poisoning complicated by lactic acidosis and pulmonary edema. Arch Intern Med 1977;137:1051–1055.
56. Grandas F, Artieda J, Obeso JA: Brief report: clinical and CT scan findings in a case of cyanide intoxication. Movement Disord 1989;4:188–193.
57. Gregorakos L, Dimopoulos G, Liberi S: Hydrogen sulfide poisoning: Management and complications. Angiology 1995;46:1123–1131.
58. Grigg B, Modeland V: The cyanide scare: A tale of two grapes. FDA Consumer 1989;July–Aug:7–11.
59. Guidotti TL: Occupational exposure to hydrogen sulfide in the sour gas industry: Some unresolved issues. Int Arch Occup Environ Health 1994;66:153–160.
60. Hall AH, Linden CH, Kulig KW, Rumack BH: Cyanide poisoning from Laetrile ingestion: Role of nitrite therapy. Pediatrics 1986;78:269–272.
61. Hall AH, Rumack BH: Hydroxocobalamin/sodium thiosulfate as a cyanide antidote. J Emerg Med 1987;5:115–121.
62. Hall AH, Rumack BH: Clinical toxicology of cyanide. Ann Emerg Med 1986;15:1067–1074.
63. Hantson P, Mahieu P, Hassoun A, Otte J: Outcome following organ removal from poisoned donors in brain death status: A report of 12 cases and review of the literature. J Toxicol Clin Toxicol 1995;33:709–712.
64. Himori N, Tanaka Y, Kurasawa M, et al: Detrorphan attenuates the behavioral consequences of ischemia and the biochemical consequences of anoxia: Possible role of *N*-methyl-*d*-aspartate receptor antagonism and ATP replenishing action in its cerebroprotecting profile. Psychopharmacology 1993;111:153–162.
65. Hoidal CR, Hall AH, Robinson MD: Hydrogen sulfide poisoning from toxic inhalations of roofing asphalt fumes. Ann Emerg Med 1986;15:826–830.
66. Horowitz BZ, Marquardt K, Swenson E: Calcium polysulfide overdose: A report of two cases. J Toxicol Clin Toxicol 1997;35:299–303.
67. Howard J, Pouw TH, Arnold J, et al: Cyanide poisonings associated with over-the-counter medication—Washington state, 1991. MMWR 1991;40:161,167–168.
68. Hume AS, Mozingo JR, McIntyre B, Ho IK: Antidotal efficacy of alpha-ketoglutaric acid and sodium thiosulfate in cyanide poisoning. J Toxicol Clin Toxicol 1995;33:721–724.
69. Isom GE, Johnson JD: Sulphur donors in cyanide intoxication. In: Ballantyne B, Marrs TC, eds: Clinical and Experimental Toxicology of Cyanides. Bristol, England, IOP Publishers, 1987, pp. 414–418.
70. Johnson JD, Conroy WG, Burris KD, Isom GE: Peroxidation of brain lipids following cyanide intoxication in mice. Toxicology 1987;46:21–28.
71. Johnson RP, Mellors JW: Arteriolization of venous blood gases: A clue to the diagnosis of cyanide poisoning. J Emerg Med 1988;6:401–404.
72. Johnson WS, Hall AH, Rumack BH: Cyanide poisoning successfully treated without "therapeutic methemoglobin levels." Am J Emerg Med 1989;7:437–440.
73. Jones AW, Lofgren A, Eklund A: Two fatalities from ingestion of acetonitrile: Limited specificity of analysis by headspace gas chromatography J Anal Toxicol 1992;16:104–106.
74. Kilburn KH: Case report: Profound neurobehavioral deficits in an oil field worker overcome by hydrogen sulfide. Am J Med Sci 1993;303:301–305.
75. Kimura K, Hasegawa M, Matsubara K: A fatal disaster case based on exposure to hydrogen sulfide concentration at the scene. Forensic Sci Int 1994;66:111–116.
76. Kirk MA, Gerace R, Kulig KW: Cyanide and methemoglobin kinetics in smoke inhalation victims treated with the cyanide antidote kit. Ann Emerg Med 1993;22:1413–1418.

77. Krieg A, Saxena K: Cyanide poisoning from metal cleaning solutions. Ann Emerg Med 1987;16:582–584.
78. Kruszyna R, Kruszyna H, Smith RP: Comparison of hydroxylamine, 4-dimethylaminophenol and nitrite protection against cyanide poisoning in mice. Arch Toxicol 1982;49:191–202.
79. Kurt TL: Chemical asphyxiants. In: Rom WN, ed: Environmental and Occupational Medicine, 2nd ed. Boston, Little Brown, 1992, pp. 539–549.
80. Kurt TL, Day LC, Reed WG, Gandy W: Cyanide poisoning from glue-on nail remover. Am J Emerg Med 1991;9: 271–272.
81. Lam de Kort W, Sangster B: Acute intoxications during work. Vet Hum Toxicol 1988;30:9–11.
82. Lambert RJ, Kindler BL, Schaeffer DJ: The efficacy of superactivated charcoal in treating rats exposed to a lethal dose of potassium cyanide. Ann Emerg Med 1988;17: 595–598.
83. Litovitz TL, Clark LR, Soloway RA: 1993 annual report of the American Association of Poison Control Centers Toxic Exposure Surveillance System. Am J Emerg Med 1994;12: 546–584.
84. Litovitz TL, Felberg L, Soloway RA, et al: 1994 annual report of the American Association of Poison Control Centers Toxic Exposure Surveillance System. Am J Emerg Med 1995;13:551–597.
85. Litovitz TL, Felberg L, White S, Klein-Schwartz W: 1995 annual report of the American Association of Poison Control Centers Toxic Exposure Surveillance System. Am J Emerg Med 1996;14:487–537.
86. Litovitz TL, Holm KC, Bailey KM, et al: 1991 annual report of the American Association of Poison Control Centers National Data Collection System. Am J Emerg Med 1992; 10:452–505.
87. Litovitz TL, Holm KC, Clancy C, et al: 1992 annual report of the American Association of Poison Control Centers Toxic Surveillance System. Am J Emerg Med 1993;11:494–555.
88. Litovitz TL, Larkin RF, Myers RAM: Cyanide poisoning treated with hyperbaric oxygen. Am J Emerg Med 1983; 1:94–101.
89. Litovitz TL, Schmitz BF, Holm KC: 1988 annual report of the American Association of Poison Control Centers national data collection system. Am J Emerg Med 1989;7: 495–545.
90. Losek JD, Rock AL, Boldt RR: Cyanide poisoning from a cosmetic nail remover. Pediatrics 1991;88:337–340.
91. Lundquist P, Rammer L, Sorbo B: The role of hydrogen cyanide and carbon monoxide in fire casualties: A prospective study. Forensic Sci Int 1989;43:9–12.
92. Maduh EU, Baskin SI: Protein kinase C modulation of rhodanese-catalyzed conversion of cyanide to thiocyanate. Res Commun Molec Pathol Pharmacol 1994;86:155–173.
93. Maduh EU, Neally EW, Song H, et al: A protein kinase C inhibitor attenuates cyanide toxicity in vivo. Toxicology 1995;100:129–137.
94. Marcus SJ: AAPCC Alert. Jan 4, 1988.
95. Messing B, Storch B: Computer tomography and magnetic resonance imaging in cyanide poisoning. Eur Arch Psych Neurol Sci 1988;237:139–143.
96. Michaelis HC, Clemens C, Kijewski H, et al: Acetonitrile serum concentrations and cyanide blood levels in a case of oral acetonitrile ingestion. J Toxicol Clin Toxicol 1991;29: 447–458.
97. Milby TH: Hydrogen sulfide intoxication. Occup Health 1961;Dec 11:431–437.
98. Moore SJ, Ho IK, Hume AS: Severe hypoxia produced by concomitant intoxication with sublethal doses of cyanide and carbon monoxide. Toxicol Appl Pharmacol 1991;109: 412–420.
99. Moore SJ, Norris JC, Walsh DA, Hume AS: Antidotal use of methemoglobin forming cyanide antagonists in concurrent carbon monoxide/cyanide intoxication. J Pharmacol Exp Ther 1987;242:70–73.
100. Nagler J, Provoost RA, Parizel G: Hydrogen cyanide poisoning: treatment with cobalt EDTA. J Occup Med 1978; 20:414–416.
101. Norris JC, Moore SJ, Hume AS: Synergistic lethality induced by the combination of carbon monoxide and cyanide. Toxicology 1986;40:121–129.
102. Norris JC, Utley WA, Hume AS: Mechanism of antagonizing cyanide-induced lethality by α-ketoglutaric acid. Toxicology 1990;62:275–283.
103. Osbern LN, Crapo RO: A report of toxic exposure to liquid manure. Ann Intern Med 1981;95:312–314.
104. Patel MN, Ardelt BK, Yim GKW, Isom GE: Cyanide induces Ca^{2+}-dependent and -independent release of glutamate from mouse brain slices. Neurosci Lett 1991;131: 42–44.
105. Patel MN, Peoples RW, Yim GKW, Isom GE: Enhancement of NMDA-mediated responses by cyanide. Neurochem Res 1994;19:1319–1323.
106. Patel MN, Yim GKW, Isom GE: *N*-Methyl-*d*-aspartate receptors mediate cyanide-induced cytotoxicity in hippocampal cultures. Neurotoxicology 1993;14:35–40.
107. Peters JW: Hydrogen sulfide poisoning in a hospital setting. JAMA 1981;246:1588–1589.
108. Petrikovics I, Pei L, McGuinn WD, et al: Encapsulation of rhodanese and organic thiosulfonates by mouse erythrocytes. Fund Appl Toxicol 1994;23:70–75.
109. Pitt BR, Radford EP, Gurtner GH, Traystman RJ: Interaction of carbon monoxide and cyanide on cerebral circulation and metabolism. Arch Environ Health 1979;34: 354–359.
110. Porter DW, Neally EW, Baskin SI: In vivo detoxification of cyanide by cystathionase gamma-lyase. Biochem Pharmacol 1996;52:941–944.
111. Rathinavelu A, Sun P, Pavlakovic G, et al: Cyanide induces protein kinase C translocation: Blockade by NMDA antagonists. J Biochem Toxicol 1994;9:235–240.
112. Ravizza A, Carugo D, Cerchlari EL: The treatment of hydrogen sulfide intoxication: Oxygen versus nitrites. Vet Hum Toxicol 1982;24:241–242.
113. Reiffenstein RJ, Hulbert WC, Roth SH: Toxicology of hydrogen sulfide. Annu Rev Pharmacol Toxicol 1992;32: 109–134.
114. Rindone JP, Sloane EP: Cyanide toxicity from sodium mitroprusside: risks and management. Ann Pharmacother 1992;26:515–519.

115. Riou B, Gerard JL, La Rochelle CD, et al: Hemodynamic effects of hydroxocobalamin in conscious dogs. Anesthesiology 1991;74:552–558.
116. Rorison DG, McPherson SJ: Acute toxic inhalations. Emerg Med Clin North Am 1992;10:409–435.
117. Rosenberg NL, Myers JA, Martin WWR: Cyanide-induced parkinsonism: Clinical, MRI, and 6-fluorodopa PET studies. Neurology 1989;39:142–144.
118. Rosenow F, Herholz K, Lanfermann H, et al: Neurological sequelae of cyanide intoxication—The patterns of clinical, magnetic resonance imaging, and positron emission tomography findings. Ann Neurol 1995;38:825–828.
119. Scolnick B, Hamel D, Woolf AD: Successful treatment of life-threatening proprionitrile exposure with sodium nitrite/sodium thiosulfate followed by hyperbaric oxygen. J Occup Med 1993;35:577–580.
120. Shragg TA, Albertson TE, Fisher CJ: Cyanide poisoning after bitter almond ingestion. West J Med 1982;136:65–69.
121. Silverman SH, Purdue GF, Hunt JL, Bost RO: Cyanide toxicity in burned patients. J Trauma 1988;28:171–176.
122. Singh BM, Coles N, Lewis P, et al: The metabolic effects of fatal cyanide poisoning. Postgrad Med J 1989;65:923–925.
123. Skene WG, Norman JN, Smith JA: Effect of hyperbaric oxygen in cyanide poisoning. In: Brown I, Cox B, eds: Proceedings of the Third International Congress on Hyperbaric Oxygen. Washington, DC, National Academy of Sciences, 1966, pp. 705–710.
124. Smilkstein MJ, Bronstein AC, Pickett HM: Hyperbaric oxygen therapy for severe hydrogen sulfide poisoning. J Emerg Med 1985;3:27–30.
125. Smith L, Kruszyna H, Smith RP: The effect of methemoglobin on the inhibition of cytochrome c oxidase by cyanide, sulfide or azide. Biochem Pharmacol 1977;26: 2247–2250.
126. Smith RP, Gosselin RE: Hydrogen sulfide poisoning. J Occup Med 1979;21:93–97.
127. Smith RP, Gosselin RE: Current concepts about the treatment of selected poisonings: Nitrite, cyanide, barium, and quinidine. Annu Rev Pharmacol Toxicol 1976;16:189–199.
128. Smith RP, Kruszyna R, Kruszyna H: Managment of acute sulfide poisoning. Arch Environ Health 1976;31: 166–169.
129. Snyder JW, Safir EF, Summerville GP: Occupational fatality and persistent neurological sequelae after mass exposure to hydrogen sulfide. Am J Emerg Med 1995;13: 199–203.
130. Stine RJ, Slosberg B, Beacham BE: Hydrogen sulfide intoxication: a case report and discussion of treatment. Ann Intern Med 1976;85:756–758.
131. Sun P, Borowitz JL, Kanthasamy AG, et al: Antagonism of cyanide toxicity by isosorbide dinitrate: Possible role of nitric oxide. Toxicology 1995;104:105–111.
132. Swanson-Biearman B, Krenzelok EP, Snyder JW, et al: Successful donation and transplantation of multiple organs from a victim of cyanide poisoning. J Toxicol Clin Toxicol 1993;31:95–99.
133. Tamulinas CB, Nizamani S, Myers M, et al: The effect of blood flow on cyanide metabolism in the isolated perfused rat liver. Fed Proc 1985;44:1796.
134. Ten Eyck RP, Schaerdel AD, Ottinger WE: Stroma-free methemoglobin solution: An effective antidote for acute cyanide poisoning. Am J Emerg Med 1985;3:519–523.
135. Ten Eyck RP, Schaerdel AD, Ottinger WE: Comparison of nitrite treatment and stroma-free methemoglobin solution as antidotes for cyanide poisoning in a rat model. J Toxicol Clin Toxicol 1985–1986;23:477–487.
136. Threshold limit values and biologic exposure indicies for 1990–1991. ACGIH 1990.
137. Trapp WG: Massive cyanide poisoning with recovery: A Boxing Day story. Can Med Assoc J 1970;102:517.
138. Turchen SG, Manoguerra AS, Whitney C: Severe cyanide poisoning from the ingestion of an acetonitrile-containing cosmetic. Am J Emerg Med 1991;9:264–267.
139. Tveldt B, Edland A, Skyberg K: Delayed neuropsychiatric sequelae after acute hydrogen sulfide poisoning: Affection of motor function, memory, vision and hearing. Acta Neurol Scand 1991;84:348–351.
140. Tveldt B, Skyberg K, Aaserud O: Brain damage caused by hydrogen sulfide: A follow-up study of six patients. Am J Ind Med 1991;20:91–101.
141. Uitti RJ, Rajput AH, Ashenhurst EM, Rozdilsky B: Cyanide-induced parkinsonism: A clinicopathologic report. Neurology 1985;35:921–925.
142. van Heijst ANP, Douze JMC, van Kesteren RG, et al: Therapeutic problems in cyanide poisoning. J Toxicol Clin Toxicol 1987;25:383–398.
143. Vesey CJ, Wilson J: Red cells. J Pharm Pharmacol 1978; 30:20–26.
144. Vick JA, Froehlich H: Treatment of cyanide poisoning. Milit Med 1991;156:330–339.
145. Vornov JJ, Tasker RC, Coyle JT: Delayed protection by MK–801 and tetrodotoxin in a rat organotypic hippocampal culture model of ischemia. Stroke 1994;25:457–465.
146. Warenycia MW, Goodwin LR, Benishin CG: Acute hydrogen sulfide poisoning. Demonstration of selective uptake of sulfide by the brainstem by measurement of brain sulfide levels. Biochem Pharmacol 1989;38:973–981.
147. Wasch HH, Estrin WJ, Yip P: Prolongation of the P–300 latency asociated with hydrogen sulfide exposure. Arch Neurol 1989;46:902–904.
148. Way JL: Cyanide intoxication and its mechanism of antagonism. Annu Rev Pharmacol Toxicol 1984;24:451–481.
149. Way JL, End E, Sheehy MH, et al: Effect of oxygen on cyanide intoxication. IV. Hyperbaric oxygen. Toxicol Appl Pharmacol 1972;22:415–421.
150. Weger NP: Treatment of cyanide poisoning with 4-dimethylaminophenol (DMAP): Experimental and clinical overview. Middle East J Anesth 1990;10:389–412.
151. Weiss LD, Van Meter KW: The applications of hyperbaric oxygen therapy in emergency medicine. Am J Emerg Med 1992;10:558–569.
152. Wesson DE, Foley R, Sabatini S, et al: Treatment of acute cyanide intoxication with hemodialysis. Am J Nephrol 1985;5:121–126.
153. Whitcraft DD, Bailey TD, Hart GB: Hydrogen sulfide poisoning treated with hyperbaric oxygen. J Emerg Med 1985;3:23–25.
154. Wilson J: Cyanide in human disease: A review of clinical and laboratory evidence. Fund Appl Toxicol 1983;3: 397–399.

ANTIDOTES IN DEPTH

Cyanide Antidotes

Cynthia K. Aaron

Cyanide is a potent intracellular poison by virtue of its affinity for the ferric form (Fe^{3+}) of many necessary enzymes including cytochrome oxidase, succinic dehydrogenase, superoxide dismutase, and others. Cyanide poisoning decreases oxygen utilization by the tissues and, if left untreated, will result in profound tissue hypoxia, acidosis, and death. For this reason, prompt recognition and treatment with the appropriate antidotes are essential.

Cyanide poisoning may result from industrial exposures (fumigation, photographic chemicals, metallurgy, electroplating, organic synthesis, fertilizers) or plant and seed ingestion,[19] Laetrile ingestion,[5,18] or iatrogenic administration (nitroprusside infusions).[16] The signs and symptoms of acute cyanide poisoning should be considered under the appropriate conditions when the patient has a continued altered mental status and acidosis. This includes a history of ingestion, nitrile exposure, or prolonged nitroprusside administration. Laboratory findings consistently demonstrate a high-anion-gap metabolic acidosis that does not improve with supportive therapy.

Cyanide poisoning may also result from smoke inhalation after combustion of materials that release hydrogen cyanide upon burning.[20] Examples include polyvinyl chloride in pipes and furniture, some organic materials, and other plastics. Diagnosis may be complicated if the patient has concomitant carbon monoxide and cyanide poisoning. The presumed carbon monoxide–poisoned patient who does not respond to 100% oxygen, has a low arteriovenous oxygen difference, and has been exposed to combustion products should be considered a possible cyanide-intoxicated person as well. Treatment is complicated by the presence of an elevated carboxyhemoglobin level.

Cyanide is believed to exert its toxicity by combining with high affinity to the iron-containing metalloenzymes while in their ferric state. The best understood mechanism involves cytochrome oxidase. Once cyanide has bound to the ferric ion, cellular respiration is halted and toxicity ensues. In the presence of nitrites, hemoglobin is reduced to methemoglobin. The methemoglobin then exerts a higher binding affinity for cyanide than that exerted by the cytochrome oxidase. Subsequently, the cyanide liberated from the cytochrome oxidases binds to methemoglobin to form cyanomethemoglobin. Cyanomethemoglobin, in the presence of sulfurtransferases, catalyzes the attachment of sulfate to cyanide and forms thiocyanate. Cyanide is also converted to thiocyanate by direct complexation with thiosulfate in the presence of sulfurtransferases. This is almost exclusively a one-way reaction and is unlikely to proceed in the reverse direction. The resultant thiocyanate is relatively nontoxic compared to cyanide and is eventually eliminated in the urine.

Administration of nitrites, used to create the methemoglobin, can cause serious impairment of oxygen delivery and oxygen utilization if the patient has an elevated carboxyhemoglobin level. In patients suffering from smoke inhalation, carbon monoxide and cyanide poisoning may coexist; treatment with nitrites may compound the problem.

Cyanide, in the presence of hydroxocobalamin, can complex to form cyanocobalamin (vitamin B_{12}). This is currently under investigation as an alternative therapy for the treatment of cyanide toxicity.

Other therapies for cyanide poisoning include the direct chelation of cyanide with dicobalt EDTA, induction of methemoglobin using the Lilly Antidote Kit, dimethylaminophenol (DMAP), hydroxylamine, or *p*-aminopropriophenone, and directly detoxifying cyanide by conversion to cyanocobalamin with hydroxocobalamin.[8] Other experimental approaches include the intravenous infusion of stroma-free methemoglobin, which directly binds free cyanide.[21,22] Nucleophiles such as alpha-ketoglutarate and dihydroxyacetone bind to cyanide, reducing its availability to cytochrome oxidase, and decrease toxicity in animal models.[14] The addition of a sulfate donor such as thiosulfate may increase the antidotal efficiency of alpha-ketoglutarate.[10] Thiosulfate, cysteine, *N*-acetylcysteine, and other sulfhydryl donors may increase the efficiency of rhodanese in detoxifying cyanomethemoglobin.[1] Thiosulfate has been used successfully by itself without the induction of methemoglobin. Other modalities under investigation include NMDA inhibitors, nitrous oxide, and antioxidant use. Standard gut decontamination with superactivated charcoal, in animal models, may bind cyanide before it can be absorbed.[12]

The only commercially available Food and Drug Administration–approved antidote in the United States is the Lilly Cyanide Kit. It contains three components: amyl nitrite pearls, a solution of 3% sodium nitrite, and 25% sodium thiosulfate. The kit has a short shelf life due to the expiration of the amyl nitrite pearls. In acute overdose, without IV access, the amyl nitrite pearls should be broken into a gauze sponge for the patient to inhale 30 seconds of each minute. In the intubated patient without IV access, the gauze can be held between the oxygen source and the endotracheal tube placed in the reservoir of an ambu bag. Enriched oxygen should be provided as soon as possible. Once IV access is obtained, sodium nitrite (10 mL of the 3% solution in the adult and 0.33 mL/kg in a child)[3] is given IV over 2–4 minutes, preferably diluted into 100–150 mL of solution. The dose must be corrected downward for children and if the patient is known to be anemic (see Table 97–2). The sodium nitrite theoretically produces a methemoglobin level of 30%. Sodium nitrite may be repeated at half the initial dose, if there is no response within 30 minutes. After the nitrite, sodium thiosulfate (50 mL of a 25% solution in an adult or 1.65 mL/kg in a child) is administered. Vasopressors may be necessary since nitrites cause vasodilation and hypotension.

Dicobalt EDTA (Kelocyanor) is an antidote currently used in Europe but not available in the United States.[9] It functions by chelating cyanide after which the complex is renally excreted. Kelocyanor is equally effective to the Lilly Kit in humans but has different side effects,[2,9,13] The initial dose is 300–600 mg given IV over 2–5 minutes. A repeat dose of 300 mg can be given if there is no clinical improvement. There is no established pediatric dose. The manufacturer suggests following the dicobalt EDTA with a dextrose infusion. Adverse effects of the antidote itself are tachypnea, cardiovascular and hemodynamic instability, seizures, gastrointestinal symptoms, angioedema, and other allergic manifestations. The advantages of dicobalt EDTA are rapid administration, rapid onset of action, effectiveness when given late in the course of the poisoning, and lack of methemoglobin formation. The antidote is not approved by the FDA for use in the United States.

Hydroxocobalamin/thiosulfate has been designated an orphan drug and is in clinical trials in the United States. It is available in France. Hydroxocobalamin (vitamin B_{12a}) loses a hydroxyl group and binds the cyanyl group from the cyanide, forming cyanocobalamin (vitamin B_{12}).[6,15,17] Cyanocobalamin is nontoxic and is renally excreted.[6] Like methemoglobin, the cyanocobalamin has a higher affinity for cyanide than the cytochrome oxidase. Approximately 50 g of hydroxocobalamin are required to bind 1 g of absorbed cyanide. Hydroxocobalamin has the ability to pass through the blood–brain barrier and directly effect central nervous system detoxification. Thiosulfate has been added to the study protocol based on the theory that cyanocobalamin may give up its cyanide to rhodanese, which then converts the cyanide to thiocyanate and regenerates the hydroxocobalamin. The initial reaction of hydroxocobalamin is rapid, whereas the rhodanese-catalyzed reaction is much slower. The addition of the thiosulfate appears to be synergistic and allows the use of less hydroxocobalmin. The current protocol calls for the infusion of 4 g hydroxocobalamin followed by 8 g of thiosulfate. Adverse reactions include a reddish discoloration of the skin and urine, anaphylactoid reactions, and other allergic phenomena.[4,8,11]

Cyanide poisoning may also result from prolonged sodium nitroprusside (SNP) infusions or SNP given to patients with renal failure. The released cyanide is transulfurated to form thiocyanate, which is then renally excreted. Thiosulfate is required to complete this transulfuration and the human body usually has adequate stores for short-term detoxification. Once thiosulfate is depleted, tissue cyanide levels increase, resulting in the diverse manifestations of cyanide toxicity. Initially there is an increase in heart rate and blood pressure, followed by hypotension and bradycardia. The patient may develop cardiac dysrhythmias and an anion-gap metabolic acidosis.[7] Patients may develop disoriention, confusion, seizures, or coma.[7]

Since the rate-limiting step in this reaction is thiosulfate availability, the provision of thiosulfate in the SNP infusion can prevent cyanide toxicity. The suggested dose is 1 g sodium thiosulfate added to each 100 mg of SNP. This mixture is stable for 7 days if protected from light. Patients may, however, develop sodium thiocyanate toxicity after prolonged (>7 days with normal renal function and 1–2 days in renal failure) SNP plus thiosulfate infusions. Treatment for thiocyanate toxicity is to discontinue the infusion and, if necessary, institute hemodialysis.[7]

References

1. Appel KE, Peter H, Bolt HM: Effect of potential antidotes on the acute toxicity of acrylonitrile. Int Arch Occup Environ Health 1981;49:157–163.
2. Bain JT, Knowles EL: Successful treatment of cyanide poisoning. Br Med J 1967;2:763.
3. Berlin CM: The treatment of cyanide poisoning in children. Pediatrics 1970;46:469–493.
4. Bismuth FC, Baud FJ, Djeghout H, et al: Cyanide poisoning from proprionitrile exposure. J Emerg Med 1987;5:191–195.
5. Braico KT, Humberg JR, Terplum KL, et al: Laetrile intoxication: Report of a fatal case. N Engl J Med 1979;300:238–240.
6. Cottrell JE, Casthely P, Brodie JD, et al: Prevention of nitroprusside-induced cyanide toxicity with hydroxocobalamin. N Engl J Med 1978;298:809–811.
7. Curry SC, Arnold-Capell P: Nitroprusside, nitroglycerine, and angiotensin-converting enzyme inhibitors. Crit Care Clin 1991;7:555–580.
8 Hall AH, Rumack BH: Hydroxocobalamin/sodium thiosulfate as a cyanide antidote. J Emerg Med 51987;115–121.
9. Hillman B, Bardhan KD, Bain JTB: The use of dicobalt edetate (Kelocyanor) in cyanide poisoning. Postgrad Med J 1974;50:171–174.
10. Hume AS, Mozingo JR, McIntyre B, Ho IK: Antidotal efficacy of alpha-ketoglutaric acid and sodium thiosulfate in cyanide poisoning. J Toxicol Clin Toxicol 1995;33:721–724.
11. Investigator's Brochure: Hydroxocobalamin/sodium thiosulfate cyanide antidote kit. Rocky Moutain Poison and Drug Center, personal communication.
12. Lambert RJ, Kindler BL, Schaeffer DJ: The efficacy of superactivated charcoal in treating rats exposed to a lethal oral

dose of potassium cyanide. Ann Emerg Med 1988;17: 595–598.
13. Naughton M: Acute cyanide poisoning. Anesth Intensive Care 1974;4:351–356.
14. Niknahad H, O'Brien PJ: Antidotal effect of dihydroxyacetone against cyanide toxicity in vivo. Toxicol Appl Pharmacol 1996;138:186–191.
15. Posner MA, Tobey RE, McElroy H: Hydroxocobalamin therapy of cyanide intoxication in guinea pigs. Anesthesiology 1976;44:330–335.
16. Posner MA, Rodman GH, Klick JM, et al: Cyanide production during nitroprusside therapy in an oliguric patient. Anesth Analg 1977;56:729–731.
17. Rose CL, Worth RM, Chen KK: Hydroxocobalamin and acute cyanide poisoning in dogs. Life Sci 1965;4:1785–1789.
18. Sadoff L, Fuchs K, Hollander J: Rapid death associated with Laetrile ingestion. JAMA 1978;239:1532.
19. Sayre JW, Kaymakeatan S: Cyanide poisoning from apricot seeds among children in central Turkey. N Engl J Med 1964;270:1113–1115.
20. Symington IS, Anderson RA, Oliver JS: Cyanide exposures in fires. Lancet 1987;2:91–92.
21. TenEyck RP, Schaerdel AD, Lynett JE, et al: Stroma-free methemoglobin solution as an antidote for cyanide poisoning: A preliminary study. J Toxicol Clin Toxicol 1983–1984; 21:343–358.
22. Ten Eyck RP, Schaerdel AD, Ottinger WE: Comparison of nitrate treatment and stroma-free methemoglobin solution as antidotes for cyanide poisoning in a rat model. J Toxicol Clin Toxicol 1985–1986;23:477–487.

CHAPTER 98

Radiation

Donald J. Pizzarello

Because emergencies involving ionizing radiation exposure are uncommon events and because there are many misconceptions about ionizing radiation and its affects on humans, there is, in the population, considerable fear of and confusion about the hazards of radiation exposure. Health professionals are no exception to this generalization. Instruction about the risks of radiation exposure are not part of the curriculum of most medical or nursing schools, and except for residents in diagnostic and therapeutic radiology, not part of the training in postgraduate medicine either. The experience with radiation for most emergency department personnel is usually limited to a nodding acquaintance with diagnostic x-ray equipment situated in the suite but generally operated in sequestered, shielded areas by specially trained professionals.

In response to the news that a potentially irradiated patient is on his way to or has appeared in an emergency department, it would not be surprising if personnel imagined such a patient presents a hazard, maybe even a serious hazard, to workers and patients in the area. They might wonder about how to protect themselves and patients from that hazard.

Questions such as these might arise. How close to the patient may attendants approach? Should the area be evacuated? Should the patient that has presented himself be isolated and attended to in a separate area? What kind of area is suitable? Should the patient on his way to the hospital be made to remain in the vehicle in which he is being carried until it can be determined how dangerous he is? How can it be determined how dangerous he is? Have the people in the vehicle with the presumably exposed person been injured because of proximity to the patient, and if so, what should be done for them upon their arrival at the emergency department?

A related set of concerns might arise as well. Is special equipment needed to handle and treat people involved in radiation incidents? What kind of equipment would it be, and where would it be found? Are there governmental or public health agencies that must or should be notified about the incident, and which ones are they?

To begin answering some of these questions it is well to start with a brief, general description and definition of the radiations under discussion in this chapter. Radiation is a general term and can be defined as energy emanating or being irradiated from a source. In this sense, heat from a fire, sound from a vibrating guitar string, light from the filament in an incandescent lamp, and radio waves from a broadcasting apparatus are all radiations. These, and others like them, are known as non-ionizing radiations and, with the exception of damage to hearing done by very loud sounds and the carcinogenic action of ultraviolet radiation, the mechanism through which most non-ionizing radiations cause biologic damage is the production of heat.

Ultraviolet radiations produce skin burns (sunburn); heat from fire, hot liquids, or other hot objects can burn tissue; ultrasound and radio frequency (microwaves) radiations produce heat in tissue that can result in damage. Heat produced by non-ionizing radiations can also be used for benefit. Diathermy, hyperthermia used in cancer therapy, and cooking with microwaves are a few examples.

The body, however, has quite efficient means of carrying off heat. Unless exposure to non-ionizing radiations produces so much heat that it overwhelms the body's capacity to dissipate it, there will be no damage. Heat damage caused by non-ionizing radiations occurs only after some threshold amount of these radiations is absorbed in the body. That threshold is crossed when more heat is produced than can be dissipated, heat builds up, and burns occur.

The carcinogenic action of ultraviolet radiations occurs through the interaction of ultraviolet radiations and DNA of skin cells, a mechanism separate from the skin-burning action of ultraviolet. This form of damage is, unfortunately, not treatable. It should be noted that the carcinogenic action of ultraviolet radiation exposure is, in normal circumstances, confined to cells of skin. The reason is that ultraviolet is not very energetic and cannot penetrate the body more deeply than the skin.

As can be inferred from the foregoing, injuries that might be brought to the emergency department produced by exposure to non-ionizing radiations are neither special nor unique. Most (except for very loud sounds) are burns and the treatment required well-known. For that reason the injuries caused by non-ionizing radiations are beyond the purview of this chapter and dealt with elsewhere.

The kind of radiations under consideration in this chapter are *ionizing* radiations. (Table 98–1 gives a listing of types, characteristics, and sources of some common ionizing radiations.) They are energy irradiated from the two major regions of atoms: atomic nuclei and atomic orbits. They include X rays, which are irradiated from atomic orbits, gamma rays, and other energetic emissions such as alpha particles, protons, neutrons, and electrons, irradiated from nuclei of radioactive atoms. When ionizing radiations pass through cells (human cells included), they disrupt the atoms in those cells in such a way as to ionize them. The process of ionization of atoms in cells caused by ionizing radiations may begin a chain of events that results in radiation damage.

It should be stressed, however, that exposure of living beings, including humans, to ionizing radiations is neither new, exceptional, nor, for that matter, necessarily dangerous. The introduction of ionizing radiation into the public consciousness by such horrific events as the atomic bombing of Hiroshima and Nagasaki and their terrible sequelae and the burning of the power reactor at Chernobyl has led to the perception on the part of many of radiation exposure as new, unnatural, and very hazardous. Without question the atomic bombings killed and injured many people, but most of this was due, not to radiation, but to fire, heat, and blast pressure generated by the bombs. At Chernobyl most injuries among the workers were the result of the fire; few were from radiation. The fallout over the Earth from the smoke raised by the Chernobyl fire contained radioactive materials and certainly people were contaminated by them. The results of that contamination will not be positively known for years, but it is unlikely that, except for those remaining near the reactor site, many detectable effects will be observed.

TABLE 98–1. SOURCES AND CHARACTERISTICS OF SOME IONIZING RADIATIONS

Radiation	Characteristics	Sources
Gamma rays	Electromagnetic (energy only, no mass or charge)	Radioactive decay
X rays	Electromagnetic	X-ray machines, radioactive decay
Beta radiation	Negative electron, particle, charge −1	Radioactive decay
	Positive electron, particle, charge +1	Radioactive decay
Alpha radiation	Doubly ionized helium, particle, charge +2	Radioactive decay of heavy, natural atoms
Protons	Hydrogen nuclei, particle, charge +1	Cosmic radiation, cyclotrons
Negative pi-mesons	Particle, variable mass, charge −1	Cosmic radiation
Neutrons	Particle, no charge	Nuclear reactors, cyclotrons, atomic bombs

The fact is that exposure to ionizing radiation is an entirely natural phenomenon. Everything on earth, living things included, is and always has been constantly irradiated. The source is the "natural background." Background radiation has three components: (1) radiations reaching Earth from outer space, the cosmos, called "cosmic radiation," (2) radiations emanating from naturally radioactive materials in the Earth's crust, "terrestrial radiation," and (3) radioactive materials within the bodies of living things. The latter is the result of the fact that plant life extracts and incorporates into itself nutrient from soil, part of which consists of radioactive elements. Plants are radioactive. Animals, including humans, eat plants and some eat other animals as well, ultimately ingesting the radioactive elements taken up by plants. In addition, there is radioactive carbon in the atmosphere. Plants fix it during photosynthesis and organisms that eat plants incorporate it. Animals, including humans, each and every one of us, are also radioactive.

Radiations from the background pass through cells of the body and could, as suggested above, disrupt atoms in those cells and ionize them. Those ionizations could lead to a chain of events that would end in damage, and, in fact, in rare instances probably do so. However, most of these ionizations have a nearly infinitely small probability of causing damage, because living matter has evolved mechanisms to protect against radiation injury (the section on the mechanisms of production of radiation damage will discuss this further). Even a moment's reflection will show this not only to be true but even to have been necessary. If there were no natural mechanisms to protect against radiation damage, it would have been very difficult for life to have evolved the complex forms it now assumes. Evolution depends on the ability to survive and adapt, accumulate a record of the past, keep what is beneficial, discard what is not. If primitive living molecules were in clear, constant, and present danger of annihilation by interaction with background radiations, the ability to accumulate a record, build on it, and adapt would be greatly impaired, and the momentum of evolution would have been slowed, perhaps nearly to the point of nonexistence.

Exposure to radiation per se, therefore, is not necessarily risky. Exposure to small amounts of radiation carries very little risk, because, among other factors elucidated in the section on mechanisms of production of radiation damage, the natural protective mechanisms are present to minimize that. Exposure to large amounts can present a hazard, because the natural defense is overwhelmed. However, the probability that people will be exposed to large doses through either unintentional or deliberate exposure is very small, indeed. Very few people have access to any radiation source at all. Most who do are people occupationally exposed and they have significant safety precautions in force that greatly reduce the chance of any except extremely small exposures.

When people are exposed to radiation and make their way to an emergency department, the overwhelming likelihood is that they will have had a very small exposure simply because it is nearly impossible to get a large one. There are several corollaries. Since their exposure is small, the risk of damage is also small. Since their exposure is small, the risk to emergency department personnel is small to nonexistent. Finally, since their exposure is small, the effects it might produce in them are generally (1) untreatable and (2) not likely to be manifest for many years, if ever.

How Is Radiation Dose Defined?

One of the important determinants of the degree of risk, kinds, seriousness, and treatability of injuries sustained by people exposed to radiation is the size of the radiation exposure and the amount of radiation energy absorbed in the body from that exposure (the dose). The word "dose," such as the dose of antibiotic appropriate to treat a particular infection or a dose of analgesic needed to control a particular level of pain, usually has a therapeutic connotation. Doses of drugs generally are administered according to a physician's prescription or, over the counter, in quantities deemed by experts effective but not harmful. Where ionizing radiation exposure is concerned, the word "dose" may be used differently. As part of a regimen of radiation therapy a physician does prescribe a particular dose of radiation to treat a particular cancer or a particular dose of radiation to alleviate pain and other symptoms of a cancer. In radiation therapy radiation "dose" has therapeutic meaning. However, in fields using or concerned with ionizing radiation other than radiation therapy, "dose" is used in connection with radiation exposure even when no therapy is involved. The radiation dose from background radiation, the dose from radiodiagnostic studies, even the dose from unintentional exposures—none of which is prescribed by a physician or has anything to do with therapy—are nonetheless called "doses." *Dose* has simply come to mean the amount of radiation to which an individual or object has been or is going to be exposed and/or the amount of radiation energy absorbed in a body or object during exposure to radiation.

There is a difference between exposure of a body or object to ionizing radiation and absorption of radiation energy within the exposed body or object. The amount of radiation to which a body or object is exposed, the amount emitted from a source and falling upon the body or object, is given in units called roentgens (abbreviated R). Thus, as an illustration, it may be said that the exposure from a particular X-ray machine at a particular distance from the X-ray generating tube in the machine is a particular number of roentgens per unit of time. That means a person standing at that distance from an X-ray machine for a certain time would be exposed, on the skin, to a particular number of roentgens of X rays. Similarly, a shipment of radioactive materials sent, for instance, to a hospital or research laboratory will have printed on the outside of its container the number of roentgens emitted per unit of time at the surface of the container or at a given distance from the surface of the container. People handling the shipment know from this how much radiation is being emitted from the box in any given unit of time and what their exposure will be.

However, the radiation energy that does harm is not the amount of radiation energy to which a person is exposed, but the fraction of exposed radiation energy absorbed in the body. A person standing in a beam of X rays may be exposed on the skin to a certain number of roentgens, and those radiations will enter his or her body. Some of the radiations will be absorbed in the body, but some will pass through. Radiations that pass through cannot do any harm. Only absorbed radiation energy has any probability of causing damage.

Absorbed radiation energy is expressed in units called rads (standing for *r*adiation *a*bsorbed *d*ose) or gray. One rad is equal to 100 ergs of radiation energy absorbed in a gram of matter (100 ergs/g equals one rad). One gray (abbreviated Gy) is equal to 100 rads. In the United States, rads are generally used to quantify the relatively small absorbed doses from diagnostic radiologic studies, from the background, and from deliberate or unintentional exposures. (See Table 98–2 for some general dose ranges resulting from background radiation and common diagnostic studies.) Gray are used to quantify the much larger absorbed doses from therapeutic radiation regimens. In Europe and other places, gray is used without regard to size of dose and rads have fallen into disuse. In this chapter, in conformity with the

TABLE 98–2. DOSE RANGES FROM BACKGROUND RADIATION AND COMMON DIAGNOSTIC STUDIES

Source	Dose[a]
Natural background (USA)	100 millirem/y total body, lungs up to 350 millirem/y depending on radon contribution (varies geographically)
Chest radiographic examination (PA and lateral plain films)	60 millirads in the collimated field[b]
Plain films of the body (eg, abdominal examination)	100–500 millirads in the collimated field[b]
Head CT	1–2 rads per slice[c]?
Body CT	1 rad per slice[c]
Flouroscopy	5 rads/min
Diagnostic nuclear medicine texts	Roughly 1 rad, total body

[a]These doses are approximations and vary according to body size, equipment, and operator.
[b]These are skin-entry doses. As described in the text, dose at depth in the body will be less.
[c]Dose is more or less the same throughout the slice. The dose per examination is about the same as the dose per slice, not the sum of all slices.

United States convention, rads will be used for most doses.

As a beam of radiations passes through a body or object, at every point along its way some of the radiations in the beam are absorbed and fewer remain; the beam is, in other words, attenuated as a function of distance of penetration. A person standing at a given distance from an X-ray machine will have the skin of the part of the body nearest the source of X rays exposed to a certain number of roentgens of radiation energy. As the beam enters and passes through the body, radiations will be absorbed by the body and the absorbed energy will be expressed in rads. At every point along the path of the X-ray beam, in every gram of tissue more and more distant from the skin surface through which the radiations entered the body, fewer and fewer X rays will be available for absorption, and therefore less and less energy absorbed. The absorbed dose (the number of rads) will drop as a function of distance from the skin surface through which the radiations entered the body. Absorbed radiation dose, therefore, can be measured and determined only at a point; that is, within given grams of tissue at particular locations in an exposed body. There is no single radiation dose from many radiation exposures, only a range of doses, the greatest being at the surface of the body through which the radiation enters, the least at the surface of the body through which the radiation leaves and a different dose in every gram of tissue between. In the instance where the whole body or a part of the body (as in computed tomography) is exposed uniformly from an external radiation source or sources, a single dose may describe reasonably well the amount of energy absorbed in all exposed parts. Also, depending upon metabolism, the ingestion of or injection with certain radioactive materials can result in relatively uniform distribution of radiation throughout the body so that all parts receive about the same dose. An example would be the distribution in the body of phosphorus-32, a radioactive isotope of phosphorus, as phosphate, or tritium, a radioactive isotope of hydrogen, as water. If eaten, drunk or injected, these materials distribute themselves more or less uniformly in the body and the absorbed radiation dose is essentially the same anywhere in the body.

As the foregoing suggests, the estimation of dose from external sources of radiation exposure is a complex matter. For simplicity's sake, the dose from diagnostic X-ray examinations or from deliberate or unintentional exposures is usually given as "the skin entry dose." The dose to tissues beneath will be less, of course, but assuming the dose to the body to be the same as the skin entry dose will overstate somewhat the dose and yield a worse-case scenario.

An exception to the convention of using skin entry dose to estimate body dose is mammography. Since, in breast, the tissue of interest and concern is ductile, mammographic dose is usually calculate as an average to ductile tissue.

Other important units are the rem (standing for *r*ad *e*quivalent *m*an) and the sievert (abbreviated Sv). These units were devised to take into account the following phenomenon. Not all radiations produce the same effects or the same level of effect with the same efficiency. That is to say, the same absorbed dose of energy (the same number of rads or Gray) absorbed from different radiations may produce different levels of effects or damage. A given number of rads of X rays, for example, produces less biologic damage (therefore carries lesser risk) than the same number of rads of alpha rays even when all other conditions are equal. Knowledge of radiation dose alone, then, may not allow the prediction of the degree of damage that radiation will do without also knowing what the radiation is and its efficiency for the production of particular radiation effects. The rem and sievert permit this.

In computing the rem, X rays have been chosen as a standard radiation and all other radiations are compared to them with respect to their efficiency or effectiveness for production of damage. The rem may be defined as follows: the dose of a radiation that produces damage *equivalent to* one rad of X rays is equal to one rem. An illustration will help. In a purely hypothetical situation suppose that it is found, experimentally, that 100 rads of X rays produces mutations in 10% of a population of a particular type of cell growing in tissue culture. It is further found that only 80 rads of alpha rays produce mutations in 10% of identical cells growing in tissue culture under identical conditions. Clearly, alpha rays are more effective at producing mutations in this cell type than are X rays, because a smaller dose produces an equivalent percentage. The alpha ray dose needed to produce this effect (80 rads) is, therefore, one rem.

It should be pointed out that the efficiency of various radiations for producing effects may differ according to the effect and to the organism that is undergoing radiation. The rem dose of the same kind of radiation may differ from tissue to tissue in the same body and from species to species.

The rem is quite useful when comparing the effect of various radiations and for expressing damage from exposure to a mixture of radiations. As examples, the dose received from background radiation is almost always given in rem, because background is a mixture of radiations; some radioactive isotopes emit more than one kind of radiation (iodine-131 emits beta and gamma radiations). People who ingest, inhale, or are injected with iodine-131 receive a mixture of radiations and their dose is best described in rem.

Another unit useful to be acquainted with is the curie. The unit defines the number of atoms undergoing radioactive disintegration, and, correspondingly, the number of radiations being emitted in given time intervals from radioactive elements. It is based on the radioactive decay rate of radium and is defined as follows: one curie is equal to 3.7×10^{10} disintegrations per second. That means, in 1 second, 3.7×10^{10} atoms are undergoing radioactive decay and emitting from a source as many ionizing radiations. (The curie is often subdivided in decimals, milli, micro, nano, and picacuries.) The curie says nothing about the kind of radiations being emitted, the type or energy, whether or not they penetrate deeply into the body, or the degree to which they are destructive. It simply tells how radioactive a source is, how much radiation is being emitted over time.

What Are the Mechanisms of Radiation Injury?

An understanding of the mechanisms by which ionizing radiations produce biologic damage elucidates the nature of radiation injuries, what might happen to people in the wake of radiation exposure, and how to treat exposed people.

Categories of Radiation Injury

Radiation injuries may be categorized according to various parameters, but a convenient classification from the point of view of mechanisms of radiation injury is stochastic and nonstochastic or deterministic.

The word *stochastic* carries the implication of randomness, which is an important property of the energy exchange between ionizing radiations and matter. Since, by definition, all ionizing radiations have enough energy to cause ionizations, they interact in living material in a random way. Any atom or molecule with which they properly interact and to which they transfer enough energy will be ionized.

The concept stochastic relates to exposure to ionizing radiation in the following way. (1) Stochastic effects occur without a threshold dose; that is, there is no dose of ionizing radiation so small that it has no probability of producing these effects in an exposed population. Therefore, any dose, irrespective of size and including the background, has some probability of producing the effect in some proportion of an exposed population. (2) The greater the dose of radiation to which a population is exposed, the greater the proportion of the population in which stochastic effects will occur. (3) Although the proportion of the population that is affected increases as the radiation dose is increased, the severity of the effects does not increase.

Carcinogenesis is presumed to be a stochastic effect of ionizing radiation. *Presumably,* there is no dose of ionizing radiation so small that it has no probability of causing cancer in some proportion of an exposed population. The greater the dose of radiation to which a population is exposed, the greater the proportion of the population that is expected to get cancer. However, the severity of the cancers produced is independent of dose. Low doses do not produce mild or weak cancers and high doses severe ones. The same kinds of cancers are produced by any dose, but the numbers increase with increasing dose.

The above makes it plain that any exposure to ionizing radiation has some probability of carrying some risk to some members of an irradiated population. What may be less obvious is that, since the energy exchange that causes the lesions leading to stochastic effects (damage to DNA) occurs at random, the effects themselves will also occur at random. The proportion of the population that will be affected from given radiation doses may eventually be accurately known, but which of the members of the population will be affected cannot be known, because the effects result from randomly occurring events.

People who have been exposed to radiation or believe they have often ask whether the radiation has hurt them. Emergency department personnel asked this question cannot give complete assurance to the patient one way or the other. Patients can be told the best estimates of risk, but they cannot be told either that they certainly will be adversely affected or that they certainly will not be adversely affected, because of the random nature of radiation injury.

Nonstochastic or deterministic effects are the opposite of stochastic ones. These effects are not believed to occur except when radiation exposure exceeds some dose characteristic for the effect. Therefore, there is a threshold dose of radiation that must be exceeded in order for them to occur. Examples include bone marrow depression, immune suppression, inhibition of fertility, skin erythema, dry and moist skin desquamation, epilation, gastrointestinal disturbances—effects that are often observed during radiation therapy. The proportion of an exposed population displaying nonstochastic effects increases as the dose, above the threshold, increases. Unlike the stochastic effects, however, the severity of the effects may increase with increasing dose (erythema, dry and moist desquamation is just such a progression).

The mechanisms of production of stochastic and nonstochastic effects differ somewhat. Stochastic effects result from DNA damage and cell killing; nonstochastic or deterministic effects are often secondary to other forms of tissue damage. The stochastic effects of greatest concern to most injured people are mutation in the germ line, which may have impact on children conceived from their irradiated gonads, in somatic cells, which may result in cancer, or on the development of children irradiated during gestation. Stochastic effects are the only injuries anticipated from exposure to small radiation doses and are the ones most commonly expected from most radiation exposures. No one can be certain if they have occurred, but if they have, they are untreatable and, at the current state of knowledge, irreversible.

Nonstochastic effects follow high doses of radiation and often result from massive cell killing or protracted inhibition of mitosis in irradiated tissues. Nonstochastic effects (some examples are given above) are often treatable, although treatment is not always neccessary, with a good expectation of recovery.

Ionization

For either category of effect, the first step is ionization. Biologic damage occurs as a result of a series of events starting at the atomic level and ending at the tissue, organ, or organism level. The first step in this series is ionization, the transfer of sufficient energy from a radiation to an orbital electron of an atom in a cell to eject the electron from the atom. The process results in the production of two ions, the residue of the atom, carrying a positive charge, and the ejected electron, carrying a negative charge. Because, by definition, all ionizing radiations have enough energy to eject orbital electrons from atoms, radiation-produced ionizations in cells occur at random. Since cells consist principally of water (about 70–80% of cells' content is water), it presents the largest cellular target for ionizing radiations; consequently, most radiation-produced ionizations occur in cellular water.

Ions, in general, are unstable and ions produced by radiation interaction are especially unstable. Instability of ions results from electrical imbalance. They have an excess of electrical charge, and this excess gives them a tendency toward some kinds of action, among them, the tendency to react chemically and combine with other atoms or molecules.

When ions are created in cells by ionizing radiations, they may react and combine with other cellular atoms or molecules and form compounds that previously did not exist. The compounds formed may range in importance from innocuous to toxic. Chance plays a great role in what happens, because the ions themselves result from chance interactions of radiation with cellular matter.

Rather than entering into chemical reactions, another possibile course of action for radiation-produced ions in cells is to undergo internal rearrangement and form free radicals. In fact, this is a very frequent occurrence. Free radicals are also unstable, but their instability results not from electrical imbalance (as is the case with ions) but because all free radicals have an electron that is unpaired for spin.

Most people are familiar with the planetary model of the atom in which electrons rotate in an orbit about a central nucleus, much as the planets rotate in orbits about the sun. What is less familiar to some, however, is that, as electrons rotate about the nucleus, they also rotate or spin about their own axes, again, similar to the axial rotation of planets in orbits. Orbital electrons are paired for spin. For each electron in an orbit rotating in one direction, there must be another rotating in the direction opposite. Occasionally, however, a situation will arise where, in an atom or molecule, there is an electron in an orbit that is unpaired for spin; there is no other electron in that orbit rotating in the opposite direction. Entities having a single, unpaired electron are free radicals. Free radicals may or may not be charged (if they are, they are also ions), and examples of uncharged free radicals abound. Hydrogen's single orbital electron is unpaired, but atomic hydrogen is not charged. It has a single proton in its nucleus that neutralizes the electron's negative charge. Similarly, since atomic nitrogen has seven electrons, one must be unpaired. It is a free radical but is not charged, because it has seven protons in its nucleus. Having an unpaired electron is an unstable condition, since in the stable condition, all electrons are paired. To achieve stability free radicals often chemically combine with other atoms or molecules and form new compounds. In cells these compounds, as those formed by the chemical reactions of ions, may range from innocuous to toxic.

Since cells are composed primarily of water and radiation-produced ionization occurs chiefly in cellular water, the free radicals hydrogen and hydroxyl derived from ionized water are the most common ones resulting from radiation exposure.

While most of the ions and free radicals produced in cells during radiation exposure are of cellular water, radiation injury is generally only indirectly the result of the ionization of or free radical formation in water. Water is indisputably of paramount importance to living cells, but individual molecules of water are generally dispensable. Water, in most cells, is present in great excess, and interactions of the ions or free radicals formed from water and the products they form are generally not important in radiation injury. Peroxides can result from ionized water or by the free radicals formed from ionized water, but the number produced, even from relatively high radiation doses, is small and easily detoxified by natural cellular processes.

A fraction of the ions caused by radiation exposure of cellular water or of the free radicals derived from those ions may not form peroxides or other compounds easily detoxified by cellular processes but, instead, chemically react with organic molecules in cells, altering their structure and, presumably, their function. There can be no cellular defense against ionization caused by radiation and, therefore, no defense against damage to organic molecules caused by these ions. However, the amount of cellular damage done this way is believed to be quite small. The reason is that radiation-produced ions are so unstable that most of them convert to free redicals before they have an opportunity to react.

Most radiation damage to organic molecules, however, is done, not by radiation-produced ions, but by radiation-produced free radicals, and there is an excellent cellular defense against this. Over the millenia of evolution, all cells have come to be equipped with molecules that preferentially interact with free radicals. When radiation produces free radicals, these compounds, known as sulfhydryls, molecules consisting of a relatively short amino acid chain, one end of which terminates in sulphur–hydrogen linkage, are highly likely to interact with them and the product produced is harmless. For this reason, sulfhydryls have come to be known as free radical "scavengers" or free radical "mops." The presence of these molecules constitutes a powerful natural protection against ionizing radiation and has almost certainly evolved to protect living things against the potentially damaging effects of natural background radiation. Sulfhydryl scavenging of free radicals is very efficient but not absolute. Some free radicals inevitably escape capture and may interact with organic molecules. When they do, they may change these molecles in such a way that whatever function they are supposed to perform for cells is lost.

The probability that significant numbers of organic molecules will be damaged by radiation exposure is dependent on radiation dose. The greater the radiation dose the more free radicals produced, and the greater the likelihood that some will escape the sulfhydryl defense.

Nearly all organic molecules in cells are present in considerable excess, and the loss of a few of them as a consequence of free radical interactions is probably meaningless. Either their place will be taken by others of the same kind or the cell may synthesize new ones to replace them.

The only organic cellular molecule not present in great excess, however, is DNA. If it is attacked by free radicals and its structure and function altered, then cells may be created that have an abnormal genome, may behave abnormally, and may even die.

The likelihood that the just-described chain of events (ionization, free radical formation, damage to DNA) will occur following exposure to electromagnetic radiation is quite small, especially when the dose is low. The reason is that the chain is much more likely to be broken at any one of its steps than it is to continue to the next step.

Water molecule ions are much more likely to recombine to form water than to go on to become free radicals. Similarly, free radicals are much more likely to recombine than to go on to attack and alter organic molecules. In addition, free radical scavengers remove many of them before they can do harm. DNA is the molecule that must be damaged before permanant cellular radiation injury occurs, but DNA is a rare molecule in cells. If free radicals are to attack organic cellular molecules, they are much more likely to attack some molecule other than DNA, because there are so many other organic molecules and so little DNA. Free radicals that combine with cellular organic molecules other than DNA cannot then go on to damage DNA and the chain is broken.

In most somatic cells much of the genome is turned off, and little of it is active. For that reason free radical attack on DNA is most likely to damage an inactive part of the genome simply because there is more inactive than active DNA. If that happens, the chain is broken.

Finally, unless active DNA in cells that have a reasonable expectation of producing many descendant cells (stem cells) is damaged, there is almost no chance that detectable radiation injury will occur. If the DNA of cells that are fully differentiated or on their way to differentiation is damaged, the result may be a few injured cells, but overwhelmed by the enormous number of normal cells in the body, they should have little impact upon the body.

Stem cells, however, comprise a very small percentage of the total number of cells in the body (some estimates put it at about 1%). Because that is true, the chances that a stem cell capable of producing many progeny will be damaged by radiation are quite small. Damage is much more likely to occur in a cell that will have no impact upon the body, and the chain will be broken.

Damage to DNA and the Mitotic Apparatus

Radiation injury is believed to result from damage to DNA and/or to the mitotic apparatus. In the case of DNA, this may happen either as the result of *direct* ionization of DNA by radiation followed by chemical reactions that change the structure of DNA or, indirectly, by interaction of DNA with free radicals created by radiation that change the structure of DNA. The latter is by far the more common mechanism.

Change in the structure of DNA may result in mutation and, if this happens to cells of the germ line in the gonads, it may have impact upon children conceived by irradiated people. Mutation, at least at the present state of knowledge, is not a reversible event, so this would not be a detectable or treatable injury in the emergency department or anywhere else. It must be stressed, however, that the probability of detectable damage occurring in offspring of irradiated people is very small, especially when the gonadal radiation dose is of the order of a few rads or even a few tens of rads. This would be the expected dose level in many if not most unintended radiation exposures since (1) people most likely to be exposed unintentionally to radiation are those working in an environment in which radiation-generating apparatuses and/or radioactive material are present and (2) the most common working environments in which these things are present are hospitals and research laboratories, where the amounts of radioactive material used and stored are quite small and in which accidental exposure to external sources of radiation (X-ray machines, linear accelerators, radioactive sources used in radiation therapy), unlikely events in the first place, are also apt to be to quite small doses.

Mutation in somatic cells (as opposed to cells of the germ line) may result in cancers years after radiation exposure. These mutations also are irreversible events, undetectable and untreatable. Again, it is worth noting that the risk of cancer following radiation doses in the range in which most unintentional exposures are likely to fall, is very small, of the order of one in a thousand to one in ten thousand, even tens of thousands.

People whose gonads have been exposed to radiation sometimes wonder whether progeny they may conceive after radiation exposure have a risk of cancer later in life. Up to now, no credible study has shown increases in cancer among progeny of people exposed to radiation.[1,2,5,8–12,14,15,20–23]

There is some probability that radiation damage of DNA can result in cell death. In theory, even the smallest dose of radiation kills some cells and it is likely that unintentional exposures, however small, kill cells. The number of cells expected to be killed by small radiation doses, the dose range in which most unintentional exposures are expected to lie, will be very small. With the possible exception of very immature stages of life (early embryonic life through the period of early major organogenesis), the loss of small numbers of cells is undetectable and very likely to be without any impact upon the body. The reason is that human bodies are composed of vast numbers of cells, almost none of which is indispensable. Loss of cells, is a natural phenomenon that occurs constantly thoughout life, and lost cells are replaced by natural processes. Examples include natural cell death (apoptosis) and cells lost to injury or wear and tear (cuts, bruises, skin scrapes, and the like). Lost cells are replaced either from stem cells in tissues and organs (the hematopoietic system, the linings of the intestines and certain glands, and the skin, as examples) or by functional cells that retain reproductive capacity and replace cells lost to natural death or injury (as in the liver).

In early embryonic life, in particular during early organogenesis, the death of a small number of cells potentially carries significance. Since the organism is composed, then, of relatively few cells, most of which are to be ancestors to very large numbers of cells in the adult body, the loss of some may leave too few to form an organism with normal anatomy and/or function. Exposure of women in early pregnancy to radiation may, therefore, carry some risk for the unborn child.

Studies of the effects of radiation on developing embryos and fetuses of lower mammals and human beings, however, reveal no significant increase in intrauterine death, malformation, or mental or growth retardation when fetal or embryonic doses have been below 10 rads or rem.[3] At the risk of being repetitive, it should be stated that, because the population most at risk of unintentional radiation exposures are hospital and research laboratory workers, most unintended exposures of pregnant women to radiation are likely to be doses well below this value. It should be noted that the embryonic or fetal dose is what is important in this instance. If the exposure is from an external source, it may be that embryonic or fetal dose is less than the dose at the mother's skin. The section on radiation dose earlier elucidates this point. Even after higher embryonic or fetal radiation doses, the probability of increases of intrauterine death (abortion), malformation, which may or may not lead to death at or around the time of birth, or retardation of growth with or without anatomic defect is small and only after fetal or embryonic doses of about 100 rads are reached does the probability of such effects become high.[13]

As in the case of adverse genetic mutations leading to detectable effects in progeny or cancer in the irradiated individual, the effects on embryo or fetus resulting from cell killing by radiation are not, at the present state of knowledge, treatable or reversible in the emergency room or elsewhere.

Unintentional radiation exposure is, for reasons already described, most likely to be to low doses and the amount of damage to DNA likely to be small. Even that, in certain types of exposure, is probably lessened by the fact that a fraction of radiation damage done to DNA is often reparable. The ratio of reparable to irreparable DNA damage done by given doses of ionizing radiation is controlled by the kind of radiation involved in the exposure. In general, electromagnetic radiations produce more reparable than irreparable DNA damage per unit of radiation dose than do charged particulate radiations, and when the electromagnetic radiation dose is small, the ratio is even more favorable to fully reparable DNA radiation damage (see Table 98–1). Consequently, even if DNA is damaged by exposure to X and gamma rays, a significant amount of the damage will be repaired, reducing risk of mutation in germ cells that may affect children conceived after radiation exposure, risk of cancer, or effects stemming from cell killing.

We may safely conclude that exposure to small radiation doses (doses up to a few tens of rads) have a very small probability of producing detectable or treatable injury. The person stuck with a needle contaminated with radioactive material or having inhaled or ingested small amounts of radioactive material or an exposure to small doses of X or gamma rays is very unlikely (1) to require any kind of treatment at all, (2) to suffer consequences later in life, or (3) pass on radiation injury to offspring.

Radiation Damage to the Mitotic Apparatus

If sufficient radiation damage is done to the mitotic apparatus, defined here as the chromosomes and mitotic spindle, detectable and potentially treatable injury is possible. Doses of a few hundred rads (200 and above) to the total body or doses of several hundred rads to parts of the body may result in injury, sometimes serious injury.

Chromosomes. Radiation damage to chromosomes may, in proliferative cells, result in cell death. It is believed to be one of the chief mechanisms through which radiation produces injuries that may require emergency treatment.

Radiation-induced chromosomal injuries may be of two kinds: those which result in abnormalities in chromosome number and those which result in abnormalities in chromosome structure.

Abnormalities in Chromosome Number. The diploid number of chromosomes in humans is 46, 44 autosomes and 2 sex chromosomes. All normal somatic cells, except mature red blood cells, must have this number. Mature red blood corpuscles have no nuclei (during maturation of red cells, the nucleus is lost) and, therefore, no chromosomes. During meiosis, the number of chromsomes is halved and resulting germ cells have the haploid number, 23, 22 autosomes and 1 sex chromosome.

Ionizing radiation can injure the mitotic spindle and/or the centromeres of chromosomes (the mitotic apparatus) in such a way that the distribution of chromosomes during cell division (either mitosis or meiosis) is abnormal. When this happens, daughter cells are produced that have too many or too few chromosomes. In somatic cells the condition of having too many or too few chromosomes (called aneuploidy) is almost invariably lethal, and cells inheriting this condition die. In this way, cells are injured during radiation exposure, but may die only if and when they divide. If cells are recruited into division soon after they have been irradiated, death occurs then, but if recruitment into division occurs a long time after irradiation, cell death may not occur for weeks, months, or even years.

Aneuploidy, as alluded to above, is apparently incompatible with life in normal somatic cells, but for some reason, it is very common in cancers. Nearly all cancer cells have abnormalities of chromosome number but, nevertheless, live and multiply. The reasons for this are unknown, yet there seems no question about the fact that abnormality in chromosome number and cancer are closely associated. Some investigators believe that abnormality in chromosome number is one of the causes of cancer but others suggest it may be the result of the changes that take place in transforming normal into malignant cells.

Aneuploidy and survival of germ cells (sperm or ova) are not always incompatible. Germ cells inheriting too few chromosomes seem inevitably to die, but those inheriting an extra chromosome can sometimes live and be successfully involved in conception. The condition of having an extra chromosome is called trisomy and is believed to result from injury to the centromere of chromosomes.

During meiosis, the centromere of a chromsosome may fail to split and, as a result, a whole chromosome fails to be included in the nucleus of one daughter while a doubled chromosome is included in the nucleus of the other. In consequence, instead of having the haploid chromosome number, 23, one cell has 22 and the other, 24. The cell lacking the chromosome usually dies, but the other may survive and become involved in fertilization. At conception it may fuse with a gamete having the haploid number (an aneuploid sperm unites with a normal ovum or the reverse), and a conceptus is formed with 47 chromosomes, one more than the normal diploid number.

In many cases these conceptuses are not viable, but in a few instances they seem to be. If trisomy occurs with chromosome 21 (an autosome), it results in the familiar condition, Down's syndrome. Other syndromes resulting from trisomy of other chromosomes are Klinefelter's and Turner's.

It must be stressed that, while ionizing radiation is known to produce trisomy in experimental animals and cells in tissue culture, there is no known, convincing correlation between any of the syndromes associated with trisomy in humans and radiation exposure.[7] Down's syndrome, the most common human condition associated with trisomy, seems most likely to be the result of accumulated damage to ova, not the result of a single insult or damaging event.

Thus, it seems very unlikely that people exposed to ionizing radiation, even relatively high radiation doses, are in danger of producing children with a syndrome caused by trisomy resulting from the exposure.

Abnormalities of Chromosome Structure. The absorption of energy from ionizing radiation can induce chemical changes in large, organic molecules that can lead to a change in their structure. When this happens in DNA, cross-linking between two DNA molecules or DNA and protein may result or the backbone of the DNA molecule (the sugar–phosphate moiety) may break. These and other structural changes can then lead to changes in and abnormalities of chromosome structure.

Chromosomes may be broken by radiation and, if the broken ends do not heal or if they rejoin inappropriately, aberrant chromosomes may result. Some aberrations do not interfere with cell division and are therefore viable and heritable. The inappropriate sequencing of genes in the genome due to incorrect rejoining of chromosome ends, or the loss of small parts of chromosomes when they are broken and lost when broken ends rejoin, do act, however, as mutations. The aberrant chromosome may not be lethal to the cell that inherits it, but the cell will not be normal either.

Other aberrations, however, do present a block to successful mitosis, and cells in which they occur die if they are recruited into division. As in the case of somatic cells with abnormal numbers of chromosomes, they may die sooner or later after radiation exposure depending on how soon after exposure they divide.

The expression of many kinds of radiation injury may either occur soon after radiation exposure or take several days to weeks before they show up, depending on two factors: (1) the number of cells sustaining lethal chromosomal injury and (2) the probability of recruitment of injured cells into mitosis. The former depends on radiation dose and the latter, the probability of recruitment into division, depends on the nature of the tissue or tissues irradiated. Given that a relatively high radiation dose has been received, in tissues in which there is rapid cell turnover—namely, tissues in which functional cells have a short life and are rapidly replaced—radiation injury will be expressed relatively soon after exposure. That is because the high dose is likely to have injured the chromosomes of many cells in the tissue and the probability of mitosis in injured cells is high. Examples of tissues of this type would be the linings of the intestines, skin, hair follicles, and bone marrow.

Even if a relatively high radiation dose has been received, however, tissue injury may not be seen for a period of time after irradiation if the tissue is one in which there is a low natural cell turnover. In such tissues the life of functional cells is long and they do not need to be replaced very often. In time, functional cells will, owing to natural aging, die. Other cells in the tissue will divide to replace them and those with lethal chromosomal damage will then die. Insufficient numbers of replacements for dying functional cells will be produced and the level of tissue function will then decline. Examples of tissues of this sort are bone, liver, and lung.

The fact that a person who has had radiation exposure and does not display detectable injury does not necessarily mean no injury has occurred. At a later time, a time dependent on radiation dose and tissue irradiated, injury may become patent, a fact health care personnel must know.

Repair of Cellular Radiation Damage. If cells are irradiated and DNA damaged, but the cells not killed, they may repair the damage. This kind of damage is termed sublethal, and what is required to repair it are time and oxygen. Given enough time and adequate oxygen, sublethal damage will be repaired completely and very often correctly.

The amount of time cells need to repair sublethal damage completely is about 6 hours; the amount of oxygen is in the range of normal venous tension, a partial pressure of about 20–40 mm Hg. Repair of sublethal damage is the principal reason for the practice of fractionated radiation therapy. The large radiation doses required to cure cancers, if given in a single, rapid exposure, exceed the radiation tolerance of normal tissues. Patients exposed to such a treatment would develop complications that result from too much killing of normal tissue, and these complications would be at an unacceptable level.

Fractionation of radiation dose, however, gives tissue time to repair cellular damage between each dose fraction and enables quite large radiation doses to be given without unacceptable complication rates. Both normal and cancer tissues repair DNA damage between dose fractions to some extent, but many cancers repair damage less efficiently than does normal tissue. This is due in part to the fact that regions of many cancers, carcinomas, in particular, have an inadequate oxygen supply and in part to less efficient enzymatic repair mechanisms in some cancer cells. The unequal rates of sublethal damage repair give an advantage to normal tissue. Between dose fractions it repairs damage more efficiently and to a greater extent than do cancers. Radiation damage accumulates in cancer cells and, during a radiation therapy regimen, more of them are killed. The therapy results in great reduction in cancer cell number and cancer size, and, in ideal circumstances, cure of the cancer without unacceptable levels of normal tissue damage.

While repair of sublethal DNA radiation damage does commonly occur, the repaired molecule may not always be identical to what it was before damage. The changed form is a mutation.

Many forms of chromosome damage are also reparable. For every observable chromosome break caused by irradiation, there were probably many more that healed. Some estimate that about 90% of chromosome breaks heal. This is because broken chromosome threads exhibit great powers of adhesion, and when breaks occur, the tendency is for broken ends to come together and stick to each other, a process known as "restitution." During the interfraction interval in radiation therapy regimens, chromosome breaks are usually repaired. However, as mentioned in the preceding section, it occasionally happens that repair is incorrect and healed chromosomes may differ from normal. These structural rearrangements can lead to cell death during cell division.

Chromosome breaks, restitution, and structural rearrangements probably occur with approximately equal frequency in normal and cancer cells. However, the more rapid cell division in cancers compared to most normal tissues leads to greater numbers of cancer cells dying because of aberrant chromosomes than those of normal tissue. This also leads to an advantage for normal tissue.

Intrastitial radiation therapy for cancers is not fractionated. A radioactive source (or number of sources) is implanted in cancers and the cancer is continuously irradiated at a relatively low dose rate. The advantage for normal tissue in this instance is that the sources are placed in such a way that the cancer receives substantially more radiation than surrounding normal tissue.

Intracavitary radiation therapy may also not be fractionated. In this technique a source of radiation is placed in a body cavity (the body of the uterus, for example) next to a cancer and the cancer is continuously irradiated at a low dose rate for as long as the source is present. Again, the advantage for normal tissue stems from dose distribution; the cancer is given substantially more than surrounding normal tissue.

Recently, a form of intracavitary radiation therapy has been introduced that is fractionated. In this technique a source of radiation that emits its radiations at a high rate is placed in a body cavity next to a cancer. The tissue is irradiated at a high rate for a short time and the source removed. The procedure is repeated at intervals until the prescribed dose is given.

This latter technique spares the patient the discomfort of the presence of an intracavitary device for long periods and other inconveniences attendant on having a source of radiation in the body over several days. It is not clear, yet, whether the newer method will have side effects that may offset its presumed advantages.

What Are the Types of Radiation Injury and What Is Their Relationship to Dose?

Low Doses

When the dose of radiation is low, in the dose range of up to about 150 rads, there is little likelihood of physical symptoms and essentially no likelihood of treatable injury. Some people experience some nausea at doses under 150 rads, but the symptom is transient and rarely very severe. The fact that no injury is noticeable does not mean nothing at all may have happened. Exposures in this dose range carry some risk of stochastic effect, which include (1) mutations in cells in the gonads, which may result in effects in the next and future generations, (2) mutations in somatic cells that result in the production of cancers, and (3) effects on babies irradiated in utero, during their mothers' pregnancy.

Unfortunately, at the current state of knowledge, no way is known of preventing or reversing stochastic effects such as radiogenic mutations, radiation-induction of cancers, or radiation-produced defects of embryonic or fetal development. Accordingly, it might be thought that there is no place for discussion of these things in a chapter of this kind. However, many people are aware that radiation exposure can injure the unborn, cause cancer or harm the germ cells and, if exposed to radiation, might ask emergency department personnel whether they may have sustained such damage. It is very important to be able to give informed answers to patients' questions on this subject (or failing that, no answer at all) at the time they are asked. Misinformation given at such a time can lead to confusion and even suspicion on the part of the patient later on. Therefore, the risk of such injuries will be briefly discussed here in an effort to equip emergency department personnel to respond better to patients' questions and concerns.

What Are the Effects of Gonadal Radiation Exposure on the Next Generation? People who have been exposed to radiation may realize that their gonads have been exposed and become concerned about conceiving children and ask about it. They may worry about the possibility of some detectable effect showing up in a child that is the result of their radiation exposure. A number of studies have dealt with this issue, but the thorough, intense, and extended study of the offspring of the survivors of the atomic bomb attacks on Hiroshima and Nagasaki probably sums the issue up best.[16–19] In spite of the fact that many of the gonadal doses to the survivors of the atomic bomb attacks were fairly high (in the several tens of rads), no effects were detected in children conceived from those gonads, a finding confirmed by nearly all other studies of this and other populations.

The individual who has received even substantial gonadal exposure and dose, then, can be assured that there is little to fear for his or her children. The probability of detectable effects are evidently very low and masked by the normal biologic variation and the natural hazards of pregnancy.

Radiation Carcinogenesis. Similarly, many people are aware of the fact that radiation can cause cancer and ask about their risk. While ionizing radiation is often perceived as being powerfully carcinogenic, in fact it is a weak carcinogen. The study of many exposed populations from the atomic bomb survivors to people in former times treated for benign diseases with X rays to people occupationally exposed to radiation suggest an estimate as follows: following an acute exposure (radiation exposure occurring in a brief period of time) of 10 rads (which would very likely be quite high for unintentional exposures), there is a population-weighted, lifetime, radiogenic mortality rate of 0.08% (0.5–1.2%).[4] Protraction of dose over time could well reduce the risk.

What Are the Effects on Developing Embryo or Fetus? The probability of a pregnant woman being involuntarily exposed is presumably extremely small but intentional irradiation is less uncommon. It can occur that a pregnant woman has come into the emergency department as the result of a separate condition (auto crash, burn, broken bone, for instance) and requires diagnostic studies including X ray, or that a woman is in the emergency department as the result of a separate condition and has X-ray examinations and reveals later that she is pregnant. The woman and/or her family or loved ones may express concern for the baby.

Ionizing radiation has also acquired a reputation as a powerful teratogen, but in fact is only very weakly teratogenic. Embryonic radiation doses of under 10 rads, well below the dose given by just about any diagnostic X ray or nuclear medicine procedure, have not been shown to have any detectable effect on development. Doses above 10 rads have increased abortion frequency in rodents irradiated in the preimplantation period, but comparable data for humans do not exist. Even doses of 25 rads during early organogenesis do not seem to have produced detectable effects in humans, and doses well above this value (100 rads or more) are needed to produce a high expectation of effect.[3,4,6,7,17]

The pregnant patient exposed to radiation intentionally as described above need have little concern about her baby, and unintentional exposures, unless they are very large, are very unlikely to be damaging either.

What Are the Effects of High Doses?

The degree of injury done by exposure to ionizing radiation is very much dependent on the amount of the body exposed. As a rule of thumb, the greater the part of the body exposed, the greater the damage or gravity of injury from any given radiation dose. A dose of only a few hundred rads (500 rads, as a reasonable approximation) given, in a single exposure, to the total body will be lethal to very nearly 100% of irradiated humans but many thousands of rads given to the restricted treatment fields during radiation therapy regimens are well tolerated. Even in the case of total-body radiation, there may be a difference in response and degree of injury between the situation where the exposure is reasonably uniform over the total body compared to where the total body is irradiated but some parts get more than others.

The symptoms of total-body radiation rarely become manifest for several hours after irradiation and may not be apparent when a patient appears in the emergency department. If the dose is high enough (the next section gives dose ranges), however, the patient should be hospitalized, as the symptoms are likely to show up and to require some form of treatment.

What Are the Effects of Total-Body Radiation? The symptoms of "radiation sickness," also called "radiation syndromes" are the result of depletion of functional cells in tissue, but the underlying cause of the syndromes caused by total-body (or nearly total-body) doses of up to about 5000 rads is the killing of stem cells.

An hour or two after exposure of a major part of the body to a dose of radiation in excess of about 50 rads, transitory symptoms, called the prodromal reaction, begin to appear. The time of onset and severity depend to some extent on individual susceptibility, but the principal influencing factor is radiation dose. The approximate doses eliciting signs and symptoms in 50% of those exposed are anorexia, 100 rads; nausea, 140 rads; vomiting, 180 rads; and diarrhea, 230 rads.

The prodromal reaction is followed by the so-called latent period, a relatively asymptomatic period, the length of which depends on the time required for development of sustained disturbances in organ function related to functional cell depletion. An exception is lethal brain damage, which presumably is not due to functional cell depletion. As dose increases, the latent period becomes shorter and may not exist after very high doses.

The main phase of radiation-induced illness returns after the latent period and, with increasing dose, death becomes more likely as an outcome and occurs sooner after irradiation.

The acute effects fall into three rather distinct subgroups or syndromes. The dose ranges given for these syndromes are, at best, estimates, since there is modest experience of exposure to high doses of radiation. The doses quoted are for single, whole-body exposures from high-energy radiation, such as X and gamma rays.

The three subgroups or syndromes, arranged in order of increasing dose, are as follows: those in which the organ system primarily responsible for death is the hematopoietic system; those in which the organ systems primarily responsible for death are the hematopoietic and gastrointestinal systems; and those in which the organ system primarily responsible for death is the cerebrovascular system.

What Are the Effects of Hematopoietic System Failure? This response and its associated mortality, known also as the bone marrow syndrome, occurs in most patients after doses of 200–1000 rads. Mean survival time of irradiated groups varies with dose, ranging from 4 to 6 weeks at the lower end of the dose range to less than 1 week at its upper limit. There is a complex of signs and symptoms, but death occurs because the bone marrow fails to produce mature functional cells for the circulating blood. Because of the short life span and rapid renewal of most peripheral blood and marrow cells, effects are dramatic. Small lymphocytes and reduced numbers are seen in a few hours. The half-life of platelets and granulocytes is 1 week, and depletion is maximal at 3 weeks. The half-life of red blood cells is about 100 days. There is thus a dynamic balance between the declining numbers of mature cells and regeneration.

Whether organisms die as a result of loss of function of bone marrow depends on whether recovery of damaged bone marrow cells occurs quickly enough for them to divide, differentiate, and replace functioning cells that are lost from irradiated individuals at about the same rate as from nonirradiated individuals. The loss of bone marrow function ultimately means the loss of an organism's ability to combat infection and loss of the ability of blood to clot, because the supply of new granulocytes and platelets is cut off. These factors are the cause of death as they lead to infection, nearly always from the organism's own intestinal flora, and the risk of hemorrhage.

What Are the Effects on the Gastrointestinal System? As dose increases to 700–1000 rads, more and more cells of the gastrointestinal tract (particularly the small intestine) become damaged by irradiation. This dose range marks the transition between the hematopoietic and gastrointestinal syndromes. For doses above 1000 rads up to about 5000 rads, gastrointestinal injury is the principal cause of death and survival time becomes much less dose dependent. Those who receive a dose large enough so that gastrointestinal damage results in death will have received far more than enough radiation to have resulted in hematopoietic death. Death from gut damage occurs, however, before the full effect of radiation on the blood-forming organs is expressed.

The mucosa of intestinal villi consists of four types of cellular compartments. At the base of the villi are the crypts of Lieberkühn, the stem-cell compartment which is a region of high mitotic activity. Somewhat higher along each villus is another region of high mitotic activity, the differentiating compartment. Near the villus tip are the functional absorptive cells, which are produced in the crypts and have differentiated in the differentiating compartment. At the tip itself, spent functional cells are extruded from the villi into the intestinal lumen. Ideally, the number of cells lost from the tip equals the number produced in the crypt.

For most mammals, after doses in the range of 1000 rads, large numbers of crypt cells and cells of the differentiating compartment are killed. Spent functional cells are nevertheless extruded from the tips of villi at approximately the same rate as in unirradiated organisms but few new ones are produced in the crypts to replace them.

In time, the continuity of the intestinal lining is breached as spent cells leave and are not replaced. Eventually, these breaches become gaps of denuded intestine. Through these gaps, intestinal flora penetrate the organism, infecting it. The lack of mature granulocytes—resulting from radiation's effect on bone marrow—permits infective organisms to spread and multiply. Also, from these gaps leakage of blood occurs, and the short supply of platelets fails to stop it.

Finally, the loss of absorptive cells seriously impairs the capacity of the distal end of the small intestine to resorb bile salts. These pass into and irritate the large intestine thus causing copious watery diarrhea.

In most mammals, death occurs between 3 and 4 days after irradiation. In humans, although data are few, this time appears to be somewhat longer and is probably related to longer transit times of crypt and villus cells in humans. Death occurs as a direct result of infection, fluid and plasma loss, and salt imbalance, all consequences of severe diarrhea and vascular collapse.

What Are the Effects on the Central Nervous System? As dose is increased from 5000 to 10,000 rads, mean survival time again becomes dose dependent (and is uniformly fatal). This is a signal that death is no longer caused by loss of gastrointestinal function. The mechanisms responsible for death are not nearly as clear as they are at lower doses. The signs and symptoms comprising this syndrome point toward the central nervous system, but there is little gross or histologic evidence of what happens. In addition to diarrhea and vomiting, which probably result from effects on the digestive tract, signs and symptoms include agitation alternating with apathy, disorientation, loss of balance, tetanic spasms, convulsions, prostration, and coma.

The time of onset depends on dose, but even during irradiation, some mammalian species display hyperactivity and irritability, occasionally alternating with spells of apathy.

As the syndrome progresses, more tremor, vomiting, watery diarrhea, and hysteria occur. Prostration and coma follow and then death occurs, usually within 1–2 days. As dose is increased from 10,000 to 50,000 rads, acute functional changes related to direct effects on the neurons occur and, at the highest dose, will produce immediate death.

Most attribute the cause of death to cerebral edema, which they believe accompanies very high irradiation doses. There is considerable evidence of infiltration of fluid, granulocytes, macrophages, and mononucleocytes into the meninges and brain. There is liquid infiltration into the choroid plexus, but the cause of these events is uncertain. Bacterial invasion seems unlikely. More likely, radiation damage to capillaries and possibly larger vessels, such as arterioles in the brain itself, causes the leakage. This fact prompts some to call this syndrome the cerebrovascular syndrome in recognition of the role of blood vessels.

Since so little is known for certain about this syndrome, explanations other than the foregoing can be devised to cover the observed facts. Some argue, for example, that extravasation of fluid and cells into the brain is the effect, not the cause, of the syndrome since much higher doses are required to produce the syndrome if the head alone is irradiated. Some feel high doses of radiation obliterate the blood–brain barrier, and numerous elements normally excluded from the brain can enter and affect it.

How Is Exposure Assessed?

The clinical symptoms of the acute radiation syndrome can serve as a guide for the assessment of the level of exposure. Nausea and vomiting due to radiation are seldom experienced unless the exposure has been at least 70–100 rads of penetrating radiation and has occurred within a few hours. The time of onset of prodromal symptoms (anorexia, nausea, and vomiting) can provide a useful clinical estimate of whole-body dose. In fact, this was the major triage mechanism used during the Chernobyl accident. A time of onset of symptoms of more than 2 hours indicates a dose less than 200 rads, whereas a time interval less than 0.5 hours indicates a dose greater than 600 rads. If the patient has been asymptomatic for 24 hours, it indicates a dose of less than 70 rads of whole-body radiation.

A primary concern should be to establish a baseline for later blood counts that will reveal the degree of injury. Thus, a complete blood count, including platelets and differential count, should be performed immediately. A determination of the absolute lymphocyte count of peripheral blood is essential since circulating lymphocytes are extremely radiosensitive and furnish the earliest and most accurate indication of radiation. Blood should also be obtained on day 1 for HLA typing of potential bone marrow transplant candidates because typing may be complicated later by radiation-induced lymphocytopenia. Blood counts should be repeated at 12, 24, and 48 hours to indicate the rate of change in the lymphocyte count with further frequent blood samples to monitor granulocyte and platelet levels since they correlate well with infection and hemorrhage. If neutron exposure is involved, there is also some urgency in obtaining a blood sample so that the radiation dose can be estimated from induced sodium-24 activity (it has a half-life of 15 hours).

Serial mitotic indices of bone marrow have also been suggested as an indicator of radiation exposure in the range of 50–200 rads. Although the number of irradiated individuals that the data are based on is small, mitotic depression appears to be dose dependent in this dose range. A mitotic index approaching zero (the normal level is approximately 9 cells per 1000) at about 4 days postexposure indicates a dose of 200 rads or more.

Sperm counts can also provide evidence that exposure exceeds 300 rads. For radiation exposure below this level, no significant change in sperm count is observed before day 45, whereas with doses of 400–600 rads, sperm count depression is observed after the first 3 weeks (probably representing death of primary spermatocytes). This has led to the recommendation that sperm counts be obtained in the first week, at day 45, and after day 60.

It can be seen that few of these procedures will be done in the Emergency Department since they are done well after exposure and/or on a continuing basis. Most treatment, if any is needed, would occur in irradiated patients who have been hospitalized.

Partial-Body Radiation

The symptoms of partial-body radiation will also be dose dependent and will represent the results of tissue damage by radiation. As in the case of total-body radiation, symptoms are most likely to develop only after appreciable threshold radiation doses are absorbed and are not likely to be manifest for some time (days, at least) after radiation exposure. An attempt to assess dose should be made, however, so that the appearance of symptoms can be anticipated and properly handled when they do appear. Table 98–3 gives a list of the kinds of damage associated with various partial-body radiation doses.

TABLE 98–3. ESTIMATES OF THRESHOLD ON NONSTOCHASTIC EFFECTS IN HUMANS, ACUTE EXPOSURE

Tissue and Effect	Total Dose Equivalent Received in a Single Brief Exposure (rads)
Testes	
Temporary sterility	15
Permanent sterility	350
Ovaries	
Sterility	250–600
Lens (cataracts)	
Detectable opacities	50–200
Visual impairment	500
Bone marrow	
Depression of hematopoiesis	50
Fatal aplasia	150–200
Skin	
Early transient erythema	200
Temporary epilation	300
Prolonged erythema	600
Permanent epilation	700
Dermal atrophy	1100
Dermal necrosis	1800

Irradiation Only or Contamination With Radioactive Material?

Exposure to ionizing radiations may occur one of three ways: (1) exposure to radiations from a source outside the body; (2) exposure to radiations from radioactive substances deposited on or taken into the body; or (3) both.

The degree to which people exposed to radiation will be a hazard to themselves and others depends on whether the person has been irradiated from a source outside the body or whether they have been contaminated by radioactive material—for example, by radioactive material deposited on the skin, or within the body (as when someone ingests, inhales, or has been injected with radioactive material), or some combination of the foregoing.

The person who has been irradiated from an external source and is *not* contaminated with radioactive material may, depending on the dose of radiation received, become very sick but poses no radiation risk to people around them or caring for them. The reason is that people who have been exposed to radiation from external sources without contamination by radioactive material do not, themselves, become radioactive or emit ionizing radiation. This may seem condescending or too elementary to have been pointed out; however, it is surprising how many people, health professionals included, have the mistaken belief that people exposed to ionizing radiation, for example, X rays during diagnostic procedures or gamma rays during treatment for cancer, become radioactive, emit radiation, and constitute a radiation hazard to those around them.

One of the first things to be done when presented with a radiation emergency is to ascertain, as far as that is possible, whether people presumed to have been exposed to radiation are contaminated. If there is no contamination, then there is no radiation hazard to anyone else. The patient will need to be evaluated and potentially treated for their radiation exposure but will expose no one else.

The determination of whether a person is contaminated may be done through the individual him- or herself or other people present at the place at which irradiation took place. If that is not possible, there are detectors (about which more will follow), which are very likely to be available in the hospital, that can be used for that purpose.

The person who is contaminated with radioactive materials *may* present a hazard to those in contact with him or her if the radioactive material is (1) on the skin, (2) being excreted in the breath or urine, feces, or sweat, (3) or in vomitus or (4) if radiations from radioactive material within the body are sufficiently energetic to escape the body and irradiate the area around the contaminated person. However, it should be stressed that the circumstances under which this might occur are likely to be very few and far between. Most people who are likely to become contaminated by radioactive materials are likely (1) to be contaminated with very small amounts, which, in many cases, will be essentially entirely contained within their bodies; (2) to be contaminated by radioisotopes whose radiations are too weak to emerge from the body and irradiate the area around them to any significant degree; and (3) to have ingested or inhaled too little radioactive material to cause vomiting or diarrhea. Vomiting may occur for reasons other than ingestion of radioactive materials, extreme fear or anxiety among them, but it would be a rare event for a person to have ingested enough radioactive material into the body to produce this reaction.

There is, therefore, a potential difference in the radiation hazard presented to others by people irradiated alone and those contaminated by radioactive materials, and there may be a difference in facilities needed to care for patients depending on whether they are or are not contaminated. The person who has only been irradiated, from the point of view of danger to emergency department personnel, will need no special facilities or equipment. He or she can be handled like any other patient. The contaminated person *may* require some facilities or equipment not ordinarily found in emergency departments. However, in many cases these are very likely to be found elsewhere in the hospital.

In most cases, then, radiation emergencies are *less*, often much less, threatening to emergency department personnel than many more familiar problems—as examples, people infected with HIV, hepatitis virus, or tubercule bacilli. What makes radiation emergencies fearsome to so many people is the lack of knowledge about radiation and its effects and lack of familiarity with such emergencies.

Radiation Injuries

As has been seen from the the introductory part of this chapter, the injuries caused by such esoteric and threatening-sounding entities as non-ionizing radiations are as ordinary and familiar as burns. Now it can be said that injuries caused by *ionizing* radiations are often not unique, either. The damage produced in and symptoms exhibited by people exposed to ionizing radiations are often also caused by other, more familiar agents, and the care involved in treating them is already well-known to emergency department personnel.

The news that someone presumably exposed to radiation is on the way to the emergency department or that someone presumably exposed to radiation is already in the area need not be a reason for fear or confusion. The likelihood is that the patient is suffering from a familiar condition or injury, caused, in this instance, by an unfamiliar source.

The following scheme suggests the appropriate reaction of the emergency department to the news that a putative radiation injury is on its way to or already in the department.

1. Determine whether there is a significant "conventional" injury (burn, cut, other wound, broken bone,

etc) in the patient. If there is, this should be treated first. As can be gleaned from the foregoing, radiation injuries rarely, if ever, need immediate attention.

2. The radiation safety department or officer should be notified and summoned.
3. Determine whether or not any radiation was actually involved in the patient's case. Radiation exposure is often suspected or imagined. As a so-called silent killer or cause of injury, people may impute radiation as a cause of physical or psychogenic illness. Questioning of the patient may be valuable in determining whether he or she has actually been near a radiation source. If contamination is suspected or possible, a radiation detector will be needed. The hospital's radiation safety office is a source of help as will be the Nuclear Medicine Department in both dose determination and detection of contamination.
4. If no radiation is involved, no further action is needed.
5. If the patient is contaminated on the surface of the skin, the best method of removal is what would be used for cleaning any skin: washing either with water or other appropriate solvent. Forceful scrubbing, which may damage the skin, is not recommended. Emergency Department personnel will be protected from radiation contamination by the use of the universal precautions currently employed in hospitals Emergency Departments.
6. If the dose evaluations indicate a small dose (up to about 25 rads), no action is likely to be needed. Symptoms are unlikely to appear, and whatever damage has been done may lead to the irreversible and untreatable changes due to mutation.
7. If the dose has fallen in a medium range (between 25 and 100 rads), the patient may exhibit some symptoms, especially if the exposure was total body. Possible hospitalization may be desirable, but no action is necessary in the Emergency Department.
8. If the dose is large (100 rads and over) hospitalization should be considered (especially in the case of total-body radiation), but except in the case of very large exposures (over 300 rads), no special action is likely to be needed in the emergency department. In the case of very large exposures, the patient may have gastrointestinal reactions that need support.
9. The containment of radioactive contamination and the cleanup of contamination should be done under the supervision of and by the Radiation Safety Department.

References

1. Baverstock KF: DNA instability, paternal irradiation and leukaemia in children around Sellafield. Int J Radiat Biol 1991;60:581–595.
2. Black D: Investigation of the Possible Increased Incidence of Cancer in West Cumbria. London, HM Stationery Office, 1984.
3. Brent RL: Radiation teratogenesis. Teratology 1980;32: 281–298.
4. Committee on the Biological Effects of Ionizing Radiations, The National Research Council: National Academy Press, Washington, DC, 1990.
5. Darby SC, Olsen JH, Doll R, et al: Trends in childhood leukemia in the Nordic countries in relation to fallout from atmospheric nuclear weapons testing. Br Med J 1992;304, 1005–1009.
6. Dekaban AS: Abnormalities in children exposed to radiation during various stages of gestation: A tentative timetable of radiation injury to the human fetus. J Nucl Med 1968;9: 471–477.
7. Denniston C: Low level radiation and genetic risk estimation in man. Annu Rev Genet 1982;16:329–355.
8. Gardner MJ: Father's occupational exposure to radiation and the raised level of childhood leukemia near the Sellafield nuclear plant. Environ Health Perspect 1991;94: 5–7.
9. Gardner MJ, Hall AJ, Downes S, et al: Follow-up study of children born elsewhere but attending schools in Seascale, West Cumbria (schools cohort). Br Med J 1987;295:819–822.
10. Gardner MJ, Hall AJ, Downes S, et al: Follow-up study of children born to mothers resident in Seascale, West Cumbria (birth cohort). Br Med J 1987;295:822–827.
11. Gardner MJ, Hall AJ, Snee MP, et al: Methods and basic data of case-control study of leukaemia and lymphoma among young people near Sellafield nuclear plant in West Cumbria. B Med J 1990;300:429–434.
12. Gardner MJ, Snee MP, Hall AJ: Results of case-control study of leukaemia and lymphoma among young people near Sellafield nuclear plant in West Cumbria. Br Med J 1990;300:423–429.
13. Goldstein L, Murphy DP: Microcephalic idiocy following radium therapy for uterine cancer during pregnancy. Am J Obstet Gynecol 1929;18:189–195; 281–283.
14. Holmes GE, Holmes FF: Pregnancy outcome of patients treated for Hodgkin's disease. Cancer 1978;41:1317–1322.
15. LeFloch O, Donaldson SS, Kaplan JS: Pregnancy following oophorectomy and total nodal irradiation in women with Hodgkin's disease. Cancer 1976;38:2263–2268.
16. Neel JV, Kato H, Schull WJ: Mortality in the children of atomic bomb survivors and controls. Genetics 1974: 311–326.
17. Otake M, Schull WJ: In utero exposure to A bomb radiation and mental retardation: A reassessment. Br J Radiol 1984; 57:409–414.
18. Satoh C, Awa AA, Neel JV, et al: Genetic Effects of Atomic Bombs. Human Genetics, Part A: The unfolding genome. New York, AR Liss, 1982, pp. 267–276.
19. Schull WJ, Otake M, Neel JV: Genetic effects of the atomic bombs: A reappraisal. Science 1981;213:1220–1227.
20. Selby PB, Russell WL: First generation litter-size reduction following irradiation of spermatogonial stem cells in mice and its use in risk estimation. Environ Mutagenesis 1985;7: 451–469.
21. Vogel F: Risk calculations for hereditary effects of ionizing radiation in humans. Hum Genet 1992;89:127–146.
22. Watson GM: Leukaemia and paternal radiation exposure. Med J Aust 1991;154:483–487.
23. Yoshimoto Y: Cancer risk among children of atomic bomb survivors: A review of RERF epidemiologic studies. JAMA 1990;264:596–600.

CHAPTER 99

Snakes and Other Reptiles

James R. Roberts and Edward J. Otten

CASE 1. A 25-year-old man exploring the mountains of Virginia was bitten on the toe by an unidentified snake when he was rock-climbing in bare feet. He did not hear a rattle and only caught a glimpse of the copper-colored snake as it crawled away. Within 10 minutes he noted mild swelling and discomfort around a single puncture wound on the top of the fourth toe.

Within 1 hour the man developed moderate throbbing pain in the entire foot, associated with paresthesias. At 2 hours a hemorrhagic blister developed at the bite site (see Color Plate Fig. 4). The swelling had progressed to the dorsum of the ankle, but he had no systemic symptoms. A friend drove him to a local hospital. At this juncture, it appeared that the snake was poisonous and envenomation had occurred.

No specific first aid was administered. The swelling did not progress past the ankle and there was no nausea, vomiting, diaphoresis, dizziness, or systemic weakness. The vital signs and a CBC and coagulation profile were normal. The patient reported only mild pain of the foot.

Because of progression of local symptoms and lack of definitive identification of the snake, the patient was admitted to the hospital. Antivenin was obtained but not administered. The foot demonstrated moderate pain and stiffness; edema reached the lower leg at 48 hours but did not progress further. No systemic symptoms developed and the laboratory profile remained normal. Minor surgical debridement of a small area of skin slough on the toe was required. The patient was discharged after 24 hours to continue extremity elevation, and outpatient physical therapy was arranged. After 10 days of a progressive decrease in swelling, the patient had full use of the foot with only minor stiffness. Within 3 weeks the stiffness had disappeared completely.

This patient suffered minimal envenomation from a copperhead. Although it would be tempting to give "prophylactic" antivenin, he lacked the physical and laboratory characteristics that typically require the use of antivenin and it could safely be withheld. Specifically, there were no signs of coagulopathy or systemic effects, conditions that would mandate antivenin.

CASE 2. A 6-year-old girl was bitten on the left ankle by a 2-foot snake in her backyard. The snake was not positively identified, but rattlesnakes (western diamondback) were known to frequent the area. The child's father reported that she complained of severe pain in the leg within 30 seconds of the bite. Within 2 minutes she became weak and diaphoretic and vomited. She appeared pale and became agitated and disoriented.

The child was immediately taken to the hospital but became more lethargic en route, a sign of serious systemic envenomation, possibly a direct intravenous envenomation.

No first aid was administered. By the time she arrived at the hospital (transportation time of 25 minutes), the child's face and lips were swollen, and generalized muscle fasciculations were noted. The initial vital signs were: palpable blood pressure, 40 mm Hg; pulse, 150 beats/min; shallow respirations at 38 breaths/min; and temperature, 97°F (36.1°C). The patient was slightly cyanotic and obtunded. The entire lower leg was swollen and two small puncture wounds were evident over the medial malleolus of the ankle, in the area of the saphenous vein. Arterial blood gas analysis revealed the following: pH, 7.12; PCO_2, 20 mm Hg; and PO_2, 130 mm Hg (while breathing oxygen at 4 L/min).

This child was seriously envenomated. In addition to the protocol described, she required the mobilization of resources to treat a life-threatening snakebite. This should include consulting with someone experienced with such cases, generally available through the regional poison center, and obtaining at least 40 vials of crotalid antivenin. The immediate onset of symptoms and the serious clinical condition supported the assumption that the child sustained serious envenomation by a rattlesnake. Direct IV envenomation was likely.

Initial therapy consisted of the placement of a thigh tourniquet (constrictor) to impede lymphatic flow and the rapid infusion of lactated Ringer's solution at two peripheral IV sites. Blood was drawn for a CBC, BUN, creatinine, electrolytes, type and cross-match, and clotting studies, including fibrinogen level. A Foley catheter was inserted and gross hematuria was noted.

The child was immediately skin-tested for sensitivity to horse serum. Within 3 minutes erythema developed at the skin test site. Although sensitivity to antivenin was suggested by the reaction, the consensus of the treating physician and a toxicology consultant was that the benefits of antivenin outweighed the risks. The decision was made to treat aggressively with antivenin. To ameliorate allergic reactions, 125 mg of methylprednisolone plus 50 mg of diphenhydramine were given IV. An infusion of 1 mg epinephrine in 1 L of 0.9% sodium chloride solution saline was prepared but not given. Broad-spectrum antibiotics and tetanus prophylaxis were given.

After fluid administration, the blood pressure was measured at 85/50 mm Hg. With continuous ECG monitoring crotalid polyvalent antivenin (Wyeth Laboratories) was administered by slow IV push, at a rate of 1 vial (diluted 1:10 with 0.9% NaCl solution) over 2 minutes. During administration of the second vial the child's blood pressure became unobtainable but quickly responded to titration of the epinephrine infusion, increasing the rate of the crystalloid infusion, and stopping the antivenin. Subsequent vials were infused more slowly (each vial over 5 minutes) and the hypotension did not return. A total of 20 vials of antivenin was given over 2 hours. The tourniquet was removed without sequelae after the antivenin was administered. The epinephrine infusion was not required after the initial hypotensive episode, but a transient episode of urticaria required an additional 25 mg of diphenhydramine IV. Significant initial laboratory values included: PT, 25 seconds (control, 12 seconds); PTT, 65 seconds (control, 25 seconds); fibrinogen, 60 mg/dL (normal, 170–410 mg/dL); platelet count, 15,000/mm^3; and leukocyte count, 28,800/mm^3. The hemoglobin/hematocrit, electrolytes, BUN, and creatinine were normal.

The child's clinical condition greatly improved over the next 8 hours. Her pulse and respirations slowed, her consciousness improved, and her blood pressure stabilized at 95/40 mm Hg. The gross hematuria cleared after the infusion of 4 units of fresh frozen plasma and 6 units of platelet concentrate. The coagulopathy completely resolved in 48 hours and no other bleeding complications were noted. The swelling about the face decreased, but she developed increased edema and hemorrhagic blisters at the site of the bite. The peripheral pulses remained intact. The leg swelled to the groin to about twice its normal size but there was no objective evidence for a compartment syndrome and gradually the edema abated.

Minor surgical debridement was required at the site of the bite. One week after therapy the child developed a low-grade fever and generalized urticaria and malaise, interpreted as serum sickness. The symptoms responded to oral prednisone and diphenhydramine and the child eventually recovered without sequelae.

The cardiovascular, respiratory, and central nervous system (CNS) depression and the significant coagulopathy that quickly followed the bite in this patient are common in severe envenomation by rattlesnakes, and the rapid use of large doses of antivenin was appropriate. The coagulopathy can develop within minutes and to a degree not suggested by other signs of envenomation. Although antivenin often corrects a minor coagulopathy, blood component replacement therapy, as administered in this case, may be required. Although the child had evidence of sensitivity to horse serum, her critical condition nonetheless mandated the use of antivenin. Prophylactic pretreatment with corticosteroids and antihistamines is frequently recommended in such cases. Epinephrine should be available to titrate as an IV infusion should anaphylaxis occur. The hypotension associated with antivenin therapy is often controlled simply by slowing the rate of infusion. In severe cases, antivenin and epinephrine can be given simultaneously (by separate IV infusions), titrating the rate of each against the clinical condition. The tourniquet was not removed until after the antivenin was infused.

Both patients developed minor morbidity at the envenomation site, but neither required extensive surgical treatment. Although the extremities manifested substantial swelling, a compartment syndrome did not develop.

It is not uncommon for patients to require local debridement, especially following rattlesnake bites. Amputation of digits and skin grafting may be required. Bleeding complications (hematuria, hematemesis, CNS hemorrhage, generalized bleeding), upper airway obstruction requiring intubation or tracheostomy, adult respiratory distress syndrome, renal failure, sepsis, or cardiac or respiratory arrest may be seen. Prolonged parethesias and stiffness of hands and feet, occasionally for months afterwards, is also occasionally noted.

What Is the Incidence of Venomous Snakebites in the United States?

Venomous snakes are found throughout the United States, except Maine, Alaska, and Hawaii. They are common in the southern and western states but rare in New England and the northern states. There are approximately 6000–8000 venomous snakebites per year, but many thousands more from nonvenomous species. Mortality from snakebite is quite rare in the United States, with estimates ranging from 5 to 15 deaths per year.[25] Mortality rates can be significantly higher in other countries. There may be as many as 27,000 rattlesnake bites and 100 fatalities per year in Mexico,[10] and thousands of deaths per year in some underdeveloped locales of India, Burma, and African countries.

Because snakes hibernate in the winter, most bites in the United States occur between May and October. Snakes may bite at night, but the most common time for envenomation is from 2 to 6 P.M.[71] Coral snakes are particularly known for their nocturnal habits. The majority of bites occur in the extremities, but bites to the face and tongue have been reported. Some religious groups in the mid- and southeastern states handle poisonous snakes (usually rattlesnakes) as a routine ceremonial practice (see Acts 28:4 and Mark 16:17–18), and envenomation is common. Children, intoxicated individuals (mostly men), snake handlers, and collectors are frequent victims. Over half of the bites occur while the individual is purposely handling a known venomous snake. There is a significant market for many illegal and dangerous reptiles, and a surprising number of individuals keep and sell venomous snakes as pets. Many specimens are exotic and highly toxic species from other countries. The striking range of a snake is approximately one half its length

TABLE 99–1. SCIENTIFIC AND COMMON NAMES OF SOME MEDICALLY IMPORTANT VENOMOUS SNAKES OF NORTH AMERICA

Scientific Name	Common Name
Crotalids: Pit Viper	
Agkistrodon contortrix contortrix	Southern copperhead
Agkistrodon contortrix laticinctus	Broad-banded copperhead
Agkistrodon contortrix mokason	Northern copperhead
Agkistrodon piscivorus conanti	Florida cottonmouth
Agkistrodon piscivorus piscivorus	Eastern cottonmouth
Agkistrodon piscivorus leucostoma	Western cottonmouth
Bothrops lanceolatus	Fer-de-lance
Rattlesnakes	
Crotalus adamanteus	Eastern diamondback
Crotalus atrox	Western diamondback
Crotalus cerastes cerastes	Mojave Desert sidewinder
Crotalus cerastes cercobombus	Sonoran Desert sidewinder
Crotalus horridus horridus	Timber
Crotalus horridus atricaudatus	Canebrake
Crotalus molossus	Northern black tailed
Crotalus ruber ruber	Red diamond
Crotalus scutulatus scutulatus	Mojave
Crotalus viridis cerberus	Arizona black
Crotalus viridis helleri	Southern Pacific
Crotalus viridis lutosus	Great Basin
Crotalus viridis nuntius	Hopi
Crotalus viridis oreganus	Northern Pacific
Crotalus viridis viridis	Prairie
Sistrurus catenatus catenatus	Eastern massasauga
Sistrurus catenatus edwardsi	Desert massasauga
Sistrurus catenatus tergeminus	Western massasauga
Sistrurus millarius millarius	Carolina pigmy
Elapids: Coral Snakes	
Micruroides euryxanthus	Sonoran
Micrurus fulvius fulvius	Eastern
Micrurus fulvius tenere	Texas

but many bites occur when snakes are purposefully held near the body.

Of the 120 species of snakes native to North America, approximately 30 species are dangerous (Table 99–1). Most of these venomous snakes are members of the Crotalidae family, which includes the rattlesnakes, copperheads, and semiaquatic water moccasins. These three snakes are also called pit vipers because of the presence of a pitlike depression of the skin behind the nostril that functions as a heat-sensing organ. The other family of venomous snakes native to the United States is Elapidae, which includes the coral snakes.

What First Aid or Field Treatment Is Appropriate for Stable Snakebite Victims?

Undue importance has been placed on the immediate prehospital care of patients with snake bites. When the patient is not in extremis and medical attention is available within a few hours, the prudent approach is a conservative one. The excitement or hysteria generated by a possible poisonous snakebite compels some caregivers to intervene quickly, often irrationally, and with unproven or harmful procedures. It is common to confuse treatment priorities and create additional morbidity with hurried or ill-conceived attempts to stop or limit "certain death" or amputation (see Color Plate Fig. 5). In reality, both death and amputation are quite rare if proper medical attention is available within a few hours. Most morbidity stems from delayed treatment, either because of inaction on the patient's part (often due to alcohol intoxication) or because of inaccessible medical care. Prehospital care should generally be limited to immobilization of the patient and rapid transport to a medical facility. Physical activity, such as walking, and elevation of an extremity should be avoided because these maneuvers may hasten systemic absorption of venom.

When the Victim Is Unstable and Medical Care Is Delayed or Inaccessible, What Treatments Are Indicated for Snakebite Victims?

A possible exception to the dictum of conservative nonintervention in the field can be invoked if deterioration is immediate, and if the victim is more than 3–4 hours from medical care and significant envenomation is certain. If there are immediate symptoms of severe envenomation, the traditional tourniquet or incision and suction may have some value and can be considered. These procedures should not be done routinely in the field and should be considered only when significant envenomation is certain. Unfortunately, this determination is often a difficult or retrospective clinical decision for most laypersons and many physicians, so there is considerable opportunity for errors in judgment.

Tourniquet/Constriction Band

Although an extremity tourniquet will decrease distal to systemic egress of venom, the true value of any intervention designed to limit the systemic absorption of venom is uncertain. A standard of care is impossible to determine because of lack of scientific proof that limiting absorption is clinically helpful and by confusion of anecdotal reports that are uncontrolled and do not consider different species and degrees of envenomation. Also there is no standardization of technique, such as amount of pressure applied, or length of tourniquet application. Suggested techniques include a simple thin tourniquet, a broad band, or wrapping an entire extremity with a compression device.

As a conservative temporizing recommendation for extremity envenomation, a wide (2–4 cm) constricting band loosely applied to limit lymphatic (but not venous) flow may be placed a few inches proximal to the bite. Although this has the theoretical disadvantage of concentrating venom in the extremity and increasing local necrosis, a device that decreases systemic absorption of venom may be beneficial in instances where systemic signs and symptoms are rapidly occurring. A properly applied lymphatic tourniquet would be appropriate treatment for the Case 2 patient but would be overtreatment for the Case 1 patient.

The specific effect of a tourniquet on the course of envenomation in humans is unknown, but animal studies suggest a possible benefit. A porcine model using *Crotalus atrox* (western diamondback rattlesnake) venom demonstrated that a constriction band tourniquet placed immediately after experimental envenomation and maintained in place for 4 hours was effective in reducing systemic venom absorption from an extremity, without increasing local swelling and local tissue injury.[6] When a blood pressure cuff was maintained to 45 mm Hg, the maximum plasma concentration of venom was reduced by 25%, and total venom absorption was reduced by 33%. This model also demonstrated that removal of the constriction band 4 hours postenvenomation did not result in a significant surge in plasma venom concentration. A sudden worsening of symptoms has been reported, however, after tourniquet removal in patients with crotalid envenomations.[33,68] Therefore, antivenin should be given before tourniquet removal to decrease toxicity from sudden systemic absorption of pooled venom. In the absence of antivenin therapy, the band should remain in place for a few hours but pressures should be checked and the constriction loosened or moved proximally if it becomes too tight due to swelling.

The difficulties of laypersons applying and monitoring a properly applied tourniquet are easy to appreciate. If a tourniquet is used in the field, a reasonable guide would be to wrap it as tight as a compression bandage would be applied for a sprained ankle, and combine the compression with immobilization. There is some evidence that a broad, firm, constrictive wrap (elastic bandage) placed over the bitten area and encircling the entire immobilized limb offers advantage over the traditional tourniquet. This wrapping procedure (the Sutherland wrap) is intended to collapse lymphatics and superficial veins to retard venom uptake and has been beneficial in the treatment of non-necrotizing elapid snakebites in Australia.[56] In a human volunteer study simulating intradermal and subcutaneous envenomation using labeled radiotracer, immediately wrapping an entire extremity with a rolled elastic bandage to a pressure of 50–70 mm Hg significantly increased transit time from periphery to the systemic circulation.[37] The benefit of this technique for the more necrotizing bite of a crotalid or for coral snake envenomations seen in the United States is unclear.

Thus, the suggested constriction band is not a true tourniquet; if it is applied properly, a finger may be easily placed between the band and the skin. A tourniquet that occludes venous or arterial flow is contraindicated and may compound the initial insult by increasing edema and aggravating ischemia.

Incision and Suction

Under field circumstances, when serious envenomation is certain, the envenomated tissue may be incised and suction applied in an effort to extract venom. Alternatively, suction may be applied without skin incision, via the puncture wounds themselves. Suction is probably of value only within the first 5–30 minutes after the bite and is generally considered only after envenomation by a rattlesnake. Other crotalids (copperheads and water moccasins) and coral snakes do not usually warrant this aggressive therapy.

Two parallel incisions, 0.5–1 cm long traversing the fang marks, should be made just deep enough to penetrate the subcutaneous fat (intramuscular envenomation is rare). Care should be taken to avoid tendons, blood vessels, or nerves, and incisions parallel to the long axis of the extremity are preferred. Cross-hatch or cruciate incisions should not be made since they offer no additional value and may increase scarring or predispose to skin necrosis. Continuous suction is applied for 20–30 minutes. The value of mouth suction is unproved and can introduce bacteria, but it may be used. Swallowed venom is not harmful since venom is not absorbed through the intact oral mucosa; however, local oral injury is possible if venom contaminates open lesions on the buccal mucosa. It has been estimated that even under ideal circumstances, incision and ideally applied suction will remove less than 20–30% of injected venom. Although it has theoretical benefit, neither a definite decrease in morbidity and mortality nor a mitigation of the severity of local or systemic symptoms has been documented with incision and suction.[62] Some authorities believe that such surgical therapy is never indicated as first aid treatment, but we believe selected patients may benefit. Cases should be individualized and clinical judgment carefully applied.

There may be some value to a commercially available plunger-type suction device (The Extractor, Sawyer Products, Long Beach, CA) that can generate up to 1 atm of negative pressure when placed over nonincised puncture wounds to extract venom.[1] In animal studies this device was reported to have removed up to 37% of radiolabeled venom when applied for 3 minutes immediately after venom injection. Like incision and suction, venom extractors are currently unproved therapy but offer some theoretical benefit if used immediately.[21,22,56,62] Simple suction cups supplied in first aid kits are worthless.

It should be stressed that tourniquets, incision and suction, and vacuum extraction should not be instituted if the patient can rapidly reach a hospital or if there are no definite signs of serious envenomation. Minor pain or swelling is not an indication for zealous field treatment. Furthermore, these treatments are never a substitute for rapid transport, in-hospital evaluation, or antivenin therapy. Incision and suction would have been overtreatment in Case 1 and would likely have been ineffective and only delayed transport of the seriously ill patient in Case 2.

The bitten area should not be placed in ice, as

cryotherapy is not effective in neutralizing venom and may compound the initial injury.[49] Minor cooling may be of some value and is not harmful, but such recommendations are difficult to quantitate and can be misinterpreted by the lay public.

What Immediate Steps Should Be Taken for Snakebite Victims When They Arrive in the Hospital?

A complete medical history, including current tetanus immunization status and sensitivity to medication and horse serum, should be obtained. Patients may be shown pictures of local snakes to make specific identification, but mistakes are common. A careful description of the bite and the extent of the local pathology should be documented, including measuring the diameter of the extremity and noting the extent of edema by marking the skin with a pen to help recognize progression of the envenomation. This evaluation should be repeated hourly. A comprehensive physical examination should be done, with emphasis on vital signs, cardiorespiratory and neurologic status, neurovascular status of the extremity, and evaluation for evidence of bleeding (in the stool, gums, or urine). A baseline complete blood count (CBC), electrolytes, urinalysis, BUN, glucose, prothrombin and partial thromboplastin times (PT/PTT), fibrinogen level, and platelet count should be obtained initially and repeated in 4–8 hours. Because venom may interfere with typing and cross-matching procedures, additional blood should be drawn since a future transfusion may be required.

Pain and anxiety should be alleviated. Tetanus prophylaxis should be addressed, and antibiotics are utilized under most circumstances, although evidence is limited. Initially the extremity should be immobilized in a well-padded splint and kept at or below heart level until it is certain that there is no systemic envenomation (see Table 99–2). If the patient remains stable, the extremity should be elevated to decrease edema. Ice should not be applied, and incision and suction or the use of a tourniquet are not indicated at this juncture. If discharged, a follow-up visit should be arranged in 48–72 hours.

Victims of proven copperhead bites should be observed for 4–6 hours and evaluated for signs of systemic

TABLE 99–2. EVALUATION AND TREATMENT OF CROTALID ENVENOMATION

Extent of Envenomation	Clinical Observations	Antivenin Recommendation	Other Treatment	Disposition
None	Fang marks may be seen, but there are no local or systemic manifestations after 6–8 h of observation.	None	Local wound care Tetanus prophylaxis Value of prophylactic antibiotic unknown	Discharge with follow-up after 6–8 h of observation[a]
Minimal	Minor local swelling and discomfort. No systemic symptoms, normal laboratory findings. No blisters, ecchymoses, or necrosis. No progression after 6 h of observation.	None	Same as above	Same as above
Moderate	Progression of swelling beyond area of bite. Moderate to severe pain. Petechiae and ecchymosis of bite area. Minor systemic symptoms, such as anxiety, nausea, tingling, may be seen. Minor laboratory value abnormalities may be noted.	5–10 vials, depending on severity	Tetanus prophylaxis Broad-spectrum antibiotics Cardiac and vital sign monitoring IV fluids Analgesics Assess for compartment syndrome, debridement as necessary Follow laboratory abnormalities	Admit for observation to monitored unit
Severe	Marked progressive swelling and pain, early blisters, ecchymoses, and necrosis. Systemic symptoms such as vomiting, fasciculations, weakness, tachycardia, hypotension, incontinence, epistaxis, hematuria, or cardiopulmonary arrest. Coagulopathy, hemolysis, renal failure.	10–40 vials	Tetanus prophylaxis, prophylactic antibiotics, cardiac and vital sign monitoring, IV fluids, analgesics, vasopressors, oxygen, monitor coagulopathy, assess for compartment syndrome, debridement as necessary	Admit to intensive care unit

[a]Admit all patients with bites from a Mojave rattlesnake because of potential for delayed toxicity.

involvement, the development of coagulation abnormalities, or progression of the local pathology. The length of observation and extent of evaluation for known copperhead bites should be individualized. In the absence of progression of local symptoms and the lack of any systemic symptoms, observation for a few hours may be sufficient. In many instances the entire care of a patient with a minimal copperhead envenomation can be accomplished in the emergency department, but a conservative approach is advised. Hospitalization, if only for further observation, would be prudent for the unreliable patient or if there are questions as to the identification of the snake or progression of symptoms. Testing for sensitivity to horse serum is not routine[65] and many do not believe that pretesting is indicated. The availability of antivenin should always be determined and at least 5 vials should be obtained on site.

How Can a Venomous Snake Be Identified?

Exact identification of a snake is often not possible unless the victim brings the offending reptile to the hospital. Ideally, the snake should be captured and killed, but this should not usually be done as it delays transport or poses an additional threat to the victim or prehospital personnel. Because of the excitement generated by the bite, the victim's identification of the snake may not be accurate. Identifying a snake by its color or markings is difficult for the novice. Knowledge of the indigenous venomous snakes is often helpful to medical personnel. Snake handlers and owners of pet snakes usually know the exact species responsible for the bite but some are reluctant to offer specific information due to fear of prosecution or confiscation of the illegal snake by authorities.

Rattlesnakes have rattles that are occasionally heard prior to a strike. Water moccasins have a distinct white mouth (cotton mouth) and white buccal mucosa. The undersurface of pit vipers has a single row of plates or scales, as opposed to the double row found on nonvenomous varieties. The venomous snakes in the United States usually have a triangular-shaped head, vertically elliptical pupils (except the coral snakes, which have round pupils, like nonvenomous snakes), and easily identifiable fangs (Fig. 99–1). Fangs are paired, needlelike structures that inject venom. Rattlesnakes have the longest fangs, reaching 3–4 cm. Fangs retract on a hingelike mechanism into the roof of the mouth. In addition to fangs, venomous snakes also have rows of small teeth. An adult snake usually has two fangs, but fangs may be single or multiple.

The fangs of coral snakes are much smaller (1–3 mm) than those of the rattlesnakes and discrete fang marks may not be obvious after envenomation. There appears to be a curious propensity of coral snakes to hang

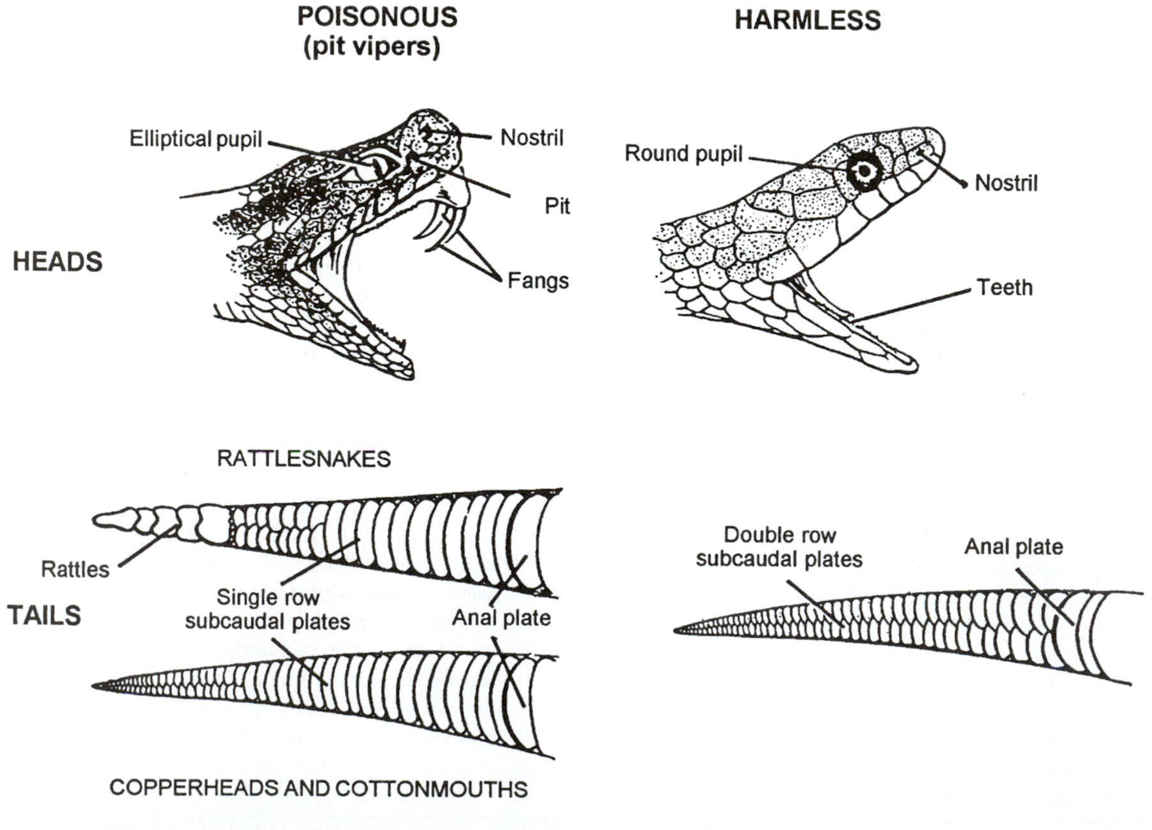

Figure 99–1. Features of pit vipers and harmless snakes. *(Modified and reprinted, with permission, from Parrish HM, Carr CA: Bites by copperheads in the United States. JAMA. 1967;201:927.)*

on to a victim or "chew" for a few seconds, and a history of this activity may help identify a coral snakebite when the offending reptile cannot be located. Removal of a coral snake from the skin has been likened to separating pieces of Velcro. Coral snakes have easily identifiable red, yellow, and black bands along the length of the body. Coral snakes and the similarly colored nonpoisonous scarlet king snake are often confused. In one report of 39 victims of coral snake bites, 9 patients were envenomated because they erroneously believed they were dealing with the nonpoisonous scarlet king snake.[44] The coral and king snake can be distinguished by the spacing of their colored rings and color of the head. Coral snakes have black snouts, whereas king snakes have red snouts. Both species have red, yellow, and black rings but in a different sequence: The red and yellow rings touch in the coral snake but in king snakes are separated by black rings ("Red on yellow kills a fellow, red on black, venom lack").

What Are the Properties of Snake Venom?

It is difficult to attribute specific pathology or pathophysiology to particular components of snake venom. Crotalid venom is a complex heterogeneous solution and suspension of various proteins, peptides, lipids, carbohydrates, and enzymes and contains RNAase and DNAase, kinins, leukotrienes, histamine, phospholipase, serotonin, hyaluronidase, acetylcholinesterase, collagenase, and metallic ions.[40,41] It has been referred to as a "mosaic of antigens." Numerous unidentified proteolytic enzymes, procoagulants and anticoagulants, cardiotoxins, hemotoxins, and neurotoxins abound in crotalid venom, making it very complex to analyze. Snake venom can simultaneously damage tissue directly, affect blood vessels and cellular elements of blood, and alter the myoneural junction and nerve transmission. Toxic components of snake venom exhibit their pathology at varying times, and some of the variation in clinical manifestations of envenomation are due not only to the specific properties of the venom but to differences in absorption rates and ability to permeate membranes and tissues. In addition, the content and potency of venom in any given snake varies with size, age, diet, climate, and time of year. Coral snake venom consists of a number of unidentified neurotoxins with curare-like effects that produce systemic neurotoxicity as opposed to local tissue injury.[59]

What Are the Characteristics of a Venomous Snakebite?

About 60% of reported venomous bites from reptiles native to the United States are rattlesnake bites.[65] Tissue destruction from rattlesnake venom may be quite significant, resulting in amputation or permanent disability (Fig. 99–2). About 40% of bites are from the copperheads and water moccasins, and fewer than 1% from the docile coral snake.[52,60] The severity and clinical manifestations of envenomation depend on a number of factors, including numbers of strikes, depth of envenomation, size of the snake, potency and amount of venom injected, size and underlying health of the victim, and location of the bite.[47] Larger snakes generally inject more venom, but the potency is species-variable. Children and small adults, as well as those with underlying medical conditions (diabetes, cardiovascular disease) are more seriously affected by envenomation.[53] Envenomation usually occurs in subcutaneous tissues, and less commonly in muscle. Systemic absorption occurs as a result of lymphatic and venous drainage of the envenomated sites. As a general rule the distance between fang marks on the skin is equal to approximately the depth of the bite, but this guideline is quite variable and has little clinical significance. Intravenous envenomation may occur, resulting in the rapid development of life-threatening complications.[18] Airway obstruction necessitating tracheal intubation has been reported after a rattlesnake bite to the face and tongue.[23,27]

Pit vipers produce a characteristic bite when they strike, and distinct fang marks can usually be identified. The small delicate fangs of coral snakes may not produce easily identifiable fang marks. Fang marks may be single, double, and occasionally multiple. Although most snakes have two fangs, the exact number of fang marks may vary because of glancing blows and/or multiple strikes. Protection by clothing or shoes can alter classical findings. The bites of rodents, lizards, and even thorn or cactus injuries can be mistaken for the bite of a poisonous snake.

Crotalid Envenomation

Crotalid (pit viper) venom is usually injected only into the subcutaneous tissue, although deeper, intramuscular (subfascial) envenomation may rarely occur. Not every bite from a venomous snake, however, results in the release of venom into the victim. So-called dry bites may occur in up to 20% of strikes,[45] although it is our experience that a true "dry bite" from a rattlesnake is quite rare. Repeat strikes may result in additional envenomation because the snake's entire supply of venom is not usually exhausted with the first attack. About 25–75% of stored venom is discharged following a rattlesnake bite, and the entire supply is replenished in 3–4 weeks.[60]

It is usually not difficult to identify serious crotalid envenomation (Fig. 99–3 and Color Plate Fig. 4). Symptoms may range from mild to severe, but the initial benign presentation of a pit viper bite may be very misleading[39] (see Tables 99–2 and 99–3). Generally, within minutes after significant envenomation from a pit viper, the area around the bite becomes swollen. Pain, often severe, quickly develops. Within minutes to hours, ecchymosis, blistering, and signs of tissue necrosis may be evident both proximal and distal to the bite. The patient may describe numbness, tingling, or other neurologic symptoms around the bite. Edema may progress to involve an entire extremity within a few hours, and systemic symptoms may develop. The local reaction to pit

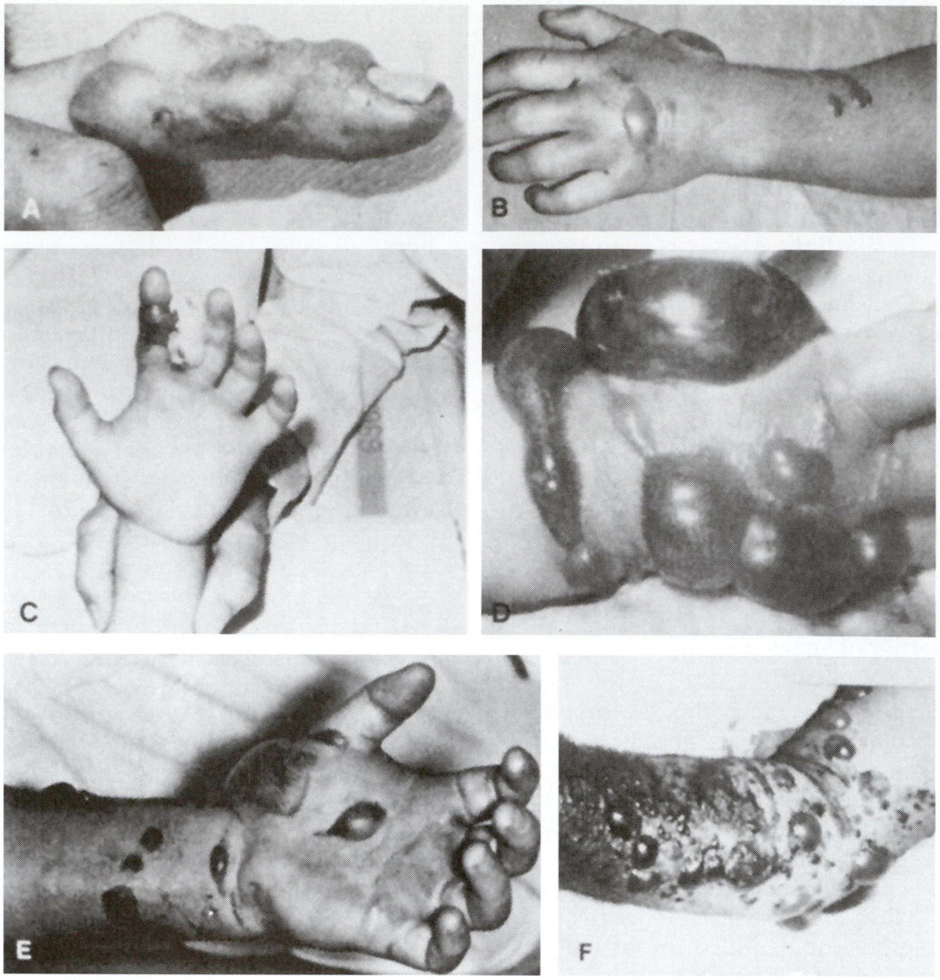

Figure 99–2. (A) Bullae filled with serous fluid 12 hours following a bite by *Crotalus atrox*. **(B)** Bullae 12 hours following a bite by an unknown rattlesnake. **(C)** Bullae containing serosanguineous fluid 24 hours following a bite by *Crotalus adamanteus*. **(D)** Bullae containing serosanguineous fluid 36 hours following a bite by *Crotalus viridis helleri*. **(E)** Bullae containing blood and serosanguineous fluid 36 hours following a bite by *Crotalus viridis oreganus*. **(F)** Bullae containing blood and serosanguineous fluid 72 hours following a bite by *Crotalus horridus*. *(Reprinted, with permission, from Russell FE: Snake Venom Poisoning. Port Washington, NY, Scholium International Inc., 1983, p. 562.)*

viper envenomation is due to altered blood vessel permeability and direct necrosis of the tissue caused by the venom. Additional tissue damage can result from the effects of ischemia, swelling, and secondary infection.

Local reaction to all rattlesnake venom is usually quite pronounced, but a potential exception to this is envenomation from the Mojave rattlesnake (*Crotalus scutulatus*), a pit viper found in Arizona and other southwestern states. Envenomation from the Mojave rattlesnake may not always produce immediate, severe local symptoms. The potent venom can produce a systemic neurotoxic syndrome (lethargy, obtundation, cranial nerve dysfunction, and respiratory paralysis) in the absence of significant local symptoms, requiring extreme caution in prognosticating lack of envenomation or when treating an apparently "benign" bite from this snake.[42] Mojave venom, unlike the venom of other rattlesnakes, does not usually produce a significant coagulopathy.[9]

Compared with the venom of rattlesnakes, the venom of water moccasins produces less-severe local and systemic pathology. Envenomation from copperheads tends to be less severe than either rattlesnake or water moccasin envenomation. Copperhead envenomation often results in only minimal edema and pain and usually requires only conservative local treatment.[70] Although the soft tissue swelling from a copperhead bite may be significant, envenomation from this snake does not usually cause a coagulopathy, systemic symptoms, or extensive tissue destruction. We have been unable to find a report of a lethal copperhead bite in the medical literature.

It is difficult to quantify crotalid envenomation initially. Envenomation is a dynamic and ever-changing process that can rapidly or unpredictably progress to serious local or systemic involvement. It may require a number of hours for the full extent of envenomation to become evident. On rare occasions symptoms may appear to be resolving, only to return minutes to hours later

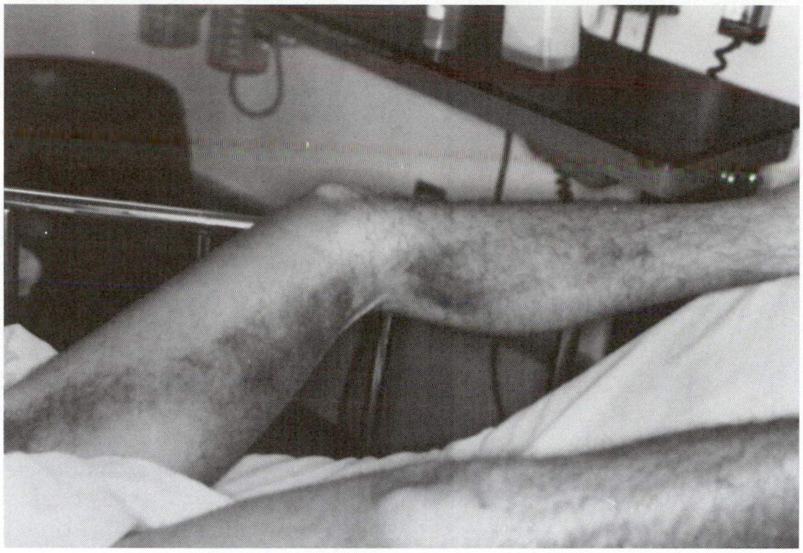

Figure 99–3. This patient's ascending subcutaneous hemorrhagic ecchymosis developing within 8 hours of a copperhead bite to the foot follows the course of lymphatic or venous drainage. Only minor discomfort was noted and there was no coagulopathy. The actual cause is unknown but this is an example of the hemorrhagic diathesis produced by crotalid envenomation. *(Reproduced, with permission, from Roberts JR, Greenberg MJI: Ascending hemorrhagic signs after a bite from a copperhead. N Engl J Med 1997;336:1262–1263.)*

with greater intensity. As a general rule, however, it may be assumed that if no symptoms develop within 6–8 hours, envenomation from a pit viper (other than Mojave rattlesnake) has not occurred (dry bite).

Rarely, patients bitten by crotalids may experience classic anaphylaxis from the venom itself that can complicate evaluation or mimic a severe systemic reaction to venom. In one report a man developed pruritus and shortness of breath, accompanied by hypotension, generalized urticaria, and wheezes immediately following a rattlesnake bite.[35] The symptoms quickly responded to standard treatment for anaphylaxis (epinephrine, antihistamines, and corticosteroids). The patient had been bitten previously and may have been sensitized at that time. Snake handlers may be sensitized through inhalation or skin contact and develop IgE antibodies to venom. Antivenin is not indicated for the treatment of anaphylaxis, but differentiating anaphylaxis from envenomation may be clinically difficult. The presence of pruritus and urticaria or wheezing, uncommon with envenomation, should suggest anaphylaxis.

Elapid Envenomation

The severe local reaction to crotalid envenomation is in contrast with the usually minor pain and clinically unimpressive local reactions seen with a coral snake bite. However, lack of local symptoms does not signify that serious envenomation has not occurred. It is difficult to judge initially which patients bitten by coral snakes will develop symptoms. About 75% of patients bitten by a coral snake are subsequently determined to have been envenomated.[44] Coral snake envenomation may be manifested by serious systemic reactions with little symptomatology at the actual site of envenomation even after an asymptomatic period of up to 12 hours. The venom of the eastern coral snake (*Micrurus fulvius*) is probably more potent than that of the Sonoran coral snake (*Micruroides euryxanthus*) or the Texas coral snake (*Micrurus tenere*).

What Are the Systemic Signs of Envenomation?

Crotalid

Most bites from pit vipers that occur on the extremities are limited to local or regional pathology, but systemic symptoms of life-threatening proportions may develop (Table 99–3). When venom is injected subcutaneously, it travels by lymphatic and superficial venous channels and spreads rather slowly to reach the general circulation. It generally requires a number of hours for subcutaneous envenomation to produce systemic symptoms, but this timetable is quite variable, occasionally occurring quite rapidly even with subcutaneous envenomation. Intravascular envenomation produces significant systemic symptoms in a matter of minutes.[18] Direct blood envenomation is probably quite rare and may account for the majority of fatalities. Bites to the head and neck may also be more dangerous than extremity bites because of the rapid absorption of venom from these highly vascular areas and because of airway compromise.

Systemic signs of pit viper envenomation are varied.

TABLE 99–3. SIGNS AND SYMPTOMS OF RATTLESNAKE ENVENOMATION (*N* = 100)

Sign or Symptom	Percent
Fang marks	100
Swelling and edema	74
Pain	65
Ecchymosis	51
Vesiculations	40
Changes in pulse rate	60
Weakness	72
Sweating and/or chills	64
Numbness or tingling of tongue and mouth or scalp or feet	63
Faintness or dizziness	57
Nausea, vomiting, or both	48
Blood pressure changes	46
Change in body temperature	31
Swelling of regional lymph nodes	40
Fasciculations	41
Increased clotting time	39
Sphering of red blood cells (spherocytes)	18
Tingling or numbness of affected part	42
Necrosis	27
Respiratory rate changes	40
Decreased hemoglobin	37
Abnormal electrocardiogram	26
Cyanosis	16
Hematemesis, hematuria, or melena	15
Glycosuria	20
Proteinuria	16
Unconsciousness	12
Thirst	34
Increased salivation	20
Swollen eyelids	2
Retinal hemorrhage	2
Blurring of vision	12
Convulsions	1
Muscle contractions	6
Increased platelets	4
Decreased platelets	42

Adapted, with permission, from Russell FE: Snake Venom Poisoning. Philadelphia, Lippincott, 1980, p. 281.

Some symptoms may be due to fear, pain, or anxiety alone. In mild cases the patient may manifest nonspecific weakness, malaise, nausea, and restlessness. More severe envenomation produces confusion, abdominal pain, vomiting, sweating, dyspnea, tachycardia, blurred vision, salivation, and an unusual or metallic taste in the mouth. Severe envenomation may induce a coagulopathy characterized by spontaneous epistaxis, hematuria, or disseminated intravascular coagulation (DIC). Neurologic symptoms, such as fasciculations, slurred speech, and seizures, may occur. Although crotalid venom may be directly nephrotoxic, renal failure is probably secondary to hemoglobinuria, myoglobinuria, or cardiovascular collapse. Multisystem failure, predominantly cardiac arrest or ARDS, may be the end result of severe envenomation.[13]

Significant crotalid envenomation may produce complex but rather dramatic hematologic abnormalities, usually a combination of hypoprothrombinemia, thrombocytopenia, fibrinolysis, and hypofibrinogenemia[5,59,64] (see Fig. 99–3). *Crotalus atrox* venom, for example, can render human blood uncoagulable. A routine coagulation profile should be obtained following envenomation by a crotalid (and repeated in 4–8 hours). A significant coagulopathy, especially thrombocytopenia, may be present with a paucity of other systemic effects, so evaluation should be routine even in the absence of signs and symptoms. Laboratory abnormalities, including prolonged PT and PTT, are frequently seen, and changes in red blood cell morphology, decreased platelet count and function, and bleeding tendencies have been well described. Coagulopathy has been attributed to a complex variety of anticoagulants, procoagulants, fibrinolysin, and hemorrhagins in crotalid venom. Overall, crotalid venom has a thrombin-like effect, but specific hematologic effects are species-dependent. Platelet consumption at the site of envenomation may occur. Patients may experience spontaneous epistaxis, hematuria, or hematemesis. An initial drop in fibrinogen levels (to near zero) and platelet count (in the 10,000–50,000/mm^3 range) are frequently seen after moderate to severe crotalid envenomation. Following the trend in these laboratory parameters is an important way to assess the progression or reversal of systemic envenomation.

A major difficulty in objectively grading the severity of crotalid envenomation, and following its progress, is that no scoring system readily fits the vagaries of envenomation. Most patients exhibit only a subset of all of the possible consequences, so all, some, or none of the anticipated signs and symptoms may develop in any given individual. In addition, some of the characteristics of envenomation (nausea, tachycardia, restlessness, tachypnea) may be related to fear, and not to envenomation. Recently a validated severity score for the objective assessment of crotalid envenomation has been developed and holds promise as a standardization tool for research and clinical evaluation.[16]

Elapid

The systemic effects of elapid envenomation are characteristically delayed for a number of hours (Table 99–4). One report described a patient who had an asymptomatic period of 13 hours followed by a sudden and precipitous deterioration severe enough to require ventilatory support.[44] The neurologic abnormalities noted included slurred speech, paresthesias, ptosis, diplopia, dysphagia, stridor, muscle weakness, fasciculations, and respiratory paralysis.[44] Coral snake envenomation results in fewer cardiovascular effects than crotalid envenomation; the major immediate cause of death is respiratory arrest. Pulmonary aspiration is a common sequela in the subacute phase. Patients can develop total-body paraly-

TABLE 99–4. SIGNS AND SYMPTOMS OF ENVENOMATION BY THE EASTERN CORAL SNAKE (*MICRURUS FULVIUS*) (*N* = 20)

Sign or Symptom	Percent
Fang marks	85
Local swelling	40
Paresthesias	35
Nausea	30
Vomiting	25
Euphoria	15
Weakness	15
Dizziness	10
Diplopia	10
Dyspnea	10
Diaphoresis	10
Muscle tenderness	10
Fasciculations	5
Confusion	5

Reprinted, with permission, from Kitchens CS, Van Mierop LHS: Envenomation by the eastern coral snake (Micrurus fulvius fulvius): A study of 39 victims. JAMA 1987;258:1615.

sis that may last 3–5 days and take weeks to resolve completely. With respiratory support, however, the paralysis is completely reversible. Primary cardiac arrest and cardiac dysrhythmias are rare, even in severely envenomated patients.

The benign local effect of coral snake envenomation can be misleading and mistakenly be equated with a dry bite. Because it is difficult to judge initially which patients are envenomated, any patient with coral snake exposure with fang marks or other evidence of skin penetration requires at least 24 hours of observation. Clinical deterioration may be totally unexpected and progress rapidly. Coral snake envenomation can be fatal, but with supportive care and antivenin therapy, patients usually recover completely. In one series, 6 of 39 patients required intubation and ventilation, but none died or suffered tissue loss or permanent neurologic sequelae.[44]

What Are the Characteristics of Nonvenomous Snakebites?

There are approximately 50,000 snakebites annually in the United States, and most (90–95%) are from nonvenomous snakes.[25] Most snakes in the United States are nonvenomous and the majority are of the Colubrid family, which are generally considered harmless to humans. However, several authors have reported toxic secretions from Duvernoy's glands in many common species, including the hognose snake, garter snake, parrot snake, banded water snake, and ringneck snake.[27,50,67] Although there have been no deaths reported, some victims have developed coagulopathies and local edema and hemorrhage that could be confused with early crotalid envenomation.[49] There is no antivenin available to treat bites from these snakes, and serious complications from nonvenomous snakebites are extremely rare.

Although Colubrids do not possess true fangs, some species, such as the common wandering garter snake (*Thamnophis* sp.) have elongated and grooved posterior maxillary teeth (a primitive rear fang) that can penetrate the skin and deliver irritating saliva into the victim via a chewing motion. Some clinicians believe that the presence of teeth marks at the bite excludes the possibility that the bite was made by a venomous snake. Although it is true that fang marks are absent following nonvenomous snakebites, venomous snakes do have teeth, and abrasions or teethmarks may be seen in conjunction with a venomous bite. This fact, along with the possibility that snakes heretofore considered nonvenomous may be dangerous, should make the clinician more cautious in diagnosing a nonvenomous bite based entirely on the presence of teeth marks.

When there is no sign of envenomation after an appropriate period of observation following a suspected nonpoisonous snakebite, attention should be focused on the basic principles of wound care. Incision and suction, excision, and wide debridement are obviously unnecessary in such bites. The wound should be treated as a contaminated puncture wound, as it may contain foreign material, especially broken teeth. Any foreign material should be removed and an appropriate dressing applied. Certain large snakes of the Biodae family (not seen in the United States, except as pets or in zoologic gardens), including boas, pythons, and anacondas, may present a special problem, since the force of contraction of their jaws may be great enough to cause severe tissue contusion or fractures (Fig. 99–4). These reptiles also have numerous large, brittle teeth that commonly are broken off and lodged in the wound when the bitten part is forcibly extricated from the snake's mouth. Usually radiographs of the bitten area are needed to exclude fracture or foreign body.

The morbidity associated with a nonvenomous snakebite is from the rare case of bony injury and wound infection. Nearly all authors recommend antibiotics for venomous snakebites, although their routine use has not been systematically analyzed. In one report no infections followed nonpoisonous snakebites in 72 patients bitten by a variety of nonpoisonous snakes indigenous to New England and imported boa constrictors and pythons.[69] Although *Clostridium tetanus* has not been isolated from the mouths of snakes, the ubiquitous nature of this organism requires prophylaxis following the recommended approach for a contaminated wound. A cogent argument can be made for administering prophylactic antibiotics in nonvenomous snakebites if tooth fragments are retained or if there is significant soft tissue contusion. A first-generation cephalosporin or antistaphylococcal penicillin given for 7–10 days should be adequate. Outpatient therapy is appropriate; the patient should be instructed with regard to wound care and to seek medical care if signs of infection occur. Minor abrasions from nonvenomous snakes require only local wound care and tetanus prophylaxis. Delayed infection should prompt an investigation for a retained foreign body, especially a tooth fragment.[31]

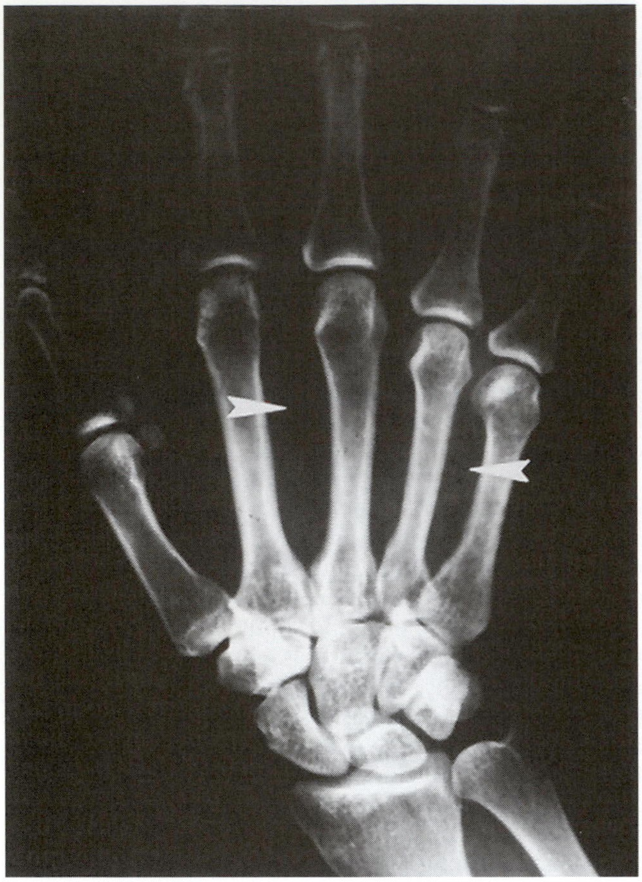

Figure 99–4. Significant local morbidity developed after the bite of a 6-foot boa constrictor. The patient had extensive soft tissue swelling and developed a gas-forming bacterial infection (note gas in interdigital spaces). Subcutaneous gas and/or crepitus following a snakebite does not always indicate a serious infection. Benign ambient air can be injected during the bite. Peroxide use and mouth suction can also introduce air into the wound. There was no fracture, but the force of the bite could have broken a metacarpal.

What Are the Objectives for Treatment of Patients With Envenomation?

The specific treatment of a patient with a snakebite is controversial, and the literature contains confusing and contradictory recommendations. Folklore and home remedies abound, but the benign natural history of many bites undoubtedly has accounted for many "miraculous cures." Many accepted treatment plans are based on anecdotal or biased information with conclusions drawn from animal studies or uncontrolled case reports. Many authors tend to be staunch advocates of their particular regimens and unwilling to accept a less rigid approach. The initial objectives are to determine the identity of the offending snake and presence or absence of envenomation, to provide basic supportive therapy, to treat the local and systemic effects of envenomation, and to limit or repair tissue loss and/or functional disability (see Table 99–2).

Two distinct therapeutic approaches are promulgated. One recommends primarily antivenin therapy, whereas the other advocates primarily a surgical approach with an emphasis on surgical debridement and early fasciotomy. Some advocate a very conservative approach that eschews both routine surgery and antivenin, citing a lack of serious morbidity in patients given symptomatic treatment and supportive care after snakebite.[4] A combination of medical therapy (mainly antivenin) and conservative surgical treatment (mainly debridement of devitalized tissue), individualized for each patient, will likely provide the best results. In general, the more rapidly treatment is instituted, the better the final outcome, but no specific standard of care exists for the institution of various interventions.

How Long Should Asymptomatic Patients Be Observed?

All patients reporting a history of snakebite should be observed for 6–8 hours if the skin is broken and the offending snake cannot be positively identified as nonpoisonous. Fang marks can be quite subtle and initially mistaken for scratches or teeth marks. Although most poisonous snakebites declare their presence by the development of significant symptomatology within a few minutes of the bite, delayed toxicity or resolution of symptoms with a serious recurrence hours later may rarely occur.[29] Delayed symptomatology has been specifically noted after the bite of coral snakes and the Mojave rattlesnake; patients possibly bitten by these snakes should be observed for 24 hours regardless of symptoms. The initial presentation of other pit viper bites may be misleading and significant worsening of a seemingly benign bite may occur as long as 8 hours after presentation,[39] but such cases are quite unusual. A prudent and conservative approach would be to observe all victims of possible crotalid bites for at least 6–8 hours and admit those with systemic symptoms at any time postenvenomation or those with progressive local symptoms. Intoxicated patients should not be allowed to sign out against medical advice. Restlessness, anxiety, abdominal pain, nausea, and tachycardia are nonspecific symptoms but could signal systemic envenomation, and they should not be routinely dismissed as being a result of fear or anxiety.

In Addition to Antivenin, What Other Treatment Modalities Should Be Considered for Envenomated Patients?

Surgical Therapies

Surgery is not a concern in the treatment of coral snakebites, and similarly copperhead and water moccasin bites rarely require aggressive therapies. There is, however, considerable controversy as to the role of surgery to treat patients who are envenomated by rattlesnakes. Some authors advocate such aggressive therapy as immediate excision of the bitten area to remove venom, extensive debridement, and the liberal use of fasciotomy to decompress an extremity.[38,70] Rattlesnake venom is clearly tissue-toxic and produces necrosis. Edema secondary to necrosis and local alterations of vascular permeability produced by venom is common and may be quite impressive. Because subfascial envenomation is uncommon, much of the edema produced by envenomation does not occur in compartmentalized areas. The early use of adequate amounts of antivenin may limit necrosis and edema. Although there is little doubt that many crotalid bites may eventually require some surgical debridement or even skin grafting, the initial routine use of tissue excision, fasciotomy, or "exploration and debridement," is not warranted. Although there are staunch advocates of this therapy, its benefits are unproven.

It is unlikely that excising tissue will halt the envenomation process significantly. With the development of techniques to monitor compartment pressures, indications for fasciotomy can be based on objective data. With noninvasive vascular arterial studies and skin temperature determinations in patients with rattlesnake envenomation, one report demonstrated that pulsatile arterial blood flow to an envenomated extremity actually increased after tissue excision, even distal to the site of envenomation.[12] Skin temperatures also usually increased, but a decrease in skin temperature was associated with vascular insufficiency. One patient in their series developed an arterial embolism, necessitating embolectomy. The authors concluded that increased tissue pressures are not severe enough to cause ischemia to an extremity in most patients bitten by a rattlesnake if antivenin and supportive care are given, and those at risk for ischemia can be identified by noninvasive techniques.

Surgical debridement of necrotic tissue and hemorrhagic blebs and blisters is usually done between the third and sixth day after envenomation. Physical therapy should be instituted early to ameliorate stiffness and decrease swelling.

Blood Products

A minor bleeding diathesis as defined by alterations in platelet count, PT/PTT, fibrin split products, and fibrinogen levels is common with crotalid envenomation, and all victims of crotalid envenomation should be evaluated for a coagulopathy, even in the absence of severe symptoms.[18,53] Coral snake venom does not alter coagulation. Crotalid-induced coagulopathy usually resolves spontaneously or is corrected with antivenin therapy, but occasionally fresh frozen plasma, cryoprecipitate, packed red blood cells, or platelet transfusions are required. The decision to administer blood products should be based on clinical condition, trend of clotting parameters, and other standard criteria for the treatment of coagulopathies. Criteria for the use of blood products appears to be quite arbitrary in clinical practice but can be associated with significant risks to the patient. Therefore it is cautioned that blood products be used only if antivenin is ineffective and for specific conditions. In general blood products should be administered if coagulation abnormalities continue to be unstable after antivenin use or if active bleeding occurs. Minor oozing or microscopic hematuria can frequently be treated with antivenin alone.

The specific mechanism by which antivenin reverses the coagulopathy is unknown, but crotalid antivenin appears to decrease platelet aggregation in vitro. Heparin does not appear to correct the coagulopathy associated with crotalid envenomation. Monitoring trends in the coagulation profile is one objective way of monitoring the seriousness of envenomation and the response to antivenin therapy.

Antibiotics

The incidence of wound infection following crotalid envenomation is quite low. In one report only 1 in 33 patients not treated with prophylactic antibiotics following a rattlesnake bite developed evidence of a wound infection, prompting the authors to conclude that routine prophylactic antibiotics are not warranted.[6] However, infection is often difficult to differentiate from envenomation, and the use of broad-spectrum antibiotics for patients with serious bites is intuitively reasonable.[8] A first-generation cephalosporin or a penicillinase-resistant penicillin should suffice. The mouths of snakes have been found to harbor various aerobic and anaerobic bacteria (Fig. 99–4).[26] *Mycobacterium* infection has been reported following snakebite.[34] Tetanus prophylaxis should be administered and hyperimmune tetanus antitoxin given if there is inadequate primary immunization or if the history is uncertain. Antibiotics are also recommended if treatment included incision, especially if mouth suction was used.

Other Considerations

There is no rationale for the use of corticosteroids or antihistamines in the routine treatment of patients with snakebite, but they are used to combat the rare case of anaphylaxis from exposure to venom or the more common acute and delayed allergic reactions to antivenin. Corticosteroids may be detrimental to local tissue in the early stages of envenomation.[11] Cardiovascular collapse is a life-threatening consequence of severe systemic envenomation and should be treated aggressively with large amounts of antivenin, invasive monitoring, and standard intensive care techniques.[13] Vasopressors may be required, and respiratory compromise should be anticipated in severe cases. Because of sudden and unpredictable respiratory paralysis associated with coral snake envenomation, tracheal intubation should be considered at the first sign of bulbar paralysis. Any patient given antivenin or with significant envenomation should be observed in an intensive care unit.

There are several reports of a beneficial effect of

high-voltage electric shock treatment for poisonous snakebites, but this approach is unproved and cannot be recommended.[17,28] Multiple treatments with hyperbaric oxygen suggest that enhanced healing of myonecrosis may occur in mice injected with *Crotalus atrox* venom. There was no effect on the edema associated with envenomation in one study and the beneficial effect was dose-dependent, and up to 10 treatments (1–1.5 hours at 2–2.75 atm) were given.[43] The mechanism of action is not known but is speculated to be related to enhanced tissue oxygenation. The effects of hyperbaric oxygen therapy of poisonous snakebites in humans is unknown; its use should be considered experimental at this time.

What Are the Special Considerations for the Management of Pregnant Patients With Snakebites?

There is scant information available on the effects of poisonous snakebites during pregnancy. If envenomation is significant, fetal morbidity, mortality, or normal delivery may occur. Three of the four pregnant women bitten by crotalids in one report delivered normal infants, but one woman suffered a spontaneous abortion within 24 hours. The mechanism of injury to the fetus from envenomation includes uterine artery hypotension and subsequent hypoxia, hemorrhagic complications, such as abruptio placenta, or uterine contractions initiated by venom.[54]

Intracranial hemorrhage and death in an infant born at 34 weeks' gestation was reported in a woman envenomated by a copperhead during week 28 of her pregnancy.[20] At the time of the bite she was given antivenin and developed hypotension treated with large doses of epinephrine. It is suggested that the alpha-adrenergic effects of epinephrine on the uterine artery, coupled with maternal hypotension, contributed more to the fetal demise than the direct effects of venom. Ephedrine (25–50 mg IV bolus) would be an appropriate alternative to epinephrine in that it spares uterine blood flow while supporting blood pressure. As in each case of snakebite, it is prudent to evaluate the need for antivenin carefully during pregnancy and to administer it only when envenomation is significant and the benefits of antivenin outweigh the possible risks from allergic reactions. Fetal monitoring should be routine following poisonous snakebite.

Can Individuals Become Immune to Snake Venom?

Handlers and collectors are at risk for multiple bites over their careers, and questions have been raised about possible immunity. No evidence was established that immunity develops as a result of repeated envenomation in one report of 14 patients with two or more bites.[55] Victims of repeat bites may actually be at greater risk for anaphylaxis because of a prior sensitization and the development of IgE antibodies to venom.

What Special Actions Should Be Taken for a Victim Bitten by an Exotic Snake?

About 3% of poisonous snakebites in the United States are from nonnative species. Many such snakes are illegally imported or stolen from zoos or pet stores. Exotic snakes (venomous snakes not native to the United States) pose a particularly difficult problem in both diagnosis and management. Many victims are collectors or researchers who can identify the offending snake. If they cannot provide identification, the local zoo, regional poison center, or herpetology society may be helpful. Once the snake has been identified, the antivenin must be obtained. Local zoos, poison centers, or collectors may have the antivenin. The American Association of Zoological Parks and Aquariums (304–242–2160) maintains the Antivenin Index, a listing of currently available antivenins for exotic snakes.

Bites from many nonnative elapidae snakes, such as mambas, kraits, cobras, and several Australian species, are associated with high morbidity and mortality rates. Bites from these snakes may not display early local or systemic signs (Table 99–2); therefore, the grading system developed for North American pit vipers is not helpful. Although local tissue destruction and edema may develop, classically it is the neurologic signs, such as ptosis, dysphagia, muscular weakness, paresis, ophthalmoplegia, and respiratory failure, that are noted, often at a delayed or advanced stage. Enzyme-linked immunosorbent assay (ELISA) techniques may be used to identify specific venom antigens in suspected exotic snakebites. This technique is not currently available in the United States but is used in Africa, Asia, and Australia.

Guidelines for the administration of antivenin for exotic snakes are not as well supported by scientific evidence as those for North American poisonous snakes. In addition, there is little standardization of the antivenin; antivenins for the same snake vary by manufacturer. Since exotic snakes are generally quite poisonous, if fang marks are present, envenomation is strongly suspected, the snake has been identified, and the specific antivenin has been obtained, many physicians believe that it is logical to proceed with antivenin administration empirically. The patient should be tested for horse serum sensitivity and the antivenin administered according to the package insert. This approach appears to lack clinical logic. Generally 4–5 vials are administered under the same guidelines given for crotalid antivenin. If the antivenin cannot be obtained, then supportive care and close in-hospital observation may be all that is possible. Local incision and suction are best avoided. Compression of an entire extremity with an elastic bandage (the Sutherland wrap) for the bite of some elapids (eg, brown snake bites) has been shown to be useful when antivenin is not available and is recommended for bites from exotic elapids. Crotalidae Polyvalent Antivenin (Wyeth) commonly used for North American pit vipers is ineffective for the bites of elapid snakes, but it is active against South American pit vipers, such as the bushmaster, cascabel, and fer-de-lance. Coral snake antivenin is active only against the eastern North American coral snake and is not effective against the western, Mexican, or South American species. It is prudent to obtain expert assistance in managing any exotic snakebite.

One report documents rather dramatic reversal of the neurotoxic effects of a monocellate cobra (*Naja kaouthia*) bite following the intravenous administration of the anticholinesterase neostigmine methyl sulfate (0.5 mg every 20 minutes for 4 doses).[24] The major neurotoxin from this snake is believed to resemble curare, causing a postsynaptic blockade of nicotinic neuromuscular receptor sites. The neurotoxicity from sea snakes and other elapids has been experimentally reversed with neostigmine.[63] Edrophonium chloride (10 mg administered intravenously with 0.5 mg of atropine) has also been suggested.

What Other Poisonous Reptiles Are Found in the United States?

In North America there are two indigenous species of venomous lizards that belong to the order Squamata, the same order as venomous snakes: the Gila monster (*Heloderma suspectum*) and the beaded lizard (*Heloderma horridum*). These lizards are found primarily in the desert areas of Arizona, southwestern Utah, southern Nevada, New Mexico, California, and Mexico. They are large, slow-moving, nocturnal thick-bodied lizards that are prized by collectors and hobbyists. Adults are 30–40 cm long and are generally shy creatures, so bites are relatively rare, being unintentional or secondary to handling. Gila monsters are known for their forceful bite and propensity to hang on tenaciously during a bite and may be difficult to disengage. Some rather unique techniques have been developed to remove a Gila monster from an extremity, including the use of chisels, screwdrivers, and crowbars, pouring gasoline or ammonia into the lizard's mouth, or holding a flame to the animals jaw. Teeth may break off in the wound.

Gila monster venom is complex, containing components similar to those of snake venoms, including numerous enzymes, hyaluronidase, phospholipase A, kallikrein, and serotonin.[30,61,66] Helothermine is a suspected toxin. Their venom delivery systems are not as efficient as those of poisonous snakes, consisting of venom glands and grooved teeth, rather than fangs. Dry bites often occur due to the ineffective mechanism of delivery. Following skin puncture and venom release, the victim experiences local tenderness and soft tissue swelling, pain, and edema; there are occasional reports of anaphylactic reactions, hypotension, angioedema of lip, tongue, and throat, respiratory depression, coagulopathy, and myocardial infarction.[57,58] Significant tissue destruction is unusual but maceration may occur, and a cyanosis or blue discoloration is noted about the wound. There is no antivenin available against lizard venom. Treatment consists of avoiding overaggressive local treatment and providing supportive care and wound care. Serious morbidity from lizard bites is unusual. The characteristics of the beaded lizard are similar, but their bites are less commonly confronted clinically.

Are There Any Other Venomous or Poisonous Animals That May Be Encountered?

It was generally believed that there are poisonous or venomous members of all classes of animal except birds. Recent discoveries in New Guinea, however, have added birds to the list.[19,36] Three avian *Pitohui* species have been found to contain homobatrachotoxin, a poison very similar to that in poison dart frogs of South America. Like the frogs, the *Pitohui* birds are conspicuous and brightly colored. There is little information available concerning the toxicity of these birds.

Several species of mammals contain venomous members. For example, the male Australian duckbilled platypus (*Ornithorhynchus anatinus*) has a hollow spur that may inject venom, and the Cuban insectivore (*Solendon paradoxes*) and North American short-tailed shrew both secrete venom from the maxillary glands and bite with the lower incisors. Envenomations from mammals are quite rare, and little is known about the specific clinical toxicity from these creatures.

Several species of amphibians, frogs, toads (*Anura*), newts, and salamanders (*Urodela*) can secrete toxins through their skins, which may be a defensive repellant or alarm mechanism.[2,7,14,15,32] These creatures are not truly venomous, for they have no specific mechanism for delivering the toxin. Most cases of toxicity involve children or pets ingesting the animals. The best-known examples are the Colombian poison dart frogs (*Phyllobates* and *Atelopus*), which secrete the toxins zetekitoxin, tetrodotoxin, and batrachotoxin.[51] Batrachotoxin irreversibly activates (depolarizes) the sodium channel and is 250 times more toxic than curare in mice. Newts of the genus *Taricha* contain the irreversible sodium channel blocking agent tetrodotoxin in their skin and internal organs. Their toxicity would be expected to be similar to that occurring with puffer fish (fugu) poisoning. Ingestion of a newt has potential adverse consequences. Treatment is supportive. The East Coast species is less toxic than the West Coast variety, the Oregon rough-skinned newt (*Taricha granulosa*). Salamanders of the genus *Salamandra* contain a very potent CNS toxin, salamandarin. Large exposures could theoretically produce neurotoxicity.

Toad species of the genus *Bufo* have been known to be abused by a curious technique of licking their skin, which contains a number of toxic substances, including biogenic amines (serotonin), steroids, and polypeptides. An LSD like high has been reported but there is considerable folklore and confusion on the exact effects.[48] Toxicity has been reported following toad licking, toad mouthing, ingestion of toads, and eating toad soup. Salivation, seizures, and cardiac dysrhythmias have been reported with ingestion of toxin from *Bufo alvarius*, the Colorado

River toad. The cane toad (*Bufo marinus*) is less toxic. Bufotalin, a cardioactive steroid toxin (bufadienolide) derived from this toad has a chemical structure very similar to that of digoxin. Some nonprescription naturopathic remedies (such as the Chinese traditional medicine Chan Su) contain derivatives of toad and frog skin. Digitalis toxicity may be associated with their chronic use.[46] A number of poisonings, some fatal, have been reported after the ingestion of a purported Chinese topical aphrodisiac ("Rock Hard," "Love Stone") containing bufotenine and a variety of cardioactive steroids found in dried toad venom. Patients presented with hyperkalemia, severe vomiting, and bradycardia and other cardiac dysrhythmias reminiscent of digoxin toxicity. Serum digoxin levels were documented by radioimmunoassay, but did not correlate with toxicity; however, treatment with digoxin Fab antibodies (Digibind) appeared to be lifesaving in some instances.[3]

The clinical toxicity associated with many of these animals has not been well delineated, and treatment consists of supportive care based on the clinical presentation rather than concentrating on the specific poison.

References

1. Bornstein AD, Russell FE, Sullivan JB: Negative pressure suction in field treatment of rattlesnake bite. Vet Hum Toxicol 1985;25:297–299.
2. Bradley SG, Klika LJ: A fatal poisoning from the Oregon rough skinned newt *(Taricha granulosa)*. JAMA 1981;246:247.
3. Brubacher JR, Ravikumar PR, Bania T, Heller MG, Hoffman RS: Treatment of toad venom poisoning with digoxin-specific Fab gragments. Chest 1996;110:1282–1288.
4. Burch JM, Agarwal R, Mattox KL, et al: The treatment of crotalid envenomation without antivenin. J Trauma 1988; 28:35–43.
5. Burgess JL, Dart RC: Snake venom coagulopathy: Use and abuse of blood products in the treatment of pit viper envenomation. Ann Emerg Med 1991;20:795–780.
6. Burgess JL, Dart RC, Egen NB, et al: Effects of constriction bands on rattlesnake venom absorption: A pharmacokinetic study. Ann Emerg Med 1992;1:1068–1093.
7. Chadwick JB: New England's venomous mammals. N Engl J Med 1969;281:274.
8. Clark RF, Selden, BS, Furbee B: The incidence of wound infection following Crotalid envenomation. J Emerg Med 1993;11:583–586.
9. Corrigan JJ, Jeter MA: Mojave rattlesnake (*Crotalus scutulatus scutulatus*) venom: In vitro effect on platelets, fibrinolysis, and fibrinogen clotting. Vet Hum Toxicol 1990;32: 439–441.
10. Cruz NS, Alvarez RG: Rattlesnake bite complications in 19 children. Pediatr Emerg Care 1994;10:30–33.
11. Cunningham ER, Sabback MS, Smith RM, et al: Snakebite: Role of corticosteroids as immediate therapy in an animal model. Am Surg 1979;45:757–759.
12. Curry SC, Kraner JC, Kunkel DB, et al: Noninvasive vascular studies in management of rattlesnake envenomation to extremities. Ann Emerg Med 1985;4:1081–1084.
13. Curry SC, Kunkel DB: Death from a rattlesnake bite. Am J Emerg Med 1985;3:227–235.
14. Daly JW: Biologically active alkaloids from poison frogs (Denodrobatidae). Toxin Rev 1982;1:33.
15. Daly JW, Myers CW, Whittaker N: Further classification of skin alkaloids from neotropical poison from Denodrobatidae, with a general survey of toxic/noxious substances in the amphibia. Toxicon 1987;25:1023–1095.
16. Dart RC, Hurlbut KM, Garcia R, Bkoren J: Validation of severity score for the assessment of crotalid snakebite. Ann Emerg Med 1996;27:321–326.
17. Dart RC, Lindsey D, Schulman A: Snakebites and shocks. Ann Emerg Med 1988;17:1262. Letter.
18. Davidson TM: Intravenous rattlesnake envenomation. West J Med 1988;148:45–47.
19. Dumbacher JP, Beehler BM, Spande TF, et al: Homobatrachotoxin in the genus *Pitohui*: Chemical defense in birds? Science 1992;258:799–801.
20. Entman SS, Moise KJ: Anaphylaxis in pregnancy. South Med J 1984;77:402.
21. Forgey WE: More on snake-venom and insect venom extractors. N Engl J Med 1993;328:516. Letter.
22. Gellert GA: Snake-venom and insect-venom extractors: An unproved therapy. N Engl J Med 1992;327:1322. Letter.
23. Gerkin R, Sergent K, Curry SC: Life-threatening airway obstruction from rattlesnake bite to the tongue. Ann Emerg Med 1987;16:813–816.
24. Gold BS: Neostigmine for the treatment of neurotoxicity following envenomation by the Asiatic Cobra. Ann Emerg Med 1996;28:87–89.
25. Gold BS, Barish RA: Venomous snakebites: Current concepts in diagnosis, treatment and management. Emerg Med Clin North Am 1992;10:249–267.
26. Goldstein EJ, Citron DM, Gonzalez H, et al: Bacteriology of rattlesnake venom and implications for therapy. J Infect Dis 1979;14:818–821.
27. Gomez HF, Davis M, Phillips S, McKinney P, Brent J: Human envenomation from a wandering garter snake. Ann Emerg Med 1994;23:1117–1118.
28. Guderian RH, MacKenzie CK, Williams JF: High voltage shock treatment for snakebite. Lancet 1986;2:229. Letter.
29. Guisto JA: Severe toxicity from crotalid envenomation after early resolution of symptoms. Ann Emerg Med 1995;26: 387–389.
30. Hendon RA, Tu AT: Biochemical characterization of the lizard toxin gilatoxin. Biochemistry 1981;20:3517–3522.
31. Herman RS: Nonvenomous snakebite. Ann Emerg Med 1988;17:1262–1263.
32. Hitt M, Ettinger DD: Toad toxicity. N Engl J Med 1986; 314:1517–1518.
33. Ho M, Warrell DA, Looareesuwan S, et al: Clinical significance of venom antigen levels in patients envenomated by the Malaysian pit viper. Am J Trop Med Hyg 1986;35: 579–587.
34. Hofer M, Hirschel B, Kirschner P, et al: Disseminated osteomyelitis from *Mycobacterium ulcerans* after a snakebite. N Engl J Med 1993;328:1007–1009.
35. Hogan DE, Dire DJ: Anaphylactic shock secondary to rattlesnake bite. Ann Emerg Med 1990;19:814–816.
36. Holloway M: Pitohui: The colorful bird that looks better than it tastes. Sci Am 1993;258:20–22.
37. Howarth DA, Southee AE, Whyte IM: Lymphatic flow rates

and first-aid in simulated peripheral snake or spider envenomation. Med J Aust 1994;161:695–699.
38. Huang TT, Lynch JB, Larson DL, et al: The use of excisional therapy in the management of snakebite. Ann Surg 1974; 179:598–607.
39. Hurlbut KM, Dart RC, Spaite D: Reliability of clinical presentation for predicting significant pit viper envenomation. Ann Emerg Med 1988;12:438.
40. Iyaniwura TT: Snake venom constituents: biochemistry and toxicology, Part 1. Vet Hum Toxicol 1991;33:468–474.
41. Iyaniwura TT: Snake venom constituents: biochemistry and toxicology, Part 2. Vet Hum Toxicol 1991;33:475–480.
42. Jansen PW, Perkin RM, VanStralen D: Mojave rattlesnake envenomation: Prolonged neurotoxicity and rhabdomyolysis. Ann Emerg Med 1992;21:322–325.
43. Kelly JJ, Sadeghani K, Gottlieb SF, et al: Reduction of rattlesnake-venom-induced myonecrosis in mice by hyperbaric oxygen therapy. J Emerg Med 1991;9:1–7.
44. Kitchens CS, Van Mierop LHS: Envenomation by the eastern coral snake (*Micrurus fulvius fulvius*). JAMA 1987;258: 1615–1618.
45. Kunkel DB, Curry SC, Vance MV, Ryan PJ: Reptile envenomations. J Toxicol Clin Toxicol 1983–84;21:503–526.
46. Kwan T, Paiusco AD, Kohl L: Digitalis toxicity caused by toad venom. Chest 1992;102:949–950.
47. Lewis JV, Portera CA: Rattlesnake bite of the face: Case report and review of the literature. Am Surg 1994;60:681–682.
48. Lyttly T, Goldstein D, Gartz J: Bufo toads and bufotenine: Fact and fiction surrounding an alleged psychedelic. J Psychoactive Drugs 1996;28:267–281.
49. McCollough N, Gennaro J: Evaluation of venomous snakebite in the southern United States. J Fla Med Assoc 1963;49:959–967.
50. McKinstry DM: Evidence of toxic saliva in some colubrid snakes of the United States. Toxicon 1978;16:523–534.
51. Myers CW, Daly JW: Dart-poison frogs. Sci Am 1983; 248:96–105.
52. Parrish HM: Incidence of treated snakebites in the United States. Public Health Rep 1966;81:269–276.
53. Parrish HM, Goldner JC, Silbert SL: Comparison between snakebites in children and adults. Pediatrics 1965;36:251.
54. Parrish HM, Khan MS: Snakebite during pregnancy. Report of four cases. Obstet Gynecol 1966;27:468–471.
55. Parrish HM, Pollard CB: Effects of repeated poisonous snakebites in man. Am J Med Sci 1959;237, 277–286.
56. Peam J, Morrison J, Charles N, et al: First aid for snakebite. Med J Aust 981;2:293–295.
57. Placentine J, Curry SC, Ryan PJ: Life-threatening anaphylaxis following Gila monster bite. Ann Emerg Med 1986; 15:147–149.
58. Preston CA: Hypotension, myocardial infarction, and coagulopathy following Gila monster bite. J Emerg Med 1989; 7:38–40.
59. Roberts JR, Greenberg JI: Ascending hemorrhagic signs after a bite from a copperhead. N Engl J Med 1997;336: 1262–1263.
60. Russell FE: Snake Venom Poisoning. Philadelphia, Lippincott, 1980.
61. Russell FE, Bogert CM: Gila monster: Its biology, venom and bite—A review. Toxicon 1981;19:341–359.
62. Russell FE, Emery JA: Incision and suction following injection of rattlesnake venom. Am J Med Sci 1961;241:160–161.
63. Sakai A, Junsuke T, Mamoru V: Efficacy of anticholinesterase against paralysis caused by postsynaptic neurotoxic snake venom. Ann Emerg Med 1995;26:712–713. Abstract.
64. Simon TL, Grace TG: Envenomation coagulopathy in wounds from pit vipers. N Engl J Med 1981;305:443–447.
65. Spaite D, Dart R, Sullivan JB: Skin testing in cases of possible crotalid envenomations. Ann Emerg Med 1988;7: 105–106.
66. Tu AT: Handbook of Natural Toxins, Vol. 5. New York, Marcel Dekker, 1991, pp. 755–776.
67. Vest DK: Toxic Duvernoy's secretions of the wandering garter snake *Thaminophis elegans vagrans*. Toxicon 1981;19: 831–839.
68. Watt CH, Genarro JF: Pit vipers in south Georgia and north Florida. Trans South Surg Assoc 1965;77:378–386.
69. Weed HG: Nonvenomous snakebite in Massachusetts: Prophylactic antibiotics are unnecessary. Ann Emerg Med 1993;22:220–224.
70. Whitley RE: Conservative treatment of copperhead snakebites without antivenin. J Trauma 1996;41:219–221.
71. Wingert WA, Chan L: Rattlesnake bites in southern California and rationale for recommended treatment. West J Med 1988;148:37–43.

ANTIDOTES IN DEPTH

Antivenin (Crotalid and Elapid)

James R. Roberts and Edward J. Otten

Although no controlled human trials have demonstrated a decrease in morbidity or mortality from poisonous snakebites with antivenin therapy, it is considered by most authorities to be a mainstay in the treatment of poisonous snakebites. Some clinicians, however, eschew its use entirely, preferring surgical therapy and/or supportive care. Those who advocate antivenin use promulgate that antivenin ameliorates tissue injury and general systemic toxicity and reverses coagulopathies from snake venom; they reference data from animal studies and human case reports. Opponents emphasize the significant potential for allergic reactions to antivenins and lack of scientific proof substantiating a change in morbidity and mortality in humans. Antivenin will no doubt continue to be the subject of debate for some time. However, based on current knowledge and clinical evidence, our opinion is that antivenin is the treatment of choice in cases of serious envenomation. Two types of antivenin are readily available to treat snakebites in the United States: crotalid and coral snake antivenin. Both are derived from horse serum. Although not yet commercially available, a refined crotalid antivenin, derived from sheep serum, holds promise as an effective and less allergenic alternative to currently available horse serum products. If clinical trials are successful, this new antivenin will likely replace the current polyvalent crotalid antivenin. Numerous antivenins exist for bites from exotic or foreign snakes, but they have limited availability and are difficult to obtain and rarely used. Since the only products that are currently available are horse serum products, this discussion will focus on the production, clinical use, and specifics of administration of this type of antivenin.

Crotalid Antivenin

Crotalidae Polyvalent Antivenin (Wyeth) is active against the venom of rattlesnakes (*Crotalus*, *Sistrurus*), water moccasins and copperheads (*Agkistrodon*), some South American pit vipers, and some Asian snakes. It is not effective for bites of exotic snakes, such as cobras and other elapididae. Antivenin is a refined and concentrated preparation of equine serum globulins (IgG) formulated into a freeze-dried powder to be reconstituted prior to use. It is a suspension of various venom-neutralizing antibodies prepared from the serum of horses that are gradually hyperimmunized against the venom of a group of pit vipers found in the Western hemisphere: *Crotalus adamanteus* (eastern diamondback rattlesnake), *Crotalus atrox* (western diamondback rattlesnake), *Crotalus durrisus terrificus* (tropical rattlesnake), and *Bothrops atrox* (fer-de-lance). These crotalids share many of the common antigens found in pit viper venom throughout the world, so the polyvalent antivenin is effective against a number of species, including all pit vipers found in the United States. Crotalid polyvalent antivenin is given to ameliorate the effects of local and systemic envenomation by pit vipers, and it is thought, by some clinicians, to be lifesaving. Numerous animal studies document a decrease in mortality and amount of tissue necrosis when antivenin is given immediately after envenomation. A delay in treatment of even a few hours lessens the beneficial effects of antivenin in animal models. Case reports and anecdotal evidence support the concept that antivenin will reverse local and systemic effects, including most coagulation defects in humans, but the specific effect of antivenin on human morbidity and mortality is not known.

Crotalid antivenin should not be given "prophylactically" to patients with minimal symptoms or to those who demonstrate no evidence of envenomation. It is prudent, however, routinely to obtain adequate supplies of antivenin for possible use should the subsequent development of symptoms warrant treatment. It is our experience that most rattlesnake bites will progress to an extent that antivenin is required. Some authors recommend the use of prophylactic antivenin in all cases of proven bites from the Mojave rattlesnake because local symptomatology may not precede systemic symptoms. Although almost all envenomated rattlesnake bites require antivenin, most patients with copperhead bites can be treated conservatively without antivenin. The severity of envenomation by water moccasins lies somewhere between that of the relatively benign copperhead and the more destructive rattlesnake.

Because it is a horse serum product, antivenin use entails a significant incidence of immediate or delayed hypersensitivity reactions,[4] including minor cutaneous hypersensitivity (urticaria), anaphylaxis, anaphylactoid reactions, and serum sickness. As the dose or rapidity of administration of antivenin is increased, the incidence of anaphylactoid reactions also increases. Because the ammonium sulfate precipitation process currently used to prepare antivenin is inefficient, the serum contains unwanted contaminants in the form of extraneous heterologous proteins (albumin, alpha and beta globulins, and IgM) in addition to the venom-specific IgG. These contaminants are largely responsible for the allergic properties of antivenin.

Anaphylactic reactions are due to the presence of circulating IgE antibodies to horse protein in the recipient's blood and from direct degranulation and histamine release from mast cells or basophils by horse proteins. Non-IgE-mediated anaphylactoid reactions are also seen. Serum sickness is due to the delayed production of antibodies by the recipient following the infusion of a relatively large dose of foreign protein (antigen excess reaction). Serum sickness often develops a few days to weeks after the administration of horse serum and is virtually certain to occur if more than 4–5 vials of antivenin are given. Fortunately, serum sickness is generally mild, easily treated, and not associated with significant chronic sequelae, although rarely immune-complex vasculitis, myocarditis, neuritis, and glomerulonephritis are noted. There are few data on the exact incidence of allergic reactions, but some form of hypersensitivity is seen in 20–40% of patients receiving antivenin[5] (see Table 99–5).

Technique of Administration

Before antivenin is administered, the patient should be asked about previous antivenin exposure or allergies. Tetanus immunoglobulin was derived from horse serum until the early 1960s; however, sensitivity to current tetanus toxoid, which is not a horse-serum-derived product, is not a contraindication to the use of antivenin.[7,8] Prior to antivenin administration the patient may be tested for sensitivity to horse serum with an intradermal (not conjunctival) skin test, although the skin test is an unreliable predictor of either immediate or delayed hypersensitivity reactions. Both false positive (about 50%) and false negative (about 20%) skin tests are encountered. Skin testing is usually done with plain horse serum provided with the antivenin by the manufacturer; more logical and clinical information may be possible if skin testing is done with the actual reconstituted antivenin although this is probably also unnecessary. The skin test is accomplished with 0.01–0.02 mL of serum injected intradermal (not subcutaneously) in the volar forearm, with a 0.9% sodium chloride solution control. A positive test is defined by the development of erythema, edema, wheal formation, or intense itching at the site within 15–30 minutes. Testing may be done with 1:10 dilution horse serum or antivenin (reconstituted and then also diluted 1:10). In one report six patients had a positive skin test but only four developed an immediate reaction to antivenin.[2] Of 20 patients with a negative skin test, 2 (10%) developed immediate hypersensitivity. Since skin testing is inaccurate, some clinicians prefer to forgo the procedure entirely.

It may be intuitively tempting to skin test all patients who potentially may require antivenin, but skin testing should be considered only if the decision has been made to administer antivenin. Patients should not be "prophylactically" tested for horse serum allergy, because the skin test may sensitize the individual to future use of horse serum products, a particular problem in snake collectors and handlers at risk for subsequent bites. Anaphylaxis and death have been reported following skin testing, emphasizing that this procedure is not innocuous.[9] In life- or limb-threatening situations the administration of antivenin to patients with a positive skin test or known allergy to horse serum is warranted. Antivenin administration may be continued in selected cases of serious envenomation even in the presence of an allergic reaction. In such cases where the skin test is positive or a reaction develops during administration of antivenin, the prophylactic or concomitant use of corticosteroids, epinephrine, and antihistamines has alleviated most of the allergic symptoms. Treatment should entail both the use of H_1 and H_2 antihistaminic receptor blockade (with 1 mg/kg IV diphenhydramine and cimetidine 300 mg IV, or ranitidine IV). In one study the cutaneous and systemic signs and symptoms of immediate hypersensitivity were all effectively treated with antihistamines and epinephrine, with no adverse sequelae.[5] Slowing the rate of infusion of the antivenin or increasing the dilution frequently lessens the severity of the allergic reaction (see Chap. 99). There is no practical way to desensitize patients to antivenin.

The routine pretreatment of all patients who receive antivenin is controversial. Most authors reserve H_1- and H_2-blocking antihistamines (diphenhydramine, 0.5–1 mg/kg IV alone, or in combination with cimetidine 300

TABLE 99–5. COMPLICATIONS OF CROTALIDAE ANTIVENIN THERAPY

Snake involved[a]	
Eastern diamondback rattlesnake	10
Cottonmouth (moccasin)	10
Copperhead	2
Unidentified	18
Number of patients treated with antivenin	26 (66%)
Average number of vials of antivenin	19.5 (range 1–119)
Incidence of immediate allergic reactions	23% (6 patients)
Cutaneous symptoms only	3 patients
Systemic reaction	3 patients
Incidence of immediate hypersensitivity	
Positive skin test	67% (4 of 6)
Negative skin test	10% (2 of 20)
Incidence of delayed reactions (serum sickness)	50% (10 of 20)
Symptoms of serum sickness	
Rash, pruritus, urticaria	100%
Fever or malaise	30%
Arthralgias	10%
Lymphadenopathy	10%
Peripheral neuritis	None
Renal failure	None

[a]Not all treated with antivenin.

Based on a retrospective study of 26 patients with crotalidae snake bites treated with antivenin. Data from Jurkovich GJ, Luterman A, McCullar K: Complication of Crotalidae antivenin therapy. J Trauma 1988;28:1032–1037.

mg every 6 hours) and corticosteroids (methylprednisolone, 1–2 mg/kg IV) for patients with a positive skin test or for those who develop a reaction during the infusion. The value of corticosteroids for the treatment of acute allergic reactions is probably limited. Anaphylaxis usually requires the cautious use of subcutaneous epinephrine (0.3–0.5 mg every 20 minutes in adults, repeated 3 times if needed) or an IV infusion of epinephrine (1 mg in 1 L of 0.9% sodium chloride solution, titrated to effect) in addition to other standard supportive measures. One report described the simultaneous use of antivenin and an epinephrine infusion in a severely envenomated patient who displayed allergy to horse serum.[7]

Reconstituted antivenin should be diluted to 1:10 to 1:100 in 0.9% sodium chloride solution and given IV. It is not given intramuscularly or directly into the area of the bite. Antivenin is initially infused slowly (25–50 mL/h), but the rate of infusion may be cautiously increased in the absence of allergic reactions. If antivenin is well tolerated, subsequent vials can be diluted 1:2 or 1:4 with 0.9% sodium chloride solution. An infusion rate of 2–10 vials/h is a general guideline, but data are lacking on the ideal protocol. In critical situations, multiple vials of crotalid antivenin have been safely given by bolus injection.[2] Antivenin should be given with constant observation of the clinical status and vital signs and with the patient on a cardiac monitor in an area where cardiopulmonary resuscitation is possible.

Recommendations for the amount of antivenin required for an envenomation are vague and varied (see Table 99–2). Children usually require more antivenin per body weight than adults, but there is no standard dose of antivenin.[2] Because of the unpredictable progression of envenomation, it is often difficult initially to estimate the total amount of antivenin required. What initially appears to be a minor bite may progress over a period of hours to become a severe local or even a systemic envenomation.

Patients with mild symptomatology should not be given antivenin. There is no justification for infusions of 1–2 vials in minor cases. At least 5–10 vials of antivenin are generally recommended initially for both adults and children in cases of moderate envenomation, but up to 30–40 vials may be required in cases of severe systemic envenomation. There are reports of patients safely receiving more than 100 vials, but such massive doses are unusual.[2] The initial dose of antivenin should be given as soon as possible, but administered cautiously, to limit reactions from rapid infusion. Antivenin may reverse a coagulopathy even if given more than 24 hours after the bite, negating the need for blood products traditionally administered for coagulation defects. In the specific case of proven rattlesnake bite, we advocate the initial use of 5 vials of antivenin in all instances where symptoms are progressive, even if they are still considered minor. This is because in our experience, once symptoms begin to progress they usually continue, and to the extent that antivenin is warranted, early treatment is likely to be more effective than late administration.

In contrast to rattlesnake bites, studies have reported that antivenin was required in only 12% of bites from copperheads and water moccasins.[10] Table 99–2 presents guidelines for estimating the degree of envenomation and the need for antivenin based on symptoms, but it is stressed that each case must be individualized, and repeat clinical examinations are needed to assess the true extent of envenomation. One problem with attempting to guide antivenin use by a grading system is that the severity of the coagulopathies seen following snakebites do not always correlate with objective signs of envenomation. In general, all of the antivenin should be given over the first 24 hours. Although its efficacy after 24 hours has been questioned, antivenin is advised in severe poisonings even after this time, especially if a coagulopathy persists. All patients who receive antivenin should be hospitalized for at least 24 hours.

There is approximately a 50% chance of developing serum sickness within 3–20 days of antivenin administration, especially if more than five vials are administered. The development of serum sickness cannot be predicted on the basis of a positive or negative skin test for horse serum sensitivity. Mild cases of serum sickness consist of urticaria, pruritus, and mild systemic symptoms, such as malaise. Occasionally arthralgias, lymphadenopathy, and fever may develop. Immune-complex glomerulonephritis, neuritis, vasculitis, or myocarditis rarely occur. The syndrome of serum sickness after antivenin use has not been well characterized or studied, but it is usually neither serious nor associated with chronic sequelae.[4] Most patients respond favorably to antihistamines or systemic corticosteroids. There is a trend toward the routine prophylactic use of corticosteroids or antihistamines to prevent serum sickness, but controlled trials are lacking. Since antihistamines and short-term steroid regimens are safe, their use can be considered following large doses of antivenin.

Elapid Antivenin

An antivenin of equine origin is available to treat envenomation by the Eastern coral snake (*Micrurus fulvius fulvius*) and Texas coral snake (*Micrurus fulvius tenere*), but none is available against the venom of the less virulent Arizona (Sonoran, *Micruroides euryxanthus*) coral snake or coral snakes found in Mexico, Central America, or South America. Deaths have not been reported after the bite of the Sonoran coral snake. In contrast to the recommendation to withhold crotalid polyvalent antivenin unless signs of significant envenomation are evident, coral snake antivenin is recommended prophylactically in any symptomatic patient and in asymptomatic cases where it is assumed or proven that the patient was bitten by a coral snake.[6] Following the bite of a coral snake, there may be little objective evidence to suggest envenomation for a number of hours, but systemic symptoms can develop insidiously. Therefore, at least 3–5 vials of coral snake antivenin are given initially and repeated on the basis of the clinical condition. The caveats for the administration of crotalid antivenin (skin testing, rate of infusion, treatment of reactions) apply to coral snake antivenin, except that usually less antivenin is required for coral snakes. Up to 10 vials may be administered, but dosing recommendations are vague.

Future Developments

Many of the clinical problems currently associated with the administration of equine-based antivenin may be eliminated in the future by the development of alternative sources for neutralizing antibodies. Less-antigenic antivenins can be produced by techniques such as an affinity purification process designed to concentrate venom-specific proteins and eliminate the unwanted and immunogenic extraneous proteins present in current equine-derived antivenins. Techniques have been developed to generate highly refined, purified, and potent antivenins derived from sheep and chickens. Ovine and avian antivenins are expected to be safer and more economical than equine antivenins. A crotalid polyvalent antivenin, derived by immunizing chickens with venom and purifying the antibodies from egg yolks, is currently undergoing development but clinical availability appears different (Wyeth-Ayerst and Ophidia Pharmaceuticals). A crotalid antivenin (CroTAb) derived from sheep and produced using the Fab technique, successful in the development of digitalis antibody fragments, is also undergoing testing. Initial clinical trials are quite promising, and the antivenin appears effective in halting progression of crotalid envenomation while greatly minimizing allergic reactions.[1,3]

References

1. Bogdan GM, McKinney P, Porter RS, et al: Clinical efficacy of two dosing regimens of affinity purified, mixed monospecific Crotalid antivenom Ovine Fab (CroTAb). Ann Emerg Med 1997;4:518. Abstract.
2. Buntain WL: Successful venomous snakebite neutralization with massive antivenin infusion in a child. J Trauma 1983; 23:1012–1014.
3. Dart RC, Seifert SA, Carroll L, et al: Mixed monospecific Crotalid antivenom Ovine Fab for the treatment of Crotalid venom poisoning. Ann Emerg Med 1997,30:33–39.
4. Howland MA, Smilkstein MJ: Primer on immunology with applications to toxicology. Contemp Manage Crit Care 1991;1:109–145.
5. Jurkovich GJ, Luterman A, McCullar K, et al: Complications of Crotalidae antivenin therapy. J Trauma 1988;28:1032–1037.
6. Kitchen CS, Mierop LHS: Envenomation by the Eastern coral snake *Micrurus fulvius fulvius*). JAMA 1987;258: 1615–1618.
7. Loprinzi CL, Hennessee J, Tamsky L, et al: Snake antivenin administration in a patient allergic to horse serum. South Med J 1983;76:501–502.
8. Otten EJ, McKimm D: Venomous snakebite in a patient allergic to horse serum. Ann Emerg Med 1983;12:624–627.
9. Spaite D, Dart R, Sullivan JB: Skin testing in cases of possible crotalid envenomations. Ann Emerg Med 1988;17:105–106.
10. White RR, Weber RA: Poisonous snakebite in central Texas: Possible indications for antivenin treatment. Ann Surg 1991;213:466–471.

CHAPTER 100

Arthropods

Neal A. Lewin

A 24-year-old man presented to the emergency department (ED) with a chief complaint of a "bite" on his right hand that occurred several hours previously. He had been unpacking crates of vegetables in his grocery store when he initially felt the bite on his hand. Within 2 hours it became painful and blistered at the site. He had seen several small brown spiders in the bottom of the empty crates.

His vital signs were: blood pressure, 130/80 mm Hg; pulse, 74 beats/min; respiration, 12 breaths/min; and temperature, 100°F (37.2°C). The only remarkable finding was a painful blister surrounded by erythema on the dorsal aspect of his right thumb. The lesion was cleaned with soap and water. Two hours later, the wound became slightly ulcerated and painful. The presumptive diagnosis of a local cutaneous reaction to a brown recluse spider bite was made based on the history and physical findings. The patient was shown a picture of the suspected spider and identified the brown recluse as his presumed attacker. The patient was to be followed by a dermatologist as an outpatient and he was told to return if systemic symptoms developed.

Most clinicians regard bites and stings as inconsequential, more of a nuisance than a threat to life. However, many serious diseases are arthropod-borne, such as encephalitis, Rocky Mountain spotted fever (RMSF), human ehrlichiosis, babesiosis, and Lyme disease. Some spiders and ticks produce neurotoxic venoms that can produce painful lesions, systemic disease, or paralysis.

This chapter highlights the significant clinical syndromes produced by bites or stings from the phylum Arthropoda, specifically the classes Arachnida (spiders, scorpions, and ticks) and Insecta (bees, wasps, hornets, and ants) (Table 100–1). Infectious diseases transmitted by arthropods are not discussed in this chapter.

Arthropoda is the largest phylum in the animal kingdom, with at least a million and a half named and half a million yet to be classified (Fig. 100–1).[36] The Arthropoda phylum includes more species than all of the other phyla combined. The majority of arthropods, fortunately, are benign and beneficial; others are dangerous as a result of their ability to cause envenomation, physical trauma, anaphylaxis to sensitizing antigens, foreign body reaction, or contact dermatitis or their actions as vectors for other disease-causing organisms.[28,29] Araneism or arachnidism is the envenomation caused by a spider bite. Most spiders are venomous, which enables them to kill their prey, but they are not aggressive toward humans unless provoked.

The order of spiders (Araneae) differs from other members of the class because of various anatomic differences best assessed by an entomologist. Simplistically, the arachnids have four pairs of legs and insects have three pairs. The arachnid's body is divided into cephalothorax, pedicle, and unsegmented abdomen. The black widow, brown recluse, and hobo spiders produce the most severe reactions.

Spiders

Approximately 200 species of spiders have been associated with significant envenomations.[28,29] Eighteen genera

TABLE 100–1. INSECTS AND OTHER ARTHROPODS THAT BITE, STING, OR NETTLE HUMANS

Arthropod	Description
Honeybee (*Apis mellifera*)	Hairy, yellowish brown with black markings
Bumble bee and carpenter bee (*Bombus* spp. and *Xylocopa* spp.)	Hairy, but larger than honeybees and colored black and yellow
Vespids (yellow jackets, hornets, paper wasps)	Short-waisted, robust black and yellow or white combination
Schecoids (thread-waisted wasps)	Threadlike waist
Nettling caterpillars (browntail, Io, hag, and buck moths, saddleback and puss caterpillars)	Caterpillar-shaped
Southern fire ant (*Solenopsis* spp.)	Ant-shaped
Spiders (*Arachnida*) black widow, brown recluse	Body with two regions, cephalothorax and abdomen; eight legs
Scorpions (*Centruroides*)	Eight-legged, crablike, stinger at the tip of the abdomen; pedipalps (pincers) highly developed (not a true insect)
Centipedes (*Chilopoda*)	Elongated, wormlike, with many jointed segments and legs; one pair of poison fangs behind head

TABLE 100–2. NORTH AMERICAN SPIDERS OF MEDICAL IMPORTANCE

Genus	Common Name
Araneus sp.[a]	Orb weavers
Argiope aurantia[a]	Orange argiope
Bothriocyrtum sp.	Trap door spider
Chiracanthium sp.[a]	Running spider
Drassodes sp.	Gnaphosid spider
Heteropoda sp.	Huntsman spider
Latrodectus sp.	Widow spider
Liocranoides sp.[a]	Running spider
Loxosceles sp.[a]	Brown, violin, or recluse spider
Lycosa sp.[a]	Wolf spider
Misumenoides sp.	Crab spider
Neoscona sp.[a]	Orb weaver
Peucetia varidans	Green lynx spider
Phidippus sp.[a]	Jumping spider
Rheostica (Aphonopelma) sp.	Tarantula
Steatoda grossa	False black widow spider
Tegenaria agrestis[a]	Hobo spider
Ummidia sp.	Trap door spider

[a]Associated with necrotic lesions.

of North America produce poisonings that require clinical intervention (Table 100–2). In one series of 600 suspected spider bites, 80% were found to be due to arthropods other than spiders, such as ticks, bugs, mites, fleas, lepidopterous insects, flies, beetles, water bugs, and *Hymenoptera*. Ten percent of the presumed bites were actually manifestations of other disorders.[28,29]

Black Widow Spider (*Latrodectus mactans*; Hourglass Spider)

The popular name "widow spider" is due to the female's practice of destroying the male after insemination.[16] There are five species of widow spiders in the United States: *Latrodectus mactans* (black widow), *Latrodectus hesperus* (Western states), *Latrodectus variolus, Latrodectus bishopi* (brown widow of the South), and *Latrodectus geometricus* (red widow of Florida). The true incidence of venomous spider bites is unknown since these bites are not reportable in any state.[2] These spiders live in temperate and tropical latitudes in stone walls, crevices, woodpiles, outhouses, barns, stables, and rubbish piles. They molt multiple times and can change colors as a result. The female is shiny, jet black, large (8–10 mm), with a rounded abdomen and a red hourglass mark on its ventral surface. The male is smaller, lighter in color, with a more elongated abdomen and fangs inadequate to envenomate humans. The female spider is most venomous and most toxic in the summer (Table 100–3). A bite by the female spider produces latrodectism. Widow spiders usually bite on unintentional skin contact.[16] A sharp pain occurs as the victim is bitten and a pair of red spots evolve at the site. The local reaction is limited (Table 100–4). The neurotoxic venom

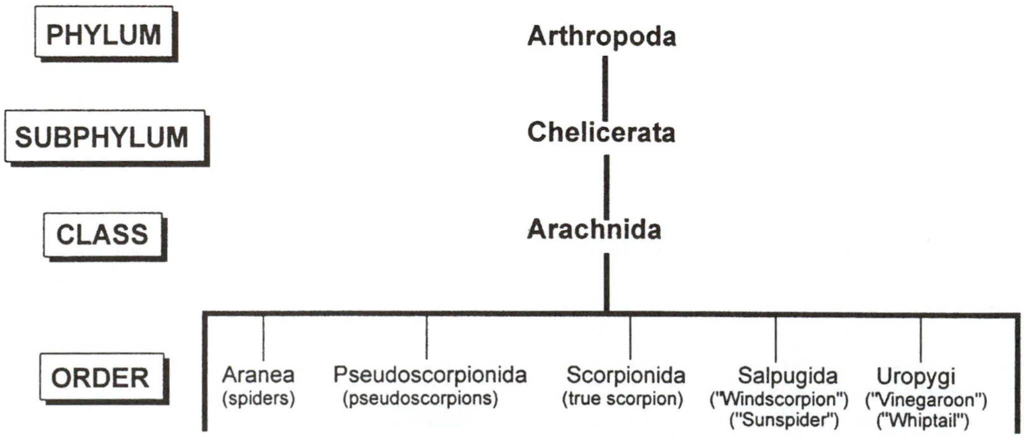

Figure 100–1. Taxonomy of the phylum Arthropoda. *(Reprinted with permission from Allen C: Arachnid envenomations. Emerg Clin North Am 1992;10:270.)*

TABLE 100–3. BROWN RECLUSE AND BLACK WIDOW SPIDERS: DIVERSE COMPARATIVE CHARACTERISTICS

	Brown Recluse (*Loxosceles*)	Black Widow (*Latrodectus*)
Description	Female—brown, 6–20 mm, violin-shaped mark on dorsum of cephalothorax; female greater toxicity than male	Female—jet black, 8–10 mm, red hourglass mark on ventral surface; female greater toxicity than male
Major venom component	Sphingomyelinase D	Alpha latrotoxin
Pathophysiology of envenomation	Vascular injury, dermonecrosis, hemolysis	Lymphatic, hematogenous spread Neurotoxicity
Epidemiology	Bites more common in warmer months N. America (southern and western states): *L. reclusa* S. America: *L. laeta, L. gaucho* Europe: *L. rufescens* Africa (Southern): *L. parrami, L. spiniceps, L. pillosa, L. bergeri* Asia/Australia: rare	Bites more common in warmer months in subtropical and temperate areas; perennial in tropics N. America: *L. mactans, L. hesperus, L. geometricus* Europe: (*L. tredecimguttatus*) Africa (southern): *L. indistinctus* Australia: *L. hasselti* Asia/S. America: rare
Clinical effects	Cutaneous Initial (0–2 h after bite): painless, erythema, edema 2–8 h: hemorrhagic, ulcerates 1 wk: eschar Months: healing	Cutaneous Initial (5 min–1 h after bite): local pain 1–2 h: puncture marks $^1/_2$ h–several hours: regional lymph nodes swollen, central blanching at bite site with surrounding erythema CVS: initial tachycardia followed by bradycardia, dysrhythmias, initial hypotension followed by hypertension GI: nausea, vomiting, mimic acute abdomen
	Hematologic: methemoglobinemia, hemolysis, thrombocytopenia, DIC	Hematologic: leukocytosis Metabolic Hyperglycemia (transient) Urinary VMA (increased) Musculoskeletal: hypertonia, abdominal rigidity, "facies latrodectismica" Neurologic CNS: psychosis, hallucinations, visual disturbance, seizures PNS: pain at the site ANS: increase in all secretions; sweating, salivation, lacrimation, diarrhea, bronchorrhea, mydriasis, miosis, priapism, and ejaculation
	Renal: renal failure 2^0 hemolysis	Renal: glomerulonephritis, oliguria, anuria Respiratory: bronchoconstriction, pulmonary edema
Treatment	1. Analgesia 2. Wound care 3. Dapsone (?) 4. Hyperbaric oxygen (?) 5. Antivenin (?) not available universally 6. Corticosteroids (?)	1. Analgesia 2. Calcium gluconate (?) 3. Muscle relaxants 4. Antivenin

produces symptoms 15 minutes to several hours later. This venom, more potent on a volume-per-volume basis than that of a pit viper, contains six active components with molecular weights of 5000–130,000 D.[2] The protein neurotoxin of the venom is alpha latrotoxin, which binds with high affinity to a specific presynapticreceptor.[19] The venom affects the motor end plates of neuromuscular synaptic membranes by the binding of gangliosides and glycoproteins at the synapses. This allows channels for sodium influx into neurons to remain open, resulting in the extensive release of acetylcholine and norepinephrine into the synapses, thereby inhibiting reuptake.[2] The result is the excessive stimulation of motor end plates as venom spreads through the lymphatic system. Muscle cramps initially occur at the site of the bite but may later involve other skeletal muscles, particularly muscles of the chest, abdomen, and face. The sweating, contorted, grimaced face is called "facies latrodectismica." The time between the bite and onset of symptoms may be 15 minutes to 6 hours. Usually the shorter the time to onset of symptoms, the more severe the envenomation. Nausea, weakness, hyperesthesias, ptosis, hyperreflexia, seizures, tremor, arthralgias, and diaphoresis are also noted.[2] Extreme restlessness occurs and recovery usually ensues within 24–48 hours, but symptoms may last several days with more severe envenomations. Death has been reported, secondary to seizures and respiratory compromise. The highest risk groups are infants, the elderly, the chronically ill, and

TABLE 100–4. SIGNS AND SYMPTOMS OF LATRODECTISM

Local
Pain at bite site, erythema, edema, urticaria, piloerection
Limb pain, local adenopathy
Systemic (general)
Facies latrodectismica: sweaty, flushed, blepharoconjunctivitis, grimaced
Pavor mortis (fear of death)
Priapism
Salivation
Urinary retention
Vomiting
Neuromuscular
Muscle cramps: thighs, abdomen, chest
Muscle rigidity, fibrillation, contractions, tremor
Cardiopulmonary
Bronchorrhea
Hypertension, tachycardia
Laboratory
Leukocytosis, hyperglycemia, elevated creatinine phosphokinase

pregnant women.[33] Laboratory data are not generally helpful in managing or predicting outcome.

Treatment. Treatment involves establishing an airway and supporting respiration and circulation if indicated. Wound evaluation and tetanus prophylaxis are essential.[39] Cold packs applied to the bite may be beneficial. Salicylates, nonsteroidal antiinflammatory agents, or opioids may be necessary for pain control. In severe envenomations, parenteral opioids may be insufficient to control pain. Traditionally, 10 mL of 10% calcium gluconate solution given intravenously (IV) has been employed to decrease cramping. It has been infused over 10 minutes and repeated at 30 minutes. A retrospective chart review of 163 patients envenomated by the black widow concluded that calcium gluconate was ineffective for pain relief, compared with a combination of IV opioids (morphine sulfate or meperidine) and benzodiazepines (diazepam or lorazepam).[6] Calcium's mechanism(s) of action remains unknown and its efficacy is anecdotal. Methocarbamol has been used as a muscle relaxant, but diazepam is more effective and also achieves sedation, anxiolytic, and amnestic effects. *Latrodectus* antivenin is rapidly effective and curative. This antivenin is effective for all species but is available as a crude hyperimmune horse serum and may cause anaphylaxis and serum sickness. The antivenin can be administered in severe reactions or to high-risk patients.[6] The usual dose is one to two vials diluted in sodium chloride solution, infused over 1 hour (see Antidotes in Depth: Antivenin [Scorpion and Spider]).

Prevention consists of destroying the spider and taking precautions in the areas spiders inhabit. Creosote can be sprayed in outdoor areas every 3 months. When working in high-risk areas, gloves, heavy garments buttoned at the wrists and collars, and shoes should be worn.

Brown Recluse Spider (*Loxosceles reclusa*; Violin or Fiddleback Spider)

This spider has a brown violin-shaped mark on the dorsum of the cephalothorax (see color plate Fig. 6). It is small (6–20 mm long), gray to orange or reddish brown, and usually found in the southern United States, living in dark areas (woodpiles, rocks, basements) (Table 100–3). It can live up to 6 months without water or food and survive temperatures from 8°C to 43°C.[30,37,40] There are 13 *Loxosceles* species in the United States, but *L. reclusa* is most common. Like the black widow spider, the female is more dangerous than the male and bites when provoked.

The clinical presentation varies from local cutaneous necrosis to systemic loxoscelism. Most victims are bitten in the morning, and spring to autumn is the peak time for envenomation. The bite, which is initially painless, blisters, bleeds, and then ulcerates 2–8 hours later (Table 100–3 and Color Plate Fig. 6). The venom is cytotoxic; purification techniques have identified eight subcomponents, including various enzymes, such as hyaluronidase, deoxyribonuclease, ribonuclease, alkaline phosphatase, lipase, and sphingomyelinase D. The sphingomyelinase D, with a MW of 32,000 D, is the primary constituent of the venom that causes tissue destruction. Sphingomyelinase also reacts with sphingomyelin in the red blood cell membrane to release choline and *N*-acylsphingosine phosphate.[41] Two cases were reported of severe intravascular hemolysis associated with a brown recluse spider bite leading to death in one of the victims.[41] Coagulation and vascular occlusion of the microcirculation occur, leading ultimately to necrosis. If untreated, the resulting lesions may enlarge for a week. By 1 week an eschar is usually present, but granulation and healing may take 2 months. Loxoscelism, which is not predicted by the extent of cutaneous reaction, includes fever, chills, nausea, morbilliform rash, arthralgias, seizures, coma, hemolysis, disseminated intravascular coagulopathy (DIC), and renal failure. Laboratory data may be remarkable for hemolysis, presence of fibrin split products, decreased fibrinogen levels, a positive D-dimer assay, increase PT and PTT, spherocytosis, Coombs-positive hemolytic anemia, thrombocytopenia, or abnormal renal and liver function tests.[2,3,8,28,29,36,40]

Treatment. Local treatment of the lesion is controversial. Probably the most prudent management of the dermonecrotic lesion is cleansing, immobilization, tetanus prophylaxis, analgesics, and antipruritics as warranted[2,8,38,39] (Table 100–5). Antibiotics should be used to treat apparent infection but should not be used prophylactically. Early excision or intralesional injection of corticosteroids appear unwarranted. Corrective surgery can be done several weeks after adequate tissue demarcation has occurred. The early use of dapsone, a leukocyte inhibitor, has been advocated by some.[24] The dosage recommended is 100 mg twice a day for 2 weeks.[25] However, prospective trials with large numbers of patients are lacking. One study compared erythromycin and dap-

TABLE 100–5. MANAGEMENT OF BROWN RECLUSE SPIDER BITE

General wound care
Clean
Tetanus prophylaxis as indicated
Immobilize and elevate bitten extremity
Apply cool compresses; avoid local heat
Local wound care
Serial observations
Natural healing by granulation
Delayed primary closure
Delayed secondary closure with skin graft
Gauze packing, if applicable
Systemic
Antipruritic/antianxiety and/or analgesic agents
Antibiotics for secondary bacterial infection
(?) Polymorphonuclear white blood cell inhibitors: dapsone, colchicine
Antivenin (experimental)
(?) Hyperbaric oxygen
Laboratory
Culture
Gram stain
Biopsy to determine etiology of lesion
G-6-PD level if dapsone therapy required

Modified, with permission, from Wasserman GS: Wound care of spider and snake envenomations. Ann Emerg Med 1988;17:1333.

sone therapy, erythromycin and antivenin therapy, and erythromycin, dapsone, and antivenin therapy.[24] Although the treatment groups were very small, all groups showed wound healing at about 20 days. Hepatitis,[27] methemoglobinemia, and hemolysis (Chap. 93) are associated with the use of dapsone, and weekly CBCs are necessary if this drug is used. A baseline glucose-6-phosphate dehydrogenase determination should be made prior to initiation of dapsone therapy.

A recent animal study evaluated the effects on the size of skin lesions induced by *Loxosceles* envenomation by treatment with hyperbaric oxygen therapy (HBO), dapsone, and HBO and dapsone. Unfortunately, the study design was limited and could find only a 100% difference in treatment groups. It was concluded that there was no clinically significant change in necrosis or induration by these treatment modalities. Further evaluation of these interventions remains appropriate.[15]

Another study using hyperbaric oxygen in the treatment of *Loxosceles*-induced necrotic lesions model revealed no clinical improvement in the size of the lesion; however, the histology of the lesions improved. Whether this is of value in humans is yet to be determined.[34]

The use of 1.2 mg of colchicine, a leukocyte inhibitor, followed at 2-hour intervals with 0.6 mg for 2 days, then 0.6 mg every 4 hours for 2 additional days has substantial potential toxicity, but has been recommended in the treatment of dermonecrotic lesions.[28,29]

Patients manifesting systemic loxoscelism or those with expanding necrotic lesions should be admitted to the hospital. All the patients should be monitored for evidence of hemolysis, renal failure, or coagulopathy. If hemoglobinuria ensues, increased IV fluids and urinary alkalinization may be used in an attempt to prevent acute renal failure. Hemolysis, if significant, can be treated with transfusions. Patients with a coagulopathy should be monitored with serial CBC, platelet count, PT, PTT, fibrin split products, and fibrinogen. Disseminated intravascular coagulopathy may require treatment, based on severity. Antivenin research has been initiated, but an antivenin is not yet commercially available.[33]

Hobo Spider (*Tegenaria agrestis*)

Healthcare providers should consider the hobo spider, formerly called the "aggressive house spider," in cases of necrotic arachnidism.[20] The hobo spider is native to Europe and was introduced to the northwestern United States in the 1920s or 1930s. These spiders build webs in wood piles, crawl spaces, basements, and moist areas. They are brown with gray markings and 7–14 mm in length. They are most abundant in the midsummer through the fall. They bite if provoked or threatened. Unlike the black widow and brown recluse spiders, the hobo males are more venomous than the females. The local effects of the hobo spider's envenomation are similar to those of the brown recluse. The initial bite is painless, but as the area of erythema expands, a blister ensues in 15–35 hours and rupture of these lesions creates an eschar-covered necrotic ulcer. Sloughing occurs and healing with a scar occurs from 45 days up to 3 years. Systemic symptoms occur consisting of nausea, vomiting, fatigue, memory loss, and visual impairment. Serious outcomes have been reported including aplastic anemia, intractable vomiting, a profuse secretory diarrhea, and death.[20]

Treatment. Treatment emphasizes local wound care, although systemic steroids for hematologic complications may be of value. Surgical graft repair for severe ulcerative lesions may be warranted when there is no additional necrosis.[20]

Funnel Web Spiders (*Atrax* and *Trechona* spp.)

The funnel web spider belongs to the family Dipluridae, suborder Mygalomorphae, and contains a potent neurotoxin. [9] The most common of these spiders, *Atrax robustus*, is found in Queensland, New South Wales, Victoria, and Tasmania.[10] Children are particularly susceptible to their effects, with death sometimes occurring within 4 hours.[14] They are large, with the female about 5 cm in length. The male's venom is more potent than the female's. *Atrax* inhabit burrows and *Hadronyche* inhabit trees. The toxin atraxotoxin is a neurotoxin causing release of acetylcholine, norepinephrine, and epinephrine at the motor end plate and autonomic nervous system. Two stages of toxicity are observed. In stage I, piloerection and widespread muscle fasciculations are seen, followed rapidly within 5 minutes by tachycardia, dysrhythmias, hypertensive crisis, coma, cholingeric crisis, apnea, and rarely pulmonary edema and metabolic acidosis. In stage II, several hours after envenomation, the adrenergic and cholinergic symptoms abate and progressive hypotension, pulmonary edema, and respiratory depression may persist.[2]

Treatment. Due to its lethality, the bite of a funnel web spider requires immediate prehospital measures, such as limb immobilization and lymphatic bandages proximal to the bite. A negative-pressure suction device is recommended after bandaging is applied.

Antivenin of rabbit origin, which is an IgG immunoglobin, is available in Australia. The antivenin is given IV, two ampules every 15 minutes, until a response is seen.[35] Atropine is used to control the bronchorrhea and salivation. Symptomatic use of muscle relaxants, sedatives, and antihypertensive agents is recommended.

Scorpions

Fortunately, these members of the class Arachnida rarely cause mortality in victims older than 6 years.[26] Approximately three to four deaths per year are reported from scorpion envenomations in the United States.[23] These stings occur predominantly in the southwestern United States. The poisonous scorpions in the United States are *Centruroides gertschii,* and the most important *Centruroides sculpturatus* (currently termed *Centruroides exilicauda).*

In general, scorpions sting only if disturbed. The site of the sting becomes slightly erythematous, with an ensuing tingling or burning, and, occasionally discoloration and necrosis (Table 100–6). The toxin consists of phospholipase, acetylcholinesterase, hyaluronidase, serotonin, and neurotoxins. Components of scorpion venom are complex and species-specific, those of the family Buthidae being most harmful to humans.[11,12,23,26]

TABLE 100–6. ENVENOMATION GRADATION FOR *CENTRUROIDES SCULPTURATUS* (BARK SCORPIONS)

Grade	Signs and Symptoms
I	Site of envenomation Pain and/or paresthesias Positive "tap test" (severe pain increase with touch or percussion)
II	As in grade I Pain and paresthesias remote from sting site (eg, paresthesias moving up an extremity, perioral "numbness")
III	One of the following: Somatic skeletal neuromuscular dysfunction: jerking of extremity(s), restlessness, severe involuntary shaking and jerking, which may be mistaken for seizures Cranial nerve dysfunction: blurred vision, wandering eye movements, hypersalivation, trouble swallowing, tongue fasciculation, upper airway dysfunction, slurred speech
IV	Both cranial nerve and somatic skeletal neuromuscular dysfunction

Modified, with permission, from Curry SC, Vance MV, Ryan PJ, et al: Envenomation by the scorpion Centruroides sculpturatus. *J Toxicol Clin Toxicol 1983–1984;21:417–449; Allen C: Arachnid envenomations. Emerg Med Clin North Am 1992;10:276.*

Venoms of the *Centruroides* genus of Arizona and Mexico are primarily neurotoxic. They affect sodium channels with prolongation of action potentials as well as spontaneous depolarization of nerves of both adrenergic and parasympathetic nervous systems.[26] Therefore, both adrenergic and cholinergic symptoms are seen: hypertension, tachycardia, seizures, hyperglycemia, and salivation, lacrimation, urination, defecation, and emesis, respectively. The genus *Tityus* of Brazil and Trinidad have caused pancreatitis.

Venoms of *Buthus* and *Parabuthus* of India and Africa possess phospholipase A, which may cause gastrointestinal (GI) and pulmonary hemorrhages and a disseminated intravascular coagulopathy.

A neurotoxin envenomation can produce severe systemic toxicity, especially in children. Symptoms include hypertension or hypotension, dysrhythmias, throat spasms, muscular fasciculations, abdominal cramps, seizures, oliguria, pulmonary edema, and respiratory collapse (Table 100–6).

Treatment

Since most envenomations produce no severe effects, local wound care is usually all that is warranted. In young children or patients who manifest severe toxicity, hospitalization may be required.

Treatment emphasizes support of the airway, breathing, and circulation. One to two grams of 10% calcium gluconate given IV may relieve muscle cramps, and diazepam can be used for seizures. A goat serum–derived antivenin is available in Arizona and has been used successfully in a limited number of severe cases.[4] This approach is not universally accepted. Proponents believe antivenin may resolve symptoms sooner, while opponents cite serum sickness as a substantial concern[4] (see Antidotes in Depth: Antivenin [Scorpion and Spider]).

A retrospective chart review of children younger than 10 years of age who experienced severe *Centruroides* scorpion envenomation found that anti-*Centruroides* antivenin resulted in rapid resolution of all symptoms in all 12 patients treated.[4] Of those treated with antivenin, 58% had a delayed rash or serum sickness.

Treatment for scorpion envenomation outside the United States should be dictated by observed toxicity and known scorpions of the geographic area. A negative-pressure suction device has been used in prehospital management to extract venom at approximately 1 atm of negative pressure. Lymphatic band tourniquets and immobilization may also be used in prehospital management.[2]

Scorpion envenomations may require atropine to counteract parasympathetic crisis; intubation and diuretics for pulmonary edema and calcium channel blockers, angiotensin converting enzyme inhibitors, beta-adrenergic antagonists, and alpha-adrenergic antagonists have been used to treat associated hypertension.[11,13]

An animal study suggested benefit from quinine and aspirin if used shortly after a scorpion envenomation.[13] It is postulated that aspirin's antiplatelet-aggregating characteristics inhibit the scorpion venom's thrombotic effect.

Quinine has diverse pharmacologic characteristics (see Chap. 44). It acts as a curarizing agent on skeletal muscle and an antihypertensive agent by its vasodilatory action. It has a membrane-stabilizing effect and decreases transmembrane sodium flux and therefore may modify permeability to sodium caused by the neurotoxins in scorpion's venom. It also has vagolytic, beta-adrenergic receptor antagonism, and antimuscarinic effects, all of which may be beneficial in treating scorpion toxicity.

Prevention

Scorpion envenomation can be prevented by wearing shoes when walking, particularly at night, owing to the nocturnal nature of the scorpions. Shoes, sleeping bag, and tent should be shaken out prior to use. Cracks and crevices should be filled, wood piles and rubbish piles eliminated, and insecticides used in infested areas. The bark scorpion (*C. sculpturatus*), which is fluorescent, can be demonstrated in the dark using a Wood's lamp.

Ticks

A progressive ascending flaccid paralysis is reported after bites from *Dermacentor andersoni, Dermacentor variabilis, Amblyomma americanum, Amblyomma maculatum,* and *Ixodes scapularis*. The paralysis is due to a neurotoxin that affects bulbar and spinal nuclei. Usually the tick must remain on the person for 5–6 days. Ticks typically attach to the scalp but can be found on any part of the body, including the ear canals and anus. Children, particularly girls, are most often affected. Mild diarrhea and lower extremity weakness may be the first manifestations, followed by absent or decreased deep tendon reflexes, which develop over the next 24–48 hours. The trunk, arms, neck, and pharynx become involved if the tick is not removed. The differential diagnosis includes Guillain-Barré syndrome, poliomyelitis, botulism, transverse myelitis, and spinal cord lesions. The cerebrospinal fluid remains normal.

Treatment is removal of the entire tick; usually symptoms improve within several hours. If more serious symptoms develop, supportive care is given as necessary. The best method for tick removal is with forceps or gloved hands.[21]

Hymenoptera: Bees, Wasps, Hornets, Yellow Jackets, and Ants

Insects of this subclass (Fig. 100–2) are of great medical importance, since bites or stings can cause acute toxic and allergic reactions that can be fatal (Table 100–7). Nearly twice as many people die in the United States as a result of hymenopterous insect bites or stings as die from poisonous snakebites.[18] Normally, the honeybee sting is manifested as localized edema without a systemic reac-

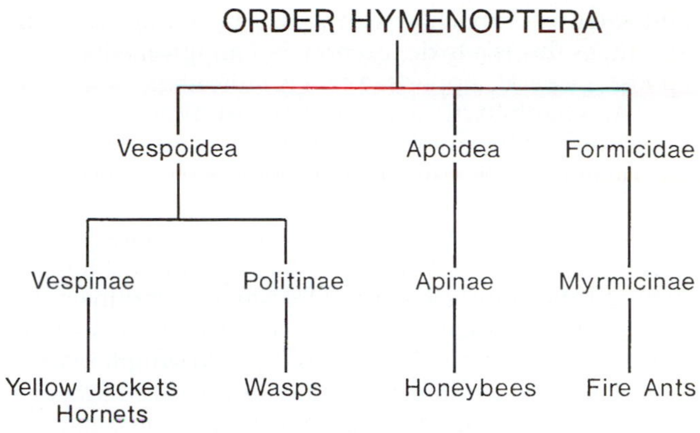

Figure 100–2. Taxonomy of Hymenoptera. *(Reproduced, with permission, from Sinkinson CA, French RS, Graft DF, eds: Individualizing therapy for Hymenoptera stings. Emerg Med Rep 1990;11:134.)*

tion. Rarely, a sting in the oropharynx can produce airway compromise. Application of ice at the site is usually sufficient to halt discomfort. The stinger should be removed by scraping, as opposed to pulling, which may release additional retained venom. Toxic reactions occur with multiple stings (greater than 500 stings is described as possibly fatal) and include GI symptoms, headache, fever, syncope and, rarely, rhabdomyolysis, renal failure,

TABLE 100–7. CLASSIFICATION OF REACTIONS TO HYMENOPTERA STING

Reaction	Clinical Presentations
Local	
Minimal	Localized pain, pruritus, swelling
	Lesion < 5 cm
	Duration several hours
Large	Localized pain and pruritus
	Contiguous swelling and erythema
	Lesion > 5 cm
	Duration 1–3 days
Systemic	
Minimal	Localized pain, pruritus, swelling
	Distant and diffuse urticaria, angioedema, pruritus, and/or erythema; conjunctivitis
	Abdominal pain, nausea, diarrhea
Severe	Dermatologic
	Local: pain, pruritus, and swelling
	Distant: urticaria, angioedema, pruritus, and/or erythema
	Gastrointestinal
	Nausea, abdominal pain, diarrhea
	Respiratory
	Nasal congestion, rhinorrhea, hoarseness, bronchospasm, stridor, tachypnea, dyspnea, cough, wheezing
	Cardiovascular
	Tachycardia, hypotension, dysrhythmias, myocardial infarction
	Miscellaneous
	Seizures, feeling of impending doom, uterine contractions

Reprinted, with permission, from Sinkinson CA, French RS, Graft DF, eds: Individualizing therapy for hymenoptera stings. Emerg Med Rep 1990;11:134.

and seizures. Bronchospasm and urticaria are typically absent, as this is a toxic reaction, not an IgE-mediated response. General supportive care is indicated.

An anaphylactic reaction may also occur and is not dependent on the number of stings. As in any anaphylactic reaction, death may ensue if the reaction is not managed properly and expeditiously. In patients who are allergic to hymenoptera venom, a wheal and flare reaction occurs at the site of the inoculum; the shorter the interval between the sting and onset of systemic symptoms, the more likely the reaction will be severe. Fatalities can occur within several minutes; even initially mild symptoms may be followed by a fulminant course. Generalized urticaria, throat and chest tightness, stridor, fever, chills, and cardiovascular collapse can ensue. Anaphylaxis is IgE-mediated. The IgE antibodies attach to tissue mast cells and basophils in an individual previously sensitized to the venom. These cells are then activated, allowing for the progression of the cascade reaction of increased vasoactive substances, such as leukotrienes, eosinophil chemotactic factor-A (ECF-A), and histamine (see Chap. 14).

Several allergens (Table 100–8) have been found in honeybee venom: phospholipase A_2, hyaluronidase, mellitin, acid phosphatase, and allergen C. There are differences in venom produced by wasps, hornets, and yellow jackets. Treatment consists of immediate airway and circulatory support, with fluid resuscitation in an attempt to reverse hypotension. Subcutaneous (1:1,000) or IV (1:100,000) epinephrine should be used, depending on the patient's blood pressure. Diphenhydramine or corticosteroids may be necessary, but these medications are secondarily important to the immediate airway and cardiopulmonary support with fluids, epinephrine, and vasopressors. A delayed reaction, characterized by fever, malaise, headache, polyarthritis, and lymphadenopathy, may first appear 1–2 weeks after the sting. Unless specifically suggested, the distant bite may be forgotten and the diagnosis of a delayed reaction missed.[1,18]

Prevention, especially in the allergic person, includes avoiding bright clothing, flowers, scented deodorants and shampoos, perfumes, and barefoot walks outdoors. An emergency kit containing a prefilled spring-loaded epinephrine syringe with careful instructions from a physician, as well as an antihistamine and an emergency alert card or tag, should be carried or worn by the sensitized individual.

Commercial preparations of venom from the honeybee, yellow jacket, white-faced hornet, yellow hornet, and wasp can be used for diagnosis and immunotherapy of patients at risk of life-threatening sting reaction. Several authors have discussed the indications and safety of immunotherapy.[17,42]

TABLE 100–8. COMPOSITION OF HYMENOPTERA VENOM

Vespid (wasps, hornets, yellow jackets)
Biogenic amines (diverse)
Phospholipase A, phospholipase B
Hyaluronidase
Antigen 5
Acid phosphatase
Mast cell degranulating peptide
Kinin
Apids (honeybees)
Biogenic amines (diverse)
Phospholipase A, phospholipase B (?)
Hyaluronidase
Acid phosphatase
Minimine
Mellitin
Apamin
Mast cell degranulating peptide
Formicids (fire ants)
Biogenic amines (diverse)
Phospholipase
Hyaluronidase
Unidentified others
Piperidines

Modified, with permission, after Sinkinson CA, French RS, Graft DF, eds: Individualizing therapy for hymenoptera stings. Emerg Med Rep 1990;11:134; King TP, Valentine MD: Allergens of hymenoptera venoms. Clin Rev Allergy 1987;5:137; Stablein JJ, Lockey RF: Adverse reactions to ant stings. Clin Rev Allergy 1987;5:161.

Fire Ants

The aggressive fire ant's venom causes necrosis at the site of their bite and sting. The venom is 95% alkaloid, with a small aqueous fraction that contains soluble proteins. Of the alkaloid, 99% is a 2,6,di-substituted piperidine that has hemolytic, antibacterial, insecticidal, and cytoxic properties. The proteins identified in the venom include a phospholipase, a hyaluronidase, and the enzyme *N*-acetyl-beta-glucosaminidase.[7,32] The sting first forms a wheal; several hours later clear vesicles develop, and pustules are noted within 12 hours. In 24 hours, the pustules umbilicate on an erythematous base. Often, healing occurs with scarring. A systemic reaction can occur, and in sensitized patients anaphylactic shock can develop.

Treatment

Local reactions require cold compresses and cleansing with soap and water. Some authors recommend topical or injected lidocaine with or without 1:100,000 epinephrine and topical vinegar and salt mixtures to decrease pain at the site of the bite and sting.[7,32] Large local reactions can be treated with oral corticosteroids, oral H_1 or H_2 antagonists, and analgesics. Secondary infections should be treated with antibiotics.

Butterflies, Moths, and Caterpillars

Butterflies and moths are insects of the order Lepidoptera. One family of butterflies and nine families of moths have a caterpillar stage that is clinically important. Some caterpillars have hollow spines containing an urticarial poison. The puss caterpillar (*Megalopyge opercularis*) is the most toxic of the caterpillars in the United States. The sting is painful, and white or red papules appear. Generalized symptoms, seizures, and shock have been reported.[22] Regional adenopathy is common with caterpillar stings. Treatment should be immediate, with removal of the embedded spines using cellophane tape and application of ice. If muscle cramps develop, 10% calcium gluconate IV is given, and topical corticosteroids can be used to decrease local inflammation.

Blister Beetles (*Tegrodera aloga*)

Blister beetles, found in the eastern United States, are from the family Epicauta. They produce a cantharidin that causes a dermatitis manifested several hours later by blisters or vesiculobullae.[5] If ingested, severe GI disturbances can occur. Treatment is supportive.

Tarantulas

Tarantulas, ancestors to the true spider, belong to the family Theraphosidae.[31] More than 40 species are found in the desert in the western United States. Tarantulas liberate urticating hairs, resulting in local histamine reactions in humans. Bites, which are rare, create a local histamine response. The venom of the *Dugesiella henzi* has been shown to contain hyaluronidase, nucleotidase (ATP), and spermine, a polyamine compound.[30]

Treatment

Treatment is supportive, with oral antihistamines, cool compresses, and analgesics given as needed. If the hairs are barbed, as in some species, they can be removed by using adhesive or cellophane tape followed by compresses or irrigation with sodium chloride solution. Topical steroids may be used.

Summary

Healthcare providers should have a good fund of knowledge regarding bites and stings by arthropods and arachnids to enable them to recognize local and systemic reactions. The treatment of arthropod-borne disease rarely entails the use of antivenins. Proper hygiene to prevent secondary infections, avoiding contact with arthropods, decreasing the arthropod population mechanically and/or chemically, and the use of repellents are all important measures to decrease morbidity from arthropods. The patient should bring the arthropod to the hospital for identification, and every attempt should be made to describe the evolution of the bite to assist in the differential diagnosis.

References

1. Abramowicz M (ed): Insect venoms. Med Lett Drug Ther 1983;25:53–54.
2. Allen C: Arachnid envenomations. Emerg Med Clin North Am 1992;10:269–298.
3. Babcock JL, Marmer DJ, Steele RW: Immunotoxicology of brown recluse spider venom. Toxicon 1986;24:783–790.
4. Bond GR: Antivenin administration for *Centruroides* scorpion sting risks and benefits. Ann Emerg Med 1992;21: 788–791.
5. Browne SG: Cantharidin poisoning due to a blister beetle. Br Med J 1960;2:1290–1291.
6. Clark RF, Wethem-Kestner S, Vance MV, Gerkin R: Clinical presentation and treatment of black widow spider envenomation: A review of 163 cases. Ann Emerg Med 1992;21: 782–787.
7. DeShazo RD, Butcher BT, Banks WA: Reactions to the stings of the imported fire ants. N Engl J Med 1990;327: 462–466.
8. Gendron BP: *Loxosceles reclusa* envenomation. Am J Emerg Med 1990;8:51–54.
9. Gertsch WJ: American Spiders, 2nd ed. New York, Van Nostrand Reinhold, 1979.
10. Gray RR: Getting to know funnel-webs. Aust Nat Hist 1981;20:256–258.
11. Gueron M, Reuben I, Sofer S: The cardiovascular system after scorpion envenomation: A review. J Toxicol Clin Toxicol 1992;30:215–258.
12. Gueron M, Sofer S: Vasodilators and calcium channel blocking agents as treatment of cardiovascular manifestations of human scorpion envenomation. Toxicon 1990;28:127–128.
13. Guieu R, Kopyan C, Rochat H: Utilization of aspirin, quinine and verapamil in the prevention and treatment of scorpion venom intoxication 1993;53:1935–1946.
14. Hartman LJ, Sutherland SK: Funnel-web spider (*Atrax robustus*) antivenin in the treatment of human envenomation. Med J Aust 1984;141:796–799.
15. Hobbs, GD, Anderson AR, Greene TJ, et al: Comparison of hyperbaric oxygen and dapsone therapy for Loxosceles envenomation. Acad Emerg Med 1996;3:758–761.
16. Kunkel DB: The sting of the arthropod. Emerg Med 1996; 28:137–141.
17. Lichtenstein LM, Valentine MD, Sobotka AK: Insect allergy: The state of the art. J Allergy Clin Immunol 1979;64:5–12.
18. Marshall TK: Wasp and bee stings. Practitioner 1957; 178:712–722.
19. Muller GJ: Black and brown widow spider bites in South Africa. S Afr Med J 1993;83:399–405.
20. Necrotic arachnidism—Pacific Northwest 1988–1995. MMWR 1996;45:433–436.
21. Needham GR: Evaluation of five popular methods for tick removal. Pediatrics 1985;75:997–1002.
22. Pinson RT, Morgan JA: Envenomation by the puss caterpillar (*Megalopyge opercularis*). Ann Emerg Med 1991;20:562–564.
23. Rachesky IJ, Banner W, Dansky J, et al: Treatments for *Centruroides exilicauda* envenomation. Am J Dis Child 1984; 138:1136–1139.
24. Rees R, Campbell D, Rieger E, King LE: The diagnosis and treatment of brown recluse spider bites. Ann Emerg Med 1987;16:945–949.

25. Rees RS, Altenbern DP, Lynch JB, et al: Brown recluse spider bites: A comparison of early surgical excision versus dapsone and delayed surgical excision. Ann Surg 1985;202:659–663.
26. Rimza ME, Zimmerman DR: Scorpion envenomation. Pediatrics 1980;66:298–301.
27. Robertson FM, Olsen SB, Jackson MR: Dapsone hepatitis following treatment of a brown recluse spider bite. Compl Surg 1992;33–35.
28. Russell FE: Venomous animal injuries. Curr Prob Pediatr 1973;3:1–47.
29. Russell FE, Gertsch WJ: Arthropod bites. Toxicon 1983;21:337–339.
30. Schanbacher FL, Lee CK, Wilson IB, et al: Composition and properties of tarantula *Dugesiella henzi* (Girard) venom. Toxicon 1973;11:21–29.
31. Schanbacher FL, Lee CK, Wilson IR, et al: Purification and characterization of tarantula *Dugesiella henzi* venom hyaluronidase. Comp Biochem Physiol 1973;44:389–396.
32. Stafford CT, Hoffman DR, Rhoades RB: Allergy to imported fire ants. South Med J 1989;82:1520–1527.
33. Stewart C, Roberge R, Lawler H, eds: Emergency management of arachnid envenomations: Spider bites and scorpion stings. Emerg Med Rep 1993;14:75–82.
34. Strain GM, Snider TG, Tedford B, et al: Hyperbaric oxygen effects on brown recluse spider (*Loxosceles reclusa*) envenomation in rabbits. Toxicon 1991;29:989–996.
35. Sutherland SK: Treatment of arachnid poisoning in Australia. Aust Fam Physician 1990;19:50–61.
36. Toewe CH: Bug bites and stings. Am Fam Physician 1980;21:90–95.
37. Trestrail JH: Poisonous spiders and spider bite poisonings: Bites and stings of poisonous insects. Unpublished monograph.
38. Verheyden CN: Snakebite and spider bite. Hosp Physician 1988;24:21–32.
39. Wasserman G: Wound care of spider and snake envenomations. Ann Emerg Med 1988;17:1331–1335.
40. Wasserman GS, Kunkel D: Venomous bites and stings. J Toxicol Clin Toxicol 1984;21:417–502.
41. Williams ST, Khare VK, Johnston GA, et al: Severe intravascular hemolysis associated with brown recluse spider envenomation. Am J Clin Pathol 1995;104:463–467.
42. Youlten LJ, Atkinson BA, Lee TH: The incidence and nature of adverse reactions to injection immunotherapy in bee and wasp venom allergy. Clin Exp Allergy 1995;25:159–165.

ANTIDOTES IN DEPTH

Antivenin (Scorpion and Spider)

Jeffrey N. Bernstein

The terms *antivenom* and *antivenin* have been used interchangeably. In various countries the term for antivenom has been based on the term for venom in the respective language of that country. In most of Europe, for example, the term *antivenin* or *antivenene* is used. Wyeth, the maker of Crotalid and Micrurus antivenom, has adopted *antivenin* as a part of the brand name for their product. Since the North American English term for animal toxin is venom, some manufacturers use the term antivenom whereas certain brand names include "antivenin" which will be used here.

The vector of envenomation in North America is typically assumed from the species of spider or scorpion known in that geographic distribution. For example, black widow type envenomations that occur in southern Arizona are presumed to be from *Latrodectus hesperus* rather than *L. mactans*. Occasionally, stings have resulted from scorpions or spiders in imported oriental rugs and fruit. The clinician must also be aware that professional and amateur entomologists may present with more exotic bites or stings. In these instances the genus of the arachnid or at least the common name is often known.

Antivenin for spiders and scorpions is prepared by immunizing animals with venom and then collecting the immune serum for administration. Monkeys, horses, goats, sheep, chicken, and rabbits have been used as sources of antivenin. The animals are placed on an immunization schedule to allow production of immunoglobulins, mostly specific IgG. Optimal antibody production typically takes about 6 weeks. The choice of animal used to make immune sera is more often dictated by the availability of a species, financial considerations, and tradition rather than on scientific modeling. Although manufacturers may state that a specific animal gives a "cleaner" (ie, less immunogenic) product, no studies have compared immune sera of different animals for human compatability or tolerance.

Centruroides sculpturatus

Centruroides species is the only scorpion of medical importance in the United States. It is indigenous to the desert southwest of Arizona but has been reported to inhabit Texas, New Mexico, California, and Nevada as well.[5] Occasionally, envenomations have occurred in nonindigenous areas of the country from "stow away" scorpions in the luggage of travelers.[15]

At one time the mortality from scorpion envenomation in this country was twice as high as that of all other venomous animals combined.[8] The two poison centers in Arizona receive between 2000 and 3000 calls annually for scorpion envenomations. While the incidence remains high, no deaths have been reported for more than 35 years. The absence of fatalities is attributable to the development of pediatric intensive care and better methods of supportive care, as well as the use of antivenin.

Antivenin for this species of scorpion was produced in Mexico, in horses, as early as the 1930s.[5] In 1947, antivenin was produced from rabbits and cats immunized with *C. sculpturatus* and *C. gertschi*.[12] The Antivenom Production Laboratory at Arizona State University (APL-ASU) began producing antivenin to *C. sculpturatus* in goats in 1965 and continues production today. No FDA approval exists for this product. Its use is restricted to the state of Arizona, where it is supplied free of charge to hospitals for compassionate use. Its transport across state lines is prohibited.

Efficacy of the APL-ASU antivenin has been demonstrated in both animals and humans.[2,3,5] In a study of 15 children below age 11 years, 12 patients receiving antivenin had resolution of neurologic, respiratory, and cardiovascular symptoms within 3 hours of initiating therapy. In those patients who did not receive antivenin therapy, symptoms lasted 15–24 hours.

With such low mortality and a relatively high incidence of hypersensitivity and serum sickness from administration of antivenin[3] there is rarely, if ever, an absolute indication for administration of scorpion antivenin. Administration of this antivenin is, therefore, reserved for the most severe scorpion envenomations, typically in children under age 6. A four-level severity grading of scorpion envenomation has been described (see Table 100–6).[5] Administration of antivenin is recommended for patients with systemic toxicity found in grades III or IV. It should be noted, however, that these same symptoms can also be successfully managed in an intensive care setting with aggressive airway management, monitoring, and benzodiazepine infusions. Geographic and financial factors also favor the administration of antivenin. Transport times to hospitals equipped for appropriate pediatric intensive care in the southwest desert are often long and may require costly air transportation. The ability to administer an effective antidote in a remote emergency department may avert the need for unnecessary expense or delay in achieving appropriate care. The decision to administer antivenin should be based on an analysis of the potential risks and benefits.

Obtaining toxicologic consultation should be considered for those not familiar with antivenin administration. Informed consent should be obtained. Prior to the administration of antivenin, an appropriate allergy history should be taken and skin testing should be performed. A history of allergy to antisera or to animal products does not contraindicate antivenin administration; however, patients or their guardians should be cautioned of possible adverse reactions.

Scorpion antivenin was formerly supplied as lyophylized serum and may occassionaly be found in hospitals in this form. Currently it is shipped from APL-ASU to the hospital as fresh immune serum. Each vial contains 5 mL of serum for use over 15–30 minutes. Experience with crotalid antivenin, however, suggests that more dilute concentrations given over a longer time period may be better tolerated by patients and may produce fewer allergic reactions. More severely envenomated patients will require faster infusion rates. Allergic reactions occur in approximately 60% of patients receiving antivenin therapy.[5]

Serum sickness, or type III hypersensitivity may occur in as many as 85% of patients.[5] Experience with crotalid antivenin suggests that the risk of serum sickness is directly correlated with the number of vials of antivenin received. Serum sickness typically occurs within 2 weeks of antivenin administration.

The Mexico-Pharma Polyvalent Scorpion Antivenom may also be effective against North American *Centruroides* stings; however, there is no known reliable repository of this antivenin in the United States.[1]

Fab has been made from immune goat serum for the treatment of *Centruriodes*.[2] No commercially available Fab exists for use in scorpion stings. A listing of scorpion antivenins available throughout the world is presented in Table 100–9.[14] Individual patient risk factors such as known sensitivity to antivenins or specific animal products and allergy to conventional medications should also be considered. Patients should be counseled on the risk to benefit ratio of the use of immune sera prior to administration.

TABLE 100–9. ANTIVENINS AVAILABLE WORLDWIDE

Scorpion	Antivenin
Androctonus	France-Pasteur Merieux Antiscorpion Venom Serum
Buthotus	Iran Scorpion antivenin
Buthus occitanus	France—Pasteur Merieux Antiscorpion Venom Serum
	Germany—Twyford Scorpion
Buthus gibbosusbrulla	Turkey Anti-Scorpion Antivenin
Centruroides (elegans, limpidus, noxius, suffusus)	Mexico—Pharma Polyvalent Scorpion Antivenin
Euscorpius (carpathicus, italicus)	Turkey Anti-Scorpion Antivenin
Leiurus quinquestreatus	France—Pasteur Merieux Antiscorpion Venom Serum
	Germany—Twyford Scorpion Antivenin
	Israel—Leiurus quinquestriatus
	Turkey Anti-Scorpion Antivenin
Mesobuthus eupeus	Iran Scorpion Antivenin
Odontobuthus doriae	Iran Scorpion Antivenin
Parabuthus species	South African Scorpion Antivenin
Scorpio maurus	Iran Scorpion Antivenin
	Turkey Anti-Scorpion Antivenin

Reprinted, with permission, from Theakston RDG, Warrell DA: Antivenoms: a list of hyperimmune sera currently available for the treatment of envenoming by bites and stings. Toxicon 1991;29: 1419–1470.

Latrodectus (mactans, hesperus, bishopi, geometricus)

Administration of antivenin for black widow spider envenomation is also somewhat controversial. Although the morbidity of black widow envenomations is high, with severe muscle pain and cramping and autonomic disturbances,[4,6] mortality is low.

Indications for antivenin administration include severe muscle cramping, hypertension, diaphoresis, nausea, vomiting, and respiratory difficulty that is not responsive to other therapy. Pregnancy has also been reported as a possible indication for antivenin administration.[11] Symptomatic treatment can almost always be accomplished with muscle relaxants and opioids alone or in combination. Some authors believe that antivenin has too high a risk to benefit ratio to justify its use.[10] In selected patients, however, the use of antivenin may reduce or eliminate the need for hospitalization, reduce pain and suffering, and shorten the course of the envenomation.

Antivenin (MSD) for black widow (*Latrodectus mactans*) is made by immunizing horses. Each vial of antivenin contains 6000 antivenin units standardized by biologic assay in mice. Since the venoms of *Latrodectus* species are virtually identical by immunologic and electrophoretic mechanisms, *Latrodectus mactans*–derived antivenin is presumed to be effective in other species of *Latrodectus* as well.[7] In a review of 163 cases of *Latrodectus* envenomation (presumed *Latrodectus hesperus*), antivenin reduced the durations of symptoms from a mean of 22 ± 24.9 hours to a mean of 9 ± 22.7 hours. Symptoms usually subside within 1–3 hours of administration of the antivenin. Hospital admission rate fell from 52% in those who were managed with opioids and muscle relaxants to 12% in those patients receiving antivenin.[4] Delayed administration of antivenin has also been shown to be effective. Antivenin has been reported to be effective when given as late as 30 hours after envenomation.[13]

Dosage of antivenin is usually the contents of one reconstituted vial (2.5 mL) diluted in 50 mL of saline for intravenous administration. Black widow antivenin can also be given IM; however, this route carries the disadvantage of slower, more erratic absorption, less control over the rate of administration, and the inability to stop administration of the drug should an allergic reaction occur.

Despite the apparent efficacy of antivenin, the decision to give horse serum for a disease with a low mortality is of great concern. Death from bronchospasm has been reported as a complication of antivenin administration, as has serum sickness.[4] Black widow antivenin is listed as a Pregnancy Category C.

Loxosceles spp.

Envenomation by the brown recluse spider, *Loxosceles reclusa,* although low in mortality, is a significant source of morbidity, particularly in the southeast United States. Antivenin to *L. reclusa* has been produced in rabbits. Efficacy of antivenin has been shown, if given prior to the onset of necrosis, usually within the first 24–48 hours.[9,11] Comparisons, however, have not revealed significant clinical differences between patients treated with antivenin as opposed to those treated with dapsone.[11] No commercially available product exists for the treatment of *Loxosceles* envenomation.

Summary

Controversy exists over the indication for antivenin administration in both spider and scorpion envenomations. Consideration should be given to the known efficacy of the antivenin, the relative morbidity and mortality of the disease, the risk of giving foreign immune sera, the level of available supportive care, the cost of supportive care, and the cost of obtaining or importing antivenin.

References

1. Antivenom Index. The American Zoo and Aquarium Association and The American Association of Poison Control Centers, 1994.
2. Bernstein JN, Dart RC, Garcia R, et al: Efficacy of antiscorpion (*Centruroides exilicauda*) Fab in a mouse model. Vet Hum Toxicol 1994;36:346. Abstract.
3. Bond RG: Antivenin administration for *Centruroides* scorpion sting: risks and benefits. Ann Emerg Med 1992;21: 788–791.
4. Clark RF, Werthern-Kestner S, Vance, MV, Gerkin R: Clinical presentation and treatment of black widow spider envenomation: a review of 163 cases. Ann Emerg Med 1992; 21:782–787.
5. Curry SC, Vance MV, Ryan PJ, et al: Envenomation by the scorpion *Centruroides sculpturatus*. J Toxicol Clin Toxicol 1983–1984;21:417–449.
6. Kobernick M: Black widow spider bite. Am Fam Physician 1984;29:241–245.
7. McCrone JD, Netzcoff ML: An immunological and electrophoretical comparison of the venoms of the North American Latrodectus spiders. Toxicon 1965;3:107–110.
8. Rachesky IJ, Banner W, Dansky J, Tong T: Treatments for *Centruroides exilicauda* Envenomation. Am J Dis Child 1984;138:1136–1139.
9. Rees R, Campbell D, Rieger E, King LE: The diagnosis and treatment of brown recluse spider bites. Ann Emerg Med 1987;16:945–949.
10. Robertson WO: Black widow spider case. Am J Emerg Med 1997;15:211.
11. Russell FE, Marcus P, Streng JA: Black widow spider envenomation during pregnancy. Toxicon 1979;17:188–189.
12. Schnur L, Schnur P: A case of allergy to scorpion antivenin. Ariz Med 1968;25:413–414.
13. Suntorntham S, Roberts JR, Nilsen GJ: Dramatic clinical response to the delayed administration of black widow spider antivenom. Ann Emerg Med 1994;24:1198–1199.
14. Theakston RDG, Warrell DA: Antivenoms: A list of hyperimmune sera currently available for the treatment of envenoming by bites and stings. Toxicon 1991;29:1419–1470.
15. Trestrail JH: Scorpion envenomation in Michigan: Three cases of toxic encounters with poisonous stow-aways. Vet Hum Toxicol 1981;23:8–11.

CHAPTER 101

Marine Envenomations

Richard S. Weisman

A 28-year-old man was stung on the lateral surface of his right hand by a lionfish when he reached into his tropical fish aquarium to adjust the aerator. Within seconds the man developed severe pain and swelling of his hand. While on route to the hospital the patient had applied an ice pack. On arrival in the emergency department he was awake, alert, and in considerable distress. His vital signs were: blood pressure 150/90 mm Hg; pulse 110 beats/min; respiratory rate 18 breaths/min; and temperature 98.6°F (37°C) (orally).

There were three small linear puncture marks, approximately 8 mm apart on the lateral surface of his right hand. The hand was swollen and erythematous but the neurovascular examination was intact.

The hand was immersed in water that had been heated to 110°F, resulting in relief of pain within 5 minutes. The pain recurred when the water cooled to room temperature. The patient received a diphtheria-tetanus toxoid vaccination. The patient was discharged 4 hours after arrival when his pain was significantly decreased and no systemic signs had developed. He was instructed to take a nonprescription analgesic for pain and to have his hand examined by his private physician the next day.

What Are the Most Common Marine Envenomations Brought to Medical Attention?

During the last decade there has been an increase in the popularity of sport diving and other water related activities resulting in an increase in marine envenomations.[27] The health care provider in an oceanside community must be prepared to care for patients with a variety of marine-related maladies ranging from dermatitis, to life-threatening allergic reactions, trauma, and envenomations.[2,8] Table 101–1 contains the most common painful marine envenomations, characteristic symptoms, and therapy.

Many creatures of the sea have improved their odds of surviving the natural evolutionary process by developing elaborate apparati to deliver a poison or venom to their prey while limiting the risk of falling victim to their predators. These venoms are often complex mixtures of high-molecular-weight proteins and low-molecular-weight compounds including histamine, bradykinin, and indole derivatives.[17,24,34,40,41] They often are capable of causing pain, degranulating mast cells, interfering with cellular transport and metabolism, disrupting neuronal transmission, and causing myocardial depression.[2]

The marine animals that are capable of causing harm to man can be divided into the vertebrates and invertebrates some of which are swimmers and some nonswimmers. The vertebrates because of their strength and mobility are capable of inflicting more structural damage than the often passive invertebrates. However, the potential morbidity and even mortality that can result from the venomous and nonvenomous invertebrates should not be underestimated.

Which Vertebrates Are Commonly Associated With Human Injuries?

The Scorpaenidae (class: Osteichthyes; order: Perciformes) are the most common vertebrates to sting man. The most dangerous members of the Scorpaenidae family, *Pterois volitans* (lionfish, turkeyfish, zebrafish, tigerfish, scorpionfish) and *Synanceja horrida* (stonefish), are almost exclusively found in the Gulf of Mexico and Pacific and Indian oceans.

TABLE 101–1. ORGANISMS RESPONSIBLE FOR PAINFUL MARINE ENVENOMATIONS

Organism	Common Signs/Symptoms	Treatment
Pterois	Pain, swelling	Hot water, analgesics, digital block
lionfish		
turkeyfish		
zebrafish		
tigerfish		
scorpionfish		
Synanceja		
stonefish	Pain, swelling, hypotension, dysrhythmias	Hot water, analgesics, digital block, antivenin
Trachinus weeverfish	Pain, swelling, nausea, edema vomiting, diaphoresis, hypotension seizures, dysrhythmias	Analgesics, digital block
Dasyatis		
Urolophus		
stingray	Pain, deep ulcerated wound, muscle cramping, weakness, hypotension, syncope, dysrhythmias, seizures	Hot water, analgesics, antibiotics
Sea Snakes		
Enhydrina schistosa	Pain, swelling, neuropathies, paralysis, respiratory failure, myonecrosis, renal failure	Analgesics, IV hydration, antivenin
Hydrophis ornatus		
H. cyanocinctus		
Lapemis hardwickii		
Pelamis platurus		
Thalassophina viperina		
Aipysurus laevis		
Coelenterata	Pain, burning, urticaria lymphadenopathy, anaphylactic reactions	5% acetic acid, remove tentacles, papain tenderizer, analgesics, antihistamines
jellyfish		
sea anemones		
corals		
hydroids		
Physalia		
Portuguese man-of-war	Pain, burning, urticaria lymphadenopathy, anaphylactic reactions	5% acetic acid, remove tentacles, papain tenderizer, analgesics, antihistamines
Millepora fire coral	Pain, burning, urticaria, intense pruritis	5% acetic acid, remove tentacles, corticosteroids
Acanthaster crown-of-thorns	Pain, erythema, nausea, vomiting, syncope, ataxia, paresthesias, muscle cramps, respiratory distress	Hot water, surgical removal of spines, analgesia
Diadema sea urchins		

In the United States, most scorpaenid stings reported to poison centers are the result of lionfish exposures in home aquaria.[25] Lionfish are among the most beautiful of reef fish. Their long curved dorsal spines are ornately covered with a lacy tissue that allows them to corner their prey before suddenly lunging at their intended target. Lionfish will normally not attack man unless they become cornered and are denied an escape route. When they are attacking, they will erect their dorsal spines and make quick thrusting jabs at their pray or an intruder. The *Pterois volitans* venom is a complex mixture of inflammatory mediators including prostaglandin $F_2\alpha$, thromboxane B_2 and prostaglandin E_2.[4] Victims will experience a severe burning pain and swelling within seconds of contact with the spines. The venom glands of the lionfish (*Pterois* species) are smaller than the glands of the stonefish (*Synanceja* species). Severe systemic cardiovascular symptoms that may occur with stonefish envenomations are less commonly observed with lionfish envenomations.

Within the Scorpaenidae family, the stonefish (*Synanceja horrida*) is most likely to be responsible for serious injury.[40] This camouflaged fish can be found in coral reefs or among the algae. Unlike most of the other venomous fish, the stonefish prefers to attack humans rather than to swim away. Stonefish venom is a high-molecular-weight (150,000 D), heat-labile, antigenic, nondialyzable protein.[41] The effect of stonefish venom appears to be a direct muscular toxicity. The pain caused by the envenomation is so excruciating that it may cause a diver to lose consciousness. The pain will continue to intensify for several hours after the initial sting. Other localized symptoms from scorpaenid envenomations may include erythema and ecchymosis, induration, hyperesthesia, anesthesia or dysesthesia of the affected limb and subsequently lymphadenopathy. Early systemic symptoms may include nausea, vomiting, diaphoresis, dyspnea, hypotension, and syncope. Later manifestations such as cardiac dysrhythmias, conduction abnormalities, myocardial ischemia, pulmonary edema, convulsions, and paralysis may develop with severe envenomations.[17]

The weeverfish (order: Perciformes; family: Trachinidae) inhabits the muddy- or sandy-bottomed bays within the temperate zones of the eastern Atlantic Ocean, Mediterranean Sea, and European coastal waters.[18] The small fish (10–50 cm) often burrows into the ocean's bottom, leaving only its head visible. Most envenomations occur when a diver or fisherman steps on the fish. The fish has sharp dorsal and opercular spines that are capable of penetrating a leather boot when thrust forward at its intended prey. Venom-containing glandular tissue surrounds the spines in a thin integumentary sheath.[11] The venom, which has not been completely characterized, consists of several peptides, high-molecular-weight proteins, mucopolysaccharides, serotonin, epinephrine, norepinephrine, and histamine.[33] Following envenomation, the victim will experience a burning or crushing pain that will increase in intensity as it spreads through the limb. The wound site will appear edematous, erythematous, and ecchymotic. The edema may involve the entire affected limb and may persist for months after the sting.[18] The systemic symptoms that have been reported with weeverfish envenomations include headache, fever, chills, nausea, vomiting, diaphoresis, hypotension, seizures, and cardiac dysrhythmias.[11]

What Is the Best Way to Relieve Pain From a Scorpaenidae Envenomation?

The intensity of pain experienced by victims of Scorpaenidae envenomations can be extremely variable and probably reflects both the amount of venom injected and the depth of the injury. The treatment of Scorpaenidae envenomations should include soaking the affected limb in water heated to 110–115°F, local wound care, tetanus prophylaxis, and supportive care for systemic symptoms. It is postulated that many of the complex venoms will denature at temperatures above 105°F.[31] If blisters form at the site of the envenomation, they should be surgically excised. The fluid aspirated from blisters following a lionfish envenomation contains high concentrations of prostaglandins F_2 and E_2 and thromboxane B_2.[4] If adequate pain relief is not obtained with immersion of the limb in water, the patient should be given a salicylate, another nonsteroidal antiinflammatory analgesic, or acetaminophen in combination with oral codeine. If pain fails to respond to an oral analgesic regimen, the patient should be given a sufficient dose of a parenteral opioid to obtain analgesia. The administration of a digital nerve block with 0.25% bupivacaine was successfully used in a patient with refractory pain.[14]

An antivenin is available from the health services departments of most of the major aquaria throughout the United States. The antivenin is most often required for stonefish envenomations where life-threatening systemic toxicity may be more common.

Why Are Stingray Envenomations so Common Along the West Coast of the United States and the Caribbean?

The stingray (class: Chondrichthyed; order: Rajiformes) is a peaceful bottom feeder that is responsible for approximately 1800 envenomations each year primarily along the West Coast of the United States.[1] Eleven different species of rays have been found in U.S. coastal waters.[30] The stingray can be distinguished from other fish by having gills exclusively located on the ventral surfaces of their bodies.[17] Stingrays tend to burrow into the sand, where careless divers may unintentionally step on them. The stingray is armed with a tail barb that will reflexively impact on anything with which it comes in contact. The long serrated spines on the dorsum of the stingray's tail can easily penetrate human flesh and produce a deep, jagged laceration, most commonly on a lower extremity.[35] Severe injuries are common, with deep ulcers at the wound site and secondary bacterial infections.[6] The bacterial flora that has been cultured from marine animals, sea water, and ocean sediment is diverse. Antibiotic therapy should address infections due to *Vibrio* species in general and *Vibrio vulnificus* specifically.[21,23] The third-generation cephalosporins are considered to be appropriate for ocean-acquired infections.[29]

The venom isolated from the stingray contains a mixture of phosphodiesterase, 5′-nucleotidase, and serotonin.[16] When experimentally administered to animals, the venom caused peripheral vasoconstriction, bradycardia, conduction abnormalities, respiratory depression, ataxia, and seizures.[34] Most victims experience severe pain and burning, which intensifies for several hours after the sting. The pain is usually out of proportion to the amount of visible tissue injury. Severe trauma may occur without venom release from the venom glands. The wound will often initially appear cyanotic or dusky and subsequently becomes erythematous, hemorrhagic, and then necrotic.[6] When systemic effects occur they may include muscle cramping, weakness, tremor, syncope, hypotension, cardiovascular collapse, convulsions, and paralysis.

Treatment consists of pain control by immersing the affected limb in hot water 110–115°F, thorough wound cleansing and debridement, tetanus prophylaxis, irrigation of the wound to remove as much venom as possible, and treatment of infection should it develop. If adequate pain relief is not obtained with immersion of the limb in water, the patient should be given a salicylate, nonsteroidal antiinflammatory analgesic, or acetaminophen in combination with oral codeine. If adequate pain relief is not obtained with these approaches, the patient should be treated as described previously for Scorpaenidae envenomations.

Do Sea Snake Bites Have Toxic Effects?

There are more than 50 species of sea snakes, making them the most common reptile found in the ocean. The large number of sea snakes makes both the taxonomy and therapeutic regimens difficult to evaluate. Sea snakes are found in the Pacific and Indian oceans commonly along the coast of Southeast Asia, the Malay Archipelago, and the Persian Gulf. There are no sea snakes in the Atlantic Ocean or Caribbean Sea. All species of sea snakes are toxic and seven have been known to be fatal to man.[1] These include: *Astrotia stokesii, Enhydrina schistosa, Hydrophis ornatus* and *H. cyanocinctus, Lapemis hardwickii, Pelamus platurus,* and *Thalassophina viperina.* Most of the snakes range from 3 to 4 feet in length, but some may be considerably longer.[28] The majority of sea snake bites do not result in envenomation because the snake's fangs are short and are easily dislodged.[13] The venom is a peripheral neurotoxin that alters sodium and chloride permeability without affecting the Na-K ATPase pump.[15] Phospholipases, nerve growth factor, capillary permeability factor, anticomplement-active factor, acetylcholinesterase, hyaluronidase, leucine aminopeptidase, 5′-nucleotidase, and several hemolytic and myotoxic compounds have been identified in the venom.[1] The symptoms occurring following an envenomation rarely result in a local reaction. Commonly 3–6 hours after envenomation the patient develops both cranial and peripheral neurologic abnormalities including paralysis and respiratory failure, myonecrosis, myoglobinuria, and renal failure.[28] The olive sea snake (*Aipysurus laevis*) differs from the others because it contains a primarily myopathic venom that causes paralysis and respiratory failure.[13]

The treatment of sea snake envenomations is similar to the care of other snake bites. Emphasis should be placed on stabilization of the patient's vital signs. Pulmonary and renal function must be carefully monitored. With any evidence of an envenomation, polyvalent sea snake antivenin should be administered (Commonwealth Serum Laboratories, Melbourne, Australia). This equine-derived immunoglobulin is prepared against two of the more common sea snakes venoms, *Enhydrina schistosa* and *Notechis scutatis*.[7] It is believed to have activity against most of the other sea snake venoms as well.

What Are the Most Common Invertebrate Envenomations?

There are approximately 9000 species in the phylum Coelenterata, of which several hundred are dangerous to man. The phylum is characterized by a unique gastrovascular cavity that has a single opening for both digestion and circulation. The Coelenterata are responsible for more marine envenomations than any other phylum.[24]

Most of the marine life within the phylum Coelenterata (jellyfish, sea anemones, corals, and hydroids) contain stinging structures called nematocysts (cnidocytes). These poisonous dartlike structures are tightly coiled and enclosed within their venom sacs. Following external contact, the nematocysts are shot out of their containment sacs, injecting their venom as they penetrate the flesh of their prey. The nematocyst venom is a complex mixture containing bradykinin, hemolysin, serotonin, histamine, prostaglandins, adenosine triphosphatase, nucleotidases, hyaluronidase, alkaline and acid proteases, alkaline and acid phosphatases, phosphodiesterases, fibrinolysin, leucine aminopeptidase, RNAase, and DNAase.[10]

Jellyfish travel in groups called smucks, which may contain more than a thousand individual jellyfish. The jellyfish has long tentacles that hang down from an air-filled pneumatophore. The tentacles contain hundreds of thousands of nematocysts, each containing a small amount of venom. Most of the members of this family are capable of incapacitating small fish or other marine life, but in humans they typically cause only a painful sting. Subsequently a severe burning sensation with resulting erythematous or violaceous lesions and regional lymph node involvement ensue. More severe envenomations may lead to ulceration with a delayed healing phase. Anaphylactoid reactions manifested as bronchospasm, dysrhythmias, hypotension, and cardiovascular collapse can occur. Erythema nodosum and arthralgias are also reported.[3] A healthy woman developed blurred vision that persisted for 8 days following a jellyfish envenomation.[9]

The larvae of the jellyfish *Linuche unguiculata* are capable of causing an atopic dermatitis after they become attached to the fibers of bathing attire.[39] This is called seabather's eruption or sea lice and is commonly reported between March and June along the southeast coast of Florida. Symptoms usually resolve spontaneously several hours to days after the development of a pruritic, erythematous maculopapular rash, limited to areas covered by bathing attire.

The Portuguese man-of-war (*Physalia*) is a well-known, pale-blue, bell-shaped inhabitant of the Floridia coast of the Atlantic and the Gulf of Mexico.[37] The Portuguese man-of-war is most commonly found close to shore between July and September. Tentacles may trail as far as 10 feet behind the body. The almost invisible tentacles contain nematocysts that can release a neurotoxic venom capable of causing excruciating pain. Subsequently, linear red papules and large erythematous welts develop. Envenomations may be accompanied by nausea, vomiting, myalgia, headache, chills, respiratory distress, and cardiovascular collapse.[22] Death may ensue if multiple stings are inflicted on the victim. Tentacles dislodged in turbulent water may remain capable of discharging nematocysts for a significant time after detachment.

Which Coelenterate Has the Greatest Potential for Morbidity and Mortality?

The sea wasp or box jellyfish (*Chironex fleckeri*) is the most venomous and deadly of all stinging marine life. It is found predominantly in the Australian and Southeast Asian waters, but can also be found in the open ocean.[36] The sea wasp like the Portuguese man-of-war often rides the current of the tide. Each box jellyfish carries enough venom to kill several adults. At least 72 fatalities have been attributed to the box jellyfish in waters off the coast of Australia and Southeast Asia,[42] and the overall fatality rate is estimated to approach 20%. The sting from a sea wasp may result in hypotension, profound muscle spasm, respiratory paralysis, and cardiac arrest. Death has occurred within 30 seconds of envenomation.[20]

How Should the Victim of a Coelenterate Envenomation Be Treated?

The treatment should include supporting vital signs, preventing worsening of the envenomation, wound care, and pain management. The area of the sting should be rinsed with 5% acetic acid (vinegar) or sea water to remove nematocysts that may be present on the surface. Although unsubstantiated, it has been suggested that fresh water or alcohol (isopropanol or ethanol) should be avoided as they may cause a discharge of the nematocysts already present on the skin surface. Alcohols also do not destroy or deactivate nematocysts and are therefore not recommended. Health care providers should wear gloves to prevent being stung by any nematocysts remaining on the victim's skin. Papain (meat tenderizer) may be effective in destroying any remaining nematocysts.[26] If tentacles remain attached to the skin, shaving cream, baking soda, or flour may be applied over the tentacles. After a few minutes, a dull knife or any available firm object (such as the side of a credit card) should be scraped across the skin to carefully dislodge the nematocysts. Pruritus may respond well to antihistamines. If adequate pain relief is not obtained after removal of the nematocycts and application of 5% acetic acid, the patient should be treated as described previously for Scorpaenidae envenomations. Tetanus prophylaxis should be assured.

A sheep-derived *Chironex* antivenin is available for victims of sea wasp envenomations (Commonwealth Serum Laboratory, Australia). The antivenin is best administered intravenously (one ampule, 20,000 units, diluted 1:5 to 1:10 in isotonic crystalloid) over a 5-minute period.[24] The antivenin may be readministered every 2 hours until there is no further progression of symptoms.

What Type of Injury Can Result from Contact with Coral?

The fire coral (*Millepora*) is not a true coral but a close relative of the fresh water *hydra* containing very powerful and deeply penetrating nematocysts with a very toxic venom. Fire coral, frequently incorrectly identified as seaweed, is most commonly found in shallow tropical waters. Contact with the fire coral may result in an immediate burning or stinging pain, urticaria and intense pruritis.[1] The wheals may take several weeks to resolve and may leave a hyperpigmented scar.

Treatment of fire coral envenomation should consist of immediate irrigation with sea water followed by rinsing with either a 5% acetic acid solution or isopropanol. Systemic corticosteroids have been used for treating the rash if it persists.[1]

Are There Toxic Octopi?

The giant monster octopus prefers to avoid humans when possible. However, when provoked this sea creature will mount an effective attack. The octopus has a distinct venom delivery system consisting of two sets of salivary glands that will release venom from a powerful parrotlike beak.

The blue-ringed octopus (*Hapalochlaena maculosus*) contains the potent neurotoxin, tetrodotoxin, as well as at least eight other neuroactive amines.[12] Symptoms from an envenomation may include local pain, a burning sensation, numbness, and ischemia while paresthesias may extend from the wound site to involve the lips and tongue. Aphonia, dysphagia, blurred vision, coma, and cardiovascular collapse may ensue. An intense autonomic ganglionic blockade may be responsible for hypotension and respiratory failure. Treatment of an octopus envenomation is symptomatic and supportive.

Control of respiration, blood pressure, and pulse must be assured. The use of a direct-acting vasopressor such as norepinephrine or phenylephrine may be needed to control blood pressure.[11] The use of hot water on the envenomated area seems to be of little benefit.[29] If adequate pain relief is not obtained with immersion of the limb in water, the patient should be treated as described previously for Scorpaenidae envenomations. Tetanus prophylaxis should be administered if immunization status is not current.

Is the Cone Shell Toxic to Man ?

The cone shell (order: Archaeogastropoda; family: Conidae), a nocturnal predatory carnivore, contains a potent neurotoxin. It has an ejectable tooth on the end of a long flexible proboscis.[19] It attacks its prey (or humans) by sinking its venomous tooth deep into the victim's flesh. Signs and symptoms developing from the poorly characterized venom include local pain, a burning sensation, numbness, ischemia, and paresthesias. Distal manifestations include paresthesias of the lips and tongue, aphonia, dysphagia, blurred vision, coma, and cardiovascular collapse. In most instances, symptoms do not progress beyond local manifestations and resolve in 6–8 hours. Treatment is supportive. Pain relief may be obtained by placing the involved area in water heated to 110–115°F. Tetanus prophylaxis should be administered as indicated.

Are Starfish and Sea Urchins a Threat to Man?

With the exception of the crown of thorns (*Acanthaster planci*), most starfish are nonvenomous, or at least not a risk for humans. A careless brush with this thorned creature can leave the diver with many very deep and painful puncture wounds and occasionally, nausea, vomiting, and muscular paralysis. The venom is composed of toxic saponins with hemolytic and anticoagulant effects and histamine-like substances.[38] Therapy is primarily symptomatic and supportive, with immersion in hot water 110–115°F and the administration of oral analgesics usually being sufficient for pain relief.[32]

Physical contact with sea urchins should be avoided. Certain nonvenomous sea urchins have very long, sharp, and brittle spines that easily penetrate flesh and tend to snap off, leaving a barbed foreign body behind. The spines of the urchin (*Diadema*) can be as long as a foot. These spines can easily advance deep into muscle and joint spaces, resulting in tissue destruction, pain, and infection.

Many species of sea urchin have venom glands located both at the ends of their spines and in pedicellariae, which are fanglike jaws located at the ends of flexible stalks used to gather food. The victim of a venomous sting will experience intense pain, erythema, and swelling. The venom is believed to be composed of steroid glycosides, hemolysins, proteases, serotonin, and cholinergic-like substances. Partial paralysis of the affected extremity has been reported with some species. Rarely, systemic symptoms may develop, including nausea, syncope, paresthesias, ataxia, muscle cramps, weakness, and respiratory distress.[5] There is no universally accepted treatment for sea-urchin spine puncture wounds. Submersing the affected area in hot water 110–115°F seems to be accepted for pain relief. The decision to remove embedded spines should be based upon their location, evident infection, or persistent pain. Removal should be attempted only after radiographic localization and may necessitate use of an operating microscope.[24]

Summary

The healthcare provider and poison center specialist should become familiar with the toxic marine life found in their geographic region. Although marine envenomations rarely result in severe morbidity, hundreds of painful envenomations may occur each day in coastal locations during certain seasons of the year. Understanding the clinical course and effective therapies for such stings can often help reduce the anxiety and painful consequences caused by these exposures.

References

1. Auerbach PS: Marine Envenomations. In: Auerbach PS, ed: Wilderness Medicine: Management of Wilderness and Environmental Emergencies, 3rd ed. New York, Macmillan, 1995, pp. 1327–1374.
2. Auerbach PS: Marine envenomations. N Eng J Med 1991;325:486–493.
3. Auerbach PS, Hays JT: Erythema nodosum following a jellyfish sting. J Emerg Med 1987;5:487–491.
4. Auerbach PS, McKinnney HE, Rees RS, Heggers JP: Analysis of vesicle fluid following the sting of the lionfish *Pterois volitans*. Toxicon 1987;25:1350–1353.
5. Baden HP, Burnett JW: Injuries from sea urchins. South Med J 1977; 23:459–460.
6. Bars P: Wound necrosis caused by the venom of stingrays. Med J Aust 1984;141:854–855.
7. Baxter EH, Gallichio HA: Protection against sea snake envenomation: Comparative potency of four antivenins. Toxicon 1976;14:347–355.
8. Brown CK, Shepherd SM: Marine trauma, envenomations and intoxications. Emerg Med Clin North Am 1992;10: 385–408.
9. Burnett HW, Burnett JW: Prolonged blurred vision following coelenterate envenomation. Toxicon 1990;28:731–733.
10. Burnett JW, Calton GJ: The chemistry and toxicology of some venomous pelagic coelenterates. Toxicon 1977;15: 177–196.
11. Cain D: Weeverfish sting: An unusual problem. Br Med J 1983;287:406.
12. Flachsenberger WA: Respiratory failure and lethal hypotension due to blue-ringed octopus and tetrodotoxin envenomations observed and counteracted in animal models. J Toxicol Clin Toxicol 1987;24:485–502.
13. Fulde GWO, Smith F: Sea snake envenomation at Bondi. Med J Aust 1984;141:44–45.
14. Garyfallou GT, Madden JF: Lionfish envenomation. Ann Emerg Med 1996;28:456–457.
15. Gerencser GA, Loo SY: Effect of *Laticauda semifasciata* (sea snake) venom on sodium transport across frog skin. Comp Biochem Physiol 1982;72A:727–730.
16. Halstead BW: Current status of marine toxicology—An overview. Colton, CA, International Biotoxicological Center, World Life Research Institute, 1980.
17. Halstead BW: Poisonous and Venomous Marine Animals of the World. Princeton, NJ, Darwin Press, 1978, pp. 1–135.
18. Halstead BW, Modglin FR: Weeverfish stings and venom apparatus of weever (Trachinus). Z Tropenmed Parasitol 1958;9:129.
19. Hinegardner RT: The venom apparatus of the cone shell. Hawaii Med J 1958;17:533–536.
20. Holmes JL: Marine stingers in far North Queensland. Aust J Dermatol 1996;37:23–26.
21. Johnson JM Becker SF, McFarland LM: *Vibrio vulnificus*: Man and the sea. JAMA 1985;253:2850–2853.
22. Kaufman MB: Portuguese man-of-war envenomation. Pediatr Emerg Care 1992;8:27–28.
23. Kelly MT, McCormick WF. Acute bacterial myositis caused by *Vibrio vulnificus*. JAMA 1981;246:72–73.
24. Kizer KW: Marine envenomations. J Toxicol Clin Toxicol 1984;21:527–555.
25. Kizer KW, McKinney HE, Auerbach PS: Scorpaenidae envenomation: A five-year poison center experience. JAMA 1985;253:807–810.
26. Loder JS: Treatment of jellyfish stings. JAMA 1973;226:1228.
27. McGoldrick J, Marx JA: Marine envenomations. J Emerg Med 1992;10:71–77.
28. Mercer HP, McGill JJ, Ibraham RA: Envenomation by sea snake in Queensland. Med J Aust 1981;1:130–132.
29. Morris JG, Tenney J: Antibiotic therapy for *Vibrio vulnificus* infection. JAMA 1985;253:1121–1122.
30. Mullaney PJ: Treatment of sting ray wounds. Clin Toxicol 1970;3:613–615.
31. Patel MR, Wells: Lionfish envenomation of the hand. J Hand Surg 1993;18:523–525.
32. Roscoe MD: Cutaneous manifestations of marine animal injuries, including diagnosis and treatment. Cutis 1977;19: 507–510.
33. Russell FE: Weeverfish sting: The last word. Br Med J 1983; 287:981–982.
34. Russell FE: Comparative pharmacology of some animal toxins. Fed Proc 1967;26:1206–1218.
35. Russell FE: Stingray injuries. Public Health Rep 1959;74: 855–859.
36. Southcott RV: Studies on Australian Cubomedusae, including a new genus and species apparently harmful to man. Aust J Mar Freshw Res 1956;7:254.
37. Stein MR, Marrachini JV, Rothschild NE: Fatal Portuguese man-of-war (*Physalia physalis*) envenomation. Ann Emerg Med 1989;18:312–315.

38. Taira E, Tananara N, Fanatsu M: Studies on the toxin in the spines of the starfish *Acanthaster planci*. 1. Isolation and properties of the toxin found in spines. Sci Bull Coll Agr Univ Ryukus 1975;22:203–212.
39. Tomchik RS, Russell MT, Szmant AM, Black NA: Clinical perspectives on seabather's eruption, also known as sea lice. JAMA 1993;269:1669–1672.
40. Wiener S: Observations on the venom of the stonefish (*Synanceja trachynis*). Med J Aust 1959;2:260–265.
41. Wiener S: The production and assay of stone-fish antivenene. Med J Aust 1959;4:715–719.
42. Williamson JA, LeRay LE, Wohlfahrt M, Fenner PJ: Acute envenomation by box jellyfish (*Chironex fleckeri*). Med J Aust 1989;141:851–853.

CHAPTER 102

Prehospital and Interhospital Principles

Neal E. Flomenbaum and Theodore I. Benzer

An advanced life support (ALS or paramedic) unit arrived at the scene of a call for a "man down" on a street corner. The two paramedics rapidly initiated the evaluation and treatment for an "unconscious patient." During the course of this treatment, 0.8 mg of naloxone was administered intravenously (IV) and within 30–60 seconds the patient regained consciousness and began fighting with the paramedics. Police at the scene helped restrain the patient temporarily, but he adamantly refused all treatment and specifically refused to get into the ambulance. The police maintained that unless the patient agreed to be treated they could not force the him to go to the hospital. After a total of 20–25 minutes at the scene, the paramedics were ready to depart. At this time the patient was somewhat drowsy, but still refused to go to the hospital.

The paramedics contacted their base station physician by telemetry for further instructions in managing this complex situation. Since the patient was now somnolent, the paramedics were instructed to carefully place him in the ambulance and transport him to the ED, monitoring his breathing pattern and refraining from administering any additional opioid antagonist unless he became apneic.

Because of the increasing availability of basic and advanced emergency medical technicians (EMTs and AEMTs) and paramedics together with easy access to regional poison centers, the management of toxicologic emergencies frequently begins in the home or on the street and continues en route to the hospital. In addition, paramedics and EMTs capable of providing high-quality care for critically ill patients have enabled many community hospitals to transfer seriously ill victims of carbon monoxide poisoning to hyperbaric oxygen facilities, victims of envenomations to antivenin treatment centers, and victims of drug overdoses and poisonings to designated poison treatment centers and other hospitals capable of providing hemodialysis and/or hemoperfusion. Appropriate pre- and interhospital care of the poisoned or overdosed patients begins with a knowledge of those aspects of management described in detail in Chapters 3 and 30. This chapter considers issues of pre- and interhospital care of the poisoned or overdosed patient. Issues involving eye, skin, and pulmonary decontamination are addressed in Chapters 3, 30, and 92. Unfortunately, there is currently a dearth of sound scientific information regarding management of poisonings and overdoses in the prehospital setting and many of the recommendations that follow have been extrapolated from similar situations that arise in the hospital setting. Hopefully this chapter will also stimulate investigators to scientifically study toxicologic management in the prehospital setting.

How Should EMTs and Paramedics Deal With the Personal Danger in Rescuing and Treating Poisoning Victims?

In this textbook overdoses and poisonings are usually considered together because, for the most part, initial clinical management is the same. Management does differ, however, with regard to diagnosis, definitive treatment, and personal safety of rescue personnel.

Victims of deliberate poisonings and patients who have taken drug overdoses with true suicidal intent are often unable or unwilling to describe accurately the extent of the ingestion or exposure (Chaps. 3 and 30). Conversely, after a suicide "gesture" the patient may deliberately exaggerate the nature of the overdose or exposure or suggest that there is a widespread danger to others.

When dealing with an actual or possible source of danger, EMTs and paramedics must protect themselves from exposure to poisons or inhalation of toxic chemicals and fumes by using appropriate protective equipment and providing adequate ventilation to enclosed places suspected of containing high concentrations of toxic gases (see Chap. 92). Many toxic gases are colorless and odorless, and some chemicals (eg, organophosphates) can be absorbed through intact skin. Paramedics and EMTs must also be aware of the danger of mouth-to-mouth resuscitation for patients suspected of having cyanide poisoning. Protocols written for prehospital personnel should include specific instructions, and ambulances must be adequately equipped (ambu bags, etc) to avoid primary or secondary poisoning of the rescuer.[1]

Overdose victims who are conscious or who have an altered level of consciousness other than coma present other difficulties in the prehospital setting: They may be combative, placing themselves and paramedics or EMTs at risk, or they may be unwilling to accept medical care, particularly transport to the hospital. Prehospital care providers must maintain their objectivity and compassion and not allow these factors to alter acceptable standards of care such that the patient is placed at greater risk.

As with all patient interactions, care must be taken to avoid blood and body fluid contamination. Patients using illicit drugs intravenously are especially prone to bloodborne infections (HIV and hepatitis), and great care must be taken to avoid contamination during treatment and handling of drug paraphernalia.

What Considerations Should Be Given to Initial Prehospital Management of a Poisoned or Overdosed Patient?

Initial control of airway, breathing, and circulation are of prime importance in managing the toxicologic emergency, as they are in treating any emergency. Prehospital personnel should be mindful that the patient's condition may deteriorate rapidly and unpredictably. For an unconscious patient, definitive control of the airway with endotracheal intubation and establishment of an IV line should be considered early in the management. A properly secured airway not only ensures adequate ventilation and oxygenation but may prevent further aspiration of gastric contents. Indications for the use of $D_{50}W$, thiamine, naloxone, and oxygen in a patient with an altered level of consciousness are generally consistent with their use in the ED as described in Chapters 3 and 30. However, the value of the empiric use of naloxone and $D_{50}W$ in the prehospital setting has been questioned in two retrospective studies; the findings are summarized in the antidote section below.[3,4]

What Is the Role of the EMT or Paramedic in Establishing a Diagnosis of Poisoning or Overdose?

One of the most important functions an EMT or paramedic can perform in managing a toxicologic emergency is to evaluate the patient's environment, to the extent permitted by the patient's condition. For example, an elderly patient brought in unconscious from home may be suffering from hypoglycemia, hyperosmolar coma, diabetic ketoacidosis, sepsis, poisoning, overdose, intoxication, and so on. However, if the EMT notices an unvented space heater in the corner of the room and reports this finding to the emergency physician, the diagnosis of carbon monoxide (CO) poisoning can be pursued expeditiously. This consideration is especially important, since oxygen administration en route may begin to treat the signs and symptoms before the patient is examined in the ED, thereby potentially obscuring the etiology of the patient's initial altered consciousness. Reporting the presence of the space heater to the local health department or Environmental Protection Agency (EPA) will allow appropriate personnel to seek out and eliminate the CO source before others die from the exposure.

In addition to noting empty pill bottles, suicide notes, or illicit drug paraphernalia found with a patient, prehospital personnel should be aware of any unusual smells, sources of toxic gases, and evidence of toxic chemicals in the patient's environment. Chemicals in the workplace, for example, may present a difficult diagnostic challenge that is made easier if the EMT notes the few *specific* chemicals that are available.

Prehospital evaluation and care should include transport to the ED of containers (labeled or not), pills and pill bottles, and any possible ingested plant material for definitive identification. Some prehospital personnel carry "patient belongings" bags in the ambulance for this purpose. If possible, animals at the scene, which may be either a source or a victim of poisoning, should be restrained or contained and transported later by appropriate personnel such as the ASPCA.

Finally, recognition of the possibility of concomitant trauma to the victim is essential for appropriate and timely management. Many overdose patients also become victims of blunt or penetrating trauma. Conversely, many trauma victims are also inebriated or overdosed on medications or drugs.

Should Gastric Decontamination Be Initiated by Paramedics?

Administration of syrup of ipecac to alert patients after a recent oral ingestion may be considered. In some types of poisoning, gastric emptying (most typically by emesis) may be possible only early in the clinical course, before the resultant toxicity precludes such intervention, as in colchicine or a heavy metal poisoning. Especially when transport time is long, syrup of ipecac may therefore have to be administered at home as directed by a regional poison center or by prehospital personnel, if it is to be administered at all. Arguments against prehospital administration of syrup ipecac include (1) a patient who starts vomiting en route to the hospital may be difficult to position properly, and (2) controlling the airway in the back of a moving ambulance may be difficult, with the added danger that the patient may lose the gag reflex prior to vomiting. Orogastric lavage, which may be an appropriate alternative, form of gastric emptying, has not gained widespread use in the prehospital setting.

Prehospital administration of activated charcoal (AC) may offer a relatively safe and attractive alternative to both emesis and lavage. Even in an area where ambulance transport time was relatively short (about 10–12 minutes on average), the authors of one pilot study were able to demonstrate that prehospital, AC could be administered in an average of 5.0 minutes from the first encounter with paramedics versus 51.4 minutes when AC was delayed until arrival in the ED.[2] Even when no form of gastric decontamination (GID) is offered prehospital, ambulance transportation to the ED by itself appears to result in decreased time to GID. In a retrospective review of 167 overdose patients receiving gastric lavage or activated charcoal, the median interval from presentation to GID was 55 minutes for patients arriving by ambulance compared to 73 minutes for the nonambulance patients.[11] The authors concluded that although ambulance-transported overdose patients waited a shorter time than nonambulance patients for GID, the delay was unacceptably long in either case. The findings of this study support the argument that some form of GID should be initiated prehospital.

It is virtually impossible to design a protocol that takes into consideration all of the factors relevant to the very large number of substances that may be involved in an overdose or poisoning. In addition, variations in transport time in different regions of the country (eg, urban vs rural) may make gastric emptying essential or lifesaving in one case and unnecessary or dangerous in another case involving the same drug or toxin.

For these reasons, EMTs and paramedics must be able to contact a physician located in a hospital ED, regional poison center, or base station telemetry unit to tailor options in gastric decontamination or gastric emptying to the individual patient. The various methods of gastric emptying and indications and contraindications for their use are described in Chapter 3. Issues regarding gastric decontamination are thoroughly discussed in Chapter 4.

TABLE 102–1. MEDICATIONS COMMONLY CARRIED BY PARAMEDICS THAT CAN ALSO BE USED AS ANTIDOTES[a,b]

Medication	Primary Use	Antidotal Use
Atropine	Bradydysrhythmias	Beta-adrenergic antagonist, calcium channel blocker, and cardiac gylcoside (digoxin) overdoses; muscarinic mushroom (clitocybe, inocybe) poisoning; organophosphate and carbamate insecticide poisoning
Benzodiazepines[c]	Seizures, severe agitation	Stimulants
Calcium chloride[d]	Hyperkalemia, hypocalcemia	Calcium channel blocker overdose (causing hypotension and bradydysrhythmias), hydrofluoric acid
Diphenhydramine	Allergic reactions	Extrapyramidal reactions from neuroleptics or antiemetics
Glucagon	Hypoglycemia (only for patients with normal liver function)	Beta-adrenergic antagonists, calcium channel blocker overdoses (larger doses of glucagon required)
Oxygen	CPR, chest pain, CHF	Carbon monoxide, cyanide, hydrogen sulfide poisoning
Sodium bicarbonate	Metabolic acidosis	(1) Cyanide, methanol, ethylene glycol (reversal of metabolic acidosis) (2) Salicylates, chlorpropamide, phenobarbital, methanol, chlorphenoxy herbicides (enhanced elimination) (3) Cyclic antidepressants, quinine, carbamazepine, type IA and IC antidysrhythmics, cocaine, some phenothiazines (reversal of type IA ECG effects)

[a]Use of medications outside of protocols may not be permissible in some areas, even with on-line medical control.

[b]Table does not include medications such as naloxone primarily intended to be used as antidotes or $D_{50}W$ and thiamine used as standard parts of (altered level of consciousness) overdose management.

[c]Usually together with hypertonic dextrose and oxygen to avoid masking hypoglycemia, hypoxia, etc.

[d]No longer recommended for routine use in cardiac arrests. (Emergency Cardiac Care Committee and Subcommittees, American Heart Association: Guidelines for cardiopulmonary resuscitation and emergency cardiac care. JAMA 1992;268:2171–2302.)

What Is the Role of Antidotal Therapy in Prehospital Care and Which Specific Antidotes Should AEMTs and Paramedics Carry?

The list of available antidotes is quite extensive when compared to a list of the medications a paramedic generally carries in the drug box and/or vehicle (see Tables 102–1 and 3–1). Several considerations must be addressed before making an antidote available for use in the prehospital setting: (1) the vast majority of poisonings and overdoses require care directed by clinical presentation as opposed to care for a known or presumed drug or toxin (Chaps. 3 and 30); (2) there are space limitations in the prehospital setting, restricting the total number of medications and the amount of equipment that can be carried; (3) antidotes that are rarely used may have to be restocked, often at considerable cost, to comply with manufacturer's expiration dates, even though the potency may not deteriorate for years afterwards (eg, the cyanide antidote kit); (4) medications that must be refrigerated or prepared (mixed) for each shift are impractical; (5) antidotes used inappropriately may be extremely toxic or lethal to a patient (eg, the cyanide antidote kit). Some prehospital care systems address this last issue by providing only nontoxic or relatively nontoxic antidotes, or the nontoxic *component(s)* of multistep antidotes such as only the sodium thiosulfate from the cyanide antidote kit.

Few organized attempts to study the use of antidotes in the prehospital setting have been conducted to date and virtually all of the studies that have been published are retrospective analyses.[2–4,8,12] One such study investigating the safety of the prehospital use of 0.4–0.8 mg of naloxone in 813 patients found it to be a safe component of paramedic treatment protocols for patients with an acute loss of consciousness.[12] However, another retrospective study of the empiric use of naloxone by paramedics in 730 patients with acute alterations in mental status found that selective administration based on the presence of pinpoint pupils, bradypnea, or circumstantial evidence of drug use identified "narcotized" patients with a sensitivity of 92% and a specificity of 76%. The authors concluded that implementing a screening strategy for naloxone use based on these historical and physical findings could reduce naloxone administration by 75% while achieving cost-savings, faster prehospital care, and less iatrogenic effects of naloxone.[3] Interestingly, these same authors reviewed 340 records retrospectively in an attempt to identify a subset of prehospital patients at risk for *hypoglycemia* by utilizing the clinical findings of tachycardia, diaphoresis, and a history of diabetes. In stark contrast to the results of their naloxone study, they found that only 76% of hypoglycemic patients were identified and with a specificity of only 54%. Thus, the prehospital use of hypertonic dextrose could only be reduced by 46% while at the same time withholding it from 25% of hypoglycemic patients. The authors concluded that selective use of $D_{50}W$ for AMS would be feasible only with concomitant field use of a rapid, accurate test of serum glucose.[4]

Uncommon or unusual poisonings present additional problems in the use of antidotes in the prehospital setting. One way of dealing with uncommon poisonings is to have protocols, treatments, and antidotes readily available for use after an identified index case or cases indicate the possibility of a large number of exposures. Examples of such poisonings include CO and cyanide exposures and lethal drugs or combinations that may affect a particular population, such as sudden widespread availability of fentanyl, unexpectedly potent opioids, or opioid substitutes and combinations.

Finally, AEMTs and paramedics should be mindful that almost all prehospital care protocols are sign- or symptom-driven; few, if any, ambulances routinely carry all available specific antidotes to treat all potential poisonings. Moreover, even when an antidote (such as glucagon) is available because the medication is also used in other ALS protocols, its dosage as an antidote may differ (see Table 102–1).[5–7] For these reasons, rather than applying a series of protocols over a prolonged period of time to treat a variety of *signs and symptoms,* AEMTs and paramedics should initiate early telemetry contact with a base station physician, and a rational decision should be made regarding any further treatment or immediate transport of the patient to a facility where a specific antidote is available.

What Is the Optimal Position for Transporting a Poisoned or Overdosed Patient?

In one attempt to identify the optimal transport position for a poisoned or overdosed patient, volunteers were given 80 mg/kg of acetaminophen to simulate an overdose, and five different (stationery) body positions commonly used in prehospital and emergency department settings were examined over a 2-hour period.[10] Although the difference did not reach statistical significance, initial drug absorption was lowest in the left lateral decubitus position, a position that also offers advantages in preventing aspiration, enhancing oropharyngeal drainage, and maximizing patient observation in an ambulance.[10]

What Is the Role of the AEMT or Paramedic in Transferring a Poisoned or Overdosed Patient for Definitive Care?

Certain poisonings and overdoses require specific treatments not available at a community hospital or not available soon enough to help a particular patient (Table 102–2). Emergency physicians must sometimes weigh the benefits and risks of transferring ill, poisoned, or overdosed patients to tertiary care centers. In general, a patient presenting with a toxicologic emergency should be moved to another facility only if the primary hospital does not have the necessary therapy and if there is no acceptable alternative treatment available.

Hyperbaric Oxygen for Carbon Monoxide Poisoning

Criteria for determining which patients may benefit from hyperbaric oxygen treatment (HBO) are discussed in detail in Chapter 96. A carbon monoxide (CO) poisoning

TABLE 102–2. PATIENTS WITH POISONING OR OVERDOSE WHO MAY REQUIRE TRANSFER TO SPECIAL TREATMENT CENTERS

Poisoning/Overdose	Type of Care
Carbon monoxide (high levels and /or serious clinical sequelae)	Hyperbaric oxygen
Snake or spider venom	Antivenin treatment
Lithium, salicylates, theophylline, methanol, or ethylene glycol	Hemodialysis and/or hemoperfusion
Acetaminophen (with significant hepatic damage)	Hepatic transplantation
Myocardial depressants (massive amounts that cannot be metabolized or dialyzed or otherwise treated; eg, lidocaine, calcium channel blockers)	Cardiopulmonary bypass
Infants with serious poisonings or drug overdoses from a variety of sources	Neonatal intensive care unit

victim should be provided with 100% oxygen while being transported to a hyperbaric chamber; assisted ventilation should be provided to any patient who is not breathing spontaneously. A physician or paramedic able to administer advanced cardiac life support should accompany the patient. Attention to the patient's ongoing cardiorespiratory needs is critical.

The safety of transferring CO-poisoned patients for HBO was addressed in a 10-year retrospective study of 297 consecutive CO-poisoned patients requiring HBO.[8] The authors concluded that CO-induced cardiac or respiratory arrests, myocardial infarctions, and worsening mental status are not likely to occur during transport to the hyperbaric chamber if they did not occur prior to the decision to perform HBO and, therefore, transfer need not be deferred for fear of these occurrences. However, dysrhythmias, hypotension, seizures, agitation, and emesis as well as repeat cardiac arrests and near arrests can occur and therefore complete preparedness for cardiac resuscitation, airway control, and volume expansion during transport was recommended.[8]

Transfer principles for referral to a hyperbaric treatment center are outlined in Table 102–3.

Hemoperfusion and/or Hemodialysis

Transferring a patient to a facility capable of hemodialysis or hemoperfusion is most commonly required for poisoning with methanol or ethylene glycol and serious overdoses of lithium, salicylates, and theophylline (see Chaps. 32, 39, 59, 64). All initial treatment should be instituted prior to, and continued during interhospital transport. Patients sick enough to require hemodialysis or hemoperfusion should ideally be transported in an advanced life-support ambulance and with an accompanying physician.

Antivenin Treatment Centers for Envenomations

Because envenomations are relatively rare and may be extremely serious or lethal, victims may require transportation to a specialty center for treatment. Table 102–4 outlines the New York City Snake Bite Protocol, which includes a section on patient transport.

TABLE 102–3. SUGGESTED PROTOCOL FOR TRANSFERRING A PATIENT TO HYPERBARIC TREATMENT

A physician at the sending facility must perform a basic physical examination and laboratory assessment including:
- History (past medical history, medications, complaints)
- COHb/arterial blood gas analysis (in carbon monoxide cases)
- Chest radiograph
- Electrocardiogram
- Blood tests—chemistry profile, toxicology tests (if applicable)
- Pregnancy test (for women of childbearing age)
- Neurologic examination (including mental status exam)
- Formal ENT examination for smoke inhalation, noting any indicators of respiratory involvement, including stridor, hoarseness, carbonaceous sputum, and singed nasal hairs

Any patient requiring transfer for hyperbaric treatment is best considered unstable; therefore, the sending institution should consider the need for physician accompaniment when indicated.

TABLE 102–4. SNAKEBITE PROTOCOL FOR NEW YORK CITY

Identification of snake

Record verbal description of snake, time of bite, description of wound(s), and signs and symptoms of envenomation.

If snake is identified as poisonous or symptoms warrant it, proceed with first-aid measures and transportation.

If snake is identified as nonpoisonous, treat as any other animal bite (tetanus prophylaxis, infection precautions, etc).

First-aid measures for poisonous snakebite to be instituted by EMS or other trained medical personnel

DO NOT EMPLOY TOURNIQUET, CUT AND SUCTION, OR CRYOTHERAPY.

If snake has been identified as an elapid (cobra, mamba, coral snake, sea snake, kreit, tiger snake, taipan), apply an Ace bandage on the affected extremity, encompassing the wound(s) and extending up the entire extremity.

Do not apply an Ace bandage if the snake has been identified as a crotalid (rattlesnake, copperhead, cottonmouth, fer-de-lance, puff adder, Gaboon viper).

Splint the affected extremity to decrease mobility in all bites.

Begin a large-bore IV in an unaffected extremity and start an infusion of 0.9% sodium chloride or lactated Ringer's solution.

Transport immediately.

EMS or 911

Ambulance unit should have a trained paramedic, capable of intubation and CPR if necessary, when transferring a patient from another hospital.

Helicopter transport is available through EMS (or 911) if deemed necessary.

Receiving hospital ED must be informed of estimated time of arrival and method of transportation.

Are There Any Legal Constraints on Transferring Poisoned or Overdosed Patients?

Incorrect interpretation of the United States Federal EMTALA and COBRA legislation[9] adopted and implemented to prevent inappropriate transfers of indigent patients (patient dumping) may hinder or prevent transporting a patient who, though medically "unstable," may nevertheless require specialized treatment or facilities. Nothing in the legislation precludes such a transfer, provided that: (1) the treatment is considered necessary, that is, the benefits of the transfer outweigh the risks; (2) the sending and receiving institutions are in agreement regarding the necessity of the transfer and the medical care being provided to accomplish it; (3) the transfer is effected in accordance with accepted medical practice; and (4) the transfer is not for economic reasons.

As with any patient transfer between institutions, care must be taken to ensure that prior to transport the patient has been medically stabilized as much as possible within the time constraints dictated by the nature of the exposure. With respect to the level of care during transport, a physician accompanying a patient would be ideal, but in most situations properly trained and qualified paramedics and a vehicle equipped to provide advanced life support may be acceptable, especially if the alternative (ie, not transporting the patient) would probably result in morbidity or mortality.

Summary

The use of $D_{50}W$, thiamine, naloxone, oxygen, activated charcoal, possibly syrup of ipecac or orogastric lavage, and benzodiazepines, as well as many other therapeutic modalities discussed elsewhere in this text, are also applicable to prehospital management. There are, however, certain unique considerations that are extremely important to keep in mind in the prehospital setting:

- Initial management should consider and eliminate any possible risk to rescue personnel at the scene.
- Without compromising patient care, paramedics and EMTs should try to note and collect evidence at the scene that may be essential in establishing a definitive diagnosis.
- Specific antidotes must be used appropriately; conversely the lack of availability of other antidotes (antivenin) or treatment (HBO) at particular hospitals must be considered in making decisions regarding the best time to initiate transport or rapid evacuation to a specialized treatment facility.
- Appropriate use of paramedics or AEMTs and well-equipped vehicles will facilitate safe transport of poisoned or overdosed patients to specialty or tertiary care centers.

Pitfalls to Avoid in Providing Prehospital Care to Victims of Poisonings or Overdoses

- Not recognizing or acting on index cases to prevent further exposures or deaths.
- Relying on sign- or symptom-driven standing protocols to treat a patient for a prolonged period of time or using standard advanced-life-support dosages of medications when only a larger dose of medication or a specific antidote, not available at the scene, will save the patient.

References

1. Berumen U Jr: Dog Poisons Man. JAMA 1983;249:353. Letter.
2. Crockett R, Krishel SJ, Manoguerra A, et al: Prehospital use of activated charcoal: A pilot study. J Emerg Med 1996;14: 335–338.
3. Hoffman JR, Schriger DL, Luo JS: The empiric use of naloxone in patients with an altered mental status: A reappraisal. Ann Emerg Med 1991;20:246–252.
4. Hoffman JR, Schriger DL, Votey SR, Luo JS: The empiric use of hypertonic dextrose in patients with altered mental status: A reappraisal. Ann Emerg Med 1992;21:20–24.
5. Nelson L: What to do when drug poisoning causes hypotension. J Crit Illness 1996;11:88–92.
6. Nelson L, Hoffman RS: Effective strategies for drug induced bradycardia and heart block. J Crit Illness 1994;9: 916–930.
7. Nelson L, Hoffman RS: What to do when drug poisoning causes tachycardia. J Crit Illness 1994;9:831–842.
8. Sloan EP, Murphy DG, Hart R, et al: Complications and protocol considerations in carbon monoxide-poisoned patients who require hyperbaric oxygen therapy: Report from a ten-year experience. Ann Emerg Med 1989;18:629–634.
9. United States Public Law 99-272. Section 9121 and 42 USC 1395 DD: cc (a) 1 (1).
10. Vance MV, Selden BS, Clark RF: Optimal patient position for transport and initial management of toxic ingestions. Ann Emerg Med 1992;21:243–245.
11. Wolsey BA, McKinney PE: Does transportation by ambulance decrease time to gastrointestinal decontamination after overdose? Acad Emerg Med 1997;4:456. Abstract.
12. Yealy DM, Paris PM, Kaplan RM, et al: The safety of prehospital naloxone administration by paramedics. Ann Emerg Med 1990;19:902–905.

CHAPTER 103

Use of the Intensive Care Unit

Mark A. Kirk

Over the past few decades, the intensive care unit (ICU) has dramatically improved survival from many serious conditions. This is the direct result of the ability to continuously monitor physiologic parameters, pay meticulous attention to supportive care, and use modern medical technology and treatment. Most critically ill poisoned patients have acutely reversible conditions that will clearly benefit from intensive care intervention.[84]

Many diseases managed in the ICU have a well-recognized clinical course with predictable complications. More than almost any other disease managed in the ICU, uncertainties typify toxicologic emergencies. A patient's history is often unreliable with regard to the kind of toxin ingested, time of ingestion, and amount ingested. The poison may have unknown or unpredictable toxic effects. The therapies, antidotes, and complications of acute poisoning may be unfamiliar to the ICU staff. These uncertainties challenge health care providers and influence decisions about admitting patients to the ICU.

Often a patient may be admitted to the ICU, not for intervention, but for observation and monitoring.[107] Of the 9.4 million reported poison exposures from 1991 to 1995, only 5% had toxic effects serious enough to be admitted to the hospital.[55–59,72] In addition, only 10–30% of those hospitalized required specific treatments or antidotes other than GI decontamination.[57,72,107] Many physicians elect to observe poisoned patients in an ICU in anticipation of possible delayed, unrecognized life-threatening toxicity. The ICU provides necessary monitoring and individual nursing care that can help in the early recognition of developing toxicity. Intensive care units allow health care providers the best opportunity to minimize morbidity and decrease mortality. However, the ICU is a major source of expensive health care that has contributed significantly to the escalation of health care costs.

It is hoped that ICU admission guidelines presented in this chapter will encourage effective use of ICU resources without compromising patient care. Effective guidelines must consider a toxin's unique characteristics, the hospital's capabilities, and all realistic alternatives for managing and observing poisoned patients without compromising care. Current medical literature allows us to develop only very general guidelines. Future clinical studies addressing the use of health care resources for the poisoned patient will allow refinement of these guidelines.

Criteria for ICU Admission

Are There Reliable Criteria to Help Select Poisoned Patients Who Require ICU Admission?

Overcrowded ICUs and escalating health care costs have been incentives to develop severity of illness models that predict the benefits of ICU care. The Acute Physiology and Chronic Health Evaluation (APACHE II), the Mortality Probability Model (MPM II), and the Simplified Acute Physiology Score (SAPS) are widely studied and generally accepted severity-of-illness models.[99] They score certain physiologic parameters and other factors in order to estimate risks and predict outcomes.[46] These models are most effective for stratifying risks in clinical research trials and comparing quality of care among ICUs. They have been applied to subgroups of patients and individual patients to determine prognosis and deter excessive use of ICU resources.

Clinical studies to validate such scoring systems have evaluated patients with a variety of medical and surgical conditions. No study has exclusively investigated patients with overdoses or even included large numbers of overdose patients.[107] Such scoring systems may be less useful for the poisoned patient because parameters that ordinarily predict clinical outcome, such as coma following cardiac arrest, are not reliable in the poisoned patient.[26,81] Severe poisoning may clinically mimic brain death.[5,78,103,106] As an example, a barbiturate overdose may result in a Glasgow Coma Scale of 3 and an isoelectric EEG. However, complete neurologic recovery may occur with only supportive care. In addition, many toxicologic emergencies occur in young patients, who are free of underlying chronic diseases. This increases the likelihood of surviving significant insults such as prolonged hypotension or hypoxia. Despite negative predictors of outcome, aggressive resuscitation efforts may be justified for the subgroup of patients who are poisoned. Specifically, prolonged cardiac resucitation should be provided for the victim of a cardiac arrest resulting from cyclic antidepressant overdoses or severe hypothermia.[74,91]

Few studies have evaluated the use of the ICU for poisoned patients.[11,26,41,43,50,95] Prospective studies have focused on mortality rates, use of resources, or types of toxins ingested whereas others have focused on a single toxin.[41,44] Most of these studies are retrospective and have relatively small study populations.[11,26,43,50,95]

A set of criteria to determine whether initial clinical assessment could identify those poisoned patients at risk of developing serious toxicity, thus needing ICU admission, was established.[11] The specific toxin ingested was not considered in defining risks. Criteria defining high-risk patients were: need for intubation; unresponsiveness to verbal stimuli; seizures; PCO_2 > 45 mm Hg; systolic blood pressure < 80 mm Hg; QRS duration ≥ 0.12 msec; or any cardiac rhythm except normal sinus, sinus tachycardia, or sinus bradycardia. Patients were classified as low-risk when none of the above criteria was present in the emergency department (ED). Retrospectively, 209 cases were analyzed using the above parameters. The most commonly ingested drugs in both the high- and low-risk groups were alcohol, cyclic antidepressants, benzodiazepines, barbiturates, phenothiazines, opioids, and aspirin. None of the 151 patients considered low-risk developed complications or required ICU interventions after admission. Of the 58 patients deemed high-risk, 35 required ICU interventions such as intubation, treatment of dysrhythmias, treatment of seizures, intravenous vasopressors, or hemodialysis/hemoperfusion. Seven patients developed high-risk complications, such as need for intubation, hypotension, and seizures after admission, but all had other high-risk criteria in the ED. The authors concluded that the clinical course of poisoned patients can be predicted during the initial 2–3 hours of observation, although toxins with delayed or prolonged toxic effects, such as sustained-release products, lithium, and oral hypoglycemic agents, were not prominent in their study population.

In their study population, 70% of the low-risk patients were admitted to the ICU for observation. Since none of these patients developed complications or required ICU intervention, the authors postulate that using these criteria would have eliminated 50% of the ICU days without compromising care.

The limitations of this study are its retrospective design, relatively small study population, and limited variety of toxin exposures. However, it does suggest that with some clinical judgment, many poisoned patients will not require ICU admission.

Ideally, clinical indicators for ICU care should be established for each toxin. Criteria cannot be generalized because of the unique clinical course of some toxins. Until more specific predictors of outcome are developed for individual toxins, nothing will be more useful than experience and good clinical judgment in predicting who may benefit from ICU admission. At present, withholding ICU care from poisoned patients based solely on a nonspecific "score" will not result in significant cost savings in the ICU but may increase the risk of morbidity and mortality.[17,48,99]

End-organ Toxicity as Basis for ICU Admission

It seems reasonable that a patient's signs and symptoms can be used to decide the need for ICU admission. Indications for ICU admission based on pathophysiologic criteria is logical. The presence of certain signs or symptoms requires ICU observation or intervention, whatever the toxic exposure. This approach is most consistent with the philosophy of "treating the patient and not the poison," and may prove most helpful for patients with polydrug ingestions.

Central nervous system (CNS) manifestations are common to many poisonings. Toxin-induced acute delirium or coma often require ICU admission, because these findings will not resolve quickly. Any comatose patient without an identifiable cause requires continued investigation in the ICU. Toxin-induced status epilepticus is best managed in the ICU.

A patient with any signs of respiratory compromise necessitates ICU admission. Toxins can harm any portion of the respiratory system from the upper airway to the alveoli. Toxins may act by several different mechanisms to produce respiratory compromise. For example, organophosphate poisoning produces respiratory compromise by CNS depression, respiratory muscle weakness, and copious pulmonary secretions. In addition, evidence of impaired oxygen-carrying capacity or tissue hypoxia requires ICU admission. Poisoning by hydrogen sulfide, cyanide, carbon monoxide, or methemoglobin inducers will impair oxygen utilization or oxygen-carrying capacity, producing tissue hypoxia.

Any evidence of cardiac toxicity, such as conduction disturbances (QRS prolongation and at times a QT segment prolongation), bradydysrhythmias, tachydysrhythmias, or hypotension requires that the patient be admitted to the ICU. Toxin-induced chest pain can be due to myocardial ischemia from exposure to toxins such as cocaine or carbon monoxide. Patients with toxin-induced chest pain should be treated with the same sense of urgency and caution as those suspected of having a myocardial infarction from any other etiology. Persistent, toxin-induced hypertension, especially with associated headache or chest pain, also requires ICU intervention.

Gastrointestinal symptoms, particularly vomiting and diarrhea, are an early manifestation of poisoning by many toxins. When symptoms are severe and persistent, significant fluid and electrolyte losses can occur. For example, a patient with a serious iron ingestion can have a GI mucosal injury, leading to vomiting, diarrhea, profound volume loss, and significant hypotension. Hepatotoxicity from poisoning or overdose usually occurs days after toxin exposure. If hepatotoxicity is evident at admission (especially with hepatic encephalopathy), ICU management is suggested.

Renal toxicity may be a direct toxic effect or a complication of other toxic manifestations, such as hypotension or rhabdomyolysis. Severe toxin-induced metabolic acidosis needs ICU intervention. Metabolic acidosis is an important clue to the presence of toxins such as ethylene glycol, methanol, and salicylates. Investigation into the cause of an unexplained acidosis should be pursued in the ICU. Persistent or refractory hypoglycemia, resulting from an oral hypoglycemic, insulin overdose, or other toxins, needs ICU admission. In addition, severe toxin-induced alterations in temperature regulation or electrolyte disturbances merit close monitoring and intervention in the ICU.

Chemical burns of the skin have complications similar to those of thermal burns. The injured dermis may be unable to prevent significant fluid losses, regulate core body temperature, and prevent infection. Besides these complications, systemic toxic effects may occur through dermal absorption. As little as 2.5% body surface area exposure to concentrated hydrofluoric acid has resulted in systemic hypocalcemia and death.[98]

End-organ toxicity is the most important reason to admit poisoned patients to the ICU. However, restricting ICU admission to those with only end-organ toxicity is inadequate. Minimally symptomatic or asymptomatic patients may require ICU admission because other factors must be considered.

What Additional Information Should Influence ICU Admission of the Poisoned Patient?

In addition to end-organ toxicity, the toxin, its treatment, and specific patient characteristics should influence ICU admission decisions.

Toxin Characteristics as Basis for ICU Admission (Table 103–1). Unique absorption, distribution, metabolism, or elimination characteristics of toxins may alter the time of onset of symptoms, duration of effects, and risk of complications. Some toxins have proven their ability to cause harm or death to humans. Well-described, expected toxic effects assist in early recognition of poisoning. For other toxins, the consequences after human exposure are not yet reported. Both the known and unknown about a toxin will assist with ICU admission decisions.

ICU admission is always warranted for patients with expected serious toxic effects from an ingested poison. This is especially true for those toxins known to be deadly, such as salicylates, cyclic antidepressants, cocaine, cyanide, and calcium channel blockers. For example, patients with salicylate poisoning who develop respiratory distress or significant metabolic derangements require close attention and aggressive treatment only available in the ICU. Strong consideration should also be given to ICU admission when signs and symptoms suggest a progression of toxicity.

Indicators of toxicity should be identified for individual toxins so that high-risk patients are closely monitored and aggressively treated. Cyclic antidepressants were studied in great detail to determine indicators of toxicity and safe disposition.[3,14,15,27,44,70,76,101] Research efforts have focused on identifying those patients at risk for serious cyclic antidepressant toxicity because cyclic antidepressants are one of the most common and lethal overdoses reported. They account for 25% of drug overdoses admitted to adult ICUs, yet there are many unnecessary admissions for trivial overdoses.[21,57] Studies concerning cyclic antidepressant overdoses suggest that patients may be safely discharged if they remain asymptomatic for a 6-hour observation period after presentation.[3,15,32,44,75,101] Studies report that prolonged QRS duration on a 12-lead ECG is predictive of serious complications such as seizures and dysrhythmias.[6,70,104] Any patient manifesting persistent tachycardia, ECG abnor-

TABLE 103–1. CRITERIA FOR ICU ADMISSION BASED ON TOXIN CHARACTERISTICS

Signs of end-organ toxicity

Selected toxins and their well-known serious toxic effects

Cardiac drugs (digitalis, beta-adrenergic antagonists, calcium channel blockers, antidysrhythmics): dysrhythmias or hypotension
Cocaine: persistent dysrhythmias, hypertension, myocardial ischemia, status epilepticus, focal neurologic deficits, hyperthermia, severe agitation
Cyclic antidepressants: QRS duration $\geq$ 0.10 sec, hypotension, lethargy, and seizures
Salicylates: altered mentation, metabolic acidosis, pulmonary edema
Theophylline: persistent GI symptoms, cardiovascular toxicity, seizures
Rattlesnake envenomation: GI symptoms, hypotension, coagulopathy

Examples of toxins characterized by prolonged absorption

Slows GI motility
Anticholinergics

Enteric-coated preparations
Salicylates

Sustained-release preparations
Theophylline
Lithium
Beta-adrenergic antagonists
Calcium channel blockers

Examples of toxins with delayed onset of toxicity

Cocaine and heroin body stuffers/body packers
Colchicine
Coral snake envenomation
Digoxin
Ergotamines
Inhalation of chlorine, phosgene, arsine, nitrogen dioxide, and sulfur dioxide gases
Lomotil (diphenoxylate and atropine)
Monoamine oxidase inhibitors
Sulfonylureas/insulin overdose
Paraquat

Toxins with unknown (uncertain) effects[a]

New products with limited toxicity information
Toxins with no human exposure data

[a]When the toxin has uncertain effects, and the patient is asymptomatic, observation may be warranted.

malities (including QRS ≥ 0.10 sec), hypotension, anticholinergic signs, or neurologic symptoms needs ICU monitoring.[15,32]

Poisoning is a dynamic disorder. The initial examination may show only mild signs of toxicity, but the patient may progress to more severe toxicity. Some toxins may have a delayed onset or an unpredictable course. An asymptomatic patient may be a "time bomb" with the potential to deteriorate rapidly. Failure to appreciate the potential for serious, delayed toxic effects could be a major pitfall in managing poisoned patients.

Certain toxins prolong GI absorption, delaying onset of toxicity. Opioids and the anticholinergic effects of drugs, such as cyclic antidepressants and antihistamines, will delay gastric emptying and prolong drug absorption.[14] In children, Lomotil (atropine and diphenoxylate) can produce delayed and prolonged coma from slowed GI motility.[64] Salicylates produce pylorospasm that delays gastric emptying.[8] Iron, theophylline, verapamil, meprobamate, and salicylates may form gastric bezoars, producing prolonged GI absorption.[4,51,73,86,94]

The type of preparation of some drugs may alter absorption and delay onset of symptoms. Sustained-release preparations enhance patient compliance by increasing dosing intervals; in overdose, enteric coatings may delay absorption and in turn delay the onset of toxicity.[22,67] One patient with an overdose of a sustained-release theophylline preparation did not attain a peak level until 26 hours after ingestion.[83] There are reports of overdoses of enteric-coated aspirin reaching peak levels at 24–36 hours after ingestion.[8,105] Cardiac dysrhythmias developed as late as 16 hours following ingestion of sustained-release verapamil in two cases.[92] Common sustained-release preparations of toxicologic importance include theophylline, phenylpropanolamine, potassium, calcium channel blockers, beta-adrenergic antagonists, and lithium.[67] Serial levels of readily measurable drugs are necessary to verify peaks and ensure that levels are decreasing. However, some do not have readily obtainable serum levels that can be monitored. In such cases, admission and observation are required. Smuggling (body packing) or hiding (body stuffing) contraband drugs in the GI tract has resulted in delayed onset of serious toxicity from ruptured bags.[65,82]

Clinical effects may be delayed when toxicity depends on alteration of enzyme functions, cellular reproduction, or metabolic function. Toxicity of monoamine oxidase inhibitors (MAOI) may not appear for more than 12 hours after an overdose but then may progress rapidly to cardiovascular collapse.[54] Because of the delay in onset of severe toxicity, even if the patient is asymptomatic, a history of MAOI ingestion mandates ICU monitoring for 24 hours. The GI toxicity of colchicine may resolve within hours of ingestion with apparent recovery, only to have multisystem organ failure occur 24–72 hours later.[7] When there is potential for serious delayed toxicity, the patient may need prolonged close monitoring.

The natural history of some toxins is unknown. New pharmaceutical and industrial products are introduced each year with little or no available data on toxic amounts and human health effects. Sometimes, animal studies provide the only known toxicologic data, or preclinical trials for new drugs may have excluded the populations at risk, such as infants, children, or the elderly. In these cases, the clinician must often make therapeutic decisions and anticipate potential toxicity with little or no reliable data. Since early recognition of serious toxicity could prevent an adverse outcome, expectant observation may be the only rational approach. For example, multiple suicidal and unintentional ingestions occurred following the introduction of fluoxetine (Prozac). Clinicians lacked experience treating overdoses of this drug and had no data regarding the natural course and toxic dose. Many appropriately admitted fluoxetine overdosed patients to the ICU to observe for toxic effects. However, now that clinicians have experience with this drug and studies are available demonstrating few severe manifestations, ICU resources are seldom needed to treat such patients.[9,16,93]

Diagnostic tests such as routine laboratory analysis, electrocardiography, and radiography should also be used as indicators of the potential for serious toxicity (see Table 103–2). These diagnostic tests may suggest the

TABLE 103–2. CRITERIA FOR ICU ADMISSION BASED ON DIAGNOSTIC TESTS[a]

Specialized tests

Significantly elevated serum drug concentrations:
- Iron, digitalis, lithium, salicylates, theophylline, ethylene glycol/methanol, isopropanol, anticonvulsants (carbamazapine, phenobarbital, valproic acid)

Serial measurements demonstrating rising serum drug concentrations:
- Lithium, salicylates, theophylline

Depressed cholinesterase activity in the presence of cholinergic symptoms

Metabolic studies

Significant electrolyte abnormalities
Hypoglycemia (persistent, refractory, or unexplained)
Significant metabolic acidosis
Hypocalcemia from hydrofluoric acid exposure

Arterial blood gas/co-oximetry

Hypoxia, hypercarbia, acidosis
Elevated methemoglobin levels refractory to methylene blue treatment
Elevated carboxyhemoglobin levels with persistent cardiovascular or CNS symptoms

Radiography

Chest radiography
- Pulmonary aspiration in patients with altered mental status, hydrocarbon ingestion
- Acute lung injury: Noncardiogenic pulmonary edema
- Cardiomegaly/volume overload/congestive heart failure
- Mediastinal widening (aortic dissection)
- Pneumothorax

Abdominal radiography
- Evidence of body packing or body stuffing
- Large amount of radiopaque pills or liquids

Electrocardiogram

AV conduction abnormalities
QRS prolongation
QT prolongation (certain circumstances)
Dysrhythmias

[a]Most often, decisions are made based on the patient's clinical status and not on a single test result. These examples involve patients at high risk of developing toxicity.

TABLE 103–3. CRITERIA FOR ICU ADMISSION BASED ON NEED FOR INVASIVE MONITORING OR INTERVENTIONS

Patients requiring intervention to maintain normal physiology
Intubation
Mechanical ventilation
Fluid resuscitation
Vasopressors
Antidysrhythmics
Hypo-/hyperthermia control
Patients needing invasive procedures or invasive monitoring
Arterial blood pressure monitoring
Arterial infusion of calcium for hydrofluoric acid burns
Cardiac pacemaker
Cardiopulmonary bypass
Continuous arteriovenous hemofiltration/continuous venovenous hemofiltration
Extracorporeal membrane oxygenation
Hemodynamic monitoring: central venous pressure, pulmonary artery catheter
Hemoperfusion/hemodialysis
Intraaortic balloon pump assistance

need for more aggressive management or careful monitoring. Elevated serum levels of some drugs indicate an increased likelihood of serious toxicity. Serial serum levels show the benefits of GI decontamination and warn of increasing potential for serious toxic effects. Relatively few patients should be admitted to the ICU based on the results of a single diagnostic test.

Treatment and Invasive Monitoring as Requirements for ICU Admission (Table 103–3). The ICU setting typically offers the most highly skilled staff and modern technology available to manage many complex medical problems. Also, it provides a ratio of nursing personnel to patients that allows for frequent or continuous monitoring of basic physiologic parameters, enabling early detection of toxicity and prevention of complications. Both invasive and noninvasive measurements of vital signs, neurologic status, and intake/output measurements, along with continuous cardiac monitoring, provide important clues to the early development of serious toxicity or complications and the need for active intervention to prevent or treat complications.

Most critically ill, poisoned patients have acute reversible conditions requiring supportive care measures (ie, ventilator support, vasopressor support, and close monitoring) that ICUs are most skilled in providing. In the 1930s, patients with barbiturate overdoses were common and mortality was greater than 20%. Treatment consisted of gastric lavage and administration of "central analeptics." In the 1950s, mortality from barbiturate overdoses decreased to less than 2%.[18] This significant decrease in mortality was attributed to therapy that focused on supportive care measures such as maintaining a patent airway, preventing hypoxia with the administration of oxygen, and treatment of shock. A study published in 1987 reported a good outcome in most of 103 critically ill overdosed patients treated with only mechanical ventilation, vasopressor support, and careful monitoring.[26] In a pediatric study, only 19 of 105 patients admitted to the ICU required specialized treatment beyond mechanical ventilation and careful monitoring.[50] Most often, supportive care measures, such as airway protection, ventilator support, vasopressor support, and close monitoring, improve the outcome of critically ill poisoned patients rather than antidotes and specialized treatments.

Invasive monitoring is routinely used in the ICU and is beneficial to some poisoned patients. Hemodynamic parameters are valuable for the patient with hypotension, intravascular volume depletion, or noncardiogenic pulmonary edema (NCPE). Intraarterial monitoring provides a more accurate and continuous record of actual blood pressure in a patient with cardiovascular compromise.[19] A pulmonary artery catheter assists fluid and inotropic therapy for patients with NCPE and toxin-induced cardiogenic pulmonary edema.

Extracorporeal methods of eliminating toxins, such as hemodialysis or hemoperfusion, are best performed in the ICU for a critically ill patient. Extracorporeal membrane oxygenation, cardiopulmonary bypass, and intraaortic balloon pump–assisted perfusion have been used successfully in resuscitating critically ill poisoned patients and are currently being evaluated on a larger scale in animal studies.[28,39,42,61,71,89]

Antidotes and specific treatments, while possibly lifesaving, are not without inherent risks. Table 103–4

TABLE 103–4. CRITERIA FOR ICU ADMISSION BASED ON USE OF ANTIDOTES AND SPECIFIC TREATMENTS

Antidotes with potential serious adverse effects
Crotalid, elapidae, or black widow spider antivenin
Deferoxamine for iron poisoning
Ethanol for methanol and ethylene glycol poisoning
Sodium nitrite for cyanide poisoning
Antidotes with a shorter duration of action than the toxin
Atropine for organophosphates
Dextrose for oral hypoglycemic agents
Flumazenil for benzodiazepines
Naloxone for opioids
Physostigmine for anticholinergics
Unconventional dosing of familiar medications
Atropine for organophosphates
Benzodiazepines for ethanol and sedative-hypnotic withdrawal
Unfamiliar medications or unusual indications for medications
Calcium for calcium channel blockers
Calcium for hydrofluoric acid burns (intra-arterial)
Digoxin-specific antibody fragments for digoxin
Glucagon for beta-adrenergic antagonists
Treatments that require time-consuming care, frequent assessment, or continuous monitoring
Aggressive GI decontamination: multiple-dose activated charcoal for theophylline poisoning, whole-bowel irrigation
Antidysrhythmics
Bronchodilators for toxic inhalant–induced bronchospasm: chlorine/chloramine gas, smoke inhalation
Frequent repetitive doses of benzodiazepines for agitation or withdrawal
Hemodialysis and hemoperfusion
Rapid warming or cooling of core body temperature
Urine alkalinization with hourly urine pH measurements
Vasopressors

outlines the rationale for administering antidotes and other specific treatments in an ICU. For example, antivenin administration for rattlesnake envenomations may cause anaphylaxis, and rapid intravenous infusion of deferoxamine for iron poisoning may cause hypotension. Because these treatments may be unfamiliar to staff and have their own inherent risks, the ICU is the most prudent environment to monitor such treatments.

In toxicologic emergencies, a familiar medication may be an antidotal therapy that requires doses that far exceed conventional regimens. High doses of atropine (hundreds of milligrams) may be necessary for the treatment of organophosphate poisoning.[24,36,52] Very high doses of epinephrine or isoproterenol may be necessary to overcome receptor antagonism from beta-adrenergic antagonists. Intravenous calcium, which is no longer a part of empiric advanced cardiac life support (ACLS) protocols, is used in reversing toxicity from calcium channel blockers,[79] and (by intra-arterial infusion) for hydrofluoric acid burns of the extremities.[102] Sodium bicarbonate as a bolus and infusion is the treatment of choice for cyclic antidepressant cardiac toxicity.[75,90] Direct vasopressors such as norepinephrine or phenylephrine may be more appropriate than the usual first-line vasopressor, dopamine, for some toxins. In addition to using drugs by unconventional methods, some familiar drugs are to be avoided in treating toxic emergencies. For example, type IA antidysrhythmics, such as procainamide and quinidine, must not be used in patients with overdoses of cardiac sodium channel antagonists, such as cyclic antidepressants, phenothiazines, and propoxyphene.

A false sense of security can result when an antidote reverses toxicity but has a shorter duration of effect than the toxin. An example is a patient, comatose from an opioid overdose, who responds to naloxone, awakens, and refuses further treatment. Toxicity may recur when naloxone's short duration of effect allows opioid toxicity to recur. These patients need for be closely observed for the possible need for readministration of the antidote.

Some treatment regimens may require inordinate amounts of nursing time that cannot realistically be provided by an ordinary hospital inpatient service, where each nurse is responsible for numerous patients. To ensure adequate monitoring and good patient care, those patients requiring extraordinary time commitments from the nursing staff should be admitted to the ICU.

Patient Factors as Criteria for ICU Admission

Patients with preexisting medical conditions may have an increased risk of developing toxicity. Many elderly patients have chronic medical problems and do not tolerate major physiologic alterations without significant compromise. For example, a patient with underlying cardiac disease may develop severe myocardial ischemia from a carbon monoxide exposure. An elderly patient with chronic salicylism is likely to have major respiratory and CNS complications.[2,100] Conditions that alter drug metabolism or elimination, such as renal or hepatic disease, may prolong toxicity or produce toxicity after lesser amounts are ingested.

Patients with physical dependency on ethanol, benzodiazepines, barbiturates, or opioids may show signs of withdrawal while hospitalized.[33] A period of abstinence during treatment for other toxicologic or psychosocial problems may result in an acute withdrawal syndrome. Often withdrawal may be the reason for admission to the hospital. Withdrawal from ethanol and sedative-hypnotics can have serious consequences and complications. Large doses of medications with respiratory depressant effects may be required to treat acute withdrawal. For all of these reasons, cases of severe withdrawal may require ICU management.

Of recognized suicide attempts, 80% are due to an overdose of medications.[69] Complications of poisoning make it difficult to assess the suicidal risks of such patients adequately. Patients have an increased rate of suicide following discharge from an ICU for drug overdose.[95] Until suicidal risks are adequately assessed, it must be assumed that the patient needs close observation. Monitoring policies for suicidal patients not on a psychiatric ward may differ among institutions. The ultimate goal of treatment for any suicidal patient is to provide a totally safe environment, which may include admitting all patients with suicidal risks to the ICU, physically or chemically restraining a ward patient, or providing a patient with one-to-one observation. In many hospitals, the ICU is the safest place, but also the most expensive place, to observe a patient with suicidal risks until it is medically safe to transfer the patient to the psychiatric service.

What Complications Prolong ICU Care of the Poisoned Patient?

Poisoning produces both anticipated and unanticipated complications that can prolong ICU care and decrease survival. Serious complications of poisoning include pulmonary compromise, rhabdomyolysis, compartment syndrome, and anoxic brain injury. Complications such as acute renal or fulminant hepatic failure may also prolong the ICU course.

Pulmonary compromise following toxic exposures may not be evident until several hours or days in the ICU. Pulmonary complications following a toxic exposure include aspiration pneumonitis, NCPE, and adult respiratory distress syndrome (ARDS). Aspiration of gastric contents is a common complication following poisoning, especially when a patient's mental status is altered and protective airway reflexes are lost.[1,37,45,88] The incidence of pulmonary aspiration in a series of 185 barbiturate overdoses increased with the increase in depth of coma.[37] Poisoned patients may aspirate spontaneously while lying unresponsive prior to being discovered, or from stomach dilation due to bag-valve-mask ventilation, or from GI decontamination procedures such as syrup of ipecac–induced emesis and orogastric lavage, or during insertion of endotracheal or nasogastric tubes.[49,66,77] Loss of airway protective reflexes allows liquid gastric contents to cause a parenchymal inflammatory reaction and ventilation–perfusion mismatch.[13] Pulmonary aspiration results in an increased risk of secondary bacterial invasion of the lungs, prolonged hypoxemia, and progression to ARDS. The mortality of aspiration pneumonitis is reported to be as high as 30–60%.[13,23]

Pulmonary toxicity may occur in the form of NCPE. It results from either a direct cellular toxic effect or a microvascular injury to the lung. Central neurogenic mechanisms may be responsible for some drug-induced pulmonary edema. Salicylates, opioids, cyclic antidepressants, carbon monoxide, sedative-hypnotics, phosgene, chlorine, nitrogen oxides, and organophosphate insecticides have been reported to produce NCPE.[25,29,31,40,85,88,97] Frequently invasive hemodynamic monitoring and other ICU interventions are necessary to manage this complex condition. It can progress to ARDS.

Besides pulmonary aspiration and NCPE, toxic inhalation, shock, respiratory failure, and sepsis are complications of poisonings that may lead to ARDS, which has a mortality as high as 50%.[10,30,68] Its treatment requires expertise and technology that are best provided in an ICU.

Drug- and toxin-induced rhabdomyolysis is a skeletal muscle injury that leaks intracellular contents into plasma.[20,34,47] It may be due to direct toxic injury to muscle cells, pressure necrosis, or excessive energy expenditure from severe agitation, seizures, or hyperthermia. Barbiturates, carbon monoxide, and cocaine are examples of toxins with a high incidence of producing rhabdomyolysis.[20] Acute renal failure, dysrhythmias from electrolyte disturbances, and disseminated intravascular coagulation complicate this condition. Ensuring adequate urine output and closely monitoring laboratory tests are best done in the ICU and may prevent serious complications.

Rhabdomyolysis may not always be generalized muscle injury but can be a local injury within a fascial compartment.[20,62] Compartment syndrome is the increased pressure within a fascial compartment that compromises distal blood flow. Irreversible muscle damage may occur within 6–12 hours. The comatose poisoned patient may develop compartment syndrome after lying on an extremity or from direct pressure injury. Commonly compartments in the hand, arm, forearm, buttocks, thigh, or leg are involved. Establishing the diagnosis requires close examination of all compartments, reassessment, serial CPK levels, and early surgical consultation for evidence of ischemia.

Poisoning causes global cerebral anoxia from prolonged shock, respiratory failure, or direct toxic/metabolic effects. Distinguishing anoxic cerebral injury from reversible encephalopathy can be difficult in poisoned patients. Coma and loss of brainstem reflexes after prolonged severe cerebral hypoxia indicates a poor prognosis.[53] In contrast, patients with reversible encephalopathy can have profound CNS depression that mimics brain death, yet recover fully.[5,74,78,91,103,106] As mentioned previously, clinical predictors of outcome may be unreliable when applied to poisoned patients; therefore, the diagnosis of brain death should be made cautiously. Often, cerebral edema is a secondary effect of global cerebral anoxia, although some toxins have direct cellular effects. Cerebral edema is a complication of acetaminophen-induced fulminant hepatic failure and a direct neuronal injury from salicylate and lead poisoning.[60,80,96] Aggressive ICU care is necessary to treat toxin-induced cerebral injuries.

When Is It Safe to Discharge a Poisoned Patient From the ICU?

Once toxicity has resolved, most patients may be safely transferred to a regular hospital ward. Patients with cyclic antidepressant overdoses have been extensively studied to determine when it is safe to discontinue monitoring. Concerns arose from case reports of patients developing sudden death as late as several days following a cyclic antidepressant overdose.[14,63,87] In most cases, delayed complications developed in the setting of continued toxicity evidenced by lethargy or sinus tachycardia. More recent studies demonstrate that dysrhythmias do not occur after signs of toxicity have resolved (ie, CNS and cardiac manifestations).[15,35,75] Current recommendations based on these studies suggest cardiac monitoring for an additional 24 hours after normalization of ECG occurs and the patient is without other signs of continued toxicity.[90] This additional period of monitoring should occur after discontinuation of all specific forms of therapy, such as serum alkalinization. Unfortunately, most toxins have not received the extensive attention given to cyclic antidepressants. Pending further research and experience, clinical judgment is the only basis for deciding when to discharge a patient from the ICU.

As previously mentioned, potentially serious toxic effects can recur while antidotes are being administered. The duration of action of the toxin may be longer than the duration of action of the specific treatment or antidote; for example, the action of naloxone is shorter than that of the opioids. In addition, the cholinergic effects of organophosphate poisoning may recur shortly after the administration of atropine. GI absorption must be terminated before the patient can be safely discharged from the ICU. Continued absorption is not likely to be clinically significant when serum drug concentrations are decreasing.

Finally, the patient's suicidal intent must be considered prior to transfer to a less closely monitored ward. A patient's transfer from the ICU can be delayed awaiting assessment of suicide risk or other important psychosocial issues. Early involvement of psychiatric services, chemical-dependency counseling, and social services can expedite ICU disposition. These providers can begin to consider disposition and treatment options, despite a medically unstable patient, by interviewing family, friends, and outpatient counselors. In addition, patients and families can benefit from their familiarity with local mental health and social support resources.

What Are the Alternatives to ICU Admission?

Often, placing patients in the ICU solely for observation is not an effective use of this expensive resource. Until further clinical studies are available to define those patients at risk, many poisoned patients will be admitted to the ICU for observation. If information about the toxin, the patient, and the capabilities of the ward are considered, many patients could safely be observed outside the ICU. Some considerations to assist with disposition decisions are presented in Table 103–5.

Alternatives to the ICU include the medical service, an intermediate care unit, a telemetry monitored bed, a medical–psychiatric service, or an ED observation unit. Capabilities for managing poisoned patients may vary considerably between institutions and in different types of patient care areas. It is essential to understand the capabilities of the unit or inpatient service where a patient is being considered for admission. If nursing staff is unfamiliar with the potential for rapid, serious deterioration of the patient or the staffing does not allow for close observation, the results could be disastrous. For example, it is unrealistic to expect a nurse to manage intravenous fluids, record hourly intake and output measurements, record frequent vital signs, and check hourly urine pH measurements for a salicylate-poisoned patient while caring for 10 other patients. Emergency department observation may be an alternative for observing and treating selected poisoned patients. Emergency department observation units exist currently in nearly one-third of EDs in the United States.[12,38] Many are capable of frequent monitoring of vital signs, continuous cardiac monitoring, and maintaining a safe environment for suicidal patients.[12,38] Patients with a low risk of serious toxicity or life-threatening complications and who require only observation are ideal candidates for ED observation units. Studies are needed to define better those patients for whom observation units can safely provide adequate care.

Toxins with a well-defined toxicity profile allow clinicians to make educated decisions regarding safe observation outside the ICU. For example, acetaminophen toxicity has a well-defined clinical course and an effective antidote. Toxicity develops slowly and is not clinically evident until several days after ingestion. Antidote administration does not require special ICU care, and the ICU can offer little to prevent hepatotoxicity. Most patients with an acetaminophen overdose can be treated outside of the ICU, providing suicide risks can be monitored and regular administration of the antidote ensured.

Many poisoned patients are placed in the ICU or remain long after toxicity has resolved because of suicide risk. Other than the ICU, many hospitals cannot provide an alternative for observing a high-risk, suicidal patient. Less costly alternatives do exist but they must assure a safe environment for suicidal patients. Suicidal patients may be safely observed in an ED observation unit, in an intermediate care unit, in a medical–psychiatric service, or with a one-on-one observer.

TABLE 103–5. CONSIDERATIONS FOR INTENSIVE CARE ADMISSION

Toxin characteristics

Does the ingested toxin have well-known serious sequelae (eg, cyclic antidepressant cardiotoxicity)?
Can the patient deteriorate rapidly from its toxic effects?
Is the onset of toxicity likely to be delayed (eg, sustained-release preparation, slowed GI motility, or delayed toxic effects)?
Does the toxin have cardiac effects that will require cardiac monitoring?
Is the amount ingested a potentially serious or potentially lethal dose?
Is the therapy unconventional (eg, large doses of atropine for treating organophosphate overdoses)?
Does the therapy have potential adverse effects?
Is there a significant risk of the unknown?
Is there insufficient literature to describe the potential human toxic effects?
Are potenially serious coingestants likely (must take into account the reliability of the history)?

Patient characteristics[a]

Does the patient have any signs of serious end-organ toxicity?
Is there progression of the end-organ toxic effects?
Are laboratory data suggestive of serious toxicity?
Are serum drug concentrations rising?
Is the patient at high risk for complications requiring ICU intervention?[11]
- Seizures
- Unresponsive to verbal stimuli
- Level of consciousness impaired to the point of potential airway compromise
- $PCO_2 > 45$ mm Hg
- Systolic blood pressure < 80 mm Hg
- Cardiac dysrhythmias
- Prolonged ECG complexes and intervals (QRS duration $\geq$ 0.10 sec, QT prolongation)

Does the patient have prexisting medical conditions that could predispose to complications?
- Chronic alcohol or drug use
- Chronic liver disease
- Chronic renal failure or insufficiency
- Heart disease
- Pregnancy

Is the patient suicidal?

Assessing the capabilities of the inpatient service/observation unit

Does the admitting team (attending, house staff, students) appreciate the potential seriousness of a toxicologic emergency?
Is the nursing staff:
- Familiar with this toxicologic emergency?
- Familiar with the potential serious complications?

Is the staffing adequate to monitor the patient?
- What is the ratio of patients to nurses?
- Are time-consuming nursing activities required (eg, hourly urine and pH assessment or whole-bowel irrigation)?

Can a safe environment be provided for a suicidal patient?
- Can a patient have suicide precautions and monitoring on a ward?
- Can a one-on-one observer be present in the room with the patient?
- Can the patient be physically restrained?

[a]A no answer to all of the questions in this section indicates ICU admission may not be required and alternatives may be considered without compromising patient safety.

Future studies must define prognostic factors for poisoning complications. Patients can then be stratified into high-risk or low-risk groups. Because of their limitations, current studies often cannot be extrapolated to individual patients or certain subgroups. Unfortunately, many current clinical guidelines for rationing care may be based on poorly tested models with no scientific basis and may be solely based on financial concerns. We must demand guidelines based on the best evidence available. The goal of these guidelines should be to provide the best care with less intensive use of health care resources.

Summary

Acute poisoning is a challenging medical problem, with an unpredictable clinical course that often requires therapy unfamiliar to medical and nursing staff. The lack of both historical data on individuals and accurate information on toxic effects to humans creates many uncertainties in management. Because the ICU offers the highest level of skilled staff and modern technology available, most seriously poisoned patients should be admitted to the ICU. Whether this is clinically justified or is an effective use of resources for a given patient is always an issue since admission of the poisoned patient continues to be based mostly on clinical judgment and the best available information.

References

1. Allen J: Aspiration pneumonitis. Clin Toxicol Rev 1984;7:1.
2. Anderson R, Potts D, Gabow P, et al: Unrecognized adult salicylate intoxication. Ann Intern Med 1976;85:745–748.
3. Banahan B, Schelkun P: Tricyclic antidepressant overdose: Conservative management in a community hospital with cost-saving implications. J Emerg Med 1990;8:451–454.
4. Bernstein G, Jehle D, Bernaski E, et al: Failure of gastric emptying and charcoal administration in fatal sustained-release theophylline overdose: Pharmacobezoar formation. Ann Emerg Med 1992;21:1388–1390.
5. Bird T, Plum F: Recovery from barbiturate overdose coma with a prolonged isoelectric electroencephalogram. Neurology 1968;18:456–460.
6. Boehnert M, Lovejoy F: Value of the QRS duration vs the serum drug level in predicting seizures and ventricular arrhythmias after an acute overdose of tricyclic antidepressants. N Engl J Med 1985;313:474–479.
7. Boehnert M, McGuigan M: Colchicine. Clin Toxicol Rev 1983;5:1.
8. Bogacz K, Caldron P: Enteric-coated aspirin bezoar: Elevation of serum salicylate level by barium study. Am J Med 1987;83:783–786.
9. Borys D, Setzer S, Ling L, et al: Acute fluoxetine overdose: A report of 234 cases. Am J Emerg Med 1992;10:115–120.
10. Bresler M, Sternbach G: The adult respiratory distress syndrome. Emerg Med Clin North Am 1989;7:419–430.
11. Brett A, Rothchild N, Gray R, et al: Predicting the clinical course in intentional drug overdose. Arch Intern Med 1987; 147:133–137.
12. Brillman J, Mathers-Dunbar L, Graff L, et al: Management of observation units. Ann Emerg Med 1995;25:823–830.
13. Bynum L, Pierce A: Pulmonary aspiration of gastric contents. Am Rev Respir Dis 1976;114:1129–1136.
14. Callaham M: Admission criteria for tricyclic antidepressant ingestion. West J Med 1982;137:425–429.
15. Callaham M, Kassel D: Epidemiology of fatal tricyclic antidepressant ingestion: Implications for management. Ann Emerg Med 1985;14:1–9.
16. Chiang W, Ford M, Wax P: Prospective evaluation of fluoxetine ingestions. Vet Hum Toxicol 1990;32:348. Abstract.
17. Civetta J: Setting objectives: Perspectives for care. In: Civetta JM, Taylor RW, Kirby RR, eds: Critical Care, 2nd ed. Philadelphia, Lippincott, 1992, pp. 13–23.
18. Clemmesen C, Nilsson E: Therapeutic trends in the treatment of barbiturate poisoning: The Scandinavian method. Clin Pharmacol Ther 1961;2:220–229.
19. Cohn JN: Blood pressure measurement in shock: Mechanism of inaccuracy in auscultatory and palpatory methods. JAMA 1967;199:972–976.
20. Curry S, Chang D, Connor D: Drug- and toxin-induced rhabdomyolysis. Ann Emerg Med 1989;18:1068–1084.
21. Dec W: Tricyclic antidepressants in the intensive care. J Intensive Care Med 1990;5:69.
22. Dederich R, Szefler S, Green E: Intrasubject variation in sustained release theophylline absorption. J Allergy Clin Immunol 1981;67:465–471.
23. Dines D, Titus J, Sessler A: Aspiration pneumonitis. Mayo Clin Proc 1970;45:347–360.
24. Du Toit P, Muller F, Van Tonder W, et al: Experience with the intensive care management of organophosphate insecticide poisoning. S Afr Med J 1981;60:227–229.
25. Duberstein J, Kaufman D: A clinical study of an epidemic of heroin intoxication and heroin-induced pulmonary edema. Am J Med 1971;51:704–707.
26. Elk J, Linton D, Potgieter P: Treatment of acute self-poisoning in a respiratory intensive care unit. S Afr Med J 1987;72:532–534.
27. Emerman CL, Connors AF, Burma GM: Level of consciousness as a predictor of complications following tricyclic overdose. Ann Emerg Med 1987;16:326–330.
28. Fell R, Gunning A, Bardhan K, et al: Severe hypothermia as a result of barbiturate overdose complicated by cardiac arrest. Lancet 1968;1:392–394.
29. Fisher C, Albertson T, Foulke G: Salicylate-induced pulmonary edema: Clinical characteristics in children. Am J Emerg Med 1985;3:33–37.
30. Fowler A, Hamman R, Zerbe G, et al: Adult respiratory distress syndrome: Prognosis after onset. Am Rev Respir Dis 1985;132:472–478.
31. Frand U, Shim C, Williams M: Heroin-induced pulmonary edema. Ann Intern Med 1972;77:29–35.
32. Frommer D, Kulig K, Marx J, et al: Tricyclic antidepressant overdose. JAMA 1987;257:521–526.
33. Fruensgaard K: Withdrawal psychosis: A study of 30 consecutive cases. Acta Psychiatr Scand 1976;53:105–118.
34. Gabow P, Kaehny W, Kelleher S: The spectrum of rhabdomyolysis. Medicine 1982;61:141–151.
35. Goldberg R, Capone R, Hunt J: Cardiac complications fol-

lowing tricyclic antidepressant overdose. JAMA 1985;254: 1772–1775.
36. Golsousidis H, Kokkas V: Use of 19,590 mg of atropine during 24 days of treatment after a case of unusually severe parathion poisoning. Hum Toxicol 1985;4:339–340.
37. Goodman J, Bischel M, Wagers P, et al: Barbiturate intoxication: Morbidity and mortality. West J Med 1976;124:179–186.
38. Graff L, Zun L, Leikin J, et al: Emergency department observation beds improve patient care: Society for Academic Emergency Medicine debate. Ann Emerg Med 1992;21: 967–975.
39. Hart L, Cobaugh D, Dean B, et al: Successful use of extracorporeal membrane oxygenation (ECMO) in the treatment of refractory respiratory failure secondary to hydrocarbon aspiration. Vet Hum Toxicol 1991;33:361. Abstract.
40. Heffner J, Sahn S: Salicylate-induced pulmonary edema. Ann Intern Med 1981;95:405–409.
41. Henderson A, Wright M, Pond SM: Experience with 732 acute overdose patients admitted to an intensive care unit over six years. Med J Aust 1993;158:28–30.
42. Hendren W, Schieber R, Garrettson L: Extracorporeal bypass for the treatment of verapamil poisoning. Ann Emerg Med 1989;18:984–987.
43. Heyman EN, LoCastro DE, Gouse LH, et al: Intentional drug overdose: Predictors of clinical course in the intensive care unit. Heart Lung 1996;25:246–252.
44. Hulten BA, Adams R, Askenasi R, et al: Predicting severity of tricyclic antidepressant overdose. J Toxicol Clin Toxicol 1992;30:161–170.
45. Jay S, Johanson W, Pierce A: Respiratory complications of overdose with sedative drugs. Am Rev Respir Dis 1975; 112:591–598.
46. Knaus W, Draper E, Wagner D, et al: APACHE II: A severity of disease classification system. Crit Care Med 1985;13: 818–829.
47. Koppel C: Clinical features, pathogenesis and management of drug-induced rhabdomyolysis. Med Toxicol 1989; 4:108–126.
48. Kruse J, Thill-Baharozian M, Carlson R: Comparison of clinical assessment with APACHE II for predicting mortality risk in patients admitted to a medical intensive care unit. JAMA 1988;260:1739–1742.
49. Kulig K, Bar-Or D, Cantrill S, et al: Management of acutely poisoned patients without gastric emptying. Ann Emerg Med 1985;14:562–567.
50. Lacroix J, Gaudreault P, Gauthier M: Admission to a pediatric intensive care unit for poisoning: A review of 105 cases. Crit Care Med 1989;17:748–750.
51. Landsman I, Bricker J, Reid B, et al: Emergency gastrotomy: Treatment of choice for iron bezoar. J Pediatr Surg 1987;22:184–185.
52. LeBlanc F, Benson B, Gilg A: A severe organophosphate poisoning requiring the use of an atropine drip. J Toxicol Clin Toxicol 1986;24:69–76.
53. Levy DE, Bates D, Caronna JJ, et al: Prognosis in nontraumatic coma. Ann Intern Med 1981;94:293–301.
54. Linden C, Rumack B, Strehlke C: Monoamine oxidase inhibitor overdose. Ann Emerg Med 1984;13:1137–1144.
55. Litovitz TL, Clark LR, Soloway RA: 1993 Annual Report of the American Association of Poison Control Centers Toxic Exposure Surveillance System. Am J Emerg Med 1994;12: 546–584.
56. Litovitz TL, Felberg L, Soloway RA, et al: 1994 Annual Report of the American Association of Poison Control Centers Toxic Exposure Surveillance System. Am J Emerg Med 1995;13:551–597.
57. Litovitz TL, Felberg L, White S, et al: 1995 Annual Report of the American Association of Poison Control Centers Toxic Exposure Surveillance System. Am J Emerg Med 1996;14:487–537.
58. Litovitz TL, Holm KC, Bailey KM, et al: 1991 Annual Report of the American Association of Poison Control Centers Toxic Exposure Surveillance System. Am J Emerg Med 1992;10:452–505.
59. Litovitz TL, Holm KC, Clancy C, et al: 1992 Annual Report of the American Association of Poison Control Centers Toxic Exposure Surveillance System. Am J Emerg Med 1993;11:494–555.
60. Manton WI, Kirkpatrick JB, Cook JP: Does the choroid plexus really protect the brain from lead? Lancet 1984; 2:351. Letter.
61. Martin T, Klain M, Molner R, et al: Extracorporeal life support vs thumper after lethal desipramine OD. Vet Hum Toxicol 1990;4:349. Abstract.
62. Matsen FA: Compartment syndrome: A unified concept. Clin Orthop 1975;113:8–14.
63. McAlpine S, Calabro J, Robinson M, et al: Late death in tricyclic antidepressant overdose revisited. Ann Emerg Med 1986;15:1349–1352.
64. McCarron M, Challoner K, Thompson G: Diphenoxylate-atropine (Lomotil) overdose in children: An update (report of eight cases and review of the literature). Pediatrics 1991;87:694–700.
65. McCarron M, Wood J: The cocaine body packer syndrome. JAMA 1983;250:1417–1420.
66. Merigian K, Woodard M, Hedges J, et al: Prospective evaluation of gastric emptying in the self-poisoned patient. Am J Emerg Med 1990;8:479–483.
67. Minocha A, Spyker D: Acute overdose with sustained release drug formulations. Med Toxicol 1986;1:300–307.
68. Montgomery A, Stager M, Carrico C, et al: Causes of mortality in patients with the adult respiratory distress syndrome. Am Rev Respir Dis 1985;132:485–489.
69. Murphy G, Wetzel R: Family history of suicidal behavior among suicide attempters. J Nerv Ment Dis 1982;170: 86–90.
70. Niemann J, Bessen H, Rothstein R, et al: Electrocardiographic criteria for tricyclic antidepressant cardiotoxicity. Am J Cardiol 1986;57:1154–1159.
71. Noble J, Kennedy D, Latimer R, et al: Massive lignocaine overdose during cardiopulmonary bypass. Br J Anesthesiol 1984;56:1439–1441.
72. Nogue S, Marruecos L, Nolla J, et al: The profile evolution of acute severe poisoning in Spain. Toxicol Lett 1992; 64–65:725–727.
73. North D: Meprobamate and bezoar formation. Ann Emerg Med 1987;16:472–473. Letter.
74. Orr D, Bramble M: Tricyclic antidepressant poisoning and prolonged external cardiac massage during asystole. Br Med J 1981;283:1107–1108.

75. Pentel P, Benowitz N: Tricyclic antidepressant poisoning: management of arrhythmias. Med Toxicol 1986;1:101–121.
76. Pentel P, Sioris L: Incidence of late arrhythmias following tricyclic antidepressant overdose. Clin Toxicol 1981;18: 543–546.
77. Pond SM, Lewis-Driver DJ, Williams GM, et al: Gastric emptying in acute overdose: A prospective randomised controlled trial. Med J Aust 1995;163:345–349.
78. Powner D: Drug-associated isoelectric EEGs. A hazard in brain death certification. JAMA 1976;236:1123.
79. Ramoska E, Spiller H, Winter H, et al: A one-year evaluation of calcium channel blocker overdoses: Toxicity and treatment. Ann Emerg Med 1993;22:196–200.
80. Reed JR, Palmisano PA: Central nervous system salicylate. Clin Toxicol 1975;8:623–631.
81. Rinaldo J, Snyder J: Survival database: Central nervous system injury. Am Rev Respir Dis 1989;140:S25–S27.
82. Roberts J, Price D, Goldfrank L: The body stuffer syndrome: A clandestine form of drug overdose. Am J Emerg Med 1986;4:22–27.
83. Robertson N: Fatal overdose from sustained-release theophylline preparation. Ann Emerg Med 1985;14:154–158.
84. Ron A, Aronne L, Kalb P, et al: The therapeutic efficacy of critical care units. Arch Intern Med 1989;149:338–341.
85. Rorison D, McPherson S: Acute toxic inhalations. Emerg Med Clin North Am 1992;10:409–435.
86. Schwartz H: Acute meprobamate poisoning with gastrotomy and removal of a drug-containing mass. N Engl J Med 1976;295:1177–1178.
87. Sedal L, Korman M, Williams P, et al: Overdosage of tricyclic antidepressants: A report of two deaths and a prospective study of 24 patients. Med J Aust 1972;2:74–79.
88. Shannon M, Lovejoy F: Pulmonary complications of severe tricyclic antidepressant ingestion. J Toxicol Clin Toxicol 1987;25:443–461.
89. Shub C, Gau G, Sidell P, et al: The management of acute quinidine intoxication. Chest 1978;73:173–178.
90. Smilkstein M: Reviewing cyclic antidepressant cardiotoxicity: Wheat and chaff. J Emerg Med 1990;8:645–648.
91. Southall D, Kilpatrick S: Imipramine poisoning: Survival of a child after prolonged cardiac massage. Br Med J 1974;4:508.
92. Spiller H, Meyers A, Ziemba T, et al: Delayed onset of cardiac arrhythmias from sustained-release verapamil. Ann Emerg Med 1991;20:201–203.
93. Spiller H, Morse S: Fluoxetine ingestion: A one year retrospective study. Vet Hum Toxicol 1990;32:153–155.
94. Sporer K, Manning J: Massive ingestion of sustained-release verapamil with a concretion and bowel infarction. Ann Emerg Med 1993;22:603–605.
95. Strom J, Thisted B, Krantz T, et al: Self poisoning treated in an ICU: Drug pattern, acute mortality and short term survival. Acta Anaesthesiol Scand 1986;30:148–153.
96. Sutherland LR, Muller P, Lewis DR: Massive cerebral edema associated with fulminant hepatic failure in acetaminophen overdose. Am J Gastroenterol 1981;76: 446–448.
97. Tafuri J, Roberts J: Organophosphate poisoning. Ann Emerg Med 1987;16:193–202.
98. Tepperman P: Fatality due to acute systemic fluoride poisoning following a hydrofluoric acid skin burn. J Occup Med 1980;22:691–692.
99. Teres D, Lemeshow S: Severity-of-illness modeling and potential applications. In: Rippe JM, Irwin RS, Fink MP, Cerra FB, eds: Intensive Care Medicine, 3rd ed. Boston, Little, Brown, 1996, pp. 2589–2598.
100. Thisted B, Krantz T, Strom J, et al: Acute salicylate self-poisoning in 177 consecutive patients treated in ICU. Acta Anaesthesiol 1987;31:312–316.
101. Tokarski G, Young M: Criteria for admitting patients with tricyclic antidepressant overdose. J Emerg Med 1988;6: 121–124.
102. Vance M, Curry S, Kunkel D, et al: Digital hydrofluoric acid burns: Treatment with intraarterial calcium infusion. Ann Emerg Med 1986;15:890–896.
103. White A: Overdose of tricylclic antidepressants associated with absent brain-stem reflexes. Can Med Assoc J 1988; 139:133–134.
104. Wolfe T, Caravati E, Rollins D: Terminal 40-ms frontal plane QRS axis as a marker for tricyclic antidepressant overdose. Ann Emerg Med 1989;18:348–351.
105. Wortzman D, Grunfeld A: Delayed absorption following enteric-coated aspirin overdose. Ann Emerg Med 1987; 16:434–436.
106. Yang K, Dantzker D: Reversible brain death: A manifestation of amitriptyline overdose. Chest 1991;99:1037–1038.
107. Zimmerman J, Knaus W, Judson J, et al: Patient selection for intensive care: a comparison of New Zealand and United States hospitals. Crit Care Med 1988;16: 318–326.

CHAPTER 104

Reproductive and Perinatal Principles

Jeffrey S. Fine

Reproductive and perinatal principles in toxicology are derived from many areas of basic science and in turn may be applied to many aspects of clinical practice. This chapter will review several principles of reproductive medicine that have implications for toxicology—the physiology of pregnancy and placental drug transfer, the effects of chemical substances on the developing fetus and the neonate, and the management of overdose in a pregnant woman.

One of the most dramatic effects of exposure to a toxin during pregnancy is the birth of a child with congenital malformations. Teratology is the science of birth defects and has classically been concerned with the study of such physical malformations. A broader view of teratology includes "developmental" teratogens—agents that induce structural malformations, metabolic or physiologic dysfunction, or psychological or behavioral alterations or deficits in the offspring, either at birth or in a defined postnatal period.[196] Only 4–6% of birth defects are related to known pharmaceutical agents or occupational and environmental exposures.[23,84,196]

Reproductive effects of toxins may occur prior to conception. Female germ cells are formed in utero; adverse effects from xenobiotic (foreign substance) exposure can theoretically occur from the time of a woman's own intrauterine development to the end of her reproductive years. An example of a drug that has had both teratogenic and reproductive effects in the same individual is diethylstilbestrol (DES), which caused vaginal and/or cervical adenocarcinoma in some women exposed in utero and also had effects on fertility and pregnancy outcome.[11,16]

Men generally receive less attention with respect to reproductive risks. Male gametes are formed after puberty; only from that time on are they susceptible to toxic injury. An example of a toxin affecting male reproduction is dibromochloropropane. Dibromochloropropane reduces spermatogenesis, with subsequent reduced fertility. In general, little is known about the sperm's contribution to teratogenesis.

Occupational exposures to reproductive toxins are potentially important but often poorly defined. It has been estimated that there are 20 million women of reproductive age in the workforce.[173] Ninety thousand chemicals are used commercially in the United States; however, only 2200 industrial and pharmaceutical agents have been specifically evaluated for reproductive toxicity. Many agents have teratogenic effects when tested in animal models, but relatively few well defined human teratogens have been identified.[201] Most tested chemicals therefore do not appear to present a human teratogenic risk, but most chemicals have not been tested. Some of the presumed safe chemicals may have other reproductive, nonteratogenic toxicity. Several excellent reviews are available.[161,196,231]

Another type of toxic exposure for a pregnant woman is the intentional overdose. Although a drug taken in overdose may have direct toxicity for the fetus, the acute toxicity to the fetus frequently results from maternal pulmonary and/or hemodynamic compromise (ie, hypoxia or shock).

Toxic exposures prior to and during pregnancy can have effects throughout gestation and may extend into and beyond the newborn period. In addition, the effects of drug administration in the perinatal period including the special case of drug delivery to an infant via the breast milk, deserve special consideration.

Which Toxins Are Pregnant Women Exposed To?

Medications, alcohol, caffeine, and nicotine, as well as drugs of abuse, are all obvious sources of xenobiotic exposure to both pregnant women and men during spermatogenesis. Thirty to 70% of pregnant women may use 3–10 different medications at some time during pregnancy—primarily analgesic, antipyretic, antimicrobial, and antiemetic agents as well as vitamins, caffeine, ethanol, and nicotine.[20,86,166,190] Some use medications to treat chronic disease; some use these agents prior to the determination of pregnancy. There is evidence that women tend to decrease their exposure to drugs once they know they are pregnant.[21,95,98]

The U.S. Food and Drug Administration (FDA) categorizes pharmaceutical agents according to potential benefits and risks for a pregnant woman and the fetus (Table 104–1). This system has been criticized as being too conservative as well as for conveying the impression that a category C drug is worse than a category B drug in pregnancy. This occurs because when there is little or no information available, the agent is by default placed into category C.[69] A modified system is in place in Europe.[194] Agents classified as FDA category X and category D drugs are listed in Tables 104–2 and 104–3, respectively. Many of these agents are known or suspected human teratogens and are more fully described in Table 104–4. Although most women are concerned about the teratogenic effects of medications, in utero exposure to therapeutic medications can have other pharmacologic effects on the newborn infant.[19,26]

In surveys regarding drug use, as many as 15–25% of pregnant women either report some licit or illicit drug use or have positive urine screens at some time during pregnancy. Ethanol and tobacco are the most common licit agents,[156] while cocaine and marijuana are the most frequently used illicit agents.[37,120] Estimates of the use of alcohol by pregnant women vary widely from 1% to 70%.[4,129,156]

TABLE 104–1. FDA USE-IN-PREGNANCY RATINGS

Category	Example	Meaning
A	Multiple vitamins	**Controlled studies show no risk.** Adequate, well-controlled studies in pregnant women have failed to demonstrate risk to the fetus.
B	Acetaminophen, penicillin	**No evidence of risk in humans.** Either animal findings show risk, but human findings do not; or, if no adequate human studies have been done, animal findings are negative.
C	Albuterol	**Risk cannot be ruled out.** Human studies are lacking, and animal studies are either positive for fetal risk or lacking as well. However, potential benefits may justify the potential risk.
D	Tetracycline	**Positive evidence of risk.** Investigational or postmarketing data show risk to the fetus. Nevertheless, potential benefits may outweigh the potential risk.
E	Isotretinoin	**Contraindicated in pregnancy.** Studies in animals or humans, or investigational or postmarketing reports have shown fetal risk that clearly outweighs any possible benefit to the patient.

Adapted, with permission, from Freidman JM: Report of the Teratology Society Public Affairs Committee symposium on FDA classification of drugs. Teratology 1993;48:5–6.

TABLE 104–2. FDA USE-IN-PREGNANCY CATEGORY X DRUGS[a]

Estrogens—possible increased risk of congenital malformations
Ethanol
Iodine (iodinated glycerol, iodine[125], iodine[131])—may cause neonatal hypothyroidism or goiter
Menadione—hemolytic anemia, kernicterus
Misoprostol—vascular disruptive phenomena
Progestogens (norethindrone, norethynodrel, norgestrel, oral contraceptives)
Quinine—malformations associated with use of toxic doses as abortifacient. Also thrombocytopenic purpura and hemolysis in a G-6-PD-deficient infant.
Retinoids (etretinate, isotretinoin, vitamin A)
Ribavirin—teratogenic or embryolethal in animal species
Temazepam—possible interaction with diphenhydramine leading to a stillbirth
Vaccines (MMR, smallpox)—small risk of congenital rubella or other fetal viral syndromes. Fetal death has been associated with smallpox vaccination.

[a]Many of these agents are known or suspected human teratogens (see Table 104–4). This is a selected list; for changes and additions, consult current drug references. Comments are included for agents not listed in Table 104–4.

Data adapted from Briggs GG, Freeman RK, Yaffe SJ; Drugs in Pregnancy and Lactation, 3rd ed. Baltimore, Williams & Wilkins, 1990.

How Do Physiologic Changes During Pregnancy Affect Drug Distribution in the Pregnant Woman?

Many physical and physiologic changes that occur during pregnancy affect both absorption and distribution of drugs in the pregnant woman and consequently affect the amount of drug delivered to the fetus.[94,145]

During pregnancy there is delayed gastric emptying, decreased gastrointestinal (GI) motility, and increased transit time through the GI tract. These changes result in delayed but more complete GI absorption of drugs and consequently lower peak plasma concentration. Since blood flow to the skin and mucous membranes is increased, absorption from dermal exposure may be increased. Similarly, absorption of inhaled agents may be increased due to increased tidal volume and decreased residual lung volume.

An increased free drug concentration in the pregnant woman may be due to several factors, such as decreased plasma albumin, increased binding competition, and decreased hepatic biotransformation during the later stages of pregnancy. Fat stores increase during the early stages of pregnancy; free fatty acids are released during the later stages and, with them, drugs that may have accumulated in the lipid compartment. The increased concentration of free fatty acids can compete with circulating free drug for binding sites on albumin.

Other factors may lead to decreased free drug concentrations. The increased fat stores as well as the increased plasma and extracellular fluid volume will lead

TABLE 104–3. FDA USE-IN-PREGNANCY CATEGORY D DRUGS[a]

Drug Category / Class / Agent	Known or Presumed Effect
Aminoglycosides	8th nerve damage, hearing loss
Anticonvulsants (bromides, hydantoins, barbiturates, oxazolidinediones, phensuximide, valproate)	See Table 104–4. Bromides are associated with possible growth retardation and malformations and neonatal bromism. There are case reports of malformations with phensuximide.
Antidepressants (amitriptyline, butriptyline, clomipramine, dibenzepin, dothiepin, imipramine, iprindole, nortriptyline, opipramol)	Occasional reports of malformations, antidepressant toxicity or withdrawal, and urinary retention. Seizures associated with clomipramine. Desipramine is Category C.
Antineoplastic agents	This group includes multiple agents, with different effects. Not all agents are definitely toxic during pregnancy but there is concern for chromosomal damage and immunosuppression with these agents.
Antithyroid (carbimazole, methimazole, propylthiouracil)	Possible aplasia cutis (carbimazole, methimazole) and other malformations, neonatal hypothyroidism and goiter.
Aspirin	Maternal—anemia, antepartum/postpartum hemorrhage, prolonged gestation, prolonged labor. May be beneficial in pregnancy-induced hypertension. Infant—hemorrhage, high doses may lead to intrauterine growth retardation and increased perinatal mortality.
Carbarsone	Contains arsenic, which has caused fetal fatalities.
Cortisone	Reports of malformations, concern about neonatal adrenal hyperplasia or insufficiency.
Coumarin derivatives/wafarin	See Table 104–4.
Diuretics (thiazides, ethacrynic acid, potassium sparing)	1st trimester use may be associated with malformations. Possible hypoglycemia, thrombocytopenia, hyponatremia, hypokalemia. Concern about the thiazide diuretics have been extended to other classes of diuretics.
Iodine-containing compounds	Hypothyroidism and goiter.
Lithium	See Table 104–4.
Methylene blue	Intraamniotic injection—methemoglobinemia, staining of fetal skin.
Nonsteroidal antiinflammatory agents	These agents generally carry a Category B designation, but there is concern when used for more than 48 h or after 34 wk gestation. Closure of ductus arteriosus with pulmonary hypertension, oligohydramnios. Most information based on indomethacin.
Opioid analgesics / anatagonists	These agents generally carry a Category B designation, but use near delivery may lead to respiratory depression; antagonists may precipitate fetal or neonatal opioid withdrawal.
Progestogens (ethisterone, ethynodiol, hydroxyprogesterone, medroxyprogesterone)	Possible association with cardiovascular malformations, hypospadias. Masculinization of the female infant.
Sedative-hypnotic agents (barbiturates, benzodiazepines, meprobamate, methaqualone)	Possible malformations, neonatal sedation or withdrawal; barbiturates have been associated with hemorrhagic disease; benzodiazepines have been associated with floppy infant syndrome. Abusable substances.
Sulfonamides and sulfa analogs	Use near term may lead to neonatal jaundice.
Sulfonylureas (acetohexamide, chlorpropamide, tolazamide, tolbutamide)	Poor control of diabetes mellitus in pregnancy. Use near term is associated with prolonged neonatal hypoglycemia.
Sympathomimetic agents (levarterenol, metaraminol)	Possible maternal hypertension, decreased uterine blood flow.
Tetracyclines	See Table 104–4.
Vitamin D and analogues	See Table 104–4.

[a]Some of these agents are known or suspected human teratogens (see Table 104–4). This is a selected list; for changes and additions, consult current drug references.
Data from Briggs GG, Freeman RK, Yaffe SJ; Drugs in Pregnancy and Lactation, 3rd ed. Baltimore, Williams & Wilkins, 1990.

to a greater volume of distribution. Increased renal blood flow and glomerular filtration may result in increased renal elimination.

Cardiac output increases throughout pregnancy, with the placenta receiving a gradually increasing proportion of total blood volume. Drug delivery to the placenta may therefore increase over the course of pregnancy.

These processes interact dynamically and it is difficult to predict their net effect. The concentration of many drugs such as lithium, gentamicin, and carbamazepine decrease during pregnancy even if the administered dose is not changed.[111]

Though not specifically related to the physiologic changes occurring during pregnancy, the fetus may be exposed to drugs and chemicals that accumulated in adipose tissue prior to pregnancy. For example, typical retinoid malformations were seen in a baby born to a woman whose pregnancy began 1 year after the drug etretinate (retinoic acid) was discontinued.[117]

TABLE 104–4. HUMAN TERATOGENS

Agent	Reported Effects	Comments
Androgens	Masculinization of female embryo: clitoromegaly with or without fusion of labia minora.	Effects are dose dependent: stimulates growth and differentiation of sex-steroid receptor-containing tissue.
Angiotensin-converting enzyme inhibitors	Fetal/neonatal death, oligohydramnios, pulmonary hypoplasia, neonatal anuria, IUGR, and skull hypoplasia.	Low risk. Effects related to chronic fetal hypotension during 2nd/3rd trimester. Risk appears to be low. If in use during early pregnancy, can be switched during 1st trimester. Does not interfere with organogenesis.[25]
Alkylating agents (busulfan, chlorambucil, cyclophosphamide, mechlorethamine)	Growth retardation, cleft palate, microphthalmia, hypoplastic ovaries, cloudy corneas, renal agenesis, malformations of digits, cardiac defects, other anomalies.	10–50% malformation rate, depending on which drug. Cyclophosphamide-induced damage requires cytochrome P450 monoxidase activation. Metabolite interacts with DNA, resulting in cell death.
Antimetabolites (aminopterin, azauridine, cytarabine, 5-FU, 6-MP, methotrexate)	Hydro/microcephaly, meningoencephalocele, anencephaly, abnormal cranial ossification, cerebral hypoplasia, growth retardation, eye, ear, and nose malformations, cleft palate, malformed extremities/fingers, reduction in derivatives of 1st branchial arch.	These folate antagonists inhibit dihydrofolate reductase, resulting in cell death. Depending on specific agent, 7–75% rate of malformation.[220]
Carbamazepine	Upslanting palpebral fissures, epicanthal folds, short nose with long philtrum, fingernail hypoplasia, developmental delay, neural tube defects (NTD)	Mechanism unknown. Risk is unknown but may be significant for minor anomalies. 1% risk for NTD. Risk is compounded with those associated with epilepsy itself.[100]
Cocaine	IUGR, microcephaly, neurobehavioral abnormalities, vascular disruptive phenomenon (limb amputation, cerebral infarction, visceral/urinary tract abnormalities).	Vascular disruptive effects due to decreased uterine blood flow and fetal vascular effects from 1st trimester through the end of pregnancy. Risk for major disruptive effects is low.
Carbon monoxide	Cerebral atrophy, mental retardation, microcephaly, convulsions, spastic disorders, intrauterine death.	With severe maternal poisoning, high risk for neurologic sequelae; no increased risk in mild unintentional exposures.
Coumarins	Fetal warfarin syndrome: nasal hypoplasia, chondrodysplasia punctata, brachydactyly, skull defects, abnormal ears, malformed eyes, CNS malformations, microcephaly, hydrocephalus, skeletal deformities, mental retardation, spasticity.	10–25% risk of malformation for exposure during 1st trimester; 3% risk of hemorrhages; 8% risk of stillbirths. Bleeding is an unlikely explanation for effects produced in the 1st trimester. CNS defects may occur during 2nd/3rd trimesters and may be related to bleeding.[99,221]
Diethylstilbestrol (DES)	Female offspring: vaginal adenosis, clear cell carcinoma, irregular menses, reduced pregnancy rates, increased rate of preterm deliveries, increased perinatal mortality and spontaneous abortion. Male offspring: cysts of epididymis, cryptorchidism, hypogonadism, diminished spermatogenesis.	DES stimulates estrogen receptor-containing tissue and may cause misplaced genital tissue, which may have a greater propensity to develop cancer. 40–70% risk of morphologic changes in vaginal epithelium. Risk of adenocarcinoma approximately 1/1000 for exposure before the 18th week. Majority of children exposed to DES in utero can conceive and deliver normal children.[11]
Ethanol	Fetal alcohol syndrome(FAS): pre/postnatal growth retardation, mental retardation, fine motor dysfunction, hyperactivity, microcephaly, maxillary hypoplasia, short palpebral fissures, hypoplastic philtrum, thinned upper lips, joint, digit anomalies.	Other effects: increased incidence of spontaneous abortion, premature delivery, and stillbirth; neonatal withdrawal. Effects may be direct cytotoxic effects of ethanol or acetaldehyde and/or indirect effects of alcoholism and other substance/tobacco use. FAS in 10–40% of offspring of alcoholic women consuming above 2 g/kg/d (6 oz/d) ethanol over the 1st trimester. Fetal alcohol effects at lower doses. There may be a threshold for effects but a safe dose has not been identified.[23,26,205]
Iodine, radioactive	Thyroid hypoplasia after the 8th week of development.	Higher doses of radioisotopes can produce cell death and mitotic delay. Tissue and organ-specific damage is dependent on the specific radioisotope, dose, distribution, metabolism, and localization.
Lead	Lower scores on developmental tests.	Higher risk when maternal lead is >10 μg/dL.
Lithium carbonate	Possible increased risk of Ebstein's anomaly.	Low risk.
Methyl mercury, mercuric sulfide	Normal appearance at birth; cerebral palsy-like syndrome after several months; microcephaly, mental retardation, cerebellar symptoms, eye/dental anomalies.	Inhibit enzymes particularly those with sulfhydryl groups. 13/220 babies born following the Minamata Bay exposure had severe disease. Mothers of affected babies consumed 9–27 ppm mercury; greater risk when ingested at 6–8 gestational months. In acute poisoning, the fetus is 4–10 times more sensitive than an adult. Pathologically there is atrophy and hypoplasia of the brain cortex and abnormalities in cytoarchitecture.[84,225]
Misoprostol	Vascular disruptive phenomenon such as limb reduction defects; mobius syndrome.	Prostaglandin analog. Effects occur after the period of early organogenesis.
Oxazolidine-2,4-diones (trimethadione, paramethadione)	Fetal trimethadione syndrome: V-shaped eyebrows, low-set ears with anteriorly folded helix, high arched palate, irregular teeth, CNS anomalies, severe developmental delay, cardiovascular, genitourinary, and other anomalies.	83% risk of at least one major malformation with any exposure; 32% die. Characteristic facial features are associated with chronic exposure.

(*continued*)

TABLE 104–4. HUMAN TERATOGENS (continued)

Agent	Reported Effects	Comments
Polychlorinated biphenyls	Cola-colored children; pigmentation of gums, nails, and groin; hypoplastic, deformed nails; intrauterine growth retardation; abnormal skull calcifications.	Cytoxic agent. Body residue can affect subsequent offspring for up to 4 years after exposure. Most cases followed high consumption of PCB-contaminated rice oil, 4–20% of offspring were affected
Penicillamine	Cutis laxa, hyperflexibility of joints.	Copper chelator—copper deficiency inhibits collagen synthesis/maturation. Few case reports; low risk.
Phenytoin	Fetal hydantoin syndrome: microcephaly, mental retardation, cleft lip/palate, hypoplastic nails/phalanges, characteristic facies—low nasal bridge, inner epicanthal folds, ptosis, strabismus hypertelorism, low-set ears, wide mouth.	Phenytoin has a direct effect on cell membranes and folate and vitamin K metabolism. Epoxide intermediate postulated as teratogenic agent. Effects seen with chronic exposure. 5–10% risk of typical syndrome, 30% risk of partial syndrome. Risk is confounded by those associated with epilepsy itself.[83]
Progestins	Masculinization of female embryo.	Stimulates or interferes with sex-steroid receptor-containing tissue. Effects only after exposure to high doses of some testosterone-derived progestins. Doses in modern oral contraceptives do not cause these effects.
Radiation (external irradiation)	Microcephaly, mental retardation, eye anomalies, growth retardation, visceral malformations.	Significant doses of radiation from diagnositic or therapeutic sources produce cell death and mitotic delay. There is no measurable risk with x-ray exposures of 5 rads or less at any stage of pregnancy.[14]
Retinoids (isotretinoin, etretinate, vitamin A)	Spontaneous abortions, micro/hydrocephalus, deformities of cranium, ears, face, heart, limbs, liver.	Retinoids can cause direct cytotoxicity and alter programmed cell death. Neural crest cells are particularly sensitive. For isotretinoin, 38% risk of malformations; 80% are CNS malformations. Topical retinoids are not considered a reproductive risk. Effects have been associated with vitamin A doses of 25,000–100,000 U/d. Exposures below 10,000 U/d present no risk to fetus.[209]
Smoking	Placental lesions, IUGR, increased postnatal morbidity and mortality.	Maternal or placental complications can result in fetal death. Nicotine can result in vascular spasm leading to placental pathology.
Streptomycin	Hearing deficiency.	Rare reports. A low-risk phenomenon that could be associated with long-duration maternal therapy during pregnancy.
Tetracycline	Yellow, gray-brown, or brown staining of deciduous teeth, hypoplastic tooth enamel.	Effects seen from 4 months of gestation on, because tetracyclines have to interact with calcified tissue. Effects in 50% of fetuses exposed to tetracycline; 12.5% exposed to oxytetracycline.
Thalidomide	Limb phocomelia, amelia, hypoplasia, congenital heart defects, renal malformations, cryptorchidism, abducens paralysis, deafness, microtia, anotia.	Approx. 20% risk when exposure to drug occurs during days 34–50 of gestation.
Valproate	Lumbosacral spina bifida with meningomyelocele; CNS defects, microcephaly, cardiac defects, narrow face with high forehead, epicanthal folds, broad low nasal bridge with short nose, long philtrum with a thin vermilion border, long thin fingers and toes.	Risk for spina bifida is approx. 1%, but the risk for facial dysmorphology may be greater. The mechanism of teratogenicity is unknown. Possible explanations include interference with glutathione, folate, or zinc metabolism, or regulation of intracellular pH. Risk is confounded by those associated with epilepsy itself.[118]
Vitamin D	Possible association with supravalvular aortic stenosis, elfin facies, and mental retardation.	Large doses of vitamin D may disrupt cellular calcium regulation. Genetic susceptibility may play a role.

Adapted, with permission, from Koren G, Nulman I: Teratogenic drugs and chemicals in humans. In: Koren G, ed: Maternal-Fetal Toxicology: A Clinician's Guide, 2nd ed. Marcel Dekker, New York, 1994; and Brent RL: The application of the principles of toxicology and teratology in evaluating the risks of new drugs for the treatment of drug addiction in women of reproductive age. NIDA Research Monograph 1995;149:130–179.

How Does the Placenta Function to Transfer Xenobiotics to the Fetus?

With respect to the transfer of chemicals from mother to fetus, the placenta functions like other lipoprotein membranes. Most xenobiotics enter the fetal circulation by passive diffusion down a concentration gradient across the placental membranes. The characteristics of a substance that favor this passive diffusion are low molecular weight, lipid solubility, neutral polarity, and low protein binding.[154] Polar molecules and ions may be transported through interstitial pores.[214]

Xenobiotics with a molecular weight greater than 1000 D do not diffuse passively across the placenta. This characteristic is used to therapeutic advantage. For example, warfarin (MW = 1000 D) easily crosses the placenta and causes specific fetal malformations.[221] However, heparin (MW = 20,000 D), which is too large to cross the placenta, is not teratogenic and is consequently the preferred anticoagulant during pregnancy. Most drugs have molecular weights between 250 and 400 D and easily cross the placenta.

Thiopental is highly lipid soluble and crosses the placenta rapidly. Fetal plasma levels reach maternal levels within a few minutes. Muscle relaxants such as vecuronium are more polar and cross the placenta slowly.[57]

Although the state of ionization is a limiting factor for diffusion, some highly charged compounds can diffuse across the placenta. Valproic acid ($pK_a = 4.7$) is nearly completely ionized at physiologic pH, yet there is rapid equilibration across the placental membrane. The small amount of drug that exists in the non-ionized form rapidly crosses the placenta; as equilibrium is reestablished a new small amount of non-ionized drug becomes available for diffusion.[155]

Fetal blood pH changes during gestation. Embryonic intracellular pH is high relative to the pregnant woman. During this developmental stage weak acids would diffuse across the placenta to the embryo and remain there because of "ion trapping." Many teratogens such as valproic acid, trimethadione, phenytoin, thalidomide, warfarin, and isotretinoin are weak acids. Ion trapping does not explain the mechanism of teratogenesis but may explain how the embryo accumulates the toxin. Late in gestation the fetal blood is 0.10–0.15 pH units more acidic than the mother's, suggesting that weakly basic drugs might concentrate in the fetus during this period.[154]

The relative concentrations of protein binding sites in the pregnant woman and fetus also have an impact on the extent of drug transfer to the fetus.[195] When maternal free fatty acid concentrations increase near term, they can displace drugs like valproic acid or diazepam from maternal protein binding sites and make the free drug available for transfer to the fetus. Fetal albumin levels increase during gestation and exceed maternal albumin concentrations at term. Since the fetus does not have high levels of free fatty acids to compete for protein binding sites, these sites are available for binding the drugs. At birth, when neonatal free fatty acid levels increase two- to threefold, they displace stored drug from the binding protein. In the cases of valproic acid and diazepam, the elevated levels of free drug have been shown to have adverse effects on the newborn infant.[73,96,155,172]

The placenta has two other functions that may affect drug presentation to the fetus: ion trapping and drug metabolism. The placenta blocks the transfer of some positively charged ions like cadmium and mercury[84] and may even accumulate them. This barrier does not protect the fetus, however, because these heavy metal ions interfere with normal placental function and may lead to placental necrosis and subsequent fetal death.[147]

The placenta contains drug-metabolizing enzymes capable of performing both phase I and phase II reactions (see Chaps. 11 and 12). However, the concentration of biotransforming enzymes in the placenta is significantly lower than in the liver and it is unlikely that the level of enzymatic activity would be protective for the fetus. Moreover, reactive intermediates that formed during these processes may be presented to the fetus. However, glutathione may also be present in the placenta and may detoxify some of these reactive intermediates.[101]

What Are the Effects of Xenobiotic Agents on the Developing Organism?

One of the basic premises of teratogenicity is that the particular toxic effects of drugs are determined by the organism's stage of development.[23,198] The fertilized ovum is thought to be resistant to toxic insult prior to implantation.[23] However, drugs and chemicals in the fallopian or uterine secretions may prevent implantation of the embryo. Drug exposure leading to cell loss or chromosomal abnormalities may also lead to a spontaneous abortion, possibly even before pregnancy has been detected. If the preimplantation embryo survives a toxic exposure, the functional cells usually proceed to normal development.[198] Teratogens that act in such a manner elicit an "all-or-none response"—the exposed embryo will either die or go on to normal development.

Teratogens behave according to a dose–response curve; as the dose of the teratogen increases, the magnitude of the response increases. For example, in experimental animals, more members of a litter will be malformed by an increased dose, or in the case of the "all or none" more members of a litter may die. However, the dose–response effect does not generally mean that a higher dose will cause worse malformations than a lower dose. Actual teratogenic effects should occur at doses that do not cause maternal toxicity because the development of maternal toxicity itself might be responsible for any observed adverse or teratogenic effects on the developing organism.

Organogenesis occurs during the embryonic stage between days 18 and 60 of gestation. Most gross malformations are determined before day 36, although genitourinary and craniofacial anomalies occur later.[23] The period of susceptibility to teratogenic effects varies for each organ system (Fig. 104–1). For instance, the palate has a very short period of sensitivity, lasting approximately 3 weeks, whereas the central nervous system (CNS) remains susceptible throughout gestation.

Theoretically, knowing the exact time of teratogen exposure during gestation should allow prediction of a teratogenic effect; this is true in animal models where dose and time can be strictly controlled. It is also true for thalidomide, where different limb anomalies are related to exposures on different days.[198] In most clinical situations, relating teratogenicity to a particular drug exposure is difficult because drugs are generally administered intermittently over a period of time or chronically, and also it is often difficult to determine the exact time of exposure relative to conception.

During the fetal period formed organs continue their cellular differentiation and grow to functional maturity. Exposure to toxic agents such as methadone or cigarettes during this period generally leads to growth retardation. Teratogenic malformations or death may still occur due to disruption or destruction of growing

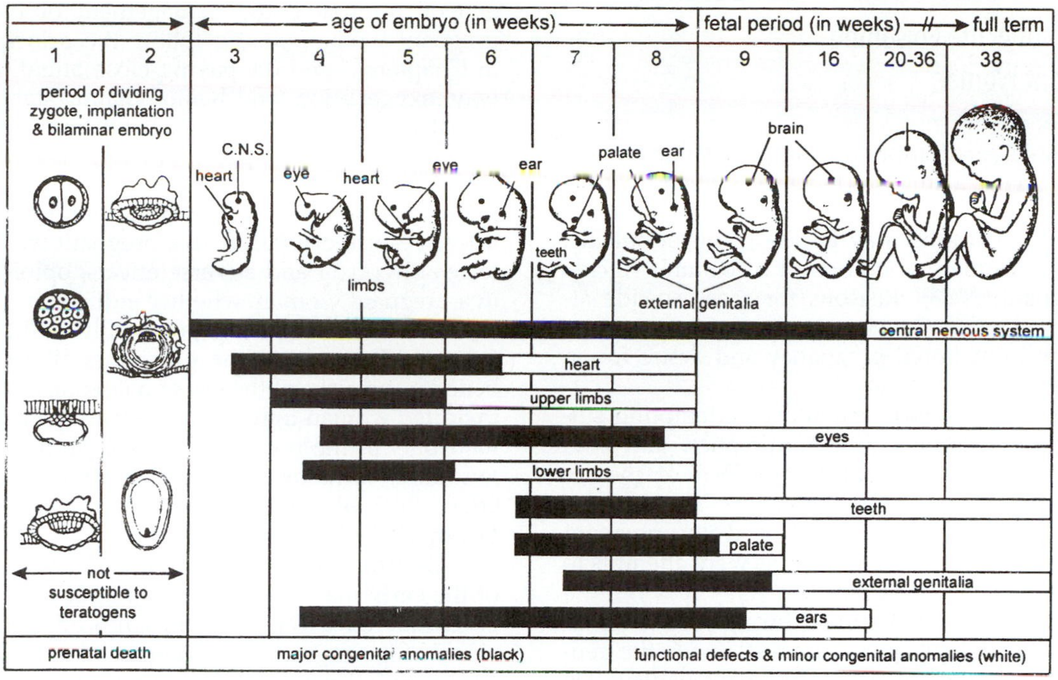

Figure 104–1. Critical periods of fetal development. *(Modified with permission from Moore KL, Persaud TVN: The Developing Human: Clinically Oriented Embryology, 5th ed. Philadelphia: Saunders, 1993.)*

organs, as has been seen with the angiotensin-converting enzyme inhibitors and cocaine.[13]

Another concern during the fetal period is the initiation of carcinogenesis (see Chap. 16). Significant cellular replication and proliferation lead to a dramatic growth in size of the organism. At the same time, development of biotransformation systems may, after the fetus is exposed to xenobiotic agents, expose the organism to reactive metabolites that might initiate tumor formation. Some tumors, like neuroblastoma, appear early in postnatal life, suggesting a prenatal origin. In pregnant rats given ethylnitrosourea during the embryonic period, lethal or teratogenic effects occur.[175] If ethylnitrosourea is administered during the fetal period, there is an increased incidence of tumors in the offspring. Clear cell vaginal and cervical adenocarcinomas are seen in the offspring of women exposed to diethylstilbesterol during pregnancy.[16]

What Are the Mechanisms of Teratogenesis?

Cytotoxicity is one mechanism of teratogenesis and is characteristic of alkylating or antineoplastic agents. Aminopterin, for example, inhibits dihydrofolate reductase activity and leads to suppression of mitosis and cell death. If exposure to a cytotoxic agent occurs very early in development, the embryo may die, whereas sublethal exposure during organogenesis may result in maldevelopment of particular structures. There is evidence that following cell death, the remaining cells in an affected region may try to repair the damage from the missing cellular elements. This "restorative growth" may lead to uncoordinated growth and exacerbate the original malformation.

In the case of the cytotoxic agents, the mechanism of action is understood, although it is not always clear why particular agents affect particular structures. With other agents, the structural effects have a clearer relationship to the site of action. For instance when glucorcorticoids are administered in large doses to experimental animals during the period of organogenesis, malformations of the palate occur. Glucocorticoid receptors are found in high concentrations in the palate of the developing embryo.[168]

Caloric deficiency is not considered teratogenic during the period of organogenesis. However, specific nutritional or vitamin deficiencies such as folate deficiency are teratogenic, at least in animal species. Aminopterin, a folate antagonist, may prevent the transfer of folate to the fetus or antagonize folate function. Alcohol affects the fetus both directly and indirectly. The craniofacial malformations seen in the fetal alcohol syndrome probably result from alcohol effects during the period of organogenesis. Growth retardation may represent direct effects on fetal growth or indirect effects resulting from maternal nutritional deficiencies.

Management of Acute Poisoning in the Pregnant Woman

Suicide and suicide attempts during pregnancy are uncommon. Each year a small number of women die during pregnancy or the postpartum period; 1–5% of these pregnancy-related deaths may be the result of suicide. Two to 12% of women who attempt or commit suicide may be pregnant.[108,162,227] Reasons for these suicide attempts include: loss of a lover, economic crisis, prior loss of children, and unwanted pregnancy and desire for an abortion.[49,125,227]

Ingestion is a common method of attempting suicide. Analgesics, vitamins, iron, antibiotics, and psychotropic medications account for 50–79% of the reported ingestions by pregnant women.[162,169] These agents are regularly prescribed for and used by pregnant women. In one series, 12% of ingestions were attempts to terminate pregnancy[162] (see Chap. 29).

Managing any acute overdose during pregnancy always raises several consequential questions: Is the general management different in the pregnant patient? Do altered metabolism and pharmacokinetics during pregnancy increase (or decrease) the woman's risk of morbidity or mortality from a drug overdose? Is the fetus at risk of intoxication from a maternal intoxication? Is there a teratogenic risk to the fetus from an acute drug overdose or intoxication? Is the use of antidotes contraindicated or modified in the pregnant patient? Should a potentially viable fetus be emergently delivered to prevent toxicity? Should abortion be recommended?

Physiologic changes during pregnancy affect pharmacokinetics, and drugs used in overdoses have altered pharmacokinetics. In any significant overdose during pregnancy, pregnancy-related alterations in pharmacokinetics are not likely to protect the woman from significant morbidity or mortality.

Although a single high-dose exposure to a drug during the period of organogenesis might mimic an experimental model to induce teratogenesis, most commonly ingested drugs do not induce physical deformities. Ethanol and many of the anticonvulsant agents are teratogenic and may be ingested in toxic doses, but their teratogenicity is probably related to chronic exposure. Acute acetaminophen intoxication in the first trimester may lead to an increased risk of spontaneous abortion,[181] suggesting a teratogenic effect similar to the all-or-none response described earlier. There is one report of multiple severe congenital malformations in the stillborn fetus of a woman who overdosed on isoniazid during the 12th week of pregnancy.[123] Since the background incidence of congenital malformations is 3–6%, it is impossible to determine for a single case whether a particular drug exposure is the etiology of any particular malformations.

In general, any condition that leads to a severe metabolic derangement in the pregnant woman is likely to have an adverse impact on the developing fetus. As a general approach, the management of overdose in a pregnant woman should follow the principles outlined in Chapters 3 and 30, paying close attention to the airway, oxygenation, and hemodynamic stability. The use of naloxone and dextrose has not been specifically assessed but should be guided by the same considerations raised in managing a nonpregnant patient with alterations in respiratory or neurologic function. Opioid-induced respiratory failure in a pregnant woman will lead to fetal hypoxia and adverse effects; opioid withdrawal in a pregnant woman, whether induced by abstinence or the use of naloxone, may potentially lead to adverse effects on the fetus or the pregnancy. Evaluation of the benefits and risks of the use of naloxone for an opioid-intoxicated woman in respiratory distress favors the use of naloxone. In the non-apneic comatose pregnant patient, low doses of naloxone, while observing for withdrawal effects, may be beneficial (see Chap. 60 and Antidotes in Depth: Opioid Antagonists).

Gastrointestinal decontamination is frequently part of the early management of acute poisoning. Pregnancy is considered a relative contraindication to the use of syrup of ipecac because it increases intrathoracic and intraabdominal pressure during vomiting; therefore, gastric lavage is a more appropriate method of gastric emptying for the pregnant patient. The usual concerns about protecting the airway apply to the pregnant patient as well.

There is no specific contraindication to the use of activated charcoal in a pregnant woman. There may be a specific role for whole-bowel irrigation in the treatment of iron overdose in pregnancy (see below).

When considering the use of antidotes, the primary concern should be for the health of the pregnant woman. Almost all antidotal agents are categorized as FDA pregnancy-risk Category C; that is, there is little information to guide use. Ethanol is a classified as Category D (positive evidence of risk) although this is related to chronic use throughout pregnancy, not as an antidote. Pyridoxine and thiamine are Category A drugs; *N*-acetylcysteine, magnesium, glucagon, and naloxone are Category B drugs.

There are no reported cases of adverse effects on the fetus by antidotal treatment of a poisoned pregnant woman. Conversely, at least in one case, withholding antidotal therapy may have contributed to both the woman's and the fetus's deaths.[137,208] In the hypothetical case of a pregnant woman poisoned with a toxic alcohol, we would support the use of ethanol until hemodialysis can be performed, although we cannot predict the specific outcome.

Acetaminophen

Acetaminophen is the most common analgesic agent used during pregnancy and is one of the most common agents ingested in overdose during pregnancy.[162,169] Most women recover from acetaminophen ingestion without adverse effects to themselves or their offspring.[30,132,143,181,184,207]

In two large series of acetaminophen overdoses in pregnancy,[143,181] 8 of 33 women who overdosed in the first trimester and continued their pregnancy experienced spontaneous abortions, most within 2 weeks of the ingestion. Six of the 8 had toxic acetaminophen levels; none received *N*-acetylcysteine (NAC) within 8 hours. Five patients with toxic levels delivered healthy term newborns. There is also one case report of a woman in the first trimester who had a toxic acetaminophen level, developed hepatotoxicity, and delivered at 31 weeks gestation.[132]

In the two large series, there were 28 second-trimester ingestions.[143,181] In this group there were two spontaneous abortions, probably not related to the ingestion, and one premature birth in a woman with a nontoxic level. There is one case report of a woman with a toxic level who received NAC and went on to deliver at term.[184] The baby's course was complicated only by hyperbilirubinemia. In another case, the woman had a toxic level and hepatotoxicity.[207] At 41 weeks, labor was induced because of maternal weight loss; the infant was irritable and developed hyperbilirubinemia, both of which resolved after several days of phototherapy.

Several cases of acetaminophen overdose in the third trimester have been reported. In the two series, 5 of 34 women delivered prematurely; 3 of the 5 had toxic acetaminophen levels.[143,181] One of these women developed severe hepatotoxicity and there was evidence of fetal distress. Labor was induced and the child had some transient neonatal problems; no acetaminophen was detected in the cord blood. One other woman in the series delivered a stillborn infant at 33 weeks' gestation, 2 days after a toxic ingestion; the fetal acetaminophen level was 330 μg/mL and the liver showed centrilobular hepatic necrosis.[181] There are also several case reports of third-trimester overdoses. One patient had a toxic acetaminophen level at 29 weeks' gestation and delivered a 1.2-kg infant 16 hours after ingestion; the cord blood acetaminophen level was 76 μg/mL, the baby was treated with exchange transfusions, and hepatotoxicity did not develop.[122] Another woman who had a toxic acetaminophen level at 27–28 weeks' gestation had fetal demise at the time of presentation; the autopsy showed panlobular lysis and the hepatic acetaminophen level was 250 μg/gm.[81] Another woman had a toxic acetaminophen level and severe hepatotoxicity at 32 weeks gestation. There was evidence of fetal distress and 84 hours after the maternal ingestion, labor was induced. The baby had transient hypoglycemia, respiratory distress, and hyperbilirubinemia, all of which could have been related to prematurity or fetal distress. Acetaminophen was not detected in the cord blood.[189] Finally, one woman with a toxic level had labor induced. The infant's Apgar scores were 5 at 1 minute and 7 at 5 minutes. Seventeen hours after ingestion both the woman and the infant had acetaminophen levels of 13 μg/mL and the infant remained asymptomatic.[115]

The ability of the fetal liver to metabolize acetaminophen to an active metabolite through the P450 pathway and detoxify that metabolite with glutathione has been demonstrated in vitro.[186] Fetal P450 activity was only 10% of adult activity and increased with increasing gestational age. This study suggests that the fetus is able to generate the toxic metabolite; the clinical cases suggest that the fetal liver is susceptible to toxicity. Whether a toxic metabolite is the mechanism of toxicity in the first trimester is unknown.

The pregnant patient with an acute toxic acetaminophen ingestion should be treated with *N*-acetylcysteine (see Chap. 31 and Antidotes in Depth: *N*-Acetylcysteine). Whether a "nontoxic" acetaminophen ingestion may still be toxic for the fetus or whether NAC administered to the mother can prevent potential fetal toxicity is unknown. In an ovine model, after a single IV dose, NAC was detected in the fetus at a level only 0–5% of the maternal level.[199] Considering the fact that two cases of fetal demise occurred after third-trimester ingestions, there has been a recommendation to induce delivery so that the neonate may receive antidotal therapy ex utero.[211] In several cases women were delivered emergently,[183,192] but whether this was responsible for good neonatal outcomes is unknown. Similarly, whether exchange transfusion was necessary or responsible for a favorable outcome in two cases where the cord blood acetaminophen level was toxic is un-known.[122,192]

Regardless of the acetaminophen level or development of hepatotoxicity, the pregnant woman may be at risk for spontaneous abortion or premature delivery within days to weeks of the ingestion and should be so cautioned when discharged.

Iron

Iron is another common ingestant during pregnancy; maternal toxicity is generally greater than fetal toxicity. In two reported cases, normal babies were delivered although the mothers died.[160,176] In another case, the mother had severe iron toxicity with acidosis, shock, renal failure, and disseminated intravascular coagulation but was not treated with deferoxamine because of concerns about its teratogenic risks. Instead the mother received an exchange transfusion followed 45 minutes later by a spontaneous abortion of the 16-week fetus.[137,208] Neonatal and cord blood iron levels were not elevated. In several cases pregnant women who had signs and symptoms of iron poisoning and elevated serum iron levels were treated with deferoxamine and delivered normal babies.[18,106,116,170,197,215]

Although the placenta transports iron to the fetus efficiently,[149] the placenta blocks the transfer of large quantities of iron. This is supported by a sheep model of iron poisoning, where only a small amount of iron was transferred across the placenta despite significantly elevated serum iron levels.[48]

Deferoxamine is the antidote for iron poisoning (see Chap. 35 and Antidotes in Depth: Deferoxamine), but it is reported to be an animal teratogen that causes skeletal deformities and abnormalities of ossification (Class C pregnancy risk according to the FDA).[164] A recent animal model observed similar effects, but only with doses of deferoxamine that caused maternal toxicity.[22] Experimentally, little transfer of deferoxamine across the placenta has been demonstrated;[48] therefore, the reported fetal effects may be secondary to chelation of essential nutrients (such as trace metals) on the maternal side of the placenta.[211]

In clinical case reports of iron overdose for which deferoxamine was used, there have been no adverse effects on the fetus, although most have been second-[106,197] or third-trimester poisonings.[18,106,116,160,170,215] In one case series of 49 patients with iron poisoning during pregnancy, 25 received deferoxamine.[142] Only one woman who received deferoxamine in the first trimester continued her pregnancy to term; she had a normal infant. One woman who recived deferoxamine at 20 weeks had a premature delivery at 24 weeks, and one other woman who received deferoxamine at 30 weeks delivered a baby at term with webbed fingers, a malformation felt to be unrelated to the intoxication or the therapy.

In support of the safety of deferoxamine in pregnancy is the fact that it has been administered without adverse effects to pregnant women with thalassemia, as part of the therapy for posttransfusion iron overload.[41,139,213,218]

Deferoxamine is probably safe for use in pregnant women. Considering the potentially fatal nature of a significant iron intoxication, deferoxamine should be administered to pregnant women with signs and symptoms of significant iron poisoning.

Serious iron intoxication is also probably one of the few specific indications for whole-bowel irrigation because iron is not adsorbed to activated charcoal (see Antidotes in Depth: Activated Charcoal). Return of pill fragments has been achieved in a pregnant woman with whole-bowel irrigation.[216]

Carbon Monoxide

Carbon monoxide is the leading cause of poisoning fatalities. In contrast to iron and most other drugs and toxins, the fetus may be at greater risk of toxicity from carbon monoxide than is the pregnant woman. There are reports of maternal and fetal deaths, maternal survival and fetal deaths, and maternal and fetal survival with adverse neonatal outcomes, primarily brain damage resembling that seen following severe cerebral ischemia.[31,47,113,130,138,151,159,230] Similar clinical effects have also been observed in animal models.[56,75,131]

The case literature suggests increased risk of poor fetal outcome with clinically severe maternal intoxication or significantly elevated carboxyhemoglobin level.[113,159] Women with minimal symptoms and/or low levels of carboxyhemoglobin have a low risk of fetal toxicity[113] but a lower limit of effects has not been specifically defined.

In animal models, under physiologic conditions the fetus has a carboxyhemoglobin concentration 10–15% higher than the mother. After exposure to carbon monoxide, the fetus achieves peak carboxyhemoglobin levels 58% higher than those achieved by the mother at steady state, and the time to peak level is also delayed compared to the mother. Similarly, the elimination of carbon monoxide occurs more slowly in the fetus than in the mother.[87,130,131] One case report describes such a phenomenon where, after 1 hour of supplemental oxygen, the maternal carboxyhemoglobin was 7% and the corrected fetal carboxyhemoglobin was 61% at the time of death in utero.[63]

Carbon monoxide leads to fetal hypoxia by several mechanisms: (1) maternal carboxyhemoglobin leads to a decrease in the oxygen content of maternal blood, and therefore less oxygen is delivered across the placenta to the fetus, which normally has an arterial PO_2 of only 20–30 mm Hg; (2) fetal carboxyhemoglobin causes a decrease in fetal PO_2; (3) carbon monoxide shifts the oxyhemoglobin dissociation curve to the left and decreases the release of oxygen to the fetal tissues (an exacerbation of the physiologic left shift found with normal fetal hemoglobin); and (4) carbon monoxide may inhibit cytochrome oxidase or other mitochondrial functions.[130,131,165]

The treatment for severe carbon monoxide poisoning is hyperbaric oxygen therapy (HBO) (see Chap. 96 and Antidotes in Depth: Hyperbaric Oxygen). Questions have been raised about the use of HBO in pregnant women because animal models suggested adverse effects of HBO on the embryo or fetus.[64,146,195,210] The applicability of the animal models to humans is difficult to assess; many of the animal models employed hyperbaric conditions of greater pressures and duration than those clinically employed for humans.

HBO has been used clinically for carbon monoxide poisoning in pregnancy with good results, although there are limited data on the long-term follow-up of the children.[28,63,70,88,113,217] One large series reported 44 women who were exposed to carbon monoxide during pregnancy and were treated with hyperbaric oxygen regardless of clinical severity or gestational age—33 had term births, 1 had a premature delivery (22 weeks after HBO in the context of maternal fever), 2 had spontaneous miscarriages (12 hours after severe intoxication and 15 days after mild intoxication), 1 delivered a child with Down's syndrome, 1 had an elective abortion, and 6 were lost to follow-up.[62] Unfortunately, the information regarding trimester of exposure, maternal carboxyhemoglobin level, and severity of symptoms is not detailed with regard to outcome. Although HBO is probably safe for pregnant women and presents little risk to the fetus, it is not clear whether HBO prevents carbon monoxide–related fetal toxicity for those at risk.

Carbon monoxide can have a severe impact on fetal health and development, and the maternal carboxyhemoglobin level may not accurately reflect the fetal carboxyhemoglobin level. Hyperbaric oxygen should therefore be considered for any pregnant women exposed to carbon monoxide, especially for women with an elevated carboxyhemoglobin level or any evidence of fetal distress. If hyperbaric oxygen therapy is not available, 100% oxygen should be administered to the mother for a period of time five times longer than the time needed for the maternal carboxyhemoglobin to return to the normal range.

What Are Some of the Toxicologic Problems in the Perinatal Period?

As many as 8% of all drug doses administered in neonatal intensive care units (NICU) are either 10 times greater or less than the dose ordered.[152] As many as 30% of newborns in NICUs may sustain adverse drug reactions, some of which may be life-threatening or fatal.[8] Physiologic differences between adults and newborn infants affect drug absorption, distribution, and metabolism;[153,171] these pharmacokinetic differences account for some cases of drug toxicity seen in the newborn infant.

Gastrointestinal (GI) absorption of drugs in the neonate is generally slower than in adults.[153,171] This delay may be related to decreased gastric acid secretion, decreased gastric emptying and transit time, and decreased pancreatic enzyme activity. The GI environment of the newborn and young infant has been postulated as one mechanism for the growth of *Clostridium botulinum* and the subsequent development of infantile botulism (see Chap. 73). Infantile botulism has been reported in infants within several weeks of birth.[92,212]

Cutaneous absorption of drugs may pose a risk for toxic exposure to the newborn.[61,193] Aniline dyes used for marking diapers have been absorbed, causing methemoglobinemia;[193] contaminated diapers were also responsible for an epidemic of mercury poisoning.[10] The absorption of hexachlorophene antiseptic wash led to neurotoxicity; marked vacuolization of myelin was seen microscopically.[119,141,203] Antiseptic ethyl alcohol has caused hemorrhagic necrosis of the skin of some premature infants. Iodine antiseptics have led to hypothyroidism in mature newborns.[32] An increased potential for absorption and toxicity has been seen following the dermal use of corticosteroids[71,191] and boric acid in children with cutaneous disorders.[60]

Other routes of exposure have led to clinical poisoning. Talcum powder has been responsible for several cases of aspiration and death.[27,150] Inhalation of mercury from incubator thermometers may be a potential risk.[5] One death has been reported following the ophthalmic instillation of cyclopentalate hydrochloride.[12]

Because of differences in total body water and fat compared to the adult, the distribution of absorbed drugs may differ in neonates. Water represents 80% of body weight in a full-term baby and 60% in an adult. About 20% of a term baby's body weight is fat, versus only 3% in a premature baby. The increased volume of water means that the volume of distribution for some water-soluble drugs, such as theophylline or phenobarbital, is increased.

Protein binding of drugs is decreased in newborns compared to adults: The concentration of proteins is lower, there are fewer receptor sites that become saturated at lower drug concentrations, and binding sites have decreased binding affinity.[171] Protein binding has potential relevance with respect to bilirubin, an endogenous metabolite that at very high concentrations can cause kernicterus; bilirubin competes with exogenously administered drugs for protein-binding sites. In vitro, certain drugs such as sulfonamides and ceftriaxone displace bilirubin from protein-receptor sites; this may increase the risk of kernicterus, although this has not been clinically demonstrated. Conversely, bilirubin, with its strong affinity for these protein-binding sites, may displace drugs such as phenobarbital or phenytoin, leading to increased plasma drug levels.

Newborn infants have decreased hepatic metabolic capacity compared to adults, and this may lead to drug toxicity. For instance, the newborn has limited ability to oxidize drugs, so theophylline is metabolized primarily to the active metabolite caffeine instead of methylxanthine and 1,3-dimethyluric acid, which are the primary inactive metabolites in the adult. In addition, immaturity of the P450 system leads to increased elimination half-lives of drugs such as phenytoin, phenobarbital, and theophylline.

The deficiency of glucuronidation is responsible for the "gray-baby syndrome" following high doses of chloramphenicol.[89] More recently, "gasping-baby syndrome" (gasping respirations, metabolic acidosis, hypotension, central nervous system depression, convulsions, renal failure, and occasionally death) was attributed to high concentrations of benzyl alcohol and benzoic acid in the plasma of affected infants.[6,29,72] Benzyl alcohol, a bacteriostatic agent, was added to intravenous flush solutions and accumulated in newborns after repetitive doses. The high concentrations of benzoic acid could not be further metabolized to hippuric acid by the immature liver (see Chaps. 54 and 105).

The umbilical vessels are a common site of vascular access in sick neonates. Because blood drains into the portal vein, it is possible that IV medications experience a "first-pass" effect, although whether this route of drug administration affects drug metabolism or clearance has not been well studied.

Most renal functions, including glomerular filtration rate and tubular secretion, are relatively immature at birth;[97] a newborn's glomerular filtration rate is approximately 30% of that of an adult. Drugs such as aminoglycoside antibiotics and digoxin are excreted unchanged by the kidney and therefore depend on glomerular filtration for clearance. Dosing of these agents in the the newborn must account for these differences.

Very little information is available to guide the clinician as to the management of drug poisoning in the newborn infant. Cutaneous absorption is probably already complete by the time toxicity is noted, although further exposure may be prevented. Gastrointestinal decontamination is not generally performed in neonates; syrup of ipecac is contraindicated and lavage or catharsis would probably lead to fluid, electrolyte, and thermoregulatory problems. Multiple-dose activated charcoal has been used in a 1.4-kg 2-week-old premature infant to treat theophylline poisoning.[200] Hemodialysis, hemoperfusion, and exchange transfusion have been used in neonates to treat drug toxicity (see Chaps. 5 and 105).

Substance Abuse in Pregnancy

One of the most complex areas of toxicology deals with the effects of substance abuse in pregnancy and whether that substance abuse has specific adverse effects during the pregnancy as well as on fetal and postnatal development. In this section we will briefly review some of the important aspects of this special topic.

Clinical research in the area of substance abuse in pregnancy is very difficult to perform. As an example, with the increased use of cocaine during the latter half of the 1980s and the first half of the 1990s, there was great interest in determining the effects of cocaine use during pregnancy. As research in this area is reviewed and evaluated, many of the critical methodologic issues related to substance abuse research have also been highlighted.[66,93,124,133,157,233]

Substance-abusing women have multiple risk factors for adverse pregnancy outcomes such as low socioeconomic status, polysubstance use, alcohol and cigarette use, sexually transmitted diseases, malnutrition, and lack of prenatal care. For instance, lack of prenatal care is highly associated with premature birth; smoking is highly associated with spontaneous abortion, growth retardation, and sudden infant death syndrome (SIDS).[105] Other factors not specifically related to substance use also have an effect on pregnancy outcome such as age, race, gravidity, and prior pregnancy outcome. Each of these factors represents a significant potential confounding variable when evaluating the effects of a particular agent such as cocaine or marijuana during pregnancy and must be controlled for in the research design.

There may be bias in the selection of study subjects. For example, if all the patients are selected from an inner-city hospital obstetric service, there is potential for overestimating the effects of the substance being studied. If cohorts are followed over a long period of time, there are frequently study subjects who fail to follow up. Are the ones who continue more motivated or do they have more problems that need attention?

Similarly, categorizing patients into substance use groups is difficult. Self-reporting of substance abuse is frequently unreliable or inaccurate, making determinations about the nature, quantity, or timing of drug use difficult. Consequently, there may be no real drug-free control groups, or patients using different drugs may be grouped together. Also any substance-abusing person is likely to be be abusing multiple substances, making categorization difficult.

When urine drug screens are used to identify drug-users, there is a high probability of false negatives because drug screens reflect only recent use. This factor is particularly important, because drug use decreases later in pregnancy and a negative urine screen may fail to identify a woman who was using drugs early in pregnancy. Testing for drugs in hair or meconium may improve the accuracy of the analysis for the entire pregnancy.[110]

Another bias involves selection of infants who are exposed to substances. Evaluating newborns who are "at-risk," show signs of "withdrawal," or have positive urine drug screens will miss some exposed infants. When research concerns the neurobehavioral development of children exposed in utero to substances, it is important the the examiners performing the evaluation be blinded to the infants' drug exposure category.

Finally, there may be a bias against publishing research that shows a negative or "not significant" effect.[112]

Alcohol

Alcohol use during pregnancy produces a constellation of fetal effects. The most severe effects are seen in the fetal alcohol syndrome (FAS), characterized by intrauterine or postnatal growth retardation, facial dysmorphogenesis, particularly microcephaly, short palpebral fissures, epicanthal folds, maxillary hypoplasia, cleft palate, hypoplastic philtrum, micrognathia, and mental retardation or behavioral abnormalities.[99] These effects are seen after consumption of the equivalent of 2–3 ounces of absolute ethanol (four to six drinks of hard liquor) per day throughout pregnancy or with frequent binge drinking.[205] The craniofacial effects probably represent early teratogenic effects on the embryo, whereas the central nervous system abnormalities and growth retardation may result from adverse effects later in gestation. Less severe effects such as milder forms of mental retardation or growth delay are termed fetal alcohol effects.

As many as 20% of women may consume some alcohol during pregnancy;[156] only 1–2% consume four or more drinks each day. The incidence of FAS is 1 per 1000 live births; 4% of women who drink heavily may give birth to children with FAS.[2] This means that several hundred children with fetal alcohol syndrome and several thousand with fetal alcohol effects will be born each year; alcohol use is considered the leading preventable cause of mental retardation in this country.[43] Although the primary determinant of fetal alcohol syndrome or effects is the level of maternal alcohol consumption, there is some evidence that paternal alcohol exposure may play a contributing role.[1]

Other effects of alcohol use during pregnancy may include an increased incidence of spontaneous abortion, premature deliveries, and stillbirths,[46,128] neonatal alcohol withdrawal,[15] and possibly carcinogenesis.[107] Infants may be irritable or hypertonic and may have problems with habituation and arousal. Long-term behavioral and intellectual effects include cognitive deficits, with decreased IQ, problems with attention, memory, and speech, hyperactivity, and dysfunctional behavior in school.[43]

The exact mechanism of these alcohol-induced effects is unknown. Possibilities include direct or indirect toxicity of ethanol or its metabolite acetaldehyde, via complex interactions with neuronal and nonneuronal brain elements and/or modulation of neurotransmitters.[174,226] One model proposes that sociobehavioral risk factors, such as drinking behavior, smoking behavior, low socioeconomic status, and cultural/ethnic influences create provocative biologic conditions such as high peak blood alcohol levels, circulating tobacco constituents, and undernutrition. These provocative factors exacerbate fetal vulnerability to alcohol-related hypoxia and free radical–induced cell damage.[3]

TABLE 104–5. SIGNS AND SYMPTOMS OF OPIOID WITHDRAWAL

W—wakefulness
I—irritability
T—tremulousness, temperature variation, and tachypnea
H—hyperactivity, high-pitched persistent cry, hyperacusis, hyperreflexia, and hypertonicity
D—diarrhea, diaphoresis, and disorganized suck
R—rub-and-scratch marks, respiratory distress, and rhinorrhea
A—apneic episodes and autonomic dysfunction
W—weight loss or failure to gain weight
A—alkalosis (respiratory)
L—lacrimation

Reprinted, with permission, from the Committee on Drugs: Neonatal drug withdrawal. Pediatrics 1983;72:895–902.

Opioids

Opioid addiction remains a significant cause of both maternal and neonatal morbidity. It is estimated that 0.2% of pregnant women use heroin or methadone[156] and up to 75,000 babies per year may be exposed to opioids in utero.[77] Pregnant opioid users have an increased risk of many medical complications of pregnancy such as hepatitis, sepsis, endocarditis, sexually transmitted diseases, and AIDS and may have an increased risk of obstetric complications such as miscarriage, premature delivery, or stillbirth.[66,76] Some of the obstetric complications may be related to associated risk factors in addition to the opioid use.

The most well-defined fetal effects are on growth.[76,233] Pregnant opioid users give birth to an increased frequency of infants with low birth weights compared to non-drug-using controls; the greatest effect is seen with heroin. Most of the infants are small for gestational age. The effect of methadone is considered to be intermediate. Women who receive low-dose methadone and good prenatal care have birth outcomes similar to nonaddicted controls, although even methadone-maintained women have a higher incidence of pregnancy-related complications than nonaddicted controls.[66]

The most significant acute neonatal complication of opioid use during pregnancy is the neonatal withdrawal syndrome (NWS), characterized by hyperirritability, GI dysfunction, respiratory distress, and vague autonomic symptoms including yawning, sneezing, mottling, and fever.[15,66] Myoclonic jerks or seizures may also signify neurologic irritability. These infants are recognizable by their extreme jitteriness, despite efforts at consolation; ecchymoses and contusions may be found on the tips of their fingers or toes from repeated trauma on the sides of the bassinet. The features of NWS are described by the mnemonic WITHDRAWAL[45] (Table 104–5). Sixty to 90% of opioid exposed offspring will show some signs of withdrawal.[66]

Some of the manifestations of the neonatal withdrawal syndrome may be due to enhanced alpha-adrenergic activity in the locus ceruleus. Firing of neurons in this region of the brain leads to NWS-like behaviors such as wakefulness and tremors; these effects are inhibited by opioid agonists. Chronic opioid administration leads to tolerance as well as an increased number of alpha$_2$-adrenergic receptors. Presumably, withdrawal of opioids causes increased stimulation of a large number of receptors in this region, leading to clinical signs of withdrawal.[15]

Withdrawal symptoms usually occur within 2 weeks of birth. Heroin withdrawal usually occurs within the first 24 hours, although methadone may cause delayed withdrawal because it has a larger volume of distribution and slower metabolism in the neonate. Withdrawal from methadone occurs when the plasma level falls below 0.06 μg/mL.[187] The time of onset and severity of symptoms may be related to whether heroin, methadone, or both were used, how much was used chronically, how much was used near the time of delivery, the character of the labor and whether analgesic or anesthetic agents were used, and the maturity, nutrition, and medical condition of the neonate.[51] The acute symptoms generally last from days to weeks but may persist for months.[15,66]

Five to 7% of babies with signs of withdrawal develop seizures, generally by 10 days after birth.[85] Seizures may be more likely after methadone than after heroin withdrawal.[232] These seizures do not necessarily imply an underlying chronic seizure disorder; in one small study, children who had withdrawal seizures were normal at a one-year follow-up.[53]

Treatment of withdrawal begins by providing a comforting environment: swaddling or tightly wrapping the infant, minimal handling or stimulation, and demand feeding. More severe symptoms may require pharmacologic therapy. One way of determining the need for therapy is based on a severity scoring scale.[65] In general, if babies are having feeding difficulties, diarrhea, significant tremors, or irritability or are crying continuously, they are candidates for pharmacologic therapy.[102]

Opioid agonists such as tincture of opium or paregoric and sedative-hypnotic agents have been used for treatment of withdrawal symptoms. Opioid agonists may be more effective at preventing withdrawal seizures from heroin or methadone than phenobarbital or diazepam.[85,103] Because sedative-hypnotic agents are commonly abused by heroin abusers or adults maintained on methadone, sedative-hypnotic withdrawal seizures may contribute to the overall abstinence symptomatology. In this setting there may be a role for phenobarbital. One of the problems with phenobarbital may be that oral dosing may lead to a delay in achieving a therapeutic level.[15,102]

Infants of opioid-using mothers are at increased risk for SIDS compared to controls.[102] The relative risk is 3.6 for methadone and 2.3 for heroin. The mechanism may be related to a decreased medullary responsiveness to CO_2 or the effect may be related to some condition of the postnatal environment.[104,219]

Although young children born to opioid users do not seem to have significant differences in behavior compared to controls, older children have increased learning problems and school dysfunction particularly related to behavior difficulties.[233]

Cocaine

Approximately 1% of pregnant women in the United States use cocaine sometime during their pregnancy.[156] The rate may be as high as 15% in certain populations,[50] and it is estimated that more than 100,000 infants born in the United States each year may be exposed to cocaine in utero.[33] The consequences of cocaine abuse during pregnancy have been extensively reviewed.[90,93,167,179]

The most commonly reported obstetric complications of gestational cocaine use are increased rates of abruptio placenta, premature delivery, and intrauterine growth retardation. Other significant perinatal effects include seizures, cerebral infarctions, and other CNS effects.[34,54,55,68,78,114] A recent meta-analysis of studies published before 1989 concluded that adverse effects on head circumference, gestational age, and birth weight were related to polysubstance abuse, but the effects could not be attributed specifically to cocaine.[133] In this analysis, no increased risk of abruptio placenta was demonstrated. However, some more recent work, which included control groups, suggests that there are significant effects on intrauterine growth and prematurity.[36,40,44,74,82,109,158,163,234] The incidence of abruptio placenta may be significant when related to acute use.[202] Most of these studies did not control for smoking and alcohol use. However, it seems that good prenatal care can mitigate many of the adverse effects.[134,178,234]

There have been reports of significant congenital malformations among infants who had been exposed to cocaine in utero, specifically genitourinary malformations,[35,38,188] cardiovascular malformations,[17,91,126,129] and limb-reduction defects.[91] Other researchers have not observed significant malformations.[39,74,80] In one large population-based study, there was no increase in the incidence of malformations.[140]

Animal models have also identified teratogenic effects of in utero cocaine exposure. Decreased maternal and fetal weight gain and an increased frequency of fetal resorption were demonstrated in rats;[62] sporadic physical anomalies have also been observed.[42] Teratogenic effects similar to those observed in humans have been reported in mice: bony defects of the skull, cryptorchidism, hydronephrosis, ileal atresia, cardiac defects, limb deformities, and eye abnormalities.[67,127,135,136,144] Cocaine has been observed to cause hemorrhage, edema, and subsequently limb-reduction defects in rats when administered during midgestation in the postorganogenic period.[222]

The perinatal effects of cocaine are probably mediated through a vascular mechanism. Cocaine administration to the pregnant ewe causes increased uterine vascular resistance, decreased uterine blood flow, increased fetal heart rate and arterial blood pressure, and decreased fetal PO_2 and O_2 content.[148,228,229] The fetal hypoxia may cause rupture of fetal blood vessels and infarction in developing organ systems such as the the genitourinary system[38,144,204] or the CNS;[34,52,223] hyperpyrexia or direct effects of cocaine in the fetus may exacerbate these effects.[24] Limb-reduction defects similar to those attributed to cocaine have been produced after clamping of the uterine vessels.[24,224]

Despite the reported malformations and a possible mechanism, neither the human epidemiology nor effects observed in animal models have identified a specific teratogenic syndrome. The risk of a significant malformation from prenatal cocaine exposure is low, but the effect, if one occurs, may be severe.[23,58]

The effects of intrauterine exposure to cocaine on neonatal, infant, and child development are not clear.[177] Initial reports described many abnormal newborn behaviors such as increased irritability and abnormal "state" functions (the ability to respond appropriately to external auditory or verbal stimuli).[59] Several controlled studies, however, failed to find significant differences in infant behaviors when evaluated with standard tests.[36,43,158,178] In one cohort of children evaluated at 3 years of age, there was no significant diffference on global measures of intellectual development between cocaine/polydrug-exposed children and nonexposed controls.[79] However, the cocaine/polydrug group did score lower on verbal-reasoning tasks. The effect of substance abuse on behavior and intellectual function becomes more difficult to evaluate as children grow older and effects of the environment have greater influence. At the same time it is possible that as children grow and are presented with more complex tasks, subtle prenatally induced neurobehavioral deficits may become apparent. Current standardized evaluation instruments may not be sensitive enough to ascertain the deficits; therefore, animal models to determine these effects are being designed.[58,206]

Breast-Feeding

Breast-feeding has become the recommended method of infant nutrition because it offers nutritional, immunologic, and psychological benefits. Many breast-feeding women may need to use prescription and nonprescription medications. Thus, along with the increase in the prevalence of breast-feeding has come concern about the possible ill effects of chemicals in the breast milk on the infant. This concern has extended to the possible exposure through breast milk to occupational and environmental chemicals.[185] The response to these concerns is determined by the answer to this question, does the risk to an infant from a chemical exposure via breast milk exceed the benefit of being breast-fed?[121]

Pharmacokinetic factors determine the extent of drug available for transfer from maternal plasma into breast milk; only free drug can traverse the mammary alveolar membrane. Most drugs are transported by passive diffusion. A few drugs, such as alcohol and lithium, are transported through aqueous-filled pores. The factors that determine how well a chemical diffuses across the membrane are similar to those for other biologic membranes like the placenta: molecular weight, lipid solubility, and degree of ionization.

Large-molecular-weight compounds, such as heparin or insulin, will not pass into breast milk. Lipid solubility is important not only for diffusion but for drug accumulation in breast milk, since milk is rich in fat, especially milk that is produced in the postcolostral period (3–4 days postpartum).

With a pH near 7.0, breast milk is slightly more acidic than plasma. Weak acids will exist to a larger extent as ionized molecules in the plasma and will not be as available for transport into milk. Weak bases will exist to a larger extent as non-ionized molecules in the plasma and will be available for transport into milk, where they will be ion-trapped. In other words, weak bases may concentrate in breast milk. Sulfacetamide (pK_a 5.4) has a concentration in plasma 10 times that in breast milk, whereas sulfanilamide (pK_a 10.4) is found in equal concentrations in both plasma and breast milk.

The net effect of these physiologic processes is expressed in the milk/plasma (M/P) drug ratio. Drugs with higher M/P ratios have greater concentration into breast milk. The milk/plasma ratio does not reflect the actual concentration of a drug in the breast milk. A drug with a high milk/plasma ratio is not necessarily found at high concentration in the breast milk. Morphine has an M/P ratio of 2.46 (is concentrated in milk), but only 0.4% of a maternal dose is excreted into the breast milk.[9] About 1–2% of a maternally administered drug dose is generally presented to the infant in breast milk.[121]

The M/P ratio has several limitations. It does not take into account differences in drug concentration that may result from: (1) repeat or chronic dosing, (2) breast-feeding at different times relative to maternal drug dosing, (3) differences in milk production during the day or even during a particular breast-feeding session, (4) the time postpartum (days, weeks, or months) when the measurement is made, or (5) maternal disease.

A spot breast milk drug concentration or a concentration estimate based on the M/P ratio allows an estimation of the quantity of drug to which an infant is exposed, assuming a constant breast-milk concentration:

$$\text{Infant Dose} = \text{Breast-Milk Concentration} \times \text{Amount Consumed}$$

The effect of this dose on the infant depends on the bioavailability of drug in breast milk, the pharmacokinetic parameters that determine drug levels in the infant, and the infant's receptor sensitivity to the drug. These parameters are often different in neonates than in adults and may lead to drug accumulation; absorption is generally greater while metabolism and clearance are generally reduced. These effects are exaggerated in premature infants (see above).[171,182] Nonetheless, the amount of most drugs delivered to infants in breast milk can probably be adequately metabolized and eliminated.[182]

Many of the considerations above are theoretical. Published guidelines about the advisability of breast-feeding during periods of maternal drug therapy are generally based on expected effects of full doses in the infant or on case reports of adverse occurrences. For this reason, the number of specifically contraindicated drugs is quite small. The recommendations of the American Academy of Pediatrics (AAP) are shown in Table 104–6. The AAP considers substance abuse a contraindication to breast-feeding, because of adverse effects on the baby as well as detrimental effects on the physical and emotional health of the mother. Although ethanol is not specifically contraindicated for the breast-feeding mother, adverse effects are noted with maternal consumption of large amounts.

The AAP recommends the temporary cessation of breast-feeding when the mother is exposed to metronidazole, an in vitro mutagen, and certain radiopharmaceuticals, specifically isotopes of copper, gallium, indium, iodine, sodium, and technetium. In these cases breast milk can be collected and stored prior to medication use for later feeding to the baby. Breast feeding is resumed when the milk is no longer radioactive, generally 1–3 days for most of the isotopes mentioned except gallium, in which radioactivity may be present for 2 weeks.

TABLE 104–6. DRUGS AND TOXINS THAT ARE CONTRAINDICATED DURING BREAST-FEEDING

Drug/Toxin	Effect
Bromocriptine	Suppresses lactation
Cyclophosphamide Cyclosporine Doxorubicin Methotrexate	Possible immune suppression, unknown effect on growth or association with carcinogenesis
Ergotamine	Vomiting, diarrhea, seizures
Lithium	Subtherapeutic levels in infant
Phenindione	Increased prothombin and partial thromboplastin time
Amphetamine Cocaine Phencyclidine Heroin Marijuana	Intoxication
Nicotine	Vomiting, diarrhea, tachycardia, shock, restlessness, decreased milk production

Adapted, with permission, from American Academy of Pediatrics Committee on Drugs: Transfer of drugs and other chemicals into human milk. Pediatrics 1994;93:137–150.

Although there are no data to specifically suggest any ill effects, the AAP suggests caution with regard to breast-feeding during the use of sedative-hypnotic, antidepressant, and neuroleptic medications. These medications modulate neurotransmitters in the central nervous system, and there is concern that these agents may have an adverse effect on the developing nervous system.

Other drugs as well as foods and environmental agents that have been found in breast milk and where some effects have been noted are listed in Table 104–7. The AAP considers some of these effects to militate against the use of the drug if possible in breast-feeding mothers, while for the others, the effects are not considered a contraindication to breast-feeding. In addition to these listed effects, there may be a small increased risk of carcinogenicity associated with exposure to some of these environmental agents through breast milk.[185]

Most pharmaceuticals do not require cessation of breast-feeding, although "compatibility" with breast-feeding is generally based on the lack of reported adverse effects, which may reflect a limited clinical experience and study of breast-feeding patients. Every exposure to a drug must be regarded as a small potential risk, and the infant should receive appropriate medical follow-up. Not all "compatible" drugs are safe in all situations. For instance, phenobarbital can produce CNS depression in the infant if the mother's serum level is in the high therapeutic or supratherapeutic range, which often occurs while dosage adjustments are being made. Such a level may or may not produce CNS depression in the mother. Nalidixic acid, nitrofurantoin, sulfapyridine, and sulfisoxazole can cause hemolysis in a breast-fed infant with glucose-6-phosphate dehydrogenase deficiency.

Decisions on breast-feeding should be made with the informed involvement of the woman, her physicians, and, when necessary, a consultant with special expertise in this field. Guidelines may be obtained from several sources.[7,26,180]

Summary

The use of medications and chemicals in the pregnant or breast-feeding woman is a complex area of medical prac-

TABLE 104–7. DRUGS, FOODS, AND ENVIRONMENTAL AGENTS THAT HAVE BEEN ASSOCIATED WITH EFFECTS ON SOME NURSING INFANTS

Use with Caution when Breast-feeding	
Drug	***Effect Described in Literature***
Aspirin	Metabolic acidosis; may affect platelet function; rash
Clemastine	Drowsiness, irritability, refusal to feed, high-pitched cry, meningismus
5-Amino salicylic acid	Diarrhea
Atenolol	Hypotension, bradycardia, cyanosis
Acebutalol	Hypotension, bradycardia, tachypnea
Phenobarbital	Sedation, infantile spasms after weaning from phenobarbital-containing milk, methemoglobinemia
Primidone	Sedation, feeding problems
Sulfisoxazole	Caution in infant with jaundice or G-6-PD deficiency, and ill, stressed, or premature infant
Sulfapyridine	Caution in infant with jaundice or G-6-PD deficiency, and ill, stressed, or premature infant
Sulfasalazine	Bloody diarrhea

Maternal Medication Usually Compatible With Breast Feeding	
Drug	***Effect Described in Literature***
Ethanol	Large doses: decreased milk ejection reflex. Infant: drowsinesss, diaphoresis, decreased growth and weight gain
Bendroflumethazide	Suppresses lactation
Bromide	Rash, weakness, absence of cry
Caffeine	Irritability, poor sleeping pattern (no effect with usual amount of caffeinated beverages)
Carbimazole	Goiter
Chloral hydrate	Sleepiness
Contraceptive pills with estrogen/ progesterone	Rare breast enlargement; decrease in milk production and protein content (not confirmed in several studies)
Danthron	Increased bowel activity
Dexbrompheniramine maleate with *d*-isoephedrine	Crying, irritability, poor sleeping pattern
Estradiol	Withdrawal vaginal bleeding
Indomethacin	Seizure
Iodine, topical	Odor of iodine on infant's skin
Iodine	Goiter
Methaprylon	Drowsiness
Nalidixic acid	Hemolysis in infant with G-6-PD deficiency
Phenytoin	Methemoglobinemia
Theophylline	Irritability

Effects of Food and Environmental Agents on Breast-feeding	
Agent	***Effect Described in Literature***
Aspartame	Caution if mother or infant has phenylketonuria
Chocolate (theobromine)	Irritability or increased bowel activity if mother consumes large amounts
Fava beans	Hemolysis in infant with G-6-PD deficiency
Hexachlorobenzene	Skin rash, diarrhea, vomiting, dark urine, neurotoxicity, death
Lead	Possible neurotoxicity
Methylmercury, mercury	Possible neurodevelopmental toxicity
Polyhalogenated biphenyls	Lack of endurance, hypotonia, sullen expressionless facies
Tetrachloroethylene	Obstructive jaundice, dark urine
Vegetarian diet	B_{12} deficiency

Adapted, with permission, from American Academy of Pediatrics Committee on Drugs: The transfer of drugs and other chemicals into human milk. Pediatrics 1994; 93:137–150.

tice and presents the clinician with potentially difficult management decisions. The previous discussion has highlighted some of the important principles of drug effects in both the pregnant woman and the fetus. Appropriate management of many of the potential problems will be facilitated by a coordinated effort of obstetricians, perinatologists, neonatologists, pediatricians, and toxicologists.

References

1. Abel EL: Paternal exposure to alcohol. In: Sonderegger TB, ed: Perinatal Substance Abuse: Research Findings and Clinical Implications. Baltimore, The Johns Hopkins University Press, 1992, pp. 132–160.
2. Abel EL: An update on incidence of FAS: FAS is not an equal opportunity birth defect. Neurotoxicol Teratol 1995; 17:437–443.
3. Abel EL, Hannigan JH: Maternal risk factors in fetal alcohol syndrome: Provocative and permissive influences. Neurotoxicol Teratol 1995;17:445–462.
4. Abel EL, Sokol RJ: Incidence of fetal alcohol syndrome and impact of FAS-related anomalies. Drug Alcohol Depend 1987;19:51–70.
5. American Academy of Pediatrics: Mercury vapor contamination of infant incubators: A potential hazard. Pediatrics 1984;67:637.
6. American Academy of Pediatrics: Benzyl alcohol: Toxic agent in neonatal units. Pediatrics 1983;72:356–358.
7. Anderson PO: Therapy review: Drug use during breast feeding. Clin Pharm 1991;10:594–624.
8. Aranda JV, Portuguez-Malavasi A, Collinge JM, et al: Epidemiology of adverse drug reactions in the newborn. Dev Pharmacol Ther 1982;5:173–184.
9. Atkinson HC, Begg EJ, Darlow BA: Drugs in human milk: Clinical pharmacokinetic considerations. Clin Pharmacokinet 1988;14:217–240.
10. Banzaw TM: Mercury poisoning in Argentine babies linked to diapers. Pediatrics 1981;67:637.
11. Barnes AB, Colton T, Gundersen J, et al: Fertility and outcome of pregnancy in women exposed in utero to diethylstilbestrol. N Engl J Med 1980;302:609–613.
12. Bauer CR, Trottier MCT, Stern L: Systemic cyclopentalate (cyclogyl) toxicity in the newborn infant. J Pediatr 1973; 82:501.
13. Beckman DA, Brent RL: Teratogenesis: Alcohol, angiotensin-converting-enzyme inhibitors, and cocaine. Curr Opin Obstet Gynecol 1990;2:236–245.
14. Bentur Y: Ionizing and nonionizing radiation in pregnancy. In: Koren G, ed: Maternal-Fetal Toxicology: A Clinician's Guide, 2nd ed. New York, Marcel Dekker, 1994, pp. 515–574.
15. Besunder JB, Blumer JL: Neonatal drug withdrawal syndromes. In: Koren G, ed: Maternal-Fetal Toxicology: A Clinician's Guide, 2nd ed. New York, Marcel Dekker, 1994, pp. 321–352.
16. Bibbo M, Gill WB, Azizi F, et al: Follow-up study of male and female offspring of DES-exposed mothers. Obstet Gynecol 1977;49:1–8.
17. Bingol N, Fuchs M, Diaz V, et al: Teratogenicity of cocaine in humans. J Pediatr 1987;110:93–96.
18. Blanc P, Hryhorczuk D, Danel I: Deferoxamine treatment of acute iron intoxication in pregnancy. Obstet Gynecol 1984;64:12S–14S.
19. Bologa M, ul Qamar I, Laila W, Koren G: Direct drug toxicity to the fetus. In: Koren G, ed: Maternal-Fetal Toxicology: A Clinician's Guide, 2nd ed. New York, Marcel Dekker, 1994, pp. 267–300.
20. Bonati M, Bortolus R, Marchetti F, et al: Drug use in pregnancy: An overview of epidemiological (drug utilization) studies. Eur J Clin Pharmacol 1990;38:325–328.
21. Bonati M, Fellin G: Changes in smoking and drinking behaviour before and during pregnancy in Italian mothers: Implications for public health intervention. Int J Epidemiol 1991;20:927–32.
22. Bosque MA, Domingo JL, Corbella J: Assessment of the developmental toxicity of deferoxamine in mice. Arch Toxicol 1995;69:467–471.
23. Brent RL: The application of the principles of toxicology and teratology in evaluating the risks of new drugs for the treatment of drug addiction in women of reproductive age. NIDA Research Monograph 1995;149:130–179.
24. Brent RL: Relationship between uterine vascular clamping, vascular disruption syndrome, and cocaine teratogenicity. Teratology 1990;41:757–760.
25. Brent RL, Beckman DA: Angiotensin-converting enzyme inhibitors, an embryopathic class of drugs with unique properties: information for clinical teratology counselors. Teratology 1991;43:543–546.
26. Briggs GG, Freeman RK, Yaffe SJ: Drugs in Pregnancy and Lactation, 3rd ed. Baltimore, Williams & Wilkins, 1990.
27. Brouillette F, Weber ML: Massive aspiration of talcum powder by an infant. Can Med Assoc J 1978;119:354–355.
28. Brown DB, Mueller GL, Golich FC: Hyperbaric oxygen treatment for carbon monoxide poisoning in pregnancy: A case report. Aviat Space Environ Med 1992;63:1011–1014.
29. Brown WJ, Buist NR, Cory-Gipson HT, et al: Fatal benzyl alcohol poisoning in a neonatal intensive care unit. Lancet 1982;1:1250. Letter.
30. Byer AJ, Trayler TR, Semmer JR. Acetaminophen overdose in the third trimester of pregnancy. JAMA 1982;247: 3114–3115.
31. Caravati EM, Adams CJ, Joyce SM, Schafer NC: Fetal toxicity associated with maternal carbon monoxide poisoning. Ann Emerg Med 1988;17:714–717.
32. Chabrolle JP, Rossier A: Goiter and hypothyroidism in the newborn after cutaneous absorption of iodine. Arch Dis Child 1978;53:495–498.
33. Chasnoff I: Drug use and women: Establishing a standard of care. Ann NY Acad Sci 1989;562:208–210.
34. Chasnoff IJ, Bussey ME, Salvich R, Stack CM: Perinatal cerebral infarction and maternal cocaine use. J Pediatr 1986;108:456–459.
35. Chasnoff IJ, Chisum GW, Kaplan WE: Maternal cocaine use during early pregnancy as a risk factor for congenital malformations. Teratology 1988;37:201–204.
36. Chasnoff IJ, Griffith DR, Freier C, Murry J: Cocaine/polydrug use in pregnancy: Two year followup. Pediatrics 1992;89:284–289.
37. Chasnoff IJ, Landress HJ, Barrett ME: The prevalence of illicit-drug or alcohol use during pregnancy and discrepan-

cies in mandatory reporting in Pinellas County, Florida. N Engl J Med 1990;322:1202–1206.
38. Chavez GF, Mulinare J, Cordero JF: Maternal cocaine use during early pregnancy as a risk factor for congenital anomalies. JAMA 1989;262:795–798.
39. Cherukuri R, Minkoff H, Feldman J, et al: A cohort study of alkaloidal cocaine ("crack") in pregnancy. Obstet Gynecol 1989;72:147–151.
40. Chouteau M, Namerow PB, Leppert P: The effect of cocaine abuse on birthweight and gestational age. Obstet Gynecol 1988;72:351–354.
41. Christiaens GCML, Rijksen G, Marx J, et al: Desferrioxamine in pregnancy. Arch Gynecol 1985;237(suppl):80. Abstract.
42. Church MW, Dintcheff BA, Gessner P. Dose-dependent consequences of cocaine on pregnancy outcome in the Long-Evans rat. Neurotoxicol Teratol 1988;10:51–58.
43. Coles CD: Impact of prenatal alcohol exposure on the newborn and the child. Clin Obstet Gynecol 1993;36: 255–256.
44. Coles CD, Platzman KA, Smith I, et al: Effects of cocaine and alcohol use in pregnancy on neonatal growth and neurobehavioral status. Neurotoxicol Teratol 1992;14: 23–34.
45. Committee on Drugs: Neonatal drug withdrawal. Pediatrics 1983;72:895–902.
46. Coustan D: Nonprescription drugs and alcohol: Abuse and effects in pregnancy. In: Reece EA, Hobbins JC, Mahoney MJ, Petrie RH, eds: Medicine of the Fetus and Mother. Philadelphia, Lippincott, 1992, pp. 317–327.
47. Cramer CR: Fetal death due to accidental maternal carbon monoxide poisoning. J Toxicol Clin Toxicol 1982;19:297–301.
48. Curry S, Bond GR, Rashke R, et al: An ovine model of maternal iron poisoning in pregnancy. Ann Emerg Med 1990; 19:632–638.
49. Czeizel A, Lendvay A: Attempted suicide and pregnancy. Am J Obstet Gynecol 1988;158:1084–1085.
50. Day NL, Cottreau CM, Richardson GA: The epidemiology of alcohol, marijuana, and cocaine use among women of child bearing age and pregnant women. Clin Obstet Gynecol 1993:36:232–245.
51. Desmond MM, Wilson GS: Neonatal abstinence syndrome: Recognition and diagnosis. Addict Dis 1975;2:113–121.
52. Dixon SD, Bejar R: Echoencephalographic findings in neonates associated with maternal cocaine an metamphetamine use: Incidence and clinical correlates. J Pediatr 1989;115:770–778.
53. Doberczak TM, Shanzer S, Cutler R, et al: One-year followup of infants with abstinence-associated seizures. Arch Neurol 1988;45:649–653.
54. Doberczak TM, Shanzer S, Senie RT: Neonatal neurologic and electroencephalographic effects of intrauterine cocaine exposure. J Pediatr 1988;113:354–358.
55. Dominguez R, Vila-Coro AA, Slopis JM, Bohan TP: Brain and ocular abnormalities in infants with in uetro exposure to cocaine and other street drugs. Am J Dis Child 1991; 145:688–695.
56. Dominick MA, Carson TL: Effects of carbon monoxide exposure on pregnant sows and their fetuses. Am J Vet Res 1983;44:35–40.
57. Douglas MJ: Perinatal physiology and pharmacology. In: Norris MC, ed: Obstetric Anesthesia. Philadelphia, Lippincott, 1993.
58. Dow-Edwards D: Comparability of human and animal studies of developmental cocaine exposure. NIDA Research Monograph 1996;164:146–174.
59. Dow-Edwards D, Chasnoff IJ, Griffith DR: Cocaine use during pregnancy: Neurobehavioral changes in the offspring. In: Sonderegger TB, ed: Perinatal Substance Abuse: Research Findings and Clinical Implications. Baltimore, The Johns Hopkins University Press, 1992, pp. 184–206.
60. Ducey J, Brooke D: Transcutaneous absorption of boric acid. Pediatrics 1953;43:644–651.
61. Elhassani HB: Neonatal poisoning: Causes, manifestations, prevention, and management. South Med J 1986;79: 1535–1543.
62. Elkharrat D, Raphael JC, Korach JM, et al: Acute carbon monoxide intoxication and hyperbaric oxygen in pregnancy. Intensive Care Med 1991;17:282–292.
62a. Fantel AG, MacPhail BJ: The teratogenicity of cocaine. Teratology 1982;26:17–19.
63. Farrow JR, Davis GJ, Toy TM, et al: Fetal death due to nonlethal maternal carbon monoxide posioning. J Forensic Sci 1990;35:1448–1452.
64. Ferm VH: Teratogenic effects of hyperbaric oxygen. Proc Soc Exp Biol Med 1964;90:854–858.
65. Finnegan LP: Neonatal abstinence. In: Nelson NM, ed: Current Therapy in Neonatal-Perinatal Medicine, 1985–1986. St Louis, Mosby, 1985, pp. 262–270.
66. Finnegan LP, Kandall SR. Maternal and neonatal effects of alcohol and drugs. In: Lowinson JH, Ruiz P, Millman RB, Langrod JG, eds: Substance Abuse: A Comprehensive Textbook, 2nd ed. Baltimore, Williams & Wilkins, 1992, pp. 628–656.
67. Finnell RH, Toloyan S, van Waes M, Kalivas PW: Preliminary evidence for a cocaine-induced embryopathy in mice. Toxicol Appl Pharmacol 1990;103:228–237.
68. Frank D, McCarten K, Cabral H, et al: Association of heavy in utero cocaine exposure with caudate hemorrhage in term newborns. Pediatr Res 1994;35:269. Abstract.
69. Friedman JM: Report of the Teratology Society Public Affairs Committee symposium on FDA classification of drugs. Teratology 1993;48:5–6.
70. Gabrielli A, Layon AJ, Gallagher TJ: Carbon monoxide intoxication during pregnancy: A case presentation and pathophysiologic discussion with emphasis on molecular mechanisms. J Clin Anesth 1995;7:82–87.
71. Gemme G, Ruffa G, Bonioli E, et al: Cushing's syndrome due to topical administration of corticosteroids. Am J Dis Child 1984;138:987–988.
72. Gershanik J, Boecler B, Ensley H, et al: The gasping syndrome and benzyl alcohol poisoning. N Engl J Med 1982;307:1384–1388.
73. Gillberg C: "Floppy infant syndrome" and maternal diazepam. Lancet 1977;2:244. Letter.
74. Gillogley KM, Evans AT, Hansen RL, et al: The perinatal impact of cocaine, amphetamine, and opiate use detected by universal intrapartum screening. Am J Obstet Gynecol 1990;163:1535–1542.

75. Ginsberg MD, Myers RE: Fetal brain injury after maternal carbon monoxide intoxication. Neurology 1976;26:15–23.
76. Glantz JC, Woods JR: Cocaine, heroin, and phencyclidine: Obstetric perspectives. Clin Obstet Gynecol 1993;36:279–301.
77. Gomby DS, Shiono PH: Estimating the number of substance-exposed infants. The future of children. Center for the Future of Children; 1:17.
78. Good WV, Ferriero DM, Golabi M, Kobori JA: Abnormalities of the visual system in infants exposed to cocaine. Ophthalmology 1992;99:341–346.
79. Griffith DR, Azuma SD, Chasnoff IJ: Three-year outcome of children exposed prenatally to drugs. J Am Acad Child Asolesc Psychiatry 1994;33:20–27.
80. Hadeed AJ, Siegel SR: Maternal cocaine use during pregnancy: Effect on the newborn infant. Pediatrics 1989;84: 205–210.
81. Haibach H, Akhter JE, Muscato MS, et al: Acetaminophen overdose with fetal demise. Am J Clin Pathol 1984;82: 240–242.
82. Handler A, Kistin N, Davis F: Cocaine use during pregnancy: Perinatal outcomes. Am J Epidemiol 1991;133: 818–825.
83. Hanson JW: Teratogen update: Fetal hydantoin effects. Teratology 1986;33:349–353.
84. Harada M: Congenital Minamata disease: Intrauterine methylmercury poisoning. Teratology 1986;123–126.
85. Herzlinger RA, Kandall SR, Vaughan HG: Neonatal seizures associated with narcotic withdrawal. J Pediatr 1977;91:638–641.
86. Heikkila AM, Erkkola RU, Nummi SE: Use of medication during pregnancy—A prospective cohort study on use and policy of prescribing. Ann Chirurg Gynaecol 1994;83: 80–83.
87. Hill EP, Hill JR, Power GG, Longo LD: Carbon monoxide exchanges between the human fetus and mother: A mathematical model. Am J Physiol 1977;232:H311–H323.
88. Hollander DI, Nagey DA, Welsch R, et al: Hyperbaric oxygen therapy for the treatment of acute carbon monoxide poisoning in pregnancy. J Reprod Med 1987;32:615–617.
89. Holt D, Harvey D, Hurley R: Chloramphenicol toxicity. Adverse Drug React Toxicol Rev 1993;12:3–95.
90. Holtzman C, Paneth N: Maternal cocaine use during pregnancy and perinatal outcomes. Epidemiol Rev 1994;16: 315–334.
91. Hoyme HE, Jones KL, Dixon SD, et al: Prenatal cocaine exposure and fetal vascular disruption. Pediatrics 1990;85: 743–747.
92. Hurst DL, Marsh WW: Early severe infantile botulism. J Pediatr 1993;122:909–911.
93. Hutchings DE: The puzzle of cocaine's effects following maternal use during pregnancy: Are there reconcilable differences? Neurotoxicol Teratol 1993;15:281–286.
94. Hytten FE: Physiologic changes in the mother related to drug handling. In: Krauer B, Krauer F, Hytten F, del Pozo E, eds: Drugs in Pregnancy. Orlando, Academic Press, 1984, pp. 7–17.
95. Ihlen BM, Amundsen A, Sande HA, Daae L: Changes in the use of intoxicants after onset of pregnancy. Br J Addict 1990;85:1627–1631.
96. Jager-Roman E, Deichl A, Jakob S, et al: Fetal growth, major malformations, and minor anomalies in infants born to women receiving valproic acid. J Pediatr 1986;108: 997–1004.
97. John EG, Guignard JP: Development of renal excretion of drugs during ontogeny. In: Polin RA, Fox WW, eds: Fetal and Neonatal Physiology. Philadelphia, Saunders, 1992, pp. 153–159.
98. Johnson SF, McCarter RJ, Ferencz C: Changes in alcohol, cigarette, and recreational drug use during pregnancy: Implications for intervention. Am J Epidemiol 1987;126: 695–702.
99. Jones KL: Smith's Recognizable Pattern's of Human Malformation, 4th ed. Philadelphia, Saunders, 1988.
100. Jones KL, Lacro RV, Johnson KA, Adams J: Pattern of malformations in the children of women treated with carbamazepine during pregnancy. New Engl J Med 1989;320: 1661–1666.
101. Juchau MR, Rettie AE: The metabolic role of the placenta. In: Fabro S, Scialli AR, eds: Drug and Chemical Action in Pregnancy. New York, Marcel Dekker, 1986, pp. 153–169.
102. Kandall SR: Treatment options for drug exposed infants. NIDA Research Monograph 1995;149:78–99.
103. Kandall SR, Doberczak TM, Mauer KR, Strashun RH, Korts DC: Opiate v CNS depressant therapy in neonatal drug abstinence syndrome. Am J Dis Child 1983;137: 378–382.
104. Kandall SR, Gaines J: Maternal substance use and subsequent sudden infant death syndrome (SIDS) in offspring. Neurotoxicol Teratol 1991;13:235–240.
105. Kandall SR, Gaines J, Habel L, et al: Relationship of maternal substance abuse to subsequent sudden infant death syndrome in offspring. J Pediatr 1993;123:120–126.
106. Khoury S, Odeh M, Oettinger M: Deferoxamine treatment for acute iron intoxication in pregnancy. Acta Obstet Gynecol Scand 1995;74:756–757.
107. Kiess W, Linderkamp O, Hadorn HB, Haas R: Fetal alcohol syndrome and malignant disease. Eur J Pediatr 1984; 143:160–161.
108. Kleiner GJ, Greston WM: Suicide during pregnancy. In: Cherry SH, Merkatz IR, eds: Complications of Pregnancy: Medical, Surgical, Gynecologic, Psychosocial, and Perinatal, 4th ed. Baltimore, Williams & Wilkins, 1991, pp. 269–289.
109. Kliegman RM, Madura D, Kiwi R, et al: Relation of maternal cocaine use to the risk of prematurity and low birth weight. J Pediatr 1994;124:751–756.
110. Koren G: Measurement of drugs in neonatal hair: A window to fetal exposure. Forensic Sci Int 1995:70:77–82.
111. Koren G: Changes in drug disposition in pregnancy and their clinical implication. In: Koren G, ed: Maternal-Fetal Toxicology: A Clinician's Guide, 2nd ed. New York, Marcel Dekker, 1994, pp. 3–14.
112. Koren G, Graham K, Shear H, et al: Bias against the null hypothesis: the reproductive hazards of cocaine. Lancet 1989;1:1440–1442.
113. Koren G, Sharav T, Pastuszak A, et al: A multicenter, prospective study of fetal outcome following accidental carbon monoxide poisoning in pregnancy. Reprod Toxicol 1991;5:397–403.

114. Kramer LD, Locke GE, Ogunyemi A, et al: Neonatal cocaine-related seizures. J Child Neurol 1990;5:60–64.
115. Kumar A, Goel KM, Rae MD: Paracetamol overdose in children. Scottish Med J 1990;35:106–107.
116. Lacoste H, Goyert GL, Goldman LS, et al: Acute iron intoxication in pregnancy. Obstet Gynecol 1992;80:500–501.
117. Lammer EJ: A phenocopy of the retinoic acid embryopathy following maternal use of etretinate that ended one year before conception. Teratology 1988;37:472. Abstract.
118. Lammer EJ, Sever LE, Oakley GP: Valproic acid. Teratology 1987;35:465–473.
119. Lampert PW, O'Brian JS, Garrett R: Hexachlorophene encephalopathy. Acta Neuropathol 1973;23:326–333.
120. Land DB, Kushner R: Drug abuse during pregnancy in an inner-city hospital: Prevalence and patterns. J Am Osteopath Assoc 1990;90:421–426.
121. Lawrence RA: Breastfeeding: A Guide for the Medical Professional, 4th ed. St Louis, Mosby, 1994, pp. 323–358.
122. Lederman S, Fysh WJ, Tredger M, et al: Neonatal paracetamol poisoning: Treatment by exchange transfusion. Arch Dis Child 1983;58:631–633.
123. Lenke RR, Turkel SB, Monsen R: Severe fetal deformities associated with ingestion of excessive isoniazid in early pregnancy. Acta Obstet Gynecol Scand 1985;64:281–282.
124. Lester BM, LaGrasse L, Freier K, Brunner S: Studies of cocaine-exposed human infants. NIDA Research Monograph 1995;149:175–209.
125. Lester D, Beck AT: Attempted suicide and pregnancy. Am J Obstet Gynecol 1988;158:1084–1085.
126. Lipshultz SE, Frassica JJ, Orav EJ: Cardiovascular abnormalities in infants prenatally exposed to cocaine. J Pediatr 1991;118:44–51.
127. Little BB, Snell LM, Klein VR, Gilstrap LC: Cocaine abuse during pregnancy: Maternal and fetal implications. Obstet Gynecol 1989;73:157–160.
128. Little BB, Snell LM, Gilstrap LC: Alcohol use during pregnancy and maternal alcoholism. In: Gilstrap LC, Little BB, eds: Drugs and Pregnancy. New York, Elsevier, 1992, pp. 367–374.
129. Little BB, Snell LM, Gilstrap LC, Grant NF, Rosenfeld CR: Alcohol abuse during pregnancy: Changes in prevalence in a large urban hospital. Obstet Gynecol 1989;74:547–550.
130. Longo LD: The biological effects of carbon monoxide on the pregnant woman, fetus and newborn infant. Am J Obstet Gynecol 1977;129:69–103.
131. Longo LD, Hill EP: Carbon monoxide uptake and elimination in fetal and maternal sheep. Am J Physiol 1977;232: H324–H330.
132. Ludmir J, Main DM, Landon MB, Gabbe SG. Maternal acetaminophen overdose at 15 weeks of gestation. Obstet Gynecol 1986;67:750–751.
133. Lutiger B, Graham K, Einarson TR, Koren G: Relationship between gestational cocaine use and pregnancy outcome: A meta-analysis. Teratology 1991;44:405–414.
134. MacGregor SN, Keith LG, Bachicha JA, et al: Cocaine abuse during pregnancy: correlation between prenatal care and perinatal outcome. Obstet Gynecol 1989;74: 882–885.
135. Mahalik MP, Gautieri RF, Mann DE: Teratogenic potential of cocaine hydrochloride in CF–1 mice. J Pharm Sci 1980; 69:703–706.
136. Mahalik MP, Hitner HW: Antagonism of cocaine-induced fetal anomalies by prazosin and diltiazem in mice. Reprod Toxicol 1992;6:161–169.
137. Manoguerra AS: Iron poisoning, report of a fatal case in an adult. Am J Hosp Pharm 1976;33:1088–1090.
138. Margulies JL: Acute carbon monoxide poisoning during pregnancy. Am J Emerg Med 1986;4:516–519.
139. Martin K: Successful pregnancy in β-thalassemia major. Aust Paediatr J 1983;19:182–183.
140. Martin ML, Khoury MJ, Cordero JF: Trends in rates of multiple vascular disruption defects, Atlanta, 1968–1989. Teratology 1992;45:647–653.
141. Martin-Boyer G, Lebretton R, Toga M, et al: Outbreak of accidental hexachlorophene poisoning in France. Lancet 1982;1:91–95.
142. McElhatton PR, Roberts JC, Sullivan FM: The consequences of iron overdose and its treatment with desferrioxamine in pregnancy. Hum Exp Toxicol 1991;10: 251–259.
143. McElhatton PR, Sullivan FM, Volans GN, Fitzpatrick R: Paracetamol poisoning in pregnancy: An analysis of the outcomes of cases referred to the teratology information service of the national poisons information service. Hum Exp Toxicol 1990;9:147–153.
144. Mehanny SZ, Abdel-Rahman MS, Ahmed YY: Teratogenic effect of cocaine and diazepam in CF–1 mice. Teratology 1991;43:11–17.
145. Metcalfe J, Stock M, Barron D: Maternal physiology during pregnancy. In: Knobil E, Neill J, eds: The Physiology of Reproduction. New York, Raven, 1988, pp. 2145–2177.
146. Miller PD, Telford IR, Haas GF: Effect of hyperbaric oxygen on cardiogenesis in the rat. Biol Neonate 1971;17: 44–52.
147. Miller RK: Placental transfer and function: The interface for drugs and chemicals in the conceptus. In: Fabro S, Scialli AR, eds: Drug and Chemical Action in Pregnancy. New York, Marcel Dekker, 1986, pp. 123–152.
148. Moore TR, Sorg J, Miller L, et al: Hemodynamic effects of intravenous cocaine on the pregnant ewe and fetus. Am J Obstet Gynecol 1986;155:883–888.
149. Moriss FH, Boyd RDH: Placental transport. In: Knobil E, Neill JD, eds: The Physiology of Reproduction, Vol. 2. New York, Raven, 1988, p. 2063.
150. Motomatsu K, Adachi H, Uno T: Two infant deaths after inhaling baby powder. Chest 1979;75:448–450.
151. Muller GL, Graham S: Intrauterine death of the fetus due to accidental maternal carbon monoxide poisoning in pregnancy. Reprod Toxicol 1991;5:397–403.
152. Murphy MG, Turner BS: Pharmacology in neonatal care. In: Merenstein GB, Gardner SL, eds: Handbook of Neonatal Intensive Care. St Louis, Mosby, 1989, p. 146.
153. Nagourney BA, Aranda JV: Physiologic differences of clinical significance. In: Polin RA, Fox WW, eds: Fetal and Neonatal Physiology. Philadelphia, Saunders, 1992, pp. 169–177.
154. Nau H: Physicochemical and structural properties regulating placental drug transfer. In: Polin RA, Fox WW, eds:

Fetal and Neonatal Physiology, Vol 1. Philadelphia, Saunders, 1992, pp. 130–141.
155. Nau H, Helge H, Luck W: Valproic acid in the perinatal period: Decreased maternal serum protein binding results in fetal accumulation and neonatal displacement of the drug and some metabolites. J Pediatr 1984;104:627–634.
156. National Institute of Drug Abuse: National Pregnancy & Health Survey: Drug Use Among Women Delivering Livebirths: 1992. National Institutes of Health, Rockville, MD, 1996.
157. Neuspiel DR: Behavior in cocaine-exposed infants and children: Association versus causality. Drug Alcohol Depend 1994;36:101–107.
158. Neuspiel DR, Hamel SC, Hochberg E, et al: Maternal cocaine use and infant behavior. Neurotoxicol Teratol 1991; 13:455–460.
159. Norman CA, Halton DM: Is carbon monoxide a workplace teratogen? A review and evaluation of the literature. Ann Occup Hyg 1990;34:335–347.
160. Olenmark M, Biber B, Dottori O, Rybo G: Fatal iron intoxication in late pregnancy. J Toxicol Clin Toxicol 1987;25: 347–359.
161. Paul M, ed: Occupational and Environmental Reproductive Hazards: A Guide for Clinicians. Baltimore, Williams & Wilkins, 1993.
162. Perrone J, Hoffman RS: Toxic ingestions in pregnancy: Abortifacient use in a case series of pregnant overdose patients. Acad Emerg Med 1997;4:206–209.
163. Petiti DB, Coleman C: Cocaine and the risk of low birth weight. Am J Public Health 1990;80:25–28.
164. Physicians' Desk Reference. Montvale, NJ, Medical Economics Data, 1997.
165. Piantadosi CA: Carbon monoxide, oxygen transport, and oxygen metabolism. J Hyperbaric Med 1987;2:27–44.
166. Piper JM, Baum C, Kennedy DL: Prescription drug use before and during pregnancy in a Medicaid population. Am J Obstet Gynecol 1987;157:148–165.
167. Plessinger MA, Woods JR: Maternal, placental, and fetal pathophysiology of cocaine exposure during pregnancy. Clin Obstet Gynecol 1993;36:267–278.
168. Pratt R, Salomon DS: Biochemical basis for the teratogenic effects of glucocorticoids. In: Juchau MR, ed: The Biochemical Basis of Chemical Teratogenesis. New York, Elsevier/North Holland, 1981, pp. 179–199.
169. Rayburn W, Aronow R, DeLancey B, Hogan MJ: Drug overdose during pregnancy: An overview from a metropolitan poison control center. Obstet Gynecol 1984;64: 611–614.
170. Rayburn WF, Donn SM, Wulf ME: Iron overdose during pregnancy. Successful therapy with deferoxamine. Am J Obstet Gynecol 1983;147:717–718.
171. Reed MD, Besunder JB: Developmental pharmacology: Ontogenic basis of drug disposition. Pediatr Clin North Am 1989;36:1053–1074.
172. Rementeria JL, Bhatt: Withdrawal symptoms in neonates from intrauterine exposure to diazepam. J Pediatr 1977;90: 123–126.
173. Reproductive Health Hazards in the Workplace. Office of Technology Assessment. Washington DC, Congress of the United States, 1985.
174. Reynolds JD, Brien JF: Ethanol neurobehavioral teratogenesis and the role of l-glutamate in the fetal hippocampus. Can J Physiol Pharmacol 1995;73:1209–1223.
175. Rice JM, Donovan PJ, Anderson LM: Mutagenesis and carcinogenesis. In: Fabro S, Scialli AR, eds: Drug and Chemical Action in Pregnancy. New York, Marcel Dekker, 1986, pp. 205–236.
176. Richards R, Brooks SEH: Ferrous sulphate poisoning in pregnancy with afibrogenaemia as a complication. West Indian Med J 1966;15:134–140.
177. Richardson GA, Day NL: Detrimental effects of prenatal cocaine exposure: Illusion or reality. J Am Acad Child Adolesc Psychiatry 1994;33:28–34.
178. Richardson GA, Day NL: Maternal and neonatal effects of moderate cocaine use during pregnancy. Neurotoxicol Teratol 1991;13:455–460.
179. Richardson GA, Day NL, McGauhey PJ: The impact of prenatal marijuana and cocaine use on the infant and child. Clin Obstet Gynecol 1993;36:302–318.
180. Rieder MJ: Drugs and breastfeeding. In: Koren G, ed: Maternal-Fetal Toxicology: A Clinician's Guide. New York, Marcel Dekker, 1990, pp. 63–85.
181. Riggs BS, Bronstein AC, Kulig K, et al: Acute acetaminophen overdose during pregnancy. Obstet Gynecol 1989;74:247–253.
182. Rivera-Calimlim L: The significance of drugs in breast milk: Pharmacokinetic considerations. Clin Perinatol 1987; 14:51–70.
183. Roberts I, Robinson MJ, Mughal MZ, et al: Paracetamol metabolites in the neonate following maternal overdose. Br J Clin Pharmacol 1984;18:201–206.
184. Robertson RG, van Cleave BL, Collins JJ: Acetaminophen overdose in the second trimester of pregnancy. J Fam Pract 1986;23:267–268.
185. Rogan WJ: Breastfeeding in the workplace. Occup Med 1986;1:411–413.
186. Rollins DE, von Bahr C, Glaumann H, et al: Acetaminophen: Potentially toxic metabolite formed by human fetal and adult liver microsomes and isolated fetal liver cells. Science 1979;205:1414–1416.
187. Rosen TS, Pippenger CE: Pharmacologic observations on the neonatal withdrawal syndrome. J Pediatr 1984;88: 1044–1048.
188. Rosenstein BJ, Wheeler JS, Heid PL: Congenital renal abnormalities in infants with in utero cocaine exposure. J Urol 1990;144:110–112.
189. Rosevear SK, Hope PL: Favourable neonatal outcome following maternal paracetamol overdose and severe fetal distress. Br J Obstet Gynaecol 1989;96:491–493.
190. Rubin PC, Craig GF, Gavin K, Sumner D: Prospective survey of use of therapeutic drugs, alcohol, and cigarettes during pregnancy. Br Med J 1986;292:81–83.
191. Ruiz-Maldonado R, Zapta G, Tamayo L, et al: Cushing's syndrome after topical application of corticosteroids. Am J Dis Child 1982;136:274–275.
192. Ruthnum P, Goel KM: ABC of poisoning: Paracetamol. Br Med J 1984;289:1538–1539.
193. Rutter N: Percutaneous drug absorption in the newborn: Hazards and uses. Clin Perinatol 1987;14:911–930.
194. Sannerstedt R, Lundborg P, Bengt R, et al: Drugs during

pregnancy: An issue of risk classification and information to prescribers. Drug Safety 1996;14:69–77.
195. Sapunar D, Saraga-Babic M, Peruzovic M, Marusic M: Effects of hyperbaric oxygen on rat embryos. Biol Neonate 1993;63:360–369.
196. Schardein JL: Chemically Induced Birth Defects. New York, Marcel Dekker, 1985.
197. Schauben JL, Augenstein WL, Cox J, Sato R: Iron posioning: report of three cases and a review of therapeutic intervention. J Emerg Med 1990;8:309–319.
198. Scialli AR, Fabro S: The stage dependence of reproductive toxicology. In: Fabro S, Scialli AR, eds: Drug and Chemical Action in Pregnancy. New York, Marcel Dekker, 1986, pp. 191–204.
199. Selden BS, Curry SC, Clark RF, et al: Transplacental transport of *N*-acetylcysteine in an ovine model. Ann Emerg Med 1991;20:1069–1072.
200. Shannon M, Amitai Y, Lovejoy FH: Multiple dose activated charcoal for theophylline poisoning in young infants. Pediatrics 1987;80:368–370.
201. Shepard TH: Catalog of teratogenic agents. Baltimore, The Johns Hopkins University Press, 1992, p. xiii.
202. Shiono PH, Klebanoff MA, Nugent RP, et al: The impact of cocaine and marijuana on low birth weight and preterm birth: A multicenter study. Am J Obstet Gynecol 1995;172: 19–27.
203. Shuman RM, Leach RW, Alvord EC: Neurotoxicity of hexachlorophene in humans. Arch Neurol 1975;32:320.
204. Slutsker L: Risks associated with cocaine use during pregnancy. Obstet Gynecol 1992;79:778–789.
205. Sokol RJ, Abel EL: Risk factors for alcohol-related birth defects: threshold, susceptibility, and prevention. In: Sonderegger TB, ed: Perinatal Substance Abuse: Research Findings and Clinical Implications. Baltimore, The Johns Hopkins University Press, 1992, pp. 90–103.
206. Spear LP: Assessment of the effects of developmental toxicants: Pharmacological and stress vulnerability of offspring. NIDA Research Monograph 1996;164:125–145.
207. Stokes IM: Paracetamol overdose in the second trimester of pregnancy. Br J Obstet Gynaecol 1984;91:286–288.
208. Strom RL, Schiller P, Seeds AF, ten Bensel R: Fatal poisoning in a pregnant female. Minn Med 1976;59:483–489.
209. Teelman K: Retinoids: Toxicology and teratogenicity to date. Pharmacol Ther 1989;40:29–43.
210. Telford IR, Miller PD, Haas GF: Hyperbaric oxygen causes fetal wastage in rats. Lancet 1969;2:220–221.
211. Tenenbein M: Poisoning in pregnancy. In: Koren G, ed: Maternal-Fetal Toxicology: A Clinician's Guide. New York, Marcel Dekker, 1990, pp. 89–114.
212. Thilo EH, Townsend SF, Deacon J: Infant botulism at 1 week of age: Report of two cases. Pediatrics 1993;92: 151–153.
213. Thomas RM, Skalicka AB: Successful pregnancy in transfusion-dependent thalassemia. Arch Dis Child 1980;55: 572–574.
214. Thornburg KL, Faber JJ: Transfer of hydrophilic molecules by placenta and yolk sac of the guinea pig. Am J Physiol 1977;233:C111–C124.
215. Turk J, Aks S, Ampuero F, Hryhorczuk D: Successful therapy of iron intoxication in pregnancy with intravenous deferoxamine and whole bowel irrigation. Vet Hum Toxicol 1993;35:441–444.
216. Van Amedyne KJ, Tenenbein M: Whole bowel irrigation during pregnancy. Am J Obstet Gynecol 1989;160:646–647.
217. Van Hoesen KB, Camporesi EM, Moon RE, et al: Should hyperbaric oxygen be used to treat the pregnant patient for acute carbon monoxide poisoning? A case report and literature review. JAMA 1989;261:1039–1043.
218. Voskaridou E, Konstantopoulous K, Kyriakou D, Loukopoulous D: Deferoxamine treatment during early pregnancy: Absence of teratogenicity in two cases. Haematologica 1993;78:183–184.
219. Ward SLD, Keens TG: Prenatal substance abuse. Clin Perinatol 1992;19:849–860.
220. Warkany J: Aminopterin and methotrexate: Folic acid deficiency. Teratology 1978;17:353–358.
221. Warkany J: Warfarin embryopathy. Teratology 1976;14:205–210.
222. Webster WS, Brown-Woodman PDC: Cocaine as a cause of congenital malformations of vascular origin: Experimental evidence in the rat. Teratology 1990;41:689–697.
223. Webster WS, Brown-Woodman PDC, Lipson AH, Ritchie HE: Fetal brain damage in the rat following prenatal exposure to cocaine. Neurotoxicol Teratol 1991;13:621–626.
224. Webster WS, Lipson AH, Brown-Woodman PDC: Uterine trauma and limb defects. Teratology 1987;35:253–260.
225. Weiss B, Doherty RA: Methylmercury poisoning. Teratology 1975;12:311–313.
226. West JR, Chen WA, Pantazis NJ: Fetal alcohol syndrome: The vulnerability of the developing brain and possible mechanisms of damage. Metabol Brain Dis 1994;9:291–322.
227. Whitlock FA, Edwards JE: Pregnancy and attempted suicide. Compr Psychiatry 1968:9:1–12.
228. Woods JR, Plessinger MA, Clark KE: Effect of cocaine on uterine blood flow and fetal oxygenation. JAMA 1987; 257:957–961.
229. Woods JR, Plessinger MA, Scott K, Miller RK: Prenatal cocaine exposure to the fetus: A sheep model for cardiovascular evaluation. Ann NY Acad Sci 1989;562:267–279.
230. Woody RC, Brewster MA: Telencephalic dysgenesis associated with presumptive maternal carbon monoxide intoxication in the first trimester of pregnancy. J Toxicol Clin Toxicol 1990;28:467–475.
231. Working PK, ed: Toxicology of the Male and Female Reproductive Systems. New York, Hemisphere, 1989.
232. Zelson C, Rubio E, Wasserman E: Neonatal narcotic addiction: 10-year observation. Pediatrics 1971;48:179–189.
233. Zuckerman B, Frank D, Brown E: Overview of the effects of abuse and drugs on pregnancy and offspring. NIDA Research Monograph 1995;149:16–38.
234. Zuckerman BS, Frank D, Hingson R, et al: Effects of maternal marijuana and cocaine use on fetal growth. N Engl J Med 1989;320:762–768.

CHAPTER 105

Pediatric Principles

Jeffrey S. Fine

Children are more frequently exposed to poisons than any other group, and poisoning is a significant cause of pediatric injury morbidity. Therefore pediatricians have been active in helping to establish and promote the field of medical toxicology as well as regional poison control centers. Although the basic approach to the medical management of toxicologic problems outlined in Chapters 3 and 30 is generally applicable to children as well as adults, there are several issues of unique concern to children when special considerations may be appropriate. This chapter provides a pediatric perspective on the application of toxicologic principles.

Epidemiology

In order to achieve a perspective on the problem of pediatric poisoning, it is necessary to understand the magnitude of the problem. When assessing the impact of a particular type of injury such as poisoning, epidemiologists examine a number of parameters to measure the effects, such as exposure, morbidity, mortality, and cost. All of these parameters are difficult to measure accurately. One of the important sources for information on the extent and effects of poisoning exposures comes from the American Association of Poison Control Centers (AAPCC). Each year the AAPCC compiles standardized data collected from poison centers throughout the United States; the 1996 annual review included information submitted by 67 poison centers. In the following discussion, comments on AAPCC data refer to cumulative information from the last five published reports covering the years 1991 to 1995.[58–60,62,63]

The AAPCC reports approximately 1.8 million potentially toxic exposures per year for children and adolescents aged 0 to 19 (0 to 17 in some of the years considered), and these pediatric exposures represent 68% of the reported poisoning exposures for all age groups. Children under the age of 6 account for 82% of all reported pediatric exposures and 56% of all reported pediatric and adult poisoning exposures. Adolescents aged 13 to 19 account for only 9% of the pediatric poisoning exposures. Females represent 57% of the reported poisoning exposures among young children and 66% of the reported exposures among adolescents.

Ninety-nine percent of the AAPCC reported poisoning exposures in children under 6 years of age are unintentional. Only 50% of the reported adolescent poisoning exposures are unintentional while 46% are intentional, frequently suicidal in nature. This high frequency of suicidal intent is also reported by others.[92] These differences between young children and adolescents are specifically reflected in the outcome of these exposures.

Table 105–1 shows the leading causes of reported exposures in children and adolescents. According to the AAPCC, approximately 55% of reported pediatric exposures in children are to nonpharmaceutical agents, substances that are commonly found around the house such as cosmetics, plants, hydrocarbons, and insecticides; while approximately 45% are to pharmaceutical agents. Table 105–1 lists the most common *reported* exposures, but these agents are not necessarily the ones that cause the most serious morbidity and mortality (see Tables 105–2 and 105–3).

Under the age of 6 months, poisoning in children is unusual but may result from inadvertent administration of an incorrect drug or drug dose by a parent,[37] intentional administration of a drug by a parent or sibling, or passive exposure, for instance to the smoke of "crack cocaine."[8] Any poisoning in a child under 1 year of age should be carefully evaluated for possible child abuse or neglect.[9]

Several characteristics associated with ingestions in toddlers differentiate them from ingestions in adolescents or adults: (1) they are without suicidal intent; (2) there is usually only one substance involved; (3) the substances are usually nontoxic; (4) the amount is usually small; and (5) children usually present for evaluation soon after the ingestion. As many as 30% of children who experience one ingestion will experience a repeat inges-

TABLE 105–1. TYPES OF SUBSTANCES MOST FREQUENTLY REPORTED TO THE AAPCC

Age < 6 y		Age 6–17 y	
Category	*Exposures[a]*	*Category*	*Exposures[a]*
Cosmetics/personal care	123,505	Analgesic agents	35,026
Cleaning substances	115,632	Cough/cold preparations	14,492
Analgesic agents	82,542	Cleaning substances	14,484
Plants	80,250	Bites/envenomations	17,081
Cough/cold preparations	73,560	Cosmetics/personal care products	11,392
Topical agents	53,335	Plants	10,730
Foreign bodies	49,864	Foreign bodies	10,136
Antimicrobials	38,715	Stimulants/street drugs	8,995
Vitamins	35,283	Food products/poisoning	8,564
GI preparations	33,492	Antimicrobials	8,148

[a]Numbers are the average of annual exposures reported by the AAPCC for 1991–1995.
Data from references 58–60, 62, and 63.

tion.[61] Children who ingest poisons may be at risk for other types of injuries.[6,30]

The peak age for childhood poisoning is between 1 and 3 years.[18] Unintentional ingestion is unusual after age 5 and may reflect mistaken consumption of a substance from a mislabeled container.[14] Between the ages of 5 and 9, poisoning may be a reflection of intrafamilial stress or suicidal intent. After age 9 and through adolescence, overdose or poisoning exposure frequently results either from a suicidal gesture or attempt, or from an adverse effect while seeking drug-induced euphoria. Unintentional poisonings are invariably preventable (see Chap. 115).

Because many children are exposed to nontoxic substances or to nontoxic amounts of toxic substances, it is not surprising that the relative number of children and adolescents who are reported to suffer significant morbidity is small (Table 105–2). However, because there are millions of exposures each year, the number of children reported by the AAPCC who suffer at least moderate effects is approximately 21,000 per year.

Although the AAPCC is not the only source for epidemiologic data, there is little detailed information available on poisoning morbidity. Estimates of the rate of emergency department visits are approximately 650 per 100,000 for children under 5 and 360 per 100,000 for adolescents.[18,32,35] The Centers for Disease Control estimate that approximately 100,000 children are seen in emergency departments each year for poisoning-related injuries and 20,000 are hospitalized.[19] Reported rates of hospitalization range from 100 to 170 per 100,000.[32,78,92]

With respect to hospitalized children exposed to drugs or toxins, adolescents are more frequently admitted than children; suicidal adolescents may suffer serious toxicity more frequently than children who do not intend to hurt themselves, although some adolescents may be admitted for psychiatric evaluation. The peak age of hospitalization for children is between 1 and 3. Hospitalized children under the age of 2 are more commonly exposed to nonpharmaceutical substances whereas children over the age of two and adolescents are more commonly exposed to pharmaceutical agents.[32,92]

Although the AAPCC does report outcome related to age, it does not generally stratify outcome with regard to age and substance. However, in an earlier multiyear review, the AAPCC did report those agents causing the greatest number of major and fatal effects in children less than 6 years old.[65] The agents that cause significant morbidity and mortality are listed in Table 105–3. Other re-

TABLE 105–2. OUTCOME OF REPORTED PEDIATRIC EXPOSURES

	Effects[a] (% of reported exposures)			
Age (y)	*Minor*	*Moderate*	*Major*	*Death*
0–5	93	1	0.05	0.003
6–12	86	2	0.1	0.005
13–19	75	7	0.7	0.04
All children and adolescents[b] (0–19)	91	2	0.1	0.006

[a]Minor = minimal signs and symptoms, often not requiring therapy; moderate = more pronounced, prolonged, or systemic signs and symptoms, often requiring therapy; major = life-threatening signs and symptoms.
[b]Percentages are based on an average of the number of effects reported by the AAPCC for 1991–1995. Column totals do not add up to 100% because not all reported exposures are fully characterized with respect to morbid effects.
Data from references 58–60, 62, and 63.

TABLE 105–3. TYPES OF SUBSTANCES RESPONSIBLE FOR SIGNIFICANT PEDIATRIC MORBIDITY AND MORTALITY

	Age <6 y				Age 13–17 y[a]	
	Major Effects[b]		*Deaths*		*Deaths*	
Category	**no.**	**(%)**	**no.**	**(%)**	**no.**	**(%)**
Cleaning substances	277	(12)	7	(6)	1	(<1)
Cardiovascular agents	182	(8)	7	(6)	12	(7)
Hydrocarbons	168	(7)	5	(4)	56	(31)
Sedative-hypnotic agents	153	(7)	2	(2)	5	(3)
Antidepressants	125	(6)	7	(6)	49	(27)
Insecticides/pesticides	122	(5)	6	(5)	0	(0)
Analgesic agents	119	(5)	8	(7)	26	(14)
Anticonvulsants	106	(5)	4	(3)	2	(1)
Bites/envenomations	100	(4)	0	(0)	0	(0)
Stimulants/street drugs	84	(4)	1	(<1)	7	(4)
Iron	85	(4)	8	(7)	2	(0)
Carbon monoxide	42	(2)	18	(15)	5	(3)
Alcohols	52	(2)	5	(4)	3	(2)
Theophylline	38	(2)	3	(2)	3	(2)
Total for listed substances	1653	(73)	81	(68)	170	(94)
Total reported[c]	2270		122		182	

[a]No specific outcome effects for this age group are reported and therefore the number of major effects cannot be calculated.
[b]Major effect = life-threatening signs and symptoms.
[c]Not all reported substances are listed and therefore columns do not add up to 100%.
Data from references 58–60, 62, 63, and 65.

ports of hospitalized patients describe a similar distribution of agents causing significant morbidity with some differences.[31,32] In Australia, for instance, quinine, digoxin, and eucalyptus oil were significant causes of hospitalization.[16]

Poison-related deaths represent approximately 2.5% of childhood and adolescent unintentional injury-related deaths annually.[74] The AAPCC reported 444 child and adolescent deaths from 1991 to 1995; these deaths represent 12% of the reported poisoning fatalities for all age groups. One hundred forty six (33%) were children aged 0 to 5, 29 (6%) were children 6 to 12, and 267 (41%) were adolescents 13 to 19 years old.

The number of children under age 5 dying from poisons is extremely low. The AAPCC reports 26 per year on average between 1985 and 1995. This is a 94% decrease from a high of 456 in 1959.[18] This dramatic decrease in poisoning mortality may be the result of improved poisoning prevention (for example, child-resistant closures) and improved medical care, or may reflect a decrease in reporting (discussed later). Fifty-seven percent of the AAPCC reported deaths in the under-5-year age group were related to unintentional ingestions and 18% were related to environmental exposures such as carbon monoxide.

The most notable difference between the toxins listed in Table 105–3 and earlier studies is that salicylates are no longer the leading cause of reported poisoning morbidity and mortality.[23,26] This change is probably related both to federal regulations requiring child-resistant closures as well as the decreased use of aspirin following the recognition of its association with Reye's syndrome in children.

There are some significant etiologic differences in Table 105–3 between children and adolescents, particularly with regard to the lethality of agents. The leading three categories/agents for children are carbon monoxide, iron, and hydrocarbons, which account for 46% of all reported poisoning deaths. The top three categories for adolescents are hydrocarbons, antidepressants (almost all tricyclics), and analgesic agents (almost equal numbers of salicylates and acetaminophen), accounting for 72% of reported poisoning deaths. Importantly, the hydrocarbon deaths in children generally result from aspiration, but almost all the adolescent deaths were due to effects related to abuse of inhaled hydrocarbons such as trichloroethane or chlorofluorocarbons. Fifty percent of AAPCC-reported adolescent deaths are deemed suicides while 32% are related to substance abuse.

Although the AAPCC data provide a remarkable amount of epidemiologic information, there are questions about accuracy.[45,95] The most serious concern is that many significant poisonings may not be reported to poison centers. For instance, physicians managing "common" toxicologic problems may not feel the need for the assistance of a local or regional poison center and may not feel compelled to participate in the reporting process (see Chap. 115). Therapeutic misadventures may also go unreported. In Rhode Island, only 45 of 369 poisoning deaths were reported to the regional poison center.[57] Some of the reasons for this discrepancy were that deaths occurred outside of, or prior to arrival at the hospital and that poisoning was not recognized as a potential reason for illness prior to death. In addition, several cases were known poison-related deaths but were not reported. In another study, half of the poison-related deaths reviewed never presented to the hospital.[92] As a comparison, the National Center for Health Statistics reports that in 1992, the last year for which information is available, there were 53 poison-related deaths for children under 5 years old, 36 for children aged 5 to 14, and 155 for adolescents aged 15 to 19.[73] For the same year, the AAPCC reports 27 deaths for children under 5, 9 for children 6 to 12, and 61 for adolescents 13 to 19 years of age.[63]

Poisoning also has an economic cost. For one 3-month period, 21 children who ingested medications were hospitalized for a total of 39 days at a cost of $95,000.[51] In a large economic analysis of the cost of injury in the United States, the cost of poisoning was $495 per child and $10,839 per adolescent or young adult injured by poisoning.[78]

Behavioral, Environmental, and Physical Issues

A simplistic approach to childhood poisonings is that unobserved toddlers exploring their environment inadvertently ingest toxins. This approach ignores the complex interaction of factors that may lead to pediatric ingestions.

One approach to understanding injury causation uses an infectious disease model where a host, an agent, and an environment are identified.[44] In the case of poisoning, the host is the child or adolescent, the agent is the particular toxin, and the environment is usually the home. This approach to injury prevention considers intervention with respect to these three factors during three time periods relative to injury occurrence—the preinjury, injury, and postinjury phases. The postinjury phase is mainly concerned with the medical management of a poisoning once it has occurred and is the focus of much of the rest of this text. Considering these factors allows us to focus on several aspects of poisoning, although it is often difficult to examine any single factor independently and the relative contribution of these factors has not been well defined.

When considering the agent, the toxin itself, there are a number of issues that affect the preinjury and injury phases. Ideally, pharmaceutical and nonpharmaceutical substances would have beneficial or useful effects without potential toxicity. Practically, however, there may be ways to reduce the toxicity of available agents. Less toxic rodenticides such as warfarin have replaced many more toxic types such as thallium or sodium monofluoroacetate. Nontoxic paradichlorobenzene mothballs have largely replaced toxic camphor-containing mothballs. Legislation has been proposed to add denatonium benzoate, an aversive bittering agent, to some liquid preparations, with the expectation that this will prevent poisoning. Some trials have shown that older children respond negatively to these agents, but that younger children may ingest one to two teaspoons of a substance before responding to the bitter flavor.[79]

The problem of unintentional ingestions is compounded by poison "look-alikes," pharmaceutical or toxic substances that resemble candy or food products.[34] Some common examples are ferrous sulfate tablets that look like M&M candies, prenatal vitamins that resemble Good and Plenty candies, and fuel oils that come in cans that resemble soft drink containers (see Color Plate Fig. 20). Many shampoos and dishwashing-detergents are given lemon or strawberry scents and have pictures of fruits on the labels. Children are not always capable of distinguishing nontoxic candies, fruits, and sodas from poison "look-alikes" and may be attracted to bright colors, pleasant smells, and appealing packages. Eliminating these "look-alikes" might prevent many unintentional ingestions.

Probably the most significant change to the physical aspect of the toxin itself has been packaging of pharmaceuticals and some other toxic substances with child-resistant-closures mandated by the Poison Prevention Packaging Act of 1972 (see Chap. 115). This legislation is credited with a significant reduction in morbidity and mortality related to poisoning from aspirin and other regulated products.[22,94] Child-resistant closures were also shown to reduce the number of toxic exposures to kerosene in South Africa.[53] There are currently proposals to regulate the packaging of iron-containing pills in an attempt to reduce iron poisoning-related deaths.[3]

Nonetheless, problems with child-resistant closures include pharmaceuticals being dispensed in nonresistant containers, resistant containers not being properly closed, and medicines being out of the resistant container for use.[17] Seventy percent of toxic pharmaceuticals may be in non-child-resistant or effectively non-child-resistant containers. Several studies have identified poor functioning of the closures when there is sticky liquid or pill residue around the top of the container or screw threads.[48,51,98]

Although child-resistant containers are a significant deterrent to unintentional ingestions in toddlers, they are not completely effective, and even without the problems noted some children can open them. The sense of security associated with these closures may lead some parents to be less compulsive with regard to safe storage. It has been recommended that for a few pharmaceuticals associated with a large number of significant poisonings (iron or antidepressant agents), a double barrier be instituted, such as a unit dose dispenser within a child-resistant container.[51]

A discussion of containers and storage naturally leads to consideration of the environment, which is particularly important in the preinjury and the injury phases. About 80% of childhood ingestions occur at home; the remainder occur at the homes of grandparents, other relatives, and friends. The medicine usually belongs either to the child or to the mother, although a significant number of medications both at home and away from home belong to a grandparent.[48,64] Grandparents, other relatives, or family friends without children regularly around the home may not receive or keep medications in child-resistant containers and may not pay attention to safe-storage recommendations.

In general, there are not significant differences in the general storage practices between the homes of children who ingest and those who do not ingest medicines.[87,98] However, medications are frequently stored in the kitchen, and are frequently ingested in the kitchen or the bedroom when they are outside their usual storage location for use.[48,98] In the kitchen, medications are in the refrigerator, on the table, or on the counter, while in the bedroom, medications are on a dresser or bedside table. A mother's purse is another common location in which to find medications.

One important caveat relates to the storage of nonpharmaceutical substances, particularly those in liquid form. Toxic materials should not be transferred to familiar containers like food jars or wine or soda bottles for storage. Both children and adults have been exposed to poisons such as sodium hydroxide or potassium cyanide stored in bottles in the refrigerator.[90]

Childhood and adolescence are times of tremendous growth and development.[99] Some of these physical and social changes place children and teenagers at increased risk for poisonings.

By 7 months of age an infant sitting up can pivot in order to grab an object; by 9 to 10 months of age most infants can creep and crawl; by 15 months of age most toddlers are walking quite competently and eagerly exploring. Between 9 and 12 months of age a child is developing a skillful pincer grasp with the thumb and forefinger that allows him or her to pick up small objects. Throughout this period, one of the child's primary sensory experiences is sucking on or gumming objects that are placed in the mouth.

The combination of three developmental skills—the ability to move around the home and go beyond the immediate view of a guardian, the ability to pick up and manipulate small objects, and the tendency of children to put things in their mouths—places them at risk for both foreign body aspiration and toxic ingestions. In addition, the fact that infants are crawling a lot and children younger than 2 are just becoming comfortable moving around in an upright position explains why they are more likely to ingest common household substances. Pharmaceutical products stored in cabinets are generally out of reach of these young children, although a 1-year old would be able to grab something from a bedside table if he or she was on the bed or pulled himself or herself up to a standing position.

As children develop socially they desire to become more like their parents and they tend to imitate behaviors, such as taking medicine or using mouthwash. Children are taught that medicine is good for them when they are sick. Many children's medicines are sweetened and flavored to make them more palatable, and in fact many parents encourage their children to take medicines by telling them "it tastes like candy." Children have also been observed "making tea" from plants or "making pizza" with mushrooms from the yard.[14]

As children become more mobile, agile, and curious, toxic substances that were previously outside their reach are now accessible, even when stored in some difficult to reach places. There is some evidence to suggest that parents underestimate the developmental skills of their children.[30] We should also reconsider the meaning of term "unintentional" with respect to childhood poisoning. The toddler quite purposefully intends to get to a pill and eat it, but the subsequent injury is unintentional.

We have tried to explain some of the reasons why a child wants to ingest a pill: because it is there, it looks like candy or food, the parent takes pills, and taking medicine is considered good for health. These reasons may not be sufficient to explain why a child does something that he or she knows should not be done. One other aspect of childhood poisoning that must be considered is the interaction between the child's temperament and his or her social environment.

Many authors have tried to identify psychosocial predictors for childhood poisoning in general and repeat poisoning in particular.[10,33,50,86] As many as 30% of children may have repeat episodes of ingestions, frequently of the same substance. Certain risk factors have been identified for single and repeated episodes of childhood poisoning such as hyperactivity, impulsive risk-taking behavior, rebelliousness, or negativistic attitude. Other factors seem to be more associated with the parents such as medical illness, depression, or social isolation. Finally, a stressful environment or major social problem may also be a contributing factor.[85,86] It is not difficult to imagine a situation where a parent is depressed, cannot give adequate attention to a demanding child, and uses antidepressant medication that is kept at the bedside. In a bid for attention or as an expression of anger or frustration, the child ingests some of the parent's medicine.

History of the Ingestion

The appropriate management of any poisoned patient is influenced by the history of the exposure. Parents or guardians who are not abusing children will generally provide information to the extent they are able. As a rule, in the case of children, the substance and time of ingestion are known although the number of pills or the volume of liquid ingested may be inaccurate. Clues to the amount ingested are the number of pills or volume of liquid in a bottle before and after an ingestion, the number of pills set out on the night table, or the area of a spot of liquid after a spill. When symptoms are suggestive of poisoning, but the history is inadequate, remember to try to get information about possible exposure outside of the home, such as with a babysitter, grandparent, friend, or other relative. About 15% of childhood poisonings occur outside the home.[48,76]

Suicidal adolescents may be unreliable when relating the history of an ingestion. When caring for these patients the clinician must utilize the history provided but should remain skeptical about the reported type and number of agents ingested as well as the time of ingestion.

In cases where a child may be the victim of abuse or intentionally poisoned by a caretaker, the healthcare provider must insure that: (1) the history of the poisoning remains consistent over time and between those people providing the details of the event, (2) the child's clinical presentation is consistent with the history of the poisoning, and (3) the child's developmental level makes him or her capable of the events described.

Gastrointestinal Decontamination

Chapter 4 is devoted to a complete discussion of gastrointestinal decontamination. In this section, we will reiterate and emphasize only a few important points.

As previously described, children frequently ingest small quantities of single agents. For most of these ingestions gastric emptying is unnecessary. Some examples of nontoxic ingestions are eating a crayon or the leaf of a jade plant, licking the cap of a household bleach container, or swallowing two adult-strength acetaminophen tablets.

Orogastric lavage is generally the preferred method of gastric emptying for most serious ingestions. Even small children can generally tolerate orogastric lavage with a large-bore 28F or 34F tube. However the smaller "large-bore" tubes may not be effective for removing large pills or fragments from the stomach of a small child. In order to use orogastric lavage safely in a child with a diminished gag reflex or in one who is comatose, the trachea should be intubated to protect the airway.

Syrup of ipecac was, until recently, considered a primary intervention for significant pediatric exposures. According to AAPCC data, syrup of ipecac was used for 13% of exposures in 1983 but only 2% of exposures in 1995.[60]

There may still be a limited role for syrup of ipecac, however, when there is ingestion of (1) a massive amount of a slow-release product whose onset of effects and toxicity will be delayed for several hours, (2) tablets that are too large to pass through an orogastric tube, or (3) medications with only limited adsorption to activated charcoal. (See Chap. 4 and Antidotes in Depth: Syrup of Ipecac.)

One special pediatric consideration is the use of syrup of ipecac at home. Parents are commonly advised to have syrup of ipecac at home so that it can be used upon the recommendation of a physician or a poison center specialist.[37] Administering syrup of ipecac at home is theoretically ideal to achieve gastric emptying within 1 hour; if syrup of ipecac is given close to the time of the ingestion, then vomiting would be expected to occur within 20 to 30 minutes, perhaps by the time the child arrives at the emergency department. Under some circumstances it may be reasonable to administer syrup of ipecac and keep the child at home (see Chap. 115).

Although children who receive syrup of ipecac at home generally do not present to hospital emergency departments for medical evaluation, the utility of the home use of syrup of ipecac is largely unproven. An attempt was made to examine this by studying children under

5 years of age who had ingested acetaminophen.[2] The use of syrup of ipecac reduced the *expected* peak acetaminophen serum level and the effect was greater if the syrup of ipecac was administered at home. A problem with this study is that what the *actual* peak levels would have been without treatment are unknown, and therefore the extent of the actual treatment effect is unknown. Questions about the home use of syrup of ipecac still remain.[36]

Activated charcoal is one of the current mainstays of poison treatment. Children generally will not drink activated charcoal willingly. Some children can be coaxed to do so if the activated charcoal is disguised in a baby bottle or soft drink container, or sweetened with juice or sorbitol. A nasogastric tube may have to be inserted to administer activated charcoal. This can be a small-bore tube because it is not intended for lavage, although the smaller the bore, the more difficult it will be to administer the thick mixture of activated charcoal. Placement of the tube, the presence of activated charcoal in the stomach, the effects of the toxin, or the previous use of syrup of ipecac may all make the child vomit. Aspiration of activated charcoal or stomach contents is a risk. In order to use activated charcoal safely in a patient who is comatose and does not have a gag reflex, the trachea should be intubated and the airway protected. For a nontoxic ingestion, even activated charcoal alone may be unnecessary.

In Scandinavia, activated charcoal is available for home use.[54] Although it would seem to have potential benefit as home therapy, activated charcoal is highly unpalatable, difficult to administer, and quite messy, and as a result has not yet achieved widespread use. Despite the fact that pediatricians have struggled to get parents to have syrup of ipecac available in the home, there is still poor compliance. If activated charcoal should replace syrup of ipecac for home therapy, it will require a substantial reeducation effort on the part of pediatricians and toxicologists.

Methods of Enhanced Elimination

For consequential poisoning with toxins such as methanol, ethylene glycol, salicylates, lithium, and theophylline, hemodialysis or activated charcoal hemoperfusion are the optimal techniques to enhance elimination. These techniques can be performed on newborns or small infants in specially equipped centers with dedicated personnel[21,68]; the primary limiting factor is the ability to obtain vascular access.[43,91] However, even large centers that routinely do pediatric hemodialysis may not be able to manage the very small infant.

Another technique frequently employed in the newborn nursery to treat polycythemia and occasionally used to enhance drug elimination is exchange transfusion. This technique might be applicable in cases where multiple-dose activated charcoal cannot be administered, the toxin is poorly adsorbed to charcoal, or access to specialized pediatric hemodialysis or hemoperfusion is not readily available. Exchange transfusion has been used successfully for salicylates[29,67] and theophylline.[7,75,83]

Another drug for which exchange transfusion may be the treatment of choice is chloral hydrate.[4] This agent is still widely used as a sedative-hypnotic agent for children undergoing diagnostic studies such as CT scans, although it is being replaced in many centers with other sedative-hypnotic agents such as midazolam that can be titrated or potentially reversed. Chloral hydrate toxicity is mediated through one of its metabolites, trichloroethanol. For a small child who receives a supratherapeutic dose and manifests toxicity, exchange transfusion may be a therapeutic alternative if hemodialysis is unavailable.

Agents That May be Toxic or Fatal in Small Quantities

When children ingest small quantities of toxic substances they potentially ingest large doses because of their small size.[52,56] There are a number of substances that may cause significant toxicity or even death with as little as one pill or one teaspoon. These substances are listed in Table 105–4.

Agents That May Have Delayed Toxicity in Children

There are several agents that warrant particular concern either because the effects may be significantly delayed or because even one tablet may lead to significant toxicity. Classic examples are atropine/diphenoxylate (Lo-

TABLE 105–4. DRUGS AND TOXINS THAT CAN CAUSE SEVERE TOXICITY TO A 10-KG CHILD AFTER A SMALL DOSE

Drug	Estimated or Reported Fatal Dose/kg	Maximum Unit Dose Available	Number of Units to Cause Toxicity
Benzocaine	10 mg	1 g/tsp	<1 tsp
Camphor	100 mg	1000 mg/tsp	1 tsp
Chloroquine	20 mg	500 mg	1 tablet
Chlorpromazine	25 mg	200 mg	1–2 tablets
Clonidine	0.01 mg	0.3 mg	1 tablet
Codeine	15 mg	60 mg	5 tablets
Desipramine	15 mg	75 mg	2 tablets
Diphenhydramine	25 mg	50 mg	5 tablets
Diphenoxylate	1.2 mg	2.5 mg	5 tablets
Ethylene glycol	1 mL	4.7 g/tsp	2 tsp
Hydroxychloroquine	20 mg	200 mg	1 tablet
Imipramine	15 mg	150 mg	1 tablet
Methanol	0.6 mL	5 g/tsp	1 tsp
Methyl salicylate	200 mg	7000 mg /tsp	< 1 tsp
Orphenadrine	25 mg	50 mg	5 tablets
Quinine	80 mg	650 mg	1–2 tablets
Theophylline	8.4 mg	500 mg	1 tablet
Thioridazine	15 mg	200 mg	1 tablet

Adapted, with permission, from Koren GK: Medications which can kill a toddler with one tablet or teaspoon. J Toxicol Clin Toxicol 1993;31:407–413.

motil)[11,25,69] and oral hypoglycemic agents such as chlorpropamide.[42,77] Both of these agents have been reported to cause serious morbidity with initial symptoms or recurrence of symptoms as late as 24 hours after ingestion.

Children who have ingested or may have ingested these medications must be admitted for observation and monitoring even if they are asymptomatic, because effects may not become apparent for 24 hours. With the advent of new slow-release formulations of calcium channel blockers and beta-adrenergic antagonists, concern for delayed toxicity has been extended to other drugs.

Agents That Have Unusual or Idiosyncratic Reactions in Children

Benzyl Alcohol: Gasping Syndrome

Benzyl alcohol is a preservative added to liquid pharmaceutical preparations; for small-volume medications administered to adults, the benzyl alcohol additive is quite safe (see Chap. 54). At toxic doses, benzyl alcohol can cause respiratory failure, vasodilation, hypotension, convulsions, and paralysis (see Chap. 64). Intravenous flush solutions containing benzyl alcohol were implicated as the cause of the "gasping syndrome" in sick newborns—severe metabolic acidosis, encephalopathy, respiratory depression, and gasping.[1] The association was made when infants with this syndrome were found to have elevated levels of benzoic acid and hippuric acid, metabolites of benzyl alcohol.[15,38] The metabolism of benzyl alcohol by the conjugation of benzoic acid with glycine to form hippuric acid may not be functional in premature infants. Benzyl alcohol administration has also been associated with kernicterus and intraventricular hemorrhage in premature infants.[46,49]

Although benzyl alcohol has been removed from many medications used in neonates, there still are preparations containing this agent.[96]

Imidazolines/Clonidine: CNS Effects

Imidazoline agents such as tetrahydrolozine, oxymetazoline, xylometazoline, and naphazoline are over-the-counter sympathomimetic agents used as nasal decongestants and conjunctival vasoconstrictors (see Chap. 34). Clonidine is an imidazoline derivative used as a antihypertensive agent (see Chap. 51). In small children, these agents can cause central nervous system depression, respiratory depression, bradycardia, miosis, and hypotension.[5,66,97] The presumed mechanism of action is through stimulation of central α_2-adrenergic receptors. Although naloxone has been reported to reverse some of the CNS effects of clonidine, there are no reports of its successful use with the other imidazoline agents (see Chap. 51).

Ethanol: Hypoglycemia

Ethanol, is the primary component of alcoholic beverages, as well as a major constituent of many liquid preparations such as mouthwash, vanilla flavoring, and perfume. Besides the well-known sedative-hypnotic effects associated with alcohol intoxication, ethanol intoxication in children is associated with hypoglycemia.[55,93] Ethanol-induced hypoglycemia may cause seizures and may exacerbate the other CNS effects induced by ethanol intoxication. The mechanism of hypoglycemia is presumed to be related to the fasting state induced by depressed consciousness in the young child with limited glycogen stores. Whether the metabolism of ethanol is specifically related to the development of hypoglycemia is unknown. There does not seem to be a blood alcohol level threshold for the development of hypoglycemia, which has been seen with blood alcohol levels as low as 20 mg/dL.[24]

Chloramphenicol: Gray Baby Syndrome

Chloramphenicol is a broad-spectrum antibiotic that has been used in pediatrics because of its activity against *Haemophilus influenzae*. Its use in the United States has largely been replaced by other antibiotics because of chloramphenicol's association with aplastic anemia. When administered at high doses, chloramphenicol can produce the "gray baby syndrome"—abdominal distension, vomiting, metabolic acidosis, progressive pallid cyanosis, irregular respirations, hypothermia, hypotension, and vasomotor collapse. Although these effects are seen primarily in premature newborn infants, they can also be seen in older children and adults (see Chap. 46).

Gray baby syndrome is associated with serum concentrations greater than 100 mg/L. Increased chloramphenicol levels may be due to (1) inadequate conjugation of chloramphenicol with glucuronic acid because of inadequate activity of glucuronyl transferase in the newborn liver and (2) decreased renal elimination of unconjugated chloramphenicol. The exact mechanism of toxicity is unknown; there has been speculation that free radicals produced during the metabolism of chloramphenicol may interfere with mitochondrial function.[47]

Problems With Drug Dosing and Administration

Because children are small, they generally require smaller amounts of drugs to achieve therapeutic plasma levels, even when the mg/kg dosing requirement is greater than for an adult. Therefore, children are particularly susceptible to therapeutic errors in drug dosing. The AAPCC reports that almost 10% of the poisoning deaths in children for 1991 to 1995 were related to therapeutic medication error or misuse.[58–60,62,63]

Dosing and drug administration errors take many forms:

1. The wrong drug is administered. In one nursery, an epidemic mimicking neonatal sepsis was caused when racemic epinephrine was inadvertently administered instead of vitamin E because both drugs were manufactured by the same company, distributed in nearly identical bottles, and stored near each other inside the nursery refrigerator.[88]
2. A drug dose is calculated incorrectly. A 1-kg prema-

ture infant required sedation for a diagnostic study. A high dose of chloral hydrate, 100 mg/kg, was calculated to be 1 g (1000 mg) instead of 100 mg. The child had a cardiopulmonary arrest and died.

3. A drug dose is calculated correctly, but written illegibly or transcribed incorrectly. When drugs require mg/kg dosing, it is easy to make decimal mistakes in the calculation or in the transcription. Clearly written orders and prescriptions are essential.
4. A drug dose is calculated and ordered correctly but the wrong dosage form is dispensed. Acetaminophen suppositories (120 mg) were ordered for a toddler but adult strength suppositories (650 mg) were distributed and administered every 4 hours. The child developed hepatotoxicity requiring hospitalization and therapy (see Chap. 31).
5. A drug dose is correctly calculated, formulated, and dispensed but the wrong dose is administered to the child.

Somewhat different errors can occur when drugs are administered intravenously:

6. Medications may be infused at an incorrect rate, either by miscalculation or through illegibility. This can be avoided by writing out the order in longhand, for example, "five milliliters per hour to deliver five milligrams per kilogram per hour."
7. Intravenous medications may be administered as a bolus rather than a slow infusion. Phenytoin, which has a recommended administration rate in adults of no more than 50 mg/min, should be infused at a rate of 1 mg/kg per minute in a child.
8. A drug meant to be administered by one route is given by another. In one case, paraldehyde was administered through an umbilical artery catheter with subsequent development of gangrene of the lower extremities followed by death.[40]

Intentional Poisoning and Child Abuse

Intentional poisoning of children is an unusual though significant form of child abuse. There are several types of intentional poisoning, some of which define pathologic characteristics of the caretaker: (1) undifferentiated child abuse, neglect, or impulsive acts under stress; (2) factitious illness (Münchausen syndrome by proxy); (3) overt parental psychosis; (4) altruistic motivation or bizarre childrearing practices; and (5) the Medea complex, or the vengeful killing of a child out of spite for one's spouse.[9,89]

Intentional poisoning is rarely suspected unless the patient dies and an autopsy is performed, a wide-ranging drug screen is ordered, or the history is bizarre enough to raise suspicions. In many cases where children were later found to be poisoned, the initial diagnoses were sepsis, meningitis, seizures, intracranial hemorrhage, gastroenteritis, apnea, apparent life-threatening events (near-miss SIDS), or metabolic derangements.[9] In addition to many pharmaceutical agents, salt, pepper, water, caffeine, ethylene glycol, herbs, plants, and traditional remedies have been used to poison children.[9,28] Although the death rate from unintentional poisoning in childhood is much less than 1%, the death rate from inflicted poisoning may be as high as 20 to 30%.[9,28,89]

Intentional poisoning may be associated with other abuse; in one report, 20% of poisoned children had evidence of physical abuse.[28] Of children presenting to the emergency department after presumed unintentional poisoning, 36% had previous emergency department visits for trauma, 7% for poisoning, 6% for both trauma and poisoning, and 1.4% for failure to thrive. At the time of the visit, only 7% were evaluated for possible abuse and 2.7% were considered neglected.[80]

Substance abuse by a parent or guardian may play a role in unintentional or intentional poisoning of children. Children have been intoxicated with cocaine by passive inhalation[8] as well as through breast milk.[20] Children have been given doses of methadone mixed in orange juice to quiet them down.[27] There are reports of babysitters blowing marijuana smoke into babies' faces to "get them high" or quiet them down.[9]

Factitious illness (Münchausen syndrome) by proxy (MSBP) is a condition where a parent, usually the mother, fabricates a history of a nonexistent disease in a child or creates the signs and symptoms of disease in a child.[71,72,81] This is usually a manifestation of the parent's complex psychiatric illness, which may include Münchausen syndrome itself.[12,41] There may be only a fine line separating MSBP from an intentional poisoning with intent to harm or kill a child. Regardless of the specific intent, this condition is considered a form of child abuse.

A child's fabricated illness can lead to multiple medical evaluations by multiple physicians, frequent hospitalizations, unnecessary surgery and diagnostic testing, and occasionally, the death of the child. Administration of exogenous drugs is frequently the mechanism of creating a particular set of signs and symptoms. Agents that have been used to create factitious illness include analgesics, antidepressants, insulin, syrup of ipecac, lomotil, phenothiazines, sedative-hypnotics, warfarin, phenolphthalein, and hydrocarbons.[82] Several warning signals are outlined in Table 105–5 that may suggest a diagnosis of MSBP.

In one illustrative case of MSBP,[39] a 29-month-old male with a previous history of appendectomy was hospitalized multiple times for vomiting, diarrhea, and dehydration. Evaluation included multiple laboratory evaluations of blood and stool, a pH probe, CT, MRI, endoscopy, and upper GI series. At the fourth admission a small bowel obstruction was identified and the child had lysis of adhesions. Nonetheless symptoms recurred every 2 to 4 months, necessitating hospitalization. The child failed to thrive and required a nasoduodenal tube for feeding, which frequently became dislodged. The child went on to have a jejunostomy tube and a permanent central venous catheter placed. Eighteen months after his initial presentation, the child presented in congestive heart failure with evidence of cardiomyopathy. A urine screen identified emetine and cephaline, components of syrup of ipecac. The child recovered, was re-

TABLE 105–5. FACTITIOUS ILLNESS (MÜNCHAUSEN SYNDROME) BY PROXY: SUGGESTIVE CHARACTERISTICS IN CLINICAL SITUATIONS

1. A persistent or recurrent illness that cannot be explained.
2. The history of disease or results of diagnostic tests are inconsistent with the general health and appearance of the child.
3. The signs and symptoms cause the clinician to remark that "I've never seen anything like this before!"
4. The signs and symptoms do not occur when the child is separated from the parent.
5. The parent is particularly attentive and refuses to leave the child's bedside even for a few minutes.
6. The parent develops particularly close relations with hospital staff.
7. The parent seems less worried about the child's condition than the physician.
8. Treatments are not tolerated—intravenous lines fall out frequently; prescribed medications lead to vomiting.
9. The proposed diagnosis is a very rare disease.
10. "Seizures" are unwitnessed by medical staff and reportedly do not respond to any treatment.
11. The parent has a complicated medical or psychiatric history.
12. The parent is or was associated with the healthcare field.

Adapted, with permission, from Meadow R: Münchausen syndrome by proxy. Arch Dis Child 1982;57:92–98.

moved from his home to protective custody, and remained asymptomatic while receiving a regular diet.

Siblings of children being poisoned may also suffer or have suffered from factitious illness. In addition, there is persistent psychological and family pathology that is manifested by the victim, the parents, and the siblings.[13,70]

Child abuse or neglect may be appropriately considered in any case of childhood intoxication. Intentional poisoning should be considered for (1) any medical case with a confusing presentation, history, or symptomatology; (2) any child with multiple presentations for a rare or unexplained medical condition; (3) any child who presents with apnea or SIDS (actual or near-miss); (4) "ingestions" in a child under 6 to 9 months of age; (5) massive ingestions by small children; (6) intoxications with substances to which a child could or would not have access; (7) ingestion of multiple substances by a small child; and (8) "accidental ingestions" in the school-age child who is at low risk for unintentional ingestions.

These considerations of child abuse notwithstanding, rare diseases do occur. One child's rare inherited metabolic disorder, methyl malonic acidemia, was misdiagnosed as ethylene glycol poisoning because the chromatographic appearance of the metabolite propionic acid was similar to that of ethylene glycol.[84]

Summary

Poisoning in childhood is common; fortunately most childhood exposures are ingestions of nonpoisonous materials or small nontoxic quantities of potentially toxic agents. When a child sustains a significant toxic exposure, management follows general toxicologic principles. Although most childhood exposures are unintentional, the clinician should be alert to the possibility of the intentional poisoning of a child with pharmaceutical or household agents.

The normal development of children puts them at risk for unintentional ingestions. A chaotic home environment or a disorganized social structure may compound these risks. Children's small size puts them at increased risk for medication dosing and dispensing errors, and their immature metabolic processes may lead to unexpected toxicity from pharmaceutical agents.

As toxicologists, we should encourage parents to provide as safe a home environment as possible to prevent unintentional ingestions, and we must encourage practitioners to exercise special vigilance when administering medications to children.

References

1. American Academy of Pediatrics: Benzyl alcohol: Toxic agent in neonatal units. Pediatrics 1983;72:356–358.
2. Amitai Y, Mitchell AA, McGuigan MA, Lovejoy FH: Ipecac-induced emesis and reduction of plasma concentrations of drugs following accidental overdose in children. Pediatrics 1987;80:364–367.
3. Anonymous: Proposed safety measures aimed at protecting children from iron posioning. Am J Hosp Pharm 1994;51:2887.
4. Anyebuno MA, Rosenfeld CR: Chloral hydrate toxicity in a term infant. Dev Pharmacol Ther 1991;17:116–120.
5. Bamshad MJ, Wasserman GS: Pediatric clonidine intoxications. Vet Hum Toxicol 1990;32:220–223.
6. Baraff LJ, Guterman JJ, Bayer MJ: The relationship of poison center contact and injury in children 2 to 6 years old. Ann Emerg Med 1992;21:153–157.
7. Barazarte V, Rodriguez Z, Ceballos S, et al: Exchange transfusion in a case of severe theophylline poisoning. Vet Hum Toxicol 1992;34:524.
8. Bateman DA, Heagarty MD: Passive freebase cocaine ("crack") inhalation by infants and toddlers. Am J Dis Child 1989;143:25–27.
9. Bays J: Child abuse by poisoning. In: Reece R, ed: Child Abuse: Medical Diagnosis and Management. Philadelphia, Lea & Feibiger, 1994 pp. 69–106.
10. Bithoney WG, Snyder J, Michalek J, Newberger EH: Childhood ingestions as symptoms of family distress. Am J Dis Child 1985;139:456–459.
11. Block SM, Dansky R, Davis MD: Lomotil poisoning in children: Two case reports. S Afr Med J 1977;51:553–554.
12. Bools CN, Neale BA, Meadow SR: Münchausen syndrome by proxy: A study of psychopathology. Child Abuse Neglect 1994;18:773–788.
13. Bools CN, Neale BA, Meadow SR: Co-morbidity associated with fabricated illness (Münchausen syndrome by proxy). Arch Dis Child 1992;67:77–79.
14. Brayden RM, MacClean WE, Bonfiglio JF, Altemeier W: Behavioral antecedents of pediatric poisonings. Clin Pediatr 1993;32:30–35.
15. Brown WJ, Buist NR, Cory-Gipson HT, et al: Fatal benzyl alcohol poisoning in a neonatal intensive care unit. Lancet 1982;1:1250.
16. Campbell D, Oates RK: Childhood poisoning—A changing

profile with scope for prevention. Med J Aust 1992;156: 238–240.

17. Centers for Disease Control. Unintentional ingestions of prescription drugs in children under five years old. MMWR 1987;36:124–126.
18. Centers for Disease Control. Update: Childhood posioning—United States. MMWR 1985; 34:117–118.
19. Centers for Disease Control: Unintentional poisoning among young children—United States. MMWR 1983;32:529–531.
20. Chasnoff IA, Lewis DE, Squires L: Cocaine intoxication in a breast-fed infant. Pediatrics 1987;80:836–838.
21. Chavers BM, Kjellstrand CM, Wiegand C, et al: Techniques for use of charcoal hemoperfusion in infants: Experience in two patients. Kidney Int 1980;18:386–389.
22. Clarke A, Walton WW: Effect of safety packaging on aspirin ingestion by children. Pediatrics 1979; 63: 687–693.
23. Craft AW: Circumstances surrounding deaths from accidental poisoning 1974–80. Arch Dis Child 1983; 58:544–546.
24. Cummins LH: Hypoglycemia and convulsions in children following alcohol ingestion. J Pediatr 1961;58:23–26.
25. Cutler EA, Barrett GA, Craven PW, Cramblett HG: Delayed cardiopulmonary arrest after Lomotil ingestion. Pediatrics 1980;65:157–158.
26. Deeths TM, Breeden JT: Poisoning in children—A statistical study of 1,057 cases. J Pediatr 1971; 78:299–305.
27. Densen-Gerber J: The forensic pathology of drug-related child abuse. Leg Med Annu 1978;135–148.
28. Dine MS, McGovern ME: Intentional poisoning of children—An overlooked category of child abuse: Report of seven cases and review of the literature. Pediatrics 1982;70:32–35.
29. Done AK, Otterness LJ: Exchange transfusion in the treatment of oil of wintergreen (methyl salicylate) poisoning. J Pediatr 1956;18:80–85.
30. Eriksson M, Larsson G, Winbladh B, Zetterstrom R: Accidental poisoning in pre-school children in the stockholm area. Act Paediatr Scand 1979; 275(suppl):96–101.
31. Fazen LE, Lovejoy FH, Crone RK: Acute poisoning in a children's hospital: A 2-year experience. Pediatrics 1986:77: 144–151.
32. Ferguson J, Sellar C, Goldacre MJ: Some epidemiological observations on medicinal and non-medicinal poisoning in preschool children. J Epidemiol Comm Health 1992;46: 207–210.
33. Flagler SL, Wright L: Recurrent poisoning in children: A review. J Pediatr Psych 1987; 12:631–641.
34. Flomenbaum NE, Howland MAH, Weissman R: Pretty poison. Emerg Med 1986;4:69–84.
35. Gallagher SS, Finison K, Guyer B, Goodenough S: The incidence of injuries among 87000 Massachusetts children and adolescents: Results of the 1980–81 statewide childhood injury prevention program surveillance system. Am J Public Health 1984; 74:1340–1347.
36. Garrettson LK: Ipecac home use: We need hope replaced with data. J Toxicol Clin Toxicol 1991;29:515–519. Editorial.
37. Gaudreault P, McCormick MA, Lacouture PG, Lovejoy FH: Poison exposures and use of ipecac in children less than 1 year old. Ann Emerg Med 1986;15:808–810.
38. Gershanik J, Boecler B, Ensley H, et al: The gasping syndrome and benzyl alcohol poisoning. N Engl J Med 1982; 307:1384–1388.
39. Goebel J, Gremse DA, Artman M: Cardiomyopathy from ipecac administration in Münchausen syndrome by proxy. Pediatrics 1993;92:601–603.
40. Gooch WM, Kennedy J, Banner W, McGuire HJ: Generalized arterial and venous thrombosis following intra-arterial paraldehyde. Clin Toxicol 1979;15:39–44.
41. Gray J, Bentovim A: Illness induction syndrome: I. A series of 41 children from 37 families identified at the Great Ormond Street Hospital for Children NHS Trust. Child Abuse Neglect 1996;20:655–673.
42. Greenberg B, Weihl C, Hug G: Chlorpropamide poisoning. Pediatrics 1968;41:145–147.
43. Gruskin AB, Baluarte HJ, Dabbagh S: Hemodialysis and peritoneal dialysis. In: Edelman CM, ed: Pediatric Kidney Disease, 2nd ed. Boston, Little,Brown, 1992, pp. 843–844.
44. Haddon W: Advances in the epidemiology of injuries as a basis for public policy. Pub Health Rep 1980;95:411–421.
45. Hamilton RJ, Goldfrank LR: Poison center data and the Pollyanna phenomenon. J Toxicol Clin Toxicol 1997;35: 21–23.
46. Hiller JL, Benda GI, Rahatzad M, et al: Benzyl alcohol toxicity: Impact on mortality and intraventricylar hemorrhage among very low birth weight infants. Pediatrics 1986;77: 500–506.
47. Holt D, Harvey D, Hurley R: Chloramphenicol toxicity. Adverse Drug React Toxicol Rev 1993;12:83–95.
48. Jacobson BJ, Rock AR, Cohn MS, et al: Accidental ingestions of oral prescription drugs: A multicenter survey. Am J Public Health 1989; 79:853–856.
49. Jardine DS, Rogers K: Relationships of benzyl alcohol to kernicterus, intraventricular hemorrhage, and mortality in preterm infants. Pediatrics 1989;83:153–160.
50. Jones J: The child accident repeater. Clin Pediatr 1980;19: 284–288.
51. King WD, Palmisano PA: Ingestion of prescription drugs by children: An epidemiologic study. South Med J 1989;82: 1468–1471.
52. Koren GK: Medications which can kill a toddler with one tablet or teaspoon. J Toxicol Clin Toxicol 1993;31:407–413.
53. Krug A, Ellis JB, Hay IY, et al: The impact of child-resistant containers on the incidence of parafin (kerosene) ingestion in children. S Afr Med J 1994; 84: 730–734.
54. Lamminpaa A, Vilska J, Hoppu K: Medical charcoal for a child's poisoning at home: Availability and success of administration in Finland. Hum Exp Toxicol 1993;12:29–32.
55. Leung AK: Ethyl alcohol ingestion in children. A 15-year review. Clin Pediatr 1986;25:617–619.
56. Liebelt EL, Shannon MW: Small doses, big problems: A selected review of highly toxic common medications. Pediatr Emerg Care 1993;9:292–297.
57. Linakis JG, Frederick KA: Poisoning deaths not reported to the regional poison control center. Ann Emerg Med 1993; 22:1822–1828.
58. Litovitz TL, Clark LR, Soloway RA: 1993 Annual report of the American Association of Poison Control Centers Toxic Exposure Surveillance System. Am J Emerg Med 1994;12: 546–584.
59. Litovitz TL, Felberg L, Soloway RA, et al: 1994 Annual report of the American Association of Poison Control Centers Toxic Exposure Surveillance System. Am J Emerg Med 1995;13:551–597.
60. Litovitz TL, Felberg L, White S, Klein-Schwartz W: 1995

Annual report of the American Association of Poison Control Centers Toxic Exposure Surveillance System. Am J Emerg Med 1996;14:487–537.

61. Litovitz TL, Flagler SL, Manoguerra AS, et al: Recurrent poisoning among paediatric poisoning victims. Med Toxicol Adverse Drug Exp 1989; 4:381–386.
62. Litovitz TL, Holm KC, Bailey KM, Schmitz BF: 1991 annual report of the American Association of Poison Control Centers National Data Collection System. Am J Emerg Med 1992; 10:452–505.
63. Litovitz TL, Holm KC, Clancy C, et al: 1992 Annual report of the American Association of Poison Control Centers Toxic Exposure Surveillance System. Am J Emerg Med 1993;11:494–555.
64. Litovitz TL, Klein-Schwartz W, Veltri JC, Manoguerra AS: Prescription drug ingestions in children: Whose drug? Vet Hum Toxicol 1986; 28:14–15.
65. Litovitz T, Manoguerra A: Comparison of pediatric poisoning hazards: An analysis of 3.8 million exposure incidents. Pediatrics 1992;89:999–1006.
66. Mahieu LM, Rooman RP, Goosens E: Imidazoline intoxication in children. Eur J Pediatr 1993;152:944–946.
67. Manikian A, Stone S, Hamilton R, et al: Exchange transfusion as an alternative to hemodialysis in severe infant salicylism. J Toxicol Clin Toxicol 1996:34:585. Abstract.
68. Mauer SM, Chavers BM, Kjellstrand CM: Treatment of an infant with severe chloramphenicol intoxication using charcoal-column hemoperfusion. J Pediatr 1980;96:136–139.
69. McCarron MM, Challoner KR, Thompson GA: Diphenoxylate-atropine (Lomotil) overdose in children: An update (report of eight cases and review of the literature). Pediatrics 1991;87:694–700.
70. McGuire TL, Feldman KW: Psychologic morbidity of children subjected to Münchausen syndrome by proxy. Pediatrics 1989;83:289–292.
71. Meadow R: Münchausen syndrome by proxy. Arch Dis Child 1982;57:92–98.
72. Meadow R: Münchausen syndrome by proxy: The hinterland of child abuse. Lancet 1977;2:343–345.
73. National Center for Health Statistics. Vital Statistics of the United States, 1992, Vol. 2, Mortality, Part A. Washington, DC, Public Health Service, 1996.
74. National Safety Council: Accident Facts, 1996 edition. Itasca, IL, National Safety Council, 1996.
75. Osborn HH, Henry G, Wax P, et al: Theophylline toxicity in a premature neonate—Elimination kinetics of exchange transfusion. J Toxicol Clin Toxicol 1993;31:639–44.
76. Polakoff JM, Lacouture PG, Lovejoy FH: The environment away from home as a source of potential poisoning. Am J Dis Child 1984; 138:1014–1017.
77. Quadrani DA, Spiller HA, Widder P: Five year retrospective evaluation of sulfonylurea ingestion in children. J Toxicol Clin Toxicol 1996;34:267–270.
78. Rice DP, MacKenzie EJ, Jones AS, et al: Cost of Injury in the United States: A Report to Congress. San Francisco, Institute for Health and Aging, University of California; and Injury Prevention Center, Johns Hopkins University, 1989.
79. Rodger GC, Tenenbein M: The role of aversive bittering agents in the prevention of pediatric poisonings. Pediatrics 1994; 93:68–69.
80. Rodgers GC, Baird J: Association between childhood poisoning and trauma and child abuse and neglect. Unpublished data cited in Bays J: Child abuse by poisoning. In: Reece R, ed: Child Abuse: Medical Diagnosis and Management. Philadelphia, Lea & Feibiger, 1994, pp. 69–106.
81. Rosenberg DA: Müchausen syndrome by proxy. In: Reece R, ed: Child Abuse: Medical Diagnosis and Management. Philadelphia, Lea & Feibiger, 1994, pp. 266–278.
82. Rosenberg DA: Web of deceit: A literature review of Münchausen syndrome by proxy. Child Abuse Negl 1987; 11:547–563.
83. Shannon M, Wernovsky G, Morris C: Exchange transfusion in the treatment of severe theophylline poisoning. Pediatrics 1992;89:145–147.
84. Shoemaker JD, Lynch RE, Hoffman JW, Sly WS: Misidentification of proprionic acid as ethylene glycol in a patient with methylmalonic acidemia. J Pediatr 1992;120:417–421.
85. Siebert R: Stress in families of children who have ingested poisons. Br Med J 1975;3:87–89.
86. Sobel R: The psychiatric implications of accidental poisoning in childhood. Pediatr Clin North Am 1970:17: 653–685.
87. Sobel R: Traditional safety measures and accidental posioning in childhood. Pediatrics 1969;44:811–816.
88. Solomon SL, Ford-Jones EL, Baker WM, et al: Medication errors with inhalant epinephrine mimicking an epidemic of neonatal sepsis. N Engl J Med 1984;310:166–170.
89. Tenenbein M: Pediatric toxicology: Current controversies and recent advances. Curr Probl Pediatr 1986;16:192–233.
90. Thompson JN: Corrosive esophageal injuries: A study of nine cases of concurrent accidental caustic ingestion. Laryngoscope 1987;97:1060–1068.
91. Tolman IJ, Done GA: Hemodialysis of the neonate weighing less than 4 kg. ANNA J 1989;16:421–424.
92. Trinkoff AM, Baker SP: Poisoning hospitalizations and deaths from solids and liquids among children and teenagers. Am J Public Health 1986; 76:657–660.
93. Vogel C, Caraccio T, Mofenson H, Hart S: Alcohol intoxication in young children. J Toxicol Clin Toxicol 1995;33:25–33.
94. Walton WW: An evaluation of the posion prevention packaging act. Pediatrics 1982; 69:363–370.
95. Weisman RS, Goldfrank LR: Poison center numbers. J Toxicol Clin Toxicol 1991;29:553–557.
96. Weissman DB, Jackson SH, Heicher DA, Rockoff MA: Benzyl alcohol administration in neonates. Anesthes Analges 1990;70:673–674.
97. Wiley JF, Wiley CC, Torrey SB, Henretig FM: Clonidine poisoning in young children. J Pediatr 1990:116:654–658.
98. Wiseman HM, Guest K, Murray VSG, et al: Accidental poisoning in childhood: A muticentre survey. 2. The role of packaging in accidents involving medications. Hum Toxicol 1987; 6:303–314.
99. Zuckerman BS, Duby JC: Developmental approach to injury prevention. Pediatr Clin North Am 1985;32:17–29.

CHAPTER 106

Geriatrics

Judith C. Ahronheim and Mary Ann Howland

The U.S. population is aging steadily: Those older than 65 years of age comprise not only an increasing proportion of the population at large (12%) but an increasing proportion of patients seen in medical practices. Patients older than 65 years of age account for 43% of emergency department visits and 48% of all critical care admissions from emergency departments.[42]

Although the elderly account for only a small minority of poisoning victims, once poisoned they have the highest mortality rate.[29–33] People age 60 and older accounted for only 3.2% of poisoning exposures from 1991 to 1995 but for 19% of deaths.[29–33]

There are several possible reasons for this vulnerability. First, there is a lack of recognition of drug toxicity in the elderly.[4] Because of pharmacokinetic and pharmacodynamic changes in the elderly, which will be discussed later, a given drug dose may produce an unexpectedly serious effect.[3] The presentation of toxicity may be atypical. Falls, a common presentation of disease in the elderly, may be the presenting sign of drug toxicity; if the patient is cognitively impaired and the fall is unwitnessed, the immediate consequences of the fall may be addressed but the cause of the fall may not be determined.[24,37,39] Drug overdose can also result in focal neurologic deficits that may be attributed solely to cerebrovascular or cardiovascular disease, and a specific insult leading to the event may remain unrecognized.[46] The drugs most commonly responsible for acute and chronic toxicity in the elderly are listed in Table 106–1.

The manifestations of drug toxicity may be delayed in the elderly. Drugs with a long half-life may not reach a steady state and hence peak action until many days after the prescription is written and drug therapy is initiated. In one case, a 78-year-old woman received a prescription for the hypnotic flurazepam (Dalmane). She experienced no obvious adverse effects during a week of taking the drug nightly, but then developed slurred speech and weakness, which resolved a few days after the drug was stopped. In some older patients flurazepam's active metabolite desalkylflurazepam has a half-life of up to 100 hours or longer, which necessitates days to achieve a steady state. When peak effects are delayed in this way, drug toxicity can easily be mistaken for non-drug-related illness.

Suicide and Intentional Poisonings

The risk of suicide by all means increases steadily with age, particularly among white males.[35] Although data for individual ethnic groups are sparse, white men have a substantially higher risk of suicide than their same age cohorts among the black population.[7,35,36] Whereas death by completed suicide is more common among men than among women, women are responsible for more suicide attempts. The male to female ratio of suicide attempts narrows with increasing age, so that in the oldest age groups men attempt suicide slightly more often than women, when all means of attempted suicide are considered.[19]

Although firearms are the most common instrument of completed suicide, and far outpace drug overdose as a cause of suicide among men over 65, among women, drug overdose is nearly as frequent, accounting for about 25% of completed suicides. When death by inhalation is included, poison exposure surpasses gunshot wounds as a cause of death by suicide among elderly women.[35] Drug overdose is an infrequent cause of death by suicide among elderly men, accounting for only about 3% of deaths. However, overdose is a common cause of suicide attempts among elderly of both sexes.[19]

Poisoning and Adverse Drug Events

Compared to younger adults, the elderly are at increased risk of unintentional poisoning and other adverse drug events. An adverse drug event (ADE) is defined as "an injury resulting from medical intervention related to a

TABLE 106–1. DRUGS MOST COMMONLY RESPONSIBLE FOR ACUTE AND CHRONIC TOXICITY IN THE ELDERLY

Acute Toxicity
- Analgesics
  - Acetaminophen
  - Opioids
  - Salicylates
- Anticholinergics
- Cardiovascular medications
  - Digoxin
  - Calcium channel blockers
- Sedative-hypnotics
- Tricyclic antidepressants

Chronic Toxicity
- Anticholinergics
- Digoxin
- Magnesium-containing antacids/laxatives
- Neuroleptics
- Salicylates
- Sedative-hypnotics
- Theophylline
- Tricyclic antidepressants

drug."[6] This definition encompasses events that result from inappropriate use of medications, such as a prescribing error, or appropriate use. Several life-threatening reactions may occur with therapeutic doses; examples include the fluoxetine-induced serotonin syndrome and the neuroleptic malignant syndrome. However, whereas those reactions are relatively unpredictable and may occur at all ages, others are more likely to occur in an aged population and are potentially avoidable if patients are carefully monitored; examples include severe bleeding due to nonsteroidal anti-inflammatory agents (NSAID gastropathy), and metformin-induced lactic acidosis.

Whereas reported poisoning exposures among the elderly are much lower than among children and younger adults,[29–33] the incidence of ADEs increases steadily with age.[9,26] Furthermore, in late life, ADEs are more likely to be serious. The incidence of serious ADEs (defined as those resulting in death, hospitalization, prolongation of hospitalization, or permanent or serious disability) increases steadily with increasing age, and is highest in people 85 years of age and older.[9] Thus, the concepts of poisoning and ADE blur in the geriatric population.

Pharmacokinetic Factors

Age-related pharmacokinetic factors are an important starting point for an overall understanding of the geriatric patient's response to the drug milieu. The most important and consistent pharmacokinetic change that occurs with aging is a decrease in renal function. Glomerular filtration rate (GFR) declines, on the average, by 50% between the ages of 30 and 80 years.[14,41] The GFR cannot be accurately predicted by serum creatinine, because muscle mass, the source of serum creatinine, declines with age, and serum creatinine may not be elevated even if GFR has undergone this age-related decline.

Because it is impractical and often difficult to measure 24-hour creatinine clearance prior to instituting therapy with an important, renally excreted drug, it is common for clinicians to estimate creatinine clearance using age-adjusted formulas or nomograms. A popular formula derived from clinical experience in hospitalized patients is fairly predictive of renal function when renal function is stable.[11] However, age-related declines in GFR are not universal, and data from longitudinal studies suggest that as many as one-third of the elderly do not experience this age-related decline.[28] Moreover, predictive formulas often overestimate actual creatinine clearance in chronically ill, debilitated elderly by as much as 20%.[15] In short, it is difficult to predict an elderly patient's ability to eliminate renally excreted drugs or drug metabolites. A practical solution would be to assume that renal function has declined and to exercise caution when prescribing maintenance doses of drugs with a narrow therapeutic-to-toxic ratio (Table 106–2). Failure to do so is an important cause of toxicity.[27]

With advancing age, there are changes in hepatic function as well. Hepatic blood flow appears to decline with age.[50] So drugs removed by hepatic extraction may be eliminated less efficiently. Enzymatic processes are variable. Hepatic conjugation does not decline significantly with age, so drugs metabolized by these processes, such as temazepam and oxazepam, do not have a prolonged elimination half-life. In contrast, hepatic oxidative enzyme activity may decline, so that drugs me-

TABLE 106–2. DRUGS WITH NARROW THERAPEUTIC-TO-TOXIC RATIO AND POTENTIAL FOR ACCUMULATION IN THE PRESENCE OF DIMINISHED RENAL FUNCTION IN THE ELDERLY

- Antimicrobial agents
  - Aminoglycosides
  - Imipenem
  - Pyrazinamide
  - Vancomycin
- Benzodiazepines with active metabolites
  - Chlordiazepoxide
  - Clorazepate
  - Diazepam
  - Flurazepam
  - Halazepam
- Digoxin
- Lithium
- Meperidine (active metabolite is normeperidine)
- Metformin
- Procainamide (active metobolite *N*-acetyl procainamide)
- Salicylates
- Sulfonylureas with active metabolites
  - Chlorpropamide
  - Acetohexamide

TABLE 106–3. DRUGS THAT MAY BE AFFECTED BY A DECREASE IN HEPATIC PERFUSION OR HEPATIC OXIDATION IN THE ELDERLY

High Hepatic Extraction	Hepatic Oxidation
Lidocaine	Chlordiazepoxide
Meperidine	Cyclic antidepressants
Metoprolol	Diazepam
Pentazocine	Quinidine
Propranolol	Theophylline
Tocainide	Thioridazine
Triazolam	Triazolam
Verapamil	

Data from Brouwer K, Dukes G, Powel J: Influence of liver function on drug disposition. In: Evans W, Schetag J, Jusko W, eds: Applied Pharmacokinetics. Vancouver, Applied Therapeutics, 1992.

tabolized by that system, such as diazepam and flurazepam, are eliminated more slowly.[20] Unlike conjugated metabolites, which tend to be inactive, products of oxidative metabolism are often active. Because these active metabolites are generally excreted by the kidney, the presence of active drug may be markedly prolonged. However, there is considerable controversy over the extent to which advanced age alters the ability of drugs to undergo hepatic metabolism, particularly oxidative processes.[48]

Age-related alterations in enzyme activity are not associated with any clinical signs or simple laboratory abnormalities, making it impossible to predict a given patient's ability to eliminate a hepatically metabolized drug. Adding to this unpredictability is the age-independent genetic variability in hepatic metabolism, the ability of microsomal oxidative enzymes to be induced or inhibited by many exogenous substances, and the possibility that advanced age may affect the inducibility or inhibition of this enzyme system. Because of these uncertainties, caution must be paid to particular drugs (Table 106–3).

Age-related alterations in body composition can affect drug disposition in later life. The fat-to-lean ratio increases with advancing age (Table 106–4).[38] Thus, highly lipid-soluble drugs tend to have an increased volume of distribution (V_d). As a result, there may be a delay before steady state is reached, and peak effect and toxicity may occur later than expected. This mechanism may be part of the reason drugs such as diazepam and flurazepam have a prolonged half-life in otherwise healthy elderly patients. In contrast to lipid-soluble drugs, substances that distribute in water, such as ethanol, have a smaller V_d; this may lead to peak effects that develop more rapidly and are more pronounced than expected.

Protein synthesis declines with age.[40] Although serum albumin remains in the normal range in the healthy elderly,[10] this age group is probably more likely to experience a rapid decrease in albumin levels when there is acute or chronic illness, or when protein intake does not keep up with demand.[51] A decline in serum protein increases the free or active fraction of drugs that are highly protein-bound. Free drug is able to travel more readily to the liver and kidney for metabolism or excretion, so that a gradual change in the serum protein level is unlikely to lead to a change in the patient's response to the drug. However, these changes may be clinically important when interpreting serum levels of highly bound drugs. Clinical laboratories measure total (free plus bound) levels of drug, but because most drug is bound, the reported value reflects mostly bound drug. Thus, the total drug concentration may lie in the therapeutic range even though the undefined unbound fraction might be high. Phenytoin, which is highly bound to albumin, serves as an illustrative example. If the serum level of phenytoin is reported as subtherapeutic, the physician might order a dose increase even though the free fraction, which was not separately determined, lies in the therapeutic range. With a dose increase, the free or active fraction of the drug may increase to toxic levels.

Basic drugs are not bound to albumin but to $alpha_1$ acid glycoprotein (AAG), an acute-phase reactant that tends to increase rather than decrease with age.[1] However, the increase attributed to age is most likely related to underlying disease. These unpredictable changes would be expected to have the reverse effect on the ratio of bound to unbound drug in any laboratory report.[47] The correlation between clinical effect and free drug lev-

TABLE 106–4. SPECIAL PHARMACOKINETIC CONSIDERATIONS IN THE ELDERLY

	Young	Elderly	Consideration
Fat (% of body weight)	15	↑(=30)	↑ V_d for drugs distributing to fat (diazepam, amitriptyline, lidocaine)
Intracellular water (% of body weight)	42	↓(=30)	↓ V_d for water-soluble drugs
Muscle (% of body weight)	17	↓(=12)	↓ V_d for drugs distributing into lean tissue (digoxin, acetaminophen, caffeine, ethanol)
Albumin (g/dL)	4	↓ With acute or chronic illness	↑ Free levels of drugs > 90% bound to albumin, especially with overdose Interpretation of serum concentration altered
$Alpha_1$-acid glycoprotein	Normal	↑	Affects distribution of basic drugs
Liver	Normal	↓ Size, possible ↓ in hepatic blood flow	Liver enzymes not predictive; drugs with high extraction (propranolol, triazolam) may increase
		↓ In oxidation (phase I reactions)	Drug accumulation (diazepam, phenytoin)
Kidney	Normal	Possible ↓ GFR	Accumulation (lithium, aminoglycosides, N-acetyl procainamide)

Data from Mayersohn M: Special pharmacokinetic considerations in the elderly. In: Evans WE, Schentag JJ, Jusko WJ, eds: Applied Pharmacokinetics: Principles of Therapeutic Drug Monitoring, 3rd ed. Vancouver, Applied Therapeutics, 1992, pp. 1–43; and Fox F, Auestad A: Geriatric emergency clinical pharmacology. Emerg Med Clin North Am 1990;8:221–239.

els requires further study, because there may be complex factors involved, including alterations in V_d and specific tissue concentrations.

The contribution of gastrointestinal absorption to drug toxicity is unknown, but absorption tends to decline modestly, if at all, with advancing age, despite age-related changes in the gastric mucosa.

What Pharmacodynamic Factors Contribute to Toxicity in the Elderly?

Pharmacodynamic factors may also affect the patient's response to a given drug. In general, age-related physiologic changes in target or nontarget organs lead to increased sensitivity of a given drug. Sensitivity to some drugs may also be decreased. For example, there is evidence that beta-adrenergic receptor sensitivity declines with aging, leading to a diminished response to both beta agonists and antagonists.[12,49] However, it is likely that most elderly do respond adequately to drugs of this category.[18] Thus, experimental findings should not lead to the belief that beta-adrenergic agents are less effective or of less potential risk.

The observation of enhanced sensitivity to drugs[21] is probably related to altered pharmacokinetics in many, if not most, cases. Proving that a patient's enhanced sensitivity is related to altered pharmacodynamics would require demonstrating that the concentration of drug at the tissue site was not increased as the result of diminished elimination.[16] However, regardless of the mechanism, it is important for practical purposes to recognize that the response to a given drug might be altered in specific ways among the elderly. These altered responses are probably due less to chronologic aging and more to an increased prevalence of disease in an aged population.[21] Examples of altered effects frequently seen among the elderly are given in Table 106–5.

Risk Factors for Adverse Events

The likelihood of experiencing an ADE increases with the increasing number of drugs prescribed for a patient.[34] Geriatric patients take more prescription and nonprescription drugs than any patient group.[9] A complicated drug regimen also increases the risk of clinically important drug interactions. Among hospitalized patients, approximately 7% of adverse drug reactions occur as a consequence of drug–drug interactions; in a chronic disease hospital, as many as 22% are due to these interactions.[8]

Drugs involved in serious interactions, such as digoxin, warfarin, and diuretics, are commonly prescribed in the elderly population. This situation is complicated by the fact that elderly patients often have multisystem disease and may visit several physicians, who prescribe medications without knowledge or attention to the remainder of the patient's drug regimen. For example, a urologist prescribed trimethoprim-sulfamethoxazole for a patient receiving warfarin prescribed by her internist; the resulting drug–drug interaction increased warfarin sensitivity and led to a severe intestinal hemorrhage. In another case, an ophthalmologist prescribed acetazolamide for a patient taking hydrochlorothiazide, prescribed by her primary care physician for systemic hypertension; this drug–drug interaction led to symptomatic hypokalemia, weakness, and a fall resulting in injury.

Concurrent disease in target or nontarget organs may alter the patient's sensitivity to a given drug.[22] This may result in a serious ADE even if the patient is given a standard or previously used dose of a drug. Coexistent disease is often subclinical, and the patient's enhanced sensitivity may not be anticipated. A patient with subclinical Alzheimer's disease whose cognitive function is overtly normal may acutely develop delirium or symptoms of dementia when given drugs that would not ordinarily be expected to have this effect. Delirium is a med-

TABLE 106–5. ALTERED DRUG RESPONSES FREQUENTLY SEEN IN THE ELDERLY

	Drug	Possible Outcome
Alteration		
Impaired baroreceptor function, venous insufficiency	Diuretics: cyclic antidepressants; methyldopa	Orthostatic hypotension
Altered temperature regulation	Phenothiazines	Hypo- or hyperthermia
Increased ADH secretion	Chlorpropamide; many others	Hyponatremia
Decreased androgenic hormones (male)	Digoxin; spironolactone	Gynecomastia
Underlying Disorder[a]		
Atrophic gastritis	Aspirin; NSAIDs	Gastric hemorrhage
Immobility; cathartic bowel	Many	Constipation
Dementia	Many	Confusion
Sinus or AV nodal disease	Digoxin; verapamil	Bradycardia
Venous insufficiency	Nifedipine	Edema
Unstable bladder	Diuretics	Incontinence
Prostatic hyperplasia	Anticholinergics; tricyclic antidepressants, disopyramide	Urinary retention
Parkinson's disease	Metoclopramide; neuroleptics	Parkinsonian symptoms

[a]May be subclinical.

Modified, with permission, from Ahronheim JC: Handbook of Prescribing Medications for Geriatric Patients. Boston, Little, Brown, 1992, p. 3.

ical emergency and an important reason for emergency department visits among the elderly.[22]

Another contributing factor is physician lack of knowledge about principles of geriatric prescribing.[17] In one recent series of hospitalized patients, failure to take into account advanced age was the most common factor associated with clinically important prescribing errors, and inattention to abnormal renal function was the second most important.[27] Inattention to risk factors can lead to disaster. Metformin, a biguanide oral hypoglycemic agent in use outside the United States for 40 years, was only recently approved for use in this country, and may produce life-threatening lactic acidosis in the presence of renal insufficiency.[23] Compounding the problem of lack of knowledge is the fact that new drugs have not often been adequately studied in the elderly.[43] Phase I studies involve only 100 normal healthy patients, phase II efficacy studies involve only approximately 200 to 300 patients, and phase III studies include approximately 1000 to 3000 patients. Reactions occurring in a small percentage of patients in a special subgroup can easily be missed during the initial investigations. Even when a substantial number of subjects older than 60 years are studied, much smaller proportions of patients older than 70 and fewer than 1% of those older than 80 may be included in clinical trials.[2] Thus, the very adults at highest risk for many forms of drug toxicity are those least often studied. Subjects undergoing drug testing are generally young and disease free, so pharmacokinetic profiles do not reflect patterns of drug disposition that might be experienced by many geriatric patients. Pharmacokinetic testing may be limited to a one-time dose, and frequently the evaluation takes place over a short period of time. On the average, approximately 5 half-lives of a drug must transpire before a steady state is reached; thus, a drug with a half-life of 24 hours may not reach a steady state for 5 days, and if elimination of the drug is prolonged by age-related factors a steady state may not be reached for substantially longer. Thus, even if subjects studied in a drug trial were elderly, the ultimate effect of that drug in the elderly subject might not be noted during the testing interval.

Death or serious morbidity due to drugs that has occurred in elderly patients might have been avoided had the responsible drugs been studied under such specialized conditions. For example, benoxaprofen, a long-acting nonsteroidal antiinflammatory agent, was responsible for several deaths from cholestatic jaundice in elderly patients. The jaundice and other serious dose-related toxicity from the drug were recognized only belatedly. Another example was the antibiotic temafloxacin. Temafloxacin was available for only 3 months before it was withdrawn after reports of 3 deaths and more than 300 cases of hypoglycemia, many of which were in elderly patients with diminished renal function. Other adverse effects of this drug included hemolytic anemia and allergic reactions with respiratory distress.

If pharmacokinetic studies identify vulnerable subgroups, a safe maximum dose could be recommended, theoretically preventing this kind of problem.[5] Because of these problems, federal regulations may be implemented that mandate targeted testing and geriatric prescribing information. In November 1990, the Food and Drug Administration proposed a modification of its labeling regulations (21 CFR 201.567) that would include specific statements regarding the amount of information about the drug in the elderly. The labeling would indicate whether the drug had been tested in a sufficient number of elderly to detect a meaningful difference from younger patients and whether any special monitoring or dosage adjustments should be made.[45]

Old drugs may also be a problem, because older individuals often have access to products that have been on their shelves for decades. In one case, a 70-year-old woman presented to the emergency department after ingesting purple oblong (coffin-shaped) tablets in a suicide attempt. She developed abdominal cramps, melena, and hematemesis within several hours. She had ingested mercuric chloride tablets, a topical antiseptic used commonly 50 years ago. In other cases, patients continue to obtain prescriptions for the same drug year after year. One example is meprobamate, a sedative-hypnotic that is still widely available, but far less often prescribed today than the benzodiazepines. Unlike benzodiazepines, meprobamate participates in pharmacokinetic drug interactions and has a narrower therapeutic-to-toxic ratio. Patients may be unwilling to change, or the physician may have readily renewed the prescription without asking, or without sufficiently reevaluating the patient. One 90-year-old woman who presented with heart block had been taking digoxin 0.25 mg for many years without a clear indication. Although her BUN and creatinine were normal, her digoxin level was elevated. A dose that might have been appropriate years before was now too high for her ability to eliminate the drug; in addition, subclinical cardiac changes might have occurred, making her more sensitive to the drug.

Additional factors may enhance the risk of unintentional poisonings in geriatric patients. Impaired vision, hearing, and memory may lead to misunderstanding or the inability to follow directions concerning the use of prescription and nonprescription drugs. Dementia is an important risk factor in unintentional poisonings. In addition to cognitive impairment, patients with dementia sometimes exhibit a variety of feeding impairments, including ingestion of inappropriate substances; this may represent reflex behavior analogous to feeding reflexes seen in young children. In one case, a 74-year-old woman with Alzheimer's disease ingested a glassful of ceramic glaze during art class in the nursing home where she lived. That substance contained 30% lead oxide, a soluble lead salt that resulted in an acute lead level of 80 mg/dL. Wandering is another behavior exhibited by patients with dementia, which can enhance risk. One 88-year-old man with dementia was brought to the emergency department in a deep stupor, which was traced to ingestion of medications that belonged to his daughter, with whom he lived. She took a variety of medications for a chronic pain syndrome, including a long-acting morphine preparation (Oramorph SR 60 mg) and diazepam (Valium 10 mg). The patient had a tendency to wander and to put everything in his mouth.

What Special Considerations Are Indicated for Management of a Geriatric Patient?

Management decisions must be made with the foregoing principles in mind. Gastrointestinal decontamination should proceed as in younger patients. Because constipation is a more frequent complaint in the elderly, if multiple-dose activated charcoal is indicated, particular attention must be paid to gastrointestinal function and motility. Cathartics or whole-bowel irrigation may be required in this patient population more than for younger patients, bearing in mind the specific precautions and contraindications listed in Chapter 30.

The presence of clinical or subclinical heart failure or renal failure increases the risk of fluid overload associated with the use of sodium bicarbonate. Monitoring must be intensive and risk-benefit analyses applied. Hemodialysis or hemoperfusion may be indicated earlier in cases where elimination of the poison is hampered by a decreased creatinine clearance or reduced endogenous clearance. Two examples are lithium or theophylline poisoning in patients with decreased renal elimination or impaired cytochrome P450 activity, respectively, due to concurrent disease or drug utilization.

In addition, patients sometimes develop withdrawal symptoms during hospitalization for their poisoning. Among the elderly, the offending drugs tend to be sedative-hypnotics, such as benzodiazepines. Because these poisonings are often unintentional and elderly patients might not be perceived as drug abusers, the physician might fail to consider the possibility of withdrawal in the differential diagnosis. A patient whose general condition appears to be improving but then begins to deteriorate should be evaluated for the possibility of sedative-hypnotic withdrawal and managed accordingly.

Strategies to limit poisonings in certain elderly are similar to those employed in young children, who are at high risk for ingesting toxic substances or pharmaceuticals prescribed for others in the household. The strategies should include the removal of potentially dangerous substances from the environment and all unnecessary drugs from the household. The physician might request that all medications be brought into the office and then limit the number of pills dispensed or accessible. It may be necessary to limit medications such as antidepressants to a 1-week supply, and administration and control should be left to a care partner.

When Should a Patient Be Admitted to the Hospital?

When geriatric patients are evaluated in the emergency department for poisonings or serious ADEs, the need for hospital admission should be guided by the same principles that would be applied to nonelderly patients. Although concerns about a very old patient's frailty might lead the admitting physician to lower the threshhold for admission, these concerns should be weighed carefully against the known hazards of hospitalization for the elderly.[13]

The physician should be alert for certain situations, however, which might mandate admission. These situations include, but are not limited to, elder abuse or neglect, unresolved acute status change, inadequate home care, unexplained fall, or overdose of medication with prolonged duration of action.

When there is concern that established caregivers at home are abusing the patient, the patient requires further observation, and hospitalization if necessary. Signs of actual physical abuse may be more obvious than signs of neglect.[25] It is not uncommon for vulnerable elderly who are physically disabled or cognitively impaired to be brought to the hospital because of presumed illness, but the source of the problem is found to be the caregiver. Sometimes the caregiver, frequently a family member, has been using the patient's funds for personal use, which often includes the purchase of illicit drugs. Sometimes the patient becomes ill because funds were diverted from the purchase of food; sometimes the patient's prescription drugs are sold on the street in exchange for illicit drugs. More direct abuse could take the form of intentional poisoning of the patient by overdose of prescription drugs.

Unresolved acute mental status change requires close observation and possible hospitalization. Elderly patients who are confused or unable to walk are sometimes mistakenly assumed to be chronically impaired. However, incomplete resolution of altered mental status or physical function should prompt careful inquiry into the patient's baseline functional status, because many very elderly patients are cognitively normal and physically robust and independent in all activities of daily living. Inability to walk or pain on weight bearing, especially when pain is in the hip, in the presence of a "negative" radiograph may mean there is an occult fracture that will only be revealed with a bone scan or MRI.

Overdose with long-acting agents requires careful monitoring. Because duration of action of certain drugs may be markedly prolonged among geriatric patients, a higher degree of vigilance is required. A classic example is the sulfonylurea agent chlorpropamide, which has a half-life of 24 to 72 hours or more, and can cause persistent hypoglycemia. Hypoglycemia leading to serious morbidity or death is an important drug-related problem among the elderly, and occurs with virtually all sulfonylurea agents,[44] although duration of hypoglycemia may vary.

Summary

Older patients account for only a small minority of poisoning victims but once poisoned, have the highest mortality rate. In addition, the elderly are more likely to experience serious adverse drug events as a consequence of appropriate or inappropriate use of medications. Attention to risk factors is essential in this vulnerable population. Important risk factors include pharmacokinetic and pharmacodynamic changes; the presence of overt or subclinical disease, including dementia; patient and physician error; suicide risk; complex therapeutic drug regimens; inadequate numbers of elderly in clinical trials; and lack of knowledge about the principles of geriatric prescribing.

References

1. Abernethy DR, Kerzner L: Age effects on alpha-1-acid glycoprotein concentration and imipramine plasma protein binding. J Am Geriatr Soc 1984;32:705–708.
2. Abrams WB: Food and Drug Administration (FDA) Guidelines for the study of drugs in elderly patients: An industry perspective. In: Inclusion of Elderly Individuals in Clinical Trials: Cardiovascular Disease and Cardiovascular Therapy as a Model. Kansas City, Marion Merrell Dow, 1993, pp. 213–217.
3. Ahronheim JC: Handbook of Prescribing Medications for Geriatric Patients. Boston, Little, Brown, 1992.
4. Anderson R, Potts D, Gabow P, et al: Unrecognized adult salicylate intoxication. Ann Intern Med 1976;85:745–748.
5. Bateman DN, Chaplin S: Adverse reactions. Br Med J 1988; 296:761–764.
6. Bates DW, Cullen DJ, Laird N: Incidence of adverse drug events and potential adverse drug events. Implications for prevention. JAMA 1995;274:29–34.
7. Blumental SJ, Kupfer DJ: Suicide Over the Life Cycle. Washington, DC, American Psychiatry Press, 1990.
8. Boston Collaborative Drug Surveillance Program. Adverse drug interactions. JAMA 1972;220:1238–1239.
9. Burke LB, Jolson H. Goetsch R, et al: Geriatric drug use and adverse drug event reporting in 1990: A descriptive analysis of the two national data bases. Annu Rev Gerontol Geriatr 1992;12:1–28.
10. Campion EW, deLabry LO, Glynn RJ: The effect of age on serum albumin in healthy males: Report from the normative aging study. J Gerontol 1988;43:M18-M20.
11. Cockcroft DW, Gault M: Prediction of creatinine clearance from serum creatinine. Nephron 1976;16:31–41.
12. Connolly MJ, Crowley JJ, Charan NB, et al: Impaired bronchodilator response to albuterol in healthy elderly men and women. Chest 1995;108:401–406.
13. Creditor MC. Hazards of hospitalization of the elderly. Ann Intern Med 1993;118:219–223.
14. Davies DF, Shock NW: Age changes in glomerular filtration rate: Effective renal plasma flow and tubular excretory capacity in adult males. J Clin Invest 1950;29:496–507.
15. Drusano GL, Muncie HL, Hoopes JM, et al: Commonly used methods of estimating creatinine clearance are inadequate for elderly debilitated nursing home patients. J Am Geriatr Soc 1988;36:437–441.
16. Feely J, Coakley D: Altered pharmacodynamics in the elderly. Clin Geriatr Med 1990;6:269–283.
17. Ferry ME, Lamy PP, Becker LA: Physicians' lack of knowledge of prescribing for the elderly: A study in primary care physicians in Pennsylvania. J Am Geriatr Soc 1985;33: 616–625.
18. Fitzergald JD: Age-related effects of beta blockers and hypertension. J Cardiovasc Pharmacol 1988;12:S83-S92.
19. Frierson RL: Suicide attempts by the old and the very old. Arch Intern Med 1991;151:141–144.
20. Greenblatt DJ, Divoll M, Harmatz JS, et al: Kinetics and clinical effects of flurazepam in young and elderly noninsomniacs. Clin Pharmacol Ther 1981;30:475–486.
21. Gurwitz JH, Avorn J. The ambiguous relation between aging and adverse drug reactions. Ann Intern Med 1991; 114: 956–966.
22. Johnson J: Delirium in the elderly. Emerg Med Clin North Am 1990;8:255–265.
23. Jurovich MR, Wooldridge JD, Force RW: Metformin-associated nonketotic metabolic acidosis. Ann Pharmacother 1997;31:53–55.
24. Kruse W: Problems and pitfalls in the use of benzodiazepines in the elderly. Drug Saf 1990;5:328–344.
25. Lachs M, Pillemer K: Abuse and neglect of elderly persons. N Engl J Med 1995;332:437–443.
26. Leape LL, Brennan TA, Laird N, et al: The nature of adverse events in hospitalized patients. Results of the Harvard medical practice study II. N Engl J Med 1991;324:377–384.
27. Lesar TS, Briceland L. Stein DS: Factors related to errors in medication prescribing. JAMA 1997;277:312–317.
28. Lindeman R, Tobin J, Shock NW: Longitudinal studies on the rate of decline in renal function with age. J Am Geriatr Soc 1985;33:278–285.
29. Litovitz TL, Clark LR, Soloway RA: 1993 Annual report of the American Association of Poison Control Centers National Data Collection System. Am J Emerg Med 1994; 13:546–515.
30. Litovitz TL, Felberg L, Soloway RA, et al: 1994 Annual report of the American Association of Poison Control Centers National Data Collection System. Am J Emerg Med 1995; 13:551–597.
31. Litovitz TL, Felberg L, White S, et al: 1995 Annual report of the American Association of Poison control Centers Toxic Exposure Surveillance System. Am J Emerg Med 1996;14: 487–537.
32. Litovitz TL, Holm KC, Bailey KM, Schmitz RF: 1991 Annual report of the American Association of Poison control Centers National Data Collection System. Am J Emerg Med 1992;10:452–505.
33. Litovitz TL, Holm KC, Clancy C, et al: 1992 Annual report of the American Association of Poison Control Centers National Data Collection System. Am J Emerg Med 1993; 11:494–555.
34. May FE, Stewart RB, Cluff LE: Drug interactions and multiple drug administration. Clin Pharmacol Ther 1977;22: 322–328.
35. Meehan PJ, Saltzman LE, Sattini RW: Suicides among older United States residents: Epidemiologic characteristics and trends. Am J Public Health 1991;81:1198–1200.
36. Monk M: Epidemiology of suicide. Epidemiol Rev 1987; 9:51–59.
37. Nelson R, Amin M: Falls in the elderly 1990. Emerg Med Clin North Am 1990;8:309–324.
38. Novak LP: Aging, total body potassium, fat-free mass, and cell mass in males and females between ages 18 and 85 years. J Gerontol 1972;27:428–443.
39. Olsky M, Murray J: Dizziness and fainting in the elderly. Emerg Med Clin North Am 1990;8:295–308.

40. Rattan SI, Derventzi A, Clark BFC: Protein synthesis, post-translational modifications, and aging. Ann NY Acad Sci 1992;663:48–62.
41. Rowe J, Andres R, Tobin J, et al: The effect of age on creatinine clearance in men: A cross-sectional and longitudinal study. J Gerontol 1976;31:155–163.
42. Sanders A: Geriatric Emergency Medicine Task Force: The care of the elderly in emergency departments: A report prepared by the Society for Academic Emergency Medicine. Geriatric Emergency Medicine Task Force, Lansing, MI, 1992.
43. Schwartz J, Temple R, Lemke J, et al: Drug testing in the elderly. Pharmacol Ther 1992;17:1715–1748.
44. Shorr RI, Ray WA, Daugherty JR, et al: Individual sulfonylureas and serious hypoglycemia in older people. J Am Geriatr Soc 1996;44:751–755.
45. Specific requirements on content and format of labeling for human prescription drugs: Proposed addition of "geriatric use" subsection on the labeling. Federal Register 1990;55: 46134–46137.
46. Svenson J: Obtundation in the elderly patient. Am J Emerg Med 1987;5:524–527.
47. Svensson CK, Woodruff MN, Baxter JR, et al: Free drug concentration monitoring in clinical practice: Rationale and current status. Clin Pharmacokinet 1986;11:450–469.
48. Vestal RE, Cusack BJ: Pharmacology and aging. In: Schneider EL, Rowe JW, eds: Handbook of the Biology of Aging, 3rd ed. San Diego, Academic Press, 1990, pp. 349–383.
49. Vestal RE, Wood AJJ, Shand DG: Reduced beta-adrenoceptor sensitivity in the elderly. Clin Pharmacol Ther 1979; 26:181–186.
50. Woodhouse KW, Wynne HA: Age-related changes in liver size and hepatic blood flow: The influence on drug metabolism in the elderly. Clin Pharmacokinet 1988;15:287–294.
51. Young VR: Amino acids and proteins in relation to the nutrition of elderly people. Age Ageing 1990;19:S10–S24.

CHAPTER 107

AIDS—Pharmacology and Toxicology

Neal A. Lewin and Kevin Smothers

Overview and Epidemiology

AIDS is the new leading cause of death of young adults worldwide. An estimated 50,000 to 61,000 new persons are infected with HIV in the United States each year, and 40 million people worldwide may be infected with HIV by the year 2000.[40] With no likelihood that a reliable cure will be identified within the near future, clinicians are facing new toxicologic issues daily: the availability of new drugs (approved and unapproved), and multidrug regimens leading to overdoses, polypharmacologic interactions, and an array of toxidromes require an in-depth understanding of the management of an intentional or unintentional overdose and the adverse effects of these therapies. As will become apparent from a review of the specific AIDS medications in this chapter, most of the known toxicity of these agents is related to their adverse effects and drug interactions. In many cases, little or nothing is known at this time about the effects of an overdose.

In order to understand the effect of the antiviral agents it is imperative to review the HIV-1 replication cycle and the potential points of inhibition by these drugs (Fig. 107–2). The first step in HIV-1 replication is the attachment of the virus envelope to the specific host-cell receptors. The surface glycoprotein gp120 (Figs. 107–1 and 107–3) attaches to CD4 molecules on the cell surfaces found on some lymphocytes and macrophages. Next, entry into the cells occurs, followed by transcription of the viral genome (viral RNA into proviral DNA) by reverse transcriptase. Integration with the host nucleus mediated by an integrase protein (see Fig. 107–3) forms a provirus. Expression of the integrated provirus produces both spliced and unspliced mRNA transcripts that encode the regulatory and structural viral proteins. Finally, new virus particles assemble and particles bud (see Fig. 107–2) through the cell membrane as mature infectious HIV-1 virus.[44]

Understanding the reproduction cycle of HIV has led to the development of pharmacologic interventions to inhibit each stage of the cycle. Thus drugs are now

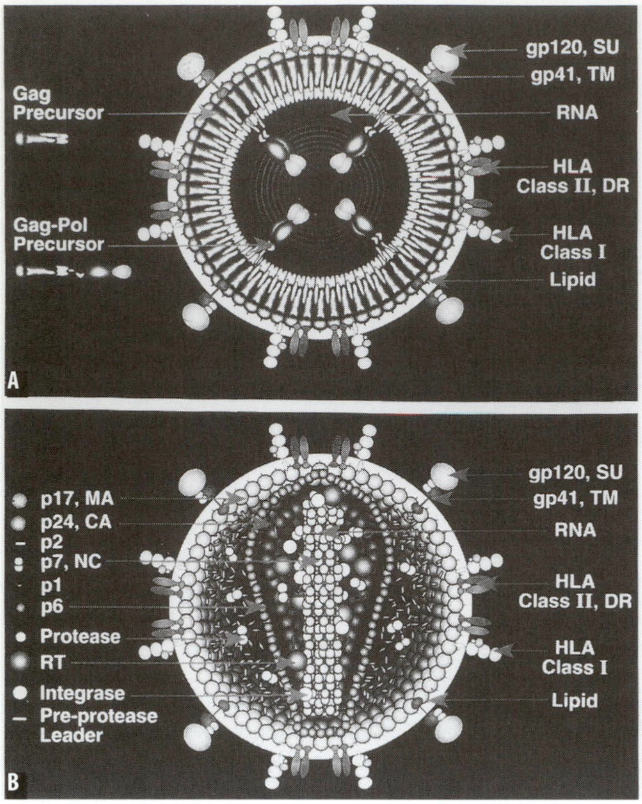

Figure 107–1. The immature **(A)** and mature **(B)** HIV particle. The virion is composed of the envelope RNA genome and structural proteins. *(Reprinted, with permission, from Infect Med 1996;13(suppl F):10–11, Copyright ©1996, SCP Communications.)*

available to inhibit viral attachment, reverse transcription, protease, and the regulatory proteins (see Fig. 107–2).[44]

How Does HIV Infection Result in a Toxicologic Problem?

A myriad of potentially useful HIV drugs in various stages of testing have become available directly to the public through a burgeoning network of buyers' clubs (Table 107–1). Several of these agents are being used in their native herbal form by patients who are unaware of which herbs they are using but who believe that medicinal herbs are less toxic than traditional therapy. (see Chap. 76).[51] As a result of these practices, untested and unapproved agents are being used widely with only limited information about toxicity.

In an effort to help seriously ill AIDS patients, the Food and Drug Administration (FDA) has made readily available many new medications to treat HIV-related problems through controlled expanded-access programs.[10] This novel approach to drug testing has shortened the time required to make potentially useful drugs available to patients.[10] Under these programs, agents still in experimental testing stages and not ready for marketing and wide distribution are made available to patients on a compassionate-use basis. Although more patients may benefit from such medication while avoiding uncontrolled uses through buyers' clubs, an anticipated short-term effect of these programs will be greater toxicity from increased use of inadequately tested agents.

Patients with HIV infection take, on average, 6 to 9 medications for the remainder of their lives, making the magnitude and extent of drug exposure in these patients substantial. Several reports show that adverse drug reactions are greatly increased with HIV infection.[13,19,43] Hypersensitivity reactions are encountered regularly. Dosing errors by patients with HIV dementia complex increase the risk of drug reactions and drug overdoses as well.

A recent study of 1450 HIV-infected patients with a CD4 count of 500 cells/mm^3 or less calculated adverse event rates from the use of AZT (ZDV), didanosine (ddI), zalcitabine (ddC), cotrimoxazole, and dapsone. The conclusions of the study were that the adverse events from these drugs were common, that serious events requiring hospitalization were rare, that adverse events rates increase progressively with a fall in CD4 count, and that race and gender may modify risk with several of these drugs (female > male with ddI and cotrimoxazole, white > black from cotrimoxazole).[70]

Most individuals infected with HIV are also emotionally affected. Depression is common, and the rate of suicide is significantly greater in persons with HIV infection than in the general population.[20,52,58] Initially there was a 17 to 35 times increased risk of suicide in persons with AIDS,[52,60] and although better treatment of the disease has decreased this risk, it is still 7 times that of the general population.[87] In a recent study of military personnel it was found that there was not a significantly increased risk of death from suicide in the months following being told of HIV results. It should be noted that this population was asymptomatic whereas previous studies have evaluated patients with active disease.[24] The overall incidence of depression in HIV infected patients is 7 to 10%, and is particularly high immediately before and after HIV testing.[3] Polypharmaceutical toxic overdose is the suicide method most often chosen, which in turn may reflect the easy access to a large number of highly toxic medications prescribed during the course of the illness.

What Effect Does HIV Infection Have on Drug Metabolism and Elimination?

HIV-infected individuals initially have normal hepatic and renal function and, therefore, normal drug metabolism and elimination. As noted previously, cells infected directly by HIV possess the CD4 receptor allowing the gp120 portion of the HIV to bind, thereby permitting viral penetration into the cell.[41] Because intestinal, hepatic, renal, and biliary cells do not possess CD4 receptors, they are not directly affected by HIV, and patients with asymptomatic HIV infection usually maintain their

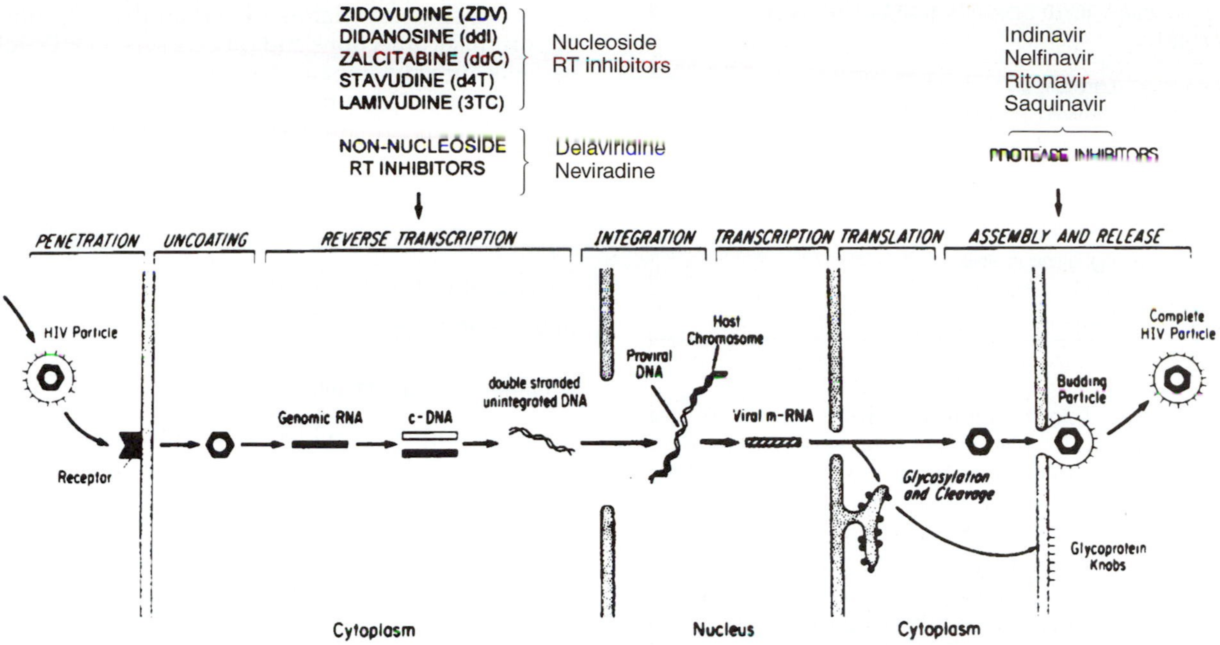

Figure 107–2. Summary of the replication cycle of HIV and potential points of inhibition by antiretroviral agents. *(Reprinted, with permission, from Threlkeld SC, Hirsch MS: Antiretroviral therapy. In: Gold JWM, Telzak EE, White DA, eds: The diagnosis and management of the HIV-infected patient, part 1. Med Clin North Am 1996;80:1264. Previously published in Hirsch M, D'Aquila R: Drug Therapy: Summary of HIV replication cycle and available antiretroviral agents. N Engl J Med 1993;328:1687. Massachusetts Medical Society.)*

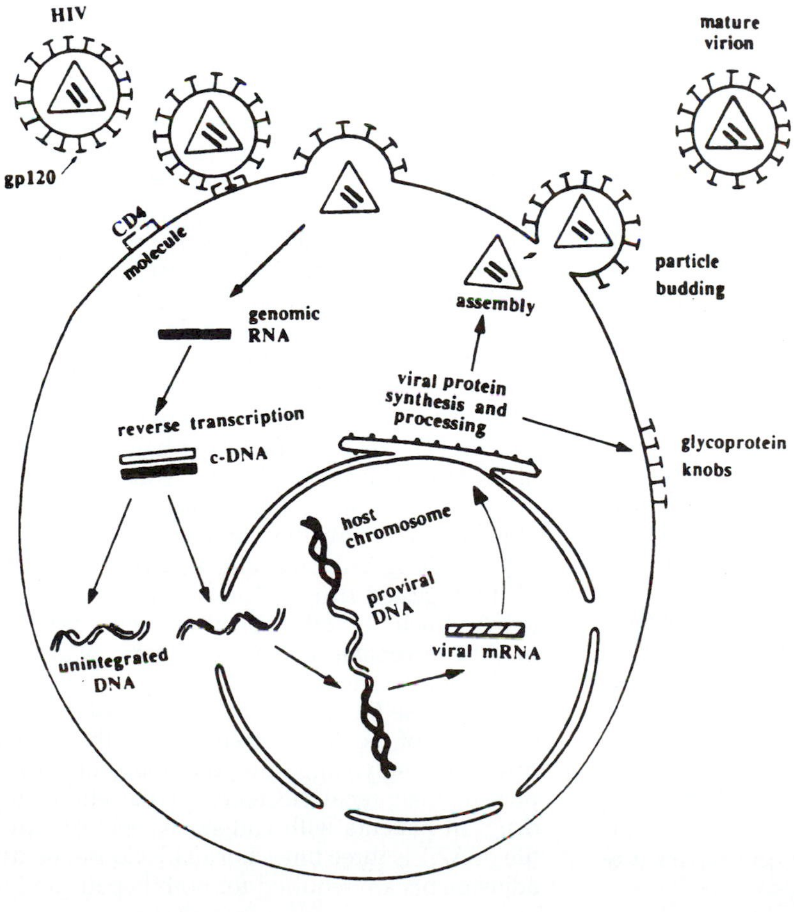

Figure 107–3. The HIV-1 replication cycle is characterized by the following stages: virus attachment, entry, reverse transcription of the viral genome, integration, gene expression, assembly, budding, and maturation. *(Reprinted, with permission, from Hardy WD: The human immunodeficiency virus. In: Gold JWM, Telzak EE, White DA, eds: The diagnosis and management of the HIV-infected patient, part 1. Med Clin North Am 1996;80:1244. Previously published in Connor RI, Ho DD: Biology and molecular biology of HIV. In: Rizzo PA, Wilfert CM, eds: Pediatric AIDS, 2nd ed. Baltimore, Williams & Wilkins, 1994, p. 97.)*

TABLE 107–1. UNAPPROVED THERAPIES AVAILABLE THROUGH BUYERS' CLUBS

Compound Q
Hypericin (Saint John's wort)
Imuthiol/dithiocarb
Isoprinosine
Marijuana
N-Acetylcysteine
Oral Interferon-alpha
Oral amphotericin B
Ribavirin

ability to metabolize and eliminate drugs. However, persons with advanced HIV infection develop altered drug pharmacokinetics resulting from the many infections, immunologic factors, and drugs that alter hepatic and renal function. HIV-associated nephropathy (HIVAN) is a syndrome characterized by massive proteinuria, hematuria, azotemia, and unusual clinical renal pathologic features; the renal insufficiency created by this syndrome may alter drug elimination.[76] HIVAN is seen in all risk groups for HIV infection: men who have sex with men (MSM), injection drug users (IDU), recipients of contaminated blood and blood products, and children born to infected mothers. The most common histopathology in HIVAN is focal and segmental glomerulosclerosis (FSGS).[76] Another cause of renal damage is electrolyte imbalance, which can result from the drugs used in HIV disease[86] (Table 107–2).

The incidence of enteropathy is high in HIV-infected patients, resulting in malabsorption of oral medications.[5,90] Diarrheal syndromes with malabsorption occur in greater than half of AIDS patients during their lifetime, and bacteria, fungi, viruses, parasites, and drugs are implicated as causative.[94] There are several-HIV related causes of impairment of hepatic function that in turn may affect drug metabolism. Interestingly, glutathione, which is important for drug metabolism and detoxification as well as combating oxidative stress, is decreased in HIV-infected cells.[92] Some HIV-infected patients are slow acetylators of certain drugs[59]; numerous opportunistic infections and cancers seen in HIV-infected patients directly impair the function of the liver and, most important, several of the treatments for HIV infection and AIDS are directly hepatotoxic and nephrotoxic. Finally, many drug–drug interactions alter metabolism (Tables 107–3 to 107–5).

TABLE 107–2. DRUG-INDUCED ELECTROLYTE DISORDERS IN HIV DISEASE

Disorder	Drug
Hyponatremia	Didanosine, itraconazole, TMP/SMX
Hypokalemia	Amphotericin B, didanosine, foscarnet, itraconazole
Hypocalcemia	Amphotericin B, foscarnet, pentamidine
Hypomagnesemia	Amphotericin B, foscarnet, pentamidine
Hypernatremia	Amphotericin B, foscarnet, rifampin
Hyperkalemia	Pentamidine, TMP/SMX
Hypercalcemia	Foscarnet
Hypophosphatemia/hyperphosphatemia	Foscarnet
Hyperuricemia	Didanosine, zalcitabine, zidovudine

TMP/SMX = Trimethoprim/sulfamethoxazole.

Modified, with permission, from Rao TK: Renal complications in HIV disease. Med Clin North Am 1996;80:1444.

Specific Antiretroviral Agents: Adverse and Overdose Effects

Inhibitors of Viral Attachment

A logical approach to block the replication cycle would be to interfere with the binding surface gp120 to cell surface CD4 molecules. The use of recombinant soluble CD4 or immunoglobulins directed at viral epitopes (antigenic determinants) has been tried, but thus far all pharmacologic agents in this category are strictly experimental. None are yet available, nor are any data on adverse effects of these experimental drugs available.[41,96]

Nucleoside Analogue Reverse Transcriptase Inhibitors

The nucleoside analogue reverse transcriptase inhibitors inhibit reverse transcription of viral RNA into proviral DNA. They are incorporated into the growing DNA strand and prevent its further replication.[39] Nucleoside analogue reverse transcriptase inhibitors include zidovudine (AZT, ZDV), zalcitabine (ddC), didanosine (ddI), stavudine, and lamivudine.

Zidovudine. Zidovudine (AZT, ZDV; Retrovir) was the first licensed antiretroviral treatment for HIV infection in the United States. It is a deoxynucleoside analog of thymidine. Cellular kinases convert zidovudine into its triphosphate form (AZTTP), which is the active intracellular compound. This triphosphate form competitively inhibits viral reverse transcriptase, thereby terminating viral DNA chain formation (see Figs. 107–2 and 107–3).

In therapeutic doses, zidovudine is rapidly absorbed from the gastrointestinal tract and reaches a peak serum concentration of 0.62 μg/mL in approximately 1 hour.[103] Zidovudine has a plasma half-life of 1.1 hours, and AZTTP has an intracellular half-life of 3 hours.[36] Zidovudine achieves high CSF concentrations (50% of plasma).[54] It is metabolized principally in the liver by glucuronide conjugation and is subject to first-pass effect, resulting in a bioavailability of approximately 60% of the ingested drug.[36] The metabolite (G-AZT) has no antiviral activity, although the glucuronidation process may be reversible and G-AZT may be reconverted to AZT. Zidovudine and G-AZT are excreted almost exclusively by the kidneys, with a mean half-life of 1 hour.[54] Only 19% of the dose is recovered in the urine as parent drug,[53] strongly suggesting that metabolism is more important than renal clearance in the elimination of the drug. In patients with end-stage renal disease the half-life of AZT is three times normal.[28] Consequently, dosage adjustments are required for both hepatic and renal dys-

TABLE 107–3. TOXICITY OF MEDICATIONS USED TO TREAT PATIENTS WITH HIV DISEASE

Drug	Organ System	Signs, Symptoms, Laboratory
Antifungal Therapy		
Amphotericin B (AmB)	Hematologic	Anemia, leukopenia, thrombocytopenia
	Renal	Azotemia,[a] renal tubular acidosis
	Miscellaneous	Fever, chills, rigors, vomiting, headache
Fluconazole (Diflucan)	Gastrointestinal	Anorexia, nausea, vomiting, hepatitis (rare)
Flucytosine (5-FC)	Hematologic	Bone marrow suppression[a]
Itraconazole (Sporanox)	Neurologic	Dizziness, headache, seizure (all rare)
	Miscellaneous	Rashes, anemia
Ketoconazole (Nizoral)	Gastrointestinal	Anorexia, nausea, vomiting
	Miscellaneous	Paresthesias, thrombocytopenia, hepatitis
Antimycobacterial Therapy		
Azithromycin	Gastrointestinal	Nausea, vomiting, diarrhea
	Miscellaneous	Hypoacusis (high doses), headache, dizziness
Clarithromycin	Gastrointestinal	Nausea, vomiting, diarrhea
	Miscellaneous	Hypoacusis (high doses), headache, dizziness
Anti-opportunistic Therapy (PCP, Toxoplasmosis, Cryptosporidiosis)		
Atovaquone (Mepron)	Miscellaneous	Rashes, anemia, leukopenia, elevated AST and ALT
Dapsone	Gastrointestinal	Anorexia, nausea, vomiting, hepatitis
	Hematologic	Methemoglobinemia
	Neurologic	Headache, nervousness, insomnia, blurred vision, paresthesias, peripheral neuropathy, psychosis
	Dermatologic	Exfoliative dermatitis,[a] toxic epidermal necrolysis, erythema multiforme
	Miscellaneous	Sore throat, fever, pallor, malaise, myalgias
Paromomycin (Humatin)	Dermatologic	Rash
	Gastrointestinal	Nausea, vomiting, diarrhea
	Neurologic	Vertigo, headache
Pentamidine (Pentam) (IV)	Cardiovascular	Hypotension, dysrhythmias (torsades de pointes), phlebitis
	Dermatologic	Rash, Stevens-Johnson syndrome
	Endocrine	Hypoglycemia[a] (early) and hyperglycemia (late), hypocalcemia, hypokalemia
	Gastrointestinal	Anorexia, nausea, vomiting, metallic taste
	Hematologic	Leukopenia, thrombocytopenia
	Renal	Azotemia,[a] renal failure (rare)
Sulfadiazine	Dermatologic	Rash,[a] Stevens-Johnson syndrome,[a] toxic epidermal necrolysis,[a] erythema multiforme[a]
	Neurologic	Headaches, depression, hallucinations, ataxia, tremor
	Renal	Crystalluria, hematuria, proteinuria, nephrolithiasis
Sulfadoxine-pyrimethamine	Hematologic	Agranulocytosis, aplastic anemia, thrombocytopenia, leukopenia
TMP-SMX (Bactrim, Septra)	Dermatologic	Rash,[a] Stevens-Johnson syndrome,[a] toxic epidermal necrolysis,[a] erythema multiforme[a]
	Gastrointestinal	Nausea, vomiting, diarrhea, hepatitis
Antiretroviral Drugs		
Protease Inhibitors		
Indinavir (Crixavan)	Gastrointestinal	Increased indirect hyperbilirubinemia
	Genitourinary	Nephrolithiasis
Ritonavir (Norvir)	Gastrointestinal	Abdominal pain, altered taste
	Neurologic	Circumoral paresthesias
	Miscellaneous	Serum lipid abnormalities
Saquinavir (Invirase)	Gastrointestinal	Elevated AST and ALT, nausea, diarrhea
	Neurologic	Headache
Nucleoside Analogue Reverse Transcriptase Inhibitors		
Didanosine (Videx)	Gastrointestinal	Diarrhea, nausea, pancreatitis[a]
	Neurologic	Peripheral neuropathy,[a] headaches
	Miscellaneous	Hyperuricemia, rash

(*continued*)

TABLE 107–3. TOXICITY OF MEDICATIONS USED TO TREAT PATIENTS WITH HIV DISEASE (continued)

Drug	Organ System	Signs, Symptoms, Laboratory
Lamivudine (3TC; Epivir)	Gastrointestinal	Abdominal pain
	Neurologic	Headache
	Miscellaneous	Cough, malaise, nasal symptoms
Stavudine (d4T; Zerit)	Neurologic	Peripheral neuropathy
Zalcitabine (ddC; Hivid)	Dermatologic	Cutaneous eruptions, nail changes, aphthous stomatitis
	Gastrointestinal	Diarrhea, nausea, pancreatitis[a]
	Hematologic	Leukopenia, thrombocytopenia
	Neurologic	Peripheral neuropathy,[a] headaches
	Miscellaneous	Fever, malaise, peripheral edema, arthralgias
Zidovudine (AZT, ZDV; Retrovir)	Dermatologic	Nail changes
	Hematologic	Anemia,[a] leukopenia,[a] thrombocytosis, macrocytosis
	Gastrointestinal	Nausea,[a] vomiting,[a] acute hepatitis
	Neurologic	Wernicke's encephalopathy, dementia, seizures, lethargy, nystagmus, insomnia, headache, mania, ataxia, polymyositis
Nonnucleoside Analogue Reverse Transcriptase Inhibitors		
Ampligen	Miscellaneous	Flulike symptoms, flushing
Foscarnet (Foscavir) (DNA polymerase inhibitor and NNRTI)	Dermatologic	Genital and oral ulcers, fixed drug eruptions (rare)
	Gastrointestinal	Nausea, vomiting
	Hematologic	Anemia (rare)
	Neurologic	Malaise, headaches, seizures, coma
	Renal	Azotemia,[a] renal failure, diabetes insipidus
	Miscellaneous	Hypocalcemia,[a] hypophosphatemia, hypokalemia, hypomagnesemia
Nevirapine	Dermatologic	Rash
	Gastrointestinal	Elevated AST and ALT
Ribavirin	Gastrointestinal	Nausea, vomiting, diarrhea
	Hematologic	Anemia (normochromic, normocytic), bone marrow suppression, aplastic anemia
	Neurologic	Fatigue, headache
Rifabutin	Gastrointestinal	Nausea,[a] vomiting,[a] diarrhea,[a] hepatotoxicity
	Hematologic	Mild neutropenia and thrombocytopenia
	Miscellaneous	Hypersensitivity reactions
Antiviral drugs		
Acyclovir (Zovirax)	Gastrointestinal	PO: Nausea, vomiting
	Neurologic	IV: Seizures, encephalopathy, coma, hallucinations
	Renal	IV: Crystalluria, acute tubular necrosis, renal failure
Cidofovir (Vistide)	Renal	Nephrotoxicity
Cytokines		
Erythropoietin	Cardiovascular	Hypotension
G-CSF	Hematologic	Thrombosis, phlebitis
GM-CSF	Miscellaneous	Fever, bone pain, myalgias, flushing
Ganciclovir (Cytovene)	Gastrointestinal	Nausea, vomiting, diarrhea, elevated AST and ALT
	Hematologic	Leukopenia,[a] anemia, thrombocytopenia
	Neurologic	Headache, dizziness, confusion, seizures
	Renal	Worsening of renal function[a]
Herbs		
Compound Q	Neurologic	Delirium,[a] dementia,[a] coma,[a] paresis,[a] myalgia
	Miscellaneous	Hypersensitivity reactions, hypoglycemia, fever
Hypericin	Dermatologic	Photosensitivity[a]
	Miscellaneous	MAO inhibitor[a]
Immunomodulators		
Disulfiram (Antabuse)	Cardiovascular	Hypotension
With alcohol[b]	Gastrointestinal	Nausea, vomiting
	Neurologic	Confusion, headache
	Miscellaneous	Facial flushing, respiratory difficulty
Dithiocarb	Gastrointestinal	Metallic taste, GI upset, hepatotoxicity
Without alcohol[b]		

(*continued*)

TABLE 107–3. TOXICITY OF MEDICATIONS USED TO TREAT PATIENTS WITH HIV DISEASE (continued)

Drug	Organ System	Signs, Symptoms, Laboratory
Interferon-alpha	Cardiovascular	Ventricular tachydysrhythmias
(Roferon-A, Intron-A)	Gastrointestinal	Nausea, vomiting
	Hematologic	Bone marrow suppression
	Neurologic	Confusion, paresthesias
	Pulmonary	Interstitial, pneumonitis
	Miscellaneous	Fever, chills, malaise
Androgen Therapy		
Fluoxymesterone	Gastrointestinal	Hepatic dysfunction
Nandrolone decanoate		Hair Loss
(Deca Durabolin)	Dermatologic	Rash with dermal preparations (patch)
		Acne
Oxymetholone	Metabolic	Lipid abnormalities
Oxandrolone	Metabolic	Lipid abnormalities
Stanozolol	Metabolic	Lipid abnormalities
Testosterone	Urologic	Increased prostate size
		Virilization
Treatment of Cachexia		
Human growth hormone	Rheumatologic	Joint pain
(Somatotropin)	Gastrointestinal	Diarrhea
Dronabinol (THC)	Neurologic	Dizziness, confusion, somnolence
Thalidomide (Synovir)	Neurologic	Worsen pre-existing neuritis
	Reproductive	Embryopathy—phocomelia
Megestrol (Megace)	Cardiovascular	Superior vena cava syndrome, fluid retention, CHF
	Endocrinologic	Glucose intolerance, Cushing's syndrome
	Gastrointestinal	Vomiting
	Neurologic	Headache, depression

[a]Significant toxicity.
[b]Metabolic toxicity.

TABLE 107–4. CLINICAL PRESENTATIONS ASSOCIATED WITH MEDICATIONS USED TO TREAT HIV DISEASE

Confusion	AZT, interferon-alpha, compound Q, acyclovir, ganciclovir
Cyanosis	Dapsone
Fever	Compound Q, G-CSF, dapsone, amphotericin B, TMP-SMX, AZT, ddI, nevirapine
Flushing	Ampligen, disulfiram (with alcohol), G-CSF
Headache	AZT, ddC, ddI, foscarnet, ribavirin, disulfiram (with alcohol), sulfadiazine, itraconazole, amphotericin, azithromycin, 3TC, interferon-alpha, saquinavir, indinavir
Hepatitis	AZT, dapsone, diflucan, ketoconazole, itraconazole, fluconazole
Pallor	AZT, interferon-alpha, ribavirin, TMP-SMX, dapsone, amphotericin B, 5 FC, foscarnet, ddC, ganciclovir
Peripheral neuropathy	AZT, ddC, ddI, dapsone, 3TC, stavudine
Rash	Zalcitabine, didanosine, foscarnet, hypericin, NAC, disulfiram, G-CSF, TMP-SMX, sulfadiazine, dapsone, pentamidine, itraconazole, ribavirin, nevirapine, delavidine
Renal colic	Sulfadiazine, TMP-SMX, indinavir
Seizures	AZT, foscarnet, acyclovir, ganciclovir, INH, interferon-alpha

AZT = zidovudine; ddC = zalcitabine; ddI = didanosine; G-CSF = growth colony stimulating factor; NAC = *N*-acetylcysteine; TMP-SMX = bactrim, Septra; 3TC = lamidivudine.

function. Zidovudine is adsorbed by activated charcoal and is dialyzable.

The dosage range of AZT is 600 to 1500 mg/d in equally divided doses every 4 or 8 hours. Lower doses are adequate for most forms of symptomatic HIV infection and cause adverse effects much less frequently.[35] Higher doses are required for the treatment of HIV dementia and immune thrombocytopenia.[49]

Although significant clinical benefits from AZT are documented, several adverse reactions, including some serious toxicity, are also reported. The most common adverse effects are nausea, myalgias, insomnia, and severe headaches.[80]

Zidovudine causes or is associated with a multitude of neuropsychiatric reactions, such as mania,[62] Wernicke's encephalopathy,[25] dementia,[16] and seizures.[46] It can cause a severe myopathy (polymyositis-like syndrome) after prolonged use secondary to myocyte mitochondrial toxicity.[4,23] Acute hepatitis[32] and nail dyschromia[30] are also reported. The majority of these effects are transient, occur only during therapy, and gradually diminish after the drug is discontinued and/or the dosage is reduced.

TABLE 107–5. HIV DRUG INTERACTIONS

	Interacting Drugs	Effect	Comments
Antifungal Drugs			
Amphotericin B (AmB)	AZT[a]	Bone marrow toxicity	Monitor CBC frequently.
	Flucytosine (5-FC)	Increased antifungal activity, increased bone marrow toxicity	Given as adjunct to AmB. Trials underway with 5-FC as adjunct to fluconazole and itraconazole. Monitor 5-FC levels weekly when used with AmB for cryptococcal meningitis. Monitor CBC.
	Nephrotoxic agents	Increased nephrotoxicity	Prehydration may reduce nephrotoxicity.
Fluconazole (Diflucan), itraconazole (Sporanox)	Hydrochlorothiazide	Decreased renal clearance of fluconazole	Co-administration results in approximately 40% increase in serum fluconazole concentrations. Clinical significance unknown.
	Hismanal	Inhibits hismanal metabolism	Avoid co-administrations.
	Phenytoin	Decreased phenytoin metabolism	Monitor phenytoin levels.
	Rifampin	Increased fluconazole metabolism	May explain apparent fluconazole failure. Increased dose of fluconazole may be required.
	Sulfonylureas	Increased hypoglycemia	Monitor blood glucose.
	Terfenadine	Inhibits terfenadine metabolism	Advoid co-administrations.
	Warfarin	Decreased warfarin metabolism	Monitor prothrombin time.
Flucytosine (5-FC)	Amphotericin B,[a] ganciclovir[a]	Increased bone marrow toxicity	Monitor 5-FC levels weekly when used with amphotericin B. Monitor CBC.
	Antacids	Decreased 5-FC absorption	Antacids should be taken at least 2 hours before 5-FC.
Ketoconazole (Nizoral)	Antacids, ddI, H_2 antagonists	Decreased ketoconazole bioavailability	Basic pH reduces ketoconazole absorption. Give ketoconazole 2 h before antacids, ddI, or H_2 antagonists.
	Hismanal	Inhibits hismanal metabolism	Avoid co-administrations.
	Isoniazid	Increased ketoconazole metabolism	Higher doses of ketoconazole may be needed.
	Phenytoin	Altered metabolism	Co-administration may cause altered metabolism of one or both drugs. Monitor serum phenytoin.
	Terfenadine[a] (Seldane); Astemizole (Hismanal)	Inhibited terfenadine metabolism	Avoid co-administration, which may result in elevated serum terfenadine and ventricular dysrhythmias.
	Warfarin	Warfarin is increased, probable inhibition of warfarin metabolism	Monitor patient and INR every 2 days. Adjust warfarin as needed.
Antimycobacterial Therapy			
Azithromycin (Zithromax), clarithromycin (Biaxin)	Antacids	Decreased azithromycin absorption	Administer these drugs at least 2 h apart.
	AZT (see AZT)		
	Carbamazepine, theophylline, ergots, warfarin	Decreased metabolism of drugs listed in Interacting Drugs for clarithromycin	Increased serum concentration of drugs listed in Interacting Drugs. Monitor levels and prothrombin time. Avoid concomitant use with ergots.
Capreomycin	Nephrotoxic agents[a]	Increased nephrotoxic and/or ototoxic effects	Monitor BUN, serum creatinine, and capreomycin levels.
	Phenothiazines	Increased risk of respiratory paralysis	Monitor respiratory function closely; if signs of respiratory distress occur, discontinue medication.
Ciprofloxacin, norfloxacin, ofloxacin (quinolone group)	Antacids, ddI, iron supplements, sucralfate, zinc	Decreased quinolone group absorption	Quinolone group form chelate complexes, decreasing absorption. Patients should take quinolones and medications listed in column 2 at least 2 hours apart.
	Theophylline	Increased serum theophylline	Ciprofloxacin can decrease metabolic clearance of theophylline; ofloxacin and temafloxacin less likely to decrease clearance. Monitor theophylline levels.
	Foscarnet	Increased risk of seizures	Monitor for seizures.
	Warfarin	Increased prothrombin time	Decreased warfarin metabolism. Monitor prothrombin time frequently.
Cycloserine	Isoniazid[a], ethionamide[a]	Increased CNS toxicity	Use cycloserine with caution in patients on INH or ethionamide.
Ethambutol	Aluminum salts	Decreased ethambutol absorption	Avoid co-administration.
Ethionamide	Cycloserine[a]	Increased CNS toxicity	Use cycloserine with caution in patients on ethionamide.

(continued)

TABLE 107–5. HIV DRUG INTERACTIONS (continued)

	Interacting Drugs	Effect	Comments
Isoniazid (INH)	Acetaminophen, carbamazepine, phenytoin	Decreased acetaminophen, carbamazepine, and phenytoin metabolism	Monitor phenytoin and carbamazepine serum levels.
	Aluminum salts	Decreased INH absorption	INH should be taken 1 hour before antacids containing aluminum.
	Corticosteroids	Increased INH metabolism	High doses of INH may be required.
	Cycloserine[a]	Increased CNS toxicity	Use cycloserine with caution in patients on INH.
	Ketoconazole	Increased metabolism	See Ketoconazole (antifungal).
	Phenytoin	Increased serum levels of phenytoin	Monitor serum levels, look for signs of phenytoin toxicity.
	Rifampin	Altered INH metabolism	Co-administration may result in increased hepatotoxicity. Monitor liver enzymes.
	Sulfonylureas	Hyperglycemia	INH may lead to loss of glucose control in patients on sulfonylureas. Monitor blood sugar.
Rifampin, rifabutin	Dapsone, fluconazole, ketoconazole, methadone, oral contraceptives, steroids, AZT, sulfonylureas	Increased metabolism of drugs listed in Interacting Drugs; rifampin may precipitate acute withdrawal when given with methadone	Rifampin and rifabutin, to a lesser extent, induce hepatic microsomal enzymes (cytochrome P450). Patients may require higher doses of drugs listed in Interacting Drugs when coadministered with rifampin or rifabutin. Consider increasing methadone dose by 10 mg every 1–2 d starting the day rifampin is added. Some patients may require a 50% dose increase. Split dosing may help.
	Beta-adrenergic antagonists	Decrease beta-adrenergic antagonists pharmacologic effect because increased hepatic metabolism from enzyme induction by rifampin	Monitor therapeutic response of beta-adrenergic antagonists—may need to increase dose of beta antagonists.
Anti-opportunistic Therapy (PCP and Toxoplasmosis Therapy)			
Atovaquone (Mepron)	Phenytoin	Possible increased phenytoin levels	Both drugs are highly protein-bound and my displace each other.
Clindamycin (Cleocin)	Kaolin-pectin	Decreased clindamycin absorption	Administer kaolin-pectin 2 hours before clindamycin. Antidiarrheal agents should not be used with clindamycin until *C. difficile* has been excluded as the cause of diarrhea.
Dapsone	AZT (ZDV)	Increased bone marrow toxicity	Monitor CBC frequently.
	ddI	Decreased dapsone absorption	Administer dapsone and ddI at least 2 hours apart.
	Probenecid	May decrease dapsone clearance	Clinical significance may be small because only 5–15% of the dapsone is excreted in the urine.
	Pyrimethamine/primaquine	Increased risk of hemolysis	Monitor CBC.
	H_2 receptor antagonists	Increased dapsone plasma concentration	Consider decreasing dapsone dosing; avoid H_2 receptor antagonists.
	Rifampin	Increased dapsone clearance	Higher doses of dapsone may be necessary.
	Trimethoprim	Decreased TMP clearance	The plasma concentration of both drugs is increased when they are used together. Consider reducing the TMP dose in patients with anemia.
Pentamidine (IV)	Foscarnet[a]	Severe hypocalcemia; may increase risk of nephrotoxicity	Strongly consider alternatives before combining these drugs. Pretherapy hydration may reduce nephrotoxicity.
Pyrimethamine	AZT	Possible increased bone marrow suppression	Increased bone marrow suppression may occur during initial pyrimethamine therapy for toxoplasmosis. Consider holding AZT when using maximum pyrimethamine doses during acute therapy. Give folinic acid with pyrimethamine.
	TMP-SMX	Anemia	See TMP-SMX entry below.
Sulfadiazine	Sulfonylureas	Increased hypoglycemia	Sulfonamides may potentiate hypoglycemic effects by displacing these agents from their protein binding sites. Monitor serum glucose.
	Warfarin	Increased prothrombin time	Sulfonamides may potentiate the effects of warfarin by displacing it from its binding sites. Monitor prothrombin time.
TMP-SMX (Bactrim, Septra)	Pyrimethamine	Megaloblastic anemia	Additive inhibition of dihydrofolate reductase. Use together in low dosages. Monitor serum iron. Give folinic acid with pyrimethamine.
	Warfarin	Increased prothrombin time	TMP-SMX inhibits warfarin metabolic clearance. Monitor prothrombin time.

(*continued*)

TABLE 107–5. HIV DRUG INTERACTIONS (continued)

	Interacting Drugs	Effect	Comments
Protease Inhibitors			
Indinavir	Amiodarone	Increased concentration of amiodarone; decreases metabolism of amiodarone	Contraindication.
Ritonavir	Astemizole	Astemizole toxicity (potential life-threatening dysrhythmias), increased concentration of antihistamines , increased cardiotoxicity	Concurrent administration is contraindicated.
Saquinavir	Cisapride	Potential life-threatening dysrhythmias, increased concentration of antihistamines, increased cardiotoxicity	Concurrent administration is contraindicated.
	Ketoconazole	Increased levels of protease inhibitors	
	Norvir (Ritonavir)	Inhibits P450 enzymes	
	Rifampin	Decreased levels of protease inhibitors	
	Terfenadine	Potential life-threatening dysrhythmias, Increased concentration of antihistamines, cardiotoxicity	Concurrent administration is contraindicated.
Antiretroviral Drugs			
Ampligen	AZT	See AZT	
	IFN-α	See Interferon-alpha	
Didanosine, (ddI; Videx)	Antacids	Bioavailability of ddI increases because of increased stomach pH	May be advantageous, must be monitored.
	Dapsone	Decreased dapsone absorption	Administer dapsone and ddI at least 2 hours apart.
	Ganciclovir	Possible increased risk of pancreatitis (dose related)	These drugs can be used together with caution.
	H_2 receptor antagonists	Decreased serum concentration of ddI and ranitidine	
	Itraconazole	Decreased itraconazole absorption	
	Indinavir	Therapeutic effect of indinavir is decreased, buffers in ddI decrease the absorption of indinavir	
	Ketoconazole	Decreased ketoconazole absorption	The buffered ddI tablets raise gastric pH to enhance ddI absorption. Ketoconazole requires an acidic pH for absorption and should be given 2 hours before ddI.
	Pentamidine,[a] (IV) ddC[a]	Increased risk of pancreatitis	IV pentamidine, ddC, and ddI cause pancreatitis; hold ddI during acute PCP treatment with pentamidine; unknown clinical significance in combination therapy with ddC and ddI.
	Quinolones, tetracyclines	Decreased quinolone/tetracycline absorption	Quinolones and tetracyclines bind to divalent cations (Al^{2+}, Mg^{2+}) in ddI buffer, decreasing their bioavailability. These antibiotics should be taken at least 2 hours before ddI.
Foscarnet (Foscavir)	Ciprofloxacin (see Ciprofloxacin)	Increased risk of seizure	
	Nephrotoxic agents[a]	Increased nephrotoxicity	Up to 50% of patients on foscarnet develop nephrotoxicity. Avoid co-administration with other nephrotoxic drugs. If co-administration is required, monitor BUN and serum creatinine 3× weekly.
	Pentamidine[a] (IV)	Hypocalcemia, nephrotoxicity	See Pentamidine under Anti-opportunistic Therapy.

(continued)

TABLE 107–5. HIV DRUG INTERACTIONS (continued)

	Interacting Drugs	Effect	Comments
Interferon-alpha	Ampligen	Increased in vitro antiretroviral activity	Clinical significance unknown.
	AZT	See AZT	
Ribavirin	AZT	See AZT	
Rifabutin	See Rifampin/rifabutin under antimycobacterial therapy		
Zidovudine (AZT, ZDV; Retrovir)	Acetaminophen, aspirin, NSAIDs	Decreased AZT metabolism, possible increased bone marrow toxicity	Although increased bone marrow toxicity has occurred rarely, acetaminophen can be given with AZT. A multicenter trial failed to support an association between anemia and ASA or NSAID use with AZT.
	Acyclovir	Increased in vitro antiretroviral activity	Clinical significance unknown. Reports of improved survival with AZT and acyclovir are unsubstantiated. There is a single case report of neurotoxicity in a patient taking both AZT and acyclovir. Most experts think these drugs can be given together safely.
	Amphotericin B[a], dapsone[a]	Increased bone marrow toxicity, may increase AZT toxicity	Monitor CBC frequently.
	Atovaquone (Mepron)	Increased AZT serum concentration; potential toxicity appears to decrease the glucuronidation of AZT	Monitor AZT during concomitant use with Mepron.
	Interferon-alpha	Increased in vitro antiretroviral activity, increased AZT-related bone marrow toxicity	
	Interferon beta	Serum AZT levels may decrease glucuronidation of AZT	Monitor. Lower dose of AZT may be needed.
	Clarithromycin	Decreased/increased AZT serum concentration, altered rate of absorption of AZT (usually increases rate of absorption of AZT)	
	Dipyridamole	Increased in vitro antiretroviral activity	Clinical significance unknown.
	Ganciclovir[a]	Increased bone marrow toxicity (neutropenia)	AZT should be held during induction therapy with ganciclovir but can be reinstituted with caution during maintenance. Hematopoietic growth factors may be necessary to treat neutropenia.
	Lamivudine	Increased AZT serum concentration	
	Methadone	Decreased AZT metabolism	No recommendation for dose change in patients on AZT and methadone; monitor for AZT toxicity when methadone is started or after methadone dose is increased.
	Phenytoin	Increased or decreased phenytoin levels, may inhibit zidovudine glucuronidation and zidovudine clearance	Monitor phenytoin levels.
	Probenecid	Decreased AZT metabolism and clearance	Clinical significance is probably small because only 19% of AZT is excreted in the urine.
	Ribavirin	Decreased in vitro antiretroviral activity, hematologic toxicity	Clinical significance unknown.
	Ritonavir	Increased AZT serum concentration	
	Sulfadiazine/ pyrimethamine	Decreased AZT clearance, increased bone marrow toxicity	AZT's half-life may double in patients receiving both agents. Clinical significance unknown. Consider holding AZT during initial therapy for toxoplasmosis and restarting when maintenance begins. Give folinic acid with pyrimethamine.

(*continued*)

TABLE 107–5. HIV DRUG INTERACTIONS (continued)

	Interacting Drugs	Effect	Comments
	TMP-SMX (Bactrim, Septra)	Possible increased anemia, neutropenia	Anemia and neutropenia are more common when AZT and high-dose TMP-SMX are combined. Consider withholding AZT during acute therapy for PCP with high-dose TMP-SMX. AZT may be taken with low-dose TMP-SMX for PCP prophylaxis.
Zalcitabine (ddC; Hivid)	Amphotericin B[a], foscarnet[a]	Decreased renal clearance of of ddC, may increase risk of pancreatitis and peripheral neuropathy	Discontinue use of ddC before starting these drugs.
	Dapsone, disulfiram, ethionamide, INH, phenytoin, ribavirin	Possible increased peripheral neuropathy	These drugs alone are associated with peripheral neuropathy; therefore do not combine them with ddC.
	ddI[a], IV pentamidine[a]	Increased pancreatitis	Do not use these drugs concomitantly with ddC.
	Probenecid	Increased risk of zalcitabine toxicity	Toxicity: peripheral neuropathy, pancreatitis, lactic acidosis, hepatomegaly, hepatic failure. Monitor patient for adverse effects of zalcitabine; if they occur, decrease zalcitabine dose.
Antiviral Drugs			
Acyclovir (Zovirax)	Interferon-alpha	Increased antiviral activity in vitro	Clinical significance unknown.
	AZT		See AZT (antiretroviral drugs).
	Probenecid	30% Decreased acyclovir clearance	Consider reducing acyclovir dose.
Ganciclovir (Cytovene)	Amphotericin B[a], antineoplastic agents[a], 5-FC	Increased bone marrow toxicity	These agents inhibit replication of rapidly dividing cells and so increase bone marrow toxicity. Monitor closely for anemia and neutropenia.
	AZT	Neutropenia	See Zidovudine under Antiretroviral Drugs.
	ddI	Pancreatitis	See ddI under Antiretroviral Drugs.
	Imipenem/cilastatin	Increased CNS toxicity	Seizures.
	Probenecid	Decreased ganciclovir clearance	Clinical significance unknown. Monitor CBC frequently.
Herbs			
Compound Q	Antiretrovirals	Increased CNS toxicity	Unknown phenomenon.
Hypericin	Sympathomimetics	Possible hypertensive crisis	Hypericin is a weak MAO inhibitor. Clinical significance is unknown. Avoid combining these drugs.
Immunomodulators			
Disulfiram (Antabuse)	Alcohol	Severe GI and CNS toxicity	Avoid concomitant use.
Dithiocarb	Phenytoin, INH, warfarin	Decreased metabolism of Interacting Drugs	Monitor phenytoin level and prothrombin. Observe for signs of INH toxicity.
Flagyl	Cisplatin	Increased toxicity of cisplatin	
Interferon-alpha (Roferon-A, Intron-A)	Cardiovascular	Ventricular tachydysrhythmias	
	Gastrointestinal	Nausea, vomiting	
	Hematologic	Bone marrow suppression	
	Neurologic	Confusion, paresthesias	
	Pulmonary	Interstitial, pneumonitis	
	Miscellaneous	Fever, chills, malaise	
N-Acetylcysteine	Disulfiram (Antabuse)	Decreased effect of tetracyclines	Unregulated form in use may be toxic.
	Dithiocarb	Decreased effect of penicillin G	

[a]Combinations with serious toxicity. This list is not exhaustive and continuous updating is essential.

Modified, with permission, from Amodio-Groton M, Currier J: HIV drug interactions. AIDS Clin Care 1992;4:25–29.

The major adverse effect of AZT is hematologic toxicity.[80,103] Initial use indicated that anemia occurred in 38% of those taking the drug, with 31% requiring transfusion.[80] Anemia is usually not seen until after 6 weeks of therapy. Approximately 16% of patients using AZT develop severe leukopenia (<500/mm^3).[80] Although the platelet count can be either increased or decreased,[80] in most cases a mild increase occurs. Limited work shows that persons with HIV-associated immune thrombocytopenia have an increase in platelets after initiating AZT therapy.[48]

Although macrocytosis usually appears early with

the use of AZT, vitamin B_{12}, folate, and erythropoietin deficiencies are rarely identified.[79,98] Zidovudine does not cause GI blood loss. Anemia is usually caused by selective red cell aplasia or hypoplasia,[101] but bone marrow aplasia of all cell lines also occurs.[37,80] Although the bone marrow effects are usually reversible after discontinuing AZT, in some cases the marrow never or only partially recovers.[37] Erythropoietin, granulocyte colony-stimulating factor (G-CSF), and granulocyte-macrophage colony-stimulating factor (GM-CSF), singly or in combination, greatly reduce the bone marrow toxicity associated with AZT.[34,68,74]

Certain drugs used in conjunction with AZT increase its toxicity (see Table 107–5).[80] When AZT is used with ganciclovir or amphotericin B, bone marrow toxicity is greatly increased. Some drugs (acyclovir, alpha interferon, dipyridamole) increase in vitro antiretroviral activity, while others (ribavirin) decrease in vitro activity. Some (acetaminophen, methadone, probenecid) decrease metabolism through competitive demand for glucuronidation, and others (probenecid, sulfadiazine) decrease renal clearance through impaired tubular excretion, but the clinical significance of these interactions is unknown. Lamivudine and Ritonavir increase the concentration of AZT when used concomitantly.

Intentional AZT overdoses are occurring with increasing frequency. In the few case reports of AZT overdose, patients ingested 3.6 to 20.0 g of drug without any long-term sequelae.[45,69,73,84,91] Transient headache, nausea, lethargy, nystagmus, mild ataxia, seizure, or no symptoms at all are reported.[45,69,73,84,91] No short-term or long-term hematologic effects were identified at 6-week follow-up.[45,73] The lethal dose of AZT in humans has not been determined. All reported cases of AZT overdose to date were managed conservatively. Current recommendations for treatment of AZT overdose include activated charcoal in addition to other standard methods of managing an acute drug overdose.

Zalcitabine. Zalcitabine (ddC, dideoxycytidine; Hivid) is approximately 10 times more potent an inhibitor of HIV replication than AZT.[104] At present ddC is recommended for combination therapy with AZT in advanced HIV infection. Zalcitabine undergoes intracellular conversion to its active form (dideoxycytidine triphosphate, ddCTP) in a manner similar to that of AZT. It is well absorbed in the GI tract, with an oral bioavailability of 70 to 80%, peak serum concentration of 0.5 μg/mL, and CSF concentration of approximately 20% of serum level.[104] The agent has a plasma half-life of approximately 1 to 2 hours and an intracellular half-life of 2 to 3 hours. It is eliminated mostly by renal clearance (70%).[104] Zalcitabine is adsorbed to activated charcoal and is probably dialyzable. The recommended dosage is 0.75 mg every 8 hours with AZT 200 mg every 8 hours.

Unlike zidovudine, ddC has little bone marrow toxicity.[104] Macrocytosis and anemia have not been encountered. Mild thrombocytopenia and leukopenia may develop.

Seventy-five percent of patients using ddC develop a transient symptom complex that appears to be a dose-related toxic effect, including cutaneous eruptions, fevers, malaise, headache, aphthous stomatitis, arthralgias, peripheral edema, nail changes, nausea, and diarrhea.[104] In most cases, these symptoms subside during therapy and do not necessitate discontinuing the drug. A severe sensory peripheral neuropathy, manifested by painful dysesthesias of the feet, develops in 30% of patients treated with ddC.[66,104] The neuropathy occurs relatively late, usually after more than 10 weeks of use, and gradually subsides after termination of therapy.[66,104] Although rare, pancreatitis, which may be fatal, has been reported in patients using ddC both alone and in combination with AZT.

Several drugs cause adverse drug interactions when used with ddC (see Table 107–5). Agents with the potential to cause peripheral neuropathy and pancreatitis should be avoided, as should drugs such as amphotericin B and foscarnet, which decrease renal clearance of ddC and may potentiate toxicity. There are no reported cases of overdose with this agent. Conservative management with activated charcoal is appropriate.

Didanosine. Didanosine (ddI, dideoxyinosine; Videx) has a mechanism of action similar to those of AZT and ddC. It is approved for use as a single agent or in combination therapy for HIV infection. Didanosine is converted intracellularly to its active form, dideoxyadenosine triphosphate (ddATP). Didanosine is very acid-labile and must be administered in a buffered form. It has an oral bioavailability of 23 to 40%, with peak plasma concentrations reached in 0.6 to 1.0 hours.[55] The mean plasma half-life of ddI is 1.5 hours[55] and the intracellular half-life of ddATP is 12 to 24 hours.[1] Didanosine penetrates the CSF at 20% of the plasma concentration. The drug is metabolized by hepatic glucuronidation and renal clearance. The recommended twice-daily dosage of ddI is weight-dependent: 300 mg for patients who weigh greater than 75 kg, 200 mg for 50 to 74 kg, and 125 mg for 35 to 49 kg.

Didanosine has a toxicity profile similar to that of ddC. The principal adverse effects are diarrhea (34%), painful sensory peripheral neuropathy (34%), and pancreatitis (9%).[55] Pancreatitis may be fatal and is associated with a prior history of pancreatitis, advanced HIV disease, and concomitant use of other medications that affect the pancreas (see Table 107–5).[55] Pancreatitis should be considered whenever a patient taking ddI develops abdominal pain, nausea, and vomiting. Asymptomatic hyperuricemia is common with higher doses and probably reflects normal metabolic degradation of the drug.[55] Headaches, rashes, and elevated hepatic aminotransferases may occur.[55] Bone marrow toxicity is not encountered with ddI usage,[55] so white blood cells, platelets, and hemoglobin tend to increase during administration. Because ddI is administered in a buffered form, it should not be administered with other drugs that bind to buffer or require an acid environment for absorption (Table 107–5). Concomitant use of ddC, IV pentamidine, and ganciclovir increases the risk of pancreatitis. There are no reported cases of overdoses. Conservative management with activated charcoal and close monitoring for evidence of pancreatitis is indicated.

Stavudine. Stavudine (2′3′-didehydro-3′-deoxythmidine; d4T; Zerit) was approved for use in the United States in 1994. This nucleoside reverse transcriptase inhibitor is currently being used in patients intolerant to AZT, ddI, or ddC, or if immunologic deterioration occurs on the regimens already outlined. Stavudine is well absorbed orally and its principal adverse reaction is peripheral neuropathy similar to ddI and ddC . No reports of overdose appear in the literature.

Lamivudine. Lamivudine (2′-deoxy-3′-thiacytidine; 3TC; Epivir) was approved for use in United States in 1995. This nucleoside reverse transcriptase inhibitor is used in combination with AZT. It is well absorbed orally and penetrates CSF similarly to ddI and ddC. Adverse effects are GI irritation, headache, fatigue, and rash.[96] No reports of overdose appear in the literature.

Nonnucleoside Analogue Reverse Transcriptase Inhibitors

Nevirapine. Nevirapine and delaviridine are presently the only nonnucleoside reverse transcriptase inhibitors (NNRTI) approved by the FDA for use in combination with other antiviral agents. The NNRTI drugs are chemically different from the five presently available nucleoside analogue RT inhibitors. The NNRTIs bind directly to the RT enzyme causing allosteric inhibition of enzyme function.[96] They have excellent bioavailability and are specific to HIV. The most common adverse reaction to these drugs is rash. Overdose with these agents has not been reported in the literature.

Foscarnet. Foscarnet (phosphonoformate; Foscavir), a pyrophosphate analog, is a viral DNA polymerase inhibitor and nonnucleoside reverse transcriptase inhibitor (NNRTI). It is active against a number of herpes viruses and retroviruses, but its greatest clinical use has been for resistant herpes simplex virus (HSV) infection and cytomegalovirus (CMV) retinitis. Foscarnet may prolong the lives of HIV-infected patients.[2] Rapid emergence of viral resistance has limited its usefulness in HIV infection. Foscarnet may have its greatest utility in combination with AZT, ddI, or ddC.[15]

Foscarnet is very poorly absorbed, with an oral bioavailability of 12 to 22%, and is poorly tolerated because of GI toxicity.[89] Consequently, IV administration is required to yield therapeutic concentrations of the drug. The plasma half-life is 3 hours and it penetrates the CSF (13 to 68% of plasma).[88] Foscarnet is cleared principally by the kidneys (80%), with 20% deposited in bone.[51] The recommended initial dose is 60 mg/kg IV every 8 hours for 2 to 3 weeks, followed by a 90 to 120 mg/kg per day maintenance dose. Foscarnet is dialyzable.

Renal toxicity is the major dose-limiting adverse effect. A decrease in creatinine clearance is common.[88] Nephrogenic diabetes insipidus[33] and acute renal failure are reported.[11] Common electrolyte abnormalities include hypocalcemia, hypophosphatemia, hypokalemia, and hypomagnesemia. Foscarnet should not be administered with IV pentamidine because of increased risk of hypocalcemia (see Table 107–5).

Fatigue, malaise, headache, nausea, and vomiting are common and are dose-related effects.[88] Severe neurotoxicity, with seizures and coma, is seen in about 10% of cases, and is directly related to overdosage and electrolyte abnormalities. Genital and oral ulceration[38] and fixed drug eruptions[18] are rare adverse effects. Bone marrow toxicity, manifested by anemia, is rarely encountered.

Several cases of unintentional overdose have resulted in renal and neurotoxicity. The majority of patients were treated supportively with hydration and replacement of electrolyte deficiencies. Hemodialysis may be of benefit, but it has yet to be tested.

Rifabutin. Rifabutin (Ansamycin), a rifamycin S derivative, is another HIV NNRTI, approved for prophylactic therapy for *Mycobacterium avium* complex (MAC) and also used in combination therapy for MAC.

Rifabutin is well absorbed from the GI tract, with peak serum levels of 0.49 μg/mL occurring 4 hours after administration.[72] The serum half-life is 16 hours; the intracellular half-life is 10 times higher.[72] Rifabutin is principally eliminated in the bile, where enterohepatic circulation results in progressive deacetylation. One of the metabolites (25-deacetylrifabutin) retains the same biologic activity as the parent drug.[72] Rifabutin is adsorbed to activated charcoal and is dialyzable. The recommended dosage of rifabutin is 300 to 450 mg/d.

Rifabutin has a relatively mild toxicity profile. Gastrointestinal upset with nausea, vomiting, and diarrhea are common. Clinically insignificant hepatotoxicity is manifest by elevated aminotransferases, bilirubin, and alkaline phosphatase. Neutropenia and thrombocytopenia may occur. Various hypersensitivity reactions (rash and fever) are reported. Rifabutin stimulates cytochrome P450 microsomal enzymes, which may increase metabolism of certain drugs (see Table 107–5).

A patient who overdoses with rifabutin should be treated supportively. Induction of emesis is usually not necessary and may be contraindicated because of the frequency of vomiting associated with overdose. Intravenous hydration and activated charcoal are the standard of care. Hemodialysis and charcoal hemoperfusion might be useful in severe overdose where supportive therapy is not adequate.

Protease (Proteinase) Inhibitors

The viral protease (proteinase) enzyme is essential for viral replication.[96] Inhibition of the protease leads to defective viral particles (see Fig. 107–2). These nonnucleoside protease inhibitors are valuable because they prevent viral replication even in chronically infected cells, and prevent cell-to-cell transmission of HIV. No intracellular processing of the drug is needed here as is the case with the nucleoside analogue RT inhibitors by cellular kinases. The four protease inhibitors currently available in the United States are saquinavir, ritonavir, indinavir, and nelfinavir.

Saquinavir. Saquinavir (Invirase) is synergistic with RT inhibitors. Saquinavir is metabolized in the liver via the cytochrome P450 oxidase system, and is excreted by renal and hepatic routes. Adverse effects include GI irritation, headache, and liver enzyme abnormalities.[96] Currently this drug is only approved in combination with RT inhibitors.

Ritonavir. Ritonavir (Norvir) has greater oral bioavailability than does saquinavir. Common adverse effects are circumoral paresthesias, nausea, diarrhea, altered taste, and liver enzyme and lipid abnormalities.[96] Inhibition of the P450 cytochrome system makes drug interactions a potential hazard.

Indinavir. Indinavir (Crixavan), like ritonavir, has good bioavailability. Adverse effects are increased indirect bilirubin and nephrolithiasis of crystallized indinivar in 2 to 5% of treated patients.[96]

Immunomodulators

Interferon-Alpha. Interferons are host cell-derived cytokines that possess broad-spectrum antiviral and immune-modulating activity. There are three classes: alpha, beta, and gamma. They inhibit viral transcription, translation, assembly, and release. They stimulate T-cell-mediated cytotoxicity, natural killer cell activity, macrophage functions, and antibody synthesis.[78] Parenteral preparations of recombinant alpha interferon (IFN-α; Roferon-A, Intron-A) are somewhat effective treatments for the early stages of AIDS-associated Kaposi's sarcoma.[56] Oral preparations have not been proven effective, although they are readily available through buyers' clubs (see Table 107–1).

Bioavailability for oral preparations of interferon-alpha is very poor. After intramuscular or subcutaneous injection, peak serum concentrations are achieved in 4 to 8 hours. The elimination half-life is approximately 3 to 5 hours. Interferon-alpha penetrates the CSF poorly and is thought to be eliminated via the kidneys.

Parenterally administered IFN-α often produces adverse effects. Many patients experience transient fever, malaise, chills, and lymphopenia. Nausea, vomiting, paresthesias, confusion, and bone marrow suppression are also common. In a recent case report, intravenous interferon-alpha caused an acute interstitial pneumonitis in a patient being treated for a recurrent multifocal hemangioendothelioma. This patient had received radiotherapy prior to the interferon-alpha therapy and it is known that IFN-α is a potent radiosensitizer. The mechanism of the pneumonitis is unknown and treatment is stopping of the interferon-alpha and supportive care.[102] The hematologic effects are dose dependent and reversible. Reversible cardiac dysfunction is also reported.[29] Interferon-alpha's bone marrow toxicity is synergistic with AZT (see Table 107–5). Overdosage is usually self-limited and should be treated supportively.

Ribavirin. Ribavirin possesses broad-spectrum antiviral activity against many RNA and DNA viruses. It inhibits HIV replication at relatively high concentrations (50 μg/mL), levels at which it can interfere with host cell RNA and DNA synthesis.[26] At present, ribavirin is approved for use only in an aerosolized form (Virazole) for the treatment of respiratory syncytial virus infections. Although there is no evidence that oral ribavirin is clinically effective in HIV infection,[81] it remains available through buyers' clubs. Ribavirin's mechanism of action is poorly understood and differs depending on the class of virus.[22] This drug appears to inhibit viral protein production by inhibiting messenger RNA and viral-coded RNA polymerases.

Ribavirin is incompletely absorbed from the GI tract, with an oral bioavailability of 45%. In oral doses of 600 to 2400 mg it reaches peak serum concentrations (5.1 to 12.6 μmol/L) in 1.5 hours.[57] Significant CSF concentration can be achieved after prolonged administration.[21] The metabolism of ribavirin is incompletely understood. Ribavirin accumulates in RBCs and achieves concentrations approximately ninefold greater than that in the serum.[57] The drug is phosphorylated to triphosphate nucleotides, which are polar and become trapped in RBCs. Renal excretion accounts for approximately one-third of the drug's elimination.[57] The serum half-life is 9 hours and the RBC half-life is 40 days.[77]

Toxicity from ribavirin is dose dependent. Low-dose (600 mg/d) ribavirin is not associated with any toxicity, even in those who are very symptomatic with HIV infection.[72] In doses approaching 2400 mg/d, however, patients may experience nausea, vomiting, fatigue, and headache.[57] The most significant toxicity seen at these or higher doses is a normochromic, normocytic anemia caused by rapid extravascular RBC clearance.[77] Very high doses can result in bone marrow suppression with resultant aplastic anemia.[77] Ribavirin has antagonistic effects on HIV replication when used in conjunction with AZT.[21] Overdoses are best treated conservatively with supportive care.

Ampligen. Ampligen is a mismatched double-stranded RNA molecule with antiviral and immune modulatory properties.[13] Ampligen belongs to the hybridon class of drugs, which are oligonucleosides that are complementary sequences to portions of the HIV genome. They affect transcription and translation by competitively inhibiting viral RNA and messenger RNA[77] and by promoting the production of interferons. Ampligen is synergistic with AZT and IFN-α.[13] Ampligen may serve a role in combination therapy with other retroviral agents.

At present there is little information on the absorption, pharmacokinetics, metabolism, elimination, and toxicity of ampligen. An IV preparation is being used in early clinical trials. In doses of 250 mg twice a week there are no reports of clinically significant toxicity.[13] Some patients may develop influenza-like symptoms and flushing.

Medicinal Herbs

Hypericin. Hypericin (pseudohypericin) is an anthraquinone dimer extracted from the plant *Hypericin triquetrifoltan* that has in vitro activity against HIV by either reverse transcriptase inhibition[85] or blockade of viral assembly or budding.[67] A herbal preparation (Saint John's wort, a combination of several herbs) is available through buyers' clubs. The amount of active hypericin in this compound is low and of doubtful efficacy.

Very little is known about the pharmacokinetics of hypericin and Saint John's wort. Photosensitization is the principal toxicity, and it can be severe. Moreover, patients are taking large doses of the herbal preparation while the full toxic effects remain unknown. Hypericin's antiretroviral activity appears to be synergistic with AZT.[67] It is a mild monoamine oxidase inhibitor,[9] and drug interactions with sympathomimetic agents are possible (see Table 107–5). For all of these reasons, this drug should not be used in combination with other drug treatments.

Trichosanthin. Trichosanthin (GLQ223) is derived from the Chinese plant *Trichosanthin kirilowii* and exhibits potent inhibitory activity against HIV through inactivation of viral ribosomes.[64] It may be efficacious.[63] Extracts are fairly easy to obtain and some patients are using these herbal preparations (known as compound Q). Trichosanthin has poor oral bioavailability and causes intense diarrhea when taken orally. It is therefore administered intramuscularly or intravenously.

The pharmacokinetics are unknown, but the toxicity profile is well reported.[50,83,97] Parenteral administration is often associated with severe neurotoxicity; approximately 24 to 72 hours after administration some patients develop an acute encephalomyelitis manifested by fever, myalgia, paresis, delirium, dementia, and coma. This syndrome is more likely to develop when GLQ223–15 is used with other antiretroviral agents and is usually self-limiting and reversible. Hypersensitivity reactions ranging from rashes to anaphylaxis are common, and premedication with prostaglandin inhibitors is usually required. Hypoglycemia also may occur.

Coma secondary to compound Q usually occurs less than 1 week after IV infusion. Whether combination therapy will result in delayed CNS toxicity has not been determined.

Immunomodulators

N-Acetylcysteine. Patients with HIV infection have a deficiency of intracellular reduced glutathione. Glutathione is important to the cell not only for clearing reactive oxygen intermediates produced during drug metabolism, but also for combating oxidative stress induced by inflammatory cytokines, normal immune responses that stimulate HIV replication.[83] Because of the high cost of prescription *N*-acetylcysteine (NAC; Mucomyst), buyers' clubs provide their own brand of NAC of unmeasured quality.

The pharmacokinetics of NAC are discussed in Chapter 31. There is little toxicity from use of the correct dose of the prescription drug. Some patients experience nausea and vomiting; rarely, fever and rash occur. Experience with the nonprescription form of NAC is limited.

Disulfiram and Dithiocarb. Dithiocarb (diethyldithiocarbamate, DTC; Imuthiol), the major metabolite of disulfiram (Antabuse), may bolster depressed immune functions in HIV-infected patients by unknown mechanisms.[47] Although no clinical trials have evaluated disulfiram, the same benefit as with DTC is postulated. The majority of patients use disulfiram because of its easy access. Some have obtained the raw chemical DTC and make DTC enteric-coated capsules or enemas.[75]

The principle toxicity from disulfiram and DTC occurs with concomitant ethanol ingestion (disulfiram or "Antabuse" reactions). The interaction causes varying degrees of facial flushing, headache, nausea, vomiting, respiratory difficulty, weakness, blurred vision, hypotension, and altered mental status (see Chap. 63).

Disulfiram treatment without alcohol use may cause drowsiness, lethargy, metallic taste, and abdominal discomfort. On very rare occasions hepatotoxicity, peripheral neuropathy, psychosis, and dementia develop.

Antivirals

Acyclovir. Acyclovir (Zovirax) is a synthetic purine nucleoside analog. It requires intracellular phosphorylation mediated by thymidine kinase to convert it to its active form, acyclovir triphosphate, which inhibits viral reverse transcriptase and thus terminates viral DNA synthesis. Acyclovir is used principally in the treatment of herpes simplex virus (HSV) and varicella-zoster virus (VZV) infections. Acyclovir is available in oral, IV, and topical preparations. It is poorly absorbed, with an oral bioavailability of approximately 15 to 30%.[27] Recommended oral doses achieve peak serum concentrations in 1.5 hours.[27] Excellent CSF concentrations (50% of serum) are achieved. It is eliminated, 90% unchanged, in the urine by glomerular filtration and tubular secretion.[101] The half-life of acyclovir is 2.5 hours with normal renal function and 20 hours with end-stage renal disease. Acyclovir is adsorbed to activated charcoal and is dialyzable. The usual dosage is 200 to 800 mg orally five times daily or 10 to 12 mg/kg IV three times daily.

Acyclovir has a relatively low toxicity at recommended doses. The most common adverse reactions are nausea, vomiting, and headache. Intravenous use may cause acute renal dysfunction and encephalopathy. Rapid IV infusion can result in acyclovir crystalluria and subsequent acute tubular necrosis and renal failure. Renal deposition is easily preventable by slow infusion over 1 hour. Encephalopathy manifests as lethargy, confusion, hallucinations, delirium, tremors, seizures, and/or coma. It is encountered with high-dose administration and generally resolves with discontinuation of the drug.[78] Probenecid decreases renal clearance of acyclovir, and acyclovir potentiates the in vitro antiviral effect of AZT. Because the toxicity from oral acyclovir is minimal, even in overdose, standard overdose management utilizing activated charcoal is recommended.

Ganciclovir. Ganciclovir (DHPG; Cytovene) is a nucleoside analog used in the treatment of serious CMV infection. It is structurally similar to acyclovir but is 50 times more active against CMV. Ganciclovir utilizes cellular kinases for conversion to its active triphosphate form, as CMV lacks the gene for thymidine kinase. Ganciclovir triphosphate acts to inhibit viral DNA replication.[31]

Ganciclovir is available orally, intravenously, intravitreally, and via a sustained release intraocular device.[97] With the usual IV dosage (5 mg/kg) the peak plasma levels are approximately 6 to 15 μg/mL and the serum half-life is 2.9 hours.[31] The drug is excreted almost entirely unmetabolized by the kidneys.[31]

Toxicity frequently limits therapy with ganciclovir. Almost all patients using the drug experience some form of hematologic toxicity.[9,17] Leukopenia often necessitates lowering the dose. Anemia and thrombocytopenia are also common.[9] Azotemia is commonly seen and requires dosage adjustments. Nausea, vomiting, abnormal liver function tests, diarrhea, confusion, seizures, headaches, and dizziness are less frequent.[31]

Adverse reactions are dose dependent and exacerbated by renal dysfunction. The toxicity from ganciclovir is usually reversible with dosage reduction or discontinuance of the drug and supportive care. There are reports that the hematologic toxicity may be fatal.[9,17] Agents such as G-CSF and GM-CSF significantly decrease the hematologic toxicity of ganciclovir.

Cytokines. Erythropoietin (EPO; Epogen, Procrit), G-CSF (Leukine, Prokine), and GM-CSF (Neupogen) are recombinant glycoproteins that stimulate hematopoietic cell growth and maturation.[65] These agents are available only in parenteral forms and are well tolerated. Erythropoietin may cause hypertension and predisposes to increased thrombosis. Use of G-CSF is associated with fever, myalgia, flushing, and phlebitis as well as mild azotemia and elevated transaminases. Use of GM-CSF may cause bone pain.

Pneumocystis carinii Pneumonia and Toxoplasmosis Therapy

Trimethoprim-Sulfamethoxazole. Trimethoprim-sulfamethoxazole (TMP-SMX, cotrimoxazole; Bactrim, Septra) is commonly used for the treatment and prophylaxis of *Pneumocystis carinii* pneumonia (PCP) and may offer prophylaxis against toxoplasmosis.[12] It is well absorbed and reaches a peak serum concentration in 1 to 4 hours. Both components are protein bound (44 and 70%, respectively). TMP-SMX is metabolized in the liver through a number of pathways and excreted via the kidneys through both glomerular filtration and tubular secretion. The serum half-life is approximately 10 hours.

There is a high incidence of adverse reactions associated with the use of TMP-SMX in HIV-infected patients. Nausea and vomiting are almost unavoidable, and virtually all HIV-infected patients who use this drug experience some degree of hypersensitivity manifested by various rashes, fever, leukopenia, thrombocytopenia, myelosuppression, nephritis, and hepatitis.[59] With high doses, TMP induces hyperkalemia due to sodium channel inhibition in the distal tubule.[14] These adverse effects are dose dependent and usually do not require discontinuance of treatment.[61] Adverse neurologic reactions rarely occur but include headaches, depression, hallucination, focal seizures, ataxia, and tremor. General toxicologic management is indicated for TMP-SMX overdose. TMP-SMX increases AZT and lamivudine levels.

Sulfadoxine-Pyrimethamine. Sulfadoxine-pyrimethamine (Fansidar) is sometimes used for PCP prophylaxis. The drug has a very prolonged half-life (7 to 9 days). Severe, potentially fatal, cutaneous reactions such as erythema multiforme, Stevens-Johnson syndrome,[71] and toxic epidermal necrolysis[77] have occurred.

Sulfadiazine, used to treat toxoplasmosis, may induce acute renal failure secondary to sulfadiazine crystalluria with stone formation. This condition is usually associated with dehydration, which is increasingly common in AIDS-related diarrheal conditions. Hypersensitivity reactions such as fever, rashes, and leukopenia are common.

Dapsone. Dapsone, used for the treatment and prophylaxis of PCP and prevention of toxoplasmosis, is associated with a number of adverse effects. Anorexia, nausea, and vomiting frequently occur. Fever, rash, and a mononucleosis-like syndrome may occur. Neurologic toxicity is manifested as headache, nervousness, insomnia, blurred vision, paresthesia, peripheral neuropathy, and psychosis.

Hemolytic anemia and methemoglobinemia are the major adverse effects of dapsone. Hemolysis occurs in the setting of G-6-PD deficiency. Dapsone-induced methemoglobinemia is the most consequential toxicity in AIDS patients who are already compromised by anemia and hypoxemia.[87] Obtaining a methemoglobin level and CBC are mandatory. Treatment with standard GI decontamination multiple-dose activated charcoal and methylene blue has been successful for methemoglobinemia (see Chap. 93).

Pentamidine. Pentamidine (Pentam) is frequently used for the treatment and prophylaxis of PCP. Toxic effects are common (approximately 50%).[6] The drug is administered parenterally and by aerosol. Inhaled pentamidine is well tolerated, although some patients develop bronchospasm, which responds well to bronchodilator agents. The vast majority of adverse effects are seen with parenteral usage.

Anorexia, nausea, metallic taste, orthostatic hypotension, hypoglycemia followed by hyperglycemia, hepatitis, dysrhythmias, azotemia, leukopenia, and thrombocytopenia are observed in various combinations in most patients.[61] Severe hypotension occurs when the drug is administered too rapidly. Torsades de pointes can occur and therefore an ECG should be obtained prior to administration of pentamidine.[100] Hypoglycemia followed by hyperglycemia is the direct result of toxic injury to the insulin-producing pancreatic islet beta cells.[6] This results in inappropriately high insulin levels and subsequent hypoglycemia. Several days to months later diabetes mellitus develops. Severe hypocalcemia results from coadministration with foscarnet. Frequently there is a mild elevation in creatinine; rarely, renal failure ensues.

In a recent case report a patient received 40 times the prescribed dose of IV pentamidine due to a pharmacy mixing error. Severe hypotension persisted and a pressor was necessary to maintain blood pressure. Charcoal hemoperfusion was performed over a 4-hour period. Pentamidine levels fell during hemoperfusion; however, reaccumulation occurred in the serum due to release of drug from tissue stores. The authors observed that the blood pressure stabilized during hemoperfusion, but state correctly that the direct contribution of this modality to clinical improvement requires further study.[99]

Atovaquone. Atovaquone (Mepron) is another drug for treatment prophylaxis for PCP[48] and toxoplasmosis.[54] The oral bioavailability is low, but administration with food greatly increases absorption. It is highly protein bound (99%) and is recirculated in the enterohepatic system with eventual fecal excretion. None of the drug is excreted by the kidneys. Toxicity is limited to mild rashes, leukopenia, anemia, and elevated transaminases.

Antifungal Drugs

Amphotericin B. Amphotericin B (AmB; Fungizone) remains an important treatment for a number of serious systemic fungal infections. Unfortunately, its administration is associated with systemic toxicity.[7] During IV administration, fevers, chills, rigors, vomiting, and headaches often occur. Premedication with hydrocortisone, NSAIDs, and diphenhydramine greatly reduces these forms of toxicity. Renal impairment is the most significant adverse effect. Azotemia, observed in approximately 80% of cases,[7] is dose dependent and reversible with dosage reduction. A type I (distal) renal tubular acidosis may occur (see Chap. 23). Amphotericin B should not be given with other nephrotoxic agents. Anemia secondary to reduced erythropoietin is common. Leukopenia and thrombocytopenia are rare. Concurrent administration with AZT results in greater bone marrow toxicity. Earlier preparations of amphotericin B were associated with ventricular fibrillation during infusion.

Flucytosine. Flucytosine (5 FC; Ancobon) is often used in conjunction with amphotericin B. The drug's principle toxicity is bone marrow suppression. Severe reversible leukopenia and anemia often limit use.

Ketoconazole. Ketoconazole (Nizoral) is an imidazole used in the treatment of mucocutaneous candidiasis and maintenance therapy for coccidioidomycosis and histoplasmosis. The drug is absorbed erratically (oral bioavailability is 75%). Absorption is impaired by antacids and H_2 blockers.[93] Ketoconazole has a short half-life (2 to 8 hours) and is highly protein bound (>90%).[93] Minimal CSF penetration limits its utility in CNS mycoses. The usual dose is 200 to 400 mg/d. Anorexia, nausea, and vomiting are the principle toxic reactions. Paresthesias, thrombocytopenia, and mild hepatitis may occur. Ketoconazole suppresses testosterone and cortisol synthesis. Isoniazid and rifampin increase ketoconazole metabolism. Ketoconazole decreases astemizole (Hismanal) and terfenadine (Seldane) metabolism, and coadministration may result in life-threatening dysrhythmias. Didanosine decreases the antifungal effect of ketoconazole. Ketoconazole increases the levels of saquinavir by threefold.

Fluconazole. Fluconazole (Diflucan) is a triazole used in the treatment of serious candida infections and CNS mycoses (cryptococcosis and coccidioidomycosis). Fluconazole has a high oral bioavailability (>90%), long serum half-life (30 hours), low protein binding (12%), and excellent CSF penetration (60 to 80%).[8] Renal excretion accounts for more than 90% of the drug's metabolism; dosage adjustments are required in patients with renal disease.[8] The usual dose is 100 to 400 mg/d.

Fluconazole is minimally toxic with standard dosing. Gastrointestinal upset, rashes, dizziness, and headache are the most common adverse reactions.[82] Rare episodes of anemia, seizures, or hepatitis are reported, but they occurr in patients with advanced HIV disease who were taking multiple drugs, and resolve with discontinuation of fluconazole.[82]

Itraconazole. Itraconazole (Sporanox) is an oral triazole used in the treatment of serious non-CNS fungal infections (histoplasmosis, blastomycosis, and coccidioidomycosis). On an empty stomach, the drug has an oral bioavailability of 85%; it is highly protein bound (>90%).[93] Absorption is impaired by antacids and H_2 blockers. Itraconazole is metabolized in the liver to inactive metabolites. It is widely distributed in the body, with therapeutic tissue levels at sites of fungal infection.[93] The standard dosage is 100 to 400 mg/d. The toxic profile is similar to that of ketoconazole. Itraconazole interferes weakly with the cytochrome P450 (CYP 3A4) enzyme system, so it will decrease the metabolism of cyclosporine, digoxin, astemizole, and terfenadine. Rifampin, phenytoin, and carbamazepine increase the elimination of itraconazole and may result in treatment failures.

Antimycobacterial Therapy

Clarithromycin. Clarithromycin (Biaxin) is a macrolide analog of erythromycin with broad-spectrum antimicrobial activity against MAC. It is used both for prophylaxis as well as in combination with other drugs in treatment of MAC. It is acid stable with an oral bioavailability of 85%.[42] The majority of the drug is metabolized by the liver to an active 14-hydroxyl metabolite. Approximately 20 to 30% of the drug is renally excreted unchanged. The parent compound and metabolite have a serum half-life of 2 to 6 hours and 2 to 9 hours, respectively.[42] The usual dose for MAC disease is 500 to 1000 mg twice a day. Clarithromycin is better tolerated than erythromycin, with less GI upset. Headache and dizziness occur rarely. Reversible dose-related hearing loss has occurred in patients treated for MAC infection. Clarithromycin, like all macrolide antibiotics except for azithromycin, inhibits cytochrome P450 hepatic metabolism and consequently decreases elimination of theophylline, carbamazepine, cyclosporine, warfarin, corticosteroids, and ergotamine. Combination with ergots may precipitate signs of ergotism (Chap. 45).

Azithromycin. Azithromycin (Zithromax) is another macrolide with a spectrum similar to that of clarithromycin. The oral bioavailability is 37%.[42] It has wide tissue distribution with very low serum concentrations, and is extensively metabolized by the liver, with only 5% excreted unchanged by the kidneys.[42] The toxicity profile and drug interactions are unlike those of clarithromycin because it does not inhibit CYP3A4.

Summary

In summary, as the pandemic continues, new drugs are being formulated and used mostly in combination. With the multiple organ system disease that HIV creates and with its effect on drug metabolism, many adverse and potentially fatal reactions have been reported. By recognizing various toxidromes and understanding management strategies, it is the hope that a decrease in morbidity and mortality will occur.

References

1. Ahluwalia G, Johnson MA, Fridland A, et al: Cellular pharmacology of the anti-HIV agent 2′,3′ dideoxyadenosine. Proceedings of the American Association of Cancer Research, New Orleans, May 1988; Baltimore, Waverly, 29 (abst):349.
2. AIDS Trials Group: Mortality in patients with the acquired immunodeficiency syndrome treated with either foscarnet or ganciclovir for cytomegalovirus retinitis. N Engl J Med 1992;326:213–220.
3. Atkinson JH, Capaldini L, Levine JF, et al: Dementia, depression and quality of life. Patient Care 1996;131–143.
4. Besson LJ, Greene JB, Louie E, et al: Severe polymyositis-like syndrome associated with zidovudine therapy of AIDS and ARC. N Engl J Med 1988;318:708. Letter.
5. Berning SE, Huitt GA, Iseman MD, et al: Malabsorption of antituberculosis medication by a patient with AIDS. N Engl J Med 1992;327:1817–1818.
6. Bouchard P, Sai P, Reach G, et al: Diabetes mellitus following pentamidine-induced hypoglycemia in humans. Diabetes 1982;31:40–45.
7. Bowler WA, Oldfield EC III: New approaches to amphotericin B administration. Infect Med 1992;9:17–23.
8. Brammer KW, Farrow PR, Faulkner JK: Pharmacokinetics and tissue penetration of fluconazole in humans. Rev Infect Dis 1990;12(suppl 3):S318-S326.
9. Buhles WC Jr, Mastre BJ, Tinker AJ, et al: Ganciclovir treatment of life- or sight-threatening cytomegalovirus infection: Experience in 314 immunocompromised patients. Rev Infect Dis 1988;10(suppl 3):S495-S506.
10. Byar DP, Schoenfeld DA, Green SB, et al: Design considerations for AIDS trials. N Engl J Med 1990;323:1343–1348.
11. Cacoub P, Deray G, Baumelou A, et al: Acute renal failure induced by foscarnet: 4 cases. Clin Nephrol 1988;29: 315–318.
12. Carr A, Tindall B, Brew BS, et al: Low dose trimethoprim-sulfmethoxazole prophylaxis for toxoplasmic encephalitis in patients with AIDS. Ann Intern Med 1992; 117:106–111.
13. Carter WA, Brodsky I, Pellegrino MG: Clinical, immunological, and virological effects of ampligen, a mismatched double stranded RNA, in patients with AIDS or AIDS-related complex. Lancet 1987;1:1286–1292.
14. Choi MJ, Fernandez PC, Patnaik A, et al: Brief report: Trimethoprim-induced hyperkalemia in a patient with AIDS. N Engl J Med 1993;328:703–704.
15. Chow YK, Hirsch MS, Merril DP, et al: Use of evolutionary limitations of HIV-1 multidrug resistance to optimize therapy. Nature 1993;361:650–654.
16. Cohn J, Shapiro C, Keyes C, Smothers K: Neurologic disease associated with zidovudine (AZT (ZDV)). Presented at the 27th ICAAC, Washington, DC 1987;abstract 381.
17. Collaborative DHPG Treatment Study Group: Treatment of serious cytomegalovirus infections with 9-(1,3-dihydroxy-2-propoxymethyl) guanine in patients with AIDS and other immunodeficiencies. N Engl J Med 1986;314: 801–805.
18. Connolly GM, Gazzard BG, Hawkins DA: Fixed drug eruption due to foscarnet. Genitour Med 1990;66:97–98.
19. Coopman SA, Johnson RA, Platt R: Cutaneous disease and drug reactions in HIV infection. N Engl J Med 1993;328: 1670–1674.
20. Cote TR, Biggar RJ, Dannenberg AL: Risk of suicide among persons with AIDS. JAMA 1992;268:2066–2068.
21. Crumpacker KS, Bubley, G, Hussey S, Connor J: Ribavirin enters cerebral spinal fluid. Lancet 1986;2:45–46.
22. Crumpacker KS, Heagy W, Bubley G, et al: Ribavirin treatment of the acquired immunodeficiency syndrome (AIDS) and acquired immunodeficiency syndrome-related complex (ARC). Ann Intern Med 1987;107:664–674.
23. Dalakas MC, Illa I, Pezeshkpour GH, et al: Mitochondrial myopathy caused by long term zidovudine therapy. N Engl J Med 1990;322:1098–1105.
24. Dannenberg AL, McNeil JG, Brundage JF, et al: Suicide and HIV infection mortality follow-up of 4147 HIV-seropositive military service applicants. JAMA 1996;276: 1743–1746.
25. Davtiyan DG, Vinters HV: Wernicke's encephalopathy in an AIDS patient treated with zidovudine. Lancet 1987; 1:919–920.
26. DeClerq E: Perspectives for the chemotherapy of AIDS. Anticancer 1987;7:1023–1038.
27. DeMiranda P, Blum MR: Pharmacokinetics of acyclovir after intravenous and oral administration. J Antimicrob Chemother 1983;12(suppl B):29–37.
28. DeRay G, Diquet B, Martinez F, et al: Pharmacokinetics of zidovudine in a patient on maintenance hemodialysis. N Engl J Med 1988;319:1606–1607.
29. Deyton LR, Walker RE, Kovacs JA, et al: Reversible cardiac dysfunction associated with interferon alfa therapy in AIDS patients with Kaposi's sarcoma. N Engl J Med 1989;321:1246–1249.
30. Don PC, Fusco F, Fried P, et al: Nail dyschromia associated with zidovudine. Ann Intern Med 1990;112:145–146.

31. Drew WL: Antiviral therapy of CMV infection. AIDS Reader 1993;3:99–104.
32. Dubin G, Braffman MN: Zidovudine-induced hepatotoxicity. Ann Intern Med 1989;110:85–86.
33. Farese RV, Schambelan M, Hollander H, et al: Nephrogenic diabetes insipidus associated with foscarnet treatment of cytomegalovirus retinitis. Ann Intern Med 1990;112:955–956.
34. Fischl M, Galpin JE, Levine JD, et al: Recombinant human erythropoietin for patients with AIDS treated with zidovudine. N Engl J Med 1990;322:1488–1493.
35. Fischl MA, Parker CB, Pettinelli C, et al: A randomized controlled trial of a reduced dose of zidovudine in patients with acquired immunodeficiency syndrome. N Engl J Med 1990;323:1009–1014.
36. Furman PA, Fyfe JA, St Clair MH, et al: Phosphorylation of 3′ azido-3′-deoxythymidine and selective interaction of the 5′-triphosphate with human immunodeficiency virus reverse transcriptase. Proc Natl Acad USA 1986;83: 8333–8337.
37. Gill PS, Rarick M, Byrnes RK, et al: Azidothymidine associated with bone marrow failure in the acquired immunodeficiency syndrome (AIDS). Ann Intern Med 1987; 107: 502–505.
38. Gilquin J, Weiss L, Kazatchkine MD: Genital and oral erosions induced by foscarnet. Lancet 1990;1:287. Letter.
39. Gold JWM: The diagnosis and management of HIV infection. In: Gold JWM, Telzak EE, White DA, eds: The diagnosis and management of the HIV-infected patient, part 1. Med Clin North Am 1996;80:1283–1307.
40. Goulvetch MN: The epidemiology of HIV and AIDS: Current trends. Med Clin North Am 1996;80:1223–1239.
41. Greene WC: The molecular biology of human immunodeficiency virus type I infection. N Engl J Med 1991;324: 308–317.
42. Guay DRP: Pharmacokinetic of new macrolides. Infect Med 1992;9 (suppl A):9–13.
43. Harb GE, Jacobson MA: Human immunodeficiency virus (HIV) infection: Does it increase susceptibility to adverse drug reactions? Drug Saf 1993;9:1–8.
44. Hardy WD: The human immunodeficiency virus. In: Gold JWM, Telzak EE, White DA, eds: The diagnosis and management of the HIV-infected patient, part I. Med Clin North Am 1996;80:1239–1263.
45. Hargreaves M, Fuller G, Costello, Gazzard B: Zidovudine overdose. Lancet 1988; 2:509. Letter.
46. Harris PJ, Caceres CA: Azidothymidine in the treatment of AIDS. N Engl J Med 1988;318:250–251. Letter.
47. Hersh EM: Dithiocarb sodium (diethyldithiocarbamate) therapy in patients with symptomatic HIV infection and AIDS. JAMA 1991;265:1538–1544.
48. Hughes W, Leoung G, Kramer F: Comparison of atovaquone (566C80) with trimethoprim-sulfamethoxazole to treat *Pneumocystis carinii* pneumonia in patients with AIDS. N Engl J Med 1993;328:1521–1527.
49. Hymes KB, Greene JB, Karpatkin S: The effect of azidothymidine on HIV-related thrombocytopenia. N Engl J Med 1988;318:516–517.
50. Kahn J, Kaplan L, Gambertoglio J, et al: A phase I study of GLQ223 in subjects with AIDS and ARC. Paper presented at the VI International Conference on AIDS, San Francisco, June, 1990.
51. Kassler WJ, Blanc P, Greenblatt R: The use of medicinal herbs by human immunodeficiency virus-infected patients. Arch Intern Med 1991;151:2281–2288.
52. Kizer KW, Green M, Perkins CI, et al: AIDS and suicide in California. JAMA 1988;260:1881.
53. Klecker RW, Collins JM, Yarchoan R, et al: Plasma and cerebrospinal fluid pharmacokinetics of 3′ azido-3′-deoxythymidine: A novel pyrimidine analogue with potential application for the treatment of patients with AIDS and related diseases. Clin Pharmacol Ther 1987;41: 407–412.
54. Kovacs JA: Efficacy of atovaquone in treatment of toxoplasmosis in patients with AIDS. Lancet 1992;2:637–638.
55. Lambert JS, Seidlin M, Reichman RC, et al: 2′, 3′-dideoxyinosine (ddI) in patients with acquired immunodeficiency syndrome or AIDS-related complex: A phase I trial. N Engl J Med 1990;322:1333–1340.
56. Lane HC, Kovacs JA, Feinberg J: Anti-retroviral effects of interferon-α in AIDS-associated Kaposi's sarcoma. Lancet 1988;2:1218–1222.
57. Laskin OL, Longstreth JA, Hart CC, et al: Ribavirin disposition in high-risk patients for acquired immunodeficiency syndrome. Clin Pharmacol Ther 1987;41:546–555.
58. Laurence J: AIDS: Evolving perspectives. AIDS Reader 1991;1:3–6.
59. Lee BL, Moore L, Wilson M, et al: Increased prevalence of slow acetylator status in patients with the acquired immunodeficiency syndrome. Abstract presented at the 93rd annual meeting of the American Society of Clinical Pharmacology and Therapeutics, Orlando, March 1992, p. 183.
60. Marzuk PM, Tierney H, Tardiff K, et al: Increased risk of suicide in persons with AIDS. JAMA 1988;259:1333–1337.
61. Masur H: Drug therapy: Prevention and treatment of *Pneumocystis* pneumonia. N Engl J Med 1992;327:1853–1860.
62. Maxwell S, Scheftner WA, Kessler HA, Busch K: Manic syndrome associated with zidovudine treatment. JAMA 1988;259:3406–3407.
63. Mayer RA, Sergios PA, Coonan K, O'Brien L: Trichosanthin treatment of HIV-induced immune dysregulation. Eur J Clin Invest 1992;22:113–122.
64. McGrath MA, Hwang KM, Caldwell SE, et al: GLQ223: An inhibitor of human immunodeficiency virus replication in acutely and chronically infected cells of lymphocyte and mononuclear phagocytes lineage. Proc Natl Acad Sci USA 1989;86:2844–2848.
65. Mcphedran P: Using hematopoietic hormones in HIV disease. AIDS Clin Care 1992;4:43–44.
66. Meng TC, Fischl MA, Boota AH, et al: Combination therapy with zidovudine and dideoxycytidine in patients with advanced human immunodeficiency virus infection. Ann Intern Med 1992;116:13–20.
67. Meruelo D, Lavie G, Lavie G: Therapeutic agents with dramatic antiretroviral activity and little toxicity at effective doses: Aromatic polycyclic diones hypericin and pseudohypericin. Proc Natl Acad Sci USA 1988;85: 5230–5234.
68. Miles SA, Mitsuya RT, Lee K, et al: Recombinant human granulocyte colony-stimulating factor increases circulating burst forming unit: Erythron and red blood cell pro-

duction in patients with severe human immunodeficiency virus infection. Blood 1990;75:2137–2142.
69. Moore EC, Cohen F, Kauffman RE, Aravind MK: Zidovudine overdose in a child. N Engl J Med 1990;322:408–409.
70. Moore RD, Fortyana I, Keruly J, et al: Adverse events from drug therapy for human immunologic virus disease. Am J Med 1996;101:34–40.
71. Navin TR, Miller KD, Satriale RF, Lobel HO: Adverse reactions associated with pyrimethamine-sulfadoxine prophylaxis for *Pneumocystis carinii* infections in AIDS. Lancet 1985;1:1332.
72. Obrien RJ, Lyle MA, Snider DE Jr: Rifabutin (ansamycin LM 427): A new rifamycin-S derivative for the treatment of mycobacterial disease. Rev Infect Dis 1987; 9:519–530.
73. Pickus OB: Overdose of zidovudine. N Engl J Med 1988; 318:1206. Letter.
74. Pluda JM, Yarchoan R, Smith PD, et al: Subcutaneous recombinant granulocyte-macrophage colony-stimulating factor used as a single agent and in an alternating regimen with zidovudine in leukopenic patients with severe human immunodeficiency virus infection. Blood 1990;76: 463–472.
75. Project Inform Fact Sheet: DTC-imuthiol (diethyldithiocarbamate). Project Inform, San Francisco, June 2, 1988.
76. Rao TK: Renal complications in HIV disease. Med Clin North Am 1996;80:1427–1451.
77. Raviglione MC, Dinan WA, Pablos-Mendez A, et al: Fatal toxic epidermal necrolysis during prophylaxis with pyrimethamine and sulfadoxine in a human immunodeficiency virus infected person. Arch Intern Med 1988;148: 2683–2685.
78. Reines ED, Gross PA: Antiviral agents. Med Clin North Am 1988;72:691–715.
79. Reiter WM, Cimoch PJ: Dapsone-induced methemoglobinemia in a patient with *P. carinii* pneumonia and AIDS. N Engl J Med 1987;317:1741–1742.
80. Richman DD, Fischl MA, Grieco MH, et al: The toxicity of azidothymidine (AZT (ZDV)) in the treatment of patients with AIDS and AIDS-related complex. N Engl J Med 1987;317:192–197.
81. Roberts RB, Jurica K, Meyer WA, et al: Phase I study of ribavirin in human immunodeficiency virus infected patients. J Infect Dis 1990;162:638–642.
82. Robinson PA, Knirsch AK, Joseph JA: Fluconazole for life-threatening fungal infections in patients who cannot be treated with conventional antifungal agents. Rev Infect Dis 1990;12(suppl 3):S349-S363.
83. Roederer M, Ela SW, Staal FJ, et al: *N*-acetylcysteine: A new approach to anti-HIV therapy. AIDS Res Hum Retroviruses 1992;8:209–217.
84. Routy JP, Prajs E, Blanc AP, et al: Seizure after zidovudine overdose. Lancet 1989;1:184–185.
85. Schinazi RF, Chu CK, Babu JR, et al: Anthraquinones as a new class of antiviral agents against human immunodeficiency virus. Antiviral Res 1990;13:265–272.
86. Schoenfeld P: HIV infection and renal disease. AIDS Clin Care 1991;3:9–11.
87. Selwyn PA, Alcabes P, Hartel D, et al: Clinical manifestations and predictors of disease progression in drug users with human immunodeficiency virus infection. N Engl J Med 1992;327:1607–1703.
88. Sjovall J, Bergdahl S, Movin G, et al: Pharmacokinetics of foscarnet and distribution to cerebrospinal fluid after intravenous infusion in patients with human immunodeficiency virus infection. Antimicrob Agents Chemother 1989;33:1023–1031.
89. Sjovall J, Karlson A, Ogenstad S, et al: Pharmacokinetics and absorption of foscarnet after intravenous and oral administration to patients with human immunodeficiency virus. Clin Pharmacol Ther 1988;44:65–73.
90. Smith PD: Gastrointestinal infections in AIDS. Ann Intern Med 1992;116:63–77.
91. Spear JB, Kessler HA, Lehrman SN, de Miranda P: Zidovudine overdosage. Ann Intern Med 1988;109:76–77.
92. Staal FJT, Ela SW, Roederer M, et al: Glutathione deficiency and human immunodeficiency virus infection. Lancet 1992;1:909–912.
93. Sugar AM, Stern JJ, Dupont B: Overview: Treatment of cryptococcal meningitis. Rev Infect Dis 1990;2(suppl 3): S338–S348.
94. Tanowitz HB, Simon D, Weiss L, et al. Gastrointestinal manifestations. In: Gold JWM, Telzak EE, White DA, eds: The diagnosis and management of the HIV-infected patient, part 1. Med Clin North Am 1996;80:1395–1414.
95. Tay-Kearney ML, Jabs DA: Ophthalmic complications of HIV Infection. In: Gold JWM, Telzak EE, White DA, eds: The diagnosis and management of the HIV-infected patient, part 1. Med Clin North Am 1996;80:1471–1492.
96. Threlkeld SC, Hirsch MS: Antiviral therapy: The epidemiology of HIV and AIDS: Current trends. In: Gold JWM, Telzak EE, White DA, eds: The diagnosis and management of the HIV-infected patient, part 1. Med Clin North Am 1996;80:1263–1283.
97. Waites L, Levin AS, Starrett BA, et al: Trichosanthin treatment of HIV disease. Paper presented at the sixth international conference on AIDS, San Francisco, June 1990.
98. Walker RE, Parker RI, Kovacs JA, et al: Anemia and erythropoiesis in patients with acquired immunodeficiency syndrome (AIDS) and Kaposi sarcoma treated with zidovudine. Ann Intern Med 1988;108:372–376.
99. Watts RG, Conte SE, Zuilinden E, et al: Effect of charcoal hemoperfusion on clearance of pentamidine after accidental overdose. J Toxicol Clin Toxicol 1997;35:89–92.
100. Wharton JM, Demopulos PA, Goldschlager N: Torsades des pointes during administration of pentamidine isothionate. Am J Med 1986;83:571–576.
101. Whitley RJ, Gnann JW Jr: Acyclovir: A decade later. N Engl J Med 1992;327:782–789.
102. Wolf Y, Haddad R, Jossopov J, et al: Alpha interferon induced severe pneumonitis. J Toxicol Clin Toxicol 1997;35: 113–114.
103. Yarchoan R, Klecker RW, Weinhold KJ, et al: Administration of 3′-azido-3′-deoxythymidine, an inhibitor of HTLV III/LAV replication, to patients with AIDS or AIDS-related complex. Lancet 1986;1:575–580.
104. Yarchoan R, Thomas RV, Allain JP, et al: Phase I studies of 2′,3′-dideoxycytidine in severe human immunodeficiency virus infection as a single agent and alternating with zidovudine (AZT). Lancet 1988;1:76–81.

CHAPTER 108

Substance Users

James E. Cisek

This chapter will focus on the assessment and management of complications arising in substance users, unrelated to the direct affects of the drugs involved. Optimal medical and psychiatric care and the initiation of preventative strategies require the healthcare provider to have a thorough understanding of all aspects of the substance user's life. The following discussion will focus on the epidemiology of substance use, and aims to further understanding of the infectious, traumatic, psychiatric, and sociologic issues unique to the substance-using population.[35]

How Can the Diagnosis of Substance Dependence/Abuse Disorders Be Established?

There are many substance users and a certain percentage of them are drug dependent. In the most recent *Diagnostic and Statistical Manual of Mental Disorders* (DSM-IV), a diagnosis of substance dependence is based on the presence of at least three symptoms (from a list of seven), occurring at any time in a 12-month period (Table 108–1).[2] This modified concept of dependence stresses the impaired control of substance use and applies to a variety of substances that do not normally produce signs of physiologic dependence (eg, anticholinergics, nonsteroidal anti-inflammatory agents).

TABLE 108–1. SUBSTANCE DEPENDENCE—DEFINED BY AT LEAST THREE OF THE FOLLOWING IN A 12-MONTH PERIOD

- Tolerance
- Withdrawal
- Administration in larger doses or over longer periods than originally intended
- Decreased control over usage
- Increased time investment in acquisition, use, or recovery from the substance
- Decreased participation in occupational, recreational, or social events
- Continued use despite social, psychological, or physical problems caused by the substance

Reprinted, with permission, from American Psychiatric Association: Diagnostic and Statistical Manual of Mental Disorders, 4th ed. Washington, D.C., APA, 1994.

Substance abuse implies a dangerous pattern of substance use and includes the inability to fulfill important roles (eg, neglect of children, absence from work), frequent use in physically hazardous environments (driving an automobile, operating a machine), recurrent substance-related legal problems, and continued use despite social problems caused or worsened by the effects of the substance.[2] Despite these rather clear definitions, there is still a great deal of controversy as to what constitutes drug use, dependence, and abuse. A high-school student who dies during her first experience with cocaine might be considered a drug user while the same student who drives her car under the influence of ethanol could be labeled as a drug abuser.

The risk analysis for single use is extensive and includes infection, injury, and end-organ toxicity such as stroke or myocardial ischemia. Individuals who use multiple times have added risks that include such entities as dependence, prostitution, criminal activities such as theft and drug sales, violence, homelessness, and lost productivity. The societal implications of these behaviors is significant; it is estimated that 21% of tax dollars in New York City are spent on problems related to substance abuse.[9]

What Is the Epidemiology of Substance Use?

It has been proposed that the proper theoretic construct should consider drug use as a communicable disease.[36,38] This is controversial, as the study of the frequency and distribution of drug use may be approached differently than that of an infectious disease or hypertension. The application of traditional epidemiologic concepts to the study of substance use should be done with great caution. The use of drugs may be prolonged, short term, or episodic, and may be associated with unique aspects of lifestyle. Data collection can be difficult because there is no universally accepted point separating "use" from "abuse." Reports of drug availability and the aggressiveness of law enforcement may vary greatly and give false impressions of the prevalence of substance use. A brief visit by a clandestine chemist to a community may be followed by a sharp rise in the synthesis and use of a "designer drug."[23]

The limitations of epidemiologic data can be appreciated by an understanding of the methods and sources of data collection. Many different methods exist to define the epidemiology of substance abuse. The Drug Abuse Warning Network (DAWN) collects data on persons presenting to emergency departments age 6 years and older.[69] In 1995, 489 hospitals participated in data collection. Data are collected by nurses or clerical personnel based upon the emergency department record and analytical drug detection. At each facility reporting data, a drug-related episode must meet all four of the following criteria:

1. The patient was treated in the hospital emergency department.
2. The presenting problem was related to drug use.
3. The case involved the nonmedical use of a legal drug or the use of an illegal drug.
4. The patient's reason for taking the substance includes dependence, suicide attempt, or mind-altering effects.

The DAWN data provide useful information on trends in morbidity and mortality associated with illicit drugs, but the data must be interpreted with caution because only episodes in which a drug is part of the presenting problem are reported. For example, an increased reporting of cocaine could mean that more cocaine users with HIV-related infections are seeking medical care rather than that more persons are using cocaine. The analysis does not indicate the nature of the relationship between drug use and the presenting problem; which of the various drugs, if any, caused the episode; or if the patient was a naive or experienced substance user. Finally, there is concern that DAWN data may underreport drug-related episodes.[6] Critically ill patients may not provide a history of drug use in the emergency department, and analytical results are often not available until the patient has left the emergency department. Records generated outside of the emergency department are excluded from review. In summary, DAWN data are valuable but the healthcare provider must understand the significant limitations.

The 1995 National Household Survey on Drug Abuse surveyed 17,747 individuals age 12 and older in households, noninstitutional group quarters (eg, shelters, rooming houses, dormitories), and civilians living on military bases.[70] The interview lasted about 1 hour and collected data on the recency and frequency of illicit drug use, opinions about drugs, problems associated with drug use, and drug abuse treatment experience. Demographic data were also collected including employment, education, income, general and mental health status, and access to health care. The information was collected on self-administered answer sheets that were returned by mail.

Other sources of data include information obtained from local and federal law enforcement agencies detailing trends in drug preferences, purity, and prices. Prescription audits establish the changes in prescribing patterns for a specific drug. Many communities perform independent local surveys to define attributes of the region that contribute to the area's rate or prevalence of substance use.

In 1995, data from DAWN and the National Household Survey on Drug Abuse revealed that an estimated 12.8 million Americans (6% of population 12 years of age and older) were current (in the month prior to the interview) illicit drug users. Though there was no change from 1994, these data reflected an approximately 50% decrease from 1979. Current drug use among youths, however, has continued to increase, with a doubling since 1992. In 1995, 11% of adolescents were current users of illicit substances.

Men have a higher rate of current illicit drug use than women (7.8 versus 4.5%). Of the 4.3 million women aged 15 to 44 who were current drug users in 1995, 38% had children living with them, including 9% with at least one child under the age of 2 years. Women of childbearing age showed a decrease in drug use during pregnancy (9.3 versus 2.3%), but this rate increases to 5.5% shortly after giving birth. There was no significant difference in rates in urban versus rural settings. The rate of current illicit drug use for blacks (7.0%) remained higher than for whites (6.0%) and Hispanics (5.1%) in 1995. The highest rates of drug use were among those individuals aged 16 to 20, with rare individuals using illicit drugs after age 50 years. Illicit drug use correlates highly with educational status, with those who had not completed high school having the highest rate of use (15.4%), while college graduates have the lowest rate of use (5.9%). In addition to education, current employment status predicts illicit drug use. In 1995, 14.3% of unemployed adults versus 5.5% of full-time employed adults used illicit drugs. The cause and effect relationship of these data is unclear.

A comparison of 1994 and 1995 data reveals no significant change in the number of cocaine users or cocaine-related episodes. In 1995, there were an estimated 1.5 million current cocaine users with 582,000 (0.3% of the population) classified as frequent cocaine users. The estimated number of occasional cocaine users declined from 7.1 million in 1985 to 2.5 million in 1995. In 1995, DAWN data indicated that cocaine-related episodes accounted for 27% of all emergency department drug-related episodes, with 54% occurring among blacks, 29% among whites, and 8% among Hispanics. Rates of current cocaine use were highest for blacks, men, and individuals aged 18 to 25.

Fourteen percent of all drug-related episodes involved heroin in 1995, with 39% among whites, 38% among blacks, and 13% among Hispanics. Since 1990, heroin-related episodes have increased by 134% for blacks and 115% for whites.

Marijuana is the most commonly used illicit drug, with 5% of the population aged 12 and older classified as current users. Since 1992, the rate of use among youth has more than doubled. It is estimated that 2.2% of the population has tried methamphetamine, and DAWN data indicate a 261 and 322% respective increase in the number of methamphetamine and amphetamine-related episodes between 1991 and 1995. In 1995, 1.2% of the population admitted to the nonmedical use of antidepressants, antipsychotics, sedatives, and analgesics. For inhalants and hallucinogens, the rate of past-month use was approximately 0.5% of the population.

Approximately 29% of all Americans are currently smoking cigarettes, and an estimated 20% of youths aged 12 to 17 were smoking in 1995. No significant differences in smoking rates exist by ethnicity. Current smokers are more likely to be involved in heavy alcohol consumption and the use of illicit drugs. An estimated 3.3% of the population used smokeless tobacco in 1995 (90% male). In 1995, 37% of adults who had not completed high school smoked, while 17% of college graduates smoked.

In 1995, approximately 52% of the population older than 12 years were current ethanol users, with 16% involved in binge drinking and 6% classified as heavy users. Individuals between the ages of 18 and 25 years were the most likely to be involved in binge (5 or more drinks at one occasion in the past month) and heavy drinking (5 or more drinks per occasion on 5 or more days in the past month). Whites have a higher rate of ethanol use and binge drinking over black individuals with no significant racial difference for heavy use. Men have greater representation in all categories of ethanol consumption. The rate of heavy alcohol use is higher among those who have not completed high school.

What Medical Problems Are Related to Adulterants, Contaminants and Routes of Administration?

In the clinical evaluation of patients who are using "street drugs," the presence of contaminants should be presumed. These may be purposely added, present as a result of the synthesis of the drug, or present as a contamination of the injection process. Common adulterants added to cocaine, heroin, and hallucinogens include any of the local anesthetics, amphetamines, phencyclidine, lysergic acid diethylamide, quinine, phenylpropanolamine, any of the sugars, corn starch, flour, inositol, talc (magnesium silicate), and sodium bicarbonate. These agents dilute the concentration of the desired drug. Some adulterants simulate the desired effects of the drug and others are added simply to increase the mass and subsequent street value of the product. Occasionally, substances are added for the purpose of inflicting physical harm (eg, strychnine, thallium).[66]

Data from crime laboratories indicates that many street drug sales involve illicit material with no mind-altering potential, sold for large sums of money to the unwary substance user. Of 614 alleged cocaine samples collected in Los Angeles County, cocaine was found to be absent in 19%, combined with stimulant substitutes in 23%, and found by itself in 58%. Fifty percent of the amphetamine samples lacked any of the alleged drug.[42]

Clandestine drug laboratories may produce an undesired chemical as a result of a sloppy synthesis. In the early 1980s, "designer" chemists produced a formulation contaminated with 1-methyl-4-phenyl-1,2,3,6-tetrahydropyridine (MPTP) while attempting to synthesize an anolog of meperidine. This contaminant caused a rapidly developing, severe form of parkinsonism characterized by hypokinesia, rigidity, tremor, and fixed posture.[8] The MPTP was metabolized by monoamine oxidase B in the substantia nigra, producing 1-methyl-4-phenylpyridinium (MPP^+) that selectively destroyed neurons in the substantia nigra (see Chap. 60).[44]

The illegal synthesis of drugs can also be associated with potential exposures to metals, caustics, and solvents. This occurs by an unintentional exposure during the synthetic process or by the injection of contaminated product. Methcathinone (CAT) is a synthetic amphetamine produced from ephedrine. In the synthesis, ephedrine is oxidized using sodium dichromate in an acid environment, and then extracted using solvents. "Green cat" was sold at a reduced price and was found to be contaminated with residual chromium salts, with the potential for chromium-induced multisystem organ failure.[23] Methamphetamine abuse was associated with an epidemic of lead poisoning when lead acetate was used in the synthetic process.[1,47] Law enforcement personnel consider all clandestine laboratories as harboring hazardous materials and proceed with great caution in their investigations.

The evaluation of the substance user with pulmonary symptoms is very complex and must include infectious and noninfectious etiologies. Barotrauma occurs in individuals while smoking cocaine and nasally insulfating cocaine and other drugs. Patients will present with cough, chest pain, and dyspnea secondary to a pneumothorax, pneumomediastinum, or pneumopericardium. Barotrauma occurs secondary to an increased intraalveolar pressure generated by the deep inhalation followed by a Valsalva maneuver and the cough provoked by the drug and heated gases. Carbonaceous sputum is quite common in individuals smoking cocaine, and is probably related to the inhalation of residue from the butane and alcohol used to ignite the drug.[30] Heroin overdose can also be associated with noncardiogenic pulmonary edema accompanied by fever and leukocytosis. This most likely is related to hypoxia and usually becomes clinically apparent within 6 hours of the intoxication, but may be delayed up to 24 hours. Starch, cotton fibers, and talc cause pulmonary granulomas when injected.[3,59,60] The nasal application of cocaine commonly leads to epistaxis and septal perforation.

Medical Illness in the Substance Abuser

The intoxicated patient's clinical manifestations are often nonspecific and could represent acute medical, surgical, psychiatric, or combined processes.[13,14,56,57,65] A thorough history and physical examination are essential because the differential diagnosis is often extensive. Medical causes must be meticulously sought prior to diagnosing a primary psychiatric disease. A psychiatric diagnosis in a substance user must often be a diagnosis of exclusion. Drug-induced agitation or coma has an extensive differential diagnosis and involves many substances that may not be reported on routine urine and serum drug screens. Without a history, it is often impossible to distinguish between a primary medical event and a drug-induced event. Even then, the primary and secondary characteristics can simulate each other. It is best to admit the patient to a medical facility and provide close observation for either clinical resolution or worsening symptomatology. The health care provider must always assume the presence of concomitant trauma and thoroughly examine the patient for subtle injuries.

What Are the Infectious Complications Associated With Substance Abuse?

The diagnosis and management of the infected substance user can be complicated by the presence of multiple medical problems and the unique psychosocial aspects of their lives. Common difficulties are the lack of a clear history, malnutrition, poverty, homelessness, concomitant HIV-1 infection, noncompliance, and associated mental illness. Parenteral drug users often purchase "street" antibiotics at the time they obtain their drugs. One study demonstrated that 18% of intravenous drug users (IVDUs) had purchased antibiotics compared to only 5% of nonparenteral drug users.[48] The self-administration of antibiotics prior to hospital arrival can make the diagnosis of an infectious process very difficult. Frequent parenteral injections, skin colonization with resistant *Staphylococcus aureus,* and the self-administration of antibiotics are important considerations in the evaluation of infectious processes. The drug itself is usually not contaminated with the causative organism.[55]

Immunologic dysfunction is probably of minor importance in the pathogenesis of infection in drug users who are not infected with HIV. There is no evidence for an impaired humoral immunity in parenteral drug users. In fact, there is evidence of a polyclonal B cell activation with IgM, the immunoglobulin most frequently elevated in IVDUs. Clinical examples of enhanced humoral response include a false-positive rheumatoid factor and Venereal Disease Research Laboratory (VDRL) test. Depressed cell-mediated immunity is common in IVDUs. In vitro lymphocyte response to mitogens is diminished by the addition of methadone, and the delayed hypersensitivity skin test is commonly absent in heroin addicts. Altered populations and functioning of helper, suppressor, and natural killer cells can be demonstrated in patients receiving methadone, but the clinical significance is uncertain as clinical infections typical of T-cell dysfunction were uncommon in drug abusers prior to the advent of the HIV virus.[7,45] The influence of cocaine on the immune response is an area of active research, with data thus far suggesting an immunosuppressive affect of cocaine and its metabolites.[4,15,16,43,63]

Infection is the most common cause of death in hospitalized parenteral drug users. Infectious complications account for 60% of hospital admissions among IVDUs, and endocarditis is associated with 5 to 8% of these episodes.[48] It is estimated that 2 cases of endocarditis will occur per 1000 IVDUs per year.[48] Infective endocarditis implies infection of the endocardial surface of the heart and the physical presence of microorganisms in the lesion. Endocarditis is of great importance given its high frequency of serious complications and significant mortality.

TABLE 108–2. CRITERIA FOR DIAGNOSIS OF ENDOCARDITIS IN PARENTERAL DRUG USERS

1. Temperature greater than or equal to 38.0°C with two positive blood cultures and vegetations on 2-D echocardiography.
2. Temperature greater than or equal to 38.0°C with new vegetations seen on 2-D echocardiography with negative blood cultures (culture-negative endocarditis).
3. Positive blood cultures with new vegetations seen on 2-D echocardiography in absence of fever.
4. Temperature greater than 38.0°C, positive blood cultures, evidence of systemic embolization or valve regurgitation, but the absence of vegetations on echocardiography.

Reprinted, with permission, from Weisse AB, Heller DR, Schimenti RJ, et al: The febrile parenteral drug abuser: A prospective study in 121 patients. Am J Med 1993;94:274–280.

The initial history and physical examination is limited in diagnosing endocarditis in the febrile IVDU. Fever is nonspecific because it may be associated with bacterial, viral, fungal, or protozan infections; reactions to injected drugs, adulterants, or contaminants; or of unknown origin. The presence of embolic phenomena and echocardiographically demonstrated vegetations are the most important predictors of endocarditis in febrile IVDUs. All IVDUs with a fever should be admitted for the evaluation of bacteremia and possible endocarditis.[72] The diagnosis of viral syndromes and other trivial illnesses cannot be established on the initial evaluation. Of all parenterally abused drugs, cocaine has the highest incidence of endocarditis.[11] Table 108–2 lists the common criteria adopted for the diagnosis of endocarditis in the IVDU.[72]

Endocarditis in the IVDU presents in a similar fashion to nonsubstance-using patients with a few exceptions. Important differences include a high incidence of right-sided endocarditis (tricuspid valve) and the absence of underlying structural heart disease in two thirds of IVDUs with endocarditis.[71] Cardiac murmurs are noted in only 35% of IVDUs with proven endocarditis.[48] Tricuspid valve involvement occurs in approximately 5% of non-IVDUs who develop endocarditis. The distribution of valvular involvement in IVDUs with endocarditis is illustrated in Table 108–3.[49] A study of 74 intravenous opioid abusers

TABLE 108–3. DISTRIBUTION OF VALVULAR INVOLVEMENT IN INTRAVENOUS DRUG USERS WITH ENDOCARDITIS

Tricuspid valve alone or in combination	52%
Aortic valve alone	19%
Mitral valve alone	11%
Aortic and mitral valves together	13%

Reprinted, with permission, from Levine D, Sobel J: Infections in Intravenous Drug Abusers. New York, Oxford University Press, 1991. Copyright 1991, Oxford University Press.

with endocarditis found the following bacterial agents: *Staphylococcus aureus,* 61%[10]; streptococci, 16%; *Pseudomonas aeruginosa,* 14%; polymicrobial, 8%; and *Corynebacterium,* 1%.[48] *S. aureus* is of endogenous origin in the majority of cases as it is infrequently isolated from street heroin or paraphernalia. Biventricular and multiple-valve disease occur more frequently with *Pseudomonas* infections. Left-sided endocarditis secondary to *P. aeruginosa* is often refractory to antibiotic therapy and has a mortality rate of 60%. Regional and transient variations occur (eg, *P. cepacia* for a few years in New York City), making it important that the clinician have knowledge of current epidemiologic trends unique to their institutions.

HIV infection predisposes the IVDU to unusual pathogens including *Corynebacterium, Neisseria* species, *Salmonella* species, and fungal infections of the endocardium.[20] Parenteral drug abuse is the most common risk factor for recurrent native-valve endocarditis. Patients frequently survive the initial infection, with subsequent infections causing more significant cardiac complications (valvular dysfunction, myocardial abscess, conduction blocks).

All IVDUs who present with fever (>38°C) should be admitted and have at least two blood samples obtained from different sites for aerobic, anaerobic, and fungal cultures (Fig. 108–1).[52,72] Empiric antibiotic therapy should consider the most common organisms and their antibiotic sensitivities in the geographic location. Initial coverage is usually directed against *S. aureus* using either nafcillin or vancomycin if methicillin-resistant organisms are common. The addition of an aminoglycoside provides synergy against *S. aureus* and may shorten the duration of therapy to 2 weeks in patients with right-sided endocarditis. The typical aminoglycoside dosing used for synergy with *S. aureus* provides little effect against *Pseudomonas,* which requires large doses (8 mg/kg) for satisfactory activity. The initial use of an aminoglycoside to provide protection against gram-negative organisms is controversial. Enterococcal endocarditis is typically treated with a combination of vancomycin and gentamycin. Enterococci that develop gentamycin resistance are commonly treated with streptomycin, and resistance to vancomycin is treated with early surgical intervention as there is no established antibiotic therapy. It is essential that antibiotic therapy is based on susceptibility data and that pharmacokinetic information is followed closely. Septic emboli are frequent after the initiation of antibiotic therapy. Vegetation size does not cor-

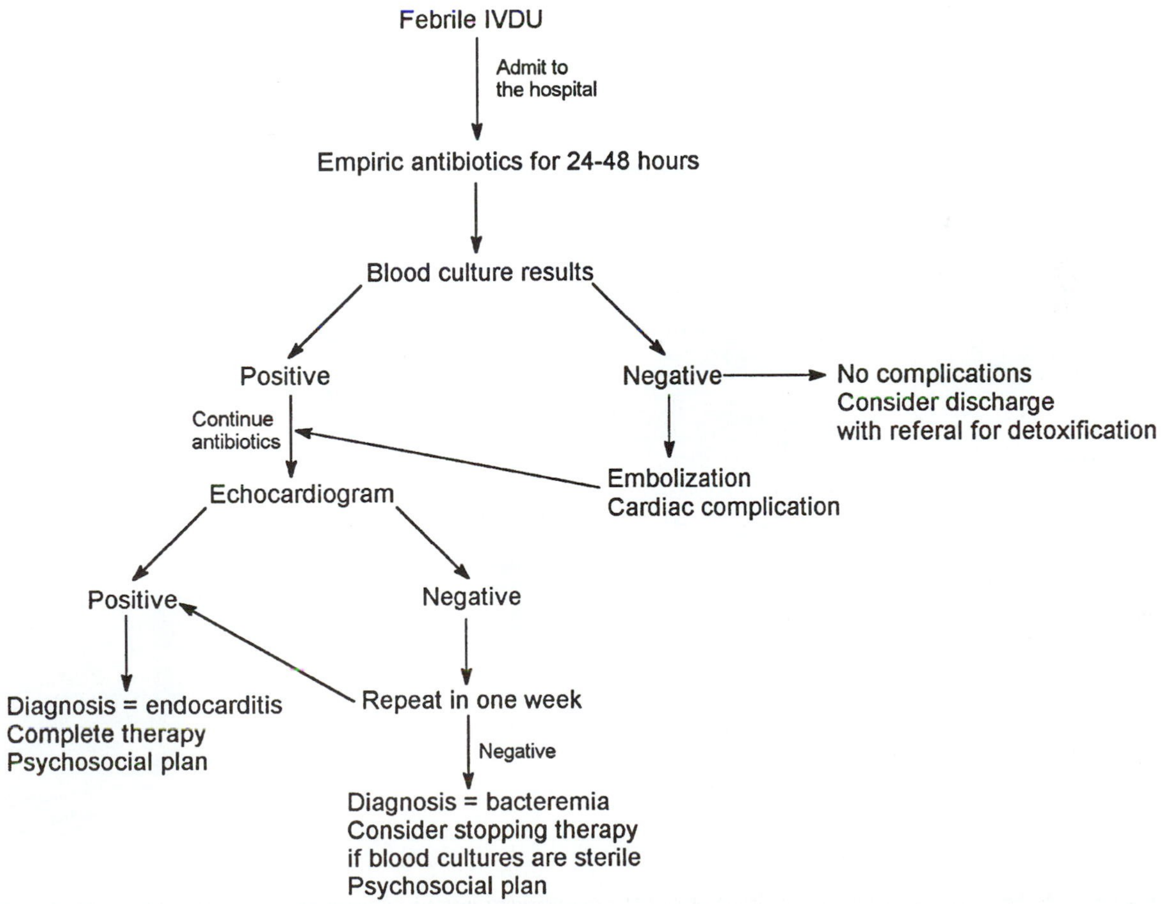

Figure 108–1. Algorithm for the evaluation of the febrile intravenous drug user.

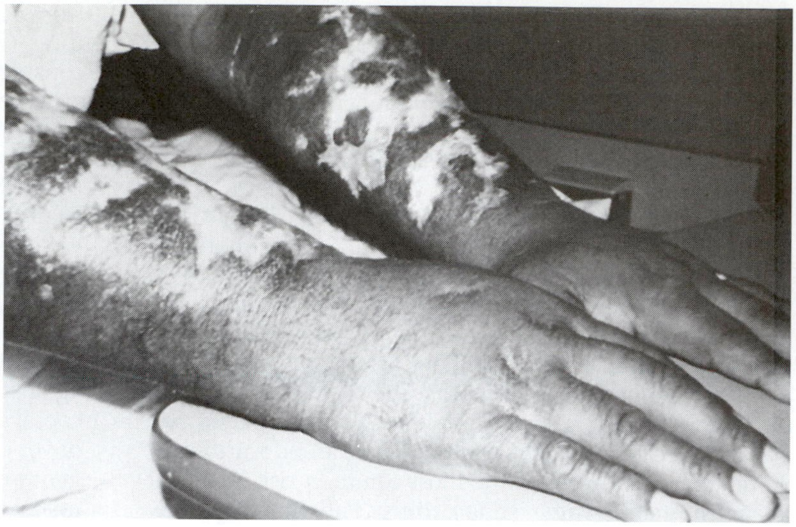

Figure 108–2. Markedly swollen hands with ulcerated cellulitic forearms in a chronic heroin abuser. The dorsum of each hand demonstrates nonpitting edema.

relate with embolization; however, vegetations greater than 2 cm are associated with a 33% mortality versus a 1.3% mortality with vegetations less than than 2 cm.[14,49]

Skin and soft tissue infection represent the most common infectious etiologies requiring hospital admission (Fig. 108–2). The infection may involve only a limited region of the epidermis and superficial dermis as in "skin popping," or may extend into a more typical abscess, cellulitis, or necrotizing fasciitis (see Color Plate Fig. 11). The infection may progress to involve the mediastinum, great vessels, muscle, or fascia and can lead to sepsis and death. Necrotizing fasciitis may present subtly with pain and hemodynamic instability disproportionate to the local process. Great care must be maintained as bullae, crepitance, and skin necrosis are late physical findings in necrotizing fasciitis. Imaging procedures such as ultrasound or computed tomography can help identify abscesses in the neck and groin if the diagnosis is uncertain. Vascular imaging prior to surgery is sometimes necessary if a pseudoaneurysm is suspected at the infected site (Fig. 108–3). Early antibiotic therapy and surgical drainage are essential.[14,49]

Suppurative thrombophlebitis is an inflammation of the vein wall due to the presence of bacteria and is fre-

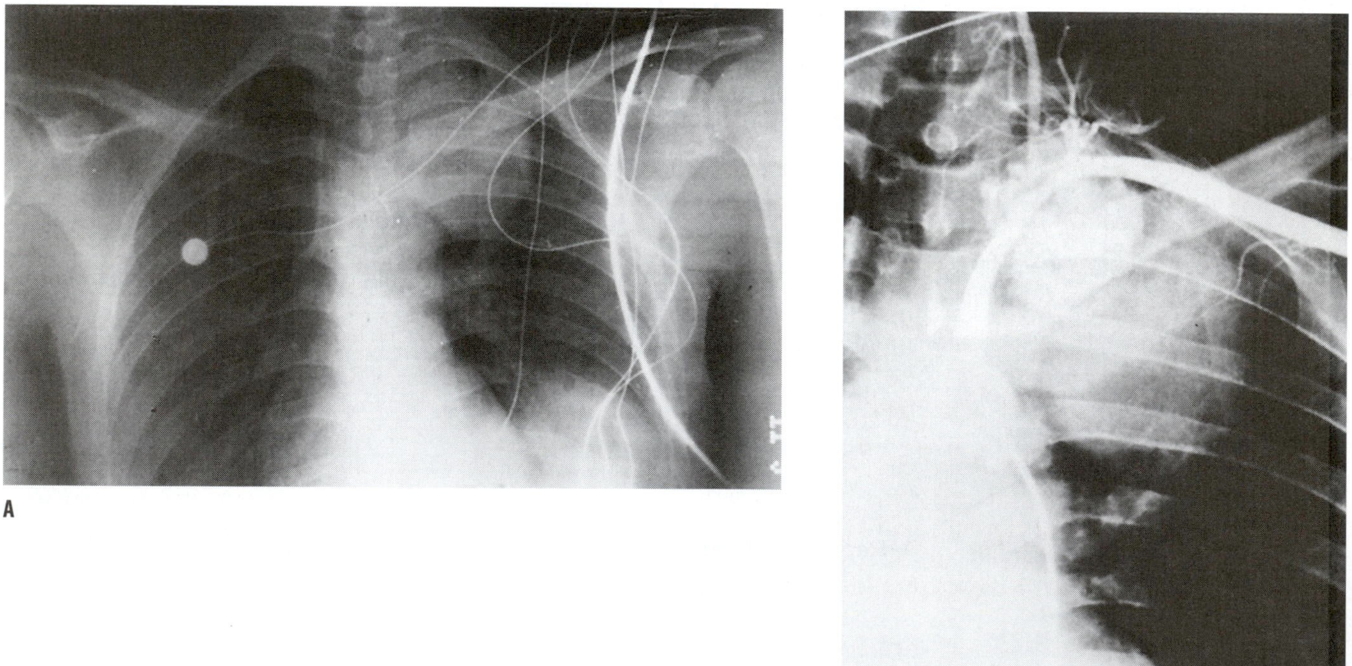

A

B

Figure 108–3. A. Chest radiograph of a young drug abuser who used the supraclavicular approach for heroin injection. The large mass in the left chest was thought to be a pseudoaneurysm. **B.** An arch aortogram performed on the patient revealed a large pseudoaneurysm and hematoma subsequent to arterial tear during attempted injection. Surgical repair was performed. *(Courtesy of Richard LeFleur, Department of Radiology, Bellevue Hospital.)*

quently associated with thrombosis. Fever, warmth, tenderness, swelling, and lymphadenopathy are common. Superficial and deep venous involvement may occur depending on the injection site (Fig. 108–4). Recurrent injections can lead to deep venous thrombosis with the potential for pulmonary emboli. Antibiotic therapy should include a semisynthetic penicillin or vancomycin. Surgery is usually required. Anticoagulants are usually contraindicated because a clear benefit has not been established and the IVDU is at great risk from complications related to anticoagulation.[14,49]

Mycotic aneurysms may occur as an isolated entity or accompany endocarditis. The femoral (most common) and neck vessels are the sites of mycotic aneurysms that occur directly during the injection of drugs. Frequent intravascular injections cause the formation of a perivascular hematoma that subsequently becomes infected by direct spread of cutaneous bacteria or overlying infections. These usually represent pseudoaneurysms as only the adventitia is involved. Involvement of the cerebral or abdominal vessels most commonly occurs during an episode of bacteremia with infection of the arterial vasa vasorum. Common clinical findings include fever, a painful pulsatile mass associated with a bruit or thrill, and ischemia distal to the mass. Early diagnosis prior to rupture is essential and commonly involves the use of ultrasound or angiography. Needle aspiration and incisions must be avoided in inguinal or neck masses prior to imaging procedures, as clinical examination may be unreliable in detecting the presence of an aneurysm. Early surgical excision is usually required as expansion and rupture is common.[14,49]

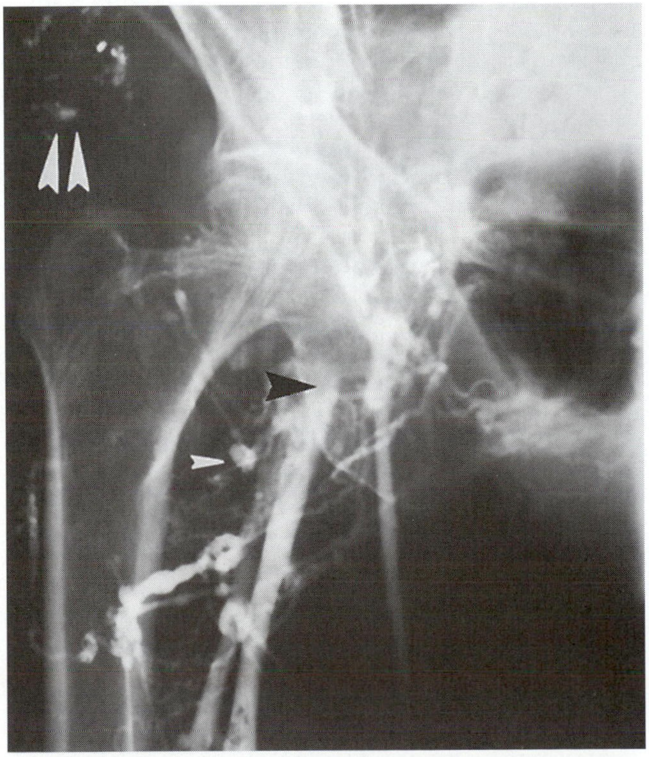

Figure 108–4. Venogram of a 50-year-old patient who routinely injected heroin into his groin. Occlusion of the femoral vein (*large arrow*) with diffuse aneurysmal dilation (*small arrow*) and extensive collaterals are shown. Incidental radiopaque materials are noted in the right buttock (*double arrow*). By history, this represents either bismuth or arsenicals he received as antisyphilitic therapy. *(Courtesy of Richard Lefleur, MD, Associate Professor of Radiology, New York University.)*

Viral hepatitis is very common in substance abusers and is acquired by needle sharing and by sexual transmission. IVDUs account for 15% of acute hepatitis B infections. Data from the United States and Europe indicate that 25 to 50% of IVDUs have antibodies against hepatitis B surface antigen.[34,62] Approximately 5 to 12% of infected patients become hepatitis B surface antigen carriers with higher percentages among those who are also HIV infected.[21] Ethanol abuse in combination with hepatitis B infection is associated with a more severe injury to the liver.

The hepatitis D virus is a co-virus that requires the presence of hepatitis B for its replication. This virus occurs in 80% of chronic carriers of hepatitis B but is present in less than 10% of IVDUs who have serum antibodies to hepatitis B surface antigen. Patients are most commonly infected with hepatitis B prior to the acquisition of hepatitis D. Simultaneous infection with both hepatitis B and D is uniquely common in IVDUs and will more likely result in fulminant hepatic failure.[46] The incidence of hepatitis C among IVDUs varies with location, but is in excess of 70% in Amsterdam and Spain.[32] Hepatitis A transmission occurs by close personal contact, the ingestion of contaminated drugs, or by intravenous injection. Virtually every form of viral hepatitis can be found in substance abusers.

Splenic abscesses are common and may be multiple and small or singular and large. Common symptoms include fever, abdominal pain, left shoulder pain, and pleuritic chest pain. Physical examination may reveal splenomegaly, left upper quadrant tenderness, and left pleural effusion. Antibiotics with percutaneous drainage or splenectomy are the mainstays of therapy.[17]

Most lung infections result from the common respiratory pathogens seen in community acquired pneumonias. Opportunistic infections must be considered if the patient is HIV infected. Primary pulmonary infections must be distinguished from septic pulmonary emboli arising from endocarditis or extremity deep venous thrombosis. Lung abscesses are common and occur through aspiration, necrotizing pneumonia, or septic emboli. Tuberculosis is common even in the non-HIV-infected patient given alcoholism, malnutrition, crowding, poor compliance with medical care, and coughing induced during the smoking and nasal insulfation of drug. Pneumonia is reported to be one of the most common causes of infection in febrile substance users. The initial antibiotic therapy must be broad based prior to definitive cultures, and the healthcare provider must always consider the possibility of multiple processes affecting the lung at the same time.[49]

Bone and joint infections are also common in parenteral drug users. The infection most commonly occurs during an episode of bacteremia, but may also develop via the spread from contiguous foci. Most joint infections involve the knee but other common sites include the sternoclavicular, manubriosternal (Fig. 108–5), costochondral (almost pathognomonic for substance use), and sacroiliac joints. Vertebral osteomyelitis commonly involves the cervical and lumbosacral spine (see Fig. 7–11 B) and may lead to epidural abscess formation with possible spinal cord compression. Patients with vertebral body infections often have an early subtle presentation and a prompt diagnosis is based on a heightened awareness in a substance user with spine pain, fevers, and/or focal neurologic deficits. A diagnostic aspiration is essential in assessing skeletal infections, as there is commonly a discrepancy between organisms causing bone and joint infections and those isolated from the blood. Specific antimicrobial therapy for 4 to 6 weeks is essential, along with frequent arthrocentesis and debridement of necrotic bone as needed.[12] The transient rheumatologic prodrome of hepatitis B antigenemia and chronic amyloidosis associated with daily parenteral drug abuse should also be considered in substance users with bone or joint pain.[37]

The evaluation of a substance user with neurologic findings is quite challenging and must involve both infectious and noninfectious etiologies. In the non-HIV-infected patient, endocarditis is the most common cause of CNS infection, which includes brain abscesses, meningitis, and subarachnoid hemorrhage from ruptured mycotic aneurysms. Mycotic aneurysms present with focal neurologic dysfunction as a result of the expanding aneurysm or subarachnoid or intracerebral hemorrhage (see Fig. 7–24). Cerebral abscesses usually result from emboli arising from the mitral or aortic valves. Cerebritis may be from a viral etiology or due or to excessive bacteremia associated with endocarditis.[49]

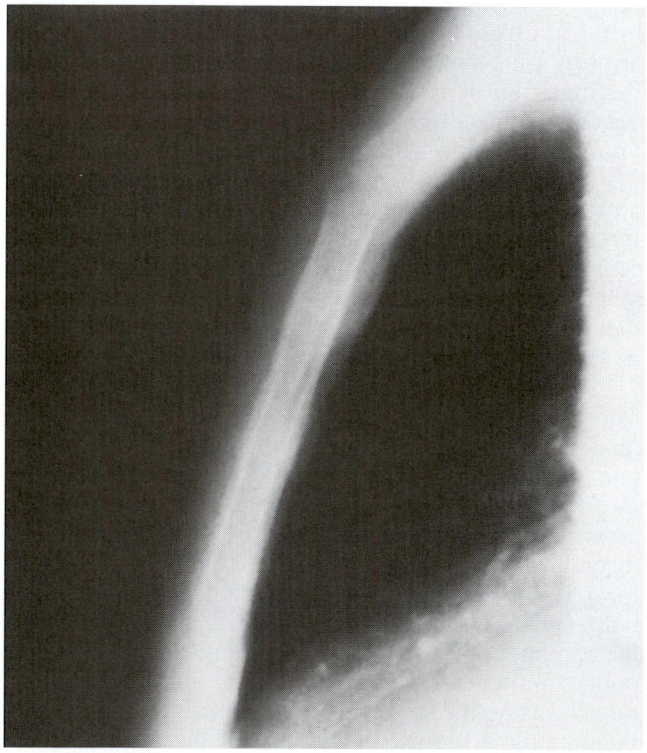

Figure 108–5. A patient with a manubriosternal osteomyelitis complicating IV drug use. He presented with chest pain and fever that developed over 2 weeks. The patient was treated with long-term antistaphylococcal penicillinase-resistant antibiotics. The manubriosternal region is also a characteristic site for osteomyelitis in parenteral drug users.

Currently, the incidence of sexually transmitted diseases (STDs) in substance abusers is increasing dramatically. Prostitution and sexual promiscuity are strongly related to drug abuse.[14,49,56] The most important organisms include HIV, penicillinase-producing strains of *Neisseria gonorrhoeae, Treponema pallidum, Haemophilus ducreyi,* and *Chlamydia trachomatis*.[27] Approximately one third of female IVDUs have a history of prostitution and 60% of IVDUs report a history of an STD.[14,49] The common practice of exchanging sex (usually unprotected) for crack cocaine has dramatically increased the incidence of all sexually transmitted diseases. The risk of transmission of HIV infection in parenteral drug abusers via the sexual route is tremendous. A 1993 Centers for Disease Control study of male IVDUs with known HIV infection revealed that 28% reported having vaginal or anal sex without a condom during the preceding 30 days, and 23% admitted to trading sex for money. Thirty-two percent had not revealed their HIV status to all partners.[18] A study of an indigent group of emergency department patients who admitted to using cocaine once each week found a syphilis rate of 28%.[24]

The health care provider must always consider the possibility of uncommon infections in the substance abuser. In the early 1970s, a group of patients acquired *Plasmodium vivax* in California by the sharing of needles.[25] Substance users risked quinine toxicity in the 1930s as the drug was added to heroin to help control malaria. The ease of travel to areas endemic with malaria makes this disease a consideration even in the United States. Historically, tetanus is the oldest infectious complication afflicting patients who use parenterally administered drugs. Tetanus and botulism[73] must be considered in substance abusers as *Clostridium* spp can grow well in facial sinuses (as with cocaine insulfation) or in extremities as a result of "skin popping" or compromised extremity perfusion.[49]

Bleach distribution and syringe exchange programs were developed in an attempt to minimize the spread of infectious diseases and have been a subject of great controversy. Results from several programs demonstrate a reduction in the transmission of hepatitis B, hepatitis C, and HIV.[22,29,32,40] Their role in decreasing the incidence of endocarditis will require further study. The healthcare provider must understand the limitations of these programs and educate each IVDU, as drug sharing can play an important role in the social organization of the drug-using culture.[28]

What Are the Traumatic Complications Commonly Associated With Substance Use?

Deaths in substance users may occur unrelated to the drug, as a result of an overdose of the drug, as a result of medical complications associated with the drug, or from drug-induced psychological responses that lead to trauma. Drug abuse increases both the incidence of trauma and the severity of each event. Benzoylecgonine was detected in 27% of all New York City residents sustaining fatal injuries and cocaine was detected in 18%. This study found that two thirds of the deaths were not from acute intoxication but resulted from homicides, suicides, automobile collisions, and falls.[5,53] A study involving six regional trauma centers demonstrated that 40% of adult trauma patients had a positive blood alcohol content on admission. Alcohol contributes to 53% of highway deaths and alcohol dependence or use is nine times higher in hospitalized trauma patients than in the general population.[68] Numerous drugs such as alcohol, marijuana, cocaine, and benzodiazepines are all demonstrated to impair driving tasks.[41] A study from Chicago demonstrated ethanol, cannabinoids, and cocaine in 53, 37, and 34%, respectively of trauma patients.[67] In a study of 231 injured patients aged 12 to 18 years, alcohol use was identified in 39%.[50,51] Even though the elderly have a lower incidence of drug-related trauma, 14% of drivers over age 60 were found to have the presence of ethanol in their blood.[33]

Numerous studies from burn centers demonstrate that substance use is commonly associated with thermal injury and that substance users have a greater percentage of burned body surface area, inhalation injury, and mortality.[31,54] Substance use is one of the most substantial risk factors for traumatic brain injury.[19] Similar relationships exist between substance abuse and hypothermia fatalities, drownings, and spinal cord injuries.[64]

A report from Chicago indicates that of 634 trauma patients admitted to a level one trauma center following trauma, 45% were considered impaired with either alcohol or drugs. Of the impaired group, only 17% were cited by police for driving under the influence.[58] These data indicate the importance of close dialogue between the healthcare provider and law enforcement to communicate possible mechanisms involved in the traumatic event.

The clinical evaluation of intoxicated patients is difficult, and thus more diagnostic testing is required to determine occult internal organ injury. Common examples include the need for a computed tomography evaluation of the brain and abdomen, as physical diagnosis is less reliable if the patient is intoxicated. Sympathomimetic agents may cause a tachycardia unrelated to blood loss and the hypertension could mask hypovolemic shock. Long bone, pelvic, and cervical spine fractures may not be perceived as painful events, mandating a low threshold for obtaining radiographs.

Routine drug testing may be important to allow for an early diagnosis of substance use and the initiation of chemical dependence treatment. One study suggested that surgical services identified alcoholism in less than 25% of affected patients and addressed the problem in less than one half of the patients detected. Chemical dependence consultation and referral for rehabilitation is critical to the management of these patients if prevention of further events is to be achieved. A number of authors suggest that patients are more amenable to a "critical intervention" and referral for rehabilitation in the posttraumatic period. Long-term survival may depend more on substance use rehabilitation than on initial trauma management.[26,61]

What Is the Relationship Between Substance Use and Other Psychiatric Illness?

Comorbidity implies the presence of two or more psychiatric disorders in the same patient. The National Institute of Mental Health's Epidemiologic Catchment Area Study remains a landmark study demonstrating the large percentage of substance users with a dual diagnosis. This study was conducted in the early 1980s and involved the interviews of more than 20,000 people in five communities in the United States. In this study, 76% of men and 65% of women demonstrated comorbidity (Table 108–4). Among prisoners, the comorbidity rates were even higher, with addictive disorders found in approximately 90% of patients with schizophrenia, antisocial personality disorders, and bipolar disorders.[39]

Studies thus far describe the incidence of comorbidity but they do not explain the reasons for the associations. It is uncertain whether the use of substances with mind-altering properties is an attempt at self-medication or whether mentally ill patients are less able to contend with the effects of substance use and thus are more likely to become dependent. The causal relationship between these disorders is complex, and further studies are neces-

TABLE 108–4. PREVALENCE OF OTHER PSYCHIATRIC DISORDERS AMONG MEN AND WOMEN IN TOTAL POPULATION DIAGNOSED AS HAVING DRUG USE-DEPENDENCE DISORDERS

	Prevalence of Other Disorders	
Specific Additional Diagnoses	***Men (%)***	***Women (%)***
Alcohol use-dependence	60	30
Antisocial personality disorder	22	10
Phobic disorders	19	29
Major depression	14	28
Dysthymla	9	12
Obsessive-compulsive disorder	6	9
Mania	5	7
Schizophrenia	5	8
Panic disorder	3	6

Reprinted, with permission, from Kandal DB: Epidemiological trends and implications for understanding the nature of addiction. In: O'Brien CP, Jaffe JH, eds: Addictive States. New York, Raven, 1992, pp. 23–40.

sary to determine whether substance abuse contributes to the risk of developing other psychiatric disorders or vice versa. It is postulated that amphetamines and lysergic acid diethylamine may induce persistent psychiatric syndromes lasting long after the drug is eliminated (post-hallucinogen perceptual disorder).

A reliable psychiatric diagnosis in substance abusers often requires a 2-week period of abstinence to eliminate the potential for concurrent intoxication or withdrawal. Several important principles must be remembered when performing a psychiatric evaluation of a substance abuser. The medical assessment must always precede the psychiatric evaluation. In most patients with a presumed dual diagnosis, inpatient care is probably the best setting and psychotropic medications are only initiated when spontaneous remission is not possible. Care must be given to identifying medical and drug-induced disease that may masquerade as psychiatric illnesses. Substance abusers are often unable to give reliable clinical information, and emphasis must be placed on analytical drug data from biologic specimens, physical examinations, laboratory testing, history from family and friends, past medical histories, and family psychiatric histories. In prescribing medication, addictive agents must be avoided once detoxification is accomplished, as these drugs may stimulate the cycle of euphoria and craving and thus jeopardize the recovery. Psychiatric and rehabilitative approaches are often conflicting in philosophy and must be carefully coordinated to optimize care.

Summary

The optimal care of substance users is quite challenging and demands a thorough understanding of all aspects of their lifestyle. The healthcare provider must approach these patients in a compassionate and nonjudgmental manner so as to gain their confidence and enhance the care rendered. It is essential to maintain a knowledge of the current patterns of substance use and to understand the many medical, surgical, and psychiatric issues these patients face as a result of their drug use. Physicians are an integral part of a team of professionals that include psychologists, home care nurses, sociologists, substance abuse counselors, individuals from law enforcement, clergy, and volunteers at various shelters. In an era of cost containment, it is essential that each provider of healthcare maintain a focus on this important group of individuals and not allow financial pressures to alter appropriate decisions.

References

1. Allcott JV, Barnhart RA, Mooney LA: Acute lead poisoning in two users of illicit methamphetamine. JAMA 1987;258:510–511.
2. American Psychiatric Association: Diagnostic and Statistical Manual of Mental Disorders, 4th ed. 1994. Washington, D.C.
3. Arnett EN, Battle WE, Russo JV, Roberts WC: Intravenous injections of talc-containing drugs intended for oral use. Am J Med 1976; 60:711–718.
4. Bayer BM, Mulroney SE, Hernandez MC, et al: Acute infusions of cocaine result in time-and dose-dependent effects on lymphocyte responses and corticosterone secretion in rats. Immunopharmacology 1995;29:19–28.
5. Blanc PD, Saxena M, Olson KR: Drug detection and trauma cause—A case control study of fatal injuries. J Toxicol Clin Toxicol 1994;32:137–145.
6. Brookoff D, Campbell EA, Shaw LM: The underreporting of cocaine-related trauma: Drug abuse warning network reports versus hospital toxicology tests. Am J Public Health 1993;83:369–371.
7. Brown SM, Stimmel B, Taub R, et al: Immunologic dysfunction in heroin addicts. Arch Intern Med 1974;134:1001–1006.
8. Burns RS, Lewitt PA, Ebert MH, et al: The clinical syndrome of striatial dopamine deficiency: Parkinsonism induced by MPTP. N Engl J Med 1985;312:1418–1421.
9. Center on Addiction and Substance Abuse at Columbia University. Substance abuse and urban America: Its impact on an American city. New York. 1996.
10. Chambers HF, Korzeniowski OM, Sande MA: *Staphylococcus* aureus endocarditis: Clinical manifestations in addicts and nonaddicts. Medicine 1983;62:170–177.
11. Chambers HF, Morris DL, Tauber MG, Modin G: Cocaine use and the risk for endocarditis in intravenous drug abusers. Ann Intern Med 1987;106:833–836.
12. Chandrasekar PH, Narula A: Bone and joint infections in intravenous drug abusers. Rev Infect Dis 1986;8:904–910.
13. Cherubin CE: The medical sequelae of narcotic addiction. Ann Intern Med 1967;67:23–33.
14. Cherubin CE, Sapira JD: The medical complications of drug addiction and the medical assessment of the intravenous drug abuser: 25 years later. Ann Intern Med 1993;119:1017–1028.
15. Chiappelli F, Frost P, Manfrini E, et al: Cocaine blunts human CD4+ cell activation. Immunopharmacology 1994;3:233–240.
16. Chiappelli F, Kung MA, Villanueva P, et al: Immunotoxicology of cocaethylene. Immunopharmacol Immunotoxicol 1995;2:399–417.
17. Chun C, Raff M, Varghese R, et al: Splenic abscess. Medicine 1980;59:50–65.
18. Continued sexual risk behavior among HIV-seropositive, drug-using men—1993. MMWR 1996;45:151–154.
19. Corrigan JD: Substance abuse as a mediating factor in outcome after traumatic brain injury. Arch Phys Med Rehabil 1995;76:302–309.
20. Currie PF, Sutherland GR, Jacob AJ, et al: A review of endocarditis in acquired immunodeficiency sydrome and human immunodeficiency virus infection. Eur Heart J 1995;16:15–18.
21. Davis G, Hoffnagle J, Waggoner J: Spontaneous reactivation of chronic hepatitis B virus infection. Gastroenterology 1985;86:230–235.
22. Des Jarlais DC, Paone D, Friedman SR, et al: Regulating controversial programs for unpopular people: Methadone maintenance and syringe exchange programs. Am J Public Health 1995;85:1577–1584.
23. Emerson TS, Cisek JE: Methcathinone: A Russian designer

amphetamine infiltrates the rural midwest. Ann Emerg Med 1993;22:1897–1903.

24. Ernst AA, Martin DH: High syphilis rates among cocaine abusers identified in an emergency department. Sex Transm Dis 1992;20:66–69
25. Friedman CT, Dover AS, Roberto RR, Kerns OA: A malaria epidemic among heroin addicts. Am J Trop Med Hyg 1973; 22:302–307.
26. Fuller MG, Diamond DL, Jordan ML, Walters MC: The role of a substance abuse consultation team in a trauma center. J Stud Alcohol 1995;56:267–271.
27. Goldsmith M: Sex tied to drugs = STD spread. JAMA 1988;260:2009–2011.
28. Grund JP, Friedman SR, Stern LS, et al: Syringe-mediated drug sharing among injecting drug users: Patterns, social context, and implications for transmission of blood-borne pathogens. Soc Sci Med 1996;42:691–703.
29. Hagan H, Jarlais DC, Friedman SR, et al: Reduced risk of hepatitis B and hepatitis C among injection drug users in the Tacoma syringe exchange program. Am J Public Health 1995;85:1531–1537.
30. Haim DY, Lippman ML, Goldberg SK, Walkenstein MD: The pulmonary complications of crack cocaine: A comprehensive review. Chest 1995;107:233–240.
31. Haum A, Perbix W, Hack HJ, et al: Alcohol and drug abuse in burn patients. Burns 1995;21:194–199.
32. Heimer R, Khoshnood K, Jariwala-Freeman B, et al: Hepatitis in used syringes: The limits of sensitivity of techniques to detect hepatitis B virus DNA, hepatitis C virus RNA, and antibodies to HBV core and HCV antigens. J Infect Dis 1996;4:997–1000.
33. Higgins JP, Wright SW, Wrenn KD: Alcohol, the elderly, and motor vehicle crashes. Am J Emerg Med 1996;14:265–267.
34. Hoffman I, Stratton J, Lemon S, et al: Hepatitis B among parenteral drug abusers—North Carolina. JAMA 1986;256: 1262–1269.
35. Hoffman RS, Goldfrank LR: The impact of drug abuse and addiction on society. Emerg Med Clin North Am. 1990;8: 467–480.
36. Hughes PH, Barker NW, Crawford MA, Jaffe JH: The natural history of a heroin epidemic. Am J Pub Health 1972;62:995–1001.
37. Jacob H, Charytan C, Rascoff JH, et al: Amyloidosis secondary to drug abuse and chronic skin suppuration. Arch Intern Med 1978:138:1150–1151.
38. Jonas S: Heroin utilization A communicable disease? NY State J Med 1972;72:1292–1299.
39. Kandal DB: Epidemiological trends and implications for understanding the nature of addiction. In: O'Brien CP, Jaffe JH, eds: Addictive States. New York, Raven, 1992, pp. 23–40.
40. Kaplan EH, Heimer R: HIV incidence among New Haven needle exchange participants: Updated estimates from syringe tracking and testing data. J Acquir Immune Decif Syndr Hum Retrovirol 1995;10:175–176.
41. Kirby JM, Maull K, Fain W: Comparability of alcohol and drug use in injured drivers. South Med J 1992;85:800–803.
42. Klatt EC, Montgomery S, Namiki T, et al: Misrepresentation of stimulant street drugs. A decade of experience in an analysis program. J Toxicol Clin Toxicol 1986;24:441–450.
43. Klein TW, Matsui K, Newton CA, et al: Cocaine suppresses proliferation of phytohemagglutinin-activated human peripheral blood T-cells. Int J Immunopharmacol 1993;1:77–86.
44. Langston JW, Ballard P, Tetrud JW, Irwin I: Chronic parkinsonism in humans due to a byproduct of meperidine analog synthesis. Science 1983; 219:979–980.
45. Layon J, Idris A, Warzynski M, et al: Altered T lymphocyte subsets in hospitalized intravenous drug abusers. Arch Intern Med 1984;144:1376–1380.
46. Lead poisoning associated with intravenous-methamphetamine use—Oregon, 1988. MMWR 1989;38:830–831.
47. Lettau L, McCarthy J, Smith M, et al: Outbreak of severe hepatitis due to delta and hepatitis B viruses in parenteral drug abusers and their contacts. N Engl J Med 1987;317: 1256–1262.
48. Levine D, Crane L, Zervos M: Bacteremia in narcotic addicts at the Detroit Medical Center. II. Infectious endocarditis: A prospective comparative study. Rev Infect Dis 1986; 8:374–396.
49. Levine D, Sobel J: Infections in Intravenous Drug Abusers. New York, Oxford University Press, 1991.
50. Loiselle JM, Baker MD, Templeton JM, et al: Substance abuse in adolescent trauma. Ann Emerg Med 1993;22:1530–1534.
51. Mannenbach MS, Hargarten SW, Phelan MB: Alcohol use among injured patients aged 12 to 18 years. Acad Emerg Med 1997;4:40–44.
52. Marantz PR, Linzer M, Feiner CJ, et al: Inability to predict diagnosis in febrile intravenous drug abusers. Ann Intern Med 1987;106:823–828.
53. Marzuk PM, Tardiff K, Leon AC, et al: Fatal injuries after cocaine use as a leading cause of death among young adults in New York City. N Engl J Med 1995;332:1753–1757.
54. McGill V, Kowal-Vern A, Fisher SG, et al: The impact of substance abuse on mortality and morbidity from thermal injury. J Trauma 1995;38:931–934.
55. Moustoukas NM, Nichols RL, Smith JW, et al: Contaminated street heroin: Relationship to clinical infections. Arch Surg 1983;118:746–749.
56. O'Connor PG, Samet JH, Stein MD: Management of hospitalized intravenous drug users: Role of the internist. Am J Med 1994;96:551–558.
57. O'Connor PG, Selwyn PA, Schottenfeld RS: Medical care for injection-drug users with human immunodeficiency virus infection. N Engl J Med 1994;331:450–459.
58. Orsay EM, Doan-Wiggins L, Lewis R, et al: The impaired driver: Hospital and police detection of alcohol and other drugs of abuse in motor vehicle crashes. Ann Emerg Med 1994;24:51–55.
59. Padley SP, Adler BD, Staples CA, et al: Pulmonary talcosis: CT findings in three cases. Radiology 1993;186:125–127.
60. Pare JP, Cote G, Fraser RS: Long-term follow-up of drug abusers with intravenous talcosis. Am Rev Resp Dis 1989; 139:233–241.
61. Parran TV, Weber E, Tasse J, et al: Mandatory toxicology testing and chemical dependence consultation follow-up in a level-one trauma center. J Trauma 1995;38:278–280.
62. Piot P, Goilav C, Kegels E: Hepatitis B: Transmission by sexual contact and needle sharing. Vaccine 1990;8S:37–40
63. Pirozhkov SV, Watson RR, Chen GJ: Ethanol enhances im-

munosuppression induced by cocaine. Alcohol 1992;6:489–494.
64. Radnitz CL, Tirch D: Substance misuse in individuals with spinal cord injury. Int J Addict 1995;30:1117–1140.
65. Selwyn PA: Illicit drug use revisited: What a long, strange trip it's been. Ann Intern Med 1993;119:1044–1045.
66. Shannon M: Clinical toxicity of cocaine adulterants. Ann Emerg Med 1988;17:1243–1247.
67. Sloan EP, Zalenski R, Smith R, et al: Toxicology screening in urban trauma patients: Drug prevalence and its relationship to trauma severity and management. J Trauma 1989;29:1647–1653.
68. Soderstrom C, Dischinger P, Smith G, et al: Psychoactive substance dependence among trauma center patients. JAMA 1992;267:2756–2759.
69. Substance Abuse and Mental Health Services Administration/Office of Applied Studies: Preliminary Estimates from the Drug Abuse Warning Network. Advanced Report 17, August 1996.
70. Substance Abuse and Mental Health Services Administration/Office of Applied Studies. Preliminary Estimates from the 1995 National Household Survey on Drug Abuse. 1996.
71. Watanakunakorn C: Changing epidemiology and newer aspects of infective endocarditis. Adv Intern Med 1977;22:21–24.
72. Weisse AB, Heller DR, Schimenti RJ, et al: The febrile parenteral drug abuser: A prospective study in 121 patients. Am J Med 1993;94:274–280.
73. Wound botulism—California 1995. MMWR 1995;44:889–892.

CHAPTER 109

Healthcare Workers

Michael I. Greenberg

The numbers and types of potential toxins that healthcare workers may be exposed to are as varied as the occupations and job categories that exist in a modern healthcare facility. Typically, the particular toxic hazards that a worker may be exposed to are more a function of the immediate work environment within the healthcare facility (eg, ICU, laboratory, ambulance) than of the job or profession itself (eg, nurse, physician, unit receptionist).

Although each category of healthcare worker may be exposed to toxins inherent to the performance of their own duties, it is important to remember that they too can be exposed to toxins that are generated or exist in areas proximate to their immediate work environment but that have nothing at all to do with the performance of their specific duties.

Why Should Toxic Hazards in Healthcare Be of Concern? What Types of Toxins Are More Likely to Be Involved in Exposures?

Hospital and healthcare workers constitute the largest single group of employees in the United States today,[22,25] and job-related health and safety issues for these employees have been ignored until recently.

Large numbers of the public pass through hospitals each year as patients, visitors, vendors, delivery personnel, and so forth. Consequently, many people may potentially be exposed to various toxic hazards within the hospital environment.

Individuals employed in healthcare occupations can be exposed to a multitude of hazardous toxins and chemicals. Certain work areas as well as specific jobs within those areas in the hospital environment have specific toxic hazards commonly associated with them. Knowing which toxins may generally be associated with specific jobs will facilitate the formulation of a differential diagnosis list for each exposed patient.

Table 109–1 lists the most common potential toxic hazards for workers in the healthcare industry. Table 109–2 cites the locations of greatest risk of exposure. These chemical hazards can be categorized as disinfectants, sterilizing agents, solvents, anesthetic agents, chemotherapeutic agents, latex-containing products, detergents, tissue fixatives, and chemical reagents. They may enter the body by dermal absorption, inhalation, ingestion, and accidental needle stick, with the most common routes being inhalation (through aerosolization) and skin absorption.

Glutaraldehyde

Because endoscopy equipment is delicate as well as heat sensitive, it cannot be sterilized by traditional means utilizing heat and pressure. The chemical glutaraldehyde is the sterilizing agent most commonly used for heat-sensitive medical equipment.[30] In the hospital glutaraldehyde is also commonly found in the histology laboratory, where it is used as a tissue fixative. Although glutaraldehyde is commonly used as a 2% solution in hospitals it may be found in formulations with concentrations as high as 50% solutions.[50] The higher the concentration of the solution, the greater the volatility at room temperature, and consequently the higher the concentration of aerosolized chemical that might exist in the ambient air.

Glutaraldehyde is chemically related to formaldehyde and can cause very similar adverse effects, including irritation of the eyes, respiratory tree, and skin.[71] It can cause sensitization resulting in allergic contact dermatitis, asthma, and asthmatic exacerbations.[29] Inhalational exposure resulting in recurrent epistaxis has also been reported.[51] In addition, fetal toxicity has been identified in certain animal studies.[13]

Prevention of toxicity is best achieved by reducing the risk of exposure. Local exhaust ventilation (even a simple shielding structure connected to duct ventilation) can be easily provided in areas where glutaraldehyde is used, although dilution of concentrated glutaraldehyde solutions should be performed in very well ventilated areas. Employees should be thoroughly educated and trained regarding the potential adverse health effects of working with glutaraldehyde. In addition, personnel

TABLE 109–1. CHEMICAL AND PHYSICAL HAZARDS FOR HEALTHCARE WORKERS

Chemical Hazards	Biomedical adhesives
Disinfectants	Methyl methacrylate
Isopropyl alcohol, iodine, betadine, chlorine, phenol	
Sterilants	***Physical Hazards***
Formaldehyde, glutaraldehyde, ethylene oxide (EtO)	Ionizing radiation
	Nonionizing radiation
	Laser hazards
	Electrocautery smoke
Solvents	
Acetone, benzoin, ethanol	***Allergic Sensitization Hazards***
Anesthetic agents	Latex (as in latex gloves)
Nitrous oxide, enflurane, halothane, isoflurane	Lab animal allergy
Chemotherapeutic agents	
Antineoplastic and cytotoxic drugs	
Pharmaceuticals	
Pentamidine, ribavirin	
Heavy Metals	
Mercury	
Detergents	
Tissue fixatives	
Laboratory reagents	

TABLE 109–2. TOXIC HAZARDS FOR HEALTHCARE WORKERS BY LOCATION

Hospital-Wide
Disinfectants
  Isopropyl alcohol, iodine, Betadine, chlorine, phenol
Sterilants
  Formaldehyde, glutaraldehyde, ethylene oxide (EtO)
Solvents
  Acetone, benzoin, ethanol
Detergents
Ionizing radiation
Latex-containing materials

Operating Rooms
Anesthetic agents
  Nitrous oxide, enflurane, halothane, isoflurane, tissue fixatives, biomedical adhesives (methacrylates), nonionizing radiation, laser hazards, electrocautery smoke

Pharmacy
  Chemotherapeutic agents, pentamidine, ribavirin

Hospital Clinical and Research Laboratories
  Tissue fixative, lab chemicals and reagents, laboratory animal allergy

Outpatient/Day Hospital Facilities
  Chemotherapeutic agents, pentamidine, ribavirin

Hospital Repair Shops
  Mercury, solvents

protective equipment in the form of respiratory and skin protection should be provided.

Formaldehyde

Formaldehyde is generally found in the hospital setting as an aqueous solution known as formalin. The most commonly encountered solution contains formaldehyde at a concentration of 37% and is used primarily as a fixative for histology specimens and as an embalming material. In addition, formaldehyde-containing, solutions are sometimes used as disinfectants. The hospital autopsy room is probably the location that can be expected to demonstrate the highest air levels of formaldehyde gas.

Significant exposure of healthcare workers to formaldehyde and formalin has occurred both by virtue of unintentional exposure during the course of working as well as by intentional ingestion.[56] Following intentional ingestions of formalin, death has been reported to occur within a matter of hours. However, if the patient survives for a period of 48 hours, recovery generally can be expected. Once ingested, formalin can create local corrosive injury in the gastrointestinal tract as metabolism of formaldehyde proceeds to generate formic acid. Elevated formate levels can be associated with circulatory collapse, severe metabolic acidosis, and the development of acute renal failure.

Following inhalational exposure to low concentrations of formaldehyde, most individuals will experience initial mucous membrane irritation manifested as conjunctivitis and sore throat. This may be followed by the development of pulmonary irritation with coughing, shortness of breath, and difficulty breathing. However, exposure to formaldehyde gas in patients who were suspected of having formaldehyde-related asthma failed to induce symptoms consistent with asthma.[40]

At high concentrations (50 to 100 ppm), pulmonary edema and death have been reported. Although formaldehyde is a proven animal carcinogen, its carcinogenicity in humans is not certain. The specific concern involves formaldehyde's affinity to chemically react with hydrogen chloride to yield bis(chloromethyl)ether, a compound that is a known pulmonary carcinogen. Similarly, there is no definitive scientific evidence linking formaldehyde to the development of chronic obstructive pulmonary disease in individuals who are clinically exposed. Several studies performed in both the United States and abroad have failed to definitively link formaldehyde to either nasal or pulmonary cancers.[3,100]

How Should Healthcare Workers Acutely or Chronically Exposed to Antineoplastic Agents Be Managed?

Although each chemotherapeutic agent may pose specific potential hazards to an individual, one important common denominator of concern is the potential for bone marrow suppression with the possible development of marrow aplasia and aplastic anemia.[10,92,97] In addition, many of these agents may have inherent carcinogenic potential of their own.[35,47–49,54,87,88,93] Obviously removal from exposure is the first essential step in treatment. However, a complete blood count should be monitored at regular intervals. No published guidelines are available for such monitoring, but the patient's psychological needs should be taken into consideration and monitoring provided that is medically prudent as well as psychologically comforting. An example is baseline values, 3 months, 6 months, 12 months, 18 months, 24 months, 30 months, and 36 months. Additional CBCs should be obtained based upon the clinical status of the patient and the best judgment of the physician.

What Are the Significant Reproductive Hazards to Which Healthcare Workers Are Exposed and How Does That Exposure Occur?

The potential reproductive risk of exposure to potential carcinogens must also be considered.[88,93] The agents that are generally considered to be significant reproductive risks for healthcare workers include inhalational anesthetic gases, antineoplastic agents, sterilizing chemicals, tissue fixatives, aerosolized antiviral agents, and ionizing radiation.

Anesthetic Agents

The first report of adverse reproductive effects related to anesthetic agents appeared in the late 1960s. Subsequently, an increased rate of teratogenic events among anesthetists was reported,[12] and in 1971 an increase in unsuccessful pregnancies among nurse anesthetists and nurses working in the operating room was noted.[23] A 16.4% increased risk of birth defects among female nurse anesthetists who continued to work while pregnant compared with those nurse anesthetists who did not continue to work while pregnant was also reported.[27] The American Society of Anesthesiologists completed a survey of anesthetists, operating room nurses, and operating room technicians with regard to work-related reproductive risks.[7] In this study of 50,000 individuals, the investigators discovered an increased (1.3 to 2.0-fold) risk of spontaneous miscarriage when compared with controls. In addition, the number of congenital abnormalities noted in these individuals was approximately double that of the unexposed females. The risk of congenital abnormalities was noted to be 1.6 times greater for nurse anesthetists. The following discussion details the reproductive risks involved with exposure to specific anesthetic agents.

Ethylene Oxide

Ethylene oxide (EtO) is one of the most significant reproductive hazards to which healthcare workers may be exposed. A gaseous chemical with an odor similar to that of ether, EtO finds its principle use in the hospital setting in the gas sterilization of medical and surgical equipment that cannot be safely sterilized by heat and moisture. It is important to note that currently, there is no acceptable substitute for EtO sterilization, and the continued use of EtO is essential for the control of nosocomial infections. Therefore, EtO continues to be widely used in hospitals around the world.

Hospital workers become exposed to EtO largely as the result of residual ethylene oxide gas that remains in and around sterilization equipment. When removed from the gas sterilizer, the material being sterilized may contain residual amounts of the gas as well. Proper gas sterilization techniques, therefore, require periods of thorough aeration in order to allow residual ethylene oxide to properly dissipate.

Inhalational exposure provides the primary means for acute exposure to ethylene oxide.[16] At low concentrations, such an exposure results primarily in irritation to mucous membranes. However, exposure to increasingly elevated concentrations of EtO can cause gastrointestinal symptoms including nausea, vomiting, and diarrhea as well as headache. Some exposed individuals have described an unusual but distinctly nonmetallic taste as well. Following substantial acute exposures, central nervous system depression can occur.[16] Such exposures may be followed by delayed symptoms including weakness, malaise, and lack of coordination. Ethylene oxide exposure-associated central nervous system dysfunction has been reported to involve deficits in cognition, memory, and psychomotor skills.[16] Cataracts have also been reported to occur following exposure to very high concentrations of EtO.[86] In addition, pulmonary edema and ECG abnormalities have been reported as late sequelae of EtO exposure.[86] Skin burns can result from dermal exposure to ethylene oxide-containing solutions, the severity and depth of which depends upon the length of exposure and concentration of the ethylene oxide solution at issue.[89]

EtO has also been classified as a human carcinogen even though its human carcinogenicity is highly controversial. EtO is, however, a proven genotoxic animal carcinogen.[20,46,80] In laboratory animals, EtO has been proven to act by alkylation of DNA and other cellular proteins.[60]

How Can Hospitals Best Protect Healthcare Workers from the Hazards Posed by EtO? The Occupational Safety and Health Administration (OSHA) released its first formal standard on occupational exposure to ethylene oxide in 1984. The publication of these standards is based on animal and human data, that exposures to EtO present a carcinogenic, mutagenic, reproductive, neurologic, and sensitization hazard to workers. This standard set the permissible exposure level (PEL) for ethylene oxide at 1.0 part per million (ppm), determined as an 8-hour time-weighted average air concentration. In addition, OSHA also established an action level (AL) for EtO of 0.5 ppm determined as an 8-hour time-weighted average. In 1988, OSHA amended the previously published standards by adding a short-term exposure limit (STEL) for EtO of 5.0 ppm, determined as a 15-minute time-weighted average.

The exposure of healthcare workers to EtO can be thought of as consisting of essentially three distinct factors: personnel practices, equipment conditions, and ventilation characteristics. Based upon an analysis of these three components, each hospital and work site must determine the strategy it will use in developing a control program that will reduce ethylene oxide exposure to the limits addressed by OSHA standards.

Several biologic markers for ethylene oxide exposure have been sought. These include finding increased numbers of hemoglobin adducts and sister-chromatid exchanges. These markers have not been demonstrated to be consistent indicators of genotoxicity or increased risk of disease. Nonetheless, these changes do appear to reflect exposure to ethylene oxide, although the clinical application of these methods is not currently available.[35]

Nitrous Oxide

Physicians, veterinarians, and dentists frequently employ nitrous oxide (N_2O) as an anesthetic agent, and along with their assistants, may be exposed to N_2O during procedures. The acute toxic effects of N_2O may be of concern in the setting of substance abuse.[94]

Nitrous oxide often is the exclusive anesthesia drug used by dentists in their office suites. The problem with use in this setting is that exposures in the private dental office tend to be somewhat more difficult to control than in other settings. The National Institute of Occupational Health and Safety (NIOSH) demonstrated exposures to N_2O as high as 300 ppm in hospital operating rooms and exposures higher than 1000 ppm of N_2O in dental operatories.[67] These extremely high levels found in dental offices occur despite the general use of highly efficient gas-scavenging systems. In addition, control of N_2O escaping into the ambient air tends to be more difficult to control during dental procedures: only the patient's nose is covered during dental anesthesia, whereas both the nose and mouth are covered during other forms of surgery. In 1977, NIOSH published a technical report entitled "Control of Occupational Exposure to N_2O in the Dental Operatory."[69,70] This report described various methods for limiting the concentration of waste N_2O in this setting. This report notes that properly operating scavenging systems can reduce N_2O concentrations in the ambient air by as much as 70%.[62]

The magnitude of the potential medical problems attributable to N_2O exposure in dental medicine alone can be put into perspective when one considers that more than 424,000 individuals (dentists, dental assistants, and dental hygienists) are involved in dentistry in the United States.[24] In addition, the American Dental Association (ADA) reported in 1983 that 35% of dentists used N_2O to control pain and anxiety in their patients.[6] The ADA 1991 Survey of Dental Practice indicated that 58% of dentists reported having N_2O anesthetic equipment, but only 64% of those practitioners also reported having a scavenging system.[6] The percentage of pediatric dentists using N_2O increased from 65% in 1980 to 88% in 1988.[32]

The fact that N_2O may adversely impact reproductive outcomes was first demonstrated in animal models. Several studies in females demonstrated adverse reproductive effects following exposure to nitrous oxide.[28,98,99]

A number of observational studies have investigated workers who were occupationally exposed to N_2O. These studies have demonstrated specific adverse effects following exposure including a reduction in overall fertility.[85] In addition, an increase in the rate of spontaneous abortions was reported along with increases in neurologic, renal, and liver disease.[25] Female dental assistants exposed to N_2O for more than 5 hours per week had a significantly increased incidence of diminished fertility in comparison with unexposed female dental assistants.[85] Exposed individuals suffered a 59% decrease in ability to conceive during any given menstrual cycle compared with unexposed controls. When an effective gas-scavenging system was in place, however, the probability of conception was essentially equal to that of the unexposed controls.[85]

OSHA does not currently have a standard for N_2O. In addition, there is currently no NIOSH recommended exposure limit intended to prevent adverse reproductive effects. However, NIOSH has recommended an exposure limit of 25 ppm as a time-weighted average for N_2O, which is intended primarily to prevent decreases in mental performance and changes in audiovisual ability, and deterioration of manual dexterity, of dental personnel who work with N_2O.[69,70]

The only organization to specifically address the protection of workers from the reproductive hazards of N_2O to date has been the American Conference of Governmental Industrial Hygienists (ACGIH). This group has recommended a threshold limit value for N_2O of 50 ppm as an 8-hour TWA.[1,2] These guidelines state that "control to this level should prevent embryo-fetal toxicity in humans and significant decrements in human psychomotor and cognitive functions or other adverse health effects in exposed personnel."[1]

Antiviral Agents

The treatment of respiratory syncytial virus in pediatric patients often involves the administration of antiviral agents delivered via aerosol. When administered either via hood, oxygen tent, or nebulizer, significant amounts of these agents may escape into the ambient room air. Consequently, nurses, respiratory therapists, visitors, physicians, and occasionally others may be exposed. One of the most commonly used antiviral agents is the synthetic nucleoside ribavirin.[42,45] Despite the fact that ribavirin has not been conclusively shown to exert adverse reproductive effects in humans, it has indeed been shown to be teratogenic in laboratory animals.[60] A recent study demonstrated that the typical in-hospital occupational exposure to ribavirin, even without the use of appropriate personal protective equipment, would not result in significant levels of ribavirin.[58] However, another study evaluated urine collected from respiratory therapists and nurses following the completion of their work shifts. This study demonstrated that despite the use of high-efficiency respirators worn by all subjects, ribavirin was detected in the urine of 11 of the 17 individuals. The urine levels of ribavirin were significantly higher for the nurses than for the respiratory therapists.[33] Hospital personnel should avoid exposure to ribavirin before and during pregnancy as well as during lactation.[102] Other potential adverse health effects referable to aerosolized ribavirin have included ocular irritation as well as contact lens damage.[34]

Another antiviral agent administered via aerosol is pentamidine, commonly used in treating *Pneumocystis carinii* pneumonia. Just as with ribavirin, this mode of drug administration can easily result in exposure to healthcare workers, patients, and visitors. One report indicated that the removal of the delivery nebulizer from the patient's mouth before it was turned off increases the ambient levels of pentamidine.[73] In addition, if the patient being treated coughs, the levels of pentamidine in the air can increase as well.[73] Another report documented the acute onset of bronchospasm in a nurse with no prior history of asthma immediately following the administration of aerosolized pentamidine to a patient.[73] Bronchospasm has also been reported in patients receiving pentamidine treatments.[33]

Additional chronic effects of occupational pentamidine exposure have been reported as well. One example of such chronic effects involves the case of respiratory technician whose carbon monoxide diffusing capacity declined significantly during the time that he worked with pentamidine aerosols.[33] Pentamidine levels have been detected in the urine of those healthcare workers who are involved in the administration of pentamidine aerosol treatments.[64] This is clear evidence of systemic absorption of pentamidine resulting from this type of inhalation exposure. Conversely, 16 healthcare workers who administered aerosolized pentamidine while working were studied and despite the fact that aerosolized pentamidine levels in the ambient air were documented to be elevated, no pentamidine was detected in the urine of any of these subjects. These investigators emphasize the importance of taking steps to minimize healthcare worker exposure to aerosolized pentamidine.[14]

What Toxic Physical Hazards Affect Healthcare Workers?

Table 109–1 lists the most common toxic physical hazards found in the hospital and health care setting. Ionizing and nonionizing radiation represent important sources of exposure hazards for healthcare workers; a complete discussion of the biophysics of these hazards can be found in Chapter 98.

Ionizing Radiation

Healthcare workers may be exposed to ionizing radiation in essentially two ways. Exposure may occur as the result of random scatter from x-ray beams, especially from portable x-ray equipment used in the emergency department,[21] operating room, and intensive care areas. Exposure can also occur as the result of gamma or beta emissions from patients who have been treated with radioactive implants or who are undergoing diagnostic procedures involving radionucleosides. Almost any hospital staff member may be at risk of exposure from these sources, but some personnel (especially nurses) seem to be at greater risk.

In a prospective study of radiation exposure in the emergency department, mean lapel and wrist dosimetry was measured during a 2-year period for emergency department personnel.[21,68] Emergency physicians demonstrated a lapel level that was approximately half that of radiology technicians. However, when wrist levels were compared, emergency physicians were found to have almost twice the exposure of radiology technicians. This may reflect direct physical involvement when, for example small children require stress films of extremities. Another study of physician exposure to ionizing radiation during trauma resuscitation revealed that significant radiation exposures can occur.[103] To obtain complete cervical spine radiography, healthcare workers may be asked to stabilize the necks.[91] When radiographic procedures are done, the use of protective garments is mandatory. Personnel positioned more than several feet from the x-ray beam will generally have relatively insignificant exposures.[43]

When an acute radiation exposure takes place, the effects are usually local and superficial, resulting in erythroderma. More significant exposure may result in radiodermatitis. More serious effects from occupational exposure are distinctly rare. The degree of risk to healthcare workers is yet to be precisely determined. Only a few studies have addressed the risk related to long-term, low-dose x-ray exposure.[9,19,101] However, several studies have identified a high prevalence of cancer of the thyroid as well as thyroid nodules resulting from occupational exposure.[11] OSHA maintains a standard for ionizing radiation-limiting radiation exposure.[78]

Nonionizing Radiation

Table 109–1 lists nonionizing radiation hazards that may be present in the healthcare work environment. One of the most common forms of nonionizing radiation is lasers.

The term "laser" is an acronym for "Light Amplification by Stimulated Emission of Radiation." The energy is a specific form of light that is produced when energy of electrical origin interfaces with a solid, liquid, or gas medium. The resultant light is a single wavelength consisting of a parallel focused high-energy beam.

Several different types of lasers are currently available for medical use, including the Nd:Yag (neodymium:yttrium-aluminum-garnet) laser, the carbon dioxide laser, the argon laser, the dye laser, and the excimer laser.[61] Lasers can be used to incise, or destroy tissue depending upon the unique physical properties of the laser beam.

When a concentrated laser beam destroys tissue, cell vaporization results and causes what is known as a "laser plume" of smoke, which is actually a complex mixture of steam, cellular debris, and smoke associated with a pungent, unpleasant odor. The odor can be so intense that the use of high-pressure extraction devices may be necessary to eliminate it from the area. Laser plume odor has been reported to be so noxious that healthcare workers have been "overcome" by the odor.[104]

Inhalational exposure to the laser "plume" during operative procedures is also of concern. Studies have attempted to determine if pathogenic organisms or even viable cells might be disseminated during the production of a laser plume. Aerosols produced from laser-treated rodents have been studied and intact cells from the laser plume were recovered. These cells proved to be culture negative for pathogens.[61] However, other investigators have recovered pathogenic bacteria from laser plume cultures.[61] These studies concluded that the laser plume could carry and disseminate pathogenic material during laser treatments. Nonetheless, there are no current recommendations addressing special precautions to be taken in this regard or regarding the advisability of pregnant individuals avoiding laser plumes. It is important to note that the smoke generated by electrocautery devices used to stop small amounts of local bleeding can also be harmful in the same way as the laser plume.

Ocular toxicity from laser exposure is an important concern. A specific period of time, measured in maximal permissible exposure times (MPEs), determines the amount of time that the eye can be safely exposed to a laser beam. All personnel working around lasers must be thoroughly knowledgeable in the proper use of eye protection during laser operations. The acute ocular injury that may result from exposure to a laser beam may be ameliorated by proper eye protective devices, although there may be ocular damage from long-term laser exposure with or without proper eye protection. Macular damage may occur in ophthalmologists who have been exposed to laser beams during operative conditions over the course of many years.[104] Several recommendations, established specifically for healthcare workers, describe steps to be taken to provide protection of the eyes from laser injury.[31]

An additional concern with regard to lasers is the potential for the development of an explosive hazard during use. Explosions have occurred when lasers caused the ignition of either anesthetic gases or bowel gases.[31] In one case report, a 41-year-old patient with carcinoma of the larynx was seriously injured when a laser ignited the patient's endotracheal tube, causing severe laryngeal and tracheal burns.[31]

Ultraviolet Light Radiation

Ultraviolet light radiation (UVLR) is a form of nonionizing radiation that may represent a health hazard to certain healthcare workers. This form of radiation ranges in wavelength from 200 to 400 nm.

Three specific "regions" exist within the UVLR spectrum that are the focus of most concern. UVLR in the "A" region (UV-A) is reported to be the most important factor in the development of cataracts following exposure, while UV-B is generally considered the most dangerous of the UVLR exposures. UV-C, on the other hand, is considered to be the most benign form of this sort of radiation and has primarily germicidal properties only. Consequently, UV-C is often used as a means of food and air sterilization. UV-C light sources can be found at entryways to operating room areas in the hospital as well as in the food service areas. To date, no firm scientific evidence has been reported to implicated UV-C radiation as a source for health problems in exposed individuals.

Mercury

Elemental mercury is widely encountered in hospital environments in various kinds of medical equipment and monitoring devices including sphygmomanometers, thermometers, and thermostats. When such equipment breaks, healthcare workers, patients, and visitors may be exposed to elemental mercury. Repairing biomedical equipment may also be a source of mercury spills.

Mercury is also used as a tissue fixative in the histology lab. Dentists can be occupationally exposed to the mercury used in dental amalgams.[36,79,82] In all of these cases, exposure is by inhalation because at room temperature mercury easily vaporizes and becomes airborne.

Acutely inhaled, mercury vapor can cause direct respiratory damage by corrosive bronchitis and potentially fatal interstitial pneumonitis. Chronic exposure to mercury results in primarily neurologic effects, which are discussed in Chapter 80.

Pharmaceuticals

Pharmaceuticals may present a significant risk to health care workers as a result of acute or chronic low-dosage exposure. As previously discussed, chemotherapeutic agents are an example. Most other pharmaceuticals are hazardous primarily by inhalational exposure and primary pulmonary toxicity. The pulmonary hazards more commonly occur where pharmaceuticals are manufactured. However, healthcare workers who administer and/or prepare these agents are also at risk of developing either asthma or other allergic manifestations. Examples of such pharmaceutical hazards include certain antibiotics and such proteolytic enzymes as pancreatic extracts and papain. Preparations involving drugs that generate dusts are a particular problem. Even the simple act of counting pills can produce small amounts of powder that may aerosolize and sensitize an individual.

Another specific problem material is psyllium, which is often found as a constituent in bulk laxatives. Psyllium is implicated in the sensitization of exposed workers and associated with the development of occupationally related asthma.[39] The problem is probably more common in chronic care facilities, where the use of laxatives is widespread. In one study, as many as 18% of healthcare workers reported allergic reactions while handling psyllium.[41] The reactions varied from mild mucosal irritation to respiratory compromise. Psyllium challenge testing to evaluate sensitization of personnel working in chronic care institutions[59] and the prevalence of asthmatic symptoms was similar to that found in workers manufacturing psyllium.

Other forms of testing workers for possible sensitization to various inhaled drugs and allergens, such as assays to measure specific hazardous drug levels or their metabolites in blood and urine, and tests measuring urine mutagenicity or cytogenetic changes, have proved inefficient and may not be accurate prognostically. Because the use of these inhalational materials may be episodic, poorly documented, and difficult to quantify, control becomes problematic. Adequate preventive measures depend on adequate reduction in exposure and many hospitals have instituted the use of "biologic safety cabinets" (BSCS) and built-in vertical air flow systems. They are widely used in the preparation of hazardous drugs. Several agencies including OSHA and the American Society of Hospital Pharmacists have published guidelines for the proper handling of these agents.[8,76]

Methacrylate Compounds

Methacrylate-containing compounds are widely used in orthopedic surgery and in dental procedures as biologic adhesives. In order to create the adhesive effect, a liquid and a powder constituent are mixed together. During the mixing process, healthcare workers may be exposed to the components.

Upper respiratory irritation and contact dermatitis—both the allergic and irritant type—may follow acute exposure to methacrylate compounds.[26,84] Sensitization to the methacrylate dusts repeatedly has resulted in asthma[15] in dental assistants and several dental patients.[4] Allergic conjunctivitis associated with occupational exposure to methacrylate has also been reported.[38] The appropriate use of exhaust systems in conjunction with adequate ventilation will minimize the possibility of significant exposures.

Chlorine gas and chloramine gas are generated when certain cleaning products are mixed together.[63] Either of these gases can produce upper respiratory irritation. In addition, if the concentrations are high enough, lower respiratory effects, such as pulmonary edema, can occur. In a review of 216 patients exposed to chlorine/chloramine gas generated by mixing home cleaning products, 200 were asymptomatic within 6 hours, 71 required emergency department care including oxygen bronchodilators and in some cases systemic steroids, and 1 required hospital admission.[65] Although the generation of chloramine gas by mixing cleaning products usually does not cause serious morbidity or mortality, it can. Such patients should be carefully assessed for underlying pulmonary pathology that might be further compromised by this exposure. Proper education of the cleaning staff as well as closer supervision would be helpful in preventing such untoward events.

How Common Is Latex Allergy and What Is Its Pathophysiology?

Approximately 2% of the general population may be affected by mild to severe allergic reactions to latex.[5] Frequency of exposure may be a factor. For example, up to 50% of children who have spina bifida reportedly experienced severe latex reactions.[55] Such children may be sensitized by frequent bladder catheterizations using rubber tubing and individuals with latex gloves. Three percent of all hospital workers experience immediate type hypersensitivity to latex, and as many as 10% of operating room nurses may react to rubber in this way.[105,106] Approximately 5% of workers involved in the manufacturing of surgical gloves and in the rubber industry also may develop an immediate-type hypersensitivity to rubber.[106]

Latex is the milk-like sappy material that emanates from the rubber tree *Hevea brasiliensis.* Adverse reactions to natural rubber products were first reported in the early 1930s and were attributed to the many compounding agents that may be added during production.[5] In fact, the hand dermatitis that occurs in reaction to latex gloves is usually due to a delayed (type IV) hypersensitivity reaction to thiurams or other additives rather than to the latex itself.[95] Because evidence for immunoglobulin (Ig) E-mediated (type 1) reactions to protein antigens in latex itself were first documented some 15 years ago, the incidence of such reactions has increased dramatically. The implementation of the "universal precautions" against infectious diseases has been identified as the key reason for this increase.[5] However, in addition to the substantial increase in the use of latex gloves by healthcare workers in order to avoid infection, the apparent antigenicity of latex products has increased as a result of changes in manufacturing process designed to increase production.[96] Although the amount of antigen present in latex gloves tends to be highly variable, factors that lower the amount of allergen in these gloves include leaching and steam sterilization. Studies have identified many possible antigens in latex. Although the cornstarch used in latex gloves is nonallergenic,[106] latex particles can be adsorbed by the starch and become aerosolized, thus increasing the possibility of airborne exposure.

The most common presenting symptoms seen in latex-sensitive healthcare workers is localized urticaria or simple dermatitis. Systemic symptoms including generalized urticaria, rhinitis, asthmatic symptoms, and generalized anaphylaxis can also develop.[5] Nonmedical hospital workers who may also be exposed to latex include kitchen workers.[5]

The clinical presentation of latex allergy can be highly variable and is largely dependent on two specific factors: the amount of antigen in the product and the form of exposure. Skin exposure to latex gloves can result in localized contact dermatitis, widespread urticaria, or both. However, both widespread urticaria and systemic anaphylaxis have been reported. The most serious reactions attributable to latex resulted from parenteral or mucosal contact.[105] Specific examples of such exposures include those that occur intraoperatively or during barium enemas, GU catheterization, and dental procedures.

IgE-mediated reactions to latex product exposure on the job have been recognized since 1988. Occupational allergy to latex antigen has been reported in surgeons, nurses, dentists, pharmacists, and radiology and other medical technicians. Recent surveys have found that 10 to 17% of all hospital personnel, 7.4% of surgeons, and 5.2 to 10.7% of operating room staff are sensitive to latex.[106]

The diagnosis of IgE-mediated allergy typically is confirmed by skin prick or radioallergosorbent testing (RAST). However, the interpretation of these tests for latex sensitivity can be problematic, as there are currently no standardized commercial extracts for skin testing available in the United States. Older RAST methods had only a 60 to 65% sensitivity, whereas newer tests have a somewhat higher sensitivity.[52]

The first approach is simply to apply the rubber material to the skin and then wait approximately 30 minutes to see if any skin reaction or other symptoms occur. Another approach is the so-called "prick test," in which a drop of fluid containing the allergen is applied to the surface of the skin at the site of a needle prick or a series of superficial skin abrasions. Although these kinds of tests tend to be the most sensitive for determining allergy to rubber, they also have the very real potential to trigger life-threatening reactions. Consequently, it is extremely important to have appropriate resuscitation equipment and drugs (including the means for airway control) readily available to treat possible anaphylactic reactions, and physicians in attendance capable of providing advanced cardiac life support, should that become necessary.

In order to prevent occupational exposure of healthcare workers, nonlatex, low antigen-containing, powder-free gloves and latex substitutes for nonglove products must be utilized. A future goal involves the production of rubber products for hospital use that have no or only very minimal allergenicity.

Another important issue to consider is the accuracy of labeling of rubber products. The removal of antioxidants and the accelerant previously used in the vulcanization process was thought to have made rubber gloves "safe for rubber-allergic persons."[96] Although gloves manufactured in this way have been labeled as protective for latex-allergic individuals, this applies mostly to people who only have delayed-type hypersensitivity dermatitis, leading to simple scaling and blisters of their hands, and not to the much more serious immediate-type hypersensitivity, which can lead to anaphylaxis. This point is illustrated by the report of a cardiac catheterization nurse who developed periorbital swelling as well as pharyngeal edema following exposure to latex in gloves that were supposedly "nonallergenic." Within approximately 90 minutes following exposure to this "safe" product, this individual required epinephrine and intravenous corticosteroid therapy.[72]

Gloves have historically been used to protect people from various hazards found in their work environment. Rubber gloves can, however, represent a substantial toxic hazard for some workers and may possibly be lethal for those with immediate-type hypersensitivity to latex. In the hospital setting, where so many individuals rely on latex gloves, a periodic review of workers' skin reactions due to exposure to rubber products is important. However, as illustrated above, it is important to be aware that workers' sensitivities to rubber products may have manifestations other than simple dermal manifestations, and workers who complain of mucosal irritation, difficulty breathing, or upper airway irritation should be evaluated promptly.

What Are the Most Important Considerations in Establishing a Latex-Safe Environment for Healthcare Workers?

When a sensitized individual is continually exposed to latex, increased sensitivity to latex usually follows and the possibility of developing permanent respiratory sequela that can become life threatening is a pressing concern. As many as 15 to 17% of healthcare workers are sensitized to latex and go on to develop occupational asthma.[5] Because there is no cure for latex-related allergy, avoidance of exposure is the most important means for preventing an allergic reaction to latex. It is important to remember that latex reactions can be minimized through early diagnosis.

Currently, there are no published guidelines for the establishment of a latex-safe environment. However, it is clear that those individuals who manifest findings consistent with anaphylaxis must be permanently removed from such exposure.[90]

Further, it is unlikely that a rubber glove proven to be completely safe will be developed for individuals who have immediate-type hypersensitivity in the near future. In some instances, vinyl gloves may be a reasonable substitute; however, they offer no protection against environmental (airborne) contamination. One recent study indicated that approximately 25% of medical personnel had demonstrable hand contamination with bacteria when wearing vinyl gloves, while only approximately 2% had hand contamination when wearing rubber-containing gloves.[72] Consequently, the use of vinyl gloves corrects the potential for exposure to one serious toxin while exposing the worker to significant risks for pathogen exposure.

Some workers may attempt to protect their hands using a vinyl glove covered by a rubber glove. This approach to "double gloving" may give the worker sufficient protection from bacterial contamination, but there is still the possibility of continued latex sensitization, airborne contamination, and possible anaphylaxis. Table 109–3 lists

TABLE 109–3. STEPS TO BE TAKEN FOR LATEX-SAFE ENVIRONMENT

1. Glove education for all employees.
2. Comprehensive employee health histories, updated periodically, including history of food sensitivity.
3. Do not rely on "hypoallergenic" claims.
4. Replace latex nose pieces and rubber dental dams.
5. Create latex safe crash carts.
6. Clean and maintain all air ducts and filters.
7. Removal of all powdered gloves is the ultimate protective strategy.

some of the measures that can be taken to implement a latex-safe environment for healthcare workers.

What Other Allergens May Cause Sensitization Illness in Healthcare Workers?

Large numbers of healthcare workers and those working in related fields (eg, pharmaceutical development) may be exposed to animal-derived allergenic materials on a regular basis. These individuals may develop what has come to be known as laboratory animal allergy (LAA), a clinical syndrome characterized by rhinitis, upper airway inflammation, and occasionally bronchospasm. It is important to note that the majority of workers suffering from LAA report symptoms associated with rhinitis and upper airway symptoms as opposed to asthmatic symptoms.[37]

Laboratory animal allergy (LAA) involves the development of a hypersensitivity reaction in association with dermal or inhalational exposure to animal allergens. LAA is an IgE-mediated reaction affecting approximately 30% of workers exposed to lab animals.[37] Exposure to animal urine and saliva seems to be an especially powerful inciting agent for the development of LAA. Although specific risk factors for the development of LAA have not been well defined, several studies have addressed this question. Surprisingly, a history of atopy was not found to increase the risk of LAA in some studies.[81] However, atopy was indeed found to be an associated risk factor in other studies.[57,81] One study found a history of allergic symptoms in 168 of 364 animal handlers.[66] There is also controversy with regard to the ability of skin prick and RAST tests to detect LAA.

To control exposure for workers, systematic surveillance for the presence of airborne allergens may be useful. One study demonstrated a strong correlation between airborne rat urinary allergen and the symptoms of LAA.[67] In another study of over 500 animal handlers, almost 25% of workers reported LAA symptoms with a substantial percentage of those reporting the need to cease working as a result of the severity of their LAA-related symptoms.[37] The latter study was unable to demonstrate a salutary effect from the use of personal protective equipment. However, this study recommends using dustless animal bedding, reducing the use of animal bedding materials, and using local exhaust ventilation (hoods) when cleaning animal cages in order to minimize the aerosolizing of allergens. In workers who have not progressed to develop asthmatic symptoms, respiratory protective devices are recommended. In 58% of workers suffering from LAA the use of PPE was reported to improve symptoms.[18] These investigators point out that the expense of more rigorous prevention of exposure is justified in light of the savings from decreased time lost from work.

What Are the Potentials for Self-Poisoning in Healthcare Workers?

Healthcare workers have relatively easy access to a wide variety of drugs, toxic laboratory chemicals, and other toxic materials. Consequently, one might expect intentional self-poisoning with these substances to be a problem. In addition, many healthcare workers have knowledge regarding the effects of these drugs and toxins. The literature supports the claim that healthcare personnel utilize different substances in suicidal gestures than does the general public: Barbiturates, carbon monoxide, cyanide, azides, and methemoglobin-forming chemicals may be more commonly used in suicidal attempts by healthcare personnel.[17] This should be kept in mind when treating a healthcare worker for an unknown overdose or poisoning.

Laboratory Chemicals and Reagents

A multitude of potentially dangerous chemicals and reagents are present in various areas of the hospital environment. For the most part, however, these materials are found in the confines of the various clinical and research lab facilities that any given hospital might house.

In general, most of these materials simply fall into the category of either being weak or strong acids or bases or organic solvents. Toxicity stems from exposure to these substances generally represented by skin burns due to accidental dermal exposures. On occassion, intentional ingestions occur and result in injury consistent with the substance ingested. The pathophysiology and treatment of these injuries are dealt with elsewhere in this book.

One specific laboratory chemical of special concern is sodium azide. This chemical is widely available in hospitals, and thus is of concern when it comes to its availability as an intentional or accidental toxicant. Sodium azide is often found as a component chemical in the fluid used to dilute blood samples prior to the use of autoanalyzer analysis. In addition, sodium azide can be found as a constituent of one of the buffering reagents used in testing for the presence of hepatitis antigen.[83]

Sodium azide exerts its toxic effects within the mitochondria, where it interferes with energy transfer by mediating the uncoupling of oxidative phosphorylation. In addition, the enzymes catalase and cytochrome oxidase are specifically inhibited by sodium azide. Although the precise mechanisms involved with sodium azide's toxicity have not yet been fully elucidated, there is some indication that cyanide may be formed in the presence of sodium azide and be responsible, in part, for some of the clinical manifestations of sodium azide toxicity.

Clinically, sodium azide intoxication may result in a wide range of effects including central nervous system effects manifested as seizures, hyporeflexia, coma, and headache. In addition, nausea, vomiting, diarrhea, and the effects of vascular smooth muscle relaxtion causing hypotension have been reported. Death may follow, and at autopsy pulmonary, cerebral, and myocardial edema with myocardial necrosis have been reported.[53]

The treatment of sodium azide intoxication is primarily aimed at providing symptomatic relief and cardiovascular support. Because clinical deterioration may be delayed following sodium azide intoxication, intensive care monitoring should be considered for a minimum of 72 hours.

What Governmental Regulations Apply to Healthcare Workers at Risk for Toxic Exposures?

Many of the chemical and physical hazards to healthcare professionals are regulated by The Occupational Safety and Health Administration. There are strict and enforceable OSHA "standards" for several chemical hazards such as formaldehyde[75] and ethylene oxide.[77] "Guidelines" expressing OSHA's opinion about the proper handling of certain specific hazards are also issued. Although not carrying the force of an OSHA standard, these guidelines are meant to disseminate information and to engender voluntary compliance. An example of such a guideline is the 1986 "Safe Handling of Anticancer or Cytotoxic Drugs," which describes the need for proper engineering controls when cytotoxic agents are handled in the healthcare setting.[74] The broadest OSHA communication is the so-called Hazard Communication Standard,[78] which requires all employers to inform their employees of the specific chemical hazards involved in their jobs. In the healthcare setting, this standard would include the preparation of drugs and medicines by pharmacists and nurses. In addition, this standard requires that employees be provided with written information (in the form of the Material Safety Data Sheet) describing the chemical hazards to which they may be exposed on the job.[44]

References

1. American Conference of Governmental Industrial Hygienists: 1994 Threshold Limit Values for Chemical Substances and Physical Agents and Biological Exposure Indices. Cincinnati, ACGIH, 1993.
2. American Conference of Governmental Industrial Hygienists: Documentation of the Threshold Limit Values and Biological Exposure Indices, 6th ed. Cincinnati, ACGIH,1992, pp. 1134–1138.
3. Acheson ED, Barnes HR, Gardner MJ, et al: Formaldehyde in the British chemical industry. Lancet 1984;1:611–616.
4. Agner T, Menne T: Sensitization to acrylates in a dental patient. Contact Dermatitis 1994;30:249–250.
5. Altman LC: Occupational exposure to latex. West J Med 1995;163:369–370.
6. American Dental Association: The 1991 survey of dental practice: General characteristics of dentists. Chicago, American Dental Association, 1992.
7. American Society of Anesthesiology Ad Hoc Committee on the Effect of Trace Anesthetics on the Health of Operating Room Personnel: Occupational Disease among operating room personnel: A national study. Anesthesiology 1974;41:321–340.
8. American Society of Hospital Pharmacists. ASHP technical assistance bulletin on handling cytotoxic and hazardous drugs. Am J Hosp Pharm 1990;47:1033–1049.
9. Anderson M, Engholm G, Ennow K, et al: Cancer risk among staff at two radiotherapy departments in Denmark. Br J Radiol 1991;64:455–460.
10. Anderson RW, Puckett WH, Dana WJ, et al: Risk of handling injectable antineoplastic agents. Am J Hosp Pharm 1982;39:1881–1887.
11. Antonelli A, Silvano G, Bianchi F: Risk of thyroid nodules in subjects occupationally exposed to radiation: A cross sectional study. Occup Environ Med 1995;52:500–504.
12. Askrog V, Harvald B. Teratogenic effects of inhalational anesthetics. Nordisk Med 1970;83:498–500.
13. Ballantyne B: Toxicology of Glutaraldehyde. Review of Studies and Human Health Effects. Danbury, CT, Union Carbide, 1995.
14. Balmes JR, Estacio PL, Quinlan P, et al: Respiratory effects of occupational exposure tom aerosolized pentamidine. J Occup Environ Med 1995;37:145–150.
15. Bardana EJ: Occupational asthma and related respiratory disorders. Dis Mon March 1995, pp. 141–200.
16. Bihari V, Srivastava AK, Gupta BN: Occupational health hazards among operating room personnel exposed to anesthetic gases: A review. J Environ Pathol Toxicol Oncol 1994;13:213–219.
17. Binder L, Fredrickson L: Poisonings in laboratory personnel and health care professionals. Am J Emerg Med 1991;9:11–15.
18. Bland SM, Levine MS, Wilson PD, et al: Occupational allergy to laboratory animals; An epidemiologic study. J Occup Med 1986;28:1151–1157.
19. Boice JD, Mandel JS, Doody MM, et al: Health survey of radiologic technologists. Cancer 1992;69:586–598.
20. Bolt HM: Quantification of endogenous carcinogens. The ethylene oxide paradox. Biochem Pharmacol 1996;52:1–59.
21. Braun BJ, Skiendzielewski JJ: Radiation exposure of emergency physicians. Ann Emerg Med 1982;11:535–540.
22. Bureau of Labor Statistics. Outlook 2000. Washington, DC, U.S. Department of Labor, Bureau of Labor Statistics, Bulletin 2352, 1990, pp. 51, 54.
23. Cohen EN, Beliville JW, Brown BW: Anesthesia, pregnancy, and miscarriage: A study of operating room nurses and anesthetists. Anesthesiology 1971;35:343–347.
24. Cohen EN, Gift HC, Brown BW, et al: Occupational disease in dentistry and chronic exposure to trace anesthetic gases. J Am Dent Assoc 1980;101:21–31.
25. Cohen JH: Occupational stress among nurse executives. Nurse Admin Q 1989;13:41–46.
26. Conde-Salazar L, Guimaraens D, Romero CV: Occupational allergic contact dermatitis from anaerobic acrylic sealants. Contact Dermatitis 1988;18:129–132.
27. Corbett TN, Cornell RG, Endres IL, et al: Birth effects among children of nurse anesthetists. Anesthesiology 1974;41:341–344.

28. Corbett TH, Cornell RG, Endres JL, Millard RI: Effects of low concentrations of nitrous oxide on rat pregnancy. Anesthesiology 1973;39:299–301.
29. Corrado OJ, Osman J, Davies RJ: Asthma and rhinitis after exposure to glutaraldehyde in endoscopy units. Hum Toxicol 1986;5:325–327.
30. Cowan RE, Manning AP, Ayliffe GA, et al: Aldehyde disinfectants and health in endoscopy units. Gut 1993;34: 1641–1645.
31. Cozine K, Rosenbaum LM, Rosenbaum SH: Laser induced endotracheal tube fire. Anesthesiology 1981;55:583–585.
32. Davis MJ: Conscious sedation practices in pediatric dentistry: A survey of members of the American Board of Pediatric Dentistry College of Diplomates. Pediatr Dent 1988; 10:328–329.
33. Decker JA, Seitz TA, Shults RA, et al: Occupational exposures to aerosolized pharmaceuticals and control strategies. Scand J Work Env Health 1992;18(suppl 2): 100–102.
34. Diamond SA, Dupuis LL: Contact lens damage due to ribavirin exposure. Drug Intell Clin Pharm 1989;23:428–425. Letter.
35. Dumont D: Risques encourus par les personnels soignants manipulant des cytostatiques. Arch Mal Prof 1989;50: 1209–1253.
36. Echeverria D, Heyer NJ, Martin MD, et al: Behavioral effect of low level exposure to elemental mercury among dentists. Neurotoxicol Teratol 1995;17:161–189.
37. Eggleston PA, Wood RA: Management of allergies to animals. Allergy Proc 1992;13:289–292.
38. Estlander T, Kanerva L, Kari O, et al: Occupational conjunctivitis associated with type IV allergy to methacrylate. Allergy 1996;51:56–59.
39. Freeman GL: Psyllium hypersensitivity. Ann Allergy 1994; 73:490–492.
40. Frigas E, Filley WV, Feed CE: Bronchial challenge with formaldehyde gas: Lack of bronchoconstriction in 13 patients suspected of having formaldehyde induced asthma. Mayo Clin Pro 1984;59:295–299.
41. Gillespie BF, Rathburn FJ: Adverse effects of psyllium. Can Med Assoc J 1994;146:16–17.
42. Gladu JM, Ecobichon DJ: Evaluation of exposure of health care personnel to ribavirin. J Toxicol Environ Health 1989; 28:1–12.
43. Grazer RE, Meislin HW, Westerman BR, et al: Exposure to ionizing radiation in the emergency department from commonly performed portable radiographs. Ann Emerg Med 1987;16:417–420.
44. Greenberg MI, Cone DC, Roberts JR: The material safety data sheet: A useful resource for the emergency physician. Ann Emerg Med 1996;27:347–352.
45. Harrison R, Bellows J, Rempel D, et al: Assessing exposures of health care personnel to aerosols of ribavirin. MMWR 1988;37:560–563.
46. Hopkins J: The carcinogenic potential of ethylene. Food Chem Toxicol 1994;32:191–193.
47. International Agency for Research on Cancer: IARC Monographs on the Evaluation of the Carcinogenic Risk to Humans, Vol. 50. Pharmaceutical Drugs. Lyon, France, IARC, 1990.
48. International Agency for Research on Cancer: IARC Monographs on the Evaluation of the Carcinogenic Risk to Humans, suppl 7. Overall Evaluations of Carcinogenicity: An Updating of IARC Monographs Vols. 1 to 42. Lyon, France, IARC, 1987.
49. International Agency for Research on Cancer: IARC Monographs on the Evaluation of the Carcinogenic Risk to Humans, Vol. 26. Some Antineoplastic and Immunosuppressive Agents. Lyon, France, IARC, 1981.
50. Jackuck SJ, Bound CL, Steel J: Occupational hazard in hospital staff exposed to 2% glutaraldehyde in an endoscopy unit. J Soc Occup Med. 1989;39:69–71.
51. Janardhanan R: Endoscopist's nose. Gastrointest Endoscp 1986;32:247.
52. Kelly KJ, Kurup VP, Reijula KE, Fink JN: The diagnosis of natural rubber latex allergy. J Allergy Clin Immunol 1994;93:813–816.
53. Klein-Schwartz W, Gorman RL, Oderda GM, et al: Three fatal sodium azide poisonings. Med Toxicol Adverse Drug Exp 1989;4:219–227.
54. Kolmodin-Hedman B. Hartvig P. Sorsa M, et al: Occupational handling of cytostatic drugs. Arch Toxicol 1983;54: 25–33.
55. Konz KR, Chia JK, Kurup VP, et al: Comparison of latex hypersensitivity among patients with neurologic defects. J Allergy Clin Immunol 1995;95:950–954.
56. Koppel C, Baudisch H, Schneider V, et al: Suicidal ingestion of formalin with fatal complications. Intensive Care Med 1990;16:212–214.
57. Lemiere C, Charpin D, Vervloet D: Is atopy a risk factor of occupational asthma? Rev Mal Respir 1995;12:231–239.
58. Linn WS, Gong H, Anderson KR, et al: Exposures of health-care workers to ribavirin aerosol: A pharmacokinetics study. Arch Environ Health 1995;50:445–451.
59. Maio JL, Cartier A, L'Archeveque J, et al: Prevalence of occupational asthma and immunologic sensitivity to psyllium among health personnel in chronic care hospitals. Am Rev Resp Dis 1990;142:1359–1366.
60. Marczynski B, Marek W, Baur X: Ethylene oxide as a major factor in DNA and RNA evolution. Med Hypotheses 1995;44:97–100.
61. Matthews J, Newsome SW, Walters NP: Aerobiology of irradiation with carbon dioxide laser. J Hosp Infect 1985;6: 230–233.
62. McGlothlin JD, Jensen PA, Cooper TC, et al: In-Depth Survey Report: Control of Anesthetic Gases in Dental Operatories at University of California at San Francisco Oral Surgical Dental Clinic, San Francisco, CA. Cincinnati, U.S. Department of Health and Human Services, Centers for Disease Control, National Institute for Occupational Safety and Health, report no. ECTB 166B-12b, 1990.
63. Minami M, Katsumata M, Miyake K, et al: Dangerous mixture of household detergents in an old-style toilet: A case report with simulation experiments of the working environment and warning of potential hazard relevant to the general environment. Hum Exp Toxicol 1992;11: 27–34.
64. Montgomery AB, Corkery KJ, Brunette ER, et al: Occupational exposure to aerosolized pentamidine. Chest 1990; 98:386–388.
65. Mrvos R, Dean BS, Krenzelok EP: Home exposures to

chlorine/chloramine gas: Review of 216 cases. South Med J 1993;86:654–657.
66. Newill CA, Eggleston PA, Prenger VL, et al: Prospective study of occupational asthma to laboratory animal allergens: Stability of airway responsiveness to methacholine challenge for one year. J Allergy Clin Immunol 1995; 95:707–715.
67. Nieuwenhuijsen MJ, Gordon S, Harris JM, et al: Variation in rat urinary aeroallergen levels explained by differences in site, task, and exposure group. Ann Occup Hyg 1995; 39:819–825.
68. National Institute for Occupational Safety and Health: Health Hazard Evaluation Report: Hennepin County Medical Center, Minneapolis, MS. Cincinnati, U.S. Department of Health and Human Services, Public Health Service, Centers for Disease Control, HETA 84BO46Bl584, 1985.
69. National Institute for Occupational Safety and Health: Control of Occupational Exposure to N_2O in the Dental Operatory. Cincinnati, U.S. Department of Health, Education, and Welfare, Public Health Service, Centers for Disease Control, DHEW (NIOSH) pub. no. 77Bl7l, 1977.
70. National Institute for Occupational Safety and Health: Criteria for a Recommended Standard: Occupational Exposure to Waste Anesthetic Gas and Vapors. Cincinnati, U.S. Department of Health, Education, and Welfare, Public Health Service, Centers for Disease Control, DHEW (NIOSH) pub. no. 77B-140, 1977.
71. Norback D: Skin and respiratory symptoms from exposure to glutaraldehyde in medical services. Scand J Work Environ Health 1988;14:366–371.
72. Olsen RJ, Lynch P, Coyle MB, et al: Examination gloves as barriers to hand contamination in clinical practice. JAMA 1993;270:350–353.
73. O'Riordan TG, Smaldone GC: Exposure of health care workers to aerosolized pentamidine. Chest 1992;101: 1494–1499.
74. OSHA Instruction. PUB 8-1.1 Guidelines for cytotoxic (antineoplastic) drugs, 1986.
75. OSHA Regulations (Standards 29 CFR) 1910.1048. Occupational Exposure to Formaldehyde, 1992.
76. OSHA Regulations (Standards-29 CFR) 1910.1003-13. Carcinogens, 1997.
77. OSHA Regulations (Standards 29 CFR) 1910.1047. Ethylene oxide, 1997.
78. OSHA Regulations (Standards 29 CFR) 1910.90. Hazard Communication Standard, 1997.
79. Pohl L, Bergman M: The dentists exposure to elemental mercury vapor during clinical work with amalgams. Acta Odontol Scand 1995;53:44–81.
80. Preston RJ, Fennell TR, Leber AP, et al: Reconsideration of the genetic risk assessment for ethylene oxide exposures. Environ Mol Mutagen 1995;26:189–202.
81. Renstrom A, Malmberg P, Larsson K, et al: Prospective study of laboratory animals allergy: Factors predisposing to sensitization and development of allergic symptoms. Allergy 1994;49:548–552.
82. Ritchie KA, MacDonald EB, Hammersley R, et al: A pilot study of the effects of low level exposure to mercury on the health of dental surgeons. Occup Environ Med 1995; 52:813–817.
83. Roberts RJ, Simmons A, Barrett DA. Accidental exposure to sodium azide. Am J Clin Pathol 1974;61:879–880.
84. Romaquera C, Vilaplana J, Grimalt F: Contact sensitization to methacrylate in a limb prosthesis. Contact Dermatitis 1989;21:125.
85. Rowland AS, Baird DD, Weinberg CR, et al: Reduced fertility among women employed as dental assistants exposed to high levels of nitrous oxide. N Engl J Med 1992; 327:993–997.
86. Sass-Kortsak AM, Purdham JT, Bozek PR, et al: Exposure of hospital operating room personnel to potentially harmful environmental agents. Am Ind Hyg Assoc J 1992;53: 203–209.
87. Schmahl D, Kaldor JM: Carcinogenicity of Alkylating Cytostatic Drugs. IARC scientific publications, no. 78. Lyon, France, International Agency for Research on Cancer, 1986.
88. Selevan SG, Lindbohm ML, Hornung RW, et al: A study of occupational exposure to antineoplastic drugs and fetal loss in nurses. N Engl J Med 1985;313:1173–1178.
89. Sexton RJ and Henson EV: Experimental ethylene oxide human skin injuries. Arch Ind Hyg Occup Med 1990;2: 549–564.
90. Shepherd GM: Safe use of latex rubber. Ann Intern Med 1995;23:234–235. Letter.
91. Singer CM, Baraff LJ, Benedict SH, et al: Exposure of emergency medicine personnel to ionizing radiation during cervical spine radiography. Ann Emerg Med 1989; 18:822–825.
92. Skov T: Handling antineoplastic drugs in the European Community countries. Eur J Cancer Prev 1993;2: 43–46.
93. Stucker I, Caillard JF, Collin R, et al: Risk of spontaneous abortion among nurses handling antineoplastic drugs. Scand J Work Environ Health 1991;16:102–107.
94. Suruda AJ, McGlothlin JD: Fatal abuse of nitrous oxide in the workplace. J Occup Med 1990;32:682–684.
95. Tomazic VJ, Withrow TJ, Hamilton RG: Characterization of the allergens in latex protein extracts. J Allergy Clin Immunol 1995;96:635–642.
96. Turjanmaa K: Allergy to natural rubber latex: A growing problem. Ann Med 1994;26:297–300.
97. Valanis B, Vollmer WM, Labuhn K, et al: Antineoplastic drug handling protection after OSHA guidelines. J Occup Environ Med 1992;34:149–155.
98. Vicira E, Cleaton-Jones JP, Austin JC, et al: Effects of low concentrations of nitrous oxide on rat fetuses. Anesth Analg 1980;59:175–177.
99. Vieira E: Effect of the chronic administration of nitrous oxide 0.5% to gravid rats. Br J Anaesthesiol 1979;51: 283–287.
100. Wald N, Ritichie C: Formaldehyde process workers and lung cancer. Lancet 1984;1:1066–1067.
101. Wang JX, lnskip PD, Boice JD, et al: Cancer incidence among medical diagnostic x-ray workers in China, 1950 to 1985. Cancer 1990;45:889–955.
102. Waskin H: Toxicology of antimicrobial aerosols: A review

of aerosolized ribavirin and pentamidine. Respir Care 1992;36:1026–1036.

103. Weiss EL, Singer CM, Benedict SH, et al: Physician exposure to ionizing radiation during trauma resuscitation: A prospective clinical study. Ann Emerg Med 1990;19: 134–138.

104. Wenig BL, Stenson KM, Wenig BM, et al: Effects of plume produced by the ND:YAG laser and electrocautery on the respiratory system. Lasers Surg Med 1993;13: 242–245.

105. Wolf BL: Anaphylactic reaction to latex gloves. N Engl J Med 1993;329:278–280.

106. Yassin MS, Lierl MB, Fischer TJ, et al: Latex allergy in hospital employees. Ann Allergy 1994;72:245–249.

CHAPTER 110

Farmers

By William J. Meggs, Ricky L. Langley, and Paul A. James

A 36-year-old mother of four lived with her family in a house across a rural road from a cotton field when she developed a complex multiorgan system illness with severe headaches, nausea, vomiting, abdominal cramps, and diarrhea. Symptoms developed one September evening after she spent 8 hours working in her garden. This patient was seen by her family physician, who entertained a variety of diagnoses, including viral syndrome, gastroenteritis, inflammatory bowel disease, brain tumor, and subarachnoid hemorrhage. Evaluation included hospitalization with a host of studies, including CT scan of the head, chemistry and hematologic profiles, and upper and lower GI series. All of these studies were normal.

Symptoms continued over the next 4 weeks, with continued headache, blurred vision, inability to read, photophobia, sensitivity to noise, dizziness, nausea, diarrhea, abdominal cramps, and pleuritic chest pain. An erythematous rash developed over her chest, neck, and hands. Symptoms of mental confusion, forgetfulness, inability to recognize friends, and problems with short-term memory developed. Her husband and children also complained of abdominal cramps and diarrhea during this period of time. One month after the onset of illness the patient asked her physician if the frequent spraying of the cotton field across the road from her house could be the cause of her illness. She reported that the day the illness started, a plane billowing spray flew so low over her yard that it passed under the power lines along her front yard. Numerous sprayings followed over the next weeks, and on one occasion the spray residue coated the exterior of her house.

The physician contacted the regional poison center by telephone after learning that the cotton field had received frequent applications of the organophosphate insecticide malathion as part of an experimental program. The regional poison center suggested a diagnosis of mild organophosphate insecticide poisoning and recommended determination of red blood cell cholinesterase levels and treatment with atropine. Pralidoxime was not recommended.

Atropine was given, but did not help her symptoms. Cholinesterase levels were in the normal range for the laboratory. Public health officials were consulted and determined malathion concentrations of 37 parts per million in the soil of her yard and terminated the spray program in late November. Control samples taken from the yards of other residents in the county had negligible malathion levels. Two years after the incident, she continued to have severe headaches, right flank pain for which she is treated by a specialist in chronic pain, mental confusion, difficulty with short-term memory, and irritability.

This case illustrates three of the toxicologic problems associated with agriculture. Rural residents can be exposed to agricultural chemicals from "drift" from the intended area of application, particularly with aerial spraying. Persons exposed to organophosphate pesticides can have a subacute syndrome that is different from the cholinergic poisoning seen with acute high doses poisonings and does not respond to atropine.[16] Individuals with both acute and subacute organophosphate pesticide poisoning can have chronic sequela of their poisoning.

Farmers, rural residents, family members of farmers including children, and visitors are at risk for exposure to many chemicals found on the contemporary farm, including pesticides, fumes, solvents, corrosive agents, fertilizers, venoms, and natural toxic aerosols (Table 110–1). A history of exposure should be taken for any person in or recently from a rural area presenting with unexplained illness, especially if symptoms are nonspecific or involve multiple organ systems. Clinicians in rural areas should be familiar with local agricultural practices. A thorough history and physical examination should be supplemented with questions about chemicals and routes of exposure. Clinicians in rural areas should educate their patients about prevention of future exposures. This chapter discusses poisonings that occur in rural areas.

What Are the Clinical Consequences of Subacute and Chronic Organophosphate Poisoning?

Farm workers, rural residents living by fields, workers in pesticide manufacturing plants, and exterminators may be chronically exposed to organophosphate pesticides. The manifestations associated with chronic exposures differ from those of acute exposures. A study of exposed orchard sprayers found headache to be the most common complaint, followed by nausea, weakness or fatigue, and chest tightness. Symptoms of abdominal pain, vertigo or incoordination, vomiting, perspiration, cough,

TABLE 110–1. TOXINS ENCOUNTERED ON THE FARM

Pesticides
Insecticides
Herbicides
Rodenticides
Fungicides
Acaracides
Fumes
Methane (decaying organic matter, compost)
Carbon dioxide (grain elevators, silos)
Carbon monoxide (combustion)
Butane, propane (bottled gas)
Hydrogen sulfide (septic tanks, liquid manure tanks)
Hydrocarbons
Gasoline
Kerosene
Motor oils
Hydraulic fluid
Plant Toxins Inducing Dermatoses
Crop dermatitis (celery, cucumber, limes)
Tobacco (cutaneous absorption of nicotine)
Poison ivy, oak, and sumac
Flowering plants (pyrethrum)
Envenomation
Inorganic Chemicals
Ammonia
Carbon monoxide
Nitrogen
Nitrous oxide
Phosphorus
Potash
Physical Toxins
Sunlight

vision disturbance, loss of appetite, dyspnea, nasal discharge, miosis, and wheezing were also reported.[58]

What Are the Chronic Sequelae of Organophosphate Poisoning?

Neuropsychiatric deficits and paralysis are reported following organophosphate poisoning.[50] The neuropsychiatric disability, verified in controlled studies,[40,48,56] is found to correlate with measures of the severity of poisoning.[56] Persistent peripheral neuropathy is also described, with decreased finger and toe vibrotactile sensitivity.[56] A study of farm workers who suffered a single acute poisoning found that poisoned workers performed poorly relative to matched controls on all neuropsychological tests, including verbal and visual attention, visual memory, visuomotor speed, sequencing and problem solving, motor steadiness, and dexterity.[48] A literature review reveals a consistent pattern of impaired vigilance and reduced concentration, reduced information processing and psychomotor speed, memory deficit, linguistic disturbances, depression, anxiety, and irritability.[15]

A controlled study of sheep farmers exposed to organophosphate pesticides in sheep dip found significantly worse performance on tests to assess sustained attention and speed of information processing relative to controls, as well as "vulnerability to psychiatric disorder" as determined by a questionnaire. Short-term memory and learning testing was not affected in this study.[57] Peripheral neuropathy was documented in chronically exposed workers in India,[16] and elevated tactile and vibratory thresholds were seen in exposed workers relative to controls.[39]

Paralysis is also reported as a complication of organophosphate poisoning. Delayed bilateral recurrent laryngeal nerve paralysis can occur 25 to 35 days after poisoning with chlorpyrifos, parathion, and methamidophos.[11] Chronic fatigue[9] and an acquired intolerance to chemicals[60] are also reported.

Are Cholinesterase Levels Helpful in These Cases?

Because organophosphates inhibit plasma and red blood cell cholinesterase, functional assays of these enzymes can be used as markers of exposure. Because of population variability, decreases in the enzyme activity from baseline measurements are of greater value than a single determination. Thus, an individual whose baseline enzyme levels are high in the normal range can become poisoned, have a decrease in enzyme level, and still remain in the normal range. Studies of exposed greenhouse workers show decreases in cholinesterase levels during seasons in which pesticides are used.[35] An Israeli study found symptoms associated with chronic exposure to organophosphate pesticides in individuals with normal cholinesterase levels.[47]

In spite of these difficulties, a decrease in cholinesterase activity from baseline in a given individual is thought to correlate with toxicity. In one study a 60% decrease in cholinesterase levels was associated with headache and mild parasympathetic symptoms.[42] A 60 to 90% decrease in levels was associated with muscle weakness, tremor, and neuropsychiatric symptoms that persisted for up to 2 weeks. A 90 to 100% reduction in levels was associated with seizures, cyanosis, pulmonary edema, respiratory failure due to muscle weakness, coma, and death.[42]

Unfortunately, serum cholinesterase levels in acute organophosphate poisoning have no long-term prognostic value. Additionally, no correlation between serum levels and the amount of atropine required or need for mechanical ventilation has been shown.[43] A study of chronically exposed workers found no correlation between symptoms and cholinesterase levels.[37]

What Is the Epidemiology of Poisonings With Agricultural Chemicals?

A study of mortality and morbidity from agricultural chemical poisonings, including horticulture, is summarized in Table 110–2.[32] Over a third of a million expo-

TABLE 110–2. SUMMARY OF EXPOSURES, HOSPITALIZATIONS, AND DEATHS FROM FARM CHEMICALS BY CAUSE, UNITED STATES 1985–1990

	Unintentional (%)	Suicide (%)	Unknown (%)	Total
Exposures	327,599 (96.9)	7848 (2.3)	2723 (0.8)	338,170
Hospitalizations	19,753 (77.7)	4458 (17.5)	1207 (4.7)	25,418
Deaths	97 (28.4)	217 (63.6)	27 (7.9)	341

Adapted, with permission, from Klein-Schwartz W, Smith GS: Agricultural and horitcultural chemical poisonings: Mortality and morbidity in the United States. Ann Emerg Med 1997;29: 232–238.

sures were reported to poison centers from 1985 to 1990, and there were over 25,000 hospitalizations during that period. Suicides represented only 2.3% of the exposures, but accounted for over 17% of the hospitalizations and approximately two thirds of the deaths. Organophosphate pesticides were the leading known cause of hospitalizations and deaths. Paraquat, diquat, chlorophenoxy compounds, chlorinated hydrocarbons, carbamates, strychnine, arsenic, and anticoagulants were also associated with deaths. This study demonstrated the importance of suicides in deaths associated with farm chemicals.

What Pulmonary Diseases in Farmers Are Due to Toxins?

A number of agricultural exposures can cause pulmonary disease. Organophosphate and carbamate insecticides affect respirations via several mechanisms. Bronchospasm and pulmonary edema result from parasympathetic stimulation. Respiratory failure can result from weakness of the muscles of respiration and central depression of the respiratory drive center.[13,51] Anhydrous ammonia is a respiratory irritant that causes pulmonary edema at high doses.[53] It is found on farms as a fertilizer where exposures most commonly occur during transfer operations. It reacts with water to form ammonium hydroxide, a strong alkali. Bronchiolitis obliterans has been reported from exposure, but most victims recover without sequelae. Fumigants such as methyl bromide and carbon disulfide can cause pulmonary edema if inhaled.[53] Certain fungicides containing arsenic may lead to the development of lung cancer.

A dose-related pulmonary fibrosis occurs from the ingestion and dermal absorption, but not inhalation, of paraquat. Type I and II alveolar epithelial cells accumulate paraquat and are destroyed, followed by inflammatory cell infiltration and hemorrhage. Fibroblast proliferation then leads to fibrosis and impaired gas exchange.

Dinitrophenol and its derivatives are used on farms as herbicides. These compounds uncouple oxidative phosphorylation, causing malaise, headache, thirst, hyperthermia, dyspnea, and respiratory failure.[53] These highly toxic compounds are absorbed through the skin and can quickly cause death.

Chlorine-containing cleaning agents can act as upper airway respiratory irritants and may cause pulmonary parenchymal damage, if the exposure is prolonged. Certain veterinary antibiotics can act as sensitizers, and farmers may develop asthmatic reactions to these compounds.

Silo filler's disease is caused by nitrogen dioxide (NO_2) in silos. Nitrates in the plants are oxidized to nitrogen dioxide and nitrogen tetroxide. This process starts shortly after filling the silo and continues for several weeks. The reddish-brown haze of nitrogen oxides in gaseous form can be seen above the silage and has a bleach-like odor. Because nitrogen dioxide is a mild irritant, farmers may be exposed for periods long enough for the gas to penetrate deep within the lungs. Nitrogen dioxide reacts with water in the airways to form nitrous (HNO_2) and nitric (HNO_3) acids, leading to chemical pneumonitis and pulmonary edema.

Symptoms range from a mild tracheobronchitis and cough to pulmonary edema and pneumonitis, with fatality rates reported as high as 30%.[41,45] Severe symptoms may present hours after exposure. Initially, patients may present with cough, shortness of breath, chest pain, nausea, vomiting, and cyanosis. Victims should be admitted to the hospital and treated with oxygen. Corticosteroids may be of benefit in some cases. Methemoglobinemia may occur from conversion of nitrogen dioxide to nitrates (see Chap. 93).

A 2 to 6-week latent phase may be followed by a sudden relapse with dyspnea, cough, fever, and pulmonary edema. These symptoms occur with the development of fibrotic, obliterative lesions of the terminal airways known as bronchiolitis obliterans. Both airway obstruction and reduced diffusion capacity are seen. The chest roentgenogram may show small opacities similar to the pattern seen with miliary tuberculosis or confluent opacities as seen with pulmonary edema. Corticosteroids are beneficial, and victims can recover without long-term pulmonary dysfunction. In a few untreated cases, pulmonary fibrosis has occurred.

What Are the Causes of Occupational Asthma Among Farmers?

Farmers are exposed to animals, plants, and chemicals that can provoke bronchospasm by allergic or other mechanisms. Animal danders, urine, saliva, and fecal proteins can all be antigenic. Contact with horses, cows, sheep, and household pets can result in hypersensitivity reactions. Farmers may develop allergy to the grain storage mite (*Glycyphagus destructor*) as demonstrated by radioallergosorbent testing.[29] Exposure to a wide variety of food antigens can trigger allergic asthma in farmers, but workers who process foods are more susceptible than farmers. Pyrethrin pesticides derived from chrysanthemum plants can also cause allergic asthma.

What Are the Consequences of Exposure to Agricultural Dusts?

Agricultural operations are the third leading cause of particulate air pollution in the United States. Inorganic dust from rock or soil is a mild irritant, but cases of silicosis have been reported in farmers.[14,54] Organic dusts may consist of animal dander, hair, feathers, urine and feces, insects or mites or their bodily components, bacteria, endotoxin, fungal spores or hyphae, mycotoxins, pollen grains, feed grains, hay, silage, and other plant products.

Grain dust is a variable mixture of organic and inorganic particles, depending on the type of grain, growing conditions, and methods of harvest, storage, and processing. Duram wheat and barley dusts are noted irritants. High moisture content and resultant spoilage increase health risks.

Clinical effects of grain dust exposure include nasal stuffiness, rhinorrhea, sore throat, acute bronchitis, asthma, chronic bronchitis, acute febrile syndrome, hypersensitivity pneumonitis, and eye and skin irritation.[13] Febrile reactions may be due to endotoxins.[44,49] Bronchitis may be caused by proteolytic enzymes produced by microbes or the total dust load. Symptoms of bronchitis are greatest in workers exposed to environments where the total dust load is greater than 5 mg/m^3. The allowable threshold limit value (TLV) in the United States is 10 mg/m^3. The proposed TLV for grain dust is 4 mg/m^3. During unloading operations, levels can greatly exceed allowable levels.

Distinctive syndromes associated with organic dust inhalation include hypersensitivity pneumonitis, organic dust toxic syndrome, and occupational asthma,[13,51] as described in Table 110–3. The time course of symptoms; the characteristics of the symptoms; and pulmonary function test results, including carbon monoxide diffusion capacity, arterial blood gas analysis, and chest roentgenogram; are important diagnostic considerations. Bronchial alveolar lavage and pulmonary biopsy are occasionally useful.

Organic dust toxic syndrome is much more common than hypersensitivity pneumonitis.[13] Prevalence estimates suggest that fewer than 8% of exposed individuals will develop hypersensitivity pneumonitis while 30 to 40% of exposed individuals may develop organic dust toxic syndrome. Thus, several individuals exposed to moldy straw or hay may develop organic dust toxic syndrome while only one or two members of an exposed group may develop hypersensitivity pneumonitis.[6,13] Antibodies are frequently measured in patients with hypersensitivity pneumonitis.[18] The demonstration of antibodies to *Saccharopolyspora rectivirgala* and other *Thermoactinomyces* species is evidence of exposure and a host reaction, but has poor predictive value for the risk of development of symptoms. Antibodies are not usually detected in the organic dust toxic syndrome. There appear to be no long-term sequelae associated with the organic dust toxic syndrome; however, restrictive lung disease may develop if a patient with hypersensitivity pneumonitis continues to be exposed. If avoidance of dust exposure is not possible, agricultural workers should use tight-fitting dust masks or respirators. If symptoms persist, it may be necessary to avoid potential agricultural work that would involve exposure to organic dust.

What Are the Respiratory Hazards of Animal Confinement Facilities?

Confinement buildings are facilities where a large number of animals are raised in small enclosed spaces. The buildings are equipped with systems for temperature, humidity, feeding, watering, and ventilation control. Close to one million persons are occupationally exposed to poultry, swine, and cattle confinement facilities in the United States.

Respiratory hazards arise from organic dust and toxic gas exposures.[12] Organic dusts are primarily from dried fecal material and feed grains. Toxic gases arise from urine and fecal degradation, incomplete combustion of fuels, and animal respiration. Over 40 different gases have been identified, but hydrogen sulfide, ammonia, methane, carbon dioxide, and carbon monoxide are those most commonly noted.

Ammonia and hydrogen sulfide can be adsorbed to dust particles that are inhaled. Bacteria and endotoxins can also be inhaled. Workers can develop symptoms within minutes of entering the confinement facility.[13,51] Symptoms of cough, runny nose, scratchy throat, eye irritation, chest tightness, wheezing, and dyspnea may occur and usually subside within 24 to 48 hours of exposure. As in the case with other chronic organic dust exposures, smokers are more likely to be affected.

Fatal exposures from high concentrations of toxic gases are reported. Deaths occur in manure pits from hy-

TABLE 110–3. RESPIRATORY DISORDERS ASSOCIATED WITH FARM TOXINS

Disease	Exposure	Onset	Symptoms	Chest Radiograph
Silo filler's disease (chemical alveolitis)	Silo gas (NO_2)	Immediate to days	Cough, dyspnea	Diffuse edema or miliary pattern
Farmer's lung (hypersensitivity pneumonitis)	Moldy hay, silage, bedding	4–8 hours	Cough, dyspnea, flu like symptoms	Diffuse nodular; patchy consolidation
Mycotoxicosis	Moldy dust	Hours	Flu like symptoms	Usually normal
Grain fever	Grain dust	Immediate to hours	Cough, flu like symptoms	Normal
Occupational asthma	Animal and plant proteins, chemicals	Immediate to hours	Bronchospasm, bronchorrhea, cough	Normal or hyperinflation

poxia due to high methane concentrations. Hydrogen sulfide is a metabolic poison similar to cyanide, and hydrogen sulfide levels in agitated manure may reach 400 to 500 ppm or more. At these levels, unconsciousness, convulsions, and sudden death may occur. The worker entering a closed space containing manure must wear a self-contained breathing apparatus. The individual should wear a life-line and should have an observer outside the tank at all times.

How Common Are Occupational Skin Diseases on the Farm?

Irritant and allergic contact dermatitis can result from a number of agents on the farm, and farming has the highest incidence of occupational skin disease among all occupations. In a survey from California in 1979, the incidence of occupational skin disease was 6.1 cases per 1000 workers per year for farmers versus 1.59 cases per 1000 workers per year for all industries.[38] Plant and animal products accounted for 63% of the cases, with poison oak accounting for 48% of the cases. Other plants (including weeds and flowers), leather, hides, fur, feathers, lumber, and wood products less commonly cause dermatitis. Agricultural chemicals caused 20% of cases; a review cited approximately 75 farm chemicals that are known to cause dermatitis.[2] Fungicides and herbicides are the most common chemical sensitizers, accounting for more than half of cases in the California study.[38] Edible food products can also cause dermatitis, with fruits and nuts causing over half of the cases associated with edible food products.[38] Vegetables are also associated with contact dermatitis, even when grown without the use of pesticides.[1] Careful history and testing may be required to distinguish the cause of dermatitis in an individual case, as both the herbicide on the plant and the plant itself may be etiologic.

Exposures to much higher concentrations of antigen are needed to initiate sensitization than are needed to produce contact dermatitis in sensitized individuals. Dilutions as low as one part per million can produce a positive patch test response in sensitized individuals.[28,40]

Skin infections must be considered in the differential diagnosis of dermatitis in farm workers, and zoonotic skin diseases are common. A number of *Trichophyton* and *Microsporium* species have nonhuman hosts including cattle, dogs, horses, sheep, pigs, and wildlife (deer and moose). These species can cause infections in humans that are generally more severe than those from anthrophilic species, with a severe pustular folliculitis and hair loss on exposed areas of the arms, head, and body in severe cases.[3]

A number of studies indicate that farmers have an increased risk of melanoma and other skin cancers that most likely relates to their increased exposure to ultraviolet radiation from sunlight.[4] Sun exposure is also associated with actinic keratosis, a carcinoma precursor.

Is There Toxicity Associated With Farm Crops?

Green tobacco sickness is an occupational illness of farm workers associated with skin contact to wet, green tobacco. More than 50% of tobacco handlers are affected to some degree. The illness is attributed to dermal absorption of nicotine, and the symptoms correlate with increased urinary levels of nicotine and cotinine.[21,22] Type of clothing worn, hydration status, previous exposures, and smoking history (ie, tolerance) affect the severity of illness. Patients report symptoms of dizziness, headache, nausea, and vomiting, which resolve with adequate hydration and observation. Prevention consists of avoiding dermal contact of any part of the body with green tobacco.[21]

What Hazards Are Associated With Veterinary Pharmaceuticals?

Hundreds of veterinary pharmaceuticals are available to treat illnesses in animals. Veterinarians frequently prescribe human medicines to treat animal diseases as well. Veterinary pharmaceuticals and animal feed additives have been involved in both unintentional and suicidal poisonings. Child-resistant packaging is not universally required for veterinary medications.

Veterinarian products have produced both toxicity and hypersensitivity in humans, and infections have resulted from human exposure to vaccines. Ultrapotent opioids may cause rapid death if injected in humans.[23,25] Antineoplastic agents may result in mutagenic or carcinogenic effects in animal handlers if appropriate precautions are not followed.[59] Waste anesthetic gases and ethylene oxide are associated with adverse health effects in physicians and may cause similar problems in veterinarians and their assistants (see Chap. 109).[46]

Animal feed additives often contain toxic metals and antibiotics that are growth promoters for animals. Unintentional poisonings from ingestion of these products has been reported. Veterinary pharmaceuticals and animal feed additives can cause systemic or dermatologic reactions in people handling these products (Tables 110–4 and 110–5).[17,61] Skin reactions can be either allergic or irritant reactions.[19]

Carbamates, organophosphates, and pyrethrum pesticides are frequently applied to animals as well as the facility housing the animal. Both systemic and dermatologic effects can occur.[24,36] Biologic agents that are used to immunize animals against infectious diseases have lead to infections of humans from unintentional needle sticks.[5,20,34] Veterinarians must comply with OSHA regulations and educate their employees of the risks associated with hazardous agents.[7,52] Pharmaceuticals with abuse potential should be stored in locked cabinets, and needles must be disposed of in a proper manner. Children must be protected from exposure to pharmaceutical products.

TABLE 110–4. VETERINARY PRODUCTS AND ANIMAL FEED ADDITIVES REPORTED TO CAUSE SYSTEMIC POISONINGS OR ADVERSE EFFECTS IN HUMANS

Acerpromazine	Flunixin meglumine
Amitraz	Levamisole
Azaperone	Methimazole
Bayo-*N*-Ox-1	Organochlorine pesticides
Berenil	Organophosphate pesticides
Brucella abortus strain 19	Penicillin
Carbamate pesticides	Phenylbutazone
Carisoprodol	Sodium monesin
Chloramphenicol	Sodium pentobarbital
Clenbuterol	Spiramycin
Closantel	T-61
Detomidine hydrochloride	Tilmicosin
Etamphylline	Xylazine

Are Chemical Injuries to the Eyes a Problem for Farmers?

There are many agents on the farm that can be dangerous to the eyes. The most serious injuries are associated with anhydrous ammonia, which can cause a severe eye injury and blindness.[27] Injury occurs rapidly due to the high solubility of ammonia, and is typical of alkaline injury. Rapid irrigation with liters of normal saline may be necessary in patients with alkaline injuries, and irrigation should begin emergently (see Chap. 26). Pesticides are usually dissolved in organic solvents, which may cause chemical burns to the eye. Inert ingredients not listed on pesticide labels may also be hazardous to the eye. Prevention consists of always wearing protective goggles when working with anhydrous ammonia, pesticides, and other liquid chemicals.

TABLE 110–5. VETERINARY PHARMACEUTICALS AND ANIMAL FEED ADDITIVES CAUSING DERMATITIS IN HUMANS

Bacitracin	Merthiolate
Benzocaine	Methylisothiazoline
Bronopol	Neomycin
Carbamates	Nitrofurazone
Chlorpromazine	Olaquindox
Chlortetracycline	Oxytetracycline
Chromate	Penethamate
Dinitolmide	Phenothiazines
3,5 Dinitro-o-toluamide	Piperazine
Ethoxyquin	Procaine
Ethylenediamine	Quindoxin
Ethylenediaminedihydroiodine	Quinoxaline
Formalin	Spiramycin
Furazolidone	Sulfacetamide
Halquinol	Sulfamethazine
Hydroquinone	Thiobendazole
Latex	Tylosin
Levamisole	Virginiamycin
Mercaptobenzothiazole	

How Can Farm Poisonings Be Prevented?

The farm presents unique challenges for prevention of poisonings (Table 110–6). Education is the most important component of a prevention program.[53] Education must focus on populations at risk, including small children and their families. Topics to be emphasized in safety education include the use of protective clothing, using appropriate equipment for applying pesticides, strict adherence to pesticide labels, knowledge of reentry times after spraying, and first aid for exposures to agricultural chemicals. Understanding the indications for using a pesticide and utilizing only those needed is an important component of safety that begins before a product is purchased. Pesticide labels are important legal documents, and farmers should be educated to read them carefully several times before use.

Protective clothing should be used by those working with chemicals, but expense and the discomfort of bulky clothing on hot summer days limit its use.[8] Understanding risks can increase compliance with recommendations for protective clothing. Research into affordable, comfortable protective clothing is ongoing. Farmers must know that contaminated protective clothing can be a source of pesticide poisoning, even after repeated laundering.[8]

During mixing and loading of pesticides, concentrated solutions are handled and the risk for pesticide poisoning is highest. Improved equipment design keeping poisonous chemicals within closed systems can decrease exposure. Minimizing the use of toxic chemicals is a strategy that can reduce poisoning while limiting adverse environmental effects. Integrated pest management, an agricultural program that emphasizes surveillance rather than routine applications of pesticides, has great potential to reduce the use of toxic chemicals in agriculture. Bioengineered strains of plants may require fewer pesticides and indirectly reduce toxic hazards in the future. An improved rural health care system is needed with access to primary care physicians who are aware of farm toxicology.

Educating farmers and their families about first aid may be life saving in emergency situations, because farms are often distant from medical facilities. Farm workers must know decontamination techniques. Res-

TABLE 110–6. PREVENTING FARM POISONINGS

- Safety programs for farmers
- Proper protective clothing when using toxic chemicals
- Closed system product and equipment designs
- Strict adherence to pesticide labels
- Reduced use of toxins by improved agricultural biotechnology and integrated pest management
- Improved rural health access to primary care physicians trained in agricultural medicine
- Emphasis on child safety

cuers must recognize that the clothing, bronchial secretions, skin, blood, and urine of victims of organophosphate poisoning can poison others secondarily, and rescuers must therefore protect themselves.

What Groups Are at Risk for Farm Poisonings?

Populations at risks for agricultural chemical poisonings may be divided into occupational and nonoccupational groups. Poisonings occur in workers at increased risk of exposure. These include handlers of pesticides: mixers, loaders, and applicators. Flaggers for aerial sprayers, and harvesters of recently sprayed produce are at increased risk. Migrant workers may camp near recently sprayed fields and have language barriers that further increase risk.

Another population that is at high risk for farm poisonings is children, especially those under 10 years old.[55] Because they are smaller, a given amount of toxin will have a greater effect. Children are curious by nature, willing to explore exciting tastes and smells on the farm. They wear minimal clothing in the summer, affording no protection from skin absorption. The skin of children is more absorbent, with a larger surface area per unit weight. The tendency of small children to place things in their mouths increases the risk of ingestion. The case of a 1-year old who was severely poisoned after hugging his father who was wearing clothing contaminated with parathion illustrates the particular vulnerability of farm children.[55] Carbon monoxide poisoning of children riding in the back of pick-up trucks is also well documented.[26] Farm families generally drink well water, and contamination of ground water with nitrates from fertilizers has led to methemoglobinemia (see Chap. 93). Infants are especially vulnerable, and fatalities have been reported in this age group.[31,33]

What Are the Unique Problems With Transportation for Victims of Agricultural Chemical Poisonings?

Agricultural chemical exposures often occur in isolated areas distant from medical resources. First-aid and decontamination supplies may not be readily available. Transportation is often by farm vehicles, and decontamination is readily forgotten, even by knowledgeable personnel. Transportation without decontamination at the scene prolongs exposure and places healthcare personnel at risk for illness. This may have dire consequences for helicopter transport.[30] Agricultural chemical exposures are sometimes complicated by major trauma, which further diverts attention from necessary decontamination. The chemicals at the scene should always be identified and communicated to the receiving hospital. Table 110–7 outlines the important considerations for transporting poisoned farm workers.

TABLE 110–7. IMPORTANT CONSIDERATIONS FOR TRANSPORTATION OF POISONED FARM VICTIMS

- Avoid contamination and poisoning of rescuers.
- Maintain ABCs.
- Initiate decontamination.
  - Remove victim from source of exposure.
  - Remove and properly dispose of any contaminated clothing.
  - Irrigate and wash with soap and water profusely.
- Identify source of chemical exposure, collect label if available.
- Optimize transportation, using helicopter transport with scene runs if possible.
- Healthcare personnel should wear protective clothing.
- Means of transportation should reflect severity of injury to patient and health risk to transport team.

What Informational Resources Are Available to the Farmer?

Healthcare providers are usually unaware of the resources available to farmers. Pesticide and agricultural chemical education is performed in each state by the Cooperative Extension System, which serves as a resource for farmers and farm families. Restricted-use pesticides require a licensed applicator who has undergone training for restricted-use pesticides. However, a farmer who undergoes certification may purchase a restricted-use pesticide, but have a farm laborer apply the chemical under his supervision. These untrained workers may be poorly supervised.

County agricultural extension agents are a useful resource, and these agents often make recommendations to farmers regarding options for pest control. The 4H Clubs provide education in health and safety to farm children. Chemical companies are another resource, especially if the chemical product is known. Chemtrac is a toll free number (800-424-9300) available to farmers to assist with questions of potential or actual toxicity and risk.

Rural healthcare providers are another resource. These practitioners often may have backgrounds in agriculture and should have more experience than their urban colleagues in addressing agricultural chemical health problems. Primary physicians for farmers and farm laborers can play a vital role in educating farmers about prevention. Unfortunately, this practice is not often emphasized in medical education.

Regional poison centers are excellent resources for assistance with toxicities. These centers are most effectively utilized if the chemical agent is known. Algorithms for patient treatment are succinct and up to date. Emergency medical technicians are another resource for farmers. First providers should be trained to minimize poisoning by initiating early decontamination while protecting themselves from exposure.

References

1. Aberer W: Occupational dermatitis from organically grown parsnip (*Pastinaca sativa*). Contact Dermatitis 1992;26:62.

2. Abrams K, Hogan DJ, Maibach HI: Pesticide-related dermatoses in agricultural workers. Occup Med 1991;6: 463–492.
3. Armstrong KR, Post K: The role of farm animals in the control of zoonotic skin diseases in man. In: Dosman JA, Crockfort DW, eds: Principles of Health and Safety in Agriculture. Boca Raton, CRC Press, 1989, pp. 288–291.
4. Blair A, Zahm SH: Cancer among farmers. Occup Med 1991;6:335–354.
5. Blasco JM, Diaz R: Brucella melitensis Rev–1 vaccine as a cause of human brucellosis. Lancet 1993;342:805.
6. Brinton WT, Vastbinder EE, Greene JW, et al: An outbreak of organic dust toxic syndrome in a college fraternity. JAMA 1987;258:1210–1212.
7. Brody MD, Shroff AA: AVMA guide to hazard communication. J Am Vet Med Assoc 1990;196:1–11.
8. Clifford NJ, Nies AS: Organophosphate poisoning from wearing a laundered uniform previously contaminated with parathion. JAMA 1989;262:3135–3136.
9. Corrigan PM, MacDonald S, Brown A, et al: Neurasthenic fatigue, chemical sensitivity and $GABA_A$ receptor toxins. Med Hypotheses 1994;43:195–200.
10. Council on Scientific Affairs, American Medical Association: Biotechnology and the American agricultural industry. JAMA 1991;265:1429–1436.
11. De Silva HJ, Sanmuganathan PS, Senanyake N: Isolated bilateral recurrent laryngeal nerve paralysis: A delayed complication of organophosphorus poisoning. Hum Exp Toxicol 1994;13:171–173.
12. Donham KJ: Hazardous agents in agricultural dusts and methods of evaluation. Am J Indust Med 1986;10: 205–220.
13. Do Pico GA: Hazardous exposure and lung disease among farm workers. Clin Chest Med 1992;13:311–328.
14. Dynnik VI, Khizhniakova LN, Baranenko AA, et al: Silicosis in tractor drivers working on sandy soils on tree farms. Gig Truda 1981;12:26–28.
15. Ecobichon DJ, Joy RM: Pesticides and Neurological Disease, 2nd ed. Boca Raton, CRC Press, 1994.
16. Ernest K, Thomas M, Paulose M, et al: Delayed effect of exposure to organophosphates. Indian J Med Res 1995;101: 81–84.
17. Falk ES, Hektoen H, Thune PO: Skin and respiratory tract symptoms in veterinary surgeons. Contact Dermatitis 1985; 12:274–278.
18. Fink JN: Hypersensitivity pneumonitis. Clin Chest Med 1992;13: 303–309.
19. Fisher A: Contact Dermatitis, 3rd ed. Philadelphia, Lea & Febiger, 1986, pp. 522–523.
20. Geller RJ: Human effects of veterinary biological products. Vet Hum Toxicol 1990;32:479–480.
21. Ghosh SK, Gokani VN, Parikh JR, et al: Protection against "green symptoms" from tobacco in Indian harvesters: A preliminary intervention study. Arch Environ Health 1987; 42:121–124.
22. Ghosh SK, Saiyed HN, Gokani VN, Thakker MU: Occupational health problems among workers handling Virginia tobacco. Int Arch Occup Environ Health 1986;58:47–52.
23. Goodrich PGE: Accidental self-injection. Vet Rec 1977: 458–459.
24. Hafer A, Langley R, Morrow WE, Tulis J: Occupational hazards reported by swine veterinarians in the United States. Swine Health Production 1996;4:128–141.
25. Haigh JC: Hazardous drugs in zoo and wildlife medicine: An update, 1989. Drugs. AAZV Annual Proceedings, Greensboro, NC, 1989, pp. 69–71.
26. Hampson NB, Norkool DM: Carbon monoxide poisoning in children riding in the back of pickup trucks. JAMA 1992; 267:538–540.
27. Helmers S, Top FH, Knapp LW: Ammonia injuries in agriculture. J Iowa Med Soc 1971;36:271–280.
28. Hogan DJ, Lane PR: Allergic contact dermatitis to a herbicide (barban). Can Med Assoc J 1986;132:285–300.
29. Iverson M, Dahl R: Allergy to storage mites in asthmatic patients and its relation to damp housing conditions. Allergy 1990;45:81–85.
30. James PA, St Clair MB: Agrichemicals complicating emergency helicopter transport of a farm worker. J Agromed 1994;1:21–27.
31. Johnson CJ, Bonrud PA, Dosch TL, et al: Fatal outcome of methemoglobinemia in an infant. JAMA 1987;257:2796–2797.
32. Klein-Schwartz W, Smith GS: Agricúltural and horitcultural chemical poisonings: Mortality and morbidity in the United States. Ann Emerg Med 1997;29:232–238.
33. Kross BC, Ayebo AD, Fuorrtes LJ: Methemoglobinemia: Nitrate toxicity in rural American. Am Fam Physician 1992;46: 183–188.
34. Kurt TL, Bost R, Gilliland M, et al: Accidental Kwell (lindane) ingestions. Vet Hum Toxicol 1986;28:552–553.
35. Lander F, Hinke K: Indoor application of anti-cholinesterase agents and the influence of personal protection on uptake. Arch Environ Contamin Toxicol 1992;22: 163–166.
36. Langley R, Pryor W, O'Brien K: Health hazards among veterinarians: A survey and review of the literature. J Agromed 1995; 2:23–52.
37. Matchaba-Hove RB, Siziya S: Organophosphate exposure in pesticide formulation and packaging factories in Harare, Zimbawe. Central Afr J Med 1995;41:40–44.
38. Mathias CGT: Epidemiology of occupational skin disease in agriculture. In: Dosman JA, Crockfort DW, eds: Principles of Health and Safety in Agriculture. Boca Raton, CRC Press, 1989, pp. 285–287.
39. McConnell R, Keifer M, Rosenstock L: Elevated quantitative vibrotactile threshold among workers previously poisoned with methamidophos and other organophosphate pesticides. Am J Indust Med 1994;25:325–334.
40. Milby TH, Epstein WL: Allergic contact sensitivity to malathion. Arch Environ Health 1964;9:434–437.
41. Morgan WK, Seaton A: Occupational Lung Diseases, 2nd ed. Philadelphia, Saunders, 1984.
42. Namba T: Cholinesterase inhibition by organophosphate compounds and its clinical effects. Bull Organisation Mondiale de la Sante 1971;44:289–307.
43. Nouira S, Abroug F, Elatrous S, et al: Prognostic value of serum cholinesterase in acute organophosphate poisoning. Chest 1994:106:1811–1814.
44. Olenchock SA, May JJ, Pratt DS, et al: Endotoxins in the Agricultural Environment. Am J Indust Med 1986;10: 325–327.

45. Parkes WR: Occupational Lung Disorders, 2nd ed. London, Butterworth, 1982, pp. 619–621.
46. Quick TA: Veterinarians should measure ethylene oxide sterilizing practices against health risks. J Am Vet Med Assoc 1990; 196:1021–1023.
47. Richter ED, Chuwers P, Levy Y, et al: Health effects from exposure to organophosphate pesticides in workers and residents in Israel. Isr J Med Sci 1992;28:584–598.
48. Rosenstock L, Keifer M, Daniell W, et al: Chronic central nervous system effects of acute organophosphate pesticide intoxication. Lancet 1991;338:223–227.
49. Rylander R, Bake B, Fischer J, et al: Pulmonary function and symptoms after inhalation of endotoxin. Am Rev Respir Dis 1989;140:981–986.
50. Savage E, Keefe T, Mounce L, et al: Chronic neurological sequela of acute organophosphate pesticide poisoning. Arch Environ Health 1988;43:38–45.
51. Schenker M, Ferguson T, Gamsky T: Respiratory risks associated with agriculture. Occup Med 1991;6:415–428.
52. Seibert PJ Jr: Hazards in the hospital. J Am Vet Med Assoc 1994; 204:352–359.
53. Shaver CS, Tong T: Chemical hazards to agricultural workers. Occup Med 1991;6:391–413.
54. Sherwin RP, Barman ML, Abraham JL: Silicate pneumoconiosis of farm workers. Lab Invest 1979; 40:576–582.
55. Shuman SH, Caldwell ST, Whitlock NH, Brittain, JA: Etiology of hospitalized pesticide poisonings in South Carolina, 1979–1982. J SC Med Assoc 1986;36:73–77.
56. Steenland K, Jenkins B, Ames RG, et al: Chronic neurological sequela to organophosphate pesticide poisoning. Am J Pub Health 1994;84:731–736.
57. Stephens R, Spurgeon A, Calvert IA, et al: Neuropsychological effects of long-term exposure to organophosphates in sheep dip. Lancet 1995;345:1135–1139.
58. Sumerford WT, Hayes WJ Jr, Johnson JM, et al: Cholinesterase response and symptomatology from exposure to organic phosphorus insectides. Arch Indust Hyg Occup Med 1953;7:383–398.
59. Swanson LV: Potential hazards associated with low-dose exposure to antineoplastic agents, part I. Evidence for concern. Compendium Small Animal 1988; 10:293–298.
60. Tabershaw IR, Cooper WC: Sequelae of acute organic phosphate poisoning. J Occup Med 1966:8:5–19.
61. Woodward KN: Hypersensitivity in humans and exposure to veterinary drugs. Vet Hum Toxicol 1991; 33:168–171.

Artists

Michael McCann

A 74-year-old woman was sent to the Emergency Department (ED) by the staff of her nursing home. The patient had a history of Alzheimer's disease and congestive heart failure and was maintained on a diuretic, digoxin, and haloperidol as needed. As part of her nursing home routine she attended regularly scheduled arts and crafts classes. On the day of admission, while in the pottery class, she was noted to take several large sips from a bottle of glaze. After witnessing this, the nursing home staff called their regional poison center and were told to refer her to the hospital because the glaze contained 40% lead.

On arrival to the ED the patient was awake and alert and offered no complaints. Her vital signs were: blood pressure, 140/90 mm Hg; pulse, 88 beats/min; respiratory rates, 12 breaths/ min; rectal temperature, 98.8°F (37.1°C). The physical examination was within normal limits except for the neurologic assessment, which revealed disorientation to time, poor recall and concentration, and a fine resting tremor. All of these were chronic, according to the nursing home.

An intravenous catheter was inserted and blood samples were obtained for CBC, electrolytes and glucose, erythrocyte protoporphyrin, and whole blood lead concentration. Urinanalysis and ECG were unremarkable, and an abdominal radiograph was obtained (Fig. 111–1).

The CBC showed a hemoglobin of 13 g/dL with normal indices, a WBC of 9000/mm^3, and a platelet count of 145,000/mm^3. Electrolytes and glucose were within normal limits.

Because of the radiographic findings, whole-bowel irrigation with PEG-ELS was administered at 2 L/h via a nasogastric tube. Serial radiographs revealed clearing of the radiopaque material over 8 hours. She remained asymptomatic throughout this period.

The next day her lead level was reported as 46 μg/dL, with an EP of 18 μg/dL. A repeat whole blood lead level, obtained as an outpatient 1 week later, was 30 μg/dL. No therapy was administered.

How Common a Problem Is the Ingestion of Ceramic Glazes?

Ingestion of ceramic glazes is the most frequent type of acute poisoning call received by the Center for Safety in the Arts (CSA) from poison control centers. These ingestions usually involve either children younger than 5 years old or the elderly. More than 10 cases of lead poisoning were reported in nursing home residents who were given lead-containing, liquid ceramic glazes in small medication cups.[34,46] The American Association of Poison Control Centers receives approximately 300 reports annually of ceramic glaze ingestion.[28–32] One resultant case of lead encephalopathy proved fatal.[26]

The major concern in all cases of ceramic glaze ingestions is whether or not the glaze contains lead. Other toxic metals might be found in small amounts (usually less than 5% by weight), but leaded glazes might contain up to 40% lead by weight. Although there are many lead-free glazes available, lead-containing glazes are still found in elementary schools, homes, nursing homes, and hospitals.

Unintentional or deliberate ingestion of art materials can also result in serious illness or even death. This happens most commonly with young children, especially by the ingestion and subsequent aspiration of hydrocarbon solvents such as turpentine or mineral spirits stored in food or drink containers. The failure to lock up art materials has resulted in many preventable toxic childhood exposures.

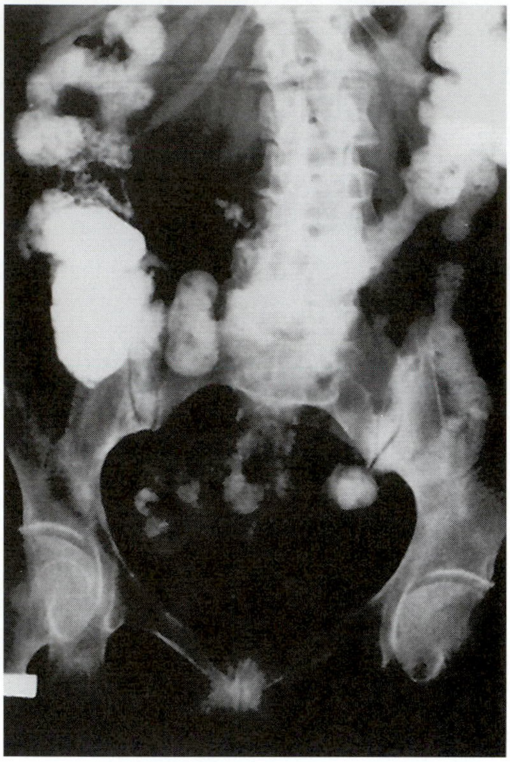

Figure 111–1. An abdominal radiograph of the patient showing the presence of the ceramic glaze containing 40% lead.

Many other arts and crafts materials contain chemicals that pose acute and/or chronic hazards from overexposure.[33] Table 111–1 lists toxic chemicals commonly found in art materials.

Acute Exposures

Acute harmful exposure to toxic chemicals in art materials can occur in several ways. Exposure to toxic chemicals from normal use of art materials without adequate precautions can result in acute illness. Use of solvents frequently results in acute poisoning from inhalation. The inhalation of methylene chloride paint stripper vapors or spray mist from a xylene-containing paint[36,44] may be fatal. Myocardial infarction may result from toluene used in silk screen printing.[47] Other examples of inhalation toxicity include metal fume fever from inhalation of fresh zinc or copper fumes from welding or foundry operations, chemical pneumonia from cadmium-containing silver solders used in jewelry making, and hydrofluoric acid burns from glass etching.

Unintentional exposures involving the mixing of two incompatible chemicals or the decomposition of chemicals can also result in acute health problems. An example is hydrogen cyanide poisoning during jewelry making from inadvertent spills of acid into gold or silver cyanide-containing electroplating baths or cyanide cleaning solutions.[27] Another example of toxicity from a chemical reaction is the decomposition of the photographic chemical, potassium ferricyanide, to hydrogen cyanide after unintentional exposure to heat, ultraviolet radiation, or acid.[19]

"Glue sniffing," the deliberate inhalation of a large concentration of solvent vapors to become intoxicated, can result in sudden death or other serious acute and chronic medical problems. This practice is especially common in adolescents and young adults. Examples include fatalities from inhalation of typewriter correction fluids containing 1,1,1-trichloroethane and/or trichloroethylene,[21] severe polyneuropathy from hexane-containing rubber cements and contact cements,[13,14,24] and fatalities or encephalopathy from toluene-containing products.[13,22] Deliberate inhalation of toluene has also caused central nervous system birth defects.[17] Many art materials contain these or similar solvents (Table 111–1).

How Can the Risks of an Acute Exposure Be Evaluated?

Factors to include in evaluating the risk to an individual who has had acute exposure to art materials are (1) the toxicity of the material, (2) the route of entry (especially the possibility of skin absorption by many solvents), (3) the dose, and (4) any pre-existing medical condition that might increase risk.

Toxicity

In theory, the label on a container should indicate whether the material is hazardous by ingestion or any other route of entry. The warnings on art materials and other consumer products are under the jurisdiction of the Consumer Products Safety Commission, which administers the Federal Hazardous Substances Act (FHSA). Until 1988, the FHSA required only acute hazard labeling on art materials.[11] The FHSA regulations currently require that the label of a hazardous consumer product contain the following: the name and place of business of the manufacturer, packer, distributor or seller; the common, usual, or chemical names of components contributing substantially to the hazard; a signal word (DANGER for products that are extremely flammable, corrosive or highly toxic, and WARNING or CAUTION for other hazardous substances); a statement of the principle hazard(s); the word POISON for highly toxic substances; precautionary measures to be taken; first-aid instructions; instructions for handling and storage, if needed; and the statement "Keep out of the reach of children," or adequate instructions to protect children if the product is intended for use by children.[11]

An art material is not considered toxic under FHSA regulations if its oral LD_{50} is greater than 5 g/kg of body weight, if its inhaled LD_{50} is greater than 20,000 ppm of air (or greater than 200 mg/L), or if its skin LD_{50} is greater than 2 g/kg, unless human experience indicates

TABLE 111–1. HAZARDS OF ART TECHNIQUES

Technique	Material/Process	Hazard
Airbrush	Pigments	Lead, cadmium, manganese, cobalt, mercury, and other metals
	Solvents	Mineral spirits, turpentine
Batik	Wax	Fire, wax, fumes
	Dyes	Dyes
Ceramics	Clay dust	Silica
	Glazes	Silica, lead, cadmium, and other toxic metals
	Slip casting	Talc, asbestiform materials
	Kiln firing	Sulfur dioxide, carbon monoxide, fluorides, infrared radiation
Commercial art	Rubber cement	*n*-Hexane, *n*-heptane, fire
	Permanent markers	Xylene, propyl alcohol
	Spray adhesives	*n*-Hexane, 1,1,1-trichloroethane, fire
	Airbrushing	See Airbrush
	Typography	See Photography
	Photostats, proofs	Alkali, propyl alcohol
Computer art	Ergonomics	Carpel tunnel syndrome, poorly designed work stations
	Video display	Glare, extremely low frequency radiation
Drawing	Spray fixatives	*n*-Hexane, other solvents
Electroplating	Gold, silver, other metals	Cyanide salts, hydrogen cyanide, acids
Enameling	Enamels	Lead, cadmium, arsenic, cobalt, and other metals
	Kiln firing	Infrared radiation
Forging	Hammering	Noise
	Hot forge	Carbon monoxide
Glassblowing	Batch process	Lead, silica, arsenic
	Furnaces	Heat, infrared radiation
	Coloring	Metal fumes
	Etching	Hydrofluoric acid, fluoride salts
	Sandblasting	Silica
Holography	Lasers	Nonionizing radiation, electrical
	Developing	Bromine, pyrogallol; see also Photography
Intaglio	Acid etching	Hydrochloric and nitric acids, nitrogen dioxide, chlorine gas
	Solvents	Alcohol, mineral spirits, kerosene
	Aquatint	Rosin dust, dust explosion
	Photoetching	Glycol ethers, xylene
Jewelry	Silver soldering	Cadmium fumes, fluoride fluxes
	Pickling baths	Acids, sulfur oxides
Lithography	Solvents	Mineral spirits, isophorone, cyclohexanone, kerosene, methylene chloride, and other solvents
	Acids	Nitric, phosphoric, hydrofluoric, hydrochloric, and others
	Talc	Asbestiform materials
	Photolithography	Dichromates
Lost wax casting	Investment	Cristobalite
	Wax burnout	Wax fumes, carbon monoxide
	Crucible furnace	Carbon monoxide, metal fumes
	Metal pouring	Metal fumes, infrared radiation, molten metal
	Sandblasting	Silica
Painting	Pigments	Lead, cadmium, mercury, cobalt, manganese compounds
	Oil, alkyd	Mineral spirits, turpentine
	Acrylic	Trace amounts of ammonia, formaldehyde
Pastels	Pigment dusts	Lead, cadmium, and mercury compounds
Photography	Developing bath	Hydroquinone, monomethyl-p-aminophenol sulfate, alkalis
	Stop bath	Acetic acid
	Fixing bath	Sulfur dioxide
	Intensifier	Dichromates, hydrochloric acid
	Toning	Selenium compounds, hydrogen sulfide, uranium nitrate, sulfur dioxide, gold salts
	Color processes	Formaldehyde, solvents, color developers
	Platinum printing	Platinum salts, lead, acids, oxalates
Relief printing	Solvents	Mineral spirits
Sculpture, clay	See Ceramics	See Ceramics

(*continued*)

TABLE 111–1. HAZARDS OF ART TECHNIQUES (continued)

Technique	Material/Process	Hazard
Sculpture, lasers	Lasers	Nonionizing radiation, electrical hazards
Sculpture, neon	Neon tubes	Mercury, electrical hazards
Sculpture, plastics	Epoxy resin	Amines, diglycidyl ethers
	Polyester resin	Styrene, methyl methacrylate, methyl ethyl ketone peroxide
	Polyurethane resins	Isocyanates, organotin compounds, amines, mineral spirits
	Acrylic resins	Methyl methacrylate, benzoyl peroxide
	Plastic fabrication	Decomposition products (carbon monoxide, hydrogen chloride, hydrogen cyanide)
Sculpture, stone	Marble	Nuisance dust
	Soapstone	Silica, talc, asbestiform materials
	Granite, sandstone	Silica
	Pneumatic tools	Vibration, noise
Silk screen printing	Pigments	Lead, cadmium, manganese, and other compounds
	Solvents	Mineral spirits, toluene, xylene
	Photoemulsions	Ammonium dichromate
Stained glass	Lead	Lead
	Soldering	Lead, zinc chloride fumes
Weaving	Loom	Ergonomic problems
	Dyeing	Dyes, acids, dichromates
Welding	Oxyacetylene	Carbon monoxide
	Arc	Ozone, nitrogen dioxide, ultraviolet and infrared radiation, electrical hazards
	Metal fumes	Copper, zinc, lead, nickel
Woodworking	Machining	Wood dust, noise, fire
	Glues	Formaldehyde, epoxy
	Paint strippers	Methylene chloride, toluene, methyl alcohol, and other solvents
	Paints and finishes	Mineral spirits, toluene, turpentine, ethyl alcohol
	Preservatives	Chromated copper, arsenate, pentachlorophenol, cresote

Reprinted, with permission, from McCann M: Artist Beware, 2nd ed. New York, Lyons & Buford, 1992.

otherwise.[11] If these conditions are not exceeded, the art material does not need a warning label unless it is chronically hazardous. There are many instances of children's art materials that contain acutely or chronically hazardous chemicals despite being labeled "nontoxic." Moreover, many of the hazard and precautionary statements on the labels are not sufficiently informative.[37]

Currently there is one industry program that has been somewhat successful in dealing with the issue of the toxicity of children's art materials. Since the 1940s, the Arts and Crafts Materials Institute (ACMI), formerly known as the Crayon, Watercolor and Craft Institute, has sponsored a certification program for children's art materials. Participating manufacturers whose products pass a review by a consulting toxicologist can place the AP (approved product) or CP (certified product) ACMI seal on the products. This program has successfully reduced the availability of toxic children's art materials.

Unfortunately, the manufacturers of children's art materials that have been involved in this program are mostly large manufacturers; conversely, most smaller manufacturers do not participate. Because of a greater concern on the hazards of art materials in the past several years, the program has been expanded. A persistent problem affecting the success of the program is the ACMI approval of art materials, such as certain oil paints, which themselves are nontoxic but require the use of toxic solvents for cleanup. If such a potentially toxic cleanup is required, these paints are not suitable for children.

Route of Exposure

In children the most common mechanism of acutely toxic exposure to art material is ingestion resulting from either deliberate ingestion of the materials or from placing contaminated hands, paint brushes, or other materials in the mouth. Ingestion of petroleum distillates such as mineral spirits, paint thinner, turpenoid, toluene, xylene, benzene, and rubber cement thinner as well as turpentine may result in chemical pneumonia if the solvent is aspirated into the lungs. The risk of aspiration increases when spontaneous or induced vomiting occurs after ingestion. Deliberate ingestion is not uncommon in the elderly or psychiatrically impaired.

In contrast to the situation with children, inhalation of art materials is the most common type of acute exposure in adults. The materials that can be inhaled include solvent and other liquid vapors, spray mists from airbrushing and aerosol spray cans, gases from the decomposition or chemical reactions of art materials, metal fumes and other fumes from vaporization of metals and other solids, and powders.

Splashing of irritating, caustic, and sensitizing chemicals can result in acute skin and eye problems. Solvents, acids, alkalis, formaldehyde, tropical woods, epoxy resins and glues, chromates and dichromates, nickel compounds, and photographic developers are among the most common offending agents.[33] Methyl ethyl ketone peroxide, a hardener used in making polyester resin sculpture, can cause blindness.[30] Some solvents found in art materials (eg, methyl alcohol, turpentine, toluene, xylene, chlorinated hydrocarbons, and glycol ethers) are easily absorbed through the skin. This route of entry should be considered in dealing with acute solvent exposure.

Dose

As is typically the case with other types of toxic exposures, the major concern with acute poisonings by art materials is how much was actually absorbed. This is especially problematic when young children put paint, ceramic glazes, or other liquids in their mouth. Often it is not known how much was actually swallowed, and assumptions must be made.

When dealing with exposure to heavy metals, another complicating factor is how much of the metal is bioavailable and actually absorbed into the bloodstream. This varies, depending on the metal and manufacturing process. Although most metallic pigments, such as cadmium sulfide pigments, are only slightly soluble in stomach acid and thus unlikely to cause acute poisoning,[45] there is concern about chronic toxicity, since the solubility of cadmium in cadmium pigments can vary extensively, depending on the source of the pigment.[42]

There is also significant confusion regarding the bioavailability of lead from lead glazes. The ceramic literature has traditionally described glazes containing lead carbonate, lead oxide, and other so-called "raw" lead compounds as hazardous. However, the same literature describes glazes based on lead frits (a glasslike substance used in glazes) as safe because the lead is in an insoluble lead silicate form, which is not absorbed. Many commercial lead glazes sold in schools contain these lead frits. Actual tests of the solubility of lead frits have shown wide variation in solubility, both in vitro and in vivo.[43] Many factors affect the solubility of the lead in these glazes, including the form of lead silicate, presence of other metals, and the manufacturing process. Because of the number of documented cases of lead poisoning that have occurred with these glazes, all ingestions of lead-containing ceramic glazes should be considered as potential lead poisoning cases.

Risk Factors

Art materials are commonly used by children in day care centers, elementary schools, and the home; by hospital patients in art and occupational therapy programs; by the disabled in schools and institutions; and by the elderly in community art centers and nursing homes. A variety of factors may make these groups more susceptible to the toxic effects of art materials, including age, medical problems, medications, and simultaneous exposure to several toxic chemicals.

Children are the most obvious high-risk group, due to their small body weight, more rapid metabolism, and other physiologic factors. Very young children deliberately swallow many substances, and older children inadvertently place their hands in their mouths. For these reasons, along with the fact that they may not understand the risks or take suitable precautions, children are at higher risk than adults for exposure to toxic chemicals.[3]

Various temporary and permanent disabilities can place children and adults at higher risk if a particular chemical targets an already compromised organ.[35] Some examples are people with epilepsy exposed to turpentine, which may result in seizures[39]; people with hepatitis exposed to organic solvents that damage the liver; asthmatics exposed to dusts, molds, spray mists, or sulfur dioxide; and people with dysrhythmias exposed to solvents such as methylene chloride, 1,1,1-trichloroethane, freon, and toluene, all of which can induce dysrhythmias. Individuals who have difficulty reading and following directions or understanding warning labels, and those individuals who have a tendency to "sniff" hazardous solvents, are all considered high-risk groups.

The alcohol content of art products may pose another potential risk. The interaction of many substances and medications with alcohol is another well established hazard, especially with respect to the central nervous system.[15] Like ethyl alcohol, many other solvents can cause CNS depression. In the presence of medications that affect the CNS, such as sedative-hypnotics, ingestion of alcohol-containing products could cause even more severe depressant effects. Of course, drinking alcoholic beverages and exposure to solvents can have similar effects and are therefore not always distinguishable clinically.

Chronic Exposures

Many art materials are associated with chronic hazards, including silicosis from crystalline silica in clay in potters[6]; mesotheliomas from asbestos in jewelers and ceramicists[9,10]; bladder cancer, leukemia, and renal cancer from asbestos in painters[38]; lead poisoning from lead and lead-containing solders in stained-glass artists[12]; renal damage from cadmium-containing silver solders in jewelers[4]; solvent-induced peripheral and central nervous system damage in silk-screen artists[40]; peripheral neuropathy from rubber cement and aerosol spray products containing *n*-hexane in art students[25]; chronic respiratory problems from sulfur dioxide and other irritants in photographers[18,23]; and chromium sensitization from the use of dichromates as a natural dye mordant in fiber artists.[5]

In the past, it was difficult to identify toxins in art materials, as the original Federal Hazardous Substances Act required label warnings only for acute hazards. Concern in the arts community about the chronic hazards of art materials during the late 1970s culminated in congressional hearings in 1980.[16] At that point, to prevent passage of a chronic hazards labeling law, art materials manufacturers developed a voluntary chronic hazards labeling standard under the auspices of the American Society of Testing and Materials.[1] Voluntary labeling adhering to this standard was acknowledged by the ACMI with their Health Label seal. Compliance with this program required labeling developed by a consultant toxicologist. The program was particularly successful for fine art painting materials, but most manufacturers of the more hazardous products, such as solvent-based silk screen printing inks, did not participate.

In the mid-1980s, California, Oregon, Tennessee, Illinois, Florida, Virginia, and Connecticut passed laws mandating chronic hazard labeling of all art materials. They also banned the use of toxic art materials in elementary schools.

Faced with variations in laws from state to state, the industry supported federal legislation, and in 1988 Congress amended the Federal Hazardous Substances Act by passing the Labeling of Hazardous Art Materials Act. This law requires art and craft manufacturers to determine the chronic hazards of their products and to place warning labels on those products. It also provided for the Consumer Products Safety Commission (CPSC) to develop criteria for evaluating chronic hazards of art materials and pre-empted state laws on art material labeling. Although the law went into effect in 1990, the final regulations were not published until 1992.[41]

The Federal labeling requirements include the following: the signal word "WARNING" if only a chronic hazard exists; a list of the possible chronic hazards; the names of chronically hazardous components; safe handling instructions; list of sensitizing components; and a source for further information. The label must also carry the statement "Conforms to ASTMA D-4236" or similar wording. As of this writing, many art materials are still not properly labeled.

One result of this law has been the development of safer art materials due to a reluctance to put cancer warnings, reproductive hazards warnings, and so forth on labels. One such change is the replacement of *n*-hexane with *n*-heptane in most brands of rubber cements, rubber cement thinners, spray adhesives, and similar products.

Accurate, acute, and chronic hazard labeling of imported art materials is a persistent problem despite the legislation, because many importers have had difficulty ascertaining the ingredients in the art materials they are importing. A 1994 recall of crayons imported from China that contained excessive lead levels illustrates this problem.[8]

Children's Art Materials

The AP/CP seal program of the ACMI has been praised by medical authorities. However, because the approval of art materials does not require long-term animal testing, there have been questions about the chronic effects of some materials.

As a result of the labeling law passed in California in 1987, the California State Department of Health Services published a list of art materials approved for use in elementary schools; the list was updated in 1988.[2] An audit of the CP/AP program demonstrated that the list did not contain many products with the AP/CP label due to differing toxicologic criteria, inadequate documentation, and differences of opinion over approving materials such as oil paints, which customarily necessitate the use of solvents.[7] Many of these problems have since been resolved, although products such as oil paints and airbrush paints are still not considered suitable for elementary school children. Unfortunately, as a result of budget cuts, the California State Department of Health Services discontinued publication of the list of approved children's art materials.

The Labeling of Hazardous Art Materials Act of 1988 requires that all chronically hazardous art materials carry a statement that such materials are inappropriate for children, and allows the CPSC to obtain a court injunction against any school purchasing these materials for use by children in grade six and below. To date, the CPSC has not yet obtained a court injunction against any school under this provision of the law; and more unfortunately, there has been little active enforcement of the law in general.

Further information on the hazards of arts and crafts materials can be obtained from the Center for Safety in the Arts gopher/web site on the Internet. The URL is http://artswire.org:70/1/csa. The Art Hazards Information Center of the Center for Safety in the Arts itself has closed because of a lack of funding.

References

1. American Society for Testing and Materials Subcommittee D-01.57 on Artist Paints and Related Materials: ASTM D-4236-83, Standard Practice for Labeling Art Materials for Chronic Health Hazards. Philadelphia, ASTM, 1984.
2. Art and Craft Materials Acceptable for Kindergarten and Grades 1–6, Updated List. Sacramento, California Department of Health Servicesm, 1988.
3. Babin A, Peltz PA, Rossol M: Children's Art Supplies Can Be Toxic. New York, Center for Safety in the Arts, 1989.
4. Baker EL, Peterson WA, Holtz JL, et al: Cadmium poisoning in jewelry workers. In: McCann M, Barazani G, eds: Health Hazards in the Arts and Crafts. Proceedings of the SOEH conference on health hazards in the arts and crafts. Washington, DC, Society for Occupational and Environmental Health, 1980, pp. 16–22.
5. Chromium sensitization in an artist's workshop. MMWR 1982;31:111–112.
6. Cone J: Silicosis in a ceramics technician. Paper presented at the first national conference on health risks in the arts, crafts and trades, Chicago, April 1981.
7. Controversy over non-toxic labels article. Art Hazards News 1989;12:1–3.
8. CPSC announces recalls of imported crayons because of lead poisoning hazard. U.S. Consumer Product Safety Commission Release #94-055, April 5, 1994.

9. Driscoll RJ, Mulligan WJ, Schultz D, Candelaria A: Malignant mesothelioma: A cluster in a native American population. N Engl J Med 1988;318:1437–1438.
10. Eichelmann A: Cancer in a ceramicist. Art Hazards News 1980;3:2.
11. Federal Hazardous Substances Act Regulations (16 CFR 1500). Fed Reg 1973;38:27012–27038.
12. Feldman R, Sedman T: Hobbyists working with lead. N Engl J Med 1975;292:929.
13. Garriot J, Petty CS: Death from inhalation abuse: Toxicological and pathological evaluation of 34 cases. Clin Toxicol 1980;16:305–315
14. Gonzalez EG, Downey JA: Polyneuropathy in a glue sniffer. Arch Phys Med Rehab 1972;53:333–337.
15. Hardman JG, Limbird LE, Molinoff PB, Ruddon RW, eds: Goodman and Gilman's The Pharmacological Basis of Therapeutics, 9th ed. New York, McGraw Hill, 1996, p. 390.
16. Hearings on HR 6977, Chronic Hazards Labeling Bill, Washington, September 15–16, 1980.
17. Hersh JH: Toluene embryopathy: Two new cases. J Med Genet 1989;26:333–337.
18. Hodgson M, Parkinson D: Respiratory disease in a photographer. Am J Ind Med 1986;9:349–354.
19. Houk C, Hart C: Hazards in a photography lab: A cyanide incident case study. J Chem Educ 1987;64:A234–A236.
20. Hubley M: Methyl ethyl ketone peroxide. Art Hazards News 1981;4:3. Letter.
21. King GS, Smialek JE, Troutman WG: Sudden death in adolescents resulting from the inhalation of typewriter correcting fluid. JAMA 1985;253:1604–1606.
22. King MD, Day RE, Oliver JS, et al: Solvent encephalopathy. Br Med J 1981; 283:663–665.
23. Kipen H, Lerman Y: Respiratory abnormalities among photographic developers: A report of these cases. Am J Ind Med 1986;9:341–347.
24. Korobkin R, Asbury AK, Sumner AJ, Nielsen SL: Glue-sniffing neuropathy. Arch Neurol 1975;32:158–162.
25. Lawsuit against art school by art student. Art Hazards News 1989;12:1.
26. Lead ingestion and ceramic glazes. MMWR 1992;41:1.
27. Letts N: Artist dies in basement cyanide accident. Art Hazards News 1991;14:1.
28. Litovitz TL, Clark LR, Soloway RA: 1993 Annual report of the American Association of Poison Control Centers Toxic Exposure Surveillance System. Am J Emerg Med 1994;12: 546–584.
29. Litovitz TL, Felberg MA, Soloway RA, et al: 1994 Annual report of the American Association of Poison Control Centers Toxic Exposure Surveillance System. Am J Emerg Med 1995;13:551–597.
30. Litovitz TL, Felberg MA, White S, Klein-Schwartz W: 1995 Annual report of the American Association of Poison Control Centers Toxic Exposure Surveillance System. Am J Emerg Med 1996;14:487–537.
31. Litovitz TL, Holm KC, Baily KM, Schmitz BF: 1991 Annual report of the American Association of Poison Control Centers National Data Collection System. Am J Emerg Med 1992;10:452–505.
32. Litovitz TL, Holm KC, Clancy C, et al: 1992 Annual report of the American Association of Poison Control Centers Toxic Exposure Surveillance System. Am J Emerg Med 1993;11:494–555.
33. McCann, M: Artist Beware, 2nd ed. New York, Lyons & Burford, 1992.
34. McCann M: Lead poisoning from pottery glazes in nursing homes. Art Hazards News 1988;11:1.
35. McCann M: Teaching art safely to the disabled. New York, Center for Safety in the Arts, 1987.
36. McCann M: Fatality from xylene spraying. Art Hazards News 1981;4:1.
37. McCann M: Labeling needs of arts and crafts materials. In: McCann M, Barazani G, eds: Health Hazards in the Arts and Crafts. Proceeding of the SOEH conference on health hazards in the arts and crafts. Washington, DC, Society for Occupational and Environmental Health, 1980, pp. 161–165.
38. Miller AB, Silverman DT, Hoover RN, Blair A: Cancer risk among artistic painters. Am J Ind Med 1986;9:281–287.
39. Nerby D: Turpentine and young children. Art Hazards News 1983;6:3. Letter.
40. Prockup L: Multifocal nervous system damage from inhalation of volatile hydrocarbons. J Occup Med 1977;19:139–140.
41. Regulations [16 CFR 1500.14(b)(8), 11500.135]. Fed Reg 1992; 46626–46674.
42. Rutter HA, Copeland G: Biological Availability of Cadmium from Cadmium Pigments: Final Report. Hazleton Laboratories America, September 16,1977.
43. Sartorelli E, Loi F, Gori R: Lead silicate toxicity: A comparison among different compounds. Environ Res 1985;36: 420–425.
44. Stewart R, Hakę C: Paint remover hazard. JAMA 1976; 235:398–401.
45. Stopford W: Bioavailability of cadmium in pigments: Testimony on OSHA cadmium standard (Docket H057A Exhibits List Ex. 14-14). April 11, 1990.
46. Vance MV, Curry SC, Bradley JM, et al: Acute lead poisoning in nursing home and psychiatric patients from the ingestion of lead-based ceramic glazes. Arch Intern Med 1990;150:2085–2092.
47. Ziem G: Silk screen printing and heart attack. Art Hazards News 1984;7:2. Letter.

CHAPTER 112

Psychosocial Principles in Assessment and Intervention

Frances A. Gautieri and Kenneth O. Brambill

The Changing Paradigm of Healthcare

Reconfiguration of healthcare services in the United States provides impetus and opportunity for emergency departments to consider their pivotal position within the integrated delivery systems that are emerging. Monolithic healthcare institutions are giving way to coordinated multifaceted programs and services in geographically dispersed sites throughout a community or region. Evolving standards of practice continue to clarify and refine requirements for development of a comprehensive and functional continuum of care, the principles of which apply in widely diverse areas across the country.[15]

The expansion of healthcare networks to include all levels of care as well as linkages to community-based mental health, substance abuse treatment, and social service agencies is of particular relevance to emergency department interdisciplinary teams in their management of toxicologic emergencies. Despite the highest levels of clinical and technological expertise applied in the diagnosis and treatment of poisoned or overdosed patients, successful outcomes may be compromised by inadequacies in aftercare and follow-up. The new paradigm brings promise as the hospital becomes part of an integrated network of community-focused health and social services systems with shared objectives that include promotion of primary care, effective case management, and continuity among multiple providers in various settings.[6]

Access issues related to managed care authorization requirements and lack of coverage notwithstanding, the improved information and referral systems of the new healthcare networks benefit patients and providers as the potential is enhanced for ensuring continuing care and follow-up services. The extent to which emergency departments take initiative in developing specialized resources and work proactively to identify unmet needs and advocate for continuing care services will be increasingly important in supporting the goal of achieving a comprehensive continuum of care.

Historical Perspective

The importance of understanding the social and community context for medical conditions and larger public health problems has been recognized in the United States for nearly a century. The rationale for a psychosocial approach in healthcare began to emerge clearly in the first decade of the 20th century as the medical profession perceived the negative and pathogenic conditions in poor, densely populated, urban areas and the correlation with the major public health issues of the time. The growing awareness of the linkage between social factors and serious health problems led to the introduction of social service workers as an extension of the hospital into the community, first in 1905 at Massachusetts General Hospital in Boston and then in 1906 at Bellevue Hospital in New York City.[9] These early outreach workers began to make home visits, educate patients and families about health and nutrition, and offer supportive counseling and concrete services to provide for basic human needs of food, clothing, and shelter in order to improve compliance with medical recommendations and attempt to ameliorate unhealthy conditions in the environment. Their reports about the conditions in which patients were living helped to heighten awareness about social problems and gain support for public health initiatives.[20]

This early emphasis on the environment or social context as a determinant of pathologic conditions was later refined to incorporate the influence of psychological factors. The term "psychosocial" came to reflect the dynamic interaction of internal and external aspects of a person's life, personality, and milieu—the person in his or her situation.[13] Emotions, feelings, developmental factors, individual coping patterns, family background, cultural differences, and socioeconomic factors came to be recognized as significant variables in patient response to illness or injury.

The importance of addressing the psychosocial needs of patients in healthcare settings was well accepted so that by 1930, there were more than 1000 hospital-based social service departments in the United States.[7] Professional social workers are present today in all areas of healthcare. The scope of their practice paralleled the growth of medical specialization while adhering to the basic generic principles of the psychosocial evaluation, planning, and intervention process. In the new healthcare environment of integrated networks and closer working relationships with community agencies, social workers may develop, implement, and facilitate the linkages necessary for continuing care and coordination of services.

The Psychosocial Approach In Emergency Medicine

As in all other areas of healthcare, it has become evident in emergency medicine that psychosocial factors are significant in etiology of illness, outcome potential, and options for prevention. Psychosocial issues are particularly compelling in the evaluation and treatment of toxicologic emergencies.

With the development of comprehensive emergency services in the 1970s, the multidisciplinary healthcare model was adopted. Many emergency departments incorporated social work as part of the basic interdisciplinary team to assist in the assessment and management of acute medical and psychiatric conditions. The liaison or emergency psychiatrist and the social worker became part of the crisis intervention team needed to care for the patient who was poisoned, drug overdosed, or manifesting a withdrawal syndrome. Emergency medicine as a specialty area of practice has grown rapidly.[19] There has been a concomitant movement toward on-site social work coverage for emergency service patients rather than on call consultation. Many large urban hospitals have moved toward 24-hour coverage by social work staff. The availability of social workers on site in emergency departments has contributed to professional credibility, enhanced team functioning, and improved services for patients and families.[14] Social workers are able to engage families and other collaterals, to identify and assess potential support systems, to assist patients in obtaining concrete services, and to make effective referrals for continuing care. However, in those settings where social workers are not part of the healthcare team, the responsibility for addressing psychosocial needs rests with the attending physician and may be assigned to another discipline based on the particular staffing structure.

The increased focus on emergency services is related to the major public health and social welfare problems that continue to escalate in volume and severity and are manifested daily by patients who appear in emergency departments. There is growing public awareness that poverty, homelessness, drug and alcohol abuse, family breakdown, child abuse and neglect, and violence are phenomena that affect all communities. Transformation of these broad social issues into acute medical or psychiatric problems as well as personal and family crises occurs in hospital emergency departments across the country, in cities, suburbs, small towns, and even rural areas, where the patient may present with an overdose, in withdrawal, or perhaps as a case of a seemingly unintentional pediatric ingestion.

Substance Abuse and Social Dysfunction

The adult substance abuser may be dysfunctional in one or several areas of his or her life.[12] Substance abuse is often accompanied by difficulties in holding a job, maintaining personal relationships, and carrying out family and child care responsibilities. It is common in hospital emergency departments to see patients from all walks of life for whom alcohol or drug abuse has precipitated a crisis. Examples of this diversity might include a wealthy businessman with family supports and solid community ties who fell while intoxicated and suffered a fracture, but sees himself as a social drinker and denies any problem with alcohol; a battered housewife, depressed and frightened, who took an overdose of barbiturates in a desperate effort to obtain relief from an intolerable situation; and a homeless man, a veteran with no current source of income, long estranged from family and friends, who has fallen into polydrug abuse that masks long-standing depression. In each of these examples attention to the psychosocial factors is critical to comprehensive case evaluation and differential treatment planning.

Social problems are often interrelated. For example, drug or alcohol use or abuse by caregivers is clearly associated with a high risk of child abuse and neglect.[4] Among women, childhood sexual abuse and domestic violence correlate with increased incidence of substance abuse.[11] Substance abuse frequently leads to placement of children.[2] Conversely, the fear of losing their children often prevents women from acknowledging substance problems and obtaining needed services.[1] It is also known that drug and alcohol abuse among adolescents and suicidal attempts in this age group usually reflect long-standing family problems and may indicate abuse and neglect, including sexual abuse.[18] As the ability to identify child abuse and neglect improves, it becomes increasingly obvious that childhood incidents, including ingestions, are often correlated with neglect by their caregivers and exacerbated by extraordinary family stress due to marital problems, joblessness, dislocation, and homelessness.

Psychosocial assessment has become an important component in the comprehensive evaluation of toxicologic emergencies and may even be required under state-mandated child protection laws in cases where there is any suspicion that a child's ingestion or an adolescent's drug use, alcohol intoxication, or suicide attempt might be related to abuse or neglect by a parent or guardian. Similarly, the overdose of an adult who has young children in his or her care raises serious questions about whether his or her drug use or abuse has caused a situation in which children are, have been, or could be endangered or neglected.

The relationship between substance abuse and maternal/child health problems has become very evident.[8] There is urgent need to develop protocols for the systematic identification of drug abuse in pregnancy and to intervene expeditiously to improve outcomes for both women and their infants. Women of childbearing age who appear in emergency departments with substance-related conditions require meticulous attention, continuity of care, and active follow-up. Encounters with the healthcare system in emergencies provide the opportunity for pregnant drug-involved women to access many other services. This is accomplished most effectively through the assistance of social work staff, who are in a unique position at the interface between the hospital and the community. They are able to address clinical as well as personal concrete needs such as food, clothing, and shelter and to help patients negotiate complex social systems.[5]

The Emergency Episode: Opportunity for Intervention

The hospital emergency department is usually the first point of entry into the healthcare system for substance abusers. Often they are assessed, treated, and released to the same environment in which their drug-taking behavior is supported and reinforced, only to return repeatedly to the emergency department with more evidence of debilitation and dysfunctional behavior. A comprehensive psychosocial approach, including early patient identification and intervention, is a prerequisite for a positive outcome for these apparently intractable, complex, and multicausal cases. Success rarely occurs following initial contact, but rather depends on a gradual, incremental process that includes ready access to a community service network, a flexible case management approach, and active follow-up.

Considerations In Emergency Care of Substance Abusers

The taking of a comprehensive substance abuse and alcohol history is of paramount importance in an emergency department because the visit often provides an excellent opportunity for a therapeutic intervention. Patients who have alcohol abuse problems remain in the hospital longer than the non-problem drinkers.[16] The numbers of emergency department visits due to heroin overdose and cocaine reaction tends to ebb and flow dependent upon the extent of problems being experienced among the heaviest users.[21] However, frequently someone who has suffered injury or assault simultaneous to intoxication or oversedation has never had the opportunity for a credible healthcare professional to help him or her examine personal behavior, and to focus on the psychosocial consequences, health issues, and treatment options related to chemical dependence. This becomes even more important when, as is sometimes the case, demographic data and psychosocial history had to be obtained from a family member or other collateral source due to incapacitation of the patient. Because information relating to drug and alcohol use carries a social stigma, interviewees often construct elaborate defenses and will invariably deny the existence of a problem. In these instances, if the interviewer has a reasonable suspicion that there is substance involvement, it is wise to offer interventive measures, referral resources, and counseling as a matter of course. Very frequently if the physician does not provide information about drinking behavior, it may not be obtained or pursued by the treatment team.[17] It is important for the patient to receive clear, unambiguous information from credible healthcare providers about the physical and social consequences of drug and alcohol consumption.[3] The emergency episode presents an opportunity for focused education and counseling that has potential for motivating the patient toward change.

Social workers who practice case finding are frequently utilized as confidants of substance users for whom they provide supportive counseling. They should not ignore anecdotal information provided during their interactions with active users about the stressors involved in that person's daily activities, around drug procurement, differential quality of available street drugs, obstacles to rehabilitation, and any new drug-taking trends which could pose health problems for the general patient population in the community.

Substance users also confront the risk of HIV. It has been widely recognized that sharing of unsterile injecting paraphernalia while using illicit substances is a principal cause of AIDS. Moreover, many cocaine users claim that cocaine is an aphrodisiac.[10] This causes chronic smokers of crack-cocaine in particular to engage in sexual practices for pay and/or pleasure, frequently ignoring the need for safety precautions to prevent AIDS and other sexually transmitted diseases. This activity is believed to be the leading cause of AIDS cases among women and heterosexual men, and through sex can lead to infection of others, such as spouses and unborn children. It is therefore important to augment screening and counseling about substance and alcohol abuse with information about AIDS and to offer referrals for HIV testing and, where possible, arrange pretest counseling within the emergency department as rapidly as possible for those who request to be tested.

The Assessment Process

Any patient who has taken an overdose of a prescribed medication, alcohol, or illicit substance, or ingested a poison, whether or not he or she manifests suicidal ideation, requires interdisciplinary assessment, support, and preliminary intervention in the emergency services setting.

Decisions about psychiatric consultation, evaluation, and treatment follow medical stabilization. However, the social worker may be needed from the point of triage to determine whether there are family or child welfare issues that require immediate attention. For example, if the patient is an unaccompanied child or adolescent, or if the patient is a parent of young children for whom care must be arranged, efforts must be initiated promptly to reach responsible family members or to seek assistance from appropriate child welfare agencies.

Patients with toxicologic emergencies are by definition high risk, based on accepted psychosocial indices (Table 112–1).

The psychosocial evaluation process is fluid and multifaceted (Table 112–2). Psychosocial assessments can be initiated through interviewing of collateral sources before a patient is physically able to respond. Delay in obtaining psychosocial information can have serious consequences, as in cases where an overdosed adult patient may have small children who were left unattended.

Psychosocial assessment includes clinical observation and interviewing of the patient and accompanying family members or friends; it may also involve contact with health or social service agencies to which the patient may be known. In cases involving young children, nonverbal modalities using play or drawings may be helpful after the situation is medically stabilized. Observation of interactions between the child and parent or caregiver, and the responses of family members to the emergency, can be helpful in understanding family dynamics. Assessment efforts are enhanced when therapeutic rapport can be established early in the contact. It is essential to adopt a sensitive, empathic approach in which the social worker clearly explains why personal and family information is needed.

In evaluating the adult overdosed or withdrawing patient, it is important to elicit information about the patient's history of drug and alcohol use and any involvement with substance abuse treatment programs, including detoxification, methadone maintenance, and drug-free modalities. Contact with current treatment programs can be very helpful in coordinating the case and should be encouraged, especially when arranging discharge plans. It is also important to differentiate, early in the contact, the adult with no children from the adult with minor children in his or her care. The psychosocial needs of an isolated, homeless, middle-aged man are very different from those of a pregnant 24-year-old woman on methadone maintenance and with two preschool children. In the latter example, the social worker's immediate focus must be on the needs of the children, pending medical stabilization of their mother. If the children are present they should be evaluated. If they are not present, their whereabouts should be determined. Any indication that they may have been left unattended requires immediate contact with local child protection authorities. In any event, the social worker's assessment must consider the impact of the woman's drug involvement on her ability to care for the children, her judgment in arranging adequate alternate child care with relatives or friends, and her own medical, counseling, and supportive service needs. The social worker should explore the family and community resources available to the patient, consult with the clinical staff of the woman's methadone treatment program, consider whether the case comes under state-mandated child protection reporting procedures, and develop a coordinated treatment plan that addresses prenatal needs in addition to a follow-up related to the patient's drug-induced emergency and the child welfare issues.

TABLE 112–1. HIGH-RISK SCREENING GUIDE FOR EMERGENCY DEPARTMENT PATIENTS

Psychosocial Assessment Is Required Whenever the Case Involves:

- Drugs or alcohol
- Suspicion of child abuse or neglect
- Domestic violence or other crime victim
- Suggestion of suicidal intent
- Psychiatric history
- Mental retardation or developmental disability
- Physical handicap, including vision or hearing impairment
- Frail or elderly
- Medical conditions with home care needs
- Patient with minor children
- Homelessness

TABLE 112–2. PSYCHOSOCIAL EVALUATION PROCESS

Assessment

Perform clinical observation/evaluation.
Interview patient and collaterals.
Obtain information on family history and current situation.
Evaluate minor children for immediate needs.
Establish drug and alcohol profile, including past treatment attempts.
Identify potential family and community support.

Interdisciplinary

Develop medical and psychosocial diagnosis.

Collaboration

Plan for intervention based on differential case needs: medical or psychiatric admission, referral for detoxification, report to Child Protective Services.

Implementation

Coordinate case.
Facilitate intervention plan and advocate for services as needed.
Refer to community agencies.
Provide concrete services: food, clothing, financial assistance, transportation.
Perform crisis counseling.
Followup.
Establish case management and follow-up plan, either directly or via community agency.

Case Examples

The following cases support the efficacy of prompt psychosocial assessment as an integral part of comprehensive medical care.

PATIENT 1. A 2-year-old boy required admission for treatment following ingestion of antidepressant medication that had been prescribed for his paternal grandmother, with whom he lived. Social work assessment initiated in the emergency service revealed a troubled family, including an absent, drug-addicted natural mother; an inconsistently involved natural father with a history of drug use and incarcerations; the paternal grandmother; a paternal uncle; and an older sibling of the patient. Interviews with the grandmother and uncle initially suggested an unintentional ingestion by an active toddler with appropriate response by the family and prompt accessing of emergency medical care. Further exploration revealed a prior admission to another hospital, due ostensibly to the child's ingestion of the grandmother's medication. This raised concerns about the adequacy of supervision in the household and need for further evaluation to develop a safe discharge plan. The case was coordinated with Child Protective Services (CPS) and a discharge plan was developed that included home visits, parenting education for the grandmother, follow-up medical care for the child, and consultation with the grandmother's mental health provider as needed. It was determined that CPS would carry primary responsibility for case management.

PATIENT 2. A 14-year-old boy ingested acetaminophen and other nonprescription drugs in an apparent suicidal gesture. Initial psychosocial assessment elicited a history of family problems and sexual identity issues. The youngster was admitted for observation and further exploration of family, school, and other potential support systems. It became clear that the one stable person in the patient's life was his maternal grandmother. She was caring and supportive but unable to manage the boy's behavior or understand his mood swings. Both the patient and his grandmother agreed to recommendations for follow-up psychotherapy and family counseling in the adolescent mental health clinic. Interdisciplinary collaboration among three hospital units—the emergency department, the inpatient service, and the outpatient clinic—made it possible to develop and implement a prompt, appropriate, and safe discharge plan.

PATIENT 3. A 77-year-old man was brought to the Emergency Department (ED) by his home health attendant after falling at home. He was immobilized on a board, unable to move his extremities, and had suffered trauma to his right eye as well as minor contusions. Medical examination revealed the patient had a biliary shunt due to a cholecystectomy and that he suffered from cirrhosis of the liver. It was also noted that he had the smell of alcohol on his breath, was disoriented, and was somewhat agitated. The patient was admitted to the alcohol detoxification unit under close medical supervision. Psychosocial assessment initiated in the ED showed the patient to be a retired hospital worker who lived with his wife and had adult children and grandchildren, and a large extended family—all of whom were very supportive. His medical condition had deteriorated following gallbladder surgery, which led to the need for a home health aide for 12 hours per day, 7 days a week. The social worker noted during hospital visits that the patient presided over his family in a patriarchal, often dictatorial manner, and gave direction to everyone with whom he came in contact. He had been a vital, active person prior to the illnesses, which now had him confined to a wheelchair, increasingly dependent upon his wife and home health aide, which he strongly resented. They were not always able to keep him away from alcohol despite its potential life-threatening impact on him in his deteriorated physical state. Prompt, effective collaboration between ED and alcoholism service teams led to appropriate care that addressed the medical, emotional, and substance abuse needs of this alcohol-dependent elderly man with depressive features whose strengths included a stable support network and health benefits. Upon discharge, he was referred to the hospital's alcohol aftercare treatment program and to the geriatric clinic for coordinated medical and psychiatric follow-up. A case conference was held with the home health agency to point out the need for vigilance because of the patient's propensity to sneak a drink of beer, and support was given to the family to reinforce the need to keep the patient engaged in pursuits not related to drinking.

PATIENT 4. A 41-year-old, single unemployed male was admitted to hospital through the ED after falling out of bed following a long bout of alcohol bingeing. He was discovered on the floor by his brother, with whom he lived. The severity of his withdrawal required intensive care before he could be safely transferred to the alcohol detoxification unit. Upon arrival on the ward, the patient stated that he had not slept in 72 hours. He constantly paced the hallways, was very tremulous, and had to be patiently counseled against leaving prematurely. Psychosocial assessment showed the patient to be the eldest of three siblings who began alcohol consumption at age 9 and was drinking problematically by age 13. During adolescence, he had been sent to a psychiatrist due to his intractable drinking problem. Nonetheless he managed to complete high school and had held restaurant jobs, the most recent one being 10 years prior to this hospital admission. The patient subsisted through the largesse of his brother, had Medicaid coverage, and had been involved in episodic outpatient alcohol treatment. Upon admission he was drinking 3 or more pints of vodka daily as well as several 16-ounce bottles of beer. The clinical impression was that of a 41-year-old, docile, chronic alcoholic, possibly with incipient organic brain damage due to long-term alcohol abuse. When medically cleared for discharge, he refused to await placement in a short-term rehabilitation program; therefore, the plan was adjusted for the patient to receive outpatient services with an active case management approach at a hospital-based alcoholism clinic.

PATIENT 5. A 26-year-old woman was brought to emergency services having ingested numerous substances including heroin, cocaine, marijuana, and alcohol. From psychosocial assessment initiated in the ED it was determined that she was also suffering from childhood sexual abuse that occurred within the family, and from current domestic violence, the result of her relationship with an abusive boyfriend. Medical problems included persistent anemia, asthma, and developmental disability. She was admitted to an inpatient unit for mentally ill chemical abusers (MICA). Relevant history included that the patient was the youngest of five siblings and lived primarily with her dysfunctional family. She received Supplemental Security Income and Medicaid. She became involved with illicit drugs at an early age and would frequently sleep in the homes of friends who also indulged in abuse of substances. She met her current boyfriend, a heavy user of alcohol and other drugs, when they both attended a sheltered workshop. He began battering her almost immediately, threatened her with weapons, and in some instances injured her so badly she required medical attention and he was placed under arrest. Several orders of protection were issued for him through the courts. The patient stated she ingested the overdose in her effort of "trying to forget," that she also tried using crack but "it made my heart beat too fast." During the course of her treatment on the substance abuse unit she repeatedly stated that upon discharge she wished to continue her relationship with her boyfriend, but wanted him to cease his battering behavior. The ED and MICA unit teams worked closely with the hospital's domestic violence coordinator in the treatment and continuing care planning for this vulnerable patient with limited functioning, numerous medical complaints, in an abusive relationship, and periodically experiencing suicidal depression and repressed rage partly due to signs and symptoms of posttraumatic stress disorder. Coordinated efforts upon discharge included follow-up case management to obtain housing with supportive services, substance abuse and mental health counseling, and attempts to engage the boyfriend in order to prevent further domestic violence. Subsequent threats by the boyfriend resulted in his incarceration due to the advocacy provided by the domestic violence coordinator who functioned as the primary case manager. The patient responded well to the clinical and supportive services and showed signs of generally improved functioning.

Good psychosocial assessments form a basis for more effective case management, especially where treatment depends on referral to community agencies for services such as drug or alcohol treatment, family counseling, child welfare services, emergency financial assistance, shelter, or home healthcare. Emergency departments that have formal or informal relationships with community service providers are better able to assure continuity of care. Regularly updated resource lists with clear referral guidelines are invaluable (Table 112–3).

The Role of the Emergency Department in the Continuum of Care

The effectiveness of a hospital ED is measured by how well individual cases are evaluated, treated, and managed and to what extent communication and coordination are maintained with other settings and organizations in the community that provide for continuing healthcare and social service needs. Efficacy is enhanced when the emergency department recognizes its strategic position in the continuum of care, seeks to develop and cultivate working relationships with a wide range of other providers, and makes reasonable efforts to formulate, implement, and follow up on continuing care plans.

The morbidity of substance abuse and its relationship to AIDS; the widespread use of drugs and alcohol at all levels of society, including women of childbearing age; the nationwide increase in neglect, maltreatment, and physical and sexual abuse of children; adolescent suicide; domestic violence; and the problems of homelessness are markers everywhere of severe societal distress. Evolving public policy and planning related to these issues will affect delivery of services to ED patients. Eligibility restrictions on medical and financial assistance deriving from the 1996 federal welfare reform legislation can be expected to erect more barriers to the goal of a comprehensive continuum of care. The challenge must be met by informed advocacy through awareness and involvement by emergency department staff at many levels beyond the care of the individual patient.

Even the best emergency care is limited in efficacy if resources for ongoing treatment and supportive services are nonexistent or inadequate. The individual who is homeless and drug dependent and must wait weeks or months for entry into an inpatient or outpatient drug treatment program will inevitably continue maladaptive behaviors, which might include the risk of HIV transmission to sexual partners and those sharing needles. Current experience demonstrates the benefit to patients of providing HIV counseling and education in the ED which is often the sole healthcare resource for this significant group of high-risk patients. The ED encounter presents an opportunity for the patient and the healthcare provider to interact at a higher level of mutual advantage and to the benefit of the community. By addressing the needs of the whole person, patterns of repeated emergencies may be interrupted. The strategic importance of the ED should not be underestimated in developing effective approaches to current social and public health problems.

TABLE 112–3. EMERGENCY DEPARTMENT BASIC RESOURCE GUIDE

Develop Resource List and Referral Protocols for the Following:

- Drug and alcohol treatment services for all modalities and levels of care: detoxification, sobering up, therapeutic communities, other residential programs, methadone maintenance, drug-free outpatient clinics, 12-step programs
- Mental health programs
- Family services agencies
- Child protective and voluntary child welfare services
- Crime victims services
- Shelters and emergency housing
- Concrete services: food, clothing, financial assistance, transportation
- Legal and advocacy services

References

1. Abbott AA: A feminist approach to substance abuse treatment and service delivery. Soc Work Health Care 1994; 19:67–83.
2. Azzi-Lessing, Olsen LJ: Substance abuse-affected families in the child welfare system: New challenges, new alliances. Soc Work 1996;41:15–23.
3. Barber J: Working with resistant drug abusers. Soc Work 1995; 40:17–23.
4. Bays J: Substance abuse and child abuse: The impact of addiction on the child. Pediatr Clin North Am 1990;37: 881–904.
5. Berger C: Cocaine and pregnancy: A challenge for health care providers. Health Soc Work 1990;15:310–316.

6. Berkman B: The emerging health care world: Implications for social work practice and education. Soc Work 1996;41: 541–551.
7. Carlton TO: Clinical Social Work in Health Settings. New York Springer, 1984, p. 4.
8. Chasnoff IJ, Schnoll SH: Consequences of cocaine and other drug use in pregnancy. In: Washton AM, Gold MS, eds: Cocaine: A Clinician's Handbook. New York. Guilford Press, 1987, pp. 241–251.
9. Friedlander WA: Social work in medical and psychiatric settings. In: Introduction to Social Welfare. Englewood Cliffs, NJ, Prentice-Hall, 1961, pp. 389–395.
10. Gold MS: Cocaine (and crack): Clinical aspects. In: Lowinson JH, Ruiz P, Millman RB, eds: Substance Abuse: A Comprehensive Textbook. Baltimore, Williams & Wilkins, 1992, p. 211.
11. Goldberg ME: Substance abusing women: False stereotypes and real needs. Soc Work 1995;40:789–798.
12. Herrington RE, Jacobson GR, Benzer DG, eds: Alcohol and Drug Abuse Handbook. St. Louis, WH Green, 1987, pp. 259–260.
13. Hollis F: Casework: A Psychosocial Therapy. New York, Random House, 1965, Chaps. 1, 10.
14. Johnson LC, Schwartz CL, Tate DS: Health care and social welfare. In: Social Welfare: A Response to Human Need. Allyn & Bacon, 1997.
15. Joint Commission on Accreditation of Health Care Organizations: 1996 Comprehensive Accreditation Manual for Hospitals, Update February 1, 1997. Continuum of Care CC–1 to CC–17.
16. McCusker J, Cherubin E, Zimberg S: Prevalence of alcoholism in general municipal hospital population. NY State J Med 1971;71:751–754.
17. Niles BL, McCrady BS: Detection of alcohol problems in a hospital setting. J Addict Behav 1991;16:223–233.
18. Riggs S, Alario AG, McHorney C: Health risk behaviors and attempted suicide in adolescents who report prior maltreatment. Pediatrics 1990;116:815–821.
19. Soskis CW: Social Work in the Emergency Room. New York, Springer, 1985, pp. 1–11.
20. Starr J: Hospital City. New York, Crown, 1957, pp. 185–193.
21. Treaster JB: Emergency hospital visits rise among drug abusers. New York Times, April 23, 1993.

CHAPTER 113

Psychiatric Principles

Evaluating and Managing Suicidal and Violent Patients

Michael H. Allen, Wendy Rives, and Mark R. Serper

Suicide

Self-destructive behavior is among the most common and challenging Emergency Department (ED) presentations. It can take the form of attempted suicide or nonlethal self-injurious behavior, also known as parasuicide. As these two clinical conditions significantly overlap, the identification of the acutely suicidal patient places an extreme burden on the physician to intervene and prevent deaths. In 1993, the last year for which statistics are available, the suicide rate in the United States was 12.4 per 100,000.[42] Suicide was the ninth leading cause of death, totaling more than 30,000 deaths per year, or one every 20 minutes.

Suicidal ideation ranges from normal thoughts to lethal intentions. Suicidal crises are heterogeneous, with suicide the final outcome of many possible psychiatric conditions and social circumstances. Self-poisoning or deliberate overdosing, is a common method of attempting suicide, but this possibility must also be differentiated from unintentional overdose, particularly in the young, the mentally retarded, the confused elderly, and the chronic drug-abusing patient. This distinction is rendered even more complex by the possibility that suicidal ideation may be deliberately concealed.

Much is known about the risk of suicide for various groups over time, but little can be said with certainty about individual patients at particular points in time. There is no typical suicidal patient who may be routinely hospitalized.

Likewise, there is no patient in distress for whom the risk of suicide is so remote that it need not be considered. There is no clinically useful test or rating scale. Hence, the assessment of the potentially suicidal patient remains a highly individualized exercise in clinical judgment.

Self-Poisoning

Suicide is discussed in terms of attempts and completions. When the term "suicide" is used alone it refers to completed suicide. The two are considered separately because those who attempt and those who complete suicide appear to constitute different groups. Those who attempt suicide are more commonly younger women with personality disorders, and self-poisoning is common in this group. Those who complete suicide, however, are more commonly older men with major depression or alcoholism, and they typically use more violent methods.

At this time firearms are the most commonly used method of suicide in both sexes. In 1993, 60.9% of suicide deaths were attributable to gunshot wounds. In males, 65% of suicides were by firearms and 15.3% were by hanging or strangulation. The methods perferred by women have shifted over time.

Self-poisoning was a very common method of suicide in the 1960s and 1970s, but it has since decreased, perhaps due in part to changing prescription practices and in part to other social changes. In 1970, 47.9% of female suicides were by poisoning compared to 34.6% in 1993. In 1993 women, like men, were most frequently the victims of self-inflicted gunshot wounds (41.9%). This decline in self-poisoning may be due to decreased use of more lethal medications such as barbiturates and monoamine oxidase inhibitors.[12]

When benzodiazepines were more tightly regulated in New York State, there was again a shift to somewhat more consequential overdoses with more dangerous nonprescription drugs.[22] However, antidepressant medications are the most common drugs implicated in suicide due to their toxicity and frequent use in some of the populations at risk.

Psychiatric Management of Self-Poisoning

Table 113–1 depicts a case of suspected self-poisoning from the starting point of prehospital care through the completion of a comprehensive assessment and treatment planning. The upper row describes the evolving clinical course of the patient while the middle row shows the progression of emergency care provided to the patient. The bottom row lists specific diagnostic and treatment goals that should be completed at various points in the patient's care.

Focused Psychiatric Assessment. Thorough psychiatric consultation is possible only when a patient is no longer intoxicated or otherwise acutely medically compromised. The determination that the patient has cleared cannot be established on the basis of blood levels but should be approached clinically. Psychiatric examination must be postponed until signs of intoxication such as somnolence, slurred speech, and ataxia are no longer present. There are several reasons for this approach.

First, the physician should not unequivocally attribute altered mental status to intoxication until signs of intoxication have passed and cognitive functions have returned to normal. Until that time, other medical conditions that might coexist with or masquerade as intoxication cannot be excluded. Second, the patient's cognitive functioning will be too impaired by the drugs and/or alcohol to provide critical historical details reliably. Third, much of what the patient reports will be ephemeral, due to the predictable, temporary effects on mood of the substances ingested. Nevertheless, at this relatively early point in the patient's course, a focused psychiatric assessment may be needed to address specific clinical concerns that can arise at this stage.

Elopement is a risk in this stage of the patient's care. Patients may have subacute residual CNS effects of the substance ingested; confusion, whether overt or subtle, fatigue, and fear can predispose patients to wandering or flight. Additionally, the patient's intentions remain unclear at this point; the question of accidental versus intentional ingestion cannot be completely resolved. For these reasons, a high level of observation should be maintained. Depending on the physical plant and personnel, it may be sufficient to place the patient in an open area in the direct line of sight of nursing staff. If such an arrangement is not possible or the patient is agitated and disruptive, it may be necessary to separate the patient. Under these circumstances, an individual aide should be assigned to observe the patient. Some form of restraint may be necessary to prevent wandering, elopement, or injury, even if the patient appears calm the majority of the time.

Aggression may arise from lingering effects of toxic ingestions, severe anxiety, and/or fear or anger at the loss of autonomy and unpleasant treatments. Although patients may respond to verbal limit setting and repeated explanations of their care, they may require sedation and/or restraint. As a general rule, unless the patient incidentally carries a diagnosis of a psychotic disorder, a benzodiazepine is the treatment of choice for the management of agitated, aggressive behavior. The specific choice of benzodiazepine and route of administration may vary according to the treatment setting. In medical emergency departments, sedation may be given via intravenous administration because of the rapid rate of onset and routine intravenous accesss for life-saving care. Diazepam has been used to treat aggression and agitation in a variety of medically ill patients, including postoperative cardiac patients, patients requiring cardioversion, and preoperative anxiety.[1,27,33] ED physicians utilize the rapidity of onset and the efficacy of diazepam in increasing doses of 5 to 10 mg IV for the treatment of aggression. Patients may require repeated administration in extreme agitation, and the interval may be within 5 to 10 minutes; careful monitoring of clinical response and respiratory function should provide for safe tranquilization. Psychiatrists in ED setting may prefer the use of lorazepam as this benzodiazepine is described in a number of clinical reports concerning rapid tranquilization.[6,17,29,30] Lorazepam, 1 to 2 mg, may be given orally or

TABLE 113–1. CASE PRESENTATION

	Case	Evolution			Disposition
Patient Course	Patient found in the community. Unresponsive.	Patient monitored in the ED. Vital signs stable. Still unresponsive.	Patient lethargic, but following commands. Answers simple questions.	Patient fully awake and alert.	Evaluation complete.
Treatment Course	Prehospital.	Triage. Medical assessment.	Observation and monitoring.	Formal psychiatric evaluation.	Treatment planning.
Physician Course	Patient identification. Search for prescription drugs, drug paraphernalia. Assessment of cardiac and respiratory functions.	Orogastric lavage, activated charcoal. Diagnostic testing (blood studies, ECG, toxicology). Contact collateral sources for history. Prior records.	Focused psychiatric assessment: elopement, aggressive behavior, decisional capacity, addressing confidentiality and immediate suicide risk.	Comprehensive psychiatric assessment: diagnostic interviewing, risk factors, future risk.	Treatments: medication, hospitalization, substance abuse, crisis intervention, family therapy.

parentally and repeated at 30 to 60 minute intervals, respectively, until the patient is calm. Haloperidol is preferred for the treatment of agitation in patients with functional psychoses. The usual dose of haloperidol is 5 mg orally or parentally given at 30 to 60 minute intervals, most patients respond after 1 to 3 doses.

Another issue that frequently emerges at this point is that of decisional capacity. Patients may request their discharge, refuse care, or become aggressive. In general, patients are presumed competent and must consent to treatment. However, they are not allowed to make poor healthcare decisions if their ability to weigh the risks and benefits of the proposed care is limited by cognitive deficits or mental illness. In the setting of intoxication, appropriate care may be provided under the doctrine of implied consent.

The emergency exception to the doctrine of informed consent may also apply in circumstances where self-injury is suspected. The emergency exception permits forcible detention, restraint, medication over objection, and necessary medical care until psychiatric assessment can be accomplished. After the management of the immediate medical emergency and resolution of intoxication, suspected self-injury is sufficient evidence of impaired decisional capacity for the emergency physician to hold a patient for further psychiatric assessment. The emergency physician should note the patient's objections in the record and indicate the basis for the determination of diminished capacity.

After the self-poisoned patient is stabilized, there may be a need for a more thorough assessment of decisional capacity; psychiatric consultation may be useful at this stage to help document the degree of impairment, determine the etiology, and predict the likely course.

Immediate Risk. After these safety considerations have been addressed, the aim of the focused psychiatric assessment moves toward a determination of immediate suicide risk. This examination should answer the following questions:

1. What is the patient's attitude toward life-saving care?
2. What are the patient's current wishes with regard to living or dying?
3. What are the patient's thoughts about his or her rescue and likely recovery?

These questions can only be answered in the course of a frank discussion between the patient and the emergency physician. Do not be concerned about "provoking" further self-injurious impulses with this vital discussion; many patients will be relieved that the caregiver is speaking directly about their distress.

Reliability and Confidentiality. Mention should be made here about the difficult issues of reliability and confidentiality with regard to gathering history. Evasiveness, lack of detail, inconsistency, and improbability taken together suggest an unreliable history. It is appropriate to confront the patient with the implausible aspects of the history they have provided and offer an opportunity to provide more useful information. This is often successful, though subsequent reports are, of course, equally suspect.

The most important step from the standpoint of both clinical care and risk management is to locate other sources of information to clarify the patient's situation. A careful review of any previous records is critical. Any pattern to a patient's presentations such as increasing frequency, more aggravated behavior, or dishevelled appearance should be noted.

Collateral contacts are another important source of information, though the level of involvement, sophistication, and reliability of the collaterals must also be taken into account. The mere fact that a person is a patient at a hospital is not considered confidential and hence the ED may make contacts that are limited to soliciting information without specific consent. An effort should be made to obtain consent for any broader discussion with family, friends, or other treaters. The patient may express concern about the ED staff contacting a family member or counselor. Any information to be imparted to third parties can be negotiated in advance with the patient. The patient may restrict consent to receiving information only and may withhold consent to impart certain information. More caution is indicated in contacting an employer. While disclosing information about the patient without his or her consent is a breach of confidentiality, a physician may do so in the interest of protecting the patient.[4]

Comprehensive Psychiatric Assessment

The comprehensive psychiatric assessment includes a characterization of the suicidal ideation present, exploration of certain so-called risk factors, and the formulation of a diagnostic impression. These three elements help to determine the attendant risk and guide treatment planning.

Characterization of Suicidal Ideation. The core of the suicide risk assessment is a detailed discussion of the patient's suicidal thoughts and urges. This must be included in every mental status examination. It is important to establish rapport and introduce the topic in an appropriate context in order to improve the patient's candor. This requires extensive time and skillful evaluation, for which there is no substitute. This approach will enhance the therapeutic quality of the interview as well as its reliability. For example, almost everyone has had some period in life when they have been discouraged. The clinician may spend a few moments talking with the patient about the point in life when he or she was most disheartened. This is done by asking the patient if he or she has been feeling "down" lately; and then, if the patient has, by asking if this is the worst the patient has ever felt. If the patient denies recent depression altogether or indicates that this is not the worst, it is helpful, for several reasons, to ask the patient to describe the point in his or her life when the patient felt worst, which may or may not be the current episode. Depression fluctuates a great deal, and characterizing the worst period assures that a prior history of major depression will not be overlooked.

At some point, the physician might ask if, during that worst period in the patient's life, the patient ever felt that perhaps things would never get better (hopelessness), that he or she could not go on (helplessness), or perhaps that he or she would be better off dead (passive suicidal ideation). If failing others was involved in the patient's demoralization (guilt), the physician might ask if the patient felt at any time as if others would be better off without him or her. These are common thoughts that most people can endorse without much difficulty and lay the groundwork for discussing more troublesome ideas in the suicidal spectrum. Ultimately, the patient must be asked directly if he or she has ever felt like "killing" himself or herself (active suicidal ideation). Nothing else will do. The more generic form, "hurting" themselves, which might seem to cover more, is in fact confusing to patients—even those who wish to die do not usually consciously intend to hurt themselves in the process. The latter is more typical of multiple suicide attempters than suicide completers.

For those patients who have felt like killing themselves at some point, the next step in this scenario might be to establish how the patient is currently, and to compare this to a prior episode(s). One dimension to assess is the progression from passive to active suicidal ideation. Suicidal feelings may take the form of a relatively inchoate wish to die, perhaps from a fatal disease or accident; and then proceed to considering various active means of hastening death. Planning might include fleeting thoughts or images of a variety of methods from which the patient recoils; to a more detailed consideration of a particular, realistic method of choice; to serious planning concerning acquisition of the means, and so-called last acts. At some point the patient goes beyond thinking to acting by hoarding pills or completing his or her will. An astute family member may observe a series of odd conversations including phone calls to distant friends and family members as the suicidal individual begins to implement the plan with a series of vague farewells. In psychological autopsy studies, approximately 50 to 70% of completed suicides gave some warning of their intention; 30 to 40% of completed suicides disclosed a direct and specific intent to kill themselves.[5,36]

Other dimensions to assess include frequency, urgency, chronicity, reactivity to positive and negative external events, and subjective distress. A schema for the detailed characterization of suicidal ideation appears in Table 113–2.

The communication of suicidal ideas either directly or indirectly should not be misconstrued as a "cry for help" and hence evidence of lower risk. Communication is probably related to the degree of preoccupation with morbid thoughts and to personality characteristics that dispose individuals to revealing their thoughts to various degrees.[23]

Multiaxial Diagnosis. Diagnostic assessment also weighs heavily in the overall risk analysis, as there is a group of treatable psychiatric disorders associated with a high risk of suicide. Psychological autopsy studies in the United States and Europe over the years have consistently revealed major psychiatric illness to be a factor in suicide, present in 93% of adult suicide cases by some reports.[35,37] In particular, prospective cohort studies and retrospective case control investigations have revealed clinical depression to dramatically increase suicide risk.[8,20,31] For affective disorders, factors correlated with acute suicidality have included current depression, severe anxiety, anhedonia, panic, insomnia, ambivalence, and acute alcohol abuse. Responsibility for child care is inversely correlated with risk, suggesting a protective effect.[14]

After affective disorders, chronic alcoholism is the most commonly reported disorder, present in about 20% of cases. Moreover, alcoholic patients who also suffer from periodic episodes of depression are at more risk for suicide than patients who present with either disorder separately. As a result, any assessment conducted on pa-

TABLE 113–2. CHARACTERIZATION OF SUICIDAL IDEATION

Dimension	Benign	Intermediate	Malignant
Onset	None	Chronic, stable	New or fluctuating
Frequency	Occasional	Daily	Constant
Persistence	Fleeting thoughts	Persistent thoughts	Preoccupation
Urgency	Disinterested	Engaged	Intense
Complexity	Simple	Some detail	Elaborate
Activity	Passive ideas	Plans without action	Action
Emotional response	Death repellent	Ambivalent	Death desirable
Circumstances	Victim identifies one clear precipitant	Several complex contributory stressors	Either noncontributory or overwhelming stressors
Alternatives	Some, realistic	Few, problematic	Seems hopeless
Insight	Recognizes remediable psychologic problem	Overvalued ideas present, temporarily reassured	Morbid delusions present, reassurance impossible
Intent	Opposed to suicide	Suicide acceptable but prefers to live	Resolutely suicidal

tients with a substance abuse history must include an examination of symptoms of major depression.[15]

Schizophrenic patients are also at increased risk for suicide compared to the general population. Approximately 10% of schizophrenic patients will commit suicide.[8] Additionally, between 5 and 18% of patients with severe borderline personality disorder (especially patients who are comorbid for depression) ultimately kill themselves.[16,40]

The ability to treat the two conditions most strongly associated with suicide—major affective disorder and alcoholism—suggests that most suicides are preventable. The possibility of preventing suicide necessitates a comprehensive psychiatric assessment to identify contributory psychiatric disorders.

Risk Factors. A complete assessment should also include an examination of risk factors. Factors have been identified empirically that place groups of individuals at high risk for suicide. Although this level of prediction is actuarial and reflective of groups rather than individuals, knowledge of probability theory is important when evaluating individual cases.[28]

Although not specifically predictive, statistically suicide is more common in men than women and in whites than in nonwhites. In 1993, there were a total of 31,102 suicides; of these 80% were males. In 1993, the age-adjusted suicide rate for males (19.9 per 100,000) was more than four times that for females (4.6 per 100,000).[42] The suicide rate for black males was 12.5 per 100,000 in 1993; the figure for white males, by contrast, was 21.4 per 100,000. Among completed suicides in women, the suicide rate for white women was 5.0 per 100,000 compared to 2.1 per 100,000 in black women. Although still constituting a minority of cases seen in emergency settings, adolescent suicide has increased drastically over the past 40 years. Suicide rates for adolescents (15 to 19 years of age) have increased since 1980 from 8.5 to 10.9 per 100,000 in 1993. In contrast, suicide rates in the elderly have decreased threefold since 1940, but still occur in disproportionately high numbers.[42]

These stark figures should be contrasted to the demographic characteristics of persons who engage in "parasuicide" or nonfatal self-destructive behavior. This later category of individuals comprises a markedly different demographic group than individuals who have died from suicide. For example, parasuicidal behavior is more common in 25 to 44-year-olds than in the elderly, and more common in women than men. Existing data also indicate that nonfatal suicide attempters are equally prevalent across racial and ethnic groups.[14,32]

However, most persons belonging to a high-risk group do not commit suicide, and some individuals with no apparent risk factors do. This type of information, then, weighs most heavily in the assessment in the absence of other more specific data, early in the hospital course or in the case of the uncooperative or hostile patient. The best foundation for treatment planning and clinical decision-making is the clinician's direct examination.

Treatment

Following the comprehensive psychiatric assessment, the next step is deciding on treatment alternatives. Any patient who has made a suicide attempt must be considered to be at risk and some further intervention is warranted. The risk of a subsequent lethal attempt is approximately 1% per year over the first 10 years. The risk is highest in the first 1 month to 1 year.

The treatment alternatives available will depend on the psychiatric sophistication of the staff available to the ED at any given time. The following section describes the commonly used interventions in the emergency department; they can be used singly or in combination.

Medications can be used acutely in the treatment of severe anxiety or psychosis; however, in the case of antidepressants, a period of weeks is required for therapeutic effect, so their immediate use is not indicated in the ED. In fact, there are concerns about prescribing medications with relatively high lethality in overdose, such as tricyclic antidepressants and monoamine oxidase inhibitors, to persons who have recently attempted suicide. However, newer antidepressants and particularly the selective serotonin reuptake inhibitors (SSRIs) can be used as first-line drugs for treatment of most depressions and they are relatively safe in overdose. A marked drop in the number of deaths per million antidepressant prescriptions was observed between 1970 and 1974 in Europe.[21] Nonetheless, the initiation of antidepressant therapy by the nonpsychiatric physician is not recommended unless a tight linkage can be made between discharge and immediate (within days) aftercare by either a community outreach team or crisis clinic.

Patients with depressive disorders may suffer from significant anxiety; also, patients with overwhelming situational stressors (job loss, new financial hardship, bereavement, divorce, etc) may have episodic anxiety or insomnia. The prescription of a short course of a benzodiazepine may provide significant relief to the patient in crisis.

After treating the patient's immediate symptoms in the emergency department, the next treatment decision is determining the setting in which further treatment may safely be provided. Not all patients with suicidal ideation or even significant attempts necessarily require hospitalization, and there is still a substantial stigma attached to psychiatric hospitalization. In general, it should be the treatment used if less restrictive measures cannot insure the patient's safety. If significant doubt exists about the safety of outpatient treatment, the patient should be held in the ED for further evaluation, admitted to a general hospital with close nursing supervision, or admitted to a psychiatric unit. "Holding beds" now available in some larger psychiatric emergency services are ideal for this purpose. Some localities may also have crisis outreach services, which follow the patient after discharge from the ED and improve appropriate monitoring and continuity of care.

Patients most likely to respond to interventions in the ED are individuals who until recently have been stable, but who, as a result of some external event, find their way of life threatened. This results in a painful state of anxiety and the mobilization of some combination of adaptive and maladaptive coping strategies. Finally, a second event, the precipitant, intensifies the anxiety to the point that the patient cannot tolerate it and is thrown into crisis. The patient then feels desperate and may be completely immobilized or vulnerable to various strong impulses including the impulse to run away, strike out at someone else, or kill themselves. Reality testing is preserved and no major psychiatric syndrome is present. The patient accurately perceives his or her situation, understands that the current reaction is a psychological problem, and is highly motivated to obtain help. The crisis may last for a matter of hours or weeks before the ED presentation and will ultimately resolve. Such patients respond well to crisis intervention and may actually undergo some positive development in the course of treatment.

By contrast, patients whose condition has been deteriorating for some time in the absence of significant stressors, and who appear on examination to be suffering from severe depressive symptoms, are unlikely to benefit rapidly from supportive techniques. If such patients present with suicidal ideation or attempts, it will be difficult, though not impossible, to manage them outside the hospital.

Outpatient settings have the advantage of maintaining the patient's functioning as much as possible. Work and child care responsibilities, financial obligations, and social relationships are not disrupted. Unnecessary regression is halted. The patient is able to assume more responsibility for his or her outcome, and independence helps preserve self-esteem. These individuals remain closer to and more engaged with the people and situations with which they must learn to cope. Their morale may be rapidly improved by the combination of support, planning and modest early treatment successes.

In some cases, though, these same factors may be disadvantageous. Routine tasks may seem overwhelming. High levels of conflict may render major relationships at least temporarily unworkable.

Inpatient settings offer the advantage of respite, high levels of structure, more intensive professional and peer support, constant supervision, and usually, more rapid pharmacologic and psychosocial intervention. The physical plant reduces, though it cannot eliminate, the possible means of suicide.

The choice of inpatient or outpatient setting will depend on the balance of strengths and weaknesses of the patient, the involvement and competence of family or friends, the availability of a therapist in the community, and the ongoing stresses in the patient's life. This decision is best made by a psychiatrist after performing his or her own examination. Many facilities will not have a psychiatrist available much of the time. However, a trained mental health professional should be on call to every emergency department. This may be a psychiatric social worker, nurse clinician, or psychologist supervised on a regular basis by a psychiatrist or with a psychiatric consultant available by phone. When such services are not available, it is appropriate to detain patients in the ED until a practitioner with specific competence is available or to transfer the patient to another facility for evaluation. Every state has laws that provide for the involuntary commitment of the mentally ill under circumstances that vary from state to state. Any acute, deliberate self-injurious behavior would generally qualify. Chronic, repetitive dangerous behavior that is not "deliberate," such as frequent unintentional opioid or sedative-hypnotic overdoses, warrant careful evaluation; but in the absence of psychiatric illness, involuntary treatment is usually not an option. The practitioner should be familiar with the criteria for commitment and the classes of healthcare providers so empowered under state law.

There are other treatment interventions that can be provided in the emergency setting; these include crisis intervention, substance abuse counseling, and family therapy. A single session in the ED may be sufficient to defuse a crisis or to spur the drug-abusing patient to seek help; alternatively, the intervention may be begun in the ED and continued in another setting.

Crisis intervention is a brief, highly focused therapy that seeks to deconstruct how a crisis occured, with an eye toward examining the patient's role. Oftentimes, patients have distorted perceptions of the crisis and a gentle "correction" of catastrophic thinking can be extremely helpful. (Here is an example. Patient: "I'm going to be broke and unemployed the rest of my life." Physician: "How did you get your last job?" Patient: "Well, I interviewed a couple of times." Physician: "So people have hired you in the past, right?") The crisis is presented to the patient as an unfortunate and perhaps tragic experience that he or she can overcome. Ideally, the patient should have a relief of symptoms and learn how crises may be avoided in the future. This intervention will likely fail in patients with severe depression because of the presence of profound hopelessness. It is best utilized for patients who give a history of high functioning just prior to the crisis.

Substance abuse treatment is ultimately an intermediate (weeks to months) to long-term (months to years) intervention. However, there are powerful initial steps that the emergency physician can take. Chief among these is confronting the patient about the medical consequences of substance use. This can take the form of discussion only, or the physician can invite the patient to examine clinical laboratory results or view remarkable radiographic findings (hepatomegaly, repeated fractures from falls, increased liver enzymes, evidence of "silent" past myocardial infarction, etc). There is little to be lost from a respectful but blunt confrontation of the patient's deterioration, and he or she may listen to a physician rather than family or friends. Peer counseling is particularly useful in addictive disorders; if possible, patients should be referred to community 12-step programs such as Alcoholics Anonymous.

Family therapy can occur as a series of sessions over the long term or can be useful in the emergency setting to defuse a crisis, reinstate social supports for the patient, or educate families about mental illness. It is most important to respect a patient's request as to the level of family involement; it may often occur in the emergency setting that patients are either too angry or ashamed to confront their families. At this point, it is prudent to defer and to assure the family that the patient is safe and that you will keep them informed as confidentiality and discretion allow.

Violence

The violent patient presents unique challenges to the emergency physician. Violent patients are difficult to treat and they tend to elicit strong negative reactions in ED personnel. In one study of violence in the ED, directors of residency programs in emergency medicine were surveyed as to the frequency of verbal threats, physical attacks, and the presence of weaponry in the area. Of the 127 institutions, 74.7% of the residency directors responded; 41 (32%) reported receiving at least one verbal threat each day; moreover, 23 (18%) reported that weapons were displayed as a threat at least once each month. Fifty-five program directors (43%) noted that a physical attack on medical staff occurred at least once a month.[24] In a second study, the authors conducted a retrospective review of university police log records and ED staff incident reports to examine the problem of violence in the ED setting. Almost 75% of the incidents occurred during the evening or night. Of the 686 episodes of violence in this study, more than 25% required physical restraint or removal from the premises; additionally, it was found that the police responded to the ED nearly twice daily.[34] These studies underscore the need for timely identification of the violent patient as well as appropriate management for this diagnostically heterogeneous group. The assessment and management of the violent patient should include provisions for patient and staff safety as well as a thorough search for the cause of violent behavior. This section will address the differential diagnosis of violent behavior, the pharmacotherapy of aggressive and/or agitated behavior, and the use of seclusion and restraint.

Stress-Vulnerability Model of Agression

There are many and varied causes of violent behavior, some more social and some more medical in nature. It is most helpful to think of violence as the outcome of a dynamic interaction between numerous factors both intrinsic and extrinsic to the individual, some of which promote and some of which ameliorate the potential for violent behavior at any given moment. This is a stress-vulnerability model. Education may provide alternatives to violence, but delirium may cause an otherwise nonviolent person to misinterpret healthcare efforts. Their education is of no benefit in the delirious state. Hence, they become violent under circumstances that would not normally be sufficient to provoke a violent outburst. Some patients, on the other hand, come from cultures in which violence is viewed positively, and these patients require little stress or provocation before responding violently.

In the ED, likely medical sources of vulnerability include metabolic derangements, drug and/or alcohol intoxication, withdrawal syndromes, seizure disorders, head trauma, psychotic states, and personality disorders. Additionally, patients with severe pain, delirium, or extreme anxiety can respond to the efforts of emergency personnel with resistance, hostility, or frank aggression.

Substance Abuse

The association between substance abuse and violence is well established. Alcohol is found in the offender, the victim, or both in one half to two third of homicides and serious assaults.[11] Substance abuse is seldom the sole cause, but may contribute to violence in a number of ways. The direct pharmacologic effects include disinhibition and misinterpretation, suspiciousness, or paranoia. Psychological effects of substance use include cultural expectations of appropriate behavior under the influence and the ability to excuse or disavow inappropriate behavior that occurs while intoxicated. Substance use then interacts with other physiologic, cognitive, psychological, situational, and cultural factors including any mental illness. A tripartite model has been described: (1) systemic violence related to drug distribution, (2) economic compulsive violence associated with the criminal activity necessary to sustain a drug habit, and (3) psychopharmacologic violence resulting from the direct effects of the particular drug.[19]

Mental Illness

The relationship between mental illness and violence is also complex. Efforts made to destigmatize mental illness have confused the issue, but it seems clear that mental illness is associated with a greater risk for violence. In one large epidemiologic study, the prevalence of violence for those with no disorder was 2%. Schizophrenia was associated with an 8% rate of violent behavior, and other mental disorders were all similar at approximately 12%. But of all respondents reporting violent behaviors, 42% had a substance use disorder. Substance use more than tripled the rate of violence for schizophrenics. For various reasons, mental illness appears to reduce the threshold for aggression; and the more comorbid conditions present, the greater the risk.[41]

However, antisocial personality is the condition most strongly associated with both substance abuse and aggression. In one study, when the history of juvenile deviance was controlled, alcohol—the drug most commonly associated with violence—accounted for only 2% of the violent behavior.

In conclusion, some aggressive behavior is attributable to the direct pharmacologic effects of substances, but probably represents a modest fraction. Substances are also a part of the setting of violent behavior in the community, a coincidental part of the lifestyle of violent individuals; and both substance use and violence are related to common underlying characteristics such as character disorder.

Assessment

The comprehensive evaluation of the violent patient should include a complete physical examination. The examination may reveal the underlying cause of the violent behavior as well as insuring the treatment of any secondary patient injuries. Laboratory analysis of blood chemistry, a complete blood count, and diagnostic imaging as guided by the examination and available clinical history may also be helpful.

Illicit drug and alcohol abuse often present with symptoms of violence. Acute intoxication with cocaine can produce extreme psychomotor agitation, delirium, and transient psychosis characterized by paranoia and hallucinations; a clinically indistinguishable syndrome can be seen following the ingestion of amphetamines. Phencyclidine intoxication is manifested by assaultiveness, muscle rigidity, dysarthria, nystagmus, autonomic instability, and ataxia. Alcohol intoxication is characterized by typical signs of cerebellar dysfunction (slurred speech, gait ataxia, and incoordination); however, persons who are intoxicated are also at risk for violent behavior. Cannabis does not typically produce violent or aggressive behavior; however, paranoia can occur with intoxication and can secondarily promote reactions of extreme fear associated with distorted perception; the same can be said for intoxication with LSD and psilocybin, particularly in the naive user.

Withdrawal syndromes from specific drugs can also promote aggressive behavior as a consequence of physical discomfort or anticipatory anxiety. Opioid withdrawal is characterized by myalgias, rhinorrhea, and piloerection; alcohol, benzodiazepines, and barbiturates share a common syndrome of autonomic hyperreactivity and subsequent delirium. Patients suffering from any of the these signs and symptoms may become aggressive, verbally abusive, or threatening; prompt recognition of these syndromes and immediate treatment can prevent some aggressive outbursts. Because drug use is often concealed, is difficult to ascertain on clinical grounds, and frequently contributes to violent behavior, urine toxicologic studies may be useful to enhance the understanding and long-range treatment of some patients.

Delirium can be a cause of aggression. Patients are often suddenly confused, frightened, or frankly psychotic as a result of impaired perception. Patients may require sedation or restraint in order to prevent injury; some guidelines for this will be presented in the next section.

Although persons suffering from psychotic disorders are not generally aggressive, there are aspects of a the psychotic state that place patients at risk for aggressive behavior. Paranoid ideation can serve to promote misperceptions of impending bodily harm ("They're trying to kill me"), sexual victimization ("Men and women are raping me"), and humiliation ("Everyone is laughing at me"). It follows that these fearful perceptions might provoke violent reactions in a patient. Hallucinations can cause aggression, either as a result of command hallucinations or due to the anxiety and irritation that patients experience with loud or persistent "voices." Persons with either borderline or antisocial personality disorder are at risk for violent acting-out as a result of poor impulse control.

Treatment

The pharmacotherapy of violent behavior seeks to quell psychomotor agitation and concomitant psychosis. As aggression derives from varied and multiple etiologies, it follows that there is much debate about the specific sedative used, the route of administration, and the dosing interval. Studies examining the treatment of aggression and/or agitation have included such diverse populations as schizophrenics, acutely intoxicated patients (alcohol), trauma patients, postoperative patients, patients in alcohol withdrawal, and patients with presumed personality disorders. Treatment settings for these studies included psychiatric inpatient units, intensive care units, and the ED.[1,9,25–27] An excellent review examined a number of these studies and found that both benzodiazepines and neuroleptics afforded relief of agitation and aggression.[13] It seems, however, that there are specific clinical situations when benzodiazepines and neuroleptics might be preferentially used. Haloperidol has been safely used in the treatment of agitation and aggression in patients with psychoses, alcohol intoxication, and delirium.[2,9,25,26] The drug can be administered orally, intravenously, or intramuscularly; dosing intervals range from 30 minutes to 2 hours. The usual regimen is 5 mg haloperidol given every 30 to 60 minutes; most patients respond after 1 to 3 doses. The dose of haloperidol needed to achieve sedation rarely exceeds a total of 50 mg. Benzodiazepines are also quite effective for tranquilization; their use has been examined in patients with psychoses, stimulant intoxication, and postoperative agitation.[1,18,29,30] Lorazepam 1 to 2 mg may be given orally or parenterally and repeated at 30 or 60-minute intervals, respectively, until the patient is calm. As diazepam is poorly absorbed from intramuscular sites, the preferred route of adminisration is intravenous or oral. Diazepam may be given 5 to 10 mg IV with repeat dosing as needed; concerns about respiratory depression mandate careful observation of patients receiving tranquilization with these agents. Diazepam may have a unique role in the treatment of agitation secondary to cocaine intoxication, as seizures may emerge in this syndrome (see Chap. 65). Neuroleptics, particularly low-potency neuroleptics, are known to lower seizure threshold in animals, so their use in patients with cocaine intoxication may be limited. Studies have examined the use of combinations of lorazepam with neuroleptics in patients with psychiatric illness and delirium; it appears that the combination of benzodiazepine and neuroleptic afforded relief of psychotic symptoms while allowing for a reduced dose of neuroleptic.[2,10,39]

Physical Restraint

Seclusion and restraint are also used in the treatment of violent behavior. Seclusion can help to diminish environmental stimuli and thereby reduce hyperreactivity; it is not commonly used in the medical ED, so its use will not be discussed in great detail here. However, a few reminders are worthwhile to mention: as seclusion is defined by a condition of very limited interactive and environmental cues, it is not indicated for patients with unstable medical conditions, delirium, dementia, self-injurious behavior (cutting, head-banging), or who are suffering extrapyramidal reactions to antipsychotic medication.[3] Restraint is used to prevent patient and staff injury. All facilities should have clear written policy guidelines for restraint that address monitoring, provisions for patient comfort, and documentation.

Training

Finally, it has been shown that training in the management of aggression helps to reduce violence and injuries through the early identification of impending episodes of violence, use of verbal techniques to defuse incidents, and appropriate physical techniques to minimize injuries in those that occur. It behooves the healthcare provider to maintain his or her skills through training and to advocate for continuing medical education on this topic at the workplace.[7]

Acknowledgment

Cherie Elfenbein, MD, contributed to this chapter in a previous edition.

References

1. Abel RM, Reis RL: Intravenous diazepam for sedation following cardiac operations: Clinical and hemodynamic assessments. Anesth Analg 1971;50:244–248.
2. Adams F: Neuropsychiatric evaluation and treatment of delirium in the critically ill cancer patient. Cancer Bull 1984;36:156–160.
3. American Psychiatric Association: Clinician Safety. Task force report no. 33. Washington, DC, American Psychiatric Association, 1992.
4. American Psychiatric Association: The Principles of Medical Ethics With Annotations Especially Applicable to Psychiatry. Washington, DC, American Psychiatric Association, 1989.
5. Barraclough B, Bunch J, Nelson B, Sainsbury P: A hundred cases of suicide: Clinical aspects. Br J Psychiatry 1974; 125: 355–373.
6. Bick PA, Hannah AL: Intramuscular lorazepam to restrain violent patients. Lancet 1986;1:206. Letter.
7. Carmel H, Hunter M: Compliance with training in managing assaultive behavior and injuries from inpatient violence. Hosp Community Psychiatry 1990;41:558–560.
8. Clayton PJ: Suicide. Psychiatr Clin North Am 1985;8: 203–214.
9. Clinton JE, Sterner S, Steimachers Z, Ruiz E: Haloperidol for sedation of disruptive emergency patients. Ann Emerg Med 1987;16:319–322.
10. Cohen S, Khan A, Johnson S: Pharmacological management of manic psychosis in an unlocked setting. J Clin Psychopharmacol 1987;7:261–264.
11. Collins JJ, Schlenger WE: Acute and chronic effects of alcohol use on violence. J Stud Alcohol 1988;49:516–522.
12. Crome P: The toxicity of drugs used for suicide. Acta Psychiatr Scand 1993;371 (suppl): 33–37.
13. Dubin W: Rapid tranquilization: Antipsychotics or benzodiazepines? J Clin Psychiatry 1988;49(suppl 12):5–12.
14. Fawcett J, Clark DC, Busch KA: Assessing and treating the patient at risk for suicide. Psychiatr Ann 1993;23:244–255.
15. Fawcett J, Scheftner WA, Fogg L, et al: Time-related predictors of suicide in major affective disorder. Am J Psychiatry 1990;144:923–926.
16. Frances A, Blumenthal S: Personality as a predictor of youthful suicide. In: Risk Factors for Youth Suicide. Report of the Secretary's Task Force on Youth Suicide, Vol. 2. Alcohol, Drug Abuse, and Mental Health Administration. DHHS pub. No. (ADM) 89–1624. Washington, DC, U.S. Government Printing Office, 1989, pp. 160–171.
17. Garza-Trevino E, Hollister LE, Overall JE, Alexander WF: Efficacy of combinations of intramuscular antipsychotics and sedative-hypnotics for control of psychotic agitation. Am J Psychiatry 1989;146:1598–1601.
18. Goldfrank LR, Hoffman RS: The cardiovascular effects of cocaine. Ann Emerg Med 1991;20:165–175.
19. Goldstein PJ: The drugs–violence nexus: A tripartite conceptual framework. J Drug Issues 1986;15:493–506.
20. Hagnell O, Lanke J, Rorsman B: Suicide rates in the Lundby study: Mental illness as a risk factor for suicide. Neuropsychobiology 1981;7:248–253.
21. Henry, JA: A fatal toxicity index for antidepressant poisoning. Acta Psychiatr Scand 1989;354:37–45.
22. Hoffman RS, Wipfler MG, Maddaloni MA, Weisman RS: The effect of the triplicate benzodiazepine prescription regulation on sedative-hypnotic overdoses. NY State J Med 1991;91:436–439.
23. Kovacs M, Beck A, Weissman A: The communication of suicidal intent. Arch Gen Psychiatry 1976;33:198–201.
24. Lavoie F, Carter G, Danzi D, Berg R: Emergency department violence in United States teaching hospitals. Ann Emerg Med 1988;17:1227–1233.
25. Lenehan G, Gastfriend DR, Stetler C: Use of haloperidol in the management of agitated or violent, alcohol-intoxicated patients in the emergency department: A pilot study. J Emerg Nurs 1985;11:72–79.
26. Lerner Y, Lwow E, Levitin A, Belmaker R: Acute high-dose parenteral haloperidol treatment of psychosis. Am J Psychiatry 1979;136:1061–1064.
27. McClish A, Andrew D, Tetreault L: Intravenous diazepam for psychiatric reactions following open heart surgery. Can Anaesth Soc J 1968;15:63–79.
28. Meehl PE: Psychodiagnosis: Selected papers. Minneapolis, University of Minnesota Press, 1973.

29. Modell JG: Further experience and observations with lorazepam in the management of behavioral agitation. J Clin Psychopharmacol 1986;6:385–387. Letter.
30. Modell JG, Lenox RH, Weiner S: Inpatient clinical trial of lorazepam for the management of manic agitation. J Clin Psychopharmacol 1985;5:109–113.
31. Monk M: Epidemiology of suicide. Epidemiol Rev 1987; 9:51–69.
32. Moscicki EK, O'Carroll P, Rae DS, et al: Suicide attempts in the epidemiologic catchment area study. Yale J Biol Med 1988;61:259–268.
33. Nutter DO, Massumi RA: Diazepam in cardioversion. N Engl J Med 1965;273:650–651.
34. Pane G, Winiarski A, Salness K: Aggression directed toward emergency department staff at a university teaching hospital. Ann Emerg Med 1991;20:283–286.
35. Rich CL, Young D, Fowler RC: San Diego suicide study, I: Young vs. old subjects. Arch Gen Psychiatry 1986;43: 577–582.
36. Robins E, Gassner S, Kayes J, et al: The communication of suicidal intent: A study of 134 consecutive cases of successful (completed) suicide. Am J Psychiatry 1959;115:724–733.
37. Robins E, Murphy GE, Wilkinson RH, et al: Some clinical considerations in the prevention of suicide based on a study of 134 successful suicides. Am J Public Health 1959;49: 888–889.
39. Salzman C, Green A, Rodriguez-Villa F, et al: Benzodiazepines combined with neuroleptics for management of severe disruptive behavior. Psychosomatics 1986; 27(suppl): 17–21.
40. Stone MH: The course of borderline personality disorder. In: Tasman A, Hales RE, Frances AJ, eds: Review of Psychiatry, Vol. 8. Washington, DC, American Psychiatric Press, 1989.
41. Swanson J, Holzer C, Ganju V, Jono R: Violence and psychiaric disorder in the community: Evidence from the Epidemiologic Catchment Area Survey. Hosp Commun Psychiatry 1990; 41:761–770.
42. U. S. Department of Commerce. Statistical Abstracts of the United States, 116th ed, 1996.

CHAPTER 114

Nursing Principles

Susan Callaghan-Montella and Barbara E. Soppet

Management of the poisoned patient requires an integrated response on the part of healthcare providers of all disciplines. This chapter offers specific considerations with regard to general management and a detailed approach to patient evaluation. The discussion is not intended to be specific only to nurses or assume that the nurse's role in care is limited to these points. The collaborative roles of all emergency care providers consistently overlap, and it is this spontaneous team response that is essential for successful resuscitation. The necessity of professional collaboration is particularly evident in the areas of assessment, physical findings, toxidrome identification, and in the implementation of all aspects of standard medical management (see Chaps. 3 and 30).

The optimal approach to the poisoned patient as a nursing process is assessment, planning, implementation, and evaluation. However, as in the medical management of the poisoned or overdosed patient (Chaps. 3 and 30), the customary sequence of evaluation must sometimes be altered to address each particular clinical situation. With respect to the patient with an altered level of consciousness, even before the full assessment is performed, the airway must be stabilized, the cervical spine protected, and supplemental oxygen, dextrose, thiamine, and naloxone must be administered. In the case of a severly agitated patient who is breathing but combative, physical and chemical restraints to assure patient and staff safety preclude a full patient assessment. Only after immediate life-threatening issues are addressed can the formal nursing process begin. If the patient arrives in the emergency department (ED) awake, alert, and oriented, the standardized clinical approach should be initiated immediately (Table 114–1).

Triage: Initial Assessment of the Patient

Often, the first healthcare professional to evaluate a patient in the ED is the triage nurse. Information crucial to diagnosis and treatment may be available only at this early encounter before the patient's consciousness becomes altered as a result of a CNS depressant. An astute, inquisitive, and intuitive triage assessment often results in initiation of the necessary therapy and avoidance of subsequent mortality and morbidity.

The triage (from the French "to sort") nurse separates the emergent and urgent patients from the nonurgent and establishes the priority of care. In doing this, the nurse must perform another vital function, which is to sort out critical information that may identify a particular toxic syndrome, thus allowing for more timely intervention. The practitioner's ability to obtain and use the vital signs, together with the information provided to the examiner's senses of sight, touch, and smell, can provide valuable clues to the nature of an ingestion.

CASE PRESENTATION. A young woman was brought to the ED by two friends who stated that she suddenly collapsed at a party approximately 20 minutes ago, and that she had been moaning in response to stimuli until arrival at the ED. The friends stated that they did not know her medical history. They described the patient as an occasional social contact and then rapidly left the ED.

Vital signs were: blood pressure, 100/60 mm Hg; pulse, 110 beats/min; respirations shallow, at 6 breaths/min. The patient's respirations were immediately assisted via bag valve mask with 100% O_2, and she was placed on a pulse oximeter and cardiac monitor. An endotracheal tube was inserted for continued airway management and respiratory therapy was called. A rectal temperature registered 101°F (38.3°C) and the patient was completely undressed for a secondary survey and IV insertion. The radiology technician was notified of the need for a portable chest radiograph to check for pathology and to verify endotracheal tube placement.

The patient appeared to be in her early to mid-20s, was disheveled, but had good personal hygiene (perfume, manicured nails, tasteful makeup) and was expensively dressed and bejeweled. She was unresponsive to all verbal stimuli and reacted to painful stimuli by withdrawing her extremities. The odor of alcohol was noted on her breath. Her pupils were equal and sluggishly reactive to light. There were no signs of chest, abdominal, or head trauma. No Battle sign, raccoon eyes, otorrhea, or rhinorrhea were noted. Her abdomen

TABLE 114–1. STANDARD NURSING CARE PLAN FOR THE POISONED PATIENT: MANAGEMENT OF THE ADULT IN THE EMERGENCY DEPARTMENT

Assessment

Objective—Triage Examination (categorize patient's emergency)

Check airway: Is it open and clear? Can patient speak, cough? Are there obvious signs of head or neck trauma?

Check breathing: Presence or absence, rate, rhythm, abnormal breath sounds?

Check circulation: Assess pulse, blood pressure, skin color and temperature, capillary refill, cutaneous moisture.

Neurologic status: Level of consciousness, pupils, movement of extremities, gag reflex.

General appearance: Dress, body size, tissue turgor, cleanliness, wounds, bruises, marks on skin, odor of breath.

Subjective—Brief History (if patient is alert and/or obtain details from those accompanying patient)

Chief complaint

Name of substance taken

Route of administration

Amount taken

Time taken

Time of onset of symptoms

Past medical history

Maintenance medications

Allergies, risk factors

Prehospital treatment initiated at the scene by EMS personnel

Intervention (Fig. 3–1)

Administer oxygen via nasal cannula or face mask (if patient is breathing), or initiate respirations with pocket mask or bag value mask with 100% oxygen (if patient is not breathing).

Stabilize neck if appropriate.

Insert oral or nasal airway as necessary.

Clear patient's secretions with suction if necessary.

Check equipment for proper functioning; assist physician with intubation.

Request chest radiograph.

Obtain vital signs, including rectal temperature; place patient on a cardiac monitor and pulse oximeter. If pulse is absent, proceed with appropriate resuscitation care plan. Remove all clothing.

Initiate IV therapy, using a macrodrip, initially, and D_5W or 0.9% sodium chloride solution.

Draw blood for serum glucose, CBC, BUN, electrolytes, ABGs, and appropriate toxicology testing. Test blood with glucose indicator strip. Beta HCG if appropriate.

Secure 12-lead ECG.

Prepare naloxone first and then D_5W and thiamine for administration.

Rapidly evaluate patient's response, neurologic status, and vital signs.

Evaluate the need for physical restraint if patient is agitated and/or uncooperative.

If Patient Is Conscious

Check gag reflex.

Prepare to administer medication to induce emesis if appropriate (Chaps. 3 and 30).

Provide fluid to drink after administration of medication.

Provide a large emesis basin and tissues.

Have functional suction unit ready.

Keep the patient in open, observable area.

Prepare activated charcoal and cathartic, if appropriate.

If Patient Is Unconscious

Protect airway with intubation, when indicated.

Prepare for gastric lavage with orogastric tube, if appropriate (Chaps. 3 and 30).

Following lavage, administer activated charcoal and a cathartic.

Consider potential need for a specific antidote.

Evaluation—Monitor

Vital signs, include repeat temperature.

Cardiac monitoring; pulse oximetry; 12-lead ECG.

Rapid head-to-toe assessment.

Response to emetic (if given) or orogastric lavage and cathartic.

Urine flow (output).

Oral and IV fluids given (input).

Emotional status—evaluate need for psychiatric consultation and/or social worker assessment if patient is stable.

Prepare patient for admission to hospital or continued observation and inform family and friends.

If patient is discharged, after medical and psychiatric clearance, provide patient and family members with discharge instructions and follow-up care; ensure, through feedback, that instructions are understood.

was soft and not distended. Physical inspection revealed no lacerations, bruises, abrasions, or hematomas, but a small, fresh puncture wound was noted at the left antecubital fossa. A search of her property identified her as M.S., age 28, single, and currently working in an advertising agency as an assistant manager of production. No medic alert bracelet, allergy, or medical information was found. The Poison Control Center was notified and all data obtained from the primary and secondary survey was related.

After intravenous administration of 100 mg of thiamine, 100 mL of $D_{50}W$, and 2 mg of naloxone, the patient began to resist ventilation and attempted to remove the endotracheal tube. The nurse calmed the patient, held her hands away from the airway, explained what had happened, and urged her to cooperate. The patient relaxed a bit and within one-half hour became lethargic, lapsing again into unconsciousness. A second dose of 0.4 mg of naloxone produced improvement in the patient's level of consciousness without producing agitation, and a continuous infusion of naloxone titrated to a therapeutic patient response was initiated to allow the patient to breathe effectively (see Chap. 60).

The patient's level of consciousness later improved, but once again the patient attempted to remove her endotracheal tube. She responded to verbal reassurances but soon thrashed about, pulling the tube and shaking her head. Although it appeared that she had become more cooperative in response to antidotal therapy, it was important to ensure that this improved level of consciousness was neither transient nor posed a threat to her overall therapy.

The first priority of the triage nurse is to initiate a primary survey and identify any immediate life-threatening problems necessitating treatment. This patient was noted to be in respiratory distress upon admission to the ED. Therefore, immediate airway management with appropriate attention to the possibility of head/cervical spine injury must be accomplished before assessment proceeds. Once airway, breathing, bleeding, and circulation are assessed and stabilized (see "General Acute Management" later in the chapter; and also Chaps. 3 and 30 and Fig. 3–1), the next task is to establish the database necessary for ongoing management of the patient. The questions that need to be asked as part of patient assessment and sequence of care are covered in the next sections.

Who Is This Patient? The patient's age, sex, general appearance, skin hygiene, mental status, physical findings, and social, family, and medical history are all potential clues to the development of a differential diagnosis, priority assessment, and plan of care.

Unfortunately, in poisoned patients, a history is not always readily available. Often the patient is unaccompanied and unable to offer details of his or her illness. Hence, prehospital teams become potential sources of very valuable data: Were there family, friends, or neighbors present? Was any important information secured from this source? What relevant prehospital clinical data are available? What was the condition at the scene? Was there a suicide note? Were there any signs of ingestion—pill bottles, "syringes," tablets, or capsules? Remember that the label may not reflect the substance that was actually in the bottle. The need to initiate therapy rapidly often precludes waiting for laboratory results. Changes in level of consciousness, associated with pupilary findings and vital signs, may represent toxidromes that alert the nurse to asssociated toxins such as opioids, sympathomimetics, cholinergics, and anticholinergics (see Chap. 17 and Table 17–2).

In the present case, no obvious means of securing a history is evident. Thus, the triage nurse must use alternative measures and a knowledge of toxidromes to develop a definitive plan of care. What precipitated this acute episode and the patient's present medical condition?

If the patient has ingested a toxic substance, what drug or substance was taken? Is there any characteristic odor that might indicate a specific ingestion or clinical condition? The odor of vomitus, sweat, and urine, as well as the color and quality of stool, can be diagnostic. Are there characteristic physical signs? Some physical symptoms may be masked by the ingestion of multiple substances, which often have opposing or confounding toxicologic effects. Is alcohol responsible for the patient's condition? Has it been ingested in addition to other substances, and can it potentiate their effects? Were any remedies initiated by the friends? Are there any diagnoses, other than a toxic ingestion, that might present in this fashion; and, if so, how must immediate management be altered? What additional tests are necessary to evaluate the patient?

In this case we only know that the patient was at a party and suddenly collapsed. No empty pill bottles, works, or drugs were found on her person. Alcohol (its congeners) was noted on her breath, and a single, fresh puncture wound is noted on her right antecubital fossa. The presence of a toxin abused intravenously, as well as alcohol, were suspected. However, these symptoms cannot be attributed to alcohol based on odor alone: a blood alcohol level is needed. In addition, the ingestion of additional substances, not readily evident but responsible for the symptoms noted, must always be anticipated. Reporting to the poison center offers a discussion with experts and clinical follow-up in cases of toxic ingestions. Collaboration with these specialists potentiates immediate patient management and clinical follow-up. The poison control staff's awareness of new trends and "fad" drugs can assist clinicians in the initial understanding and management.

Where Did the Exposure Occur? Is the time of the ingestion known? Was the patient at home, alone, or at a social gathering? Was the ingestion taken in a secluded or hidden place? Such information may reveal whether there was a purpose to the patient's exposure. Was it an intentional or unintentional exposure? A toxic ingestion taken in a secluded hotel room should suggest the possibility of a suicide attempt, which would necessitate additional clinical interventions, both acute and long term. A positive pregnancy test in a patient of childbearing age may be a determining factor in decisions about specific supportive measures. Is a pregnancy responsible for the ED presentation or is it a coincidental finding? Does the pregnancy contraindicate any otherwise routine therapies?

This ingestion occurred at a party, where, according to friends, the patient collapsed just minutes prior to her arrival in the ED. The puncture wound on her arm was still fresh, probably having been inflicted recently. Although the possibility of depression and intentional overdose were not excluded, the patient's participation at a party and the rapid departure by her friends pointed more to the possibility of substance abuse.

When Did the Exposure Occur? It is necessary to determine how much time has elapsed since the exposure and how much of the drug can be expected to be absorbed. These factors affect general management (eg, gastric lavage and activated charcoal or activated charcoal alone) as well as decisions regarding toxin-specific antidotes or tertiary care procedures (eg, hemoperfusion and hemodialysis).

The time of year and climatic conditions must be noted, especially in the case of patients found on the street. Environmental conditions can rapidly alter thermoregulation in the drug-overdosed patient. Hypothermia or hyperthermia require a comprehensive care plan. The need for a rectal temperature is therefore an integral part of admission vital signs. If the patient's temperature is at either extreme of a traditional thermometer, there is a suspicion of hypothermia or hyperthermia, or the patient is agitated or uncooperative, a thermocouple (or other indwelling temperature device that can monitor the extremes of temperature of 60 to 120°F [15.5 to 48.9°C]) should be used. Both hypothermia and hyperthermia may cause an altered mental status and may prevent a response or signs of a response to appropriate therapeutics. In addition, the patient's temperature may provide clues to the possibility of a pre-existing or concommittant disease process that must be considered in developing a plan of care.

How Did This Emergency Occur? What route of exposure was used? Was it a planned event or unintentional due to ignorance or impaired judgment? Was this event a manifestation of chronic abuse? What implements were used? Were any other substances taken that might potentiate the effects of the toxic substances?

Because this patient had an injection site, it was assumed the route of poisoning was intravenous, but this did not preclude the presence of additional substances or additional quantities of the same substance absorbed via another route. The odor of alcohol implicated at least a second substance. The fact that the patient was at a party, and in view of a continuing high incidence of substance abuse, there was a significant suspicion of polypharmaceutical drug abuse. No information was available with regard to the patient's premorbid psychological state.

Given the patient's obtunded condition, an episode of significant bradypnea, and the additional data secured by objective assessment, the patient must be triaged as emergent to the critical care area to be managed as a toxic exposure.

General Acute Management: Planning and Intervention

The nursing and medical roles in this phase of care are quite similar and interdependent, and thus the nurse should be reasonably comfortable with the recognition of common toxic syndromes so as to anticipate tasks of care and facilitate their delivery. The nurse must coordinate the patient's immediate physical care as it relates to immediate survival as well as overall well-being (Tables 114–1 and 114–2). Priority must be given to life-threatening aspects. Assessment, plan implementation/intervention, and evaluation may, therefore, be applied in a systematic manner to both immediate and ongoing therapy considerations. (Nursing care interventions for emergency management: A quick reference tool may be found in Table 114–3.)

The first therapeutic consideration is airway management. Patients with suspected toxic ingestion who enter the hospital with respiratory compromise, initially require assisted ventilation. The American Heart Association's guidelines suggest that mouth-to-mask or bag valve mask techniques be used to minimize any possibility of infectious disease contamination. Whenever possible, two people should be present, one controlling ventilation with the bag and the other maintaining head position and face-mask seal. An oxygen reservoir and 100% oxygen should be attached to the bag. Patients with opioid overdoses frequently respond to naloxone prior to intubation, and management of the airway with mouth-to-mask or bag valve mask devices may be all that is required until an improved level of consciousness is achieved. For patients who do not require intubation, oral airways are tolerated only by unconscious patients lacking a gag reflex. Nasal airways should be used in conscious patients who require an airway but have an intact gag reflex.

For a conscious but lethargic patient who needs only supplemental oxygen, many types of airway adjuncts are available. It is important not to confuse the nonrebreathing mask, delivering 95 to 100% oxygen, with the rebreather mask, which delivers an FIO_2 of only 50 to 60%. Awareness of the idiosyncrasies of various types of Venturi masks and the manufacturer's recommendations for assembly eliminate unnecessary confusion under emergent circumstances. Some patients may tolerate nasal cannulas better than face masks, because they are less confining, but "mouth breathers" fare better clinically with masks.

When a nurse receives a patient who is intubated and being ventilated via bag valve mask, tube placement and the presence of breath sounds should be verified. Reassessment includes vital signs, pulse oximetry, level of consciousness, cardiovascular and neurologic status, the need for ongoing ventilatory support, and the approach to maintaining adequate circulation. The patient must then be undressed completely and a rapid head-to-toe assessment performed. The presence of a gag reflex, speech quality, recall of events, and emotional state are evaluated. Pupil size and reactivity, extraocular movements, and the presence of nystagmus, tremors, weakness, paralysis, and paresthesias should be noted as well as any other physical findings.

Frequently injected substances potentially responsible for the patient's level of unconsciousness include heroin and cocaine. Heroin could certainly be responsible for this patient's near respiratory arrest but would not fully explain the temperature of 38.3°C and the tachycardia without suggesting other concomitant drug use or complications, such as aspiration pneumonitis, endocarditis, or a mixed heroin-cocaine overdose.

Cocaine, on the other hand, is often associated with hyperthermia, atrial and ventricular dysrhythmias, as well as acute myocardial infarction. Cardiac monitoring in this patient is essential, with monitor rate alarms set and functioning. Heart rate as part of a toxidrome, can offer a valuable clue to the identification of the ingested substance. After immediate life-threatening measures have been completed, a 12-lead ECG should be done to search for dysrhythmias and/or conduction abnormali-

TABLE 114–2. EXAMPLES OF NURSING DIAGNOSES IN TOXICOLOGIC EMERGENCIES

Fear	Ineffective breathing pattern
Infection	Injury
Altered body temperature	Poisoning
Altered bowel elimination	Aspiration
Fluid volume deficit	Violence
Decreased cardiac output	Sensory/perceptual alteration
Altered tissue perfusion	Self-esteem disturbance
Impaired gas exchange	Ineffective coping
Ineffective airway clearance	

TABLE 114–3. ALPHABETIC TOOL TO ASSIST IN ASSESSMENT AND STABILIZATION OF THE PATIENT WITH A TOXICOLOGIC EMERGENCY

Airway and Antidote	Control airway using C-spine precautions as needed. Consider need for immediate and specific antidote by history or examination (eg, naloxone, cyanide antidote kit, removal and/or irrigation of noxious, topical agents).
Breathing and Behavior Control	Place on O_2 (mask or bag-valve-mask as needed). Does behavior warrant either physical or chemical restraint? Are there contraindications?
Circulation and Coma Antidotes	Check pulse; start CPR if absent. Start IV. Place on cardiac monitor and pulse oximetry. Administer ($D_{50}W$, thiamine, and naloxone) only if indicated.
Drug Elimination	Decontaminate. Emesis or orogastric lavage if indicated. Administer activated charcoal and cathartic as needed. Continue irrigation for topical contamination. Consider specific antidote, if not already initiated.
Expose, Examine, Evaluate	Perform a quick examination after completely undressing the patient.
Fluid Management	Is the patient in need of a fluid bolus? Are there any specific drips that should be initiated (eg, naloxone or sodium bicarbonate)?
Get Vital Signs and Diagnostic Tests	Obtain a complete set of vital signs including core temperature to rule out hypo/hyperthermia. Obtain routine bloodwork and U/A, and consider blood and urine for toxicology testing. Obtain ABG, ECG, and chest radiograph. Consider other radiographs or tests that may be needed to exclude injury or other complications (eg, C-spine radiograph, carboxyhemoglobin level).
Head-to-Toe and History	Look for hidden clues. Do a complete and thorough reevaluation of the patient. Obtain a detailed history from ambulance personnel or significant other.
Initiate Consultation	Contact psychiatric or social service consults. Consider other specialty consultations as necessary.

ties. When frequent blood pressure evaluation is necessary an external blood pressure monitor should be considered if an arterial line has not been inserted. Assisted ventilation must also be provided due to the patient's respiratory depression and the strong clinical suspicion of opioid overdose. Respiratory therapy should be notified to provide continuous ventilatory support and ongoing monitoring of ventilation–perfusion adequacy.

Once an IV has been established and fluid replacement initiated, specific management may necessitate IV medication administration. Many nurses develop shortcuts to calculate IV fluid infusion time and flow rates. We recommend preprinted readily accessible IV drip tickets in the ED for frequently used IV drips. These precalculated dose charts also serve as markers on the IV bottles. Infusion pumps that automatically deliver precalculated doses in a predetermined time frame are ideal for use in a busy ED.

As thiamine, 50% dextrose, and naloxone are administered intravenously, documentation of the patient's response to therapy and anticipation of the need for further interventions and complications of care become the priorities of the nurse. Acutely, a depressed sensorium secondary to hypoglycemia or opioid overdose may respond to these antidotes ($D_{50}W$ and naloxone, respectively), whereas a patient with Wernicke's encephalopathy will have an immediate biochemical benefit and a delayed clinical response to thiamine. When and how the patient responds, as well as the duration of the response, yield clues to the etiology of the obtundation and thus to further management strategies. If the only etiology is an injected opioid, then an immediate response to naloxone is anticipated, varying in intensity from slow, appropriate movement to violent thrashing, associated with retching and coughing around the endotracheal tube. The nurse must be alert to these possibilities to prevent the patient from tube dislocation, self-inflicted injury, and in the case of the nonintubated patient, aspiration. The nurse then reevaluates any change in status to determine whether additional therapies are appropriate or whether some previous interventions may be discontinued (Table 114–4).

In the poisoned or overdosed patient with respiratory and/or cardiovascular compromise, intravenous insertions can be difficult. Naloxone—as well as atropine, epinephrine, and lidocaine—can be administered via the endotracheal tube if necessary, as they are well absorbed through the tracheobronchial tree.

An additional consideration is that an opioid is not the only substance responsible for the patient's CNS depression; other substances present could continue to cause CNS depression, and therefore any additional substances present in the GI tract may need to be evacuated or adsorbed to prevent absorption. Coexisting illnesses or injuries can also complicate management decisions. Consideration must be given to whether additional diagnostic studies, such as a head CT, might provide further information significant for the treatment plan.

text continues on page 1799

TABLE 114–4. ANTIDOTES FOR GENERAL MANAGEMENT

Poison: Acetaminophen

Antidote

N-Acetylcysteine (NAC, Mucomyst)

Action

Detoxifies toxic metabolite (enhances glutathione synthesis) early and mediates inflammatory response late (>24 h) after ingestion.

Nursing Considerations

Unpleasant odor. Should be diluted to a 5% concentration from a 20% solution, by a 1:3 ratio with water, fruit juice, or carbonated beverage. Must be used within 1 h of dilution. After opening, can be stored in refrigerator for 96 h. Repeat dose if vomiting occurs within 1 h of administration. May try antiemetic (Metoclopramide) or NG tube for persistent vomiting. If repeat-dose activated charcoal indicated for coingestant separate by at least 1–2 h.

Poison: Acetylcholinesterase Inhibitors (organophosphate pesticides and carbamate insecticides)

Antidote

Atropine

Action

Antagonist to acetylcholine; blocks muscarinic and CNS manifestations.

Nursing Considerations

If patient is placed on a drip, use 20-mL vials. Hundreds of mg may be used in massive poisoning. Maximal oxygenation should be achieved before atropine administration to avoid risk of ventricular tachydysrhythmias associated with atropine. This may not be achievable, however, without atropine, when copious secretions and bronchospasm are present. Tachycardia is not a contraindication (may be due to hypoxia and autonomic stimulation). Heart rate may actually slow as oxygenation improves, although increases of 10–20 beats/min are not uncommon. Has no effect on skeletal muscle weakness or paralysis. Pupillary dilation is an early response and is not a therapeutic endpoint.

Poison: Acetylcholinesterase Inhibitors (organophosphate pesticides and carbamate insecticides)

Antidote

Pralidoxime chloride (2-PAM-chloride, Protopam)

Action

Restores acetylcholinesterase activity and detoxifies remaining organophosphate molecules.

Nursing Considerations

Protect the airway! After regaining consciousness, patients may become agitated. Transient dizziness and blurred vision may be related to rate of infusion. Avoid rapid IV bolus; respiratory and cardiac arrest may occur. Reduce rate or stop infusion if hypotension occurs. Rarely used alone. Works synergistically with atropine. Avoid dermal contact with the patient. Wash all dermal exposures with copious amounts of water. Wear protective clothing (gloves, gown). Dispose of contaminated clothing and leather.

Poison: Alcoholism / Malnutrition

Antidote

Thiamine hydrochloride

Action

Facilitates aerobic metabolism of glucose to ATP, linking glycolysis to the Krebs cycle. Also has a role in maintaining normal neuronal conduction.

Nursing Considerations

Given in conjunction with $D_{50}W$ to treat or to avoid development of Wernicke's encephalopathy in adults and adolescents. Thiamine is not routinely administered to children, unless they are malnourished.

Poison: Anticholinergics (eg, antihistamines, atropine, scopolamine, and some plants and mushrooms)

Antidote

Physostigmine sulfate

Action

Reverses coma, seizures, and severe myoclonic and choreoathetoid activity from anticholinergic poisons.

Nursing Considerations

Use only clear, colorless solutions. IM route is unacceptable due to erratic absorption. Establish airway, ventilation, and hemodynamic stabilization first. Patient should have a narrow QRS complex on both ECG and current monitor strip. Excessive use or too rapid administration may cause SLUDGE, bronchorrhea, seizures, bradycardia, and respiratory depression. Have atropine on hand, equal to one-half the dose of physostigmine given, to reverse cholinergic activity.

Poison: Anticoagulants (warfarin, superwarfarins)

Antidote

Vitamin K_1 (Mephyton, aquamephyton, konakion)

Action

Required for blood clotting; reverses anticoagulant deficiency, and is indicated for long-term control of bleeding.

(*continued*)

TABLE 114–4. ANTIDOTES FOR GENERAL MANAGEMENT (continued)

Nursing Considerations

Unless patient is critically ill, give by other means than IV route. IV route may cause anaphylactoid reaction and in a rare instance, death. Dilute only in D_5W, NS, or D_5NS, preservative-free solutions and infuse slowly to decrease risk of anaphylactoid reactions. Use oral preparations for long-term care. If more than 5 mL of the drug is required, the SC route cannot be used.

Poison: Arsenic

Antidote

2,3-dimercaprol (British-anti-lewisite, BAL)

Action

Heavy metal chelator.

Nursing Considerations

Contact of drug with skin may cause reactions. May also cause pain or abscess at injection site; rotate sites. Prolonged use of BAL may cause chelation of essential metals—monitor these levels (eg, copper). Maintaining alkaline urine may protect kidney from damage; monitor I&O. Has many adverse affects including hypertension, fever, diaphoresis, nausea, vomiting, headaches, salivation and lacrimation, and burning feeling of lips, mouth, and throat.

Poison: Beta-Adrenergic Antagonists, Calcium Channel Blockers, Sulfonylureas

Antidote

Glucagon

Action

Glucagon is a polypeptide hormone that stimulates the mobilization of glycogen. Normally, hypoglycemia stimulates glucagon release and intracellular glycogen is broken down to meet the energy needs of the body. It is also postulated that glucagon, by increasing cyclic AMP levels, is able to increase inotropic and chronotropic activity of the heart, thus antagonizing beta adrenergic antagonist effects on the heart.

Nursing Considerations

Glucagon is packaged as a powder with a phenol-based (2 mg/mL) diluent. An initial bolus dose of 50 μg/kg of glucagon is recommended and infused over 1 minute. Additional bolus or infusion doses may be necessary. Watch total phenol load in administering additional quantities. Dilute any additional vials with sterile water, not the phenol diluent. Watch for hypersensitivity, generalized allergic reactions. Nausea and vomiting can occur. Monitor cardiac status and vital signs for changes induced by inotropic and chronotropic effects. Glucagon may induce hyperglycemia and/or hypokalemia. Check electrolytes and watch for ECG changes or problems related to electrolyte shifts.

Poison: Cyanide

Antidote

Cyanide antidote kit (amyl nitrite pearls, 3% sodium nitrite, and 25% sodium thiosulfate)

Action

Nitrite-induced methemoglobinemia bind with cyanide to make cyanomethemoglobin. With the addition of thiosulfate and the enzyme rhodanese, the cyanomethemoglobin is converted to methemoglobin and thiocyanate, the latter being excreted in the urine.

Nursing Considerations

Check expiration dates of kit components (amyl nitrite has shortest shelf life). Sodium nitrite intravenously is preferable to the amyl nitrite for immediate use. For adults, 10 mL of a 3% sodium nitrite solution is administered intravenously followed by 50 mL of 25% aqueous solution of sodium thiosulfate in the same line. Amyl nitrite pearls are used as an immediate measure until the IV insertion necessary for sodium nitrite. The pearls are crushed into a piece of gauze and inhaled. If IV insertion is delayed, a new amyl nitrite pearl should be used every 3 min due to rapid dissipation. In the case of an unconscious patient, the amyl nitrite-soaked gauze is placed in the reservoir of the bag valve mask. Maintain airway control, watch for nitrite-induced hypotension, and continue appropriate supportive therapy. Have vasopressors available. Creation of thiocyanate in the presence of renal failure may cause abdominal pain, vomiting, and CNS dysfunction. Pulse oximetry may be unreliable as a measurement due to the creation of methemoglobin, which compromises the oxygen-carrying capacity of hemoglobin. Administration of 100% oxygen treats patient hypoxia and potentiates action of antidotes. Check the package insert for dosing of nitrites in children and for those with anemia.

Poison: Digoxin

Antidote

Digibind (Digoxin-specific antibody fragments)

Action

Binds both digoxin and digitoxin, effectively reducing the amount of free drug available in the circulation and allowing for excretion in the urine.

Nursing Considerations

Dosing of antibodies depends on ingested dose and total body load. Each vial (38 mg) will bind 0.5 mg of digoxin. (Total body load and dosing calculations are discussed in text.) The required amount is reconstituted with 4 mL of sterile water as a bolus dose intravenously, or in more stable clinical situations, administered over 30 min. Children require additional dilution. Use immediately or within 4 h with refrigeration. Monitor vital signs and cardiac rhythm! Until free digoxin levels decrease, patients may manifest nausea, vomiting, and dizziness. Cardiac abnormalities include SA node block, ventricular dysrhythmias, bradycardias, and/or ventricular tachycardias caused by rentrant excitation. Observe for any potential allergic reactions.

(*continued*)

TABLE 114–4. ANTIDOTES FOR GENERAL MANAGEMENT (continued)

Poison: Ethylene glycol

Antidote

Calcium chloride, calcium gluconate

Action

Combats systemic hypocalcemia caused when metablosim of ethylene glycol produces oxalic acid, which combines with systemic calcium and precipitates in the brain, kidneys, etc.

Nursing Considerations

Calcium chloride is never given intramuscularly or subcutaneously. Parenteral use is IV only. Avoid extravasation of calcium preparations. Calcium gluconate is preferred. Administer slowly—rapid infusion causes vasodilation, nausea/vomiting, dysrhythmias, bradycardia, syncope, shortened QT intervals on EKG, and may cause cardiac arrest. Place patient on cardiac monitor. Monitor patient's vital signs carefully.

Poison: Hydrofluoric Acid

Antidote

Calcium chloride, calcium gluconate

Action

Combats tissue destruction and hypocalcemia caused by complexation of fluoride with calcium.

Nursing Considerations

Intravenous calcium considerations are as noted in ethylene glycol. For hydrofluoric acid burns, infiltration of the affected tissues with calcium gluconate is recommended until pain subsides. Recurrence of pain requires subcutaneous or intra-arterial dosing of calcium gluconate. *Topical treatment* of hydrofluoric acid burns is accomplished by the mixing of calcium with K-Y jelly to make a calcium paste, which is applied to the affected area. Burns of the hand may be treated by filling a surgical glove with the paste and placing it on the hand.

Poison: Hypoglycemic Agents, Ethanol

Antidote

Dextrose

Action

Increases glucose availability for metabolism.

Nursing Considerations

Should be considered in any patient with altered mental status. Whenever possible rapid bedside glucose level determination should be done. $D_{50}W$ is available in 50 to 100-mL prefilled syringes (25 g per 50 mL); a large volume and viscous, often messy, and difficult (slow) to administer. Children require more dilute solutions; 20–25% concentrations. All individuals should be given doses of 0.5–1 g/kg.

Poison: Iron

Antidote

Deferoxamine

Action

Chelates excessive iron.

Nursing Considerations

Dosing may be IM or IV depending on degree of toxicity. Severe toxicity requires intravenous dosing at 15 mg/kg/h reconstituted in D_5W, lactated Ringer's solution or normal saline to a maximum of 6–8 g/d. Dosing should continue as long as patient is ill, urine remains red-orange color, or both. Note patient's vital signs. High doses and rapid rates of infusion can cause hypotension; hypersensitivity can manifest as urticaria. Prolonged use of intravenous form may contribute to ARDS. *Intramuscular dosing causes pain and induration at site.* Rotate sites of injection; reconstitute until completely dissolved with 2 mL sterile water. Solution will remain stable for 1 week at room temperature. Oral dose is not FDA approved and is not recommended.

Poison: Methemoglobinemia

Antidote

Methylene blue

Action

Methylene blue is reduced to leukomethylene, which in turn reduces methemoglobin to hemoglobin. The presence of methylene blue enhances this chemical reaction and makes it the treatment of choice in methemoglobinemia.

Nursing Considerations

Methemoglobin has a greater affinity for oxygen, and does not allow dissociation of oxygen to the tissues. Pulse oximetry is helpful in detection but is not a true measure of clinical status. Although oxygen saturation will register below normal, it often does not reflect severely toxic levels. The oxygen saturation will fall to approximately 85% but not continue to fall despite additional rise in levels. Arterial oxygen levels of blood gases (PO_2) are normal. Blood gases reflect measurements of partial pressure, not oxygen-carrying capacity. Don't depend on ABGs to detect hypoxemia. Don't rely on pulse oximetry to convey severity of symptoms. Give methylene blue 1% solution as soon as possible at 1–2 mg/kg; which for a 70-kg person is 70–140 mg or 7–14 mL of the 1% solution. This should be given slowly intravenously over 5 min. Pain at the site of infusion can be minimized with slow infusion and by following with a flush of saline. Patient's urine will become greenish blue. Pulse oximetry measurement will fall abruptly.

(*continued*)

TABLE 114–4. ANTIDOTES FOR GENERAL MANAGEMENT (continued)

Poison: Opioids

Antidote

Naloxone

Action

Competes with opioids at the receptor sites; reverses respiratory depressant effects; and improves blood pressure and CNS effects of opioids.

Nursing Considerations

Patients withdrawing from opioids exhibit nausea, vomiting, agitation, restlessness, diaphoresis, abdominal pain, piloerection. Careful attention must be paid to issues of airway protection and patient safety. Concentrations of naloxone may vary with manufacturer. Available also in neonatal concentration, but this preparation has no use in the ED for treatment of drug overdoses. Prepackaged bolus doses containing 2 mg facilitate rapid titration from 0.1–2.0 mg in opioid dependent patients and appropriate use for management of the suspected opioid overdose.

Poison: Phenobarbital, Salicylates, Tricyclic Antidepressants, Chlorpropamide, Chlorphenoxy Herbicides, Quinidine, Procainamide, Encainide, Methotrexate, Flecainide, Amantadine, Phenothiazines, Carbamazepine, Propoxyphene, and Cocaine

Antidote

Sodium bicarbonate

Action

Give 1–2 mEq/kg of sodium bicarbonate as a bolus. Place 2–3 ampules (88–132 mEq) of sodium bicarbonate in 1 L of D_5W. IV should run at 1.5–2 times the maintenance fluid range (alkalinizes serum and urine). Maintain urine pH at 7.5–8.0. Maintain serum pH between 7.50 and 7.55.

Nursing Considerations

Alkalemia, hypokalemia and decreased ionized calcium occur with bicarbonate therapy. Monitor pH (blood and urine) and electrolytes closely and replace as needed. Observe patient's neurologic studies. Hyperosmolality, hypernatremia, and paradoxical CSF acidosis may occur. Give patients supplemental oxygen to decrease tissue hypoxia. Sodium bicarbonate causes precipitation of calcium salt and may inactivate catecholamines. Use separate IV access.

Poison: Snake and Spider Envenomations

Antidote

Antivenins

Action

Neutralization of target toxin.

Nursing Considerations

Beware: High incidence of hypersensitivity reactions including urticaria, anaphylaxis, and serum sickness. Allergic reaction development is directly proportional to rate and amount of antivenin administered. Keep diphenhydramine and epinephrine readily available. Get a good history of allergies and previous antivenin exposure. Skin testing for sensitivity prior to administration is controversial. Antivenin is given slow intravenously. Initial vial should be diluted 1:10–1:100 in 0.9% sodium chloride and administered slowly (approximately 50 mL/h). In the absence of an allergic reaction, subsequent vials may be reconstituted 1:2 or 1:4 and infusion rates may be judiciously increased and titrated to patient response/reaction.

Activated charcoal is administered via orogastric tube and naloxone infusion is hung for continuous administration. The nursing considerations for the commonest antidotes used in the emergency setting are presented in Table 114–4. A more in-depth discusison of these agents is presented in the individual "Antidotes in Depth" as well as throughout the text.

Orogastric lavage is described in detail in Chapter 30 and Table 30–1. The goal is to create a siphon effect and ensure uninterrupted flow. A large enough orogastric hose (40F) with multiple distal and lateral openings should be used. Nasogastric tubes are not adequate for overdose management (except liquids). After passage of the orogastric tube, patients are placed in the left lateral decubitus position for administration of saline, drainage, and subsequent administration of activated charcoal.

Lavage tubes are now available with special ports on them for a more efficient, cleaner method of medication administration, which is especially desirable when giving activated charcoal. Lavage tubes with pre-established bite blocks are also available if preferred.

Patients who are alert and have an intact gag reflex may choose to drink the activated charcoal. Because activated charcoal is unattractive in appearance, some clinicians prefer to administer it to the patient in an opaque cup (or prepackaged opaque plastic bottle) with an opaque flexible straw. When a cup is used, it should be held away from the patient to conceal the appearance. A washcloth should be provided to wipe the patient's face when the emergency situation has passed, as activated charcoal will transiently discolor the skin. (For dosing of activated charcoal, see Chap. 30 and Table 30–2.)

Magnesium or sorbitol cathartics (see Chap. 30 and Table 30–3) are given simultaneously with activated charcoal, orally or via orogastric tube. The nurse should be prepared to handle the resultant diarrhea with a bedpan and wash basin. Should the patient be discharged soon after cathartic administration, he or she should be advised to expect (copious) black diarrhea due to the rapid transit of activated charcoal.

In adults if the syrup of ipecac is indicated (Table 30–4), it should be administered followed by no less than 200 to 300 mL of water. The patient should be provided with a large receptacle for vomiting (a small emesis basin is inadequate) and must be observed at all times. The nurse should never close a curtain around the patient and leave him or her unattended.

During gastric decontamination, the role of the nurse includes the continuous monitoring and reassessment of the patient's clinical status, anticipating changes that might occur in response to or in spite of therapy. Verification of the initial placement of the orogastric tube as well as continued patency and accuracy of placement is essential to avoid aspiration. In lavaging children and agitated patients, additional assistance may be necessary to minimize trauma during insertion and to avoid complications associated with the hose being dislodged from the esophagus. In cases where the patient is obtunded, endotracheal intubation may offer protection of the airway and prevent aspiration from tube displacement or post therapy vomiting.

Even the patient with a normal level of consciousness necessitates continuous monitoring of vital signs and ventilatory status. Serial neurologic and pulmonary evaluation must be done and clearly documented. Patients who are combative must be prevented from terminating any essential aspect of care prematurely.

If the patient can understand and is willing to accept a reasonable explanation for the discomfort associated with therapy, reassurance and explanation may be all that is necessary to regain patient compliance. On the other hand, patients who are disoriented or refuse to accept a reasonable explanation for essential therapy must be protected from potential risks associated with unplanned withdrawal of therapy. It is mandatory that a patient whose impaired capacity to make a decision is secondary to a drug or toxic effect (or hypoxia, etc) not be permitted to terminate care, as it is likely to adversely effect outcome.

Although universal precautions should be used for all patients being cared for in the hospital, today we feel the need to emphasize the use of measures to avoid contamination from the poisoned patient. Parenteral drug abuse is known to cause both HIV infection and hepatitis. Substance abuse, usually injecting drug use, is known to increase the risk for tuberculosis. Healthcare workers may also risk danger from exposure to toxic topical substances, when decontaminating a patient (see Chaps. 107 and 108).

For these reasons, the resuscitation team should apply gowns, gloves, masks, and protective eyewear before approaching the patient. Needleless devices, and needles with shields or retraction devices, should be used whenever possible, for both drug administration and any arterial or venous puncture. Irrigation and lavage equipment with splashguards should be considered.

How Should the Agitated Patient Be Restrained?

Overdosed or poisoned patients who have an altered consciousness, who become agitated and uncooperative, or who exhibit violent behavior due to poisoning often require the application of physical restraints until their condition stabilizes and they are capable of understanding the intervention. All efforts at verbal reassurance, using staff members who may have developed a rapport with the patient, must be employed. If this fails, and the impaired patient continues to refuse and thwart convential care, physical restraint may be necessary as a primary therapy or until chemical restraint can be administered safely. Basic patient care objectives are to protect the patient from self-injury and to protect others from injury by the patient. Restraints should be used only when there is no other alternative.

The decision to physically restrain a patient must be made only after all other attempts at calming the patient have failed and there is a true threat to patient (pulling out an intravenous line or endotracheal tube) or staff safety. Verbal and social interaction may help to diffuse a potentially volatile situation, allowing the patient to maintain some control in his or her care. A skilled interviewer must recognize the patient's feelings of powerlessness, fear, misunderstanding, and in some cases, embarrassment or anger. Identify these feelings, tell the patient you understand, and offer to provide information to allay the patient's concerns.

If the patient continues to pose a threat to himself or herself or others, the clinician must impose limits and inform the patient that such behavior cannot be tolerated. It may be suggested that the patient's inability to maintain a peaceful and cooperative demeanor may necessitate the summoning of "a specially trained crisis group" that will assist in regaining control. At this point, sometimes the mere presence of an organized group of individuals will help the patient rethink his or her behavior and reestablish self-control.

If all of these measures fail, and physical restraint becomes necessary, clear, objective documentation of the events leading to physical restraint must be entered in the chart. Knowledge of certain toxidromes will alert the clinician to substances that increase the likelihood for violent behavior. The patient's medical condition—including alertness, orientation, and thought process—should be noted, along with a detailed description of the measures used to secure the patient's cooperation prior to the application of physical restraints. A physician's written order must be present on the chart, though in an emergency situation a verbal order may be acceptable if a written order is recorded immediately after the crisis intervention has been performed.

Clinical staff and security personnel expected to participate as members of the restraint team should be given formal training in technique and philosophy. This preparation also allows for clear definition and understanding of roles and responsibilities prior to mobilization for crisis intervention. A team approach to the application of restraints, with a team leader in control, is essential. If possible, a team of five staff members should be gathered. Each of the first four is responsible for one extremity and the fifth, who assumes the role of leader, is positioned at the patient's head. The team leader is critical and should be the staff member most experienced in crisis intervention techniques and restraint application.

It is important to ensure that all potentially dangerous items (keys, shoes, pens, pins, stethoscopes) are taken away from the patient and not immediately accessible to the patient. The team leader secures the patient's head by grasping the forehead with one hand and securing the chin with the other (Fig. 114–1). This immobilizes the patient's head, minimizing the leverage he or she could gain by lifting the head, shoulders, and chest. The leader should speak calmly to the patient, explaining the necessity for the procedure and requesting his or her help.

The other members must be agile and secure in their approach. The team members' strength is not as important as proper hand placement and technique. The limb should be grasped firmly, with one hand just above the joint and one hand immediately below, so as to immobilize elbows and knees in extension, thus restricting movement (Fig. 114–2). Pressure directly on the joint should be avoided, as it is painful and will initiate a response from the patient that may inhibit successful restraint. In addition, such pressure may cause injury.

The restraints should be applied sequentially, starting with the upper extremities, so that the other limbs remain well immobilized while each is being restrained. The lower extremities are bound together to create three-point restraint. Initiating restraint with the arms prevents the patient from attempting to vault off the stretcher with only his or her feet restrained and potentially incurring head and facial trauma. If a sixth team member is available, he or she may apply the restraints while the others continue to secure the limbs. Otherwise, the team leader should identify which limb to restrain and direct specific team members to assist each other. The team

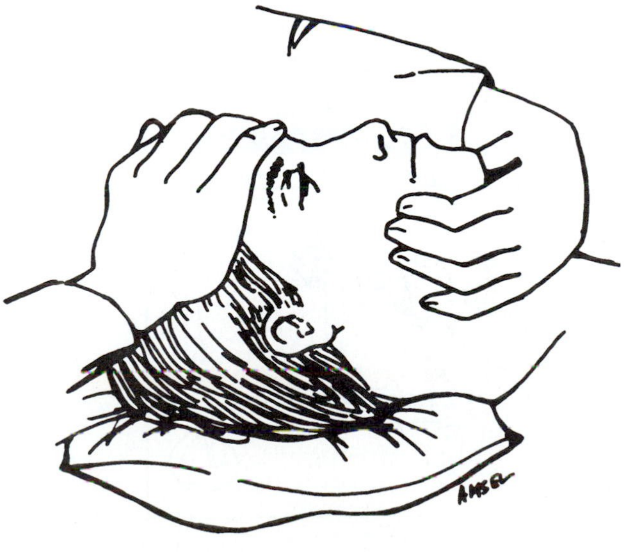

Figure 114–1. Appropriate approach by the team leader to secure the patient's head by grasping the forehead with one hand and securing the chin with the other.

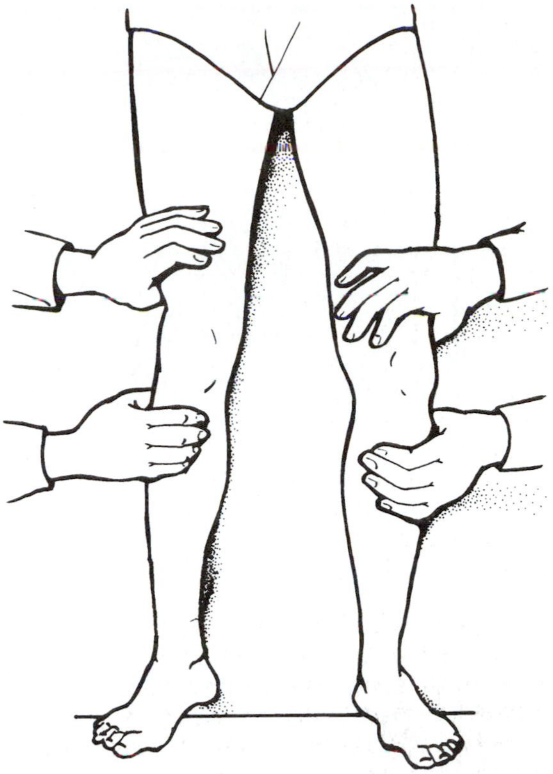

Figure 114–2. Appropriate approach to limb restraint, using one hand just proximal and one hand just distal to the joint. This immobilizes both elbows and knees in extension and effectively restricts movement.

leader must take note of any individual who is unable to control his or her assigned limb or who should be given additonal assistance. Throughout this effort, the team leader must constantly reassure the patient in a calm, firm manner and maintain a secure hold on the patient's head and chin.

Many institutions continue to use metal or leather restraints. We feel that particularly in an emergency situation, these types of restraints increase the risk of injury to a patient's extremities. Although some institutions use lamb's wool and roller gauze, in the setting of the ED, we feel that this method is only acceptable as an interim measure as this form of restraint is not secure enough to sustain continued, safe, control of the agitated patient. We suggest the use of cloth restraints with padded centers, which allow for both flexibilty and security without patient injury. A hitch knot (as described by Cassidy J: Scouting Book of Knots, Klutz Press, 1989) should be slipped over the extremity, but direct pressure should not be placed over any joint (Fig. 114–3). The ends of each restraint should be securely fastened to a nonmovable part of the stretcher with a slip knot, which allows rapid removal of the restraint if necessary. The loose ends of each restraint must be tucked under the mattress, well out of reach of the patient (Fig. 114–4).

After the restraints are secured (Fig. 114–5), each limb should be checked for discoloration and any compromise of pulse and capillary refill. The clinician must

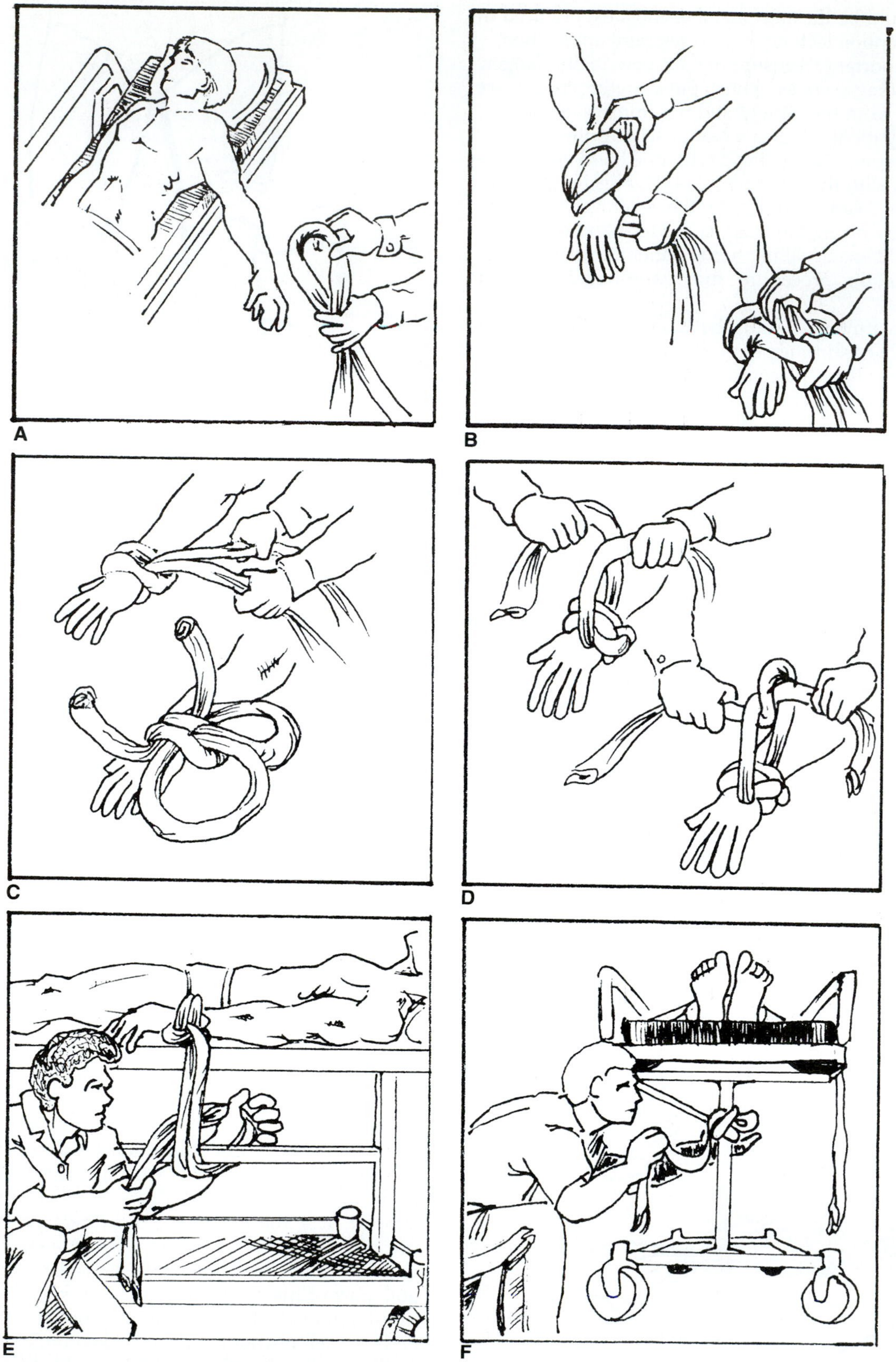

Figure 114–3. Restraints must have a padded center. A hitch knot is slipped over the extremity. The sequence of securing the extremity applies no direct pressure over the joint.

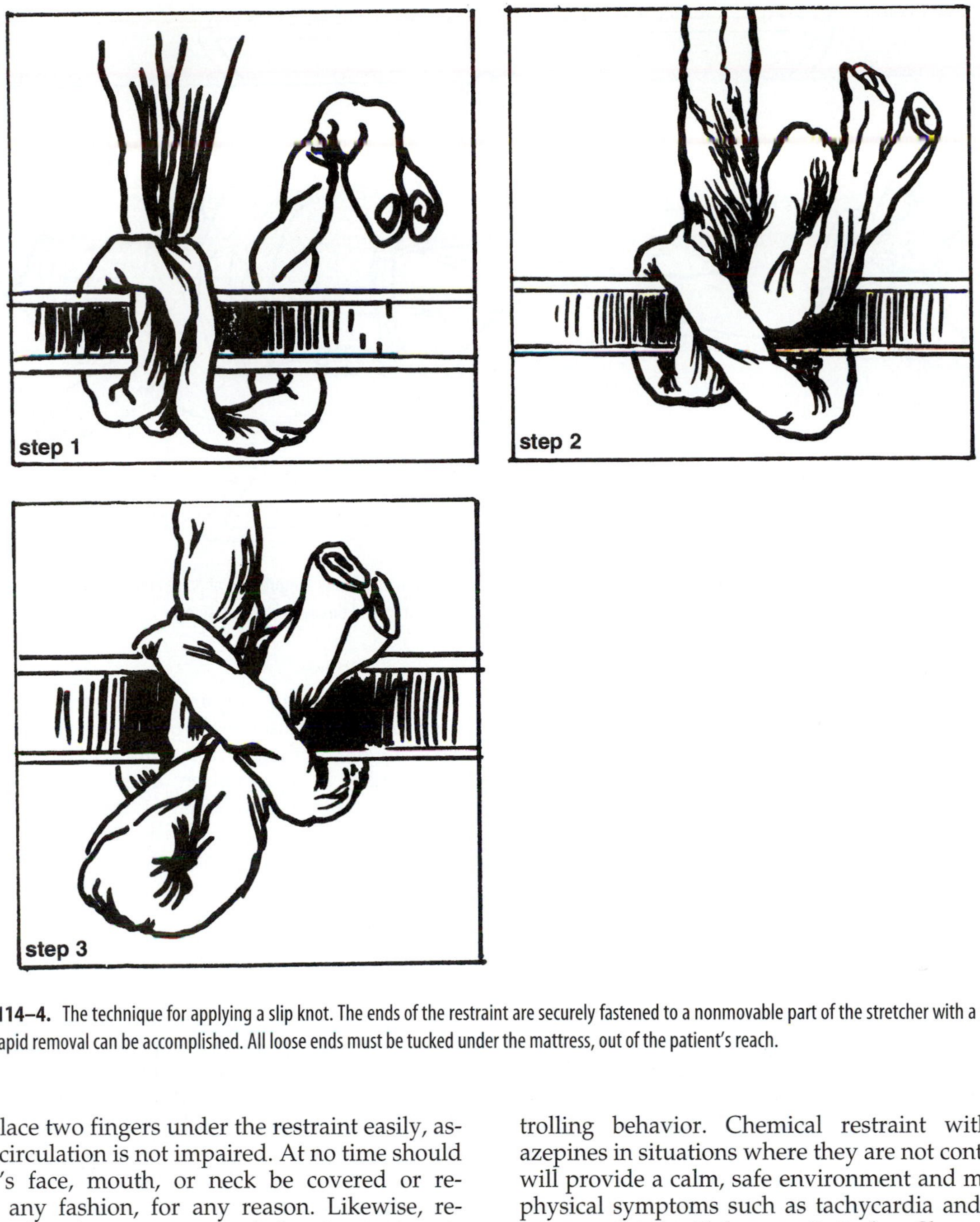

Figure 114–4. The technique for applying a slip knot. The ends of the restraint are securely fastened to a nonmovable part of the stretcher with a slip knot so that rapid removal can be accomplished. All loose ends must be tucked under the mattress, out of the patient's reach.

be able to place two fingers under the restraint easily, assuring that circulation is not impaired. At no time should the patient's face, mouth, or neck be covered or restrained in any fashion, for any reason. Likewise, restraint of the chest is not recommended, as it may impair respirations; however, a chest support may be applied so as to prevent the patient from sliding off the end of the stretcher. If a support is applied, a slip knot should be fastened loosely so as not to restrict movement completely and/or apply any pressure to the axillae. The patient should be told why the restraints were applied, and what change in behavior is expected to allow him or her to regain independent responsibility and thus minimize the length of time that the restraints stay in place.

Once the environment is made safer for the patient and staff, chemical restraint should be considered. Patients under the influence of drugs and/or alcohol are often incapable of making conscious decisions and controlling behavior. Chemical restraint with benzodiazepines in situations where they are not contraindicated will provide a calm, safe environment and minimize the physical symptoms such as tachycardia and hyperthermia associated with hyperactivity (see Chaps. 65 and 70).

A note should be made in the patient chart that three-point restraints were applied because of a specific patient behavior. The patient's initial response to the intervention and current condition must be noted. Continued observation must then be part of the care plan. The restraints should be checked on a periodic basis to assure that the patient remains protected, that clinical needs are being met, and that circulation and pulse remain intact.

Patients presenting with altered mental status often arrive with concomitant trauma, compartment syndromes, and/or decubiti secondary to immobility. Accurate observation and intervention to prevent further injury is of key importance, especially in cases where

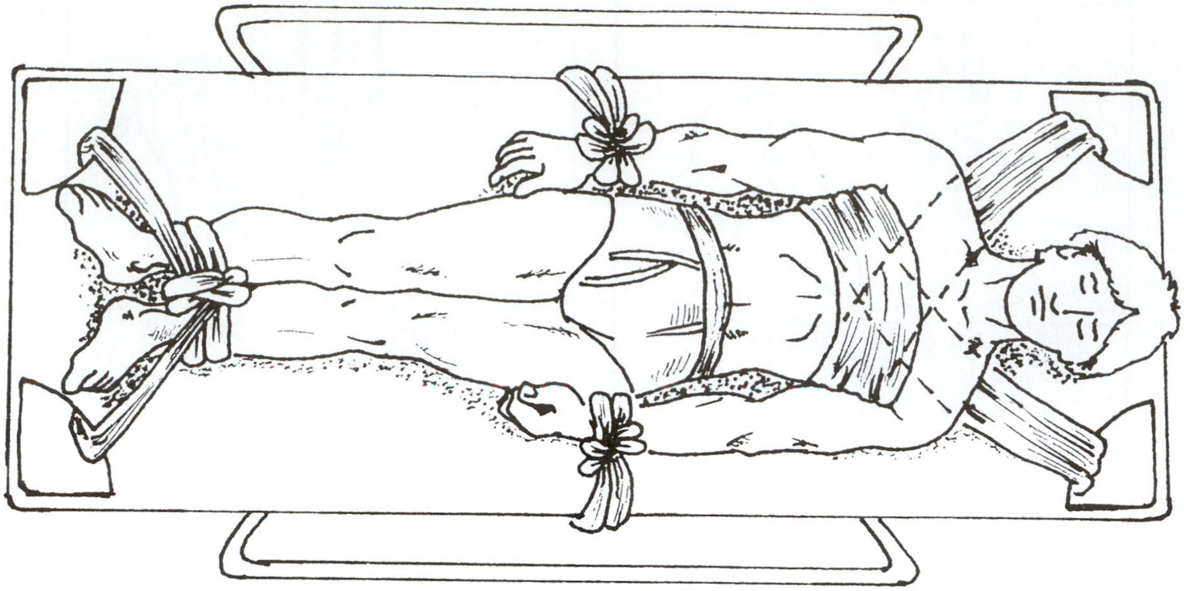

Figure 114–5. When the restraints are secured, each limb must be checked for discoloration and any compromise of pulse and capillary refill. The clinician must be able to place two fingers under the restraint. The patient's face, mouth, and neck must not be covered or restrained.

restraint may further immobilize the patient. Documentation of conditions as pre-existing will avoid labeling the condition as iatrogenic later in the management course. In addition, the patient's mental status should be periodically reevaluated and documentation should be placed in the chart as to the need for continued restraint and/or to allow for the initiation of alternative measures.

A restraint flow sheet should be developed to satisfy documentation requirements and to also serve as a clinical reminder to fulfill the patients basic personal needs at regular intervals. A regularly scheduled systematic retrospective review of the data with corrective recommendations should be part of the ED's Quality Performance Program.

If data secured during treatment suggest any suspicion of self-destructive or suicidal behavior, the patient should be placed on a 1:1 suicide watch until further psychiatric evaluation can be acomplished. This requires that the individual be placed under the direct observation of one staff member who then documents on an hourly basis (at a minimum) as to the patient's behavior, comments, and actions. A full psychiatric evaluation should be done as soon as the patient is alert and coherent enough to answer questions and discuss the events leading up to hospitalization (see Chap. 113). Removal of the patient's clothing and property and dressing the patient in a hospital gown may also act as a deterrent to patient elopement.

Disposition: Acute and Long Term

Continued reassessment of the patient's condition yields information that will constitute the nursing documentation of the patient's ongoing status and ultimate disposition. The nurse must begin planning for disposition very early in the patient's care. Immediately following the acute phase of intervention, attention must be given to notification of the individual's family. In the case of a patient who is responsible for the care of children, careful consideration must be made as to the children's safety and welfare. In the case of a substance-abusing parent, the social services staff must be notified to assure an immediate home assessment and follow-up after hospitalization (see Chap. 112). The patient's property must be secured and protected, even if the patient is not admitted. Caution must be exercised while undressing patients. Searching pockets and property can yield dangerous items such as needles, syringes, knives, razor blades, and drugs, which pose a threat to staff safety. Gloves should always be worn and illicit items should be turned over to security personnel.

Familiarity with the pattern of toxicologic symptoms allows the nurse to suspect a likely toxin. Consideration of the clinical manifestations of the particular substance(s) allows the nurse to anticipate not only ongoing care needs but also those that will affect the patient at the time of discharge.

Patients not requiring medical admission to the hospital must be alert and communicative before psychiatric consultation is recommended. Referral sources for rehabilitation of substance users should be available if requested by the patient. Finally, clear, concise, specific discharge instructions must be given to the patient. Details of these instructions must be noted, and a signature indicating patient understanding must be entered on the chart. In many cases, duplicate instruction sheets are used to minimize omissions and standardize the individual effort. A copy is given to the patient for reference on discharge and a signed copy attached to the permanent record. This level of documentation is particularly important in verifying the patient's capacity to understand, especially in a previously impaired patient. This is important not only from a medical-legal point of view but also from a quality management perspective.

Discharge Instructions

Each patient to be discharged should have individualized instructions. Considerations when giving the instructions include the patient's level of comprehension (including any potential language barrier) and the caregiver's level of comprehension, if the patient's care is to be entrusted to another. Social factors—such as whether the patient has a home, whether the patient is pregnant, whether the patient is responsible for living children and, if so, whether he or she is able to provide necessary care—must be considered in the discharge plan. Before release from the institution the patient must be provided with clothing appropriate for the weather. Family contact may be necessary or, in some institutions, the social service division may have developed resources in this area. Instruction with regard to poison prevention must be given both verbally and in written format. This is paramount, especially in cases where poisoning was unintentional. Follow-up must be arranged and stressed with the patient and caregiver. Hospital-based quality assurance mechanisms for recall must be in place and readily activated in the event that the patient fails to follow up as instructed All teaching issues should be rediscussed with the patient on discharge. Questions addressed during an earlier phase of treatment, when the patient may have had an altered sensorium, must be readdressed to potentiate understanding. Psychiatric consultation prior to discharge is essential in any case where destructive behavior is suspected in conjunction with the ingestion.

Documentation

Staffing deficiencies, particularly in EDs, have made ongoing documentation extremely difficult, especially when patients remain many hours prior to a final disposition. The use of checklists optimizes continued periodic documentation and minimizes the need for extensive, detailed notes.

Evaluation of the Poisoned Patient and the Quality of Care Rendered

The evaluation of care entails an appraisal not only of the nursing care received by the patient but also of the overall quality of care. The assessment of the patient's physical and emotional status and evaluation of the patient's response to the nursing care plan are measured in terms of desired patient outcomes, based on an established standard of care. Specific desired patient outcomes can also be based on the individual nursing diagnoses (see Table 114–2). For a diagnosis of ineffective airway clearance, the expected outcome of effective gas exchange would be evidenced by a PO_2 value greater than 80 mm Hg on room air, for example. In altered tissue perfusion, the presence of strong palpable pulses demonstrates adequate circulatory function. Ongoing reassessment of the patient's vital signs and neurologic status is essential to evaluate the patient's response to therapy.

The second part of the process, evaluation of the overall quality of care, is an assessment of the nurse's adherence to the care plan and to the nursing standard of care. Regulatory agencies mandate that written care plans and measurable nursing standards be developed, and that adherence to the established standard be documented in both prospective and retrospective audits. To meet this requirement, care must be taken to ensure that the standard of care is meaningful and functional for the staff nurse. Once the standard guidelines have been established, an evaluation tool should be generated to test whether or not the set criteria have been met. This quality management program may be complex.

Emergency patients do not necessarily have a clearly defined diagnosis. Many patients present with an array of complaints; others are unable to give any history. A poisoned patient may initially have to be placed into a more generic category (eg, unconscious patient) until a specific diagnosis is confirmed. This problem-oriented approach may necessitate multiple interventions to define the appropriate management strategy.

The ED is not a controlled environment. Few options are available (eg, ambulance diversion, supplemental staff) to bring order out of chaos when overcrowding occurs. The variation in occupancy of the ED as well as patient acuity greatly affects the quality and thoroughness of patient care given. When a care plan or standard is established, it must be flexible enough to be useful and valid whether the ED is peaceful or exceedingly busy, and it must be independent of the patient's severity of illness.

Many patient interventions must be accomplished in a relatively brief period of time. Outcome is often measured by an analysis of short-term goals. In many hospitals, however, admitted patients may be delayed for prolonged periods of time in the ED, or kept in observation units. Under these circumstances new and different standards may therefore be indicated.

Because emergent patients continually arrive without warning, achieving a standard such as the measurement of vital signs every 4 hours becomes a difficult task. However, a standard should not simply be monitored. A mechanism must also be established whereby noncompliance can be addressed and corrective actions implemented. Once corrective actions are initiated, their effectiveness must also be evaluated. Standards must not only be flexible and measurable, but also the personnel responsible for initiating corrective action must have the ultimate authority with the staff for interpreting and implementing the standard in the plan of care.

Finally, the principles of the standardized care plan (suggested in Table 114–1) must be routinely assessed

NURSING CHART AUDIT
EMERGENCY DEPARTMENT TREATMENT—ADULT
GENERAL ADULT TREATMENT

PRIORITIES AND EXAM

- ☐ Checked patient for ABCs
- ☐ Cleared airway and ventilated with BVM if not breathing or severe respiratory depression
- ☐ C-spine immobilzed if indicated
- ☐ ET tube inserted if CNS depression makes it tolerable
- ☐ Nasal O_2 if patient is awake but lethargic
- ☐ IV established
- ☐ History (from patient, family, friends) obtained if possible
- ☐ Nursing assessment performed - head to toe
  1. Vital signs (BP ______ T ______ P ______ RR ______)
  2. Neurologic check: verbal and motor response, pupils
  3. Evidence of head trauma
  4. Odor of breath
  5. Neck evaluation for tenderness, trauma, venous distension, tracheal position
  6. Chest evaluation—breath sounds, chest rise, sign of injury
  7. Abdominal evaluation—appearance, tenderness, bowel sounds and masses
  8. Extremities—movement, sensation, color, pulses, skin temperature, capillary refill, puncture marks, scars, deformities
- ☐ Bloods drawn for CBC, electrolytes, glucose, toxicology tests, and ABGs
- ☐ Urine obtained for toxicology screen

IMMEDIATE TREATMENT

- ☐ Orders written by MD and signed by RN
- ☐ 100 mL of $D_{50}W$ IV
- ☐ Naloxone 2 mg IV (given first if opioid suspected)
- ☐ Thiamine 100 mg IV
- ☐ Seizures controlled with diazepam/other agents if indicated

REMOVING INGESTANTS (when indicated)

- ☐ Ipecac 30 mL followed by several glasses of water (unless contraindicated) for awake patient
- ☐ Cuffed endotracheal intubation followed by lavage with saline via orogastric tube if patient is obtunded, comatose, or lacks a gag reflex

ADSORPTION OF INGESTANTS AFTER (OR IN PLACE OF) EMESIS OR LAVAGE

- ☐ Oral activated charcoal. 1.0 g/kg or 10 x the amount of drug, if quanity known (whichever is greater)

CATHARSIS

- ☐ Sorbitol 70%, 50 mL: magnesium citrate, 10 oz. or magnesium sulfate 30 g, if indicated

☐ SPECIFIC ANTIDOTES INDICATED AND GIVEN?

☐ INTAKE MONITORED–IV, PO, NG?

☐ OUTPUT MONITORED–URINE, EMESIS (LAVAGE), STOOL?

CONSULTATION

- ☐ Psychiatry called
- ☐ Social services called
- ☐ Poison Center called
- ☐ Medical toxicologist called

DISPOSITION

- ☐ Treated and released in <24 h
- ☐ Treated and released in >24 h
- ☐ Transferred to psychiatric unit
- ☐ Admitted
- ☐ Other

FOLLOW-UP PLAN

- ☐ Medical
- ☐ Psychiatric
- ☐ Social Services

DISCHARGE INSTRUCTIONS—IF INDICATED

- ☐ Specific instructions documented
- ☐ Documentation of patient understanding

COMMENTS

CHART NUMBER ____________________ DATE OF VISIT ____________________

Figure 114–6. Example of a retrospective chart audit.

and reevaluated. This audit analyzes both the conscious and unconscious patient in one plan. We suggest that the standard quality management project be as simple as possible without compromising standards. This allows staff participation in the project to be less tedious and a positive personal learning experience.

Using this chart audit, a threshold for performance can be established. Any value falling below this threshold requires further evaluation because the established standard of care is unmet. Specific objective criteria should be developed for each problematic area; the data collected can then be evaluated and corrective action initiated. Constant reevaluation should continue until the threshold is met. Figure 114–6 is suggested as an objective retrospective chart audit.

Acknowledgment

The graphics for this chapter were done by William P. Callaghan.

CHAPTER 115

Certified Poison Information Centers and the Role of Poison Prevention

Richard S. Weisman

The primary functions of poison centers in the United States are to provide recommendations for the management of poisoning to both the public and healthcare professionals, and to increase the awareness of poisoning risks and prevention strategies. Other major functions of the poison center include the collection of epidemiologic data; toxicosurveillance for the emergence of new public health risks; promotion of preventive devices such as safety closures, cabinet locks, and aversive taste additives; provision of assistance to public health agencies involved with hazardous materials; and training of physicians, nurses, and pharmacists involved with the care of poisoned patients.[3,17,22,26,27]

Management and Treatment Recommendations for the Public and for Health Professionals

Immediate telephone access to credible treatment advice and product information after a poisoning exposure, regardless of financial status, is the most essential component of the U.S. poison center system.[24] Poison center staff routinely triage poisoning exposures requiring hospital care and those that can be handled safely at home, provide patient-specific treatment recommendations or basic information about poisons, and facilitate efficient use of the medical care system.[5] Through the use of triage protocols and extensive training, the poison information specialist can make appropriate cost-effective decisions for each call.[19] The center provides consultation to those patients who can manage their own care or the care of a family member at home without involvement of the prehospital system or health care facilities and when necessary can help the patient to receive care through various outpatient clinics, crisis intervention units, and when needed hospital emergency departments.[5]

In 1988, Louisiana was forced to close the State Regional Poison Center. During the year that the poison center was closed, the cost of emergency medical services for poisoning in Louisiana increased by more than $1.4 million. This additional expenditure represented an increase of more than three times the cost of operating the poison center.[10]

The American Association of Poison Control Centers (AAPCC) certified poison centers can provide treatment recommendations and guidance to both the public and healthcare providers. To provide the highest level of care for the victim of poisoning, many levels of professional support may be needed. Each exposure may require between one and five follow-up calls to assess the impact of the exposure and make additional recommendations.[11] Consultation provided by the poison information specialists allow more than 72% of poisoning exposures received by a center to be safely managed at home without additional healthcare costs.[12–16,21,22]

Nationally, approximately 13% of exposure calls to the poison center system are from physicians or healthcare facilities.[12–16,21] Poison centers centralize costly information and toxicology resources, making them available to healthcare professionals throughout their regions and avoiding unnecessary duplication of resources.[17]

What Are the Qualifications of the Personnel Who Staff American Association of Poison Control Centers Certified Poison Centers?

Medical Director

The medical director should be board certified in medical toxicology by the American Board of Medical Speciaties.[1] In the absence of this certification, the medical director must be board certified in internal medicine, pediatrics, family medicine, or emergency medicine and be able to clearly demonstrate ongoing interest and expertise in toxicology as evidenced by publications, research, and meeting attendance. The medical director must have a medical staff appointment at a comprehensive poison treatment facility and must be involved in the management of poisoned patients. The medical director should devote at least 50% of his or her professional activities to toxicology. In addition to clinical, academic teaching, and research activities, the medical director must formally commit at least 10 hours per week to poison center operational activities, involving staff training, development of medical guidelines, and quality assurance.[1]

Managing Director

The managing director of a regional poison center must be a registered nurse, pharmacist, or physician or hold a degree in a health science discipline.[1] This individual may also be the medical director. This individual should be certified or eligible for certification as a medical toxicologist by the American Board of Medical Specialties for physicians or by the American Board of Applied Toxicology for nonphysicians. In the absence of certification, the managing director must be able to demonstrate ongoing interest and expertise in toxicology as evidenced by publications, research, and meeting attendance. The managing director must be able to demonstrate full-time commitment to poison center related activities, including the areas of medical toxicology, education, research, and administration.[1]

Specialists in Poison Information

Specialists in poison information must be registered nurses, pharmacists, or physicians, or be currently certified by the AAPCC as a specialist in poison information.[1] Specialists in poison information must be qualified to understand and interpret standard poison information resources and to transmit that information in a logical, concise, and understandable way to both healthcare professionals and the public. All specialists in poison information must complete a training program approved by the medical director and must be certified by the AAPCC as a specialist in poison information within two examination administrations of their initial eligibility for the certification process. Specialists in poison information must spend an annual average of 16 hours per week in poison center related activities, including providing telephone consultation, teaching, public education, or in poison center operations. Poison information specialists must dedicate 100% of their job effort to poison center activities and cannot be simultaneously working in another area of the hospital or institution.[1]

In the United States there are presently 45 poison information centers that are meeting the certification criteria of the AAPCC and approximately 40 centers that are working to achieve this goal. The centers that are not certified most often have deficiencies in either the number or the qualifications of their staff, are not operational 24 hours a day, or are unable to submit data to the national database.

Credibility of the poison center system as a nucleus for a region's toxicology services is linked to a center's rapport with regional or local healthcare organizations.[6] The effective exchange of information between the poison center system and healthcare facilities can help improve the outcome of a poisoning exposure. In a study comparing advice provided by emergency department personnel or poison center personnel, the recommendations that were provided by the emergency department personnel were often inaccurate and inconsistent.[28]

Public Prevention and Promotion

Public awareness of the services offered by a poison center is critical in attaining recommended penetrance levels in communities. Penetrance is defined as the number of exposures reported to a poison center per 1000 population. The current minimum AAPCC requirement for penetrance is 5 exposures per 1000 population.[1] Centers with well-developed public awareness programs and acceptance by their communities have achieved 20 exposures per 1000 population.[7] Outreach and poison prevention activities are required to be conducted by the poison center's public and professional education staff.[1] The poison centers that have achieved the greatest success in regional awareness frequently target prevention campaigns in both high-risk areas and regions with low call-to-population ratios.

Nearly 40% of poisoning exposures reported to the AAPCC during the past 5 years have occurred in children under 3, and 54% occurred in children younger than 6. The poison information system focuses considerable effort on the prevention of childhood poisonings.[12–16,21] Prevention and outreach activities are often integrated into classroom and day care curricula and into courses for new parents. Pediatricians, community health educators, and parent-teacher's associations often work closely with poison centers to assist with poison prevention activities.[18]

What Are Some Common Strategies Advocated by Poison Centers to Prevent Poisonings?

1. Locks must be applied to all medicine cabinets that are within reach. In the absence of a lock, the more toxic

medications and pharmaceuticals should be stored on the highest shelves. All vitamins commonly found on the kitchen or dining room tables, should be made inaccessible to children. Medications should never be left in the glove compartment of the family car. Spot checks should be made frequently to return all products to their proper storage places.

2. All medications and toxic substances should be kept in their original containers. Medications often resemble candy and toxins may ressemble drinks (see Color Plate Fig. 20). Any container other than the original with its correct product labeling leads to confusion for both children and adults. Milk bottles, soft drink bottles, and even baby bottles have been used to store toxic substances such as paint thinners and insecticides and have led to catastrophic exposures. Food and drink containers should never be used for the excess of a toxic substance, which should preferably be discarded in an environmentally sound manner. In addition, no inadequately sealed or incorrectly labeled containers should ever be used for storage.
3. Parents should buy or accept medication only if it is in a child-proof container. If an adult has difficulty with a child-proof container, "new child resistant, adult friendly" packaging is available.[4]
4. Medication should be considered as medicine, not a plaything and certainly not candy. A child should be told why and for how long the medication must be taken. Adults should not take their medications in front of children. This will limit exposure to drug-taking role models that may become objects of imitative behavior.
5. Household cleaning products should be stored in a high, locked cabinet rather than under the kitchen sink, as is commonly done. Safety latches should be placed on all kitchen and bathroom drawers and cabinets containing hazardous substances including cleaning products, personal health care products, and medications.
6. Syrup of ipecac and activated charcoal should be readily available in the home for use if directed by a poison information specialist or physician.
7. Unused portions of prescription medications should be discarded by flushing them down the toilet at the completion of drug therapy.
8. It should be anticipated that about 10% of children who have ingested a poison will do so again within a year.[9]

Data Collection and Toxicosurveillance

The American Association of Poison Control Centers developed the National Data Collection Program for poisonings in 1984. In 1992, the system was revised, expanded, and renamed the Toxic Exposure Surveillance System (TESS). The TESS data include epidemiologic data about each exposure reported to a poison center. The data are used to focus prevention education, guide clinical research, and direct training.[17] The surveillance system is instrumental in identifying hazards and poisoning trends and in reporting hazards to regulatory agencies and other centers in the system. The Consumer Products Safety Commission relies heavily on the poison center data system to identify new poison hazards and to monitor compliance with child-resistant packaging regulations.[24] TESS data have prompted product reformulations, repackaging, recalls, and the removal of products from the marketplace. Examples of recent public health problems that have been recognized with TESS data are the health problems resulting from Wilson's Leather Protector and iron ingestion in children.[24] The data also form the basis for postmarketing surveillance of newly released drugs and products. Most products that have recently become available over the counter and no longer require a prescription, have been carefully evaluated by the FDA using TESS data. Repeated experience in treating many of the same types of exposures enables centers within the poison information system to develop and refine triage and treatment protocols. Participation in the TESS project is required for all poison centers certified by the AAPCC.[1]

Interaction With Public Safety Officials

Involvement in the management of occupational and hazardous materials exposures requires a poison center to work closely with local emergency-response facilities (HAZMAT units) and to identify risks within a community.[20] During the 1980s, the percentage of reports of occupational exposures to poison centers nearly doubled. Although this may reflect an increase in reporting, it more likely indicates a need for treatment and prevention services for occupational and hazardous materials exposures. The poison center can play a crucial role as information resource on the possible health hazards and medical effects of chemicals released into communities during hazardous material accidents.

Professional Education

Toxicology fellowship programs, which give special training to physicians and clinical pharmacists in the diagnosis and treatment of poisoned, overdosed, and occupationally exposed patients, are integral parts of many U.S. poison center systems.[2] Having specially trained physicians or pharmacists available to assist with the care of difficult cases referred to a poison center and to treat patients referred to an affiliated emergency department, enhances patient care. In addition, students of medicine, nursing, and pharmacy, as well as physicians in residency training, often participate in on-site rotations at poison control centers. The training opportunities result in a greater number of healthcare providers, many of whom are primary healthcare providers and emergency physicians, with added expertise in the management of poisoned, overdosed, and occupationally exposed patients.

What Is the History of Poison Centers in the United States?

The first poison center in the United States was established in Chicago in 1953, after the American Academy of Pediatrics Committee on Accident Prevention brought national attention to the fact that unintentional poisoning was a leading cause of injury in young children.[23] Within a short time the success of the Chicago center was replicated in several other cities around the country. The benefits of these new centers were heralded by pediatrics groups, public health agencies, hospitals, and community organizations. In 1958, the American Association of Poison Control Centers was founded to foster the exchange of experience and scientific data and to foster a closer working relationship.[8] As a result of the organization's efforts, important legislative initiatives occured. Among the legislation were the Federal Hazardous Substance Labelling Act of 1960, the Child Protection Act of 1966, and the Poison Prevention Packaging Act of 1970. The number of centers in the Unites States grew steadily to a peak of 661 in 1978, when it began to decline.[25] A more complete discussion of poison centers in the United States can be found in Chapter 1.

Early centers were often based in emergency departments or hospital pharmacies and were staffed by emergency department nurses, pediatric residents, or hospital pharmacists with no special training in toxicology and limited information resources.[25] By the late 1970s with financial assistance from the Emergency Medical Services Systems Act of 1973, efforts to improve the quality of poison information services in the United States were underway. These efforts led to the development of national standards for poison centers and a certification process to assure compliance with these standards.

The early 1980s were characterized by a rapid decline in the number of poison centers, as small local services coalesced to serve larger regions. The trend toward regionalization meant that benefits were provided to a wider community—extending well beyond the revenue base of the sponsoring institutions. In most instances, the decline in numbers led to an improvement in the quality of services, including better economies of scale and an increase in call volume. These larger certified centers had a dedicated healthcare professional staff, 24-hour service, extensive on-site resources, medical toxicologist backup, comprehensive regional poison prevention programs, education programs for area health professionals, and poison hazard surveillance programs. By 1983, the number of U.S. poison information centers had dropped to 395, and it has continued to decline.[17] With this decline, the percentage of the population served by a certified poison center has also dropped. Today only 60% of the United States is served by a poison center meeting minimum quality standards. Efforts by the Centers for Disease Control's Injury Prevention and Control Division and the Bureau of Maternal and Child Health's Emergency Medical Services for Children, to obtain partial federal funding for poison centers are presently underway, and may ultimately help to both stabilize and improve the quality of services offered by poison centers.

References

1. American Association of Poison Control Centers: Criteria for Certification as a Regional Poison Control Center, October 1991. Previously Published in Vet Hum Toxicol 1978;20: 117–118.
2. Anonymous: Fellowship programs in medical toxicology. Ann Emerg Med 1995;26:728–732.
3. Berning CK, Griffith JF, Wild JE: Research on the effectiveness of denatonium benzoate as a deterrent to liquid detergent ingestion in children. Fundam Appl Toxicol 1982;2: 44–48.
4. Brown A: Importance of child-resistant packaging. Poison Prevention Week Council, press conference, March 12, 1996, Washington, DC.
5. Chaffee-Bahamon C, Lovejoy FH: Effectiveness of a regional poison control center in reducing excess emergency room visits for children's poisoning. Pediatrics 1983;72: 164–169.
6. Chaffee-Bahamon C, Lovejoy FH: Patterns in hospitals' use of a regional poison information center. Am J Pub Health 1983;73:396–400.
7. Felberg L, Litovitz TL, Soloway RA, Morgan J: State of the nation's poison centers: 1994 American Association of Poison Control Centers survey of U.S. poison centers. Vet Human Toxicol 1996;38:214–219.
8. Grayson R: The poison control movement in the United States. Ind Med Surg 1962;31:296–297.
9. Jacobziner H: Causation, prevention and control of accidental poisoning. JAMA 1959;171:1769–1777.
10. King WD, Palmisano PA: Poison control centers: Can their value be measured? South Med J 1991;84:722–726.
11. Litovitz TL: Poison center operations: The necessity of follow-up. Ann Emerg Med 1982;11:348–352.
12. Litovitz TL, Clark LR, Soloway RA: 1993 Annual report of the American Association of Poison Control Centers Toxic Exposure Surveillance System. Am J Emerg Med 1994;12: 546–584.
13. Litovitz TL, Felberg L, Soloway RA, et al: 1994 Annual report of the American Association of Poison Control Centers Toxic Exposure Surveillance System. Am J Emerg Med 1995;13:551–597.
14. Litovitz TL, Felberg L, White S, Klein-Schwartz W: 1995 Annual report of the American Association of Poison Control Centers Toxic Exposure Surveillance System. Am J Emerg Med 1996;14:487–537.
15. Litovitz TL, Holm KC, Bailey KM, Schmidtz BF: 1991 Annual report of the American Association of Poison Control Centers, National Data Collection System. Am J Emerg Med 1992;10:452–505.
16. Litovitz TL, Holm KC, Clancy C, et al: 1992 Annual report of the American Association of Poison Control Centers Toxic Exposure Surveillance System. Am J Emerg Med 1993;11:494–555.
17. Litovitz T, Kearney TE, Holm K, et al: Poison control centers: Is there an antidote for budget cuts? Am J Emerg Med 1994;12:585–599.
18. Lovejoy FH, Robertson WO, Woolf AD: Poison centers, poi-

son prevention and the pediatrician. Pediatrics 1994;94: 220–224.

19. Miller T: Government Financial Options to Preserve and Expand Poison Control Centers: A Report to Congress. Submitted by the Department of Health and Human Services to the 103rd Congress, September 1995.
20. Mrvos R, Dean BS, Krenzelok EP: A poison center's emergency response plan. Vet Hum Toxicol 1998;30:138–140.
21. Normann SA, Schauben JL: Florida poison information network: Saving lives and money. J Fla Med Assoc 1994;81: 741–744.
22. Payne HAS, Smalley HM, Tracey MJ: Denatonium benzoate as a bitter aversive additive in ethylene glycol and methanol-based automotive products. Society of Automotive Engineers Technical Paper Series, 1993;pp. 125–131.
23. Press E, Mellins RB: A poisoning control program. Am J Pub Health 1954;44:1515–1525.
24. Report of the Poison Control Center Leadership Group. Published in part in Vet Hum Toxicol 1996;38: 50–53.
25. Scherz RG, Robertson WO: The history of poison control centers in the United States. Clin Toxicol 1978;12:291–296.
26. Temple AR: Testing of child-resistant containers. Clin Toxicol 1978;12:357–366.
27. Waltar WW: An evaluation of the poison prevention packaging act. Pediatrics 1982;69:363–370.
28. Wigder HN, Erickson T, Morse T, Saporta V: Emergency department poison advice telephone calls. Ann Emerg Med 1995;25:349–352.

CHAPTER 116

Risk Management and Legal Principles

Walter LeStrange and Kevin Porter

The use of emergency services has increased dramatically since the early 1970s. Although patterns of use show that patients with nonurgent medical problems account for a significant amount of the increase in usage,[7] the number of toxicologic emergencies increased steadily in the 1980s and continues to rise today. This is especially true in large urban emergency departments (EDs). This chapter is concerned with the medical-legal management of patients who present to an ED with an organic impairment, that is, manifested by a relatively recent deterioration in the level of cognitive or behavioral function caused by the effects of drugs or alcohol.

Patients suffering toxicologic emergencies require immediate care, yet they are often unable to give consent because their impaired consciousness prevents them from making decisions. Treating patients who present with an acute organic impairment manifested by confusion and irrational, or even dangerous, behavior, is extremely difficult. Emergency physicians must recognize the medical-legal problems created when the impaired patient refuses treatment or admission to the hospital and insists on leaving against medical advice.

No clear guidelines are available to the physician confronted with a toxicologic emergency. The law relating to these issues is unsettled nationally and varies from state to state. The emergency physician must become familiar with the legal requirements of informed consent and the essential management necessary to avoid liability for negligence and abandonment. Of particular concern are the risk management and liability issues that relate to the patient who attempts to leave the ED while impaired. The legal requirements of informed consent in emergency settings, the duty to treat, medical malpractice, battery, and negligence are examined. Guidelines based on generally accepted common law principles, as well as New York State case law and statutes, are suggested for developing appropriate patient care plans and departmental policies.

Informed Consent

A patient who understands the risks and benefits of medical treatment is afforded a legally enforceable right to accept or refuse any treatment that is proposed, by reference to constitutionally protected rights of privacy and control of one's body. In addition, when a determination is made that a patient is capable of consenting to or refusing treatment, the law requires that adequate information be disclosed to patients so that they may comprehend (1) the potential risks and benefits associated with receiving the treatment recommended, in order to make an informed consent to treatment; (2) the potential risks of not receiving treatment, in order to make an informed refusal; and (3) possible alternative treatments and their potential risks. Personal autonomy and self-determination are the two basic principles that provide the foundation for the modern doctrine of informed consent, which requires the practitioner "to disclose to the patient such alternatives thereto and the reasonably foreseeable risks and benefits involved as a reasonable medical, dental, or pediatric practitioner under similar circumstances would have disclosed, in a manner permitting the patient to make a knowledgeable evaluation."[13]

An early landmark case in the evolution of the doctrine of informed consent to treatment is Schloendorff v. Society of New York Hospital (1914), which upheld the right of individuals to self-determination and, therefore, the right to consent to or refuse any proposed treatment. The "emergency doctrine" was first enunciated in the Schloendorff decision to address aspects of the doctrine of informed consent that are problematic when patients are deemed not capable of participating in the consent process. Justice Cardozo's decision in Schloendorff stated:

> Every human being of adult years and sound mind has a right to determine what shall be done with his own

> body and a surgeon who performs an operation without his patient's consent commits an assault, for which he is liable in damages, except in cases of emergency where the patient is unconscious and where it is necessary to operate before consent can be obtained.[14]

In the matter of Storar (1981), the Court of Appeals held the right of a competent individual to refuse medical assistance as a matter of law in New York.[5] Section 2504 of the New York State Public Health Law gives physicians the authority to treat patients without consent if "the person is in immediate need of medical attention and an attempt to secure consent would result in delay of treatment which would increase the risk to the person's life or health."[12] As currently formulated, Section 2504 is interpreted to apply under special circumstances. Exceptions to idealized informed consent and the right to refuse treatment include the cases of minors and victims of emergencies for whom delays in treatment, while consent is being obtained, would seriously compromise the patient's clinical condition.[1]

The New York State Public Health Law provides basic guidelines describing the extent of disclosure requirements for a patient. However, disclosure of pertinent information is frequently not possible in the provision of emergency care to the organically impaired patient who has limited or no decision-making capacity.

Often the physician's well-intended efforts to communicate treatment information to the impaired patient prove ineffectual and present the practitioner with a medical-legal dilemma. The physician is unable to discuss in a legally meaningful way the implication of the proposed treatment with the impaired patient; however, there is a duty to treat patients who present with the potential for permanent disability or life-threatening conditions. In these situations, consent on the part of the impaired patient is considered to be implied and emergency treatment should be provided. Support for this view of implied consent is a general tenet of tort law.[11] Implied consent is manifest by patient action and determined by the emergency nature of the patient's condition and capacity to consent.

Patient Refusal and Implied Consent

PATIENT 1. A 34-year-old man was brought to the ED alert and oriented after ingesting 40 to 50 aspirin tablets (325 mg each). He was fully cognizant of the physician's intent to treat him and initially refused treatment. However, very soon after arrival, his level of consciousness deteriorated and the physician initiated emergency management, including the use of restraints to allow orogastric lavage to be performed with limited patient resistance.

This case raises two important issues. First, the practitioner must question whether or not the patient, although "alert and oriented," is initially capable of making a decision for himself. Given the history of abnormal behavior manifested by an apparent deliberate overdose ingestion, a reasonable argument could be made that the patient's judgment is so impaired that his initial refusal of treatment should not be honored. This conclusion must be supported by specific documentation in the medical record of the nature of the ingestion, specific statements suggesting suicidal ideations or attempts (if any), and the patient's statements and behavior. Where available, a written psychiatric consultation should be obtained. If psychiatric consultation is not immediately available, the emergency physician should use whatever mental health resources are available (eg, social worker) to assist in evaluating the suicidal risks of the patient.

Second, this case illustrates how the doctrine of implied consent can be applied to a difficult clinical situation. Patients who present with an altered consciousness are presumed under law to have consented to necessary treatment. The law further assumes that the patient would have consented to the indicated treatment if conscious and able to communicate with his or her physician. The 34-year-old man in this case developed an altered level of consciousness and required immediate intervention, potentially to save his life. By using the legal assumptions in the doctrine of implied consent, the emergency physician is able lawfully to intervene on the patient's behalf without any consequential risk of potential liability for assault and battery.

Documentation describing the patient's altered level of consciousness would be particularly critical in support of the physician's determination that the patient's condition was emergent and justifies the physician's invocation of a specific duty to treat the patient which arises under the law of implied consent.

By altering the facts of this case, a more complex ethical problem may confront the physician. Assume that the same patient was witnessed to have ingested these pills and remains fully cognizant with no observable deterioration, and that the patient adamantly refuses any medical intervention and desires to leave the ED. What course of action should the emergency physician follow?

Under such circumstances, a strong argument can nevertheless be made mandating immediate patient care intervention. The medical record should document any statements or actions by the patient suggesting impaired judgment. Further, an accurate and detailed description of this suicidal act should be recorded, and the source of this information (family, police, friends) noted in the ED record. If the patient persists in his refusal to accept intervention, the application of physical restraints may be necessary and should be considered. Such a patient could also benefit from psychiatric consultation, and the hospital chaplain might be utilized as an additional resource in this situation.

After restraints are applied correctly (Chap. 114), all appropriate medical intervention—including induction of emesis, orogastric lavage, or the use of activated charcoal—can be initiated. To obtain maximal legal protection, the emergency physician must document the reasons for intervention in the specific factual manner described.

Forcible Restraint of the Impaired Patient

PATIENT 2. A 31-year-old woman who reportedly injected heroin was brought to the ED by emergency medical service (EMS) and became apneic within a few seconds of arrival. Upon administration of 2 mg of naloxone IV the patient regained consciousness and demanded immediate release. The patient was fully alert and oriented, with no evidence of hypoxia or other clinical signs to suggest impaired judgment at this time. Routine evaluation of the patient's belongings revealed a small glassine envelope of white powder.

There is fairly good support from statutes and case law granting a hospital the right to retain and physically restrain a person who is dangerously disturbed, at least for a short time pending evaluation and emergency intervention.[4] This case represents a different and frequent problem that arises when a patient is brought to an ED in an obviously incapacitated or dangerously unstable clinical condition due to the ingestion of pharmacologic or toxicologic agents, and after partial recovery demands to be released from the hospital. In most states, legal precedents for such a situation have yet to be formally established by either written statutes or reported case law.

However, reasonably clear guidelines for the management of such impaired patients have evolved from legal precedents governing appropriate medical assessment, from risk management considerations, and from the predictability of patient injury in the event of premature discharge.

A staff decision to allow a treated or partially treated patient with a drug overdose who subsequently becomes alert to return to the community must be based on a medical assessment encompassing a number of factors. The initial concern is the patient's capacity to comprehend. Before the patient can be permitted to leave the hospital, he or she would have to be determined capable of understanding the information presented and have neither a medical nor a psychiatric problem preventing her from making a voluntary decision.

In patient 2, such an assessment cannot be limited to an evaluation of the patient's statements at the time she is momentarily oriented and "apparently capable" due to the administration of naloxone. In a situation such as this, patients appear to be alert, demand to be released from the ED, and may even be willing to sign the "Against Medical Advice" waiver that is a part of the ED record in many hospitals. Under these circumstances, it must be determined whether the ED staff has a legal duty to prevent such an individual from leaving before the toxic metabolic condition has been completely stabilized.

Common ED practice and sound legal principles suggest that both the hospital and its staff have a duty to prevent such a person from leaving, if the duration of the effect of the involved drugs or toxins is characteristically longer than the expected duration of the antidote's effect. Patient 2 was brought to the ED in a comatose state after the injection of heroin. Naloxone treatment rendered her temporarily awake and alert. She would not be allowed to leave on demand, because the emergency physician can predict with reasonable medical certainty what will happen to the patient in the near future—recurrence of coma or apnea (see Antidotes in Depth: Opioid Antagonists).

If this patient is permitted to leave, her welfare will be at risk. Such a person could collapse while driving an automobile or lose consciousness in a location where no medical attention is available. If a physician makes a judgment that such an event is probable or likely, he or she has a duty to inform the individual of the life-threatening nature of the condition and then, if necessary, retain the patient in the hospital until the decision to offer medical clearance is well established.

The patient in such a situation should be retained in the ED, even if appropriately applied physical restraints are required. Liability is further reduced when the chart substantiates the medical judgment on which the decision to use restraint and retain the patient was based. Such documentation should specifically note the likely relapse of the patient into a symptomatic state and should further state that such an occurrence could place the patient and others in a life-threatening situation. If such documentation is clearly entered on the medical record, legal challenge to the decision to restrain the patient would have very little chance of success. Sound risk management supports treatment and detainment, rather than permitting premature release of the patient. Releasing a seriously intoxicated patient prematurely exposes the physician and hospital to a claim of negligence on the grounds of failure to foresee a likely and harmful event.

Risk Management Consideration and Documentation

PATIENT 3. 6:05 PM. A 28-year-old woman was brought to the ED by the police. The police believed she might be a body packer.

6:10 PM. The triage nurse helped the patient onto a stretcher and brought her to the treatment area. The physician was summoned to see the patient. Her vital signs are blood pressure, 130/70 mm Hg; pulse, 78 beats/min; respiratory rate, 24 breaths/min; temperature, 36.7°C (98°F).

As the physician initiated the examination the patient became combative and uncooperative. The physician verbally ordered that the patient be restrained. The patient was placed on 40% oxygen via face mask, cardiac monitoring was begun, and an intravenous line was started with D_5W at 125 mL/h; 100 mL of $D_{50}W$ and 100 mg of thiamine were then given IV. Orogastric lavage was performed, followed by the administration of 50 g of activated charcoal.

7:10 PM. The patient's vital signs were blood pressure, 120/70 mm Hg; pulse, 82 beats/min; respiratory rate, 24 breaths/min. The patient was noted to be stable and moved to the observation unit. Oxygen and cardiac monitoring were discontinued. No further orders were written, and the patient remained restrained.

11:15 PM. The vital signs were blood pressure, 110/60 mm Hg; pulse, 92 beats/min; respiratory rate, 18 breaths/min. A nurse's note stated that the patient was resting comfortably.

11:50 PM. The initial physician completed his shift and was replaced at midnight by another physician. The first physician informed his replacement that the patient was stable and resting in the holding area.

4:20 AM. The patient was found unresponsive, with agonal respirations. She was hypotensive and had no palpable radial pulse. She felt very hot to the touch and had a rectal temperature of 108°F (42.2°C). Resuscitative efforts were initiated but unsuccessful.

4:50 AM. The patient was pronounced dead.

Several important risk management questions frequently arise in medical malpractice litigation involving the ED. To prove that a case constitutes medical malpractice, a plaintiff's attorney must show clear and convincing evidence of a departure from good practice by the physician. The attorney must further demonstrate that the negligent act or omission by the physician proximately caused the patient's injury. Courts have held that where "there is substantial probability that [if] the [defendant's] negligent conduct caused the resulting injury that sufficient evidence has been developed against [the] physician."[18]

The problem issues that can develop regarding the ED record are numerous, but they can be minimized if the practitioner is cognizant of risk management principles. When the attorney for the patient (plaintiff's attorney) introduces evidence to prove a case, the central document in the medical malpractice trial is likely to be the ED record. Thus, every entry in that record is scrutinized with great care by both parties (plaintiff and defendants), and the importance of completing it with knowledge of risk management implications should be a concern for all emergency physicians.

The emergency physician is required to write a medical record that will amply support the basis for his or her judgment. If the physician chooses to only write a summary statement on the ED record without noting supporting clinical data or patient history, then any claim against him or her alleging failure to diagnose will be extremely difficult, if not impossible, to defend. One of the basic elements of the defense in a medical malpractice case is that the physician's judgment was appropriate, given the clinical facts and the patient's history available at that time. Therefore, emergency physicians who do not record supporting clinical data and history deprive themselves of a strong "medical judgment" defense.

Inappropriate entries or markings on the medical record can weaken the defense in a liability case. For example, if the emergency physician or nurse totally obliterates an oxygen (PO_2) value, an attorney representing a patient may suggest to the jury that the obliteration was done intentionally to conceal clinical data harmful to the position of the defense. If a physician must correct a prior entry made on the ED record, the preferable method is to draw a single line through the value or word to be changed and insert the correct information directly above and to initial the correction. Dating the correction also precludes potential difficult questions in a courtroom setting. By following these suggestions, the emergency physician avoids any accusations that he or she intentionally concealed an error in judgment (Fig. 116–1).

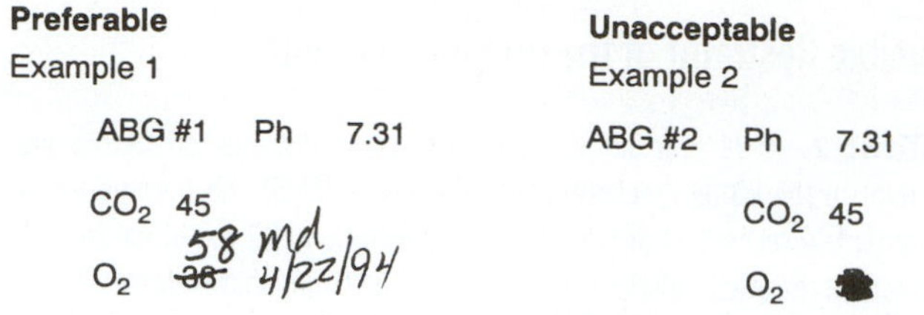

Figure 116–1. An example of the preferred and unacceptable procedures for correcting an error in the medical record.

A frequent claim is that the patient was improperly monitored or abandoned. For patient 3, although the chart appears to document repeated vital signs at appropriate intervals, the temperature is not noted after the first set until the patient is moribund, nor is mention made again of the continued use of restraints and the patient's condition with regard to the need for these restraints. Quality assurance reviews of ED records very often demonstrate inadequate charting by physicians and nurses monitoring patients with long-term ED stays (greater than 8 hours). Any lapse of (approximately) 4 hours or longer after initial physician and nursing assessment with no clinical notation as to patient status creates a potential risk management problem. The plaintiff's attorney would use such a record to develop the theory that no care whatsoever was given to the patient during this time interval and that the patient was abandoned.

Notations on the record with regard to monitoring are considered inadequate if they offer no insight into the patient's clinical status. Thus, any monitoring note for a patient who must be retained in the ED for a lengthy evaluation must include specific clinical data and observations (laboratory results, radiographic findings, hemodynamic changes, and infusion of medications and solutions). Both of these risk management deficiencies would undoubtedly be highlighted by a plaintiff's expert at trial (frequently a physician board-certified in emergency medicine and/or medical toxicology).

Any documentation supporting the restraint of a patient against his or her will due to impairment must include a clinical description to support such a forcible impediment to the patient's right to liberty and freedom of movement. Such a clinical description would include the patient's manifestation of agitation and uncooperative behavior. The chart should refer to the specific uncooperative acts of the patient and, most important, should comment on the difficulties in providing care to the patient owing to the patient's actions. If such documentation is present, a theory of negligence against the emergency physician for inappropriate restraints would be virtually impossible to set forth with any degree of success.

Physicians who order restraints for patients in the ED need to use caution in the language used to describe patients. If the physician's note states that a patient is "a chronic drunk and obnoxious" it could damage the support for the use of restraints. As a general rule, all professionals in the ED setting should describe patient behavior and lifestyles in objective and concrete terms, to depict a compassionate and professional manner. An alternative and more appropriate description of a comparable patient would describe a patient with a "history of alcohol abuse, who is uncooperative and combative." Poorly written physician notes can become an issue in a medical malpractice action, and a plaintiff's attorney could focus on the derogatory nature of a statement such as the original description. This could suggest a less-than-caring attitude by the doctor toward the patient. Such an appeal criticizing the ethical and social consciousness of the physician could very likely be seized upon by a jury and result in a punitive verdict against the physician.

To summarize, the best course for the emergency physician in managing a difficult overdose situation where legal principles may appear initially to be at odds with proper management is a well-documented ED record consistent with the risk management principles set forth.

Blood Alcohol and Evidence Collection

PATIENT 4. A 41-year-old male automobile driver was brought to the ED from a motor vehicle crash in which two other motorists were killed. The patient had no physical injuries and was brought to the hospital because he refused a breathalizer test at the scene. On arrival, he was alert and oriented, responded appropriately to all commands, and demonstrated a normal gait and motor function.

The police officers accompanying the patient informed the ED staff that he was suspected of driving while intoxicated and might be charged with vehicular homicide. The officers requested that the emergency physician draw blood for an alcohol concentration. The patient refused to allow ED staff to draw blood for an alcohol determination.

Pertinent questions with regard to this case are:

1. Can blood be drawn against a patient's will?
2. If the blood is drawn, can the physician be accused by the patient of assault and battery?
3. Do law officers have the right to demand that ED staff obtain specimens against a patient's wishes?
4. If the patient were obtunded, could an alcohol concentration be obtained without consent? What are the legal implications?
5. If specimens are obtained for legal proceedings, what is the appropriate chain for evidence collection?

Numerous states have policies that encourage taking a blood alcohol concentration if a patient is arrested and suspected of driving a motor vehicle while impaired. In New York State, Section 1194 of the Vehicle and Traffic Law states: "Any person who operates a motor vehicle is considered to have consented to a chemical test of breath, blood, urine or saliva for the purpose of determining alcoholic and/or drug content, provided that such test is administered at the direction of a police officer."[16]

This case raises several potential constitutional questions of significant magnitude. Defendants in criminal trials have claimed that a compulsory blood test under similar circumstances violates the Fifth Amendment privilege against self-incrimination. It has been argued that a compulsory blood test against the wishes of a patient infringes on the constitutionally protected concerns for human dignity and privacy, as expressed in the Fourth Amendment of the Constitution. However, in Schmerber v. California, the U.S. Supreme Court stated that blood may be taken from a patient against his or her will if done so in the context of a lawful arrest. In explaining its decision, the Court stated:

> In the case of a conscious individual, a chemical test can be administered since he is deemed to have given his consent when he used the highway. It is not necessary that a person be given the opportunity to revoke his consent. The only reason the opportunity is given is to eliminate the need for the use of force by police officers if an individual in a drunken condition should refuse to submit to the test.[15]

To determine whether blood can be drawn against the patient's will, the ED staff must become familiar with the specific requirements of the motor vehicle law in the state where the crash took place. Many states allow a patient to refuse a blood alcohol test, in circumstances similar to those involving patient 4.

As a general rule, emergency physicians and nurses cannot be compelled to take a specimen from a patient/driver who refuses such a test under state law. If this case occurred in New York State, the patient would have been informed by the arresting police officer that his license to drive would be immediately suspended if he refused to undergo a blood alcohol test. The patient's license could be suspended for as long as 16 days after arraignment. The patient would then be entitled to a hearing concerning the suspension of his license.[17] This statutory approach to dealing with the impaired driver of a motor vehicle is consistent with the motor vehicle law of many state statutes.

The emergency physician should consider the potential for a lawsuit alleging assault and battery under comparable circumstances. If the patient consented to the blood test, any action alleging assault and battery would be unsuccessful. However, if the patient arrived obtunded, confused, or comatose, a serious question would arise as to whether or not he or she could consent to a blood alcohol test requested by a police officer.

A resolution to this dilemma is provided in the case of People v. Kates, in which the court was confronted with a disoriented person recently involved in a fatal motor vehicle crash. The court suggested that the combination of probable cause, the circumstances of the patient's condition, and a reasonable examination procedure permitted the performance of a blood alcohol test without the patient's consent.[10] The court expressly stated that performing the test under these circumstances did not violate the patient's constitutional rights. It is suggested that the emergency physician should review with hospital counsel the local state law governing compulsory testing at the request of a police officer when there is an indication of suspected criminal behavior. The laws vary from state to state, and the examples in this discussion refer specifically to the approach currently followed in New York State.

Evidence Collection

Once the blood specimen is obtained, another significant medical-legal task confronts the entire ED staff. Compliance with the chain of evidence approach can eliminate the risk of nonadmissability of a specimen in a later criminal proceeding.

In cases where laboratory results are likely to be used in a legal discussion of criminal conduct, it is essential to establish the appropriate chain of evidence. It is essential that the laboratory specimens be processed in a meticulous fashion. This toxicologic assay may or may not support the defendant's charge of driving while intoxicated.

First, the specimen must be obtained in full view of a witness. Second, if the hospital laboratory is used to analyze the specimen, it is prudent to alert the laboratory that the specimen is likely to become evidence in a criminal trial. Accordingly, every processing step for that specimen, beginning with the act of collection, each individual test done on the specimen, and transport to and from the laboratory must be documented with the name of the person performing the task. The "chain of evidence" requires that each step in the processing and transport of the specimen be documented without a break in the custody of the specimen. These same requirements apply to a specimen for a toxicologic analysis that may be sent outside the primary hospital. To ensure the chain of custody from the hospital to the outside laboratory, prudent practice would suggest sending the specimens in a clearly labeled package and obtaining a receipt from the laboratory.

Some practitioners have questioned the legality of blood alcohol concentrations when these tests are drawn for some other clinical use. For example, seriously traumatized victims commonly have blood alcohol concentrations drawn to exclude a cause of an altered level of consciousness and altered level of perception. In these cases, the legality of the laboratory value can be questioned. It should be noted that the entire medical record can be introduced as evidence if it is deemed relevant by the court. However, without a chain of evidence, an attorney can challenge the validity of a blood alcohol concentration, especially when it was obtained for another clinical use or was considered a routine part of ED trauma assessment.

Furthermore, the outside laboratory should be called prior to delivery of the specimen and instructed to document each step in the performance of the required test. Usually, the police department will sign for and assume responsibility of all such specimens taken to an outside laboratory.

Discharging Patients With Elevated Blood Alcohol Levels

Most legal authorities would agree that the legal limit of a blood alcohol concentration is 100 mg/dL. This guideline is appropriate to assess legal blood alcohol concentrations but is not an accurate parameter to determine clinical intoxication or impairment. There are patients who chronically abuse alcohol, develop tolerance, and may have baseline alcohol concentrations several times the legal level, yet clinically they may not be considered impaired or intoxicated. Although these patients would be considered legally intoxicated, they are clinically sober. In cases where such patients are awaiting discharge from an ED, their blood alcohol concentrations should not be used as the criterion for delaying discharge. Although a concentration may exceed the legal limits, if the patient is not clinically impaired, discharge should not be delayed. If the patient is known to be operating a motor vehicle it would be prudent to obtain assistance for him or her (family, friend, or taxi) to limit the use of the motor vehicle.

The decision to discharge a patient under these circumstances should be based on sound clinical grounds. To minimize the liability associated with this decision, the physician should carefully document the patient's condition. He or she should test the patient's motor function and ability to reason. A detailed discharge summary must document results that reflect the patient's competency. It is also advised that the physician counsel and caution the patient regarding the health implications of the elevated blood alcohol concentration and risk to self and others in the operation of any type of motor vehicle. The physician should initiate the social and psychologic support necessary for the patient to seek alcohol detoxification. Obviously, this conversation should be documented. Following these recommendations minimizes the legal liability of the emergency physician and hospital. The potential for any successful litigation against these parties is significantly reduced on the grounds of comparative negligence.

Risk Management Considerations for Patient Triage, Discharge, and Transfer

PATIENT 5. A 26-year-old male intravenous drug user (IVDU) was brought to the ED after falling in the street and bumping his head. The odor of alcohol was noted on the patient's breath. He was alert and oriented and denied any loss of consciousness. The patient was evaluated by the triage nurse and then by the physician. A complete physical examination, including a detailed neurologic examination, was performed. The entire examination was normal and the patient was released.

What Are the Essential Components of Triage That Minimize Potential Risk Management Problems?

Beginning with the initial contact at triage, medical personnel must be extremely observant in evaluating the victim of a head injury. This task is more difficult and more important if the patient has potentially abused illicit drugs, alcohol, or medications. The assessment should be initiated by obtaining a past medical history, including medical problems, allergies, and immunizations. The history of alcohol or substance abuse (acute and chronic) should also be obtained to determine the potential impact on the patient's clinical presentation, particularly neurologic findings.

The patient's chief complaint should be solicited and documented in his or her own words. A subjective interpretation of a patient's complaints, particularly in this setting, should be avoided; similarly, a presumptive diagnosis should not be made. Sound medical and legal principles governing triage establish that the nurse and physician must objectively describe findings based on observations and assessment. If the patient was brought by ambulance, the report of prehospital personnel should be incorporated into the triage notes. In situations similar to patient 5, careful assessment and documentation of mental status is critical, since the history offered (IVDU) and the clinical findings (odor of alcohol) are highly suggestive of acute and chronic substance abuse.

The final component of triage is assessing and recording vital signs. Vital signs should be documented in the appropriate area of the chart, and the time should be noted accordingly. For patients not immediately triaged to a patient care area, vital signs must be retaken at fixed intervals. At these times, patients should also be reassessed, and any change in the clinical condition should be noted. If any deterioration or suspicion of significant changes in the patient's condition occurs, the patient may need to be recategorized and "up-triaged." Patients may also improve, and recategorization may occur for this reason as well.

In triage, patients are categorized as emergent (any life-threatening condition, must be evaluated immediately); urgent (less acute, not life-threatening but may become life-threatening); or nonurgent (no immediate threat) to determine the priority of care (Chap. 114).[8] If patients are not examined in the appropriate order, a note should be entered on the chart to justify this and to describe the patient's condition at the time of reevaluation.

Occasionally, the triage person needs to provide treatment to the emergent patient (eg, oxygen therapy, hemorrhage control, insertion of an airway). In this instance, documentation of emergency interventions and their outcome is required. Careful documentation of immediate interventions provides important information essential to ongoing emergency care and may also be valuable to the defense of a civil lawsuit.

How Can the ED Practitioner Reduce the Legal Risks Associated With Patient Discharge?

Detailed criteria for release from an ED serve to protect patients from injury due to premature discharge and also greatly reduce the risk of liability. These criteria are particularly important for a patient whose mental status might be impaired from alcohol or drug abuse. Sample criteria include giving the patient and/or family members written discharge instructions. These instructions should advise the patient to return to the ED should any abnormal symptoms appear. Well-drafted instructions should also inform the patient of any activities to perform and/or avoid at home (eg, rest, elevation, and ice). Verbal instructions should also include follow-up information regarding prescriptions (eg, adverse effects, impact on driving, medicating schedule). These instructions should also emphasize the goal of sobriety and support for detoxification. Documentation that written and verbal instructions were given and that the patient understood these instructions are obligatory for the ED practitioner with sound risk management training.

The ED staff should obtain the patient's signature, with date and time. This practice creates an inference in court that the patient received discharge instructions. However, in cases of head injury and/or intoxication, discharge is recommended only when the patient is accompanied by family or friends. In these cases, the accompanying individuals should also sign the chart, demonstrating that instructions were understood. The chart should clearly state the relationship of the family member or friend to the patient.

Finally, in any situation where the ED staff suspect that drugs were ingested, psychiatric consultation is strongly recommended. Whether the intoxication was a conscious intentional act or unintentional, psychiatric consultation is indicated to ensure safe risk management practices. By so doing, the emergency physician will obtain another objective professional assessment of the patient's ability to make basic decisions about his or her care and plan for future behavioral changes.

What Potential Legal Liabilities Are Associated With Patient Transfer and Refusal to Treat?

"Patient dumping" increased dramatically as a phenomenon in the 1980s. Patient dumping occurs when a hospital that is capable of providing emergency medical care to a particular patient turns the individual away because of the patient's inability to pay. Congress enacted the Consolidated Omnibus Budget Reconciliation Act (COBRA), which encompassed the Emergency Medicine Treatment and Active Labor Act (EMTALA) in 1985. This statute was intended to create significant penalties for hospitals and physicians who discharge patients solely for financial reasons.

The statute also focuses on patient transfers from EDs to other institutions. It states that "if an individual patient has an emergency medical condition that has not been stabilized, it is unlawful to transfer the patient unless a number of conditions are met." These conditions are as follows:

1. The physician must certify in writing that it is his or her professional opinion that the anticipated medical benefits of transfer outweigh the risks.

2. The patient must consent to transfer.
3. The transferring hospital must assure adequate medical treatment during the transfer to minimize the risks to the patient or fetus.
4. The receiving facility must be notified prior to the transfer, agree to accept the patient, and have the capability to treat the patient.
5. Adequate medical information, such as a copy of the medical records and/or a well-prepared interinstitutional transfer form, must accompany the patient.

Sanctions under COBRA can be severe. If a physician authorizes an inappropriate transfer, fines up to $50,000 can be assessed for each violation. Such an action could conceivably be found to be "gross and flagrant," and the physician could be excluded from the Medicare and state Medicaid programs. An institution held responsible for a pattern of inappropriate transfers could be suspended or terminated from the Medicare program for a violation of any COBRA requirement.[6] Therefore, the guidelines concerning documentation of triage decisions, discharge, and transfer must be followed without any deviation to ensure that the acts of an individual will not lead to any institutional or individual liability.

Legal Considerations for Poison Centers and Information Specialists

PATIENT 6. The local poison center received a call from concerned parents regarding the acute ingestion of a full bottle of liquid Tylenol by their child. The parents were advised by an information specialist to administer 30 mL of syrup of ipecac to induce vomiting. Three days later the baby lapsed into coma and the parents called the 911 emergency number. An ambulance arrived and transported the child to the local hospital. The child suffered irreversible liver damage. Action was subsequently brought against the local poison center, alleging inappropirate advice and failure to recommend transport to a hospital.

Does Telephone Contact With a Poison Information Specialist Create a Duty of Care Recognizable by Law?

As a general rule, any physician who decides to treat a patient enters into a physician–patient relationship that creates well-established legal duties. Courts have ruled that the physician–patient encounter need not be a face-to-face interaction to have legal consequences. For example, the absence of physical contact between a physician and patient as in the practice of radiologists and pathologists does not preclude a patient from asserting that a duty of care exists.[2] More particularly, and quite relevant to the practice of a poison center, a New York State court ruled that an initial telephone call from a patient to a physician can be sufficient basis to hold that physician responsible for inappropriate advice or a significant error in judgment.[9]

Given the legal precedents previously stated, it is eminently clear that patient contact with a poison information specialist is a sufficient foundation for a subsequent legal action if inappropriate advice was given. In this case, a medical toxicologist could criticize the advice given to the parents. In particular, the recommendation apparently failed to include a directive to seek immediate emergency assistance. The advice to give the child syrup of ipecac was appropriate, but the failure to recommend emergency transport rendered the totality of the advice given substandard and less than the applicable duty of care.

What Standards of Care Are Applicable to Poison Information Specialists?

Any discussion of the standard of care to which a poison information specialist should be held would be misleading without mentioning several operational aspects of most poison centers. The specialist would be required to have rapid and accurate access to a standard information resource system, such as Poisindex, a computerized information source that is updated quarterly and contains both basic information and recommendations to deal with most encountered toxic ingestions. Advice that differs significantly from an existing protocol or standard of care would be subject to critical review in a civil lawsuit. If a patient were to bring an action, the negligence theory against the poison center might rely particularly on deviations from the standard recommendations.

It would be inaccurate to suggest, however, that the duty of care owed by a poison information specialist can be measured only by how closely the advice given compares with the standard resources. Frequently, a specialist may encounter situations that cannot be managed in accordance with an information system alone, and the poison information specialist may have to seek counsel from a doctor of pharmacy or physician consultant working with the poison center. If this were to occur, any subsequent legal proceeding would also review carefully the content of the input given by the consultant as to its accuracy and appropriateness to the underlying toxicologic problem.

What Practices Can Be Incorporated by Regional Poison Centers to Reduce Potential Liabilities?

It is clear that a poison center has some inherent risks of potential liability. To minimize the risk of liability and civil actions against a poison center, it is suggested that quality assurance and risk management programs be given high priority. This is usually the case with regional poison centers. Daily physician audits of poison information specialist care should be done. This interaction enhances care and ensures patient safety in each individual case, as well as establishing a higher general standard.

The medical toxicologist and clinical pharmacist responsible for supervising the poison information specialist must be able to assess adequately the competence and capability of the poison center staff, thereby making individual recommendations, corrective actions, and suggestions to involved members.

Both individual case audits and departmental committee review of complicated toxic ingestions should address the quality of poison information specialist documentation. The medical toxicologist must assess the adequacy of the patient history obtained and should pay particular attention to the written documentation of advice given. If a lawsuit ensues, the most likely area of dispute will be with regard to what was actually said to the patient.

In a case similar to that of patient 6, a patient might be told to seek immediate emergency help from a physician or ambulance service and choose not to follow this advice, to his or her detriment. The failure of the poison information specialist to document such advice meticulously could lead to a significant credibility issue in subsequent litigation. If the patient's lawyer knew that such specific documentation were lacking, then a likely claim in the lawsuit would be that the advice was not actually given. This risk management advice with regard to critical patient information is equally applicable to the poison information specialist.

Implications of Living Wills, Do-Not-Resuscitate Orders, Advanced Directives, and Physician-Assisted Suicide for Patients With Drug Overdose or Toxic Ingestion

PATIENT 7. A 75-year-old man was brought to the ED by EMS. He was unresponsive and reported to have ingested a large quantity of phenobarbital. The patient was well known to the medical center staff and had been previously diagnosed as having metastatic prostate cancer. It was also suspected that he had a living will and explicitly refused advanced life support and resuscitation.

On arrival in the ED, the patient was hypotensive with a blood pressure of 80/40 mm Hg, a pulse of 80 in normal sinus rhythm, a respiratory rate of 4 breaths/min, and a rectal temperature of 96°F (35.6°C). He was immediately given naloxone, dextrose, and thiamine without response; an endotracheal tube was then inserted and he was ventilated on 100% oxygen. Orogastric lavage was performed and activated charcoal was instilled prior to removal of the lavage hose. Despite being given 2 liters of lactated Ringer's solution, his systolic blood pressure remained at 80 mm Hg and he was started on a dopamine infusion. Neurologic examination at the time revealed fixed and dilated pupils with absent corneal and occulocephalic reflexes. The patient was transferred to the MICU for further management.

Pertinent questions with regard to this case are (1) whether this patient should be resuscitated and (2) the implication of a living will in a patient who has intentionally ingested a drug overdose.

An advanced directive, a living will, or a healthcare proxy (a document that transfers to an agent the right to make life and death decisions for an impaired patient) is considered to be legally binding when a patient presents with symptoms from a naturally occurring disease process. It is not the intent of any state to use these documents to assist a patient who has attempted to commit suicide. Such a view would be considered violative of public policy.

A decision in this instance cannot be made simply by reference to the patient's intentions as individually expressed in a living will or through a designated agent in the healthcare proxy. The regulatory authorities in most states (living will and healthcare proxy statutes are regulated by state health departments) would probably indicate that the patient should be resuscitated in this situation due to the society's position that a physician should not assist in a suicide attempt. The American Medical Associations's Ethical Guidelines take a similar position.

In view of the current debate in the medical, legal, and ethical literature with regard to euthanasia in controlled and state-approved circumstances, the approach in this hypothetical case may very well be different in several years. This area of law and ethics is evolving at a rapid and variable pace throughout the individual states. The issue of physician-assisted suicide and the circumstances under which it is permissible was left ambiguous by a 1997 United States Supreme Court decision. Ethicists have taken strong positions on both sides of this controversial issue and a clear understanding of the controlling law in this area will have to await several forays in the legal reviews. Accordingly, this is an issue that ED practitioners will have to monitor closely as individual state governments and health departments create regulations. One of the arguments asserted by those in the medical community supporting physician-assisted suicide is that patients experiencing extreme suffering with no possible amelioration by medical means are a protected class and should be granted equal protection under the constitution. Whether or not this view will prevail is highly uncertain at this time. It is recommended that EDs routinely incorporate discussions of these issues into their educational programs.

Intoxication and Patient Confidentiality

PATIENT 8. A 52-year-old man was seen by his general practitioner during his lunch hour for the complaint of recurring headaches. The patient was the local school bus driver in a small rural community. The physician believed the patient was intoxicated and noted the odor of alcohol on his breath. The patient was well known and respected throughout the community. The physician confronted the patient with his suspicion, and the patient adamantly denied alcohol use. The physician requested permission to draw blood tests, including a blood alcohol level. The patient refused. He stated that he would sue the physician if he reported his suspicions.

Pertinent questions with regard to this question are as follows.

1. Would the release of information regarding the physician's suspicions constitute a violation of patient confidentiality?
2. Do the facts of this case present a public policy exception to the patient's rights of confidentiality in light of the general societal need to protect the safety of passengers and children?

This case presents a dilemma that occasionally confronts every practitioner. As a first point it must be emphasized that any release of patient information to an individual or agency not involved in the patient's care (school authority or supervisors) would clearly be a technical violation of the normal patient confidentiality requirements. However, the facts in any particular case may create an exception to the normal rules governing the release of patient information. In this case a convincing and compelling argument could be made that public policy mandates practitioners to advise school authorities of the bus driver's potentially intoxicated condition in the interest of preserving life and safety of children who would ride on his bus on that same day or in the future.

If the bus driver chooses to bring a lawsuit against the practitioner and hospital on the grounds that he had lost his job due to the unauthorized release of medical information, such a case could be well defended with the public policy arguments just given. There is little likelihood of success of such a lawsuit. These principles would apply to any scenario involving an individual who is responsible for public safety (eg, train conductor, airline pilot, police officer).

A more complicated situation arises if the patient is not intoxicated but the physician smells the odor of alcohol on the patient's breath. In this case the physician may be less willing to report his or her suspicion because of the seriousness of the accusation and the degree of uncertainty regarding the extent of alcohol use. Despite this dilemma, the highest ethical standards suggest that the physician has a duty to protect society and to report his or her suspicions to the appropriate authority.

Implications for Emancipated Minors, Child Abuse and Neglect, and the Unborn Fetus

PATIENT 9. A 17-year-old female presented to the ED for altered mental status. Physical examination revealed an obviously pregnant young woman with a blood pressure of 150/100 mm Hg, pulse of 140 beats/min, respiratory rate of 30 breaths/min, and rectal temperature of 101°F (38.3°C). Her skin was diaphoretic and her pupils were 6 to 7 mm and reactive to light. The remainder of her evaluation was unremarkable except for a 28-week size uterus with strong fetal heart tones. After receiving 20 mg of Valium IV, her vital signs normalized and she admitted to frequent crack cocaine use. She had no prenatal care, was not married, and her two-year-old child had been brought in from home by the police for evaluation.

The ED received a telephone call from the patient's grandmother (the legal guardian) inquiring about her condition. The patient indicated that she did not want her grandmother to know about her admission or pregnancy.

Pertinent question for this case are the following.

1. Can the physician accept the patient's wishes not to inform the grandmother of her medical condition?
2. Is the patient an emancipated minor capable of making her own consent for treatment?
3. What is the responsibility of the ED staff when confronted with a patient refusal to obtain social service help for his or her child?
4. Can the hospital and the ED staff compel this patient to go for routine prenatal care in the obstetrical clinic?

Many states have guidelines that protect the confidentiality of adolescent patients seeking obstetrical and gynecologic healthcare. Despite the wishes of this young patient to keep her status confidential, a delicate balance must be considered when the emergency physician is confronted with an impaired adolescent who is pregnant and the mother of a small child. In such an example, societal concerns and sound hospital policy suggest that the grandmother would have to be fully informed of the patient's medical condition. There are several reasons for this conclusion, and one controlling factor in this decision is the state's interest in insuring the protection of a small child. When balanced against this overriding ethical concern, the patient's desire for confidentiality cannot be met.

The legal doctrine of emancipated minor varies somewhat in different states, but the general definition is consistent and quite similar throughout the United States. If an adolescent patient lives apart from her parental home, and is pregnant, then such a grouping of factual elements would constitute emancipated minor status in virtually all states. If this patient was not impaired due to cocaine, then she would have a legal right to make decisions about her healthcare in all respects. However, the ingestion of crack cocaine permitted the ED staff to treat her despite protestation because of her present inability to fully comprehend the implications of her actions. As noted in Chapter 113, the patient's impairment must be documented as to specific clinical symptoms.

Child abuse and neglect statutes require the ED staff (often as a mandated reporter) to inform the designated state authorities when they suspect child abuse or neglect. If the 2-year-old were permitted to leave the ED under the care of this young patient/mother, the expanded definition of neglect in most state statutes would preclude disposition at stage of care. The appropriate course of action for the ED staff includes coordinating a number of steps to provide maximum support for this potentially imperiled child.

A social worker should assist with an assessment of the home situation. It is often beneficial if the social worker (a child abuse specialist) speaks to the state authorities in addition to the ED staff. In this example, a possible resolution that is minimally disruptive to the child's well-being would be placement with the grandmother. This would only be done after approval from the state child abuse authority.

If the hospital and ED staff seek to compel this patient to go to outpatient visits in the obstetrical clinic, some form of court intervention would have to be sought. As a rule, the courts have been reluctant on the grounds of abuse and neglect to compel care to a fetus, despite harmful behavior by the mother to the prospects for the child. However, a case plan that includes close follow-up of the adolescent mother's condition by an in-hospital child abuse interdisciplinary team in conjunction with a child welfare agency that has jurisdictional responsibility for the adolescent's care is probably the optimal method to achieve a coordinated solution to this difficult ethical and medical problem. There are times when a court order is not effective and a more appropriate solution may be the intervention of a child welfare agency.

The Jehovah's Witness Refusal to Accept Treatment and the Relationship to Toxicologic Care

A comprehensive review of medical-legal issues should always include a discussion of the care of the patient who is also a Jehovah's Witness. Although religious and legal issues rarely are relevant in toxicologic emergencies, the rights of a patient who is also a Jehovah's Witness is a subject worthy of a detailed discussion. This analysis may allow for a thoughtful review of toxicologic issues. The most common scenario involving a patient who is also a Jehovah's Witness is refusal by the patient to receive transfusions of any blood or blood products. Three variations of this scenario have been discussed in legal briefs.

1. A conscious patient who understands the risks and benefits of medical treatment requires emergency transfusions. The patient refuses all transfusions and risks death as a consequence.
2. An unconscious patient arrives in an ED and requires emergency blood transfusions to sustain life. Family members accompanying the patient inform the staff that the patient is a Jehovah's Witness and they refuse to consent to any blood transfusions.
3. The parents of a child requiring emergency transfusions to sustain life refuse to allow blood to be given to their child on the grounds of religious beliefs.

A serious legal and ethical dilemma is confronted when an individual who understands the risks and benefits of medical treatment refuses the treatment necessary to save his or her life. Numerous cases have decided this issue. The courts generally agree that a competent individual has a constitutional right to refuse medical treatment. Refusal to accept life-saving treatments, or in this case blood transfusions, is supported by the fact that every individual is entitled to bodily integrity and privacy. An important note is that this constitutional right exists irrespective of the individual's religious belief. In fact, in the landmark case of Fosmire v. Nicoleau, New York's highest court, the State Court of Appeals, ruled definitively that the state's interest in preserving an individual's life cannot override the individual's right to refuse life-saving medical treatments.[3]

A variation of this case caused the courts to struggle with the question of how to deal with the parent of a small child who refuses blood transfusions for himself or herself. In these cases, the court has decided to protect the rights of the parent even when the individual has responsibility for minors or children. In most cases, the individual's rights to refuse treatment is protected under the First Amendment if it is linked to a religious objection or can be linked to the fundamental right of privacy.

The most complicated scenario involving patients who are also Jehovah's Witnesses is when the patient is unconscious and requires emergency blood transfusions and accompanying family members refuse to sign consent for transfusions. Under these circumstances the physician must immediately determine whether the patient's illness is emergent (life threatening), urgent, or nonurgent (not life threatening). In emergent cases, particularly when there is inadequate time to make a detailed assessment, the physician has a duty to treat the patient immediately. This premise is identical to the principles of implied consent discussed for patient 7. Immediate action rarely creates any significant liability, whereas delays and deliberations associated with negative outcomes can have enormous liability. If the case is not emergent, the emergency physician should verify the family's request, provided that this delay will not jeopardize the patient's condition. The family should be given an opportunity to provide clear and convincing evidence that the patient would have refused transfusions or other medical interventions.

A separate issue arises in cases of minors or children as to whether a competent guardian or parent can exercise the right to refuse medical treatment for the child. In a case such as this, virtually all states invoke the parens patriae doctrine, which permits the state to protect its citizens who are unable to protect themselves. This doctrine has been upheld in multiple cases of Jehovah's Witnesses' patients who have not been permitted to refuse the transfusion of blood products for their children.

In terms of practical management, the emergency physician must be mindful of several steps in the communication process when administering transfusions to a child. The parents or guardians must be told that a transfusion(s) is anticipated and that the hospital will proceed on the basis of state law. A progress note must be entered into the chart documenting the time of transfusion, the medical necessity of the transfusion, and the conversations with the parents. A court order to administer blood transfusions to a child in a life-threatening circumstance is not required, and this should not delay emergency treatment.

It is strongly recommended that any emergency physician confronted with a life-threatening refusal of blood products by a patient who is also a Jehovah's Witness work closely with the hospital's risk management staff. Legal advice should always be sought to ensure that all risk management concerns are addressed.

References

1. Borak J, Veilleux S: Informed consent in emergency settings. Ann Emerg Med 1984; 13:731–735.
2. Capuano v. Jacobs, 33A.D., 2d. 743, 305 N.Y. State, 2d 837 (1960).
3. Fosmire v. Nicoleau, A.D., 2d. 876, 551 N.Y. State (1990).

4. Gonzalez v. State, 110 A.D., 2d. 810, 488 N.Y. 2d. 231, 67 N.Y. 2d. 647 (1985).
5. In the Matter of Storar, 52 N.Y. 2d 363, 377 (1981).
6. Krugh T: Medical COBRA: The federal anti-dumping act. For the Defense, June 1992:14–16.
7. Makadon HJ, Gerson S, Ryback R: Managing the care of the difficult patient in the emergency unit. JAMA 1984;252: 2585–2588.
8. New York City Health and Hospitals Corporation, Bellevue Hospital Center: Policy and Procedure Manual for Emergency Services, 1993.
9. O'Neil v. Montefiore Hospital, 11A.D., 2d 132, 202 N.Y. State, 2d 436 (1960).
10. People v. Kates, 444 N.Y. Suppl. 2d 446, 53 N.Y. 2d. 590 (1981).
11. Prosser WL: The Law of Torts. St. Paul, West, 1984.
12. Public Health Law Section 2504(4). McKinney's Consolidated Laws of New York Annotated book 44, public health law sections 2100–3399. St. Paul, West, 1985.
13. Public Health Law, Section 2805 (d) (1). McKinney's Consolidated Laws of New York Annotated, book 44, public health saw sections 2100–3399. St. Paul, West, 1985.
14. Schloendorff v. Society of New York Hospital, 211 N.Y. 125, 105 N.E. 92, 93 (1914).
15. Schmerber v. California, 384 US 757, 16L ed 2d. 908, 86 Sct 1826 (1966).
16. Vehicle and Traffic Law, section 1194 (2) (a), McKinney's Consolidated Laws of New York Annotated, book 62A, vehicle and traffic law sections 600–end. St. Paul, West, 1970.
17. Vehicle and Traffic Law, Section 1194 (2) (b), McKinney's Consolidated Laws of New York, Annotated, book 62A, vehicle and traffic law sections 600–end. St. Paul, West, 1970.
18. Vialva v. City of New York, 118 A.D., 2d. 701, 499 N.Y. 2d. 977 (2nd Dept. 1986).

CHAPTER 117

Principles of Research Design

Eddy A. Bresnitz

A 37-year-old woman presented to the emergency department (ED) complaining of progressive generalized muscle aches and weakness for 2 months. Additional symptoms included mouth ulcers, abdominal discomfort, a rapid heartbeat, and a 10-kg weight loss. She had a history of allergic rhinitis but had been otherwise healthy. Initial physical examination revealed normal vital signs, diffuse muscle tenderness and weakness, flushing of the skin, a puffy face, and oral ulcers. Laboratory data were remarkable for an elevated white blood cell count of 11,900/mm^3 with 42% eosinophils and mildly elevated liver function tests; serum albumin, total protein, creatine kinase, creatinine, and erythrocyte sedimentation rate were normal.

She was referred to the medical clinic, where she was evaluated for her marked eosinophilia, which had increased to 45% 1 month later. Extensive laboratory evaluation effectively excluded the possibility of neoplasm, parasitic infection, generalized infection, or an autoimmune process. Liver enzymes increased slightly. A muscle biopsy showed normal muscle cells with a perimysial infiltrate of eosinophils.

A careful drug history indicated that the woman began taking 2 g of L-tryptophan nightly for insomnia 8 weeks prior to the onset of her symptoms. She was not taking any other medications.

This case represents one of the first descriptions of what proved to be a nationwide epidemic of L-tryptophan-associated eosinophilic-myalgia syndrome (EMS).[16] The clinical staff initially evaluating this patient could not be sure that the drug was related to the patient's symptoms, especially since tryptophan had been used for many years as a dietary supplement. They had to assess her complaints as best they could without knowing the appropriate management of the problem. How could they be sure that any treatment they prescribed was appropriate for this situation? How could they decide whether this was an uncommon reaction to a commonly used drug? Answers to these questions are derived from epidemiologic and toxicologic research. With continual additions being made to cumulative knowledge, medical toxicologists are confronted daily with the task of reading and evaluating the clinical literature.

This chapter outlines the principles of assessing causation in disease-exposure associations; choosing or evaluating the appropriateness of the research design; and evaluating the validity of a particular research study. For a comprehensive review of the steps in assessing a particular study design, the interested reader is referred to a series of articles that address in more detail many of the issues discussed in this chapter.[10]

What Are the Basic Principles of Determining That a Particular Toxic Exposure Causes a Specific Syndrome or Disease?

In both experimental and nonexperimental (observational) research, the statistical association of an "exposure," be it a risk factor or a therapy, with an outcome, such as a disease, in any *one* study does not prove necessarily that a causal relationship exists. This association may occur because of (1) bias in the selection of study subjects or in the measurements of exposure and outcome, (2) indirect association through a variable that is associated with both the disease and the exposure (a confounding variable), (3) chance association, and (4) true causal association.[13] Even one well-designed study does not necessarily prove that an exposure and outcome are causally related. Scientists usually apply several criteria in the assessment of causal relationships.

Hill outlined the criteria by which scientists and clinicians assess true causation in any disease–exposure association (Table 117–1).[17] These principles can also be used to evaluate therapeutic measures in the treatment of disease. However, these principles should be used to assess true causation only if they are applied to studies that are both reliable and valid. In a reliable study, the results are consistent and reproducible but not necessarily valid. A valid study accurately measures the outcome of interest. For example, a laboratory test may consistently produce values of an electrolyte that are 20 mg/dL over the true value. These results would be reliable but invalid.

TABLE 117–1. CRITERIA TO ASSESS CAUSATION

- Strength of the disease–exposure association
- Consistency of the association in different places under different circumstances
- Specificity of the association
- Temporality
- Dose–response effect
- Supporting experimental evidence
- Biologic plausibility
- Coherence with other clinical or biologic observations

Hill's first criterion, the strength of a disease–exposure association, can be measured by the magnitude of the *relative risk* (also called the odds ratio). This is the ratio of the incidence of disease in the group exposed to a risk factor, compared to the incidence of disease in the control group (the group not exposed to the risk factor). For example, when we say that people exposed to asbestos are five times as likely to contract lung cancer in their lifetime as are people who have not been exposed to asbestos, we are saying that the relative risk of this disease is 5. Similarly, initial studies of patients with EMS indicated that they were many more times as likely to have ingested L-tryptophan-containing products (LTCPs) compared to healthy controls.[2]

Hill's second criterion for judging the true relationship between a disease and an exposure is the *consistency* of the observed association. A causal association is more likely if the association has been reproduced in different studies using different research designs in different groups of people in different geographic locations. An excellent illustration of consistency is the relationship between smoking and lung cancer. The surgeon general's original report on the association of smoking and lung cancer was based on 29 retrospective and 7 prospective studies, all finding approximately the same magnitude of association.[27] In the case of EMS, there have been numerous reports of the syndrome occurring in geographically diverse groups of individuals worldwide, most of whom ingested LTCPs that were produced by a single manufacturer in Japan.[1,20]

A meta-analysis attempts to combine studies of the same design to achieve greater statistical power in assessing disease–exposure relationships.[11] For example, during the 1980s, several epidemiologic studies showed an inconsistent relationship between the risk of breast cancer and alcohol consumption. Separate meta-analyses of case-control and cohort studies done to date revealed a 40 to 70% increased risk of breast cancer in women who drank 1 oz (30 mL) of absolute alcohol daily.[23] There was also strong evidence for a dose–response relationship between exposure and disease.

The specificity of an association is another important criterion for judging causality. *Specificity* refers to the association of an exposure with one specific disease. The association of adenocarcinoma of the vagina in women and exposure to diethylstilbestrol in their mothers while in utero[15] is a good example of the specificity of a disease–exposure association.

The fourth criterion relates to *temporality*. In essence, it means an exposure must precede a disease before it can be concluded that the association is causal. The risk of EMS was temporally linked to changes in the fermentation and production process used to produce L-tryptophan at a single Japanese manufacturing plant. Specifically, using the case-control method (described later), investigators linked the use of less powdered activated carbon in the purification process and a change to a new bacterial strain in the fermentation process to the risk of disease.[1,20]

Two very strong arguments for causality are the presence of a *dose–response effect* and a decreased risk of disease with removal of exposure. The toxic oil syndrome epidemic in Spain illustrates these points well.[21] Over a 2-month period in 1981, approximately 20,000 people developed a syndrome consisting of pulmonary infiltration, eosinophilia, and neuromuscular problems. About 450 people died. Different hypotheses were proposed early in the epidemic. Eventually, the suspected source was identified as adulterated rapeseed oil that had been sold illicitly as olive oil. There was a clear dose–response relationship: Those who used more oil were more likely to become ill. When the oil was confiscated, the only people who continued to become ill were those who had withheld some of the oil from the government. Although the exact chemical substance that caused the syndrome was not identified, the causal relationship between the oil and the syndrome was clearly established by the dose–response association and by the decreased risk of disease on elimination of the exposure.

The EMS was similar in these respects to the toxic oil syndrome. For example, in one study of patients in a South Carolina psychiatric practice, the risk of the development of EMS was directly related to daily dose of the L-tryptophan, whose origin was a contaminated lot from the manufacturer.[19] Thirteen percent of 38 persons taking 250 to 1500 mg of L-tryptophan developed EMS, compared to 50 percent of 38 persons taking greater than 4000 mg daily. Intermediate daily doses resulted in intermediate risks. When the Food and Drug Administration recalled tryptophan in mid-fall 1989, reported cases of EMS decreased from a high of almost 300 cases in October 1989 to no cases in June 1990.[28]

Biologic plausibility is another important factor for establishing causal associations. Identification of a contaminant substance, 1,1′-ethylidenebis tryptophan or EBT, in the tryptophan in the case lots that were strongly associated with disease onset, supported the hypotheses of a contaminant-induced disease.[1,20] In addition, rats fed implicated tryptophan developed changes in their fascia and perimysium similar to the histopathology of human EMS victims.[8]

In summary, the cause and effect relationship between EMS and ingestion of LTCP are supported by a high relative risk, a consistent pattern of disease onset with drug ingestion, a similar syndrome in those ingesting the contaminated drug, a temporal pattern to the rise and fall of the epidemic, a clear dose–response pattern, and identification of a suspected agent.

Not all of these criteria need be present to conclude that a causal association exists between a disease and an exposure.[12] However, the more criteria that are present, the more likely an association is truly causal and not secondary to bias, confounding, or chance.

What Are the Basic Research Designs Available to Study Clinical Problems?

Experimental Design

Table 117–2 lists the various research designs available to study clinical problems. The randomized clinical trial (RCT) is the best design for inferring causal relationships. The strength of this design stems from the randomization of study subjects into treatment (exposure) and control groups. Assuming successful randomization—that is, balancing the groups on risk factors and potential confounders—the difference in outcome between the groups is solely dependent on the exposure or treatment of interest. Masking (blinding) of study subjects, investigators, and assessors of outcome is a design factor that strengthens this method of investigating.

For example, Chapter 67 discusses several therapeutic measures that have been proposed to treat phencyclidine (PCP) toxicity. There is controversy, for example, on the use of phenothiazines to control agitation. Proponents and opponents of this therapeutic modality would best resolve their dispute by conducting an RCT to assess the issue. Patients with PCP toxicity could be randomized into phenothiazine, diazepam, or haloperidol treatment groups to assess which drug is more efficacious in achieving sedation with the least adverse effects.

Despite the strength of the RCT, there are many situations in which it would be unethical to do a study by exposing patients to a potential risk factor. For example, in 1984 a cotton manufacturer proposed waiving the cotton dust standard in a southern state so the company could assess a theory that byssinosis was caused by certain bacteria, and not by high concentrations of cotton dust.[9] Clearly, this would not be an ethical design to test such an hypothesis.

Observational Design

There are many nonexperimental (observational) study designs that are either descriptive or analytic in approach.[22] Descriptive studies, which define the characteristic of a patient or group of patients, include case reports, case series, and incidence studies. Population-based mortality studies (as opposed to hospital-based autopsy series) are examples of incidence studies.

TABLE 117–2. RESEARCH DESIGNS

Randomized clinical trial (RCT)	Cross-sectional study
Cohort study	Case series
Case-control study	Case report

An analytic study tests a specific hypothesis that relates a disease to one or more exposures. Disease is related to exposure for *each* individual in the study. Cross-sectional, case-control, and cohort studies are examples of analytic studies.

The cross-sectional study is often used to estimate the prevalence of disease in a population. It is usually the first step in the investigation of an epidemic. This design was used to investigate the outbreak of hexachlorophene poisoning in children that occurred in France during 1972.[24] The initial epidemic curve revealed a well-defined outbreak of fever, encephalopathy, and diaper rash in a limited geographic area in France. Interviews with the victims' parents revealed that most had used the same baby powder, which was subsequently found to be contaminated with hexachlorophene. This is an excellent example of the use of epidemiologic methods to identify an unknown toxin exposure. The establishment of causality in this case was relatively easy. Early studies in the EMS epidemic were also cross-sectional in nature and readily suggested L-tryptophan as the likely cause of the outbreak.[20] Other situations are often more difficult.

To establish a causal association between a disease and an exposure, the logical sequence of studies progresses from the case report, to the case series, to the prevalence study, to the incidence study, to the case-control study, to the cohort study, and finally to the clinical trial. To illustrate this sequence, consider the ongoing investigation of the AIDS epidemic. In 1981, the first studies on AIDS were reported by the Centers for Disease Control (CDC).[5] They consisted of case reports and case series. Subsequently, the CDC reported many more cases and calculated prevalence and incidence rates that were clearly of significant magnitude. At the same time the CDC was calculating these rates, it was performing the initial case-control studies to assess potential risk factors for disease.[4] Using this method, representative cases were compared to a control group of individuals who were unaffected by AIDS. The proportion of cases with the exposure(s) in question were compared to the proportion of controls with the same exposure(s). The advantages and disadvantages of the case-control design are listed in Table 117–3.

When the etiology of a disease is unknown, as initially in the AIDS epidemic, an exploratory study is done to assess multiple hypotheses. If several potential risk factors are suggested by an initial study, a separate and more detailed study of these risk factors is done. In the case of AIDS it seemed initially that only homosexuals were at risk. Indeed, for a brief time the disease was named GRID, for gay-related immunodeficiency disease.[26] Looking for causative agents in this population focused attention on the use of amyl and butyl nitrite (see Chap. 93). However, a subsequent exploratory study[18] showed that homosexuals with AIDS were no more likely to use butyl nitrite or any illicit drugs than were homosexuals without AIDS. It was apparent after several such exploratory studies that hemophiliacs and Haitians seemed at increased risk for the development of AIDS but this was also disproven (see Chap. 107).[29]

TABLE 117–3. ADVANTAGES AND DISADVANTAGES OF THE CASE-CONTROL METHOD

Advantages	Disadvantages
1. Well suited to the study of rare disease or those with long latency.	1. Relies on recall or records for information on past exposures.
2. Relatively quick to mount and conduct.	2. Validation of information is difficult or sometimes impossible.
3. Relatively inexpensive.	3. Control of extraneous variables may be incomplete.
4. Requires comparatively few subjects.	4. Selection of an appropriate comparison group may be difficult.
5. Existing records can occasionally be used.	5. Rates of disease in exposed and unexposed individuals cannot be determined.
6. No risks to subjects.	6. Method relatively unfamiliar to the medical community and difficult to explain.
7. Allows study of multiple potential causes of a disease.	7. Detailed study of mechanism is rarely possible.

Reprinted, with permission, from Schlesselman JJ, Stolley PD: Planning and conducting a study. In: Schlesselman JJ, ed: Case-Control Studies. New York, Oxford University Press, 1982, p. 18. Copyright 1982, Oxford University Press.

In case-control studies, the outcome measure used to assess the existence of an increased risk of disease is the odds ratio, which is a reasonable estimate of the relative risk. When the odds ratio is greater than 1, the risk of disease among those exposed is said to be elevated when compared to those who are unexposed. Homosexuals, for example, initially were found to have a 100-fold increase in risk for developing AIDS compared to heterosexuals. In contrast, there was no increase in the odds ratio in people who used amyl nitrite (poppers), one of the factors initially proposed as the cause of the disease. More recently, the risk of HIV infection among homosexuals has begun to plateau (in concert with increases in condom use during sex) in contrast to a rise in risk among heterosexuals as the virus becomes more prevalent in this population.[6]

The approach in assessing a causal relationship between a suspected toxin and a new clinical syndrome is similar to the study of a new infectious agent. As mentioned earlier, Japanese investigators used the case-control method to establish a link between changes in the manufacturing process of L-tryptophan and the risk of EMS.[1,20]

Once the data from the early case-control studies on AIDS became available, there was enough evidence to suggest that the disease was transmitted by a parenteral route or by sexual contact.[3] The CDC then began a cohort study to further elucidate the risk factors for AIDS among healthcare workers who are at increased risk of contamination by blood and other body fluids from HIV-infected individuals.

In the cohort design, two groups of individuals, one with and one without a common exposure, are compared for various outcomes of interest that may develop over time. The groups can be assembled and studied prospectively, as in the case of Framingham cohorts assembled to study the incidence of cardiovascular disease. Alternatively, the groups (or cohorts) can be assembled retrospectively from available records; this is often done in occupational epidemiologic studies. For example, the associations between exposure to asbestos, radon, nickel, arsenic, and chromium and the development of lung cancer were all established via historical (retrospective) cohort studies.

In the cohort method, the population at-risk—those with at least a minimal exposure to the substance in question—is identified. Death and/or disease rates are determined for this cohort for varying periods of time following exposure. These rates are then compared to the death/disease rates for some standard, presumably unexposed, population. Then a ratio of mortality rates (the standardized mortality ratio; SMR) is calculated. Hypothesis testing can then be done to determine whether the difference in mortality rates between the exposed and unexposed populations is statistically significantly different. Alternatively, a confidence interval around the estimate of the mortality rate can be calculated. If the confidence interval includes the null (no effect) value (100 for the SMR), the investigator can conclude that the null hypothesis of no association between disease and exposure cannot be rejected. Table 117–4 lists the advantages and disadvantages of the cohort method.

TABLE 117–4. ADVANTAGES AND DISADVANTAGES OF THE COHORT METHOD

Advantages	Disadvantages
1. In principle, provides a complete description of experience subsequent to exposure, including rates of progression, staging of disease, and natural history.	1. Requires large numbers of subjects to study rare diseases.
2. Allows study of multiple potential effects of a given exposure, thereby obtaining information on potential benefits as well as risks.	2. Potentially long duration of follow-up.
3. Allows for the calculation of rates of disease in exposed and unexposed individuals.	3. Current practice, usage, or exposure to study factors may change, making findings irrelevant.
4. Permits flexibility in choosing variables to be systematically recorded.	4. Relatively expensive to conduct.
5. Allows for thorough quality control in measurement of study variables.	5. Control of extraneous variables may be incomplete.
	6. Detailed study of mechanism is rarely possible.

Reprinted, with permission, from Schlesselman JJ, Stolley PD: Planning and conducting a study. In: Schlesselman JJ, ed: Case-Control Studies. New York, Oxford University Press, 1982, p. 18. Copyright 1982, Oxford University Press.

In the case of AIDS, the National Institute of Allergy and Infectious Diseases conducted a prospective cohort study of asymptomatic HIV-negative healthcare workers who were exposed to HIV-positive individuals through needle punctures and other exposures.[14] The seroconversion rate in this exposed cohort was compared to the rate of seroconversion in workers contaminated with blood from HIV-negative patients to assess the risk of infection in exposed hospital workers. Seroconversion occurred in 1 of 179 workers (0.56%) parenterally exposed to blood from an HIV-infected patient and none of the workers exposed otherwise over a 6-year period.

The major difference between a cohort study and a randomized clinical trial is that in the former, study subjects are not assigned to an exposure group but are only observed for a particular outcome. Because of this, investigators using this method must ensure that the analysis adjusts for any discrepancies between the study groups. That is, the two groups must be similar in the prevalence of confounders or variables, such as age, that may affect outcome. In a randomized clinical trial, the randomization process is supposed to balance the group for various baseline physiologic measurements and confounders. The investigator is obligated to verify, however, that the randomization procedure accomplished its goal. If it did not, the analysis must be adjusted for the imbalance. Adjustment procedures include standardization, stratification, and various regression techniques. These methods are outlined in Table 117–5.

Figure 117–1 summarizes the major differences between the case-control and the cohort methods. The former identifies patients by disease, and the latter identifies patients by exposure. Tables 117–3 and 117–4, respectively, list the advantages and disadvantages of each method.

TABLE 117–5. METHODS FOR CONTROLLING CONFOUNDING

Restriction	When selecting participants for a study, limit their range of characteristics.
Matching	For each patient in one group, select one or more patients with the same characteristics (except the one under study) for a comparison group.
Stratification	Compare rates within subgroups (strata) of patients with otherwise similar risks.
Standardization	Mathematically adjust crude rates so that for the groups being compared, equal weight is given to strata of similar risk.
Multivariate adjustment	Adjust for differences in a large number of factors related to outcome, using mathematical techniques.
Assuming the worst	When a factor cannot be controlled, examine the consequences of an unlikely (or worst possible) maldistribution between groups.
Randomization	Assign patients to groups in a way that gives each patient an equal chance of falling into one or the other group.

Reprinted, with permission, from Fletcher RH, Fletcher SW, Wagner EH: Clinical Epidemiology: The Essentials. Baltimore, Williams & Wilkins, 1982.

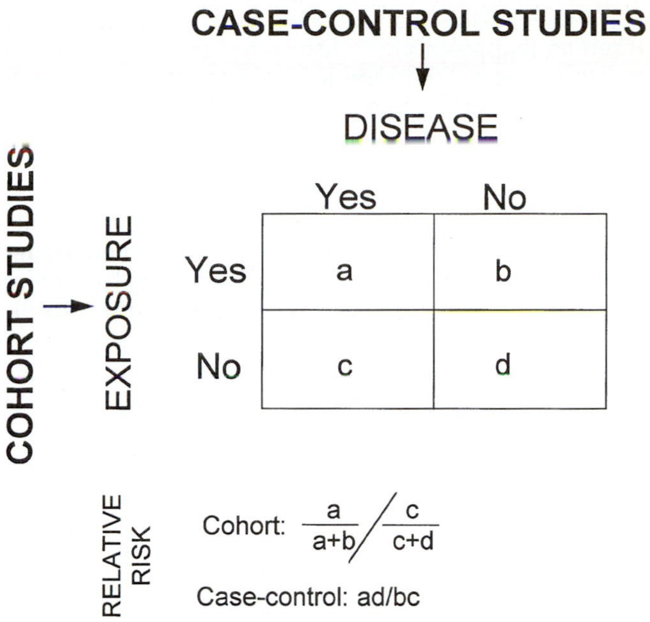

Figure 117–1. Design of case-control and cohort studies.

What Methodologic Criteria Must Be Considered in the Evaluation of Any Study?

Each of these designs has its own strengths and limitations. In addition, there are certain basic concepts that affect the internal validity of any study. *Bias* and *confounding* are the two major errors that may jeopardize validity.

An association between an exposure and an outcome may be due to bias, confounding, chance, or true causality. Bias is a systematic *error* that results in an overestimate or underestimate of the true value of some outcome measure. A confounder is a variable associated with both an outcome and an exposure. A confounding variable may bias a study because of the variable's differential distribution between the exposed group and the control group. These two factors should be considered during each of the four major phases of a study: design, data collection, analysis, and reporting.

There are two major categories of bias: selection (ascertainment) bias and information bias. Types of selection bias include biases secondary to the selective referral of patients, the drop-out of patients from a study, the different methods of disease detection in the study and control groups, and the use of volunteers in a study.

Information bias may occur when (1) patients are incorrectly classified according to disease or exposure, (2) laboratory tests are incorrectly interpreted, and (3) recall of historical information is poor or incomplete. Selection bias often occurs in the design phase of a study; information bias occurs in the data collection phase.

Biases in the analysis phase of a study may occur when an inappropriate statistical test is used to test the null hypothesis. For example, a very common mistake is the use of multiple *t*-tests to compare study groups when a repeated measures test, such as the analysis of variance, is most appropriate. The use of an inappropriate test may not only be too conservative in testing a hypothesis, but it also may present completely fallacious results because many statistical tests are based on underlying mathematical assumptions that must be fulfilled before they can be applied. Sackett reviewed the numerous biases that can affect a study.[25]

Confounding is a problem (not an error) that frequently can be anticipated in a study if enough is known about the disease in question. The investigator and the reader must always be alert for this type of problem. Drug abuse studies are particularly prone to confounding because of the high incidence of multiple drug abuse and the similarity of effects of many agents. An example of confounding may occur in a study of the relationship between smoking marijuana and loss of lung function. Smoking tobacco is a potential confounder. We know that smoking tobacco is associated with both smoking marijuana and pulmonary function loss. The careful investigator must adjust for this confounder by one of several methods listed in Table 117–5. For example, if the study and control groups are stratified on average cigarette consumption, the relative risk of a specified loss of forced expiratory volume in 1 second (FEV_1) in marijuana users compared to nonusers may be estimated, independent of cigarette intake.

Another type of confounding that may occur, especially in clinical drug trials, is confounding by indication for therapy. In a therapeutic trial the investigator must ensure an equal distribution of people with different diseases, or stages of disease, in both the treatment and control groups. If this is not done, the treatment group may include more patients who have a more favorable outcome than are included in the control group. If so, the treatment group will tend to have a better outcome, perhaps falsely attributed to the therapy being evaluated. For example, in a randomized clinical trial to assess the efficacy of phenothiazines in the treatment of PCP toxicity, it would be important that both the treatment and control groups had patients with similar levels of psychiatric dysfunction.

Another common error that occurs in both experimental and observational research is the failure to assess the power of a negative study. The power of a study is the ability to detect a significant difference in outcome between the study and control groups when such a difference actually exists. The statement that there is no effect is usually based on a hypothesis test that failed to reject the null hypothesis of no association between the drug and the effect(s). This is not the same as saying there is no effect. The investigators must make a statement about the likelihood of finding a significant effect in the study.

For example, if (1) a study has a sufficient number of people to detect an a priori specified outcome; and (2) the study fails to reject the null hypothesis at a specified level of significance (for example, less than 0.05); and (3) the probability of failing to reject the null hypothesis when the alternate hypothesis is true is 20%, then the investigator can state that the study had an 80% chance (power) of detecting the a priori specified outcome if that outcome was the true state of affairs in the underlying population. Power tables[7] and nomograms[30] are available to make these calculations relatively easy. It is important to remember that a negative study using a small number of patients does not necessarily mean no effect.

In summary, bias and confounding frequently affect the outcome of a study. The vigilant investigator and the cautious reader must consider the many biases that may occur during any step of a study.[25] Although confounding should be anticipated during the design phase of a study, the search for potential confounders must continue right through the analysis phase.

Healthcare providers must understand the issues outlined in this chapter to keep up with the literature effectively. New proposed therapies should be assessed rigorously before application in the clinical setting. Emergency department personnel should be always vigilant for unusual reactions to new drugs. The practice of modern medical toxicology requires a thorough knowledge of the principles and limitations of medical research.

Epidemiologic Research Terms

Association

Association is the degree of statistical dependence between two or more events or variables. *Events* are said to be associated when they occur more frequently together than one would expect by chance. Associated *variables* are those in which knowledge of a subject's value on one conveys information about his or her likely position on the other. Association of either sort does not imply a causal relationship. Statistical significance testing enables us to determine how unlikely it would be to observe the sample relationship by chance if in fact no association exists in the population that was sampled.

Bias

Bias is any effect at any stage of investigation or inference tending to produce results that depart systematically from the true values (to be distinguished from random error). The term does not necessarily carry an imputation of prejudice or other subjective influence, such as the experimenter's desire for a particular outcome. This differs from conventional usage, in which bias refers to a partisan point of view.

Case-Control Study

A case-control study (also called case comparison study, case history study, case referent study, retrospective study, or trohoc study) starts with the identification of persons with the disease (or other outcome variable) of interest, and a suitable control (comparison, reference) group of persons without the disease. The relationship of an attribute to the disease is examined by comparing the diseased and nondiseased with regard to how frequently the attribute is present or, if quantitative, the levels of the attribute, in each of the groups.

Causation

Causation is a particular type of association involving a true causal link between variables or events. A cause is termed *necessary* when it must always precede the effect. This effect need not be the sole result of the one cause. A cause is termed *sufficient* when it inevitably initiates or produces the effect. Any given cause may be necessary, sufficient, neither, or both.

Cohort

A cohort is that component of the population born during a particular period and identified by period of birth, so that its characteristics (eg, causes of death and numbers still living) can be ascertained as it enters successive time and age periods. The term has broadened, however, to describe any designated group of persons who are followed or traced over a period of time, as in *cohort study* (prospective study).

Cohort Study

The cohort study (also called concurrent, follow-up incidence, longitudinal, and prospective study) is a method of epidemiologic study in which subsets of a defined population can be identified who are, have been, or in the future may be exposed or not exposed, or exposed in different degrees, to a factor or factors hypothesized to influence the probability of occurrence of a given disease or other outcome. The alternative terms for a cohort study describe an essential feature of the method, which is observation of the population for a sufficient number of persons-years to generate reliable incidence or mortality rates in the population subsets. This generally implies study of a large population, study for a prolonged period (years), or both.

Confounding

Confounding is a situation in which the relationship between an independent and a dependent variable is distorted by the association of both with a third (confounding) variable. Often it refers to the distortion of the apparent effect of an exposure on risk brought about by the association with other factors that can influence the outcome.

Cross-Sectional Study

A cross-sectional study (also called disease frequency survey, prevalence study) examines the relationship between diseases (or other health-related characteristics) and other variables of interest as they exist in a defined population at one particular time. The presence or absence of disease and the presence or absence of the other variables (or, if they are quantitative, their level) are determined in each member of the study population or in a representative sample at one particular time.

Information Bias

Information bias (also called observational bias) is a flaw in measuring exposure or outcome that results in differential quality (accuracy) of information between compared groups.

Null Hypothesis

In simplest terms, the null hypothesis states that the independent variable(s) under study has (have) no association with, or effect on, the dependent or outcome variable(s). The truth of this hypothesis is determined by calculating the probability that the apparent association or effect (that seen in the sample) would have arisen by chance if the null hypothesis were true. By convention, a probability (p value) ≤ 0.05 is taken as grounds for rejecting the null hypothesis in favor of a true effect or association.

Power

Power is the relative frequency with which a true association or effect of a specified magnitude would be detected by the proposed study.

Randomized Controlled Trial

A randomized controlled trial (RCT) is an epidemiologic experiment in which subjects in a population are randomly allocated into groups that receive different experimental, preventive, or therapeutic procedures, maneuvers, or interventions. In some studies one of the groups may receive no treatment or an inactive one (a placebo). The results are assessed by rigorous comparison of rates of disease, death, recovery, or other appropriate outcomes in the study groups.

Relative Risk

The ratio of the incidence rate of disease or death among those exposed to that among those unexposed is the relative risk (also called risk ratio and closely related to odds ratio).

Reliability

Reliability is the degree of stability exhibited when a measurement is repeated under identical conditions. Reliability refers to the degree to which the results obtained by a measurement procedure can be replicated. Lack of reliability may arise from divergences between observers or instruments of measurement.

Selection Bias

Selection bias refers to error due to systematic differences in characteristics between those who are selected for study and those who are not. Examples include hospital cases or cases under a physician's care, excluding patients who die before hospital admission because the course of their disease is so acute, those not sick enough to require hospital care, or those excluded by distance, cost, or other factors. Selection bias also invalidates generalizable conclusions from surveys that would include only volunteers from a healthy population.

Validity

Validity is an expression of the degree to which a measurement measures what it purports to measure.

References

1. Belongia EA, Hedberg CW, Gleich GJ, et al: An investigation of the cause of the eosinophilia-myalgia syndrome associated with tryptophan use. N Engl J Med 1990;323: 357–365.
2. Centers for Disease Control: Eosinophilia-myalgia syndrome and L-tryptophan-containing products—New Mexico, Minnesota, Oregon, and New York. MMWR 1989;38: 785–788.
3. Centers for Disease Control: Antibodies to a retrovirus etiologically associated with acquired immunodeficiency syndrome (AIDS) in populations with increased incidence of the syndrome. MMWR 1984;33:377–379.
4. Centers for Disease Control: Task force on Kaposi's sarcoma and opportunistic infections: Epidemiologic aspects of the current outbreak of Kaposi's sarcoma and opportunistic infections. N Engl J Med 1982;306:248–252.
5. Centers for Disease Control: Kaposi sarcoma and pneumocystis pneumonia among homosexual men: New York City and California. MMWR 1981;30:305–308.
6. Centers for Disease Control and Prevention: Projections of the number of persons diagnosed with AIDS and the number of immunosuppressed HIV-infected persons, United States, 1992–1994. MMWR 1992;41:5–13.
7. Cohen J: Statistical Power Analysis for the Behavioral Sciences. New York, Academic Press, 1977.
8. Crofford LJ, Rader JI, Dalakas MC, et al: L-tryptophan implicated in human eosinophila-myalgia syndrome causes facsiitis and perimyositis in the Lewis rat. J Clin Invest 1990; 86:1757–1763.
9. Dan River cancels variance request. Occup Health Saf 1984; 53:10.
10. Department of Clinical Epidemiology and Biostatistics, McMaster University Health Sciences Center: How to read clinical journals. Can Med Assoc J 1981;124:555, 703, 869, 985, 1156.
11. Dickersin K, Berlin JA. Meta-analysis: State-of-the-science. Epidemiol Rev 1992;14:154–176.
12. Dinman B, Sussman NB: Uncertainty, risk and the role of epidemiology in public policy development. J Occup Med 1983;25:511–516.
13. Fletcher RH, Fletcher SW, Wagner EH: Clinical Epidemiology: The Essentials, 2nd ed. Baltimore, Williams & Wilkins, 1988.
14. Henderson DK, Fahey BJ, Willy M, et al: Risk for occupational transmission of human immunodeficiency virus type 1 (HIV–1) associated with clinical exposures. Ann Intern Med 1990;113:740–746.
15. Herbst AL, Ulfelder H, Poskanzer DC: Adenocarcinoma of the vagina: Association of maternal stilbestrol therapy with tumor appearance in young women. N Engl J Med 1971; 284:878–881.
16. Hertzman PA, Blevins WL, Mayer J, et al: Association of the eosinophilia-myalgia syndrome with the ingestion of tryptophan. N Engl J Med 1990;322:869–873.
17. Hill AB: The environment and disease: Association or causation? Proc Royal Soc Med 1965;58:295.
18. Jaffe HW, Choi K, Thomas PA, et al: National case control study of Kaposi's sarcoma and *Pneumocystis carinii* pneumonia in homosexual men. 1: Epidemiologic results. Ann Inter Med 1983;99:145–151.
19. Kamb ML, Murphy JJ, Jones JL, et al: Eosinophilic-myalgia syndrome in L H tryptophan-exposed patients. JAMA 1992;267:77–82.
20. Kilbourne EM: Eosinophilia-myalgia syndrome: Coming to grips with a new illness. Epidemiol Rev 1992;14: 16–36.
21. Kilbourne EM, Rigau-Perez JH, Heath CW, et al: Clinical epidemiology of toxic-oil syndrome: Manifestations of a new illness. N Engl J Med 1983;309:1408–1414.
22. Kleinbaum DG, Kupper LL, Morgenstern H: Epidemiology Research Principles and Quantitative Methods. Belmont, CA, Lifetime Learning Publications, 1982.
23. Longnecker MP, Berlin JA, Orza MJ, Chalmers TC: A meta-analysis of alcohol consumption in relation to risk of breast cancer. JAMA 1988;260:652–656.
24. Martin-Bouyer G, Lebreton R, Toga M, et al: Outbreak of accidental hexachlorophene poisoning in France. Lancet 1982;1:91–95.
25. Sackett DL: Bias in analytic research. J Chron Dis 1979;32: 51–63.
26. Shilts R: And the Band Played On: Politics, People, and the AIDS Epidemic. New York, St. Martin's Press, 1987.
27. Smoking and Health: Report of the Advisory Committee to the Surgeon General of the Public Health Service. U.S. Department of Health, Education, and Welfare, Public Health Service, Centers for Disease Control, PHS pub. no. 1103, 387, 1964.
28. Swygert LA, Maes EF, Sewell LE, et al: Eosinophilic-myalgia syndrome: Results of national surveillance. JAMA 1990; 264:1698–1703.
29. U.S. Public Health Service: AIDS Update. FDA Drug Bulletin. U.S. Department of Health and Human Services, Public Health Service, Food and Drug Administration (HFW-42), 1983, 13:9.
30. Young MF, Bresnitz EA, Strom BL: Sample size nomograms for interpreting negative clinical studies. Ann Intern Med 1983; 99:248–251.

Index

Page numbers followed by f and t indicate figures and tables, respectively. Page numbers in **boldface** type, preceded by **cp** indicate Color Plates (e.g., **cp3** indicates Color Plate 3). Main headings in SMALL CAPS represent pharmaceutical trade names.

A

B

C

D

E

F

G

H

I

J

K

M

N

O

P

Q

R

S

T

U

V

W